Walsh and Hoyt's
Clinical
Neuro-Ophthalmology

Volume One

Sixth Edition

Walsh and Hoyt's
Clinical
Neuro-Ophthalmology

Sixth Edition

Neil R. Miller, MD

Professor of Ophthalmology, Neurology, and
  Neurosurgery
Frank B. Walsh Professor of Neuro-Ophthalmology
Director, Neuro-Ophthalmology and Orbital Units
Wilmer Eye Institute
Johns Hopkins Hospital
Baltimore, Maryland

Nancy J. Newman, MD

LeoDelle Jolley Professor of Ophthalmology
Professor of Ophthalmology and Neurology
Instructor in Neurological Surgery
Director, Neuro-Ophthalmology Unit
Emory University School of Medicine
Atlanta, Georgia
Lecturer in Ophthalmology
Harvard Medical School
Boston, Massachusetts

Valérie Biousse, MD

Cyrus H. Stoner Professor of Ophthalmology
Associate Professor of Ophthalmology and Neurology
Emory University School of Medicine
Atlanta, Georgia

John B. Kerrison, MD

Assistant Professor of Ophthalmology, Neurology, and
  Neurosurgery
Wilmer Eye Institute
Johns Hopkins Hospital
Baltimore, Maryland

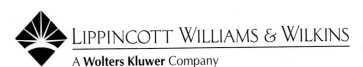

LIPPINCOTT WILLIAMS & WILKINS
A **Wolters Kluwer** Company
Philadelphia • Baltimore • New York • London
Buenos Aires • Hong Kong • Sydney • Tokyo

Acquisitions Editor: Jonathan Pine
Developmental Editor: Grace Caputo and Stacey Sebring
Project Manager: David Murphy
Manufacturing Manager: Ben Rivera
Production Services: Maryland Composition, Inc.
Printer: Maple Press

530 Walnut Street
Philadelphia, Pennsylvania 19106 USA

351 West Camden Street
Baltimore, Maryland 21201-2436 USA

The publisher is not responsible (as a matter of product liability, negligence or otherwise) for any injury resulting from any material contained herein. This publication contains information relating to general principles of medical care which should not be constructed as specific instruction for individual patients. Manufacturer's product information should be reviewed for current information, including contraindications, dosages, and precautions.

Printed in the United States of America

Library of Congress Cataloging-in-Publication Data

Walsh and Hoyt's clinical neuro-ophthalmology.—6th ed. / [editors,
  Neil R. Miller et al.]
    p.   cm.
    Includes bibliographical references and index.
    ISBN 0-7817-4811-9 (v. 1)—ISBN 0-7817-4812-7 (v. 2)—
  ISBN 0-7817-4813-5 (v. 3)—ISBN 0-7817-4814-3 (set)
    1. Neuroophthalmology.   2. Eye—Diseases.   I. Title: Clinical
neuroophthalmology.
  II. Miller, Neil R.   III. Walsh, Frank Burton, 1896–
  IV. Hoyt, William Fletcher, 1926–
    [DNLM: 1. Eye Diseases.   2. Neurologic Manifestations.
    WW 140 W223 2005]
    RE725.W348 2005
    617.7—dc22   2004021741

The publishers have made every effort to trace copyright holders for borrowed material. If they have inadvertently overlooked any, they will be pleased to make the necessary arrangements at the first opportunity.

To purchase additional copies of this book, call our customer service department at (800) 638-3030 or fax orders to (301) 824-7390. For other book services, including chapter reprints and large quantity sales, ask for the Special Sales department.

For all other calls originating outside of the United States, please call (301) 714-2324.

Visit Lippincott Williams & Wilkins on the Internet: http://www.lww.com. Lippincott Williams & Wilkins customer service representatives are available from 8:30 am to 6:30 pm, EST, Monday through Friday, for telephone access.

Dedication

To Our Families

Preface

It goes without saying (but I will say it anyway) that times have changed since Dr. Frank B. Walsh wrote the first edition of this text in 1947. The first two editions, each a single volume, were written by Dr. Walsh alone and primarily related his personal experiences and those of his colleagues. In 1969, he and Dr. William F. Hoyt, wrote the third edition—a three-volume masterpiece of ophthalmology, neurology, neurosurgery, and general medicine with extensive illustrations and references. In 1978, I was asked to write the next edition. That 4th edition consisted of five volumes and took 14 years to produce, with the volumes published sequentially between 1982 and 1996. Inevitably, the material was destined to become outdated, even during the production of the edition. Thus, for the next edition, it was clear that a single-authored text was no longer feasible, and I asked my friend and colleague, Dr. Nancy J. Newman, to co-edit a multi-authored edition. Sixty contributors updated the material from the 4th edition and, in some cases, completely wrote or rewrote their chapters. They brought a depth of understanding and a wealth of knowledge to the 5th edition that could not possibly be accomplished with single or dual au-thorship. The publication of this 5-volume work occurred in the nearly record time of 2 years.

It is now time for a 6th edition and for this, Dr. Newman and I have invited two associate editors, Dr. Valérie Biousse and Dr. John B. Kerrison, to assist. In addition, because of the explosion of information available on the world-wide web and search engines such as Pub Med and OVID, the four of us decided to reduce the size of the text to make it more manageable and more accessible for the reader, while at the same time maintaining the high quality of the previous editions, including an up-to-date set of references. Once again, we called upon 60 of our trusted colleagues to help us achieve this goal, and they have risen to the task. With their help, we have produced a three-volume 6th edition that is about 2000 pages shorter than the previous edition, but maintains the high-quality illustrations, personal observations, and both new and old references that characterized the previous editions of this text. We hope our readers will enjoy the new edition and that it will provide them with a useful resource for teaching, research, and the best possible patient care.

Neil R. Miller, MD FACS

Acknowledgements

The editors would first like to thank each of the authors who contributed to this text. It is only through their dedication and hard work that this text could be produced. We also appreciate the hard work and expertise of the terrific staff at LWW and Maryland Composition, particularly Stacey Sebring, Grace Caputo, Joyce Murphy, Jonathan Pine, Scott Lavine, and Heidi Pongratz. They and others spent many long hours crafting this text.

Melissa Surbaugh provided superb editorial assistance for the chapters edited by Drs. Newman and Biousse, whereas Drs. Miller and Kerrison were aided by the extraordinary editorial skills of Drs. Richard Levy and Aarup Kubal. Michael McIlwaine and other members of the Photography department of the Wilmer Eye Institute provided rapid and superb photographic assistance for many of the chapters.

Drs. Miller and Kerrison thank their past chairman, Morton F. Goldberg, MD, for his unwavering support during the initial phases of this project, and their current chairman, Peter J. McDonnell, MD, who continues the Wilmer tradition of excellence. Dr. Kerrison would like to thank Neil R. Miller, MD, Nancy J. Newman, MD, Irene H. Maumenee, MD, William R. Green, MD, and Donald J. Zack, MD, PhD for their continual support and encouragement. Above all, Dr. Kerrison wishes to express his awe and gratitude to the Lord, who makes all things worthwhile.

Drs. Newman and Biousse would like to personally thank Thomas M. Aaberg, MD, for continuing to foster an unparalleled academic environment at Emory University. A special thanks also from Dr. Newman to Simmons Lessell, MD, and from Dr. Biousse to her mentors Marie-Germaine Bousser, MD, Nancy J. Newman, MD, and Monique Schaison, MD.

Finally, Dr. Miller would like to thank Carol Miller, RD, MEd for 25 years of editorial and photographic assistance.

Contributors

Madhu R. Agarwal, MD
Assistant Professor of Ophthalmology
Division of Neuro-Ophthalmology and Orbital Surgery
Loma Linda University Medical Center
Loma Linda, California
Clinical Instructor of Ophthalmology
Doheny Eye Institute
University of Southern California Keck School of
    Medicine
Los Angeles, California

Anthony C. Arnold, MD
Professor and Chief
Neuro-Ophthalmology Division
Jules Stein Eye Institute
Department of Ophthalmology
University of California-Los Angeles
Los Angeles, California

Laura J. Balcer, MD, MSCE
Associate Professor of Neurology and Ophthalmology
University of Pennsylvania
Neuro-Ophthalmologist
Hospital of the University of Pennsylvania
Scheie Eye Institute
Philadelphia, Pennsylvania

Jason J. S. Barton, MD, PhD, FRCP(C)
Associate Professor of Neurology
Harvard Medical School
Adjunct Professor of Bioengineering
Boston University
Director of Neuro-Ophthalmology
Beth Israel Deaconess Medical Center
Boston, Massachusetts

Ghassan K. Bejjani, MD
Clinical Assistant Professor of Neurosurgery
University of Pittsburgh School of Medicine
Pittsburgh, Pennsylvania

M. Tariq Bhatti, MD
Assistant Professor of Ophthalmology, Neurology, and
    Neurosurgery
University of Florida College of Medicine
Ophthalmology Consultant
Malcolm Randall Veterans Administration Medical Center
Gainesville, Florida

Valérie Biousse, MD
Cyrus H. Stoner Professor of Ophthalmology
Associate Professor of Ophthalmology and Neurology
Emory University School of Medicine
Atlanta, Georgia

Mark S. Borchert, MD
Associate Professor of Ophthalmology and Neurology
University of Southern California Keck School of
    Medicine
Division Head
Department of Ophthalmology
Childrens Hospital of Los Angeles
Los Angeles, California

Paul W. Brazis, MD
Professor of Neurology
Consultant in Neurology and Neuro-ophthalmology
Mayo Clinic-Jacksonville
Jacksonville, Florida

Michael C. Brodsky, MD
Professor of Ophthalmology and Pediatrics
University of Arkansas for Medical Sciences
Chief of Pediatric Ophthalmology
Arkansas Childrens Hospital
Little Rock, Arkansas

Preston C. Calvert, MD
Assistant Professor of Neurology
Johns Hopkins University School of Medicine
Baltimore, Maryland
Attending Physician in Neurology
Fairfax Hospital
Fairfax, Virginia

David Alston Chesnutt, MD
Clinical Assistant Professor of Ophthalmology
Duke University Eye Center
Attending Surgeon in Ophthalmology Service
Durham Veterans Administration Medical Center
Durham, North Carolina

Kimberley P. Cockerham, MD
Associate Professor of Ophthalmology
University of California-San Francisco
San Francisco, California

Wayne T. Cornblath, MD
Clinical Professor of Ophthalmology and Visual Science
  and Neurology
University of Michigan
Ann Arbor, Michigan

Kathleen B. Digre, MD
Professor of Neurology and Ophthalmology
Moran Eye Center
University of Utah
Departments of Neurology and Ophthalmology
University of Utah Hospital
Salt Lake City, Utah

Robert A. Egan, MD
Associate Professor of Ophthalmology, Neurology, and
  Neurosurgery
Casey Eye Institute
Oregon Health and Science University
Portland, Oregon

Eric R. Eggenberger, DO
Professor of Neurology and Ophthalmology
Department of Neurology and Ophthalmology
Michigan State University
East Lansing, Michigan

Rod Foroozan, MD
Assistant Professor of Ophthalmology
Baylor College of Medicine
Houston, Texas

Deborah I. Friedman, MD
Associate Professor of Ophthalmology and Neurology
University of Rochester
Rochester, New York

Benjamin M. Frishberg, MD
Associate Clinical Professor of Neuroscience
University of California-San Diego
Department of Neurology
Scripps Memorial Hospital
La Jolla, California

Steven L. Galetta, MD
Van Meter Professor of Neurology
Professor of Neurology and Ophthalmology
University of Pennsylvania Medical Center
Chief, Division of Neuro-Ophthalmology
Philadelphia, Pennsylvania

John W. Gittinger, Jr., MD
Professor of Ophthalmology and Neurology
Boston University School of Medicine
Residency Program Director for Ophthalmology
Boston Medical Center
Boston, Massachusetts

Robert A. Goldberg, MD, FACS
Professor of Ophthalmology
Chief, Orbital and Ophthalmic Plastic Surgeon Division
Jules Stein Eye Institute
University of California-Los Angeles
Los Angeles, California

Karl C. Golnik, MD
Associate Professor of Ophthalmology, Neurology,
  Neurosurgery
University of Cincinnati
Cincinnati Eye Institute
Cincinnati, Ohio

Lynn K. Gordon, MD, PhD
Assistant Professor of Ophthalmology
Jules Stein Eye Institute
Chief, Ophthalmology Section
Greater Los Angeles Veterans Affairs Health Care System
Los Angeles, California

Steven R. Hamilton, MD
Clinical Associate Professor of Ophthalmology and
  Neurology
University of Washington
Neuro-Ophthalmic Consultants Northwest
Seattle, Washington

Thomas R. Hedges III, MD
Professor of Ophthalmology and Neurology
Tufts University
Director of Neuro-Ophthalmology
Tufts New England Medical Center
Boston, Massachusetts

Paul N. Hoffman, MD, PhD
Research Associate of Ophthalmology and Neurology
Wilmer Ophthalmological Institute
The Johns Hopkins School of Medicine
Baltimore, Maryland

Daniel M. Jacobson
deceased

Chris A. Johnson, PhD
Director of Diagnostic Research in Ophthalmology
Devers Eye Institute
Legacy Health Systems
Portland, Oregon

Randy Kardon, MD, PhD
Professor of Ophthalmology and Visual Science
University of Iowa College of Medicine
Director of Neuro-Ophthalmology
University of Iowa Hospital and Clinics and Veterans
  Administration
Iowa City, Iowa

Barrett Katz, MD, MBA
Professor of Ophthalmology, Neurology, and
   Neurosurgery
Weill Medical College of Cornell University and New
   York-Presbyterian Hospital
Vice President for Medical Affairs
Eyetech Pharmaceuticals, Inc.
New York, New York

David I. Kaufman, DO
Professor and Chair
Department of Neurology and Ophthalmology
Michigan State University
East Lansing, Michigan
Director of Clinical Neurosciences
Sparrow Health Systems
Lansing, Michigan

Aki Kawasaki, MD, MER
Mantre d'Enseignement et de Recherche of
   Ophthalmology
University of Lausanne
Medecin Associee in Neuro-Ophthalmology
Hopital Ophtalmique Jules Gonin
Lausanne, Switzerland

Christopher Kennard, PhD, FRCP, FMedSci
Head, Department of Visual Neuroscience
Faculty of Medicine
Imperial College London
Charing Cross Hospital
London, United Kingdom

John S. Kennerdell, MD
Professor of Ophthalmology
Drexel University College of Medicine
Philadelphia, Pennsylvania
Chairman of Ophthalmology
Allegheny General Hospital
Pittsburgh, Pennsylvania

John B. Kerrison, MD
Assistant Professor of Ophthalmology, Neurology, and
   Neurosurgery
Wilmer Eye Institute
Johns Hopkins Hospital
Baltimore, Maryland

Andrew G. Lee, MD
Professor of Ophthalmology, Neurology, and
   Neurosurgery
University of Iowa Hospitals and Clinics
Iowa City, Iowa

R. John Leigh, MD
Blair-Daroff Professor of Neurology
Case Western Reserve University
Staff Neurologist
Louis Stokes Veterans Affairs Medical Center
Cleveland, Ohio

Robert L. Lesser, MD
Clinical Professor of Ophthalmology and Visual Science,
   and Neurology
Yale University School of Medicine
New Haven, Connecticut
Clinical Professor of Neurology and Neurosurgery
University of Connecticut School of Medicine
Farmington, Connecticut

Leonard A. Levin, MD, PhD
Associate Professor of Ophthalmology and Visual
   Sciences, Neurology, and Neurological Surgery
University of Wisconsin
Madison, Wisconsin

Grant T. Liu, MD
Professor of Neurology and Ophthalmology
University of Pennsylvania School of Medicine
Hospital of the University of Pennsylvania
Children's Hospital of Philadelphia
Scheie Eye Institute
Philadelphia, Pennsylvania

Joseph C. Maroon
Professor of Neurosurgery
Heindl Scholar
Tristate Neurosurgical Associates
University of Pittsburgh Medical Center
Pittsburgh, Pennsylvania

Neil R. Miller
Professor of Ophthalmology, Neurology, and
   Neurosurgery
Frank B. Walsh Professor of Neuro-Ophthalmology
Director, Neuro-Ophthalmology and Orbit Units
Wilmer Eye Institute
Johns Hopkins Hospital
Baltimore, Maryland

Mark L. Moster, MD
Professor of Neurology
Thomas Jefferson School of Medicine
Chairman, Division of Neuro-Ophthalmology
Albert Einstein Medical Center
Instructor, Neuro-Ophthalmology
Wills Eye Institute
Philadelphia, Pennsylvania

Golnaz Moazami
Assistant Clinical Professor of Ophthalmology
Edward S. Harkness Eye Institute
Columbia University
New York, New York

Parashkev Nachev, MRCP
Clinical Research Fellow of Visual Neuroscience
Faculty of Medicine
Imperial College London
London, United Kingdom

Nancy J. Newman, MD
LeoDelle Jolley Professor of Ophthalmology
Professor of Ophthalmology and Neurology
Instructor in Neurological Surgery
Director, Neuro-Ophthalmology Unit
Emory University School of Medicine
Atlanta, Georgia
Lecturer in Ophthalmology
Harvard Medical School
Boston, Massachusetts

Steven A. Newman, MD
Professor of Ophthalmology
University of Virginia
Director, Neuro-Ophthalmology
University of Virginia
Charlottesville, Virginia

David E. Newman-Toker, MD
Assistant Professor of Neurology and Ophthalmology
The Johns Hopkins University School of Medicine
Active Staff in Neurology
Johns Hopkins Hospital
Baltimore, Maryland

Paul H. Phillips, MD
Associate Professor of Ophthalmology
University of Arkansas for Medical Sciences
Department of Ophthalmology
Arkansas Childrens Hospital
Little Rock, Arkansas

Howard D. Pomeranz, MD, PhD
Associate Professor of Ophthalmology, Neurology, and
  Neurosurgery
University of Minnesota Medical School
Minneapolis, Minnesota

Valerie Purvin, MD
Clinical Professor of Ophthalmology and Neurology
Indiana University Medical Center
Chief, Neuro-Ophthalmology Service
Midwest Eye Institute
Methodist Hospital
Indianapolis, Indiana

Michael X. Repka, MD
Professor of Ophthalmology and Pediatrics
The Johns Hopkins School of Medicine
Department of Ophthalmology
The Johns Hopkins Hospital
Baltimore, Maryland

Joseph F. Rizzo III, MD
Associate Professor of Ophthalmology
The Massachusetts Eye and Ear Infirmary
Harvard Medical School
Director, Center for Innovative Visual Rehabilitation
Boston Veterans Administration Hospital
Boston, Massachusetts

Matthew Rizzo, MD
Professor of Neurology, Engineering, and Public Policy
Director, Division of Neuroergonomics
Carver College of Medicine
University of Iowa
Iowa City, Iowa

Janet C. Rucker, MD
Assistant Professor of Neurology
Case Western Reserve University
Staff Neurologist
University Hospitals
Cleveland, Ohio

Alfredo A. Sadun, MD, PhD
Thornton Chair
Professor of Ophthalmology and Neurological Surgery
Doheny Eye Institute
University of Southern California Keck School of
  Medicine
Los Angeles, California

Jane C. Sargent, MD
Professor of Clinical Neurology and Clinical Surgery
University of Massachusetts Medical School
Department of Neurology
University of Massachusetts Memorial Medical Center
Worcester, Massachusetts

James A. Sharpe, MD, FRCP(C)
Professor of Neurology
University of Toronto
Director of Neuro-Ophthalmology and Neuro-Otology
  Center
University Health Network
Toronto, Ontario, Canada

Barry Skarf, MD, PhD
Adjunct Associate Professor of Ophthalmology
University of Toronto
Toronto, Ontario, Canada
Director of Neuro-ophthalmology service
Henry Ford Hospital
Detroit, Michigan

Craig H. Smith, MD
Clinical Professor of Neurology, Medicine, and
  Ophthalmology
University of Washington
President, MS Hub Medical Group
Seattle, Washington

Kenneth David Steinsapir, MD
Assistant Clinical Professor of Ophthalmology
Jules Stein Eye Institute
David Geffen School of Medicine at the University of
  California-Los Angeles
Los Angeles, California

Prem S. Subramanian, MD, PhD
Assistant Professor of Surgery
Division of Ophthalmology
Uniformed Services University of the Health Sciences
Bethesda, Maryland
Director, Neuro-Ophthalmology
Walter Reed Army Medical Center
Washington, District of Columbia

Gregory P. Van Stavern, MD
Assistant Professor of Ophthalmology and
    Neurology
Wayne State University
Director of Neuro-Ophthalmology
Kresge Eye Institute
Detroit, Michigan

Michael S. Vaphiades, DO
Associate Professor of Ophthalmology, Neurology, and
    Neurosurgery
University of Alabama at Birmingham
Birmingham, Alabama

Nicholas J. Volpe, MD
Adele Niessen Associate Professor of Ophthalmology
    and Neurology
University of Pennsylvania School of Medicine
Vice Chairman, Residency Program Director
Scheie Eye Institute
Philadelphia, Pennsylvania

Michael Wall, MD
Professor of Neurology & Ophthalmology
University of Iowa College of Medicine
Veterans Administration Hospital
Iowa City, Iowa

Joel M. Weinstein, MD
Clinical Associate Professor of Ophthalmology & Visual
    Sciences and Neurology
University of Wisconsin
University of Wisconsin Hospital
Madison, Wisconsin

Jacqueline M. S. Winterkorn, MD, PhD
Clinical Professor of Ophthalmology and Neurology &
    Neuroscience
Weill Medical College of Cornell University
Attending in Ophthalmology and Neurology
The New York Presbyterian Hospital
New York, New York

Agnes M. F. Wong, MD, PhD, FRCSC
Assistant Professor of Ophthalmology and Neurology
University of Toronto
UHN-Toronto Western Hospital, and The Hospital for
    Sick Children
Toronto, Ontario, Canada
Assistant Professor (adjunct) of Ophthalmology and
    Visual Sciences
Washington University
St. Louis, Missouri

Rochelle S. Zak, MD
Clinical Instructor
Department of Neurology in Psychiatry
Weill Cornell Medical College
New York-Presbyterian Hospital
New York, New York

David S. Zee, MD
Professor of Neurology and Ophthalmology
The Johns Hopkins University School of Medicine
Baltimore, Maryland

Contents

Volume I

Section I: The Visual Sensory System

Section II: The Autonomic Nervous System

Section III: The Ocular Motor System

Section IV: The Eyelid

Section V: Facial Pain and Headache

Section VI: Nonorganic Disease

Volume II
Section VII: Tumors

Section VIII: The Phacomatoses

Section IX: Vascular Disease

Volume III
Section X: Degenerative and Metabolic Diseases

Section XI: Infectious, Inflammatory, and Demyelinating Diseases

SECTION I:
The Visual Sensory System

Nancy J. Newman, section editor

Each human optic nerve contains about 1.2 million axons, representing about 40% of all fibers entering or leaving the central nervous system (CNS). When the rods and cones are added to this number, the total number of sensory units that forward visual information to the brain is increased by a factor of 80. That number is increased further when one considers the millions of axons that transmit information from the lateral geniculate body to the striate cortex and from the striate cortex to other parts of the CNS. Thus, any physician who evaluates patients with disorders of vision must have knowledge of the embryology, anatomy, and physiology of the visual sensory system. This information is covered in the first chapter of this section. The second chapter describes the principles and techniques of examination of the visual sensory system. The ophthalmoscopic recognition and differential diagnosis of swelling or pallor of the optic disc and their distinction from congenital disc anomalies are of fundamental importance not only to the ophthalmologist but also to the neurologist, neurosurgeon, and other physicians. Chapters 3–11 are devoted to the symptoms, signs, pathogenesis, and various etiologies of both anterior (with optic disc swelling) and retrobulbar (with an initially normal disc) optic neuropathies and optic atrophy and to their differentiation from congenital disc anomalies. Knowledge of the various disorders that affect the optic chiasm, tracts, radiations, and striate cortex are also important to the physician dealing with patients complaining of visual dysfunction, as is an understanding of the so-called "central" (also called "higher") disorders of visual function. The last two chapters of this section deal with the features of such disorders.

CHAPTER 1

Embryology, Anatomy, and Physiology of the Afferent Visual Pathway

Joseph F. Rizzo III

The brain devotes more cells and connections to vision than any other sense or motor function. This chapter presents an overview of the development, anatomy, and physiology of this extremely complex but fascinating system. Of necessity, the subject matter is greatly abridged, although special attention is given to principles that relate to clinical neuro-ophthalmology.

Light initiates a cascade of cellular responses in the retina that begins as a slow, graded response of the photoreceptors and transforms into a volley of coordinated action potentials at the level of the retinal ganglion cells (RGCs), the axons of which form the optic nerve. The outflow of visual signals from photoreceptors is parsed into parallel pathways that are distributed to the diencephalon, midbrain, lateral geniculate body, primary visual cortex, and beyond. These pathways are broadly divided into three major streams—the parvocel-

lular, magnocellular, and koniocellular pathways—each of which contributes to visual processing at the primary visual cortex. Beyond the primary visual cortex, two streams of information flow develop: the dorsal stream, primarily for detection of where objects are and for motion perception, and the ventral stream, primarily for detection of what objects are (including their color, depth, and form). At every level of the visual system, however, information among these "parallel" pathways is shared by intercellular, thalamic-cortical, and intercortical connections. The mechanisms by which the visual system uses these data streams to create vision remain mysterious and are beyond the current grasp of technology, although recent multichannel recordings within associative visual cortices are providing insights into how complex visual scenes are assembled by the brain.

RETINA

EMBRYOLOGY OF THE EYE AND RETINA

The sensory retina is a part of the central nervous system (CNS). The retina develops from the *optic cup*, a structure formed by the invagination of the lateral walls of the *optic vesicles*, which emerge as outpouchings of the prosencephalon during the third week of gestation (1–3) (Fig. 1.1). The invagination is dependent upon a temporally specific association of the developing optic vesicle with the overlying prelens ectoderm (4). The outer wall of the optic cup becomes the retinal pigment epithelium (RPE), while the inner wall mostly develops into the sensory retina (3).

Several highly conserved genes contribute to the formation of the eye and retina (5). The optic cup and optic stalk express *Pax-2* and *Pax-6*, which belong to a family of transcription factors involved in the regulation of early development. *Pax-2* expression occurs in cells that will form the optic fissure (which develops at the future site of the optic nerve head) and the optic stalk (which becomes the optic nerve) (6). Pax-6 expression occurs in cells that will become the neural retina (and most of the eye except the cornea and lens) (7).

The general principles of retinal development are as follows (2,8). Ganglion cells develop first, at the seventh week of gestation. Amacrine and horizontal cells develop next. Connections among amacrine cells and RGCs create a nascent inner nuclear layer (INL), at which time bipolar and Müller cells differentiate. Cones, which appear before rods, develop around the same time as the horizontal cells, but both cones and rods do not mature until after connections within the inner retina begin to form. Maturation of the photoreceptors leads to formation of the outer plexiform layer (OPL), which establishes connections among photoreceptors and horizontal and bipolar cells (Fig. 1.2). Each Müller cell may be the kernel of a functionally intertwined "columnar unit"—each Müller cell (in the rabbit) ensheathes a collection of rods, bipolar cells, and amacrine cells, with each cell class having a precisely maintained ratio to Müller cells across the retina (9).

Generation of cells from the neuroepithelial (or neuroblastic) layers is followed by their differentiation, and most differentiated cells then migrate through the developing retina. RGCs migrate inward, leaving in their wake an acellular region that is developing into an expanded inner plexiform layer (IPL) (Fig. 1.3). Simultaneously, horizontal cells migrate inward and combine with cells of the inner neuroblastic layer to form the INL. Photoreceptors remain stationary. Determination of cell number for each cell class is controlled by expression of the homeodomain protein *Prox 1*, which regulates the timing at which dividing cells become quiescent (10). Fibroblastic growth factors and hedgehog (Hh) proteins also are important for retinal development and RGC axon guidance (11). N-cadherin plays a crucial role in the

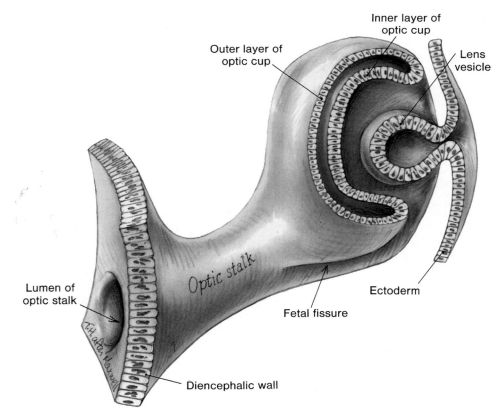

Figure 1.1. The formation of the optic vesicle and cup in a 7.5-mm (5-week) human embryo. Note that the stalk has two separate regions, a distal invaginated, crescent-shaped segment and a proximal noninvaginated circular segment. The lens vesicle is formed by an invagination of the pre-lens ectoderm, which in turn prompts the invagination of the optic cup. (Redrawn from Hamilton WJ, Boyd JD, Mossman HW. Human Embryology. Baltimore, Williams & Wilkins, 1962.)

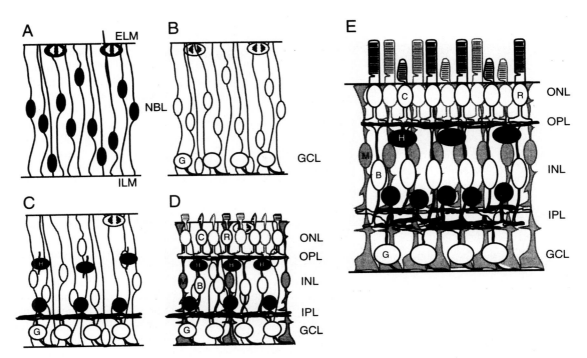

Figure 1.2. Basic structure and temporal order of cell differentiation of the vertebrate retina. *A*, The neural retina begins as a sheet of neuroepithelial cells (NBL, neuroblastic layer) with processes that contact the internal (ILM) and external (ELM) limiting membranes. *B*, Ganglion cells (G) are the first cell type to differentiate and migrate toward the ILM to form the ganglion cell layer (GCL). *C*, Amacrine cells (A) and horizontal cells (H) differentiate next. Cone photoreceptors are born at this stage but do not differentiate until later. The first network of connections, between amacrine cells and ganglion cells, is established as a continuous inner plexiform layer (IPL) across the retina. *D*, In the inner nuclear layer (INL), bipolar cells (B) and Müller cells (M) are generated and differentiate. At this stage, both cone (C) and rod (R) photoreceptors composing the outer nuclear layer (ONL) begin to mature, bearing few outer segments or discs. The outer plexiform layer (OPL) emerges, and connections between photoreceptors, horizontal cells, and bipolar cells are formed. Cell genesis (mainly rods) continues at this stage but to a greatly reduced degree. *E*, At maturity, all cell types are present, connections in both plexiform layers are established, and photoreceptor outer segments are well developed. (From Chalupa LM, Werner JS, eds. The Visual Neurosciences. Cambridge, MA, MIT Press, 2004:78.)

development of lamination within the retina (12). RGCs may regulate the ultimate number of amacrine cells by secreting brain-derived neurotrophic factor (13).

RGC axonal guidance is partially directed by *EphA* receptor tyrosine kinases (14). EphA receptors are expressed on all RGC axons, but only temporal axons have receptors with high ligand sensitivity. The differential (i.e., temporal versus nasal) sensitivity is determined by varying degrees of phosphorylation of the EphA receptor, which (in the chick) is controlled by relatively greater expression of *ephrin-A6* in the nasal retina (15). The relatively low state of phosphorylation of EphA receptors on temporal axons increases their sensitivity, which allows them to respond to low concentrations of ephrin-A ligands at the tectal termination zone. Proper topography at the tectum is also at least partially controlled by variable expression of ephrin-A at that location (16). Neuronal activity (via *N*-methyl-D-aspartate [NMDA] receptors) and expression of nitric oxide also contribute to topographic precision (17–19). Embryonic spontaneous activity of RGCs, which is regulated by γ-aminobutyric acid (GABA) receptor activity, specifically GABA, receptorac-

tivity, influences a competitive selection process that determines the final number of RGCs and their pattern of synaptic arrangement at their termination sites (20). Apoptosis eliminates noncompetitive RGCs (21).

BASIC ANATOMY AND PHYSIOLOGY

Retinal Pigment Epithelium

The RPE is a monolayer of cells whose development in lower vertebrates involves expression of Hh proteins (Fig. 1.3). Peripherally, in the homologous zone of the pigmented ciliary epithelium in mammals, expression of Hh proteins is associated with the presence of retinal stem cells that retain a capacity to differentiate into any type of retinal neuron, which has therapeutic implications (22).

The RPE has several functions. It (*a*) regenerates chromophore; (*b*) provides trophic support for photoreceptors; (*c*) is a transport barrier between the choriocapillaris and the sensory retina; (*d*) participates in ocular immune responses; (*e*) binds reactive oxygen species; and (*f*) absorbs excess radiation with their melanin granules. These granules can

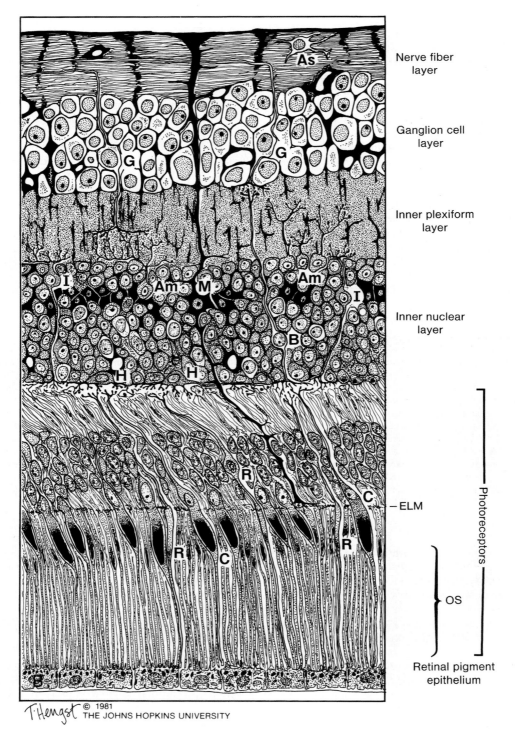

Figure 1.3. Cellular components of the fully developed primate retina, showing cellular relationships and major synaptic interactions. OPL, outer plexiform layer; ONL, outer nuclear layer; ELM, external limiting membrane; OS, outer segment; As, astrocyte; G, ganglion cell; Am, amacrine cell; I, interplexiform cell; H, horizontal cell; B, bipolar cell; c, cone; R, rod; M, Müller cell. The photoreceptor nuclei lie in the ONL, and a large stretch of the photoreceptors consists of their outer segments, which lie proximal (i.e., nearer to the retinal pigment epithelium) to their nuclei. The outer segments contain chromophore, which captures the energy from incoming light and initiates the ionic exchange that hyperpolarizes the photoreceptors. The inner segments of photoreceptors (not labeled) are the segments between the outer segments and the nucleus that contain a high concentration of mitochondria and endoplasmic reticulum.

bind photosensitizing drugs, like hydroxychloroquine, and cause blindness by interfering with the ability of the RPE to support the photoreceptors (23). RGCs are also damaged by hydroxychloroquine, although presumably by some other mechanism.

Eyes of almost any species detect light in basically the same manner. The process begins when rhodopsin molecules located on the horizontal discs of the outer segment of photoreceptors (Fig. 1.4) capture photons, which causes isomerization of 11-*cis*-retinal to all-*trans*-retinal (24,25). This reaction initiates the phototransduction cascade that ultimately influences the propagation of nerve impulses through the retina. Regeneration of 11-*cis*-retinal, which is necessary to maintain the responsiveness of photoreceptors to light, is performed by the RPE (Fig. 1.5). Interphotoreceptor retinol binding protein (IRBP) contributes to this process by binding retinols and retinals (which alone are highly insoluble) and escorting them to and from the RPE (26,27). Generation of the 11-*cis* chromophore in vertebrates requires the enzyme *RPE65*. Mutations in RPE65 cause Leber congenital amau-

rosis (LCA), the most common inherited form of childhood blindness. Gene therapy in the RPE65 null mutation dog model has produced some recovery of vision, which is the first molecular genetic therapeutic success for blindness (28). In total, six genes preferentially expressed in the retina or RPE account for half of all LCA cases (29). The metabolic strategies used to regenerate 11-*cis* chromophore are remarkably conserved across species, but only for rods. Cones regenerate their respective photopigments by interactions with Müller (not RPE) cells (30). However photopigment regeneration is achieved, sluggishness in doing so interferes with vision by causing an abnormally prolonged recovery of central vision following exposure to bright light, as is often reported by patients with a maculopathy.

Sensory Retina and Glial Cells

The human retina contains over 110 million neurons, among which are approximately 55 cell types that use at least 10 neurotransmitters (31–33). The functions of about

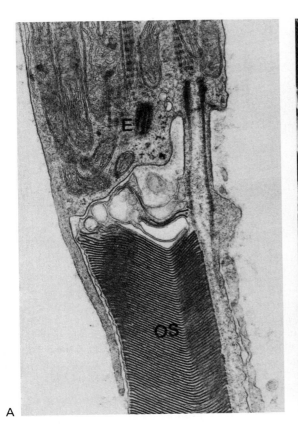
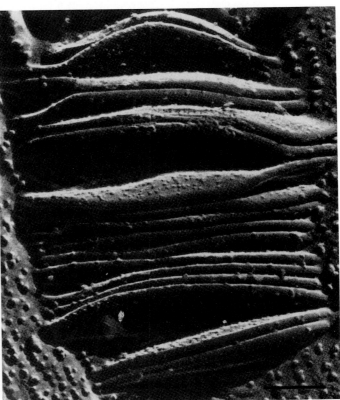

A   B

Figure 1.4. *A,* Electron micrograph of a rod, showing the outer segment (OS) connected to the ellipsoid (E). Note the horizontal disc membranes, which represent the bulk of the outer segment, and the numerous mitochondria within the ellipsoid portion of the inner segment. *B,* A portion of amphibian rod outer segment showing a stack of disc membranes. The segment was treated with low salt to strip away the plasma membrane, rapidly frozen, etched to expose the disc surfaces, and unidirectionally shadowed with a mixture of platinum and carbon. The small bumps scattered across the cytoplasmic surface of each membrane are transducin molecules. Bar = 0.1 μm. (*A,* From Hogan MJ, Alvarado JA, Weddell JC. Histology of the Human Eye: An Atlas and Textbook. Philadelphia, WB Saunders, 1971. *B,* From Roof D, Heuser J. Surfaces of rod photoreceptor disk membranes: integral membrane components. J Cell Biol 1982;95:487–500.)

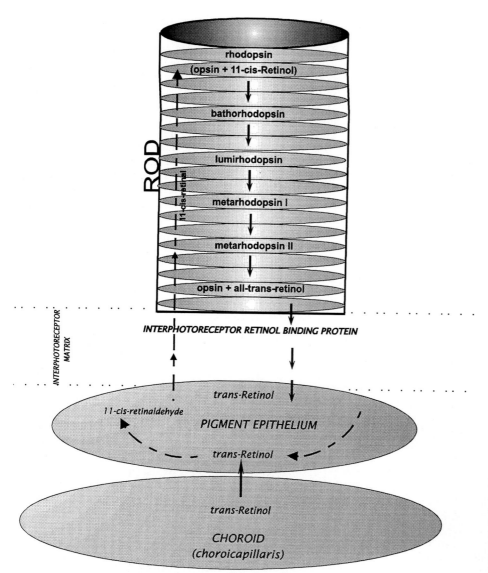

Figure 1.5. Phototransduction cascade. Junction of rod, retinal pigment epithelium, and choroid shows the interrelationship among those structures required to regenerate photopigment. *Trans*-retinol is carried by the blood to the choriocapillaris, where it can then enter the retinal pigment epithelium and contribute to the cycle.

22 of these cells are known or reasonably well appreciated. This base of knowledge makes the retina the best-understood area of the more complex regions of the brain (34).

Most architectural schemas fail to represent the intricacy of the retina because retinal function depends on a variety of factors, including the region of the retina being illuminated, the characteristics of the light stimulus, and the state of light adaptation. For instance, colors of short wavelength are relatively more apparent when viewed under dim rather than bright light because of the shift toward rod function in the scotopic state (i.e., the Purkinje shift). Given this complexity, one might imagine that a large number of symptoms would result from dysfunction of these many cell types. On the contrary, most clinically recognized diseases of the retina are limited to dysfunction of either photoreceptors or RGCs. Undoubtedly, new patterns of visual loss secondary to mal-function of other retinal neurons will be recognized in the future.

The retina contains six classes of neurons that are arranged into three parallel layers (Table 1.1), except in the perifovea, where the retina thins to a single layer. The retina also contains three types of glial cells—astrocytes and Müller cells, and a smaller number of microglia.

Photoreceptors

The photoreceptors are the primary sensory transducers of the visual system. Photoreceptor pigments respond to wavelengths of light (400–700 nm) that are not absorbed by the optical media and hence reach the retina. Most vertebrate eyes contain two types of photoreceptors, rods and cones. A small number of RGCs also contain an opsin and are capable of responding to light (discussed later).

Table 1.1
Cellular Organization of the Retina

Cell Layer	Neuronal and Glial Nuclei
Outer nuclear layer	Photoreceptors
Inner nuclear layer	Horizontal cells
	Bipolar cells
	Interplexiform cells
	Amacrine cells
	Müller cells
Ganglion cell layer	Ganglion cells
	Displaced amacrine cells
	Astrocytes

Rods contain rhodopsin, a molecule that is composed of the apoprotein, opsin, and 11-*cis*-retinal (35). A rod (and cone) "*Rim*" protein, which is encoded by the *ABCA4* gene, is the transmembrane transporter of vitamin A intermediates needed for the visual cycle. Mutations in this gene produce Stargardt macular dystrophy and fundus flavimaculatus (36). Once in the extracellular space, vitamin A intermediates are shuttled by the IRBP to the RPE (discussed previously).

Rhodopsin is present in very high concentrations within the membranes of the outer segment discs (Fig. 1.4), which are oriented vertically to maximize capture of incident photons. The efficiency of this system is so great that single photons can initiate the phototransduction cascade (37), although in the dark-adapted (i.e., the most sensitive) state, about five photons are needed to induce light perception. Photon capture causes phosphorylation of rhodopsin. This step, which initiates the phototransduction cascade, can be modulated by recoverin, a 23-kD intracellular protein that inhibits rhodopsin kinase, which in turn inhibits the phosphorylation of rhodopsin. Antibodies to recoverin, which may push the photoreceptors into a persistent state of hyperpolarization (because of prolonged phosphorylation of rhodopsin), may be found in association with apoptosis-induced photoreceptor death in patients with small cell carcinoma who develop cancer-associated retinopathy (38,39).

Activation of the phototransduction cascade causes an intracellular decline in the guanosine cyclic monophosphate (cGMP) concentration within rod outer segments, followed by closure of the cGMP-gated cation channel and cessation of inflow of the extracellular cations that generate the "dark current." The resultant hyperpolarization decreases neurotransmitter (i.e., glutamate) release at the synaptic terminal (Fig. 1.6). The decline in cGMP after light exposure is caused by activation of rod outer segment phosphodiesterase (PDE), specifically *PDE-6*. Inhibition of PDE, as occurs with sildenafil (which mainly inhibits PDE-5, but also weakly inhibits PDE-6), increases the cGMP concentration, which opens sodium channels and depolarizes the rods. This effect may account for the transient disturbance of color (typically blue-yellow) vision reported by some users of sildenafil (40,41).

Vitamin A is used in phototransduction and photopigment regeneration. Vitamin A must be replenished from the circulation, and failure to do so can result in retinopathy. Since rods are predominately affected in vitamin A deficiency retinopathy, nyctalopia is usually the initial visual symptom. The retinopathy of vitamin A deficiency is reversible if treatment is prompt enough. Hypovitaminosis A is a leading cause of blindness in developing countries, but it also occurs in developed countries in patients with malabsorption syndromes, liver disease, or restrictive diets (42–44). A wide range of genetic mutations that interfere with vitamin A (i.e., all-*trans* retinol) metabolism may cause blindness (45).

Cones also contain 11-*cis*-retinal but have different apoproteins than rods. Variation of the opsin moiety produces three spectral response curves that correspond to the blue, green, and red cones, which are more appropriately called short (S-), medium (M-), and long (L-) wavelength cones to emphasize that their responsiveness spans across a portion of the visible spectrum. The amino acid sequences of rhodopsin and the three cone pigments have been characterized (46). Antibodies to the three cone pigments have revealed mosaics for each photoreceptor class in the primate retina. Human cone mosaics can be noninvasively visualized in a living eye (47).

Congenital dyschromatopsia is usually caused by loss or significant alteration in the red or green photopigment gene(s), which are located on the X chromosome and which are 98% homologous with one another (46). Anomalous trichromacy, a more minor defect, is caused by gene hybridization. Among individuals with "normal" color vision, there is a surprisingly large variation in performance (7–8 nm range in peak spectral responsiveness), presumably due to polymorphic variations in human M- and L-cone pigments (48) and variation in the relative number of M- and L-cones (49).

Humans have a cone-to-rod ratio of approximately 1 : 20, with each retina containing 92 million rods and 4.6 million cones, on average. Rods are absent or only rarely present in the fovea (Fig. 1.7) and are in highest density in an elliptical ring that passes through the optic nerve. Fifty percent of cones in the human retina are located within the central 30 degrees of the visual field (50), an area that roughly corresponds to the size of the macula. There is an age-related decline in the number of rods in human retina, with an annual loss of about 0.2–0.4% (51). The age effect upon cones is less clear (52).

The human fovea matures anatomically just prior to 4 years of age (53). By this time, the outer segments of the foveal cones attain a width of only 1.0 μm, which permits very high spatial resolution (i.e., acuity). The high density of foveal cones poses a structural problem because the cone synaptic terminals, known as pedicles, and the RGCs to which they connect have larger diameters than the cone inner segments. Thus, each foveal ganglion cell soma is displaced from the cone that provides its input. This resulting horizontal displacement occurs via the *nerve fiber layer of Henle*, an elongation of photoreceptors between their nuclei and their synaptic terminals (Fig. 1.7). Deposition of hard exudates within the Henle layer produces the clinical sign of a "macular star."

As described previously, retinal neurons mature at different times, influencing the timing of their respective synaptic

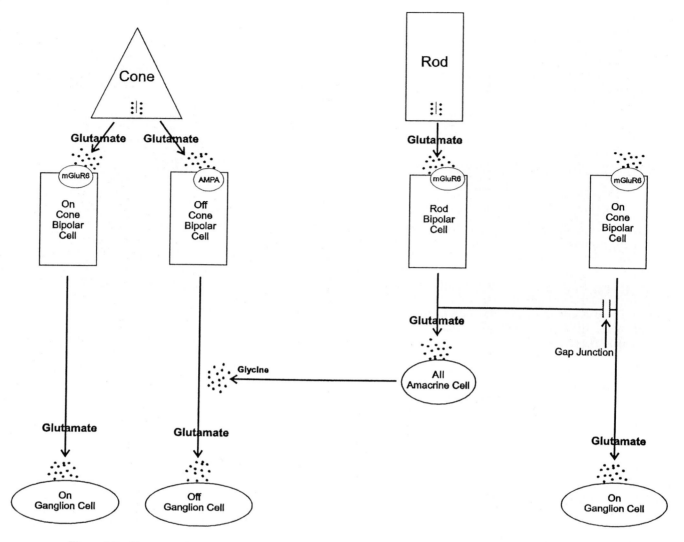

Figure 1.6. Neurotransmitters used by retinal neurons of the rod and cone pathways. The neurotransmitters are released within the outer and inner plexiform layers. The mGluR6 and AMPA receptors (see text) of the bipolar cells are also depicted. The former uses a G protein to control the intracellular concentration of cGMP that, in turn, regulates the Na^+-Ca^{2+}-cGMP-gated ion channel.

connections. There is a prodigious expansion of synapses for several years after birth, which doubles the width of the IPL between birth and adulthood. The human foveal outflow pathway (cones to ganglion cells) develops more quickly, with synapses being established possibly as early as midgestation (54). During the period of synaptogenesis, widespread neuronal death can occur if there is significant exposure to ethanol because of disruption of glutamate and GABA neurotransmitter systems (55). The complex process of retinal development does not occur without flaws, in that seemingly misplaced cones and cone bipolar and horizontal cells are not infrequently observed in the retina (56,57).

The normal delay in achieving adult visual performance for spatial resolution and various other tasks may extend to 3 years postpartum (58) and is probably related to both reti-

nal and central factors (59). An abnormal delay in achieving normal vision occurs in patients with delayed maturation of the visual system, which results from excessively slow myelination along the afferent visual pathway (60).

The synaptic terminals of photoreceptors contain ribbon synapses, which are specialized synaptic features found only in the retina and pineal gland. Ribbon synapses guide synaptic vesicles to preferred sites on the presynaptic membrane in preparation for their release. Photoreceptor synapses usually exist as a triad, which comprises one bipolar and two horizontal cells. Gap junctions are ion channels through which pass ions and molecules without typical synaptic specializations. Gap junctions, which are formed by alignment of two connexin hexamers, create a cellular syncytium. Gap junctions normally exist between adjacent photoreceptors and are

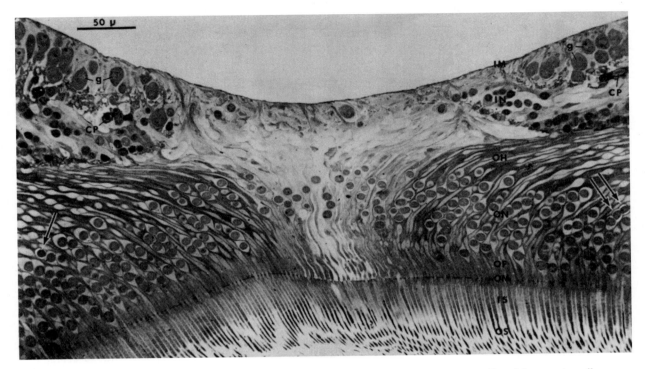

Figure 1.7. Section through center of fovea. Nuclei of rod receptor cells are indicated by *arrows*. Remaining receptor cells are foveal cone cells. Os, outer nuclear layer; of, outer cone fiber; oh, outer fiber layer of Henle; in, inner nuclear layer; ip, inner plexiform layer; g, ganglion cell; cp, capillary; im, internal limiting membrane; is, inner segment; om, outer limiting membrane; on, outer nuclear layer (reduced from ×400). (From Yamada E. Some structural features of the fovea centralis in the human retina. Arch Ophthalmol 1969;82:151–159.)

typically present near their synaptic terminals. Gap junctions also occur between horizontal cells, between amacrine cells, and between bipolar and amacrine cells.

Photoreceptor terminals contain dystrophin, the cytoskeletal protein that is a product of the Duchenne muscular dystrophy (DMD) gene. Patients with DMD can have an abnormal electroretinogram (ERG) that reveals abnormal transmission between photoreceptors and ON-bipolar cells. The role of dystrophin in the retina is not known, although there are three isoforms distributed widely on neurons, blood vessels and Müller cell end-feet, where dystrophin influences the formation of potassium channels (61,62).

Horizontal Cells

Photoreceptors and horizontal and bipolar (discussed later) cells synapse in the OPL (Fig. 1.8). Humans have two types of horizontal cells, both of which have axons. The HI cell, the smaller of the two, makes dendritic contact with cones and axonal contact with rods, whereas both ends of the HII cell synapse with cones. Both horizontal cell types appear to contact all three types of cones, which suggests that color input to horizontal cells is not spectrally selective (63), although in macaque monkeys specific contact occurs between horizontal cells and blue cones (64). Horizontal cells provide an inhibitory feedback to cones via hemi-channels (i.e., one part of a normally dual component gap junc-

tion), through which electrical current alters the release of glutamate by modulating the calcium channels of cones (65).

Given the length and small diameter of the HII axon, it is unlikely that the cell body and axon terminal of the same cell influence one another electrically (66). On the other hand, the axon of the HII cell can extend several millimeters, which presumably allows this cell to influence signal transmission over a very wide area. The presence of gap junctions, which permit electrical potentials to spread among cells, probably further extends the effective reach of horizontal cells. An increase in extracellular dopamine or nitric oxide, as occurs in the light-adapted state, closes gap junctions between horizontal cells. Constraining the horizontal spread of electrical signals between horizontal cells may be one mechanism by which central acuity is enhanced under photopic conditions. The interplexiform cell (discussed later) may be the source of dopamine in the OPL.

Horizontal cells may provide the anatomic substrate for the concentric, circular, antagonistic, center-surround response characteristics of RGCs and bipolar cells. Specifically, the response of RGC to light that falls within the center of its receptive field (which matches the dendritic arbor of the cell) is opposite to that which occurs if the same light stimulus falls within its "surround" (i.e., that portion of the receptive field concentric to but beyond the center). The antagonistic center-surround response property emphasizes contrast within the visual scene by generating marked

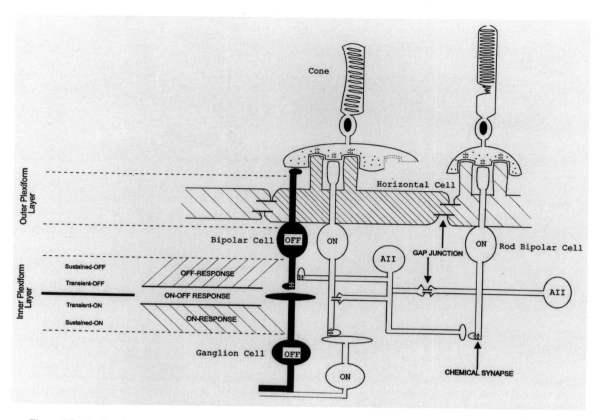

Figure 1.8. Rod and cone through pathways to the retinal ganglion cells. The photoreceptor synaptic terminals (i.e., the cone pedicles and rod spherules) have flat and invaginating surfaces upon which bipolar and horizontal cells make contact within the outer plexiform layer. AII amacrine cells and bipolar cells contact one another within the inner plexiform layer, which is subdivided into zones that contain synapses of either ON center or OFF center cells. In particular, the OFF zone, which is closer to the photoreceptors, is known as sublamina *a*, and the ON zone, which is nearer to the vitreous, is known as sublamina *b*. Sites of chemical (i.e., ribbon) synapses and gap junctions between cells are labeled or indicated by symbols (=, gap junction; *four small circles, two on each side of a small line,* chemical synapse); AII, AII amacrine cell.

differences in the responsiveness of cells at precise points across the retina (Fig. 1.9). Enhanced contrast improves spatial resolution, which underlies the routine use of high-contrast charts to measure the best-corrected acuity of patients. In the macaque, the HI cell, which is not highly electrically coupled to other HI cells, has a relatively small receptive field that may form the "surround" of foveal midget cell outflow (67), which provides the greatest spatial resolution in the retina. The center-surround profile is maintained, although altered somewhat, at the dorsal lateral geniculate nucleus (dLGN) (discussed later).

Bipolar Cells

Bipolar cells receive input from photoreceptors and provide output to amacrine and RGCs. There are roughly 17 types of bipolar cells, which can be broadly divided into ON and OFF cells, midget cells, and diffuse cells. Some receive input solely from rods (i.e., rod bipolar cells), whereas others receive input solely from cones (i.e., cone bipolar cells). There is only one type of rod bipolar cell, which begins at invaginations of the rod synaptic terminal (i.e., spherule) and

extends to sublamina *b* of the IPL to synapse exclusively with an AII amacrine cell (discussed later) (Fig. 1.8). The rod pathway, therefore, is formed by sequential connections from rods to rod bipolar cells to AII amacrine cells to RGCs.

Two main types of cone bipolar cells can be distinguished by whether they make an invaginating or a flat synapse at the photoreceptor terminal. These synaptic structures correspond to the IPL termination site of the cells' dendrites. Invaginating cone bipolar cells terminate more vitreally in the IPL within sublamina *b*, whereas flat cone bipolar cells terminate more proximally in sublamina *a*. This anatomic segregation is of fundamental importance in that bipolar cells whose processes ramify in sublamina *b* produce more action potentials when their receptive field centers are stimulated with light (i.e., ON cells). Conversely, bipolar cells whose dendrites ramify in sublamina *a* become more quiet when their receptive field centers are covered with light (i.e., OFF cells) (Fig. 1.8).

The midget outflow pathway provides the most spatially detailed visual profile. Midget cells dominate the center of the retina but are also present peripherally (68,69). Centrally, the midget system is organized such that each M or L cone

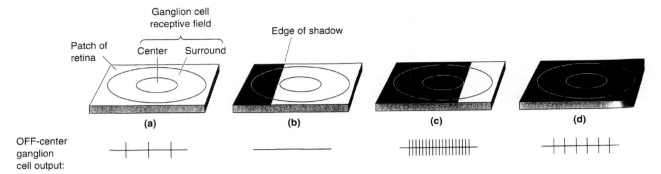

Figure 1.9. Center-surround organization of retinal ganglion cell receptive fields, and the resultant output of a ganglion cell in response to a light-dark border falling within its receptive field. Depicted is an OFF center ganglion cell, which responds most vigorously when a dark spot precisely fills its receptive field center. The responsiveness of the cell is diminished by darkness that covers its surround. The output in (*a*) is the resting, basal level of spontaneous action potentials, which are a characteristic feature of all retinal ganglion cells. In (*b*), the output is decreased because the darkness falls only across the inhibitory surround. In (*c*), the responsiveness is greatly enhanced because darkness fills the excitatory center of this OFF cell. In (*d*), the cellular output is above the basal level of activity because the receptive field center is filled by darkness, despite the fact that the entire surround is also covered by darkness. (From Bear MF, Connors BW, Paradiso MA. Neuroscience. Exploring the Brain. 2nd ed. Baltimore, Lippincott Williams & Wilkins, 2001:306.)

contacts one ON and one OFF center bipolar cell, and each bipolar cell contacts only one cone. In the fovea, OFF RGCs receive input from only one (OFF) bipolar cell, whereas ON RGCs may receive input from up to three (ON) bipolar cells, although at the synaptic level only one bipolar cell dominates. This organizational pattern shifts across the retina. In the parafovea, *all* midget RGCs receive input from only one midget bipolar cell, although more peripherally they receive input from up to four bipolar cells (69). In the periphery, midget bipolar cells can receive input from up to 12 cones. In contrast, in the peripheral retina one RGC may receive input from up to 1,500 rods through bipolar cells (70).

The ON signal in the blue (i.e., short wavelength) pathway does not pass through a midget bipolar cell; rather, a special S-cone ON bipolar cell receives ON input from S-cones. In the fovea, the dendritic arbor of this bipolar cell is so small that it receives input from only one S-cone. Each S-cone also contacts an OFF midget bipolar cell (71). The blue pathway also uses a special RGC—the small, bistratified cell (discussed later).

The major excitatory neurotransmitter in the retina is glutamate. Photoreceptors are hyperpolarized by light, which decreases their release of glutamate. Reduced glutamate concentration within the OPL causes two opposing effects on bipolar cells (Fig. 1.6). For OFF center bipolar cells, decreased glutamate at their ionotrophic (i.e., ion-exchanging) alpha-amino-3-hydroxy-5-methyl-4 isoxazole propionic acid (AMPA) glutamate receptors hyperpolarizes the cell, thus conserving the sign of the response with respect to the photoreceptor. ON center bipolar cells, however, possess a different receptor, a metabotropic glutamate receptor (mGluR6) that drives ion exchange via a second messenger system. The metabotropic receptor becomes active by changing its conformation after binding to glutamate. Decreased glutamate concentration, therefore, reduces the activity of the mGluR6 receptor, which increases the intracellular con-

centration of cGMP; this, in turn, opens cation channels that depolarize the cell. As such, release of glutamate by photoreceptors initiates two opposing but parallel signals to the inner retina (72). These ON and OFF bipolar responses are matched to two RGCs of the same physiologic type. Rod bipolar cells also have a metabotropic receptor; hence, they become depolarized when rods are activated by light.

Bipolar cells may be the target of a paraneoplastic immune attack in some patients with cutaneous malignant melanoma (73). The primary physiologic impact is loss of the scotopic b-wave of the ERG, similar to that seen in patients with congenital stationary night blindness (74). The persistence of the scotopic a-wave in eyes in this melanoma-associated retinopathy (MAR) indicates that the rods are responsive to light, whereas loss of the b-wave is evidence of a blocked transmission distal to the rod synapses. Selective immunohistochemical staining suggests that the signal blockage is caused by dysfunction of rod bipolar cells. MAR patients also exhibit abnormal ERG cone "ON" responses, which suggests that the primary deficit may be generalized dysfunction of depolarizing ("ON") bipolar cells (75,76). Antibipolar cell antibodies have also been found in a patient with a paraneoplastic retinopathy secondary to colon cancer (77).

Amacrine Cells

Amacrine cells were named in the belief that they lacked axons, which is now recognized not to be universally true. Unlike axons of RGCs, amacrine cell axons, when present, do not enter the optic nerve. There are 26–40 types of amacrine cells (71,78), most of which have somas that lie at the inner border of the INL, although some somas are "displaced" into the ganglion cell layer. In the peripheral retina, the spatial density of amacrine cells within the ganglion cell layer can exceed that of RGCs. Some amacrine cells are interneurons between bipolar and RGCs. Others connect to fellow amacrine cells, forming a lateral pathway within the IPL reminiscent of horizontal cells that ramify within the OPL. These different subtypes can be differentiated according to various criteria, including the shape of the cell, the zone or zones in which their dendrites ramify within the IPL, and their neurotransmitter(s) (Fig. 1.10).

The most numerous amacrine cell is the AII cell, which is an integral part of the rod pathway. Outflow of rod bipolar cells is entirely to sublamina *b* of the IPL, which indicates that rod outflow is entirely ON in nature. The AII cell receives and then transmits this ON rod signal to one cone ON and one cone OFF center bipolar cell. Both cone bipolar cells transmit their signals to RGCs of the same physiologic type (Fig. 1.8). Rods, therefore, influence both ON and OFF pathways, despite having only one of the two bipolar cell types found in the cone pathway. This architecture is an apparent conservation of resources for the highly preponderant rod pathway that contains roughly 92 million rods (versus 5 million cones) in humans.

"Starburst" amacrine cells exist as equal populations of ON and OFF varieties (79). These cells have several interesting features. Starburst cells release acetylcholine in response to light stimulation and also have the capacity to generate GABA, although they do not release GABA in response to light (80). Acetylcholine also "leaks" out of the cell in darkness, a phenomenon of unknown significance that is similar to the leakage of acetylcholine that occurs at the neuromuscular junction (81). Starburst cells are presynaptic to three cell types: amacrine cells, bipolar cells, and dendrites of "direction-selective" RGCs (82). The role of starburst cells in motion detection is revealed by the fact that they do not develop in mouse embryos that are genetically modified so as not to develop extraocular muscles (83).

An odd-shaped, polyaxonal amacrine cell (with a small dendritic field but many widely ramifying axons) has recently been recognized as playing an important role in distinguishing movement of an image against a stationary background. It is biologically important to distinguish such *relative* movement from the type of global movement of the visual scene that occurs during saccades and microsaccades. The "suppression" of vision during a saccade was believed to be a cortical phenomenon. However, the discovery of the polyaxonal amacrine cell indicates that visual suppression during some eye movements begins in the retina. This function is accomplished with a specialized RGC that responds only when movement has a different trajectory across the center versus surround of its receptive field (i.e., relative movement) (84,85).

Nitric oxide synthase (NOS) is found in some amacrine cells, but its function is unknown. It has been observed that release of nitric oxide is associated with neuronal injury (via a second messenger) and that upregulation of NOS-containing retinal cells occurs following reperfusion of the retina after a period of induced ischemia (86), perhaps because of excessive glutamate stimulation caused by the ischemia. Further, degeneration of RGCs following axotomy may be secondary to upregulation of NOS (87). Generation of nitric oxide, however, does not necessarily injure neurons; for instance, the endothelial isoform of nitric oxide is protective.

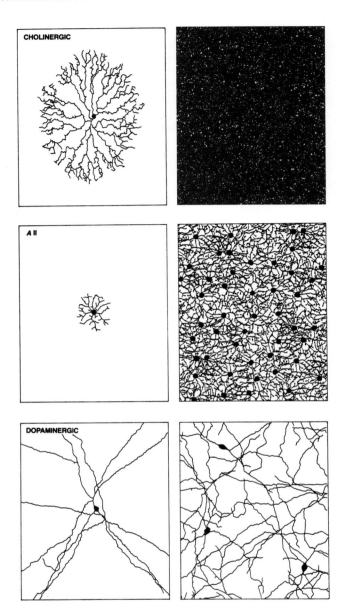

Figure 1.10. Mosaics of various anatomically distinct amacrine cells showing their different dendritic patterns. Three cell types are shown, all in flat view. Individual cells are at the *left;* the drawings at the *right* were synthesized on the basis of average cell shape and density and show an approximation of the mosaic that would result if all the cells of that particular class were seen simultaneously. *Top,* Cholinergic amacrine cells are numerous, and their branching dendrites form an almost uninterrupted meshwork. *Center,* the mosaic of AII amacrine cells is sparser, and there is more space among their dendrites. *Bottom,* Dopaminergic amacrine cells are sparser still. (From Masland RH. The functional architecture of the retina. Sci Am 1986;255:102–111.)

A dopaminergic amacrine cell has been identified in the retinas of all species that have been appropriately examined (88). Dopaminergic amacrine cells have far-reaching dendrites that contact cone bipolar cells (Fig. 1.10); however, they also synapse with AII and other amacrine cells that are part of the rod pathway. Thus, the dopaminergic amacrine cell contributes to both rod and cone outflow pathways. Retinal dopamine also plays a role in light adaptation. Dopamine, which is released during light exposure, uncouples gap junctions in horizontal cells. In this way, dopamine acts as a neuromodulator in that it can affect the function of nearby neurons in the absence of synaptic connections to those neurons. Dopamine also can be neuroprotective, given its ability to inhibit NOS-induced glutamate toxicity (89). Dopaminergic amacrine cells spontaneously generate action potentials in a rhythmic fashion, at least in vitro (90,91). These rhythmic potentials emanate specifically from interplexiform neurons, which have their cell bodies in the IPL and extend their axons to the OPL, and thus convey information opposite to the direction of normal retinal outflow (92–96). Dopaminergic neurons in the midbrain also show spontaneous action potentials.

A clinical form of amacrine cell blindness may occur following endoscopic surgery of the prostate gland. This condition apparently occurs from the toxic effects of the irrigating solution—usually isotonic glycine—on the visual sensory pathway. The finding of an abnormal ERG (i.e., large amplitude a-wave; reduced amplitude and loss of oscillatory potentials of the b-wave) coupled with the fact that glycine is an inhibitory neurotransmitter normally present in the inner retina suggests that amacrine cells are the likely targets of this toxicity (97,98).

Glial Cells

Müller Cell

The primary glial cell of the retina is the Müller cell. Somas of Müller cells are located in the IPL, but their processes extend throughout the retina (Fig. 1.3). The apical processes form the outer limiting membrane by making junctional complexes with one another and with photoreceptors. On the vitreal side, apposed Müller cell end-feet form the inner limiting membrane. Lateral extensions from Müller cells (*a*) contact neurons, (*b*) form synapses with dendrites within the plexiform layers and with axons within the nerve fiber layer (NFL), and (*c*) contribute to the blood–retinal barrier by their contact with blood vessels. Müller cells also provide trophic support for blood vessels within the inner retina through release of vascular endothelial growth factor (VEGF) (99).

Müller cells metabolize glucose to lactate, which is released and used by photoreceptors for oxidative phosphorylation. The need for energy is signaled by neuronal (i.e., photoreceptor and bipolar) release of glutamate, which is aggressively taken up by Müller cells (100). Once absorbed, glutamate is detoxified by conversion to glutamine, which is then recycled by photoreceptors to glutamate for subsequent release (101). Müller cells provide nourishment to neurons while protecting them by absorbing excess glutamate and nitric oxide (102,103). The ability of Müller cells to uptake glutamate (and GABA) rapidly also probably reduces the synaptic noise that would otherwise be present with any lingering concentrations of these neurotransmitters.

The radial architecture of Müller cells provides guidance during retinal development for migrating neurons and formation of interneuronal connections (104). The ability of Müller cells to generate adenosine triphosphate (ATP) from glycolysis frees them from the need to generate energy from oxygen, which is thus spared for use by neurons (105).

Müller cells have high-affinity potassium channels, permitting low-resistance entry of extracellular potassium even at the normally high resting electrical potential of the cell. These channels allow Müller cells to serve as a sink for the elevated levels of extracellular potassium that arise following activation of ON bipolar cells in response to light. The Müller cells then release the absorbed potassium at their endfeet. This cycling of potassium generates an electrical current that is the substrate of the ERG b-wave (Fig. 1.11). Oguchi's disease, a form of congenital stationary night blindness, is one of a small number of diseases that manifest the Mizuo phenomenon, in which the retina develops a golden metallic sheen when light-adapted. Although the mechanism of this phenomenon is not known, one hypothesis asserts that the sheen relates to an abnormally high extracellular potassium concentration that is a consequence of decreased absorption by Müller cells (106). Müller cells are also thought to be the source of the negative component and proximal slow component of the ERG c-wave (107).

Blindness may result from a (35-kD) antibody directed against Müller cells. In the one reported case, which occurred in the absence of a known malignancy, slowly progressive blindness developed over several years. The ERG showed greatly reduced b-wave amplitudes (photopic greater than scotopic), perhaps from deficient uptake of potassium by Müller cells (108).

Most remarkably, there is growing evidence that glial cells can be progenitors for neurons (109). At least in the chick retina, fully developed and functional Müller cells can become neurons (110). A similar phenomenon has not yet been identified in non-avian retina.

Astrocytes and Oligodendrocytes

Astrocytes are found only on the vitreal side of the retina, within the nerve fiber and ganglion cell layers, but only in species that have a retinal vasculature (111). Two types of retinal astrocytes develop from stem cells in the optic nerve, and each type preferentially contacts either nerve fiber bundles or blood vessels (112). These astrocytes migrate from the optic nerve and serve as a retinal angiogenic factor by secreting VEGF adjacent to developing blood vessels. VEGF production is induced by hypoxia (secondary to neuronal metabolism), which entices growth of the blood vessels. The newly formed blood vessels release oxygen, which encourages the astrocytes to remain mobile and stay just ahead of the wave of the developing vasculature (113).

During retinal development, astrocyte precursor cells around the optic nerve head express the *Pax2* gene. A *Pax2* gene defect is found in some patients with optic nerve colobomas, which suggests that abnormal development of the lineage or function of astrocytes may be responsible (114). Astrocytes also are a controlling influence for synapse formation. In fact, few neuronal synapses form in the absence of glia. The astrocyte mediator of synapse formation appears

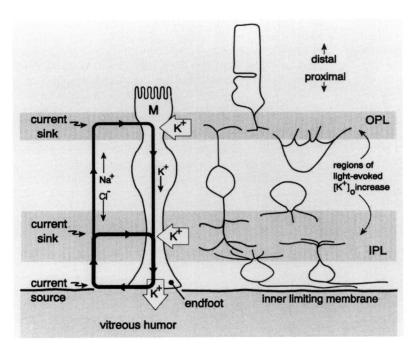

Figure 1.11. Müller cell regulation of potassium ions and generation of the ERG b-wave in the amphibian retina. Depolarizing neurons within the retina release potassium ions (K^+) upon stimulation with light, resulting in an increase in potassium $[K^+]_o$ in the inner (IPL) and outer (OPL) plexiform layers. The increase in $[K^+]_o$ causes an influx of K^+ into Müller cells (M) and a simultaneous efflux of K^+ from their end-feet (*white arrows*). These K^+ fluxes establish a radially oriented flow of current within the retina (*solid lines*) that results in the transfer of K^+ from the retina to the vitreous. The flow of current generates a vitreous-positive potential, the ERG b-wave. (From Albert DM, Jakobiec FA. Principles and Practice of Ophthalmology. Philadelphia, WB Saunders, 1994:406.)

to be cholesterol, which is transported by apolipoprotein E. Neurons take up apolipoprotein E molecules, which is associated with expanded synaptogenesis (115,116).

Astrocytes, like Müller cells, also may protect neurons by taking up glutamate. In certain circumstances, however, astrocytes may mediate neuronal injury by release of stored glutamate via hemi-channels. The ability of astrocytes to release glutamate has the potential to affect synaptic transmission (117). Astrocytes also communicate among themselves, even at extended distances, via release of ATP, which causes an increase in calcium in neighboring glia that prompts ATP release from those cells, and so on. Astrocytes also have the ability to modulate neuronal synapses (118).

Oligodendrocytes migrate into the optic nerve from the brain during embryonic development and usually do not extend past the lamina cribrosa in primates (119). However, the presence of myelinated nerve fibers in the retinas of about 0.5% of normal persons indicates that migration across the lamina cribrosa does occasionally occur. Rarely, especially in patients with neurofibromatosis, myelination in the retina may appear to increase during childhood (120).

A new class of glial cells, called synantocytes, have been discovered. These cells, which are ubiquitous, specifically contact neurons at their synapses and at nodes of Ranvier (121). The role of these cells is not well understood, but they are in an advantageous position to monitor neuronal activity and potentially detect altered function.

Retinal Microglia

Microglial cells enter the retina from the bloodstream as macrophages during mid-embryogenesis. In human retinas, quiescent microglia exist throughout much of the retina, although they are more common near inner retinal blood vessels (122). Retinal microglia become activated after section of the optic nerve (123) and in association with a variety of retinal degenerations (124). Activated microglia may secrete molecules that kill retinal neurons (124). In glaucoma, microglia in the optic nerve head become activated and migrate into the peripapillary chorioretinal region, which becomes increasingly atrophic as the disease progresses (125).

Retinal Ganglion Cells

Adult humans have, on average, 1.2 million RGCs (126,127). This is the residual number following loss of 50–90% of the population originally present early in development (128,129). RGC attrition is effected by apoptosis. A similar, massive loss of neurons occurs throughout the brain during early development. Across individuals there is marked variability in the final RGC number (127,130). Whatever that final number, roughly 70% of RGCs will subserve the central 30 degrees of the visual field. Some RGCs are "displaced" into the INL, and the RGC layer contains "displaced" amacrine cells. In fact, displaced amacrine cells account for 3–80% of neurons in the RGC layer, depending upon eccentricity (127). Astrocytes, endothelial cells, and pericytes are also found in the ganglion cell layer. The distribution of RGCs with respect to the Goldmann visual field map is shown in Fig. 1.12.

The fate determination that leads to creation of an RGC is not sufficient for axonal generation. Axons are generated only after exposure to glial cells and neurotrophic factors. A complex orchestration of molecular factors and physiologic activity is also required to ensure proper growth and direction of RGC axons to their targets. There is also evidence that RGCs secrete their own neurotrophic factors to help sustain themselves, perhaps even bolstering their ability to

GOLDMANN VISUAL FIELD OVERLAY
For Distribution of Human Retinal Ganglion Cells

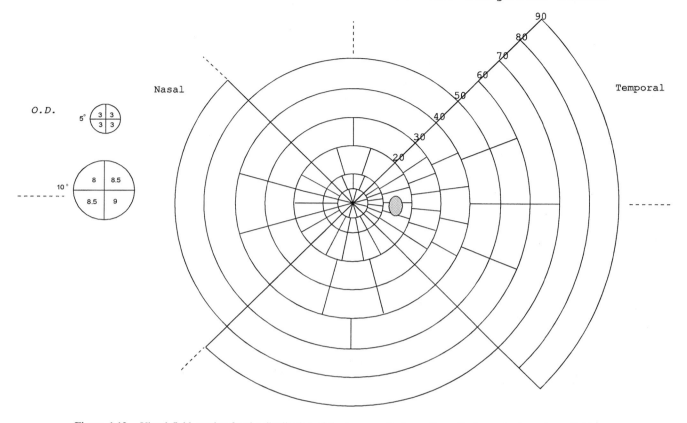

Figure 1.12. Visual field overlay for the distribution of the human retinal ganglion cells for perimetry using a Goldmann perimeter. Each sector of the map equals 1% of the total number of cells. An inset (*left*) has been provided to assist in counting of boxes when a field defect involves the central region. The blind spot is included for orientation only and should not influence the counting of boxes when field defects involve the peripapillary region. The *hatched lines* extending from the meridia in the nasal quadrants are a reminder that a relatively small number of ganglion cells (less than 1%) are present beyond the superior, inferior, and nasal borders of the map. (Map constructed by Rizzo JF and Castelbuono AC using original data from Curcio CA, Allen KA. Topography of ganglion cells in human retina. J Comp Neurol 1990;300:5–25.)

withstand axonal injury (126). The possible clinical significance of neurotrophic factors on RGC survival is revealed by the report of a deficiency in retrograde transport of brain-derived neurotrophic factor (BDNF) and upregulation of the BDNF receptor (TrkB) at the optic nerve head in a glaucoma model (131,132).

Dendrites of RGCs branch in well-defined strata within the IPL, and the specific region of stratification varies with the particular cell type. As noted above, ON center and OFF center ganglion cells have dendrites that terminate in either the *b* or *a* sublamina of the IPL, respectively (Fig. 1.8). Axons of RGCs terminate in the dLGN, hypothalamus, pretectum, or midbrain. In the primate, there may be 15–20 more subpopulations of RGCs (71,133,134). Each RGC type has a specific anatomy (Fig. 1.13), and for many a specific physiology (i.e., "form matches function") has been identified (Fig. 1.14).

RGCs have traditionally been divided into two main types

based on cell size (71) (Table 1.2). Of these, the most numerous are small cells known as "beta" or "P" (for parvocellular) cells, which as their name implies, synapse in the parvocellular layers of the dLGN. A much smaller population, perhaps 5–10% of primate RGCs, are large cells known as "alpha," "parasol," or "M" (for magnocellular) cells, which synapse in the magnocellular layers of the dLGN. These cell types, which are divided equally between ON and OFF varieties, are the best-studied RGCs. It has generally been assumed that collectively these populations represent 85–90% of all primate RGCs. Recently it has been reported that a small cell type (i.e., a "local edge detector" cell) may be the most common RGC in the rabbit (133), although it is not yet known whether this finding will hold for primates.

The smallest RGCs are the κ, koniocellular, or K cells, so named because the cell bodies are small enough to resemble small particles of dust (from the Greek word *konis*) (135) (Table 1.2). These cells are a mixed population with the

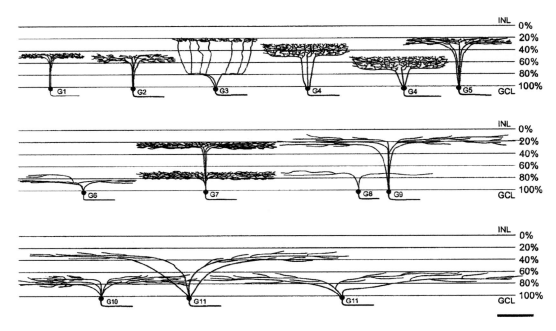

Figure 1.13.   The branching and level of stratification for 11 types of ganglion cells identified in rabbit retina. Several labeling methods were used to identify these cell types, and it is likely that these representations constitute most ganglion cell types in the rabbit retina. The cell types with a known physiologic response profile are as follows: G1, local edge detector; G4, either an ON or OFF brisk sustained; G6, uniformity detector; G7, ON-OFF direction selective; G10, ON direction selective; G11, either an ON or OFF brisk transient. Cells with both ON and OFF varieties (i.e., G4 and G11) ramify in one of two sublaminae within the inner plexiform layer. Ramification nearer the ganglion cell layer (i.e., in sublamina *b*) is associated with ON responsiveness. INL, inner nuclear layer; GCL, ganglion cell layer. Numbers to the right indicate depth within the inner plexiform layer. Scale bar = 100 μm. (From Rockhill RL, et al. The diversity of ganglion cells in a mammalian retina. J Neurosci 2002;22:3831–3843.)

common features of a small cell body and wide, diffusely branching dendrites (136), although some have a larger soma (137). These diverse anatomic traits suggest that the κ cell class includes more than one physiologic type of cell.

A few RGCs exit the afferent visual pathway via the posterior aspect of the optic chiasm and terminate in one of several areas of the hypothalamus, one of which is the suprachiasmatic nucleus that regulates circadian rhythms (138,139). Retinohypothalamic cells can survive and regulate circadian rhythms even when retinal or optic nerve disease causes

complete loss of conscious vision (140). The majority of cells in the retinohypothalamic pathway begin not at the level of photoreceptors, but rather with a small population of RGCs that respond to light (Fig. 1.15). This light-responsiveness is conferred by melanopsin, a recently described, novel opsin-like protein (141–145). Roughly 30% of the melanopsin-containing RGCs receive input from rods and cones, and thus presumably are activated directly (via their own melanopsin) and indirectly (via synaptic input from bipolar cells) by light (146).

Table 1.2

Equivalent Anatomic Nomenclature and Associated Physiologic Properties of Some Retinal Ganglion Cell Types

Anatomic Reference[a]	Cell Size/Dendritic Field Size	Physiologic Reference	Concentric Center/Surround	Linear/ Nonlinear	Sustained/ Transient
Beta; Pβ; P; Parvo-	Medium/narrow and dense	X	+	Linear	Sustained
Alpha; Pα; M-; Magno	Large/wide and dense	Y	+	Non-linear	Transient
Gamma; koniocellular; K-	Most have small somas and/wide but sparse dendrites. Some have larger somas.	Mixed types/some W	Most	Either	Either
Delta	Medium/wide, moderately dense	Mixed types/some W	Most	Either	Either

[a] The nomenclature can be confusing since multiple names are used to define the same cell types. For instance, The P in the Pβ or Pα nomenclature is a reference to primate. The P- and M-cell nomenclature refers to whether the cell terminates in the parvocellular or magnocellular region of the dorsal lateral geniculate nucleus.

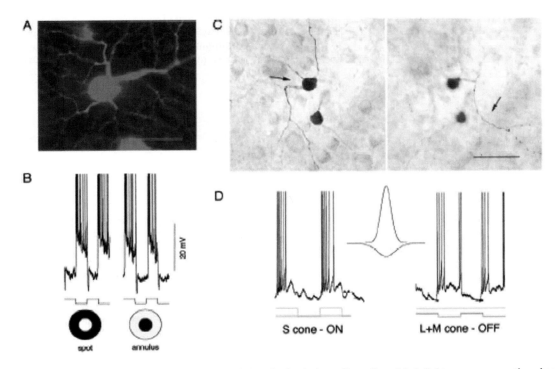

Figure 1.14. Correlation between morphology of photostained retinal ganglion cells and their light response properties when recorded in vitro. *A* and *B,* Aspects of the spatial and temporal response properties of an OFF-center parasol ganglion cell photostained prior to intracellular penetration and voltage recording. *A,* In vitro photomicrograph of recorded cell taken after recording was complete and electrode was withdrawn from cell. Dendritic field diameter equals 240 μm. Scale bar = 50 μm. *B,* Intracellular recording in response to a spot or annulus centered on receptive field shows OFF-center (*left trace*), ON surround (*right trace*) light response; square wave below voltage trace shows time course of 2-Hz modulated stimulus; icons situated below trace illustrate spatial configuration of stimulus. When the light stimulus is turned on (indicated by the upward direction of the square wave trace shown below the physiologic recording), the bright spot of light placed in the center of the receptive field of this OFF cell (*left*) results in dramatic reduction of recorded activity. By comparison, stimulating this same cell with a bright annulus in the surround of its receptive field (*right*) produces a dramatic increase in firing rate. This response profile reveals the antagonistic, center-surround organization that is characteristic of most retinal ganglion cells. *C and D,* Morphology and light response of a large field bistratified cell. *C,* Photomicrograph of a darkly stained cell that was retrogradely labeled by tracer injections placed in the lateral geniculate nucleus and then processed for histochemistry after labeling with horseradish peroxidase immunoreaction. On the left, the soma (*arrow*) and inner dendrites are shown; on the right, a slightly different focal plane shows the outer dendrites (*arrow*) of the same cell. Dendritic field diameter equals 415 μm. Scale bar = 50 μm. *D,* The cell shown in *C* gave an ON response to 1-Hz square wave chromatic stimuli modulated to isolate S cones (*left trace*) and an OFF response to stimuli modulated to isolate L and M cones (*right trace*). A difference of Gaussian model fit to spatial frequency response data (not shown) was used to construct the one-dimensional center and surround receptive field profiles shown in the middle insert. The model gives a Gaussian receptive field diameter of 510 μm. (Modified from Dacey DM, et al. Fireworks in the primate retina: In vitro photodynamics reveals diverse LGN-projecting ganglion cell types. Neuron 2003; 37:15–27.)

Most RGCs that contain melanopsin mRNA project to each suprachiasmatic nucleus and to the contralateral pretectal area via collaterals, which allow one cell to provide input to two locations (142,147). Roughly 20% of these special RGCs innervate the intergeniculate leaflet (see dLGN, below). The olivary pretectal nuclei and superior colliculi also receive input from melanopsin-containing RGCs. These latter inputs to noncircadian centers suggest that these cells serve broader roles (145), perhaps by providing information about the mean retinal illumination that may contribute to control of sleep–wake cycles and influence pupillary light reflexes (147,148). The relationship of these cells to the pre- viously identified biplexiform (or interplexiform) RGCs, which stretch into the OPL and receive input directly from rods, is not known (71). However, the fact that biplexiform cells bypass the middle retinal circuitry suggests they influence functions that depend upon ambient light intensity, like circadian rhythms and pupillary light reflexes.

A subset of motion-detecting cells known as *object motion cells* respond differently depending on whether object motion is similar to or different from the background (84). In other words, these cells are quiet if an object moves "in sync" with the background but fire when "local" motion differs from the background (also see polyaxonal amacrine

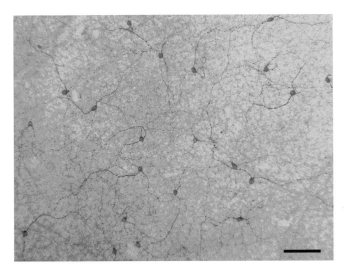

Figure 1.15. Melanopsin immunoreactivity is found in a subset of retinal ganglion cells constituting the retinohypothalamic tract. This is a photomicrograph of a flat-mounted rat retina that reveals a subpopulation of retinal ganglion cells that contain melanopsin immunoreactivity in the plasma membrane of the soma and dendritic processes, which forms an extensive photoreceptive network. Scale bar = 100 μm. (From Hannibal J, Fahrenkrug J. Melanopsin: a novel photopigment involved in the photoentrainment of the brain's biological clock? Ann Med 2002;34:401–407.)

cell, above). This response property may form (or contribute to) cognitive inattention to visual input during saccadic or microsaccadic eye movements. These cells have been identified in a mammalian retina but not yet in primates, although the requisite neuronal architecture is present in primates.

Some RGCs respond preferentially to short wavelengths. One such cell (i.e., "small, bistratified" cell) has a small soma with (relatively wide, similar to parasol cells) dendritic arbors that ramify in both the ON and OFF sublaminae of the IPL. The ON input derives from "blue" cones (via 2 or 3 S-cone bipolar cells); the OFF input derives from M- and L-cones. These cells are therefore sensitive to blue and yellow colors. Collectively these cells constitute perhaps 10% of the color-sensitive RGCs.

Retinal Ganglion Cell Physiology

Most RGCs share some fundamental physiologic properties (149,150) (Table 1.2). First, RGCs have a concentric and antagonistic center-surround organization, a property that probably derives from lateral inhibition of horizontal and, possibly, amacrine cells (151). Second, most RGCs respond in an ON or OFF manner to change in luminosity or spectral distribution of light within their receptive field centers, which correspond to a particular depth of the dendritic arbor that ramifies in either sublamina *a* (i.e., OFF) or sublamina *b* (i.e., ON) of the IPL (152). The precise depth within the IPL differs for the major RGC classes (e.g., M versus P cells). This physiologic dichotomy of ON and OFF pathways, which requires postnatal visual stimulation for

their development (153), is not one of symmetric opposition. ON pathways introduce a tonic inhibition of OFF cells at mean luminances and a phasic inhibition of the OFF pathway in response to increases of incident light (154). As such, the pathways are not truly "parallel" in that there are significant asymmetries, with a unidirectional inhibition of the ON system onto the OFF system.

Third, the responses to light of most RGCs are either sustained or transient (155,156). Transient responses are believed to result from feedback synapses within the IPL that alter the sustained responses typical of the outer retina. Cells with sustained responses also show linearity of spatial summation (i.e., the response magnitude is proportional to the area of illumination within the receptive field center). Generally, cells classified anatomically as P cells have a sustained (i.e., X-cell) response profile, whereas M cells have a transient (i.e., Y-cell) response profile (Table 1.2). Lastly, RGCs maintain a continuous spontaneous discharge, which requires considerable energy but provides a dynamic range of response for either increases or decreases in the level of illumination for each cell type. In other words, even an ON RGC can signal a response to decreased light in the center of its receptive field by reducing its spontaneous firing rate. However, the dynamic range of its response to lowered illumination is substantially less than it can achieve to increased illumination, for which its dynamic range of response is vastly greater. OFF RGCs have a higher spontaneous firing rate than ON cells, which may contribute to the physiologic segregation of these cell types at the dLGN (discussed later).

P cells are color-opponent (i.e., the center of the receptive field is maximally responsive to either red or green light, whereas the inverse is true for the surround), have small receptive fields, and have low sensitivity to contrast in the visual scene (155,157). Color-opponency is generated by connections at both the OPL and IPL (158). P cells are probably the major afferent input to the brain for central (e.g., Snellen) acuity, color vision, and fine stereopsis (159).

M cells are spectrally "broad-band." In other words, their peak responsiveness at a given intensity of light is not determined by the wavelength, a property that derives from the combined input from all three cone types. M cells also have much larger receptive fields and are more responsive to luminance contrast than P cells (152,157). Most M cells respond nonlinearly to light. In other words, their activity increases in response to *changes* in the visual scene, rather than responding proportionately to the intensity and duration of the stimulating light.

Lesions of the "M" retinogeniculate pathway in monkeys impair high-temporal-frequency flicker and motion perception (159). It might therefore be assumed that the increased sensitivity of M cells to luminance contrast would permit selective testing of these cells in patients with optic neuropathies. Selective lesions to the M-cell pathway in monkeys, however, do not degrade performance on tests of contrast sensitivity (160). This apparent paradox can be explained by the preponderance of P cells. Although P cells are individually less responsive to contrast than M cells, their total number is much greater than M cells (perhaps an 8:1 ratio).

Thus, patients with a neurologic decrement in contrast sensitivity probably have P- and M-cell dysfunction.

As suggested above, cells that conform to the κ morphology (i.e., K cells) are physiologically diverse. These cells may or may not have concentric center-surround receptive field organization, may have sustained or transient changes in firing rate, and may be ON center or OFF center responsive (161). Some κ cells are part of a third physiologic class of RGCs called W cells, which have large receptive fields, slow onset latency, and slow axonal conduction velocity. At the level of the dLGN, K cells receive direct input from the superficial layers of the superior colliculus, which is not provided to M or P cells. In addition, many K cells project indirectly to the dorsal visual pathway (discussed later). These features suggest that some K cells contribute information about eye movements, since both the superior colliculus and dorsal median visual area are preferentially driven by motion.

Some W cells are direction-selective cells. One such cell type is the ON center *direction selective cell*, which transiently increases its firing rate when a stimulus enters its receptive field from a specific direction. These cells receive their primary input from ''starburst'' cholinergic amacrine cells (discussed previously). Another type of direction-selective W cell responds when a stimulus enters (ON) or leaves (OFF) its receptive field. As might be expected (Figs. 1.8 and 1.13), such cells have bistratified dendritic arborization within the IPL.

Retinal Ganglion Cell Axons

As mentioned above, RGCs are the first retinal neurons to develop. The extension and guidance of their axons are complex phenomena directed by growth factors. Both attractive and repulsive molecules are present in the developing retina and optic nerve head, and RGC axons express receptors for those molecules that participate in the growth process (162).

RGC axonal sprouts are repulsed from penetrating into the retina, perhaps by Müller cell somata (which conversely encourage growth of RGC dendrites). Axonal repulsion may be performed by ephrin-A5, one of many ligands for receptor tyrosine kinases of the ''Eph'' family (163). (Other ligands of this family are involved in axonal termination in the midbrain; discussed later.) With molecular guidance, the axons move toward the vitreal surface and then bend toward the optic nerve when they contact the end-feet of the developing Müller cells (164). The axons travel within fascicles toward the optic nerve head with remarkable, although not perfect, precision. Their journey across the retina is probably influenced by several factors, although laminin (especially laminin-1) may be particularly instrumental. RGC axons express integrins, which are the receptors for laminin. At the optic nerve head, the guidance molecule netrin-1 influences axonal bending into the optic nerve head (ONH) (165). Deficiency of netrin-1 is a cause of optic nerve hypoplasia in humans.

The first RGCs develop in the dorsotemporal quadrant, near the optic nerve stalk. The axons that sprout thereafter within this quadrant can take advantage of cues from the previously established axons for guidance toward the optic nerve head. Epithelial cells in the optic stalk give rise to glial cells in the optic nerve and other cells that line the fissure (Fig. 1.1). The latter cells express the transcription factor *Pax-2*. Failure to express Pax-2 prevents closure of the optic nerve fissure and causes failure of axons to leave the retina (6). Pax-2 deficiency is a cause of optic nerve head coloboma and optic nerve hypoplasia in humans (166).

RGCs have relatively long axons, which are entirely dependent upon their soma for tropic support. An axon is a dynamic structure that requires nearly constant repair of its membranes, a process that includes bidirectional transport of proteins, enzymes, and subcellular components (including mitochondria) to, and detritus from, sites up to the synapse. Axonal velocities are somewhat bimodal and range from fast (i.e., hundreds of millimeters per day) to slow (less than 10 mm/day) speeds. At least five classes of proteins are transported at different velocities within RGCs, and these relationships vary during development (167).

Slow anterograde transport, which largely carries components like cytoskeletal proteins that remain within the cell, constitutes the bulk (about 85%) of all transport. Fast anterograde transport is used to carry neurotransmitter-containing vesicles. Molecular transport is aided by repetitive to-and-fro realignment of kinesin, a protein ''molecular motor'' with a globular head that reacts with microtubules, structures that serve as internal guidewires for transport within the axon. Transport speed for neurofilaments, the most significant cytoskeletal protein, is slowed by increased C-terminal phosphorylation, which may dissociate neurofilament molecules from kinesin. Rapid axonal transport may be predominately impaired in axons that project to the magnocellular layers of the dLGN in instances of chronic (but not acute) elevation of intraocular pressure (168). Retrograde transport, which is less well understood, proceeds at roughly half the maximum velocity of anterograde transport. Axonal transport, whether anterograde or retrograde, is highly energy dependent. The ATP needed to sustain transport is supplied by mitochondria that are distributed along the axon.

The common defect in pathologic swelling of the optic disc from almost any etiology is disruption of anterograde axonal transport of RGCs at the lamina cribrosa. Experimentally induced ischemia of the anterior optic nerve of monkeys disrupts both fast and slow anterograde axonal transport (169,170). Slow anterograde transport can be selectively disrupted in experimental optic nerve crush injury (171). Anterograde axonal transport also can be disrupted by increased or decreased intraocular pressure, increased intracranial pressure (172–175), and possibly decreased energy reserves secondary to mitochondrial dysfunction (176). Disruption of axonal transport may contribute to the death of RGCs. Following severe injury, some RGCs can regenerate, but the potential is quite limited (177,178). Generally, the larger RGCs are more capable of surviving axotomy and regenerating their axons (179).

Membranes of RGC axons contain many ionic channels. The voltage-dependent sodium channel (Na_v) is the most important channel with respect to generation of action potentials. Na$_v$ channels exist in very high density at the axonal hillock and nodes of Ranvier. The normal complement and localization of channel isoforms along axons are altered with demyelination, which presumably accounts for some of the disability that occurs in multiple sclerosis (180,181).

Bifurcation of RGC axons has been well documented, especially for cells that terminate in the hypothalamus and that also may send an axonal branch to the intergeniculate leaflet of the thalamus (145,147,182). In the cat, axonal bifurcation occurs for all three major physiologic classes of RGCs (i.e., X, Y, and W cells). Such bifurcations have not been documented in humans but have been discovered in many areas of the monkey brain (183).

A superficial plexiform layer located between the ganglion cell layer and the traditional nerve fiber layer is present in some mammalian retinas. The layer is composed of processes of M RGCs and some amacrine cells. This arrangement provides the potential for local feedback loops (184).

Nerve Fiber Layer

The NFL is composed of RGC axons, astrocytes, components of Müller cells, and rare efferent fibers to the retina whose function is unknown (185,186). The NFL is thinnest in the peripheral retina and thickest adjacent to the superior and inferior margins of the optic disc, where it measures about 200 μm in humans. The temporal and nasal NFL adjacent to the optic disc is about one-tenth as thick (187). NFL thickness declines with age, which can be demonstrated noninvasively with optical coherence tomography (188).

The gross organization of the NFL bears several distinctive features. First, peripheral RGC axons from the temporal retina arch around the papillomacular bundle, which contains nerve fibers originating from RGCs in the foveal area. This pattern is dictated by the relatively early formation of the central retina. Second, a demarcation on the temporal side of the fovea called the temporal raphe separates superior and inferior axons out to the far periphery of the retina (189). This raphe therefore creates a physiologic separation between the superior and inferior regions of the nasal visual field (which is monitored by the retina temporal to the fovea). Third, fibers from the nasal aspect of the optic disc are organized radially as they approach the optic nerve head (Fig. 1.16).

The demarcation between temporal and nasal retina (and thus the visual field) is a vertical line that passes through the fovea—not the optic disc. Generally, RGC axons nasal to the fovea decussate within the optic chiasm, whereas axons temporal to the fovea remain ipsilateral. However, at a cellular level in monkeys, some RGC axons temporal to the fovea cross within the chiasm, whereas some nasal axons remain uncrossed (190–194). This overlap, which is more significant in the peripheral retina (192,193), if present in humans would not necessarily disrupt the demarcation between nasal and temporal hemifields. A RGC located on one side of the fovea does not necessarily receive input from a photoreceptor located on the same side of the fovea. The relatively larger width of the cone pedicle compared to the foveal cone soma forces a lateral displacement of cone pedicles via the

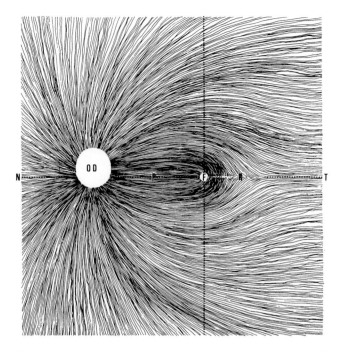

Figure 1.16. Retinal nerve axons as they extend from the ganglion cells to the disc. The axons arising from ganglion cells in the nasal macula project directly toward the optic disc (OD) and compose part of the papillomacular bundle (P). Axons from ganglion cells of the temporal macula have a slight arching pattern around the nasal macular axons. They form the remainder of the papillomacular bundle. Axons from nonmacular ganglion cells that are nasal to the fovea (F) have a straight or gently curved course to the optic disc, whereas axons from ganglion cells temporal to the fovea must arch around the papillomacular bundle and enter the disc at its superior and inferior poles. The superior and inferior portions of the temporal retina are delineated by an anatomic landmark, the temporal raphe (R). The *dotted lines* delineate the nasal (N), temporal (T), superior, and inferior portions of the retina. Consider that the temporal and nasal parts of the retina are defined by a vertical line through the fovea, not the OD. (Redrawn from Hogan MJ, Alvarado JA, Weddell JE. Histology of the Human Eye. An Atlas and Textbook. Philadelphia, WB Saunders, 1971.)

nerve fiber layer of Henle (discussed previously). This lateral shifting could theoretically connect photoreceptors on one side of the vertical meridian to RGCs on the opposite side (195). This seemingly awry anatomy would not necessarily disrupt visual field topography, since the determinant for visuospatial localization is based upon the position of the photoreceptor and not the RGC soma. Nonetheless, some degree of imprecision between nasal and temporal hemifields can be observed by visual field testing, especially more peripherally (196), even when the scanning laser ophthalmoscope is used to precisely control the position of the stimulus on the retina.

Within the NFL, axons from central RGCs are more superficial than those from more peripheral RGCs. To achieve this arrangement, fibers from central RGCs extend upward between fibers of more peripheral RGCs (197) (Fig. 1.17). Near the disc margin, most axons from peripheral RGCs are relatively deep within the NFL and more peripheral at the

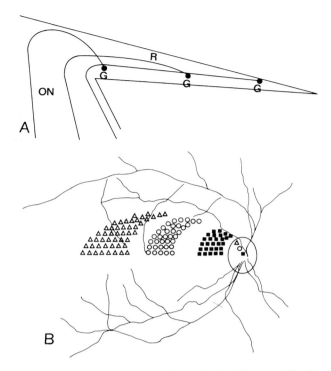

Figure 1.17. The three-dimensional organization of the nerve fiber layer in the primate retina and optic disc. *A,* Anterior-posterior organization of axons projecting from ganglion cells (G) located in peripheral, middle, and peripapillary retina (R) into the optic nerve (ON). Lamination of axons within retina is speculative. Only half of retina and optic nerve are represented, as if displayed in standard horizontal section. *B,* Horizontal topography of axon bundles from the arcuate fibers (i.e., those that course around the papillomacular bundle) as they project into the anterior portion of the optic nerve head. Peripherally located ganglion cells project to the peripheral aspect of the optic nerve (*triangles*), centrally located ganglion cells to the midperipheral aspect of the optic nerve (*circles*), and peripapillary ganglion cells to the center of the nerve (*squares*). (From Minkler DS. The organization of nerve fiber bundles in the primate optic nerve head. Arch Ophthalmol 1980;98:1630–1636.)

optic nerve head (197). Despite this general plan, near the optic disc there is significant intermingling of fibers (198).

Macula

Numerous anatomic specializations contribute to the higher spatial resolution afforded by the macula. The most significant factor is the especially high density of photoreceptors, particularly cones (50). At the fovea, cones have a center-to-center separation of only 2 μm. The foveal pit (Fig. 1.7) enhances spatial fidelity by reducing the amount of tissue through which light must pass to reach the cones. The relatively high density of centrally placed rods (but not cones) and RGCs is related to the greater density of ocular melanin, although not in a dose-dependent fashion (199). This observation provides a theoretical basis for the poor vision of albinos. Melanin also plays a critical role in axonal direction at the chiasm (discussed later). The lack of blood vessels in the central macula (i.e., the foveal avascular zone)

and possibly the presence of xanthophyll within the macula, which absorbs shorter wavelengths of light and thus reduces chromatic aberration, also contribute to the high spatial resolution provided by the central retina.

Retinal Blood Vessels

The human retina receives its essential nutrients, oxygen and glucose, from both the retinal and the choroidal circulations. The border between these circulations is near the OPL (200). The choroidal circulation supplies the photoreceptors, whereas the retinal arteries supply the inner retina, except within the foveal avascular zone. The degree to which the inner retina is vascularized appears to correlate best with the degree of oxidative metabolic demand rather than with the thickness of the retina (201). Astrocytes in the developing retina are extremely sensitive to hypoxia, which prompts release of VEGF. The release of VEGF just ahead of the advancing edge of the developing retinal vasculature promotes further extension of the vasculature into the more peripheral retina (202). Amacrine cells and RGCs synthesize and express VEGF, which presumably helps to secure a viable blood supply. Müller cells also provide a similar trophic support via VEGF (99).

Retinal blood vessels are barrier vessels, analogous to the blood–brain barrier elsewhere in the CNS. These vessels are impermeable to particles larger than 20 Å (203). Astrocytes and pericytes almost certainly play a role in maintaining low capillary permeability within the NFL, whereas Müller cells probably play a similar role more deeply within the retina. The blood–retinal barrier is also maintained by chemical factors (204).

Autoregulation of retinal (and choroidal) blood vessels may be at least partially controlled chemically by hormonal products of the local vascular endothelium, including vasodilators such as nitric oxide and prostaglandins, and vasoconstrictors, particularly endothelin and the products of the renin-angiotensin system that are produced and released via angiotensin-converting enzyme located on the endothelial cell membrane (205). Additionally, adenosine and α_1-adrenergic receptors mediate vasodilation and vasoconstriction, respectively. Amacrine cells contact retinal vessels and may also influence autoregulation.

Retinal blood vessels impede light transmission through the retina and produce "angioscotomas." This highly local-

Table 1.3
Retinal Neurons and Some of Their Associated Neurotransmitters

Cell Type	Neurotransmitter
Photoreceptors	Glutamate
Horizontal cells	GABA
Bipolar cells	
ON-center (depolarizing)	Glutamate
OFF-center (hyperpolarizing)	Glutamate
Interplexiform cells	Dopamine, GABA
Amacrine cells	Acetylcholine glycine, GABA
	peptides, dopamine

Table 1.4
Primary Projection Pathways from the Retina

Retinal Outflow	Site of Termination	Function
Parvocellular	Layers 3–6 of dLGN	Fine spatial detail Color vision
Magnocellular	Layers 1–2 of dLGN	Contrast sensitivity Motion detection
Koniocellular	Intercalated layers of dLGN Pregeniculate complex	Contribute information about eye motion Manifests saccade-related activity and influences activity in the 6 primary laminae, especially for the M-pathway
Gamma cell	Pre-tectal nuclei	Pupillomotor function
Melanopsin-containing retinal ganglion cells	Intergeniculate leaflet Hypothalamus	"Phase shifting" of circadian cycle Regulation of circadian cycle

This table is meant to convey only general patterns of information flow and function. This list of retinal outflow cell types descriptions of function are not complete .

ized visual depravation causes a rewiring of connections between the dLGN and the primary visual cortex. The corresponding areas of the visual cortex are relatively less active, as revealed by "shadows" in the cytochrome oxidase staining pattern (206).

Retinal Neurotransmitters

A review of neurotransmitters in the retina is beyond the scope of this chapter. Table 1.3 provides a list of known neurotransmitters for the major classes of retinal cells, and Figure 1.6 shows some of the neurotransmitters used by the intraretinal cone and rod through pathways.

OVERVIEW OF RETINAL OUTFLOW: PARALLEL PATHWAYS

There is a complex orchestration of neuronal responses evoked by light stimulation of the retina. Light causes the photoreceptors to hyperpolarize, which decreases the release of glutamate from both rod and cone synaptic terminals. Horizontal cells then become hyperpolarized, which suppresses the light response of the photoreceptors. Rod and cone out flows generally diverge, although gap junctions between them are believed to provide a signal path from rods to cones under mesopic or photopic conditions. Under scotopic conditions, rod signals are transmitted to the rod bipolar cells via a sign-inverting signal that depolarizes the bipolar cells. The signal is then carried via rod bipolar cell to sublamina b of the IPL, where there is a sign-conserving synapse onto AII amacrine cells. (Rod bipolar cells do not make direct contact with RGCs.) AII amacrine cells have gap junctions with depolarizing cone bipolar cells and also make a sign-inverting glycinergic synapse onto hyperpolarizing cone bipolar cells, which terminate in sublamina a of the IPL, where they contact OFF center RGCs.

Cone output in the central retina uses the "midget" system. A sign-conserving synapse using the AMPA glutamate receptor is made on a cone-hyperpolarizing (OFF center) bipolar cell, and a sign-conserving synapse that uses the mGluR6 receptor is made with a cone-depolarizing (ON center) bipolar cell. The two bipolar cells terminate in sublamina a and sublamina b of the IPL, respectively, where they contact OFF center (sublamina a) or ON center (sublamina b) RGCs. Amacrine cells have a complex influence on RGCs, with both diffuse and highly local control and both excitatory and inhibitory effects. Various qualitative aspects of vision (e.g., spatial detail, color, contrast, motion detection) proceed to the brain through the optic nerve in parallel (Table 1.4), although there are physiologic interactions across the "parallel" pathways at the retina, dLGN, and cortex.

OPTIC NERVE

EMBRYOLOGY

The optic nerve develops in the substance of the optic stalk (1,2,207,208). This stalk, which becomes apparent at the fourth week of gestation, has a wide circular lumen that is continuous with the cavity of the forebrain at one end and the optic vesicle at the other (Fig. 1.1). Its walls are composed of a single layer of undifferentiated epithelial cells. The optic stalk and vesicle both invaginate; in the stalk this produces a shallow depression ventrally. The lumen of the stalk shrinks as the stalk lengthens.

A proliferation of glial cells on the developing optic disc produces the Bergmeister papilla. This structure later becomes atrophic as its blood supply withers when the hyaloid artery involutes. The degree of atrophy determines the size of the optic nerve head cup: more complete atrophy produces a deeper cup. With minimal atrophy, glial remnants remain on the surface of the optic disc. A Bergmeister papilla can persist as glial sheaths of the proximal segments of retinal arteries.

At 8 weeks, two glial cell populations develop from two cell lines of the primitive neuroepithelium of the optic stalk and ventral forebrain. One cell line produces type 1 astrocytes. The second cell line originates from the oligodendrocyte type 2 astrocyte (also known as the oligodendrocyte precursor cell), which produces both oligodendrocytes and type 2 astrocytes. The size of the astrocytic populations depends upon signaling from RGCs, which express Hh protein, which in turn induces expression of the Pax2 gene, which is expressed in the neuroepithelial precursor cells (114,209). Mutations of the Pax2 gene are associated with optic nerve coloboma, which suggests that disordered astrocytic development may cause this defect. Partitioning of the glial populations is influenced by local biochemical cues. For instance, astrocytes within the optic nerve avoid the chiasm because of the presence of netrin-1 and semaphorin 3a (210,211). The functions of astrocytes are described above. Within the optic nerve, astrocytes also participate in the formation of connective tissue septae (see later).

Neuroepithelial cells within the ventral forebrain, also responding to an Hh protein, migrate into the developing optic nerve and express different genes that direct neuroepithelial cells to become oligodendrocytes, which is the first step toward the myelination of axons (210). Migration to distant targets (i.e., here, into the optic nerve) is characteristic of the development of oligodendrocyte populations elsewhere in the CNS. The differentiation of glial cell populations also is influenced by exposure to extrinsic factors that influence the redox state of the precursor cells. In general, greater oxidation encourages differentiation (212).

Myelination, which begins centrally during embryogenesis, gradually extends up to the lamina cribrosa and invests almost all optic nerve fibers at or shortly after birth, and then ceases. In about 1% of patients, however, oligodendrocytes enter or are already present within the eye during embryogenesis and produce intraocular myelination that usually affects the NFL adjacent to the optic disc (213). The ''stop'' signal that (typically) prevents migration of oligodendrocytes into the retina may be related to transient expression of netrin-1 and increased concentration of tenascin-C (214).

Myelination is also dependent upon connexins, which promote gap junction formation (215). Both astrocytic and oligodendrocytic populations are linked by gap junctions, which create a functional syncytium (216,217). Abnormal connexin protein can cause peripheral nervous system dysmyelination, as is seen in Charcot-Marie-Tooth disease. The role that connexins might play with respect to RGC axons is not known. Myelin speeds the transmission of impulses but is not essential for some visual system functions, as is evident in newborns, in whom myelination may not be completed for 2–4 years after birth (120,218,219). In general, the thickest myelin sheaths are found around the thickest axons (i.e., those of ''M'' RGCs), endowing them with the fastest conduction velocities of 1.3–20 m/sec (220).

The optic nerve increases both in diameter and length during gestation and through early adolescence (221–223). By the beginning of the second decade, the diameter of the intraocular portion of the optic nerve is 2 mm, while that of the extraocular portion of the nerve is 3–4 mm, the difference resulting largely from the formation of myelin sheaths. The optic nerve diameter increases even beyond this time (224). The adult length of the nerve is 40–50 mm, with most

of the variation occurring intracranially. A discussion of optic nerve axon number is provided above.

GENERAL ANATOMY

The optic nerve can be separated into four sections: the intraocular, intraorbital, intraosseous, and intracranial portions (Fig. 1.18). The intraocular segment of the optic nerve (i.e., the ONH) is primarily formed by coalescence of RGC axons, with the addition of three nonneural elements: astrocytes, capillary-associated cells, and fibroblasts. The ONH is a major zone of transition because the nerve fibers (*a*) pass from an area of relatively high intraocular pressure to the lower-pressure zone of the retro-orbital segment of the optic nerve, which is (usually) equivalent to the intracranial pressure; (*b*) leave the blood supply of the central retinal artery to receive blood from branches of the posterior ciliary and ophthalmic arteries; (*c*) make a 90-degree turn and enter the tight confines of the lamina cribrosa; and (*d*) become myelinated just behind the lamina cribrosa (Fig. 1.19).

The lamina cribrosa is a specialized arrangement of glial columns and connective tissue plates that form 200–300 holes through which all optic nerve axons pass (225,226) (Figs. 1.20 and 1.21). The fenestrations of the lamina cribrosa form a tight seal that shields the relatively high intraocular pressure from the retrolaminar tissues (227,228). Cells within the lamina cribrosa and the ONH astrocytes secrete neurotrophin and glial cell-line–derived neurotrophic factor (GDNF), which suggests they may be important in maintaining the health of the nearby axons, although it is not yet known whether RGC axons express GDNF receptors (229,230). However, alterations in the structure of the lamina cribrosa may damage neurons. For instance, elevated intraocular pressure induces (*a*) changes in the extracellular matrix that cause posterior displacement of the lamina cribrosa; (*b*) changes in the pore size of the lamina cribrosa; (*c*) a higher translaminar pressure gradient; and (*d*) astrocytes to elaborate nitric oxide, which kills neurons (231–236). Similarly, elevated intracranial pressure, which is transmitted along the perineural subarachnoid space to the ONH (237), can displace the lamina cribrosa anteriorly, which also can damage axons (238).

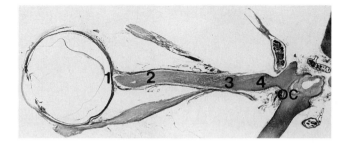

Figure 1.18. Histologic section showing the four topographic divisions of the normal optic nerve (1, intraocular; 2, intraorbital; 3, intracanalicular; 4, intracranial) and optic chiasm (OC). (From Hogan MJ, Zimmerman LE. Ophthalmic Pathology. An Atlas and Textbook. Philadelphia, WB Saunders, 1962.)

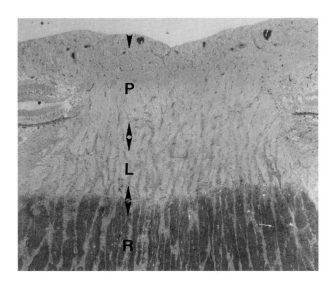

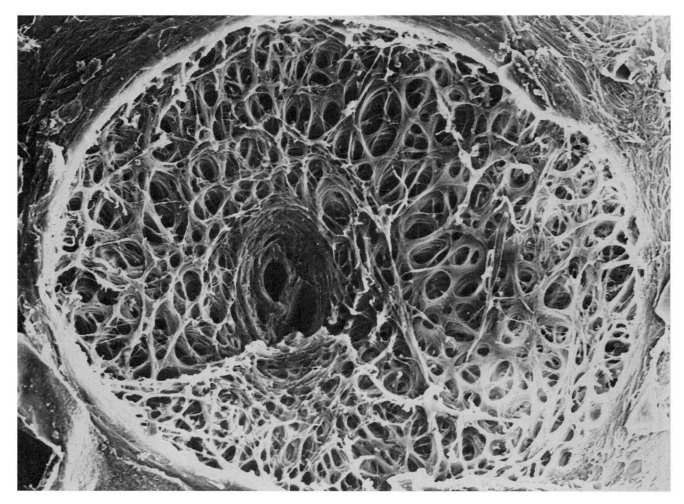

Figure 1.19. Light photomicrograph showing architectural arrangement of the prelaminar (P), laminar (L), and retrolaminar (R) portions of the optic nerve. The retrolaminar segment of the optic nerve is darker because of the presence of myelin. Note the abrupt transition between myelinated and unmyelinated segments of the optic nerve, which occurs just posterior to the lamina cribrosa. (Courtesy of Dr. H. A. Quigley.)

Figure 1.20. Scanning electron micrograph of the lamina cribrosa, viewed from the vitreous cavity.

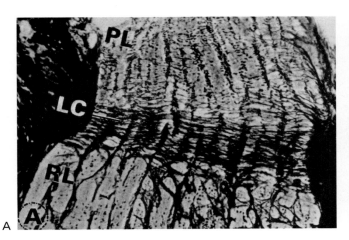 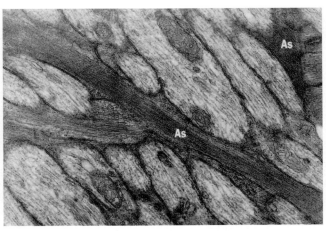

Figure 1.21. Histology of the optic nerve head at the laminar cribrosa. *A,* Longitudinal section of the optic nerve head and adjacent retrolaminar segment of the optic nerve in rhesus monkeys. LC, lamina cribrosa; PL, prelaminar region; RL, retrolaminar region. *B,* Transmission electron micrograph of optic nerve axons (lighter cells) of lamina choroidalis. Axons make intimate contact with astrocytic processes (As), which are the dark cells that are filled with intermediate filaments and interconnect with each other. Magnification ×13,000. (*A,* Hayreh SS. From Anterior Ischemic Optic Neuropathy. New York, Springer-Verlag, 1975:4. *B,* From Kline LD, ed. Optic Nerve Disorders. American Academy of Ophthalmology Monograph, 1996:5.)

The extracellular space is relatively small compared to the total tissue volume of the ONH (173). However, diffusion of ions, molecules, or fluid within the extracellular space may alter axonal function (239). Normally, free diffusion of molecules within the intravascular spaces of the ONH is limited by tight junctions between capillary endothelial cells. Further, free diffusion of molecules to the subretinal space is constrained by tight junctions between specialized cells located at the point of contact between the medial edge of the retina and the perineural RPE (240). However, there is no impediment to intercellular molecular diffusion at the ONH surface, and thus fluid can move from choroid to the optic nerve extracellular space or between the vitreous and the cerebrospinal fluid (CSF) through the ONH.

The clinical appearance of the ONH varies with the size of the scleral canal and the angle at which the optic nerve exits the eye. A larger scleral canal is associated with a larger physiologic cup size (241). A relatively small optic nerve cup is generally associated with a smaller scleral canal. Patients with a small cup-to-disc ratio are prone to develop nonarteritic, anterior ischemic optic neuropathy (242–244). There is a positive correlation between the size of the ONH and the number of photoreceptors, RGC axons, and retinal surface area (245–247).

A tilted ONH is a common feature of myopia. In this condition, the optic nerve fibers exit the sclera at an acute angle temporally and a turn of more than 90 degrees nasally. This anomaly is also associated with a slightly recessed temporal, perineural border of the RPE, which produces a temporal crescent. Also, there is ectasia of the inferonasal fundus, which often accounts for the relative depression of superotemporal isopters on visual field testing of myopic patients. Stimuli presented superotemporally may fall short of the retinal focal plane in myopic eyes, which retards their recognition and produces an apparent depression of the visual field. Alternatively, visual field defects may result from neural and not optical factors, owing to a partially hypoplastic nerve as an associated finding of the titled disc syndrome (248).

The orbital segment of the optic nerve is about 25 mm long and is lax in its course, which allows the eye to move fully without creating tension on the optic nerve (249) (Fig. 1.22). This redundancy also provides an allowance of up

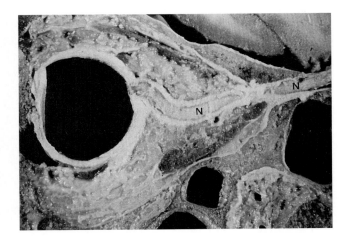

Figure 1.22. Sagittal section through a normal orbit showing the optic nerve (N). The length of the nerve within the orbit appears to exceed the distance from the posterior aspect of the globe to the apex of the orbit. The intraorbital and intracanalicular portions of the nerve are covered by leptomeninges, the dural sheath of which is continuous with the periorbita lining the inner surface of the orbital walls and the dura lining the base of the skull. (From Unsöld R, DeGroot J, Newton TH. Images of the optic nerve: anatomic-CT correlation. AJR Am J Roentgenol 1980; 135:767–773.)

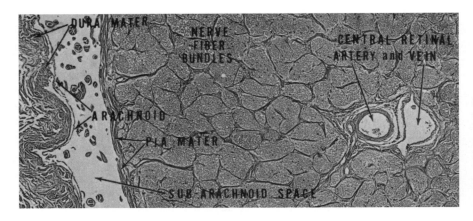

Figure 1.23. Cross-section of human optic nerve. Bundles of nerve fibers are divided into bundles by connective tissue septa that are continuous with both the connective tissue of the pia mater and the adventitia of the central retinal vessels. Small, penetrating blood vessels and capillaries within the connective tissue septae are the dominant source of nourishment to the axons along the orbital segment of the optic nerve.

to 9 mm of proptosis before the optic nerve becomes fully stretched. The orbital segment of the optic nerve expands to ~4.5 mm from 3 mm because of the addition of myelin to most axons (225) (Fig. 1.20). Bundles of nerve fibers are surrounded by connective tissue septa containing small arterioles, venules, and capillaries (Fig. 1.23). With the exception of the central retinal artery (CRA), there are few vessels larger than capillaries within this portion of the optic nerve. At the orbital apex, the ophthalmic artery lies below and lateral to the optic nerve. The inferior division of the oculomotor nerve, the abducens nerve, and the ciliary ganglion are all located lateral to the optic nerve (Fig. 1.24).

The intracanalicular (intraosseous) segment of the optic nerve exits the orbit through the optic foramen, which is the anterior opening of the optic canal in the orbital apex. The 10-mm-long canal, which widens toward the intracranial end, is formed by the union of the lesser wings of the sphenoid bone (250–252) (Fig. 1.25). The thickness of the bony optic canal wall varies from medial to lateral, and anterior to posterior. The medial wall, which is thinnest in the mid-canal, separates the optic nerve from the sphenoid and posterior ethmoid sinuses. Inferolaterally, the optic canal is separated from the superior orbital fissure by a bony ridge, the optic strut. Anomalies of the optic canals may occur, including its absence (253,254).

Each optic canal runs posteriorly and medially at an angle

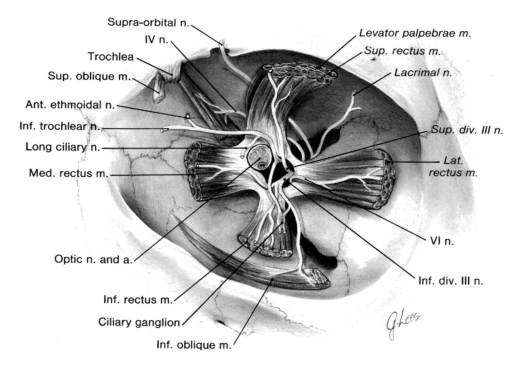

Figure 1.24. View of the posterior orbit showing the relationship of the optic nerve to the ocular motor nerves and extraocular muscles. The ophthalmic artery lies immediately below the optic nerve. (Redrawn from Wolff E. Anatomy of the Eye and Orbit. 6th ed. Philadelphia, WB Saunders, 1968.)

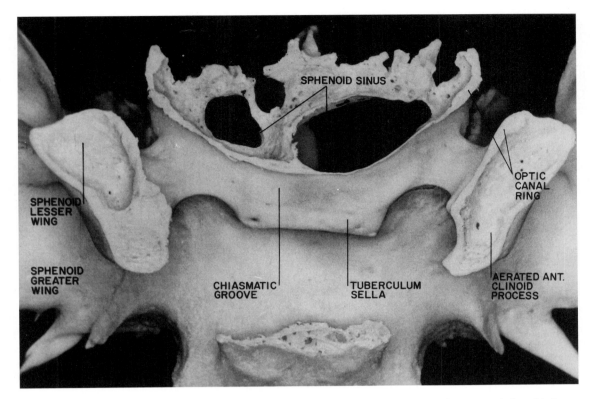

Figure 1.25. Horizontally sectioned sphenoid bone demonstrates tapering of optic canals as they approach the orbit (best seen on the right). The optic ring is formed by dense bone that surrounds the distal segment of the optic canal. The roof of both optic canals has been removed. (From Maniscalco JE, Habal MB. Microanatomy of the optic canal. J Neurosurg 1978; 48:402–406.)

of about 35 degrees with the midsagittal plane (Fig. 1.26). The intracanalicular optic nerve is tightly fixed within the optic canal, which is lined with dura mater (Fig. 1.27). This tight packing of the nerve within the canal may predispose the optic nerve to percussive trauma from a blow to the frontotemporal region of the skull (i.e., indirect traumatic optic neuropathy), even sometimes following seemingly insignificant trauma. Each canal transmits the optic nerve, the ophthalmic artery, some filaments of the sympathetic carotid plexus, and the orbital extension of the cranial leptomeninges. Above each optic canal is a plate of bone that separates it from the frontal lobe of the brain. Medially, the sphenoid sinus and the posterior ethmoidal air cells border the canal.

Anatomic variations of the canalicular region include absence of bone (255), protrusion of the optic canal into the sphenoid sinus (256), and pneumosinus dilatans, which is an expansion of the paranasal sinuses without erosion of adjacent bone. Development of pneumosinus dilatans may be associated with an adjacent optic nerve sheath meningioma (257–260). Lack of a bony partition from the sinuses can permit spread of sinus infection to the optic nerve (256,261).

The intracranial segment of the optic nerve exits under a firm fold of dura mater. The optic nerves, which are somewhat flattened immediately after emerging from the canal, extend posteriorly, superiorly, and medially to join at the

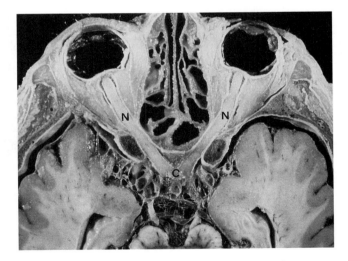

Figure 1.26. Axial section of normal optic nerves (N) showing relationships to other orbital and intracranial structures. The intraorbital and intracanalicular portions of the nerve are covered by a dural sheath that is continuous with the periorbita lining the inner surface of the orbital walls and the dura lining the base of the skull. C, optic chiasm. (From Unsöld R, DeGroot J, Newton TH. Images of the optic nerve: anatomic-CT correlation. AJR Am J Roentgenol 1980;135:767–773.)

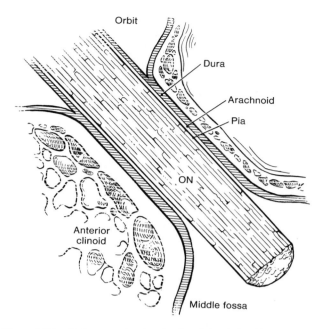

Figure 1.27. Optic nerve sheaths, showing their relationship to the optic nerve (ON) and to the surrounding sphenoid bone. The dura is tightly adherent to the bone within the optic canal. Within the orbit it divides into two layers: one remains as the outer sheath of the optic nerve, and the other becomes the orbital periosteum (periorbita). Intracranially, the dura leaves the optic nerve to become the periosteum of the sphenoid bone.

optic chiasm. The length of the intracranial optic nerve varies considerably, from 3 to 16 mm (262). Proximally, the gyrus recti of the frontal lobes lie above the optic nerves. The olfactory tract is separated from the optic nerve by the anterior cerebral and anterior communicating arteries. The internal carotid arteries lie lateral to the optic nerves (255,263–266).

OPTIC NERVE BLOOD SUPPLY

Most of the optic nerve receives its blood from branches of the ophthalmic artery (OA), which is the first major branch of the internal carotid artery (ICA). The OA arises typically just above the exit of the ICA from the cavernous sinus (265,267). The OA then passes through the optic canal below the optic nerve (Fig. 1.24), although the artery is separated from the nerve by a dural sheath. Within the orbit, the ophthalmic artery gives rise to two or three posterior ciliary arteries (PCAs) and the CRA, which pierces the optic nerve approximately 12 mm behind the globe and then runs anteriorly within the optic nerve (Fig. 1.28).

The blood supply to the optic nerve differs significantly depending upon which segment is considered. Although there is considerable variability in the pattern of blood supply to the optic nerve, the following generalizations follow from studies of large numbers of humans (268). The blood supply to the most superficial aspect of the ONH is from branches of the CRA (Fig. 1.29). The blood supply to the region around the lamina cribrosa derives from the short PCAs or

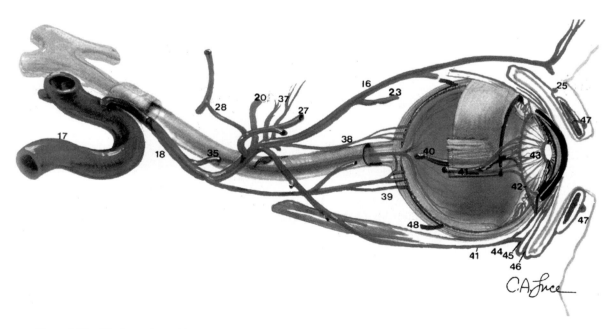

Figure 1.28. The internal carotid artery blood supply to the orbit and eye, with emphasis on the ophthalmic artery and its major branches. Key for arteries: 16, frontal branch; 17, internal carotid; 18, ophthalmic; 20, posterior ethmoidal branch of the ophthalmic; 25, superior peripheral arcade; 27, lacrimal; 28, recurrent meningeal; 35, central retinal; 37, muscular branches for the superior rectus, superior oblique, and levator palpebrae muscles; 38, medial posterior ciliary; 39, short ciliary; 40, long ciliary; 41, anterior ciliary; 42, greater circle of the iris; 43, lesser circle of the iris; 44, episcleral; 45, subconjunctival; 46, conjunctival; 47, marginal arcade; 49, medial palpebral; 48, vortex vein. (From BM Zide, GW Jelks. Surgical Anatomy of the Orbit. New York: Raven Press, 1985.)

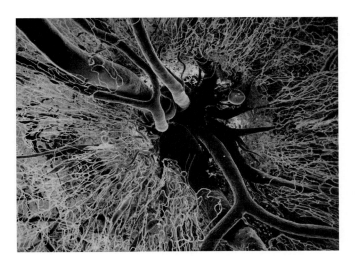

Figure 1.29. Scanning electron micrograph showing intraocular vasculature of the optic disc. Note central retinal artery, central retinal vein, and numerous capillary-sized vessels. (Courtesy of Dr. H. A. Quigley.)

circle of Zinn-Haller. More specifically, the prelaminar region is derived mostly from the peripapillary, short PCAs via the choroid (Figs. 1.30 to 1.32). The laminar supply is usually more directly from the short posterior ciliary arteries or the circle of Zinn-Haller (265,267,269–276). This circle, when present, lies within the sclera and surrounds the optic nerve at the neuro-ocular junction. It receives blood from four to eight PCAs, choroidal feeder vessels, and the perineural, pial arterial network (272,273,277–279). The vessels entering the circle of Zinn-Haller do not always form a com-

plete ring, which should not necessarily imply there is an incomplete functional anastomosis. The radial branches from the circle of Zinn-Haller that supply the laminar optic disc are autoregulated (275,280). The venous drainage of the ONH is primarily via the central retinal venous system.

The blood supply to the orbital segment of the optic nerve is almost entirely from PCAs via the pial network (Fig. 1.30). The plethora of pial vessels that surround and enter the optic nerve proper within the septae (Fig. 1.23) presumably explains the relative resilience of the intraorbital segment of the optic nerve to ischemia. Branches of the internalized CRA also may contribute to the optic nerve blood supply (115,267,269–276,281). At the orbital apex, collateral circulation from the external carotid artery via the middle meningeal artery may contribute substantially to the optic nerve blood supply (269,270). Orbital vessels can be seen with magnetic resonance imaging (MRI) (282).

The blood supply to the intracanalicular segment of the optic nerve lies within a watershed zone. Here there are contributions anteriorly from collateral branches of the ophthalmic artery and posteriorly from pial vessels arising from the ICA and superior hypophyseal arteries (269,270,283).

The blood supply to the intracranial segment of the optic nerve derives from several sources, including the ICA, the superior hypophyseal arteries, the A1 segment of the anterior cerebral artery, and the anterior communicating artery (263–265,283,284) (Fig. 1.33).

The blood vessels of the optic nerve generally have been believed to have a blood–brain barrier. Recently, however, human prelaminar microvessels have been shown to lack a characteristic biochemical marker of a blood–brain barrier. Despite the presence of tight junctions, these vessels are

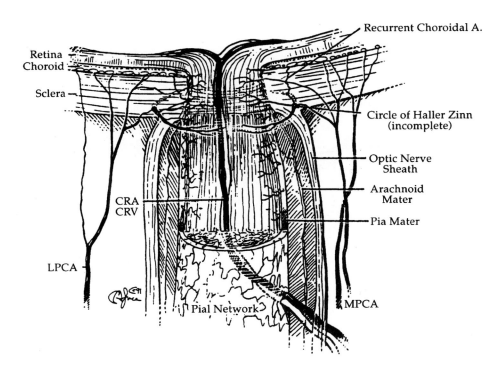

Figure 1.30. The blood supply to the proximal optic nerve and choroid arises from the branches of the medial (MPCA) and lateral (LPCA) posterior ciliary arteries, the incomplete circle of Zinn-Haller, the pial network, and recurrent choroidal arteries. The posterior ciliary arteries send branches to the circle of Zinn-Haller and the pial network. The central retinal artery (CRA) provides minute branches to the optic nerve capillaries as it passes anteriorly to supply the retina. The central retinal vein (CRV) parallels the course of the CRA. (From Kupersmith MJ. Neurovascular Neuro-Ophthalmology. New York, Springer-Verlag, 1993.)

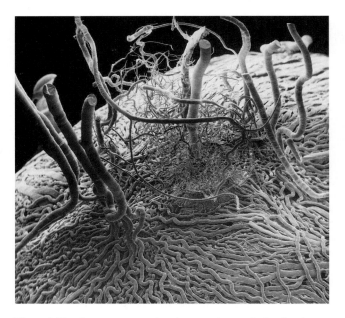

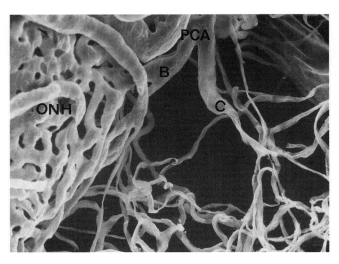

Figure 1.32. High-power scanning electron micrograph showing a posterior ciliary artery (PCA) with separate branches to the choroid (C) and to the optic nerve head (B). ONH, optic nerve head. (Courtesy of Dr. H. A. Quigley.)

Figure 1.31. Low-power scanning electron micrograph showing the vasculature of the posterior aspect of the globe as viewed from behind the globe. The posterior ciliary arteries (long and short) are visualized, as are their branches to the choroid and optic nerve head. (From Risco JM, Grimson BS, Johnson PT. Angioarchitecture of the ciliary artery circulation of the posterior pole. Arch Ophthalmol 1981;99:864–868.)

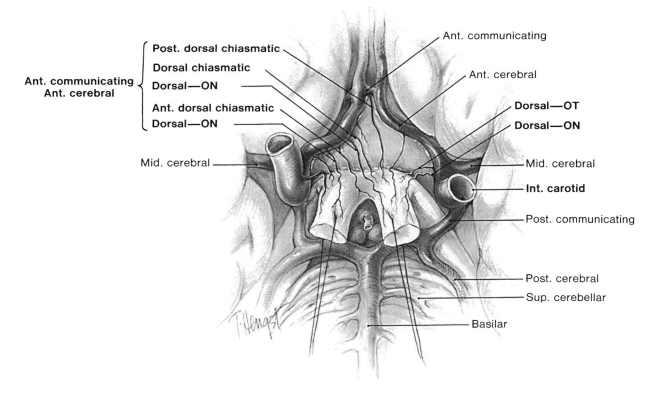

Figure 1.33. Blood supply to the dorsal aspect of the optic chiasm and intracranial optic nerves. ON, optic nerve; OT, optic tract. (From Wollschlaeger P, Wollschlaeger G, Ide C, et al. Arterial blood supply of the human optic chiasm and surrounding structures. Ann Ophthalmol 1971;3:862–869.)

abnormally permeable, perhaps because of active transendothelial, pinocytotic vesicular transport (285). This permeability may explain the very early hyperfluorescence of the ONH seen in fluorescein angiography, a finding previously ascribed to diffusion of dye from the adjacent choroid.

OPTIC NERVE SHEATHS

The leptomeninges that surround the optic nerve—the dura mater, arachnoid, and pia mater—are continuous with the leptomeninges of the brain (Figs. 1.27 and 1.34). Embryologically, the meninges develop from different sources: the dura from mesenchyme, and the arachnoid and pia largely from ectoderm. The dura mater near the globe splays out slightly and fuses with the sclera surrounding the optic nerve. At the apex of the orbit, the dura fuses with the periosteum and annulus of Zinn, then passes through the foramen, where it merges with the intracranial dura that lines the base of the skull. Thus, the intracranial portion of the optic nerve is surrounded only by pia mater. Normal human optic nerves have a sparse population of mast cells in their dura mater (much less so in the arachnoid). These cells become more numerous and can be found in the optic nerve parenchyma in injured eyes, although it is not known whether they can incite injury to the optic nerve or are merely epiphenomenal to the primary disease (286).

The arachnoid that surrounds the optic nerve consists of a trabeculum of collagenous and elastic fibers that is identical with arachnoid tissue elsewhere in the CNS. Delicate trabeculae connect the arachnoid with the dura and underlying pia. Mesothelial cells line the subarachnoid and subdural spaces and can give rise to laminated and often calcified psammoma bodies. Arachnoidal villi are present in the optic nerve sheaths (287). The perineural subarachnoid space is quite small, holding approximately 0.1 mL of fluid. This space is continuous with the intracranial subarachnoid space, and there is a rough equivalence between subarachnoid and CSF pressure (237). Variations in partitioning of the perineural subarachnoid space may explain the variable presence of papilledema among patients with increased intracranial pressure (288).

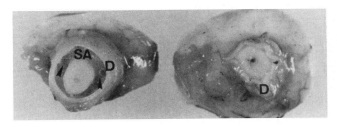

Figure 1.34.   Transverse section through the optic nerves of a patient with optic atrophy. The dura mater (D) and arachnoid of the left optic nerve are distended and show the delicate subarachnoid trabeculae stretched between the arachnoid and the pia (*arrowheads*). SA, distended subarachnoid space. The sheaths of the right optic nerve are folded around the nerve so that neither the arachnoid trabeculae nor the pia are visible. (From Lindenberg R, Walsh FB, Sacks JG. Neuropathology of Vision: An Atlas. Philadelphia, Lea & Febiger, 1973.)

The pia mater is a very thin and delicate membrane that adheres to the surface of the optic nerve. The pia, which is the most vascular sheath covering the optic nerve, invests capillaries as they enter the substance of the nerve to create fibrovascular septa within the optic nerve (Fig. 1.23).

OPTIC NERVE AXONS

Nerve fibers represent roughly 90% of the tissue of the ONH (173). The topography of the fibers at the ONH is described above (Fig. 1.17). The right-angle turn of the axons at the ONH is associated with an increased concentration of mitochondria in the prelaminar region (227,289). This accumulation of mitochondria, which had been thought to result from mechanical stricture of axons as they pass through the lamina cribrosa, may more likely reflect metabolic differences between unmyelinated and myelinated segments of the optic nerve (290). Unmyelinated nerves require more energy to conduct impulses than myelinated axons, which (mostly) only need to employ energy demanding voltage-gated channels at the nodes of Ranvier. Mitochondrial accumulation at the ONH can be induced by elevated intraocular pressure, which decreases the expression of microtubule-associated protein 1, which disrupts axonal ultrastructure and transport (289).

RGC axons express numerous types of ionic channels. Voltage-gated sodium channels are located at nodes of Ranvier at 25 times the concentration found along myelin-covered axonal segments. The high density of sodium channels at the nodes is guided by a protein secreted by oligodendrocytes. The voltage-gated sodium channels permit the rapid influx of sodium ions that depolarizes the cell, which can lead to generation of an action potential. By contrast, voltage-gated potassium channels (of which there are at least four types) permit the efflux of potassium ions to repolarize a cell after an action potential has been generated. The potassium channels are located mainly at juxtaparanodal regions where the axon is covered by compact myelin sheaths, which produce tight axoglial contact. A molecular cue for potassium channel development has not been identified (291). Voltage-gated sodium and voltage-gated potassium channels, therefore, are segregated along an axon. Their respective distributions change after a demyelinating injury.

The axons within the optic nerve are extensions from a diverse collection of RGC types. As such, the optic nerve is a conduit for parallel paths that transmit visual information to the brain. A review of afferent pathway physiology is presented above and below.

Adult humans have, on average, 1.2 million RGCs (126,127,246,292–297). The axonal diameters have two peaks (0.7 and 1.5 μm), which presumably correlate with the large (i.e., M-) and small (i.e., P-) RGC classes (246,292,297). A few centrifugal fibers that originate in the brain are present in the optic nerve, even in humans (298–301). In the rat, cell bodies of origin for these efferent fibers have been identified in the suprachiasmatic nucleus, which suggests they might participate in circadian rhythm physiology (302).

The arrangement of fibers in the ONH and distal optic

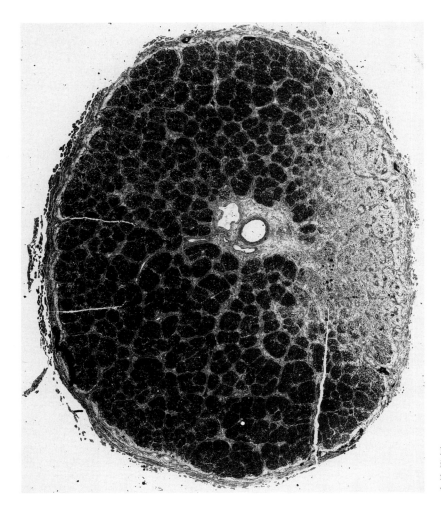

Figure 1.35. Cross-section of the anterior optic nerve in a patient with atrophy of the papillomacular bundle from toxic optic neuropathy. The atrophy is confined to a wedge-shaped sector in the temporal portion of the nerve.

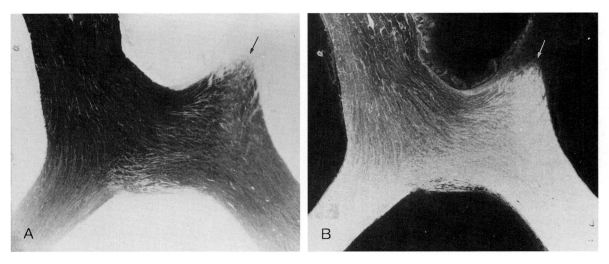

Figure 1.36. Light-field (*A*) and dark-field (*B*) autoradiographs of a horizontal section through the optic chiasm of a macaque monkey. The right eye was enucleated 4 years earlier, at which time the left eye was injected with [H³]proline. *A*, Under lightfield illumination, the labeled left optic nerve appears dark. Label extends into the distal portion of the atrophic right optic nerve (*arrow*), producing Wilbrand's knee. *B*, Under dark-field illumination, the radioactive label from the left eye appears bright. Note the extension of label representing Wilbrand's knee into the distal aspect of the atrophic right optic nerve. (Courtesy of Dr. Jonathan Horton.)

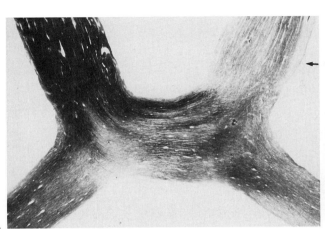
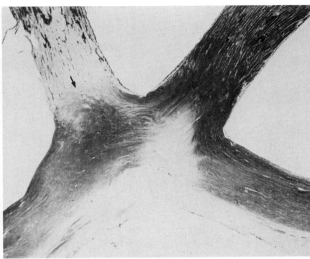

Figure 1.37. Wilbrand's knee in human tissue. *A,* Woelcke myelin stain of a horizontal section through the optic chiasm from a patient whose left eye was enucleated 5 months before death. There is reduced myelin staining in the left optic nerve (*arrow*), but there is no evidence of Wilbrand's knee. *B,* Woelcke myelin stain of a horizontal section through the optic chiasm from a patient whose right eye was enucleated 2 years before death. There is more pronounced atrophy of the right optic nerve, and a small Wilbrand's knee is evident (*arrow*). (Courtesy of Dr. Jonathan Horton.)

nerve corresponds generally to their distribution in the retina. The outflow from the papillomacular bundle is positioned temporally within the anterior optic nerve (Fig. 1.35), then gradually moves centrally in the more posterior optic nerve (303–305). Intracranially, the axons partially lose their retinotopy because of the decussation of some axons (306). The macular projection does not have a precise localization in the posterior nerve (307).

Historically, a Wilbrand's knee was believed to exist at the junction of the optic nerve and chiasm, where a small number of inferonasal retinal axons were believed to cross into the opposite optic nerve and pass anteriorly for a few

millimeters, then turn back posteriorly to enter the chiasm (308,309). The "knee" is now believed to be an artifact (310). A "knee" can be created by removal of one eye (310). Apparently, the gliotic reaction secondary to optic nerve atrophy over a period of years distorts the anterior chiasm, pulling some axons into an aberrant location (Figs 1.36 and 1.37). Thus, a "knee" is not present normally. A paradox therefore exists, given that visual field defects produced by compressive lesions at the anterior chiasm often include a contralateral, superotemporal field depression (i.e., junctional scotoma), which heretofore was explained by the presence of a "knee."

OPTIC CHIASM

EMBRYOLOGY

The optic chiasm is a commissure formed by converging optic nerves anteriorly and diverging optic tracts posteriorly (Fig. 1.38). During development, the chiasmal anlage separates from the floor of the third ventricle, maintaining contact only at the boundary between its posterior aspect and the anterior-inferior wall of the third ventricle (Fig. 1.39).

The location of the chiasm is established by the first RGC fibers that arrive, which occurs between the fourth and sixth week of development. The next fundamental step is the proper routing of the incoming axons. Numerous factors contribute to the directional preferences of the arriving axons (311,312) (Fig. 1.40). Glia within the optic nerve and some highly conserved molecules are believed to be instrumental to the process (306,313–318). For instance, *Zic2* is expressed early in retinal development in the cells that will project ipsilaterally, and thus Zic2 may endow these cells with response properties that influence their trajectory at the

chiasm. The differential spatial and temporal expression of the *Pax2* gene by the growing axons and the sonic Hh gene at the developing chiasm are also likely relevant to the formation of the decussation (319). Specialized glial cells in the developing diencephalon extend their radial processes, which physically interact with the incoming axons (306). These glial cells express *Eph/ephrinA* molecules, which influence the growth of axons within the chiasm (see also the section on the retina). Metalloproteases, which modulate the interaction of local environmental cues with growth cones extending from the distal axons, also seem to be relevant for proper wiring (320). Axons that remain uncrossed tend to reach the chiasm before those that will cross, which might expose the different populations to time-varying changes in the local environment (321,322).

The decision point is apparently not binary for these incoming axons. Real-time video microscopy has revealed that axons move through the chiasm in a pulsed, saltatory fash-

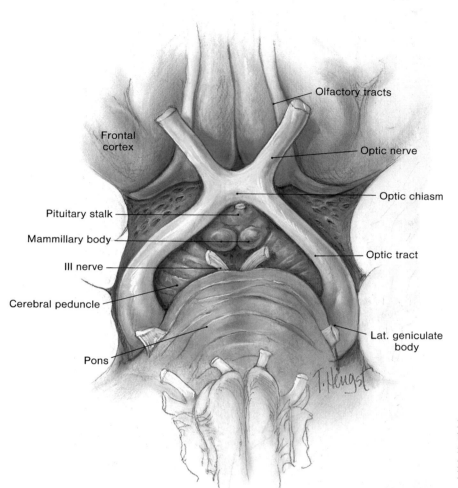

Figure 1.38. The optic chiasm viewed from below. Note relationships of the mammillary bodies, oculomotor nerves (III nerve), and cerebral peduncles to the chiasm. (Redrawn from Pernkopf E. In: Ferner HA, ed. Atlas of Topographical and Applied Human Anatomy. Vol 1. Philadelphia, WB Saunders, 1963.)

ion. All axons that approach the chiasmal midline display especially long pauses in activity, with ameboid movements of their growth cones, which assume a more complex morphology than is typical of advancing axons (323,324). Following this complex orchestration near the end of 3 months of gestation, an adult-like hemidecussation is established.

The shape of the developing optic chiasm differs from that of the mature chiasm. The evolution in shape partly relates to the shift from a lateral to eventually a frontal position of the eyes in the head. In the second half of gestation the gross anatomic changes include (*a*) progressive narrowing of the angle between the two optic nerves to about 45 degrees, without a corresponding change in the angle formed by the optic tracts; (*b*) separation of the chiasm from the diaphragma sellae and pituitary gland with development of the chiasmatic cistern; (*c*) progressive elevation of the chiasm above the optic foramina; and (*d*) thinning of attachments of the chiasm to the floor of the third ventricle.

Rarely, a chiasm does not form, and this can occur despite normal development of the fovea (325,326). Malformation

of the fovea *and* chiasm occurs in patients with albinism. Deficient melanin production leads to an abnormally small uncrossed projection, perhaps because of the timing of RGC development (discussed previously) rather than to some influence at the chiasm per se (312). In particular, albino mice have fewer Zic2-positive retinal neurons than their pigmented counterparts, which (given the putative role of Zic2 described above) may explain the diminished ipsilateral projection (327). The disordered chiasmal projection in albinos can be recognized by MRI, which can reveal a smaller chiasmal width and a relatively wide angle between the optic nerves and the optic tracts (328).

GROSS ANATOMY OF THE CHIASM AND PERICHIASMAL REGION

The optic chiasm has a transverse diameter of 10–20 mm, an anteroposterior width of 4–13 mm, and thickness of 3–5 mm (262,329). The optic chiasm is covered, except where attached to the brain, by arachnoid and pia mater, the latter

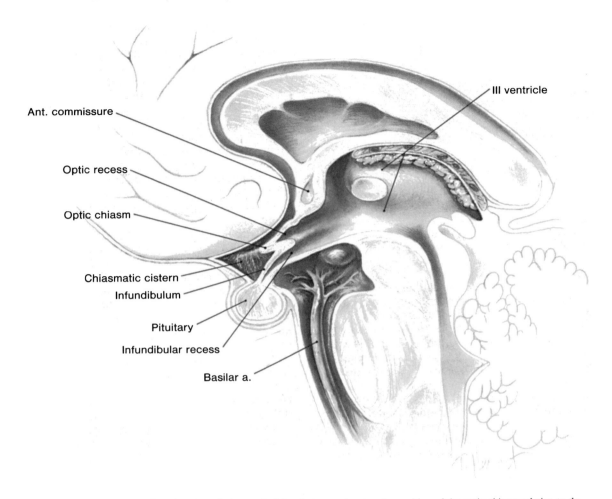

Figure 1.39. Midsagittal section through the cerebral hemispheres, showing the position of the optic chiasm relative to the third ventricle and basal cisterns. (Redrawn from Pernkopf E. In: Ferner HA, ed. Atlas of Topographical and Applied Human Anatomy. Vol 1. Philadelphia, WB Saunders, 1963.)

being continuous with the pia of the optic nerves and part of the optic tracts. The optic chiasm is in direct contact with CSF anteriorly within the subarachnoid space, and posteriorly within the third ventricle (Fig. 1.39 and 1.41), features easily visualized with MRI (Fig. 1.42).

Inferiorly, the optic chiasm lies over the body of the sphenoid bone, typically above the diaphragma sellae and (paradoxically) only rarely within the sulcus chiasmatis (330) (Fig. 1.25). The relative position of the chiasm over the sella turcica is variable. The chiasm is (*a*) above the tuberculum sellae (i.e., "prefixed") in 12%; (*b*) above the diaphragma sellae in 79%; and (*c*) above the dorsum sellae (i.e., "postfixed") in 4% of cases (264,330) (Fig. 1.41). In patients with brachycephaly, the chiasm typically is more rostral and dorsal than in dolichocephaly. This variability of position partially accounts for the variable patterns of visual field defects seen in patients with upwardly expanding pituitary adenomas.

The intracranial optic nerves do not lie on a horizontal plane; rather, they rise upward from the optic canals at an

angle of 15–45 degrees (331). The chiasm lies above the diaphragma sellae, the dural covering of the sella turcica, by approximately 10 mm (332–335) (Fig. 1.43). The sphenoid sinuses lie under the chiasm only when they extend far back into the body of the sphenoid bone. In one third of adults, an arachnoid membrane extends outward from the infundibulum to fuse with arachnoid around the carotid arteries and the inferior surface of the chiasm (336).

The shape of the pituitary gland varies considerably among individuals. The width of the gland is typically greater than or equal to its depth or length. The lateral and superior margins of the gland are more variable in shape because they are not confined within bone. Rarely, the pituitary gland protrudes inferiorly into the sphenoid sinus (264).

Superiorly, the lamina terminalis, which defines the anterior end of the diencephalon, extends upward from the chiasm to the anterior commissure. The A2 segments of the anterior cerebral arteries pass medially and upward above the optic chiasm. The anterior cerebral and anterior communicating arteries may be situated above the chiasm or the

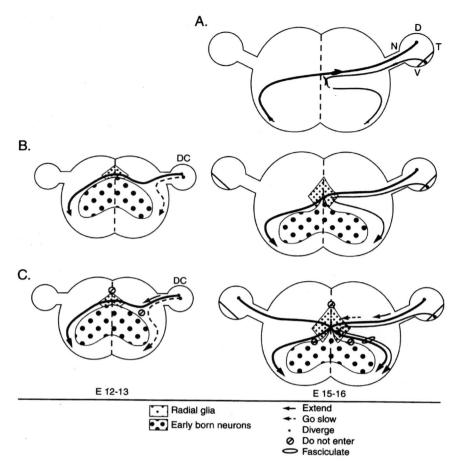

Figure 1.40. Trajectory of retinal ganglion cell axons during early and late phase of chiasm formation. Horizontal view of axon growth and cells of the ventral diencephalon during the early (E12–E13) and later (E15–E16) phases of axon growth. Specialized radial glia (*small dots*) form palisades on either side of the midline and express RC2 as well as *Slit2* (rostrally), EphA and EphB receptors, and NrCAM. The early-born neurons (*large dots*) express CD44 and SSEA-1 as well as ephrinAs, Slit 1, Robo1 and Robo2, and disulfated proteoglycans. *Slit1* is expressed dorsal to and around the optic nerve as it enters the brain and more weakly by the CD44/SSEA neurons. *Slit2* is strongly expressed in the preoptic region directly dorsal and anterior to the chiasm. *A*, At E15–E16, during the major phase of retinal axon divergence, growth cones have different forms depending on their locale and behavior. Crossing (*thick line*) and uncrossed (*thin line*) fibers have slender streamlined growth cones in the optic nerve and optic tract. Near the midline, all axons pause and have more spread forms. Uncrossed growth cones extend along the midline in highly complex shapes before turning back to the ipsilateral optic tract. *B*, In the early phase of retinal axon growth, the first-born uncrossed retinal axons from the dorsocentral retina (DC) enter the ipsilateral optic tract directly, quite far from the midline. In contrast, in the later period, uncrossed axons travel toward the midline and diverge from crossing axons within the radial glial palisade. Crossed axons at both ages traverse the midline close to the rostral tip of the early-born neurons. All retinal axons at both ages grow around the contours of the early-born neurons. *C*, Maneuvers of retina axons with respect to the resident cells of the optic chiasm. DC, dorsocentral; D, dorsal; V, ventral; N, nasal; T, temporal. (From Mason C, Erskine L. The development of retinal decussations. In: Chalupa LM, Werner JS, eds. The Visual Neurosciences. Cambridge, MA, MIT Press, 2004:97.)

optic nerves, or they may rest directly on these structures (Fig. 1.44). The junction of the anterior communicating artery with the A1 segments usually occurs above the chiasm rather than the optic nerves (263). Laterally, the ICAs emerge from the cavernous sinuses and approach the posterior optic nerves and sides of the chiasm. Occasionally, the ICAs contact and compress these structures. Posteriorly, the chiasm is bounded by the third ventricle, which explains

the vulnerability of the chiasm to compression or infiltration by lesions within the ventricle or even an expanded ventricle.

ORGANIZATION OF NERVE FIBERS WITHIN THE OPTIC CHIASM

Several generalizations can be made about the topography of fibers passing through the chiasm, although much of our knowledge in this regard derives from nonhuman primates.

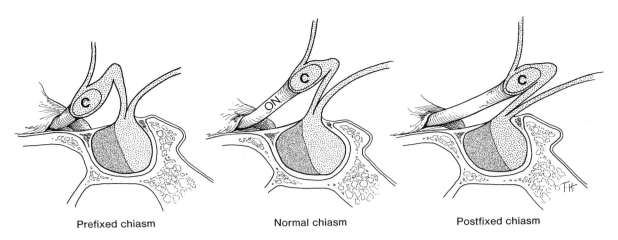

Prefixed chiasm   Normal chiasm   Postfixed chiasm

Figure 1.41. Three sagittal sections of the optic chiasm and sellar region showing the positions of a prefixed chiasm above the tuberculum sellae (*left*), a normal chiasm above the diaphragma sellae (*center*), and a postfixed chiasm above the dorsum sellae (*right*). The W-shaped clear zone behind the chiasm is the anterior aspect of the third ventricle. (Redrawn from Rhoton AL Jr, Harris FS, Renn WH. Microsurgical anatomy of the sellar region and cavernous sinus. In: Glaser JS, ed. Neuro-Ophthalmology Symposium of the University of Miami and the Bascom Palmer Eye Institute. St Louis, CV Mosby, 1977:75–105.)

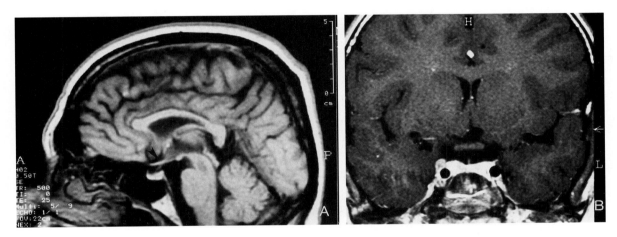

Figure 1.42. MRIs of the normal optic chiasm. *A,* Noncontrast T1-weighted image shows position of the optic chiasm in sagittal section. Note the angle made by the incline of the intracranial portion of the optic nerve as it approaches the chiasm (*arrowhead*). *B,* T1-weighted image after contrast administration shows the position of the body of the chiasm in coronal section.

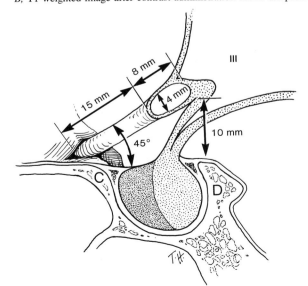

Figure 1.43. Relationships of the optic nerves and optic chiasm to the sellar structures and 3rd ventricle (III); C, anterior clinoid; and D, dorsum sellae. (Redrawn from Glaser JS. Neuro-ophthalmology. Hagerstown, MD, Harper & Row, 1978.)

39

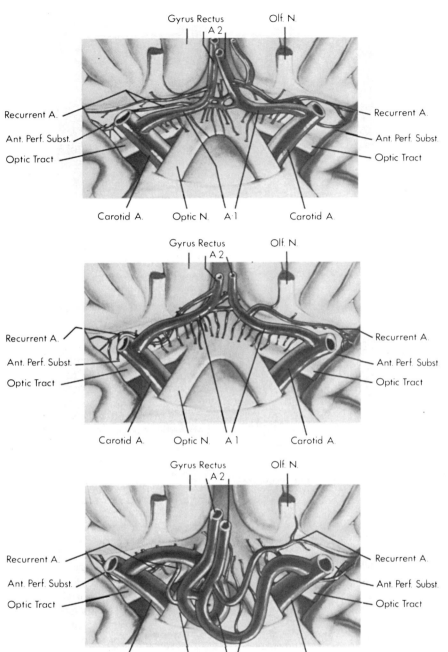

Figure 1.44. Anterior views of the A1 and proximal A2 segments of the anterior cerebral arteries, anterior communicating arteries, and recurrent arteries, showing variations in their relationship to the intracranial optic nerves and optic chiasm. Gyri recti and olfactory nerves are located superiorly. (From Perlmutter D, Rhoton AL Jr. Microsurgical anterior cerebral–anterior communicating–recurrent artery complex. J Neurosurg 1976; 45:259–272.)

First, the proportion of crossed fibers is always greater than the uncrossed population, typically with a ratio of roughly 53:47 in humans (293). Second, retinal fibers projecting to the ipsilateral dLGN come only from the temporal retina, whereas fibers projecting to the contralateral dLGN come only from the nasal retina. The separation between crossed and uncrossed fibers begins just as the fibers reach the chiasm. Uncrossed fibers, both dorsal and ventral, maintain their relative position through the lateral chiasm and pass directly into the ipsilateral optic tract (310). Crossed fibers

from the dorsal retina project more caudally in the chiasm than crossed fibers of the ventral retina. An exception to these principles occurs for fibers that project to the superior colliculi, which project from throughout the retinae (337). Third, macular projections are both crossed and uncrossed and constitute a large percentage of the chiasmal fibers. Macular fibers are more concentrated dorsally and centrally and are generally not present in the inferior rostral and caudal regions of the chiasm (68,307,329,338). Fourth, retinohypothalamic axons exit the chiasm posteriorly (without entering the tracts) to reach the hypothalamus. Finally, some retinal fibers, especially those of melanopsin-containing RGCs (discussed previously), bifurcate and project to two central sites after they emerge from the chiasm.

BLOOD SUPPLY

The distal optic nerves, optic chiasm, and proximal optic tracts pass below the anterior communicating artery and anterior cerebral arteries and above the posterior communicating arteries, PCAs, and basilar artery (339) (Figs. 1.33 and 1.44). The chiasm obtains blood from branches of all of these surrounding vessels. There is considerable interindividual variation in the blood supply of the chiasm (329). In general, the chiasmal blood supply comes from a dorsal and ventral group of feeder vessels. The dorsal supply derives from branches of the ICA, usually via superior hypophyseal arteries, the A1 and occasionally the A2 segments of the anterior cerebral artery, and the anterior communicating artery. Branches from more distal stretches of the anterior cerebral artery typically supply some of the dorsal chiasm (265,340). The ventral supply derives from branches of the posterior communicating artery, PCA, and basilar artery (339). The superior hypophyseal artery, a branch of the ICA, often provides blood to the ventral chiasm (284). There is often significant collateralization among these vessels (341), which explains the utter rarity of chiasmal infarction.

OPTIC TRACT

The optic tract, which is fully formed by the 13th week of gestation, is the segment of the afferent visual pathway between the chiasm and dLGN. From their origin, the optic tracts diverge in front of the interpeduncular space and wind laterally above the uncus and then around the internal cap-sule to reach the dLGN (Figs. 1.38, 1.45, and 1.46). Unlike the intracranial optic nerves, the optic tracts are firmly attached to the brain throughout their course by glial cells.

Each tract contains crossed and uncrossed fibers, most of which synapse in the dLGN. A few tract fibers turn medially

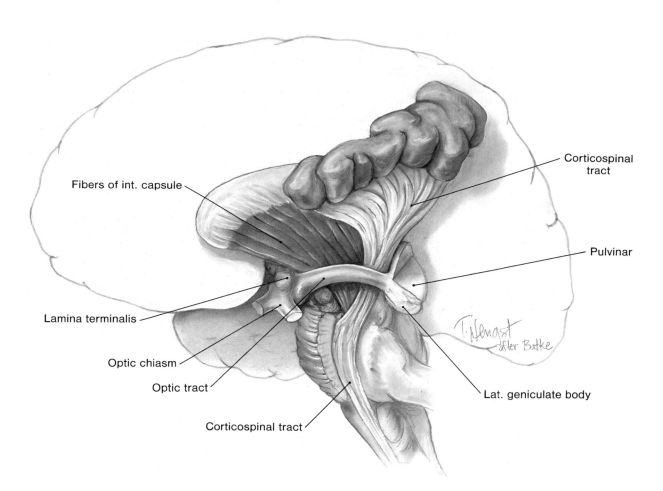

Figure 1.45. The optic tracts and lateral geniculate body viewed in sagittal section. Note the relationship of the optic tract to the internal capsule and corticospinal tract. The pulvinar is just medial to the lateral geniculate body. (Redrawn from Pernkopf E. Atlas of Topographical and Applied Human Anatomy. Vol 1. Philadelphia, WB Saunders, 1963.)

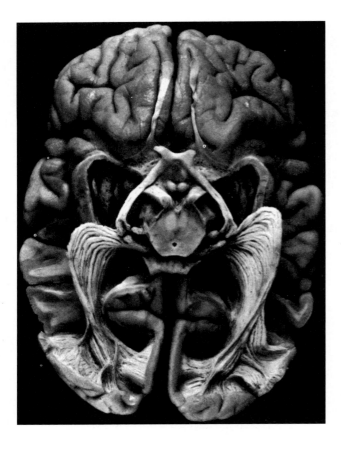

Figure 1.46. Anatomy of the optic tracts and optic radiations. Appearance of the visual sensory pathway in axial section, viewed from below. Note the position of the optic tracts as they originate from the optic chiasm and diverge to end at the lateral geniculate nuclei. The optic radiations extend as fan-shaped structures from the lateral geniculate nuclei to the visual cortices. A large proportion of fibers in the radiations are feedback fibers projecting from the visual cortices to the lateral geniculate nuclei and other deep structures. (From Ghuhbegovic N, Williams TH. The Human Brain: A Photographic Guide. Hagerstown, MD, Harper & Row, 1980.)

before reaching the dLGN to terminate in the pretectal nuclei of the rostral midbrain, where they influence the pupillomotor light reflex. A few of these fibers, whose function is not known, enter the medial geniculate body.

The optic tract fibers rotate their topographic axes with respect to the fibers that enter the tracts. The superior retinal fibers rotate laterally in the tract, and the ventral fibers rotate to a medial position (342,343). The macular fibers shift slightly to the dorsolateral position, whereas the peripheral fibers from the upper and lower retinas are situated dorsomedially and ventrolaterally, respectively. Within the

tracts, there is a partial rearrangement of fibers based upon the functional class of cells. The larger axons of the M-RGCs (discussed previously) are generally more superficial, and the smaller fibers of the P-RGCs are nearest to the pia mater (343,344).

The major blood supply to the optic tract comes from the anterior choroidal artery, a branch of the ICA (345,346). Other arteries often contribute to the blood supply. A dorsal and a ventral "artery of the optic tract" may arise directly from the internal carotid artery (341). The posterior communicating artery may also supply branches to the tract (347).

LATERAL GENICULATE NUCLEUS

The lateral geniculate nucleus (LGN) develops from the lateral wall of the diencephalon, which gives rise to the thalamic, hypothalamic, and habenular nuclei. The LGN is the first of the habenular nuclei to appear, which occurs at the eighth week of gestation as RGC axons arrive (348–351). Myelination of the optic tract begins only after the axonal connections to the LGN have been established. Myelination of the pregeniculate visual pathway begins at the LGN at the fifth month of gestation, then moves rostrally. Lamination of the LGN does not develop until the following month.

ANATOMIC AND FUNCTIONAL ORGANIZATION

The LGN is the principal thalamic visual center linking the retina and the visual cortical areas V1 and to a lesser

extent V2. Each LGN is an oval structure situated in the posterior thalamus, below and lateral to the pulvinar (Fig. 1.45). There is considerable variability in the structure of the LGN (352,353), which is also true for the striate cortex (354).

Dorsal to the LGN are the white matter tracts of the acoustic radiations that connect the medial geniculate nucleus to the transverse convolution of Heschl, which is the primary hearing cortex. Dorsolateral to the LGN are the fibers of the optic radiations (Figs. 1.46 and 1.47). Optic and acoustic radiations both pass through the temporal isthmus, the narrow bridge that connects the deep nuclei of the brain to the temporal lobe. The LGN can be visualized by MRI (355).

The LGN contains three substructures: the dorsal nucleus

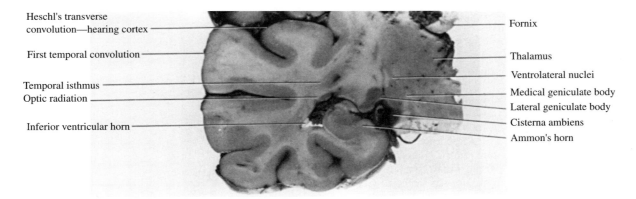

Heschl's transverse
convolution—hearing cortex

First temporal convolution

Temporal isthmus
Optic radiation

Inferior ventricular horn

Fornix

Thalamus

Ventrolateral nuclei

Medical geniculate body

Lateral geniculate body

Cisterna ambiens

Ammon's horn

Figure 1.47. Axial section of brain demonstrating lateral geniculate body and surrounding structures. (From Lindenberg R, Walsh FB, Sacks JG. Neuropathology of Vision: An Atlas. Philadelphia, Lea & Febiger, 1973.)

(dLGN), the pregeniculate complex, and the intergeniculate leaflet (IGL). Development of the dLGN occurs in three phases: (*a*) initial segregation of eye-specific laminae, (*b*) initial segregation of cell-specific (P- versus M-RGCs) and ON and OFF laminae, and (*c*) refinement of the receptive fields for all cells that synapse in the dLGN (Fig. 1.48). The first two processes are completed prior to visual experience, whereas the latter is completed with the addition of visual experience (356). How are some of these primary anatomic characteristics established without visual experience?

The dLGN, which is the largest of the three subunits, receives the great majority of retinothalamic and corticothalamic input and is the interconnection for the conscious (i.e., retinocalcarine) pathway. The dLGB has six laminae, with laminae 2, 3, and 5 (with numbering beginning ventrally) receiving input solely from the ipsilateral eye and laminae 1, 4, and 6 receiving input solely from the contralateral eye. This laminar segregation evolves from an earlier developmental stage in which projections from both eyes completely overlap. Refinement of this laminar organization, which requires at least weeks of visual experience after birth to develop (357), is created by comparison of the relative activity among axonal terminals arriving at the dLGN (358).

Relative synchrony among axons increases the probability those synapses will strengthen and be retained. The discovery of spontaneous, slow (i.e., one or two times per minute) "waves" of retinal activity that are present only during early development have been considered the likely force that drives eye-specific lamination in the dLGN. These waves, initiated by the "starburst" amacrine cells (359) (discussed previously), are synchronized within each retina but desynchronized between the two retinas. Incoming retinogeniculate fibers are therefore divided into those with one or the other firing pattern. Adjacent fibers with more similar wave patterns are more likely to be retained, while those with more dissimilar patterns are more likely to be eliminated. These waves persist through the development of eye-specific laminae and then segregation of ON and OFF laminae (360), and may participate in constructing the retinotopic maps to various brain termination sites (361). More recent and some-

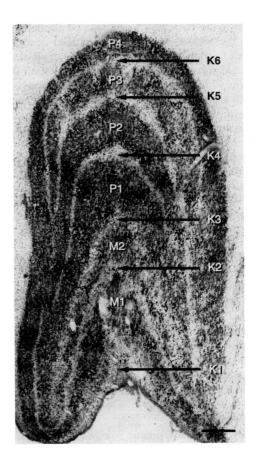

Figure 1.48. A coronal section through the lateral geniculate nucleus of a macaque monkey showing the parvocellular (P), magnocellular (M), and koniocellular (K) layers. At this plane there are four P layers, two M layers, and six K layers. Laminae 1, 4, and 6 receive input from the contralateral eye; laminae 2, 3, and 5 receive input from the ipsilateral eye. The thin layers ventral to each of the six primary lamina to which the K-retinal ganglion cells project are known as "intercalated" or interlaminar layers. Scale bar = 500 μm. (From VA Casagrande, JM Ichida. The lateral geniculate nucleus. In: Kaufman PL, Alm A, eds. Adler's Physiology of the Eye. 10th ed. St Louis, Mosby, 2003:657.)

what contradictory evidence regarding the developmental role of the spontaneous waves derives from experimental ablation selectively of the starburst amacrine cells, which eliminates retinal waves but does not disrupt eye-specific lamination of the dLGN, although elimination of all activity certainly does (362).

Laminar segregation extends beyond eye-specific input. Layers 1 and 2 receive input exclusively from M-RGCs and contain relatively large somas, and are therefore referred to as magnocellular layers. Layers 3–6 receive input exclusively from P-RGCs and contain relatively small somas, and are therefore referred to as parvocellular layers (363). Each M cell innervates many more relay cells in the dLGN than do P cells, such that the total number of relay cells in the dLGN devoted to M- or P-cell input is roughly equal, even though there are roughly eight times as many incoming P-RGCs. There is also a small input from K-RGCs, which synapse in thin *intercalated laminae* that lie ventral to each of the primary lamina (Figs. 1.48 to 1.50).

Following the eye-specific and M- versus P-specific organization, there is a further separation of each lamina into ON and OFF sublaminae (364). This separation also appears

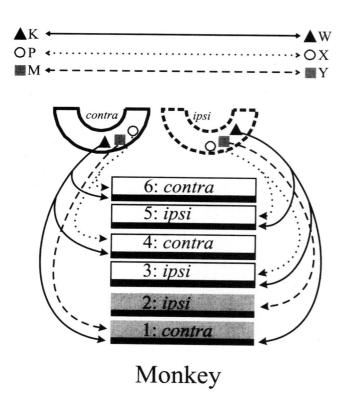

Figure 1.49. Eye-specific and functional-specific laminar organization of the lateral geniculate nucleus in the macaque monkey. Projections from the contralateral and ipsilateral eyes are shown with respect to parvo (P), magnocellular (M), and koniocellular (K) retinal ganglion cell axons. The abbreviations W, X, and Y refer to physiologic criteria, and the abbreviations K, P, and M refer to morphologic criteria, used to classify retinal ganglion cells (see text for details). (From Sherman SM, Guillery RW. The visual relays in the thalamus. In: Chalupa LM, Werner JS, eds. The Visual Neurosciences. Cambridge, MA, MIT Press, 2004:567.)

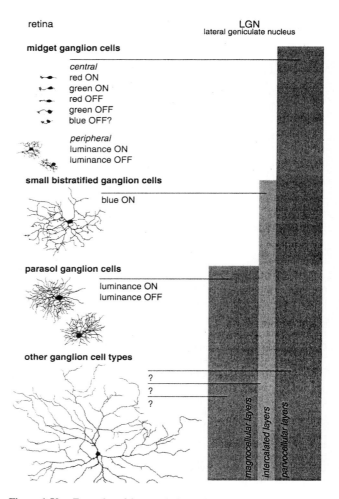

Figure 1.50. Examples of the morphology of some of the common retinal ganglion cell types in the primate retina, together with their projection targets in the lateral geniculate nucleus and some of their physiological properties. (From DM Dacey. Parallel pathways for spectral coding in the primate retina. Annu Rev Neurosci 2000;23:743–755.)

to be related to a competitive process. OFF cells have significantly higher spontaneous mean firing rates than ON cells, and thus these cell types can be distinguished by comparison of their relative activities during development (365).

The pregeniculate nucleus, which is part of the ventral thalamus, is actually a collection of nuclei known as the pregeniculate complex (PrGC). The PrGC is a relatively thin (partially) multilayered structure that extends over the medial and lateral aspects of the dLGN. The PrGC receives input from the retina, striate, and extrastriate cortices and has extensive connections with the superior colliculus (SC) and pretectal nucleus of the optic tract (NOT) (366) (Fig 1.51). Neurons of the PrGC in primates manifest saccade-related activity, which can be modulated by visual input (367). This visuosensory input alters the firing rate and sensitivity of neurons in the six primary laminae, especially for the M-pathway (368,369). This saccadic influence presumably contributes to the "suppression" of visual awareness during saccades.

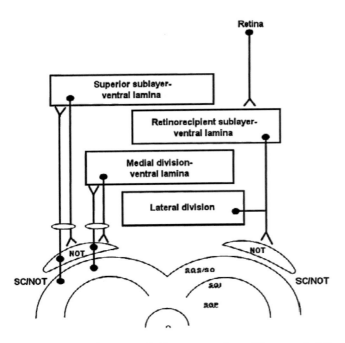

Figure 1.51. The afferent and efferent connections of the pregeniculate nuclear complex (PrGC) subnuclei. The restriction of retinal input to a single subnucleus is evident. Neurons in the retinorecipient sublayer and the lateral subdivision of the ventral lamina project to the superior colliculus (SC) and pretectal nucleus of the optic tract (NOT). The superior sublayer and the medial division of the PrGC are reciprocally connected with the SC/NOT. (From Livingston CA, Mustari MJ. Brain Res 2000;876:166–179.)

The IGL is a relatively thin cellular layer that separates the dLGN from the PrGC. In rats, the majority of input to the IGL is from melanopsin-containing RGCs, 20% of which send axons to the IGL (147). The IGL is believed to control circadian ''phase-shifting'' but may influence other aspects of photoperiodic control (i.e., regulation of circadian period and phase angle) via its photic and nonphotic output through the geniculohypothalamic tract (370).

Organization of Afferent Input

Each dLGN receives a precise retinotopic map from the contralateral visual hemifield. The macular fibers terminate within the center region over the caudal three quarters of the nucleus that includes all six laminae (371,372) (Fig. 1.52). There is a 90-degree counterclockwise rotation (as if viewed from the incoming side) of the retinotopic orientation, such that the axons from the superior retina lie laterally and those from the inferior retina lie medially (Fig. 1.53). All fibers rotate to the position they had assumed in the proximal optic tract as they exit the dLGN along its superoposterior margin. The mature dLGN usually has a monocular segment, a small ventral region with one M- and one P-cell layer, and a segment with four layers (371).

The corticothalamic pathway is the major source of nonretinal input. This pathway is oriented topographically such that regions in the striate cortex representing a particular retinal location project to cells in the dLGN that also represent that location. This spatial fidelity is maintained for the physiologically distinct classes of parvocellular and magnocellular LGN layers, which may be independently modulated by separate populations of cortical layer 6 neurons (373,374).

Other afferent input comes from the brain stem, including the SC, the parabigeminal nucleus (at least in the cat), several pretectal nuclei, and caudal midbrain and rostral pontine regions. Inputs from the SC and parabigeminal nucleus are concentrated within the interlaminar zones (375). The parabrachial nucleus, locus ceruleus, and dorsal raphe nucleus send cholinergic, noradrenergic, and serotonergic projections, respectively, to the dLGN (376). These projections modulate function in different ways. For example, serotonergic axons appear to have a diffuse neuromodulatory role in dLGN transmission, whereas cholinergic connections from the parabrachial region provide selective synaptic input to specific postsynaptic elements.

Organization of Efferent Output

Dorsal LGN cells send their main axons almost exclusively to the striate cortex, where they terminate primarily within granular layer 4 (discussed later). Geniculocalcarine projections from the parvocellular layers of the dLGN terminate mainly within the lower portion of layer 4 (i.e., layer 4C), with some terminating higher in layer 4A (discussed previously) (374,377,378). The projections from magnocellular cells also terminate in layer 4C (379,380). The magnocellular and parvocellular pathways also send collaterals to layer 4A, which sends retinotopic collaterals back to the dLGN. The koniocellular laminae send afferents to layers 1 and 3 of the striate cortex (135,380–382). The efferent projections from the dLGN are far more limited than the afferent (retinogeniculate and corticogeniculate) input.

PHYSIOLOGY

Relay Neurons

Dorsal LGN relay neurons are those that receive input from RGCs and project to the visual cortices, almost exclusively to area V1. The receptive field properties of these relay neurons are similar to those of the RGCs that supply their afferent input, although the surround properties of dLGN relay neurons are generally stronger (383) (Table 1.5). Early in development, there are imprecisions in the anatomic and physiologic matching of retinal inputs and geniculate relay neurons. The establishment of proper interconnections is then molded by Hebbian influences, which is to say that synapses with coordinated activity are more likely to survive. Visual experience after birth contributes to a pruning of the input pathways and their alignment with the relay neurons. Eventually, Hebbian principles create a spatially and physiologically precise arrangement of retinothalamic connections. Merger of this neuronal substrate with other afferent inputs, mostly from area V1, yields the mature profile of thalamocortical response properties.

Dorsal LGN relay cells have (*a*) circular receptive-field centers with an antagonistic surround; (*b*) receptive-field

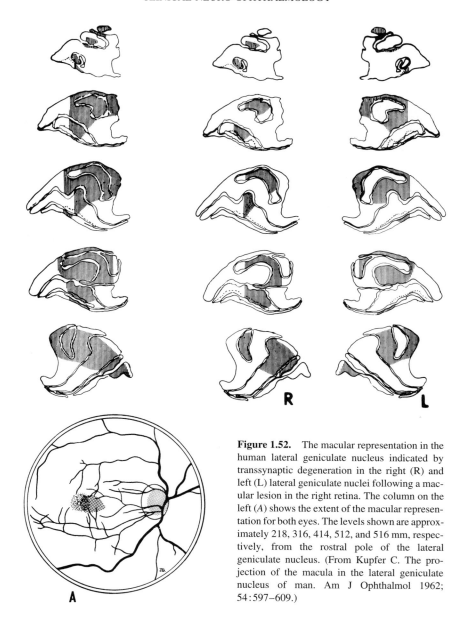

Figure 1.52. The macular representation in the human lateral geniculate nucleus indicated by transsynaptic degeneration in the right (R) and left (L) lateral geniculate nuclei following a macular lesion in the right retina. The column on the left (*A*) shows the extent of the macular representation for both eyes. The levels shown are approximately 218, 316, 414, 512, and 516 mm, respectively, from the rostral pole of the lateral geniculate nucleus. (From Kupfer C. The projection of the macula in the lateral geniculate nucleus of man. Am J Ophthalmol 1962; 54:597–609.)

centers that enlarge with increasing eccentricity within the visual field; and (*c*) the same ON and OFF dichotomy found in RGCs (discussed previously) (383). Dorsal dLGN neurons also display orientation selectivity, which is not found in RGCs. This orientation selectivity, a fundamental property of area V1 neurons, might be related to the shapes of the dendritic arbors of dLGN relay cells (384,385).

The surround antagonism of dLGN relay neurons is stronger than that of the RGCs that synapse with these neurons. This enhanced surround response is believed to result from (feedforward and feedback) inhibition upon the dLGN, primarily from the visual cortex (386,387). The corticogeniculate pathways that influence the spatial, temporal, and gating responses of dLGN neurons are both excitatory and inhibitory (388–390).

Another distinction of dLGN physiology is reduced re-

sponsiveness to visual contrast. RGCs respond to increasing stimulus intensity (or contrast) with a monotonic increase in their firing rate. Thus, the frequency of a RGC response codes the stimulus intensity. However, dLGN relay cells respond less vigorously than RGCs for the same intensity stimulus (391), which reduces the likelihood of signal transmission to the visual cortex. This "nonlinear gain control" may protect cells in the striate cortex from response saturation. This response attenuation may relate to the organization of having several dLGN relay cells provide input to one striate cortical cell: any decrease in individual cell responsiveness can be balanced by the influence of a local population of neurons that collectively exert a stronger input to the cortex.

Many dLGN cells exhibit responses to more complex stimuli than RGCs. Roughly 40% of dLGN cells are sensi-

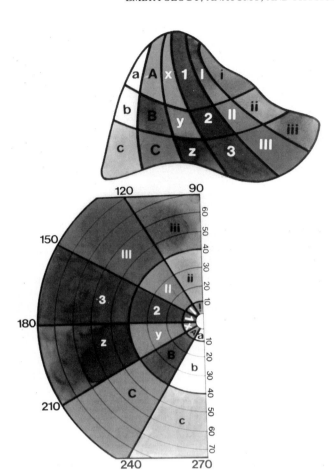

Figure 1.53. Representation of the visual field in the lateral geniculate nucleus (LGN) in humans. *Top,* The right LGN in coronal section from behind. *Bottom,* The left homonymous hemifield separated into specific sectors designated by numbers (*top*) and letters (*bottom*). The numbers and letters on the LGN correspond to the projection of the similarly numbered and lettered sectors of the visual hemifield. Central vision is represented by cells located superiorly in the LGN, peripheral vision by cells located inferiorly. The upper quadrant of the visual field is represented in the lateral portion of the LGN, the lower portion of the visual field in the medial portion of the LGN. The horizontal meridian is roughly a vertical curved line through the midportion of the LGN. A consecutive series of numbers or letters (i.e., i, ii, iii; 1, 2, 3; or A, B, C) indicates a sector of the visual field; corresponding symbols from adjoining series of numbers or letters (e.g., ii, II, 2 or y, B, b) indicate an arc in the visual field. (From Shacklett DE, O'Connor PS, Dorwart H, et al. Am J Ophthalmol 1984;98:283–290.)

Table 1.5
Overview of Physiological Response Properties Along the Afferent Visual Pathway

Response Properties	Outer Retina	Retinal Ganglion Cells	Dorsal Lateral Geniculate Nucleus	Primary Visual Cortex
Graded responses	+			
Sustained responses		+	+	+ (simple and complex cells)
Transient responses		+	+	+ (simple and complex cells)
Circular receptive fields		+	+	
Linear receptive fields				+ (much larger surround zone compared to RGCs or dLGN cells)
Antagonistic surround responses		+	Stronger than retinal ganglion cells	Substantially larger
On vs off		+	+	+
Binocular response cells				+ (the majority of cells in layers 2, 3, 5, and 6)
Responses to horizontal and vertical disparity				+
Orientation selectivity			+	+
Motion sensitive responses		Relatively small population(s)		Complex cells (relatively large population)
Sensitive to direction of moving stimulus		Small number	20%	
Response to contrast		Strong	Weaker	
Responses influenced by eye movement; auditory and tactile stimuli			+	

dLGN, dorsal lateral geniculate nucleus; RGCs, retinal ganglion cells.

tive to orientation, and 20% are sensitive to the direction of a moving stimulus (392). Auditory and tactile stimuli, stretching of eye muscles (393), and saccadic eye movements also influence dLGN responses (394).

There are different types of relay neurons for both of the major retinal outflow pathways. For the M-cell pathway, there are two types of relay neurons and one type of interneuron. For the P-cell pathway, there is one type of relay neuron and one type of interneuron (395).

Information Transfer

Perception and visual behavior do not result from activation of single neurons. Rather, the brain receives input from populations of afferent neurons, which must then be "processed" to create vision as we experience it. Visual signals leaving the eye are the primary input to the visual brain, but action potentials from RGCs do not necessarily reach the visual cortex. The dLGN imposes significant influences on what information is transmitted to the striate visual cortex.

This influence on information transfer at the dLGN is dependent upon at least three factors: retinal input, local interneurons, and subcortical and cortical afferent input. The relative dominance of these factors is revealed by the fact that more than 80% of synapses within the dLGN are not from the retina, but from local interneurons and other afferent sources. All of these afferent inputs converge upon the dLGN relay neurons.

The retinogeniculate pathway is excitatory to dLGN relay neurons, which substantially outnumber the incoming RGC axons (396). The retinal input is spatially divergent in that most relay neurons receive strong input from one or two RGCs, with additional weaker input from several other RGCs (397). The input from the dLGN to the primary visual cortex, however, is convergent. This architecture allows a cluster of RGCs to strongly influence a small number of dLGN relay neurons, which strongly influence the responses of the smaller number of cortical neurons upon which they converge.

Any visual stimulus alters activity among a population of RGCs. The incoming signals from these cells will more likely effect transmission through the dLGN if the afferent signals come from cells with substantial receptive field overlap and similar physiology (397). Nearly coincident firing of adjacent retinogeniculate neurons strongly increases transmission efficiency through the dLGN (398). Higher-frequency action potentials have a greater chance of exciting dLGN relay neurons and thus are more likely to influence the signals sent to the visual cortex.

As stated above, dLGN relay neurons have relatively strong, antagonistic surround responses. More diffuse retinal illumination is more likely to activate these receptive field surrounds, which decreases transmission efficiency to the cortex. Viewed in another way, the dLGN sharpens the spatial detail of percepts by increasing the likelihood that smaller attributes of a stimulus will reach the cortex.

The influence of local interneurons within the dLGN on information transfer is especially strong. Interneurons represent a substantial proportion (25–35%) of all dLGN neurons (399). Incoming RGC axons synapse on the interneurons,

which release GABA and inhibit the relay neurons. The inhibition of relay neurons decreases their transmission ratio of visual signals from the retina to the visual cortex (Fig. 1.54).

Afferent input from area V1 of the visual cortex is retinotopically organized with respect to the dLGN cells. This corticogeniculate feedback pathway, which is substantially larger than the geniculate-cortical pathway, utilizes glutamate and aspartate as neurotransmitters, thus imparting an excitatory influence onto the dLGN (400). This excitation increases the firing rate and transmission efficiency of dLGN neurons (401). The same corticogeniculate pathway passes through the perigeniculate nucleus and synapses onto neurons that send inhibitory input via the same neurons within the dLGN (Figs. 1.55 and 1.56). This feedforward influence is thought to account for the bias for dLGN neurons to transmit impulses generated by relatively long lines that exceed a critical threshold for length. This response property, which is quite different from the preferred circular response properties of the RGCs that provide input to the dLGN, is shaped by feedback connections from the primary visual cortex, which responds very strongly to linear stimuli and only weakly to circular stimuli. Other elements of the cortical-geniculate feedback pathway are inhibitory. In general, the magnocellular pathway is more significantly affected by cortical influences than is the parvocellular pathway (390).

Some brain stem pathways globally influence dLGN responses through sparse but diffuse connections. One pathway is a serotonergic, primarily inhibitory connection from the raphe nucleus (402). Another is a noradrenergic, excitatory influence from the locus ceruleus (403). There are also cholinergic inputs from several brain stem afferent pathways that provide a relatively strong excitation directly onto dLGN relay cells (404), although this same pathway inhibits

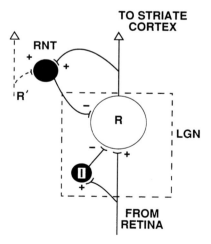

Figure 1.54. Synaptic contacts within the lateral geniculate nucleus (LGN) between retinal afferents and LGN relay cells (R), feedforward interneurons (I), and feedback cells in the reticular nucleus of the thalamus (RNT). GABA-ergic inhibitory neurons are indicated in *black*. The *dashed line* making a synapse onto the RNT cell represents collateral inputs from other relay cells (R′) that is adjacent to the LGN relay cell in the center of the diagram. (From Casagrande VA, Norton TT. Lateral geniculate nucleus: a review of its physiology and function. In: Leventhal AG, ed. The Neural Basis of Visual Function. Boca Raton, CRC Press, 1991:46.)

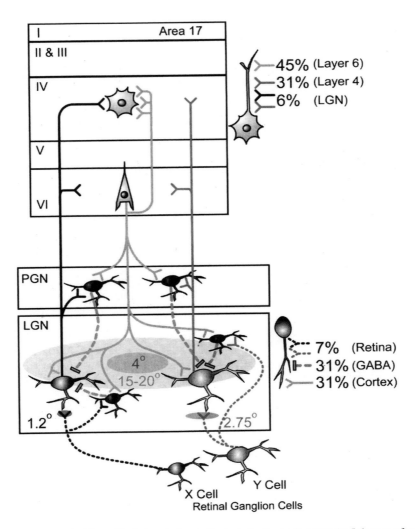

Figure 1.55. Geniculate-cortical loop. *Shaded ovals* denote the typical retinotopic extent (at 5 degrees of eccentricity from the area centralis) of the axonal arborizations of X and Y retinal ganglion cell axons and corticofugal axons. Two dimensions are given for feedback axons: the smaller dimension depicts the typical spread for the dense central core projection, while the larger dimension depicts the overall coverage of the axonal arborization. Percentages to the right of the drawing summarize the contribution of synaptic contacts from retinal axons, corticofugal feedback axons, and inhibitory interneurons that synapse on lateral geniculate nucleus relay cells, as well as the contributions from geniculate axons, layer 6 collaterals, and layer 4 connections that synapse on spiny stellate cells in layer 4 of the cortex. (From Sillito AM, Jones HE. Feedback systems in visual processing. In: Chalupa LM, Werner JS, eds. The Visual Neurosciences. Cambridge, MA, MIT Press, 2004:610.)

dLGN interneurons (405). Afferents from the SC and pretectal nuclei provide excitatory input, enhancing information transfer through the dLGN (400,401).

Collectively, the gating of activity at the dLGN presumably influences the level of cognitive attention to visual stimuli, which varies greatly with the level of alertness. Apropos to this role in attention, en route to the dLGN the corticofugal pathway passes through and provides input to the thalamic reticular nucleus, which drapes the lateral aspect of the dLGN. The thalamic nucleus contains GABA-ergic neurons, from which enlarge strong reciprocal connections with the dLGN.

BLOOD SUPPLY

The dLGN has a dual blood supply. The anterior hilus, together with the anterior and lateral aspects of the nucleus, is usually supplied by branches of the anterior choroidal artery, which arises from the ICA. The remainder of the dLGN receives blood from the lateral choroidal artery, which arises from the posterior cerebral artery (346,406–409). Both arteries probably supply the area of the macular representation. Distinct visual field defects occur with compromise of either of these vascular distributions (410) (see Chapter 12).

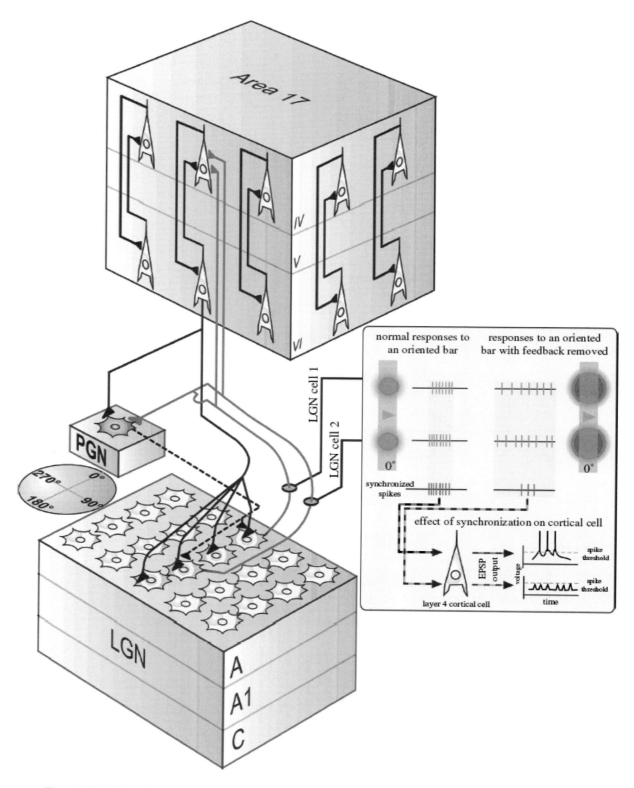

Figure 1.56. Schematic organization that summarizes the notion that feedback-linked surround antagonism leads to greater synchronization of firing of relay cells in the lateral geniculate nucleus to coherent contours, which thus increases the probability of transmission of this visual input arriving at the lateral geniculate nucleus to layer 4 neurons in the striate cortex. (From Sillito AM, Jones HE. Corticothalamic interactions in the transfer of visual information. Philosophical Trans R Soc Lond B 2002;357:1739–1752.)

POSTGENICULATE VISUAL SENSORY PATHWAYS

EMBRYOLOGY

The telencephalon develops at about 6 weeks of gestation from the most anterior aspect of the prosencephalon as bilateral evaginations, the walls of which develop into the cerebral hemispheres. The superior portions of the walls develop into the pallium, or primordium of the cerebral cortex. In humans, the largest portion of the pallium is the neopallium, from which arise the visual cortices.

Cortical differentiation begins as a migration of cells from the mantle zone into the marginal zone to form a superficial cortical layer, which begins at 8 weeks of gestation. This migration, which is complete shortly thereafter, occurs first in the olfactory cortex, then the somatic sensory cortex, and lastly in the frontal and visual cortices. Programmed cell death occurs in the human cerebral cortex, just as it does in the optic nerve (discussed earlier) (411). The number of neurons initially increases, peaking at about 28 weeks of gestation, and then progressively declines by about 70% around the time of birth (412).

Myelination of the visual pathways does not begin until the entire pathway has developed. Myelination of the postgeniculate visual sensory pathway begins at birth and generally is complete by the fourth month of life, although the occipital poles may not be fully myelinated until the twelfth month (218,219). Myelination begins at the occipital poles and progresses anteriorly.

ANATOMY OF THE OPTIC RADIATIONS

The optic radiations, also called the geniculocalcarine tract, extend from the dLGN to the primary visual cortex (V1, striate cortex, Brodmann area 17) in the occipital lobe (Fig. 1.46). The optic radiations are separated into three bundles that occupy the external sagittal stratum: the upper, lower, and central bundles (413). The upper and central bundles pass posteriorly through the temporal and parietal lobes to reach the occipital lobes. The lower bundle (i.e., Meyer's loop) initially courses anteriorly, superior to and around the

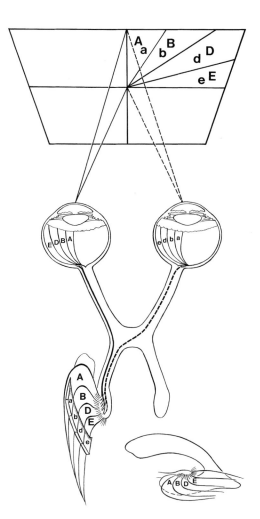

Figure 1.58.   The representation of the inferior retinal quadrants in the temporal lobe portion of the optic radiation in humans, based on studies of patients who have undergone temporal lobectomy. The tip of the temporal horn is not surrounded by the optic radiation. Further, although the distribution from each retina extends anteriorly to an equal degree, the representation of the ipsilateral retina lies lateral to that from the contralateral retina. The macular fibers at all levels are considered to lie mesial to the fibers representing the peripheral retina. (Redrawn from Van Buren JM, Baldwin M. The architecture of the optic radiation in the temporal lobe of man. Brain 1958;81:15–40.)

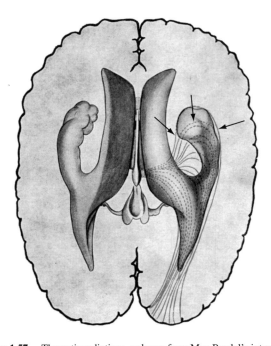

Figure 1.57.   The optic radiations, redrawn from Max Brodel's interpretation of the geniculocalcarine radiation in humans. Meyer's loop is that portion of the optic radiation that projects anteriorly (*arrows*) before then turning back to extend toward the primary visual cortex. (From Cushing H. Distortions of the visual fields in cases of brain tumor: the field defects produced by temporal lobe lesions. Brain 1922;44:341–396.)

temporal horn of the lateral ventricle (414) (Figs. 1.57 and 1.58). This bundle then turns laterally and posteriorly to reach the striate cortex. The central bundle, which is the largest, transmits the macular projection in a base-out wedge configuration (Fig. 1.59). The upper and lower bundles transmit information about the lower and upper regions of the visual field, respectively.

Damage to Meyer's loop causes a partial, superior homon-

ymous quadrantanopia. There is conflicting evidence regarding the congruity of such field defects, with numerous opinions for both incongruity (415,416) and congruity (417–421). Variable anatomy may account for some of the discrepancy of visual field findings. There is some consensus that (*a*) projections of central vision are positioned laterally at the anterior aspect of the radiations and then move to a more intermediate zone, and (*b*) fibers subserving peripheral vision initially are medial and then extend posteriorly to the upper and lower edges of the radiations (353,418,422,423) (Fig. 1.58). MRI can reveal the topographic pattern of fiber degeneration following cortical injury (424).

The location of optic radiation fibers subserving the temporal crescent, the unpaired nasal fibers (discussed later), is uncertain. In general, however, the projection from the inferior visual field of the monocular crescent travels in the upper quadrant of the superior radiation, and vice versa (425). These fibers converge in the most anterior part of the striate cortex to occupy less than 10% of the total surface of the striate cortex (426). The counterclockwise rotation of fibers that occurs in the dLGN (discussed previously) is rectified within the 2–3 mm anterior to the visual cortex. The medial dLGN fibers pass downward to reach the inferior bank of the occipital cortex to serve the superior visual field, while the lateral dLGN fibers pass upward (353,422). There is no interhemispheric crossing of the optic radiations (338, 427,428).

BLOOD SUPPLY

The superior portion of the optic radiation is supplied primarily by branches from the inferior division of the middle cerebral artery. The inferior portion of the radiation receives blood mainly from the PCA. The PCA dominates the blood supply to the optic radiation more posteriorly (Fig. 1.60).

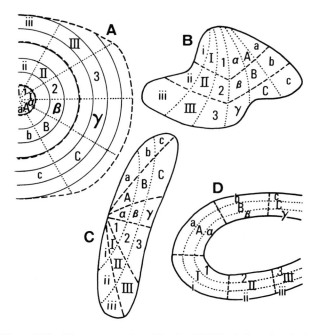

Figure 1.59. The representation of the visual field in the lateral geniculate body and the optic radiations. In the representation of the visual field (*A*), the different parts of the upper quadrant are indicated by numbers and the lower by letters. In both quadrants, each series runs from center to periphery, so that any one series (e.g., i, ii, iii) indicates a sector, whereas the corresponding symbols from adjoining series (e.g., i, 1, I) indicate an arc of the visual field. Radii dividing the visual field are represented by *dotted lines* and linear arcs by *dashed lines*. In the lateral geniculate body (*B*), central vision is represented in cells lying superiorly and peripheral vision in cells lying inferiorly. The upper quadrant of the visual field is represented laterally, the lower medially, and the horizontal meridian approximately vertically. In the anterior radiation (*C*), the orientation of fibers has turned counterclockwise through almost a right angle. The fibers representing central vision are now spread out over a large part of the lateral aspect of the visual radiation, although they tend to concentrate on its intermediate part. In contrast, the fibers of peripheral vision are spread out over the medial aspect of the visual radiation and tend to concentrate at the upper and lower margins and to thin out over the intermediate part. The horizontal meridian, therefore, is represented more or less horizontally in the intermediate part of the radiation at this point. In the posterior radiation (*D*), the fibers of central vision have come to occupy the whole of the intermediate part of the radiation and lie lateral to the posterior horn of the lateral ventricle as they pass back to the posterior pole of the occipital lobe. The fibers of peripheral vision have become concentrated at the margins of the radiation, at the two ends of the horseshoe-shaped structure. At this location the fibers are entering the anterior part of the striate cortex. (Redrawn from JMK Spalding. Wounds of the visual pathway: I. The visual radiation. J Neurol Neurosurg Psychiatry 1952;15:99–107.)

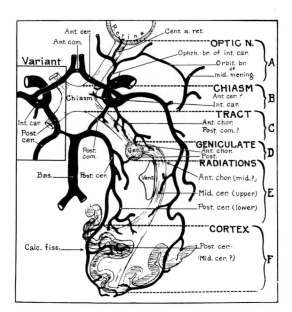

Figure 1.60. Blood supply of the visual sensory system. (From Walsh FB, Smith GW. J Neurosurg 1952;9:517–537.)

CORTICAL VISUAL AREAS

CORTICAL AREA V1

Anatomy

In the human, the primary visual cortex is situated along the superior and inferior banks of the calcarine fissure, corresponding to area 17 of Brodmann (Fig. 1.61). This area often is called the striate cortex because of a prominent white band of myelinated fibers known as the stria of Gennari, which forms horizontal connections within the cortex. The striate cortex envelops the posterior pole of the hemisphere, extending laterally about 1.5 cm. Rostrally and medially, V1 extends anteriorly beyond the juncture of the parieto-occipital and calcarine fissures, especially ventrally (427,429,430). The optic radiations from the dLGN provide the main afferent connections to area V1. The three main outflow pathways from the retina—parvocellular, magnocellular, and koniocellular (discussed previously)—remain distinct at the dLGN, but there is some convergence of these outflow in area V1 (431,432). There are also inputs to area V1 from the pulvinar and other cortical regions.

V1 represents about 3.5% of the cortical area of the brain. There is considerable variability in the configuration of the calcarine fissure and the distribution of the striate cortex, even within an individual. The surface covered by the visual projection area varies among individuals 2.5–3-fold, with a range of 15–45 cm^2. There is even considerable variability of the area of exposed striate cortex (3.6–13 cm^2) (427,430,433). These estimates indicate that on average 67% of the striate cortex is buried in the calcarine fissure or its accessory sulci. The striate cortex does not always reach the occipital pole, and the calcarine fissure is sometimes crossed by other gyri (430). An average neuron in macaque striate cortex receives approximately 2,300 synapses (1,400 in layer 4Cβ and 2,800 in layers 2 and 3; discussed later) (434). There are approximately 150,000 cells/mm^3 in visual cortex.

Visual cortical neurons are separated into two main morphologies (pyramidal and nonpyramidal), which forms the basis for the histologic segregation of the visual cortex into six laminae (435,436) (Fig. 1.62). Layer 1, the most superficial layer, contains few neurons and is composed mostly of fibrillary astrocytes with some microglia and oligodendrocytes. Layer 2 contains small pyramidal cells, many with short axons or axons that ascend and split within layer 1 (437).

Layer 3, which is indistinctly separated from layer 2, is traditionally defined as containing mostly medium-sized and small pyramidal cells, with granule cells more deeply. A more recent interpretation further divides layer 3 into four subregions: 3A, 3Bα, 3Bβ, and 3C (438,439) (Fig. 1.62). Large pyramidal cells of 3A project to V2 in the monkey (437) (Fig. 1.63). Cells in 3Bβ project to area V2, while those in 3C project both to V2 and MT (discussed later). An appealing feature to this newer schema (which has not yet been widely adopted) is that layer 3 is the primary projection layer from area V1 to the associative visual cortices. In the macaque, layer 3 receives input from the intercalated layers of the dLGN (135) (Figs. 1.48 and 1.50). Projections from layer 3 of area V1 to cortical area V2 arise from "interpatches," whereas projections to area MT arise from both interpatches and patches (i.e., more darkly staining cyto-

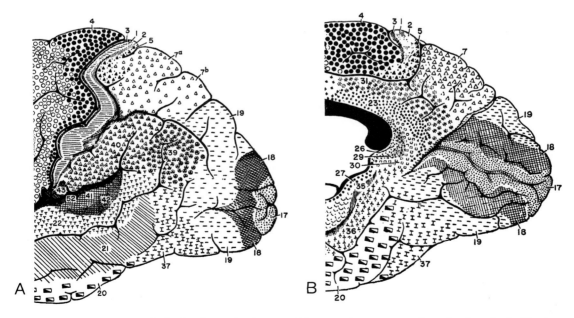

Figure 1.61. The areas occupied by the primary visual cortex and the extrastriate areas, according to Brodmann's classification. *A*, Lateral surface; *B*, Mesial surface. (From Lindenberg R, Walsh FB, Sacks JG. Neuropathology of Vision: An Atlas. Philadelphia, Lea & Febiger, 1973.)

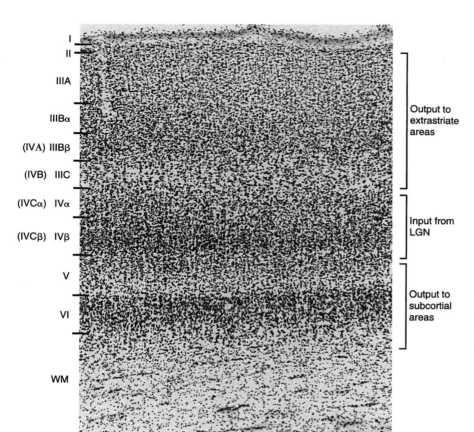

Layers labeled (left side): I, II, IIIA, IIIBα, (IVA) IIIBβ, (IVB) IIIC, (IVCα) IVα, (IVCβ) IVβ, V, VI, WM

Brackets (right side): Output to extrastriate areas; Input from LGN; Output to subcortical areas

Figure 1.62. Nissl-stained section through area V1 of macaque monkey. The layers are numbered according to a recent modification of Hässler's nomenclature. The more traditional Brodmann's nomenclature is shown in parentheses. As indicated by the brackets, layer IV receives the main input from the lateral geniculate nucleus, the layers above IV send projections to other cortical areas, and the layers below IV send projections to subcortical areas. A subdivision of layer 4 known as layer 4ctr (i.e., center) which lies between layers 4α and 4β is not shown. WM, white mater. (From Casagrande VA, Ichida JM. The primary visual cortex. In: Kaufman PL, Alm A, eds. Adler's Physiology of the Eye. 10th ed. St Louis, Mosby, 2003:672.)

chrome oxidase regions). Layer 3 can be considered the point at which the dorsal and ventral steams of information begin to diverge to different cortical regions (discussed later).

Layer 4 is a relatively large lamina that is the primary recipient area of the geniculate-calcarine projection, which mostly synapses on stellate cells that have a uniform, radial topography. A recent revision of visual cortical architecture divides layer 4 into three zones: 4α, 4ctr, and 4β (438,439) (Figs. 1.62 and 1.63). Using this new schema, layer 4 does not send axons outside of area V1; rather, layer 4 forms a host of intracortical connections to areas, like layer 3, which then project to associative visual cortices. The traditionally described layer 4A, which contains large stellate cells with axons that descend to deeper laminae or enter the subcortical white matter, expresses in humans monoclonal staining patterns not found in nonhuman primates, which suggests evolution of an enhanced interneuronal population (440).

The traditional layer 4B, recently considered to be 3C, contains mostly granule cells and has the stria of Gennari. The neurons of layer 4B, which predominantly receive input from the "M" pathway via layer 4α (new classification), are mostly tuned for orientation, although a smaller population of cells are direction-selective (377,441–443). These cells project mostly to area MT. Pyramidal cells in layer 3C receive M- and P-cell input and project mainly to area V2 (444,445); (446–448). Parvocellular input from the dLGN is to layers 4β and 4ctr (449).

Layer 5 contains pyramidal cells of various sizes, including the giant pyramidal cells of Meynert. Layer 5 (in the monkey) projects to the SC and pulvinar nucleus (444). Layer 6 contains medium-sized neurons (450–452), most of which project as a feedback pathway to the dLGN (discussed previously) (444,453,454). Layer 6 of macaque consists of three sublayers, only two of which project to the dLGN. The upper tier projects exclusively to parvocellular layers, while the lower tier projects to parvocellular and magnocellular layers of the dLGN (454).

The majority of striate cortical cells receive their (suprathreshold) excitatory input from either the "P" or "M" pathway via the dLGN. This description of parallel inputs, however, too greatly simplifies the reality. In macaque monkeys, a substantial proportion (at least 25%) of area V1 neurons receive convergent input from two dLGN outflow pathways, usually the "M" and "P" pathways, and possibly from the koniocellular projections as well (431). This type of area V1 neuron, which responds to both color and luminance (i.e., black-white, contrast-sensitive cells), may provide boundary cues between differently colored regions. Other neurons in V1 that respond purely to color are not very sensitive to spatial localization and therefore may provide information about fluctuation of color within a particular region (455).

The primary projections of area V1 are to areas V2 or MT. Uncommonly but notably, some V1 "manifold"neu-

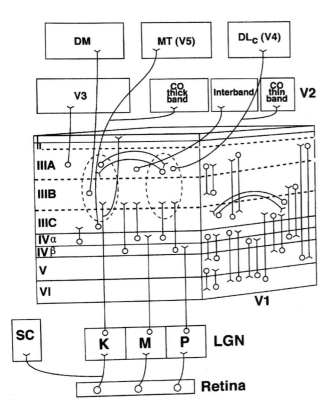

Figure 1.63. Some of the main intrinsic and extrinsic connections of V1 in primates. No effort is made to define the strength of connections or to indicate true axon collaterals or species-unique features. Feedback connections to V1 and the lateral geniculate nucleus (LGN), as well as connections between extrastriate areas, are not shown. The major input to V1 is from the dorsal LGN, which arrives via three pathways: the koniocellular (K), magnocellular (M), and parvocellular (P) pathways. The retina also projects to other targets, one of which, the superior colliculus (SC), is shown. Within V1, cell layers are heavily interconnected, not only by some of the axonal pathways shown but also by dendritic arbors (not shown). The main ipsilateral connections to extrastriate cortex exit from layer III. In layer IIIA, the cells within cytochrome oxidase (CO)–rich blobs (indicated by *dotted ovals;* see text), and CO-poor interblobs send information to different target cells within bands of V2. In layer IIIB, cells within CO blobs send projections to the dorsomedial area (DM) of the cortex. Cells that lie under the CO blobs in layer IIIC send information to the middle temporal area (MT), also called cortical area V5. Although connections between V1 and V3 have been documented, it is not known from which layer/module these connections arise. A subdivision of layer 4 known as layer 4ctr (i.e., center) which lies between layers 4α and 4β, is not shown. DL$_c$ (V4), dorsolateral caudal (cortical area V4). (From Casagrande VA, Ichida JM. The primary visual cortex. In: Kaufman PL, Alm A eds. Adler's Physiology of the Eye. 10th ed. St Louis, Mosby, 2003:675.)

rons project to both sites (448). The MT projecting axons come from "patch" areas, which provide koniocellular system input to area MT (448). In general, the receptive field widths of outwardly projecting cells from the striate cortex are smaller than those of cells that project to the striate cortex (456). This observation suggests that the striate cortex is organized partly to enhance detection of fine spatial detail.

Most cortical outputs from other brain regions project to the superficial layers of the striate cortex, which then connect to (traditional) layer 4. Feedback projections, on the other hand, emerge more deeply within the striate cortex and extend to either layers 1 or 6 (457). Feedback projections are typically more divergent, partly because of their use of manifold neurons (discussed previously) that project to two sites, and they arise from widespread areas, including limbic-associated cortices. Thus, the patterns of interconnections are complex and not well appreciated (458,459). Nonetheless, the sheer number and extent of feedback connections indicate their probable importance in the process of creating vision. For example, feedback connections may enhance attention or synchronize responses that bind different features of an image (460–462).

Physiology

The physiology of the striate cortex initially was defined in the cat, which led to the recognition of distinctive response properties of simple and complex cells (383,463–465). Subsequent work in monkeys revealed significant differences from the cat (379,465–474), including identification of a third cortical neuron, the end-stopped cell. In general, the receptive field properties of cortical neurons are quite different and more complicated than the circular receptive field properties found in the retina and dLGN (Table 1.5). This might seem counterintuitive, given that there is a monosynaptic connection between the geniculate afferent and layer 4 neurons with area V1. This intricacy of feedforward and intracortical and intercortical connections to area V1 presumably accounts for this more intricate physiology (475). Comparisons of some response properties across the various visual cortical areas are shown in Table 1.6.

The receptive fields of simple cells, like retinal and dLGN cells, show either ON or OFF responses, each with an antagonistic surround. Unlike RGCs, however, receptive field centers of simple cells are linear rather than circular, which explains the high sensitivity of these cells to long, narrow slits of light. Simple cells also are orientation-selective—that is, they respond best to a line oriented at a particular angle (Fig. 1.64). The response of simple cells increases in proportion to the stimulus length, up to the limit of the receptive field. Adjacent columns of simple cells show a progressive shift in their preferred orientation. In the monkey, simple cells are almost entirely in (traditional) layer 4, with a few cells in layer 6.

Complex cells are orientation-selective and motion-sensitive. Complex cells respond inconsistently to stationary stimuli but fire vigorously to a moving stimulus oriented at preferred angles. The responses are direction-specific and are also influenced by the stimulus speed (Fig. 1.65). Like simple cells, the response of complex cells is proportionate to stimulus size up to the limit of the receptive field. Like RGCs and dLGN cells, both simple and complex cells have spatial and temporal responses that can be either sustained or transient (476–478). Complex cells, which greatly outnumber simple cells, are found above and below (traditional) layer 4, but only rarely in layer 4.

Table 1.6
General Summation of Certain Features of Visual Cortical Areas

Cortical Area	Some Specialized Response Properties or Cell Types	General Comments
V1	• Simple cells • Complex cells • End-stopped cells	• Receives almost all of the cortical afferent input from the dLGN • "Cortical magnification" of dLGN input is substantial • Some convergence of the P-, M- and K-cell input • Response properties in general are more complicated than dLGN relay neurons • Primary projections are to V2 and MT • Some cells respond to first order motion
V2	• Most neurons are orientation selective • Half of the neurons are color selective • "Depth cells" respond to retinal disparity • Many neurons respond to more than one visual feature, which suggests convergence of input • Directionally selective cells are sparse (motion information may largely bypass V2)	• Largest extrastriate visual cortical area • First location along visual pathway at which there is a convergence of input from retina and pulvinar • Most of the V1 afferent input is sent to V2 before being distributed elsewhere • Further increase in cortical magnification from V1 to V2 • Receptive fields are larger than V1 • Assessment of retinal disparity may be an important feature • Some cells respond to first order motion • Projects to V3 (mainly), V4 and V5 ipsilaterally; V2 contralaterally
V3/V3A	• 76% of neurons are strongly orientation selective • 40% of neurons are strongly direction selective • Most neurons are optimized for stimulus speed direction • 50% of neurons are color sensitive • Most neurons are binocularly driven • 33% of V3A neurons may respond to light even with complete ablation of V1	• Area 3d has more connections with V1 than any other area, but these are less numerous than V1 to V2 connections • Relatively small area • Likely receives nonretino-calcarine input from pulvinar • Receptive fields larger than V2 • V3d and V3v respond to second order motion • Projects primarily to pulvinar and midbrain • Anatomical subdivisions are controversial
V4	• Neurons respond primarily to shape, color, and texture of visual stimulus • Most neurons show preference for near objects • 50% of neurons are color opponent • Few neurons are orientation or direction selective	• Receptive fields are larger than V3, which are larger than more proximal visual cortices • Major projection to IT, but significant projection to posterior parietal cortex • Neurons code shape in reference to boundary features of objects • May play a role in visual discrimination tasks
TE	• 33% of neurons selectively respond to 3D object shape	• Lies at end of ventral stream of visual information • May play a role in identification of visually complex objects • Strong output to medial temporal region, perhaps important to establish visual memory
V5 (MT)	• 90% of neurons are direction selective • 33% of neurons are direction selective for patterns of movement • Area MST contains neurons that specialize in processing "motion in depth," which may permit estimation of one's direction of movement in an environment	• Smallest of the named visual areas • Receives direct but sparse, high velocity input from V1; also receives input from V2, V3d, V3v, MST • Dense intracortical branching may amplify incoming signals • Ablation of V1 does not eliminate activity, even direction selectivity • May be primary cortical area for motion processing, especially of motion *patterns*; also responds to first and second order motion
V6	• Cells respond nearly identically to those of V6A to orientation and direction of movement of visual stimuli • Like neurons of V6A, the response of neurons is affected by eye movements	• Poorly understood • Receives input from V2 • Has large receptive fields • May function in mapping of relative spatial relationships • Responds strongly to motion • Does not contain a conventional retinotopic map • Strongly interconnected to V6A
V6A	• Contains cells that do not respond to visual stimuli but respond to intentional arm movements • "Real-position" cells that represent orientation with respect to craniotopic receptive fields • Response of neurons is affected by eye movements	• Much larger receptive fields than V6 • Retinotopy is relatively coarse • May function to help guide skeletomotor activity into extrapersonal space

The descriptions in this table are meant to serve as a superficial overview of the purported function of these areas. Any notion that specific visual cortical areas perform only certain highly specific tasks should be carefully scrutinized.

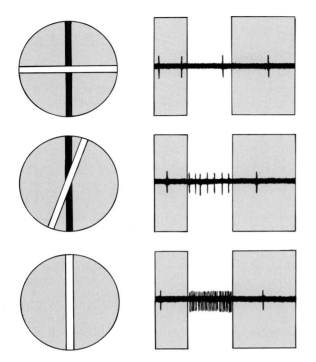

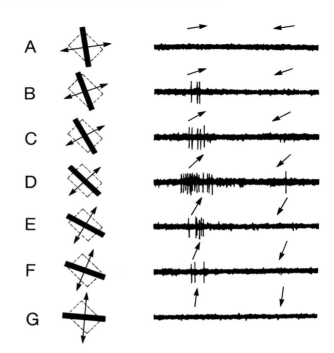

Figure 1.64. Simple cortical cell with preferred axis of orientation. Stimulus is white bar of varying orientation shown on representation of receptive field at *left*. A horizontal stimulus (*top*) falls on excitatory and inhibitory regions, and therefore no response is evident in the recording from the cell (shown on *right*). A stimulus that is tilted slightly off vertical (*middle row*) produces a weak response. When stimulus is vertical (*bottom*), however, the stimulus is entirely in the excitatory region of field and the response is vigorous. (From D Hubel. The visual cortex of the brain. Sci Am 1963; 209:54–62.)

Figure 1.65. Receptive field of a complex cell from the monkey striate cortex. Outline of receptive field is shown by the *dashed lines*. Orientations of black bar stimulus are shown on the *left*, and responses to that particular orientation are shown on the *right*. *Arrows* indicate direction of bar movement. (From DH Hubel, TN Wiesel. Receptive fields and functional architecture of monkey striate cortex. J Physiol [Lond] 1968;195:215–243.)

End-stopped cells (once called hypercomplex cells) also respond proportionately to the length of a stimulus, but they are novel in that their response *decreases* when the stimulus length reaches the boundary of the activating portion of the receptive field (Figs. 1.66). This effect results from an inhibitory surround. Unlike the simple and complex cells, stimulation exclusively within the antagonistic zone of an end-stopped cell does not alter the cell's responsiveness. End-stopped cells are located above and below (traditional) layer 4. In the cat, these cells are also found in areas V2 and V3.

The antagonistic surrounds of these cortical cells are substantially larger than those of RGCs or dLGN neurons. These relatively large surrounds are thought to result from feedback from other cortical areas, especially from V2, V3, and V5 (475).

Each of these striate cells is arranged in columns, within which the cells show a consistent preference for stimulus orientation and have very similar receptive fields (379,468–470,479,480) (Fig. 1.67). Adjacent columns, separated by about 50 μm in the monkey, contain cells with sequential shifts of about 10 degrees in the preferred orientations. Therefore, approximately 1 mm in linear dimension contains 18 orientation columns and subserves all possible linear orientations. In a rare opportunity to correlate neuronal

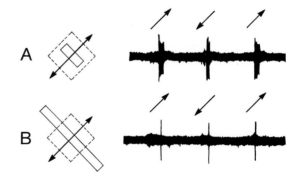

Figure 1.66. End-stopped cell recorded in area 17 of the monkey. Activating region of receptive field is outlined by the *broken line* on the *left*. Stimulus, in this instance a moving slit of white light, is represented by the *solid rectangles,* and responses to movements in directions indicated by *arrows* are shown on the *right*. *A*, The stimulus is contained within the activating region. *B*, The stimulus extends into antagonistic regions on either side. In the latter case the response is substantially reduced because the stimulus exceeded a critical length and entered an antagonistic surround region. (From DH Hubel, TN Wiesel. Receptive fields and functional architecture of monkey striate cortex. J Physiol [Lond] 1968;195:215–243.)

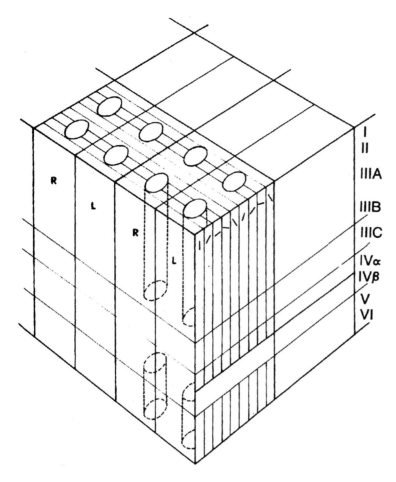

I
II
IIIA
IIIB
IIIC
IVα
IVβ
V
VI

Figure 1.67. Modular organization of the primary visual cortex (area V1). Each module (or hypercolumn) consists of two ocular dominance columns (representing right [R] and left [L] eyes), a series of orientation columns (representing 180 degrees of rotation), and cytochrome oxidase blobs (*dotted columns*; representing color information). This schematic uses the traditional designation for the cortical layers. (From Livingstone MS, Hubel DH. Anatomy and physiology of a color system in the primate visual cortex. J Neurosci 1984;4:309.)

activity and perceptual behavior, improved performance on psychophysical tests of orientation selection in monkeys has been correlated with training-induced refinement of orientation tuning of individual striate neurons (481).

A full set of orientation columns defines the spatial extent of a pixel for one eye, which is referred to as an ocular dominance column (discussed later). An immediately adjacent ocular dominance column is present for the fellow eye. A hypercolumn is a pair of ocular dominance columns, each with its full set of orientation columns and cytochrome oxidase blobs (379) (Fig. 1.67). There are several hundred hypercolumns throughout the striate cortex.

Binocularity and Ocular Dominance Columns

The primary visual cortex integrates visual information from both eyes. Although the ''simple'' cells of the striate cortex can receive input from either one eye or both, the complex and end-stopped cells receive only binocular input, which is nearly identical from each eye. Given the respective locations of these cells (discussed previously), almost all cells in layer 4C are monocular, whereas over half of the cells in layers 2, 3, 5, and 6 are binocular. Specialized cells that respond to horizontal disparity of a visual stimulus are present within the foveal representation of V1, and within

the parafoveal representations of V1 and V2 in monkeys. Within this parafoveal response zone, roughly 20% of the cells respond solely to vertical disparity, and they do so with a higher spatial resolution than cells that respond to horizontal disparity (482). This tighter monitoring of vertical interocular disparity might account for the relatively uncommon occurrence of congenital vertical strabismus in the primary position.

Adjacent columns of eye-specific input form the ocular dominance columns (468,472,483–485) (Fig. 1.68). These columns are roughly 0.4 mm wide in the macaque monkey (379,486–488). The columns can be visualized with cytochrome oxidase (CO), a marker for areas of high metabolic activity within mitochondria and the neuropil in general. By removing visual input from one eye, obvious differences can be seen in CO staining among adjacent ocular dominance columns. The positive staining regions contain blobs, oval-shaped regions of greater staining, organized in rows aligned within ocular dominance columns (Figs. 1.69 and 1.70). Ocular dominance columns are found mostly in primates, including humans (483,489,490). The blobs are most evident in (traditional) layers 4A, 4C, and 6, which are those that receive ''M'' and ''P'' afferent input from the dLGN (Fig. 1.70).

Ocular dominance columns begin to form in the monkey in the last month of gestation, prior to visual experience, and they are nearly developed at birth (491,492). Deprivation amblyopia (created by closing the palpebral fissure of one eye) in cats and monkeys causes shrinkage of ocular dominance columns from that eye (493,494). In humans, however, neither anisometropic nor strabismic amblyopia alters the width of ocular dominance columns (495,496), which suggests that deprivation amblyopia is caused by a different mechanism. In fact, the molecular basis for deprivation amblyopia has recently been shown to result from changes in the postsynaptic NMDA glutamate receptor. The retinal activity from the ''weak'' eye does not drive the visual cortex as strongly as the normally sighted eye. This imbalance initiates a cascade of biochemical changes, beginning with altered phosphorylation of specific AMPA receptors, which leads to a decrease in the surface expression of the synaptic

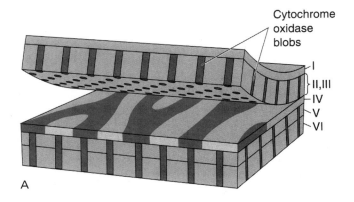

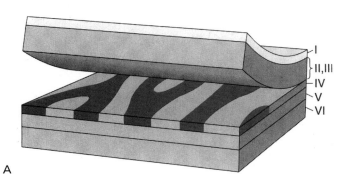

A

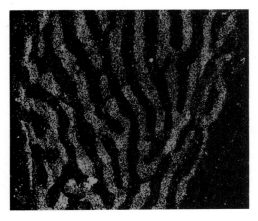

B

Figure 1.68. Ocular dominance columns in striate cortex. *A,* Organization of ocular dominance columns in layer IV of the striate cortex of a macaque monkey. The distribution of lateral geniculate nucleus (LGN) axons serving one eye is darkly shaded. In cross-section, these eye-specific zones appear as patches, each about 0.5 mm wide, in layer IV. When the superficial layers are peeled back, allowing a view of the ocular dominance columns in layer IV from above, these zones take on the appearance of zebra stripes. *B,* An autoradiograph of a histologic section of layer IV viewed from above. Two weeks prior to the experiment, one eye of this monkey was injected with radioactive praline. In the autoradiograph, the radioactive LGN terminals appear bright on a dark background. (From LeVay S, Wiesel TN, Hubel DH. The development of ocular dominance columns in normal and visually deprived monkeys. J Comp Neurol 1980;191:1–51.)

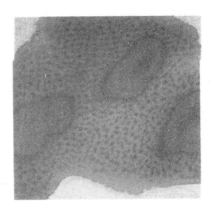

B

Figure 1.69. Distribution of the enzyme cytochrome oxidase in the cells of the striate cortex. *A,* The organization of cytochrome oxidase blobs in striate cortex of a macaque monkey. *B,* A photograph of a histologic section of layer III, stained for cytochrome oxidase and viewed from above. (From Bear MF, Connors BW, Paradiso MA. Neuroscience: Exploring the Brain. Philadelphia, Lippincott Williams & Wilkins, 2001:330.)

glutamate receptor and therefore to decreased transmission across the synapse (497). By this same mechanism, monocular deprivation can alter the relative sizes of ocular dominance columns, even in adult mice (498). Of further clinical significance is the observation that decreases in CO activity within the striate columns are induced by panretinal laser photocoagulation in monkeys (499).

Some Psychophysical Aspects

The majority of the human striate cortex represents only the central portion of the visual field. In fact, the central 10 degrees of the visual field is subserved by at least 50–60% of the striate cortex, and the central 30 degrees is represented by about 80% of the cortex (Fig. 170a) (426,500). The large area that is devoted to central vision explains the fact that the pattern-reversal visual evoked potential is essentially a reflection of macular activity (501). In the striate cortex, the area devoted to a square degree of the fovea is almost 1,000 times greater than that devoted to the same amount of area from the far peripheral (60 degrees from fixation) retina. The cortical representation of the macula is large enough to

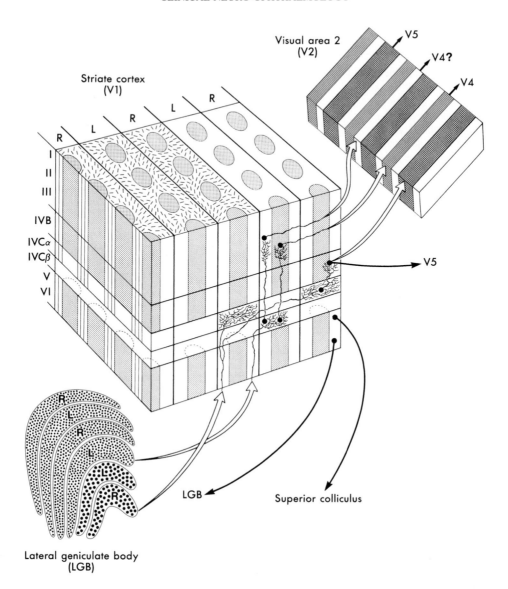

Figure 1.70. Magnocellular (originating from *large dots*) and parvocellular (originating from *small dots*) pathways from the lateral geniculate body extending through areas V1 and V2 to eventually reach areas V4 and V5. Each module of striate cortex contains a few complete sets of ocular dominance columns (R and L), orientation columns, and about a dozen cytochrome oxidase-positive blobs (*stippled cylinders*). The orientation columns, depicted with *hashmarks* on the cortical surface, extend through all layers except 4Cβ. Their borders are not discrete. The magnocellular stream courses through layer 4C to layer 4B and then to dark thick stripes in area V2 and to area V5. The parvocellular stream courses through layer 4Cβ to layers 2 and 3. Cells within the cytochrome oxidase blobs project to dark thin stripes in area V2, whereas cells within interblob regions project to pale thin stripes in V2. Both dark and pale thin stripes in area V2 probably project to area V4 and other regions. Layers 5 and 6 in area V1 send projections to the superior colliculus and the lateral geniculate body, respectively. The koniocellular pathway is not shown. (From JC Horton. The Central Visual Pathways. In: Hart WM Jr. Adler's Physiology of the Eye. 9th ed. St Louis, CV Mosby, 1992:751.)

straddle the vascular territories of the PCA and middle cerebral artery (MCA), which might explain the phenomenon of macular sparing that may occur in patients with visual field defects secondary to occipital lobe injury.

Color information is transmitted to the primary visual cortex along parallel pathways. In macaque monkeys, red-green afferent channels terminate in layer 4Cβ and blue/yellow afferent channels terminate exclusively in layers 3B and 4A. The "blue OFF" cells terminate in layer 4A, while the "blue ON" cells terminate in layers 4A and lower layer 2/3 (502). Color-selective cells in the striate cortex have been believed to terminate mostly within the CO blobs (503–507) (Fig. 1.70). Although not yet resolved, recent data reveal that color patches in striate cortex only loosely correlate with the loca-

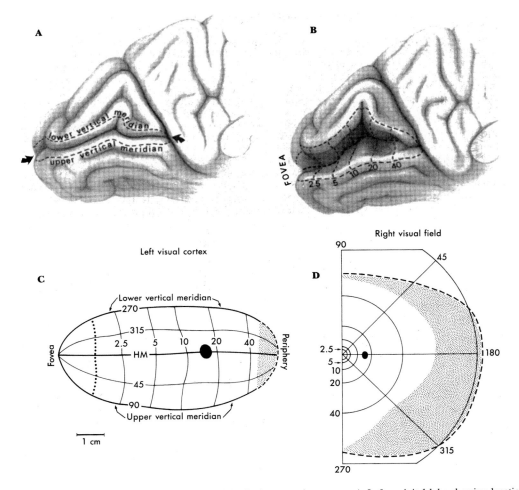

Figure 1.70a   The representation of the visual field in the human striate cortex. *A*, Left occipital lobe showing location of striate cortex within the calcarine fissure (*between arrows*). The boundary (*dashed line*)between the striate cortex (area V1) and the extrastriate cortex contains the representation of the vertical meridian. *B*, View of the striate cortex after opening the lips of the calcarine fissure. The *dashed lines* indicate the coordinates of the visual field map. The representation of the horizontal meridian runs approximately along the base of the calcarine fissure. The *vertical dashed lines* mark the isoeccentricity contours from 2.5 to 4.0. Striate cortex wraps around the occipital pole to extend about 1 cm onto the lateral convexity where the fovea is represented. *C*, Schematic map showing the projection of the right visual hemifield upon the left visual cortex by transposing the map illustrated in *B* onto a flat surface. The *row of dots* indicates approximately where striate cortex folds around the tip of the occipital lobe. The *black oval* marks the region of the striate cortex corresponding to the blind spot of the contralateral eye. *HM*, horizontal meridian. *D*, Right visual hemifield plotted with a Goldman perimeter. The *strippled region* corresponds to the monocular temporal crescent, which is mapped within the most anterior 8–10% of the striate cortex. (From Horton JC, Hoyt WF. The representation of the visual field in human striate cortex. A revision of the classic Holmes map. Arch Ophthalmol 1991;109:816–824.)

tion or size of CO blobs. Further, color-selective patches may be poorly correlated with the location of ocular dominance and orientation columns. Further, in squirrel monkeys at least, there is a tremendous variability in the expression of ocular dominance columns (206). These observations call into question the validity or consistency of the ocular dominance and hypercolumn organizational schema (508).

Nonetheless, color cells that do terminate within CO blobs are grouped together by wavelength sensitivity, such that individual blobs appear to process only one class of color opponency (509). Although color-sensitive cells are present

in the striate cortex, the extrastriate cortex (discussed later) is a more color-dominant area. There are light-driven cells within CO blobs that are neither orientation- nor wavelength-selective but that respond to high-spatial-frequency contrast gratings (510).

Blood Supply

The striate cortex benefits from a rich anastomotic network between terminal branches of the MCA and PCA, particularly at the occipital pole. The primary branches of the

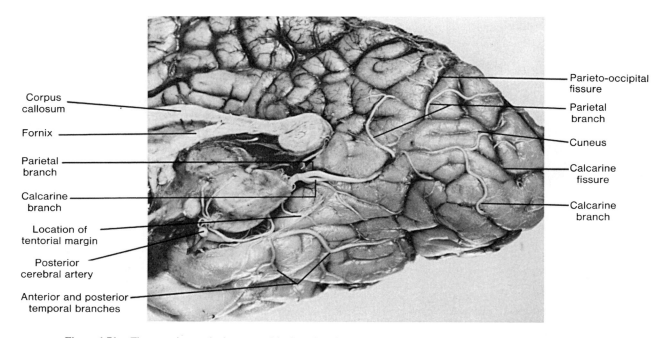

Figure 1.71. The posterior cerebral artery and its branches that supply the striate cortex. (From Lindenberg R, Walsh FB, Sacks JG. Neuropathology of Vision. Philadelphia, Lea & Febiger, 1973.)

MCA that serve the primary visual cortex are the occipital branches. The primary branches of the PCA that serve the visual cortex are the parieto-occipital (superiorly), calcarine (centrally), and posterior temporal (inferiorly) branches (511–517) (Figs. 1.60 and 1.71).

CORTICAL AREA V2

In the human, area V2 (corresponding to area 18 of Brodmann) is within the occipital lobe, adjacent to area V1 (518,519) (Figs. 1.72 and 1.73). Area V2, the largest of the extrastriate visual areas, is the first region along the afferent visual pathway at which there is a convergence of input from the retina and pulvinar (Fig. 1.74). Although these inputs terminate in different areas, the dense network of local interconnections in layer 2/3 may integrate them. Most retino-

calcarine input to area V1 passes to area V2 before being distributed elsewhere (520,521). There is a further increase in "cortical magnification" from V1 to V2 (522,523).

As described above, area V1 shows two distinct modules: blobs and orientation columns (Fig. 1.70). The output from area V1 to V2 is primarily via two paths—either from the patch or interpatch areas related to CO staining (524). Within area V2, most neurons are orientation-selective, and half are color-selective (525,526). Information from the two eyes has converged by the time it reaches area V2, and "depth cells" within the thick stripe regions respond to retinal spatial disparity (522,527,528). In fact, assessment of retinal disparity may be one of the more significant roles of area V2. These various functions are segregated in three distinct area V2 modules: pale, thin, and thick CO-staining regions (Figs. 1.63, 1.70, and 1.75). Cells within cytochrome "patches"

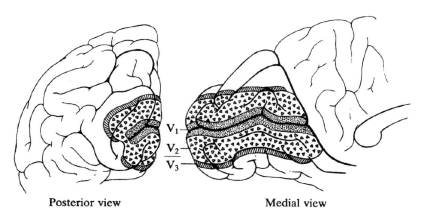

Posterior view   **Medial view**

Figure 1.72. Arrangement of V1, V2, and V3 along the medial and posterior occipital surface. Most of V1 is buried within the calcarine fissure. Considerable variation occurs among individuals in the relative position and size of different cortical visual areas. (From Horton JC, Hoyt WF. Quadrantic visual field defects. A hallmark of lesions in extrastriate [V2/V3] cortex. Brain 1991;114:1703–1718.)

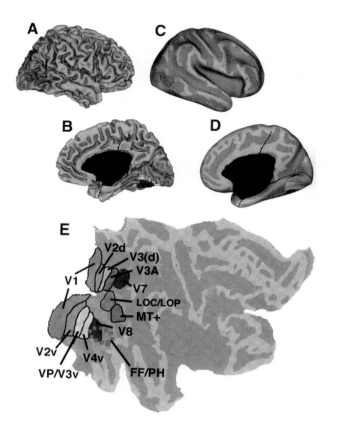

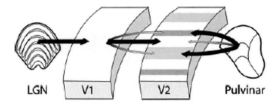

Figure 1.74. How projections from primary visual cortex (V1) and the pulvinar converge in the cortical visual area V2. As indicated by *black arrows*, the projections from V1 to V2 are richest to pale stripes, whereas those from the pulvinar are strongest to thick and thin stripes. This segregation is far from absolute, as shown by *gray arrows* indicating weaker projections. The strongest projections from V1 and the pulvinar are interdigitated in V2. LGN, lateral geniculate nucleus. (From Sincich LC, Horton JC. Pale cytochrome oxidase stripes in V2 receive the richest projection from macaque striate cortex. J Comp Neurol 2002;447:18–33.)

Figure 1.73. Identified visual areas on the Human.colin surface-based atlas. The boundary of MT+ on the atlas map was estimated by projecting the motion-related activation foci tabulated by Van Essen and Drury (1997) onto the atlas surface. The visuotopic map from Figure 5A of Tootel and Hadjikhani (2001) was then registered to the atlas using the V1/V2 boundary and the posterior boundary of MT+ as landmarks. Additional areas LO and V7 were drawn manually onto the atlas, based respectively on the studies of Tootel and Hadjikhani (2001) and Press et al. (2001). *A,* Lateral view. *B,* Medial view. *C,* Inflated (i.e., the cortex is shown as a flat surface without the normal indentations of the sulci) lateral view. *D,* Inflated medial view. *E,* Flat magnified view. The red dotted contour represents the main cluster activation focus center involved in face and place analysis. The abbreviations indicate areas of striate and extrastriate cortex: FF, fusiform face area; LOP, lateral occipital parietal; PH, parahippocampal place area; VP, ventral posterior area. (From Van Essen DC. Organization of visual areas in macaque and human cerebral cortex. In: Chalupa LM, Werner JS, eds. The Visual Neurosciences. Cambridge, MA, MIT Press, 2004:610.)

of V1 send their axons to thin V2 stripes; cells between cytochrome V1 patches ("interpatches") send their axons to pale and thick stripes of area V2 (524). In area V2, the thin, pale, and thick CO bands are primarily responsive to color, orientation, and retinal disparity, respectively (529) (Fig. 1.70). Each of these zones contains smaller compartments, each with functional distinctions (523). The dark (thin and thick) zones receive significant input from the pulvinar (530).

Many area V2 cells respond to more than one visual feature, which suggests that some degree of visual integration occurs in V2 (Table 1.6). For instance, color cells with com-

plex responses (e.g., binocular color cells with orientation selectivity) are found in area V2 (523,531,532). There are also cells with mixed color and disparity functions. The two "interpatch" projections (one from layer 4B and one from layer 2/3 of area V1) are composed primarily of M- and P-cell input, respectively, from area V1. But some interpatch afferents project to the same V2 stripes. This suggests that M and P outflow is merged at V2 and then distributed to both dorsal and ventral streams via V3 (discussed later) (524).

Compared to V1, receptive fields are larger in V2, and cells can respond to lower spatial frequencies. However, directionally selective cells are sparse in area V2, which suggests that motion information bypasses V2 en route to area V5 (discussed later). Some cell columns are arranged in a highly ordered fashion, with the orientation of cells in adjacent columns differing by small but constant amounts. Occasionally, the shift in orientation between neighboring columns is abrupt and appears random in direction and variable in size (523).

Area V2 is intimately related with area V3 on the same side of the brain, and also projects ipsilaterally to V4 and V5. Area V2 projects contralaterally via the corpus callosum to the fellow area V2. This callosal connection integrates roughly half of V2 from each side and connects topographically opposite halves of the homonymous visual field between the vertical meridian and the 45-degrees isopolar line (533) (Fig. 1.76). The connections between areas V1 and V2 occur between cells at the same cortical depth (with the greatest input coming from layer 4) and are retinotopically organized (Fig. 1.77). Area V2 projects to and receives input from prefrontal, sensory, motor, and auditory association areas; the insula; and, by multisynaptic pathways, the anterior temporal lobe. Area V2 contributes corticotectal and corticomesencephalic fibers to the superior colliculi that may function in initiation of slow vertical or oblique eye movements.

The clinical consequences of lesions restricted to area V2 in humans is unclear. In monkey, cell body-specific (i.e., axonal sparing) lesions of V2 produce no decrement in visual acuity or contrast sensitivity, although complex spatial func-

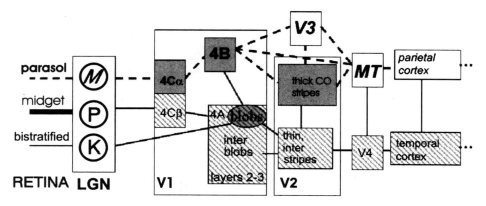

Figure 1.75. A simplified connectivity diagram of the magnocellular (M), parvocellular (P), and koniocellular (K) pathways in the primate visual system. The magnodominant (''where'') stream is marked in *dashed lines* and *bold italics*; the ventral (''what'') stream is indicated by *solid lines* and *faint stripes*. (From Kaplan E. The M, P, and K pathways of the primate visual system. In: Chalupa LM, Werner JS eds. The Visual Neurosciences. Cambridge, MA, MIT Press, 2004:486.)

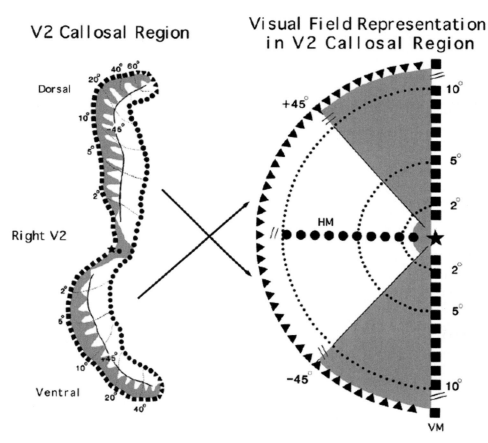

Figure 1.76. Correlating the callosal pattern and the visual field map in area V2. The *left* panel shows the overall pattern of callosal connections (in *gray*) in dorsal and ventral halves of right area V2 superimposed to mapping data of V2 taken from Gattass et al. (1981), Van Essen et al. (1986), and Rosa et al. (1988). Posterior is to the left. The symbols in the topographic map correspond with those in the left visual hemifield represented in the *right* panel. The arrows between left and right panels indicate that dorsal and ventral V2 represent lower and upper visual field quadrants, respectively. The posterior border of V2 represents the vertical meridian (*black squares*); the striate cortex would then be to the left of the black squares. The anterior border represents the horizontal meridian (*large dots*), the uppermost and lowermost regions of V2 represent peripheral fields (*triangles*), and the fovea representation is in the middle of V2 (*star*). Isoeccentricity lines are represented with small dots, isopolar contours with thin lines. The shaded area in the hemifield corresponds approximately to the extent of the visual field represented in the callosally connected region in V2. (From Abel PL et al. Organization of callosal linkages in visual area V2 of macaque monkey. J Comp Neurol 2000;428:278–293.)

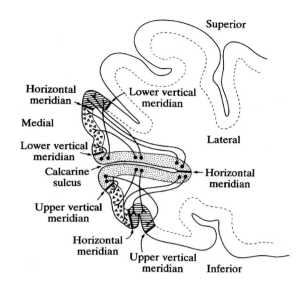

Figure 1.77. Schematic coronal section through right occipital lobe showing connections from V1 (*stippled area*) to V2/V3 (*small triangles* and *hatched lines*, respectively). Projections pass between common retinotopic coordinates. In V1, the horizontal meridian is represented along the base of the calcarine sulcus. Fibers coursing in the white matter of the upper and lower calcarine banks serve the lower and upper visual quadrants, respectively. For simplicity, feedback pathways from V2/V3 to V1 and the projection between V2 and V3 are omitted. The ventral V1 to V3 pathway is doubtful (Van Esen et al. [1986]). (From Horton JC, Hoyt WF. Quadrantic visual field defects. A hallmark of lesions in extrastriate [V2/V3] cortex. Brain 1991;114:1703–1718.)

tions (e.g., orientation of lines or detection of texture) are abolished. In humans, lesions of V2 and V3 produce homonymous quadrantanopias (534). Loss of visual field along the horizontal meridian is explained by the mutual alignment of the representation of the horizontal visual field meridian at the intersection of V2 and V3 (Fig. 1.78). Human lesions of V2 may cause selective impairment of the perception of the direction of first-order motion (i.e., spatial and temporal variation of luminance in a scene), even with an intact area MT (discussed later) (535).

CORTICAL AREAS V3 AND V3A

The most detailed information regarding the organization of the visual cortices comes from monkeys, and this body of information provides moderate detail on only three areas: V1, V2, and MT (discussed later). The current frontier of study is of area V3, for which there are good anatomic data of its interconnections but only recently a compelling picture of its retinotopy. Area V3d (i.e., dorsal) has more connections with V1 than any other area, although these are less numerous than the connections between areas V1 and V2. Area V3, which is relatively small (i.e., roughly half the width of V2) is located adjacent to the boundary between areas 18 and 19 of Brodmann (area V3 is not synonymous with area 19 of Brodmann, which occupies a large area laterally where it surrounds area V2).

The anatomy of the visual cortices just lateral and rostral

to area V2 (including area V3) is highly controversial (Fig. 1.79). One current opinion is that macaque and owl monkeys have both a dorsal and ventral area V3 (i.e., area V3d and V3v) that are physically discontinuous (536). This view contrasts with the view that the absence of connections between V1 and a ventral V3 area indicates that there is no V3v (537). With this interpretation, the ventral area of V3 is referred to as VP (i.e., ventroposterior) (538). A third opinion is that there is little or no area V3 in macaque monkeys, but rather an area V6 (discussed later) that abuts the rostral border of area V2 (539). However they are referred to, the area contiguous but peripheral to V2 is heavily myelinated, and there is strong immunoreactivity for the antibody CAT-301 within the area referred to as V3d. Functional MRI data from humans, however, suggest that there is one functionally similar although physically discontinuous area V3 (540). Nonetheless, the weight of evidence from animal experimentation favors the notion that V3d and V3v are functionally distinct (discussed later).

A definite retinotopy exists for area V3, with the border between areas V2 and V3 sharing the representation of the horizontal meridian of the visual field (541–543) (Figs. 1.78 and 1.80). Topographically, areas V2 and V3 are mirror images of one another (536). The fovea is represented where the upper and lower fields of areas V2 and V3 are juxtaposed (544). Area V3 projects primarily to the pulvinar and the midbrain. Area V3 also has CO staining patterns, but these are relatively weak and variable.

Within area V3, 76% of neurons are strongly orientation-selective, whereas 40% are strongly direction-selective. Most V3 neurons are optimized for stimulus speed discrimination, with half of the cells being optimized for stimulus movement of 16 degrees per second, which gives this area a strong sensitivity for motion detection, like area V5 (discussed later) (526,545,546). Functional MRI in humans reveals that the V3 complex is activated strongly by second-order motion (i.e., contrast or frequency modulation, not luminance modulation) (540). Additionally, roughly half of area V3d neurons are color-sensitive (546), which is similar to area V3v (alternatively referred to as VP) (547). Most area V3 neurons are binocularly driven.

One interpretation of the anatomy of area V3 is that its two divisions—V3d and V3v or VP—are differentially involved in partitioning visual information. Area V3d may be part of the dorsal stream that specializes in motion detection. Area V3d may be part of the ventral stream that specializes in form recognition (discussed later). Neurons in both V3d and V3v have response properties similar to those found in V2 (i.e., they respond to color, object, motion, and space), although V3v neurons are more wavelength-selective and less directionally selective than those in V3d. Interestingly, the representation of each V3 area is only for one quadrant of the visual field (e.g., V3d represents only the contralateral, inferior visual field) (537,538).

Complete damage to V1 quiets all V2 and nearly V3 neuronal responses to visual stimuli. However, roughly one third of the area V3A (i.e., the adjoining cortex just rostral to V3) neurons may respond to photic stimuli even with complete ablation of V1 or V2 (548,549). Area V5 also re-

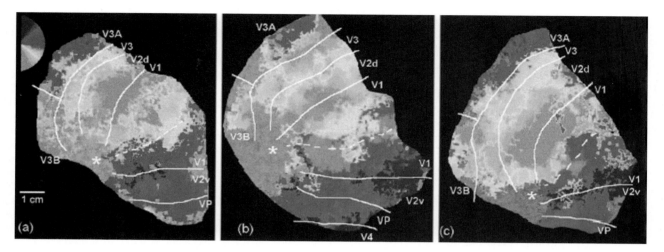

Figure 1.78. Maps of the posterior cortex of three subjects obtained by simulating a flattening of the gray matter. The left hemisphere is shown in all cases; similar results were obtained in the right hemispheres. Overlaid on the map is a pseudocolor representation of the phase of the fundamental component of the activation time course elicited by a rotating, flickering checkerboard (*inset, upper left*). The variations in gray reflect visual field position (key in *a*) and show a smooth progression through the visual field within each visual area, with a reversal of the direction of change at each cortical boundary. Estimates of the locations of various boundaries are indicated. The *dotted white line* shows the approximate location of the fundus of the calcarine sulcus. The approximate position of the occipital pole is marked with a *star*. (From Smith AT, et al. The processing of first- and second-order motion in human visual cortex by functional magnetic resonance imaging [fMRI]. J Neurosci 1998; 18:3816–3830.)

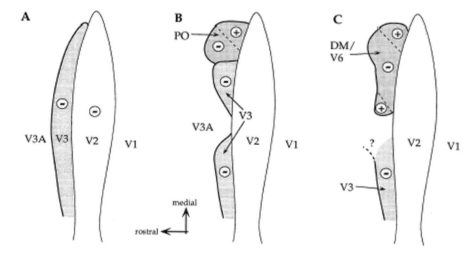

Figure 1.79. Three views of the organization of dorsal extrastriate cortex in the macaque. Each diagram is an unfolded view of the cortex of the left hemisphere. *A,* An early opinion of the organization (e.g., Van Essen and Zeki [1978]), which proposed that a striplike V3, containing a representation of the lower quadrant (−), formed the rostral border of dorsal V2. *B,* Revised view based on the studies of Gattass et al. (Colby et al. [1988]; Gattass et al. [1988]; Neuenschewander et al. [1994]). In this construct, the lower-quadrant representation in area V3 is discontinuous. Moreover, V3 does not extend as far medially as shown in *A*. Instead, another area (PO), which represents the periphery of both quadrants, is present medial to V3. *C,* A more current interpretation based on the results of Galletti et al. (1999) in the macaque, and Rosa and Schmid (1995) in the marmoset. Area PO, together with the medial island of V3 and an adjacent part of V3A, forms a complete representation of the visual field, named V6 or DM. This area contains a continuous representation of the lower quadrant and a split representation of the upper quadrant (+). Area V3 does not extend medially as far as proposed by earlier studies. (From Rosa MGP, Tweedale R. The dorsomedial visual areas in New World and Old World monkeys: homology and function. Eur J Neurosci 2001; 13:421–427.)

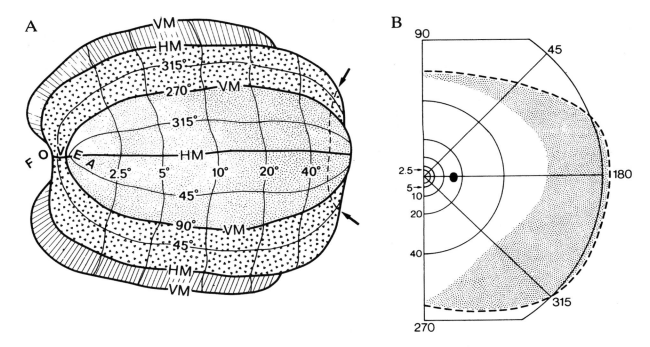

Figure 1.80. *A*, Artificially flattened map showing retinotopic organization of V1 (*stippled area*), V2 (*small triangles*), and V3 (*hatched lines*) in the left occipital lobe. *B*, Right visual field coordinates corresponding to map in *A*. The monocular temporal crescent (*stippled area*) is represented within a small area at the rostral end of striate cortex (border between binocular and monocular field runs between arrows in *A*). V2 and V3 are split along the representation of the horizontal meridian into separate dorsal and ventral halves. More than half of visual cortex is devoted to processing the central 10 degrees of vision. (From Horton JC, Hoyt WF. Quadrantic visual field defects: a hallmark of lesions in extrastriate [V2/V3] cortex. Brain 1991; 114:1703–1718.)

mains visually responsive without input from V1, although more weakly than V3A. The retained responsiveness of these extrastriate cortices even without input from area V1 is evidence that they receive input from other than the retinocalcarine pathway. The most likely alternative pathway is probably dominated by input from the pulvinar. Any such nonretinocalcarine pathway provides a neuroanatomic basis for the (admittedly controversial) clinical phenomenon of "blindsight" (see Chapter 13).

DORSAL AND VENTRAL VISUAL STREAMS

Two major streams of information flow are believed to exist from the V1 and V2 areas to other visual association cortices in primates: the dorsal and ventral pathways (Fig. 1.81). The dorsal pathway, which is divided into dorsomedial and dorsolateral sectors, is believed to be primarily concerned with where objects are and how they could be manipulated. The ventral pathway is believed to be primarily concerned with form (i.e., "what") detection, although detection of "second-order" motion (i.e., spatiotemporal scene variation of contrast, depth, etc., but not luminance) or "biologic motion" (discussed later) may be impaired with lesions to this pathway (550). The dorsal and ventral information streams do not have precise anatomic boundaries.

The area of visual cortex just rostral to V3 has been variably referred to as area V3A, V6, or DM (i.e., dorsal median,

a term used in New World monkeys). Area 6, as it will be called here, is located between areas V3 and V4, in the lunate and parieto-occipital sulci (Fig. 1.73). Area 6 has reciprocal connections with areas V1, V2, V3, MT, MST, and other sensorimotor areas (551). As such, area V6 is in a position to distribute visual information from area V1 throughout the sensorimotor cortices of the parietal lobe, and thus assist in coordination of visuomotor tasks (Fig. 1.82). Area V6 has a retinotopy that is distinct among visual cortices—there is a physical discontinuity between central and peripheral vision for the upper quadrant only (539). Most cells in V3 and V6 are binocularly driven. The receptive fields of cells are larger in areas V3 and V6 than in area V2. There is a similarity of responses among cells within V6 and the medial part of V3, which has contributed to the controversy over regional boundaries (539) (Fig. 1.79). The medial extrastriate cortex in and around the V6 area is one of the major afferent inputs from the cortex to the pontine nuclei (552). Area V6 is heavily myelinated, as is area 5 (discussed later).

The area just dorsal to V6 in macaque is known as V6A. Area V6 and V6A are strongly interconnected (553), although their physiologic properties are quite different. Most significantly, V6A contains some cells that do not respond to visual stimuli; "real-position" cells that represent orientation with respect to craniotopic receptive fields; and cells with much larger receptive fields than area V6, among other

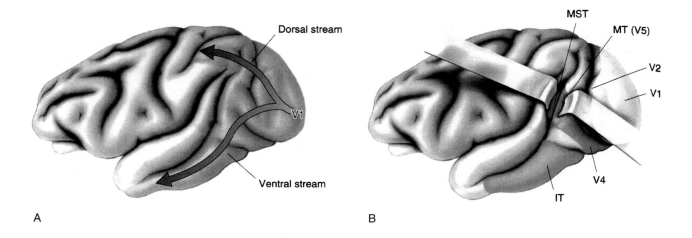

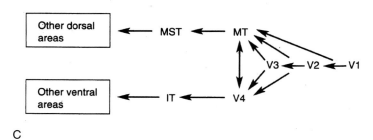

Figure 1.81. Beyond striate cortex in the macaque brain. *A*, Dorsal and ventral visual processing streams. *B*, Extrastriate visual areas. *C*, Flow of information in the dorsal and ventral streams. (From Bear MF, Connors BW, Paradiso MA. Neuroscience: Exploring the Brain. 2nd ed. Philadelphia, Lippincott Williams & Wilkins, 2001:338.)

properties. The nonvisual neurons are activated by intentional arm movements into peripersonal space, even in the dark (554). There are some physiologic similarities between V6 and V6A in that these two areas respond nearly identically to orientation and direction of movement of visual stimuli, and their cells are similarly affected by eye movement (i.e., gaze activity). The retinotopy in area V6A is coarser than the more proximal visual cortical areas.

Area 6A receives input from both of the better-characterized motion-sensitive areas V6 and MT (discussed later). Given this input, the function of area V6A is believed to help guide skeletomotor activity into extrapersonal space (555). Lesions of area V6A in monkeys cause specific deficits in reaching, wrist orientation, and grasping and a reluctance to move (556). Disruption of V6A or nearby areas may explain the inability of patients with Balint syndrome to accurately reach out to objects that they can see and describe (557) (see Chapter 13).

CORTICAL AREA V5

Area V5 is also referred to as MT because of its location in the caudal third of the middle temporal gyrus of the owl monkey (558). Area 5 is the smallest of the named visual areas. V5 in humans is an oval area, located 5–6 cm anterior and dorsal to the foveal V1–V2 border, at the junction of Brodmann areas 19 and 37 (Fig. 1.73). Area V5 receives direct but relatively sparse inputs from striate cortex (specifically from layers 4B and 6 to layers 3, 4, and 6)

(544,558–560) and from area V2 (specifically to layers 1, 2, and 4) (561). The sparseness of input from these areas does not necessarily imply that V5 has any less significant functional impact. Consider the following: The area V1 neurons that project to MT have very large receptive fields and the highest velocity compared to other paths of outflow from V1. Area MT also receives input from V3d, V3v, MST, and the pulvinar. There may also be considerable amplification of incoming signals in area V5 because of very dense intracortical branching and the relatively large, excitatory postsynaptic densities that are present in this area (562). Blocking input from area V1 impairs but does not eliminate activity in MT, and in this situation even direction selectivity of the neurons is retained (although it is more crude than normal) (549,563). Activity in MT is abolished when both the SC (with input via the pulvinar) and area V1 are damaged (563).

Positron emission tomography (PET) and functional MRI have demonstrated the presumptive location of area V5 in humans by having subjects view an array of moving stimuli (564–567). The location of area V5 varies by as much as 27 mm in the left hemisphere and 18 mm in the right but is consistently located ventrolaterally, just posterior to the junction of the ascending limb of the inferior temporal sulcus and the lateral occipital sulcus. Area V5 has a columnar organization for direction specificity similar to area V1 (568).

Ninety percent of neurons within area V5 are direction-selective (526,569,570). Although this property is common among complex cells of the magnocellular pathway in area

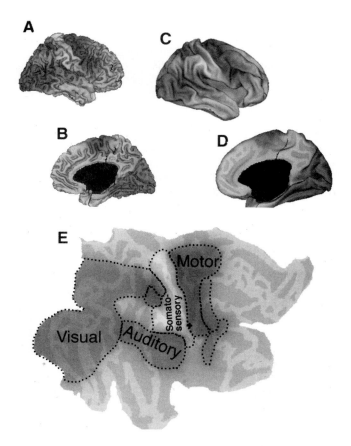

Figure 1.82. Functional magnetic resonance imaging (fMRI) representations of the proximity of various sensory and motor cortices in the human brain. The visual cortex and other functional modalities are mapped onto a surface-based atlas of human cerebral cortex. The atlas was generated from a high-resolution structural MRI volume provided by A. Toga (Case Human.colin) using SureFit and Caret software. *A*, Modality assignments were based on (*A*) stereotactic mapping of fMRI volume data on the atlas surface from the studies of Corbetta et al. (1998), Lewis and DeYoe (2000), and Lewis et al. (2001); (*B*) stereotactic projection of published Talairach coordinates of activation focus centers (Ishai et al. [1999]; Kanwisher et al. [1997]; Van Essen and Drury [1997]); and (*C*) manually transposed boundaries related to local geographic and/or functional landmarks from surface maps published by Burton and Sinclair (2000), Press et al. (2001), and Tootel and Hadjikhani (2001). (From Van Essen DC. Organization of visual areas in macaque and human cerebral cortex. In: Chalupa LM, Werner JS, eds. The Visual Neurosciences. Cambridge, MA, MIT Press, 2004.)

data in humans (discussed later). PET scanning, however, has shown that many areas in the human brain, including bilateral foci at the border between Brodmann areas 19 and 37, a V1/V2 focus, and foci in the cuneus, cerebellum, and cortical vestibular areas, are also involved with visual motion perception (573). In fact, motion perception can occur even with disruption of the magnocellular system (i.e., the retinal outflow pathway concerned with motion detection) at the level of the dLGN (574).

Nonetheless, it is generally considered that the magnocellular pathway is the primary conduit for motion processing. The heavily myelinated outflow from area V1 to area V5 within the dorsal stream delivers very rapid visual input to the parietal lobe, even before an object is precisely fixated. This extraordinary response time may be important for generating visual attention to a visual stimulus (575). The clinical relevance of area MT neurons is revealed by the extremely close match between the response rates of directionally selective neurons in MT to the psychophysical response rates of monkeys when they discriminate the direction of moving visual stimuli (576). This direction response property is fairly modest for most individual area MT neurons, but it seems likely that information from many neurons is pooled, given that so many of the neurons respond similarly. Area MST lies close to area V5, from which it receives significant input. Area MST contains neurons that behave indistinguishably from those in area V5 (577), but also may specialize in processing "motion in depth," which permits an estimation of one's direction of movement within an environment (578). Lesions of area V1 produce the same effect upon areas MT and MST (579). In one human, blindness caused by a (subtotal) lesion of the primary visual cortex was associated with functional MRI activity within the blind visual field that was confined to the dorsal pathway, which reveals the presence of an alternative path to the dorsal stream from areas other than area V1 (580).

Functional MRI studies have revealed significant insights into the motion processing streams in humans. For instance, areas V1 and V2 respond well to all motion stimuli. Areas 3d and 3v show much greater responsiveness for second-order (contrast or flicker modulation, with luminance held constant) versus first-order (spatiotemporal changes in luminance) motion than is found in areas V1 or V2. Area V5 participates in both types of motion processing (540). Another newly recognized area for motion processing is known as area V3B (referred to previously as KO, for kinetic occipital).

Damage to area V5 in monkeys produces deficits for ocular pursuit of moving targets and for adjusting the amplitude of a saccadic eye movement in response to target motion, although saccades to stationary targets are unaffected (581). The threshold for direction discrimination also increases (582). The significance of area V5 for motion detection in humans has been revealed with transcranial magnetic stimulation, which was to reversibly inactivate areas V1 and V5 (583). The speed of a moving object had been reported to influence the patterns of induced cortical activity in that relatively fast visual motion would activate area V5 before area V1 (584), although this finding was not corroborated by a

V1 and in some cells in areas V2, V3, V3A, and V4 (526,571), area V5 appears to be the primary cortical region for processing the direction of stimulus movement. The input to MT from area V1 is directionally selective and appears to convey motion of individual regions within a visual scene rather than motion of the entire scene (i.e., "global motion") (572). Area MT may perform a higher-order analysis of motion by extracting patterns of movement from the specific data that it receives from each pixel of visual space. Approximately one third of MT neurons are directionally selective for patterns of movement. To a lesser extent, area V3 may perform similar tasks, as is suggested by the functional MRI more recent study in monkeys with unilateral area V1 lesions (579).

The ability of humans to detect visual motion even in areas rendered "blind" by a lesion of area V1 (i.e., blindsight) is consistent with the presence of parallel pathways for motion detection (585–591). The availability of more than one pathway for motion detection makes it challenging to find patients with complete blindness to moving visual stimuli (i.e., cerebral akinetopsia) (592). Extensive bilateral lesions of the dorsolateral visual association cortices that spare areas area V1 can produce severe deficits in motion detection (593), although by more sophisticated testing such a patient may be shown to retain the ability to perceive global coherent motion and discriminate motion direction, although with less sensitivity than normal when there is background noise in the visual scene (594). These motion deficits, however, almost never occur in pure isolation. Deficits in speed and motion direction discrimination have also been reported in humans with more restricted lesions involving the lateral occipital areas, possibly more specifically at area V5 (595,596).

There is evidence for two dorsal pathways for motion processing: a medial and lateral pathway. The dorsomedial pathway includes area V6; the dorsolateral pathway includes area MT as well as the parietal-insular vestibular cortex. This distinction has been demonstrated by functional MRI studies in humans in which area V6 is activated mostly by wide-field coherent motion, while area MT is activated primarily by movement within a limited area of the visual field or by differential movement in different areas of the visual field (597). These two pathways may provide information about self-motion through the dorsomedial pathway and object motion through the dorsolateral pathway (598). This distinction is reminiscent of the newly described RGC type known as the *object motion cell*, which responds differently depending on whether object motion is similar to or different from the background (discussed previously) (84).

Clinical manifestations related to these two dorsal pathways have been defined. Humans with lesions of area V6 experience difficulty with postural adjustments and walking (599), possibly because V6 may be important in determining the direction and speed of one's own body motion through an environment. In distinction, perception of "biologic motion" (i.e., perception of motion created by lights to the major joints and head of a human who is walking but whose form is otherwise not evident) has been shown by functional MRI to activate both dorsal and ventral streams of visual outflow. Perception of biologic motion may depend upon information processing in both dorsal pathways, the confluence of which is at the superior temporal sulcus (STS) (600). Patients with bilateral lesions of the ventral visual pathways can see and describe motion, which distinguishes them from patients with cerebral akinetopsia, but they have difficulty recognizing moving (even very familiar) faces, persons, or objects. These patients report no difficulty with stationary visual stimuli (601).

CORTICAL AREA V4

Visual detection of the shape of an object requires the integration of neuronal responses from pixels of the visual scene that encompass the object of regard. The visual integration to determine "form" seems to occur within the ventral visual pathway, which derives from input primarily from areas V1 and V2. An intermediate step along the ventral pathway occurs at area V4, which in humans is located in the lingual and fusiform gyri, with a caudal region that extends into area 18 of Brodmann (602) (Figs. 1.73, 1.75, and 1.80). Area V4 receives projections from the CO-rich thin stripes and the CO-poor interstripe regions of V2 (537). Area V4 contains a complete topographic representation of the contralateral visual field (542,603). The receptive fields of V4 are larger than those of V3 (542), which are in turn larger than the more proximal visual cortices. The major projection of V4 is to IT (i.e., inferotemporal cortex, discussed later), but there is also a significant projection to the posterior parietal cortex.

Area V4 neurons respond primarily to the shape, color, and texture of a visual stimulus (Fig. 1.83). Area V4 neurons receive input from both P- and M-retinofugal pathways (604), perhaps via a subset of area V1 neurons that receive convergent input from these pathways (431). Inactivation of either the P or M pathway moderately but equivalently reduces the responsiveness of V4 neurons (604). A prevalence of area V4 neurons show preferences for objects that are relatively near (605). Few V4 neurons are orientation- or direction-sensitive (526).

In monkeys, half of area V4 neurons have color-opponent properties (570,602,606–608). Cerebral dyschromatopsia may occur in humans following damage to an area of visual cortex anterior and inferior to the primary visual cortex, which has been presumed to be the homolog of area V4 in monkeys (609) (see Chapter 13). Bilateral removal of area V4 in monkeys, however, does not disrupt the ability to discriminate between rows of colored or gray stimuli. Although in this experimental paradigm there are deficiencies in color performance, the color impairment is no more severe than for discrimination of gray tones (610). This seeming inconsistency is probably explained by the fact that human diseases that affect area V4 (mainly strokes and tumors) produce less specific cortical injury and tend to include underlying white matter. The human case with perhaps the most selective, bilateral lesions of area V4 had severe color blindness and pattern perception loss with prosopagnosia, although there was normal luminance detection thresholds, spatial contrast sensitivity, stereopsis, motion processing, and flicker perception (611).

Area V4 neurons code shape in reference to the boundary features of objects. Their responses vary with respect to the location and angulation of contour features within the image of the object. Recent experimentation has provided a compelling insight into how an image might be created. The shape of an object can be predicted by assimilating the peaks of activity across a population of area V4 neurons, each of which responds maximally to specific structural elements of the object (612). These results suggest that the brain uses a "parts-based" representation method, rather than the alternative notion of a "holistic" representation, where neurons would be most responsive to the form of the entire object. Area V4 neurons are not only tuned to one particular geome-

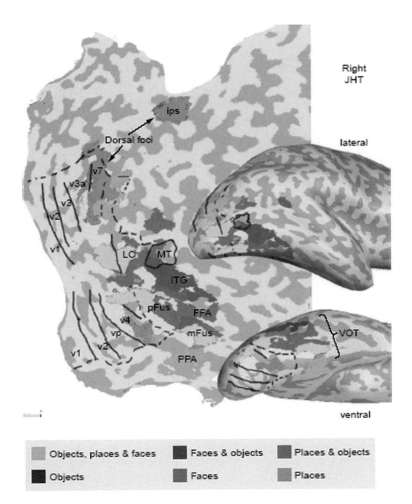

Figure 1.83. Functional magnetic resonance imaging (fMRI) maps that reveal activation of specific cortical regions in response to a variety of visual stimuli in humans. The images are "inflated" (i.e., the cortical sulci are eliminated by digitally expanding the sulci to present a flattened cortical surface). The large cortical map (*left*) is a flattened, lateral and ventral view of the upper and lower visual cortical pathways of the right hemisphere. The two smaller cortical maps on the right are the inflated (but not flattened) views of the lateral (*top right*) and ventral (*bottom right*) posterior right hemisphere that were combined to form the larger flattened map. Certain cortical regions are more strongly activated by either images of objects, faces, or places. (From Grill-Spector K. The neural basis of object perception. Curr Opin Neurobiol 2003;13:159–166.)

try but rather respond to a wide variety of shapes, although their strongest response is for a particular boundary shape located at a specific position within the object (613). In addition to this presumed capability to extract object shape, area V4 neurons may also convey information about the location of the object in visual field space.

Area V4 may also be important for responding to targets within a field of similar stimuli that have relatively low contrast, smaller size, or slower motion (614). Preliminary inferences about the role of area V4 for these types of functional tasks come from single cell recordings that have shown increased activity of V4 neurons when unique features of stimulus embedded within other similar stimuli were being discriminated (615,616). The evidence of impaired clinical function comes from ablation studies in monkeys. In rhesus monkeys, V4 ablation creates significant visual deficits when multiple stimuli are presented but permits normal performance when the same stimuli are presented individually (617). In macaque monkeys, ablation of V4 produces severely disrupted form and shape discrimination, mildly reduced luminance and red-green contrast sensitivity, and an inability to learn hue and luminance matching (although the monkeys retained the matching skills if they had been previously learned). Area V4, therefore, may play a generic role in visual discrimination tasks including color, pattern, luminance, texture, rate of movement, and size when many relatively similar objects are viewed. Chronic lesions of area V4 in monkeys, however, produce relatively little or no deficit for motion-, color-, or luminance-defined contours, although there are significant deficits for contours defined by texture and for illusory contours. Perhaps area V4 plays only a minor role in color and luminance perception and motion detection, or perhaps there is sufficient plasticity following a chronic injury to area V4 that these visual functions can be subserved in other ways (618).

The effect of disrupting the major retinocalcarine pathways differs for various extrastriate cortices. For area V4, inactivation of either the parvocellular or magnocellular layers causes a moderate reduction of visual responses (604). For area V5, inactivation of the magnocellular area of the dLGN produces greatly reduced responses, whereas few neurons are affected by parvocellular blockade (619). Presumably area V4, but not V5, receives strong input from both the magnocellular and parvocellular subdivisions of the dLGN.

Perceptual learning has been shown to modify the re-

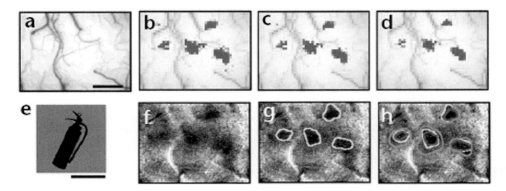

Figure 1.84. Demonstration from the inferotemporal cortex of a macaque monkey that a spatially complex visual stimulus (like the fire extinguisher shown in *e*) activates combinations of discontinuous, cellular modules. Each module responds to specific visual features of the stimulus, and in combination, the perception of the object is created. This experiment used an intrinsic signal imaging technique to detect local modulation of light absorption changes in area TE. *a,* Surface view of the exposed portion of dorsal area TE. *b–d,* Active regions, elicited by the visual stimulus shown in *e*, in which the reflection change elicited by the stimulus was significantly greater than that elicited by the control. *f,* A filtered differential image showing local increase in absorption. *g,* Extracted active spots outlined by connecting pixels with half the peak absorption value. *h,* Active spots outlined by different thresholds, one third, one half, and two thirds of the peak absorption value. Scale bars = 1.0 mm (*a–d, f–h*); 10 degrees (*e*). These results argue against the concept that object recognition results from activation of a combination of cells specific for each type of stimulus. (From Tsunoda K et al. Complex objects are represented in macaque inferotemporal cortex by the combination of feature columns. Nature Neurosci 2001;4:832–838.)

sponse properties of neurons in area V4. In macaque monkeys, the process of learning to discriminate the orientation of a visual stimulus has been correlated with the development of stronger and more narrowly tuned responses of area V4 neurons. This is the first demonstration that training to perform a complex task modifies neuronal responses related to that task (620).

AREA TE

The end of the ventral pathway for form recognition occurs at the anterior region of the inferotemporal cortex, area TE, which is the last area that is exclusively visual along this pathway. Area TE may play a role in the visual identification of complex objects. Unlike almost all other visual cortical areas that maintain a precise retinotopic organiza-

tion, visual stimuli elicit responses within area TE from several clusters of neurons that are not physically contiguous. Recognition of an object may derive from activation of specific combinations of cortical columns, each of which responds to different spatial aspects of the object shape; they tend to respond best to less spatially complicated objects (621) (Fig. 1.84). The complexity of the object shape may be derived by assessing the combinations of activated and nonactivated neuronal regions. For instance, some objects with relatively simple geometries activate a larger number of cortical columns within area TE than some more complex visual stimuli. There are other less common neurons in area TE that respond more specifically to objects of a particular shape or object class. For instance, some area TE cells are especially well tuned for faces or hands, while others are

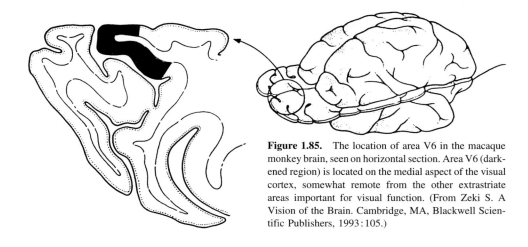

Figure 1.85. The location of area V6 in the macaque monkey brain, seen on horizontal section. Area V6 (darkened region) is located on the medial aspect of the visual cortex, somewhat remote from the other extrastriate areas important for visual function. (From Zeki S. A Vision of the Brain. Cambridge, MA, Blackwell Scientific Publishers, 1993:105.)

tuned for more general images of the human body (622,623) (Fig. 1.83). Generally, however, object recognition in area TE probably relates to the patterns of activity of multiple columns of cells, rather than the responses of individual cells. Recognition of complex object shape may be facilitated in area TE by a substantial population of neurons (roughly one third of the total number) that selectively respond to three-dimensional object shapes (624). Area TE has strong connections to the medial temporal region, which may provide a substrate to form visual memories (625).

CORTICAL AREA V6

Area V6, which is located medially in the parietal cortex adjacent to area V3A (Fig. 1.85), is poorly understood (see the previous section on Area V3 for discussion of controversy in naming this and related areas). Area V6 receives input from V2, has large receptive fields, and is thought to function in the mapping of relative spatial relationships (626). Adjacent cells within area V6 respond to stimuli that are located in a similar area of the visual field, although V6 does not have a conventional retinotopic map.

OTHER CEREBRAL AREAS CONTRIBUTING TO VISUAL PERCEPTION

Many areas of the brain other than those listed in Table 1.6 contribute to the analysis of vision. Neurons in the SC are special in their ability to respond to stimuli from different sensory inputs (627). These multisensory neurons have overlapping receptive fields for input from, for instance, simultaneous visual and auditory input. The SC in the monkey contains cells in its superficial layers that fire in response to visual stimulation and may play a role in localization of targets in space (628–632). The SC contains fixation, burst, and build-up cells. Monkeys can quickly learn to make accurate saccades into a hemifield made ''blind'' by ablation of area V1, but lose the ability to do so if their SC is then destroyed (590). The SC projects to pulvinar, which projects to area MT and to all other visual cortical regions (633) (Fig. 1.86). Isolated SC lesions in humans do not cause lasting visual deficits.

Neuronal responses to visual stimuli are typically enhanced by visual attention to the object. Effects of attention may be mediated partly by widespread influences on neuronal activity. For instance, activation of the frontal eye fields increases the gain of neuronal responses in area V4 (634). Activation of the occipital cortex results in distribution of visual information widely over temporal, parietal, and frontal lobes. Excitatory activity can spread from the occipital cortex to the frontal lobes in just over 20 msec (635).

Extensive interconnections exist among cortical areas and from cortical areas to deeper structures. In humans there are 25 neocortical areas that predominantly or exclusively subserve vision, and 7 other areas have some visual function (636). All corticocortical connections among visual areas appear to be reciprocal and are linked retinotopically (637).

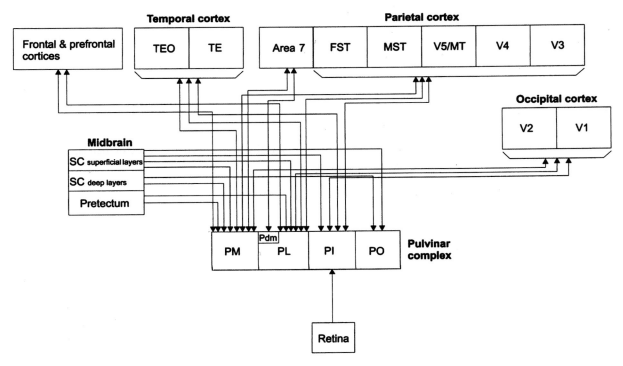

Figure 1.86.   Main efferent and afferent connections of the primate pulvinar. PM, medial pulvinar; PL, lateral pulvinar; PI, inferior pulvinar; PO, oral (i.e., anterior) pulvinar; SC, superior colliculus. (From Casanova C. The visual functions of the pulvinar. In: Chalupa LM, Werner JS, eds. The Visual Neurosciences. Cambridge, MA, MIT Press, 2004:594.)

Cortical feedback to deeper centers is essential for their proper function. In particular, cortical feedback must be established before the multisensory neurons of the SC can perform properly, which does not occur until some months after birth, at least in monkeys (627). The extensive cortical feedback from area V1 to the dLGN is topographically reciprocal (373) and can serve to optimize neuronal response and transmission properties of the dLGN (638).

REFERENCES

1. Mann I. Development of the Human Eye. New York, Grune & Stratton, 1964.
2. Ozanics VK, Jakobiec F. Prenatal development of the eye and its adnexa. In: Ocular Anatomy, Embryology, and Teratology. Philadelphia, Harper & Row, 1982:12–96.
3. Cohen A. The retina. In: Adler's Physiology of the Eye. St Louis, CV Mosby, 1992:579–615.
4. Hyer J, et al. Optic cup morphogenesis requires pre-lens ectoderm but not lens differentiation. Dev Biol Sci 2003;259:351–363.
5. Cook T. Cell diversity in the retina: more than meets the eye. Bioessays 2003;25:921–925.
6. Nornes HO, et al. Spatially and temporally restricted expression of Pax2 during murine neurogenesis. Development 1990;109:797–809.
7. Walther C, Gruss P. Pax-6, a murine paired box gene, is expressed in the developing CNS. Development 1991;113:1435–1449.
8. Duke-Elder S. Congenital deformities. In: System of Ophthalmology. Vol 3, Pt 2. St Louis, CV Mosby, 1963:661.
9. Reichenbach A, et al. Development of the rabbit retina. V. The question of 'columnar units.' Brain Res Dev Brain Res 1994;79:72–84.
10. Dyer MA, et al. Prox1 function controls progenitor cell proliferation and horizontal cell genesis in the mammalian retina. Nat Genet 2003;34:53–58.
11. Russell C. The roles of hedgehogs and fibroblast growth factors in eye development and retinal cell rescue. Vision Res 2003;43:899–912.
12. Masai I, et al. N-cadherin mediates retinal lamination, maintenance of forebrain compartments and patterning of retinal neurites. Development 2003;130:2479–2494.
13. Cusato K, et al. Cell death in the inner nuclear layer of the retina is modulated by BDNF. Brain Res Dev Brain Res 2002;139:325–330.
14. Marcus RC, et al. Eph family receptors and their ligands distribute in opposing gradients in the developing mouse retina. Dev Biol Sci 1996;180:786–789.
15. Menzel P, et al. Ephrin-A6, a new ligand for EphA receptors in the developing visual system. Dev Biol Sci 2001;230:74–88.
16. Yates PA, et al. Topographic-specific axon branching controlled by ephrin—as is the critical event in retinotectal map development. J Neurosci 2001;21:8548–8563.
17. Ernst AF, Jurney WM, McLoon SC. Mechanisms involved in development of retinotectal connections: roles of Eph receptor tyrosine kinases, NMDA receptors and nitric oxide. Prog Brain Res 1998;118:115–131.
18. Wu HH, et al. The role of nitric oxide in development of topographic precision in the retinotectal projection of chick. J Neurosci 2001;21:4318–4325.
19. Ruthazer ES, Akerman CJ, Cline HT. Control of axon branch dynamics by correlated activity in vivo. Science 2003;301:66–70.
20. Sernagor E, Young C, Eglen SJ. Developmental modulation of retinal wave dynamics: shedding light on the GABA saga. J Neurosci 2003;23:7621–7629.
21. Nucci C, et al. Apoptosis in the mechanisms of neuronal plasticity in the developing visual system. Eur J Ophthalmol 2003;13(Suppl 3):S36–43.
22. Perron M, et al. A novel function for Hedgehog signalling in retinal pigment epithelium differentiation. Development 2003;130:1565–1577.
23. Weiner A, et al. Hydroxychloroquine retinopathy. Am J Ophthalmol 1991;112:528–534.
24. Rando R, Bernstein P, Barry R. New insights into the visual cycle. In: Osborn N, Chader G, eds. Progress in Retinal Research. Oxford, Pergamon Press, 1991:161–178.
25. Saari JC. Biochemistry of visual pigment regeneration: the Friedenwald lecture. Invest Ophthalmol Vis Sci 2000;41:337–348.
26. Chader GJ. Interphotoreceptor retinoid-binding protein (IRBP): a model protein for molecular biological and clinically relevant studies. Friedenwald lecture. Invest Ophthalmol Vis Sci 1989;30:7–22.
27. Bridges C, et al. Transport, utilization, and metabolism of visual cycle retinoids in the retina and pigment epithelium. In: Osborn N, Chader G, eds. Progress in Retinal Research. Oxford, Pergamon Press, 1983:137–162.
28. Acland GM, et al. Gene therapy restores vision in a canine model of childhood blindness. Nat Genet 2001;28:92–95.
29. Cremers FP, van den Hurk JA, den Hollander AI. Molecular genetics of Leber congenital amaurosis. Hum Mol Genet 2002;11:1169–1176.
30. Gonzalez-Fernandez F. Evolution of the visual cycle: the role of retinoid-binding proteins. J Endocrinol 2002;175:75–88.
31. Kolb H, Linberg KA, Fisher SK. Neurons of the human retina: a Golgi study. J Comp Neurol 1992;318:147–187.
32. Vaney DI. Retinal neurons: cell types and coupled networks. Prog Brain Res 2002;136:239–254.
33. Masland RH. The fundamental plan of the retina. Nat Neurosci 2001;4:877–886.
34. Masland RH. Neuronal diversity in the retina. Curr Opin Neurobiol Sci 2001;11:431–436.
35. Stryer L. The molecules of visual excitation. Sci Am 1987;257:42–50.
36. Koenekoop RK. The gene for Stargardt disease, ABCA4, is a major retinal gene: a mini-review. Ophthalmol Genet 2003;24:75–80.
37. Baylor DA. Photoreceptor signals and vision. Proctor lecture. Invest Ophthalmol Vis Sci 1987;28:34–49.
38. Ohguro H, Nakazawa M. Pathological roles of recoverin cancer-associated retinopathy. Adv Exp Med Biol Sci 2002;514:109–124.
39. Shiraga S, Adamus G. Mechanism of CAR syndrome: anti-recoverin antibodies are the inducers of retinal cell apoptotic death via the caspase 9- and caspase 3-dependent pathway. J Neuroimmunol 2002;132(1–2):72–82.
40. Gabrieli CB, et al. Subjective visual halos after sildenafil (Viagra) administration: electroretinographic evaluation. Ophthalmology 2001;108:877–881.
41. McCulley TJ, et al. Acute effects of sildenafil (Viagra) on blue-on-yellow and white-on-white Humphrey perimetry. J Neuroophthalmol 2000;20:227–228.
42. Newman NJ, et al. Clinical and subclinical ophthalmic findings with retinol deficiency. Ophthalmology 1994;101:1077–1083.
43. Anastasi M, Lauricella M, Ponte F. Surgical therapy for obesity can induce a vitamin A deficiency syndrome. Doc Ophthalmol 1995;90:143–155.
44. Lesser RL, Brodie SE, Sugin SL. Mastocytosis-induced nyctalopia. J Neuroophthalmol 1996;16:115–119.
45. Thompson DA, Gal A. Vitamin A metabolism in the retinal pigment epithelium: genes, mutations, and diseases. Prog Retin Eye Res 2003;22:683–703.
46. Nathans J, Thomas D, Hogness DS. Molecular genetics of human color vision: the genes encoding blue, green, and red pigments. Science 1986;232:193–202.
47. Pallikaris A, Williams DR, Hofer H. The reflectance of single cones in the living human eye. Invest Ophthalmol Vis Sci 2003;44:4580–4592.
48. Jacobs GH. Photopigments and seeing: lessons from natural experiments: the Proctor lecture. Invest Ophthalmol Vis Sci 1998;39:2204–2216.
49. Dacey DM. Parallel pathways for spectral coding in primate retina. Annu Rev Neurosci 2000;23:743–775.
50. Curcio CA, et al. Human photoreceptor topography. J Comp Neurol 1990;292:497–523.
51. Panda-Jonas S, Jonas JB, Jakobczyk-Zmija M. Retinal photoreceptor density decreases with age. Ophthalmology 1995;102:1853–1859.
52. Curcio CA, et al. Aging of the human photoreceptor mosaic: evidence for selective vulnerability of rods in central retina. Invest Ophthalmol Vis Sci 1993;34:3278–3296.
53. Hendrickson AE, Yuodelis C. The morphological development of the human fovea. Ophthalmology 1984;91:603–612.
54. van Driel D, Provis JM, Billson FA. Early differentiation of ganglion, amacrine, bipolar, and Muller cells in the developing fovea of human retina. J Comp Neurol 1990;291:203–219.
55. Tenkova T, et al. Ethanol-induced apoptosis in the developing visual system during synaptogenesis. Invest Ophthalmol Vis Sci 2003;44:2809–2817.
56. Gunhan E, van der List D, Chalupa LM. Ectopic photoreceptors and cone bipolar cells in the developing and mature retina. J Neurosci 2003;23:1383–1389.
57. Wassle H, et al. The mosaic of horizontal cells in the macaque monkey retina: with a comment on biplexiform ganglion cells. Vis Neurosci 2000;17:591–608.
58. Mohn G, van Hof-van Duin J. Development of spacial vision. In: Dillon C, ed. Vision and Visual Development, Spacial Vision. Vol 10. London, Pergamon Press, 1991.
59. Curcio CA, Hendrickson A. Organization and development of the primate photoreceptor mosaic. In: Osborn N, Chader G, eds. Progress in Retinal Research. Oxford, Pergamon Press, 1991:89–120.
60. Pinckers A, Cruysberg J, Renier W. Delayed myelination of the optic nerve and pseudo optic atrophy of Beauvieux. Neuroophthalmology 1993;13:165–170.
61. Ueda H, Baba T, Ohno S. Current knowledge of dystrophin and dystrophin-associated proteins in the retina. Histol Histopathol 2000;15:753–760.
62. Connors NC, Kofuji P. Dystrophin Dp71 is critical for the clustered localization of potassium channels in retinal glial cells. J Neurosci 2002;22:4321–4327.
63. Dacheux RF, Raviola E. Physiology of HI horizontal cells in the primate retina. Proc R Soc Lond B Biol Sci 1990;239:213–230.
64. Goodchild AK, Chan TL, Grunert U. Horizontal cell connections with short-wavelength-sensitive cones in macaque monkey retina. Vis Neurosci 1996;13:833–845.
65. Kamermans M, et al. Hemichannel-mediated inhibition in the outer retina. Science 2001;292:1178–1180.
66. Dacheux RF, Raviola E. Horizontal cells in the retina of the rabbit. J Neurosci 1982;2:1486–1493.
67. Packer OS, Dacey DM. Receptive field structure of H1 horizontal cells in macaque monkey retina. J Vis 2002;2:272–292.
68. Polyak S. The retina. In: The Anatomy and the Histology of the Retina in Man, Ape, and Monkey, Including the Consideration of Visual Function, the History of Physiological Optics and the Histological Laboratory Technique. Chicago, University of Chicago Press, 1941.
69. Kolb H, Marshak D. The midget pathways of the primate retina. Doc Ophthalmol 2003;106:67–81.

70. Sterling P, et al. Microcircuitry and functional architecture of the cat retina. Trends Neurosci 1986;9:186–192.

71. Rodiek R. The primate retina. In: Steklis H, Erwin J, eds. Comparative Primate Biology. New York, AR Liss, 1988:203–278.

72. DeVries SH, Baylor DA. Synaptic circuitry of the retina and olfactory bulb. Cell 1993;72(Suppl):139–149.

73. Milam AH, et al. Autoantibodies against retinal bipolar cells in cutaneous melanoma-associated retinopathy. Invest Ophthalmol Vis Sci 1993;34:91–100.

74. Berson EL, Lessell S. Paraneoplastic night blindness with malignant melanoma. Am J Ophthalmol 1988;106:307–311.

75. Alexander KR, et al. 'On' response defect in paraneoplastic night blindness with cutaneous malignant melanoma. Invest Ophthalmol Vis Sci 1992;33:477–483.

76. Lei B, et al. Human melanoma-associated retinopathy (MAR) antibodies alter the retinal ON-response of the monkey ERG in vivo. Invest Ophthalmol Vis Sci 2000;41:262–266.

77. Jacobson DM, Adamus G. Retinal anti-bipolar cell antibodies in a patient with paraneoplastic retinopathy and colon carcinoma. Am J Ophthalmol 2001;131:806–808.

78. MacNeil MA, Masland RH. Extreme diversity among amacrine cells: implications for function. Neuron 1998;20:971–982.

79. Masland RH, Mills JW, Hayden SA. Acetylcholine-synthesizing amacrine cells: identification and selective staining by using radioautography and fluorescent markers. Proc R Soc Lond B Biol Sci 1984;223:79–100.

80. O'Malley DM, Sandell JH, Masland RH. Co-release of acetylcholine and GABA by the starburst amacrine cells. J Neurosci 1992;12:1394–1408.

81. Masland RH, Cassidy C. The resting release of acetylcholine by a retinal neuron. Proc R Soc Lond B Biol Sci 1987;232:227–238.

82. Yamada ES, et al. Synaptic connections of starburst amacrine cells and localization of acetylcholine receptors in primate retinas. J Comp Neurol 2003;461:76–90.

83. Kablar B. Determination of retinal cell fates is affected in the absence of extraocular striated muscles. Dev Dyn 2003;226:478–490.

84. Olveczky BP, Baccus SA, Meister M. Segregation of object and background motion in the retina. Nature 2003;423:401–408.

85. Roska B, Werblin F. Rapid global shifts in natural scenes block spiking in specific ganglion cell types. Nat Neurosci 2003;6:600–608.

86. Cheon EW, et al. Nitric oxide synthase expression in the transient ischemic rat retina: neuroprotection of betaxolol. Neurosci Lett 2002;330:265–269.

87. Lee EJ, et al. Neuronal nitric oxide synthase is expressed in the axotomized ganglion cells of the rat retina. Brain Res 2003;986(1–2):174–180.

88. Dacey DM. The dopaminergic amacrine cell. J Comp Neurol 1990;301:461–489.

89. Yamauchi T, et al. Inhibition of glutamate-induced nitric oxide synthase activation by dopamine in cultured rat retinal neurons. Neurosci Lett 2003;347:155–158.

90. Feigenspan A, et al. Spontaneous activity of solitary dopaminergic cells of the retina. J Neurosci 1998;18:6776–6789.

91. Raviola E. A molecular approach to retinal neural networks. Funct Neurol 2002;17:115–119.

92. Boycott BB, et al. Interplexiform cells of the mammalian retina and their comparison with catecholamine-containing retinal cells. Proc R Soc Lond B Biol Sci 1975;191:353–368.

93. Oyster CW, Takahashi ES. Interplexiform cells in rabbit retina. Proc R Soc Lond B Biol Sci 1977;197:477–484.

94. Hashimoto Y, Abe M, Inokuchi M. Identification of the interplexiform cell in the dace retina by dye-injection method. Brain Res 1980;197:331–340.

95. Hedden WL Jr, Dowling JE. The interplexiform cell system. II. Effects of dopamine on goldfish retinal neurones. Proc R Soc Lond B Biol Sci 1978;201:27–55.

96. Dowling JE, Ehinger B. The interplexiform cell system. I. Synapses of the dopaminergic neurons of the goldfish retina. Proc R Soc Lond B Biol Sci 1978;201:7–26.

97. Creel DJ, Wang JM, Wong KC. Transient blindness associated with transurethral resection of the prostate. Arch Ophthalmol 1987;105:1537–1539.

98. Barletta JP, Fanous MM, Hamed LM. Temporary blindness in the TUR syndrome. J Neuroophthalmol 1994;14:6–8.

99. Famiglietti EV, et al. Immunocytochemical localization of vascular endothelial growth factor in neurons and glial cells of human retina. Brain Res 2003;969(1–2):195–204.

100. Poitry S, et al. Mechanisms of glutamate metabolic signaling in retinal glial (Muller) cells. J Neurosci 2000;20:1809–1821.

101. Tsacopoulos M, et al. Trafficking of molecules and metabolic signals in the retina. Prog Retin Eye Res 1998;17:429–442.

102. Garcia M, Vecino E. Role of Muller glia in neuroprotection and regeneration in the retina. Histol Histopathol 2003;18:1205–1218.

103. Kawasaki A, Otori Y, Barnstable CJ. Muller cell protection of rat retinal ganglion cells from glutamate and nitric oxide neurotoxicity. Invest Ophthalmol Vis Sci 2000;41:3444–3454.

104. Sharma RK, Johnson DA. Molecular signals for development of neuronal circuitry in the retina. Neurochem Res 2000;25(9–10):1257–1263.

105. Winkler BS, et al. Energy metabolism in human retinal Muller cells. Invest Ophthalmol Vis Sci 2000;41:3183–3190.

106. de Jong P, et al. Mizuo phenomenon in X-linked retinoschisis: pathogenesis of the Mizuo phenomenon. Arch Ophthalmol 1991;109:1104–1108.

107. Hanitzsch R, Lichtenberger T. Two neuronal retinal components of the electroretinogram c-wave. Doc Ophthalmol 1997;94:275–285.

108. Peek R, et al. Muller cell-specific autoantibodies in a patient with progressive loss of vision. Invest Ophthalmol Vis Sci 1998;39:1976–1979.

109. Barres BA. A new role for glia: generation of neurons! Cell 1999;97:667–670.

110. Fischer AJ, Reh TA. Potential of Muller glia to become neurogenic retinal progenitor cells. Glia 2003;43:70–76.

111. Schnitzer J. Astrocytes in the guinea pig, horse, and monkey retina: their occurrence coincides with the presence of blood vessels. Glia 1988;1:74–89.

112. Ogden TE. Nerve fiber layer astrocytes of the primate retina: morphology, distribution, and density. Invest Ophthalmol Vis Sci 1978;17:499–510.

113. Zhang Y, et al. Tissue oxygen levels control astrocyte movement and differentiation in developing retina. Brain Res Dev Brain Res 1999;118(1–2):135–145.

114. Chu Y, Hughes S, Chan-Ling T. Differentiation and migration of astrocyte precursor cells and astrocytes in human fetal retina: relevance to optic nerve coloboma. FASEB J 2001;15:2013–2015.

115. Barres BA, Smith SJ. Neurobiology: cholesterol: making or breaking the synapse. Science 2001;294:1296–1297.

116. Ullian EM, et al. Control of synapse number by glia. Science 2001;291:657–661.

117. Ye ZC, et al. Functional hemichannels in astrocytes: a novel mechanism of glutamate release. J Neurosci 2003;23:3588–3596.

118. Fields R. The other half of the brain. Sci Am 2004;290:55–61.

119. Small RK, Riddle P, Noble M. Evidence for migration of oligodendrocyte–type-2 astrocyte progenitor cells into the developing rat optic nerve. Nature 1987;328:155–157.

120. Ali BH, et al. Progression of retinal nerve fiber myelination in childhood. Am J Ophthalmol 1994;118:515–517.

121. Butt AM, et al. Synantocytes: new functions for novel NG2 expressing glia. J Neurocytol 2002;31(6–7):551–565.

122. Chen L, Yang P, Kijlstra A. Distribution, markers, and functions of retinal microglia. Ocul Immunol Inflamm 2002;10:27–39.

123. Schnitzer J, Scherer J. Microglial cell responses in the rabbit retina following transection of the optic nerve. J Comp Neurol 1990;302:779–791.

124. Gupta N, Brown KE, Milam AH. Activated microglia in human retinitis pigmentosa, late-onset retinal degeneration, and age-related macular degeneration. Exp Eye Res 2003;76:463–471.

125. Neufeld AH. Microglia in the optic nerve head and the region of parapapillary chorioretinal atrophy in glaucoma. Arch Ophthalmol 1999;117:1050–1056.

126. Isenmann S, Kretz A, Cellerino A. Molecular determinants of retinal ganglion cell development, survival, and regeneration. Prog Retin Eye Res 2003;22:483–543.

127. Curcio CA, Allen KA. Topography of ganglion cells in human retina. J Comp Neurol 1990;300:5–25.

128. Provis JM, et al. Human fetal optic nerve: overproduction and elimination of retinal axons during development. J Comp Neurol 1985;238:92–100.

129. Sturrock RR. Changes in the number of axons in the human embryonic optic nerve from 8 to 18 weeks gestation. J Hirnforsch 1987;28:649–652.

130. Masland RH, Rizzo JF III, Sandell JH. Developmental variation in the structure of the retina. J Neurosci 1993;13:5194–5202.

131. Quigley HA, et al. Retrograde axonal transport of BDNF in retinal ganglion cells is blocked by acute IOP elevation in rats. Invest Ophthalmol Vis Sci 2000;41:3460–3466.

132. Pease ME, et al. Obstructed axonal transport of BDNF and its receptor TrkB in experimental glaucoma. Invest Ophthalmol Vis Sci 2000;41:764–774.

133. Rockhill RL, et al. The diversity of ganglion cells in a mammalian retina. J Neurosci 2002;22:3831–3843.

134. Dacey DM, et al. Fireworks in the primate retina: in vitro photodynamics reveals diverse LGN-projecting ganglion cell types. Neuron 2003;37:15–27.

135. Hendry SH, Yoshioka T. A neurochemically distinct third channel in the macaque dorsal lateral geniculate nucleus. Science 1994;264:575–577.

136. Boycott BB, Wassle H. The morphological types of ganglion cells of the domestic cat's retina. J Phys Sci 1974;240:397–419.

137. Stone J, Clarke R. Correlation between soma size and dendritic morphology in cat retinal ganglion cells: evidence of further variation in the y-cell class. J Comp Neurol 1980;192:211–217.

138. Sadun AA, et al. A retinohypothalamic pathway in man: light mediation of circadian rhythms. Brain Res 1984;302:371–377.

139. Moore RY, Speh JC, Card JP. The retinohypothalamic tract originates from a distinct subset of retinal ganglion cells. J Comp Neurol 1995;352:351–366.

140. Czeisler CA, et al. Suppression of melatonin secretion in some blind patients by exposure to bright light. N Engl J Med 1995;332:6–11.

141. Freedman MS, et al. Regulation of mammalian circadian behavior by non-rod, non-cone, ocular photoreceptors. Science 1999;284:502–504.

142. Gooley JJ, et al. Melanopsin cells of origin of the retinohypothalamic tract. Nat Neurosci 2001;4:1165.

143. Berson DM, Dunn FA, Takao M. Phototransduction by retinal ganglion cells that set the circadian clock. Science 2002;295:1070–1073.

144. Hattar S, et al. Melanopsin-containing retinal ganglion cells: architecture, projections, and intrinsic photosensitivity. Science 2002;295:1065–1070.

145. Morin LP, Blanchard JH, Provencio I. Retinal ganglion cell projections to the hamster suprachiasmatic nucleus, intergeniculate leaflet, and visual midbrain: bifurcation and melanopsin immunoreactivity. J Comp Neurol 2003;465:401–416.

146. Belenky MA, et al. Melanopsin retinal ganglion cells receive bipolar and amacrine cell synapses. J Comp Neurol 2003;460:380–393.
147. Gooley JJ, et àl. A broad role for melanopsin nonvisual photoreception. J Neurosci 2003;23:7093–7106.
148. Lucas RJ, et al. Diminished pupillary light reflex at high irradiances in melanopsin-knockout mice. Science 2003;299:245–247.
149. Benardete EA, Kaplan E. The receptive field of the primate P retinal ganglion cell, I: Linear dynamics. Vis Neurosci 1997;14:169–185.
150. Benardete EA, Kaplan E. The receptive field of the primate P retinal ganglion cell, II: Nonlinear dynamics. Vis Neurosci 1997;14:187–205.
151. Mangel SC, Miller RF. Horizontal cells contribute to the receptive field of ganglion cells in the rabbit retina. Brain Res 1987;414:182–186.
152. Wassle H, Boycott BB, Illing RB. Morphology and mosaic of on- and off-beta cells in the cat retina and some functional considerations. Proc R Soc Lond B Biol Sci 1981;212:177–195.
153. Tian N, Copenhagen DR. Visual stimulation is required for refinement of ON and OFF pathways in postnatal retina. Neuron 2003;39:85–96.
154. Zaghloul KA, Boahen K, Demb JB. Different circuits for ON and OFF retinal ganglion cells cause different contrast sensitivities. J Neurosci 2003;23:2645–2654.
155. Enroth-Cugell C, Robson JG. Functional characteristics and diversity of cat retinal ganglion cells. Basic characteristics and quantitative description. Invest Ophthalmol Vis Sci 1984;25:250–267.
156. Maguire G, Lukasiewicz P, Werblin F. Amacrine cell interactions underlying the response to change in the tiger salamander retina. J Neurosci 1989;9:726–735.
157. Perry VH, Cowey A. The morphological correlates of X- and Y-like retinal ganglion cells in the retina of monkeys. Exp Brain Res 1981;43:226–228.
158. Kolb H. Anatomical pathways for color vision in the human retina. Vis Neurosci 1991;7(1–2):61–74.
159. Schiller PH, Logothetis NK, Charles ER. Role of the color-opponent and broad-band channels in vision. Vis Neurosci 1990;5:321–346.
160. Schiller PH, Logothetis NK, Charles ER. Functions of the colour-opponent and broad-band channels of the visual system. Nature 1990;343:68–70.
161. Stanford LR. W-cells in the cat retina: correlated morphological and physiological evidence for two distinct classes. J Neurophysci 1987;57:218–244.
162. Stuermer CA, Bastmeyer M. The retinal axon's pathfinding to the optic disk. Prog Neurobiol Sci 2000;62:197–214.
163. Orioli D, Klein R. The Eph receptor family: axonal guidance by contact repulsion. Trends Genet 1997;13:354–359.
164. Stier H, Schlosshauer B. Axonal guidance in the chicken retina. Development 1995;121:1443–1454.
165. Deiner MS, et al. Netrin-1 and DCC mediate axon guidance locally at the optic disc: loss of function leads to optic nerve hypoplasia. Neuron 1997;19:575–589.
166. Sanyanusin P, et al. Mutation of the PAX2 gene in a family with optic nerve colobomas, renal anomalies and vesicoureteral reflux. Nat Genet 1995;9:358–364.
167. Willard M, Simon C. Modulations of neurofilament axonal transport during the development of rabbit retinal ganglion cells. Cell 1983;35(2 Pt 1):551–559.
168. Dandona L, Hendrickson A, Quigley HA. Selective effects of experimental glaucoma on axonal transport by retinal ganglion cells to the dorsal lateral geniculate nucleus. Invest Ophthalmol Vis Sci 1991;32:1593–1599.
169. Levy NS. The effect of interruption of the short posterior ciliary arteries on slow axoplasmic transport and histology within the optic nerve of the rhesus monkey. Invest Ophthalmol 1976;15:495–499.
170. McLeod D, Marshall J, Kohner EM. Role of axoplasmic transport in the pathophysiology of ischaemic disc swelling. Br J Ophthalmol 1980;64:247–261.
171. McKerracher L, et al. Selective impairment of slow axonal transport after optic nerve injury in adult rats. J Neurosci 1990;10:2834–2841.
172. Anderson DR, Hendrickson A. Effect of intraocular pressure on rapid axoplasmic transport in monkey optic nerve. Invest Ophthalmol 1974;13:771–783.
173. Minckler D, Tso M, Zimmerman L. A light microscopic, autoradiographic study of axoplasmic transport in the optic nerve head during ocular hypotony, increased intraocular pressure and papilledema. Am J Ophthalmol 1976;82:741–755.
174. Tso MO, Hayreh SS. Optic disc edema in raised intracranial pressure. IV. Axoplasmic transport in experimental papilledema. Arch Ophthalmol 1977;95:1458–1462.
175. Radius RL. Pressure-induced fast axonal transport abnormalities and the anatomy at the lamina cribrosa in primate eyes. Invest Ophthalmol Vis Sci 1983;24:343–346.
176. Rizzo JF III. Adenosine triphosphate deficiency: a genre of optic neuropathy. Neurology 1995;45:11–16.
177. So KF, Aguayo AJ. Lengthy regrowth of cut axons from ganglion cells after peripheral nerve transplantation into the retina of adult rats. Brain Res 1985;328:349–354.
178. Carter DA, Bray GM, Aguayo AJ. Regenerated retinal ganglion cell axons can form well-differentiated synapses in the superior colliculus of adult hamsters. J Neurosci 1989;9:4042–4050.
179. Maki H, et al. Axons of alpha ganglion cells regenerate faster than other types into a peripheral nerve graft in adult cats. J Neurosci Res 2003;72:218–226.
180. Rasband MN, et al. Dysregulation of axonal sodium channel isoforms after adult-onset chronic demyelination. J Neurosci Res 2003;73:465–470.
181. Craner MJ, et al. Abnormal sodium channel distribution in optic nerve axons in a model of inflammatory demyelination. Brain 2003;126(Pt 7):1552–1561.

182. Pickard GE. Bifurcating axons of retinal ganglion cells terminate in the hypothalamic suprachiasmatic nucleus and the intergeniculate leaflet of the thalamus. Neurosci Lett 1985;55:211–217.
183. Bullier J, Kennedy H. Axonal bifurcation in the visual system. Trends Neurosci 1987;10:205–210.
184. Wieniawa-Narkiewicz E, Hughes A. The superficial plexiform layer: a third retinal association area. J Comp Neurol 1992;324:463–484.
185. Honrubia FM, Elliott JH. Efferent innervation of the retina. I. Morphologic study of the human retina. Arch Ophthalmol 1968;80:98–103.
186. Honrubia FM, Elliott JH. Efferent innervation of the retina. II. Morphologic study of the monkey retina. Invest Ophthalmol 1970;9:971–976.
187. Radius RL. Thickness of the retinal nerve fiber layer in primate eyes. Arch Ophthalmol 1980;98:1625–1629.
188. Alamouti B, Funk J. Retinal thickness decreases with age: an OCT study. Br J Ophthalmol 2003;87:899–901.
189. Vrabec F. The temporal raphe of the human retina. Am J Ophthalmol 1966;62:926–938.
190. Stone J, Leicester J, Sherman SM. The naso-temporal division of the monkey's retina. J Comp Neurol 1973;150:333–348.
191. Stone J. The naso-temporal division of the cat's retina. J Comp Neurol 1966;126:585–600.
192. Bunt AH, Minckler DS. Foveal sparing. New anatomical evidence for bilateral representation of the central retina. Arch Ophthalmol 1977;95:1445–1447.
193. Bunt AH, Minckler DS. Displaced ganglion cells in the retina of the monkey. Invest Ophthalmol Vis Sci 1977;16:95–98.
194. Leventhal AG, Ault SJ, Vitek DJ. The nasotemporal division in primate retina: the neural bases of macular sparing and splitting. Science 1988;240:66–67.
195. Schein SJ. Anatomy of macaque fovea and spatial densities of neurons in foveal representation. J Comp Neurol 1988;269:479–505.
196. Younge BR. Midline tilting between seeing and nonseeing areas in hemianopia. Mayo Clin Proc 1976;51:562–568.
197. Minckler DS. The organization of nerve fiber bundles in the primate optic nerve head. Arch Ophthalmol 1980;98:1630–1636.
198. Ogden TE. Nerve fiber layer of the owl monkey retina: retinotopic organization. Invest Ophthalmol Vis Sci 1983;24:265–269.
199. Donatien P, Aigner B, Jeffery G. Variations in cell density in the ganglion cell layer of the retina as a function of ocular pigmentation. Eur J Neurosci 2002;15:1597–1602.
200. Alder VA, Cringle SJ. Vitreal and retinal oxygenation. Graefes Arch Clin Exp Ophthalmol 1990;228:151–157.
201. Snodderly DM, Weinhaus RS, Choi JC. Neural-vascular relationships in central retina of macaque monkeys (Macaca fascicularis). J Neurosci 1992;12:1169–1193.
202. Provis JM. Development of the primate retinal vasculature. Prog Retin Eye Res 2001;20:799–821.
203. Henkind P, Hanson R, Szalay J. Ocular circulation. In: Duane T, Jaeger E, eds. Biomedical Foundations of Ophthalmology. Vol 2. Philadelphia, Harper & Row, 1985:17.
204. Holash JA, Stewart PA. The relationship of astrocyte-like cells to the vessels that contribute to the blood-ocular barriers. Brain Res 1993;629:218–224.
205. Brown SM, Jampol LM. New concepts of regulation of retinal vessel tone. Arch Ophthalmol 1996;114:199–204.
206. Adams DL, Horton JC. Capricious expression of cortical columns in the primate brain. Nat Neurosci 2003;6:113–114.
207. O'Rahilly R. The prenatal development of the human eye. Exp Eye Res 1975;21:93–112.
208. Rhodes RH. Development of the optic nerve. In: Jakobiec FA, ed. Ocular Anatomy, Embryology, and Teratology. Philadelphia, Harper & Row, 1982:601–638.
209. Dakubo GD, et al. Retinal ganglion cell-derived sonic hedgehog signaling is required for optic disc and stalk neuroepithelial cell development. Development 2003;130:2967–2980.
210. Tsai HH, Miller RH. Glial cell migration directed by axon guidance cues. Trends Neurosci 2002;25:173–176.
211. Sugimoto Y, et al. Guidance of glial precursor cell migration by secreted cues in the developing optic nerve. Development 2001;128:3321–3330.
212. Noble M, et al. Redox state as a central modulator of precursor cell function. Ann NY Acad Sci 2003;991:251–271.
213. Straatsma BR, et al. Myelinated retinal nerve fibers. Am J Ophthalmol 1981;91:25–38.
214. Kiernan BW, et al. Tenascin-C inhibits oligodendrocyte precursor cell migration by both adhesion-dependent and adhesion-independent mechanisms. Mol Cell Neurosci 1996;7:322–335.
215. Menichella DM, et al. Connexins are critical for normal myelination in the CNS. J Neurosci 2003;23:5963–5973.
216. Quigley HA. Gap junctions between optic nerve head astrocytes. Invest Ophthalmol Vis Sci 1977;16:582–585.
217. Butt AM, Ransom BR. Visualization of oligodendrocytes and astrocytes in the intact rat optic nerve by intracellular injection of lucifer yellow and horseradish peroxidase. Glia 1989;2:470–475.
218. Yakovlev P, Lecours AR. The myelogenetic cycles of regional maturation of the brain. In: Minkowski A, ed. Regional Development of the Brain in Early Life. Oxford, Blackwell, 1967:3–70.
219. Brody BA, et al. Sequence of central nervous system myelination in human

infancy. I. An autopsy study of myelination. J Neuropathol Exp Neurol 1987; 46:283–301.

220. Ogden TE, Miller RF. Studies of the optic nerve of the rhesus monkey: nerve fiber spectrum and physiological properties. Vision Res 1966;6:485–506.

221. Sylvester PE, Ari K. The size and growth of the human optic nerve. J Neurol Neurosurg Psychiatry 1961;24:45–49.

222. Takayama S, et al. Immunohistochemical study on the developing optic nerves in human embryos and fetuses. Brain Dev 1991;13:307–312.

223. Rimmer S, et al. Growth of the human optic disk and nerve during gestation, childhood, and early adulthood. Am J Ophthalmol 1993;116:748–753.

224. Cavallotti C, et al. Age-related changes in the human optic nerve. Can J Ophthalmol 2002;37:389–394.

225 Anderson DR. Ultrastructure of human and monkey lamina cribrosa and optic nerve head. Arch Ophthalmol 1969;82:800–814.

226. Jonas JB, et al. Morphometry of the human lamina cribrosa surface. Invest Ophthalmol Vis Sci 1991;32:401–405.

227. Minckler DS, McLean IW, Tso MO. Distribution of axonal and glial elements in the rhesus optic nerve head studied by electron microscopy. Am J Ophthalmol 1976;82:179–187.

228. Morgan WH, et al. The influence of cerebrospinal fluid pressure on the lamina cribrosa tissue pressure gradient. Invest Ophthalmol Vis Sci 1995;36:1163–1172.

229. Lambert W, et al. Neurotrophin and neurotrophin receptor expression by cells of the human lamina cribrosa. Invest Ophthalmol Vis Sci 2001;42:2315–2323.

230. Wordinger RJ, et al. Cells of the human optic nerve head express glial cell line-derived neurotrophic factor (GDNF) and the GDNF receptor complex. Mol Vis 2003;9:249–256.

231. Quigley HA, Addicks EM. Regional differences in the structure of the lamina cribrosa and their relation to glaucomatous optic nerve damage. Arch Ophthalmol 1981;99:137–143.

232. Hollander H, et al. Evidence of constriction of optic nerve axons at the lamina cribrosa in the normotensive eye in humans and other mammals. Ophthalmic Res 1995;27:296–309.

233. Nickells RW. Retinal ganglion cell death in glaucoma: the how, the why, and the maybe. J Glaucoma 1996;5:345–356.

234. Hernandez MR, Ye H. Glaucoma: changes in extracellular matrix in the optic nerve head. Ann Med 1993;25:309–315.

235. Tezel G, Trinkaus K, Wax MB. Alterations in the morphology of lamina cribrosa pores in glaucomatous eyes. Br J Ophthalmol 2004;88:251–256.

236. Neufeld AH, Liu B. Glaucomatous optic neuropathy: when glia misbehave. Neuroscientist 2003;9:485–495.

237. Liu D, Michon J. Measurement of the subarachnoid pressure of the optic nerve in human subjects. Am J Ophthalmol 1995;119:81–85.

238. Morgan WH, et al. Optic disc movement with variations in intraocular and cerebrospinal fluid pressure. Invest Ophthalmol Vis Sci 2002;43:3236–3242.

239. Hayreh SS. Fluids in the anterior part of the optic nerve in health and disease. Surv Ophthalmol 1978;23:1–25.

240. Tso MO, Shih CY, McLean IW. Is there a blood-brain barrier at the optic nerve head? Arch Ophthalmol 1975;93:815–825.

241. Robin AL, et al. An analysis of visual acuity, visual fields, and disk cupping in childhood glaucoma. Am J Ophthalmol 1979;88:847–858.

242. Doro S, Lessell S. Cup-disc ratio and ischemic optic neuropathy. Arch Ophthalmol 1985;103:1143–1144.

243. Beck RW, Servais GE, Hayreh SS. Anterior ischemic optic neuropathy. IX. Cup-to-disc ratio and its role in pathogenesis. Ophthalmology 1987;94:1503–1508.

244. Burde RM. Optic disk risk factors for nonarteritic anterior ischemic optic neuropathy. Am J Ophthalmol 1993;116:759–764.

245. Quigley HA, Coleman AL, Dorman-Pease ME. Larger optic nerve heads have more nerve fibers in normal monkey eyes. Arch Ophthalmol 1991;109:1441–1443.

246. Jonas JB, et al. Human optic nerve fiber count and optic disc size. Invest Ophthalmol Vis Sci 1992;33:2012–2018.

247. Panda-Jonas S, et al. Retinal photoreceptor count, retinal surface area, and optic disc size in normal human eyes. Ophthalmology 1994;101:519–523.

248. Brazitikos PD, et al. Threshold perimetry in tilted disc syndrome. Arch Ophthalmol 1990;108:1698–1700.

249. Unsold R, DeGroot J, Newton TH. Images of the optic nerve: anatomic-CT correlation. AJR Am J Roentgenol 1980;135:767–773.

250. Maniscalco JE, Habal MB. Microanatomy of the optic canal. J Neurosurg 1978;48:402–406.

251. Slavin K, et al. Optic canal: microanatomic study. Skull Base Surg 1994;4:136–144.

252. Chou PI, Sadun AA, Lee H. Vasculature and morphometry of the optic canal and intracanalicular optic nerve. J Neuroophthalmol 1995;15:186–190.

253. Le Double A. Traite des Variations des Os du Crane le l'Homme. Paris, Vigot Freres, 1908:400.

254. Kommerell L, Wallow IH. Physiological variations in X-ray appearance of the optic foramen. Mod Probl Ophthalmol 1975;14:103–109.

255. Renn WH, Rhoton AL Jr. Microsurgical anatomy of the sellar region. J Neurosurg 1975;43:288–298.

256. Dessi P, et al. Protrusion of the optic nerve into the ethmoid and sphenoid sinus: prospective study of 150 CT studies. Neuroradiology 1994;36:515–516.

257. Spoor T, Kennerdell J, Maroon J. Pneumosinus dilatans, Klippel-Trenauay Weber syndrome, and progressive visual loss. Ann Ophthalmol 1981;13:105–108.

258. Hirst LW, Miller NR, Allen GS. Sphenoidal pneumosinus dilatans with bilateral optic nerve meningiomas. Case report. J Neurosurg 1979;51:402–407.

259. Hirst LW, et al. Sphenoid pneumosinus dilatans. A sign of meningioma originating in the optic canal. Neuroradiology 1982;22:207–210.

260. Miller NR, et al. Pneumosinus dilatans: a sign of intracranial meningioma. Surg Neurol 1996;46:471–474.

261. Zhaboedov GD, Skripnikov NS. [Clinical importance of the topographic anatomical interrelationships of the optic nerve canal and paranasal sinuses]. Vestn Oftalmol 1979:60–63.

262. Whitnall S, ed. An Anatomy of the Human Orbit and Accessory Organs of Vision. 2nd ed. London, Oxford University Press, 1932.

263. Perlmutter D, Rhoton AL Jr. Microsurgical anatomy of the anterior cerebral-anterior communicating-recurrent artery complex. J Neurosurg 1976;45:259–272.

264. Rhoton AL, Jr, Harris FS, Renn WH. Microsurgical anatomy of the sellar region and cavernous sinus. In: Smith J, ed. Neuro-Ophthalmology. Vol 9. St Louis, CV Mosby, 1977:54–85.

265. Gibo H, Lenkey C, Rhoton AL Jr. Microsurgical anatomy of the supraclinoid portion of the internal carotid artery. J Neurosurg 1981;55:560–574.

266. Rhoton AL Jr. Microsurgical anatomy. In: Landolt A, Vance M, Reilly P, eds. Pituitary Adenomas. New York, Churchill Livingstone, 1996:241–282.

267. Hayreh SS, Dass R. The ophthalmic artery: I. Origin and intra-cranial and intra-canalicular course. Br J Ophthalmol 1962;46:65–98.

268. Hayreh SS. Inter-individual variation in blood supply of the optic nerve head. Its importance in various ischemic disorders of the optic nerve head, and glaucoma, low-tension glaucoma and allied disorders. Doc Ophthalmol 1985;59:217–246.

269. Hayreh SS. Arteries of the orbit in the human being. Br J Surg 1962;50:938–953.

270. Hayreh SS. The ophthalmic artery. Br J Ophthalmol 1962;46:212–247.

271. Hayreh SS, Dass R. The ophthalmic artery: II. Intra-orbital course. Br J Ophthalmol 1962;46:165–185.

272. Lieberman MF, Maumenee AE, Green WR. Histologic studies of the vasculature of the anterior optic nerve. Am J Ophthalmol 1976;82:405–423.

273. Zhao Y, Li FM. Microangioarchitecture of optic papilla. Jpn J Ophthalmol 1987;31:147–159.

274. Olver JM, Spalton DJ, McCartney AC. Microvascular study of the retrolaminar optic nerve in man: the possible significance in anterior ischaemic optic neuropathy. Eye 1990;4(Pt 1):7–24.

275. Cioffi GA, van Buskirk EM. Microvascular study of the anterior optic nerve. Surv Ophthalmol 1994:107–117.

276. Onda E, et al. Microvasculature of the human optic nerve. Am J Ophthalmol 1995;120:92–102.

277. Hayreh SS. Anatomy and physiology of the optic nerve head. Trans Am Acad Ophthalmol Otolaryngol 1974;78:240–254.

278. Risco JM, Grimson BS, Johnson PT. Angioarchitecture of the ciliary artery circulation of the posterior pole. Arch Ophthalmol 1981;99:864–868.

279. Hayreh SS. Blood supply of the optic nerve head. Ophthalmologica 1996;210:285–295.

280. Komai K, et al. Vasomotor nerves of vessels in the human optic nerve. Acta Ophthalmol Scand 1995;73:512–516.

281. Olver JM, Spalton DJ, McCartney AC. Quantitative morphology of human retro-laminar optic nerve vasculature. Invest Ophthalmol Vis Sci 1994;35:3858–3866.

282. Ettl A, et al. High-resolution magnetic resonance imaging of neurovascular orbital anatomy. Presented at the 14th meeting of the European Society of Ophthalmic Plastic and Reconstructive Surgery, Utrecht, The Netherlands, 1996.

283. van Overbeeke J, Sekhar L. Microanatomy of the blood supply to the optic nerve. Orbit 2003;22:81–88.

284. Krisht AF, et al. The microsurgical anatomy of the superior hypophyseal artery. Neurosurgery 1994;35:899–903.

285. Hofman P, et al. Lack of blood-brain barrier properties in microvessels of the prelaminar optic nerve head. Invest Ophthalmol Vis Sci 2001;42:895–901.

286. Levin LA, Albert DM, Johnson D. Mast cells in human optic nerve. Invest Ophthalmol Vis Sci 1993;34:3147–3153.

287. Shanthaveerappa TR, Bourne GH. Arachnoid villi in the optic nerve of man and monkey. Exp Eye Res 1964;10:31–35.

288. Killer HE, et al. Architecture of arachnoid trabeculae, pillars, and septa in the subarachnoid space of the human optic nerve: anatomy and clinical considerations. Br J Ophthalmol 2003;87:777–781.

289. Ou B, Ohno S, Tsukahara S. Ultrastructural changes and immunocytochemical localization of microtubule-associated protein 1 in guinea pig optic nerves after acute increase in intraocular pressure. Invest Ophthalmol Vis Sci 1998;39:963–971.

290. Bristow EA, et al. The distribution of mitochondrial activity in relation to optic nerve structure. Arch Ophthalmol 2002;120:791–796.

291. Baba H, et al. Completion of myelin compaction, but not the attachment of oligodendroglial processes triggers K(+) channel clustering. J Neurosci Res 1999;58:752–764.

292. Sadun AA. Discussion of the effect of age on normal human optic nerve fiber number and diameter. Ophthalmology 1989;96:31–32.

293. Kupfer C, Chumbley L, Downer JC. Quantitative histology of optic nerve, optic tract and lateral geniculate nucleus of man. J Anat 1967;101:393–401.

294. Potts AM, et al. Morphology of the primate optic nerve. I. Method and total fiber count. Invest Ophthalmol 1972;11:980–988.

295. Balazsi AG, et al. The effect of age on the nerve fiber population of the human optic nerve. Am J Ophthalmol 1984;97:760–766.

296. Johnson B, Miao M, Sadun AA. Age-related decline of human optic nerve axon populations. Age 1987;10:5–9.

297. Mikelberg FS, et al. The normal human optic nerve. Axon count and axon diameter distribution. Ophthalmology 1989;96:1325–1328.

298. Cowan W. Centrifugal fibres to the avian retina. Br Med Bull 1970:112–118.

299. Sacks JG, Lindenberg R. Efferent nerve fibers in the anterior visual pathways in bilateral congenital cystic eyeballs. Am J Ophthalmol 1969;68:691–695.

300. Reperant J, Gallego A. [Centrifugal fibers in the human retina]. Arch Anat Microsc Morphol Exp 1976;65:103–120.

301. Wolter JR. Centrifugal nerve fibers in the adult human optic nerve: 16 days after enucleation. Trans Am Ophthalmol Soc 1978;76:140–155.

302. Schutte M. Centrifugal innervation of the rat retina. Vis Neurosci 1995;12:1083–1092.

303. Hoyt WF, Tudor RC. The course of parapapillary temporal retinal axons through the anterior optic nerve. A Nauta degeneration study in the primate. Arch Ophthalmol 1963;69:503–507.

304. Hoyt WF. Anatomic considerations of arcuate scotomas associated with lesions of the optic nerve and chiasm. A nauta axon degeneration study in the monkey. Bull Johns Hopkins Hosp 1962;111:57–71.

305. Hoyt WF, Luis O. Visual fiber anatomy in the infrageniculate pathway of the primate. Arch Ophthalmol 1962;68:94–106.

306. Marcus RC, et al. Retinal axon divergence in the optic chiasm: uncrossed axons diverge from crossed axons within a midline glial specialization. J Neurosci 1995;15(5 Pt 2):3716–3729.

307. Hoyt WF, Luis O. The primate optic chiasm: details of visual fiber organization studied by silver impregnation techniques. Arch Ophthalmol 1963;70:69–85.

308. Wilbrand H. Schema des Verlaufs der Sehnervenfasern durch das Chiasma. Z Aufenheilkd 1926;59:135–144.

309. Breen LA, Quaglieri FC, Schochet SS Jr. Neuro-anatomical feature photo. Optic nerve. J Clin Neuroophthalmol 1983;3:283–284.

310. Horton JC. Wilbrand's knee of the primate optic chiasm is an artefact of monocular enucleation. Trans Am Ophthalmol Soc 1997;95:579–609.

311. Oster SF, Sretavan DW. Connecting the eye to the brain: the molecular basis of ganglion cell axon guidance. Br J Ophthalmol 2003;87:639–645.

312. Jeffery G. Architecture of the optic chiasm and the mechanisms that sculpt its development. Physiol Rev 2001;81:1393–1414.

313. Marcus RC, Mason CA. The first retinal axon growth in the mouse optic chiasm: axon patterning and the cellular environment. J Neurosci 1995;15:6389–6402.

314. Guillery R, Mason CA, Taylor J. Developmental determinants at the mammalian optic chiasm. J Neurosci 1995;15:4727–4737.

315. Stoeckli ET, Landmesser LT. Axon guidance at choice points. Curr Opin Neurobiol Sci 1998;8:73–79.

316. Sretavan DW, et al. Disruption of retinal axon ingrowth by ablation of embryonic mouse optic chiasm neurons. Science 1995;269:98–101.

317. Plump AS, et al. Slit1 and Slit2 cooperate to prevent premature midline crossing of retinal axons in the mouse visual system. Neuron 2002;33:219–232.

318. Rasband K, Hardy M, Chien CB. Generating X: formation of the optic chiasm. Neuron 2003;39:885–888.

319. Torres M, Gomez-Pardo E, Gruss P. Pax2 contributes to inner ear patterning and optic nerve trajectory. Development 1996;122:3381–3391.

320. Webber CA, et al. Metalloproteases and guidance of retinal axons in the developing visual system. J Neurosci 2002;22:8091–8100.

321. Colello RJ, Guillery RW. Observations on the early development of the optic nerve and tract of the mouse. J Comp Neurol 1992;317:357–378.

322. Meissirel C, Chalupa LM. Organization of pioneer retinal axons within the optic tract of the rhesus monkey. Proc Natl Acad Sci USA 1994;91:3906–3910.

323. Bovolenta P, Mason C. Growth cone morphology varies with position in the developing mouse visual pathway from retina to first targets. J Neurosci 1987;7:1447–1460.

324. Godement P, Wang LC, Mason CA. Retinal axon divergence in the optic chiasm: dynamics of growth cone behavior at the midline. J Neurosci 1994;14(11 Pt 2):7024–7039.

325. Apkarian P, et al. Non-decussating retinal-fugal fibre syndrome. An inborn achiasmatic malformation associated with visuotopic misrouting, visual evoked potential ipsilateral asymmetry and nystagmus. Brain 1995;118(Pt 5):1195–1216.

326. Korff CM, et al. Isolated absence of optic chiasm revealed by congenital nystagmus, MRI and VEPs. Neuropediatrics 2003;34:219–223.

327. Herrera E, et al. Zic2 patterns binocular vision by specifying the uncrossed retinal projection. Cell 2003;114:545–557.

328. Schmitz B, et al. Configuration of the optic chiasm in humans with albinism as revealed by magnetic resonance imaging. Invest Ophthalmol Vis Sci 2003;44:16–21.

329. Hoyt WF. Correlative functional anatomy of the optic chiasm. Clinical Neurosurg 1969;17:189–208.

330. Schaeffer JP. Some points in the regional anatomy of the optic pathway, with special reference to tumors of the hypophysis cerebri; and resulting ocular changes. Anat Rec 1924;28:243–279.

331. Dubois-Poulsen A. Le Champ Visuel: Topographie Normale et Pathologique de ses Sensibilities. Paris, 1952.

332. Walker A. The neurosurgical evaluation of the chiasmal syndromes. Am J Ophthalmol 1962;54:563–581.

333. Traquair H. The antomical relations of the hypophysis and the chiasma. Ophthalmoscope 1916;14:562–563.

334. Cope V. The pituitary fossa and the methods of surgical approach thereto. Br J Surg 1916–1917;4:107–144.

335. de Schweinitz G. Concerning certain ocular aspects of the pituitary body disorders, mainly, exclusive of the usual central and peripheral hemianopic field defects. The Bowman Lecture Trans Ophthalmol Soc U K 1923;43:12–109.

336. Lindgren E. Radiologic examination of the brain and spinal cord. Acta Rad Sci 1957;16(Suppl 151):1–147.

337. Wassle H, Illing RB. The retinal projection to the superior colliculus in the cat: a quantitative study with HRP. J Comp Neurol 1980;190:333–356.

338. Polyak S. Projection of the retina upon the cerebral cortex, based upon experiments with monkeys. In: Proceedings of the Association for Research in Nervous and Mental Diseases. Baltimore, Williams & Wilkins, 1934:535–557.

339. Bergland R, Ray BS. The arterial supply of the human optic chiasm. J Neurosurg 1969;31:327–334.

340. Perlmutter D, Rhoton AL Jr. Microsurgical anatomy of the distal anterior cerebral artery. J Neurosurg 1978;49:204–228.

341. Wollschlaeger PB, et al. Arterial blood supply of the human optic chiasm and surrounding structures. Ann Ophthalmol 1971;3:862–864.

342. Torrealba F, et al. Studies of retinal representations within the cat's optic tract. J Comp Neurol 1982;211:377–396.

343. Reese BE, Cowey A. Fibre organization of the monkey's optic tract: I. Segregation of functionally distinct optic axons. J Comp Neurol 1990;295:385–400.

344. Reese BE. The distribution of axons according to diameter in the optic nerve and optic tract of the rat. Neuroscience 1987;22:1015–1024.

345. Carpenter MB, Noback CR, Moss ML. The anterior choroidal artery; its origins, course, distribution, and variations. AMA Arch Neurol Psychiatry 1954;71:714–722.

346. Fujii K, Lenkey C, Rhoton AL Jr. Microsurgical anatomy of the choroidal arteries: lateral and third ventricles. J Neurosurg 1980;52:165–188.

347. Walsh FB, Smith GW. The ocular complications of carotid angiography; the ocular signs of thrombosis of the internal carotid artery. J Neurosurg 1952;9:517–537.

348. O'Rahilly R, et al. Computer ranking of the sequence of appearance of 100 features of the brain and related structures in staged human embryos during the first 5 weeks of development. Am J Anat 1984;171:243–257.

349. O'Rahilly R, et al. Computer ranking of the sequence of appearance of 73 features of the brain and related structures in staged human embryos during the sixth week of development. Am J Anat 1987;180:69–86.

350. O'Rahilly R, et al. Computer ranking of the sequence of appearance of 40 features of the brain and related structures in staged human embryos during the seventh week of development. Am J Anat 1988;182:295–317.

351. Muller F, O'Rahilly R. The human brain at stages 21–23, with particular reference to the cerebral cortical plate and to the development of the cerebellum. Anat Embryol (Berl) 1990;182:375–400.

352. Hickey TL, Guillery RW. Variability of laminar patterns in the human lateral geniculate nucleus. J Comp Neurol 1979;183:221–246.

353. Connolly M, van Essen D. The representation of the visual field in parvocellular and magnocellular layers of the lateral geniculate nucleus in the macaque monkey. J Comp Neurol 1984;226:544–564.

354. Van Essen DC, Newsome WT, Maunsell JH. The visual field representation in striate cortex of the macaque monkey: asymmetries, anisotropies, and individual variability. Vision Res 1984;24:429–448.

355. Horton JC, et al. Arrangement of ocular dominance columns in human visual cortex. Arch Ophthalmol 1990;108:1025–1031.

356. Sernagor E, Grzywacz NM. Influence of spontaneous activity and visual experience on developing retinal receptive fields. Curr Biol Sci 1996;6:1503–1508.

357. Williams AL, Jeffery G. Growth dynamics of the developing lateral geniculate nucleus. J Comp Neurol 2001;430:332–342.

358. Stellwagen D, Shatz CJ. An instructive role for retinal waves in the development of retinogeniculate connectivity. Neuron 2002;33:357–367.

359. Feller MB, et al. Requirement for cholinergic synaptic transmission in the propagation of spontaneous retinal waves. Science 1996;272:1182–1187.

360. Wong RO, Meister M, Shatz CJ. Transient period of correlated bursting activity during development of the mammalian retina. Neuron 1993;11:923–938.

361. Simon DK, et al. N-methyl-D-aspartate receptor antagonists disrupt the formation of a mammalian neural map. Proc Natl Acad Sci USA 1992;89:10593–10597.

362. Huberman AD, et al. Eye-specific retinogeniculate segregation independent of normal neuronal activity. Science 2003;300:994–998.

363. von Noorden G, Middleditch P. Histological observations in the normal monkey lateral geniculate nucleus. Invest Ophthalmol Vis Sci 1975;14:55–58.

364. Leamey CA, Ho-Pao CL, Sur M. Role of calcineurIn activity-dependent pattern formation in the dorsal lateral geniculate nucleus of the ferret. J Neurobiol Sci 2003;56:153–162.

365. Myhr KL, Lukasiewicz PD, Wong RO. Mechanisms underlying developmental changes in the firing patterns of ON and OFF retinal ganglion cells during refinement of their central projections. J Neurosci 2001;21:8664–8671.

366. Livingston CA, Mustari MJ. The anatomical organization of the macaque pregeniculate complex. Brain Res 2000;876(1–2):166–179.

367. Buttner U, Fuchs AF. Influence of saccadic eye movements on unit activity in simian lateral geniculate and pregeniculate nuclei. J Neurophys Sci 1973;36: 127–141.

368. Burr DC, Morrone MC, Ross J. Selective suppression of the magnocellular visual pathway during saccadic eye movements. Nature 1994;371:511–513.

369. Reppas JB, Usrey WM, Reid RC. Saccadic eye movements modulate visual responses in the lateral geniculate nucleus. Neuron 2002;35:961–974.

370. Harrington ME. The ventral lateral geniculate nucleus and the intergeniculate leaflet: interrelated structures in the visual and circadian systems. Neurosci Biobehav Rev 1997;21:705–727.

371. Brouwer B, Zeeman W. The projection of the retina in the primary optic neuron in monkeys. Brain 1926;49:1–35.

372. Kupper C. The projection of the macula in the lateral geniculate nucleus of man. Am J Ophthalmol 1962;54:597–609.

373. Ichida JM, Casagrande VA. Organization of the feedback pathway from striate cortex (V1) to the lateral geniculate nucleus (LGN) in the owl monkey (*Aotus trivirgatus*). J Comp Neurol 2002;454:272–283.

374. Lund JS, et al. The origin of efferent pathways from the primary visual cortex, area 17, of the macaque monkey as shown by retrograde transport of horseradish peroxidase. J Comp Neurol 1975;164:287–303.

375. Harting J, Casagrande VA, Weber J. The projection of the primary superior colliculus upon the lateral geniculate nucleus: autoradiographic demonstration of interlaminar distribution of tectogeniculate axons. Brain Res 1978;150:93–199.

376. Hughes HC, Mullikin WH. Brainstem afferents to the lateral geniculate nucleus of the cat. Exp Brain Res 1984;54:253–258.

377. Hubel DH, Wiesel TN. Laminar and columnar distribution of geniculo-cortical fibers in the macaque monkey. J Comp Neurol 1972;146:421–450.

378. Lund JS. Organization of neurons in the visual cortex, area 17, of the monkey (*Macaca mulatta*). J Comp Neurol 1973;147:455–496.

379. Hubel DH, Wiesel TN, Ferrier lecture. Functional architecture of macaque monkey visual cortex. Proc R Soc Lond B Biol Sci 1977;198:1–59.

380. Nealey T, Maunsell J. Magnocellular and parvocellular contributions to the responses of neurons in macaque striate cortex. J Neurosci 1994;5:2069–2079.

381. Diamond I, et al. Laminar organization of geniculocortical projections on *Galago senegalensis* and *Autus trivirgatus*. J Comp Neurol 1985;242:584–610.

382. Celesia GG, DeMarco PJ Jr. Anatomy and physiology of the visual system. J Clin Neurophys Sci 1994;11:482–492.

383. Hubel DH, Wiesel TN. Integrative action in the cat's lateral geniculate body. J Phys Sci 1961;155:385–398.

384. Shou T, Leventhal AG. Orientation sensitivity in the cat's lateral geniculate nucleus (LGN). Soc Neurosci Abst 1988;14:309.

385. Smith EL III, et al. Orientation bias of neurons in the lateral geniculate nucleus of macaque monkeys. Vis Neurosci 1990;5:525–545.

386. Singer W. Control of thalamic transmission by corticofugal and ascending reticular pathways in the visual system. Physiol Rev 1977;57:386–420.

387. Eysel UT, Pape HC, Van Schayck R. Excitatory and differential disinhibitory actions of acetylcholine in the lateral geniculate nucleus of the cat. J Phys Sci 1986;370:233–254.

388. Murphy PC, Duckett SG, Sillito AM. Feedback connections to the lateral geniculate nucleus and cortical response properties. Science 1999;286:1552–1554.

389. Worgotter F, et al. The influence of corticofugal feedback on the temporal structure of visual responses of cat thalamic relay cells. J Phys Sci 1998;509(Pt 3): 797–815.

390. Webb BS, et al. Feedback from V1 and inhibition from beyond the classical receptive field modulates the responses of neurons in the primate lateral geniculate nucleus. Vis Neurosci 2002;19:583–592.

391. Kaplan E, Purpura K, Shapley R. Contrast affects the transmission of visual information through the mammalian lateral geniculate nucleus. J Physiol (London) 1987;391:267–288.

392. Xu X, et al. Are primate lateral geniculate nucleus (LGN) cells really sensitive to orientation or direction? Vis Neurosci 2002;19:97–108.

393. Lal R, Friedlander MJ. Gating of retinal transmission by afferent eye position and movement signals. Science 1989;243:93–96.

394. Bartlett JR, et al. Mesencephalic control of lateral geniculate nucleus in primates. 3. Modifications with state of alertness. Exp Brain Res 1973;18:214–224.

395. Liu S, Wong-Riley M. Quantitative light- and electron-microscopic analysis of cytochrome-oxidase distribution in neurons of the lateral geniculate nucleus of the adult monkey. Vis Neurosci 1990;4:269–287.

396. Levick WR, Cleland BG, Dubin MW. Lateral geniculate neurons of cat: retinal inputs and physiology. Invest Ophthalmol 1972;11:302–311.

397. Usrey WM, Reppas JB, Reid RC. Specificity and strength of retinogeniculate connections. J Neurophys Sci 1999;82:3527–3540.

398. Alonso JM, Usrey WM, Reid RC. Precisely correlated firing in cells of the lateral geniculate nucleus. Nature 1996;383:815–819.

399. Sherman SM, Koch C. The control of retinogeniculate transmission in the mammalian lateral geniculate nucleus. Exp Brain Res 1986;63:1–20.

400. Casagrande VA, Norton TT. Lateral geniculate nucleus: a review of its physiology and function. In: Leventhal AG, ed. The Neural Basis of Visual Function. Boca Raton, CRC Press, 1991:41–84.

401. Posner MI. Orienting of attention. Q J Exp Psychol 1980;32:3–25.

402. Wilson JR, Hendrickson AE. Serotonergic axons in the monkey's lateral geniculate nucleus. Vis Neurosci 1988;1:125–133.

403. Rogawski MA, Aghajanian GK. Activation of lateral geniculate neurons by locus coeruleus or dorsal noradrenergic bundle stimulation: selective blockade by the alpha 1-adrenoceptor antagonist prazosin. Brain Res 1982;250:31–39.

404. Francesconi W, Muller CM, Singer W. Cholinergic mechanisms in the reticular control of transmission in the cat lateral geniculate nucleus. J Neurophys Sci 1988;59:1690–1718.

405. Cucchiaro J, Ulrich D, Sherman S. Parabrachial innervation of the cat's dorsal lateral geniculate nucleus: an electron microscopic study using the tracer *Phaseolus vulgaris* levoagglutinin (PHA-L). J Neurosci 1988;8:4576–4588.

406. Abbie A. The blood supply of lateral geniculate body with note on morphology of choroidal arteries. J Anat 1933;67:491–521.

407. Collette JM, Francois J, Neetens A. Vascularization of the optic pathway. IV. Optic tract and external geniculate body. Br J Ophthalmol 1956;40:341–354.

408. Fujino,T. [The blood supply of the lateral geniculate body]. Nippon Ganka Gakkai Zasshi 1961;65:1428–1443.

409. Fujino T. The blood supply of the lateral geniculate body. Acta Soc Ophthalmol Jpn 1962;16:24–33.

410. Frisen L, Holmegaard L, Rosencrantz M. Sectorial optic atrophy and homonymous, horizontal sectoranopia: a lateral choroidal artery syndrome? J Neurol Neurosurg Psychiatry 1978;41:374–380.

411. Burek MJ, Oppenheim RW. Programmed cell death in the developing nervous system. Brain Pathol 1996;6:427–446.

412. Rabinowicz T, et al. Human cortex development: estimates of neuronal numbers indicate major loss late during gestation. J Neuropathol Exp Neurol 1996;55: 320–328.

413. Meyer A. The connections of the occipital lobes and the present status of the cerebral visual affections. Trans Assoc Am Physicians 1907;22:7–15.

414. Ebeling U, Reulen HJ. Neurosurgical topography of the optic radiation in the temporal lobe. Acta Neurochir (Wien) 1988;92(1–4):29–36.

415. Marino R Jr, Rasmussen T. Visual field changes after temporal lobectomy in man. Neurology 1968;18:825–835.

416. Tecoma ES, et al. Frequency and characteristics of visual field deficits after surgery for mesial temporal sclerosis. Neurology 1993;43:1235–1238.

417. Traquair H. An Introduction to Clinical Perimetry. St Louis, CV Mosby, 1940.

418. Spalding J. Wounds of the visual pathway: II The visual radiation. J Neurol Neurosurg Psychiatry 1952;15:99–107.

419. Hughes B. The Visual Fields: A Study of the Applications of Quantitative Perimetry to the Anatomy and Pathology of the Visual Pathways. Oxford, Blackwell Scientific Publications, 1954.

420. Falconer MA, Wilson JL. Visual field changes following anterior temporal lobectomy: their significance in relation to Meyer's loop of the optic radiation. Brain 1958;81:1–14.

421. Wendland J, Nerenberg S. The geniculo-calcarine pathway in the temporal lobe. Univ Minn Med Bull 1960;31:482.

422. Nelson R, Kolb H. A17: a broad-field amacrine cell in the rod system of the cat retina. J Neurophys Sci 1985;54:592–614.

423. Senoh K, Naito J. A WGA-HRP study of the fiber arrangement in the cat optic radiation: a demonstration via three-dimensional reconstruction. Exp Brain Res 1991;87:473–483.

424. Savoiardo M, et al. The effects of wallerian degeneration of the optic radiations demonstrated by MRI. Neuroradiology 1992;34:323–325.

425. Bender M, Strauss I. Defects in visual field of one eye only in patients with a lesion of one optic radiation. Arch Ophthalmol 1937;17:765–787.

426. Horton JC, Hoyt WF. The representation of the visual field in human striate cortex. A revision of the classic Holmes map. Arch Ophthalmol 1991;109: 816–824.

427. Putnam T. Studies of the central visual connections. General relationship between external geniculate body, optic radiation and visual cortex in man. Arch Neurol Psychiatr 1926;16:566–596.

428. Putnam T. Studies on the central visual connections II. A comparative study of the form of the geniculo-striate visual system of mammals. Arch Neurol Psychiatr 1926;17:285–300.

429. Polyak S. The Vertebrate System, ed. H. Kluver. Chicago, University of Chicago Press, 1958.

430. Stensaas SS, Eddington DK, Dobelle WH. The topography and variability of the primary visual cortex in man. J Neurosurg 1974;40:747–755.

431. Vidyasagar TR, et al. Convergence of parvocellular and magnocellular information channels in the primary visual cortex of the macaque. Eur J Neurosci 2002; 16:945–956.

432. Callaway EM. Local circuits in primary visual cortex of the macaque monkey. Annu Rev Neurosci 1998;21:47–74.

433. Filimonoff I. Uber die variabilitat der grosshirnrindenstrukter. Regio occipitalis beim erwachsenen menschen. J Pshchol Neurol 1932;44:1–96.

434. O'Kusky J, Colonnier M. A laminar analysis of the number of neurons, glia, and synapses in the adult cortex (area 17) of adult macaque monkeys. J Comp Neurol 1982;210:278–290.

435. Saint Marie RL, Peters A. The morphology and synaptic connections of spiny stellate neurons in monkey visual cortex (area 17): a Golgi-electron microscopic study. J Comp Neurol 1985;233:213–235.

436. Levitt JB, Yoshioka T, Lund JS. Intrinsic cortical connections in macaque visual area V2: evidence for interaction between different functional streams. J Comp Neurol 1994;342:551–570.

437. Braak H. On the striate area of the human isocortex. A Golgi and pigment architectonic study. J Comp Neurol 1976;166:341–364.

438. Boyd JD, Mavity-Hudson JA, Casagrande VA. The connections of layer 4 subdivisions in the primary visual cortex (V1) of the owl monkey. Cereb Cortex 2000; 10:644–662.
439. Kaas JH, Collins CE. The organization of sensory cortex. Curr Opin Neurobiol Sci 2001;11:498–504.
440. Preuss TM, Coleman GQ. Human-specific organization of primary visual cortex: alternating compartments of dense Cat-301 and calbindin immunoreactivity in layer 4A. Cereb Cortex 2002;12:671–691.
441. Lund JS, Boothe R. Interlaminar connections and pyramidal neuron organization in the visual cortex, area 17 of the macaque monkey. J Comp Neurol 1975;159: 305–334.
442. Boothe R, et al. A quantitative investigation of spine and dendrite development of neurons in visual cortex (area 17) of Macaca nemestrina monkeys. J Comp Neurol 1979;186:473–490.
443. Fitzpatrick D, Lund JS, Blasdel GG. Intrinsic connections of macaque striate cortex: afferent and efferent connections of lamina 4C. J Neurosci 1985;5: 3329–3349.
444. Lund JS, et al. The origin of efferent pathways from the primary visual cortex, area 17, of the macaque monkey as shown by retrograde transport of horseradish peroxidase. J Comp Neurol 1976;164:287–304.
445. Maunsell J, van Essen D. The connections of the middle temporal visual are in the macaque and its relationship to a hierarchy of cortical visual areas. J Neurosci 1983;3:2563–2586.
446. Sawatari A, Callaway EM. Convergence of magno- and parvocellular pathways in layer 4B of macaque primary visual cortex. Nature 1996;380:442–446.
447. Rockland KS. Laminar distribution of neurons projecting from area V1 to V2 in macaque and squirrel monkeys. Cereb Cortex 1992;2:38–47.
448. Sincich LC, Horton JC. Independent projection streams from macaque striate cortex to the second visual area and middle temporal area. J Neurosci 2003;23: 5684–5692.
449. Yoshioka T, Hendry SH. Compartmental organization of layer IVA in human primary visual cortex. J Comp Neurol 1995;359:213–220.
450. Bolton J. The Brain in Health and Disease. London, Edward Arnold Publishers, Ltd, 1914.
451. von Economo C, Koskinas G. Die Cytoarchitektonik der hirnrinde des Erwachsenen. Wien, Springer-Verlag, 1925.
452. Hines M. Recent contributions to localization of vision in the central nervous system (review). Arch Ophthalmol 1942;28:913–937.
453. Garey LJ, Powell TP. An experimental study of the termination of the lateral geniculo-cortical pathway in the cat and monkey. Proc R Soc Lond B Biol Sci 1971;179:41–63.
454. Fitzpatrick D, et al. The sublaminar organization of corticogeniculate neurons in layer 6 of macaque striate cortex. Vis Neurosci 1994;11:307–315.
455. Shapley R, Hawken M. Neural mechanisms for color perception in the primary visual cortex. Curr Opin Neurobiol Sci 2002;12:426–432.
456. Snoddely DM, Gur M. Organization of striate cortex of alert, trained monkeys (Macaca fascicularis): ongoing activity, stimulus selectivity, and widths of receptive field activating regions. J Neurophys Sci 1995;74:2100–2125.
457. Rockland KS, Pandya DN. Laminar origins and terminations of cortical connections of the occipital lobe in the rhesus monkey. Brain Res 1979;179:3–20.
458. Rockland K. The organization of feedback connections from area V2 to V1. Cereb Cortex 1994;10:261–300.
459. Rockland KS, Van Hoesen GW. Direct temporal-occipital feedback connections to striate cortex (V1) in the macaque monkey. Cereb Cortex 1994;4:300–313.
460. Crick F. The Astonishing Hypotheses; The Scientific Search for the Soul. New York, Charles Scribner, 1994.
461. Gray CM, McCormick DA. Chattering cells: superficial pyramidal neurons contributing to the generation of synchronous oscillations in the visual cortex. Science 1996;274:109–113.
462. Miyashita Y. How the brain creates imagery: projection to primary visual cortex. Science 1995;268:1719–1720.
463. Hubel DH, Wiesel TN. Receptive fields of single neurones in the cat's striate cortex. J Phys Sci 1959;148:574–591.
464. Hubel DH, Wiesel TN. Receptive fields of cells in striate cortex of very young, visually inexperienced kittens. J Neurophys Sci 1963;26:994–1002.
465. Hubel DH, Wiesel TN. Anatomical demonstration of columns in the monkey striate cortex. Nature 1969;221:747–750.
466. Hubel DH, Wiesel TN. Receptive fields of optic nerve fibres in the spider monkey. J Phys Sci 1960;154:572–580.
467. Hubel DH, Wiesel TN. Effects of varying stimulus size and color on single lateral geniculate cells in Rhesus monkeys. Proc Natl Acad Sci USA 1966;55: 1345–1346.
468. Hubel DH, Wiesel TN. Receptive fields and functional architecture of monkey striate cortex. J Phys Sci 1968;195:215–243.
469. Hubel DH, Wiesel TN. Sequence regularity and geometry of orientation columns in the monkey striate cortex. J Comp Neurol 1974;158:267–293.
470. Hubel DH, Wiesel TN. Uniformity of monkey striate cortex: a parallel relationship between field size, scatter, and magnification factor. J Comp Neurol 1974; 158:295–305.
471. Wiesel TN, Hubel DH, Lam DM. Autoradiographic demonstration of ocular-dominance columns in the monkey striate cortex by means of transneuronal transport. Brain Res 1974;79:273–279.
472. Hubel DH, Freeman DC. Projection into the visual field of ocular dominance columns in macaque monkey. Brain Res 1977;122:336–343.
473. Hubel DH, Wiesel TN, Stryker MP. Orientation columns in macaque monkey visual cortex demonstrated by the 2-deoxyglucose autoradiographic technique. Nature 1977;269:328–330.
474. Hubel DH, Wiesel TN, Stryker MP. Anatomical demonstration of orientation columns in macaque monkey. J Comp Neurol 1978;177:361–380.
475. Levitt JB, Lund JS. The spatial extent over which neurons in macaque striate cortex pool visual signals. Vis Neurosci 2002;19:439–452.
476. Ikeda H, Wright MJ. Evidence for "sustained" and "transient" neurones in the cat's visual cortex. Vision Res 1974;14:133–136.
477. Ikeda H, Wright MJ. Spatial and temporal properties of sustained and "transient" neurons in area 17 of the cat's visual cortex. Exp Brain Res 1975;22: 363–383.
478. Ikeda H, Wright MJ. Retinotopic distribution, visual latency and orientation tuning of sustained and transient cortical neurones in area 17 of the cat. Exp Brain Res 1975;22:385–398.
479. Hubel DH, Wiesel TN. Receptive fields, binocular interaction and functional architecture in the cat's visual cortex. J Phys Sci 1962;160:106–154.
480. Hubel DH, Wiesel TN, LeVay S. Functional architecture of area 17 in normal and monocularly deprived macaque monkeys. Cold Spring Harb Symp Quant Biol 1976;40:581–589.
481. Schoups A, et al. Practising orientation identification improves orientation coding in V1 neurons. Nature 2001;412:549–553.
482. Durand JB, et al. Neurons in parafoveal areas V1 and V2 encode vertical and horizontal disparities. J Neurophys Sci 2002;88:2874–2879.
483. Horton JC, Hedley-Whyte ET. Mapping of cytochrome oxidase patches and ocular dominance columns in human visual cortex. Philos Trans R Soc Lond B Biol Sci 1984;304:255–272.
484. LeVay S, et al. The complete pattern of ocular dominance stripes in the striate cortex and visual field of the macaque monkey. J Neurosci 1985;5:486–501.
485. Livingstone MS. Ocular dominance columns in New World monkeys. J Neurosci 1996;16:2086–2096.
486. Sokoloff L. Influence of functional activity on local cerebral glucose utilization. In: Ingvar D, Lassen N, eds. Brain Work. The Coupling of Function, Metabolism and Blood Flow in the Brain. New York, Academic Press, 1975:385.
487. Sokoloff L. Measurement of local glucose utilization and its use in mapping local functional activity in the central nervous system. In: The 4th World Congress of Psychiatric Surgery, 1977, Madrid.
488. Obermeyer K, Blasdel G. Geometry of orientation and ocular dominance columns in monkey striate cortex. J Neurosci 1993;13:4129.
489. Horton JC, Hubel DH. Regular patchy distribution of cytochrome oxidase staining in primary visual cortex of macaque monkey. Nature 1981;292:762–764.
490. Horton JC. Cytochrome oxidase patches: a new cytoarchitectonic feature of monkey visual cortex. Philos Trans R Soc Lond B Biol Sci 1984;304:199–253.
491. Rakic P. Prenatal genesis of connections subserving ocular dominance in the rhesus monkey. Nature 1976;261:467–471.
492. Rakic P. Prenatal development of the visual system in rhesus monkey. Philos Trans R Soc Lond B Biol Sci 1977;278:245–260.
493. Wiesel TN, Hubel DH. Single-cell responses in striate cortex of kittens deprived of vision in one eye. J Neurophys Sci 1963;26:1003–1017.
494. Des Rosiers MH, et al. Functional plasticity in the immature striate cortex of the monkey shown by the [14C]deoxyglucose method. Science 1978;200:447–449.
495. Horton JC, Hocking DR. Pattern of ocular dominance columns in human striate cortex in strabismic amblyopia. Vis Neurosci 1996;13:787–795.
496. Horton JC, Stryker MP. Amblyopia induced by anisometropia without shrinkage of ocular dominance columns in human striate cortex. Proc Natl Acad Sci USA 1993;90:5494–5498.
497. Heynen A, et al. Molecular mechanism for loss of visual cortical responsiveness following breif monocular deprivation. Nat Neurosci 2003;8:854–862.
498. Sawtell NB, et al. NMDA receptor-dependent ocular dominance plasticity in adult visual cortex. Neuron 2003;38:977–985.
499. Matsubara JA, et al. The effects of panretinal photocoagulation on the primary visual cortex of the adult monkey. Trans Am Ophthalmol Soc 2001;99:33–43.
500. McFadzean R, et al. Representation of the visual field in the occipital striate cortex. Br J Ophthalmol 1994;78:185–190.
501. Yiannikas C, Walsh JC. The variation of the pattern shift visual evoked response with the size of the stimulus field. Electroencephalogr Clin Neurophys Sci 1983; 55:427–435.
502. Chatterjee S, Callaway EM. Parallel colour-opponent pathways to primary visual cortex. Nature 2003;426:668–671.
503. Lennie P, Krauskopf J, Sclar G. Chromatic mechanisms in striate cortex of macaque. J Neurosci 1990;10:649–669.
504. Michael CR. Color-sensitive complex cells in monkey striate cortex. J Neurophys Sci 1978;41:1250–1266.
505. Michael CR. Color vision mechanisms in monkey striate cortex: dual-opponent cells with concentric receptive fields. J Neurophys Sci 1978;41:572–588.
506. Michael CR. Color-sensitive hypercomplex cells in monkey striate cortex. J Neurophys Sci 1979;42:726–744.
507. Michael CR. Columnar organization of color cells in monkey's striate cortex. J Neurophys Sci 1981;46:587–604.
508. Landisman CE, Ts'o DY. Color processing in macaque striate cortex: relation-

ships to ocular dominance, cytochrome oxidase, and orientation. J Neurophys Sci 2002;87:3126–3137.

509. Ts'o DY, Gilbert CD. The organization of chromatic and spatial interactions in the primate striate cortex. J Neurosci 1988;8:1712–1727.

510. Tootell RB, et al. The representation of the ipsilateral visual field in human cerebral cortex. Proc Natl Acad Sci USA 1998;95:818–824.

511. Beauvieux J. La pseudo-atrophie optique des nouveau-nes (Dysgenesie myelinique des voies optiques). Ann Ocul 1926;163:881–921.

512. Polyak S. The Vertebrate Visual System, ed. H. Kluver. Chicago, University of Chicago Press, 1958.

513. Smith CG, Richardson WF. The course and distribution of the arteries supplying the visual (striate) cortex. Am J Ophthalmol 1966;61:1391–1396.

514. Hoyt WF, Margolis M. Arterial supply of the striate cortex: angiographic changes with occlusion of the posterior cerebral artery. Excerpta Med Int Congr 1970:1323–1332.

515. Hoyt WF, Newton TH. Angiographic changes with occlusion of arteries that supply the visual cortex. Aust NZ J Med 1970;71:310–317.

516. Newton TH, Potts D. Radiology of the Skull and Brain. St Louis, CV Mosby, 1974:2.

517. Zeal A, Rhoton A, Microsurgical anatomy of the posterior cerebral artery. J Neurosurg 1978;48:534–559.

518. Brodmann K. Individuelle variationen der sehsphare und ihre bedeutung fur die klinik der hinterhauptschusse. Allgz Psychiatr (Berlin) 1918;74:564–568.

519. Brodmann K. Vergleichende Localisationslehre der Grosshirnrinde in ihren Prinzipien Dargestellt auf Grund des Zellenbaues. Leipzig, Barth, 1909.

520. Livingstone MS, Hubel DH. Connections between layer 4B of area 17 and the thick cytochrome oxidase stripes of area 18 in the squirrel monkey. J Neurosci 1987;7:3371–3377.

521. Casagrande VA, Kaas J. The afferent, intrinsic, and efferent connections of primary visual cortex in primates. Cereb Cortex 1994;10:201–259.

522. Roe AW, Ts'o DY. Visual topography in primate V2: multiple representation across functional stripes. J Neurosci 1995;15(5 Pt 2):3689–3715.

523. Ts'o DY, Roe AW, Gilbert CD. A hierarchy of the functional organization for color, form and disparity in primate visual area V2. Vision Res 2001;41(10–11):1333–1349.

524. Sincich LC, Horton JC. Divided by cytochrome oxidase: a map of the projections from V1 to V2 in macaques. Science 2002;295:1734–1737.

525. Gegenfurtner KR, Kiper DC, Fenstemaker SB. Processing of color, form, and motion in macaque area V2. Vis Neurosci 1996;13:161–172.

526. Zeki SM. Uniformity and diversity of structure and function in rhesus monkey prestriate visual cortex. J Phys Sci 1978;277:273–290.

527. Hubel DH, Wiesel TN. Stereoscopic vision in macaque monkey. Cells sensitive to binocular depth in area 18 of the macaque monkey cortex. Nature 1970;225:41–42.

528. Thomas OM, Cumming BG, Parker AJ. A specialization for relative disparity in V2. Nat Neurosci 2002;5:472–478.

529. Vanduffel W, et al. The organization of orientation selectivity throughout macaque visual cortex. Cereb Cortex 2002;12:647–662.

530. Sincich LC, Horton JC. Pale cytochrome oxidase stripes in V2 receive the richest projection from macaque striate cortex. J Comp Neurol 2002;447:18–33.

531. Baizer JS, Robinson DL, Dow BM. Visual responses of area 18 neurons in awake, behaving monkey. J Neurophys Sci 1977;40:1024–1037.

532. Hubel DH, Livingstone MS. Complex-unoriented cells in a subregion of primate area 18. Nature 1985;315:325–327.

533. Abel PL, O'Brien BJ, Olavarria JF. Organization of callosal linkages in visual area V2 of macaque monkey. J Comp Neurol 2000;428:278–293.

534. Horton JC, Hoyt WF. Quadrantic visual field defects. A hallmark of lesions in extrastriate (V2/V3) cortex. Brain 1991;114(Pt 4):1703–1718.

535. Vaina LM, et al. A lesion of cortical area V2 selectively impairs the perception of the direction of first-order visual motion. Neuroreport 2000;11:1039–1044.

536. Lyon DC, Kaas JH. Evidence for a modified V3 with dorsal and ventral halves in macaque monkeys. Neuron 2002;33:453–461.

537. Nakamura H, Le WR, Wakita M, et al. Projections from the cytochrome oxidase modules of visual area V2 to the ventral posterior area in the macaque. Exp Brain Res 2004;155:102–110.

538. Felleman DJ, Burkhalter A, Van Essen DC. Cortical connections of areas V3 and VP of macaque monkey extrastriate visual cortex. J Comp Neurol 1997;379:21–47.

539. Rosa MG, Tweedale R. The dorsomedial visual areas in New World and Old World monkeys: homology and function. Eur J Neurosci 2001;13:421–427.

540. Smith AT, et al. The processing of first- and second-order motion in human visual cortex assessed by functional magnetic resonance imaging (fMRI). J Neurosci 1998;18:3816–3830.

541. Lyon DC, et al. Optical imaging reveals retinotopic organization of dorsal V3 in New World owl monkeys. Proc Natl Acad Sci USA 2002;99:15735–15742.

542. Gattass R, Sousa AP, Gross CG. Visuotopic organization and extent of V3 and V4 of the macaque. J Neurosci 1988;8:1831–1845.

543. Rosa MG, et al. "Third tier" ventral extrastriate cortex in the New World monkey, *Cebus apella*. Exp Brain Res 2000;132:287–305.

544. Zeki SM. Representation of central visual fields in prestriate cortex of monkey. Brain Res 1969;14:271–291.

545. Adams DL, Zeki S. Functional organization of macaque V3 for stereoscopic depth. J Neurophyssci 2001;86:2195–2203.

546. Gegenfurtner KR, Kiper DC, Levitt JB. Functional properties of neurons in macaque area V3. J Neurophys Sci 1997;77:1906–1923.

547. Burkhalter A, et al. Anatomical and physiological asymmetries related to visual areas V3 and VP in macaque extrastriate cortex. Vision Res 1986;26:63–80.

548. Girard P, Salin PA, Bullier J. Visual activity in areas V3a and V3 during reversible inactivation of area V1 in the macaque monkey. J Neurophys Sci 1991;66:1493–1503.

549. Rodman HR, Gross CG, Albright TD. Afferent basis of visual response properties in area MT of the macaque. I. Effects of striate cortex removal. J Neurosci 1989;9:2033–2050.

550. Vaina LM, Soloviev S. First-order and second-order motion: neurological evidence for neuroanatomically distinct systems. Prog Brain Res 2004;144:197–212.

551. Galletti C, et al. The cortical connections of area V6: an occipito-parietal network processing visual information. Eur J Neurosci 2001;13:1572–1588.

552. Brodal P. The corticopontine projection in the rhesus monkey. Origin and principles of organization. Brain 1978;101:251–283.

553. Galletti C, et al. Functional demarcation of a border between areas V6 and V6A in the superior parietal gyrus of the macaque monkey. Eur J Neurosci 1996;8:30–52.

554. Fattori P, et al. 'Arm-reaching' neurons in the parietal area V6A of the macaque monkey. Eur J Neurosci 2001;13:2309–2313.

555. Shipp S, Blanton M, Zeki S. A visuo-somatomotor pathway through superior parietal cortex in the macaque monkey: cortical connections of areas V6 and V6A. Eur J Neurosci 1998;10:3171–3193.

556. Battaglini PP, et al. Effects of lesions to area V6A in monkeys. Exp Brain Res 2002;144:419–422.

557. Rizzo M, Vecera S. Psychoanatomical substrates of Balint's syndrome. J Neurol Neurosurg Psychiatry 2002;72:162–178.

558. Allman JM, Kass JH. A representation of the visual field in the caudal third of the middle temporal gyrus of the owl monkey (*Aotus trivirgatus*). Brain Res 1971;31:85–105.

559. Cragg BG. The topography of the afferent projections in the circumstriate visual cortex of the monkey studied by the Nauta method. Vision Res 1969;9:733–747.

560. Shipp S, Zeki S. The organization of connections between areas V5 and V1 in macaque monkey visual cortex. Eur J Neurosci 1989;1:309–1332.

561. Verson JC, Martin KA. Connection from cortical area V2 to MT in macaque monkey. J Comp Neurol 2002;443:56–70.

562. Verson JC, et al. The connection from cortical area V1 to V5: a light and electron microscopic study. J Neurosci 1998;18:10525–10540.

563. Rodman HR, Gross CG, Albright TD. Afferent basis of visual response properties in area MT of the macaque. II. Effects of superior colliculus removal. J Neurosci 1990;10:1154–1164.

564. Watson JD, et al. Area V5 of the human brain: evidence from a combined study using positron emission tomography and magnetic resonance imaging. Cereb Cortex 1993;3:79–94.

565. Zeki S, Watson JD, Frackowiak RS. Going beyond the information given: the relation of illusory visual motion to brain activity. Proc R Soc Lond B Biol Sci 1993;252:215–222.

566. Rakic P, Lidow MS. Distribution and density of monoamine receptors in the primate visual cortex devoid of retinal input from early embryonic stages. J Neurosci 1995;15(3 Pt 2):2561–2574.

567. Tootell RB, et al. Functional analysis of human MT and related visual cortical areas using magnetic resonance imaging. J Neurosci 1995;15:3215–3230.

568. Albright TD, Desimone R, Gross CG. Columnar organization of directionally selective cells in visual area MT of the macaque. J Neurophys Sci 1984;51:16–31.

569. Dubner R, Zeki SM. Response properties and receptive fields of cells in an anatomically defined region of the superior temporal sulcus in the monkey. Brain Res 1971;35:528–532.

570. Zeki SM. Cells responding to changing image size and disparity in the cortex of the rhesus monkey. J Phys Sci 1974;242:827–841.

571. Felleman DJ, Van Essen DC. Receptive field properties of neurons in area V3 of macaque monkey extrastriate cortex. J Neurophys Sci 1987;57:889–920.

572. Movshon JA, Newsome WT. Visual response properties of striate cortical neurons projecting to area MT in macaque monkeys. J Neurosci 1996;16:7733–7741.

573. Dupont P, et al. Many areas in the human brain respond to visual motion. J Neurophys Sci 1994;72:1420–1424.

574. Merigan WH, Byrne CE, Maunsell JH. Does primate motion perception depend on the magnocellular pathway? J Neurosci 1991;11:3422–3429.

575. Anderson SJ, et al. Localization and functional analysis of human cortical area V5 using magneto-encephalography. Proc R Soc Lond B Biol Sci 1996;263:423–431.

576. Britten KH, et al. A relationship between behavioral choice and the visual responses of neurons in macaque MT. Vis Neurosci 1996;13:87–100.

577. Celebrini S, Newsome WT. Neuronal and psychophysical sensitivity to motion signals in extrastriate area MST of the macaque monkey. J Neurosci 1994;14:4109–4124.

578. Britten KH, van Wezel RJ. Electrical microstimulation of cortical area MST biases heading perception in monkeys. Nat Neurosci 1998;1:59–63.

579. Azzopardi P, et al. Response latencies of neurons in visual areas MT and MST of monkeys with striate cortex lesions. Neuropsychologia 2003;41:1738–1756.

580. Baseler HA, Morland AB, Wandell BA. Topographic organization of human visual areas in the absence of input from primary cortex. J Neurosci 1999;19: 2619–2627.

581. Newsome WT, et al. Deficits in visual motion processing following ibotenic acid lesions of the middle temporal visual area of the macaque monkey. J Neurosci 1985;5:825–840.

582. Newsome WT, Pare EB. A selective impairment of motion perception following lesions of the middle temporal visual area (MT). J Neurosci 1988;8:2201–2211.

583. Beckers G, Zeki S. The consequences of inactivating areas V1 and V5 on visual motion perception. Brain 1995;118(Pt 1):49–60.

584. Ffytche DH, Guy CN, Zeki S. The parallel visual motion inputs into areas V1 and V5 of human cerebral cortex. Brain 1995;118(Pt 6):1375–1394.

585. Poppel E, et al. Residual visual function after brain wounds involving the central visual pathways in man. Nature 1973;243:295–296.

586. Weiskrantz L, et al. Visual capacity in the hemianopic field following a restricted occipital ablation. Brain 1974;97:709–728.

587. Perenin MT, Jeannerod M. Residual vision in cortically blind hemifields. Neuropsychologia 1975;13:1–7.

588. Barbur JL, Harlow AJ, Weiskrantz L. Spatial and temporal response properties of residual vision in a case of hemianopia. Philos Trans R Soc Lond B Biol Sci 1994;343:157–166.

589. Weiskrantz L, Barbur JL, Sahraie A. Parameters affecting conscious versus unconscious visual discrimination with damage to the visual cortex (V1). Proc Natl Acad Sci USA 1995;92:6122–6126.

590. Mohler CW, Wurtz RH. Role of striate cortex and superior colliculus in visual guidance of saccadic eye movements in monkeys. J Neurophys Sci 1977;40: 74–94.

591. Cowey A, Stoerig P. Blindsight in monkeys. Nature 1995;373:247–249.

592. Zeki S. Cerebral akinetopsia (visual motion blindness). A review. Brain 1991; 114(Pt 2):811–824.

593. Zihl J, von Cramon D, Mai N. Selective disturbance of movement vision after bilateral brain damage. Brain 1983;106(Pt 2):313–340.

594. Rizzo M, Nawrot M, Zihl J. Motion and shape perception in cerebral akinetopsia. Brain 1995;118(Pt 5):1105–1127.

595. Plant GT, Nakayama K. The characteristics of residual motion perception in the hemifield contralateral to lateral occipital lesions in humans. Brain 1993;116(Pt 6):1337–1353.

596. Plant GT, et al. Impaired visual motion perception in the contralateral hemifield following unilateral posterior cerebral lesions in humans. Brain 1993;116(Pt 6): 1303–1335.

597. Previc FH, et al. Functional imaging of brain areas involved in the processing of coherent and incoherent wide field-of-view visual motion. Exp Brain Res 2000;131:393–405.

598. Previc FH. The neuropsychology of 3-D space. Psychol Bull 1998;124:123–164.

599. Heide W, et al. Optokinetic nystagmus, self motion sensation and their after-effects in patients with occipito-parietal lesions. Clin Vis Sci 1990;5:145–156.

600. Vaina LM, et al. Functional neuroanatomy of biological motion perception in humans. Proc Natl Acad Sci USA 2001;98:11656–11661.

601. Cowey A, Vaina LM. Blindness to form from motion despite intact static form perception and motion detection. Neuropsychologia 2000;38:566–578.

602. Zeki S. A century of cerebral achromatopsia. Brain 1990;113(Pt 6):1721–1777.

603. Van Essen DC, Maunsell JH, Bixby JL. The middle temporal visual area in the macaque: myeloarchitecture, connections, functional properties and topographic organization. J Comp Neurol 1981;199:293–326.

604. Ferrera VP, Nealey TA, Maunsell JH. Responses in macaque visual area V4 following inactivation of the parvocellular and magnocellular LGN pathways. J Neurosci 1994;14:2080–2088.

605. Rosenbluth D, Allman JM. The effect of gaze angle and fixation distance on the responses of neurons in V1, V2, and V4. Neuron 2002;33:143–149.

606. Zeki SM. Cortical projections from two prestriate areas in the monkey. Brain Res 1971;34:19–35.

607. Zeki SM. Colour coding in rhesus monkey prestriate cortex. Brain Res 1973; 53:422–427.

608. Zeki SM. Functional organization of a visual area in the posterior bank of the superior temporal sulcus of the rhesus monkey. J Phys Sci 1974;236:549–573.

609. Green GJ, Lessell S. Acquired cerebral dyschromatopsia. Arch Ophthalmol 1977;95:121–128.

610. Heywood CA, Gadotti A, Cowey A. Cortical area V4 and its role in the perception of color. J Neurosci 1992;12:4056–4065.

611. Rizzo M, et al. A human visual disorder resembling area V4 dysfunction in the monkey. Neurology 1992;42:1175–1180.

612. Pasupathy A, Connor CE. Population coding of shape in area V4. Nat Neurosci 2002;5:1332–1338.

613. Pasupathy A, Connor CE. Shape representation in area V4: position-specific tuning for boundary conformation. J Neurophys Sci 2001;86:2505–2519.

614. Schiller PH, Lee K. The role of the primate extrastriate area V4 in vision. Science 1991;251:1251–1253.

615. Motter BC. Neural correlates of attentive selection for color or luminance in extrastriate area V4. J Neurosci 1994;14:2178–2189.

616. Motter BC. Neural correlates of feature selective memory and pop-out in extrastriate area V4. J Neurosci 1994;14:2190–2199.

617. Schiller PH. Effect of lesions in visual cortical area V4 on the recognition of transformed objects. Nature 1995;376:342–344.

618. De Weerd P, Desimone R, Ungerleider LG. Cue-dependent deficits in grating orientation discrimination after V4 lesions in macaques. Vis Neurosci 1996;13: 529–538.

619. Maunsell JH, Nealey TA, DePriest DD. Magnocellular and parvocellular contributions to responses in the middle temporal visual area (MT) of the macaque monkey. J Neurosci 1990;10:3323–3334.

620. Yang T, Maunsell JH. The effect of perceptual learning on neuronal responses in monkey visual area V4. J Neurosci 2004;24:1617–1626.

621. Tsunoda K, et al. Complex objects are represented in macaque inferotemporal cortex by the combination of feature columns. Nat Neurosci 2001;4:832–838.

622. Desimone R, et al. Stimulus-selective properties of inferior temporal neurons in the macaque. J Neurosci 1984;4:2051–2062.

623. Downing PE, et al. A cortical area selective for visual processing of the human body. Science 2001;293:2470–2473.

624. Janssen P, Vogels R, Orban GA. Macaque inferior temporal neurons are selective for disparity-defined three-dimensional shapes. Proc Natl Acad Sci USA 1999; 96:8217–8222.

625. Erickson CA, Desimone R. Responses of macaque perirhinal neurons during and after visual stimulus association learning. J Neurosci 1999;19:10404–10416.

626. Fattori P, Galletti C, Battaglini PP. Parietal neurons encoding visual space in a head-frame of reference. Boll Soc Ital Biol Sper 1992;68:663–670.

627. Wallace MT, Stein BE. Onset of cross-modal synthesis in the neonatal superior colliculus is gated by the development of cortical influences. J Neurophys Sci 2000;83:3578–3582.

628. Humphrey NK. Responses to visual stimuli of units in the superior colliculus of rats and monkeys. Exp Neurol 1968;20:312–340.

629. Schiller PH, Koerner F. Discharge characteristics of single units in superior colliculus of the alert rhesus monkey. J Neurophys Sci 1971;34:920–936.

630. Wurtz RH, Goldberg ME. Superior colliculus cell responses related to eye movements in awake monkeys. Science 1971;171:82–84.

631. Goldberg ME, Wurtz RH. Activity of superior colliculus in behaving monkey. II. Effect of attention on neuronal responses. J Neurophys Sci 1972;35:560–574.

632. Munoz DP, Wurtz RH. Role of the rostral superior colliculus in active visual fixation and execution of express saccades. J Neurophys Sci 1992;67: 1000–1002.

633. Stepniewska I, Qi HX, Kaas JH. Do superior colliculus projection zones in the inferior pulvinar project to MT in primates? Eur J Neurosci 1999;11:469–480.

634. Moore T, Armstrong KM. Selective gating of visual signals by microstimulation of frontal cortex. Nature 2003;421:370–373.

635. Foxe JJ, Simpson GV. Flow of activation from V1 to frontal cortex in humans. A framework for defining ''early'' visual processing. Exp Brain Res 2002;142: 139–150.

636. Felleman DJ, Van Essen DC. Distributed hierarchical processing in the primate cerebral cortex. Cereb Cortex 1991;1:1–47.

637. Symonds LL, Rosenquist AC. Corticocortical connections among visual areas in the cat. J Comp Neurol 1984;229:1–38.

638. Sillito AM, Jones HE. Corticothalamic interactions in the transfer of visual information. Philos Trans R Soc Lond B Biol Sci 2002;357:1739–1752.

Principles and Techniques of the Examination of the Visual Sensory System

Michael Wall and Chris A. Johnson

HISTORY
CLINICAL EXAMINATION
    Refraction and Visual Acuity
    Stereoacuity
    Color Vision and Brightness Comparison
    Visual Field Examination
    Photo Stress Test
    Pulfrich Phenomenon
    Pupillary Examination
    Fundus Examination
    Other Procedures

PSYCHOPHYSICAL TESTS
    Visual Acuity
    Contrast Sensitivity
    Perimetry and Visual Field Testing
    Color Vision
    Dark Adaptation
ELECTROPHYSIOLOGIC TESTS
    Electroretinogram (ERG)
    Electro-Oculogram (EOG)
    Other Retinal Potentials
    Visual-Evoked Potential

Despite advances in neurodiagnostic imaging and other techniques, examination of the afferent visual sensory system is still the core of the neuro-ophthalmologic examination. This chapter describes the most common subjective and objective tests used in the afferent visual system examination. In addition, recent developments in perimetry, clinical psychophysics, and electrophysiology are discussed.

We begin with an overview of the basic neuro-ophthalmologic examination of the afferent visual sensory system. Next, key visual functions (visual acuity, contrast sensitivity, perimetry, new visual field tests, color vision, and dark adaptation) associated with the afferent system are discussed along with their physiologic and psychophysical principles.

Examples of the various concepts and test procedures are presented, where appropriate. Electrophysiologic tests (i.e., electroretinography, electrooculography, visual-evoked potentials) that may be helpful in assessing the afferent system are also described.

Evaluation of the afferent system begins with a thorough medical history, followed by an ophthalmologic examination, evaluation of selected psychophysical visual functions (acuity, stereoacuity, color vision, visual fields, contrast sensitivity, etc.) and relevant ancillary test procedures. Once the examiner has performed these functions, it should be possible to provide a diagnosis, or at least a differential diagnosis, for the etiology of an afferent visual system deficit.

HISTORY

An examination of patients experiencing dysfunction of the afferent visual system begins with a history of the details of the visual loss. This thorough history is often the most important part of the evaluation, because it determines the initial strategy for differential diagnostic evaluation and examination. It is essential to establish if the visual loss is monocular or binocular, if its location is central, peripheral, altitudinal, or hemianopic, and if the onset of the loss is gradual, sudden, or intermittent along with any associated symptoms.

It is also important to ask about photopsias (visual phenomena such as flashing black squares, flashes of lights, or showers of sparks), distortions in vision (metamorphopsia or micropsia), and positive scotomas. A positive scotoma is one that is seen by the patient, like the purple spot that is often seen after a flash bulb goes off, whereas a negative scotoma refers to a non-seeing area of the visual field. Metamorphopsia, micropsia, and positive scotomas often occur in patients with maculopathies, whereas photopsias may be present in patients with retinal disease, optic nerve dysfunction, or cerebral dysfunction from migraine and other vascular disorders.

CLINICAL EXAMINATION

Clinical evaluation of the afferent visual system for each eye incorporates the items in Table 2.1, which can be performed in the office. This section presents a brief discussion of each component, with a more detailed discussion of several visual function tests (visual acuity, contrast sensitivity, color vision, perimetry, and visual field testing) and ancillary procedures (dark adaptation and clinical electrophysiology) presented later in this chapter. Other aspects of the clinical examination are covered in subsequent chapters of this book.

The first goal for the neuro-ophthalmology examination is to determine if the visual loss is caused by a disorder anterior to the retina (ocular media), in the retina, in the optic nerve, in the optic chiasm, in the retrochiasmal pathways, or is nonorganic (i.e., hysteria or malingering). The second goal is to establish a differential and working diagnosis. By examining various parameters of afferent visual function, the examiner can frequently make a determination as to the anatomic site of the afferent system abnormality and the most probable cause or causes.

REFRACTION AND VISUAL ACUITY

A thorough refraction is an essential part of all clinical neuro-ophthalmologic examinations. Identification of a previously undetermined refractive error, corneal pathology, or a subtle lens problem can prevent initiation of an expensive and time-consuming evaluation. It is essential to have the best refraction possible when measuring visual acuity to distinguish whether visual acuity loss is caused by optical factors or damage to neural elements in the visual system. Refractive problems can not only cause loss of visual acuity but may also produce symptoms such as monocular diplopia. A cycloplegic refraction is important, not only to obtain the correct refraction, but also to observe the red reflex through the retinoscope as a means of identifying corneal irregularities and lens opacities that may not be as apparent with a slit lamp examination. Visual acuity measurements obtained with the patient viewing through a pinhole can also help identify problems with the optics of the eye. In many instances, it is useful to dilate the patient in conjunction with the use of a pinhole to maximize the likelihood of finding a clear pinhole region around an opacity. Improvement of visual acuity with the use of a pinhole indicates that the cause of the visual loss is optical in nature.

Small degrees of visual acuity loss can be due to large losses in neuronal function. Frisén and Frisén (1) estimated that 20/20 visual acuity requires no more than 44% of the normal quantity of foveolar, neuro-retinal channels. Since 20/15 acuity is the population norm up to age 50, asymmetry of best corrected visual acuity of 20/20 to 20/15 can indicate substantial damage to the prechiasmal afferent system.

The Potential Acuity Meter (PAM), which utilizes the pinhole principle, can be helpful (2). Keratoconus and surface irregularities of the cornea can be diagnosed by improvement in visual acuity with the use of a hard contact lens. A Placido's disk, keratometry readings, or corneal topography maps can also help to identify corneal surface irregularities and associated problems.

Subtle central vision loss can often be identified by the use of low contrast visual acuity charts or contrast sensitivity measurements. In addition, low luminance visual acuity can be compared with similar measures made under standard lighting conditions. von Noorden and Burian (3) and Glaser and Goodwin (4) reported that placing a 2.0 log unit neutral density filter before the eye (i.e., producing a 100-fold reduction in the luminance of the visual acuity chart) causes a normal eye to be reduced from 20/20 to 20/40 visual acuity (a factor of 2 or 0.3 logMAR). Patients with optic nerve conduction abnormalities, such as optic neuritis or multiple

---

Table 2.1
Components of the Clinical Neuro-Ophthalmologic Examination

  I. REFRACTION
     Retinoscopy
     Keratometry
     Manifest refraction
     Cycloplegic refraction
 II. VISUAL FUNCTION
     Visual acuity (distance and near)
     Stereoacuity
     Color vision, color comparison
     Brightness comparison
     Photo stress test
     Pulfrich phenomenon
     Visual fields
     Confrontation fields
     Amsler grid
     Tangent screen
     Manual kinetic perimetry (Goldmann perimeter)
     Automated static perimetry
III. PUPILS
     Size
     Direct and consensual response
     Accommodation response
     Afferent pupillary defect
 IV. CRANIAL NERVES I, III, IV, V, VI, VII, VIII
  V. EXOPHTHALMOMETRY
 VI. EXTERNAL AND ANTERIOR SEGMENT
     External examination
     Slit lamp examination
     Applanation tonometry
VII. FUNDUS
     Optic nerve head and nerve fiber layer appearance
     Macula and retinal vessels
     Peripheral retina

sclerosis with optic atrophy, have a disproportionately greater reduction in visual acuity (e.g., from 20/30 down to 20/200) when the neutral density filter is placed before the affected eye. Other anomalies such as amblyopia do not demonstrate this disproportionate drop in visual acuity with the neutral density filter.

Another low-contrast visual acuity test that also uses low background luminance levels is the SKILL (Smith-Kettlewell Institute Low Luminance) test, which has been used to evaluate patients with optic neuritis, children with amblyopia, and the reading abilities of younger and older individuals (5–9).

Measuring visual acuity in children requires skill, patience, and an enthusiastic attitude. By creating a friendly, relaxed environment for the child in which vision testing is presented as a game, the chances of success will be greater. A system of positive rewards, ranging from a verbal "Hooray!" or "That's Terrific!" to the use of mechanical animal toys and projected cartoons, is essential (Fig. 2.1). A video demonstration of many techniques for evaluating children and infants is available from the American Academy of Ophthalmology (10).

During any neuro-ophthalmologic examination, it is essential to measure not only distance visual acuity but also near visual acuity. In some instances (e.g., an in-hospital consultation on a patient who is unable to come to the examination room), near visual acuity is the only measurement

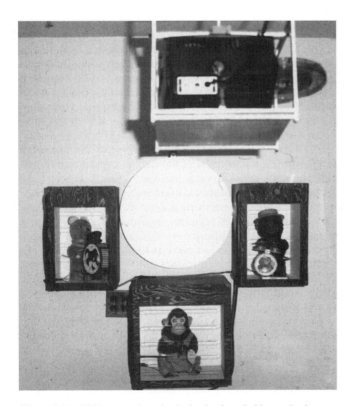

Figure 2.1. Wall-mounted mechanical animals and video projection system for providing fixation targets and "rewards" for pediatric patients during the examination.

that is possible. Near visual acuity measurements can be performed with any of the standard near acuity cards, which are held at 13–14 inches from the eyes with the patient wearing an appropriate near refractive correction. In patients with normal visual function, there is little or no difference between distance and near visual acuity. A discrepancy between near and distance visual acuity suggests several possible etiologies. Patients with cataracts often perform better on near acuity than distance acuity. Young patients with head trauma may complain of reading problems from loss of accommodation, resulting in poorer near acuity than distance acuity. Patients with nonorganic loss of vision may not understand the relationship between near and distance acuity and may provide inconsistent responses with the two measurements (11). One must be careful, however, to ensure that optical factors (e.g., cataract, accommodation loss) are not responsible for the differences.

STEREOACUITY

Stereoacuity requires good visual acuity in both eyes and normal cortical development. As such, stereoacuity can be helpful in establishing if a patient has visual loss from congenital amblyopia or monofixation syndrome, as well as verifying the extent of any monocular visual acuity loss. Using the Titmus Stereo Tester, Donzis and coworkers (12) measured stereoacuity in 30 normal observers with good binocular function and visual acuity. Stereoacuity was 40 seconds of arc or better when both eyes had 20/20 visual acuity. They then placed plus lenses before one eye and published a nomogram that relates visual acuity to stereoacuity. This provides a useful reference for cross-checking mild losses of monocular visual acuity, especially when nonorganic visual loss is suspected (11) (see Chapter 27). Random dot stereogram tests can also be helpful in identifying patients with good binocular visual acuity.

COLOR VISION AND BRIGHTNESS COMPARISON

Color vision testing, using pseudoisochromatic plates, the Farnsworth 100 Hue and D-15 tests, or the Lanthony 15 Desaturated D-15 panel can be helpful in detecting subtle signs of optic neuropathy or macular disease. While it has been proposed that *acquired* color vision loss respects color vision axes, more often than not, this does not hold. On the other hand, *congenital* loss respects these axes with red/green deficits occurring in approximately 8% of the male population and in 0.4% of females (13) (Table 2.2). Congenital blue/yellow deficits are much less common, occurring in 0.005% of the population. Nevertheless, both types of congenital color vision deficits need to be distinguished from acquired color vision loss. A comparison of color vision between the two eyes can be helpful, because both the type and severity of congenital color vision deficits are the same for each eye, a situation that is often not true for acquired color vision loss. In addition, congenital color vision deficits are stable over time and are almost always red/green deficits.

A comparison of the saturation of colors, between eyes and across the vertical midline, can sometimes identify subtle optic nerve dysfunction or chiasmal lesions. The same is

Table 2.2
Approximate Incidence of Congenital Color Vision Deficiencies

Type	Incidence (%)
Red-green (females)	0.4%
Red-green (males)	8%
Anomalous trichromacy	
Protanomalous (red)	1%
Deuteranomalous (green)	5%
Dichromacy	
Protanopia (red)	1%
Deuteranopia	1%
Blue-yellow (tritan)	0.005%
Monochromacy (achromats)	0.003%

Adapted from Pokorny et al., 1979, Table 7.1.

true for brightness comparisons between the two eyes and across the vertical midline. Glaser and Goodwin (4) emphasized the use of subjective color and brightness comparisons in the assessment of presumed unilateral or asymmetric optic neuropathy. Although such tests can be used to corroborate other evidence of optic neuropathy, subjective brightness differences between the two eyes as an isolated finding with an otherwise normal examination should be treated with caution.

VISUAL FIELD EXAMINATION

Examination of the visual field is one of the fundamental portions of the afferent system evaluation. A variety of visual field test procedures can be employed, including confrontation fields, the Amsler grid, the tangent (Bjerrum) screen, manual kinetic testing using a Goldmann perimeter, and automated static perimetry. When evaluating a patient with an afferent system deficit, it is important to keep in mind the advantages and disadvantages of the various procedures.

Confrontation visual fields should be part of every afferent system examination. Although testing by confrontation may lack the sophistication of modern techniques, it is the most flexible form of visual field testing, can be performed almost anywhere, and may be the only form of visual field testing that is possible. In skilled hands, confrontation testing can provide information equivalent to that obtained with more extensive forms of visual field testing, although only 1/3 of optic nerve-related defects are detected by this method (14).

The Amsler grid can be useful in identifying patients with retinal pathology. Amsler grid testing is performed at 30 cm, where each 5-mm square subtends 1° of visual angle (total extent is 20° diameter, or 10° radius). The patient is shown the Amsler grid with a black background and is told to look at the center spot and report if there is absence or distortion of the central fixation spot, if any portions of the Amsler grid are missing, and if any of the lines are wavy or bent (metamorphopsia). This type of image distortion is usually indicative of macular disease (Fig. 2.2A), whereas inability to see the central fixation point may indicate a central scotoma (Fig. 2.2B).

Tangent screen testing permits evaluation of the central

30° radius of the visual field. A 1-meter tangent screen can be placed on the wall of an examining room for easy use. It can provide more detailed, quantitative visual field information than that afforded by confrontation field testing. In the hands of a skilled perimetrist, the tangent screen examination may provide information that is equal to or better than that obtained with automated perimetric test procedures.

Sophisticated, quantitative evaluations can be achieved with kinetic testing on the Goldmann perimeter, which provides greater flexibility through close interaction between the patient and the perimetrist to obtain the most accurate responses from the patient. In children, the elderly, or patients with dementia, this may be the only form of quantitative visual field test that can be performed. The Goldmann perimeter also makes it possible to evaluate efficiently the far peripheral visual field beyond a radius of 30°. In some instances, this information can be useful in determining the extent of visual field loss and in establishing a differential diagnosis. The major disadvantages of this form of perimetry include the lack of standards and normative values and the high dependence on the skills of the perimetrist.

Automated perimetry is the most popular form of visual field testing. The major advantages of automated perimetry include standardized test procedures, age-related normal population values, and statistical analysis procedures for evaluating the data. Its major disadvantages include long testing times, high variability in areas of visual loss, inflexibility, and learning and fatigue effects.

PHOTO STRESS TEST

The differentiation between unilateral retinal disease and retrobulbar optic neuropathy may be aided using the photo stress recovery test described by Glaser et al. (15). This test is based on the principle that visual pigments bleach when exposed to an intense light source, resulting in a transient state of sensitivity loss and reduced central visual acuity. Recovery of retinal sensitivity is dependent upon regeneration of visual pigments, which is determined by the anatomic and physiologic apposition of the photoreceptors and retinal pigment epithelium. It is independent of neural mechanisms (16). Diseases that produce visual loss by damaging the photoreceptors or the adjacent retinal pigment epithelium cause a lag in regeneration of pigment, resulting in a delay in visual recovery following light stress.

The photo stress test is performed by determining best-corrected visual acuity, shielding one eye, and then asking the patient to look directly at a bright focal light held 2 to 3 cm from the eye for about 10 seconds. The time needed to return to within one line of best-corrected visual acuity level is called the photo stress recovery time (PSRT). In the study by Glaser et al. (15), PSRT in 179 normal eyes averaged 27 seconds with a standard deviation of 11 seconds. Ninety-nine percent of the normal eyes had a PSRT of 50 seconds or less. In 63 eyes with macular disease, PSRT was significantly prolonged, even when the retina appeared to be relatively normal. PSRT was relatively normal in 20 eyes with optic neuropathies. The photo stress test is especially useful in the differential diagnosis of subtle macular disease

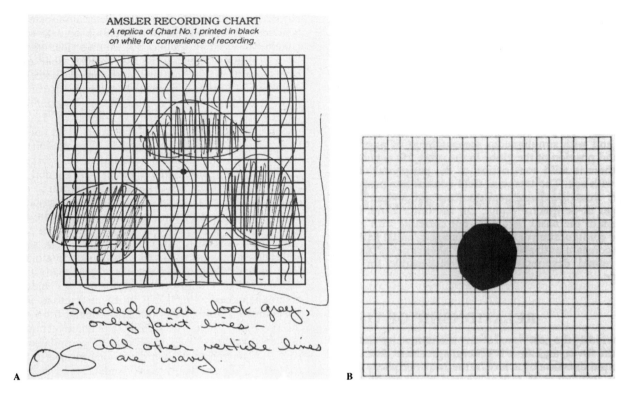

Figure 2.2. Amsler grid defects. *A,* Metamorphopsia and paracentral scotomas in a patient with a maculopathy. *B,* A small central scotoma in a patient with optic neuritis.

from subtle optic neuropathies. It may also be abnormal with severe carotid stenosis and borderline ocular perfusion.

PULFRICH PHENOMENON

In 1922, Pulfrich reported that when a small target oscillating in a frontal plane is viewed binocularly with one eye covered with a filter to reduce light intensity, the target appears to move in an elliptic path, rather than a to-and-fro path (17). When the filter is placed over the right eye, the rotation appears counterclockwise; if it is placed over the left eye, the rotation appears clockwise. The explanation for this stereo phenomenon is that the covered eye is more weakly stimulated than the uncovered eye, resulting in a delay in the transmission of visual signals to the striate cortex. This disparity in latency between eyes results in a difference in the apparent position of the target in the two eyes, thereby producing a retinal disparity cue underlying the stereoscopic effect. The magnitude of the effect is determined by the velocity of the target, the difference in retinal illumination between the two eyes, the level of retinal illumination, and the distance of the observer from the target (18).

Because optic nerve damage results in delayed transmission of impulses to the occipital cortex, patients with unilateral or markedly asymmetric optic neuropathy sometimes observe the Pulfrich phenomenon under natural viewing conditions without a filter in front of one eye (19–23). This can present difficulties for the patient driving an automobile,

mobility over uneven terrain, or with recreational activities such as tennis, volleyball, and baseball. The Pulfrich phenomenon has a similar clinical implication as a relative afferent pupillary defect.

PUPILLARY EXAMINATION

Examination of the pupils is an essential part of the afferent system evaluation. Pupil size for each eye should be noted, as should the magnitude and latency of the direct and consensual responses to light and near stimulation. The presence of a relative afferent pupil defect (RAPD) is the hallmark of a unilateral afferent sensory abnormality or bilateral asymmetric visual loss (24–26). The etiology is usually an optic neuropathy, but other abnormalities such as a central retinal artery occlusion, retinal detachment, or a large macular scar may be responsible (24–27). In the case of a retrobulbar optic neuropathy with a relatively normal-appearing fundus examination, the RAPD may be the only objective sign of anterior visual pathway dysfunction. Cataracts, refractive errors, and nonorganic visual loss do not cause a RAPD. A patient with a dense strabismic or anisometropic amblyopia (visual acuity of 20/200 or worse) may demonstrate a mild RAPD, but the clinical history will be of a long-standing visual deficit rather than a progressive or sudden onset of visual loss (28,29). Fineberg and Thompson (30) recommended quantifying the RAPD by placing graded neutral density filters over the normal or lesser affected eye until the RAPD can no longer be appreciated. The amount of neutral density filter needed is proportional to the amount of visual field loss present.

FUNDUS EXAMINATION

A fundus examination is essential for evaluating the macula, retina, nerve fiber layer, and optic nerve. This can be performed by several methods, including direct ophthalmoscopy and indirect ophthalmoscopy with a 20-diopter handheld lens. Examination of the macula with a 78- or 90-diopter handheld lens or a corneal contact lens viewed through a slit lamp may identify the cause of visual loss as being from retinal dysfunction rather than neuro-ophthalmologic disease.

Performing a fundus examination on infants and young children can be a challenge. In preparation for the examination, the parents should bring an assortment of treats for young children and plenty of feeding bottles for infants. It is best to leave the room after performing the afferent system and motility evaluations, allowing a nurse or technician to administer dilating drops to preserve your rapport with the child. In the case of infants, it is best to ask the parents to withhold a feeding bottle until you return to the room. Most infants will readily accept a bottle at this point and will be cooperative during a cycloplegic refraction and dilated fundus examination. The soporific effect of the cycloplegic drops may also cause them to fall asleep.

After completing the cycloplegic refraction, the physician should perform a dilated fundus examination using both a handheld direct ophthalmoscope and a 20-diopter lens in conjunction with an indirect ophthalmoscope, using a low level of illumination for both assessments. A lid speculum is not necessary for most pediatric neuro-ophthalmologic examinations, because the macula and optic disc are the primary areas of interest. If a child becomes uncooperative, it may be necessary for the parents to hold the child in a "lockdown" position (one parent holding the arms outstretched over the ears with the other parent holding the feet) to complete the examination. This is a stressful and difficult situation for all concerned, and all rapport with the child is gone when this occurs. If it is not possible to perform an adequate dilated examination of the infant or child, it may be necessary to conduct an evaluation with light sedation.

OTHER PROCEDURES

Other tests beyond a conventional office examination may be needed to establish the site of the pathology in the afferent visual system. Fluorescein angiography and indocyanine green angiography (ICG) may be necessary to identify retinal pathology. An electroretinogram (ERG), focal or maculoscope ERG, pattern ERG (PERG), dark adaptation, visual-evoked potential (VEP), multifocal ERG, multifocal VEP, or a combination of these tests may be needed to establish the locus of the afferent system disorder. Finally, neuroimaging with magnetic resonance (MR) imaging or computed tomographic (CT) scanning may be needed to establish the anatomic site of the afferent system abnormality.

PSYCHOPHYSICAL TESTS

Light represents a very small portion of the electromagnetic spectrum (wavelengths between 400 and 700 nm), is emitted by natural and artificial sources, and is reflected by objects in the environment, thereby serving as the stimulus for vision. Light entering the eye is first refracted by the tear film, cornea, and lens to form an inverted image on the retina. Photoreceptors convert this light energy into electric signals that are subsequently processed by neural elements in the retina, optic nerve, and higher visual centers of the brain. The relationship between the physical properties of light and perceptual and behavioral responses is known as **visual psychophysics,** which serves as the foundation for the clinical assessment of visual function.

A variety of specialized neural mechanisms are responsible for encoding motion, form, color, depth and other fundamental properties of the visual image (31–36), with new information about neural processing of visual information accumulating rapidly. Beginning at the ganglion cell level, there are three major visual processing streams whose pathways run in parallel. Ganglion cells that project to the parvocellular layers of the lateral geniculate nucleus (P-cells) are most prevalent in central vision, tend to have smaller diameter axons with lower conduction velocities, and are most effectively stimulated by low temporal frequencies and high spatial frequencies (31–34). Some P-cells respond most effectively to chromatic information whereas others have achromatic responses to luminance and contrast. The P-cell pathway appears to be primarily involved in the processing of color, form, acuity, and related functions (31–34).

Ganglion cells that project to the magnocellular layers of the lateral geniculate nucleus (M-cells) are distributed rather uniformly throughout the visual field, tend to have larger-diameter axons and higher conduction velocities, and are most effectively stimulated by high temporal frequencies and low spatial frequencies (31–34). The M-cell pathway appears to be primarily involved in the processing of motion, high-frequency flicker, and related functions. These major pathways can be further divided into more specific subgroups with distinct response properties. The M-cell and P-cell dichotomy carries through to higher visual centers, with specific projections to a large number of cortical sites that have highly specialized functions (35), although there is considerable overlap of these pathways at the cortical level (see Chapter 1). A third group of ganglion cells (37) project to the koniocellular (K-cell) intralaminer layers of the lateral geniculate nucleus and are believed to be involved in the processing of blue-yellow opponent color information.

Because these subpopulations of neural elements have such distinct response characteristics to particular visual attributes, it is possible to design psychophysical tests that isolate (or at least are dominated by) the activity of specific visual mechanisms. These psychophysical tests can thus serve as probes to evaluate different neural populations throughout the visual pathways. Early detection of eye disease, differential diagnosis of various ocular and neurologic disorders, and monitoring the efficacy of therapeutic regimens are just a few of the purposes that psychophysical tests can subserve in a clinical setting. This section provides a brief overview of some of the more common psychophysical test procedures that can be used in the clinical evaluation of patients.

VISUAL ACUITY

The most common measurement of visual function in a clinical setting is visual acuity. It is the primary method of assessing the integrity of the optics of the eye and the neural mechanisms subserving the fovea. Visual acuity is used to monitor central visual function in patients, is an essential part of clinical refraction procedures, and is important to the patient for reading (38,39), face recognition (40), and other tasks involving fine visual detail. Visual acuity is specified in terms of the visual angle subtended by the finest spatial detail that can be identified by the observer. The physical size of an object and its distance from the observer determines its visual angle.

There are three basic types of visual acuity measurements: detection acuity, resolution acuity, and identification acuity. Detection acuity is the smallest stimulus object or pattern of elements (the minimum angle of detection) that can be distinguished from a uniform field and it is primarily limited by stimulus contrast. The optics of the eye are the main factors limiting detection acuity for normal human foveal vision, producing an attenuation of contrast for small stimuli imaged on the retina (41). Resolution acuity is the smallest spatial detail that can be discriminated to permit one stimulus pattern to be distinguished from another (e.g., distinguishing horizontal from vertical stripes), and it is usually measured by grating patterns of alternating light and dark lines of varying widths. Resolution acuity also is limited by contrast.

Identification acuity, the measure used for clinical purposes, is the smallest spatial detail that can be resolved in order to recognize objects (e.g., letters of the alphabet). It is specified in terms of the Minimum Angle of Resolution (MAR), logMAR, or values such as Snellen notation or metric equivalents based on MAR. Table 2.3 presents a comparison of the various methods of designating visual acuity. For clinical visual acuity charts, the MAR is the angle subtended by the thickness or stroke of a letter, with the overall height and width of the letter typically being five times larger than the thickness. Figure 2.3 presents an example of a typical

Table 2.3
Visual Acuity Notation Systems

Distance (feet)	Snellen	Ditance (meters)	Metric	MAR (minutes)	LogMAR	Cycles/ Degree
10	20/10	3.0	6/3	0.50	−0.3	60.0
12	20/12	3.6	6/3.8	0.60	−0.2	50.0
16	20/16	4.8	6/4.8	0.80	−0.1	38.0
20	20/20	6.0	6/6	1.00	0.0	30.0
25	20/25	7.5	6/7.5	1.25	0.1	24.0
30	20/30	9.0	6/9	1.50	0.2	20.0
40	20/40	12.0	6/12	2.00	0.3	15.0
50	20/50	15.0	6/15	2.50	0.4	12.0
60	20/60	18.0	6/18	3.00	0.5	10.0
80	20/80	24.0	6/24	4.00	0.6	7.5
100	20/100	60.0	6/60	5.00	0.7	6.0
200	20/200	120.0	6/120	10.0	1.0	3.0
400	20/400	240.0	6/240	20.0	1.3	1.5

MAR = minimum angle of resolution.

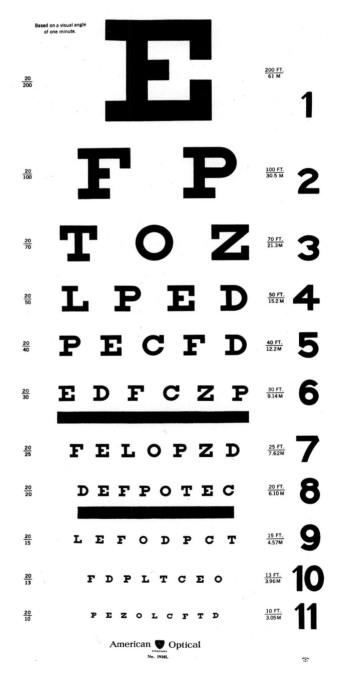

Figure 2.3. An example of a standard eye chart for visual acuity testing.

eye chart used for clinical evaluation of visual acuity. This design is essentially the same as that introduced by Snellen in 1862, and the most common form of reporting visual acuity is still in terms of "Snellen notation," consisting of a fraction in which the numerator is the testing distance (20 feet or 6 meters) and the denominator is the distance at which a "normal" observer is able to read the letter (42). By definition, a visual acuity of 20/20 (6/6) refers to a MAR of one minute of arc letter thickness. A 20/60 (6/18) visual acuity letter therefore has a thickness corresponding to 3 minutes of arc and is 15 minutes of arc high and wide. The standard of 20/20 for "normal" vision was developed more than 100 years ago, and with today's high contrast eye charts and better light sources, normal best-corrected visual acuity for persons under the age of 50 is 20/16 or better (43) (Fig. 2.4).

Another type of visual acuity chart is known by various names, including the Early Treatment for Diabetic Retinopathy Study (ETDRS) chart, the Bailey-Lovie chart, and the logMAR chart (44,45) (Fig. 2.5). This chart has several advantages over the standard Snellen chart. First, the letters used are equally detectable for normal observers. Second, each line has an equal number of letters. Third, the spacing between letters is proportional to the letter size. Fourth, the change in visual acuity from one line to another is in equal logarithmic steps. Fifth, better specification of visual acuity with either Snellen notation, MAR or logMAR values can be achieved. Also, new methods of scoring responses can be implemented that produce greater sensitivity and reliability (46,47).

The measurement of visual acuity in special populations (e.g., young children and physically challenged persons) is not always possible with a standard letter chart. Testing of central visual function of infants begins with an assessment of how well the infant fixes and follows the examiner's face, a small toy, or other objects of interest. For older children, the "Tumbling E Cube" can be used for visual acuity testing. This cube is a white block with black E letters of different sizes on each of its sides. By rotating the cube, an individual E can be presented in four different orientations to test the patient's ability to distinguish the direction of the E. The cube can be placed at various distances from the patient, and different-sized E targets can be evaluated to make a determination of visual acuity. The Tumbling E Cube thus relies on a child's ability to orient the hand according to the direction of the E. For older children the "E game" can be performed using a projected "E" acuity chart. The "HOTV" test, a simplification of the older Sheridan-Gardiner test (48), involves matching each test letter to one of four letters (H, O, T, or V) printed on a card held by the child. Some visual acuity tests use pictures or symbols (49). These may be more reliable than the HOTV test. The most popular of the picture visual acuity tests are the Allen Cards (50). Projector slides with the familiar cake, bird, telephone, and other pictures are also available. Other devices like the B-VAT vision tester can generate many random sequences of characters and figures to avoid memorization by the child.

"Preferential-looking" techniques, oculomotor responses such as optokinetic nystagmus, and electrophysiologic measures such as the VEP can also be used to estimate visual acuity (51–54). In addition, a number of eye charts and behavior test procedures can be used to assess visual acuity in nonverbal or physically challenged patients (55). These tests utilize patterned stimuli and caricatures of faces (e.g., Mr. Happy Face) or common objects with "critical detail" (e.g.,

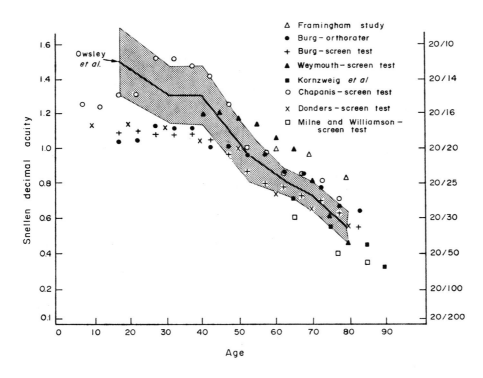

Figure 2.4. Population normal scores for visual acuity across ages (43). Note that normal visual acuity is 20/16 or better up to age 50.

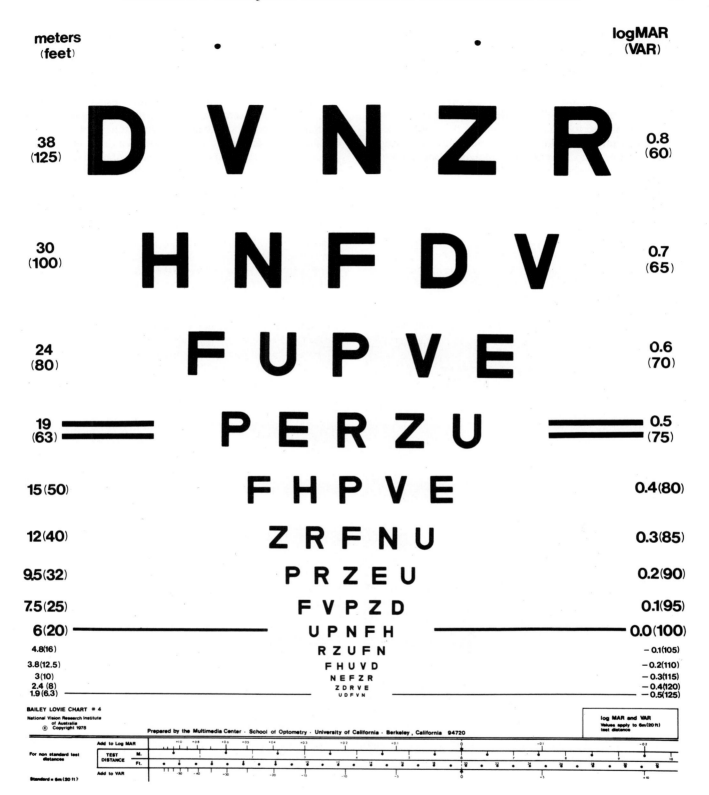

Figure 2.5. An example of the Bailey-Lovie logMAR visual acuity chart.

Cheerios) that can be used to obtain an indication of the individual's level of visual acuity.

Visual acuity measurements in children present special problems, in part because the child wants to do well and please the examiner. It is therefore important for the examiner to ensure that the non-tested eye is properly occluded to avoid peeking (Fig. 2.6). The examiner must work quickly, may need to use more than one procedure to establish visual acuity capabilities, and should continually provide positive feedback to the child to maintain cooperation.

In patients suspected of having nonorganic visual loss, several additional methods of assessing visual acuity may be useful (11). The Tumbling E cube can be used as a cross-check of the eye chart visual acuity determination (e.g., a patient that can see the 20/200 E on the eye chart at 20 feet

should be able to see an E that is five times smaller at a distance of 4 feet, because they subtend the same visual angle). By moving the cube from one distance to another, the consistency of visual acuity responses can be ascertained. If this is done quickly, it is extremely difficult for a patient with nonorganic visual loss to maintain consistent responses (i.e., select appropriate target sizes for different distances to maintain a constant visual angle). Often the patient will pick the same physical target size, irrespective of the distance at which it is presented (11).

A helpful device that can be used to test patients with suspected nonorganic monocular visual acuity loss is a cross-Polaroid projection chart (the American Optical Vectograph Project-O-Chart slide). This consists of a projector eye chart that is combined with polarizing material. The left or right

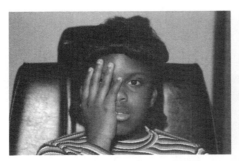
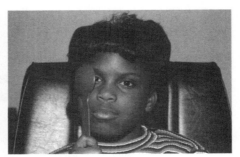
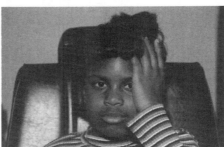
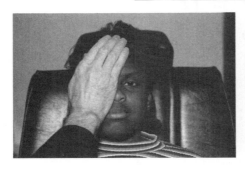
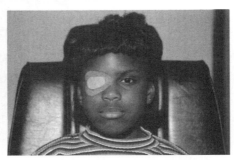

Figure 2.6. Peeking techniques that may be used by children whose visual acuity is being tested and techniques to avoid this problem. *Top left,* the examiner is attempting to test vision in the left eye. The child is supposed to be covering the right eye with her fingers, but the fingers are spread, allowing her to view with the right eye. *Top right,* the examiner is attempting to test vision in the left eye. The child is supposed to be covering the right eye with an occluder but is holding the occluder to one side, allowing her to view with the right eye. *Middle,* the examiner is attempting to test vision in the right eye. The child is supposed to be covering the left eye with the palm of her hand but is holding the hand to one side, allowing her to view with the right eye. *Bottom left,* the examiner uses his or her own hand to occlude one of the child's eyes. In this way, the examiner can be certain that the child is viewing with only one eye. *Bottom right,* using a patch to occlude one eye is the optimum technique for testing monocular visual function.

half of the eye chart is projected through horizontally polarized material, and the other half is projected through vertically polarized material. The patient views the chart wearing a pair of glasses with polarized material that has different orientations over the two eyes (e.g., horizontal left eye polarization, vertical right eye polarization). Thus, one eye sees only the left half of the eye chart, and the other eye sees only the right half. The chart is viewed by the patient with both the "good" eye and the "bad" eye open. Patients with nonorganic visual loss in one eye will often read all of the eye chart, even though the "good" eye can only see half of the chart. Another portion of the American Optical Vectograph slide has randomly arranged visual acuity letters (ranging from 20/20 to 20/40) that can be seen with the left eye only, the right eye only, or with both eyes. This is especially useful in patients with nonorganic monocular visual acuity loss.

In normal observers, visual acuity is highest for the foveal region and decreases rapidly with increasing visual field eccentricity (Fig. 2.7). Randall et al. (56) evaluated visual acuity from the fovea out to 20° along the horizontal meridian of 27 normal subjects and compared their results with data obtained from 30 subjects with central scotomas of varying sizes. The results from the patients with central scotomas were similar to those of normal observers viewing the stimuli at an eccentricity corresponding to the edge of a patient's scotoma. For example, visual acuity dropped from approximately 20/20 to 20/40 at an eccentricity of 2.5° nasal to the fovea and was reduced to 20/120 for an eccentricity of 10° from the fovea (Fig. 2.8).

In many instances, central visual field loss and reduced visual acuity appear to be closely related. However, visual acuity can also be reduced when there is generalized depression of the central visual field and no scotoma is apparent. There are also several conditions for which the visual field

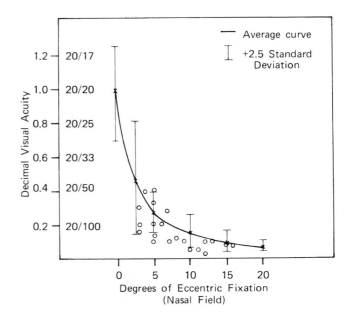

Figure 2.8. The relationship of visual acuity and visual field in patients with experimental (x) and actual (o) central scotomas. (From Randall HG, Brown J, Sloan LL. Peripheral visual acuity. Arch Ophthalmol 1966; 75:500–504.)

may be at or near normal sensitivity, but visual acuity may be dramatically reduced. These conditions include refractive errors, corneal surface irregularities, cataract, retinal edema or serous detachment, and amblyopia. Frisén (57) noted that patients with a "median chiasmal syndrome" have subnormal visual acuity despite perimetric evidence of disturbed conduction only in crossing fibers (temporal field defects). The explanation for these findings is unclear but probably emphasizes the relative insensitivity of conventional visual field testing for some forms of damage to the visual system.

CONTRAST SENSITIVITY

Visual acuity defines the smallest spatial detail that can be resolved for high-contrast stimuli, but it does not specify the responses of the visual system to objects of different sizes and contrasts. Measurement of the spatial contrast sensitivity function (CSF) is necessary to obtain this information. The CSF is most commonly determined by measuring contrast thresholds for sinusoidal gratings, an alternating pattern of light and dark bars with luminance that varies sinusoidally in a direction perpendicular to orientation of the grating. The size of the grating is specified according to spatial frequency, which is the number of cycles (pairs of light and dark bars) of the grating pattern per degree of visual angle. Typically, between 3 and 10 spatial frequencies from 0.5 to 30 cycles per degree are measured for the CSF. Contrast is defined by the luminance of the peaks (Lmax) and troughs (Lmin) of the sinusoidal grating, according to the equation:

$$Contrast = \frac{Lmax - Lmin}{Lmax + Lmin}$$

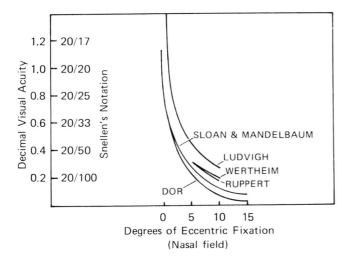

Figure 2.7. Reduction in visual acuity with visual field eccentricity. The graph presents a composite of results obtained by various investigators. (From Randall HG, Brown J, Sloan LL. Peripheral visual acuity. Arch Ophthalmol 1966;75:500–504.)

Contrast can vary from a minimum of 0 for a uniform field (Lmax = Lmin) to a maximum of 1 (Lmin = 0). A contrast threshold is the minimum amount of contrast needed to detect the presence of the grating, and contrast sensitivity is the reciprocal of the contrast threshold (sensitivity = 1/threshold).

There are several advantages of using sinusoidal gratings to evaluate the CSF. First, blur does not change the shape or appearance of sinusoidal gratings, other than to reduce contrast. Second, the CSF provides a means of characterizing the overall response properties of the visual system to a wide variety of visual images. The CSF may be considered the visual counterpart of an audiogram (58). The audiogram specifies the minimum amount of sound energy necessary to detect pure tones (temporal sinusoidal waveforms) for various frequencies of pitch. This information can then be used to determine an individual's ability to hear complex sounds. In a similar fashion, the spatial CSF for vision makes it possible to determine an individual's ability to process spatial information from complex visual scenes. Fourier analysis demonstrates that any complex waveform can be decomposed into a series of sine waves of various frequencies, amplitudes, and phase (position) relationships (59). Thus, any complex visual scene can be broken down into a specific combination of sinusoidal distributions of light of different spatial frequencies, amplitudes, and phases in the vertical and horizontal dimensions. It should be emphasized, however, that the CSF describes the behavior of the visual system at **threshold** contrast levels, which is not completely representative of the visual system's characteristics for processing suprathreshold contrast information (60).

A number of factors influence the measurement of the normal CSF, including background adaptation luminance (61–63), stimulus size (64,65), visual field eccentricity (66–68), pupil size (69,70), temporal characteristics (62,71), stimulus orientation (72,73), and various optical factors such as defocus, dioptric blur, diffusive blur, and astigmatism (70,71). The CSF can be used to evaluate optical properties of the human eye, including refractive error and defocus (70,71), corneal disease (74), cataract (75), refractive surgery (76), intraocular lenses (77), and the normal aging properties of the optics of the eye (78,79). Contrast sensitivity deficits sometimes occur in patients with normal visual acuity and optical conditions that produce subtle changes in the quality of their vision.

CSF losses occur in patients with retinal conditions such as diabetic retinopathy (80), age-related macular degeneration (81), and a variety of other disorders. Foveal contrast

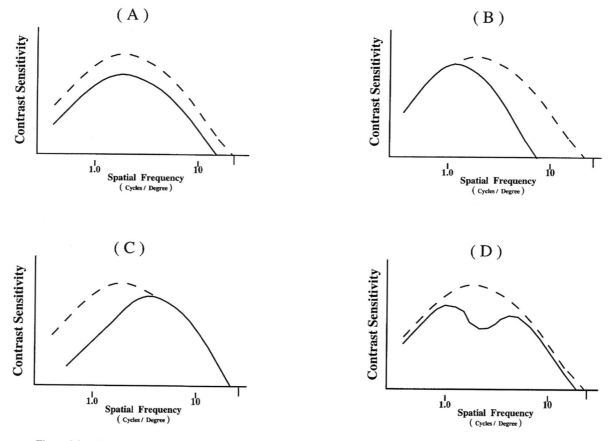

Figure 2.9. Examples of the various types of contrast sensitivity loss: generalized depression (*A*); high spatial frequency loss (*B*); low spatial frequency loss (*C*); middle spatial frequency loss (*D*).

sensitivity deficits also occur in patients with glaucoma (82–84).

From a neuro-ophthalmologic standpoint, measurement of the CSF can reveal subtle deficits in patients with optic neuritis and multiple sclerosis (85,86) *as well as* in patients with a variety of other optic neuropathies and cerebral abnormalities (86–89), amblyopia (90), and other conditions such as Alzheimer's disease (91) and Parkinson's disease (86).

In general, the CSF is clinically useful for detecting early or subtle visual loss (especially when visual acuity is normal), making comparisons between the two eyes, or for monitoring the progression or improvement of visual function. One of the shortcomings of the CSF, however, is that sensitivity losses have little specificity for differential diagnostic purposes. The main patterns of contrast sensitivity loss are (*a*) generalized contrast sensitivity loss at all spatial frequencies; (*b*) greater high spatial frequency contrast sensitivity loss; (*c*) greater low spatial frequency contrast sensitivity loss; and (*d*) a "notch" produced by contrast sensitivity loss for a particular group of spatial frequencies (Fig. 2.9). Generalized and high-frequency contrast sensitivity deficits are by far the most common patterns of loss across a wide variety of pathologic ocular conditions.

The CSF can be measured in infants and young children using either electrophysiologic or behavior techniques (92) and can provide valuable clinical information about the functional visual status in such individuals. The CSF also may be helpful in predicting the performance for various daily tasks, such as the identification of distant objects (93), reading highway signs (94) and books (95), recognizing faces (96), and mobility (97). Thus, the CSF is not only useful for revealing subtle visual deficits associated with ocular disorders but is also helpful in identifying problems that a patient is likely to encounter during daily activities.

Contrast sensitivity may be measured with wall charts in a manner similar to the way in which visual acuity is typically measured. One of these methods uses the Vistech chart (98). This chart has a series of five rows (A–E), each with a different spatial frequency. Each row consists of a group of nine circular targets containing a sinusoidal grating that is either vertical, tilted to the left, or tilted to the right. From the left side of the chart to the right, there is a successive reduction in the contrast of the grating. Patients are positioned 10 feet from the chart and are asked to read each row from left to right by indicating the orientation of the grating.

A second method of testing contrast sensitivity utilizes the typical letter charts for testing visual acuity, but there is a low contrast between the letters and the background. Regan and Neima (99,100) developed a series of visual acuity charts at several different contrast levels. Although normal observers show a small reduction in visual acuity for low contrast targets (about two lines), patients with early or subtle abnormalities sometimes demonstrate quite profound reductions in visual acuity for low contrast targets compared with high contrast letters. Thus, this approach to contrast sensitivity testing can reveal mild disturbances of visual sensory function not detectable by standard visual acuity testing. The advantage of a low contrast acuity chart is that it uses a test procedure that is highly familiar to most patients and clinicians.

A third method of testing contrast sensitivity using a chart was introduced by Pelli et al. (101) and is called the Pelli-Robson chart (Fig. 2.10). The Pelli-Robson chart consists of letters of a fixed size that vary in contrast. Each line consists of six letters, with the three left-most and three right-most letters having the same amount of contrast. The patient reads the chart in a manner similar to a standard visual acuity chart, and the minimum contrast at which the letters can be detected is recorded. This method of testing contrast sensitivity is highly reproducible (102) and is capable of detecting disturbances in visual function that are not evident with standard visual acuity testing. The Optic Neuritis Treatment Trial (103) used the Pelli-Robson charts for evaluation of contrast sensitivity as an outcome measure for comparison of treatment groups.

The use of sinusoidal gratings versus low contrast letters for the measurement of contrast sensitivity is controversial. A number of arguments support each approach (104–106). It is also important to note that different results are sometimes obtained by the two procedures. Under certain stimulus conditions, normal observers can demonstrate different contrast sensitivity characteristics for gratings versus letters (107), and patients with certain visual disorders can also produce different contrast sensitivity values for gratings versus letters under standard clinical testing conditions (108).

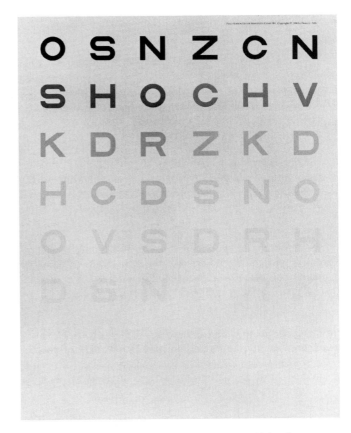

Figure 2.10. The Pelli-Robson contrast sensitivity chart.

PERIMETRY AND VISUAL FIELD TESTING

General Principles

Perimetry and visual field testing have been clinical diagnostic test procedures for more than 150 years. Although instrumentation and testing strategies have changed dramatically over this time, the basic principle underlying conventional perimetry has remained the same. Detection sensitivity is determined for a number of locations throughout the visual field using a small target presented against a uniform background. The loss of sensitivity at various visual field locations serves as a noninvasive marker for identifying pathology or dysfunction of the visual pathways. The ability of perimetry to provide helpful clinical information has been responsible for its long-term use as a diagnostic procedure. Because perimetry can provide information about both the likely anatomic locus and disease process or processes for afferent system abnormalities, it remains a vital part of the neuro-ophthalmologic evaluation.

Perimetry and visual field testing fulfill several important diagnostic functions:

1. **Early detection of abnormalities.** Because many ocular and neurologic disorders are initially expressed as sensitivity loss in the peripheral visual field, perimetry is an important factor in identifying early signs of afferent system dysfunction. Perimetry is typically the only clinical procedure that evaluates the status of the afferent visual pathways for locations outside the macular region.
2. **Differential diagnosis.** The spatial pattern of visual field deficits and comparison of patterns of visual field loss between the two eyes also provide valuable differential diagnostic information. Not only can this information be helpful in defining the location of damage along the visual pathways, it can also assist in identifying the specific type of disease that has caused the damage.
3. **Monitoring progression and remission.** The ability to monitor a patient's visual field over time is important for verifying a working diagnosis, establishing whether a condition is stable or progressive, and evaluating the effectiveness of therapeutic interventions.
4. **Revealing hidden visual loss.** Perhaps the most important role subserved by perimetry is the ability to find afferent visual pathway loss that may not be apparent to the patient. Changes in foveal visual function are typically symptomatic. Peripheral vision loss, on the other hand, can often go unnoticed, especially if it is gradual and monocular. Visual field screening of 10,000 California driver's license applicants was performed, and nearly 60% of individuals with peripheral visual field loss were unaware that they had any vision problem (109). Paradoxically, even though a patient may be unaware of peripheral visual field loss, it can significantly affect the performance of daily activities such as driving (109–112), orientation, and mobility (97).

Perimetry and visual field testing are therefore important in identifying visual abnormalities that might not otherwise be detected by either a history or other parts of a standard eye examination.

In this section, we present a brief description of the psychophysical basis for perimetry, the various methods for performing visual field testing, and some helpful guidelines for interpreting test results. It is not intended to be a comprehensive treatment of perimetry, however, and the interested reader is directed to several excellent sources for a more detailed account of perimetric techniques and other related topics (113–124).

Some form of visual field testing should be performed on all patients, particularly those at greater risk of having visual field loss: (a) patients over the age of 60; (b) individuals with high myopia, elevated intraocular pressure, diabetes, vascular disease, systemic disease, family history of glaucoma or other eye disease, or other risk factors for development of ocular or neurologic disorders; (c) individuals with visual symptoms or complaints, but minimal findings on their eye examination; and (d) individuals with significant problems involving orientation and mobility, balance, driving, night vision and related activities. It is not feasible or necessary to perform a long quantitative visual field examination on all patients. However, a confrontation visual field or brief tangent screen evaluation should be performed as part of a standard neuro-ophthalmologic examination. When more sensitive measurements of the visual field are needed, automated static perimetry or manual kinetic perimetry can be performed.

Manual perimetry with the Goldmann perimeter has many advantages. Since the perimetric stimulus presentation is done by a human, subjects can be cheered on or cajoled into performing. When the perimetrist senses subject fatigue, a rest break is given. Unlike the fixed, 6° spaced grid of conventional automated perimetry, Goldmann perimetry has custom test point locations along with improvisation of strategies based on coexisting findings. Specific exploration strategies can be used for individual concerns. This allows for much more accurate mapping of defect shape. This can be invaluable for the topographic localization of visual field defects. However, manual perimetry is less sensitive than conventional automated perimetry and it may be more time-consuming. Its most severe limitation, though, is that many perimetrists are not adequately trained (125). This may be worse than no perimetry at all.

Automated perimetry has had a dramatic impact on improving the quality of care for patients with ocular disorders. Automatic calibration of instruments, standardized test procedures, high sensitivity and specificity, reliability checks (''catch trials''), and quantitative statistical analysis procedures are some of the many advantages of this method of perimetry; however, there are also disadvantages of automated perimetry, including prolonged test time, increased cognitive demands, fatigue, and lack of flexibility for evaluating difficult patient populations. We believe that there is no single method of visual field testing that is best for all circumstances and all patients. Automated perimetry is but one of many tools that the clinician can use to evaluate peripheral visual function, and the various forms of visual field testing should be regarded as **complementary** techniques, the utility and appropriateness of which are determined by the clinical circumstances and the question that is being addressed. There is no single method of data representation, analysis procedure, visual field index, or other method of evaluating visual field data that provides all of the essential clinical information. It is important to consider all of the information available, including reliability characteristics and the subjective clinical interpretation of the visual field. In addition, it should be kept in mind that although the test may be automated, the patient is not. It is unreasonable to begin an automated visual field test, leave a patient alone in a dark room, and expect the patient to remain alert, energetic, attentive, interested, and to maintain proper alignment and fixation throughout the test procedure. Some patients require periodic rest breaks, encouragement, and personal contact to perform visual field examinations in a reliable manner. It is also important to insure that proper test conditions, refractive characteristics, and other factors have been properly established before initiating the examination. Visual field testing can be a powerful clinical diagnostic tool when these factors are kept in mind.

Psychophysical Basis For Perimetry and Visual Field Testing

The primary psychophysical concept underlying perimetry and visual field testing is the increment or differential light threshold. The increment threshold (Weberian contrast) is the minimum amount of light that must be added to a stimulus (gdL) to make it just detectable from the background (L). At very low background luminances, the amount of light needed to detect a stimulus is constant. At higher background luminances, the increment threshold increases in direct proportion to the background luminance, e.g., a doubling of the background luminance requires a doubling of the stimulus luminance for detection. This relationship, which holds over a large range of background luminance levels, is known as Weber's law, in honor of the German scientist who initially described it (126).

The standard background luminance used by most perimetric devices is 31.5 apostilbs (asb), or 10 cd/m^2. This is in the range of background luminance levels for which Weber's law is valid. There are several advantages to the use of this background luminance level: (a) it is close to the ambient lighting conditions found in offices and waiting rooms, requiring a minimal amount of adaptation time; (b) the background luminance is one that is comfortable for most patients; (c) patients have the least amount of response variability at this background luminance; and (d) factors affecting the amount of light reaching the retina (pupil size changes, ocular media transmission loss, etc.) have an equal effect on the background and stimulus luminance. Thus, over the range of background illuminances for which Weber's law holds, these changes in retinal illumination will not affect the increment threshold measure.

Increment threshold determinations are usually made at a number of visual field locations during quantitative perimetry. For a normal visual field, the increment threshold varies as a function of visual field location. Visual field results are

usually represented in terms of sensitivity, the reciprocal of threshold (sensitivity = 1/threshold). At the 31.5 asb background luminance, the fovea has the highest sensitivity and is able to detect both the dimmest and the smallest targets. Sensitivity drops rapidly between the fovea and 3° decreases gradually out to 30°, and then drops off more rapidly again beyond 50° (Fig. 2.11). The characteristic three-dimensional representation of the visual field sensitivity profile is often called the "hill of vision" or an "island of vision in a sea of blindness." In addition to eccentricity-dependent changes in the slope of the visual field profile, the temporal visual field (to the right of the foveal peak) extends farther than the nasal visual field, and the inferior visual field extends farther than the superior visual field. The location of the blind spot, approximately 15° temporal to the foveal peak, is indicated in most representations by a darkened vertically oval area.

Visual field sensitivity can be affected by many different stimulus attributes, including background luminance

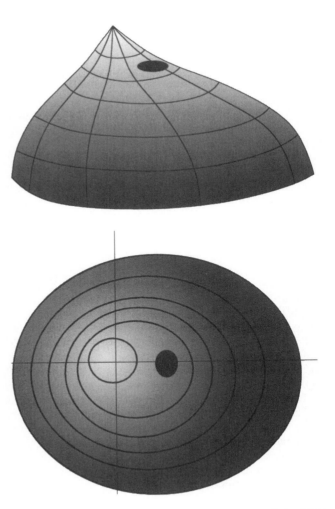

Figure 2.11. Three-dimensional representation of the normal visual field represented as a hill of vision. Sensitivity is plotted as a function of visual field eccentricity.

(113,115,127), stimulus size (113,115,128–130), stimulus duration (113,115,131), chromaticity (132–136), and other factors (113,115). Of these parameters, stimulus size is the most important for clinical perimetry. Next to stimulus luminance, it is the most common method of adjusting the detectability of perimetric stimuli. Not only does a change in stimulus size affect the overall sensitivity to light, but the slope of the sensitivity profile is also changed (113,115). Small targets produce steeper sensitivity profiles, and larger targets result in a flatter sensitivity profile, especially for the central 30–40° eccentricity. Response variability is also reduced as stimulus size is increased (130).

Certain patient characteristics that are not associated with ocular or neurologic pathology can also influence the increment or differential light threshold. Blur and refractive error (137), media opacities such as cataract (138), ptosis (139), and pupil size (140,141) can affect visual field sensitivity characteristics. In addition, procedural circumstances related to trial lens rim obstructions (142), fixation instability (143), response errors (144–146), and other artifacts of testing can produce the appearance of visual field loss or can obscure visual field deficits that are actually present.

Cognition, attention, and other higher-order functions in patients undergoing visual field testing can influence visual field sensitivity, as well as attention, practice, and learning (147–151). Fatigue effects can reduce visual field sensitivity (152–154), particularly after the test procedure has taken more than 5–7 minutes of testing. Patients with visual field loss typically demonstrate greater fatigue effects than those with normal perimetric function, and this may be especially true for some conditions such as optic neuritis (155,156).

Techniques For Perimetry and Visual Field Testing

Visual field examinations have been conducted for over 150 years and, as a consequence, a variety of procedures and techniques have been developed. Perimetry and visual field test procedures may be categorized in several different ways: (a) the amount of information obtained by the test, i.e., screening versus quantitative; (b) the type of stimulus used to perform the test (kinetic, static, or suprathreshold static); and (c) the manner in which the test is administered (manually vs. computer-driven). There are both advantages and disadvantages for each method. Automated perimetry, for example, provides greater standardization, calibration, and statistical analysis of results than manual visual field testing, but it is less efficient, less flexible, and too demanding for some patients. Kinetic perimetry, when performed appropriately, is a more efficient method of performing an evaluation of the full visual field than static perimetry and the technique can yield exquisite information about defect shape, but the technique varies from one test to another. Quantitative procedures provide a better ability to detect subtle anomalies and monitor changes over time, but they are more time-consuming than screening procedures and may cause fatigue in some patients.

Confrontation Visual Fields

Confrontation visual field examination is rapid, reliable, and easy to perform. It is tailored to the clinical situation.

Most examiners test patients monocularly using double simultaneous finger counting to survey the visual field for any dense quadrantic defect. Finger counting is followed by a test of the central visual field to evaluate for the presence of relative visual field defects. One such test is to have the subject look at the examiner's face and report any difference from the expected. Another is to use two red objects and compare perception of the two eyes or parts of the visual field. Unfortunately, for optic nerve-related visual field defects, finger confrontation identifies only about 10% of defects while bedside color techniques yield defects in about one-third of patients with abnormalities on formal perimetry (157). Color confrontation techniques fare better with chiasmal defects, detecting about three-quarters of patients (157). Even by combining seven confrontation visual field tests, only about half of perimetrically identified defects are found (158). Therefore, formal perimetry is usually necessary when the patient has visual loss not explained by a general ophthalmologic examination.

Confrontation visual field techniques for infants and children can be quite challenging (Fig. 2.12). Because of their adaptive abilities, children may demonstrate good mobility skills and fool the examiner as to the extent of visual field loss. For infants and young children, a visually mediated startle response can be used to detect hemianopic defects and other substantial defects in the peripheral field. A child who sees a startle stimulus will look in that direction. For older children, finger mimicking or a "Simon says" game can be used to evaluate the peripheral visual field. The child mimics the examiner by holding up the same number of fingers he or she observes. "Finger puppet perimetry" can be performed, with one puppet used to direct central fixation and the other puppet used as a peripheral stimulus for saccadic eye movements. A story with dialogue between the puppets is used to redirect attention from one puppet to the other.

In many instances, simultaneous comparison of color saturation or brightness of stimuli between hemifields or between the two eyes is useful in distinguishing subtle anomalies. When the stimuli are presented in a double simultaneous fashion to the right and left of fixation, it is possible to detect homonymous defects. Subtle deficits across the vertical midline can be detected by asking the patient to indicate which of the two test objects is clearer or brighter. In addition, double simultaneous presentation can be used to detect the phenomenon of visual extinction—the lack of awareness of an object in a seeing area of the visual field when other seeing areas of the visual field are stimulated simultaneously. Confrontation visual field testing is also useful in evaluating patients suspected of having nonorganic visual field loss (11).

The obvious advantages of confrontation visual field testing include its simplicity, flexibility, speed of administration, and ability to be performed in any setting, including at the bedside. The disadvantages of confrontation visual field testing include the lack of standardization, the qualitative nature of the results, and the limited ability to detect subtle deficits and monitor progression or remission of visual loss. Because it is quick and easy to perform, confrontation visual

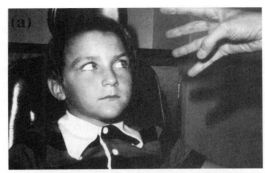

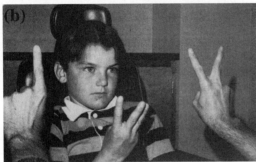

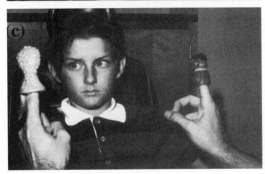

Figure 2.12. Examples of confrontation visual field testing in children using the startle response (*a*); finger counting (*b*); and finger puppets (*c*).

field should be performed on all patients, regardless of their visual complaints.

Amsler Grid

Mark Amsler developed a series of charts, specifically designed to qualitatively analyze the disturbances of visual function which accompany the beginning and evolution of maculopathies. The charts are a series of lined and patterned grids that test the central visual field within 10° of fixation when the plates are held at 1/3 of a meter from the eyes (159). Each square of the grid subtends 1° of visual angle, making the ability to define the location of small defects rather easy. The patient is asked to fixate a central spot on the grid, using one eye at a time, and is asked if he or she can see the spot. If not, the patient's finger can be placed on the center to help fixation. The patient is then asked to point out any regions in which the lines are missing, blurred, distorted, bent, or irregular.

This technique is well known to ophthalmologists who routinely examine patients with known or suspected macular disease, because Amsler grids can be used to identify and plot small scotomas and other visual field defects that occur with macular scars, mild macular degeneration, central serous chorioretinopathy, and related disorders. It is perhaps less well recognized that small central or paracentral scotomas that occur with optic nerve disease can also be identified with these plates. The Amsler grid (Fig. 2.2) is particularly useful for identifying small central scotomas and other subtle central visual disturbances that are difficult to detect with more sophisticated automated and manual perimeters. Here, patients report missing areas rather than metamorphopsia. The grid can be dimmed in various ways to increase the sensitivity of detection of these small scotomas (160). The Amsler grid is very quick and easy to administer. Its main disadvantages are related to the qualitative, subjective nature of the information derived from the test.

Tangent (Bjerrum) Screen

The central visual field can be studied in detail using a tangent or Bjerrum screen. The screen is made of black felt or other black matte material and can be mounted on the wall or hung from the ceiling. The screen has several concentric circles and radial lines imprinted on it to provide a reference for the examiner. A dark wand with circular targets of various sizes and colors mounted on the end is used to examine the central visual field, usually within 30° of fixation. In its most common application, testing is performed at a distance of 1 meter, and a light source is employed to provide a relatively uniform illumination of 7 foot-candles on the screen. Targets are specified in terms of their diameter, their color, and the testing distance in millimeters. For example, a 1-mm-diameter white target used with the patient located 1 meter from the tangent screen would be designated as 1/1000W, and a 5-mm red target used with the patient located 2 meters from the screen would be designated as 5/2000R.

A kinetic technique is usually performed to test the visual field during a tangent screen examination. The patient fixates a central target, and a stimulus is slowly moved from the periphery towards the center of the screen along a particular meridian until the patient reports detection of the stimulus. By repeating this procedure along different meridians, a contour of equal sensitivity—an **isopter**—can be plotted (Fig. 2.13). The use of several different target sizes generates several different isopters and creates a map of visual field sensitivity. Scotomas, areas of low sensitivity or non-seeing areas surrounded by normal visual field regions, are also plotted. A well-performed kinetic tangent screen examination can detect subtle defects and provide quantitative information for the central visual field that is comparable to that obtained by more sophisticated automated procedures.

Suprathreshold static visual field screening can also be accomplished with the tangent screen. Using targets that are white on one side and black on the other, the wand can be rotated to present and then extinguish the stimulus at key locations throughout the visual field. The target size employed is typically one that can be readily detected by per-

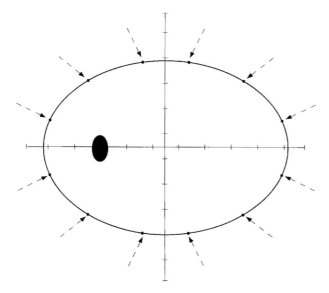

Figure 2.13. An example of an isopter generated by kinetic perimetric testing. (From Johnson CA. Perimetry and visual field testing. In Zadnik K, ed. The Ocular Examination. Philadelphia, WB Saunders, 1996.)

sons with normal visual fields. In this manner, it is possible to quickly determine whether or not visual field abnormalities are present.

The main advantages of the tangent screen are its flexibility (i.e., variable distance from the patient, different colored

objects, single versus multiple stimuli used simultaneously), speed, and ease of use. Varying the distance of the patient from the screen can be helpful in differentiating organic from nonorganic constriction of the visual field (Fig. 2.14). The main disadvantages are the strong dependence of results on the skill and technique of the perimetrist, the lack of standardization, difficulty in monitoring the patient's fixation while performing the visual field examination, and the need to establish age-related population norms.

Goldmann Manual Projection Perimeter

The Goldmann perimeter is a white hemispheric bowl of uniform luminance (31.5 asb) onto which a small bright stimulus is projected. It is generally used to perform kinetic perimetry, although static and suprathreshold static perimetry can also be tested with this perimeter. Unlike the Amsler grid and tangent screen, the Goldmann perimeter can be used to evaluate the entire visual field. With one eye occluded, the patient fixates a small target in the center of the bowl, and the perimetrist monitors eye position by means of a telescope. A particular stimulus size and luminance is projected onto the bowl, the target is moved from the far periphery toward fixation at a constant rate of speed, typi-

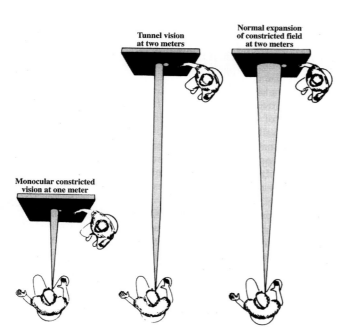

Figure 2.14. A demonstration of physiologically invalid tunnel vision ("tubular vision") associated with nonorganic visual field loss, and the normal cone-shaped expansion of the normal visual field as testing distance is increased. (From Beck RW, Smith CH. The neuro-ophthalmologic examination. Neurol Clin 1983;1:807–830.)

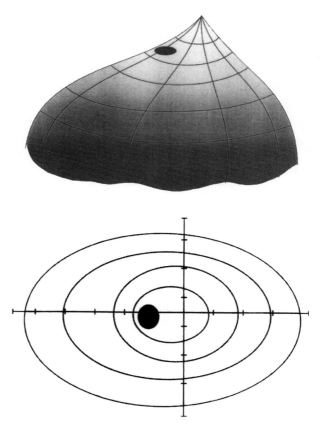

Figure 2.15. Representation of kinetic perimetry results (*below*) compared with three-dimensional hill of vision (*above*). (From Johnson CA. Perimetry and visual field testing. In Zadnik K, ed. The Ocular Examination. Philadelphia, WB Saunders, 1996.)

cally 4–5° per second (161), and the patient is instructed to press a response button when he or she first detects the stimulus. The location of target detection is noted on a chart, and the process is repeated for different meridians around the visual field. Isopters and scotomas are plotted in a manner similar to that described for the tangent screen examination, except that both the target size and luminance can be adjusted to vary stimulus detectability. This process produces a two-dimensional representation of the hill of vision that is basically a topographical contour map of the eye's sensitivity to light (Fig. 2.15). Kinetic testing (at least 1 or 2 isopters) on the Goldmann perimeter can be performed in cooperative children as young as 5 or 6 years of age.

Static Perimetry

Static perimetry uses a stationary target, the luminance of which is adjusted to vary its visibility. Although it can be performed manually using either the Goldmann or Tübinger

perimeters, it is most often performed with an automated perimeter such as the Humphrey Field Analyzer or the Octopus perimeter. Measurements of the increment threshold are obtained at a variety of visual field locations that are usually arranged in a grid pattern or along meridians. A bracketing or staircase procedure may be used to measure threshold sensitivity, although new techniques such as SITA (162–164) and ZEST (165–167) use Bayesian forecasting methods.

The **SITA** method uses two maximum likelihood visual field models: normal and glaucoma. The likelihood of a set of data is the probability of obtaining that set of data, given the chosen probability distribution model (in this case either a normal or glaucoma model). The models are based on the fact that the slope of the frequency-of-seeing curves (variability) increases with threshold. Figure 2.16 shows the two models. Log likelihood is on the y-axis and threshold (intensity) on the x-axis. At the beginning of the test, there is a

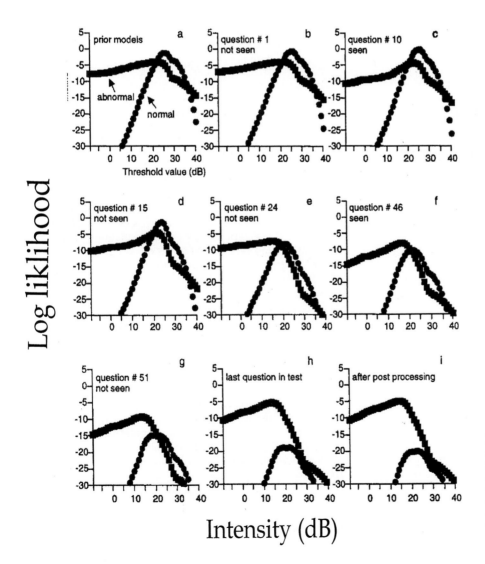

Figure 2.16. Visual field models for normal and glaucoma test results and their change during the perimetry test using SITA. As the test continues, the maximum likelihood model is updated based on the results at the tested location and surrounding correlated locations. In this example, the glaucoma model gradually becomes the most likely model at the end of the test.

likelihood that the test location results are either normal or abnormal. As the test continues, the model is updated until the threshold is estimated with the given level of confidence. To reduce test time, the SITA-FAST algorithms interrupt the threshold even earlier. However, this reduction in test time is at the expense of accuracy and variability.

Introduction of the SITA algorithm resulted in a 50% reduction in test time. Thresholds are 1 to 2 db higher than with the use of the full staircase (full threshold) method. The shortening of test time is likely the result of a combination of less patient fatigue and interruption of the staircase procedure before threshold is reached. The algorithm has been so successful in cutting down test time that full threshold testing has largely been replaced. However, the efficacy of SITA for serial examinations to detect change has not yet been validated.

The presentation of visual field sensitivity for grid patterns is typically a gray scale representation (Fig. 2.17A), rather than the three-dimensional ''hill of vision'' that is produced during kinetic perimetry. Areas of high sensitivity near the peak of the hill of vision are denoted by lighter shading and areas of low sensitivity by dark shading. Determinations

along meridians are usually represented by a sensitivity profile plot (Fig. 2.17B).

The major advantages of automated static perimetry are standardization of test conditions, quantitative visual field measurements, a normative database, statistical analysis procedures, and automatic calibration. The major disadvantages include a lengthy amount of time required for testing, limited flexibility, the need for additional testing space, and a high variability in areas of visual field damage.

Both static and kinetic perimetry are quantitative procedures that require a considerable amount of testing time. **Suprathreshold static perimetry** is a procedure that is faster than quantitative techniques and is typically used for screening purposes. There are a number of variations in test procedures, strategies, and theoretical bases for suprathreshold static perimetry (113,123,168). The basic technique, however, is that stimuli that can be easily detected by persons with normal peripheral vision are presented at specific locations throughout the visual field. These locations are selected to evaluate areas that are frequently affected by various ocular or neurologic disorders that damage the visual pathways (e.g., glaucoma, chiasmal tumors). Locations at which the target is seen are denoted by one symbol and locations where the target is not seen are denoted by another.

Interpretation of Visual Field Information

A large amount of visual field information is derived from perimetric testing, especially from automated perimetry. Test conditions and stimulus parameters used, indicators of patient reliability and cooperation, physiologic factors (pupil size, refractive state, visual acuity, etc.), summary statistics and visual field indices, and other items are presented in conjunction with sensitivity values for various locations in the patient's visual field. Visual field sensitivity can also be represented in many different forms (numerical values, deviations from normal, gray scale representations, probability plots, etc.). The following discussion presents a brief overview of the various types of information provided on the final printed outputs. Because of its current popularity and widespread use, this discussion and most of the examples are derived from automated static perimetry. However, some examples of kinetic testing using the Goldmann perimeter are presented for certain clinical cases, especially for situations in which kinetic testing provides more information about visual field status.

There is no single type of data representation or item of visual field information that provides a sufficient or complete description of visual field properties. All of the available information from the output needs to be evaluated in order to properly interpret the results. Just as the results from individual components of a standard eye exam need to be combined to render an appropriate impression and diagnosis, consideration of all of the individual components of perimetry must be considered in order to properly appreciate the findings.

Graphic Representation of Visual Field Data

In most instances, the numeric representation of visual field information, whether by means of summary values such

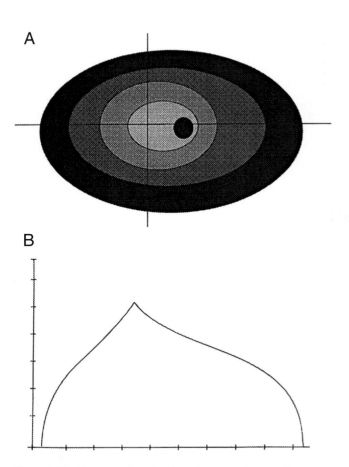

Figure 2.17. Representation of static perimetry results according to gray scale (A) and profile sensitivity plots (B).

as visual field indices or by sensitivity values for individual visual field locations, is difficult to interpret. A graphic representation of visual field data makes it easier to evaluate, particularly for detecting specific patterns of visual field loss or for assessing progression or other visual field changes over time. There are three primary methods of graphically representing visual field data: isopter/scotoma plots, profile plots, and gray scale plots (Fig. 2.18).

Ancillary

Several important pieces of information that should be checked on each visual field examination are the position of the eyelids, the refractive correction used for testing, pupil size, and visual acuity. Ptosis can produce a superior visual field defect that may be minimal or significant (Fig. 2.19A). High refractive corrections (greater than 6-diopter spherical equivalent) can sometimes produce trial lens rim artifacts (Fig. 2.19B). When a patient's spherical equivalent correction for perimetric testing exceeds 6 diopters, it is advisable

to use a soft contact lens correction that is appropriate for the testing distance to avoid lens rim artifacts. Proper near refractive corrections that are appropriate for the near testing distance of the perimeter bowl and the patient's age must be used to minimize the likelihood of refraction scotomas and sensitivity reductions from blur (Fig. 2.19C). Small pupils (less than 2 mm diameter) can produce spurious test results, especially in older persons who may have early lenticular changes. If pupil size is small, the patient should be dilated to 3 mm or greater (Fig. 2.19D). Finally, the patient's visual acuity can also provide useful information when assessing generalized visual field sensitivity loss and the potential sources responsible for the loss.

Reliability Indices

The quality of information obtained from perimetry and visual field testing depends on a patient's cooperation, willingness, and ability to respond in a reliable fashion and maintain a consistent response criterion. It is important to have

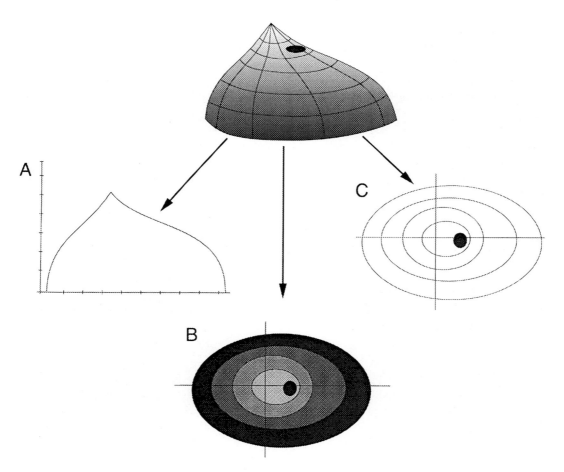

Figure 2.18.   A comparison of the various graphic methods of representing visual field data: profile plot (*A*); gray scale plot (*B*); isopter/scotoma plot (*C*).

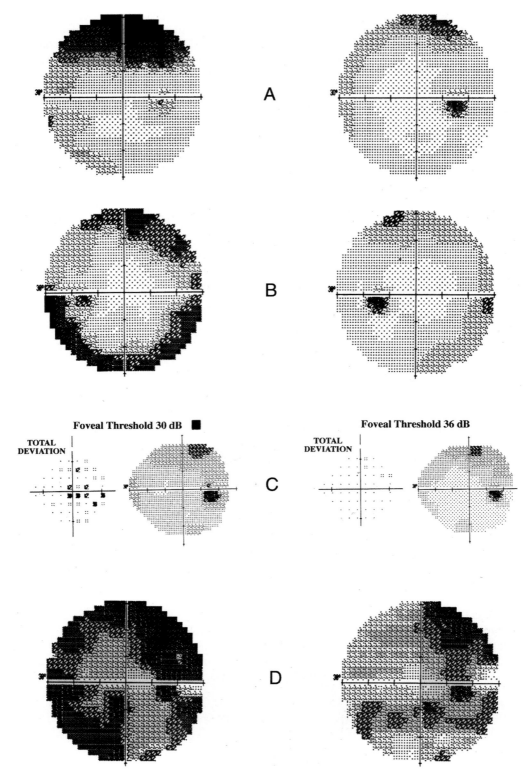

Figure 2.19. Influences on visual field test results. *A,* An example of visual field results for ptosis before (*left*) and after (*right*) taping up the upper lid and brow. *B,* Example of trial lens rim artifact (*left*) and its disappearance (*right*) after realigning the patient. *C,* Refractive error introduced by improper lens correction (*left*) and results after proper lens was employed (*right*). *D,* Visual field results obtained in the same eye with a 1 mm (*left*) and a 3 mm (*right*) pupil diameter.

an assessment of patient reliability and consistency in order to properly evaluate the significance of visual field information. With manual perimetry, it is possible to monitor the patient's fixation behavior directly by means of a telescopic viewer. The use of "catch" trials has been as an index of patient response reliability. False-positive errors (responses when no stimulus is presented) and false-negative errors (failure to respond to a stimulus presented in a region previously determined to be able to detect equal or less detectable targets) can be monitored throughout the test procedure.

Automated test procedures not only have the capability of monitoring false-positive errors, false-negative errors, and fixation behavior in the same manner as described above, but also can obtain an assessment of response fluctuation by retesting a sample of visual field locations. Also, indirect indicators of fixation accuracy (e.g., whether or not a patient responds to a target presented to the physiologic blind spot) can be monitored. An additional advantage of automated test procedures is that these **reliability indices** (false positives, false negatives, fixation losses, short-term fluctuations) can be immediately compared with those of age-adjusted normal control subjects, thereby providing an indication as to whether or not the patient's reliability parameters are within normal population characteristics.

Some of the reliability indices for automated perimetry are not always accurate indicators of a patient's true performance. For example, false-negative rates are correlated with visual field deficits, i.e., there is an increase in false-negative responses with increased field loss (144). Thus, high false-negative rates may be more indicative of disease severity than of unreliable patient responses. Excessive fixation losses can be caused by factors such as mislocalization of the blind spot during the initial phases of testing, misalignment or head tilt of the patient midway through testing, or inattention on the part of the technician administering the visual field examination. Also, one should be careful not to consider reliability indices as a replacement for technician interaction and monitoring of patients. Some patients are uncomfortable when left alone in a darkened room during automated perimetry testing. In addition, misalignment of the patient, drowsiness, and related factors can occur during testing and go undetected if the patient is not adequately monitored. It is important to remember that it is the test procedure that is automated, not the patient.

Although reliability indices are helpful in determining if the visual field is accurate, they are not sufficient to eliminate the possibility that a visual field defect is nonorganic in nature. It has been shown that both patients and otherwise normal subjects can "fool" the automated perimeter, producing a variety of abnormal fields despite maintaining reliability indices that are within normal limits (169–171).

Visual Field Indices

A distinct advantage afforded by automated perimeters is the ability to provide summary statistics, usually called **visual field indices**. The Mean Deviation (MD) on the Humphrey Field Analyzer and the Mean Defect (MD) on the Octopus perimeters refer to the average deviation of sensitivity at each test location from age-adjusted normal population values. They provide an indication of the degree of generalized or widespread loss in the visual field. The Pattern Standard Deviation (PSD) on the Humphrey Field Analyzer and the Loss Variance (LV) on the Octopus perimeter present a summary measure of the average deviation of individual visual field sensitivity values from the normal slope after correcting for any overall sensitivity differences, i.e., MD. They represent the degree of irregularity of visual field sensitivity about the normal slope and therefore indicate the amount of localized visual field loss, because scotomas produce significant departures from the normal slope of the visual field. Corrected Pattern Standard Deviation (CPSD) and Corrected Loss Variance (CLV) take into account the patient's short-term fluctuation (STF) during testing. STF is derived by testing a sample of ten locations twice to determine the average deviation of repeated measures. This correction minimizes the influence of patient variability on the local deviation measures. Note that CPSD and STF are not evaluated by the SITA test algorithm.

Probability Plots

Another advantage of automated static perimetry is that a patient's test results are compared with age-adjusted normal population values. Thus, it is possible to determine the amount of deviation from normal population sensitivity values on a point by point basis for all visual field locations tested. A useful means of expressing this information is by means of **probability plots**. The Humphrey Field Analyzer has two methods of presenting this type of information. One is called the "Total Deviation Plot" and the other is called the "Pattern Deviation Plot." For the Total Deviation Plot, each visual field location has one of a group of different symbols indicating whether the sensitivity is within normal limits, or is below the 5, 2, 1, or 0.5% of normal limits, respectively. In other words, visual field locations or indices that have a probability corresponding to p less than 1% mean that this value is observed less than 1% of the time in a normal population of the same age. This provides an immediate graphic representation of the locations that are abnormal and the degree to which they vary from normal levels.

The Pattern Deviation Plot is similar to the Total Deviation Plot, except that the determinations are performed after the average or overall sensitivity loss has been subtracted, thereby revealing specific locations with **localized** deviations from normal sensitivity values. The value of these representations is twofold. First, they provide an immediate indication of the locations with sensitivity loss. Second, the comparison of the Total and Pattern Deviation Plots provides a clear indication of the degree to which the loss is diffuse or localized. If the loss is predominantly diffuse, the abnormal locations will appear on the Total Deviation Plot, but all or most of these locations will be within normal limits on the Pattern Deviation Plot (Fig. 2.20*A*. If the deficit is predominantly localized, the Total and Pattern Deviation Plots will

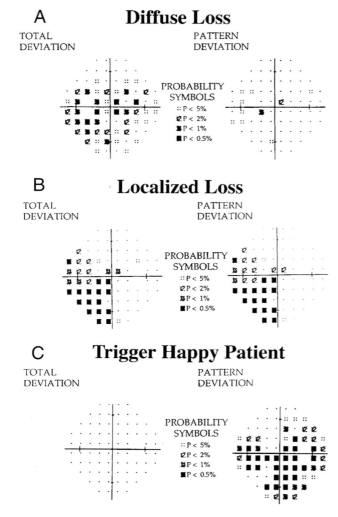

Figure 2.20. Examples of diffuse loss (*A*), localized loss (*B*), and "trigger happy" (*C*) patient results as they are depicted on the Total Deviation and Pattern Deviation probability plots for the Humphrey Field Analyzer.

look almost identical (Fig. 2.20*B*). The degree of similarity between the Total and Pattern Deviation Plots thus gives an indication of the proportion of loss that is diffuse and localized. In a few instances, the Total Deviation Plot may appear to be normal, but the Pattern Deviation Plot reveals a number of abnormal locations (Figs. 2.20*C* and 2.21). This occurs when the patient's measured sensitivity is significantly better than normal, and it is most often caused by a patient who presses the response button too often ("trigger happy").

Progression of Visual Field Loss

The determination of whether a patient's visual field improves, worsens, or remains stable over time is the most difficult aspect of visual field interpretation. Although there are several quantitative analysis procedures available for evaluating visual field progression, none of them enjoys

complete acceptance by the clinical ophthalmic community (172). Nevertheless, the use of quantitative statistical analysis procedures may be helpful in monitoring a patient's visual field status.

There are several important factors to consider when evaluating a patient's visual field status over time. First, it is necessary to examine the test conditions that were present for each visual field examination. If different test strategies, target sizes or other test conditions are different from one examination to another, it is difficult to compare the results, because the type of test procedure and the stimulus size (and characteristics) can significantly alter the appearance of the visual field (Figs. 2.22 and 2.23). Second, it is important to determine if there are any differences in patient conditions from one visual field to another. If there are meaningful differences in pupil size, refractive corrections, visual acuity, time of day, or other factors (e.g., upper lid taped on one occasion and not on another occasion), this can have a dramatic effect on the visual field results obtained on different visits (Fig. 2.19). Third, unless the visual field changes are dramatic, it is important to base judgments of visual field progression or stability on the basis of the entire series of visual fields that are available. It is not possible to distinguish subtle visual field changes from long-term variation on the basis of two visual fields (e.g., comparing the current visual field to the previous visual field). In particular, patients with moderate to advanced visual field loss can sometimes exhibit considerable variations from one visual field to another. Also, factors such as fatigue and experience can produce significant differences in visual field characteristics (147–154). If it is suspected that a change in visual field loss has occurred, it is best to repeat the examination on a separate visit to confirm the suspected change. Depending on which part of the sequence and which eye is examined, any two successive visual fields can reflect apparent improvement, progression, or stability of the visual field.

Five-Step Approach to Visual Field Interpretation

One of the common errors that occur in visual field interpretation is the lack of attention to details and specific patterns of visual field loss before obtaining a global evaluation of the visual field. To avoid this tendency, we suggest a simple five-step approach to visual field interpretation:

1. Determine if the visual field is normal or abnormal for each eye separately. Automated perimetry results provide assistance with this task, because they show both point-by-point and summary comparisons of the patient's test results with age-matched normal population values. If both eyes are normal, both in terms of statistical comparison and clinical assessment, then further evaluation is not necessary. However, subtle visual field loss can sometimes be present despite visual field indices that are within normal limits. Perhaps the most common of these occurrences are the subtle vertical steps in the superior visual field that may reflect an early bitemporal chiasmal lesion.

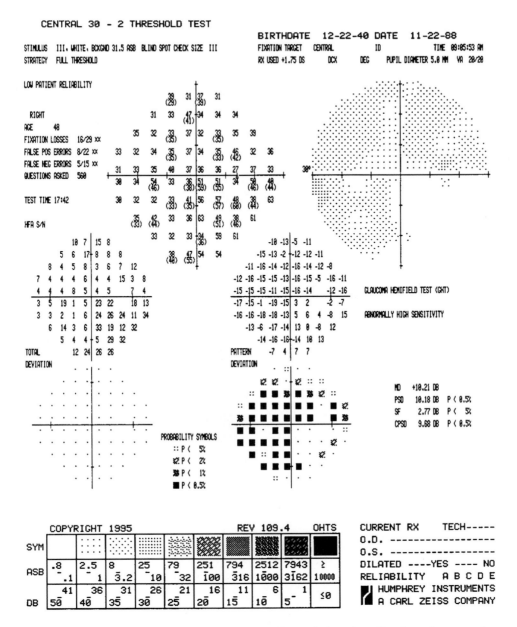

CENTRAL 30 - 2 THRESHOLD TEST

STIMULUS III, WHITE, BCKGND 31.5 ASB BLIND SPOT CHECK SIZE III
STRATEGY FULL THRESHOLD

BIRTHDATE 12-22-40 DATE 11-22-88
FIXATION TARGET CENTRAL ID TIME 09:05:53 AM
RX USED +1.75 DS DCX DEG PUPIL DIAMETER 5.0 MM VA 20/20

LOW PATIENT RELIABILITY

RIGHT

AGE 48
FIXATION LOSSES 16/29 xx
FALSE POS ERRORS 8/22 xx
FALSE NEG ERRORS 5/15 xx
QUESTIONS ASKED 560

TEST TIME 17:42

HFA S/N

GLAUCOMA HEMIFIELD TEST (GHT)

ABNORMALLY HIGH SENSITIVITY

TOTAL DEVIATION

PATTERN DEVIATION

MD +10.21 DB
PSD 10.18 DB P < 0.5%
SF 2.77 DB P < 5%
CPSD 9.68 DB P < 0.5%

PROBABILITY SYMBOLS
:: P < 5%
P < 2%
P < 1%
■ P < 0.5%

	COPYRIGHT 1995					REV 109.4			OHTS
SYM									
ASB	.8 .1	2.5 1	8 3.2	25 10	79 32	251 100	794 316	2512 1000	7943 3162	≥ 10000
DB	41 50	36 40	31 35	26 30	21 25	16 20	11 15	6 10	1 5	≤0

CURRENT RX TECH-----
O.D. -------------------
O.S. -------------------
DILATED ----YES ---- NO
RELIABILITY A B C D E
HUMPHREY INSTRUMENTS
A CARL ZEISS COMPANY

Figure 2.21. An example of automated static perimetry results from a ''trigger happy'' patient who presses the response button too often and inappropriately.

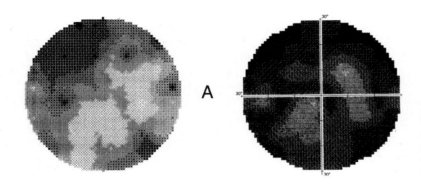

A

Figure 2.22. Examples of different fields obtained when patients with a field defect are tested with different strategies on an automated perimeter or with different perimeters. *A*, A patient with an optic neuropathy who was tested on two different automated perimeters. Note marked difference in results. *(Figure continues.)*

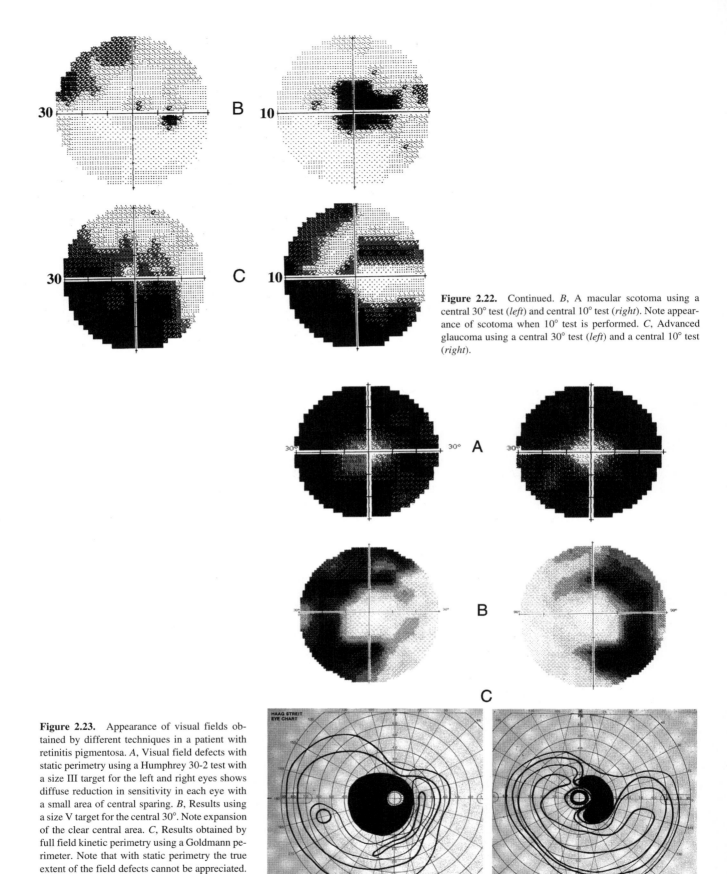

Figure 2.22. Continued. *B*, A macular scotoma using a central 30° test (*left*) and central 10° test (*right*). Note appearance of scotoma when 10° test is performed. *C*, Advanced glaucoma using a central 30° test (*left*) and a central 10° test (*right*).

Figure 2.23. Appearance of visual fields obtained by different techniques in a patient with retinitis pigmentosa. *A*, Visual field defects with static perimetry using a Humphrey 30-2 test with a size III target for the left and right eyes shows diffuse reduction in sensitivity in each eye with a small area of central sparing. *B*, Results using a size V target for the central 30°. Note expansion of the clear central area. *C*, Results obtained by full field kinetic perimetry using a Goldmann perimeter. Note that with static perimetry the true extent of the field defects cannot be appreciated. With kinetic perimetry the scotomatous nature of the defects can be appreciated.

2. If one or both visual fields are abnormal, examine the ancillary information to determine if proper test conditions were employed, the appropriate near correction was used (based on the patients' age, distance refraction, and whether or not they were cyclopleged), and the pupil size was sufficiently large. Also, check for patterns of visual field loss that are indicative of a trial lens rim artifact, a droopy upper eyelid, or other nonpathologic conditions that may account for the visual field loss. Fatigue, drowsiness, and related conditions can also produce apparent visual field loss. It is crucial that the person who performs the perimetric testing, especially with automated perimetric tests, be attentive to these factors. A surprising number of visual field deficits can be attributed to nonpathologic influences.

3. Determine if the visual field is abnormal in both eyes or

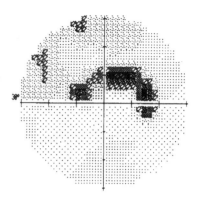

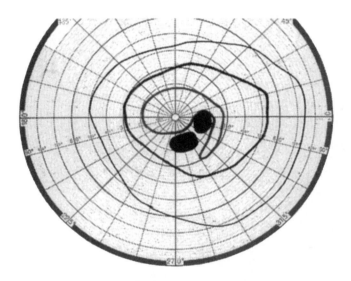

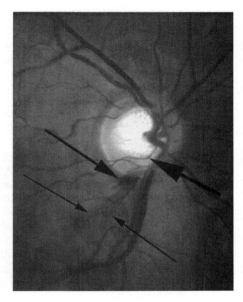

Figure 2.25. Humphrey visual field (*top*) and corresponding fundus photo (*bottom*) from a patient with low tension glaucoma in the right eye. Note moderate cupping (*large arrow*), small peripapillary nerve fiber layer hemorrhage (*medium arrow*), and wedge-shape nerve fiber layer defect (*thin arrows*) that corresponds to the superior arcuate field defect detected by perimetry.

in only one eye. If the visual field is abnormal in only one eye, the defect is almost always caused by a disorder anterior to the optic chiasm (Figs. 2.24–2.27). If the visual field of both eyes is abnormal, it means that the deficit is at or posterior to the optic chiasm (Figs. 2.28–2.30) **or** that the patient has bilateral intraocular or optic nerve disease (Figs. 2.31–2.33).

4. Determine the general location of the visual field loss for each eye independently. Specifically, determine if the visual field loss is in the superior or inferior hemifield, the nasal or temporal hemifield, or the central portion of the field. This is especially important for the nasal and temporal hemifield assessment. If the loss is extensive, determine where the **greatest** amount of visual field loss is present. If the visual field loss is bitemporal and respects the vertical midline, then a chiasmal locus should

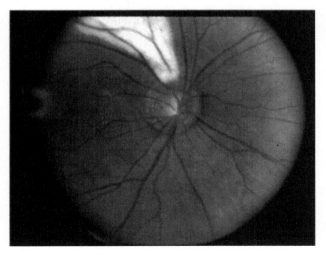

Figure 2.24. Monocular field loss in a patient with myelinated nerve fibers in the right eye. Kinetic visual field testing, performed on the Tübinger perimeter (*top*), shows an inferior arcuate scotoma that corresponds to the area of myelinated nerve fibers in the superior arcuate region (*bottom*).

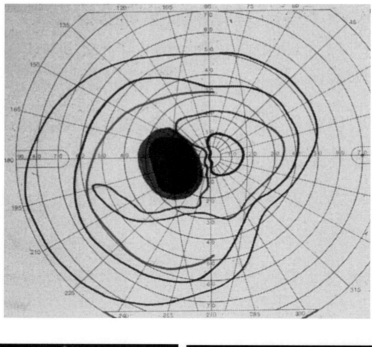

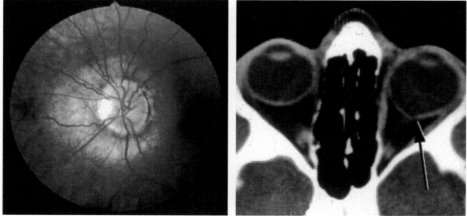

Figure 2.26. Unilateral visual field defect in the left eye of a patient with a peripapillary staphyloma. *Top,* Visual field of the left eye shows marked enlargement of the physiologic blind spot. *Bottom left,* Appearance of left ocular fundus. *Bottom right,* Axial computed tomographic scan shows ovoid enlargement of posterior aspect of the left globe (*arrow*). The patient's visual acuity in this eye was 20/20.

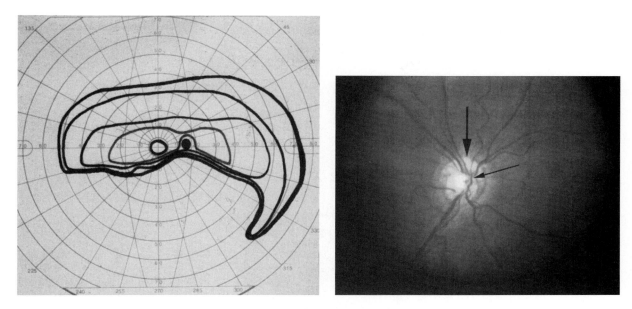

Figure 2.27. Unilateral visual field defect in a patient with segmental hypoplasia of the right optic nerve. Visual acuity was 20/20 in the eye. *Left,* Kinetic perimetry using a Goldmann perimeter shows marked inferior altitudinal defect that does not obey the horizontal midline. Note preservation of the central field to small isopters. *Right,* Fundus photograph shows absence of the upper part of the disc substance. The *thin arrow* indicates the location of the optic disc and the *thick arrow* indicates the scleral crescent.

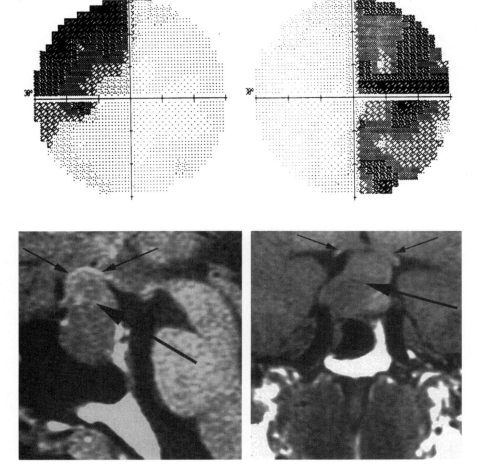

Figure 2.28. Bilateral visual field defect in a patient with a tumor in the region of the optic chiasm. *Top,* Static perimetry reveals a bilateral temporal hemianopia, worse in the right eye (*right*). *Bottom,* Sagittal (*left*) and coronal (*right*) T1-weighted magnetic resonance images show a large mass in the sella turcica with suprasellar extension (*large arrows*). The mass compresses and elevates the optic chiasm (*small arrows*).

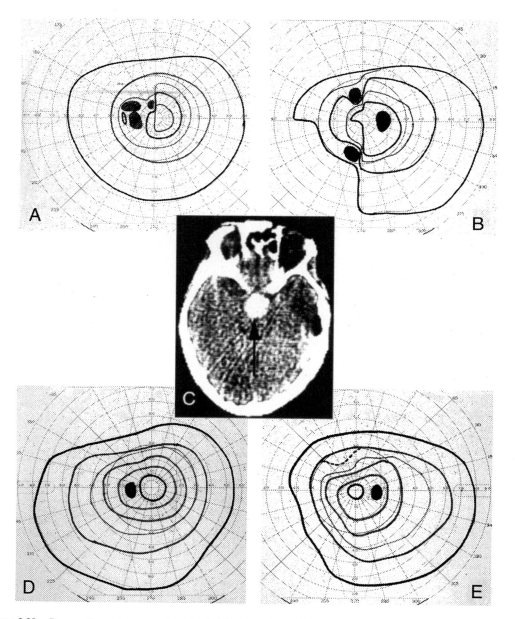

Figure 2.29. Preoperative and postoperative visual fields in a patient with a craniopharyngioma. *A and B*, Kinetic perimetry reveals an incomplete incongruous left homonymous hemianopia. *C*, Axial computed tomographic scan shows an enhancing lesion in the suprasellar region. *D and E*, Marked improvement in visual fields following removal of the tumor. The homonymous field defect resulted from compression of the right optic tract by the mass.

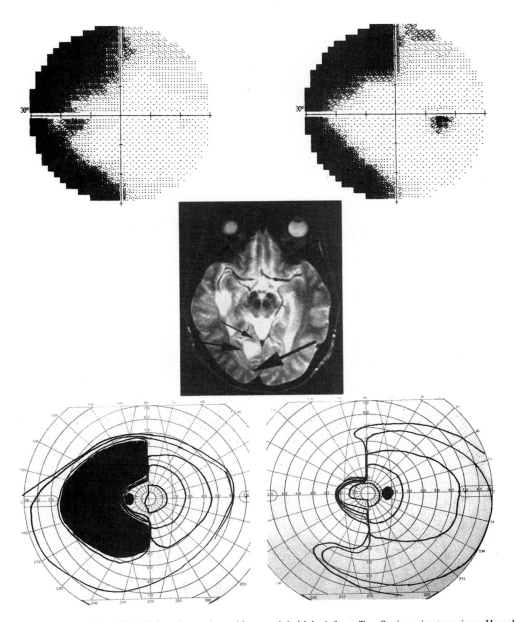

Figure 2.30.   Bilateral visual field defects in a patient with an occipital lobe infarct. *Top,* Static perimetry using a Humphrey visual field analyzer shows a left homonymous field defect with macular sparing. *Middle,* T2-weighted axial magnetic resonance image shows a hyperintense region consistent with an infarct (*medium arrow*) in the right occipital lobe. Note normal appearance of the posterior aspect of the right occipital lobe (*thick arrow*), corresponding to the macular sparing. In addition, the deep portion of the calcarine fissure (*thin arrow*), which has only monocular representation and is responsible for the temporal crescent, also appears normal. *Bottom,* Kinetic perimetry confirms a left homonymous hemianopia with macular sparing and sparing of the temporal crescent of the visual field of the left eye.

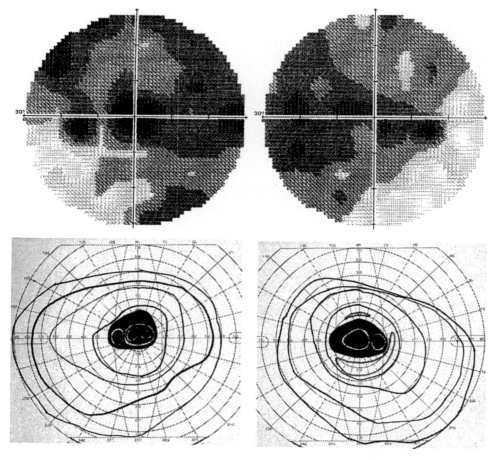

Figure 2.31.   Bilateral visual field defects in a patient with a progressive retinal cone dystrophy. *Top,* Static perimetry shows dense central field defects with extension toward the periphery. *Bottom,* Kinetic perimetry demonstrates dense central scotomas with sparing of the peripheral visual field of both eyes.

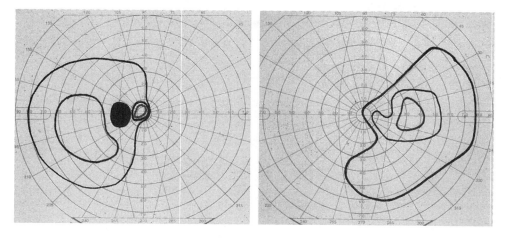

Figure 2.32.   Bilateral visual field defects in a patient with pseudotumor cerebri. Kinetic perimetry demonstrates complete loss of the nasal visual field of both eyes, with involvement of the temporal fields as well. *(Figure continues.)*

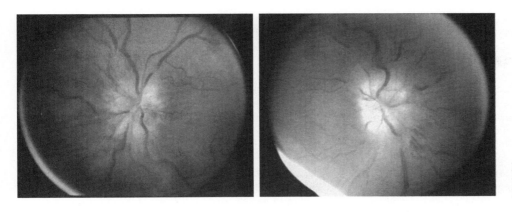

Figure 2.32. Continued. Fundus photographs show bilateral chronic papilledema with early atrophy.

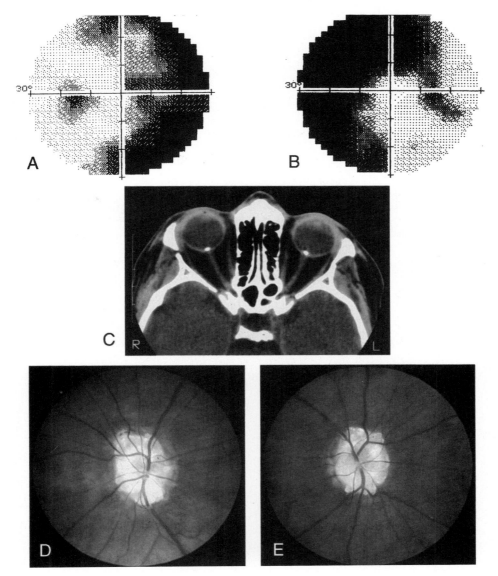

Figure 2.33. Bilateral visual field defects in a patient with bilateral optic disc drusen. *A and B*, Static perimetry reveals significant nasal field loss in both eyes. *C*, Axial computed tomographic scan set at bone window density shows calcified drusen. *D and E*, Fundus photographs show extensive optic disc drusen. Note absence of visible nerve fiber layer and constriction of retinal arteries.

be strongly suspected, especially if the deficit is in the superior temporal quadrant in each eye (Fig. 2.34). If the visual field loss is nasal in one eye and temporal in the other eye (i.e., homonymous), then a retrochiasmal location should be suspected (Fig. 2.35). Binasal defects or a nasal deficit in only one eye should generate a suspicion of glaucoma, various nonglaucomatous optic neuropathies, or certain types of retinal disorders (Figs. 2.36 and 2.37). A central deficit in one or both eyes may indicate a macular disorder (especially if the visual field defect does not connect to the blind spot) or an optic neuropathy (Figs. 2.38 and 2.39). With this simple step, a **global** view of visual field properties is generated, and a hierarchy of potential locations of damage along the visual pathway and probable disease entities is hypothesized.

5. Look at the specific shapes, patterns, and features of the visual field loss (Figs. 2.40–2.43 and Table 2.4). Does the defect respect either the horizontal or vertical meridians? What is the shape of the deficit (arcuate, oval, circular, pie-shaped, irregular)? Does the deficit ''point'' to the blind spot or to fixation? If there is visual field loss in both eyes, is it congruous or incongruous, symmetric between the two eyes, or asymmetric? Do the edges of the defect have a steep or a gradual sloping profile? These and other specific features of the visual field should provide confirmatory information for the location of the damage determined by Step 4 or allow one to differentiate among several possible alternative locations. However, it should not be used as the initial basis for generating a hypothesis about location of damage. Attention to

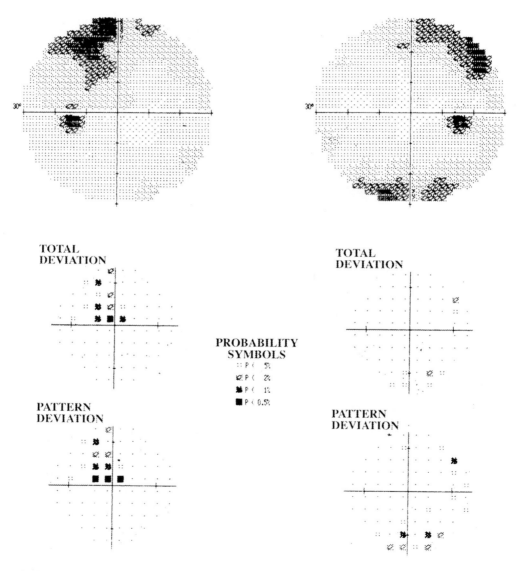

Figure 2.34.   Mild superior bitemporal field defect in a patient with 20/20 vision in both eyes. The gray scale representation demonstrates the superior temporal deficit respecting the vertical meridian in both eyes, although the probability plots do not show the deficit in the right eye. The patient was found to have a pituitary adenoma.

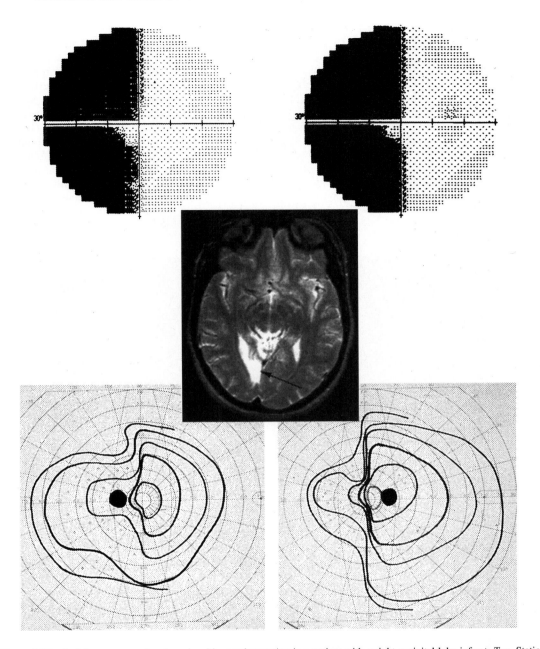

Figure 2.35.   Left homonymous hemianopia with macular sparing in a patient with a right occipital lobe infarct. *Top,* Static perimetry demonstrates a dense left homonymous hemianopia with about 5° of inferior macular sparing. Note marked congruity of the field defects in the two eyes. *Bottom,* Kinetic perimetry reveals that the homonymous field defect has both absolute and relative features. The congruous nature of the defects is apparent, at least with small isopters. *Middle,* Axial T1-weighted magnetic resonance shows hyperintensity in right occipital lobe, consistent with the congruous homonymous visual field defect.

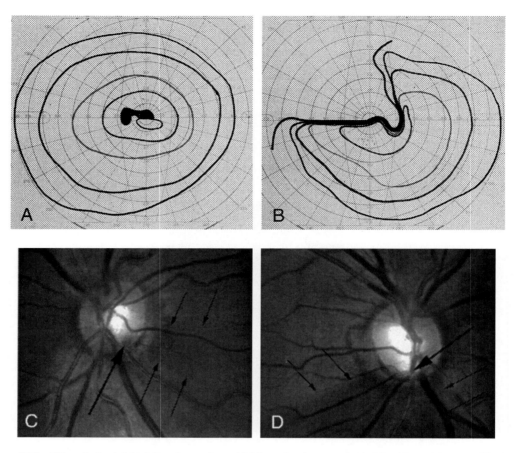

Figure 2.36. Bilateral visual field defects in a patient with bilateral optic nerve pits and focal loss of the nerve fiber layer. *A,* Kinetic perimetry in left eye shows small superior arcuate defect encroaching on fixation. *B,* Kinetic perimetry in right eye shows large superior nasal/arcuate defect. *C,* Fundus photograph of left eye shows a small inferotemporal optic pit (*large arrow*) and loss of nerve fiber layer in the inferior arcuate region (*small arrows*). *D,* Fundus photograph of the right eye shows an inferior pit (*large arrow*) associated with a broad region of nerve fiber loss in the inferior and inferotemporal region (*small arrows*).

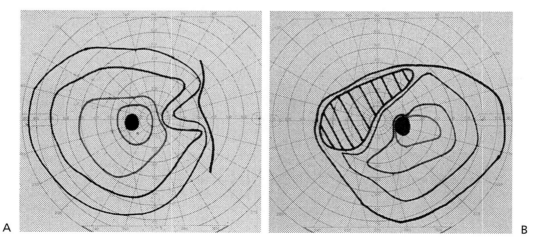

Figure 2.37. Bilateral visual field defects in a patient with postpapilledema optic atrophy. *A and B,* Kinetic perimetry shows mild loss of the nasal visual field in the left (*A*) and right (*B*) eyes. Note that most of the field loss is relative. (*Figure continues.*)

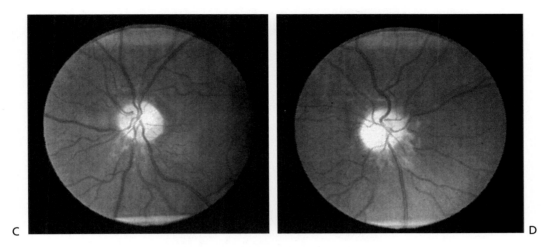

Figure 2.37. Continued. *C and D*, Fundus photographs show moderate postpapilledema optic atrophy.

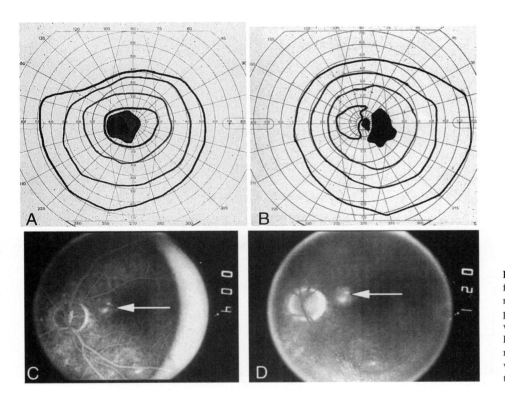

Figure 2.38. Bilateral visual field defects in a patient with bilateral central serous chorioretinopathy. *A and B*, Kinetic perimetry reveals bilateral central defects with normal peripheral fields. *C and D*, Early (*C*) and late (*D*) fluorescein angiography shows leakage of dye consistent with central serous chorioretinopathy in the posterior pole of the left eye (*arrows*).

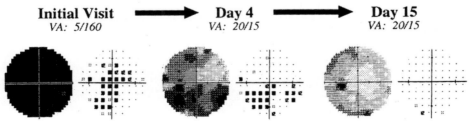

Figure 2.39. Improvement in a visual field defect as detected by static perimetry in a patient with optic neuritis over a 15-day period. Note marked clearing of the defect. (From Keltner JL, Johnson CA, Spurr JO, et al. Visual field profile of optic neuritis: One year followup in the Optic Neuritis Treatment Trial. Arch Ophthalmol 1994;112:946–953.)

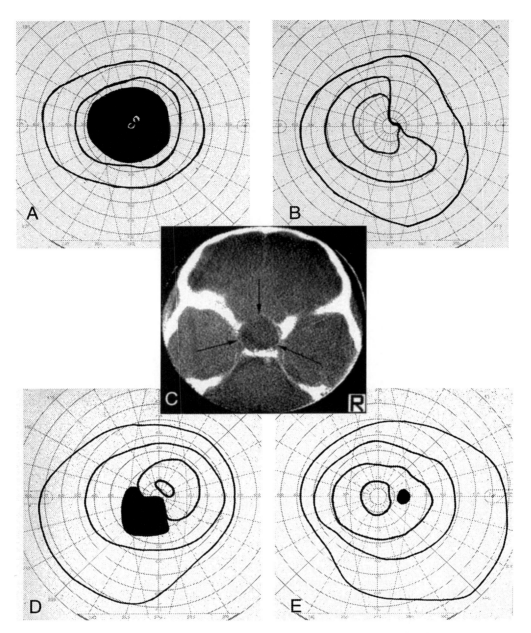

Figure 2.40.   Visual field defects indicating an anterior chiasmal mass in a 7-year-old child with decreased vision in the left eye. *A*, Kinetic perimetry in the left eye reveals a dense central scotoma with constriction of the peripheral field. *B*, Kinetic perimetry in the right eye reveals a supertemporal field defect (junctional scotoma of Traquair). *C*, Axial computed tomographic scan shows a large circular lesion in the suprasellar region (*arrows*). At surgery, a craniopharyngioma was found and removed. *D*, After surgery, kinetic perimetry shows substantial improvement in the visual field of the left eye. *E*, Kinetic perimetry in the right eye reveals a normal visual field.

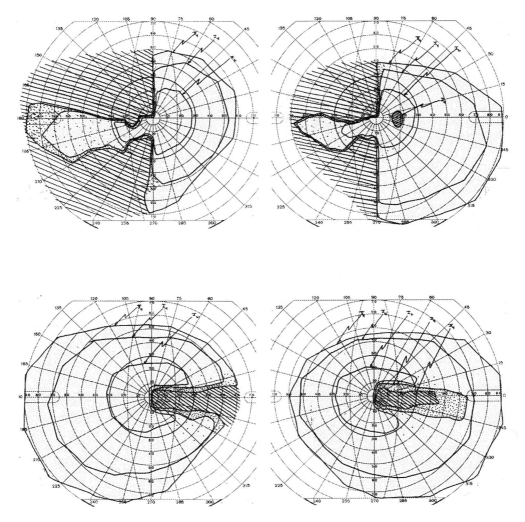

Figure 2.41. Two examples of visual field deficits produced by lesions of the lateral geniculate body (LGB). *Top,* Kinetic perimetry from a patient who experienced a stroke reveal a left quadruple sectoranopia from damage to the LGB in the territory of the distal anterior choroidal artery. *Bottom,* Right homonymous horizontal sectoranopia with metastatic cancer to the LGB in the region supplied by the lateral choroidal artery. (Courtesy of Dr. William T. Shults.)

specific features of the visual field before getting a global view of the visual field from Step 4 may lead to misinterpretation of visual field information.

The approach to visual field interpretation outlined above is not intended to cover all possible scenarios but is rather meant as a guide to identify most kinds of visual field deficits and to avoid many of the common pitfalls. Once the pattern and degree of visual field loss has been established, a differential diagnosis needs to be determined. If there is doubt about the validity of visual field results, the test should be repeated when the patient is well-rested. Pathologic visual field changes usually are replicable, whereas nonpathologic visual field changes typically are not. If there is concern about fatigue affecting visual field results, a shorter test procedure should be employed.

New Perimetry Tests

Automated perimetry has enhanced the clinical utility of visual field testing by providing standardized procedures, quantitative measures, normative population characteristics, immediate statistical analyses, new graphic representations of data, and many other desirable features. However, the basic test procedures have essentially remained the same for more than 150 years. Usually, a small white stimulus is presented on a uniformly illuminated adapting background, and the detection threshold of the stimulus is determined at various locations throughout the visual field.

In order to improve sensitivity of visual field testing, several test procedures have been modified for use in perimetry. Although the tests vary widely in terms of the visual functions that they measure, they have a common objective: by creating a unique stimulus display, these tests attempt to

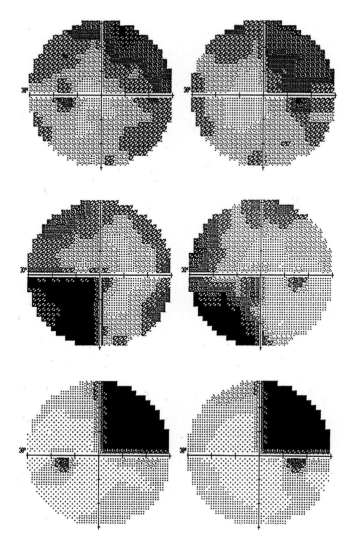

Figure 2.42. Visual field defects caused by postgeniculate lesions in the temporal (*top*), parietal (*middle*), and occipital (*bottom*) lobes as defined by static perimetry. *Top,* Right incomplete incongruous homonymous hemianopia, denser above, from left temporal lobe lesion. *Middle,* Left incomplete incongruous homonymous hemianopia, denser below, from lesion of the right parietal lobe. *Top,* Right congruous superior quadrantanopia from lesion of the inferior aspect of the left occipital lobe.

isolate (or strongly bias) threshold responses to be mediated by a specific subpopulation of neural mechanisms, instead of the wide range of neural mechanisms stimulated by conventional perimetry.

These test procedures have several theoretical advantages. First, because these tests are designed to target specific visual mechanisms, their response properties bear a strong linkage to the underlying physiology and anatomy of the visual pathways. Second, if certain diseases cause selectively greater amounts of damage to some visual mechanisms than others, these new test procedures may be able to detect early losses or changes in visual function that may not otherwise be noticed with conventional perimetry. Finally, because

Table 2.4
Differential Diagnosis of Visual Field Deficits

I. GENERAL DEPRESSION
    A. Cataract (diffuse depression from cataracts may improve with dilation)
    B. Corneal disease (shows no improvement with dilation)
    C. Other media opacities
    D. Some optic neuropathies
II. ENLARGED BLIND SPOT
    A. Optic nerve disease
       1. Papilledema and big blind spot syndrome
       2. Drusen of the optic nerve head
       3. Congenital optic nerve lesion (coloboma, staphyloma)
       4. Optic neuritis
    B. Retinal disease
       1. Multiple evanescent white dot syndrome (MEWDS)
       2. Acute zonal occult outer retinopathy (AZOOR)
    C. High myopia
III. ARCUATE, ALTITUDINAL, NASAL STEP, NASAL DEPRESSION
    A. Optic nerve disease
       1. Glaucoma
       2. Papilledema
       3. Drusen of the optic nerve head
       4. Other optic neuropathies (AION, optic neuritis, etc.)
    B. Branch artery occlusion
IV. CROSSES THE VERTICAL AND HORIZONTAL MERIDIANS
    A. Retinal disease
       1. Ring scotomas, peripheral depression, "scalloped" field loss
    B. Optic neuropathy
       1. Generalized depression, sparing of central vision
    C. Fatigue, poor testing ability
       1. Fatigue in conjunction with visual pathology
    D. Malingering
       1. Peripheral depression, square visual fields, spiraling or crossed isopters, inconsistent patterns of loss
V. CENTRAL OR CENTROCECAL DEFECTS
    A. Maculopathy (visual acuity often more affected than visual field)
    B. Optic neuropathies of all types
VI. BITEMPORAL DEFECTS
    A. Superior bitemporal defects (pituitary adenoma)
    B. Inferior bitemporal defects (craniopharyngioma, hypothalamic tumor)
VII. HOMONYMOUS HEMIANOPSIA
    A. Complete homonymous hemianopsia
       1. Retrochiasmal defect with no further localizing value
    B. Tongue- or keyhole-shaped homonymous defect, or remaining visual field
       1. Lateral geniculate lesion
    C. Incongruous homonymous hemianopsia (anterior optic tract, radiations)
       1. Optic tract
       2. Temporal lobe ("pie in the sky" defect)
       3. Parietal lobe ("pie on the floor" defect)
    D. Highly congruous homonymous hemianopsia
       1. Occipital lobe lesion
          a. "Cookie cutter" punched-out lesion
          b. Macular sparing
          c. Temporal crescent
          d. Statokinetic dissociation

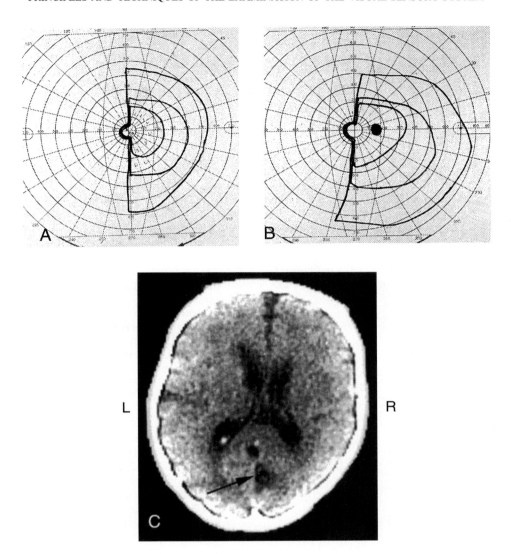

Figure 2.43. Complete homonymous hemianopia with macular sparing from an occipital lobe lesion. *A and B,* Kinetic perimetry shows a complete left homonymous hemianopia with about 5° of macular sparing. *C,* Axial computed tomographic scan shows a small low-density area, consistent with an infarct, in the right occipital lobe (*arrow*), with sparing of the occipital tip.

these test procedures are designed to isolate specific subpopulations of neural mechanisms, they eliminate much of the redundancy and overlap that is normally present in the visual pathways. By reducing this redundancy, it becomes easier to detect early, subtle losses or changes in visual function, even if these losses are not selective (173).

In this section, we briefly describe five perimetry tests that appear to have the greatest potential for clinical utility in neuro-ophthalmologic diagnosis: Short Wavelength Automated Perimetry [SWAP], High-Pass Resolution Perimetry (HRP), Flicker Perimetry, Motion and Displacement Perimetry, and Frequency Doubling Perimetry.

Short Wavelength Automated Perimetry (SWAP)

Short Wavelength Automated Perimetry [SWAP] utilizes a bright yellow background and a large short-wavelength

(''blue'') stimulus to isolate and measure the sensitivity of short-wavelength chromatic mechanisms. The bright yellow background depresses the sensitivity of middle (''green'') and long (''red'') wavelength mechanisms, thereby allowing the sensitivity of the short-wavelength system to be measured using a large blue target. The test is available on several automated projection perimeters and can utilize the same test strategies, target presentation patterns, and other parameters that are employed in conventional automated perimetry (174–177). The test procedure is commercially available for the Humphrey Field Analyzer, which provides a statistical analysis procedure and age-related normative database for interpreting results. The SITA strategy is also available for SWAP (178).

A number of longitudinal and cross-sectional investigations have established that SWAP is not only an early indicator of damage from glaucoma but that it also detects visual field defects that are not determined by conventional automated perimetry (174–177). About 5–20% of glaucoma suspects with normal visual fields when tested by conventional automated perimetry have localized deficits when testing with SWAP. In addition, SWAP deficits are present in 35–40% of high-risk glaucoma suspects compared with about 8% of low-risk glaucoma suspects. Longitudinal investigations demonstrate that SWAP is able to predict the onset and location of subsequent glaucomatous visual field loss by conventional perimetry 3–5 years before its occurrence. SWAP is also able to predict subsequent progression of glaucomatous visual field loss (Fig. 2.44). However, its high variability limits its ability to detect progression (176).

SWAP is also useful for patients with neuro-ophthalmologic disorders. Keltner and Johnson (179) studied 40 patients with various neuro-ophthalmologic disorders. In some instances, SWAP deficits were present in eyes with normal visual fields obtained with conventional automated perimetry. In cases in which visual field loss was evident for conventional automated perimetry, the SWAP deficit was more extensive (Figs. 2.45 and 2.46).

High-Pass Resolution Perimetry (HRP)

High-pass resolution perimetry (HRP) was developed by Frisén (180,181) and consists of a series of "ring" targets of varying size that are generated on a video monitor by performing a "high pass" spatial frequency filtering of a target incorporating a light circular center and a dark annular surround (Fig. 2.47). The average luminance of the ring stimulus is equal to the background. This combination creates a vanishing optotype. The special property of a vanishing optotype is that detection and resolution occur at approximately the same threshold. The ring test is believed to predominantly test the function of parvocellular mechanisms that are responsible for the processing of fine detail, form vision, and related spatial vision functions (181).

Sample et al. (182) reported a 67% agreement between HRP and the Humphrey Field Analyzer in a group of normal persons, ocular hypertensives, and patients with primary open-angle glaucoma. In patients with visual field defects detected with both tests, there was a 92% agreement in the location of the deficit. Lachenmayr et al. (183,184) reported that HRP was significantly less sensitive in detecting early glaucomatous visual field loss than either conventional automated perimetry or flicker perimetry (see later).

Evaluations of HRP in patients with neuro-ophthalmologic disorders are encouraging (180–182,185–192). For example, Wall et al. (188) found that in patients with pseudotumor cerebri, HRP had slightly lower sensitivity and slightly higher specificity than automated perimetric testing using a Humphrey Field Analyzer, although the differences were not statistically significant. Wall (187) also reported that HRP was useful for evaluating patients with optic neuritis and was especially sensitive in revealing subtle deficits in the fellow "uninvolved" eyes of optic neuritis patients.

Most importantly, the ring test has been shown to have low retest variability (188,193). Chauhan and coworkers have shown that the ring test can detect visual field progression in glaucoma significantly earlier than conventional automated perimetry.

The main advantages of HRP are its relatively quick examination time, the interactive feedback the test procedure provides to patients, excellent patient ergonomics, low retest variability, and the high degree of patient preference for HRP over conventional perimetric techniques. The main disadvantages are its greater susceptibility to blur, and alignment problems (e.g., lens rim artifacts).

Flicker Perimetry

Another psychophysical procedure that shows promising initial results for detecting and evaluating subtle visual loss is the detection of flicker. The rationale underlying flicker perimetry testing is that high temporal frequencies of flicker preferentially stimulate ganglion cells that project to the magnocellular layers of the lateral geniculate body. M-cell

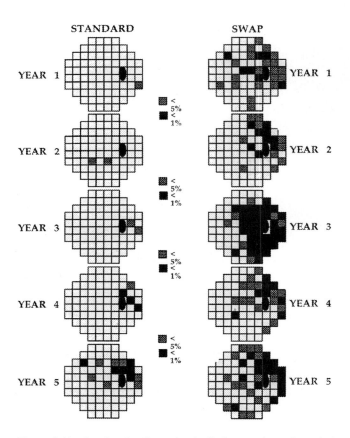

Figure 2.44. Results of a 5-year longitudinal comparison of standard white-on-white perimetry (*left*) and short wavelength automated perimetry [SWAP] (*right*) in an ocular hypertensive patient who converted to glaucoma. Note that the SWAP deficit was present before the standard visual field loss, and predicted its development and location several years later. (From Johnson CA, Adams AJ, Casson EJ, et al. Blue-on-yellow perimetry can predict the development of glaucomatous visual field loss. Arch Ophthalmol 1993;111:645–650.)

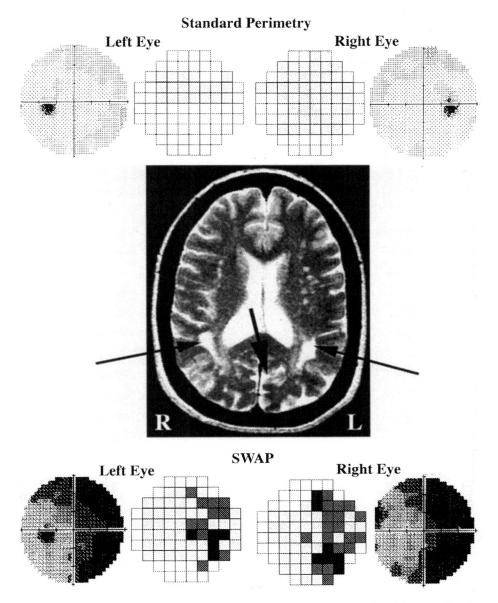

Figure 2.45. Gray scale and total deviation plots for standard automated perimetry (*top*) and short wavelength automated perimetry [SWAP] (*bottom*) for an asymptomatic patient with multiple white matter abnormalities on magnetic resonance imaging (*thick and thin arrows*). The standard visual fields are normal, whereas SWAP reveals a right homonymous hemianopia, probably related to the white matter lesions in the left occipital lobe (*large arrow*). (From Keltner JL, Johnson CA. Short wavelength automated perimetry [SWAP] in neuro-ophthalmologic disorders. Arch Ophthalmol 1995;113:475–481.)

fibers primarily consist of large-diameter ganglion cell axons that may be preferentially damaged in glaucoma. Thus, by presenting a stimulus that preferentially stimulates this group of nerve fibers, mild glaucomatous deficits may be more readily detected. Flicker perimetry is effective in detecting mild glaucomatous visual field loss. Indeed, in some ocular hypertensives, flicker deficits are found in locations within the visual field in which there were normal responses when tested using conventional automated perimetry. In addition, this form of perimetry seems to have predictive value in

distinguishing which ocular hypertensives with normal visual fields will develop glaucomatous visual field loss within several years (194). Thus, flicker perimetry seems to be a useful adjunct to conventional automated perimetry, especially for detecting early glaucomatous losses.

Flicker sensitivity has several desirable features as a clinical diagnostic test procedure. Unlike many psychophysical tests, flicker detection thresholds are relatively unaffected by moderate amounts of blur, light scatter, and other forms of image degradation (195). Thus, optical factors such as

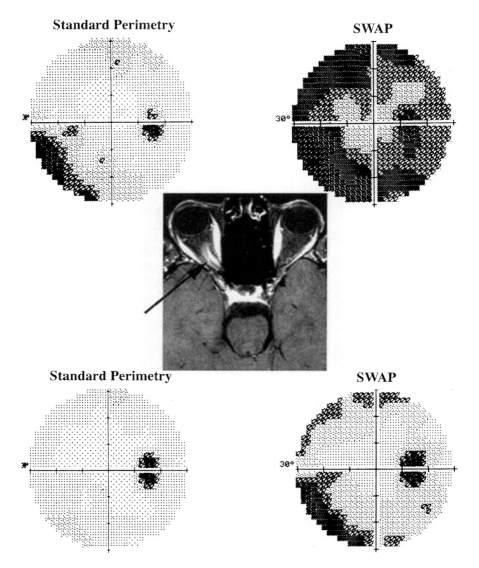

Figure 2.46. Pretreatment (*top*) and posttreatment (*bottom*) standard visual fields (*left*) and Short Wavelength Automated Perimetry [SWAP] fields (*right*) in a patient with a right optic nerve sheath meningioma. Standard perimetry shows a minimal inferonasal defect in the visual field of the right eye (*top left*), whereas SWAP shows an extensive reduction in sensitivity (*top right*). *Middle,* T1-weighted axial MR image after intravenous injection of paramagnetic contrast material shows enlargement and enhancement of the posterior portion of the right optic nerve (*arrow*). Following radiation treatment, standard automated perimetry is normal (*bottom left*), but SWAP shows a persistent nasal step (*bottom right*). (From Keltner JL, Johnson CA. Short wavelength automated perimetry [SWAP] in neuro-ophthalmologic disorders. Arch Ophthalmol 1995;113:475–481.)

cataract, refractive error, and media opacities do not influence flicker sensitivity as much as they affect visual acuity and related psychophysical tests. The primary disadvantage of flicker sensitivity is that specialized equipment must be used. Most automated projection perimeters and other clinical instruments are not easily modified to perform this type of visual field testing.

Motion Perimetry

The ability to detect motion or small displacements of a stimulus at various locations in the visual field can be adapted for use as a perimetric test procedure. As with high temporal frequency flicker, the rationale underlying this test procedure is that motion is preferentially detected by M-cell mechanisms, which may be more susceptible to glaucomatous damage. Thresholds for detection of motion may therefore reveal early glaucomatous defects in localized visual field locations.

Two different approaches have been used to evaluate motion sensitivity of the visual field. The first method measures the minimum displacement of a small target superimposed on a uniform background that can be detected as movement

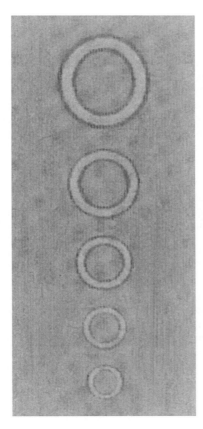

Figure 2.47. High-pass resolution perimetry targets. (From Frisén L. High pass resolution perimetry: Recent developments. In Heijl A, ed. Perimetry Update 1988/1989. Amsterdam, Kugler and Ghedini, 1989:383–392.)

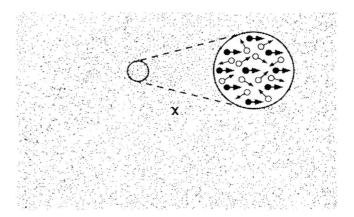

Figure 2.48. An example of the video stimuli used to determine motion and coherence thresholds for motion perimetry. (From Wall M, Ketoff KM. Random dot motion perimetry in patients with glaucoma and in normal subjects. Am J Ophthalmol 1995;120:587–596.)

(196–199). Motion displacement thresholds are then determined for a number of visual field locations in a manner similar to traditional static perimetry. In this way, motion sensitivity can be determined for small localized regions of the visual field. The second method presents a large display of small dots that are moving in random directions (Brownian-like motion). A stimulus is produced by briefly moving a small group of dots in the same direction (coherence). The patient's task is to detect this coherent direction of dot motion. A ''motion coherence'' threshold is determined by varying the percentage of dots within the small group that are moving in the same direction (200,201), or by keeping coherence constant and changing the size of the patch of coherent motion (202–204) (Fig. 2.48). This test evaluates large visual field regions but requires the combined input from a population of cells to be able to detect motion. Other versions of this test limit the size of the stimulus so that more localized regions of the visual field can be tested (202,203,205).

Studies of motion and displacement threshold perimetry indicate that motion sensitivity is abnormal in glaucoma patients, and that motion thresholds are sometimes able to detect subtle glaucomatous losses that are not evident with conventional automated perimetry (196–199,202,204,206).

Longitudinal studies are needed to verify the clinical significance of these findings and those of Wall and Montgomery (203) that motion perimetry is able to detect localized visual field defects in patients with idiopathic intracranial hypertension (see Chapter 5).

Motion and displacement perimetry have several desirable characteristics as clinical diagnostic test procedures. Motion detection is a very robust visual function, being only modestly affected by such factors as contrast, luminance, adaptation level, and target size (207). In addition, motion detection, like flicker sensitivity, is very resistant to the effects of cataract, refractive error, and other forms of image degradation (199). The dynamic stimulus range for motion is also very large, especially for displacement of a single small target.

Frequency Doubling Perimetry

When a low spatial frequency sinusoidal grating (less than 1 cycle/degree) undergoes high temporal frequency counterphase flicker (greater than 15 Hz), the grating appears to have twice its real spatial frequency (i.e., there appear to be twice as many light and dark bars in the grating) (Fig. 2.49). This phenomenon, called **the frequency doubling effect**, was first described by Kelly (208,209). Because the frequency doubling stimulus incorporates a low spatial frequency and a high temporal frequency, it is ideally suited for stimulation of M-cell mechanisms and has been adapted for use as a screening test for glaucoma by Maddess and Henry (210). Johnson and Samuels (211) modified the original test procedure to perform frequency doubling perimetry of localized visual field regions. In its initial form, frequency doubling perimetry evaluated 17 visual field locations (four per visual field quadrant, each 10° in diameter, plus a stimulus presented to the central 5° of the visual field) throughout the central 20° radius of the visual field. In its current form (the Humphrey Matrix FDT perimeter), 54 and 72 test locations matching the 24–2 and 30–2 grids of conventional

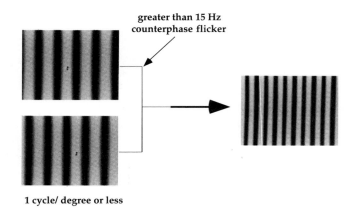

greater than 15 Hz counterphase flicker

1 cycle/ degree or less

Figure 2.49. Schematic representation of the stimulus used in frequency doubling perimetry.

automated perimetry are utilized. A contrast threshold is obtained for detection of the frequency-doubled stimuli at each visual field location. The sensitivity and specificity of frequency doubling perimetry are similar to those of conventional automated perimetry for detection of glaucomatous visual field loss (sensitivity and specificity of 95% or better) (211–213) (Fig. 2.50). In addition, results obtained in patients with nonglaucomatous optic neuropathies suggest that frequency doubling perimetry is also useful for evaluation of such patients (213, 214). Commercial versions of the frequency doubling perimetry test developed by Welch Allyn, Inc. (Skaneateles, NY) is available from Carl Zeiss Meditec (Dublin, CA).

Frequency doubling perimetry has several advantages as a clinical diagnostic tool. First, it is a rapid test. Second,

patients prefer the test to conventional automated perimetry. Third, it has low test-retest variability. Fourth, the equipment is small and portable and does not require a special room with controlled lighting. Fifth, it is unaffected by blur of up to 3 diopters for FDT using the 24–2 pattern and 6–7 diopters for the initial version with larger stimuli. Finally, patients can wear their normal spectacle correction to take the test, even if they have a bifocal added. The primary disadvantage of frequency doubling perimetry is that it is affected by cataract, as are all tests of contrast sensitivity.

COLOR VISION

A comprehensive discussion of color vision is beyond the scope of this chapter. Instead, we will limit our discussion of this subject to an overview of normal color vision and its underlying physiologic mechanisms, congenital and acquired color vision deficiencies, the use and interpretation of common clinical color vision tests, and the diagnostic value of color vision testing in ophthalmic and neurologic disorders. Several excellent sources are available (13, 215,216) for those interested in a more thorough discussion of color vision, the history of color vision research, and a detailed account of color vision deficiencies in specific ocular disorders. In particular, the book by Kaiser and Boynton (216) contains an especially interesting chapter pertaining to the history of color vision.

General Principles of Color Testing

From a clinical diagnostic standpoint, it is important to distinguish whether a color vision deficiency is congenital or acquired (Table 2.5). Congenital color vision deficits are usually easy to classify using standard clinical color vision tests because color discrimination is usually impaired for a

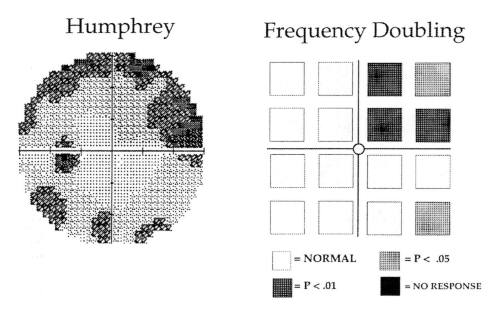

= NORMAL   = P < .05

= P < .01   = NO RESPONSE

Figure 2.50. Comparison of results obtained for the Humphrey Field Analyzer and frequency doubling perimetry in a patient with glaucomatous visual field loss.

Table 2.5
Differences Between Congenital and Acquired Color Defects

Cogenital	Acquired
Usually color vision loss in specific spectral regions.	Often no specific spectral region of color discrimination loss.
Less marked dependence of color vision on target size and illuminance.	Marked dependence of color vision on target size and illuminance.
Characteristic results obtained on various clinical color vision tests.	Conflicting or variable results may be obtained on various clinical color vision tests.
Many object colors are named correctly, or predictable errors are made.	Some object colors are named incorrectly.
Both eyes are usually affected to the same degree.	The two eyes are often affected to different degrees.
Usually there is no other visual complaint or problems.	Often there are additional visual complaints, reduced visual acuity or visual field loss.
The deficit does not change appreciably over time.	The defect may show clear progression or remission of color discrimination loss.
Are almost always red/green deficits and are mostly found in males.	Are often blue or blue-yellow deficits.

Adapted from Pokorny J, Smith VC, Verriest G, et al., eds. Congenital and Acquired Color Vision Defects. New York, Grune & Stratton, 1979, Table 4.1.

specific region of the visual spectrum, and the deficits are long-standing, stable, symmetric in the two eyes, and unassociated with other visual symptoms or complaints. In patients with acquired color vision loss, however, color discrimination may be impaired throughout the visual spectrum or along a specific axis, and the deficits may be mild or severe, of sudden onset, asymmetric, and often associated with other visual symptoms or complaints.

Table 2.6 presents a list of color vision deficits associated with various ocular and neurologic disorders. Additional information may be found in Pokorny et al. (13).

Investigations of acquired color vision losses in retinal and

optic nerve disease, using specialized laboratory techniques, suggest that although many optic nerve and retinal diseases affect more than just a single opponent pathway, the magnitude of loss in such disorders is often greater in one of the opponent channels than in any of the others (224–227). Cerebral dyschromatopsias are uncommon, but result in severe color vision loss, sometimes producing a total achromatopsia (vision in black and white only) (228).

It should be emphasized that **color comparison tests**, although only qualitative in nature, can provide valuable information concerning subtle visual anomalies. Using pages from the pseudoisochromatic plates, colored bottle caps, or other brightly colored objects, comparisons of color appearance can be very effective in detecting subtle differences between the two eyes. The brightness or saturation of the colored objects may be less in one eye, making the object's color appear to be dim or washed out. Similarly, comparisons within the same eye across the vertical and horizontal midline, or between central vision and the mid-periphery can detect subtle differences in color appearance that are indicative of an early visual disturbance.

Table 2.6
Acquired Color Vision Deficits Associated with Eye Disease

Condition	Color Vision Defect
Glaucoma	B-Y
Retinal detachment	B-Y
Pigmentary degeneration of retina (including RP)	B-Y
Age-related macular degeneration	B-Y
Myopic retinal degeneration	B-Y
Chorioretinitis	B-Y
Retinal vascular occlusion	B-Y
Diabetic retinopathy	B-Y
Hypertensive retinopathy	B-Y
Papilledema	B-Y
Methyl alcohol poisoning	B-Y
Dominant hereditary optic atrophy	B-Y
Central serous retinopathy	B-Y
Optic neuritis	R-G
Tobacco-alcohol (ETOH) or toxic amblyopia	R-G
Leber's optic atrophy	R-G
Lesions of the optic nerve and posterior pathways	R-G
Papillitis	R-G
Stargardt's disease	R-G
Best's disease	R-G
Juvenile macular degeneration	R-G or B-Y

Adapted from Adams AJ, Verdon WA, Spivey BE. Color vision. In: Tasman W, Jaeger EA, eds. Duane's Foundations of Clinical Ophthalmology. Vol 1, Chap 52, pp 1–43, Philadelphia, JB Lippincott, 1996.

Normal Color Vision Mechanisms

Beginning approximately 200 years ago, a controversy existed concerning the mechanisms underlying normal color vision. The trichromatic theory of color vision, usually attributed to Young (217) and Helmholtz (218), was that there were three different receptors that were maximally sensitive to wavelengths in different regions of the visual spectrum, with sensitivity peaks at short (blue), middle (green), and long (red) wavelengths, respectively. Although maximally sensitive to a specific part of the spectrum, each of these receptor types has some degree of sensitivity to wavelengths throughout most of the visual spectrum. An efficient means of uniquely signaling thousands of different colors is achieved by examining the ratio of excitation of the three receptors. A large amount of psychophysical evidence was accumulated in support of the trichromatic theory of color vision.

An alternate view of color vision, the opponent-process

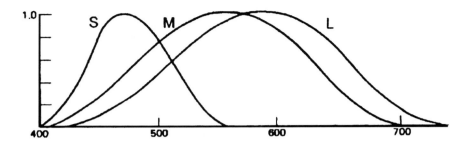

Figure 2.51. Schematic representation of the absorption spectra of the three major cone types associated with human color vision. S, short wavelength (blue) cone; M, middle wavelength (green) cone; L, long wavelength (red) cone. (From Kaiser PK, Boynton RM. Human Color Vision. Washington DC, Optical Society of America, 1996.)

theory was proposed by Hering (219), who believed that there were two chromatic mechanisms (red-green and blue-yellow) and one achromatic mechanism (black-white) that paired sensations in an opposing or antagonistic manner. Much of the evidence he provided to support this theory was observational. For example, after prolonged viewing of a bright red stimulus, a neutral color would appear to be green. Surrounding a neutral color with a large blue annulus would cause it to appear yellow. In addition, some color combinations would give rise to the appearance of both components (e.g., blue-green or red-yellow), but there was never the appearance of yellow-blue or red-green. The opponent process theory was proposed as a means of accounting for the six distinct color sensations (blue, green, yellow, red, black, and white) proposed by Hering (219).

There is abundant psychophysical and physiologic evidence supporting both theories (13,215,216). Initially, visual stimuli are processed by three types of cone photoreceptors, one with peak sensitivity in the short wavelength region (approximately 440 nm), one with peak sensitivity in the middle wavelength region (approximately 530–540 nm), and one with peak sensitivity in the long wavelength region (approximately 560–580 nm) (Fig. 2.51). The output from the three cone photoreceptors is then transmitted to neurons in the inner retina that process information according to two opponent chromatic mechanisms (yellow-blue and red-green) and one achromatic mechanism (black-white), in accordance with the opponent process theory (Fig. 2.52). Although there is additional spatial and temporal processing of this information at different levels of the visual pathways, this opponent coding of chromatic information is carried through to the higher visual centers.

Clinical Tests of Color Vision

A wide variety of color vision tests are available clinically. Because most of them were designed to evaluate congenital red-green color vision deficiencies, many do not permit adequate testing of blue-yellow deficits or optimal characterization of acquired color vision losses. A number of techniques can be used to evaluate acquired color vision deficiencies (220–222), but most of them are not available for routine clinical use.

As with any test of visual function, it is important that the testing conditions are standardized and are performed in the proper manner. Each of the clinically available color vision tests comes with a set of detailed instructions for administering the test and interpreting the results. These in-

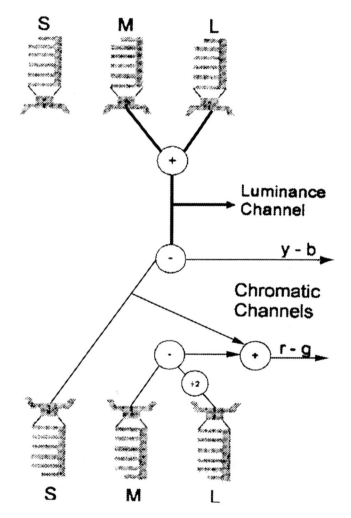

Figure 2.52. An illustration of a simple model for obtaining opponent process responses from the three cone types. Interactions within the inner retina transform trichromatic photoreceptor responses into center-surround opponent responses at the retinal ganglion cell level. An achromatic (black-white) luminance channel is activated by the summed input from middle (M) and long (L) wavelength cones. The red-green (r-g) spectrally opponent pathway is activated by the difference in output by the M and L cones. The yellow-blue (y-b) spectrally opponent pathway by the difference in output by the short wavelength (S) cones and by the summed output of the M and L cones (the luminance channel). (From Kaiser PK, Boynton RM. Human Color Vision. Washington, DC, Optical Society of America, 1996.)

structions should be judiciously followed, because erroneous results can sometimes be obtained if the tests are not properly administered.

An important factor for all clinical color vision test procedures is the use of proper lighting, both in terms of having an adequate amount of light for the test and having a light source with the proper spectral distribution. Most color vision tests specify that testing should be performed under daylight illumination. Because natural daylight varies in spectral distribution and intensity, it is not a reliable source. Instead, a standardized daylight lighting source (Illuminant C) is preferred. This is usually provided by a Macbeth Easel Lamp, which consists of a tungsten filament bulb that is located behind a light blue glass filter. The filtered light provides an appropriate source of Illuminant C for color vision testing. Because of the high cost of the Macbeth Easel Lamp, an alternative approach consists of using a specialized fluorescent bulb such as the Verilux daylight F15 T8 VLX (or an equivalent fluorescent tube with a high color rendering index) placed in a desk lamp (13).

Pseudoisochromatic Plates

Pseudoisochromatic plates are the most common color vision tests employed clinically. A number of pseudoisochromatic plate tests are available, although the Ishihara and Hardy-Rand-Rittler are the most commonly used versions in a clinical setting. Each of these tests consists of a series of plates that contain colored dots of varying size and brightness. The tests are designed so that humans with normal color vision will see numbers, shapes, or letters as a consequence of grouping certain colored dots together to form a figure. Depending on how the particular test is designed, those with color deficiencies will either be unable to see the figure because the figure dots are confused with the background dots, or they will see a figure different from that seen by persons with normal color vision. The variation in size and brightness of the dots is used to ensure that recognition of figures is made on the basis of color discrimination and not other cues.

The main advantages of color vision tests using pseudoisochromatic plates are that they are quick and easy to perform and therefore are an excellent screening procedure for distinguishing between normal color vision and any type of color vision abnormality. The disadvantages of pseudoisochromatic plate tests are that they have rather limited ability to classify color vision deficits and determine their severity, and they have little or no ability (depending on the particular test) to test for blue-yellow color vision deficits.

Farnsworth Panel D-15 Test

The Farnsworth Panel D-15 test is a color arrangement test consisting of 15 caps that form a color circle covering the visual spectrum. A reference cap is permanently fixed in the arrangement tray; the other 15 caps are placed in a scrambled order in front of the patient. The patient's task is to select the cap that is closest in hue to the reference cap and place it next to the reference cap in the tray. The patient is then asked to continue to place the caps in the tray, one at a time, so that they are arranged in an orderly transition of hue. Once all the caps are in the tray, the patient has an opportunity to make any final changes in the order of caps. The caps are designed so that persons with normal color vision or very mild color vision deficits (e.g., mild anomalous trichromacy) will arrange the caps in a perfect color circle. Patients with moderate to severe protan (red), deutan (green), or tritan (blue) color vision deficits will confuse colors across the color circle, so that the arrangement contains misplaced caps. The specific arrangement indicates the type of color deficiency (Fig. 2.53). The Panel D-15 test does not indicate the degree of color deficiency, other than to separate color normals and mild anomalous trichromats from those with moderate to severe color vision deficiencies. A desaturated D-15 test has been developed and validated

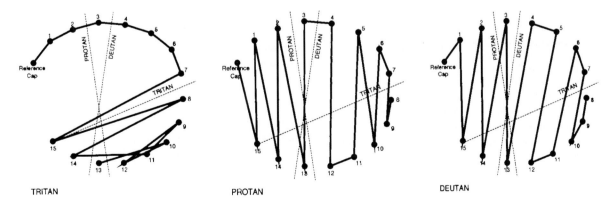

Figure 2.53. Examples of tritan (blue), protan (red), and deutan (green) color vision deficiencies as determined by the Farnsworth Panel D-15 Test. (From Elliott DB. Supplementary clinical tests of visual function. In Zadnik K, ed. The Ocular Examination. Philadelphia, WB Saunders, 1996.)

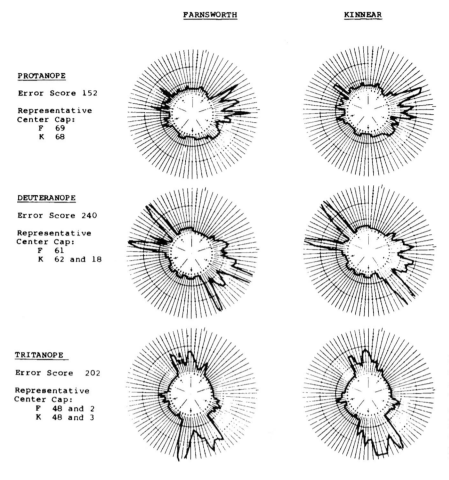

FARNSWORTH   KINNEAR

PROTANOPE

Error Score 152

Representative
Center Cap:
    F   69
    K   68

DEUTERANOPE

Error Score 240

Representative
Center Cap:
    F   61
    K   62 and 18

TRITANOPE

Error Score 202

Representative
Center Cap:
    F   48 and 2
    K   48 and 3

Figure 2.54. Examples of tritan (blue), protan (red), and deutan (green) color vision deficiencies as determined by the Farnsworth-Munsell 100 Hues Test. The figures on the *left* depict the results scored according to the method originally described by Farnsworth, whereas the figures on the *right* depict a modified scoring system. (From Kinnear PR. Proposals for scoring and assessing the 100-Hue test. Vision Res 1970;10:423–433.)

by Lanthony (13), and it detects milder color vision deficiencies.

Farnsworth-Munsell 100 Hues Test

The Farnsworth-Munsell 100 Hues test permits both classification of the type of color vision deficiency and its severity. Since Farnsworth determined that 15 of the original caps were too difficult for most normals the test now consists of **85** colored caps that are arranged in roughly equal small steps around the color circle. Interestingly, Nichols and coworkers (223) have shown that at least two more caps in the blue range are too difficult for many normals.

The caps are divided into four boxes, and arrangements of caps are performed one box at a time. In each box, there are two reference caps, one at each end, that are permanently attached to the box. The other caps are taken out of the box, scrambled, and placed before the patient. The patient is then asked to arrange the caps so that there is an orderly transition in hue from one reference cap to another. As with the Panel D-15 test, the Farnsworth-Munsell 100 Hues test is designed so that certain caps will be confused by persons with both congenital and acquired color deficiencies. The caps are

numbered on the back, and scoring is determined by the arrangement of the caps in the box. Depending on the type of color deficiency, specific caps across the color circle will be confused, resulting in greater arrangement errors in those locations. In this manner, the type of color vision deficit can be classified (Fig. 2.54). In addition to classification of the color deficiency, its severity can be quantified by determining an overall error score for arrangement errors. Thus, it is possible to quantify the degree of color vision deficiency and monitor progression and remission of acquired color losses. Normative values for different age groups are also available for the Farnsworth-Munsell 100 Hues test (13). There is evidence that certain types of optic neuropathies, including optic neuritis, can be diagnosed reliably using only 21 of the 85 chips (chips 22–42) in the set (223).

Other Color Vision Test Procedures

A number of instruments can be used to test color vision tests other than those described above, including the Nagel anomaloscope, the Pickford-Nicholson anomaloscope, lantern tests, the Lovibond Color Vision Analyzer, and the Chromagraph (13, 215). However, because these devices are not often used for routine clinical testing, their availability is limited. The reader interested in these additional color vision tests is directed to the aforementioned reference sources.

ELECTROPHYSIOLOGIC TESTS

Frequently, the physician is confronted with a patient who has unexplained loss of vision and an apparently normal fundus examination. Because electrophysiologic testing often provides diagnostic clues as to the etiology of the unexplained visual loss, it should be part of the neuro-ophthalmologic examination in selected patients. Electrophysiology provides an objective method for evaluating the function of the visual system from the retina to the visual cortex. Several electrodiagnostic methods can be used to evaluate the status of individual components of the afferent visual pathways (Table 2.7). The reader interested in a more detailed account of retinal and optic nerve electrophysiology is directed to the excellent chapter by Berson in *Adler's Physiology of the Eye* (229), as well as to several additional resource texts (229–233). This section is largely based on material from Berson (229) and Fishman and Sokol (232).

ELECTRORETINOGRAM (ERG)

Historical Overview

The Swedish physiologist Holmgren reported in 1865 that in vertebrates and higher invertebrates, an alteration in the electric potential occurred when light fell on the retina. Dewar (234) subsequently recorded this electric response and called it the electroretinogram. Einthoven and Jolly (235) identified three main components of the ERG: (*a*) an early cornea-negative ''a-wave''; (*b*) a cornea-positive ''b-wave''; and (*c*) a slower, usually cornea-positive ''c-wave''

(Fig. 2.55). Granit (236) identified three fundamental processes that he called P-I, P-II, and P-III from the ERG of a cat. He proposed that these components interact to produce the ERG waveform, with the P-II giving rise to the leading edge of the a-wave, P-II and P-III interacting to produce the b-wave, and the interaction of P-I and P-III producing the c-wave.

The consequence of the pioneering work of Granit (236) was a continuing search for the retinal generators that are responsible for the P-I, P-II, and P-III. Tomita (237,238) reported that the ERG components of the frog could be localized in the retina by depth recording with microelectrodes, and that the retinal components corresponded to those waveforms that were recorded at the cornea. Brown and Wiesel (239) demonstrated that part of the a-wave was generated in a layer external to that responsible for the b-wave, and these investigators also found that maximum responses for the a-, b-, and c-waves occurred in different retinal layers. Subsequently, Brown and Watanabe (240) recorded a large a-wave in the fovea of the monkey; in the periphery, the a-wave was much smaller and the b-wave was relatively larger. Their findings provided evidence that the photoreceptor layer was responsible for the a-wave. Murakami and Kaneko (241) divided the P-III into a distal component in the receptor layer that correlated with the onset of the a-wave (242) and a proximal component generated by the inner nuclear layer. Armington et al. (243) identified two components of the a-wave recorded under dark-adapted (scotopic) conditions. The a_s component had the spectral sensitivity of the rod system and was depressed by light adaptation, whereas the a_p component had the spectral sensitivity of the cone system and was relatively unaffected by light adaptation. It is now generally accepted that the leading edge of the a-wave of the human ERG is generated by the rods and cones in the

Table 2.7
Isolation of Components of the Afferent Visual Pathways Using Electrophysiology

Anatomical Structure	Technique
Retinal pigment epithelium	Electro-oculogram
	Electroretinogram (flash ERG)
	c-wave
Photoreceptors	
Rods	Rod-flash ERG (scotopic) a-wave
Cones	Cone-flash ERG (photopic) a-wave
	30 Hz flicker ERG
Middle retinal layers	Scotopic threshold response
	Flash ERG b-wave
	Oscillatory potentials
	Pattern ERG (P50)
Ganglion cell layer	Pattern ERG (N95)
Macula or other local region	Focal ERG
	30 Hz flicker ERG
Optic tract, radiations, and cortex	VEP

From Weisinger HS, Vingrys AJ, Sinclair AJ, 1996c, Table 1.

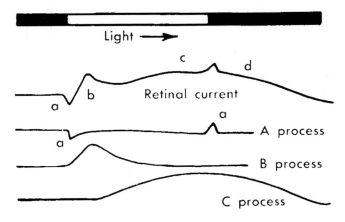

Figure 2.55. Einthoven and Jolly's separation of retinal responses into three components or processes. (Courtesy of Adrian and Mathews, 1927.)

photoreceptor layer of the retina and that this can be modeled by the photochemical events involved in the process of phototransduction (243, 244).

The cellular origin of the b-wave is less clear. Henkes (245) and Gouras and Carr (246) studied the ERG following central retinal artery occlusion, which leaves the photoreceptor response intact because this layer receives its blood supply from the choroidal vasculature, not the retinal vessels. Under these conditions, the b-wave was eliminated, whereas a modified a-wave was preserved. Hashimoto et al. (247) showed that responses similar in waveform to the b-wave were present when microelectrodes were placed on opposite sides of the inner nuclear layer. Subsequent studies by Miller and Dowling (248) showed that the b-wave potential and the potential recorded from Müller cells are similar across 5–6 log units of intensity, suggesting that Müller cell currents subserve the b-wave. Stockton and Slaughter (249) showed that the ON-bipolar cells are the source of the potassium ion fluxes that create the Müller cell currents and are therefore the generators of the P-II portion of the ERG.

Rod and cone contributions to the ERG response were initially reported by Adrian (250, 251). Photopic (cone) stimulus conditions resulted in small b-waves with short latency, whereas stimulation using scotopic (rod) conditions produced relatively large b-waves with longer latency (Fig. 2.56). The peak sensitivity of the ERG b-wave under complete dark adaptation conditions is approximately 504 nm, and the spectral sensitivity approximates the rhodopsin absorption spectrum. Under conditions of steady white light adaptation sufficient to eliminate rod contribution to the ERG, the peak sensitivity of the ERG b-wave shifts from 504 nm to approximately 555 nm, consistent with the photopic (cone) system (252). The photopic b-wave can be further separated into three distinct responses, depending on the wavelength of the light stimulus (253,254). The spectral sensitivity curves of these three ERG-derived mechanisms approximate the cone pigment absorption data from microspectrophotometric measurements of individual cones (255,256). Thus, it would appear that ERG b-waves provide some measure of cone and rod system activity in primates.

Microelectrode studies, as well as observations of the effects of various retinotoxic agents, have helped define the cellular origin of the c-wave. In the cat, c-wave polarity becomes reversed when a microelectrode penetrates the ''R membrane'' of the retinal pigment epithelium (238). A modified c-wave was also recorded intracellularly from retinal pigment epithelium by Steinberg et al. (257). These findings indicate that the retinal pigment epithelium must be present to generate the c-wave. However, because the spectral sensitivity of the dark-adapted c-wave corresponds to the absorption spectrum of rhodopsin and not to that of melanin contained in the retinal pigment epithelium, the photoreceptors must also contribute to this response (258, 259).

Separation of Rod and Cone ERG Components

The rod and cone components of the ERG may be separated on the basis of their respective spectral sensitivities by

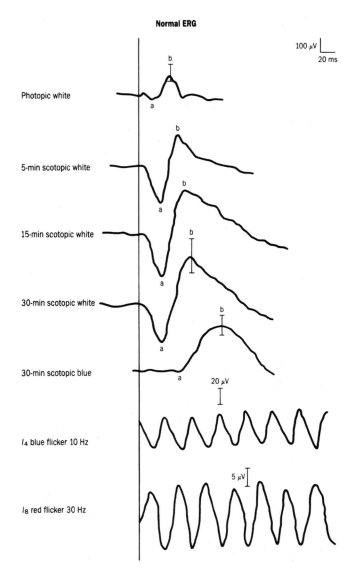

Figure 2.56. Normal electroretinographic response under photopic and scotopic conditions. Cone responses are generally isolated using photopic adaptation conditions and 30-Hz flicker. Rod responses are isolated after 30 minutes of dark adaptation with a low luminance short-wavelength stimulus either as a single flash or with 10-Hz flicker. A dark-adapted scotopic white flash measures a combined rod-cone response. (From Fishman GA, Sokol S. Electrophysiologic Testing in Disorders of the Retina, Optic Nerve, and Visual Pathway. San Francisco, American Academy of Ophthalmology, 1990.)

altering the retinal state of adaptation or by using different flicker rates for the stimulus. Although the rods are more sensitive than the cones across most of the visible spectrum, this difference decreases with increasing wavelength so that it is possible to isolate a cone response if the stimulus wavelength is greater than 680 nm. The rod contribution to the ERG can be separated by recording from a dark-adapted subject and stimulating with a short wavelength or long wavelength light that has been scotopically matched for their luminances.

ERGs are often described as having photopic (light-adapted) and scotopic (dark-adapted) responses. ERG waveforms obtained from relatively intense white stimuli usually represent contributions from both the rod and cone systems (mixed response), whereas scotopic ERGs to relatively dim blue light can be generated by the rods alone. Photopic ERGs obtained on an adapting background represent responses from the cone system. The wavelength, intensity, and temporal properties of the stimulus, as well as the state of retinal adaptation are all important in separating rod and cone system contributions (229,261). To successfully separate rod and cone responses, it is important to carefully control the stimulus conditions used to obtain these measures in order to ensure that rod and cone responses have been adequately isolated. International standards for ERG testing are available (262). These standards should be considered to be a minimum clinical protocol, and some physicians may wish to perform more extensive evaluations by determining a complete intensity–response relationship to achieve greater information about the nature of the retinal response (263).

By stimulating the eye in the presence of a background light sufficient to eliminate the rod response, it is possible to obtain a reasonably isolated cone response (264) (Fig. 2.57). The cone and rod ERG responses have temporal aspects that are dependent on stimulus intensity and state of retinal adaptation. Dim, short wavelength light elicits slow, small responses from the rod system, and more intense light

stimuli result in faster and larger responses. Flickering stimuli presented at 25 to 30 flashes per second (25–30 Hz) isolate cone responses, because the rod system is unable to follow a flickering stimulus above 20 Hz (265–268). The ERG elicited with a white stimulus of high luminance after 30 minutes of dark adaptation has both rod and cone components. The major contributor to both the increased amplitude and implicit time is the rod component. However, an isolated rod response can be evoked by a low-intensity short wavelength (blue) stimulus (232).

Oscillatory Potentials

In normal persons, low-amplitude rapid oscillations are superimposed on the ascending limb of the b-wave (269). These are called the **oscillatory potentials** (OPs). Special recording procedures are required to isolate the OPs (229). Bandpass filtering over 70–300 Hz will extract these oscillations from the underlying a- and b-waves (Fig. 2.57), and they can then be quantified by giving their summed and rectified amplitudes. OPs are thought to reflect activity in the inner retinal layers. They are of clinical importance because they are often absent in patients with diabetic retinopathy and other diseases that are associated with ischemia of the inner retina (229,270).

Testing Conditions and Interpretation

One of the major advances in ERG technology was the development of low impedance, user-friendly electrodes.

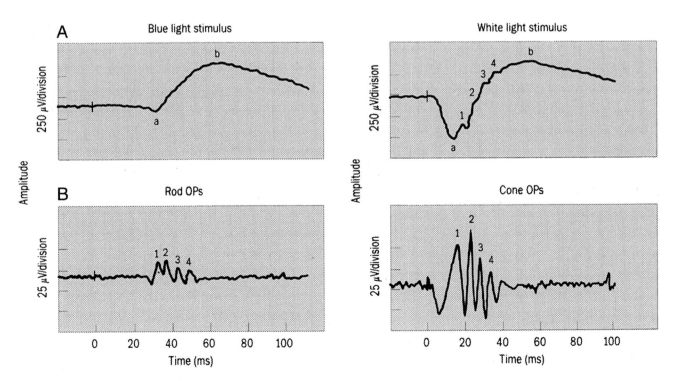

Figure 2.57. Rod (*top left*) and cone (*top right*) electroretinographic waveforms and corresponding oscillatory potentials (*bottom*) extracted from the ascending limb of the b-wave. (From Fishman GA, Sokol S. Electrophysiologic Testing in Disorders of the Retina, Optic Nerve, and Visual Pathway. San Francisco, American Academy of Ophthalmology, 1990.)

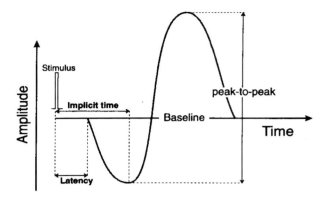

Figure 2.58. Amplitude, latency, and implicit time measurements for the standard single flash electroretinogram. (From Weisinger HS, Vingrys AJ, Sinclair AJ, et al. Electrodiagnostic methods in vision. I. Clinical application and measurement. Clin Exp Optom 1996;79:50–61.)

Riggs (271) discovered that a stable electric connection with the cornea could be achieved with a silver disc electrode mounted in a scleral contact lens. The electrode made contact with a physiologic saline solution between it and the cornea when the contact lens was placed on the cornea. A modified version of the Riggs scleral electrode is the Burian-Allen electrode, which contains a silver annulus implanted into a plastic (hard) contact lens that is placed on a topically anesthetized cornea. The contact lens is insulated and kept separate from a lid speculum that is used to keep the eyelids open during testing. Physiologic saline solution is necessary to improve electrical contact and minimize impedance. If the speculum is impregnated with silver granules, it can serve as an inactive electrode, permitting a difference potential to be measured. This is called a bipolar electrode (272). Difference potentials have the benefit of affording better signals by removing noise common to both the active and inactive electrodes by means of a differencing process. Bipolar electrodes produce high-quality signals, because the active and inactive electrodes are close to each other.

ERG Waveform and Factors Affecting It

The ERG is described by the temporal characteristics and amplitudes of the recorded waveform (Fig. 2.58). The tem-

poral aspects of the waveform can be described by the latency and implicit times. Latency refers to the time between stimulus onset and response onset, whereas implicit time refers to the time needed for the response to reach maximum amplitude. Waveform amplitudes are measured from the baseline (which is usual for the a-wave) or as a peak-to-peak comparison (which is usual for the b-wave). The b-wave/a-wave ratio can be used as an index of inner to outer retinal function.

The ERG can be affected by a number of additional factors. The implicit time of the waveform does not mature until 4–6 months of age (273), and the amplitude may be reduced until 1 year of age (274). The ERG may be greater in women than in men (274,275) and may be reduced in myopes with more than 6 D of refractive error (275,276). There may be as much as a 13% reduction in ERG amplitude in the morning, which corresponds to the time of the maximal photoreceptor disk shedding (277). Systemic drugs and anesthetics may also alter the ERG (278–280).

Use of the Electroretinogram

An ERG can provide important information about a number of retinal disorders that may simulate neuro-ophthalmologic problems. A number of different conditions can affect retinal function and produce an abnormal ERG; however, there are a limited number of patterns that the ERG waveform can exhibit in normal and diseased retinas (Fig. 2.59). Nevertheless, ERG can be used to diagnose such disorders as congenital stationary night blindness, congenital achromatopsia, retinitis pigmentosa (rod-cone dystrophy), retinitis pigmentosa sine pigmenta, cone-rod dystrophy, cone dystrophy, cancer-associated retinopathy (CAR syndrome) (281–283), and melanoma-associated retinopathy (MAR syndrome) (284,285) (Figs. 2.60–2.63). An ERG is also useful for diagnosis of toxic retinopathies (232).

The pattern electroretinogram (PERG) is produced by a phase-reversing patterned stimulus (checkerboard or grating) that maintains a constant average luminance. When the pattern reverses once or twice per second, an isolated response is obtained, whereas a steady-state signal is generated when faster reversal rates (greater than 9 Hz) are used. Signal averaging techniques are employed to record the small signals. The isolated PERG has three components: (*a*) a nega-

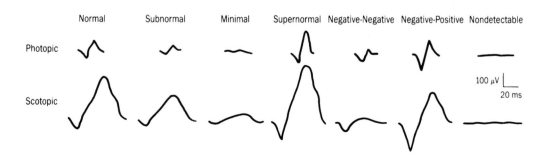

Figure 2.59. Examples of the different patterns of normal and abnormal photopic and scotopic electroretinographic responses that can be obtained in patients with retinal diseases. (From Fishman GA, Sokol S. Electrophysiologic testing in Disorders of the Retina, Optic Nerve, and Visual Pathway. San Francisco, American Academy of Ophthalmology, 1990.)

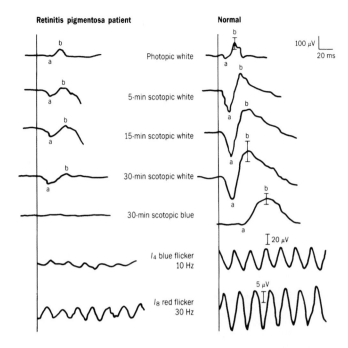

Figure 2.60. An example of electroretinogram (ERG) recordings from a patient with autosomal-dominant retinitis pigmentosa (*left*) compared with normal ERG responses (*right*). (From Fishman GA, Sokol S. Electrophysiologic Testing in Disorders of the Retina, Optic Nerve, and Visual Pathway. San Francisco, American Academy of Ophthalmology, 1990.)

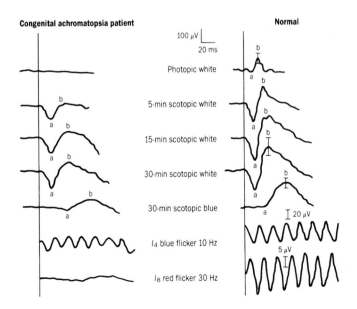

Figure 2.61. Electroretinographic (ERG) recordings from a patient with congenital achromatopsia (*left*) compared with normal ERG responses (*right*). (From Fishman GA, Sokol S. Electrophysiologic Testing in Disorders of the Retina, Optic Nerve, and Visual Pathway. San Francisco, American Academy of Ophthalmology, 1990.)

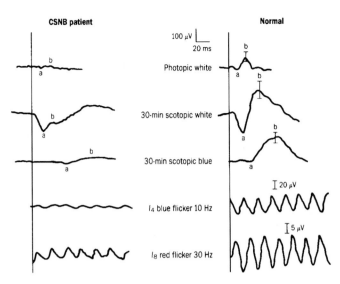

Figure 2.62. Electroretinogram (ERG) from a patient with congenital stationary night blindness (*left*) compared with normal ERG (*right*). Note enhanced a-wave. (From Fishman GA, Sokol S. Electrophysiologic Testing in Disorders of the Retina, Optic Nerve, and Visual Pathway. San Francisco, American Academy of Ophthalmology, 1990.)

tive lobe at about 30 msec called N1 or N30; (*b*) a positive lobe at about 50 msec called P1 or P50; and (*c*) a second negative lobe at about 95 msec called N2 or N95. In normal observers, the PERG waveforms are symmetric between eyes and have an amplitude ratio of about 0.8–0.9. It is believed that the N2 reflects ganglion cell activity and the P1 reflects outer retinal function. The PERG is abnormal in a variety of retinal and optic nerve diseases (261,278–280).

Multifocal ERG Mapping Techniques (Topographical ERG)

Sutter and colleagues (286,287) developed a method of simultaneously recording ERG signals from a large (up to 256) number of retinal locations. These investigators used a binary m-sequence procedure that simultaneously tests a large number of small retinal areas by multiplexing their responses onto a single signal derived from the cornea. After processing of the signal, the net result is an ERG map of the central visual field (Fig. 2.64). This **topographical ERG** is able to detect localized abnormalities in a variety of retinal diseases, including age-related macular degeneration, macular holes, retinitis pigmentosa, branch retinal artery occlusion, and other retinal conditions (287,288). The test has great utility for evaluation of patients with disease of the retina and a normal or near normal retinal examination. It may also be useful in optic neuropathies. A commercial system is available for clinical use.

ELECTRO-OCULOGRAM (EOG)

In 1848, Dubois-Reymond reported that a difference in electric potential of about 6 microvolts was present between the cornea and the back of the eye (229). It was subsequently

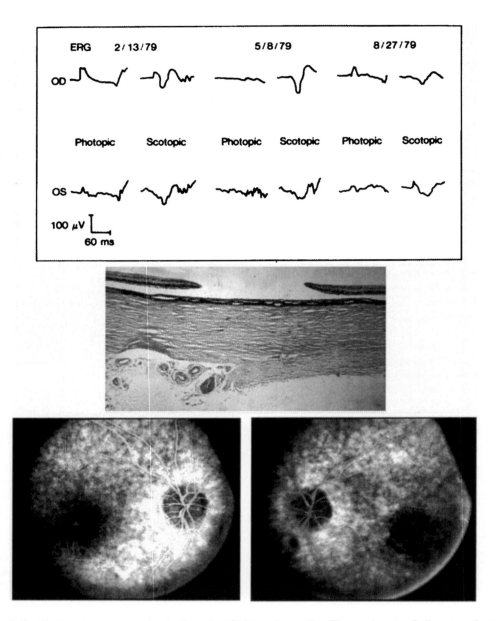

Figure 2.63. Findings in cancer-associated retinopathy (CAR) syndrome. *Top,* Electroretinogram findings over 6 months. Note progressive loss of both photopic and scotopic responses in both eyes. *Bottom,* Fluorescein angiograms of the right (*left*) and left (*right*) fundi show mottling of the retinal pigment epithelium in both eyes and a macular hole in the right eye. *Middle,* Histopathology reveals the macular hole in the right eye and almost complete absence of photoreceptors. (Adapted from Thirkill CE, Roth AM, Keltner JL. Cancer-associated retinopathy. Arch Ophthalmol 1987;105:372–375.)

appreciated that the human eye acts as a dipole, with the cornea positive with respect to the retina. If two electrodes are placed near the inner and outer canthi respectively, movement of the eye will produce a change in the potential measured between the two electrodes, with the electrode closest to the cornea being more positive. A recording of this potential change produced by movement of the eye is called the electro-oculogram (289). The EOG consists of two different potentials, one that is sensitive to light, and the other that is insensitive to light (Fig. 2.65).

Under typical recording conditions, the EOG is measured under conditions of dark adaptation after prior exposure to a pre-adapting illumination (289). The patient is asked to make saccades every second between two stimuli (usually LEDs) spaced approximately 30° apart that are alternately illuminated (Fig. 2.65). These saccadic eye movements produce the change in potential that comprises the EOG signal, with the average of several saccades being taken as the potential at that time. The light-insensitive potential (also called the standing potential) decreases slightly over a period

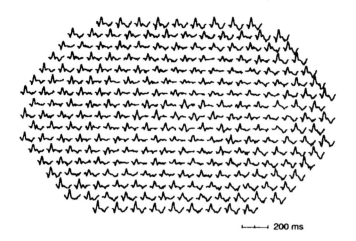

Figure 2.64. Example of a topographic electroretinogram obtained at 255 locations throughout the central 30° of the visual field. (From Sutter EE, Tran D. The field topography of ERG components in man. I. The photopic luminance response. Vision Res 1992;32:433–446.)

of 8 or 9 minutes, at which time the lowest potential recorded in the dark-adapted state can be measured (the dark trough). Following reexposure to light, the potential gradually increases and reaches its peak in another 10 to 15 minutes (the light peak). The amplitude of the light peak is approximately twice that of the dark trough (light rise of the EOG) in normal persons. Because the standing potential can vary considerably, in part related to the placement of the electrodes, the EOG is most appropriately represented as a ratio of the light peak to the dark trough. This ratio is called the **Arden ratio** and is typically greater than 1.8 in normal persons. The International Society for Clinical Electrophysiology of Vision (ISCEV) standards have been established for EOG testing (290).

Clinical studies suggest that the retinal pigment epithelium is probably responsible for generating the EOG. Microelectrode investigations revealed a large direct current (DC) component of the EOG just distal to the outer margin of the outer nuclear layer of the retina (239). The light-sensitive, large, slow, cornea-positive component must depend upon the activity of the photoreceptors and on cells in the inner nuclear layers of the retina, because it is induced by light

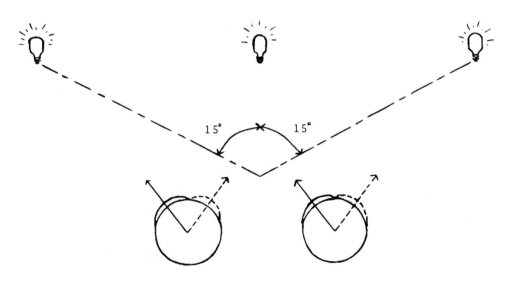

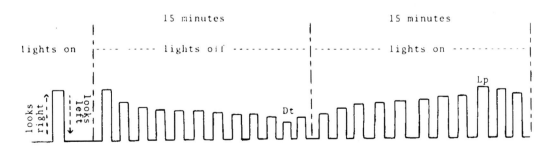

Figure 2.65. The electro-oculogram (EOG). *Top,* Method of obtaining the EOG. The patient looks from right to left, and the movement produces an electric potential. *Bottom,* The EOG signal with dark and light adaptation. Dt, dark trough; Lp, light peak. (Courtesy of Dr. G.A. Fishman, 1982.)

and can be eliminated by central retinal artery occlusion (247).

Based on studies of the action spectrum of the EOG in both dark-adapted and light-adapted states, as well as the observation that human subjects without rod function may have a large, light rise response, this response is thought to represent both rod and cone activity. The light-insensitive potential of the EOG provides a way to measure the function of the pigment epithelium without having to stimulate the photoreceptors (291). The EOG probably should not be used in patients with poor fixation because their poor ability to make accurate saccades can affect the outcomes. In the early stages of retinitis pigmentosa, the light rise of the EOG is reduced, but the standing potential is normal even at a time when the ERG is abnormal or even nondetectable (229). In advanced retinitis pigmentosa, the standing potential of the EOG becomes reduced.

The EOG has limited usefulness in the diagnosis of visual dysfunction. It can help to distinguish the dominant type of stationary night blindness from the recessive type (229) as well as from Stargardt's disease and Best's disease (see below). In chloroquine retinopathy, the EOG is abnormal in the advanced stages when large areas of retinal pigment epithelium are abnormal, but in the very early stage, the EOG is normal (292,293).

When the EOG is abnormal, the ERG is also usually abnormal. There are four exceptions, however, in which patients may have a normal or nearly normal ERG with an abnormal EOG light-rise to dark-trough ratio. The conditions are (a) butterfly-shaped pigment dystrophy of the fovea (294); (b) Stargardt's disease (fundus flavimaculatus) (294); (c) advanced drusen (295); and (d) vitelliform dystrophy or Best's disease (296,297). The EOG is probably most useful in vitelliform macular dystrophy because the EOG is abnormal even in the presence of a normal ERG. In addition, abnormal EOGs may be found in asymptomatic "carriers" who have no abnormalities visible in the fundus (289,298). Thus, the EOG can serve as a genetic marker to identify this autosomal-dominant disease in families with skipped generations (229). From a neuro-ophthalmologic standpoint, the EOG is more important for the recording and analysis of ocular motor function than in diagnosing causes of visual loss.

OTHER RETINAL POTENTIALS

There are several retinal potentials other than the ERG and EOG (e.g., early receptor potentials, oscillatory potentials, the scotopic threshold response) that can be measured under specific test conditions, but they are more commonly used for clinical research studies than for routine clinical evaluation of patients and are therefore not discussed further in this chapter. The interested reader is directed to several excellent sources (229,299–304) for descriptions of these techniques and the waveforms generated.

VISUAL-EVOKED POTENTIAL (VEP)

Until the early 1960s, the electroencephalogram (EEG) was the main technique available for clinical evaluation of electric activity of the human cortex. It was subsequently determined that if the spontaneous occipital EEG was recorded while brief flashes of light were presented to an eye, changes would result in the occipital potential. These changes were called the **visual-evoked potential**, visual-evoked response (VER), or the visual-evoked cortical potential (VECP). The VEP is simply a gross electric potential of the visual cortex in response to visual stimulation. Unlike the alpha rhythm that can be recorded from most regions of the cortex, the VEP is limited mainly to the occipital region of the brain. In addition, although the EEG contains signals with amplitudes generally between 20 and 100 microvolts and occasionally larger, the amplitude of VEP is between 1 and 20 microvolts. Because the VEP amplitude is considerably smaller than the EEG, a major problem that existed for many years was that of extracting the VEP from the background EEG. Initially, van Balen and Henkes (305) used time-locked signal averaging techniques to separate light-evoked responses, based on the assumption that by repetitively stimulating the occipital cortex, one can produce a consistent wave form that can be distinguished from the nonspecific EEG wave produced by the rest of the brain. Another technique involved obtaining a difference potential between two cortical locations—one in which the signal included both the VEP and the EEG (active electrode: occipital lobe) and the other in which the signal had only the EEG and no or very little VEP (inactive electrode: EEG only). This technique allowed extraction of the VEP even when there was a substantial EEG component.

Although the VEP can easily be measured, the portion or portions of the brain responsible for its generation are unclear. Jeffreys and Axford (306,307) studied the first two components of the human VEP (which they called C.I and C.II). These investigators concluded that the first component originated in striate cortex from surface negative cortical activity, whereas the second component originated from extrastriate cortex on the outer surface of the occipital lobes. Streletz et al. (308) emphasized a positive correlation of unilateral occipital lobe lesions, homonymous visual field loss, and VEP abnormalities, but Cohn (309) reported that the VEP to light stimulation in monkeys was initially attenuated after ablation of the occipital cortex and then returned to normal 3 weeks later despite persistence of visual deficits. Bodis-Wollner et al. (310) described normal VEPs to both flash and pattern stimuli in a patient in whom CT scanning suggested bilateral destruction of areas 18 and 19 with preservation of area 17. Clearly, the VEP is dependent on the integrity of the entire visual pathway, although it remains to be seen whether or not its components can truly be separated into anatomic correlates (311). The precise origin and pathways through which the VEP is mediated are still in question. Nevertheless, the clinical importance of the VEP rests on its usefulness as a relatively objective determinant of the integrity of the visual pathways. Numerous reviews of the VEP are available and should be consulted by the interested reader (312–318).

Methodology

The VEP is measured by placing scalp electrodes over the occipital region (Oz) of both hemispheres, with reference

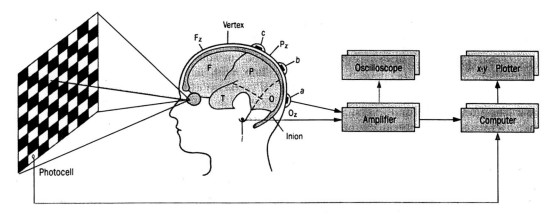

Figure 2.66. Method for generating and recording the visual-evoked potential (VEP). (From Fishman GA, Sokol S. Electrophysiologic Testing in Disorders of the Retina, Optic Nerve, and Visual Pathway. San Francisco, American Academy of Ophthalmology, 1990.)

electrodes attached to the ear (Fig. 2.66). The patient then views the display; typically a xenon-arc photostimulator for flash VEPs and a television screen or computer video display with checkerboard patterned stimuli for pattern VEPs. Recordings of the VEP may be made from either hemisphere with one or both eyes fixating. Typically, 100 to 150 stimulus presentations are generated, and time-locked signal averaging procedures are used to extract the VEP waveform from the spontaneous EEG activity. The amplitude and latency of the waveform are then measured. A flash stimulus is generally used only when no response is produced using a pattern stimulus. Thus, patients with extremely poor acuity, dense media opacities, poor fixation and infants are most commonly tested with flash VEP. In most patients, however, a pattern stimulus is preferred for obtaining the VEP, because of the greater clinical utility and more reliable waveform generated with this stimulus. Rather than bright flashes of light, a repetitive pattern of light and dark areas (checkerboards, bar gratings) are phase-reversed every 1 or 2 seconds. The pattern VEP is primarily generated from the central 5° of the visual field. Indeed, when the central 3° is occluded (Fig. 2.67, *middle*), there is a dramatic reduction in the amplitude of the pattern VEP, and the waveform almost completely disappears when the central 9° is occluded (Fig. 2.67, *bottom*). These findings are consistent with the findings of Horton and Hoyt (319), who estimated that the central 10° of the visual field are represented by at least 50–60% of the posterior striate cortex and that the central 30° is represented by about 80% of the cortex (see Chapters 1 and 12).

The VEP appears different for stimuli that reverse contrast (ON-OFF-ON) compared with those that abruptly come on (onset) and then go off (offset). Why these differences occur is not clear, but they may reflect the fact that these different onset modalities tap discrete cortical processes (i.e., contrast versus luminance). Most clinical laboratories use contrast-reversal patterns.

The amplitude of the pattern VEP is affected by a number of different factors. The size of the stimulus pattern can affect the amplitude of the VEP signal (Fig. 2.68), as can the rate of alternation of the pattern. At low rates of alternation (1–2 reversals per second), the waveform typically contains two negative (N1, N2) and two positive (P1, P2) potentials. This is called the "transient" pattern VEP and is the most commonly used procedure for routine clinical purposes. As the rate of alternation is increased (more than six

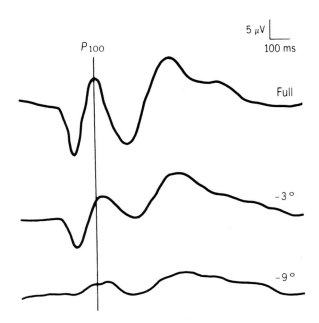

Figure 2.67. Visual-evoked potential waveforms. *Top,* From stimulation of the central 30° visual field. *Middle,* With the central 3° occluded. *Bottom,* With the central 9° occluded. Note that the majority of the waveform is subserved by the central 9° of the visual field. This is consistent with the observations of Horton and Hoyt (319) that the central 10° of the visual field are represented by at least 50–60% of the posterior striate cortex. (From Fishman GA, Sokol S. Electrophysiologic Testing in Disorders of the Retina, Optic Nerve, and Visual Pathway. San Francisco, American Academy of Ophthalmology, 1990.)

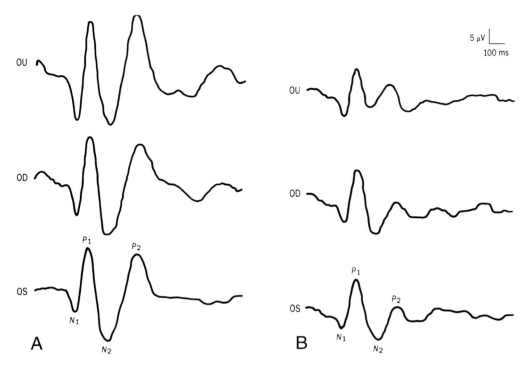

Figure 2.68. Transient visual-evoked response waveforms for small (12 minutes of arc) (*A*) and large (48 minutes of arc) (*B*) checkerboard stimuli. Note difference in size of waveforms. (From Fishman GA, Sokol S. Electrophysiologic Testing in Disorders of the Retina, Optic Nerve, and Visual Pathway. San Francisco, American Academy of Ophthalmology, 1990.)

reversals per second), the response is not able to fully recover between presentations, and only the initial portions of the waveform are observed, similar to the waveforms obtained for ERG with rapidly flickering stimuli. This is called the "steady-state" VEP. In addition, Celesia and Daly (320) found that the latencies of the first major positive and negative components of the VEP become increasingly delayed with increasing age in adults. Latency of the response is indirectly related to stimulus intensity, but amplitude tends to reach maximum at only moderate stimulus intensities and varies with electrode placement, scalp thickness, etc. Infants and young children have quite variable waveforms and prolonged latencies (52,321–323). The VEP also varies with stimulus size and frequency, attention, mental activity, pupil size, fatigue, state of dark adaptation, color of the stimulus, background illumination, and the emotional content of the stimulus (313–315,318,324,325). All of these factors emphasize the importance of using standardized and optimized test conditions (including the best refractive correction) for clinical VEP testing, as well as establishing age-related normative standards for the procedures employed for each laboratory.

Analysis of the VEP waveform is rather complex. For transient pattern VEPs, the amplitude and latency of the N1, P1, and N2 components are typically measured (Figs. 2.67 and 2.68). For steady-state VEPs, the amplitude and phase of the waveform are measured. The latencies of the pattern VEP are quite consistent both within and among observers,

although the amplitudes vary considerably from one person to another. The most useful clinical features of the VEP are therefore the latency of its major components and a comparison of the symmetry of the amplitudes between eyes and between hemispheres in the same person. van Dijk (326) presented an excellent discussion of the pitfalls associated with VEP testing, and many other authors have emphasized the importance of optimized and standardized test conditions (327–329).

Visual-Evoked Potential in Clinical Ophthalmology and Neuro-Ophthalmology

The VEP represents sensory activity in the visual pathways, beginning at the retina and ending at the occipital cortex. A summary of the changes observed in VEP recordings from different visual disorders was published by Sokol and Fishman (330) and are reproduced in Table 2.8. As can be seen from the table, the VEP can be useful in differentiating among retinal, optic nerve, and cortical diseases (331–335). It may also be helpful in determining if an infant or young child has intact vision (336) and if a patient has nonorganic visual loss (337). In general, the VEP should be evaluated for latency, amplitude, waveform, and morphology. The latency and amplitude can be quantified, but waveform morphology is more of a subjective interpretation.

Although the clinical utility and differential diagnostic capabilities of the VEP are limited, there are numerous set-

Table 2.8
Visual-Evoked Potential Abnormalities

Disorder	Amplitude	Latency	Morphology
Optic nerve and visual pathway			
Optic neuritis	A/N	+++	N
Ischemic optic neuropathy	−−	+	A
Toxic amblyopia	−	N	A
Dominant optic atrophy	−	N/+	?
Leber's optic atrophy	−−	+	A
Optic nerve hypoplasia	−−	+	A
Glaucoma	N/−	N/−	N
Optic disc drusen	−	+	A
Papilledema	N/−	N/+	N/A
Tumors (anterior pathway)	−	+	A
Neurologic disorders			
Multiple sclerosis	N/−	+++	N/A
Vitamin B_{12} deficiency	N	+	N
Congenital nystagmus	−	+	A
Parkinson's disease	N/−	N/++	N
Migraine	N	+	N/A
Down syndrome	−	N	?
Cortical blindness	N/−	N	N
Occipital lobe lesion	−	+	A
Huntington's chorea	−	N	A
Friedreich's ataxia	−	++	A
Hereditary spastic ataxia	N	N/+	N
Nonspecific rec. ataxia	N	N	N
Charcot-Marie-Tooth	?	+	N
Phenylketonuria	N	+	N

N = normal, A = abnormal, ? = information not available, +(−) = mild increase (decrease), ++(−−) = moderate increase (decrease), +++(−−−) = severe increase (decrease).
From Sokol and Fishman, 1990, Table 3.1.

tings in which the VEP can be quite helpful (see above and Table 2.8). In conjunction with retinal electrophysiologic responses, the status of visual function from retina to cortex can be evaluated. The VEP and ERG are usually performed separately; however, Hirose et al. (338) developed a system that allows simultaneous recording of both the ERG and VEP with *focal photic* stimulation of the retina under direct observation of the fundus.

Celesia and Daly (339) used computer analysis to evaluate several parameters of the visual-evoked response generated by both flash and pattern-reversal stimulation. These investigators selected for analysis: (*a*) peak latency of the first negative wave; (*b*) interocular difference of peak latency for the first negative wave; (*c*) peak latency of the first positive wave; (*d*) interocular difference of peak latency for the first positive wave; and (*e*) critical frequency of photic driving. They studied 194 subjects and concluded that measurement and computer analysis of these five parameters, which they called "visual electroencephalographic computer analysis" or "VECA," was a more reliable and sensitive method of detecting both clinical and subclinical optic neuropathies than routine evaluation of the VEP.

Multifocal VEP

Many attempts have been made to investigate visual field function using evoked potentials to visual stimuli. A major

breakthrough occurred when Sutter and coworkers used a 60−sector scaled checkerboard set of patches that subserves the central 22°. The stimuli are presented in a pseudo-random m-sequence (340,341). Using these sequences with cross-correlation techniques, electrical responses to pattern reversal stimuli can be extracted from occipital scalp recordings.

In 30 patients with established glaucoma, Klistorner and Graham demonstrated a good concordance of visual field defects found by conventional automated perimetry and with mfVEP (342). Both the number and location of the defects were highly correlated between the two tests. An excellent general review of this technique is provided by Hood (343).

Wall and colleagues (344) tested normals and patients with three types of neuro-ophthalmologic disease: demyelinating optic neuropathies, nondemyelinating optic neuropathies, and homonymous hemianopias. They found that in nondemyelinating optic neuropathies mfVEP results correlate very well with perimetry. In demyelinating optic neuropathies, the mfVEP showed defects when conventional automated perimetry was normal. The mfVEP failed to detect perimetrically obvious homonymous hemianopia in three of five subjects tested. The test does perform well in patients with nonorganic visual loss as long as they look at the stimulus display. This new technique is early in its development. It may become a more clinically useful test in time.

Simultaneous Recording of the Visual-Evoked Potential and PERG

Simultaneous recording of PERG and VEP was found by Kaufman and Celesia (345) to be helpful in the diagnosis of neuro-ophthalmologic disorders (Fig. 2.69). The PERG and pattern VEP can be used to assess the onset of the electrical activity traveling from the retina to the visual cortex to determine retino-cortical transit time (RCT). RCT is defined as the time between the peak latency of the b-wave of the PERG and either the N1 or P1 potential of the pattern VEP. Kaufman and Celesia (345) investigated simultaneous

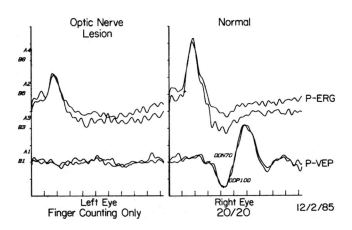

Figure 2.69. Simultaneous recordings of pattern electroretinogram (P-ERG) and pattern visual-evoked potential (P-VEP) in a patient with a left optic nerve lesion and a normal right eye. Note abnormalities in both studies. (Courtesy of Dr. David I. Kaufman.)

PERG and pattern VEP responses in 27 patients with maculopathies, optic atrophy, and MS. Three patterns of abnormalities were reported: (*a*) prolonged PERG, VEP, and RCT latencies were found in early maculopathies; (*b*) normal PERGs in conjunction with prolonged VEP and RCT latencies were found in optic nerve lesions without optic atrophy, probably indicating the presence of a demyelinating lesion of the optic nerve; and (*c*) very small or absent PERGs and VEPs in more advanced maculopathy and optic atrophy cases. Froelich and Kaufman (346) reported that simultaneous recording of PERG and pattern VEP was useful in distinguishing between patients with acute optic neuritis (n = 16) and nonarteritic anterior ischemic optic neuropathy (n = 13). The N95 component of the PERG was reduced in the anterior ischemic optic neuropathy patients, but was normal in the optic neuritis patients. The P50 component was normal in both patient groups. The combined PERG and VEP can also be used to diagnose other forms of optic neuropathy (347) and to detect nonorganic visual loss (348).

ACKNOWLEDGMENTS   Supported in part by a VA Merit Review (M.W.), and a National Eye Institute Research Grant qEY-03424 (C.A.J.).

REFERENCES

1. Frisén L, Frisén M. Micropsia and visual acuity in macular edema. A study of the neuro-retinal basis of visual acuity. Albrecht Von Graefe's Archiv fur Klinische und Experimentelle Ophthalmologie 1979;210:69–77.
2. Minkowski JS, Palese M, Guyton DL. Potential acuity meter using a minute aerial pinhole aperture. Ophthalmology 1983;90:1360–1368.
3. von Noorden GK, Burian HM. Visual acuity in normal and amblyopic patients under reduced illumination. I. Behavior of visual acuity with and without a neutral density filter. Arch Ophthalmol 1959;61:533–535.
4. Glaser JS, Goodwin JA. Neuro-ophthalmologic examination: The visual sensory system. In Tasman W, Jaeger EA, eds. Duane's Clinical Ophthalmology. Vol 2, Chap 2. Philadelphia, JB Lippincott, 1996:1–23.
5. Long DT, Beck RW, Moke PS, et al. The SKILL Card test in optic neuritis: experience of the Optic Neuritis Treatment Trial. Smith Kettlewell Institute Low Luminance Optic Neuritis Study Group. Neuroophthalmology 2001;21:124–131.
6. Leguire LE, Suh S, Rogers GL, Bremer DL. SKILL card results in amblyopic children. J Pediatr Ophthalmol Strabismus 1994;31:256–261.
7. Lott LA, Schneck ME, Haegerstrom-Portnoy G, Brabyn JA, Gildengorin GL, West CG. Reading performance in older adults with good acuity. Optom Vis Sci 2001;78:316–324.
8. Haegerstrom-Portnoy G, Brabyn JA, Schneck ME, Jampolsky A. The SKILL card. An acuity test of reduced luminance and contrast. Smith Kettlewell Institute Low Luminance. Invest Ophthalmol Vis Sci 1997;38:207–218.
9. Kulp MT, Schmidt PP. Visual predictors of reading performance in kindergarten and first grade children. Optom Vis Sci 1996;73:255–262.
10. Keltner JL, Wand M, Van Newkirk MR. Techniques for the Basic Ocular Examination (Video). San Francisco, American Academy of Ophthalmology, 1989.
11. Keltner JL, May WN, Johnson CA, et al. The California syndrome: Functional visual complaints with potential economic impact. Ophthalmology 1985;92:427–435.
12. Donzis PB, Rappazzo JA, Burde RM, Gordon M. Effect of binocular variations of Snellen's visual acuity on Titmus stereoacuity. Arch Ophthalmol 1983;101:930–932.
13. Pokorny J, Smith VC, Verriest G, et al. eds. Congenital and Acquired Color Vision Defects. New York, Grune & Stratton, 1979.
14. Trobe JD, Acosta PC, Krischer JP, Trick GL. Confrontation visual field techniques in the detection of anterior visual pathway lesions. Ann Neurol 1981;10:28–34.
15. Glaser JS, Savino PJ, Sumers KD, et al. The photostress recovery test: A practical adjunct in the clinical assessment of visual function. Am J Ophthalmol 1977;83:255–260.
16. Brindley GS. Physiology of the Retina and Visual Pathways. Baltimore, Williams & Wilkins, 1970.
17. Pulfrich C. Die Stereoskopie im Dienste der isochromen und heterochromen Photometrie. Naturwissenschaften 1922;10:533–564.
18. Lit A. The magnitude of the Pulfrich stereo-phenomenon as a function of target velocity. J Exp Psychol 1960;59:165–175.
19. Grimsdale H. A note on Pulfrich's phenomenon with a suggestion on its possible clinical significance. Br J Ophthalmol 1925;9:63–65.
20. Frisén L, Hoyt WF, Bird AC, et al. Diagnostic uses of the Pulfrich phenomenon. Lancet 1973;2:385–386.
21. Burde RM, Gallin PF. Visual parameters associated with recovered retrobulbar optic neuritis. Am J Ophthalmol 1975;79:1034–1037.
22. Rushton D. Use of the Pulfrich pendulum for detecting abnormal delay in the visual pathway in multiple sclerosis. Brain 1975;98:283–296.
23. Slagsvold JE. Pulfrich pendulum phenomenon in patients with a history of acute optic neuritis. Acta Ophthalmol 1978;56:817–826.
24. Levatin P. Pupillary escape in disease of the retina or optic nerve. Arch Ophthalmol 1959;62:768–779.
25. Thompson HS. Afferent pupillary defects: Pupillary findings associated with the afferent arm of the pupillary light reflex arc. Am J Ophthalmol 1966;62:860–873.
26. Thompson HS. Pupillary signs in the diagnosis of optic nerve disease. Trans Ophthalmol Soc UK 1976;96:377–381.
27. Newsome DA, Milton RC, Gass JDM. Afferent pupillary defect in macular degeneration. Am J Ophthalmol 1981;92:396–402.
28. Greenwald MJ, Folk ER. Afferent pupillary defects in amblyopia. J Pediatr Ophthalmol Strabis 1983;20:63–67.
29. Portnoy JZ, Thompson HS, Lennarson L, et al. Pupillary defects in amblyopia. Am J Ophthalmol 1983;96:609–614.
30. Fineberg E, Thompson HS. Quantitation of the afferent pupillary defect. In Smith L, ed. Neuro-Ophthalmology Focus. New York, Masson, 1979:25–29.
31. Lennie P. Parallel visual pathways: A review. Vis Res 1980;20:561–594.
32. Livingstone M, Hubel D. Psychophysical evidence for separate channels for the perception of form, color, movement and depth. J Neurosci 1987;7:3416–3468.
33. Livingstone M, Hubel D. Segregation of form, color, movement and depth: Anatomy, physiology and perception. Science 1988;240:740–749.
34. Shapley R. Visual sensitivity and parallel retinocortical channels. Annu Rev Psychol 1990;41:635–658.
35. van Essen DC, Anderson CH, Felleman DJ. Information processing in the primate visual system: An integrated systems perspective. Science 1992;255:419–423.
36. Merigan WH, Maunsell JH. How parallel are the primate visual pathways? Ann Rev Neurosci 1993;16:369–402.
37. Dacey DM, Packer OS. Color coding in the primate retina: diverse cell types and cone-specific circuitry. Curr Opin Neurobiol 2003;13:421–427.
38. Goodrich GL, Apple LE, Frost A, et al. A preliminary report on experienced closed-circuit television users. Am J Optom Physiol Opt 1976;53:7–15.
39. Bullimore MA, Bailey IL, Wacker RT. Contrast sensitivity and functional performance in low vision. Invest Ophthalmol Visual Sci 1990;31(Suppl):598.
40. Bullimore MA, Bailey IL, Wacker AT. Face recognition in age-related maculopathy. Invest Ophthalmol Visual Sci 1991;32:2020–2029.
41. Thibos LN, Bradley A. New methods for discriminating neural and optical losses of vision. Optom Vis Sci 1993;70:279–287.
42. Snellen H. Probebuchstaben zur Bestimmung der Sehscharfe. Utrecht, PW van de Weijer, 1862.
43. Owsley C, Sekuler R, Siemsen R. Contrast sensitivity throughout adulthood. Vis Res 1983;23:689–699.
44. Bailey IL, Lovie JE. New design principles for visual acuity letter charts. Am J Optom Physiol Opt 1976;53:740–745.
45. Ferris FL III, Kassoff A, Bresnick GH, et al. New visual acuity charts for clinical research. Am J Ophthalmol 1982;94:91–96.
46. Bailey IL, Bullimore MA, Raasch TW, et al. Clinical grading and the effect of scaling. Invest Ophthalmol Vis Sci 1991;32:422–432.
47. Bailey IL. New procedures for detecting early vision losses in the elderly. Optom Vis Sci 1993;48(70):299–305
48. Friendly DS. Preschool visual acuity screening tests. Trans Am Ophthalmol Soc 1978;76:383–480.
49. Hered RW, Murphy S, Clancy M. Comparison of the HOTV and Lea Symbols charts for preschool vision screening. J Pediatr Ophthalmol Strabismus 1997;34:24–28.
50. Greenwald MJ, Parks MM. Amblyopia. In Tasman W, Jaeger EA, eds. Duane's Clinical Ophthalmology, Vol I, Chap 10. Philadelphia, JB Lippincott, 1996:1–22.
51. Dobson V, Teller DY. Visual acuity in human infants: A review and comparison of behavioral and electrophysiological studies. Vision Res 1978;18:1469–1483.
52. Norcia AM, Tyler CW. Spatial frequency sweep VEP: Visual acuity during the first year of life. Vision Res 1985;25:1399–1408.
53. Fern KD, Manny RE. Visual acuity of the preschool child: A review. Am J Optom Physiol Opt 1986;63:319–345.
54. Preston KL, McDonald M, Sebris SL, et al. Validation of the acuity card procedure for assessment of infants with ocular disorders. Ophthalmology 1987;94:644–653.
55. Haegerstrom-Portnoy G. New procedures for evaluating vision functions of special populations. Optom Vis Sci 1993;70:306–314.
56. Randall HG, Brown DJ, Sloan LL. Peripheral visual acuity. Arch Ophthalmol 1966;75:500–504.
57. Frisén L. The neurology of visual acuity. Brain 1980;103:639–670.

58. Ginsberg AP. Spatial filtering and vision: Implications for normal and abnormal vision. In Proenza LM, Enoch JM, Jampolsky A, eds. Clinical Applications of Visual Psychophysics. Cambridge UK, Cambridge University Press 1981: 70–106.

59. Campbell FW, Robson JG. Application of Fourier analysis to the visibility of gratings. J Physiol 1968;197:551–566.

60. Hess RF, Bradley A. Contrast perception above threshold is only minimally impaired in human amblyopes. Nature 1980;287:463–464.

61. Van Nes FL, Koenderink JJ, Nas H, et al. Spatial modulation transfer in the human eye. J Opt Soc Am 1967;57:1082–1088.

62. Kelly DH. Adaptation effects on spatiotemporal sine-wave thresholds. Vision Res 1972;12:89–101.

63. Koenderink JJ, Bouman MA, Bueno de Mesquita AE, et al. Perimetry of contrast detection thresholds of moving spatial sine wave patterns. IV. The influence of mean retinal illuminance. J Opt Soc Am 1978;68:860–865.

64. Hoekstra J, Van der Groot DP, van den Brink G, et al. The influence of the number of cycles upon the visual contrast threshold for spatial sine wave patterns. Vision Res 1974;14:365–368.

65. Koenderink JJ, Bouman MA, Bueno de Mesquita AE, et al. Perimetry of contrast detection thresholds of moving spatial sine wave patterns. III. The target extent as a sensitivity controlling parameter. J Opt Soc Am 1978;68:854–860.

66. Daitch JM, Green DG. Contrast sensitivity of the human peripheral retina. Vision Res 1969;9:947–952.

67. Koenderink JJ, Bouman MA, Bueno de Mesquita AE, et al. Perimetry of contrast detection thresholds of moving spatial sine wave patterns. I. The near peripheral visual field (eccentricity 0–8 deg). J Opt Soc Am 1978;68:845–849.

68. Koenderink JJ, Bouman MA, Bueno de Mesquita AE, et al. Perimetry of contrast detection thresholds of moving spatial sine wave patterns. II. The far peripheral visual field (eccentricity 0–50 deg). J Opt Soc Am 1978;68:850–854.

69. Westheimer G. Pupil size and visual resolution. Vision Res 1964;4:39–45.

70. Campbell FW, Green DC. Optical and retinal factors affecting visual resolution. J Physiol 1965;181:576–593.

71. Henning GB. Spatial-frequency tuning as a function of temporal frequency and stimulus motion. J Opt Soc Am 1988;5:1362–1373.

72. Campbell FW, Kulikowski JJ, Levinson J. The effect of orientation on the visual resolution of gratings. J Physiol 1966;187:427–436.

73. Zemon V, Gutowski W, Horton T. Orientational anisotropy in the human visual system: An evoked potential and psychophysical study. Int J Neurosci 1983;19:259–286.

74. Hess RF, Garner LF. The effect of corneal edema on visual function. Invest Ophthalmol Visual Sci 1977;16:5–13.

75. Hess RF, Woo G. Vision through cataracts. Invest Ophthalmol Visual Sci 1978;17:428–435.

76. Krasnov MM, Avetisov SE, Makashova NV, et al. The effect of radial keratotomy on contrast sensitivity. Am J Ophthalmol 1988;105:651–654.

77. Hess RF, Woo GC, White PD. Contrast attenuation characteristics of iris clipped intraocular lens implants in situ. Br J Ophthalmol 1985;69:129–135.

78. Owsley C, Sekuler R, Siemsen D. Contrast sensitivity throughout adulthood. J Optom Soc Am 1983;23:689–699.

79. Whitaker D, Elliott DB. Simulating age-related optical changes in the human eye. Doc Ophthalmol 1992;82:307–316.

80. Trick GL, Burde RM, Gordon MO. The relationship between hue discrimination and contrast sensitivity deficits in patients with diabetes mellitus. Ophthalmology 1988;95:693–698.

81. Sjöstrand J, Frisén L. Contrast sensitivity in macular disease: A preliminary report. Acta Ophthalmol 1977;55:507–514.

82. Arden GB, Jacobson JJ. A simple grating test for contrast sensitivity. Preliminary results indicate value in screening for glaucoma. Invest Ophthalmol Visual Sci 1978;17:23–32.

83. Atkin A, Bodis-Wollner I, Wolkstein M, et al. Abnormalities of central contrast sensitivity in glaucoma. Am J Ophthalmol 1979;88:205–211.

84. Wood JM, Lovie-Kitchin JE. Evaluation of the efficacy of contrast sensitivity measures for the detection of early primary open-angle glaucoma. Optom Vis Sci 1992;69:175–181.

85. Regan D, Silver R, Murray TJ. Visual acuity and contrast sensitivity in multiple sclerosis: Hidden visual loss. Brain 1977;100:563–579.

86. Storch RL, Bodis-Wollner I. Overview of contrast sensitivity and neuro-ophthalmic disease. In Nadler MP, Miller D, Nadler DJ, eds. Glare and Contrast Sensitivity for Clinicians. New York, Springer-Verlag, 1990:85–112.

87. Bodis-Wollner I, Diamond SP. The measurement of spatial contrast sensitivity in cases of blurred vision associated with cerebral lesions. Brain 1976;99:695–710.

88. Bulens C, Meerwaldt JD, van der Wildt GJ, et al. Spatial contrast sensitivity in unilateral cerebral ischemic lesions involving the posterior visual pathway. Brain 1989;112:507–528.

89. Wall M. Sensory visual testing in idiopathic intracranial hypertension: Measures sensitive to change. Neurology 1990;40:1859–1864.

90. Hess RF. Application of contrast-sensitivity techniques to the study of functional amblyopia. In: Proenza LM, Enoch JM, Jampolsky A, eds. Clinical Applications of Visual Psychophysics. Cambridge UK, Cambridge University Press, 1981.

91. Cronin-Golomb A, Rizzo JF, Corkin S, et al. Visual function in Alzheimer's disease and normal aging. Ann NY Acad Sci 1991;640:28–35.

92. Swanson WH, Birch EE. Infant spatiotemporal vision: Dependence of spatial contrast sensitivity on temporal frequency. Vision Res 1990;30:1033–1048.

93. Ginsberg AP, Evans DW, Sekule R, et al. Contrast sensitivity predicts performance in aircraft simulators. Am J Optom Physiol Opt 1982;59:105–109.

94. Evans DW, Ginsberg AP. Contrast sensitivity predicts age-related differences in highway sign discriminability. Human Factors 1985;27:637–642.

95. Leat SJ, Woodhouse JM. Reading performance with low vision aids: Relationship with contrast sensitivity. Ophthalmic Physiol Opt 1993;13:9–16.

96. Owsley C, Sloane ME. Contrast sensitivity, acuity and the perception of "real-world" targets. Br J Ophthalmol 1987;71:791–796.

97. Marron JA, Bailey IL. Visual factors and orientation-mobility performance. Am J Optom Physiol Opt 1982;59:413–426.

98. Ginsberg AP. A new contrast sensitivity vision test chart. Am J Optom Physiol Opt 1984;61:403–407.

99. Regan D, Neima D. Low-contrast letter charts in early diabetic retinopathy, ocular hypertension, glaucoma and Parkinson's disease. Br J Ophthalmol 1981;68:885–889.

100. Regan D, Neima D. Low-contrast letter charts as a test of visual function. Ophthalmology 1983;90:1192–1200.

101. Pelli DG, Robson JG, Wilkins AJ. The design of a new letter chart for measuring contrast sensitivity. Clin Vision Sci 1988;2:187–199.

102. Rubin GS. Reliability and sensitivity of clinical contrast sensitivity tests. Clin Vision Sci 1988;2:169–177.

103. Optic Neuritis Study Group. The clinical profile of optic neuritis: Experience of the Optic Neuritis Treatment Trial. Arch Ophthalmol 1991;109:1673–1678.

104. Leguire LE. Do letter charts measure contrast sensitivity? Clin Vision Sci 1991;6:391–400.

105. Pelli DG, Robson JG. Are letters better than gratings? Clin Vision Sci 1991;6:409–411.

106. Regan D. Do letter charts measure contrast sensitivity? Clin Vision Sci 1991;6:401–408.

107. Herse PR, Bedell HE. Contrast sensitivity for letter and grating targets under various stimulus conditions. Optom Vis Sci 1989;66:774–781.

108. White JM, Loshin DS. Grating acuity overestimates Snellen acuity in patients with age-related maculopathy. Optom Vis Sci 1989;66:751–755.

109. Johnson CA, Keltner JL. Incidence of visual field loss in 20,000 eyes and its relationship to driving performance. Arch Ophthalmol 1983;101:371–376.

110. Hedin A, Lovsund P. Effects of visual field defects on driving performance. Doc Ophthalmol 1987;49:541–548.

111. Szlyk JP, Alexander KR, Severing K, et al. Assessment of driving performance in patients with retinitis pigmentosa. Arch Ophthalmol 1992;110:1709–1713.

112. Szlyk JP, Brigell M, Seiple W. Effects of age and hemianopic visual field loss on driving. Optom Vis Sci 1993;70:1031–1037.

113. Aulhorn E, Harms H. Visual Perimetry. In Jameson D, Hurvich LM, eds.Visual Psychophysics: Handbook of Sensory Physiology. Vol VII, Chap 4. New York, Springer-Verlag, 1972.

114. Greve EL. Single and Multiple Stimulus Static Perimetry: The Two Phases of Perimetry. The Hague, Dr. W Junk Publishers, 1973.

115. Tate GW, Lynn JR. Principles of Quantitative Perimetry: Testing and Interpreting the Visual Field. New York, Grune & Stratton, 1977.

116. Drance SM, Anderson DL. Automated Perimetry in Glaucoma: A Practical Guide. New York, Grune & Stratton, 1985.

117. Anderson DR. Perimetry with and without Automation. St Louis, CV Mosby, 1987.

118. Anderson DR, Patella VM. Automated Static Perimetry. St Louis, CV Mosby, 1999.

119. Langerhorst CT. Automated Perimetry in Glaucoma. Amsterdam, Kugler, 1988.

120. Frisén L. Clinical Tests of Vision. New York, Raven Press, 1990.

121. Harrington DO, Drake MV. The Visual Fields: Text and Atlas of Clinical Perimetry. St Louis, CV Mosby, 1990.

122. Lieberman MF, Drake MV. Computerized Perimetry: A Simplified Guide. Thorofare NJ, Slack, 1992.

123. Henson DB. Visual Fields. New York, Oxford University Press, 1993.

124. Choplin NT, Edwards RP. Visual Field Testing with the Humphrey Field Analyzer. Thoroughfare NJ, Slack, 1995.

125. Trobe JD, Acosta PC, Shuster JJ, Krischer JP. An evaluation of the accuracy of community-based perimetry. Am J Ophthalmol 1980;90:654–660.

126. Boring, EG. A History of Experimental Psychology. New York, Appleton-Century-Crofts, 1950.

127. Johnson CA, Keltner JL, Balestrery FG. Static and acuity profile perimetry at various adaptation levels. Doc Ophthalmol 1981;50:371–388.

128. Johnson CA, Keltner JL, Balestrery FG. Effects of target size and eccentricity on visual detection and resolution. Vision Res 1978;18:1217–1222.

129. Uyama K, Matsumoto C, Okuyama S, et al. Influence of the target size on the sensitivity of the central visual field in patients with early glaucoma. In Perimetry Update 1992/1993. Amsterdam, Kugler, 1993;381–386.

130. Wall M, Kutzko KS, Chauhan BC. Variability in patients with glaucomatous optic nerve damage is reduced using size V stimuli. Invest Ophthalmol Vis Sci 1997;38:426–435.

131. Pennebacker GE, Stewart WC, Stewart JA, et al. The effect of stimulus duration

upon the components of fluctuation in static automated perimetry. Eye 1992;6: 353–355.

132. Hedin A, Verriest G. Is clinical color perimetry useful? Doc Ophthalmol 1980; 26:161–184.

133. Hart WM, Kosmorsky G, Burde RM. Color perimetry of central scotomas in diseases of the macula and optic nerve. Sixth International Visual Field Symposium, Santa Margherita Ligure 1984. Dordrecht, The Netherlands, Dr W Junk, 1985:239–246.

134. Hansen E, Olsen BT, Tomaki R, et al. A modification of the Goldmann perimeter designed for color perimetry. In Seventh International Visual Symposium, Amsterdam, September 1996. Dordrecht, The Netherlands, Martinus Nijhoff, 1987.

135. Kitahara K, Kandatsu A, Tamaki R, et al. Spectral sensitivities on a white background as a function of retinal eccentricity. In Seventh International Visual Symposium, Amsterdam, September 1996. Dordrecht, The Netherlands, Martinus Nijhoff, 1987.

136. Flanagan JG, Hovis JK. Colored targets in the assessment of differential light sensitivity. In Perimetry Update 1988/1989. Amsterdam, Kugler, 1989;67–76.

137. Fankhauser F, Enoch JM. The effects of blur on perimetric thresholds. Arch Ophthalmol 1962;68:120–131.

138. Budenz DL, Feuer WJ, Anderson DR. The effect of simulated cataract on the glaucomatous visual field. Ophthalmology 1993;100:511–517.

139. Meyer DR, Stern JH, Jarvis JM, et al. Evaluating the visual field effects of blepharoptosis using automated static perimetry. Ophthalmology 1993;100: 651–658.

140. Mikelberg FS, Drance SM, Schulzer M, et al. The effect of miosis on visual field indices. In Greve EL, Heijl A, eds. Seventh International Visual Symposium, Amsterdam, September 1996. Dordrecht, The Netherlands, Martinus Nijhoff 1987:645–650.

141. Lindenmuth KA, Skuta GL, Rabani R, et al. Effects of pupillary constriction on automated perimetry in normal eyes. Ophthalmology 1989;96:1298–1301.

142. Zalta AH. Lens rim artifact in automated threshold perimetry. Ophthalmology 1989;96:1302–1311.

143. Demirel S, Vingrys AJ. Fixational instability during perimetry and the blindspot monitor. In Mills RP, ed. Perimetry Update 1992/1993. Amsterdam, Kugler 1993:515–520.

144. Katz J, Sommer A. Reliability indexes of automated perimetric tests. Arch Ophthalmol 1988;106:1252–1254.

145. Johnson CA, Nelson-Quigg JM. A prospective three year study of response properties of normals and patients during automated perimetry. Ophthalmology 1993;100:269–274.

146. Vingrys AJ, Demirel S. The effect of fixational loss on perimetric thresholds and reliability. In Mills RP, ed. Perimetry Update 1992/1993. Amsterdam, Kugler, 1993:521–526.

147. Wild JM, Dengler-Harles M, Searle AE, et al. The influence of the learning effect on automated perimetry in patients with suspected glaucoma. Acta Ophthalmol 1989;67:537–545.

148. Werner EB, Krupin T, Adelson A, et al. Effect of patient experience on the results of automated perimetry in glaucoma suspect patients. Ophthalmology 1990;97:44–48.

149. Guttridge NM, Allen PM, Rudnicka AR, et al. Influence of learning on the peripheral field as assessed by automated perimetry. In Mills RP, Heijl A, eds. Perimetry Update 1990/1991. Amsterdam, Kugler & Ghedini, 1991:567–576.

150. Saarinen J, Julesz B. The speed of attentional shifts in the visual field. Proc Natl Acad Sci 1991;88:1812–1814.

151. Searle AET, Shaw DE, Wild JM, et al. Within and between test learning and fatigue effects in normal perimetric sensitivity. In Perimetry Update 1990/1991. Amsterdam, Kugler and Ghedini, 1991:533–538.

152. Langerhorst CT, van den Berg TJTP, Veldman E, et al. Population study of global and local fatigue with prolonged threshold testing in automated perimetry. In Greve EL, Heijl A, eds. Seventh International Visual Symposium, Amsterdam, September 1996. Dordrecht, The Netherlands, Martinus Nijhoff, 1987: 657–662.

153. Johnson CA, Adams CW, Lewis RA. Fatigue effects in automated perimetry. Appl Opt 1988;27:1030–1037.

154. Hudson C, Wild JM, Searle AET, et al. The magnitude and locus of perimetric fatigue in normals and ocular hypertensives. In Perimetry Update 1992/1993. Amsterdam, Kugler, 1993:503–507.

155. Sunga RN, Enoch JM. Further perimetric analysis of patients with lesions of the visual pathways. Am J Ophthalmol 1970;70:403–423.

156. Enoch JM. Quantitative layer-by-layer perimetry. Invest Ophthalmol Vis Sci 1978;17:208–257.

157. Trobe JD, Acosta PC, Krischer JP, Trick GL. Confrontation visual field techniques in the detection of anterior visual pathway lesions. Ann Neurol 1981;10: 28–34.

158. Pandit RJ, Gales K, Griffiths PG. Effectiveness of testing visual fields by confrontation. Lancet 2001;358:1339–1340.

159. Amsler M. Quantitative and qualitative vision. Trans Ophthalmol Soc UK 1949; 69:397–410.

160. Wall M, May DR. Threshold Amsler grid testing in maculopathies. Ophthalmology 1987;94:1126–1133.

161. Johnson CA, Keltner JL. Optimal rates of movement for kinetic perimetry. Arch Ophthalmol 1987;105:73–75.

162. Bengtsson B, Olsson J, Heijl A, Rootzen H. A new generation of algorithms for computerized threshold perimetry, SITA. Acta Ophthalmol Scand 1997;75: 368–375.

163. Bengtsson B, Heijl A, Olsson J. Evaluation of a new threshold visual field strategy, SITA, in normal subjects. Swedish interactive thresholding algorithm. Acta Ophthalmol Scand 1998;76:165–169.

164. Bengtsson B, Heijl A. Comparing significance and magnitude of glaucomatous visual field defects using the SITA and Full Threshold strategies. Acta Ophthalmol Scand 1999;77:143–146.

165. King-Smith PE, Grigsby SS, Vingrys AJ, et al. Efficient and unbiased modifications of the QUEST threshold method: theory, simulations, experimental evaluation and practical implementation. Vision Res 1994;34:885–912.

166. Turpin A, McKendrick AM, Johnson CA, Vingrys AJ. Performance of efficient test procedures for frequency doubling technology (FDT) perimetry in normal and glaucomatous eyes. Invest Ophthalmol Vis Sci 2002;43:709–715.

167. Turpin A, McKendrick AM, Johnson CA, Vingrys AJ. Properties of perimetric threshold estimates from Full Threshold, ZEST and SITA-like strategies as determined by computer simulation. Invest Ophthalmol Vis Sci 2003;44:4787–4795.

168. Johnson CA. The test logic of automated perimetry. ACTA:XXIV International Congress of Ophthalmology. Philadelphia, JB Lippincott, 1983:151–155.

169. Glovinsky Y, Quigley HA, Bissett RA, et al. Artificially produced quadrantanopsia in computed visual field testing. Am J Ophthalmol 1990;110:90–91.

170. Stewart JF. Automated perimetry and malingerers. Can the Humphrey be outwitted? Ophthalmology 1995;102:27–32.

171. Thompson JC, Kosmorsky GS, Ellis BD. Fields of dreamers and dreamed-up fields: Functional and fake perimetry. Ophthalmology 1996;103:117–125.

172. Spry PGD, Johnson CA. Identification of progressive glaucomatous visual field loss. Surv Ophthalmol 2002;47:158–173.

173. Johnson CA. Selective versus nonselective losses in glaucoma. J Glaucoma 1994;3(Suppl 1):S32–S44.

174. Johnson CA, Brandt JD, Khong AM, et al. Short-wavelength automated perimetry in low-, medium-, and high-risk ocular hypertensives: Initial baseline results. Arch Ophthalmol 1995;113:70–76.

175. Wild JM, Moss ID, Whitaker D, et al. The statistical interpretation of blue-on-yellow visual field loss. Invest Ophthalmol Vis Sci 1995;36:1398–1410.

176. Wild JM. Short wavelength automated perimetry. Acta Ophthalmol Scand 2001; 79:546–559.

177. Sample PA, Johnson CA, Hagerstrom-Portnoy G, et al. The optimum parameters for Short-Wavelength Automated Perimetry. J Glaucoma 1996;5:375–383.

178. Bengtsson B. A new rapid threshold algorithm for short-wavelength automated perimetry. Invest Ophthalmol Vis Sci 2003;44:1388–1394.

179. Keltner JL, Johnson CA. Short Wavelength Automated Perimetry [SWAP] in neuro-ophthalmologic disorders. Arch Ophthalmol 1995;113:475–481.

180. Frisén L. A computer graphics visual field screener using high pass spatial frequency resolution targets and multiple feedback devices. In: Greve EL, Heijl A, eds. Seventh International Visual Symposium, Amsterdam, September 1996. Dordrecht, The Netherlands, Martinus Nijhoff 1987:446.

181. Frisén L. High pass resolution perimetry: Recent developments. In Perimetry Focus 1988/1989. Amsterdam, Kugler & Ghedini, 1989:383–392.

182. Sample PA, Ahn DS, Lee PC, et al. High-pass resolution perimetry in eyes with ocular hypertension and primary open-angle glaucoma. Am J Ophthalmol 1992; 113:309–316.

183. Lachenmayr BJ, Drance SM, Douglas GR, et al. Light-sense, flicker and resolution perimetry in glaucoma: A comparative study. Graefe's Arch Clin Exp Ophthalmol 1991;229:246–251.

184. Lachenmayr BJ, Drance SM, Chauhan BC, et al. Diffuse and localized glaucomatous field loss in light-sense, flicker and resolution perimetry. Graefe's Arch Clin Exp Ophthalmol 1991;229:267–273.

185. Dannheim F, Abramo F, Verlohr D. Comparison of automated conventional and spatial resolution perimetry in glaucoma. In Perimetry Update 1988/1989. Amsterdam, Kugler, 1989:383–392.

186. Bynke H. Evaluation of high-pass resolution perimetry in neuro-ophthalmology. In Mills RP, Heijl A, eds. Perimetry Update 1990/1991. Amsterdam, Kugler 1991:143–149.

187. Wall M. High-pass resolution perimetry in optic neuritis. Invest Ophthalmol Vis Sci 1991;32:2525–2529.

188. Wall M, Conway MD, House PH, et al. Evaluation of sensitivity and specificity of spatial resolution and Humphrey automated perimetry in pseudotumor cerebri patients and normal subjects. Invest Ophthalmol Vis Sci 1991;32:3306–3312.

189. Lindblom B, Hoyt WF. High-pass resolution perimetry in neuro-ophthalmology. Ophthalmology 1992;99:700–705.

190. Chauhan BC, LeBlanc RP, McCormick TA, et al. Correlation between the optic disc and results obtained with conventional, high-pass resolution and pattern discrimination perimetry in glaucoma. Can J Ophthalmol 1993;28:312–316.

191. Chauhan BC, Mohandas RN, Whelan JH, et al. Comparison of high-pass resolution perimetry and pattern discrimination perimetry to conventional perimetry in glaucoma. Can J Ophthalmol 1993;28:306–311.

192. Wanger P, Martin-Boglind LM. High-pass resolution perimetry: Comparison

between mean dB score and neural capacity in glaucoma diagnosis and followup. In Perimetry Update 1992/1993. Amsterdam, Kugler, 1993:415–418.

193. Chauhan BC, House PH, LeBlanc RP, et al. Comparison of conventional and high-pass resolution perimetry in a prospective study of patients with glaucoma and healthy controls. Arch Ophthalmol 1999;117:24–33.

194. Casson EJ, Johnson CA, Shapiro LR. Longitudinal comparison of temporal-modulation perimetry with white-on-white and blue-on-yellow perimetry in ocular hypertension and early glaucoma. J Optom Soc Am 1993;10:1792–1806.

195. Lachenmayr BJ, Gleissner M. Flicker perimetry resists retinal image degradation. Invest Ophthalmol Vis Sci 1992;33:3539–3542.

196. Fitzke FW, Poinoosawmy D, Ernst W, et al. Peripheral displacement thresholds in normals, ocular hypertensives and glaucoma. In: Greve EL, Heijl A, eds. Seventh International Visual Symposium, Amsterdam, September 1986. Dordrecht, The Netherlands, Martinus Nijhoff, 1987:447–452.

197. Fitzke FW, Poinoosawmy D, Nagasubramanian S, et al. Peripheral displacement thresholds in glaucoma and ocular hypertension. In Perimetry Update 1988/1989. Amsterdam, Kugler, 1989:399–405.

198. Poinoosawmy D, Wu JX, Fitzke FW, et al. Discrimination between progression and non-progression visual field loss in low tension glaucoma using MDT. In Perimetry Update 1992/1993. Amsterdam, Kugler, 1992:109–114.

199. Johnson CA, Marshall D, Eng C. Displacement threshold perimetry in glaucoma using a Macintosh computer system and a 21-inch monitor. In: Perimetry Update 1994/1995. Amsterdam, Kugler, 1995:103–110.

200. Silverman SE, Trick GL, Hart WM Jr. Motion perception is abnormal in primary open-angle glaucoma and ocular hypertension. Invest Ophthalmol Vis Sci 1990;31:722–729.

201. Bullimore MA, Wood JM, Swenson K. Motion perception in glaucoma. Invest Ophthalmol Vis Sci 1993;34:3526–3533.

202. Wall M, Ketoff KM. Random dot motion perimetry in patients with glaucoma and in normal subjects. Am J Ophthalmol 1995;120:587–596.

203. Wall M, Montgomery EB. Using motion perimetry to detect visual field defects in patients with idiopathic intracranial hypertension: A comparison with conventional automated perimetry. Neurology 1995;45:1169–1175.

204. Wall M, Jennisch CS, Munden PM. Motion perimetry identifies nerve fiber bundlelike defects in ocular hypertension. Arch Ophthalmol 1997;115:26–33.

205. Wojciechowski R, Trick GL, Steinman SB. Topography of the age-related decline in motion sensitivity. Optom Vis Sci 1995;72:67–74.

206. Joffe KM, Raymond JE, Crichton A. Motion coherence perimetry in glaucoma and suspected glaucoma. Vision Res 1997;37:955–964.

207. Johnson CA, Scobey RP. Foveal and peripheral displacement thresholds as a function of stimulus luminance, line length and duration of movement. Vision Res 1980;20:709–715.

208. Kelly DH. Frequency doubling in visual responses. J Optom Soc Am 1966;56:1628–1633.

209. Kelly DH. Nonlinear visual responses to flickering sinusoidal gratings. J Optom Soc Am 1981;71:1051–1055.

210. Maddess T, Henry GH. Performance of nonlinear visual units in ocular hypertension and glaucoma. Clin Vis Sci 1992;7:371–383.

211. Johnson CA, Samuels SJ. Screening for glaucomatous visual field loss with frequency doubling perimetry. Invest Ophthalmol Vis Sci 1997;38:413–425.

212. Cello KE, Nelson-Quigg JM, Johnson CA. Frequency Doubling Technology (FDT) perimetry as a means of detecting glaucomatous visual field loss. Am J Ophthalmol 2000;129:314–322.

213. Anderson AJ, Johnson CA. Frequency-doubling technology perimetry. Ophthalmol Clin North Am 2003;16:213–225.

214. Wall M, Neahring RK, Woodward KR. Sensitivity and specificity of frequency doubling perimetry in neuro-ophthalmic disorders: a comparison with conventional automated perimetry. Invest Ophthalmol Vis Sci 2002;43:1277–1283.

215. Adams AJ, Verdon WA, Spivey BE. Color vision. In: Tasman W, Jaeger EA, eds. Duane's Foundations of Clinical Ophthalmology, Vol I, Chap 52. Philadelphia, JB Lippincott, 1996:1–43.

216. Kaiser PK, Boynton RM. Human Color Vision. Washington DC, Optical Society of America, 1996.

217. Young T. On the theory of light and colors. Philos Trans R Soc Lond 1802;92:12.

218. Helmholtz HLF. On the theory of compound colors. Phil Mag 1852;4:519–534.

219. Hering E. Outlines of a theory of the light sense. (Translated by Hurvich and Jameson.) Cambridge, MA, Harvard University Press, 1964.

220. Gunduz K, Arden GB, Perry S, et al. Color vision defects in ocular hypertension and glaucoma: Quantification with a computer driven color television system. Arch Ophthalmol 1988;106:929–935.

221. King-Smith PE. Psychophysical methods for the investigation of acquired color vision deficiencies. In Cronley-Dillon JR, ed. Vision and Visual Dysfunction. Vol 7. New York, Macmillan Press, 1991:38–55.

222. Yu TC, Falcao-Reis F, Spileers W, et al. Peripheral color contrast: A new screening test for preglaucomatous visual loss. Invest Ophthalmol Vis Sci 1991;32:2779–2789.

223. Nichols BE, Thompson HS, Stone EM. Evaluation of a significantly shorter version of the Farnsworth-Munsell 100-Hue Test in patients with three different optic neuropathies. J Neuroophthalmol 1997;17:1–6.

224. Adams AJ. Chromatic and luminosity processing in retinal disease. Am J Optom Physiol Opt 1982;59:954–960.

225. Dain SJ, Rammohan KW, Benes SC, et al. Chromatic, spatial and temporal losses of sensitivity in multiple sclerosis. Invest Ophthalmol Vis Sci 1990;31:548–558.

226. Grigsby SS, Vingrys AJ, Benes SC, et al. Correlation of chromatic, spatial and temporal sensitivity in optic nerve disease. Invest Ophthalmol Vis Sci 1991;32:3252–3262.

227. Billock VA, Vingrys AJ, King-Smith PE. Opponent-color detection threshold asymmetries may result from reduction of ganglion cell populations. Vis Neurosci 1994;11:99–109.

228. King-Smith PE. Cortical color defects. In Drum B, Verriest G, eds. Color Deficiencies, IX. The Hague, Dr W Junk, 1989:131–143.

229. Berson EL. Electrical phenomena in the retina. In Hart WM Jr, ed. Adler's Physiology of the Eye. 9th ed. St Louis, CV Mosby, 1992:641–707.

230. Regan D. Human Brain Electrophysiology. Evoked Potentials and Evoked Magnetic Fields in Science and Medicine. New York, Elsevier, 1989.

231. Carr RE, Siegal IM. Electrodiagnostic Testing of the Visual System: A Clinical Guide. Philadelphia, FA Davis, 1990.

232. Fishman GA, Sokol S. Electrophysiologic Testing in Disorders of the Retina, Optic Nerve, and Visual Pathway. San Francisco, American Academy of Ophthalmology 1990:1–142.

233. Heckenlively JR, Arden G. Principles and Practice of Clinical Electrophysiology of Vision. St Louis, CV Mosby, 1991.

234. Dewar J. The physiological action of light. Nature 1877;15:433.

235. Einthoven W, Jolly WA. The form and magnitude of the electrical response of the eye to stimulation by light at various intensities. Q J Exp Physiol 1908;1:373.

236. Granit R. Sensory Mechanisms of the Retina. London, Oxford University Press, 1947.

237. Tomita T. Studies on the intraretinal action potential. I. Relation between the localization of micro-pipette in the retina and the shape of the intraretinal action potential. Jpn J Physiol 1950;1:110–117.

238. Tomita T. Electrophysiological study of the mechanisms subserving color coding in the fish retina. Cold Spring Harbor Symp Quant Biol 1965;30:559–566.

239. Brown KT, Wiesel TN. Localization of origins of electroretinogram components by intraretinal recording in the intact cat eye. J Physiol 1961;158:257–280.

240. Brown KT, Watanabe K. Isolation and identification of a receptor potential from pure cone fovea of the monkey retina. Nature 1962;193:958–960.

241. Murakami M, Kaneko A. Subcomponents of PIII in cold-blooded vertebrate retina. Nature 1966;210:103–104.

242. Brown KT, Watanabe K, Murakami M. The early and late receptor potentials of monkey cones and rods. Cold Spring Harb Symp Quant Biol 1965;30:457–482.

243. Armington JC, Johnson EP, Riggs LA. The scotopic a-wave in the electrical response of the human retina. J Physiol 1952;118:289–298.

244. Lamb TD, Pugh EN. A quantitative account of the activation steps involved in phototransduction in amphibian photoreceptors. J Physiol 1992;449:719–758.

245. Breton ME, Schueller AW, Lamb TD, et al. Analysis of the ERG a-wave amplification and kinetics in terms of the G-protein cascade of phototransduction. Invest Ophthalmol Vis Sci 1994;35:295–310.

246. Henkes HE. Electroretinography in circulatory disturbances of the retina. Arch Ophthalmol 1954;51:42–53.

247. Gouras P, Carr RE. Light-induced DC responses of monkey retina before and after central retinal artery interruption. Invest Ophthalmol 1965;4:310–317.

248. Hashimoto Y, Murakami M, Tomita T. Localization of the ERG by aid of histological method. Jpn J Physiol 1961;11:62–70.

249. Miller RF, Dowling JE. Intracellular responses of the Müller (glial) cells of mudpuppy retina: Their relation to b-wave of the electroretinogram. J Neurophysiol 1970;33:323–341.

250. Stockton RA, Slaughter MM. B-wave of the electroretinogram: A reflection on ON bipolar cell activity. J Gen Physiol 1989;93:101–122.

251. Adrian ED. Electric responses of the human eye. J Physiol 1945;84:84–104.

252. Adrian ED. Rod and cone components in the electric response of the eye. J Physiol 1946;105:24–37.

253. Johnson EP, Cornsweet TN. Electroretinal photopic sensitivity curves. Nature 1954;174:614–615.

254. Padmos P, van Norren D. Cone spectral sensitivity and chromatic adaptation as revealed by human flicker electroretinography. Vision Res 1971;11:27–42.

255. Mehaffey L, Berson EL. Cone mechanisms in the electroretinogram of the cynomolgus monkey. Invest Ophthalmol 1974;13:266–273.

256. Brown PK, Wald G. Visual pigments in single rods and cones of the human retina. Science 1964;144:45–52.

257. Marks WB, Dobelle WH, MacNichol EJ Jr. Visual pigments of single primate cones. Science 1964;143:1181–1183.

258. Steinberg RH, Schmidt R, Brown KT. Intracellular responses to light from cat pigment epithelium: Origin of the electroretinogram c-wave. Nature 1970;227:728–730.

259. Granit R, Munsterhjelm A. The electrical response of dark-adapted frog's eyes to monochromatic stimuli. J Physiol 1937;88:436–458.

260. Dodt E. Ein Doppelinterferenzfilter—Monochromator besonders hoher Leuchtdichte. Bibl Ophthalmol 1957;48:32–37.

261. Carr RE. Electroretinography. In Tasman W, Jaeger EA, eds. Duane's Clinical Ophthalmology, Vol II, Chap 103. Philadelphia, JB Lippincott, 1996:1–15.

262. Marmor MF, Arden GB, Sven Erik GN, et al. Standard for clinical electro-retinography. Arch Ophthalmol 1989;107:816–819.

263. Johnson MA, Marcus S, et al. Neovascularization in central retinal vein occlusion: Electroretinographic findings. Arch Ophthalmol 1988;106:348–352.

264. Gouras P. Relationships of the electrooculogram to the electroretinogram. In The Clinical Value of Electroretinography. ISCERG Symposium, Ghent 1966. Basel, S Karger, 1967:66–73.

265. Hecht S. Rods, cones and the chemical basis of vision. Physiol Rev 1937;17: 239–290.

266. Dodt E, Wadensten L. The use of flicker electroretinography in the human eye. Acta Ophthalmol 1954;32:165–180.

267. Dodt E. Cone electroretinogram by flicker. Nature 1957;168:783–786.

268. Goodman G, Bornschein H. Comparative electroretinographic studies in congenital night blindness and total color blindness. Arch Ophthalmol 1957;58: 174–182.

269. Wachtmeister L. On the oscillatory potentials of the human electroretinogram in light and dark adaptation. Acta Ophthalmol Suppl 1973;116:1–32.

270. Bresnick GH, Korth K, Groo A, et al. Electroretinographic oscillatory potentials predict progression of diabetic retinopathy. Arch Ophthalmol 1984;102: 1307–1311.

271. Riggs LA. Continuous and reproducible records of the electrical activity of the human retina. Proc Soc Exp Biol Med 1941;48:204–207.

272. Lawwill T, Burian HM. A modification of the Burian-Allen contact lens electrode for human electroretinography. Am J Ophthalmol 1966;61:1506–1509.

273. Kriss A, Jeffrey B, Taylor D. The electroretinogram in infants and young children. J Clin Neurophysiol 1992;9:373–393.

274. Zeidler I. The clinical electroretinogram. IX. The normal electroretinogram—value of the b-potential in different age groups and its difference in men and women. Acta Ophthalmol 1959;37:294–301.

275. Vainio-Mattila B. The clinical electroretinogram. II. The difference between the electroretinogram in men and women. Acta Ophthalmol 1951;29:25–32.

276. Pallin O. The influence of axial length of the eye on the size of the recorded b-potential in the clinical single-flash electroretinogram. Acta Ophthalmol 1969; 47:1–47.

277. Birch DG, Berson EL, Sandberg MA. Diurnal rhythm of the human rod ERG. Invest Ophthalmol Vis Sci 1984;25:236–238.

278. Weisinger HS, Vingrys AJ, Sinclair AJ, et al. Electrodiagnostic methods in vision. I. Clinical application and measurement. Clin Exp Optom 1996;79: 50–61.

279. Weisinger HS, Vingrys AJ, Sinclair AJ, et al. Electrodiagnostic methods in vision. II. Origins of the flash ERG. Clin Exp Optom 1996;79:62–72.

280. Weisinger HS, Vingrys AJ, Sinclair AJ, et al. Electrodiagnostic methods in vision. III. Clinical electrophysiology. Clin Exp Optom 1996;79:73–85.

281. Keltner JL, Roth AM, Chang RS. Photoreceptor degeneration: Possible autoimmune disease. Arch Ophthalmol 1983;101:564–569.

282. Thrikill CE. Cancer-associated retinopathy: The CAR syndrome. Neuroophthalmology 1994;14:297–323.

283. Thirkill CE, Roth AM, Keltner JE. Cancer-associated retinopathy. Arch Ophthalmol 1987;105:372–375.

284. Kim RY, Retsas S, Fitzke FW, et al. Cutaneous melanoma–associated retinopathy. Ophthalmology 1994;101:1837–1843.

285. Weinstein JM, Kelman SE, Bresnick GH, et al. Paraneoplastic retinopathy associated with antiretinal bipolar cell antibodies in cutaneous malignant melanoma. Ophthalmology 1994;101:1236–1243.

286. Sutter EE, Tran D. The field topography of ERG components in man. I. The photopic luminance response. Vision Res 1992;32:433–446.

287. Bearse MA, Sutter EE. Imaging localized retinal dysfunction with the multifocal electroretinogram. J Optom Soc Am 1996;13:634–640.

288. Kondo M, Miyake Y, Horiguchi M, et al. Clinical evaluation of multifocal electroretinogram. Invest Ophthalmol Visual Sci 1995;36:2146–2150.

289. Arden GB, Barrada A, Kelsey JH. New clinical test of retinal function based upon the standing potential of the eye. Br J Ophthalmol 1962;46:449–467.

290. Marmor MF, Holder GE, Seeliger MW, Yamamoto S. Standard for clinical electroretinography (in press).

291. Krill AE. The electroretinogram and electrooculogram: Clinical application. Invest Ophthalmol 1970;9:600–617.

292. Gouras P, Gunkel RD. The EOG in chloroquine and other retinopathies. Arch Ophthalmol 1963;70:629–639.

293. Okun E, Gouras P, Bernstein H, et al. Chloroquine retinopathy: A report of eight cases with ERG and dark-adaptation findings. Arch Ophthalmol 1963;69: 59–71.

294. Deutman AF, van Blommestein JD, Henkes HE, et al. Butterfly-shaped pigment dystrophy of the fovea. Arch Ophthalmol 1970;83:558–569.

295. Krill AE, Klien BA. Flecked retina syndrome. Arch Ophthalmol 1965;74: 496–508.

296. Francois J, de Rouck A, Fernandez-Sasso D. Electro-oculography in vitelliform degeneration of the macula. Arch Ophthalmol 1967;77:726–733.

297. Deutman AF. Electro-oculography in families with dystrophy of the fovea. Arch Ophthalmol 1969;81:305–316.

298. Cross HE, Bard L. Electro-oculography in Best's macular dystrophy. Am J Ophthalmol 1974;77:46–50.

299. Berson EL, Goldstein EB. Recovery of the human early receptor potential during dark adaptation in hereditary retinal disease. Vision Res 1970;10:219–226.

300. Berson EL, Goldstein EB. The early receptor potential in dominantly inherited retinitis pigmentosa. Arch Ophthalmol 1970;83:412–416.

301. Sieving PA, Frishman LJ, Sternberg RH. Scotopic threshold response of proximal retina in cat. J Neurophysiol 1986;56:1049–1061.

302. Aylward GW. The scotopic threshold response in diabetic retinopathy. Eye 1989; 3:626–637.

303. Aylward GW, Vaegan Billson FA. The scotopic threshold response in man. Clin Vis Sci 1989;4:373.

304. Sieving PA. Retinal ganglion cell loss does not abolish the scotopic threshold response (STR) of the cat and human ERG. Clin Vis Sci 1991;6:149–158.

305. van Balen ATM, Henkes HE. Recording of the occipital lobe response in man after light stimulation. Br J Ophthalmol 1960;44:449–460.

306. Jeffreys DA, Axford JG. Source locations of pattern-specific components of human visual-evoked potentials. I. Component of striate cortical origin. Exp Brain Res 1972;16:1–21.

307. Jeffreys DA, Axford JG. Source locations of pattern-specific components of human visual-evoked potentials. II. Component of extrastriate origin. Exp Brain Res 1972;16:22–40.

308. Streletz LJ, Bae SH, Roeshman RM, et al. Visual-evoked potentials in occipital lobe lesions. Arch Neurol 1981;38:80–85.

309. Cohn R. Visual-evoked responses in the brain-injured monkey. Arch Neurol 1969;21:321–329.

310. Bodis-Wollner I, Atkin A, Raab E, et al. Visual association cortex and vision in man: Pattern-evoked occipital potentials in a blind boy. Science 1977;198: 629–631.

311. Valberg A, Rudvin I. Possible contributions of magnocellular and parvocellular pathway cells to transient VEPs. Vis Neurosci 1997;14:4–11.

312. Vaughn HG, Katzman R. Evoked response in visual disorders. Ann NY Acad Sci 1964;112:305–319.

313. Regan D. Evoked Potentials in Psychology, Sensory Physiology and Clinical Medicine. London, Chapman & Hall, 1972.

314. Regan D. Rapid objective refraction using evoked brain potential. Invest Ophthalmol Vis Sci 1973;12:669–679.

315. Regan D. Recent advances in electrical recording from the human brain. Nature 1975;253:401–407.

316. Sokol S. The visually-evoked potential: Theory, techniques, and clinical applications. Surv Ophthalmol 1976;21:18–44.

317. Weinstein GW. Clinical aspects of the visually-evoked potential. Trans Am Ophthalmol Soc 1977;75:627–673.

318. Glaser JS, Laflamme P. The visual-evoked response: Methodology and application in optic nerve disease. In Thompson HS, ed. Topics in Neuro-Ophthalmology. Baltimore, Williams & Wilkins 1979:199–218.

319. Horton JC, Hoyt WF. The representation of the visual field in human striate cortex. Arch Ophthalmol 1991;109:816–824.

320. Celesia GG, Daly RF. Effects of aging on visual-evoked responses. Arch Neurol 1977;34:403–407.

321. Marg E, Freeman DN, Peltzman P, et al. Visual acuity development in human infants: Evoked potential measurements. Invest Ophthalmol Vis Science 1976; 15:150–153.

322. Sokol S. Measurement of infant visual acuity from pattern reversal evoked potentials. Vision Res 1978;18:33–39.

323. Sokol S, Dobson V. Pattern reversal visually-evoked potential. Invest Ophthalmol Vis Sci 1976;15:58–62.

324. Hawkes CH, Stow B. Pupil size and the pattern-evoked visual response. J Neurol Neurosurg Psychiatry 1981;44:90–91.

325. Korth M, Nguyen NX. The effect of stimulus size on human cortical potentials evoked by chromatic patterns. Vision Res 1997;37:649–657.

326. van Dijk JG. Pitfalls, fallacies and false positive rates. Clin Neurol and Neurosurg 1992;94(Suppl):S161–164.

327. Harding GF. Flash-evoked cortical and subcortical potentials in neuro-ophthalmology. Acta Neurol Belg 1985;85:150–165.

328. Hammond SR, Yiannikas C. Contribution of pattern reversal foveal and half-field stimulation to analysis of VEP abnormalities in multiple sclerosis. Electroencephalogr Clin Neurophysiol 1986;64:101–118.

329. Hughes JR, Stone JL, Fino JJ, et al. Usefulness of different stimuli in visual-evoked potentials. Neurology 1987;37:656–662.

330. Fishman GA, Sokol S. Electrophysiologic Testing in Disorders of the Retina, Optic Nerve, and Visual Pathway. San Francisco, American Academy of Ophthalmology, 1990.

331. Zeese JA. Pattern visual-evoked responses in multiple sclerosis. Arch Neurol 1977;34:314–316.

332. Neetens A, Hendrata Y, van Rompaey J. Pattern and flash-evoked responses in disseminated and selective optic pathway damage. Trans Ophthalmol Soc UK 1979;99:103–110.

333. Nikoskelainen E, Falck B. Do visual-evoked potentials give relevant information to the neuro-ophthalmological examination in optic nerve lesions? Acta Neurol Scand 1982;66:42–57.

334. Taylor MJ, McCulloch DL. Prognostic value of VEPs in young children with acute onset of cortical blindness. Pediatr Neurol 1991;7:111–115.

335. Brigell M, Kaufman DI, Bobak P. The pattern visual-evoked potential: A multi-center study using standardized techniques. Doc Ophthalmol 1994;86:65–79.

336. Taylor MJ, McCulloch DL. Visual-evoked potentials in infants and children. J Clin Neurophysiol 1992;9:357–372.

337. Towle VL, Sutcliffe E, Sokol S. Diagnosing functional visual deficits with the P300 component of the visual-evoked potential. Arch Ophthalmol 1985;103: 47–50.

338. Hirose T, Miyake Y, Hara A. Simultaneous recording of electroretinogram and visual-evoked response. Arch Ophthalmol 1977;95:1205–1208.

339. Celesia GG, Daly RF. Visual electroencephalographic computer analysis (VECA). Neurology 1977;27:637–641.

340. Sutter EE. The fast m-transform: a fast computation of cross-correlations with binary m-sequences. Soc Ind Appl Math 1991;20:686–694.

341. Baseler HA, Sutter EE, Klein SA, Carney T. The topography of visual evoked response properties across the visual field. Electroencephalogr Clin Neurophysiol 1994;90:65–81.

342. Klistorner A, Graham SL. Objective perimetry in glaucoma. Ophthalmology 2000;107:2283–2299.

343. Hood DC, Greenstein VC. Multifocal VEP and ganglion cell damage: Applications and limitations for the study of glaucoma. Progr Retinal Eye Res 2003; 22:201–251.

344. Wall M, Woodward K, Sleep T. The Multifocal VEP. In Optic Neuropathies and Homonymous Hemianopias. Perimetry Update 2002/2003, in press.

345. Kaufman DI, Celesia GG. Simultaneous recording of pattern electroretinogram and visual-evoked responses in neuro-ophthalmologic disorders. Neurology 1985;35:644–651.

346. Froehlich J, Kaufman DI. The pattern electroretinogram: N95 amplitudes in normal subjects and optic neuritis patients. Electroencephalogr Clin Neurophysiol 1993;88:83–91.

347. Scholl GB, Song HS, Winkler DE, et al. The pattern visual-evoked potential and pattern electroretinogram in drusen-associated optic neuropathy. Arch Ophthalmol 1992;110:75–81.

348. Rover J, Bach M. Pattern electroretinogram plus visual-evoked potential: A decisive test in patients suspected of malingering. Doc Ophthalmol 1987;66: 245–251.

CHAPTER 3

Congenital Anomalies of the Optic Disc

Michael C. Brodsky

OPTIC NERVE HYPOPLASIA
EXCAVATED OPTIC DISC ANOMALIES
    Morning Glory Disc Anomaly
    Optic Disc Coloboma
    Peripapillary Staphyloma
    Megalopapilla
    Optic Pit
    Papillorenal Syndrome (the "Uncoloboma")
CONGENITAL TILTED DISC SYNDROME
OPTIC DISC DYSPLASIA

CONGENITAL OPTIC DISC PIGMENTATION
AICARDI SYNDROME
DOUBLING OF THE OPTIC DISC
OPTIC NERVE APLASIA
MYELINATED (MEDULLATED) NERVE FIBERS
PSEUDOPAPILLEDEMA
    Pseudopapilledema Associated with Optic Disc Drusen
    Anomalous Disc Elevation without Either Visible or Buried
    Drusen

Certain general principles are particularly useful in the evaluation and management of patients with anomalous optic discs.

1. Children with bilateral optic disc anomalies generally present in infancy with poor vision and nystagmus; those with unilateral optic disc anomalies generally present during their preschool years with sensory esotropia.
2. CNS malformations are common in patients with malformed optic discs. Small discs are associated with a variety of malformations of the cerebral hemispheres, pituitary infundibulum, and midline intracranial structures (septum pellucidum, corpus callosum). Large optic discs of the morning glory configuration are associated with the transsphenoidal form of basal encephalocele, whereas colobomatous optic discs may be associated with a systemic anomalies and a variety of syndromes.
3. Any structural ocular abnormality that reduces visual acuity in infancy may lead to superimposed amblyopia (1). A trial of occlusion therapy may be warranted in young children with unilateral optic disc anomalies and decreased vision (2).
4. Anomalous optic discs (particularly excavated optic disc anomalies and pseudopapilledema with or without optic disc drusen) may produce episodes of transient visual loss (3–6).

OPTIC NERVE HYPOPLASIA

Optic nerve hypoplasia is an anomaly that, until recently, escaped the scrutiny of even the most meticulous observers (7). It was not until the late 1960s that its clinical description became commonplace. Optic nerve hypoplasia is now unquestionably the most common optic disc anomaly encountered in ophthalmologic practice. The dramatic increase in prevalence of optic nerve hypoplasia primarily reflects its greater recognition by clinicians. Many cases of optic nerve hypoplasia that previously went unrecognized or were misconstrued as congenital optic atrophy are now correctly diagnosed. In addition, some investigators believe that parenteral drug and alcohol abuse, which have become more widespread in recent years, may also be contributing to an increasing prevalence of optic nerve hypoplasia (8,9).

Ophthalmoscopically, the hypoplastic disc appears as an abnormally small optic nerve head (10–14) (Fig. 3.1A). It may appear gray or pale in color and is often surrounded by a yellowish mottled peripapillary halo, bordered by a ring of

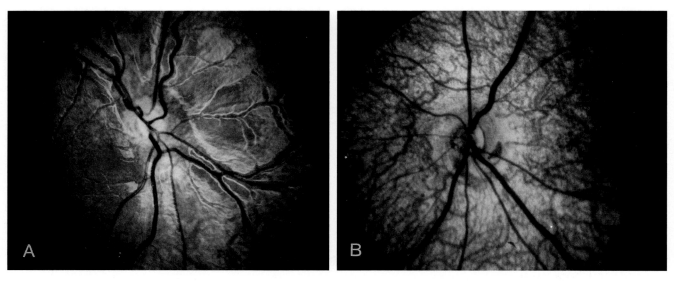

Figure 3.1. Optic nerve hypoplasia. *A,* The disc is small and pale but the retinal vessels are of normal size. *B,* The disc is small and surrounded by a rim of variably pigmented tissue.

increased or decreased pigmentation (dubbed the "double-ring" sign), which facilitates recognition of the anomaly (15) (Fig. 3.1*B*). Optic nerve hypoplasia is often associated with selective tortuosity of the retinal veins. This finding can be particularly helpful in establishing the diagnosis in infants with nystagmus (16).

Optic nerve hypoplasia is characterized histopathologically by a subnormal number of optic nerve axons with normal mesodermal elements and glial supporting tissue (17,18). The double-ring sign correlates to a normal junction between the sclera and lamina cribrosa, which corresponds to the outer ring, and the termination of an abnormal extension of retina and pigment epithelium over the lamina cribrosa, which corresponds to the inner ring (17,18) (Fig. 3.2).

Visual acuity in optic nerve hypoplasia ranges from 20/20 to no light perception, and affected eyes show localized visual field defects, often combined with generalized constriction (19–25). Because visual acuity is determined primarily by the integrity of the papillomacular nerve fiber bundle, it does not necessarily correlate with the overall size of the disc. The strong association of astigmatism with optic nerve hypoplasia warrants careful attention to correction of refractive errors (26).

Unilateral optic nerve hypoplasia has recently been implicated in the pathogenesis of amblyopia (27). Using optic disc photographs corrected for magnification, Lempert found smaller optic discs and smaller axial lengths in amblyopic eyes compared to their fellow eyes and suggested that vision impairment in presumed amblyopia may be caused by optic nerve hypoplasia with relative microphthalmos (27). Archer noted that a small optic disc area could be associated with amblyopia by being correlated with hyperopia and anisometropia rather than being the cause of the decreased vision (28). Archer stated that small eyes may have small optic discs, and either the small optic nerves or the associated

hyperopia or anisometropia could be causative (29). Lempert addressed this issue in a subsequent study which showed that, even when axial length was factored into the calculation, the optic disc areas of eyes with hyperopic strabismus with and without amblyopia were disproportionately and markedly reduced when compared with hyperopic eyes without amblyopia or esotropia (29).

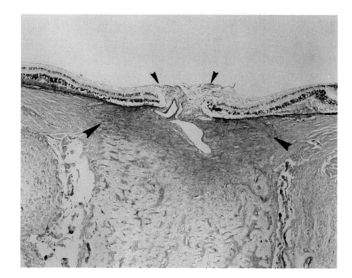

Figure 3.2. Pathology of optic nerve hypoplasia. Section through center of optic disc shows junction of sclera and lamina cribrosa (*large arrowheads*) delineating outer ring and extension of retina and retinal pigment epithelium overlying the lamina cribrosa on both sides. Termination of retina and retinal pigment epithelium (*short arrowheads*) marks inner ring or hypoplastic nerve head. (From Mosier MA, Lieberman MF, Green WR, et al. Hypoplasia of the optic nerve. Arch Ophthalmol 1978;96:1437–1442.)

Except when amblyopia develops in one eye, visual acuity usually remains stable throughout life. However, Taylor (30) has documented mild optic nerve hypoplasia in patients with congenital suprasellar tumors. Such tumors can slowly enlarge to produce acquired visual loss. Spandau et al. (31) recently reported bilateral visual loss in an elderly patient with severe optic nerve hypoplasia in both eyes. The authors attributed this phenomenon to normal axonal loss superimposed upon a critically low retinal nerve fiber count with no compensatory reserve.

Although moderate or severe optic nerve hypoplasia can be recognized ophthalmoscopically, the diagnosis of mild hypoplasia is problematic in infants and small children whose visual acuity cannot be quantified with accuracy (32). Several techniques have been devised to measure fundus photographs of the optic disc directly in an attempt to apply quantitative criteria to the diagnosis of optic nerve hypoplasia. Jonas et al. (33) defined ''microdiscs'' statistically as the mean disc area minus two standard deviations (33). In their study of 88 patients, the mean optic disc area measured 2.89 mm^2 and the diagnosis of a microdisc corresponded to a disc area smaller than 1.4 mm^2. Romano et al. (34) advocated the simple method of directly measuring the optic disc diameter using a hand ruler and a 30° transparency (both under magnification) and concluded that a horizontal disc diameter of less than 3.4 mm constitutes optic nerve hypoplasia. This quick and simple technique is limited to eyes with minimal spherical refractive error. Zeki et al. (35) calculated the disc-to-macula/disc diameter ratio and found, in 95% of normals, that the ratio was greater than 2.94, in contrast to an average of 2.62 for the group with optic nerve hypoplasia. Calculation of this ratio has the important advantage of eliminating the magnification effect of high refractive errors (myopic refractive errors can make a hypoplastic disc appear normal in size, whereas hyperopic refractive errors can make a normal disc appear abnormally small). Borchert et al. (32) found a bimodal distribution in the ratio of the horizontal disc diameter to the disc-macula distance, with a ratio of greater than 0.3 separating eyes with good acuity from those with poor acuity.

Although the technique described by Zeki et al. (35) is especially useful in patients with high refractive errors, the notion that one can establish an unequivocal dividing line between the normal and hypoplastic disc is inherently flawed (36), because large optic discs can be axonally deficient (14,37), and small optic discs do not preclude normal visual function. Theoretically an extremely small disc is associated with a diminution in axons, but this reasoning has limited applications with regard to mild or borderline cases. Other variables must be considered, including the size of the central cup, the percentage of the nerve occupied by axons (as opposed to glial tissue and blood vessels), and the cross-sectional area and density of axons. Furthermore, segmental forms of optic nerve hypoplasia (see below) may affect a sector of the disc without producing a diffuse diminution in size. As such, it would seem prudent to reserve the diagnosis of optic nerve hypoplasia for patients with small optic discs who have reduced vision or visual field loss with corresponding nerve fiber bundle defects.

Electroretinography is normal in the majority of patients with optic nerve hypoplasia (38). However, a subgroup have decreased amplitudes, suggesting coexistent retinal dysgenesis (39,40). Visual-evoked responses (VER) vary from normal to extinguished (38,39). Some patients with poor vision have normal flash VEP latencies, probably resulting from the normal transmission speed of residual axons (32).

Optic nerve hypoplasia is frequently associated with other CNS anomalies. Septo-optic dysplasia (de Morsier syndrome) refers to the constellation of small anterior visual pathways, absence of the septum pellucidum, and thinning or agenesis of the corpus callosum (41). The clinical association of septo-optic dysplasia and pituitary dwarfism was documented by Hoyt et al. in 1970 (42). Subsequent studies demonstrated deficiencies of other anterior pituitary hormones as well as diabetes insipidus in patients with septo-optic dysplasia (43–57). Growth hormone deficiency is the most common endocrinologic deficiency associated with optic nerve hypoplasia, but hypothyroidism, hypocortisolism, diabetes insipidus, and hyperprolactinemia may also occur (58–63). Children with an intact septum pellucidum and optic nerve hypoplasia may still have endocrinologic deficiency (64). Parents should be asked about previous episodes of hypoglycemia in the neonatal period or during periods of illness (which suggest hypocortisolism), and neonatal jaundice (which suggests hypothyroidism) (8,65,66). Conversely, newborn infants with hypoglycemia and cholestasis should probably be screened for optic nerve hypoplasia (67). Growth hormone deficiency may not be clinically apparent within the first 3–4 years of life because high prolactin levels can stimulate normal growth over this period (68). Puberty may be precocious or delayed in children with hypopituitarism (49,69). Anterior pituitary hormone deficiencies may evolve over time in some patients; thus, longitudinal reevaluation and periodic monitoring of anterior pituitary hormone function are indicated in children with posterior pituitary ectopia (66,70). Estimates of the prevalence of pituitary hormone deficiency in children with septo-optic dysplasia are as high as 62% (56), but these clinical reports are strongly skewed toward cases with endocrinologic manifestations, and the true prevalence is probably closer to 15% (64,71).

Children with septo-optic dysplasia and corticotropin deficiency are at risk for sudden death during febrile illness (72). This clinical deterioration appears to be caused by an impaired ability to increase corticotropin secretion to maintain blood pressure and blood sugar in response to the physical stress of infection. These children may have coexistent diabetes insipidus that contributes to dehydration during illness and hastens the development of shock. Some also have hypothalamic thermoregulatory disturbances signaled by episodes of hypothermia during well periods and high fevers during illnesses, which may predispose to life-threatening hyperthermia. Children with septo-optic dysplasia who are at risk for sudden death usually have had multiple hospital admissions for viral illnesses. These viral infections can precipitate hypoglycemia, dehydration, hypotension, or fever of unknown origin (72). Because corticotropin deficiency represents the preeminent threat to life in children with septo-optic dysplasia, a complete anterior pituitary hormone evaluation, including provocative serum cortisol testing and assessment for diabetes insipidus, should be performed in children who have clinical symptoms (history of hypoglycemia, dehydration, or hypothermia) or neuroimaging signs (absent pituitary infundibulum with or without posterior pituitary ectopia) of pituitary hormone deficiency. Sherlock and McNicol (73) noted that subclinical hypopituitarism can manifest as acute adrenal insufficiency following surgery under general anesthesia and suggested that it may be prudent to empirically treat children who have optic nerve hypoplasia with perioperative intravenous corticosteroids.

Magnetic resonance imaging is the optimal noninvasive neuroimaging modality for delineating associated CNS malformations in patients with optic nerve hypoplasia (74). MR imaging provides high-contrast resolution and multiplanar imaging capability, allowing the anterior visual pathways to be visualized as distinct, well-defined structures (74). In optic nerve hypoplasia, coronal and sagittal T1-weighted MR images consistently demonstrate thinning and attenuation of hypoplastic prechiasmatic intracranial optic nerves (Fig. 3.3). Coronal T1-weighted MR imaging in bilateral optic nerve hypoplasia shows diffuse thinning of the optic chiasm (Fig. 3.3*B*) in patients with bilateral optic nerve hypoplasia, and focal thinning or absence of the side of the chiasm corresponding to the hypoplastic nerve in unilateral optic nerve hypoplasia. When MR imaging shows a decrease in intracranial optic nerve size accompanied by other features of septo-optic dysplasia, a presumptive diagnosis of optic nerve hypoplasia can be made (74).

The notion of septo-optic dysplasia as a distinct nosologic entity has been overturned because MR imaging has fre-

quently demonstrated structural abnormalities involving the cerebral hemispheres and the pituitary infundibulum (9,64). Cerebral hemispheric abnormalities, which are evident on MR imaging in approximately 45% of patients with optic nerve hypoplasia, may consist of hemispheric migration anomalies (Fig. 3.4) such as schizencephaly, cortical heterotopia, polymicrogyria, as well as evidence of intrauterine or perinatal hemispheric injury such as periventricular leukomalacia, encephalomalacia, or porencephaly (75–83). Midline fusion of the cerebral hemispheres (holoprosencephaly) (84) and cerebellar hemispheres (85) is also occasionally seen. Barkovich (86) questioned whether those forms of septo-optic dysplasias with central holoventricles and no hemispheric malformations represent the mildest end of the spectrum of holoprosencephaly. Optic nerve hypoplasia may also accompany other intracranial anomalies including anencephaly (87,88), hydranencephaly (89–91), and transsphenoidal encephalocele (92). The association of optic nerve hypoplasia with periventricular leukomalacia presents an interesting diagnostic challenge. In 1995, Jacobson et al. recognized that periventricular leukomalacia produces a unique form of bilateral optic nerve hypoplasia characterized by an abnormally large optic cup and a thin neuroretinal rim contained within a normal-sized optic disc (Fig. 3.5) (93). They attributed this morphologic characteristic to intrauterine injury to the optic radiations with retrograde transsynaptic degeneration of retinogeniculate axons after the scleral canals had established normal diameters. Unlike other forms of optic nerve hypoplasia, the pseudoglaucomatous optic hypoplasia of periventricular leukomalacia is not associated

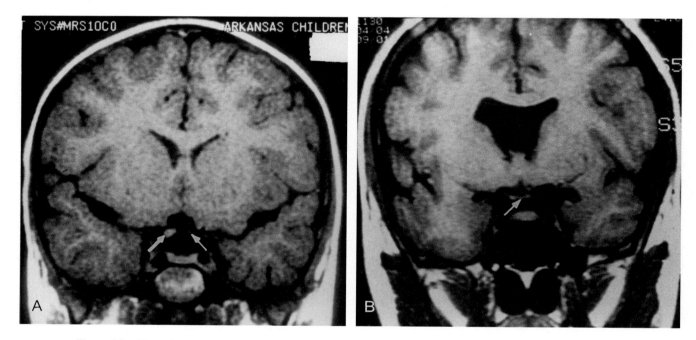

Figure 3.3. Magnetic resonance imaging in optic nerve hypoplasia. *A,* Left optic nerve hypoplasia. *Thick arrow* denotes normal right optic nerve. *Thin arrow* denotes hypoplastic intracranial prechiasmatic optic nerve. *B,* Bilateral optic nerve hypoplasia. *Arrow* denotes hypoplastic chiasm. (From Brodsky MC, Glasier CM, Pollock SC, et al. Optic nerve hypoplasia: Identification by magnetic resonance imaging. Arch Ophthalmol 1990;108:562–567.)

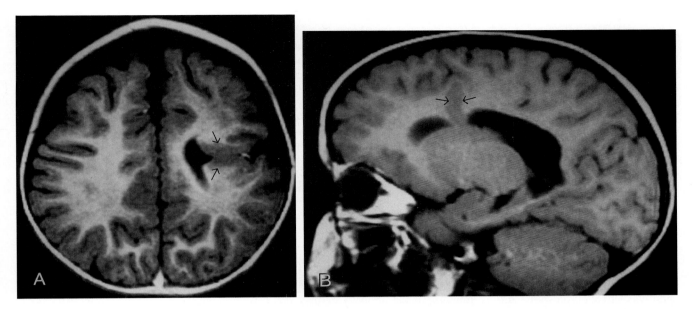

Figure 3.4. Cerebral hemispheric abnormalities commonly associated with optic nerve hypoplasia. *A,* Schizencephaly. The schizencephalic cleft (*arrows*) consists of an abnormal band of dysmorphic gray matter in the left cerebral hemisphere extending from the cortical surface to the lateral ventricle. *B,* Cortical heterotopia. An abnormal area of gray matter (*black arrows*) in the deep white matter, indents the ventricular lumen. (From Brodsky MC, Glasier CM, Pollock SC, et al. Optic nerve hypoplasia: Identification by magnetic resonance imaging. Arch Ophthalmol 1990;108:562–567.)

with endocrinologic deficiency. The large optic cups can simulate glaucoma, but the history of prematurity, normal intraocular pressure, and characteristic symmetrical inferior visual field defects all serve to distinguish periventricular leukomalacia from glaucomatous optic atrophy (94). Whether this anomaly warrants classification as a prenatal form of optic atrophy because of its normal optic disc diameter remains controversial (94).

Evidence of perinatal injury to the pituitary infundibulum (seen on MR imaging as posterior pituitary ectopia) is found in approximately 15% of patients with optic nerve hypoplasia (64). Normally, the posterior pituitary gland appears bright on T1-weighted images (Fig. 3.6*A*), probably because of the phospholipid membrane component of its hormone-containing vesicles (95). In posterior pituitary ectopia, MR imaging demonstrates absence of the normal posterior pituitary bright spot, absence or attenuation of the pituitary infundibulum, and an ectopic posterior pituitary bright spot where the upper infundibulum is normally located (Fig. 3.6*B*) (9,64,66). It is unknown whether posterior pituitary ectopia results from defective neuronal migration during embryogenesis (66), or from a perinatal injury to the hypophyseal-portal system, which causes necrosis of the infundibulum (96,97). In a retrospective study, Phillips et al. found posterior pituitary ectopia and/or absence of the pituitary infundibulum in 23 of 26 cases of optic nerve hypoplasia and congenital hypopituitarism, versus none of the 41 cases with normal endocrinologic function (97). The finding of posterior pituitary ectopia implicates the pituitary infundibulum as one site of structural derangement in children with septo-optic dysplasia and panhypopituitarism (98). Signs of hypo-

thalamic dysgenesis, including absence of hypothalamic nuclei, neuronal loss, and gliosis have also been found at necropsy in children with septo-optic dysplasia and hypopituitarism. These findings suggest that a central hypothalamic insufficiency may coexist in some cases (48,49,52, 83,99).

In a child with optic nerve hypoplasia, posterior pituitary ectopia is virtually pathognomonic of anterior pituitary hormone deficiency with normal posterior pituitary function, while absence of a normal or ectopic posterior pituitary bright spot predicts coexistent antidiuretic hormone deficiency (i.e., diabetes insipidus) (57,66). Cerebral hemispheric abnormalities are highly predictive of neurodevelopmental deficits (64). Absence of the septum pellucidum alone does not portend neurodevelopmental deficits or pituitary hormone deficiency (100). Thinning or agenesis of the corpus callosum is predictive of neurodevelopmental problems only by virtue of its frequent association with cerebral hemispheric abnormalities. The finding of unilateral optic nerve hypoplasia does not preclude coexistent intracranial malformations (64). MR imaging thus provides critical prognostic information regarding the likelihood of neurodevelopmental deficits and pituitary hormone deficiency in the infant or young child with *unilateral* or *bilateral* optic nerve hypoplasia (64).

Numerous environmental factors that are detrimental to the fetus are sporadically associated with optic nerve hypoplasia. These include maternal insulin-dependent diabetes mellitus (23,101–104), fetal alcohol syndrome (107), maternal ingestion of quinine (105), anticonvulsants (106), illicit drugs (61,62,107), and fetal or neonatal infection with cyto-

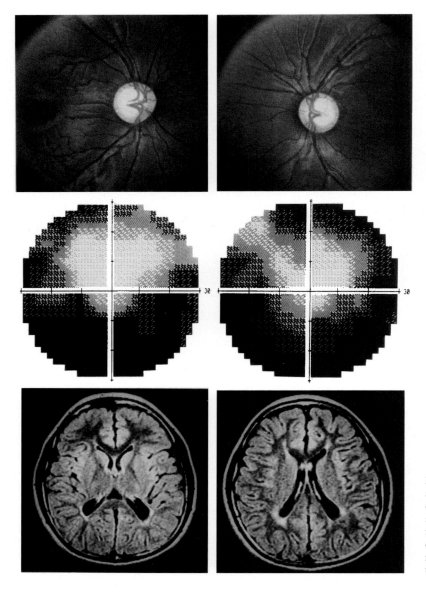

Figure 3.5. Pseudoglaucomatous optic nerve hypoplasia associated with periventricular leukomalacia. *Top,* Both optic discs are normal in size with large cups. *Middle,* Visual fields show bilateral constriction with symmetrical inferior depression that spares fixation. *Bottom,* Magnetic resonance imaging shows high signal intensity in the optic radiations and contiguous enlargement of the posterior ventricles.

megalovirus (108,109) or hepatitis B virus (109). Optic nerve hypoplasia occurs with increased frequency in first-born children of young mothers (110–113). The majority of cases are sporadic, although a handful of familial cases have been reported in siblings (21,114–116). The growing list of systemic and ocular disorders associated with optic nerve hypoplasia includes frontonasal dysplasia (92,117), aniridia (118), fetal alcohol syndrome (107), Dandy-Walker syndrome (116), Kallmann syndrome (119), Delleman syndrome (120), Duane syndrome (121), Klippel-Trenaunay-Weber syndrome (122,123), Goldenhar syndrome (124), linear nevus sebaceous syndrome (125), Meckel syndrome (126), hemifacial atrophy (13), blepharophimosis (127), osteogenesis imperfecta (128), chondrodysplasia punctata (129–131), Aicardi syndrome (82,132–134), Apert syndrome (135), Potter syndrome (136), chromosome 13q− (137), trisomy 18 (138), neonatal isoimmune thrombocyto-

penia (139), and bilateral microphthalmos (140). A purported association between optic nerve hypoplasia and albinism (141) is controversial because high-resolution MR imaging of the intracranial optic nerves in human albinos shows no diminution in size (36). Kottow (142) described unilateral optic nerve hypoplasia in three patients with ipsilateral congenital retinal arteriovenous malformations and no evidence of cutaneous or intracranial involvement.

Some forms of optic nerve hypoplasia are segmental. A superior segmental optic hypoplasia with an inferior visual field defect occurs in children of insulin-dependent diabetic mothers (Fig. 3.7) (23,102–104). In a prospective study of children of diabetic mothers, Landau et al. (143) found an 8.8% prevalence of superior segmental optic hypoplasia. Despite the multiple teratologic effects of maternal diabetes early in the first trimester (144), superior segmental hypoplasia is usually diagnosed in patients with no other systemic

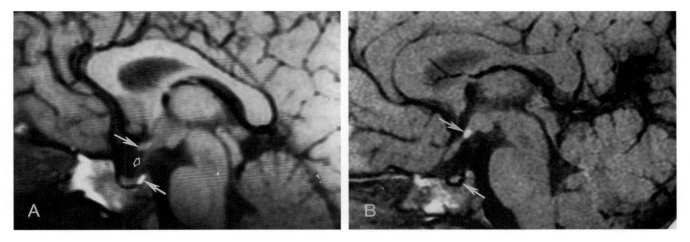

Figure 3.6. Posterior pituitary ectopia. *A,* MR image demonstrating the normal hyperintense signal of the posterior pituitary gland (*lower arrow*), normal pituitary infundibulum (*open arrow*), optic chiasm (*upper arrow*). *B,* MR image demonstrating posterior pituitary ectopia that appears as an abnormal focal area of increased signal intensity at the tuber cinereum (*upper arrow*). Note absence of the pituitary infundibulum and absence of the normal posterior pituitary bright spot (*lower arrow*). (From Brodsky MC, Glasier CM, Pollock SC, et al. Optic nerve hypoplasia: Identification by magnetic resonance imaging. Arch Ophthalmol 1990;108:562–567.)

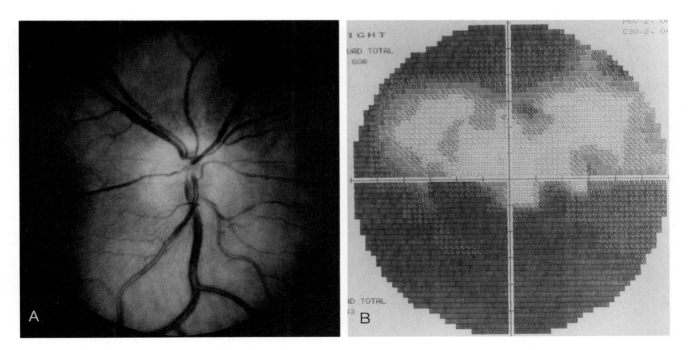

Figure 3.7. Superior segmental optic hypoplasia in a child whose mother had adult-onset diabetes mellitus. *A,* Right optic disc demonstrating an abnormal superior entrance of the central retinal artery, relative pallor of the superior disc, and a superior peripapillary halo. The superior nerve fiber layer is absent, while the inferior nerve fiber layer is clearly seen. *B,* Humphrey visual field in superior segmental hypoplasia showing a nonaltitudinal inferior visual field defect with milder superior depression. (From Brodsky MC, Schroeder GT, Ford R. Superior segmental optic hypoplasia in identical twins. J Clin Neuroophthalmol 1993;13:152–154.)

anomalies (145). Kim et al. (104) noted that the inferior visual field defects in superior segmental optic hypoplasia differ from typical nerve fiber bundle defects, and suggested that a regional impairment in retinal development could play a role in the pathogenesis. Hashimoto et al. (146) documented superior segmental optic hypoplasia in four Japanese patients whose mothers were not diabetic, demonstrating that this anomaly is not pathognomonic for maternal diabetes.

The teratologic mechanism by which insulin-dependent diabetes mellitus selectively interferes with the early gestational development of superior retinal ganglion cells or their axons is unknown (147). Mice lacking EphB receptor guidance proteins exhibit specific guidance defects in axons originating from the dorsal or superior part of the retina (148). Developmental mechanisms that control the expression of axon guidance molecules along the dorsal-ventral axis of the retina may eventually explain this segmental optic hypoplasia (148).

Congenital lesions of the retina, optic nerve, chiasm, tract, or retrogeniculate pathways are associated with segmental hypoplasia of the corresponding portions of each optic nerve (149,150). Hoyt et al. (151) coined the term "homonymous hemioptic hypoplasia" to describe the asymmetric form of segmental optic nerve hypoplasia seen in patients with unilateral congenital hemispheric lesions affecting the postchiasmal afferent visual pathways. In this setting, the nasal and temporal aspects of the optic disc contralateral to the hemispheric lesion show segmental hypoplasia and loss of the corresponding nerve fiber layers (Fig. 3.8). This anomaly may be accompanied by a central band of horizontal pallor

across the disc. The ipsilateral optic disc may range from normal in size to frankly hypoplastic (149). Homonymous hemioptic hypoplasia in retrogeniculate lesions results from transsynaptic degeneration of the optic tract (78,149,151).

The term "optic nerve hypoplasia" implies that the nerve is deficient in axons because of a primary failure of these axons to develop. Initial investigators understandably attributed optic nerve hypoplasia to a primary failure of retinal ganglion cell differentiation at the 13- to 15-mm stage of embryonic life (4–6 weeks' gestation) (11). However, Mosier et al. (17) noted that third-order retinal neurons (i.e., ganglion cells) arise from the same precursor cells as amacrine and horizontal cells, and injury to the stem cells would be unlikely to affect only one of the differentiated cell types.

At least two distinct mechanisms appear to be operative in the embryogenesis of optic nerve hypoplasia. Recent experiments have shown that a deficiency of axon guidance molecules at the optic disc can lead to optic nerve hypoplasia. Netrin-1 is an axon guidance molecule that is involved in the development of spinal commissural axons and is expressed by neuroepithelial cells at the developing optic nerve head. Retinal ganglion cells in vitro respond to netrin-1 as a guidance molecule. Mice with a targeted deletion of the netrin-1 gene exhibit pathfinding errors at the optic disc, where retinal ganglion cells fail to exit into the optic nerve and instead grow inappropriately into the other side of the retina. As a result of this aberrant pathfinding, these mice exhibit optic nerve hypoplasia (152,153). In addition to defects in optic nerve formation, the lack of netrin-1 function

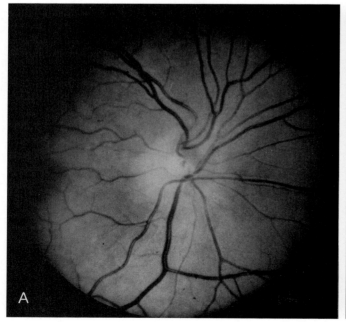 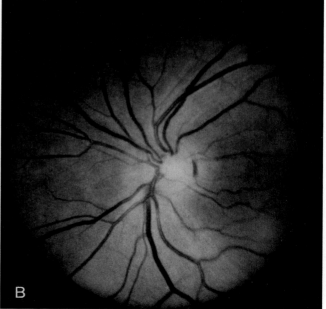

Figure 3.8. Homonymous hemioptic hypoplasia in a patient with a right occipital porencephalic cyst. Both optic discs are hypoplastic (*A and B*). The left optic disc shows some loss of disc substance and peripapillary nerve fiber layer nasally and temporally. (From Novakovic P, Taylor DSI, Hoyt WF. Localizing patterns of optic nerve hypoplasia-retina to occipital lobe. Br J Ophthalmol 1988;72:176–182.)

during development also results in abnormalities in other parts of the CNS, such as agenesis of the corpus callosum, and cell migration and axonal guidance defects in the hypothalamus (154). Thus, elimination of specific axon guidance molecules during development of the mouse nervous system results in a phenotype that bears striking resemblance to septo-optic dysplasia (153).

The timing of coexistent CNS injuries would suggest that some cases of optic nerve hypoplasia result from intrauterine destruction of a normally developed structure (i.e., an encephaloclastic event), whereas others represent a primary failure of axons to develop (8,55,155,156). In human fetuses, Provis et al. (157) found a peak of 3.7 million axons at 16–17 weeks of gestation, with a subsequent decline to 1.1 million axons by the 31st gestational week (see Chapter 1). This massive degeneration of supernumerary axons, termed "apoptosis," occurs as part of the normal development of the visual pathways and may serve to establish the correct topography of the visual pathways (8). Toxins or associated CNS malformations could augment the usual processes by which superfluous axons are eliminated from the developing visual pathways (8,9,55,64,149). Taylor (30) documented mild optic nerve hypoplasia in patients with congenital suprasellar tumors, suggesting that the space-occupying effects of these lesions can directly interfere with the normal migration of optic axons to their target sites. Prenatal hemispheric

injuries or malformations that injure the optic radiations can lead to retrograde transsynaptic degeneration and segmental hypoplasia of both optic nerves (64,81,149,151). These latter lesions clearly cannot be reconciled with a deficiency of axon guidance molecules at the optic disc (64,93,94,156, 158,159).

Reported cases of optic nerve hypoplasia in siblings (115,160) are sufficiently rare that parents of a child with optic nerve hypoplasia can reasonably be assured that subsequent siblings are at little or no additional risk. While genetic mutations in the human netrin-1 and DCC genes have not been described, homozygous mutations in the *Hesx1* gene have been identified in two siblings with optic nerve hypoplasia, absence of the corpus callosum, and hypoplasia of the pituitary gland (161). Five additional mutations in *Hesx1* have recently been observed in children with sporadic pituitary disease and septo-optic dysplasia (162). Mutations have clustered in the DNA-binding region of the protein consistent with a presumed loss in protein function. Formal examination of homeobox genes with expression patterns similar to *Hesx1,* such as *Six3* and *Six6,* may yield additional genes responsible for both sporadic and familial septo-optic dysplasia (163). Optic nerve hypoplasia may accompany other ocular malformations in patients with mutations in the PAX6 gene (164).

EXCAVATED OPTIC DISC ANOMALIES

Excavated optic disc anomalies include optic disc coloboma, morning glory disc anomaly, peripapillary staphyloma, megalopapilla, and optic pit. Recently, two new excavated optic disc anomalies have been associated with periventricular leukomalacia (see above) and the "vacant optic disc" associated with papillorenal syndrome. In the morning glory disc anomaly and peripapillary staphyloma, an excavation of the posterior globe surrounds and incorporates the optic disc, while in the other conditions, the excavation is contained within the optic disc. Pollock (165) has detailed the clinical features that distinguish the excavated optic disc anomalies. He emphasized that the terms "morning glory disc," "optic disc coloboma," and "peripapillary staphyloma" are often transposed in the literature, causing tremendous confusion regarding their diagnostic criteria, associated systemic findings, and pathogenesis. From his analysis, it is clear that optic disc colobomas, morning glory optic discs, and peripapillary staphylomas are distinct anomalies, each with its own specific embryologic origin, and not simply clinical variants along a broad phenotypic spectrum.

MORNING GLORY DISC ANOMALY

The morning glory disc anomaly is a congenital, funnel-shaped excavation of the posterior fundus that incorporates the optic disc (165). It was so-named by Kindler (166) because of its resemblance to the morning glory flower. Ophthalmoscopically, the disc is markedly enlarged, orange or pink in color, and may appear to be recessed or elevated centrally within the confines of a funnel-shaped peripapillary

excavation (167–173) (Fig. 3.9). A wide annulus of chorioretinal pigmentary disturbance surrounds the disc within the excavation. A white tuft of glial tissue overlies the central portion of the disc. The blood vessels appear increased in number and often arise from the periphery of the disc (165). They often curve abruptly as they emanate from the disc, then run an abnormally straight course over the peripapillary retina. It is often difficult to distinguish arterioles from venules. Close inspection may reveal the presence of peripapillary or arteriovenous communications that can be confirmed by fluorescein angiography (174,175). The macula may be incorporated into the excavation (165,174). Computed tomographic (CT) scanning shows a funnel-shaped enlargement of the distal optic nerve at its junction with the globe (Fig. 3.10) (176–178). Additional findings may include diffuse thickening with increased or decreased radiodensity of the orbital optic nerve, cavum vergae, and, most notably, transsphenoidal encephalocele (179).

The morning glory disc anomaly usually occurs as a unilateral condition, but several bilateral cases have been reported (174). Visual acuity usually ranges from 20/200 to finger counting, but cases with 20/20 vision as well as no light perception have been reported. Unlike optic disc colobomas, which have no racial or gender predilection, morning glory discs are more common in females and rare in African Americans (165,172,180). With rare exceptions (164,181), the morning glory disc anomaly is not part of a genetic disorder (165). However, Holmström and Taylor (182) documented the association of morning glory disc anomaly with ipsilateral orofacial hemangioma. Metry et al. (183) sug-

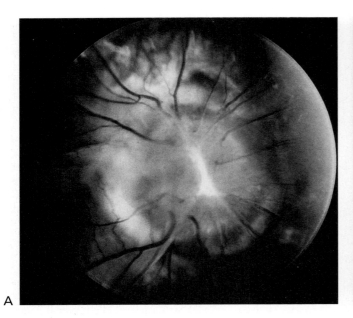
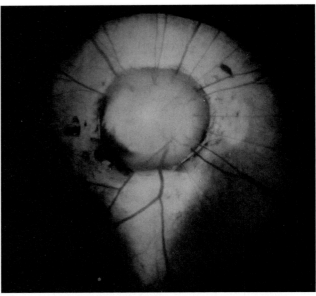

A   B

Figure 3.9. Morning glory disc anomaly. *A,* The optic disc shows the classic features of the morning glory syndrome: An enlarged, funnel-shaped, excavated and distorted optic disc that is surrounded by an elevated annulus of chorioretinal pigmentary disturbance. *B,* In another case of morning glory syndrome, a large optic disc is surrounded by an annular zone of pigmentary disturbance and a V-shaped zone of infrapapillary depigmentation. The retinal vessels appear increased in number, appear to emerge from the disc periphery, and have an abnormally straight radial configuration. A tuft of white glial overlies the center of both optic discs.

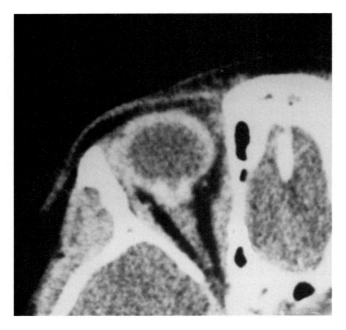

Figure 3.10. CT scan of morning glory disc anomaly. Note calcified funnel-shaped enlargement of the distal optic nerve at its junction with the globe. (From Brodsky MC. Congenital optic disk anomalies. Surv Ophthalmol 1994;39:89–112.)

gested that this association falls within the spectrum of the PHACE syndrome (**p**osterior fossa malformations, large facial **h**emangiomas, **a**rterial anomalies, **c**ardiac anomalies and aortic coarcation, and **e**ye anomalies), which occurs only in girls. Recent findings of ipsilateral intracranial vascular dysgenesis in such patients support this contention (184). Atypical morning glory disc anomalies have also rarely been reported in patients with neurofibromatosis 2 (185).

The association of morning glory disc anomaly with the transsphenoidal form of basal encephalocele is well established (174,177,186–191). The finding of V- or tongue-shaped infrapapillary depigmentation adjacent to a morning glory disc anomaly or other optic disc malformation (Fig. 3.9*B*) is highly associated with transsphenoidal encephalocele (92), although transsphenoidal encephalocele is also well-documented in the absence of this unique infraperipapillary retinal malformation (117). Transsphenoidal encephalocele is a rare midline congenital malformation in which a meningeal pouch, often containing the chiasm and adjacent hypothalamus, protrudes inferiorly through a large, round defect in the sphenoid bone (Fig. 3.11). Patients with this occult basal meningocele have a wide head, flat nose, mild hypertelorism, a midline notch in the upper lip, and sometimes a midline cleft in the soft palate (Fig. 3.12*A*). The meningocele protrudes into the nasopharynx, where it may obstruct the airway. Symptoms of transsphenoidal encephalocele in infancy include rhinorrhea, nasal obstruction, mouth-breathing, or snoring (186,192,193). These symptoms may be overlooked unless the associated morning glory

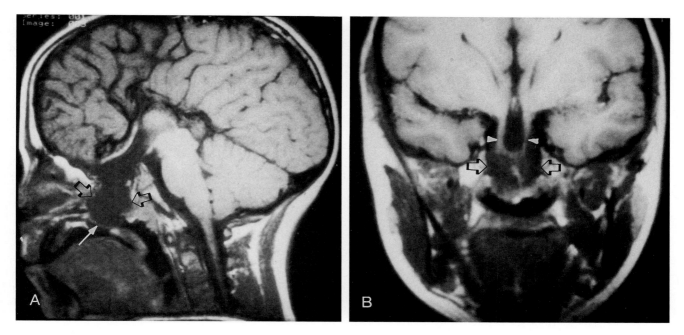

Figure 3.11. MR imaging in transsphenoidal encephalocele. *A,* Sagittal MR image shows an encephalocele (delimited by *open arrows*) extending down through the sphenoid bone into the nasopharynx with impression on the hard palate (*white arrow*). *B,* Coronal MR image shows the third ventricle and hypothalamus (*white arrowheads*) extending inferiorly into the encephalocele (delimited inferiorly by *open arrow*). (From Brodsky MC. Congenital optic disk anomalies. Surv Ophthalmol 1994;39:89–112. Courtesy of A. James Barkovich, MD.)

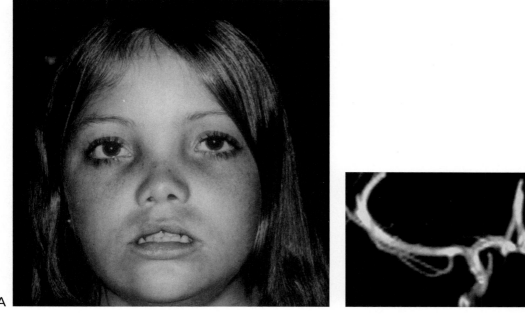

Figure 3.12. *A,* Photograph of a child with transsphenoidal encephalocele. Note hypertelorism, depressed nasal bridge, and subtle midline upper lip defect. *B,* MR angiography in a different patient with a morning glory disc anomaly. Note decrease in caliber of the left internal carotid artery with focal narrowing of the distal portion (*long arrow*), and narrowing of the bifurcation into middle and anterior cerebral arteries. The increased size of the lenticulostriate arteries (*short arrow*) produce a moyamoya appearance. (*A,* From Brodsky MC, Hoyt WF, Hoyt CS, et al. Atypical retinochoroidal coloboma in patients with dysplastic optic discs and transsphenoidal encephalocele. Arch Ophthalmol 1995;113:624–628. *B,* From Wisotsky BJ, Magat-Gordon CB, Puklin JE. Vitreopapillary traction as a cause of elevated optic nerve head. Am J Ophthalmol 1998;126:137–139.)

disc anomaly or the characteristic facial configuration are recognized. A transsphenoidal encephalocele may appear clinically as a pulsatile posterior nasal mass or as a "nasal polyp" high in the nose, and surgical biopsy or excision of the lesion can have severe and even lethal consequences (186). Associated brain malformations include agenesis of the corpus callosum and posterior dilatation of the lateral ventricles. Absence of the chiasm is seen in approximately one-third of patients at surgery or autopsy. Most of the affected children have no overt intellectual or neurologic deficits, but hypopituitarism is common (186,192,194,195). Surgery is contraindicated for transsphenoidal encephalocele because herniated brain tissue may include vital structures such as the hypothalamic-pituitary system, optic nerves and chiasm, and anterior cerebral arteries, and because of the high postoperative mortality, particularly in infants.

In 1985, Hansen et al. documented the association of morning glory disc anomaly with hypoplasia of the ipsilateral intracranial vasculature (196). With the advent of MR angiography, numerous reports have found ipsilateral intracranial vascular dysgenesis (hypoplasia of the carotid arteries and major cerebral arteries with or without Moyamoya syndrome), in patients with morning glory disc anomaly (Fig 3.12B). These reports underscore the need for MR angiography in the neurodiagnostic evaluation of patients with morning glory disc anomaly (197–199). The coexistence of these intracranial vascular anomalies supports the Dempster hypothesis that the morning glory disc anomaly results from a primary vascular dysgenesis that occurs in the context of a regional mesodermal dysgenesis (200).

Patients with a morning glory disc anomaly may experience both transient visual loss (3) and permanent visual loss later in life. Serous retinal detachments occur in 26–38% of eyes with morning glory optic discs (172,180,201). These detachments typically originate in the peripapillary area and extend through the posterior pole, occasionally progressing to total detachments (202). Although retinal tears are rarely evident, several reports identified small retinal tears adjacent to or overlying the optic nerve in patients with morning glory disc-associated retinal detachments (202–205). In other cases with acquired visual loss, there is nonattachment and radial folding of the retina within the excavated zone (165). The sources of subretinal fluid may be multiple (206). Brown and Brown (207) reported successful retinal reattachment with pars plana vitrectomy, laser photocoagulation, and intravitreal gas injection. Irvine et al. (206) reported a patient with a morning glory disc-associated retinal detachment, who was treated with optic nerve sheath fenestration followed by gas injection into the vitreous cavity. Following the procedure, gas bubbled out through the dural window, suggesting a connection between the vitreous cavity and the subarachnoid space through the anomalous disc. Chang et al. (208) also reported resolution of a morning glory-associated serous retinal detachment following optic nerve sheath fenestration. Bartz-Schmidt and Hermann (209) noted subretinal leakage of gas injected into the vitreous following vitrectomy for a complete retinal detachment in as eye with a morning glory anomaly, thereby demonstrating a direct communication between the vitreous cavity and the subretinal

space, which may have resulted from surgical removal of tractional glial tissue overlying the disc. Spontaneous resolution of morning glory-associated retinal detachments have also been reported (180).

Several authors have documented contractile movements in a morning glory optic disc (165,210–212). Pollock (165) attributed the contractile movements in his case to fluctuations in subretinal fluid volume, altering the degree of retinal separation within the confines of the excavation. Graether (3) described a patient with a morning glory disc anomaly in whom episodes of amaurosis were accompanied by transient dilation of the retinal veins in an eye with a morning glory disc. Subretinal neovascularization may occasionally develop within the circumferential zone of pigmentary disturbance adjacent to a morning glory disc (213,214).

The embryologic defect leading to the morning glory disc anomaly is widely disputed (177). Histopathologic reports have, unfortunately, lacked clinical confirmation (215–218). Some authors hypothesized that the morning glory disc anomaly results from defective closure of the embryonic fissure and is but one phenotypic form of a colobomatous (i.e., embryonic fissure-related) defect (176,219). Others interpreted the clinical findings of a central glial tuft, vascular anomalies, and a scleral defect, together with the histologic findings of adipose tissue and smooth muscle within the peripapillary sclera in presumed cases of the morning glory disc to signify a primary mesenchymal abnormality. These researchers suggested that the associated midfacial anomalies in some patients further support the concept of a primary mesenchymal defect, since most of the cranial structures are derived from mesenchyme (177). Dempster (200) has attempted to reconcile these two views by proposing that the basic defect is mesodermal but that some clinical features of the defect result from a dynamic disturbance between the relative growth of mesoderm and ectoderm. Pollock (165) has argued that the fundamental symmetry of the fundus excavation with respect to the disc implicates an anomalous funnel-shaped enlargement of the distal optic stalk at its junction with the primitive optic vesicle, as the primary embryologic defect.

OPTIC DISC COLOBOMA

The term "coloboma," of Greek derivation, means curtailed or mutilated (220,221). It is used only with reference to the eye. According to Mann (220), colobomas of the optic disc result from incomplete or abnormal coaptation of the proximal end of the embryonic fissure. Liebrich (222) is credited with the first ophthalmoscopic description of an isolated optic disc coloboma, and Coats discussed the subject in detail in 1908, adding clinical and pathologic data on cases from his own experience to the three cases already in the literature at that time. Subsequent reports presented similar examples of isolated optic disc coloboma (223–226).

Optic disc coloboma is characterized by a sharply delimited, glistening white, bowl-shaped excavation that occupies an enlarged optic disc (Fig. 3.13). The excavation is decentered inferiorly, reflecting the position of the embryonic fissure relative to the primitive epithelial papilla (165). The

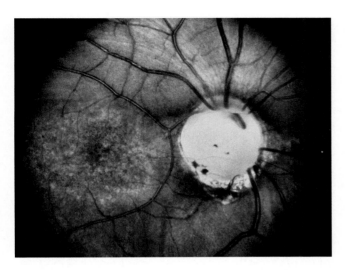

Figure 3.13. Coloboma of the optic disc in an eye with an old serous macular detachment. The disc is enlarged. A deep white excavation occupies most of the disc but spares its superior aspect. Note absence of inferior retinal nerve fiber layer and pigment epithelial disturbance in the macula. The patient had a large superior, altitudinal visual field defect.

inferior neuroretinal rim is thin or absent, while the superior neuroretinal rim is relatively spared. Rarely, the entire disc appears excavated; however, the colobomatous nature of the defect can still be appreciated ophthalmoscopically because the excavation is deeper inferiorly (165). The defect may extend further inferiorly to include the adjacent choroid and retina, in which case microphthalmia is frequently present (227). Iris and ciliary colobomas often coexist. Axial CT scanning shows a crater-like excavation of the posterior globe at its junction with the optic nerve (176,219). Colobomatous malformations of the optic disc produce an inferior segmental hypoplasia of the optic nerve, with a C-shaped or quarter-moon-shaped neuroretinal rim confined to the superior aspect of the optic disc (Fig. 3.13) (228). Colobomas constitute the most common segmental form of optic nerve hypoplasia encountered in clinical practice (228). Coronal T1-weighted MR imaging confirms that the intracranial portion of the optic nerve is reduced in size (228). The nosological overlap between colobomatous derangement of the optic nerve and segmental hypoplasia reflects the early timing of colobomatous dysembryogenesis which results in primary failure of inferior retinal ganglion cells to develop.

Visual acuity, which depends primarily upon the integrity of the papillomacular bundle, may be mildly to severely decreased and is difficult to predict from the appearance of the disc. Unlike the morning glory disc anomaly, which is usually unilateral, optic disc colobomas occur unilaterally or bilaterally with approximately equal frequency (165). As with uveal colobomas, isolated optic disc colobomas may be sporadic or inherited (230–235). Ocular colobomas may be accompanied by other systemic anomalies (236–239), in genetic disorders such as the CHARGE association (240–243), Walker-Warburg syndrome (240), Goltz focal dermal hypoplasia (240,244), Aicardi syndrome (82,106),

Goldenhar sequence (245,246), and linear sebaceous nevus syndrome (240,244). Optic disc coloboma has recently been linked to a mutation of the PAX6 (164).

Optic disc coloboma may be accompanied by other ocular malformations. For example, large orbital cysts can communicate with atypical dark excavations of the disc that may be colobomatous in nature (151,223,229,247). Villalonga Gornés et al. (247) photographically documented an eye with an orbital cyst in which spontaneous closure of a large inferior papillary excavation transformed the colobomatous disc into a morning glory anomaly! Theodossiadis et al. (248) described a unique case of an optic disc coloboma that was associated with a small disc and numerous retinal venous malformations. Biedner et al. (249) found a macular hole in a myopic patient with an optic disc coloboma. Although peripapillary subretinal neovascularization, which may complicate chorioretinal colobomas, has been reported in two patients with optic disc colobomas (214,250), these optic disc anomalies were, in fact, a morning glory anomaly and an optic pit.

Histopathologic examination in optic disc coloboma demonstrates intrascleral smooth muscle strands oriented concentrically around the distal optic nerve (251,252). Presumably, this pathologic finding accounts for the contractility of the optic disc seen in rare cases of optic disc coloboma (253). Heterotopic adipose tissue is also present within and adjacent to some optic disc colobomas (251,252). Eyes with an isolated optic disc coloboma can develop a serous macular detachment (Fig. 3.13) (in contrast to the rhegmatogenous retinal detachments that complicate retinochoroidal colobomas) (254,255). In a clinicopathologic study of an optic disc coloboma and associated macular detachment in a rhesus monkey, Lin et al. (254) noted disruption of the intermediary tissue of Kuhnt with diffusion of retrobulbar fluid from the orbit into the subretinal space. The nonrhegmatogenous detachment can be treated in a variety of ways, including occlusion of the affected eye, bed rest, corticosteroids, vitrectomy, scleral buckling procedures, gas-fluid exchange, and photocoagulation (207,255,256). Schatz and McDonald (255) advocated waiting 3 months before treating coloboma-associated macular detachments because spontaneous reattachment may occur (256).

Unfortunately, many uncategorizable dysplastic optic discs (discussed later) are indiscriminately labeled as optic disc colobomas. This practice complicates the nosology of coloboma-associated genetic disorders. It is therefore crucial that the diagnosis of optic disc coloboma be reserved for discs that show an inferiorly decentered, white-colored excavation, with minimal peripapillary pigmentary changes. For example, the purported association between optic disc coloboma and basal encephalocele (186,257,258) is deeply entrenched in the literature; however, a critical review reveals only two photographically documented cases (258,259). In striking contrast to the numerous well-documented reports of morning glory optic discs occurring in conjunction with basal encephaloceles, cases of optic disc coloboma with basal encephalocele are actually conspicuous by their absence.

Early in the century, von Szily, in his monumental study

Table 3.1
Ophthalmoscopic Findings That Distinguish the Morning Glory Disc Anomaly from Optic Disc Coloboma

Morning Glory Disc	Optic Disc Coloboma
Optic disc lies within the excavation	Excavation lies within the optic disc
Symmetrical defect (disc lies *centrally* within the excavation	Asymmetrical defect (excavation lies *inferiorly* within the disc)
Central glial tuft	No central glial tuft
Severe peripapillary pigmentary disturbance	Minimal peripapillary pigmentary disturbance
Anomalous retinal vasculature	Normal retinal vasculature

of colobomas, stated ''with certainty'' that ''all the true morphological malformations of the optic disc, including true colobomas . . . are only different manifestations of the same developmental anomaly, namely a different form and degree of malformation of the primitive or epithelial optic papilla'' (187,260). However, the ophthalmoscopic features of optic disc coloboma are most consistent with a primary structural dysgenesis of the proximal embryonic fissure, as opposed to an anomalous dilation confined to the distal optic stalk in the morning glory disc anomaly (Table 3.1) (165,261). The profound differences in associated ocular and systemic findings between the two anomalies (Table 3.2) lend further credence to this hypothesis. Anomalous optic discs with overlapping features of the morning glory disc anomaly and optic disc coloboma are occasionally seen (235,262). These ''hybrid'' anomalies could easily represent instances of early embryonic injury affecting both the proximal embryonic fissure and the distal optic stalk. Their existence should not obscure the fact that colobomatous and morning glory optic discs appear as clinically distinct anomalies in most cases. The concept of ''an optic disc coloboma with a morning glory configuration'' should be abandoned.

PERIPAPILLARY STAPHYLOMA

Peripapillary staphyloma is an extremely rare, usually unilateral anomaly, in which a deep fundus excavation sur-

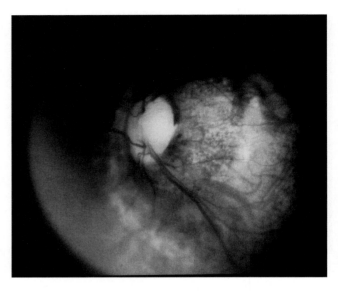

Figure 3.14. Peripapillary staphyloma. The optic disc is situated within a bowl-shaped excavation.

rounds the optic disc (Fig. 3.14) (263,264). In this condition, the disc is seen at the bottom of the excavated defect and may appear normal or show temporal pallor (165,265). The walls and margin of the defect may show atrophic changes in the retinal pigment epithelium (RPE) and choroid (265). Unlike the morning glory disc anomaly, there is no central glial tuft overlying the disc, and the retinal vascular pattern remains normal, apart from reflecting the essential contour of the lesion (165). The staphylomatous excavation in peripapillary staphyloma is also notably deeper than that seen in the morning glory disc anomaly. Several cases of contractile peripapillary staphyloma have been documented (265–268). Seybold and Rosen (269) described a patient who had transient visual obscurations in an eye with an atypical peripapillary staphyloma.

Visual acuity is usually markedly reduced in eyes with a peripapillary staphyloma, but cases with nearly normal acuity have also been reported (270). Affected eyes are usually emmetropic or slightly myopic, and eyes with decreased vision frequently have centrocecal scotomas (264). Although peripapillary staphyloma is clinically and embryologically distinct from morning glory optic disc, these conditions are frequently transposed in the literature (3,210,271). Table 3.3

Table 3.2
Associated Ocular and Systemic Findings That Distinguish the Morning Glory Disc from Isolated Optic Disc Coloboma

Morning Glory Disc	Optic Disc Coloboma
More common in females; rare in blacks	No sex or racial predilection
Rarely familial	Often familial
Rarely bilateral	Often bilateral
No iris, ciliary, or retinal colobomas	Iris, ciliary, and retinal colobomas common
Rarely associated with multisystem genetic disorders	Often associated with multisystem genetic disorders
Basal encephalocele common	Basal encephalocele rare

Table 3.3
Ophthalmoscopic Findings That Distinguish Peripapillary Staphyloma from the Morning Glory Disc Anomaly

Peripapillary Staphyloma	Morning Glory Disc
Deep, cup-shaped excavation	Less depth, funnel-shaped excavation
Relatively normal, well-defined optic disc	Grossly anomalous, poorly defined optic disc
Absence of glial and vascular anomalies	Central glial bonquet, anomalous vascular pattern

contrasts the ophthalmoscopic features that distinguish these two anomalies.

Although peripapillary staphyloma is usually unassociated with systemic or intracranial disease, it has been reported in association with transsphenoidal encephalocele (272), PHACE syndrome (184,273), linear nevus sebaceous syndrome (274), and 18q− (de Grouchy) syndrome (275).

The fairly normal appearance of the optic disc and retinal vessels in eyes with a peripapillary staphyloma suggests that the development of these structures is complete before the staphylomatous process begins (165). Pollock (165) has argued that the clinical features of peripapillary staphyloma are most consistent with diminished peripapillary structural support, perhaps resulting from incomplete differentiation of sclera from posterior neural crest cells in the 5th month of gestation.

MEGALOPAPILLA

This congenital anomaly was first described by Kraupa (276) and has since been reported in numerous other individuals (187,277–286). In 1950, Franceschetti and Bock originally applied the term megalopapilla to signify enlargement of the optic disc without additional structural abnormalities. Since that time, megalopapilla has become a generic term that connotes an abnormally large, excavated optic disc that lacks the numerous anomalous features of the morning glory disc anomaly, the inferior displacement of a coloboma, or the striking cilioretinal circulation of the papillorenal syndrome (see below). In its current usage, megalopapilla comprises two phenotypic variants. The first is a common variant in which an abnormally large optic disc (greater than 2.1 mm in diameter) retains an otherwise normal configuration (264,278). This form of megalopapilla is usually bilateral

and is often associated with a large cup-to-disc ratio, which almost invariably raises the diagnostic consideration of normal-tension glaucoma (Fig. 3.15A). However, the optic cup is usually round or horizontally oval with no vertical notching or encroachment, so that the quotient of horizontal to vertical cup-to-disc ratio remains normal, in contradistinction to the decreased quotient that characterizes glaucomatous optic atrophy (33). Because the axons are spread over a larger surface area, the neuroretinal rim may also appear pale, mimicking optic atrophy (286). Less commonly, the normal optic cup is replaced by a grossly anomalous noninferior excavation that obliterates the adjacent neuroretinal rim (Fig. 3.15B), as described in a large autosomal-dominant pedigree by Slusher et al. (287). The inclusion of this rare variant under the rubric of megalopapilla serves the nosologically useful function of distinguishing it from a colobomatous defect with the latter's attendant systemic implications. Cilioretinal arteries are common in eyes with megalopapilla (33). A high prevalence of megalopapilla was observed in natives of the Marshall Islands (288).

Two reports documented large optic discs in patients with optic nerve hypoplasia associated with a congenital homonymous hemianopia (37,289). This rare combination of findings suggests that a prenatal loss of optic nerve axons leading to optic nerve hypoplasia does not always alter the genetically predetermined size of the scleral canals (37).

Visual acuity is usually normal with megalopapilla, but it may be mildly decreased. The visual field is also usually normal, except for an enlarged blind spot, allowing the examiner to rule out normal-tension glaucoma or compressive optic atrophy. Colobomatous discs are distinguished from megalopapilla by their predominant excavation of the inferior optic disc. Aside from glaucoma and optic disc coloboma, the differential diagnosis of megalopapilla includes

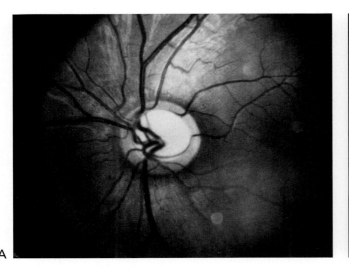
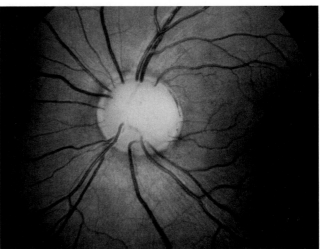

A   B

Figure 3.15. Megalopapilla. *A,* A common variant of megalopapilla in which an abnormally large optic disc contains a large central cup. Unlike glaucomatous optic atrophy, the cup is horizontally oval with an intact neuroretinal rim, and there is no nasalization of vessels at the point of origin. *B,* An uncommon variant of megalopapilla in which an anomalous superior excavation obliterates much of the temporal neuroretinal rim. (From Brodsky MC. Congenital optic disk anomalies. Surv Ophthalmol 1994;39:89–112.)

orbital optic glioma, which in children can cause progressive enlargement of a previously normal-sized optic disc (290).

Pathogenetically, most cases of megalopapilla may simply represent a statistical variant of normal. However, it is likely that megalopapilla occasionally results from altered migration of optic axons early in embryogenesis, as evidenced by two reports of megalopapilla in patients with anterior encephaloceles (187,291). Nevertheless, the rarity of an association between megalopapilla and CNS abnormalities suggests that neuroimaging is unwarranted in a patient with megalopapilla, unless midline facial anomalies (e.g., hypertelorism, cleft palate, cleft lip, depressed nasal bridge) coexist.

OPTIC PIT

An optic pit is a round or oval, gray, white, or yellowish depression in the optic disc (Fig. 3.16A). Wiethe (292) first described two black depressions with an olive-gray tint within the optic disc of a 62-year-old woman. Early investigators labeled these depressions as colobomas, crater-like holes, congenital holes, and congenital pits (293). Reis (294) estimated the frequency of optic pits to be approximately 1 in 11,000—a figure later confirmed by Kranenburg (295). Numerous reports of familial optic pits suggest an autosomal-dominant mode of transmission (296–298).

Optic pits commonly affected the temporal portion of the optic disc but may be situated in any sector (207). Such temporally located pits are often accompanied by adjacent peripapillary pigment epithelial changes. One or two cilioretinal arteries emerge from the bottom or the margin of the pit in more than 50% of cases (264,299). Although optic pits are typically unilateral, bilateral pits are seen in 15% of cases (264). In unilateral cases, the affected disc is slightly larger than the normal disc. Visual acuity is typically normal unless there is fluid within or beneath the macula (see below). Although visual field defects are variable and often correlate poorly with the location of the pit, the most common defect appears to be a paracentral arcuate scotoma connected to an enlarged blind spot (293,295). Optic pits do not portend additional CNS malformations, although rare exceptions exist (300). Acquired depressions in the optic disc that are indistinguishable from optic pits are said to occur in normal-tension glaucoma (301).

Serous macular elevations develop in 25–75% of eyes with optic pits (Fig. 3.16B) (293,295,302,303). Optic pit-associated maculopathy generally becomes symptomatic in the third and fourth decades of life. Vitreous traction on the margins of the pit and tractional changes in the roof of the pit may be the inciting events that ultimately lead to late-onset macular detachment (299,303,304).

All optic pit-associated macular elevations were once thought to be caused by serous detachments. Lincoff et al. (305), however, proposed that careful stereoscopic examination of the macula in conjunction with kinetic perimetry demonstrates the following progression of events:

1. A schisis-like inner layer retinal separation initially forms in direct communication with the optic pit, producing a mild, relative, centrocecal scotoma.
2. An outer layer macular hole develops beneath the boundaries of the inner layer separation and produces a dense central scotoma.
3. An outer layer retinal detachment develops around the macular hole, presumably from influx of fluid from the inner layer separation. This outer layer detachment ophthalmoscopically resembles an RPE detachment but fails to hyperfluoresce on fluorescein angiography.
4. The outer layer detachment may eventually enlarge and

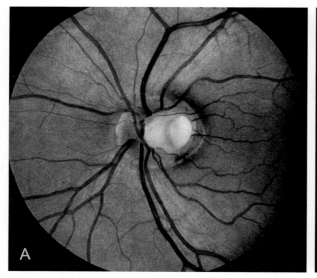
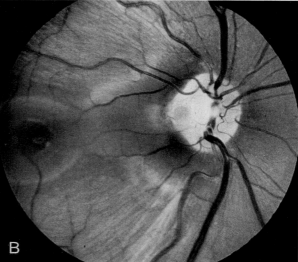

Figure 3.16. Optic pit. *A,* Oval white excavation occupies the temporal portion of the disc. *B,* Grayish temporal optic disc with adjacent retinoschisis cavity (*large arrows*), serous macular detachment (*small arrows*) and outer layer hole (*open arrow*).

obliterate the inner layer separation. At this stage, it is no longer ophthalmoscopically or histopathologically distinguishable from a primary serous macular detachment.

Optical coherence tomography confirms the presence of an inner layer retinal separation in communication with the optic pit in eyes with serous macular detachments (306–308). Figure 3.16*B* depicts the retinal findings that can be observed in the evolution of an optic pit-associated macular detachment. The finding of a sensory macular detachment in histopathologically studied eyes with optic pits presumably represents the end stage of this sequence of events. Whether or not this sequence of events leads to all optic pit-associated macular detachments is unclear.

The risk of optic pit-associated macular detachment is greater in eyes with large optic pits and in eyes with temporally located pits (293). Spontaneous reattachment occurs in approximately 25% of cases (213,293). Sugar's (302) early report of spontaneous resolution of most optic pit-associated macular detachments with good visual recovery differs from the experience of most subsequent investigators, who reported permanent visual loss in untreated patients, even when spontaneous reattachment occurred (213,309). Bed rest and bilateral patching have led to retinal reattachment in some patients, presumably by decreasing vitreous traction (255,310). Laser photocoagulation to block the flow of fluid from the pit to the macula is usually unsuccessful, perhaps because of the inability of laser photocoagulation to seal a retinoschisis cavity (255,303,305,309–312). Vitrectomy with internal gas tamponade and laser photocoagulation were shown to produce long-term improvement in acuity in several independent studies (207,255,305,310,311, 313–315). The initial intent of this treatment was to compress the retina at the edge of the disc to enhance the effect of laser treatment (316). However, Lincoff et al. (316) have postulated that internal gas tamponade functions to mechanically displace subretinal fluid away from the macula, allowing a shallow, inner-layer separation to persist, which is associated with a mild scotoma and relatively good visual acuity. Based upon clinical and perimetric observations following treatment, Lincoff et al. (316) concluded that laser photocoagulation probably does not contribute to the success of this procedure. Perhaps because of age-related differences in vitreopapillary traction, optic pit-associated serous maculopathy in children may have a tendency toward spontaneous resolution (317,318).

The source of intraretinal fluid in eyes with optic pits is controversial. Possible sources include vitreous cavity via the pit, the subarachnoid space, blood vessels at the base of the pit, and the orbital space surrounding the dura (254,264,303,319). Although fluorescein angiography shows early hypofluorescence of the pit, followed in many cases by late hyperfluorescent staining (293,303,311,320), optic pits do not generally leak fluorescein and there is no extension of fluorescein into the subretinal space toward the macula (319,321). The finding of late hyperfluorescent staining correlates strongly with the presence of cilioretinal arteries emerging from the pit (299). Careful slit-lamp biomicros-

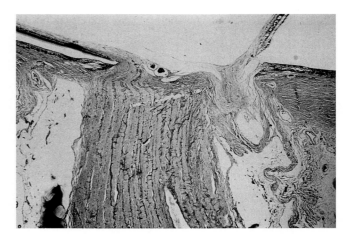

Figure 3.17. Histologic appearance of optic pit.

copy often reveals a thin membrane overlying the pit (293) or a persistent Cloquet's canal, terminating at the margin of the pit (322). Brown et al. (323) documented active flow of fluid from the vitreous cavity through the pit to the subretinal space in collie dogs, but this mechanism has never been conclusively demonstrated in humans.

Histologically, optic pits consist of herniations of dysplastic retina into a collagen-lined pocket extending posteriorly, often into the subarachnoid space, through a defect in the lamina cribrosa (Fig. 3.17) (264,304). Friberg and McLellan (324) demonstrated a pulsatile communication of fluid between the vitreous cavity and a retrobulbar cyst through an optic pit. Rarely, macular holes can develop in eyes with optic pits or optic disc colobomas and lead to rhegmatogenous retinal detachment (249,325).

Although most researchers view optic pits as the mildest variant in the spectrum of optic disc colobomas (179, 206,254,255,293,295,301,309,319,321,326,327), this widely accepted hypothesis is probably untenable for the following reasons:

1. Optic pits are usually unilateral, sporadic, and unassociated with systemic anomalies. Colobomas are bilateral as often as unilateral, commonly autosomal dominant, and may be associated with a variety of multisystem disorders.
2. It is rare for optic pits to coexist with iris or retinochoroidal colobomas.
3. Optic pits usually occur in locations unrelated to the embryonic fissure.

PAPILLORENAL SYNDROME (THE "UNCOLOBOMA")

The papillorenal syndrome, also previously known as renal-coloboma syndrome, was first described by Rieger in 1977 (328). This syndrome was initially considered to be a rare autosomal-dominant disorder consisting of bilateral optic disc anomalies associated with hypoplastic kidneys

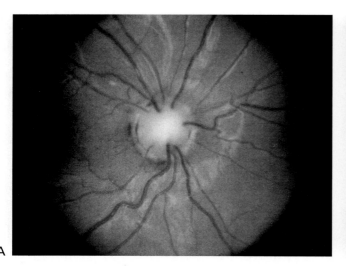
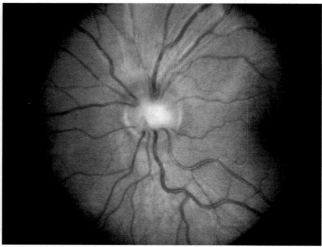

Figure 3.18. Papillorenal syndrome. Both optic discs show a central excavation with multiple cilioretinal arteries in place of the normal central retinal circulation. This 9-year-old girl with chronic renal failure had 20/20 acuity in each eye. Renal biopsy showed interstitial fibrosis. (Photographs courtesy of Erika M. Levin, M.D.)

(329). Associated retinal detachments were described, as was eventual renal failure. In 1995, Sanyanusin et al. discovered mutations in the developmental gene PAX2, the human homologue of the mouse gene Pax2 in two affected families (330). Schimmenti et al. (331) identified three additional families with PAX2 mutations with similar ophthalmologic features and a wider spectrum of renal abnormalities, which may include hypoplasia, variable proteinuria, vesiculoureteral reflux, recurrent pyelonephritis, microhematuria, echogenicity on ultrasound, or high resistance to blood flow on Doppler ultrasound (331).

Parsa et al. have since determined that the papillorenal syndrome is characterized by a distinct optic disc malformation that bears no relationship to coloboma (329,332,333). In this syndrome, the excavated optic disc is normal in size, and may be surrounded by variable pigmentary disturbance. Unlike in colobomatous defects, the excavation is centrally positioned. According to Parsa et al., the defining feature is the presence of multiple cilioretinal vessels which emanate from the periphery of the disc, and variable attenuation or atrophy of the central retinal vessels (Fig. 3.18) (329). Color Doppler imaging has confirmed the absence of central retinal circulation in patients with papillorenal syndrome (329). Visual acuity is usually 20/20 but may occasionally be severely diminished (329,334) secondary to choroidal and reti-

nal hypoplasia and, in some cases, to later-onset serous retinal detachments. Peripheral visual field defects corresponding to areas of retinal hypoplasia are often present. The central optic disc excavation and peripheral field defects can simulate coloboma as well as normal tension glaucoma. Follow-up examination has shown renal disease in some patients who were originally reported as having isolated familial autosomal dominant "coloboma." (333).

Parsa et al. have attributed this malformation to a primary deficiency in angiogenesis involved in vascular development (329). In these patients, there is a failure of the hyaloid system to convert to normal central retinal vessels. The absence of a well-defined central retinal artery or vein in several adult mammalian species including lemurs and cats, suggests that this malformation could be considered analogous to an evolutionary regression to a feline pattern of circulation (329). Since ocular tissues and renal cortex are the most highly perfused tissues of the body, both develop a significant portion of their vasculature by means of angiogenesis (budding) in addition to vasculogenesis (329). These tissues may thus be particularly susceptible to anomalies in vascular development resulting in hypoplasia or anomalies of associated structures (329). Many patients with papillorenal syndrome have no detectable mutations in the PAX2 gene (329,334).

CONGENITAL TILTED DISC SYNDROME

The tilted disc syndrome is a nonhereditary, usually bilateral condition in which the superotemporal optic disc is elevated and the inferonasal disc is posteriorly displaced, resulting in an oval-appearing optic disc, with its long axis obliquely oriented (Fig. 3.19). This configuration is accompanied by *situs inversus* of the retinal vessels, congenital

inferonasal conus, thinning of the inferonasal RPE and choroid, and bitemporal hemianopia that does not respect the vertical midline (335). Histopathologically, the optic nerve enters at an extremely oblique angle, the superior or superotemporal portion of the disc is elevated, and there is posterior ectasia of the inferior or inferonasal fundus and optic disc

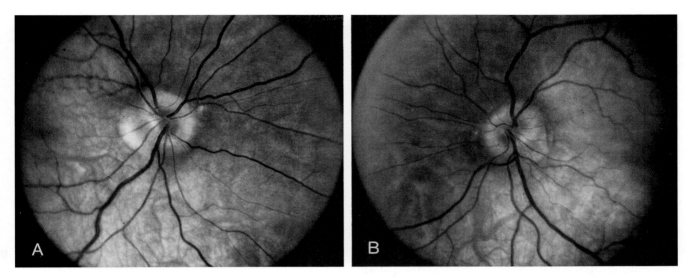

Figure 3.19.   Congenital tilted disc syndrome. Both optic discs are oval with relative elevation of the superior-temporal portion compared to the inferior-nasal portion. This elevation is often mistaken for true disc swelling. Note situs inversus of the vessels and inferior retinochoroidal hypopigmentation.

(Figs. 3.20 and 3.21). Affected patients often have myopic astigmatism, with the plus-axis oriented parallel to the ectasia. The ocular imagery resulting from a tilted retina creates a type of curvature of field that may subjectively simulate astigmatic blur (336). Flüeler and Guyton (336) demonstrated that the astigmatic retinoscopic reflex in the tilted disc syndrome cannot result from the retinal tilt, since only a minute area of the tilted retina is viewed during retinoscopy. The tilted disc syndrome has been described in detail as such by several authors (335,337–342). In retrospect, however, early descriptions of congenital crescent, congenital conus, situs inversion of the disc, optic disc dysversion,

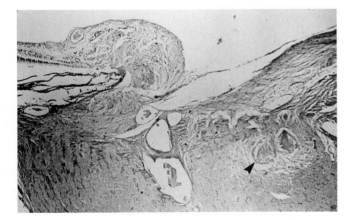

Figure 3.20.   Histologic appearance of a tilted optic disc. The nerve enters the eye at an extremely oblique angle. Also note elevation of the superior (*left*) portion of the disc as compared with the inferior (*right*) portion of the disc. A small area of optic nerve infarction is present just posterior to the lamina cribrosa (*arrowhead*).

and ''Fuchs coloboma'' probably are descriptions of this condition in its full or partial form. The inferior crescent is created by a disparity between the size of the retinal and scleral openings. According to Dorrell (340), the retinal opening is usually circular in shape, whereas the outline of the scleral canal is contracted across one segment, so that it conforms to a stirrup or D-shape. In some eyes, the entire disc assumes a D-shape. The congenital tilted disc syndrome is bilateral in about 80% of cases (343). The cause of the tilted disc syndrome is unknown, but the inferonasal or inferior location of the excavation suggests a pathogenetic relationship to retinochoroidal coloboma (319).

Familiarity with the tilted disc syndrome is crucial for the ophthalmologist, since affected patients may present with bitemporal hemianopia, suggesting a chiasmal syndrome (335,337–339,344,345). The bitemporal hemianopia in patients with tilted discs, however, is typically incomplete and confined primarily to the superior quadrants. It is, in fact, a refractive scotoma, secondary to regional myopia localized to the inferonasal retina (Fig. 3.22) Unlike the visual field loss that results from damage to the optic chiasm, the field defects seen in the tilted disc syndrome fail to respect the vertical meridian on both kinetic and static perimetry. Furthermore, the superotemporal depression on Goldmann perimetry is selectively detected with mid-sized isopters, whereas the large and small isopters give fairly normal results because the ectasia that occurs in such cases is confined to the midperipheral fundus (Fig. 3.22) Despite the regional retinal ectasia, recent topography studies have suggested that an irregular corneal curvature underlies the associated astigmatism (346,347). Repeat perimetry with a spectacle lens in place to correct myopic astigmatism may reduce or eliminate the superotemporal defect, confirming its refractive nature (348). In some cases, retinal sensitivity may be de-

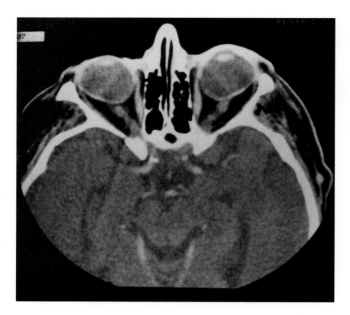

Figure 3.21. CT scan showing ectasia of the lower nasal aspect of globes in a patient with the congenital tilted disc syndrome. The nasal aspects of both globes protrude posteriorly. (From Brodsky MC. Congenital optic disk anomalies. Surv Ophthalmol 1994;39:89–112.)

or optic nerve hypoplasia. In some cases, elevation of the superior-temporal portion of the disc mimics optic disc swelling (319,340,351).

The congenital retinal malformation in tilted disc syndrome may influence the development of acquired retinal diseases. For example, the chorioretinal degenerative changes within the ectatic inferonasal sector of retina may predispose to macular subretinal neovascularization (352,353). Numerous reports suggest that associated anomalies at the junction of the staphyloma (354) or at the junction of between peripapillary retina and the altered disc margin (355,356) may play a role in the pathogenesis of serous macular detachments (354–356). Central serous papillopathy occurs in eyes with tilted discs or the full tilted disc syndrome. On the other hand, the inferonasal ectasia may also exert a regional protective effect against background diabetic retinopathy because of increased oxygenation from the choroid to the thin ectatic retina (357).

It should be emphasized that a true bitemporal hemianopia may occur in patients with the tilted disc syndrome who also harbor a congenital suprasellar tumor (30). As with optic nerve hypoplasia, these two seemingly disparate lesions may reflect the disruptive effect of a suprasellar lesion on the migration of optic axons during embryogenesis (30, 358,359). This sinister association mandates neuroimaging in any patient with a tilted disc syndrome whose bitemporal hemianopia either respects the vertical meridian or fails to preferentially involve the midperipheral isopter on kinetic perimetry. Margolis and Siegel (291) also documented the tilted disc syndrome in patients with craniofacial anomalies, including Crouzon's disease and Apert's disease.

Tilted discs without retinal ectasia occur in patients with transsphenoidal encephalocele (92,272), congenital tumors

creased in the area of the ectasia, and the defect thus persists to some degree despite appropriate refractive correction (335,340,342,349). Brazitikos et al. (350) demonstrated that other quadrants also show mildly decreased sensitivities on threshold perimetry and suggested that the tilted disc syndrome may actually include some degree of diffuse retinal

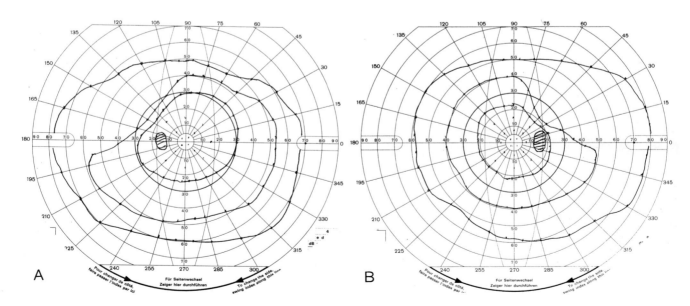

Figure 3.22. Kinetic perimetry demonstrates a supertemporal visual field defect in both left (*A*) and right (*B*) eyes. Note that the defect is confined to the midperipheral isopter that does not respect the horizontal meridian.

of the anterior visual pathways (30), X-linked congenital stationary night blindness (360,361), Ehlers-Danlos syndrome (type III), and familial dextrocardia (362). Rothkoff and Biedner (363) reported a patient who had bilaterally tilted discs, facial hemiatrophy, and congenital horizontal gaze paralysis.

OPTIC DISC DYSPLASIA

Optic disc dysplasia is a term that connotes a markedly deformed optic disc that fails to conform to any recognizable diagnostic category (Fig. 3.23). The distinction between an nonspecifically "anomalous" disc and a "dysplastic" disc is somewhat arbitrary and based primarily upon the severity of the lesion. For instance, in the past, the term "optic disc dysplasia" was applied to cases that are now identified as the morning glory disc anomaly or papillorenal syndrome (187,364). Conversely, many dysplastic optic discs have been indiscriminately labeled as optic disc colobomas. New variants of optic disc dysplasia continue to be recognized (365,366).

Dysplastic optic discs in patients with transsphenoidal encephalocele (188,367) tend to be associated with a discrete infrapapillary zone of V- or tongue-shaped retinochoroidal depigmentation (Figs. 3.9 and 3.24) (92). These juxtapapillary defects differ from typical retinochoroidal colobomas, which widen inferiorly and are not associated with basal encephalocele. Unlike the typical retinochoroidal coloboma, this distinct juxtapapillary defect is associated with minimal scleral excavation and no visible disruption in the integrity of the overlying retina. In patients with anomalous or dysplastic optic discs, the finding of a V- or tongue-shaped retinochoroidal defect should prompt neuroimaging to look for transsphenoidal encephalocele (92).

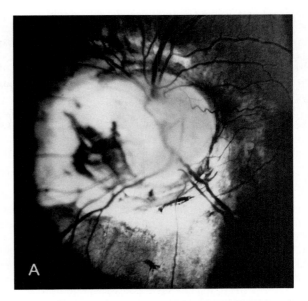

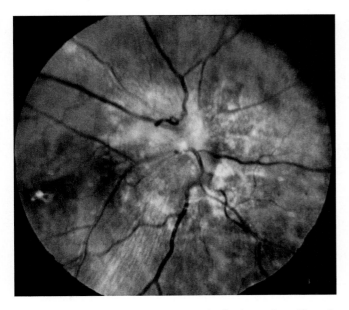

Figure 3.23. Optic disc dysplasia. The optic disc is grossly malformed, and the retinal vessels emerge from the region of the disc in an anomalous pattern.

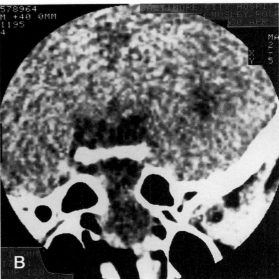

Figure 3.24. Optic disc dysplasia and transsphenoidal encephalocele. *A,* Enlarged dysplastic optic disc with peripapillary pigmentary disturbance and tongue-shaped area of inferior depigmentation. Optic disc dysplasia with peripapillary pigmentary disturbance. *B,* Computed tomographic scan shows transsphenoidal encephalocele.

CONGENITAL OPTIC DISC PIGMENTATION

Congenital optic disc pigmentation is a condition in which melanin deposition anterior to or within the lamina cribrosa imparts a slate-gray appearance to the entire optic disc. True congenital optic disc pigmentation is extremely rare, but it has been described in a child with an interstitial deletion of chromosome 17 (368), in Aicardi syndrome (244), and in optic nerve hypoplasia (Fig. 3.25) (368,369). Congenital optic disc pigmentation is compatible with good visual acuity but may be associated with coexistent optic disc anomalies that decrease vision (368). Silver and Sapiro (370) demonstrated that, in developing mice and rats, a transient zone of melanin in the distal developing optic stalk influences migration of the earliest optic nerve axons. The effects of abnormal pigment deposition on optic nerve embryogenesis could explain the frequent coexistence of congenital optic disc pigmentation with other anomalies, particularly optic nerve hypoplasia.

The majority of patients with gray optic discs do not have congenital optic disc pigmentation. For reasons that are poorly understood, optic discs of infants with delayed visual maturation and albinism often have a diffuse gray tint when viewed ophthalmoscopically. In these conditions, the gray tint usually disappears within the first year of life without visible pigment migration (371). Beauvieux (372,373) observed gray optic discs in premature infants and in albinotic infants who were apparently blind but who later developed good vision as the gray color disappeared. He attributed the gray appearance of these neonatal discs to delayed optic nerve myelination with preservation of the "embryonic tint." It should be noted, however, that gray optic discs may also be seen in normal neonates and are usually a nonspecific finding of little diagnostic value, except when accompanied by other clinical signs of delayed visual maturation or albinism. Myelinated peripapillary nerve fibers may impart a gray cast to the optic disc (374), as may pseudopapilledema associated with buried drusen (368,375). A grayish cast to the optic discs was described in three patients with Pelizaeus-Merzbacher disease (376), in an infant with maple syrup urine disease (377), and in a child with partial trisomy 10q syndrome (378).

Optically gray optic discs and congenital optic disc pig-

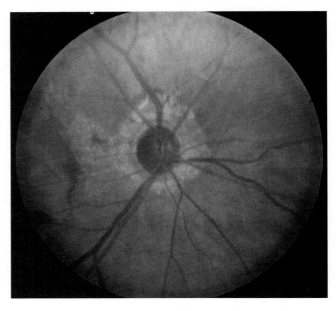

Figure 3.25. Congenital optic disc pigmentation. Entire disc is gray, and the disc is hypoplastic with a surrounding zone of depigmentation, suggesting migration of peripapillary pigment onto the disc.

mentation can usually be distinguished ophthalmoscopically, because melanin deposition in true congenital optic disc pigmentation is often discrete, irregular, and granular in appearance (368). True optic disc pigmentation may also be acquired, as in cases of melanocytoma or malignant melanoma of the optic nerve head. Sobanski (379) documented acquired pigmentation of the optic disc following a scleral buckling procedure. Hoyt and Beeston (374) photographed acquired pigmentation of the optic disc following retrobulbar amputation for optic glioma. Taylor and Ffytche (380) described a patient who developed an area of optic disc pigmentation associated with a visual field defect following an episode of presumed optic neuritis associated with chickenpox.

AICARDI SYNDROME

Aicardi syndrome is a congenital cerebroretinal disorder of unknown etiology. Its salient clinical features are infantile spasms, agenesis of the corpus callosum, a modified form of the electroencephalographic pattern termed hypsarrhythmia, and a pathognomonic optic disc appearance consisting of multiple depigmented "chorioretinal lacunae" clustered around the disc (82,106) (Fig. 3.26). Histologically, chorioretinal lacunae consist of well-circumscribed, full-thickness defects limited to the retinal pigment epithelium and choroid. The overlying retina remains intact but is often histologically abnormal (82).

Congenital optic disc anomalies, including optic disc coloboma, optic nerve hypoplasia, and congenital optic disc pigmentation, may accompany chorioretinal lacunae (82,134).

Other ocular abnormalities include microphthalmos, retrobulbar cyst, pseudoglioma, retinal detachment, macular scar, cataract, pupillary membrane, iris synechiae, iris coloboma, and persistent hyperplastic primary vitreous (106,134). The most common systemic findings associated with Aicardi syndrome are vertebral malformations (fused vertebrae, scoliosis, spina bifida) and costal malformations (absent ribs, fused or bifurcated ribs) (106,134,381). Other systemic findings in Aicardi syndrome include muscular hypotonia, microcephaly, dysmorphic facies, cleft lip and palate, auditory disturbances, and auricular anomalies (134,382,383). Aicardi syndrome has also been associated with choroid plexus papilloma (382,384).

Severe mental retardation is present in almost all cases

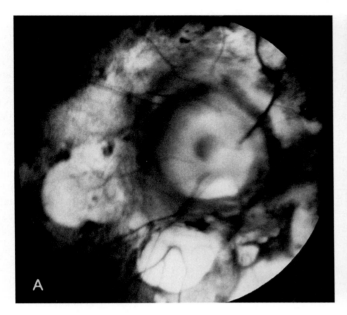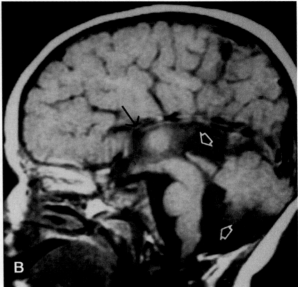

Figure 3.26. Aicardi syndrome. *A,* An enlarged, malformed optic disc is surrounded by numerous, well-circumscribed, chorioretinal lacunae. *B,* Sagittal MR image demonstrating agenesis of the corpus callosum (*upper solid arrow* denotes normal position of the corpus callosum), an arachnoid cyst in the region of the quadrigeminal cistern (*open arrows*) and hypoplasia of the cerebellar vermis with cystic dilatation of the 4th ventricle (Dandy-Walker variant). (*A,* From Carney SH, Brodsky MC, Good WV, et al. Aicardi syndrome: More than meets the eye. Surv Ophthalmol 1993;37:419–424.)

(82,134). Aicardi syndrome is associated with decreased life expectancy, but some patients survive into their teenage years. Menezes et al. (385–387) retrospectively reviewed ocular and neurologic findings in 14 girls with Aicardi syndrome and found that the size of the largest chorioretinal lacuna correlated significantly with neurologic outcome, whereas age at presentation, type, and severity of seizures did not. Rosser et al. (388) found the neurodevelopmental prognosis of Aicardi syndrome to be extremely poor, with most children having seizures that are intractable despite therapy, and 91% attaining milestones no higher than 12 months. Ganesh et al. (389) have proposed that a persistence of fetal vasculature between gestational weeks 9 and 12 may provide a unifying hypothesis for the embryogenesis of Aicardi syndrome, based on the presence of associated intraocular malformations such as microphthalmos, persistent pupillary membrane, persistent hyperplastic primary vitreous, vascular loops on the optic disc, and epiretinal glial tissue. Since callosal development and neuronal migration occur concurrently during this period of gestation, this mechanism would also explain the associated callosal agenesis and neuronal migration defects within the brain.

Central nervous system anomalies in Aicardi syndrome include agenesis of the corpus callosum, cortical migration anomalies (pachygyria, polymicrogyria, cortical heterotopias), and multiple structural CNS malformations (cerebral hemispheric asymmetry, Dandy-Walker variant, colpocephaly, midline arachnoid cysts) (Fig. 3.26) (390–393).

Neuropathologic specimens show a characteristic profile, consisting of unlayered polymicrogyria, subcortical or periventricular heterotopias, and agenesis of the corpus callosum (394–396). This complex cerebral malformation suggests a problem in nerve cell proliferation and migration (396). An overlap between Aicardi syndrome and septo-optic dysplasia has been recognized in several patients (82,134).

Aicardi syndrome is thought to result from an X-linked mutational event that is lethal in males (134,397). Parents should therefore be asked about a previous history of miscarriages. In 1986, Chevrie and Aicardi suggested that all cases of Aicardi syndrome represent fresh gene mutations because no cases of affected siblings had been reported (134), however, a report of Aicardi syndrome in two sisters challenges this notion that Aicardi syndrome always results from a de novo mutation in the affected infant and suggests that parental gonadal mosaicism for the mutation may be an additional mechanism of inheritance (398). With rare exceptions (399,400), cytogenetic testing with special attention to the X chromosome gives normal results in Aicardi syndrome (401). One girl reported as having Aicardi syndrome with a balanced X/3 translocation had no chorioretinal lacunae (402). Although early infectious CNS insults could lead to severe CNS anomalies, tests for infective agents are consistently negative. No teratogenic drug or other toxin has yet been associated with Aicardi syndrome. Based on the pattern of cerebroretinal malformations in Aicardi syndrome, it is speculated that an insult to the CNS must occur between the 4th and 8th week of gestation (134).

DOUBLING OF THE OPTIC DISC

Doubling of the optic discs is a rare anomaly in which two optic discs are seen ophthalmoscopically and presumed to be associated with a duplication or separation of the distal optic nerve into two fasciculi (403). Collier (404) described a case and reviewed eight such reports in the literature. Although these anomalies varied considerably, most had a "main" disc and a "satellite" disc, each with its own vascular system (Fig. 3.27). Most cases occur unilaterally and are associated with decreased acuity in the affected eye (403). Since Collier's report, several other cases have been reported which appear to represent "pseudodoubling" of the optic disc (403,405–411).

Documented separation of the optic nerve into two or more strands is rare in humans but common in some lower vertebrates (403). A handful of autopsy cases document sep-

aration of various portions of an intracranial or orbital optic nerve into two strands as an incidental finding (412–416). This anomaly was also visualized by Sourdille during an enucleation (407). The majority of clinical reports antedate the use of high-resolution neuroimaging and have relied upon the roentgenographic demonstration of two optic nerves in the same orbit, the results of fluorescein angiography, synchronous pulsations of each major disc artery, dual blind spots, and angioscotomas to provide indirect evidence of double optic nerves (403). More commonly, an apparent doubling of the optic disc results from focal juxtapapillary retinochoroidal colobomas, which may display abnormal vascular anastomoses with the optic disc (403). Neuroimaging should allow in vivo confirmation of true optic nerve diastasis.

OPTIC NERVE APLASIA

Optic nerve aplasia is a rare nonhereditary malformation, that is seen most often in a unilaterally malformed eye of an otherwise healthy person (18,417–425). In its current usage, the term implies complete absence of the optic nerve (including the optic disc), retinal ganglion and nerve fiber layers, and optic nerve vessels (426). Histopathologic examination usually demonstrates a vestigial dural sheath entering the sclera in its normal position, as well as retinal dysplasia with rosette formation (Fig. 3.28) (423). Some early reports of optic nerve aplasia actually described patients with severe hypoplasia at a time when the latter entity was not clearly recognized (422).

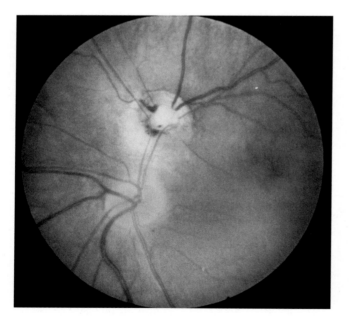

Figure 3.27. Doubling of the optic disc. Note "main" disc and "satellite" disc. (From Donoso LA, Magaragal LE, Eiferman RA. Ocular anomalies simulating double optic discs. Can J Ophthalmol 1981;16:84–87. Photograph courtesy of Larry A. Donoso.)

Ophthalmoscopically, optic nerve aplasia may take on any of the following appearances (7):

1. Absence of a normally defined optic nerve head or papilla in the ocular fundus, without central blood vessels and with an absence of macular differentiation;
2. A whitish area corresponding to the optic disc, without central vessels or macular differentiation;
3. A deep avascular cavity in the site corresponding to the optic disc, surrounded by a whitish annulus.

Visual fields are normal in the unaffected eye (427). Fluorescein angiography shows absent retinal blood vessels in the affected eye and normal retinal circulation in the opposite eye (7,422,427). The electroretinographic waveform (ERG) may be flat; if present, the a- and b-waves are diminished (7,422,427). CT scanning may show the globe and bony orbit to be smaller than normal (426). In addition, MR imaging may show isolated absence of the optic nerve on the affected side (426,427). The cause of optic nerve aplasia is unknown. Chromosome studies were normal in all cases studied by Howard et al. (427).

Optic nerve aplasia seems to fall within a malformation complex that is fundamentally distinct from that seen with optic nerve hypoplasia, as evidenced by the proclivity of optic nerve aplasia to occur unilaterally and its frequent association with malformations that are otherwise confined to the affected eye (microphthalmia, malformations in the anterior chamber angle, hypoplasia or segmental aplasia of the iris, cataracts, persistent hyperplastic primary vitreous, anterior colobomas, macular staphyloma, retinal dysplasia, or pigmentary disturbance) (7,425,427,428). However, when optic nerve aplasia occurs bilaterally, it is usually associated with severe and widespread congenital CNS malformations (426,427,429,430). An animal model of unilateral optic nerve aplasia was induced in rat fetuses by folic acid deficiency, in rat offspring by x-ray irradiation, and in rabbit fetuses by actinomycin D treatment (431).

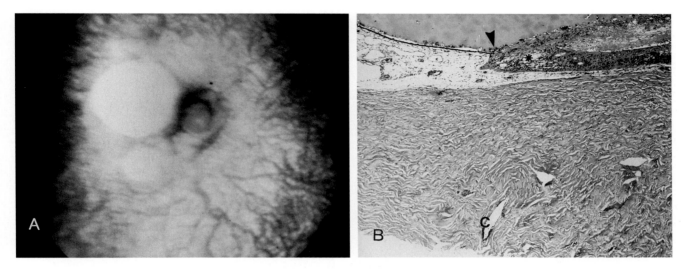

Figure 3.28. Optic nerve aplasia. *A,* Note absence of optic disc and retinal vessels. *B,* Histologic appearance of optic nerve aplasia. The edge of the choroid and retinal pigment epithelium is marked by an *arrowhead.* Fibroglial tissue (*asterisk*) occupies the colobomatous area. A ciliary vessel (C) traverses the sclera, but optic nerve tissue is absent. (*A,* From Little LE, Whitmore PV, Wells TW Jr. Aplasia of the optic nerve. J Pediatr Ophthalmol 1976;13:84–88. *B,* From Hotchkiss ML, Green WR. Optic nerve aplasia and hypoplasia. J Pediatr Ophthalmol Strabismus 1979;16:225–240.)

In patients with unilateral optic nerve aplasia, the intracranial course of the ''intact'' optic nerve may vary. Hoff et al. (432) reported on a patient with unilateral anophthalmos with optic nerve aplasia associated with a congenital giant suprasellar aneurysm. The remaining optic nerve was identified at craniotomy as passing posteriorly as a single cord to form an optic tract with no adjoining chiasm. Hotchkiss and Green (18) provided necropsy findings from a patient with a Hallerman-Streiff-like syndrome and left optic nerve aplasia in whom the lateral geniculate bodies and optic tracts appeared grossly normal bilaterally, even though the optic chiasm was formed from a single optic nerve on the right side. Margo et al. (426) described a patient with unilateral optic nerve aplasia and microphthalmos in whom MR imaging demonstrated true unilateral optic nerve aplasia, hemichiasmal hypoplasia on the affected side, but bilateral optic tracts. VEPs were increased over the occipital lobe contralateral to the intact optic nerve, suggesting chiasmal misdirection of axons from the temporal retina of the normal eye, as seen in albinos.

MYELINATED (MEDULLATED) NERVE FIBERS

Myelination of the anterior visual system begins centrally at the lateral geniculate body at 5 months of gestation. It proceeds distally and reaches the chiasm by 6–7 months of gestation, the retrobulbar optic nerve by 8 months, and the lamina cribrosa at term; although in some cases myelination may continue for a short time after birth. Normally, myelin does not extend intraocularly; however, intraocular myelination of retinal nerve fibers occurs in 0.3–0.6% of the population by ophthalmoscopy and in 1% by postmortem examinations (433). Straatsma et al. (434) studied both eyes from 3,968 consecutive autopsy cases and found 37 eyes from 32 patients with myelinated retinal nerve fibers. In this series, males and females were equally affected, and in most eyes (81%), myelination was continuous with the optic disc. The majority of the patients had normal visual acuity, although four patients with unilateral myelinated nerve fibers had ipsilateral anisometropic myopia, strabismus, and amblyopia (435). The explanation for the occurrence of intraocular myelination is unknown. Oligodendrocytes, which are responsible for myelination of the CNS, are not normally present in the human retina, but histologic studies confirm their presence in some areas of myelinated nerve fibers, and their absence in other areas (434).

Ophthalmoscopically, myelinated nerve fibers usually appear as white striated patches at the upper and lower poles of the optic disc (Fig. 3.29). In these locations, they may impart a gray appearance to the optic disc, and they may also simulate papilledema, both by elevating the adjacent portions of the disc and by obscuring the disc margin and underlying retinal vessels (436). Distally, they have an irregular fan-shaped appearance that facilitates their recognition. Small slits or patches of normal-appearing fundus color are occasionally visible within areas of myelination. Myelinated nerve fibers are bilateral in 17–20% of cases and, clinically, they are discontinuous with the optic nerve head in 19%. Isolated patches of myelinated nerve fibers are occasionally found in the peripheral retina (Fig. 3.29).

Leys et al. (437) described seven patients who had retinal vascular abnormalities within areas of myelinated nerve fibers. These abnormalities ranged from mild telangiectasis to frank neovascularization, with or without obstruction of the capillary network and signs of branch artery and vein

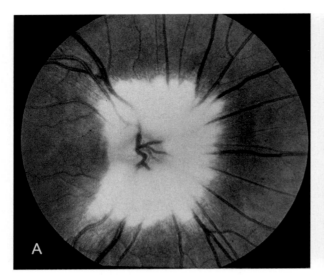
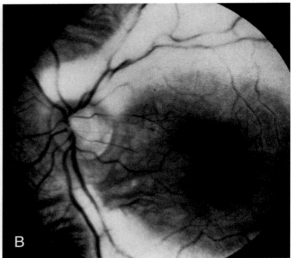

Figure 3.29.   Myelinated nerve fibers. *A,* The optic disc is surrounded by myelinated, feathery nerve fibers. *B,* Myelinated nerve fibers extend superiorly and inferiorly from the optic disc along the arcuate nerve fiber bundles.

occlusion. Vitreous hemorrhage occurred in the four youngest patients. This report, together with a similar one by Tabassian et al. (438) would suggest that the retinal vessels within patches of myelinated nerve fibers should be carefully examined for occult microvascular abnormalities.

Myelinated retinal nerve fibers do not usually reduce visual acuity; however, relative scotomas may be charted if a sufficient number of myelinated fibers are present. The scotomas are invariably smaller than the size of the myelinated patch would suggest. Because myelinated fibers are usually adjacent to the optic disc, the blind spot is often enlarged in such patients. When the nerve fibers surround the macula, there may be a ring scotoma, and isolated patches in the retinal periphery may produce isolated peripheral scotomas. If the macula is affected, there may be a central scotoma, but this is exceedingly rare. In a single instance, Walsh and Hoyt (439) observed a pronounced defect in visual acuity as a result of myelinated fibers. In that case, the entire fundus except for a small area temporal to the disc contained myelinated nerve fibers.

The pathogenesis of myelinated nerve fibers remains largely speculative, but Williams (436) questioned whether a defect in the lamina cribrosa may allow oligodendrocytes to gain access to the retina and produce myelin there. It is known that animals with little or no evidence of lamina cribrosa tend to have deep physiologic cups and extensive myelination of retinal nerve fibers, whereas animals with a well-developed lamina cribrosa tend to show fairly flat nerve heads and no myelination of retinal nerve fibers. In eyes with remote, isolated peripheral patches of myelinated nerve fibers, an anomaly in the formation or timing of formation of the lamina cribrosa could permit access of oligodendrocytes to the retina. These cells may then migrate through the nerve fiber layer until they find a region of lower nerve fiber layer density, where they proceed to myelinate some axons (436).

Extensive unilateral (or rarely bilateral) myelination of nerve fibers can be associated with high myopia and severe amblyopia. Unlike other forms of unilateral high myopia that characteristically respond well to occlusion therapy, the amblyopia that occurs in children with myelinated nerve fibers is notoriously refractory to this treatment (440). In such patients, myelination surrounds most or all of the circumference of the disc. Additionally, the macular region (although unmyelinated) usually appears abnormal, showing a dulled reflex or pigment dispersion (441). Hittner et al. (441) found the appearance of the macula to be the best direct correlate of response to occlusion therapy.

Myelinated nerve fibers occur in association with the Gorlin syndrome (multiple basal cell nevi) (442). This autosomal-dominant disorder can often be recognized by the finding of numerous tiny pits in the hands and feet, which produce a ''sandpaper'' irregularity. Multiple cutaneous tumors develop in the second to third decades, but they may occasionally develop in the first few years of life. When present in childhood, these lesions remain quiescent until puberty, when they increase in number and demonstrate a more rapid and invasive growth pattern (443). Additional features include jaw cysts (which are found in approximately 70% of patients and often appear in the first decade of life), and mild mental retardation (443). Rib anomalies (bifid ribs, splaying, synostoses, and partial agenesis) are found in approximately 50% of patients. Facial abnormalities include hypertelorism, prominent supraorbital ridges, frontoparietal bossing, a broad nasal root, and mild mandibular prognathism (443). Ectopic calcification, especially of the falx cerebri, is an almost constant finding (442). Medulloblastomas develop in some patients. Gorlin syndrome should be considered in children with myelinated nerve fibers and cutaneous lesions because small lesions can be treated with curettage, electrophotocoagulation, cryosurgery, and topical

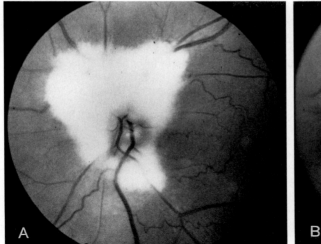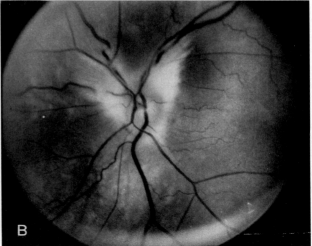

Figure 3.30. Disappearance of myelinated nerve fibers following an acute optic neuropathy. *A,* Prior to visual symptoms, patient has 20/25 visual acuity with an enlarged blind spot. Myelinated nerve fibers completely surround the disc. *B,* Seven years later, after an acute optic neuropathy, there is marked disappearance of intraocular myelin. Visual acuity is 20/300 and there are superior and inferior arcuate defects. (From Schachat AP, Miller NR. Atrophy of myelinated nerve fibers after acute optic neuropathy. Am J Ophthalmol 1981;92:854–856.)

chemotherapy to forestall the development of more aggressive and invasive lesions (443).

Myelinated nerve fibers may be familial, in which case the trait is usually inherited in an autosomal-dominant fashion (220,444). Isolated cases of myelinated nerve fibers may also occur in association with abnormal length of the optic nerve (oxycephaly) (445), defects in the lamina cribrosa (tilted disc) (446), anterior segment dysgenesis (436,441), and neurofibromatosis type 2 (447). Although myelinated nerve fibers are purported to be associated with neurofibromatosis, many authorities believe that this association is fortuitous, and we agree.

Traboulsi et al. (448) described an autosomal-dominant vitreoretinopathy associated with myelination of the nerve fiber layer. The condition is characterized by congenitally poor vision, bilateral extensive myelination of the retinal nerve fiber layer, severe degeneration of the vitreous, high myopia, a retinal dystrophy with night blindness, reduction of the electroretinographic responses, and limb deformities.

Rarely, areas of myelinated nerve fibers may be acquired after infancy and even in adulthood (1). Trauma to the eye (a blow to the eye in one patient and an optic nerve sheath fenestration in the other) seems to be a common denominator in these cases (449,450). Williams (436) suggested that sufficient damage to the lamina cribrosa may permit oligodendrocytes to enter the retina, whereupon they move to the nearest area of fairly loose nerve fibers and myelinate them. Aaby and Kushner (451) photographically documented progression of myelinated nerve fibers in children. Conversely, myelinated nerve fibers disappear as a result of tabetic optic atrophy (452), pituitary tumor (453), glaucoma (454), central retinal artery occlusion (455), branch retinal artery occlusion (456), and various optic neuropathies (Fig. 3.30) (457,458).

PSEUDOPAPILLEDEMA

Anomalous optic disc elevation (pseudopapilledema) may bear a striking resemblance to true optic disc swelling and therefore represents a primary diagnostic consideration in the patient referred for papilledema (374). In most instances, a patient is noted to have elevated optic discs or blurred disc margins during the course of a routine examination. The diagnostic uncertainty and alarm created by this finding overshadows the fact that the patient has no other signs or symptoms of increased intracranial pressure. Many patients with pseudopapilledema are referred for neuro-ophthalmologic evaluation only after being subjected to neuroimaging, lumbar puncture, and extensive laboratory studies.

Once the diagnosis of pseudopapilledema is established, pseudopapilledema associated with optic disc drusen must be distinguished from other local causes of pseudopapilledema, such as hyaloid traction on the optic disc (459), epipapillary glial tissue, myelinated nerve fibers, scleral infiltration, vitreopapillary traction (6), and high hyperopia (244,375,460). In the patient with additional systemic disorders, consideration must be given to the possibility that pseudopapilledema may be related to an underlying genetic disorder. Systemic disorders that include pseudopapilledema are Down syndrome (461), Alagille syndrome (arteriohepatic dysplasia) (462), Kenny syndrome (hypocalcemic dwarfism) (410), linear nevus sebaceous syndrome (463), and Leber's hereditary optic neuropathy. Awan (464) described an association between orbital hypotelorism and pseudopapilledema with situs inversus of the vessels.

PSEUDOPAPILLEDEMA ASSOCIATED WITH OPTIC DISC DRUSEN

The word drusen, of Germanic origin, originally meant tumor, swelling, or tumescence (4). According to Lorentzen (4), the word was used in the mining industry approximately 500 years ago to indicate a crystal-filled space in a rock. Drusen of the optic disc were first described clinically by Liebreich in 1868. Other terms for these lesions include *hyaline bodies* and *colloid bodies* of the optic disc (465–467).

Epidemiology

Lorentzen (4) reported a prevalence of optic drusen of 3.4 per 1,000 in a clinical study of 3,200 individuals. This prevalence increased by a factor of 10 in family members of patients with disc drusen. The prevalence of drusen in autopsy series varies between 0.41% (468) and 2.0% (469). Rosenberg et al. (470) examined 98 patients with disc elevation and ophthalmoscopic evidence of buried drusen. Their ages ranged from 7 to 73 years, with a mean age of 22 years. Males and females were equally affected. Visible drusen were bilateral in approximately two-thirds of cases, whereas pseudopapilledema associated with buried drusen was bilateral in 86% of cases. These findings were in accordance with previous clinical studies (4,471,472). Erkkila (473,474) found a high prevalence of clumsiness, learning disabilities, and neurologic problems in a Finnish population of children with drusen, but subsequent studies have not substantiated these findings. The early notion that pseudopapilledema associated with disc drusen tend to develop primarily in hyperopic eyes has also been dispelled; Hoyt and Pont (475) found an equal number of hyperopes and myopes in their study of 28 patients with pseudopapilledema, and Rosenberg et al. (470) found a distribution of refractive error among their pseudopapilledema patients (both with and without visible drusen) identical with that present in the general population; François (476–478), and later Lorentzen (479), determined that familial drusen are transmitted as an autosomal-dominant trait, and subsequent studies have confirmed the familial nature of this anomaly (475,480,481). The low prevalence of disc drusen in African Americans (470,475) may be attributable to racial variation in optic disc size (482).

Natural History

The evolution of disc drusen is a dynamic process that continues throughout life. It is rare to see visible drusen or significant optic disc elevation in an infant. During childhood, the affected optic disc begins to appear "full" and acquires a tan, yellow, or straw color (483,484). In a retrospective study of 40 children, Hoover et al. (484) first noted drusen at a mean age of 12.1 years and found that visual field defects are commonly detectable in the second decade of life. Gradually, buried drusen impart a scalloped appearance to the margin of the disc and produce subtle excrescences on the disc surface that tend to predominate nasally (4,204). They later enlarge and calcify, and become more visible on the disc surface (485–487). As they enlarge they sometimes deflect retinal vessels overlying the disc (486). In adulthood, the optic disc elevation diminishes, the disc gradually becomes pale, the nerve fiber layer thins, and discrete slits appear (483,488). This evolution reflects a slow attrition of optic axons over decades. Despite this progression, most patients remain asymptomatic and retain normal acuity. The finding of disc elevation without visible drusen in children of parents with florid drusen attests both to the dynamic nature of this anomaly and to its heredofamilial character.

Ophthalmoscopic Appearance of Visible Drusen

When a beam of light from a direct or scanning laser ophthalmoscope or a slit lamp is directed on a portion of the elevated disc, drusen appear as round, slightly irregular excrescences that are present within and occasionally around

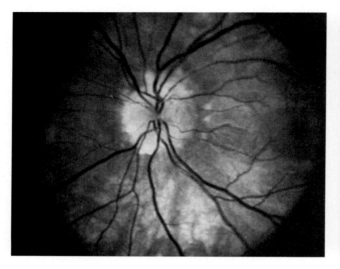 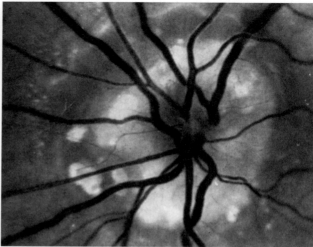

Figure 3.31. Visible disc drusen. Note multiple white nodules lining the periphery of the discs and abnormal branching of retinal vessels.

the disc (Fig. 3.31) (479,489). Surface drusen may be scattered or form conglomerates that cover part or all of the disc. Surface drusen affecting only a portion of the disc are usually concentrated nasally and are most conspicuous at the periphery of the disc. Superficial drusen reflect whitish yellow light, are globular, and vary in size from minute dots to granules 2 or 3 times the diameter of a retinal vessel. When illuminated directly drusen glow brightly at their edges, and uniformly but less intensely at their center. In indirect light, the side of a drusen that is away from the light appears as a dark crescent in contrast to its glowing central region. Deeply situated drusen lack sharp margins, but they may still be illuminated when indirect lighting is used.

Ophthalmoscopic Appearance of Buried Disc Drusen

Drusen buried within the tissue of the disc produce moderate elevation of the surface of the disc, as well as blurring of its margins with the following features (Fig. 3.32):

1. The anomalously elevated disc is not hyperemic, and there are no dilated capillaries on its surface.
2. Despite extreme elevation of the disc, the surface arteries are not obscured.
3. The physiologic cup is absent in the anomalously elevated disc.
4. Anomalously elevated discs are smaller than normal (490,491).
5. The most elevated portion of the disc is usually the central area from which the vessels emerge.
6. In a large percentage of cases, there are anomalous vascular patterns on the disc surface, including an increased number of otherwise normal vessels, abnormal arterial

and venous branchings, increased tortuosity, vascular loops, and cilioretinal arteries (4,474,476,477,492,493).
7. Elevation is confined to the optic disc and does not extend to the peripapillary nerve fiber layer, which may retain its normal linear pattern of light reflexes (494) or show abnormalities indicative of nerve fiber atrophy (349,495).
8. The anomalously elevated disc usually has an irregular border with pigment epithelial defects being present, giving the border a ''moth-eaten'' appearance.

Distinguishing Pseudopapilledema Associated with Buried Drusen from Papilledema

The distinction between pseudopapilledema associated with buried drusen and papilledema (or other forms of optic disc swelling) can be difficult (Fig. 3.33), but several clinical signs are particularly helpful (Table 3.4). In papilledema, the disc swelling extends into the peripapillary retina and obscures the peripapillary retinal vasculature. In pseudopapilledema, there is a discrete, sometimes grayish or straw-colored elevation of the disc without obscuration of vessels or opacification of peripapillary retina. Hoyt and Knight (494) emphasized the graying or muddying of the peripapillary nerve fiber layer that occurs with swelling of the optic disc from papilledema or other causes. In pseudopapilledema associated with buried drusen, light reflexes of the peripapillary nerve fiber layer appear sharp, and the elevated disc is often haloed by a crescentic peripapillary ring of light that reflects from the concave internal limiting membrane surrounding the elevation (Fig. 3.32). This crescentic light reflex is absent in papilledema, because of diffraction of light from distended peripapillary axons (494,496–498). Individ-

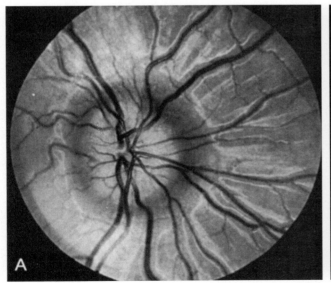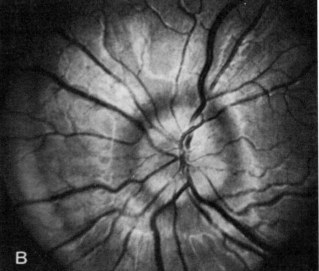

Figure 3.32. Buried disc drusen. Both optic discs have a similar appearance, with absence of the central cup, and an increased number of retinal vessels with an anomalous branching pattern. The disc elevation does not obscure the overlying vessels. Although no discrete drusen are seen, there is a subtle nodularity of the disc margin.

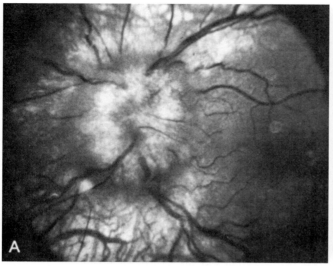
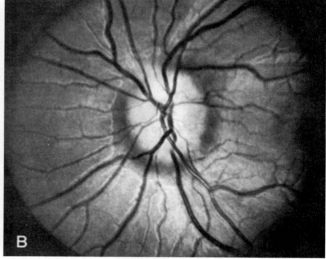

Figure 3.33. Comparison of papilledema and pseudopapilledema with buried drusen. *A,* Papilledema. The disc is elevated and hyperemic. There is distortion of the normal linear light reflexes from the peripapillary nerve fiber layer and obscuration of large vessels as they cross the disc surface. *B,* Pseudopapilledema. The disc is elevated but shows no hyperemia, disruption of the nerve fiber layer reflexes, or obscuration of vessels.

ual flame-shaped, subretinal, or sub-RPE hemorrhages are occasionally seen in the peripapillery region in eyes with optic disc drusen, but exudates, cotton wool spots, hyperemia of the disc, and venous congestion are conspicuously absent (4,493,497).

Ancillary Studies

The differentiation between papilledema and pseudopapilledema caused by buried drusen is frequently aided by ancil-

lary studies. It is common for children who carry the diagnosis of papilledema to arrive for consultation with their "negative" CT scan in hand, only to observe calcification of the optic discs upon review of the scan. Both CT scanning and ultrasonography readily demonstrate such calcification within the elevated optic disc (Figs. 3.34 and 3.35). Opinions

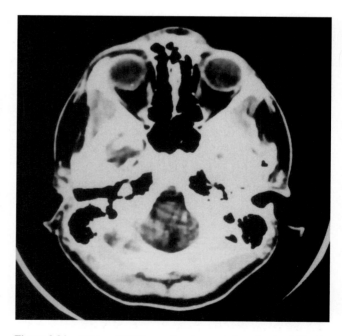

Figure 3.34. "Normal" CT scan showing posterior scleral calcification corresponding to optic disc drusen. (From Brodsky MC, Baker RS, Hamed LM. Pediatric Neuroophthalmology. New York, Springer-Verlag, 1996. Photograph courtesy of Stephan C. Pollock, MD.)

Table 3.4
Ophthalmoscopic Features Useful in Differentiating Optic Disc Edema from Pseudopapilledema Associated with Buried Drusen

Optic Disc Edema	Pseudopapilledema with Buried Drusen
Disc vasculature obscured at disc margins	Disc vasculature remains visible at disc margins
Elevation extends into peripapillary retina	Elevation confined to optic disc
Graying and muddying of peripapillary nerve fiber layer	Sharp peripapillary nerve fiber
Venous congestion	No venous congestion
± exudates	No exudates
Loss of optic cup only in moderate to severe disc edema	Small cupless disc
Normal configuration of disc vasculature despite venous congestion	Increased major retinal vessels with early branching
No circumpapillary light reflex	Crescentic circumpapillary light reflex
Absence of spontaneous venous pulsations	Spontaneous venous pulsations may be present or absent

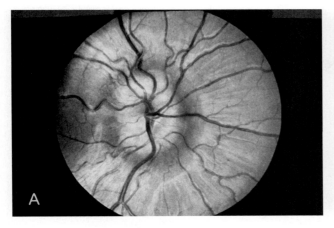
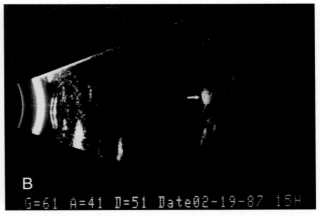

Figure 3.35. Ultrasonography in a patient with deep (buried) optic disc drusen. *A*, Appearance of the right optic disc. *B*, B-scan ultrasonography, high gain, shows that the area of disc elevation is clearly seen as a focal area of brightness that persists when reflections from the remainder of the posterior segment of the eye are no longer visible (*arrow*). This finding is consistent with the appearance of calcified drusen. (Courtesy of Cathy DiBernardo, RN, RMDS.)

differ as to which imaging modality is preferable (25,499–505). Kurz-Levin and Landau (506) found B-scan ultrasonography to be superior to either CT scanning or photography to look for autofluorescence in the detection of disc drusen.

Special photographic techniques may also be useful in identifying superficial or buried optic disc drusen. Monochromatic (red-free) photography may highlight the glistening drusen against the intact or atrophic nerve fiber layer. Photographs taken with the filters normally used for fluorescein photography in place, but without injection of fluorescein show that superficial disc drusen often demonstrate the phenomenon of autofluorescence (Fig. 3.36) (349,507,508). Fluorescein angiography can also facilitate the differentiation between true papilledema and pseudopapilledema. After intravenous fluorescein injection, drusen exhibit a true nodular hyperfluorescence corresponding to the location of the visible drusen (467,508). The late phases may be characterized by minimal blurring of the drusen that either fade or maintain fluorescence (i.e., stain) (467,508). Unlike in papilledema, however, there is no visible leakage along the major vessels (476,480,509). Fluorescein angiography may also disclose venous anomalies (venous stasis, venous convolutions, and retinociliary venous communications) and staining of the peripapillary vein walls in eyes with optic disc drusen (508,510). Electrophysiologic studies may show abnormalities but add little to the diagnostic evaluation of pseudopapilledema (495,511–513).

Patients with pseudopapilledema are not immune to the neurologic and ophthalmologic disorders of the general population (125,514). We have observed concomitant papilledema, anterior optic neuritis, and anterior ischemic optic neuropathy in patients with anomalously elevated discs. In all cases, however, the history was typical of either increased intracranial pressure or an optic neuropathy, and obvious disc swelling was present. Of the 142 patients with pseudopapilledema studied by Rosenberg et al. (470), 2 patients had concomitant papillitis, 2 patients had intracranial neoplasms, and 1 patient had pseudotumor cerebri. Not surprisingly, patients with optic disc drusen and progressive visual loss can also have pituitary tumors (515–519), meningiomas (349,520–523), craniopharyngiomas (524), ophthalmic artery aneurysms (525), cerebral abscesses (526), and other intracranial masses (262,519,527,528), but no significant relationship between drusen and any of these lesions has ever been established.

There is absolutely no evidence that patients with optic disc drusen are at increased risk to develop an intracranial mass later in life. Recognition of papilledema in eyes with disc drusen is confounded by the fact that globular intrapapillary masses that are indistinguishable from hyaline bodies can develop in patients with chronic papilledema (522). Unlike disc drusen, however, these lesions disappear following regression of papilledema (522,529).

Complications Associated With Pseudopapilledema and Disc Drusen

Visual Field Defects

Peripheral visual field defects develop in 71–75% of eyes with disc drusen (460,471,476,477,495,530). In most cases, the asymptomatic nature of the defects reflects the insidious attrition of optic nerve fibers over decades. Nevertheless, a minority of patients experience episodes of sudden, step-like visual field loss (77,460,476,477). Mustonen (477) found visual field defects in 38.9% of eyes with pseudopapilledema and 73.4% of eyes with visible drusen. Savino et al. (460) found visual field defects in 21% of eyes with pseudopapilledema without visible drusen, and 71% of eyes with visible drusen. These visual field defects fall into three general categories: (*a*) nerve fiber bundle defects; (*b*) enlargement of the blind spot; and (*c*) concentric visual field constriction. Several studies using kinetic perimetry described inferonasal steps as the most common nerve fiber bundle defect, but both arcuate defects and sector defects may also occur (4,460,465, 479,495,530,531). Lansche and Rucker (530) and François

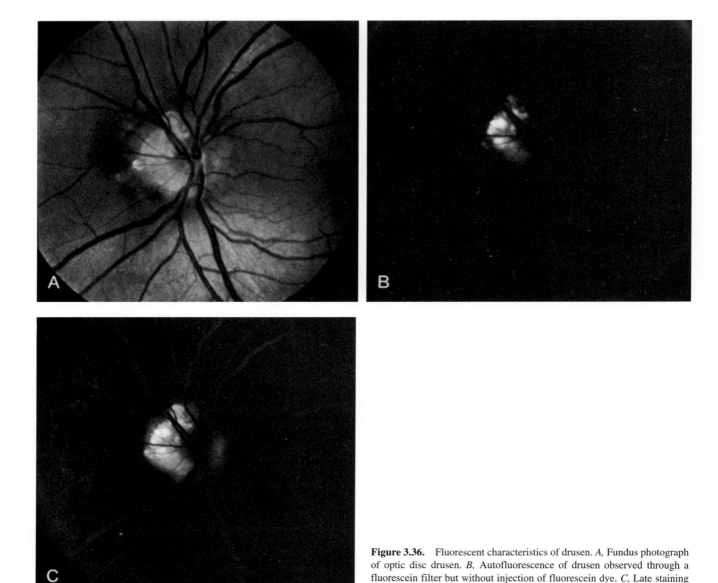

Figure 3.36. Fluorescent characteristics of drusen. *A,* Fundus photograph of optic disc drusen. *B,* Autofluorescence of drusen observed through a fluorescein filter but without injection of fluorescein dye. *C,* Late staining of drusen after fluorescein angiogram.

and Verriest (471) emphasized the slowly progressive nature of many of the defects. Although concentric constriction of the visual field is usually a chronic process, some patients experience sudden severe visual field constriction with and without preservation of central vision (532–534). These patients often have no disc swelling or retinal edema to suggest an ischemic process. A relative afferent pupillary defect may result from unilateral or asymmetric visual field loss in the absence of central acuity loss (477,535).

The pathogenesis of visual field loss in patients with disc drusen could involve one or more of the following mechanisms:

1. Impaired axonal transport in an eye with a small scleral canal leading to gradual attrition of optic nerve fibers; (483,536);

2. Direct compression of prelaminar nerve fibers by drusen; and/or;

3. Ischemia within the optic nerve head (77).

At the heart of the controversy is whether drusen produce damage to nerve fibers through direct axonal or vascular compression, or whether they are merely an epiphenomenon of a chronic low-grade axonal stasis that produces a slowly progressive diminution in optic axons (375). Several studies have been unable to correlate the location of visible disc drusen with the location of field defects (4,537). Stevens and Newman (495) found no correlation between the degree of nerve fiber layer damage and the degree of visual field abnormality in eyes with disc drusen. These results do not rule out the possibility that axonal compression could result from drusen that lie just above the lamina cribrosa rather than those that are superficial and easily seen.

Central Visual Loss

Idiopathic central visual loss is a rare but well-documented complication of disc drusen (77,496,538–540) that should be considered only when no other causes can be identified (521). In such cases, central visual loss usually follows a series of episodic, step-like events that progressively diminish the peripheral visual field. Beck et al. (77) described four patients with reduced central acuity resulting from optic disc drusen. The authors emphasized that this rare phenomenon remains a diagnosis of exclusion that should be considered when visual loss is acute and nonprogressive, stepwise in a nerve fiber bundle distribution, or not produced until visual field constriction is severe.

Prepapillary or Peripapillary Hemorrhages

Prepapillary or peripapillary hemorrhages may develop in eyes with disc drusen (497,519,531,538,541–548). Sanders et al. (538) divided hemorrhages associated with optic drusen into three groups:

1. Small superficial hemorrhages on the optic disc;
2. Large hemorrhages on the disc, extending into the vitreous; and
3. Deep peripapillary hemorrhages extending from the optic disc under the peripapillary retina (Fig. 3.37).

Large superficial hemorrhages may rarely extend into the vitreous. In our experience, subretinal and subpigment epithelial hemorrhages, although uncommon, are much more

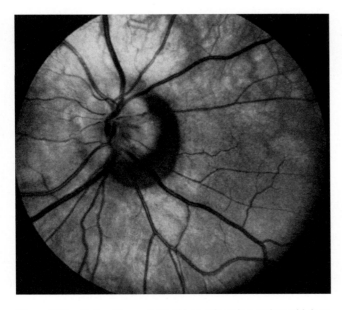

Figure 3.37. Peripapillary subretinal hemorrhage in a patient with intrapapillary drusen. Note the difference between this type of hemorrhage and the superficial nerve fiber layer hemorrhages seen with optic disc swelling.

frequent in patients with optic disc drusen than are superficial (flame-shaped), subhyaloid, or vitreous hemorrhages. Splinter hemorrhages associated with optic disc drusen tend to be single and prepapillary in location, in contrast to the multiple nerve fiber layer hemorrhages that characterize papilledema (497). Deep peripapillary hemorrhages may be subretinal or subpigment epithelial and are typically circumferentially oriented around the disc (470,474,538,548).

Even in severe cases, most patients with optic disc drusen and hemorrhages recover normal or near-normal vision. Whether or not these hemorrhages can be caused by compression of thin-walled veins by conglomerates of drusen or by erosion of the vessel wall by the sharp edge of the drusen (510) remains unsettled. Wise et al. (549) postulated that enlarging disc drusen could result in circulatory compromise and local hypoxia, which might stimulate the growth of new vessels between the RPE and Bruch's membrane. Peripapillary pigmentary disruption may remain following resolution of subretinal hemorrhage. Subretinal hemorrhage may also occur in severe papilledema, but its occurrence in mild papilledema is rare and should suggest the possibility of disc drusen (497). A subgroup of patients can develop a serous maculopathy without hemorrhage, which can tent the temporal peripapillary retina into striate folds (548).

Ischemic Optic Neuropathy

Ischemic optic neuropathy may occur as a single episode or as successive episodes of discrete visual loss over years (374,550,551). Karel et al. (510) reported ischemic optic neuropathy associated with the abrupt onset of arcuate field defects and segmental disc pallor in three young patients with optic disc drusen. Michaelson et al. (552) described bilateral visual loss that was precipitated by systemic hypotension from peritoneal dialysis in a patient with disc drusen. Newman and Dorrell (553) described anterior ischemic optic neuropathy in a 13-year-old boy with disc drusen.

Retinal Vascular Occlusions

Retinal vascular occlusions occur in patients with optic disc drusen (554–559). Drusen-associated retinal arterial and venous occlusions tend to occur in young adults (5) but may rarely be seen in children (560). Retinal vascular occlusions that occur in eyes with disc drusen could result from:

1. Vascular crowding secondary to the small scleral canal size in eyes with drusen;
2. Anomalous optic disc vasculature that may make it more susceptible to the effects of disrupted hemodynamics; or
3. Mechanical displacement of the prelaminar vasculature by hard, unyielding drusen (5,561).

Transient Visual Loss

Transient visual loss occurred in 8.6% of the patients with disc drusen in Lorentzen's study (5). Sadun et al. (562) proposed that such visual loss occurs because both papilledema and anomalous elevation of the optic discs produce increased interstitial pressure and decreased perfusion pressure in the intraocular portion of the optic nerve. Thus, minor fluctuations in arterial, venous, or cerebrospinal fluid pressure result in brief but critical decrements in perfusion, leading to transient obscurations of vision. Katz and Hoyt (6) attributed mild visual disturbances to vitreopapillary traction in a group of young myopic Asians whose optic discs were mildly dysplastic and slightly elevated. These patients manifested intrapapillary and subretinal peripapillary hemorrhages, with incomplete posterior vitreous detachment. Rarely, transient visual loss may be a harbinger of retinal vascular occlusion in patients with disc drusen (5).

Peripapillary Subretinal Neovascularization

Peripapillary subretinal neovascularization is a rare but well-documented complication in eyes with disc drusen. Henkind et al. (563) and Wise et al. (549) emphasized that temporary or permanent visual loss can occur in patients with optic disc drusen who develop subpigment epithelial hemorrhages from subretinal neovascularization (Fig. 3.38). In severe cases, this complication may simulate a juxtapapillary mass lesion or a neuroretinitis (375,547,564). Harris et al. (547) found subretinal neovascularization in seven eyes of 57 patients with optic disc drusen. These investigators emphasized that hemorrhages occurring in the absence of choroidal vascularization produced no symptoms and resolved without sequelae, whereas hemorrhages arising from choroidal neovascularization commonly produced visual symptoms. Six of the seven eyes with neovascularization retained visual acuities of 20/40 or better. Based upon these findings, Harris et al. (547) recommended observation rather than laser photocoagulation for peripapillary choroidal neovascularization associated with disc drusen. Saudax et al. (565) reported an 8-year-old girl with a peripapillary subretinal membrane that extended from the inferotemporal disc to the macula and produced a serous hemorrhagic maculopathy. In one case, surgical excision of a peripapillary subretinal neovascular membrane produced marked improvement in vision (566).

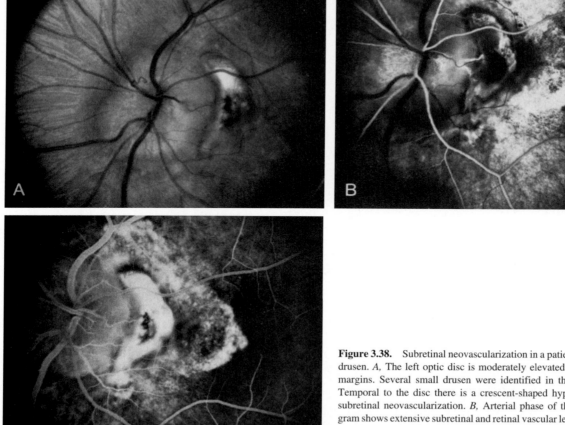

Figure 3.38.   Subretinal neovascularization in a patient with intrapapillary drusen. *A,* The left optic disc is moderately elevated and has blurred disc margins. Several small drusen were identified in the center of the disc. Temporal to the disc there is a crescent-shaped hyperpigmented area of subretinal neovascularization. *B,* Arterial phase of the fluorescein angiogram shows extensive subretinal and retinal vascular leakage from abnormal vessels. Note that there is no leakage from the disc vessels. *C,* In the arteriovenous phase of the fluorescein angiogram, there is diffuse staining of the optic disc and there is both staining of and leakage of dye from the area of subretinal neovascularization.

Peripapillary Central Serous Choroidopathy

Peripapillary central serous choroidopathy was documented in an eye with disc drusen (567). Fluorescein angiography showed a bright hyperfluorescent spot superonasal to the disc. The detachment resolved following focal laser photocoagulation of the RPE defect.

Histology of Optic Disc Drusen

Drusen of the optic disc were first described histologically by Müller (568). Several investigators subsequently performed histopathologic examinations on optic disc drusen and found that they consist of homogenous, globular concretions, often collected in larger, multilobulated agglomerations (Fig. 3.39) (467–469,561,569–571). Individual druse usually exhibit a concentrically laminated structure, that is not encapsulated and contains no cells or cellular debris (4). Drusen are often most concentrated within the nasal portion of the disc. The common finding of prelaminar spongiotic edema may contribute to the optic disc elevation seen clinically (561). Optic disc axons are atrophic adjacent to large accumulations of drusen, whereas axons that are not adjacent to the drusen are normal (4,467–469). Drusen take up calcium salts and must be decalcified before being cut into sections for histopathologic study. According to most investigators, drusen are composed predominantly of a mucoprotein matrix with significant quantities of acid mucopolysaccharides, small quantities of ribonucleic acid and, occasionally, iron. In addition, Friedman et al. (467,469) found that drusen stain positively for amino acids and calcium but negatively for amyloid. Boyce et al. (468) found Bodian's stain for the presence of nerve fibers to be positive in the two cases that they studied in this fashion; however, specific stains, including the Nauta-Gygax stain for degenerating axon terminals and Guillery's stain for degenerating nerve fibers were negative in the same cases. Drusen are insoluble in most of the common solvents, including absolute ethanol, ether, chloroform, xylene, acetic acid, hydrochloric acid, nitric acid, sulfuric acid, potassium hydroxide, and sodium hydroxide.

Pathogenesis of Optic Disc Drusen

The primary pathology of optic disc drusen may be an inherited dysplasia of the optic canal, or the optic disc and its vasculature, which predisposes to the formation of optic disc drusen (572). Mullie and Sanders (490) suggested that the primary developmental expression of the genetic trait for drusen may be a smaller-than-normal scleral canal (482). After formation of the optic stalk is complete, mesenchymal elements from the sclera invade the glial framework of the primitive lamina, reinforcing it with collagen (490). An abnormal encroachment of sclera, Bruch's membrane, or both, upon the developing optic stalk would narrow the exit space of optic axons from the eye (490,561). The small optic disc size and absence of a central cup in affected eyes are consistent with the mechanism of axonal crowding. The clinical and histopathologic observation that drusen are often first detected at the margins of the optic disc suggests that the rigid edge of the scleral canal may be an aggravating factor in producing a relative mechanical interruption of axonal transport (490). The lower prevalence of optic disc drusen in African Americans, who have a larger disc area with less potential for axonal crowding, is also consistent with the notion that axonal crowding is a fundamental anatomic substrate for disc drusen (482).

In 1962, Seitz and Kersting first proposed that drusen may be the product of long-term pathologic alterations in the retinal nerve fibers. In 1968, Seitz again proposed this idea and concluded from a series of histochemical studies that drusen originate from axoplasmic derivatives of disintegrating nerve fibers. Seitz (573) also suggested that drusen form by a slow degenerative process rather than by a rapid one. Sacks et al. (574) advanced an alternative hypothesis that the tendency to develop optic nerve drusen results, at least in part, from a congenitally abnormal disc vasculature that allows transudation of plasma proteins which in turn

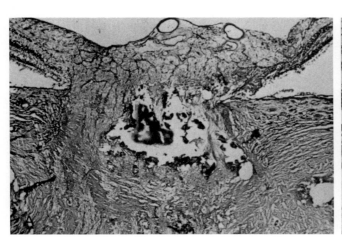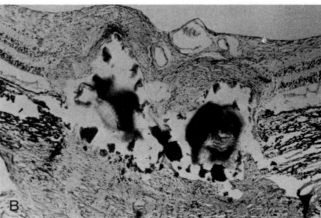

Figure 3.39. Histopathology of drusen. Intrapapillary drusen are seen as irregular dark masses within the substance of the prelaminar optic nerve head. Note the diffuse elevation of the optic disc.

serve as a nidus for the deposition of extracellular materials. The axonal degeneration theory of Seitz and Kersting (571) is supported by the findings of Spencer (483,575) and Tso (536). Spencer (483,575) has proposed that alteration in axonal transport might be the basic pathogenetic mechanism for formation of drusen in the optic nerve. Tso (536) studied 18 cases of optic disc drusen ultrastructurally and proposed that abnormal axonal metabolism leads to intracellular mitochondrial calcification. Some axons then rupture; mitochondria are extruded into the extracellular space; and calcium continues to be deposited in the extracellular mitochondria. Small calcified microbodies are then produced, and calcium continues to deposit on the surface of these nidi to form drusen.

Systematic Associations With Optic Disc Drusen

Retinitis Pigmentosa

Retinitis pigmentosa—globular excrescences of the optic nerve head—are occasionally seen in patients with this condition (576–579). Spencer (483) emphasized that although the drusen associated with retinitis pigmentosa may arise within the optic disc, they more often lie just off the disc margin in the superficial retina (Fig. 3.40). In such cases, the disc is not elevated or anomalous but appears waxy yellow. These drusen increase in size, leading some authors to conjecture that they may be hamartomas rather than drusen (367,580);

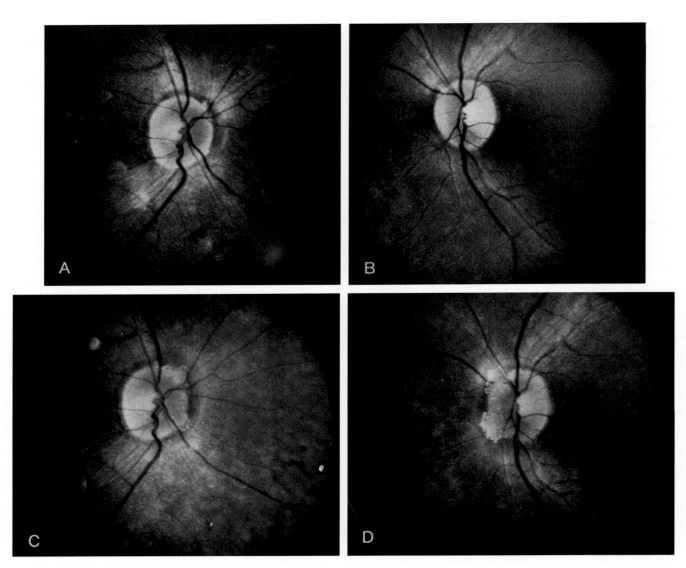

Figure 3.40. Development of drusen in a patient with retinitis pigmentosa. *A,* The right optic disc is fairly normal. Small drusen bodies can be appreciated at 2 and 5 o'clock at the disc margin. *B,* The left optic disc showed drusen only at 10 o'clock at the disc margin when the patient was first examined. *C and D,* Four years later, the entire nasal margin of the disc is surrounded by drusen and the left disc shows marked drusen formation from 7 to 11 o'clock.

however, histopathologic examination indicates that the globular excrescences of the optic nerve in retinitis pigmentosa are drusen and not astrocytic hamartomas (581). Patients with syndromes that include pigmentary retinopathy may also have optic disc drusen. Shiono et al. (582) described optic disc ''mulberry'' tumors that were presumed to be drusen in two children with Usher syndrome, and Edwards et al. (583) reported photographically apparent optic disc and peripapillary drusen in 24 of 151 patients (16%) with Usher syndrome. Sebag et al. (584) documented histopathologically giant intrapapillary drusen in a patient with Alström syndrome. Young and Small (585) noted disc drusen in a patient with pigmented paravenous retinochoroidal atrophy.

Children with retinitis pigmentosa and buried drusen may present with optic disc elevation and be thought to have neurologic disease (586). The combination of vitreous cells with optic disc elevation may mimic uveitis in children with early retinitis pigmentosa. In this setting, the finding of attenuated retinal arterioles provides an important (and easily overlooked) clue to the diagnosis, which can be established by electroretinography (586).

Angioid Streaks

Initial observations suggested that the association of disc drusen with angioid streaks was unique to patients with pseudoxanthoma elasticum (587–590). Subsequent studies indicate a primary association between disc drusen and angioid streaks irrespective of systemic disease (504,591,592). Mansour (592) reviewed ophthalmoscopic photographs from 110 patients with angioid streaks and found disc drusen in five cases (4.5% versus the reported incidence by Lorentzen of 0.34%), two of whom had pseudoxanthoma elasticum. Mansour (592) noted that Bruch's membrane becomes mineralized with elastin in eyes with angioid streaks and suggested that elastin mineralization and adherence of abnormal glycosaminoglycans to elastic fibers (as seen in the dermis in patients with pseudoxanthoma elasticum) may also affect the lamina cribrosa. Crowding of the laminar portion of the optic nerve and secondary alteration in axonal transport would result. Coleman et al. (590) described a patient in whom disc drusen were the earliest clinical manifestation of pseudoxanthoma elasticum. Using ultrasonography, Pierro et al. (504) found disc drusen in 21% of patients with pseudoxanthoma elasticum and 25% of patients with angioid streaks with no pseudoxanthoma elasticum.

Megalencephaly

In 1960, Riley and Smith (593) described a syndrome of macrocephaly, multiple hemangiomata, and pseudopapilledema. Dvir et al. (594) described pseudopapilledema in a child with macrocephaly, lipoangiomatosis, and pigmentation. This child may have had a variant of the Riley-Smith syndrome. Paes-Alves et al. (595) described pseudopapilledema in three Brazilian patients with mixed deafness and congenital anomalies of the face, ears, hands, and feet, who appeared to show an autosomal recessive inheritance pattern. Hoover et al. (484) found megalencephaly in 3 of 40 children with pseudopapilledema and cautioned that such children can be misdiagnosed as having hydrocephalus.

Migraine Headaches

Migraine headaches are said to occur with increased frequency in patients with disc drusen (202,596). Newman et al. (5) pointed out that the concurrence of migraine and optic disc drusen probably reflects the frequent and often expedited referral of patients with headache and elevated discs for specialty evaluation.

ANOMALOUS DISC ELEVATION WITHOUT EITHER VISIBLE OR BURIED DRUSEN

Not all anomalously elevated optic discs develop drusen. As noted above, the morning glory syndrome is associated with disc elevation; the superotemporal portion of a tilted optic disc is usually elevated; and dysplastic discs may show some degree of elevation. In addition, hypoplastic discs may have some elevation that seems out of proportion to the size of the disc. Such discs are often described as ''crowded'' to distinguish them from discs that are truly swollen. In addition, vitreopapillary traction can produce optic disc elevation (6,597). B-scan ultrasonography and optical coherence tomography allow confirmation of vitreopapillary traction (597).

REFERENCES

1. Kushner BJ. Functional amblyopia associated with abnormalities of the optic nerve. Arch Ophthalmol 1985;102:683–685.
2. Yang LLH, Lambert SR. Reappraisal of occlusion therapy for severe structural abnormalities of the optic disc and macula. J Pediatr Ophthalmol Strabismus 1995;32:37–41.
3. Graether JM. Transient amaurosis in one eye with simultaneous dilatation of retinal veins. Arch Ophthalmol 1963;70:342–345.
4. Lorentzen SE. Drusen of the optic disc. Dan Med Bull 1967;14:293–298.
5. Newman ND, Lessell S, Brandt EM. Bilateral central retinal artery occlusions, disc drusen, and migraine. Am J Ophthalmol 1989;107:236–240.
6. Katz B, Hoyt WF. Intrapapillary and peripapillary hemorrhage in young patients with uncomplicated posterior vitreous detachment: Signs of vitreopapillary traction. Ophthalmology 1995;102:349–354.
7. Blanco R, Salvador F, Galan A, et al. Optic nerve aplasia: Report of three cases. J Pediatr Ophthalmol Strabismus 1992;29:228–231.
8. Lambert SR, Hoyt CS, Narahara MH. Optic nerve hypoplasia. Surv Ophthalmol 1987;32:1–9.
9. Brodsky MC. Septo-optic dysplasia: A reappraisal. Semin Ophthalmol 1991;6: 227–232.
10. Ridley H. Aplasia of the optic nerves. Br J Ophthalmol 1938;22:669–671.
11. Scheie HG, Adler FH. Aplasia of the optic nerve. Arch Ophthalmol 1941;26: 61–70.
12. Whinery RD, Blodi FC. Hypoplasia of the optic nerve: A clinical and histopathological correlation. Trans Am Acad Ophthalmol Otolaryngol 1963;67:733–738.
13. Edwards WC, Layden WE. Optic nerve hypoplasia. Am J Ophthalmol 1970;70: 950–959.
14. Manor RS, Korczyn AD. Retinal red-free light photographs in two congenital conditions: A case of optic hypoplasia and a case of congenital hemianopia. Ophthalmologica 1976;173:119–127.
15. Hoyt CS, Billson FA. Maternal anticonvulsants and optic nerve hypoplasia. Br J Ophthalmol 1978;62:3–6.
16. Hellström A, Wiklund L-M, Svensson E, et al. Optic nerve hypoplasia with isolated tortuosity of the retinal veins. Arch Ophthalmol 1999;117:880–884.
17. Mosier MA, Lieberman MF, Green WR, et al. Hypoplasia of the optic nerve. Arch Ophthalmol 1978;96:1437–1442.
18. Hotchkiss ML, Green WR. Optic nerve aplasia and hypoplasia. J Pediatr Ophthalmol Strabismus 1979;16:225–240.
19. Schwarz O. Ein fall von mangelhafter bildung (hypoplasie) beider sehnerven. Albrecht von Graefes Arch Ophthalmol 1915;90:326–328.
20. Cords R. Einseitige kleinheit der papille. Klin Monatsbl Augenheilkd 1923;71: 414–418.

21. Missiroli G. Una nuova sindrome congenita a carattere famigliare: Ipoplasia del nervo ottico ed emianopsia binasale. Boll Ocul 1947;26:683–698.
22. Gardner HB, Irvine AR. Optic nerve hypoplasia with good visual acuity. Arch Ophthalmol 1972;88:255–258.
23. Petersen RA, Walton DS. Optic nerve hypoplasia with good visual acuity and visual field defects: A study of children of diabetic mothers. Arch Ophthalmol 1977;95:254–258.
24. Bjork A, Laurell C-G, Laurell U. Bilateral optic nerve hypoplasia with normal visual acuity. Am J Ophthalmol 1978;86:524–529.
25. Frisén L, Holmegaard L. Spectrum of optic nerve hypoplasia. Br J Ophthalmol 1978;62:7–15.
26. Zeki SM. Optic nerve hypoplasia and astigmatism: a new association. Br J Ophthalmol 1990;74:297–299.
27. Lempert P. Optic nerve hypoplasia and small eyes in presumed amblyopia. J AAPOS 2000;4:258–266.
28. Archer SM. Amblyopia? J AAPOS 2000;4:257.
29. Lempert P. Axial length-disc area ratio in esotropic amblyopia. Arch Ophthalmol 2003;121:821–824.
30. Taylor D. Congenital tumors of the anterior visual pathways. Br J Ophthalmol 1982;66:455–463.
31. Spandau UHM, Jonas JB, Gass A. Progressive visual loss in optic nerve hypoplasia and bilateral microdiscs. Arch Neurol 2002;59:1829–1830.
32. Borchert M, McColloch D, Rother C, Stout AU. Clinical assessment, optic disk measurements, and visual-evoked potential in optic nerve hypoplasia. Am J Ophthalmol 1995;120:605–612.
33. Jonas JB, Koniszewski G, Naumann GO. "Morning Glory Syndrome" and "Handmann's Anomaly in Congenital Macropapilla. Extreme variants of confluent optic pits." Klin Monatsbl Augenheilkd 1989;195:371–374.
34. Romano PE. Simple photogrammetric diagnosis of optic nerve hypoplasia. Arch Ophthalmol 1989;107:824–826.
35. Zeki SM, Dudgeon J, Dutton GN. Reappraisal of the ratio of disc to macula/disc diameter in optic nerve hypoplasia. Br J Ophthalmol 1991;75:538–541.
36. Brodsky MC. Congenital optic disk anomalies. Surv Ophthalmol 1994;39:89–112.
37. Ragge N, Hoyt WF, Lambert SR. Big discs with optic nerve hypoplasia. J Clin Neuroophthalmol 1991;11:137.
38. Sprague JB, Wilson WB. Electrophysiologic findings in bilateral optic nerve hypoplasia. Arch Ophthalmol 1981;99:1028–1029.
39. Janáky M, Deák A, Pelle Z, et al. Electrophysiologic alterations in patients with optic nerve hypoplasia. Doc Ophthalmol 1994;86:247–257.
40. Cibis GW, Fitzgerald KM. Optic nerve hypoplasia in association with brain anomalies and an abnormal electroretinogram. Docum Ophthalmol 1994;86:11–22.
41. de Morsier G. Etudes sur les dysraphies crânio-encéphaliques. III. Agénésis du septum lucidum avec malformation du tractus optique. La dysplasie septo-optique. Schweiz Arch Neurol Psychiatr 1956;77:267–292.
42. Hoyt WF, Kaplan SL, Grumback MM, et al. Septo-optic dysplasia and pituitary dwarfism. Lancet 1970;2:893–894.
43. Ellenberger C Jr, Runyan TE. Holoprosencephaly with hypoplasia of the optic nerves, dwarfism, and agenesis of the septum pellucidum. Am J Ophthalmol 1970;70:960–967.
44. Billson F, Hopkins IJ. Optic hypoplasia and hypopituitarism. Lancet 1972;1:905.
45. Brook CGD, Sanders MD, Hoare RD. Septo-optic dysplasia. Br Med J 1972;3:811–813.
46. Harris RJ, Haas L. Septo-optic dysplasia with growth hormone deficiency (De Morsier syndrome). Arch Dis Child 1972;47:973–976.
47. Davis GV, Shock JP. Septo-optic dysplasia associated with see-saw nystagmus. Arch Ophthalmol 1975;93:137–139.
48. Patel H, Wjtze WJ, Crichton JU, McCormick A, Robinson G, Dolman C. Optic nerve hypoplasia with hypopituitarism: Septo-optic dysplasia with hypopituitarism. Am J Dis Child 1975;129:175–180.
49. Huseman CA, Kelch RP, Hopwood NJ, et al. Secual precocity in association with septo-optic dysplasia and hypothalamic hypopituitarism. J Pediatr 1978;92:748–753.
50. Lovrencic MK, Oberiter V, Banovac ZR, Schmutzer L, Petek M. Pituitary function in a patient with septo-optic dysplasia and pituitary dwarfism (Kaplan-Grumbach-Hoyt syndrome). Eur J Pediatr 1978;129:47–53.
51. Rush JA, Bajandas FJ. Septo-optic dysplasia (de Morsier syndrome). Am J Ophthalmol 1978;86:202–205.
52. Wilson PW, Easley RB, Bolander FF, et al. Evidence for a hypothalamic defect in septo-optic dysplasia. Arch Intern Med 1978;138:1276–1277.
53. Kingham JD, Fox MJ. Bilateral optic nerve hypoplasia with unilateral retinal vessel abnormality. Ann Ophthalmol 1980;12:377–380.
54. Krause-Brucker W, Gardner DW. Optic nerve hypoplasia associated with absent septum pellucidum and hypopituitarism. Am J Ophthalmol 1980;89:113–120.
55. Skarf B, Hoyt CS. Optic nerve hypoplasia in children. Arch Ophthalmol 1984;102:255–258.
56. Morishima A, Aranoff GS. Syndrome of septo-optic dysplasia: The clinical spectrum. Brain Dev 1986;8:233–239.
57. Sorkin JA, Davis PC, Meacham LR, et al. Optic nerve hypoplasia: Absence of posterior pituitary signal on magnetic resonance imaging correlates with diabetes insipidus. Am J Ophthalmol 1996;122:717–723.
58. Benoit Gonin J-J, David M, Feit J-P, et al. La dysplasie septo-optique avec deficit en hormone antidiuretique et insufficisance surrenale centrale. Nouv Presse Med 1978;7:3327–3331.
59. Stewart C, Mastro-Magana M, Sherman J, et al. Septo-optic dysplasia and median cleft face syndrome in a patient with isolated growth hormone deficiency and hyperprolactinemia. Am J Dis Child 1983;137:484–487.
60. Arslanian SA, Rothfus WE, Foley TP, Becker DJ. Hormonal, metabolic, and neuroradiologic abnormalities associated with septo-optic dysplasia. Acta Endocrin 1984;139:249–254.
61. Izenberg N, Rosenblum M, Parks JS. The endocrine spectrum of septo-optic dysplasia. Clin Pediatr 1984;23:632–636.
62. Margalith D, Tze WJ, Jan JE. Congenital optic nerve hypoplasia with hypothalamic-pituitary dysplasia. AJDC 1985;139:361–366.
63. Hoyt CS, Billson FA. Optic nerve hypoplasia: Changing perspectives. Aust New Zealand J Ophthalmol 1986;14:325–331.
64. Brodsky MC, Glasier CM. Optic nerve hypoplasia: Clinical significance of associated central nervous system abnormalities on magnetic resonance imaging. Arch Ophthalmol 1993;11:66–74.
65. Costello JM, Gluckman JM. Neonatal hypopituitarism: A neurological perspective. Dev Med Child Neurol 1988;30:190–199.
66. Ultmann MC, Siegel SF, Hirsch WL, et al. Pituitary stalk and ectopic hyperintense T-1 signal on magnetic resonance imaging: Implications for anterior pituitary dysfunction. AJDC 1993;147:647–652.
67. Fahnehjelm KT, Fischler B, Jacobson L, Nemeth A. Optic nerve hypoplasia in cholestatic infants: a multiple case study. Acta Ophthalmological Scand 2003;81:130–137.
68. Costin G, Murphree AL. Hypothalamic pituitary dysfunction in children with optic nerve hypoplasia. AJDC 1985;143:249–254.
69. Hanna CE, Mandel SH, LaFranchi SH. Puberty in the syndrome of septo-optic dysplasia. AJDC 1989;143:186–189.
70. Crowne EC, Shalet SM. Adult panhypopituitarism presenting as idiopathic growth hormone deficiency in childhood. Acta Pediatr Scand 1991;80:255–258.
71. Acers TE. Optic nerve hypoplasia: Septo-pituitary-optic dysplasia syndrome. Tr Am Ophthalmol Soc 1981;79:425–457.
72. Brodsky MC, Conte FA, Taylor D, et al. Sudden death in septo-optic dysplasia: Report of five cases. Arch Ophthalmol 1997;15:66–70.
73. Sherlock DA, McNicol LR. Anaesthesia and septo-optic dysplasia. Anaesthesia 1987;42:1302–1305.
74. Brodsky MC, Glasier CM, Pollock SC, et al. Optic nerve hypoplasia: Identification by magnetic resonance imaging. Arch Ophthalmol 1990;108:562–567.
75. Greenfield PS, Wilcox LM, Weiter JJ, et al. Hypoplasia of the optic nerve in association with porencephaly. J Pediatr Ophthalmol Strabismus 1980;17:75–80.
76. Chuang SH, Fitz CR, Chilton SJ, et al. Schizencephaly: spectrum of CT findings in association with septo-optic dysplasia. Radiology 1984;153:118.
77. Beck RW, Corbett JJ, Thompson HS, et al. Decreased visual acuity from optic disc drusen. Arch Ophthalmol 1985;103:1155–1159.
78. Hoyt WF. Congenital occipital hemianopia. Neuroophthalmol Jpn 1985;2:252–259.
79. Barkovich AJ, Norman D. Anomalies of the corpus callosum. Correlation with further anomalies of the brain. AJNR 1988;9:493–501.
80. Kuban KC, Teele RL, Wallman J. Septo-optic-dysplasia-schizencephaly: Radiographic and clinical features. Pediatr Radiol 1989;19:145–150.
81. Ragge NK, Barkovich AJ, Hoyt WF, et al. Isolated congenital hemianopia caused by prenatal injury to the optic radiation. Arch Neurol 1991;48:1088–1091.
82. Carney SH, Brodsky MC, Good WV, et al. Aicardi syndrome: More than meets the eye. Surv Ophthalmol 1993;37:419–424.
83. Coulter CL, Leech RW, Schaefer GB, et al. Midline cerebral dysgenesis, dysfunction of the hypothalamic-pituitary axis, and fetal alcohol effects. Arch Neurol 1993;50:771–775.
84. Kobori JA, Herrick MK, Urich H. Arhinencephaly: The spectrum of associated malformations. Brain 1987;110:237–260.
85. Michaud J, Mizrahi EM, and Urich H. Agenesis of the vermis with fusion of the cerebellar hemispheres, septo-optic dysplasia, and associated anomalies. Acta Neuropathol 1982;56:161–166.
86. Barkovich A, Fram EK, Norman D. Septo-optic dysplasia: MR imaging. Radiology 1989;171:189–192.
87. Mayou MS. The condition of the retina and optic nerves in anencephaly. Trans Ophthalmol Soc UK 1904;24:150–161.
88. Boniuk V, Ho PK. Ocular findings in anencephaly. Am J Ophthalmol 1979;88:613–617.
89. Crome L, Sylvester PE. Hydranencephaly (hydrencephaly). Arch Dis Child 1958;33:235–245.
90. Muir CS. Hydranencephaly and allied disorders. Arch Dis Child 1959;34:231–246.
91. Manschot WA. Eye findings in hydranencephaly. Ophthalmologica 1971;162:151–159.
92. Brodsky MC, Hoyt WF, Hoyt CS, et al. Atypical retinochoroidal coloboma in patients with dysplastic optic discs and transsphenoidal encephalocele. Arch Ophthalmol 1995;113:624–628.

93. Jacobson L, Hellstrom A, Flodmark O. Large cups in normal-sized optic discs. Arch Ophthalmol 1997;115:1263–1269.

94. Brodsky MC. Periventricular leukomalacia: An intracranial cause of pseudoglaucomatous cupping. Arch Ophthalmol 2001;119:626.

95. Kucharczyk W, Lenkinski R, Kucharczyk J, Henkelman RM. The effect of phospholipid vesicles on the NMR relaxation of water: An explanation for the MR appearance of the neurohypophysis? AJNR 1990;11:693–700.

96. Kelly WM, Kucharczyk W, Kucharczyk J, et al. Posterior pituitary ectopia: An MR feature of pituitary dwarfism. Am J Neuroradiol 1988;9:453–460.

97. Phillips PH, Spear C, Brodsky MC. Magnetic resonance diagnosis of congenital hypopituitarism in children with optic nerve hypoplasia. J AAPOS 2001;5:275–280.

98. Kaufman LM, Miller MT, Mafee MF. Magnetic resonance imaging of pituitary stalk hypoplasia: a discrete midline anomaly associated with endocrine abnormalities in septo-optic dysplasia. Arch Ophthalmol 1989;107:1485–1489.

99. Roessmann U, Velasco ME, Small EJ, et al. Neuropathology of ''septo-optic dysplasia'' (de Morsier syndrome) with immunohistochemical studies of the hypothalamus and pituitary gland. J Neuropathol Exp Neurol 1987;46:597–608.

100. Williams J, Brodsky MC, Griebel M, et al. Septo-optic dysplasia: Clinical significance of an absent septum pellucidum. Dev Med Child Neurol 1993;35:490–501.

101. Donat JFG. Septo-optic dysplasia in an infant of a diabetic mother. Arch Neurol 1981;38:590–591.

102. Nelson M, Lessell S, Sadun AA. Optic nerve hypoplasia and maternal diabetes mellitus. Arch Neurol 1986;43:20–25.

103. Petersen RA, Holmes LB. Optic nerve hypoplasia in infants of diabetic mothers. Arch Ophthalmol 1986;104:1587.

104. Kim RY, Hoyt WF, Lessell S, et al. Superior segmental optic hypoplasia: A sign of maternal diabetes. Arch Ophthalmol 1989;107:1312–1315.

105. McKinna AJ. Quinine induced hypoplasia of the optic nerves. Can J Ophthalmol 1966;1:261–263.

106. Hoyt CS, Billson F, Ouvrier R, et al. Ocular features of Aicardi's syndrome. Arch Ophthalmol 1978;96:291–295.

107. Stromland K. Ocular abnormalities in the fetal alcohol syndrome. Acta Ophthalmol 1985;63:7–47.

108. Hittner JM, Desmond MM, Montgomery JR. Optic nerve manifestations of cytomegalovirus infection. Am J Ophthalmol 1976;81:661–665.

109. Margalith D, Jan JE, McCormick AQ, et al. Clinical spectrum of congenital optic nerve hypoplasia: Review of 51 patients. Dev Med Child Neurol 1984;26:311–322.

110. Elster AB, McAnarney ER. Maternal age re: Septo-optic dysplasia. J Pediatr 1979;94:162–163.

111. Lippe B, Kaplan SA, LaFranchi S. Septo-optic dysplasia and maternal age. Lancet 1979;2:92–93.

112. van Dyk HJL, Morgan KS. Optic nerve hypoplasia and young maternal age. Am J Ophthalmol 1980;89:879.

113. Robinson GC, Conry RF. Maternal age and congenital optic nerve hypoplasia: A possible clue to etiology. Devel Med Child Neurol 1986;28:294–298.

114. Kytila J, Miettinen P. On bilateral aplasia of the optic nerve. Acta Ophthalmol 1961;39:416–419.

115. Hackenbruch Y, Meerhoff E, Besio R, et al. Familial bilateral optic nerve hypoplasia. Am J Ophthalmol 1975;79:314–320.

116. Benner JD, Preslan MW, Gratz E, et al. Septo-optic dysplasia in two siblings. Am J Ophthalmol 1990;109:632–637.

117. Hodgkins P, Lees M, Lawson J, et al. Optic disc anomalies in frontonasal dysplasia. Br J Ophthalmol 1998;82:290–293.

118. Layman PR, Anderson DR, Flynn JT. Frequent occurrence of hypoplastic optic disks in patients with aniridia. Am J Ophthalmol 1974;77:513–516.

119. Levine LM, Bhatti MT, Mancuso AA. Septo-optic dysplasia with olfactory tract and bulb hypoplasia. J AAPOS 2001;5:398–399.

120. Brodsky MC, Harper RA, Keppen LD, et al. Anophthalmia in Delleman syndrome. Am J Med Genet 1990;37:157–158.

121. Denslow GT, Sims M. Duane's retraction syndrome associated with optic nerve hypoplasia. J Pediatr Ophthalmol Strabismus 1980;17:26–28.

122. Rathbun JE, Hoyt WF, Beard C. Surgical management of obitofrontal varix in Klippel-Trenaunay-Weber syndrome. Am J Ophthalmol 1970;70:109–112.

123. O'Connor PS, Smith JL. Optic nerve variant in the Klippel-Trenaunay-Weber syndrome. Ann Ophthalmol 1978;10:131–134.

124. Margolis S, Aleksic S, Charles N, et al. Retinal and optic nerve findings in the Goldenhar-Gorlin syndrome. Ophthalmology 1984;91:1327–1333.

125. Katz B, Van Patten P, Rothrock JF, et al. Optic nerve head drusen and pseudotumor cerebri. Arch Neurol 1988;45:45–47.

126. Macrae DW, Howard RO, Albert DM, et al. Ocular manifestations of the Meckel syndrome. Arch Ophthalmol 1972;88:106–113.

127. Chesmire KJ, Witkop GS. Optic nerve hypoplasia and angle dysgenesis in a patient with blepharophimosis syndrome. Am J Ophthalmol 1994;117:676–677.

128. Kreibig W. Uber aplasie und hypoplasie der papilla nervi optici. Klin Monatsbl Augenheilkd 1959;135:212–223.

129. van Balen A, Santens P. Chondrodystrophia calcificans congenita. J Pediatr Ophthalmol 1968;5:151–156.

130. Billson FA, Hoyt CS. Optic nerve hypoplasia in chondrodysplasia punctat. J Pediatr Ophthalmol 1977;14:144–147.

131. Lloyd L, Buncic JR. Hypoplasia of the optic nerve and disc. In Smith JL, ed, Neuro-Ophthalmology Focus 1980. New York, Masson, 1979:85–96.

132. Harcourt RB. Developmental abnormalities of the optic nerve. Trans Ophthalmol Soc UK 1976;96:395–398.

133. Weleber RG, Lovrien EW, Isom JB. Aicardi's syndrome: Case report, clinical features, and electrophysiologic studies. Arch Ophthalmol 1978;96:285–290.

134. Chevrie JJ, Aicardi J. The Aicardi syndrome. In Pedley TA, Meldrum BS, eds. Recent Advances in Epilepsy. New York, Churchill Livingstone, 1986:189–210.

135. Teng R-J, Wang P-J, Wang T-R, Shen Y-Z. Apert syndrome associated with septo-optic dysplasia. Pediatr Neurol 1989;5:384–389.

136. Brownstein S, Kirkham TH, Kalousek DK. Bilateral renal agenesis with multiple congenital ocular anomalies. Am J Ophthalmol 1976;82:770–774.

137. Weichselbaum RR, Zakov ZN, Albert DM, et al. New findings in the chromosome 13 long-arm deletion syndrome and retinoblastoma. Ophthalmology 1979;86:1191–1201.

138. Calderone JP, Chess J, Borodic G, et al. Intraocular pathology of trisomy 18 (Edward's syndrome): Report of a case and review of literature. Br J Ophthalmol 1983;67:162–169.

139. Davidson JE, McWilliam RC, Evans TJ, et al. Porencephaly and optic hypoplasia in neonatal thrombocytopenia. Arch Dis Child 1989;64:858–860.

140. Gündüz K, Günalp I, Saatçi I. Septo-optic dysplasia associated with bilateral complex microphthalmos. Ophthalmic Genet 1996;17:109–113.

141. Spedick MJ, Beauchamp GR. Retinal vascular and optic nerve abnormalities in albinism. J Pediatr Ophthalmol Strabismus 1986;23:58–62.

142. Kottow MH. Congenital malformations of the retinal vessels with primary optic nerve involvement. Ophthalmologica 1978;176:86–90.

143. Landau K, Bajka JD, Kirchschlager BM. Topless optic disks in children of mothers with Type 1 diabetes mellitus. Am J Ophthalmol 1998;125:605–611.

144. Hod M, Diamant YZ. The offspring of a diabetic mother: Short- and long-range implications. Isr J Med Sci 1992;28:81–86.

145. Brodsky MC, Schroeder GT, Ford R. Superior segmental optic hypoplasia in identical twins. J Clin Neuroophthalmol 1993;13:152–154.

146. Hashimoto M, Ohtsuka K, Nakagawa T, Hoyt WF. Topless optic disk syndrome without maternal diabetes mellitus. Am J Ophthalmol 1999;128:111–112.

147. Brodsky MC, Glasier CM, Creel DJ. Magnetic resonance imaging of the visual pathways in human albinos. J Pediatr Ophthalmol Strabismus 1993;30:382–385.

148. Birgbauer E, Cowan CA, Sretavan DW, Henkemeyer M. Kinase independent function of EphB receptors in retinal axon pathfinding to the optic disc from dorsal but not ventral retina. Development 2000;127:1231–1241.

149. Novakovic P, Taylor DSI, Hoyt WF. Localizing patterns of optic nerve hypoplasia-retina to occipital lobe. Br J Ophthalmol 1988;72:176–182.

150. Margo CE, Hamed LM, McCarty J. Congenital optic tract syndrome. Arch Ophthalmol 1991;109:1120–1122.

151. Hoyt WF, Rios-Montenegro EN, Behrens MM, Eckelhoff RJ. Homonymous hemioptic hypoplasia: Fundoscopic features in standard and red-free illumination in three patients with congenital hemiplegia. Br J Ophthalmol 1972;56:537–545.

152. Deiner MS, Kennedy TE, Fazeli A, et al. Netrin-1 and DCC mediate axon guidance locally at the optic disc: Loss of function leads to optic nerve hypoplasia. Neuron 1997;19:575–589.

153. Oster SF, Sretavan DW. Connecting the eye to the brain: the molecular basis of ganglion cell axon guidance. Brit J Ophthalmol 2003;87:639–645.

154. Deiner MS, Sretavan DW. Altered midline axon pathways and ectopic neurons in the developing hypothalamus of netrin-1 and DCC deficient mice. J Neurosci 1999;19:9900–9912.

155. Zaias B, Becker D. Septo-optic dysplasia: developmental or acquired abnormality? A case report. Trans Am Neurol Assoc 1978;103:273–277.

156. Hoyt CS, Good WV. Do we really understand the difference between optic nerve hypoplasia and atrophy? Eye 1992;6:201–204.

157. Provis JM, Van Driel D, Billson FA, et al. Human fetal optic nerve: Overproduction and elimination of retinal axons during development. J Comp Neurol 1985;238:92–100.

158. Hatten ME, Mason CA. Mechanisms of glial guided neuronal migration in vitro and in vivo. Experientia 1990;46:907–916.

159. Barkovich AJ, Lyon G, Evrard PL. Formation, maturation, and disorders of white matter. AJNR 1992;13:447–461.

160. Brenner JD, Preslan MW, Gratz E, et al. Septo-optic dysplasia in two siblings. Am J Ophthalmol 1990;109:632–639.

161. Dattani M, Martinez-Barbera JP, Thomas PQ, et al. Mutations in the homeobox gene HESX1/Hesx1 associated with septo-optic dysplasia in human and mouse. Nat Genet 1998;19:125–133.

162. Dattani M, Martinez-Barbera JP, Thomas PQ, et al. Molecular genetics of septo-optic dysplasia. Horm Res 2000;53(Suppl 1):26–33.

163. Bennett JL. Developmental neurogenetics and neuro-ophthalmology. J Neuro-ophthalmol 2003;22:286–296.

164. Azuma N, Yamaguchi Y, Handa H, et al. Mutations of the PAX6 gene detected in patients with a variety of optic nerve malformations. Am J Hum Genet 2003;72:1565–1570.

165. Pollock S. The morning glory disc anomaly: Contractile movement, classification, and embryogenesis. Doc Ophthalmol 1987;65:439–460.

166. Kindler P. Morning glory syndrome: Unusual congenital optic disk anomaly. Am J Ophthalmol 1970;69:376–384.

167. Hamada S, Ellsworth RM. Congenital retinal detachment and the optic disk anomaly. Am J Ophthalmol 1971;71:460–464.

168. Krause U. Three cases of the morning glory syndrome. Acta Ophthalmol 1972; 50:188–198.

169. Jensen PE, Kalina RE. Congenital anomalies of the optic disk. Am J Ophthalmol 1976;82:27–31.

170. Steahly LP. A colobomatous optic disc anomaly and associated retinal detachment. J Pediatr Ophthalmol 1977;14:103–105.

171. Bruner H-J, Fechner PU. Uber das morning glory-syndrom. Klin Monatsbl Augenheilkd 1978;172:114.

172. Steinkuller PG. The morning glory disc anomaly. Case report and literature review. J Pediatr Ophthalmol Strabismus 1980;17:81–87.

173. Jonas JB, Zach FM, Gusek GC, et al. Pseudoglaucomatous physiologic optic cups. Am J Ophthalmol 1989;107:137–144.

174. Beyer WB, Quencer RM, Osher RH. Morning glory syndrome: A functional analysis including fluorescein angiography, ultrasonography, and computerized tomography. Ophthalmol 1982;89:1362–1364.

175. Brodsky MC, Wilson RS. Retinal arteriovenous communications in the morning glory disc anomaly. Arch Ophthalmol 1995;113:410–411.

176. Mafee MF, Jampol LM, Langer BG, et al. Computed tomography of optic nerve colobomas, morning glory anomaly, and colobomatous cyst. Radiol Clin North Am 1987;25:693–699.

177. Traboulsi EI, O'Neill JF. The spectrum in the morphology of the so-called "morning glory disc anomaly." J Pediatr Ophthalmol Strabismus 1988;25: 93–98.

178. Murphy BL, Griffin JF. Optic nerve coloboma (morning glory syndrome): CT findings. Radiology 1994;191:59–61.

179. Okada K, Sakata H, Shirane M, et al. Computerized tomography of two patients with morning glory syndrome. Hiroshima J Med Sci 1994;43:111–113.

180. Haik BG, Greenstein SH, Smith ME, et al. Retinal detachment in the morning glory syndrome. Ophthalmology 1984;91:1638–1647.

181. Nucci P, Mets MB, Gabianelli EB. Trisomy 4q with morning glory anomaly. Ophthalmic Pediatr Genet 1990;2:143–145.

182. Holmström G, Taylor D. Capillary haemangiomas in association with morning glory disc anomaly. Acta Ophthalmol Scand 1998;76:613–616.

183. Metry DW, Dowd CF, Barkovich AJ, Frieden IJ. The many faces of PHACE syndrome. J Pediatr 2001;139:117–123.

184. Kniestedt C, Brodsky MC, North P. Infantile orofacial hemangioma with ipsilateral peripapillary excavation in girls: A variant of the PHACE syndrome. Arch Ophthalmol 2004, In press.

185. Brodsky MC, Landau K, Wilson RS, Boltshauser E. Morning glory disc anomaly in neurofibromatosis type 2. Arch Ophthalmol 1999;117:839–841.

186. Pollock JA, Newton TH, Hoyt WF. Transsphenoidal and transethmoidal encephaloceles: A review of clinical and roentgen features in 8 cases. Radiology 1968; 90:442–453.

187. Goldhammer Y, Smith JL. Optic nerve anomalies in basal encephalocele. Arch Ophthalmol 1975;93:115–118.

188. Koenig SP, Naidich TP, Lissner G. The morning glory syndrome associated with sphenoidal encephalocele. Ophthalmology 1982;89:1368–1372.

189. Caprioli J, Lesser RL. Basal encephalocoele and morning glory syndrome. Br J Ophthalmol 1983;67:349–351.

190. Hope-Ross M, Johnston SS. The morning glory syndrome associated with sphenoethmoidal encephalocele. Ophthal Pediatr Genet 1990;2:147–153.

191. Itakura T, Miyamoto K, Uematsu Y, et al. Bilateral morning glory syndrome associated with sphenoid encephalocele. J Neurosurg 1992;77:949–951.

192. Diebler C, Dulac O. Cephalocoeles: Clinical and neuroradiological appearance. Neuroradiology 1983;25:199–216.

193. Yokota A, Matsukado Y, Fuwa I, et al. Anterior basal encephalocele of the neonatal and infantile period. Neurosurgery 1986;19:468–478.

194. Eustis HS, Sanders MR, Zimmerman T. Morning glory syndrome in children. Arch Ophthalmol 1994;112:204–207.

195. Moroika M, Marubayashi T, Masumitsu T, et al. Basal encephaloceles with morning glory syndrome and progressive hormonal and visual disturbances: case report and review of the literature. Brain Devel 1995;17:196–201.

196. Hansen MR, Price RL, Rothner AD, Tomsak RL. Developmental anomalies of the optic disc and carotid circulation: A new association. J Clin Neuro-ophthalmol 1985;5:3–8.

197. Massaro M, Thorarensen O, Liu GT, et al. Morning glory disc anomaly and Moyamoya vessels. Arch Ophthalmol 1998;116:253–254.

198. Komiyama M, Yasui T, Sakamoto H, et al. Basal meningocele, anomaly of optic disc and panhypopituitarism in association with Moyamoya disease. Pediatr Neurosurg 2000;33:100–104.

199. Bakri SJ, Skier D, Masaryk T. Ocular malformations, Moyamoya disease, and midline cranial defects: A distinct syndrome. Am J Ophthalmol 1999;127: 356–357.

200. Dempster AG, Lee WR, Forrester JV, McCreath GT. The "morning glory syndrome." A mesodermal defect? Ophthalmologica 1983;187:222–230.

201. Takida A, Hida T, Kimura C, et al. A case of bilateral morning glory syndrome with total retinal detachment. Foliathalmologica Japonica 1981;32:1177–1182.

202. von Fricken MA, Dhungel R. Retinal detachment in the morning glory syndrome: Pathogenesis and management. Retina 1984;4:97–99.

203. Akiyama K, Azuma N, Hida T, et al. Retinal detachment in morning glory syndrome. Ophthalmic Surg 1984;15:841–843.

204. Harris MJ, De Bustros S, Michels RG, et al. Treatment of combined traction-rhegmatogenous retinal detachment in the morning glory syndrome. Retina 1984; 4:249–252.

205. Coll GE, Chang S, Flynn TE, et al. Communication between the subretinal space and the vitreous cavity in the morning glory syndrome. Graefe's Arch Clin Exp Ophthalmol 1994;233:441–443.

206. Irvine AR, Crawford JB, Sullivan JH. The pathogenesis of retinal detachment with morning glory disc and optic pit. Retina 1986;6:146–150.

207. Brown GC, Brown MM. Repair of retinal detachment associated with congenital excavated defects of the optic disc. Ophthalmic Surg 1995;26:11–15.

208. Chang S, Haik BG, Ellsworth RM, et al. Treatment of total retinal detachment in morning glory syndrome. Am J Ophthalmol 1984;97:596–600.

209. Bartz-Schmidt KU, Heimann K. Pathogenesis of retinal detachment associated with morning glory disc. Int Ophthalmol 1995;19:35–38.

210. Sugar HS, Beckman H. Peripapillary staphyloma with respiratory pulsations. Am J Ophthalmol 1969;68:895–897.

211. Vuori M-L. Morning glory disc anomaly with pulsating peripapillary staphyloma. A case history. Acta Ophthalmol 1987;65:602–606.

212. Chuman H, Nao-i N, Sawada A. A case of morning glory syndrome associated with contractile movement of the optic disc and subretinal neovascularization. J Jpn Ophthalmol 1996;100:705–709.

213. Sobol WM, Bratton AR, Rivers MB, et al. Morning glory disk syndrome associated with subretinal neovascularization. Am J Ophthalmol 1990;110:93–94.

214. Dailey JR, Cantore WA, Gardner TW. Peripapillary choroidal neovascular membrane associated with an optic disc coloboma. Arch Ophthalmol 1993;111: 441–442.

215. Pedler C. Unusual coloboma of the optic nerve entrance. Br J Ophthalmol 1961; 45:803–807.

216. Rack JH, Wright GF. Coloboma of the optic nerve entrance. Br J Ophthalmol 1966;50:705–709.

217. Cogan DG. Coloboma of optic nerve with overlay of peripapillary retina. Br J Ophthalmol 1978;62:347–350.

218. Manschot WA. Morning glory syndrome: a histopathological study. Br J Ophthalmol 1990;74:56–58.

219. Gardner TW, Zaparackas ZG, Naidich TP. Congenital optic nerve colobomas: CT demonstration. J Comp Assist Tomog 1984;8:95–102.

220. Mann I. Developmental Abnormalities of the Eye. Ed 2. Philadelphia, JB Lippincott, 1957:74–91.

221. Pagon RA. Ocular coloboma. Surv Ophthalmol 1981;25:223–236.

222. Coats G. The pathology of coloboma at the nerve entrance. R Lond Ophthalmol Hosp Rep 1908;17:178–224.

223. Calhoun FP. Bilateral coloboma of the optic nerve associated with holes in the disc and a cyst of the optic nerve sheath. Arch Ophthalmol 1930;3:71–79.

224. Lyle D. Coloboma of the optic nerve. Am J Ophthalmol 1932;15:347–349.

225. Adler F. Bilateral partial colobomata of the optic nerve. Am J Ophthalmol 1937; 20:777–791.

226. Steinberg T. Coloboma of the optic nerve. Am J Ophthalmol 1943;26:846–849.

227. François J. Colobomatous malformations of the ocular globe. Int Ophthalmol Clin 1968;8:797–816.

228. Brodsky MC. Magnetic resonance imaging of colobomatous optic hypoplasia. Brit J Ophthalmol 1999;83:755–756.

229. Slamovits TL, Kimball GP, Friberg TR, et al. Bilateral optic disc colobomas with orbital cysts and hypoplastic optic nerves and chiasm. J Clin Neuro-ophthalmol 1989;9:172–177.

230. Weyert F. Zur hereditat der opticus-colobome. Klin Monatsbl Augenheilkd 1890;28:325–331.

231. Hoeve J. Colobom am sehnerveneintritt mit normaler sehscharfe. Arch Augenheilkd 1907;57:13–20.

232. Crampton G. Two cases of binocular coloboma of the optic nerve in the same family. Ophthalmol Rec 1913;22:377–378.

233. Heine L. Angeborene gesichtsfelddefekte (amotio, glaukom, embolie vortauschend). Arch Augenheilkd 1927;98:108–120.

234. Sandvig K. Pseudoglaucoma of autosomal dominant inheritance. Acta Ophthalmol 1961;39:33–43.

235. Savell J, Cook JR. Optic nerve colobomas of autosomal-dominant heredity. Arch Ophthalmol 1976;94:395–400.

236. Nicholson DH, Goldberg MF. Ocular abnormalities in the de Lange syndrome. Arch Ophthalmol 1966;76:214–220.

237. Yanoff M, Rorke LB, Niederer BS. Ocular and cerebral abnormalities in chromosome 18 deletion defect. Am J Ophthamol 1970;70:391–402.

238. Drews RC, Pico G. Heterochromia associated with coloboma of the iris. Am J Ophthalmol 1971;72:827.

239. Drews RC. Heterochromia iridum with coloboma of the optic disc. Arch Ophthalmol 1973;90:437.

240. Pagon RA, Graham JM, Zonana J, et al. Coloboma, congenital heart disease, and choanal atresia with multiple anomalies: CHARGE association. J Pediatr 1981;99:233–237.

241. Chestler RJ, France TD. Ocular findings in the CHARGE syndrome. Ophthalmology 1988;95:1613–1619.

242. Risse JF, Guillaume JB, Boissonnot M, et al. Un syndrome polymalformatif inhabituel: 1. Association charge; morning glory syndrome. Unilateral Ophtalmologie 1989;3:196–198.
243. Russell-Eggitt IM, Blake KD, Taylor DSI, et al. The eye in the CHARGE association. Br J Ophthalmol 1990;74:421–426.
244. Taylor D. Optic nerve. In Pediatric Ophthalmology. Cambridge MA, Blackwell Scientific 1990:441–466.
245. Limaye SR. Coloboma of the iris and choroid and retinal detachment in oculoauricular dysplasia (Goldenhar's syndrome). Eye Ear Nose Throat Monthly 1972;51:28–31.
246. Warburg M. Update of sporadic microphthalmos and coloboma. Ophthalmic Pediatr Genet 1992;13:111–122.
247. Villalonga Gornés PAV, Galan Terraza A, Gil-Gibernau JJ. Ophthalmoscopic evolution of papillary colobomatous malformations. J Pediatr Ophthalmol Strabismus 1995;32:20–25.
248. Theodossiadis GP, Damanakis AG, Theodossiadis PG. Coloboma of the optic disk associated with retinal vascular abnormalities. Am J Ophthalmol 1995;120:798–800.
249. Biedner B, Klemperer I, Dagan M, et al. Optic disc coloboma associated with macular hole and retinal detachment. Ann Ophthalmol 1993;25:350–352.
250. Yedavally S, Frank RN. Peripapillary subretinal neovascularization associated with coloboma of the optic nerve. Arch Ophthalmol 1993;111:552–553.
251. Font RL, Zimmerman LE. Intrascleral smooth muscle in coloboma of the optic disc. Am J Ophthalmol 1971;72:452–457.
252. Willis R, Zimmerman LE, O'Grady R, et al. Heterotopic adipose tissue and smooth muscle in the optic disc, association with isolated colobomas. Arch Ophthalmol 1972;88:139–146.
253. Foster JA, Lam S. Contractile optic disc coloboma. Arch Ophthalmol 1991;109:472–473.
254. Lin CCL, Tso MOM, Vygantas CM. Coloboma of the optic nerve associated with serous maculopathy: A clinicopathologic correlative study. Arch Ophthalmol 1984;102:1651–1654.
255. Schatz H, McDonald HR. Treatment of sensory retinal detachment associated with optic nerve pit or coloboma. Ophthalmology 1988;95:178–186.
256. Bochow TW, Olk RJ, Knupp JA, Smith ME. Spontaneous reattachment of a total retinal detachment in an infant with microphthalmos and an optic nerve coloboma. Am J Ophthalmol 1991;112:347–349.
257. Lewin ML, Schuster MM. Transpalatal correction of basilar meningocele with cleft palate. Arch Surg 1965;90:687–693.
258. Streletz LJ, Schatz NJ. Transsphenoidal encephalocele associated with colobomas of the optic disc and hypopituitary dwarfism. In Smith JL, Glaser JS, eds. Neuro-Ophthalmology Symposium of the University of Miami and the Bascom Palmer Eye Institute. Vol 7. St Louis, CV Mosby, 1973:78–86.
259. Corbett JJ, Savino PJ, Schatz NJ, et al. Cavitary developmental defects of the optic disc: Visual loss associated with optic pits and colobomas. Arch Neurol 1980;37:210–213.
260. Von Szily A. Die Ontogenese der idiopathiachen (erbbildlichen Spaltbildungen des Auges des Mikrophthalmus und der Orbitalcysten. Z Anat Entwicklungsgesch 1924;74:1–230.
261. Brodsky MC. Morning glory disc anomaly or optic disc coloboma. Arch Ophthalmol 1994;112:153.
262. Rosenberg LF, Burde RM. Progressive visual loss caused by an arachnoidal brain cyst in a patient with an optic nerve coloboma. Am J Ophthalmol 1988;106:322–325.
263. Singh D, Verma A. Bilateral peripapillary staphyloma (ectasia). Ind J Ophthalmol 1978;25:50–51.
264. Brown G, Tasman W. Congenital Anomalies of the Optic Disc. New York, Grune & Stratton, 1983:31–215.
265. Wise JB, Maclean AL, Gass JDM. Contractile peripapillary staphyloma. Arch Ophthalmol 1966;75:626–630.
266. Konstas P, Katikos G, Vatakas LC. Contractile peripapillary staphyloma. Ophthalmologica 1971;172:379–381.
267. Kral K, Svarc D. Contractile peripapillary staphyloma. Am J Ophthalmol 1971;71:1090–1092.
268. Cennamo G, Sammartino A, Fioretti F. Morning glory syndrome with contractile peripapillary staphyloma. Br J Ophthalmol 1983;67:346–348.
269. Seybold ME, Rosen PN. Peripapillary staphyloma and amaurosis fugax. Ann Ophthalmol 1977;9:139–141.
270. Caldwell JBH, Sears ML, Gilman M. Bilateral peripapillary staphyloma with normal vision. Am J Ophthalmol 1971;71:423–425.
271. Donaldson DD, Bennett N, Anderson DR, et al. Peripapillary staphyloma. Arch Ophthalmol 1969;82:704–705.
272. Hodgkins P, Lees M, Lawson J, et al. Optic disc anomalies and frontonasal dysplasia. Brit J Ophthalmol 1998;82:290–293.
273. Kirath H, Bozkurt B, Mocan C. Peripapillary staphyloma associated with orofacial capillary hemangioma. Ophthalmic Genetics 2001;22:249–253.
274. Sherman AR. Teratoid tumor of conjunctiva and other developmental anomalies with naevus verrucosus of scalp. Report of a case. Arch Ophthalmol 1943;29:441–445.
275. Izquierdo NJ, Maumenee IH, Traboulsi EI. Anterior segment malformations in 18q- (de Grouchy) syndrome. Ophthal Pediatr Genet 1993;14:91–94.
276. Kraupa E. Beitrage zur morphologie des augenhintergrundes. III. Klin Monatsbl Augenheilkd 1921;67:15–26.
277. Bock R. Une nouvelle anomalie congénitale: La mégalopapille. Confin Neurol 1949;9:407–408.
278. Franceschetti A, Bock RH. Megalopapilla: A new congenital anomaly. Am J Ophthalmol 1950;33:227–235.
279. Malbran JL, Roveda JM. Megalopapilla. Arch Oftal B Aires 1951;26:331–335.
280. Badtke G. Über die grossenanomaliender papilla nervi optici, unter besonderer berucksichtigung der schwarzen megalopapille. Klin Monatsbl Augenheilkd 1959;135:502–510.
281. Collier M, Adias L. Les anomalies congénitales des dimensions papillaires. Clin Oftalmol 1960;2:1–23.
282. Streiff B. Uber megalopapille. Klin Monatsbl Augenheilkd 1961;139:824–827.
283. Amalric P, Bessou P, Farenc M. A propos d'un cas de mégapapille unilatérale. Bull Soc Ophtalmol Fr 1964;64:1083–1085.
284. Watanabe C. Giant optic disc. Ophthalmology (Tokyo) 1966;8:596–599.
285. Gruner H-J, Fechner PU. Die megalopapille, eine seltene kongenitale anomalie. Klin Monatsbl Augenheilkd 1977;171:611–612.
286. Bynke H, Holmdahl G. Megalopapilla: A differential diagnosis in suspected optic atrophy. Neuroophthalmology 1981;2:53–57.
287. Slusher MM, Weaver RG, Greven CM, et al. The spectrum of cavitary optic disc anomalies in a family. Ophthalmology 1989;96:342–347.
288. Maisel JM, Pearlstein CS, Adams WH, et al. Large optic discs in the Marshallese population. Am J Ophthalmol 1989;107:145–150.
289. Manor RS, Kesler A. Optic nerve hypoplasia, big discs, large cupping, and vascular malformation embolized: 22 years of follow-up. Arch Ophthalmol 1993;111:901–902.
290. Grimson BS, Perry DD. Enlargement of the optic disk in childhood optic nerve tumors. Am J Ophthalmol 1984;97:627–631.
291. Margolis S, Siegel IM. The tilted disc syndrome in craniofacial diseases. In Smith JL, ed. Neuro-Ophthalmology Focus 1980. New York, Masson, 1979:97–116.
292. Wiethe T. Ein fall von angeborener difformitat der sehnervenpapille. Arch Augenheilkd 1882;11:14–19.
293. Brown GC, Shields JA, Goldberg RE. Congenital pits of the optic nerve head. II. Clinical studies in humans. Ophthalmology 1980;87:51–65.
294. Reis W. Eine wenig bekannte typische missbildung am sehnerveneintritt: Unschriebene grubenbildung aufder papilla n. optici. Z Augenheilkd 1908;19:505–528.
295. Kranenburg EW. Crater-like holes in the optic disc and central serous retinopathy. Arch Ophthalmol 1960;64:912–924.
296. Stefko ST, Campochiaro P, Wang P, et al. Dominant inheritance of optic pits. Am J Ophthalmol 1997;124:112–113.
297. Ragge NK. Dominant inheritance of optic pits. Am J Ophthalmol 1998;125:124–125.
298. Jonas JB, Freisler KA. Bilateral congenital optic nerve head pits in monozygotic twins. Am J Ophthalmol 1997;124:844–845.
299. Theodossiadis GP, Kollia AK, Theodossiadis PG. Cilioretinal arteries in conjunction with a pit of the optic disc. Ophthalmologica 1992;204:115–121.
300. Van Nouhuys JM, Bruyn GW. Nasopharyngeal transsphenoidal encephalocele, crater-like hole in the optic disc and agenesis of the corpus callosum pneumoencephalographic visualization in a case. Psychiatr Neurol Neurochir 1964;67:243–258.
301. Javitt JC, Spaeth GL, Katz LJ, et al. Acquired pits of the optic nerve. Ophthalmology 1990;97:1038–1044.
302. Sugar HS. Congenital pits of the optic disc and their equivalents (congenital colobomas and coloboma-like excavations) associated with submacular fluid. Am J Ophthalmol 1967;63:298–307.
303. Bonnet M. Serous macular detachment associated with optic nerve pits. Arch Clin Exp Ophthalmol 1991;229:526–532.
304. Ferry AP. Macular detachment associated with congenital pit of the optic nerve head. Arch Ophthalmol 1963;70:346–357.
305. Lincoff H, Lopez R, Kreissig I, et al. Retinoschisis associated with optic nerve pits. Arch Ophthalmol 1988;106:61–67.
306. Krivoy D, Gentile R, Liebmann JM, et al. Imaging congenital optic disc pits and associated maculopathy using optical coherence tomography. Arch Ophthalmol 1996;114:165–170.
307. Lincoff H, Schiff W, Krivoy D, Ritch R. Optical coherence tomography of optic pit maculopathy. Am J Ophthalmol 1996;122:264–266.
308. Rutledge BK, Pulafito CA, Duker JS, et al. Optical coherence tomography of macular lesions associated with optic nerve head pits. Ophthalmology 1996;103:1047–1053.
309. Gass JDM. Serous detachment of the macula: Secondary to congenital pit of the optic nervehead. Am J Ophthalmol 1969;67:821–841.
310. Cox MS, Witherspoon D, Morris RE, et al. Evolving techniques in treatment of macular detachment caused by optic nerve pits. Ophthalmology 1988;95:889–896.
311. McDonald HR, Schatz H, Johnson RN. Treatment of retinal detachment associated with optic nerve pits. Int Ophthalmol Clin 1992;32:35–42.
312. Lee KJ, Peyman GA. Surgical management of retinal detachment associated with optic nerve pit. Int Ophthalmol 1993;17:105–107.

313. Alexander TA, Billson FA. Vitrectomy and photocoagulation in the management of serous detachment associated with optic nerve pits. Aust J Ophthalmol 1984; 12:139–142.

314. Bartz-Schmidt KU, Heimann K, Esser P. Vitrectomy for macular detachment associated with optic nerve pits. Internat Ophthalmol 1996;19:323–329.

315. Hoerauf H, Schmidt-Erfurth U, Laqua H. Clinical findings after vitrectomy for retinal detachment associated with an optic disc pit. Klin Monatsbl Augenheilkd 1996;209:238–243.

316. Lincoff H, Yannuzzi L, Singerman L, et al. Improvement in visual function after displacement of the retinal elevation emanating from optic pits. Arch Ophthalmol 1993;111:1071–1079.

317. Yuen CHW, Kaye SB. Spontaneous resolution of serous maculopathy associated with optic disc pit in a child: A case report. J AAPOS 2002;6:330–331.

318. Brodsky MC. Congenital optic pit with serous maculopathy in childhood. J AAPOS 2003;7:150.

319. Apple DJ, Rabb MF, Walsh PM. Congenital anomalies of the optic disc. Surv Ophthalmol 1982;27:3–41.

320. Chang M. Pits and crater-like holes of the optic disc. Ophthalmic Semin 1976; 1:21–61.

321. Rubenstein K, Ali M. Complications of optic disc pits. Trans Ophthalmol Soc UK 1978;98:195–200.

322. Akiba J, Kakehashi A, Hikichi T, et al. Vitreous findings of optic nerve pits and serous macular detachment. Am J Ophthalmol 1993;116:38–41.

323. Brown BC, Shields JA, Patty BE, et al. Congenital pits of the optic nerve head. I. Experimental studies in collie dogs. Arch Ophthalmol 1979;97:1341–1344.

324. Friberg TR, McClellan TG. Vitreous pulsations, relative hypotony, and retrobulbar cyst associated with a congenital optic pit. Am J Ophthalmol 1992;114: 767–768.

325. Theodossiadis G. Evolution of congenital pit of the optic disc and macular detachment in photocoagulated and non-photocoagulated eyes. Am J Ophthalmol 1977;84:620–631.

326. Sugar HS. Congenital pits of the optic disc with acquired macular pathology. Am J Ophthalmol 1962;53:307–311.

327. Ribeiro-da-Silva J, Castanheira-Dinis A, Agoas V, Dodinho-de-Matos J. Congenital optic disc deformities. A clinical approach. Ophthalmic Pediatr Genet 1985;5:67–70.

328. Rieger G. Zum Krankheitsbild der Handmannschen Sehnerven-anomalie: "Windenblüten"-("Morning Glory"-) Syndrom? Klin Monatsbl Augenheilkd 1977; 170:697–706.

329. Parsa CF, Silva ED, Sundin OH, et al. Redefining papillorenal syndrome: An underdiagnosed cause of ocular and renal morbidity. Ophthalmology 2001;108: 738–749.

330. Sanyanusin P, Schimmenti LA, McNoe A, et al. Mutation of the PAX2 gene in a family with optic nerve colobomas, renal anomalies, and vesiculouretral reflux. Nat Genet 1995;9:358–364.

331. Schimmenti LA, Cunliffe HE, McNoe LA, et al. Further delineation of renal-coloboma syndrome in patients with extreme variability of phenotype and identical PAX2 mutations. Am J Hum Genet 1997;60:869–878.

332. Parsa CF, Cheeseman EW, Maumenee IH. Demonstration of exclusive cilioretinal vascular system supplying the retina in man: Vacant discs. Trans Am Ophthalmol Soc 1998;96:106–109.

333. Parsa CF, Goldberg MF, Hunter DGP. Papillorenal ("renal coloboma") syndrome. Am J Ophthalmol 2002;134:301–302.

334. Dureau P, Attie-Bitach T, Salomon R, et al. Renal coloboma syndrome. Ophthalmology 2001;108:1912–1916.

335. Young SE, Walsh FB, Knox DL. The tilted disc syndrome. Am J Ophthalmol 1976;82:16–23.

336. Flüeler UR, Guyton DL. Does a tilted retina cause astigmatism? The ocular imagery and the retinoscopic reflex resulting from a tilted retina. Surv Ophthalmol 1995;40:45–50.

337. Rucker CW. Bitemporal defects in the visual fields resulting from developmental anomalies of the optic disks. Arch Ophthalmol 1946;35:546–554.

338. Graham MV, Wakefield GJ. Bitemporal visual field defects associated with anomalies of the optic discs. Br J Ophthalmol 1973;57:307–314.

339. Manor RS. Temporal field defects due to nasal tilting of discs. Ophthalmologica 1974;168:269–281.

340. Dorrell D. The tilted disc. Br J Ophthalmol 1978;62:16–20.

341. Mimura O, Shiraki K, Shimo-oku M. Fundus controlled perimetry in the tilted disc syndrome. Jpn J Ophthalmol 1980;24:105–111.

342. Shiraki K, Mimura O, Shimo-oku M. The tilted disc syndrome. Acta Soc Ophthalmol Japonicae 1980;84:529–536.

343. Bonamour MG. Dysversion of disc. Bull Soc Ophtalmol Fr 1956;56:756.

344. Riise D. Visual field defects in optic disc malformation with ectasia of the fundus. Acta Ophthalmol 1966;48:906–918.

345. Smith JL, McCrary JA. Recent advances in optic nerve disease. In Smith FL, ed. Neuro-Ophthalmology Symposium of the University of Miami and the Bascom Palmer Eye Institute. Vol 5. Hallandale, FL, Huffman Publishing Co, 1970: 17–21.

346. Jonas JB, Kling F, Gründler AE. Optic disc shape, corneal astigmatism and amblyopia. Ophthalmology 1997;104:1934–1937.

347. Banu B, Murat I, Gedik S, et al. Topographical analysis of corneal astigmatism in patients with tilted disc syndrome. Cornea 2002;21:458–462.

348. Behrens-Baumann W, Lauritzen K. Fundus heterotopicus: Eine leicht zu Ubersehende Fehlbildung. Klin Monatsbl Augenheilkd 1992;200:278–283.

349. Miller NR, Fine SL. The ocular fundus in neuro-ophthalmologic diagnosis. In Sights and Sounds in Ophthalmology. Vol. 3. St Louis, CV Mosby, 1977.

350. Braziticos PD, Safran AB, Simona F, Zulauf M. Threshold perimetry in the tilted disc syndrome. Arch Ophthalmol 1990;108:1698–1700.

351. Sowka J, Aoun P. Tilted disc syndrome. Optometry Visual Science 1999;76: 618–623.

352. Stur M. Congenital tilted disk syndrome associated with parafoveal subretinal neovascularization. Am J Ophthalmol 1988;105:98–99.

353. Giuffre' G. Angioid streaks and associated lesions: Ophthalmoscopic and fluorescein angiographic interpretation. J Fr Ophtalmol 1986;9:811–824.

354. Cohen SY, Quentel G, Guiberteau B, et al. Macular serous retinal detachment cased by subretinal leakage in tilted disc syndrome. Ophthalmology 1998;105: 1831–1834.

355. Tosti G. Serous macular detachment and tilted disc syndrome. Ophthalmology 1999;106:1453–1454.

356. Brodsky MC. Central serous papillopathy. Brit J Ophthalmol 1999;83:878.

357. Malinowski SM, Pulido JS, Flickinger RR. The protective effect of the tilted disc syndrome in diabetic retinopathy. Arch Ophthalmol 1996;114:230–231.

358. Keane JR. Suprasellar tumors and incidental optic disc anomalies: Diagnostic problems in two patients with hemianopic temporal scotomas. Arch Ophthalmol 1977;95:2180–2183.

359. Osher RH, Schatz NJ. A sinister association of the congenital tilted disc syndrome with chiasmal compression. In Smith JL, ed. Neuro-Ophthalmology Focus 1980. New York, Masson, 1979:117–123.

360. Hittner HM, Borda RP, Justice J. X-linked recessive congenital stationary night blindness, myopia, and tilted discs. J Pediatr Ophthalmol Strabismus 1981;18: 15–20.

361. Heckenlively JR, Martin DA, Rosenbaum AL. Loss of electroretinographic oscillatory potentials, optic atrophy, and dysplasia in congenital stationary night blindness. Am J Ophthalmol 1983;96:526–534.

362. Fishman J, Spaier AH, Cohen MM. Familial dextrocardia, divergent strabismus, and situs inversus of optic disc. Am J Med Sci 1976;271:225–231.

363. Rothkoff L, Biedner B. Congenital horizontal gaze paralysis, facial hemiatrophy, and situs inversus of the optic disc: A case report. Acta Ophthalmol 1979;57: 1091–1095.

364. Handmann M. Erbliche, vermutlich angeborene zentrale gliose entartung des sehnerven mit besonderer beteilgung der zentralgefasse. Klin Monatsbl Augenheilkd 1929;83:145.

365. Barroso LHL, Ragge NK, Hoyt WF. Multiple cilioretinal arteries and dysplasia of the optic disc. J Clin Neuroophthalmol 1991;11:278–279

366. Hegab S, Sheriff SM. Retinal dysplasia involving the optic disc and retina. J Pediatr Ophthalmol Strabismus 1994;31(2):107–109.

367. De Bustros S, Miller NR, Finkelstein D, et al. Bilateral astrocytic hamartomas of the optic nerve heads in retinitis pigmentosa. Retina 1983;3:21–23.

368. Brodsky MC, Buckley EG, Rosell-McConkie A. The case of the gray optic disc! Surv Ophthalmol 1989;33:367–372.

369. Acers TE. Congenital Abnormalities of the Optic Nerve and Related Forebrain, pp. 16–17. Philadelphia, Lea & Febiger, 1983.

370. Silver J, Sapiro J. Axonal guidance during development of the optic nerve: The role of pigmented epithelia and other factors. J Comp Neurol 1981;202:521–538.

371. Halbertsma KTA. Pseudo-atrophy of the optic nerve in infant 2 months old. Ned Tijdschr Geneeskd 1937;81:1230–1236.

372. Beauvieux J. La pseudo-atrophie dés nouveau-nes (dysgénésie my-élinique des voies optiques). Ann Ocul (Paris) 1926;163:881–921.

373. Beauvieux J. La cécité apparente chez le nouveau-né: La pseudoatrophie grise du nerf optique. Arch Ophthalmol (Paris) 1947;7:241–249.

374. Hoyt WF, Beeston D. The Ocular Fundus in Neurologic Disease. St Louis, CV Mosby, 1966.

375. Brodsky MC, Baker RS, Hamed LM. Pediatric Neuroophthalmology. New York, Springer-Verlag, 1996.

376. Hall SM, Beauchamp GR, Rothner AD. Pelizaeus-Merzbacher disease. Presented to the American Association for Pediatric Ophthalmology & Strabismus, 13th Ann Meet. March 15–19, 1987. Scottsdale, AZ.

377. François P, Fontaine G, Farriaux J-P, et al. Syndrome de Beauvieux (papille grise) au cours d'une amino-acidopathie rare: La Leucinose. Bull Soc Ophtalmol Fr 1968;68:584–589.

378. Neely K, Mets MB, Wong P, et al. Ocular findings in partial trisomy 10q syndrome. Am J Ophthalmol 1988;106:82–87.

379. Sobanski J. Eine schiefergraue sehnerven papille. Klin Monatsbl Augenheilkd 1939;102:704–706.

380. Taylor DSI, Ffytche TJ. Optic disc pigmentation associated with a field defect following chickenpox. J Pediatr Ophthalmol 1976;13:80–83.

381. Altinbasak S, Baytok V, Yalaz M, et al. The Aicardi syndrome. A case report and review of the literature. Turkish J Pediatr 1993;35:305–312.

382. Hamano K, Matsubara T, Shibata S, et al. Aicardi syndrome accompanied by auditory disturbance and multiple brain tumors. Brain Dev 1991;13:438–441.

383. Umansky WS, Neidich JA, Schendel SA. The association of cleft lip and palate with Aicardi syndrome. Plast Reconstructr Surg 1994;93:595–597.

384. Tagawa T, Mimaki T, Ono J, et al. Aicardi syndrome associated with an embryonal carcinoma. Pediatr Neurol 1989;5:45–47.

385. Menezes AV, MacGregor DL, Buncic JR. Aicardi syndrome: Natural history and possible predictors of severity. Pediatr Neurol 1994;11:313–318.

386. Negi VS, Sarin K, Daga MK, et al. A rare case of Aicardi syndrome. JAPI 1994; 42:919–920.

387. Menezes AV, Lewis TL, Buncic JR. The role of ocular involvement in the prediction of visual development and clinical prognosis in Aicardi syndrome. Brit J Ophthalmol 1996;80:805–811.

388. Rosser TL, Acosta MT, Packer RJ. Aicardi syndrome: spectrum of disease and long-term prognosis in 77 females. Pediatr Neurol 2002;77:343–346.

389. Ganesh A, Mitra S, Koul RL, Venugopalan P. The full spectrum of persistent fetal vasculature in Aicardi syndrome: An integrated interpretation of ocular malformations. Br J Ophthalmol 2000;84:227–228.

390. Igidbashian V, Mahboubi S, Zimmerman RA. Clinical Images: CT and MR findings in Aicardi syndrome. J Comp Assist Tomogr 1987;11:357–358.

391. Baieri P, Markl A, Thelen M, et al. MR imaging in Aicardi syndrome. AJNR 1988;9:805–806.

392. Gloor P, Pulido JS, Judisch GF. Magnetic resonance imaging and fundus findings in a patient with Aicardi's syndrome. Arch Ophthalmol 1989;107:922–923.

393. Hall-Craggs MA, Harbord MG, Finn JP, et al. Aicardi syndrome: MR assessment of brain structure myelination. AJNR 1990;11:532–536.

394. de Jong JGY, Delleman JW, Houben M, et al. Agenesis of the corpus callosum, infantile spasms, ocular anomalies (Aicardi's syndrome). Clinical and pathologic findings. Neurology 1976;26:1152–1158.

395. Ferrer I, Cusi MV, Liarte A, et al. A Golgi study of the polymicrogyric cortex in Aicardi syndrome. Brain Dev 1986;8:518–525.

396. Billette de Villemeur T, Chiron C, Robain O. Unlayered polymicrogyria and agenesis of the corpus callosum: A relevant association? Acta Neuropathol 1992; 83:265–270.

397. Neidich JA, Nussbaum RL, Packer RJ, et al. Heterogeneity of clinical severity and molecular lesions in Aicardi syndrome. J Pediatr 1990;116:911–917.

398. Molina, JA, Mateos F, Merino M, et al. Aicardi syndrome in two sisters. J Pediatr 1989;115:282–283.

399. Donnenfeld AE, Graham JM, Packer RJ, et al. Microphthalmia and chorioretinal lacunae in a girl with an Xp22.2–pter deletion and partial 3p trisomy. Am J Med Genet 1990;37:182–186.

400. Ohtahara S, Ohtsuka Y, Yamatogi Y, et al. Prenatal etiologies of West syndrome. Epilepsia 34:716–722, 1993.

401. Nielsen KB, Anvret M, Flodmark O, et al. Aicardi syndrome: Early neuroradiological manifestations and results of DNA studies in one patient. Am J Med Genet 1991;38:65–68.

402. Ropers HH, Zuffardi O, Bianchi E, Tiepolo L. Agenesis of corpus callosum, ocular and skeletal anomalies (X-linked dominant Aicardi's syndrome) in a girl with balanced X/3 translocation. Hum Genet 1982;61:364–368.

403. Donoso LA, Magargal LE, Eiferman RA, Meyer D. Ocular anomalies simulating double optic discs. Can J Ophthalmol 1981;16:87.

404. Collier M. Les doubles papilles optiques. Bull Mem Soc Fr Ophtalmol 1958; 71:328–352.

405. Bonamour MG. A propos des "double papille." Bull Soc Ophtalmol Fr 1964; 64:802–805.

406. von Bajan M, Holmay O. Doppelte sehnervenscheibe bei einem jugendlichen. Klin Monatsbl Augenheilkd 1967;151:207–210.

407. Lamba PA. Doubling of the papilla. Acta Ophthalmol 1969;47:4–9.

408. Aouchiche M, Boyer R, Fetchi A. A propos du diagnostic, des doubles papille. Bull Mem Soc Ophtalmol Fr 1971;84:625–635.

409. Straburzynski J. Double optic disc in patient with Marfan's syndrome. Klin Oczna 1972;42:913–915.

410. Boynton JR, Pheasant TR, Johnson BL, Levin DB, Streeten BW. Ocular findings in Kenny's syndrome. Arch Ophthalmol 1979;97:896–900.

411. Schmidt D, Mathieu M, Schumacher M. Seltene retinale anomalie: Die doppelte papille. Klin Monatsbl Augenheilkd 2003;220:276–280.

412. Snead CM. Congenital division of the optic nerve at the base of the skull. Arch Ophthalmol 1915;44:418–120.

413. Fuchs E. Über den anatomischen Befund einiger angeborener Anomalien der Netzhaut und des Sehnerven. Albrecht Von Graefes Arch Opthalmol 1917;93: 1.

414. Slade HW, Weekley RD. Diastasis of the optic nerve. J Neurosurg 1957;14: 571–574.

415. Collier M. Communications sur le sujet du rapport les doubles papilles optiques. Bull Soc Ophtalmol Fr 1958:328–252.

416. Orcutt JC, Bunt AH. Anomalous optic discs in a patient with a Dandy-Walker cyst. J Clin Neuro Ophthalmol 1982;2:43–47.

417. von Graefe A. Ganzliches fehlen der netzhautgefasse. Albrecht von Graefes Arch Ophthalmol 1854;1:403–404.

418. Retze G. Einige interessante spiegelfalle. Beitrage Augenheilkd Band V. Heft 1902;47:832–845.

419. Meissner W. Ein kolobom der aderhaut und netzhaut mit aplasie des sehnerven. Albrecht von Graefes Arch Ophthalmol 1911;79:308–328.

420. Krauss W. Kongenitale hochgradige veranderungen an der sehnerveneintrittsstelle. Klin Monatsbl Augenheilkd 1920;64:125–126.

421. Renelt P. Beitrag zur eichten papillenaplasie. Albrecht von Graefes Arch Ophthalmol 1972;184:94–98.

422. Little LE, Whitmore PV, Wells TW Jr. Aplasia of the optic nerve. J Pediatr Ophthalmol 1976;13:84–88.

423. Weiter JJ, McLean IW, Zimmerman LE. Aplasia of the optic nerve and disk. Am J Ophthalmol 1977;83:569–576.

424. Yanoff M, Rorke LB, Allman MI. Bilateral optic system aplasia with relatively normal eyes. Arch Ophthalmol 1978;96:97–101.

425. Ginsberg J, Bove KE, Cuesta MG. Aplasia of the optic nerve with aniridia. Ann Ophthalmol 1980;12:433–439.

426. Margo CE, Hamed LM, Fang E, et al. Optic nerve aplasia. Arch Ophthalmol 1992;110:1610–1613.

427. Howard MA, Thompson JT, Howard RO. Aplasia of the optic nerve. Transact Am Acad Ophthalmol 1993;91:276–281.

428. Recupero SM, Lepore GF, Plateroti R, et al. Optic nerve aplasia associated with macular 'atypical coloboma.' Acta Ophthalmol 1994;72:768–770.

429. Storm RL, PeBenito R. Bilateral optic nerve aplasia associated with hydranencephaly. Ann Ophthalmol 1984;16:988–992.

430. Barry DR. Aplasia of the optic nerves. Int Ophthalmol 1985;7:235–242.

431. Shibuya K, Tajima M, Yamate J. Unilateral optic nerve aplasia in an F344 rat with special reference to pathomorphological changes of the optic nerve pathways. J Vet Med Sci 1992;54(3):571–574.

432. Hoff J, Winestock D, Hoyt WF. Giant suprasellar aneurysm associated with optic stalk agenesis and unilateral anophthalmos. J Neurosurg 1975;43:495–498.

433. Duke-Elder S. ed. Congenital deformities. In System of Ophthalmology. Vol 3, Part 2. St Louis, CV Mosby, 1963:661.

434. Straatsma BR, Foos FY, Heckenlively JR, et al. Myelinated retinal nerve fibers. Am J Ophthalmol 1981;91:25–38.

435. Straatsma BR, Heckenlively JR, Foos RY, et al. Myelinated retinal nerve fibers associated with ipsilateral myopia, amblyopia, and strabismus. Am J Ophthalmol 1979;88:506–510.

436. Williams TD. Medullated retinal nerve fibers: Speculations on their cause and presentation of cases. Am J Optometry Physiol Opt 1986;63:142–151.

437. Leys AM, Leys ML, Hooymans JMM, et al. Myelinated nerve fibers and retinal vascular abnormalities. Retina 1996;16:89–96.

438. Tabassian AR, Reddy CV, Folk JC. Retinal vascular abnormalities associated with myelinated nerve fibers. Invest Ophthalmol Visc Sci 1995;36(ARVO Suppl):594.

439. Walsh FB, Hoyt WF. Clinical Neuro-Ophthalmology, Ed 3, Vol 1. Baltimore, Williams & Wilkins, 1969:667.

440. Ellis GS, Frey T, Gouterman RZ. Myelinated nerve fibers, axial myopia, and refractory amblyopia: An organic disease. J Pediatr Ophthalmol Strabismus 1987;24:111–119.

441. Hittner HM, Kretzer FL, Antoszyk JH, et al. Variable expressivity of autosomal dominant anterior segment mesenchymal dysgenesis in six generations. Am J Ophthalmol 1982;93:57–70.

442. De Jong PTVM, Bistervels B, Cosgrove J, et al. Medullated nerve fibers: A sign of multiple basal cell nevi (Gorlin's) syndrome. Arch Ophthalmol 1985; 103:1833–1836.

443. Kronish JW, Tse DT. Basal cell nevus syndrome. In Gold DH, Weingeist TA, eds. The Eye in Systemic Disease. Philadelphia, JB Lippincott, 990:583–585.

444. François J. Myelinated nerve fibers. In Heredity in Ophthalmology, St Louis, Mosby-Year Book, 1961:494–496.

445. Bertelsen TI. The premature synostosis of the cranial sutures. Acta Ophthalmol 1958;51(Suppl):65.

446. Cockburn DM. Tilted disc and medullated nerve fibers. Am J Optom Physiol Opt 1982;59:760–761.

447. Goldsmith J. Neurofibromatosis associated with tumors of the optic papilla. Arch Ophthalmol 1949;41:718–729.

448. Traboulsi EI, Lim JI, Pyeritz R, et al. A new syndrome of myelinated nerve fibers vitreoretinopathy and skeletal malformations. Arch Ophthalmol 1993;111: 1543–1545.

449. Kushner BJ. Optic nerve decompression: Presumed postoperative development of medullated nerve fibers. Arch Ophthalmol 1979;97:1459–1461.

450. Baarsma GS. Acquired medullated nerve fibers. Brit J Ophthalmol 1980;64:651.

451. Aaby AA, Kushner BJ. Acquired and progressive myelinated nerve fibers. Arch Ophthalmol 1985;103:542–544.

452. Wagenmann A. Schwund markhaltiger nervenfasern in der retina in folge von genuiner sehnervenatrophie bei tabes dorsalis. Graefes Arch Clin Exp Ophthalmol 1894;40:250–258.

453. Sachsalber A. Schwund markhaltiger nervenfasern in der netzhaut bei intzundlicher atrophie des sehnerven infolge eines tumor cerebri. Z Augenheilkd 1905; 13:739–750.

454. Fuchs A. Diseases of the Fundus Oculi, London, Lewis, 1951:14.

455. Bachmann R. Schwund markhaltiger nervenfasern in der netzhaut nach embolie der art centralis retinae. Albrecht von Graefes Arch Ophthalmol 1922;107:10.

456. Teich SA. Disappearance of myelinated retinal nerve fibers after a branch retinal artery occlusion. Am J Ophthalmol 1987;103:835–836.

194 CLINICAL NEURO-OPHTHALMOLOGY

457. Sharpe JA, Sanders MD. Atrophy of myelinated nerve fibers in the retina in optic neuritis. Br J Ophthalmol 1975;59:229–232.
458. Schachat AP, Miller NR. Atrophy of myelinated nerve fibers after acute optic neuropathy. Am J Ophthalmol 1981;92:854–856.
459. Kilty LA, Hiles DA. Unilateral posterior lenticonus with posterior hyaloid remnant. Arch Ophthalmol 1993;116:104–106.
460. Savino PJ, Glaser JS, Rosenberg MA. A clinical analysis of pseudo-papilledema. II. Visual field defects. Arch Ophthalmol 1979;97:71–75.
461. Catalano RA, Simon JW. Optic disc elevation in Down syndrome. Am J Ophthalmol 1990;10:28–32.
462. Brodsky MC, Cunniff G. Ocular anomalies in the Alagille syndrome. Ophthalmology 1993;100:1767–1774.
463. Campbell SH, Patterson A. Pseudopapilloedema in the linear naevus syndrome. Br J Ophthalmol 1992;76:372–374.
464. Awan KJ. Hypotelorism and optic disc anomalies: An ignored ocular syndrome. Ann Ophthalmol 1977;9:771–777.
465. Rucker CW. Defects in visual fields produced by hyaline bodies in optic disks. Arch Ophthalmol 1944;32:56–59.
466. Petersen HP. Colloid bodies with defects in field of vision. Acta Ophthalmol 1957;35:243–272.
467. Friedman DH, Beckerman B, Gold DH, et al. Drusen of optic disc. Surv Ophthalmol 1977;21:375–390.
468. Boyce SW, Platia EV, Green WR. Drusen of the optic nerve head. Ann Ophthalmol 1978;10:695–704.
469. Friedman DH, Gartner S, Modi SS. Drusen of the optic disc: A retrospective study in cadaver eyes. Br J Ophthalmol 1975;59:413–421.
470. Rosenberg MA, Savino PJ, Glaser JS. A clinical analysis of pseudo-papilledema. I. Population, laterality, acuity, refractive error, ophthalmoscopic characteristics, and coincident disease. Arch Ophthalmol 1979;97:65–70.
471. François J, Verriest G. Les druses de la papille. Ophthalmologica 1958;136:289–325.
472. Pietruschka G, Priess G. Zur klinischen bedeutung und prognose der drusenpapille. Klin Monatsbl Augenheilkd 1973;162:331–341.
473. Erkkila H. Optic disc drusen in children. Albrecht von Graefes Arch Klin Exp Ophthalmol 1974;189:1–7.
474. Erkkila H. Optic disc drusen in children. Acta Ophthalmol 1977;129:7–44.
475. Hoyt WF, Pont ME. Pseudopapilledema: Anomalous elevation of optic disk. Pitfalls in diagnosis and management. JAMA 1962;181:191–196.
476. Mustonen E. Pseudopapilloedema with and without verified optic disc drusen. A clinical analysis. I. Acta Ophthalmol 1983;61:103 /–1056.
477. Mustonen E. Pseudopapilloedema with and without verified optic disc drusen. A clinical analysis. II. Visual fields. Acta Ophthalmol 1983;61:1057–1066.
478. François J. L'hérédité en ophtalmologie. Paris, Masson, 1958:509–602.
479. Lorentzen SE. Drusen of the optic disk, an irregularly dominant hereditary affection. Acta Ophthalmol 1961;39:626–643.
480. Singleton EM, Kinsbourne M, Anderson WB Jr. Familial pseudopapilledema. S Med J 1973;66:796–802.
481. Mamalis N, Mortenson S, Digre B, et al. Congenital anomalies of the optic nerve in one family. Ann Ophthalmol 1992;24:126–131.
482. Mansour AM, Hamed LM. Racial variation of optic nerve disease. Neuro-ophthalmology 1991;11:319–323.
483. Spencer WH. Drusen of the optic disk and aberrant axoplasmic transport. Am J Ophthalmol 1978;85:1–12.
484. Hoover DL, Robb RM, Petersen RA. Optic disc drusen and primary megalencephaly. J Pediatr Ophthalmol Strabismus 1989;26:81–85.
485. Frisén L, Scholdstrom G, Svendsen P. Drusen in the optic nerve head: Verification by computerized tomography. Arch Ophthalmol 1978;96:1611–1614.
486. Mustonen E, Alanko HI, Nieminen H. Changes in optic disc drusen. Demonstration by stereophotographs and electronic subtraction. Acta Ophthalmol 1982;60:3–15.
487. Miller NR. Appearance of optic disc drusen in a patient with anomalous elevation of the optic disc. Arch Ophthalmol 1986;104:794–795.
488. Mustonen E, Nieminen H. Optic disc drusen—a photographic study. II. Retinal nerve fibre layer photography. Acta Ophthalmol 1982;60:859–872.
489. Morimura Y, Hirakata A, Maeda T. A case of bilateral superficial optic disc drusen. Folia Ophthalmol Jpn 1996;47:1115–1119.
490. Mullie MA, Sanders MD. Scleral canal size and optic nerve head drusen. Am J Ophthalmol 1985;99:356–359.
491. Jonas JB, Gusek GC, Guggenmoss-Holzmann I, et al. Variability of the Real Dimensions of Normal Human Optic Discs. Graefes Arch Clin Exp Ophthalmol 1988;226:332–336.
492. Erkkila H. The central vascular pattern of the eyeground in children with drusen of the optic disk. Albrecht von Graefes Arch Klin Exp Ophthalmol 1976;199:1–10.
493. Borruat FX, Sanders MD. Anomalies et complications vasculaires dans les drusen du nerf Optique. Klin Monatsbl Augenbeiled 1996;208:294–296.
494. Hoyt WF, Knight CL. Comparison of congenital disc blurring and incipient papilledema in red-free light–photographic study. Invest Ophthalmol 1973;12:241–247.
495. Stevens RA, Newman NM. Abnormal visual-evoked potentials from eyes with optic nerve head drusen. Am J Ophthalmol 1981;92:857–862.
496. Knight CL, Hoyt WF. Monocular blindness from drusen of the optic disk. Am J Ophthalmol 1972;73:890–892.
497. Hitchings RA, Corbett JJ, Winkleman J, et al. Hemorrhages with optic disc drusen. Arch Neurol 1976;33:675–677.
498. Miller NR, George TW. Monochromatic (red-free) photography and ophthalmoscopy of the peripapillary retinal nerve fiber layer. In Smith JL, ed. Neuro-Ophthalmology Focus 1980. New York, Masson, 1979:43–51.
499. Ramirez H, Blatt ES, Hibri NS. Computed tomographic identification of calcified optic disc drusen. Radiology 1983;148:137–139.
500. Bec P, Adam P, Mathis A, et al. Optic nerve head drusen: High resolution computed tomographic approach. Arch Ophthalmol 1984;102:680–682.
501. Irnberger T. Diagnosis and differential diagnosis of drusen of the optic papilla with special reference to computed tomography. Fortschritte auf dem Gebiete der Rontgenstrahlen und der Nuklearmedizin. 1984;141:136–139.
502. Chercota V. Computed tomographic aspects of drusen of the optic papilla. Oftalmologia 1994;38:234–238.
503. McNicholas MM, Power WJ, Griffin JF. Sonography in optic disk drusen: imaging clinical role in diagnosis when funduscopic findings are normal. AJR 1994;162:161–163.
504. Pierro L, Brancato R, Minicucci M, et al. Echographic diagnosis of drusen of the optic nerve head in patients with angioid streaks. Ophthalmologica 1994;108:239–242.
505. Kheterpal S, Good PA, Beale DJ, et al. Imaging of optic disc drusen: a comparative study. Eye 1995;9:67–69.
506. Kurz-Levin M, Landau K. A comparison of imaging techniques for diagnosing drusen of the optic nerve head. Arch Ophthalmol 1999;117:1045–1049.
507. Kelley JS. Autofluorescence of drusen of the optic nerve head. Arch Ophthalmol 1974;92:263–264.
508. Mustonen E, Nieminen H. Optic disc drusen—a photographic study. I. Autofluorescence pictures and fluorescein angiography. Acta Ophthalmol 1982;60:849–858.
509. Sanders MD, Ffytche TJ. Fluorescein angiography in the diagnosis of drusen of the disc. Trans Ophthalmol Soc UK 1967;87:457–468.
510. Karel I, Otradovec J, Peleska M. Fluorescein angiography in circulatory disturbances in drusen of the optic disc. Ophthalmologica 1972;164:449–462.
511. Mustonen E, Sulg I, Kallanranta T. Electroretinogram (ERG) and visual evoked response (VER) studies in patients with optic disc drusen. Acta Ophthalmol 1980;58:539–549.
512. Vieregge P, Rosengart A, Mehdorn E, et al. Drusen papilla with vision disorder and pathologic visual evoked potentials. Nervenarzt 1990;61:364–368.
513. Scholl GB, Song HS, Winkler DE, Wray SH. The pattern visual evoked potential and pattern electroretinogram in drusen-associated optic neuropathy. Arch Ophthalmol 1992;110:75–81.
514. Mustonen E, Kallanranta T, Toivakka E. Neurological findings in patients with pseudopapilloedema with and without verified optic disc drusen. Acta Neurol Scandinavia 1983;68:218–230.
515. Rath W. Beitrag zur symptomenlehre der geschwulst der hypophysis cerebri. Albrecht von Graefes Arch Ophthalmol 1888;34:81–130.
516. Lauber H. Drusen des sehnerven. Z Augenhilkd 1913;19:201.
517. Lauber H. Klinische und anatomische untersuchugen uber drusen im sehnervenkopf. Albrecht von Graefes Arch Ophthalmol 1921;105:567–589.
518. Steifel JW, Smith JL. Hyaline bodies (drusen) of the optic nerve and intracranial tumor. Arch Ophthalmol 1961;65:814–816.
519. Mustonen E. Optic disc drusen and tumours of the chiasmal region. Acta Ophthalmol 1977;55:191–200.
520. Harms H. Fall von drusenpapillen. Klin Monatsbl Augenheilkd 1960;136:122.
521. Rucker CW, Kearns TP. Mistaken diagnosis in some cases of meningioma. Am J Ophthalmol 1961;51:15–19.
522. Okun E. Chronic papilledema simulating hyaline bodies of the optic disc. Am J Ophthalmol 1962;53:922–927.
523. Ben Zur PH, Lieberman TW. Drusen of the optic nerves and meningioma: A case report. Mt Sinai Med J 1972;39:188–196.
524. Kurus I. Zur definition der drusenpapille. Ber Dtsch Ophthalmol Ges 1955;59:46–47.
525. Cunningham RD, Sewell JJ. Aneurysm of the ophthalmic artery with drusen of the optic nerve head. Am J Ophthalmol 1971;72:743–745.
526. François P. Les verrucosités hyalines de la papille. Ann Oculis. 1949;182:249–278.
527. Fejer J. Uber die drusen des sehnervenkopfes. Albrecht von Graefes Arch Ophthalmol 1909;72:454–455.
528. Chambers JW, Walsh FB. Hyaline bodies in the optic discs: Report of ten cases exemplifying importance in neurologic diagnosis. Brain 1951;74:95–108.
529. Carter JE, Merren MD, Byrne BM. Pseudodrusen of the optic disc. Papilledema simulating buried drusen of the optic nerve head. J Clin Neuro-ophthalmol 1989;9:273–276.
530. Lansche RK, Rucker CW. Progression of defects in visual fields produced by hyaline bodies in optic disks. Arch Ophthalmol 1957;58:115–121.
531. Reese AB. Relation of drusen of the optic nerve to tuberous sclerosis. Arch Ophthalmol 1940;24:369–371.
532. Miller NR. Sudden visual field constriction associated with optic disc drusen. J Clin Neuroophthalmol 1993;13:14.

533. Moody TA, Irvine AR, Cahn PH, et al. Sudden visual field constriction associated with optic disc drusen. J Clin Neuroophthalmol 1993;13:8–13.
534. Berman EL. Sonography in optic disk drusen. Am J Roentgenol 1995;164:770–771.
535. Barry WE, Tredici TJ. Drusen of the optic disc with visual field defect and Marcus Gunn pupillary phenomenon (Aeromedical consultation service case report). Aerospace Med 1972;43:203–206.
536. Tso MOM. Pathology and pathogenesis of drusen of the optic nervehead. Ophthalmology 1981;88:1066–1080.
537. Pollack IP, Becker B. Hyaline bodies (drusen) of the optic nerve. Am J Ophthalmol 1962;54:651–654.
538. Sanders MD, Gay AJ, Newman M. Hemorrhagic complications of drusen of the optic disc. Am J Ophthalmol 1971;71:204–217.
539. Bishara S, Feinsod M. Visual evoked response as an aid in diagnosing optic nerve head drusen: Case report. J Pediatr Ophthalmol Strabismus 1980;17:396–398.
540. Fanti A, Gatti M, Tosti G, et al. Central vision impairment from optic disk drusen in the young. Metab Pediatr Systemic Ophthalmol 1990;13:85–87.
541. Gallais MP. Pseudo-stase papillaire avec corps hyalins. Rev Otoneuroophthalmol 1952;24:369–371.
542. Brégeat P. L'Oedeme Papillaire. Paris, Masson, 1956.
542a. Brodrick JD: Drusen of the disc and retinal haemorrhages. Br J Ophthalmol 1973;57:299–306.
543. Otradovec J, Vladykova J. Kotazce hemorrhagii venostazy us drusove papily. Sb Lek 1970;72:202–212.
544. Mooney D. Bilateral haemorrhages associated with disc drusen. Trans Ophthalmol Soc UK 1973;93:739–743.
545. Saraux H, Nou B, Audrain G, Offret H. Formes hemorrhagiques des verrucosites hyalines de la papille. J Ophtalmol Fr 1980;3:647–651.
546. Taglioni M, Lemoine L, Sourdille P. Druses de la papille avec hemorrhagies. J Ophtalmol Fr 1980;3:583–587.
547. Harris MJ, Fine SL, Owens S. Hemorrhagic complications of optic nerve drusen. Am J Ophthalmol 1981;92:70–76.
548. Rubenstein K, Ali M. Retinal complications of optic disc drusen. Brit J Ophthalmol 1982;66:83–95.
549. Wise GN, Henkind P, Alterman M. Optic disc drusen and subretinal hemorrhage. Trans Am Acad Ophthalmol Otolaryngol 1974;78:212–219.
550. Gittinger JW, Lessell S, Bondar RL. Ischemic optic neuropathy associated with disc drusen. J Clin Neuroophthalmol 1984;4:79–84.
551. Sarkies NJ, Sanders MD. Optic disc drusen and episodic visual loss. Br J Ophthalmol 1987;71:537–539.
552. Michaelson C, Behrens M, Odel J. Bilateral anterior ischaemic optic neuropathy associated with optic disc drusen and systemic hypotension. Brit J Ophthalmol 1989;73:762–764.
553. Newman WD, Dorrell ED. Anterior ischemic optic neuropathy associated with disc drusen. J Neuroophthalmol 1996;16:7–8.
554. Purcell JJ Jr, Goldberg RE. Hyaline bodies of the optic papilla and bilateral acute vascular occlusions. Ann Ophthalmol 1974;6:1069–1076.
555. ten Doesschate MJ, Manschot WA. Optic disc drusen and central retinal vein occlusion. Docum Ophthalmol 1985;59:27–31.
556. Lodato G. Hemorrhagic complications in drusen of the optic papilla. J Fr Ophtalmologie 1986;9:567–572.
557. Masuyama Y, Kodama Y, Matsuura Y, et al. Clinical studies on the occurrence and the pathogenesis of optociliary veins. J Clin Neuro Ophthalmology 1990;10:1–8.
558. Chern S, Magargal LE, Annesley WH. Central retinal vein occlusion associated with drusen of the optic disc. Ann Ophthalmol 1991;23:66–69.
559. Austin JK. Optic disc drusen and associated venous stasis retinopathy. J Am Optom Assoc 1995;66:91–5.
560. Gifford H. An unusual case of hyaline bodies in the optic nerve. Arch Ophthalmol 1895;24:395.
561. Giarelli L, Ravalico G, Saviano S, et al. Optic nerve head drusen: Histopathological considerations—clinical features. Metab Pediatr Systemic Ophthalmol 1990;13:88–91.
562. Sadun AA, Currie JN, Lessell S. Transient visual obscurations with elevated optic discs. Ann Neurol 1984;6:489–494.
563. Henkind P, Alterman M, Wise GN. Drusen of the optic disc and subretinal and subpigment epithelial hemorrhage. In Cant JS, ed. The Optic Nerve. London, Henry Kimpton, 1972:281.
564. Brown SM, Del Monte MA. Choroidal neovascular membrane associated with optic nerve head drusen in a child. Am J Ophthalmol 1996;121:215–216.
565. Saudax E, Martin-Beuzart S, Lesure P, et al. Subretinal neovascular membrane and drusen of the optic disk. J Fr Ophtalmologie 1990;13:219–222.
566. Sullu Y, Yildiz L, Erkan D. Submacular surgery for choroidal neovascularization secondary to optic nerve drusen. Am J Ophthalmol 2003;136:367–370.
567. Moisseiev J, Cahane M, Treister G. Optic nerve head drusen and peripapillary central serous chorioretinopathy. Am J Ophthalmol 1989;108:202–203.
568. Müller, H. Anatomische beitrage zur ophthalmologie. Part 8. Albrecht von Graefes Arch Ophthalmol 1858;4:1–40.
569. Tobler T. Uber kalkdrusen in der papille des nervus opticus und uber kombination derselben mit zystoider entartung der macula lutea. Z Augenheilkd 1922;47:215–230.
570. Samuels B. Drusen of the optic papilla: A clinical and pathologic study. Arch Ophthalmol 1941;25:412–423.
571. Seitz R, Kersting G. Die drusen der sehnervenpapille und des pigmentepithels. Klin Monatsbl Augenheilkd 1962;140:75–88.
572. Antcliff R, Spalton DJ. Are optic disc drusen inherited? Ophthalmology 1999;106:1278–1281.
573. Seitz R. Die intraokularen drusen klin monatsbl augenheilkd. 1968;152:203–211.
574. Sacks JG, O'Grady RB, Choromokos E, et al. The pathogenesis of optic nerve drusen: A hypothesis. Arch Ophthalmol 1977;95:425–428.
575. Spencer WH. In Discussion of Tso MOM: Pathology and pathogenesis of drusen of the optic nervehead. Ophthalmology 1981;88:1079–1080.
576. Morton AS, Parsons JH. Hyaline bodies at the optic disc. Trans Ophthalmol Soc UK 1903;23:135–153.
577. Oliver GH. Hyaline bodies at the optic disc in a case of retinitis pigmentosa. Ophthalmoscope 1913;11:716–718.
578. Walker CH. Diseases of the retina and optic nerve: A case of hyaline bodies at the disc. Trans Ophthalmol Soc UK 1915;35:366–370.
579. Robertson DM. Hamartomas of the optic disk with retinitis pigmentosa. Am J Ophthalmol 1972;74:526–531.
580. Pillai S, Limaye SR, Saimovici LB. Optic disc hamartoma associated with retinitis pigmentosa. Retina 1983;3:24–26.
581. Puck A, Tso MOM, Fishman GA. Drusen of the optic nerve associated with retinitis pigmentosa. Arch Ophthalmol 1985;103:231–234.
582. Shiono T, Noro M, Tamai M. Presumed drusen of the optic nerve head in siblings with Usher syndrome. Jpn J Ophthalmol 1991;35:300–305.
583. Edwards A, Grover S, Fishman GA. Frequency of photographically apparent optic disc and parapapillary nerve fiber layer drusen in Usher syndrome. Retina 1996;16:388–392.
584. Sebag J, Albert DM, Craft JL. The Alström syndrome: Ophthalmic histopathology and retinal ultrastructure. Brit J Ophthalmol 1984;68:494–501.
585. Young WO, Small KW. Pigmented paravenous retinochoroidal atrophy (PPRCA) with optic disc drusen. Ophthalmol Pediatr Genet 1993;1:23–29.
586. Heidemann DG, Beck RW. Retinitis pigmentosa. A mimic of neurological disease. Surv Ophthalmol 1987;32:45–51.
587. Lorentzen SE. Drusen of the optic disc. A clinical and genetic study. Acta Ophthalmol 1966;90(Suppl):1–181.
588. Erkkila H, Raitta C, Niemi KM. Ocular findings in four siblings with pseudoxanthoma elasticum. Acta Ophthalmol 1983;61:589–599.
589. Gass JMD. Stereoscopic Atlas of Macular Diseases: Diagnosis and Treatment. Vol 2. St Louis, CV Mosby, 1987:103–106, 470–475, 746–751.
590. Coleman K, Hope-Ross M, McCabe M, et al. Disk drusen and angioid streaks in pseudoxanthoma elasticum. Am J Ophthalmol 1991;112:166–170.
591. Giuffre' G. Chorioretinal degenerative changes in the tilted disc syndrome. Int Ophthalmol 1991;15:1–7.
592. Mansour AM. Is there an association between optic disc drusen and angioid streaks? Graefes Arch Clin Exp Ophthalmol 1992;230:595–596.
593. Riley HD, Smith RW. Macrocephaly, pseudopapilledema, and multiple hemangiomata. Pediatrics 1960;26:293–300.
594. Dvir M, Beer S, Aladjem M. Heredofamilial syndrome of mesodermal hamartomas, macrocephaly, and pseudopapilledema. Pediatrics 1988;81:287–290.
595. Paes-Alves AF, Azevedo ES, Sousa MDGF, et al. Autosomal recessive malformation syndrome with minor manifestation in the heterozygotes: A preliminary report of a possible new syndrome. Am J Med Genet 1991;41:141–152.
596. Webb NR, McCrary JA. Hyaline bodies of the optic disc and migraine. In Smith JL, ed. Neuro-Ophthalmology Update. New York, Masson, 1977:155–162.
597. Wisotsky BJ, Magat-Gordon CB, Puklin JE. Vitreopapillary traction as a cause of elevated optic nerve head. Am J Ophthalmol 1998;126:137–139.

CHAPTER 4

Topical Diagnosis of Acquired Optic Nerve Disorders

Alfredo A. Sadun and Madhu R. Agarwal

DISTINGUISHING AN OPTIC NEUROPATHY FROM RETINAL DISEASE

Severe optic neuropathies associated with syndromes and producing profound losses of optic nerve functions may be obvious. However, mild optic neuropathies may only produce subtle impairments of visual function and be difficult to diagnose. When the optic discs appear normal and the visual field defects do not have a classical pattern, distinguishing such a mild optic neuropathy from retinal disease may be difficult. For example, optic neuritis can be an easy diagnosis, but when it produces very mild loss of vision, it may be easily confused with central serous retinopathy. Both occur in young adults and can present as acute, painless, mild monocular visual loss. The relative absence of fundus findings in such patients further challenges the clinician in sorting out the differential diagnosis. However, since optic nerve disease may be the harbinger of intracranial pathology, and both optic nerve and retinal diseases are often amenable to a variety of therapeutic modalities, it is important for the clinician to make the early and accurate distinction between an optic neuropathy and macular or other retinal disease.

The most common optic neuropathies in adults are optic neuritis and nonarteritic anterior ischemic optic neuropathy. The cell that is injured in these disorders, or in any optic neuropathy, is the retinal ganglion cell. Often, its axon undergoes degeneration and then anterograde degeneration results in optic atrophy. Retinal diseases may arise from a variety of lesions of the outer or inner retina or choroid and significant improvement in visual function is often possible.

Retinal diseases may be divided into two main groups: (*a*) those affecting the detecting apparatus, i.e., the receptor cells and their synapses; and (*b*) those affecting the conducting apparatus, i.e., the ganglion cell and nerve fiber layer. In many cases, the diagnosis is obvious from the appearance of the affected region of the retina. In other cases, however, it may be possible to diagnose retinal dysfunction from other aspects of the clinical examination. Patients with ''unexplained visual loss'' may, in fact, have a disorder of the retina that may not be obvious during a clinical examination. Indeed, even when the examination of the ocular fundus is performed with a 90-diopter hand-held lens, or direct ophthalmoscope, a retinal disorder may be missed.

DIFFERENTIATION BY HISTORY

It is important to elicit from the patient the timing (tempo) of the visual loss, including the onset and course of each of the symptoms. For example, optic neuritis often develops over a few days, stabilizes and then shows improvement over a period of weeks. Anterior ischemic optic neuropathy begins suddenly with little by way of progression or resolution thereafter (1). Central serous retinopathy, by comparison, often comes on more insidiously.

The nature of the visual loss needs to be characterized in the history as well. Loss of visual acuity from optic nerve disease is usually perceived as a darkening. Patients may

Table 4.1
Distinguishing Optic Neuropathies and Maculopathies

Features	Optic Nerve	Macula
Presenting deficit	Central dark cloud	Distortions
Pain (rarely)	Sometimes with eye movement	Rarely
Refractive error	Unchanged	Sometimes hyperopia
Visual acuity	Variable	Markedly impaired
Afferent pupillary defect	Present	Absent
Color vision	Very reduced	Slightly reduced
Brightness sense	Very reduced	Variable
Amsler grid	Scotoma	Metamorphopsia

describe this as a black, gray, or brown patch or more generally as a generalized dimness across portions of the visual field (1). There is darkening, or desaturation of colors and a loss of color contrast. Patients may see worse when the lighting is hazy. Some optic neuropathies produce phosphenes (positive visual phenomenon, often in the form of bright spots or sparkles). Pain, especially with eye movements, is part of the presentation of several optic neuropa-

thies (Table 4.1). By comparison, patients with retinal disease, especially maculopathies, most often note metamorphopsia in the central visual field (2). Objects look distorted and straight lines become irregularly curved. Micropsia (seeing everything slightly minimized) is more common than macropsia. Patients with retinal disease that involves the macula also complain of mild photophobia or glare. Instead of seeing a central patch that is too dim, as in optic neuropa-

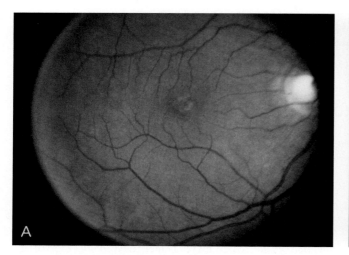

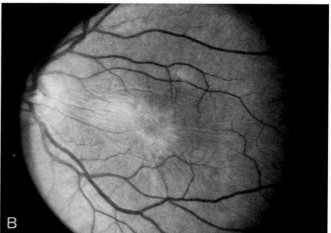

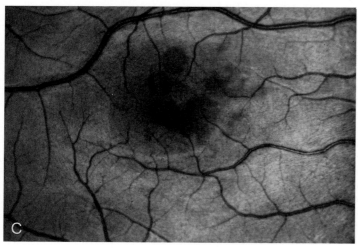

Figure 4.1. Subtle macular lesions causing visual loss. *A*, Pigment changes in right macula of a patient with "unexplained" central visual loss. *B*, Epiretinal membrane in the left macula of a patient complaining of blurred vision in the eye. *C*, Changes in the right macula of a patient who complained of decreased central vision in the eye after blunt ocular trauma. It was initially suspected that he had a traumatic optic neuropathy or was malingering.

thies, such patients often note a zone that appears as too bright (3).

DIFFERENTIATION BY PHYSICAL EXAMINATION

Visual acuity is nearly always impaired in macular disease and often in optic neuropathies. The issue often comes to the extent of loss of vision in comparison to the three common measures of optic nerve function. This optic nerve triad consists of the relative afferent pupillary defect (APD), color vision and brightness sense (4–6). An APD is seen when the consensual pupillary response is greater than the direct pupillary response. This is noted qualitatively, or it can be quantitated with the use of neutral density filters (5). Color vision is best assessed with a Farnsworth-Munsell 100-hue (FM-100) test (6). However, shorter and more convenient tests are often performed, such as the D-15 which is the desaturated form of the FM-100, or the use of pseudoisochromatic plates of the A-O or Ishihara type. A third sensitive measure of optic nerve function is noting the change in brightness sense. This can be performed subjectively or with some quantitative objectivity through the use of a device that uses cross-polarizing filters to diminish light transmission as a match of the perceived brightness-sense disparity (3). In optic neuropathies, these three measures of optic nerve function are usually greatly diminished in proportion to the loss of visual acuity. While there might be some slight loss of these functions in retinal disease as well, this is usually in the setting of a profound loss of visual acuity (Table 4.1).

Visual Acuity

Central vision may or may not be affected by disease that damages the retina. Disorders that cause dysfunction only of extramacular retina typically are unassociated with a reduction in central acuity, whereas macular disorders and disorders that damage the entire retina invariably reduce central vision. Most disorders that affect the macula are easily detected by a careful funduscopic examination, particularly when the macula is examined with a slit lamp biomicroscope using a corneal contact lens, a 78- or 90-diopter handheld lens. Nevertheless, some disorders, such as central serous chorioretinopathy, cystoid macular edema, and epiretinal membrane formation (surface wrinkling retinopathy, cellophane maculopathy) can easily be overlooked (Fig. 4.1). In other diseases that affect the macula, such as macular cone dystrophy, there are often no changes that can be observed in the macula, even though the patient has decreased central vision and a visual field defect. In such cases, the diagnosis of retinal disease may be suspected if there is associated metamorphopsia (an irregularity or distortion in the appearance of viewed objects), photophobia, nyctalopia (night blindness), or hemeralopia (the inability to see as distinctly in a bright light as in a dim one). These symptoms occur much more often in patients with ocular disease than in patients with neurologic disease (7–12). Photophobia should be obvious during the examination. Evidence of metamorphopsia may be detected in patients with and without the complaint of distortion of objects by using an Amsler grid

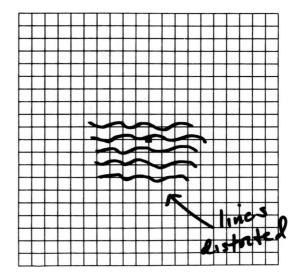

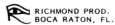

RICHMOND PROD.
BOCA RATON, FL.

Figure 4.2. Distortion of lines on Amsler grid in a patient with unilateral visual loss. The patient had central serous chorioretinopathy.

(Fig. 4.2). The results of a photostress test usually are abnormal in such patients (13–15), as are the results of fluorescein angiography, focal electroretinography (16–19), or both.

Color Vision

Color vision is often but not always abnormal in patients with retinal disease. For instance, patients with central serous chorioretinopathy and epiretinal membrane formation rarely have any significant dyschromatopsia, whereas patients with macular cone or cone-rod dystrophies usually do (20); such patients may even develop difficulties with color vision as the initial sign of the disease (21). In such cases, the correct diagnosis is not made until other studies such as photostress testing, fluorescein angiography, or electroretinography are performed. Retinal disorders are more likely to produce either generalized loss of color vision or a blue-yellow dyschromatopsia (22–24), but there are sufficient exceptions that make the pattern of color vision loss an unreliable diagnostic criterion.

Afferent Pupillary Defect

A relative afferent pupillary defect can be detected clinically as well as with neutral density filters in patients with unilateral or asymmetric retinal disease. In most cases, the retinal disease is severe, affects most of the retina or the entire macula, and is obvious during a funduscopic examination (25–27). If a relative afferent pupillary defect is observed in a patient with decreased visual acuity associated with some macular drusen, central serous chorioretinopathy, cystoid macular edema, an epiretinal membrane, or a normal-appearing fundus, a lesion affecting the optic nerve should be suspected.

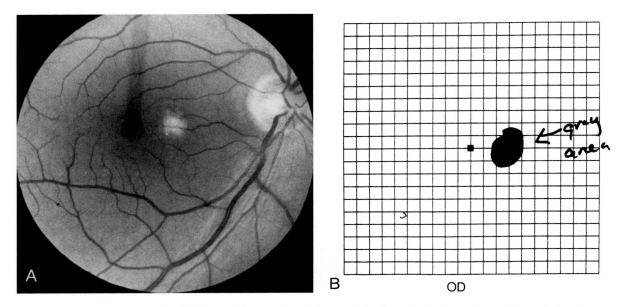

Figure 4.3. Variation in visual fields caused by posterior pole lesions. *A*, Small chorioretinal scar in the papillomacular bundle adjacent to right fovea. Because this lesion is located in the deep retina at the level of the photoreceptors and retinal pigment epithelium, it produces only a small central scotoma (*B*).

DIFFERENTIATION BY VISUAL FIELD

Peripheral Retina

When the photoreceptors are affected, the defect in the visual field corresponds to the retinal defect in position, shape, extent, and intensity (28). When the ganglion cell or nerve fiber layer is damaged, however, the field defect does not conform to the size and shape of the lesion but rather to the field represented by the ganglion cells whose fibers are damaged. Thus, a small lesion situated close to the optic disc that damages only photoreceptors usually causes a small scotoma, whereas a lesion of the same size that damages the ganglion cells and nerve fibers in the same area may result in an extensive defect in the visual field (Fig. 4.3). Conversely, a small lesion in the periphery that damages only a few fibers transmitting impulses from widely separated ganglion cells may produce such a small field defect that it may be difficult or even impossible to detect.

Diseases that cause photoreceptor damage usually produce a greater loss of the visual field when it is tested with blue stimuli than when it is tested with red stimuli (28). This observation is useful because the situation is reversed in disorders that damage the conducting apparatus of the retina. In lesions of the ganglion cells, retinal nerve fiber layer, and optic nerve, there usually is a more pronounced loss of the visual field for red than for blue.

If a lesion superotemporal or inferotemporal to the optic disc damages peripheral visual fibers, the field defect is arcuate in shape because the fibers from peripheral ganglion cells arch around the papillomacular bundle (Fig. 4.4). The field defect is, of course, situated nasal to the blind spot. If the lesion is nasal to the optic disc, it damages a nasal bundle. The resultant field defect is temporal and fan-shaped, be-

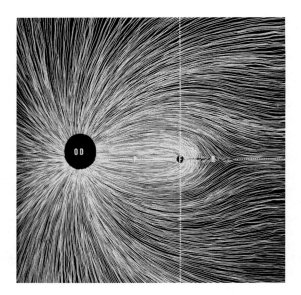

Figure 4.4. Anatomy of the retinal nerve fiber layer and retinal origin of arcuate visual field defect produced by a chorioretinal scar. *A*, Drawing of the normal pathway of retinal nerve fiber layer axons. The axons that originate from ganglion cells superior, inferior, and nasal to the optic disc (OD) take a fairly straight course to the disc, as do the axons in the papillomacular bundle (P) that originate from ganglion cells nasal to the fovea (F) but temporal to the disc. The courses of axons from peripheral ganglion cells temporal to the disc are arched. N, nasal retina; R, horizontal raphe; T, temporal retina. The *dotted lines* delineate the nasal, temporal, superior, and inferior portions of the retina. (Redrawn from Hogan MJ, Alvarado JA, Weddell JE. Histology of the Human Eye: An Atlas and Textbook. Philadelphia, WB Saunders, 1971.)

cause fibers from ganglion cells located nasal to the optic disc take a direct path to the disc.

An arcuate defect in the visual field may indicate a defect in the nerve fiber layer. When such a retinal lesion is present, it usually can be identified by ophthalmoscopic examination. Because of the anatomy of the temporal raphe that separates fibers from ganglion cells located above the horizontal midline from those from ganglion cells below the horizontal midline, there is often a sharp dividing line between the area

of the scotoma and the functioning upper or lower field. This is particularly evident in large arcuate scotomas, so much so that visual fields performed on tangent screen or by automated static perimetry may suggest complete loss of the superior or inferior hemifield unless the entire field is tested (Fig. 4.5).

Retinal photoreceptors (by way of intermediaries) project to ganglion cells, and the axons of the ganglion cells comprise the nerve fiber layer which, in turn, makes up the optic

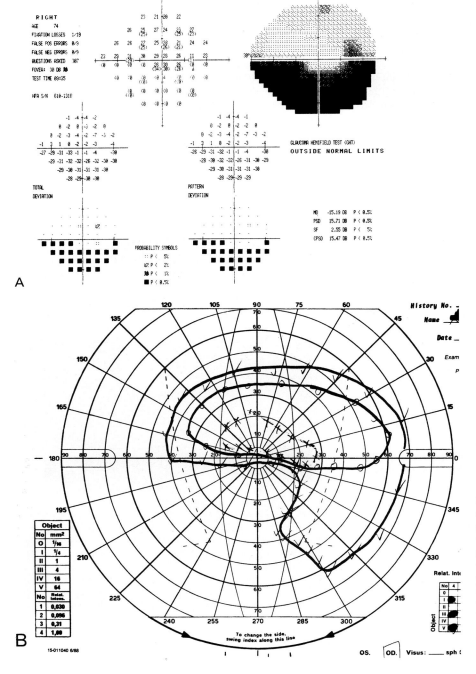

Figure 4.5. Arcuate visual field defect that appears altitudinal when only the central field is tested. The patient was a 74-year-old man who experienced an attack of nonarteritic anterior ischemic optic neuropathy. Visual acuity was 20/30 in the affected right eye. *A,* Static perimetry demonstrates a ''complete'' inferior altitudinal defect. *B,* Kinetic perimetry shows that the defect identified on static perimetry is actually a scotoma. The actual field defect is arcuate in nature, and the remaining field is larger than might have been expected from the results of static perimetry.

nerve. Clearly, then, any visual field defect that can be produced by a retinal lesion can also be produced by a lesion of the optic nerve (29). Ophthalmoscopic evidence pointing to the retina as the site of the lesion is conclusive, but, as noted in the section below, lack of an ophthalmoscopically visible retinal abnormality does not necessarily indicate that the retina is not the site of the lesion.

Central Retina

Most visual field defects in the central fields that are caused by retinal lesions are associated with ophthalmoscopically visible changes. In patients with macular lesions, the field defects are those already described as resulting from lesions of the receptor cells; that is, the field defect occupies an area consistent with the size of the lesion. However, some macular lesions that produce a central scotoma cannot be easily detected by ophthalmoscopy. In most of these cases, small lesions of the retina or retinal pigment epithelium may be diagnosed using red-free ophthalmoscopy, slit lamp biomicroscopy with a contact lens or a 90- or 78-diopter hand-held lens, fluorescein angiography, or a combination of these techniques. In other cases, the diagnosis cannot be made without a focal electroretinogram (ERG).

Multifocal ERG (mfERG) relies on multiple samples of ERG responses from different parts of the retina. Computed localization is made by Fourier transform analysis (30–32). Like a visual field, this technology can map out retinal impairments (33). Furthermore, an optic nerve head component (ONHC) can be dissected out through an algorithm that takes into account the distance from the optic disc (34). This new methodology has much promise in the diagnosis of regional retinal diseases.

Of course, not all monocular field defects are caused by organic retinal or optic nerve lesions. Patients with nonor-

ganic disease can produce spurious central, paracentral, and even quadrantanopic and hemianopic field defects, regardless of whether they are tested with kinetic or static perimetric techniques (35–41). It should also be emphasized that a spurious central or paracentral scotoma may be charted if the central field of an eye with a high refractive error or under a cycloplegic is plotted without correction for the refractive error (42).

Symptoms of metamorphopsia or micropsia are caused by distortion or displacement of the retinal photoreceptors. Metamorphopsia is usually caused by a distortion of the normal alignment of the photoreceptors. When there is increased separation among cones (and among rods to a lesser extent because of the central position of the lesion), there is an apparent decrease in the size of objects (micropsia). The foveal cones are already so close to each other that it is unlikely that an apparent increase in the size of objects (macropsia) can occur from further crowding together of these cells.

Changes in the apparent size of viewed objects usually result from primary retinal damage. Such symptoms may also be described by patients with acquired cerebral disorders that affect perception (e.g., migraine) (43–45), although the phenomenon should occur in both eyes simultaneously in that setting. One case of micropsia associated with myasthenia gravis has been reported in which the authors postulated that the symptom was caused by overconvergence (46,47).

Cecocentral Scotomas

Damage to the papillomacular area of the retina results in a central scotoma that connects to the physiologic blind spot; this is a cecocentral scotoma (Fig. 4.6). A cecocentral scotoma may result from damage to the papillomacular bundle

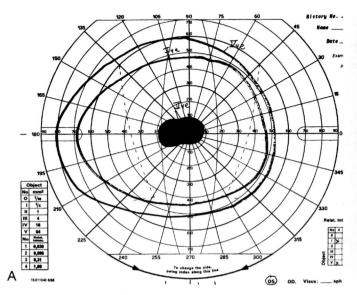
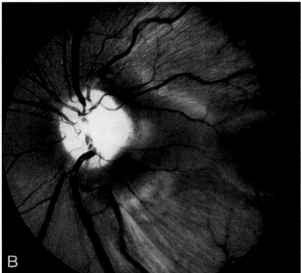

Figure 4.6. Cecocentral scotoma caused by a lesion in the papillomacular bundle. *A,* The patient has a small cecocentral scotoma in the visual field of the left eye. *B,* There is a serous detachment of the retina in the papillomacular bundle of the left eye, associated with a temporal optic pit.

alone or may occur in conjunction with peripheral contraction of the visual field (48).

Arcuate (Nonglaucomatous) Defects

An arcuate visual field defect usually results from damage to retinal nerve fibers or ganglion cells in the superior or inferior arcuate nerve fiber bundles. In such cases, there is a central field defect that is not circular but instead is limited above or below by the horizontal meridian. This visual field defect may occur in patients with occlusion of the blood supply of the superior or inferior portion of the macula or in patients with glaucoma (49). In both settings, the scotoma is associated with normal visual acuity, since it does not completely affect the macula. Virtually any lesion, whether ischemic, inflammatory, infiltrative, or compressive, can cause an arcuate field defect and, as noted above, may be located in either the retina or the optic nerve.

A roughly circular pericentral scotoma may be observed in patients with macular or papillomacular disease. Such a scotoma, when unilateral, always indicates damage to the macula. When bilateral pericentral scotomas are present, there is usually bilateral macular disease; however, bilateral "pericentral" scotomas can develop from lesions that damage the posterior aspects of both occipital poles. When such lesions occur bilaterally at the occipital tips, bilateral "central" scotomas occur. Actually, these visual field defects are bilateral homonymous scotomas, and kinetic or static perimetry will generally disclose a vertical step between the two hemianopic scotomas, indicating their true nature (50) (Fig. 4.7).

Annular or ring scotomas occur in a variety of conditions, most notably in patients with various pigmentary retinopathies. Ring scotomas may also occur in patients with open angle glaucoma, but in such cases, the ring is actually caused by the coalescence of upper and lower arcuate scotomas originating from the physiologic blind spot and extending across the vertical midline into the nasal visual field (51). Rarer causes of annular or ring scotomas include retinitis, choroiditis, blinding by diffuse light, retinal migraine, mal-

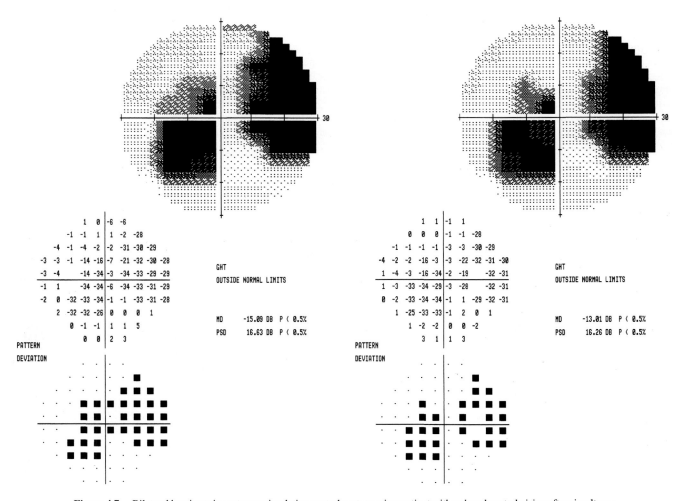

Figure 4.7. Bilateral hemianopic scotomas simulating central scotomas in a patient with reduced central vision after simultaneous bilateral occipital lobe infarctions.

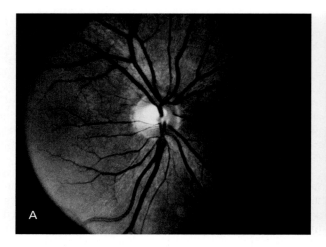
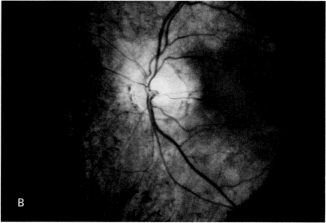

Figure 4.8. Optic atrophy in unilateral retinitis pigmentosa. *A,* The right optic disc is normal. Note healthy color of the disc and normal-appearing peripapillary retinal nerve fiber layer. *B,* The left optic disc is pale. Note marked pigmentary change in the posterior pole, as well as marked narrowing of the retinal arteries. (Courtesy of Dr. Daniel Finkelstein.)

nutrition, and myopia (52). Similar defects may be seen in various optic neuropathies, particularly those caused by ischemia, compression, and inflammation. The width of such scotomas varies within wide limits, but the ring is rarely less than 5–6° in width, and may be much wider. Occasionally, ring or annular scotomas are found in patients with nonorganic visual loss. In such patients, the scotomas are typically very narrow.

A ring scotoma can be detected in most types of pigmentary retinopathy (e.g., retinitis pigmentosa) if the visual field is carefully examined. In some cases, however, the periph-

eral field is so contracted and central vision so reduced that the ring scotoma may not be detected even when careful perimetry is performed. A ring scotoma may also persist after incomplete resolution of a preexisting central scotoma in patients with retinal or optic nerve disease.

In general, a unilateral temporal or nasal hemianopia that respects the vertical midline is either nonorganic or caused by dysfunction of the optic nerve (see below). Nevertheless, a unilateral temporal hemianopia rarely can be caused by sectoral retinitis pigmentosa (53).

The optic nerve is composed primarily of axons whose

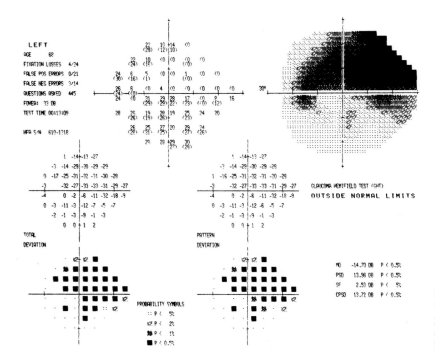

Figure 4.9. Arcuate visual field in a 68-year-old woman with open-angle glaucoma. Static perimetry, using a Humphrey perimeter to perform a 24-2 Threshold Test, reveals a superior arcuate defect located within the central 30° from fixation.

cell bodies are the ganglion cells of the retina. Any retinal disorder that directly or indirectly damages the ganglion cells or their axons in the retinal nerve fiber layer will produce optic atrophy. Loss of the nerve fiber layer and optic atrophy are not uncommon in patients with various photoreceptor dystrophies and degenerations, particularly those affecting the cones (20,54–60) (Fig. 4.8).

Glaucomatous Optic Neuropathy

The visual field defects in chronic open angle glaucoma occur from damage to nerve fiber bundles at the level of the lamina within the optic nerve head (61). This damage seems to occur focally in its initial stages and is thus expressed in the visual field as isolated scotomas appearing between 5° and 30° from fixation in the arcuate or Bjerrum area (51,62–64) (Fig. 4.9). About two-thirds of these isolated paracentral or arcuate scotomas are accompanied by a depression in sensitivity in the upper or lower half of the field. This loss of sensitivity appears initially as a step in a plotted isopter, usually at the nasal, horizontal meridian (the nasal step of Rönne) (28,65) (Fig. 4.10). One-third of early

paracentral scotomas that occur in patients with chronic open angle glaucoma have no associated nasal step and, even less frequently, a nasal step is present without a paracentral scotoma. As damage proceeds, the paracentral scotoma becomes deeper, wider, or both, and new scotomas may develop in the same arcuate region. As these defects coalesce, they take on an arching shape between the nasal horizontal meridian and the blind spot. Isolated enlargement or elongation of the blind spot is a relatively nonspecific finding and is not considered diagnostic for glaucomatous damage, although it may indicate a general depression in visual sensitivity. Defects in the field temporal to the blind spot occur in early glaucomatous damage, but are much less frequent (66). As arcuate scotomas enlarge and affect both the upper and lower regions, they may meet at the horizontal meridian and produce a ring-shaped scotoma, as noted above. Further damage results in the breaking out of the scotoma to the peripheral field, so-called "baring" to the periphery. Thus, patients with advanced glaucoma may retain only the central 5° and a temporal island of vision.

Although the visual field defects that occur in chronic

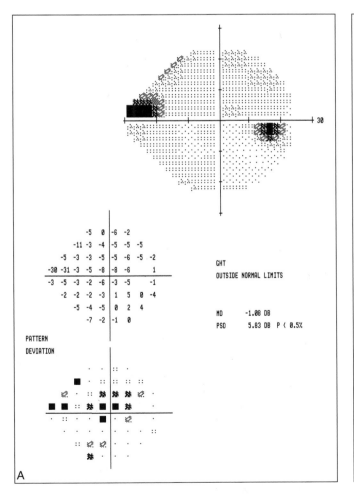

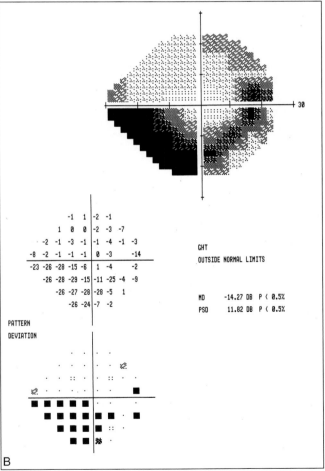

Figure 4.10. Field changes in various patients with glaucomatous optic neuropathy. *A,* Superior nasal step in right eye. *B,* Inferior arcuate field defect in right eye. *(Figure continues.)*

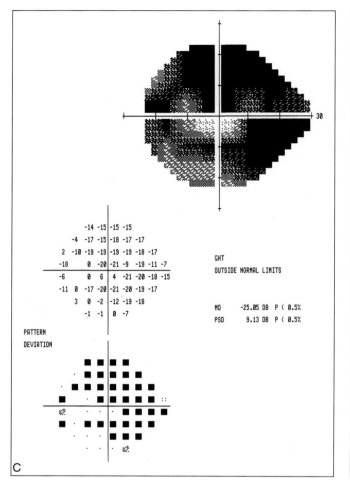

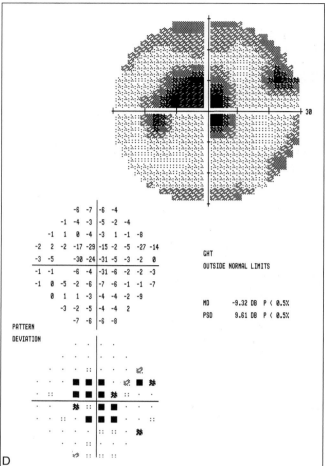

Figure 4.10. Continued. *C*, Progression of inferior and superior arcuate defects in left eye. *D*, Central field loss in left eye. In the cases in which central field loss is seen in glaucoma, the horizontal meridian is usually respected, as in this case.

open angle glaucoma may be identical with defects that result from various types of nonglaucomatous optic neuropathy, the differentiation between glaucoma and nonglaucomatous optic neuropathy is made by history and examination. Most patients with chronic open angle glaucoma develop loss of visual field long before they experience loss of central vision, although exceptions indeed occur. Color vision deficits are typically of the blue-yellow type (67–80) but again, exceptions regularly occur, and red-green deficits are not uncommon (81). A relative afferent pupillary defect is not uncommon in cases of unilateral or asymmetric glaucoma (82–86).

Patients with glaucoma develop visual field defects only after there is extensive damage to the optic disc. The ophthalmoscopic appearance of such a disc is typical: in nearly every such case, there is substantial cupping of the disc with the remaining neuroretinal rim appearing relatively normal, without evidence of pallor, and with diffuse thinning of the retinal nerve fiber layer (Fig. 4.11*A* and *B*). This is in contrast to other types of optic nerve diseases producing similar visual field defects, in which the optic disc may appear normal

(Fig. 4.11*C*), diffusely or sectorally pale without enlargement in the size of the cup (Fig. 4.11*D*), or pale with substantial cupping but also with pallor of the remaining neuroretinal rim (Fig. 4.11*E*) (87–91). Thus, when the optic disc and retinal nerve fiber layer findings are considered in a patient with various visual field defects, it is rarely difficult to differentiate glaucoma from other diseases producing such defects.

The Blind Spot

The blind spot also plays a role in the interpretation of the visual field. It represents the negative scotoma that is the projection of the optic disc. The optic disc is located nasal to the fovea, and its center is slightly above it. Thus, the blind spot is temporal to the point of fixation, and its center is slightly below it.

The dimensions of the blind spot have already been noted; however, it is important to be aware that the blind spot has both an absolute and a relative portion. The relative portion is a band, about 1° in width, that surrounds the absolute

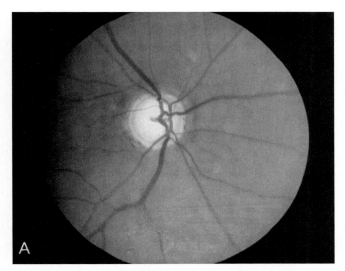

Figure 4.11. Appearance of optic disc in patient with glaucomatous field loss, compared with varied appearances of optic discs with nonglaucomatous field loss. *A*, Right optic disc in an eye with glaucomatous field loss. Note moderate cupping with preservation of normal color of remaining neuroretinal rim. *B*, In another patient with glaucoma, the right optic disc is markedly cupped, but the remaining neuroretinal rim (from about 12 to 7 o'clock) retains its normal color. *C*, In a patient with 20/20 visual acuity and visual field loss similar to that seen in glaucoma, the right optic disc is normal in appearance. The patient had experienced an attack of retrobulbar neuritis several days earlier. *D*, Appearance of left optic disc in a patient with good visual acuity but significant visual field loss in the left eye after an attack of optic neuritis. Note diffuse pallor of the disc without obvious cupping. *E*, Appearance of the left optic disc after an attack of anterior ischemic optic neuropathy in the setting of temporal arteritis. The disc is diffusely pale and cupped. Note that the remaining neuroretinal rim, particularly temporally, is as pale as the cupped portion of the disc.

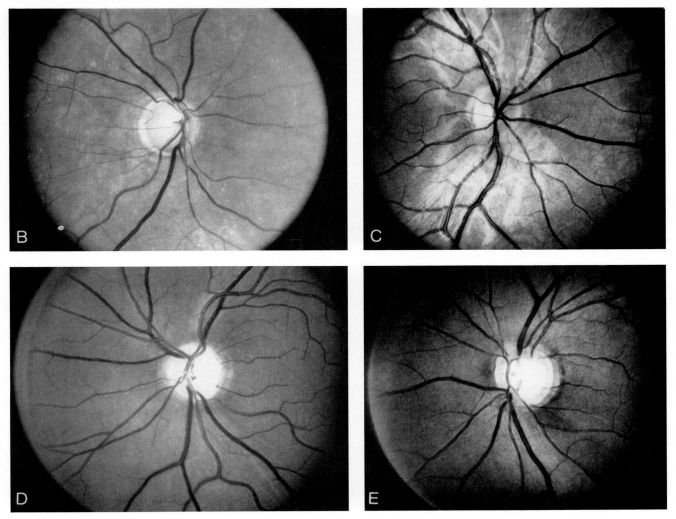

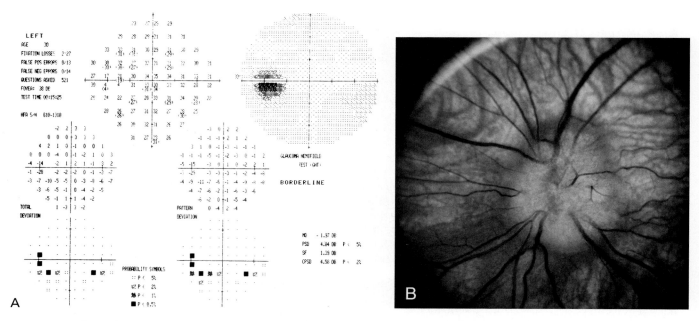

Figure 4.12. *A*, Enlargement of the blind spot in a 30-year-old obese woman with headaches. *B*, Appearance of left optic disc, showing chronic swelling. An evaluation revealed increased intracranial pressure.

scotoma. In this band, white objects of 1–2 mm can be seen when a subject is tested at 2 meters (28). This zone of relative scotoma is caused by the gradual rather than abrupt termination of the retina at the edge of the optic disc (28), and in it metamorphopsia can often be demonstrated (92).

Undoubtedly, then, the blind spot becomes larger when small or less bright test objects are used to test the visual field. It has also been demonstrated that the size of the blind spot depends in part on the surrounding illumination. It is smaller when the visual field is tested with high degrees of illumination than when testing is performed in dim light. Finally, the size of the blind spot is smaller when it is tested centripetally than when it is tested centrifugally (93).

The blind spot becomes enlarged from peripapillary reti-nal dysfunction. This dysfunction can occur because the peripapillary retina is diseased, as occurs in patients with the so-called ''big blind spot syndrome'' (94) and related disorders such as acute zonal occult outer retinopathy (AZOOR) and the multiple evanescent white dot syndrome (MEWDS) (95–99), or because expansion of the optic disc tissue encroaches on the peripapillary retina, as occurs in optic disc swelling and in pseudopapilledema (Fig. 4.12).

Because both true optic disc swelling and pseudopapille-dema are often associated with a variable degree of enlarge-ment of the blind spot, the size of the blind spot is rarely a crucial factor in determining the presence or absence of disc swelling or in differentiating acquired disc swelling from congenital elevation of the optic disc.

OPTIC ATROPHY

Optic atrophy is not a disease. It is a nonspecific morpho-logic end point of disease—any disease—that causes damage to ganglion cells and axons of the optic nerve. The term ''optic atrophy'' is, therefore, a pathologic generalization applied to an appearance due to degeneration of axons in the anterior visual system. Although the pathologist can de-termine optic atrophy by direct observation of histopatho-logic changes in the optic nerve, the clinical diagnosis of atrophy is usually based on ophthalmoscopic abnormalities of color and structure of the optic disc with associated changes in the retinal vessels and nerve fiber layer, and de-fective visual function that can be localized to the optic nerve.

Both the pathologic and ophthalmoscopic features of optic atrophy are discussed in this section, but a listing of all causes of optic atrophy is not attempted. These disorders are discussed in detail elsewhere in this text.

NONPATHOLOGIC PALLOR OF THE OPTIC DISC

The determination of disc pallor requires familiarity with normal disc color. The temporal side of the normal disc usually has less color than its nasal side. The degree of this temporal pallor is primarily related to the size of the physio-logic cup, and to the thin translucent character of the tem-poral nerve fiber layer.

The normal physiologic cup may vary in size. When it extends almost to the temporal edge of the disc, the temporal side of the disc is pale. Sometimes the temporal margins of large physiologic cups are steep-walled. When the margins slope gradually downward from the margin of the disc, the crescent of sclera adjacent to the temporal, and occasionally to the inferior margin of the disc, is visible and appears mottled grayish white. This crescent, known as a temporal or sometimes inferior conus, is exposed by retraction of the dark retinal pigment epithelium from the disc margin and enhances the whitish appearance of such a disc.

Marked recession or excavation of a physiologic cup creates a central area of pallor. The retinal vessels are partially obscured as they ascend through a thin rim of neural tissue that borders the excavation. It is difficult to distinguish this cup from a glaucomatous cup. The pallor of the floor of a physiologic cup comes from the glistening whiteness of the lamina cribrosa, a connective and elastic tissue structure with small sieve-like openings through which axonal bundles pass. Because the openings are irregular, direct light entering them is reflected in many directions, and the holes appear as yellow/white ovals or dots. When this dotting is seen, it signifies that there is no abnormal opaque connective tissue present over the surface of the cribriform plate.

A white-appearing disc is common in an eye with axial myopia. Because the optic nerve enters the globe obliquely, the contents of the disc, including the nerve fibers and the retinal vessels, are displaced nasally. The physiologic cup is shallow, and its extension to the temporal margin produces relative temporal pallor that is often exaggerated by a temporal conus.

In infants, ophthalmoscopic examinations are more difficult. Opening the lids against squeezing may increase the intraocular pressure and that may artifactually add to the appearance of optic disc pallor.

A brighter, whiter ophthalmoscope bulb may give the illusory impression of disc whiteness. Similarly, true pallor of an optic disc may be overlooked when the light source has become weak and yellow. The color of the disc changes with the color temperature of the light source (100) and the age of the lens (101,102). Sorensen (103) examined the color of the optic discs of 200 normal subjects using a slit lamp and contact lens. His findings are in agreement with those of others (102,104,105) that optic disc color depends on the incident light on the disc.

PATHOLOGY OF OPTIC ATROPHY

The optic nerve axons arise from the ganglion cells located in the retina. Hence damage to such axons may occur at several locations: (*a*) from disease within the eye that damages the ganglion cells, the retinal nerve fiber layer, or the optic disc; (*b*) from disease within or surrounding the intraorbital, intracanalicular, or intracranial portions of the optic nerve; (*c*) from intracranial diseases of the optic chiasm, optic tracts, or lateral geniculate body (LGB); and (*4*) from diseases of the retrogeniculate pathways that produce trans-synaptic (transneuronal) degeneration. Such precesses may be focal, multifocal, or diffuse. They may destroy axons directly or by effects on the blood supply. Focal disruption at any place along an axon causes degeneration of the entire axon and its cell body, the retinal ganglion cell. When large numbers of axons undergo such degeneration, gross shrinkage or atrophy of the optic nerve becomes evident (Fig. 4.13).

When an axon is irreversibly damaged, it undergoes either

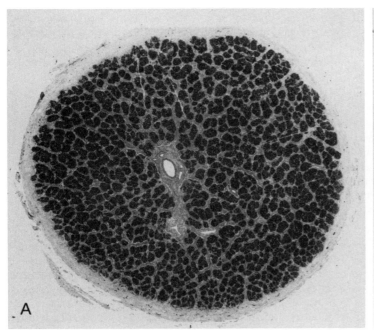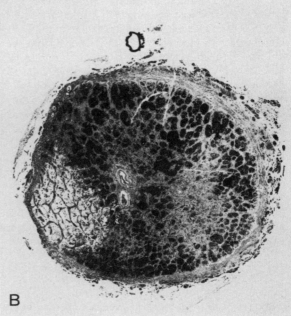

Figure 4.13. Histopathologic appearance of optic atrophy. *A*, Cross section of normal optic nerve stained with myelin. *B*, Cross section of atrophic optic nerve photographed at same magnification to show extensive shrinkage. This nerve is about one-third the diameter of the specimen seen in *A*. (Courtesy of Dr. Harry A. Quigley.)

anterograde or retrograde degeneration. Anterograde degeneration proceeds posteriorly along the axon that has been separated from its cell body, whereas retrograde degeneration occurs in the proximal segment of the axon that remains in contact with the cell body.

Anterograde (Wallerian) Ascending Degeneration of Axons

When an axon of the central nervous system is severed, its distal (ascending) segment, being separated from its cell body, quickly degenerates and disappears, and its investing myelin sheath undergoes a slower breakdown into simpler lipids that are eventually catabolized. This process is called **anterograde** or **Wallerian** degeneration (106).

Axons in the optic nerve undergo Wallerian degeneration at a rate proportional to their thickness. Large axons show varicosities as early as 30 hours from the time of severance from the cell body. Within 4–8 days, they break up into shorter oval or spherical fragments that progressively disintegrate and disappear. In medium-sized myelinated fibers, the axon is still in the varicose or beaded stage at the end of a week and it finally breaks up from the second week onward. In small-caliber fibers, the process is slower, with many axons showing little change during the first 10 days. Changes in their myelin sheaths correspond to the changes in the axon. Breakdown of myelin into simpler lipids occurs over the subsequent weeks and spherules of myelin may be present indefinitely (107,108). By the end of the fourth month, most or all of the broken down myelin has been engulfed and removed by phagocytic microglia. These microglia appear around degenerating fibers by the fourth day and increase in numbers during the next two weeks, with their cytoplasm filling with fine fatty droplets. These phagocytes absorb the large amount of lipid that is produced as myelin breakdown occurs. The lipid-laden microglia (Gitterzells) migrate to blood vessel walls where, from the third month onward, they crowd the adventitial spaces. Leukocytes are rarely present in Wallerian degeneration.

An essential feature of Wallerian degeneration is the swelling and degeneration of the axon terminals in the lateral geniculate bodies. This consists of globular thickening or swelling of the terminals of visual axons that can be identified within layers of the geniculate body as early as 24 hours after a lesion of the axon (109). Wallerian degeneration and the optic pallor it produces can only be observed clinically when this dying-back reaches the axons within the eye (110–115).

Retrograde (Descending) Degeneration of Axons

Anterograde degeneration begins and becomes virtually complete within 7 days after injury; however, the portion of the axon still connected to the cell body, and the cell body itself, can remain normal in appearance for up to 3–4 weeks. During this time, orthograde axonal transport continues. Eventually, however, the entire remaining structure (the cell body and axon from the point of injury) degenerates by retrograde degeneration so that by about 6–8 weeks after severe optic nerve injury, no affected ganglion cells remain viable.

Retrograde degeneration is relatively independent of the distance of the injury from the ganglion cell body. Damage to the retrobulbar portion of the optic nerve, the optic chiasm, and the optic tract all cause pathologic and visible degeneration of the ganglion cell bodies at about the same time (116–118).

After an optic nerve is severed, bulbous axonal swellings (Cajal end bulbs) can be seen at the anterior cut ends of the fibers. A few additional swellings on the posterior end of the severed nerve provide evidence of centrifugal axons in the optic nerve (119,120). This has been confirmed by ultrastructured analysis of optic nerves in humans with complete loss of retinal ganglion cell bodies due to Leber's hereditary optic neuropathy (121). These fibers, about 1,000 in number, may have a vasomotor function and may represent melatonin-containing cells that subserve circadian rhythm (122).

Regeneration of axons in the optic nerve in human and nonhuman primates is quite limited and abortive. By about 2 months, all sectional optic nerve fibers degenerate (123,124). Various purported neurotrophic factors can extend but not preserve indefinitely retinal ganglion cells from retrograde degeneration (125–128).

Remyelination does occur after injury to the optic nerve. Bunge et al. (129) and Bornstein et al. (130) first showed that CNS tissue in various species, including primates, has the capacity to reform myelin following experimental primary demyelination as long as the axon itself is intact. Other investigators subsequently confirmed these initial observations (131–140). This remyelination results from the activity of uninjured, injured but surviving, and newly generated oligodendroglia (141). This has also been demonstrated in optic neuropathies such as Leber's hereditary optic neuropathy (142–144).

In multiple sclerosis (MS) and other immune-mediated disorders, remyelination occurs both in and at the edges of plaques (137,138,140,145). Restoration of conduction by remyelination may thus play a role in the characteristic remissions of MS.

Remyelination probably plays a larger role in the recovery from acute and chronic compressive lesions of the CNS than it does in the recovery from primary demyelinating disease (138,139). Acute experimental compression of the spinal cord is accompanied by secondary demyelination that is followed almost immediately by remyelination that occurs even though the nerve is still compressed (132–136,146). Thus, even nerves within the CNS that have been chronically compressed have the potential to begin conducting impulses as soon as the compression is relieved, as long as there has not been severe irreversible damage to the axons themselves. This phenomenon may explain the progressive improvement in vision that is often seen after removal of compressive lesions of the optic nerves and chiasm that have produced profound visual loss. Likewise, it may explain why the degree of visual recovery depends to a large extent on the duration of visual symptoms, the severity of preoperative visual loss, and the presence or absence of optic atrophy (147–150).

Primate retinal ganglion cells show no detectable regeneration after injury. These cells are capable of developing an axon in embryologic life; but it remains hotly debated as to whether the adult primate ganglion cell fails to receive a signal for regeneration, is actively inhibited from regeneration, or has lost this ability.

Transsynaptic (transneuronal) degeneration is a phenomenon by which a neuron on one side of a synapse degenerates as a consequence of the loss of a neuron on the other side. This is more likely to occur in the anterograde direction and when the lesion occurs in the immature brain (151). Transneuronal degeneration is a well-established phenomenon in the cells of the LGB following destruction of parts of the retina or the optic nerve (152–157). Van Buren (158) performed a right-sided occipital lobectomy on an adolescent macaque monkey and examined the eyes 4 years later. He found a striking loss of ganglion cells in the corresponding right halves of the retinas and also noted subtle changes in the bipolar cells of the retina. These observations were subsequently confirmed by other investigators working with developing monkeys (159,160). Wilbrand and Saenger (161) thought that retrograde transsynaptic degeneration occurred most often in patients with occipital lobe damage *in utero* or during early infancy, and this has been confirmed pathologically (156).

It has been suggested that transsynaptic degeneration may occur in mature adult primate visual systems if enough time has elapsed. Weller and Kaas (160) reported loss of retinal ganglion cells in adult monkeys with striate cortex lesions, but the changes were less severe than in developing monkeys. Weller et al. (162) were unable to produce similar changes in the adult prosimian primate, *Galago,* so there appears to be major species differences. Retrograde transsynaptic degeneration probably is not clinically significant in human adults. (163). However, histological evidence of retrograde degeneration in the human visual system exists. Van Buren (164) described three cases of metastatic cancer affecting the occipital lobes in which histopathological evidence of degeneration was found in the lateral geniculate nuclei and retinas in all three cases. In addition, Beatty et al. (165) used paraphenylene diamine to stain degenerated optic nerve axons and axon terminals in a patient who had unilateral removal of the striate cortex 40 years before necropsy and showed histologic evidence of retrograde transsynaptic degeneration of retinal ganglion cells in both eyes.

PATHOGENESIS OF ACQUIRED OPTIC DISC PALLOR

Loss of function within the CNS is consistently associated with a reduction of blood supply to the affected tissue, regardless of the primary pathogenetic process. When the optic nerve degenerates, its blood supply is reduced, and smaller vessels that have been recognizable in the normal nerve are no longer visible. Optic atrophy reflects this reduction of blood supply and also the formation of reactive glial tissue. Quigley and Anderson (166) performed histopathologic studies on monkey eyes with descending optic atrophy and suggested that the factors important for the normal pink appearance of the optic disc were its thickness and the cytoarchitecture of fiber bundles passing between glial columns

containing capillaries. They postulated that the transparent nerve fibers act as fiberoptic pathways in conducting light. The light diffuses among adjacent columns of glial cells and capillaries and acquires the pink color of the capillaries. The axon bundles of an atrophic optic disc have been destroyed, and the remaining astrocytes are arranged at angles to the entering light. Thus, little light passes into the disc substance to traverse the capillaries The light reflected from opaque glial cells does not pass through capillaries, remains white, and the optic disc appears pale. In some areas, loss of tissue also allows light to pass directly to the opaque scleral lamina, and this adds to the white color of the disc.

Other explanations for optic disc pallor include the paucity of capillaries and astroglial proliferation. However, Henkind et al. (167) as well as Quigley and Anderson (166) observed that despite optic atrophy, disc capillaries are still present and appear to be functional. In addition, Hayreh (168) showed that small blood vessels can be demonstrated in pale discs by fluorescein angiography.

OPHTHALMOSCOPIC FEATURES OF OPTIC ATROPHY

The evaluation of optic disc color is a routine but often challenging problem. This seemingly simple task has many pitfalls. Estimating the lack of color in an optic disc is difficult to assess, record, compare, and describe. The normal color of the optic disc is dependent upon its composition and the relationship of the components to each other and to the light that is reflected or refracted from the disc surface. Because the neural elements are gray, the pink color of the disc is also related to its blood vessels .

Pallor of the optic disc has often been graded as mild, moderate, or severe; however, such distinctions are subjective and unreliable. More objective evaluation of the pale optic disc can be obtained by detailed observation of its configuration and neural tissue; its veins, arteries, and capillaries; and the peripapillary retinal nerve fiber layer that surrounds it.

Schwartz et al. (169) suggested that pallor of the optic disc be assessed with color fundus photographs from which enlarged, high-contrast black and white prints are made. The measure of color contrast for estimating the degree of optic disc pallor was studied by other investigators (170–174). Sorensen (175) estimated the degree of optic atrophy by color contrast and quantitated the degree of atrophy by microdensitometry in the blue (470 nm) and in the red (640 nm) regions. This technique has proven to be of limited value to most clinicians. Red-free nerve fiber layer photography is both useful as well as practical. Newer technologies such as Optical Cohenence Tomography (OCT) or Gdx, which measure the polarization of light produced by nerve fiber layer microtubuoles, have also proven useful.

Appearance of the Atrophic Optic Disc with Special Reference to Vasculature

Pallor of the optic disc may be diffuse or confined to one sector (Fig. 4.14). Kestenbaum (176) introduced a "capillary number test" in which the small vessels at the margins of

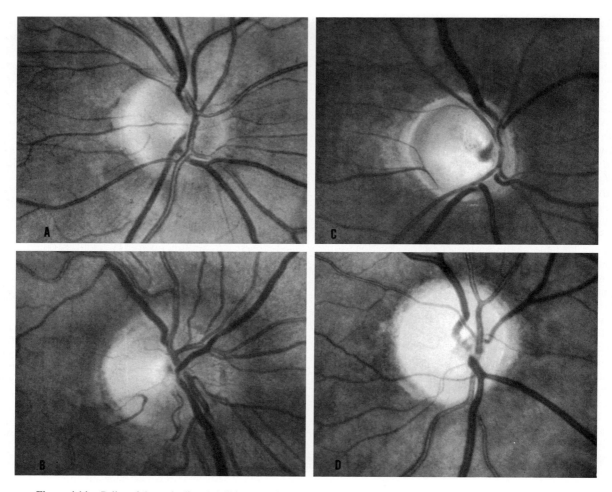

Figure 4.14. Pallor of the optic disc. *A,* Mild temporal pallor in a patient with multiple sclerosis but who denied acute optic neuritis. *B,* Temporal pallor in a patient with toxic amblyopia. *C,* Pallor with glaucomatous cupping. Note preservation of small nasal neuroretinal rim. *D,* Diffuse pallor in a patient with retrograde (descending) optic atrophy from the effects of an intracranial mass. (From Hoyt WF, Beeston D. The Ocular Fundus in Neurologic Disease. St Louis, CV Mosby, 1966.)

an optic disc are observed and counted using an ophthalmoscope. There are usually about 10 such vessels, but Kestenbaum (176) found that the number of visible vessels was decreased in patients with diffuse optic atrophy. Kant (177) performed the capillary number test on the optic discs of 125 eyes. Forty-nine of the optic discs were said to have had normal optic discs by other criteria, whereas the remaining 76 eyes had atrophic discs. The Kestenbaum count can also be used to measure hyperemia of the optic disc when the number of visible vessels exceeds 12.

Appearance of the Atrophic Optic Disc with Respect to Cupping

In the early stages of atrophy, the optic disc loses its reddish hue, and the substance of the disc slowly disappears, leaving a pale, shallow concave meniscus, the exposed lamina cribrosa (Fig. 4.15). In the end stages of the atrophic process, retinal vessels of normal caliber still emerge centrally through the otherwise avascular disc. In many cases,

the changes that develop during the progression to atrophy do not result in a significant change in the central cup of the optic disc. In some cases, however, pathologic optic disc cupping develops in patients with normal intraocular pressures and optic atrophy from various causes, including ischemia, compression, inflammation, hereditary disorders, and trauma (87,91,178–183). There has been significant controversy as to whether the cupping in such cases is equivalent to that seen with glaucoma. Both Quigley and Anderson (182) and Radius and Maumenee (183) concluded that the cupping seen in nonglaucomatous optic neuropathies, such as the arteritic variety of anterior ischemic optic neuropathy, was quite distinct from that seen in glaucoma. Trobe et al. (87) asked three ophthalmologists experienced in assessing optic discs to evaluate stereo fundus photographs of 29 eyes with nonglaucomatous optic atrophy associated with cupping. Thirteen of the discs (44%) were misdiagnosed as showing glaucomatous cupping by at least one observer. Trobe et al. (87) also analyzed various morphologic features

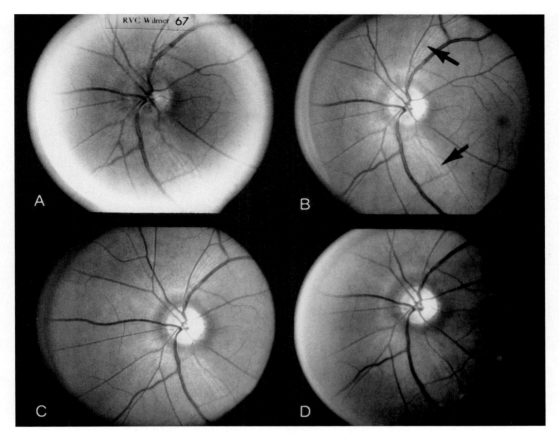

Figure 4.15. Development of pallor of the optic disc in a patient with retrograde (descending) optic atrophy. *A*, The optic disc is normal in the early stage of the process. *B*, With time, the optic disc loses its reddish hue, and the substance of the disc slowly disappears, leaving a pale, shallow concave meniscus, the exposed lamina cribrosa. As these changes occur, the peripapillary retinal nerve fiber layer begins to show defects that appear as dark linear striations (*arrowheads*). *C*, With more time, the disc becomes more diffusely pale, and the peripapillary nerve fiber layer becomes less visible. *D*, In the end stage of the atrophic process, retinal vessels of normal caliber still emerge centrally through the otherwise avascular-appearing disc, and the peripapillary retinal nerve fiber layer is no longer visible. (From Miller NR, Fine SL. The Ocular Fundus in Neuro-Ophthalmologic Diagnosis: Sights and Sounds in Ophthalmology. Vol 3. St Louis, CV Mosby, 1977.)

of the optic disc in patients with both glaucomatous and nonglaucomatous cupping and concluded that pallor of the neuroretinal rim was 94% specific for nonglaucomatous atrophy and cupping, whereas focal or diffuse obliteration of the neuroretinal rim with preservation of color of any remaining rim tissue was 87% specific for glaucoma. Thinning of the neuroretinal rim was more common in glaucomatous cupping than in nonglaucomatous cupping, but not significantly.

There is occasional confusion between glaucomatous and nonglaucomatous optic neuropathy that occurs in patients with pathologic cupping and pallor of the optic disc (88–90). However careful clinical examination invariably results in the correct diagnosis. Glaucomatous visual field defects occur only after extensive cupping is present, and visual acuity loss usually occurs even later. In such cases, there is usually absence of at least a portion of the neuroretinal rim,

and any remaining rim tissue has a normal color (Fig. 4.16). In nonglaucomatous optic neuropathies, significant loss of visual acuity, color vision, and field often occurs in combination with little or only mild cupping. In addition, the optic discs in such cases rarely have any areas in which the neuroretinal rim is completely absent, and the remaining rim is often pale (87). The appearance of the neuroretinal rim is a crucial factor in determining whether cupping is caused by glaucomatous or nonglaucomatous optic nerve damage.

Evaluation of the Peripapillary Retinal Nerve Fiber Layer in the Diagnosis of Optic Atrophy

Focal destruction of nerve fiber bundles occur in diseases that affect the inner retinal layers, optic disc, retrobulbar optic nerve, or a combination of these structures. Hoyt et al. (184) first called attention to the ophthalmoscopic appearance of such defects. These authors emphasized that the nor-

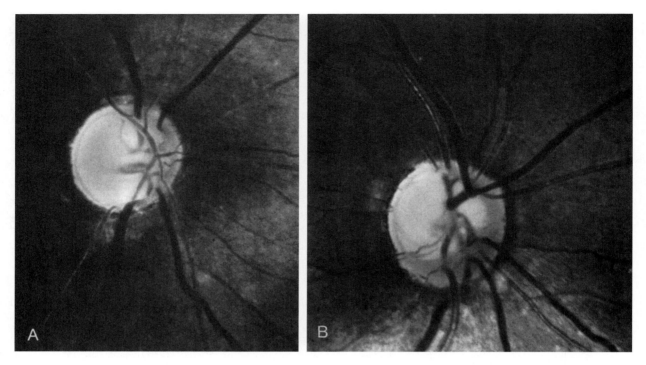

Figure 4.16. Optic disc cupping in glaucomatous and nonglaucomatous optic atrophy. *A*, Glaucomatous cupping. Note pallor and thinning of the neuroretinal rim. *B*, Nonglaucomatous cupping. This patient had sudden loss of the inferior visual field associated with optic disc swelling. When the swelling subsided, the superior-temporal portion of the disc was pale and deeply cupped. Note thinning and pallor of the neuroretinal rim.

mal appearance of the peripapillary retinal nerve fiber layer consists of fine curvilinear striations that overlie the retinal vessels, causing them to be seen slightly out of focus (Fig. 4.17).

Early focal loss of axons is represented by the development of dark slits or wedges in the peripapillary retinal nerve fiber layer (184,185). These slits or bands appear darker or redder than the adjacent normal tissue in which the normal linear or curvilinear nerve fiber layer striations can easily be seen (186) (Figs. 4.18A and B). The slit defects are most easily identified in the superior and inferior arcuate regions where the nerve fiber layer is particularly thick. With increasing distance from the disc, the defects gradually lose contrast and cannot be identified. When only a few nerve fiber bundle defects are present, they can be identified only by the appearance of a dark, linear, arching region among the lighter, linear nerve fiber reflexes; however, when multiple nerve fiber bundle defects are present they impart a ''raked'' appearance to the nerve fiber layer.

Multiple nerve fiber bundle defects may coalesce to produce a large wedge pattern (Fig. 4.18C–E). This pattern may also occur when a large region of nerve fiber layer is simultaneously damaged (e.g., after ischemic optic neuropathy). Within the wedge, the entire retina takes on a flat granular appearance with no striations (Figs. 4.18E and F). In addition, vessels in this area, being denuded of their surrounding nerve fiber covering, appear darker than normal and stand out sharply in relief.

Diffuse thinning of the nerve fiber layer around the optic disc is difficult to recognize in the early stages. In more advanced stages, signs of atrophy include decreased opacity of the arcuate fiber bundles, enhanced linear highlights on large and small retinal blood vessels, reduced caliber of blood vessels, and pallor of the optic disc with fewer detectable disc capillaries (Fig. 4.18F). Diffuse thinning of the nerve fiber layer may accompany focal atrophy (slit defects).

To view such abnormalities the illumination of the ophthalmoscope must be sufficiently bright. In addition, Hoyt (187,188) and others (100,189–205) have stressed the advantage in visualization of the nerve fiber layer provided by red-free light. Lundstrom and Frisén (117) and Lundstrom (206) assessed atrophy of the nerve fiber layer in the manner described above and found a fairly high degree of correlation among observers. In addition, Quigley and Addicks (207) demonstrated that clinical detection of nerve fiber layer atrophy is possible in nonhuman primates, but only after loss of 50% of the neural tissue in a given area. The detectability of nerve fiber layer atrophy is directly affected both by the pattern of nerve fiber loss as well as by the zone of the retina in which the loss has occurred. Computer densitometry has been used Lundstrom and Eklundh (208) to evaluate progressive nerve fiber layer atrophy, as have other methods of assessing the thickness of the retinal nerve fiber layer (197,205,209–215). None of these methods of analysis has yet been shown as practical for the clinician (216).

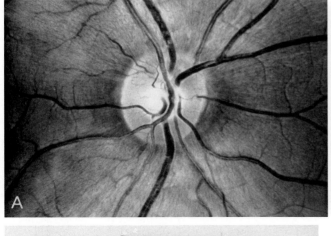

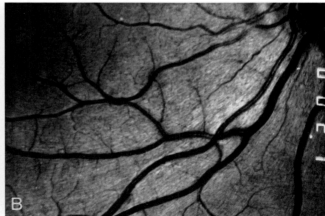

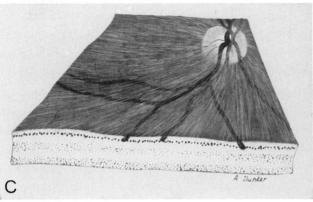

Figure 4.17. Appearance of the normal peripapillary retinal nerve fiber layer. *A,* Normal nerve fiber layer in the right ocular fundus of a patient with no visual complaints and a normal ocular examination. Note fine, linear, and curvilinear striations emanating from all parts of the optic disc and representing light reflexes from bundles of nerve fibers. *B,* Normal nerve fiber layer in the inferior arcuate region of the right eye from another patient. Again, note fine curvilinear striations. Both photographs were obtained using a monochromatic red-free (540 nm) filter. *C,* Artist's drawing of normal peripapillary retinal nerve fiber layer (Schematic illustrations from Miller NR, Fine SL. The Ocular Fundus in Neuro-Ophthalmologic Diagnosis: Sights and Sounds in Ophthalmology. Vol 3. St Louis, CV Mosby, 1977.)

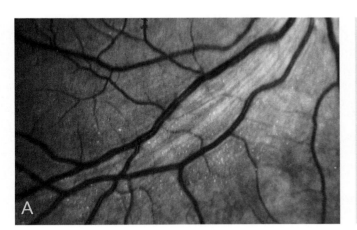

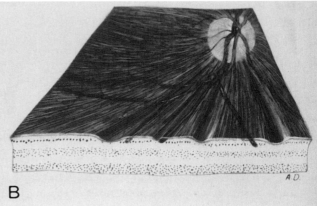

Figure 4.18. Appearance of atrophy of the peripapillary retinal nerve fiber layer. *A,* Monochromatic red-free photograph shows mild nerve fiber bundle defects in the inferior arcuate fiber bundle. They are seen as thin dark streaks interrupting the normal linear light reflexes. *B,* Artist's drawing of the thin defects in the peripapillary retinal nerve fiber layer that occur in patients with mild optic neuropathies. *(Figure continues.)*

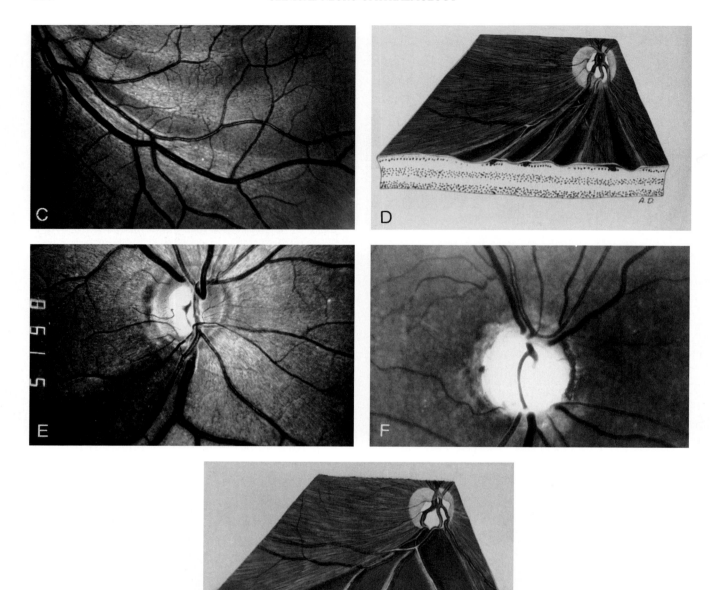

Figure 4.18. Continued. *C,* Monochromatic red-free photograph shows two large defects in the peripapillary retinal nerve fiber layer in the inferior arcuate region of the left eye in a patient with radiation-induced optic neuropathy. Compared with *A,* the defects in this photograph are darker, wider, and more distinct from the surrounding nerve fiber layer. *D,* Artist's drawing of moderate defects in the peripapillary retinal nerve fiber layer. Note that the darker appearance results both from widening and deepening of the defects. *E,* Monochromatic red-free photograph shows a single broad defect in the peripapillary retinal nerve fiber layer in the inferior arcuate region of the right eye in a patient with early glaucoma and inferior extension of the optic cup. The defect is dark and quite distinct from the otherwise normal peripapillary nerve fiber layer. Note the granular appearance of the fundus within the defect caused by loss of the axons. The vessels crossing the defect are seen more clearly than are other vessels for the same reason. *F,* Complete loss of the peripapillary retinal nerve fiber layer in a patient with severe glaucoma. No linear striations can be seen; the peripapillary region has a distinct granular appearance; and the retinal vessels are seen clearly because of absence of overlying nerve fibers. *G,* Artist's drawing of complete loss of the nerve fiber layer in a large sector. Note draping of the inner limiting membrane over the retinal vessels.

Retinal Vascular Changes Associated with Optic Atrophy

In most cases of optic atrophy, the retinal arteries are narrowed or attenuated (217,218). In some instances, the narrowing is minor in nature; however, in others, such as in severe nonarteritic anterior ischemic optic neuropathy, the vessels may be focally narrowed or completely obliterated (217). Not all cases of optic atrophy are associated with retinal vascular changes, however. Henkind et al. (219) found normal-sized vessels in a trypsin digest of the retina of an eye that had been blind for 4 months following arteritic anterior ischemic optic neuropathy (AION). This finding is consistent with the finding of Rader et al. (217) that eyes with arteritic AION are least likely to have significant narrowing of retinal arteries, compared with eyes with most other types of optic neuropathies. Kurz et al. (220) reported the case of a 33-year-old man with a gunshot injury to the head, resulting in no light perception, absence of pupillary reactions to direct light, and diffuse, severe optic atrophy. Remarkably, on postmortem examination, the retinal vascular pattern in both eyes was completely normal.

Landers et al. (221) studied five patients with unilateral optic atrophy. Two of these patients had experienced orbital trauma; one had an orbital granuloma and two had intracranial lesions in the region of the optic chiasm. None of these patients had any changes in the retinal vasculature of the affected eye when compared with the vasculature of the unaffected eye by clinical observation, color fundus photography, and fluorescein angiography. Henkind et al. (222), performed unilateral optic nerve transection without damage to the intraocular circulation in 13 cats. These investigators performed fluorescein angiography, trypsin digestion, and histologic preparation of the retinas of all animals and found no changes in the retinal circulation or angioarchitecture. Apparently, if optic atrophy is from damage to the retrolaminar optic nerve, the retinal vessels are often unaffected. Eyes with retinal vascular changes associated with optic atrophy presumably have suffered an additional insult in addition to loss of the retinal ganglion cells.

DIFFERENTIAL DIAGNOSIS OF OPTIC ATROPHY

When optic atrophy is complete, it is often impossible to determine its etiology solely from its appearance. Trobe et al. (223) viewed 163 color fundus stereophotographs of nine disease entities: glaucoma, central retinal artery occlusion, ischemic optic neuropathy, anterior and retrobulbar optic neuritis, compressive optic neuropathy, traumatic optic neuropathy, Leber's hereditary optic neuropathy, and autosomal dominant optic neuropathy. The atrophy caused by glaucoma, central retinal artery occlusion, and ischemic optic neuropathy was diagnosed by at least one of five observers with an accuracy above 80%; however, the other conditions were correctly identified with less than 50% accuracy. Retinal arteriolar attenuation and sheathing were most helpful in differentiating central retinal artery occlusion and ischemic optic neuropathy from other entities.

Temporal pallor is the most common expression of seg-

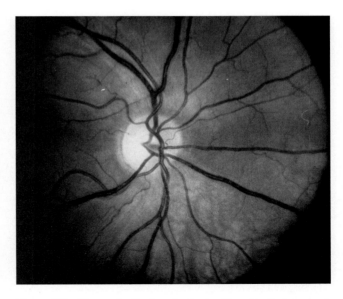

Figure 4.19. Temporal pallor in optic atrophy. The patient had previously experienced an attack of acute retrobulbar optic neuritis in the right eye. She initially had visual acuity of 20/200 in the eye, but the vision improved over several months to 20/25. The fundus photograph shows temporal pallor of the right optic disc.

mental optic atrophy (Fig. 4.19). The white area, which generally extends from the temporal edge of the disc to the central vessels, may appear totally devoid of capillaries. Margins of this white area tend to blend gradually with the reddish-yellow color of the surrounding disc tissue. However, sharply demarcated wedge-shaped temporal pallor is a consequence of specific lesions to the papillomacular bundle that usually occur in the retina between the macula and the disc. Temporal pallor is usually caused by optic neuropathies that selectively affect central vision and field, sparing the peripheral field. Such optic neuropathies include toxic and nutritional optic neuropathies, hereditary optic neuropathies, and optic neuritis. When superior or inferior disc pallor is present, an ischemic etiology is more likely.

The specific organization of the retinal nerve fiber layer results in specific patterns of nerve fiber layer and optic atrophy in patients with visual loss from optic chiasmal and retrochiasmal-pregeniculate lesions. In patients with chiasmal lesions, for example, temporal field defects are mirrored by loss of fibers from ganglion cells nasal to the fovea. The atrophy is most impressive directly nasal and temporal to the disc, since the superior and inferior arcuate nerve fiber bundles are composed of fibers from ganglion cells both temporal and nasal to the fovea. Thus, the arcuate bundles are relatively spared compared with other areas. The optic pallor is thus primarily nasal and temporal with sparing superiorly and inferiorly. This "band" or "bow tie" atrophy is characteristic of temporal field loss (Fig. 4.20). Patients with optic chiasmal syndromes and bitemporal hemianopic field defects develop "band" optic atrophy (187,188,191, 224–226) (see Chapter 12).

In patients with congenital or neonatally acquired homon-

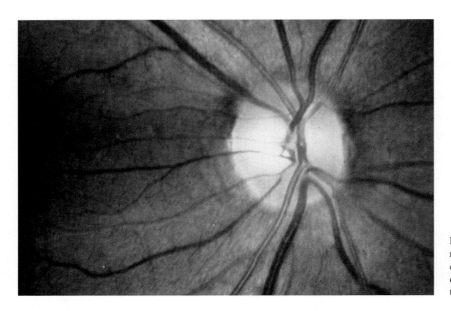

Figure 4.20. "Band" or "bowtie" atrophy of the right optic disc in a patient with a temporal hemianopia caused by a pituitary adenoma. Note horizontal band of atrophy across the right disc, with preservation of the superior and inferior portions of the disc.

ymous hemianopia, or in patients with pregeniculate homonymous hemianopias, the eye contralateral to the lesion shows the pattern of nerve fiber and optic nerve atrophy described above with temporal field loss. The eye ipsilateral to the lesion has a complete nasal field loss with loss of ganglion cells temporal to the fovea. Because the nerve fibers from these ganglion cells primarily comprise the superior and inferior arcuate bundles, these regions show extensive loss of nerve fibers; nonetheless the disc atrophy is generalized. The characteristic features of the fundi of such individuals are thus a "bow tie" or "band" atrophy in the contralateral eye and a relative absence of the superior and inferior arcuate nerve fiber bundles in the ipsilateral eye (187,188,191,225, 227,228).

In conclusion, the extent of pathologic pallor of the optic disc cannot be directly equated with visual function. Further-

more, judgment of optic disc atrophy must be made in the context of optic nerve function. Careful testing of visual acuity, contrast sensitivity, and color vision, as well as quantitative perimetry, examination of the pupils, and electrophysiologic studies must be taken into consideration. In the absence of visual impairment, an optic disc that appears to be pale is most likely reflecting physiologic rather than pathologic changes. Conversely, an optic disc occasionally appears normal despite severe and even long-standing visual acuity or field loss caused by optic nerve dysfunction. In most of these cases, careful evaluation of the optic disc as well as the peripapillary retinal nerve fiber layer will provide evidence of retinal nerve fiber atrophy, either too focal or too mild and diffuse to produce obvious optic pallor. Nevertheless, there are rare patients with clinical and electrophysiologic evidence of chronic optic nerve dysfunction who exhibit a normal-appearing optic disc and nerve fiber layer.

TOPICAL DIAGNOSIS OF OPTIC NERVE LESIONS

The diagnosis of an optic neuropathy depends upon the constellation of signs and symptoms including history of visual loss (rapid vs. slow onset, progressive vs. stable), the presence or absence of other neurologic or ocular signs (relative afferent pupillary defect, acquired color deficit, visual field loss, ocular motor paresis, proptosis, optociliary shunt veins, optic disc swelling, optic pallor), and, occasionally, the results of electrophysiologic testing (187,188,229–233).

Indeed, the optic disc has only two main ways to respond to the many pathologic processes that may affect the optic nerve. It can swell, or it can remain normal in appearance. If the pathologic process causes irreversible damage to the optic nerve, the disc will eventually become pale (see above).

OPTIC DISC SWELLING

Swelling of the optic disc occurs when there is obstruction of axonal transport at the level of the lamina cribrosa. This

may result from compression, ischemia, inflammation, metabolic, or toxic disturbances. In some cases, infiltration of the proximal portion of the disc by inflammatory or malignant processes causes an appearance that is indistinguishable from true swelling. In other cases, congenital anomalies of the optic disc produce an appearance that mimics swelling of the optic disc.

True Optic Disc Swelling

Papilledema

Patients with increased intracranial pressure may develop optic disc swelling. This condition is called **papilledema**. The symptoms and signs in patients with papilledema generally are those typically associated with raised intracranial pressure, including headache, nausea, vomiting, and pulsatile tinnitus. Visual symptoms in such patients include transient obscurations of vision and diplopia. Loss of central vision, dyschromatopsia, a relative afferent pupillary defect, and visual field defects other than enlargement of the blind spot caused by the swollen disc are uncommon in patients with acute papilledema unless the lesion causing the increased intracranial pressure also directly damages the visual sensory system in some way or there are hemorrhages or exudates in the macula.

The optic disc swelling in papilledema is usually bilateral and symmetric, but it may be asymmetric or even unilateral. It may be very mild or extremely severe (Fig. 4.21) Although some physicians believe they can diagnose papilledema from the appearance of the optic disc, patients with a typical "choked disc" suggestive of papilledema may, in fact, have inflammatory or ischemic disc swelling (Fig 4.22).

There are ten cardinal signs of papilledema. The five mechanical signs are (a) anterior extension of the optic nerve head; (b) blurring of the disc margins; (c) loss of the physiologic cup; (d) edema of the nerve fiber layer; and (e) retinal or choroidal folds. The five vascular signs are (a) hyperemia of the optic disc; (b) venous dilation and tortuousity; (c) peripapillary flame-shaped hemorrhages; (d) peripapillary exudates; and (e) nerve fiber layer infarcts. Papilledema is further discussed in Chapter 5.

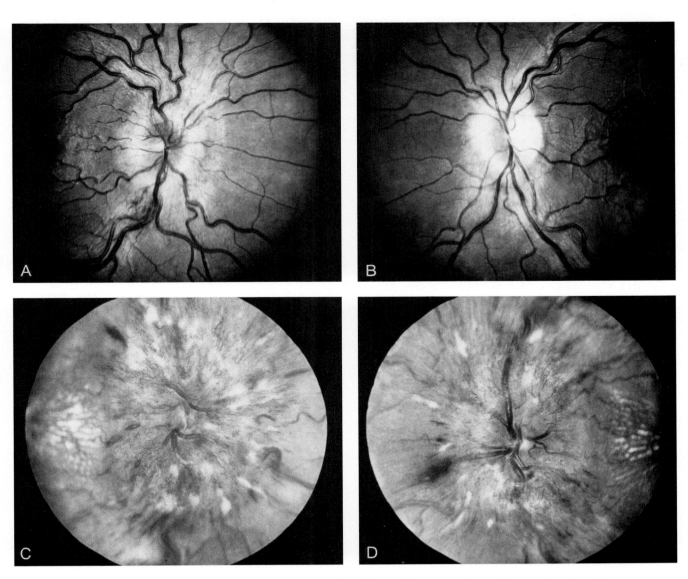

Figure 4.21. Variability in severity of papilledema. *A and B*, Mild papilledema in a 14-year-old boy with hydrocephalus caused by congenital aqueductal stenosis. The right disc (*A*) is somewhat more hyperemic and swollen than the left (*B*). *C and D*, Severe papilledema in a 32-year-old woman with pseudotumor cerebri. Note numerous hemorrhages and nerve fiber layer infarcts surrounding the markedly swollen right (*C*) and left (*D*) optic discs as well as other cardinal signs. Also note hard exudates (lipid) in both maculae.

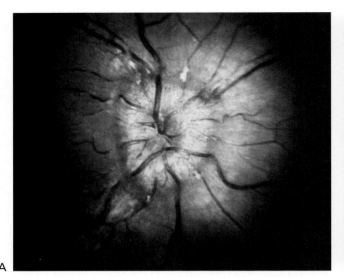

A

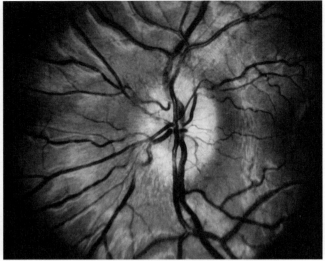

B

Figure 4.22.   The appearance of a "choked disc" caused by papilledema compared with a "choked disc" in a patient with anterior optic neuritis. *A*, Right optic disc in a young woman with papilledema. There is moderate swelling of the disc, which is surrounded by several intraretinal hemorrhages and soft exudates. *B*, Left optic disc in a patient with anterior optic neuritis. The disc is moderately swollen, and there are mild circumferential retinal folds temporal to the disc. Note that both optic discs appear similar in appearance. It is impossible to determine the cause of optic disc swelling in most cases withhout clinical correlation.

Ischemic Optic Neuropathy

Ischemia that affects the prelaminar portion of the optic nerve will produce swelling of the optic disc. This condition, called **anterior ischemic optic neuropathy** (AION), is characterized by the sudden, monocular, and usually painless occurrence of visual loss associated with a relative afferent pupillary defect and the development of a visual field defect that is most often altitudinal or arcuate in nature. The loss of vision usually occurs over several hours to several days. It then stabilizes and remains stable in most cases; however, about 40% of patients with the nonarteritic form of the condition who have worse than 20/60 vision will improve spontaneously within 6 months. AION occurs most often in patients over 50 years of age, many of whom have underlying systemic vasculopathies, such as systemic hypertension, diabetes mellitus, and giant cell arteritis. The optic disc swelling that occurs in AION may be hyperemic or pallid and is usually accompanied by one or more flame-shaped hemorrhages near the margins of the swollen disc (Fig. 4.23). When the swelling is pallid, visual loss is usually very severe and incapable of improving. Patients with nonarteritic AION invariably have a congenitally small optic disc with an absent or small central cup (Fig. 4.24), and this congenital abnormality is thought to be a major risk factor for the development of the disorder. Patients with arteritic AION, on the other hand, may have congenitally small or normally developed optic discs. Thus, if a patient with AION has a normal optic disc in the opposite eye, one should be suspicious the AION is arteritic in origin. Further discussion of ischemic optic neuropathy is in Chapter 7.

Optic Neuritis

Inflammation of the proximal portion of the optic nerve will produce swelling of the optic disc. This condition, called **anterior optic neuritis** or **papillitis**, is characterized by the sudden occurrence of visual loss, usually in one eye and usually associated with pain around or behind the eye. The pain is often exacerbated by eye movement. The appearance of the optic disc ranges from very mild to severe swelling (Fig. 4.25). Vitreous cells may be present, particularly overlying the swollen disc, but peripapillary hemorrhages are rarely seen.

In most cases of anterior optic neuritis, vision continues to decline for several hours to several days. It then stabilizes and, after several days to several weeks, begins to improve.

Anterior optic neuritis typically occurs in young adults and is most often caused by demyelination, although it may also develop in patients with a variety of systemic disorders, such as Lyme disease, sarcoidosis, and syphilis. In demyelinating optic neuritis, vitreous cells are almost always absent, whereas they are more likely to be present and significant in patients with underlying systemic inflammatory or infectious disease. Patients who develop optic neuritis that is unassociated with a systemic inflammatory or infectious disorder have an increased risk of having white matter lesions on MR imaging and of developing clinical evidence of multiple sclerosis (MS).

Neuroretinitis, is characterized ophthalmoscopically by optic disc swelling associated with a macular star figure composed of lipid exudates in Henle's nerve fiber layer (234,235) (Fig. 4.26). This form of optic neuritis is almost never caused by demyelination and occurs most often in the

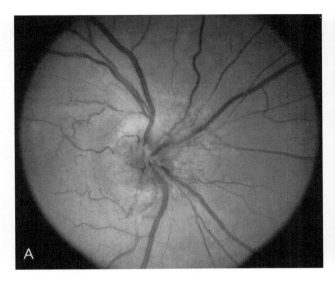
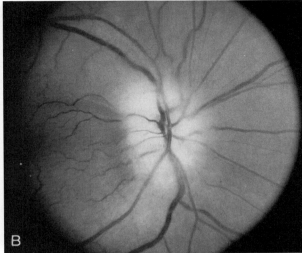

Figure 4.23. Optic disc swelling in anterior ischemic optic neuropathy. *A*, Hyperemic swelling. *B*, Pallid swelling. Eyes with pallid disc swelling usually have worse visual function than eyes with hyperemic disc swelling.

setting of cat scratch disease or in association with other systemic infectious diseases, such as Lyme disease, sarcoidosis, syphilis, toxoplasmosis, and tuberculosis. Optic neuritis is further discussed in Chapter 6.

Compressive Optic Neuropathy

Compression of the proximal portion of the optic nerve may produce optic disc swelling. The compression may be caused by a tumor, such as a glioma, meningioma, or schwannoma. In other cases, enlargement of structures nor-

mally in the orbit, such as the extraocular muscles in dysthyroid ophthalmopathy, causes optic nerve compression. Patients in whom such compression occurs initially may have no visual complaints and may have few signs of optic nerve dysfunction. Alternatively, they may complain of insidious and slowly progressive visual loss. In such cases, there is invariably some degree of dyschromatopsia, a relative afferent pupillary defect, and a defect in the visual field of the affected eye. The optic disc is generally only mildly to moderately swollen and hyperemic (Fig. 4.27). Peripapillary hemorrhages are usually absent, but chorioretinal striae are

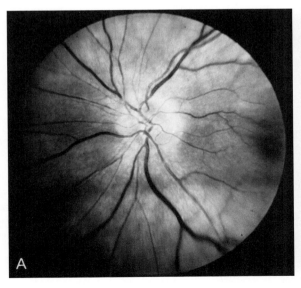
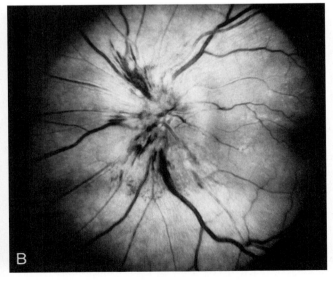

Figure 4.24. The "disc at risk" in nonarteritic anterior ischemic optic neuropathy (NAION). *A*, Small left optic disc with no cup in a patient who had experienced an attack of NAION in the right eye several months earlier. *B*, NAION characterized by hyperemic disc swelling and peripapillary hemorrhages in the same eye several months later.

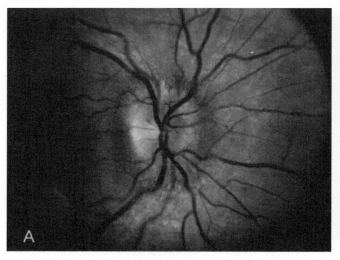

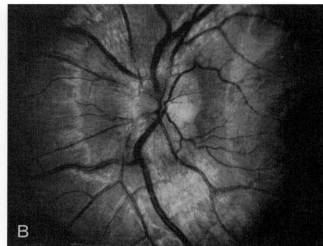

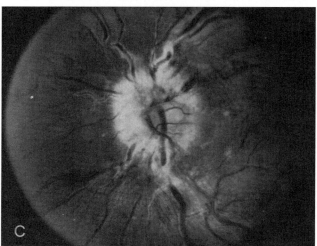

Figure 4.25. Variability in appearance of the optic disc in patients with anterior optic neuritis. *A,* Mild swelling of right optic disc in a 13-year-old girl with acute loss of vision in the right eye, a central visual field defect, and an ipsilateral relative afferent pupillary defect. *B,* Moderate swelling of the left optic disc in a 20-year-old woman with a similar history. *C,* Severe swelling with exudates and sheathing in a 25-year-old man with syphilis.

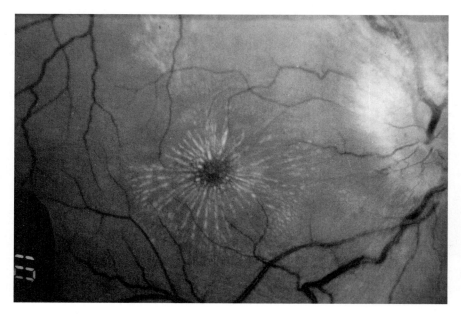

Figure 4.26. Neuroretinitis. The patient was a young woman who developed acute visual loss in the right eye while visiting Connecticut. The right optic disc is swollen, and there is a star figure composed of lipid (hard exudate) in the macula. An evaluation revealed serologic evidence of Lyme disease. Neuroretinitis is not associated with the subsequent development of MS, but is most often caused by an underlying systemic infection, such as cat-scratch disease, Lyme disease, syphilis, or sarcoidosis.

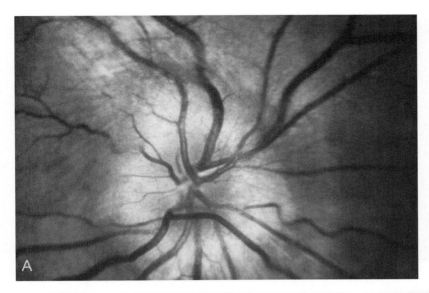

Figure 4.27. Optic disc swelling from compression of the anterior portion of the orbital optic nerve. *A*, Right optic disc of a 25-year-old man who noted mildly decreased vision in the right eye. Visual acuity was 20/25 and there was an ipsilateral relative afferent pupillary defect. The optic disc is moderately swollen. *B*, Noncontrast CT scan, coronal view, shows that the mass compresses the nasal and superior portions of the optic nerve, displacing it downward. *C*, Noncontrast CT scan, axial view, shows a well-circumscribed orbital mass compressing the optic nerve. Note distortion and irregularity of the nerve. The patient's vision returned to normal, and the optic disc swelling resolved after the mass was removed.

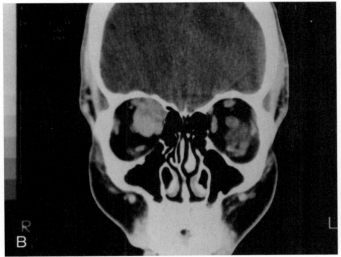

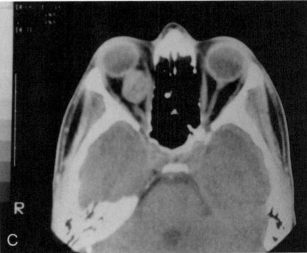

present in some cases, particularly when the compressive lesion is adjacent to the globe (Fig. 4.28). The diagnosis of anterior compressive optic neuropathy is usually made by ultrasonography or neuroimaging of the orbit. More discussion of compressive optic neuropathies is in Chapter 8.

Toxic and Metabolic Optic Neuropathies

Toxic and metabolic disorders rarely cause swelling of the optic disc. In such cases, the swelling is usually bilateral and mild (Fig. 4.29). Central vision is often reduced, with visual loss progressing slowly over several weeks to months, and color vision is almost always markedly abnormal, regardless of the level of central vision. Bilateral symmetry of visual impairment reflects the symmetry of the systemic metabolic process. Bilateral central or cecocentral scotomas are the rule, in some cases being associated with mild to severe constriction of the peripheral visual field. In many but not all cases, eliminating the source of the toxicity or

reversing the metabolic abnormality is associated with some degree of recovery of visual function. Chapter 10 further details toxic optic neuropathies.

Hypotony

Intraocular **hypotony** may induce optic disc swelling. It is well known that following a penetrating wound of the eye or following an operation in which the wound is not tightly closed, there may be development of disc swelling. In addition, blunt trauma to the eye may result in damage to the ciliary body and reduction of aqueous humor formation with subsequent development of hypotony and disc swelling despite the absence of globe rupture (236) (Fig. 4.30). In such cases, the hypotony resolves spontaneously as does the disc swelling. Although visual acuity is impaired in such cases, the visual disturbance appears to be related primarily to increased corneal thickness from the hypotony rather than to a true optic neuropathy.

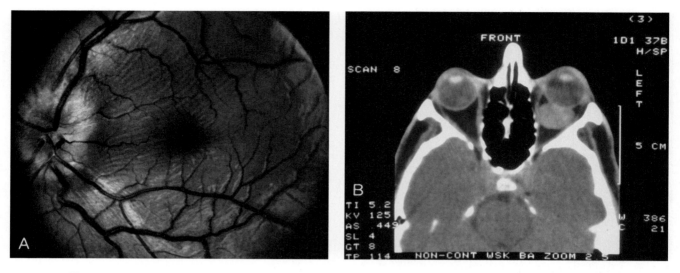

Figure 4.28. Chorioretinal striae associated with optic disc swelling in a patient with a left orbital hemangioma. *A,* Left optic disc is swollen and hyperemic. Note curvilinear chorioretinal striae radiating from the temporal and superior aspects of the disc. *B,* Noncontrast computed tomographic scan, axial view, shows a well-circumscribed mass compressing the posterior aspect of the left globe.

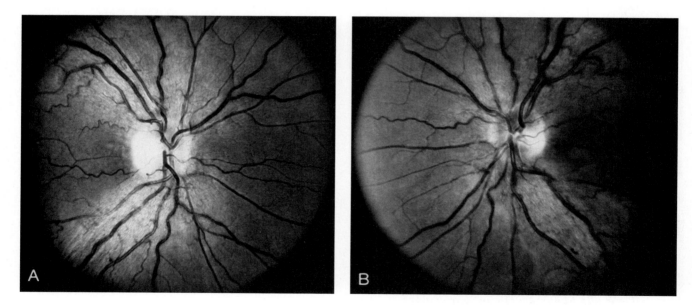

Figure 4.29. Optic disc swelling in nutritional optic neuropathy. The patient was a 34-year-old alcoholic man who had a poor diet and who developed progressive loss of vision in both eyes. Visual acuity was 20/200 OU, and there were bilateral cecocentral scotomas. The concentration of folic acid in the patient's red blood cells was low. *A,* The right optic disc is pale temporally and hyperemic nasally. There is atrophy of the papillomacular bundle. *B,* The left optic disc is hyperemic and mildly swollen. An assay of the patient's blood for mitochondrial mutations of Leber's optic neuropathy was negative. The patient's vision improved and the disc swelling resolved after he reduced his alcohol intake, improved his diet, and was treated with vitamin supplements that included folic acid.

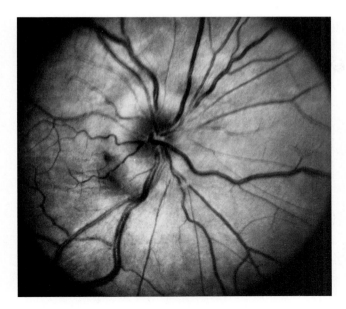

Figure 4.30. Optic disc swelling in hypotony. The patient was a 43-year-old woman who developed hypotony in the right eye after a glaucoma filtering operation. Note moderate swelling and hyperemic of the right optic disc. The appearance of this disc is similar to that which may occur in papilledema, anterior optic neuritis, and other conditions that produce optic disc swelling.

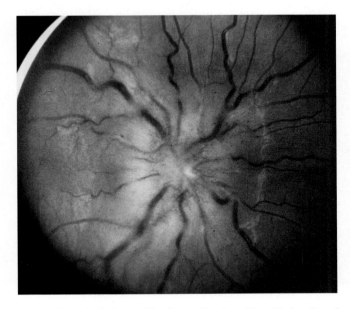

Figure 4.31. Optic disc swelling from infiltration of the orbital portion of the optic nerve. The patient was an 11-year-old boy with acute lymphocytic leukemia that was thought to be in remission when he developed mild blurred vision in the right eye. Note moderate swelling of the right optic disc, associated with dilation of small disc vessels. Malignant cells were detected in the patient's cerebrospinal fluid. The disc swelling resolved and visual acuity improved after radiation therapy.

As with other forms of disc swelling, the pathophysiology of disc swelling in patients with ocular hypotony appears to be blockage of axonal transport at the lamina cribrosa (237,238,239).

Infiltrative Optic Neuropathy

Infiltration of the proximal portion of the optic nerve by tumor or inflammatory cells can produce an appearance similar to true swelling of the optic disc (Fig. 4.31). The disc changes may be asymptomatic or associated with variable visual loss, dyschromatopsia, and a visual field defect. The infiltration may be unilateral or bilateral, and a relative afferent pupillary defect may be present if the infiltration is unilateral or bilateral but asymmetric. Infiltration of the optic nerve occurs most frequently in patients with malignant tumors, such as leukemia, lymphoma, and various carcinomas that spread to the central nervous system (CNS), but it may also occur in patients with systemic inflammatory disorders, including sarcoidosis, tuberculosis, and syphilis. Further discussion of infiltrative optic neuropathy is in Chapter 8.

Anomalous Elevation of the Optic Disc

Anomalous elevation of the optic disc (pseudopapilledema) may bear a striking resemblance to true optic disc swelling and thus represents a major pitfall in neuro-ophthalmologic diagnosis. Congenital elevation of the optic disc may be caused by drusen that are visible with an ophthalmoscope, by drusen that are invisible by ophthalmoscopic examination (''buried'' drusen), by an oblique entrance of the optic disc into the eye (the ''tilted'' optic disc), or simply by abnormal development of tissue without any other associated abnormalities.

Optic disc drusen are structures that may occur within the substance of the optic nerve anterior to the lamina cribrosa. They probably result from abnormal axon metabolism that leads to calcification of intracellular mitochondria (240–243). Superficial drusen reflect whitish-yellow light, are globular, and vary in size from minute dots to granules 2–3 times the diameter of a retinal vessel. Although they may be scattered, they tend to form conglomerates that may fill the entire disc. When the drusen are visible over only a portion of the disc, they are most often concentrated nasally and are usually most conspicuous at the periphery of the disc. Visual field defects may occur and are often peripheral in nature. Photographs taken with the filters normally used for fluorescein photography, but without injection of fluorescein (hence blocking the blue light used for illumination) have shown that superficial disc drusen often demonstrate the phenomenon of autofluorescence (225,244). The autofluorescence is at a longer wavelength which can get through the barrier filter. Diagnosis can be confirmed by ultrasonography and computed tomographic (CT) scanning. Optic disc drusen are further discussed in Chapter 3.

Tilted Optic Disc

In eyes with a congenitally **tilted optic disc**, the optic nerve enters the eye at an extremely oblique angle. This oblique entrance produces a unique ophthalmoscopic ap-

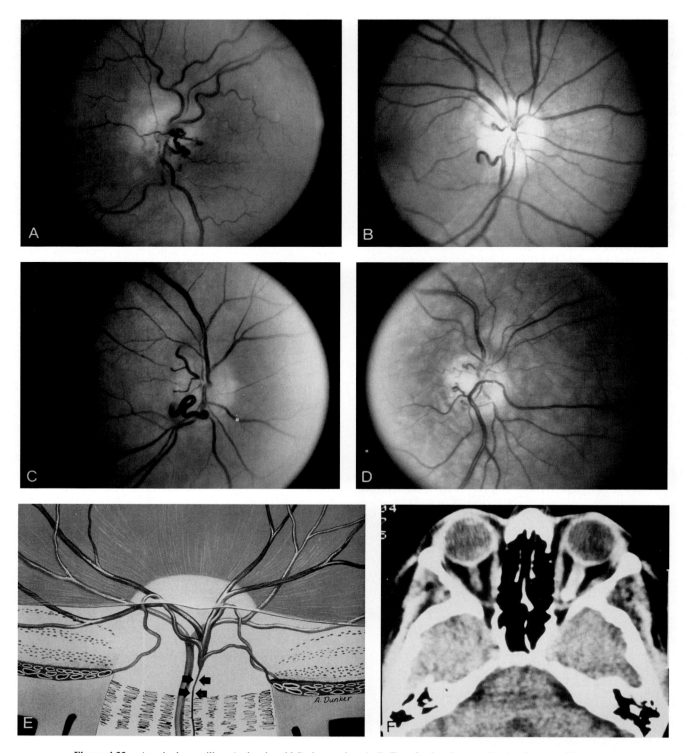

Figure 4.32. Acquired optociliary (retinochoroidal) shunt veins. *A–D*, Four fundus photographs showing optociliary shunt veins in patients with optic atrophy from chronic compression of the optic nerves. Note varying size of the vessels, which are shunting venous blood from the retinal to the choroidal circulation so that it can exit the eye via the vortex veins to the superior and inferior ophthalmic veins rather than via the central retinal vein. *E*, Artist's drawing of retinochoroidal shunt veins that enlarge in the setting of chronic compression of the optic nerve. *F*, Computed tomographic scan, axial view, shows the appearance of a left optic nerve sheath meningioma in the patient whose fundus appearance is shown in *A*. Note that the nerve is thickened and brighter than the opposite optic nerve. (Schematic drawing from Miller NR, Fine SL. The Ocular Fundus in Neuro-Ophthalmologic Diagnosis: Sights and Sounds in Ophthalmology. Vol 3. St Louis, CV Mosby, 1977.)

pearance characterized by (*a*) an oval disc with a depression on one side, usually inferiorly, and an elevation on the other, usually superiorly; (*b*) a peripapillary crescent, usually inferior; and (*c*) an oblique direction of retinal vessels, usually emerging from the superior–temporal portion of the disc and sweeping nasally across the disc before turning temporally. In extreme cases, all of these features are obvious; however, in milder cases, only one or two of the features are apparent.

Patients with congenitally tilted optic discs usually have normal visual acuity, although they often have myopic astigmatism, and normal color vision. Visual field testing, on the other hand, may reveal an asymptomatic temporal field defect that either crosses or does not reach the vertical midline. Further discussion of tilted discs can be found in Chapter 3.

SYNDROMES OF UNILATERAL OPTIC NERVE DYSFUNCTION

Although the appearance of the optic disc alone is usually insufficient to permit an accurate diagnosis of the cause of an optic neuropathy, the consideration of a complete history and a meticulous examination can often provide an accurate diagnosis of an acquired optic neuropathy.

Optociliary Shunts and the Syndrome of Chronic Optic Nerve Compression

Chronic optic nerve compression may cause a specific syndrome characterized by progressive loss of vision, optic disc swelling that is accompanied by optic atrophy, and the appearance of dilated venous channels called optociliary shunt veins. These shunt veins are new potential connections between the retinal and choroidal venous circulations. Chronic compression of the optic nerve, particularly when the lesion is within the orbit, causes these veins to enlarge and shunt blood from the retinal to the choroidal venous circulation, thus allowing the retinal venous blood to bypass the obstructed central retinal vein and exit the orbit via the choroidal circulation, vortex veins, and ophthalmic veins (245) (Fig. 4.32). *Sphenorbital* meningiomas most commonly cause this syndrome, although it may also be caused by chronic papilledema (246–249), arachnoid cysts of the optic nerve (250), craniopharyngioma (251), and probably any cause of chronic congestion of the anterior optic nerve. Acquired optociliary shunt veins also develop in patients after central retinal vein occlusion and in patients with orbital vascular malformations (252).

Prechiasmal Optic Nerve Compression Syndrome

This syndrome is characterized by slowly progressive monocular dimming of vision with near-normal acuity (initially), poor color vision, a relative afferent pupillary defect, and a normal-appearing optic disc (253). In such patients, there are generally subtle central or arcuate visual field defects that can be detected by careful tangent screen examination and that are themselves slowly progressive. Neuroimag-

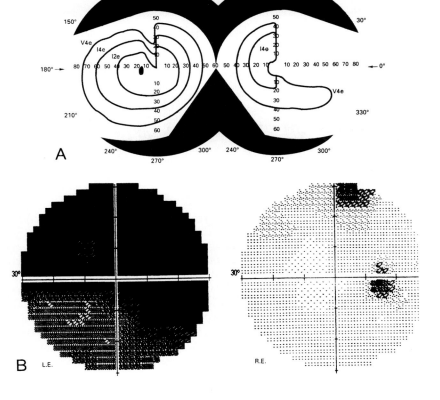

Figure 4.33. Two examples of the syndrome of the distal optic nerve (anterior chiasmal syndrome). *A*, Kinetic perimetry in a patient with a decreased vision in the right eye from a pituitary adenoma shows a dense temporal defect with a central scotoma in that eye. In addition, however, there is a superior temporal defect in the visual field of the contralateral eye. *B*, Static perimetry in another patient with loss of vision in the left eye from a pituitary adenoma shows almost complete loss of the central field in that eye as well as a small superior temporal defect in the visual field of the right eye.

ing in such patients almost always detects a compressive lesion.

Distal Optic Nerve Syndrome (Distal Optic Neuropathy; Anterior Optic Chiasm Syndrome)

The particular fiber anatomy at the optic nerve/chiasm junction provides another opportunity for anatomic diagnosis. Traquair (28) termed this region the anterior angle of the optic chiasm. The crossed and uncrossed fibers are separated at this level but are quite compact, and a small lesion affecting either the crossed or the uncrossed fibers can produce a unilateral hemianopic defect. Traquair (28) called such a defect a "junctional scotoma." In such cases, it is not uncommon to find an asymptomatic scotoma in the upper temporal field of the **opposite** eye (Fig. 4.33). This scotoma results from damage to ventrally located fibers originating from ganglion cells located inferior and nasal to the fovea that, upon reaching the distal end of the optic nerve, are thought to loop anteriorly as much as 4mm, but more probably only about 1–2 mm into the contralateral optic nerve (Fig. 4.34). This loop, called **Wilbrand's knee** is vulnerable to damage from lesions that damage the distal aspect of an optic nerve (254) (Fig. 4.35). Horton (255) has argued that Wilbrand's knee is not a true anatomic structure under normal circumstances; rather, it is an artifact that develops when there is distortion from chronic atrophy of the ipsilateral optic nerve. This may well be the case, but Wilbrand's knee exists from a clinical standpoint, and the concept of an optic neuropathy in one eye with a superior temporal defect in the visual field of the opposite eye remains important in the topical diagnosis of unilateral optic neuropathy.

As mentioned, Traquair (28) used the term "junctional scotoma" to refer to the temporal hemianopic scotoma produced by damage to nasal fibers of the intracranial optic nerve at its junction with the optic chiasm. Thus, the term was used when a strictly unilateral visual field defect was present, and the assumption was made that the lesion was near the optic chiasm. However, it has become common practice to use the term "junctional scotoma" to refer not to the field defect in the affected eye but rather to the superior temporal field defect seen in the **opposite** or unaffected eye. In this setting, the location of the lesion is definite rather than assumed.

Most monocular temporal field defects, whether quadrantanopic or hemianopic, are caused by damage to the distal optic nerve near the optic chiasm. However, such defects can also be produced voluntarily by normal subjects and by malingerers with no organic disease (35,37,38,41). The detection of a monocular defect in the temporal visual field that respects the vertical midline should establish that a lesion of the distal optic nerve is present and the patient needs neuroimaging; however, such a lesion is not always present.

Foster Kennedy Syndrome

Intracranial lesions that exert direct pressure on one optic nerve often lead to unilateral optic atrophy. As these lesions enlarge, they may eventually produce increased intracranial pressure. Because the compressed optic nerve is already atro-

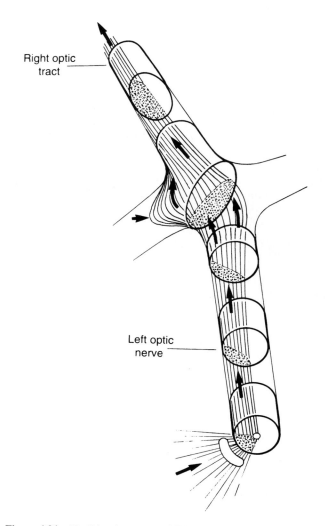

Figure 4.34. Traditional anatomy of Wilbrand's knee. Artist's drawing shows visual fiber projections from the upper and lower nasal quadrants of the retina of the left eye. Note that the fibers from the superior quadrant pass directly into the contralateral (right) optic tract (*arrows*), whereas fibers from the inferior quadrant pass for a short distance into the distal portion of the contralateral optic nerve (*short arrowhead*) before proceeding into the optic tract. (Redrawn from Hoyt WF, Luis O. Visual fiber anatomize in the infrageniculate pathways of the primate; uncrossed and crossed retinal quadrant fiber projections studied with Nauta silver stain. Arch Ophthalmol 1962;68:94–106.)

phic, the increased intracranial pressure produces papilledema only in the contralateral eye (dead axons do not swell). Ipsilateral optic atrophy and contralateral papilledema, often associated with anosmia, are the hallmarks of the so-called **Foster Kennedy syndrome** (256). This is seen with frontal lobe tumors and olfactory groove meningiomas; however, François and Neetens (257) have also described the syndrome in patients with optochiasmatic arachnoiditis and atherosclerosis of an internal carotid artery. Huber (7) reported that in his series, 68% of cases of Foster Kennedy syndrome were caused by tumor, whereas 32% were caused by other disorders.

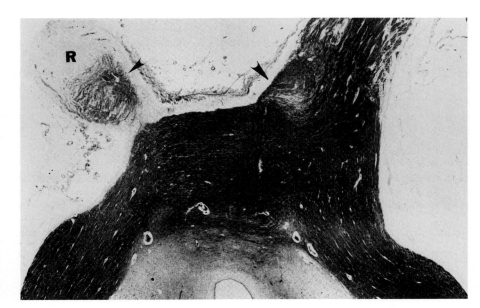

Figure 4.35. Traditional anatomy of Wilbrand's knee. A section through the optic nerves, optic chiasm, and optic tracts of a 43-year-old man who died after coronary bypass surgery, and who had loss of vision in the right eye shortly after birth, reveals a loop or "knee" of stained fibers (*small arrowhead*) in the otherwise unstained right optic nerve (R) at its junction with the optic chiasm. There is also mild pallor in the corresponding area of the normal left optic nerve (*large arrowhead*). (Section stained with Luxol fast blue.) Note alternative explanation in text. (From Breen LA, Quaglieri FC, Schochet SS Jr. J Clin Neuroophthalmol 1983;3:283–284.)

This syndrome of optic atrophy in one eye and papilledema in the other eye has been shown to be falsely localizing in some cases, with the optic atrophy on the side contralateral to the tumor (258). Indeed, a true Foster Kennedy syndrome is rare (7). Optic atrophy on one side and optic disc swelling on the other may result from asymmetric optic nerve compression from an intracranial mass in the absence of increased intracranial pressure (259). Furthermore, it is much more common to see optic atrophy on one side with optic disc swelling on the opposite side in cases of bilateral nonsimultaneous anterior ischemic optic neuropathy or anterior optic neuritis (pseudo-Foster Kennedy syndrome). In such cases, the symptoms and signs are profoundly different and should cause no difficulty in diagnosis.

BILATERAL LESIONS OF THE OPTIC NERVES

The visual fields of both eyes may be altered by a single lesion posterior to the optic chiasm, by a single lesion affecting the chiasm itself, or by bilateral optic nerve lesions. In the majority of cases, the distinction between a single chiasmal or retrochiasmal lesion and lesions of both optic nerves is not difficult. Bilateral central, cecocentral, and arcuate defects all suggest dysfunction of both optic nerves. Ring scotomas do the same when there is no visible retinal abnormality to account for them. Bitemporal visual field defects are usually produced by a single lesion affecting the optic chiasm, whereas homonymous visual field defects are invariably produced by a single lesion affecting the visual sensory pathway posterior to the optic chiasm. Bilateral altitudinal field defects usually are caused by bilateral retinal or optic nerve lesions, although, rarely, they may be caused by bilateral postgeniculate lesions as well (see Chapter 12).

Bilateral Superior or Inferior (Altitudinal) Hemianopia

A unilateral visual field defect in which all or most of the upper or lower portion of the field is abnormal is always caused by a lesion of the retina or optic nerve. Similarly, bilateral visual field defects of this type usually represent bilateral lesions damaging the retinas or optic nerves. In many of these cases, one eye is affected before the other. In such cases, the pathology is typically ischemia, and most patients have an underlying systemic vasculopathy, such as giant cell arteritis, diabetes mellitus, or systemic hypertension that has caused nonsimultaneous bilateral ischemic optic neuropathy (260). In other cases, acute hemorrhage with resultant anemia; acute intraoperative, postoperative, or spontaneous hypotension; or a combination of these phenomena may cause a simultaneous bilateral ischemic optic neuropathy (261–263).

Rarely, a large prechiasmal lesion compresses both optic nerves, producing bilateral altitudinal field defects. Schmidt and Buhrmann (264) reviewed their experience with intracranial mass lesions in the chiasmal region that produced such defects. In most cases, the etiology was a pituitary adenoma that compressed the inferior aspects of both optic nerves, producing bilateral superior altitudinal defects. In other cases, however, compression of the optic nerves from below elevates them against the dural shelves extending out from the intracranial end of the optic canals (Fig. 4.36). Pressure from the dura against the superior aspects of the nerves subsequently produces bilateral inferior altitudinal defects.

Bilateral altitudinal visual field defects may also result from bilateral symmetric damage to the postchiasmal visual pathways. Bilateral occipital lesions (usually traumatic or ischemic, but occasionally inflammatory) may produce bilateral inferior or, somewhat less frequently, superior hemianopias (265–268) (see Chapter 12).

Some patients with bilateral optic neuropathies, particularly those who develop bilateral simultaneous or nonsimultaneous anterior ischemic optic neuropathy, develop a superior altitudinal defect in one eye and an inferior altitudinal

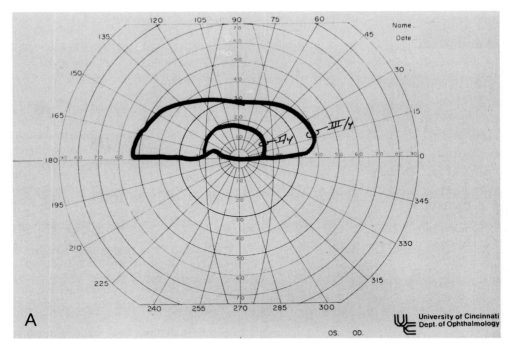

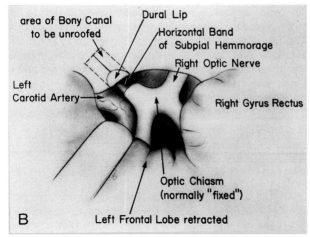

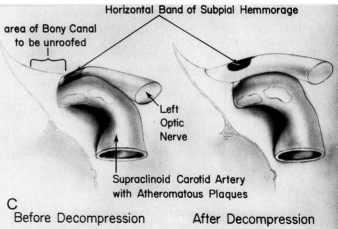

Figure 4.36. Upward displacement of the intracranial portions of the optic nerves from below, causing compression of the superior aspects of the nerves against the dural folds at the intracranial ends of the optic canals. Such compression explains how intracranial lesions that compress the optic nerves from below can nevertheless produce inferior visual field defects. *A*, Inferior altitudinal defect in the visual field of the left eye of a 66-year-old man with progressive visual loss in the eye. Arteriography demonstrated dolichoectasia of the supraclinoid portion of the left internal carotid artery. The patient underwent an exploratory craniotomy. *B*, Artist's drawing of intraoperative findings. Left optic nerve is pushed upward by the dolichoectatic atheromatous artery. The superior aspect of the optic nerve is compressed against the dural shelf of the optic canal, causing a horizontal band of subpial hemorrhage. *C*, Artist's drawing shows relationship of left optic nerve and carotid artery before and after unroofing of optic canal. Before unroofing (*left*), there is compression and upward displacement of the optic nerve against the dural shelf, producing subpial hemorrhage. After unroofing (*right*), the nerve is no longer compressed. The area of hemorrhage on the superior aspect of the nerve, corresponding to the inferior visual field defect, can be clearly seen. (Courtesy of Dr. Joel G. Sacks.)

defect in the other, the so-called **bilateral "checker board" altitudinal hemianopia**. Such patients may experience, in addition to the loss of visual acuity, color vision, and visual field, binocular diplopia caused by decompensation of a preexisting vertical or horizontal phoria. The problems encountered by these patients result from loss of the normal partial overlap of the superior or inferior fields of the two eyes. This overlap normally permits fusion of images and helps to stabilize ocular alignment in patients with vertical or horizontal phorias. Because their remaining visual fields do not overlap, patients with a superior hemianopia in one eye and an inferior hemianopia in the other do not have a physiologic linkage between the two remaining altitudinal hemifields. In such patients, a preexisting minor phoria becomes a tropia because of vertical or horizontal separation or overlap of the two nonoverlapping hemifields (269). These patients complain of diplopia and may have difficulty reading because of doubling or inability to see printed letters or words. This condition, called the "hemifield slide phenomenon" (270) (Fig. 4.37), was initially described in patients with bitemporal hemianopic field defects (271–274), and it is in such patients that it most often occurs (see Chapter 12).

Unilateral and Bilateral Nasal Hemianopia

As mentioned above, most organic nasal visual field defects are actually arcuate in nature. In some cases, however, a true unilateral hemianopia or bilateral nasal hemianopias may develop, with the defects having no connection to the blind spot and respecting the vertical meridian. Such field defects are rarely caused by direct damage to the lateral aspects of the optic chiasm. Rather, they result from damage to the temporal aspects of one or both optic nerves (28).

A unilateral nasal hemianopia has been reported by several investigators (275,276). Amyot (277) and Cox et al. (278) described cases with unilateral nasal hemianopia from suprasellar aneurysms, whereas Meadows (279) described a patient with a unilateral nasal hemianopia from a pituitary adenoma compressing the lateral aspect of one optic nerve. Two other cases of unilateral nasal hemianopia were reported by Schlossberg (280) and Huber (7), but neither of these authors reported the complete ophthalmologic findings in their patients.

Binasal hemianopia is an exceedingly infrequent visual field defect that can be explained only by damage to the temporal fibers of the two optic nerves. A clear-cut bilateral nasal hemianopia with the vertical meridians passing through the points of fixation is infrequent (281). O'Connell and Du Boulay (282) described three patients with "binasal hemianopia," each of whom had an intracranial tumor that had grown between the intracranial optic nerves, pushing them laterally against the anterior cerebral or internal carotid arteries. However, the field defects described in these patients (282) were, in fact, arcuate in nature and did not respect the vertical midline.

Numerous authors have described bilateral nasal field defects in patients with a variety of intracranial lesions, including pituitary tumors (283,284), meningiomas (284), dolichoectatic internal carotid arteries (284), optochiasmatic arachnoiditis (284–287), and primary empty sella syndrome (288) (Fig. 4.38).

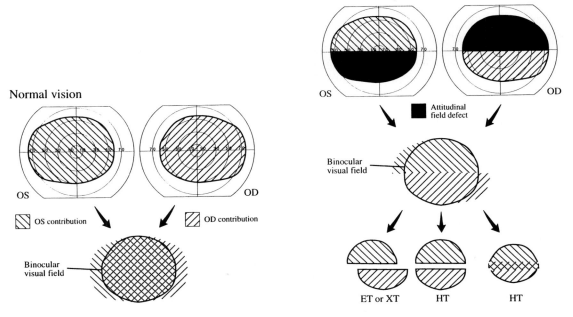

Figure 4.37. Hemifield slide phenomenon from bilateral optic neuropathy. Artist's drawing shows that such defects can produce a vertical or horizontal hemifield slide phenomenon from loss of overlapping portions of the visual fields. Affected patients may complain of vertical, horizontal, or diagonal diplopia.

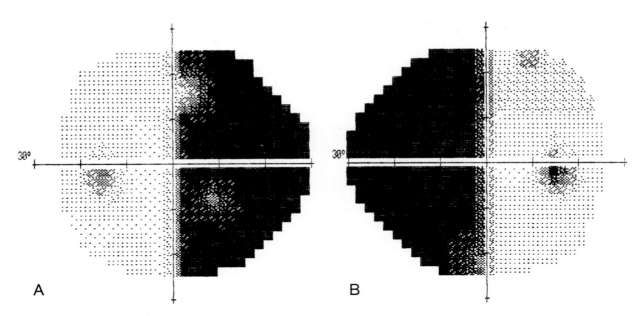

Figure 4.38. Bilateral complete nasal hemianopia in a 34-year-old woman with a suprasellar aneurysm that displaced both optic nerves laterally against the supraclinoid portion of the internal carotid arteries. The field defect resolved after clipping of the aneurysm. *A,* Visual field of the left eye. *B,* Visual field of the right eye.

Bilateral nasal field defects also occur in patients with both primary hydrocephalus and with hydrocephalus caused by intracranial tumors. In such cases, enlargement of the 3rd ventricle pushes the optic chiasm forward, causing lateral displacement of the chiasm and optic nerves against the supraclinoid portion of the internal carotid arteries (285,287). Interestingly, most of the nasal defects resulting from intracranial optic nerve damage affect the inferior, rather than the superior, visual field. Hoyt (289) speculated that the areas most susceptible to pressure from intracranial lesions are those where the intrinsic capillary network first collapses. The fact that none of the cases reported by Manor et al. (284) improved following decompression may be taken as indirect evidence for a vascular etiology for these particular field defects as opposed to a direct block of axoplasmic transport from pressure alone. Bilateral irregular nasal field defects are often associated with drusen of the optic disc but such defects, as in those commonly seen in glaucoma, do not obey the vertical midline and are often arcuate in nature.

REFERENCES

1. Glaser JS. Neuro-Ophthalmology. Ed 2. Philadelphia, JB Lippincott, 1990: 115–117.
2. Fine AM, Elman MJ, Ebert JE, et al. Earliest symptoms caused by neovascular membranes in the macula. Arch Ophthalmol 1986;104:513–514.
3. Sadun AA, Lessell S. Brightness-sense and optic nerve disease. Arch Ophthalmol 1985;103:39–43.
4. Sadun AA. Differentiation of optic nerve from retinal macular disease. In Ophthalmology. Ed 2. St Louis, Mosby, 2003:1253–1254.
5. Fineberg E, Thompson HS. Quantitation of the afferent pupillary defect. In Smith JL, ed. Neuro-Ophthalmology Focus. New York, Masson, 1979:25–29.
6. Hart WM Jr. Acquired dyschromatopsias. Surv Ophthalmol 1987;32:10–31.
7. Huber A. Eye Signs and Symptoms in Brain Tumors. Ed 3. Blodi FC, ed. St Louis, CV Mosby, 1976:12.
8. Safran AB, Kline LB, Glaser JS. Positive visual phenomena in optic nerve disease: Photopsias and photophobia. In Glaser JS, ed. Neuro-Ophthalmology. Vol 10. St Louis, CV Mosby, 1980:225–231.
9. Cummings JL, Gittinger JW Jr. Central dazzle: A thalamic syndrome? Arch Neurol 1981;38:372–374.
10. Brau RH, Lameiro J, Llaguno AV, et al. Metamorphopsia and permanent cortical blindness after a posterior fossa tumor. Neurosurgery 1986;19:263–266.
11. Young WB, Heros DO, Ehrenberg BL, et al. Metamorphopsia and palinopsia: Association with periodic lateralized epileptiform discharges in a patient with malignant astrocytoma. Arch Neurol 1989;46:820–822.
12. Seron X, Matagine F, Coyette F, et al. Étude d'un cas de métamorphopsie limitée aux visages et à certains objects familiers. Rev Neurol 1995;151:691–698.
13. Severin SL, Tour RL, Kershaw RW. Macular function and the photostress test. 1. Arch Ophthalmol 1967;77:2–7.
14. Severin SL, Tour RL, Kershaw RH. Macular function and the photostress test. 2. Arch Ophthalmol 1967;77:163–167.
15. Glaser JS. Office and laboratory testing of visual function. Trans Am Acad Ophthalmol Otolaryngol 1977;83:797–804.
16. Sandberg MA, Jacobson SG, Berson EL. Foveal cone electroretinograms in retinitis pigmentosa and juvenile macular degeneration. Am J Ophthalmol 1979; 88:702–707.
17. Sandberg MA, Hanson AH, Berson EL. Foveal and parafoveal cone electroretinograms in juvenile macular degeneration. Ophthalmic Pediatr Genet 1983;3: 83–87.
18. Fish GE, Birch DG. The focal electroretinogram in the clinical assessment of macular disease. Ophthalmology 1989;96:109–114.
19. Matthews GP, Sandberg MA, Berson EL. Foveal cone electroretinograms in patients with central visual loss of unexplained etiology. Arch Ophthalmol 1992; 110:1568–1570.
20. Krill AE, Deutman AF, Fishman M. The cone degenerations. Doc Ophthalmol 1973;35:1–80.
21. Mäntyjärvi MI. Color vision defect as first symptom of progressive rod cone dystrophy. J Clin Neuroophthalmol 1990;10:266–270.
22. Goodman G, Ripps H, Siegel IM. Cone dysfunction syndromes. Arch Ophthalmol 1963;70:214–231.
23. François J, De Rouck A, Verriest G, et al. Progressive generalized cone dysfunction. Ophthalmologica 1974;169:255–284.
24. Pinckers AJLG, Pokorny J, Smith VC, et al. Classification of abnormal color vision. In Pokorny J, Smith VC, Verriest G, Pinckers AJLG, eds. Congenital and Acquired Color Vision Defects. New York, Grune & Stratton, 1979:71–82.
25. Newsome DA, Milton RC, Gass JDM. Afferent pupillary defect in macular degeneration. Am J Ophthalmol 1981;92:396–402.
26. Servais GE, Thompson HS, Hayreh SS. Relative afferent pupillary defect in central retinal vein occlusion. Ophthalmology 1986;93:301–303.
27. Folk JC, Thompson HS, Farmer SG, et al. Relative afferent pupillary defect in eyes with retinal detachment. Ophthalmic Surg 1987;18:757–759.
28. Traquair HM. An Introduction to Clinical Perimetry. Ed 6. London, Kimpton, 1949.

29. Harrington DO. Differential diagnosis of the arcuate scotoma. Invest Ophthalmol 1969;8:96–105.

30. Hood DC. Assessing retinal function with the multifocal technique. Prog Retin Eye Res Sep 2000;19:607–646.

31. Sutter E. The interpretation of multifocal binary kernels. Doc Ophthalmol 2000; 100(2–3):49–75.

32. Sutter EE. Imaging visual function with the multifocal m-sequence technique. Vision Res 2001;41:1241–1255.

33. Gerth C, Sutter EE, Werner JS. MfERG response dynamics of the aging retina. Invest Ophthalmol Vis Sci 2003;44:4443–4450.

34. Hood DC, Bearse MA Jr, Sutter EE, et al. The optic nerve head component of the monkey's (Macaca mulatta) multifocal electroretinogram. Vision Res 2001; 41:2029–2041.

35. Keane JR. Hysterical hemianopia: The ''missing half'' field defect. Arch Ophthalmol 1979;97:865–866.

36. Ellenberger C Jr. Tunnel vision. Neurology 1984;34:129.

37. Gittinger JW Jr. Functional monocular temporal hemianopsia. Am J Ophthalmol 1986;101:226–231.

38. Glovinsky Y, Quigley HA, Bissett RA, et al. Artificially produced quadrantanopsia in computed visual field testing. Am J Ophthalmol 1990;110:90–91.

39. MacLeod JDA, Manners RM, Heaven CJ, et al. Visual field defects: How easily can they be fabricated using the automated perimeter? Neuroophthalmology 1994;14:185–188.

40. Stewart JFG. Automated perimetry and malingers: Can the Humphrey be outwitted? Ophthalmology 1995;102:27–32.

41. Thompson JC, Kosmorsky GS, Ellis BD. Fields of dreamers and dreamed up fields: Functional and fake perimetry. Ophthalmology 1996;103:117–125.

42. Havener WH, McReynolds WU. False scotomas associated with high uncorrected refractive errors. Arch Ophthalmol 1952;48:616–619.

43. Wilson SAK. Dysmetropsia and its pathogenesis. Trans Ophthalmol Soc UK 1916;36:412–444.

44. Gloning I, Gloning K, Hoff H. Neuropsychological Symptoms and Syndromes in Lesions of the Occipital Lobe and the Adjacent Areas. Paris, Gauthier Villars, 1968.

45. Cohen L, Gray F, Meyrignac C, Dehaene S, Degos JD. Selective deficit of visual size perception: Two cases of hemimicropsia. J Neurol Neurosurg Psychiatry 1994;57:73–78.

46. Michaeli Cohen A, Almog Y, Loewenstein A, et al. Presumed ocular myasthenia and micropsia: A case report. J Neuroophthalmol 1996;16:18–20.

47. Burde RM. Editorial comment. J Neuroophthalmol 1996;16:21–22.

48. Shaw HE, Smith JL. Cecocentral scotomas: Neuro-ophthalmologic considerations. In Smith JL, ed. Neuro-Ophthalmology Focus, 1980. New York, Masson, 1979:165–174.

49. Birchall CH, Harris GS, Drance SM, et al. Visual field changes in branch retinal ''vein'' occlusion. Arch Ophthalmol 1976;94:747–754.

50. Halpern JI, Sedler RR. Traumatic bilateral homonymous hemianopic scotomas. Ann Ophthalmol 1980;12:1022–1026.

51. Aulhorn E, Harms H. Early visual field defects in glaucoma. In Glaucoma Symposium, Tutzing Castle, 1966. Karger, Basel, 1967:151–166.

52. Stoll MR. Pericentral ring scotoma. Arch Ophthalmol 1950;43:66–91.

53. Johnson LN, Rabinowitz YS, Hepler RS. Hemianopia respecting the vertical meridian and with fovial sparing from retinal degeneration. Neurology 1989; 39:872–873.

54. Sloan LL, Brown DJ. Progressive retinal degeneration with selective involvement of the cone mechanism. Am J Ophthalmol 1962;54:629–641.

55. Krill AE. The electroretinographic and electrooculographic findings in patients with macular lesions. Trans Am Acad Ophthalmol Otolaryngol 1966;70: 1063–1083.

56. Krill AE. Cone degenerations. In Krill's Hereditary Retinal and Choroidal Diseases, Vol II. Hagerstown MD, Harper & Row, 1977:421–487.

57. Newman NM, Stevens RA, Heckenlively JR. Nerve fibre layer loss in diseases of the outer retinal layer. Br J Ophthalmol 1987;71:21–26.

58. Weleber RG, Eisner A. Cone degeneration (''bull's eye dystrophies'') and color vision defects. In Newsome DA, ed. Retinal Dystrophies and Degeneration. New York, Raven Press, 1988:233–256.

59. Newman NJ, Slavin M, Newman SA. Optic disc pallor: A false localizing sign. Surv Ophthalmol 1993;37:273–282.

60. Ninomiya T, Yamazaki H, Munakata S, et al. A case of congenital stationary night blindness with optic disc pallor. Folia Ophthalmol Jpn 1996;47:519–522.

61. Quigley HA, Green WR. The histology of human glaucoma cupping and optic nerve damage: Clinicopathologic correlation in 21 eyes. Ophthalmology 1979; 10:1803–1827.

62. Drance SM. The early field defect in glaucoma. Invest Ophthalmol 1969;8: 84–91.

63. Werner EB, Drance SM. Early visual field disturbances in glaucoma. Arch Ophthalmol 1977;95:1173–1175.

64. Morin JD. Changes in the visual fields in glaucoma: Static and kinetic perimetry in 2000 patients. Trans Am Ophthalmol Soc 1979;77:622–642.

65. Rönne H. The focal diagnostic of the visual path. Acta Ophthalmol 1938;16: 446–453.

66. Brais P, Drance SM. The temporal field in chronic simple glaucoma. Arch Ophthalmol 1972;88:518–522.

67. François J, Verriest G. Les dyschromatopsies acquises dans le glaucoma primaire. Ann Ophtalmol 1959;192:191–199.

68. Grützner P, Schleicher S. Acquired colour vision defects in glaucoma patients. Mod Probl Ophthalmol 1972;11:136–140.

69. Austen DJ. Acquired color vision defects in patients suffering from chronic simple glaucoma. Trans Ophthalmol Soc UK 1974;94:880–883.

70. Fishman GA, Krill AE, Fishman M. Acquired colour defects in patients with open angle glaucoma and ocular hypertension. Mod Probl Ophthalmol 1974;13: 335–338.

71. Kalmus H, Luke J, Svedburgh D. Impairment of colour vision in patients with ocular hypertension and glaucoma. Br J Ophthalmol 1974;58:922–926.

72. Poinoosawmy D, Nagasubramanian S, Gloster J. Colour vision in patients with chronic simple glaucoma and ocular hypertension. Br J Ophthalmol 1980;64: 852–857.

73. Drance SM. Early disturbances of colour vision in chronic open angle glaucoma. Doc Ophthalmol 1981;26:155–159.

74. Airaksinen PJ, Lakowski R, Drance SM, et al. Color vision and retinal nerve fiber layer in early glaucoma. Am J Ophthalmol 1986;101:208–213.

75. Stamper RL. Psychophysical changes in glaucoma. Surv Ophthalmol 1989; 33(Suppl):309–318.

76. Bartos D. Color vision in glaucoma. Cesk Oftalmol 1990;46:194–207.

77. Jonas JB, Zäch F M. Farbsehstörungen bei chronischem Offenwinkelglaukom. Fortschr Ophthalmol 1990;87:255–259.

78. Huang S, Wu L, Wu DZ. The color vision in patients with optic neuritis and chronic open angle glaucoma. Eye Science 1991;7:92–94.

79. Korth M, Nguyen NX, Junemann A, et al. Blau selektiver VEP Test fur die Glaukomdiagnostik. Klin Monatslbl Augenheilkd 1993;203:324–328.

80. Koseki N, Yamagami J, Araie M, et al. A study of parafoveal color vision in normal tension and primary open angle glaucoma eyes. Nippon Ganka Gakkai Zasshi 1993;97:526–531.

81. Sample PA, Boynton RM, Weinreb RN. Isolating the color vision loss in primary open angle glaucoma. Am J Ophthalmol 1988;106:686–691.

82. Levitan P, Prasloski PF, Collen MF. The swinging flashlight test in multiphasic screening for eye disease. Can J Ophthalmol 1973;8:356–360.

83. Kaback MB, Burde RM, Becker B. Relative afferent pupillary defect in glaucoma. Am J Ophthalmol 1976;81:462–468.

84. Prywes AS. Unilateral afferent pupillary defects in asymmetric glaucoma. Arch Ophthalmol 1976;94:1286–1288.

85. Kohn AN, Moss AP, Podos SM. Relative afferent pupillary defects in glaucoma without characteristic field loss. Arch Ophthalmol 1979;97:294–296.

86. Brown RH, Zillis JD, Lynch MG, et al. The afferent pupillary defect in asymmetric glaucoma. Arch Ophthalmol 1987;105:1540–1543.

87. Trobe JD, Glaser JS, Cassady JC, et al. Nonglaucomatous excavation of the optic disc. Arch Ophthalmol 1980;98:1046–1050.

88. Kuppersmith MJ, Krohn D. Cupping of the optic disc with compressive lesions of the anterior visual pathway. Ann Ophthalmol 1984;16:948–953.

89. Kalenak JW, Kosmorsky GS, Hassenbusch SJ. Compression of the intracranial optic nerve mimicking unilateral normal pressure glaucoma. J Clin Neuroophthalmol 1992;12:230–235.

90. Bianchi Marzoli S, Rizzo JF, Brancato R, et al. Quantitative analysis of optic disc cupping in compressive optic neuropathy. Ophthalmology 1995;102:436–440.

91. Nicolela MT, Drance SM. Various glaucomatous optic nerve appearances: Clinical correlations. Ophthalmology 1996;103:640–649.

92. Brøns J. The blind spot of Mariotte: Its ordinary imperceptibility or filling in and its facultative visibility. Acta Ophthalmol 1939;17(Suppl 17):1–348.

93. Berens C. Examination of the blind spot of Mariotte. Trans Am Ophthalmol Soc 1923;21:271–290.

94. Fletcher WA, Imes RF, Goodman D, et al. Acute idiopathic blind spot enlargement: A big blind spot syndrome without optic disc edema. Arch Ophthalmol 1988;106:44–49.

95. Gass JDM. Retinal causes of the big blind spot syndrome. J Clin Neuroophthalmol 1989;9:144–145.

96. Hamed L, Glaser JS, Gass JDM, et al. Protracted enlargement of the blind spot in multiple evanescent white dot syndrome occurring in the same patients. Arch Ophthalmol 1989;107:194–198.

97. Wakakura M, Furuno K. Bilateral slowly progressive big blind spot syndrome. J Clin Neuroophthalmol 1989;9:141–143.

98. Dodwell DG, Jampol LM, Rosenberg M, et al. Optic nerve involvement associated with multiple evanescent white dot syndrome. Ophthalmology 1990;97: 862–868.

99. Reddy CV, Brown J Jr, Folk JC, et al. Enlargement of the blind spot in multiple evanescent white dot syndrome and multifocal choroiditis. Ophthalmology 1994; 101(Suppl):95.

100. Miller NR, George TW. Monochromatic photography and ophthalmoscopy of the peripapillary retinal nerve fiber layer. Invest Ophthalmol 1978;17: 1121–1124.

101. Said FS, Weale RA. The variation with age of the spectral transmissivity of the living human crystalline lens. Gerontologica 1959;3:213–231.

102. Snydacker D. The normal optic disc: Ophthalmoscopic photographic studies. Am J Ophthalmol 1964;58:958–964.
103. Sorensen PN. The colour of the optic disc variation with location of illumination. Acta Ophthalmol 1980;58:1005–1010.
104. Kronfeld PC. The optic nerve. In Symposium on Glaucoma: Transactions of the New Orleans Academy of Ophthalmology, St Louis, CV Mosby, 1967:62–73.
105. Schwartz B. Cupping and pallor of the optic disc. Arch Ophthalmol 1973;89: 272–277.
106. Duchen LW. General pathology of neurons and neuroglia. In Adams JH, Duchen LW, eds. Greenfield's Neuropathology. Ed 5. New York, Oxford University Press, 1992:1–68.
107. Sadun AA, Schaechter JD. Tracing axons in the human brain: A method utilizing light and TEM techniques. J Electron Microsc Tech 1985;2:175–186.
108. Johnson BM, Sadun AA. Ultrastructural and paraphenylene studies of degeneration in the primate visual system: Degenerative remnants persist for much longer than expected. J Electron Microsc Tech 1988;8:179–183.
109. Blackwood W, McMenemey WH, Meyer A, et al. Greenfield's Neuropathology. Baltimore, Williams & Wilkins, 1963:19–32.
110. Hoyt WF. Anatomic considerations of arcuate scotomas associated with lesions of the optic nerve and chiasm: A Nauta axon degeneration study in the monkey. Bull Johns Hopkins Hosp 1962;111:57–71.
111. Hoyt WF, Luis O. Visual fiber anatomy in the infrageniculate pathway of the primate; uncrossed and crossed retinal quadrant fiber projections studied with Naura silver stain. Arch Ophthalmol 1962;68:94–106.
112. Hoyt WF, Tudor RC. The course of peripapillary temporal retinal axons through the anterior optic nerve. A Nauta degeneration study in the primate. Arch Ophthalmol 1963;69:503–507.
113. Anderson DR. Ascending and descending optic atrophy produced experimentally in squirrel monkeys. Am J Ophthalmol 1973;76:693–711.
114. Radius RL, Anderson DR. Retinal ganglion cell degeneration in experimental optic atrophy. Am J Ophthalmol 1978;86:673–679.
115. Radius RL, Anderson DR. The course of axons through the retina and optic nerve head. Arch Ophthalmol 1979;97:1154–1158.
116. Kupfer C. Retinal ganglion cell degeneration following chiasmal lesions in man. Arch Ophthalmol 1963;70:256–260.
117. Lundstrom M, Frisén L. Evolution of descending optic atrophy: A case report. Acta Ophthalmol 1975;53:738–746.
118. Quigley HA, Davis EB, Anderson DR. Descending optic nerve degeneration in primates. Invest Ophthalmol Vis Sci 1977;16:841–849.
119. Wolter JR. The centrifugal fibers in the human optic tract, chiasm, optic nerve and retina. Trans Am Ophthalmol Soc 1965;63:678–707.
120. Wolter JR. Centrifugal fibers in the adult human optic nerve 16 days after enucleation. Trans Am Ophthalmol Soc 1978;76:140–151.
121. Carelli V, Ross-Cisneros FN, Sadun AA. Optic nerve degeration and mitochondrial dysfunction: genetic and acquired optic neuropathies. Neurochem Internat 2002;40:573–584.
122. Wee R, Van Gelden RN. Sleep disturbances in young subjects with visual dysfunction. Ophthalmology 2004;111:297–303.
123. Cone W, MacMillan JA. The optic nerve and papilla. In Penfield W, ed. Cytology and Cellular Pathology of the Nervous System. Vol 2. New York, Paul B. Hoeber, 1932:837–901.
124. Wolter JR. Regenerative potentialities of the centrifugal fibers in the human optic nerve. Arch Ophthalmol 1960;64:697–707.
125. Lam T. Targeting the apoptotic pathway for neuroprotection. In Neuroprotection: Implications for Eye Disease. Doheny Eye Institute, 2002:30–32.
126. Wheeler LA. Alpha-2 agonists. Neuroprotection and glaucoma. In Neuroprotection: Implications for Eye Disease. Doheny Eye Institute, 2002:25–27.
127. McKinnon SJ. Gene threapy using caspase inhibitors prevents optic nerve loss in experimental rat glaucoma. In Neuroprotection: Implications for Eye Disease. Doheny Eye Institute, 2002:40–42.
128. Sadun AA. Apoptosis and the retinal ganglion cell. In Neuroprotection: Implications for Eye Disease. Doheny Eye Institute, 2002:16–19.
129. Bunge MB, Bunge RP, Ris H. Ultrastructural study of remyelination in an experimental lesion in adult cat spinal cord. J Biophys Biochem Cytol 1961;10:67–94.
130. Bornstein MB, Appel SH, Murray MR. The application of tissue culture to the study of experimental "allergic" encephalomyelitis: Demyelination and remyelination. In Jacob H, ed. Proceedings of the IVth International Congress of Neuropathology. Vol 2. Stuttgart, Thieme, 1962:279–282.
131. Bunge RP. Glial cells and the central myelin sheath. Physiol Rev 1968;48: 197–251.
132. Gledhill RF, Harrison BM, McDonald WI. Pattern of remyelination in the CNS. Nature 1973;244:443–444.
133. Gledhill RF, Harrison BM, McDonald WI. Demyelination and remyelination after acute spinal cord compression. Exp Neurol 1973;38:472–487.
134. Harrison BM, Gledhill RF, McDonald WI. Remyelination after transient compression of the spinal cord. Proc Aust Assoc Neurol 1975;12:117–122.
135. Gledhill RF, McDonald WI. Morphological characteristics of central demyelination and remyelination: A single fibre study. Ann Neurol 1977;1:552–560.
136. Harrison BM, McDonald WI. Remyelination after transient experimental compression of the spinal cord. Ann Neurol 1977;1:542–551.
137. Prineas JW, Connell F. Remyelination in multiple sclerosis. Ann Neurol 1979; 5:22–31.
138. Ludwin SK. Remyelination in demyelinating diseases of the central nervous system. Crit Rev Neurobiol 1987;3:1–28.
139. Hirano A. Review of the morphological aspects of remyelination. Dev Neurosci 1989;11:112–117.
140. Prineas JW, Barnard RO, Kwon EE, et al. Multiple sclerosis: Remyelination of nascent lesions. Ann Neurol 1993;33:137–151.
141. Herndon RM, Price DL, Weiner LP. Regeneration of oligodendroglia during recovery from demyelinating disease. Science 1977;195:693–694.
142. Sadun AA. Mitochondrial optic neuropathies. J Neurol Neurosurg Psych 2002; 72:423–425.
143. Sadun AA, Carelli V. Mitochondrial function and dysfunction within the optic nerve. Arch Ophthalmol 2003;121:1342–1343.
144. Sadun AA. Acquired mitochondrial impairment as a cause of optic nerve disease. Trans Am Soc 1998;96:881–923.
145. Rodriguez M. Mechanisms of virus induced demyelination and remyelination. Ann NY Acad Sci 1988;540:240–251.
146. Clifford Jones RE, Landon DN, McDonald WI. Remyelination during optic nerve compression. J Neurol Sci 1980;46:239–243.
147. Kayan A, Earl CJ. Compressive lesions of the optic nerves and chiasm: Pattern of recovery of vision following surgical treatment. Brain 1975;98:13–25.
148. Rosenberg LF, Miller NR. Visual results after microsurgical removal of meningiomas involving the anterior visual system. Arch Ophthalmol 1984;102: 1019–1023.
149. Symon L, Rosenstein J. Surgical management of suprasellar meningioma. Part 1: The influence of tumor size, duration of symptoms, and microsurgery on surgical outcome in 101 consecutive cases. J Neurosurg 1984;61:633–641.
150. Marcus M, Vitale S, Calvert PC, et al. Visual results after transsphenoidal removal of pituitary tumors. Aust NZ J Ophthalmol 1991;19:111–118.
151. Beatty R, Sadun AA, et al. Direct demonstration of transsynaptic degeneration in the human visual system: a comparison of retrograde and anterograde changes. J Neurol Neurosurg Psych 1982;45(2):143–146.
152. Brouwer B, Zeeman WPC. The projection of the retina in the primary optic neuron of monkeys. Brain 1926;49:1–35.
153. Le Gros Clark WE. A morphologic study of the lateral geniculate body. Br J Ophthalmol 1932;16:264.
154. Polyak S. The nervous system. In Maximow A, Bloom W, eds. Textbook of Histology. Ed 3. Philadelphia, WB Saunders, 1938:173.
155. Fulton JF. Physiology of the Nervous System. Ed 2. London, Oxford University Press, 1943:38.
156. Haddock JN, Berlin L. Transsynaptic degeneration in the visual system: Report of a case. Arch Neurol Psychiatr 1950;64:66–73.
157. Juba A, Szatmari A. Uber seltene hirnanatomische befune in fallen von einseitiger peripherer blindheit. Klin Monatsbl Augenheilkd 1937;99:173.
158. Van Buren JM. The Retinal Ganglion Cell Layer. Springfield IL, Charles C Thomas, 1963a:102–121.
159. Cowey A. Atrophy of retinal ganglion cells after removal of striate cortex in a rhesus monkey. Perception 1974;3:257–260.
160. Weller RE, Kaas JH, Wetzel AB. Evidence for the loss of X cells of the retina after long term ablation of the visual cortex in monkeys. Brain Res 1980;160: 134.
161. Wilbrand H, Saenger A. Die Erkrankungen des Opticusstammes. In Die Neurologie des Auges. Vol 5. Wiesbaden, JF Bergmann, 1913.
162. Weller RE, Kaas JH, Ward J. Preservation of retinal ganglion cells and normal patterns of retinogeniculate projections in prosimian primates with long term ablations of striate cortex. Invest Ophthalmol Vis Sci 1981;20:139–148.
163. Miller NR, Newman SA. Transsynaptic degeneration. Arch Ophthalmol 1981; 99:1654.
164. Van Buren JM. Transsynaptic retrograde degeneration in the visual system of primates. J Neurol Neurosurg Psychiatry 1963;26:402–409.
165. Beatty RM, Sadun AA, Smith LEH, et al. Direct demonstration of transsynaptic degeneration in the human visual system: A comparison of retrograde and anterograde changes. J Neurol Neurosurg Psychiatry 1982;45:143–146.
166. Quigley HA, Anderson DR. The histologic basis of optic disc pallor. Am J Ophthalmol 1977;83:709–717.
167. Henkind P, Bellhorn R, Rabkin M, et al. Optic nerve transection in cats. 2. Effects on vessels of optic nerve head and lamina cribrosa. Invest Ophthalmol Vis Sci 1977;16:445–447.
168. Hayreh SS. Colour and fluorescence of the optic disc. Ophthalmologica 1972; 165:100–108.
169. Schwartz B, Reinstein NM, Lieberman DM. Pallor of the optic disc: Quantitative photographic evaluation. Arch Ophthalmol 1973;89:278–286.
170. Bock RH. Zur klinischen messung der papillenfarbe. Ophthalmologica 1950; 120:174–177.
171. Gloster J. The colour of the optic disc. Doc Ophthalmol 1969;26:155–163.
172. Berkowitz JS, Balter S. Colorimetric measurement of the optic disc. Am J Ophthalmol 1970;69:385–386.
173. Davies EWG. Quantitative assessment of colour of the optic disc by a photographic method. Exp Eye Res 1970;9:106–113.

174. Gloster J, Parry DG. Use of photographs for measuring cupping in the optic disc. Br J Ophthalmol 1974;58:850–862.

175. Sorensen PN. The pallor of the optic disc. A quantitative photographic assessment by purple filter. Acta Ophthalmol 1979;57:718–724.

176. Kestenbaum A. Clinical Methods of Neuro-Ophthalmologic Examination, New York, Grune & Stratton, 1946:81.

177. Kant A. The ophthalmoscopic evaluation of optic atrophy. Am J Ophthalmol 1949;32:1479–1486.

178. Dalsgaard Nielsen E. Glaucoma like cupping of the optic disc and its etiology. Acta Ophthalmol 1937;15:151–178.

179. Blazar HA, Scheie HG. Pseudoglaucoma. Arch Ophthalmol 1950;44:499–513.

180. Miller S. The enigma of glaucoma simplex. Trans Ophthalmol Soc UK 1972;92:563–584.

181. Portney GL, Roth AM. Optic cupping caused by an intracranial aneurysm. Am J Ophthalmol 1977;84:98–103.

182. Quigley HA, Anderson DR. Cupping of the optic disc in ischemic optic neuropathy. Trans Am Acad Ophthalmol Otolaryngol 1977;83:755–762.

183. Radius RL, Maumenee AE. Optic atrophy and glaucomatous cupping. Am J Ophthalmol 1978;85:145–153.

184. Hoyt WF, Schlicke B, Eckelhoff RJ. Fundoscopic appearance of a nerve fibre bundle defect. Br J Ophthalmol 1972;56:577–583.

185. Sommer A, Miller NR, Pollack I, et al. The nerve fiber layer in the diagnosis of glaucoma. Arch Ophthalmol 1977;95:2149–2156.

186. Jonas JB, Schiro D. Localized retinal nerve fiber layer defects in nonglaucomatous optic nerve atrophy. Graefe's Arch Clin Exp Ophthalmol 1994;232:759–760.

187. Hoyt WF. Fundoscopic changes in the retinal nerve fibre layer in chronic and acute optic neuropathies. Trans Ophthalmol Soc UK 1976;96:368–371.

188. Hoyt WF. Ophthalmoscopy of the retinal nerve fiber layer in neuro-ophthalmologic diagnosis. Aust J Ophthalmol 1976;4:14–34.

189. Hoyt WF, Knight CL. Comparison of congenital disc blurring and incipient papilledema in red free light—a photographic study. Invest Ophthalmol 1973;12:241–247.

190. Miller NR, George TW. Monochromatic (red free) photography and ophthalmoscopy of the peripapillary retinal nerve fiber layer. In Smith JL, ed. Neuro-Ophthalmology Focus 1980. New York, Masson, 1979:43–51.

191. Frisén L. Ophthalmoscopic evaluation of the retinal nerve fiber layer in neuroophthalmologic disease. In Smith JL, ed. Neuro-Ophthalmology Focus 1980. New York, Masson, 1979:53–67.

192. Tagami Y. Atrophy of maculopapillar bundles in recovered optic neuropathies. Jpn J Ophthalmol 1979;23:301–309.

193. Enoksson P, Nordell S. Retinal nerve fibre degeneration in optic glioma. Neuroophthalmology 1980;1:3–10.

194. Manor RS, Schleinn N, Yassur Y, et al. Narrow band (540 nm) green light stereoscopic photography of the surface details of the peripapillary retina. Am J Ophthalmol 1981;91:774–780.

195. Sommer A, D'Anna SA, Kues HA, et al. High resolution photography of the retinal nerve fiber layer. Am J Ophthalmol 1983;96:535–539.

196. Airaksinen PJ, Drance SM, Douglas GR, et al. Diffuse and localized nerve fiber loss in glaucoma. Am J Ophthalmol 1984;98:566–571.

197. Peli E, Hedges TR, Schwartz B. Computerized enhancement of retinal nerve fiber layer. Acta Ophthalmol 1986;64:113–122.

198. Pollock SC, Miller NR. The retinal nerve fiber layer. Int Ophthalmol Clin 1986;26:201–221.

199. Kanatani I, Mizokami K. Clinical evaluation of retinal nerve fiber layer atrophy. Acta Soc Ophthalmol Jpn 1987;91:1154–1159.

200. Jonas JB, Nguyen NX, Naumann GOH. The retinal nerve fiber layer in normal eyes. Ophthalmology 1989;96:627–632.

201. Barry CJ, Cooper RL, Eikelboom RH. Simplification of unsharp masking in retinal nerve fibre layer photography. Aust N Z J Ophthalmol 1990;18:411–420.

202. Bartz Schmidt KU, Schmitz Valckenberg P. Diagnostische Hinweise bei Optikuskrankungen mit Hilfe der retinalen Nervenfaserphotographie. Fortschr Ophthalmol 1990;87:467–470.

203. Muntean P. RNFS (Retinale Nervenfaserschichte) bei Neuritis retrobulbaris. Fortschr Ophthalmol 1991;88:401–403.

204. Sommer A, Katz J, Quigley HA, et al. Clinically detectable nerve fiber layer atrophy precedes the onset of glaucomatous field loss. Arch Ophthalmol 1991;109:77–83.

205. Niessen AGJE, van den Berg TJTP, Langerhorst CT, et al. Grading of retinal nerve fiber layer with a photographic reference set. Am J Ophthalmol 1995;120:577–586.

206. Lundstrom M. Atrophy of optic nerve fibres in compression of the chiasm: Observer variation in assessment of atrophy. Acta Ophthalmol 1977;55:217–226.

207. Quigley HA, Addicks EM. Quantitative studies of retinal nerve fiber layer defects. Arch Ophthalmol 1982;100:807–814.

208. Lundstrom M, Eklundh J-O. Computer densitometry of retinal nerve fibre atrophy: A pilot study. Acta Ophthalmol 1980;58:639–644.

209. Caprioli J, Miller JM. Measurement of relative nerve fiber layer surface height in glaucoma. Ophthalmology 1989;96:633–641.

210. Takamoto T, Schwartz B. Photogrammetric measurement of nerve fiber layer thickness. Ophthalmology 1989;96:1315–1319.

211. Weinreb RN, Dreher AW, Coleman A, et al. Histopathologic validation of Fourier ellipsometry measurements of retinal nerve fiber layer thickness. Arch Ophthalmol 1990;108:557–560.

212. Zinser G, Harbarth U, Schroder H. Formation and analysis of three dimensional data with the laser tomographic scanner. In Nasemann JE, Burk ROW, eds. Scanning Laser Ophthalmoscopy and Tomography. Munich, Quintessenz, 1990:243–252.

213. Miglior S, Rossetti L, Brigatti L, et al. Reproducibility of retinal nerve fiber layer evaluation by dynamic scanning laser ophthalmoscopy. Am J Ophthalmol 1994;118:16–23.

214. Caprioli J, Prum B, Zeyen T. Comparison of methods to evaluate the optic nerve head and nerve fiber layer for glaucomatous change. Am J Ophthalmol 1996;121:659–667.

215. Schuman JS, Pedut Kloizman T, Hertzmark E, et al. Reproducibility of nerve fiber layer thickness measurements using optical coherence tomography. Ophthalmology 1996;103:1889–1898.

216. Sommer A. Retinal nerve fiber layer. Am J Ophthalmol 1995;120:665–667.

217. Rader J, Feuer WJ, Anderson DR. Peripapillary vasoconstriction in the glaucomas and the anterior ischemic optic neuropathies. Am J Ophthalmol 1994;117:72–80.

218. Papastathopoulos KI, Jonas JB. Focal narrowing of retinal arterioles in optic nerve atrophy. Ophthalmology 1995;102:1706–1711.

219. Henkind P, Charles NC, Pearson J. Histopathology of ischemic optic neuropathy. Am J Ophthalmol 1970;69:78–90.

220. Kurz GH, Ogata J, Gross EM. Traumatic optic pathways degeneration: Antegrade and retrograde. Br J Ophthalmol 1971;55:233–242.

221. Landers MB III, Bradbury MJ, Sydnor CF. Retinal vascular changes in retrograde optic atrophy. Am J Ophthalmol 1978;86:177–181.

222. Henkind P, Gould H, Bellhorn RW. Optic nerve transection in cats. 1. Effect on the retinal vessels. Invest Ophthalmol 1975;14:610–613.

223. Trobe JD, Glaser JS, Cassady JC. Optic atrophy: Differential diagnosis by fundus observation alone. Arch Ophthalmol 1980;98:1040–1045.

224. Lundstrom M, Frisén L. Atrophy of optic nerve fibres in compression of the chiasm: Degree and distribution of ophthalmoscopic changes. Acta Ophthalmol 1976;54:623–640.

225. Miller NR, Fine SL. The ocular fundus in neuro-ophthalmologic diagnosis. In Sights and Sounds in Ophthalmology. Vol 3. St Louis, CV Mosby, 1977:50–53.

226. Unsöld R, Hoyt WF. Band atrophy of the optic nerve. Arch Ophthalmol 1980;98:1637–1638.

227. Hoyt WF, Rios Montenegro EN, Behrens MM, et al. Homonymous hemioptic hypoplasia: Fundoscopic features in standard and red free illumination in three patients with congenital hemiplegia. Br J Ophthalmol 1972;56:537–545.

228. Hoyt WF, Kommerell G. Der Fundus oculi bei Homonymer Hemianopie. Klin Monatsbl Augenheilkd 1973;162:456–464.

229. Halliday AM. Visually evoked responses in optic nerve disease. Trans Ophthalmol Soc UK 1976;96:372–376.

230. Harms H. Role of perimetry in assessment of optic nerve function. Trans Ophthalmol Soc UK 1976;96:363–367.

231. Thompson HS. Pupillary signs in the diagnosis of optic nerve disease. Trans Ophthalmol Soc UK 1976;96:377–381.

232. Aroichane M, Pieramici DJ, Miller NR, et al. A comparative study of Hardy Rand Rittler and Ishihara colour plates for the diagnosis of nonglaucomatous optic neuropathy. Can J Ophthalmol 1996;31:350–355.

233. Lueck CJ. Investigation of visual loss: Neuro-ophthalmology from a neurologist's perspective. J Neurol Neurosurg Psychiatry 1996;60:275–280.

234. Hamard P, Hamard H, Nigohou S. Leber's idiopathic stellate neuroretinitis: Apropos of 9 cases. J Fr Ophtalmol 1994;17:116–123.

235. Wang AG, Liu JH, Lin CL, et al. Macular star in optic neuropathy. Ann Ophthalmol 1995;27:107–112.

236. Collins ET. Intra-ocular tension. I. The sequelae of hypotony. Trans Ophthalmol Soc UK 1917;37:281–308.

237. Minckler DS, Tso MOM. Experimental papilledema produced by cyclocryotherapy. Am J Ophthalmol 1976;82:577–589.

238. Minckler DS, Tso MOM, Zimmerman LE. A light microscopic, autoradiographic study of axoplasmic transport in the optic nerve head during ocular hypotony, increased intraocular pressure, and papilledema. Am J Ophthalmol 1976;82:741–757.

239. Minckler DS, Bunt AH. Axoplasmic transport in ocular hypotony and papilledema in the monkey. Arch Ophthalmol 1977;95:1430–1436.

240. Seitz R, Kersting G. Die Drusen der Sehnervenpapille und des pigmentephitiels. Klin Monatsbl Augenheilkd 1962;140:75–88.

241. Spencer WH. Drusen of the optic disk and aberrant axoplasmic transport. Am J Ophthalmol 1978;85:1–12.

242. Spencer WH. Pathology and pathogenesis of drusen of the optic nervehead (discussion). Ophthalmology 1981;88:1079–1080.

243. Tso MOM. Pathology and pathogenesis of drusen of the optic nervehead. Ophthalmology 1978;88:1066–1078.

244. Kelley JS. Autofluorescence of drusen of the optic nerve head. Arch Ophthalmol 1974;92:263–264.

245. Frisén L, Hoyt WF, Tengroth BM. Optociliary veins, disc pallor and visual loss. Acta Ophthalmol 1973;51:241–249.

246. Sanders MD. A classification of papilloedema based on a fluorescein angiographic study of 69 cases. Trans Ophthalmol Soc UK 1969;89:177–192.

247. Hedges TR. Papilledema: Its recognition and relation to increased intracranial pressure. Surv Ophthalmol 1975;19:201–223.

248. Henkind P, Benjamin JV. Vascular anomalies and neoplasms of the optic nerve head. Trans Ophthalmol Soc UK 1976;96:418–423.

249. Hoyt WF, Beeston D. The Ocular Fundus in Neurologic Disease. St Louis, CV Mosby, 1966.

250. Miller NR, Green WR. Arachnoid cysts involving a portion of the intraorbital optic nerve. Arch Ophthalmol 1975;93:1117–1121.

251. Weiter JJ. Retinociliary vein associated with a craniopharyngioma. Ann Ophthalmol 1979;11:751–754.

252. Kollarits CR, Lubow M, Johnson JC. Visual loss and perioptic vascular malformations in the eye and orbit. Am J Ophthalmol 1976;82:237–240.

253. Knight CL, Hoyt WF, Wilson CB. Syndrome of incipient prechiasmal optic nerve compression: Progress towards early diagnosis and surgical management. Arch Ophthalmol 1972;87:1–11.

254. Breen LA, Quaglieri FC, Schochet SS Jr. Neuro-anatomical feature photo. J Clin Neuroophthalmol 1983;3:283–284.

255. Horton JC. Wilbrand's knee of the optic chiasm is an artifact of long-term monocular enucleation. Paper presented at the Meeting of the North American Neuro-Ophthalmology Society, Snowbird, Utah, February 10–11, 1996.

256. Kennedy F. Retrobulbar neuritis as an exact diagnostic sign of certain tumors and abscesses in the frontal lobe. Am J Med Sci 1911;142:355–368.

257. François J, Neetens A. Le syndrome de Foster Kennedy et son étiologie. Ann Oculist 1955;188:219–253.

258. David M, Sourdille G. Sur la valeur localisatrice des signes dits de compression directe due nerf optique, en particulier du syndrome de Foster Kennedy dans les tumeurs cérébrales. J Ophthalmol 1942;1:215–232.

259. Watnick RL, Trobe JD. Bilateral optic nerve compression as a mechanism for the Foster Kennedy syndrome. Ophthalmology 1989;96:1793–1798.

260. Boghen DR, Glaser JS. Ischemic optic neuropathy. Brain 1975;98:699–708.

261. Grüber H. Bilaterale untere hemianopsie. Klin Monatsbl Augenheilkd 1980;177:706–709.

262. Johnson MW, Kincaid MC, Trobe JD. Bilateral retrobulbar optic infarctions after blood loss and hypotension: A clinicopathologic study. Ophthalmology 1987;94:1577–1584.

263. Brown RH, Schauble JF, Miller NR. Anemia and hypotension as contributors to perioperative loss of vision. Anesthesiology 1994;80:6–11.

264. Schmidt D, Buhrmann K. Inferior hemianopia in parasellar and pituitary tumors. In Glaser JS, Smith JL, eds. Neuro-Ophthalmology. Vol 9. St Louis, CV Mosby, 1977:236–247.

265. Holmes G. Disturbances of vision by cerebral lesions. Br J Ophthalmol 1918;2:353–384.

266. Berkley WL, Bussey FR. Altitudinal hemianopia. Report of two cases. Am J Ophthalmol 1950;33:593–600.

267. Bogousslavsky J, Miklossy J, Deruaz JP, et al. Lingual and fusiform gyri in visual processing: A clinico-pathologic study of superior altitudinal hemianopia. J Neurol Neurosurg Psychiatry 1987;50:607–614.

268. Vighetto A, Grochowicki M, Aimard G. Altitudinal hemianopia in multiple sclerosis. Neuroophthalmology 1991;11:25–27.

269. Borchert MS, Lessell S, Hoyt WF. Hemifield slide diplopia from altitudinal visual field defects. J Neuroophthalmol 1996;16:107–109.

270. Kirkham TH. The ocular symptomatology of pituitary tumours. Proc R Soc Med 1972;65:517–518.

271. Kubie LS, Beckmann JW. Diplopia without extraocular palsies, caused by heteronymous defects in the visual fields associated with defective macular vision. Brain 1929;52:317–333.

272. Bardram MT. Oculomotor pareses and nonparetic diplopia in pituitary adenomata. Acta Ophthalmol 1949;27:225.

273. Chamlin M, Davidoff LM, Feiring EH. Ophthalmologic changes produced by pituitary tumors. Am J Ophthalmol 1955;40:353–368.

274. Elkington SG. Pituitary adenoma: Preoperative symptomatology in a series of 260 patients. Br J Ophthalmol 1968;52:322–328.

275. von Graefe A. Ein Fall von linksseitigem Gesichtsfelddefect des rechten Auges Dtsch Med Wochenschr. 1897;23:197.

276. Dubois-Poulsen A. Le Champ Visuel. Paris, Mason, 1952:921–922.

277. Amyot R. Rupture d'un aneurysme de la carotide interne; hemianopsie nasale, unilaterale; hemiplegie croisee par spasme de la carotide. Union Med Canada 1959;88:825–830.

278. Cox TA, Corbett JJ, Thompson HS, et al. Unilateral nasal hemianopia as a sign of intracranial optic nerve compression. Am J Ophthalmol 1981;92:230–232.

279. Meadows SP. Unusual clinical features and modes of presentation in pituitary adenoma, including pituitary apoplexy. In Smith JL, ed. Neuro-Ophthalmology. Vol 4. St Louis, CV Mosby, 1968:178–189.

280. Schlossberg FR. Aneurysm of the anterior cerebral artery. Arch Ophthalmol 1959;62:894.

281. Pilley SFJ, Thompson HS. Binasal field loss and "prefixation blindness." In Glaser JS, Smith JL, eds. Neuro-Ophthalmology. Vol 8. St Louis, CV Mosby, 1975:277–284.

282. O'Connell JEA, Du Boulay FPGH. Binasal hemianopia. J Neurol Neurosurg Psychiatry 1973;36:697–709.

283. Best F. Die Augenveränderungen bei den organischen nichtenzündlichen Erkrankungen des Zentralnervensystems. In Schieck F, Brückner A, eds. Kurzes Handbuch der Ophthalmologie. Vol 6. Berlin, Julius Springer, 1931:476–668.

284. Manor RS, Ouaknine GE, Matz S, et al. Nasal visual field loss with intracranial lesions of the optic nerve pathways. Am J Ophthalmol 1980;90:1–10.

285. Lutz A. Über einige weitere Fälle von binasaler Hemianopsie. (Bericht über eine neue eigene Beobachtung unter spezieller Berücksichtigung der Pupillenreaktion,) Graefe's Arch Ophthalmol 1930;125:103–124.

286. Kyrieleis W. Die Augenveränderungen bei den entzündlichen Erkrankungen des Zentralnervensystems. In Schieck F, Brückner A, eds. Kurzes Handbuch der Ophthalmologie. Vol 6. Berlin, Julius Springer, 1931:669–799.

287. François J. L'hemianopsie binasle. Ophthalmologica 1947;113:321–334.

288. Charteris DG, Cullen JF. Binasal field defects in primary empty sella syndrome. J Neuroophthalmol 1996;16:110–114.

289. Hoyt WF. The human optic chiasm: A neuroanatomical review of current concepts, recent investigations and unsolved problems. In Smith JL, ed. The University of Miami Neuro-Ophthalmology Symposium. Springfield, Charles C Thomas, 1964:1–47.

Papilledema

Deborah I. Friedman

TERMINOLOGY

Papilledema is one of the most alarming signs in clinical medicine. Papilledema specifically refers to swelling of the optic disc resulting from increased intracranial pressure (ICP). The term ''papilledema'' is often loosely applied to any type of swelling of the optic disc regardless of the etiology (1). Although the literal interpretation of ''papilledema'' encompasses optic nerve head swelling from any cause, the term has evolved to connote a particular, ingrained meaning to ophthalmologists, neurologists, and neurosurgeons. Therefore, other forms of disc swelling caused by local or systemic processes should be designated in general terms as ''optic disc edema'' and referenced to the presumed etiology (i.e., anterior ischemic optic neuropathy, optic nerve meningioma, etc.).

Confusion in the English terminology dates back to the 1800s, when Hughlings Jackson and others of his time called all cases of optic disc swelling ''optic neuritis,'' even though they were aware that not all cases of ''optic neuritis'' were inflammatory (2). Although Parsons first used the term ''papilledema'' in 1908 to refer to optic disc swelling associ-

ated with increased ICP, few authors followed his lead (3). For instance, Foster Kennedy's classic monograph regarding frontal lobe tumors that cause optic atrophy in one eye from compression by the tumor and optic disc swelling in the other from increased ICP is entitled ''Retrobulbar neuritis as an exact diagnostic sign of certain tumors and abscesses in the frontal lobe'' (4).

The first detailed morphologic studies of optic disc swelling performed in 1911 provided definitive descriptions of the noninflammatory ''passive edema'' associated with normal visual acuity that was encountered in patients with increased ICP (5). The term ''papilledema'' distinguished these cases from those with ''optic neuritis,'' the optic disc swelling associated with visual loss and presumably caused by local or systemic inflammation. Other nomenclature has been used over time, including ''noninflammatory papilledema'' for optic disc swelling from increased ICP, ocular hypotony, orbital masses, and ischemia, as well as ''inflammatory papilledema'' for optic disc swelling from demyelination, infection, and inflammation. These obsolete terms are not clinically useful. When reviewing the medical literature one should be aware that there is a tendency for some authors to call all cases of optic disc swelling, regardless of the etiology, papilledema,

and for others to diagnose papilledema on insufficient grounds. In this chapter, the term "papilledema" refers to optic disc swelling associated with and caused by *proven* increased ICP.

MEASUREMENTS OF INTRACRANIAL PRESSURE

Normal cerebrospinal fluid (CSF) pressure in adults, measured by lumbar puncture with the patient in the lateral decubitus position, varies between 80 and 200 mm of water. Contrary to popular belief, CSF pressure is not dependent on weight or height (6) (Figure 5.1), although pressure readings may be spuriously elevated when the patient coughs, strains, or holds his or her breath during the procedure. Measurements between 201 and 249 mm water are not diagnostic and those greater than 250 mm water are elevated. Normal values have not been well established in children but are generally accepted to be 200 mm water or less. Additionally, ICP in normal persons and in patients with increased ICP can vary widely from one moment to the next (Fig. 5.2). Adson and Lillie (7) introduced a needle into the lateral ventricle of a patient with a glioma of the frontal lobe and made continuous readings of the ICP at hourly intervals for 4 days and recorded variations in pressure that ranged from 130 to 980 mm of water! Fifty years later, Gucer and Viernstein (8) implanted a small epidural pressure sensor in four patients with pseudotumor cerebri (PTC) and continuously monitored the patients before and after medical and surgical treatment. ICP before treatment showed irregular variations ranging from 50 to 500 mm of water over a 24-hour period. Their findings support the claim of Ford and

Murphy in 1939 that "one determination of intracranial pressure in a case of disease of the central nervous system (CNS) is no more instructive than one determination of a patient's temperature during the course of a fever" (9).

In addition to situational and and temporal variations in ICP, one must be aware of other factors in the assessment of ICP. Lumbar CSF pressure is often lower than the true ICP in patients with infratentorial tumors that block communication between the ventricular system and the spinal subarachnoid space (10). However, papilledema is occasionally found with low intrathecal pressure, regardless of the tumor location (11,12).

Lumbar puncture (LP) is generally a safe procedure, but in certain situations it carries significant risk. Except under extraordinary circumstances, a neuroimaging study (computed tomography or magnetic resonance imaging) should always be performed prior to the LP to make sure there is no mass effect in the brain. Removal of fluid from the spinal canal may allow the compressed brain to shift downward and to impact at the tentorial incisura or the foramen magnum, often with fatal results. LP occasionally induces an acquired Chiari malformation that may be reversible (13,14). Post-LP headaches may occur in up to 40% of patients after a lumbar tap. The symptoms of having low CSF pressure mimic those of increased ICP with visual disturbances and diplopia from VI, III, or IV nerve paresis (15). Despite the devastating consequences of brain herniation, the incidence is actually quite low, even when a mass lesion is present. A large series of diagnostic LP in 129 patients with unequivocal papilledema or intracranial hypertension from a variety

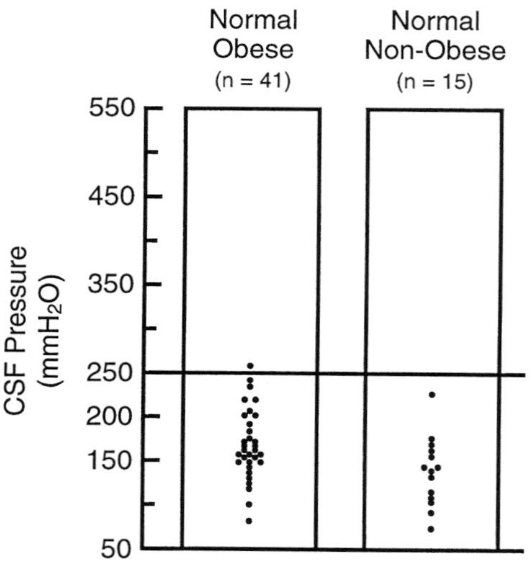

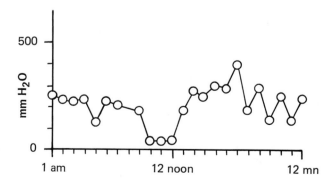

Figure 5.1. Range of normal cerebrospinal fluid pressure in nonobese and obese adults. Note that normal intracranial pressure does not exceed 250 mm of water. (From Corbett JJ, Mehta MP. Cerebrospinal fluid pressure in normal obese subjects and patients with pseudotumor cerebri. Neurology 1983;33:1386-1388,)

Figure 5.2. Intracranial pressure (ICP) recorded by epidural sensor over 24 hours. The intracranial pressure shows great variability ranging from 50 to 400 mm of water. (Redrawn from Gucer G, Viernstein L. Long-term intracranial pressure recording in the management of pseudotumor cerebri. J Neurosurg 1978;49:256-263.)

of causes had only one complication (16). A review by the same authors of 418 additional cases of papilledema from mass lesions and increased ICP verified by lumbar puncture found only five complications (1.2%) (16).

In cases where the physician cannot decide if the elevation of the optic disc is true papilledema or pseudopapilledema (see Chapter 3), computed tomography (CT) scanning or magnetic resonance imaging (MRI) can be obtained immediately to determine if an intracranial mass is present or the ventricles are enlarged. The LP may then be performed if needed, and a decision can be made regarding the need for further diagnostic testing.

OPHTHALMOSCOPIC APPEARANCE

There are several classification systems for papilledema. One system describes the disc appearance according to the duration of papilledema: (a) early; (b) fully developed; (c) chronic; and (d) atrophic (17,18). However, for medical decision making, the Frisén grading system (Table 5.1) is most useful as it classifies the papilledema grade by severity (19).

Table 5.1
Papilledema Grading System (Frisén Scale)

Stage 0 – Normal Optic Disc
    Blurring of nasal, superior and inferior poles in inverse proportion to disc diameter
    Radial nerve fiber layer (NFL) without NFL tortuosity
    Rare obscuration of a major blood vessel, usually on the upper pole
Stage 1 – Very Early Papilledema
    Obscuration of the nasal border of the disc
    No elevation of the disc borders
    Disruption of the normal radial NFL arrangement with grayish opacity accentuating nerve fiber layer bundles
    Normal temporal disc margin
    Subtle grayish halo with temporal gap (best seen with indirect ophthalmoscopy)
    Concentric or radial retrochoroidal folds
Stage 2 – Early Papilledema
    Obscuration of all borders
    Elevation of the nasal border
    Complete peripapillary halo
Stage 3 – Moderate Papilledema
    Obscurations of all borders
    Increased diameter of optic nerve head
    Obscuration of one or more segments of major blood vessels leaving the disc
    Peripapillary halo–irregular outer fringe with finger-like extensions
Stage 4 – Marked Papilledema
    Elevation of the entire nerve head
    Obscuration of all borders
    Peripapillary halo
    Total obscuration on the disc of a segment of a major blood vessel
Stage 5 – Severe Papilledema
    Dome-shaped protrusions representing anterior expansion of the optic nerve head
    Peripapillary halo is narrow and smoothly demarcated
    Total obscuration of a segment of a major blood vessel may or may not be present
    Obliteration of the optic cup

(Frisén L. Swelling of the optic nerve head: A staging scheme. J Neurol Neurosurg Psychiatry 1982;45:13–18.)

STAGES OF PAPILLEDEMA

Normal Optic Disc (Frisén Stage 0)

Stereoscopic viewing of a normal optic disc often reveals mild nasal elevation of the nerve fiber layer, owing to the increased density of nerve fibers representing the temporal visual field. With the direct ophthalmoscope the nasal disc margin may appear indistinct compared to the temporal disc rim. The vessels are generally seen coursing across the optic nerve head, although, rarely, a portion of a major vessel may be obscured in the upper pole.

Very Early Papilledema (Frisén Stage 1)

The early phase of papilledema consists of the incipient disc changes that occur before the development of obvious disc swelling. Papilledema may be difficult to detect at this stage. Several features have been described, including hyperemia of the optic disc, blurring of the peripapillary retinal nerve fiber layer, swelling of the optic disc, blurring of the disc margins, peripapillary flame-shaped hemorrhages, and absent spontaneous venous pulsations (20) (Fig. 5.3A). None of these features are reliable indicators of very early papilledema.

The term "hyperemia" has been used to indicate a reddish discoloration of the optic nerve head as well as increased vascularity of the optic disc. As the natural disc color is quite variable, reliance on this sign is often misleading. True "hyperemia," or increased vascularity, develops as a result of dilation of capillaries on the surface of the disc in early papilledema; however, it is unclear whether the hyperemia always precedes actual disc swelling (21,22). Stereoscopic color photography and fluorescein angiography of experimentally produced papilledema in monkeys showed that hyperemia of the disc as well as capillary dilatation and development of microaneurysms on the disc surface appear *after* disc swelling and blurring of the peripapillary retinal nerve fiber layer (22).

The detection of early papilledema is enhanced by bright direct ophthalmoscopes and handheld 90- or 78-diopter lenses using slit lamp biomicroscopy. Incorporating a red-free filter accentuates subtle changes in the peripapillary retinal nerve fiber layer that may be observed in early papilledema. During this stage, there may be disruption of the normal radial nerve fiber layer arrangement with grayish opacity accentuating nerve fiber bundles. A subtle grayish halo may be visible with the indirect ophthalmoscope (19). In eyes with early papilledema, the peripapillary retina loses its su-

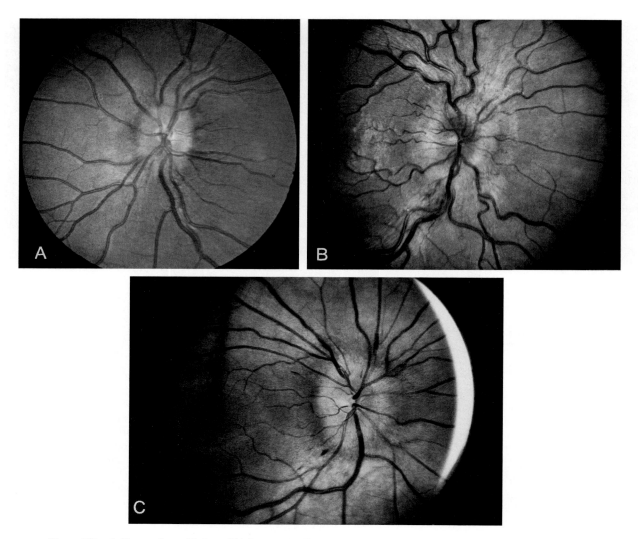

Figure 5.3. *A,* Very early papilledema (Frisén stage 1). The disc shows slight hyperemia and blurring of the peripapillary nerve fiber layer at the superior and inferior poles of the disc. *B,* Early papilledema (Frisén stage 2). This disc is hyperemic and mildly swollen. Note the inferior peripapillary nerve fiber hemorrhages. *C,* The disc is moderately swollen (Frisén stage 3) with obscuration of all borders, a peripapillary halo, and several small "splinter" hemorrhages adjacent to the disc margins at 7 and 10 o'clock.

perficial linear and curvilinear light reflexes and appears deep red and without luster (23) (Fig. 5.4*A*).

The absence of spontaneous retinal venous pulsations is thought by some investigators to be an early sign of papilledema. According to several authors, pulsations cease when ICP exceeds about 200 mm of water (24–26). Thus, if spontaneous venous pulsations are present, ICP should be below this figure. However, as noted above, marked fluctuations in ICP can occur in patients with increased ICP (8,27,28), and in such patients, the ICP may occasionally drop into the normal range. A patient could therefore have increased ICP but be examined at a time when ICP was transiently reduced at the trough of a pressure wave, at which time spontaneous venous pulsations might be observed. In addition, spontaneous venous pulsations occur in only about 80% of normal

subjects (8,29,30). Thus, 20% of patients with normal ICP also lack spontaneous venous pulsations. For these reasons, the absence of spontaneous venous pulsations does not always support a diagnosis of papilledema. The observation of spontaneous venous pulsations suggests only that the ICP is probably below 200–250 mm of water at that moment.

Early Papilledema (Frisén Stage 2)

Early papilledema is characterized by obscuration of the optic disc borders, elevation of the nasal border and a complete peripapillary halo (Figs. 5.3*B* and 5.5). Using stereoscopic color photography and fluorescein angiography, Hayreh and Hayreh concluded that the first sign of raised ICP is swelling of the optic disc (21,22). In 32 animals with

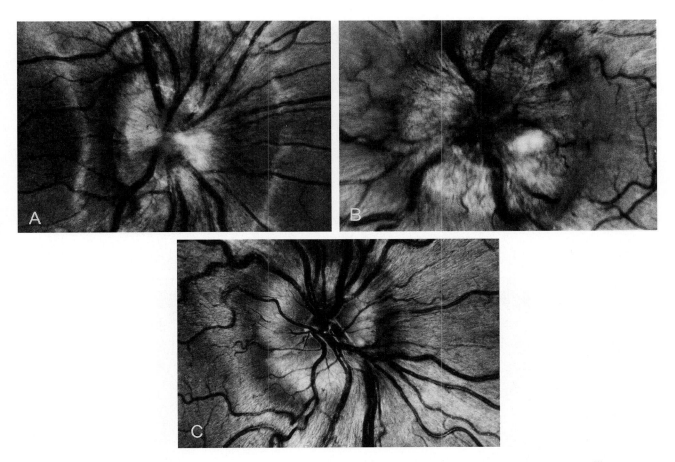

Figure 5.4. Red-free photographs showing nerve fiber layer in papilledema and in pseudopapilledema. *A,* Moderate papilledema (Frisén stage 3). The nerve fiber layer has mild distortion of light reflexes and a ''muddy'' appearance obscuring small vessels traversing the disc margin. *B,* Marked papilledema (Frisén stage 4). The reflexes from the peripapillary retinal nerve fiber layer are completely distorted and blurred. Note the dilated disc capillaries. *C,* Pseudopapilledema. Although the disc is moderately elevated, the surface vessels appear normal and the nerve fiber layer reflexes are sharply defined. Superficial drusen are visible between 3 and 4 o'clock.

papilledema produced by a balloon introduced into the subarachnoid space, the swelling did not affect the entire disc simultaneously or to an equal degree. Instead, it appeared first at the lower pole, then at the upper pole, and later at the nasal and temporal portions of the disc. The investigators could visualize this early swelling only with stereoscopic photography and not by direct ophthalmoscopy (21,22). Slit lamp biomicroscopy is especially helpful in this circumstance.

''Blurring of the disc margins'' is a nebulous description that is neither specific nor helpful. Numerous congenital anomalies of the optic disc are associated with indistinct disc margins. Moreover, interpretation of a ''blurred'' disc margin is often impossible using the direct ophthalmoscope. Unless it is accompanied by other more definitive signs of papilledema, this sign has limited clinical utility.

In summary, the diagnosis of early papilledema cannot and should not be made on the basis of a single finding. Often, the disc appearance is suggestive of papilledema but

there is lingering uncertainty of the diagnosis. If clinically prudent, serial observations may be made in order to establish a diagnosis. In the setting of a potentially serious condition the diagnosis must be established by other means, including ultrasonography, fluorescein angiography, CT scanning, MR imaging, or lumbar puncture (see below).

Moderate Papilledema (Frisén Stage 3)

As the severity of papilledema increases, the margins of the optic disc become obscured and elevated. The diameter of the optic nerve head increases, often resulting in enlargement of the physiologic blind spot. The optic cup may still be preserved at this stage. An important finding is that the edematous, opaque nerve fiber layer obscures one or more segments of major blood vessels leaving the disc (19). The gray peripapillary halo becomes more apparent and may have an irregular outer fringe with finger-like extensions conforming to the nerve fiber layer (Fig. 5.3C).

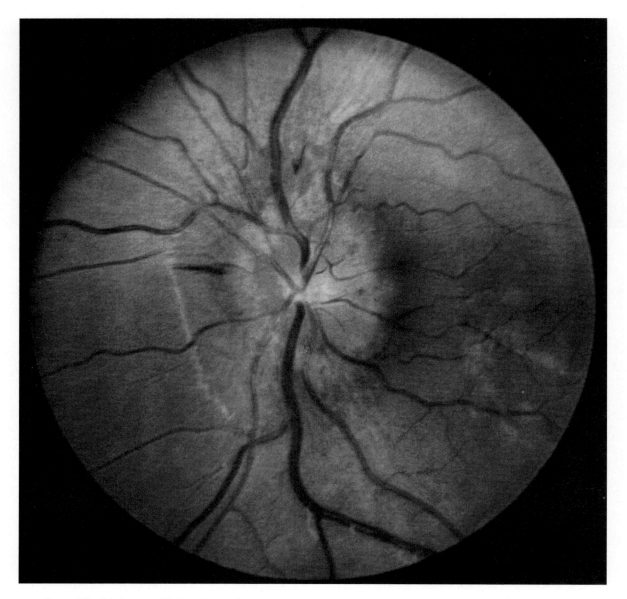

Figure 5.5. Moderate papilledema. Two splinter hemorrhages can be seen in the nerve fiber layer adjacent to the disc margin at 9 o'clock and 12 o'clock. Gray edema surrounds the disc, and the optic cup is partially obliterated by hyperemic disc tissue. Both veins and venules are engorged. (From Hoyt WF, Beeston D. The Ocular Fundus in Neurologic Disease. St Louis, CV Mosby, 1966.)

Marked Papilledema (Frisén Stage 4)

Marked papilledema is characterized by elevation of the entire optic nerve head. The optic cup is often obliterated. There is obscuration of all the borders of the nerve with a prominent peripapillary halo. Edema and infarction of the nerve fiber layer cause total obscuration on the disc of a segment of a major blood vessel. The retinal veins are often engorged and tortuous (Fig. 5.6A and B).

Severe Papilledema (Frisén Stage 5)

Severe, acute or subacute, papilledema is present when the optic nerve protrudes anteriorly with a dome-shaped con-

figuration. The optic cup is obliterated and the peripapillary halo is narrow and smoothly demarcated. Often, there are no appreciable landmarks to distinguish the optic nerve head from the surrounding retina. Obscuration of segments of major blood vessels may or may not be present (Figs. 5.7–5.9).

OTHER SIGNS OF PAPILLEDEMA

Other signs of papilledema may contribute to visual impairment but are often not helpful in determining the severity of papilledema. One may observe flame-shaped, nerve fiber layer hemorrhages, that may increase in number as the ICP

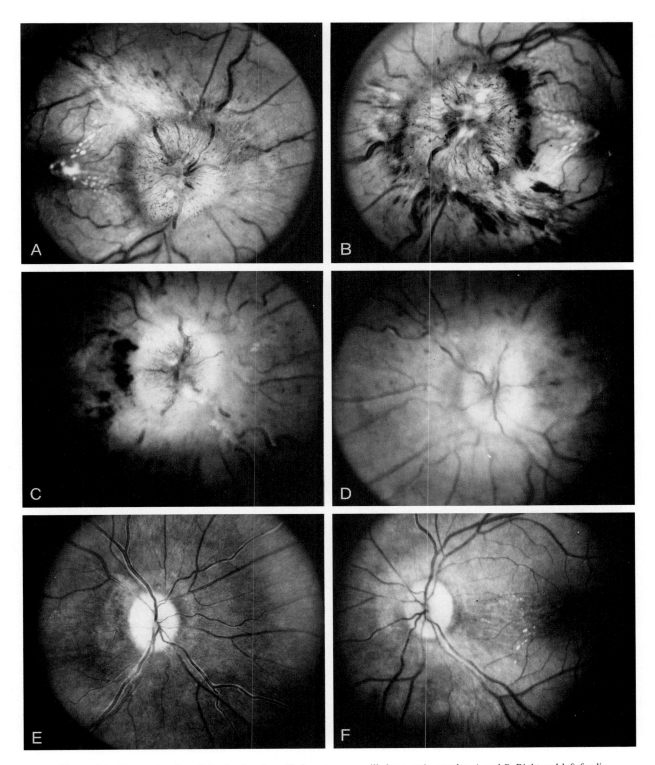

Figure 5.6. Progression from fully developed papilledema to postpapilledema optic atrophy. *A and B*, Right and left fundi showing severe papilledema. Note the obscuration of major vessels traversing the disc margin, and the extensive peripapillary hemorrhages and exudates, including star figure of lipid in the maculae. *C and D*, Two weeks later, both optic discs are less swollen but pale. The hemorrhages and exudates are resolving but the vessels crossing the disc are still partially obscured by the edematous nerve fiber layer. *E and F*, Four months later, both optic discs are diffusely pale; the retinal vessels are sheathed; and the nerve fiber layer is absent.

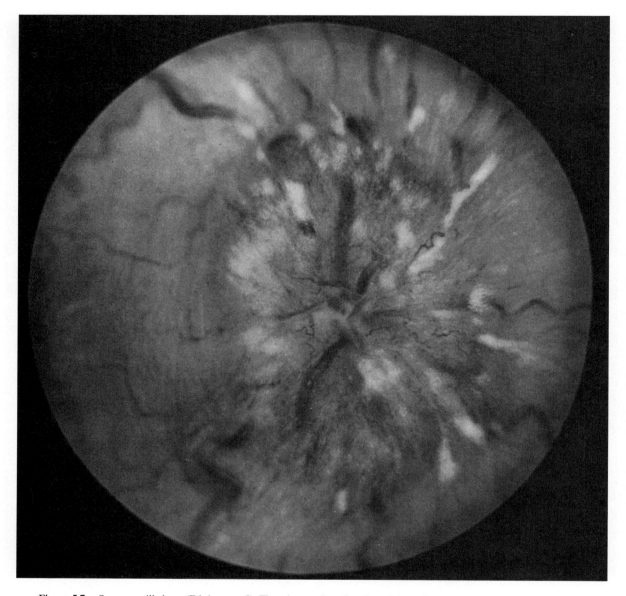

Figure 5.7. Severe papilledema (Frisén stage 5). There is complete elevation of the optic disc with obliteration of the optic cup. The major vessels are obscured as they cross the disc margin. There are white "fleck" exudates (small infarcts) among the nerve fibers, retinal wrinkling, and intraretinal exudates in the macular area (on the *left*). Note the corkscrew-like venules on the surface of the swollen tissue. (From Hoyt WF, Beeston D. The Ocular Fundus in Neurologic Disease. St Louis, CV Mosby, 1966.)

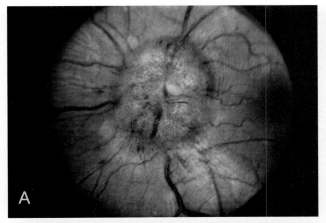

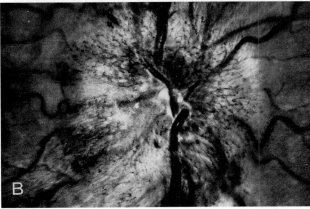

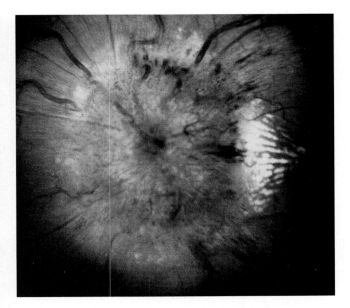

Figure 5.9. Macular star figure in fully developed papilledema. The incomplete star in the papillomacular bundle is characteristic but occasionally a complete star figure is seen.

Figure 5.8. Severe papilledema (Frisén stage 5) with marked dilation of disc vessels and formation of microaneurysms. This nerve is the same Frisén stage as the optic disc in Figure 5.7 as hemorrhages and exudates are not used in the Frisén classification scheme. *A,* Fundus photograph; *B,* Red-free photograph.

increases. There may also be cotton wool spots (focal retinal infarcts) and tortuous vessels on or surrounding the disc (Fig. 5.7). In severe cases, circumferential retinal folds (Paton's lines) often develop; linear or curvilinear choroidal folds may be observed (31–34) (Fig. 5.10). Choroidal folds from increased intracranial pressure often result in acquired, progressive hyperopia (32–34). Hard exudates and hemorrhages may occur in the peripapillary region and in the macula, producing decreased central vision (35,36) (Figs. 5.9 and 5.11*C*). Because nerve fibers in the macula have a radial orientation, hemorrhages and exudates in this region can assume a fan or star shape. Since vascular compromise on and around the optic disc is responsible for these macular changes, the star figure in such cases is usually asymmetric, being more prominent on the nasal side of the fovea toward the disc.

Hemorrhages are frequently present with papilledema, although they are not incorporated into the Frisén staging system. Nerve fiber layer hemorrhages are the most common and indicate that the edema is acute to subacute (Figs. 5.8 and 5.9). A small nerve fiber layer hemorrhage in the peri-

papillary region may be an extremely important sign of early papilledema. Such a hemorrhage appears as a thin, radial streak on the disc or near its margins and is presumably caused by rupture of a distended capillary within or surrounding the disc (Fig. 5.5). Although peripapillary nerve fiber layer hemorrhages can be detected by routine direct ophthalmoscopy, they are often more apparent with the magnification provided by slit lamp biomicroscopy using a hand-held or contact lens.

When the increase in ICP is rapid, subhyaloid hemorrhages may be present in addition to the more common intraretinal hemorrhages (Fig. 5.12). These hemorrhages may break into the vitreous in some cases (37). Among 402 patients with papilledema from various causes, 14 (4%) had severe posterior pole hemorrhages or prominent subhyaloid and vitreous bleeding (38). In these patients, the subhyaloid and vitreous hemorrhages were thought to have resulted from forward dissection of severe peripapillary hemorrhage, whereas scattered posterior pole hemorrhages were believed to represent central retinal vein compromise from optic disc swelling (38). Rarely patients with papilledema develop macular and peripapillary subretinal neovascularization, especially when the papilledema is chronic (39–41) (Fig. 5.11). The presence of peripheral retinal hemorrhages in addition to hemorrhages in the posterior pole suggests extensive retinal venous congestion produced by significantly elevated ICP (42). In moderate to severe papilledema, the retinal veins are frequently engorged and tortuous. This feature is often helpful in distinguishing papilledema from local causes of optic disc edema.

CHRONIC PAPILLEDEMA

When papilledema persists, hemorrhages and exudates slowly resolve, and the disc develops a rounded appearance

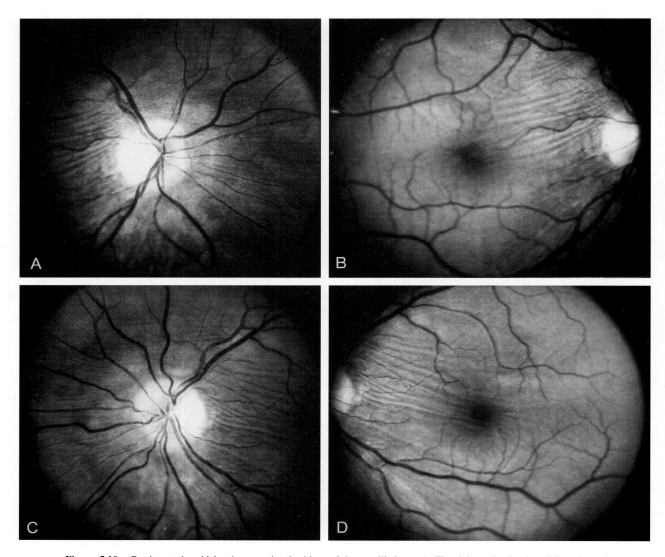

Figure 5.10. Persistent choroidal striae associated with resolving papilledema. *A*, The right optic disc is mildly pale and minimally swollen. Curvilinear striae extend toward the macula. *B*, Striae extend into the right macula. *C*, The left optic disc is also mildly pale and minimally swollen. Striae are present in the papillomacular region. *D*, The striae extend into the left macula.

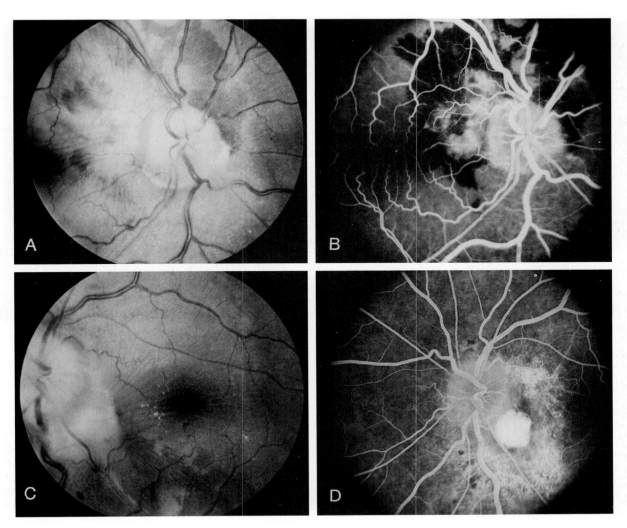

Figure 5.11. Subretinal neovascularization in chronic papilledema. *A*, Right eye shows a marked subretinal neovascular membrane superotemporal to the optic disc with subretinal hemorrhage, serous subretinal fluid, and retinal striae. *B*, Late stage fluorescein angiogram of right eye reveals marked staining of subretinal neovascular membrane and hyperfluorescence of the disc. *C*, Left eye with elevated disc and an inferior-temporal subretinal neovascular membrane with surrounding hemorrhage, hard exudate, and retinal striae. *D*, Fluorescein angiogram of the left eye shows the residual subretinal neovascular membrane with a surrounding area of mottled disruption of the retinal pigment epithelium. (From Morse PH, Leveille AS, Antel JP, et al. Bilateral juxtapapillary subretinal neovascularization associated with pseudotumor cerebri. Am J Ophthalmol 1981; 91:312–317.)

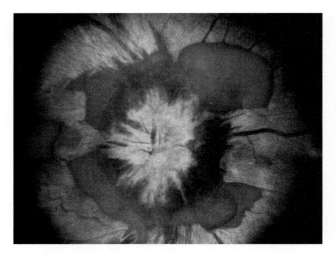

Figure 5.12. Subhyaloid hemorrhage with papilledema. The patient had a severe, subarachnoid hemorrhage from an intracranial aneurysm.

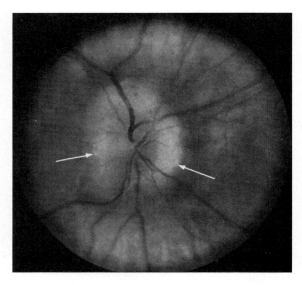

Figure 5.14. Drusen-like bodies (*arrows*) in chronic atrophic papilledema. (From Hoyt WF, Beeston D. The Ocular Fundus in Neurologic Disease. St Louis, CV Mosby, 1966.)

(20) (Fig. 5.13). The central cup, which may be retained in the acute phase of papilledema, ultimately becomes obliterated. Over a period of months, the initial disc hyperemia changes to a milky gray appearance, with hard exudates becoming apparent in the superficial disc substance. These exudates resemble optic disc drusen (Fig. 5.14) and may result in a misdiagnosis of pseudopapilledema (43,44) (Fig. 5.4C).

Most patients with chronic papilledema have evidence of nerve fiber layer atrophy (45). The appearance of the atrophy ranges from slit-like defects to diffuse loss. Nerve fiber layer atrophy can be best appreciated by viewing through the red-free filter of a direct ophthalmoscope or slit lamp biomicroscope.

Occasionally, papilledema persists for a long period of time without significant visual symptoms (46). This situation

occurs primarily in patients with pseudotumor cerebri (PTC) but may also be observed in patients with intracranial tumors.

POSTPAPILLEDEMA ATROPHY

With time, untreated papilledema subsides, the disc becomes atrophic, and the retinal vessels become narrow and sheathed (20). In such cases, the nerve fiber layer can no longer be visualized by either direct ophthalmoscopy or slit lamp biomicroscopy (45). Some patients have persistent pigmentary changes or choroidal folds in the maculae (20,47,48) (Fig. 5.15). If the papilledema has been particularly severe, these changes may resemble those caused by a hamartoma of the pigment epithelium (49).

The time required for papilledema to evolve into optic atrophy depends upon many factors, including the severity and constancy of the increased intracranial pressure (ICP). Atrophic changes can appear within weeks or days following the initial observation of acute papilledema in some cases, particularly if the rise in ICP is rapid, severe, and sustained. In such cases, the disc appearance may rapidly progress to fully developed papilledema and then to postpapilledema optic atrophy without ever having gone through a stage of chronic papilledema. In still other cases, many months or even years may elapse before atrophy develops. In such cases, the appearance of the fundus is typically that of chronic papilledema that gradually melts away into atrophy. Finally, there are patients who appear to have stable chronic papilledema for many months to years until, for unclear reasons, they rapidly develop optic atrophy.

In some cases, as papilledema evolves from the fully developed stage to the chronic stage and then to the atrophic stage, optociliary shunt veins develop and then disappear (50–53). These vessels, which are pre-existing veins that

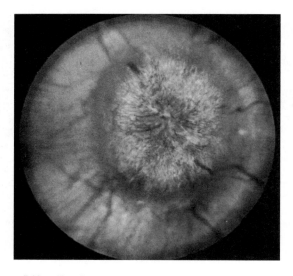

Figure 5.13. Chronic, severe papilledema. Note round compact appearance of the optic disc and lack of hemorrhages.

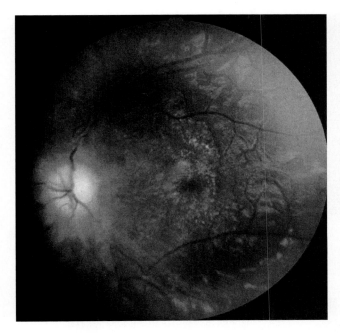

Figure 5.15. Postpapilledema optic atrophy and pigmentary changes in the macula in a patient who previously had severe papilledema. The gliotic changes of the nerve fiber layer give the disc margin a "dirty" appearance. Note pallor of left optic disc, narrowed sheathed retinal vessels, and extensive pigmentary changes in left macula.

connect the retinal and choroidal venous circulations (53), enlarge because the increased ICP either directly compresses the central retinal vein or indirectly compresses it by compressing the optic nerve (Fig. 5.16). In either case, the vessels shunt venous blood from the retinal to the choroidal venous circulations. Therefore, blood exits the eye and orbit via the vortex veins to the superior and inferior ophthalmic veins, bypassing the obstructed central retinal vein. At this stage, patients usually have significant visual field defects, diminished color vision, and variably reduced visual acuity (see below). Optociliary shunt veins may disappear after the ICP is surgically lowered or following optic nerve sheath decompression surgery (54,55) (Fig. 5.17).

Optic atrophy that results from chronic papilledema has a specific pattern of axonal loss. Loss of peripheral axons with sparing of central axons has been demonstrated in several postmortem studies (56,57). Good central visual acuity despite severe papilledema and optic atrophy is found in most patients with chronic papilledema.

UNILATERAL OR ASYMMETRIC PAPILLEDEMA

Papilledema is usually bilateral and relatively symmetric in the two eyes. In some instances, it is strictly unilateral or at least much more pronounced in one eye than in the other (58–60) (Figs. 5.18 and 5.19). Some patients may have had preexisting atrophy before the development of increased ICP (the pseudo-Foster Kennedy syndrome; see below and in Chapter 4). If there are not enough viable nerve fibers, papilledema cannot occur ("dead axons don't swell"). However,

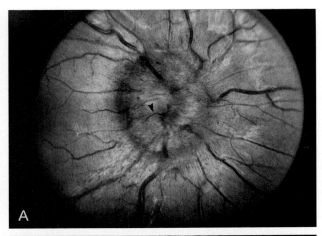

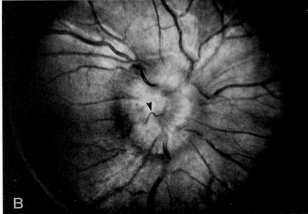

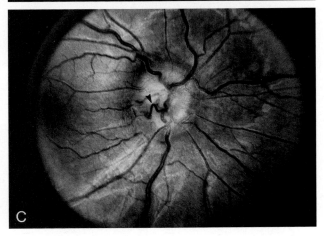

Figure 5.16. Development of optociliary shunt veins in a patient with chronic papilledema from pseudotumor cerebri. *A,* Marked (Frisén stage 4) papilledema. Note the small vessel located on the surface of the disc at 8 o'clock (*arrowhead*). *B,* As disc swelling resolves, the previously noted vessel becomes more apparent (*arrowhead*). *C,* Disc swelling has almost completely resolved. The vessel at 8 o'clock appears larger than previously, and clearly represents a retinal-choroidal shunt (*arrowhead*).

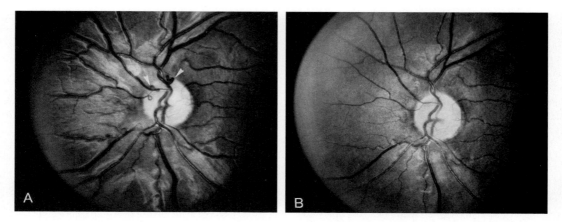

Figure 5.17. Disappearance of optociliary shunt veins in a patient with postpapilledema optic atrophy after intracranial decompression for sclerosteosis. *A,* Preoperative appearance of left optic disc shows shunt vessels at 10 and 12 o'clock (*arrowheads*). *B,* Postoperative photograph of left disc shows disappearance of shunt veins. (From Stein SA, Witkop C, Hill S, et al. Sclerosteosis: Neurogenetic and pathophysiologic analysis of an American kinship. Neurology 1983;33:267–277.)

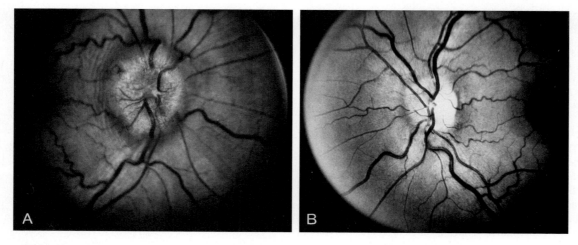

Figure 5.18. Unilateral papilledema in a 34-year-old woman with pseudotumor cerebri. *A,* The right optic disc shows fully developed papilledema. *B,* The left optic disc is normal.

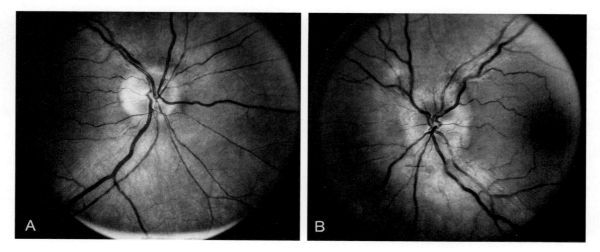

Figure 5.19. Asymmetric papilledema in a 35-year-old man with pseudotumor cerebri. *A,* The right optic disc is minimally hyperemic and swollen (Frisén stage 1). *B,* Frisén stage 3 papilledema of the left optic disc.

if sufficient nerve fibers remain, papilledema may develop even though the optic disc is pale. A particularly interesting pattern of papilledema can occur in patients with optic atrophy from previous damage to the optic chiasm or optic tract. In such patients, an eye with a temporal hemianopia and atrophy of nasal fibers has band atrophy with preservation of the majority of the upper and lower (temporal) arcuate fibers. When papilledema develops, the swelling is thus confined to the superior and inferior poles of the disc. In an eye with a nasal hemianopia, atrophy of temporal fibers has occurred, and most of the swelling is confined to the nasal portion of the disc (61). This specific pattern of papilledema also occurs in patients with congenital hemioptic hypoplasia who develop increased ICP (62).

In the Foster Kennedy syndrome (see Chapter 4) patients with frontal lobe or olfactory groove tumors develop the triad of (*a*) optic atrophy in one eye; (*b*) papilledema in the other eye; and (*c*) anosmia (Fig. 5.20). The optic nerve

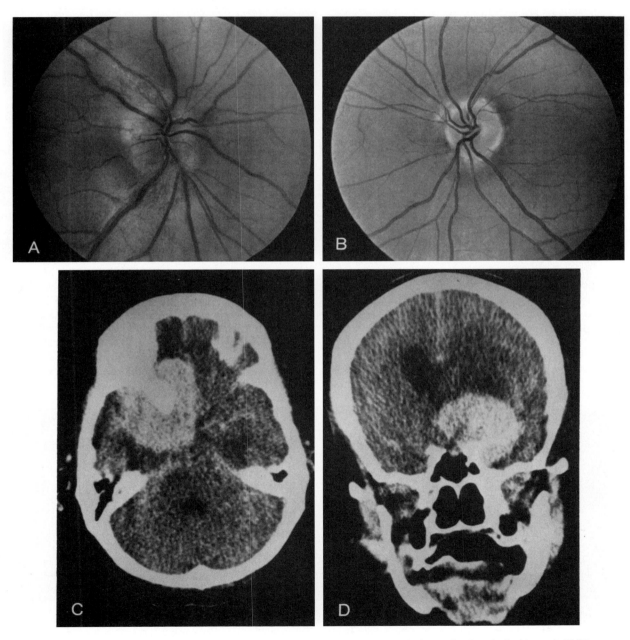

Figure 5.20. Foster Kennedy syndrome. *A*, The right optic disc shows mild papilledema. Visual acuity in this eye is 20/20. There is slight enlargement of the blind spot on visual field testing. *B*, The left disc is pale with vision of hand motions. *C and D*, Computed tomographic scan in axial (*C*) and coronal (*D*) planes shows large right sphenoid ridge meningioma.

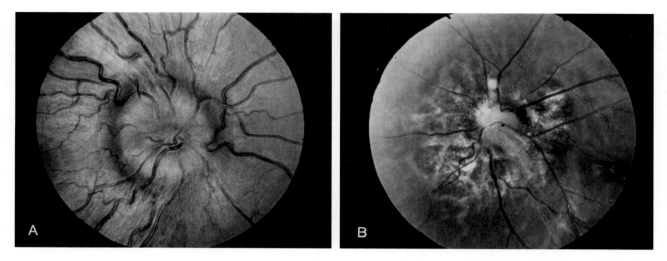

Figure 5.21. Unilateral papilledema with contralateral optic disc dysplasia. This 25-year-old woman had pseudotumor cerebri. *A,* The right optic disc shows marked (Frisén stage 4) papilledema. *B,* The left optic disc is markedly dysplastic and definite papilledema cannot be identified.

ipsilateral to the tumor is generally atrophic because of compression. A rise in CSF pressure in the optic nerve sheath is a prerequisite condition for development of papilledema (63,64). Optic nerve compression prevents elevated intrasheath pressure and produces ipsilateral atrophy of optic nerve fibers. Similarly, patients with unilateral optic disc dysplasia may develop papilledema only on the side of the previously normal disc (Fig. 5.21).

When unilateral papilledema occurs in a patient with an apparently normal optic disc on the opposite side, it often results from some congenital anomaly of the optic nerve sheath that prevents transmission of pressure to the optic nerve head on the side where the papilledema is absent (65). Neuroimaging and ultrasonography in such patients reveal *bilateral* dilation of the optic nerve sheaths (59,66) (Fig.

5.22), suggesting that pressure is transmitted at least to the globe. The anatomic arrangement of the venous sinuses may contribute to unequal or unilateral papilledema in patients with previously normal optic discs, particularly in the setting of venous sinus thrombosis (67,68). Lastly, a difference in the lamina cribrosa between the two optic discs producing reduced transmission of the ICP to the optic nerve in the scleral canal has been postulated (60). If congenital anomalies of the optic nerve sheaths or venous sinuses cause absence of ipsilateral papilledema, they may also explain the absence, asymmetry or unilaterality of papilledema in at least some patients with significantly elevated ICP (69).

In most patients with apparent unilateral papilledema, careful observation of the ''normal'' optic disc often discloses minimal hyperemia, a blurred nerve fiber layer, or disc

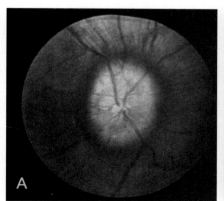
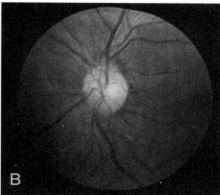
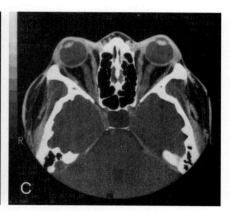

Figure 5.22. Bilaterally enlarged optic nerve sheaths in a patient with unilateral papilledema. The patient was a 32-year-old woman with pseudotumor cerebri. *A,* The right optic disc is moderately swollen (Frisén stage 3) with a well-developed peripapillary halo. *B,* The left optic disc is normal. *C,* Computed tomographic scan, axial view, after intravenous injection of contrast material, shows bilateral symmetric dilation of the optic nerve sheaths. (From Strominger MB, Weiss GB, Mehler MF. Asymptomatic unilateral papilledema in pseudotumor cerebri. J Clin Neuroophthalmol 1992;12:238–241.)

swelling that is easily overlooked in the face of significant papilledema on the opposite side (70) (Fig. 5.19). Careful stereoscopic ophthalmoscopy and fluorescein angiography may be necessary to detect subtle papilledema. Nevertheless, purely unilateral papilledema has been described with PTC, cerebral tumors, abscesses, intracranial hemorrhage caused by aneurysm, aqueductal stenosis, and traumatic brain injury (58,71–74). In a series of 1,346 neurosurgical patients with papilledema admitted to the State Hospital of Copenhagen over a 15-year period, 25 cases (1.8%) revealed unilateral papilledema with a normal contralateral optic disc (72); 17 patients had papilledema ipsilateral to the lesion; 7 patients had contralateral papilledema; and 1 patient had a midline tumor.

Papilledema that is unilateral, or at least more pronounced on one side, may be of significance in many cases of intracranial mass lesions, particularly abscesses, where the papilledema is usually ipsilateral to the lesion (72).

In summary, unilateral optic disc swelling is unlikely to be true papilledema. More frequently, it is caused by local pathology (e.g., inflammation, ischemia, or compression of the optic nerve within the orbit). When an optic disc is significantly atrophic or anomalous, it may not develop papilledema, or papilledema will develop only in the regions of functioning axons. Most patients with ''unilateral'' optic disc swelling in the setting of increased ICP actually have bilateral asymmetric papilledema, but truly unilateral edema does infrequently occur.

DIAGNOSIS

The most important method of diagnosing papilledema is careful ophthalmoscopic examination, assessing the features described above. An examination that includes red-free ophthalmoscopy (23) and slit lamp biomicroscopy with a hand-held or contact lens is usually sufficient to determine whether papilledema is present. If the diagnosis remains uncertain several options are available. Fluorescein angiography is often used to confirm early papilledema (50,75–82). The test itself is easily performed in an outpatient setting: 5 ml of 10% fluorescein sodium are rapidly injected into a superficial arm vein. Alternatively fluorescein can be given orally (83). The passage of dye through retinal vessels is then observed and photographed at rapid intervals, with a cobalt blue filter interposed in front of the light source to visualize the fluorescence of the dye. Even if photographic facilities are lacking, the examiner can observe the ocular fundus using an indirect ophthalmoscope or a slit lamp with a hand-held or contact lens with the correct filter in place.

According to most investigators, the earliest frames of the fluorescein angiogram in patients with early papilledema show disc capillary dilation, dye leakage, and microaneurysm formation, whereas later frames show leakage of dye beyond the disc margins (Fig. 5.23). Unfortunately, the above findings do not always correctly identify true papilledema (50,79). Some authors claim that fluorescein angiography may not show any abnormalities until optic disc swelling is of a ''mild to moderate degree'' (22). Nevertheless, one study reviewed the fluorescein angiograms of 100 patients with possible papilledema and found that in all cases of true papilledema, the retinal angiograms showed a combination of either excess early and late disc fluorescence or excess disc vascularity with late fluorescence (81).

If it is available, orbital echography is extremely useful in cases of questionable papilledema. This sensitive test reliably determines if the diameter of the optic nerve is increased and, if so, whether or not the increase is caused by CSF surrounding the nerve. It can also easily detect buried optic disc drusen. Thus, by performing A- and B-scan ultrasonography with a 30° test when indicated, the examiner can determine not only if an optic disc is truly swollen but if there is increased ICP (84,85). Coexisting optic disc drusen and papilledema from PTC (86,87) create diagnostic confusion

that may be resolved with ultrasonography. CT scanning can be used to determine if there are buried drusen causing an appearance mimicking papilledema, and both CT scanning and MR imaging can be used to detect evidence of an intracranial mass or hydrocephalus.

High resolution MRI of the orbits shows characteristic changes of the optic nerves and posterior globe in papilledema. In papilledema, the subarachnoid space becomes distended, the nerve sheath widens and there is flattening of the posterior sclera (88,89). The prelaminar optic nerve may enhance and protrude anteriorly (88).

Confocal scanning laser tomography (CSLT; Heidelberg Retinal Tomography) of normal optic nerves demonstrates gradually increasing retinal surface elevation from the center of the disc to the disc margin, with a steeper contour nasally than temporally (90). The retinal surface area over the optic disc is diffusely displaced anteriorly in patients with active papilledema from PTC, and significantly different from control optic nerves in all locations. Compared to controls, patients with clinically resolved papilledema show anterior displacement of the optic nerve head in all areas except nasally. Another study comparing B-scan ultrasonography to CSLT found a positive correlation (R = .62) between the two modalities in papilledema from idiopathic intracranial hypertension, although there was much higher agreement (R = .84) for optic nerve cupping (85). This may be attributable to a difference in reference planes used in each method. Ultrasound measures the maximum elevation from the optic disc to the lamina cribrosa; since the lamina is not recognizable with papilledema, the distance is measured from the disc to the retinal surface. Multiple measurements may be required to achieve optimal accuracy with CLST in edematous optic nerves (91), but this new modality is promising for quantitative evaluation of papilledema (90). In clinical practice, the diagnosis of papilledema may elude even the most experienced examiners. One study assessed the ability of various medical specialists to identify papilledema and pseudopapilledema using stereophotographic slides (92). Under such ideal circumstances, even the neuro-ophthalmologic ''experts'' who pre-screened the study slides did not achieve a perfect score! However, neuro-ophthalmologists and ophthalmologists were more accurate than family physicians,

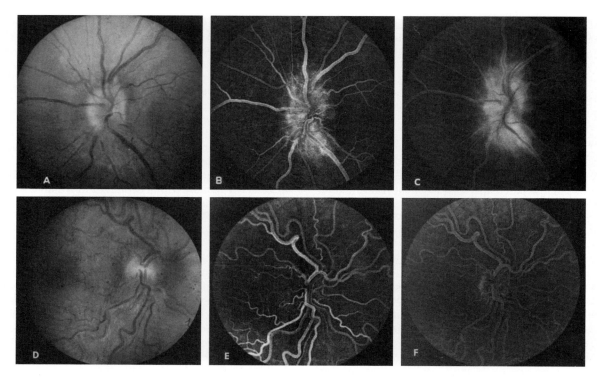

Figure 5.23. Fluorescein angiogram of mild papilledema (*A–C*) and pseudopapilledema (*D–F*). *A,* Reproduction of color photograph of the left fundus showing indistinct disc margins and an incomplete peripapillary halo (Frisén stage 2). No hemorrhages are visible. *B,* In arteriovenous phase, fluorescein angiogram shows early leakage of dye into peripapillary region. *C,* Ten minutes after fluorescein injection, angiogram shows residual hyperfluorescence of disc and surrounding region. *D,* Optic disc shows tortuous vessels, indistinct disc margins and mild elevation. *E,* Fluorescein angiogram in early arteriovenous phase shows no disc fluorescence or leakage into the peripapillary region. *F,* Eight minutes after fluorescein injection shows no evidence of disc leakage or hyperfluorescence. (Courtesy of Dr. Michael Sanders.)

neurologists, and neurosurgeons in identifying papilledema and pseudopapilledema (92). Family physicians were as good as or better than neurologists and neurosurgeons in identifying acute and chronic papilledema, but had difficulty distinguishing between papilledema and pseudopapilledema. One would expect that the detection rate among all specialists would decline under many less ideal circumstances, e.g., using direct ophthalmoscopy through an undilated pupil.

Finally, if the diagnosis of papilledema remains uncertain, the ICP can be measured directly by lumbar puncture. This procedure should only be performed after neuroimaging has been performed to determine that no intracranial mass is present.

DIFFERENTIAL DIAGNOSIS

The differential diagnosis of papilledema (with normal visual acuity and bilaterality) includes anomalous elevation of one or both optic discs and true optic disc swelling caused by some etiologies other than increased ICP (Table 5.2). In most cases, the patients have no neurologic or systemic symptoms or signs referable to increased ICP, and this lack of manifestations should help the physician focus on other possibilities. When the patient does have other complaints,

such as headaches, however, the differentiation of papilledema from other causes of optic disc elevation becomes more complex.

Anomalous elevation of the optic discs is probably caused most often by buried optic disc drusen; however, hypoplastic discs may be anomalously elevated, and tilted optic discs often show elevation of their superior and nasal portions. In addition, some optic discs are anomalously elevated but do not contain drusen, nor are they small or tilted. In all cases,

Table 5.2
Differential Diagnosis of Papilledema

Anomalously elevated optic disc
  With and without buried drusen
  Tilted optic disc
  Hypoplastic optic disc
Intraocular inflammation
Asymptomatic nonarteritic anterior ischemic optic neuropathy (e.g., diabetic "papillopathy")
Hypertensive disc edema
Optic neuritis, optic perineuritis (perioptic neuritis)
Infiltrative optic neuropathy (e.g., from leukemia)
Compressive optic neuropathy (e.g., from optic nerve sheath meningioma)

a careful ophthalmoscopic examination combined with ultrasonography should differentiate anomalously elevated optic discs from true optic disc swelling. Anomalous optic discs are discussed in Chapter 3 of this text.

True optic disc swelling that mimics papilledema may be caused by inflammatory, vascular or infiltrative disease. Inflammatory conditions are generally accompanied by other evidence of inflammation such as aqueous or vitreous cells, and sheathing of retinal vessels. Retinal vascular disturbances can also produce optic disc swelling. In this circumstance, correct diagnosis may not be possible without performing appropriate neuroimaging and a lumbar puncture. Patients with optic perineuritis (perioptic neuritis) have optic disc swelling that is also indistinguishable from papilledema unless there is associated intraocular inflammation.

Nonarteritic anterior ischemic optic neuropathy (NAION) can mimic papilledema, particularly when it is asymptomatic. The sectoral nature of the disc swelling, and the pattern of visual field loss in NAION generally distinguish it from true papilledema. Rare patients with anterior optic neuritis have normal central visual acuity; however, such patients invariably complain of pain on eye movement and decreased vision, and other tests of visual function in such patients (e.g., contrast sensitivity, color vision, visual fields) usually reveal an abnormality inconsistent with papilledema (93). Unlike papilledema and NAION, nerve fiber layer hemorrhages are very uncommon in optic neuritis (94). Finally, optic discs infiltrated by inflammatory or neoplastic cells may appear similar to papilledema. The diagnosis in such cases can usually be made by neuroimaging, with or without a lumbar puncture.

COURSE

The rapidity of developing papilledema depends to a large extent on the etiology and degree of the increased ICP. Experimental models using inflatable balloons in the subarachnoid space of monkeys showed papilledema in 30% of the animals in 24 hours, in 50% after 2 days, and in 90% after 5 days when papilledema was assessed using direct ophthalmoscopy, stereoscopic photography, and fluorescein angiography (21,22). Most of the animals developed papilledema from the surgery even prior to the balloon being inflated (21) and papilledema took 1 to 3 weeks to re-develop after the postoperative edema resolved and the balloon was inflated (21). Clinical experience with humans suggests that the development of optic disc edema may be protracted. The largest study investigating this process was performed in 37 patients with acutely elevated ICP from cerebral hemorrhage or trauma receiving continuous ICP monitoring (95). Using both direct and indirect ophthalmoscopy, no papilledema was observed in the 13 patients with mildly elevated ICP (20–30 mm Hg) and only two patients had venous congestion by day six. In seven patients with ICP ranging from 30–70 mm Hg, papilledema developed in one patient with a subarachnoid hemorrhage who developed fatal cerebral edema and carotid artery distribution infarction postoperatively. No optic disc or fundus abnormalities were seen in the other six patients. Within the first three days of developing transient increased ICP (prior to successful treatment), none of 17 patients had papilledema. This experience suggests that clinically detectable papilledema is not usually present with acute elevations of ICP, and may take over a week to develop.

Cases have been reported of papilledema within 2 to 4 hours after intracranial hemorrhage (96). Fulminant, hemorrhagic papilledema was also seen within 5 to 8 hours in the context of other conditions (metastatic frontal lobe tumor, epidural hematoma) (97). In addition, minimal papilledema may exist and suddenly become fully developed in several hours in certain settings, such as encephalitis in the setting of a cerebral abscess (98,99). Occasionally, a paradoxic development or progression of papilledema several days to a week after normalization of increased ICP may occur (100).

Papilledema usually produces swelling of the inferior and superior poles of the optic disc prior to the nasal and temporal poles (21). Blurring of the disc margins by direct ophthalmoscopy is only apparent after optic disc elevation occurs (21).

Fully developed papilledema may resolve completely within hours, days, or weeks, depending on the way in which ICP is lowered (Fig. 5.24). In monkeys with experimental intracranial hypertension produced by an inflatable balloon, papilledema disappeared within 2 weeks after the intracranial pressure was abruptly normalized (21). In humans, papilledema can resolve 6-8 weeks after a successful craniotomy to remove a brain tumor or after subtemporal decompression for PTC (101). Optic disc edema may improve in less than a week following optic nerve sheath decompression surgery (102), but the time course to complete resolution is uncertain. Papilledema from PTC generally takes two or more months to resolve (103).

In most cases, retinal venous as well as disc capillary dilations begin to regress as soon as ICP is lowered to a normal level. During the next few days to weeks, presumably because of the change in hemodynamics at the disc, new hemorrhages may appear; however, these are of no significance and they disappear within a short time. Gradually, disc hyperemia and elevation resolve. The last abnormalities to disappear are blurring of the disc margins and abnormalities of the peripapillary retinal nerve fiber layer. In some cases, as noted above, papilledema resolves into optic atrophy. Optic atrophy following papilledema is sometimes referred to as "secondary" or "dirty" optic atrophy. Unlike the crisp optic disc margin seen in optic atrophy following other types of optic neuropathy, there may be extensive sheathing of vessels and gliosis following papilledema, suggesting that the optic nerve axons died "after a struggle." However, in many cases, the atrophy is indistinguishable from that caused by inflammation, vascular disease, or trauma (104). In other cases, the papilledema never completely resolves despite normalization of the ICP.

VISUAL PROGNOSIS

Establishing the visual prognosis in a patient with papilledema is often impossible. Generally, the more severe the

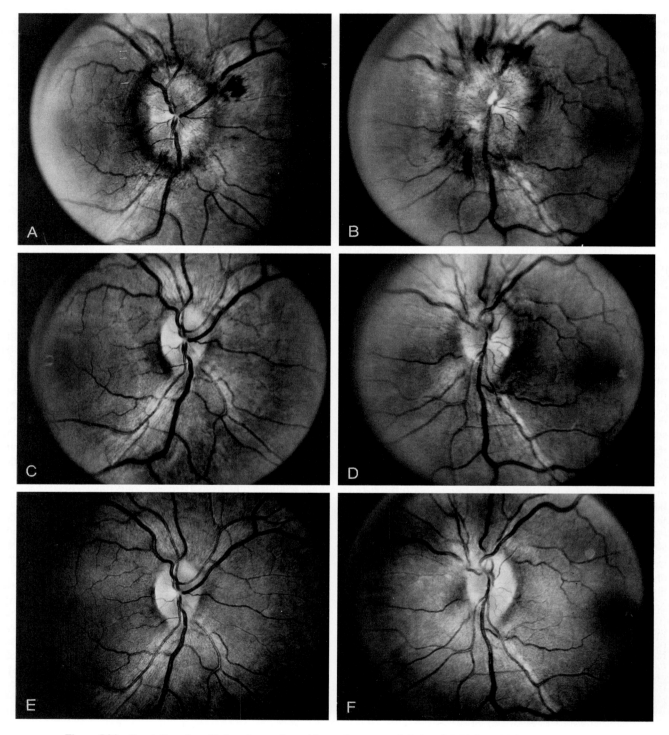

Figure 5.24.   Resolution of papilledema in a patient with pseudotumor cerebri. *A and B*, Right and left optic discs prior to treatment. *C and D*, One month after beginning treatment with dehydrating agents, much of the disc swelling has resolved in both eyes, and no hemorrhages are evident. *E and F*, Three months after beginning treatment, both discs show complete resolution of swelling and now appear normal.

papilledema, the worse the visual prognosis (105). An ominous sign is narrowing of the retinal arteries, which often occurs with sheathing. In this setting, irreversible damage to the optic nerve tissue has already occurred, as is the case when there is loss of the peripapillary retinal nerve fiber layer. Disc pallor that becomes evident while papilledema is still present is also an indication of poor visual prognosis (105), even if ICP is lowered immediately, because the pallor is caused by loss of axons. Most patients with these changes have clinical evidence of visual dysfunction, including decreased color vision, visual field defects, and abnormal contrast sensitivity. Loss of visual acuity may be the last visual parameter to be affected, much as in patients with chronic open angle glaucoma. It is our experience that once there is visual acuity decline or significant visual field deficits the visual prognosis is extremely tenuous. On the other hand, severe venous engorgement, retinal hemorrhages, and hard and soft exudates have no prognostic significance.

PAPILLEDEMA AND AGE

Papilledema may be observed at any age. Not only is there no upper age limit, but there is abundant evidence that papilledema also occurs frequently in infants and children. This phenomenon is remarkable because we explain the absence of papilledema in most cases of congenital hydrocephalus on the basis of expansibility of the skull. If this were true, one would expect a lower prevalence of papilledema in infants and children with intracranial tumors. Nevertheless, there are many reports of papilledema or post-papilledema optic atrophy in children and in infants under two years of age (9,106–108). Walsh reviewed the case records of the pediatrics department of the Johns Hopkins Hospital from 1928 to 1944 and found 18 cases of cerebral tumor in children 3 years of age or younger (26); 13 patients (72%) had papilledema. The youngest patient was 3 months old and had a cerebellar medulloblastoma. Thus, the distensibility of an infant's skull may not prevent an increase in pressure within the optic nerve sheaths.

PATHOLOGY

The essential histological features of papilledema are optic disc edema, neuronal swelling, venous and capillary dilatation, an abnormal protrusion of the optic nerve head toward the vitreous, lateral displacement of the adjacent retina, and folds of the posterior retinal layers (Fig. 5.25) (5,109). The physiologic optic cup is generally preserved (109). The separation of the swollen optic disc from the adjacent retina is typically sharp and has the form of an S-shaped curve.

Compression, detachment, and lateral displacement of the peripapillary retina appear to be the major reasons that the blind spot increases in size in patients with papilledema (110,111); however, the blind spot may be enlarged even when there is no obvious retinal displacement or detachment. In this setting, the enlarged blind spot represents a refractive scotoma caused by acquired peripapillary hyperopia from elevation of the retina by peripapillary subretinal fluid (112). A blind spot that is enlarged by this mechanism can be reduced to near normal size by the use of progressively stronger plus lenses (112). The neuronal swelling in papilledema is more extensive peripherally, accounting for the visual field constriction. Vascular interruption at the annulus of Zinn produces the typical arcuate and inferonasal visual field defects (111,113).

Hemorrhages may overlie and obscure the optic disc and may occur in all layers of the peripapillary retina, occasionally extending into the vitreous or into the adjacent subretinal space. Focal necroses of nerve fibers are frequent, most often occurring in the lateral outpouchings of the nerve substance adjacent to the retina. The small vessels of the optic disc often appear prominent with abnormally plump and proliferative endothelial cells (1). The substance of the prelaminar portion of the optic nerve is clearly swollen, but does not ordinarily show any increase in cellularity until secondary gliosis occurs. By light microscopy, the swelling takes the form of vacuoles (21). The swelling does not extend to the postlaminar optic nerve which usually appears normal unless secondary optic atrophy has occurred. The perineuronal spaces are often distended, with stretching of the delicate arachnoidal strands that bridge the subarachnoid space (Fig. 5.26).

Electron microscopic studies indicate that most of the increase in tissue elevation that occurs in papilledema results from intra-axonal swelling and not from extracellular edema (114). The swelling is most marked in the superficial optic nerve head, where some of the axons increase to 10 to 20 times their normal diameter (21,115). The intra-axonal swelling is accompanied by an increase in mitochondria, disorganization of neurofilaments, and the accumulation of dense intracellular membrane-enclosed bodies. With severe papilledema, cytoid bodies are especially apt to occur in those portions of the optic disc that bulge laterally toward the adjacent retina. These cytoid bodies and resultant necroses appear to result from strangulation of the angulated nerve fibers. Although interstitial fluid is present in the region of degenerating fibers (116,117), it is insufficient to account for the large increase in the mass of the optic disc that occurs in fully developed papilledema. Electron microscopy demonstrates that what appear to be free intra-axonal spaces by light microscopy are actually swollen axons (Fig. 5.27). The findings noted above in humans also occur in rhesus monkeys with experimentally produced papilledema (21,118).

PATHOGENESIS

Any unifying mechanism for papilledema must account for (*a*) transient unilateral or bilateral visual obscurations; (*b*) edema localized to the optic nerve head; (*c*) flattening of the posterior sclera as demonstrated by neuroimaging techniques, and (*d*) venous distension and cessation of venous pulsations (111). Various hypotheses have been proposed over the years, including direct infiltration of the optic nerve head by CSF (119,120), obstruction of posterior flow of intraocular fluid (121), inherent turgescence of prelaminar nerve substance (122), swelling of glia (123), absence of the

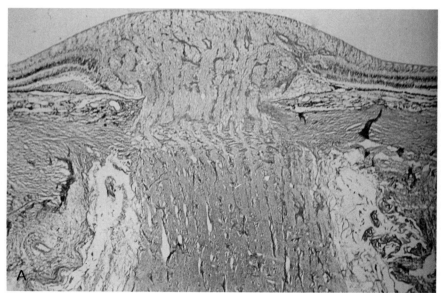

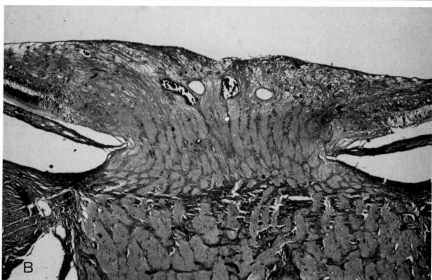

Figure 5.25. Histological appearance of papilledema by light microscopy. *A and B*, Both photographs show axonal swelling limited to the prelaminar portion of the optic nerve. The peripapillary retina is pushed laterally. Note small collection of subretinal fluid in the peripapillary region.

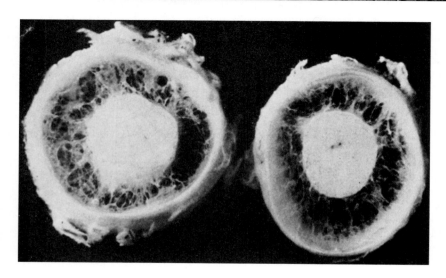

Figure 5.26. Gross pathologic appearance of orbital optic nerves, subarachnoid space, and optic nerve sheaths in chronic papilledema. Note marked distention and stretching of the delicate arachnoid trabeculations that bridge the subarachnoid space around the nerves. (From Cogan DG. Neurology of the Visual System, Ed 6. Springfield, IL, Charles C Thomas, 1966.)

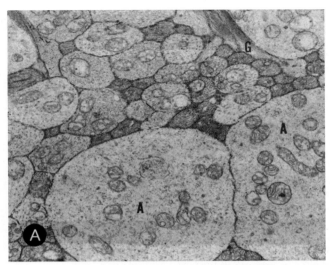

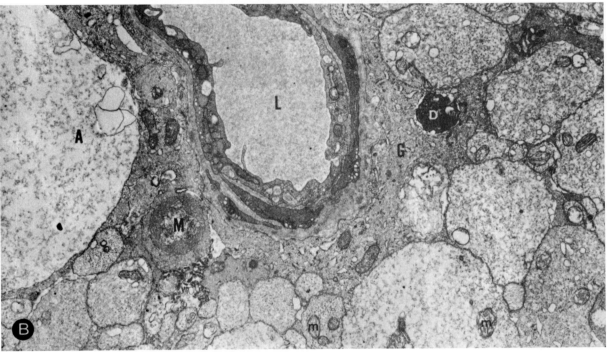

Figure 5.27. Ultrastructural appearance of papilledema. *A*, Most of the axons in the immediately prelaminar portion of the optic nerve are swollen (A) and show disruption of their neurotubules and swelling of the mitochondria. Some of the axons remain normal in size and structure. Glial elements (G) in this region are not swollen. *B*, Another section of the prelaminar portion of the optic nerve head demonstrates axonal swellings of varying severity. Some axons are mildly swollen, whereas others show hydropic degeneration (A). One axon contains giant mitochondria (M), whereas in other axons, the mitochondria are normal in size (m). A dense body (D) is present in the cytoplasm of a perivascular glial cell (G). L, lumen of a blood vessel. (From Tso MOM, Hayreh SS. Optic disc edema in raised intracranial pressure. III. A pathologic study of experimental papilledema. Arch Ophthalmol 1977;95:1448–1457.)

restraining influence of Müller cells in the peripapillary retina (124), disequilibrium of hydrostatic pressure in the tissue and bloodstream (125), and compression of the central retinal vein as it traverses the subarachnoid space (125) or cavernous sinus (126) with elevated central venous pressure (111).

An animal model of experimental papilledema, developed in the 1960s, provided a means to test most of the theories regarding the pathogenesis of papilledema. Increased ICP has been produced in monkeys by cranial irradiation (127) and by the introduction of an inflatable balloon into the subarachnoid space (63,128,129). Using these models, there are some general points of agreement regarding the pathogenesis of papilledema. First, papilledema occurs only when there is patency of the subarachnoid space surrounding the optic nerve and intracranial structures (116,130,131). Blockage of these spaces by adhesions or tumor prevents papilledema from occurring on the side of the obstruction. Second, papilledema does not occur when antecedent optic atrophy has destroyed most or all of the nerve fibers. Finally, and most important, axonal transport is clearly abnormal in patients with papilledema as well as in patients with disc swelling from all other causes (e.g., ischemia, inflammation, hypotony).

Orthograde transport is studied using autoradiography by injecting labeled amino acids (usually leucine or proline) into the vitreous cavity. Both the fast (± 400 mm/day) and slow (± 1 mm/day) components of axon transport accumulate in the regions of the lamina cribrosa of monkeys with experimentally produced increased ICP and papilledema (132,133) (Fig. 5.28). The stagnant axoplasmic flow results in the swelling of axons seen by electron microscopy (118). Several studies confirm that eyes with optic disc swelling from increased ICP as well as other causes have stasis of both fast and slow axonal transport (115,133–136).

The role of central retinal venous pressure in papilledema is controversial. If the CSF pressure in the optic nerve sheath constantly fluctuates, as it does in the brain, the sheath, like the spinal dural sac, could function as an expansion vessel (111). Unlike the extradural veins of the spinal sac, the central retinal vein is located within the subarachnoid space. With markedly elevated ICP, the venous pressure in the optic nerve sheath could be double that of the eye, accounting for the loss of spontaneous venous pulsations and the presence

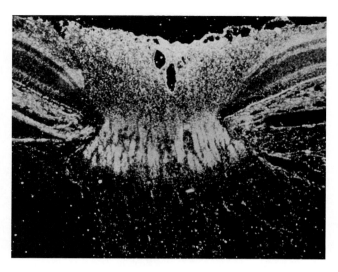

Figure 5.28. Blockage of axon transport in papilledema. Phase contrast photomicrograph shows accumulation of axonal products (seen as white material) in the region of the lamina cribrosa.

of choroidal folds, acquired hypermetropia, shortening of the globe on MRI scanning, and forward bowing of the lamina cribrosa (111). However, experimental compression of the central retinal vein at its site of exit from the optic nerve does not produce optic disc edema (137). Similarly, monkeys exposed to raised CSF pressure for up to 2 hours showed increased ophthalmic vein pressure but not disc edema (138). Concurrent impaired perfusion of the neurons traversing the lamina cribrosa (the arteriolar branches of the circle of Zinn) may be the final critical factor required to produce the vascular changes at the optic disc and impaired axoplasmic flow in papilledema (111,139).

Research to date suggests that there are three components required for the development of papilledema: increased and fluctuating pressure in the distal optic nerve sheath; elevated central retinal venous pressure; and impaired perfusion of the nerve fibers traversing the lamina cribrosa (111). Despite the findings described above, numerous questions still exist regarding the pathogenesis of papilledema (140).

SYMPTOMS AND SIGNS

Both nonvisual and visual symptoms occur in patients with papilledema. As a general rule, the nonvisual symptoms are more severe and bothersome to the patient, although visual symptoms can be both distressing and indicative of impending permanent visual dysfunction.

NONVISUAL MANIFESTATIONS

Headache

Headache is often the first symptom of increased ICP, although there may be a considerable increase in ICP without headache. The characteristics of headaches with increased

ICP are nonspecific. They are usually global and aching (''tension type''), but may be unilateral and throbbing (''migrainous''). The headache may be constant or intermittent. Neither the severity of the headache nor its location has any value in determining whether an intracranial mass is present and, if so, its location. The typical ''brain tumor headache'' that is worst upon awakening is only present in about one-third of patients with tumors and does not correlate with the presence of increased ICP (141). Headaches associated with increased ICP often worsen during a Valsalva maneuver (coughing, straining, etc.). The headache associated with increased ICP may be caused by stretching of the meninges or from distention of cerebral veins.

Nausea, Vomiting, and Photophobia

Nausea and vomiting are frequently associated with significantly increased ICP. Photophobia is commonly present and is occasionally the presenting symptom of intracranial hypertension.

CSF Rhinorrhea

Spontaneous CSF rhinorrhea is most commonly seen in patients with a mass lesion, congenital anomaly or previous trauma (142). This phenomenon has also been reported with PTC and in patients with a CSF fistula that is usually located in the region of the cribriform plate (143).

VISUAL MANIFESTATIONS

Early papilledema is usually asymptomatic. Even well-developed papilledema may produce minimal or no symptoms. Sometimes the only abnormality found on careful testing is mild to moderate enlargement of the physiologic blind spot. Other patients may be aware of their physiologic blind spot, and describe a negative scotoma in the temporal field of vision of one or both eyes. Still other patients have variable loss of visual acuity, visual field, or both.

Coexisting retinal or vitreous hemorrhages or exudates may reduce central acuity (37) (Fig. 5.29). For example, sudden monocular blindness from a subretinal neovascular membrane has been reported as the first symptom of PTC (144). When papilledema is caused by an intracranial mass, decreased acuity or a visual field defect in one or both eyes may occur by several mechanisms, including direct compression of a portion of the visual sensory pathway (e.g., compression of the occipital lobe by a meningioma, producing a homonymous field defect), indirect compression of part of the pathway via a secondary effect on surrounding brain (e.g., gyrus rectus compression of the optic nerves producing a bilateral optic neuropathy in a patient with a frontal lobe tumor), and infiltration of a part of the pathway (e.g., infiltration of the optic chiasm by a germinoma, producing a bitemporal hemianopia).

Transient Visual Obscurations

As papilledema worsens, patients may experience brief, transient obscurations of vision. During these episodes, vision may vary from mild blurring to complete blindness. Some patients describe a rapid gray-out of vision, whereas others experience positive visual phenomena, such as photopsias and phosphenes that obscure their vision. In all cases, however, recovery of vision is invariably rapid and complete (17,145). The obscurations may affect either eye or both eyes simultaneously (146). They usually last only a few seconds, although attacks lasting several hours rarely occur (17,145,147–149). The episodes may occur up to 20–30 times a day, and are often precipitated by changes in posture, particularly from a bent-over position (146). There may be gaze-evoked amaurosis, a phenomenon that is also observed by patients with orbital lesions that compress the optic nerve (150) (see Chapter 4). Transient obscurations of vision are often worrisome to the patient but they do not predict visual outcome (105,151).

Although transient obscurations were once thought to occur most frequently with lesions in the posterior fossa, particularly cerebellar tumors (145,148), they occur more in patients with PTC than in patients with intracranial mass lesions. They are most likely attributable to transient compression or ischemia of the optic nerve, as they are identical to those that occur in patients with unilateral meningiomas of the optic nerve sheath (see Chapter 8).

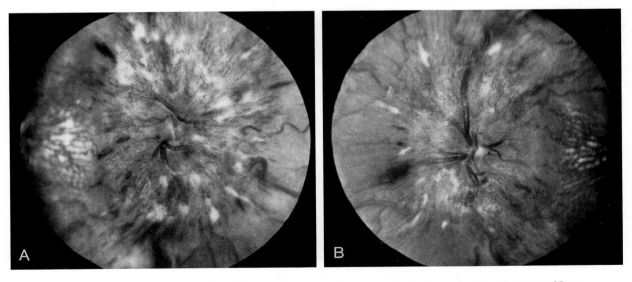

Figure 5.29. Papilledema associated with bilateral visual loss related to macular hard exudate. The patient was a 35-year-old woman with headaches and decreased vision in both eyes. Visual acuity was 20/50 OU. Visual fields showed marked enlargement of the blind spots. Both optic discs are severely swollen (Frisén stage 5). *A and B.* There are numerous hemorrhages and soft exudates on and surrounding the discs, and there is a star figure composed of hard exudate (lipid) in the maculae.

Visual Field Defects

Concentric enlargement of the blind spot is the most common—and frequently the only—visual field defect in patients with papilledema (152). Compression, detachment, and lateral displacement of the peripapillary retina appear to be the major reasons that the blind spot increases in size in patients with papilledema (110); however, the blind spot may be enlarged even when there is no obvious retinal displacement or detachment. In this setting, the enlarged blind spot represents a refractive scotoma caused by acquired peripapillary hyperopia that, in turn, results from elevation of the retina by peripapillary subretinal fluid (153).

Uhthoff (154) described the various types of visual field

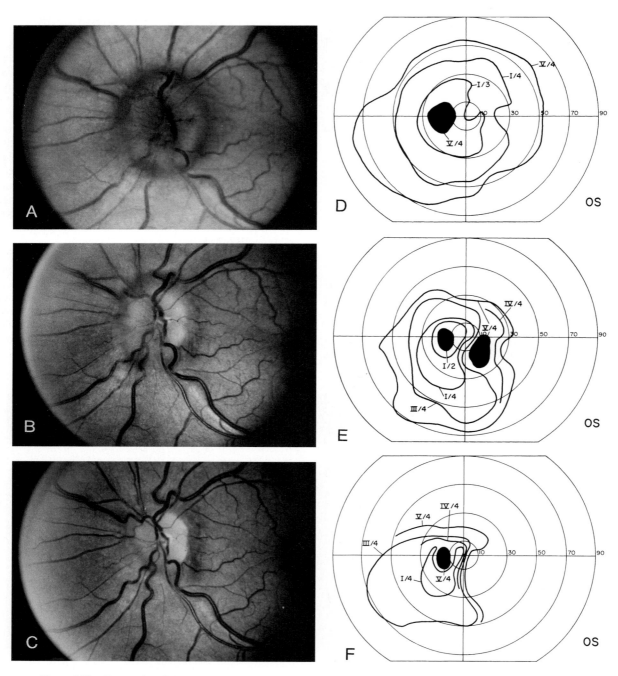

Figure 5.30. Progression of visual field defect in a patient with chronic papilledema. *A–C*, Progression of chronic papilledema to optic atrophy. *D–F*, Progression of the visual field defects. Note progressive loss of nasal and superotemporal fields and associated constriction with preservation of visual acuity.

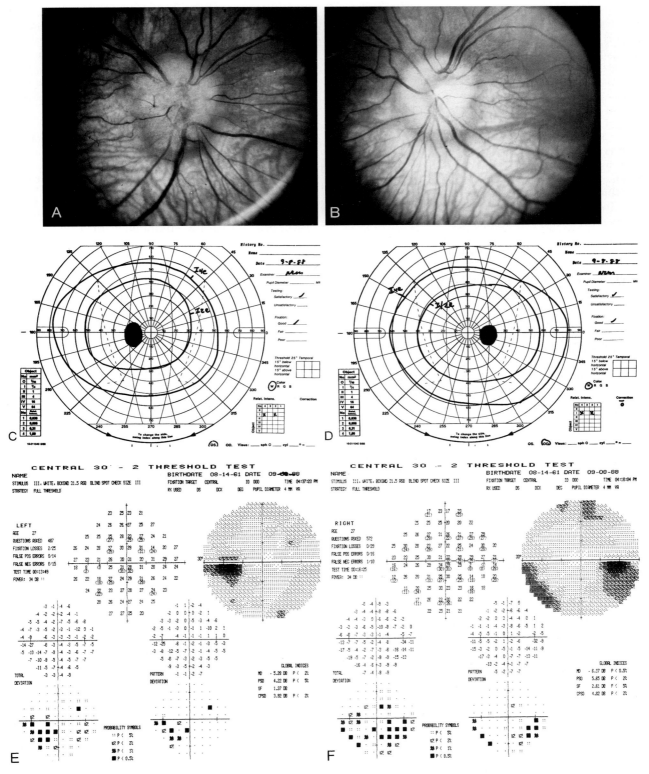

Figure 5.31. Difference in sensitivity of kinetic versus static perimetry in chronic papilledema. *A and B*, Right and left optic discs show chronic papilledema. *C and D*, Kinetic perimetry shows no abnormalities except for mildly enlarged blind spots. *E and F*, Static perimetry in the same patient shows nasal steps, inferior arcuate defects, and reduction in sensitivity in both eyes.

defects in papilledema, including enlargement of the blind spot (30%), concentric constriction (29%), and complete blindness (25%), with the rest of the defects divided among homonymous hemianopia and central and arcuate scotomas. In chronic papilledema, the inferior nasal quadrant is most often affected (155). Dense paracentral scotomas may be found in the Bjerrum area, and may progress to form ring scotomas (155). Visual acuity usually deteriorates late in the course of the disease. The defects can be reversed if ICP is lowered before chronic papilledema develops (156). As with loss of visual acuity, loss of visual field is usually slow and progressive. Sudden loss of visual field suggests a superimposed local cause, such as ischemia (113).

Automated static perimetry confirms that early visual field defects in eyes with papilledema are not uncommon and are often present when standard kinetic perimetry gives normal results (157–159). These early defects are generally arcuate scotomas or nasal steps. Constriction of the visual fields may occur with high-grade papilledema or as a late sign of papilledema during the chronic stage as it progresses to optic atrophy. The field defects are usually worse nasally than temporally (160) (Figs. 5.30 and 5.31). Thus, in advanced papilledema, only a temporal island of vision may remain before progressing to complete blindness. The slowly progressive visual field defects in chronic papilledema are similar to those seen in glaucoma, suggesting that there may be a common pathogenetic mechanism in the two conditions (155), or a similar vulnerability of specific nerve fibers to different insults.

Loss of Central Vision

Patients with papilledema caused by intracranial mass lesions or meningitis (septic, aseptic, carcinomatous, and lymphomatous) can lose central vision acutely or progressively from the effects of the underlying process on the optic nerves. In other cases, permanent loss of central vision results from the nonspecific effects of increased ICP on the optic nerve and begins with visual field constriction that is slowly progressive. In this setting, loss of central acuity usually is a late phenomenon, although it may occur over several weeks in cases with markedly increased ICP (161). When acute loss of vision occurs in patients with papilledema, local causes are generally responsible (161,162). Central vision loss may be produced by hemorrhages or exudates in the maculae. Ischemic optic neuropathy or retinal vascular occlusions may be related to the underlying process (e.g., a coagulopathy) or to the rapid rate at which the ICP has risen (163–167). Rare patients, many of them children, seem to have a fulminant course characterized by a rapid progression from normal vision to profound and permanent visual loss (162,168,169).

Other Abnormalities in Visual Sensory Function

As in other optic neuropathies, papilledema may be associated with nonspecific abnormalities of visual sensation that can be detected when specific tests are performed. For example, patients with visual acuity of 20/20, a full visual field, and normal color perception may nevertheless have abnormal contrast sensitivity (170–174). Visual evoked potentials do not become abnormal until marked visual loss has occurred and have no role in the diagnosis or monitoring of visual function with papilledema (171,175).

Diplopia

The most common cause of diplopia from increased ICP is a lateral rectus palsy, as one or both abducens nerves are compressed against one of the transverse branches of the basilar artery at the base of the skull (176,177). Infrequently, trochlear nerve palsies occur in patients with increased ICP, presumably from compression of either the dorsal midbrain or the nerves themselves, by a ballooned suprapineal recess (178,179). Trochlear nerve palsies may be mistaken for a "skew deviation" if quantitative testing of eye movements or a Bielschowsky head tilt test is not performed, although true skew deviation can also occur in patients with increased ICP (168,180,181). Oculomotor nerve palsy is distinctly uncommon as a non-localizing sign of increased ICP (168,182). Intracranial hypertension occasionally presents with global ophthalmoparesis that resolves as the ICP is normalized (183).

ETIOLOGY

GENERAL CONSIDERATIONS

The craniospinal cavity is an almost rigid bony enclosure completely filled by tissue, CSF, and circulating blood. Within this enclosure, CSF is constantly produced at the rate 500 ml/day, or 0.35 ml/minute (184). Almost all of the production is by the choroid plexus within the lateral ventricles, although the choroid plexuses of the 3rd and 4th ventricles and the ependymal lining of the ventricular system also contribute a small amount. The secretion of CSF is related to sodium transport in the brush border of the choroid plexus epithelium, and is dependent on sodium-potassium-activated ATPase as well as the enzyme carbonic anhydrase (184).

CSF flows from the lateral ventricles through the interventricular foramina into the 3rd ventricle and mixes with the CSF produced in that ventricle. The CSF then flows through the cerebral aqueduct (of Sylvius) into the 4th ventricle, and out into the subarachnoid space through the foramina of Luschka and Magendie. In the subarachnoid space, CSF flows rostrally from the posterior fossa through the lower ventral basal cisterns and tentorial notch to reach the interpeduncular and chiasmatic cisterns. The CSF then flows dorsally through the communicating cisterns to reach the dorsal cisterns, and lateral and superiorly from the chiasmatic cistern into the cisterns of the Sylvian fissure. From the cisterns and Sylvian fissures, CSF moves outward and superiorly over the cerebral convexities where it is absorbed.

The chief route of absorption of CSF in the brain is passively through the arachnoid granulations that protrude into the venous sinuses and diploic veins. These vessels drain to the internal jugular vein and other extracranial veins. CSF is also absorbed in the spinal sac.

Many factors influence CSF formation, including toxins, medications, and neurotransmitters. Cholera toxin increases CSF production (185,186), while serotonin, sympathomimetic drugs, acetazolamide, furosemide, vasopression, dopamine D1 receptor antagonists, atrial naturetic hormone, hyperosmolar agents and hypothermia decrease CSF formation (184,187). Corticosteroids seem to have no effect on CSF production but lower intracranial pressure by a different mechanism (184). There is likely a feedback mechanism of increased ICP on CSF production but it is not well elucidated (188).

The Monro-Kellie hypothesis (189,190), states that the volume of blood, brain and CSF within the cranial cavity must be in equilibrium, and a change in the volume of one component must be offset by a reciprocal change in another. However, within this rigid system, there is an elastic element of the spinal dural sac and the vascular channels (191). Under appropriate circumstances, as little as 80 cc of rapidly added volume (CSF, blood, edema, tissue, etc.) will raise ICP to a level incompatible with life (189). Given the intracranial compartmental equilibrium, increased ICP occurs by several mechanisms:

An increase in the total amount of intracranial tissue by a space-occupying lesion;

An increase in intracranial tissue volume by focal or diffuse cerebral edema;

A decrease in total volume within the cranial vault by thickening of the skull;

Blockage of the flow of CSF within the ventricular system (obstructive or noncommunicating hydrocephalus) or within the arachnoid granulations (nonobstructive or communicating hydrocephalus);

Reduced absorption of CSF from obstruction or compromise of venous outflow both intracranially and extracranially; and/or

Increased production of CSF by an intracranial tumor at a rate that precludes adequate absorption for maintenance of normal ICP (192,193).

CONDITIONS ASSOCIATED WITH PAPILLEDEMA

Tumors

Intracranial masses such as tumors produce increased ICP through most of the mechanisms mentioned above. They may act solely as space-occupying lesions; they may produce focal or diffuse cerebral edema, and they may block the outflow of CSF by direct compression of CSF drainage pathways or by infiltration of the arachnoid villi or the cerebral venous sinuses. Other potential mechanisms are the production of increased protein or blood products that secondarily block the arachnoid villi, and by directly producing CSF.

Papilledema does not develop in every patient with a cerebral tumor. Several large studies found papilledema in 60–80% of patients with cerebral tumors (194–198). Tumors that are situated below the tentorium (infratentorial) are more likely to produce papilledema than those situated above it (supratentorial). Supratentorial tumors rarely cause primary obstruction to the flow of CSF through the aqueduct

of Sylvius, but may produce papilledema by deflection of the falx and pressure upon the great vein of Galen (199). Tumors below the tentorium usually produce papilledema by obstruction of the aqueduct. Nevertheless, some infratentorial masses do not obstruct the aqueduct but still produce papilledema, perhaps related to elevation of the tentorium with pressure on the vein of Galen or on other cerebral venous sinuses (165,197–200). Both central and transtentorial herniation syndromes may cause papilledema.

Brain tumors in certain locations may produce papilledema without lateralizing or localizing signs, particularly if they are supratentorial and situated within the nondominant hemisphere or within one of the lateral ventricles (201). Moreover, not all intracranial tumors cause a pressure rise sufficient to produce papilledema (202).

Papilledema may be dependent not only on tumor location but also on the type and growth rate of the tumor. For example, gliomas may produce papilledema in three-quarters of cases, whereas meningiomas produce papilledema in less than half (203). Papilledema was observed in 50% of patients with rapidly growing glioblastomas, while 65% of those patients with slowly progressive benign astrocytomas and meningiomas demonstrated papilledema (204). Papilledema was present in 61% of patients with cerebral metastases (204). These data raise the possibility that papilledema may develop more frequently in those patients with slowly progressive tumors rather than those with malignant and rapidly growing masses (204).

Papilledema may occur with other intracranial masses, such as hamartomas (205), teratomas, parasitic lesions such as cysticercus cysts (206), abscesses, hematomas, aneurysms, and granulomas, usually in association with sarcoidosis, tuberculosis, or syphilis.

Arteriovenous Malformation (AVM)

AVMs need not rupture to produce papilledema (176,207–213). The mechanism producing increased ICP is likely from direct shunting of arterial blood from AVMs into the cerebral venous system, elevating the cerebral venous pressure and decreasing CSF resorption (209,214–217). Additionally, there may be venous sinus thrombosis or direct venous sinus compression from the AVM causing increased ICP (209). Both intracerebral and dural-based AVMs involving the transverse sinus are associated with papilledema (218). Treatment may include surgery, embolization or shunt placement to lower the intracranial pressure (209,217).

Aqueductal Stenosis

Aqueductal stenosis often presents in childhood. It may be congenital, in which case it may or may not be associated with a Chiari malformation, or it may be acquired from intracranial infections such as toxoplasmosis or mumps ependymitis (219). Presentation in infancy is accompanied by macrocephaly. Adults may have headaches, dorsal midbrain syndrome, meningitis, hemorrhage, endocrine disturbances from compression of the pituitary gland, seizures, gait disturbances, and CSF rhinorrhea (220,221). Occasionally aqueductal stenosis produces unilateral ocular symptoms and optic disc edema (58).

Intracranial Hemorrhage

Papilledema occurs in patients with both acute and chronic subdural hematoma but is more commonly observed in the acute phase (204,222,223). The converse is true with epidural hematoma, when the papilledema may develop many weeks after the injury, particularly when the hematoma is located at the vertex causing compression of the superior sagittal sinus (224–226).

In almost all cases, subarachnoid hemorrhage produces papilledema either by blocking CSF flow within the ventricular system or by blocking CSF absorption at the arachnoid granulations. The site of the hemorrhage may be intracranial or spinal (227). In one series of 192 patients with ruptured intracranial aneurysms, papilledema was found in 16% (228). The presence of papilledema was not related to gender, age, or site of the aneurysm. In seven cases, the papilledema was unilateral, and it was ipsilateral to the lesion in six of these cases. Other investigators report the incidence of papilledema in patients with aneurysmal subarachnoid hemorrhage as 10–24% (229,230). It may be present within several hours after the hemorrhage (154,231), or develop only after several weeks of increased ICP (232).

Infections

Although papilledema is uncommon in patients with a cerebral hemispheric **abscess**, abscesses in the occipital lobe frequently produce pronounced papilledema (204), and chronic brain abscesses are associated with papilledema more frequently than acute abscesses (99,233). There is no definite relationship between the size of the abscess and the severity of the papilledema. Unilateral papilledema caused by a brain abscess may have localizing value. Cerebellar abscesses are not likely to produce papilledema, perhaps because of more rapid surgical intervention or hastened mortality compared to supratentorial hemispheric lesions (98).

The etiology of ICP in patients with **meningitis** or **encephalitis** is usually diffuse cerebral edema. However, the reported frequency of papilledema with meningitis is fairly small, and the papilledema tends to be mild and transient. Only 2.5% of patients had papilledema in one study of 2,178 cases of meningitis (234) and other large series of syphilitic meningitis showed a similar incidence of papilledema (235,236). Papilledema was more likely to occur in patients with tuberculous meningitis (25% of cases) than in any other type of bacterial meningitis (234).

Among 80 patients with clinical signs of aseptic meningitis, 17 had optic disc swelling (237). The disc swelling was associated with moderate elevation of the discs, minimal venous congestion, and small peripapillary hemorrhages. In slightly more than half of the patients, there was confirmed increased ICP. In the others, it is likely that the disc swelling was caused by an optic perineuritis (see Chapter 6). All patients recovered completely in 6–12 months. A retrospective review of 100 patients hospitalized with a definite or probable diagnosis of viral meningitis, encephalitis, or meningoencephalitis found six patients with disc swelling, two of whom had increased ICP (238). In the four other patients, the CSF was under normal pressure but pleocytosis was present,

suggesting that the disc swelling was caused by inflammation rather than increased ICP.

Papilledema may occur with any form of meningoencephalitis. Many viral encephalidites are associated with papilledema (239,240), including herpes simplex and herpes zoster encephalitis (241,242), measles encephalitis (243), California encephalitis (244), lymphocytic choriomeningitis (245), infectious mononucleosis (246), and coxsackie B2, B4, and B5 meningoencephalitis (247,248). However, papilledema uncommonly occurs with encephalitis caused by rubella, mumps and varicella (249). Patients with poliomyelitis may develop increased ICP during both the acute and convalescent phases of the disease, and papilledema may develop in such cases (250–253). Generally, there is an elevated CSF protein with a moderate lymphocytic or mixed pleocytosis. Papilledema is rare in subacute sclerosing panencephalitis as the disease is slowly progressive and not generally associated with increased ICP (254,255). Papilledema in syphilis and tuberculosis may result from meningoencephalitis, obstruction of CSF flow or mass effect.

Psittacosis presented with increased ICP and papilledema in a 46-year-old man who developed headache, malaise, weight loss, sweats, and anorexia (256). Central nervous system involvement of Whipple's disease has also been associated with papilledema and increased ICP (257,258).

Papilledema occurs occasionally in Reye syndrome, an encephalopathy that follows a viral illness and occurs in children between ages 1 and 15 years (259,260), associated with fever and vomiting followed by convulsions and coma. Fatty infiltration and inflammation of the liver, kidney, and pancreas occur, and the mortality rate is 10% (259). In all patients, acute noninflammatory encephalopathy is confirmed by increased ICP, normocellular CSF, and diffuse cerebral edema. Although the fundi are normal in most cases, papilledema has been reported in rare instances (259,260).

Noninfectious Inflammatory Disorders

Sarcoidosis affecting the CNS occurs in about 5% of cases, mimicking practically any intracranial mass lesion (261,262); see (Chapter 59). Granulomas may develop in the meninges, causing nodular masses or, more commonly, an adhesive meningitis, or they may develop within brain parenchyma. The papilledema that occurs in sarcoidosis is usually associated with an aseptic meningitis, obstructed CSF flow or mass effect (263). Occasionally, however, sarcoidosis is associated with a true PTC syndrome; i.e., there is no evidence of a mass lesion, the ventricles are normal in size, the ICP is elevated, and the CSF contains no cells and has a normal concentration of glucose and protein. Some of these cases may be caused by dural venous sinus thrombosis (264). In other cases, the etiology is unclear. PTC associated with sarcoidosis often responds to treatment with systemic corticosteroids.

Behçet's disease is a multisystemic, recurrent, inflammatory disorder affecting the eyes, skin, mucosa, joints, vascular system, gastrointestinal tract, and nervous system (265). The disc swelling often seen in patients with Behçet's disease is usually associated with intraocular inflammation.

However, Behçet's syndrome has been associated with papilledema from dural venous sinus thrombosis and thrombophlebitis (266–270). The PTC syndrome with papilledema is the most common presentation of dural venous sinus thrombosis in Behçet's disease (265,270,271) and is an important diagnostic consideration in atypical patients with PTC. The MRI scan is abnormal in almost all cases of Behçet's disease affecting the brain, revealing contrast-enhancing lesions in the basal ganglia or diencephalon, small scattered periventricular or white matter lesions, or dural sinus occlusion (265).

Papilledema and the PTC-like syndrome was reported in a patient with familial Mediterranean fever, an inherited inflammatory disease of unknown cause (272).

In almost all CNS infections and inflammations, swelling of the optic disc may occur without elevated ICP, presumably from inflammation of the optic nerve. Many times the disc swelling is termed "papilledema" (240) even though the ICP is normal, because the discs are swollen and the patients have normal visual function. In other cases, the diagnosis of papilledema is made on clinical grounds alone, without measurement of ICP. However, some patients have both increased ICP and a substantial inflammatory reaction in the CSF. In this situation, differentiating between papilledema and optic perineuritis is impossible because, in both conditions, there is normal visual function. Only when a lumbar puncture is performed in a patient with a CNS infection and disc swelling, and the CSF is found to be under normal pressure with an increased protein and a pleocytosis, can the true inflammatory etiology of the disc swelling be ascertained.

Neoplastic Infiltrating Disorders

Increased ICP, often associated with papilledema, occurs in patients with **diffuse spread of tumors** throughout the CNS. These tumors include carcinomas, lymphomas, and leukemias (273,274). The increased pressure is usually caused by tumor cells that either obstruct CSF outflow across the arachnoid villi or CSF flow in the basal cisterns.

While most intracranial gliomas occur as solid mass lesions within the brain, in rare cases, the entire brain is infiltrated by a glioma—**gliomatosis cerebri**. The MRI usually shows multifocal lesions (275), but occasionally the diffusely infiltrated brain may present with normal neuroimaging and normal CSF contents (276). The most common presenting symptoms are headaches, seizures, mental status and cognitive changes, and hemiparesis (275). Papilledema may be present in one-third of patients at diagnosis (275). Such patients may initially be thought to have PTC, until further growth of tumor cells occurs, and the true diagnosis becomes evident.

Leptomeningeal gliomatosis affecting the spinal cord can also cause increased ICP and papilledema (277,278). Patients with this condition have a diffuse CNS glioma that is confined to the leptomeninges and that is thought to originate from a heterotopic glial nest in the subarachnoid space (279). The initial manifestations are headache, papilledema, and evidence of aseptic meningitis. Tumor cells are almost always found in the CSF.

Trauma

Papilledema occurs in 20–30% of persons who have suffered severe cranial injuries, both with and without an associated skull fracture (280). In most of these cases, the increased ICP is caused by a severe subarachnoid hemorrhage or a significant intracerebral, subdural, or epidural hematoma. In other cases, however, the increased ICP is caused by diffuse or localized cerebral edema (280). Papilledema that develops in patients after head trauma is usually mild and may develop immediately, several days after the injury, or up to 2 weeks later (281). Among 15 patients evaluated by a neuro-ophthalmologist after blunt head trauma, papilledema was recognized immediately in 1 patient, during the first week in 10 patients, and not until the second week in 4 patients (282). A sudden, severe, but transient increase in ICP is postulated to be responsible for the immediate development of papilledema, whereas sustained but mild to moderately elevated ICP accounts for papilledema that appears during the first week after injury (282). Papilledema during the second week or later results from impaired CSF absorption and consequent communicating hydrocephalus or delayed focal or diffuse cerebral swelling.

Just as not all patients with increased ICP from an intracranial mass develop papilledema, not all patients with increased ICP after head trauma develop papilledema, especially in the acute period (95). Thus, the absence of papilledema in a patient with head trauma does not exclude the presence of increased ICP.

Spinal Cord Lesions

The association of increased ICP and papilledema with tumors in the spinal canal is an unusual but well-documented phenomenon (283–287). Most of these tumors are intradural; however, extradural spinal tumors can also cause increased ICP associated with papilledema (288,289). In some cases, the tumors are located in the high cervical region, and the explanation for the increased ICP is thought to be upward swelling of the tumor with compression of the cerebellum and obstruction of CSF flow through the foramen magnum (106,290). This mechanism seems unlikely in the majority of cases, however, because over 50% of spinal cord lesions associated with papilledema are ependymomas or neurofibromas, usually in the thoracic and lumbar regions (291). These tumors can produce extremely high concentrations of protein in the CSF, and therefore the likely cause of increased ICP and papilledema is via defective CSF absorption that results from blockage of the arachnoid granulations by protein. In other cases, recurrent subarachnoid hemorrhage, which occurs commonly from bleeding from the surface of ependymomas, may also cause lowered CSF absorption from blockage of the arachnoid villi by blood or blood products. Other mechanisms for the production of increased ICP in patients with spinal cord tumors are probable but have yet to be elucidated.

Papilledema may occasionally be present in patients with spinal cord pathology other than malignancy, presumably by a similar mechanism. It has been reported in a patient with a herniated thoracic disc, resolving postoperatively

(292). The authors postulated that the papilledema in this patient was caused either by chronic epidural venous congestion from pressure of the extradural herniated disc producing a partial subarachnoid block, or by an associated aseptic meningitis and an elevated CSF protein.

Demyelinating Disorders

Papilledema is an uncommon complication of the **Guillain-Barré syndrome** (GBS) and its pathogenesis remains uncertain (293–295). Denny-Brown postulated that papilledema was a consequence of abnormal protein that interfered with the absorption of CSF (296). Six years later, Joynt described cerebral edema with normal CSF absorption in patients with GBS (297). Subsequently, evidence was submitted supporting both theories, as well as invoking a partial venous sinus thrombosis (298–300); the mechanism may be multifactorial.

GBS usually is a monophasic illness, with a rapid initial onset, progressive weakness and other neurologic manifestations over 1–4 weeks, and partial or complete recovery over subsequent months. However, a small percentage of patients with an otherwise typical episode of acute GBS subsequently relapse, have a protracted onset, or slowly improve and then worsen over weeks to months. The chronic and relapsing form of GBS was first defined largely by its responsiveness to systemic corticosteroids (301). This disorder, now known as **chronic inflammatory demyelinating polyneuropathy** (CIDP), is distinguished from acute GBS by: (*a*) a longer progression (2–3 months) before plateau; (*b*) a tendency for the illness to be less severe than the typical acute disease; (*c*) fluctuations in the severity of symptoms over many years; (*d*) greater elevations in CSF protein concentration; (*e*) more profoundly slowed motor nerve conduction velocities indi-

cating axonal loss; and (*f*) a frequent association with systemic diseases such as systemic lupus erythematosus and Hodgkin's disease (300,302).

Increased ICP, often associated with papilledema, occurs more often in patients with CIDP than in patients with acute GBS, and appears to result from the markedly increased protein concentration that is one of the laboratory hallmarks of the disease (303) (Fig. 5.32).

Papilledema occurs in a small percentage of patients with myelinoclastic diffuse sclerosis (**Schilder disease**). Cerebral edema from the numerous acute demyelinating brain lesions may mimic the clinical presentation of a neoplasm, abscess or PTC (304). In the majority of cases, optic neuritis is also present from demyelination of the optic nerves (see Chapter 60). Disc edema in multiple sclerosis most commonly reflects optic nerve demyelination and inflammation, rather than increased intracranial hypertension. Bilateral, simultaneous anterior optic neuritis may be difficult to distinguish clinically from acutely elevated ICP (305). The reported association between papilledema and increased intracranial pressure in a few patients with multiple sclerosis may be coincidental (306).

Inborn Errors of Metabolism

Hydrocephalus is a known complication of the inherited disorders of lysosomal multienzymes called the **mucopolysaccharidoses** (MPS) (307) and papilledema occurs in some of these cases (308–311). Increased ICP in patients with the systemic mucopolysaccharidoses probably results from an obstruction to the distal circulation of CSF over the cerebral convexities, in the arachnoid villi, or both, by the deposition of mucopolysaccharide in the meninges, leading to delayed CSF absorption.

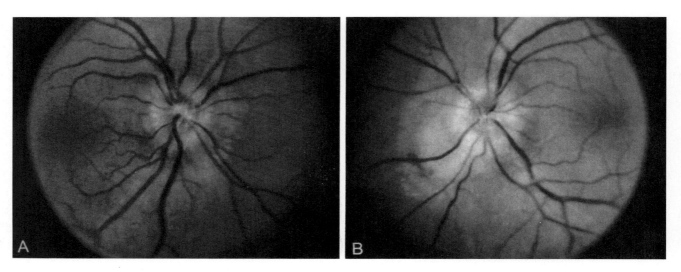

Figure 5.32. Papilledema in chronic inflammatory demyelinating polyneuropathy (CIDP). The patient was a 44-year-old man with well-documented CIDP who was being treated with low-dose systemic corticosteroids when he developed mild headaches but no visual symptoms. Visual acuity was 20/20 OU; color vision was normal; and visual fields were full. *A*, The right optic disc is mildly hyperemic and swollen (Frisén stage 2). *B*, The left optic disc is mildly hyperemic and swollen (Frisén stage 2). Brain neuroimaging was normal. A lumbar puncture showed increased intracranial pressure with a moderately increased concentration of protein. No specific treatment was given, and the papilledema gradually resolved over about 6 months.

Citrullinemia is caused by deficient activity of argininosuccinate synthetase, a urea-cycle enzyme. Hyperammonemia is usually present in this disorder (312,313). Citrullinemia may present acutely in neonates, subacutely in children, or as a late-onset condition in young adults. The late-onset type (Type II) may be associated with increased ICP and papilledema (314). Affected patients experience lethargy or recurrent episodes of syncope. Neuroimaging shows small ventricles and changes consistent with cerebral edema (312). CSF pressure is elevated, but the CSF contains no cells and normal concentrations of protein and glucose. Most patients in whom late-onset citrullinemia occurs have a peculiar fondness for beans, peanuts, and meat. Although the findings in late-onset citrullinemia associated with papilledema suggest a diagnosis of pseudotumor cerebri, i.e., no intracranial mass lesion, small ventricles, increased ICP, normal CSF content (see below), affected patients have evidence of an encephalopathy and thus do not strictly meet the diagnostic criteria for PTC (315).

Anomalies of the Cranium

The intracranial vault may become smaller in certain types of **craniosynostoses**. Of 171 patients with premature synostosis of the cranial sutures, the vast majority (91%) had simple cranial synostosis (oxycephaly, scaphocephaly, trigonocephaly, or plagiocephaly), whereas the remainder had dysostosis craniofacialis (Crouzon's syndrome) or acrocephalosyndactyly (Apert's syndrome) (316). Twenty-six of these patients (15%) had papilledema (316). When patients with simple cranial stenosis, which is almost never associated with papilledema, were excluded, however, the incidence of papilledema increased to 40%. In another large case series, ophthalmoscopic evaluations were performed in 122 children with craniosynostoses who then underwent monitoring of ICP revealing 15 patients (12%) with papilledema and 4 patients with optic atrophy (317). The patients with papilledema had higher ICP, were older, and were more likely to have craniofacial syndromes than patients without papilledema (317). The authors concluded that the presence of papilledema in a young child with craniosynostosis reliably indicates increased ICP, but its absence does not exclude increased ICP.

Papilledema that occurs in patients with craniosynostoses is often chronic by the time it is detected, possibly because such patients may not undergo a careful examination of the ocular fundi unless they complain of visual disturbances (154,316,318). Almost 50% of patients with craniosynostosis and papilledema eventually develop severe reduction of vision or blindness in both eyes (195). In one study of 31 patients with postpapilledema optic atrophy, 52% had visual acuity of 20/60 or better in both eyes, 29% had acuity of 20/60 or better in one eye, and only 19% had visual acuity less than 20/60 in both eyes (316).

Papilledema in craniosynostosis usually develops before the age of 10 years (317,319) but a patient with oxycephaly was observed to developed papilledema at 53 years of age (317,320,321). Papilledema occurs not only in patients with primary craniosynostosis (322) but also in patients with hypophosphatasia (323), sclerosteosis (324), progressive diaphyseal dysplasia (324) and idiopathic acroosteolyses (Hedju-Cheney syndrome) (325).

Plasma Cell Dyscrasias

POEMS syndrome (Crow-Fukase syndrome) is an unusual multisystem disorder that is characterized by polyneuropathy (**P**), organomegaly (**O**), endocrinopathy (**E**), monoclonal gammopathy (**M**), and skin changes (**S**) (326–328). Polyneuropathy is frequently the initial and most disabling problem. It is usually associated with electrophysiological and histological evidence of mixed demyelination and axon degeneration (328). Enlarged organs include the liver, spleen, and kidneys (328). Common endocrine abnormalities are diabetes mellitus, hypothyroidism, hypogonadism, hypocortisolism, and gynecomastia in men (328). Polycythemia is often present. Common skin findings include diffuse hyperpigmentation, peripheral edema, hypertrichosis, skin thickening similar to that observed in scleroderma, hyperhidrosis, and clubbing of the fingers (328,329). Additional systemic features include osteosclerotic bone lesions, lymphadenopathy, and peripheral edema.

Over 50% of patients with the POEMS syndrome develop papilledema (327,328,330) that may occur with or without increased ICP (331,332). The disc swelling in most of these cases results from altered capillary permeability in the optic disc or from the effects of an associated infiltrative orbitopathy.

The POEMS syndrome is usually associated with a plasma cell dyscrasia, such as myeloma, plasmacytoma, or monoclonal gammopathy of undetermined significance. A monoclonal immunoglobulin, inflammatory cytokines, vascular endothelial growth factor and human herpes virus-8 are implicated in its pathogenesis (333). The monoclonal protein component, present in most cases, may be IgG gamma, IgM gamma, gamma light chain, or others (328). Clinical improvement following treatment of the plasmacytoma or solitary bone lesion associated with an M component suggests that a tumor product may be the cause of the condition (328).

Patients with **multiple myeloma** can develop increased intracranial pressure and papilledema from CNS involvement (334,335). The PTC syndrome was described in patients with multiple myeloma who had no other features of the POEMS syndrome (see above) or generalized hyperviscosity (336). The mechanism of the raised ICP in these patients is unclear.

Toxins

Lead has both direct and indirect effects on the nervous system. At levels above 4 μM the blood brain barrier is damaged, leading to severe cerebral edema and increased ICP (337,338). Lead encephalopathy in children is characterized by lethargy, anorexia and irritability, progressing over weeks to clumsiness, ataxia then stupor, coma, and seizures (338). Lead toxicity continues to be a public health problem, particular in the inner city, from the ingestion of lead-based paint chips (pica). Exposure to lead dust during the renovation or restoration of older homes is another source of toxicity.

Hyperthyroidism

Optic disc swelling in hyperthyroidism is usually due to compression or ischemia of the optic nerves caused by dysthyroid orbitopathy. Nevertheless, true papilledema can oc-cur in association with hyperthyroidism without dysthyroid orbitopathy (339–341). One patient had communicating hydrocephalus and papilledema associated with severe thyrotoxicosis; the ICP and papilledema fluctuated proportionate to her serum thyroid hormone levels (340). Increased cerebral blood volume during thyrotoxicosis was proposed as the cause of the hydrocephalus (340).

PSEUDOTUMOR CEREBRI (IDIOPATHIC INTRACRANIAL HYPERTENSION)

DEFINITION

The pseudotumor cerebri syndrome was first described by Quincke in 1897 (342). The terminology used historically in the literature gives a sense of the various conditions associated with pseudotumor cerebri (PTC): toxic hydrocephalus (343), otitic hydrocephalus (344), hypertensive meningeal hydrops (345), pseudoabscess (7), ICP without brain tumor (27), brain swelling of unknown cause (346,347), and papilledema of indeterminate etiology (348). The most popular and enduring term ''pseudotumor cerebri'' was first used in 1914 (349). Noting that the condition was not caused by a tumor or malignancy, Foley introduced the term ''benign intracranial hypertension'' in 1955 (350). However, the term ''benign'' also implies a favorable process or the absence of harm. As significant visual morbidity may result from PTC, the use of the prefix ''benign'' was challenged (351) and is no longer considered acceptable terminology. The disorder is most correctly termed idiopathic intracranial hypertension (IIH) or intracranial hypertension from a secondary cause, depending upon whether or not an etiology is identified. The older term, PTC, describes the clinical syndrome without reference to the underlying cause.

EPIDEMIOLOGY

PTC affects infants, children and young adults but rarely has onset over age 45 years (161,169,352–357). The idiopathic form (IIH) is typically a disorder of obese females of childbearing age. The incidence of PTC varies throughout the world. Two studies in the United States estimated the incidence at approximately 0.9 per 100,000 in the general population with a female:male ratio of 8:1 (358,359). The incidence rises to 3.5 per 100,000 in women aged 20 to 44 years, and further increases to 13 per 100,000 in women who are 10% over ideal weight, and 19 per 100,000 in women who are 20% over ideal weight (358). The incidence in Benghazi, Libya was 2.2 per 100,000 in the general population, 4.3 per 100,000 in women, and 21.4 per 100,000 in women aged 15-44 years who were 20% over ideal weight (360). In Israel, whose population is a mixture of people originating from various Eastern and Western countries, the incidence was similar to that in western populations with a preponderance of obese women (361).

DIAGNOSIS

The diagnostic criteria for IIH are: (*a*) symptoms and signs solely attributable to increased ICP; (*b*) elevated CSF pressure; (*c*) normal CSF composition; (*d*) normal neuroimaging studies; and (*e*) no other etiology of intracranial hypertension identified (315,362). Each of these criteria are discussed below.

Symptoms and Signs

Occasionally, PTC is asymptomatic and discovered during a routine ophthalmic examination when papilledema is found (363). However, the most common symptom is headaches, occurring in approximately 90% of cases (362,364–366). The character of the headache is not specific but it is usually different from previous headaches and is severe (367). It most commonly is bifrontal or generalized, pressure-like, and often associated with neck pain (367). The headache is usually daily but may be intermittent. Many patients have migrainous features including unilateral pain, nausea, vomiting, photophobia and phonophobia. It may awaken the patient from sleep or resemble a ''brain tumor headache'' that is worse in the morning, and aggravated when cerebral venous pressure is increased by Valsalva maneuvers (coughing, sneezing, etc.).

The second most common symptom of PTC is transient visual loss. Typical transient obscurations of vision (TOV) are reported by approximately 70% of patients (367). They may be unilateral or bilateral, usually last less than a minute, and are often precipitated by a change in posture (e.g., bending over, arising from a stooped position) or rolling the eyes. In some patients TOVs occur 20 to 30 times daily. The visual loss may be partial or complete. TOVs indicate the presence of optic disc edema and are not, in isolation, an ominous symptom if the vision returns to normal interictally. They likely reflect transient ischemia to the optic nerve head caused by papilledema.

While TOV are common and generally not worrisome, a smaller percentage of patients will complain of visual loss. They may notice an enlarged physiologic blind spot, describing a dark spot in the temporal visual field. Tunnel vision and central visual loss may occur (362,367). With severe disease, ischemic optic neuropathy ensues, producing rapid, severe and often irreversible visual loss (113). Visual loss in PTC may also arise from macular hemorrhages, exudates, pigment epithelial changes, retina striae, choroidal folds, subretinal neovascularization or retinal artery occlusion (41,48,144,166,368).

Diplopia, observed by approximately 40% of patients, is usually horizontal resulting from unilateral or bilateral abducens nerve paresis, a nonlocalizing feature of increased intracranial pressure (362,367). Rarely, there is vertical diplopia from trochlear nerve paresis, oculomotor nerve paresis, or skew deviation (168,179–181,369).

Intracranial noises (pulsatile tinnitus) are also common but must be queried for as patients seldom volunteer this symptom. Often described as a whooshing sound, "hearing my heartbeat in my head" or high-pitched noises, they are thought to reflect flow disturbances within the cerebral venous system (366,367,370). They may be unilateral or bilateral and are often more prominent at night.

Focal neurologic deficits in patients with PTC are extremely uncommon, and their occurrence should make one consider alternative diagnoses (371). Nevertheless, isolated unilateral and bilateral facial paresis (171,372–376), hemifacial spasm (377,378), trigeminal sensory neuropathy (379), hearing loss (380), hemiparesis, ataxia, paresthesias, mononeuropathy multiplex (381), arthralgias, and both spinal and radicular pain (382) have been reported in patients with PTC (383,384). Patients with chronic PTC are more likely to be anxious or depressed than age- and weight-matched control subjects (385). Cognitive deficits are less well substantiated and may be a manifestation of headache-related concentration difficulties, depression, or anxiety (386,387).

Papilledema is the diagnostic hallmark of PTC and is present in almost all patients (362,366,367). The papilledema of PTC is identical with that which occurs in patients with other causes of increased ICP and may be asymmetrical or, occasionally, unilateral (60). PTC without papilledema has been reported but it is uncommon and the diagnosis should be made with caution (69,388–390). Occasionally, continuous CSF pressure monitoring may be needed to confirm the diagnosis (391). Although there is a correlation between visual loss and high-grade papilledema, the appearance of the optic disc does not predict visual loss (105,392). There is no correlation between severity of optic disc swelling and age, race, or body weight in patients with PTC (393).

As with papilledema from other causes, loss of central visual acuity is uncommon in PTC. One prospective study showed Snellen visual acuity worse than 20/20 in approximately 15% of patients at presentation (367). Visual acuity is relatively insensitive to visual loss in PTC and should not be relied upon as the sole indicator of visual function (158). Color vision testing and visual evoked potentials are similarly insensitive (171). In general, early central acuity loss, particularly if it is rapidly progressing, is a worrisome sign.

Postpapilledema optic atrophy occurs in untreated or inadequately treated patients after a variable period of time, usually over several months, but occasionally within weeks of the onset of symptoms. Some patients have persistent chronic papilledema without visual deterioration or optic atrophy. Postpapilledema optic atrophy in patients with PTC usually develops symmetrically, but just as papilledema may be asymmetric, so postpapilledema optic atrophy can be asymmetric. Some patients develop a pseudo-Foster Kennedy syndrome characterized by postpapilledema optic atrophy in one eye and papilledema in the other (394).

Visual field testing, by either automated static or manual (Goldmann) perimetry, reveals enlargement of the physiologic blind spot in virtually all patients with PTC who have papilledema (158). Other common visual field defects include inferonasal loss (nasal step) and generalized constriction of the visual field. Central, paracentral, arcuate and altitudinal scotomas may occur (158,367). Abnormalities of ocular motility include unilateral or bilateral abducens paresis (362,367) or, uncommonly, trochlear nerve paresis, oculomotor nerve paresis or skew deviation (168,179–181,369). Global ophthalmoparesis or ophthalmoplegia may be present, and resolves as the intracranial pressure normalizes (183).

Cerebrospinal Fluid Examination

A CSF examination is required for the diagnosis of PTC to confirm an elevated opening pressure and exclude a malignant, infectious or inflammatory process that might simulate PTC. Normal lumbar CSF pressure in adults is 200 mm water or less. For the diagnosis of PTC, the CSF opening pressure should be 250 mm of water or greater. Values between 201–249 are not diagnostic (6). In prepubertal children, a value over 200 mm water is likely abnormal. Because CSF pressure normally fluctuates, multiple CSF pressure measurements or prolonged CSF pressure monitoring is sometimes required, depending on the clinical circumstance (395). In obese patients, the LP may be technically challenging to perform. To ensure accuracy, the lumbar CSF pressure must be measured with the patient in the lateral decubitus position, relaxed with the legs partially extended. The pressure may be artifactually elevated if the patient is crying, performing a Valsalva maneuver or is in severe pain (396). It is recommended that the CSF from the initial LP be analyzed for glucose, protein, cell count, cytology, and atypical infections (e.g., syphilis, *Cryptococcus*, fungus). The CSF contents should be normal in PTC; the protein is generally in the normal to low-normal range (397,398).

Neuroimaging Studies

The rationale for neuroimaging studies in patients with suspected PTC is twofold:

1. Prior to obtaining the cerebrospinal fluid, a brain imaging study is required to exclude a condition that would put the patient at risk of herniation, such as a tumor producing hydrocephalus or mass effect; and
2. To assure that there is no secondary cause of increased ICP.

The recommended type of study has been modified with advances in neuroimaging technology. While a plain CT scan is generally adequate to ensure that the patient is not at risk for having a lumbar puncture, the resolution of this study is insufficient to exclude posterior fossa abnormalities, isodense lesions not associated with ventriculomegaly, gliomatosis cerebri, meningeal abnormalities or venous sinus thrombosis. Thus, MRI is recommended for most patients. For those patients who are not "typical," such as slim individuals, children and men, contrast-enhancement and MR venography should also be considered (315). If the patient's body habitus exceeds the capacity of the MR gantry, a CT scan with contrast should be obtained; catheter angiography with venous phase sequences may also be needed in such patients if venous sinus thrombosis is suspected.

The brain MRI is normal in PTC. The ventricular size should be normal for the patient's age (399). An asymptomatic empty sella which results from chronically increased ICP may be present in over half of cases (400–403). Other radiographic evidence of increased ICP, best visualized on orbital images, includes dilation of the perineuronal subarachnoid space surrounding the optic nerves, protrusion of the optic papilla into the posterior aspect of the globe and flattening of the posterior sclerae (88,404–406). A small percentage of patients of patients have a Chiari type 1 malformation. In addition, orbital echography may be useful to differentiate pseudopapilledema from optic nerve head drusen and to identify the edematous optic nerve sheath using a 30° test (see above) (84,85,407).

Secondary Causes

IIH is a diagnosis of exclusion that occurs primarily in young obese women, and occasionally obese men, with no evidence of any underlying disease (362,366,408,409). The PTC syndrome may be associated with a number of different conditions. The suspicion of a secondary cause is heightened in prepubertal children, men, nonobese women and otherwise typical patients with rapidly progressive visual loss that does not respond to treatment. The secondary causes of PTC include: (a) obstruction or impairment of cerebral venous drainage; (b) endocrine and metabolic dysfunction; (c) exposure to exogenous drugs and other substances; (d) withdrawal of certain drugs; and (e) systemic illnesses (351, 357,409,410). It is important to realize that, although many conditions have been reported with PTC, relatively few are likely to be true associations. Tables 5.3–5.6 list associated conditions; the best-substantiated and most frequently observed ones are discussed in the text.

Obstruction or Impairment of Intracranial Venous Drainage

Uncompensated obstruction of cerebral venous drainage may result in increased ICP and papilledema without enlargement of the ventricles and with otherwise normal CSF (68,411–417) (Table 5.3). The obstruction is most often caused by compression or thrombosis, with the superior sagittal and transverse (lateral) sinuses most often affected (see Chapter 45). As previously discussed, tumors that obstruct the superior sagittal sinus are usually extra-axial masses, such as meningiomas and vascular lesions (165,418). The transverse sinus may be occluded by acoustic neuromas, meningiomas, and metastatic tumors (165,419).

Septic thrombosis of the transverse sinus tends to occur in the setting of acute or chronic otitis media, with extension of the infection to the mastoid air cells and then to the adjacent lateral sinus (412,420). In such cases, papilledema usually occurs early and tends to be bilateral and symmetric (421). A similar appearance occurs in patients with septic thrombosis of the superior sagittal sinus, a much less common condition. Septic thrombosis of the cavernous sinus

Table 5.3

Etiologies of Obstruction/Impairment of Cerebral Venous Drainage Associated with Pseudotumor Cerebri

Obstruction of superior sagittal sinus
  Primary hematologic
    Activated protein C deficiency (427,438)
    Essential thrombocythemia (434,436)
    Factor V Leiden mutation (424)
    Idiopathic thrombocytopenic purpura (430)
    Paroxysmal nocturnal hemoglobinuria (683,684)
    Prothrombin gene 20210GA transition (425,426)
    Thrombocytopenic purpura (430)
  Systemic conditions associated with coagulopathy
    Behçet's disease (266–268,271,685)
    Cancer (439,686)
    Neurosarcoidosis (264)
    Pregnancy (433)
    Renal disease (495,687)
    Systemic lupus erythematosus (101,435,573–576,688,689)
    Trichinosis (690)
  Surgical/traumatic (440)
  Tumors
    Extravascular
    Intravascular (418)
Obstruction of transverse sinus
  Dural arteriovenous fistula (165,210,211,215)
  Hematologic (see above)
  Infection (mastoiditis) (412,420)
  Tumors (extravascular) (419)
Occlusion of internal jugular vein (441–444,686)
  Iatrogenic
    Indwelling catheter (416)
    Surgery/traumatic (441–444)
  Tumors
    Intravascular
    Extravascular

may also be associated with papilledema, although the disc swelling develops late.

Aseptic thrombosis usually occurs in the nonpaired sinuses of both adults and children, with the superior sagittal sinus most frequently affected (422,423). It is sometimes accompanied by pronounced engorgement of the vessels of the scalp, retina, and conjunctiva in addition to papilledema. Many of these patients have a coagulopathy from a primary hematologic disorder such as factor V Leiden mutation (424), prothrombin gene 20210GA transition (424–426), activated protein C resistance (427), essential thrombocythemia (428) or, rarely, anti-anticardiolipin antibodies (429) and thrombocytopenic purpura (430). Venous sinus thrombosis is also associated with systemic conditions (e.g., renal disease, pregnancy, cancer), medication (oral contraceptives), or systemic inflammatory or infectious diseases (e.g., systemic lupus erythematosus, Behçet's disease, trichinosis, sarcoidosis) (264,268,269,430–439).

PTC was reported in a patient after surgical ligation of the dominant sigmoid sinus to treat long-standing pulsatile tinnitus (440). Ligation of one jugular vein (if it is the principal vein draining the intracranial area) or both jugular veins may produce papilledema. In most instances, occlusion of the jugular veins occurs during radical neck dissection for regional tumors (441–444); in other cases, the veins become thrombosed from the effects of indwelling catheters (416). The papilledema in such cases usually does not appear for a week or two. It is virtually always bilateral and severe; however, it typically resolves in 2–3 months as collateral venous drainage from the head develops to meet the demands of cerebral blood flow.

Endocrinologic and Metabolic Conditions

Obesity is the most common finding in patients with PTC (362,445–448); one case-control study found obesity and recent weight gain significantly more prevalent in PTC patients compared to control subjects (449). Many of these patients also have irregular menses, likely a co-morbidity of obesity rather than an effect of increased ICP (450). The female gender predilection in adolescents and adults with PTC also suggests a hormonal component. PTC in children affects prepubertal boys and girls equally and without regard to body habitus (103,451,452). After puberty, the female predominance and association with obesity emerge as factors for idiopathic PTC (451,453,454).

PTC has been associated with numerous forms of endocrine and metabolic dysfunction (Table 5.4) but no specific endocrinologic disturbances are evident (447). Plasma and urinary levels of adrenal steroids in females and urinary gonadotrophins in males are normal (362,364). Plasma renin activity and aldosterone levels at baseline, following plasma volume contraction by furosemide, and after dexamethasone therapy in six women with PTC were within normal range (455). In women, PTC is associated with idiopathic orthostatic edema, a condition characterized by abnormal retention of sodium, water or both (456). Such patients have symptoms and signs of peripheral edema that may worsen during menses, when fluid retention is most common (456,457).

Although there is no increased incidence of PTC during pregnancy compared to nongravid young women of similar ages (433), PTC may occur or recur during pregnancy (458–462). The risk of visual loss in pregnant women with PTC is no greater than in those who are not pregnant (433). There is no contraindication to pregnancy among women with PTC; the management of PTC during pregnancy is discussed below.

Papilledema occurs in patients with both primary and secondary hypoparathyroidism (354,463–466). ^{131}I-RISA scanning demonstrated a marked reduction of CSF absorption in a patient with primary hypoparathyroidism, papilledema and seizures that returned to normal after correction of the patient's hypocalcemia (467). It is possible that hypocalcemia in patients with hypoparathyroidism leads to an increase in intracellular sodium and water that, in turn, interferes with transport of CSF through the arachnoid granulations (468).

Medications and Other Exogenous Agents

Patients who are exposed to, or ingest, a variety of substances can develop PTC (Table 5.5). For some of these substances, the association between exposure or ingestion and the development of PTC is well documented in numerous reports and investigations; for others, however, a causative relationship is supported by only a single case report and is tenuous at best (409).

Even when a patient is taking a drug that is known or suspected to cause PTC, one should not necessarily assume that the drug is the sole cause of the condition. For example, patients may have idiopathic PTC or a real tumor (276) that is brought to medical attention or worsens when a particular medication is used.

Several antibiotics have been associated with the development of PTC. The most well-known of these drugs are the tetracyclines. Tetracycline can produce the syndrome in infants (469,470), children (471,472), and young and older adults (473–477). PTC has also been infrequently associated with minocycline (478–482) and, rarely, with doxycycline (483–485). In infants, the condition manifests itself as bulging of the fontanelles and occasionally by spreading of sutures. Irritability, drowsiness, feeding disturbances, and

---

Table 5.4

Endocrine and Metabolic Disturbances Associated with Pseudotumor Cerebri

Addison's disease (691)
Hypoparathyroidism (354,464,466,467)
Obesity (idiopathic) (447,449)
Orthostatic edema (456)
Turner's syndrome (585,692)

Table 5.5

Exogenous Substances Whose Exposure or Ingestion Has Been Associated with Pseudotumor Cerebri

Amiodarone (524–527)
Antibiotics
   Tetracycline (469–471,475)
   Minocycline (478,479,481,482,693)
   Doxycycline (483–485)
   Nalidixic acid (486–488)
Beta-human chorionic gonadotropin hormone withdrawal (536,537)
Chlordecone (Kepone) (539)
Corticosteroids withdrawal (355,490–496)
Danazol administration (528,529) or withdrawal (530)
Growth hormone (516–520)
Isotretinoin (509,510)
Lead (338)
Leuprolide acetate (Lupron) (531,532)
Levonorgesterol implants (Norplant) (521–523)
Lithium carbonate (533,534)
Oxytocin (intranasal)
Quinagolide (535)
Retinoids
   Vitamin A (501–504,506–508,694–705)
   Isotretinoin (509,538,706,707)
   All-*trans*-retinoic acid (511–514)
Thyroid hormone (708,709)

vomiting are common, although some infants are asymptomatic. There is no correlation between the onset of the syndrome and either the dosage of the drug or the length of therapy, and the reaction has been observed within weeks of starting the medication (481). Older children and adults have manifestations more consistent with typical PTC. Tetracycline is no longer recommended for use in young children because of permanent tooth discoloration, so tetracycline-induced PTC is most frequently encountered in adolescents and young adults who are treated for acne. Cessation of tetracycline administration causes regression of symptoms, although intracranial pressure-lowering therapies may be needed in the short term, as permanent visual deficits may occur. Although no longer used, nalidixic acid has also been associated with PTC (486–488).

Corticosteroids are frequently used to treat increased ICP in patients with brain tumors and may be given acutely to lower the ICP in patients with PTC. Thus, it seems contradictory that corticosteroids may be associated with the development of PTC. Nonetheless, chronic functional suppression of the adrenal cortex with systemic corticosteroid therapy has been recognized as a cause of PTC since the late 1950s (489). Subsequently, it was recognized that regardless of their underlying condition, patients with steroid-induced PTC had certain features of Cushing's syndrome (490). Within days or weeks after a change in the dosage or type of steroid, and sometimes associated with an intercurrent infection, the patients complained of headache, often accompanied by nausea and vomiting, less commonly by diplopia, and occasionally drowsiness or stupor. Examination of the fundi revealed bilateral papilledema, usually low-grade and often without hemorrhage (490–492). Whereas corticosteroids initially lower ICP, their withdrawal may prompt a rebound increase in the ICP and produce PTC (355,493–495). There is only one report of papilledema associated with topical steroid treatment in a child being treated for severe eczema (496).

Although there are isolated reports of PTC in patients taking oral contraceptives (497–499) or estrogen replacement after hysterectomy (500), this association is likely coincidental. One would imagine an epidemic of PTC if this relationship was causal, given the number of women worldwide using these medications.

Hypervitaminosis A is another well-recognized cause of PTC. Daily ingestion of 100,000 or more units of vitamin A may, within a few months, produce increased intracranial pressure. In infants and small children, the condition is characterized by anorexia, lethargy, and an increasing head circumference (501–503). Older children and adults develop PTC (504–506). Other manifestations of hypervitaminosis A may be present, such as fissuring of the angles of the lips, loss of hair, migratory bone pain, hypomenorrhea, hepatosplenomegaly, and dryness, roughness, and desquamation of the skin.

The diagnosis of PTC caused by hypervitaminosis A is usually straightforward, providing the physician knows that the patient is ingesting excessive amounts of vitamin A, either as the vitamin itself or in calf, bear, chicken or shark liver (507). Reduction of the excessive vitamin intake is associated with resolution of all symptoms and signs, although Morrice et al. emphasized that resolution of disc swelling may take 4 to 6 months (508). Other systemic retinoids may produce PTC, such as isotretinoin (509,510) and all-*trans* retinoic acid (511–514). Rarely, PTC is caused by vitamin A deficiency (515).

Other substances associated with the development of PTC include supplemental growth hormone (516–520), levon-orgestrel implants (Norplant) (521–523), amiodarone (524–527), danazol administration and withdrawal (528–530), leuprolide acetate (Lupron—a gonadotropin-releasing hormone) (531,532), lithium carbonate (533,534), and quinagolide (a nonergot-derived dopamine agonist) (535). It has also been reported following treatment with declining levels of exogenous beta human chorionic gonadotropin (536,537).

Patients who develop drug-induced PTC are not necessarily susceptible to PTC when they take another drug that is known to induce the condition. On the other hand, some patients develop PTC when they are taking more than one implicated medication, most commonly for the treatment of acne vulgaris (538). Therefore, appropriate caution and monitoring is advised if attempting to administer another potentially causative agent in a patient who has a history of drug-induced PTC.

Chlordecone (Kepone) is an organochlorine insecticide associated with PTC (539). The capacity for CSF absorption as assessed by graded saline infusions into the subarachnoid space was found to be impaired in three patients with elevated blood, serum and adipose levels of chlordecone (539). One effect of chlordecone in experimental animals is inhibition of Na-K-ATPase, a major component of the cellular sodium transport system (540). Because inhibition of this system may cause cellular edema, interference with this enzyme may contribute to edema within subarachnoid villi in patients intoxicated with chlordecone.

Systemic Illnesses

Vitamin D deficiency produces nutritional rickets and can be associated with PTC in infants and young children (541,542). In developed countries, the child at special risk is an exclusively breast-fed child of a strict vegan mother (357). This form of PTC resolves slowly.

Many systemic disorders have been reported in associated with PTC but most of them do not cause a true PTC syndrome (Table 5.6). Although they produce papilledema with normal ventricular size and increased intracranial pressure, they are generally associated with fever, other neurologic deficits, altered mental status, seizures or abnormal cerebrospinal fluid.

Hematologic Disorders

The association of PTC with anemia is tenuous as some of the reported cases had other co-morbid conditions, such as obesity. Anemia was not shown to be a risk factor for PTC in case-control studies (366,449). Papilledema is a rare finding in patients with anemia from iron deficiency or, rarely, vitamin B12 deficiency, hemolytic anemia, megalo-

Table 5.6
Systemic Illnesses Associated with Pseudotumor Cerebri

Anemia (543–545)
Chronic respiratory insufficiency (551)
Pickwickian syndrome (562,564)
Obstructive sleep apnea (561,563,565)
Hyperthyroidism (339,341)
Polyangiitis overlap syndrome (578)
Psittacosis (256)
Renal disease (495,687)
Sarcoidosis (263,710)
Systemic lupus erythematosus (101,573,574,576,689,711)
Thrombocytopenic purpura
Vitamin D deficiency (541,542)

blastic anemia, or aplastic anemia (543–546). Almost all of the patients are women under age 45, and most have systemic manifestations of anemia, including fatigue and dyspnea (543). The presenting symptoms of PTC are headaches, with or without or diplopia, and the exam reveals optic disc and retinal hemorrhages. The mechanism may be a related to a hypercoagulable state in cases of iron defiency anemia, venous sinus thrombosis, or increased blood volume (543). Most patients reported to date have recovered promptly after treatment of their anemia.

PTC occurs in association with two forms of thrombocytopenic purpura, both of which are associated with decreased platelet survival: immune idiopathic thrombocytopenic purpura (ITP) and nonimmune thrombotic thrombocytopenic purpura (TTP). ITP may be acute or chronic. Acute ITP occurs most often in children, usually after an upper respiratory tract infection, whereas chronic ITP occurs most often in women between 20 and 45 years of age. The etiology of this condition is a spontaneously appearing antibody that damages the platelets, causing them to be removed from the circulation by the reticuloendothelial system. PTC in this setting may be associated with cerebral venous sinus thrombosis (430). TTP occurs abruptly in previously healthy people (547). It is characterized by severe thrombocytopenia, hemolytic anemia, fever, renal dysfunction, and CNS disturbances. Papilledema and increased ICP occur rarely in TTP (548,549).

Chronic Respiratory Insufficiency and Hypercapnia

Chronic respiratory insufficiency of various etiologies may produce the PTC syndrome. Affected patients have chronic hypercapnia, with retention of carbon dioxide (CO_2), reduced blood oxygen (O_2) levels, polycythemia, increased venous pressure, and increased ICP (550). In most cases of increased ICP related to pulmonary insufficiency, the pulmonary dysfunction is caused by primary pulmonary disease (551–554). One of the earliest reports in 1933 described a 34-year-old miner with severe pulmonary emphysema who initially developed bilateral disc swelling and venous congestion and who eventually became blind from optic atrophy (555). Increased ICP was subsequently described with emphysema, the Pickwickian syndrome, systemic myopa-

thies, and obstructive sleep apnea (556,557). Studies of the pH and pCO_2 levels in arterial blood gases and CSF were performed over a 3-month period in a patient with chronic respiratory insufficiency and optic disc swelling (558). The authors concluded that respiratory acidosis causes an accumulation of CO_2 in brain tissue, reflected by inversion of the normal CO_2 tension ratio between CSF and arterial blood. This, in turn, causes dilation of cerebral capillaries and increases intracranial blood volume.

The Pickwickian syndrome develops when extreme obesity produces hypoventilation and a typical cardiopulmonary syndrome (559). The obesity causes diminished vital capacity, polycythemia, and cyanosis. Severe drowsiness is common, and many patients have obstructive sleep apnea (OSA) (560–562). OSA may be underrecognized in obese patients with PTC and is diagnosed using overnight polysomnography. Continuous ICP monitoring in an obese man with OSA and papilledema showed increased ICP during sleep only, with normal CSF values recorded while he was awake (563). The nocturnal rise in ICP correlated with a 20–52% drop in oxygen saturation. This finding suggests that increased ICP may be missed in patients with OSA if the LP is performed during the daytime. Clinical and necropsy findings were described in another patient who weighed 330 pounds (564). The patient had marked bilateral optic disc swelling; the retinal veins were dilated, tortuous, and had a blue-black appearance. A lumbar puncture revealed an opening pressure of 480 mm of water with normal CSF contents. Pulmonary function studies showed a combination of hypoxemia and hypercapnia. At autopsy, the cerebral vessels were dilated, but the dural sinuses were patent. Cut sections of the brain showed diffuse congestion and vascular engorgement with small ventricles.

The optic disc swelling that is seen in patients with chronic respiratory disease is likely true papilledema associated with cerebral edema and increased ICP. In some patients, however, disc swelling occurs in the absence of increased ICP, presumably from a local tissue response to changes in blood viscosity and venous pressure (565). When disc swelling is secondary to local causes, it is usually not severe (566). The most prominent features are dilation and tortuosity of retinal vessels, with the fundus having a cyanotic appearance. When increased ICP is present, papilledema may be minimal or severe. The disc swelling and fundus abnormalities usually resolve rapidly once respiratory acidosis and hypoxia are treated (563,566).

Other neurologic manifestations of respiratory failure include somnolence, asterixis, other movement disorders, and in severe cases, coma (567). Supportive respiratory therapy and prompt treatment of the acute physiologic, metabolic, and electrolyte abnormalities can significantly prolong survival and improve the quality of survival time in patients with respiratory failure who have papilledema or other neurologic complications (551,568).

Hypertension

Optic disc swelling occurs in some patients with severe hypertension (569). Some of these patients have neurologic symptoms of an encephalopathy; others do not. Among the patients with evidence of an encephalopathy, almost all have increased ICP caused by cerebral edema. In addition, some patients without symptoms of encephalopathy have evidence of cerebral edema by neuroimaging and increased ICP on lumbar puncture. In patients with optic disc swelling associated with normal ICP, the swelling may be caused by breakdown of the blood-retinal barrier, or it may represent hypertensive retinopathy or an anterior ischemic optic neuropathy (570,571). Coexisting systemic hypertension confers a poor visual prognosis in patients with PTC (105,572).

Vasculitis

The PTC syndrome may occur in patients with systemic lupus erythematosus (101,573,574). In some of these cases, the pathogenesis is occlusion of one of the dural venous sinuses, usually the superior sagittal sinus (435,575). In other cases, the pathogenesis is unclear (576). The condition usually resolves with corticosteroid treatment suggesting that inflammation and tissue necrosis in the region of the arachnoid villi interferes with CSF absorption, raising the ICP. In other patients, fluctuating corticosteroid dosage and the weight gain associated with corticosteroid use may be contributory.

PTC was described as the presenting sign of the polyangiitis overlap syndrome, a disorder with a conglomerate of features that intersect several vasculitic syndromes, particularly Churg-Strauss syndrome and polyarteritis nodosa (577). A 9-year-old girl presenting with PTC as the cardinal manifestation of the polyangiitis overlap syndrome has been reported. The child died despite treatment with high-dose systemic corticosteroids (578). At postmortem examination, cerebral edema was present, but the dural sinuses were patent. Two primary mechanisms by which vasculitis causes PTC were postulated: (a) the vasculitis may affect the cerebral venous sinuses and produce thrombosis; or (b) inflammation and tissue necrosis in the region of the arachnoid villi could interfere with CSF absorption (578).

Renal Failure

Renal failure is uncommonly associated with PTC. Reports suggest that coexisting renal failure may be associated with more aggressive intracranial hypertension that causes visual loss and is often refractory to treatment (293,572,579). The cause of PTC in patients with renal failure is probably multifactorial. Some patients are obese, an important association in PTC. Fluid overload, increased cerebral blood flow and hypervitaminosis A may also be contributory.

Familial Pseudotumor Cerebri

The occurrence of PTC in multiple family members is well recognized (351,476,580) (Fig. 5.33). In some families, the affected members are all obese but no definitive common metabolic or endocrinologic abnormalities have been found.

COMPLICATIONS

The natural history of PTC is unknown. In some cases it is a self-limited condition; in others, the ICP remains ele-vated for many years, even if systemic and visual symptoms resolve. The feared complication of PTC is permanent visual loss. In one long-term study performed prior to the era of modern neuroimaging, 57 patients with a diagnosis of PTC were followed for 5–41 years (572). Severe visual impairment occurred in one or both eyes in 14 patients (26%), and in 7 patients the visual loss occurred months to years after initial symptoms appeared. In over 80% of the patients in this study, CSF pressure remained elevated, regardless of the treatment the patients had received. PTC may recur years after successful treatment, sometimes resulting in visual loss (165,167). The effects of even self-limited PTC on the visual system may be catastrophic. PTC produces significant visual impairment in approximately 25% of patients (151,350,357, 581,582) and permanent visual field abnormalities in most patients (156,158,367).

PATHOPHYSIOLOGY

The etiology of increased ICP in patients with idiopathic PTC is uncertain (583,584). A unifying theory must explain several features of IIH: (a) the predilection for obese women of childbearing age; (b) lack of ventriculomegaly; and (c) clinically identical syndrome produced by other etiologies, such as cerebral venous sinus thrombosis and medications. Several mechanisms are postulated to account for the disruption in CSF homeostasis, including increased CSF production and decreased CSF absorption.

Why is the disorder more common in overweight women? Some authors have suggested that extraovarian estrogen may produce the menstrual irregularities in some of the obese young women with PTC (585). After finding that the concentration of estrone in the CSF of obese women was higher than normal, it was postulated that estrone stimulates the secretory cells of the choroid plexus to produce more CSF than can be absorbed at normal CSF pressures (586). However, others could not confirm this finding and indeed found that the concentration of estrogen in the CSF of 15 patients with PTC, 8 of whom were obese women, was undetectable (587).

What is the primary pathology of PTC? Most evidence points to decreased absorption of CSF (362,588,589) with increased cerebral blood volume (590). ICP is normally maintained by a compliance factor arising from distention of meningeal membranes and compression of vascular volume, and a resistance factor that modulates CSF volume by venting CSF through the arachnoid granulations into the cerebral venous system (591). Fifty percent of CSF is below the foramen magnum and almost half is absorbed in the spinal sac (111,590). In the intracranial compartment, infusion studies indicate that resistance factors are quickly exceeded (591). With increased CSF volumes, a point is eventually reached where compliance mechanisms fail and a small increase in volume results in a large increased in ICP (592,593).

Some authors speculate that within the cranium, there may be increased cerebral venous pressure, reversing the normal gradient between sinus and subarachnoid space, or an increase in the resistance to flow of CSF across the arachnoid villi (362,364). Others postulate that an abnormality in the

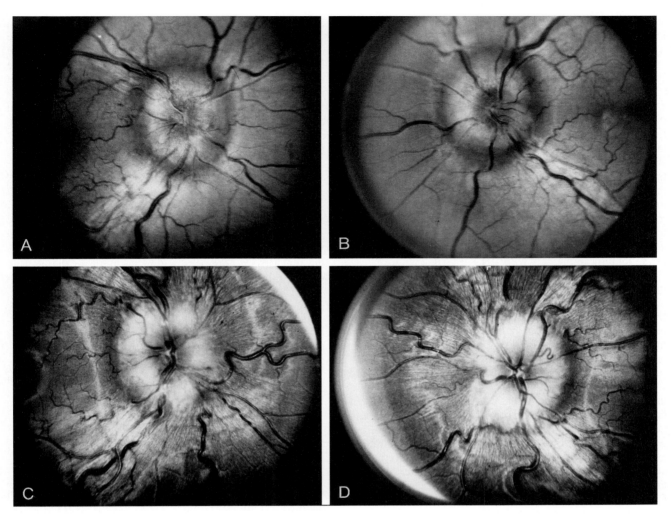

Figure 5.33. Familial pseudotumor cerebri. *A and B*, Right and left optic discs, respectively, in a 45-year-old man with pseudotumor cerebri. *C and D*, Right and left optic discs, respectively, in his 18-year-old daughter who also had pseudotumor cerebri.

cerebral microvasculature is responsible for an elevated cerebral blood volume and that the intracranial hypertension in patients with IIH can be explained only by tissue swelling from an increase in total water content (590).

Why is there no ventricular enlargement? Measurements of ICP, conductance to CSF outflow, and cerebral blood flow in 14 patients with PTC suggest that patients with PTC have both a defect in CSF absorption and an increased cerebral volume associated with a noncompliant ventricular system that resists dilation (594). The presence of cerebral edema could also account for the lack of ventriculomegaly. Some MRI studies have shown white matter signal changes consistent with increased water content in patients with PTC (595,596) while others have not (400,597). An initial report of a pathology specimen examined from subtemporal decompression suggested that edema might be present (347) but reexamination of the pathologic material and evidence from two other cases refuted the presence of interstitial edema (598).

It is possible that the increased pressure and cerebral blood volume is reflected primarily within the venous system, as it is distensible, rather than the ventricles. Venous hypertension has been proposed as a unifying hypothesis to explain PTC syndromes (599,600). Manometry has shown elevated cerebral venous pressure in patients with PTC (599). Cerebral venography and manometry demonstrated venous hypertension in the superior sagittal sinus and proximal transverse sinus, but not in the distal transverse sinus, of all patients with idiopathic PTC but not in the patients with minocycline-induced PTC (601). The possibility of focal stenosis or thrombosis of the venous sinuses was raised. Subsequent studies showed a reciprocal relationship between CSF pressure and pressure in the superior sagittal sinus and transverse sinuses in patients with IIH (600). That is, removal of CSF from the cervical region resulted in a decline of venous pressure. The investigators postulated that the increased venous pressure was a result of compression from raised ICP rather than a primary venous occlusive process. Lateral sinus stenting in 12 patients produced a reduction in torcular and jugular bulb pressure in all cases that was not necessarily accompanied by clinical improvement (602).

The association between venous hypertension and PTC syndrome seen with venous sinus thrombosis has prompted investigations looking for a hypercoaguable state in patients with idiopathic and secondary PTC. Initial studies suggested that anticardiolipin antibodies were more common in patients with PTC than would be expected in the general population (603,604). Subsequently, a prospective case-control study evaluated subjects for the factor V Leiden mutation, the prothrombin G20210A allele, homocysteine, antithrombin III, protein C, activated protein C resistance, protein S, lupus anticoagulant, anticardiolipin antibodies, liver and thyroid functions, urea, glucose, electrolytes, lipid levels, prothrombin time, activated partial thromboplastin time, and derived fibrinogen (605). There was no evidence of familial thrombophilia in patients with IIH.

Can the conditions known to produce the PTC syndrome provide any clues to the pathogenesis of the disorder? Hypervitaminosis A is perhaps the best studied of these associations, as PTC may develop with the use of vitamin A and other retinoids. Vitamin A, in the form of retinol, is carried in the serum by retinol-binding protein (RBP) (606). This protein is normally excreted by the kidney; however, in the setting of renal failure, or when the capacity for hepatic storage or binding to RBP is exceeded, the concentration of the protein in the serum rises, as do the concentrations of both bound and unbound vitamin A (579,606,607). Although bound retinol is nontoxic, unbound retinyl esters cause hypervitaminosis A (607,608). Excessive retinol and retinyl esters disrupt the integrity of cell membranes. Retinol is actively transported across the blood-brain barrier by transthyretin (previously called prealbumin) in a complex with RBP and is found in human choroid plexus epithelium. It is also transported to endothelial cells in the microvasculature of the brain (609,610). The effect on choroid plexus transport may be impairing CSF outflow or producing a toxic effect on CSF absorption (607,610,611).

One study demonstrated that serum retinol levels were higher in IIH patients than in control subjects, and were not correlated to body mass index, diet, or age (612). No difference was found in retinyl ester concentration or retinyl ester levels. Another study found no significant difference in serum retinol and RBP levels between IIH patients and controls subjects overall (613). However, some of the IIH patients had markedly elevated RBP levels whereas none of the control subjects did (613). Examination of vitamin A in the cerebrospinal fluid showed significantly higher CSF vitamin A levels in some IIH patients that were not associated with increased ICP, body mass index, age, or gender (609).

IIH in women is associated with idiopathic orthostatic edema, a condition characterized by excessive sodium and/or water retention, particularly in the upright posture (456). The pathogenesis of both disorders has been linked to a vascular etiology and abnormal vasopressin regulation. Orthostatic edema is generally attributed to an incompetent precapillary sphincter causing increased vascular permeability and transudation (614). Urinary excretion of vasopressin (AVP) is excessive in patients with orthostatic edema in the upright posture (614). High levels of vasopressin are found in the CSF of patients with PTC (587,615–617). The role of AVP in the CSF is to regulate brain water content and it raises intracranial pressure by increasing water transudation from cerebral capillaries in the choroid plexus epithelium and the arachnoid villi (618). Although there does not seem to be a significant component of cerebral edema in PTC, the excessive fluid may be absorbed by the venous system, accounting for the venous hypertension described above.

The high association of anxiety and depression in PTC patients compared to age- and weight-matched control subjects (385) raises the possibility of a common neurotransmitter derangement. Serotonin and norepinephrine are associated with these mood disorders and CSF homeostasis. Serotonin, implicated in depression and anxiety, is found in the highest concentrations within the brain in the choroid plexus, and serotonin receptors play a role in CSF production (619). Administration of 5-hydroxytryptamine intrathecally, or intraventricular or intravenous infusion of norpinephrine, produce a dose-related decrease CSF production of 30–50% in rabbits (186,187). Neurotransmitter levels in PTC patients have not been studied.

Despite the progress in our understanding of IIH, Fishman's comment that there are ''more speculations than data available'' remains applicable (584).

MONITORING

Since the major morbidities of PTC are visual loss and headaches, a team approach to management is necessary. The tempo of visual loss in patients with PTC may be rapid or slowly progressive. Most visual defects associated with papilledema are reversible if ICP is lowered before there is severe visual loss or optic nerve ischemia (105,156). Thus, it is imperative that patients be monitored by an ophthalmologist who can assess the best corrected visual acuity, optic nerve functions, visual fields by quantitative static or kinetic perimetry, and the severity of papilledema (157,367). Patients with papilledema most often develop progressive loss of visual function in a manner similar to that which occurs in chronic open angle glaucoma. Loss of central vision is usually a late phenomenon, whereas visual field defects, usually arcuate scotomas and nasal steps, are an early finding (157).

Although all patients with papilledema should be tested to determine if there is a relative afferent pupillary defect (RAPD), papilledema tends to be a bilateral and fairly symmetric in this condition (see above). Thus, when present in a patient with papilledema, a RAPD is a cause for concern as it indicates more damage to the retina or optic nerve of the affected eye with the RAPD. The absence of a RAPD, however, cannot be taken as evidence that there is no optic nerve damage from increased ICP (620). In addition to standard clinical testing, stereo color photographs of the optic discs obtained on a regular basis are helpful to provide the examiner with objective evidence of the appearance of the optic discs. Alternatively, scanning laser tomography of the discs can be performed (90,621).

The intervals between clinical assessments of patients with papilledema must be individualized. At disease onset, some patients will require an evaluation every 1–2 weeks until a pattern of progression or stability is established. Other patients are examined every 1–3 months, and patients with stable vision from papilledema may only be examined every 4–12 months. Most patients may be monitored clinically by following their visual status. Monitoring the status of the ICP by lumbar puncture is not necessary on a routine basis. Once it is established that the neuroimaging studies are normal, subsequent scans are not helpful to assess the patient's progress unless another condition, such as venous sinus thrombosis, is suspected.

TREATMENT

Most patients with PTC will require co-management from more than one physician. A neurologist, ophthalmologist, primary care physician and neurosurgeon may be involved in the patient's care. The primary responsibility for coordinating the patient's treatment is generally relegated to the neurologist or neuro-ophthalmologist; good communication between providers is crucial for a successful outcome. The approach to treatment depends on several factors:

The presence and degree of symptoms such as headache;
The degree of visual loss at presentation;
The rate of progression of visual loss;
The presence of an identifiable underlying etiology (e.g., medication induced PTC);
The detection of factors known to be associated with a poorer visual prognosis (e.g., high-grade papilledema with macular edema, venous sinus thrombosis, systemic hypertension);
Pregnancy.

Regardless of the etiology, the primary goals of treatment are to preserve vision and alleviate symptoms. The treatment of PTC in adults and children is similar. Both medical and surgical treatments are used, often in combination. No single treatment is completely effective in this regard (151, 388,622). Current practice patterns regarding the management of PTC are based largely on case series and clinical experience; there are no randomized trials prospectively assessing the effectiveness of treatment in this disorder. Additionally, PTC is considered an ''off label'' usage for all medications currently prescribed to treat the disorder.

Medical Treatment

Medical therapy is most appropriate when the primary problem is headache in the setting of good vision. In asymptomatic patients with papilledema, close observation of visual function without specific therapy may be employed once an underlying etiology is excluded. If a secondary cause is identified, it should be treated appropriately. For example, implicated exogenous agents should be discontinued. Al-though treating the underlying condition usually produces improvement, it may also be necessary to employ other medical and surgical treatments specifically directed at controlling ICP (417).

Treatment Related to Obesity

Weight loss is advised for obese patients based on retrospective analyses indicating that a modest degree of weight loss (approximately 6% of body weight) correlates with a reduction in papilledema (623–625). Weight reduction should be considered a long-term management solution and is not useful as a sole treatment modality for patients with acute visual loss. When possible, the weight loss should be achieved through a combination of diet and exercise prescribed by a registered dietician or nutritionist setting realistic goals. Many women with idiopathic PTC also have orthostatic edema and have excessive sodium or water retention (456). In such patients, decreasing the food intake while increasing water consumption, as is commonly employed in weight reduction plans, may be counterproductive, and sodium restriction is often helpful (456). When weight loss efforts fail, bariatric surgery may be considered. Such surgery is generally successful in producing weight reduction (626), although significant complications exist, including anastomotic leaks, small bowel obstruction, malabsorption syndromes and gastrointestinal bleeding. Normalization of ICP and resolution of papilledema have been reported after bariatric surgery in retrospective case series (626,627).

Obese patients with PTC from hypoxia and hypercapnia (i.e., the Pickwickian syndrome, obstructive sleep apnea) may respond not only to weight loss but also to low flow oxygen and positive airway ventilation using either continuous positive airway pressure (CPAP) or bilevel positive airway pressure (bi-PAP) (568,628). Often there is a rapid improvement in headaches once CPAP or bi-PAP is initiated.

Medications to Lower the Intracranial Pressure

Carbonic anhydrase, present in the choroid plexus, has a major role in the secretion of CSF. Carbonic anhydrase inhibitors decrease production of CSF, resulting in decreased sodium ion transport across the choroidal epithelium (184,629,630). They also have a mild diuretic effect. The most commonly used agent is acetazolamide (Diamox) (631–633). Reduced ICP may be observed in patients with idiopathic PTC treated with intravenous acetazolamide within several hours (8). In adults, acetazolamide is started at a dose of 1 gm per day, given in divided doses of either 250 mg qid or 500 mg Sequels™ bid. Theoretically, the dose can be increased up to a maximum of 4 gm per day. The effective dose is 1–4 grams daily, but maximum dose is often limited by side effects, which include paresthesias of the extremities, lethargy, and altered taste sensation (8,631). These side effects can be reduced but not eliminated by using Sequels, if available (634). Alternatively, methazolamide (Neptazane) may be used and is sometimes better tolerated than acetazolamide.

Other diuretics are used to treat PTC (635), including furosemide and chlorthalidone (456,579,632). Spironolactone and triamterene may be considered in patients who are allergic to carbonic anhydrase inhibitors and other sulfonamide containing diuretics. Combining diuretics, or using them with carbonic anhydrase inhibitors, may produce hypokalemia and should be done with extreme caution.

Although systemic corticosteroids are clearly beneficial in the treatment of PTC associated with various systemic inflammatory disorders, such as sarcoidosis and systemic lupus erythematosus, they are not generally recommended for routine use in PTC. Corticosteroids lower the ICP acutely but their withdrawal leads to a rebound increase in ICP. Moreover, their long-term side effects (weight gain, fluid retention) are undesirable in the population most affected by PTC. Corticosteroids are reserved for the urgent treatment patients with impending or progressive visual loss while arranging a definitive surgical procedure (410,636).

Headache Management

For patients in whom headache is the main problem, techniques of headache management are employed as in patients with frequent migraines or tension-type headaches. There are many prophylactic medications that may be helpful, although some of them have the potential to cause weight gain (e.g., sodium valproate, tricyclic antidepressants), or fluid retention (e.g., calcium channel blockers). Early experience with topiramate has been promising; it effectively prevents headaches, has mild carbonic anhydrase activity and commonly produces weight loss (637). Many patients with PTC experience other types of headaches unrelated to their intracranial pressure (638). The frequent use of analgesics is discouraged, as analgesic induced headaches may develop.

Repeated Lumbar Punctures

Lumbar punctures are sometimes useful to relieve the increased ICP of idiopathic PTC. The rationale behind the procedure is uncertain. Repeated LPs are traumatic for the patient and often technically difficult to perform but they are useful in selected individuals with intermittent symptom exacerbations. They are also one of the preferred treatments of PTC during pregnancy. Some clinicians favor a "high volume" LP, removing 20 ml or CSF or more, but patients may develop low pressure headaches after this procedure. Another approach is to lower the pressure into the normal range (target range for closing pressure 140–180 mm water), which generally affords relief while lessening the likelihood of post-LP headache.

Surgical Procedures

Surgery is employed when patients initially present with severe optic neuropathy or when other forms of treatment have failed to prevent visual loss. It is not recommended for the treatment of headaches alone. Historically, subtemporal decompression was performed but it has been replaced by a shunting procedure or optic nerve sheath decompression (ONSD). The decision of whether to proceed with a shunt versus ONSD depends largely on the local resources available. Although one may argue that shunting treats the primary pathology, the risks and benefits to each procedure must be considered for each patient. Sometimes more than one type of surgical procedure is necessary (167,639). Neither procedure is generally employed until there is convincing evidence of an optic neuropathy that accounts for the lack of improvement or continued visual deterioration in some patients undergoing technically "successful" surgery. There are no studies comparing ONSD and shunting. Meta-analysis of either condition is confounded by differences in surgical technique and outcomes assessment, the retrospective nature of the data, and underreporting of adverse events.

Cerebrospinal Fluid Diversion Procedures

Ventriculoperitoneal shunting is quite effective in lowering intracranial pressure in patients with PTC but this procedure can be difficult unless a stereotactic method is used, because the ventricles in patients with PTC are normal in size, not enlarged (640–642). Thus, most neurosurgeons prefer the lumboperitoneal shunt, in which a silicone tube is placed percutaneously between the lumbar subarachnoid space and the peritoneal cavity (643). Most patients treated with a shunt experience rapid normalization of ICP and resolution of papilledema, often with improvement in visual function after shunting (644–648). However, the shunts tend to obstruct over time, and over half of patients ultimately require one or more shunt revisions, often within months after their initial insertion (647–649). Complications of the shunt procedure include spontaneous obstruction of the shunt, usually at the peritoneal end, excessively low pressure, infection, radiculopathy, and migration of the tube, resulting in abdominal pain (645,649–652). Some patients also develop a Chiari malformation after lumboperitoneal shunting that may or may not be symptomatic (647). Although the risks of shunting are generally minor, fatal tonsillar herniation after shunting in PTC has been reported (13). Many of the complications from lumboperitoneal shunts can be avoided by using a programmable valve. Alternatively, ventriculoperitoneal shunting or cisterna magna shunting (589), can be performed, but those procedures are technically more difficult.

Optic Nerve Sheath Decompression

Optic nerve sheath decompression (ONSD) was first used to treat papilledema in increased ICP in 1872 (653). Subsequent investigators employed modifications of de Wecker's technique and found it to be at least transiently effective (654,655). In 1964, Hayreh employed the technique on monkeys to demonstrate that papilledema could be relieved by reducing the CSF pressure within the subarachnoid space of the optic nerve (63). Both lateral (656–658) and medial (64,659) approaches are used, incorporating the operating microscope.

A successful optic nerve sheath fenestration results in resolution of papilledema on the operated side and, occasionally, on the other, with bilateral improvement in visual function in many cases (392,622,660–669). The procedure immediately reduces pressure on the nerve by creating a filtration apparatus that controls the intradural pressure surrounding the orbital segment of the optic nerve (102). Although patients sometimes relate that it reduces headaches, there is probably little effect on ICP in most cases (670). Two studies found no postoperative changes in ICP following ONSD and concluded that the decrease in papilledema and the visual improvement occurred from a local decrease in optic nerve sheath pressure rather than from a generalized decrease in ICP (670,671). However, a third study showed persistently decreased CSF pressure after ONSD as assessed by repeated lumbar punctures for three years following ONSD (672). The mechanism of long-term effectiveness from ONSD may be fibrous scar formation between the dura and optic nerve blocking creating a barrier to protect the anterior optic nerve from the intracranial CSF pressure.

The risks of optic nerve sheath fenestration, although low, are nevertheless significant. They include transient (673,674) or permanent (675,676) loss of vision from vascular occlusion, diplopia, and infection (392,663,664,673,677). Some patients will require a repeat procedure as vision may worsen months to years later (666,678). Nevertheless, most adults and children have stabilization or improvement of vision following optic nerve sheath fenestration (679,680).

SPECIAL CIRCUMSTANCES

Pregnancy

Women who develop PTC during pregnancy are diagnosed and treated similarly to nonpregnant women. Most women do well, with little or no permanent visual loss (675,676,681). There is no contraindication to pregnancy in women with a history of PTC and no special provisions are required for delivery unless other medical complications are present. The majority of patients may be managed with careful neuro-ophthalmic follow-up and repeated lumbar punctures. Acetazolamide may be used after 20 weeks gestation. Caloric restriction, thiazide diuretics and tricyclic antidepressants are generally avoided. If vision deteriorates, corticosteroids may be used. ONSD or lumboperitoneal shunting may be performed if needed, although there is a theoretical risk of shunt malfunction from peritoneal catheter obstruction as the uterus enlarges (681). PTC arising in the postpartum period or following fetal loss should raise the suspicion of cerebral venous sinus thrombosis (682) .

Fulminant PTC

There is a small subgroup of patients with PTC who experience a rapid onset of symptoms and precipitous visual decline. They often have significant visual field loss, central visual acuity loss, and marked papilledema at presentation. Macular edema or ophthalmoparesis may also be present. A progressive or "malignant" course requires rapid and aggressive treatment. A multidisciplinary physician team and one or more surgical procedures are usually required, and may still be unsuccessful in preserving vision. Other therapeutic measures include intravenous corticosteroids, intravenous acetazolamide, and insertion of a lumbar drain. Cerebral venous sinus thrombosis is an important diagnostic consideration in these patients.

REFERENCES

1. Cogan DG, Kuwabara T. Papilledema. Exp Eye Res 1977;25(Suppl):419–433.
2. Jackson JH. Observations on defects of sight in brain disease. R Lond Ophthalmol Hosp Rep 1863;4:10–19.
3. Parsons JH. The Pathology of the Eye. New York, GP Putnam's Sons, 1908.
4. Kennedy F. Retrobulbar neuritis as an exact diagnostic sign of certain tumors and abscesses in the frontal lobe. Am J Med Sci 1911;142:355.
5. Paton L, Holmes G. The pathology of papilloedema. A histological study of 60 eyes. Brain 1911;33:289–432.
6. Corbett JJ, Mehta MP. Cerebrospinal fluid pressure in normal obese subjects and patients with pseudotumor cerebri. Neurology 1983;33:1386–1388.
7. Adson AW. Pseudobrain abscess. Surg Clin North Am 1924;4:503–512.
8. Gucer G, Viernstein L. Long-term intracranial pressure recording in the management of pseudotumor cerebri. J Neurosurg 1978;49:256–263.
9. Ford FR, Murphy EL. Increased intracranial pressure: clinical analysis of the causes and characteristics of several types. Bull Johns Hopkins Hosp 1939;64:369–398.
10. Hodgson J. Combined ventricular and lumbar puncture in diagnosis of brain tumor: further studies. JAMA 1928;90:1524–1526.
11. Leinfelder P. Choked discs and low intrathecal pressure occurring in brain tumor. Am J Ophthalmol 1943;26:1294–1298.
12. Ayer JB. Cerebrospinal fluid (lumbar) in brain tumor. Analysis of 67 cases of tumor and cysts of the brain. JAMA 1928;90:1521–1524.
13. Sullivan HC. Fatal tonsillar herniation in pseudotumor cerebri. Neurology 1991;41:1142–1144.
14. Evans RW. Complications of lumbar puncture. Neurol Clin 1998;16:83–105.
15. Horton JC, Fishman RA. Neurovisual findings in the syndrome of spontaneous intracranial hypotension from dural cerebrospinal fluid leak. Ophthalmology 1994;101:244–251.
16. Korein J, Cravioto H, Leicach M. Reevaluation of lumbar puncture: A study of 129 patients with papilledema or intracranial hypertension. Neurology 1959;9:290–297.
17. Jackson JH. On the routine use of the ophthalmoscope in cases of cerebral disease. Med Times Gaz 1871;I:627–629.
18. Hoyt WF, Beeston D, eds. The Ocular Fundus in Neurologic Disease. St Louis, CV Mosby, 1966.
19. Frisén L. Swelling of the optic nerve head: A staging scheme. J Neurol Neurosurg Psychiatry 1982;45:13–18.
20. Neetens A, Smets RM. Papilledema. Neuroophthalmology 1989;9:81–101.
21. Hayreh MS, Hayreh SS. Optic disc edema in raised intracranial pressure. I. Evolution and resolution. Arch Ophthalmol 1977;95:1237–1244.
22. Hayreh SS, Hayreh MS. Optic disc edema in raised intracranial presure. II. Early detection with fluorescein fundus angiography and stereoscopic color photography. Arch Ophthalmol 1977;95:1245–1254.
23. Hoyt WF, Knight CL. Comparison of congenital disc blurring and incipient papilledema in a red-free light—a photographic study. Invest Ophthalmol 1973;12:241–247.
24. Kahn EA, Cherry GR. The clinical importance of spontaneous retinal venous pulsations. Univ Mich Med Bull 1950;16:305–308.
25. Williamson-Noble FA. Venous pulsation. Trans Ophthalmol Soc UK 1952;72:317–326.
26. Walsh FB, Hoyt WF. In Clinical Neuro-Ophthalmology. Ed 3. Baltimore, Williams & Wilkins, 1969:588.
27. Dandy W. Intracranial pressure without brain tumor: Diagnosis and treatment. Ann Surg 1937;106:492–513.
28. Lundberg N. Continuous recording and control of ventricular fluid pressure in neurosurgical practice. Acta Psychiatr Scand 1960;36(Suppl 149):1–193.
29. Lorentzen SE. Incidence of spontaneous venous pulsations in the retina. Acta Ophthalmol 1970;48:765–776.
30. Levin BE. The clinical significance of spontaneous pulsations of the retinal vein. Arch Neurol 1978;35:37–40.
31. Nettleship E. Peculiar lines in the choroid in a case of post-papillitic atrophy. Trans Ophthalmol Soc UK 1884;4:167–168.
32. Bird AC, Sanders MD. Choroidal folds in association with papilloedema. Br J Ophthalmol 1973;57:89–97.
33. Jacobson DM. Intracranial hypertension and the syndrome of acquired hyperopia with choroidal folds. J Neuroophthalmol 1995;15:178–185.
34. Griebel SR, Kosmorsky GS. Choroidal folds associated with increased intracranial pressure. Am J Ophthalmol 2000;129:513–516.
35. Miller NR, Fine SL. The Ocular Fundus in Neuro-Ophthalmologic Diagnosis: Sights and Sounds in Ophthalmology. St Louis, CV Mosby, 1976.
36. Carter SR, Seiff SR. Macular changes in pseudotumor cerebri before and after optic nerve sheath fenestration. Ophthalmology 1995;102:937–941.
37. Watson AP, Sanford-Smith JH. Spontaneous vitreous hemorrhage in a young patient with benign intracranial hypertension. Neuroophthalmology 1986;6:153–158.
38. Keane JR. Papilledema with unusual ocular hemorrhages. Arch Ophthalmol 1981;99:262–263.
39. Jamison RR. Subretinal neovascularization and papilledema associated with pseudotumor cerebri. Am J Ophthalmol 1978;85:78–81.

40. Akova YA, Kansu T, Yazar Z, et al. Macular subretinal neovascular membrane associated with pseudotumor cerebri. J Neuro-ophthalmol 1994;14:193–195.

41. Pollack SC. Acute papilledema and visual loss in a patient with pseudotumor cerebri. Arch Ophthalmol 1987;105:752–753.

42. Galvin R, Sanders MD. Peripheral retinal hemorrhages with papilloedema. Br J Ophthalmol 1980;64:262–266.

43. Carter JE, Merren MD, Byrne BM. Pseudodrusen of the optic disc: Papilledema simulating buried drusen of the optic nerve head. J Clin Neuroophthalmol 1989; 9:273–276.

44. Okun E. Chronic papilledema simulating hyaline bodies of the optic disc. Am J Ophthalmol 1962;53:922–927.

45. Hedges TR III, Legge RH, Peli E, et al. Retinal nerve fiber layer changes and visual field loss in idiopathic intracranial hypertension. Ophthalmology 1995; 102:1242–1247.

46. Fischer F. Zur frage sog. permanenter stauungspapille. Klin Mbl Augenheilk 1939;102:656–663.

47. Gittinger JW Jr., Asdourian GK. Macular abnormalities in papilledema from pseudotumor cerebri. Ophthalmology 1989;96:192–194.

48. Morris AT, Saunders MD. Macular changes resulting from papilloedema. Br J Ophthalmol 1980;64:211–216.

49. Hrisomalos NF, Mansour AM, Jampol LM, et al. ''Pseudo''-combined hemartoma following papilledema. Arch Ophthalmol 1987;105:1634–1635.

50. Sanders MD. A classification of papilloedema based on a fluorescein angiographic study of 69 cases. Trans Ophthalmol Soc UK 1969;89:177–192.

51. Hedges T. Papilledema: Its recognition and relation to increased intracranial pressure. Surv Ophthalmol 1975;19:201–223.

52. Henkind P, Benjamin J. Vascular anomalies and neoplasms of the optic nerve head. Trans Ophthalmol Soc UK 1976;96:418–423.

53. Eggers HM, Sanders MD. Acquired optociliary shunt vessels in papilloedema. Br J Ophthalmol 1980;64:267–271.

54. Perlmutter JC, Klingele TG, Hart WM Jr, et al. Disappearing opticociliary shunt vessels and pseudotumor cerebri. Am J Ophthalmol 1980;89:703–707.

55. Stein SA, Witkop C, Hill S, et al. Sclerosteosis: Neurogenetic and pathophysiologic analysis of an American kinship. Neurology 1983;33:267–277.

56. Levin PS, Newman SA, Quigley HA, et al. A clinicopathologic study of optic neuropathies associated with intracranial mass lesions with quantification of remaining axons. Am J Ophthalmol 1983;95:295–306.

57. Gu XZ, Tsai JC, Wurdemen A, et al. Pattern of axonal loss in long-standing papilledema due to idiopathic intracranial hypertension. Curr Eye Res 1995;14: 173–180.

58. Moster ML, Slavin M, Wall M. Unilateral disk edema in a young woman. Surv Ophthalmol 1995;39:409–416.

59. Strominger MB, Weiss GB, Mehler MF. Asymptomatic unilateral papilledema in pseudotumor cerebri. J Clin Neuroophthalmol 1992;12:238–241.

60. Sanders MD, Sennhenn R. Differential diagnosis of unilateral oedema. Trans Ophthalmol Soc UK 1980;100:123–131.

61. Paul TO, Hoyt WF. Funduscopic appearance of papilledema with optic tract atrophy. Arch Ophthalmol 1976;94:467–468.

62. Hoyt WF, Rios-Montenegro EN, Behrens MM, et al. Homonymous hemioptic hypoplasia. Br J Ophthalmol 1972;56:537–545.

63. Hayreh SS. Pathogenesis of oedema of the optic disc. Br J Ophthalmol 1964; 48:522–543.

64. Smith JL, Hoyt WF, Newton TH. Optic nerve sheath decompression for relief of chronic monocular choked disc. Am J Ophthalmol 1969;68:633–639.

65. Lepore FE. Unilateral and highly asymmetric papilledema in pseudotumor cerebri. Neurology 1992;42:676–678.

66. Muci-Mendoza R. Unilateral and asymmetric optic disk swelling with intracranial abnormalities. Am J Ophthalmol 1984;97:253.

67. Gibbs FA. Intracranial tumor with unequal choked disc: Relationship between the side of greater choking and the position of the tumor. Arch Neurol Psychiatr 1932;27:828–835.

68. Woodhall B. Variations of the cranial venous sinuses in the region of the torcular Herophili. Arch Surg 1936;33.

69. Lipton HL, Michelson PE. Pseudotumor cerebri syndrome without papilledema. JAMA 1972;220:1591–1592.

70. Sedwick L, Burde RM. Unilateral and asymmetric optic disk swelling with intracranial abnormalities. Am J Ophthalmol 1983;96:484–487.

71. Kirkham TH, Sanders MD, Sapp GA. Unilateral papilledema in benign intracranial hypertension. Can J Ophthalmol 1973;8:533–538.

72. Bruntse E. Unilateral papilloedema in neurosurgical patients. Acta Ophthalmol 1970;48:759–764.

73. Sher NA, Wirtschafter J, Shapiro SK, et al. Unilateral papilledema in ''benign'' intracranial hypertension (pseudotumor cerebri). JAMA 1983;250:2346–2347.

74. Huna-Baron R, Landau K, Rosenberg M, Warren FA, Kupersmith MJ. Unilateral swollen disc due to increased intracranial pressure. Neurology 2001;56: 1588–1590.

75. Barrios RR. Fluorescein angioretinography as a diagnostic method for papilloedema. Acta Neurol Lat Am 1963;9:213–221.

76. David NJ, Heyman S, Hart LM. Fluorescence photography of retinal vessels and optic discs in papilledema. Trans Am Neurol Assoc 1963;88:155–158.

77. Miller SJ, Sanders MD, Tftyche T. Fluorescein fundus photography in the detection of early papilloedema and its differentiation from pseudopapilloedema. Lancet 1965;2:651–654.

78. Blair CJ, Walsh FB. Papilloedema, optic neuritis, and pseudopapilloedema. Trans Am Acad Ophthalmol Otolaryngol 1969;73:914–920.

79. Bynke HG, Åberg L. Differentiation of papilloedema from pseudopapilloedema by fluorescein ophthalmoscopy. Acta Ophthalmol 1970;48:752–758.

80. Heydenreich A, Lemke L, Jutte A. Differential diagnose von papillenveranderungen mit fluorescein. Klin Mbl Augenheilk 1973;163:131–139.

81. Cartlidge NE, Ng RC, Tilley PB. Dilemma of the swollen optic disc: A fluorescein retinal angiography study. Br J Ophthalmol 1977;61:385–389.

82. Kottow M. Fluoreszenzangiographische differentialdiagnose der randunscharfen papille. Klin Mbl Augenheilk 1980;177:696–705.

83. Ghose S, Nayak BK. Role of oral fluorescein in the diagnosis of early papilloedema in children. Br J Ophthalmol 1987;71:910–915.

84. Salgarello T, Tamburrelli C, Falsini B, et al. Optic nerve diameters and perimetric thresholds in idiopathic intracranial hypertension. Br J Ophthalmol 1996; 80:509–514.

85. Tamburrelli C, Salgarello T, Caputo CG, Giudiceandrea A, Scullica L. Ultrasonographic evaluation of optic disc swelling: comparison with CSLO in idiopathic intracranial hypertension. Invest Ophthalmol Vis Sci 2000;41:2960–2966.

86. Katz B, Van Patten P, Rothrock JF. Optic nerve head drusen and pseudotumor cerebri. Arch Neurol 1988;45:45–47.

87. Reifler DM, Kaufman DI. Optic disk drusen and pseudotumor cerebri. Am J Ophthalmol 1988;106:95–96.

88. Brodsky MC, Vaphiades M. Magnetic resonance imaging in pseudotumor cerebri. Ophthalmology 1998;105:1686–1693.

89. Mashima Y, Oshitari K, Imamura Y, et al. High-resolution magnetic resonance imaging of the intraorbital optic nerve and subarachnoid space in patients with papilledema and optic atrophy. Arch Ophthalmol 1996;114:1197–1203.

90. Trick GL, Vesti E, Tawansy K, Skarf B, Gartner J. Quantitative evaluation of papilledema in pseudotumor cerebri. Invest Ophthalmol Vis Sci 1998;39: 1964–1971.

91. Weinreb RN, Lusky M, Bartsch D-U, Morsman D. Effect of repetitive imaging on topographic measurements of the optic nerve head. Arch Ophthalmol 1993; 111:636–638.

92. Johnson LN, Hepler RS, Bartholomew MJ. Accuracy of papilledema and pseudopapilledema detection: a multispecialty study. J Fam Pract 1991;33:381–386.

93. Keltner JL, Johnson CA, Spurr JO, et al. Comparison of central and peripheral visual field properties in the optic neuritis treatment trial. Am J Ophthalmol 1999;128:543–553.

94. Optic Neuritis Study Group. The clinical profile of optic neuritis: Experience of the Optic Neuritis Treatment Trial. Arch Ophthalmol 1991;109:1673–1678.

95. Steffen H, Eifert B, Aschoff A, Kolling GH, Völcker HE. The diagnostic value of optic disc evaluation in acute elevated intracranial pressure. Ophthalmology 1996;103:1229–1323.

96. Pagani LF. The rapid appearance of papilledema. J Neurosurg 1969;30:247–249.

97. Glowacki J. Acute papilledema. Bull Pol Med Sci Hist 1962;5:15–16.

98. Coleman CC. Brain abscess: A review of 28 cases with comment on the ophthalmologic observations. JAMA 1930;95:568–572.

99. Lillie WI. The clinical significance of choked discs produced by abscess of the brain. Surg Gynecol Obstet 1928;47:405–406.

100. Levatin P, Raskin R. Delayed appearance of papilledema. Can J Ophthalmol 1973;8:451–455.

101. Bettman JW Jr, Daroff RB, Sanders MD, et al. Papilledema and symptomatic intracranial hypertension in systemic lupus erythematosus. Arch Ophthalmol 1968;80:180–193.

102. Hamed LM, Tse DT, Glaser JS, Frazier Byrne S, Schatz NJ. Neuroimaging of the optic nerve after fenestration for management of pseudotumor cerebri. Arch Ophthalmol 1992;110:636–639.

103. Cinciripini GS, Donahue S, Borchert MS. Idiopathic intracranial hypertension in prepubertal pediatric patients: characteristics, treatment and outcome. Am J Ophthalmol 1999;127:178–182.

104. Trobe JD, Glaser JS, Cassady JC. Optic atrophy. Arch Ophthalmol 1980;98: 1040–1045.

105. Orcutt JC, Page NGR, Sanders MD. Factors affecting visual loss in benign intracranial hypertension. Ophthalmology 1984;91:1303–1312.

106. Newman EW. Ocular signs of intracranial disease in children and juveniles. Am J Ophthalmol 1938;21:286–292.

107. Rand CW, van Wagenen RJ. Brain tumors in childhood. J Pediatr 1935;6: 322–339.

108. Gross SW. Tumors of the brain in infancy. Am J Dis Child 1934;48:739–763.

109. Samuels B. The histopathology of papilloedema. Tran Ophthalmol Soc UK 1938; 57:529–556.

110. Zimmerman LE. Histology and general pathology of the optic nerve: Symposium on diseases of the optic nerve. Trans Am Acad Ophthalmol Otolaryngol 1956; 60:14–30.

111. Sanders MD. The Bowman Lecture. Papilloedema: 'The pendulum of progress'. Eye 1997;11:267–294.

112. Corbett JS, Nerad JA, Tse DT, et al. Results of optic nerve sheath fenestration

for pseudotumor cerebri: The lateral orbitotomy approach. Arch Ophthalmol 1980;106:1391–1397.

113. Green GJ, Lessell S, Lowenstein JL. Ischaemic optic neuropathy in chronic papilledema. Arch Ophthalmol 1980;98:502–504.

114. Tso MO, Fine BS. Electron microscopic study of human papilledema. Am J Ophthalmol 1976;82:424–434.

115. Minckler DS, Tso MO. A light microscopic autoradiographic study of axoplasmic transport in the normal rhesus optic nerve head. Am J Ophthalmol 1976;82:1–15.

116. Hayreh SS. Blood supply of the optic nerve head and its role in optic atrophy, glaucoma, and oedema of the optic disc. Br J Ophthalmol 1969;53:721–748.

117. Schutta HS, Hedges TR. Fine structure observations on experimental papilledema in the rhesus monkey. J Neurol Sci 1971;12:1–14.

118. Tso MO, Hayreh SS. Optic disc edema in raised intracranial pressure. III. A pathologic study of experimental papilledema. Arch Ophthalmol 1977;95:1448–1457.

119. Schieck F. Uber die entstehungsart der stauungspapille. Verh Phys Med Gesamte 1926;51:121.

120. Fry WE. The pathology of papilledema. An examination of 40 eyes with special reference to compression of the central retinal vein. Am J Ophthalmol 1931;14:874–883.

121. Hogan MJ, Zimmerman LE. Ophthalmic Pathology. Philadelphia, Saunders, 1987.

122. van Heuven JA, Fischer PF. The water-binding of the optic nerve and its sheaths. Br J Ophthalmol 1936;20:204.

123. Rosomoff HL, Zugibe FT. Distribution of intracranial contents in experimental edema. Arch Neurol 1963;9:26–34.

124. Duke-Elder S. System of Ophthalmology. St Louis, CV Mosby, 1933.

125. Hedges TR, Weinstein JD. The hydrostatic mechanism of papilledema. Trans Am Acad Ophthalmol Otolaryngol 1968;72:741–750.

126. von Graefe A. Uber neuroretinitis and gewisse falle fulminierender erblindung. Graefe's Arch Ophthalmol 1866;12 (part 2):114–149.

127. Caviness WF, Tanaka A, Hess KH. Delayed brain swelling and functional derangement after x-radiation of the right visual cortex in the macaca mulatta. Radiat Res 1975;57:104–120.

128. Hedges TR, Weinstein JD, Crystle CD. Orbital vascular response to acutely increased intracranial pressure in the rhesus monkey. Arch Ophthalmol 1964;1242–1247.

129. Hayreh SS. Pathogenesis of oedema of the optic disc. Doc Ophthalmol 1968;24:289–411.

130. Hayreh SS, Dass R. The ophthalmic artery. I. Origin and intra-cranial course. Br J Ophthalmol 1962;46:65–98.

131. Ernest JT, Potts AM. Pathophysiology of the distal portion of the optic nerve. I. Tissue pressure relationships. Am J Ophthalmol 1968;66:373–387.

132. Taylor AC, Weiss P. Demonstration of axonal flow by the movement of tritium-labeled protein in mature optic nerve fibers. Proc Natl Acad Sci USA 1965;54:1521–1527.

133. Tso MO, Hayreh SS. Optic disc edema in raised intracranial pressure: IV. Axoplasmic transport in experimental papilledema. Arch Ophthalmol 1977;95:1458–1462.

134. Minckler DS, Tsai JC, Zimmerman LE. A light microscopic, autoradiographic study of axoplasmic transport in the optic nerve head during ocular hypotony, increased intraocular pressure, and papilledema. Am J Ophthalmol 1976;82:741–757.

135. Minckler DS, Bunt AH. Axoplasmic transport in ocular hypotony and papilledema in the monkey. Arch Ophthalmol 1977;95:1430–1436.

136. Anderson DR, Hendrickson A. Effect of intraocular pressure on rapid axoplasmic transport in monkey optic nerve. Invest Ophthalmol Vis Sci 1974;13:771–783.

137. Hayreh SS. Optic disc edema in raised intracranial pressure. V. Pathogenesis. Arch Ophthalmol 1977;95:1553–1565.

138. Hayreh SS, Edwards J. Ophthalmic arterial and venous pressure. Br J Ophthalmol 1971;55:649–663.

139. Primrose J. Pathogenesis of papilledema. Doc Ophthalmol 1976;40:391–408.

140. Primrose J. Pathogenesis of optic disc swelling. Br J Ophthalmol 1979;63:211–212.

141. Forsyth PA, Posner JB. Headaches in patients with brain tumors: A study of 111 patients. Neurology 1993;43:1678–1683.

142. Bjerre P, Lindholm J, Glydensted C. Pathogenesis of nontraumatic cerebrospinal fluid rhinorrhea. Acta Neurol Scand 1982;66:180–192.

143. Clark D, Bullock P, Hui T, et al. Benign intracranial hypertension: A cause of CSF rhinorroea. J Neurol Neurosurg Psychiatry 1994;57:847–849.

144. Troost BT, Sufit RL. Sudden monocular visual loss in pseudotumor cerebri. Arch Neurol 1979;36:440–442.

145. Paton L. Optic neuritis in cerebral tumours. Trans Ophthalmol Soc UK 1908;28.

146. Cogan DG. Blackouts not obviously due to carotid occlusion. Arch Ophthalmol 1961;66:180–187.

147. West S. Sequel of a case of optic neuritis, with numerous sudden, short attacks of complete blindness. Trans Ophthalmol Soc UK 1883;3:136–138.

148. Paton L. Optic neuritis in cerebral tunours and its subsidence after operation. Trans Ophthalmol Soc UK 1905;28:112–144.

149. de Schweinitz GE. The relation of cerebral decompression to the relief of the ocular manifestations of increased intracranial tension. Ann Ophthalmol 1911;20:271–284.

150. Pascual J, Combarros O, Berciano J. Gaze-evoked amaurosis in pseudotumor cerebri. Neurology 1988;38:1654–1655.

151. Rush JA. Pseudotumor cerebri: Clinical profile and visual outcome in 63 patients. Mayo Clin Proc 1980;55:541–546.

152. Knapp H. The channel by which, in cases of neuroretinitis, the exudation proceeds from the brain into the eye. Trans Am Ophthalmol Soc 1870;1:118–120.

153. Corbett JJ, Jacobson DM, Mauer RC, et al. Enlargement of the blind spot caused by papilledema. Am J Ophthalmol 1988;105:261–265.

154. Uhthoff W. Ophthalmic experiences and considerations on the surgery of cerebral tumors and lower skull: The Bowman lecture. Trans Ophthalmol Soc UK 1914;34:47–123.

155. Grehn F, Knorr-Held S, Kommerell G. Glaucomatous-like visual field defects in chronic papilledema. Graefe's Arch Ophthalmol 1981;21:99–109.

156. Wall M, Hart WM Jr, Burde RM. Visual field defects in idiopathic intracranial hypertension (pseudotumor cerebri). Am J Ophthalmol 1983;96:654–669.

157. Wall M, Conway MD, House PH, et al. Evaluation of sensitivity and specificity of spatial resolution and Humphrey automated perimetry in pseudotumor cerebri patients and normal subjects. Invest Ophthalmol Vis Sci 1991;32:3306–3312.

158. Wall M, George D. Visual loss in pseudotumor cerebri: Incidence and defects related to visual field strategy. Arch Neurol 1987;44:170–175.

159. Gruber H, Czech T. Computerperimetrie zur Verlaufskontrolle der Opticusneuropathie bei Pseudotumor Cerebri. Klin Mbl Augenheilk 1990;196:214–215.

160. Duke-Elder S, Scott GI. Neuro-Ophthalmology. In Duke-Elder S, ed. System of Ophthalmology. St Louis, CV Mosby, 1971;60.

161. Baker RS, Carter DC, Hendrock EB, Buncic JR. Visual loss in pseudotumor cerebri of childhood: A follow-up study. Arch Ophthalmol 1985;103:1681–1686.

162. Kidron D, Pomeranz S. Malignant pseudotumor cerebri: Report of two cases. J Neurosurg 1989;71:443–445.

163. Baker RS, Buncic JR. Sudden visual loss in pseudotumor cerebri due to central retinal artery occlusion. Arch Neurol 1984;41:1274–1276.

164. Gutgold-Glen H, Kattah JC, Chavis RM. Reversible visual loss in pseudotumor cerebri. Arch Ophthalmol 1984;102:403–406.

165. Repka MX, Miller NR. Papilledema and dural sinus obstruction. J Clin Neuroophthalmol 1984;4:247–250.

166. Lam BL, Siatkowski RM, Fox GM, et al. Visual loss in pseudotumor cerebri from branch retinal artery occlusion. Am J Ophthalmol 1992;113:334–336.

167. Liu GT, Volpe NJ, Schatz NJ, et al. Severe sudden visual loss caused by pseudotumor cerebri and lumboperitoneal shunt failure. Am J Ophthalmol 1996;122:129–131.

168. Baker RS, Buncic JR. Vertical ocular motility disturbances in pseudotumor cerebri. J Clin Neuroophthalmol 1985;5:41–44.

169. Lessell S, Rosman NP. Permanent visual impairment in childhood pseudotumor cerebri. Arch Neurol 1986;43:801–804.

170. Wall M. Contrast sensitivity in pseudotumor cerebri. Ophthalmology 1986;93:4–7.

171. Verplanck M, Kaufman DI, Parsons T, et al. Electrophysiology versus psychophysics in the detection of visual loss in pseudotumor cerebri. Neurology 1988;38:1789–1792.

172. Buncic JR, Tytla M. Spatial contrast sensitivity impairment in optic nerve head swelling. Neuroophthalmology 1989;9:293–298.

173. Grochowicki M, Vighetto A, Pissavin C. Pseudotumor cerebri: Longitudinal study using contrast sensitivity and automated static perimetry. Neuroophthalmology 1990;10:97–108.

174. Wall M. Sensory visual testing in idiopathic intracranial hypertension: Measures sensitive to change. Neurology 1990;40:1859–1864.

175. Falsini B, Tamburrelli C, Porciatti V, et al. Pattern electroretinograms and visual evoked potentials in idiopathic intracranial hypertension. Ophthalmologica 1992;205:194–203.

176. Cushing H, Bailey P. Tumors Arising from the Blood Vessels of the Brain. 1928; Sect. 74.

177. Keane JR. Bilateral sixth nerve palsy. Arch Neurol 1976;33:681–683.

178. Cobbs WH, Schatz NJ, Savino PJ. Midbrain eye signs in hydrocephalus. Ann Neurol 1978;4:172.

179. Halpern JI, Gordon WH Jr. Trochlear nerve palsy as a false localizing sign. Ann Ophthalmol 1981;12:53–56.

180. Keane JR. Ocular skew deviation: Analysis of 200 cases. Arch Neurol 1975;32:185–190.

181. Merikangas JR. Skew deviation in pseudotumor cerebri. Ann Neurol 1978;4:583.

182. McCammon A, Kaufman HH, Sears ES. Transient oculomotor paralysis in pseudotumor cerebri. Neurology 1981;31:182–184.

183. Friedman DI, Forman S, Levi L, et al. Unusual ocular motility disturbances with increased intracranial pressure. Neurology 1998;50:1893–1896.

184. Fishman RA. Anatomical aspects of the cerebrospinal fluid. In Fishman R, ed. Cerebrospinal Fluid in Diseases of the Nervous System. Philadelphia, W.B. Saunders, 1992:20–21.

185. Epstein MH, Feldman MH, Brusilow SW. Cerebrospinal fluid production: stimulation by cholera toxin. Science 1977;196:1012–1013.

186. Lindvall-Axelsson M, Mather C, Nilsson C, Owman C. Effect of 5-hydroxytryptamine on the rate of cerebrospinal fluid production in rabbit. Exp Neurol 1988; 99:362–368.

187. Lindvall M, Edvinsson L, Owman C. Effect of sympathomimetic drugs and corresponding receptor antagonists on the rate of cerebrospinal fluid production. Exp Neurol 1979;64:132–145.

188. Welch K. The principles of physiology of the cerebrospinal fluid in relation to hydrocephalus including normal pressure hydrocephalus. In Friedlander WJ, ed. Advances in Neurology. Current Reviews. New York, Raven Press, 1975: 247–332.

189. Robertson DN, Dinsdale HB. The Nervous System. Baltimore, Williams & Wilkins, 1972.

190. Kellie G. An account of the appearances observed in the dissection of two or three individuals presumed to have perished in the storm of the 3rd, and whose bodies were discovered in the vicinity of Leith on the morning of the 4th, November 1821 with some reflections on the pathology of the brain. Trans Edinb Med Chir Soc 1824;1:84–169.

191. Weed LH. Positional adjustments of the pressure of the cerebro-spinal fluid. Phys Rev 1933;13:80–102.

192. Bezeaud D, Vadot E. Aspects étiologiques actuels des oedèmes papillaires. Bull Soc Ophtalmol Fr 1990;90:409–411.

193. Andeweg J. Concepts of cerebral venous drainage and the aetiology of hydrocephalus. J Neurol Neurosurg Psychiatry 1991;54:830–831.

194. Paton L. Papilledema and optic neuritis: A retrospect. Trans Sect Ophthalmol Am Med Assoc 1935;30:98–119.

195. Uhthoff W. Die augenveraderungen bei den erkrankungen des gihirnes. In Graefe-Saemish, ed. Handbuch der Gesamten Augenheilkunde. Wilhelm Engelman, 1915:1143,1430.

196. Van Wagenen WP. The incidence of intracranial tumors without ''choked disc'' in one year's series of cases. Am J Med Sci 1928;176:346–366.

197. Tönnis W. Pathophysiologie und klinik der intracraniellen drucksteigerung. In Olivecrona H, Tönnis W, eds. Handbuch der Neurochirurgie. Berlin, Julius Springer, 1959.

198. Petrohelos MA, Henderson JW. The ocular findings of intracranial tumor. Trans Am Acad Ophthalmol 1950;55:89–98.

199. Stopford JSB. Increased intracranial pressure. Brain 1928;51:485–507.

200. Petrohelos MA, Henderson JW. The ocular findings of intracranial tumor. Am J Ophthalmol 1951;34:1387–1394.

201. Berg L, Rosomoff HL, Aronson V, et al. Investigation of the syndrome of increased intracranial pressure without localizing signs. Trans Am Neurol Assoc 1954;79:131.

202. Van Crevel H. Absence of papilledema in cerebral tumours. J Neurol Neurosurg Psychiatry 1975;38:931–933.

203. Hartmann E, Guillaumat L. Aspect du fond d'oeil dans les tumeurs intracraniennes: Etude stastique. Ann Oculist (Paris) 1938;175:717–737.

204. Huber A, ed. Eye Signs and Symptoms in Brain Tumors. Ed 3. St Louis, CV Mosby, 1976.

205. Dabenzies OH, Walsh FB, Hayes GJ. Papilledema with hamartoma of the hypothalamus. Arch Ophthalmol 1961;65:174–180.

206. Keane JR. Neuro-ophthalmologic signs and symptoms of cysticercosis. Arch Ophthalmol 1982;100:1445–1448.

207. Dandy WE. Arteriovenous aneurysm of the brain. Arch Surg 1928;17:190–243.

208. Forman AR, Luessenhop AJ, Limaye SR. Ocular findings in patients with arteriovenous malformations of the head and neck. Am J Ophthalmol 1975;79: 626–633.

209. Lamas E, Lobato RD, Esparza J, et al. Dural posterior fossa AVM producing raised sagittal sinus pressure. J Neurosurg 1977;46:804–810.

210. Takahashi T, Okukubo K, Tagami Y, et al. A case of dural arteriovenous malformation with papilledema. Neuroophthalmology 1983;3:199–204.

211. Regolo P, Bianchi S, Righi C, et al. Dural artero-venous fistulas (AVFs): A possible cause of pseudotumor cerebri in men. J Neurol Sci 1996;39:101.

212. Rozot P, Berrod JP, Bracard S. Stase papillaire et fistule durale. J Fr Ophtalmol 1991;14:13–19.

213. Letessier J-B, Courthéoux O, Sautreuil B, et al. Fistule durale complexe du sinus latérale a symptomatologie opthalmologique prédominante. Bull Soc Ophtalmol Fr 1991;91:295–301.

214. Barrow DL. Unruptured cerebral arteriovenous malformations presenting with intracranial hypertension. Neurosurgery 1988;23:484–490.

215. Gelwan MJ, Choi IS, Berenstein A, et al. Dural arteriovenous malformations and papilledema. Neurosurgery 1988;22:1079–1084.

216. Chimowitz MI, Little JR, Awad IA, et al. Intracranial hypertension associated with unruptured cerebral arteriovenous malformations. Ann Neurol 1990;27: 474–479.

217. Weisberg LA, Pierve JF, Jabbari B. Intracranial hypertension resulting from a cerebral vascular malformation. South Med J 1977;70:624–626.

218. Kuhner A, Krastel A, Stoll W. Arteriovenous malformations of the transverse dural sinuses. J Neurosurg 1976;45:12–19.

219. Lahat E, Aladjem M, Schiffler J, et al. Hydrocephalus due to bilateral obstruction

220. Corbett J. Neuro-ophthalmologic complications of hydrocephalus and shuntng procedures. Semin Neurol 1986;6:111–123.

221. Chahlavi A, El-Babaa SK, Luciano MG. Adult-onset hydrocephalus. Neurosurg Clin N Am 2001;12:753–760.

222. Kunkel PA, Dandy WE. Subdural hematoma: Diagnosis and treatment. Arch Surg (Chicago) 1939;38:24–54.

223. Govan CD, Walsh FB. Symptomatology of subdural hematoma in infants and in adults. Arch Ophthalmol 1947;37:701–715.

224. Askenasy HM, Kosary IZ, Braham J, et al. An insidiously developing form of fronto-polar extradural haematoma. Neurchirurgia (Stuttg) 1962;4:206–211.

225. El Ladki S, Segal A, Bernard M-H, et al. Hématome extra-dural chronique du vertex révélé par un oedème de stase bilatéral. Bull Soc Ophtalmol Fr 1992;92: 331–335.

226. Stevenson GC, Brown HA, Hoyt WF. Chronic venous epidural hematoma at the vertex. J Neurosurg 1964;21:887–891.

227. Luxon L, Harrison MJG. Subarachnoid hemorrhage and papilledema due to a cervical neurilemoma. J Neurosurg 1978;48:1015–1018.

228. Fahmy JA. Papilledema associated with ruptured intracranial aneurysms. Acta Ophthalmol 1972;50:793–802.

229. Griffith JQ, Jeffers WE, Fry WE. Papilledema and subarachnoid hemorrhage: Experimental and clinical study. Arch Int Med 1938;61:880.

230. Dandy WE. Intracranial Arterial Aneurysm. Ithaca NY, Comstock Publishing Co., 1944.

231. Tureen L. Lesions of the fundus associated with brain haemorrhage. Arch Neurol Psychiatr 1938;42:664–678.

232. Paton L. Diseases of the nervous system: Ocular symptoms in subarachnoid haemorrhage. Trans Am Soci UK 1924;44:110–126.

233. Weber G. Der Hirnabszess. Stuttgart, G Theime Verlag KG, 1957.

234. Hanna LS, Girgis NI, Yassin MMW, et al. Incidence of papilloedema and optic atrophy in meningitis. Jpn J Ophthalmol 1981;25:69–73.

235. Drake RL. Ocular syphilis. III. Review of the literature and report of a case of acute syphilitic meningitis and meningoencephalitis with special reference to papilledema. Arch Ophthalmol 1933;9:234–243.

236. Studer A, Leuenberger AE. Die Differentialdiagnose des Papillenödems bei Lues. Klin Mbl Augenheilk 1983;183:391–392.

237. Pedersen E. Papilledema in encephalitis. Arch Neurol 1965;13:403–408.

238. Silverstein A. Papilledema with acute viral infections of the brain. Mt Sinai Med J 1974;41:435–443.

239. Miller JD, Ross CAC. Encephalitis. A four year survey. Lancet 1968;1: 1121–1126.

240. Silverstein A. Papilledema associated with acute viral infections of the brain. Mt Sinai J Med 1974;41:435–443.

241. Applebaum E, Kreps SI, Sunshine A. Herpes zoster encephalitis. Am J Med 1962;32:25–31.

242. Mearza AA, Chan JH, Gair E, Jagger J. Herpes zoster ophthalmicus presenting as contralateral disc swelling. Eye 2000;14(Pt. 2):251–252.

243. Applebaum E, Dolgopol VB, Dolgin J. Measles encephalitis. Am J Dis Child 1949;77:25–48.

244. Cramblett HG, Stegmiller H, Spencer C. California encephalitis virus infections in children. JAMA 1966;198:128–132.

245. Dimsdale H. Acute encephalomyelitis of viral origin. In Modern Trends in Neurology (Second Series). London, Butterworth, 1957:185.

246. Silverstein A, Steinberg N, Nathanson M. Nervous system involvement in infectious mononucleosis. Arch Neurol 1972;26:353–358.

247. Wooley CF. Intracranial hypertension associated with recovery of a Coxsackie virus from the cerebrospinal fluid. Neurology 1960;10:572–574.

248. Lods F. A proposo d'un cas d'oedème papillaire au cours d'une meningoencephalite a Coksakie B2. Bull Soc Ophtalmol Fr 1971;71:725–726.

249. Cifarelli PS, Freireich AW. Rubella encephalitis. NY State J Med 1966;66: 1117–1122.

250. Ayer JB, Trevett LD. Acute poliomyelitis with choked discs: Note on prolonged observation of the spinal fluid and the use of the respirator. Arch Neurol Psychiatr 1934;31:396–402.

251. Weiman CG, McDowell FH, Plum F. Papilledema in poliomyelitis. Arch Neurol Psychiatr 1951;66:722–727.

252. Murray RG, Walsh FB. Ocular abnormalities in poliomyelitis and their pathogenesis. Can Med Assoc J 1954;70:141–147.

253. Gass HH. Papilledema and pseudotumor cerebri following poliomyelitis. Arch Ophthalmol 1957;93:640–646.

254. Green SH, Wirtschafter JD. Ophthalmoscopic findings in subacute sclerosing panencephalitis. Br J Ophthalmol 1973;57:780–787.

255. Kirkpatrick BV, David RB. Subacute sclerosing panencephalitis. J Pediatr Ophthalmol 1973;10:74–76.

256. Prevett M, Harding AE. Intracranial hypertension following psittacosis. J Neurol Neurosurg Psychiatry 1993;56:425–426.

257. Knox DL, Bayless TM, Pittman FE. Neurologic disease in patients with treated Whipple's disease. Medicine 1976;55:467–476.

258. Switz DM, Casey TR, Bogaty GV. Whipple's disease and papilledema. Arch Int Med 1969;123:74–77.

of the foramen of Monro: A ''possible'' late complication of mumps encephalitis. Clin Neurol Neurosurg 1996;95:151–154.

259. Massey JY, Roy H, Bornhofen JH. Ocular manifestations of Reye syndrome. Arch Ophthalmol 1974;91:441–444.
260. Smith P, Green WR, Miller NR, et al. Central retinal vein occlusion in Reye's syndrome. Arch Ophthalmol 1980;98:1256–1260.
261. Newman LS, Rose CS, Maier LA. Medical progress: Sarcoidosis. N Engl J Med 1997;336:1224–1234.
262. Scott TF. Neurosarcoidosis: Progress and clinical aspects. Neurology 1993;43:8–12.
263. Corbett AJ, Pollack M. Identical twins with papilloedema and cranial nerve palsies. J Neurol Neurosurg Psychiatry 1979;42:764–766.
264. Byrne JV, Lawton CA. Meningeal sarcoidosis causing intracranial hypertension secondary to dural sinus thrombosis. Br J Radiol 1983;56:755–757.
265. Akman-Demir G, Serdaroglu P, Tasçi B, et al. Clinical patterns of neurological involvement in Behçet's disease: Evaluation of 200 patients. Brain 1999;122:2171–2181.
266. Masheter HC. Behçet's syndrome complicated by intracranial thrombophlebitis. Proc R Soc Med 1959;52:1039–1040.
267. Kalbian VV, Challis MT. Behçet's disease: Report of 12 cases with three manifesting as papilledema. Am J Med 1970;49:823–829.
268. Harper CM, O'Neill BP, O'Duffy JD, et al. Intracranial hypertension in Behçet's disease: Demonstration of sinus occlusion with use of digital subtraction angiography. Mayo Clin Proc 1985;60:419–422.
269. El Ramahi KM, Al-Kawi MZ. Papilloedema in Behçet's disease: Value of MRI in diagnosis of dural sinus thrombosis. J Neurol Neurosurg Psychiatry 1991;54:826–829.
270. Pamir MN, Kansu T, Erbengi A, Zileli T. Papilledema in Behcet's syndrome. Arch Neurol 1981;38:643–645.
271. Graham EM, Al-Askar AF, Sanders MD, et al. Benign intracranial hypertension in Behçet's syndrome. Neuroophthalmology 1980;1:73–76.
272. Gökalp HZ, Basaya MK, Aydin V. Pseudotumor cerebri with familial Mediterranean fever. Clin Neurol Neurosurg 1992;94:261–263.
273. Brown JL, Anderson SF, Townsend JC, et al. Papilledema secondary to metastatic prostate disease. J Am Optom Assoc 1994;65:585–595.
274. Wolfe GI, Galetta SK, Mollman JE. Spontaneous remission of papilledema and sixth nerve palsy in acute lymphoblastic leukemia. J Neuroophthalmol 1994;14:91–94.
275. Vates GE, Chang S, Lamborn KR, Prados M, Berger MS. Gliomatosis cerebri: A review of 22 cases. Neurosurgery 2003;53:261–271.
276. Aroichane M, Miller NR, Eggenberger ER. Glioblastoma multiforme masquerading as pseudotumor cerebri: A case report. J Clin Neuroophthalmol 1993;13:105–112.
277. Baborie A, Dunn EM, Bridges LR, Bamford JM. Primary diffuse leptomeningeal gliomatosis predominantly afffecting the spinal cord: case report and review of the literature. J Neurol Neurosurg Psychiatry 2001;70:256–258.
278. Kobayashi M, Hara K, Nakatsukasa M, et al. Primary spinal leptomeningeal gliomatosis presenting visual disturbance as the initial symptom: Case report. Acta Neurochir 1996;138:480–481.
279. Cooper IS, Kernohan JW. Heterotopic glial nests in subarachnoid space: Histopathologic characteristics, mode of origin and relation to meningeal gliomas. J Neuropathol Exp Neurol 1951;10:16–29.
280. Courville CB. Pathology of the Central Nervous System: A Study Based Upon a Survey of Lesions Found in a Series of 15,000 Autopsies. Mountain View, CA, Pacific Press Publishing Association, 1931.
281. Wertheimer P, Wertheimer J, Laptas C, et al. Semeiological significance of papilledema during cranial trauma. Bull Soc Ophtalmol Fr 1963;76:275.
282. Selhorst JB, Gudeman SK, Butterworth JF IVth, et al. Papilledema after acute head injury. Neurosurgery 1985;16:357–363.
283. Arseni C, Maretsis M. Tumors of the lower spinal cord associated with increased intracranial pressure and papilledema. J Neurosurg 1967;27:105–110.
284. Nicola GC, Nizzoli V. Increased intracranial pressure and papilloedema associated with spinal tumors. Neurochirurgica 1969;12:138–144.
285. Raynor RB. Papilledema associated with tumors of the spinal cord. Neurology 1969;19:700–704.
286. Ammerman BJ, Smith DR. Papilledema and spinal cord tumors. Surg Neurol 1975;3:55–57.
287. Tankak K, Waga S, Shimosaka S. Papilledema and spinal cord tumors. Surg Neurol 1988;29:462–466.
288. Mittal MM, Gupta NC, Sharma ML. Spinal epidural meningioma associated with increased intracranial pressure. Neurology 1970;20:818–820.
289. Schijman E, Zuccaro G, Monges JA. Spinal tumors and hydrocephalus. Childs Brain 1981;8:401–405.
290. Davis TK. Double papilledema caused by blocking of cord at fourth cervical vertebra greatly relieved by operation. Arch Neurol Psychiatr 1923;9:245–246.
291. Celli P, Cervoni L, Morselli E, et al. Spinal ependymomas and papilledema: Report of 4 cases and review of the literature. J Neurol Sci 1993;37:97–102.
292. Michowiz SD, Rappaport HZ, Shaked I, et al. Thoracic disc herniation associated with papilledema: case report. J Neurosurg 1984;61:1132–1134.
293. Ford FR, Walsh FB. Guillain-Barré syndrome (acute infective polyneuritis) with increased intracranial pressure and papilledema: Report of 2 cases. Bull Johns Hopkins Hosp 1943;73:391–395.
294. Popek K. Recurrent Guillain-Barré syndrome with recurrent papilledema. Cesk Neurol 1957;20:380–393.
295. Sullivan RL Jr, Reeves AG. Normal cerebrospinal fluid protein, increased intracranial pressure, and the Guillain-Barré syndrome. Ann Neurol 1977;1:108–109.
296. Denny-Brown DE. The changing pattern of neurological medicine. N Engl J Med 1952;246:839–846.
297. Joynt RJ. The mechanism of production of papilledema in the Guillain-Barré syndrome. Neurology 1958;8:8–12.
298. Morley JB, Reynolds EG. Papilloedema and the Landry-Guillain-Barré syndrome. Brain 1966;89:205–222.
299. Davidson DLW, Jellinek EG. Hypertension and papilloedema in the Guillain-Barré syndrome. J Neurol Neurosurg Psychiatry 1977;40:144–148.
300. Ropper AH, Marmarou A. Mechanism of pseudotumor in Guillain-Barré syndrome. Arch Neurol 1984;41:259–261.
301. Austin JH. Recurrent polyneuropathies and their corticosteroid treatment: With five-year observations of placebo-controlled case treated with corticotropin, cortisone, and prednisone. Brain 1958;81:157–192.
302. Mendell JR. Chronic inflammatory demyelinating polyradiculoneuropathy. Annu Rev Med 1993;44:211–219.
303. Fantin A, Feist RM, Reddy CV. Intracranial hypertension and papilloedema in chronic inflammatory demyelinating polyneuropathy. Br J Ophthalmol 1993;77:193.
304. Kotil K, Kalayci M, Koseoglu T, Turgrul A. Myelinoclastic diffuse sclerosis (Schilder's disease): report of a case and review of the literature. Br J Neurosurgery 2002;16:516–519.
305. McCrary J, Demer J, Friedman D, Mawad M. Computed tomography and MRI in the diagnosis of inflammatory disease of the optic nerve. Surv Ophthalmol 1987;31:352–355.
306. Newman NJ, Selzer KA, Bell RA. Association of multiple sclerosis and intracranial hypertension. J Neuroophthalmol 1994;14:189–192.
307. Pshezhetsky AV, Ashmarina M. Lysosomal multienzyme complex: biochemistry, genetics and molecular pathophysiology. Prog Nucleic Acid Res Mol Biol 2001;69:81–114.
308. Shinnar S, Singer HS, Valle D. Acute hydrocephalus in Hurler's syndrome. Am J Dis Child 1982;136:556–557.
309. Sheridan MM, Johnston I. Hydrocephalus and pseudotumor cerebri in the mucopolysaccharidoses. Childs Nerv Syst 1994;10:148–150.
310. Goldberg MF, Scott CI, McKusick VA. Hydrocephalus and papilledema in the Maroteaux-Lamy syndrome (Mucopolysaccharidosis type VI). Am J Ophthalmol 1970;69:969–975.
311. Beck M. Papilloedema in association with Hunter's syndrome. Br J Ophthalmol 1983;67:174–177.
312. Chen YF, Huang YC, Liu HM, Hwu WL. MRI in a case of adult-onset citrullinemia. Neuroradiology 2001;43:845–847.
313. Wilson CJ, Lee PJ, Leonard JV. Plasma glutamine and ammonia concentrations in ornithine carbamoyltransferase deficiency and citrullinaemia. J Inherit Metab Dis 2001;24:691–695.
314. Hayasaka S, Tabata K, Ohmura M, et al. Papilloedema in late-onset cirtullinemia: Report of a second case. Graefe's Arch Clin Exp Ophthalmol 1984;221:262–264.
315. Friedman DI, Jacobson DM. Diagnostic criteria for idiopathic intracranial hypertension. Neurology 2002;59:1492–1495.
316. Bertelsen TI. The premature synostosis of the cranial sutures. Acta Ophthalmol 1958;51(Suppl):1–176.
317. Tuite GF, Chong WK, Evanson J, et al. The effectiveness of papilledema as an indicator of raised intracranial pressure in children with craniosynostosis. Neurosurgery 1996;38:272–278.
318. Dollfus H, Vinikoff L, Renier D, et al. Insidious craniosynostosis and chronic papilledema in childhood. Am J Ophthalmol 1996;122:910–911.
319. Uhthoff W. Zur pathogenese der sehstorungen bei schadeleformitat. Berlin Ophthalmol Gesellsch Heidelberg 1910;36:140.
320. Jensch PA. Zur genealogie und klinik des turmschadels. Arch Psychiatr 1942;114:444.
321. Nager FR, de Raynier PJ. Das gehororgan be angeborenen kopfmissbidungen. Prac Otorhinolaryng 1948;10(Suppl 2):1.
322. David LR, Velotta E, Weaver RG Jr, Wilson JA, Argenta LC. Clinical findings precede objective diagnostic testing in the identification of increased ICP in syndromic craniosynostosis. J Craniofac Surg 2002;13:676–680.
323. Brenner RL, Smith JL, Cleveland WW, et al. Eye signs of hyphosphatasia. Ophthalmology 1969;81:614–617.
324. Beighton P, Durr L, Harrersma H. The clinical features of sclerosteosis. Ann Intern Med 1976;84:393–397.
325. Golnik KC, Kersten RC. Optic nerve head swelling in the Hadju-Cheney syndrome. J Neuroophthalmol 1998;18:60–65.
326. Crow RS. Peripheral neuritis in myelomatosis. Br Med J 1956;2:802–804.
327. Bardwick PA, Zvaifler NJ, Gill GN, et al. Plasma cell dyscrasia with polyneuropathy, organomegaly, endocrinopathy, M protein and skin changes: The POEMS syndrome. Medicine 1980;59:311–322.
328. Soubrier MJ, Dubost J-J, Sauvezie BJM, et al. POEMS Syndrome: A study of 25 cases and a review of the literature. Am J Med 1994;97:543–553.

329. Piette WW. Myeloma, paraproteinemias, and the skin. Med Clin North Am 1986;70:155–176.
330. Sasaki A, Kogure M, Shimomura M, et al. A case of Crow-Fukase syndrome associated with empty sella. Folia Ophthalmol Jpn 1995;46:324–328.
331. Bourdette DN, Rosenberg NL. Infiltrative orbitopathy, optic disk edema, and POEMS. Neurology 1984;34:532–533.
332. Spielmann AC, Angioi-Duprez K, Dorvaux V, et al. Oedème papillaire et syndrome POEMS. J Fr Ophthalmol 1996;19:467–469.
333. Munteanu GH, Munteanu M, Budau M. Papilloedema and POEMS syndrome. Oftalmologia 2001;53:35–44.
334. Sugita K, Kayama T, Ohwada K, et al. A case of multiple myeloma showing intracranial hypertension due to a large cranial mass lesion. No To Shinkei 1986;38:6259.
335. Collier A, Ashworth B. Multiple plasmacytoma presenting as raised intracranial pressure. J Neurol Neurosurg Psychiatry 1987;50:495–496.
336. Wasan H, Mansi JL, Benjamin S, et al. Myeloma and benign intracranial hypertension. BMJ 1992;304:685.
337. Blackman SS. The lesions of lead encephalitis in children. Bull Johns Hopkins Hosp 1937;61:1–61.
338. Lidsky TI, Schneider JS. Lead neurotoxicity in children: basic mechanisms and clinical correlates. Brain 2003;126:5–19.
339. Dickman MS, Somasundaram M, Brzozowski L. Pseudotumor cerebri and hyperthyroidism. NY State J Med 1980;80:1118–1120.
340. Stern BJ, Gruen R, Koeppel J, et al. Recurrent thyrotoxicosis and papilledema in a patient with communicating hydrocephalus. Arch Neurol 1984;41:65–67.
341. Bettman JW Jr, Daroff RB, Sanders MD, Hoyt WF. Edema of the optic disc in hyperthyroidism without exophthalmos: A fluorescein angiographic study of its resolution. Am J Ophthalmol 1968;66:714–719.
342. Quincke H. Uber meningitis serosa und verewandte zustande. Deutsche Zeitschrift fur Nervenheilkunde 1897;9:149–168.
343. McAlpine D. Toxic hydrocephalus. Brain 1937;60:180–203.
344. Symonds CP. Otitic hydrocephalus. Neurology 1952;6:681–685.
345. Davidoff LM, Dyke CG. Hypertensive meningeal hydrops: Syndrome frequently following infection in middle ear or elsewhere in body. Am J Ophthalmol 1937;20:908–927.
346. Sahs AL, Joynt RJ. Brain swelling of unknown cause. Neurology 1956;6:791–803.
347. Sahs AL, Hyndman OR. Intracranial hypertension of unknown cause: Cerebral edema. Arch Surg 1939;38:429–434.
348. Yaskin JC, Groff RA, Shenkin HA. Severe bilateral papilledema of indeterminate etiology with report of 12 cases. Confin Neurol 1949;9:108–112.
349. Warrington WB. Intracranial serous effusions of inflammatory origin: Meningitis ependymitis serosa—meningism—with note on "pseudo-tumors" of the brain. Q J Med 1914;7:93–118.
350. Foley J. Benign forms of intracranial hypertension: "Toxic" and "otitic hydrocephalus." Brain 1955;78:1–41.
351. Bucheit WA, Burton C, Haag B, et al. Papilledema and idiopathic intracranial hypertension. N Engl J Med 1969;280:938–942.
352. Bandyopadhyay S, Jacobson DM. Clinical features of late life-onset pseudotumor cerebri fulfilling the Modified Dandy Criteria. J Neuroophthalmol 2002;22:9–11.
353. Rose A, Matson DD. Benign intracranial hypertension in children. Pediatrics 1967;39:227–237.
354. Grant DN. Benign intracranial hypertension: A review of 79 cases in infancy and childhood. Arch Dis Child 1971;46:651–655.
355. Weisberg LA, Chutorian AM. Pseudotumor cerebri of children. Am J Dis Child 1977;131:1243–1248.
356. Baker RS, Baumann RJ, Buncic JR. Idiopathic intracranial hypertension (pseudotumor cerebri) in pediatric patients. Pediatr Neurol 1989;5:5–11.
357. Lessell S. Pediatric pseudotumor cerebri (idiopathic intracranial hypertension). Surv Ophthalmol 1992;37:155–166.
358. Durcan FJ, Corbett JJ, Wall M. The incidence of pseudotumor cerebri. Population studies in Iowa and Louisiana. Arch Neurol 1988;45:875–877.
359. Radhakrishanan K, Ahlskog JE, Cross SA, Kurland LT, O'Fallon WM. Idiopathic intracranial hypertension (pseudotumor cerebri): Descriptive epidemiology in Rochester, Minn, 1976–1990. Arch Neurol 1993;50:78–80.
360. Radhakrishanan K, Sridharan R, Askhok PP, et al. Pseudotumor cerebri: incidence and pattern in north-eastern Libya. Acta Neurologica 1986;25:117–124.
361. Kesler A, Gadoth N. Epidemiology of idiopathic intracranial hypertension in Israel. J Neuroophthalmol 2001;21:12–14.
362. Johnston IH, Paterson A. Benign intracranial hypertension. I. Diagnosis and prognosis. Brain 1974;97:289–300.
363. Winner P, Bello L. Idiopathic intracranial hypertension in a young child without visual symptoms or signs. Headache 1996;36:574–576.
364. Johnston I, Paterson S. Benign intracranial hypertension. II. Cerebrospinal fluid pressure and circulation. Brain 1974;97:301–312.
365. Wall M, Giuseffi V, Rojas PB. Symptoms and disease associations in pseudotumor cerebri: A case-control study. Neurology 1989;39:210.
366. Giuseffi V, Wall M, Spiegel PZ, et al. Symptoms and disease associations in idiopathic intracranial hypertension (pseudotumor cerebri): A case-control study. Neurology 1991;41:239–244.
367. Wall M, George D. Idiopathic intracranial hypertension: A prospective study of 50 patients. Brain 1991;114:155–180.
368. Akova YA, Kansu T, Yazar Z, et al. Macular subretinal neovascular membrane associated with pseudotumor cerebri. J Neuroophthalmol 1994;14:193–195.
369. Rowe FJ. Ocular motility disturbances in benign intracranial hypertension. Br Orthop J 1996;53:22–24.
370. Felton WL, Sismanis A. Otologic aspects of idiopathic intracranial hypertension in patients with and without papilledema. Neuroophthalmology 1996;16(Suppl):279.
371. Corbett JJ. Problems in the diagnosis and treatment of pseudotumor cerebri. Can J Neurol Sci 1983;10:221–229.
372. Kiwak LJ, Levine SE. Benign intracranial hypertension and facial diplegia. Arch Neurol 1984;41:787–788.
373. Davie C, Kennedy P, Katifi HA. Seventh nerve palsy as a false localising sign. J Neurol Neurosurg Psychiatry 1992;55:510–511.
374. Selky AK, Dobyns WB, Yee RD. Idiopathic intracranial hypertension and facial diplegia. Neurology 1994;44:357.
375. Capobianco DJ, Brazis PW, Cheshire WP. Idiopathic intracranial hypertension and seventh nerve palsy. Headache 1997;37:286–288.
376. Chutorian AM, Gold AP, Braun CW. Benign intracranial hypertension and Bell's palsy. N Engl J Med 1977;296:1214–1215.
377. Selky AK, Purvin VA. Hemifacial spasm: An ususual manifestation of idiopathic intracranial hypertension. J Neuroophthalmol 1994;14:196–198.
378. Benegas NM, Volpe NJ, Liu GT, et al. Hemifacial spasm and idiopathic intracranial hypertension. J Neuroophthalmol 1996;16:70.
379. Davenport RJ, Will RG, Galloway PJ. Isolated intracranial hypertension presenting with trigeminal neuropathy. J Neurol Neurosurg Psychiatry 1994;57:381–386.
380. Dorman PJ, Campbell MJ. Hearing loss as a false localising sign in raised intracranial pressure. J Neurol Neurosurg Psychiatry 1995;58:516.
381. Jöbges EM, Johannes S, Schubert M, et al. Mononeuropathia multiplex and idiopathic intracranial hypertension. Clin Neurol Neurosurg 1996;98:37–39.
382. Bortoluzzi M, Di Lauro L, Marini G. Benign intracranial hypertension with spinal and radicular pain. J Neurosurg 1982;57:833–836.
383. Round R, Keane JR. The minor symptoms of increased intracranial pressure: 101 patients with benign intracranial hypertension. Neurology 1988;38:1461–1464.
384. Zachariah SB, Jiminez L, Zachariah B, et al. Pseudotumor cerebri with focal neurological deficit. J Neurol Neurosurg Psychiatry 1990;53:360–361.
385. Kleinschmidt JJ, Digre KB, Hanover R. Idiopathic intracranial hypertension: Relationship to depression, anxiety, and quality of life. Neurology 2000;54:319–324.
386. Soelberg Sørensen P, Thomsen AM, Gjerris F. Persistent disturbances of cognitive functions in patients with pseudotumor cerebri. Acta Neurol Scand 1986;73:264–268.
387. Kaplan CP, Miner ME, McGregor JM. Pseudotumor cerebri: Risk for cognitive impairment? Brain Injury 1997;11:293–303.
388. Boddie HG, Banna M, Bradley WG. "Benign" intracranial hypertension. Brain 1974;97:313–326.
389. Wang S-J, Silberstein SD, Patterson S, Young WB. Idiopathic intracranial hypertension without papilledema: A case-control study in a headache center. Neurology 1998;51:245–249.
390. Huff AL, Hupp SL, Rothrock JF. Chronic daily headache with migrainous features due to papilledema-negative idiopathic intracranial hypertension. Cephalalgia 1996;16:451–452.
391. Spence JD, Amacher AL, Willis NR. Benign intracranial hypertension without papilledema: Role of 24-hour cerebrospinal fluid pressure monitoring in diagnosis and management. Neurosurgery 1980;34:1509–1511.
392. Sergott RC, Savino PJ, Bosley TM. Modified optic nerve sheath decompression provides long-term visual improvement for pseudotumor cerebri. Arch Ophthalmol 1988;106:1384–1390.
393. Mansour AM, Zatorski J. Analysis of variables for papilledema in pseudotumor cerebri. Ann Ophthalmol 1994;26:172–174.
394. Torun N, Sharpe JA. Pseudotumor cerebri mimicking Foster Kennedy syndrome. Neuroophthalmology 1996;16:55–57.
395. Ecker A. Irregular fluctuation of elevated cerebrospinal fluid pressure. Arch Neurol Psychiatry 1955;74:641–649.
396. Khandhar S, Friedman DI. Cerebrospinal fluid measurements in patients experiencing severe, benign headaches. Headache 2003;43:553–554.
397. Chandra V, Bellue SN, Anderson RJ. Low CSF protein concentration in idiopathic pseudotumor cerebri. Ann Neurol 1986;14:1127–1130.
398. Johnston PK, Corbett JJ, Maxner CE. Cerebrospinal fluid protein and opening pressure in idiopathic intracranial hypertension (pseudotumor cerebri). Neurology 1991;41:1040–1042.
399. Jacobson DM, Karanjia PN, Olson KA, et al. Computed tomography ventricular size has no predictive value in diagnosing pseudotumor cerebri. Neurology 1990;40:1454–1455.
400. Silbergleit R, Junck L, Gebarski SS, Hatfield MK. Idiopathic intracranial hypertension (pseudotumor cerebri): MR imaging. Neuroradiology 1989;170:207–209.
401. Foley KM, Posner JB. Does pseudotumor cerebri cause the empty sella syndrome? Neurology 1975;25:565–569.

402. De Vries-Knoppert WAEJ. Primary empty sella syndrome and benign intracranial hypertension. Doc Ophthalmol 1986;61:319–325.
403. Weisberg LA, Housepain EM, Saur DP. Empty sella syndrome as complication of benign intracranial hypertension. J Neurosurg 1975;43:177–180.
404. Gass A, Barker GJ, Riordan-Eva P, et al. MRI of the optic nerve in benign intracranial hypertension. Neuroradiology 1996;38:769–773.
405. Jinkins JR, Zthale S, Xiong A, et al. MR of the optic papilla protrusion in patients with high intracranial pressure. AJNR 1996;17:665–668.
406. Manfré L, Lagalla R, Mangiameli A, et al. Idiopathic intracranial hypertension: Orbital MRI. Neuroradiology 1995;37:459–461.
407. Shuper A, Snir M, Barash D, et al. Ultrasonography of the optic nerves: clinical application in children with pseudotumor cerebri. J Pediatrics 1997;131:734–740.
408. Digre KB, Corbett JJ. Pseudotumor cerebri in men. Arch Neurol 1988;45:866–872.
409. Digre KB, Corbett JJ. Idiopathic intracranial hypertension (pseudotumor cerebri): A reappraisal. Neurologist 2001;7:2–67.
410. Friedman DI. Papilledema and pseudotumor cerebri. Neurol Clin 2001;14:129–147.
411. Byers RK, Haas GM. Thrombosis of the dural venous sinuses in infancy and in childhood. Am J Dis Child 1933;45:1161–1183.
412. Greer M. Benign intracranial hypertension. I. Mastoiditis and lateral sinus obstruction. Neurology 1962;12:472–476.
413. Greer M. Benign intracranial hypertension in children. Pediatr Clin North Am 1967;14:819–830.
414. Purvin VA, Trobe JD, Kosmorsky G. Neuro-ophthalmic features of cerebral venous obstruction. Arch Neurol 1995;52:880–885.
415. Biousse V, Ameri A, Bousser M-G. Isolated intracranial hypertension as the only sign of cerebral venous thrombosis. Neurology 1999;53:1537–1542.
416. Lam BL, Schatz NJ, Glaser JS, Bowen BC. Pseudotumor cerebri from cranial venous obstruction. Ophthalmology 1992;99:706–712.
417. Horton JC, Seiff SR, Pitts LH, et al. Decompression of the optic nerve sheath for vision-threatening papilledema caused by dural sinus occlusion. Neurosurgery 1992;31:203–212.
418. Wen DY, Hardten DR, Wirtschafter JD, et al. Elevated intracranial pressure from cerebral venous obstruction by Masson's vegetant intravascular hemangioendothelioma. J Neurosurg 1991;75:787–790.
419. Truong DD, Holgate RC, Hsu CY, et al. Occlusion of the transverse sinus by meningioma simulating pseudotumor cerebri. Neuroophthalmology 1987;7:113–117.
420. Lenz RP, McDonald GA. Otitic hydrocephalus. Laryngoscope 1984;94:1451–1454.
421. Dill JL, Crowe SJ. Thrombosis of the sygmoid or lateral sinus: Report of thirty cases. Arch Surg 1934;29:705–722.
422. Castillok IG, Foroozan R, Sergott RC. A sticky situation. Surv Ophthalmol 2002;47:491–499.
423. Bergui M, Bradac GB. Clinical picture of patients with cerebral venous thrombosis and patterns of dural sinus involvement. Cerebrovasc Dis 2003;16:211–216.
424. Weib M, Junge-Hulsung J, Mehraein S, Ziemer S, Einhaupl KM. Hereditary thrombophilia with ischemic stroke and sinus thrombosis: Diagnosis, therapy and meta-analysis. Nervenarzt 2000;71:936–945.
425. Reuner KH, Ruf A, Grau A, et al. Prothrombin gene G20210 to A transition is a risk factor for cerebral venous thrombosis. Stroke 1998;29:1765–1769.
426. van Krimpen J, Leebeek FW, Dippel DW, Gomez Garcia E. Prothrombin gene variant (G20210A) in a patient with cerebral venous sinus thrombosis. Clin Neurol Neurosurg 1999;101:53–55.
427. Provenzale JM, Barboriak DP, Ortel TL. Dural sinus thrombosis associated with activated protein C resistance: MR imaging findings and proband identification. AJR 1998;170:499–502.
428. Alper C, Berrak SG, Ekinci G, Canpolat C, Erzen C. Sagittal sinus thrombosis associated with thrombocytopenia: a report of two patients. Pediatr Neurol 1999;21:573–575.
429. Ishihara K, Arai D, Ichikawa H, Kawamura M. A case of cerebral deep venous and venous sinus thromboses with anti-cardiolipin antibody. No To Shinkei 2003;55:71–76.
430. Furuta M, Satoh S, Toriumi T, et al. An autopsy case of cerebral sinus thrombosis which showed papilledema and was accompanied by idiopathic thrombocytopenic purpura. Acta Soc Ophthalmol Jpn 1991;95:199–203.
431. Gettelfinger DM, Kokmen E. Superior sagittal sinus thrombosis. Arch Neurol 1977;34:2–6.
432. Sigsbee B, Deck M, Posner J. Nonmetastatic superior sagittal sinus thrombosis complicating systemic cancer. Neurology 1979;29:139–146.
433. Digre KB, Varner MV, Corbett JJ. Pseudotumor cerebri and pregnancy. Neurology 1984;34:721–729.
434. Mitchell D, Fisher J, Irving D, et al. Lateral sinus thrombosis and intracranial hypertension in essential thrombocythaemia. J Neurol Neurosurg Psychiatry 1986;49:218–219.
435. Shiozawa S, Yoshida M, Kobayashi K, et al. Superior sagittal sinus thrombosis and systemic lupus erythematosis. Ann Neurol 1986;20:272.
436. Esack A, Thompson G, Burmester H. Benign intracranial hypertension and essential thrombocythaemia. J Neurol Neurosurg Psychiatry 1989;52:914–922.
437. Mokri B, Jack CR Jr, Petty GW. Pseudotumor syndrome associated with cerebral venous sinus occlusion and antiphospholipid antibodies. Stroke 1993;24:469–472.
438. Confavreux C, Brunet P, Petiot P, et al. Congenital protein C deficiency and superior sagittal sinus thrombosis causing isolated intracranial hypertension. J Neurol Neurosurg Psychiatry 1994;57:655–657.
439. Mones RJ. Increased intracranial pressure due to metastatic disease of venous sinuses. Neurology 1965;15:1000–1007.
440. Lam BL, Schatz NJ, Glaser JS, et al. Pseudotumor cerebri from cranial venous obstruction. Ophthalmology 1992;99:706–712.
441. Blervacque A, Béal F, Malbrel P. Papilledema after an operation at the level of the neck. Bull Soc Ophthalmol Fr 1965;65:135–136.
442. Fitz-Hugh GS, Robins RB, Craddock WD. Increased intracranial pressure complicating unilateral neck dissection. Laryngoscope 1966;76:893–906.
443. Tobin HA. Increased cerebrospinal fluid pressure following unilateral radical neck dissection. Laryngoscope 1971;82:817–820.
444. De Vries WAEJ, Balm AJM, Tiwari RM. Intracranial hypertension following neck dissection. J Laryngol Otol 1986;100:1427–1431.
445. Davidoff LM. Pseudotumor cerebri: Benign intracranial hypertension. Neurology 1956;6:605–615.
446. Patterson R, DePasquale N, Mann S. Pseudotumor cerebri. Medicine 1961;40:85–99.
447. Greer M. Benign intracranial hypertension. VI. Obesity. Neurology 1965;15:382–388.
448. Wilson DH, Gardner WJ. Benign intracranial hypertension with particular reference to its occurrence in fat young women. Can Med Assoc J 1966;95:102–105.
449. Ireland B, Corbett JJ. The search for causes of idiopathic intracranial hypertension. Arch Neurol 1990;47:315–320.
450. Greer M. Benign intracranial hypertension. V. Menstrual dysfunction. Neurology 1964;14:668–673.
451. Balcer LJ, Liu GT, Forman S, et al. Idiopathic intracranial hypertension: Relation of age and obesity in children. Neurology 1999;52:870–872.
452. Gordon K. Pediatric pseudotumor cerebri: Descriptive epidemiology. Can J Neurol Sci 1997;24:219–221.
453. Greer M. Benign intracranial hypertension. IV. Menarche. Neurology 1964;14:569–573.
454. Tessler Z, Biender N, Yassur Y. Papilloedema: Benign intracranial hypertension in menarche. Arch Ophthalmol 1985;17:76–77.
455. Chen KFC, Kurtzman N, Frenkel M. Plasma renin activity and aldosterone determination in patients with pseudotumor cerebri. Ann Ophthalmol 1979;11:563–565.
456. Friedman DI, Streeten DHP. Idiopathic intracranial hypertension and orthostatic edema may share a common pathogenesis. Neurology 1998;50:1099–1104.
457. McCullagh EP. Menstrual edema with intracranial hypertension (pseudotumor cerebri): Report of a case. Cleve Clin Q 1941;8:202–212.
458. Greer M. Benign intracranial hypertension. III. Pregnancy. Neurology 1963;13:670–672.
459. Nickerson CW, Kirk RF. Recurrent pseudotumor cerebri in pregnancy: Report of 2 cases. Obstet Gynecol 1965;26:811–813.
460. Meythaler H, Meythaler-Radeck B. Zur frage des pseudotumors cerebri. Klin Mbl Augenheilk 1973;163:200–204.
461. Koontz WL, Hebert WNP, Cefalo RC. Pseudotumor cerebri in pregnancy. Obstet Gynecol 1983;62:324–327.
462. Kassam SH, Hadi HA, Fadel HE, et al. Benign intracranial hypertension in pregnancy: Current diagnostic and therapeutic approach. Obstet Gynecol Surv 1983;38:314–321.
463. Levy HA. Unusual clinical manifestations of chronic hypoparathyroidism. Med Clin North Am 1947;31:243–253.
464. Mortell EJ. Idiopathic hypoparathyroidism with mental deterioration: Effect of treatment on intellectual function. J Clin Endocrinol 1946;6:266–274.
465. Grant DK. Papilledema and fits in hypoparathyroidism. Q J Med 1953;22:243–259.
466. Palmer RF, Searles HH, Boldrey EB. Papilledema and hypoparathyroidism simulating brain tumor. J Neurosurg 1959;16:378–384.
467. Sambrook MA, Hill LF. Cerebrospinal fluid absorption in primary hypoparathyroidism. J Neurol Neurosurg Psychiatry 1977;40:1015–1017.
468. Baker BF, Blaustein MP, Hodgkin AL, et al. The influence of calcium on sodium efflux in squid axon. J Physiol 1969;200:431–458.
469. O'Doherty NJ. Acute benign intracranial hypertension in an infant receiving tetracycline. Dev Med Child Neurol 1965;7:677–680.
470. Olson CA, Riley HD Jr. Complications of tetracycline therapy. J Pediatr 1966;68:783–791.
471. Giles CL, Soble AR. Intracranial hypertension and tetracycline therapy. Am J Ophthalmol 1971;72:981–982.
472. Maroon JC, Mealy J Jr. Benign intracranial hypertension. Sequel to tetracycline therapy in a child. JAMA 1971;216:1479–1480.
473. Stuart BH, Litt IF. Tetracycline-induced intracranial hypertension in an adolescent: A complication of systemic acne therapy. J Pediatrics 1978;92:679–680.

474. Ohlrich GD, Ohlrich JG. Papilloedema in an adolescent due to tetracycline. Med J Australia 1977;1:334–335.

475. Köch-Weser J, Gilmore EB. Benign intracranial hypertension in an adult after tetracycline therapy. JAMA 1967;200:169–171.

476. Gardner K, Cox T, Digre K. Idiopathic intracranial hypertension associated with tetracycline use in fraternal twins: Case report and review. Neurology 1995;45:6–10.

477. Xenard L, George J-L, Maalouf T, et al. Les effets indésirables ptentiels des tétracyclines: A propos de deux observations. Bull Soc Ophtalmol Fr 1996;96:154–157.

478. Le Bris P, Glacet-Bernard A, Coscas G, et al. Oedème papillaire dû à la minocycline. J Fr Ophtalmol 1988;11:681–684.

479. Lander CM. Minocycline-induced benign intracranial hypertension. Clin Exp Neurol 1989;26:161–167.

480. Donnet A, Dufour H, Graziani N, Grisoli F. Minocycline and benign intracranial hypertension. Biomed Pharmacother 1992;46:171–172.

481. Chiu AM, Chuenkongkaew WL, Cornblath WT, et al. Minocycline treatment and pseudotumor cerebri syndrome. Am J Ophthalmol 1998;126:116–121.

482. Beran RG. Pseudotumor cerebri associated with minocycline therapy for acne. Med J Australia 1980;1:323–324.

483. Granholm L. Papilloedema in treatment with doxycycline. Lakartidningen 1976;73:3447.

484. Friedman DI, Gordon LK, Egan RA, et al. Doxycycline and intracranial hypertension. Neurology 2004;62:2297–2299.

485. Lochhead J, Elston JS. Doxycycline induced intracranial hypertension. Br Med J 2003;326:641–642.

486. Boreus LO, Sundstrom B. Intracranial hypertension in a child during treatment with nalidixic acid. Br Med J 1967;2:744–745.

487. Cohen DN. Intracranial hypertension and papilledema associated with nalidixic acid therapy. Am J Ophthalmol 1973;76:680–682.

488. Mukherjee A, Dutta B, Lahiri M, et al. Benign intracranial hypertension after nalidixic acid overdose in infants. Lancet 1990;335:1602.

489. Dees SC, McKay HW Jr. Occurrence of pseudotumor cerebri during treatment of children with asthma by adrenal steroids. Pediatrics 1959;23:1143–1151.

490. Walker AE, Adamkiewitz JJ. Pseudotumor cerebri associated with prolonged corticosteroid therapy. JAMA 1964;188:779–784.

491. Cohn GA. Pseudotumor cerebri in children secondary to administration of adrenal steroids. J Neurosurg 1963;20:784–786.

492. Greer M. Benign intracranial hypertension. II. Following corticosteroid therapy. Neurology 1963;13:439–441.

493. Neville BGR, Wilson J. Benign intracranial hypertension following corticosteroid withdrawal in childhood. Br Med J 1970;3:554–556.

494. Liu GT, Kay MD, Bienfang DC, Schatz NJ. Pseudotumor cerebri associated with corticosteroid withdrawal in inflammatory bowel disease. Am J Ophthalmol 1994;117:352–357.

495. Fukuda S, Kogure M, Ohsawa M. A case of pseudotumor cerebri after renal transplantation. Folia Ophthalmol Jpn 1990;41:1850–1857.

496. Wigglesworth R. Pituitary-adrenal function after topical steroids. Lancet 1967;2:1209.

497. Arbenz JP, Wormser P. Pseudotumor cerebri by sex hormones. Schweiz Med Wochenschr 1965;95:1954–1956.

498. Cogan DG. Oral contraceptives having neuro-ophthalmic complications. Arch Ophthalmol 1965;73:461–462.

499. Walsh FB. Oral contraceptives and neuro-ophthalmologic interest. Arch Ophthalmol 1965;74:628–640.

500. Longueville E, Dautheribes M, Williamson W, et al. L'hypertension intra-cranienne dite aigue bégnigne iatrogène: A propos d'un cas. Bull Soc Ophtalmol Fr 1990;90:1009–1012.

501. Marie J, See G. Acute hypervitaminosis A of the infant. Its clinical manifestation with benign acute hydrocephaly and pronounced bulge of the fontanel: A clinical and biologic study. Am J Dis Child 1954;73:731–736.

502. Persson B, Tunell R, Ekengren K. Chronic vitamin A intoxication during the first half year of life: Description of 5 cases. Acta Paediatr Scand 1965;54:49–60.

503. Manhoney CP, Margolis T, Knauss TA, et al. Chronic vitamin A intoxication in infants fed chicken liver. Pediatrics 1980;65:893–896.

504. Gerber A, Raab AR. Vitamin A poisoning in adults. With a description of a case. Am J Med 1954;16:729–745.

505. Spector RH, Carlisle J. Pseudotumor cerebri caused by a synthetic vitamin A preparation. Neurology 1984;34:1509–1511.

506. Marcus DF, Turgeon P, Aaberg TM, et al. Optic disk findings in hypervitaminosis A. Ann Ophthalmol 1985;17:397–402.

507. Selhorst JB, Waybright EA, Jennings S, Corbett JJ. Liver lover's headache; pseudotumor cerebri and vitamin A intoxication. JAMA 1984;252:3364.

508. Morrice G Jr, Havener WH, Kapetansky F. Vitamin A intoxication as a cause of pseudotumor cerebri. JAMA 1960;173:1802–1805.

509. Fraunfelder FW, Fraunfelder FT, Corbett JJ. Isotretinoin usage and intracranial hypertension. Ophthalmology 2004;111:1275–1279.

510. Fraunfelder FW, Fraunfelder FT, Edwards R. Ocular side effects possibly associated with isotretinoin usage. Am J Ophthalmol 2001;132:299–305.

511. Sano F, Tsuji K, Kunika N, et al. Pseudotumor cerebri in a patient with acute promyelocytic leukemia during treatment with all-trans retinoic acid. Int Med 1998;37:546–549.

512. Tiamkao S, Sirijirachai C. Pseudotumor cerebri caused by all-trans-retinoic acid. J Med Asso Thailand 2000;83:1420–1423.

513. Decaudin D, Adams D, Naccache P, Castagna L, Munck JN. Maintained all-trans retinoic acid therapy with pseudotumor cerebri despite aggreved symptoms. Leuk Lymphoma 1997;27(3–4):373–374.

514. Visani G, Manfroi S, Tosi P, et al. All-trans-retinoic acid and pseudotumor cerebri. Leuk Lymphoma 1996;23:437–442.

515. Kasarskis EJ, Bass NH. Benign intracranial hypertension induced by deficiency of vitamin A during infancy. Neurology 1982;32:1292–1295.

516. Blethen SL. Complications of growth hormone therapy in children. Curr Opin Pediatr 1995;7:466–471.

517. Grancois I, Castells I, Silberstein J, Casaer P, deZegher F. Empty sella, growth hormone deficiency and pseudotumour cerebri: Effect of initiation, withdrawal and resumption of growth hormone therapy. Eur J Pediatr 1997;156:69–70.

518. Malozozwski S, Tanner LA, Wysowski DK, Fleming GA, Stadel BV. Benign intracranial hypertension in children with growth hormone deficiency treated with growth hormone. J Pediatr 1995;126:996–999.

519. Rogers AH, Rogers GL, Bremer DL, McGregor ML. Pseudotumor cerebri in children receiving recombinant human growth hormone. Ophthalmology 1999;106:1186–1190.

520. Price DA, Clayton PE, Lloyd IC. Benign intracranial hypertension induced by growth hormone treatment. Lancet 1995;345(458–459).

521. Wysowski DK, Green L. Serious adverse events in Norplant users reported to the Food and Drug Administration's MedWatch spontaneous reporting system. Obstet Gynecol 1995;85:538–542.

522. Alder J, Fraunfelder F, Edwards R, et al. Levonorgestrel implants and intracranial hypertension. N Engl J Med 1995;332:1720–1721.

523. Sunku AJ, O'Duffy AE, Swanson JW. Benign intracranial hypertension associated with levonorgestrel implants. Ann Neurol 1993;34:299.

524. Bourruat F-X, Regli F. Pseudotumor cerebri as a complication of amiodarone therapy. Am J Ophthalmol 1993;116:776–777.

525. Fikkers BG, Bogousslavsky J, Regli F, et al. Pseudotumor cerebri with amiodarone. J Neurol Neurosurg Psychiatry 1986;49:606.

526. Van Zandijcke M, Dewachter A. Pseudotumor cerebri and amiodarone. J Neurol Neurosurg Psychiatry 1986;49:1463–1464.

527. Grogan WA, Narkun DM. Pseudotumor cerebri with amiodarone. J Neurol Neurosurg Psychiatry 1987;50:651.

528. Hamed LM, Glaser JS, Schatz NJ, et al. Pseudotumor cerebri induced by danazol. Am J Ophthalmol 1989;107:105–110.

529. Shah A, Roberts R, McQueen IN, et al. Danazol and benign intracranial hypertension. Br Med J 1989;294:1323.

530. Fanous M, Hamed LM, Margo CE. Pseudotumor cerebri associated with danazol withdrawal. JAMA 1991;266:1218–1219.

531. Arber N, Fadila R, Pinkhas J, et al. Pseudotumor cerebri associated with leuprorelin acetate. Lancet 1990;335:668.

532. Fraunfelder FT, Edwards R. Possible ocular adverse effects associated with leuprolide injections. JAMA 1995;273:773–774.

533. Saul RF, Hamburger HA, Selhorst JB. Pseudotumor cerebri secondary to lithium carbonate. JAMA 1985;253:2869–2870.

534. Lobo A, Pilek E, Stokes PE. Papilledema following therapeutic dosages of lithium carbonate. J Nerv Ment Dis 1978;166:526–529.

535. Atkin SL, Masson EA, Blumhardt LD, et al. Benign intracranial hypertension associated with the withdrawal of a non-ergot dopamine agonist. J Neurol Neurosurg Psychiatry 1994;57:371–372.

536. March LF, Morgan DAL, Jefferson D. Benign intracranial hypertension during chemotherapy for testicular teratoma. Br J Radiol 1988;61:692.

537. Haller JS, Meyer DR, Cromie W, et al. Pseudotumor cerebri following beta-human chorionic gonadotropin hormone treatment for undescended testicles. Neurology 1993;43:448–449.

538. Lee AG. Pseudotumor cerebri after treatment with tetracycline and isotretinoin for acne. Cutis 1995;55:165–168.

539. Sandborn GE, Selhorst JB, Calabrese VP, et al. Pseudotumor cerebri and insecticide intoxication. Neurology 1979;29:1222–1227.

540. Desaiah D, Mehendale H, Ho I. Kepone inhibition of mouse brain synaptosomal ATPase activities. Toxicol Appl Pharmacol 1978;45:268–269.

541. DeJong AR, Callahan CA, Weiss JL. Pseudotumor cerebri and nutritional rickets. Eur J Pediatr 1985;143:219–220.

542. Hochman HI, Majlszenkier JD. Cataracts and pseudotumor cerebri in an infant with vitamin D-deficient rickets. J Pediatr 1977;90:252–254.

543. Biousse V, Rucker JC, Vignal C, et al. Anemia and papilledema. Am J Ophthalmol 2003;135:437–446.

544. Taylor JP, Galetta SL, Asbury AK, Volpe NJ. Hemolytic anemia presenting as idiopathic intracranial hypertension. Neurology 2002;59:960–961.

545. van Gelder T, van Gemert HMA, Tjiong HL. A patient with megaloblastic anaemia and idiopathic intracranial hypertension: Case history. Clin Neurol Neurosurg 1991;93:321–322.

546. Nazir SA, Siatkowski RM. Pseudotumor cerebri in idiopathic aplastic anemia. JAAPOS 2003;7:71–74.

547. Ridolfi R, Bell WR. Thrombotic thrombocytopenic purpura: Report of 25 cases and a review of the literature. Medicine 1981;60:413–428.

548. Watkins CH, Wagener HP, Brown RW. Cerebral symptoms accompanied by choked optic discs in types of blood dyscrasia. Am J Ophthalmol 1941;24:1374–1383.

549. Nover A. Papilledema in blood and vascular disease. Fortschr Neurol Psychiatr 1963;31:267–274.

550. Imari AJ. Papilledema in cor pulmonale. Dis Chest 1962;41:671–675.

551. Stephens PM, Austen F, Knowles JH. Prognostic significance of papilledema in course of respiratory insufficiency. JAMA 1963;183:161–164.

552. Freedman BJ. Papilloedema, optic atrophy, and blindness due to emphysema and chronic bronchitis. Br J Ophthalmol 1963;47:290–294.

553. Westlake EK, Kaye M. Raised intracranial pressure in emphysema. Br Med J 1954;1:302–304.

554. Miller A, Bader RA, Bader ME. The neurologic syndrome due to marked hypercapnia with papilledema. Am J Med 1962;33:309–318.

555. Cameron AJ. Marked papilledema in pulmonary emphysema. Br J Ophthalmol 1933;17:167–169.

556. Buschbaum HW, Martin WA, Turino GM, et al. Chronic alveolar hypoventilation due to muscular dystrophy. Neurology 1968;18:319–327.

557. O'Halloran HS, Berger JR, Baker RS, Lee WB, Pearson PA, Ryan S. Optic nerve edema as a consequence of respiratory disease. Neurology 1999;53:2204–2205.

558. Manfredi F, Merwarth CR, Buckley CE III, et al. Papilledema in chronic respiratory acidosis. Am J Med 1961;30:175–180.

559. Dickens C. The Pickwick Papers. New York, EP Dutton, 1937.

560. Wolin MJ, Brannon SL, Kay MD, et al. Disk edema in an overweight woman. Surv Ophthalmol 1995;39:307–314.

561. Kirkpatrick PJ, Meyer T, Sarkies N, et al. Papilloedema and visual failure in a patient with nocturnal hypoventilation. J Neurol Neurosurg Psychiatry 1994;57:1546–1547.

562. Sharp JT, Barrocas M, Chokroverty S. The cardio-respiratory effects of obesity. Clin Chest Med 1980;1:103–118.

563. Purvin VA, Kawasaki A, Yee RD. Papilledema and obstructive sleep apnea. Arch Ophthalmol 2000;118:1626–1630.

564. Meyer JS, Gotham J, Tazaki Y, et al. Cardiorespiratory syndrome of extreme obesity with papilledema. Neurology 1961;11:950–958.

565. Bucci FA, Krohel GB. Optic nerve swelling secondary to the obstructive sleep apnea syndrome. Am J Ophthalmol 1988;105:428–430.

566. Spalter HF, Bruce GM. Ocular changes in pulmonary insufficiency. Trans Am Acad Ophthalmol 1964;68:661–676.

567. Kilburn KH. Neurologic manifestations of respiratory failure. Arch Intern Med 1965;116:409–415.

568. Strollo PJ5 Jr, Rogers RM. Obstructive sleep apnea. N Engl J Med 1996;334:99–104.

569. Wall M, Breen L, Winterkorn J. Optic disk edema with cotton-wool spots. Surv Ophthalmol 1995;39:502–508.

570. Hayreh SS. Classification of hypertensive fundus changes and their order of appearance. Ophthalmologica 1989;198:247–269.

571. Hayreh SS, Servais GE, Virdi PS. Fundus lesions in malignant hypertension. Ophthalmology 1986;93:74–87.

572. Corbett JJ, Savino PJ, Thompson HS, et al. Visual loss in pseudotumor cerebri. Follow-up of 57 patients from 5 to 41 years and a profile of 14 patients with permanent severe visual loss. Arch Neurol 1982;39:461–474.

573. Silverberg DH, Laties AM. Increased intracranial pressure in disseminated lupus erythematosis. Arch Neurol 1973;29:88–90.

574. Carlow TJ, Glaser JS. Pseudotumor cerebri syndrome in systemic lupus erythematosus. JAMA 1974;228:197–200.

575. Kaplan RE, Springate JE, Feld LG, et al. Pseudotumor cerebri associated with cerebral venous sinus thrombosis, internal jugular vein thrombosis, and systemic lupus erythematosus. J Pediatr 1985;107:266–268.

576. Li EK, Ho PCP. Pseudotumor cerebri in systemic lupus erythematosis. J Rheumatol 1989;16:113–116.

577. Leavitt RY, Fauci AS. Polyangiitis overlap syndrome: Classification and prospective clinical experience. Am J Med 1986;81:79–85.

578. Frohman LP, Joshi VV, Wagner RS, et al. Pseudotumor cerebri as a cardinal sign of the polyangiitis overlap syndrome. Neuroophthalmology 1991;11:337–345.

579. Guy J, Johnston PK, Corbett JJ, et al. Treatment of visual loss in pseudotumor cerebri associated with dementia. Neurology 1990;40:28–32.

580. Bynke G, Bynke H, Ljunggren B. Familial idiopathic intracranial hypertension and variegate porphyria: Is there any connection? Neuroophthalmology 1994;14:153–165.

581. Smith JL. Pseudotumor cerebri. Tran Am Acad Ophthalmol 1958;62:432–439.

582. Lavenstein B, Frey T. Benign intracranial hypertension: Atypical features and new risks. Ann Neurol 1987;22:453–454.

583. Donaldson JO. Pathogenesis of pseudotumor cerebri syndromes. Neurology 1981;31:877–880.

584. Fishman RA. The pathophysiology of pseudotumor cerebri: An unsolved puzzle. Arch Neurol 1984;41:257–258.

585. Donaldson JO, Binstock ML. Pseudotumor cerebri in an obese woman with Turner syndrome. Neurology 1981;31:758–760.

586. Donaldson JO, Horak E. Cerebrospinal fluid oestrone in pseudotumor cerebri. J Neurol Neurosurg Psychiatry 1982;45:734–736.

587. Solberg Sørensen P, Gjerris F, Svenstrup B. Endocrine studies in patients with pseudotumor cerebri: Estrogen levels in blood and cerebrospinal fluid. Arch Neurol 1986;43:902–906.

588. Bercaw GL, Greer M. Transport of intrathecal I-131 RISA in benign inracranial hypertension. Neurology 1970;20:787–790.

589. Johnston IH, Sheridan MM. CSF shunting from the cisterna magna: a report of 16 cases. Br J Neurosurgery 1993;7:39–44.

590. Raichle ME, Grubb RL Jr, Phelps ME, et al. Cerebral hemodynamics and metabolism in pseudotumor cerebri. Ann Neurol 1978;4:104–111.

591. Mann JD, Butler AB, Rosenthal JE, Maffeo CJ, Johnson RN, Bass NH. Regulation of intracranial pressure in rat, dog, and man. Ann Neurol 1978;3:156–165.

592. Löfgren J, Swetnow NN. Cranial and spinal components of the cerebrospinal fluid pressure-volume curve. Acta Neurol Scand 1973;49:599–612.

593. Jones HC, Lopman BA. The relation between CSF pressure and ventricular dilatation in hydrocephalic HTx rats. Eur J Pediatr Surg 1998;8(Suppl. 1):55–58.

594. Gjerris F, Soelberg Sørensen P, Vorstrup S, et al. Intracranial pressure, conductance to cerebrospinal fluid outflow, and cerebral blood flow in patients with benign intracranial hypertension (pseudotumor cerebri). Ann Neurol 1985;17:158–162.

595. Moser FG, Hilal SK, Abrams G, Bello JA, Schipper H, Silver AJ. MR imaging of pseudotumor cerebri. Am J Radiol 1988;150:903–909.

596. Sørensen PS, Thomsen C, Gjerris F, et al. Increased brain water content in pseudotumor cerebri measured by magnetic imaging of the brain water self diffusion. Neurol Res 1989;11:160–164.

597. Connolly MB, Farrell K, Hill A, Flodmark O. Magnetic resonance imaging in pseudotumor cerebri. Dev Med Child Neurol 1992;34:1091–1094.

598. Wall M, Dollar JD, Sadun AA, et al. Idiopathic intracranial hypertension. Lack of histological evidence for cerebral edema. Arch Neurol 1995;52:141–145.

599. Karahalios DG, Rekate HL, Khayata MH, Apostolides PJ. Elevated intracranial venous pressure as a universal mechanism in pseudotumor cerebri of varying etiologies. Neurology 1996;46:198–202.

600. King JO, Mitchell PJ, Thomson KR, Tress BM. Manometry combined with cervical puncture in idiopathic intracranial hypertension. Neurology 2002;58:26–30.

601. King JO, Mitchell PJ, Thomson KR, et al. Cerebral venography and manometry in idiopathic intracranial hypertension. Neurology 1995;45:2224–2228.

602. Higgins JNP, Cousins C, Owler BK, Sarkies N, Pickard JD. Idiopathic intracranial hypertension: 12 cases treated by venous sinus stenting. J Neurol Neurosurg Psychiatry 2003;74:1662–1666.

603. Kesler A, Ellis MG, Reshef T, Gadoth F. Idiopathic intracranial hypertension and anticardiolipin antibodies. J Neurol Neurosurg Psychiatry 2000;68:379–380.

604. Leker RR, Steiner I. Anticardiolipin antibodies are frequently present in patients with idiopathic intracranial hypertension. Arch Neurol 1998;55:817–820.

605. Backhouse OC, Johnson MH, Jamieson DR, et al. Familial thrombophilia and idiopathic intracranial hypertension. Neuroophthalmology 2001;25:135–141.

606. Smith FR, Goodman DS. The effects of diseases of the liver, thyroid and kidneys on transport of vitamin A in human plasma. J Clin Invest 1971;50:2426–2436.

607. Goodman DS. Vitamin A in health and disease. N Engl J Med 1984;310:1023–1031.

608. Smith FR, Goodman DS. Vitamin A transport in vitamin A toxicity. N Engl J Med 1976;294:435–443.

609. Warner JEA, Bernstein PS, Yemelyanov A, et al. Vitamin A in the cerebrospinal fluid of patients with and without idiopathic intracranial hypertension. Ann Neurol 2002;52:647–650.

610. McDonald PN, Bok D, Ong DE. Localization of cellular retinol-binding protein and retinol-binding protein in cells comprising the blood-brain barrier of rat and human. Proc Natl Acad Sci USA 1990;87:4265–4269.

611. Fishman R. Polar bear liver, vitamin A, aquaporins, and pseudotumor cerebri. Ann Neurol 2002;52:531–533.

612. Jacobson DM, Berg R, Wall M, et al. Serum vitamin A concentration is elevated in idiopathic intracranial hypertension. Neurology 1999;53:1114–1118.

613. Selhorst JB, Kulkanthrakorn K, Corbett JJ, Leira EC, Chung SM. Retinol-binding protein in idiopathic intracranial hypertension (IIH). J Neuroophthalmol 2000;20:250–252.

614. Streeten DHP. In Orthostatic Disorders of the Circulation: Mechanisms, Manifestations and Treatment. New York, Plenum, 1987:18,19,74,101–108, 117–119.

615. Seckl J, Lightman S. Cerebrospinal fluid neurohypophysial peptides in benign intracranial hypertension. J Neurol Neurosurg Psychiatry 1988;51:1538–1541.

616. Sørenson PS, Gjerris F, Hammer M. Cerebrospinal fluid vasopressin and increased intracranial pressure. Neurology 1982;3:1255–1259.

617. Sørenson PS, Hammer M, Gjerris F. Cerebrospinal fluid vasopressin in benign intracranial hypertension. Ann Neurol 1984;15:435–440.

618. Raichle ME, Grubb RL Jr. Regulation of brain water permeability by centrally released vasopressin. Brain Res 1978;143:191–194.

619. Lindvall-Axelsson M, Nilsson C, Owman C, Svensson P. Involvement of 5-HT1c receptors in the production of CSF from the choroid plexus. In Seylaz J,

MacKenzie ET, eds. Neurotransmission and Cerebrovascular Function. I. Amsterdam, Elsevier, 1989:237–240.

620. Frenkel REP. Evaluation of the relative afferent pupillary defect in pseudotumor cerebri in regard to surgical intervention. Arch Ophthalmol 1989;107:634–635.

621. Rohrschneider K, Burk ROW, Völcker HE. Papillenschwellung: Ferlaufsbeobachtung mittels Laser-Scanning-Tomographie. Fortschr Ophthalmol 1990;87:471–474.

622. Sedwick L, Boghen D, Moster ML. How to handle the pressure or too much of a good thing. Surv Ophthalmol 1996;40:307–311.

623. Kupersmith MJ, Gamell L, Turbin R, Spiegel P, Wall M. Effects of weight loss on the course of idiopathic intracranial hypertension in women. Neurology 1998;50:1094–1098.

624. Johnson LN, Krohel GB, Madsen RW, March GA. The role of weight loss and acetazolamide in the treatment of idiopathic intracranial hypertension (pseudotumor cerebri). Ophthalmology 1998;105:2313–2317.

625. Newberg B. Pseudotumor cerebri treated by the rice reduction diet. Arch Int Med 1974;133:802–807.

626. Amaral JF, Tsiaris W, Morgan T, et al. Reversal of benign intracranial hypertension by surgically induced weight loss. Arch Surg 1987;122:946–949.

627. Sugarman HJ, Felton WL, Salvant JB, Sismanis A, Kellum JM. Effects of surgically induced weight loss on idiopathic intracranial hypertension in morbid obesity. Neurology 1995;45:1655–1659.

628. Reeves-Hoche MK, Hudgel DW, Meck R, et al. Continuous versus bilevel positive airway pressure for obstructive sleep apnea. Am J Respir Crit Care Med 1995;151:443–449.

629. Tschirgi RD, Frost RW, Taylor JL. Inhibition of cerebrospinal fluid formation by a carbonic anhydrase inhibitor, 2-acetyl-1,3,4-thiadiazole-5-sulfonamide (Diamox). Proc Soc Exp Biol Med 1954;87:373–376.

630. Davson H, Luck CP. The effect of acetazolamide on the chemical composition of the aqueous humor and cerebrospinal fluid of some mammalian species and on the rate of turnover of ^{24}Na in these fluids. J Physiol 1957;137:279–283.

631. Tomsak RL, Niffenegger AS, Remler BF. Treatment of pseudotumor cerebri with Diamox (acetazolamide). J Clin Neuroophthalmol 1988;18:93–98.

632. Schoeman JF. Childhood pseudotumor cerebri: Clinical and intracranial pressure response to acetazolamide and furosemide treatment in a case series. J Child Neurol 1994;9:130–134.

633. Maren TH, Robinson B. The pharmacology of acetazolamide as related to cerebrospinal fluid and the treatment of hydrocephalus. Johns Hopkins Hosp Bull 1960;106:1–24.

634. Lichter PR. Reducing side effects of carbonic anhydrase inhibitors. Ophthalmology 1981;88:266–269.

635. Jefferson A, Clark J. Treatment of benign intracranial hypertension by dehydrating agents with particular reference to the measurement of the blindspot area as a means of recording improvement. J Neurol Neurosurg Psychiatry 1976;39:627–639.

636. Liu GT, Glaser JS, Schatz N. High-dose methylprednisolone and acetazolamide for visual loss in pseudotumor cerebri. Am J Ophthalmol 1994;118:88–96.

637. Friedman DI, Eller PE. Topiramate for treatment of idiopathic intracranial hypertension. Headache 2003;43:592.

638. Friedman DI, Rausch EA. Headache diagnoses in patients with treated idiopathic intracranial hypertension. Neurology 2002;58:1551–1553.

639. Kelman SE, Sergott RC, Cioffi GA, et al. Modified optic nerve decompression in patients with functioning lumboperitoneal shunts and progressive visual loss. Ophthalmology 1991;98:1449–1453.

640. Tulipan N, Lavin PJM, Copeland M. Stereotactic ventriculoperitoneal shunt for idiopathic intracranial hypertension: Technical note. Neurosurgery 1998;43:175–176.

641. Howard J, Appen R. Ventriculoperitoneal shunting for pseudotumor cerebri. Invest Ophthalmol Vis Sci 2002;43(E[abstr]):2461.

642. Bynke G, Bynke H, Nordström CH. Treatment of pseudotumor cerebri with ventriculoperitoneal shunting. Neuroophthalmology 1996;16 (Suppl):273.

643. Spetzler RF, Wilson CB, Schulte R. Simplified percutaneous lumboperitoneal shunting. Surg Neurol 1977;7:25–29.

644. McGreal DA. Observations on the management of pseudotumor cerebri. Arch Neurol 1986;43:168.

645. Johnston I, Besser M, Morgan M. Cerebrospinal fluid diversion in the treatment of benign intracranial hypertension. J Neurosurg 1988;69:195–202.

646. Cornblath WT, Miller NR. Pseudotumor cerebri treated with lumbo-peritoneal shunt. Ann Neurol 1989;26:183.

647. Eggenberger ER, Miller NR, Vitale S. Lumboperitoneal shunt for the treatment of pseudotumor cerebri. Neurology 1996;46:1524–1530.

648. Burgett RA, Purvin VA, Kawasaki A. Lumboperitoneal shunting for pseudotumor cerebri. Neurology 1997;49:734–739.

649. Rosenberg ML, Corbett JJ, Smith C, et al. Cerebrospinal diversion procedures for pseudotumor cerebri. Neurology 1993;43:1071–1072.

650. Johnston I, Paterson A, Besser M. The treatment of benign intracranial hypertension: A review of 134 cases. Surg Neurol 1981;16:218–224.

651. Chumas PD, Kulkarni AV, Drake JM, et al. Lumboperitoneal shunting: A retrospective study in the pediatric population. Neurosurgery 1993;32:376–383.

652. Alleyne CH Jr, Shutter LA, Colohan ART. Cranial migration of a lumboperitoneal shunt catheter. So Med J 1996;89:634–636.

653. de Wecker L. On incision of the optic nerve in cases of neuroretinitis. Int Ophthalmol Congr Rep 1872;4.

654. Kafka H. Optikusscheiden trepanation bei stauungspapille. Z Augenheilk 1928;64:103.

655. Carter RB. Operation of opening the sheath of the optic nerve for the relief of pressure. Br Med J 1889;1:399.

656. Davidson SI. A surgical approach to plercephalic disc oedema. Trans Ophthalmol Soc UK 1969;89:669–690.

657. Anderson RL, Flaharty RM. Treatment of pseudotumor cerebri by primary and secondary optic nerve sheath decompression (letter). Am J Ophthalmol 1992;113:599–600.

658. Tse DT, Nerad JA, Andersen JW. Optic nerve sheath fenestration in pseudotumor cerebri: A lateral orbitotomy approach. Arch Ophthalmol 1988;106:1458–1462.

659. Galbraith JEK, Sullivan JH. Decompression of the perioptic meninges for relief of papilledema. Am J Ophthalmol 1973;76:687–692.

660. Burde RM, Karp JS, Miller R. Reversal of visual deficit with optic nerve decompression in long-standing pseudotumor cerebri. Am J Ophthalmol 1974;77:770–772.

661. Bilson FA, Hudson RL. Surgical treatment of chronic papilloedema in children. Br J Ophthalmol 1975;59:92–95.

662. Knoght RSG, Fielder AR, Firth JL. Benign intracranial hypertension: Visual loss and optic nerve sheath fenestration. J Neurol Neurosurg Psychiatry 1986;49:243–250.

663. Corbett JJ, Nerad JA, Anderson RL. Results of optic nerve sheath fenestration for pseudotumor cerebri. Arch Ophthalmol 1988;106:1391–1397.

664. Keltner JL. Optic nerve sheath decompression. How does it work? Has its time come? Arch Ophthalmol 1988;206:1365–1369.

665. Pearson PA, Baker RS, Khorram D, et al. Evaluation of optic nerve sheath fenestration in pseudotumor cerebri using automated perimetry. Ophthalmology 1991;98:99–105.

666. Spoor TC, Ramocki JM, Madion MP, Wilkinson MJ. Treatment of pseudotumor cerebri by primary and secondary optic nerve sheath decompression. Am J Ophthalmol 1991;112:177–185.

667. Berman EL, Wirtschafter JD. Improvement of optic nerve head appearance after surgery for pseudotumor cerebri. JAMA 1992;267:1130.

668. Kelman SE, Heaps R, Wolf A, et al. Optic nerve sheath decompression improves visual function in patients with pseudotumor cerebri. Neurosurgery 1992;30:391–395.

669. Acheson JF, Green WT, Sanders MD. Optic nerve sheath decompression for the treatment of visual failure in chronic raised intracranial pressure. J Neurol Neurosurg Psychiatry 1994;57:1426–1429.

670. Kaye AH, Galbraith JEK, King J. Intracranial pressure following optic nerve decompression for benign intracranial hypertension. J Neurosurg 1981;55:453–456.

671. Jacobson EE, Johnston IH, McCluskey P. The effects of optic nerve sheath decompression on cerebrospinal fluid dynamics. Neuroophthalmology 1996;16(Suppl):290.

672. Nguyen R, Carta A, Geleris A, Sadun AA. Long-term effect of optic sheath decompression on intracranial pressure in pseudotumor cerebri. Invest Ophthalmol Vis Sci 1997;38:S388.

673. Brodsky MC, Rettele GA. Protracted postsurgical blindness with visual recovery following optic nerve sheath fenestration. Arch Ophthalmol 1998;116:107–108.

674. Flynn WJ, Westfall CT, Weisman JS. Transient blindness after optic nerve sheath fenestration. Am J Ophthalmol 1994;117:678–679.

675. Digre KB, Varner MW, Corbett JJ. Pseudotumor cerebri and pregnancy. Neurology 1984;34:721–729.

676. Huna-Baron R, Kupersmith MJ. Idiopathic intracranial hypertension in pregnancy. J Neurol 2002;249:1078–1081.

677. Mauriello JA, Shaderowfsky P, Gizzi M, et al. Management of visual loss after optic nerve sheath decompression in patients with pseudotumor cerebri. Ophthalmology 1995;102:441–445.

678. Spoor TC, McHenry JG. Long-term effectiveness of optic nerve sheath decompression for pseudotumor cerebri. Arch Ophthalmol 1993;111:632–635.

679. Kellen RI, Burde RM. Optic nerve decompression. Arch Ophthalmol 1987;105:889.

680. Lee AG, Patrinely JR, Edmond JC. Optic nerve sheath decompression in pediatric pseudotumor cerebri. Ophthal Surg Lasers 1998;29:514–517.

681. Shapiro S, Yee R, Brown H. Surgical management of pseudotumor cerebri in pregnancy: Case report. Neurosurgery 1995;37:829–831.

682. McDonnell GV, Patterson VH, McKinstry S. Cerebral venous thrombosis occurring during an ectopic pregnancy and complicated by intracranial hypertension. Br J Clin Pract 1997;51:194–197.

683. Aktan S, Sansu T, Kansu E, et al. Papilledema in paroxysmal nocturnal hemoglobinuria. J Clin Neuroophthalmol 1984;4:47–48.

684. Hauser D, Barzilai N, Zalish M, et al. Bilateral papilledema with retinal hemorrhages in association with cerebral venous sinus thrombosis and paroxysmal nocturnal hemoglobinuria. Am J Ophthalmol 1996;122:592–593.

685. Kalbian VV, Challis MT. Behcet's Disease: Report of twelve cases with three manifesting as papilledema. Am J Med 1970;49:823–829.

686. Graus F, Slatkin NE. Papilledema in the metastatic jugular foramen syndrome. Arch Neurol 1983;40:816–818.
687. Koller EA, Stadel BV, Malozowski SN. Papilledema in 15 renally compromised patients treated with growth hormone. Pediatr Nephrol 1997;11:451–454.
688. Kan L, Sood SK, Maytal J. Pseudotumor cerebri in Lyme disease: A case report and literature review. Pediatr Neurol 1998;18:439–441.
689. Horoshovski D, Amital H, Katz M, et al. Pseudotumor cerebri in SLE. Clin Rheum 1995;14:708–710.
690. Evans RW, Patten BM. Trichinosis associated with superior sagittal sinus thrombosis. Ann Neurol 1982;11:216–217.
691. Walsh FB. Papilledema associated with increased intracranial pressure in Addison's disease. Arch Ophthalmol 1952;47:86.
692. Sybert VP, Bird TD, Salk DJ. Pseudotumor cerebri and Turner syndrome. J Neurol Neurosurg Psychiatry 1985;48:164–166.
693. Monaco F, Agnetti V, Mutani R. Benign intracranial hypertension after minocycline therapy. Eur Neurol 1978;17:48–49.
694. Lombaert A, Carton H. Benign intracranial hypertension due to A-hypervitaminosis in adults and adolescents. Eur Neurol 1976;14:340–350.
695. Feldman MH, Schlezinger NS. Benign intracranial hypertension associated with hypervitaminosis A. Arch Neurol 1970;22:1–7.
696. Josephs HW. Hypervitaminosis A and carotenemia. Am J Dis Child 1944;67:33–43.
697. Knudson AG, Rothman PE. Progress in pediatrics: Hypervitaminosis A. Am J Dis Child 1953;85:316–334.
698. Lewis JM, Cohlan SQ. Comparative toxicity of aqueous and oily preparations of vitamin A. Pediatrics 1952;9:589–596.
699. Baqui AH, de Francisco A, Arifeen SE, Siddique AK, Sack RB. Bulging fontanelle after supplementation with 25,000 IU of vitamin A in infancy using immunization contacts. Acta Paediatr 1995;84:863–866.
700. Rodahl K, Moore T. The vitamin A content and toxicity of polar bear and seal liver. Biochem J 1943;37:166–169.
701. Amrani Y, Terriza F, Moreno C, Casado A. Pseudotumor cerebri caused by vitamin A excess due to intake of milk enriched with A and D vitamins. Revista de Neurologia 1996;24:1304–1305.
702. Misbah SA, Peiris JB, Atukorala TM. Ingestion of shark liver associated with pseudotumor cerebri due to acute hypervitaminosis A. J Neurol Neurosurg Psychiatry 1984;47:216.
703. Dhiravibulya K, Ouvrier R, Johnston I, Procopis P, Antony J. Benign intracranial hypertension in childhood: A review of 23 patients. J Paediatr Child Health 1991;27:204–207.
704. Alemeyehu W. Pseudotumor cerebri (toxic effect of the ''magic bullet''). Ethiop Med 1995;33:265–270.
705. Sharieff GQ, Hanten K. Pseudotumor cerebri and hypercalcemia resulting from Vitamin A toxicity. Ann Emerg Med 1996;27:518–521.
706. Bigby M, Stern RS. Adverse reactions to isotretinoin. A report for the Adverse Reaction Reporting System. J Am Acad Dermatol 1988;18:543–552.
707. Caffery BE, Josephson JE. Ocular side effects of isotretinoin therapy. J Am Optom Assoc 1988;59:221–223.
708. Campos SP, Olitsky S. Idiopathic intracranial hypertension after L-thyroxine therapy for acquired hypothyroidism. Clin Pediatr 1995;34:334–337.
709. Raghavan S, DiMartino-Nardi J, Saenger P, et al. Pseudotumor cerebri in an infant after L-thyroxine therapy for transient neonatal hypothyroidism. J Pediatr 1997;130:478–480.
710. Pelton RW, Lee AG, Orengo-Nania SD, et al. Bilateral optic disk edema caused by sarcoidosis mimicking pseudotumor cerebri. Am J Ophthalmol 1999;127:229–230.
711. Green L, Vinker S, Amital H, et al. Pseudotumor cerebri in systemic lupus erythematosis. Semin Arthritis Rheum 1995;25:103–108.

Optic Neuritis

Craig H. Smith

Optic neuritis is a term used to refer to inflammation of the optic nerve. When it is associated with a swollen optic disc, it is called papillitis or anterior optic neuritis. When the optic disc appears normal, the term *retrobulbar optic neuritis* or *retrobulbar neuritis* is used. In the absence of signs of multiple sclerosis (MS) or other systemic disease, the optic neuritis is referred to as monosymptomatic or idiopathic, or as a clinically isolated syndrome. The pathogenesis of isolated optic neuritis is presumed to be demyelination of the optic nerve, similar to that seen in MS. It is likely that most cases of isolated acute optic neuritis are a *forme fruste* of MS. Optic neuritis, as a harbinger of a more diffuse demyelinating process, merits careful attention to an exact diagnosis and a thorough consideration of treatment paradigms.

Optic neuritis does not always present as acute loss of vision. It may develop as insidious progressive or nonprogressive visual dysfunction, and it may even be asymptomatic. Patients with asymptomatic optic neuritis have electrophysiologic evidence of optic nerve dysfunction and may also have subtle clinical evidence of optic nerve damage if appropriate clinical studies are performed.

Optic neuritis can be caused by disorders other than MS and related demyelinating diseases. In addition, two unusual variants of optic neuritis can occur. *Neuroretinitis* is a term used to describe inflammatory involvement of both the intra-ocular optic nerve and the peripapillary retina. In addition to optic disc swelling, eyes with neuroretinitis show extensive retinal edema, vitreal inflammatory changes, hemorrhages, and hard exudates (lipid) in the macula in a star-shaped pattern. *Optic perineuritis*, also called perioptic neuritis, describes inflammatory involvement of the optic nerve sheath without inflammation of the nerve itself. Patients with this condition have optic disc swelling that may be unassociated with any visual complaints. In such cases, visual acuity is normal in the affected eye, and there is no visual field defect except for an enlarged blind spot. The disc swelling thus may be difficult to differentiate from papilledema, particularly when it is bilateral, without performing neuroimaging studies and lumbar puncture (discussed later).

Most of this chapter deals with acute demyelinating optic neuritis, occurring in isolation, in association with MS, or in association with other demyelinating diseases. The later sections of the chapter discuss other forms of demyelinating optic neuritis, optic neuritis caused by processes other than MS and related disorders, and the variants of optic neuritis: neuroretinitis and perioptic neuritis. Our knowledge of the immunopathogenesis and clinical aspects of optic neuritis has taken huge steps with the information provided by the Optic Neuritis Treatment Trial (ONTT) and ancillary development of the genetic and neuroimmunologic basis of MS.

IDIOPATHIC AND PRIMARY DEMYELINATING OPTIC NEURITIS

Despite remarkable advances in neuroimaging and electrophysiologic testing, the diagnosis of optic neuritis remains basically a clinical one. Nettleship (1) first described a syndrome characterized by "failure of sight limited to one eye, often accompanied by neuralgic pain about the temple and orbit and by pain in moving the eye; many recover but permanent damage and even total blindness may ensue; there is at first little, sometimes no, ophthalmoscopic change, but the disc often becomes more or less atrophic in a few weeks." Nettleship (1) also emphasized the tendency for the orbital pain to antedate the loss of vision and for the maximum visual field defect to be central in nature. Subsequently, Parinaud (2), Uhthoff (3), Buzzard (4), and Gunn (5) described similar patients.

Optic neuritis usually is a primary demyelinating process. It almost always occurs as an isolated phenomenon or in patients who either have, or will develop, MS. Patients in whom optic neuritis occurs as an isolated phenomenon have a higher risk of developing MS at some later date than the normal population. Optic neuritis is also part of the demyelinating syndrome called "neuromyelitis optica" or "Devic's disease," and it occasionally occurs in two other primary demyelinating diseases: myelinoclastic diffuse sclerosis (encephalitis periaxialis diffusa, Schilder's disease) and encephalitis periaxialis concentrica (concentric sclerosis of Baló). There are three forms of primary demyelinating optic neuritis: acute, chronic, and subclinical.

ACUTE IDIOPATHIC DEMYELINATING OPTIC NEURITIS

Acute demyelinating optic neuritis is by far the most common type of optic neuritis throughout the world. It is also the type that is best known and understood. Although the clinical syndrome of acute optic neuritis has been well recognized for many years, much information about optic neuritis was obtained from the ONTT (6–26), a multicenter controlled clinical trial funded by the National Eye Institute of the National Institutes of Health in the United States. This trial was the first in the field of MS research to look rigorously at a treatment outcome as well as to define metrics of outcome. The ONTT enrolled 455 patients with acute unilateral optic neuritis. Although the primary objective of the trial was to assess the efficacy of corticosteroids in the treatment of optic neuritis, the trial also provided invaluable information about the clinical profile of optic neuritis, its natural history, and its relationship to MS.

Entry criteria in the ONTT included a clinical syndrome consistent with unilateral optic neuritis (including a relative afferent pupillary defect and a visual field defect in the affected eye), visual symptoms of 8 days or less, no previous episodes of optic neuritis in the affected eye, no previous corticosteroid treatment for optic neuritis or MS, and no evidence of a systemic disease other than MS as a cause for the optic neuritis. Patients were randomly assigned to one of three treatment groups: (a) oral prednisone (1 mg/kg/d) for 14 days; (b) intravenous methylprednisolone sodium succinate (250 mg QID for 3 days) followed by oral prednisone (1 mg/kg/d) for 11 days; or (c) oral placebo for 14 days. Each regimen was followed by a short oral taper.

Measurement of visual function was made at study entry, at seven follow-up visits during the first 6 months, yearly for 4 years, then at 5 and 10 years (as the Longitudinal Optic Neuritis Study [LONS]). Data collected at the 6-month follow-up visit served as the primary measure of visual outcome. Both the rate of visual recovery and long-term visual outcome were assessed by four measures:

1. Snellen acuity with a retroilluminated Bailey-Lovie chart at 4 meters
2. Color vision with the Farnsworth-Munsell 100-hue test
3. Contrast sensitivity with the Pelli-Robson chart
4. Perimetry with the Humphrey Field Analyzer (program 30-2) and Goldmann perimeter

A standardized detailed neurologic examination was performed at study entry, after 6 months, after 1 year, yearly for 4 years, and then at 5 and 10 years (in the LONS). Additional examinations were performed when patients developed new neurologic symptoms during the first 5 years, and brain magnetic resonance imaging (MRI) was obtained on all patients at 10 years who had initially had a normal brain MRI. Clinically definite multiple sclerosis (CDMS) was diagnosed when a patient developed new neurologic symptoms attributable to demyelination in one or more regions of the central nervous system (CNS), other than new optic neuritis in either eye, occurring at least 4 weeks after the optic neuritis at study entry and lasting more than 24 hours, with abnormalities documented on neurologic examination.

Demographics

Much of the following information on demographics, long-term risk of MS development, and visual outcome in optic neuritis comes from the ONTT/LONS. The annual incidence of acute optic neuritis has been estimated in population-based studies to be 1–5 per 100,000 (27–33). In Olmstead County, Minnesota, where the Mayo Clinic is located and where extensive and accurate studies of the incidence of various diseases have been performed, the incidence rate is estimated to be 5.1 per 100,000 person-years and the prevalence rate 115 per 100,000 (33).

Most patients with acute optic neuritis are between the ages of 20 and 50 years, with a mean age of 30–35 years. Females are affected more commonly than males. In the ONTT, 77% of the patients were female, 85% were Caucasian, and the mean age was 32 ± 7 years. Nevertheless, optic neuritis can occur at any age. It is well described in children in the first and second decades of life (34–38), and it can occur in adults in the sixth and seventh decades (39).

Symptoms

The two major symptoms in patients with acute optic neuritis are loss of central vision and pain in and around the affected eye. Other symptoms are much less common.

Loss of Central Vision

Loss of central visual acuity is the major symptom in most cases of acute optic neuritis, being reported by over 90% of patients (7). Loss of vision is usually abrupt, occurring over several hours to several days. Progression for a longer period of time can occur but should make the clinician suspicious of an alternative disorder. The degree of visual loss varies widely. In some cases visual acuity is minimally reduced; in others there is complete blindness with no perception of light. Most patients describe diffuse blurred vision, although some state that blurring is predominantly central. The visual loss is monocular in most cases, but in a few patients, particularly in children, both eyes are simultaneously affected.

Loss of Visual Field

Not all patients with acute optic neuritis complain of loss of central vision. Some complain of loss of peripheral vision, usually in a particular area of the visual field, such as the inferior or superior region, often to one side. Such patients may deny loss of central acuity and may be found to have 20/20 or better vision in the affected eye (40).

Ocular or Orbital Pain

Pain in or around the eye is present in more than 90% of patients with acute optic neuritis. It is usually mild, but it may be extremely severe and may even be more debilitating to the patient than the loss of vision. It may precede or occur concurrently with visual loss; usually is exacerbated by eye movement; and generally lasts no more than a few days (7,39,41–44). In the ONTT, pain was reported by 92% of patients, of whom 87% indicated that it was worsened by eye movement. Rose (45) theorized that the pain is caused by inflammation or swelling in the optic nerve sheaths that are innervated by small branches of the trigeminal nerve; however, Swartz et al. (46) hypothesized that the pain is initiated by inflammation of the optic nerve in the apex of the orbit, where the extraocular muscles are firmly attached to the sheaths of the nerve. In support of this hypothesis, Lepore (47) reported that among 101 eyes with optic neuritis, pain was more commonly present with retrobulbar neuritis than with papillitis; however, in the ONTT, pain was present in 93% of the 295 eyes with retrobulbar neuritis and in 90% of the 162 eyes with papillitis. The presence of pain is a helpful feature to differentiate it from nonarteritic anterior ischemic optic neuropathy (AION), particularly when it is severe and when it occurs or worsens during movement of the eyes. Swartz et al. (46) reported that the incidence of pain in patients with AION was only 12%, compared with a frequency of pain of 92% in the patients enrolled in the ONTT. Gerling et al. (48) reported a similar figure and also found that pain tended to be described as much more severe by patients with optic neuritis compared with patients with AION, and that patients with AION rarely experienced pain on movement of the eyes.

Positive Visual Phenomena

Patients with optic neuritis may experience positive visual phenomena, called photopsias, in addition to pain and visual blurring, both at the onset of their visual symptoms and during the course of the disorder. These phenomena are spontaneous flashing black squares, flashes of light, or showers of sparks (39,49,50). These visual phenomena may be precipitated by eye movement (44,50) or certain sounds (51,52). Positive visual phenomena were reported by 30% of the patients in the ONTT.

Signs

Examination of a patient with acute optic neuritis reveals evidence of optic nerve dysfunction. Visual acuity is reduced in most cases. Contrast sensitivity and color vision are impaired in almost all cases. The reduction in contrast sensitivity often parallels the reduction in visual acuity (53), although in some cases it is much worse (7). The reduction in color vision is often much worse than would be expected from the level of visual acuity (54,55). Visual field loss can vary from mild to severe. A relative afferent pupillary defect is present and detectable with a swinging flashlight test in almost all unilateral cases. When such a defect is not present, either there is a coexisting optic neuropathy in the fellow eye or the visual loss in the affected eye is not caused by optic neuritis or any other form of optic neuropathy. Patients with optic neuritis also can be shown to have a reduced sensation of brightness in the affected eye simply by asking them to compare the brightness of a light shined in one eye and then another or by performing more complex testing with a flickering light, the frequency of which can be varied between 50 and 0 Hz (56–58).

Slit-lamp biomicroscopy in eyes with demyelinating optic neuritis is almost always normal. There may be a few cells in the vitreous overlying the optic disc, but there is rarely any significant cellular reaction. In eyes with anterior optic neuritis (papillitis) from causes other than demyelination, such as sarcoidosis, tuberculosis, syphilis, or Lyme disease, a significant vitritis may be present (discussed later). The optic disc in optic neuritis may appear normal (retrobulbar neuritis) or swollen (papillitis), and if the patient has experienced a previous clinical or subclinical attack of optic neuritis in the eye, the disc may appear pale. Both the swelling and the pallor are nonspecific findings in optic neuritis, and neither is useful in distinguishing demyelinating optic neuritis from the optic neuritis that may accompany other inflammatory or infectious diseases.

Visual Acuity

The severity of visual acuity loss varies from a mild reduction to no light perception. In the ONTT, baseline visual acuity was ≥ 20/20 in 11%, 20/25 to 20/40 in 25%, 20/50 to 20/190 in 29%, 20/200 to 20/800 in 20%, finger counting in 4%, hand motion in 6%, light perception in 3%, and no light perception in 3% (7).

Color Vision

Color vision is almost always abnormal in patients with optic neuritis and is usually more severely affected than visual acuity itself. Thus, testing of color vision may be particu-

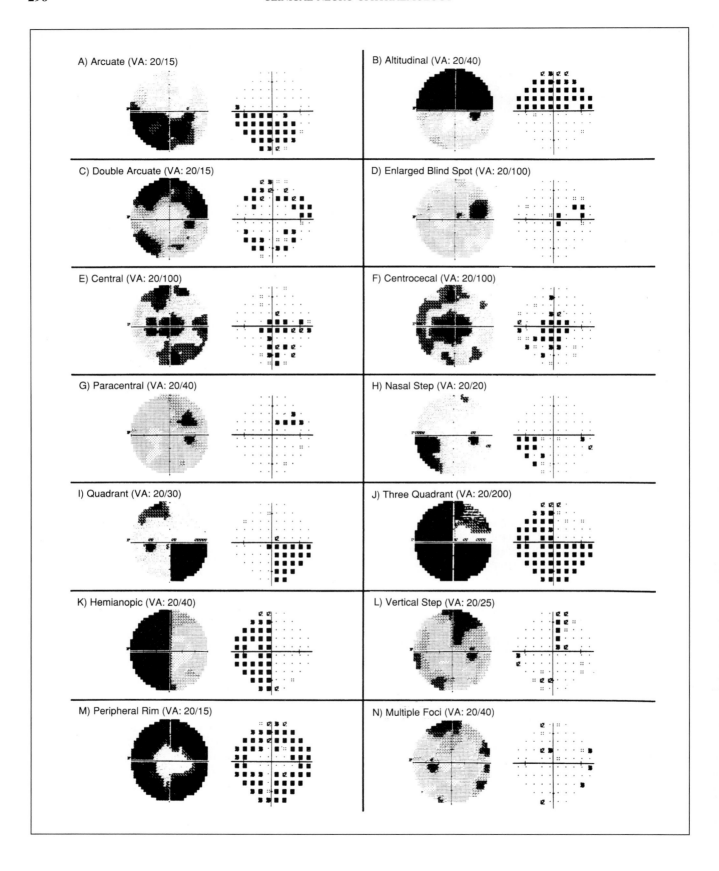

A) Arcuate (VA: 20/15)

B) Altitudinal (VA: 20/40)

C) Double Arcuate (VA: 20/15)

D) Enlarged Blind Spot (VA: 20/100)

E) Central (VA: 20/100)

F) Centrocecal (VA: 20/100)

G) Paracentral (VA: 20/40)

H) Nasal Step (VA: 20/20)

I) Quadrant (VA: 20/30)

J) Three Quadrant (VA: 20/200)

K) Hemianopic (VA: 20/40)

L) Vertical Step (VA: 20/25)

M) Peripheral Rim (VA: 20/15)

N) Multiple Foci (VA: 20/40)

larly helpful in diagnosing optic neuritis in patients with minor visual loss.

Ishihara pseudoisochromatic color plates can detect color vision defects in eyes with retrobulbar optic neuritis and normal-appearing optic discs and can detect evidence of optic nerve dysfunction in the eyes of patients with MS in whom retrobulbar neuritis is suspected. Another type of color plates, the Hardy-Rand-Rittler (HRR) pseudoisochromatic plates, was first printed in 1954 and was used by Steinmetz and Kearns (59) at the Mayo Clinic to detect acquired color vision defects in patients with presumed retrobulbar optic neuritis. Rosen (60) published the results of a study of 272 patients with MS tested with HRR plates and found that 100% of eyes with ophthalmoscopic evidence of definite optic disc pallor (n = 24) and 46% of eyes with possible pallor (n = 39) had abnormal color vision when tested with these plates. Based on these findings, he emphasized the usefulness of HRR plates in the early diagnosis of demyelinating optic neuritis and in the diagnosis of MS itself. Some patients with optic neuritis can see none or only some of the figures with the affected eye but all of the figures with the fellow eye. Other patients may see all of the figures correctly with each eye; however, when the patient is asked to look at a single plate, first with one eye and then with the other, he or she will note a striking difference in color and brightness between the two eyes. Although patients may have congenitally defective color vision, the pattern of color defects found in patients with congenital color blindness is much different from that of acquired color defects from optic neuropathy (60).

A more sensitive test of color vision, the Farnsworth-Munsell 100-Hue test, has been recommended for detection of various optic neuropathies, including optic neuritis (61–63). In the ONTT, Ishihara color plates were abnormal in the affected eye in 88%, whereas the Farnsworth-Munsell 100-Hue test was abnormal in 94% (7).

Visual Field

Griffith (64) and Gunn (65) considered the central field to be always affected in patients with optic neuritis, and both Berliner (66) and Carroll (67) recorded typical central and paracentral defects in their patients, although Carroll (67) recorded a few cases with an associated peripheral constriction or with extensions of a central defect to the periphery. Central or paracentral scotomas, with and without peripheral extension, represented over 90% of field defects in the cases reported by Marshall (68), and Hyllested and Moller (69) found such defects in 98.5% of their cases. Thus, the typical visual field defect in optic neuritis has always been thought to be a central scotoma (70). It has subsequently become clear, however, that virtually any type of field defect can occur in an eye with optic neuritis, including an arcuate defect, a cecocentral scotoma, a superior or inferior altitudinal defect, and a temporal or nasal hemianopic defect. Among 100 patients with optic neuritis, Chamlin (71) found 44 patients with arcuate defects and 4 patients with peripheral defects. Perkin and Rose (39) found only 31% of their patients to have pure central defects alone. Vighetto et al. (72) reported similar results. Patients with optic neuritis may also simply have diffuse loss of sensitivity throughout the visual field. Among 415 patients in the ONTT with baseline visual acuity of hand motions or better, the predominant pattern of visual field loss was found to be focal in 52% and diffuse in 48% (73). Focal nerve fiber bundle type defects (altitudinal, arcuate, and nasal step) were present more frequently (20%) than pure central or cecocentral defects (8%). Other types of defects were present in 24% of patients, including hemianopic defects in 5% (73) (Fig. 6.1).

Pupillary Reaction

Despite reports to the contrary (74), a relative afferent pupillary defect is almost always present in patients with acute optic neuritis, whether anterior or retrobulbar (75–78). The only exception to this rule is the patient who has suffered a previous attack of optic neuritis in the fellow eye or who has subclinical (asymptomatic) optic neuritis in the fellow eye (discussed later). In such a case, damage to the optic nerve in the fellow eye may offset the damage from acute optic neuritis in the affected eye (even when there is asymmetry of visual function by clinical testing), and there will be no evidence of a relative afferent pupillary defect. In cases of apparent acute optic neuritis in which no relative afferent pupillary defect is detected by a swinging flashlight test, the use of neutral density filters may uncover such a defect (see Chapter 15).

Ophthalmoscopic Appearance

In most series, about 20–40% of patients with acute optic neuritis have some degree of disc swelling (3,39,68,69,74, 79–83). In the ONTT, optic disc swelling was observed in 35% of the patients (7). The optic disc may be slightly or markedly blurred (Fig. 6.2). At times, the disc swelling is so severe that it mimics the ''choked disc'' seen in patients with papilledema (Fig. 6.3). The degree of disc swelling does not correlate with the severity of either visual acuity or visual field loss (39). Disc or peripapillary hemorrhages are uncommon in eyes with acute optic neuritis, as opposed to AION, in which they more frequently accompany disc swelling. In the ONTT, disc or peripapillary hemorrhages were present in 6% of patients (7).

Figure 6.1. Visual field defects in acute optic neuritis. Fourteen types of localized monocular visual field defects that may occur in acute optic neuritis, as defined by static perimetry as performed with a Humphrey automated perimeter using a 30-2 program incorporating the full-threshold test strategy, a 31.5-apostilb background, and size III targets for the test and blind spot checks. The foveal threshold and fluctuation tests were turned on. Central, cecocentral, arcuate, altitudinal, quadrantic, and even hemianopic defects may develop. VA, visual acuity. (From Keltner JL, Johnson CA, Spurr JO, et al. Baseline visual field profile of optic neuritis. The experience of the optic neuritis treatment trial. Optic Neuritis Study Group. Arch Ophthalmol 1993;111:231–234.)

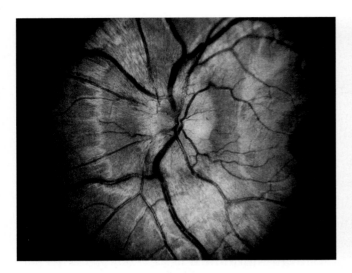

Figure 6.2. Anterior optic neuritis. There is significant swelling and hyperemia of the disc with dilated surface capillaries.

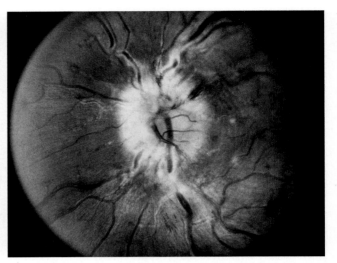

Figure 6.4. Anterior optic neuritis with venous sheathing. The patient was a 45-year-old man with sudden onset of reduced central vision in his left eye. Visual acuity was 8/200 with a large central scotoma.

In some patients with anterior optic neuritis, a few vitreous cells may be observed, particularly in the vitreous overlying the optic disc. When the cellular reaction is extensive, etiologies other than MS should be considered (discussed later). Similarly, when macular or peripapillary hard exudates accompany the disk swelling, other conditions such as neuroretinitis should be considered (discussed later). Sheathing of retinal veins may occur in acute optic neuritis caused by certain conditions, including MS and sarcoidosis (84,85) (Fig. 6.4).

Most patients with idiopathic or demyelinating acute optic neuritis have a normal optic disc in the affected eye, unless they have had a previous attack of acute optic neuritis or

have an ongoing chronic optic neuritis. With time, the optic disc becomes pale, even as the visual acuity and other parameters of vision improve (Fig. 6.5). The pallor may be diffuse or localized to a particular portion of the disc, most often the temporal region.

Other Tests of Optic Nerve Function

The results of other tests of optic nerve function, including contrast sensitivity (86), visual evoked potential (VEP), and other psychophysical tests, are almost always abnormal in patients with acute optic neuritis. For example, contrast sensitivity was abnormal in the affected eye at baseline in 98% of patients in the ONTT. Nevertheless, these tests rarely need be performed for diagnosis if other parameters are carefully evaluated. On the other hand, Froehlich and Kaufman (87) found that pattern electroretinography was useful in distinguishing anterior optic neuritis from AION. These authors reported that the amplitude of the N95 peak was abnormally reduced for every eye affected with AION, whereas it remained normal in eyes with acute anterior optic neuritis.

Visual Function in the Fellow Eye

Numerous studies have reported that asymptomatic visual dysfunction may be detected in the fellow eyes of a patient with acute unilateral optic neuritis (86–90). In the ONTT, abnormalities in the fellow eye were found on measurement of visual acuity in 13.8%, contrast sensitivity in 15.4%, color vision in 21.7%, and visual field in 48.0% of patients (7,11). Most of the fellow eye deficits resolved over several months, suggesting that such abnormalities may be caused by subclinical acute demyelination in the fellow optic nerve.

Diagnostic, Etiologic, and Prognostic Studies

Studies in patients with presumed acute optic neuritis are usually performed for one of three reasons:

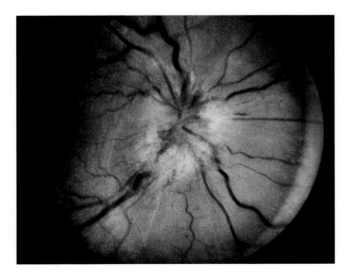

Figure 6.3. Severe optic disc swelling mimicking papilledema. Note hyperemia and elevation of the disc and several peripapillary retinal hemorrhages.

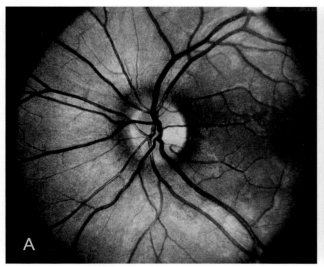 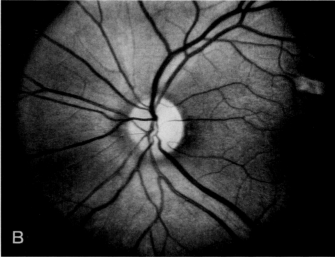

Figure 6.5. Optic atrophy after acute, retrobulbar optic neuritis. *A,* In acute phase, visual acuity in the left eye is 20/300 with a central scotoma, but the optic disc is normal. *B,* Three months later, visual acuity has returned to 20/30 but the optic disc is pale, particularly temporally, and there is mild nerve fiber layer atrophy.

1. To determine whether the cause of the acute optic neuropathy is something other than inflammation, particularly a compressive lesion
2. To determine whether a cause other than demyelination is responsible for the optic neuritis
3. To determine the visual and subsequent neurologic prognosis of optic neuritis; whether the patient will develop a more generalized demyelinating process.

Diagnostic Studies

The major concern of the physician who is evaluating a patient with acute visual loss and evidence of a unilateral optic neuropathy is whether the optic neuropathy truly is optic neuritis or is an acute manifestation of compression of the optic nerve by an intraorbital, intracanalicular, or intracranial mass. To eliminate this possibility, physicians typically perform neuroimaging studies, both computed tomographic (CT) scanning and magnetic resonance (MR) imaging, in such patients. In fact, neither study is probably warranted in patients with a typical history and findings suggesting optic neuritis.

With the widespread availability of MR imaging, CT scanning has little or no role in the evaluation of patients with presumed optic neuritis. Before MR imaging was available, CT scanning was used to detect causes of optic neuropathy other than inflammation, with positive results only occasionally. CT scanning reveals diffuse enlargement of the optic nerve in some cases of typical optic neuritis (91). The finding of an enlarged optic nerve by CT scanning in a patient with symptoms and signs most consistent with optic neuritis should not deter the physician from making that diagnosis.

MR imaging is more sensitive than CT scanning in detecting lesions that compress the optic nerve in patients with presumed optic neuritis; however, the usefulness of MR imaging in detecting such lesions in patients with presumed acute optic neuritis is minimal. Among 455 patients enrolled in the ONTT with a presumptive diagnosis of acute optic neuritis, only 2 patients (0.4%) were found to have a compressive lesion that was responsible for the acute visual loss (7). One patient had an intracranial aneurysm that was not identified at the time of the initial MR imaging but that subsequently produced visual loss in the opposite eye. This, as well as worsening of the patient's visual acuity in the initially affected eye, led to a second MR study that identified the aneurysm (92). In the second patient, a pituitary adenoma was detected by initial MR imaging; however, it may be assumed that this lesion would have been diagnosed within several weeks by neuroimaging had such imaging not been performed initially, since it is likely that the patient's vision would not have improved over several weeks, as would be expected in a patient with true acute optic neuritis (discussed previously).

MR imaging can also detect demyelinating lesions of the optic nerve in patients with optic neuritis. Such lesions are seen as foci, sometimes quite extensive, of enhancement in various locations along the nerve (Fig. 6.6). Unfortunately, the appearance of these lesions is nonspecific, and a similar appearance can be observed in patients with infectious optic neuritis and radiation-induced optic neuropathy.

Although it would seem that the use of CT scanning or MR imaging to detect either a demyelinating optic nerve lesion or a compressive lesion causing acute visual loss in a patient whose symptoms suggest optic neuritis is unwarranted from the standpoint of both yield and cost effectiveness, there are more compelling reasons to obtain neuroimaging in this patient population. MR imaging should, as

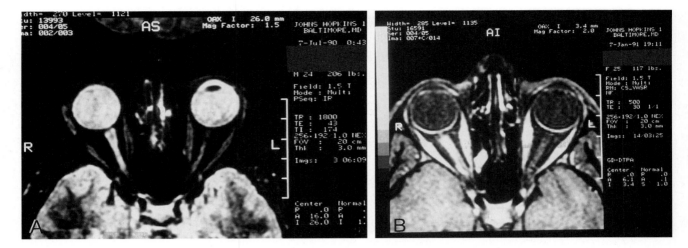

Figure 6.6. MR imaging of the optic nerve in acute demyelinating optic neuritis. *A,* Unenhanced proton density-weighted axial MR image in a 24-year-old man with right optic neuritis shows diffuse hyperintensity of the right optic nerve. *B,* T1-weighted axial MR image after intravenous injection of paramagnetic contrast material in a 25-year-old woman with right optic neuritis shows marked thickening and enhancement of the orbital portion of the right optic nerve.

noted below, be carried out primarily to look at the potential for future development of a more widespread demyelinating process in patients with a typical demyelinating optic neuritis; doing so assists clinicians in deciding on the potential use of immunomodulatory therapy.

Etiologic Studies

Although systemic and local infectious and inflammatory disorders can cause acute optic neuritis, the vast majority of patients with optic neuritis caused by such disorders can be identified simply by performing a thorough history. In patients without a history of (or consistent with) syphilis, sarcoidosis, Lyme disease, systemic lupus erythematosus, and so forth, the likelihood of such a condition being responsible for optic neuritis is low. In the ONTT, a comprehensive medical history was obtained from all patients, who then underwent blood testing for connective tissue disease (antinuclear antibody assay [ANA]) and syphilis (fluorescent treponemal antibody adsorbent test for syphilis [FTA-ABS]), and a chest radiograph to evaluate for sarcoidosis or tuberculosis (7). A lumbar puncture was optional. The key findings from this testing were as follows:

1. The ANA was positive in a titer less than 1:320 in 13% and 1:320 or more in 3%. Only one patient developed a diagnosable connective tissue disease in the first 2 years of follow-up. Visual and neurologic outcomes were no different in this subgroup.
2. The FTA-ABS was positive in six patients (1.3%), but none had active syphilis.
3. The chest radiograph did not reveal evidence of sarcoidosis or tuberculosis in any patient (8).
4. Analysis of cerebrospinal fluid (CSF) did not yield any unsuspected information in the 131 patients in whom it was performed (93).

We believe that neither serologic nor CSF studies are warranted in a patient with presumed acute optic neuritis, unless the history or examination suggests that the patient has an underlying systemic or local infection or inflammation or the patient's course does not follow that of typical optic neuritis (7).

For many years it has been postulated that a virus may play a role in the pathogenesis of MS. Numerous studies have also addressed this issue in patients with optic neuritis. Link et al. (94) found a marked increase in hemolysis-inhibiting measles virus antibody titers in the serum of patients with optic neuritis and oligoclonal immunoglobulin IgG, whereas Arnason et al. (95) were unable to find any difference in titers of hemagglutination-inhibiting measles virus antibody in patients with optic neuritis, compared with a normal population. Nikoskelainen et al. (74) studied both types of antibody in 33 patients with isolated optic neuritis and found elevated titers of both.

Antibodies against viruses other than measles have been studied in patients with optic neuritis. Nikoskelainen et al. (74) studied varicella-zoster, mumps, Coxsackie A3 and B5, polio 3, ECHO 6, cytomegalovirus, parainfluenza 1, Epstein-Barr virus, influenza A and B viruses, adenovirus, and herpes simplex antibody levels. No significant difference in viral titers was found among patients with optic neuritis, a control population, and a population with other neurologic disorders. These investigators performed serial estimations of titers in 17 patients over a period of several months and failed to find any changes in the levels. The role of a virus in the development of optic neuritis remains uncertain.

MR imaging can identify areas of inflammation within the optic nerve, thus supporting a diagnosis of optic neuritis (96–99). The most important application of MR imaging in patients with optic neuritis, however, is the identification of signal abnormalities in the white matter of the brain, usually in the periventricular region, consistent with demyelination.

Numerous studies have reported the prevalence of such abnormalities in patients with clinically isolated optic neuritis. Two or more lesions on brain MR imaging of patients with isolated optic neuritis were reported by Miller et al. (96) in 64% of 53 patients less than 50 years old who were scanned 1–40 weeks after onset. Frederiksen et al. (100) reported abnormal MR imaging in 62% of 50 patients aged 12–53 years scanned after 3–49 days, and Jacobs et al. (101) observed such abnormalities in 40% of 48 patients aged 12–61 years scanned between 3 weeks and 7 years after the onset of acute visual loss. In the ONTT, only 27% of patients had two or more signal abnormalities at least 3 mm in size (7,12), a lower percentage than reported in most other studies. The presence of multiple lesions on MR imaging in the periventricular or other white matter in the brain of a patient with presumed acute optic neuritis suggests that not only is the diagnosis of optic neuritis correct but also that the cause of the optic neuritis is demyelination.

Prognostic Studies

A substantial percentage of patients with isolated optic neuritis develop MS within months to years after the onset of the optic neuritis (discussed later). It would be helpful if there were certain studies that could be performed in a patient with isolated optic neuritis, as with any clinically isolated syndrome, that would allow the physician to accurately predict the chance of the patient developing MS. To this end, many investigators have performed serologic, CSF, and neuroimaging studies in an attempt to detect a correlation between the results of such studies and the eventual development of MS in patients with isolated optic neuritis. We will now explore that relevant information, much of which has come from the ONTT.

CSF STUDIES

The role of CSF analysis in the evaluation of patients with monosymptomatic optic neuritis is not clear. Although the presence of oligoclonal banding in the CSF is associated with the development of CDMS (102–104), the powerful predictive value of brain MR imaging for MS has reduced the role of lumbar puncture in the evaluation of a patient with optic neuritis. Whether CSF analysis can add to the predictive ability of brain MR imaging has not been definitively determined; however, results of the ONTT have helped elucidate this issue (discussed later).

Immunologic abnormalities in the CSF are common in patients with optic neuritis. Frederiksen et al. (103) reported that CSF abnormalities were present in 79% of 45 patients with isolated optic neuritis. A pleocytosis was present in 38%, increased IgG index in 36%, and oligoclonal bands in 69%. Söderström (105) reported that oligoclonal IgG bands were present in 69% of patients with optic neuritis. Other studies have reported similar results, with cell counts exceeding 4–5/mm³ in 15–51%, elevated protein concentration in 12–49%, elevated globulin in 18–40%, and oligoclonal bands in 17–51% (39,94,106–109). Rudick et al. (110) reported that free kappa-light chains in the CSF may be present in patients with optic neuritis.

In the ONTT, 131 patients underwent a lumbar puncture. Eighty-three of the patients had no clinical signs of MS at the time of optic neuritis and underwent the lumbar puncture within 24 hours of study entry (93). A pleocytosis of more than six white blood cells was present in 36% of patients; elevated levels of myelin basic protein (MBP) were present in 18%; the IgG ratio was increased in 22%; IgG synthesis was increased in 44%; oligoclonal bands were present in 50%; and kappa-light chains were present in 27%.

The predictive value of CSF oligoclonal banding for the development of CDMS within 5 years after optic neuritis was assessed in 76 patients enrolled in the ONTT (93). The presence of oligoclonal bands was associated with the development of CDMS ($P = 0.02$). However, the results suggest that CSF analysis is useful in the risk assessment of optic neuritis patients only when brain MR imaging is normal; it is not of predictive value when brain MR imaging lesions are present at the time of optic neuritis.

Of the 131 patients who had CSF testing in the ONTT cohort, 76 patients without a clinical diagnosis of probable or definite MS at trial entry who had a lumbar puncture and nonenhanced brain MR imaging performed within 24 hours of enrollment were then evaluated at 5 years into the study. The demographic characteristics of the 76 patients in this cohort were similar to the remaining ONTT patients: average age was 33 ± 7 years, 80% were female, and 91% were Caucasian. Oligoclonal band testing was performed at a local clinic laboratory for 26 of the patients and at a central laboratory for 50 (111). Brain MR imaging scans were graded by a previously published protocol (12). Neurologic examinations were performed at baseline, after 6 months, at 1 year, and yearly thereafter for 5 years. A demyelinating attack was defined as a patient-reported episode of symptoms attributable to acute demyelination in one or more regions of the CNS lasting more than 24 hours and separated from a previous attack by at least 4 weeks (112). Patients were diagnosed as having CDMS when a second attack (in addition to the optic neuritis at the time of study entry) was confirmed by an examination that detected a new neurologic abnormality. Recurrent episodes of optic neuritis in either eye were not considered in the diagnostic criteria for MS.

CDMS developed within 5 years in 22 (29%) of the 76 patients: in 16 (42%) of the 38 patients with oligoclonal bands present and in 6 (16%) of the 38 patients without bands (odds ratio [OR] = 3.88; 95% confidence interval [CI] = 1.18, 13.86; $P = 0.02$). Among the 54 patients not classified as having CDMS, 5-year follow-up was complete for 50 (93%).

The predictive value of CSF oligoclonal band assessment for the development of CDMS over and above that of brain MR imaging was apparent only among patients with no brain MR imaging lesions at study entry. Among the 39 patients with normal brain MR imaging, CDMS developed in 3 of 11 (27%) patients with oligoclonal bands present but in only 1 of 28 (4%) without oligoclonal bands. In contrast, among the 37 patients with abnormal brain MR imaging, CDMS developed in 13 of 27 (48%) with oligoclonal bands and in 5 of 10 (50%) without oligoclonal bands.

Brain MR imaging has been demonstrated to be a strong

predictor of CDMS among patients with monosymptomatic optic neuritis. In the ONTT, there was a 51% 5-year incidence of CDMS in patients who had abnormal brain MR imaging at the time of optic neuritis compared with a 16% incidence in those with normal brain MR imaging (22). These results indicated that performing a lumbar puncture to detect oligoclonal bands is not of added value for predicting the 5-year risk of CDMS in patients who have abnormal brain MR imaging at the time of development of monosymptomatic optic neuritis. However, the results suggested that oligoclonal band testing may be helpful in the risk assessment of optic neuritis patients with normal brain MR imaging.

That the value of CSF analysis would depend on the brain MR imaging findings is not surprising. Patients with abnormal brain MR imaging already have morphologic evidence of disseminated disease, and as such it is expected that most of these patients will eventually develop additional neurologic events sufficient for a diagnosis of CDMS. Therefore, there is no reason to expect that a CSF analysis would be predictive of MS among these patients. The group of patients with optic neuritis and normal brain MR imaging likely includes a subset of those destined to have MS and a subset of those who may have optic neuritis unassociated with MS. Among these patients, the finding of oligoclonal bands in the CSF does appear to increase the likelihood that CDMS ultimately will be diagnosed. Additionally and perhaps more importantly, the absence of oligoclonal bands in the CSF makes the development of CDMS within 5 years unlikely.

Although the number of patients whose CSF was studied in the ONTT was too small for definitive conclusions to be made with regard to the role of CSF analysis in the evaluation of patients with optic neuritis, the results suggest that a lumbar puncture has limited value in patients with typical monosymptomatic optic neuritis who have demyelinative changes on brain MR imaging. However, CSF analysis may help predict the development of CDMS when such MR imaging changes are not present. With longer follow-up of this cohort, a more definitive statement on the value of CSF analysis in the MR-normal patients will be possible.

IMMUNOLOGIC STUDIES

Nyland et al. (109) studied T and B lymphocytes in the blood and CSF of 10 patients with acute optic neuritis (3 with anterior optic neuritis and 7 with retrobulbar optic neuritis). These investigators found that although the percentage of T lymphocytes in the patients' blood was significantly decreased compared with controls, absolute numbers of T lymphocytes, and both relative and absolute B-lymphocyte concentrations, were not significantly different from controls. However, the percentage of T lymphocytes in the CSF of the 10 patients was significantly elevated compared with control subjects.

Frick and Stickl (113) reported that the presence of MBP in the CSF of a patient with otherwise isolated optic neuritis and no history of previous neurologic symptoms or signs nevertheless is highly predictive of the development of MS in the future, a conclusion supported by the findings of Söderström et al. (114) of anti-MBP and anti-MBP peptide antibody-secreting cells in the CSF of patients with both acute optic neuritis and MS. The presence of multiple oligoclonal bands in the CSF of a patient with isolated optic neuritis also seems to be highly predictive of the future development of MS (94,115–118). Finally, Deckert-Schlüter et al. (119) detected increased concentrations of several different cytokines in the serum, CSF, or both of 20 patients with isolated optic neuritis who eventually developed MS, and Link et al. (120) reported similar results. The presence of these substances suggests an activation of the T lymphocytes of the immune system both within and outside the CNS and suggests that either their presence alone or their particular concentration may be used to predict the ultimate development of MS in these patients.

GENETIC STUDIES

There is considerable evidence that genetic factors play a role in the development of MS (121). This is based on the familial incidence of the disease (122), twin studies (123), and HLA typing patterns (108,124–127). Because T cells bind antigen only in association with a cell surface molecule encoded by the major histocompatibility complex (MHC), genes encoded by the MHC, and class II MHC genes in particular, have long been considered as candidate susceptibility loci in MS (128,129). Although an overrepresentation of A3, B7, and DR2 alleles is common in MS patients of Northern European ancestry (124,130), other MHC alleles may be present in other ethnic groups with MS. Indeed, association studies suggest that specific DR- or DQ-related restriction fragment length polymorphisms (RFLP) influence susceptibility in some patients (131–133).

Having stated that various HLA haplotypes are found with increased frequency in patients with MS compared with controls, we must also state that HLA type does not seem to strongly influence the risk of MS in patients with isolated optic neuritis (134). Hely et al. (135) reported that the relative risk for MS in patients with optic neuritis was 2.7 for those with the DR2 haplotype, 4.8 for those with the B7/DR2 type, 1.4 for those with DR3, and 0.2 for patients with the DR4 haplotype. Francis et al. (130) compared the frequency of HLA types in optic neuritis patients who developed MS compared with those who did not. HLA DR2 was present in 57% of the 58 patients who developed MS compared with 44% of those who did not. DR3 was present in 36% and 16% of the two groups, respectively ($P < 0.05$). DR2 and DR3 together were present in 14% of the MS group and 2% of the non-MS group (relative risk = 6.7; $P < 0.05$). Sandberg-Wollheim et al. (102) found that MS developed in 42% of 45 patients with optic neuritis who had the HLA DR2 haplotype and in 34% of 41 patients without this haplotype.

Among 33 patients with optic neuritis, 23 with isolated spinal cord syndromes, and 14 with an isolated brain stem disturbance, Kelly et al. (127) reported that clinical MS developed within a mean follow-up period of 5.3 years in 67% of 30 DRB1*1501-positive patients compared with 38% of 40 negative patients; 62% of DQA1*0102-positive patients compared with 32% of negative patients; and 67% of DQB1*0602-positive patients compared with 35% of negative patients. Patients who did not progress to MS appeared to be similar to the controls. The predictive value of HLA typing in relation to brain MR imaging also was evaluated in this study. MR imaging was found to be a much stronger indicator of risk than HLA, but the combination of MR imaging and HLA haplotype DRB1*1501 increased the predictive ability. Compston et al. (125) found that positive typing for the HLA BT101, winter onset of the initial attack of optic neuritis in BT101-positive patients, and recurrent attacks of optic neuritis were associated with an increased incidence of MS.

A substantial body of data indicates that MS is a complex genetic disorder (136). This complexity may reflect polygenic inheritance (e.g., multiple susceptibility genes in a given individual), locus heterogeneity (e.g., different genes in different patients), and possibly etiologic heterogeneity as well (e.g., more than one underlying cause). To date, the most consistently observed genetic influence on MS arises from a gene or genes linked to the MHC at chromosome 6p21 and associated with haplotypes of DR2 (molecular designation DRB1*1501, DQA1*0102, DQB1*0602) (136). Several exceptions exist to the general finding of the DR2 association with MS, most notably MS in Asians (137) and MS in Sardinians (138). A recent genetic analysis of the MHC in an American MS population reported that linkage was confined to DR2-positive multiplex families; thus, locus heterogeneity exists in MS, with one DR2-associated form and one or several others unassociated with DR2 (139).

The association of the HLA-DR2 allele with brain MR imaging signal abnormalities and with the development of MS was assessed in 178 patients enrolled in the ONTT. HLA haplotype DR2 was present in 85 (48%) of the 178 patients. Its presence was associated with increased odds of probable or definite MS at 5 years (OR = 1.92, 95% CI 1.01–3.67, P = 0.04). The association was most apparent among patients with signal abnormalities on baseline brain MR imaging (140).

A high prevalence of DR2 was present in the ONTT cohort of patients with acute unilateral optic neuritis. This finding is consistent with earlier studies of HLA genes in which the DR2 association was nearly as strong for optic neuritis as for MS (141). The ONTT also confirmed that DR2 is associated with evolution of optic neuritis to MS, as reported in some but not all earlier reports (141). The predictive power of HLA typing in optic neuritis was weak compared with abnormal MR imaging, an expected observation considering the relatively high prevalence of DR2 in healthy Caucasians, and the specificity of MR imaging abnormalities for MS. Unexpected was the strong association observed between DR2 and MS among optic neuritis patients with abnormal baseline MR imaging, and the absence of this association in patients whose MR imaging was normal. Although derived from a relatively small number of observations, which limits the statistical power, this nevertheless suggests that multifocal disease at onset may be influenced by the HLA status of the individual, specifically by DR2 itself or by another gene in linkage disequilibrium with DR2.

Disease heterogeneity is an important emerging concept in MS. Neuropathologic studies support the concept that more than one form of MS exists, defined by whether the oligodendrocyte or the myelin sheath is the initial target of injury, and by whether evidence of antibody-mediated tissue damage is present (142,143). One clinical example of a restricted variant of MS is primary progressive MS, which in Caucasians is characterized by common occurrence in men, little inflammation, few cerebral lesions, frequent spinal cord disease, and a prominent axonal pathology (144). In another example, two clinical forms of MS have been described in Japan. The first, a disseminated disorder with widespread brain lesions detected by MR imaging, resembles MS in Caucasians and is associated with DR2. The second, a relapsing-remitting or progressive disorder with predominant spinal cord and optic nerve involvement, is not DR2 associated (137). Thus, at least in some situations, DR2-negative individuals may have a propensity to develop topographically restricted forms of demyelinating disease.

A better understanding of the predictive value of these and other serum and CSF findings for the development of MS awaits further development in the arenas of neuroimmunology and the genetics of demyelinating disease. Nevertheless, there appear to be certain serologic and CSF risk factors that increase the likelihood that a patient with isolated optic neuritis will eventually develop MS.

MR IMAGING

In the previous sections, we emphasized that MR imaging in patients with presumed acute optic neuritis is probably not warranted with respect to the identification of a lesion that is compressing the optic nerve and producing a compressive optic neuropathy that is mimicking optic neuritis. Similarly, one does not necessarily need to perform MR imaging to confirm a diagnosis of optic neuritis. On the other hand, it is certainly clear that the results of MR imaging correlate with the eventual development of MS.

The presence of multiple lesions in the periventricular and other white matter on MR imaging, a phenomenon noted in 30–70% of patients with isolated optic neuritis (7,12,145, 146), appears to be the most significant risk factor associated with an increased likelihood of developing MS (13,103,147, 148). MS was reported by Jacobs et al. (101) to have developed in 6 of 23 patients (26%) with abnormal brain MR imaging, compared with only 3 of 25 patients (12%) with a normal scan within a mean follow-up of 4 years. Martinelli et al. (149) diagnosed MS in 7 of 21 patients (33%) with isolated optic neuritis and an abnormal MR scan compared with none of 16 patients with optic neuritis and a normal scan within a mean follow-up of 2.7 years. Frederiksen et al. (100) diagnosed MS in 7 of 30 (23%) patients with optic neuritis and an abnormal MR scan compared with none of 20 patients with optic neuritis and a normal scan within mean follow-up of 0.9 years. Finally, Morrisey et al. (150) reported the development of MS in 23 of 28 (82%) optic neuritis patients with an abnormal scan compared with only 1 of 16 (6%) patients with a normal scan over a mean follow-up of 5.5 years. The study by Morrisey et al. (150) is particularly important because it suggested that with sufficiently long follow-up, most, if not all, patients with acute optic neuritis who have silent brain MR imaging signal abnormalities ultimately develop additional clinical manifestations sufficient for a diagnosis of definite MS. Among patients with isolated optic neuritis in the ONTT, the cumulative percentage developing MS within 4 years of the onset of the optic neuritis was about 13% in patients with normal MR imaging, 35% in patients with only one or two lesions, and 50% in patients with more than two lesions (20). By 10 years, patients who had one or more typical MR lesions had a 56% risk and those with no baseline lesions had a 22% risk (23) (Fig. 6.7). Higher numbers of lesions did not increase the risk of MS.

MR imaging has taken on an increasingly important role in the diagnosis and monitoring of patients with MS (151). Current MS diagnostic criteria following a monosymptomatic presentation incorporate changes in serial MR findings as documentation of dissemination in time (152). Accordingly, the long-term MR characteristics of monosymptomatic optic neuritis patients not developing MS on clinical grounds are of great interest. Continued follow-up of the cohort of participants enrolled in the ONTT has provided the opportunity to evaluate brain MR scans 10 to 14 years after optic neuritis in patients who have not developed CDMS. The objective of this study was to determine the proportion of such patients who manifest new brain MR lesions on follow-up scans (26).

In the ONTT, among 61 patients with normal baseline MR scan who had not developed clinical evidence of MS after 10 years, 27 (44%) exhibited at least one new lesion of more than 3 mm on follow-up brain MR scans (23,26). Subclinical demyelination is the most logical explanation for the new MR findings within this relatively young population, although for some of the patients it is possible that the lesions

were present at the time of the initial scan but were not detected due to the scan technique. On the other hand, the fact that 34 patients (56%) did not develop clinical signs or MR evidence of demyelination after 10 years suggests that there are many cases of optic neuritis that may be unrelated to MS.

Among the 35 patients whose baseline MR scan showed at least one T2 lesion measuring at least 3 mm, 26 (74%) developed at least one new lesion larger than 3 mm on follow-up imaging in the absence of a clinical diagnosis of MS (26). This phenomenon merely underscores the well-known dissociation between MR findings and clinical expression of MS. The fact that an abnormal baseline MR scan was more likely to show additional lesions than a normal baseline MR scan emphasizes the predictive value of the initial scan. The presence of even a single lesion predicted the development of further lesions. However, the development of new lesions does not necessarily indicate that the patient will develop clinical signs of MS even after 10 years.

Among the 12 patients with only punctate T2 hyperintensities on baseline imaging, 9 (75%) exhibited changes on long-term MR scanning, a frequency similar to that in the patients with at least one lesion measuring more than 3 mm on the baseline MR scan (26). This finding suggests that a focal signal abnormality of any size may predict that additional signal abnormalities will occur in this population.

The data from the ONTT follow-up patients have several limitations. MR technology continues to advance, and multicenter, serial MRI studies are often forced to compare images obtained with different magnets, field strengths, and protocols. Repositioning error on serial imaging is also a source of potential difference between baseline and follow-up MR scans. The use of magnets with higher field strength and smaller slice thickness scans at follow-up may have overestimated MR changes over time. However, changes in these parameters appear to affect the assessment of lesion volume more than lesion numbers. The addition of good-quality spinal cord imaging may also increase the percentage of patients with asymptomatic demyelinating lesions. Imaging confined to the brain would, therefore, underestimate the total burden of T2 changes over time. It is possible that not all the T2 MR changes over time were the result of demyelination. Vasculopathic risk factors such as advanced age, diabetes, and hypertension may contribute to T2 MR lesions, but this seems unlikely to explain a significant portion of the change observed in this relatively young cohort. Despite the limitations on interpretation of the results imposed by the differences in MR technique from baseline to follow-up scans in the ONTT cohort studied, it is important to recognize that these differences affect only the incidence of new lesions and not the observed proportion of patients who have remained lesion-free after 10 years.

The ONTT experience is unique in reporting the long-term MR changes following monosymptomatic optic neuritis in the absence of the development of clinical signs of MS. The results support the notion that not all cases of monosymptomatic optic neuritis are related to MS, since a subset of patients manifested neither clinical signs nor MR evidence of demyelination after more than 10 years of follow-up (23,26). In addition, the results indicate that MR signal ab-

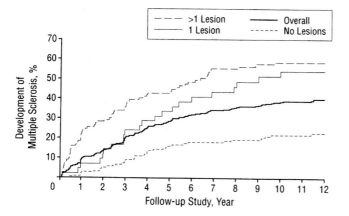

Figure 6.7. The cumulative probability of multiple sclerosis was statistically significantly higher in patients with one or more lesions seen on the baseline MR scan of the brain than in patients with no brain lesions ($P < 0.001$, log rank test) but was not significantly different between patients with a single brain lesion and patients with multiple lesions ($P = 0.22$, log-rank test). (From Optic Neuritis Study Group. High- and low-risk profiles for the development of multiple sclerosis within 10 years after optic neuritis: experience of the optic neuritis treatment trial. Arch Ophthalmol 2003;121:944–949.)

normalities may accumulate without causing any clinical manifestations of MS, even when the patient is followed for over a decade. Although treatment decisions should take this fact into account, it should be emphasized that MS is a life-long disease, and the majority of disability is encountered following 10–15 years of disease involvement.

VITREOUS FLUOROPHOTOMETRY

Braude et al. (153) evaluated vitreous fluorophotometry in six patients with acute retrobulbar optic neuritis. These investigators found an acute increase in posterior vitreous fluorophotometric readings in one or both eyes of all six patients. They speculated that the abnormally high vitreous fluorophotometric findings in the patients are caused by an increased permeability of the blood–ocular barrier, presumably the result of inflammation in the retrolaminar portion of the optic nerve and possibly in the posterior pole vasculature. As with other tests that have been suggested as aids in the diagnosis of optic neuritis, further testing is necessary to determine the accuracy and clinical usefulness of this procedure.

Treatment

In 1949, Hench et al. (154) described the beneficial effects of systemic corticosteroids in the treatment of rheumatoid arthritis. Following this report, physicians began to consider other disorders, including optic neuritis, that might respond to similar treatment or to treatment with adrenocorticotrophic hormone (ACTH). The first systematic attempt to address this issue was a double-blind prospective study of the treatment of 50 patients with acute retrobulbar neuritis with either ACTH or placebo (155,156). The study showed that the group treated with ACTH recovered vision faster, but at 1 year the mean visual acuities in the two groups were not significantly different from each other.

In the Cooperative Multiple Sclerosis Study (157), there were 41 cases in which optic neuritis was the primary manifestation of MS for which patients were entered into the study. The 22 patients treated with ACTH improved faster than the 19 patients treated with placebo, but there was no long-term follow-up. Bowden et al. (158) performed a prospective clinical trial in 54 patients with acute optic neuritis. The study showed no benefit on visual acuity of ACTH compared with placebo in these patients.

Gould et al. (159) performed a prospective single-blind controlled clinical trial in which 74 patients with optic neuritis either received a retrobulbar injection of triamcinolone or were randomized to a control group that received no treatment. Visual acuity in the affected eyes of the treated patients improved faster than did visual acuity in the affected eyes of patients who received no treatment, but there was no difference in mean visual acuity between the two groups after 6 months. Trauzettel-Klosinski et al. (160) subsequently performed a study in which 50 patients with acute optic neuritis were randomized to receive either oral corticosteroids or placebo. There was a suggestion of a slightly more rapid recovery of vision in the patients treated with steroids compared with patients in the placebo group, but there was no

difference in vision between groups at 12 months. In the meantime, Spoor (161) and Spoor and Rockwell (162) described rapid recovery of vision in two small series of patients with optic neuritis treated with intravenous methylprednisolone.

As noted previously, patients with acute optic neuritis who enrolled in the ONTT were randomized to one of three treatment groups: (*a*) oral prednisone (1 mg/kg/day) for 14 days; (*b*) intravenous methylprednisolone sodium succinate (250 mg qid for 3 days followed by an oral prednisone 1 mg/kg/day) for 11 days; and (*c*) oral placebo for 14 days. Each regimen was followed by a short oral taper (6,8). Most patients in all three treatment groups had a good recovery of vision (8). After 6 months of follow-up, the median visual acuity in each group was 20/16, and less than 10% of the patients in each group had visual acuity of 20/50 or worse. One year after the onset of visual symptoms, there was no significant difference in mean visual acuity, color vision, contrast sensitivity, or visual field (by mean deviation) among the three groups (14,15). On the other hand, patients treated with the regimen of intravenous methylprednisolone followed by oral prednisone recovered vision considerably faster than patients treated with oral placebo (8) (Fig. 6.8). The benefit of this treatment regimen was greatest in the first 15 days of follow-up and decreased subsequently.

Patients treated with oral prednisone alone did not recover vision any faster and had no better vision at the end of a 6-month follow-up period than patients treated with oral placebo (8). Unexpectedly, patients treated with oral prednisone alone had an increased rate of recurrent attacks of optic neuritis in the previously affected eye and an increased rate of new attacks of optic neuritis in the fellow eye compared with patients in the other two groups (8) (Fig. 6.9). Thus, oral prednisone in a dose of 1 mg/kg/day did not speed recovery of vision compared with no treatment, did not improve ultimate visual acuity compared with no treatment, and produced a higher rate of recurrent and new attacks of optic neuritis than no treatment.

The ONTT also evaluated the rate of development of clinical MS in the three treatment groups and found that the patients treated with the intravenous followed by oral corticosteroid regimen had a reduced rate of development of clinically definite MS during the first 2 years (13,19). The benefit of treatment was seen only in patients who had significantly abnormal brain MR imaging at the onset of the optic neuritis. The 2-year risk of MS was too low in those with normal brain MR imaging to assess the value of treatment in such patients. The clinical benefit of the intravenous treatment lessened over time, such that at 3 years of follow-up there was no significant difference in the rate of development of MS among treatment groups.

In the acute phase of optic neuritis, no treatment other than corticosteroids or related agents such as ACTH have been shown to be efficacious; however, intravenous immunoglobulin (IVIg) has been demonstrated in animals to promote remyelination of the CNS in experimental allergic encephalomyelitis (163–165) and in Theiler's virus model of MS (166–169).

In a small pilot study, it was suggested that IVIg may

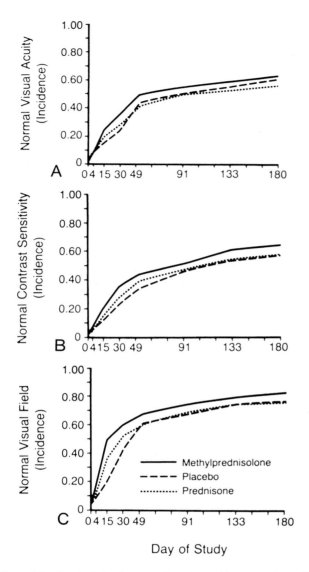

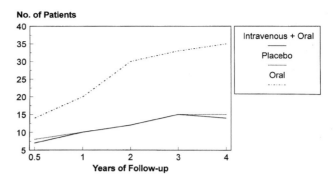

Figure 6.9. Incidence of recurrent attacks of optic neuritis in the previously affected eye and new attacks of optic neuritis in the fellow eye of patients enrolled in the Optic Neuritis Treatment Trial and Longitudinal Optic Neuritis Study by treatment groups. Patients treated with oral prednisone alone, in a dose of 1 mg/kg/day for 14 days, had a much higher incidence of such attacks than patients given oral placebo or patients treated with intravenous methylprednisolone in a dose of 250 mg q6h for 3 days, followed by an 11-day course of oral prednisone in a dose of 1 mg/kg/day.

Figure 6.8. Speed of visual recovery in patients with acute optic neuritis treated with intravenous high-dose methylprednisolone (1 g/day for 3 days), followed by a 2-week course of oral prednisone (1 mg/kg/day) (*solid line*), compared with patients treated with oral prednisone alone (*dotted line*) and untreated patients (given placebo) (*dashed line*) in the Optic Neuritis Treatment Trial. Improvement in visual acuity (*A*), contrast sensitivity (*B*), and visual field (*C*) occurred more rapidly in patients treated with the intravenous regimen than in patients given either low-dose oral prednisone or in untreated patients. (From Beck RW, Cleary PA, Anderson MM Jr, et al. A randomized, controlled trial of corticosteroids in the treatment of acute optic neuritis. The Optic Neuritis Study Group. N Engl J Med 1992; 326:581–588.)

have some benefit in patients with resolved optic neuritis who have significant residual visual deficits (170). Noseworthy et al. (171) looked at whether IVIg reverses chronic visual impairment in MS patients with optic neuritis. In a double-blind, placebo-controlled phase II trial, 55 patients with persistent acuity loss after optic neuritis were randomized to receive either IVIg 0.4 g/kg daily for 5 days followed by three single infusions monthly for 3 months, or placebo. The trial was terminated by the National Eye Institute because of negative results when 55 of the planned 60 patients had been enrolled. Fifty-two patients completed the scheduled infusions, and 53 patients completed 12 months of follow-up. Analysis of these data indicated that a difference between treatment groups was not observed for the primary outcome measure, improvement in logMAR visual scores at 6 months ($P = 0.766$). Exploratory secondary analyses suggested that IVIg treatment was associated with improvement in visual function (including logMAR visual scores at 6 months and visual fields at 6 and 12 months) in patients with clinically stable MS during the trial. It was the conclusion of the investigators that IVIg administration does not reverse persistent visual loss from optic neuritis to a degree that merits general use.

On the basis of the above data, we believe there is no treatment for acute demyelinating optic neuritis that can improve the ultimate visual prognosis compared with the natural history of the disorder (9,10,20,21). A short course of intravenous methylprednisolone (250 mg every 6 hours for 72 hours) followed by a 2-week course of oral prednisone given orally (11 days of 1 mg/kg/day followed by a 3-day taper) may result in an increase in the speed of recovery of vision by 2–3 weeks compared with no treatment when the steroids are begun within 1–2 weeks of the onset of visual loss (8,172), but the ultimate visual function at 1 year will be the same as it would have been if no treatment were given (14). The use of oral corticosteroids alone, when given to patients with acute optic neuritis at a dosage of 1 mg/kg/day, not only does not improve visual outcome or speed recovery but is also associated with a significantly higher incidence of recurrent attacks of optic neuritis in the same eye and new attacks in the contralateral eye than in patients who either are not treated or receive intravenous corticosteroids before a short oral course of steroids (8). In view of these findings, we and others believe it is inappropriate to treat any patient with acute demyelinating optic neuritis with oral corticosteroids alone at this dosage (8–10,20,21). It is possible that a high dose of prednisone, given orally, might have the same effect as intravenously administered methylprednisolone.

Visual Prognosis

The natural history of acute demyelinating optic neuritis is to worsen over several days to 2 weeks, and then to improve. The improvement initially is fairly rapid. It then levels off, but further improvement can continue to occur 1 year after the onset of visual symptoms (14,18,39,41,82) (Fig. 6.10). Among patients enrolled in the ONTT who received placebo, visual acuity began to improve within 3 weeks of onset in 79% and within 5 weeks in 93%. For most patients in this study, recovery of visual acuity was nearly complete by 5 weeks after onset (8,14). The mean visual acuity 12 months after an attack of otherwise uncomplicated optic neuritis is 20/15, and less than 10% of patients have permanent visual acuity less than 20/40 (14). Other parameters of visual function, including contrast sensitivity, color perception, and visual field, improve in conjunction with improvement in visual acuity (16,41,55,173–175).

The visual improvement that occurs in patients with acute optic neuritis tends to do so regardless of the degree of visual

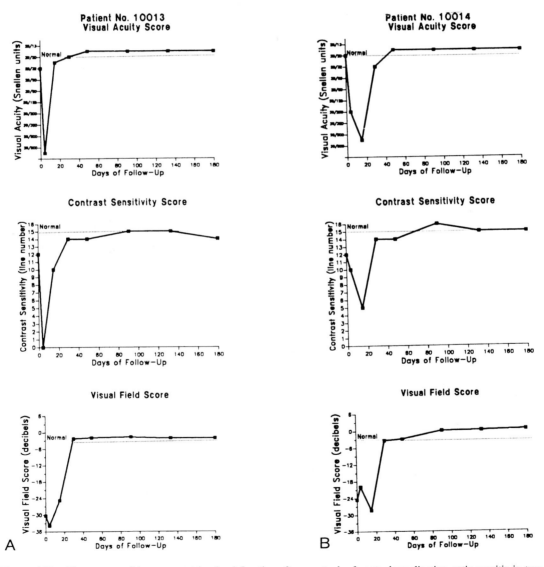

Figure 6.10. Time course of improvement in visual function after an attack of acute demyelinating optic neuritis in two different patients, neither of whom was treated with systemic corticosteroids. Note the rapid drop in visual function over several days followed shortly thereafter by concomitant improvement in visual acuity, contrast sensitivity, and visual field. Improvement in visual function initially was rapid but then leveled off.

loss, although there is some correlation between the severity of visual loss and the degree of eventual recovery. Factors such as age, gender, optic disc appearance, and pattern of the initial visual field defect do not appear to have any appreciable effect on the visual outcome (18,39,82,176). Bradley and Whitty (82) evaluated 73 patients with acute optic neuritis and found that among patients with initial visual acuity of 20/200 or worse, about 60% had acuity of 20/30 or better at 6 months compared with about 70% in patients whose initial visual acuity was better than 20/200. Cohen et al. (51) found that in 24 patients with acute unilateral optic neuritis and initial visual acuity worse than 20/200, the visual acuity remained at that level in only 9 eyes. Slamovits et al. (177) reported that of 12 patients with acute optic neuritis whose vision became reduced to no light perception, all 12 showed some improvement; indeed, visual acuity improved to 20/40 or better in 8 and 20/20 or better in 5. Of 167 eyes of patients enrolled in the ONTT in which the baseline visual acuity was 20/200 or worse, only 10 (6%) had this level of vision or worse 6 months later (8,15). Of 28 patients whose initial visual acuity in the affected eye was light perception or no light perception, 18 (64%) recovered to 20/40 or better (8,15).

Even though the overall prognosis for visual acuity after an attack of acute optic neuritis is extremely good, some patients have persistent severe visual loss after a single episode of optic neuritis (8,14,15,41,178,179). Even those patients with improvement in visual function to ''normal'' may complain of movement-induced photopsias and may have persistent visual deficits when tested using more sensitive clinical, electrophysiologic, or psychophysical tests (58,60, 180–194).

Continued follow-up of the cohort of patients who were enrolled in the ONTT has provided a unique opportunity to assess the long-term course of vision following an episode of acute optic neuritis. In most patients, once visual acuity stabilized after the initial episode of optic neuritis (as determined from the acuity measurement 1 year after the episode), it remained remarkably stable for more than 10 years (24). After 10 years, 69% of patients had acuity of 20/20 or better in each eye, whereas 1% were worse than 20/200 in both eyes. As was reported after 5 years of follow-up, visual function was worse in those patients with MS than in those without MS (22,24). Further attacks of optic neuritis in either eye occurred in 35% of all patients and were twice as common among patients diagnosed with MS at baseline or who developed MS during the follow-up period. As a group, the ONTT patients had lower (worse) quality of life scores as measured on the National Eye Institute Visual Function Questionnaire (NEI-VFQ) compared with a reference group (24). A reduction in NEI-VFQ scores was strongly related to a measured reduction in visual acuity and to the presence of MS. Among patients with acuity in each eye of 20/20 or better and among patients who did not have MS, the scores were quite similar to the reference group.

There are few long-term follow-up data in the literature for comparison with the results of the ONTT. The finding that after more than 10 years of follow-up 86% of the affected eyes had visual acuity of 20/25 or more and 91% had acuity of 20/40 or more (24) is comparable to that of Bradley and Whitty (82), who reported that 86% of 66 patients were 20/25 or more (mean follow-up after episode of optic neuritis of 10.2 years, range 6 months to 20 years), and Cohen (51), who reported that 82% of 60 patients had visual acuity of 20/40 or more (mean follow-up 7.1 years after optic neuritis, range 5–12 years). The 10-year ONTT recurrence rate of 35% is similar to that reported by Cohen (42%) (51) but higher than that reported in other studies with extended follow-up such as those by Bradley and Whitty (18%) (82), Hutchinson (24%) (83), and Rodriguez (16%) (33).

Over time, some attrition of the original ONTT cohort has occurred. This has more impact on the vision assessment than it does on the neurologic assessment, since for the latter the investigators were able in many cases to determine whether MS had developed through either phone contact with the patient or medical records, whereas the former requires the completion of specific visual function tests. Patients who were no longer being followed in the cohort had slightly worse baseline acuity in the affected eye both at baseline and at the time of the last completed visit. The ONTT reported vision results for the patients completing the examination are likely to be slightly biased toward those with better vision. The results of the ONTT can be used by clinicians to advise patients that the long-term visual prognosis is good following an episode of optic neuritis. Follow-up of this cohort will continue with the support of the National Eye Institute, and patients will be examined again in 2006 (24).

Residual Visual Deficits After Resolution of Optic Neuritis

Following an attack of acute optic neuritis, disturbances in visual acuity (15–30%), contrast sensitivity (63–100%), color vision (33–100%), visual field (62–100%), stereopsis (89%), light brightness sense (89–100%), pupillary reaction to light (55–92%), optic disc appearance (60–80%), and the VEP (63–100%) may all persist. Kirkham and Coupland (195) examined 93 patients with previously diagnosed optic neuritis and submitted the results of several diagnostic tests in these patients to linear stepwise multiple regression analysis. The analysis indicated that the most common findings after an attack of acute optic neuritis were optic atrophy, defective color vision, and a prolonged pupil cycle time. Other findings in these patients included a relative afferent pupillary defect, an abnormal response to the Pulfrich test, and an abnormal VEP.

Visual Acuity

Most patients recover to normal or near-normal visual acuity. Bradley and Whitty (82) found that 50% of patients recovered vision to 20/30 or better within 1 month of initial visual loss, and 75% recovered to 20/30 or better within 6 months. In the series reported by Perkin and Rose (39), 87% of patients with optic neuritis recovered vision better than 20/40, and only 8% had vision worse than 20/200 after a minimum follow-up period of 6 months. In the ONTT, after 12 months of follow-up visual acuity was more than 20/20 in 69%, 20/40 or more in 93%, and 20/200 or less in only 3%. The results in each treatment group were similar (14).

Color Vision

Persistent disturbances of color vision are present in a high percentage of eyes with otherwise resolved optic neuritis. Wybar (196), for instance, found disturbances of color vision in 56% of 25 cases of resolved optic neuritis using Ishihara pseudoisochromatic plates, whereas Lynn (197) reported a figure of 84% among 143 cases. Burde and Gallin (181) reported an abnormal Farnsworth-Munsell 100-Hue color test in three of nine eyes in which visual acuity had recovered to normal after an attack of retrobulbar neuritis. Griffin and Wray (63) tested 30 eyes with resolved retrobulbar neuritis that recovered visual acuity to 20/40 or better. Color vision testing using Ishihara pseudoisochromatic plates was abnormal in 15 of 22 patients tested, and assessment of color vision using the Farnsworth-Munsell 100-Hue test revealed abnormalities in all 30 patients. Perkin and Rose (39) reported finding defects in color vision in 50% of 112 eyes with resolved optic neuritis. Kirkland and Coupland (195) found that defective color vision was one of the most common findings in eyes with a history of well-documented acute optic neuritis. Fleishman et al. (90) tested 27 patients with resolved optic neuritis and found abnormalities in 34% of eyes tested with Ishihara color plates and 63% of eyes tested with the Farnsworth-Munsell 100-Hue test. In the ONTT, color vision measured by the Farnsworth-Munsell 100-Hue test was normal within 6 months in only 60% of patients (8). In our experience, the percentage of eyes with color vision disturbances is related in large part to the sensitivity of the test that is used to detect such defects.

Visual Field

Residual visual field defects are usually present in eyes after resolution of acute optic neuritis, even when visual acuity has returned to 20/20 or better. Using a Friedman Visual Field Analyzer, Bowden et al. (158) found defects in 67% of 35 eyes tested; Van Dalen and Greve (198) in 86% of 14 eyes; and Perkin and Rose (39) in 72% of 120 eyes. Nikoskelainen (107) performed kinetic perimetry using a Goldmann perimeter and found abnormalities in the visual field in 62% of 167 eyes that had experienced an attack of acute optic neuritis. Burde and Gallin (181) reported normal kinetic perimetry but abnormal static perimetry in each of nine eyes with a good recovery of visual acuity following an attack of acute retrobulbar optic neuritis. Fleishman et al. (90) reported visual field defects in 26% of eyes that had normal visual acuity after an attack of acute optic neuritis. Among patients enrolled in the ONTT, the mean deviation of the visual field performed using a Humphrey Field Analyzer was abnormal at 6 months in 32% (8).

Contrast Sensitivity

Contrast sensitivity provides a measure of the ability of an eye to detect a difference in luminosity between an object and its background. Numerous studies using various methods of measuring contrast sensitivity have shown that contrast sensitivity remains abnormal regardless of the degree of visual recovery in most eyes after resolution of acute optic neuritis. Arden and Gucukoglu (86) reported abnormal contrast sensitivity using hand-held grating plates in 70% of 57 eyes with resolved optic neuritis, and both Zimmern et al. (199) and Sjöstrand and Abrahamsson (200) reported abnormal contrast sensitivity in 100% of eyes with 20/20 visual acuity after an attack of acute optic neuritis. Using an automated system, Sanders et al. (53) found abnormal contrast sensitivity over a wide range of spatial frequencies in 63% of 64 eyes with resolved optic neuritis. In this study, the subjective visual complaints of the patients correlated better with impaired contrast sensitivity than with any other measure of visual function, including visual acuity, color vision, and visual field. Beck et al. (88) reported abnormal contrast sensitivity in 78% of 51 eyes with recovered optic neuritis. Among 33 of these eyes with visual acuity of 20/25 or better, contrast sensitivity was still abnormal in 67%. Fleishman et al. (90) found abnormalities in contrast sensitivity in 75% of 27 eyes with recovered optic neuritis and good visual acuity. Drucker et al. (201) tested 25 eyes with good visual acuity (20/30 or better) following optic neuritis with the Regan Low Contrast Letter Chart. Contrast sensitivity was abnormal (defined as two standard deviations below the normal group mean determined as part of the study) in 84% of the affected eyes. In the ONTT, contrast sensitivity measured with the Pelli-Robson chart was abnormal at 6 months in 56% (8).

Contrast sensitivity is often abnormal in cases of MS in which there has not been overt acute optic neuritis (202,203) and in some fellow eyes in cases of apparent unilateral optic neuritis (53,86,88). These findings suggest that these eyes have subclinical optic nerve demyelination that was not necessarily detected by testing of other types of visual function.

Stereopsis

Stereopsis is a binocular function that is defined as the ability to discern a separation in the distance of two static objects. Patients with reduced stereopsis often complain of a loss of depth perception. Friedman et al. (204) tested stereopsis using the Titmus test in patients with various optic neuropathies and found that it was worse relative to the reduction in visual acuity in most of these patients. In the 13 patients they tested with visual acuity of 20/40 or better, 11 had stereopsis worse than predicted by the level of acuity. Fleishman et al. (90) found stereopsis to be reduced in 89% of 19 patients with a history of unilateral optic neuritis and in 75% of 8 patients with a history of bilateral optic neuritis.

Light-Brightness Sense

Patients often complain that vision appears dimmer in one eye compared with the other after resolution of optic neuritis. Sadun and Lessell (205) developed an instrument that could quantify this reduction in brightness. Among 15 patients with acute unilateral optic neuritis of less than 3 months' duration, 12 of whom had recovered visual acuity to 20/20 in the affected eye, all noted a reduction in perceived light brightness in the previously affected eye compared with the unaffected eye. Fleishman et al. (90) found light brightness to be reduced in a high percentage (89%) of patients with resolved unilateral optic neuritis.

Pupillary Reaction

Many patients with unilateral acute optic neuritis have a persistent relative afferent pupillary defect on the affected side, even when excellent recovery of vision has occurred. In the ONTT, 54% of the patients without a past history of optic neuritis in the fellow eye had a relative afferent pupillary defect 6 months after the onset of visual symptoms (8).

Burde and Gallin (181) detected a relative afferent pupillary defect in five of nine eyes following a good recovery from acute unilateral optic neuritis. Using pupillometry, Ellis (77) found a relative afferent pupillary defect in each of 13 patients with resolved optic neuritis. All of the 13 eyes also had a persistent reduction in the amplitude of the VEP. Perkin and Rose (39) noted a relative afferent pupillary defect in 55% of 139 eyes after acute optic neuritis, Bynke et al. (206) in 41% of 31 patients. Cox et al. (78) detected a relative afferent pupillary defect by the swinging flashlight test in 92% of 50 patients with resolved optic neuritis.

Optic Disc Appearance

Optic disc pallor is almost always present when visual recovery has been incomplete and is often present even when recovery has been excellent (Figs. 6.5 and 6.11). The pallor is usually temporal, but it may be generalized. Wybar (196) noted optic disc pallor in 67% of 33 eyes with resolved optic neuritis, whereas Lynn (197) reported it in 80% of 160 eyes, Bowden et al. (158) in 70% of 54 eyes, Nikoskelainen (107)

in 60% of 167 eyes, Burde and Gallin (181) in 5 of 9 eyes, and Perkin and Rose (39) in 62% of 165 eyes. In the ONTT, 63% of patients had evidence of optic disc pallor at 6 months (8).

Perhaps more common than optic atrophy is the development of defects in the retinal nerve fiber layer after an attack of acute optic neuritis (207). Most patients develop such defects, which may be diffuse, localized to the papillomacular bundle, or isolated defects in the arcuate regions.

Visual Evoked Potentials (VEPs)

The VEP is an electroencephalographic recording over the occipital lobe in response to visual stimulation. It is occasionally used as an objective measure of conduction in the afferent visual system (see Chapter 2). After resolution of acute optic neuritis, most patients have a prolonged latency, indicating impaired optic nerve conduction. Shahrokhi et al. (208) reported an abnormal VEP in 95% of 58 eyes with resolved optic neuritis, Bynke et al. (206) in 71% of 42 cases, and Wutz et al. (209) in each of 19 patients. In cases of optic neuritis with visual recovery to 20/40 or better, Griffin and Wray (63) reported an abnormal VEP in 93% of 30 eyes, Arden and Gucukoglu (86) in 63% of 24 eyes. Halliday et al. (210) and Asselman et al. (211) found abnormal visual evoked potentials in all 24 and 15 cases, respectively, of resolved optic neuritis occurring in patients with MS. Halliday et al. (212) reported that when visual acuity returned to 20/20, the amplitude of the VEP often was normal, but the latency was virtually always still abnormal.

Subjective Visual Complaints

Despite the often-excellent measured recovery of visual function after an attack of acute optic neuritis, many patients

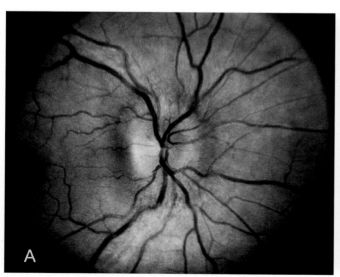 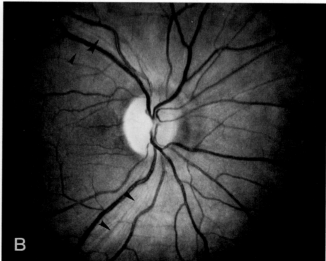

Figure 6.11. Optic atrophy after acute, anterior optic neuritis. *A,* Mild optic disc swelling. Visual acuity is 20/400, and there is a central scotoma in the right eye. *B,* Two months after initial visual loss, disc swelling has resolved. Visual acuity has returned to 20/20, but the optic disc now shows temporal pallor, and there are defects in the peripapillary retinal nerve fiber layer (*arrowheads*).

still complain of difficulties with vision. As noted above, it is important to realize that many patients with optic neuritis whose visual acuity returns to normal (20/20 or better) nevertheless have clinical and laboratory evidence of significant optic nerve dysfunction (89,90,135), particularly when using tests of color vision (60,107,197) or measuring the VEP (206,208,211,212). Such patients will state that their vision is "not right" or that it remains "fuzzy." This difficulty with fine visual function may cause disability in some patients with resolution of optic neuritis who try to return to vocations requiring detailed visual function.

In the ONTT, a questionnaire was completed after 6 months by 382 of the patients (213). Persistent visual symptoms were reported by 56% of the patients. Among the 215 patients who perceived their vision in the eye affected by optic neuritis to be somewhat or much worse than before optic neuritis, visual acuity was nevertheless normal in 66%, contrast sensitivity in 30%, color vision in 55%, and the mean deviation of the visual field in 58%.

One cause of symptoms in these patients is probably related to subtle abnormalities in the visual field that may be difficult to detect with standard static perimetry in which patients experience abnormally rapid disappearance of focal visual stimuli and abnormally rapid fatigue in sensitivity. Patients in whom such abnormalities are present typically complain that when they look at something, it appears as if they have "holes" in their field of vision. If they continue concentrating on the object, some holes fill in, whereas new holes appear elsewhere in the field. Ellenberger and Ziegler (183) called this phenomenon the "Swiss cheese" visual field. It occurs not only in optic neuritis but also in other types of optic neuropathy.

Uhthoff's Symptom

Following an episode of optic neuritis, some patients describe transient visual blurring during exercise, during a hot bath, or during emotional stress (3,214–216). This phenomenon, called Uhthoff's symptom, is most common in patients with other evidence of MS but is also experienced by otherwise healthy patients after optic neuritis, by patients with Leber's optic neuropathy (217), and by patients with optic neuropathies from other causes (218). Some patients with Uhthoff's symptom note that their visual symptoms improve in colder temperatures or when drinking cold beverages. Indeed, we have a patient who reported that she kept ice and ice water at her bedside at all times. Whenever she wanted to read something or see clearly at distance, she would place an ice cube in her mouth or drink the ice water. She would then see clearly for several minutes or longer. On examination, her visual acuity improved from 20/400 to 20/40 in both eyes about 2 minutes after she placed an ice cube in her mouth. Scholl et al. (219) reported that when Uhthoff's symptom was present following optic neuritis, MR imaging of the brain was more likely to be abnormal and MS was more likely to develop. Uhthoff's symptom was reported after 6 months by about 10% of patients enrolled in the ONTT (213).

Although the patient studied by Goldstein and Cogan (216) developed visual blurring during exercise despite a stable body temperature, most investigators agree that Uhthoff's symptom is most often associated with an elevation of body temperature (220). Two major hypotheses regarding this phenomenon are that elevation of body temperature interferes directly with axon conduction and that a rise in body temperature releases a chemical substance that interferes with conduction. Although several studies appear to demonstrate humoral factors capable of blocking nerve conduction (221–224), Zweifach (225) examined three patients with Uhthoff's symptom and found that blood removed from the patients at the time of maximal visual loss and readministered in the normothermic state did not reproduce the symptom. Tasaki (226) postulated a safety factor for nerves that he defined as the ratio of the action current generated by the nerve impulse to the minimum amount of current needed to maintain conduction; if the safety factor is decreased by injury, disease, or pharmacologic insult, a small additional insult could be sufficient to block conduction. Davis (227) and Rasminsky (228), using severely demyelinated peripheral nerve fibers, found that reversible conduction block can be induced by increasing the temperature as little as 0.5°C. Increased temperature increases the threshold for excitation for a nerve and also decreases the duration of the action, presumably reducing the safety factor in the nerve. It is likely that this direct temperature effect explains Uhthoff's symptom in most cases (229); however, although temperature elevation may be the primary factor responsible for Uhthoff's symptom, it may not be the only factor. Persson and Sachs (230) studied the effects of physical exercise on the pattern-reversal VEP in patients with MS, with and without a history of Uhthoff's symptom, and in normal subjects. These investigators found that physical effort produced a short-lasting reduction in the amplitude of the VEP and in the visual acuity of patients with MS with a history of Uhthoff's symptom; however, there was no significant change observed in the already prolonged latency of VEP. In patients with MS without a history of Uhthoff's symptom, and in normal subjects, neither visual acuity nor any aspect of the VEP was affected. The authors interpreted their results as an indication that Uhthoff's symptom results from a reversible conduction block in impulse transmission by demyelinated nerve fibers, supporting the work of Davis (227) and of Rasminsky (228); however, changes in oral temperature were very slight or nil in these patients. Selhorst et al. (231) studied the monocular pattern-reversal VEP in four patients with MS, well-compensated optic neuritis, and Uhthoff's symptom during and after peddling a lightly loaded ergometer bicycle. These investigators found no change in either oral or tympanic membrane temperature at a time when visual acuity became reduced and the VEP showed absence or reduction in amplitude of the P2 wave. Because all patients studied showed a slight decline in venous pH and a rise in lactic acid, Selhorst et al. (231) postulated that the demyelinated nerves may be susceptible not only to temperature changes but also to metabolic changes in the environment. Uhthoff's symptom can occur not only in patients who have experienced an attack of acute optic neuritis but also in patients who have chronic or subclinical optic neuritis (discussed later).

Neurologic Prognosis

Both retrospective and prospective studies have been performed in an effort to determine the prognosis for the development of MS in patients who experience an attack of acute optic neuritis (232). Retrospective studies provide figures ranging from 11.5% to 85% in both adults (28,32,82,83,118, 197,315) and children (35,233–235). The marked discrepancy in these figures may result from biases common to almost all retrospective studies, including criteria for diagnosis of MS and optic neuritis, the nature and length of follow-up, and the care with which neurologic and visual testing was performed. Most prospective studies seem to support higher figures, indicating that the risk of developing MS in patients who experience an attack of acute optic neuritis is only about 30% in patients followed 5–7 years after the attack of optic neuritis (51,135) but eventually increases to about 75% in women and 34% in men with longer follow-up (102,130,236). Rodriguez et al. (33) reported that among 95 incident cases of optic neuritis occurring in Olmstead County, the estimated risk of MS was 39% by 10 years, 49% by 20 years, 54% by 30 years, and 60% by 40 years. Again, the risk of MS was higher in women than in men in this study. The reason for the apparent difference in neurologic prognosis between women and men is unclear, particularly since there seems to be no difference in the clinical disease or its course between the two sexes (10). The average time interval from an initial attack of optic neuritis until other symptoms and signs of MS develop varies considerably; however, most authors find that the majority of persons who develop MS after an attack of optic neuritis do so within 7 years of the onset of visual symptoms (32,96,102,236). Even patients who live in tropical and subtropical regions of the world have a substantial risk of developing MS after an attack of isolated optic neuritis (237), although this risk may be lower in Japan (238) and in some Latin American countries (239). It therefore seems appropriate to consider most cases of optic neuritis a limited form of MS (240) and to counsel patients appropriately (147,241–243).

As noted above, there appear to be certain risk factors that increase the likelihood that a patient with isolated optic neuritis will eventually develop MS. Compston et al. (125) found that positive typing for HLA BT101, winter onset of the initial attack of optic neuritis in BT101-positive patients, and recurrent attacks of optic neuritis were associated with an increased incidence of MS. Frick and Stickl (113) reported that the presence of MBP in the CSF of a patient with otherwise isolated optic neuritis and no history of previous neurologic symptoms or signs nevertheless is highly predictive of the development of MS in the future, a conclusion supported by the findings of Söderström et al. (114) of anti-MBP and anti-MBP peptide antibody-secreting cells in the CSF of patients with both acute optic neuritis and MS. Multiple oligoclonal bands in the CSF of a patient with isolated optic neuritis also seems to be highly predictive of the future development of MS (94,115–118).

Among patients with isolated optic neuritis enrolled in the ONTT, a positive family history of MS, a history of previous neurologic symptoms, and a history of a previous attack of optic neuritis in the fellow eye increased the risk of the development of MS; however, at least one lesion in the periventricular white matter on MR imaging, a phenomenon noted in 30–70% of patients with isolated optic neuritis (7,12,145, 146), was the most significant risk factor associated with an increased likelihood of developing MS (13,23).

Deckert-Schlüter et al. (119) detected increased concentrations of several different cytokines in the serum, CSF, or both of 20 patients with isolated optic neuritis who eventually developed MS, and Link et al. (120) reported similar results. The presence of these substances suggests an activation of the T lymphocytes of the immune system both within and outside the CNS, and suggests that either their presence alone or their particular concentration may be used to predict the eventual development of MS in these patients.

Some authors believe that patients in whom optic neuritis is the initial manifestation of MS tend to have a more benign course than patients in whom MS presents with no visual symptoms and signs (51,82,244–247). Other investigators, however, have found no difference in the eventual outcome of the disease (248–251).

In the ONTT (23), the 10-year risk of MS was 38%. Patients (n = 160) with one or more typical lesions on the baseline brain MR scan had a risk of 56%; those with no lesions (n = 191) had a risk of 22% ($P < 0.001$). The presence of more than one lesion did not appreciably increase that risk (23–26). Even when brain MR lesions were present, over 40% of patients did not develop clinical MS after 10 years. The 10-year risk of development of MS, based strictly on conventional clinical criteria, was 38%, compared with a 5-year risk of 30% (22–26). Thus, although these patients continued to develop MS with each passing year, most did so within the first 5 years after the initial episode of optic neuritis. These results have applicability not only to optic neuritis but also to patients presenting with a first demyelinating event of the brain stem or spinal cord because the three presentations share a common pathogenesis and have been reported to have similar risks for MS (83). The finding, in the ONTT cohort of patients, of a 38% 10-year risk of MS after optic neuritis is similar to that of several prior reports (33,102,236) and lower than that of other reports (83,130,252), all of which had smaller sample sizes. Differences in risk estimates across studies can also be attributed to differences in patient inclusion criteria, retention rates, and diagnostic criteria for MS.

The most potent predictor of MS in the ONTT was the presence of white matter lesions on the baseline brain MR scan (23). The presence of one such lesion at least 3 mm in diameter more than doubled the 10-year risk of MS (from 22% to 56%). However, the presence of one or more lesions did not signify that the patient was destined to develop MS. Among patients with brain MR lesions, the 10-year probability of remaining free of MS was 44%. Conversely, the absence of brain MR lesions did not eliminate the risk of developing MS; in the absence of any lesions, the 10-year probability of MS was 22%.

There are certain gender and optic disc appearance characteristics that help predict whether a patient with optic neuritis

Table 6.1

Gender and Optic Disc Appearance Combined as Predictors of Multiple Sclerosis in Patients with No Brain Lesions on MR Imaging at Study Entry

	N	Number Developing Multiple Sclerosis	10-Year Risk of Multiple Sclerosis[a]	Hazard Ratio (95% CI)[b]
Female				
Disc normal	85	26	31%	1.0
Disc edema	57	9	16%	0.42 (0.20–0.89)
Male				
Disc normal	25	3	15%	0.36 (0.11–1.19)
Disc edema	24	1	5%	0.14 (0.02–1.00)

[a] Kaplan-Meier estimate of cumulative probability.
[b] From proportional hazards model.
(From Optic Neuritis Study Group. Long-term brain MRI changes after optic neuritis in patients without clinically definite multiple sclerosis. Arch Neurol 2004 [in press].)

will subsequently develop MS (Table 6.1) (26). In the ONTT, among patients with one or more brain MR lesions, no demographic characteristics or clinical features of the optic neuritis were useful in further defining the risk (23–26). But among patients without brain MR lesions, the risk was three times lower in males than in females, consistent with the well-documented lower prevalence of MS in males than in females and consistent with studies conducted prior to the availability of brain MR imaging. The risk was also lower when the optic neuritis was associated with a swollen rather than a normal optic disc. Among females with no brain MR lesions, those with optic disc edema had a risk of MS that was half as great as those without optic disc edema. The risk of MS when no baseline brain MR lesions were present was zero among the small group of patients who had any one of the following findings: no light perception vision in the affected eye, optic fundus findings including severe optic disc edema, peripapillary hemorrhages, retinal exudates, or the absence of periocular pain (24–26). Thus, when there are no brain MR lesions, the presence of any of these clinical features appears to predict a very low risk of MS. In patients who bear these atypical features, the optic neuritis may not be part of a multifocal demyelinating CNS illness.

The difference in the risk profile between patients with and without brain MR lesions is not surprising (24–26). Patients with MR lesions already have imaging evidence of disseminated disease, the pathogenesis of which is almost certainly related to MS. Therefore, there is no reason to expect to be able to identify true risk factors for future development of MS. On the other hand, the group of patients with optic neuritis and a normal brain MR scan likely includes a subgroup destined to have MS and another subgroup not destined to have MS.

With regard to the predictive role of MR lesions, the only study comparable to the ONTT (252,253) enrolled 131 patients with an acute demyelinating event in which optic neuritis constituted half of the cohort. Ten-year follow-up was achieved in 81 (62%) patients and 12- to 16-year follow-up

in 72 (55%). After 10 years, MS was present in 83% of those with entry MR lesions and in 11% of those without entry MR lesions. Differences between these results and the ONTT may be related to the former study's smaller sample size and lower follow-up rate. That study found, as the ONTT/LONS did, that once there is at least one MR lesion, an increasing number of lesions does not appreciably amplify the long-term risk of MS.

The eligibility criteria of the ONTT/LONS were sufficiently broad that the results should be applicable to most patients presenting with optic neuritis as a first demyelinating event. Having incomplete data for 13% of the original cohort was unlikely to be a source of appreciable bias. However, because the patients with incomplete follow-up had a lower prevalence of brain MR scans with one or more lesions than did the patients with complete follow-up, the computed 10-year risk of MS could be a slight overestimate.

The results of the ONTT/LONS long-term follow-up are important to the clinician in several respects (23,650). First, they reaffirm the prognostic value of a brain MR scan performed at the time of a first episode of optic neuritis. The presence of a single brain MR white matter lesion of at least 3 mm in diameter markedly increases the risk of developing MS; higher numbers of lesions do not appreciably increase that risk. Second, they establish that even when MR lesions are present, clinically defined MS does not develop within 10 years in over 40% of patients. Third, the results highlight the importance of an ophthalmologic examination for patients whose brain MR scan is normal, because ophthalmoscopy can identify features (severe optic disc swelling, hemorrhages, and exudates) associated with a very low risk of developing MS. This natural history information is a critical input for estimating a patient's 10-year MS risk and for weighing the benefit of initiating prophylactic treatment at the time of optic neuritis or other first demyelinating events in the CNS.

Recurrent Optic Neuritis

Patients in whom idiopathic acute optic neuritis occurs, whether anterior or retrobulbar, may experience a recurrence in the eye at a later date or may experience a similar attack in the fellow eye. Recurrent attacks occurred in 11.3% of the patients reported by Marshall (68), in 14% of the patients studied by Classman and Phillips (254), in 20.6% of the patients in the series reported by Lynn (197), in 24% of Hutchinson's patients (83), and in 16.7% of the patients studied by Perkin and Rose (39). The 10-year ONTT recurrence rate of 35% was similar to that reported by Cohen (42%) but higher than that reported in other studies with extended follow-up such as those by Bradley and Whitty (18%), Hutchinson (24%), and Rodriguez (16%). Although it has been believed that the likelihood of visual acuity returning to normal decreases with each recurrence (83,197), the experience of the ONTT has shown that long-term visual function is generally good despite this recurrence rate.

Management Recommendations for Patients with Presumed Acute Optic Neuritis

In a patient with typical features of optic neuritis, a clinical diagnosis can be made with a high degree of certainty without the need for ancillary testing. Brain MR imaging is a powerful predictor of the long-term probability of MS (for at least the first 10 years); this information, as outlined above, when coupled with clinical trial outcomes suggesting significant efficacy of early immunomodulatory therapy in patients with clinically isolated demyelinating syndromes and abnormal MR scans, should be helpful to clinicians in planning long-term therapy as prophylaxis.

Based on the results of the ONTT, it is reasonable to consider treatment with intravenous methylprednisolone, 250 mg q6h for 3 days or 1 g/day in a single dose × 3 days, followed by a 2-week course of oral prednisone, 1 mg/kg/day, with a rapid taper for patients with acute optic neuritis, particularly if brain MR imaging demonstrates multiple signal abnormalities in the periventricular white matter consistent with MS, or if a patient needs to recover vision faster than the natural history of the condition. Since the potential beneficial effects on the visual and neurologic courses are short term and not lasting, prescribing no treatment is also a reasonable approach. However, oral prednisone alone in standard dosages (e.g., less than 1 mg/kg/day) should be avoided. As noted above, the visual recovery is excellent without treatment and the long-term vision is not any better when corticosteroids are prescribed.

Pathology

There is little material available regarding the pathologic findings in the optic nerves of patients with acute isolated optic neuritis. What pathology exists has been in optic nerves from patients with acute MS and shows active demyelinating plaques similar to those in the brain (255–258). In such plaques, the inflammatory response is marked by perivascular cuffing, T cells, and plasma cells. Initially there is swelling of nerve tissue in the area of demyelination, following which the myelin sheaths begin to break down into fat droplets. As degeneration proceeds, the nerve fibers themselves are destroyed, with the degeneration occurring in both the proximal and distal segments. As the inflammatory reaction subsides, fat-laden macrophages become numerous, and there is glial proliferation. Gartner (259) examined 14 eyes from 10 patients in whom a diagnosis of MS had been made clinically and confirmed at postmortem examination. An attack of optic neuritis had been diagnosed during life in only two of the cases, and all cases were in an advanced state of the disease by the time of their death. Gartner (259) found only optic atrophy, predominantly in the temporal portion of the nerve. Although the papillomacular bundle was primarily affected, the peripheral fibers were also damaged. There was an increase in cellularity of the nerve, especially with respect to glial cells. The surface of the optic discs showed extensive gliosis, and the blood vessels on and near the disc were thickened and sclerosed. The retina showed atrophy of the nerve fibers and ganglion cells, most readily observed at the macula. de Preux and Mair (260) described the ultrastructure of the optic nerves of a patient who developed Schilder's disease and bilateral demyelinating optic neuritis. Both nerves contained areas of complete, as well as partial, demyelination. No oligodendrocytes were present in the areas of complete demyelination, and the naked axons contained swollen, vacuolated mitochondria in these areas. There were some oligodendrocytes in areas of partial demyelination, and axon architecture was maintained in these regions. In all areas, there was an excess of fibrous astrocytes.

Several experimental animal models of demyelinating optic neuritis can be produced for study of pathologic changes and other features of the condition. Rao et al. (261) produced experimental allergic optic neuritis in guinea pigs by sensitization with isogenic spinal cord emulsion in complete Freund's adjuvant. The optic neuritis produced in this manner has two major forms: (*a*) a ''retrobulbar'' form, with a diminished pupillary response to light despite a normal-appearing retina and optic disc, and (*b*) a ''neuroretinitis,'' with a diminished pupillary response associated with hyperemia and swelling of the optic disc and edema of the peripapillary retina. Histopathologic study of animals with retrobulbar neuritis reveals a mononuclear cell infiltrate localized to the retrobulbar portion of the optic nerve and chiasm with multiple foci of axial and periaxial demyelination. Similar pathologic changes are present in animals with experimental neuroretinitis, but in these animals, the lesions are located just behind the lamina cribrosa, with marked swelling of axons in the prelaminar portion of the optic nerve, identical with that seen in human disc swelling. In addition, Hayreh et al. (262) observed acute optic neuritis with variable degrees of optic disc swelling in adult rhesus monkeys with experimental allergic encephalomyelitis. Histopathologic examination of the optic nerves of these animals revealed inflammatory infiltrates, extensive demyelination, and axon degeneration, without inflammation in the retina or optic nerve head. Okamoto (263) observed macrophages in the subarachnoid space in rabbits with experimental allergic optic neuritis. He suggested that these macrophages may digest the myelin debris in the subpial spaces of the affected optic nerves. It is likely that these models will facilitate future studies of pathogenetic mechanisms of demyelinating diseases of the human optic nerve (264).

Sergott et al. (265) injected the serum from 17 patients with MS and 3 patients with isolated optic neuritis into the optic nerves of guinea pigs. These investigators then sacrificed the animals and examined the optic nerves. They found demyelination in the optic nerves injected with the serum from 12 of the 17 MS patients and in the optic nerves injected with serum from all 3 of the optic neuritis patients. There were areas in which axons were relatively spared within the areas of demyelination, similar to those seen in the brains of patients with MS.

It is believed that demyelination of nerve fibers leads to complete conduction block, slowing of conduction, or a failure to transmit a rapid train of impulses (256,266,369).

Relationship of Optic Neuritis to MS

Optic neuritis occurs in about 50% of patients with MS and in about 20% it is the presenting sign (39). Available evidence suggests that the pathogenesis of isolated optic neuritis is no different than that of MS in general. In fact, a strong case can be made for optic neuritis being a *forme fruste* of MS, based on similarities between the two in incidence, CSF findings, histocompatibility data, results of MR imaging, and family history as well as other features (240). For instance, both isolated optic neuritis and MS are more common in northern latitudes and in females compared with males. Immunologic changes in the CSF similar to those in MS may also occur in optic neuritis (267) (discussed previously). Feasby and Ebers (115) found that 75% of 36 patients with isolated optic neuritis had abnormalities on somatosensory evoked potentials, brain stem evoked potentials, or CSF protein electrophoresis, and Sanders et al. (251) found that 67% of 30 patients had similar abnormalities. As noted above, 25–60% of patients with isolated optic neuritis have changes in the brain on MR imaging consistent with areas of demyelination. Ebers et al. (268) described 10 patients with isolated optic neuritis who had a family member with MS, which also suggests an etiologic association between the two, and similar HLA types (108,125) are also present in both optic neuritis and MS.

Although Kurland et al. (269) did not find age at onset of optic neuritis to be a risk factor in the eventual development of MS, and Hely et al. (135) reported that there was no difference in the age range of those patients with optic neuritis who developed MS compared with those who did not, most studies indicate that the younger the age at which optic neuritis develops, the greater the risk for the development of MS. Bradley and Whitty (82) first suggested that the risk of MS increased with increasing age, but they did not provide any supportive data. Kahana et al. (30), however, reported that 39% of patients who were less than 39 years old when they had an initial attack of optic neuritis eventually developed MS, compared with 21% of patients who eventually developed MS after they developed optic neuritis when they were older than 40. Mapelli et al. (270) reported similar findings. These investigators reported that 31% of 26 patients who were less than 40 years of age when they experienced a first attack of optic neuritis eventually developed MS, compared with only 14% of 14 patients who were older than 40 years of age when they experienced their first attack. Rizzo and Lessell (236) reported that the relative risk for MS increased by 1.7 for each decade less than 54 years. Like Bradley and Whitty (82), Sandberg-Wollheim et al. (102) suggested that younger age at onset of optic neuritis was a risk factor in the development of MS but provided no supportive data. Age at onset was not found to be statistically related to ultimate development of MS in the ONTT/LONS (24–26).

There is some controversy as to whether gender is a risk factor for the development of MS after optic neuritis. Some investigators report no difference in the incidence of MS after optic neuritis (30,82,237,270). Rodriguez et al. (33) also found no gender differences in their study: 38% of 26 men and 40% of 66 women developed MS at 10 years after onset of optic neuritis. On the other hand, Hely et al. (135) reported that the relative risk of MS was almost three times greater in women compared with men. Rizzo and Lessell (236) reported that MS developed in 69% of 47 women and 33% of 20 men within 14.9 years of their initial attack of optic neuritis, and Sandberg-Wollheim et al. (102) reported

that 46% of 54 females and 28% of 32 men developed MS within a mean of 12.9 years after their attack. In the ONTT with 10 years of follow-up, no gender difference in risk for development of MS was observed (23) when the presenting MR scan was found to be abnormal. In contrast, among the 191 patients without MR lesions, certain features did alter the risk of MS (Table 6.1), with the risk of MS lower in males than in females.

Kurland et al. (269) found no difference between whites and nonwhites in his comparison of United States servicemen, but this study had low power to observe such a difference if, indeed, one existed. Alter et al. (271) compared the Asian and Caucasian populations in Hawaii and found no significant differences in the rate of development of MS after optic neuritis between the two races. Although the 2-year data from the ONTT suggested that Caucasians are at higher risk than African-Americans (13), results from this study at 10 years had insufficient statistical significance to comment on this variable. Among Caucasians in the study, 14% of 331 developed MS within 2 years compared with 5% of 58 non-Caucasians, most of whom were African-American. This difference was still present at 4-year follow-up (20).

Kurland et al. (269) found neither birthplace nor residence to be a risk factor for MS in a study of U.S. veterans with optic neuritis, but the study by Kahana et al. (30) of optic neuritis in Israel found that MS developed in 23% of 35 patients born in Europe, 32% of 25 patients born in Asia or Africa, and 44% of 25 patients born in Israel. There is increasing epidemiologic evidence suggesting that the place of residence in regard to distance from the equator during the first 15 years of life is a major risk factor for the development of MS after optic neuritis. Indeed, it seems clear that persons who migrate from one country or region to another during childhood (i.e., under 15 years of age) take on the risk of the country of destination (272–274). It is less clear whether persons who migrate later in life retain the risk of their country of origin or take on the risk of their new place of residence.

Kurland et al. (266) and Bradley and Whitty (82) reported that season of onset of optic neuritis was not a risk factor for the subsequent development of MS but provided no data. Sandberg-Wollheim et al. (102), however, reported that MS developed in 43% of 42 patients with onset of optic neuritis between October and March, compared with 29% of 44 patients with onset of optic neuritis between April and September.

There are few data available on the features of optic neuritis that relate to the subsequent risk of MS. Kurland et al. (266) did not find any aspects of optic neuritis to be risk factors; however, Bradley and Whitty (82), without any supporting data, reported that optic disc appearance and severity of visual loss were not risk factors for MS but that the presence of pain and a typical visual field defect were risk factors. Kahana et al. (30) found that MS developed in only 13% of 45 patients with anterior optic neuritis, compared with 60% of 30 patients with retrobulbar optic neuritis.

Data from the ONTT confirm the findings of Kahana et al. (30) that the presence of severe disc swelling reduces the likelihood that MS will develop, particularly when the patient also has normal brain MR imaging (13,23–26). In the ONTT, among the 22 patients with severe disc swelling and normal brain MR imaging at baseline, none developed clinical signs of MS in 10 years of follow-up. In patients of both genders without brain MR lesions, MS did not develop in any patients whose visual loss was painless (n = 18) or total (no light perception, n = 6) or in those who had ophthalmoscopic findings of severe disc swelling (n = 22), hemorrhage of the optic disc or surrounding retina (n = 16), or retinal exudates (n = 8) (Table 6.1). In the 191 patients without MR lesions, the risk of MS was lower when the optic disc was swollen (anterior optic neuritis, papillitis) than when it was not swollen (retrobulbar neuritis). Among females, the risk of MS was halved when optic disc swelling was present. Among males, only 1 of 24 patients with optic disc swelling developed MS. One hundred seventy-nine of the 191 patients with no brain MR lesions had no prior history of neurologic symptoms or optic neuritis in the fellow eye and would be considered to have monofocal optic neuritis; their 10-year risk of MS was 20%.

In most series, adult patients with bilateral simultaneous optic neuritis are said to have the same risk of developing MS as patients with unilateral optic neuritis (82,269,275); however, Hutchinson (83) found an increased incidence of MS in patients who developed bilateral optic neuritis either simultaneously or whose second eye became affected within 2 weeks of the first eye. In the ONTT/LONS, when the criteria for MS were expanded to include the occurrence of optic neuritis in the fellow eye, the 10-year risk of MS was 45%: 31% in patients with no baseline brain MR lesions and 60% in patients with one or more lesions (23). Most authors believe that ultimate visual acuity after optic neuritis has no bearing on the subsequent development of MS (23–26, 39,82).

Although it might be expected that recurrent optic neuritis would increase the risk for MS, the reports on this provide mixed results, with some authors reporting an increased risk (33,83,102,267) and others not (130,236). Data from the ONTT data do not show a strong relationship between recurrent optic neuritis and the early development of MS (13,20,23–26).

Evidence of immunologic dysfunction (e.g., oligoclonal banding) in the CSF is common in patients with MS. Whether the presence of these abnormalities in patients with clinically isolated optic neuritis increases the risk that such patients will develop MS in the future is controversial (discussed previously). Nikoskelainen et al. (267) studied 48 patients with isolated optic neuritis, 27 (56.3%) of whom developed probable MS during a 7- to 10-year follow-up. Although increased relative IgG, abnormal electrophoresis, or an abnormal ratio of measles antibody titer in the serum compared with the CSF at the time of presentation correlated with the development of clinical signs of disseminated disease, 6 of 11 (54.5%) patients with normal CSF values on every laboratory study developed MS. Stendahl-Brodin and Link (117) reported that 9 of 11 (81.8%) patients with isolated optic neuritis but with abnormal CSF developed MS within a mean follow-up of 11 years. During this period only 1 of 19 (5.3%) similar patients with normal CSF developed

MS. Anmarkrud and Slettnes (118) reported that 15 of 19 (78.9%) patients with optic neuritis who had abnormal CSF but only 1 of 10 (10%) patients with optic neuritis and normal CSF developed MS within a mean follow-up of 5.8 years. Sandberg-Wollheim et al. (102) reported that 26 of 55 (47.3%) patients with optic neuritis who had abnormal CSF and 7 of 31 (22.6%) patients with normal CSF developed MS over a mean follow-up of 12.9 years. These studies indicate that 25–50% of patients with isolated acute optic neuritis and abnormal CSF remain free of neurologic manifestations of MS for many years (if not for life), whereas 10–50% of patients with optic neuritis and normal CSF nevertheless develop other manifestations of MS during the same period. In view of these findings, it seems likely that CSF abnormalities alone are not a primary risk factor in determining whether a patient with acute optic neuritis eventually develops clinical evidence of disseminated demyelination.

No long-term study has evaluated the added value of the detection of CSF abnormalities in conjunction with MR imaging of the brain; however, data from the ONTT suggest that the presence of CSF abnormalities has little predictive value for the development of MS over and above the powerful predictive value of MR imaging (discussed previously) (13,93,276,277).

The predictive value of CSF oligoclonal banding for the development of CDMS within 5 years after optic neuritis was assessed in 76 patients enrolled in the ONTT. In the patients followed in the ONTT for 5 years, the following findings were noted:

1. Oligoclonal bands were present in 50% of the patients (73% of the 37 patients with abnormal brain MR and 28% of the 39 patients with normal brain MR).
2. CDMS developed within 2 years in 29% of the 38 with oligoclonal bands and in 5% of the 38 patients without oligoclonal bands ($P = 0.015$).
3. The association of oligoclonal bands and the development of CDMS was attenuated when adjusted for brain MRI (P [adjusted for MRI] = 0.09).
4. There were 11 patients with normal brain MR scans who had oligoclonal bands, two of whom had developed CDMS by 2 years (93).

CDMS developed within 5 years in 22 (29%) of the 76 patients: in 16 (42%) of the 38 patients with oligoclonal bands present and in 6 (16%) of the 38 patients without bands (OR = 3.88; 95% CI = 1.18, 13.86; $P = 0.02$). Among the 54 patients not classified as CDMS, 5-year follow-up was complete for 50 (93%). The predictive value of CSF oligoclonal band assessment for the development of CDMS over and above that of brain MR imaging was apparent only among patients with no brain MR lesions at study entry. Among the 39 patients with normal brain MR imaging, CDMS developed in 3 of 11 (27%) patients with oligoclonal bands present but in only 1 of 28 (4%) without oligoclonal bands ($P = 0.06$). In contrast, among the 37 patients with abnormal brain MR imaging, CDMS developed in 13 of 27 (48%) with oligoclonal bands and in 5 of

10 (50%) without oligoclonal bands ($P = 1.00$). The positive predictive value of oligoclonal bands was 42% and the negative predictive value was 84%. Among the 39 patients with normal brain MR imaging, the positive and negative predictive values were 27% and 96%, respectively, whereas among the 37 patients with abnormal brain MR imaging, the values were 48% and 50%, respectively.

Brain MR imaging has been demonstrated to be a strong predictor of CDMS among patients with monosymptomatic optic neuritis. In the ONTT there was a 51% 5-year incidence of CDMS in patients who had abnormal brain MR imaging at the time of optic neuritis compared with a 16% incidence in those with normal brain MR scans (22). These results indicate that performing a lumbar puncture to detect oligoclonal bands is not of added value for predicting the five-year risk of CDMS in patients who have abnormal brain MR scans at the time of development of monosymptomatic optic neuritis. However, the results suggest that oligoclonal band testing may be helpful in the risk assessment of optic neuritis patients with normal brain MR scans.

That the value of CSF analysis would depend on the brain MR findings was not felt to be surprising (277). Patients with abnormal brain MR scans already have morphologic evidence of disseminated disease, and as such it is expected that most of these patients will eventually develop additional neurologic events sufficient for a diagnosis of CDMS. Therefore, there is no reason to expect that a CSF analysis would be predictive of MS among these patients. The group of patients with optic neuritis and normal brain MR imaging likely includes a subset of those destined to have MS and a subset of those who may have optic neuritis unassociated with MS. Among these patients, the finding of oligoclonal bands in the CSF does appear to increase the likelihood that CDMS ultimately will be diagnosed. Additionally and perhaps more importantly, the absence of oligoclonal bands in the CSF makes the development of CDMS within 5 years unlikely. Although the number of patients in the ONTT was too small for definitive conclusions with regard to the role of CSF analysis in the evaluation of patients with optic neuritis, according to the authors the results suggested that a lumbar puncture has limited value in patients with typical monosymptomatic optic neuritis who have demyelinative changes on brain MR imaging (277).

CHRONIC DEMYELINATING OPTIC NEURITIS

It was once stated that for all intents and purposes chronic optic neuritis does not occur. The reason for this dogmatic statement was that too many patients with mass lesions compressing the intracranial portion of the optic nerve were being diagnosed as having chronic optic neuritis, leading to delayed treatment of the underlying lesion with resultant permanent visual loss. Thus, the statement that chronic optic neuritis was never a tenable diagnosis was made in an effort to raise the consciousness of the majority of physicians to look for another, potentially treatable, cause of unilateral progressive optic neuropathy.

In fact, chronic optic neuritis not only occurs but is not uncommon. In any group of patients with MS, one can find numerous patients who have no history of acute visual loss (painful or otherwise) but who nevertheless complain that the vision in one or both eyes is not normal and who have evidence of unilateral or bilateral optic nerve dysfunction (198,254,278–285). Such patients may complain of a static disturbance of vision, a slowly progressive loss of vision in one or both eyes, or, occasionally, a stepwise loss of vision unassociated with periods of recovery.

Some patients with MS complain of blurred or distorted vision even though visual acuity is 20/20 or better in both eyes. Such patients often are found to have evidence of chronic optic neuritis by clinical testing (e.g., color vision, visual fields, ophthalmoscopy) (Fig. 6.12), electrophysiologic testing (visual evoked responses), psychophysical testing (e.g., contrast sensitivity), or a combination of these methods (202,286–289). Regan et al. (202), for example, used sine wave gratings to test contrast sensitivity for narrow, broad, and intermediate-width bars in a group of 48 patients with MS and resolved optic neuritis. These investigators found that in 20 of the 48 patients with MS in whom Snellen acuity fell within normal limits, contrast sensitivity to gratings of broad and/or intermediate bar width was abnormally low, whereas sensitivity to narrow bars was normal.

Most patients with chronic unilateral or bilateral demyelinating optic neuritis develop visual symptoms after other signs and symptoms of MS have developed, and this is why the percentage of patients with MS and evidence of chronic progressive optic neuritis increases the longer the patients are followed (278,281). Nevertheless, slowly progressive visual loss or complaints of blurred or distorted vision are the first symptoms of the underlying neurologic disease in some patients (278,281). We are unaware of any treatment for chronic progressive demyelinating optic neuritis.

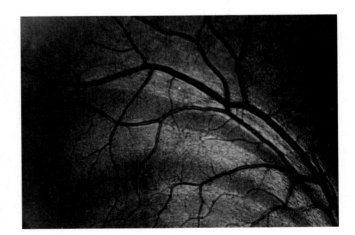

Figure 6.12. Retinal nerve fiber bundle defects in the right eye of a patient with bilateral chronic optic neuritis in the setting of multiple sclerosis. The patient had never experienced any episodes of acute loss of vision. Instead, she stated that her vision was slightly blurred and had been slowly worsening for the past 6–8 months. Visual acuity was 20/20 OU; however, color vision was slightly diminished in both eyes when tested using Hardy-Rand-Rittler pseudoisochromatic plates. Visual fields were normal by kinetic perimetry. There was no relative afferent pupillary defect. Both optic discs were mildly pale.

ASYMPTOMATIC (SUBCLINICAL) DEMYELINATING OPTIC NEURITIS

A substantial percentage of patients with MS have clinical or laboratory evidence of optic nerve dysfunction even though they have no visual complaints and believe their vision to be normal (194,198,282,283,285,290–292). The Optic Neuritis Study Group (7,11) found that 48% of patients with apparently unilateral optic neuritis and no history of previous optic neuritis in the contralateral eye nevertheless had an abnormal visual field unexplained by intraocular pathology in their asymptomatic, fellow eye. A substantial percentage of these eyes also had disturbances of visual acuity, color vision, and contrast sensitivity. These findings are consistent with the pathologic finding of demyelination in the optic nerves in patients who never had visual complaints during life (293). Miller (294) reported having evaluated a 21-year-old woman who came to the Wilmer Eye Institute for a routine examination. Visual acuity was correctable to 20/15 OU, color vision was normal, and kinetic perimetry was normal in both eyes using both a tangent (Bjerrum) screen and a Goldmann perimeter. Ophthalmoscopy revealed normal-appearing optic discs and peripapillary nerve fiber layer with no evidence of atrophy; however, the patient had a definite right relative afferent pupillary defect. It was decided to perform a CT scan. Shortly after the patient received an intravenous injection of contrast, she experienced a seizure and then had cardiorespiratory arrest from which she could not be resuscitated. Postmortem examination revealed no brain neuropathologic findings; however, the right optic nerve showed several small areas of demyelination and secondary atrophy consistent with a previous attack of subclinical optic neuritis (Fig. 6.13). Although this patient had no evidence of MS, this case emphasizes that patients with and without evidence of MS may experience an attack of subclinical optic neuritis.

Evidence for optic neuritis in a patient who is visually asymptomatic may be clinical, electrophysiologic, psychophysical, or a combination of these (40,188,291,292). A careful clinical examination may reveal that despite having visual acuity of 20/20 or better, the patient has a subtle disturbance of color perception when tested with color plates, the Farnsworth-Munsell 100-Hue test, or some other method (8,60,126,187,188,190,295,296). There may be subtle visual field defects in one or both eyes detected using automated perimetry (194,297,298). A relative afferent pupillary defect may be present (299), or the patient may have subtle optic nerve or nerve fiber layer atrophy (191,286,300–302) (Fig. 6.14). In some cases, MR imaging shows enhancement of the optic nerve in question (Fig. 6.15).

Visually asymptomatic patients suspected of having or known to have MS may be shown to have disturbances of the visual sensory pathways by electrophysiologic testing. VEPs seem to be a particularly sensitive indicator of optic nerve and other visual sensory pathway disturbances in such patients (40,188,190,191,210,289,291,292,296,303–305).

Psychophysical tests of visual function, such as contrast sensitivity using a Pelli-Robson chart, Arden gratings, oscilloscope screen projections, or similar techniques, may reveal abnormalities in patients with MS and other disorders who are visually asymptomatic (40,58,189,192,202,283,287,289, 291,292,306,307). Some psychophysical tests, such as measurements of sustained visual resolution (308) and assessment of chromatic, luminance, spatial, and temporal sensitivity (309–313), give similar results but are too complex

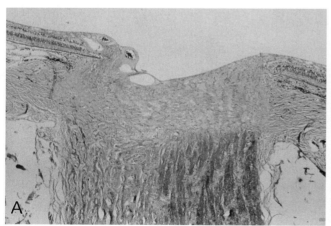
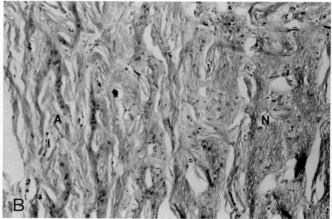

Figure 6.13. Pathology of probable subclinical optic neuritis. The patient was a 21-year-old woman with no previous history of systemic disease, neurologic disease, ocular disease, or trauma who was noted during a routine eye examination to have a right relative afferent pupillary defect. The patient had no visual complaints once her refractive error was corrected, and she had visual acuity of 20/15 OU, normal color perception in both eyes, using Hardy-Rand-Rittler pseudoisochromatic plates, and normal visual fields by kinetic perimetry. The patient subsequently suffered a fatal cardiac arrest during CT scanning, possibly related to a toxic reaction to contrast material. A, Section through the right optic disc and anterior portion of the right optic nerve shows segmental optic atrophy. Masson trichrome. B, Higher-power view of the right optic nerve shows the atrophic area (A) adjacent to normal nerve fiber bundles (N). Masson trichrome.

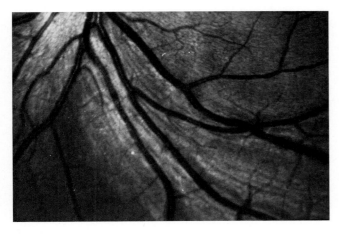

Figure 6.14. Retinal nerve fiber bundle defects in the asymptomatic eye of a patient with multiple sclerosis. Note numerous curvilinear dark streaks in the inferior arcuate nerve fiber bundle of the left eye.

and time-consuming to be of use in screening patients in clinical practice. Other tests, such as assessing the presence or absence of the Pulfrich phenomenon (314), and the "flight of colors" test (316–319), give little more information than one can obtain by an otherwise complete clinical and electrophysiologic examination.

NEUROMYELITIS OPTICA (DEVIC'S DISEASE)

The association of acute or subacute loss of vision in one or both eyes caused by acute optic neuropathy preceded or followed within days to weeks by a transverse or ascending myelitis was initially described by Allbutt (320) and later by Devic (321). Devic called the condition neuromyelitis optica, but it subsequently became known as "Devic's dis-

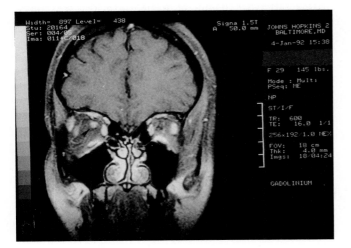

Figure 6.15. MR imaging in subclinical optic neuritis. T1-weighted coronal MR image after intravenous injection of paramagnetic contrast material in a 29-year-old woman with a history of left optic neuritis but no visual symptoms or signs of optic neuropathy in the right eye shows enhancement of the orbital portion of the right optic nerve (*arrowhead*).

ease" through the efforts of his pupil, Gault (322), who devoted his thesis to the subject.

Devic's disease (neuromyelitis optica [NMO]) is an idiopathic inflammatory demyelinating disease of the CNS, characterized by attacks of optic neuritis and myelitis. The co-occurrence of optic neuritis and myelitis is seen in patients with MS, acute disseminated encephalomyelitis, systemic lupus erythematosus (SLE), and Sjögren's syndrome; it can also occur in association with viral and bacterial infections (Table 6.2). Often, however, no underlying cause can be found. NMO may occur as a monophasic illness that is either fulminant and fatal or associated with varying degrees of recovery. A polyphasic course, characterized by relapses and remissions, also occurs (323).

Although Devic's disease has been acknowledged as a unique type of optic neuritis for over 130 years, only recently has the pathologic appearance of this unique form of demyelinating process been more clearly elucidated. Much debate has revolved around whether NMO is a distinct disease, and what its relationship is to MS and other autoimmune disorders.

Epidemiology

NMO constitutes less than 1% of demyelinating disease in Western countries (324,325) and may be more prevalent than typical MS in Japan (326–329). NMO occurs primarily in children and young adults (330–336), but all ages may be affected, and the condition has been described in patients over 60 years of age (331,337,338). Both sexes are equally affected. It does not seem to be inherited, although McAlpine (339) reported its occurrence in monozygotic twins. Although most patients who develop this condition are otherwise healthy, NMO has been reported in patients with SLE (340,341), pulmonary tuberculosis (342–344), and after chickenpox (345,346). Hainfellner et al. (347) reported the case of a previously healthy 40-year-old woman who developed both NMO and myelinoclastic diffuse sclerosis (Schilder's disease; discussed later). This case gives some credence to those who believe that both disorders are variants of MS.

Table 6.2
Neuromyelitis Optica and Associated Systemic Diseases

Autoimmune disorders
Systemic lupus erythematosus (340,341,526–530,635)
Sjögren's syndrome (636–639)
P-ANCA (640,641)
Anticardiolipin antibody syndrome (642,643)
Mixed connective tissue disease (644,645)
Infectious disease
Tuberculosis (343,344,646)
Viral
   HIV (511)
   Varicella-zoster virus (345,346,369,647)
   Epstein-Barr virus (370)
Toxins
Clioquinol (648–650)

Pathology

The brain, optic nerves, and spinal cord are affected by scattered lesions of demyelination that principally affect the white matter but may also affect the gray matter (348). In some cases, the cerebral cortex is only slightly affected or completely spared (349); however, the optic nerves and the spinal cord are invariably damaged (350). Both optic nerves are affected, although the degree of demyelination may be symmetric or asymmetric. Mandler et al. (349) described the pathologic findings in five cases of ''neuromyelitis optica'' and found unilateral demyelination in three of the five cases. All of these cases also showed evidence of a severe necrotizing myelopathy with thickening of blood vessel walls and absence of lymphocytic infiltration or demyelination in the spinal cord. In view of these unusual findings, we would question the diagnosis of NMO in these patients.

The spinal cord is extensively affected in all cases of NMO (350). Liquefaction and formation of cavities are common. There is widespread destruction of myelin sheaths, and axis cylinders may also be destroyed. There may be small areas of perivascular lymphocytes in both brain and spinal cord. Formation of glial tissue occurs in mild or moderately severe cases; however, it is not present or is minimal in fulminating, rapidly fatal cases.

Walsh (351) studied a patient with presumed NMO in whom scattered areas of destroyed tissue were present throughout the subcortex with more pronounced lesions in the occipital lobes, particularly in the region of the calcarine fissure. Small areas of demyelination were present in the basal ganglia, in the region of the red nucleus, and in perivascular locations throughout the mesencephalon. The optic nerves showed extensive demyelination, as did the optic chiasm. The spinal cord was most severely affected, with the lesions increasing in severity as they passed down the cord (352). Rare patients with NMO have pathologic evidence of a demyelinating peripheral neuropathy (353).

Although some investigators believe that NMO is simply a rare and aggressive variant of MS (329,347,354–356), there are several important differences in the pathologic findings in the two conditions (357,358). First, the cerebellum is almost never affected in patients with NMO, whereas it is frequently affected in MS. Second, excavation of affected tissue with formation of cavities is rare in MS but common in NMO, where there is often liquefaction of tissue. Third, gliosis is characteristic of MS but is almost always absent or minimal in NMO. Fourth, the arcuate fibers located in the cerebral subcortex are relatively unaffected in patients with NMO but are severely damaged in most patients with MS.

Lassmann et al. (359) proposed a classification for MS lesions based on molecular histopathologic findings from diagnostic biopsies and autopsies. The patterns I–IV of demyelination and inflammation are not closely linked to specific relapsing-remitting or progressive disease courses but may help us to understand the underlying immunologic and neurodegenerative mechanisms involved in lesion formation. These patterns may also be defining in the pathophysiologic process underlying NMO.

Although serologic and clinical evidence of B-cell autoimmunity has been observed in a high proportion of patients with NMO, the mechanisms that result in selective localization of inflammatory demyelinating lesions to the optic nerves and spinal cord are unknown. Lucchinetti et al. (360) provided detailed molecular studies on 82 lesions from nine autopsy cases of NMO using a similar classification, pathologically, as in their paper on the classification of MS lesions (359). Demyelinating activity in the lesions was immunocytochemically classified as early active (21 lesions), late active (18 lesions), inactive (35 lesions), or remyelinating (8 lesions) by examining the antigenic profile of MDPs with macrophages. The pathology of the lesions was analyzed using a broad spectrum of immunologic and neurobiologic markers, and lesions were defined on the basis of myelin protein loss, the geography and extension of plaques, the patterns of oligodendrocyte destruction, and the immunopathologic evidence of complement activation. The pathology was identical in all nine patients. Extensive demyelination was present across multiple spinal cord levels, associated with cavitation, necrosis, and acute axonal pathology (spheroids), in both gray and white matter. They found a pronounced loss of oligodendrocytes within the lesions. The inflammatory infiltrates in active lesions were characterized by extensive macrophage infiltration associated with large numbers of perivascular granulocytes and eosinophils and rare CD3 + and CD8 + T cells. A pronounced perivascular deposition of immunoglobulins (mainly IgM) and complement C9 neo-antigen in active lesions was associated with prominent vascular fibrosis and hyalinization in both active and inactive lesions. Lucchinetti et al. concluded that the extent of complement activation, eosinophilic infiltration, and vascular fibrosis observed in these Devic NMO cases was more prominent compared with that in prototypic MS, and that this supported a role for humoral immunity in the pathogenesis of NMO. Further, they felt that therapeutic strategies designed to limit the deleterious effects of complement activation, eosinophil degranulation, and neutrophil/macrophage/microglial activation were worthy of further investigation.

The animal model for MS, experimental autoimmune encephalomyelitis (EAE), may be of help in understanding which immunologic effector mechanisms, in particular autoantibodies, contribute to the pathogenesis of NMO. Augmentation of demyelination in EAE in the Lewis rat by circulating antibodies directed toward myelin oligodendrocyte glycoprotein (MOG) was described in the late 1980s (361). Since then a wide array of experimental models have focused on MOG as autoantigen and generated variants of EAE in rats and mice that more closely mimic the complex of pathologies seen in MS (362).

All the salient immunopathologic features of NMO are reproduced in Brown Norway (BN) rats immunized with MOG (363). MOG-induced EAE in this strain follows a fulminant clinical course associated with widespread demyelination and axonal injury. The lesion distribution also exhibits a preference for the optic tract and spinal cord similar to that seen in NMO. More importantly, the inflammatory infiltrate contains large numbers of eosinophils and demyelination is associated with complement deposition. Recruitment of eosinophils into the CNS was not seen in demyelinating lesions induced by the cotransfer of MOG-specific antisera and encephalitogenic Th-1 MOG-specific T cells in BN rats, suggesting that eosinophil recruitment was dependent on a MOG-specific Th-2 T-cell response. However, it was not possible to identify a clear highly polarized MOG-specific Th-2 T-cell response. In particular, no enhanced secretion of the classical Th-2–associated cytokine IL-4 was observed and the MOG-specific antibody response included both Th-1–associated (IgG2b) and Th-2–associated (IgG1 and IgE) isotypes.

These findings demonstrate that even in inbred strains with a high susceptibility for Th-2–driven autoimmune responses, it is difficult to disentangle the effector pathways involved in lesion formation and ultimately tissue destruction. Cree (323) suggested that all we know about the molecular basis for the induction of this NMO disease model is that while the eosinophilic component is controlled by non-MHC genes, the intensity and pathogenicity of the antigen-specific autoimmune response is determined by multiple genes within the MHC. Cree further queried whether the susceptibility to NMO in humans is determined by a similar interplay between ''background'' and MHC loci. Just why the immune system in NMO selectively attacks the optic tract and spinal cord while sparing the brain remains speculative. Because these regions of the CNS are not thought to possess a different repertoire of glial cells or myelin proteins, the selective attack may be the result of differences in the structure/stability of the blood–brain barrier or subtle regional differences in the ability of the CNS to process and present antigen to T cells (323,360,363).

Clinical Manifestations

The primary features of NMO are visual loss caused by damage to the anterior visual sensory pathways and paraplegia caused by damage to the spinal cord. Other visual and neurologic manifestations are much less common.

Prodrome

Approximately one third of NMO patients develop a mild febrile illness several days or weeks before the onset of visual or neurologic manifestations of the disease (323, 336,364). Typical manifestations of this prodrome include sore throat, headache, and fever (365–367). In rare cases, there is a clear history of an antecedent viral illness, such as mumps (368), varicella (369), or infectious mononucleosis (370). The patient reported by Ko et al. (366) had high titers of antibodies against Epstein-Barr virus in her serum. A patient reported by Kline et al. (371) developed typical neuromyelitis optica 11 days after receiving a vaccination with attenuated live rubella virus.

In children, NMO is frequently preceded by infection (72%); these cases typically have a monophasic course and many have a complete recovery (336). Speculation exists regarding whether pediatric NMO should be considered a variant of acute disseminating encephalomyelitis due to the association with preceding infection, monophasic course, and generally good outcome in children (336,372).

Loss of Vision

Visual loss in patients with neuromyelitis optica almost always is bilateral (323,330,331,336), although unilateral cases have been reported (323,336,349). One eye usually is affected first, but the second eye typically is affected within hours, days, or rarely weeks after onset (364). The loss of vision is typically rapid and usually severe. It is not uncommon for complete blindness to develop. The rapid, bilateral loss of vision that occurs in patients with NMO is in sharp contrast to the loss of vision in optic neuritis, which tends to be unilateral and not as severe, and to the loss of vision in Leber's hereditary optic neuropathy, which tends to be more slowly progressive. Pain in or about the eye precedes the loss of vision in a few cases, again distinguishing the condition from optic neuritis, in which pain is an almost universal feature (discussed previously). It is not currently possible to predict whether a patient presenting with optic neuritis or myelitis will develop NMO. However, the abrupt onset of a severe bilateral optic neuritis alerts one to the possible development of subsequent myelitis.

Since the foci of demyelination that affect the optic nerves are irregular and occur in a variety of different locations, the visual field defects that occur are similarly variable. In many instances, vision is so poor when the patient is first examined that it is impossible to plot the field defect. Nevertheless, central scotomas seem to be the most common defect observed, with some patients developing concentric contraction of one or both fields.

The ophthalmoscopic appearance of the optic discs varies considerably in patients with NMO. Most patients have mild swelling of both optic discs (330,336,365). Some patients, however, have substantial disc swelling that may be associated with dilation of retinal veins and extensive peripapillary exudates, and others have normal-appearing optic discs. With time, many patients develop pallor of the discs regardless of their initial appearance (Fig. 6.16). In some of these cases, there is slight narrowing of retinal vessels.

Some recovery of vision usually occurs in patients with NMO (323,331,332). Walsh stated that he had observed only one case of total permanent blindness among 12–15 cases (373), and Jeffery and Buncic (336) reported return of visual acuity to 20/20 in all 17 affected eyes of nine patients whom they studied. Visual acuity usually begins to improve within 1 week after visual symptoms begin, with maximum improvement occurring within several weeks to months. The peripheral fields usually begin to recover before there is noticeable improvement in the central-field defects. Nevertheless, some patients have severe and permanent visual loss in both eyes. Khan et al. (367), for example, reported the case of a 27-year-old pregnant woman who developed bilateral optic neuritis first in the right eye and 2 months later in the left eye. The visual function remained stable over the next several months. The patient then developed an acute transverse myelitis. On examination, she had no light percep-

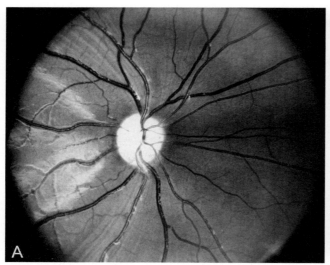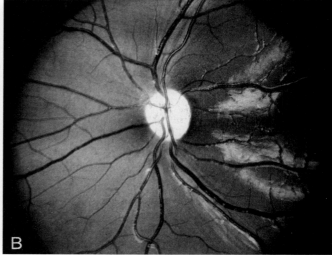

Figure 6.16. Ophthalmoscopic appearance in neuromyelitis optica (Devic's disease). The patient was a 13-year-old girl who developed transverse myelitis, followed several months later by bilateral visual loss. Visual acuity decreased to 20/400 OD and hand motions at 2 feet OS over 72 hours. The pupils were sluggishly reactive to light, and both optic discs appeared normal. The patient was treated with intravenous corticosteroids and gradually recovered both neurologic and visual function. Visual acuity eventually stabilized at 20/40 OD and 20/70 OS associated with small cecocentral scotomas. The ophthalmoscopic appearance of the right and left ocular fundi, *A* and *B* respectively, shows symmetric pallor of the optic discs associated with atrophy of the retinal nerve fiber layer, especially in the papillomacular bundles.

tion in the right eye and only bare light perception in the left eye. There was no improvement in visual acuity over the subsequent 3 months.

There is some controversy about the relationship of visual loss to the onset of paraplegia. Most authors have reported that loss of vision precedes the onset of paraplegia in most cases (374); however, others have found that paraplegia usually precedes loss of vision (375). A similar controversy relates to whether one can diagnose NMO in a patient with bilateral severe optic neuritis without clinical evidence of spinal cord dysfunction. Although we agree that spinal cord damage in such cases could be minimal and subclinical, we would be averse to diagnosing "neuromyelitis optica sine myelitis" unless other studies such as MR imaging showed clear evidence of demyelinating lesions of the spinal cord.

Paraplegia

Paraparesis, which rapidly progresses to paraplegia, may precede or follow the loss of vision in patients with NMO (330). As noted above, the experience of some authors is that the visual loss occurs first (373,374), whereas that of other authors is that paraplegia occurs initially (375) and may be mistakenly assumed to be caused by an infarct or tumor of the spinal cord (376) until appropriate neuroimaging studies are performed. Regardless of which manifestation develops first, the interval between manifestations may be days, weeks, or months (349). In some cases, the blindness and paraplegia occur simultaneously. Hershewe et al. (332) suggested that a diagnosis of NMO should not be made unless the interval between the onset of visual loss and paraplegia is 2 months or less.

The onset of paraplegia, like that of visual loss, usually is sudden and severe, and it may be associated with a mild fever. Some patients develop an ascending paralysis that simulates the Guillain-Barré syndrome; however, the presence of associated sensory symptoms should be sufficient to eliminate Guillain-Barré syndrome from consideration (see Chapter 61). The paraplegia of NMO varies in different cases. Paraplegia in flexion, paraplegia in extension, and paraplegia with loss of all deep tendon (muscle stretch) reflexes may occur. There may be severe root pains, and urinary retention may be present or develop shortly after the onset of motor weakness. Ascending paralysis may paralyze respiration and cause death at an early stage of the disease. Most patients with NMO recover to some extent but have some residual paraparesis, and some have persistent and complete paralysis. The subsequent recovery of neurologic function, particularly in children suspected of having Devic's syndrome, should alert the clinician regarding the diagnosis of possible acute disseminated encephalomyelitis.

Laboratory Studies and Neuroimaging

During the active stage of NMO, the CSF usually shows evidence of an inflammatory process. There often is a mild lymphocytic pleocytosis (323,332,338,364,366,378), although Walsh (351) reported a case in which there were 1,000 white blood cells/mm^3. The concentration of protein in the CSF may be increased, but intrathecal synthesis of IgG is not increased, and oligoclonal bands are rarely detected (378). The glucose concentration in the CSF invariably is normal. Rare cases have been recorded in which there has been evidence of increased intracranial pressure (379).

Chou et al. (380) reported a patient with NMO whose CSF contained antibody to glial fibrillary acidic protein (GFAP). The patient's serum did not contain this antibody, and it was therefore postulated by these authors that the antibody was being synthesized in the CNS.

Neuroimaging rarely shows intracranial lesions in patients with NMO (323). The spinal cord, however, may show changes consistent with demyelination (323,332,338,349, 381), typically with areas of increased signal intensity spanning several sections of the spinal cord on T2-weighted images and with gadolinium enhancement (382). Cord swelling, in our experience, has been significant enough to be mistaken for an intrinsic cord tumor. Orbital MR imaging may demonstrate enlarged optic nerves with abnormal signal (Fig. 6.17) (381).

Recent interest has centered on serologic markers with myelin-specific antigens, which might identify patients with NMO. Weinshenker (383) analyzed sera from 101 patients with potential NMO on clinical grounds. The detection rate of NMO-IgG was 26/48 (54.2%) for patients with definite or probable NMO (using the most stringent clinical diagnostic criteria that require longitudinally extensive cord lesions), 13/33 (39.4%) for high-risk patients, and 0/20 (0%) for those with MS. Three high-risk patients seropositive for NMO-

IgG had recurrent, longitudinally extensive myelitis and subsequently developed clinically definite NMO. It was their feeling that the autoantibody NMO-IgG represents a potential biologic marker of NMO, and the presence or absence of this marker might help distinguish clinically defined NMO from typical MS. Their finding that seropositive high-risk patients later developed clinically definite NMO was quite striking. When positive, this autoantibody might allow early diagnosis and initiation of treatment in cases of definite NMO and in patients at high risk to convert to NMO. These findings may extend the spectrum of NMO to include some patients with recurrent optic neuritis or longitudinally extensive transverse myelitis.

Lennon (384) looked at sera from patients with definite NMO (48), MS (20), and numerous control disorders, including paraneoplastic vision loss (16), Sjögren's syndrome (10), vasculitides (10), and myasthenia gravis (10). The assay was indirect immunofluorescence with a standard composite substrate of mouse brain, gut, and kidney; sera were preabsorbed with liver extract. IgG in 26 (54%) of 48 patients with NMO yielded a distinctive staining pattern (NMO-IgG) associated with capillaries throughout the cerebellar cortex and midbrain, and with pia and a subpial mesh (prominent in midbrain). The capillary pattern was not seen

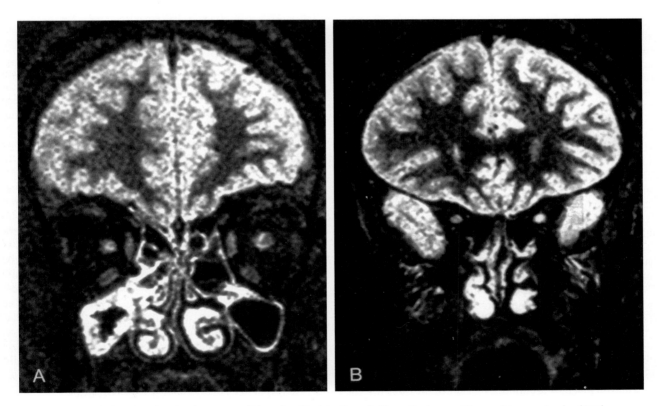

Figure 6.17. Neuroimaging in neuromyelitis optica (Devic's disease). The patient was a 39-year-old man who developed loss of vision in the left eye 4 days after developing paraparesis. *A,* Unenhanced proton density-weighted coronal MR image performed several hours after the onset of visual symptoms shows enlargement of the left optic nerve. *B,* Unenhanced proton density-weighted coronal MR image at a slightly different setting shows marked hyperintensity of the left optic nerve. (From Barkhof F, Scheltens P, Valk J, et al. Serial quantitative MR assessment of optic neuritis in a case of neuromyelitis optica, using Gadolinium-''enhanced'' STIR imaging. Neuroradiology 1991;33:70–71.)

in gut mucosa, kidney, or liver, and NMO-IgG was not noted in any other study group, but it was identified incidentally in seven patients among thousands whose sera were submitted to Mayo Clinics Neuroimmunology Laboratory for paraneoplastic Ab service testing. Their histories revealed that one had definite NMO, three were at high risk for NMO (i.e., compatible findings but not fulfilling stringent criteria for definite NMO classification), one had new-onset myelopathy, one had unclassified steroid-responsive CNS inflammatory disorder, and one had gastroesophageal cancer and akathisia.

Lennon et al. (384) believed that the novel autoantibody NMO-IgG appears to bind selectively to an element associated with CNS capillaries, pia, and subpia. They felt that it held promise as a tool for serologic diagnosis of NMO at an early stage and for advancing the classification and therapy of related disorders. Given the above discussions, this autoantibody merits investigation as a candidate effector of NMO, which recent immunohistochemical studies suggest has a humoral and complement-mediated basis targeting CNS perivascular regions.

Genetics

Kuroiwa et al. (385) found several patterns that distinguish MS in Asia from MS in Western countries. Visual impairment, often accompanied by other manifestations of NMO, was more frequently seen in Asian populations. Shibasaki et al. (386) found that visual loss at the onset of neurologic symptoms and severe visual deficits were more frequent in Japanese patients. These clinical differences between Eastern and Western cases of MS have led to a hypothesis that clinical phenotypes of Asian-type MS may be due to immunogenetic variation. Kira et al. (137) studied the HLA locus in a series of Japanese patients with MS and found that, unlike in Western MS, the DR2-associated DRB1*1501 and DRB5*0101 alleles were not associated with NMO; rather, DPA1*0202 and DPB1*0501 alleles were associated with the NMO phenotype in Japanese patients but not with healthy control subjects or Japanese patients with typical MS (387). The HLA alleles with the strongest association with Western-type MS in Japanese patients were found to be DRB1*1501 and DRP1*0301 (323).

Of interest, the clinical course of MS in Japan may be changing: fewer patients present with Asian-type (opticospinal) MS and relatively more present with Western-type MS (388). This may, however, be due to an increased awareness of Asian cultures to the more subtle forms of Western-type MS.

Diagnosis

It may be impossible to differentiate between NMO and MS on clinical grounds alone, and some authors believe, as noted above, that they are simply variants of the same disease (323,329,337,354–356,573). Indeed, review of the literature suggests that some cases diagnosed as NMO are, in fact, MS (323,389). Nevertheless, not only are there important pathologic differences and differences in the CSF findings between the two diseases (discussed previously), but also there are important clinical differences between these two

disorders. First, NMO is not uncommon in the first decade of life, whereas MS rarely occurs in patients under 10 years of age. Second, the occurrence of bilateral optic neuritis associated with myelitis is rarely recorded in cases of pathologically proven MS. Third, bilateral blindness is extremely unusual in MS but is the rule in NMO. Also, and as reviewed above, the neurogenetic, serologic, and neuroimaging findings specific to NMO will likely allow better determination of this condition in the future as these modalities of testing become more widely available.

Treatment

There is no specific treatment for NMO, although as noted above one should consider the implications of the immunopathophysiology in rendering early and perhaps selective treatment based on considerations of the uniqueness of this disease process. Supportive care is crucial to ensure survival in patients with severe myelitis. The use of intravenous corticosteroids may lessen the severity of the attack and increase the speed of recovery of both visual and motor function (323,332,366). Frohman et al. (390) reported the case of a 15-year-old boy who developed typical NMO when he was 12 years old. His vision recovered, but he experienced recurrent attacks of bilateral, simultaneous optic neuritis over the next 3 years and became steroid dependent. Administration of IVIg allowed discontinuation of steroids without further ophthalmologic or neurologic deterioration or recurrent disease.

Despite our limitations in understanding the genetics, immunology, and cellular biology of NMO, the findings of Lucchinetti et al. are of substantial therapeutic importance (362). As noted above, NMO is associated with clearly defined MR and CSF abnormalities that should allow us to identify these patients rapidly. With the recent knowledge that humoral effector mechanisms have a central role in NMO, acute therapeutic interventions may focus on interrupting antibody/complement-dependent effector mechanisms. This could include plasmapheresis in cases where glucocorticosteroids are ineffective (391), IVIg, or complement inhibitors such as soluble CR-1. Long-term immunotherapy of NMO may be more problematic as drugs such as glatiramer acetate have the potential to augment Th-2-type responses (392). In patients with NMO, it may be worthwhile to consider treatment with highly active immunosuppressants such as mitoxantrone early in disease, reducing the immunotherapeutic regimen as soon as the patient has achieved stabilization or remission.

Prognosis

The mortality rate in patients with NMO was reported in the past to be as high as 50% (374,393); however, improvements in supportive care have greatly reduced this rate, and we would estimate that death occurs in less than 10% of cases (323,364).

As noted above, most patients experience some degree of recovery of both visual and motor function (323,332,364,

366). The recovery is rarely complete but may be substantial, particularly as regards vision (333). Visual recovery usually occurs within several weeks to months after the onset of visual loss; however, Walsh and Hoyt (377) evaluated a patient whose visual acuity decreased to 20/400 OU and remained at this level for 2 years. Four years later, vision in the right eye was still 20/400, but vision in the left eye had improved to 20/30. We wonder if this was a true case of NMO or perhaps could have been a case of Leber's optic neuropathy with other neurologic manifestations and late recovery, as has been reported in patients with the some of the mitochondrial mutations (394). Some patients who experience an attack of NMO, however, never recover visual function and are left with severe bilateral visual loss.

NMO tends to occur as a single episode without recurrences, unlike MS. Nevertheless, occasional recurrences of both visual loss and paraplegia, both separate and simultaneous, have been documented (323,330,364,390).

OPTIC NEURITIS IN MYELINOCLASTIC DIFFUSE SCLEROSIS (ENCEPHALITIS PERIAXIALIS DIFFUSA, SCHILDER'S DISEASE)

In 1912, Schilder reported the case of a 12-year-old girl who experienced rapidly progressive mental deterioration associated with signs of increased intracranial pressure and death within 19 weeks. Postmortem examination disclosed large, well-demarcated areas of demyelination in the white matter of both cerebral hemispheres and a number of smaller demyelinating foci that resembled the typical plaques of MS. There was a prominent inflammatory reaction in both types of lesions with relative sparing of axon cylinders. Because of the similarities of the pathologic changes in this case to those of MS, Schilder called this disease "encephalitis periaxialis diffusa" to contrast it with the term "encephalitis periaxialis scleroticans" that had previously been used by Marburg (395) to describe a case of acute MS. Unfortunately, Schilder subsequently used the same term for two other completely different conditions (396,397). One seems to have been a case of adrenoleukodystrophy and the other a case of subacute sclerosing panencephalitis (398). These later reports seriously confused the subject for many years, and cases of adrenoleukodystrophy are still often called "Schilder's disease" (399). Nevertheless, if one separates the hereditary metabolic dystrophies and the various childhood disorders of cerebral white matter that have been called "Schilder's disease," there remains a characteristic group of cases that do indeed correspond to Schilder's original description (400,401). These latter cases, often referred to as myelinoclastic diffuse sclerosis, are nonfamilial, do not follow an obviously viral exanthem, and are not characterized pathologically by inclusion bodies or viral particles in the CNS. Throughout the remainder of this section, we will call this condition "myelinoclastic diffuse sclerosis."

The characteristic lesion in patients with myelinoclastic diffuse sclerosis is a large, sharply outlined, asymmetric focus of demyelination with severe, selective myelinoclasia that often affects an entire lobe or cerebral hemisphere

(350,402–406). There is typically extension across the corpus callosum and damage to the opposite hemisphere. Both hemispheres are symmetrically affected in some cases. Careful examination of the optic nerves, brain stem, cerebellum, and spinal cord often discloses typical discrete lesions consistent with MS, and histopathologic examination of both large and small foci reveals the characteristic features reminiscent of MS, including fibrillary gliosis with formation of giant multinucleated or swollen astrocytes and perivascular cuffing with inflammatory infiltrates containing plasma cells. The axons themselves may show little damage.

Both the clinical and histopathologic features of myelinoclastic diffuse sclerosis disease suggest that it is closely related to MS and probably is a variant of it, as Schilder originally proposed (407). The occurrence of myelinoclastic diffuse sclerosis in a patient who also had neuromyelitis optica (Devic's disease; discussed previously) lends credence to this philosophy (347).

Myelinoclastic diffuse sclerosis occurs most often in children and young adults (400,402,405,408,409,651), but it occasionally occurs in older persons (404,410). It is characterized by a progressive course that may be steady and unremitting or punctuated by a series of episodes of rapid worsening (398).

A change in personality may be the first evidence of the disease. Irritability, peevishness, unprovoked laughter or crying, and general apathy may also be present. Cortical blindness may also be an early feature of the disease, particularly in adults. Central deafness may also occur. Other manifestations include dementia, homonymous visual field defects, varying degrees of hemiparesis or quadriparesis often culminating in plegia, and pseudobulbar palsy. The brain stem and cerebellum are affected in some cases, and in such cases, nystagmus, intention tremor, scanning speech, and spastic paraplegia of spinal origin may develop.

The ocular symptoms that develop in patients with myelinoclastic diffuse sclerosis depend on the location of the lesions. As noted above, they may occur early in the course of the disease or later. Berliner (66) reviewed 35 cases of this disorder and found evidence of visual loss in 21 (60%). In 16 of the 21 cases (75%), visual loss occurred late in the disease.

Most patients who develop visual loss in this condition do so from damage to the postchiasmal visual pathways, producing homonymous hemianopic or quadrantic visual field defects or cortical blindness (402,411). Occasional patients develop demyelination in the optic chiasm, producing bitemporal field defects. Other causes of visual difficulties in patients with myelinoclastic diffuse sclerosis include papilledema (412,413), damage to association areas of the cerebral cortex, and optic neuritis.

The frequency with which optic neuritis occurs in patients with myelinoclastic diffuse sclerosis is unclear, but it seems to be less frequent than in patients with MS. Berliner (66) was able to document only two cases, although Ford (413) remarked that he had observed examples of both anterior and retrobulbar optic neuritis in the condition. Such patients invariably develop optic atrophy if they survive long enough.

Nover (414) described a case of myelinoclastic diffuse sclerosis in which the ophthalmoscopic appearance of the fundus resembled retinitis punctata albescens. Accumulations of abnormal material were present on the inner aspect of the internal limiting membrane. It is unclear to us whether this was a true case of encephalitis periaxialis diffusa and whether the retinal findings were truly related to the underlying neurologic disease.

The CSF may show changes similar to those seen in typical MS (discussed previously). The intracranial pressure usually is normal, but in some patients the CSF is under increased pressure. The protein content of the CSF is usually slightly increased, and there may be a mild lymphocytic pleocytosis. The IgG content is often increased, as is the CSF IgG index (411). Oligoclonal bands may be present, and MBP is not only present but also extremely elevated (411). Neuroimaging studies show large, multifocal areas of extensive demyelination (404,405,409,415–419). In some cases, these lesions are similar in appearance to tumors or abscesses (411,417–419).

The diagnosis of myelinoclastic diffuse sclerosis may be suspected when a child or young adult develops evidence of a subacute or chronic progressive neurologic disease with neuroimaging and laboratory evidence of focal hemispheric demyelinating disease but without adrenal dysfunction or abnormal long chain fatty-acid components of serum cholesterol esters (409). Most patients do not have evidence of peripheral nerve damage; however, Szabo and Hegedus (420) described a case of otherwise typical myelinoclastic diffuse sclerosis in which there was evidence of a mild peripheral neuropathy. The diagnosis may be confirmed by brain biopsy (402,404,405,410,411,417,419).

Most patients with myelinoclastic diffuse sclerosis follow a progressive unremitting course that ends in death within a few months or years. A few cases have been reported in which there was temporary or permanent spontaneous improvement (413,418), and rare patients have been reported to survive for a decade or longer (420). Some patients have improved after being treated with systemic corticosteroids administered orally or intravenously (404,405,409,411,421). The patient reported by Lana-Peixoto and dos Santos experienced improvement in vision from hand motions in each eye to 20/20. Konkol et al. (422) reported improvement in an 8-year-old boy after intravenous administration of ACTH and cyclophosphamide. Patients who improve clinically generally show disappearance or shrinkage of the lesions seen on neuroimaging studies.

ENCEPHALITIS PERIAXIALIS CONCENTRICA (CONCENTRIC SCLEROSIS OF BALÓ)

Encephalitis periaxialis concentrica was first described by Marburg (395) in 1906 and later by Baló (423,424) in 1927 and 1928. Since then, more than 40 case reports have appeared in the literature (425–429). The disease clinically resembles myelinoclastic diffuse sclerosis but differs from it pathologically.

Encephalitis periaxialis concentrica usually is characterized clinically by a relatively rapid course during which patients develop a variety of neurologic symptoms and signs separated in both space and time, including visual loss and diplopia. As in encephalitis periaxialis diffusa, the visual loss that occurs in most patients with encephalitis periaxialis concentrica is usually caused by damage to postgeniculate visual pathways and is characterized by homonymous field defects or cortical blindness; however, a patient reported by Currie et al. (430), who initially had a left homonymous hemianopsia, eventually developed complete blindness associated with pupils that were nonreactive to light and optic discs that were markedly pale.

The pathologic changes in the disease described by Baló consist of alternating bands of demyelination and preserved myelin in a series of concentric rings in the cerebral white matter (348,350,406,424,430,431). The occurrence of lesions in this pattern has suggested to some investigators that there is centrifugal diffusion of some factor that is damaging to myelin (427); however, Moore et al. (429) performed a complete histologic and ultrastructural examination of neural tissue obtained from a 54-year-old woman with the disease and concluded that the predominant feature of the bands of myelin is remyelination. These authors suggest that the lesion originates as a small focus of acute demyelination around a perivascular inflammatory cuff and that the concentric bands are actually alternating areas of demyelination and remyelination. The remyelination occurs at the outer rim of the initial demyelinated area. Further demyelination then occurs external to the area of remyelination, and remyelination then occurs along the outer rim of this second area of demyelination. In this way, successive concentric rings of demyelination and remyelination are produced. The findings of Moore et al. (429) have not been corroborated by other investigators (431). Some patients with otherwise typical encephalitis periaxialis concentrica have not only pathologic changes consistent with the disease but also lesions typical of acute MS (429,431), suggesting that the former disease may actually be a variant of the latter.

Neuroimaging studies initially may be normal in patients with encephalitis periaxialis concentrica; however, eventually both CT scanning and MR imaging show multiple lesions consistent with demyelination (432,433). Similarly, analysis of the CSF at an early stage of the disease may reveal normal findings, but later analysis may show mild to moderate pleocytosis, increased protein, an increased IgG index, and multiple oligoclonal bands (430). The diagnosis can be made with certainty only by a stereotactic biopsy of affected brain (432,433).

Without treatment, encephalitis periaxialis concentrica usually progresses inexorably and is invariably fatal within a few weeks to a year. Treatment with systemic corticosteroids, however, may result in both immediate and long-term improvement in neurologic symptoms and signs. Early diagnosis thus is extremely important, and stereotactic biopsy seems to be an acceptable method of achieving this goal (432,433).

CAUSES OF OPTIC NEURITIS OTHER THAN PRIMARY DEMYELINATION

In a few cases, a primary demyelinating process in the optic nerve or the CNS is not the cause of unilateral or bilateral anterior or retrobulbar optic neuritis. Instead, the condition develops in the setting of, or as the presenting manifestation of, an underlying systemic infection.

OPTIC NEURITIS FROM VIRAL AND BACTERIAL DISEASES

Parainfectious optic neuritis typically follows the onset of a viral or, less often, a bacterial infection by 1 to 3 weeks (37,434,435). It is more common in children than in adults and is thought to occur on an immunologic basis, producing demyelination of the optic nerve. The optic neuritis may be unilateral, but it is often bilateral. The optic discs may appear normal or swollen. Swelling of the peripapillary retina may be observed in patients with anterior optic neuritis. If a star figure composed of lipid exudates develops in the macula of the affected eye, the condition is called ''neuroretinitis'' (discussed later). If there is evidence of optic disc swelling but no evidence of optic nerve dysfunction, and the intracranial pressure is normal, the inflammation is assumed to be affecting the periphery of the nerve and is called ''perioptic neuritis'' or ''optic perineuritis'' (discussed later).

Parainfectious optic neuritis, whether viral or bacterial, may occur in patients with no evidence of neurologic dysfunction or in association with a meningitis, meningoencephalitis, or encephalomyelitis. When neurologic manifestations are present, patients have typical abnormalities in the CSF. Patients with encephalitis usually have disturbances on electroencephalography and also may have changes in the brain seen by neuroimaging, whereas patients with encephalomyelitis may show such changes in both the brain and the spinal cord.

Visual recovery following parainfectious optic neuritis is usually excellent without treatment. Whether corticosteroids hasten recovery in patients with postviral optic neuritis is unknown, but this treatment is reasonable to consider, particularly if visual loss is bilateral and severe.

Optic neuritis may occur in association with infections by a large number of both DNA and RNA viruses, including adenovirus (436,437), Coxsackie virus (438,439), cytomegalovirus (440), hepatitis A (441), hepatitis B (442,443), human herpesvirus type 4 (Epstein-Barr virus) (444–448), human immunodeficiency virus (HIV) type 1 (449,450), measles (451–455), mumps (456–458), rubeola, rubella (459), and varicella zoster (in chicken pox [460,461] and in herpes zoster [462,463]). The neuro-ophthalmologic significance of these and other viruses is discussed in detail in Chapters 57 and 58.

Bacterial infections can produce optic neuritis. Some bacterial infections in which anterior or retrobulbar optic neuritis may occur include anthrax (464), β-hemolytic streptococcal infection (465), brucellosis (466,467), cat scratch disease (39,468,469,470), meningococcal infection (471), pertussis (472), tuberculosis (473–477), typhoid fever (478,479), and Whipple's disease (480). The neuro-ophthalmologic signifi-

cance of these and other bacteria is discussed in detail in Chapter 49.

OPTIC NEURITIS AFTER VACCINATION

Although there is extensive anecdotal evidence of optic neuritis occurring following vaccinations, the actual evidence of a demyelinating event following vaccination is limited. In this section we first review the anecdotal information regarding optic neuritis and vaccinations; we then will explore the evidence-based medicine surrounding the relationship of vaccinations to demyelinating events in general.

Optic neuritis has been reported to occur after vaccinations against both bacterial and virus infections (38). Most cases are bilateral, and both anterior and retrobulbar forms of optic neuritis may occur. Optic neuritis may develop after vaccinations with bacillus Calmette Guérin (BCG) (481), hepatitis B virus (482,483), rabies virus (484–486), tetanus toxoid (487), and variola virus (488). The use of a combined smallpox, tetanus, and diphtheria vaccine was associated with a bilateral anterior optic neuritis in a 7-year-old child who eventually recovered completely (489), and a similar case was reported in association with combined measles, mumps, and rubella vaccination (490). Influenza vaccine is commonly associated with the development of optic neuritis. Perry et al. (491) reported a patient with bilateral anterior optic neuritis that occurred 6 days following vaccination with bivalent influenza vaccine. Ray and Dreizen (492) described a similar case. Cangemi and Bergen (493) reported a previously healthy man who developed a unilateral optic neuritis with disc swelling, 3 weeks after inoculation with 200 units of A-New Jersey swine influenza and 200 units of A-Victoria influenza whole-virus vaccine. Although most cases of postvaccination optic neuritis appear to be of the anterior variety, unilateral retrobulbar neuritis has been reported 3 weeks following a swine influenza vaccination (494).

Despite the previous anecdotal reports, the evidence-based medicine that vaccination may precipitate the onset of MS or lead to relapses is simply not present. Confavreux et al. (495) conducted a case-crossover study to assess whether vaccinations increase the risk of relapse in MS. The subjects included 643 patients included in the European Database for Multiple Sclerosis who had a relapse between 1993 and 1997. The index relapse was the first relapse confirmed by a visit to a neurologist and preceded by a relapse-free period of at least 12 months. Information on vaccinations was obtained in a standardized telephone interview and confirmed by medical records. Exposure to vaccination in the 2-month risk period immediately preceding the relapse was compared with that in the four previous 2-month control periods for the calculation of relative risks, which were estimated with the use of conditional logistic regression. Of these patients with relapses of MS, 15% reported having been vaccinated during the preceding 12 months. The reports of 94% of these vaccinations were confirmed. Of all the patients, 2.3% had been vaccinated during the preceding 2-month risk period, compared with 2.8–4.0% who were vaccinated during one or more of the four control periods. The relative risk of relapse associated with exposure to any vaccination during the previous 2 months was 0.71 (95% CI, 0.40–1.26). There was no increase in the specific risk of relapse associated with tetanus, hepatitis B, or influenza vaccination (range of relative risks, 0.22–1.08). Analyses based on risk periods of 1 and 3 months yielded similar results. These authors concluded that vaccination does not appear to increase the short-term risk of relapse in MS.

To further evaluate the association between vaccination and onset of MS or optic neuritis, DeStefano et al. (496) looked at a case-control study involving cases of MS or optic neuritis among adults 18–49 years of age. Data on vaccinations and other risk factors were obtained from computerized and paper medical records and from telephone interviews in three health maintenance organizations. Four hundred forty case subjects and 950 control subjects matched on health maintenance organization, sex, and date of birth were assessed. They noted the onset of first symptoms of demyelinating disease at any time after vaccination and during specified intervals after vaccination (less than year, 1–5 years, and more than 5 years). Cases and controls had similar vaccination histories. The odds ratios (95% CI), adjusted for potential confounding variables, of the associations between ever having been vaccinated and risk of demyelinating disease (MS and optic neuritis combined) were 0.9 (0.6–1.5) for hepatitis B vaccine; 0.6 (0.4–0.8) for tetanus vaccination; 0.8 (0.6–1.2) for influenza vaccine; 0.8 (0.5–1.5) for measles, mumps, rubella vaccine; 0.9 (0.5–1.4) for measles vaccine; and 0.7 (0.4–1.0) for rubella vaccine. The results were similar when MS and optic neuritis were analyzed separately. There was no increased risk according to timing of vaccination. It was the conclusion in this case-control study that vaccination against hepatitis B, influenza, tetanus, measles, or rubella is not associated with an increased risk of MS or optic neuritis.

It would appear that there are two primary issues regarding the relationship between vaccinations and MS: Does the vaccination precipitate the first attack of MS? Does it increase the short- or long-term risk in patients with known disease? It would appear from the preceding studies that vaccinations do not precipitate the seminal event in MS. The second question is more difficult to answer. Acute disseminated encephalomyelitis (ADEM), a monophasic and multifocal illness of the white and gray matter, has been observed following various viral or bacterial infections as well as vaccine injections for diseases such as pertussis, tetanus, and yellow fever. The similarities between ADEM and EAE are suggestive of an immunologic process. In addition to the dramatic presentation of ADEM, more limited white matter involvement, such as optic neuritis or myelitis, has been reported following vaccine injections and has occasionally been counted as the first attack of MS. In France, 25 million inhabitants, almost half of the population, were vaccinated against hepatitis B (HB) between 1991 and 1999 (497). Several hundred cases of an acute central demyelinating event following HB vaccination were reported to the pharmacovigilance unit, leading to a modification of vaccination policy in the schools and the initiation of several studies designed to examine the possible

relationship between the vaccine and the central demyelinating events. The results of these studies failed to establish the causality of the HB vaccine. Nevertheless, molecular mimicry between HB antigen(s) and one or more myelin proteins, or a nonspecific activation of autoreactive lymphocytes, could constitute possible pathogenetic mechanisms for these adverse neurologic events.

Although demyelinating events might in fact be precipitated by vaccinations, the chance of this occurring is low, and the risk to the patient with MS is minimal compared with the potential risk to the MS patient of disease state worsening due to an infectious disease.

OPTIC NEURITIS IN SARCOIDOSIS

Granulomatous inflammation of the optic nerve may occur in sarcoidosis, producing a typical anterior or retrobulbar optic neuritis (498–502). In some cases, the optic neuritis occurs during the disease; in others, it is the presenting manifestation. Clinical findings may be indistinguishable from those of demyelinating optic neuritis. However, the optic disc may have a characteristic lumpy, white appearance, which suggests a granulomatous etiology, and there may be an inflammatory reaction in the vitreous. Pain, common in a demyelinating optic neuritis, is often absent in the optic neuropathy of sarcoidosis.

Unlike primary demyelinating optic neuritis, which does not respond dramatically to systemic corticosteroids (discussed previously), the optic neuritis associated with sarcoidosis is usually extremely sensitive to steroids. In most cases, recovery of vision is rapid after treatment is instituted, although vision may decline again once steroids are tapered or stopped. Indeed, it must be emphasized that rapid recovery of vision with corticosteroid treatment and subsequent worsening when the steroids are tapered is atypical for demyelinating optic neuritis and suggests an infiltrative or nondemyelinating inflammatory process, such as sarcoidosis.

Patients with possible sarcoid optic neuritis should undergo an evaluation that includes a careful history and physical examination, a chest radiograph, serum chemistries, an assay for angiotensin converting enzyme (ACE) in the serum and CSF, a gallium scan, and in some cases bronchoscopic lavage or biopsy of skin, conjunctiva, lung, liver, or other organs looking for noncaseating granulomas. Sarcoidosis and related conditions are discussed in detail in Chapter 59.

SYPHILIS

Optic neuritis from syphilis is not rare (503–505), but it is particularly common in patients also infected with HIV (506–509) (see Chapters 56 and 58). The optic neuritis of syphilis can be unilateral or bilateral and anterior or retrobulbar. When the condition is anterior, there is usually some cellular reaction in the vitreous, which serves to distinguish it (and other systemic inflammatory diseases that cause anterior optic neuritis) from demyelinating optic neuritis, in which the vitreous usually is clear (discussed previously).

The diagnosis of syphilis is established using a variety of serologic and CSF assays. Treatment with intravenous penicillin produces visual recovery in many cases; however, the disease may be difficult to cure, particularly in patients who are HIV positive or who have the acquired immune deficiency syndrome (AIDS).

Syphilis can cause both neuroretinitis and optic perineuritis (discussed later). Syphilis is discussed in detail in Chapter 56.

OPTIC NEURITIS IN HIV-POSITIVE PATIENTS AND PATIENTS WITH AIDS

Many infectious agents that do not normally cause optic neuritis can do so in patients who are immunocompromised from drugs or disease. Such optic neuritis is particularly common in patients who are infected with HIV and in patients with AIDS (510,511).

Optic neuritis, both anterior and retrobulbar, is an occasional finding in HIV-infected patients with cryptococcal meningitis, cytomegalovirus infection, herpesvirus infections, syphilis, tuberculous meningitis, and a variety of fungal infections (440,507,510,511–517). Rare patients with toxoplasmosis may also develop optic neuritis (518,519). In some cases, such infections cause neuroretinitis, whereas in others, optic perineuritis occurs.

Some patients with AIDS develop optic neuritis that is probably caused by infection of the optic nerve by HIV itself (449). Infection with HIV and AIDS are discussed in detail in Chapter 58.

OPTIC NEURITIS IN SYSTEMIC LUPUS ERYTHEMATOSUS (SLE) AND OTHER VASCULITIDES

Patients with SLE, polyarteritis nodosa, and other vasculitides can experience an attack of what seems clinically to be typical acute optic neuritis (520). This phenomenon occurs in about 1% of patients with SLE (521–531). In rare cases, the optic neuropathy is the presenting sign of the disease. The pathogenesis is not a true infection or inflammation of the nerve tissue itself but is related to ischemia, which may produce demyelination alone, axonal necrosis, or a combination of the two.

The clinical profile of optic neuropathy in SLE and other vasculitides actually can take several forms in addition to an acute anterior or retrobulbar optic neuropathy associated with pain. Patients may present with symptoms and signs that suggest a retrobulbar or anterior ischemic optic neuropathy, or they may have slowly progressive loss of vision that suggests a compressive lesion.

The diagnosis of SLE or other vasculitides as a cause of optic neuropathy is established by identification of systemic symptoms and signs of the disease as well as by serologic testing. Treatment with either intravenous or oral corticosteroids may be indicated in this condition.

The term ''autoimmune optic neuritis'' has been suggested for cases of optic neuritis in which there is both serologic evidence of vasculitis, such as a positive ANA, but no signs of systemic involvement other than the optic neuropathy; and progressive visual loss that tends to be responsive to treatment with systemic corticosteroids and that is often steroid dependent (i.e., vision worsens when steroids are

tapered) (531,532,532a). It is interesting that among patients enrolled in the ONTT, 3% had a positive ANA titer greater than 1:320 (7). Only one of these patients developed other evidence of connective tissue disease during the first 2 years of follow-up. In addition, patients with a positive ANA (regardless of the titer) who were treated with placebo had the same visual outcome as those treated with intravenous methylprednisolone (8). SLE and other vasculitides that produce neuro-ophthalmologic manifestations are discussed in detail in Chapter 44.

LYME DISEASE

Optic neuritis can occur in patients with Lyme borreliosis (Lyme disease) (533–536). This disorder is a spirochetal infection that is transmitted through the bite of an infected tick. It can produce a multitude of ocular and neurologic findings, including both anterior and retrobulbar optic neuritis. The diagnosis of Lyme disease is made by serologic detection of infection or by finding the organism or its nucleic acid in the serum or CSF. Treatment with antibiotics is usually effective, particularly in the early stages of the disease. As with other systemic infectious processes that can cause optic neuritis, Lyme disease can also cause neuroretinitis (discussed later). Lyme disease is discussed in detail in Chapter 56.

SINUS DISEASE

In the pre-antibiotic era, spread of infection from the paranasal sinuses to the optic nerve was not unusual. However, this is a rare occurrence now, and most cases of sinusitis in patients with optic neuritis are fortuitous. Nevertheless, some patients with acute severe sinusitis develop a secondary optic neuritis from spread of infection. When the infection originates from the ethmoid or maxillary sinuses, there generally are obvious signs of orbital inflammation; however, spread of infection from the sphenoid sinus to the posterior optic nerve in the apex of the orbit or within the optic canal can be silent except for the loss of vision. Aspergillosis and other fungal infections are considerations in this clinical setting (537,538). Neuroimaging techniques, particularly CT scanning and MR imaging, generally can be used to diagnose paranasal sinus disease.

Even when sinus disease is present in the setting of optic neuritis, one must be wary of attributing the optic neuritis to this cause. Obviously, those patients with retrobulbar neuritis and supportive sinusitis with signs of orbital inflammation should be actively treated not only to eradicate the infection but also for the possible beneficial effects of treatment on the optic neuritis; however, in our opinion, operative intervention in patients with radiologic evidence of sinus disease that normally would not call for medical or surgical therapy is unwarranted.

MISCELLANEOUS CAUSES OF OPTIC NEURITIS

Optic neuritis has been reported to occur rarely in many conditions other than bacterial or viral infections, including acute posterior multifocal placoid pigment epitheliopathy

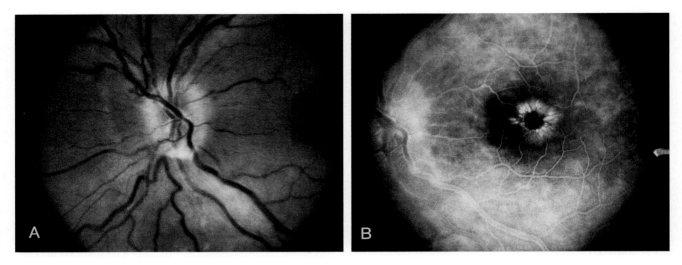

Figure 6.18. Optic disc swelling in a patient with pars planitis (chronic cyclitis). The patient was initially believed to have papilledema. *A,* The left optic disc is hyperemic and slightly swollen. The hazy appearance is due to the presence of vitreous cells. *B,* Fluorescein angiogram of the left macula shows cystoid macular edema, characteristic of this disorder. The opposite eye had a similar ophthalmoscopic appearance.

(504,539), after a bee sting (540–543), Behçet's disease (544), birdshot retinochoroidopathy (545), Creutzfeldt-Jakob disease (546,547), cysticercosis (548), familial Mediterranean fever (549), Guillain-Barré syndrome (550–553), inflammatory bowel disease (554–559), intraocular nematode infection (504,560,561), presumed histoplasmosis (562,563), Reiter's syndrome (564,565), toxocariasis (566), toxoplasmosis associated with or unassociated with AIDS (567,568), and *Mycoplasma pneumoniae* infection (569–572). As is true for optic neuritis associated with bacterial or viral infections, some of these cases are isolated, whereas others are associated with other evidence of CNS dysfunction.

Intraocular inflammation alone may cause optic disc swelling; however, in such cases, visual acuity is usually not significantly affected from damage to the optic nerve (504,573–575) (Fig. 6.18). In such patients, visual acuity is limited only by the degree of vitreous inflammation or by

secondary changes that occur in the macula (e.g., cystoid edema). Perhaps the most common form of disc swelling that occurs as part of an ocular inflammatory syndrome is that which occurs after cataract extraction and is associated with moderately decreased visual acuity and cystoid macular edema: the Irvine-Gass syndrome (576–578).

As mentioned above, the presence of uveitis and other symptoms of intraocular inflammation in a patient with acute anterior optic neuritis should alert the examiner to search for an associated intraocular or systemic disease.

Hanna and Girgis (579) found a 1.5% prevalence of optic atrophy in 2,178 patients after meningitis. Although postpapilledema optic atrophy accounted for some of these cases, primary optic atrophy, presumably the result of an associated optic neuritis, was much more frequent. In this study, optic atrophy occurred more frequently after tuberculous meningitis than after bacterial meningitis, including meningococcal, pneumococcal, and purulent meningitis of unknown etiology.

BILATERAL OPTIC NEURITIS

In adults, bilateral simultaneous acute optic neuritis, particularly that associated with MS, is uncommon but well described. Adie (80) found only one case of bilateral optic neuritis in his series of 70 adult patients, and other authors (66,580) agreed with him that both simultaneous and early consecutive cases were exceedingly rare (Fig. 6.19). However, reports indicate that the incidence of bilateral simultaneous acute optic neuritis in patients with MS is 10–75% (68,82,83,197,581). Morrissey et al. (275) performed a retrospective analysis of the causes of bilateral simultaneous acute optic neuritis in 23 adults and found that 5 of the patients (22%) had developed clinical evidence of MS. In many of these series, the time interval between attacks in the two eyes is not stated. Bradley and Whitty (82) separated

their cases into those that were unilateral (71%), those that were bilateral and simultaneous (7%), those that were bilateral and nonsimultaneous but occurred within 3 months of each other (12%), and those that occurred more than 3 months apart (12%). These authors found no significant differences in rate and degree of recovery between bilateral and unilateral cases, regardless of the time interval between the attacks. The studies of Rischbieth (582) and of Hutchinson (83) seem to support this view.

In the ONTT, approximately 48% of patients with involvement of one eye had some other definable visual field involvement of the contralateral eye, suggesting that optic neuritis is quite frequently present bilaterally from the onset (11).

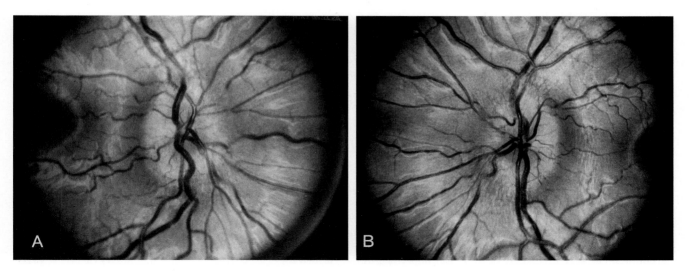

Figure 6.19. Bilateral anterior optic neuritis. The patient is a 19-year-old girl who suffered bilateral visual loss 2 weeks following a flulike illness. Both optic discs show moderate swelling without hemorrhages. Visual acuity is 20/400 in the right eye and 20/300 in the left eye, and there are bilateral central scotomas. Visual acuity returned to normal within 6 weeks, and disc swelling completely resolved.

In contrast to adults, acute optic neuritis is quite often bilateral and simultaneous in children. In such cases, it is often presumed to be related to a viral infection (discussed later).

OPTIC NEURITIS IN CHILDREN

Optic neuritis in children has several unique characteristics that distinguish it from optic neuritis in adults. First, it is more often anterior. Second, it is more often a bilateral simultaneous condition. Third, it often seems to occur within 1–2 weeks after a known or presumed viral infection. Fourth, it is less often associated with the development of MS. Finally, it is often steroid sensitive and steroid dependent.

Kennedy and Carroll (35) examined 30 children with idiopathic optic neuritis. The youngest child was 4 years old, and the mean age of the group was 9.5 years. These investigators found disc swelling in more than 70% of children (as opposed to a prevalence of 20–40% in adults). In addition, over 50% of the children whom Kennedy and Carroll (35) studied had bilateral disease, a significantly higher frequency than in adults. Most of the patients in this series had central scotomas and visual acuity less than 20/200, with only one patient having visual acuity better than 20/50. Despite the poor initial visual acuity in these patients, the visual prognosis in children with optic neuritis appears to be quite good. Kennedy and Carroll (35) performed follow-up examinations on 19 of their 22 children with idiopathic anterior optic neuritis. Fifteen of the children recovered completely, two had moderate return of vision, and only two children had no significant improvement. Of three children with acute retrobulbar optic neuritis and normal optic discs at the time of visual loss, two had a complete recovery, although the third child had only a moderate return of vision and suffered a second attack of visual loss 4 years later from which she never recovered. No further information was given by these authors regarding final visual acuity or fields in these pa-

tients. Eight of the patients with idiopathic optic neuritis in this study developed MS over a mean follow-up period of 8 years.

Kriss et al. (37) studied 39 children with optic neuritis. After a mean follow-up of 8.8 years (range 3 months to 29 years), MS had developed in six (15%). The visual prognosis was reported to be excellent. Riikonen (38) reported on 18 children with optic neuritis. A vaccination preceded the development of optic neuritis in 6 of the 18 (33%) and a bacterial or viral infection preceded it in 10 (55.6%). Eight of the 18 (44.4%) children developed MS during the study.

Nakao et al. (583) found 9 cases of optic neuritis in children among 201 cases (5%) of optic neuritis evaluated at Osaka University Medical School in Japan. In all nine cases, the optic neuritis was bilateral and associated with severe visual loss. Optic disc swelling was present in most of the children, several of whom had associated upper respiratory tract infections, meningitis, or encephalitis. All were treated with systemic corticosteroids, and all experienced improvement in vision.

Hierons and Lyle (34) collected data on 13 cases of bilateral optic neuritis in children under the age of 13, 10 of whom were girls. Five of the patients had a history of specific exanthem or an indeterminate febrile illness before visual symptoms began, and all but one patient made a good visual recovery. Only one patient developed MS over a mean follow-up period of 4 years.

Meadows (36) reviewed 35 cases of bilateral optic neuritis in children, most between the ages of 5 and 12. Over a follow-up period of 3–18 years, 12 of the patients were lost to examination, but of the remaining 21, none developed MS. Although Meadows (36) referred to his cases as examples of ''retro-bulbar neuritis,'' he stated that in the ''vast majority of cases seen during the early acute phase, the optic discs were abnormal,'' with the abnormality varying from mild blurring of the disc margins to marked swelling of the disc with peripapillary hemorrhages.

Keast-Butler and Taylor (584) described four cases, and Cohen et al. (585) and Rollinson (586) reported isolated cases, of bilateral optic neuritis with disc swelling in children. None of the children experienced any preceding exanthema, and all patients recovered excellent vision, even though the patient reported by Cohen et al. (585) had no perception of light in either eye at one point during her hospital course.

Farris and Pickard (435) described six children who developed acute simultaneous bilateral optic neuritis. Five of the six children had recently experienced a brief upper respiratory or gastrointestinal illness, presumed to be viral in nature. Five of the six patients also demonstrated marked neurologic deficits, including seizures and cerebellar dysfunction. Lumbar puncture was abnormal in three of the six patients. All patients were treated with a course of intravenous methylprednisolone, ranging from 1–2 mg/kg/day, and each patient experienced a rapid and nearly complete recovery of vision during treatment.

Koraszewska-Matuszewska et al. (587) reported a large series of optic neuritis in childhood. These investigators reviewed the records from 110 children, aged 2–18 years (mean 13 years) with optic neuritis. Sixty percent of the children had bilateral simultaneous optic neuritis. Children younger than 14 years of age tended to have anterior optic neuritis, whereas retrobulbar neuritis was more common in children over 14 years old. In younger patients, the cause of the inflammation seemed to be viral infections or chronic focal infection. Older children often had underlying neurologic disease. The use of systemic steroids resulted in improvement of visual acuity in about 75% of cases and improvement or normalization of the visual field in over 50% of cases, regardless of whether the optic neuritis was of the anterior or retrobulbar variety. Normal visual function was regained in about 50% of the children during a follow-up period of 3 years. These children tended to be those with the least severe visual loss during the acute phase of the optic neuritis.

Good et al. (588) reviewed the records of 10 children with optic neuritis in whom recovery of vision was poor or incomplete. These investigators found that in all cases, the condition had been bilateral. Optic disc swelling had been present in 7 of the 10 cases (70%), and 70% of the cases had been preceded by a viral illness. Five of the 10 children (50%) had developed evidence of MS.

Brady et al. (589) evaluated the presenting features, neuroimaging findings, CSF abnormalities, associated systemic disease, and visual outcome in children with optic neuritis. A retrospective analysis was performed on all patients who were seen at Baylor College of Medicine with optic neuritis during a 6-year period from 1991 to 1997. The degree of initial visual loss, subsequent visual recovery, and associated disease were reviewed. MR images and CSF findings were also analyzed. Twenty-five patients (39 eyes) 21 months of age to 18 years of age were included in the study, with a mean follow-up of 11 months. Fourteen patients (56%) had bilateral optic neuritis, and 11 patients (44%) had unilateral disease. Thirty-three of 39 eyes (84%) had visual acuity of 20/200 or less at presentation. Twenty-one of 25 patients (84%) were given intravenous methylprednisolone (10–30 mg/kg/day). Thirty of 39 eyes (76%) recovered 20/40 visual acuity or better. Three of 39 eyes (7%) recovered vision in the 20/50 to 20/100 range. Six of 39 eyes (15%) recovered vision of 20/200 or less. Twenty-three of 25 patients (92%) underwent MR imaging of the brain. A normal MR image of the brain was associated with recovery of 20/40 or better visual acuity in six of six affected eyes (100%). Seven patients were 6 years of age or younger at presentation. Six of these seven (85%) had bilateral disease, and 12 of 13 (92%) affected eyes recovered 20/40 visual acuity or better. Eighteen patients were 7 years of age or older at presentation. Eight of these 18 (44%) had bilateral disease, and 10 of 18 patients (56%) had unilateral disease. Eighteen of 26 affected eyes (50%) recovered 20/40 visual acuity or better. These authors concluded that pediatric optic neuritis is usually associated with visual recovery; however, a significant number (22%) remain visually disabled. A normal MR image of the brain may be associated with a better outcome. Younger patients were more likely to have bilateral disease and a better visual prognosis.

Morales et al. (590) reviewed all charts of patients less than 15 years of age who presented with optic neuritis to the Bascom Palmer Eye Institute or the Miami Children's Hospital between 1986 and 1998. Fifteen patients were identified. There was a slight female predilection in the study group (60%), with a mean age of 9.8 years at presentation. A preceding febrile illness within 2 weeks of visual symptoms was reported in 66% of patients. Initial visual acuity ranged from 20/15 to no light perception. Involvement was bilateral in 66% of patients, and disc swelling was present in 64% of involved eyes. Of the patients who underwent MR imaging, 33% had focal demyelinating lesions in the brain, and 63% of affected nerves were enlarged or enhanced with gadolinium. Eleven patients were treated with intravenous steroids. Final visual acuity was 20/40 or more in 58.3% of eyes. Thirty percent of the patients had vision of finger counting or worse. Four (26%) patients developed MS. The mean age of patients with MS was 12 years, compared with 9 years in children who did not develop MS. Patients with unilateral involvement had an excellent visual prognosis (100% more than 20/40) but a higher rate of development of MS (75%). Two patients had positive serology for Lyme disease. It was their conclusion that optic neuritis presents differently in children than in adults. Children typically have bilateral involvement with papillitis following an antecedent viral illness. Although visual prognosis is poorer in children than adults, the development of MS is less common in children. Children who present with unilateral involvement have a better visual prognosis; however, they also develop MS at a greater frequency than children with bilateral involvement. Patients who developed MS were, on aver-

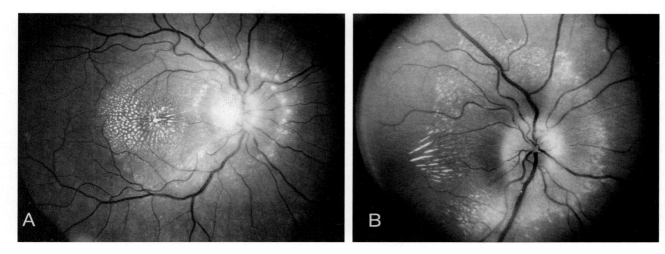

Figure 6.20. Neuroretinitis. *A,* The right optic disc is swollen; there is peripapillary edema; and there is a star figure composed of hard exudate in the macula. This is a form of optic neuritis that is not associated with multiple sclerosis. *B,* In another case, the star figure is incomplete and located nasal but not temporal to the fovea. Note the extensive transudate surrounding the swollen optic disc. (Courtesy of Dr. J.M. Christiansen.)

age, older at presentation with optic neuritis than those who did not develop MS.

We have been impressed with the tendency for optic neuritis in children, whether unilateral or bilateral, to be quite responsive to treatment with systemic corticosteroids and, more importantly, to be quite steroid sensitive. We have seen several children, primarily those with anterior optic neuritis, experience relapses of their condition, some of them quite severe, when steroids were rapidly tapered. It is our policy to evaluate all patients with optic neuritis less than 15 years of age with MR imaging and a lumbar puncture. Unless there

is a contraindication to doing so, we then treat these children with intravenous methylprednisolone 1–2 mg/kg/day for 3–5 days. We do not use an oral corticosteroid taper in these patients.

Gass (469) and Rush (591) emphasized that both children and adults can develop acute, usually unilateral, visual loss associated with an ophthalmoscopic picture of disc swelling, peripapillary exudative retinal detachment, and a macular star figure (Fig. 6.20). This type of ophthalmoscopic appearance has been called neuroretinitis (discussed later).

NEURORETINITIS

In 1916, Theodore Leber described a condition characterized by acute unilateral visual loss associated with an exudative maculopathy consisting of hard exudates arranged in a star figure around the fovea. Leber (592) believed that the condition was a primary retinal process and called it a "stellate maculopathy." The condition subsequently became known as Leber's stellate maculopathy (593) until 1977, when Gass (469) reported that patients with the condition showed swelling of the optic disc before and often concurrent with the appearance of the star figure. The optic disc swelling then resolved, leaving the maculopathy as the primary or sole ophthalmoscopic abnormality. Gass (469) performed fluorescein angiography in several of the patients with this condition and showed that there was no leakage from retinal vessels surrounding the macula. He thus concluded that the condition was not a primary maculopathy, but rather a form of optic neuritis. Because the condition affected both the optic nerve and the retina, he called it neuroretinitis. Gass (469) emphasized that the condition occurred commonly in children and young adults, up to 50%

of whom had an antecedent viral illness, usually affecting the respiratory tract, a few weeks before the onset of visual symptoms. It has subsequently become clear that some cases of neuroretinitis are associated with particular infectious diseases, whereas others occur as apparently isolated phenomena (594,595). In the latter setting, the condition is called Leber's idiopathic stellate neuroretinitis (594,596–599).

Neuroretinitis affects persons of all ages, although it occurs most often in the third and fourth decades of life. There is no sex predilection. The condition usually is painless, but some patients complain of an aching sensation behind the affected eye or eyes, and the discomfort occasionally worsens with eye movements. Affected patients complain of visual blurring that progresses as the maculopathy evolves. Visual acuity at the time of initial examination may range from 20/20 to light perception. We have never seen a patient who lost all perception of light during this condition. Color vision is variably affected, and we have the impression that the degree of color deficit is usually significantly worse than the degree of visual loss would suggest. The most common field defect is a cecocentral scotoma, but central scotomas, arcuate defects, and even altitudinal defects may be present, and the peripheral field may be nonspecifically constricted. A relative afferent pupillary defect is present in most patients, unless the condition is bilateral, in which case even patients with clinically asymmetric visual loss may have no evidence of a relative afferent pupillary defect. The degree of disc swelling ranges from mild to severe, depending in part on the point in time at which the patient is first examined. In severe cases, splinter hemorrhages may be present. Segmental disc swelling has been reported but is uncommon. A macular star figure composed of lipid (hard exudates) may not be present when the patient is examined soon after visual symptoms begin, but it becomes apparent within days to weeks and tends to become more prominent even as the optic disc swelling is resolving (469,504,594,595) (Fig. 6.21).

Small, discrete chorioretinal lesions may occur in idiopathic cases in both symptomatic and asymptomatic eyes (594–596,600). Posterior inflammatory signs consisting of vitreous cells and venous sheathing, as well as occasional anterior chamber cell and flare, may occur in patients with neuroretinitis. Fluorescein angiography in patients with acute neuroretinitis demonstrates diffuse disc swelling and leakage of dye from vessels on the surface of the discs (469). The retinal vessels may show slight staining in the peripapillary region; however, the macular vasculature is entirely normal. Chorioretinal lesions, when present, show late hyperfluorescence and exhibit progressive scarring on follow-up examinations (594,595).

Neuroretinitis is a self-limited disorder. With time, usually over 6–8 weeks, the optic disc swelling resolves, and the appearance of the disc becomes normal or nearly so

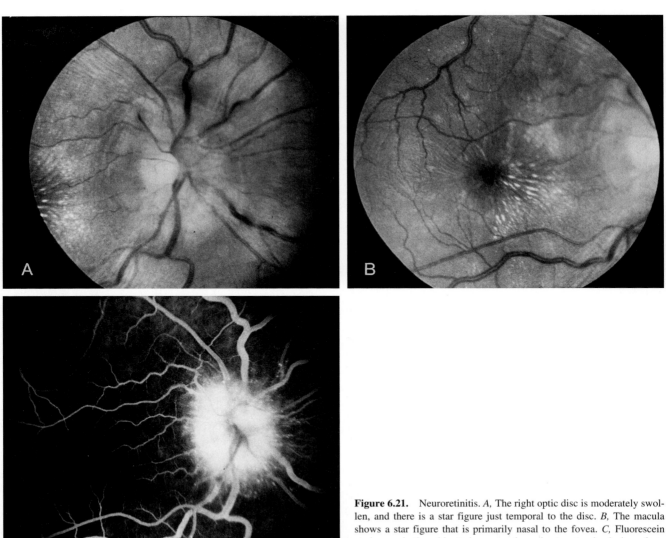

Figure 6.21. Neuroretinitis. *A,* The right optic disc is moderately swollen, and there is a star figure just temporal to the disc. *B,* The macula shows a star figure that is primarily nasal to the fovea. *C,* Fluorescein angiogram in the mid-arteriovenous phase shows extensive leakage from the optic disc but no retinal vascular abnormality in the macula or papillomacular bundle.

(469,504,594,595). The macular exudates progress over about 7–10 days. They then remain stable for several weeks before gradual resolution occurs. Resolution may take 6–12 months, but the lipid eventually completely disappears. Most patients ultimately recover good visual acuity, although some complain of persistent metamorphopsia or nonspecific blurred vision from mild disruption of the macular architecture despite disappearance of the macular exudates. Ophthalmoscopy and fluorescein angiography usually reveal defects in the retinal pigment epithelium of the macula in such cases. Rare patients develop moderate to severe visual loss, and we have seen one patient who had bilateral loss of vision down to 20/400 OU. Such patients invariably have evidence of optic atrophy.

Most patients who develop neuroretinitis do not experience a subsequent attack in the same eye, and only a few patients who have experienced an attack in one eye subsequently develop a similar attack in the fellow eye. Nevertheless, we have examined several patients who had recurrent episodes of neuroretinitis in one or both eyes. Such patients almost always suffer significant visual loss associated with optic atrophy and permanent macular pigmentary disturbances.

Neuroretinitis is thought to be an infectious or immune-mediated process that may be precipitated by a number of different agents. A common association is with an antecedent viral syndrome, suggesting a possible viral etiology for up to 50% of cases; however, viruses are rarely cultured from the CSF of such patients, and serologic evidence of a concomitant viral infection is usually lacking (469,594,595). One case of neuroretinitis associated with herpes simplex encephalitis was reported by Johnson and Wisetzley (601), as was a case of bilateral neuroretinitis associated with serologic evidence of hepatitis B virus infection (602). Foster et al. (311) reported a case of neuroretinitis that occurred in association with mumps in a young man, and Margolis et al. (603) reported the occurrence of an ''arcuate neuroretinitis'' associated with optic disc swelling in a patient with the acute retinal necrosis syndrome, a condition thought to be caused by one or more of the herpes viruses (see Chapter 57).

Neuroretinitis may occur in patients with evidence of infectious disease caused by organisms other than viruses. Gass (469) described neuroretinitis associated with cat-scratch disease, a systemic infection caused by the bacterium *Bartonella henselae* (see Chapter 49). Since then, numerous similar cases of neuroretinitis have been described in patients with clinical manifestations consistent with cat scratch disease (470,594,600,604), some of whom have had positive cat scratch antigen and antibody testing (604–606). In our experience, cat scratch disease is the most common infectious process associated with neuroretinitis. The vitreoretinal manifestations include anterior uveitis, vitritis, pars planitis, focal retinal vasculitis, a characteristic retinal white spot syndrome, *Bartonella* retinitis, branch retinal arteriolar or venular occlusions, focal choroiditis, serous retinal detachments, and peripapillary angiomatous lesions. The pattern of ocular disease in AIDS-associated *B. henselae* infections is poorly delineated; unusual manifestations include conjunctival and retinal bacillary angiomatosis.

Other common infections that cause neuroretinitis are the spirochetes. Neuroretinitis frequently occurs in patients with secondary and tertiary (late) syphilis. It may develop in patients with secondary syphilis as part of the syndrome of syphilitic meningitis (607). In such cases, it is usually bilateral and associated with evidence of meningeal irritation and multiple cranial neuropathies. It may also occur as an isolated phenomenon in patients with secondary syphilis, in which case it is often associated with uveitis and may be either unilateral or bilateral (607–614). Neuroretinitis occasionally occurs in patients with late syphilis, usually in patients with meningovascular neurosyphilis (607). The condition is indistinguishable from that which occurs in patients with secondary syphilis.

Lyme disease is another spirochete that is associated with neuroretinitis. Almost all cases occur in patients with stage II Lyme disease (534,617). Like the neuroretinitis that occurs in syphilis, the neuroretinitis of Lyme disease may be unilateral or bilateral; when bilateral, it is usually simultaneous and symmetric. Also like the neuroretinitis of syphilis, the neuroretinitis that occurs in Lyme disease may recover spontaneously but also resolves rapidly once the patient is treated with appropriate antibiotics (607).

Leptospira were identified in the CSF in one of three patients with neuroretinitis who all had unilateral visual loss and bilateral small, deep, intraretinal lesions consistent with septic retinitis (594). The patient in whom the leptospira were detected had no evidence of leptospirosis. No infectious agent was identified in blood or CSF in the remaining two patients.

Patients with toxoplasmosis, toxocariasis, and histoplasmosis may develop an acute anterior optic neuritis that, in rare cases, may be associated with a macular star figure (560,566,568,618–621). Whether such conditions are truly examples of neuroretinitis is unclear. We believe that any presumed or known inflammatory or infectious optic neuropathy that is characterized by optic disc swelling and the eventual development of a macular star figure should be defined as neuroretinitis; thus, these cases would fit that description. On the other hand, there are noninfectious and noninflammatory conditions that should not be called neuroretinitis even though they are characterized by optic disc swelling that may on occasion be associated with the development of a macular star figure. These mimicking conditions include papilledema, anterior ischemic optic neuropathy, and infiltration of the optic disc by tumor. Systemic hypertension may cause both optic disc swelling and a macular star figure, but fluorescein angiography in such cases shows leakage from macular vessels. A similar phenomenon may occur in the condition called diffuse unilateral subacute neuroretinitis, thought to be caused by one or more types of helminths (see Chapter 51).

One condition that is not associated with neuroretinitis is MS. One might assume that since neuroretinitis is a form of optic neuritis, the likelihood of developing MS after an attack of neuroretinitis would be as high as it seems to be after an attack of straightforward optic neuritis. In fact, although the rate of development of MS after an attack of anterior or retrobulbar optic neuritis is substantial (discussed previously), there is no increased tendency for patients who experience an attack of neuroretinitis to develop MS (622), and the rate of development of MS in such patients is the same as that in the normal population, about 6–80 per 100,000. Thus, the designation of an attack of acute optic neuropathy as an episode of neuroretinitis rather than anterior optic neuritis substantially alters the systemic prognosis in the patient being evaluated.

Investigation into the etiology of neuroretinitis should be done systematically. A careful history is crucial and should include questioning regarding sexually transmitted diseases, skin rashes, and viral exanthema. Complete physical and ocular examinations are also essential, and a neurologic examination may be required.

Patients with cat scratch fever usually have a history of contact with a cat. They complain of malaise, fever, muscle aches, and headache. Examination typically reveals local lymphadenopathy. Rare patients also have symptoms of arthritis, hepatitis, meningitis, or encephalitis.

Patients with secondary or tertiary syphilis usually provide a history of previous sexual contact, and they may have had a chancre in the past. They may also complain of arthralgias and myalgias, and some have symptoms of meningitis or encephalopathy. Many of these patients have been treated for syphilis or some other sexually transmitted disease in the past.

Patients with stage II Lyme disease usually live or work in an endemic area and may even give a history of a tick bite within the last 6 months. They often have cutaneous, cardiac, or neurologic manifestations in addition to visual complaints. The most common cutaneous manifestation is a solitary red or violaceous abnormality that ranges in size from a small nodule to a plaque several centimeters in diameter. The lesion is called a ''lymphocytoma'' or ''lymphadenosis benigna cutis.'' It may appear at the site of the tick bite or remote from it. Typical remote sites are the earlobe in children and the nipple in adults. Cardiac manifestations occur in about 5–8% of patients with stage II Lyme disease. Neurologic manifestations occur in 10–15% of cases of stage II Lyme disease and include meningitis, myelitis, encephalitis, cranial neuropathies, meningoradiculitis, and peripheral neuropathies. Some patients with neuroretinitis caused by Lyme disease have other ocular disturbances, including unilateral or bilateral granulomatous iridocyclitis, choroiditis, pars planitis, vitritis, and panophthalmitis. Intraocular vascular disturbances, such as retinal perivasculitis, branch retinal artery occlusion, recurrent vitreous hemorrhage, sheathing of retinal vessels, and intraretinal hemorrhages, are also common in such patients. Fluorescein angiography may reveal areas of nonperfusion in one or both eyes in such patients.

Specific patients may require lumbar puncture, MR imaging or CT scanning, and serologic tests for syphilis, Lyme disease, toxoplasmosis, histoplasmosis, or toxocariasis, whereas others should undergo antibody testing for cat scratch disease. The use of molecular biologic techniques to identify viral nucleic acids in various body tissues and fluids may eventually result in identification of specific viruses that cause the condition in otherwise normal persons or in persons who have recently suffered what seems to be a viral illness. At this time, however, we cannot recommend that such techniques be used on a regular basis, since they are both time-consuming and expensive and the therapeutic implications may be nil. Patients in whom neuroretinitis is accompanied by diffuse retinal or choroidal lesions suggesting septic retinitis or choroiditis may require a complete evaluation for systemic infection (600).

Treatment of neuroretinitis depends on whether there is an underlying infectious or inflammatory condition that requires therapy. *B. henselae* is the principal cause of cat scratch disease (623,624). The availability of specific serologic investigations has allowed the recognition of a spectrum of ocular cat scratch disease syndromes that previously were ill defined and considered idiopathic. The benefit of antimicrobial therapy for cat scratch disease in immunocompetent individuals has been difficult to establish, partly because most infections are self-limited. Empirically, azithromycin, ciprofloxacin, rifampin, parenteral gentamicin, and trimethoprim-sulfamethoxazole are the best therapeutic choices to minimize damage to the eye. Such treatment is almost always associated with improvement of the associated neuroretinitis, although whether the neuroretinitis would resolve spontaneously without treatment is unknown (470,600,623,624). Patients with neuroretinitis who are found to have secondary or late syphilis should be treated with intravenous penicillin as recommended by the Centers for Disease Control and Prevention (625), and patients with neuroretinitis that occurs in the setting of Lyme disease should also be treated with appropriate antibiotics, such as ceftriaxone, amoxicillin, or tetracycline (534). Patients in whom neuroretinitis is found to be associated with evidence of toxoplasmosis, toxocariasis, or histoplasmosis should likewise undergo treatment specific for their underlying systemic disease.

Patients with presumed viral or idiopathic neuroretinitis may or may not require treatment. Some authors advocate the use of systemic corticosteroids or ACTH to treat isolated neuroretinitis, but there is no definite evidence that such treatment alters either the speed of recovery of the condition or the ultimate outcome. Interestingly, Weiss and Beck (600) reported a case of idiopathic neuroretinitis that did not respond to treatment with oral prednisone but that improved rapidly and dramatically when intravenous corticosteroids were given.

As noted above, the ultimate prognosis for most cases of Leber's idiopathic neuroretinitis is excellent. Most patients achieve good visual recovery, although a subgroup of patients develop optic atrophy and poor vision. These patients typically have very poor visual acuity from the beginning of the process, significant visual field loss at presentation, and a marked, relative afferent pupillary defect if the condition is unilateral or asymmetric (595). Nevertheless, even patients who present with profound loss of visual function may recover normal or near-normal vision over time. Recurrent neuroretinitis may occur in rare cases (626).

OPTIC PERINEURITIS (PERIOPTIC NEURITIS)

Perioptic neuritis is a condition in which only the periphery of the optic nerve is inflamed. Edmunds and Lawford (627) initially described optic perineuritis as occurring in two forms: exudative and purulent. The exudative form, representing a localized, nonsuppurative pachymeningitis, occurs infrequently, most often in association with syphilis,

sarcoidosis, and viral encephalitides (628–632). The purulent form, actually a leptomeningitis, arises as an extension from the cerebral meninges. Pathologically, the pia and arachnoid are infiltrated by polymorphonuclear leukocytes that are also found free in the subarachnoid space surrounding the optic nerve (Fig. 6.22). From the leptomeninges, the

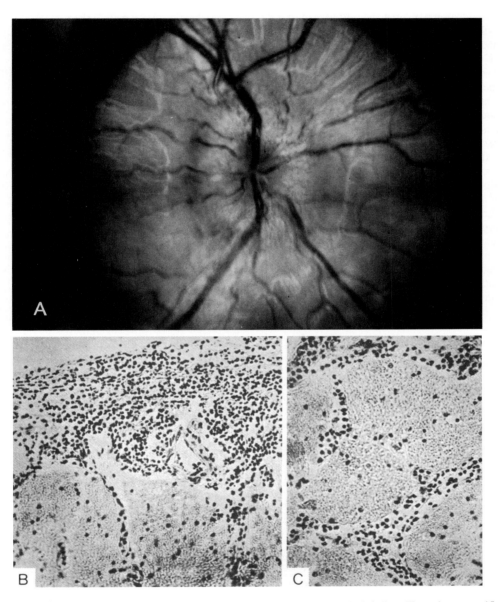

Figure 6.22. Optic perineuritis. *A,* The optic disc is hyperemic and swollen (as was the left disc). The patient was a 15-year-old boy complaining of a headache and stiff neck. He had a moderate fever. Visual acuity was 20/15 in both eyes, color vision was normal, and visual fields were full. The patient was believed to have papilledema. A lumbar puncture, however, revealed normal intracranial pressure, an increased concentration of protein in the CSF, and a significant CSF lymphocytosis. *B,* Histologic appearance of optic perineuritis in a case of fatal meningitis. Polymorphonuclear leukocytes (PMNs) are infiltrating the leptomeninges surrounding the optic nerve and are present in the subarachnoid space. *C,* Magnified view of affected area of peripheral optic nerve. PMNs extend from the pia in the septal system deep into the nerve. There is no invasion of the nerve tissue, however. (Specimen courtesy of Dr. S.T. Orion.)

infiltration may spread into the substance of the optic nerves without at first affecting the nerve fibers themselves.

Purvin et al. (633) reviewed the medical records of 14 patients with optic perineuritis who were seen in two neuro-ophthalmology clinics. The patients ranged in age from 24 to 60 years; 5 were older than 50 years. All patients had visual loss, eye pain, or both. The visual acuity was 20/20 or better in 8 of the 15 eyes. The results of visual field testing were normal in two eyes, and a paracentral scotoma or an arcuate defect was seen in seven. MR imaging demonstrated circumferential enhancement around the optic nerve, sometimes with intraorbital extension. Response to corticosteroids was dramatic; however, four patients had a relapse with lowering of the dose. The authors concluded that in contrast to those with optic neuritis, patients with optic perineuritis are often older at onset and are more likely to show sparing of central vision. MR imaging demonstrates enhancement around, rather than within, the optic nerve. Response to corticosteroids is more dramatic than in patients with optic neuritis, and patients are more likely to experience recurrence after stopping treatment.

In many cases of optic perineuritis, there are neither ocular symptoms nor signs other than disc swelling, usually bilateral. Apparently, the absence of visual dysfunction occurs because the infiltration is loose and disorganized. When vitreous cells are present, the differentiation from papilledema is easy; however, when there are no intraocular signs of inflammation, it may be necessary to perform neuroimaging and a lumbar puncture for diagnosis. Enlargement of the optic nerve sheath on CT scan may simulate optic nerve sheath meningioma (634), but advanced MR imaging is definitive (633).

REFERENCES

1. Nettleship E. On cases of retro-ocular neuritis. Trans Ophthalmol Soc UK 1884; 4:186–226.
2. Parinaud H. Trouble oculaires de la sclérose en plaques. J Sante 1884;3:3–5.
3. Uhthoff W. Untersuchungen uber die bei der multiplen herdsklerose vorkommenden augenstorungen. Arch Psychiatr Nervenkr 1890;21:55–116, 303–410.
4. Buzzard T. Atrophy of the optic nerve as a symptom of chronic disease of the central nervous system. Br Med J 1893;2:779–784.
5. Gunn RM. In discussion on retro-ocular neuritis. Trans Ophthalmol Soc UK 1897;17:107–217.
6. Beck RW, Optic Neuritis Study Group. The Optic Neuritis Treatment Trial. Arch Ophthalmol 1988;106:1051–1053.
7. Optic Neuritis Study Group. The clinical profile of acute optic neuritis: experience of the Optic Neuritis Treatment Trial. Arch Ophthalmol 1991;109: 1673–1678.
8. Beck RW, Cleary PA, Anderson MM Jr, et al. A randomized, controlled trial of corticosteroids in the treatment of acute optic neuritis. N Engl J Med 1992; 326:581–588.
9. Beck RW, Optic Neuritis Study Group. The Optic Neuritis Treatment Trial: implications for clinical practice. Arch Ophthalmol 1992;110:331–332.
10. Beck RW, Optic Neuritis Study Group. Corticosteroid treatment of optic neuritis: a need to change treatment practices. Neurology 1992;42:1133–1135.
11. Beck RW, Kupersmith MJ, Cleary PA, et al. Fellow eye abnormalities in acute unilateral optic neuritis: experience of the Optic Neuritis Treatment Trial. Ophthalmology 1993;100:691–698.
12. Beck RW, Arrington J, Murtagh FR, et al. Brain MRI in acute optic neuritis: experience of the Optic Neuritis Study Group. Arch Neurol 1993;8:841–846.
13. Beck RW, Cleary PA, Trobe JD, et al. The effect of corticosteroids for acute optic neuritis on the subsequent development of multiple sclerosis. N Engl J Med 1993;329:1764–1769.
14. Beck RW, Cleary PA, Optic Neuritis Study Group. Optic Neuritis Treatment Trial: one-year follow-up results. Arch Ophthalmol 1993;111:773–775.
15. Beck RW, Cleary PA, Optic Neuritis Study Group. Recovery from severe visual loss in optic neuritis. Arch Ophthalmol 1993;111:300.
16. Beck RW, Diehl L, Cleary PA, et al. The Pelli-Robson letter chart: normative data for young adults. Clin Vis Sci 1993;8:207–210.
17. Cleary PA, Beck RW, Anderson MM Jr, et al. Design, methods and conduct of the Optic Neuritis Treatment Trial. Control Clin Trials 1993;14:123–142.
18. Beck RW, Cleary PA, Backlund JC, et al. The course of visual recovery after optic neuritis: experience of the Optic Neuritis Treatment Trial. Ophthalmology 1994;101:1771–1778.
19. Beck RW. The Optic Neuritis Treatment Trial: three-year follow-up results. Arch Ophthalmol 1995;113:136–137.
20. Beck RW, Trobe JD, Optic Neuritis Study Group. What have we learned from the Optic Neuritis Treatment Trial? Ophthalmology 1995;102:1504–1508.
21. Beck RW, Trobe JD, Optic Neuritis Study Group. The Optic Neuritis Treatment Trial: putting the results in perspective. J Neuroophthalmol 1995;15:131–135.
22. Optic Neuritis Study Group. The five-year risk of multiple sclerosis after optic neuritis. Experience of the Optic Neuritis Treatment Trial. Neurology 1997;49: 1404–1413.
23. Optic Neuritis Study Group. High- and low-risk profiles for the development of multiple sclerosis within 10 years after optic neuritis. Arch Ophthalmol 2003; 121:944–949.
24. Optic Neuritis Study Group. Visual function more than 10 years after optic neuritis: experience of the Optic Neuritis Treatment Trial. Am J Ophthalmol 2004;137:77–83.
25. Optic Neuritis Study Group. Neurologic impairment 10 years after optic neuritis. Arch Neurology 2004 (in press).
26. Optic Neuritis Study Group. Long-term brain MRI changes after optic neuritis in patients without clinically definite multiple sclerosis. Arch Neurology 2004 (in press).
27. Alter M, Leibowitz U, Speer J. Risk of multiple sclerosis related to age at immigration in Israel. Arch Neurol 1996;15:234–237.
28. Percy AK, Nobrega FT, Kurland LT. Optic neuritis and multiple sclerosis: an epidemiologic study. Arch Ophthalmol 1972;87:135–139.
29. Wikström J. The epidemiology of optic neuritis in Finland. Acta Neurol Scand 1975;52:167–178.
30. Kahana E, Alter M, Feldman S. Optic neuritis in relation to multiple sclerosis. J Neurol 1976;213:87–95.
31. Haller P, Patzold U, et al. Optic neuritis in Hanover: an epidemiologic and serogenetic study. In: Bauer HJ, Poser S, Ritter G, eds. Progress in Multiple Sclerosis Research. New York, Springer, 1980:546–548.
32. Kinnunen E. The incidence of optic neuritis and its prognosis for multiple sclerosis. Acta Neurol Scand 1983;68:371–377.
33. Rodriguez M, Siva A, Cross SA, et al. Optic neuritis: a population-based study in Olmsted County, Minnesota. Neurology 1995;45:244–250.
34. Hierons R, Lyle TK. Bilateral retrobulbar optic neuritis. Brain 1959;82:56–67.
35. Kennedy C, Carroll FD. Optic neuritis in children. Arch Ophthalmol 1960;63: 747–755.
36. Meadows SP. Retrobulbar and optic neuritis in childhood and adolescence. Trans Ophthalmol Soc UK 1969;89:603–638.
37. Kriss A, Francis DA, Cuendet F, et al. Recovery after optic neuritis in childhood. J Neurol Neurosurg Psychiatry 1988;51:1253–1258.
38. Riikonen R. The role of infection and vaccination in the genesis of optic neuritis and multiple sclerosis in children. Acta Neurol Scand 1989;80:425–431.
39. Perkin GD, Rose FC. Optic Neuritis and Its Differential Diagnosis. Oxford, UK, Oxford Medical Publications, 1979.
40. Kupersmith MJ, Nelson JI, Seiple WH, et al. The 20/20 eye in multiple sclerosis. Neurology 1983;33:1015–1020.
41. Celesia GG, Kaufman DI, Brigell M, et al. Optic neuritis: a prospective study. Neurology 1990;40:919–923.
42. Francis DA. Demyelinating optic neuritis: clinical features and differential diagnosis. Br J Hosp Med 1991;45:376–379.
43. Compston A. Cellular organization of the optic nerve and the implications for optic neuritis. Eye 1992;6:123–128.
44. McDonald WI, Barnes D. The ocular manifestations of multiple sclerosis. 1. Abnormalities of the afferent visual system. J Neurol Neurosurg Psychiatry 1992; 55:747–752.
45. Rose FC. The aetiology of optic neuritis. In: Cant JS, ed. The Optic Nerve. St Louis, CV Mosby, 1972:217–217.
46. Swartz NG, Beck RW, Savino PJ, et al. Pain in anterior ischemic optic neuropathy. J Neuroophthalmol 1995;15:9–10.
47. Lepore FE. The origin of pain in optic neuritis: determinants of pain in 101 eyes with optic neuritis. Arch Neurol 1991;48:748–749.
48. Swartz NG, Beck RW, Savino PJ, et al. Pain in anterior ischemic optic neuropathy. J Neuroophthalmol 1995;15:9–10.
49. Traquair HM. Toxic amblyopias, including retrobulbar neuritis. Trans Ophthalmol Soc UK 1930;17:107–217.
50. Davis FA, Bergen D, Schauf C, et al. Movement phosphenes in optic neuritis: a new clinical sign. Neurology 1976;26:1100–1104.
51. Cohen M, Lessell S, Wolf P. A prospective study of the risk of developing multiple sclerosis in uncomplicated optic neuritis. Neurology 1979;19:208–213.
52. Page NGR, Bolger JP, Sanders MD. Auditory evoked phosphenes in optic nerve disease. J Neurol Neurosurg Psychiatry 1982;45:7–12.

53. Sanders EA, Volkers AC, Van der Poel JC, et al. Spatial contrast sensitivity function in optic neuritis. Neuroophthalmology 1984;4:255–259.
54. Tsukamoto M, Adachi-Usami E. Color vision in multiple sclerosis with optic neuritis. Acta Soc Ophthalmol Jpn 1987;91:613–621.
55. Ménage MJ, Papakostopoulos D, Hart JCD, et al. The Farnsworth-Munsell 100 hue test in the first episode of demyelinating optic neuritis. Br J Ophthalmol 1993;77:68–74.
56. Trauzettel-Klosinski S, Aulhorn E. Measurement of brightness sensation caused by flickering light: a simple and highly specific test for assessing the florid stage of optic neuritis. Clin Vis Sci 1987;2:63–82.
57. Stellberger C, Wetzel W, Duncker G. Comparison between the flicker test procedures of Aulhorn and of Dölle in the diagnosis of optic neuritis. Graefes Arch Clin Exp Ophthalmol 1993;231:692–696.
58. Woung L-C, Wakakura M, Ishikawa S. Critical flicker frequency in acute and recovered optic neuritis. Jpn J Ophthalmol 1993;37:122–129.
59. Steinmetz R, Kearns TP. H-R-R pseudoisochromatic plates: as a diagnostic aid in retrobulbar neuritis of multiple sclerosis. Am J Ophthalmol 1956;41:833–837.
60. Rosen JA. Pseudoisochromatic visual testing in the diagnosis of disseminated sclerosis. Trans Am Neurol Assoc 1965;90:283–284.
61. Marre M. The investigation of acquired color deficiencies. Second Congress of the International Color Association, University of York, July 2–6, 1973. London, Adam Hilger Publishers, 1973.
62. Trusiewicz D. Farnsworth 100-hue test in diagnosis of ethambutol-induced damage to optic nerve. Ophthalmology 1975;171:425–431.
63. Griffin JF, Wray SH. Acquired color vision defects in retrobulbar neuritis. Am J Ophthalmol 1978;86:193–201.
64. Griffith AH. In discussion on retro-ocular neuritis. Trans Ophthalmol Soc UK 1897;17:107–217.
65. Gunn RM. Discussion on retro-ocular neuritis. Br Med J 1904;2:1285–1287.
66. Berliner MD. Acute optic neuritis in demyelinating diseases of the nervous system. Arch Ophthalmol 1935;13:83–98.
67. Carroll FD. Retrobulbar optic neuritis: observations on one hundred cases. Arch Ophthalmol 1940;24:44–54.
68. Marshall D. Ocular manifestations of multiple sclerosis and relationship to retrobulbar neuritis. Trans Am Ophthalmol Soc 1950;48:487–525.
69. Hyllested K, Moller P. Follow-up patients with a history of optic neuritis. Acta Ophthalmol 1961;39:655–662.
70. Miller NR. Walsh and Hoyt's Clinical Neuro-Ophthalmology, 4th ed, vol 1. Baltimore, Williams & Wilkins, 1982:228.
71. Chamlin M. Visual field changes in optic neuritis. Arch Ophthalmol 1953;50:699–713.
72. Vighetto A, Grochowicki M, Aimard G. Altitudinal hemianopia in multiple sclerosis. Neuroophthalmology 1991;11:25–27.
73. Keltner JL, Johnson CA, Spurr JO, et al. Baseline visual field profile of optic neuritis: the experience of the Optic Neuritis Treatment Trial. Arch Ophthalmol 1993;111:231–234.
74. Nikoskelainen E, Nikoskelainen J, Salmi AA, et al. Virus antibody levels in serum specimens from patients with optic neuritis and from matched controls. Acta Neurol Scand 1975;51:333–346.
75. Stanley JA, Baise G. The swinging flashlight test to detect minimal optic neuropathy. Arch Ophthalmol 1968;80:769–771.
76. Thompson HS. Pupillary signs in the diagnosis of optic nerve disease. Trans Ophthalmol Soc UK 1976;96:377–381.
77. Ellis CK. The afferent pupillary defect in acute optic neuritis. J Neurol Neurosurg Psychiatry 1979;42:1008–1017.
78. Cox TA, Thompson HS, Corbett JJ. Relative afferent pupillary defects in optic neuritis. Am J Ophthalmol 1981;92:685–690.
79. Paton J. Papilloedema in disseminated sclerosis. Trans Ophthalmol Soc UK 1914;34:252–261.
80. Adie WJ. The aetiology and symptomatology of disseminated sclerosis. Br Med J 1932;2:997–1000.
81. Benedict WL. Multiple sclerosis as an etiologic factor in retrobulbar neuritis. Arch Ophthalmol 1942;28:988–995.
82. Bradley WG, Whitty CM. Acute optic neuritis: its clinical features and their relation to prognosis for recovery of vision. J Neurol Neurosurg Psychiatry 1967;30:531–538.
83. Hutchinson WM. Acute optic neuritis and the prognosis for multiple sclerosis. J Neurol Neurosurg Psychiatry 1976;39:283–289.
84. Lightman S, McDonald WI, Bird AC, et al. Retinal venous sheathing in optic neuritis: its significance for the pathogenesis of multiple sclerosis. Brain 1987;110:405–414.
85. Birch MK, Barbosa S, Blumhardt LD, et al. Retinal venous sheathing and the blood-retinal barrier in multiple sclerosis. Arch Ophthalmol 1966;114:34–39.
86. Arden GB, Gucukoglu AG. Grating test of contrast sensitivity in patients with retrobulbar neuritis. Arch Ophthalmol 1978;96:1626–1629.
87. Froehlich J, Kaufman DI. Use of pattern electroretinography to differentiate acute optic neuritis from acute anterior ischemic optic neuropathy. Electroencephalograph Clin Neurophysiol 1994;92:480–486.
88. Beck RW, Ruchman MC, Savino PJ, et al. Contrast sensitivity measurements in acute and resolved optic neuritis. Br J Ophthalmol 1984;68:756–759.
89. Sanders EA, Volkers AC, Van der Poel JC, et al. Estimation of visual function after optic neuritis: a comparison of clinical tests. Br J Ophthalmol 1986;70:918–924.
90. Fleishman JA, Beck RW, Linares OA, et al. Deficits in visual function after resolution of optic neuritis. Ophthalmology 1987;94:1029–1035.
91. Howard CW, Osher RH, Tomsak RL. Computed tomographic features in optic neuritis. Am J Ophthalmol 1980;89:699–702.
92. Miller NR, Savino PJ, Schneider T. Rapid growth of an intracranial aneurysm causing apparent retrobulbar optic neuritis. J Neuroophthalmol 1995;15:212–218.
93. Rolak LA, Beck RB, Paty DW, et al. Cerebrospinal fluid in acute optic neuritis: Experience of the Optic Neuritis Study Group. Neurology 1996;46:368–372.
94. Link H, Norrby E, Olsson J-E. Immunoglobulins and measles antibodies in optic neuritis. N Engl J Med 1973;289:1103–1107.
95. Arnason BW, Fuller TC, Lehrich J, et al. Histocompatability types and measles antibodies in multiple sclerosis and optic neuritis. J Neurol Sci 1974;22:419–428.
96. Miller DH, Ormerod IEC, McDonald WI, et al. The early risk of multiple sclerosis after optic neuritis. J Neurol Neurosurg Psychiatry 1988;51:1569–1571.
97. Guy J, Mancuso A, Quisling RG, et al. Gadolinium-DPTA-enhanced magnetic resonance imaging in optic neuropathies. Ophthalmology 1990;97:592–600.
98. Youl BD, Turano G, Miller DH, et al. The pathophysiology of acute optic neuritis: an association of gadolinium leakage with clinical and electrophysiological deficits. Brain 1991;114:2437–2450.
99. Guy J, Mao J, Bidgood WD Jr, et al. Enhancement and demyelination of the intraorbital optic nerve: fat suppression magnetic resonance imaging. Ophthalmology 1992;99:713–719.
100. Frederiksen JL, Larsson HBW, Henriksen O, et al. Magnetic resonance imaging of the brain in patients with acute monosymptomatic optic neuritis. Acta Neurol Scand 1989;80:512–517.
101. Jacobs L, Munschauer FE, Kaba SE. Clinical and magnetic resonance imaging in optic neuritis. Neurology 1991;41:15–19.
102. Sandberg-Wollheim M, Bynke H, Cronqvist S, et al. A long-term prospective study of optic neuritis: evaluation of risk factors. Ann Neurol 1990;27:386–393.
103. Frederiksen JL, Larsson HBW, Oleson J. Correlation of magnetic resonance imaging and CSF findings in patients with acute monosymptomatic optic neuritis. Acta Neurol Scand 1992;86:317–322.
104. Tourtellotte WW, Tumani H. Multiple sclerosis. Cerebrospinal fluid. In: Raine CS, McFarland HF, Tourtellotte WW, eds. Multiple Sclerosis: Clinical and Pathogenetic Basis. London, Chapman and Hall, 1997:57–59.
105. Söderström M, Lindqvist M, Hiller J, et al. Optic neuritis: findings on MRI, CSF examination and HLA class II typing in 60 patients and results of a short-term follow-up. J Neurol 1994;241:391–397.
106. Sandberg M, Bynke H. Cerebrospinal fluid in 25 cases of optic neuritis. Acta Neurol Scand 1973;49:442–452.
107. Nikoskelainen E, Irjala K, Salmi TT. Cerebrospinal fluid findings in patients with optic neuritis. Acta Ophthalmol 1975;53:105–119.
108. Sandberg-Wollheim M, Platz P, Ryder LP, et al. HL-A histocompatibility antigens in optic neuritis. Acta Ophthalmol 1975;52:161–166.
109. Nyland H, Naess A, Slagsvold JE. Lymphocyte subpopulations in peripheral blood and cerebrospinal fluid from patients with acute optic neuritis. Acta Ophthalmol 1980;58:411–417.
110. Rudick RA, Jacobs L, Kinkel PR, et al. Isolated idiopathic optic neuritis: analysis of free kappa-light chains in cerebrospinal fluid and correlation with nuclear magnetic resonance findings. Arch Neurol 1986;43:456–458.
111. Staugaitis S, Shapshak P, Tourtellotte W, et al. Isoelectric focusing of unconcentrated cerebrospinal fluid: application to ultrasensitive analysis of oligoclonal immunoglobulin-G. Electrophoresis 1985;6:287–291.
112. Poser CM, Paty D, Scheinberg L, et al. New diagnostic criteria for multiple sclerosis: guidelines for research protocols. Ann Neurol 1983;13:227–231.
113. Frick E, Stickl H. Optic neuritis and multiple sclerosis: an immunological study. Eur Neurol 1980;19:185–191.
114. Söderström M, Link H, Xu Z, et al. Optic neuritis and multiple sclerosis: anti-MBP and anti-MBP peptide antibody-secreting cells are accumulated in CSF. Neurology 1993;43:1215–1222.
115. Feasby TE, Ebers GC. Risk of multiple sclerosis in isolated optic neuritis. Can J Neurol Sci 1982;9:269.
116. Link H, Stendahl-Brodin L. Optic neuritis and multiple sclerosis. N Engl J Med 1983;308:1294–1295.
117. Stendahl-Brodin L, Link H. Optic neuritis: oligoclonal bands increase the risk of multiple sclerosis. Acta Neurol Scand 1983;67:301–304.
118. Anmarkrud N, Slettnes ON. Uncomplicated retrobulbar neuritis and the development of multiple sclerosis. Acta Ophthalmol 1989;67:306–309.
119. Deckert-Schlüter M, Schlüter D, Schwendemann G. Evaluation of IL-2, sIL2R, IL-6, TNF-α, and IL-1β in serum and CSF of patients with optic neuritis. J Neurol Sci 1992;113:50–54.
120. Link J, Söderström M, Kostulas V, et al. Optic neuritis is associated with myelin basic protein and proteolipid protein reactive cells producing interferon-gamma, interleukin-4, and transforming growth factor-beta. J Neuroimmunol 1994;49:9–18.
121. Oksenberg JR, Seboun E, Hauser SL. Genetics of demyelinating diseases. Brain Pathol 1996;6:289–302.

122. Spielman RS, Nathanson N. The genetics of susceptibility to multiple sclerosis. Epidemiol Rev 1982;4:45–65.
123. Ebers GC, Bulman DE, Sadovnick AD, et al. A population-based study of multiple sclerosis in twins. N Engl J Med 1986;315:1638–1642.
124. Sandberg-Wollheim M. Studies on the cerebrospinal fluid in relation to clinical course in 61 patients. Acta Neurol Scand 1975;52:167–178.
125. Compston DA, Batchelor JR, Earl CJ, et al. Factors influencing the risk of multiple sclerosis developing in patients with optic neuritis. Brain 1978;101: 495–511.
126. Matthews WB, Acheson ED, Batchelor JR, et al, eds. McAlpine's Multiple Sclerosis. Edinburgh, Churchill Livingstone, 1985.
127. Kelly MA, Cavan DA, Penny MA, et al. The influence of HLA-DR and -DQ alleles on progression to multiple sclerosis following a clinically isolated syndrome. Hum Immunol 1993;37:185–191.
128. Tiwari JL, Terasaki PI. HLA and Disease Associations. New York, Springer-Verlag, 1985.
129. Hauser SL, Fleischnick E, Weiner HL, et al. Extended major histocompatibility complex haplotypes in patients with multiple sclerosis. Neurology 1989;39: 275–277.
130. Francis DA, Compston DAS, Batchelor JR, et al. A reassessment of the risk of multiple sclerosis developing in patients with optic neuritis after extended follow-up. J Neurol Neurosurg Psychiatry 1987;50:758–765.
131. Marcadet A, Massart C, Semana G, et al. Association of class II HLA-DQB chain DNA restriction fragments with multiple sclerosis. Immunogenetics 1985; 22:93–96.
132. Olerup O, Hillert J, Frederickson S, et al. Primary chronic progressive and relapsing/remitting multiple sclerosis: two immunogenetically distinct disease entities. Proc Natl Acad Sci USA 1989;86:7113–7117.
133. Vartdal F, Sollid LM, Vandvik B, et al. Patients with multiple sclerosis carry DQB1 genes which encode shared polymorphic amino acid sequences. Hum Immunol 1989;25:103–110.
134. Hillert J, Käll T, Olerup O, et al. Distribution of HLA-Dw2 in optic neuritis and multiple sclerosis indicates heterogeneity. Acta Neurol Scand 1996;94:161–166.
135. Hely MA, McManis PG, Doran TJ, et al. Acute optic neuritis: a prospective study of risk factors for multiple sclerosis. J Neurol Neurosurg Psychiatry 1986; 49:1125–1130.
136. Oksenberg JR, Seboun E, Hauser SL. Genetics of demyelinating diseases. Brain Pathol 1996;6:289–302.
137. Kira J, Kanai T, Nishimura Y, et al. Western versus Asian types of multiple sclerosis: two immunogenetically and clinically distinct patient groups. Ann Neurol 1996;40:569–574.
138. Muntoni F, Murru MR, Costa G, et al. Different HLA-DR2-DQW1 haplotypes in Sardinian and northern Italian populations: implications for multiple sclerosis susceptibility. Tissue Antigens 1991;38:34–36.
139. Haines JL, Terwedow HA, Burgess K, et al. Linkage of the MHC to familial multiple sclerosis suggests genetic heterogeneity. Multiple Sclerosis Genetic Group. Hum Mol Genet 1998;7:1229–1234.
140. Hauser SL, Oksenberg JR, Lincoln R, et al. Interaction between HLA-DR2 and abnormal brain MRI in optic neuritis and early MS. Neurology 2000;54: 1859–1861.
141. Soderstrom M, Ya-Ping J, Hillert J, Link H. Optic neuritis: prognosis for multiple sclerosis from MRI, CSF, and HLA findings. Neurology 1998;50:708–714.
142. Ozowa K, Suchanek G, Breitschopf H, et al. Patterns of oligodendroglia pathology in multiple sclerosis. Brain 1994;117:1311–1322.
143. Genain CP, Cannella B, Hauser SL, Raine CS. Identification of autoantibodies associated with tissue damage in multiple sclerosis. Nat Med 1999;5:170–175.
144. Thompson AJ, Polman CH, Miller DH, et al. Primary progressive multiple sclerosis. Brain 1997;120:1085–1096.
145. Jacobs L, Kinkel PR, Kinkel WR. Silent brain lesions in patients with isolated idiopathic optic neuritis: a clinical and nuclear magnetic resonance imaging study. Arch Neurol 1986;43:452–455.
146. Hornabrook RSL, Miller DH, Newton MR, et al. Frequent involvement of the optic radiation in patients with acute isolated optic neuritis. Neurology 1992; 42:77–79.
147. Frederiksen J, Larsson HBW, Olesen J, et al. MRI, VEP, SEP and biothesiometry suggest monosymptomatic acute optic neuritis to be a first manifestation of multiple sclerosis. Acta Neurol Scand 1991;83:343–350.
148. Frederiksen J, Larsson HBW, Nordenbo AM, et al. Plaques causing hemianopsia or quadrantanopsia in multiple sclerosis identified by MRI and VEP. Acta Ophthalmol 1991;69:169–177.
149. Martinelli V, Comi G, Filippi M, et al. Paraclinical tests in acute-onset optic neuritis, basal data and results of a short follow-up. Acta Neurol Scand 1991; 84:231–236.
150. Morrissey SP, Miller DH, Kendall BE, et al. The significance of brain magnetic resonance imaging abnormalities at presentation with clinically isolated syndromes suggestive of multiple sclerosis. Brain 1993;116:135–146.
151. Frohman EM, Goodin DS, Calabresi PA, et al. The utility of MRI in suspected MS: report of the Therapeutics and Technology Assessment Subcommittee of the American Academy of Neurology. Neurology 2003;61:602–611.
152. McDonald WI, Compston A, Edan G, et al. Recommended diagnostic criteria for multiple sclerosis: guidelines from the International Panel on the Diagnosis of Multiple Sclerosis. Ann Neurol 2001;50:121–127.
153. Braude LS, Cunha-Vaz JG, Frenkel M. Diagnosing acute retrobulbar neuritis by vitreous fluorophotometry. Am J Ophthalmol 1981;91:764–773.
154. Hench PS, Kendall EC, et al. The effect of a hormone of the adrenal cortex (17-hydroxy-11-dehydrocorticosterone: compound E) and of pituitary adrenocorticotrophic hormone on rheumatoid arthritis. Proc Staff Meet Mayo Clin 1949;24: 181–197.
155. Rawson MD, Liversedge LA, Goldfarb G. Treatment of acute retrobulbar neuritis with corticotrophin. Lancet 1966;2:1044–1046.
156. Rawson MD, Liversedge LA. Treatment of retrobulbar neuritis with corticotrophin. Lancet 1969;2:222.
157. Cooperative study in the evaluation of therapy in multiple sclerosis: ACTH vs. placebo-final report. Neurology 1970;20:1–59.
158. Bowden AN, Bowden PMA, Friedmann AI, et al. A trial of corticotrophin gelatin injection in acute optic neuritis. J Neurol Neurosurg Psychiatry 1974;37: 869–873.
159. Gould ES, Bird AC, Leaver PK, et al. Treatment of optic neuritis by retrobulbar injection of triamcinolone. Br Med J 1977;1:1495–1497.
160. Trauzettel-Klosinski S, Axmann D, Aulhorn E, et al. The Tubingen study on optic neuritis treatment: a prospective, randomized and controlled trial. Clin Vision Sci 1993;8:385–394.
161. Spoor TC. Treatment of optic neuritis with megadose corticosteroids. J Clin Neuroophthalmol 1986;6:137–143.
162. Spoor TC, Rockwell DL. Treatment of optic neuritis with intravenous megadose corticosteroids: a consecutive series. Ophthalmology 1988;95:131–134.
163. Raine CS, Traugott U. Chronic relapsing experimental autoimmune encephalomyelitis: ultrastructure of the central nervous system of animals treated with combination of myelin components. Lab Invest 1982;48:275–284.
164. Traugott U, Stone SH, Raine CS. Chronic relapsing experimental autoimmune encephalomyelitis treatment with combinations of myelin components promotes clinical and structural recovery. J Neurol Sci 1982;56:65–73.
165. Raine CS, Traugott R, Traugott U, et al. Oligodendrocyte proliferation and enhanced CNS remyelination after therapeutic manipulation of chronic relapsing EAE. Ann NY Acad Sci 1988;540:712–714.
166. Rodriguez M, Lennon VA, Benveniste EN. Remyelination by oligodendrocytes stimulated by antiserum to spinal cord. J Neuropathol Exp Neurol 1987;46: 84–95.
167. Rodriguez M, Lennon VA. Immunoglobulins promote remyelination in the central nervous system. Ann Neurol 1990;27:12–17.
168. Miller DJ, Sanborn KS, Katzmann JA, et al. Monoclonal autoantibodies promote central nervous system repair in an animal model of multiple sclerosis. J Neurosci 1994;14:6230–6238.
169. van Engelen BGM, Miller DJ, Pavelko KD, et al. Promotion of remyelination by polyclonal immunoglobulin and IVIg in Theiler's virus induced demyelination and in MS. J Neurol Neurosurg Psychiatry 1994;57(Suppl):65–68.
170. van Engelen BG, Hommes OR, Pinckers A, et al. Improved vision after intravenous immunoglobulin in stable demyelinating optic neuritis. Ann Neurol 1992; 32:834–835.
171. Noseworthy JH, O'Brien PC, Petterson TM, et al. A randomized trial of intravenous immunoglobulin in inflammatory demyelinating optic neuritis. Neurology 2001;12;56:1514–1522.
172. Scorolli L, Martini E, Scorolli L, et al. Metilprednisolone in bolo endovenoso nel trattamento delle manifestazioni oculari della sclerosi multipla. Ann Ottalmol Clin Oculist 1991;117:165–171.
173. Serra A. Some temporal aspects of colour discrimination in multiple sclerosis. Doc Ophthalmol 1982;33:445–451.
174. Plant GT, Hess RF. Regional threshold contrast sensitivity within the central visual field in optic neuritis. Brain 1987;110:489–515.
175. Keltner JL, Johnson CA, Spurr JO, et al. Visual field profile of optic neuritis: one-year follow-up in the Optic Neuritis Treatment Trial. Arch Ophthalmol 1994;112:946–953.
176. Sandberg HO. Acute retrobulbar neuritis: a retrospective study. Acta Ophthalmol 1972;50:3–8.
177. Slamovits TL, Rosen CE, Cheng KP, et al. Visual recovery in patients with optic neuritis and visual loss to no light perception. Am J Ophthalmol 1991; 111:209–214.
178. Mathot E, Segal A, Bour T, et al. A propos d'un cas de nevrite optique retrobulbaire siderante bilaterisee sur sclerose en plaques. Bull Soc Ophtalmol Fr 1988;88:1449–1450.
179. Saraux H, Nordmann JPh, Denis Ph. Les formes atypiques des névrites optiques de la sclérose en plaques. J Fr Ophtalmol 1991;14:235–244.
180. Heron JR, Regan D, Milner BA. Delay in visual perception in unilateral optic atrophy after retrobulbar neuritis. Brain 1974;97:69–78.
181. Burde RM, Gallin PF. Visual parameters associated with recovered retrobulbar optic neuritis. Am J Ophthalmol 1975;79:1034–1037.
182. Galvin RJ, Regan D, Heron JR. Impaired temporal resolution of vision after acute retrobulbar neuritis. Brain 1976;99:255–268.
183. Ellenberger C Jr, Ziegler T. The Swiss cheese visual field or time-varying abnormalities of vision after ''recovery'' from optic neuritis. In: Smith JL, ed. Neuro-Ophthalmology Focus 1980. New York, Masson, 1979:175–179.

184. Hess RF, Plant GT. The effect of temporal frequency variation on threshold contrast sensitivity deficits in optic neuritis. J Neurol Neurosurg Psychiatry 1983; 46:322–330.
185. Medjbeur S, Tulunay-Keesey U. Spatiotemporal responses of the visual system in demyelinating diseases. Brain 1985;108:123–138.
186. Plant GT, Hess RF. Temporal frequency discrimination in optic neuritis and multiple sclerosis. Brain 1985;108:647–776.
187. Frederiksen J, Larsson H, Olesen J, et al. Evaluation of the visual system in multiple sclerosis. II. Colour vision. Acta Neurol Scand 1986;74:203–209.
188. Engell T, Trojaborg W, Raun NE. Subclinical optic neuropathy in multiple sclerosis: a neuro-ophthalmological investigation by means of visually evoked response, Farnsworth-Munsell 100 hue test and Ishihara test and their diagnostic value. Acta Ophthalmol 1987;65:735–740.
189. Nordmann J-P, Saraux H, Roullet E. Contrast sensitivity in multiple sclerosis: a study of 35 patients with and without optic neuritis. Ophthalmologica 1987; 195:199–204.
190. MacFadyen DJ, Drance SM, Chisholm IA, et al. The Farnsworth-Munsell 100-hue color vision score and visual evoked potentials in multiple sclerosis. Neuro-ophthalmology 1988;8:289–298.
191. MacFadyen DJ, Drance SM, Douglas GR, et al. The retinal nerve fiber layer, neuroretinal rim area and visual evoked potentials in MS. Neurology 1988;38: 1353–1358.
192. Honan WP, Heron JR, Foster DH, et al. Visual loss in multiple sclerosis and its relation to previous optic neuritis, disease duration and clinical classification. Brain 1990;113:975–987.
193. Regan D, Kothe AC, Sharpe JA. Recognition of motion-defined shapes in patients with multiple sclerosis and optic neuritis. Brain 1991;114:1129–1155.
194. Ciancaglini M, Thomas A, D'Aurelio AP, et al. Difetti perimetrici affetti da sclerosi multipla con o senza storia di neurite ottica retrobulbare. Ann Ottalmol Clin Oculist 1993;119:637–640.
195. Kirkham TH, Coupland SG. Multiple regression analysis of diagnostic predictors in optic nerve disease. Can J Neurol Sci 1981;8:67–72.
196. Wybar KC. The ocular manifestations of disseminated sclerosis. Proc Roy Soc Med 1952;45:315–319.
197. Lynn BH. Retrobulbar neuritis: a survey of the present condition of cases occurring over the last fifty-six years. Trans Ophthalmol Soc UK 1959;79:701–716.
198. Van Dalen JTW, Greve EL. Visual field defects in multiple sclerosis. Neuroophthalmology 1981;2:93–104.
199. Zimmern RL, Campbell FW, Wilkinson IM. Subtle disturbances of vision after optic neuritis elicited by studying contrast sensitivity. J Neurol Neurosurg Psychiatry 1979;42:407–412.
200. Sjöstrand J, Abrahamsson M. Suprathreshold vision in acute optic neuritis. J Neurol Neurosurg Psychiatry 1982;45:227–234.
201. Drucker MD, Savino PJ, Sergott RC, et al. Low-contrast letter charts to detect subtle neuropathies. Am J Ophthalmol 1988;105:141–145.
202. Regan D, Silver R, Murray TJ. Visual acuity and contrast sensitivity in multiple sclerosis: hidden visual loss. Brain 1977;100:563–579.
203. Kupersmith MJ, Seiple WH, Nelson JI, et al. Contrast sensitivity loss in multiple sclerosis. Invest Ophthalmol Vis Sci 1984;25:632–639.
204. Friedman JR, Kosmorsky GS, Burde RM. Stereoacuity in patients with optic nerve disease. Arch Ophthalmol 1985;103:37–38.
205. Sadun AA, Lessell S. Brightness-sense and optic nerve disease. Arch Ophthalmol 1985;103:39–43.
206. Bynke H, Rosen I, Sandberg-Wollheim M. Correlation of visual evoked potentials, ophthalmological and neurological findings after unilateral optic neuritis. Acta Ophthalmol 1980;58:673–687.
207. Hoyt WF, Schlicke B, Eckelhoff RJ. Funduscopic appearance of a nerve-fiber bundle defect. Br J Ophthalmol 1972;56:577–583.
208. Shahrokhi F, Chiappa KH, Young RR. Pattern shift visual evoked responses: two hundred patients with optic neuritis and/or multiple sclerosis. Arch Neurol 1978;35:64–71.
209. Wutz W, Bartl G, Hiti H, et al. Verlaufsbeobachtungender neuritis retrobulbaris: Vergleichende psychophysische und electroophthalmologische befunde. Klin Monatsbl Augenheilkd 1980;177:689–695.
210. Halliday AM, McDonald WI, Mushin J. Delayed pattern evoked responses in optic neuritis in relation to visual acuity. Trans Ophthalmol Soc UK 1973;93: 315–324.
211. Asselman P, Chadwick DW, Marsden CD. Visual evoked responses in the diagnosis and management of patients suspected of multiple sclerosis. Brain 1975; 98:261–282.
212. Halliday AM, McDonald WI, Mushin J. Delayed visual evoked response in optic neuritis. Lancet 1972;1:982–985.
213. Cleary PA, Beck RW, Bourque LB, et al. Visual symptoms after optic neuritis: results from the Optic Neuritis Treatment Trial. J Neuroophthalmol 1997;17: 18–23.
214. Franklin CR, Brickner RM. Vasospasm associated with multiple sclerosis. Arch Neurol Psychiatr 1947;58:125–162.
215. McAlpine D, Compston N. Some aspects of the natural history of disseminated sclerosis. Q J Med 1952;21:135–167.
216. Goldstein JE, Cogan DG. Exercise and the optic neuropathy of multiple sclerosis. Arch Ophthalmol 1964;72:168–170.
217. Smith JL, Hoyt WF, Susac JO. Ocular fundus in acute Leber optic neuropathy. Arch Ophthalmol 1973;90:349–354.
218. Nelson D, Jeffreys WH, McDowell F. Effect of induced hyperthermia on some neurological diseases. Arch Neurol Psychiatr 1958;79:31–39.
219. Scholl GB, Song H-S, Wray SH. Uhthoff's symptom in optic neuritis: relationship to magnetic resonance imaging and development of multiple sclerosis. Ann Neurol 1991;30:180–184.
220. Guthrie TC. Visual and motor changes in patients with multiple sclerosis. Arch Neurol Psychiatr Nervenkr 1951;21:55–116.
221. Bornstein MD, Crain SM. Functional studies of cultured brain tissue as related to demyelinative disorders. Science 1965;148:1242–1244.
222. Cerf JA, Carels G. Multiple sclerosis: serum factor producing reversible alteration in bioelectric responses. Science 1966;152:1066–1068.
223. Crain SM, Bornstein MB. Depression of complex bioelectric discharges in cerebral tissue cultures by thermolabile complement dependent serum factors. Exp Neurol 1975;49:330–338.
224. Sell FJ, Leiman AL, Kelly JM. Neurolectric blocking factors in multiple sclerosis and normal human sera. Arch Neurol 1976;33:418–422.
225. Zweifach PH. Studies of hyperthermia in optic neuropathy. Arch Ophthalmol 1978;96:1831–1834.
226. Tasaki I. Nervous Transmission. Springfield, IL, Charles C Thomas, 1953.
227. Davis FA. Pathophysiology of multiple sclerosis and related clinical implications. Mod Treat 1970;7:890.
228. Rasminsky M. The effects of temperature on conduction in demyelinated single nerve fibers. Arch Neurol 1973;28:287–292.
229. Bode DD. The Uhthoff phenomenon. Am J Ophthalmol 1978;85:721–722.
230. Persson HE, Sachs E. Visual evoked potentials elicited by pattern reversal during provoked visual impairment in multiple sclerosis. Brain 1981;104:369–382.
231. Selhorst JB, Saul RF, Waybright EA. Optic nerve conduction: opposing effects of exercise and hyperventilation. Trans Am Neurol Assoc 1981;106:101–105.
232. Kurtzke JF. Optic neuritis or multiple sclerosis. Arch Neurol 1985;42:704–710.
233. Kennedy C, Carter S. Relation of optic neuritis to multiple sclerosis in children. Pediatrics 1961;28:377–387.
234. Riikonen R, Donner M, Erkkilä H. Optic neuritis in children and its relationship to multiple sclerosis: a clinical study of 21 children. Dev Med Child Neurol 1988;30:349–359.
235. O'Duffy AE, Kiers L, Gomez MR, et al. Acute optic neuritis in childhood: a long-term follow-up. Ann Neurol 1993;34:273.
236. Rizzo JF, Lessell S. Risk of developing multiple sclerosis after uncomplicated optic neuritis: a long-term prospective study. Neurology 1988;38:185–190.
237. Landy PJ. A prospective study of the risk of developing multiple sclerosis in optic neuritis in a tropical and sub-tropical area. J Neurol Neurosurg Psychiatry 1983;46:659–661.
238. Isayama Y, Takahashi T, Shimoyoma T, et al. Acute optic neuritis and multiple sclerosis. Neurology 1982;32:73–76.
239. Alvarez G, Cárdenas M. Multiple sclerosis following optic neuritis in Chile. J Neurol Neurosurg Psychiatry 1989;52:15–117.
240. Ebers GC. Optic neuritis and multiple sclerosis. Arch Neurol 1985;42:702–704.
241. Beck RW. What to tell the patient with optic neuritis about multiple sclerosis. II. When to withhold. Surv Ophthalmol 1991;36:48–49.
242. Frenkel M, Lim JI, Hillman DS. What to tell the patient with optic neuritis about multiple sclerosis. III. The patient's right to know. Surv Ophthalmol 1991;36: 49–50.
243. Slamovits TL, Macklin R. What to tell the patient with optic neuritis about multiple sclerosis. Surv Ophthalmol 1991;36:47–48.
244. McAlpine D. The benign form of multiple sclerosis. Brain 1961;86:186–203.
245. Fog T, Linneman F. The course of multiple sclerosis. Acta Neurol Scand 1970; 47(Suppl):46.
246. Nikoskelainen E, Riekkinen P. Retrospective study of 117 patients with optic neuritis. Acta Ophthalmol Suppl 1974;123:202–204.
247. Wikström J, Poser S, Ritter G. Optic neuritis as an initial symptom in multiple sclerosis. Acta Neurol Scand 1980;61:178–185.
248. Leibowitz U, Alter M, Halpern L. Clinical studies of multiple sclerosis in Israel. IV. Optic neuritis and multiple sclerosis. Arch Neurol 1966;14:459–466.
249. Leibowitz U, Kahana E, Alter M. Multiple sclerosis in immigrant and native populations of Israel. Lancet 1969;2:1323–1325.
250. Leibowitz U, Alter M. Clinical factors associated with increased disability in multiple sclerosis. Acta Neurol Scand 1970;46:53–70.
251. Sanders EA, Reulen JPH, Hogenhuis LA. Central nervous system involvement in optic neuritis. J Neurol Neurosurg Psychiatry 1984;47:241–249.
252. O'Riordan JI, Thompson AJ, Kingsley, et al. The prognostic value of brain MRI in clinically isolated syndromes of the CNS: a 10-year-year follow-up. Brain 1998;121:495–503.
253. Brex PA, Ciccarelli O, O'Riordan JI, et al. A longitudinal study of abnormalities on MRI and disability from multiple sclerosis. N Engl J Med 2002;346:158–164.
254. Schlossman A, Phillips C. Optic neuritis in relation to demyelinating diseases. Am J Ophthalmol 1954;37:487–494.
255. Lumsden GE. The neuropathology of multiple sclerosis. In: Vinken PJ, Bruyn GW, eds. Handbook of Clinical Neurology. Amsterdam, North Holland, 1970: 217–309.
256. McDonald WI. Pathophysiology in multiple sclerosis. Brain 1974;97:179–196.

257. Prineas J. Pathology of the early lesion in multiple sclerosis. Hum Pathol 1975; 6:531–554.

258. Traugott U, Reinherz EL, Raine CS. Multiple sclerosis: distribution of T cell subjects within active chronic lesions. Science 1985;219:308–310.

259. Gartner S. Optic neuropathy in multiple sclerosis: optic neuritis. Arch Ophthalmol 1953;50:718–726.

260. de Preux J, Mair WGP. Ultra-structure of the optic nerve in Schilder's disease, Devic's disease and disseminated sclerosis. Acta Neuropathol 1974;30:225–242.

261. Rao NA, Tso MOM, Zimmerman EL. Experimental allergic optic neuritis in guinea pigs: preliminary report. Invest Ophthalmol Vis Sci 1977;16:338–342.

262. Hayreh SS, Massanari RM, Yamada T, et al. Experimental allergic encephalomyelitis. I. Optic nerve and central nervous system manifestations. Invest Ophthalmol Vis Sci 1981;21:256–269.

263. Okamoto N. Macrophages in the subarachnoid space in experimental allergic optic neuritis. Jpn J Ophthalmol 1981;25:38–46.

264. Rao NA. Demyelinating optic neuritis. Comp Pathol Bull 1979;2:3–4.

265. Sergott RC, Brown MJ, Polenta RM, et al. Optic nerve demyelination induced by human serum: patients with multiple sclerosis or optic neuritis and normal subjects. Neurology 1985;35:1438–1442.

266. Davis FA, Schauf C. Pathophysiology of multiple sclerosis. In: Multiple Sclerosis Research: Proceedings of a Joint Conference Held by the Medical Research Council and the Multiple Sclerosis Society of Great Britain and Northern Ireland. London, Her Majesty's Stationary Office, 1975.

267. Nikoskelainen E, Frey H, Salmi AA. Prognosis of optic neuritis with special reference to cerebrospinal fluid immunoglobulins and measles virus antibodies. Ann Neurol 1981;9:545–550.

268. Ebers GC, Cousin HK, Feasby TE, et al. Optic neuritis in familial MS. Neurology 1981;31:1138–1142.

269. Kurland LT, Beebe GW, Kurtzke JF, et al. Studies on the natural history of multiple sclerosis: 2. The progression of optic neuritis to multiple sclerosis. Acta Neurol Scand 1966;42(Suppl 19):157–176.

270. Mapelli G, de Palma P, Sebastiani A, et al. Risk of multiple sclerosis in optic neuritis: a prospective study. Acta Neurol 1986;8:619–625.

271. Alter M, Good J, Okihiro M. Optic neuritis in Orientals and Caucasians. Neurology 1973;23:631–639.

272. Alter M, Halpern L, Kurland LT, et al. The prevalence of multiple sclerosis in Israel among immigrants and native inhabitants. Arch Neurol 1962;7:253–263.

273. Dean G, Kurtzke JF. On the risk of multiple sclerosis according to age of immigration to South Africa. Br Med J 1971;3:725–729.

274. Kurtzke JF, Beebe GW, Norman JE Jr. Epidemiology of multiple sclerosis in US veterans. I. Race, sex and geographic distribution. Neurology 1979;29:1228–1235.

275. Morrissey SP, Borruat FX, Miller DH, et al. Bilateral simultaneous optic neuropathy in adults: clinical, imaging, serological, and genetic studies. J Neurol Neurosurg Psychiatry 1995;58:70–74.

276. Jacobs L, Kaba S, Miller C, et al. Correlation of clinical, magnetic resonance imaging, and cerebrospinal fluid findings in optic neuritis. Ann Neurol. 1997; 41:393–398.

277. Cole SR, Beck RW, Moke PS, et al. The predictive value of CSF oligoclonal banding for MS 5 years after optic neuritis. Neurology 1998;51:885–887.

278. Müller R. Studies on disseminated sclerosis with special reference to symptomatology, course and prognosis. Acta Med Scand 1949;133(Suppl 222):1–214.

279. Scott GI. Ophthalmic aspects of demyelinating diseases. Proc R Soc Med 1961; 54:38–42.

280. Ashworth B. Chronic retrobulbar and chiasmal neuritis. Br J Ophthalmol 1967; 51:598–702.

281. Kahana E, Leibowitz U, Fishback N, et al. Slowly progressive and acute visual impairment in multiple sclerosis. Neurology 1973;23:729–733.

282. Patterson VH, Heron JR. Visual field abnormalities in multiple sclerosis. J Neurol Neurosurg Psychiatry 1980;43:205–208.

283. Patterson VH, Foster DH, Heron JR, et al. Multiple sclerosis: luminance threshold and measurements of temporal characteristics of vision. Arch Neurol 1981; 38:687–689.

284. Ormerod IEC, McDonald WI. Multiple sclerosis presenting with progressive visual failure. J Neurol Neurosurg Psychiatry 1984;47:943–946.

285. Ashworth B. Chronic demyelinating optic neuritis: a reappraisal. Neuroophthalmology 1987;7:75–79.

286. Frisén L, Hoyt WF. Insidious atrophy of retinal nerve fibers in multiple sclerosis: funduscopic identification of patients with and without visual complaints. Arch Ophthalmol 1974;92:91–97.

287. Regan D, Bartol S, Murray TJ, et al. Spatial frequency discrimination in normal vision and in patients with multiple sclerosis. Brain 1982;105:735–754.

288. Raymond J, Regan D, Murray TJ. Abnormal adaptation of visual contrast sensitivity in multiple sclerosis patients. Can J Neurol Sci 1981;8:227–234.

289. Della Sala S, Comi G, Martinelli V, et al. The rapid assessment of visual dysfunction in multiple sclerosis. J Neurol Neurosurg Psychiatry 1987;50:840–846.

290. Soderstrom M. Multiple sclerosis: rationale for early treatment. Neurol Sci 2003; 24:S298–S300.

291. Ashworth B, Aspinall PA, Mitchell JD. Visual function in multiple sclerosis. Doc Ophthalmol 1990;73:209–224.

292. van Diemen HAM, Lanting P, Koetsier JC, et al. Evaluation of the visual system in multiple sclerosis: a comparative study of diagnostic tests. Clin Neurol Neurosurg 1992;94:191–195.

293. Ulrich J, Groebke-Lorenz W. The optic nerve in multiple sclerosis. A morphological study with retrospective clinico-pathological correlations. Neuroophthalmology 1983;3:149–159.

294. Miller NR. Walsh and Hoyt's Clinical Neuro-Ophthalmology, 4th ed. Baltimore, Williams & Wilkins, 1995:4314.

295. Menabue R, Nichelli P, Bellei S. Exposure times for color discrimination in the parafoveal field: a new procedure to detect subtle visual dysfunction in multiple sclerosis patients. J Neurol Neurosurg Psychiatry 1986;49:400–404.

296. Pinckers A, Cruysberg JRM. Colour vision, visually evoked potentials, and lightness discrimination in patients with multiple sclerosis. Neuroophthalmology 1992;12:251–256.

297. Meienberg O, Flammer J, Ludin H-P. Subclinical visual field defects in multiple sclerosis: demonstration and quantification with automated perimetry, and comparison with visually evoked potentials. J Neurol 1982;227:125–133.

298. Marra G, Ciasca S, Ratiglia R, et al. Confronto tra le alterazioni del campo visivo in soggetti affetti da sclerosi multipla con e senza pregresse neuriti ottiche. Boll Oculist 1989;68:249–252.

299. Cox TA. Relative afferent pupillary defects in multiple sclerosis. Can J Ophthalmol 1989;24:207–210.

300. Feinsod M, Hoyt WF. Subclinical optic neuropathy in multiple sclerosis: how early VER components reflect axon loss and conduction defects in optic pathways. J Neurol Neurosurg Psychiatry 1975;38:1109–1114.

301. Elbol P, Work K. Retinal nerve fiber layer in multiple sclerosis. Acta Ophthalmol 1990;68:481–486.

302. Honan WP, Baranyovits PR, Heron JR. Retinal nerve fiber layer atrophy in multiple sclerosis. Neuroophthalmology 1992;12:11–15.

303. Ellenberger C Jr, Ziegler T. Visual evoked potentials and quantitative perimetry in multiple sclerosis. Ann Neurol 1977;1:561–564.

304. Matthews WB, Acheson ED, Batchelor JR, et al, eds. McAlpine's Multiple Sclerosis. Edinburgh, Churchill Livingstone, 1985.

305. Wright CE, Drasdo N, Harding GFA. Pathology of the optic nerve and visual association areas: information given by the flash and pattern visual evoked potential, and the temporal and spatial contrast sensitivity function. Brain 1987;110: 107–120.

306. Travis D, Thompson P. Spatiotemporal contrast sensitivity and colour vision in multiple sclerosis. Brain 1989;112:283–303.

307. Ashworth B, Aspinall PA. A longitudinal study of visual function in multiple sclerosis: with a note on the Cambridge grating test. Neuroophthalmology 1993; 13:135–142.

308. Ogden NA, Raymond JE, Seland TP. Visual accommodation and sustained visual resolution in multiple sclerosis. Invest Ophthalmol Vis Sci 1992;33: 2744–2753.

309. Galvin RJ, Heron JR, Regan D. Subclinical optic neuropathy in multiple sclerosis. Arch Neurol 1977;34:666–670.

310. Daley ML, Swank RL, Ellison CM. Flicker fusion thresholds in multiple sclerosis: a functional measure of neurological damage. Arch Neurol 1979;36: 292–295.

311. Foster RE, Lowder CY, Meisler DM, et al. Mumps neuroretinitis in an adolescent. Am J Ophthalmol 1990;110:91–93.

312. Dain SJ, Rammahan KW, Benes SC, et al. Chromatic, spatial, and temporal losses of sensitivity in multiple sclerosis. Invest Ophthalmol Vis Sci 1990;31: 548–558.

313. Porciatti V, Sartucci F. Retinal and cortical evoked responses to chromatic contrast stimuli: specific losses in the eyes of patients with multiple sclerosis and unilateral optic neuritis. Brain 1996;119:723–740.

314. Pulfrich C. Die stereoskopie im Dienste der isochromen und heterochromen Photometrie. Naturwissenschaften 1922;10:553–761.

315. Rushton D. Use of the Pulfrich pendulum for detecting abnormal delay in the visual pathway in multiple sclerosis. Brain 1975;98:283–296.

316. Feldman L, Todman L, Bender B. ''Flight of colours'' in lesions of the visual system. J Neurol Neurosurg Psychiatry 1974;37:1265–1272.

317. Swart S, Millac P. A comparison of flight of colours with visually evoked responses in patients with multiple sclerosis. J Neurol Neurosurg Psychiatry 1980;43:550–551.

318. Rolak LA. The flight of colors test in multiple sclerosis. Arch Neurol 1985;42: 759–760.

319. Larsson H, Frederiksen J, Stigsby B, et al. Evaluation of visual pathways in multiple sclerosis. I. After-images compared to visual evoked potentials. Acta Neurol Scand 1986;74:195–202.

320. Allbutt TC. On the ophthalmoscopic signs of spinal disease. Lancet 1870;1: 76–78.

321. Devic E. Myélite subaigue compliquée de névrite optique. Bull Med Paris 1894; 8:1033–1034.

322. Gault F. De la neuromyélite optique aigue. Thesis, University of Lyon, 1894, Serre 1, No. 981, Lyon.

323. Cree BAC, Goodin DS, Hauser SL. Neuromyelitis optica. Semin Neurol 2002; 22:105–122.

324. Shibasaki H, Kuroda Y, Kuroiwa Y. Clinical studies of multiple sclerosis in

Japan: classical multiple sclerosis and Devic's disease. J Neurol Sci 1974;23: 215–222.

325. Pálffy G. Multiple sclerosis in Hungary, including the Gypsy. In: Kuroiwa Y, Kurland LT, eds. Multiple Sclerosis, East and West. Fukuoka, Kyushu University Press, 1982:149–158.

326. Kuroiwa Y. Multiple sclerosis and allied demyelinating encephalomyelitis in Japan. In: Bammer HG, ed. Zunkuft der Neurologie. Stuttgart, Thieme, 1967: 70–84.

327. Kuroiwa Y, Shibasaki H. Clinical studies of multiple sclerosis in Japan. I. A current appraisal of 83 cases. Neurology 1973;23:609–617.

328. Kuroiwa Y, Igata A, Itahara K, et al. Nationwide survey of multiple sclerosis in Japan: clinical analysis of 1,084 cases. Neurology 1975;25:845–851.

329. Shibasaki H, Kuroda Y, Kuroiwa Y. Clinical studies of multiple sclerosis in Japan: classical multiple sclerosis and Devic's disease. J Neurol Sci 1974;23: 215–222.

330. Stansbury FC. Neuromyelitis optica (Devic's disease): presentation of five cases, with pathologic study, and review of literature. Arch Ophthalmol 1949;42: 292–335, 465–501.

331. Scott GI. Neuromyelitis optica. Am J Ophthalmol 1952;35:755–764.

332. Hershewe GL, Corbett JJ, Thompson HS. The NANOS Devic's Study Group. Presented at the North American Neuro-Ophthalmology Society Meeting, Steamboat Springs, CO, Feb. 4–8, 1990.

333. Ramelli GP, Deonna T, Roulet E, et al. Transverse myelitis and optic neuromyelitis in children: apropos of 3 case reports. Schweiz Rundsch Med Prax 1992;81: 661–663.

334. Igarashi Y, Oyachi H, Nakamura Y, et al. Neuromyelitis optica. Ophthalmology 1994;208:226–229.

335. Jain S, Hiran S, Sarma PS. Devic's disease. J Assoc Phys India 1994;42:166.

336. Jeffery AR Buncic JR. Pediatric Devic's neuromyelitis optica. J Pediatr Ophthalmol Strabismus 1996;33:223–229.

337. Filley CM, Sternberg PE, Norenberg MD. Neuromyelitis optica in the elderly. Arch Neurol 1984;41:670–672.

338. Barbieri F, Buscaino GA. Neuromyelitis optica in the elderly. Acta Neurol 1989; 11:247–251.

339. McAlpine D. Familial neuromyelitis optica: its occurrence in identical twins. Brain 1938;61:430–448.

340. April RS, Vansonnenberg E. A case of neuromyelitis optica (Devic's syndrome) in systemic lupus erythematosus: clinicopathologic report and review of the literature. Neurology 1976;26:1066–1070.

341. Kinney EL, Berdoff RL, Rao NS, et al. Devic's syndrome and systemic lupus erythematosus: a case report with necropsy. Arch Neurol 1979;36:643–644.

342. Tommasi M, Lecuire J, Masquin A, et al. Étude anatomoclinique d'une neuromyélite optique de Devic, d'évolution artificiellement prolongée. Rev Neurol 1966; 114:378–381.

343. Barbizet J, Degos JD, Meyrignac C. Neuromyélite optique aiguë associée à une tuberculose pulmonaire aiguë. Rev Neurol 1980;136:303–309.

344. Silber MH, Willcox PA, Bowen RM, et al. Neuromyelitis optica (Devic's syndrome) and pulmonary tuberculosis. Neurology 1990;40:934–938.

345. Al-Deeb SM, Yaqub BA, Khoja WO. Devic's neuromyelitis optica and varicella. J Neurol 1993;240:450–451.

346. Ahasan H, Jafiqueuddin AK, Chowdhury MA, et al. Neuromyelitis optica (Devic's disease) following chicken pox. Trop Doc 1994;24:75–76.

347. Hainfellner JA, Schmidbauer M, Schmutzhard E, et al. Devic's neuromyelitis optica and Schilder's myelinoclastic diffuse sclerosis. J Neurol Neurosurg Psychiatry 1992;55:1194–1196.

348. Raine CS. Demyelinating diseases. In: Davis RL, Robertson DM, eds. Textbook of Neuropathology. 2nd ed. Baltimore, Williams & Wilkins, 1991:535–620.

349. Mandler RN, Davis LE, Jeffery DR, et al. Devic's neuromyelitis optica: a clinicopathologic study of 8 patients. Ann Neurol 1993;34:162–168.

350. Allen IV, Kirk J. Demyelinating diseases. In: Adams JH, Duchen LW, eds. Greenfield's Neuropathology, 5th ed. New York, Oxford University Press, 1992: 447–520.

351. Walsh FB. Neuromyelitis optica: an anatomical-pathological study of one case; clinical studies of three additional cases. Bull Johns Hopkins Hosp 1935;56: 183–210.

352. Walsh FB, Hoyt WF. Clinical Neuro-Ophthalmology, 3rd ed. Baltimore, Williams & Wilkins, 1969:996–997.

353. Aimoto Y, Ito K, Morwaka F, et al. Demyelinating peripheral neuropathy in Devic disease. Jpn J Psychiatry Neurol 1991;45:861–864.

354. Cloys DE, Netsky MG. Neuromyelitis optica. In: Vinken PJ, Bruyn GW, eds. Handbook of Clinical Neurology. New York, Elsevier North Holland, 1970: 426–436.

355. Oppenheimer DR. Demyelinating diseases. In: Blackwood W, Corsellis JA, eds. Greenfield's Neuropathology, 3rd ed. London, Edward Arnold, 1976:470–484.

356. Poser CM. Neuromyelitis optica. In: Baker AB, Baker LH, eds. Clinical Neurology. Philadelphia, JB Lippincott, 1981:70.

357. Hassin GB. Neuroptic myelitis versus multiple sclerosis: a pathologic study. Arch Neurol 1937;34:1083–1099.

358. Kohut H, Richter RB. Neuro-optic myelitis: a clinicopathological study of two related cases. J Nerv Ment Dis 1945;101:99–114.

359. Lassmann H, Bruck W, Lucchinetti C. Heterogeneity of multiple sclerosis pathogenesis; implications for diagnosis and therapy. Trends Mol Med 2001;7: 115–121.

360. Lucchinetti CF, Mandler RN, McGavern D, et al. A role for humoral mechanisms in the pathogenesis of Devic's neuromyelitis optica. Brain 2002;125:1450–1461.

361. Linington C, Bradl M, Lassmann H, et al. Augmentation of demyelination in rat acute allergic encephalomyelitis by circulating mouse monoclonal antibodies directed against a myelin/oligodendrocyte glycoprotein. Am J Pathol 1988;130: 443–454.

362. Gold R, Linington C. Devic's disease: bridging the gap between laboratory and clinic. Brain 2002;125:1425–1427.

363. Stefferl A, Brehm U, Storch M, et al. Myelin oligodendrocyte glycoprotein induces experimental autoimmune encephalomyelitis in the "resistant" Brown Norway rat: disease susceptibility is determined by MHC and MHC-lined effects on the B cell response. J Immunol 1999;163:40–49.

364. Whitham RH, Brey RL. Neuromyelitis optica: two new cases and review of the literature. J Clin Neuroophthalmol 1985;5:263–269.

365. Zangemeister WH, Mueller-Jensen A. Neuromyelitis optica: clinical and neurophysiological features. Neuroophthalmology 1984;4:81–88.

366. Ko FJ, Chiang CH, Jong YJ, et al. Neuromyelitis optica (Devic's disease): report of one case. Acta Paediatr Sinica 1989;30:428–431.

367. Khan MA, Mahar PS, Raghuraman VU. Neuromyelitis optica (Devic's disease). Br J Clin Pract 1990;44:667–668.

368. Kuroiwa Y, Igata A, Itahara K, et al. Nationwide survey of multiple sclerosis in Japan: clinical analysis of 1,084 cases. Neurology 1975;25:845–851.

369. Chusid MJ, Williamson SJ, Murphy JV, et al. Neuromyelitis optica (Devic disease) following varicella infection. J Pediatr 1979;95:737–738.

370. Williamson PM. Neuromyelitis optica following infectious mononucleosis. Proc Aust Assoc Neurol 1975;12:153–155.

371. Kline LB, Margulies SL, Oh SJ. Optic neuritis and myelitis following rubella vaccination. Arch Neurol 1982;39:443–444.

372. Breukelman AJ, Polman CH, de Slegte RG, et al. Neuromyelitis optica (Devic's syndrome); not always multiple sclerosis. Clin Neurol Neurosurg 1988;90: 357–360.

373. Walsh FB, Hoyt WF. Clinical Neuro-Ophthalmology, 3rd ed. Baltimore, Williams & Wilkins, 1969:997.

374. Goulden C. Optic neuritis and myelitis. Trans Ophthalmol Soc UK 1914;34: 229–252.

375. Beck GM. A case of diffuse myelitis associated with optic neuritis. Brain 1927; 50:687–702.

376. Markham JW, Otenasek FJ. Neuromyelitis optica simulating spinal cord tumor: report of a case with review of nine additional cases. Arch Neurol Psychiatry 1954;72:758–763.

377. Walsh FB, Hoyt WF. Clinical Neuro-Ophthalmology, 3rd ed. Baltimore, Williams & Wilkins, 1969:998.

378. Piccolo G, Franciotta DM, Camana C, et al. Devic's neuromyelitis optica: long-term follow-up and serial CSF findings in two cases. J Neurol 1990;237: 262–264.

379. Keefe RJ. Neuromyelitis optica with increased intracranial pressure. Arch Ophthalmol 1957;57:110–111.

380. Chou C-HJ, Chou FC-H, Tourtellotte WW, et al. Devic's syndrome: antibody to glial fibrillary acidic protein in cerebrospinal fluid. Neurology 1984;34:86–88.

381. Barkhof F, Scheltens P, Valk J, et al. Serial quantitative MR assessment of optic neuritis in a case of neuromyelitis optica, using gadolinium-"enhanced" STIR imaging. Neuroradiology 1991;33:70–71.

382. Filippi M, Rocca MA, Moiola L, et al. MRI and magnetization transfer imaging changes in the brain and cervical cord of patients with Devic's neuromyelitis optica. Neurology 1999;53:1705–1710.

383. Weinshenker BG, Wingerchuk DM, Lucchinetti CF, et al. A marker autoantibody discriminates neuromyelitis optica from multiple sclerosis. American Academy of Neurolology Poster S65.005, 2003.

384. Lennon VA, Lucchinetti CF, Weinshenker BG. Identification of a marker autoantibody of neuromyelitis optica. American Academy of Neurolology Poster, 2003.

385. Kuroiwa Y, Hung TP, Landsborough D, et al. Multiple sclerosis in Asia. Neurology 1977;7:188–192.

386. Shibasaki H, McDonald WI, Kuroiwa Y. Racial modification of clinical picture of multiple sclerosis: comparison between British and Japanese patients. J Neurol Sci 1981;49:253–271.

387. Yamasaki K, Horiuchi I, Minohara M, et al. HLA-DPB1*0501-associated optic-ospinal multiple sclerosis: clinical, neuroimaging and immunogenetic studies. Brain 1999;111:1689–1696.

388. Nakashima I, Fujihara K, Takase S, et al. Decrease in multiple sclerosis with acute transverse myelitis in Japan. Tohoku J Exp Med 1999;188:89–94.

389. Banerjee A, Bishop A, Elliott P. A case of neuromyelitis optica (Devic's disease). Practitioner 1989;23:202–203.

390. Frohman LP, Cook SD, Bielory L. Dysgammaglobulinemia in steroid-dependent optic neuritis: response to gamma globulin treatment. J Clin Neuroophthalmol 1991;11:241–245.

391. Keegan M, Pineda AA, McClelland RL, et al. Plasma exchange for severe attacks of CNS demyelination: predictors of response. Neurology 2002;58:143–146.

392. Duda PW, Schmied MC, Cook SL, et al. Glatiramer acetate (Copaxone®) in-

duces degenerate, TH2-polarized immune responses in patients with multiple sclerosis. J Clin Invest 2000;105:967–976.

393. Fralick FB, DeJong RN. Neuromyelitis optica. Am J Ophthalmol 1937;20: 1119–1124.

394. Johns DR, Heher KL, Miller NR, Smith KH. Leber's hereditary optic neuropathy: clinical manifestations of the 14484 mutation. Arch Ophthalmol 1993;111: 495–498.

395. Marburg O. Die sogenannte ''akute multiple Sklerose'' (Encephalomyelitis periaxialis scleroticans). Jahrb Psychiatr Neurol 1906;27:211–312.

396. Schilder P. Zur Frage der Encephalitis periaxialis diffusa (sogenannte diffuse Sklerose). Ztschr Neurol Psychiatr 1913;15:359–376.

397. Schilder P. Die Encephalitis periaxialis diffusa (nebst Bemerkungen uber die Apraxie des Lidschlusses). Arch Psychiatr Nervenkr 1924;71:327–336.

398. Adams RD, Victor M. Principles of Neurology, 4th ed. New York, McGraw-Hill, 1989:908–909.

399. Barness LA, Chandra S, Kling P, et al. Progressive neurologic deterioration in a nine-year-old white male. Am J Med Gen 1990;37:489–503.

400. Poser CM. Diffuse-disseminated sclerosis in the adult. J Neuropathol Exp Neurol 1957;16:61–78.

401. Martin J-J, Guazzi G-C. Schilder's diffuse sclerosis. Dev Neurosci 1991;13: 267–273.

402. Case Records of the Massachusetts General Hospital: Case 6-1962. N Engl J Med 1962;266:191–196.

403. Allen IV. Demyelinating diseases. In: Adams JH, Corsellis JAN, Duchen LW, eds. Greenfield's Neuropathology, 4th ed. New York, John Wiley & Sons, 1984: 338–384.

404. Dresser LP, Tourian AY, Anthony DC. A case of myelinoclastic diffuse sclerosis in an adult. Neurology 1991;41:316–318.

405. Eblen F, Poremba M, Grodd W, et al. Myelinoclastic diffuse sclerosis (Schilder's disease): Cliniconeurologic correlations. Neurology 1991;41:589–591.

406. Schmidt RE. Demyelinating diseases. In: Nelson JS, Parisi JE, Schochet SS Jr, eds. Principles and Practice of Neuropathology. St Louis, CV Mosby, 1993: 361–397.

407. Schilder P. Zur Kenntnis der sogennanten diffusen Sklerose. Ztschr Ges Neurol Psychiatr 1912;10:1–606.

408. Zeman W, Whieldon JA. Clinical considerations in ''Schilder's disease.'' Am J Dis Child 1962;104:635–643.

409. Poser CM, Goutières F, Carpentier MA, Aicardi J. Schilder's myelinoclastic diffuse sclerosis. Pediatrics 1986;77:107–112.

410. Sedwick LA, Klingele TG, Burde RM, et al. Schilder's (1912) disease: total cerebral blindness due to acute demyelination. Arch Neurol 1986;43:85–87.

411. Lana-Peixoto MA, dos Santos EC. Schilder's myelinoclastic diffuse sclerosis. J Clin Neuroophthalmol 1989;9:236–240.

412. Ford FR, Bumstead JH. Encephalitis periaxialis diffusa of Schilder: report of 2 cases with anatomical findings. Bull Johns Hopkins Hosp 1929;44:443–458.

413. Ford FR. Diseases of the Nervous System in Infancy, Childhood and Adolescence, 5th ed. Springfield, IL, Charles C Thomas, 1966:197–205.

414. Nover A. Über Netzhautveränderungen bei Schilderscher Enzephalitis. Klin Monatsbl Augenheilkd 1955;127:294–302.

415. Sagar HJ, Warlow CP, Shelton PWE, et al. Multiple sclerosis with clinical and radiological features of cerebral tumors. J Neurol Neurosurg Psychiatry 1982; 45:802–808.

416. Harpey JP, Fenault F, Foncin JF, et al. Démyélinisation aiguë pseudotumorale à poussées régressives. Arch Fr Pediatr 1983;40:407–409.

417. Mehler MF, Rabinowich L. Inflammatory myelinoclastic diffuse sclerosis. Ann Neurol 1988;23:413–415.

418. Barth PG, Derix MMA, de Krom MCTFM, et al. Schilder's diffuse sclerosis: case study with three years' follow-up and neuro-imaging. Neuropediatrics 1989; 20:230–233.

419. Mehler MF, Rabinowich L. Inflammatory myelinoclastic diffuse sclerosis (Schilder's disease): Neuroradiologic findings. AJNR Am J Neuroradiol 1989; 10:176–180.

420. Szabo P, Hegedus K. Myelinoclastic diffuse sclerosis: a case report. Acta Morphol Hung 1990;38:109–117.

421. DiMario FJ Jr, Berman PH. Multiple sclerosis presenting at 4 years of age: clinical and MRI correlations. Clin Pediatr 1988;27:32–37.

422. Konkol RJ, Bousounis D, Kuban KC. Schilder's disease: additional aspects and a therapeutic option. Neuropediatrics 1987;18:149–152.

423. Baló J. A leukoenkephalitis periaxialis concentricaról. Magy Orvosi Arch 1927; 28:108–124.

424. Baló J. Encephalitis periaxialis concentrica. Arch Neurol Psychiatry 1928;19: 242–264.

425. Bleiker H. Genuine Epilepsie und Konzentrische Sklerose. Schweiz Arch Neurol Psychiatr 1967;100:387–398.

426. Duma D, Papilian VV, Serban M. Recherches histochimiques dan certaines encéphalomyélites démyélinisantes primitives. Rev Roum Neurol 1965;2: 139–154.

427. Courville CB. Concentric sclerosis. In: Vinken PJ, Bruyn GW, eds. Handbook of Clinical Neurology. Amsterdam, North-Holland, 1970:9:437–451.

428. Harper CG. Diagnostic dilemma: acute central nervous system disorder mimicking stroke. Med J Aust 1981;1:136–138.

429. Moore GRW, Neumann PE, Suzuki K, et al. Balo's concentric sclerosis: new observations on lesion development. Ann Neurol 1985;17:604–611.

430. Currie S, Roberts AH, Urich H. The nosological position of concentric lacunar leucoencephalopathy. J Neurol Neurosurg Psychiatry 1970;33:131–137.

431. Yao D-L, Webster HD, Hudson LD, et al. Concentric sclerosis (Baló): morphometric and in situ hybridization study of lesions in six patients. Ann Neurol 1994;35:18–30.

432. Garbern J, Spence AM, Alvord EC Jr. Balo's concentric demyelination diagnosed premortem. Neurology 1986;36:1610–1614.

433. Nandini M, Gourie-Devi M, Shankar SK, et al. Balo's concentric sclerosis diagnosed intravitam on brain biopsy. Clin Neurol Neurosurg 1993;95:303–309.

434. Selbst RG, Selhorst JB, Harbison JW, et al. Parainfectious optic neuritis: report and review following varicella. Arch Neurol 1983;40:347–350.

435. Farris BK, Pickard DJ. Bilateral postinfectious optic neuritis and intravenous steroid therapy in children. Ophthalmology 1990;97:339–345.

436. Benkö E, Sipos I. Einige Fälle von Opticus-Neuritis als Begleiterscheinung der Kerato-conjunctivitis epidemica. Ophthalmology 1963;146:83–86.

437. Manor RS, Cohen S, Ben-Sira I. Bilateral acute retrobulbar optic neuropathy associated with epidemic keratoconjunctivitis in a compromised host. Arch Ophthalmol 1986;104:1271–1272.

438. Audry-Chaboud D, Durnas R, Audry F, et al. Coxsackie B virus neuropapillitis. Rev Otoneuroophtalmol 1981;53:473–482.

439. Spalton DJ, Murdoch I, Holder GE. Coxsackie B5 papillitis. J Neurol Neurosurg Psychiatry 1989;52:1310–1311.

440. Gross JG, Sadun AA, Wiley CA, et al. Severe visual loss related to isolated peripapillary retinal and optic nerve head cytomegalovirus infection. Am J Ophthalmol 1989;108:691–698.

441. Walsh FB, Hoyt WF. Clinical Neuro-Ophthalmology, 3rd ed. Baltimore, Williams & Wilkins,1969:136.

442. Galli M, Morelli R, Casellato A, et al. Retrobulbar optic neuritis in a patient with acute type B hepatitis. J Neurol Sci 1986;72:195–200.

443. Achiron LR. Postinfectious hepatitis B optic neuritis. Optomet Vis Sci 1994; 71:53–56.

444. Ashworth J, Motto S. Infectious mononucleosis complicated by bilateral papilloretinal edema: report of a case. N Engl J Med 1947;237:544–545.

445. Karpe G, Wising P. Retinal changes with acute reduction of vision as initial symptoms of infectious mononucleosis. Acta Ophthalmol 1948;26:19–23.

446. Bonynge TW, Von Hagen KO. Severe optic neuritis in infectious mononucleosis: report of a case. JAMA 1952;148:933–934.

447. Frey T. Optic neuritis in children: infectious mononucleosis as an etiology. Doc Ophthalmol 1973;34:183–188.

448. Jones J, Gardner W, Newman T. Severe optic neuritis in infectious mononucleosis. Ann Emerg Med 1988;17:361–364.

449. Newman NJ, Lessell S. Bilateral optic neuropathies with remission in two HIV-positive men. J Clin Neuroophthalmol 1992;12:1–5.

450. Sweeney BJ, Manji H, Gilson RJC, et al. Optic neuritis and HIV-1 infection. J Neurol Neurosurg Psychiatry 1993;56:705–707.

451. Walsh FB, Ford FR. Central scotomas: their importance in topical diagnosis. Arch Ophthalmol 1940;24:500–534.

452. Strom T. Acute blindness as post-measles complication. Acta Paediatr 1953;42: 60–65.

453. Tyler HR. Neurological complications of rubeola. Medicine 1957;36:147–167.

454. Srivastava SP, Neman HV. Optic neuritis in measles. Br J Ophthalmol 1963; 47:180–181.

455. Hayden M. Erblindung beider augen nach masernerkrankung. Klin Monatsbl Augenheilkd 1970;156:539–543.

456. Woodward JH. The ocular complications of mumps. Ann Ophthalmol 1907;16: 7–38.

457. Swab CM. Encephalitic optic neuritis and atrophy due to mumps: report of a case. Arch Ophthalmol 1938;19:926–929.

458. Strong LE, Henderson JW, Gangitano JL. Bilateral retrobulbar neuritis secondary to mumps. Am J Ophthalmol 1974;78:331–332.

459. Connolly JH, Hutchinson WM, Allen IV, et al. Carotid artery thrombosis, encephalitis, myelitis and optic neuritis associated with rubella virus infections. Brain 1975;98:583–594.

460. Miller DH, Kay R, Schon F, et al. Optic neuritis following chickenpox in adults. J Neurol 1986;233:182–184.

461. Purvin V, Hrisomalos N, Dunn D. Varicella optic neuritis. Neurology 1988;38: 501–503.

462. Gündüz K, Özdemir O. Bilateral retrobulbar neuritis following unilateral herpes zoster ophthalmicus. Ophthalmology 1994;208:61–64.

463. Deane JS, Bibby K. Bilateral optic neuritis following herpes zoster ophthalmicus. Arch Ophthalmol 1995;113:972–973.

464. Colarizi A, Panico E. Atrofia secondaria del nervo ottico consecutiva a infezione carbonchiosa. Bull Acad Med Roma 1933;59:399–408.

465. Smallberg GJ, Sherman SH, Pezeshkpour GH, et al. Optic neuropathy due to brain abscess. Am J Ophthalmol 1976;82:188–192.

466. Abd Elrazak M. Brucella optic neuritis. Arch Intern Med 1991;151:776–778.

467. McLean DR, Russell N, Khan MY. Neurobrucellosis: clinical and therapeutic features. Clin Infect Dis 1992;15:582–590.

468. Sweeney VP, Drance SM. Optic neuritis and compressive neuropathy associated with cat scratch disease. Can Med Assoc J 1970;103:1380–1381.

469. Gass JDM. Diseases of the optic nerve that may simulate macular disease. Trans Am Acad Ophthalmol Otolaryngol 1977;83:766–769.

470. Brazis PW, Stokes HR, Ervin FR. Optic neuritis in cat scratch disease. J Clin Neuroophthalmol 1986;6:172–174.

471. Miller NR. Walsh and Hoyt's Clinical Neuro-Ophthalmology, 4th ed. Baltimore, Williams & Wilkins, 1995:2895–2896.

472. Miller HG, Staton JB, Gibbons JL. Parainfectious encephalomyelitis and related syndromes: a critical review of the neurological complications of certain specific fevers. QJ Med 1956;25:427–505.

473. Groenouw A, Uhthoff W. Beziehungen der allgemeinleiden und organerkrankungen zu veranderungen und krankheiten des sehorganes. Leipzig, Springer Verlag, 1911.

474. Lamb HD. A case of tuberculous papillitis with anatomic findings. Am J Ophthalmol 1937;20:390–396.

475. Boke W. Neuritische sehnerveneranderungen bei der meningitis tuberculosa. Klin Monatsbl Augenheilkd 1955;126:678–683.

476. Mooney AJ. Some ocular sequelae of tuberculous meningitis. Am J Ophthalmol 1956;41:753–768.

477. Miller BW, Frenkel M. Report of a case of tuberculous retrobulbar neuritis and osteomyelitis. Am J Ophthalmol 1971;71:751–756.

478. Bajpai PC, Dikshit SK. Bilateral optic neuritis and encephalitis accompanying typhoid. J Indian Med Assoc 1958;30:54–57.

479. Glander VR, Illert H. Amaurose und Hemiparese nach Typhus abdominalis bei einem 3 jährigen Kinde. Arch Kinderheilkd 1958;158:164–170.

480. Sanders MD. Gastrointestinal and ocular disease. In: Mausolf FA, ed. The Eye and Systemic Disease. St Louis, CV Mosby, 1980:345.

481. Yen M-Y, Liu J-H. Bilateral optic neuritis following bacille Calmette-Guérin (BCG) vaccination. J Clin Neuroophthalmol 1991;11:246–249.

482. Shaw FE Jr, Graham DJ, Guess HA, et al. Postmarketing surveillance for neurologic adverse events reported after hepatitis B vaccination: experience of the first three years. Am J Epidemiol 1988;127:337–352.

483. Berkman N, Banzarti T, Dhaoui R, et al. Neuropapillite bilatérale avec décollement séreux du neuroépithélium, au décours d'une vaccination contre l'hépatite B. Bull Soc Ophtalmol Fr 1996;96:187–190.

484. Cormack HS, Anderson LP. Bilateral papillitis following antirabic inoculation: recovery. Br J Ophthalmol 1934;43:167–168.

485. Consul BN, Purohit GK, Chhabra HN. Antirabic vaccine optic neuritis. Indian J Med Sci 1968;22:630–632.

486. Chayakul V, Ishikawa S, Chotibut S, et al. Convergence insufficiency and optic neuritis due to anti-rabic inoculation. Jpn J Ophthalmol 1875;19:307–314.

487. Topaloglu H, Berker M, Kansu T, et al. Optic neuritis and myelitis after booster tetanus toxoid vaccination. Lancet 1992;339:178–179.

488. Wagener HP. Edema of the optic disks in cases of encephalitis. Am J Med Sci 1952;223:205–215.

489. McReynolds WU, Havener WH, Petrohelos MA. Bilateral optic neuritis following smallpox vaccination and diphtheria-tetanus toxoid. Am J Dis Child 1953;86:601–603.

490. Kazarian E, Gager W. Optic neuritis complicating measles, mumps, and rubella vaccination. Am J Ophthalmol 1978;86:544–547.

491. Perry HD, Mallen FJ, Grodin RW, et al. Reversible blindness in optic neuritis associated with influenza vaccination. Ann Ophthalmol 1979;11:545–550.

492. Ray CL, Dreizin IJ. Bilateral optic neuropathy associated with influenza vaccination. J Neuroophthalmol 1996;16:182–184.

493. Cangemi FE, Bergen RL. Optic atrophy following swine flu vaccination. Ann Ophthalmol 1980;12:857–863.

494. Bienfang DC, Kantrowitz FG, Noble JL, et al. Ocular abnormalities after influenza immunization. Arch Ophthalmol 1977;95:1649.

495. Confavreux C, Suissa S, Saddier P, et al. Vaccinations and the risk of relapse in multiple sclerosis. N Engl J Med 2001;344:319–326.

496. DeStefano F, Verstraeten T, Jackson LA, et al. Vaccinations and risk of central nervous system demyelinating diseases in adults. Arch Neurol 2003;60:504–509.

497. Gout O. Vaccinations and multiple sclerosis. Neurol Sci 2001;22:151–154.

498. Gould H, Kaufman HE. Sarcoid of the fundus. Arch Ophthalmol 1961;65:453–456.

499. Hart WM Jr, Burde RM. Optic disk edema in sarcoidosis. Am J Ophthalmol 1979;88:769–771.

500. Spalton DJ, Sanders MD. Fundus changes in histologically confirmed sarcoidosis. Br J Ophthalmol 1981;65:348–358.

501. Beardsley TL, Brown SVL, Sydnor CF, et al. Eleven cases of sarcoidosis of the optic nerve. Am J Ophthalmol 1984;97:62–77.

502. Graham EM, Ellis CJK, Sanders MD, et al. Optic neuropathy in sarcoidosis. J Neurol Neurosurg Psychiatry 1986;49:756–763.

503. Sloan LL, Woods AC. Perimetric studies in syphilitic optic neuropathies. Arch Ophthalmol 1938;20:201–254.

504. Miller NR, Fine SL. The Ocular Fundus in Neuro-Ophthalmologic Diagnosis: Sights and Sounds in Ophthalmology. St Louis, CV Mosby, 1977.

505. Weinstein JM, Lexow SS, Spickard A. Acute syphilitic optic neuritis. Arch Ophthalmol 1981;99:1392–1395.

506. Carter JB, Hamill RJ, Matoba AY. Bilateral syphilitic optic neuritis in a patient with a positive test for HIV: case report. Arch Ophthalmol 1987;105:1485–1486.

507. Zambrano W, Perez GM, Smith JL. Acute syphilitic blindness in AIDS. J Clin Neuroophthalmol 1987;7:1–5.

508. Becerra LI, Ksiazek SM, Savino PJ, et al. Syphilitic uveitis in human immunodeficiency virus-infected and noninfected patients. Ophthalmology 1989;96:1727–1730.

509. Katz DA, Berger JR. Neurosyphilis in acquired immunodeficiency syndrome. Arch Neurol 1989;46:895–898.

510. Winward KE, Hamed LM, Glaser JS. The spectrum of optic nerve disease in human immunodeficiency virus infection. Am J Ophthalmol 1989;107:373–380.

511. Blanche P, Diaz E, Gombert B, et al. Devic's neuromyelitis optica and HIV-1 infection. J Neurol Neurosurg Psychiatry 2000;68:795–796.

512. Grossniklaus HE, Frank KE, Tomsak RL. Cytomegalovirus retinitis and optic neuritis in acquired immune deficiency syndrome: report of a case. Ophthalmology 1987;94:1601–1604.

513. Grossniklaus HE, Specht CS, Allaire G, et al. *Toxoplasma gondii* retinochoroiditis and optic neuritis in acquired immune deficiency syndrome: report of a case. Ophthalmology 1990;97:1342–1346.

514. Litoff D, Catalano RA. Herpes zoster optic neuritis in human immunodeficiency virus infection. Arch Ophthalmol 1990;108:782–783.

515. Golnik KC, Newman SA, Wispelway B. Cryptococcal optic neuropathy in the acquired immune deficiency syndrome. J Clin Neuroophthalmol 1991;11:96–103.

516. Friedman DI. Neuro-ophthalmologic manifestations of human immunodeficiency virus infection. Neurol Clin 1991;9:55–72.

517. Nichols JW, Goodwin JA. Neuro-ophthalmologic complications of AIDS. Semin Ophthalmol 1992;7:24–29.

518. Holland GN, Engstrom RE Jr, Glasgow BJ, et al. Ocular toxoplasmosis in patients with the acquired immunodeficiency syndrome. Am J Ophthalmol 1988;106:653–657.

519. Falcone PM, Notis C, Merhige K. Toxoplasmic papillitis as the initial manifestation of acquired immunodeficiency syndrome. Ann Ophthalmol 1993;25:56–57.

520. Ohnuma I, Yamaguchi K, Takahashi S. Retrobulbar neuritis in a patient with mixed connective tissue disease. Folia Ophthalmol Jpn 1996;47:828–831.

521. Fulford KWM, Catterall RD, Delhanty JJ, et al. A collagen disorder of the nervous system presenting as multiple sclerosis. Brain 1972;95:373–386.

522. Hackett ER, Martinez RD, Larson PF, et al. Optic neuritis in systemic lupus erythematosus. Arch Neurol 1974;31:9–11.

523. Shepherd DI, Downie AW, Best PV. Systemic lupus erythematosus and multiple sclerosis. Arch Neurol 1974;30:423–426.

524. Jabs DA, Miller NR, Newman SA, et al. Optic neuropathy in systemic lupus erythematosus. Arch Ophthalmol 1986;104:564–568.

525. Kinney EL, Berdoff RL, Rao NS, et al. Devic's syndrome and systemic lupus erythematosus: a case report with necropsy. Arch Neurol 1979;36:643–644.

526. Oppenheimer S, Hoffbrand BI. Optic neuritis and myelopathy in systemic lupus erythematosus. Can J Neurol Sci 1986;13:129–132.

527. Tola MR, Granieri E, Caniatti L, et al. Systemic lupus erythematosus presenting with neurological disorders. J Neurol 1992;239:61–64.

528. Cordeiro ME, Lloyd ME, Spalton DJ, et al. Ischaemic optic neuropathy, transverse myelitis and epilepsy in an antiphospholipid positive patient with systemic lupus erythematosus. J Neurol Neurosurg Psychiatry 1994;57:1142–1143.

529. Bonnet F, Mercie P, Morlat P, et al. Devic's neuromyelitis optica during pregnancy in a patient with systemic lupus erythematosus. Lupus 1999;8:244–247.

530. Giorgi D, Balacco Gabrieli C, Bonomo L. The association of optic neuropathy with transverse myelitis in systemic lupus erythematosus. Rheumatology (Oxf) 1999;38:191–192.

531. Dutton JJ, Burde RM, Klingele TC. Autoimmune retrobulbar optic neuritis. Am J Ophthalmol 1982;94:11–17.

532. Kupersmith MJ, Burde RM, Warren FA, et al. Autoimmune optic neuropathy: evaluation and treatment. J Neurol Neurosurg Psychiatry 1988;51:1381–1386.

532a. Kidd D, Burton B, Plant GT, et al. Chronic relapsing inflammatory optic neuropathy (CRION). Brain 2003;126:276–284.

533. Winward KE, Smith JL, Culbertson WW, et al. Ocular Lyme borreliosis. Am J Ophthalmol 1989;108:651–657.

534. Lesser RL, Kornmehl EW, Pachner AR, et al. Neuro-ophthalmologic manifestations of Lyme disease. Ophthalmology 1990;97:699–706.

535. Winterkorn JMS. Lyme disease: Neurologic and ophthalmologic manifestations. Surv Ophthalmol 1990;35:191–204.

536. Jacobson DM, Marx JJ, Dlesk A. Frequency and clinical significance of Lyme seropositivity in patients with isolated optic neuritis. Neurology 1991;41:706–711.

537. Spoor TC, Hartel WC, Harding S, et al. Aspergillosis presenting as a corticosteroid-responsive optic neuropathy. J Clin Neuroophthalmol 1982;2:103–107.

538. Weinstein JM, Sattler FA, Towfighi J, et al. Optic neuropathy and paratrigeminal syndrome due to *Aspergillus fumigatus*. Arch Neurol 1982;39:582.

539. Kirkham TH, Ffytche T, Sanders MD. Placoid pigment epitheliopathy with retinal vasculitis and papillitis. Br J Ophthalmol 1972;56:875–880.

540. Goldstein NP, Rucker CW, Woltman HW. Neuritis occurring after insect stings. JAMA 1960;173:1727–1730.

541. Singh I, Chaudhary U. Bilateral optic neuritis following multiple wasp stings. J Indian Med Assoc 1986;84:251–252.

542. Song HS, Wray SH. Bee sting optic neuritis: a case report with visual evoked potentials. J Clin Neuroophthalmol 1991;11:45–49.

543. Berrios RR, Serrano LA. Bilateral optic neuritis after a bee sting [letter]. Am J Ophthalmol 1994;117:677–678.

544. Colvard DM, Robertson DM, O'Duffy JD. The ocular manifestations of Behçet's disease. Arch Ophthalmol 1977;95:1813–1817.

545. Ryan SJ, Maumenee AE. Birdshot retinochoroidopathy. Am J Ophthalmol 1980;89:31–45.

546. Lesser RL, Albert DM, Bobowick AR, et al. Creutzfeldt-Jakob disease and optic atrophy. Am J Ophthalmol 1979;87:317–321.

547. Roth AM, Keltner JL, Ellis WG, et al. Virus-simulating structures in the optic nerve head in Creutzfeldt-Jakob disease. Am J Ophthalmol 1979;87:827–833.

548. Bawa YS, Wahi PL. Cysticercosis cellulosae of the optic disc with generalized cysticercosis. Br J Ophthalmol 1962;46:753–755.

549. Lossos A, Eliashiv S, Ben-Chetrit E, et al. Optic neuritis associated with familial Mediterranean fever. J Clin Neuroophthalmol 1993;13:141–143.

550. Vlodarczyk S. Un cas de syndrome de Guillain-Barré avec névrite optique retro-bulbaire. Neurol Pol 1949;23:110–115.

551. Mouren P, Vital-Berard P, Poinso Y, et al. Névrite optique retro-bulbaire au cours d'un syndrome de Guillain-Barré. Rev Otoneuroophthalmol 1971;43:216–221.

552. Nikoskelainen E, Riekkinen P. Retrobulbar neuritis as an early symptom on Guillain-Barré syndrome. Acta Ophthalmol 1972;50:111–115.

553. Behan PO, Lessell S, Roche M. Optic neuritis in the Landry-Guillain-Barré-Strohl syndrome. Br J Ophthalmol 1976;60:58–59.

554. Ellis PP, Gentry JH. Ocular complications of ulcerative colitis. Am J Ophthalmol 1964;58:779–785.

555. Macoul KL. Ocular changes in granulomatous ileocolitis. Arch Ophthalmol 1970;84:95–97.

556. Knox DL. Optic nerve manifestations of systemic diseases. Trans Am Acad Ophthalmol Otolarnygol 1977;83:743–750.

557. Knox DL, Bayless TM. Gastrointestinal and ocular disease. In: Mausolf FA, ed. The Eye and Systemic Disease. St Louis, CV Mosby, 1980:333–344.

558. Sedwick LA, Klingele TG, Burde RM, et al. Optic neuritis in inflammatory bowel disease. J Clin Neuroophthalmol 1984;4:3–6.

559. Hutnik CML, Nicolle DA, Canny CLB. Papillitis: a rare initial presentation of Crohn's disease. Can J Ophthalmol 1996;31:373–376.

560. Bird AC, Smith JL, Curtin VT. Neomatode optic neuritis. Am J Ophthalmol 1970;69:72–77.

561. Phillips CI, Mackenzie AD. Toxocara larval papillitis. Br Med J 1973;1:154–155.

562. Husted RC, Shock JP. Acute presumed histoplasmosis of the optic nerve head. Br J Ophthalmol 1975;59:409–412.

563. Beck RW, Sergott RC, Barr CC, et al. Optic disc edema in the presumed ocular histoplasmosis syndrome. Ophthalmology 1984;91:183–185.

564. Duke-Elder S. Diseases of the outer eye. In: System of Ophthalmology. London, Henry Kimpton, 1965:1:527–532.

565. Bietti GB, Bruna F. An ophthalmic report on Behçet's disease. In: Monacelli M, Nazzaro P, eds. Symposium on Behçet's Disease. Basel, S Karger, 1966:79–110.

566. Cox TA, Haskins GE, Gangitano JL, et al. Bilateral *Toxocara* optic neuropathy. J Clin Neuroophthalmol 1983;3:267–274.

567. Willerson D, Aaberg TM, Reeser F, et al. Unusual ocular presentation of acute toxoplasmosis. Br J Ophthalmol 1977;61:693–698.

568. Folk JC, Lobes LA. Presumed toxoplasmic papillitis. Ophthalmology 1984;91:64–67.

569. Rothstein TL, Kenny GE. Cranial neuropathy, myeloradiculopathy, and myositis: complications of *Mycoplasma pneumoniae* infection. Arch Neurol 1979;36:476–477.

570. Salzman MB, Sood SK, Slavin ML, et al. Ocular manifestations of *Mycoplasma pneumoniae* infection. Clin Infect Dis 1992;14:1137–1139.

571. Nadkarni N, Lisak RP. Guillain-Barré syndrome (GBS) with bilateral optic neuritis and white matter disease. Neurology 1993;43:842–843.

572. Sheth RD, Goulden KJ, Pryse-Phillips WE. The focal encephalopathies associated with *Mycoplasma pneumoniae*. Can J Neurol Sci 1993;20:319–323.

573. Porsaa K. Papilledema in iridocyclitis. Acta Ophthalmol 1944;21:316–329.

574. Kimura SJ, Hogan MJ. Chronic cyclitis. Arch Ophthalmol 1964;71:193–201.

575. Tillmann W, Ufermann K. Papillenschwellng bei uveitis. Klin Monatsbl Augenheilkd 1972;161:42–46.

576. Irvine SR. A newly defined vitreous syndrome following cataract surgery. Am J Ophthalmol 1953;36:599–619.

577. Gass JDM, Norton EWD. Cystoid macular edema and papilledema following cataract extraction. Arch Ophthalmol 1966;76:646–661.

578. Norton AL, Brown WJ, Carlson M, et al. Pathogenesis of aphakic macular edema. Am J Ophthalmol 1975;80:96–101.

579. Hanna LS, Girgis NI. Incidence of papilloedema and optic atrophy in meningitis. Jpn J Ophthalmol 1981;25:69–73.

580. McIntyre HD, McIntyre AP. Prognosis of multiple sclerosis. Arch Neurol Psychiatr 1943;50:431–438.

581. White DN, Wheelan L. Disseminated sclerosis: a survey of patients in the Kingston, Ontario, area. Neurology 1959;9:256–272.

582. Rischbieth RC. Retrobulbar neuritis in the State of South Australia. Proc Aust Assoc Neurol 1968;5:573–575.

583. Nakao Y, Omoto T, Shimomura Y. Optic neuritis in children. Folia Ophthalmol Jpn 1983;34:496–498.

584. Keast-Butler J, Taylor D. Optic neuropathies in children. Trans Ophthalmol Soc UK 1980;100:111–118.

585. Cohen G, Gitter K, Baber BW. Reversible bilateral simultaneous papillitis with no light perception. Ann Ophthalmol 1976;8:583–586.

586. Rollinson RD. Bilateral optic neuritis in childhood. Med J Aust 1977;2:50–51.

587. Koraszewska-Matuszewska B, Samochowiec-Donocik E, Rynkiewicz E. Optic neuritis in children and adolescents. Klin Oczna 1995;97:207–210.

588. Good WV, Muci-Mendoza R, Berg BO, et al. Optic neuritis in children with poor recovery of vision. Aust NZ J Ophthalmol 1992;20:319–323.

589. Brady KM, Brar AS, Lee AG, Coats, et al. Optic neuritis in children: clinical features and visual outcome. J AAPOS 1999;3:98–103.

590. Morales DS, Siatkowski RM, Howard CW, et al. Optic neuritis in children. J Pediatr Ophthalmol Strabismus 2000;37:254–259.

591. Rush JA. Idiopathic optic neuritis of childhood. J Pediatr Ophthalmol Strabismus 1981;18:39–41.

592. Leber T. Pseudoneuritic retinal disease, stellate retinitis: the angiopathic retinal affections after severe skull injury. Graefe-Saemisch Handb Ges Augenheilkd 1916;7:1319.

593. Francois J, Verriest G, DeLaey J. Leber's idiopathic stellate retinopathy. Am J Ophthalmol 1969;68:340–345.

594. Dreyer RF, Hopen G, Gass DM, et al. Leber's idiopathic stellate neuroretinitis. Arch Ophthalmol 1984;102:1140–1145.

595. Maitland CG, Miller NR. Neuroretinitis. Arch Ophthalmol 1984;102:1146–1150.

596. Carroll DM, Franklin RM. Leber's idiopathic stellate retinopathy. Am J Ophthalmol 1982;93:96–101.

597. Neetens A, Smets RM. Leber's neurogenic stellate maculopathy. Neuroophthalmology 1987;7:315–328.

598. Guillaume J-B, Risse JF, Rovira JC. Neurorétinite aigue: discussion nosologique à propos d'un cas chez un adulte jeune. Bull Soc Ophtalmol Fr 1991;91:39–42.

599. King MN, Cartwright MJ, Carney MD. Leber's idiopathic neuroretinitis. Arch Ophthalmol 1991;23:58–60.

600. Weiss AH, Beck RW. Neuroretinitis in childhood. J Pediatr Ophthalmol 1989;26:198–203.

601. Johnson BL, Wisetzley HM. Neuroretinitis associated with herpes simplex encephalitis in an adult. Am J Ophthalmol 1977;83:481–489.

602. Farthing CF, Howard RS, Thin RN. Papillitis and hepatitis B. Br Med J 1986;292:1712.

603. Margolis T, Irvine AR, Hoyt WF, et al. Acute retinal necrosis syndrome presenting with papillitis and acute neuroretinitis. Ophthalmology 1988;95:937–940.

604. Ulrich GG, Waecker NJ Jr, Meister SJ, et al. Cat scratch disease associated with neuroretinitis in a 6-year-old girl. Ophthalmology 1992;99:246–249.

605. Bar S, Segal M, Shapira R, et al. Neuroretinitis associated with cat scratch disease. Am J Ophthalmol 1990;110:703–705.

606. Chrousos GA, Drack AV, Young M, et al. Neuroretinitis in cat scratch disease. J Clin Neuroophthalmol 1990;10:92–94.

607. Arruga J, Valentines J, Mauri F, et al. Neuroretinitis in acquired syphilis. Ophthalmology 1985;92:262–270.

608. Fewell AG. Unilateral neuroretinitis of syphilitic origin with a striate figure in the macula. Arch Ophthalmol 1932;8:615.

609. Folk JC, Weingeist TA, Corbett JJ, et al. Syphilitic neuroretinitis. Am J Ophthalmol 1983;95:480–496.

610. Veldman E, Bos PJM. Neuroretinitis in secondary syphilis. Doc Ophthalmol 1986;64:23–29.

611. McLeish WM, Pulido JS, Holland S, et al. The ocular manifestations of syphilis in the human immunodeficiency virus type 1–infected host. Ophthalmology 1990;97:196–203.

612. Ninomiya H, Hamada T, Akiya S, et al. Three cases of acute syphilitic neuroretinitis. Folia Ophthalmol Jpn 1990;41:2088–2094.

613. Halperin LS. Neuroretinitis due to seronegative syphilis associated with human immunodeficiency virus. J Clin Neuroophthalmol 1992;12:171–172.

614. Graveson GS. Syphilitic optic neuritis. J Neurol Neurosurg Psychiatry 1950;13:216–224.

615. Bialiasiewicz AA, Huk W, Druschky KF, et al. *Borrelia burgdorferi*-Infektion mit beidseitiger Neuritis nervic optici und intrazerebralen Demyelinisierungsherden. Klin Monatsbl Augenheilkd 1989;195:91–94.

616. Schönherr U, Wilk CM, Lang GE, et al. Intraocular manifestations of Lyme borreliosis. Presented at the Fourth International Conference on Borreliosis, Stockholm, Sweden, June 18–21, 1990.

617. Schönherr U, Lang GE, Meythaler FH. Bilaterale Lebersche Neuroretinitis stellata bei *Borrelia burgdorferi*-Serokonversion. Klin Monatsbl Augenheilkd 1991;198:44–47.

618. Manschot WA, Daamen CBF. Congenital ocular toxoplasmosis. Arch Ophthalmol 1965;74:48–54.

619. Brown GC, Tasman WS. Retinal arterial obstruction in association with presumed *Toxocara canis* neuroretinitis. Ann Ophthalmol 1981;13:1385–1387.

620. Moreno RJ, Weisman J, Waller S. Neuroretinitis: an unusual presentation of ocular toxoplasmosis. Ann Ophthalmol 1992;24:68–70.

621. Fish RH, Hoskins JC, Kline LB. Toxoplasmosis neuroretinitis. Ophthalmology 1993;100:1177–1182.

622. Parmley VC, Schiffman JS, Maitland CG, et al. Does neuroretinitis rule out multiple sclerosis? Arch Neurol 1987;44:1045–1048.

623. Ormerod LD, Dailey JP. Ocular manifestations of cat-scratch disease. Curr Opin Ophthalmol 1999;10:209–216.

624. Conrad DA. Treatment of cat-scratch disease. Curr Opin Pediatr 2001;13:56–59.

625. Centers for Disease Control. 1989 Sexually transmitted diseases treatment guidelines. MMWR 1989;38(Suppl 8):9.

626. Purvin VA, Chioran G. Recurrent neuroretinitis. Arch Ophthalmol 1994;112:365–371.

627. Edmunds W, Lawford JB. Examination of optic nerve from a case of amblyopia in diabetes. Trans Ophthalmol Soc UK 1883;3:160–162.

628. Silverstein A. Papilledema with acute viral infections of the brain. Mt Sinai Med J 1974;41:425–443.

629. Kline LB, Jackson WB. Syphilitic optic perineuritis and uveitis. In: Smith JL, ed. Neuro-ophthalmology Focus 1980. New York, Masson, 1979:77–84.

630. Rush JA, Ryan EJ. Syphilitic optic perineuritis. Am J Ophthalmol 1981;91:404–406.

631. McBurney J, Rosenberg ML. Unilateral syphilitic optic perineuritis presenting as the big blind spot syndrome. J Clin Neuroophthalmol 1987;7:167–169.

632. Toshniwal P. Optic perineuritis with secondary syphilis. J Clin Neuroophthalmol 1987;7:6–10.

633. Purvin V, Kawasaki A, Jacobson DM. Optic perineuritis: clinical and radiographic features. Arch Ophthalmol 2001;119:1299–1306.

634. Dutton JJ, Anderson RL. Idiopathic inflammatory perioptic neuritis simulating optic nerve sheath meningioma. Am J Ophthalmol 1985;100:424–430.

635. Gibbs AN, Moroney J, Foley-Nolan D, et al. Neuromyelitis optica (Devic's syndrome) in systemic lupus erythematosus: a case report. Rheumatology (Oxf) 2000;41:470–471.

636. Moll JW, Markusse HM, Pijnenburg JJ, et al. Antineuronal antibodies in patients with neurologic complications of primary Sjögren's syndrome. Neurology 1993;43:2574–2581.

637. Manley G, Wong E, Dalmau J, et al. Sera from some patients with antibody-associated paraneoplastic encephalomyelitis/sensory neuronopathy recognize the Ro-52K antigen. J Neurooncol 1994;19:105–112.

638. Vitali C, Bombardieri S, Moutsopoulos HM, et al. Assessment of the European classification criteria for Sjögren's syndrome in a series of clinically defined cases: results of a prospective multicentre study. The European Study Group on Diagnostic Criteria for Sjögren's Syndrome. Ann Rheum Dis 1996;55:116–121.

639. Mochizuki A, Hayashi A, Hisahara S, et al. Steroid-responsive Devic's variant in Sjögren's syndrome. Neurology 2000;54:1391–1392.

640. Fukazawa T, Hamada T, Kikuchi S, et al. Antineutrophil cytoplasmic antibodies and the optic-spinal form of multiple sclerosis in Japan. J Neurol Neurosurg Psychiatry 1996;61:203–204.

641. Harada T, Ohashi T, Harada C, et al. A case of bilateral optic neuropathy and recurrent transverse myelopathy associated with perinuclear anti-neutrophil cytoplasmic antibodies (p-ANCA). J Neuroophthalmol 1997;17:254–256.

642. Fukazawa T, Moriwaka F, Mukai M, et al. Anticardiolipin antibodies in Japanese patients with multiple sclerosis. Acta Neurol Scand 1993;88:184–189.

643. Karussis D, Leker RR, Ashkenazi A, et al. A subgroup of multiple sclerosis patients with anticardiolipin antibodies and unusual clinical manifestations: do they represent a new nosological entity? Ann Neurol 1998;44:629–634.

644. Weiss TD, Nelson JS, Woolsey RM, et al. Transverse myelitis in mixed connective tissue disease. Arthritis Rheum 1978;21:982–986.

645. Flechtner KM, Baum K. Mixed connective tissue disease: recurrent episodes of optic neuropathy and transverse myelopathy: successful treatment with plasmapheresis. J Neurol Sci 1994;126:146–148.

646. Hughes RA, Mair WG. Acute necrotic myelopathy with pulmonary tuberculosis. Brain 1977;100:223–228.

647. Doutlik S, Sblova O, Kryl R, et al. Neuromyelitis optica as a parainfectious complication of varicella. Cesk Neurol Neurochir 1975;38:238–242.

648. Tateishi J, Ikeda H, Saito A, et al. Myeloneuropathy in dogs induced by iodoxyquinoline. Neurology 1972;22:702–709.

649. Tateishi J, Kuroda S, Saito A, et al. Experimental myelo-optic neuropathy induced by clioquinol. Acta Neuropathol (Berl) 1973;24:304–320.

650. Donati E, Bargnani C, Besana R, et al. Subacute myelo-optic neuropathy (SMON) induced by antituberculous treatment in uraemia. Funct Neurol 1990;5:151–154.

651. Afifi AK, Follett KA, Greenlee J, et al. Optic neuritis: a novel presentation of Schilder's disease. J Child Neurol 2001;16:693–696.

652. Levin LA, Lessell S. Risk of multiple sclerosis after optic neuritis. JAMA 2003;290:403–404.

CHAPTER 7

Ischemic Optic Neuropathy

Anthony C. Arnold

ANTERIOR ISCHEMIC OPTIC NEUROPATHY (AION)
   Arteritic Anterior Ischemic Optic Neuropathy (AAION)
   Nonarteritic Anterior Ischemic Optic Neuropathy (NAION)
POSTERIOR ISCHEMIC OPTIC NEUROPATHY
ISCHEMIC OPTIC NEUROPATHY IN SETTINGS OF
   HEMODYNAMIC COMPROMISE
   Spontaneous or Traumatic Hemorrhage

Perioperative
Hypotension
RADIATION OPTIC NEUROPATHY
ISCHEMIC OPTIC DISC EDEMA WITH MINIMAL
   DYSFUNCTION
   Pre-AION Optic Disc Edema
   Diabetic Papillopathy

Ischemic syndromes of the optic nerve (ischemic optic neuropathy [ION]) are classified according to (*a*) the location of the ischemic damage of the nerve and (*b*) the etiologic factor, if known, for the ischemia. *Anterior* ischemic optic neuropathy (AION) includes syndromes involving the optic nerve head, with visible optic disc edema. *Posterior* ischemic optic neuropathy (PION) incorporates those conditions involving the intraorbital, intracanalicular, or intracranial portions of the optic nerve, with no visible edema of the optic disc. While several specific etiologic factors have been identified in ION, the most critical for initial management is the vasculitis of giant cell, or temporal, arteritis (GCA); therefore, ION is typically classified as either *arteritic* (usually due to GCA) or *nonarteritic*. Nonarteritic ION is most often idiopathic, but specific etiologies such as systemic hypotension and radiation injury have been identified. Finally, several syndromes of optic disc edema with relatively mild dysfunction, including preinfarct optic disc edema and diabetic papillopathy, are presumed to represent optic nerve ischemic edema with dysfunction that is not detectable, mild, or reversible.

ANTERIOR ISCHEMIC OPTIC NEUROPATHY (AION)

AION typically presents with the rapid onset of painless unilateral visual loss developing over hours to days. An altitudinal visual field defect (typically inferior) is the most common pattern of loss (Fig. 7.1 but arcuate scotomas, cecocentral defects, and generalized depression are also frequently seen (Fig. 7.2). Visual acuity is decreased if the field defect involves fixation but may be normal if an arcuate pattern spares the central region. The pupil in the affected eye is sluggishly reactive, with a relative afferent pupillary defect present unless pre-existing or concurrent optic neuropathy in the fellow eye makes its pupillary response equally sluggish. The optic disc is edematous at onset; the edema may be pallid, but it is not uncommon to see disc hyperemia, particularly in the nonarteritic form (Fig. 7.3). The disc most often is diffusely swollen, but a segment of more prominent edema is frequently present (Fig. 7.4). Flame hemorrhages are commonly located adjacent to the disc, and peripapillary retinal arteriolar narrowing may occur

(Fig. 7.5). Retinal arteriolar emboli are only rarely associated.

ARTERITIC ANTERIOR ISCHEMIC OPTIC NEUROPATHY (AAION)

Demographics

Although it often produces a severe and devastating optic neuropathy, GCA is the cause for AION in a relatively small minority (5.7%) (1) of cases, with an estimated annual incidence in the United States of 0.57 per 100,000 over age 60 (2). AION is, however, the most common cause of visual loss in GCA (3–5), accounting for 71–83% of cases (6,7), with retinal artery occlusion, choroidal ischemia, and PION less common. The mean age of onset for AAION is 70 years (1), with only rare occurrence under age 60. GCA occurs more frequently in women and with increasing age (8,9). It is most common in Caucasians and is unusual in African-

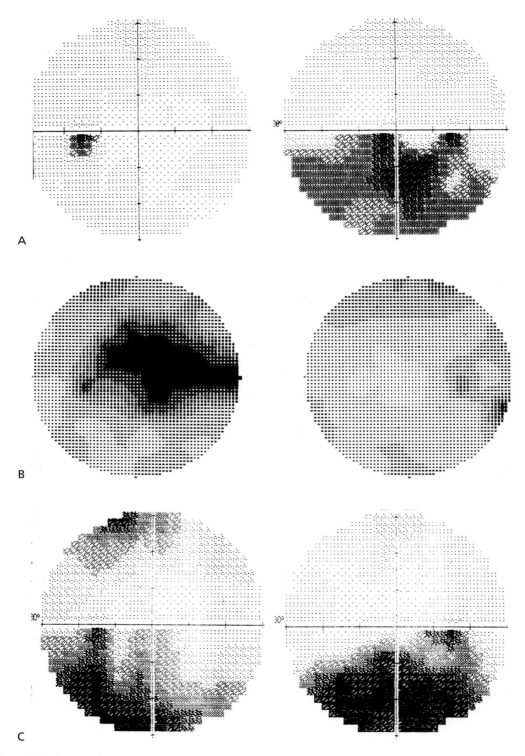

Figure 7.1. Automated quantitative perimetry in AION. Broad arcuate (altitudinal) defect (*A*) is most common, with central (*B*) and less severe arcuate (*C*) defects also frequently noted.

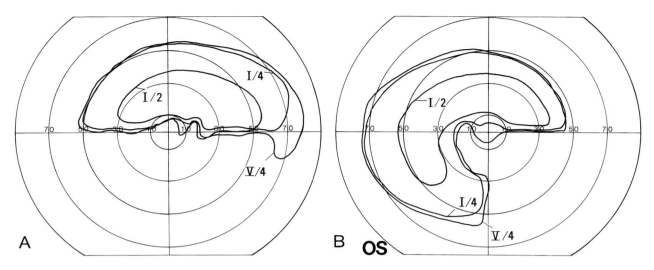

Figure 7.2. Goldmann perimetry, showing common visual field defects in anterior ischemic optic neuropathy. *A,* Altitudinal defect. *B,* Broad arcuate defect.

American and Hispanic patients (2). Liu et al. reviewed 121 consecutive temporal artery biopsies, assessing the rate of positive biopsies by ethnic background: 19/66 (29%) of Caucasian patients had positive biopsies, compared with 0/40 Hispanic patients and 0/6 African-Americans (10).

Clinical Manifestations

AAION usually occurs in association with other systemic symptoms of the disease. Headache is the most common symptom, while jaw claudication and temporal artery or scalp tenderness are the most specific for the disorder (11–13) (see also Chapter 44). The headache is often severe, constant, and disabling. True jaw claudication, with muscular cramping and fatigue progressing with continued chewing activity, has high specificity for temporal arteritis, although it has also been reported in amyloidosis (14). Claudication may also occur in muscles of the neck or tongue. The syndrome of polymyalgia rheumatica (PMR), including malaise, anorexia, weight loss, fever, proximal joint arthralgia and myalgia, is frequently reported. PMR with hematologic inflammatory markers, but without temporal artery or ocular involvement, may lead to arteritis in some cases. One series indicated that 15.8% of PMR patients eventually developed GCA with visual loss (15). In contrast, so-called occult GCA, without overt systemic symptoms and

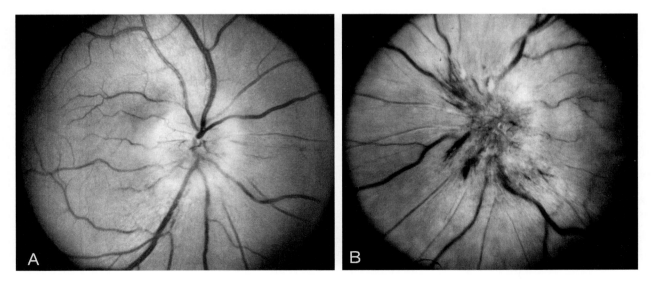

Figure 7.3. Ophthalmoscopic appearance of nonarteritic anterior ischemic optic neuropathy. *A,* Pallid swelling of the optic disc associated with a few small flame-shaped hemorrhages at the disc margin. *B,* Hyperemic swelling of the optic disc associated with numerous hemorrhages and a few soft exudates.

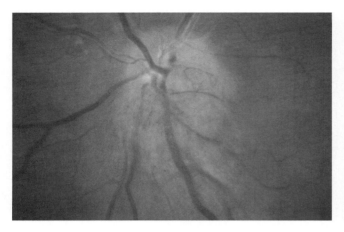

Figure 7.4.   Segmental optic disc edema in AION. The optic disc is edematous, with more prominent involvement inferiorly.

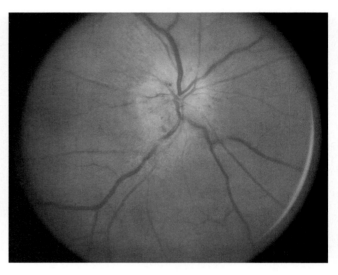

Figure 7.5.   Parapapillary retinal arteriolar narrowing in AION. The vessels are focally attenuated overlying the disc, widening as they course toward the retinal periphery.

sometimes without abnormal blood testing, may occur (16,17). In Hayreh's recent report, 21.2% of patients with GCA and visual loss had no systemic symptoms of the disease (17).

In addition to systemic symptoms, certain associated local signs may aid in the diagnosis of AAION. Induration of the temporal region, decreased or absent temporal artery pulse, and cordlike firmness or nodularity of the temporal artery all may be seen. Ischemic scalp necrosis has been documented in GCA, and it may masquerade as herpes zoster dermatitis, with facial pain and even a vesicular reaction of the affected skin (18). A wide variety of additional signs relating to vasculitic ischemia of the central nervous system have been reported; these include mental status alterations (19), brain stem and cerebellar syndromes (20), and damage to the retrochiasmal afferent visual pathways, with corresponding visual field defects (20).

AAION typically presents with severe visual loss (visual acuity less than 20/200 in 57.8% to 76.5% of cases [6,7, 21,22], frequently hand motion or worse) developing rapidly

over hours to days (Table 7.1). Twenty-one percent of cases in one series had no light perception (6). While the initial presentation is often unilateral, bilateral simultaneous AION is more commonly arteritic than nonarteritic, and its occurrence raises suspicion for GCA. The persistent visual loss of AAION is preceded in 7–18% (6,7,20,23) of cases by transient visual loss similar to that of carotid artery disease, although the episodes may be of shorter duration; these are only rarely associated with the nonarteritic form of AION and are highly suggestive of arteritis. The pallid type of optic disc edema (Fig. 7.6) is seen more frequently in the arteritic than in the nonarteritic form (24,25); chalk-white pallor with edema is seen in severe cases and is highly unusual in nonarteritic ION (NAION). Cotton-wool patches (Fig. 7.7) indicative of concurrent retinal ischemia may be seen (26). Retinal

Table 7.1
Ischemic Optic Neuropathies

	Arteritic	Nonarteritic	Diabetic Papillopathy	Posterior
Age	Mean 70 yr	Mean 60 yr	Variable (<50)	Variable
Gender	F > M	F = M	F = M	F = M
Associated symptoms	Headache, jaw claudication, transient visual loss	Usually none	Usually none	None unless arteritic or postoperative
Visual acuity	<20/200 in >60%	>20/60 in >50%	>20/40 in >75%	Usually poor
Disc	Pale swelling common	Pale or hyperemic	Hyperemia, telangiectasia	Normal
	Cup normal + choroid ischemia	Cup small	Cup small	Variable
ESR	Mean 70 mm/hr	Usually normal	Usually normal	Elevated if arteritic
FA	Disc delay	Disc delay	Disc delay	Not studied
	Choroid delay			
Natural history	Rarely improve	16–42.7% improve	Resolves 2–10 mo	Rarely improves
	Fellow eye 54–95%	Fellow eye 12–19%	Bilateral 40%	Bilateral >60%
Treatment	Systemic steroids	None proven	None proven	Steroids if arteritic

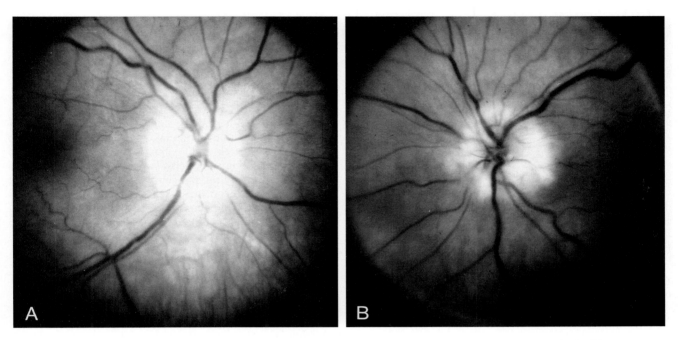

Figure 7.6. Bilateral simultaneous anterior ischemic optic neuropathy in a patient with GCA and no light perception in either eye. The right and left optic discs show markedly pale swelling.

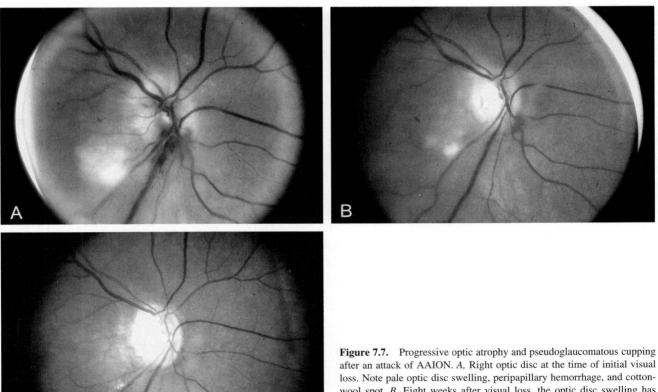

Figure 7.7. Progressive optic atrophy and pseudoglaucomatous cupping after an attack of AAION. *A,* Right optic disc at the time of initial visual loss. Note pale optic disc swelling, peripapillary hemorrhage, and cotton-wool spot. *B,* Eight weeks after visual loss, the optic disc swelling has resolved, and both the hemorrhage and the cotton-wool spot are resolving. Note narrowing of retinal vessels. *C,* Four months after visual loss, the optic disc is pale and now has a large cup. The retinal vessels, especially the arteries, are markedly narrowed.

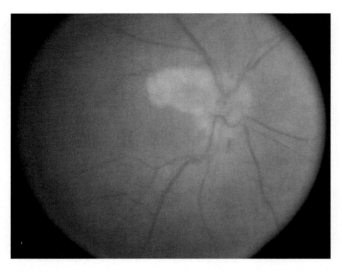

Figure 7.8. AAION with associated cilioretinal artery occlusion. In addition to the optic disc edema, there is a focus of retinal edema in the distribution of the cilioretinal artery.

arterial occlusion may occur simultaneously with the optic neuropathy (6). In Hayreh's series (23), cilioretinal artery occlusion occurred in 21.2%; this is a very unusual occurrence in NAION and is highly suggestive of GCA (Fig. 7.8). Peripapillary choroidal ischemia may be associated with the optic neuropathy, producing edema deep to the retina adjacent to the optic disc and exacerbating the visual loss (27,28). It may also occur in a more widespread area, with or without optic disc involvement (27,29). The optic disc of the fellow eye in AAION most frequently is of normal diameter, with

a normal physiologic cup (30,31), as opposed to that in NAION, which tends to be small in diameter, with little or no physiologic cup (31) (see below).

Pathophysiology

Histopathologic studies in AAION demonstrate vasculitis of the short posterior ciliary vessels supplying the optic nerve head, in addition to variable involvement of the superficial temporal, ophthalmic, choroidal, and central retinal arteries (32–37). Infiltration of the short posterior ciliary arteries by chronic inflammatory cells, with segmental occlusion of multiple vessels by inflammatory thickening and thrombus (Fig. 7.9), has been documented (32,33,37). Autopsy studies have demonstrated ischemic necrosis predominantly involving the laminar and retrolaminar portions of the optic nerve supplied by these vessels and their distal tributaries (32, 34,35).

Fluorescein angiographic data support involvement of the short posterior ciliary arteries in AAION. Delayed filling of the optic disc and adjacent choroid (Fig. 7.10) is consistently noted (24,28,38–41). Extremely poor or absent filling of the choroid has been suggested as one useful factor in distinguishing arteritic from nonarteritic AION. Mack et al. (29) reported mean choroid perfusion time (from first appearance to filling) of 69 seconds in patients with AAION, compared with 5.5 seconds in NAION; Siatkowski et al. (25) confirmed this finding with slightly different parameters, mean time from injection to choroid filling measuring 29.7 seconds in AAION compared with 12.9 seconds in NAION.

Differential Diagnosis

The acute onset of severe visual loss in the setting of headache and optic disc edema, particularly when bilateral,

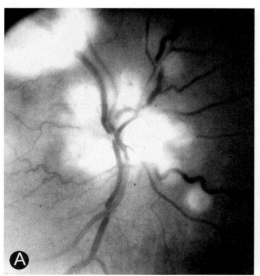
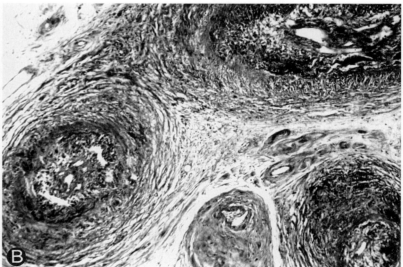

Figure 7.9. Pathophysiology of AION in GCA. *A,* The right optic disc shows pale swelling with extension of edema into the peripapillary retina. *B,* Section through several short posterior ciliary arteries shows that they contain a granulomatous inflammation in their walls with fragmentation of the internal elastic lamina and subendothelial aggregation of giant cells. The lumens are markedly narrowed or occluded. (Courtesy Dr. I. H. L. Wallow.)

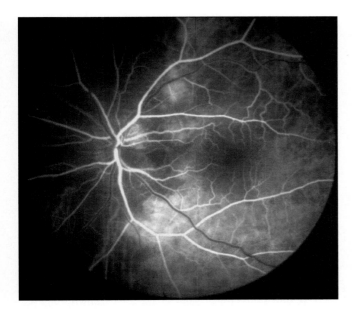

Figure 7.10. Fluorescein angiography in AAION. The optic disc and adjacent choroid show marked filling delay.

requires consideration of alternate diagnoses, including acute optic neuropathy secondary to chronic papilledema (with or without intracranial mass), infiltrative optic neuropathy, and meningeal carcinomatosis involving the optic nerves. In cases of suspected AAION with negative workup or atypical course, neuroimaging should be performed to evaluate for intracranial mass or visible meningeal thickening and enhancement, and lumbar puncture should be considered to assess for evidence of elevated intracranial pressure or malignant cells.

Clinical Course

If untreated, AAION results in severe damage of the affected optic nerve. Recovery of useful vision after initial involvement is unusual, even with prompt therapy. In cases with unilateral presentation, estimates for development of AAION in the fellow eye without therapy range from 54% to 95% (6,42–44). Time to second eye involvement varies greatly, but it may occur within hours to days. The optic disc edema typically resolves over 4–8 weeks, with resultant optic atrophy and generalized attenuation of retinal arterioles. Excavation of the optic disc (Fig. 7.7) occurs frequently after AAION (40,45–49) but is unusual in NAION. Danesh-Meyer et al. (48) reported optic disc cupping in 92% of 92 patients with AAION versus 2% of 102 patients with NAION. The excavation may be severe, mimicking glaucomatous damage. Hayreh and Jonas (49) noted lack of increase in peripapillary atrophy associated with the cupping after AAION, in contrast to glaucoma. The severity of the optic atrophy seen after AAION also differentiates it from glaucomatous excavation.

Diagnostic Confirmation

The most important initial step in the management of AION is the assessment for evidence of GCA. A tentative diagnosis may be made on the basis of advanced age and typical clinical symptoms in conjunction with elevation of the erythrocyte sedimentation rate (ESR). Most cases of active GCA show markedly elevated ESRs (mean 70 mm/hr, often above 100 mm/hr). When the level is not extremely high, however, interpretation of the value becomes more difficult, as normative data are imprecise. As a rule, we recommend the clinically useful guideline that the upper level of normal, in mm/hr, is calculated by dividing patient age by 2 in males and patient age plus 10 by 2 in females (50). However, by these criteria, the level may be normal in up to 22% of patients with GCA (5,51). Conversely, the ESR rises with age, and levels above the listed upper limit of normal for the laboratory are common (up to 40% over 60 mm/hr) in patients over 70 without arteritis (52). In the Ischemic Optic Neuropathy Decompression Trial (IONDT), 9% of patients with NAION had ESR levels over 40 mm/hr, with a range of 0–115 (53). Moreover, the test is nonspecific, elevation confirming only the presence of any active inflammatory process or other disorder affecting red cell aggregation. In studies of temporal artery biopsy-negative cases with such elevation, the most common associated diseases have been occult malignancy (most frequently lymphoma) in 18–22%, other inflammatory disease in 17–21%, and diabetes in 15–20% (54,55). In these cases initially suspected of being GCA, internal medicine consultation to rule out other systemic diseases is essential.

Additional blood abnormalities are common in GCA and may have prognostic value. Measurement of C-reactive protein, levels of which do not rise with age or anemia, may increase diagnostic accuracy and are currently recommended in conjunction with the ESR (56). Hayreh et al. (69) reported that a specificity of 97% for GCA was attained for AION patients with ESR levels above 47 mm/hr and C-reactive protein above 2.45 mg/dL (normal less than 0.5) from their laboratory. We currently recommend simultaneous measurement of both parameters in suspected cases of AAION. Fibrinogen is commonly elevated and may supplement C-reactive protein levels in increasing accuracy over the use of ESR alone (57,58). Thrombocytosis is seen in up to 50% of patients with GCA; its presence has been shown to be a marker for positive temporal artery biopsy (59) and may be a predictor of visual loss (60,61). Liozon et al. (61) assessed 174 patients with GCA, correlating thrombocytosis with the development of permanent visual loss. Of 20 patients with permanent visual loss due to AAION, 13 (65%) had thrombocytosis. This feature may have implications for therapy (see below).

Giant cell arteritis is confirmed by a positive temporal artery biopsy, which is strongly recommended in any case of suspected arteritic AION. The certainty of biopsy-proven GCA provides support for long-term systemic corticosteroid therapy, which often is required for up to a year and may be associated with severe systemic complications. It also makes later decisions regarding the risk/benefit ratio of prolonged therapy more clearcut. A negative biopsy, however, does not rule out GCA. A false-negative biopsy may result from (a) discontinuous arterial involvement ("skip lesions") (62–65), undetected in 4–5% due to insufficient length (minimum 3–6 cm recommended) of specimen or insufficiently detailed step-sectioning; (*b*) unilateral involvement with biopsy of the uninvolved temporal artery; (*c*) improper handling of specimens; or (*d*) review by a pathologist inexperienced in the diagnosis of acute and healed arteritis.

The false-negative error rate for unilateral temporal artery biopsy has previously been estimated at 5–11% (66–68). Hayreh et al. (69) more recently prospectively studied 76 patients who underwent contralateral biopsy due to high clinical suspicion after initially negative biopsy; 7 (9.2%) had evidence of active inflammation in the second biopsy. Boyev et al. (70) reviewed bilateral biopsy results for concordance in 186 cases of suspected GCA. Identical diagnoses were obtained in 176, an overall concordance rate of 97%. Six of the remaining 10 cases had useful biopsy results from each side, all demonstrating discordance (3%); 5 of the 6 were eventually diagnosed with GCA based on clinical evidence. Most (150) of the cases involved bilateral simultaneous biopsies, but 36 were sequential, more directly addressing the issue of the value of a second (contralateral) biopsy after an initially negative one; of these, only 1 (2.8%) showed discordance. Danesh-Meyer et al. (71) performed a similar retrospective study of 91 bilateral biopsies, the majority simultaneous, finding concordance in 90 (99%); it is unclear whether the discordant case involved sequential biopsies. They performed a meta-analysis of previous reports that yielded an overall discordance rate of 4%. Pless et al. (72) reviewed 60 bilateral biopsies, 31 of which were simultaneous, finding discordance in 13.4% overall but only 5% in sequential cases in which the initial result was negative. Hall et al. (73) found a similar rate.

While the overall discordance rate for bilateral biopsies is low (1–3% in the largest series), there is substantial variation, even in major academic institutions with experienced pathologists, with rates as high as 13.4%. In the critical subset of patients who undergo contralateral biopsy after an initially negative result (a sample biased toward the positive based on clinical parameters raising suspicion for GCA), studies with the greatest number of patients suggest a slightly higher discordance (2.8–9.2%), but the difference is small. The data all suggest some degree of increased accuracy from bilateral biopsies, and considering the severe consequences of missed diagnosis, the relatively low risk of procedural complications, and the benefit of biopsy proof in the long-term management of these patients, we consider bilateral biopsy in all cases. Expert opinion varies, however, as to preference for bilateral simultaneous biopsies versus immediate sequential biopsies (with negative initial frozen-section analysis) versus delayed sequential biopsies (with negative initial permanent section analysis) if clinical suspicion for GCA is high.

Therapy

If GCA is suspected, therapy should be instituted immediately, as patients are at high risk for further visual loss in the affected eye, involvement of the fellow eye, and systemic complications of vasculitis, including stroke and myocardial infarction. Initial treatment should not await diagnostic confirmation by temporal artery biopsy. Although chronic systemic corticosteroid therapy has been reported to reduce positive biopsy results in GCA from 60% to 20% (74), delay of 7–10 days has no significant effect on the results, and in some cases active inflammation may be detected after longer therapy (75). High-dose intravenous methylprednisolone at 1 g/day for the first 3–5 days is most often recommended, particularly when the patient is seen in the acute phase, since this mode of therapy produces higher blood levels of medication more rapidly than oral therapy (76,77). As these patients are often elderly with multiple and complex medical problems, we routinely provide inpatient therapy under the supervision of an internist.

Liu et al. (6) reported improvement of visual loss in AAION in 39% of those treated initially with intravenous therapy, compared with 28% in those treated orally alone. Hayreh et al. (78) similarly suggested a better visual outcome with intravenous administration, although Cornblath et al. (79) have raised questions regarding the advantages of this mode of therapy. Oral prednisone at doses of at least 1 mg/kg/day is recommended after intravenous therapy (or initially if the intravenous route is not used) and is tapered slowly, monitoring for control of systemic symptoms and ESR level; therapy is usually maintained for at least 4–6 months, often up to a year. Systemic symptoms typically subside within a week, a response so characteristic that if it is absent, an alternate disease process should be strongly considered. Alternate-day corticosteroid therapy is inadequate for GCA. Hunder et al. (66) compared alternate-day to daily therapy in GCA, finding that both systemic symptoms and ESR were incompletely suppressed on alternate-day therapy; one patient in this treatment group suffered recurrent transient visual loss, while none in the daily groups had similar symptoms.

Some degree of visual recovery in the affected eye may be obtained on therapy but is not generally anticipated. Reports of visual improvement on corticosteroids vary widely with regard to delay to therapy, dosage, and parameters for visual recovery. Aiello et al. (7) reported improvement of vision in 5 of 34 patients (15%), while Liu et al. (6) noted it in 14 of 41 (34%). Foroozan et al. (80) reported improvement in visual acuity in 5 of 39 eyes (13%), although visual fields remained severely constricted. Hayreh et al. (78) studied 114 eyes in 84 patients for evidence of visual improvement, finding only 5 eyes (4%) with both improved visual acuity and central visual field after therapy.

The major goal of therapy, other than prevention of systemic vascular complications, is to prevent contralateral visual loss. Untreated, fellow eye involvement occurs in 50–95% (42,81), often within weeks. With therapy, Aiello et al. (7) found that 2/24 (6.3%) patients with AAION developed such involvement, at 4 days and 1 month after initiation of therapy; Liu et al. (6) detected fellow-eye AAION on therapy in 3 cases. While corticosteroid therapy reduces the risk of further visual loss, it is not uniformly effective (82); breakthrough involvement of an affected eye while on therapy occurred in 9–17% (6,7). Liu et al. (6) found six cases developing AAION while on systemic corticosteroid therapy for systemic symptoms alone, without previous visual loss. The risk of recurrent or contralateral optic nerve involvement with tapering of medications has been reported at 7% (6).

Thrombocytosis in GCA and its possible predisposition to visual loss suggests the possibility that antiplatelet therapy may be of benefit in conjunction with corticosteroids. Nesher et al. (83) reviewed 175 cases with GCA for evidence of cranial ischemic complications (predominantly AION and stroke), comparing those with and without low-dose aspirin therapy for other conditions. At presentation, 3 (8%) of the aspirin-treated cases had cranial ischemic complications, compared with 40 (29%) of the non-aspirin-treated cases ($P = 0.01$). During follow-up of at least 3 months on steroid therapy, cranial ischemic complications developed in 3% of the aspirin-treated cases versus 13% on steroids alone ($P = 0.02$). Further study may confirm a benefit for low-dose aspirin or other antiplatelet therapy in GCA.

Other Vasculitides

Arteritic conditions other than GCA may cause AION, including herpes zoster (84,85), relapsing polychondritis (86,87), rheumatoid arthritis (88,89), Takayasu's arteritis (90), and connective tissue disorders such as periarteritis nodosa, systemic lupus erythematosus (91,92), and allergic granulomatosis (Churg-Strauss angiitis) (93,94). The clinical picture is typically that of sudden unilateral or bilateral visual loss, often central, and sometimes accompanied by pain, with minimal recovery. Fibrinoid necrosis of the arterioles and secondary myelin and axonal loss has been demonstrated in multiple cases (91). Crompton et al. (89) documented necrotizing lymphocytic vasculitis and perivasculitis affecting the posterior ciliary arteries, in a case of AION in rheumatoid arthritis.

Goldstein and Wexler (95) reported the histopathologic findings in a patient with periarteritis nodosa who had sudden bilateral visual loss and pale optic discs. They described mononuclear cell infiltration of the posterior ciliary arteries, necrosis and infiltration of some choroidal arteries, and infiltration and atrophy of the optic nerves. Although the patient was not examined at the time of visual loss, it is likely that the process was a bilateral simultaneous AION. AION has also been described in two patients with Behçet's disease (96) and in a patient with Crohn's disease (97), presumably from posterior ciliary arteritis.

The term ''autoimmune optic neuropathy'' (98,99) has been used to describe patients with nonspecific symptoms of connective tissue disease, frequently insufficient to confirm a specific diagnosis such as lupus, who develop acute optic neuropathy, either anterior or posterior (retrobulbar). The syndrome is atypical for optic neuritis in that pain is not a consistent feature, and visual recovery is variable. Steroid dependence, with improvement on therapy but recurrence on tapering, is common. Immunosuppressive therapy may be required. Histopathologic studies have not been documented, but it has been postulated that vasculitis of the ciliary arteries results in optic nerve ischemia in these cases.

NONARTERITIC ANTERIOR ISCHEMIC OPTIC NEUROPATHY (NAION)

Demographics

Most (94.7%) cases of AION are nonarteritic (1) NAION is the most common acute optic neuropathy in patients over 50 years of age, with an estimated annual incidence in the United States of 2.3–10.2 per 100,000 population (2,100), accounting for at least 6,000 new cases annually. The prevalence of NAION in the Medicare Database has been reported at 0.30% (101). The disease occurs with significantly higher frequency in the white population than in black or Hispanic individuals (2). There is no gender predisposition (1,21,22, 53,102). The mean age at onset in most studies ranges from 57–65 years (1,21,22,102). In the IONDT, mean age was 66 years, probably somewhat biased by the exclusion criterion for patients under 50 (53).

Clinical Presentation

NAION presents with loss of vision occurring over hours to days, often described as blurring, dimness, or cloudiness in the affected region of the visual field, most often inferiorly. Although Hayreh et al. (103) reported that visual loss was most frequently reported upon awakening, this feature was not confirmed in the IONDT (53). NAION typically presents without pain, although some form of periocular discomfort has been reported in 8–12% (21,104,105); in the IONDT, 10% reported minor ocular discomfort (53). In contrast to patients with optic neuritis, those with NAION usually do not report pain with eye movement. Headache and other symptoms associated with GCA are absent. Episodes of transient visual loss as seen in GCA are rare, but vague intermittent symptoms of blurring, shadows, or spots were reported in 5% of patients in the IONDT (53). The initial course may be static, with little or no fluctuation of visual level after initial loss, or progressive, with either episodic, stepwise decrements or steady decline of vision over weeks prior to eventual stabilization. The progressive form has been reported in 22–37% of nonarteritic cases (21,104,106, 107), 29% in a limited group of patients with visual acuity better than 20/64 in the IONDT (53).

NAION usually presents with less severe visual loss than AAION, with visual acuity better than 20/200 in 58–61.2% of patients (21,22,104) (Table 7.1). In the IONDT, 49% had initial visual acuity of at least 20/64, 66% better than 20/200 (53). Color vision loss in NAION tends to parallel visual acuity loss, as opposed to that in optic neuritis, in which color loss is often disproportionately greater than visual acuity loss. Visual field defects in NAION may follow any pattern related to optic nerve damage, but altitudinal loss, usually inferior, occurs in the majority, ranging from 55–80% of reported cases (21,22,104,108,109).

The optic disc edema in NAION may be diffuse or segmental, hyperemic or pale, but pallor occurs less frequently than in the arteritic form. A focal region of more severe swelling is often seen and may display an altitudinal distribution, but it does not consistently correlate with the sector of visual field loss (110). In the IONDT, 25% of patients demonstrated sectoral disc edema (53). Diffuse or focal telangiectasia of the edematous disc (Fig. 7.11) may be present, occasionally prominent enough to resemble a vascular mass (pseudohemangioma) (111). Peripapillary retinal hemorrhages are common, seen in 72% in the IONDT (53). Retinal exudates are unusual, but both soft and hard exudates may

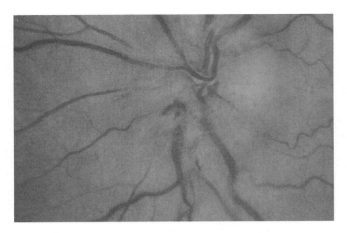

Figure 7.11. Focal optic disc surface vascular telangiectasia in NAION.

occur (7% in the IONDT) (53). A partial or complete macular star pattern of exudate, as seen in neuroretinitis, is occasionally seen (Fig. 7.12). The retinal arterioles are focally narrowed in the peripapillary region (Fig. 7.5) in up to 68% of cases (112). The optic disc in the contralateral eye is typically small in diameter (113,114) and demonstrates a small or absent physiologic cup (31,115–117) (Fig. 7.13A). The disc appearance in such fellow eyes has been described as the "disc at risk," referring to structural crowding of the axons at the level of the cribriform plate, associated mild disc elevation, and disc margin blurring without overt edema (118).

Histopathology and Pathophysiology

NAION is presumed to result from circulatory insufficiency within the optic nerve head, but the specific location of the vasculopathy and its pathogenetic mechanism remain unproven.

Location of Vasculopathy

There has been no definite histopathologic documentation of the vasculopathy resulting in NAION. Implication of both the posterior ciliary arteries and the choroid has been based on indirect evidence. Recent data suggest that vasculopathy within the paraoptic branches of the short posterior ciliary arteries may play a major role.

There are few histopathologically studied cases of typical NAION. Eight cases of nonarteritic optic nerve head infarction have been reported. Three of these cases were atypical forms, associated with internal carotid occlusion, multiple embolic lesions, and severe acute blood loss, rather than classic idiopathic NAION (36,119–124). The short posterior ciliary arteries were described only in an atypical case in which emboli within them produced optic disc infarction, and in which the central retinal and pial arteries were also involved with emboli (121). Tesser et al. indicated that the optic disc infarct studied in their case did not follow a specific vascular territory (124). Knox et al. (125) reported a series of 193 eyes with a histopathologic diagnosis of ischemic optic neuropathy, but those with typical NAION were not identifiable due to lack of clinical information. No confirmation of lipohyalinosis or other occlusive process or inflammation within the optic disc vascular supply was documented in these or other cases. The available evidence does, however, highlight one important fact: the infarctions were predominantly located in the retrolaminar region of the optic nerve head (Fig. 7.14), with extension to the lamina and prelaminar layer in some. This pattern suggests that the vasculopathy responsible for NAION does not lie within the

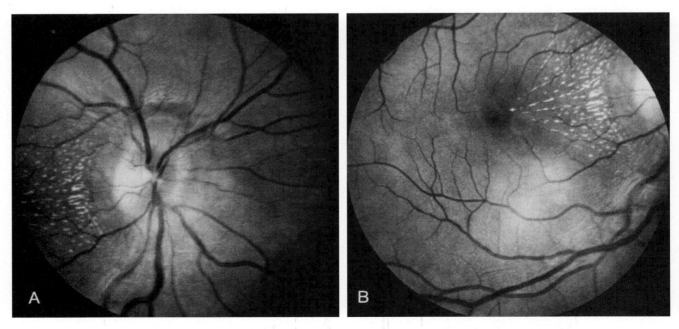

Figure 7.12. AION with partial macular star formation in the papillomacular nerve fiber layer.

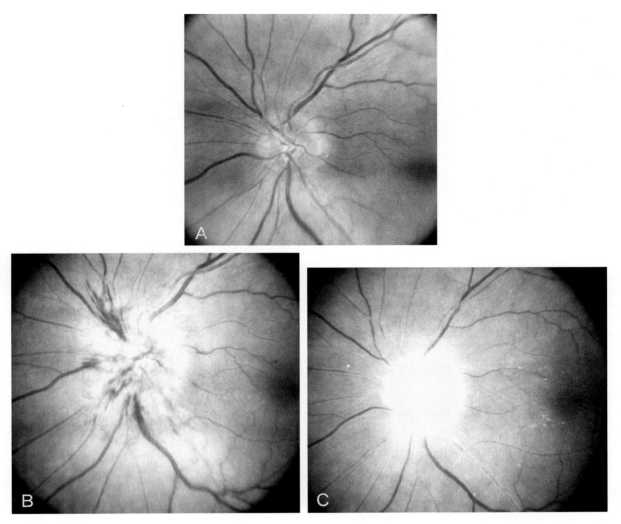

Figure 7.13. Development of optic atrophy after AION. *A,* Appearance of the left optic disc before visual symptoms in the left eye. The patient subsequently developed decreased vision in the left eye associated with an inferior altitudinal field defect. *B,* The left optic disc is swollen and hyperemic. There are numerous flame-shaped, peripapillary, intraretinal hemorrhages. *C,* Two months later, the left optic disc is diffusely pale, the retinal arteries are narrowed, and the nerve fiber layer is no longer visible.

choroidal circulation, since the contribution of the choroid to the optic nerve head vascular supply is to the more anterior laminar and prelaminar layers.

Olver et al. (126) and Onda et al. (127) have demonstrated in autopsy eyes that the optic disc is supplied by a partial or complete vascular circle (corresponding to prior descriptions of the circle of Zinn-Haller) derived from the short posterior ciliary arteries (Fig. 7.15). This vascular supply may demonstrate distinct upper and lower halves consistent with the altitudinal damage of the nerve head commonly seen in NAION. These studies also demonstrated the separation of the paraoptic branches of the short posterior ciliary arteries (optic nerve head supply) from the choroidal branches. Both studies concluded that the choroidal circulation provides only a minor contribution to the optic nerve head blood supply. Although no such studies have been per-

formed specifically in cases of NAION, these data also speak against a substantial role of the choroid in NAION pathogenesis.

In the acute phase of NAION, fluorescein angiography shows delayed filling of the prelaminar layers of the edematous optic disc. This is the most compelling in vivo evidence of optic disc circulatory impairment in NAION (38–40,110). In studies by Arnold and Hepler (110), delayed prelaminar optic disc filling (more than 5 seconds later than choroid and retinal vasculature) was demonstrable in 76% of subjects with acute NAION (Fig. 7.16). This feature was seen in no normal controls or subjects with nonischemic optic disc edema (128), suggesting that the delayed filling represents a primary ischemic process rather than a mechanical process secondary to obstruction from the disc edema itself. The overlying disc surface vasculature, derived from the retinal

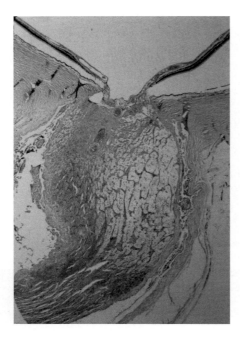

Figure 7.14. Histopathology of AION. Infarct is located in the retrolaminar portion of the optic nerve. (Courtesy of David L. Knox, MD)

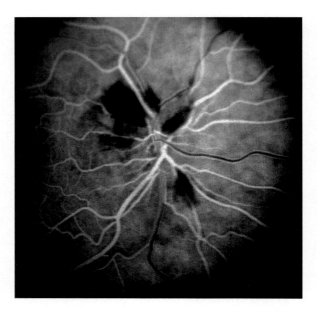

Figure 7.16. Fluorescein angiography in NAION. Optic disc filling is delayed.

arterial circulation, showed sectoral dilation and early fluorescein filling (Fig. 7.17) in 54% of cases (110). It has been postulated that this focal vascular dilation, may be analogous to the "luxury perfusion" seen at the junction of perfused and nonperfused regions in cerebral infarctions and could

be a manifestation of shunting to relatively spared regions of the disc in NAION (110,118,129).

Arnold and Hepler (110) and Siatkowski et al. (25) both found that segmental parapapillary choroidal filling delay (more than 5 seconds) was not a consistent feature in NAION (Fig. 7.18) (46%, versus 58% in normal controls). Additionally, segments of disc and adjacent choroidal filling were poorly correlated; disc filling delay was commonly seen adjacent to normally filling choroidal segments, and vice versa. Similar findings have been reported with indocyanine green

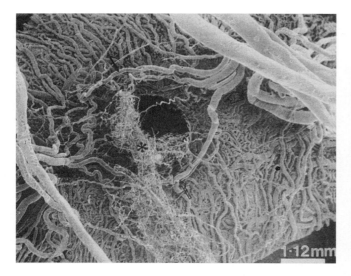

Figure 7.15. Scanning electron photomicrograph of the vasculature of the posterior globe. Superior and inferior anastomoses from the medial and lateral short posterior ciliary arteries suggest a possible anatomic correlation for the altitudinal pattern of optic nerve damage in NAION. (From Olver JM, Spalton DJ, McCartney ACE. Microvascular study of the retrolaminar optic nerve in man: the possible significance in anterior ischemic optic neuropathy. Eye 1990;4:7–24.)

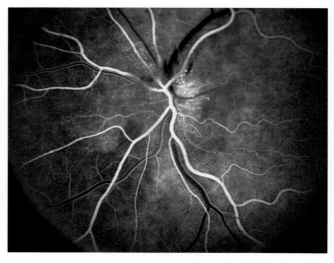

Figure 7.17. Segmental early hyperfluorescence in NAION, correlating with focal disc surface telangiectasia. (From Arnold AC, Hepler RS. Fluorescein angiography in acute anterior ischemic optic neuropathy. Am J Ophthalmol 1994;177:222–230.)

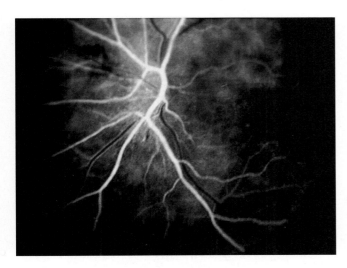

Figure 7.18. Normal parapapillary choroidal filling in NAION. Optic disc filling is delayed. (From Arnold AC, Hepler RS. Fluorescein angiography in acute anterior ischemic optic neuropathy. Am J Ophthalmol 1994;177:222–230.)

(ICG) studies of the choroidal flow, which show substantial slowing in AAION but not in NAION (130,131). These data speak against a proximal vascular occlusion in the short posterior ciliary arteries, which would produce delay in both optic disc and choroidal filling, and against a choroidal origin, which would produce consistently delayed choroidal filling. They are consistent with flow impairment at the level of the paraoptic branches of the short posterior ciliary arteries described by Olver et al. (126) and Onda et al. (127).

The significance of the location of the optic disc within the choroidal watershed zone between territories supplied by the posterior ciliary artery branches has been controversial (110,132–136). Hayreh (135,136) reported its presence in a substantial number of patients with NAION; he suggested that with impaired perfusion pressure within the distribution of a posterior ciliary artery, such a disc is at risk for infarction. Arnold and Hepler (110), however, reported significant (more than 5 seconds) delayed filling of a vertical watershed zone encompassing at least a quadrant of the optic disc in 42% of normal controls versus 27% of patients with NAION. Filling of the optic disc located within these zones, either in normals or in NAION, did not correlate with adjacent choroidal filling, again consistent with a separate source of flow to the optic disc (i.e., the paraoptic branches of the short posterior ciliary arteries). While impaired flow within the posterior ciliary artery system might produce hypoperfusion of the disc, the data suggest that distal flow impairment within the paraoptic branches is the critical feature, rather than disc location within a watershed zone.

Although carotid occlusive disease occasionally results in optic nerve ischemia, most often in the setting of more general ocular ischemia and occasionally with associated cerebral ischemia, the vast majority of cases of NAION are unrelated to carotid disease. Fry et al. (137) performed carotid duplex scans in 15 patients with NAION, 11 with transient monocular blindness (TMB), and 30 age-matched controls. Mean stenosis was not significantly worse in NAION patients (19%) than controls (9%), while those with TMB demonstrated a significantly worse mean of 77%. Two of 15 patients with NAION had stenosis of more than 30%, compared with 5 of 30 controls and 10 of 11 with TMB. Muller et al. (138) did not find hemodynamically significant stenosis in any of 17 subjects with NAION.

Pathogenetic Mechanism

The mechanisms involved in the development of optic disc ischemia in NAION similarly remain unclear. Whether ischemia results from local arteriosclerosis with or without thrombosis, embolization from a remote source, generalized hypoperfusion, vasospasm, failure of autoregulation, or some combination of these processes is not known. While structurally small, "crowded" optic discs are associated with NAION, the mechanism by which this contributes to ischemia has not been elucidated. The role of additional factors such as nocturnal hypotension and sleep apnea is unproven. Multiple risk factors for vasculopathy and coagulopathy have been associated with NAION, but conclusive large-scale epidemiologic studies have not been performed.

No studies have documented features of the optic disc vasculature in NAION in a systematic way. As noted above, isolated histopathologic studies have commented on the lack of inflammation within the visible vessels within the disc. Emboli have rarely been documented. No studies of the short posterior ciliary vessels have been performed to assess for arteriosclerotic change or thrombosis.

VASOSPASM AND IMPAIRED AUTOREGULATION

Whatever the cause for impaired blood flow in the optic nerve vasculature, persistent hypoperfusion may require impairment in the normal autoregulatory mechanisms of the optic nerve head. Flow is normally maintained constant with variations in perfusion pressure, intraocular pressure, and metabolic conditions (including tissue oxygen and CO_2 levels) by factors that vary resistance to flow. Autonomic input to vessels and vasoactive substances (e.g., vasoconstrictor, endothelins [ET], and vasodilator, nitric oxide) released in response to metabolic influences or mechanical deformation of vascular smooth muscle contribute to the regulation of blood flow in response to these external influences. These autoregulatory mechanisms may be reduced by arteriosclerosis, vasospasm, or medications, including beta-blockers and other antihypertensive medications. Intravenous and intravitreal infusions of ET-1 in rabbits have resulted in decreased optic nerve head blood flow. Strenn et al. (139) showed a decrease in blood flow measured by laser Doppler flowmetry (LDF) after ET-1 administration, reversed by the calcium channel blocker nifedipine. Oku et al. (140) produced chronic optic disc ischemia in rabbits by repeated intravitreal injections of ET-1.

Hayreh (141,142) has postulated that endogenous serotonin, released with platelet aggregation stimulated at atherosclerotic plaque, may play a role in the development of ischemic optic nerve damage via its role in vasoconstriction of arterioles and resultant impaired autoregulation, possibly mediated by endothelial-derived vasoactive agents, including endothelins. He has reported serotonin-induced vasoconstriction in the central retinal artery and posterior cerebral arteries in atherosclerotic monkeys, reversed by discontinuing the atherogenic diet (141).

DISC STRUCTURE

The optic discs in patients with NAION are typically small in diameter, with small or absent cups, suggesting that "crowding" plays a role in pathogenesis, although the precise mechanism remains unclear (113–117). The discs in AAION are usually normal in diameter and cup size (113); more severe vasculopathy in GCA probably is responsible for the development of ischemia without the contribution of disc crowding. Possible contributory mechanical effects of structural crowding in NAION include:

1. Chronic mechanical obstruction to axoplasmic flow, with resultant intracellular axonal swelling, particularly at the most crowded region, the cribriform plate
2. Secondary compression and further microcirculatory compromise in the laminar region due to additional axoplasmic stasis from subclinical ischemia created by basic vasculopathy
3. Decreased return of neurotrophins due to mechanical axoplasmic flow obstruction after ischemia, with resultant additional ganglion cell death
4. Abnormally stiff (less compliant) cribriform plate in addition to small size, and exaggerating factors 1–3

The structure of the optic disc as a relatively inflexible region encompassing the axons of the optic nerve has been implicated in two histopathologic studies. Tesser et al. (124) reported that the infarct documented in their case did not follow a specific vascular territory, suggesting a compartment syndrome as a mechanism. Knox et al. (125) reviewed the histopathologic features in 193 eyes classified as having optic nerve ischemia (without clinical correlation) in the Eye Pathology Laboratory of the Wilmer Eye Institute and accessioned from 1951–1998. Sixty-nine eyes (36%) demonstrated cavernous degeneration within the laminar region. Those cases in which there was substantial compression of the adjacent axons by the expanding mucopolysaccharide cavern (Fig. 7.19) lend support to the compartment syndrome as a mechanism in at least a portion of NAION cases.

NOCTURNAL HYPOTENSION

It is clear that acute severe systemic hypotension, particularly associated with anemia, can produce optic nerve ischemia (see below). Hayreh has proposed that less severe nocturnal systemic hypotension may play a role in the development of NAION, stating that the relative hypotension that normally occurs with sleep may chronically compromise optic disc circulation, particularly in patients with an exaggerated nocturnal "dip" or in patients, such as those with systemic hypertension, in whom optic disc circulation auto-

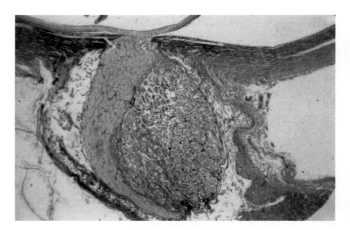

Figure 7.19. Cavernous degeneration in infarct of the optic nerve in NAION. Note the distortion of the adjacent axons. (From Knox DL, Kerrison JB, Green WR. Histopathologic studies of ischemic optic neuropathy. Trans Am Ophth Soc 2000;98:203–222.)

regulatory mechanisms are impaired (103,143). This effect might be worsened with aggressive antihypertensive therapy, particularly if administered at night, by exacerbating the nocturnal pressure drop. Hayreh et al. (103) performed 24-hour ambulatory blood pressure monitoring in 52 subjects with NAION, compared with 19 cases of primary open angle glaucoma (POAG) and 65 cases of normal tension glaucoma (NTG). Mean decreases in systolic and diastolic blood pressure of 25.3% and 31.2%, respectively, were noted in NAION. As no controls were monitored, it remains unclear whether this represents an exaggerated nocturnal drop in pressure. In general, no significant differences in pressure decrease were observed among NAION, NTG, and POAG; however, the 31.2% diastolic decrease in NAION was significantly less ($P = 0.004$) than the 36.0% figure for NTG. In patients with NAION with systemic hypertension on medication, nighttime blood pressure figures were significantly lower in those with visual field deterioration (progressive NAION, 25 of 42 patients). A subsequent report (143) from these authors included a total of 114 NAION, 131 NTG, and 30 POAG subjects, presumably incorporating the prior study. From the total data, the authors implied that nocturnal systemic hypotension played a significant role in the development of NAION in certain susceptible subjects.

In contrast, Landau et al. (144) performed 24-hour ambulatory blood pressure monitoring in 24 subjects with NAION and 24 age-, disease-, and medication-matched controls. Mean decreases of 11% systolic and 18% diastolic were measured in NAION, compared with 13% and 18%, respectively, in controls, showing no significant difference. They did, however, see mildly lower mean daytime pressures in NAION than controls, averaging 5–7 mm Hg; the largest difference was noted in the morning, indicating a slower morning rise in pressure in NAION subjects when compared with normal controls. The conflicting data from these two groups leave the role of nocturnal hypotension in NAION unresolved (145,146). We do, however, discuss with our patients and their physicians the possible accentuation of nocturnal hypotension by nighttime use of antihypertension medications; consideration of dosing other than at bedtime is recommended.

SLEEP APNEA SYNDROME

The sleep apnea syndrome (SAS) has been associated in some cases with optic disc edema, presumably the result of occult elevations in intracranial pressure. Occasional optic nerve damage was documented, but whether it resulted from chronic papilledema, the hypoxemia of SAS, or both was unclear. In 1998, Mojon et al. (147) reported seven patients with SAS evaluated for visual field loss, finding four with arcuate defects; all patients had normal optic disc appearance. In 2002, these authors compared 17 consecutively seen NAION patients to 17 age- and sex-matched controls for evidence of SAS (148). Diagnostic criteria for SAS were met in 71% of the NAION patients versus 18% of controls. Additionally, elevation of C-reactive protein, increasingly implicated as a predictor for cardiovascular disease, has been associated with SAS. Shamsuzzaman et al. (149) suggested that the chronic hypoxia occurring with repeated apneic episodes stimulates C-reactive protein. These studies are preliminary and involve small patient numbers, with insufficient data from which to draw conclusions.

VASCULOPATHIC AND COAGULOPATHIC RISK FACTORS

NAION has been reported in association with many conditions that may predispose to decreased optic nerve head perfusion via microvascular occlusion. Several cross-sectional case series have estimated the prevalence of systemic diseases that might predispose to vasculopathy in patients with NAION (1,21,22,53,102,150–152). Systemic hypertension was documented in 34–49.4% of patients (47% in the IONDT) (53); however, in several of the studies that compared these figures to matched population data from the National Health Survey, statistical significance was reached only in the younger age group, 45–64 years (1,22). Hayreh et al. (102), in contrast, found a significantly increased prevalence in all age groups. Diabetes was reported in 5–25.3% (24% in the IONDT) (53), with statistically significant increased prevalence in all ages in all but one study. Diabetes was associated with the development of NAION at a younger age in most series as well. In these series, the association of NAION with other cardiovascular events such as stroke and myocardial infarction was inconsistent. While the incidence of prior or subsequent cerebrovascular or cardiovascular events was not increased in the reports of Boghen and Glaser (21) or Repka et al. (22), Guyer et al. (1) found both events were more common than in the normal population, and in the studies of Hayreh et al. (102) and Sawle et al. (152), late cerebrovascular disease was increased.

Some investigators have identified an association between subcortical and periventricular white matter lesions observed with magnetic resonance (MR) imaging (as a marker for small vessel cerebrovascular disease) and NAION. Patients with hypertension, diabetes mellitus, cardiovascular disease, and cerebrovascular disease have an increased prevalence of such lesions, which are believed to represent focal perivascular ischemic demyelination and gliosis (153,154). Jay and Williamson (155) found no such association in 9 patients with NAION compared with 11 controls, but Arnold et al. (156) reported a significant increased number of lesions in 13 NAION patients compared with 16 controls. Both studies suffered from small sample size and questionable statistical analyses, and no firm conclusions regarding this possible association can be drawn.

Recent studies have addressed additional vasculopathic risk factors. Jacobson et al. (157) performed a case-control study in NAION, addressing hypertension and diabetes along with smoking and hypercholesterolemia in 51 patients compared with two separate control groups. While hypertension was found in 57% of patients, it was not found to be significantly more prevalent than controls in any age group; however, diabetes, found in 34%, was a significant risk factor in all age groups. Neither hypercholesterolemia nor smoking demonstrated significant risk. The 61-patient case-control study of Salomon et al. (158) also confirmed diabetes but not hypertension as a risk factor; hypercholesterolemia was found to be significant, while smoking was not. Two other case-control studies of risk factors (159,160) have addressed the issues of hyperlipidemia and smoking; hypercholesterolemia was a significant risk in both, while hypertriglyceridemia and smoking were linked in a limited number studied. A large-scale (137 cases) but uncontrolled study by Chung et al. (161) concluded that smoking was a significant risk factor on the basis that smokers developed NAION at a significantly younger age than nonsmokers. Deramo et al. (162) recently reported a series of 37 patients with NAION presenting before the age of 50, in which mean serum cholesterol level was significantly elevated when compared with age- and gender-matched controls (235.4 versus 204.0 mg/dL).

Elevated plasma homocysteine levels have been associated with an increased risk of premature ischemic events (peripheral vascular disease, stroke, myocardial infarction) in patients younger than 50. The prevalence of hyperhomocysteinemia in the general population is estimated at 5%, a figure that increases to 20–30% in nondiabetic stroke or myocardial infarction patients younger than 55. The mechanism of vasculopathy related to hyperhomocysteinemia is unclear. While some severe cases are related to an inherited deficiency of methylenetetrahydrofolate reductase (MTHFR), resulting in decreased conversion of homocysteine to methionine, in others, poor intake or absorption of common vitamins B6, B12, and folic acid may impair the breakdown of homocysteine.

Reports have linked central retinal artery and vein occlusion in younger patients to elevated blood levels of homocysteine, but the relation to NAION remains unclear. Kawasaki et al. (163) reported hyperhomocysteinemia in 2/17 cases of NAION under age 50, while Biousse et al. (164) reported normal values in 14/14 patients with a mean age of 43 years. Pianka et al. (165) reported elevated levels in 45% of 40 NAION patients (mean age 66 years) versus 9.8% of controls, and Weger et al. (166) also reported mean elevation (11.8 versus 9.8 μmol/L) in 59 NAION patients versus controls. The clinical significance of these statistically significant findings is uncertain, limited by small patient numbers and widely varying results (0/14 in Biousse et al. [164] to 45% in Pianka et al. [165]).

Isolated reports have documented prothrombotic risk factors in patients with NAION, but a larger-scale recent study by Salomon et al. (158) has not confirmed an association. They evaluated risk factors for thrombosis, including lupus anticoagulants, anticardiolipin antibodies, prothrombotic polymorphisms (factor V Leiden), and deficiencies of protein C and S and antithrombin III in a series of 61 patients with NAION versus 90 controls. No correlation with any of these factors was detected. Similarly, Salomon et al. (167) found no association of angiotensin-converting enzyme and angiotensin II type 1 receptor polymorphisms with NAION. Salomon et al. (168) recently compared 92 consecutive patients with NAION to 145 controls for evidence of platelet glycoprotein polymorphisms. They found a statistically significant association with the VNTR B allele in NAION versus controls; second eye involvement was more frequent and earlier in onset in those with the polymorphism. These data suggest that previously undetected prothrombotic conditions may be linked to the development of NAION; further investigation is required to definitively establish these and other associations.

OTHER ASSOCIATIONS

NAION has been associated infrequently with a multitude of additional factors and disorders that may be causative, either due to optic disc structure or other features that might affect optic disc perfusion pressure. These include hyperopia, optic disc drusen, elevated intraocular pressure, cataract surgery, migraine, embolism, and medications.

NAION in patients with optic disc drusen has been described in anecdotal reports (169–173). Purvin et al. (174) recently reviewed the clinical presentation in 24 eyes of 20 patients with NAION occurring in the presence of optic disc drusen. No unusual features were present aside from the substantially lower age group involved (mean 49.4 years, range 18–69). Vasculopathic risk factors were present in 50%. While it is reasonable to attribute early development of NAION in this patient group to an exaggerated contribution of optic disc "crowding" due to the drusen, it remains unclear as to why it remains a relatively rare occurrence.

Some investigators have reported an association of elevated intraocular pressure (IOP) and glaucoma with NAION (175–178). Tomsak and Remler (176) described five patients with "discs at risk" who had mild elevations of IOP at the time they developed NAION. Katz et al. (177) determined that the mean peak diurnal IOP was greater in a group of 16 NAION patients compared with 15 controls. These authors suggested that since perfusion pressure in the optic nerve is a balance between systemic blood pressure and IOP, a transient rise in IOP could result in ischemia to the optic nerve head from a fall in perfusion pressure below some critical level.

More recent and larger-scale investigations have not confirmed this association. Kalenak et al. (179) found no difference in IOP between 45 NAION patients and 45 controls. Hayreh et al. (143) performed IOP diurnal curves on patients with open angle glaucoma, normal tension glaucoma, and NAION and found no IOP elevation in the NAION patients compared with the other two groups. Chung et al. (161) found a mean IOP of 16.2 mm Hg in 137 patients with NAION, a value no higher than that expected in the general population; only 11 (8%) patients had a documented IOP above 21 mm Hg. The role of chronically elevated IOP in the pathogenesis of NAION hence remains unclear.

The role of acute elevation of IOP has also been considered. Slavin and Margulis (180) described a case of NAION 2.5 weeks following angle closure attacks in each eye. Arnold et al. (181) reported a case of NAION 1 week following ocular pneumoplethysmography, in which IOP is transiently elevated to levels near 130 mm Hg. Lee et al. (182) reported four cases of optic neuropathy associated with laser in situ keratomileusis (LASIK), in which IOP may be elevated up to 230 mm Hg during the vacuum phase. Two showed optic disc edema and two did not; all noted visual loss within hours to 3 days after the procedure and developed subsequent optic atrophy without visual recovery. The patients were presumed to have suffered ischemic optic neuropathy. Cameron et al. (183) described a patient who developed bilateral optic neuropathy after LASIK, although the clinical features may have represented a glaucomatous process. These cases are few in number, particularly in view of the large volume of LASIK procedures performed, and a definite causal association has not been established.

Two patients described by Gartner (184) developed an anterior optic neuropathy within 2 weeks of cataract surgery. Hayreh (185) described 11 patients who developed anterior optic neuropathy within 1–3 weeks after uncomplicated cataract extraction. Hayreh suggested that the condition may occur from a rise in IOP in the immediate postoperative period, but this concept was challenged by Serrano et al. (186), who reported several cases in which there was no evidence of increased IOP during or after surgery. A case of NAION developing after secondary intraocular lens implant has also been reported (187). McCulley et al. (188) reviewed 5,787 cases of cataract extraction over a 5-year period, finding 3 cases of NAION occurring within 1 year of the procedure (29, 36, and 117 days), an estimated 6-month incidence of 51.8/100,000, significantly higher than the reported overall incidence. Two of the three patients had prior NAION in the fellow eye, and as did Hayreh, the authors suggested that there may be an increased risk for NAION after cataract surgery in the second eye. The association of NAION and cataract extraction was supported by a subsequent study by McCulley et al. (189), in which the temporal association of 18 cases of NAION occurring within 1 year following cataract surgery was compared with a uniform distribution; the finding that all 18 cases occurred within 6 months after surgery was statistically significant for an association.

NAION occurs in patients with migraine and, as in those with optic disc drusen, tends to develop at an earlier age. No systematic study has been performed, but reported patients were predominantly below age 50 at onset, many in their 20s (190–193). Visual loss occurred during or immediately following an episode of cephalgia. The mechanism of vasculopathy has been postulated to be vasospasm. Katz and Bamford (192) and Kupersmith et al. (194) suggested that beta-blocking agents may potentiate this vasospastic effect in patients with complicated migraine, recommending avoidance of this class of drugs in this patient group.

Embolism to the optic disc blood supply is felt to contribute only rarely to the development of NAION. As the microvasculature of this region is supplied by both the short posterior ciliary artery and choroidal systems and is not primarily an end-arterial circulation, as is the retinal vasculature, it is likely that extensive embolization would be required for significant optic nerve damage. Confirmation of embolic NAION is dependent upon histopathologic study or evidence of simultaneous retinal embolization and NAION. A small number of case reports have confirmed its rare occurrence (121,195–197).

Two medications have been associated with the development of NAION (interferon-alpha and sildenafil), although the number of cases is insufficient to confirm a definite causative effect. A third, amiodarone, has been linked to NAION but probably produces a toxic optic neuropathy that mimics it.

Interferon-alpha is a glycoprotein with antiviral, antitumor, and antiangiogenic effects used as adjuvant therapy for malignancies, including melanoma, leukemia, and lymphoma, and for chronic hepatitis C. Ischemic retinopathy has been described with its use (198). Several reports (199–203) confirm the development of NAION, usually bilateral, sequential, and temporally associated with the institution of interferon therapy; recurrences with restarting the medication have also been described. The clinical course is variable, with some patients showing improvement with discontinuance of therapy. Possible pathogenetic mechanisms include interferon-induced systemic hypotension or immune complex deposition within the optic disc circulation.

Sildenafil is a commonly used therapy for erectile dysfunction that may produce systemic hypotension; the therapeutic dose may reduce systemic blood pressure by at least 10 mm Hg. Pomeranz et al. (204) reviewed the five cases of NAION reported in association with the use of sildenafil through 2002 (205,206). The patients ranged in age from 42–69, and four had no known vasculopathic risk factors. The optic discs in each case showed the typical "crowded" configuration commonly seen in NAION; one patient had prior NAION in the fellow eye. The onset of visual loss was within 3 hours of medication use in three cases. The postulated mechanism in these cases has been systemic hypotension in patients with structurally predisposed optic discs, possibly complicated by an exaggerated nocturnal dip in blood pressure. While the number of cases is extremely small, particularly considering the widespread use of the drug, the authors suggest that the drug may be contraindicated in patients with prior NAION, and that this group of patients should be counseled regarding the risk of developing NAION with further use. Additional data are required for definitive recommendations in this regard.

Amiodarone is in widespread use as a cardiac antiarrhythmic agent and has been associated with the development of optic neuropathy (207–213). Macaluso et al. (214) summarized the data from 73 patients, including 16 published case reports and 57 patients with information recorded in the National Registry of Drug-Induced Ocular Side Effects, with optic neuropathy associated with amiodarone use. They emphasized that these patients with significant cardiovascular disease have risk factors for NAION and that many cases of optic neuropathy with amiodarone use may be typical NAION unrelated to the drug. A syndrome more consistent with medication toxicity, including insidious bilateral onset, generalized rather than altitudinal visual field loss, and chronic optic disc edema persisting months after onset of visual loss, was suggested as more likely to represent the optic neuropathy related to amiodarone use. Limited visual recovery occurred in most cases after discontinuance of medication. Ultrastructural study of the optic nerves after amiodarone use has shown evidence of impaired axoplasmic flow, possibly responsible for chronic metabolic optic disc dysfunction and swelling (215). Nagra et al. (216) reported three cases in which optic disc edema persisted more than 4 months after discontinuing the medication, with slow, partial recovery of visual field loss. The small number of cases precludes definitive conclusions; it remains to be seen whether, as in the case of certain antineoplastic agents such as cisplatinum and BCNU, there may be a medication-induced microvasculopathy—hence an amiodarone-induced NAION.

CELLULAR MECHANISMS

Recent advances in the understanding of ischemic central nervous system damage have raised new questions regarding the pathogenesis of neuronal damage in both the arteritic and nonarteritic forms of AION (217). Neurotrophin deprivation in retinal ganglion cells after ischemic insult may play a significant role in cell death (218,219). Secondary neuronal degeneration in cells adjacent to infarcted tissue may develop as a result of a toxic environment produced by the dying cells (220). Such deterioration may be mediated by processes including excitatory amino acid (especially glutamate) toxicity, bursts of reactive oxygen species (including lipid peroxidation), intracellular calcium influx, and apoptosis (221–223). Experimental models of optic nerve injury have been shown to be associated with elevated levels of glutamate in the overlying vitreous (224). Levin et al. (123) have shown evidence of apoptosis in the ganglion cells in a case of NAION. Thus, ischemia-induced cell death may result in release of glutamate, with further cell damage and death by excitotoxic induction of apoptosis. The specific role each of these mechanisms may play in the development and clinical course of AION, however, remains unproven.

A unique animal model for optic nerve ischemia, which may provide a means to further study these aspects, has recently been developed in rodents. Bernstein et al. (225) selectively thrombosed the surface microvascular supply of the optic nerve, using a photoablative technique. After intravenous infusion of the photosensitizing agent rose bengal, the optic nerve was exposed to a laser source, producing photoactivation of the intravascular agent, with selective damage of the endothelium by the superoxide radicals created in the exposed region, with resultant thrombosis. Cellular responses, including alterations in ganglion cell histopathology, retinal gene and protein expression, were studied and are consistent with other models of ischemic neuronal injury. While the mechanism of production of ischemic injury in this model differs from typical NAION, it nevertheless provides insight into the cellular mechanisms involved with ischemic damage to ganglion cells and may be instrumental in testing future hypotheses for neuroprotective therapy in NAION.

Clinical Course

Untreated, NAION generally remains stable, most cases showing no significant improvement or deterioration over time (21,22,104,106–108,152,226,227). Even in the so-called progressive form, further deterioration after reaching the low point of visual function within 1–2 months is rare (21,228–230). Recent studies, however, indicate that spontaneous improvement of visual acuity is not unusual. Recovery of at least 3 Snellen acuity lines has been reported in 13% (152) to 42.7% (in the IONDT [231]) of patients (104,106,107,152), including up to 30.3% of those considered progressive (107,229,232). Visual acuity at 6 months was 20/200 or worse in 52% of the randomized (initial visual acuity 20/64 or worse) patients in the IONDT (231). Other studies, which include patients with better initial acuity, have reported 31–41% of patients with final visual acuity 20/200 or worse and 21–53% of patients having vision 20/200 or better (21,22,106,108,109,233). Limited quantitative visual field studies regarding the natural history of NAION are available. Arnold and Hepler (106) confirmed a 24% rate of improvement in mean sensitivity by at least 2 dB; perimetric data from the IONDT are under analysis.

After stabilization of vision, usually within 2 months, recurrent or progressive visual loss in an affected eye is extremely unusual and should prompt evaluation for another cause of optic neuropathy. Repka et al. (22) reported recurrent episodes in only 3 of 83 (3.6%) patients. Hayreh (234) reviewed 829 eyes in 594 consecutive patients with NAION for evidence of recurrent events in the same eye occurring at least 2 months after initial onset. Recurrence was documented in only 53 eyes (6.4%). A syndrome of recurrent episodes in young patients, often below age 35, has been described by several authors (232,235,236). In the study by Hayreh et al. (234), however, the greatest number of patients with recurrence were 45–64 years of age.

The optic disc becomes visibly atrophic, either in a sectoral (Fig. 7.20) or diffuse pattern (Fig. 7.21), usually within 4–6 weeks. Persistence of edema past this point should prompt consideration of an alternate diagnosis. Eventual involvement of the contralateral eye has been reported in 24% (24) to 39% (237), with varying follow-up (22,42,233). Beck et al. (238), however, systematically reviewed 431 patients with NAION, finding a substantially lower 5-year risk of 12–19%. Similarly, in the IONDT (239), the only large study with prospective follow-up, fellow-eye involvement at a me-

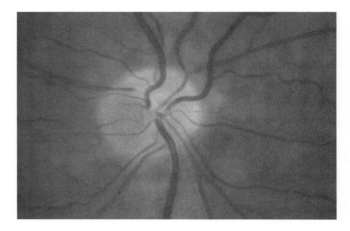

Figure 7.20. Sectoral optic atrophy after NAION.

dian follow-up of 5 years was 14.7%. A history of diabetes and baseline visual acuity of 20/200 or worse in the study eye, but not age, sex, aspirin use, or smoking were significantly associated with new NAION in the fellow eye.

Comparisons of the degree of optic nerve dysfunction and visual loss between the two involved eyes in bilateral cases have been inconclusive. Boone et al. (233) found similar degrees of loss, while WuDunn et al. (237) did not. The IONDT found second-eye visual acuity within three lines of the first in approximately half of patients (239). Final fellow-eye visual acuity was significantly worse in those patients with new fellow-eye NAION whose baseline study eye visual acuity was 20/200 or worse.

Occurrence in the second eye produces the clinical appearance of the "pseudo-Foster Kennedy syndrome," in which the previously affected disc is atrophic and the currently involved nerve head is edematous (Fig. 7.22). Significantly impaired visual function in the eye with disc edema distinguishes this condition from the true Foster Kennedy syndrome, in which disc edema is due to elevated intracranial pressure and therefore does not produce visual loss acutely in the edematous eye.

Differential Diagnosis

NAION must be differentiated from idiopathic optic neuritis, syphilitic or sarcoid-related optic nerve inflammation, particularly in patients under 50 years of age; infiltrative optic neuropathies, anterior orbital lesions producing optic nerve compression; and idiopathic forms of optic disc edema, including diabetic papillopathy. Optic neuritis may resemble ischemia with regard to rate of onset, pattern of visual field loss, and optic disc appearance; however, in most cases, the patient's younger age, pain with eye movement, and character of the disc edema (diffuse and hyperemic without hemorrhages, rather than pale or segmental) make distinction clear. Occasionally, ancillary testing such as fluorescein angiography, ultrasonography, or MR imaging of the optic nerve may be helpful in differentiation. Fluorescein angiography often shows delayed optic disc filling in optic

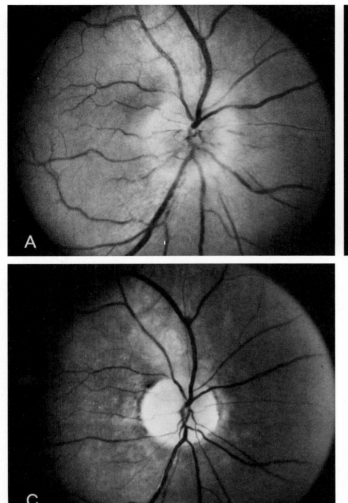

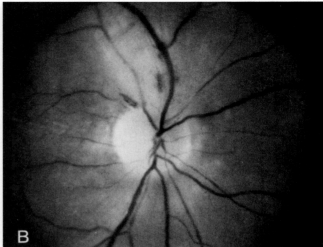

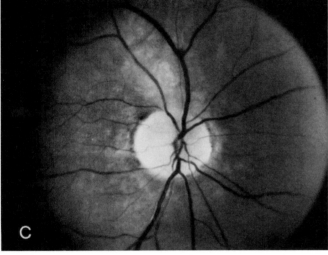

Figure 7.21. Resolution of anterior ischemic optic neuropathy. *A,* In the acute phase of visual loss, the left optic disc is hyperemic and swollen. *B,* Two weeks after the onset of visual loss, the temporal portion of the disc has become pale. The nasal disc is still slightly swollen, and there are a few small, nerve fiber layer hemorrhages. Note the apparent narrowing of retinal arteries and arterioles. *C,* Two months after visual loss, the disc is generally pale, with loss of the nerve fiber layer and apparent narrowing of retinal arteries and arterioles.

disc ischemia, whereas filling is normal in papillitis (240). Ultrasonography and MR imaging are typically normal in NAION. Intraorbital optic nerve swelling and enhancement are frequently seen on MR with inflammation and infiltration. Increased optic nerve diameter and a positive 30-degree test for perineural fluid may be seen on ultrasound in optic nerve inflammation. Optic nerve inflammation associated with syphilis or sarcoidosis often is associated with other intraocular inflammatory signs, which should prompt further testing. Orbital lesions producing disc edema usually are associated with gradually progressive visual loss, but occasionally onset is more rapid. The detection of subtle signs of orbital disease, including mild proptosis, lid or eye movement abnormalities, or the persistence of optic disc edema past the usual 4–6 weeks in NAION, may indicate the need to perform neuroimaging to detect orbital inflammation or tumor (such as optic nerve sheath meningioma). In the great majority of cases, however, such testing is not required. Diabetic papillopathy typically does not produce a significant afferent pupillary defect or visual field loss (discussed later).

Diagnostic Testing

In patients with a typical presentation of NAION, without symptoms or signs to suggest GCA, and with normal ESR and C-reactive protein levels, we do not routinely perform additional testing. Evaluation by a primary care physician for evidence and control of risk factors such as hypertension, diabetes, and hyperlipidemia is essential. Neuroimaging is not performed unless the patient presents with substantial pain or follows an atypical course, such as prolonged optic disc edema or continued progressive or recurrent visual loss more than 2 months after initial presentation. The value of additional testing for vasculopathic and prothrombotic risk factors remains unclear. Carotid studies are not routinely performed unless prominent pain or other signs of orbital ischemia are present (see above). For NAION in the typical age group, we do not routinely assess homocysteine levels, but in patients under 50, we proceed with this testing since elevated levels are amenable to therapy. We do not test for prothrombotic risk factors unless there is other evidence of personal or familial thrombosis, and we do not screen for

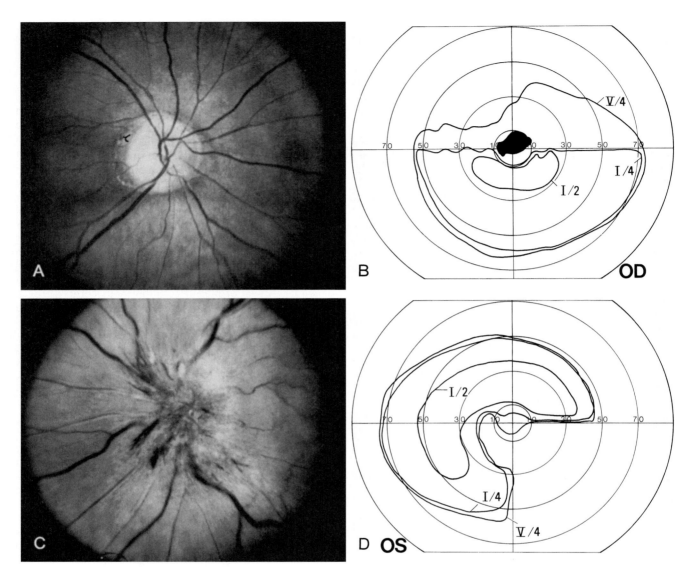

Figure 7.22.   Pseudo-Foster Kennedy syndrome in a patient with bilateral, nonsimultaneous AION. *A,* The right optic disc is pale, and the arteries are narrowed. *B,* The right visual field shows a relative, superior altitudinal defect with a central scotoma. *C,* The left optic disc is hyperemic and swollen with numerous superficial retinal hemorrhages and several soft exudates. *D,* The left visual field shows a complete, inferior arcuate defect. The patient gave a history of sudden visual loss in the right eye followed 3 months later by sudden visual loss in the left eye. Visual acuity was 20/400 in the right eye and 20/50 in the left eye.

vasculitides other than GCA unless there is clinical evidence for them. In patients with substantial hyperhomocysteinemia, we recommend vitamin supplementation (B6, B12, folic acid) and continued monitoring for evidence of systemic vasculopathy by an internist, although the value of lowering homocysteine levels for reduction of vascular events is unproven. A large-scale international study (Vitamins to Prevent Stroke [VITATOPS] [241]) is in progress to evaluate the effect of such multivitamin therapy in reducing the risk of stroke and other serious vascular events in hyperhomocysteinemic patients at risk.

Therapy

There is no proven effective therapy for NAION. Early medical therapies attempted included anticoagulants (242,243), diphenylhydantoin for its effect in improving conduction in hypoxic neurons (244–246), sub-Tenon injections of vasodilators (243,247–249), intravenous IOP-lowering agents and vasopressor agents (norepinephrine) to improve the gradient of nerve head perfusion pressure to IOP (250,251), thrombolytic agents and stellate ganglion block (252), oral corticosteroids in an attempt to decrease neuronal edema and any secondary damage related to it (38–40,

145,108,249), aspirin (253), and heparin-induced low-density lipoprotein/fibrinogen precipitation or hemodilution (254). None has been proved effective.

More recently applied nonsurgical modalities include hyperbaric oxygen and levodopa/carbidopa. Arnold et al. (255) treated 22 eyes in 20 patients with acute NAION using hyperbaric oxygen at 2.0 atmospheres twice a day for 10 days, comparing visual outcome to 27 untreated controls; no beneficial effect was found. Johnson et al. (256) reported 18 patients with NAION treated with a 3-week course of levodopa/carbidopa within 45 days of visual loss, compared with 19 historical untreated controls. At 6 months, 10 of 13 (76.9%) treated versus 3 of 10 (30%) controls improved at least 3 lines in Snellen visual acuity testing. The study was limited by small numbers and possible confounding factors, and results have not been corroborated by other investigators (257–259). This therapeutic modality remains unproven.

The IONDT studying optic nerve sheath decompression surgery for NAION was based on the beneficial effect of the surgery in the optic neuropathy of elevated intracranial pressure (260–262) and the postulate that reduction of perineural subarachnoid cerebrospinal fluid pressure could improve local vascular flow or axoplasmic transport within the optic nerve head, thus reducing tissue injury in reversibly damaged axons. Several earlier studies had suggested a beneficial effect in the progressive form of NAION (230,263,264). Recruitment for the IONDT was ceased after 2 years, with 119 treated and 125 untreated patients, when data analysis revealed no significant benefit for treatment (improvement in visual acuity by at least 3 lines was 32.6% in treated patients versus 42.7% in untreated patients) (231). Moreover, the treatment group showed a statistically significantly greater risk for worsening by 3 lines or more (23.9% among treated patients versus 12.4% in untreated patients) (231). By the criteria used in the trial for progressive NAION, there was no beneficial effect in this subgroup. The 24-month follow-up data from the study confirmed the initial 6-month report (227). This technique is not currently recommended for the treatment of NAION.

Transvitreal optic neurotomy has been proposed as a therapy for both central retinal vein occlusion (265) and NAION (266). The procedure involves a pars plana vitrectomy and induced posterior vitreous detachment, associated with a stab incision at the nasal margin of the optic disc, with the purpose of opening the scleral canal and relieving compression of an edematous optic nerve. If a compartment syndrome is at least a component of the pathophysiology of NAION, then such a procedure in theory could break the cycle of edema and vascular compression. Soheilian et al. (266) reported the results of transvitreal neurotomy performed in seven cases of NAION with severe visual loss (visual acuity range counting fingers to 20/800) and onset prior to surgery ranging from 15–90 days. Improvement of visual acuity was noted in six patients with a final range of counting fingers to 20/60. This study was limited by several factors, including small patient numbers, sample bias (i.e., severe visual loss with difficulty accurately measuring pre- and postoperative visual levels), and delayed onset of therapy. The authors emphasized the experimental nature of this procedure and recommended a randomized clinical trial prior to considering this approach.

Advances in the understanding of cellular mechanisms of retinal ganglion cell and optic nerve axonal damage in ischemic injury may point to new directions in therapy (267). Studies in traumatic optic neuropathy postulate an ischemic component, with secondary effects such as lipid peroxidation resulting in excess free radical production and further tissue damage (220–223,268). Very high doses of intravenous methylprednisolone have been shown to be beneficial for acute spinal cord injury and may be beneficial in optic neuropathy as well, based on an antioxidant effect rather than direct anti-inflammatory activity (269). The beneficial effects of neuroprotective agents in animal models of retinal ganglion cell damage and optic neuropathy have recently been reported (221,223). By intervening in such processes as excitatory amino acid toxicity, intracellular calcium ion influx, reactive oxygen species bursts, and apoptosis (222), these agents may have future applicability to the treatment of AION. A trial of megadose intravenous corticosteroids, at the level used in the NASCIS Trials (269) for presumed oxygen free radical scavenging neuroprotective effect, has been considered.

Yoles et al. (223) reported a beneficial effect of the alpha-adrenergic agonist brimonidine in the rat crush model of optic neuropathy, with an effective time window of 24–48 hours after injury. Kent et al. (270) studied the intravitreal levels attained after topical administration of brimonidine, finding adequate levels to activate peripapillary retinal ganglion cell adrenergic receptors. Based on this and other data, a national multicenter clinical trial of topical brimonidine for NAION administered during the 48 hours following acute visual loss (NPION Trial) was begun in 2000. Recruitment difficulties with the required 48-hour time window to therapy prevented completion of the trial. A similar study with a 7-day window (BRAION Trial) was performed in Europe (271). Fazzone and Kupersmith (272) treated 14 patients with NAION, using topical brimonidine one drop two to four times/day, comparing visual outcome to 17 historical controls. They found a trend to worse visual outcome with treatment at 8–12 weeks. The study was limited by small patient numbers, low doses, and delay to treatment but raised questions as to effectiveness of this mode of therapy. This prompted early termination of the BRAION trial.

Prevention

There is no proven prophylactic measure for NAION. Although aspirin has a proven effect in reducing stroke and myocardial infarction in patients at risk, published data regarding its role in decreasing the severity of optic neuropathy (253) and the incidence of fellow-eye involvement after the initial episode have been controversial. Kupersmith et al. (273) retrospectively reviewed a series of 131 patients with NAION for the effect of aspirin use (65–1,300 mg more than twice a week) on the development of fellow-eye involvement. They found an incidence of 17.5% in treated patients versus 53.5% in untreated patients, 68.8% of which occurred during the first year. Minimum follow-up was 2 years. In a similar retrospective study of 52 patients by Salomon et al. (274), fellow-eye involvement was detected in 8 of 16 (50%) untreated patients versus 3 of 8 (38%) patients treated with an aspirin dosage of 100 mg/day and 5 of 28 (18%) treated with 325 mg/day. In contrast, a larger retrospective review by Beck et al. (238) studied 431 patients with NAION for second-eye involvement with and without aspirin use. The 5-year risk for fellow-eye involvement was calculated at 12–19%, depending on the analysis method, and no long-term benefit for aspirin use was found (238,275). The 5-year cumulative probability risk for fellow-eye NAION after the initial episode was 17% among treated patients versus 20% among untreated patients.

In consideration of a national multicenter clinical trial of aspirin for NAION prophylaxis, plans for the trial were abandoned because the rate of second-eye involvement was too low to make development of a controlled study practical. Criticisms of the studies that show beneficial prophylactic effects focus on the unusually high rates of untreated fellow-eye involvement of 50–53.5%, compared with the rates of 12–19% at 5 years found by Beck et al. and confirmed at 14.7% in the follow-up phase of the IONDT (239). Aspirin was not found to be beneficial in the IONDT, but the study design was not optimal for this evaluation. Although beneficial long-term effects remain unproven for NAION, many experts recommend the use of aspirin after an initial episode, if only for its role in decreasing risk for stroke and myocardial infarction in this vasculopathic population group.

The risk for subsequent stroke, myocardial infarction, and death in patients with NAION has been incompletely studied. Early studies indicated no statistically significant increase in cerebrovascular events (21,22,150), but later studies by Guyer et al. (1), Sawle et al. (152), and Hayreh et al. (102) indicated an increased risk (only for patients with both hypertension and diabetes in the series of Hayreh et al). Guyer et al. (1) and Sawle at al. (152) also reported an increase in frequency of myocardial infarction in patients with NAION, not confirmed by other studies. Sawle et al. (152) reported increased mortality. These issues remain unclear, requiring a large-scale population study for answers.

Based on the postulated role of crowding of optic nerve head axons in the development of NAION, peripheral retinal laser photocoagulation has been suggested in an attempt to ''decompress'' the nerve by producing a controlled degree of axonal dropout and optic atrophy (118,276). This action theoretically could prevent or delay the occurrence of an acute ischemic event that would create more severe visual loss. No controlled studies of this technique have been performed.

POSTERIOR ISCHEMIC OPTIC NEUROPATHY

Although the anterior form of ION is far more common than the posterior variety, ischemia of the retrobulbar portions of the optic nerve occurs in many settings, both arteritic and nonarteritic. Ischemia can independently affect the posterior portion of the optic nerve because of the distinct and separate arterial supplies of the anterior and posterior portions of the optic nerve. The anterior optic nerve is supplied by the short posterior ciliary artery and choroidal circulations, while the retrobulbar optic nerve is supplied intraorbitally by a pial plexus arising from the ophthalmic artery, and intracranially by branches of the ipsilateral internal carotid, anterior cerebral, and anterior communicating arteries.

Posterior ischemic optic neuropathy (PION) is a syndrome of acute visual loss with characteristics of optic neuropathy without initial disc edema and marked by the subsequent development of optic atrophy. Occasionally, a small amount of disc edema appears within the first week or so after acute visual loss, presumably as a result of propagation of swelling forward along the course of the optic nerve from the point of original ischemia. The diagnosis of PION is most often made in one of the following settings (277):

1. GCA (Fig. 7.23) (3,32,278) or rarely other vasculitides such as herpes zoster, polyarteritis nodosa, or lupus erythematosus. Indeed, evaluation for GCA is essential in cases without other apparent cause and should be the primary consideration with this presentation in the elderly, with urgent ancillary testing as described earlier for AION (see above).
2. Nonarteritic PION in a population of patients with similar demographics to those patients with NAION (277)
3. Related to surgery (coronary artery bypass and lumbar spine procedures most frequently reported), or severe bleeding, or hypotension (as seen in cases of gastrointestinal hemorrhage or trauma; see below)

The differential diagnosis includes compressive and infiltrative optic neuropathies, although the onset in PION is typically more abrupt. In most cases, neuroimaging is indicated to rule out these possibilities. NAION typically shows no enhancement of the optic nerves on MR, presumably due to limitation to the optic nerve head. PION also typically shows no abnormalities of the optic nerve, except in cases of GCA PION in which enhancement has been demonstrated and must be differentiated from other causes, such as inflammation and infiltration (279,280).

Recently, Sadda et al. (277) reported a multicenter, retrospective review covering 22 years, revealing 72 patients with PION, classifying them into the three groups: perioperative PION, arteritic PION, and nonarteritic PION. The nonarteritic group accounted for 38 of the 72 patients, exhibited similar risk factors, and followed a clinical course precisely like that of NAION. In contrast to perioperative and arteritic PION, which were characterized by severe visual loss with little or no recovery, nonarteritic PION was less severe and showed improvement in 34% of patients. It is important to recognize this nonarteritic form in patients with acute optic neuropathy but no optic disc edema, a scenario that may be mistaken for optic neuritis. Such patients, as in some patients with AION and disc edema, particularly those with ischemic white matter lesions on MR imaging, might be incorrectly

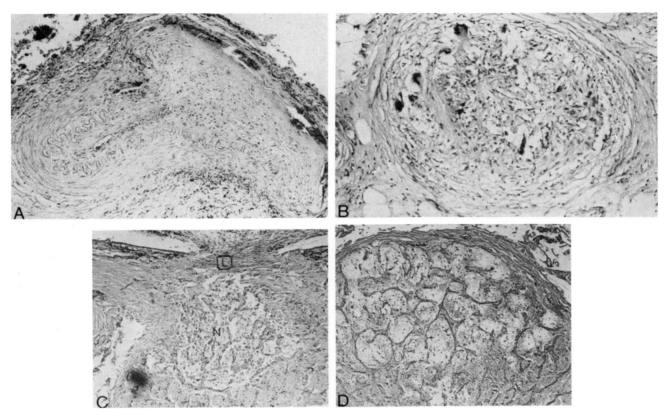

Figure 7.23. Pathology of PION in a patient with GCA. *A,* The right ophthalmic artery near its origin from the internal carotid artery shows intimal thickening with narrowing of the lumen. Numerous chronic inflammatory cells, including giant cells, surround the artery and infiltrate its wall. *B,* A short posterior ciliary artery is occluded by a marked granulomatous inflammation. Note numerous multinucleated giant cells. Many short posterior ciliary arteries in both orbits were occluded or narrowed by granulomatous inflammation. *C,* Longitudinal section through the proximal portion of the right optic nerve shows a well-defined zone of ischemic necrosis (N) immediately behind the lamina cribrosa (L). *D,* Cross-section through the ischemic zone shows complete destruction of the nerve fiber and glial elements with preservation of the fibrovascular pial septae. (From Spencer WH, Hoyt WF. A fatal case of giant cell arteritis (temporal or cranial arteritis) with ocular involvement. Arch Ophthalmol 1960;64:862–867.)

started on immunomodulatory therapy to reduce the risk of multiple sclerosis (281). PION differs from optic neuritis by its occurrence in older age groups and its lack of pain on eye movements.

ISCHEMIC OPTIC NEUROPATHY IN SETTINGS OF HEMODYNAMIC COMPROMISE

Systemic hypotension, blood loss, and anemia may produce optic nerve ischemia (36,282–285). The most commonly reported causes of blood loss associated with ION are (*a*) spontaneous gastrointestinal or uterine bleeding and (*b*) surgically induced hemorrhage, related most frequently to cardiac bypass or lumbar spine procedures. Less often, hypotensive episodes in the setting of chronic anemia without blood loss (as in chronic hemodialysis) may result in ION.

The optic neuropathy that occurs in these settings is typically bilateral, although unilateral cases occur. Visual loss is often severe. AION (with optic disc edema) accounts for the majority of cases (286), although PION is not infrequent. Visual loss may occur immediately after the episode or may be delayed as much as 2–3 weeks in cases of AION. Hayreh

(284) has postulated that delayed visual loss is caused by vasoconstriction in the ciliary artery system secondary to activation of the renin-angiotensin pathway as a late response to blood loss.

SPONTANEOUS OR TRAUMATIC HEMORRHAGE

Patients in whom visual loss occurs after spontaneous hemorrhage are usually 40–60 years old and debilitated. Most of these patients have experienced repeated episodes of bleeding, but cases following a single episode of massive hemorrhage with secondary hypotension have been reported (285). The visual loss is usually bilateral, but it may affect both eyes asymmetrically or be unilateral (282–285). The severity of visual loss ranges from mild or transient blurred vision in one eye to irreversible total blindness in both eyes (285). Both AION and PION have been reported in this setting, although AION is more common (284,285).

About 50% of patients who experience ION after an acute spontaneous hemorrhage experience some recovery of vision, but only 10–15% recover completely (282–287). The source of bleeding seems to be irrelevant, although the most frequent sites are the gastrointestinal tract in men and the uterus in women. Presencia et al. (288) reported that in most documented cases of bilateral blindness related to systemic blood loss, the hemoglobin measures less than 5.0 g/dL at the time of visual loss. Other authors have reported higher hemoglobin levels and emphasize the importance of both anemia and hypotension in the pathogenesis of optic nerve infarction (285). Hayreh (284) speculated that blood loss alone, with or without arterial hypotension, can cause an increase in the release of endogenous vasoconstrictor agents that can lead to direct vasoconstriction and occlusion of optic nerve head capillaries, resulting in AION.

PERIOPERATIVE

ION occurs in the setting of various surgical interventions, most commonly cardiopulmonary bypass (176,289–297), and lumbar spine surgery (286,298–,303). Other cases include abdominal procedures (282–284,287,288), hip incision and drainage (295), cholecystectomy (282), and parathyroidectomy (291).

In 1994, Katz et al. (286) reviewed the literature to date on perioperative ION and found 30 well-documented cases, most of which were of the anterior variety. Most cases occurred after coronary bypass surgery, but several occurred after back surgery in which there was no evidence of orbital or ocular compression. All were associated with hypotension, anemia, or both, although control values corresponding to similar procedures in patients who did not suffer ION were not provided. Among the four patients whose hemogram was reported, the mean hemoglobin level decreased from 14.3 to 8.3 g/dL (a 42% decrease) in the perioperative period. The distinguishing feature of the reviewed cases of ION associated with back surgery was the deliberate reduction of intraoperative blood pressure to reduce bleeding. All but two of the patients were over 40 years of age, and most had typical vascular risk factors for ION, including hypertension, coronary artery disease, diabetes mellitus, and a history of smoking. In 18 of 30 cases, both eyes were affected. Visual acuities were worse than 20/100 in over 50%, and substantial recovery of vision was unusual. Optic disc swelling was present at the time of initial visual loss in most cases, but it was delayed in appearance by several days in others. In most cases, the optic nerve was the only site of infarction by both clinical and imaging criteria, underscoring the apparent selective vulnerability of the optic nerve in this setting.

Brown et al. (304) reported on six patients who developed ION in the postoperative period as a result of anemia and hypotension, three of whom had AION. The condition was bilateral in two of the AION patients and unilateral in one. All of the AION patients had features consistent with the "disc at risk" seen in cases of typical NAION. All three

patients had hemoglobin counts less than 8.0 g/dL over periods of time ranging from 30 minutes to 72 hours, and all experienced episodes of decreased mean blood pressure ranging from 24–46% of preoperative levels over 15- to 120-minute periods. Based on these cases, the authors concluded that although severe anemia alone may not cause ION, even a short episode of hypotension in an already anemic patient may predispose to ION-induced vision loss.

Brown et al. (304) and Lee (298) emphasized that the acquired immunodeficiency syndrome (AIDS) epidemic has resulted in the establishment of low absolute thresholds for blood transfusion in the perioperative period. These authors point out that patients who are not transfused until their hemoglobin reaches very low levels may be at risk for developing both AION and PION related to a combination of anemia and hypotension intraoperatively or during the immediate postoperative period.

Nuttall et al. (305) assessed risk factors for ION after cardiopulmonary bypass, identifying 17 cases in 27,915 surgical procedures (0.06%). Involvement was bilateral in 53%, anterior in 71%. The presence of atherosclerotic vascular disease and a minimum postoperative hemoglobin were significantly associated with postoperative ION, although not uniformly present. Minimum hemoglobin of 8.5 g/dL was present in 76.5% of ION patients versus 41.2% of controls.

Lumbar spine surgery may carry an increased risk for postoperative ION, usually PION, compared with other surgeries. In 1997, Myers et al. (301) reviewed 37 cases of visual loss following spinal surgery, finding 8 with AION and 14 with PION. Average operative time was 410 minutes, with blood loss of 3,500 mL and a mean drop in systolic blood pressure from 130 to 77 mm Hg; none of these figures differed significantly from a matched group of operated patients without visual loss. Of the 28 patients with postoperative PION in Sadda et al.'s (277) series, 14 (50%) followed spinal surgery. Dunker et al. (306) examined seven cases of postoperative PION, five of which followed lumbar spine surgery. Contributing factors were thought to include prolonged intraoperative hypotension (diastolic range 40–60 mm Hg), blood loss (1.2–16 L) with anemia and hypovolemia, and prolonged prone, face-dependent positioning with subsequent orbitofacial vascular congestion and edema.

It is important to distinguish visual loss from postoperative ION with associated facial edema from the prolonged prone position from those cases of visual loss secondary to direct compression of the eye from malpositioning. In the latter cases (307–309), which have been termed the "head-rest syndrome," direct compression results in orbital ischemia, with severe orbital congestion, ecchymoses, and most often central retinal artery occlusion.

The purposeful maintenance of relative systemic hypotension to control intraoperative hemorrhage and the prolonged prone position may be significant features in the development of some cases of perioperative ION, although it remains a rare occurrence in a common surgical procedure. Lee (310) summarized the multiple possible contributing features and the complex nature of adjusting operative procedures to prevent ION. While aggressive fluid replacement and transfusion of blood products seem appropriate in cases where deficiencies are detected, there are no controlled studies of these interventions, and no therapy has been proven to significantly improve visual outcome in perioperative ION. To help understand the multiple and likely complicated interacting factors underlying perioperative ION, the American Society of Anesthesiologists (ASA) established the international ASA Postoperative Visual Loss (POVL) Registry in 1999 with the goal of acquiring a large database with detailed information on patient characteristics and perioperative conditions (311–313). Preliminary results confirm that at least two thirds of cases are associated with spine surgery and that ION can occur even with the head suspended in Mayfield tongs with no external compression of the eyes and face. Indeed, perioperative ION can occur in young patients, with relatively short prone durations, with little blood loss, a normal hematocrit, and without hypotension. Clearly there is more we need to learn regarding the cause of this potentially devastating disorder.

HYPOTENSION

ION related to hypotension most often presents in patients with chronic renal failure and dialysis. Haider et al. (314) found 4 cases of AION in a series of 60 patients undergoing dialysis over a 2-year follow-up. The hypotension may be acute, temporally associated with the dialysis procedure, or it may be chronic. Most patients also are chronically anemic. The accelerated diffuse vasculopathy that occurs in this disease may predispose to the development of ION, as may previous chronic hypertension, with possible arteriosclerosis and impaired autoregulation of the optic disc vascular supply.

The term "uremic optic neuropathy" has been applied to cases of acute optic nerve dysfunction and disc edema in patients with renal failure. Knox et al. (315) reported substantial visual improvement in five of six patients who underwent immediate dialysis and corticosteroid therapy, postulating that correction of the uremia reversed a metabolic optic neuropathy. Saini et al. (316) reported a similar case of improvement on dialysis. However, Hamed et al. (317) reported three cases of optic neuropathy in patients with uremia, two of which did not improve on dialysis; one of these was severely hypertensive with elevated intracranial pressure, and the other showed more typical features of AION. The third patient was presumed to suffer desferrioxamine

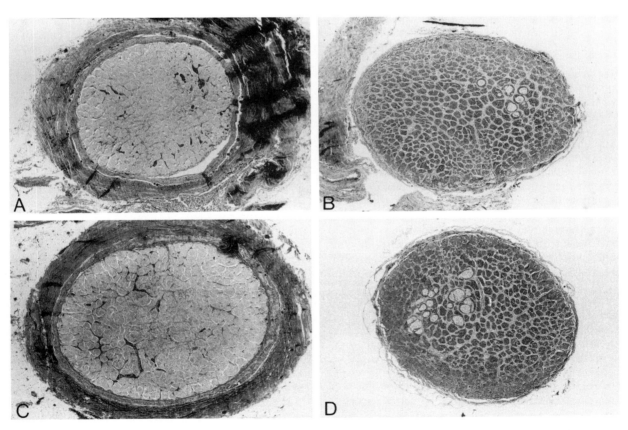

Figure 7.24. Histopathologic appearance of the optic nerves in PION. *A,* Cross-section of the right optic nerve about 2 cm posterior to the globe shows complete infarction. *B,* Cross-section of the right optic nerve about 3 cm posterior to the globe shows only a few isolated infarcted nerve fiber bundles. *C,* Cross-section of the left optic nerve about 3 cm posterior to the globe shows complete infarction. *D,* Cross-section of the left optic nerve about 3.5 cm posterior to the globe shows only a few individual infarcted nerve fiber bundles. (From Johnson MW, Kincaid MC, Trobe JD. Bilateral retrobulbar optic nerve infarctions after blood loss and hypotension. Ophthalmology 1987;94:1577–1584.)

toxicity and recovered vision after discontinuing the therapy. The authors stressed the heterogeneity of optic neuropathy in this patient group. Servilla et al. (318) reported a case of typical AION in a uremic patient, which occurred following an acute hypotensive episode (blood pressure 40/0 mm Hg) during hemodialysis. Jackson et al. (319), Michaelson et al. (320), and Basile et al. (321) also reported cases believed secondary to hypotensive episodes. Connolly et al. (322) described three patients with presumed AION in patients with chronic renal failure, hypotension, and anemia, aged 25, 26, and 39 years. Acute hypotension was a precipitating factor in all cases; volume replacement was associated with improvement of vision, in one eye from no light perception to 20/40. The authors emphasized that visual loss from hypotension-induced ischemia in this setting may respond to rapid volume replacement and restoration of normotension. Further study is required to corroborate these findings.

Johnson et al. (285) concluded that visual loss from hypotension may be of three types:

1. Sustained and profound hypotension in a nonanemic patient without arteriolar sclerosis causes watershed white and gray matter infarction in parietal and occipital lobes. The optic nerves tend to be spared.
2. Brief hypotension in an anemic patient with arterioscle-

rotic risk factors is mild enough to spare the hemispheric watershed regions but severe enough to cause juxtalaminar optic nerve infarction that produces a clinical (and pathologic) picture consistent with NAION.
3. Hypotension in an anemic patient without arteriosclerotic risk factors predisposes the patient to PION that is caused by infarction in the posterior orbital portion of the optic nerve (Fig. 7.24), where pial end vessels are subject to compression from hypoxic edema.

Although in theory this ischemia helps sort through the various proposed pathogenetic mechanisms, there is great overlap among cases of ION related to hemodynamic compromise, with multiple potential factors, some yet to be elucidated. Several cases of AION resulting from rapid correction of malignant hypertension have been reported (322–325). Two of the four children reported by Taylor et al. (325) experienced limited recovery of vision following the development of AION during treatment of accelerated hypertension, but it is unclear whether this improvement was related to any specific therapy that the children received. The pathogenesis of AION that occurs in this setting is likely related to impaired autoregulation of the nutrient vessels supplying the optic nerve head and to reduction in perfusion pressure, leading to ischemia.

RADIATION OPTIC NEUROPATHY

Radiation optic neuropathy (RON) is thought to be an ischemic disorder of the optic nerve that usually results in irreversible severe visual loss months to years after radiation therapy to the brain and orbit. It is most often a retrobulbar process. RON occurs most frequently after irradiation of paranasal sinus and other skull base malignancies, but it may develop after radiation treatment for pituitary adenomas, parasellar meningiomas, craniopharyngiomas, frontal and temporal gliomas, and intraocular tumors (326–330). In a series of 219 patients (328) treated for nasal and paranasal malignancies between 1969 and 1985, 19 patients with optic nerve or chiasmal radionecrosis were identified. It has also been reported after low-dose radiation therapy for dysthyroid orbitopathy, although only in patients with diabetes mellitus.

The pathogenesis of delayed radionecrosis in the central nervous system is not fully understood. At one time it was thought to be primarily vascular damage with subsequent neuronal injury (331); however, it may be that both direct effects to replicating glial tissue and secondary effects from damage to vascular endothelial cells are important in the pathogenesis of this condition (332,333). Somatic mutations in the glial cells induced by ionizing radiation are thought to result in genetically incompetent cells that are metabolically deficient. Over time, these cells gradually increase, producing demyelination and neuronal degeneration. A similar process may occur in vascular endothelial cells, eventually resulting in vascular occlusion and necrosis. This model is consistent with the observed long latent period of delayed radionecrosis, because both the glial and endothelial cells have a slow cellular turnover rate. It is also consistent with the observation of direct neuronal demyelination and degen-

eration prior to the development of any vascular changes (334). Pathologic specimens of optic nerves with RON show ischemic demyelination, reactive astrocytosis, endothelial hyperplasia, obliterative endarteritis, and fibrinoid necrosis (326,335–339).

Both the total dose of radiation given and the daily fractionation size are important factors in determining the risk of delayed radiation necrosis in the central nervous system. Most investigators agree that a maximum total dose of 5,000 centigray (cGy) in fractions under 200 cGy provides an acceptable low risk (340–343), except perhaps in patients with diabetes mellitus and in patients receiving chemotherapy (341,344). The cumulative doses of radiation therapy reported in patients with RON range from 2,400 cGy (345) to 12,500 cGy (346); however, over 75% of the reported cases of RON have received a total dose of more than 5,000 cGy (329). The risk of RON thus appears to increase significantly at doses over 50 Gy. Jiang et al. (328), in a retrospective study of 219 patients receiving radiation therapy for cancers of the paranasal sinuses and nasal cavity, found no cases of RON when the dose was under 50 Gy. In contrast, the 10-year actuarial risk for RON after doses of 50–60 Gy and 61–78 Gy was 5% and 30%, respectively. Parsons et al. (347) demonstrated no risk of RON in doses of 59 Gy or less. However, among nerves that received doses of 60 Gy or greater, the dose per fraction was more important than the total dose in producing RON. The 15-year actuarial risk of RON was 11% when fraction size was less than 1.9 Gy, compared with 47% when fraction size was 1.9 Gy or more. The data obtained by Parsons et al. (347) also suggested an increased risk of RON with increasing age. Goldsmith et al.

(348) found that a cumulative dose of 54 Gy delivered at 18 Gy/day carried a very low risk of RON. Young et al. (349), by correlating dosimetric measurements with gadolinium-enhanced MR images, concluded that the tolerance level of the optic nerve is 50–55 Gy.

Both Jiang et al. (328) and Parsons et al. (347) noted that in contrast to patients irradiated for paranasal and oral cavity tumors, patients irradiated for pituitary tumors can develop RON after doses ranging from 42 to 50 Gy (338,340,350). They theorized that optic nerve compression and vascular compromise lower the optic nerve threshold to injury from radiation. Similarly, patients who have received chemotherapy in conjunction with radiation therapy and those with growth hormone-secreting pituitary adenomas are also reportedly at higher risk for RON, even at lower cumulative doses (345,350–354). In some cases, the dose actually delivered to the optic nerves is higher than desired because of improper calibration or equipment malfunction. Consequently, RON should be considered even in situations where ''safe'' doses of radiation therapy have supposedly been administered.

The syndrome typically presents with acute, painless visual loss in one or both eyes. Visual loss in one eye may be rapidly followed by visual loss in the fellow eye. Episodes of transient visual loss may precede the onset of RON by several weeks (355). The onset of visual symptoms associated with RON may be as short as 3 months or as long as 8 years after radiation therapy, but most cases occur within 3 years after radiation, with a peak at 1.5 years (326,327,354, 356,357). Visual acuity loss ranges widely (329), and progression of visual loss over weeks to months is common. Spontaneous visual recovery is unusual. Final vision is no light perception in 45%, with a total of 85% of reported eyes with RON having final visual acuity of 20/200 or worse (329).

The affected optic disc is often pale initially, related to prior damage from tumor with possible superimposed radiation injury; less frequently it is edematous. Cases with disc edema at onset often have associated radiation retinopathy, with cotton-wool patches, hard exudates, and retinal hemorrhages, secondary to irradiation of intraocular or orbital structures. The visual field may show altitudinal loss or a central scotoma. A junctional syndrome with an optic neuropathy and contralateral temporal hemianopia may occur in patients with damage to the distal optic nerve (358). Patients with radionecrosis of the optic chiasm typically develop a bitemporal hemianopia that initially may suggest recurrence of the tumor for which the patient was initially irradiated (355,357), but superimposed optic neuropathy may involve the nasal visual fields as well.

The differential diagnosis of RON includes recurrence of the primary tumor, secondary empty sella syndrome with optic nerve and chiasmal prolapse (359), arachnoiditis (360,361), and radiation-induced parasellar tumor (326,362). These conditions typically present with slowly progressive visual loss rather than the rapid onset of RON.

The diagnosis of RON is generally suspected from the clinical setting and may be confirmed in most cases with neuroimaging. CT scanning is typically normal (326). MR imaging is the diagnostic procedure of choice to distinguish tumor recurrence from RON (349,354,357,358,363,364). The development of the fat-saturation techniques and the use of paramagnetic contrast solutions allow detailed imaging of the chiasm and the intracranial and orbital portions of the optic nerves. In RON, the unenhanced T1- and T2-weighted images may show no abnormality, but on T1-weighted enhanced images, there is marked enhancement of the optic nerves, optic chiasm, and even the optic tracts in some cases (Fig. 7.25). The enhancement usually resolves in several months, at which time visual function usually stabilizes. Occasionally, enhancement may even precede visual loss.

Treatment for RON is controversial. Although delayed radionecrosis in the central nervous system can be treated with some success with systemic corticosteroids, which are effective in reducing tissue edema and may have some beneficial effect on demyelination (365), their use in RON, in oral or intravenous form, has produced disappointing results. Among 16 reported cases treated with steroids alone, only 2 improved (326,347,352,355,357,363,366,367). Similarly, the use of anticoagulation to reverse or stabilize central nervous system radionecrosis (368) does not appear to provide significant benefit in patients with RON (369,370).

Hyperbaric oxygen therapy is used in the treatment of radionecrosis of bone and following irradiation in poorly healing wounds in oral and maxillofacial surgery (358, 371,372). At 2.0 atmospheres, the level of dissolved oxygen in blood may be raised 14-fold, thus extending the oxygen diffusion distance in ischemic tissue and enabling limited correction of local hypoxia (371). Hyperbaric oxygen therapy enhances fibroblastic activity, collagen synthesis, and neovascularization in irradiated tissues (372). To the extent that RON is an ischemic process, hyperbaric oxygen therapy has a theoretical basis for effectiveness, but clinical results are not uniform (373).

Guy and Schatz (355) first reported visual improvement in RON in two patients whose treatment with hyperbaric oxygen was initiated within 72 hours of onset of visual symptoms. The treatment protocol consisted of 14 daily 2-hour sessions at 2.8 atmospheres. In one patient, visual acuity improved from 20/50 to 20/20; the improvement was maintained over a 9-month follow-up period. Visual acuity in the second patient initially improved from counting fingers to 20/40 after 2 days of treatment, but it then deteriorated to 20/300 over 2 weeks and did not improve despite continued hyperbaric oxygen therapy. Two other patients treated more than 2 weeks after the onset of visual loss showed no response. Roden et al. (327) reported no improvement in 13 patients with RON treated with hyperbaric oxygen, 11 of whom were also given systemic corticosteroids; however, treatment was initiated in these patients no earlier than 2 weeks and as late as 12 weeks after the onset of visual loss. Hyperbaric oxygen therapy at 2.0 atmospheres was administered daily, ranging from a total of 18–160 hours per patient. Subsequent reports showed no significant improvement in visual function in patients with RON (374) until Borruat et al. (358) reported the case of a patient who initially lost vision to 20/70 in the left eye, associated with an inferior nasal field defect. The fellow eye was initially normal; how-

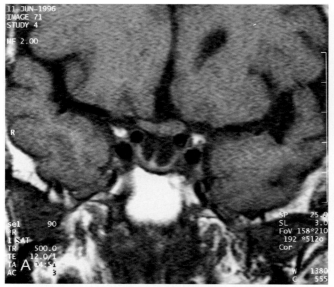

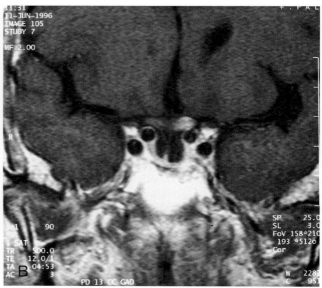

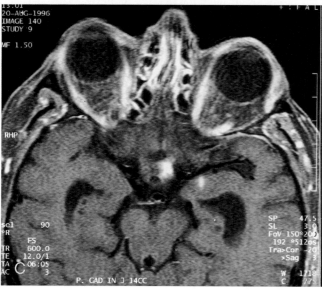

Figure 7.25. Radiation optic neuropathy in a 65-year-old woman who had undergone transsphenoidal resection of a nonsecreting pituitary macroadenoma followed by radiation therapy totalling 5,500 cGy 18 months earlier. *A*, T1-weighted MR image, coronal view, shows enlargement of the left side of the optic chiasm. *B*, T1-weighted MR image, coronal view, after intravenous injection of paramagnetic contrast material, shows enhancement of the enlarged region. *C*, T1-weighted MR image, axial view, after intravenous injection of paramagnetic contrast material, shows enhancement and enlargement of the distal portion of the left optic nerve and the left side of the optic chiasm. (Courtesy of Dr. Neil R. Miller.)

ever, 15 days later, vision in the left eye declined to no light perception, and the right eye developed marked temporal field loss. Hyperbaric oxygen therapy was initiated along with intravenous steroid therapy. Two weeks later, the visual field loss in the left eye had significantly improved, although vision in the right eye was light perception.

Borruat et al. (373) subsequently reviewed the rationale for, and results of, treatment of RON with hyperbaric oxy-

gen. These investigators concluded that hyperbaric oxygen should be started as early as possible after the onset of visual loss, even if there is a possibility that the visual loss is caused by some other process, such as recurrent tumor. From available data, visual improvement has been documented with therapy only in those treated within 72 hours. There are no good data for therapy begun 4–14 days after visual loss; after 2 weeks, therapy is most likely ineffective.

ISCHEMIC OPTIC DISC EDEMA WITH MINIMAL DYSFUNCTION

PRE-AION OPTIC DISC EDEMA

Patients may develop disc swelling from NAION before they have any visual symptoms (38,375,376). In such cases, the patient may be thought to have papilledema or a com-

pressive optic neuropathy from an orbital mass. Often, however, the asymptomatic disc swelling is noted in the fellow eye of a patient with a history of a previous attack of NAION, and the diagnosis is less confusing. Boghen and Glaser (21) reported one patient who at the time of presentation with

NAION had disc swelling in the asymptomatic contralateral eye, which lost vision 2 weeks later. Likewise, Hayreh (377) described four patients with bilateral NAION, all of whom initially had visual loss in one eye and asymptomatic optic disc swelling in the fellow eye. Several weeks later, the patients developed visual symptoms in the second eye. Others have described similar patients (232,378). Almog and Goldstein (379) reviewed a series of 23 cases of asymptomatic optic disc edema in vasculopathic patients (19 patients were diabetic). In 9 eyes, overt AION developed, within a mean interval of 16.8 weeks, while in 25 eyes, disc edema resolved over a mean of 15.5 weeks. On the basis of vasculopathic risk factors, lack of evidence for other causes of disc edema, evidence of AION in the fellow eye, and the later development in some patients of AION in the asymptomatically edematous eye, the disc edema has been presumed ischemic in origin.

DIABETIC PAPILLOPATHY

Clinical Presentation

Early reports of diabetic papillopathy described the acute onset of unilateral or bilateral optic disc edema in young, type I diabetics, without the usual defects in visual field and pupillary function associated with NAION or optic neuritis (380–384). Disc edema was prolonged in these cases, but vision generally was preserved. A recent report added a substantial number of older patients with type II diabetes (385). Overall, fewer than 100 total cases have been reported, and the specific criteria for diagnosis have been vague, especially regarding the allowable degree of optic nerve dysfunction and the corresponding differentiation from mild NAION.

The currently accepted criteria for the diagnosis of diabetic papillopathy include:

1. Presence of diabetes (approximately 70% type I, 30% type II).
2. Optic disc edema (unilateral in roughly 60%, bilateral in 40%).
3. Absence of substantial optic nerve dysfunction (at most a minor relative afferent pupillary defect; no more than mild generalized depression or enlarged blind spot on visual fields, specifically no central, cecocentral, or altitudinal visual field defect). Visual acuity levels may vary, since coexisting maculopathy is a common confounding feature, but over 75% of reported cases measured 20/40 or better at onset.
4. Lack of evidence for ocular inflammation or elevated intracranial pressure.

Although younger patients predominate (most of those reported have been under age 50), patients with diabetic papillopathy may be of any age and typically present either with no visual complaints or with vague, nonspecific visual disturbance such as mild blurring or distortion; transient visual obscurations have rarely been reported. Pain is absent, as are other ocular or neurologic symptoms.

The involved optic disc(s) may demonstrate either nonspecific hyperemic edema or, in about half of cases, marked dilation of the inner optic disc surface microvasculature (Fig. 7.26). Pale swelling has typically been a criterion for exclusion, because it suggested AION. The surface telangiectasia is prominent enough in some cases to be mistaken for optic disc neovascularization (NVD). The dilated optic nerve surface vasculature of diabetic papillopathy may be distinguished from NVD by the following characteristics:

1. Generally radial distribution of the dilated vessels in diabetic papillopathy, as opposed to the random branching pattern of neovascularization.

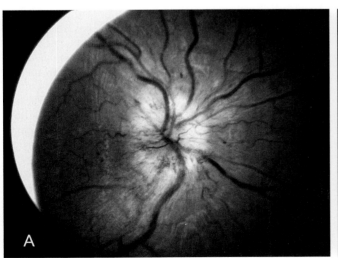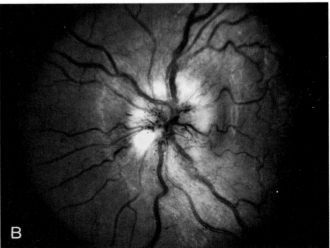

Figure 7.26. Appearance of diabetic papillopathy. The patient was an 18-year-old man with juvenile diabetes mellitus who was noted to have optic disc swelling during a routine eye examination. He had no visual complaints. Note dilated telangiectatic vessels mimicking neovascularization on the surface of both the right (*A*) and left (*B*) optic discs. (Courtesy of Dr. Neil R. Miller.)

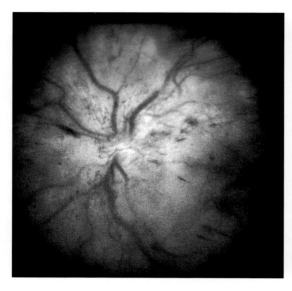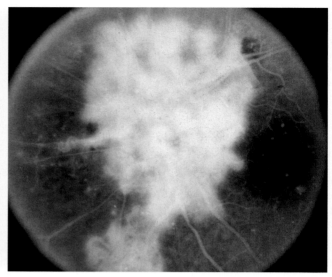

Figure 7.27. Fluorescein angiography in diabetic papillopathy (left) versus optic disc neovascularization (right). Leakage overlying the disc and vessels occurs primarily in neovascularization.

2. Limitation of the telangiectatic vessels to the disc surface in diabetic papillopathy, as opposed to proliferation into the vitreous cavity with neovascular fronds.
3. Limitation of fluorescein dye leakage to the disc substance and peripapillary retina, demonstrating late "shadowing" of the retinal vessels in diabetic papillopathy, as opposed to leakage anteriorly into the vitreous from neovascular tissue, with obscuration of the retinal vessels (Fig. 7.27).

True disc neovascularization is occasionally superimposed on the edema of diabetic papillopathy (Fig. 7.28).

Diabetic retinopathy is usually (more than 80% of reported cases) present at the time of onset of papillopathy, varying in severity and associated with macular edema in

about 25% of cases. The fellow eye frequently demonstrates a "crowded" optic disc with a small cup/disc ratio similar to the configuration seen in patients with NAION (385).

The pathogenesis of diabetic papillopathy is unproven. Early investigators postulated either a toxic effect on the optic nerve secondary to abnormal glucose metabolism or an inner disc surface vascular disturbance, with resultant microvascular leakage into the disc (380,381). The most commonly proposed theory suggests it to be a mild form of NAION, with reversible ischemia of both the prelaminar and inner surface layers of the optic nerve head (383). Ischemic optic disc edema may occur with irreversible dysfunction (infarction in NAION), with no dysfunction (pre-NAION optic disc edema without visual loss), or with varying degrees of reversible dysfunction (spontaneous recovery in NAION [377]). Diabetic papillopathy fits this category as well. The prominent surface telangiectasia seen in many cases is reminiscent of a similar phenomenon seen focally on the disc in NAION (110,111) and may represent vascular shunting from prelaminar ischemic vascular beds. The frequent occurrence of a "crowded" optic disc in the fellow eye (385), as in NAION, supports an ischemic mechanism as well. Fluorescein angiographic sequences of optic disc filling are similar to those in NAION (386), suggestive of impaired optic disc perfusion. Hayreh (387) has recently summarized his data corroborating an ischemic etiology for diabetic papillopathy and suggesting that it is indeed the same entity as NAION. We believe that it is most likely an ischemic syndrome, although the clinical course is often quite distinct from typical NAION.

Conditions that may simulate diabetic papillopathy include papilledema (elevated intracranial pressure), optic disc neovascularization, malignant hypertension, papillitis, and NAION. Symptoms of elevated intracranial pressure usually distinguish papilledema, but in patients with suspected bilat-

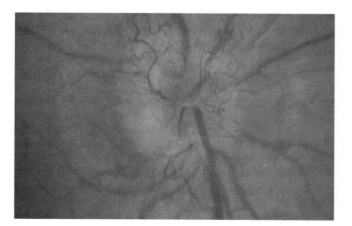

Figure 7.28. Diabetic papillopathy (left) with superimposed optic disc neovascularization (right). Note the random branching pattern of the neovascular vessels.

eral diabetic papillopathy, even without such symptoms, neuroimaging and lumbar puncture must be considered. Disc edema related to systemic hypertension does not typically demonstrate prominent telangiectasia and is usually associated with hypertensive retinopathy; blood pressure measurement is important in suspected cases. Papillitis and NAION both demonstrate significant optic nerve dysfunction, as evidenced by a relative afferent pupillary defect, visual acuity, and visual field loss.

Untreated, the optic disc edema of diabetic papillopathy gradually resolves over a period of 2–10 months, leaving minimal optic atrophy in about 20% of cases. The long-term visual prognosis for patients with diabetic papillopathy, however, is limited by the associated diabetic retinopathy. Bayraktar et al. (388) identified 4 of 24 eyes (16%) progressing to proliferative retinopathy on an average follow-up of 25.6 months. Proliferative changes, with attendant complications, have developed in approximately 25% of our cases. Ho et al. (389) reported two cases in which florid optic disc neovascularization developed within 3 months of diabetic papillopathy. Although systemic and periocular (390) corticosteroids have been used in isolated cases, there is no proven therapy for this disorder.

REFERENCES

1. Guyer DR, Miller NR, Auer CL, Fine SL. The risk of cerebrovascular and cardiovascular disease in patients with anterior ischemic optic neuropathy. Arch Ophthalmol 1985;103:1136–1142.
2. Johnson LN, Arnold AC. Incidence of nonarteritic and arteritic anterior ischemic optic neuropathy: population-based study in the State of Missouri and Los Angeles County, California. J Neuroophthalmol 1994;14:38–44.
3. Cohen DN, Damaske MM. Temporal arteritis: a spectrum of ophthalmic complications. Ann Ophthalmol 1975;7:1045–1054.
4. Graham E. Survival in temporal arteritis. Trans Ophthalmol Soc UK 1980;100:108–110.
5. Keltner JL. Giant cell arteritis: signs and symptoms. Ophthalmology 1982;89:1101–1110.
6. Liu GT, Glaser JS, Schatz NJ, Smith JL. Visual morbidity in giant cell arteritis. Ophthalmology 1994;101:1779–1785.
7. Aiello PD, Trautmann JC, McPhee TJ, et al. Visual prognosis in giant cell arteritis. Ophthalmology 1993;100:550–555.
8. Machado EBV, Michet CJ, Hunder G, et al. Temporal arteritis: clinical and epidemiological features from a community-based study, 1950–1985. Ann Neurol 1987;22:148.
9. Machado EBV, Michet CJ, Ballard DJ, et al. Trends in incidence and clinical presentation of temporal arteritis in Olmstead County, Minnesota, 1950–1985. Arthritis Rheum 1988;31:745–749.
10. Liu NH, LaBree LD, Feldon SE, et al. The epidemiology of giant cell arteritis. Ophthalmology 2001;108:1145–1149.
11. Hedges TR III, Gieger GL, Albert DM. The clinical value of negative temporal artery biopsy specimens. Arch Ophthalmol 1983;101:1251–1254.
12. Roth AR, Milsow L, Keltner JL. The ultimate diagnoses of patients undergoing temporal artery biopsies. Arch Ophthalmol 1984;102:901–903.
13. Chmelewski WL, McKnight KM, Agudelo CA, Wise CM. Presenting features and outcomes in patients undergoing temporal artery biopsy. Arch Intern Med 1992;152:1690–1695.
14. Gertz MA, Kyle RA, Griffing WL, Hunder GG. Jaw claudication in primary systemic amyloidosis. Medicine 1986;65:173–179.
15. Jones JG, Hazleman BL. Prognosis and management of polymyalgia rheumatica. Ann Rheum Dis 1981;40:1–5.
16. Simmons RJ, Cogan DG. Occult temporal arteritis. Arch Ophthalmol 1962;68:8–18.
17. Hayreh SS, Podhajsky PA, Zimmerman B. Occult giant cell arteritis: ocular manifestations. Am J Ophthalmol 1998;125:521–526.
18. Dudenhoefer EJ, Cornblath WT, Schatz MP. Scalp necrosis with giant cell arteritis. Ophthalmology 1998;105:1875–1878.
19. Pascuzzi RM, Roos KL, Davis TE Jr. Mental status abnormalities in temporal arteritis: a treatable cause of dementia in the elderly. Arthritis Rheum 1989;32:1308–1311.
20. Caselli RJ, Hunder GG, Whisnant JP. Neurologic disease in biopsy-proven giant cell (temporal) arteritis. Neurology 1988;38:352–359.
21. Boghen DR, Glaser JS. Ischaemic optic neuropathy: the clinical profile and natural history. Brain 1975;98:689–708.
22. Repka MX, Savino PJ, Schatz NJ, Sergott RC. Clinical profile and long-term implications of anterior ischemic optic neuropathy. Am J Ophthalmol 1983;96:478–483.
23. Hayreh SS, Podhajsky PA, Zimmerman B. Ocular manifestations of giant cell arteritis. Am J Ophthalmol 1998;125:509–520.
24. Hayreh SS. Anterior ischemic optic neuropathy: differentiation of arteritic from non-arteritic type and its management. Eye 1990;4:25–41.
25. Siatkowski RM, Gass JDM, Glaser JS, et al. Fluorescein angiography in the diagnosis of giant cell arteritis. Am J Ophthalmol 1993;115:57–63.
26. Melberg NS, Grand MG, Dieckert JP, et al. Cotton-wool spots and the early diagnosis of giant cell arteritis. Ophthalmology 1995;102:1611–1614.
27. Slavin ML, Barondes MJ. Visual loss caused by choroidal ischemia preceding anterior ischemic optic neuropathy in giant cell arteritis. Am J Ophthalmol 1994;117:81–86.
28. Quillen DA, Cantore WA, Schwartz SR, et al. Choroidal nonperfusion in giant cell arteritis. Am J Ophthalmol 1993;116:171–175
29. Mack HG, O'Day J, Currie JN. Delayed choroidal perfusion in giant cell arteritis. J Clin Neuroophthalmol 1991;11:221–227.
30. Jonas JB, Gabriele GC, Naumann GOH. Anterior ischemic optic neuropathy: nonarteritic form in small and giant cell arteritis in normal sized optic discs. Int Ophthalmol 1988;12:119–125.
31. Beck RW, Servais GE, Hayreh SS. Anterior ischemic optic neuropathy. IX. Cup-to-disc ratio and its role in pathogenesis. Ophthalmology 1987;94:1503–1508.
32. Spencer WH, Hoyt WF. A fatal case of giant-cell arteritis (temporal or cranial arteritis) with ocular involvement. Arch Ophthalmol 1960;64:862–867.
33. MacFaul PA. Ciliary artery involvement in giant cell arteritis. Br J Ophthalmol 1967;51:505–512.
34. Henkind P, Charles NC, Pearson J. Histopathology of ischemic optic neuropathy. Am J Ophthalmol 1970;69:78–90.
35. MacMichael IM, Cullen JF. Pathology of ischaemic optic neuropathy. In: Cant JS, ed. The Optic Nerve, Proceedings of the Second William MacKenzie Memorial Symposium. London, Henry Kimpton, 1972:108–116.
36. Rootman J, Butler D. Ischaemic optic neuropathy: a combined mechanism. Br J Ophthalmol 1980;64:826–831.
37. Crompton JL, Iyer P, Begg MW. Vasculitis and ischaemic optic neuropathy associated with rheumatoid arthritis. Aust J Ophthalmol 1980;8:219–230.
38. Sanders MD. Ischaemic papillopathy. Trans Ophthalmol Soc UK 1971;91:369–386.
39. Eagling EM, Sanders MD, Miller SJH. Ischaemic papillopathy: clinical and fluorescein angiographic review of forty cases. Br J Ophthalmol 1974;58:990–1008.
40. Hayreh SS. Anterior ischaemic optic neuropathy. II. Fundus on ophthalmoscopy and fluorescein angiography. Br J Ophthalmol 1974;58:964–980.
41. Slavin ML, Barondes MJ. Visual loss caused by choroidal ischemia preceding anterior ischemic optic neuropathy in giant cell arteritis. Am J Ophthalmol 1994;117:81–86.
42. Beri M, Klugman MR, Kohler JA, Hayreh SS. Anterior ischemic optic neuropathy. VII. Incidence of bilaterality and various influencing factors. Ophthalmology 1987;94:1020–1028.
43. Miller NR, Keltner JL, Gittinger JW, et al. Giant cell (temporal) arteritis. The differential diagnosis. Surv Ophthalmol 1979;23:259–263.
44. Graham E. Survival in temporal arteritis. Trans Ophthalmol Soc U K 1980;100:108–110.
45. Quigley H, Anderson DR. Cupping of the optic disc in ischemic optic neuropathy. Trans Am Acad Ophthalmol Otolaryngol 1977;83:755–762.
46. Sebag J, Thomas JV, Epstein DL, et al. Optic disc cupping in arteritic anterior ischemic optic neuropathy resembles glaucomatous cupping. Ophthalmology 1986;93:357–361.
47. Orgul S, Gass A, Flammer J. Optic disc cupping in arteritic anterior ischemic optic neuropathy. Ophthalmologica 1994;208:336–338.
48. Danesh-Meyer HV, Savino PJ, Sergott RC. The prevalence of cupping in end-stage arteritic and nonarteritic anterior ischemic optic neuropathy. Ophthalmology 2001;108:593–598.
49. Hayreh SS, Jonas JB. Optic disc morphology after arteritic anterior ischemic optic neuropathy. Ophthalmology 2001;108:1586–1594.
50. Miller A, Green M, Robinson D. Simple rule for calculating normal erythrocyte sedimentation rate. Br J Med 1983;286:266.
51. Wong RL, Korn JH. Temporal arteritis without an elevated erythrocyte sedimentation rate. Case report and review of the literature. Am J Med 1986;80:959–964.
52. Sharland DE. Erythrocyte sedimentation rate: the normal range in the elderly. J Am Geriatr Soc 1980;28:346–348.
53. Ischemic Optic Neuropathy Decompression Trial Research Group. Characteristics of patients with nonarteritic anterior ischemic optic neuropathy eligible for the Ischemic Optic Neuropathy Decompression Trial. Arch Ophthalmol 1996;114:1366–1374.
54. Hedges TR III, Gieger GL, Albert DM. The clinical value of negative temporal artery biopsy specimens. Arch Ophthalmol 1983;101:1251–1254.
55. Roth AR, Milsow L, Keltner JL. The ultimate diagnoses of patients undergoing temporal artery biopsies. Arch Ophthalmol 1984;102:901–903.

56. Kyle V, Cawston TE, Hazelman BL. Erythrocyte sedimentation rate and C reactive protein in the assessment of polymyalgia rheumatic/giant cell arteritis on presentation and during follow up. Ann Rheum Dis 1989;48:667–671.

57. Bates JH, Tomsak RL, Spedick MJ, et al. Serum fibrinogen concentration in the diagnosis and management of biopsy-proven giant-cell arteritis. Ophthalmology 1989;96(Suppl):105.

58. Holdstock G, Mitchell JRA. Erythrocyte sedimentation rate before and after invitro defibrination: a rapid and simple method for increasing its specificity. Lancet 1977;2:1314–1316.

59. Foroozan R, Danesh-Meyer H, Savino PJ, et al. Thrombocytosis in patients with biopsy-proven giant cell arteritis. Ophthalmology 2002;109:1267–1271.

60. Krishna R, Kosmorsky GS. Implications of thrombocytosis in giant cell arteritis. Am J Ophthalmol 1997;124:103.

61. Liozon E, Herrmann F, Ly K, et al. Risk factors for visual loss in giant cell (temporal) arteritis: a prospective study of 174 patients. Am J Med 2001;111: 211–217.

62. Klein RG, Campbell RJ, Hunder GG, Carney JA. Skip lesions in temporal arteritis. Mayo Clin Proc 1976;51:504–509.

63. Albert DM, Ruchman MC, Keltner JL. Skip lesions in temporal arteritis. Arch Ophthalmol 1976;94:2072–2077.

64. Brownstein S, Nicolle DA, Codere F. Bilateral blindness in temporal arteritis with skip areas. Arch Ophthalmol 1983;101:388–391.

65. McDonnell PJ, Moore GW, Miller NR, et al. Temporal arteritis: a clinicopathologic study. Ophthalmology 1986;93:518–530.

66. Hunder GG, Sheps SG, Allen GL, Joyce JW. Daily and alternate-day corticosteroid regimens in treatment of giant cell arteritis: comparison in a prospective study. Ann Intern Med 1975;82:613–618.

67. Klein RG, Campbell RJ, Hunder GG, et al. Skip lesions in temporal arteritis. Mayo Clin Proc 1976;51:504–510.

68. Hedges TR III, Gieger GL, Albert DM. The clinical value of negative temporal artery biopsy specimens. Arch Ophthalmol 1983;101:1251–1254.

69. Hayreh SS, Podhajsky PA, Raman R, et al. Giant cell arteritis: validity and reliability of various diagnostic criteria. Am J Ophthalmol 1997;123:285–296.

70. Boyev LR, Miller NR, Gree WR. Efficacy of unilateral versus bilateral temporal artery biopsies for the diagnosis of giant cell arteritis. Am J Ophthalmol 1999; 128:211–215.

71. Danesh-Meyer HV, Savino PJ, Eagle RC Jr, et al. Low diagnostic yield with second biopsies in suspected giant cell arteritis. J Neuroophthalmol 2000;20: 213–215.

72. Pless M, Rizzo JF, Lamkin JC, et al. Concordance of bilateral temporal artery biopsy in giant cell arteritis. J Neuroophthalmol 2000;20:216–218.

73. Hall JK, Volpe NJ, Galetta SL, et al. The role of unilateral temporal artery biopsy. Ophthalmology 2003;110:543–554.

74. Allison MC, Gallagher PJ. Temporal artery biopsy and corticosteroid treatment. Ann Rheum Dis 1984;43:416–417.

75. To KW, Enzer YR, Tsiaras WG. Temporal artery biopsy after one month of corticosteroid therapy. Am J Ophthalmol 1994;117:265–267.

76. Model DG. Reversal of blindness in temporal arteritis with methyl-prednisolone. Lancet 1978;1:340.

77. Rosenfeld SI, Kosmorsky GS, Klingele TG, Burde RM. Treatment of temporal arteritis with ocular involvement. Am J Med 1986;80:143–145.

78. Hayreh SS, Zimmerman B, Kardon RH. Visual improvement with corticosteroid therapy in giant cell arteritis: report of a large study and review of literature. Acta Ophthalmol Scand 2002;80:355–367.

79. Cornblath WT, Eggenberger ER. Progressive visual loss from giant cell arteritis despite high-dose intravenous methylprednisolone. Ophthalmology 1997;104: 854–858.

80. Foroozan R, Deramo VA, Buono LM, Recovery of visual function in patients with biopsy-proven giant cell arteritis. Ophthalmology 2003;110:539–542.

81. Miller NR, Keltner JL, Gittinger JW. Giant cell (temporal) arteritis. The differential diagnosis. Surv Ophthalmol 1979;23:259–263.

82. Myles AB, Perera T, Ridley MG. Prevention of blindness in giant cell arteritis by corticosteroid treatment. Br J Rheumatol 1992;31:103–105.

83. Nesher G, Berkun Y, Mates M, et al. Low-dose aspirin and prevention of cranial ischemic complications in giant cell arteritis. Arthritis Rheum 2004;50: 1332–1337.

84. Kattah JC, Kennerdell JS. Orbital apex syndrome secondary to herpes zoster ophthalmicus. Am J Ophthalmol 1978;85:378–382.

85. Borruat FX, Herbort CP. Herpes zoster ophthalmicus: anterior ischemic optic neuropathy and acyclovir. J Clin Neuroophthalmol 1992;12:37–40.

86. Isaak BL, Liesegang TJ, Michet CJ Jr. Ocular and systemic findings in relapsing polychondritis. Ophthalmology 1986;93:681–689.

87. Massry GG, Chung SM, Selhorst JB. Optic neuropathy, headache, and diplopia with MRI suggestive of cerebral arteritis in relapsing polychondritis. J Neuroophthalmol 1995;15:171–175.

88. McGavin DDM, Williamson J, Forrester JV, et al. Episcleritis and scleritis: a study of their clinical manifestations and association with rheumatoid arthritis. Br J Ophthalmol 1976;60:192–226.

89. Crompton JL, Iyer P, Begg MW. Vasculitis and ischaemic optic neuropathy associated with rheumatoid arthritis. Aust J Ophthalmol 1980;8:219–230.

90. Leonard TJK, Sanders MD. Ischaemic optic neuropathy in pulseless disease. Br J Ophthalmol 1983;67:389–392.

91. Hackett ER, Martinez RD, Larson PF, et al. Optic neuritis in systemic lupus erythematosus. Arch Neurol 1974;31:9–11.

92. Jabs DA, Miller NR, Newman SA, et al. Optic neuropathy in systemic lupus erythematosus. Arch Ophthalmol 1986;104:564–568.

93. Weinstein JM, Chui H, Lane S, et al. Churg Strauss syndrome (allergic granulomatous angiitis). Arch Ophthalmol 1983;101:1217–1220.

94. Kattah JC, Chousos GA, Katz PA, et al. Anterior ischemic optic neuropathy in Churg-Strauss syndrome. Ophthalmology 1994;44:2200–2202.

95. Goldstein I, Wexler D. Bilateral atrophy of the optic nerve in periarteritis nodosa. Arch Ophthalmol 1937;18:767–773.

96. Scouras J, Koutroumanos J. Ischaemic optic neuropathy in Behçet's syndrome. Ophthalmologica 1976;173:11–18.

97. Heuer DK, Gager WE, Reeser FH. Ischemic optic neuropathy associated with Crohn's disease. J Clin Neuroophthalmol 1982;2:175–181.

98. Kupersmith MJ, Burde RM, Warren FA, et al. Autoimmune optic neuropathy: evaluation and treatment. J Neurol Neurosurg Psychiatr 1988;51:1381–1386.

99. Kidd D, Burton B, Plant GT, et al. Chronic relapsing inflammatory optic neuropathy (CRION). Brain 2003;126:276–284.

100. Hattenhauer MG, Leavitt JA, Hodge DO, et al. Incidence of nonarteritic anterior ischemic optic neuropathy. Am J Ophthalmol 1997;123:103–107.

101. Gordon LK, Yu F, Coleman AL, et al. Medicare database analysis of prevalence and risk factors for ischemic optic neuropathy. Ophthalmology 2003;110(Suppl): 238.

102. Hayreh SS, Joos KM, Podhajsky PA, Long CR. Systemic diseases associated with nonarteritic anterior ischemic optic neuropathy. Am J Ophthalmol 1994; 118:766–780.

103. Hayreh SS, Podhajsky P, Zimmerman MB. Role of nocturnal arterial hypotension in optic nerve head ischemic disorders. Ophthalmologica 1999;213:76–96.

104. Rizzo JF, Lessell S. Optic neuritis and ischemic optic neuropathy: overlapping clinical profiles. Arch Ophthalmol 1991;109:1668–1672.

105. Swartz NG, Beck RW, Savino PJ, et al. Pain in anterior ischemic optic neuropathy. J Neuroophthalmol 1995;15:9–10.

106. Arnold AC, Hepler RS. Natural history of nonarteritic anterior ischemic optic neuropathy. J Neuroophthalmol 1994;14:66–69.

107. Yee RD, Selky AK, Purvin VA. Outcomes of optic nerve sheath decompression for nonarteritic ischemic optic neuropathy. J Neuroophthalmol 1994;14:70–76.

108. Hayreh SS, Podhajsky P. Visual field defects in anterior ischemic optic neuropathy. Doc Ophthalmol Proc Ser 1979;19:53–71.

109. Traustason OI, Feldon SE, Leemaster JE, et al. Anterior ischemic optic neuropathy: classification of field defects by Octopus automated static perimetry. Graefes Arch Clin Exp Ophthalmol 1988;226:206–212.

110. Arnold AC, Hepler RS. Fluorescein angiography in acute anterior ischemic optic neuropathy. Am J Ophthalmol 1994;117:222–230.

111. Smith JL. Pseudohemangioma of the optic disc following ischemic optic neuropathy. J Clin Neuroophthalmol 1985;5:81–89.

112. Rader J, Feuer WJ, Anderson DR. Peripapillary vasoconstriction in the glaucomas and the anterior ischemic optic neuropathies. Am J Ophthalmol 1994; 117:72–80.

113. Jonas JB, Gusek GC, Naumann GO. Anterior ischemic optic neuropathy: nonarteritic form in small and giant cell arteritis in normal-sized optic discs. Int Ophthalmol 1988;12:119–125.

114. Mansour AM, Shoch D, Logani S. Optic disk size in ischemic optic neuropathy. Am J Ophthalmol 1988;106:587–589.

115. Feit RH, Tomsak RL, Ellenberger C. Structural factors in the pathogenesis of ischemic optic neuropathy. Am J Ophthalmol 1984;98:105–108.

116. Beck RW, Savino PJ, Repka MX, et al. Optic disc structure in anterior ischemic optic neuropathy. Ophthalmology 1984;91:1334–1337.

117. Doro S, Lessell S. Cup disc ratio and ischemic optic neuropathy. Arch Ophthalmol 1985;103:1143–1144.

118. Burde RM. Optic disk risk factors for nonarteritic anterior ischemic optic neuropathy. Am J Ophthalmol 1993;116:759–764.

119. Cogan DG. Neurology of the Visual System. Springfield, IL, Charles C Thomas, 1966:186.

120. Knox DL, Duke JR. Slowly progressive ischemic optic neuropathy: a clinicopathologic case report. Trans Am Acad Ophthalmol Otolaryngol 1971;75: 1065–1068.

121. Lieberman MF, Shahi A, Green WR. Embolic ischemic optic neuropathy. Am J Ophthalmol 1978;86:206–210.

122. Quigley HA, Miller NR, Green WR. The pattern of optic nerve fiber loss in anterior ischemic optic neuropathy. Am J Ophthalmol 1985;100:769–776.

123. Levin LA, Louhab A. Apoptosis of retinal ganglion cells in anterior ischemic optic neuropathy. Arch Ophthalmol 1996;114:488–491.

124. Tesser RA, Niendorf ER, Levin LA. The morphology of an infarct in nonarteritic anterior ischemic optic neuropathy. Ophthalmology 2003;110:2031–2035.

125. Knox DL, Kerrison JB, Green WR. Histopathologic studies of ischemic optic neuropathy. Trans Am Ophthalmol Soc 2000;98:203–222.

126. Olver JM, Spalton DJ, McCartney ACE. Microvascular study of the retrolaminar optic nerve in man: the possible significance in anterior ischemic optic neuropathy. Eye 1990;4:7–24.

127. Onda E, Cioffi GA, Bacon DR, et al. Microvasculature of the human optic nerve. Am J Ophthalmol 1995;120:92–102.

128. Arnold AC, Badr M, Hepler RS. Fluorescein angiography in nonischemic optic disc edema. Arch Ophthalmol 1996;114:293–298.

129. Friedland S, Winterkorn JMS, Burde RM. Luxury perfusion following anterior ischemic optic neuropathy. J Neuroophthalmol 1996;16:163–171.

130. Valmaggia C, Speiser P, Bischoff P, et al. Indocyanine green versus fluorescein angiography in the differential diagnosis of arteritic and nonarteritic anterior ischemic optic neuropathy. Retina 1999;19:131–134.

131. Oto S, Yilmaz G, Cakmakci S, Aydin P. Indocyanine green and fluorescein angiography in nonarteritic anterior ischemic optic neuropathy. Retina 2002;22:187–191.

132. Feldon SE. Anterior ischemic optic neuropathy: trouble waiting to happen. Ophthalmology 2000;106:651–652.

133. Hayreh SS. Anterior ischemic optic neuropathy: trouble waiting to happen [letter]. Ophthalmology 2000;107:407–409.

134. Feldon SE. Anterior ischemic optic neuropathy: trouble waiting to happen [author's reply]. Ophthalmology 2000;409–410.

135. Hayreh SS. The blood supply of the optic nerve head and the evaluation of it: myth and reality. Progr Retin Eye Res 2001;20:563–593.

136. Hayreh SS. Blood flow in the optic nerve head and factors that may influence it. Progr Retin Eye Res 2001;20:595–624.

137. Fry CL, Carter JE, Kanter MC, et al. Anterior ischemic optic neuropathy is not associated with carotid artery atherosclerosis. Stroke 1993;24:539–542.

138. Muller M, Kessler C, Wessel K, et al. Low-tension glaucoma: a comparative study with retinal ischemic syndromes and anterior ischemic optic neuropathy. Ophthalmic Surg 1993;24:835–838.

139. Strenn K, Matulla B, Wolzt M, et al. Reversal of endothelin-1-induced ocular hemodynamic effects by low-dose nifedipine in humans. Clin Pharmacol Ther 1998;63:54–63.

140. Oku H, Sugiyama T, Kojima S, et al. Experimental optic cup enlargement caused by endothelin-1-induced chronic optic nerve head ischemia. Surv Ophthalmol 1999;44(Suppl 1):S74–S84.

141. Hayreh SS, Piegors DJ, Heisted DD. Serotonin-induced constriction of ocular arteries in atherosclerotic monkeys. Arch Ophthalmol 1997;115:220–228.

142. Hayreh SS. Retinal and optic nerve head ischemic disorders and atherosclerosis: role of serotonin. Progr Retin Eye Res 1999;18:191–221.

143. Hayreh SS, Zimmerman MB, Podhajsky P, et al. Nocturnal arterial hypotension and its role in optic nerve head and ocular ischemic disorders. Am J Ophthalmol 1994;117:603–624.

144. Landau K, Winterkorn JMS, Mailloux LU, et al. 24-hour blood pressure monitoring in patients with anterior ischemic optic neuropathy. Arch Ophthalmol 1996;114:570–575

145. Hayreh SS, Zimmerman MB, Podhajsky P, et al. Nonarteritic anterior ischemic optic neuropathy: role of nocturnal hypotension [letter]. Arch Ophthalmol 1997;115:942–943.

146. Landau K, Winterkorn JMS, Napolitano B. Nonarteritic anterior ischemic optic neuropathy: role of nocturnal hypotension [reply to letter]. Arch Ophthalmol 1997;115:943–945.

147. Mojon DS, Hedges TR 3rd, Ehrenberg B, et al. Association between sleep apnea syndrome and nonarteritic anterior ischemic optic neuropathy. Arch Ophthalmol 2002;120:601–605.

148. Mojon DS, Mathis J, Zulauf M, et al. Optic neuropathy associated with sleep apnea syndrome. Ophthalmology 1998;105:874–877.

149. Shamsuzzaman AS, Winnicki M, Lanfranchi P, et al. Elevated C-reactive protein in patients with obstructive sleep apnea. Circulation 2002;105:2462–2464.

150. Ellenberger C Jr, Keltner JL, Burde RM. Acute optic neuropathy in older patients. Arch Neurol 1973;8:18–185.

151. Moro F, Doro D, Mantovani E. Anterior ischemic optic neuropathy and aging. Metab Pediatr Syst Ophthalmol 1989;12:46–57.

152. Sawle GV, James CB, Ross Russell RW. The natural history of nonarteritic anterior ischaemic optic neuropathy. J Neurol Neurosurg Psychiatry 1990;53:830–833.

153. Awad IA, Spetzler RF, Hodak JA, et al. Incidental subcortical lesions identified on magnetic resonance imaging in the elderly. I. Correlation with age and cerebrovascular risk factors. Stroke 1986;17:1083–1089.

154. Awad IA, Johnson PC, Spetzler RF, et al. Incidental subcortical lesions identified on magnetic resonance imaging in the elderly: II. Postmortem pathological correlations. Stroke 1986;17:1090–1097.

155. Jay WM, Williamson MR. Incidence of subcortical lesions not increased in nonarteritic ischemic optic neuropathy on magnetic resonance imaging. Am J Ophthalmol 1987;104:398–400.

156. Arnold AC, Hepler RS, Hamilton DR, et al. Magnetic resonance imaging of the brain in nonarteritic ischemic optic neuropathy. J Neuroophthalmol 1995;15:158–160.

157. Jacobson DM, Vierkant RA, Belongia EA. Nonarteritic anterior ischemic optic neuropathy. A case-control study of potential risk factors. Arch Ophthalmol 1997;115:1403–1407.

158. Salomon O, Huna-Baron R, Kurtz S, et al. Analysis of prothrombotic and vascular risk factors in patients with nonarteritic anterior ischemic optic neuropathy. Ophthalmology 1999;106:739–742.

159. Giuffre G. Hematological risk factors for anterior ischemic optic neuropathy. Neuroophthalmology 1990;10:197–203

160. Talks SJ, Chong NH, Gibson JM, et al. Fibrinogen, cholesterol, and smoking as risk factors for non-arteritic anterior ischaemic optic neuropathy. Eye 1995;9:85–88.

161. Chung SM, Gay CA, McCrary JA. Nonarteritic anterior ischemic optic neuropathy. The impact of tobacco use. Ophthalmology 1994;101:779–782.

162. Deramo VA, Sergott RC, Augsburger JJ, et al. Ischemic optic neuropathy as the first manifestation of elevated cholesterol levels in young patients. Ophthalmology 2003;110:1041–1045.

163. Kawasaki A, Purvin VA, Burgett RA. Hyperhomocysteinaemia in young patients with non-arteritic anterior ischaemic optic neuropathy. Br J Ophthalmol 1999;83:1287–1290.

164. Biousse V, Kerrison JB, Newman NJ? Is non-arteritic anterior ischaemic optic neuropathy related to homocysteine? Br J Ophthalmol 2000;84:554.

165. Pianka P, Almog Y, Man O, et al. Hyperhomocysteinemia in patients with nonarteritic anterior ischemic optic neuropathy, central retinal artery occlusion, and central retinal vein occlusion. Ophthalmology 2000;107:1588–1592.

166. Weger M, Stanger O, Deutschmann H, et al. Hyperhomocysteinemia, but not MTHFR C677T mutation, as a risk factor for non-arteritic anterior ischaemic optic neuropathy. Br J Ophthalmol 2001;85:803–806.

167. Salomon O, Dardik R, Steinberg DM. The role of angiotensin converting enzyme and angiotensin II type 1 receptor gene polymorphisms in patients with nonarteritic anterior ischemic optic neuropathy. Ophthalmology 2000;107:1717–1720.

168. Salomon O, Rosenberg N, Steinberg DM, et al. Nonarteritic anterior ischemic optic neuropathy is associated with a specific platelet polymorphism located on the glycoprotein Ib-alpha gene. Ophthalmology 2004;111:184–188.

169. Cohen DN. Drusen of the optic disc and the development of field defects. Arch Ophthalmol 1971;85:224–226.

170. Karel I, Otradovec J, Peleska M. Fluorescence angiography in circulatory disturbances in drusen of the optic disk. Ophthalmologica 1972;164:449–462.

171. Gittinger JW Jr., Lessell S, Bondar RL. Ischemic optic neuropathy associated with optic disc drusen. J Clin Neuroophthalmol 1984;4:79–84.

172. Newman WD, Dorrell ED. Anterior ischemic optic neuropathy associated with disc drusen. J Neuroophthalmol 1996;16:7–8.

173. Liew SC, Mitchell P. Anterior ischaemic optic neuropathy in a patient with optic disc drusen. Aust NZ J Ophthalmol 1999;27:157–160.

174. Purvin V, King R, Kawasaki A, Yee R. Anterior ischemic optic neuropathy in eyes with optic disc drusen. Arch Ophthalmol 2004;122:48–53.

175. Begg IS, Drance SM, Sweeney VP. Ischaemic optic neuropathy in chronic simple glaucoma. Br J Ophthalmol 1971;55:73–90.

176. Tomsak RL, Remler BF. Anterior ischemic optic neuropathy and increased intraocular pressure. J Clin Neuroophthalmol 1989;9:116–118.

177. Katz B, Weinreb RN, Wheeler DT. Anterior ischemic optic neuropathy and intraocular pressure. Br J Ophthalmol 1990;74:99–102.

178. Katz B. Anterior ischemic optic neuropathy and intraocular pressure. Arch Ophthalmol 1992;110:596–597.

179. Kalenak JW, Kosmorsky GS, Rockwood EJ. Nonarteritic anterior ischemic optic neuropathy and intraocular pressure. Arch Ophthalmol 1991;109:660–661.

180. Slavin ML, Margulis M. Anterior ischemic optic neuropathy following acute angle-closure glaucoma. Arch Ophthalmol 2001;119:1215.

181. Arnold AC. Anterior ischemic optic neuropathy following ocular pneumoplethysmography. J Clin Neuroophthalmol 1987;7:58–59.

182. Lee AG, Kohnen T, Ebner R, et al. Optic neuropathy associated with laser in situ keratomileusis. J Cataract Refract Surg 2000;26:1581–1584.

183. Cameron BD, Saffra NA, Strominger MB. Laser in situ keratomileusis-induced optic neuropathy. Ophthalmology 2001;108:660–665.

184. Gartner S. Optic neuritis and macular edema following cataract extraction. Eye Ear Nose Throat Monthly 1964;43:45–49.

185. Hayreh SS. Anterior ischemic optic neuropathy: IV. Occurrence after cataract extraction. Arch Ophthalmol 1980;98:1410–1416.

186. Serrano LA, Behrens MM, Carroll FD. Postcataract extraction ischemic optic neuropathy. Arch Ophthalmol 1982;100:1177–1178.

187. Spedick MJ, Tomsak RL. Ischemic optic neuropathy following secondary intraocular lens implantation. J Clin Neuroophthalmol 1984;4:255–257.

188. McCulley TJ, Lam BL, Feuer WJ. Incidence of nonarteritic anterior ischemic optic neuropathy associated with cataract extraction. Ophthalmology 2001;108:1275–1278.

189. McCulley TJ, Lam BL, Feuer WJ. Nonarteritic anterior ischemic optic neuropathy and surgery of the anterior segment: temporal relationship analysis. Am J Ophthalmol 2003;136:1171–1172.

190. McDonald WI, Sanders MD. Migraine complicated by ischaemic papillopathy. Lancet 1971;2:521–523.

191. Weinstein JM, Feman SS. Ischemic optic neuropathy in migraine. Arch Ophthalmol 1982;100:1097–1100.

192. Katz B, Bamford CR. Migrainous ischemic optic neuropathy. Neurology 1985;35:112–114.

193. Katz B. Bilateral sequential migrainous ischemic optic neuropathy. Am J Ophthalmol 1985;99:489.

194. Kupersmith MJ, Warren FA, Hass WK. The non-benign aspects of migraine. Neuroophthalmology 1987;7:1–10.

195. Burde RM, Smith ME, Black JT. Retinal artery occlusion in the absence of a cherry red spot. Surv Ophthalmol 1982;27:181.

196. Tomsak RL. Ischemic optic neuropathy associated with retinal embolism. Am J Ophthalmol 1985;99:590–592.

197. Portnoy SL, Beer PM, Packer AJ, et al. Embolic anterior ischemic optic neuropathy. J Clin Neuroophthalmol 1989;9:21–25.

198. Esmaeli B, Koller C, Papadopoulos N, Romaguera J. Interferon-induced retinopathy in asymptomatic cancer patients. Ophthalmology 2001;108:858–860.

199. Purvin VA. Anterior ischemic optic neuropathy secondary to interferon alfa. Arch Ophthalmol 1995;113:1041–1044.

200. Norcia F, Di Maria A, Prandini F, et al. Natural interferon therapy: optic nerve ischemic damage? Ophthalmologica 1999;213:339–340.

201. Lohmann CP, Kroher G, Bogenrieder T, et al. Severe loss of vision during adjuvant interferon alfa-2b treatment for malignant melanoma. Lancet 1999;353:1326.

202. Gupta R, Singh S, Tang R, et al. Anterior ischemic optic neuropathy caused by interferon alpha therapy. Am J Med 2002;112:683–684.

203. Vardizer Y, Linhart Y, Loewenstein A, et al. Interferon-alpha-associated bilateral simultaneous ischemic optic neuropathy. J Neuroophthalmol 2003;23:256–259.

204. Pomeranz HD, Smith KH, Hart WM Jr, et al. Sildenafil-associated nonarteritic anterior ischemic optic neuropathy. Ophthalmology 2002;109:584–587.

205. Egan RA, Pomeranz HD. Sildenafil (Viagra) associated anterior ischemic optic neuropathy. Arch Ophthalmol 2000;118:291–292.

206. Cunningham AV, Smith KH. Anterior ischemic optic neuropathy associated with Viagra. J Neuroophthalmol 2001;21:22–25.

207. Gittinger JW Jr, Asdourian GK. Papillopathy caused by amiodarone. Arch Ophthalmol 1987;105:349–351.

208. Feiner LA, Younge BR, Kazmier FJ, et al. Optic neuropathy and amiodarone therapy. Mayo Clin Proc 1987;62:702–717.

209. Nazarian SM, Jay WM. Bilateral optic neuropathy associated with amiodarone therapy. J Clin Neuroophthalmol 1988;8:25–28.

210. Garrett SN, Kearney JJ, Schiffman JS. Amiodarone optic neuropathy. J Clin Neuroophthalmol 1988;8:105–110.

211. Sedwick LA. Getting to the heart of visual loss: when cardiac medication may be dangerous to the optic nerves. Surv Ophthalmol 1992;36:366–372.

212. Palimar P, Cota N. Bilateral anterior ischaemic optic neuropathy following amiodarone. Eye 1998;12:894–896.

213. Seemongal-Dass RR, Spencer SR. Bilateral optic neuropathy linked with amiodarone. Eye 1998;12:474–477.

214. Macaluso DC, Shults WT, Fraunfelder FT. Features of amiodarone-induced optic neuropathy. Am J Ophthalmol 1999;127:610–612.

215. Mansour AM, Puklin JE, O'Grady R. Optic nerve ultrastructure following amiodarone therapy. J Clin Neuroophthalmol 1988;8:231–237.

216. Nagra PK, Foroozan R, Savino PJ, et al. Amiodarone-induced optic neuropathy. Br J Ophthalmol 2003;87:420–422.

217. Nickells RW. Retinal ganglion cell death in glaucoma: the how, the why, the maybe. J Glaucoma 1996;5:345–356.

218. Quigley HA, McKinnon SJ, Zack DJ, et al. Retrograde axonal transport of BDNF in retinal ganglion cells is blocked by acute IOP elevation in rats. Invest Ophthalmol Vis Sci 2000;41:3460–3466.

219. Mansour-Robaey S, Clarke DB, Wang YC, et al. Effects of ocular injury and administration of brain-derived neurotrophic factor on survival and regrowth of axotomized retinal ganglion cells. Proc Natl Acad Sci USA 1994;91:1632–1636.

220. Sucher NJ, Lipton SA, Dreyer EB. Molecular basis of glutamate toxicity in retinal ganglion cells. Vision Res 1997;37:3483–3493.

221. Levin LA, Clark JA, Johns LK. Effect of lipid peroxidation inhibition on retinal ganglion cell death. Invest Ophthalmol Vis Sci 1996;37:2744–2749.

222. Levin LA, Louhab A. Apoptosis of retinal ganglion cells in anterior ischemic optic neuropathy. Arch Ophthalmol 1996;114:488–491.

223. Yoles E, Wheeler LA, Schwartz M. Alpha2-adrenoreceptor agonists are neuroprotective in a rat model of optic nerve degeneration. Invest Ophthalmol Vis Sci 1999;40:65–73.

224. Vorwerk CK, Zurakowski D, McDermott LM, et al. Effects of axonal injury on ganglion cell survival and glutamate homeostasis. Brain Res Bull 2004;62:485–490.

225. Bernstein SL, Guo Y, Kelman SE, et al. Functional and cellular responses in a novel rodent model of anterior ischemic optic neuropathy. Invest Ophthalmol Vis Sci 2003;44:4153–4162.

226. Movsas T, Kelman SE, Elman MJ, et al. The natural course of non-arteritic ischemic optic neuropathy. Invest Ophthalmol Vis Sci 1991;42(Suppl):951.

227. Ischemic Optic Neuropathy Decompression Trial Research Group. Twenty-four month update. Arch Ophthalmol 2000;118:793–798.

228. Borchert M, Lessell S. Progressive and recurrent nonarteritic anterior ischemic optic neuropathy. Am J Ophthalmol 1988;106:443–449.

229. Kline LB. Progression of visual defects in ischemic optic neuropathy. Am J Ophthalmol 1988;106:199–203.

230. Sergott RC, Cohen MS, Bosley TM, Savino PJ. Optic nerve sheath decompression may improve the progressive form of ischemic optic neuropathy. Arch Ophthalmol 1989;107:1743–1754.

231. Ischemic Optic Neuropathy Decompression Trial Research Group. Optic nerve decompression surgery for nonarteritic anterior ischemic optic neuropathy (NAION) is not effective and may be harmful. JAMA 1995;273:625–632.

232. Borchert M, Lessell S. Progressive and recurrent nonarteritic anterior ischemic optic neuropathy. Am J Ophthalmol 1988;106:443–449.

233. Boone I, Massry GG, Frankel RA, et al. Visual outcome in bilateral nonarteritic anterior ischemic optic neuropathy. Ophthalmology 1996;103:1223–1228.

234. Hayreh SS, Podhajsky PA, Zimmerman B. Ipsilateral recurrence of nonarteritic anterior ischemic optic neuropathy. Am J Ophthalmol 2001;132:734–742.

235. Beck RW, Savino PJ, Schatz NJ, et al. Anterior ischaemic optic neuropathy. Recurrent episodes in the same eye. Br J Ophthalmol 1983;67:705–709.

236. Hamed LM, Purvin V, Rosenberg M. Recurrent anterior ischemic optic neuropathy in young adults. J Clin Neuroophthalmol 1988;8:239–246.

237. WuDunn D, Zimmerman K, Sadun AA, et al. Comparison of visual function in fellow eyes after bilateral nonarteritic anterior ischemic optic neuropathy. Ophthalmology 1997;104:104–111.

238. Beck RW, Hayreh SS, Podhajsky PA, et al. Aspirin therapy in nonarteritic anterior ischemic optic neuropathy. Am J Ophthalmol 1997;123:212–217.

239. Newman NJ, Scherer R, Langenberg P, et al. The fellow eye in NAION: report from the Ischemic Optic Neuropathy Decompression Trial follow-up study. Am J Ophthalmol 2002;134:317–328.

240. Arnold AC, Badr M, Hepler RS. Fluorescein angiography in nonischemic optic disc edema. Arch Ophthalmol 1996;114:293–298.

241. VITATOPS Trial Study Group. The VITATOPS (Vitamins to Prevent Stroke) Trial: rationale and design of an international, large, simple, randomised trial of homocysteine-lowering multivitamin therapy in patients with recent transient ischaemic attack or stroke. Cerebrovasc Dis 2002;13:120–126.

242. Lasco F. Les affections vasculaires du nerf optique et leurs manifestations clinique. Ophthalmologica 1961;142:429–445.

243. Saraux H, Murat JP. Les pseudo papillites d'origine vasculaire. Ann Ocul 1967;200:1–19.

244. Keltner JL, Becker B, Gay AJ, et al. Effect of diphenylhydantoin in ischemic optic neuritis. Trans Am Ophthalmol Soc 1972;70:113–128.

245. Burde RM. Ischemic optic neuropathy. In: Smith JL, Glaser JS, eds. Neuro-ophthalmology Symposium of the University of Miami and the Bascom Palmer Eye Institute, vol 7. St Louis, CV Mosby, 1973:38–62.

246. Ellenberger C Jr, Burde RM, Keltner JL. Acute optic neuropathy: treatment with diphenylhydantoin. Arch Ophthalmol 1974;91:435–438.

247. Francois J, Verriest G, Neetens A, et al. Pseudo-papillitis vascularis. Ann Ocul 1962;195:830–885.

248. Calmettes L, Deodati F, Bechac G. Pseudo-papillite vasculaire. Rev Otoneuroophtalmol 1963;35:64–65.

249. Bonamour G. A propos de "pseudo-papillites vasculaires." Bull Soc Ophtalmol Fr 1966;66:846–850.

250. Kollarits CR, McCarthy RW, Corrie WS, et al. Norepinephrine therapy of ischemic optic neuropathy. J Clin Neuroophthalmol 1981;1:283–288.

251. Smith JL. Norepinephrine therapy of ischemic optic neuropathy. J Clin Neuroophthalmol 1981;1:289–290.

252. Kajiwara K, Tsubota K, Hara Y. High-dose urokinase thrombolysis and stellate ganglion block for anterior ischemic neuropathy. Fola Ophthalmol Jpn 1990;41:59–64.

253. Botelho PJ, Johnson LN, Arnold AC. The effect of aspirin on the visual outcome of nonarteritic anterior ischemic optic neuropathy. Am J Ophthalmol 1996;121:450–451.

254. Maas A, Walzl M, Jesenik F, et al. Application of HELP in nonarteritic anterior ischemic optic neuropathy: a prospective, randomized, controlled study. Graefes Arch Clin Exp Ophthalmol 1997;235:14–19.

255. Arnold AC, Hepler RS, Lieber M, Alexander JM. Hyperbaric oxygen therapy for nonarteritic anterior ischemic optic neuropathy. Am J Ophthalmol 1996;122:535–541.

256. Johnson LN, Guy ME, Krohel GB, et al. Levodopa may improve vision loss in recent-onset, nonarteritic anterior ischemic optic neuropathy. Ophthalmology 2000;107:521–526.

257. Hayreh SS. Does levodopa improve visual function in NAION? Ophthalmology 2000;107:1434–1438.

258. Cox TA. Does levodopa improve visual function in NAION? Ophthalmology 2000;107:1431.

259. Beck RW. Does levodopa improve visual function in NAION? Ophthalmology 2000;107:1431–1434.

260. Brourman ND, Spoor TC, Ramocki JM. Optic nerve sheath decompression for pseudotumor cerebri. Arch Ophthalmol 1988;106:1378–1383.

261. Sergott RC, Savino PJ, Schatz NJ. Modified optic nerve sheath decompression provides long-term visual improvement for pseudotumor cerebri. Arch Ophthalmol 1988;106:1384–1390.

262. Corbett JJ, Nerad JA, Tse DT, Anderson RL. Results of optic nerve sheath fenestration for pseudotumor cerebri: the lateral orbitotomy approach. Arch Ophthalmol 1988;106:1391–1397.

263. Spoor TC, Wilkinson MJ, Ramocki JM. Optic nerve sheath decompression for the treatment of progressive nonarteritic ischemic optic neuropathy. Am J Ophthalmol 1991;111:724–728.

264. Kelman SE, Elman MJ. Optic nerve sheath decompression for nonarteritic ante-

rior ischemic optic neuropathy improves multiple visual function measurements. Arch Ophthalmol 1991;109:667–671.

265. Opremcak EM, Bruce RA, Lomeo MD, et al. Radial optic neurotomy for central retinal vein occlusion: a retrospective pilot study of 11 consecutive cases. Retina 2001;21:408–415.

266. Soheilian M, Koochek A, Yazdani S, Peyman GA. Transvitreal optic neurotomy for nonarteritic anterior ischemic optic neuropathy. Retina 2003;23:692–697.

267. Arnold AC, Levin LA. Treatment of ischemic optic neuropathy. Semin Ophthalmol 2002;17:39–46.

268. Steinsapir KD, Goldberg RA. Traumatic optic neuropathy. Surv Ophthalmol 1994;38:487–518.

269. Bracken MB, Shepard MJ, Holford TR, et al. Administration of methylprednisolone for 24 or 48 hours or tirilazad mesylate for 48 hours in the treatment of acute spinal cord injury. Results of the Third National Acute Spinal Cord Injury Randomized Controlled Trial. National Acute Spinal Cord Injury Study. JAMA 1997;277:1597–1604.

270. Kent AR, Nussdorf JD, David R, et al. Vitreous concentration of topically applied brimonidine tartrate 0.2%. Ophthalmology 2001;108:784–787.

271. Wilhelm B, Zrenner E. Naion as a model disease for testing neuroprotective interventions: the BRAION Multicenter Study. Neuroophthalmology 2001;25:50.

272. Fazzone HE, Kupersmith MJ, Leibmann J. Does topical brimonidine tartrate help NAION? Br J Ophthalmol 2003;87:1193–1194.

273. Kupersmith MJ, Frohman L, Sanderson M, et al. Aspirin reduces the incidence of second eye NAION: a retrospective study. J Neuroophthalmol 1997;17:250–253.

274. Salomon O, Huna-Baron R, Steinberg DM, et al. Role of aspirin in reducing the frequency of second eye involvement in patients with non-arteritic anterior ischaemic optic neuropathy. Eye 1999;13:357–359.

275. Beck RW, Hayreh SS. Role of aspirin in reducing the frequency of second eye involvement in patients with non-arteritic anterior ischaemic optic neuropathy. Eye 2000;14:118.

276. Behrens MM, Odel JG. Other optic nerve disorders. In: Lessel S, Van Dalen JTW, et al. Current Neuro-ophthalmology, vol 3. St Louis, Mosby Year Book, 1991:35–50.

277. Sadda SR, Nee M, Miller NR, et al. Clinical spectrum of posterior ischemic optic neuropathy. Am J Ophthalmol 2001;132:743–750.

278. Hayreh SS. Posterior ischemic optic neuropathy. Ophthalmologica 1981b;182:29–41.

279. Lee AG, Eggenberger ER, Kaufman DI, et al. Optic nerve enhancement on magnetic resonance imaging in arteritic ischemic optic neuropathy. J Neuroophthalmol 1999;19:235–237.

280. Lopez JM, Nazabal ER, Muniz AM, et al. Detection of posterior ischemic optic neuropathy due to giant cell arteritis with magnetic resonance imaging. Eur J Neurol 2001;46:109–110.

281. Horton JC. Mistaken treatment of anterior ischemic optic neuropathy with interferon beta-1a. Ann Neurol 2002;52:129.

282. Chisholm IA. Optic neuropathy of recurrent blood loss. Br J Ophthalmol 1969;53:289–295.

283. Klewin KM, Appen RE, Kaufman PL. Amaurosis and blood loss. Am J Ophthalmol 1978;86:669–672.

284. Hayreh SS. Anterior ischemic optic neuropathy: VIII. Clinical features and pathogenesis of post hemorrhagic amaurosis. Ophthalmology 1987;94:1488–1502.

285. Johnson MW, Kincaid MC, Trobe JD. Bilateral retrobulbar optic nerve infarctions after blood loss and hypotension. Ophthalmology 1987;94:1577–1584.

286. Katz DM, Trobe JD, Cornblath WT, et al. Ischemic optic neuropathy after lumbar spine surgery. Arch Ophthalmol 1994;112:925–931.

287. Lazaro EJ, Cinotti AA, Eichler PN, et al. Amaurosis due to massive gastrointestinal hemorrhage. Am J Gastroenterol 1971;55:50–53.

288. Presencia AC, Hernandez AM, Guia ED. Amaurosis following blood loss. Ophthalmologica 1985;191:119–122.

289. Sweeney PJ, Breuer AC, Selhorst JB, et al. Ischemic optic neuropathy: a complication of cardiopulmonary bypass surgery. Neurology 1982;32:560–562.

290. Breuer AC, Furlan AJ, Hanson MR, al et. Central nervous system complications of coronary bypass graft surgery: a prospective analysis of 421 patients. Stroke 1983;14:682–687.

291. Jaben SL, Glaser JS, Daily M. Ischemic optic neuropathy following general surgical procedures. J Clin Neuroophthalmol 1983;3:239–244.

292. Shaw PJ, Bates D, Cartlidge NEF, et al. Early neurological complications of coronary artery bypass surgery. Br Med J 1985;291:1384–1387.

293. Alpert JN, Pena Y, Leachman DR. Anterior ischemic optic neuropathy after coronary bypass surgery. Tex Med 1987;83:45–47.

294. Larkin DFP, Wood AE, Neligan M, et al. Ischaemic optic neuropathy complicating cardiopulmonary bypass. Br J Ophthalmol 1987;71:344–347.

295. Rizzo JF III, Lessell S. Posterior ischemic optic neuropathy during general surgery. Am J Ophthalmol 1987;103:808–811.

296. Tice DA. Ischemic optic neuropathy and cardiac surgery. Ann Thorac Surg 1987;44:677.

297. Shahian DM, Speert PK. Symptomatic visual deficits after open heart surgery. Ann Thorac Surg 1989;48:275–279.

298. Lee AG. Ischemic optic neuropathy following lumbar spine surgery. Case report. J Neurosurg 1995;83:348–349.

299. Dilger JA, Tetzlaff JE, Bell GR, et al. Ischaemic optic neuropathy after spinal fusion. Can J Anaesth 1998;45:63–66.

300. Alexandrakis G, Lam BL. Bilateral posterior ischemic optic neuropathy after spinal surgery. Am J Ophthalmol 1999;127:354–355.

301. Myers MA, Hamilton SR, Bogosian AJ, et al. Visual loss as a complication of spine surgery: a review of 37 cases. Spine 1997;22:1325–1329.

302. Williams EL. Postoperative blindness. Anesthesiol Clin North Am 2002;20:605–622.

303. Murphy MA. Bilateral posterior ischemic optic neuropathy after lumbar spine surgery. Ophthalmology 2003;110:1454–1457.

304. Brown RH, Schauble JF, Miller NR. Anemia and hypotension as contributors to perioperative loss of vision. Anesthesiology 1994;80:222–226.

305. Nuttall GA, Garrity JA, Dearani JA, et al. Risk factors for ischemic optic neuropathy after cardiopulmonary bypass: a matched case/control study. Anesth Analg 2001;93:1410–1416

306. Dunker S, Hsu HY, Sebag J, et al. Perioperative risk factors for posterior ischemic optic neuropathy. J Am Coll Surg 2002;194:705–710.

307. Hollenhorst RW, Svien HJ, Benoit CF. Unilateral blindness occurring during anesthesia for neurosurgical operations. Arch Ophthalmol 1954;52:819–830.

308. Hoski JJ, Eismont FJ, Green BA. Blindness as a complication of intraoperative positioning: A case report. J Bone Joint Surg [Am] 1993;75:1231–1232.

309. Wolfe SW, Lospinuso MF, Burke SW. Unilateral blindness as a complication of patient positioning for spinal surgery: a case report. Spine 1992;17:600–605.

310. Lee AG. PION after lumbar spine surgery [letter]. Ophthalmology 2004;111:612.

311. Roth S, Thisted RA, Erickson JP, et al. Eye injuries after non-ocular surgery: a study of 60,965 anesthetics from 1988–1992. Anesthesiology 1996;85:1020–1027.

312. Roth S, Barach P. Post-operative visual loss: no answers—yet [editorial view]. Anesthesiology 2001;95:575–577.

313. Cheng MA, Sigurdson W, Tempelhoff R, et al. Visual loss after spine surgery: a survey. Neurosurgery 2000;46:625–630.

314. Haider S, Astbury NJ, Hamilton DV. Optic neuropathy in uraemic patients on dialysis. Eye 1993;7:148–151.

315. Knox DL, Hanneken AM, Hollows FC, et al. Uremic optic neuropathy. Arch Ophthalmol 1988;106:50–54.

316. Saini JS, Jain IS, Dhar S, et al. Uremic optic neuropathy. J Clin Neuroophthalmol 1989;9:131.

317. Hamed LM, Winward KE, Glaser JS, et al. Optic neuropathy in uremia. Am J Ophthalmol 1989;108:30–35.

318. Servilla KS, Groggel GC. Anterior ischemic optic neuropathy as a complication of hemodialysis. Am J Kidney Dis 1986;8:61–63.

319. Jackson TL, Farmer CKT, Kingswood C, et al. Hypotensive ischemic optic neuropathy and peritoneal dialysis. Am J Ophthalmol 1999;128:109–111.

320. Michaelson C, Behrens M, Odel J. Bilateral anterior ischaemic optic neuropathy associated with optic disc drusen and systemic hypotension. Br J Ophthalmol 1989;73:762–764.

321. Basile C, Addabbo G, Montanaro A. Anterior ischemic optic neuropathy and dialysis: role of hypotension and anemia. J Nephrol 2001;14:420–423.

322. Connolly SE, Gordon KB, Horton JC. Salvage of vision after hypotension induced ischemic optic neuropathy. Am J Ophthalmol 1994;117:235–242.

323. Cove DH, Seddon M, Fletcher RF, et al. Blindness after treatment for malignant hypertension. Br Med J 1979;2:245.

324. Pryor JS, Davies PD, Hamilton DV. Blindness and malignant hypertension. Lancet 1979;2:803.

325. Taylor D, Ramsay J, Day S, et al. Infarction of the optic nerve head in children with accelerated hypertension. Br J Ophthalmol 1981;65:153–160.

326. Kline LB, Kim JY, Ceballos R. Radiation optic neuropathy. Ophthalmology 1985;92:1118–1126.

327. Roden D, Bosley TM, Fowble B, et al. Delayed radiation injury to the retrobulbar optic nerves and chiasm. Ophthalmology 1990;97:346–351.

328. Jiang GL, Tucker SL, Guttenberger R, et al. Radiation-induced injury to the visual pathway. Radiother Oncol 1994;30:17–25.

329. Arnold AC. Radiation optic neuropathy. Presented at North American Neuro-Ophthalmology Society Meeting, at Tucson, Arizona, 1995.

330. Guy J, Schatz NJ. Radiation-induced optic neuropathy. In: Tusa RJ, Newman SA, eds. Neuro-Ophthalmological Disorders. New York, Marcel Dekker, 1995:437–450.

331. Pennybacker J, Russell DS. Necrosis of the brain due to radiation therapy. J Neurol Neurosurg Psychiatry 1948;11:183–198.

332. Fike JR, Gobbell GT. Central nervous system radiation injury in large animal models. In: Gutin PH, Leibel SA, Sheline GE, eds. Radiation Injury to the Central Nervous System. New York, Raven Press, 1991:113–136.

333. Van der Kogel AJ. Central nervous system radiation injury in small animal models. Gutin PH, Leibel SA, Sheline GE, eds. Radiation Injury to the Central Nervous System. New York, Raven Press, 1991:91–112.

334. Zeman W, Samorajski T. Effects of irradiation on the nervous system. In: Berdjis

CC, ed. Pathology of Irradiation. Baltimore, Williams & Wilkins, 1971: 213–277.

335. Crompton MR, Layton DD. Delayed radiation necrosis of the brain following therapeutic x-radiation to the pituitary. Brain 1961;84:86–101.

336. Ghatak NR, White BE. Delayed radiation necrosis of the hypothalamus: report of a case simulating craniopharyngioma. Arch Neurol 1969;21:425–430.

337. Ross HS, Rosenberg S, Friedman AH. Delayed radiation necrosis of the optic nerve. Am J Ophthalmol 1973;76:683–686.

338. Harris JR, Levene MB. Visual complications following irradiation for pituitary adenomas and craniopharyngiomas. Radiology 1976;120:167–171.

339. Husain MM, Garcia JH. Cerebral ''radiation necrosis'': vascular and glial features. Acta Neuropathol 1976;36:381–385.

340. Aristizabal S, Caldwell WL, Avila J. The relationship of time dose fractionation factors to complications in the treatment of pituitary tumours by irradiation. Int J Radiat Oncol Biol Phys 1977;2:667–673.

341. Sheline GE, Wara WM, Smith V. Therapeutic irradiation and brain injury. Int J Radiat Oncol Biol Phys 1980;6:1215–1228.

342. Marks SC, Jaques DA, Hirata RM, et al. Blindness following bilateral radical neck dissection. Head Neck 1990;12:342–345.

343. Kun LE. The brain and spinal cord. In: Cox JD, ed. Moss' Radiation Oncology. Rationale, Technique, Results. St Louis, Mosby, 1994:737–781.

344. Polak BCP, Wijngaarde R. Radiation retinopathy in patients with both diabetes mellitus and ophthalmic Graves' disease. Orbit 1995;14:71–74.

345. Fishman ML, Bean SC, Cogan DG. Optic atrophy following prophylactic chemotherapy and cranial radiation for acute lymphocytic leukemia. Am J Ophthalmol 1976;82:571–576.

346. Buys NS, Kerns TC Jr. Irradiation damage to the chiasm. Am J Ophthalmol 1957;44:483–486.

347. Parsons JT, Bova FJ, Fitzgerald CR, et al. Radiation optic neuropathy after megavoltage external beam irradiation: analysis of time dose factors. Int J Radiation Oncology Biol Phys 1994;30:755–763.

348. Goldsmith BJ, Rosenthal SA, Wara WM, et al. Optic neuropathy after irradiation of meningioma. Radiology 1992;185:71–76.

349. Young WC, Thornton AF, Gebarski SS, et al. Radiation-induced optic neuropathy: correlation of MR imaging and radiation dosimetry. Radiology 1992;185: 904–907.

350. Atkinson AB, Allen IV, Gordon DS, et al. Progressive visual failure in acromegaly following external pituitary irradiation. Clin Endocrinol 1979;10:469–479.

351. Peck FC Jr, McGovern ER. Radiation necrosis of the brain in acromegaly. J Neurosurg 1966;25:536–542.

352. Schatz NJ, Smith JL. Non-tumor causes of the Foster Kennedy syndrome. J Neurosurg 1967;27:37–44.

353. Brown GC, Shields JA, Sanborn G, et al. Radiation optic neuropathy. Ophthalmology 1982;89:1489.

354. Guy J, Mancuso A, Beck R, et al. Radiation-induced optic neuropathy: a magnetic resonance imaging study. J Neurosurg 1991;74:426–432.

355. Guy J, Schatz NJ. Hyperbaric oxygen in the treatment of radiation-induced optic neuropathy. Ophthalmology 1986;93:1083–1088.

356. Warman R, Glaser JS, Quencer RM. Radionecrosis of optic hypothalamic glioma. Neuroophthalmology 1989;9:219–226.

357. Zimmerman CF, Schatz NJ, Glaser JS. Magnetic resonance imaging of radiation optic neuropathy. Am J Ophthalmol 1990;110:389–394.

358. Borruat FX, Schatz NJ, Glaser JS, et al. Visual recovery from radiation-induced optic neuropathy. J Clin Neuroophthalmol 1993;13:98–101.

359. Olson DR, Guiot G, Derome P. The symptomatic empty sella: prevention and correction via the transsphenoidal approach. J Neurosurg 1972;37:533–537.

360. Spaziante R, de Divitus E, Stella L, et al. The empty sella. Surg Neurol 1981; 16:418–426.

361. Kaufman B, Tomsak RL, Kaufman BA, et al. Herniation of the suprasellar visual system and third ventricle into empty sellae: morphologic and clinical considerations. AJNR Am J Neuroradiol 1989;10:65–76.

362. Bernstein M, Lapernere N. Radiation-induced tumors of the nervous system. In: Gutin PH, Leibel SA, Sheline GE, eds. Radiation Injury to the Central Nervous System. New York, Raven Press, 1991:455–472.

363. Hudgins PA, Newman NJ, Dillon WP, et al. Radiation-induced optic neuropathy: Characteristic appearances on gadolinium enhanced MR. AJNR Am J Neuroradiol 1992;13:235–238.

364. McClellan RL, El Gammal T, Kline LB. Early bilateral radiation-induced optic neuropathy with follow-up MRI. Neuroradiology 1995;37:131–133.

365. Gutin PH. Treatment of radiation necrosis of the brain. In: Gutin PH, Leibel SA, Sheline GE, eds. Radiation Injury to the Central Nervous System. New York, Raven Press, 1991:271–282.

366. Martins AN, Johnston JS, Henry JM, et al. Delayed radiation necrosis of the brain. J Neurosurg 1977;47:336–345.

367. Tachibana O, Yamaguchi N, Yamashima T, et al. Radiation necrosis of the optic chiasm, optic tract, hypothalamus, and upper pons after radiotherapy for pituitary edema, detected by gadolinium-enhanced, T1-weighted magnetic resonance imaging: Case report. Neurosurgery 1990;27:640–643.

368. Glantz MJ, Burger PC, Friedman AH, et al. Treatment of radiation-induced nervous system injury with heparin and warfarin. Neurology 1994;44:2020–2027.

369. Landau K, Killer HE. Radiation damage. Neurology 1996;46:889.

370. Barbosa AP, Carvalho D, Marques L, et al. Inefficiency of the anticoagulant therapy in the regression of the radiation-induced optic neuropathy in Cushing's disease. J Endocrinol Invest 1999;22:301–305.

371. Bassett BE, Bennett PB. Introduction to the physical and physiological bases of hyperbaric therapy. In: Davis JC, Hunt TK, eds. Hyperbaric Oxygen Therapy Bethesda, Undersea Medical Society, 1977:11–24.

372. Marx RE, Johnson RP. Problem wounds in oral and maxillofacial surgery: the role of hyperbaric oxygen. In: Davis JC, Hunt TK, eds. Problem Wounds: The Role of Oxygen. New York, Elsevier Science, 1988:65–124.

373. Borruat FX, Schatz NJ, Glaser JS, et al. Radiation optic neuropathy: report of cases, role of hyperbaric oxygen therapy, and literature review. Neuroophthalmology 1996;16:255–266.

374. Liu JL. Clinical analysis of radiation optic neuropathy. Chinese J Ophthalmol 1992;28:86–88.

375. Georgiades G, Konstas P, Stangos N. Réflexions issues de l'étude de nombreux cas de pseudo papillite vasculaire. Bull Soc Ophtalmol Fr 1966;79:505–536.

376. Foulds WS. Visual disturbances in systemic disorders: optic neuropathy and systemic disease. Trans Ophthalmol Soc UK 1969;89:125–146.

377. Hayreh SS. Anterior ischemic optic neuropathy: V. Optic disc edema as early sign. Arch Ophthalmol 1981;99:1030–1040.

378. Miller N. Walsh and Hoyt's Clinical Neuro-Ophthalmology, 4th ed, vol 1. Baltimore, Williams & Wilkins, 1982:215.

379. Almog Y, Goldstein M. Visual outcome in eyes with asymptomatic optic disc edema. J Neuroophthalmol 2003;23:204–207.

380. Lubow M, Makley TA. Pseudopapilledema of juvenile diabetes mellitus. Arch Ophthalmol 1971;85:417–422.

381. Appen RE, Chandra SR, Klein R, Myers FL. Diabetic papillopathy. Am J Ophthalmol 1980;90:203–209.

382. Barr CC, Glaser JS, Blankenship G. Acute disc swelling in juvenile diabetes. Clinical profile and natural history of 12 cases. Arch Ophthalmol 1980;98: 2185–2192.

383. Hayreh SS, Zahoruk RM. Anterior ischemic optic neuropathy. VI. In juvenile diabetics. Ophthalmologica 1981;182:13–28.

384. Pavan PR, Aiello LM, Wafai MZ, et al. Optic disc edema in juvenile-onset diabetes. Arch Ophthalmol 1980;98:2193–2195.

385. Regillo CD, Brown GC, Savino PJ, et al. Diabetic papillopathy: patient characteristics and fundus findings. Arch Ophthalmol 1995;113:889–895.

386. Vaphiades M. The disk edema dilemma. Surv Ophthalmol 2002;47:183–188.

387. Hayreh SS. Diabetic papillopathy and nonarteritic anterior ischemic optic neuropathy [letter]. Surv Ophthalmol 2002;47:600–601.

388. Bayraktar Z, Alacali N, Bayraktar S. Diabetic papillopathy in type II diabetic patients. Retina 2002;22:752–758.

389. Ho AC, Maguire AM, Yannuzzi LA, et al. Rapidly progressive optic disk neovascularization after diabetic papillopathy. Am J Ophthalmol 1995;120:673–675.

390. Mansour AM, El-Dairi MA, Shehab MA, et al. Periocular corticosteroids in diabetic papillopathy. Eye 2004 (E publication ahead of print).

CHAPTER 8

Compressive and Infiltrative Optic Neuropathies

Nicholas J. Volpe

COMPRESSIVE OPTIC NEUROPATHIES WITH OPTIC DISC
   SWELLING (ANTERIOR COMPRESSIVE OPTIC
   NEUROPATHIES)
   Orbital Inflammatory Syndrome
   Thyroid Eye Disease
   Meningiomas

COMPRESSIVE OPTIC NEUROPATHIES WITHOUT OPTIC
   DISC SWELLING (RETROBULBAR COMPRESSIVE OPTIC
   NEUROPATHIES)
VISUAL RECOVERY FOLLOWING DECOMPRESSION
INFILTRATIVE OPTIC NEUROPATHIES
   Tumors
   Inflammatory and Infectious Infiltrative Optic Neuropathies

---

COMPRESSIVE OPTIC NEUROPATHIES WITH OPTIC DISC SWELLING (ANTERIOR COMPRESSIVE OPTIC NEUROPATHIES)

Compressive lesions within the orbit, the optic canal and, rarely, intracranially, may result in disc swelling (Fig. 8.1). Most compressive optic neuropathies, whether they result from orbital or intracranial lesions, are not associated with optic disc swelling. However tumors, infections, and inflammations, and even adnexal structures that have become swollen or enlarged by disease, can all cause an optic neuropathy associated with optic disc swelling.

Within the orbit, mass lesions that compress the proximal optic nerve and produce optic disc swelling include optic gliomas (1–8), meningiomas (4,7,9–18), hamartomas (e.g., hemangiomas, lymphangiomas), choristomas (e.g., dermoid cysts), malignancies (e.g., carcinoma, lymphoma, sarcoma, multiple myeloma) (19–22) and arachnoid cysts of the optic nerve sheath (23,24) (although some of these cysts may be associated with optic nerve sheath menigiomas at the orbital apex (25,26). Additionally, inflammatory disorders such as idiopathic orbital inflammatory syndrome and thyroid ophthalmopathy can result in compressive optic neuropathies with disc edema.

In most cases of anterior compressive optic neuropathy, there is progressive visual loss associated with proptosis; however, in many patients, visual acuity remains near normal, visual field loss is mild (blind spot enlargement and mild generalized constriction) and there is virtually no external evidence of orbital disease despite obvious disc swelling.

This clinical picture is particularly common in patients with orbital hemangiomas adjacent to the optic nerve and in patients with primary optic nerve meningiomas (4,7,11, 13–18). In such patients, careful testing of color vision may reveal subtle defects. Computerized perimetry may show enlarged blind spot or reduction of the mean deviation and there may occasionally be a relative afferent pupillary defect. When other signs of orbital disease are not present (e.g., proptosis, limitation of ocular motility, orbital congestion) these patients may be thought to have unilateral papilledema from increased intracranial pressure. Although it is obvious that patients with slowly progressive, unilateral visual loss and proptosis associated with disc swelling should undergo evaluation for a possible orbital lesion, patients with unilateral optic disc swelling without signs of intraocular inflammation and *without* visual loss should also undergo such an evaluation, particularly when there are no systemic or neurologic symptoms or signs of increased intracranial pressure. Orbital disease is the most common cause of unilateral disc swelling without visual loss since truly unilateral papilledema is rare (27).

In addition to proptosis, congestion, and limitation of ocular motility, patients with orbital disease may develop various folds or striae that occur either at the posterior pole, adjacent to the optic disc (Fig. 8.2), or elsewhere in the fundus if the orbital compressive lesion contacts the globe.

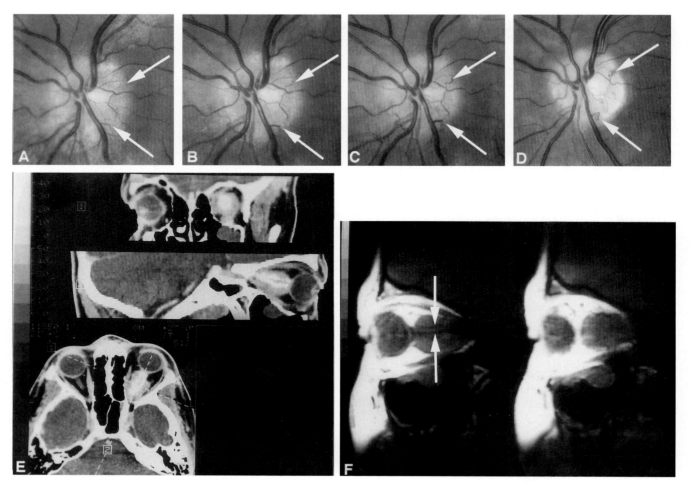

Figure 8.1.   Disc swelling and optociliary shunt veins in a patient with optic nerve sheath meningioma. *A–D,* Progressive development of optociliary shunt veins (*arrows*) from the stage of chronic disc swelling (*A*), through intermediate stages of shunt vein formation (*B and C*), to the final stage of optic atrophy with fully formed optociliary shunts (*D*). Neuroimaging with computed tomographic (CT) scanning and magnetic resonance (MR) imaging provides complementary information. Calcified psammoma bodies in the tumor produce a well-delineated "tram-track" sign in the contrast-enhanced, reconstructed CT images (*E*), whereas MR imaging with surface coil (T1-weighted, without fat suppression or enhancement) (*F*) clearly defines the nerve surrounded by tumor (*arrows*).

These folds may be horizontal or vertical and generally result from indentation of the globe by the lesion itself or secondarily by the optic nerve (28–30).

Transient monocular visual loss occurs commonly in patients with orbital lesions(4,13,31–38). The visual loss occurs only in certain positions of gaze, and vision immediately clears when the direction of gaze is changed. It has been assumed that either gaze dependency, direct pressure on the optic nerve, or interruption of the blood supply is the explanation for this phenomenon. Knapp et al. (39) demonstrated the latter with color Doppler imaging in a 13-year-old girl with a left intraconal mass. Abduction of the affected eye was associated with gaze-evoked amaurosis and a dramatic reduction in central retinal artery blood flow that returned to normal two months after removal of the lesion (an orbital varix), by which time the girl was asymptomatic. Gaze

evoked amaurosis has also been reported to occur in association with secondary lesions invading the orbit (38). Body position associated transient visual obscurations as occur in patients with papilledema also may occur in patients with unilateral disc swelling from a compressive lesion.

Computed tomographic (CT) scanning (40–53), magnetic resonance (MR) imaging (54–59), and ultrasonography (60–69) have revolutionized the diagnosis of orbital lesions. CT scanning, MR imaging, and ultrasonography are rapid, safe, and accurate methods of determining the presence of an orbital lesion, its location, and occasionally, its identity (66,70–73). CT scanning and MR imaging offer superior topographic depiction (size, shape, and location) of lesions (74), whereas standardized echography provides supplementary information that often helps in refinement of the differential diagnosis (66,69). CT scanning is particularly useful

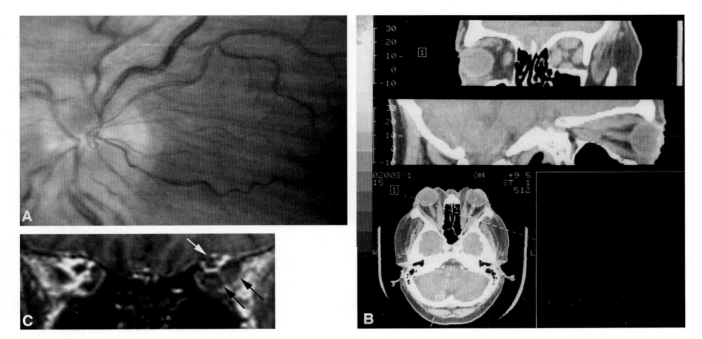

Figure 8.2. Optic disc swelling and choroidal folds in thyroid eye disease. *A,* The left optic disc shows mild hyperemia, swelling, and blurring of the peripapillary retinal nerve fiber layer at the upper and lower poles. Horizontal chorioretinal folds extend across the posterior pole toward the macula. *B,* Coronal and off-axis sagittal reconstructed computed tomographic scans show greatly enlarged extraocular muscles surrounding the optic nerve within the orbit. Note that the muscles actually appear to be in contact with the nerve. *C,* Coronal T1-weighted, enhanced MRI scan showing enlarged extraocular muscles (*black arrows*) crowding the optic nerve (*white arrow*).

for imaging bone, calcium, and metallic foreign bodies (75) (suspicion of the last being a contraindication for the use of MR imaging), whereas MR imaging excels at defining inflammatory and intrinsic disease of the visual pathway and parasellar area. MR imaging is particularly suited to imaging the intracanalicular optic nerve, as it is not affected by partial volume averaging from adjacent bone as is CT scanning (76). With the use of fat-saturation techniques and intravenous injection of paramagnetic substances such as gadolinium-diethylene-triamine-pentaacetic acid (gadolinium-DTPA), demarcation of optic nerve sheath meningiomas can be optimized (54,55). Plain skull radiographs should no longer play a role in the evaluation of patients with unexplained visual loss (77).

ORBITAL INFLAMMATORY SYNDROME

Inflammatory conditions involving the orbit, including abscesses and the nonspecific condition called idiopathic inflammatory pseudotumor or idiopathic orbital inflammatory syndrome, may also cause anterior compression of the proximal optic nerve and secondary disc swelling that can be confused with primary optic nerve tumors (78,79). Associated posterior scleritis may also cause disc swelling. Affected patients usually experience acute or subacute visual loss, pain, proptosis, and congestion associated with the optic disc swelling, possibly with retinal vein occlusion. The presence of an orbital process is rarely in question. Infre-

quently, meningiomas of the orbital apex produce a similar clinical picture (80). CT scanning and MR scanning usually show thickening and enhancement of normal tissues or a mass lesion. Ultrasound can be very helpful in the identification of posterior scleritis and thickening of Tenon's capsule and the sclera. The pain and rapid evolution of symptoms generally distinguish orbital inflammatory disease from the more indolent course characteristic of most orbital tumors. Most of these patients respond rapidly to systemic steroid treatment.

THYROID EYE DISEASE

Approximately 6% of patients with thyroid eye disease develop evidence of a compressive optic neuropathy, some associated with optic disc swelling (Fig. 8.2) (81). Dysthyroid optic neuropathy is a compressive optic neuropathy caused by pressure on the optic nerve by enlarged extraocular muscles. In such patients, congestive symptoms almost always precede visual loss, which is usually bilateral, symmetric, and gradual in onset. Of the 36 eyes of 21 patients with dysthyroid optic neuropathy examined by Trobe et al. (82), 12 (33%) had mild to marked disc swelling. Presenting visual acuities were 20/60 or worse in these patients, who usually had central scotomas, often combined with arcuate defects. Kennerdell et al. (83) emphasized the compressive etiology of the optic neuropathy in their report of the CT findings in seven patients with dysthyroid optic neuropathy, four of whom had evidence of optic disc swelling. In all cases, there was moderate to severe enlargement of the extraocular muscles at the orbital apex (Fig. 8.2). Direct measurement of orbital pressure and tissue compliance through manometry demonstrates higher orbital tissue tension and lower orbital compliance in patients with thyroid eye disease (84). Optic neuropathy can even occur as a late complication several years after initial presentation without evidence of progressive orbitopathy or recurrent inflammation (85).

Treatment options for thyroid-associated compressive optic neuropathy include intravenous or oral steroids and orbital decompression which can be accomplished successfully via a transantral (86), endoscopic (87), or transcaruncular approach (88). Combined approaches allowing endoscopic decompression of the medial wall and orbital apex and subciliary approaches to the orbital floor may be most effective (89–92). Radiation therapy may also be effective (93), but its effects are often delayed and therefore more acutely effective treatments with steroids or surgery should be given in conjunction with radiation. Visual evoked potentials have also been shown to be abnormal in patients with thyroid eye disease without symptoms or measurable optic nerve dysfunction and useful in monitoring and detecting treatment effects in thyroid patients (94–97). Most patients (90%) improve and maintain excellent vision. A subset of patients require additional interventions including repeat orbital surgery, steroid treatment or radiation, and a small percentage (5%) develop permanent visual disability (86,98,99).

MENINGIOMAS

Anterior compressive optic neuropathy may result from primary optic nerve sheath meningiomas (ONSM) (see Chapter 30). The tumors arise from meningiothelial cells in the arachnoid villi. Optic nerve sheath meningiomas surround the optic nerve and result in impaired axonal transport (leading to disc swelling) and also interfere with the pial blood supply to the optic nerve. The tumor occurs most commonly in middle-aged women and is usually unilateral (100). Patients present with slowly progressive vision loss, mild proptosis, double vision, transient visual obscurations, and gaze-evoked amaurosis (13,15,16,100). Examination reveals a color vision defect, afferent pupillary defect, and visual field defects including central scotomas, enlarged blind spots, and generalized constriction. The optic nerve appears abnormal with either optic atrophy and or with disc edema (13,15,16,100). Optociliary collateral vessels (see below) may be present and are seen in both swollen and atrophic nerves (101).

Neuroimaging (CT or MRI) demonstrates focal or diffuse, tubular or fusiform, optic nerve enlargement (Fig. 8.1) (100). MRI is often diagnostic, showing the tumor to be separate from the optic nerve proper on coronal views, allowing distinction from gliomas (Fig. 8.3). MRI is particularly good at imaging the intracanalicular optic nerve, and delineating the extent of intracranial extension of the ONSM (54,55,102). This kind of tumor is typically isointense with brain on T1 and T2 images and smoothly enhances with

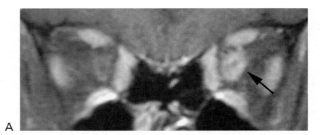

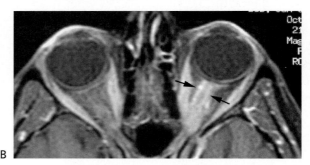

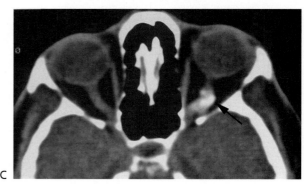

Figure 8.3. Neuroimaging in optic nerve sheath meningioma. *A,* Coronal T1-weighted, enhanced orbital image with fat saturation demonstrating enlarged and enhancing optic nerve sheath (*arrow*). *B,* Axial T1-weighted, enhanced, fat-saturated image demonstrating a left optic nerve sheath meningioma with linear enhancment (*arrows*) along the optic nerve sheath. *C,* Axial orbital CT scan demonstrating calcification (*arrow*) of an optic nerve sheath meningioma.

gadolinium. The imaging appearance of fusiform enlargement can be similar to that of optic nerve glioma but "kinking" (see later) is not seen with meningiomas. On CT, calcification (Fig. 8.3) can be seen in one third of patients as linear bright lines extending over the length of the optic nerve (tram track sign) (4,13,14,100). Clinical findings and neuroimaging generally establish the diagnosis and biopsy is almost never needed. However, the radiographic appearance of diffuse optic nerve enlargement or sheath thickening is also seen in patients with optic neuritis (103), optic perineuritis(104), sarcoidosis involving the meninges (105), orbital inflammatory syndrome (particularly the sclerosing variety) (79), metastases (106–108), and lymphomatous and carcinomatous meningitis. Clinically these conditions can usually be distinguished by a much more rapid presentation and associated pain as well as associated systemic symptoms. In the rare equivocal case, biopsy is only recommended in an eye with poor vision, after a systemic work up and serial lumbar punctures exclude inflammatory disorders and neoplasms, and after steroids fail to improve vision.

Growth of ONSM is usually indolent over many years. Growth rate may increase with pregnancy (109). Intracranial extension of optic nerve sheath meningioma with involvement of the chiasm and adjacent structures is quite rare. Bilateral cases occur in neurofibromatosis type II (110). Prospective clinical trial data are not available for comparison of available treatments. Natural history data suggest that patients can remain stable or improve over several years (100). In a series of 16 patients followed for a mean time of 6 years (2–18 years) without treatment, Egan and Lessell (111) re-

ported that none of the patients developed other neurologic sequelae of their tumor, four patients remained stable, and three actually improved based on visual acuity and visual field criteria.

Radiation therapy (50–55 Gy) is the best treatment available for patients with optic nerve sheath meningioma (11,112–120). In the largest series to date, Andrews and associates reported the results of fractionated stereotactic radiotherapy in 30 patients with ONSM (113). Vision was preserved in 92% of patients and improved visual acuity or visual fields were noted in 42%, compared to only 16% of patients with preserved vision in an historical control group (Fig. 8.4). Becker and associates (114) and Pitz and associates (120) reported similar results in two different studies

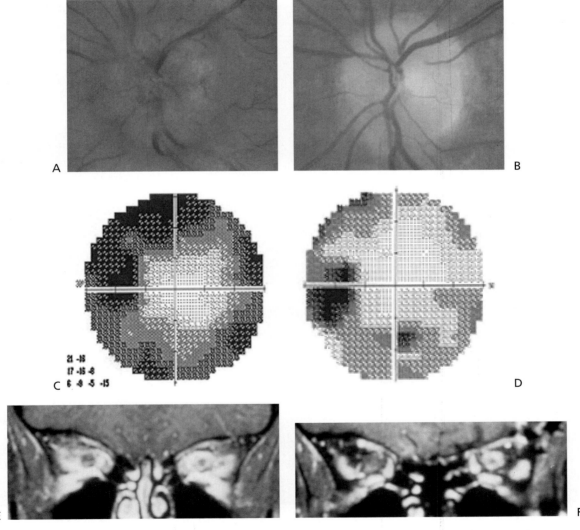

Figure 8.4. Successful treatment of optic nerve sheath meningioma with radiation treatment. The patient presented at age 39 with transient visual obscurations and blurred vision in the left eye and had optic disc swelling (*A*), reduced acuity to 20/60, and significant visual field loss including blind spot enlargement and constriction (*C*). She was found on MRI scan (*E*) to have an optic nerve sheath meningioma. Nine years after radiation therapy the visual acuity improved and remained at 20/25, the optic disc was mildly pale (*B*), the visual field (*D*) improved, and the MRI scan (*F*) showed a stable appearance.

of 15 ONSM patients. Stable visual acuity and fieldswere noted for 3 years in 29 of 30 patients treated with stereotactic radiotherapy. Narayan and associates (121) reported stability or improvement over an average of about a 4-year follow-up in 12 of 14 patients treated with three-dimensional conformal radiation. Turbin and associates (122) reviewed their series of 64 patients with ONSM who were either observed or treated with radiation and/or surgery and found that radiation alone was superior, had the least complications, best visual outcome, and least progression on MRI.

Alternatively, if visual function is excellent then observation alone is reasonable, and radiation therapy is initiated when progression is documented (100,111). Surgical excision of these lesions to improve vision is usually not possible because of the tumor involvement of the pial blood supply to the optic nerve. Portions of the tumor are occasionally removed to treat blind or uncomfortable eyes (proptosis), to decompress associated mass effect, or reduce the risk of intracranial extension. In patients with intracranial extension, surgery and radiation have been tried. Surgical results are poor, although radiation has been shown to be of some benefit (123).

Patients with meningiomas confined entirely to the optic canal may occasionally present with blurred vision and optic disc swelling (112). The mechanism by which disc swelling occurs in such cases is not clear, but it presumably results from direct compression of the optic nerve with blockage of axonal transport. Less common than optic disc swelling from an intracanalicular lesion is optic disc swelling from compression of the *intracranial portion* of the optic nerve. Tomsak et al. (124) reported a patient who developed blurred vision in the left eye associated with an inferior-temporal visual field defect, an ipsilateral relative afferent pupillary defect, and a mildly swollen, hyperemic optic disc associated with peripapillary exudates and choroidal folds. The patient was ultimately found to harbor a carotid ophthalmic aneurysm that compressed the intracranial portion of the left optic nerve superior-medially against the intracranial aspect of the optic canal.

Intracranial lesions, particularly sphenoid wing meningiomas, not infrequently extend through the optic canal, compressing the intracranial, intracanalicular, and intraorbital optic nerve in the process. Optic disc changes, from swelling to pallor, may be minimal in such cases, even when the lesion is quite large (Fig. 8.5).

In many patients with chronic compression of the intracanalicular or intraorbital optic nerve, a specific clinical triad develops. This triad consists of visual loss, optic disc swell-

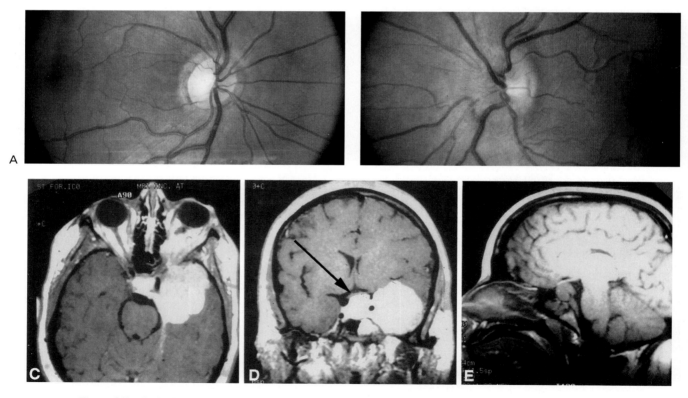

Figure 8.5. Optic disc swelling in a patient with a large meningioma with intraorbital, intracanalicular, and intracranial components. The patient was a 21-year-old woman who experienced reduced vision in the left eye during pregnancy. *A,* Normal right optic disc. *B,* Mild swelling of left optic disc. *C,* T1-weighted axial magnetic resonance image obtained after intravenous injection with gadolinium-DTPA shows large mass involving the left sphenoid wing and posterior orbit. Although both coronal (*D*) and sagittal (*E*) images clearly show compression of the optic chiasm by the tumor (*arrow*), the resulting visual field defect was purely unilateral, affecting only the left eye.

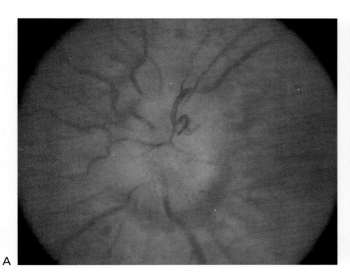

A

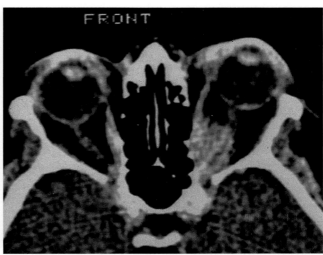

B

Figure 8.6. Left optic disc swelling in a patient with an orbital meningioma. *A*, Disc swelling is associated with the development of an optociliary shunt or collateral vessel seen at 1 o'clock position. *B*, Axial enhanced CT scan showing the large lesion compressing and surrounding the optic nerve.

ing that evolves into optic atrophy, and the appearance of optociliary (retinochoroidal) shunt veins (Figs. 8.1 and 8.6). The optociliary veins overlie the optic disc and peripapillary region and shunt venous blood between the retinal and choroidal venous circulations (125–130). The vessels may occur as congenital anomalies, in which case they are associated with normal visual acuity and shunt blood from the choroid to the retina (128–131). When they occur with chronic optic nerve compression, however, they are generally associated with severe visual loss and disc swelling or optic atrophy and they shunt blood from the retina to the choroid. The common denominator in such cases appears to be prolonged compression of the optic nerve with gradual compression and obstruction of the central retinal vein.

The normal route of retinal venous blood flow is through the central retinal vein directly to the cavernous sinus.

Chronic obstruction of the central retinal vein presumably results in dilation of a previously existing system that shunts blood to the choroid, allowing it to leave the eye via the vortex veins (132–134). These veins drain directly into the superior and inferior ophthalmic veins that anastomose with the facial and angular veins and with the pterygoid venous plexus. Thus, an outlet is provided for retinal venous blood other than via the central retinal vein to the cavernous sinus. This clinical picture has been described most frequently in patients with spheno-orbital meningiomas (12,135–138), but it also occurs in patients with optic nerve gliomas (139,140), chronic papilledema (141–144), craniopharyngioma (145), sarcoidosis (146), and other rare causes of optic nerve compression (23,147).

However, the most common cause of retinochoroidal shunt vessels is central retinal vein occlusion.

COMPRESSIVE OPTIC NEUROPATHIES WITHOUT OPTIC DISC SWELLING (RETROBULBAR COMPRESSIVE OPTIC NEUROPATHIES)

The importance of early diagnosis of compressive lesions that affect the retrobulbar portions of the optic nerve and do not cause optic disc swelling cannot be overemphasized. Early decompression of the optic nerves or chiasm may result in significant return of visual function (148,149), whereas misdiagnosis may result in progressive visual failure and irreversible visual loss, neurologic dysfunction, or death. Unfortunately, intracranial, intracanalicular, and occasionally, posterior orbital compressive lesions, usually do not produce disc swelling or significant neurologic or systemic manifestations. Thus, by the time such lesions cause visible optic pallor, significant damage to the optic nerve has often already occurred, preventing return of visual function even with otherwise successful decompression. The physician managing a patient with unexplained unilateral visual loss therefore must be aware of the characteristic his-

tory and early findings in patients with a retrobulbar compressive optic neuropathy.

In most cases of prechiasmal optic nerve compression, progressive dimming of vision is noted at an early stage. Painless, slowly progressive visual dimming should be the first warning that a compressive lesion of the optic nerve or chiasm is present. Such patients may have normal or near normal visual acuity, but they complain of "foggy," "dim," or "blurred" vision. Although these patients may read the 20/25 or the 20/20 Snellen letters with the affected eye, they do so slowly and with great difficulty compared with the opposite eye. Patients with aneurysms, mucoceles, pituitary apoplexy, and fibrous dysplasia may have a more rapidly progressive and painful course that can initially be confused with optic neuritis (discussed later).

Patients with unilateral visual complaints from compression of the optic nerve usually have some type of visual field defect, particularly when tested with automated perimetry, but the nature of the defect does not, in itself, suggest the etiology of the visual loss. Compression of the optic nerve may produce *any* type of field defect, including an altitudinal, arcuate, hemianopic, central, or cecocentral scotoma. These same defects can be caused not only by other types of optic neuropathies but also by intraocular disorders, including cataract and macular disease.

By far, the two most striking abnormalities that are present in a patient with a retrobulbar compressive optic neuropathy are unilateral dyschromatopsia (as detected using pseudoisochromatic color plates or simple red objects) and an ipsilateral relative afferent pupillary defect. The afferent defect is obvious even when visual acuity is minimally reduced and provides the observer with absolute evidence that the visual difficulty is caused by something other than a simple refractive error, incipient cataract, or minimum macular disease. Once a relative afferent pupillary defect is detected in a patient with an apparently normal fundus who is complaining of progressive dimming of vision, compression must be ruled out by whatever neuroimaging studies are available and is best suited to the task. CT scanning and MR imaging have dramatically improved the potential to diagnose retrobulbar compressive optic neuropathies and, when used in the appropriate manner, are the best screening tests to use in this setting (74,150–159) (Fig. 8.7).

Prior to the era of modern neuroimaging, many authors concluded that even if neuroradiologic diagnostic procedures fail to demonstrate a lesion, neurosurgical exploration is advisable in patients with unilateral progressive vision loss (160–162). However, with continuing advances in neuroimaging, including the use of paramagnetic substances such as gadolinium-DTPA, orbital fat suppression, MR angiography, and thin section CT scanning, it is a rare lesion that escapes detection. When modern neuroimaging techniques have been carefully tailored to the clinical problem at hand, have been properly performed, and are correctly interpreted, but are nevertheless unrevealing, *observation* rather than

neurosurgical intervention is more apt to serve the patient's best interests. Reports supporting the concept of optic nerve compression by adjacent doliochoectatic internal carotid arteries add weight to such an approach (159,163–165). Rarely does a patient require exploratory craniotomy to define the cause of compressive optic neuropathy, although decompression of the optic canal may be therapeutic in selected cases (166).

Despite the almost universal availability of CT scanning and MR imaging, it is astonishing that patients with progressive visual loss continue to be diagnosed as having macular degeneration, cataract, or "chronic optic neuritis." Certainly, chronic optic neuritis occurs and may produce slowly progressive visual loss in one or both eyes; however, chronic optic neuritis is a diagnosis of *exclusion*. This diagnosis should not be made in any patient until neuroimaging studies have been performed and have failed to detect a compressive lesion of the optic nerve. Even then, the diagnosis of chronic optic neuritis must be made with caution and follow-up imaging studies must be obtained and rigorously interpreted (167). Most cases of delayed diagnosis of compression of the anterior visual system are caused by failure to perform color vision or visual field testing, a less than careful examination of the opposite "normal" eye, failure to test for a relative afferent pupillary defect, and the necessity to obtain adequate and appropriate neuroimaging studies which are accurately interpreted (75,168).

The optic disc of a patient with a compressive optic neuropathy may appear normal or show a variable degree of pallor. Asymmetric cupping of the optic disc is not usually a prominent feature, but it may occur and be quite prominent in some patients (Fig. 8.8) (49,169–171). In such cases, the visual loss may be thought to have resulted from glaucoma, particularly when there is an arcuate defect (171).

Bianchi-Marzoli et al. (170) analyzed the occurrence of optic disc cupping (as measured by cup:disc areas) in eyes with compressive optic neuropathy. They used highly reproducible planimetric measurement techniques applied to stereoscopic disc photographs. These investigators found con-

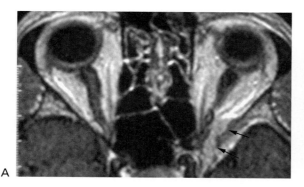
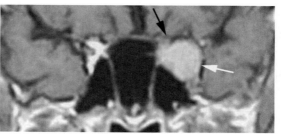

A   B

Figure 8.7.   MRI scanning in the diagnosis of retrobulbar compressive optic neuropathies. Both patients presented with slowly progressive vision loss over months with normal appearing optic nerves. *A,* Axial T1-weighted, enhanced, fat-saturated MRI scan demonstrating a subtle (*arrows*) meningioma at the orbital apex compressing the optic nerve. *B,* Coronal T1-weighted, enhanced MRI scan of a different patient demonstrating contact between meningioma (*white arrow*) and optic nerve (*black arrow*).

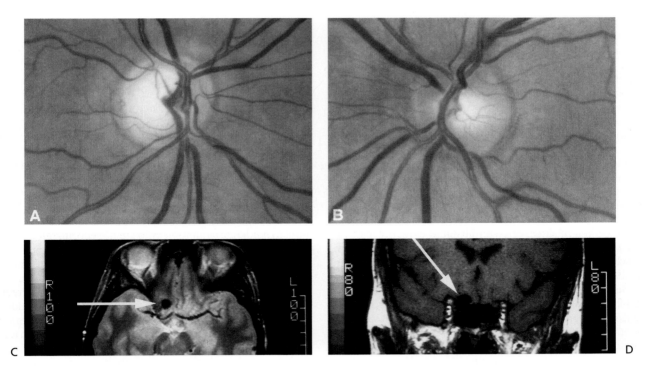

Figure 8.8. Optic disc cupping in a patient with aneurysmal compression. The patient was a 55-year-old woman who suddenly lost the inferior field in the right eye after suffering mild head trauma in a motor vehicle accident 8 days earlier. *A,* Cupped and pale right optic disc. *B,* Normal left optic disc. *C and D,* Magnetic resonance images, axial *C* and coronal *D* views, revealing flow void (*arrows*) in a carotid-ophthalmic aneurysm that is compressing the right optic nerve.

vincing evidence of acquired enlargement of the ipsilateral cup in patients with unilateral optic nerve compression.

Compressive lesions of the anterior visual pathways are important in the differential diagnosis in patients with "normal tension glaucoma," particularly if there is pallor beyond cupping, atypical rate of progression, or atypical visual field defects. Ahmed et al. (172) found compressive lesions in 4 (6.5%) of 62 consecutive patients thought to have normal pressure glaucoma. Portney and Roth (173) performed a pathologic examination of the optic nerve from a patient with progressive cupping of the optic disc caused by aneurysmal optic nerve compression. The specimen demonstrated loss of axons and glial tissue in the nerve head. It is unclear how neural compression results in loss of glial tissue in the disc of some patients and why significant cupping is such an uncommon accompaniment of compressive optic neuropathy. Optic atrophy in one eye and disc swelling in the other (Foster Kennedy syndrome) may result from asymmetric optic nerve compression (174) or from the more traditional explanation of tumor-induced direct optic nerve compression in one eye and papilledema from increased intracranial pressure in the other (see Chapter 4).

As noted above, virtually any field defect may be present in patients with a compressive optic neuropathy. Central, paracentral, cecocentral, arcuate, altitudinal, nasal, or temporal hemianopic defects, as well as diffuse depression of the visual field, have all been described in patients with compressive lesions (175–188). Although a hemianopic

field defect, a central scotoma that breaks out into the periphery, or a "junctional" scotoma in the superior temporal field of the opposite eye strongly suggest a compressive lesion, it is the *insidious, progressive* nature of the symptoms that is most often the critical feature of the compressive process.

Treatment of retrobulbar optic nerve compressive lesions must be tailored to the specific disease process and patient. Generally compression of the optic nerve must be relieved either by removal of the lesion surgically or by reducing its size with medical therapy. In addition, both intracranial and extracranial optic canal decompression may also be necessary and additive for lesions affecting the optic canal (166,189). Spontaneous improvement in visual acuity and visual field defects have been reported in patients with orbital apex lesions (190).

Causes of retrobulbar optic nerve compression include intraorbital and intracranial benign and malignant tumors (148,191–204), aneurysms (205–221) (Figs. 8.8 and 8.9), inflammatory lesions, particularly of the paranasal sinuses (222–235), primary bone disease (e.g., osteopetrosis, fibrous dysplasia, craniometaphyseal dysplasia, Paget's disease) (236–247), orbital fractures (248,249), optic canal invasion by rhabdomyosarcoma (250), dolichoectatic intracranial vessels (165,251–254), congenital and acquired hydrocephalus (255–259), thyroid eye disease (82,260–263), and orbital hemorrhage, whether spontaneous (264–266), traumatic (267–270), iatrogenic (271–274), or associated with

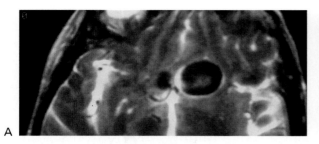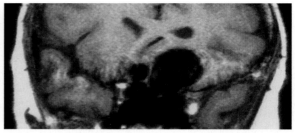

Figure 8.9. Bilateral carotid-ophthalmic aneurysms producing bilateral retrobulbar compressive optic neuropathies. Axial (*A*) and coronal (*B*) magnetic resonance images show bilateral giant carotid-ophthalmic aneurysms that produced slowly progressive visual loss in both eyes. An ophthalmologist, internist, and psychiatrist had all ascribed the loss of vision to conversion-hysteria.

orbital, paranasal sinus, or systemic diseases (275,276). Anterior visual system compression has also been reported from such disparate causes as intranasal balloon catheters placed for treatment of severe epistaxis (277), errant placement of intraventricular catheters (278,279), downward displacement of gyrus rectus in patients with meningiomas of the anterior falx cerebri (280), basal encephalocele (281), hypertrophic cranial pachymeningitis (282), renal osteodystrophy leading to calvarial hypertrophy (283), and fat packing after transsphenoidal hypophysectomy (284,285).

Meningiomas, pituitary tumors, and aneurysms are the most commonly identified lesions causing retrobulbar compressive optic neuropathy without disc swelling. Often there is associated chiasmal visual dysfunction. These lesions are discussed more extensively elsewhere in this text (see Chapters 28, 30, 31, and 41) but certain features of their presentation are worth mentioning in this discussion.

Meningiomas arising from the planum sphenoidale or olfactory groove may involve the intraorbital or intracanalicular optic nerve. Tumors in this area can grow to a large size without causing any other neurologic symptoms. Patients with olfactory groove meningiomas may present with papilledema from mass effect or retrobulbar compressive optic neuropathy and further review may reveal anosmia from compression of the olfactory nerve and abnormal behavior associated with frontal lobe dysfunction. To compress the superior aspect of the intracranial optic nerve these tumors must grow posteriorly over the planum sphenoidale. This results in compression of one optic nerve leading to unilateral optic atrophy as well as intracranial pressure elevation leading to contralateral papilledema (Foster Kennedy syndrome). Suprasellar and tuberculum sellae meningiomas more commonly cause chiasmal syndromes but can cause isolated involvement of the prechiasmatic intracranial optic nerve. Parasellar, and sphenoid wing meningiomas can also cause optic neuropathy, but because of a more lateral location generally present with cranial nerve palsies and eye movement abnormalities. Neuroimaging of patients with menigiomas reveals a lesion which is isointense with brain, smoothly enhancing, often with a dural tail (Fig. 8.5), and is usually sufficient to make the diagnosis of skull-based meningiomas, obviating the need for biopsy. The clinical course is usually one of insidious progression, although occasional patients remain stable for years. Patients with only

mild to moderate symptoms who are not good surgical candidates can be observed with serial visual fields and MRI scans. Treatment generally includes surgery and radiation therapy when vision loss is significant (see above).

The intracranial optic nerve is near the anterior cerebral artery, the anterior communicating artery, the ophthalmic artery, and the supraclinoid portion of the internal carotid artery. Aneurysms arising from the carotid ophthalmic junction, ophthalmic artery, and the supraclinoid carotid artery can all present with unilateral retrobulbar compressive optic neuropathy or chiasmal syndrome. Patients often have fluctuating visual symptoms, perhaps related to aneurysm size and flow changes. Aneurysms in the supraclinoid region classically present with a nasal scotoma which can be bilateral if there is sufficient compression of the optic nerves and chiasm shifting them toward the other carotid artery. The diagnosis is usually easily made with MRI and MRA, but conventional angiography remains the gold standard. The natural history of these lesions is generally unfavorable and therefore treatment is generally recommended with endovascular or neurosurgical intervention (see Chapter 41).

Rarely fusiform aneurysms or ectatic dilation of the carotid artery may also compress the intracranial optic nerve or chiasm (see above). This has been suggested as a possible cause of optic neuropathy in elderly patients and is thought to possibly have a role in the pathogenesis of some cases of low tension glaucoma (163,171). Jacobson et al. (286) demonstrated that contact between the carotid artery and optic nerve or chiasm is seen in 70% of asymptomatic patients suggesting that this may be a coincidental finding in patients with unexplained optic neuropathy.

The **sudden onset of unilateral visual loss**, combined with signs of retrobulbar optic nerve dysfunction, usually suggests a diagnosis of optic neuritis or ischemic optic neuropathy. In rare instances, however, compressive lesions may produce acute monocular visual loss, presumably from hemorrhage or from sudden interruption of the vascular supply to the optic nerve, and thereby mimic optic neuritis or ischemic optic neuropathy (167,287). This phenomenon probably occurs most frequently in patients with pituitary apoplexy (288), but it has also been reported in patients with pituitary tumors and meningiomas during pregnancy (289) and in otherwise healthy patients upon awakening (290). Stern and Ernest (291) reported the sudden onset of monocu-

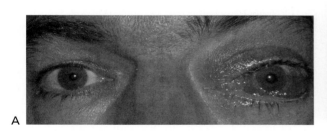
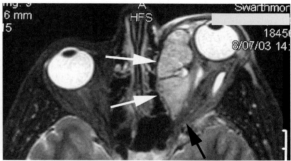

Figure 8.10. Clinical photograph (*A*) and MRI scan in patient that presented with sudden vision loss secondary to a hemorrhage in a preexisting lymphangioma. The axial T1–weighted, enhanced image (*B*) demonstrates a large tumor (*white arrows*) with heterogeneous signal that can be seen to stretch and compress the optic nerve (*black arrow*).

lar visual loss in a patient with a ruptured ophthalmic artery aneurysm and Melen et al. (292) reported sudden monocular visual loss in a 13-year-old boy with fibrous dysplasia. Dolman et al. (270) reported five patients who experienced rapidly evolving visual loss in the setting of rapidly progressive proptosis from such disparate causes as orbital hemorrhage, subperiosteal abscess, and orbital cellulitis. In all cases, there was optic nerve traction with dramatic tenting of the posterior globe that was demonstrated by orbital neuroimaging studies (Fig. 8.10).

The combination of ocular pain and unilateral visual loss, simulating retrobulbar neuritis, has been observed in cases of anterior communicating artery aneurysms, pituitary adenoma (293,294), aneurysm (295,296), craniopharyngioma (297), and in patients with mucoceles or pyoceles of the paranasal sinuses, particularly the sphenoid sinus (229,235). In other cases, patients with sudden retrobulbar optic neuropathies from compressive lesions have initially improved when treated with systemic corticosteroids. In such cases, visual function invariably worsens as soon as steroids are tapered. Lesions that have caused this syndrome include pituitary adenoma, craniopharyngioma, plasmacytoma, and medulloblastoma (168,298–300).

The current practice of obtaining MR imaging in patients with suspected optic neuritis as a means of determining which patients are at high risk for developing multiple sclerosis should lessen the frequency of such delays in diagnosis of these optic neuritis imposters.

VISUAL RECOVERY FOLLOWING DECOMPRESSION

In 1915, Cushing and Walker (301) analyzed 81 cases of chiasmal compression and showed that restoration of visual function was not only possible following surgical decompression but it began within days after surgery. Pennybacker (302) also described a dramatic response to surgical treatment in patients with loss of vision from pituitary adenoma and commented on the possibility of full recovery within a few days postoperatively. In a recent series of 27 patients undergoing decompression of the optic nerve, 47% showed improvement which, in two-thirds of the patients happened almost immediately (303). Zevgaridis and associates reported on 65 patients with meningiomas in the sellar region, and found that 39 (65%) of patients had improved vision after surgery on long-term follow-up (average 5 years) (204). Favorable prognostic indicators included younger age, shorter duration of symptoms and an intact arachnoid membrane around the lesion. Li et al. (189) reported on 30 patients with biopsy proven tumors and optic nerve compression that underwent optic canal decompression via an external ethmoidectomy approach, with 20 (67%) demonstrating improved visual function. ''Medical decompression'' of the optic nerve with bromocriptine in patients with prolactin-secreting pituitary tumors has yielded similar improvements in visual function (304). On the other hand, patients undergoing surgery for aneurysms involving the anterior visual path-

ways may experience sudden and severe vision loss presumed secondary to either optic nerve manipulation or ischemia (305,306).

Although it is not surprising that prompt decompression may restore visual function in patients rendered suddenly blind by pituitary apoplexy (307,308), it is not intuitively obvious that patients who have lost all light perception for days or weeks can occasionally experience dramatic visual recovery following decompression surgery (309,310). Kayan and Earl (311) examined 11 patients with compressive lesions of the intracranial optic nerves and chiasm, 7 of whom had complete or nearly complete visual recovery with decompression. All of these patients experienced their recovery within 15 days, with 5 patients recovering within 5 days. One patient had no change in visual acuity or visual fields following surgery. Subsequent authors reported similar results in patients with both pituitary adenomas and meningiomas (148,149). With increasing use of the transsphenoidal technique for removal of pituitary tumors and improvements in anesthesia for patients undergoing neurosurgical procedures, it has become possible to evaluate patients several hours after they have undergone decompression of the intracranial optic nerves or optic chiasm. Miller (312) found that patients with pituitary adenomas who have normal fundi (as well as many who have mild disc pallor and loss of the nerve fiber layer) invariably experience impressive return of visual acuity and visual field that can be detected almost immediately after they awaken from anesthesia. In most other cases of optic nerve compression in which adequate decompression has been obtained, patients are aware of improvement within several days. Many patients achieve maximum recovery by the time they are discharged from the hospital 5–10 days after surgery; others experience improvement during this period but continue to improve over the subsequent weeks to months (303). Other investigators have reported similar findings (313–315). Although there are patients who do not improve dramatically immediately after decompression surgery but do improve gradually several months following surgery, such patients are increasingly rare and are primarily those with preoperative hydrocephalus or postoperative cerebral edema. As in the cases reported by Kayan and Earl (311), Miller (312) found no correlation between the rapidity of visual loss and the rapidity of visual return. Tumor volume has also proved to be a poor predictor of the extent of visual recovery, both for pituitary adenomas and suprasellar meningiomas (316,317).

Visual loss in patients with compressive optic neuropathies is unlikely to be caused by vascular insufficiency, as has been postulated in the past (318), but by demyelination insufficient to cause cell death. Gledhill and McDonald (319), as well as Harrison and McDonald (320), demonstrated remyelination following the demyelination that occurs with acute compression of the cat spinal cord. Clifford-Jones et al. (321) described remyelination of demyelinated fibers of the cat optic nerve after *chronic compression*. Since remyelination is capable of restoring the ability of previously demyelinated central fibers to conduct trains of impulses at physiologic frequencies (322,323), and since impaired conduction in demyelinated axons is likely to contribute to the visual loss commonly produced by tumors compressing the anterior visual system, the observation of Clifford-Jones et al. (321) that remyelination occurs in the anterior visual system (at least in cats) is of extreme importance.

McDonald (297) provided a lucid summary of this work and described the neurophysiology underlying the visual symptoms of anterior visual pathway compression. According to McDonald (297), there are three stages of visual recovery after decompression of the anterior visual pathway. Relief of visual pathway compression is initially followed by *rapid recovery* of some vision within minutes to hours. McDonald likened this recovery to the relief of conduction block after an arm or leg "goes to sleep." This initial recovery is followed by *delayed recovery* of additional function over weeks to months. This improvement may be related to progressive remyelination of previously compressed demyelinated axons. Finally, there is an even longer period of improvement, taking many months to years. The mechanism by which this *late recovery* occurs is unknown.

Several authors have suggested that measurement of visual evoked potentials in patients undergoing neurosurgical decompression of the anterior visual system may be advantageous not only in assessing the adequacy of the procedure but also in aiding the surgeon with respect to the extent of surgery and in warning of excessive manipulation of the optic nerve (324–328). Other investigators, however, have found the results to be unreliable because the latency and configuration of the visual evoked potential wave forms are adversely affected by direct pharmacologic effects of the anesthetics, and intraoperative changes in latency and amplitude have shown little correlation with postoperative visual function change (329–332). These drawbacks have prevented the technique from being widely used.

INFILTRATIVE OPTIC NEUROPATHIES

The optic nerve can become infiltrated by tumors and by various inflammatory processes (Table 8.1). Such processes typically produce one of three clinical pictures: (*a*) optic disc elevation or swelling with evidence of an optic neuropathy; (*b*) optic disc elevation or swelling with no evidence of optic nerve dysfunction; and (*c*) a normal-appearing optic disc associated with evidence of an optic neuropathy.

Infiltration of the proximal portion of the optic nerve, either anterior or just posterior to the lamina cribrosa, produces elevation and swelling of the optic disc. When the prelaminar portion of the nerve is infiltrated, the elevation of the disc is caused by the infiltrative process and is not true disc swelling. When the retrolaminar portion of the nerve is infiltrated, the disc elevation is caused by true swelling of the disc, and the appearance is indistinguishable from the disc swelling caused by such diverse entities as increased intracranial pressure, ischemia, and inflammation.

The disc elevation observed in patients with infiltrative processes of the optic nerve, whether true swelling or an infiltrative process, may be associated with other signs of optic nerve dysfunction. In such cases, there is variable loss of visual acuity and color vision, a visual field defect that can be of any type, and a relative afferent pupillary defect when the infiltration is unilateral or asymmetric. In other cases, however, the disc elevation is asymptomatic, and there is no clinical evidence of an optic neuropathy, although electrophysiologic testing, such as visual evoked responses, may be abnormal. The more distal (posterior) the infiltrative process, the less likely it is that any change will be noted in the optic disc. In such cases, the optic nerve initially appears normal, and the clinical picture is that of a retrobulbar optic neuropathy.

Table 8.1 lists both common and uncommon processes that infiltrate the optic nerve. The most common lesions that infiltrate the optic nerve are tumors and inflammatory/infectious processes. Tumors may be primary or secondary. Primary tumors are far more common than are secondary ones. The most common inflammatory disorder is sarcoidosis; the most common infectious agents are opportunistic fungi.

TUMORS

Primary Tumors

Primary tumors that infiltrate the nerve include optic gliomas, astrocytic hamartomas, gangliogliomas, capillary and

Table 8.1
Lesions that Infiltrate the Optic Nerve

Primary Tumors
    Optic glioma
    Benign/malignant ganglioglioma
    Malignant teratoid medulloepithelioma
    Capillary hemangioma
    Cavernous hemangioblastoma
    Other
Secondary Tumors
    Metastatic carcinoma
    Nasopharyngeal carcinoma and other contiguous tumors
    Lymphoreticular tumors
    Lymphoma
    Leukemia
    Other
Infections and Inflammation
    Sarcoidosis
    Idiopathic perioptic neuritis
    Bacteria
    Virus
    Fungi

cavernous hemangiomas, hemangioblastomas, and melanocytomas.

Optic Nerve Glioma

The most common lesion that infiltrates the optic nerve is the optic glioma (1,333,334), although the most common tumors to affect the pediatric orbit are vascular tumors (335) (Fig. 8.11) (see Chapter 28). Optic pathway gliomas represent 1% of all intracranial tumors, 1.5–3.5% of all orbital tumors, and 65% of all intrinsic optic nerve tumors (336,337). Gliomas confined to the optic nerve constitute about 25% of all optic pathway gliomas, with the remainder infiltrating the optic chiasm and optic tracts in addition to one or both optic nerves (333). In the first decade of life

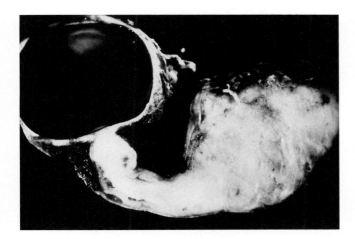

Figure 8.11. Optic nerve glioma. The optic nerve is diffusely enlarged. (Courtesy of Dr. William R. Green.)

70% of patients with optic pathway gliomas develop visual symptoms or signs, and 90% of the lesions are detected by the second decade (338–342). Some studies suggest no particular sex predilection for these tumors (333,343) and others point to a slight female predilection (338).

Patients with gliomas confined to the optic nerve have three clinical presentations that are determined in part by the location, size, and extent of the tumor (344). When the glioma is confined to the orbital portion of the nerve or the bulk of the lesion is within the orbit, the patient typically develops proptosis associated with evidence of an anterior optic neuropathy (loss of visual acuity and color vision, a visual field defect, a relative afferent defect, and a swollen optic disc) (2,345). Whether the optic disc swelling that is observed in such patients results from infiltration alone, vascular insufficiency, or compression by the arachnoidal proliferation or extension of the tumor outside the pia-arachnoid of the nerve that may accompany such lesions is unclear (346).

Another mechanism that may be responsible for disc swelling in such patients is secondary obstruction of the cerebrospinal fluid (CSF) space surrounding the orbital portion of the optic nerve by the tumor (333). Patients with gliomas that both infiltrate and compress the optic nerve can eventually develop optociliary shunt vessels–congenital venous channels that enlarge in the setting of chronic compression of the optic nerve and that shunt blood from the retinal to the choroidal circulations (see above) (Fig. 8.12). The increased volume of the optic nerve pressing on the globe and shortening it may induce hyperopia. In such a case, retinal striae may be seen (342) (Fig. 8.13A and B). In rare cases the tumor directly infiltrates the optic disc and swelling and infiltration of the surrounding retina is seen ophthalmoscopically (Fig. 8.13C).

When the tumor is located posteriorly in the orbit, and especially when the process begins in, or is limited to the intracanalicular or intracranial portions of the nerve, the presentation is that of a slowly progressive or relatively stable retrobulbar optic neuropathy (347–352). In most of these cases, the optic disc on the affected side is pale when the patient is first assessed, and the disc does not appear to have been previously swollen. Such patients do not typically have proptosis; if they do, it is usually less than 3 mm. Pain is not a feature of the clinical presentation of optic nerve gliomas, unless they suddenly hemorrhage (342,353).

With the widespread availability of neuroimaging, particularly MR imaging, and the increasing tendency of physicians to screen patients with neurofibromatosis type 1 (NF-1) radiologically, more patients with asymptomatic, presumed optic gliomas are being identified. Such patients have no visual complaints and may or may not have evidence of visual dysfunction (e.g., an asymptomatic visual field defect or a relative afferent pupillary defect) on careful testing, although most have abnormal visual evoked responses to pattern stimuli. Many patients first come to medical attention because they develop a sensory strabismus (2,333). In other patients, the tumor displaces the globe, producing a primary strabismus. Such patients may have variable visual loss that is caused not by the tumor per se but by strabismic ambly-

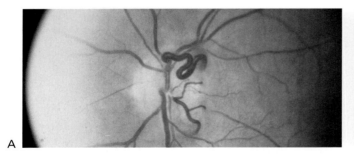
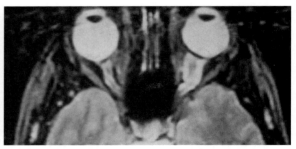

Figure 8.12. Optociliary shunt vessels in a patient with an optic nerve glioma. *A,* The left optic disc is pale and mildly swollen. There are optociliary shunt vessels on its surface. *B,* T2-weighted MR image, axial view, shows diffuse enlargement of the orbital portion of the left optic nerve. The patient was initially thought to have an optic nerve sheath meningioma. Note the ''pseudo-CSF sign'' caused by extension of the tumor into the subdural space around the intraorbital optic nerve.

opia. The diagnosis in such cases may be suspected when color vision is less severely affected than is visual acuity.

Patients with optic nerve gliomas may have stable and even normal visual acuity for many years (354–356). In some cases, however, there is slowly progressive visual loss, and in rare cases there is sudden and profound visual loss that simulates that of acute optic neuritis (357). Overall, when initially confined to the optic nerve, gliomas are associated with a 5% mortality rate, although with hypothalamic involvement mortality increases to 50% (333).

The diagnosis of an optic nerve glioma should be suspected in any young child who develops or is found to have

decreased vision with evidence of an anterior or retrobulbar optic neuropathy or who has asymptomatic optic disc swelling or pallor, particularly if the child has the stigmata of NF-1. Both CT scanning and MR imaging can be used to identify the lesion, which typically appears as a fusiform enlargement of the orbital portion of the optic nerve, with or without concomitant enlargement of the optic canal (358,359) (Figs. 8.12*B* and 8.14). In other cases, the nerve is diffusely enlarged, thus mimicking a meningioma (360).

MR imaging is generally better at defining the extent of an optic nerve glioma than is CT scanning (361). On MR imaging, optic gliomas typically have normal to slightly pro-

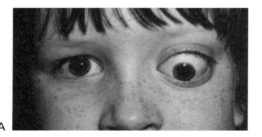

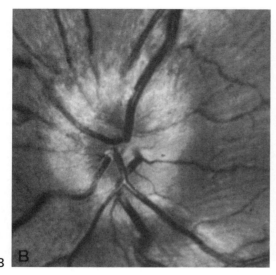

Figure 8.13. Optic nerve glioma producing proptosis, optic disc swelling, and chorioretinal striae. *A,* The left eye is proptotic and displaced inferiorly. *B,* The left optic disc is swollen, and chorioretinal striae are present. *C,* In a different patient the tumor can be seen to invade the optic nerve head and surrounding retina. (Courtesy of Dr. Grant T. Liu.)

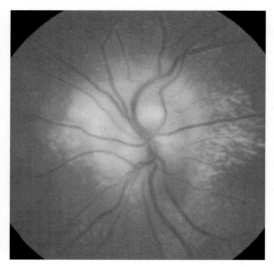

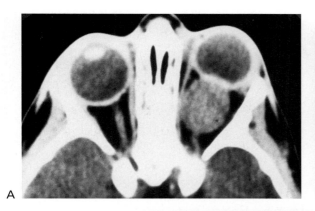
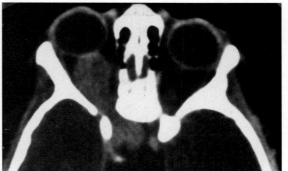
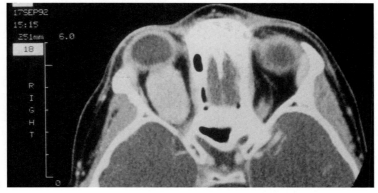

Figure 8.14. Neuroimaging in three patients with optic nerve gliomas. *A*, CT scan, axial view, shows fusiform enlargement of the orbital portion of the left optic nerve. The enlargement begins at the globe and continues for about three fourths the length of the nerve. Note normal size nerve at orbital apex. *B*, CT scan, axial view, after intravenous injection of contrast material in another patient shows fusiform enlargement and enhancement of the entire optic nerve within the right orbit. *C*, CT scan, axial view, in a third patient shows fusiform enlargement of the right optic nerve within the orbit, with extension of the enlarged nerve through an enlarged optic canal and intracranially.

longed T1 relaxation times and are isointense or hypointense to normal brain on T1-weighted images. Many of these tumors also have a prolongation of the T2 relaxation times. The T2-weighted images are better at assessing the extent of the tumor than are T1-weighted images (361). Although gliomas of the optic nerve may show minimal enhancement after intravenous injection of a paramagnetic contrast material, the enhancement is not nearly as pronounced as is typically seen with a meningioma (362).

Two important signs help differentiate optic nerve gliomas from other lesions. One is an unusual "kinking" of the optic nerve within the orbit (Fig. 8.15). This is seen almost exclusively in patients with neurofibromatosis type 1. The other is a double-intensity tubular thickening of the nerve, best seen on MR images. This sign is called the "pseudo-CSF" signal because the increase in T2 signal surrounding the nerve may be misinterpreted as a CSF signal (363) (Fig. 8.16). The genesis of this signal is perineural arachnoidal gliomatosis that occurs in optic nerve gliomas in patients with NF-1 (364,365). Cystic components to the tumor are more common in non-NF-1-associated glioma (359). Kinking of the nerve and the pseudo-CSF signal are often seen together.

A review of 2,186 published cases reveals that approximately 29% of optic pathway gliomas occur in the setting of NF-1 (333). Therefore, any patient found to harbor an optic pathway glioma should be assessed for evidence of NF-1, and patients with cutaneous lesions consistent with NF-1 should be screened for optic pathway gliomas and other intracranial lesions that occur in patients with neurofibromatosis. Indeed, Listernick et al. (366) performed neuroimaging on 176 children with NF-1 and found that 15% of those who were visually asymptomatic harbored an optic pathway glioma. Creange et al. (367) found 20 (13%) of 158 patients with NF-1 to have an optic pathway tumor. The sporadic, non-NF-1-associated form of the tumor tends to present at an earlier age, more often involves and or spreads to the chiasm with associated hydrocephalus, and may behave more aggressively (338,359,368,369).

Gliomas that affect the optic nerve may occasionally be confined to the optic disc. Most of these rare lesions occur in patients with NF-1. They may cause a change in the appearance of the optic disc that simulates true swelling (370,371). In most cases, however, the normal features of the optic disc are obscured by a mass of whitish, gray, or yellow tissue that projects from and above the disc surface

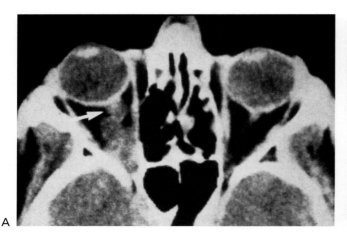
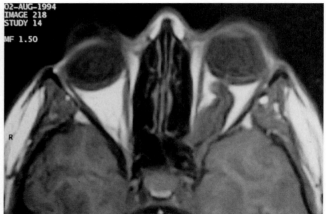

Figure 8.15. Kinking of the optic nerves in patients with neurofibromatosis type 1 and an optic nerve glioma. *A,* Axial CT scan shows "kinking" (*arrow*) of an enlarged optic nerve within the right orbit. *B,* Axial T1 weighted MRI scan demonstrating kinking of the left optic nerve. This sign is pathognomonic of an optic nerve glioma. (*B,* Courtesy of Dr. Grant T. Liu.)

(Fig. 8.17*A*). Visual acuity in patients with gliomas of the optic disc is variably affected.

Optic nerve gliomas are not hamartomas but are, in fact, true neoplasms (372,373) with a potential for significant visual morbidity and a small but significant mortality (5,374). Most of these tumors, regardless of their localization or extent within the nerve, are of the juvenile pilocytic variety and have a benign appearance on microscopy (Fig. 8.17).

Less common features include capillary proliferation, tissue necrosis with hemorrhage, glial giant cells, and even mitotic figures (342,353,375). A reactive leptomeningeal hyperplasia occurs around some of these lesions, both within the orbit and within the optic canal. This can lead to the erroneous diagnosis of optic nerve meningioma if only the superficial aspect of the nerve is biopsied (376). In one series, certain immunohistologic features were found to predict aggressive

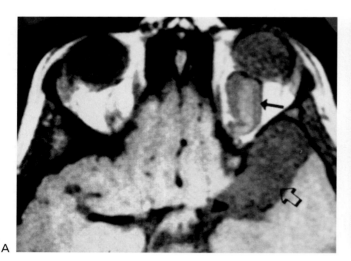
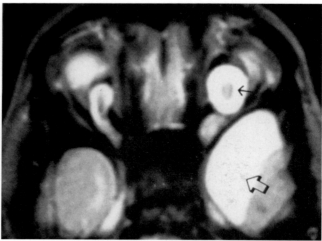

Figure 8.16. The pseudo-CSF sign in a patient with neurofibromatosis type 1 and bilateral optic nerve gliomas. *A,* T1-weighted MR image, axial view, shows that the orbital portion of the left optic nerve consists of a fusiform area of low intensity (*closed arrow*) surrounding a core of high signal intensity. An arachnoid cyst (*open arrow*) occupies the left anterior cranial fossa. Note that the peripheral (outer) tumor signal is isointense to the CSF in the cyst. The tumor is kinked posteriorly. The right optic nerve glioma cannot be seen on this image. *B,* T2-weighted MR image, axial view, shows a donut-shaped signal of high intensity (*dark arrow*) surrounding an inner circle of low signal intensity in the left orbit. This image represents a tangential cut through the superior aspect of the upwardly kinked tumor. In the right orbit, a linear area of high signal intensity surrounds a central core of low signal intensity. Note that the outer signal within both tumors is isointense to CSF within the arachnoid cyst (*open arrow*). (From Brodsky MC. The "pseudo-CSF" signal of orbital optic glioma on magnetic resonance imaging: A signature of neurofibromatosis. Surv Ophthalmol 1993;36:213–218.)

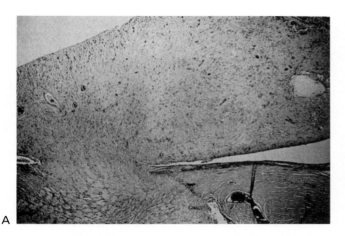

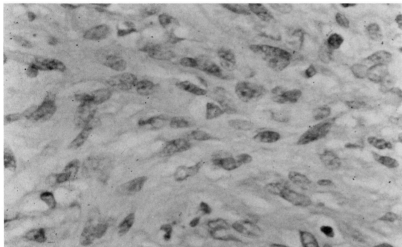

Figure 8.17. Histologic appearance of an optic disc glioma. *A*, At lower power, the disc is elevated and infiltrated with numerous astrocytes. *B*, At higher magnification optic nerve gliomas can be seen to be composed of large, benign-appearing astrocytes. (*A*, Courtesy of Dr. William R. Green.)

behavior (373). Gliomas that occur in patients with NF-1 show the unique feature of extension of tumor into the subarachnoid and dural spaces surrounding the nerve, whereas gliomas that occur in patients without neurofibromatosis produce diffuse enlargement of the nerve without extension into the subdural or subarachnoid space (364,377) (Fig. 8.18).

The treatment of optic nerve gliomas is controversial. These tumors when confined to the optic nerve generally have a more favorable prognosis than tumors presenting with or ultimately involving the chiasm, hypothalamus, and retrochiasmal visual pathways (352,368). The natural history of these benign lesions is generally good, with long-term useful visual function and few, if any, neurologic complications (369,378). Most optic nerve gliomas do not change substantially in size or shape over many years (366). Some, however, rapidly enlarge and extend along the nerve to the chiasm and even into the 3rd ventricle (379) (see below). Others suddenly expand from intraneural hemorrhage. Conversely, rare lesions exhibit spontaneous regression (380–382). Spontaneous and significant improvement of vision and reduction of lesion size has been reported in patients with optic

and chiasmal gliomas (380–383). The natural history and prognosis may be better in patients with NF-1-associated tumors (338,359,369,383).

In younger children, an optic nerve tumor can be amblyogenic. In young children with monocular vision loss from an optic pathway tumor, part-time occlusion therapy (patching) of the unaffected eye is recommended (384). Some gliomas, however, enlarge and cause progressive visual loss in one or both eyes. Lesions may even extend into the hypothalamus and 3rd ventricle and lesions that involve the postchiasmal visual pathways often have a greater effect on vision (352,385,386). There has been only one well-documented case of an optic nerve glioma presenting without radiographic demonstration of chiasmal or hypothalamic involvement which subsequently extended posteriorly (379); however this case was evaluated only with CT scanning. Patients with optic nerve glioma with unequivocal sparing of the chiasm at presentation (evaluated with modern gadolinium-enhanced MRI, with thin, high resolution sections) who later develop chiasmal involvement are exceedingly unusual. However, in a study of 106 patients with unilateral gliomas initially confined to the orbit at study entry, local progression

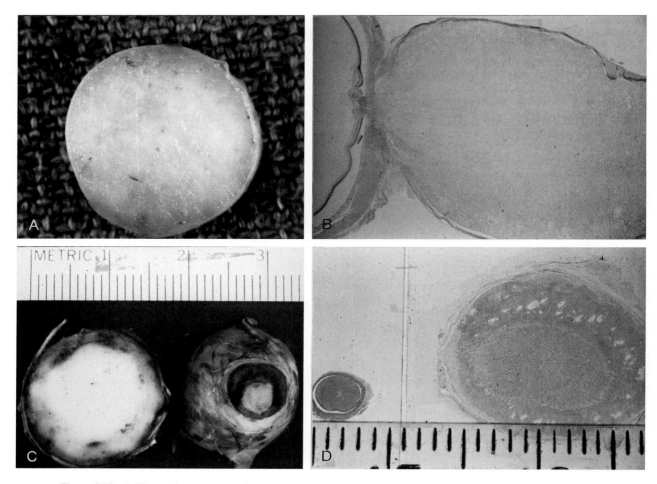

Figure 8.18.   Difference in appearance of optic nerve gliomas in patients with and without neurofibromatosis type 1 (NF-1). *A*, In a patient without NF-1, gross appearance of an optic nerve glioma in cross section shows that the nerve is diffusely enlarged. There is no extension of tumor into the subarachnoid or subdural spaces. *B*, Longitudinal histologic section through an optic nerve glioma in another patient without NF-1 also shows diffuse enlargement of the nerve without extension of tumor into the subarachnoid or subdural space. *C*, In a patient with NF-1 and an optic nerve glioma, gross appearance of the affected nerve in cross section shows that the nerve is infiltrated and enlarged by tumor. Note, however, that the tumor also extends into the subdural and subarachnoid spaces, where it appears necrotic and hemorrhagic. *D*, Histologic cross sections comparing a normal optic nerve (*left*) with an optic nerve glioma in another patient with NF-1 (*right*) show marked enlargement of the affected nerve as well as extension of tumor into the subarachnoid and subdural spaces.

occurred in 20% of untreated patients, 29% following incomplete surgical resection, and 2.3% following apparent complete excision (387). The possibility of intracranial extension exists in any given patient and for this reason patients are followed with serial neuro-ophthalmic examinations and MRI scanning.

Patients with optic nerve gliomas are generally not treated with either chemotherapy or radiation therapy unless there is clear evidence of progression with the lesion extending into the optic chiasm, opposite optic nerve, or hypothalamus (2,349,369,388,389). Radiation therapy is probably effective in improving vision and disease-specific survival probability in gliomas of the anterior visual pathway that are clearly progressing clinically (368,390). Because of the risk of radiation to the developing brain, chemotherapy is the first-

line treatment in a child under age six, while radiation of the optic nerve tumor would be the primary option in an older child.

It must be remembered that radiation therapy can have significant side effects, particularly in children. These include developmental delay, vasculitis, moya-moya disease, leukoencephalopathy, radionecrosis of the temporal lobes, endocrinopathies, behavior disturbances, and the induction of secondary malignancies (391–393). Fractionated stereotactic radiotherapy is effective and may be associated with less morbidity and pituitary gland dysfunction (394). Surgical resection is generally reserved for those patients who are already blind when first seen; for patients with severe proptosis; and for patients whose lesions seem to be threatening the optic chiasm but that have not yet reached it

(333,358,383,395–397) (Fig. 8.19). No clinical trials have been performed to indicate if removal of an apparently unilateral optic nerve glioma is associated with a better visual and neurologic prognosis than no treatment at all.

The efficacy of chemotherapeutic agents in the treatment of optic nerve gliomas is unclear. Most investigators agree that the drugs are never curative; however, they may stabilize or reduce the growth rate and progression of visual manifestations of the tumor and thus delay the need for radiation therapy, particularly in young children (374,398).

Most gliomas that infiltrate the optic nerve or chiasm are, as noted above, benign juvenile pilocytic astrocytomas; however, some are malignant (399–403). Malignant optic gliomas almost always occur in adults and produce one of two clinical pictures. When the tumor initially affects the intracranial optic nerves or chiasm, there is rapidly progressive visual loss associated with optic discs that initially appear normal but that rapidly become atrophic (404,405). The visual loss in these cases is often bilateral and simultaneous, but it may initially begin in one eye and may be mistaken for retrobulbar optic neuritis, particularly when there is associated pain (402). When the malignant glioma initially affects the proximal portion of the intraorbital optic nerve, there is acute loss of vision associated with optic disc swelling and the ophthalmoscopic appearance of a central retinal vein occlusion (402). The prognosis in almost all cases of malignant optic glioma is poor, regardless of treatment with radiotherapy or chemotherapy. Most patients become completely blind within several months after the onset of symptoms, and most die within 6–12 months.

Other Primary Tumors

Tumors primarily composed of mature ganglion cells may occur in both the peripheral nervous system and the central nervous system (CNS). **Ganglion cell tumors** of the CNS are less common than their peripheral counterparts and there are two main types. Ganglioneuromas (also called gangliocytomas) are composed predominantly of mature ganglion cells supported by a stroma of spindle cells and containing calcospherites, whereas gangliogliomas are composed of a mixture of mature ganglion cells and mature glial cells and are thus true mixed neurogliogenic tumors (406–409). These two types of tumor represent extremes of the spectrum of tumors containing mature ganglion cells, and there are many tumors that must be considered transition forms between them. Ganglion cell tumors occur most frequently in children and young adults (409,410). Nevertheless, the age range is broad—from several months (337,410,411) to 80 years of age (412). They occur with equal frequency in males and females.

The most common location of ganglion cell tumors is the floor of the 3rd ventricle, where they produce symptoms and signs related to dysfunction of the hypothalamus or pituitary gland, including precocious puberty, diabetes insipidus, acromegaly, and panhypopituitarism. In rare instances, the gangliogliomas originate within the substance of the optic chiasm or intracranial portion of the optic nerves, and thus may be mistaken for a typical ''optic glioma'' (413). Cases of gangliogliomas infiltrating one or both optic nerves and the anterior visual pathways have been reported (414–419).

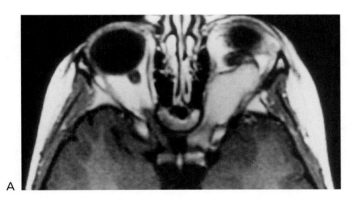

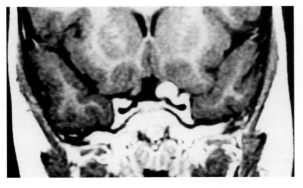

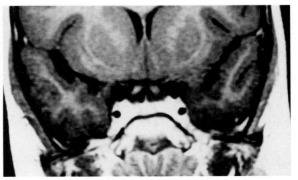

Figure 8.19. Left optic glioma near the optic chiasm in a 6-year-old boy without neurofibromatosis type 1. *A*, T1-weighted MR image, axial view after intravenous injection of paramagnetic contrast material shows that the glioma extends through the optic canal up to the optic chiasm. *B*, T1-weighted enhanced MR image, coronal view, shows enlargement and enhancement of the intracranial portion of the left optic nerve. *C*, T1-weighted enhanced MR image, coronal view, 3 mm *posterior* to the view seen in *B* shows that the left optic nerve just anterior to the optic chiasm is normal in size and does not enhance, suggesting that the tumor has not yet reached this site. This is the type of patient who might be considered a candidate for excision of the tumor.

Lu et al. (420) and Shuangshoti et al. (417) reported the MR characteristics of a ganglioglioma which had no distinguishing features and simply appeared as a fusiform dilation of the right optic nerve with enhancement in one patient and a circumscribed cystic lesion with an enhancing mural nodule in another. The lesion has been identified in a patient with NF-1 (416).

Liu et al. (421) described chiasmatic infiltration by a ganglioglioma in three patients. In one of the patients, the tumor had originated in the temporal lobe and spread to the chiasm. In a second patient who presented with a bitemporal field defect, the tumor appeared to have originated within the chiasm. The third patient had a ganglioglioma that originated within the chiasm and extended to both optic tracts. The patient was almost completely blind, having only a small left homonymous island of vision remaining. All of these patients had optic atrophy.

The microscopic appearance of the ganglion cell tumor varies according to the extent to which neuronal and glial elements participate in the neoplastic process (416). The pure ganglioneuroma is moderately cellular tumor in which the cells are clearly neuronal in origin but are often abnormal in appearance. In pure ganglioneuromas, the glial element consists of a scanty stroma of spindle cells; but in gangliogliomas there is clear evidence of neoplastic astrocytic proliferation. Gangliogliomas thus contain glial cells that show histologic differentiation that parallels that of neurons. The degree of differentiation may be so great that such tumors may initially be thought to represent pleomorphic fibrillary astrocytomas until careful examination reveals their true composition.

Most ganglion cell tumors, whether ganglioneuromas or gangliogliomas, generally have a good prognosis as they behave biologically as low-grade astrocytomas; however, the survival rates may be somewhat lower for patients with chiasmatic infiltration (422). In addition, some of these tumors do have malignant features. In these tumors, the malignant elements are usually glial rather than neuronal (423,424), and metastases may occur (337,425).

Astrocytic hamartomas can infiltrate the optic disc. In most cases, they protrude above or overlie the surface of the affected disc. They initially have a grayish or grayish-pink appearance, but they later develop a glistening, yellow, mulberry appearance (Fig. 8.20). Although this latter appearance is similar to that of optic disc drusen, drusen are located within the substance of the disc, whereas astrocytic hamartomas overlie the disc (Fig. 8.21).

The appearance of an astrocytic hamaratoma is also similar to that of an endophytic or regressing retinoblastoma; however, astrocytic hamartomas do not exhibit the same rapid growth characteristics as a retinoblastoma. They also tend to be more yellow and glistening than retinoblastomas (426). The visual function in an eye with an astrocytic hamartoma of the optic disc is usually normal. Some eyes, however, develop a serous detachment of the retina or vitreous hemorrhage, resulting in variable loss of vision (427). Spontaneous regression of such lesions may occur (428).

Astrocytic hamartomas are composed almost entirely of acellular laminated calcific concretions. In many specimens, these concretions are interspersed among areas composed of large glial cells (429). Most astrocytic hamartomas occur in patients with tuberous sclerosis or NF-1 (430). In about 30% of cases, however, the patient has no evidence of any of the phacomatoses or of any other systemic disorder.

Both **capillary and cavernous hemangiomas** can occur within the substance of the optic disc (371,431–434). In addition, cavernous hemangiomas can develop at any location in the optic nerve and in the optic chiasm (196, 435–440). Capillary hemangiomas may be endophytic or exophytic. The endophytic type appears as a circular, reddish, slightly elevated mass internal to the disc vasculature and is represented histologically by a capillary hemangioma lying immediately beneath the internal limiting membrane (Fig. 8.22). These lesions may be a manifestation of von

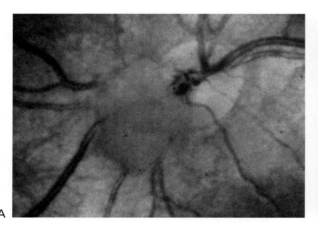

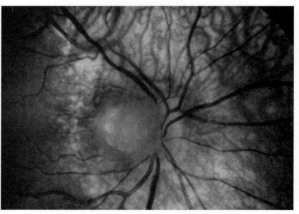

A   B

Figure 8.20. Astrocytic hamartoma of the optic disc. *A,* Before significant calcification, the lesion appears as a pinkish gray mass rising above the disc. *B,* When calcification occurs, small globular clusters can be observed within the mass. Eventually, the entire mass may become calcified.

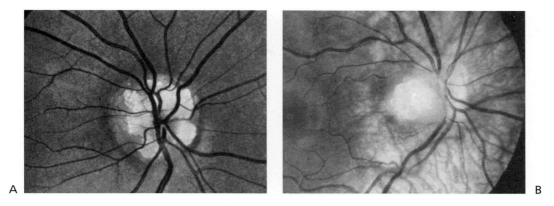

Figure 8.21.   Difference in ophthalmoscopic appearance of optic disc drusen and astrocytic hamartoma of the optic disc. *A,* Optic disc drusen are located within the substance of the disc *beneath* the vessels. *B,* Astrocytic hamartomas are located *above* the optic disc, thus obscuring the vessels.

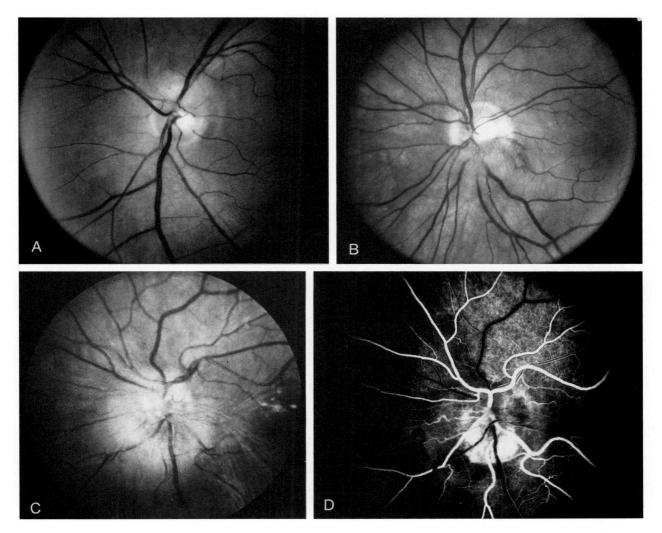

Figure 8.22.   Endophytic capillary angioma. *A–C,* The lesion appears as a circular, reddish, slightly elevated mass internal to the disc vasculature. *D,* Fluorescein angiography of lesion seen in *C* shows intense staining and leakage from vessels at inferior aspect of disc.

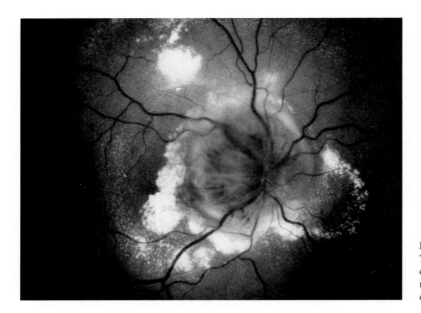

Figure 8.23. Exophytic capillary angioma of the optic disc. This lesion appears as diffuse blurring and elevation of the disc, often associated with a variable degree of serous detachment of the peripapillary sensory retina and a ring of lipid deposition. (Courtesy of Dr. Andrew Schachat.)

Hippel-Lindau disease (441), or they may occur as an isolated phenomenon. The exophytic type of capillary hemangioma is typically seen as blurring and elevation of the disc margin, often associated with a variable degree of serous detachment of the peripapillary sensory retina and a ring of lipid deposition (442) (Fig. 8.23). This lesion is often misdiagnosed as unilateral papilledema or papillitis, but fluorescein angiography clearly demonstrates the vascular anomaly (371,432,442–444), as does ultrasonography. These tumors may also occur as part of von Hippel-Lindau disease. Rarely, exophytic capillary angiomas are bilateral. In such instances, they are often misdiagnosed as papilledema; but again, fluorescein angiography and ultrasonogra-

phy are invaluable in making the correct diagnosis. Capillary angiomas do not occur within the substance of the optic nerve or chiasm.

Cavernous hemangiomas consist of large-caliber vascular channels. When these lesions occur as isolated masses within the orbit, they are well circumscribed and encapsulated. Within the eye, however, their appearance is that of a cluster of small purple blobs located within and above the substance of the optic disc (433,445–449) (Fig. 8.24). The blood flow within the vessels in cavernous hemangiomas is extremely slow, indicating that this lesion is more isolated from the general circulation than its capillary counterpart. Cavernous hemangiomas of the optic disc are usually unilateral. They

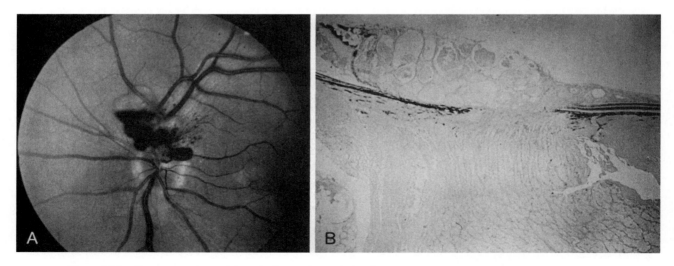

Figure 8.24. Cavernous angioma of the optic disc. *A,* Note "cluster of grapes" appearance of lesion. *B,* Histologic appearance of a cavernous angioma showing multiple dilated vessels *above* and *adjacent* to the disc surface. (From Davies WS, Thumin M. Cavernous hemangioma of the optic disc and retina. Trans Am Acad Ophthalmol Otolaryngol 1956;60:217–218. AFIP Acc. 219953.)

occur more commonly in females than in males, with an irregularly autosomal-dominant inheritance pattern. The lesion is almost always asymptomatic, with visual acuity being normal and visual fields showing only a variably enlarged blind spot; however, rare cases have been reported in which there has been vitreous hemorrhage (384). Although these lesions have been considered not to grow, Kushner et al. (384) documented growth of a cavernous hemangioma of the optic disc in two patients followed for 5 to10 years. Cavernous hemangiomas, unlike capillary hemangiomas, can occur within the optic nerves, optic chiasm, or optic tracts (196,439) (Fig. 8.25). Similar lesions can occur in the retrolaminar portion of the optic nerve (437), in the intracanalicular portion of the optic nerve (435), and in the intracranial portion of the optic nerve (438,440).

In some cases, the lesion itself causes slowly progressive loss of vision. In most cases, however, visual loss is rapidly progressive and occurs because of hemorrhage into the surrounding tissue (450,451). Regli et al. reviewed 28 cases and pointed out that these lesions typically occur in the third or fourth decade and have a triad of (*a*) sudden headache; (*b*) an acute change in visual acuity; and (*c*) a significant defect in the visual field. Interestingly, up to one third of the previously reported patients had episodes of transient visual loss that had been previously diagnosed as optic neuritis. Cavernous hemangiomas are not associated with von Hippel-Lindau disease; however, they are often associated with similar lesions of the skin and brain. In contrast to the benign nature of the ocular lesion, associated CNS vascular hamartomas may produce convulsions, intracranial hemorrhage, cranial nerve palsies, and multiple neurologic deficits.

Not all vascular lesions within the substance of the optic nerve are benign. Kerr et al. (452) described the case of a 27-year-old woman with von Hippel-Lindau disease who experienced progressive visual loss in the right eye. She had a small capillary angioma of the right optic disc and a vascular mass of the intracranial portion of the right optic nerve

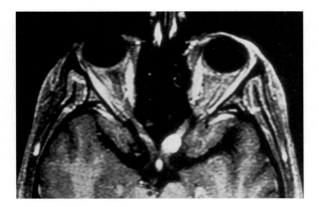

Figure 8.25. Neuroimaging appearance of cavernous angioma of the optic nerve. The patient was a 23-year-old woman with progressive loss of vision in the left eye and evidence of a retrobulbar optic neuropathy. T1-weighted MR image, axial view, after intravenous injection of contrast material shows hyperintense enhancing lesion within the intracranial portion of the left optic nerve.

that was found to be a hemangioblastoma. These authors reviewed 11 previously reported cases of **optic nerve hemangioblastoma**. Five tumors were located within the orbit and frequently produced proptosis (453,454), while four tumors were strictly intracranial, and two involved both the intracranial and intraorbital portions of the optic nerve.

The typical patient presents with progressive visual loss and evidence of an optic neuropathy that may be anterior or retrobulbar, depending on the location of the lesion, and may be bilateral (452,455,456). The degree of visual loss is variable, and any type of visual field defect may be present. There is always a relative afferent pupillary defect. The affected portion of the optic nerve is enlarged and has a fusiform appearance mimicking an optic nerve glioma on neuroimaging (454,456) (Fig. 8.26). Kerr et al. (452) emphasized that hemangioblastomas of the optic nerve, like their counterparts elsewhere in the CNS, usually have a plane of section that permits surgical removal without sacrificing the entire optic nerve.

Histologically, optic nerve hemangioblastomas are composed of a highly vascular matrix with intervascular stromal cells containing abundant, clear, foamy cytoplasm. Ultrastructurally, the spaces are lined with endothelium and occasional pericytes and lipid-containing stromal cells in the intervascular regions. Only 30% of these lesions are associated with the von Hippel-Lindau disease; however, partial expression of genetic disorders is being documented with increasing frequency, and many of the other lesions associated with von Hippel-Lindau disease may not become apparent for a number of years, especially because the previously documented cases were reported in individuals ranging in age from 15 to 44 years. Furthermore, the investigation of family members in some of these cases may have been incomplete, leading to the erroneous conclusion that the disorder was not familial.

Melanocytomas are intraocular tumors that typically occur within the substance of the optic disc (457–459). Clinically, these lesions are elevated masses that are gray to dark black in color and are located eccentrically on the disc (Fig. 8.27). About 90% are two disc diameters or less, and the majority are less than 2 mm in height (459). Swelling of the disc occurs in about 25% of cases and is thought to be caused by a disturbance of axoplasmic flow secondary to chronic compression. Vascular sheathing may be seen in 30% of eyes, and subretinal fluid is observed in approximately 10% of patients. A nevus may be seen adjacent to a melanocytoma in up to 50% of cases (458). Constriction of the visual field may also occur in patients with a melanocytoma of the optic disc (355,460). Osher et al. (461) studied 20 patients with optic disc melanocytomas; 14 of the patients had visual acuity of 20/20 or better, and all patients had visual acuity of 20/50 or better. Only 5 of the patients studied were aware of any visual distortion, but 18 of the 20 patients had abnormal visual fields. Three of these patients had minimal blind spot enlargement; the remaining 15 patients had markedly enlarged blind spots, of whom 10 also had relative or absolute arcuate scotomas. Six of these 10 patients had a relative afferent pupillary defect. However, not all patients with a melanocytoma have good visual acuity. Some patients de-

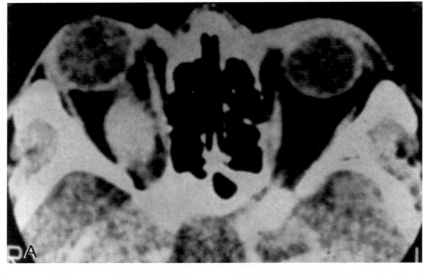

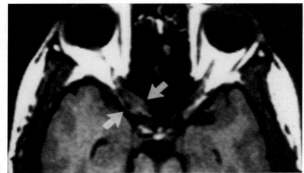

B

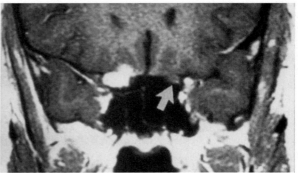

C

Figure 8.26. Neuroimaging appearance of hemangioblastomas of the optic nerve. *A,* In a 37-year-old man with von Hippel-Lindau disease. CT scan, axial view, after intravenous injection of iodinated contrast material shows that the right optic nerve has an enhancing fusiform appearance similar to that of an optic nerve glioma. The diagnosis was established at surgery. *B,* In a 40-year-old woman, T1-weighted MR image, axial view, shows enlargement of the intracanalicular portion of the right optic nerve (*arrows*). *C,* In the same patient as *B,* T1-weighted MR image, coronal view after intravenous injection of paramagnetic contrast material shows enlarged, enhancing right optic nerve within the optic canal. Note normal sized optic nerve on left (*arrow*) (*A,* From Tanaka E, Kimura C, Inoue H, et al. A case of intraorbital hemangioblastoma of the optic nerve. Folia Ophthalmol Jpn 1984;35:1390–1395. *B and C,* From Kerr J, Scheithauer BW, Miller GM, et al. Hemangioblastoma of the optic nerve: Case report. Neurosurgery 1995;36:573–579.)

velop an associated central retinal artery occlusion, central retinal vein occlusion (462), and some develop ischemic necrosis of the tumor and surrounding neural tissue (463–465). The underlying mechanism in both settings is believed to be compression of large and small vessels of the disc and spontaneous improvement of vision can occur if infarction of the melanocytoma allows decompression of the remaining nerve fibers(466).

A case of apparent neuroretinitis with recovery of vision was reported by Garcia-Arumi et al. (467) in a patient with a melanocytoma. The disorders may have been coincidental rather than directly related; however, it is possible that an infarction of the tumor could have caused leakage into the retina, clinically mimicking the ophthalmoscopic appearance of neuroretinitis.

Histologically, melanocytomas are composed of two types of cells (468). The predominant cells are plump polyhedral nevus cells containing numerous giant melanosomes. These cells show advanced differentiation and appear to be metabolically inactive. The second cell type is a smaller, lightly pigmented, spindle-shaped cell that is more metabolically active.

Melanocytomas are benign tumors that do not require therapy. The majority are likely congenital but development of this lesion has been described in an adult (469). Joffe et al. obtained follow-up data of 1 year or more in 27 patients with optic disc melanocytomas (459). No change in the appearance of the lesion had occurred in 22 of the eyes, but 4 lesions showed a slight increase in size over a period varying from 5 to19 years. None of the patients showed any changes

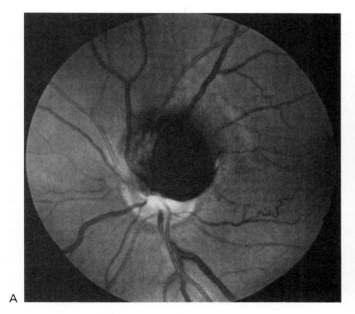
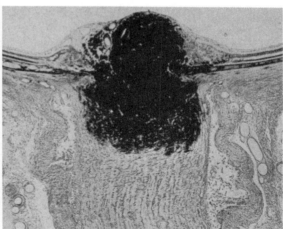

A B

Figure 8.27. *A,* Melanocytoma of the optic disc. The optic disc is almost completely obscured by an elevated black mass. The mass is much darker than a malignant melanoma. *B,* Histologic appearance of an optic disc melanocytoma. Note significant disc elevation. (From Hogan MJ, Zimmerman LE. Ophthalmic Pathology: An Atlas and Textbook, Ed 2. Philadelphia, WB Saunders, 1962:610.)

suggestive of malignant transformation, although a case of melanoma occurring within a melanocytoma has been reported (470).

The deep black appearance of melanocytomas generally allows them to be differentiated not only from optic disc swelling, but also from other lesions that infiltrate the optic disc, particularly malignant melanomas. Nevertheless, the distinction can be difficult in rare cases (471,472), particu-

larly when the lesion is not changing in size or shape (473) (Fig. 8.28). Ocular coherence tomography may ultimately prove to be a useful tool in the distinct of melanocytoma from melanoma (474).

Green et al. (475) reported the unique case of a 6-year-old girl who developed pain, proptosis, and progressive loss of vision in the right eye. The eye was subsequently enucleated, at which time it was noted that the optic nerve was

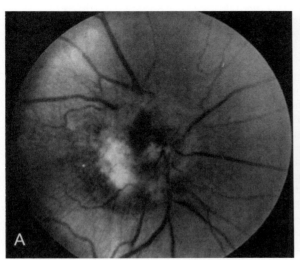
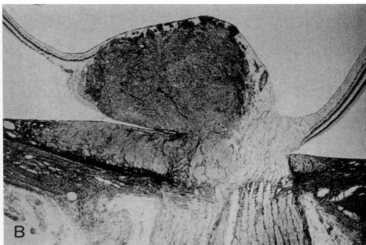

A B

Figure 8.28. Malignant melanoma of the choroid invading the optic disc. *A,* The disc tissue is elevated and shows areas of pigmentation with partial obscuration of vessels and blurring of disc margins. *B,* Histologic appearance of a juxtapapillary malignant melanoma invading the optic nerve.

infiltrated by a **malignant teratoid medulloepithelioma**. The patient subsequently underwent craniotomy and removal of the entire right optic nerve.

Secondary Tumors

The most common secondary tumors that infiltrate the optic nerve are metastatic and locally invasive carcinomas and various lymphoreticular malignancies, particularly lymphoma and leukemia.

Metastatic and Locally Invasive Tumors

The optic nerve may be the site of metastasis from distant tumors or of spread of tumor from a contiguous structure. Metastases can reach the optic nerve by one of four routes: from the choroid; by vascular dissemination; by invasion from the orbit; and from the CNS (346,476–479). Regardless of the mode of spread, the substance of the nerve is affected more often than the sheath. In one large series reported by Shields et al., metastases to the optic disc occurred in 30 (4.5%) of 660 patients with ocular metastases (480). The disease occurs more frequently in women.

Patients with metastases to the optic nerve usually have evidence of an optic neuropathy. The visual loss is usually severe, but relatively normal vision may be present in the early stages. Any type of field defect may be present. A relative afferent pupillary defect is usually present unless the patient has bilateral optic nerve metastases or the opposite retina or optic nerve has previously been damaged by some other condition. When the metastasis is located in the prelaminar or immediately retrolaminar portion of the optic nerve, the optic disc is usually swollen; a yellow-white mass can be seen to protrude from the surface of the nerve (Fig. 8.29) and clumps of tumor cells can occasionally be seen in the vitreous overlying the disc (107,478,481,482). A juxtapapillary choroidal component is frequently seen. A central retinal occlusion occurs in up to 50% of eyes. When the metastasis is to the posterior aspect of the orbital portion of the optic nerve or to the intracanalicular or intracranial portions of the nerve, the optic disc initially appears normal.

The most common metastatic tumors to the optic nerve are adenocarcinomas, primarily because these are the most common metastatic tumors to all parts of the body. In women, carcinomas of the breast and lung are the most common tumors, whereas carcinomas of the lung and bowel are most common in men (478,480,483–486). Other tumors that can metastasize to the optic nerve include carcinomas of the stomach (487), pancreas, uterus, ovary, prostate, kidney, larynx (488), and tonsillar fossa. Shields et al. (480) reported that in 6 of 30 (20%) patients the primary tumor was unknown. Fine needle aspiration can occasionally be used to establish the diagnosis (480). Skin cancers, malignant melanoma, and mediastinal tumors also may metastasize to one or both optic nerves. Isolated metastases to the optic nerve of intracranial tumors, such as medulloblastomas, may rarely occur (489,490).

Most patients with metastatic tumor to the optic nerve already have a known diagnosis of a primary carcinoma with other evidence of metastases at the time that visual loss occurs. This makes the diagnosis relatively straightforward, whereas most patients with a tumor that spreads contiguously to the optic nerve are not known to harbor a tumor when they first experience loss of vision. Nevertheless, any person with known cancer in another part of the body, with or without other evidence of metastases, who develops an optic neuropathy should be suspected of having cancer as the cause until proven otherwise. Similarly, any patient with a basal skull tumor who develops an optic neuropathy should be assumed to have spread of tumor to the optic nerve, unless there has been previous radiation therapy to the region, in which case the possibility of radiation-induced optic neuropathy must also be considered (see Chapter 7).

Contiguous spread of primary tumors from the paranasal sinuses, brain, and adjacent intraocular structures to the optic nerve occurs much less often than does metastasis to the nerve (491). A unique case of an esthesioneuroblastoma presenting with unilateral blindness in an 11-year-old girl was reported by Berman et al. (492). Initially, the child was thought to have suffered from a postviral demyelinating lesion; however, when vision failed to improve, MR imaging was performed and revealed a lesion in the ethmoid and sphenoid sinuses that pathologically was an esthesioneuroblastoma. Adenoid cystic carcinoma of the lacrimal gland has been reported to cause a steroid responsive optic neuropathy that simulated an orbital inflammatory syndrome (493).

Rarer than cases of metastatic or locally invasive tumors of the optic nerve, are cases of "tumor within a tumor" or so-called "collision tumors." Arnold et al. (494) documented a case of an adenocarcinoma of the lung metastatic to an optic nerve meningioma. These authors reviewed the available literature on this phenomenon and documented 46 previously reported cases. Renal cell carcinoma seems to be the best recipient or host tumor to "attract" other cancers, with lung carcinoma being the most common primary tumor to metastasize to the site.

Because of its close anatomic association with the paranasal sinuses, the optic nerve is frequently infiltrated or compressed by cancer that arises in the sinuses or the nasopharynx (495). In most cases, the tumor invades the posterior orbit or cavernous sinus, producing a syndrome that is characterized by loss of vision, diplopia, ophthalmoparesis, and trigeminal sensory neuropathy (496). Brain invasion can result in the Foster Kennedy syndrome (497). Prasad and Doraisamy (498) reported five patients with nasopharyngeal cancers that infiltrated the optic nerve. In three of these patients, the tumor reached the nerve by extending through the roof of the fossa of Rosenmuller. In another patient, the spread was extracranial via the pterygopalatine fossa and the posterior ethmoid sinus. In the fifth patient, the route of spread could not be determined.

Neuroimaging should be performed in all patients suspected of having infiltration of the optic nerve by cancer. CT scanning typically shows an enhancing nerve that may or may not be enlarged (Fig. 8.30). On MR imaging, either a circumscribed area of optic nerve enlargement is identified (499) or, more commonly, the nerve is usually diffusely enlarged similar to a meningioma (107,108,486) or may show varying T1 and T2 values that are presumed to be related

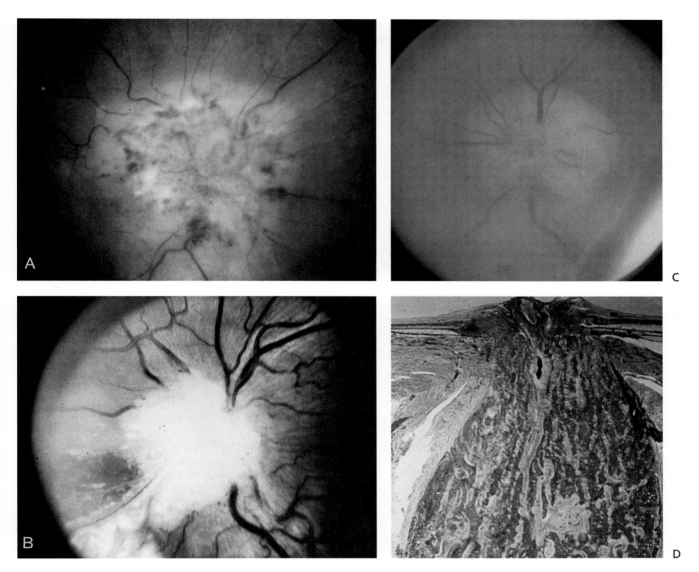

Figure 8.29.   Metastatic adenocarcinoma to the optic disc. *A*, Breast carcinoma in a 47-year-old woman. Entire optic disc is infiltrated by a large mass of yellow-white tissue. Note loss of normal disc architecture. There were numerous malignant cells in the vitreous. *B*, Lung carcinoma in a 56-year-old man. Note white mass protruding from disc surface. *C*, Breast carcinoma in a 60-year-old woman. Note the massive infiltration and elevation of disc and surrounding retina. *D*, Appearance at autopsy of optic nerve infiltration by adenocarcinoma of the lung.

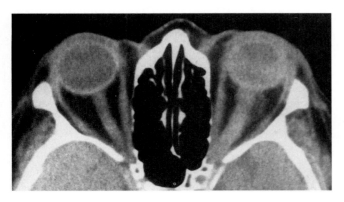

Figure 8.30.   Neuroimaging appearance of infiltration of optic nerve by metastatic carcinoma. CT scan, axial view, in a 56-year-old woman with small-cell carcinoma of the lung and progressive loss of vision in the left eye associated with a massive retinal infiltrate with nasal retinal detachment reveals that the orbital portion of the left optic nerve is diffusely enlarged. (From Allaire GS, Corriveau C, Arbour J-D. Metastasis to the optic nerve: Clinicopathological correlations. Can J Ophthalmol 1995;30:306–311.)

to associated hemorrhage or exudates. Tumors with a tendency to metastasize to bone, such as prostate and carcinoma, can present with optic canal involvement and a retrobulbar optic neuropathy (500).

Most metastatic optic nerve tumors show at least temporary response to radiation therapy. Some, however, do not (499,501). Tumors that spread contiguously to the optic nerve from the base of the skull or paranasal sinuses are typically less radiosensitive than metastatic tumors and also tend to be less responsive to chemotherapy. A mean survival of 13 months was reported by Shields et al. (480) for their 30 patients with optic disc metastases.

Meningeal tumor cuffing or direct infiltration of the optic nerve can cause loss of vision in the setting of meningeal spread of carcinoma (502–504). This phenomenon is called **carcinomatous meningitis** or **meningeal carcinomatosis** (the latter being the preferred term because it does not imply an inflammatory process). The optic neuropathy that occurs in the setting of meningeal carcinomatosis is usually associated with a ''diagnostic quartet'' that consists of (a) headaches typical of raised intracranial pressure; (b) blindness; (c) sluggish or absent pupillary reflexes; and (d) normal-appearing optic discs (505).

The frequency of optic nerve involvement in patients with carcinomatosis of the meninges is unclear. Katz et al. (506) reviewed 39 cases from the literature and indicated that visual loss occurred in 30–40% of patients with this disorder. This figure agrees with that of Fischer-Williams et al. (507); however, Little et al. (508) and Olson et al. (509) found evidence of involvement of the optic nerves in only about 15% of cases of meningeal carcinomatosis in their series. Patients who develop meningeal carcinomatosis with visual loss may do so after the primary lesion, usually in the lung or breast, has already been diagnosed. In other cases, visual loss may occur coincident with other signs of chronic meningitis (510) or as an isolated finding as the first sign of disease (511). Although blindness may begin in one eye, both eyes are usually affected within a short period of time. In rare instances, visual loss remains strictly unilateral (512). A similar presentation has been described in patients with germinomas and vision loss resulting from secondary optic nerve seeding through the CSF (513).

Histopathologic examination of cases with meningeal carcinomatosis and blindness generally shows marked cuffing of the subarachnoid space of the optic nerve by sheets of malignant cells, with little invasion of the nerves themselves. Thus, in some cases, there is true infiltration, whereas in other cases, the lesion is more compressive than infiltrative.

Lymphoreticular Tumors

CNS involvement in non-Hodgkin's **lymphoma** (NHL) is unusual, but it occurs in about 10% of cases (514). Of these, 5% (or a total of 0.5% of patients with NHL) will have infiltration of the optic nerve at some time during the course of their disease (515). Isolated optic nerve infiltration can also be the sole manifestation of recurrent non-Hodgkin's lymphoma (516). Infiltration of the optic nerve in Hodgkin's disease is even less common. Nevertheless, infiltration of the retrobulbar optic nerve and optic chiasm occurs in patients with both Hodgkin's disease and NHL (517–538). In most of these cases, the infiltration occurs from spread of CNS tumor; however, Park and Goins (539) reported a patient with Hodgkin's disease in whom there was infiltration of the optic nerve, apparently from extension of tumor from the adjacent maxillary and sphenoid sinuses. Patients with systemic lymphoma and orbital mass lesions may also develop a compressive optic neuropathy (540).

In many cases of lymphomatous infiltration of the anterior visual sensory pathway, the patient is known to have NHL or Hodgkin's disease at the time visual signs and symptoms develop, and the diagnosis is not in doubt (522). In other cases, however, the visual loss is the presenting sign of the disease (517,521,529,541) or an isolated manifestation of disease recurrence (531).

The symptoms and signs of patients with lymphomatous infiltration of the anterior visual system depend on the location and extent of the lesion. In some cases, the visual loss is insidious in onset and slowly progressive (534). In other cases, the visual loss is acute and mimics optic neuritis or ischemic optic neuropathy (521,531,533). Secondary retinal vein and retinal artery occlusions have been described in conjunction with lymphomatous infiltration of the optic nerve (516,538). Successful treatment has been described with steroids, chemotherapy, and radiation therapy.

The appearance of optic nerve or chiasm infiltration by lymphoma is nonspecific. The infiltrated structure is enlarged and reveals increased density on CT scanning; it enhances after intravenous injection of iodinated contrast material. The same structure can be iso-, hyper-, or hypointense on T1-weighted MR images; is hyperintense on T2-weighted MR images; and enhances after intravenous injection of paramagnetic contrast material (Fig. 8.31).

Angioimmunoblastic lymphadenopathy is a proliferative disease of the lymphoid system from which a malignant lymphoma may arise, and for which the etiology is unknown. Matthews et al. (527) reported the case of a patient with this condition who developed a retrobulbar optic neuropathy from infiltration of the nerve by lymphoma cells.

Multiple myeloma, **lymphomatoid granulomatosis**, and **Langerhans cell histiocytosis** can all produce an optic neuropathy (518,542–546). In some of these cases, the optic neuropathy, which may be of the anterior or retrobulbar variety, appears to be produced by infiltration of the nerve (547) rather than from compression (548,549). Bourdette and Rosenberg (550) reported the case of a patient with polyneuropathy, organomegaly, endocrinopathy, monoclonal gammopathy, and skin changes (POEMS syndrome) who developed an infiltrative orbitopathy characterized in part by enlargement of the blind spot in the visual field of the eye on the affected side. Although it was unclear if the optic nerves were infiltrated or compressed by myeloma cells, the condition improved after the patient was treated with systemic corticosteroids. Galetta et al. (551) and Anthony (552) reported patients who developed an optic neuropathy in the setting of reactive lymphohistiocytosis associated with lymphoma or pseudolymphoma syndrome secondary to the use of diphenylhydantoin. Pless et al. (546) reported a patient

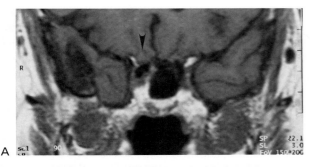

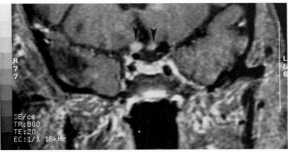

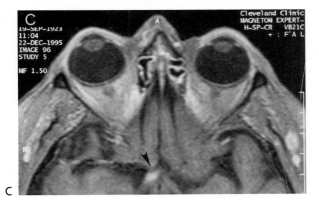

Figure 8.31. Neuroimaging appearance of infiltration of the left optic nerves by a B-cell lymphoma.

with extranodal Rosai Dorfman disease (sinus histiocytosis without diffuse lymphadenopathy) who developed a compressive optic neuropathy from an orbital apex lesion associated with uveitis and skin nodules.

Leukemia is a well-described cause of infiltrative optic neuropathy (553–568). In some of the patients, visual acuity is lost abruptly, whereas in others, there is a gradual progression of visual loss over days, weeks, or months. In still others, the disc appears swollen, but there is no evidence of visual dysfunction. Most patients with leukemic infiltration of the optic nerve are known to have leukemia at the time the visual loss occurs or the patient is found to have asymptomatic disc swelling; however, in some cases, as occurs in patients with lymphomatous infiltration of the optic nerve (see above), the optic neuropathy is the first evidence of the disease (558,569). Allen and Straatsma (553) studied the

globes of 76 patients who died of various neoplastic processes of the reticuloendothelial system. The patients ranged in age from 11 months to 80 years. These authors found infiltration of the optic disc in five patients with leukemia. Three of the patients had acute lymphocytic leukemia; one had acute myelogenous leukemia; and one had monocytic leukemia. In addition, Allen and Straatsma (553) studied 10 optic nerves in which there was retrolaminar infiltration. Five of the patients had acute lymphocytic leukemia; two had monocytic leukemia; one had acute myelogenous leukemia; one had erythroleukemia; and one had chronic lymphocytic leukemia (CLL). Clinically, these patients were said to have ''blurring of the optic nerve head margins (or) frank papilledema.'' However, Allen and Straatsma did not attempt to distinguish between the clinical picture seen in patients with infiltration of the optic disc and that seen in patients with retrolaminar infiltration.

Eichholtz (570) reported 11 patients with lymphoproliferative disorders, primarily leukemia, who developed optic disc swelling. In 9 eyes of 6 patients, visual acuity was 20/200 or worse. Visual acuity improved markedly after orbital irradiation in four of five patients. Rosenthal et al. (571) reported five children with leukemia who had infiltration of the optic nerve (one of whom was the original patient reported by Ellis and Little (572)). All of the patients had a form of acute lymphoblastic leukemia, and in four of the five patients, optic nerve involvement appeared between 7 and 20 months after their systemic disease had been diagnosed. These authors were the first to emphasize the two distinct clinical patterns of infiltration: (*a*) infiltration of the optic disc; and (*b*) infiltration of the immediate retrolaminar portion of the proximal optic nerve.

In leukemic infiltration of the optic disc, the features of the disc are obscured by a whitish fluffy infiltrate that is often associated with true disc swelling and peripapillary hemorrhage (Fig. 8.32). The visual acuity in such patients is minimally affected, unless the infiltration or associated edema and hemorrhage extends into the macula. Chalfin et al. (573) reported an excellent example of this condition. The patient had acute myelocytic leukemia and experienced sudden decreased vision in the right eye down to light perception. Ophthalmoscopy revealed a well-circumscribed, white, fairly avascular mass that both infiltrated and obscured the optic disc and macula. Postmortem examination revealed that the mass originated from the optic disc and that there was massive infiltration of the disc with leukemic cells with minimal extension of small clusters of cells to the laminar and retrolaminar optic nerve and retina. A similar case reported by Ellis and Little (572) noted the presence of a clinic picture suggestive of papilledema (high opening pressure and good visual function) in a patient with leukemia who was subsequently found on postmortem to have leukemic infiltration of the optic nerve extending into the adjacent retina and overlying vitreous.

According to Rosenthal et al. (571), infiltration of the proximal optic nerve just posterior to the lamina cribrosa usually produces markedly decreased visual acuity associated with true optic disc swelling (Fig. 8.33). Such patients

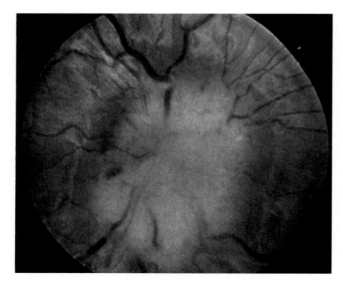

Figure 8.32. Leukemic infiltration of the optic disc mimicking optic disc swelling in a child with acute lymphocytic leukemia. The child was thought to be in remission at the time the abnormality was discovered. The disc is whitish gray and markedly elevated with obscuration of vessels. Visual acuity was 20/25.

have a variety of visual field defects, and a relative afferent pupillary defect is invariably present unless the infiltration is bilateral and symmetric. In addition, there are often peripapillary and peripheral retinal hemorrhages (571). Neuroimaging in such cases typically reveals a diffusely en-

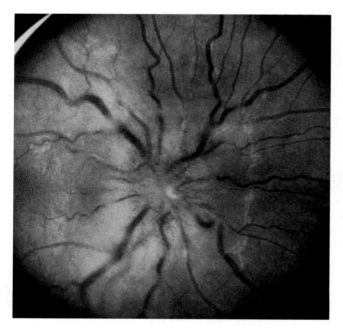

Figure 8.33. Optic disc swelling in a child with acute leukemia. The disc is swollen and hyperemic. Visual acuity was 20/80, and there was a central scotoma. The patient was thought to have leukemic infiltration of the proximal retrobulbar portion of the optic nerve.

larged optic nerve that usually enhances after intravenous injection of contrast material (565). In other patients there may be a paucity of findings on both ophthalmoscopy and MR imaging (562,568).

Ridgway et al. (574) examined 657 children with acute leukemia and found optic nerve infiltration in 29 (4.4%). As in the patients described by Rosenthal et al. (571), most of the patients had decreased vision, blurred optic discs and, rarely, eye pain. All but one of the patients had evidence of CNS leukemia. Charif Chefchaouni et al. (566) reported on 196 children treated for leukemia and found 12 with ocular, orbital, or optic nerve involvement. Two of these 12 had optic nerve infiltrative lesions with the others having either orbital or anterior segment involvement. Murray et al. (575) discussed the difficulties involved in identifying the etiology of elevated, pale, swollen optic discs in patients with leukemia and reported the clinical features in three such patients.

The response of leukemic infiltration of the optic nerve to radiation therapy is usually rapid and dramatic. In almost all cases, visual function returns to normal or near normal, and the disc elevation, if present, resolves (571). Even though some patients do not respond to this treatment (576,577), radiation therapy is the treatment of choice for optic nerve infiltration in the setting of acute leukemia (561,564,578). In addition, Brown et al. (557) successfully treated a patient with an infiltrative optic neuropathy in the setting of acute promyelocytic leukemia with transretinoic acid. This form of acute leukemia results from a chromosome translocation that is associated with the retinoic acid receptor gene (579), and transretinoic acid works by stimulating the terminal differentiation of the malignant cells so that they become normal lymphoid cells.

It must be emphasized that swelling of the optic disc can occur in patients with acute leukemia when CNS involvement by the disease results in increased intracranial pressure. Optic disc swelling and neovascularization also occur as a local phenomenon in the setting of the diffuse retinopathy of acute leukemia (571,580). Thus, one must consider a number of pathologic mechanisms in addition to infiltration in any patient with acute leukemia and apparent optic disc swelling. Additionally, myeloproliferative disorders associated with extramedullary hematopoiesis have been reported to cause both an enhancing lesion of the orbital apex and canal resulting in an orbital apex syndrome (581) and a compressive optic neuropathy from skull base involvement (582).

The acute leukemias are responsible for most of the reported cases of infiltrative optic neuropathies caused by lymphoreticular disorders; however, patients with chronic forms of leukemia may also develop optic nerve infiltration. In a review of autopsy material from the Massachusetts General Hospital, Cramer et al. (583) found a high percentage of asymptomatic CNS involvement in patients with CLL. In addition, they documented 4 cases of infiltrative optic neuropathy among 21 reported cases of CNS CLL. Patients with optic nerve infiltration in the setting of CLL and other chronic leukemias have a more indolent clinical course than patients with the acute leukemias. Visual loss is less severe, and retinal changes of the type seen in acute leukemia are rare. Optic disc swelling, however, is indistinguishable from that which occurs in patients with infiltration in the setting of acute leukemia.

INFLAMMATORY AND INFECTIOUS INFILTRATIVE OPTIC NEUROPATHIES

The intraocular, intraorbital, intracanalicular, and intracranial segments of the optic nerve can all be infiltrated by inflammatory and infectious processes. The most common inflammatory process that produces an infiltrative optic neuropathy is sarcoidosis. The most common infectious processes that produce an infiltrative optic neuropathy are syphilis, tuberculosis, and opportunistic fungal infections, such as cryptococcosis. These conditions are all discussed in greater detail in other chapters in this text.

Sarcoidosis

Optic nerve dysfunction probably is the most common neuro-ophthalmologic manifestation of sarcoidosis (584–592). The optic nerve may be affected at any time during the course of the disease and may be the site of its initial presentation in up to 70% of patients (592–594). Women are affected more commonly than men. Sarcoidosis may affect the optic nerve in several different ways. It may produce papilledema, a compressive anterior or retrobulbar optic neu-

ropathy with disc pallor, an ischemic optic neuropathy, or anterior or retrobulbar optic neuritis (592). Optic disc pallor is the most common finding. The optic neuritis results from granulomatous infiltration of the optic disc, anterior orbital, posterior orbital, intracanalicular, or intracranial portions of the nerve, or a combination of these. In some cases, more than one process may be responsible. It is noteworthy that the vast majority of patients do not have associated uveitis at the time of presentation with optic neuropathy. In Frohman et al.'s series (592,595) approximately 70% of patients had elevated angiotensin-converting enzyme (ACE) levels, abnormal chest x-rays, and abnormal MR imaging of the anterior visual pathways. Over 90% had abnormal gallium scans. Pleocytosis or increased spinal fluid protein was noted in 88% of patients.

Granulomatous infiltration of the optic disc may or may not be associated with evidence by neuroimaging or ultrasonography of diffuse enlargement of the orbital portion of the optic nerve (586,591,596–609). The optic disc in such cases usually is markedly elevated, either diffusely or sectorally (Figs. 8.34 and 8.35), and it often has a solid or nodular appearance that can best be demonstrated using ultrasonography (69,610). There may be dilated vessels resembling neovascularization on the surface of the disc (601,611–613).

The appearance of optic disc infiltration by sarcoid granulomas may mimic that of papilledema, except that this condi-

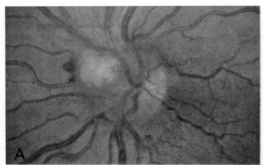

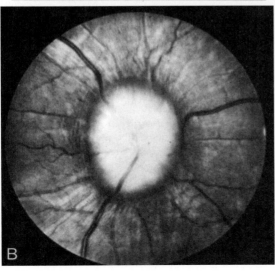

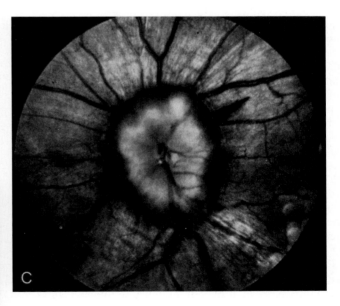

Figure 8.34. Sarcoid granulomas infiltrating the optic disc. *A*, In a 25-year-old woman with visual acuity of 20/20 OU there is a small elevated yellow-white mass overlying the nasal portion of the left optic disc. A small hemorrhage is just nasal to the mass. (From Laties AM, Scheie HG. Evolution of multiple small tumors in sarcoid granuloma of the optic disk. Am J Ophthalmol 1972;74:60–66.) *B*, In another patient, the entire disc is infiltrated by granulomas. Note diffuse symmetric elevation of the disc substance. *C*, In a third patient, a multinodular granuloma has infiltrated the left optic disc. (From Jampol LM, Woodfin W, McLean EB. Optic nerve sarcoidosis. Arch Ophthalmol 1972;87:355–360.)

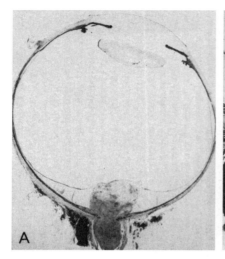

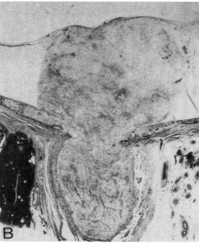

Figure 8.35. Pathology of granulomatous infiltration of the left optic disc in sarcoidosis. The eye was enucleated after the patient developed painful glaucoma. *A*, Axial section through the left globe shows a mass occupying the optic disc and protruding into the eye. (Hematoxylin and eosin ×2.5.) *B*, High-power view shows that the normal architecture of the disc has been replaced by granulomatous inflammation. (Hematoxylin and eosin ×5.) (From Beardsley TL, Brown SVL, Sydnor CF, et al. Eleven cases of sarcoidosis of the optic nerve. Am J Ophthalmol 1984;97:62–77.)

tion is more often unilateral than bilateral, and it is usually associated with decreased vision, slit-lamp biomicroscopic and ophthalmoscopic evidence of intraocular inflammation, neuroimaging evidence of an intracranial process affecting the base of the skull, or a combination of these. When the process is bilateral, however, the disc swelling may easily be mistaken for papilledema (614), even though diagnostic studies are nonconfirmatory. James et al. (615), for example, described four patients with sarcoidosis who developed "papilledema" during the course of their disease. However, lumbar puncture in three of the four patients revealed *normal* intracranial pressure, suggesting that the optic disc swelling in these cases was caused by inflammation of the intraocular or anterior orbital portions of the optic nerves and not by increased intracranial pressure. Peripapillary choroidal granulomas (without phlebitis or vitritis) (Fig. 8.36) secondary to sarcoidosis can present with vision loss and visual field defects and be difficult to distinguish from direct optic nerve involvement. This can be complicated by peripapillary choroidal neovascularization (616,617).

When the proximal portion of the intraorbital optic nerve is infiltrated by granulomatous inflammation in patients with sarcoidosis, the condition typically presents as an acute, subacute, or rarely, chronic optic neuritis. The patient typically experiences progressive loss of vision, decreased color vision, and a worsening visual field defect. A relative afferent pupillary defect is present unless there is also a contralateral optic neuropathy. The optic disc is swollen. This condition may be impossible to differentiate clinically from demyelinating optic neuritis and even from certain causes of compressive optic neuropathy, particularly optic nerve sheath meningioma. Even ultrasonography, which reveals enlargement of the orbital portion of the nerve in almost all cases, and neuroimaging, which shows enlargement and enhancement of the orbital portion of the optic nerve (Fig. 8.37) cannot establish the diagnosis with certainty. In some cases, the diagnosis is made by finding clinical, radiographic, or laboratory evidence of sarcoidosis. MRI findings can mimic those seen in multiple sclerosis, metastatic tumors, astrocy-

tomas, and menigiomas (618). In other cases, the diagnosis is not confirmed until a biopsy of the nerve is performed (591).

The posterior retrobulbar or intracanalicular portion of the optic nerve is occasionally affected by sarcoid (619). In such cases, the patient develops acute or, more often, progressive loss of vision associated with evidence of an optic neuropathy. The optic disc in such cases is normal but gradually becomes pale if no treatment is given. The neuroimaging appearance is variable. The posterior orbital portion of the optic nerve may be enlarged and may enhance after contrast injection on both CT scanning and MR imaging (Fig. 8.38). Isolated optic nerve sheath enhancement may also be seen on MR imaging (620).

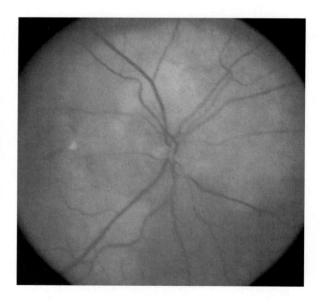

Figure 8.36. Fundus photograph of a patient with sarcoidosis who presented with decreased vision and blindspot enlargement. There was no vitritis or phlebitis. Diffuse, nodular, yellow, peripapillary subretinal granuloma are seen and the optic disc margins are obscured.

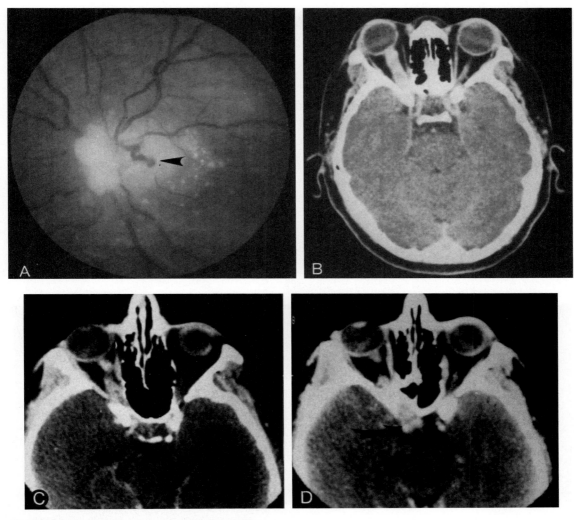

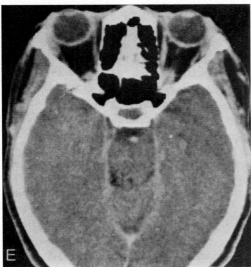

Figure 8.37. CT scanning of optic nerve sarcoidosis. *A*, Bilobed mass projecting from the medial aspect of the left optic disc in a patient with sarcoidosis. Note optociliary shunt vessel (*arrowhead*). *B*, CT scan, axial view, after intravenous injection of contrast material shows diffuse thickening and enhancement of the orbital portion of the left optic nerve. *C*, CT scan, axial view, after intravenous injection of contrast in another patient with painless progressive loss of vision in the right eye and biopsy proven sarcoidosis shows diffuse enlargement and enhancement of the *orbital* portion of the right optic nerve. Note the "kinking" of the nerve, similar to that seen in patients with optic nerve glioma in the setting of neurofibromatosis type 1. *D*, CT scan, axial view, after intravenous contrast enhancement at a slightly higher plane in the same patient as *C* shows intracranial extension of the optic nerve lesion (*arrow*). *E*, sarcoidosis at left orbital apex minimizing an apex meningioma on axial CT scanning. (*A* and *B*, from Lustgarden JS, Mindel JS, Yablonski ME, et al. An unusual presentation of isolated optic nerve sarcoidosis. J Clin Neuroophthalmol 1983;3:13–18.) (*C* and *D*, from Jordan DR, Anderson RL, Nerad JA, et al. Optic nerve involvement as the initial manifestation of sarcoidosis. Can J Ophthalmol 1988;23:232–237.)

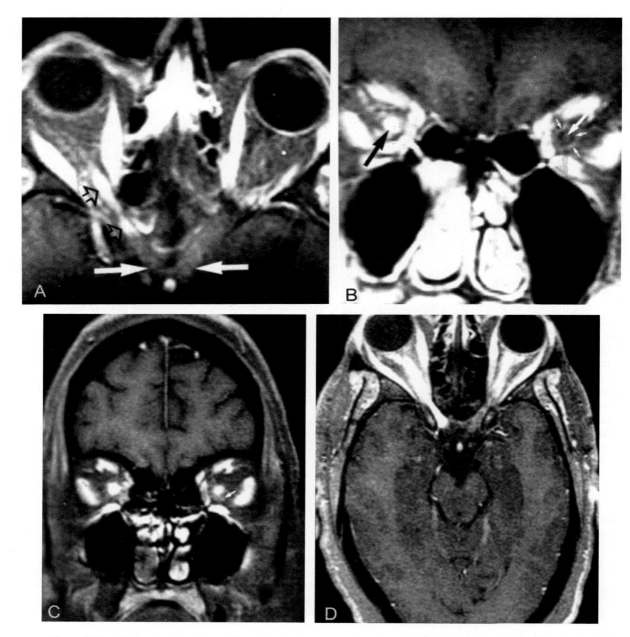

Figure 8.38. MR imaging in patients with sarcoidosis of the optic nerves. *A*, T1-weighted, fat-suppressed MR image, axial view, after intravenous injection of paramagnetic contrast material in a 52-year-old woman with progressive loss of vision in the right eye shows irregular enhancement of the right optic nerve near the apex of the orbit and within the optic canal (*open arrows*). The intracranial portions of the optic nerves and the optic chiasm do not enhance and appear normal in size and shape (*solid arrows*). *B*, Enhanced, T1-weighted, fat-suppressed MR image, coronal view, in the same patient shows enlargement and abnormal enhancement of the orbital portion of the right optic nerve (*black arrow*). The left optic nerve is normal in size and does not enhance (*large white arrow*); however, there is mild enhancement of its leptomeningeal sheath (*small white arrows*). A biopsy of the right nerve revealed noncaseating granulomas. *C*, Enhanced, T1-weighted, fat-suppressed MR image, coronal view, in another patient with sarcoidosis and progressive bilateral loss of vision with evidence of bilateral optic neuropathies reveals enlargement and abnormal enhancement of the orbital portions of both optic nerves. The right optic nerve is slightly larger than the left. Note mild enhancement of the leptomeningeal sheath of the left optic nerve (*arrow*). *D*, Enhanced, T1-weighted, fat-suppressed MR image, axial view, in the same patient shows enlargement and abnormal enhancement of both optic nerves throughout the orbits, with extension through the optic canal on the right side. (From Engelken JD, Yuh WTC, Carter KD, et al. Optic nerve sarcoidosis: MR findings. AJNR 1992;13:228–230.)

Because of the predilection of neurosarcoidosis to affect the basal meninges, the intracranial portion of one or both optic nerves and the optic chiasm may occasionally be affected by the disease, producing a variety of patterns of visual loss (621,622). In some patients, loss of vision occurs as an isolated phenomenon, either simultaneously in both eyes or in one eye followed within days to weeks by loss of vision in the other eye (594). In other patients, visual loss is associated with evidence of hypothalamic dysfunction, hypothalamic hypopituitarism (particularly gonadotropin failure), or both (228,622–624).

Aszkanazy (625) reported two patients with bitemporal hemianopia. One showed granulomatous infiltration of the optic chiasm, the prechiasmal region, and the base of the brain at autopsy. The other had a sarcoid granuloma that extended from the chiasm into the 3rd ventricle. Morax (597) described a sarcoid granuloma that infiltrated both optic nerves and the optic chiasm, producing severe bilateral loss of vision.

Tang et al. (623) described four patients with sarcoidosis who had visual findings similar to those reported by Decker et al. (228). All four had profound loss of vision in one eye with a temporal field defect in the contralateral eye. Neuroimaging studies showed no abnormalities in one patient (case 1) who was treated with prednisone with recovery of normal visual function in her previously better eye. In a second patient (case 3), radiographic studies demonstrated enlargement of the right optic canal with enlargement of the optic chiasm and the intracranial portion of the right optic nerve. The patient eventually underwent a craniotomy, at which time the right optic nerve and the optic chiasm were indeed found to be enlarged. A biopsy from the region revealed evidence of granulomatous infiltration consistent with sarcoidosis. The other two patients (cases 2 and 4) had evidence of a suprasellar mass by neuroimaging studies that was found to be a mass of granulomatous tissue consistent with sarcoidosis by craniotomy in one case and autopsy in the other.

Perioptic Neuritis

Dutton and Anderson (626) reported on four patients with unilateral progressive loss of vision who were thought to

have optic nerve meningiomas based on clinical presentations and imaging studies, but who were ultimately diagnosed by pathologic examination as having a perioptic inflammatory process (two with active inflammation and two with only fibrotic changes). These patients had no signs or symptoms of a systemic process. They ranged in age from 22 to 57 years; 3 were female and 1 was male. Three of these patients had experienced orbital pain. All four had cecocentral scotomas, and one also had significant peripheral constriction. MRI scanning generally showed enhancement of the optic nerve sheath as opposed to the nerve itself (Fig. 8.39) (627).

Similar cases were reported by other investigators (49,627–630). Purvin et al. (627) reported 14 patients and noted a wide age range and varying levels of visual function. Patients responded to steroids, although some had recurrence when steroid doses were reduced. Paracentral scotoma and arcuate defects were the most common visual field defects. This entity also occurs in patients with infections, especially syphilis which must be excluded (104,631), and has been described in a patient who simultaneously had neuroretinitis (632). The use of enhanced, fat-suppressed MR images has significantly increased the ability to visualize inflammatory perineuritis (633). This technique is not specific for inflammatory perineuritis, but in the appropriate clinical setting, the finding of an enhancing lesion on T1-weighted, fat-suppressed images is highly suggestive of this disorder.

Infectious Disorders

According to Paufique and Etienne (634), Cruveilhier described the first case of tuberculoma involving the optic nerve in 1862. Since this time, approximately 15 cases have been reported (635,636). In some cases, the tuberculoma is adjacent to the optic nerve and is part of a dense adhesive arachnoiditis that may or may not be separable from the surrounding structures (637). In other cases, however, the inflammatory tissue may actually invade the nerve (635,638) or be completely contained within the intracranial portion of the optic nerve (636).

It may be inferred from the documented intracranial and intracanalicular optic nerve invasion by tuberculomas and

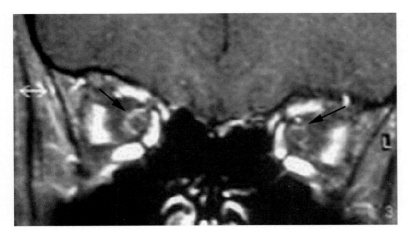

Figure 8.39. Axial T1-weighted, fat-suppressed, enhanced MRI scan of optic perineuritis. Optic nerve sheath enhancement (*arrows*) is seen bilaterally.

sarcoid granulomas that syphilitic gummas may act in a similar fashion although this has not been reported. Indeed, retrobulbar optic neuritis occurs in patients with syphilis (639,640), and gummas within the optic disc have been described (641–644). It thus seems likely that similar involvement of the intracranial and intracanalicular portions of the optic nerve must also occur. Viral diseases can produce an infiltrative process of the optic nerve. Marmor et al. (645), for example, reported a patient with systemic lymphoma who developed a unilateral optic neuropathy associated with optic disc swelling. The patient subsequently died, and postmortem examination revealed that the optic disc was infiltrated by cytomegalovirus.

Kupfer and McCrane (646) demonstrated invasion of the anterior visual system by cryptococcal organisms in the setting of fatal cryptococcal meningitis in three patients. These investigators suggested that visual loss in such instances is related to visual system invasion rather than to increased intracranial pressure with papilledema. Presumably, other organisms causing both acute and chronic meningitis cause visual loss in a similar manner.

Because of the large number of persons with the acquired immune deficiency syndrome (AIDS) in the United States and around the world, the incidence of infectious optic neuropathies continues to rise. In most of these cases, an opportunistic fungus is responsible, with *Cryptococcus neoformans* being the most common fungus. A pathologically documented case of bilateral cryptococcal optic nerve infiltration in a patient with AIDS who presented with sudden blindness was reported by Cohen and Glasgow (647). At postmortem examination, the intracanalicular portion of the right optic nerve was infiltrated by numerous organisms consistent with *C. neoformans,* and the left optic nerve contained numerous organisms throughout its orbital and canalicular portions.

Cases of pathologically verified cryptococcal optic neuropathy similar to that reported by Cohen and Glasgow (647) have been reported where the visual loss has progressed over a period of months rather than days (648–651). Likewise, numerous other authors have reported patients with presumed cryptococcal optic neuropathy but in whom clinicopathologic correlation was lacking (652–658). It is likely that crytococcus can cause a syndrome of vision loss associated with elevated intracranial pressure and papilledema, without direct optic nerve infiltration as well (659,660). Favorable visual outcomes can be achieved with treatments including lumbar puncture, steroids, antifungal agents, diuretics, and optic nerve sheath fenestration (660,661). Toxoplasmosis can also infiltrate the optic nerve head without associated chorioretinitis or vitritis and cause a presentation similar to ischemic optic neuropathy (662).

REFERENCES

1. Hoyt WF, Baghdassarian SA. Optic glioma of childhood: Natural history and rationale for conservative management. Br J Ophthalmol 1969;53:793–798.
2. Miller NR, Iliff WJ, Green WR. Evaluation and management of gliomas of the anterior visual pathways. Brain 1974;97:743–754.
3. Wright JE, McDonald WI, Call NB. Management of optic nerve gliomas. Br J Ophthalmol 1980b;64:545–552.
4. Jakobiec FA, Depot MJ, Kennerdell JS, et al. Combined clinical and computed tomographic diagnosis of orbital glioma and meningioma. Ophthalmology 1984; 91:137–155.
5. Alvord ECJ, Lofton S. Gliomas of the optic nerve or chiasm: Outcome by patients' age, tumor site, and treatment. J Neurosurg 1988;68:85–98.
6. Appleton RE, Jan JE. Delayed diagnosis of optic nerve glioma: A preventable cause of visual loss. Pediatr Neurol 1989;5:226–228.
7. Dutton JJ, Anderson RL. Optic nerve gliomas and meningiomas. Neurol Clin 1991;9:163–177.
8. Dunn DW, Purvin V. Optic pathway gliomas in neurofibromatosis. Dev Med Child Neurol 1990;32:820–824.
9. Spencer WH. Primary neoplasms of the optic nerve and its sheaths: Clinical features and current concepts of pathogenetic mechanisms. Trans Am Ophthalmol Soc 1972;70:490–528.
10. Wright JE. Primary optic nerve meningiomas: Clinical presentation and management. Trans Am Acad Ophthalmol Otolaryngol 1977;83:617–625.
11. Wright JE, Call NB, Liaricos S. Primary optic nerve meningioma. Br J Ophthalmol 1980;64:553–558.
12. Alper MG. Management of primary optic nerve meningiomas. J Clin Neruoophthalmol 1981;1:101–117.
13. Sibony PA, Krauss HR, Kennerdell JS, et al. Optic nerve sheath meningiomas. Ophthalmology 1984;91:1313–1326.
14. Sibony PA, Kennerdell JS, Slamovits TL, et al. Intrapapillary refractile bodies in optic nerve sheath meningioma. Arch Ophthalmol 1985;103:383–385.
15. Sarkies NJ. Optic nerve sheath meningioma: Diagnostic features and therapeutic alternatives. Eye 1987;1:597–602.
16. Wright JE, McNabb AA, McDonald WI. Primary optic nerve sheath meningioma. Br J Ophthalmol 1989a;73:960–966.
17. Clark WC, Theofilos CS, Fleming JC. Primary optic nerve sheath meningiomas: Report of nine cases. J Neurosurg 1989;70:37–40.
18. Dutton JJ, Anderson RL. Optic nerve sheath meningiomas. Surv Ophthalmol 1992;37:167–183.
19. Smith EG. Unilateral papilledema: Its significance and pathologic physiology. Arch Ophthalmol 1939;21:856–873.
20. Harris GJ. Bilateral blindness due to orbital lymphoma. Ann Ophthalmol 1981; 13:427–430.
21. Kattah JC, Chrousos GC, Roberts J, et al. Metastatic prostate cancer to the optic canal. Ophthalmology 1993;100:1711–1715.
22. Kazim M, Kennerdell JS, Rothfus W, et al. Orbital lymphangioma. Correlation of magnetic resonance images and intraoperative findings. Ophthalmology 1992; 99:1588–1594.
23. Miller NR, Green WR. Arachnoid cysts involving a portion of the intraorbital optic nerve. Arch Ophthalmol 1975;93:1117–1121.
24. Saari M, Mustonen E, Palva A, et al. Arachnoid cyst of the intraorbital portion of the optic nerve with unilateral disc edema and transient shallowing of the anterior chamber. Acta Ophthalmol 1977;55:959–964.
25. McNab AA, Wright JE. Cysts of the optic nerve: Three cases associated with meningioma. Eye 1989;3:355–359.
26. Lindblom B, Norman D, Hoyt WF. Perioptic cyst distal to optic nerve meningioma: MR demonstration. AJNR 1992;13:1622–1624.
27. Miller NR. Neuro-ophthalmology of orbital tumors. Clin Neurosurg 1985;32: 459–473.
28. Newell FW. Choroidal folds. Am J Ophthalmol 1973;75:930–942.
29. Cangemi FE, Trempe CL, Walsh JB. Choroidal folds. Am J Ophthalmol 1978; 86:380–378.
30. De La Paz MA, Boniuk M. Fundus manifestations of orbital disease and treatment of orbital disease. Surv Ophthalmol 1995;40:3–21.
31. Unsold R, Hoyt WF. Blickinduzierte monokulare Obskurationen bei orbitalem Hamangiom. klin Monatsbl Augenheilkd 1979;174:715–721.
32. Wilkes SR, Trautmann JC, DeSanto LW, et al. Osteoma: An unusual cause of amaurosis fugax. Mayo Clin Proc 1979;54:258–260.
33. Brown GC, Shield JA. Amaurosis fugax secondary to presumed cavernous hemangioma of the orbit. Ann Ophthalmol 1981;13:1205–1209.
34. Hamton GR, Krohel GB. Gaze-evoked blindness. Ann Ophthalmol 1983;15: 73–76.
35. Manor RS, Ben Sira I, Odel JG, et al. Amaurosis fugax at downward gaze. Surv Ophthalmol 1987;31:411–416.
36. Orcutt JC, Tucker WH, Mills RP, et al. Gaze-evoked amaurosis. Ophthalmology 1987;94:213–218.
37. Manor RS, Yassur Y, Hoyt WF. Reading-evoked visual dimming. Am J Ophthalmol 1996;121:212–214.
38. Otto CS, Coppit GL, Mazzoli RA, et al. Gaze-evoked amaurosis: a report of five cases. Ophthalmology 2003;110:322–326.
39. Knapp MP, Flaharty PM, Sergott RC, et al. Gaze-induced amaurosis from central retinal artery compression. Ophthalmology 1992;99:238–240.
40. Gawler J, Sanders MD, Bull JED, et al. Computer assisted tomography in orbital disease. Br J Ophthalmol 1974;58:571–587.
41. Grove ASJ. Orbital trauma and computed tomography. Ophthalmology 1980; 87:403–411.
42. Wright JE, Lloyd GAS, Ambrose J. Computerized axial tomography in the detection of orbital space-occupying lesions. Am J Ophthalmol 1975;80:78–84.

43. Trokel SL, Hilal SK. Computerized tomography of orbit and optic nerve lesions. In JL S, ed. Neuro-Ophthalmology Update. New York, Masson, 1977:111–118.
44. Van Damme W, Kosmann P, Wackenheim C. A standardized method for computed tomography of the orbits. Neuroradiology 1977;13:139–140.
45. Weisberg LA, Jacobs LD. Orbital computed tomography: An overview. J Clin Exp Ophthalmol 1978;1:13–28.
46. Hilal SK. Computed tomography of the orbit. Ophthalmology 1979;86:864–870.
47. Hoyt WF. Coronal sections in the diagnosis of orbital disease. In Thompson HSDR, Frisén L, et al., eds. Topics in Neuro-Ophthalmology. Baltimore, Williams & Wilkins, 1979:369–371.
48. Trokel SL, Hilal SK. CT scanning in orbital diagnosis. In Thompson HSDR, Frisén L, et al., eds. Topics in Neuro-Ophthalmology. Baltimore, Williams and Wilkins, 1979:336–346.
49. Trokel SL, Hilal SK. Submillimeter resolution CT scanning of orbital diseases. Ophthalmology 1980;412–417.
50. Grove ASJ, New PFJ, Momose KJ. Computerized tomographic (CT) scanning for orbital evaluation. Trans Am Acad Ophthalmol Otolaryngol 1975;79:137–149.
51. Cabanis EA, Pineau H, Iba-Zizen MT, et al. CT scanning in the "neuro-ocular" plane: The optic pathways as a "new" cephalic plane. Neuroophthalmology 1981;1:237–252.
52. Johns TT, Citrin CM, Black J, et al. CT evaluation of perineural orbital lesions: Evaluation of the "tram-track" sign. AJNR 1984;5:587–590.
53. Fletcher WA, Imes RK, Hoyt WF. Chiasmal gliomas: Appearance and long-term changes demonstrated by computerized tomography. J Neurosurg 1986;65:154–159.
54. Lindblom B, Truwit CL, Hoyt WF. Optic nerve sheath meningioma: Definition of intraorbital, intracanalicular, and intracranial components with magnetic resonance imaging. Ophthalmology 1992b;99:560–566.
55. Zimmerman CF, Schatz NJ, Glaser JS. Magnetic resonance imaging of optic nerve meningiomas: Enhancement with gadolinium-DTPA. Ophthalmology 1990;97:585–591.
56. Atlas SW, Grossman RI, Hackney DB, et al. STIR MR imaging of the orbit. AJR 1988;151:1025–1030.
57. Daniels DL, Herfkins R, Gager WE, et al. Magnetic resonance imaging of the optic nerves and chiasm. Radiology 1984;152:79–83.
58. Haik BG, Saint Louis L, Bierly J, et al. Magnetic resonance imaging in the evaluation of optic nerve gliomas. Ophthalmology 1987;94:709–717.
59. Klemm M, Guthoff R, Zanella F. Meningioma of the optic nerve sheath: Diagnostic problems despite use of modern imaging procedures. Klin Monatsbl Augenheilkd 1992;200:39–42.
60. Coleman DJ, Jack RL, Franzen LA. High resolution B-scan ultrasonography of the orbit. II. Hemangiomas of the orbit. Arch Ophthalmol 1972;88:368–374.
61. Coleman DJ, Jack RL, Franzen LA. High resolution B-scan ultrasonography of the orbit. III. Lymphomas of the orbit. Arch Ophthalmol 1972;88:375–379.
62. Coleman DJ, Jack RL, Franzen LA. High resolution B-scan ultrasonography of the orbit. IV. Neurogenic tumors of the orbit. Arch Ophthalmol 1972;88:380–384.
63. Coleman DJ, Jack RL, Franzen LA. High resolution B-scan ultrasonography of the orbit. V. Eye changes of Graves' disease. Arch Ophthalmol 1972;88:465–471.
64. Coleman DJ, Jack RL, Franzen LA. High resolution B-scan ultrasonography of the orbit. VI. Pseudotumors of the orbit. Arch Ophthalmol 1972;88:472–480.
65. Coleman DJ, Jack RL, Franzen LA. High resolution B-scan ultrasonograpphy of the orbit. I. The normal orbit. Arch Ophthalmol 1972;88:358–367.
66. Byrne SF. Standardized echography in the differentiation of orbital lesions. Surv Ophthalmol 1984;29:226–228.
67. Skalka HW. Ultrasonography of the optic nerve. Neuroophthalmology 1981;1:261–272.
68. Li KC, Poon PY, Hinton P, et al. MR imaging of orbital tumors with CT and ultrasound correlations. J Comput Assist Tomogr 1984;8:1039–1047.
69. Gans MS, Byrne SF, Glaser JS. Standardized A-scan echography in optic nerve disease. Arch Ophthalmol 1987;105:1232–1236.
70. Dallow RL. Reliability of orbital diagnostic tests: Ultrasonography, computerized tomography, and radiography. Ophthalmology 1978;85:1218–1228.
71. Dallow RL, Momose KJ, Weber AL, et al. Comparison of ultrasonography, computerized tomography (EMI scan) and radiographic techniques in evaluation of exophthalmos. Trans Am Acad Ophthalmol Otolaryngol 1976;81:305–322.
72. Hilal SK, Trokel SL, Coleman DJ. High resolution computerized tomography and B-scan ultrasonography of the orbit. Trans Am Acad Ophthalmol Otolaryngol 1974;81:607–617.
73. Hodes BL, Weinberg P. A combined approach for the diagnosis of orbital disease. Arch Ophthalmol 1977;95:781–788.
74. Slamovits TL, Gardner TA. Neuro-imaging in neuro-ophthalmology. Ophthalmology 1989;96:555–568.
75. Trobe JD, Gebarski SS. Looking behind the eyes: The proper use of modern imaging. Arch Ophthalmol 1993;111:1185–1186.
76. Rubenstein M, Wirtschafter JD. The role of medical imaging in the practice of neuro-ophthalmology. Radiol Clin North Am 1987;25:863–876.
77. Moseley IF. The plain radiograph in ophthalmology: A wasteful and potentially dangerous anachronism. Proc R Soc Med 1991;84:76–80.

78. Jakobiec FA, Jones JS. Orbital Inflammations. In Jones ISJF, ed. Diseases of the Orbit. Hagerstown, Harper & Row, 1979.
79. Thorne JE, Volpe NJ, Wulc AE, et al. Caught by a masquerade: Sclerosing orbital inflammation. Surv Ophthalmol 2002;47:50–54.
80. Wroe SJ, Thompson AJ, McDonald WI. Painful intraorbital meningiomas. J Neurol Neurosurg Psychiatr 1991;54:1009–1010.
81. Bartley GB. The epidemiologic characteristics and clinical course of ophthalmopathy associated with autoimmune thyroid disease in Olmsted County, Minnesota. Trans Am Ophthalmol Soc 1994;92:477–588.
82. Trobe JD, Glaser JS, Laflamme P. Dysthyroid optic neuropathy. Arch Ophthalmol 1978a;96:1199–1209.
83. Kennerdell JS, Rosenbaum AE, El-Hoshy MH. Apical optic nerve compression of dysthyroid optic neuropathy on computed tomography. Arch Ophthalmol 1981;99:807–809.
84. Riemann CD, Foster JA, Kosmorsky GS. Direct orbital manometry in patients with thyroid-associated orbitopathy. Ophthalmology 1999;106:1296–1302.
85. Chou PI, Feldon SE. Late onset dysthyroid optic neuropathy. Thyroid 1994;4:213–216.
86. Girod DA, Orcutt JC, Cummings CW. Orbital decompression for preservation of vision in Graves' ophthalmopathy. Arch Otolaryngol Head Neck Surg 1993;119:229–233.
87. Asaria RH, Koay B, Elston JS, et al. Endoscopic orbital decompression for thyroid eye disease. Eye 1998;12(Pt 6):990–995.
88. Chang EL, Bernardino CR, Rubin PA. Transcaruncular orbital decompression for management of compressive optic neuropathy in thyroid-related orbitopathy. Plast Reconstr Surg 2003;112:739–747.
89. Neugebauer A, Nishino K, Neugebauer P, et al. Effects of bilateral orbital decompression by an endoscopic endonasal approach in dysthyroid orbitopathy. Br J Ophthalmol 1996;80:58–62.
90. Schaefer SD, Soliemanzadeh P, Della Rocca DA, et al. Endoscopic and transconjunctival orbital decompression for thyroid-related orbital apex compression. Laryngoscope 2003;113:508–513.
91. Graham SM, Brown CL, Carter KD, et al. Medial and lateral orbital wall surgery for balanced decompression in thyroid eye disease. Laryngoscope 2003;113:1206–1209.
92. Graham SM, Carter KD. Combined endoscopic and subciliary orbital decompression for thyroid-related compressive optic neuropathy. Rhinology 1997;35:103–107.
93. Rush S, Winterkorn JM, Zak R. Objective evaluation of improvement in optic neuropathy following radiation therapy for thyroid eye disease. Int J Radiat Oncol Biol Phys 2000;47:191–194.
94. Salvi M, Spaggiari E, Neri F, et al. The study of visual evoked potentials in patients with thyroid-associated ophthalmopathy identifies asymptomatic optic nerve involvement. J Clin Endocrinol Metab 1997;82:1027–1030.
95. Setala K, Raitta C, Valimaki M, et al. The value of visual evoked potentials in optic neuropathy of Graves' disease. J Endocrinol Invest 1992;15:821–826.
96. Spadea L, Bianco G, Dragani T, et al. Early detection of P-VEP and PERG changes in ophthalmic Graves' disease. Graefes Arch Clin Exp Ophthalmol 1997;235:501–505.
97. Tsaloumas MD, Good PA, Burdon MA, et al. Flash and pattern visual evoked potentials in the diagnosis and monitoring of dysthyroid optic neuropathy. Eye 1994;8(Pt 6):638–645.
98. Hutchison BM, Kyle PM. Long-term visual outcome following orbital decompression for dysthyroid eye disease. Eye 1995;9(Pt 5):578–581.
99. McNab AA. Orbital decompression for thyroid orbitopathy. Aust NZ J Ophthalmol 1997;25:55–61.
100. Saeed P, Rootman J, Nugent RA, et al. Optic nerve sheath meningiomas. Ophthalmology 2003;110:2019–2030.
101. Muci-Mendoza R, Arevalo JF, Ramella M, et al. Optociliary veins in optic nerve sheath meningioma. Indocyanine green videoangiography findings. Ophthalmology 1999;106:311–318.
102. Mafee MF, Goodwin J, Dorodi S. Optic nerve sheath meningiomas. Role of MR imaging. Radiol Clin North Am 1999;37:37–58.
103. Cornblath WT, Quint DJ. MRI of optic nerve enlargement in optic neuritis. Neurology 1997;48:821–825.
104. Frohman L, Wolansky L. Magnetic resonance imaging of syphilitic optic neuritis/perineuritis. J Neuroophthalmol 1997;17:57–59.
105. Ing EB, Garrity JA, Cross SA, et al. Sarcoid masquerading as optic nerve sheath meningioma. Mayo Clin Proc 1997;72:38–43.
106. Arnold AC, Hepler RS, Badr MA, et al. Metastasis of adenocarcinoma of the lung to optic nerve sheath meningioma. Arch Ophthalmol 1995;113:346–351.
107. Backhouse O, Simmons I, Frank A, et al. Optic nerve breast metastasis mimicking meningioma. Aust NZ J Ophthalmol 1998;26:247–249.
108. Hashimoto M, Tomura N, Watarai J. Retrobulbar orbital metastasis mimicking meningioma. Radiat Med 1995;13:77–79.
109. Roelvink NC, Kamphorst W, van Alphen HA, et al. Pregnancy-related primary brain and spinal tumors. Arch Neurol 1987;44:209–215.
110. Cunliffe IA, Moffat DA, Hardy DG, et al. Bilateral optic nerve sheath meningiomas in a patient with neurofibromatosis type 2. Br J Ophthalmol 1992;76:310–312.

111. Egan RA, Lessell S. A contribution to the natural history of optic nerve sheath meningiomas. Arch Ophthalmol 2002;120:1505–1508.

112. Kennerdell JS, Maroon JC. Intracanalicular meningioma with chronic optic disc edema. Ann Ophthalmol 1975;7:507–512.

113. Andrews DW, Faroozan R, Yang BP, et al. Fractionated stereotactic radiotherapy for the treatment of optic nerve sheath meningiomas: preliminary observations of 33 optic nerves in 30 patients with historical comparison to observation with or without prior surgery. Neurosurgery 2002;51:890–904.

114. Becker G, Jeremic B, Pitz S, et al. Stereotactic fractionated radiotherapy in patients with optic nerve sheath meningioma. Int J Radiat Oncol Biol Phys 2002; 54:1422–1429.

115. Lee AG, Woo SY, Miller NR, et al. Improvement in visual function in an eye with a presumed optic nerve sheath meningioma after treatment with three-dimensional conformal radiation therapy. J Neuroophthalmol 1996;16:247–251.

116. Moyer PD, Golnik KC, Breneman J. Treatment of optic nerve sheath meningioma with three-dimensional conformal radiation. Am J Ophthalmol 2000;129: 694–696.

117. Liu JK, Forman S, Hershewe GL, et al. Optic nerve sheath meningiomas: visual improvement after stereotactic radiotherapy. Neurosurgery 2002;50:950–955; discussion 955–957.

118. Miller NR. Radiation for optic nerve meningiomas: is this the answer? Ophthalmology 2002;109:833–834.

119. Miller NR. The evolving management of optic nerve sheath meningiomas. Br J Ophthalmol 2002;86:1198.

120. Pitz S, Becker G, Schiefer U, et al. Stereotactic fractionated irradiation of optic nerve sheath meningioma: a new treatment alternative. Br J Ophthalmol 2002; 86:1265–1268.

121. Narayan S, Cornblath WT, Sandler HM, et al. Preliminary visual outcomes after three-dimensional conformal radiation therapy for optic nerve sheath meningioma. Int J Radiat Oncol Biol Phys 2003;56:537–543.

122. Turbin RE, Thompson CR, Kennerdell JS, et al. A long-term visual outcome comparison in patients with optic nerve sheath meningioma managed with observation, surgery, radiotherapy, or surgery and radiotherapy. Ophthalmology 2002; 109:890–899; discussion 899–900.

123. Kupersmith MJ, Warren FA, Newall J, et al. Irradiation of meningiomas of the intracranial anterior visual pathway. Ann Neurol 1987;21:131–137.

124. Tomsak RL, Costin JA, Hanson, M. Carotid-ophthalmic artery aneurysm presenting as unilateral disc edema with choroidal folds. In: Lawton Smith J, ed. Neuro-ophthalmology Focus 1980. New York: Masson, 1979:181–187.

125. Masuyama Y, Kodama Y, Matsuura Y, et al. Clinical studies on the occurrence and the pathogenesis of opticociliary veins. J Clin Neuroophthalmol 1990;10:1–8.

126. Boschetti NV, Smith JL, Osher RH, et al. Fluorescein angiography of opticociliary shunt vessels. J Clin Neuroophthalmol 1981;1:9–30.

127. Tsukahara S, Kobayashi S, Nakagawa F, et al. Opticociliary veins associated with meningioma of the optic nerve sheath. Ophthalmologica 1980;181:188–194.

128. Elschnig A. Ueber Opticociliare Gefasse. klin Monatsbl Augenheilkd 1898;36: 93–96.

129. Irvine AR, Shorb SR, Morris BW. Opticociliary veins. Trans Am Acad Ophthalmol Otolaryngol 1977;83:541–546.

130. Braun C. Ein Beitrag zur kenntnis Optikocilarer gefasse. klin Monatsbl Augenheilkd 1905;43:579–588.

131. Anderson SF, Townsend JC, Selvin GJ, et al. Congenital opticociliary shunt vessels. J Am Optom Assoc 1991;62:109–115.

132. Anderson DR. Vascular supply to the optic nerve of primates. Am J Ophthalmol 1970;70:341–351.

133. Hayreh SS. Blood supply of the optic nerve head and its role in optic atrophy, glaucoma and edema of the optic disc. Br J Ophthalmol 1969;53:721–728.

134. Hayreh SS, van Heuven WAJ, Hayreh MS. Experimental retinal vascular occlusion. I. Pathogenesis of central retinal vein occlusion. Arch Ophthalmol 1978; 96:311–323.

135. Frisen L, Hoyt WF, Tengroth BM. Opticociliary veins, disc pallor and visual loss. Acta Ophthalmol 1973;51:241–249.

136. Rodrigues MM, Savino PJ, Schatz NJ. Speno-orbital meningioma with opticociliary veins. Am J Ophthalmol 1976;81:666–670.

137. Hollenhorst RWJ, Hollenhorst RW, MacCarty CS. Visual prognosis of optic nerve sheath meningiomas producing shunt vessels on the optic disk. Mayo Clin Proc 1978;53:84–92.

138. Zakka KA, Summerer RW, Yee RD, et al. Opticociliary veins in a primary optic nerve sheath meningioma. Am J Ophthalmol 1979;87:91–95.

139. Henkind P, Benjamin JV. Vascular anomalies and neoplasms of the optic nerve head. Trans Ophthalmol Soc UK 1976;96:418–423.

140. Hoyt WF, Beeston, D. The Ocular Fundus in Neurologic Disease. St Louis, CV Mosby, 1966.

141. Sanders MD. A classification of papilloedema based on fluorescein angiographic study of 69 cases. Trans Ophthalmol Soc UK 1969;89:177–192.

142. Hedges TR. Papilledema: Its recognition and relation to increased intracranial pressure. Surv Ophthalmol 1975;19:201–223.

143. Eggers HM, Sander MD. Acquired opticociliary shunt veins in papilloedema. Br J Ophthalmol 1980;64:267–271.

144. Miller NR, Solomon S. Retinochoroidal (opticociliary) shunt veins, blindness and

145. Weiter JJ. Retinociliary vein associated with craniopharyngioma. Ann Ophthalmol 1979;13:751–754.

146. Mansour AM. Sarcoid optic disc edema and optociliary shunts. J Clin Neuroophthalmol 1986;6:47–52.

147. Kollarits CR, Lubow M, Johnson JC. Visual loss and perioptic vascular malformations in the eye and orbit. Am J Ophthalmol 1976;82:237–240.

148. Rosenstein J, Symon, L. Surgical management of suprasellar meningioma: Part 2, Prognosis for visual function following craniotomy. J Neurosurg 1984;61: 642–648.

149. Marcus M, Vitale S, Calvert PC, et al. Visual parameters in patients with pituitary adenoma before and after transsphenoidal surgery. Aust NZ J Ophthalmol 1991; 19:111–118.

150. Naheedy MH, Haag JR, Azar-Kia B, et al. MRI and CT of sellar and parasellar disorders. Radiol Clin North Am 1987;25:819–847.

151. Eidelberg D, Newton MR, Johnson G, et al. Chronic unilateral optic neuropathy: A magnetic resonance study. Ann Neurol 1988;24:3–11.

152. Haik BG, Zimmerman R, Saint Louis L. Gadolinium-DTPA enhancement of an optic nerve and chiasmal meningioma. J Clin Neuroophthalmol 1989;9:122–125.

153. Spalton DJ, Tonge KA. The role of MRI scanning in neuro-ophthalmology. Eye 1989;3:651–662.

154. Hupp SL, Kline LB. Magnetic resonance imaging of the optic chiasm. Surv Ophthalmol 1991;36:207–216.

155. Nadalo LA, Easterbrook J, McArdle CT, et al. The neuroradiology of visual disturbances. Neurol Clin 1991;9:1–31.

156. Kraus DH, Lanzieri CF, Wanamaker JR, et al. Complementary use of computed tomography and magnetic resonance imaging in assessing skull base lesions. Laryngoscope 1992;102:623–629.

157. Weber AL. Comparative assessment of diseases of the orbit using computed tomography and magnetic resonance imaging. Isr J Med Sci 1992;28:153–160.

158. Hodgson TJ, Kingsley DPE, Moseley IF. The role of imaging in the follow up of meningiomas. J Neurol Neurosurg Psychiatr 1995;59:545–547.

159. Golnik KC, Hund PW, Stroman GA, et al. Magnetic resonance imaging in patients with unexplained optic neuropathy. Ophthalmology 1996;103:515–520.

160. Little HL, Chambers JW, Walsh FB Unilateral intracranial optic nerve involvement. Arch Ophthalmol 1965.

161. Susac JO, Smith JL, Walsh FB. The impossible meningioma. Arch Neurol 1977; 34:36–38.

162. White DW. Progressive visual loss. Am J Ophthalmol 1972;74:752.

163. Gutman I, Melamed S, Ashkenazi I, et al. Optic nerve compression by carotid arteries in low tension glaucoma. Graefes Arch Clin Exp Ophthalmol 1993;231: 711–717.

164. Rafael H. Optic nerve compression by a dolichoectatic internal carotid artery: case report. Neurosurgery 1998;42:1196–1197.

165. Unsold R, Hoyt WF. The concept of optic nerve compression by dolichoectatic arteries revisited: The literature and why it became forgotten. In Unsold RSW, ed. Compressive Optic Nerve Lesions at the Optic Canal. Berlin, Springer-Verlag, 1989:35–37.

166. Guyer DR, Miller NR, Long DM, et al. Visual function following optic canal decompression via craniotomy. J Neurosurg 1985;62:631–638.

167. Lee AG, Lin DJ, Kaufman M, et al. Atypical features prompting neuroimaging in acute optic neuropathy in adults. Can J Ophthalmol 2000;35:325–330.

168. Pruett RC, Wepsic JG. Delayed diagnosis of chiasmal compression. Am J Ophthalmol 1973;76:229–236.

169. Kupersmith MJ, Krohn, D. Cupping of the optic disc with compressive lesions of the anterior visual pathway. Ann Ophthalmol 1984;16:948–953.

170. Bianchi-Marzoli S, Rizzo JF 3rd, Brancato R, Lessell S. Quantitative analysis of optic disc cupping in compressive optic neuropathy. Ophthalmology 1995; 102:436–440.

171. Kalenak JW, Kosmorsky GS, Hassewnbusch SJ. Compression of the intracranial optic nerve mimicking unilateral normal-pressure glaucoma. J Clin Neruoophthalmol 1992;12:230–235.

172. Ahmed II, Feldman F, Kucharczyk W, et al. Neuroradiologic screening in normal-pressure glaucoma: study results and literature review. J Glaucoma 2002; 11:279–286.

173. Portnoy GL, Roth AM. Optic cupping caused by an intracranial aneurysm. Am J Ophthalmol 1977;84:98–103.

174. Watnick RL, Trobe JD. Bilateral optic nerve compression as a mechanism for the Foster Kennedy syndrome. Ophthalmology 1989;96:1793–1798.

175. Knight CL, Hoyt WF, Wilson CB. Syndrome of incipient prechiasmal optic nerve compression. Arch Ophthalmol 1972;87:1–11.

176. O'Connell JEA, DuBoulay EPGH. Binasal hemianopia. J Neurol Neurosurg Psychiatr 1973;36:697–709.

177. Trobe JD. Chromophobe adenoma presenting with a hemianopic temporal arcuate scotoma. Am J Ophthalmol 1974;77:388–392.

178. Gregorius FK, Hepler RS, Stern WE. Loss and recovery of vision with suprasellar meningiomas. J Neurosurg 1975;42:69–75.

179. Frisen L, Sjostrand S, Norrsell K, et al. Cyclic compression of the intracranial nerve: Patterns of visual failure and recovery. J Neurol Neurosurg Psychiatr 1976;39:1109–1113.

optic atrophy: A nonspecific sign of chronic optic nerve compression. Aust NZ J Ophthalmol 1991;19:105–109.

180. Schmidt D, Buhrmann K. Inferior hemianopia in parasellar and pituitary tumors. In Glaser JS, ed. Neuro-Oophthalmology. Vol. 9. St Louis, CV Mosby, 1977: 236–247.

181. Enoksson P, Johansson JO. Altitudinal field defects and retinal nerve fibre degeneration in optic nerve lesions. Acta Ophthalmol 1978;56:957–968.

182. Trobe JD, Glaser JS. Quantitative perimetry in compressive optic neuropathy and optic neuritis. Arch Ophthalmol 1978;96:1211–1216.

183. Manor RS, Quaknine GE, Matz S, et al. Nasal visual field loss with intracranial lesions of the optic nerve pathways. Am J Ophthalmol 1980;90:1–10.

184. Cappaert WE, Kiprov RV. Craniopharyngioma presenting as unilateral central visual loss. Am J Ophthalmol 1981;13:703–704.

185. Trobe JD, Tao AH, Schuster JJ. Perichiasmal tumors: Diagnostic and prognostic features. Neurosurgery 1984;15:391–399.

186. Gutman I, Behrens M, Odel J. Bilateral central and centrocaecal scotomata due to mass lesions. Br J Ophthalmol 1984;68:336–342.

187. Slavin ML. Acute, severe, symmetric visual loss with cecocentral scotomas due to olfactory groove meningioma. J Clin Neuroophthalmol 1986;6:224–227.

188. Hershenfeld SA, Sharpe JA. Monocular temporal hemianopia. Br J Ophthalmol 1993;77:424–427.

189. Li KK, Lucarelli MJ, Bilyk JR, et al. Optic nerve decompression for compressive neuropathy secondary to neoplasia. Arch Otolaryngol Head Neck Surg 1997; 123:425–429.

190. Pless M, Lessell S. Spontaneous visual improvement in orbital apex tumors. Arch Ophthalmol 1996;114:704–706.

191. Chamlin M, Davidoff LM, Fiering EH. Ophthalmologic changes produced by pituitary tumors. Am J Ophthalmol 1955;40:353–368.

192. Stern WE. Meningiomas in the cranio-orbital junction. J Neurosurg 1973;38: 428–437.

193. Karp LA, Zimmerman LE, Borit A, et al. Primary intraorbital meningiomas. Arch Ophthalmol 1974;91:24–28.

194. Burnbaum MD, Harbison JW, Selhorst JB, et al. Blue-domed cyst with optic nerve compression. J Neurol Neurosurg Psychiatr 1978;41:987–991.

195. Trobe JD, Glaser JS, Post JE, et al. Bilateral optic canal meningiomas: A case report. Neurosurgery 1978b;3:68–74.

196. Klein LH, Fermaglich J, Kattah J, et al. Cavernous hemangioma of optic chiasm, optic nerves and right optic tract. Virchow's Arch Pathol Anat 1979;383: 225–231.

197. Safran AB, Safran E, Glaser JS, et al. Adenomes, pituitaries et meningiomes supra-sellaires. Neurochirurgie 1980;26:39–45.

198. Carlin L, Biller J, Laster DW, et al. Monocular blindness in nasopharyngeal cancer. Arch Neurol 1981;38:600.

199. Harper D. An intracranial mass lesion (cavernous angioma compressing the intracranial optic nerve). Presented at the 13th Ann. Frank B. Walsh Soc Meet. February 27–28, 1981.

200. Harbison JW, Lessell S, Selhorst JB. Neuro-ophthalmology of sphenoid sinus carcinoma. Brain 1984;107:855–870.

201. Rutka JD, Sharpe JA, Resch L, et al. Compressive optic neuropathy and ependymoma of the 3rd ventricle. J Clin Neuroophthalmol 1985;5:194–198.

202. Sharpe JA. Visual dysfunction with basal skull tumours. Can J Neurol Sci 1985; 12:332–335.

203. Gum KB, Frueh BR. Transantral orbital decompression for compressive optic neuropathy due to sphenoid ridge meningioma. Ophthal Plast Reconstr Surg 1989;5.

204. Zevgaridis D, Medele RJ, Muller A, et al. Meningiomas of the sellar region presenting with visual impairment: impact of various prognostic factors on surgical outcome in 62 patients. Acta Neurochir (Wien) 2001;143:471–476.

205. Jefferson G. Compression of the chiasm, optic nerves and optic tracts by intracranial aneurysms. Brain 1937;60:444–497.

206. Walsh FB. Visual field defects due to aneurysms at the circle of Willis. Arch Ophthalmol 1964;71:49–61.

207. Berson EL, Freeman MI, Gay AJ. Visual field defects in giant suprasellar aneurysms of internal carotid. Arch Ophthalmol 1966;76:52–58.

208. Cullen JF, Haining WM, Crombie AL. Cerebral aneurysms presenting with visual field defects. Br J Ophthalmol 1966;50:251–256.

209. Raitta C. Ophthalmic artery aneurysm. Br J Ophthalmol 1968;52:707–709.

210. Rubenstein MK, Wilson G, Levin DC. Intraorbital aneurysms of the ophthalmic artery. Arch Ophthalmol 1968;80:42–44.

211. Arseni C, Ghitescu M, Cristescu A, et al. Intrasellar aneurysms simulating hypophyseal tumors. Eur Neurol 1970;3:321–329.

212. Durston JHJ, Parsons-Smith BG. Blindness due to aneurysm of anterior communication artery. Br J Ophthalmol 1970;54:170–176.

213. Guidetti B, LaTorre E. Carotid-ophthalmic aneurysms. Acta Neurochir 1970; 22:289–304.

214. Kothandaram P, Dawson BH, Kruyt R. Carotid-ophthalmic aneurysms. J Neurosurg 1971;34:544–548.

215. Sengupta RP, Gryspeerdt GL, Hankinson J. Carotid-ophthalmic aneurysms. J Neurol Neurosurg Psychiatr 1976;39:837–853.

216. Raymond LA, Tew J. Large suprasellar aneurysms imitating pituitary tumour. J Neurol Neurosurg Psychiatr 1978;41:83–87.

217. Hahn YS, McLone DG. Traumatic bilateral ophthalmic artery aneurysms: A case report. Neurosurgery 1987;21:86–89.

218. Misra M, Mohanty AB, Rath S. Giant aneurysm of the internal carotid artery presenting features of retrobulbar neuritis. Ind J Ophthalmol 1991;1:28–29.

219. Miller NR, Savino PJ, Schneider T. Rapid growth of an intracranial aneurysm causing apparent retrobulbar optic neuritis. J Neuroophthalmol 1995;15: 212–218.

220. Bakker SL, Hasan D, Bijvoet HW. Compression of the visual pathway by anterior cerebral artery aneurysm. Acta Neurol Scand 1999;99:204–207.

221. Ernemann U, Freudenstein D, Pitz S, et al. Intraorbital aneurysm of the ophthalmic artery: a rare cause of apex orbitae compression syndrome. Graefes Arch Clin Exp Ophthalmol 2002;240:575–577.

222. Everberg G. Retrobulbar neuritis due to cyst of sphenoid sinus. Acta Otolaryngol 1955;45:492–497.

223. Waldman AL, Merrell R, Daroff RB, et al. Mucocele of the sphenoid sinus: A benign imitator. Br J Ophthalmol 1967;51:674–678.

224. Crivelli G, Riviera LC,. Unilateral blindness from aspergilloma at the right optic foramen. J Neurosurg 1970;33:207–211.

225. Nugent GR, Sprinkle P, Bloor BM. Sphenoid sinus mucoceles. J Neurosurg 1970;32:443–451.

226. Hakuba A, Katsuyama J, Matsuoka Y, et al. Sphenoid sinus mucoceles: Report of two cases. J Neurosurg 1975;43:368–373.

227. Alper MG. Mucoceles of the spenoid sinus: Neuro-ophthalmic manifestations. Trans Am Ophthalmol Soc 1976;74:53–81.

228. Decker RE, Mardayat M, Marc J, et al. Neurosarcoidosis with computerized tomographic visualization and transsphenoidal excision of a supra- and intrasellar granuloma. J Neurosurg 1979;50:814–816.

229. Imachi J, Tajino M, Okamoto N, et al. Rhinogenous retrobulbar neuritis: Pathogenic problems and case reports. Neuroophthalmology 1981;1:273–280.

230. Rothstein J, Maisel RH, Berlinger NT, et al. Relationship of optic neuritis to disease of the paranasal sinuses. Laryngoscope 1984;94:1501–1508.

231. Yue CP, Mann KS, Chan FL. Optic canal syndrome due to posterior ethmoid sinus mucocele. J Neurosurg 1986;65:871–873.

232. Newton N, Baratham G, Sinniah R, et al. Bilateral compressive optic neuropathy secondary to bilateral sphenoethmoidal mucoceles. Ophthalmologica 1989;198: 13–19.

233. Hao SP. Mucocele of the sphenoid sinus with acute bilateral blindness: Report of a case. J Formosan Med Assoc 1994;93:519–521.

234. Brown P, Demaerel P, Revesz T, et al. Neuro-ophthalmological presentation of non-invasive aspergillus sinus disease in the nonimmunocompromised host. J Neurol Neurosurg Psychiatry 1994;57:234–237.

235. Kitagawa K, Hayasaka S, Shimizu K, et al. Optic neuropathy produced by a compressed mucocele in an Onodi cell. Am J Ophthalmol 2003;135:253–254.

236. Mori PA, Holt JF. Cranial manifestations of familial metaphyseal dysplasia. Radiology 1956;66:335–343.

237. Calderon M, Brady HR. Fibrous dysplasia of bone with bilateral optic foramina involvement. Am J Ophthalmol 1969;68:513–515.

238. Aasved H. Osteopetrosis from the ophthalmological point of view. A report of two cases. Acta Ophthalmol (Copenh) 1970;48:771–778.

239. Puliafito CA, Wray SH, Murray JE, et al. Optic atrophy and visual loss in craniometaphyseal dysplasia. Am J Ophthalmol 1981;92:696–701.

240. Eretto P, Krohel GB, Shihab ZM, et al. Optic neuropathy in Paget's disease. Am J Ophthalmol 1984;97:505–510.

241. Al-Mefty O, Fox JL, Al-Rodhan N, et al. Optic nerve decompression in osteopetrosis. J Neurosurg 1988;68:80–84.

242. Weisman JS, Hepler RS, Vinters HV. Reversible visual loss caused by fibrous dysplasia. Am J Ophthalmol 1990;110:244–249.

243. Stretch JR, Poole MD. Pneumosinus dilatans as the aetiology of progressive blindness. Br J Plast Surg 1992;45:469–473.

244. Daly BD, Chow CC, Cockram CS. Unusual manifestations of craniofacial fibrous dysplasia: clinical, endocrinological and computed tomographic features. Postgrad Med J 1994;70:10–16.

245. Caldemeyer KS, Smith RR, Edwards-Brown MK Familial hypophosphatemic rickets causing ocular calcification and optic canal narrowing. AJNR 1995;16: 1252–1254.

246. Grimm MA, Hazelton T, Beck RW, et al. Postgadolinium enhancement of a compressive neuropathy of the optic nerve. Am J Neuroradiol 1995;16:779–781.

247. Messaoud R, Zaouali S, Ladjimi A, et al. Compressive optic neuropathy caused by fibrous dysplasia. J Fr Ophtalmol 2003;26:631–636.

248. Lipkin AF, Woodson GE, Miller RH. Visual loss due to orbital fracture: The role of early reduction. Arch Otolaryngol Head Neck Surg 1987;113:81–83.

249. Jordan DR, White GL, Anderson RL, et al. Orbital emphysema: A potentially blinding complication following orbital fractures. Ann Emerg Med 1988;17: 853–855.

250. Mullaney PB, Nabi NU, Thorner P, et al. Ophthalmic involvement as a presenting feature of nonorbital childhood parameningeal embryonal rhabdomyosarcoma. Ophthalmology 2001;108:179–182.

251. Walsh FB, Gass JDM. Concerning the optic chiasm: Selected pathologic involvement and clinical problems. Am J Ophthalmol 1960;50:1031–1047.

252. Mitts MG, McQueen JD. Visual loss associated with fusiform enlargement of the intracranial portion of the internal carotid artery. J Neurosurg 1965;23:33–37.

253. Matsuo K, Kobayashi S, Sugita, K. Bitemporal hemianopsia associated with

sclerosis of the intracranial internal carotid arteries. J Neurosurg 1980;53: 566–569.

254. Slavin ML. Bitemporal hemianopsia associated with dolichoectasia of the intracranial carotid arteries. J Clin Neuroophthalmol 1990;10:80–81.

255. Laurence KM, Coates S. The natural history of hydrocephalus: Detailed analysis of 182 unoperated cases. Arch Dis Child 1962;37:345–362.

256. Tamler E. Primary optic atrophy: From acquired dilation of the 3rd ventricle. Am J Ophthalmol 1964;57:827–828.

257. Lorber J, Zachary RB. Primary congenital hydrocephalus: Long-term results of controlled therapeutic trial. Arch Dis Child 1968;43:516–527.

258. Calogero JA, Alexander E Jr. Unilateral amaurosis in a hydrocephalic child with an obstructed shunt. J Neurosurg 1971;34:236–240.

259. Kirkham TH. Optic atrophy in the bobble-head doll syndrome. J Pediatr Ophthalmol 1977;14:299–301.

260. Mourits MP, Koornneef L, Wiersinga WM, et al. Orbital decompression for Graves' ophthalmopathy by inferomedial, by inferomedial plus lateral, and by coronal approach. Ophthalmology 1990;97:636–641.

261. Carter KD, Frueh BR, Hessburg TP, et al. Long-term efficacy of orbital decompression for compressive optic neuropathy of Graves' eye disease. Ophthalmology 1991;98:1435–1442.

262. Kazim M, Trokel S, Moore S. Treatment of acute Graves' orbitopathy. Ophthalmology 1991;98:1443–1448.

263. Wenz R, Levine MR, Putterman A, et al. Extraocular muscle enlargement after orbital decompression for Graves' ophthalmopathy. Ophthal Plast Reconstr Surg 1994;10:34–41.

264. Carrion LT, Edwards WC, Perry LD. Spontaneous subperiosteal orbital hematoma. Ann Ophthalmol 1979;11:1754–1757.

265. Amrith S, Baratham G, Khoo CY, et al. Spontaneous hematic cysts of the orbit presenting with acute proptosis. A report of three cases. Ophthal Plast Reconstr Surg 1990;6:273–277.

266. Moorthy RS, Yung CW, Nunery WR, et al. Spontaneous orbital subperiosteal hematomas in patients with liver disease. Ophthal Plast Reconstr Surg 1992;8: 150–152.

267. Markovits AS. Evacuation of orbital hematoma by continuous suction. Ann Ophthalmol 1977;9:1255–1258.

268. Gillum WN, Anderson RL. Reversible visual loss in subperiosteal hematoma of the orbit. Ophthalmic Surg 1981;12:203–209.

269. Kersten RC, Rice CD. Subperiosteal orbital hematoma: Visual recovery following delayed drainage. Ophthalmic Surg 1987;18:423–427.

270. Dolman PJ, Glazer LC, Harris GJ, et al. Mechanisms of visual loss in severe proptosis. Ophthal Plast Reconstr Surg 1991;7:256–260.

271. Long JC, Ellis PP. Total unilateral visual loss following orbital surgery. Am J Ophthalmol 1971;71:218–220.

272. Nicholson DH, Guzak SV Jr. Visual loss complicating repair of orbital floor fractures. Arch Ophthalmol 1971;86:369–375.

273. Moser MH, DiPirro E, McCoy FJ. Sudden blindness following blepharoplasty. J Plast Reconstr Surg 1973;51.

274. Levine MR, Bynton J, Tenzel RR, et al. Complications of blepharoplasty. Ophthalmic Surg 1975;6:53–57.

275. Sugita K, Hirota T, Iguchi I, et al. Transient amaurosis under decreased atmospheric pressure with sphenoidal sinus dysplasia. J Neurosurg 1977;46:111–114.

276. Krohel GB, Wright JE. Orbital hemorrhage. Am J Ophthalmol 1979;88: 254–258.

277. Sadowsky AE, Leavenworth N, Wirtschafter JD. Compressive optic neuropathy induced by intranasal balloon catheter. Am J Ophthalmol 1985;99:487–489.

278. Coppeto JR, Gahn NG. Bitemporal hemianopic scotoma: A complication of intraventricular catheter. Surg Neurol 1977;8:361–362.

279. Slavin ML, Rosenthal AD. Chiasmal compression caused by a catheter in the suprasellar cistern. Am J Ophthalmol 1988;105:560–561.

280. Klingele TG, Gado MH, Burde RM, et al. Compression of the anterior visual system by the gyrus rectus. J Neurosurg 1981;55:272–275.

281. Hershewe GL, Corbett JJ, Ossoinig KC, et al. Optic nerve compression from a basal encephalocele. J Neuroophthalmol 1995;15:161–165.

282. Feringa ER, Weatherbee L. Hypertrophic granulomatous cranial pachymeningitis causing progressive blindness in chronic dialysis patient. J Neurol Neurosurg Psychiatr 1975;38:1170–1176.

283. Schmidt RH, Rietz LA, Patel BC, et al. Compressive optic neuropathy caused by renal osteodystrophy. Case report. J Neurosurg 2001;95:704–709.

284. Slavin ML, Lam BL, Decker RE, et al. Chiasmal compression from fat packing after transsphenoidal resection of intrasellar tumour in two patients. Am J Ophthalmol 1993;115:368–371.

285. McHenry JG, Spoor TC. Chiasmal compression from fat packing after transsphenoidal resection of intrasellar tumor in two patients. Am J Ophthalmol 1993; 116:253.

286. Jacobson DM, Warner JJ, Broste SK. Optic nerve contact and compression by the carotid artery in asymptomatic patients. Am J Ophthalmol 1997;123: 677–683.

287. Lin MC, Bee YS, Sheu SJ. A suprasellar meningioma simulating atypical retrobulbar optic neuritis. J Chin Med Assoc 2003;66:689–692.

288. Robinson JL. Sudden blindness with pituitary tumors. J Neurosurg 1972;36: 83–85.

289. Enoksson P, Lundberg N, Sjostedt S, et al. Influence of pregnancy on visual fields in suprasellar tumours. Acta Psychiatr Neurol Scand 1961;36:524–538.

290. Schlezinger NS, Alpers BJ, Weiss BP. Suprasellar meningiomas associated with scotomatous field defects. Arch Ophthalmol 1946;35:624–642.

291. Stern WE, Ernest JT. Intracranial ophthalmic artery aneurysm. Am J Ophthalmol 1975;80:203–206.

292. Melen O, Weinberg PE, Kim KS, et al. Fibrous dysplasia of bone with acute visual loss. Ann Ophthalmol 1980;12:734–739.

293. Kelly R. Lesions of the optic chiasm due to compression. Trans Ophthalmol Soc UK 1962;82:149–164.

294. Burke WJ. Optic neuritis. Proc Aust Assoc Neurol 1968;5:243–245.

295. Ringel RA, Brick JF. Carotid-ophthalmic artery aneurysm masquerading as optic neuritis. J Neurol Neurosurg Psychiatr 1986;49:460.

296. Miller NR, Savino PJ, Schneider T. Rapid growth of an intracranial aneurysm causing apparent retrobulbar optic neuritis. J Neuroophthalmol 1995;15: 212–218.

297. McDonald WI. The 1981 Silversides Lecture: The symptomatology of tumours of the anterior visual pathways. Can J Neurol Sci 1982;9:381–390.

298. Kamin DF, Hepler RS. Solitary intracranial plasmacytoma mistaken for retrobulbar neuritis. Am J Ophthalmol 1972;73:584–586.

299. Kennerdell JS, Janetta PJ, Johnson BL. A steroid-sensitive solitary intracranial plasmacytoma. Arch Ophthalmol 1974;93:393–398.

300. Hirst LW, Miller NR, Udvarhelyi G, et al. Medulloblastoma causing a steroid-responsive optic neuropathy. Am J Ophthalmol 1980;89:437–442.

301. Cushing H, Walker CB. Distortion of the visual fields in cases of brain tumour. IV. Chiasmal lesions with special reference to bitemporal hemianopsia. Brain 1915;37:341–400.

302. Pennybacker J. The treatment of pituitary tumours. Proc R Soc Med 1961;54: 619–621.

303. Sleep TJ, Hodgkins PR, Honeybul S, et al. Visual function following neurosurgical optic nerve decompression for compressive optic neuropathy. Eye 2003; 17:571–578.

304. Wass JAH, Williams J, Charlesworth M, et al. Bromocriptine in the management of large pituitary tumours. Br J Ophthalmol 1982;284:1908–1911.

305. Rizzo JF 3rd. Visual loss after neurosurgical repair of paraclinoid aneurysms. Ophthalmology 1995;102:905–910.

306. Kang S, Yang Y, Kim T, et al. Sudden unilateral blindness after intracranial aneurysm surgery. Acta Neurochir (Wien) 1997;139:221–226.

307. Tasdemiroglu E, Zuccarello M, Tew JM Jr. Recovery of vision after transcranial decompression of pituitary apoplexy characterized by third ventricular hemorrhage. Neurosurgery 1993;32:121–123.

308. Parent AD. Visual recovery after blindness from pituitary apoplexy. Can J Neurol Sci 1990;17:88–91.

309. Striph GG, Slamovits TL, Burde RM. Visual recovery following prolonged amaurosis due to compressive optic neuropathy. J Clin Neuroophthalmol 1984;4: 189–195.

310. Tajima A, Ito M, Ishii M. Complete recovery from monocular blindness caused by aneurysmal compression to optic nerve: Report of two cases. Neurol Med Chir 1993;33:19–23.

311. Kayan A, Earl CJ. Compressive lesions of the optic nerves and chiasm. Brain 1975;98:13–28.

312. Miller NR. Clinical neuro-ophthalmology. In Walsh and Hoyt's. Clinical Neuro-Ophthalmology. Ed 4, Vol. 1. Baltimore, Williams & Wilkins, 1982b:285.

313. Cohen AR, Cooper PR, Kupersmith MJ, et al. Visual recovery after transsphenoidal removal of pituitary adenomas. Neurosurgery 1985;17:446–452.

314. Harris PE, Afshar F, Coates P, et al. The effects of transsphenoidal surgery on endocrine function and visual fields in patients with functionless pituitary tumours. Q J Med 1989;71:417–427.

315. Mohr G, Hardy J, Comtois R, et al. Surgical management of giant pituitary adenomas. Can J Neurol Sci 1990;17:62–66.

316. Rosenberg LF, Miller NR. Visual results after microsurgical removal of meningiomas involving the anterior visual system. Arch Ophthalmol 1984;102: 1019–1023.

317. Hudson H, Rissell C, Gaudeman WJ, Feldon SE. Pituitary tumor volume as a predictor of postoperative visual field recovery: Quantitative analysis using automated static perimetry and computed tomography morphometry. J Clin Neuroophthalmol 1991;11:280–283.

318. Hughes EBC. Blood supply of the optic nerves and chiasma and its clinical significance. Br J Ophthalmol 1958;42:106–125.

319. Gledhill RF, McDonald WI. Morphological characteristics of central demyelination and remyelination: A single fibre study. Ann Neurol 1977;1:552–560.

320. Harrison BM, McDonald WI. Remyelination after transient experimental compression of the spinal cord. Ann Neurol 1977;1:542–551.

321. Clifford-Jones RE, Landon DN, McDonald WI. Demyelination during optic nerve compression. J Neurol Sci 1980;46:37–40.

322. Smith KJ, Blakemore WF, McDonald WI. The restoration of conduction by central remyelination. Brain 1981;104:383–404.

323. Smith KJ, Blakemore WF, McDonald WI. Central remyelination restores secure conduction. Nature 1979;280:395–396.

324. Wright JE, Arden G, Jones BR. Continuous monitoring of the visually evoked

response during intraorbital surgery. Trans Ophthalmol Soc UK 1973;93: 311–314.

325. Feinsod M, Selhorst JB, Hoyt WF, et al. Monitoring optic nerve function during craniotomy. J Neurosurg 1976;29–31.

326. Albright AL, Sclabassi RJ. Cavitron ultrasonic surgical aspirator and visual evoked potential monitoring for chiasmal gliomas in children: Report of two cases. J Neurosurg 1985;63:138–140.

327. Costa e Silva I, Wang AD, Symon L. The application of flash visual evoked potentials during operations on the anterior visual pathways. Neurol Res 1985; 7:11–16.

328. Harding GF, Bland JD, Smith VH. Visual evoked potential monitoring of optic nerve function during surgery. J Neurol Neurosurg Psychiatr 1990;53:890–895.

329. Cedzich C, Schramm J, Fahlbusch R. Are flash-evoked visual potentials useful for intraoperative monitoring of visual pathway function? Neurosurgery 1987; 21:709–715.

330. Cedzich C, Sshramm J, Mengedoht CF, et al. Factors that limit the use of flash visual evoked potentials for surgical monitoring. Electroencephalogr Clin Neurophysiol 1988;71:142–145.

331. Cedzich C, Schramm J, Fahlbusch R. Monitoring of flash visual evoked potentials during neurosurgical operations. Int Anesthesiol Clin 1990;28:165–169.

332. Wang AD, Costa e Silva I, Symon L, et al. The effects of halothane on somatosensory and flash evoked potentials during operations. Neurol Res 1985;7: 58–62.

333. Dutton JJ, Anderson RL. Gliomas of the anterior visual pathway. Surv Ophthalmol 1994;38:427–452.

334. Lindegaard J, Heegaard S, Prause JU. Histopathologically verified non-vascular optic nerve lesions in Denmark 1940–1999. Acta Ophthalmol Scand 2002;80: 32–37.

335. Kodsi SR, Shetlar DJ, Campbell RJ, et al. A review of 340 orbital tumors in children during a 60-year period. Am J Ophthalmol 1994;117:177–182.

336. Reese AM. Tumors of the Eye. Ed 3. Hagerstown, Harper and Row, 1976: 148–154.

337. Russell DC, Rubinstein LJ. Pathology of Tumors of the Nervous System. Ed 4. Baltimore, Williams and Wilkins, 1977.

338. Czyzyk E, Jozwiak S, Roszkowski M, et al. Optic pathway gliomas in children with and without neurofibromatosis 1. J Child Neurol 2003;18:471–8.

339. Bucy PC, Russell JR, Whitsell FM. Surgical treatment of tumors of the optic nerve. Arch Ophthalmol 1950;44:411–418.

340. Mohan H, Sen DK. Astrocytoma of the optic nerve. Br J Ophthalmol 1970;53: 284–286.

341. Eggers H, Jackobiec FA, Jones IS. Optic nerve gliomas. In Jones IS, Jakobiec FA, eds. Diseases of the Orbit. Hagerstown, Harper & Row, 1979:417–443.

342. Eggers H, Jackobiec FA, Jones IS. Optic nerve gliomas. In Tasman WJE, ed. Duane's Clinical Ophthalmology. Vol. 2. Philadelphia. JB Lippincott, 1994: 1–17.

343. Wilson WB. Optic nerve gliomas: Treatment differences for the benign and malignant varieties. In Tusa RJNS, ed. Neuro-Ophthalmological Disorders: Diagnostic Work-up and Management. New York, Marcel Dekker, 1995:163–172.

344. Wiskoff J. Management of optic pathway tumors of childhood. Pediatr Neurooncol 1991;3:791.

345. Lloyd LA. Gliomas of the optic nerve and chiasm in childhood. Trans Am Ophthalmol Soc 1973;71:488–535.

346. Spencer WH. Optic nerve extension of intraocular neoplasms. Am J Ophthalmol 1975;80:465–471.

347. MacCarty CS, Boyd AS Jr, Childs DS Jr. Tumors of the optic chiasm. J Neurosurg 1970;33:439–444.

348. Bynke H, Kagstrom E, Tjernstrom K. Aspects on the treatment of gliomas of the anterior visual pathway. Acta Ophthalmol 1977;55:269–280.

349. Lowes M, Bojsen-Moller M, Vorre P, et al. An evaluation of gliomas of the anterior visual pathways: A 10-year survey. Acta Neurochir 1978;43:201–216.

350. Packer RJ, Siegel KR, Sutton LN, et al. Leptomeningeal dissemination of primary central nervous system tumors of chldhood. Ann Neurol 1985;18:217–221.

351. Lourie GL, Osborne DR, Kirks DR. Involvement of posterior visual pathways by optic nerve gliomas. Pediatr Radiol 1986;16:271–274.

352. Balcer LJ, Liu GT, Heller G, et al. Visual loss in children with neurofibromatosis type 1 and optic pathway gliomas: relation to tumor location by magnetic resonance imaging. Am J Ophthalmol 2001;131:442–445.

353. Charles NC, Nelson L, Brookner AR, et al. Pilocytic astrocytoma of the optic nerve with hemorrhage and extreme cystic degeneration. Am J Ophthalmol 1981; 92:691–695.

354. Glaser JS, Hoyt WF, Corbett J. Visual morbidity with chiasmal glioma: Long-term studies of visual fields in treated and untreated cases. Arch Ophthalmol 1971;85:3–12.

355. Spencer WH. Primary neoplasms of the optic nerve and its sheath. Clinical features and current concepts of pathogenetic mechanisms. Trans Am Acad Ophthalmol Otolaryngol 1972;70:490–528.

356. Goodman SJ, Rosenbaum AL, Hasso A, et al. Large optic nerve glioma with normal vision. Arch Ophthalmol 1975;93:991–995.

357. Pfaffenbach DD, Kearns TP, Hollenhorst RW. An unusual case of optic nerve chiasmal glioma. Am J Ophthalmol 1972;74:523–525.

358. Wright JE, McDonald WI, Call NB. Management of optic nerve gliomas. Br J Ophthalmol 1980;64:545–552.

359. Kornreich L, Blaser S, Schwarz M, et al. Optic pathway glioma: correlation of imaging findings with the presence of neurofibromatosis. Am J Neuroradiol 2001;22:1963–1969.

360. Liauw L, Vielvoye GJ, de Keizer RJ, et al. Optic nerve glioma mimicking an optic nerve meningioma. Clin Neurol Neurosurg 1996;98:258–261.

361. Brown EW, Riccardi VM, Mawad M, et al. MR imaging of the optic pathways in patients with neurofibromatosis. AJNR 1987;8:1031–1036.

362. Hendrix LE, Kneeland JB, Houghton VM, et al. MR imaging of optic nerve lesions: Value of gadopentate dimeglumine and fat-suppression technique. AJNR 1990;11:749–754.

363. Brodsky MC. The "pseudo-CSF" signal of orbital optic glioma on magnetic resonance imaging: A signature of neurofibromatosis. Surv Ophthalmol 1993; 36:213–218.

364. Stern J, Jakobiec FA, Houspian EM. The architecture of optic nerve gliomas with and without neurofibromatosis. Arch Ophthalmol 1980;98:505–511.

365. Imes RK, Hoyt WF. Magnetic resonance imaging signs of optic nerve gliomas in neurofibromatosis 1. Am J Ophthalmol 1991;111:729–734.

366. Listernick R, Charrow J, Greenwald M, et al. Natural history of optic pathway tumors in children with neurofibromatosis type 1: A longitudinal study. J Pediatr 1994;125:63–66.

367. Creange A, Zeller J, Rostaing-Rigattieri S, et al. Neurological complications of neurofibromatosis type 1 in adulthood. Brain 1999;122 (Pt 3):473–481.

368. Jenkin D, Angyalfi S, Becker L, et al. Optic glioma in children: surveillance, resection, or irradiation? Int J Radiat Oncol Biol Phys 1993;25:215–225.

369. Tow SL, Chandela S, Miller NR, et al. Long-term outcome in children with gliomas of the anterior visual pathway. Pediatr Neurol 2003;28:262–270.

370. Saran N, Winter FC. Bilateral gliomas of the optic discs. Arch Ophthalmol 1967; 64:607–612.

371. Nicholson DH, Guzak SV Jr. Tumors of the optic disc. Trans Am Acad Ophthalmol Otolaryngol 1977;83:751–754.

372. Burnstine MA, Levin LA, Louis DN, et al. Nucleolar organizer regions in optic gliomas. Brain 1993;116(Pt 6):1465–1476.

373. Cummings TJ, Provenzale JM, Hunter SB, et al. Gliomas of the optic nerve: histological, immunohistochemical (MIB-1 and p53), and MRI analysis. Acta Neuropathol (Berl) 2000;99:563–570.

374. Janss AJ, Grundy R, Cnaan A, et al. Optic pathway and hypothalamic/chiasmatic gliomas in children younger than age 5 years with a 6-year follow-up. Cancer 1995;75:1051–1059.

375. Anderson DR, Spencer WH. Ultrastructural and histochemical observations of optic nerve gliomas. Arch Ophthalmol 1970;83:324–335.

376. Borit A, Richardson EP Jr. The biological and clinical behavior of pilocytic astrocytomas of the optic pathways. Brain 1982;105:161–187.

377. Marquardt MD, Zimmerman LE. Histopathology of meningiomas and gliomas of the optic nerve. Hum Pathol 1982;13:226–235.

378. Gayre GS, Scott IU, Feuer W, et al. Long-term visual outcome in patients with anterior visual pathway gliomas. J Neuroophthalmol 2001;21:1–7.

379. McDonnell P, Miller NR. Chiasmatic and hypothalmic extension of optic nerve glioma. Arch Ophthalmol 1983;101:1412–1415.

380. Brzowski AE, Bazan C, Mumma JV, et al. Spontaneous regression of optic glioma in a patient with neurofibromatosis. Neurology 1992;42:679–681.

381. Liu GT, Lessell S. Spontaneous visual improvement in chiasmal gliomas. Am J Ophthalmol 1992;114:193–201.

382. Parsa CF, Hoyt CS, Lesser RL, et al. Spontaneous regression of optic gliomas: thirteen cases documented by serial neuroimaging. Arch Ophthalmol 2001;119: 516–529.

383. Astrup J. Natural history and clinical management of optic pathway glioma. Br J Neurosurg 2003;17:327–335.

384. Kushner MS, Jampol LM, Haller JA. Cavernous hemangioma of the optic nerve. Retina 1994;14:359–361.

385. Laue L, Comite F, Hench K, et al. Precocious puberty associated with neurofibromatosis and optic glioma. Am J Dis Child 1985;139:1097–1100.

386. Brauner R, Malandry F, Rappaport R, et al. Growth and endocrine disorders in optic glioma. Eur J Pediatr 1990;149:825–828.

387. Gliomas NASGfO. Tumor spread in unilateral optic glioma. Neurofibromatosis 1989;1:1–12.

388. Oxenhandler DC, Sayers MP. The dilemma of childhood optic gliomas. J Neurosurg 1978;48:34–41.

389. Klug GL. Gliomas of the optic nerve and chiasm in children. Neuroophthalmology 1982;2:217–223.

390. Erkal HS, Serin M, Cakmak A. Management of optic pathway and chiasmatic-hypothalamic gliomas in children with radiation therapy. Radiother Oncol 1997; 45:11–15.

391. Kingsley DPE, Kendall BE. CT of the adverse effects of therapeutic radiation of the central nervous system. AJNR 1981;2:453–460.

392. Imes RK, Hoyt WF. Childhood chiasmal gliomas: Update on the fate of the patients in the 1969 San Francisco Study. Br J Ophthalmol 1986;70:179–182.

393. Kovalic JJ, Grigsby PW, Shephard MD, et al. Radiation therapy for gliomas of the optic nerve and chiasm. Int J Rad Oncol Biol Phys 1990;18:927–932.

394. Debus J, Kocagoncu KO, Hoss A, et al. Fractionated stereotactic radiotherapy (FSRT) for optic glioma. Int J Radiat Oncol Biol Phys 1999;44:243–248.

395. Gaini SM, Tomei G, Arienta C, et al. Optic nerve and chiasmal gliomas in children. J Neurosurg Sci 1982;26:33–39.

396. Redfern RM, Scholtz CL. Long term survival with optic nerve glioma. Surg Neurol 1980;14:371–375.

397. Glaser JS, Hoyt WF, Corbett J. Gliomas of the anterior visual pathways in childhood: rationale for conservative management. In Brockhurst RJBS, Hutchinson BT, et al., eds. Controversy in Ophthalmology. Philadelphia, WB Saunders, 1977:897–909.

398. Chamberlain MC, Grafe MR. Recurrent chiasmatic-hypothalamic glioma treated with oral etoposide. J Clin Oncol 1995;13:2072–2076.

399. Rudd A, Rees JE, Kennedy P, et al. Malignant optic nerve gliomas in adults. J Clin Neuroophthalmol 1985;5:238–243.

400. Taphoorn MJ, de Vries-Knoppert WA, Ponssen H, et al. Malignant optic glioma in adults. Case report. J Neurosurg 1989;70:277–279.

401. Millar WS, Tartaglino LM, Sergott RC, et al. MR of malignant optic glioma of adulthood. Am J Neuroradiol 1995;16:1673–1676.

402. Hoyt WF, Meshel LG, Lessell S, et al. Malignant optic glioma of adulthood. Brain 1973;96:121–133.

403. Mattson RH, Peterson EW. Glioblastoma multiforme of the optic nerve. JAMA 1966;196:799–800.

404. Spoor TC, Kennerdell JS, Zorub D, et al. Progressive visual loss due to glioblastoma: Normal neuroroentgenographic studies. Arch Neurol 1981;38:196–197.

405. Spoor TC, Kennerdell JS, Martinez AJ, et al. Malignant gliomas of the optic nerve pathways. Am J Ophthalmol 1980;89:284–292.

406. Courville CB. Ganglioglioma: Tumor of the central nervous system. Review of the literature and report of two cases. Arch Neurol Psychiatr 1930;24:439–491.

407. Courville CB, Anderson FM. Neurogliogenic tumors of the central nervous system: Report of two additional cases of ganglioglioma of the brain. Bull Los Angeles Neurol Soc 1941;6:154–176.

408. Bailey P, Beiser H. Concerning gangliogliomas of the brain. J Neuropathol Exp Neurol 1947;6:24–34.

409. Demierre B, Stichnoth FA, Hori A, et al. Intracerebral ganlioglioma. J Neurosurg 1986;65:177–182.

410. Kalyan-Raman UP, Olivero WC. Ganglioglioma: A correlative clinicopathological and radiological study of ten surgically treated cases with followup. Neurosurgery 1987;20:428–433.

411. Hall WA, Yunis EJ, Albright AL. Anaplastic ganglioglioma in an infant: Case report and review of the literature. Neurosurgery 1986;19:1016–1020.

412. Johannsson J, Rekate H, Roessmann U. Gangliogliomas: Pathological and clinical correlation. J Neurosurg 1981;54:58–63.

413. Cogan DG, Poppen JL, Hicks SP. Ganglioglioma of chiasm and optic nerves. Arch Ophthalmol 1961;65:481–482.

414. Gritzman MCD, Snyckers FD, Proctor NSF. Ganglioglioma of the optic nerve: A case report. S Afr Med J 1983;63:863–865.

415. Rodriguez LA, Edwards MSB, Levin VA. Management of hypothalamic gliomas in children: An analysis of 33 cases. Neurosurgery 1990;26:242–247.

416. Meyer P, Eberle MM, Probst A, et al. Ganglioglioma of optic nerve in neurofibromatosis type 1. Case report and review of the literature. Klin Monatsbl Augenheilkd 2000;217:55–58.

417. Shuangshoti S, Kirsch E, Bannan P, et al. Ganglioglioma of the optic chiasm: case report and review of the literature. Am J Neuroradiol 2000;21:1486–1489.

418. Sugiyama K, Goishi J, Sogabe T, et al. Ganglioglioma of the optic pathway. A case report. Surg Neurol 1992;37:22–25.

419. Liu GT, Galetta SL, Rorke LB, et al. Gangliogliomas involving the optic chiasm. Neurology 1996;46:1669–1673.

420. Lu WY, Goldman M, Young B, et al. Optic nerve ganglioglioma. J Neurosurg 1993;78:979–982.

421. Liu GT, Galetta SL, Rorke LB, et al. Gangliogliomas involving the optic chiasm. Neurology 1996;46:1669–1673.

422. Burger PC, Scheithauer BW, Bogel FS. Surgical Pathology of the Nervous System and Its Coverings. Ed 3. New York, Churchill Livingstone, 1991:271.

423. Russell DC, Rubinstein LJ. Ganglioglioma: A case with long history and malignant evolution. J Neuropathol Exp Neurol 1962;21:185–193.

424. Christensen E. Nerve cell tumors (central and peripheral). In: Minckler J, ed. Pathology of the Nervous System. Vol. 2. New York, McGraw-Hill, 1971:2081–2093.

425. Wahl RW, Dillard SH Jr. Multiple ganglioneuromas of the central nervous system. Arch Pathol 1972;94:158–164.

426. Shields JA, Shields CL Differential diagnosis of retinoblastoma. In: Shields J, Shields CL, eds. Intraocular Tumors: A Text and Atlas. Philadelphia, WB Saunders, 1992:225.

427. Atkinson A, Sanders MD, Wong V. Vitreous hemorrhage in tuberous sclerosis. Br J Ophthalmol 1973;57:773–779.

428. Song S, Seo MS. Spontaneous regression of a solitary astrocytoma of the optic disk. Retina 2002;22:502–503.

429. Hogan MJ, Zimmerman LE. Ophthalmic Pathology: An Atlas and Textbook. Ed 2. Philadelphia, WB Saunders, 1962:607–608.

430. Ulbright TM, Fulling KH, Helveston EM. Astrocytic tumors of the retina: Differentiation of sporadic tumors from phakomatosis-associated tumors. Arch Pathol Lab Med 1984;108:106–163.

431. Oosterhuis JA, Rubinstein K. Haemangioma of the optic disc. Ophthalmologica 1972;164:362–374.

432. Gass JDM. Cavernous hemangioma of the retina: A neuro-ocular-cutaneous syndrome. Am J Ophthalmol 1971;71:799–814.

433. Drummond JW, Hall DL, Steen WH Jr, et al. Cavernous hemangioma of the optic disc. Ann Ophthalmol 1980;12:1017–1018.

434. Pierro L, Guarisco L, Zagnanelli E, et al. Capillary and cavernous hemangioma of the optic disc: Echographic and histological findings. Acta Ophthalmol 1992a; 204(Suppl):102–106.

435. Mouillon M, Romanet JP, Hermann M, et al. Hemangiome caverneux du nerf optique intra-canalaire. Bull Soc Ophtalmol Fr 1984;84:875–879.

436. Mohr G, Hardy J, Gauvin, P. Chiasmal apoplexy due to ruptured cavernous hemangioma of the optic chiasm. Surg Neurol 1985;24:636–640.

437. Margo CE, Kincaid MC. Angiomatous malformation of the retrolaminar optic nerve. J Pediatr Opthalmol Strabismus 1988;25:37–39.

438. Maruoka N, Yamakawa Y, Shimauchi, M. Cavernous hemangiomas of the optic nerve: Case report. J Neurosurg 1988;69:292–294.

439. Hassler W, Zentner J, Petersen, D. Cavernous angioma of the optic nerve: Case reort. Surg Neurol 1989a;31:444–447.

440. Hassler W, Zentner J, Wilhelm, H. Cavernous angiomas of the visual pathways. J Clin Neuroophthalmol 1989b;9:160–164.

441. Gass JDM. Differential Diagnosis of Intraocular Tumors. St Louis, CV Mosby, 1974:282–287.

442. Gass JDM, Braunstein R. Sessile and exophytic capillary angiomas of the juxtapapillary retina and optic nerve head. Arch Ophthalmol 1980;98:1790–1797.

443. Schindler RF, Sarin LK, MacDonald PR. Hemangiomas of the optic disc. Can J Ophthalmol 1975;10:305–318.

444. Gass JDM. Treatment of retinal vascular anomalies. Trans Am Acad Ophthalmol Otolaryngol 1977;83:432–442.

445. Niccol W, Moore RF. A case of angiomatosis retinae. Br J Ophthalmol 1934; 18:454–457.

446. Klein M, Goldberg MF, Collier, E. Cavernous hemangioma of the retina: Report of four cases. Am J Ophthalmol 1975;7:1213–1221.

447. Lewis RA, Cohen MH, Wise GN. Cavernous hemangioma of the retina and optic disc: A report of three cases and a review of the literature. Br J Ophthalmol 1975;59:422–434.

448. Colvard DM, Robertson DM, Trautman JC. Cavernous hemangioma of the retina. Arch Ophthalmol 1978;96:2042–2044.

449. Irene R, Martin Z, Peter T, et al. Kavernores Hamangiom de Papille: Klinische und echographische Befunde. klin Monatsbl Augenheilkd 1996;209:380–382.

450. Maitland CG, Abiko S, Hoyt WF, et al. Chiasmal apoplexy: Report of four cases. J Neurosurg 1982;56:118–122.

451. Hwang JF, Yau CW, Huang JK, et al. Apoplectic optochiasmal syndrome due to intrinsic cavernous hemangioma. J Clin Neuroophthalmol 1993;13:232–236.

452. Kerr J, Scheithauer BW, Miller GM, et al. Hemangioblastoma of the optic nerve: Case report. Neurosurgery 1995;36:573–579.

453. Tanaka E, Kimura C, Inoue H, et al. A case of intraorbital hemangioblastoma of the optic nerve. Folia Ophthalmol Jpn 1984;35:1390–1395.

454. Nerad JA, Kersten RC, Anderson RL. Hemangioblastoma of the optic nerve: Report of a case and review of literature. Ophthalmology 1988;95:398–402.

455. In S, Miyagi J, Kojho N, et al. Intraorbital optic nerve hemangioblastoma with von Hippel-Lindau disease. J Neurosurg 1982;56:426–429.

456. Ginzburg BM, Montanera WJ, Tyndel FJ, et al. Diagnosis of von Hippel-Lindau disease in a patient with blindness resulting from bilateral optic nerve hemangioblastomas. AJR Am J Roentgenol 1992;159:403–405.

457. Zimmerman LE, Garron LK. Melanocytoma of the optic disc. Int Ophthalmol Clin 1962;2:431–440.

458. Shields JA. Melanocytoma of the optic nerve head: A review. Int Ophthalmol Clin 1978;1:31–37.

459. Joffe L, Shields JA, Osher RH, et al. Clinical and follow-up studies of melanocytomas of the optic disc. Trans Am Acad Ophthalmol Otolaryngol 1979;86:1067–1078.

460. Balestrazzi E. Melanocytoma of the optic disc. Ophthalmologica 1973;166:289–292.

461. Osher R, Shields JA, Layman PR. Pupillary and visual field evaluation in patients with melanocytoma of the optic disc. Arch Ophthalmol 1979;97:1096–1099.

462. Shields JA, Shields CL, Eagle RC Jr, et al. Central retinal vascular obstruction secondary to melanocytoma of the optic disc. Arch Ophthalmol 2001;119:129–133.

463. Zimmerman LE. Melanocytes, melanocytic nevi, and melanocytoma. Invest Ophthalmol Vis Sci 1965;4:11–41.

464. Shuey RM, Blacharski PA. Pigmented tumor and acute visual loss. Surv Ophthalmol 1988;33:121–126.

465. Usui T, Shiramashi M, Kurosawa A, et al. Visual disturbance in patients with melanocytoma of the optic disk. Ophthalmologica 1990;201:92–98.

466. Wiznia RA, Price J. Recovery of vision in association with a melanocytoma of the optic disc. Am J Ophthalmol 1974;78:236–238.

467. Garcia-Arumi J, Salvador F, Corcostegui B, et al. Neuroretinitis associated with melanocytoma of the optic disc. Retina 1994;14:173–176.

468. Juarez CP, Tso MOM. An ultrastructural study of melanocytomas (magnocellular nevi) of the optic disk and uvea. Am J Ophthalmol 1980;90:48–62.

469. Shields JA, Shields CL, Piccone M, et al. Spontaneous appearance of an optic disk melanocytoma in an adult. Am J Ophthalmol 2002;134:614–615.
470. Meyer D, Ge J, Blinder KJ, et al. Malignant transformation of an optic disk melanocytoma. Am J Ophthalmol 1999;127:710–714.
471. Erzurum SA, Jampol LM, et al. Primary malignant melanoma of the optic nerve simulating a melanocytoma. Arch Ophthalmol 1992;110:684–686.
472. Loeffler KU, Tecklenborg H. Melanocytoma-like growth of a juxtapapillary malignant melanoma. Retina 1992;12:29–34.
473. DePotter P, Shields CL, Eagle RC, et al. Malignant melanoma of the optic nerve. Arch Ophthalmol 1996;114:608–612.
474. Antcliff RJ, Ffytche TJ, Shilling JS, et al. Optical coherence tomography of melanocytoma. Am J Ophthalmol 2000;130:845–847.
475. Green WR, Iliff WJ, Trotter RR Malignant teratoid medulloepithelioma of the optic nerve. Arch Ophthalmol 1974;91:451–454.
476. Ginsberg J, Freemond AS, Calhoun JB. Optic nerve involvement in metastatic tumors. Ann Ophthalmol 1970;2:604–617.
477. Ferry AP, Font LR. Carcinoma metastatic to the eye and orbit: A clinicopathologic study of 227 cases. Trans Am Acad Ophthalmol Otolaryngol 1974;72:877–895.
478. Arnold AC, Hepler RS, Foos RY. Isolated metastasis to the optic nerve. Surv Ophthalmol 1981;26:75–83.
479. Christmas N, Mead MD, Richardson EP, et al. Secondary optic nerve tumors. Surv Ophthalmol 1991;36:196–206.
480. Shields JA, Shields CL, Singh AD. Metastatic neoplasms in the optic disc: The 1999 Bjerrum Lecture: Part 2. Arch Ophthalmol 2000;118:217–224.
481. Gallie BL, Graham JE, Hunter WS. Optic nerve head metastasis. Arch Ophthalmol 1975;93:983–986.
482. Zappai RJ, Smith ME, Gay AJ. Prostatic carcinoma metastatic to the optic nerve and choroid. Arch Ophthalmol 1972;87:642–645.
483. Cherington FJ. Metastatic adenocarcinoma of the optic nerve head and adjacent retina. Br J Ophthalmol 1961;45:227–230.
484. Ferry AP. Metastatic adenocarcinoma of the eye and ocular adnexae. Int Ophthalmol Clin 1967;35:615–658.
485. Ring HG. Pancreatic carcinoma with metastasis to the optic nerve. Arch Ophthalmol 1967;77:798–800.
486. Newman NJ, Grossniklaus HE, Wojno TH. Breast carcinoma metastatic to the optic nerve. Arch Ophthalmol 1996;114:102–103.
487. Sung JU, Lam BL, Curtin VT, et al. Metastatic gastric carcinoma to the optic nerve. Arch Ophthalmol 1998;116:692–693.
488. Adachi N, Tsuyama Y, Mizota A, et al. Optic disc metastasis presenting as an initial sign of recurrence of adenoid cystic carcinoma of the larynx. Eye 2003;17:270–272.
489. Garrity JA, Herman DC, DiNapoli RP, et al. Isolated metastasis to optic nerve of medulloblastoma. Ophthalmology 1989;96:207–210.
490. Hirst LW, Miller NR, Kumar AJ, et al. Medulloblastoma causing a corticosteroid-responsive optic neuropathy. Am J Ophthalmol 1980;89:437–442.
491. DePotter P, Shields JA, Shields CL, et al. Unusual MRI findings in metastatic carcinoma to the choroid and optic nerve: A case report. Int Ophthalmol 1992;16:39–44.
492. Berman EL, Chu A, Wirshafter JD, et al. Esthesioneuroblastoma presenting as a sudden unilateral blindness. J Clin Neuroophthalmol 1992;12:31–36.
493. Lee AG, Phillips PH, Newman NJ. Neuro-ophthalmologic manifestations of adenoid cystic carcinoma. J Neuroophthalmol 1997;17:183–188.
494. Arnold AC, Hepler RS, Badr MA, et al. Metastasis of adenocarcinoma of the lung to optic nerve sheath meningioma. Arch Ophthalmol 1995;113:346–351.
495. Dawes JDK. Malignant disease of the nasopharynx. J Laryngol Otol 1969;83:211–238.
496. Matz GJ, Conner GH. Nasopharyngeal cancer. Laryngoscope 1968;78:1763–1767.
497. Zohdy G, Ghabra M, Zonogue C. Nasopharyngeal carcinoma: A cause of Foster Kennedy syndrome. Eye 1994;8:364–367.
498. Prasad U, Doraisamy S. Optic nerve involvement in nasopharyngeal carcinoma. Eur J Surg Oncol 1991;17:526–540.
499. Mansour AM, Dinowitz K, Chaliijub G, et al. Metastatic lesion of the optic nerve. J Clin Neuroophthalmol 1993;13:102–104.
500. Kattah JC, Chrousos GC, Roberts J, et al. Metastatic prostate cancer to the optic canal. In: Ophthalmology. Vol 100. 1993:1711–1715.
501. Allaire GS, Corriveau C, Arbour JD. Metastasis to the optic nerve: Clinicopathological correlations. Can J Neurol Sci 1995;30:306–311.
502. Terry TL, Dunphy EB. Metastatic carcinoma in both optic nerves simulating retrobulbar neuritis. Arch Ophthalmol 1933;10:611–614.
503. Danis P, Brilhaye-van Geertruyden M. Nevrite optique retrobulbaire bilaterale par metastases cancereuses dans les gaines arachnoidiennes. Acta Neruol Psychiart Belg 1952;52:345–358.
504. Ing EB, Augsburger JJ, Eagle RC. Lung cancer with visual loss. Surv Ophthalmol 1996;40:505–510.
505. McFadzean R, Brosnahan D, Doyle D, et al. A diagnostic quartet in leptomeningeal infiltration of the optic nerve sheath. J Clin Neuroophthalmol 1994;14:175–182.
506. Katz JL, Valsamis MP, Jampel RS. Ocular signs in diffuse carcinomatosis. Am J Ophthalmol 1961;52:681–690.
507. Fischer-Williams M, Bosanquet FD, Daniel PM Carcinomatosis of the meninges: A report of three cases. Brain 1955;78:42–58.
508. Little JR, Dale AJD, Okazak H. Meningeal carcinomatosis. Arch Neurol 1974;30:138–143.
509. Olson ME, Chernik NL, Posner JB. Infiltration of the leptomeninges by systemic cancer. Arch Neurol 1974;30:122–137.
510. Appen RE, de Venecia G, Selliken JH, et al. Meningeal carcinomatosis with blindness. Am J Ophthalmol 1978;86:661–665.
511. Susac JO, Smith JL, Powell JO. Carcinomatous optic neuropathy. Am J Ophthalmol 1973;76:672–679.
512. Walshe FMR. Meningitis carcinomatosa. Br J Ophthalmol 1923;7:113–123.
513. Nakajima T, Kumabe T, Jokura H, et al. Recurrent germinoma in the optic nerve: report of two cases. Neurosurgery 2001;48:214–217; discussion 217–218.
514. Lester EP, Ultman JE. Lymphoma. In Williams WJBE, Erslev AJ, eds. Hematology. New York, McGraw-Hill, 1990:1067–1089.
515. MacIntosh F, Colby TV, Podolsky WJ, et al. Central nervous system involvement in non-Hodgkin's lymphoma: An analysis of 105 cases. Cancer 1982;49:586–596.
516. Lee LC, Howes EL, Bhisitkul RB. Systemic non-Hodgkin's lymphoma with optic nerve infiltration in a patient with AIDS. Retina 2002;22:75–79.
517. Miller NR, Illif WJ. Visual loss as the initial symptom in Hodgkin's disease. Arch Ophthalmol 1975;93:1158–1161.
518. Kansu T, Orr LS, Savino PF, et al. Optic neuropathy as initial manifestation of lymphoreticular diseases: A report of five cases. In Lawton Smith J, ed. Neuro-Ophthalmology Focus 1980. New York, Masson, 1979:125–136.
519. Kattah JC, Suski ET, Killen JY, et al. Optic neuritis and systemic lymphoma. Am J Ophthalmol 1980;89:431–436.
520. Kay MC. Optic neuropathy secondary to lymphoma. J Clin Neuroophthalmol 1986;6:31–34.
521. Kline LB, Garcia JH, Harsh GR 3rd. Lymphomatous optic neuropathy. Arch Ophthalmol 1984;102:1655–1657.
522. Lanska DJ, Lanska MJ, Tomsak RL. Unilateral optic neuropathy in non-Hodgkin's lymphoma. Neurology 1987;74:60–66.
523. Bullock JD, Yanes B, Kelly M, et al. Non-Hodgkins lymphoma involving the optic nerve. Ann Ophthalmol 1979;11:1477–1480.
524. Scarpatetti A, Schmid L, Zollinger, U. Infiltrative Optikusneuropathie bei Non-Hodgkin-Lymphom. klin Monatsbl Augenheilkd 1982;180:146–150.
525. Yen MY, Liu JH. Malignant lymphoma involving the optic nerve head and the retina. Ann Ophthalmol 1985;17:697–700.
526. Howard RS, Duncombe AS, Owens C, et al. Compression of the optic chiasm due to a lymphoreticular malignancy. Postgrad Med J 1987;63:1091–1093.
527. Mattews JH, Smith NA, Foroni, L. A case of angioimmunoblastic lymphadenopathy associated with long spontaneous remission, retrobulbar neuritis, a clonal rearrangement of the T-cell receptor gamma chain gene and an unusual marrow infiltration. Eur J Haematol 1988;41:295–301.
528. Guyer DR, Green WR, Schachat AP, et al. Bilateral ischemic optic neuropathy and retinal vascular occlusions associated with lymphoma and sepsis. Ophthalmology 1990;97:882–888.
529. McFadzean RM, McIlwaine G, McLellan D. Hodgkin's disease at the optic chiasm. J Clin Neuroophthalmol 1990;10:248–254.
530. Neetens A, Clemens A, van den Ende P, et al. Nevrite optique dans le lymphome non Hodgkinien. klin Monatsbl Augenheilkd 1992;200:525–528.
531. Siatkowski RM, Lam BL, Schatz NJ, et al. Optic neuropathy in Hodgkin's disease. Am J Ophthalmol 1992;114:625–629.
532. Noda S, Hayasaka S, Setogawa, T. Intraocular lymphoma invades the optic nerve and orbit. Ann Ophthalmol 1993;25:30–34.
533. Strominger MB, Schatz NJ, Glaser JS. Lymphomatous optic neuropathy. Am J Ophthalmol 1993;110:774–776.
534. Zaman AG, Graham EM, Sanders MD. Anterior visual system involvement in non-Hodgkin's lymphoma. Br J Ophthalmol 1993;77:184–187.
535. Yamamoto N, Kiyosawa M, Kawasaki T, et al. Successfully treated optic nerve infiltration with adult T-cell lymphoma. J Neuroophthalmol 1994;14:81–83.
536. Brazis PW, Menke DM, McLeish WM, et al. Angiocentric T-cell lymphoma presenting with multiple cranial nerve palsies and retrobulbar optic neuropathy. J Neuroophthalmol 1995;15:152–157.
537. Dunker S, Reuter U, Rosler A, et al. Optic nerve infiltration in well-differentiated b-cell lymphoma. Ophthalmologica 1996;93:351–353.
538. Fierz AB, Sartoretti S, Thoelen AM. Optic neuropathy and central retinal artery occlusion in non-Hodgkin lymphoma. J Neuroophthalmol 2001;21:103–105.
539. Park KL, Goins KM. Hodgkin's lymphoma of the orbit associated with acquired immunodeficiency syndrome. Am J Ophthalmol 1993;116:111–112.
540. Esmaeli B, Ahmadi MA, Manning J, et al. Clinical presentation and treatment of secondary orbital lymphoma. Ophthal Plast Reconstr Surg 2002;18:247–253.
541. Henchoz L, Borruat FX, Gonin J, et al. Bilateral optic neuropathy as the presenting sign of systemic non-Hodgkin's lymphoma. Klin Monatsbl Augenheilkd 2003;220:189–192.
542. Langdon HM. Multiple myeloma and bilateral sixth nerve paralysis and left retrobulbar neuritis. Trans Ophthalmol Soc UK 1939;37:223–229.
543. Clarke E. Cranial and intracranial myelomas. Brain 1954;77:61–79.
544. Gudas PPJ. Optic nerve myeloma. Am J Ophthalmol 1971;71:1085–1089.
545. Goldberg S, Mahadevia P, Lipton M, et al. Sinus histiocytosis with massive

lymphadenopathy involving the orbit: reversal of compressive optic neuropathy after chemotherapy. J Neuroophthalmol 1998;18:270–275.

546. Pless M, Chang BM. Rosai-Dorfman disease. Extranodal sinus histiocytosis in three co-existing sites: A case report. J Neurooncol 2003;61:137–141.

547. Lieberman FS, Odel J, Hirsh J, et al. Bilateral optic neuropathy with IgG kappa multiple myeloma improved after myeloablative chemotherapy. Neurology 1999;52:414–416.

548. Mansour AM, Salti HI. Multiple myeloma presenting with optic nerve compression. Eye 2001;15:802–804.

549. Hogan MC, Lee A, Solberg LA, et al. Unusual presentation of multiple myeloma with unilateral visual loss and numb chin syndrome in a young adult. Am J Hematol 2002;70:55–59.

550. Bourdette DN, Rosenberg NL. Infiltrative orbitopathy, optic disc edema, and POEMS. Neurology 1984;34:532–533.

551. Galetta SL, Stadtmauer EA, Hicks DG, et al. Reactive lymphohistiocytosis with recurrence in the optic chiasm. J Clin Neuroophthalmol 1991;11:25–30.

552. Anthony JJ. Malignant lymphoma associated with hydantoin drugs. Arch Neurol 1970;22:450–454.

553. Allen RA, Straatsma BR. Ocular involvement in leukemia and allied disorders. Arch Ophthalmol 1961;66:490–508.

554. Rodgers R, Weiner M, Friedman AH. Ocular involvement in congenital leukemia. Am J Ophthalmol 1986;101:730–732.

555. Nygaard R, Garwicz S, Haldorsen T, et al. Second malignant neoplasms in patients treated for childhood leukemia. Acta Pediatr Scand 1991;80:1220–1228.

556. Wallace RT, Shields JA, Shields CL, et al. Leukemic infiltration of the optic nerve. Arch Ophthalmol 1991;109:1027.

557. Brown DM, Kimura AE, Ossoing KC, et al. Acute promyelocytic infiltration of the optic nerve treated by oral trans-retinoic acid. Ophthalmology 1992;99:1463–1467.

558. Costagliola C, Rinaldi M, Cotticelli L, et al. Isolated optic nerve involvement in chronic myeloid leukemia. Leuk Res 1992;16:411–413.

559. Horton JC, Garcia EC, Becker EK. Magnetic resonance imaging of leukemic invasion of the optic nerve. Arch Ophthalmol 1992;110:1207–1208.

560. Pierro L, Guarisco L, Zagnanelli E, et al. Ocular involvement in acute lymphoblastic leukemia: An echographic study. Int Ophthalmol 1992b;16:159–162.

561. Shibasaki HS, Hayasaka S, Noda S, et al. Radiotherapy resolves leukemic involvement of the optic nerves. Ann Ophthalmol 1992;24:395–397.

562. Camera A, Piccirillo G, Cennamo G, et al. Optic nerve involvement in acute lymphoblastic leukemia. Leuk Lymphoma 1993;11:153–155.

563. Sayli B, Cemeroglu AP, Tuncer AM, et al. Acute lymphoblastic leukemia following optic glioma treated by radiotherapy and surgery. Acta Paediatr 1993;82:327–328.

564. Kaikov Y. Optic nerve head infiltration in acute leukemia in children: an indication for emergency optic nerve radiation therapy. Med Pediatr Oncol 1996;26:101–104.

565. Madani A, Christophe C, Ferster A, et al. Peri-optic nerve infiltration during leukemic relapse: MRI diagnosis. Pediatr Radiol 2000;30:30–32.

566. Charif Chefchaouni M, Belmekki M, Hajji Z, et al. Ophthalmic manifestations of acute leukemia. J Fr Ophtalmol 2002;25:62–66.

567. Iwami T, Nishida Y, Mukaisho M, et al. Central retinal artery occlusion associated with leukemic optic neuropathy. J Pediatr Ophthalmol Strabismus 2003;40:54–56.

568. Schocket LS, Massaro-Giordano M, Volpe NJ, et al. Bilateral optic nerve infiltration in central nervous system leukemia. Am J Ophthalmol 2003;135:94–96.

569. Mayo GL, Carter JE, McKinnon SJ. Bilateral optic disk edema and blindness as initial presentation of acute lymphocytic leukemia. Am J Ophthalmol 2002;134:141–142.

570. Eichholtz W. Papillenschwellungen bei leukamien und verwandten prozessen. Ophthalmologica 1975;170:494–504.

571. Rosenthal AR, Egbert PR, Wilbur JR, et al. Leukemic involvement of the optic nerve. J Pediatr Ophthalmol Strabismus 1975;12:84–93.

572. Ellis W, Little HL. Leukemic infiltration of the optic nerve head. Am J Ophthalmol 1973;75:867–871.

573. Chalfin AL, Nash BM, Goldstein JH. Optic nerve head involvement in lymphocytic leukemia. J Pediatr Ophthalmol Strabismus 1973;10:39–43.

574. Ridgway EW, Jaffe N, Walton DS. Leukemic ophthalmopathy in children. Cancer 1976;38:1744–1749.

575. Murray KH, Paolino F, Goldman JM, et al. Ocular involvement in leukemia. Lancet 1977;1:829–831.

576. Brown GC, Shield JA, Augsburger JJ, et al. Leukemic optic neuropathy. Int Ophthalmol 1981;3:111–116.

577. Nikaido H, Mishima H, Ono H, et al. Leukemic involvement of the optic nerve. Am J Ophthalmol 1988;105:294–298.

578. Yamamoto N, Kiyosawa M, Kawasaki T, et al. Successfully treated optic nerve infiltration with adult T-cell lymphoma. J Neuroophthalmol 1994;14:81–83.

579. Biondi A, Rambaldi A, Alcalay M, et al. RAR-alpha rearrangements as a gentic marker for diagnosis and monitoring in acute promyelocytic leukemia. Blood 1991;77:1418–1422.

580. Wiznia RA, Rose A, Levy AL. Occlusive microvascular retinopathy with optic disc and retinal neovascularization in acute lymphocytic leukemia. Retina 1994;14:253–255.

581. Pless M, Rizzo JF 3rd, Shang J. Orbital apex syndrome: a rare presentation of extramedullary hematopoiesis: case report and review of literature. J Neurooncol 2002;57:37–40.

582. Aarabi B, Haghshenas M, Rakeii V. Visual failure caused by suprasellar extramedullary hematopoiesis in beta thalassemia: Case report. Neurosurgery 1998;42:922–925; discussion 925–926.

583. Cramer SC, Glapsy JA, Efird JT, et al. Chronic lymphocytic leukemia and the central nervous system. Neurology 1996;46:19–25.

584. Alajouanine T, Ferey D, Houdart R, et al. Forme Neuro-oculaire pure de la maladie de Besnier-Boeck-Schaumann: Amblyopie rapide par atteinte successive des deux nerfs optiques a un an de distance. Rev Neurol 1952;86:225–257.

585. Statton R, Blodi FC, Hanigan J. Sarcoidosis of the optic nerve. Arch Ophthalmol 1964;71:834–836.

586. Kelley JS, Green WR. Sarcoidosis involving the optic nerve head. Arch Ophthalmol 1973;89:486–488.

587. Caplan L, Corbett J, Goodwin J, et al. Neuro-ophthalmologic signs in the angitic form of neurosarcoidosis. Neurology 1983;33:1130–1135.

588. Graham EM, Ellis CJK, Sanders MD, et al. Optic neuropathy in sarcoidosis. J Neurol Neurosurg Psychiatr 1986;49:756–763.

589. Galetta SL, Schatz NJ, Glaser JS. Acute sarcoid optic neuropathy with spontaneous recovery. J Clin Neuroophthalmol 1989;9:27–32.

590. Sharma OP, Sharma AM. Sarcoidosis of the nervous system: A clinical approach. Arch Intern Med 1991;151:1317–1321.

591. Beck AD, Newman NJ, Grossniklaus HE, et al. Optic nerve enlargement and chronic visual loss. Surv Ophthalmol 1994;38:555–566.

592. Frohman LP, Guirgis M, Turbin RE, et al. Sarcoidosis of the anterior visual pathway: 24 new cases. J Neuroophthalmol 2003;23:190–197.

593. Jordan DR, Anderson RL, Nerad JA, et al. Optic nerve involvement as the initial manifestation of sarcoidosis. Can J Neurol Sci 1988;23:232–237.

594. DeBroff BM, Donahue SP. Bilateral optic neuropathy as the initial manifestation of systemic sarcoidosis. Am J Ophthalmol 1993.

595. Frohman LP, Grigorian R, Bielory L. Neuro-ophthalmic manifestations of sarcoidosis: clinical spectrum, evaluation, and management. J Neuroophthalmol 2001;21:132–137.

596. Reis W, Rothfeld, J. Tuberkulide des Sehnerven als Komplikation von Hautsarkoiden vom Typus Darier-Roussy. Graef'es Arch Clin Exp Ophthalmol 1931;126:357–366.

597. Morax PV. Les localisations neuro-oculaires de la reticulo-endotheliose de Besnier-Boeck-Schaumann. Ann Ocul 1956;189:73–91.

598. Ingestad R, Stigmar G. Sarcoidosis with ocular and hypothalamic-pituitary manifestations. Acta Ophthalmol 1971;49:1–10.

599. Jampol LM, Woodfin W, McLean EB. Optic nerve sarcoidosis. Arch Ophthalmol 1972;87:355–360.

600. Brownstein S, Jannotta FS. Sarcoid granulomas of the optic nerve and retina: Report of a case. Can J Neurol Sci 1974;9:372–378.

601. Turner RG, James DG, Friedmann AL, et al. Neuro-ophthalmic sarcoidosis. Br J Ophthalmol 1975;59:657–663.

602. Burns CL. Unusual ocular presentation of sarcoidosis. Ann Ophthalmol 1976;8:69–71.

603. Gass JDM, Olson CL. Sarcoidosis with optic nerve and retinal involvement. Arch Ophthalmol 1976;94:945–950.

604. Lustgarden JS, Mindel JS, Yablonski ME, et al. An unusual presentation of isolated optic nerve sarcoidosis. J Clin Neuroophthalmol 1983;3:13–18.

605. Beardsley TL, Brown SVL, Sydnor CF, et al. Eleven cases of sarcoidosis of the optic nerve. Am J Ophthalmol 1984;97:62–77.

606. Karma A, Mustonen EM. Optic nerve involvement in sarcoidosis. Neuroophthalmology 1985.

607. Katz B, Newman S, Wall M. Disc edema, transient obscurations of vision, and a temporal fossa mass. Surv Ophthalmol 1991;36:133–139.

608. Yohai RA, Bullock JD, Margolis JH. Unilateral optic disc edema and a contralateral temporal fossa mass. Am J Ophthalmol 1993;115:261–262.

609. Mafee MF, Dorodi S, Pai E. Sarcoidosis of the eye, orbit, and central nervous system: Role of MR imaging. Radiol Clin North Am 1999;37:73–87.

610. Farr AK, Jabs DA, Green WR. Optic disc sarcoid granuloma. Arch Ophthalmol 2000;118:728–729.

611. Noble KG. Ocular sarcoidosis occurring as a unilateral optic disk vascular lesion. Am J Ophthalmol 1979;105:294–298.

612. Doxanas M, Kelley JS, Prout TE. Sarcoidosis with neovascularization of the optic nerve head. Am J Ophthalmol 1980;90:347–351.

613. Moritera T, Sunakawa M, Arai M, et al. Optic nerve involvement in sarcoidosis. Acta Soc Ophthalmol Jpn 1986;90:1196–1202.

614. Pelton RW, Lee AG, Orengo-Nania SD, et al. Bilateral optic disk edema caused by sarcoidosis mimicking pseudotumor cerebri. Am J Ophthalmol 1999;127:229–230.

615. James DG, Zatouroff MA, Trowell J, et al. Papilloedema in sarcoidosis. Br J Ophthalmol 1967;51:526–529.

616. Cheung CM, Durrani OM, Stavrou P. Peripapillary choroidal neovascularization in sarcoidosis. Ocul Immunol Inflamm 2002;10:69–73.

617. Cook BE Jr, Robertson DM. Confluent choroidal infiltrates with sarcoidosis. Retina 2000;20:1–7.

618. Pickuth D, Heywang-Kobrunner SH. Neurosarcoidosis: Evaluation with MRI. J Neuroradiol 2000;27:185–188.

619. Rush JA. Retrobulbar optic neuropathy in sarcoidosis. Ann Ophthalmol 1980; 12:390–394.

620. Carmody RF, Mafee MF, Goodwin JA, et al. Orbital and optic pathway sarcoidosis: MR findings. Am J Neuroradiol 1994;15:775–783.

621. Engelken JD, Yuh WTC, Carter KD, et al. Optic nerve sarcoidosis: MR findings. AJNR 1992;13:228–230.

622. Sahel J, Flament J, Bucheit F, et al. La sarcoidose des voies optiques. Ophthalmologica 1986;224:219–224.

623. Tang RA, Grotta JC, Lee F, et al. Chiasmal syndrome in sarcoidosis. Arch Ophthalmol 1983;101:1069–1073.

624. Case Records of the Massachusetts General Hospital: Case 10–1991. N Engl J Med 1991;324:677–687.

625. Aszkanazy CL. Sarcoidosis of the central nervous system. J Neuropathol Exp Neurol 1952;11:392–400.

626. Dutton JJ, Anderson RL. Idiopathic inflammatory perioptic neuritis simulating optic nerve sheath meningioma. Am J Ophthalmol 1985;100:424–430.

627. Purvin V, Kawasaki A, Jacobson DM. Optic perineuritis: clinical and radiographic features. Arch Ophthalmol 2001;119:1299–1306.

628. Rush JA, Kennerdell JS, Martinez AJ. Primary idiopathic inflammation of the optic nerve. Am J Ophthalmol 1982;93:312–316.

629. Kennerdell JS, Dresner SC. The non-specific orbital inflammatory syndromes. Surv Ophthalmol 1984;29:93–103.

630. Fay AM, Kane SA, Kazim M, et al. Magnetic resonance imaging of optic perineuritis. J Neuroophthalmol 1997;17:247–249.

631. Gartaganis S, Georgiou S, Monastirli A, et al. Asymptomatic bilateral optic perineuritis in secondary syphilis. Acta Derm Venereol 2000;80:75–76.

632. Wals KT, Ansari H, Kiss S, et al. Simultaneous occurrence of neuroretinitis and optic perineuritis in a single eye. J Neuroophthalmol 2003;23:24–27.

633. Tien RD, Hesselink JR, Szumowski J. MR fat suppression combined with Gd-DTPA enhancement in optic neuritis and perineuritis. J Comput Assist Tomogr 1991;15:223–227.

634. Paufique L, Etienne R. Le Tuberculome du chiasma. Bull Mem Soc Fr Ophthalmol 1952;65:97–109.

635. Schlernitzauer DA, Hodges FJ 3rd, Bagan M. Arch Ophthalmol 1971;85:75–78.

636. Lana-Peixoto MA, Bambirra EA, Pittella JE. Optic nerve tuberculoma. Arch Neurol 1980;37:186–187.

637. Feld AP, Sicard, J. Sur deux cas de tubercule du chiasma. Rev Neurol 1947; 79:664–666.

638. Iraci G, Giordano R, Gerosa M, et al. Tuberculoma of the anterior optic pathways. J Neurosurg 1980;52:129–133.

639. Langenbeck K. Neuritis retrobulbaris und allgemeiner-krankugen. Graefes Arch Clin Exp Ophthalmol 1914;87:226–279.

640. Sloan LL, Woods AC. Perimetric studies in syphilitic optic neuropathies. Arch Ophthalmol 1938;20:201–253.

641. Verhoeff FH. Ein fall von syphilom des optikus und der papille mit spirochaten-befund. klin Monatsbl Augenheilkd 1910;48:315–321.

642. Stoewer P. Zwei seltene falle luetischer papillen-und netzhaurterkrangkung. Z Augenheilkd 1924;52:76–78.

643. Schieck F, Bruckner, A. Kurzes Handbuch der Ophthalmologie. Berlin, Julius Springer, 1931.

644. Koff R. Gumma of the optic papilla. Am J Ophthalmol 1939;22:663–665.

645. Marmor MF, Egbert PR, Egbert BM, et al. Optic nerve head involvement with cytomegalovirus in an adult with lymphoma. Arch Ophthalmol 1978;96: 1252–1254.

646. Kupfer C, McCrane E. A possible cause of decreased vision in cryptococcal meningitis. Invest Ophthalmol 1974;13:801–804.

647. Cohen DB, Glasgow BJ. Bilateral optic nerve cryptococcosis in sudden blindness in patients with acquired immune deficiency syndrome. Ophthalmology 1993; 100:1689–1694.

648. Okun E, Butler WT. Ophthalmologic complications of cryptococcal meningitis. Arch Ophthalmol 1964;71:52–57.

649. Ofner S, Baker RS. Visual loss in cryptococcal meningitis. J Clin Neuroophthalmol 1987;7:45–48.

650. Tan CT. Intracranial hypertension causing visual failure in cryptococcus meningitis. J Neurol Neurosurg Psychiatr 1988;52:944–946.

651. Lipson BD, Freeman WR, Beniz J, et al. Optic neuropathy associated with cryptococcal arachnoiditis in AIDS patients. Am J Ophthalmol 1989;107: 523–527.

652. Giberson TP, Kalyan-Raman K. Cryptococcal meningitis: Initial presentation of acquired immunodeficiency syndrome. Ann Emerg Med 1987;16:802–804.

653. Holland GN, Kreiger AE. Neuroophthalmology of acquired immunodeficiency syndrome. New York, Raven Press, 1988.

654. Maruki C, Nakano H, Shimoji T, et al. Loss of vision in cryptococcal optochiasmatic arachoiditis and optocurative surgical exploration: Case report. Neurol Med Chir 1988;28:695–697.

655. Li PK, Lai KN. Amphotericin B induced ocular toxicity in cryptococcal meningitis. Br J Ophthalmol 1989;73:397–398.

656. Winward KE, Hamed LM, Glaser JS. The spectrum of optic nerve disease in human immunodeficiency virus infection. Am J Ophthalmol 1989;107:373–380.

657. Golnik KC, Newman SA, Wispelway B. Cryptococcal optic neuropathy in the acquired immune deficiency syndrome. J Clin Neuroophthalmol 1991;11: 96–103.

658. Johnston CEL, Foster O, et al. Raised intracranial pressure and visual complications in AIDS patients with cryptococcal meningitis. J Infect 1992;24:185–189.

659. Cremer PD, Johnston IH, Halmagyi GM. Pseudotumour cerebri syndrome due to cryptococcal meningitis. J Neurol Neurosurg Psychiatry 1997;62:96–98.

660. Ferreira RC, Phan G, Bateman JB. Favorable visual outcome in cryptococcal meningitis. Am J Ophthalmol 1997;124:558–560.

661. Garrity JA, Herman DC, Imes R, et al. Optic nerve sheath decompression for visual loss in patients with acquired immunodeficiency syndrome and cryptococcal meningitis with papilledema. Am J Ophthalmol 1993;116:472–478.

662. Banta JT, Davis JL, Lam BL. Presumed toxoplasmosic anterior optic neuropathy. Ocul Immunol Inflamm 2002;10:201–211.

CHAPTER 9

Traumatic Optic Neuropathies

Kenneth D. Steinsapir and Robert A. Goldberg

CLASSIFICATION	PATHOGENESIS
EPIDEMIOLOGY	Injury Mechanisms
CLINICAL ASSESSMENT	PHARMACOLOGY
History	Experimental
Examination	Clinical Experience
Visual Evoked Potential	MANAGEMENT
Visual Field	Early Studies
Imaging	Megadose Steroids
Differential Diagnosis	Surgical Considerations
PATHOLOGY	

CLASSIFICATION

Optic nerve injuries are classically divided into direct and indirect injuries. Direct injuries are open injuries where an external object penetrates the tissues to impact the optic nerve. Indirect optic nerve injuries occur when the force of collision is imparted into the skull and this energy is absorbed by the optic nerve. The prognostic value in knowing that an injury was direct or indirect is unclear. Historically, direct optic nerve injury is associated with a poor visual outcome. It may be safe to classify an optic nerve injury as direct if orbital imaging reveals a bullet at the orbital apex, but this provides no insight into the cellular injury mechanism. The classification does not illuminate whether the nerve is severed with no hope of recovery or only mildly injured with significant recovery potential. This becomes important as strategies for treating nerve injuries evolve.

Optic nerve injuries are also classified anatomically. Injuries that occur anterior to where the central retinal artery enters the optic nerve produce abnormalities in the retinal circulation in association with visual loss (1,2) (Fig. 9.1).

Disturbances in retinal circulation can be associated with orbital hemorrhages that compromise the optic nerve. Avulsions of the optic nerve from the globe produce a distinct picture with a partial ring of hemorrhage at the optic nerve head (3) (Fig. 9.2). In contrast, posterior optic nerve injuries occur posterior to the site where the central retinal artery enters the optic nerve. The most common site of indirect optic nerve injury is the bony optic canal, referred to as an intracanalicular injury (4,5). The intracranial optic nerve is the next most common site of injury (6). Chiasmal injuries can be diagnosed on the basis of visual field changes when this test can be obtained (7). Chiasmal injuries are associated with a high incidence of diabetes insipidus, reported to be 37% in one series (8). Neuroimaging is usually able to separate intracanalicular injuries from orbital injuries occurring posterior to where the central retinal artery enters the optic nerve. Orbital optic nerve injuries can be associated with intrasheath hemorrhage, which anecdotally have benefited from clot drainage (9).

EPIDEMIOLOGY

Traumatic optic neuropathy occurs in association with high momentum deceleration injuries. Optic nerve injury is often associated with midface trauma. Table 9.1 lists the most common causes of traumatic optic neuropathy. Motor vehicle and bicycle accidents are the most frequent cause, accounting for 17–63% of cases, depending on the series. Motorcycle accident victims may be particularly vulnerable to traumatic optic neuropathy. A consecutive series of 101

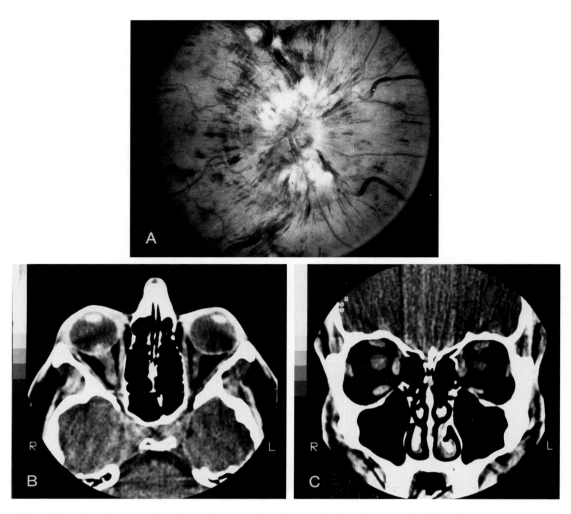

Figure 9.1.   Central retinal vein occlusion in a case of anterior (proximal) optic neuropathy. The patient was a 24-year-old man who was struck in the right eye while playing basketball and who immediately experienced loss of vision in the eye. Visual acuity was light perception OD and 20/15 OS. *A,* Ophthalmoscopic appearance of right ocular fundus reveals moderate swelling of the optic disc. The disc is surrounded by hemorrhage and soft exudates. The retinal veins are dilated and tortuous. *B,* Computed tomographic (CT) scan, axial view, shows moderate enlargement of the orbital portion of the right optic nerve. *C,* CT scan, coronal view, shows enlargement of right optic nerve compared with left nerve. Note small areas of increased density, consistent with hemorrhage, with the enlarged nerve. (Courtesy of Dr. Neil R. Miller.)

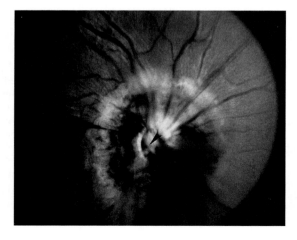

Figure 9.2.   Traumatic avulsion of the optic disc. Note ring of hemorrhage around the optic disc. The site of avulsion is clearly visible as a crescentic dark area at the temporal portion of the disc *(arrowhead).* (Courtesy of Dr. Neil R. Miller.)

Table 9.1
Etiology of Traumatic Optic Neuropathy

First Author	Cases	Motor Vehicle	Bicycle	Fall	Assualt	Other
Nau (22)	18	7 (39%)	2 (11%)	5 (28%)	1 (6%)	3 (17%)
Bodin (188)	6	1 (17%)	3 (50%)	2 (33%)	–	–
Millesi (189)	29	18 (62%)	–	6 (21%)	5 (17%)	–
Seiff (11)	36	15 (42%)	–	13 (36%)	4 (11%)	4 (11%)
Anderson (178)	7	3 (43%)	1 (14%)	2 (12%)	–	–
Matsuzaki (174)	33	20 (60%)	–	7 (21%)	4 (12%)	2 (6%)
Joseph (179)	14	2 (14%)	3 (21%)	4 (29%)	3 (21.4%)	2 (14%)
Spoor (13)	21	9 (43%)	–	3 (14%)	4 (19%)	5 (24%)
Kountakis (190)	34	18 (51%)	1 (3%)	9 (26%)	5 (15%)	–
Lubben (194)	65	15 (23%)	15 (23%)	–	7 (11%)	33 (51%)
Total	263	107 (41%)	23 (9%)	52 (20%)	33 (13%)	51 (19%)

patients with head trauma after a motorcycle accident found 18 cases of traumatic optic neuropathy (18%) (10). Falls are the next most common cause, producing 14–50% of cases. Traumatic optic neuropathy has also resulted from frontal impact by falling debris (11,12), assault (11), stab wounds (13), gun shot wounds (13,14), skateboarding (11), bottle-cork injuries (15), following seemingly trivial injuries (3,16), and following endoscopic sinus surgery (17–20). Iatrogenic optic nerve trauma with visual loss is rare following elective LeFort I osteotomy. When it does occur, it may be related to uncontrolled and unpredictable pterygomaxillary disjunction with propagation of the fractures into the optic canal (22).

Optic nerve injury is usually associated with concomitant multi-system trauma or serious brain injury. Loss of consciousness is associated with traumatic optic neuropathy in 40–72% of cases (11,21–23). The incidence of indirect trau-matic optic neuropathy has been defined in the past as a subpopulation of individuals with head trauma (4,24). In a large study of maxillofacial trauma patients, traumatic optic neuropathy occurred in 2.5% of patients with midface fracture (25). The percentage of patients with light perception and no light perception vision following traumatic optic neuropathy varies from 43% (13,26) to 78% (27) (Table 9.2). However, recent studies have higher percentages of patients with more subtle forms of traumatic optic neuropathy (11,13,26). Patients with mild forms of traumatic optic neuropathy were probably not identified in the older series

Optic nerve injury following orbital hemorrhage defines an important subset that does not fit well into the classic delineation of direct and indirect optic nerve injuries (28,29). The mechanism of neuropathy is an orbital compartment syndrome resulting in elevated orbital pressure compromis-

Table 9.2
Frequency of Improvement Over Initial Visual Acuity by Series in Chronological Order

First Author	Cases	Initial Visual Acuity				Treatment
		No Light Perception		Light Perception or Better		
		Total	Improved[a]	Total	Improved[a]	
Hooper (191)	58	14	3	–	–	–
Hughes (5)	90	51	14	39	NA	–
Edmund (192)	22	17	4	5	NA	Surgery
Anderson (178)	7	3	1	1	1	Surgery/corticosteroids
Matsuzaki (174)	33	8	0	25	14	Surgery/corticosteroids
Fujitani (175)	113	37	7	76	53	Surgery/corticosteroids
Seiff (11)	36	18	7	18	11	Observation/corticosteroids
Joseph (179)	14	5	3	9	8	Surgery/corticosteroids
Spoor (13)	22	8	5	14	14	Surgery/corticosteroids
Mauriello (57)	23	1	2	11	10	Surgery/corticosteroids
Chou (193)	58	32	13	26	15	Surgery/corticosteroids
Kountakis (190)	34	11	8	23	16	Surgery/corticosteroids
Lubben (194)	65	21	10	25	23	Surgery/corticosteroids
Wang (27)	61	48	13	13	13	Surgery/corticosteroids
Totals	636	274	90 (33%)	285	178 (62%)	

Articles listed represent those series where sufficient visual acuity data was published to permit this analysis.
[a] Visual improvement was defined as any improvement in visual function according to the authors of each listed article.

ing the circulation to the optic nerve. Orbital hemorrhage may occur spontaneously following thrombolytic therapy, in association with surgery, childbirth, and in the presence of sickle cell disease as well as known coagulopathies (30–36). In one report, a subperiosteal orbital hematoma with visual compromise occurred due to a subgaleal hemorrhage in a child following hair pulling (37). The best-studied group of patients with orbital hemorrhage are those undergoing retrobulbar injection of anesthetic for ophthalmic surgery. The prevalence of an orbital hemorrhage following a retrobulbar block is 0.44–3% (38–41). When orbital hemorrhage occurs following a retrobulbar block, it is generally recognized and readily managed with little impact on visual outcome.

Although rare, direct optic nerve injury from a retrobulbar needle has been reported (42,43). When retrobulbar hemorrhage occurs in association with trauma, the risk of visual loss is much greater. Hemorrhage following blepharoplasty is also a recognized cause of potential visual loss (44). Orbital hemorrhage is associated with alloplastic repair of orbital fractures (45,46). Blood can be dispersed in the orbit, in the subperiosteal space, and in the optic nerve sheath, or result in a hematic cyst (47,48). Imaging studies can help localize the hemorrhage (49–51).

Orbital emphysema is generally a benign condition. However, air can become trapped in the orbit due to a ball-valve mechanism typically following orbital fracture. Compressive optic neuropathy and visual loss can result (52). Vomiting and nose blowing in the setting of orbital fracture may be associated with optic nerve compromise when air is forced into the orbit (53). Optic neuropathy in conjunction with simultaneous tension orbital emphysema and pneumocephalus following blunt trauma has been reported (54). Orbital emphysema with visual loss has also been reported in one patient following the use of a high-speed air-cooled drill in the dental setting (55).

CLINICAL ASSESSMENT

Traumatic optic neuropathy remains a clinical diagnosis. By definition, there must be a history of trauma. Associated loss of consciousness is common. A diagnosis of optic nerve trauma should not be made in the presence of normal vision and normal pupillary function. Following trauma, respiratory and cardiovascular resuscitation are the first priority. Every case of optic nerve injury, however mild, represents head trauma. Therefore care of these patients usually occurs in a team setting involving emergency physicians, trauma surgeons, head and neck surgeons, neurosurgeons, and ophthalmologists. Under these circumstances, the initial ophthalmic examination may be limited by other clinical considerations. The ophthalmic assessment should be completed at the earliest opportunity.

HISTORY

Clinical evaluation of a patient with visual loss following trauma should begin with as complete a history as possible. If the patient is unconscious, the history should be obtained from significant others when present. Witnesses at the scene, including responding emergency personnel, may provide an understanding of the mechanism of injury. The possibility of exposure to hazardous materials should be considered. An ocular history must be explored to rule out visual loss prior to the injury. A detailed medical, drug, and drug allergy history is also necessary. Open injury creates a risk for tetanus, and the patient's tetanus immunization status should be investigated.

EXAMINATION

Visual Acuity

Visual acuity following indirect optic nerve trauma is often significantly reduced. Each patient in Hughes' series of 56 cases presented with no light perception (5). All 46 patients described by Turner also presented with no light perception on the side with optic nerve injury (4). In Hooper's series, 14 of 21 patients presented with no light perception (56). In the series reported by Edmund, 17 of 22 patients presented with no light perception (21). While vision better than 20/400 is not inconsistent with traumatic optic neuropathy, it is unusual in older reported cases.

As can be seen from Table 9.2, recent reports contain larger numbers of patients with visual acuity of better than 20/200 in the affected eye. In the past, patients with minor decreases in visual function may have gone undetected. Commonly, patients with traumatic optic neuropathy will have vision that is 20/400 or less in the affected eye. However, the clinician must maintain a high index of suspicion to avoid missing more subtle cases of traumatic optic neuropathy. Delayed visual loss is reported to be as high as 10% in some series (23,57).

Pupillary Reflexes

In cases of unilateral traumatic optic neuropathy, the presence of an afferent pupillary deficit is a necessary condition for the diagnosis of traumatic optic neuropathy. Afferent pupillary defects can be quantitated using photographic neutral density filters (58). These filters are calibrated in log units that measure the reduction in transmitted light. The lenses can be stacked to produce an additive effect in front of the normal eye until the reduction in light reaching the normal eye matches the reduction caused by the relative afferent pupillary defect. When the input in both sides is equal, the afferent pupillary defect will be neutralized. The log unit reduction in light reaching the good eye is a measure of the afferent pupillary defect. Afferent pupillary deficits of greater than 2.1 log units are predictive of poor visual prognosis (59).

Biomicroscopy and Fundoscopy

A complete and thorough examination of the eye and ocular adnexa is essential following trauma. Palpation of the orbital rim can identify step-off fractures. Periorbital swelling may mask the presence of proptosis. Resistance to retropulsion of the globe followed by tonometry can rapidly identify an orbit that is tense from a retro-orbital hemorrhage. Lid swelling can increase the difficulty of the ocular examination necessitating an assistant to retract the eyelids. Evidence of a penetrating ocular injury should be sought. Blunt injury to the iris may result in a hyphema or angle recession. The force of trauma may dislocate the lens.

Posteriorly, blood in the vitreous may obscure the fundus. If the patient is neurologically unstable, the treating neurosurgeon or trauma surgeon should be consulted prior to dilating the eyes. If a dilated examination is performed, to avoid confusion the time of dilation and the type of agents used must be documented both in the nursing and physician notes, and posted prominently at the bedside. Only short-acting agents should be used. When intracranial pressure is monitored invasively, pupillary response may not be critical. However, a dilated fundus exam to rule out retinal disinsertion and tears may need to be deferred until the patient is neurologically stable.

An adequate fundus examination will include assessment of abnormalities of the retinal circulation. Partial and complete avulsion of the optic nerve head produces a ring of hemorrhage at the site of injury or the appearance of a deep round pit (3,60). Anterior injuries between the globe and where the central retinal vessels enter the optic nerve produce disturbances in the retinal circulation including venous obstruction and traumatic anterior ischemic optic neuropathy (1,61). Hemorrhages in the optic nerve sheath posterior to the origin of the central retinal vessels may leave the circulation of the retina intact, but produce optic nerve head swelling (62). Frank papilledema may be seen in the setting of raised intracranial pressure despite the presence of traumatic optic neuropathy (63). The presence of choroidal rupture or *commotio retinae* may explain visual loss. Clinical judgment must be exercised to decide if these conditions are consistent with an afferent pupillary defect. The presence of decreased visual acuity and an afferent pupillary defect in the absence of intraocular pathology should suggest a posterior orbital, intracanalicular or intracranial optic nerve injury.

VISUAL EVOKED POTENTIAL

The visual evoked potential (VEP) may be of use in the unresponsive patient suspected of having traumatic optic neuropathy (22,64,65). This is especially true in possible bilateral cases where an afferent pupillary deficit may not be evident. An unresponsive patient with midface fractures and other than normal pupillary responses warrants a VEP investigation. Generally, the actual clinical utility of VEP is limited logistically. A VEP may not be available at the bedside, when the information is most critical, and moving the patient to the evoked potential laboratory may not be possible. In addition, the test requires a highly qualified technician who may not be available after hours. The VEP is useful only when it is not recordable—in which case the chance of visual recovery is very unlikely (22,66,67). The VEP can frequently be abnormal but recordable in an amaurotic eye immediately following optic nerve trauma with subsequent extinction (22). It is thought that the false-positive VEP may

be due to a limited number of still intact axons that are able to conduct.

VISUAL FIELD

Visual fields can be obtained only when sufficient vision is present following optic nerve trauma. The visual field, by virtue of the retinotopic organization of the optic nerve, provides an understanding of the localization of optic nerve damage. Within the canal, the pial penetrating vessels that provide blood to the optic nerve are subject to shearing forces at the moment of injury. Since the superior portion of the optic nerve is most tightly bound within the canal, these pial vessels are thought to be the most susceptible to shearing forces. Partial avulsion of the optic nerve at the globe produces visual field deficits that correspond to the site of avulsion. However, there is no pathognomonic visual field loss diagnostic of optic nerve trauma. Visual field testing is useful in documenting the return of visual function following injury (68). As a practical matter, confrontational visual fields may be the only type of visual field available at the bedside. Recording the ability to count fingers, detect hand motion, or light in each quadrant may crudely quantitate this. Ambulatory patients should be considered for formal visual field testing.

IMAGING

The superior imaging afforded by computed tomography and magnetic resonance imaging has made plain films and hypoclinoidal tomograms obsolete. Manfredi and coworkers reviewed the medical records of 379 patients with facial fractures (69). Twenty-one patients lost all vision in one eye (6%) and 3 of these 21 lost vision in both eyes; 12 of the 21 patients with visual loss had CT scans of the head as part of the initial assessment and of these 12, visual loss was attributed to traumatic globe injuries in 7 cases. CT scans in the remaining 5 patients demonstrated a fracture through the optic canal. The fracture may injure the optic nerve directly or it may serve as a marker of the severity of force transferred into the optic nerve (Fig. 9.3). Seiff et al. reported CT results of nine patients with traumatic optic neuropathy (70). Six of the nine patients demonstrated fractures of the optic canal. Fractures were present in adjacent structures but not extending into the optic canal in two additional patients. In a follow-up study, canal fractures were found in 16 of 36 patients and fractures of the bones adjacent to the optic canal, but not involving the optic canal, in an additional 10 of 36 patients (11). However, 63% of the patients with canal fractures presented with no light perception compared with a 40% incidence of no light perception when there was no fracture or the fracture did not extend to the optic canal.

CT scanning in the setting of traumatic optic neuropathy has demonstrated specific pathology implicated in the compromise of optic nerve function including optic nerve sheath hematoma and presumed arachnoid cyst (9,71,72). While CT scanning is clearly superior to magnetic resonance imaging (MRI) in delineating fractures of bone, MRI is superior to CT scanning in its ability to image soft tissue. Often both CT and MRI are required to fully evaluate a particular clinical situation (62,73) (Fig. 9.4). As a note of caution, MRI should

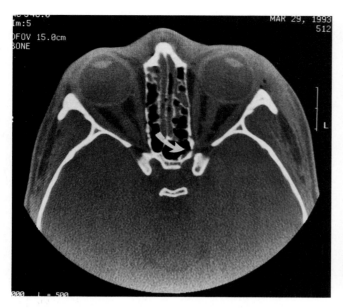

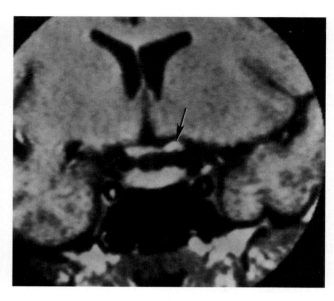

Figure 9.3. Preoperative axial CT scan of the head at the level of the optic canal. Arrow indicates an optic canal fracture in the left lateral sphenoid wall. (Courtesy of Robert A. Goldberg, MD.)

Figure 9.4. Coronal MRI of the brain at the head at the level of the optic chiasm. Arrow indicates hemorrhage in the optic nerve sheaths. (From Crowe NW, Nickles TP, Troost T, Elster AD. Intrachiasmal hemorrhage: A cause of delayed post-traumatic blindness Neurology 1989;39:863–865.)

be performed only after a metallic orbital or intraocular foreign body has been ruled out by CT scan or conventional x-ray. MR imaging is useful in assessing chiasmal trauma (74).

DIFFERENTIAL DIAGNOSIS

Causes of visual loss following trauma, other than traumatic optic neuropathy, must be considered. With a thorough history and complete ocular examination, the differential diagnosis of visual loss with disturbed pupillary function can be rapidly narrowed. An optic nerve injury can accompany other ocular injuries. If the obvious ocular injuries do not account for the loss of vision and altered pupillary function, traumatic optic neuropathy should be suspected. Traumatic

optic neuropathy can follow trivial head injuries (16,75). One must also be wary of visual loss that is merely coincidental to trauma. Monocular visual loss may not be noticed until the individual has occasion to close the uninvolved eye. In this setting the patient may attribute the visual loss to a recent traumatic event. Deciding if the visual loss is coincidental or caused by recent trauma may be difficult. Any process that can result in visual loss may be coincidentally associated with a traumatic incident such as decompensation of a vascular aneurysm, orbital or optic nerve inflammation, anterior ischemic optic neuropathy, or acute sinus disease with orbital involvement. A traumatic cavernous sinus fistula is usually accompanied by numerous orbital findings, permitting easy differentiation from traumatic optic neuropathy (76).

PATHOLOGY

Pringle conducted 174 autopsies on patients who were left unconscious from the time of head injury until death (77). In 16 cases, blood was found in the optic nerve sheath, leading him to hypothesize that indirect injury to the optic nerve was caused by hemorrhage compressing the optic nerve. These observations are also supported by the work of Hughes who explored six nerves in five patients (5).

Crompton reported the visual lesions from a series of 84 autopsies performed soon after closed head trauma (6). Optic nerve dural sheath hemorrhages were present in 69 of 84 cases (83%). Interstitial optic nerve hemorrhages were present in 30 of 84 patients (36%). The interstitial hemorrhage was present in the optic canal in 20 of these 30 cases. Shearing lesions and ischemic necrosis were present in 37 of 84 cases (44%) and the intracanalicular optic nerve was in-

volved in 30 of 37 cases. Significantly, the intracranial optic nerve also demonstrated shearing lesions and ischemic necrosis in 20 of these 37 cases. In Turner's series, skull fractures were present in 27 of 46 cases of optic nerve injury. Only four patients demonstrated an abnormality of the optic canal suggesting, at least on the basis of plain film radiographs, the rarity of canal fractures (56). More recently, studies utilizing computerized tomography suggest a 50% incidence of sphenoid fractures in cases of traumatic optic neuropathy (11). However, these studies also demonstrate the important point that traumatic optic neuropathy can occur in the absence of an optic canal fracture.

Studies using laser interferometry suggest that forces applied to the frontal bone are transferred and concentrated in the area of the optic canal (78) (Figs. 9.5 and 9.6). The entire

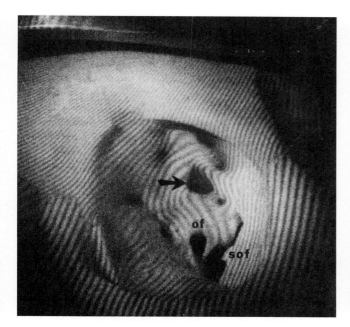

Figure 9.5. Photograph of a holographic interferogram with static loading over the glabella. *Arrow* indicates region of maximal deformation. The optic foramen *(of)* and the superior orbital fissure *(sof)* are also indicated. (From Gross CE, et al. Evidence of orbital deformation that may contribute to monocular blindness following minor frontal head trauma. J Neurosurg 1981;55:963–966.)

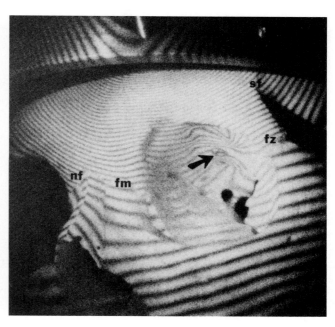

Figure 9.6. Photograph of a holographic interferogram with static loading over the medial brow showing stress lines concentrated in the left orbital roof *(arrow)*. The nasofrontal *(nf)*, frontomaxillary *(fm)*, frontozygomatic *(fz)*, and sphenofrontal sutures are indicated. (From Gross CE, et al. Evidence of orbital deformation that may contribute to monocular blindness following minor frontal head trauma. J Neurosurg 1981;55:963–966.)

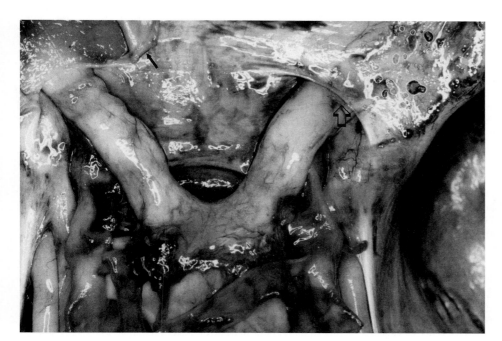

Figure 9.7. Dissection of the intracranial optic nerves and chiasm. *Open arrow* indicates the falciform dural fold in close association to the optic nerve as it enters the optic canal. The *closed arrow* indicates where the falciform dural fold has been reflected exposing the underlying sphenoid bone. (From Gossman MD, Roberts DM, Barr CC. Ophthalmic aspects of orbital injury. Clin Plast Surg 1992;19:71–85.)

force of deceleration can be loaded into the facial bones over milliseconds. Elastic deformation of the sphenoid results in the transfer of force into the intracanalicular optic nerve, where it is tightly bound causing contusion necrosis of the nerve by disrupting axons and vasculature (79). The location of a fracture is determined by the elastic limit of the involved bone. Thinner bone is more likely to deform. In contrast, thick bone is inelastic and more likely to fracture (78,80). Fractures of the canal occur, but injury of the optic nerve by displaced bone fragments appears to be infrequent (68). The intracranial optic nerve can also be injured against the falciform dural fold which overlies the sphenoid plane or where the nerve becomes fixed entering the intracranial opening of the optic foramen (6) (Fig. 9.7). Walsh hypothesized that swelling of the optic nerve within the bony canal may make the intracanalicular portion of the nerve suscepti-ble to ischemic injury (81). At present there is little information on optic nerve swelling within the optic canal (82). However, optic nerve swelling may be less significant than thought, and there is evidence that astrocytic swelling in the optic nerve is less significant than in brain injury (83).

Partial and complete avulsions of the optic nerve from the globe result from violent rotations of the globe (3). Traumatic avulsion of the optic nerve can follow self-inflicted injury, so-called autoenucleation or oedipism (84,85) or from other types of penetrating orbital injury (86). The transfer of damaging force to the optic nerve following direct injury does not imply that the nerve has been severed or precludes visual recovery (14,87). Therefore, a direct optic nerve injury may irreversibly injure a portion of the involved nerve but leave other areas with the potential for visual recovery.

PATHOGENESIS

INJURY MECHANISMS

Optic nerve injury mechanisms are thought of as primary and secondary (81). Primary mechanisms result in permanent injury to the optic nerve axons at the moment of impact. Walsh felt that primary injury resulted in mechanical shearing of the optic nerve axon and vasculature. In contrast, secondary mechanisms cause damage to the optic nerve subsequent to the force of impact. He suggested that these mechanisms included ongoing vasospasm and swelling of the optic nerve within the confines of the nonexpansile optic canal leading to worsening ischemia and further loss of axons that possessed the potential for recovery immediately following impact (79).

Experimental studies of optic nerve injury and CNS trauma support the distinction between primary and secondary injury mechanisms. These studies have used different injury methods depending on the purpose of the study (88–95). Following a severing or severe crush injury of a mammalian optic nerve, individual axons demonstrate considerable variation in their rate of Wallerian degeneration (96). Ultrastructural changes can be seen as early as 4 hours in some axons with the early formation of "retraction balls." However, normal appearing axons can be found out to 21 days. Axonal size does not appear to determine the rate of degeneration (96). Following optic nerve transection, significant descending degeneration of the retinal ganglion cells does not occur until approximately 3 weeks following injury, with maximal loss by 6 weeks (90). This corresponds to clinical observations (97–99).

There is evidence that the somas of injured and presumably uninjured adjacent neurons undergo apoptotic degeneration. This type of degeneration has been documented following ischemic optic neuropathy, experimental glaucoma, and optic nerve injury (100–102). Apoptosis, or so-called programmed cell death, encompasses a variety of secondary injury mechanisms leading to further axonal death following the initial injury. It is hoped that apoptotic cell loss can be interrupted by appropriate treatment which preserves axons that might otherwise be lost.

Ischemia is perhaps the most important aspect of secondary injury following trauma. Partial ischemia and reperfusion of transiently ischemic regions generate oxygen free radicals resulting in reperfusion damage (103,104,122,123). Until recently there was only indirect evidence for oxygen free radical damage such as reduced concentrations of ascorbic acid, alpha-tocopherol, and reduced ubiquinones following ischemia (105–107). However, $PGF_{2\alpha}$ administered via a microdialysis fiber to the rat spinal cord has been shown to directly increase extracellular levels of hydroxyl radical and malondialdehyde, which are both by-products of lipid peroxidation. Further, methylprednisolone directly blocks the release of $PGF_{2\alpha}$ following spinal cord injury and the subsequent rise levels of hydroxyl radical and malondialdehyde (108). The cell membranes of axons are composed of high concentrations of polyunsaturated lipids. The release of oxygen free radicals that follows trauma or ischemia results in the peroxidation of these lipids damaging the neural membrane. This process is thought to play a central role in cell death following ischemia or traumatic injury (109,110).

Arachidonic acid released from damaged cells is metabolized to thromboxane, PGE_1, $PGF_{2\alpha}$, hydroperoxides, and oxygen free radicals (111–113). Thromboxane induces platelet adhesion and microvascular sludging (114,115). Direct thrombin inhibition has been shown to be neuroprotective following optic nerve injury (116). Treatment with cyclooxygenase inhibitors or antioxidants also limits the severity of hypoperfusion that follows brain and spinal cord injury (117).

Several other potential mechanisms exist that can give rise to oxygen free radical production following trauma or ischemia, including the production of xanthine oxidase and the release of elemental iron from hemorrhage (118,119). The superoxide ion (O_2^-) and hydrogen peroxide (H_2O_2) are coupled to iron, which serves as a redox metal to produce the hydroxyl radical ($^{\cdot}OH$) or the feryl ion (Fe^{III}-OH), which can the oxidize a large variety of compounds including lipids (120).

Bradykinin and kallidin are agents that are activated following injury and play an important role in free radical production, alterations in intracellular calcium regulation, and the release of arachidonic acid from neurons (121). The kinins are activated by kallikrein enzymes. At the time of tissue injury the intrinsic coagulation cascade is activated with exposure of blood to collagen and basement membrane (122). Kallikrein, activated by this cascade, coverts high- and low-molecular-weight kininogens to bradykinin and kallidin, respectively. The kinins mediate early inflammation resulting in smooth muscle contraction, venous constriction, dilatation of arterioles with resulting edema, and stimulation of nociceptive receptors (123–126). Bradykinin binds to cell membrane receptors activating phospholipid metabolism (127–129). The effect of these cellular changes results in the release of arachidonic acid from the neuron (130,131). Once bradykinin has initiated the release of arachidonic acid from neurons, the resulting prostaglandins, oxygen containing free radicals, and lipid peroxides produce a loss of cerebrovascular autoregulation (103,132,133).

Following brain and spinal cord injury, there is also an indiscriminate release of excitatory amino acids that can open ligand-gated ion channels resulting in the accumulation of excessive intracellular calcium (134–136). Intracellular calcium acts as a metabolic toxin leading to cell death. Excess calcium binds to mitochondrial membranes disrupting electron transport and inhibiting ATP production (137–139). Elevated levels of intracellular calcium adversely affect enzymes that control glycolysis and activate neutral proteases and phospholipase (140–142). Activated phospholipase A_2 releases arachidonic acid which can be converted to leukotrienes and prostaglandins (143). The reader is referred to several recent reviews that discuss potential neuroprotective strategies (144–146). It has been suggested that the decreased blood flow and tissue glial swelling associated with injury and ischemia may serve to limit the influx of calcium into the injured region. At the same time the autodestructive processes that occur in irreparably injured neurons precipitate excess calcium ions creating a focal calcium sink. This last mechanism may be adaptive to limit secondary damage to adjacent axons with the potential for recovery (147).

The early events of CNS injury are associated with the release of mediators of inflammation that are chemoattractive for polymorphic neutrophils and macrophages. In CNS trauma the blood-brain barrier is significantly disrupted permitting the passage of these cells. Inflammatory cells have been found to be a prominent feature in an experimental animal model of optic nerve injury (148). Neutrophils appear to play an important role in the acute inflammatory damage that follows limb reperfusion injuries (149,150). Inducible nitric oxide synthase (iNOS) is not normally present in the normal retina; however, following experimentally induced retinal ischemia, polymorphonuclear leukocytes containing iNOS can be found in the retinal ganglion cell layer. Treatment with specific inhibitors of iNOS have been shown to be neuroprotective against the loss of retinal ganglion cells that follows retinal ischemia (151). In the first 1–2 days after injury, polymorphic neutrophils predominate but are replaced by macrophages that reach a peak at 5–7 days after injury. Macrophages are implicated in delayed tissue damage in experimental spinal cord injury models (152). There is recent evidence that T-cell-mediated immunity may also serve to limit excitatory amino acid toxicity in CNS injury (153).

PHARMACOLOGY

EXPERIMENTAL

Over the past thirty years, research in acute spinal cord trauma has demonstrated a pharmacology for very high doses of corticosteroids that is distinct from the pharmacology of steroids in the doses more typically encountered in clinical practice (154,155). In the doses usually encountered in clinical practice, corticosteroids are thought to act by decreasing the rate of protein synthesis. Receptor proteins in the cytosol mediate this action (156). In lymphocytes, this steroid-receptor complex stimulates the synthesis of an inhibitory protein (157). In addition, glucocorticoids inhibit the release of arachidonic acid from phospholipids, decreasing the production of prostaglandin endoperoxides and thromboxane (158).

Following experimental spinal cord injury, the untreated, contused segment of spinal cord demonstrates an increase in fluorescent lipid peroxidation products and concentrations of cyclic GMP, a sensitive indicator of lipid peroxidation (154). In similarly injured animals treated with 30–60 mg/ kg doses of intravenous methylprednisolone 30 minutes after injury there is a significant decrease in fluorescent lipid peroxidation products compared to untreated injured controls. Treatment with 15–30 mg/kg doses of methylprednisolone prevents the increase in cyclic GMP noted after injury without treatment. Methylprednisolone in this dose range prevents free radical pathology (105). Animals treated with 30 mg/kg doses of methylprednisolone following spinal cord trauma maintain normal spinal cord blood flow, preventing ischemia (159,160).

These studies demonstrate a biphasic dose response to methylprednisolone in a range of doses much higher than usual clinical usage. There appears to be a distinct pharmacology for massive doses of steroids (30 mg/kg). The most important of these effects appears to be as an antioxidant limiting free radical pathology (159). Very high doses of steroids may be required because one molecule of antioxidants is used for each free radical produced (105). Limiting lipid peroxidation that results from free radical formation protects the neural tissue from the secondary effects of trauma (154). Following injury, the production of prostaglandins $PGF_{2\alpha}$ and thromboxane (161) results in worsening vasoconstriction, ischemia, disturbances in cellular metabolism, and disruptions of neurofilaments (162). Cats with contusion injury to the spinal cord treated within the 15–30 mg/ kg range demonstrate improved neurophysiologic recovery (162,163).

CLINICAL EXPERIENCE

The application of corticosteroids to the treatment of brain and spinal cord trauma is based on the demonstrated efficacy of treating edema associated with brain tumors (164,165). However, translating the success of treating experimental spinal cord and brain trauma to the clinical setting represents a decade of frustration. Until the results of the second National Acute Spinal Cord Injury Study (NASCIS II) in 1990 (166), the value of methylprednisolone treatment was questioned (167). The first National Acute Spinal Cord Injury Study (NASCIS I) compared the effect of "high dose" methylprednisolone therapy (1 gram bolus followed by 1 gram per day for the next 10 days) to "standard dose" therapy (100 mg initial bolus followed by 100 mg per day for the next 10 days) (168). The high dose treatment in this protocol for a 70-kg adult equates to 14 mg/kg of methylprednisolone in a 24-hour period. This study failed to demonstrate a beneficial effect of the higher dose of methylprednisolone and lacked a placebo control.

The NASCIS II (166) was a multicenter, randomized, double blind, placebo-controlled study involving patients with acute spinal cord injury. Patients enrolled in the study were randomized to one of three treatment arms within 12 hours of injury. The treatment arms consisted of placebo, naloxone, and methylprednisolone. Naloxone, an opiate receptor partial agonist that has been effective in limiting neurologic injury in animals, was administered in an initial bolus of 5.4 mg/kg and then at a continuous infusion rate of 4.0 mg/kg/hr. Methylprednisolone was administered with an initial dose of 30 mg/kg followed by a continuous infusion at 5.4 mg/kg/hr. These treatments were provided for 24 hours. Patients were assessed neurologically by evaluating pinprick, light touch, and motor function; neurologic scores were assigned based on these evaluations.

For the purposes of the study, patients were assessed initially, at 6 weeks, and at 6 months. This study showed that treatment with methylprednisolone within 8 hours of injury at the therapeutic dose suggested by the animal spinal injury studies resulted in a significant improvement in motor and sensory function compared to placebo-treated patients. Patients treated with naloxone and patients treated with either drug more than 8 hours after injury did not demonstrate an improvement in neurologic scores compared to placebo-treated patients. Post-hoc analysis of the NASCIS II data suggests that methylprednisolone treatment initiated more than 8 hours after injury was detrimental (169). In this study, patients treated with methylprednisolone did have a higher rate of infection (7.1%) than patients treated with naloxone (3.3%) and those receiving placebo (3.6%), but this difference was not statistically significant. The success of methylprednisolone for the treatment of spinal cord injury encouraged ophthalmologists to empirically adopt this treatment for optic nerve trauma.

MANAGEMENT

The management of traumatic optic neuropathy should be guided by the Hippocratic adage to do no harm. Almost all case reports and most case series of traumatic optic neuropathy present treated cases. The older series are biased toward cases with severe visual loss. Contemporary studies contain much larger numbers of patients with mild optic nerve injuries. Consequently it is very difficult to use the retrospective data in the literature to characterize the natural history of traumatic optic neuropathy, making meaningful meta-analysis difficult (170). Without an accurate knowledge of the natural history of this injury, measuring the beneficial effect of a medical, surgical or combined approach is very difficult. This section will critically review the studies that are in the literature and summarize what is currently known concerning the clinical management of traumatic optic neuropathy.

EARLY STUDIES

Early reports concerning surgical decompression suggested it to be of little value in treating traumatic optic neuropathy (56,77,171). In these cases decompression was performed transcranially. Hooper (56) operated on five patients with traumatic optic neuropathy. Two patients recovered vision, but only one patient had optic canal decompression. Hughes (5) explored 8 cases in his series of 90 patients, with no visual improvement (5). Edmund and Godtfredsen operated on 6 patients in their series of 22 patients (21). The vision of only one patient improved following surgery, changing from no light perception to light perception. Based on this experience and the available pathologic material, Walsh felt that visual recovery was unlikely if amaurosis occurred at the moment of impact and advised against surgi-

cal intervention. He also cautioned against operating on unconscious patients. However, in cases of delayed visual loss, Walsh suggested that surgical decompression might be more promising (79).

Early papers from Japan reported that traumatic optic neuropathy was both more common in Japan and more responsive to surgical intervention (172,173). This experience has not been repeated in subsequent series from Japan. Matsuzaki et al. reported a series of 33 patients with traumatic optic neuropathy (174). Eleven patients received surgical decompression of the optic canal and 22 were managed medically. They found optic canal fractures in 51% of patients. Patients who presented with no light perception failed to demonstrate visual improvement, irrespective of treatment. Of the 11 cases receiving optic canal decompression, 8 surgeries were performed transcranially and in 3 cases the canal was decompressed transethmoidally. Vision following surgery improved in 36% of cases. Patients who were managed medically tended to have much better initial visual acuity. Medical treatment included prednisone 40–100 mg per day for 5–7 days, mannitol for 5 days, and urokinase 12,000 units per day when perineural hematoma was suspected. In medically treated patients, 50% of the individuals had improved vision.

Fujitani and coworkers reported a 16-year series of 110 cases of traumatic optic neuropathy (175). In their series, 43 patients were managed medically with corticosteroids and 70 eyes underwent transethmoidal optic canal decompression. Medical treatment consisted of oral prednisone 60 mg tapered over 2 weeks. Patients in the series after 1972 who failed to respond underwent surgical decompression. The rate of visual improvement in the medically treated cases was 44.2% (19/43). Nine eyes had an initial visual acuity of no light perception. These eyes failed to improve with medical management. Overall, eyes treated within 3 weeks of injury had a 57% rate of improvement. In cases where treatment was initiated more than 3 weeks following injury, only 15% (2/13) improved.

Seventy optic nerves underwent surgical decompression and canal fractures were found in 25% of cases at the time of surgery. The overall rate of improvement in these cases was 47.7% (33/70). Among patients undergoing surgery, 28 eyes had an initial visual acuity of no light perception. Visual improvement was seen in 7 of 28 cases (25%). Optic canal decompression was performed in 38 cases within 3 weeks with a 45% rate of improvement (17/38). In 32 eyes where vision failed to improve with medical management, surgical decompression was performed after 3 weeks. In these cases 16 of 32 eyes (50%) demonstrated improved vision after surgery. In four cases, surgery was not performed until 3 months after injury. Despite this delay, three cases improved after surgery. The results of these two series are more consistent with the Western experience.

The widespread introduction of orbital imaging and neuroimaging has provided a more accurate method for assessing the mechanisms of visual loss. This has led to a much more specific anatomical approach in planning surgical intervention. Imaging can identify pathology that when addressed surgically may result in visual improvement (9). Computed tomography has also demonstrated impingement of the optic nerve by bone fragments. Anecdotally, visual recovery has followed surgical reduction of such bone fragments (72).

The management of orbital hemorrhage that creates a compressive orbitopathy is well defined and relatively incontrovertible. The initial diagnosis is clinical. Patients present with a history of trauma. Vision may be extremely poor due to optic nerve embarrassment or compromise of retinal perfusion. Proptosis will be present and the intraocular pressure may be significantly elevated. Initial treatment is canthotomy and cantholysis to permit expansion of the orbital contents. If this does not provide sufficient relief, orbital decompression may be necessary to provide sufficient space for orbital soft tissue expansion (176,177). These initial maneuvers should be followed by orbital imaging to rule out a subperiosteal hemorrhage or other pathology which may explain the basis of visual compromise. The role for anterior segment paracentesis in the treatment of orbital hemorrhage is limited. The use of steroids to treat optic nerve compromise following orbital hemorrhage is unsettled.

MEGADOSE STEROIDS

Anderson et al. introduced the use of high dose corticosteroids for the treatment of traumatic optic neuropathy based on salutary effects of corticosteroids in the treatment of experimental CNS injury (178). They proposed a treatment protocol formulated on their experiences in treating seven patients with traumatic optic neuropathy with a combination of corticosteroids and surgery. They advised initial treatment with corticosteroids (dexamethasone, 3–5 mg/kg/day). Surgery was advocated in cases of delayed visual loss that fail to improve with treatment and in cases with initial visual improvement followed by worsening of vision despite treatment. Three of six patients had return of vision on high dose corticosteroids. Four of their patients underwent transethmoid-sphenoid optic canal decompression. Postoperatively, vision returned in only one case. Since this study, subsequent studies have combined corticosteroid treatment with surgical intervention, making it difficult to determine the therapeutic value of a particular treatment. Additionally, the percentage of patients with no light perception vision in these studies is smaller that earlier studies (Table 9.2). This most likely reflects the greater awareness of the condition and more aggressive recruitment of patients compared to earlier studies. This difference in recruitment biases these studies to better outcomes irrespective of treatment when comparison is made to earlier studies.

Seiff's study of high dose corticosteroid treatment of patients with indirect optic nerve trauma was a nonconsecutive nonrandomized retrospective series of 36 patients (11). Prior to 1983 his patients with traumatic optic neuropathy were not treated with corticosteroids. Therefore his study essentially compares the outcome of patients with traumatic optic neuropathy seen prior to 1983 with those seen after 1983. Fifteen patients did not receive corticosteroids. Twenty-one patients received dexamethasone (1 mg/kg/day). Therapy was initiated within 48 hours. If no improvement was seen within 72 hours the corticosteroids were stopped. If improvement occurred, treatment was continued until visual improvement leveled off. Steroids were then tapered off over several days. Visual improvement was seen in 13 of 21 treated patients (62%) and 5 of 15 untreated patients (33%), but this difference was not found to be significant. This study reported that treated patients recovered more vision and at a faster rate than untreated patients, and that the difference was significant. However, these conclusions are probably not meaningful. The two groups differed in initial visual acuity. The untreated group actually had much better overall vision, decreasing the opportunity for visual recovery. Four of 15 patients in the untreated group had vision that was 20/50 or better in the affected eye and 11 of 14 had vision of count fingers or worse; in contrast, all of the affected eyes in the treated group had a visual acuity of 20/200 or worse, which suggests that the two groups are probably not comparable. Additionally, as noted in the discussion of what constitutes high dose steroids, 1 mg/kg/day of dexamethasone is unlikely to provide an antioxidant effect.

Spoor and coworkers presented an uncontrolled, nonconsecutive, retrospective study of 21 patients (22 eyes) with traumatic optic neuropathy studied at two centers (13). Eight patients at one center received dexamethasone (20 mg every 6 hours, IV) and 13 patients at the second center received methylprednisolone (30 mg/kg loading followed by 15.0 mg/kg every 6 hours, IV). Treatment was initiated at a mean of 4.2 days following injury in the methylprednisolone group and 17 hours in the dexamethasone group. The authors reported that 7 of 9 eyes in the dexamethasone group and 12 of 13 patients in the methylprednisolone group improved.

The study suffers from being uncontrolled and nonconsecutive. It is not possible to draw conclusions about the efficacy of corticosteroid treatment in the management of traumatic optic neuropathy based on this study. It is interesting that the methylprednisolone-treated patients appeared to do as well as dexamethasone-treated patients, despite the fact that as a group the methylprednisolone patients had treatment started 3 days later than the dexamethasone treated individuals.

Joseph and coworkers reported a series of 14 patients with traumatic optic neuropathy managed with transethmoidal-sphenoidal optic canal decompression (179). This was also a nonconsecutive retrospective study. The patients in this series were treated with dexamethasone both before and after surgery. The interval between injury and surgery varied from one to five days. Patients who were comatose and patients with "local ocular lesions" were excluded from the study. There was no morbidity or mortality associated with the surgeries. Overall, 11 of 14 patients demonstrated visual improvement, including 3 of 5 patients who had a preoperative visual acuity of no light perception in the injured eye. Despite the lack of nonsurgical control patients, these investigators felt strongly that surgical decompression helped their patients. They proposed that patients with indirect traumatic optic neuropathy be immediately treated with both dexamethasone and surgical optic canal decompression if there is no contra-indications for surgery and no ocular injuries that might preclude visual recovery. They do not recommend surgery if more than seven days have past since the injury.

The retrospective series presented by Mauriello and coauthors included 23 patients with vision loss after trauma (57). All patients were seen at the same trauma center and treated within 48 hours. All patients received an initial loading dose of methylprednisolone (1 gram IV) followed by methylprednisolone 250 mg IV every 6 hours for 72 hours. Orbital hemorrhages with elevated intraocular pressure were treated with immediate lateral canthotomy. Orbital computed tomography was performed to identify "surgically treatable pathology."

The authors presumed that optic nerve sheath enlargement represented intrasheath hemorrhage. Patients who failed to respond to the steroids were considered for optic nerve sheath decompression if the sheath was distended, or for transcranial optic canal decompression if "the optic canal or optic nerve appeared compressed by bone spicules." Only 2 of 23 had initial vision that was 20/200 or better. Nine of 16 patients who only received steroids improved. The authors note that three of the nine patients who improved in this group had immediate canthotomy to treat an orbital hemorrhage. Three of the 23 patients additionally had optic nerve sheath decompression and one improved. Four patients had combined optic nerve sheath decompression and transcranial optic canal decompression. Three out of four of these patients had bilateral injuries. Visual improvement could be documented in only two out of seven eyes. Additional small case series have not greatly contributed to expand our understanding of treating traumatic optic neuropathy. Some of these studies are summarized in Table 9.2.

In November 1993, a conference was held at the Massachusetts Eye and Ear Infirmary on Extracranial Optic Nerve Decompression (Extracranial Optic Canal Decompression, November 6–7, 1993, Boston). At this meeting it was clear that the Second National Acute Spinal Cord Injury Study (NASCIS II) data had a significant impact on how clinicians thought about treating traumatic optic neuropathy. In developing The International Optic Nerve Trauma Study, it was felt unethical to have a placebo control and the results of the NASCIS II study were used in making this case. The International Optic Nerve Trauma Study was initially conducted as a randomized controlled pilot study to assess recruitment feasibility. However, recruitment was insufficient and the study was converted to a comparative, nonrandomized interventional study (23). A total of 133 patients met criteria for inclusion and analysis. There were three treatment arms: untreated patients, steroid treatment, and surgery with or without steroids. The authors concluded that there was no clear benefit for either corticosteroid therapy or optic canal decompression. The study has some significant limitations, but it represents the largest, most unbiased study of traumatic optic neuropathy to date. Further, it will take considerable effort to mount a better study because traumatic optic neuropathy, while a dramatic and vexing clinical problem, is relatively rare.

Critical review of the traumatic optic neuropathy literature does not provide statistical evidence to conclude that either surgery, corticosteroids, or a combination of corticosteroids is more beneficial than no treatment; yet the International Optic Nerve Trauma Study was organized with a strong bias that these treatments are beneficial. All but 9 out of 133 patients enrolled in the International Optic Nerve Trauma Study received surgery or corticosteroids within 7 days of treatment. Despite a strong bias toward treatment, no treatment benefit was found.

Mounting evidence, including the International Optic Nerve Trauma Study, raises significant questions regarding the potential benefits of corticosteroids in the treatment of traumatic optic neuropathy. First, there are no statistically valid studies supporting the use of corticosteroids in the treatment of traumatic optic neuropathy. The value of corticosteroids in the treatment of CNS injury varies by anatomic region and injury circumstance. As noted above, analysis of the NASCIS II data demonstrated that methylprednisolone treatment initiated more than 8 hours after spinal cord injury is detrimental (169). Treatment with glucocorticoids have been shown to exacerbate ischemic-induced hippocampal excitotoxicity (180,181). Even in the absence of ischemia, glucocorticoids can induce apoptosis in the hippocampus (182).

Additionally, there are now two lines of experimental evidence that suggest methylprednisolone is harmful for injured optic nerves. Steinsapir and coworkers conducted a study using a moderate crush injury to optic nerves of male rats. Thirty minutes after injury, animals received one of five intravenous treatments: saline; or methylprednisolone 30 mg/kg, 60 mg/kg, 90 mg/kg, or 120 mg/kg. Treatment was repeated at 6-hour intervals for three additional treatments. Animals were allowed to recover for 6 weeks at which time they were sacrificed and the remaining axons in the injured nerves were counted. The saline-treated animals retained the greatest number of axons and there appeared to be a dose dependent decline in residual axons with increasing doses of methylprednisolone. Axon counts (means + s.e.m.) were as follows:

Saline = 16,670 ± 8,900 (n = 5);
Methylprednisolone 30 mg/kg = 8,098 ± 4,741 (n = 5);
Methylprednisolone 60 mg/kg = 6,925 ± 6,517 (n = 4);
Methylprednisolone 90 mg/kg = 2,663 ± 2,653 (n = 4);
Methylprednisolone 120 mg/kg = 6,149 ± 3,487
    (n = 6).

The data revealed that saline-treated animals retained more axons than those administered methylprednisolone ($p < .02$) (183). In this study, methylprednisolone exacerbated axonal loss following optic nerve trauma.

The second line of evidence comes from work on an experimental model of multiple sclerosis. Diem and coinvestigators looked at the effect of high dose methylprednisolone on experimental autoimmune optic neruritis (184). In this study, methylprednisolone significantly increased apoptotic retinal ganglion cell loss. As of the writing of this chapter, these results were too new to have been investigated clinically. However, such a study will need to be mounted given that methylprednisolone therapy continues to be used to treat optic neuritis (185–187).

Given the lack of clinical evidence that corticosteroids are beneficial in the treatment of traumatic optic neuropathy, combined now with two lines of experimental evidence that methylprednisolone is harmful to the injured optic nerve, clinicians should consider abandoning the routine use of megadose corticosteroids for the treatment of traumatic optic neuropathy. Our best evidence is inconclusive so there can be no standard of care regarding a "best practice." In the setting of severe visual loss, there is often a perceived need to take heroic actions such as using megadose steroids or performing optic canal decompression. Informed consent must address the likelihood that megadose steroids may actually worsen the visual outcome. Clinicians who feel compelled to treat traumatic optic neuropathy with megadose steroids because they are beneficial in spinal cord trauma, should keep in mind that methylprednsiolone when administered more than 8 hours after spinal cord injury was harmful to outcome (169).

Further, clinical studies under the auspices of an institutional review board should strongly shift away from the bias that methylprednisolone is beneficial for optic nerve trauma. It can now be argued that it is unethical to enroll patients into a megadose corticosteroid for optic nerve trauma treatment study without some new experimental evidence showing a benefit in an animal model of optic nerve trauma. This standard was not imposed when organizing the International Optic Nerve Trauma Study.

SURGICAL CONSIDERATIONS

Surgical intervention for traumatic optic neuropathy also remains empirical. Crompton's study suggests that a large percentage of intracanalicular injuries take place at the falciform dural fold (6). This is a location that will not benefit from optic canal decompression. However, it is possible that subsets of injuries might benefit from surgical intervention. For example, reduction of bone fragments impinging on the optic nerve is a compelling reason for surgical intervention, especially in cases of delayed visual loss, although these may represent untreatable injuries (68). The hypothesis that reducing the canal fracture benefits the injured nerve remains untested. The fracture may just be residual evidence of the forces imparted into the nerve at the moment of impact; lifting these fragments of bone may not provide any therapeutic benefit.

Case reports and small series demonstrate visual improvement following evacuation of intraoptic nerve sheath hematomas, or subperiosteal hematomas causing optic nerve embarrassment (9,188). These examples provide only limited experience on which to base recommendations for surgery for individual patients. Intracanalicular optic nerve injury is the most common form of traumatic optic neuropathy. Not surprisingly, decompression of the optic canal is the most commonly reported surgical intervention. Theoretically, opening the canal to provide room for the optic nerve to swell into should be beneficial. However, the International Optic Nerve Trauma Study failed to demonstrate a beneficial effect for surgical decompression. This study had significant limitations and it is possible that the study did not have the power to identify a small beneficial effect for a subsets of patients. Consequently, it is difficult to advocate a set of best practices based on this study. Certainly in the case of orbital hemorrhage causing optic nerve compromise, there is little controversy regarding the need to provide immediate surgical relief of the compressive orbitopathy.

Lubben and coworkers reported their experience with surgical decompression within hours of trauma (188). As many of their cases had relatively good visual acuities before surgery and their series also included comatose patients, it is difficult to evaluate the relative success of their approach. However, it is reasonable to expect that if surgery is to be of benefit, then performing it earlier may decrease secondary axonal loss. An orbitotomy provides the best access for the evacuation of an optic nerve sheath hematoma, reduction of a depressed lateral orbital wall fracture that compromises the optic nerve, or drainage of a subperiosteal hematoma with posterior compression of the optic nerve. Consequently an accurate anatomical diagnosis must be made to plan appropriate surgical intervention. Walsh's admonition (81) against operating on the unconscious patient will continue to have validity until clear evidence establishes the value of surgical intervention. Given the uncertain benefit of these procedures, the patient and their significant others need to be thoughtfully counseled regarding surgery.

REFERENCES

1. Hedges TR, Gragoudas ES. Traumatic anterior ischemic optic neuropathy. Ann Ophthalmol 1981;13:625–628.
2. Wyllie AM, McLeod D, Cullen JF. Traumatic ischaemic optic neuropathy. Br J Ophthalmol 1972;56:851–853.
3. Park JH, Frenkel M, Dobbie JG et al. Evulsion of the optic nerve. Am J Ophthalmol 1971;72:969–971.

4. Turner JWA. Indirect injury of the optic nerves. Brain 1943;66:140–151.
5. Hughes B. Indirect injury of the optic nerves and chiasma. Bull Johns Hopkins Hosp 1962;111:98–126.
6. Crompton MR. Visual lesions in closed head injury. Brain 1970;93:785–792.
7. Heinz GW, Nunery WR, Grossman B. Traumatic chiasmal syndrome associated with midline basilar skull fracture. American J Ophthalmol 1994;117:90–96.
8. Hassan A, Crompton JL, Sandhu A. Traumatic chiasmal syndrome: A series of 19 patients. Clin Experiment Ophthalmol 2002;30:273–280.
9. Guy J, Sherwood M, Day AL. Surgical treatment of progressive visual loss in traumatic optic neuropathy: Report of two cases. J Neurosurg 1989;70:799–801.
10. Keane JR. Neurologic eye signs following motorcycle accidents. Arch Neurol 1989;46:761–762.
11. Seiff SR. High dose corticosteroids for treatment of vision loss due to indirect injury to the optic nerve. Ophthalmic Surg 1990;21:389–395.
12. Obenchain TG, Killeffer FA, Stern WE. Indirect injury of the optic nerves and chiasm with closed head injury: Report of three cases. Bull Los Angeles Neurol Soc 1973;38:13–20.
13. Spoor TC, Hartel WC, Lensink DB et al. Treatment of traumatic optic neuropathy with corticosteriods. Am J Ophthalmol 1990;110:665–669.
14. Feist RM, Kline LB, Morris RE et al. Recovery of vision after presumed direct optic nerve injury. Ophthalmology 1987;94:1567–1569.
15. Cavallini GM, Lugli N, Campi L et al. Bottle-cork injury to the eye: A review of 13 cases. Eur J Ophthalmol 2003;13:287–291.
16. Sullivan G, Helveston EM. Optic atrophy after seemingly trivial trauma. Arch Ophthalmol 1969;81:159–161.
17. Maniglia AJ. Fatal and major complications secondary to nasal sinus surgery. Laryngoscope 1989;99:276–283.
18. Dunya IM, Salman SD, Shore JW. Ophthalmic complications of endoscopic ethmoid surgery and their management. Am J Otolaryngol 1996;17:322–331.
19. Rose C, Rose GE, Lenthall R et al. Major orbital complications of endoscopic sinus surgery. Br J Ophthalmol 2001;85:598–603.
20. Graham SM, Nerad JA. Orbital complications in endoscopic sinus surgery using powered instrumenation. Laryngoscope 2003;113:874–878.
21. Edmund J, Godtfredsen E. Unilateral optic atrophy following head injury. Acta Ophthalmol 1963;41:693–697.
22. Nau HE, Gerhard L, Foerster M et al. Optic nerve trauma: Clinical, electrophysiological and histological remarks. Acta Neurochir (Wien) 1987;89:16–27.
23. Levin LA, Beck RW, Joseph MP et al. The treatment of traumatic optic neuropathy: The international optic nerve trauma study. Ophthalmology 1999;106:1268–1277.
24. Russell WR. Injury to cranial nerves including the optic nerves and chiasma. In Brock S, ed. Injuries of the Skull, Brain and Spinal Cord. London, Bailliere, 1940:113–122.
25. Al-Qurainy A, Stassen LFA, Dutton GN et al. The characteristics of midfacial fractures and the association with ocular injury: a prospective study. Br J Oral Maxillofacial Sur 1991;29:291–301.
26. Lessell S. Indirect optic nerve trauma. Arch Ophthalmol 1989;107:382–386.
27. Wang BH, Robertson BC, Girotto JA et al. Traumatic Optic Neuropathy: A review of 61 patients. Plast Reconstr Surg 2001;107:1655–1664.
28. Hislop WS, Dutton GN. Retrobulbar hemorrhage: Can blindness be prevented? Injury 1994;25:663–665.
29. Polito E, Leccisotti A. Diagnosis and treatment of orbital hemorrhagic lesions. Ann Ophthalmol 1994;26:85–93.
30. Atalla ML, McNab AA, Sullivan TJ et al. Nontraumatic subperiosteal orbital hemorrhage. Ophthalmology 2001;108:183–189.
31. Oruc S, Sener EC, Akman A et al. Bilateral orbital hemorrhage induced by labor. Eur J Ophthalmol 2001;11:77–79.
32. Leong JK, Ghabrial R, McCluskey PJ et al. Orbital hemorrhage complication following postoperative thrombolysis. Br J Ophthalmol 2003;87:655–656.
33. Curran EL, Flemming JC, Rice K et al. Orbital compression syndrome in sickle cell disease. Ophthalmology 1997;104:1610–1615.
34. Guirgis MF, Segal WA, Leuder GT. Subperiosteal orbital hemorrhage as initial manifestation of Christmas disease (factor IX deficiency). Am J Ophthalmol 2002;133:584–585.
35. Ganesh A, William RR, Mitra S et al. Orbital involvement in sickle cell disease: A report of five cases and review of literature. Eye 2001;15:774–780.
36. White WL, Mundis RJ. Delayed obital hemorrhage after cataract surgery in a patient with an acquired factor VIII inhibitor. Am J Ophthalmol 2001;132:785–786.
37. Yip CC, McCulley TJ, Kersten RC et al. Proptosis after hair pulling. Ophthal Plast Reconstr Surg 2003;19:154–155.
38. Edge KR, Martin J, Nicoll V. Retrobulbar hemorrhage after 12,500 retrobulbar blocks. Anesthes Analg 1993;76:1019–1022.
39. Conni RJ, Osher RH. Retrobulbar hemorrhage. Ophthalmology 1991;98:1153–1155.
40. Ruben S. The incidence of complications with retrobulbar injection of anaesthetic for ophthalmic surgery. Acta Ophthalmologica 1992;70:836–838.
41. Kallio H, Paloheimo M, Maunuksela EL. Haemorrhage and risk factors associated with retrobulbar/peribulbar block: A prospective study in 1,383 patients. Br J Anaesth 2000;85:708–711.
42. Klein ML, Jampol LM, Condon PE et al. Central retinal artery occlusion without

43. retrobulbar hemorrhage after retrobulbar anaesthesia. Am J Ophthalmol 1982;93:573–577.
43. Morgan CM, Schatz H, Vine AK et al. Ocular complications associated with retrobulbar injections. Ophthalmology 1988;95:660–665.
44. Gausas RE. Complications of blepharoplasty. Facial Plast Surg 1999;15:243–253.
45. Custer PL, Lind A, Trinkaus KM. Complications of supramid orbital implants. Ophthal Plast Reconstr Surg 2003;19:62–67.
46. Gilhotra JS, McNab AA, McKelvie P et al. Late orbital haemorrhage around alloplastic orbital floor implants: a case series and review. Clin Exp Ophthalmol 2003;30:352–355.
47. Goldberg SH, Sassani JW, Parnes RE. Traumatic intraconal hematic cyst of the orbit. Arch Ophthalmol 1992;110:378–380.
48. Wolter JR, Leenhouts JA, Coulthard SW. Clinical picture and management of subperiosteal hematoma of the orbit. J Pediatric Ophthalmol 1976;13:136–138.
49. Tonami H, Kuginuki Y, Okimura T et al. MRI of subperiosteal hematoma of the orbit. J Comput Assist Tomogr 1994;18:549–551.
50. Udstuen GJ, Claar JM. Imaging of acute head injury in the adult. Semin Ultrasound CT MR 2001;22:135–147.
51. Davis PC, Newman NJ. Advances in neuroimaging of the visual pathways. Am J Ophthalmol 1996;121:690–705.
52. Jordan DR, White GL, Thiese SM. Orbital emphysema: A potentially blinding complication following orbital fractures. Ann Emerg Med 1988;17:853–855.
53. Carter KD, Nerad JA. Fluctuating visual loss secondary to orbital emphysema. Am J Ophthalmol 1987;104:664–665.
54. Wood BJ, Mirvis SE, Shanmuganathan K. Tension pneumocephalus and tension orbital emphysema following blunt trauma. Ann Emerg Med 1996;28:446–449.
55. Buckley MJ, Turvey TA, Schumann SP et al. Orbital emphysema causing vision loss after a dental extraction. J Am Dental Assoc 1990;120:421–424.
56. Hooper RS. Orbital complications of head injury. Br J Surg 1951;39:126–138.
57. Mauriello JA, DeLuca J, Krieger A et al. Management of traumatic optic neuropathy: A study of 23 patients. Br J Ophthalmol 1992;76:349–352.
58. Thompson HS. Afferent pupillary defects. Am J Ophthalmol 1966;62:860–873.
59. Alford MA, Nerad JA, Carter KD. Predictive value of the initial quantified relative afferent pupillary defect in 19 consecutive patients with traumat optic neuropathy. Ophthal Plast Reconstr Surg 2001;17:323–327.
60. Hillman JS, Myska V, Nissim S. Complete avulsion of the optic nerve. Br J Ophthalmol 1975;59:503–509.
61. Hupp SL, Buckley EG, Byrne SF et al. Posttraumatic venous obstructive retinopathy associated with enlarged optic nerve sheath. Arch Ophthalmol 1984;102:254–256.
62. Crowe NW, Nickles TP, Troost T et al. Intrachiasmal hemorrhage: A cause of delayed post-traumatic blindness. Neurology 1989;39:863–865.
63. Manor RS, Cohen S, Svetliza E et al. Papilledema in traumatic lesion of optic nerve with amaurosis. J Clin Neuroophthalmol 1986;6:100–105.
64. Feinsod M, Rowe H, Auerbach E. Changes in the electroretinogram in patients with optic nerve lesions. Doc Ophthalmol 1971;29:169–200.
65. Feinsod M, Auerbach E. Electrophysiological examinations of the visual system in the acute phase after head injury. Eur Neurol 1973;9:56–64.
66. Jayle GE, Tassy AF. Prognostic value of the electroretinogram in severe recent ocular trauma. Br J Ophthalmol 1970;54:51–58.
67. Mahapatra AK. Visual evoked potentials in optic nerve injury. Does it merit a mention? Acta Neurochir 1991;112:47–49.
68. Kennerdell JS, Amsbaugh GA, Myers EN. Transantral-ethmoidal decompression of optic canal fracture. Arch Ophthalmol 1976;94:1040–1043.
69. Manfredi SJ, Mohammad RR, Sprinkle PS et al. Computerized tomographic scan findings in facial fractures associated with blindness. Plast Reconst Surg 1981;68:479–490.
70. Seiff SR, Berger MS, Guyon J et al. Computed tomographic evaluation of the optic canal in sudden traumatic blindness. Am J Ophthalmol 1984;98:751–755.
71. Knox BE, Gates GA, Berry SM. Optic nerve decompression via the lateral facial approach. Laryngoscope 1990;100:458–462.
72. Lipkin AF, Woodson GE, Miller RH. Visual loss due to orbital fracture. The role of early reduction. Arch Otolaryngol Head Neck Surg 1987;113:81–83.
73. Takehara S, Tanaka T, Uemura K et al. Optic nerve injury demonstrated by MRI with STIR sequences. Neuroradiology 1994;36:512–514.
74. Arkin MS, Rubin PA, Bilyk JR et al. Anterior chiasmal optic nerve avulsion. Am J Neuroradiol 1996;17:1777–1781.
75. Purvin V. Evidence of orbital deformation in indirect optic nerve injury. Weight lifter's optic neuropathy. J Clin Neuroophthalmol 1988;8:9–11.
76. Keane JR, Talla A. Posttraumatic intracavernous aneurysm: Epistaxis with monocular blindness preceded by chromatopsia. Arch Ophthalmol 1972;87:701–705.
77. Pringle JH. Atrophy of the optic nerve following diffused violence to the skull. Br Med J 1922;2:1156–1157.
78. Gross CE, DeKock JK, Panje WR et al. Evidence for orbital deformation that may contribute to monocular blindness following minor frontal head trauma. J Neurosurg 1981;55:963–966.
79. Walsh FB, Hoyt WF. Clinical Neuro-Ophthalmology. Ed 3, Vol. 3. Baltimore, Williams & Wilkins, 1969:2380.

80. Spetzler RF, Spetzler H. Holographic interferometry applied to the study of the human skull. J Neurosurg 1980;52:825–828.
81. Walsh FB. Pathological: clinical correlations. I. Indirect trauma to the optic nerves and chiasm. II. Certain cerebral involvements associated with defective blood supply. Invest Ophthalmol 1966;5:433–449.
82. Spoor TC, McHenry JG. Management of traumatic optic neurpathy. J Craniomaxillofac Trauma 1996;2:14–26.
83. Maxwell WL, Irvine A, Watt C et al. The microvascular response to stretch injury in the adult guinea pig visual system. J Neurotrauma 1991;8:271–279.
84. Aung T, Yap E, Fam HB et al. Oedipism. Aust NZ J Ophthalmol 1996;24:153–157.
85. Krauss HR, Yee RD, Foos RY. Autoenucleation. Surv Ophthalmol 1984;29:179–187.
86. Morris WR, Osborn FD, Fleming JC. Traumatic evulsion of the globe. Ophthal Plast Reconstr Surg 2002;18:261–267.
87. Spoor TC, Mathog RH. Restoration of vision after optic canal decompression: Letter. Arch Ophthalmol 1986;104:804–806.
88. Anderson DR. Ascending and descending optic atrophy produced experimentally in squirrel monkeys. Am J Ophthalmol 1973;76:693–711.
89. Yew DT, Li WWY. Early patterns of neuronal degeneration in the retina of the goldfish after optic nerve sectioning. Acta Morphol Neerl Scand 1986;24:123–132.
90. Quigley HA, Davis EB, Anderson DR. Descending optic nerve degeneration in primates. Invest Ophthalmol Visual Sci 1977;16:841–849.
91. Stevenson JA. Growth of retinal ganglion cell axons following optic nerve crush in adult hamsters. Exp Neurol 1987;97:77–89.
92. Cho EYP, So KF. Regrowth of retinal ganglion cell axons into a peripheral nerve graft in the adult hamster is enhanced by a concurrent optic nerve crush. Exp Brain Res 1989;78:567–574.
93. Selles-Navarro I, Ellezam B, Fajardo R et al. Retinal ganglion cell and nonneuronal cell responses to a microcrush lesion of adult rat optic nerve. Exp Neurol 2001;167:282–289.
94. Sautter J, Schwartz M, Duvdevani R et al. GM1 ganglioside treatment reduces visual deficits after graded crush of the rat optic nerve. Brain Res 1991;565:23–33.
95. Klocker N, Zerfowski M, Gellrich NC et al. Morphological and functional analysis of an incomplete CNS fiber tract lesion: Graded crush of the rat optic nerve. J Neurosci Meth 2001;110:147–153.
96. Hasegawa M, Rosenbluth J, Ishise J. Nodal and paranodal structural changes in mouse and rat optic nerve during Wallerian degeneration. Brain Res 1988;452:345–357.
97. Lundstrum M, Frisen L. Evolution of descending optic atrophy: A case report. Acta Ophthalmol 1975;53:738–746.
98. Medeiros FA, Moura FC, Vessani RM et al. Axonal loss after traumatic optic neuropathy documented by optical coherence tomography. Am J Ophthalmol 2003;135:406–408.
99. Miyahara T, Kurimoto Y, Kurokawa T et al. Alterations in retinal nerve fiber layer thickness following indirect traumtic optic neuropathy detected by nerve fiber analyzer, GDx-N. Am J Ophthalmol 2003;136:361–364.
100. Levin LA, Louhab A. Apoptosis of retinal ganglion cells in anterior ischemic optic neuropathy. Arch Ophthalmol 1996;114:488–491.
101. Garcia-Valenzuela E, Gorczyca W, Darzynkiewicz Z et al. Apoptosis in adult retinal ganglion cells after axotomy. J Neurobiol 1994;25:431–438.
102. Levkovitch H, Quigley HA, Kerrigan-Baumrind LA et al. Optic nerve transection in monkeys may result in secondary degeneration of retinal ganglion cells. Invest Ophthalmol Vis Sci 2001;42:957–982.
103. Flamm ES, Demopoulos HB, Seligman ML et al. Free radicals in cerebral ischemia. Stroke 1978;9:445–447.
104. Hall ED, McCall JM, Means ED. Therapeutic potential of the lazaroids (21-aminosteroids) in acute central nervous system trauma, ischemia and subarachnoid hemorrhage. Adv Pharmacol 1994;28.
105. Demopoulos HS, Flamm ES, Seligman ML et al. Further studies on free-radical pathology in the major central nervous system disorders: Effect of very high doses of methylprednisolone on the functional outcome, morphology, and chemistry of experimental spinal cord impact injury. Can J Physiol Pharmacol 1982;60:1415–1424.
106. Demopoulos HB, Flamm E, Seligman M et al. Oxygen free radicals in central nervous system ischemia and trauma. In Autor AP, ed. Pathology of Oxygen. New York, Academic Press, 1982:127–155.
107. Cristofori L, Tavazzi B, Gambin R et al. Early onset of lipid peroxidation after human traumatic brain injury: A fatal limitation for the free radical scavenger pharmacological therapy? J Investig Med 2001;49:450–458.
108. Liu D, Li L, Augustus L. Prostaglandin release by spinal cord injury mediates production of hydroxyl radical, malondialdehyde and cell death: A site of neuroprotective action of methylprednisolone. J Neurochem 2001;77:1036–1047.
109. Demopoulos HB, Flamm ES, Pietronigro DD et al. The free radical pathology and the microcirculation in the major central nervous system disorders. Acta Physiol Scand 1980;492(suppl):91–119.
110. Hanwehr RV, Smith M, Siesjo BK. Extra- and intracellular pH during near-complete forebrain ischemia in the rat. J Neurochem 1986;46:331–339.
111. Gaudet RJ, Levine L. Transient cerebral ischemia and brain prostaglandins. Biochem Biophys Res Commun 1979;86:893–901.
112. Kukreja RC, Kontos HA, Hess ML et al. PGH synthetase and lipoxygenase generate superoxide in the presence of NADH or NADPH. Circ Res 1986;59:612–619.
113. Phillis JW, O'Regan MH. The role of phospholipases, cyclooxygenases, and lipoxygenages in cerebral ischemic/traumatic injuries. Crit Rev Neurobiol 2003;15:61–90.
114. Gryglewski RJ, Buntin S, Moncada S et al. Arterial walls are protected against deposition of platelet thrombi by a substance (prostaglandin X) which they make from prostaglandin endoperoxides. Prostaglandin 1976;12:685–713.
115. Moncada S, Gryglewski S, Bunting S et al. A lipid peroxide inhibits the enzyme in blood vessel microsomes that generates from prostaglandin endoperoxides, the substance (prostaglandin X) which prevents platelet aggregation. Prostaglandins 1976;12:715–735.
116. Freidmann I, Yoles E, Schwartz M. Thrombin attenuation is neuroprotective in the injured rat optic nerve. J Neurochem 2001;76:641–649.
117. Wei EP, Kontos HA, Dietrich WD et al. Inhibition by free radical scavengers and by cyclooxygenase inhibitors of pial arteriolar abnormalities from concussive brain injuries in cats. Cir Res 1981;48:95–103.
118. McCord JM. Oxygen derived free radicals in postischemic injury. N Engl J Med 1985;312:159–163.
119. Lewen A, Matz P, Chan PH. Free radical pathways in CNS injury. J Neurotrauma 2000;17:871–890.
120. Gutteridge JMC. Iron promoters of the Fenton reaction and lipid peroxidation can be released from hemoglobin by peroxides. FEBS Lett 1986;201:291–295.
121. Rodell TC. The kallikrein/kinin system and kinin antagonists in trauma. Immunopharmacology 1996;33:279–283.
122. Erdos EG, Miwa I. Effect of endotoxin shock on the plasma kallikrein-kinin system of the rabbit. Fed Proc 1968;27:92–95.
123. Aksoy MO, Harakal C, Smith JB et al. Mediation of bradykinin-induced contraction in canine veins via thromboxane/prostaglandin endoperoxide receptor activation. Br J Pharmacol 1990;99:461–466.
124. Hori Y, Katori M, Harada Y et al. Potentiation of bradikinin-induced nociceptive response by arachidonate metabolites in dogs. Eur J Pharmacol 1986;132:47–52.
125. Northover AM. Modification by some antagonists of the shape changes of venous endothelial cells in response to inflammatory agents in vitro. Agents Action 1990;29:184–188.
126. Wahl M, Gorlach C, Hortobagyi T et al. Effects of bradykinin in the cerebral circulation. Acta Physiol Hung 1999;86:155–160.
127. Francel P, Dawson G. Bradykinin induces the biphasic production of lysophosphatidyl inositol and diacylglycerol in a dorsal root ganglion x neurotumor hybrid cell line, F-11. Biochem Biophys Res Commun 1988;152:724–731.
128. Gammon CM, Allen AC, Morell P. Bradykinin stimulates phosphoinositide hydrolysis and mobilization of arachidonic acid in dorsal root ganglion neurons. J Neurochem 1989;53:95–101.
129. Yano K, Higashida H, Inoue R et al. Bradykinin-induced rapid breakdown of phosphatidylinositol 4,5-biphosphate in neuroblastoma X glioma hybrid NB 108–15 cells. J Biol Chem 1984;259:10201–10207.
130. Gecse A, Mezei Z, Telegdy G. The effect of bradykinin and its fragments on the arachidonate cascade of brain microvessels. Adv Exp Med Biol 1989;247A:249–254.
131. Castillo MR, Babson JR. Ca(2+)-dependent mechanisms of cell injury in cultured cortical neurons. Neuroscience 1998;86:1133–1144.
132. Anderson DK, Means ED. Iron-induced lipid peroxidation in spinal cord: Protection with mannitol and methylprednisolone. Free Radical Biol Med 1985;1:59–64.
133. Yamamoto M, Shima T, Uozumi T et al. A possible role of lipid peroxidation in cellular damages caused by cerebral ischemia and the protective effect of alphatocopherol administration. Stroke 1983;14:977–982.
134. Cotman CW, Iverson LL. Excitatory amino acids in the brain: Focus on NMDA receptors. TINS 1987;10:263–265.
135. Hablitz JJ, Langmoen IA. Excitation of hippocampal pyramidal cells by glutamate in the guinea-pig and rat. J Physiol 1982;325:317–331.
136. Mayer ML, Westbrook GL. Cellular mechanisms underlying excitotoxicity. TINS 1987;10:59–61.
137. Rehncrona S, Abdul-Rahman A, Siesjo BK. Recovery of brain mitochondrial function in the rat after complete and incomplete cerebral ischemia. Stroke 1979;10:437–446.
138. Rottenberg H, Marbach M. Regulation of Ca2+ transport in brain mitochondia. II. The mechanism of adenine nucleotides enhancement of Ca2+ uptake and retention. Biochim Biophys Acta 1990;1016:87–98.
139. Vink R, Head VA, Rogers PJ et al. Mitochondrial metabolism following traumatic brain injury in rats. J Neurotrauma 1990;7:21–27.
140. Anderson DK, Means ED, Waters TR. Spinal cord energy metabolism in normal and post laminectomy cats. J Neurosurg 1980a;52:387–391.
141. Anderson DK, Means ED, Waters TR et al. Spinal cord energy metabolism following compression trauma to the feline spinal cord. J Neurosurg 1980b;53:375–380.
142. Bralet J, Beley P, Jemaa R et al. Lipid metabolism, cerebral metabolic rate, and

some related enzyme activities after brain infarction in rats. Stroke 1987;18: 418–425.

143. Demediuk P, Daly MP, Faden AI. Effect of impact trauma on neurotransmitter and nonneurotransmitter aminoacids in rat spinal cord. J Neurochem 1989;52: 1529–1536.

144. Miller NR. Optic nerve protection, regeneration, and repair in the 21st century: LVIII Edward Jackson Memorial Lecture. Am J Ophthalmol 2001;132:811–818.

145. Bleich S, Romer K, Wiltfang J et al. Glutamate and the glutamate receptor system: A target for drug action. Int J Geriatr Psychiatry 2003;18:S33–40.

146. Faden AI. Neuroprotection and traumatic brain injury: Theoretical option or realistic proposition. Curr Opin Neurol 2002;15:707–712.

147. Young W. Role of calcium in central nervous system injuries. J Neurotrauma 1992;9(suppl 1): S9–S25.

148. Steinsapir KD, Hovda DA, Goldberg RA. Experimental model of traumatic optic neuropathy. Invest Ophthalmol Vis Sci 1992;33:1226.

149. Korthius RJ, Granger DN, Townsley MI et al. The role of oxygen-derived free radicals in ischemia-induced increases in canine skeletal muscle vascular permeability. Circ Res 1985;57:599–609.

150. Korthuis RJ, Grisham MB, Granger DN. Leukocyte depletion attenuates vascular injury in postischemic skeletal muscle. Am J Physiol 1988;245:H823–H827.

151. Neufeld AH, Kawai S, Das S et al. Loss of retinal ganglion cells following retinal ischemia: The role of inducible nitric oxide synthase. Exp Eye Res 2002; 75:521–528.

152. Giulian D, Chen J, Ingenman JE et al. The role of mononuclear phagocytes in wound healing after traumatic injury to adult mammalian brain. J Neurosci 1989; 9:4416–4429.

153. Schori H, Yoles E, Schwartz M. T-cell-based immunity counteracts the potential toxicity of glutamate in the central nervous system. J Neuroimmunol 2001;119: 199–204.

154. Hall ED, Braughler JM. Glucocorticoid mechanisms in acute spinal cord injury: A review and therapeutic rationale. Surg Neurol 1982;18:320–327.

155. Hall ED, Braughler JM, McCall JM. New pharmacological treatment of acute spinal cord trauma. J Neurotrauma 1988;5:81–89.

156. Ballard PL, Baxter JD, Higgins SJ et al. General presence of glucocorticoid receptors in mammalian tissues. Endocrinology 1974;94:998–1002.

157. Makman MH, Duorkin B, White A. Evidence for induction by cortisol in vitro of a protein inhibitor of transport and phosphorylation in rat thymocytes. Proc Natl Acad Sci USA 1971;68:1269–1273.

158. Gryglewski RJ, Panczenko B, Korbut R et al. Corticosteroids inhibit prostaglandin release from perfused mesenteric blood vessels of rabbit and from perfused lungs of sensitized guinea pig. Prostaglandins 1975;10:343–355.

159. Braughler JM, Hall ED. Effects of multidose methylprednisolone sodium succinate on injured cat spinal cord neurofilament degradation and energy metabolism. J Neurosurg 1984;61:290–295.

160. Young W, Flamm ES. Effects of high-dose corticosteroid therapy on blood flow, evoked potentials, and extracellular calcium in experimental spinal cord injury. J Neurosurg 1982;57:667–673.

161. Anderson DK, Saunders RD, Demediul P et al. Lipid hydrolysis and peroxidation in injured spinal cord: Partial protection with methylprednisolone or vitamin E and selenium. CNS Trauma 1985;2:257–267.

162. Hall ED, Braughler JM. Role of lipid peroxidation in post-traumatic spinal cord degeneration: A review. CNS Trauma 1984;3:281–294.

163. Braughler JM, Hall ED, Means ED et al. Evaluation of an intensive methylprednisolone sodium succinate dosing regimen in experimental spinal cord injury. J Neurosurg 1987;67:102–105.

164. Galicich JH, French LA. The use of dexamethasone in the treatment of cerebral edema resulting from brain tumors and brain surgery. Am Pract 1961;12: 169–174.

165. Maxwell RE, Long DM, French LA. The effects of glucocorticoids on experimental cold-induced brain edema. Gross morphologic alteration and vascular permeability changes. J Neurosurg 1971;34:477–487.

166. Bracken MB, Shepard MJ, Collins WF et al. A randomized, controlled trial of methylprednisolone or naloxone in the treatment of acute spinal-cord injury. Results of the Second National Acute Spinal Cord Injury Study. N Engl J Med 1990;322:1405–1411.

167. Faden AI, Jacobs TP, Patrick DH et al. Megadose corticosteroid therapy following experimental spinal injury. J Neurosurg 1984;60:712–717.

168. Bracken MB, Collins WF, Freeman DF et al. Efficacy of methylprednisolone in acute spinal cord injury. JAMA 1984;251:45–52.

169. Bracken MB, Holford TR. Effects of timing of methylprednisolone or naloxone administration on recovery of segmental and long-tract neurologic function in NASCIS II. J Neurosurg 1993;79:500–507.

170. Cook MW, Levin LA, Joseph MP et al. Traumatic optic neuropathy. A meta-analysis. Arch Otolaryngol Head Neck Surg 1996;122:389–392.

171. Lillie WI, Adson AW. Unilateral central and annular scotoma produced by callus from fracture extending into optic canal. Arch Ophthalmol 1934;12:500–508.

172. Fukado Y. Results in 400 cases of surgical decompression of the optic nerve. Mod Prob Ophthalmol 1975;14:474–481.

173. Niho S, Niho M, Niho K. Decompression of the optic canal by the transethmoidal route and decompression of the superior orbital fissure. Can J Ophthalmol 1970; 5:22–40.

174. Matsuzaki H, Kunita M, Kawai K. Optic nerve damage in head trauma: Clinical and experimental studies. Jpn J Ophthalmol 1982;26:447–461.

175. Fujitani T, Inoue K, Takahashi T et al. Indirect traumatic optic neuropathy: Visual outcome of operative and nonoperative cases. Jpn J Ophthalmol 1986; 30:125–134.

176. Krausen AS, Ogura JH, Burde RM et al. Emergency orbital decompression: a reprieve from blindness. Otolaryngol Head Neck Surg 1981;89:252–256.

177. Liu D. A simplified technique of orbital decompression for severe retrobulbar hemorrhage. Am J Ophthalmol 1993;116:34–37.

178. Anderson RL, Panje WR, Gross CE. Optic nerve blindness following blunt forehead trauma. Ophthalmology 1982;89:445–455.

179. Joseph MP, Lessell S, Rizzo J et al. Extracranial optic nerve decompression for traumatic optic neuropathy: see comments. Arch Ophthalmol 1990;108: 1091–1093.

180. Roy M, Sapolsky RM. The exacerbation of hippocampal excitotoxicity by glucocorticoids is not mediated by apoptosis. Neuroendocrinology 2003;77:24–31.

181. Dinkel K, MacPherson A, Sapolsky RM. Novel glucocorticoid effects on acute inflammation in the CNS. J Neurochem 2003;84:705–716.

182. Haynes LE, Griffiths MR, Hyde RE et al. Dexamethasone induces limited apoptosis and extensive sublethal damage to specific subregions of the striatum and hippocampus: implications of mood disorders. Neuroscience 2001;104: 57–69.

183. Steinsapir KD, Goldberg RA, Sinha S et al. Methylprednisolone exacerbates axonal loss following optic nerve trauma in rats. Restor Neurol Neurosci 2000; 17:157–163.

184. Diem R, Hobom M, Maier K et al. Methylprednisolone increases neuronal apoptosis during autoimmune CND inflammation by inhibition of an endogenous neuroprotective pathway. J Neurosci 2003;23:6993–7000.

185. Beck RW, Cleary PA, Trobe JD et al. The effect of corticosteroids for acute optic neuritis on the subsequent development of multiple sclerosis. The Optic Neuritis Study Group. N Engl J Med 1993;329:1764–1769.

186. Optic Neuritis Study Group. The 5-year risk of MS after optic neuritis. Experience of the optic neuritis treatment trial. Neurology 1997;49:1404–1413.

187. Beck RW, Trobe JD, Moke PS et al. High- and low-risk profiles for the development of multiple sclerosis within 10 years after optic neuritis: Experience of the optic neuritis treatment trial. Arch Ophthalmol 2003;121:1039–1040.

188. Bodian M. Transient loss of vision following head trauma. NY State J Med 1964;64:916–920.

189. Millesi W, Hollmann K, Funder J. Traumatic lesion of the optic nerve. Acta Neurochir (Wien) 1988;93:50–54.

190. Kountakis SE, Maillard AA, El-Harazi SM et al. Endoscopic optic nerve decompression for traumatic blindness. Otolaryngol Head Neck Surg 2000;123: 34–37.

191. Hooper RS. Orbital compications of head injury. Br J Surg 1951;39:126–138.

192. Edmund J, Godtfredsen E. Unilateral optic nerve atrophy following head injury. Acta Ophthalmol 1963;41:693–697.

193. Chou PI, Sadun AA, Chen YC et al. Clinical experiences in the management of traumatic optic neuropathy. Neuroophthalmology 1996;16:325–336.

194. Lubben B, Stoll W, Grenzebach U. Optic nerve decompression in the comatose and conscious patients after trauma. Laryngoscope 2001;111:320–328.

CHAPTER 10

Toxic and Deficiency Optic Neuropathies

Paul H. Phillips

Physicians have known for centuries that the anterior visual pathways are vulnerable to damage from nutritional deficiency and chemicals. The resulting disorders share many signs and symptoms, and several appear to have a multifactorial etiology in which both undernutrition and toxicity play a role. In light of these facts, it is reasonable to group them together. Although evidence for the localization of the primary lesions is lacking in many of the so-called toxic and nutritional "amblyopias," they are generally assumed to be optic neuropathies and that is the rubric under which they are considered here.

ETIOLOGIC CRITERIA

Although certain optic neuropathies have an obvious toxic or nutritional etiology, the toxic or nutritional basis of others is merely presumptive, and the attribution may ultimately prove false. It is also likely that a few of the optic neuropathies now considered idiopathic or ascribed to some other etiology, actually result from toxicity or nutritional deficiency. The proliferation of drugs and the introduction of new chemicals into the workplace and environment guarantee that additional toxic optic neuropathies will be identified. For medical and legal reasons, physicians must be alert to the possibility, both in sporadic cases of visual loss and in epidemics of visual loss, that intoxication or nutritional deficiency are factors.

NUTRITIONAL OPTIC NEUROPATHIES

Proving a nutritional basis for an optic neuropathy is by no means a simple task. The first criterion is that the patient be nutritionally deficient and has been so sufficiently long to deplete nutrients. Evidence from epidemics indicates that this requires months (see below). The reports of large numbers of cases of visual loss after economic and political upheavals suggest the possibility of a nutritional etiology. The patient should show evidence of undernutrition, usually manifested in such obvious forms as weight loss and wasting. Victims of nutritional optic neuropathy, however, are not necessarily emaciated. Other signs such as peripheral neuropathy, keratitis, or the cutaneous and mucous membrane stigmata of the avitaminoses are useful, when present.

There is an important exception to the foregoing statements. The optic neuropathy of pernicious anemia or dietary vitamin B_{12} deficiency can occur in seemingly healthy individuals without obvious symptoms or signs of nutritional deficiency (see following).

It should go without saying that the symptoms and signs should be those typical of nutritional optic neuropathy and that other disorders should be considered and eliminated by appropriate investigations. Both in individual cases and in epidemics, it is especially important to establish if the patient has been exposed to substances toxic to the visual pathways. In such cases, intoxication may be the alternative explanation or be a cofactor. The absence of an optic neuropathy in well-nourished individuals in the same environment, and recovery of vision in patients with restitution of an improved diet, strongly support, but do not prove, a nutritional basis. Supporting laboratory evidence for the diagnosis of nutritional optic neuropathy can be obtained in the form of direct or indirect vitamin assays, serum protein concentrations, and antioxidant levels (1,2).

Identifying the specific nutritional deficiency responsible for an optic neuropathy is very difficult. Undernourished individuals are rarely deficient in only one nutrient; multiple deficiencies are the rule. Even if a specific deficiency is identified in a patient with loss of vision, it does not prove that the deficiency caused the visual loss. Nor does recovery when the deficient nutrient is resupplied establish that the resupplied nutrient affected the cure. With the exception of vitamin B_{12} (which only rarely becomes deficient for dietary reasons), no specific nutrient deficiency has been conclusively proved to cause optic neuropathy in humans. At the present state of knowledge, one can only speculate about which specific deficiencies can cause or contribute to nutritional optic neuropathy.

TOXIC OPTIC NEUROPATHIES

The primary issue in patients suspected of having a toxic optic neuropathy is whether or not they were exposed to a substance that has been proved to damage the optic nerve by the same route of exposure. Visual loss may occur from either acute or chronic intoxication depending upon the agent, but there should not be a long interval between the cessation of the exposure and the onset of symptoms. The patient must have symptoms and signs that are compatible with a toxic optic neuropathy and typical of those in other patients proved to have suffered loss of vision from the same agent. Of course, the symptoms cannot have preceded the exposure.

The response of patients to rechallenge is helpful in evaluating the validity of presumed intoxications and in helping to establish the cause of the patient's optic neuropathy. If a patient who has recovered vision following cessation of exposure to a drug or chemical loses vision again when reexposed, the recurrent loss of vision tends to verify the neurotoxic nature of the agent and the toxic etiology of the visual loss. Epidemiologic data, especially those showing correlation of changing disease incidence when and where specific drugs or chemicals are introduced or withdrawn, can also prove quite useful.

Confirmatory evidence of exposure from laboratory tests or from associated nonvisual symptoms is desirable. Nontoxic disorders must be considered in the diagnosis of these patients and should be ruled out with appropriate investigations.

Animal models can help to validate the optic nerve toxicity of putative intoxicants. Despite such problems as species variation in susceptibility and difficulty in measuring visual function in animals, some useful models are available.

CLINICAL CHARACTERISTICS OF NUTRITIONAL AND TOXIC OPTIC NEUROPATHIES

Individuals of all ages, races, places, and economic strata are vulnerable to the toxic and nutritional deficiency optic neuropathies. Certain groups are at higher risk because they are under treatment with drugs, because of occupational exposure, or because of habits such as smoking and drinking. Nutritional deficiency optic neuropathy is more likely to occur in the economically disadvantaged and during times of war and famine. The value of taking a thorough history, including dietary intake, exposure to drugs, use of tobacco, and social and occupational background is obvious.

The symptoms and signs of nutritional and toxic optic neuropathy are similar and resemble those of most of the other optic neuropathies, primarily those that occur bilaterally and simultaneously. No single characteristic or combination of characteristics is pathognomonic.

Toxic and nutritional optic neuropathies are not painful. Thus, one should inquire carefully about this symptom since the presence of pain would suggest some other diagnosis.

Dyschromatopsia is present early and may be the initial symptom in observant patients. Some patients notice that certain colors, such as red, are no longer as bright and vivid as previously. Others experience a general loss of color perception.

Patients with nutritional or toxic optic neuropathies often initially notice a blur, fog or cloud at the point of fixation, following which the visual acuity progressively declines. The rate of decline can be quite rapid. Although vision can decrease to any level, total blindness or vision limited to light perception is unusual in cases of nutritional optic neuropathy, even if the patient is neglected. With the exception of methanol, which typically produces complete or nearly complete blindness, visual loss less than 20/400 is unusual in the toxic optic neuropathies. Bilaterality is the rule, although in the early stages, one eye may be affected before the other becomes symptomatic. Profound loss of vision in one eye with completely normal findings in the other eye should cast doubt on the diagnosis of a toxic or nutritional optic neuropathy.

Patients with toxic or nutritional optic neuropathies typically have central or centrocecal scotomas with sparing of the peripheral visual field (Fig.10.1). Some perimetrists claimed that centrocecal scotomas with "nuclei" between fixation and the physiologic blind spot were the hallmark of toxic optic neuropathy, especially the variety blamed on tobacco (3). There are many who doubt this, and most authorities now recognize that both central and centrocecal

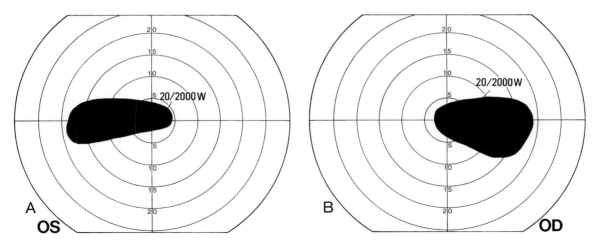

Figure 10.1.   Visual fields of a patient with a bilateral toxic optic neuropathy caused by chloramphenicol. Note cecocentral scotomas in the visual fields of the left *(A)* and right *(B)* eyes. The peripheral fields were normal.

scotomas may be encountered in either disorder (4–7). Some patients have a central scotoma in one eye and a centrocecal scotoma in the fellow eye. The anatomic basis of the centrocecal scotoma has yet to be established (8). Peripheral constriction and altitudinal visual field loss are rare.

Because of the symmetric and bilateral visual impairment in toxic and nutritional optic neuropathies, a relative afferent pupillary defect is not a common finding in affected patients. When the patient is blind or nearly so, as a consequence of methanol poisoning, the pupillary light response will be absent or weak and the pupils will be dilated. Otherwise the pupils are likely to have relatively normal responses to light and near stimulation.

In the early stages of toxic and nutritional deficiency optic neuropathy, the disc may be normal, slightly hyperemic, or swollen (Fig. 10.2). Disc hemorrhages may be present in eyes with hyperemic discs, but they are usually small (9,10). Optic atrophy develops after a variable interval (Fig.10.3).

Electrophysiologic examinations of patients with toxic or nutritional optic neuropathies may reveal changes in the electroretinogram (ERG), visual evoked potential (VEP), or both. Ikeda et al. (11) found a reduced amplitude of the VEP and of the cone functions in the ERG. There is no tendency for the P100 wave of the VEP to be delayed, however, except in pernicious anemia (12,13).

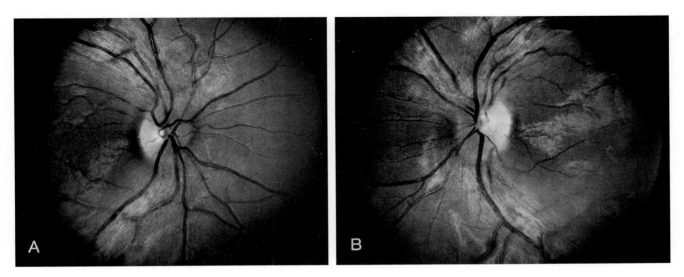

Figure 10.2.   Appearance of optic discs in a patient with bilateral toxic optic neuropathy from chloramphenicol. Note that right *(A)* and left *(B)* discs are hyperemic and somewhat swollen nasally. There is already mild pallor of the temporal portions of both optic discs, associated with early loss of the nerve fiber layer in the papillomacular bundle of both eyes.

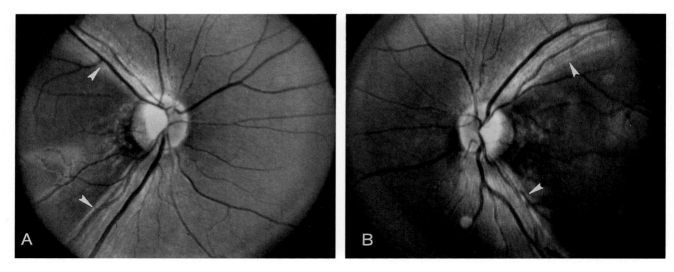

Figure 10.3. Appearance of optic discs in a patient with bilateral optic neuropathy in the setting of poor nutrition and alcohol abuse. Note extent of loss of nerve fiber layer from the papillomacular bundle *(arrowheads)* and marked temporal disc pallor. Visual acuity was 20/400 in both eyes, and there were bilateral central scotomas.

DIFFERENTIAL DIAGNOSIS

When an individual complains of bilateral visual loss that refraction cannot correct, and has an otherwise normal examination, there are many diagnostic possibilities in addition to the toxic and nutritional optic neuropathies. Certain maculopathies can present in this guise (14–20). With time, the fundus will show abnormalities, but until then, fluorescein angiography or focal electroretinography may be the only means of establishing the nature of the lesion (20). Full field electroretinography may not reveal the defect.

One should be alert to the possibility of a conversion disorder or malingering in cases of bilateral visual loss. The absence of optic atrophy is an important clue when the visual loss is long standing. In the acute phase, the characteristics of the visual field defects may help the clinician recognize that the loss of vision is nonorganic. The visual field defects in the toxic and nutritional optic neuropathies are typically central or centrocecal. Such defects are exceptional in patients with a conversion reaction or who are malingering (21). In conversion reaction and malingering, the visual fields are usually constricted and may show spiraling or have a tubular configuration.

Dominantly inherited (Kjer's) and mitochondria inherited (Leber's) optic neuropathies can be confused with nutritional optic neuropathy if no other family members are known to be affected. The confusion is most likely to occur in patients who are first evaluated late in their course. Kjer's disease progresses more slowly than the nutritional and toxic optic

neuropathies, and optic atrophy is an early finding (22). In Leber's optic neuropathy, the onset of visual loss is not infrequently symmetric or nearly so, and this disorder must therefore be considered in any patient in whom a toxic or nutritional optic neuropathy is thought to be present (23–27). Appropriate testing for mitochondrial DNA mutations may be required in some cases (see Chapter 11).

It can be tragic to mistake a compressive or infiltrative lesion of the optic chiasm for nutritional or toxic optic neuropathy. There are few instances in which one should be so confident of the diagnosis of toxic or nutritional optic neuropathy that neuroimaging is omitted. Centrocecal scotomas and the bitemporal visual field defects of chiasmal disease resemble each other, and there are many examples of bilateral central and even centrocecal scotomas from tumors (28–37).

If a demyelinating, inflammatory, or infectious optic neuritis begins simultaneously in both eyes, there may be confusion with the toxic and nutritional optic neuropathies. The visual field defects are similar, but there is pain in about 90% of cases of optic neuritis. In some cases, magnetic resonance (MR) imaging will indicate the nature of the lesion. In others, however, it may be necessary to examine the cerebrospinal fluid, perform specific tests for syphilis, sarcoidosis, or systemic vasculitis, and perform a complete neurologic examination.

EVALUATION

In most cases, analysis of the symptoms and signs obtained from a detailed history and physical examination will establish the diagnosis of a toxic or nutritional optic neuropathy. As stated above, it is prudent to obtain neuroimaging

unless one is absolutely confident of the diagnosis. MR imaging before and after intravenous injection of gadolinium-diethylenetriamine-pentaacetic acid (gadolinium-DTPA) with special attention to the optic nerves and optic chiasm, is the optimum investigation in most cases. A vitamin B_{12} level should be determined to identify pernicious anemia, and red blood cell folate levels provide one marker of general nutritional status (1).

When a specific intoxicant is suspected, one should try to identify the toxin or its metabolites in the patient's tissues or fluids. The advice of a toxicologist is invaluable in such instances. In cases of suspected intoxication, one should attempt to evaluate or obtain information about other persons who have had similar exposure. The resulting information has potential public health implications and can help to validate the toxicity of chemicals not previously recognized as dangerous to the human optic nerve.

SPECIFIC NUTRITIONAL OPTIC NEUROPATHIES

EPIDEMIC NUTRITIONAL OPTIC NEUROPATHY

The most useful observations regarding nutritional optic neuropathy have come not from sporadic cases encountered in practice, but rather from epidemics during war and famine. Two well-documented epidemics afflicted Allied prisoners of war of the Japanese during World War II (38–45) and Cubans in the early 1990s (46–50). The characteristics of the disorder in those two populations are reasonably consistent and are described as follows (51).

The symptoms developed in an undernourished population after four or more months of food deprivation (51). Among prisoners of war, vision loss occurred sooner in those who were undernourished at the time they were first incarcerated. Only a minority of people at risk developed loss of vision, and the occurrence of visual loss did not appear to correlate very well with the severity of malnutrition. In some cases, a superficial keratopathy was a prelude to the visual loss, but visual loss developed both with and without a preceding keratopathy (51). The visual loss was symmetric and often appeared suddenly. In up to one-quarter of cases the visual nadir was reached in one day. Vision plateaued after one month in the remainder. At the time of visual loss, many victims also had pain or sensory loss in their extremities. There was a high incidence of bilateral sensorineural hearing loss. The fundi were usually normal at first, but a minority had peripapillary hemorrhages associated with mild optic disc hyperemia and swelling. Optic atrophy was a late development. The visual field defects were central or centrocecal. Most abnormalities could be reversed with improved nutrition.

Pathologic information on nutritional optic neuropathies is scarce. Fisher (52) described the results of postmortem examinations on repatriated Allied prisoners. He found atrophy of the papillomacular bundle and lesions in the fasciculus gracilis of the spinal cord. Smiddy and Green (53) reviewed the records of civilian patients in whom atrophy in the papillomacular bundle was found at autopsy. They concluded that malnutrition, associated with alcoholism, was common.

In 1992 and 1993, an epidemic of optic neuropathy and peripheral neuropathy similar to that reported among prisoners of war occurred in Cuba (47–49,54–59). The epidemic began in the province of Pinar del Río, located at the northwestern tip of Cuba and gradually spread southeastern. More than 50,000 persons were affected with bilateral optic neuropathy, sensory and dysautonomic peripheral neuropathy, sensory myelopathy, spastic paraparesis, or sensorineural deafness in various combinations. Slightly more than half of the affected persons had evidence of optic neuropathy, which occurred as a painless rapid loss of vision in both eyes associated with marked dyschromatopsia, central or centrocecal scotomas, and normal appearing optic discs. Patients who did not recover vision (discussed later) developed temporal pallor of the optic discs, associated with marked loss of the nerve fiber layer in the papillomacular bundle (Fig. 10.4). The majority of cases occurred in people between 25–64 years old, and with a predominance of males being among those with optic nerve disease. The relative low incidence of disease in persons outside this age range is likely secondary to the extra rations of food provided to children and older persons (60). Partial and complete recovery occurred following treatment with parenteral and oral vitamins (61). In addition, supplementation of the general population with B-complex vitamins and vitamin A since 1993 coincided with a dramatic decrease in new cases of the condition (49).

Although the loss of vision in the epidemic cases was undoubtedly caused by malnutrition, it is impossible to identify a specific deficient nutrient that caused either of the epidemics (51). Malnourished individuals have multiple deficiencies. Clinical and laboratory data make it unlikely that nutritional deficiency was the sole factor. Systematic investigation of Cuban epidemic optic neuropathy and controls showed an increased risk associated with tobacco use and cassava consumption and a decreased risk associated with high serum levels of antioxidant carotenoids, ingestion of B vitamins, and ingestion of animal products (49). Physical labor also seemed to be a risk factor among the prisoners of war. In any case, the conclusion that epidemic cases of nutritional optic neuropathy (and probably sporadic cases as well) are the result of some multifactorial etiology is inescapable.

The treatment of nutritional optic neuropathy is improved nutrition and, unless the vision loss is extensive, there is an excellent prospect for recovery or at least improvement.

VITAMIN B_{12} DEFICIENCY

Although the role of vitamin B_{12} in the maintenance and function of the nervous system has yet to be explained, depletion of the nutrient almost invariably leads to neurologic dysfunction. The body's nutritional requirements must be met entirely by food (particularly meat and dairy products). The abundant stores, particularly in the liver, are redistributed so gradually that it takes years for poor intake to cause disease. However, a poor diet is rarely the cause of vitamin B_{12} deficiency and when it is, it is found only in strict vegans (62). Impaired absorption because of diphyllobothriasis (63),

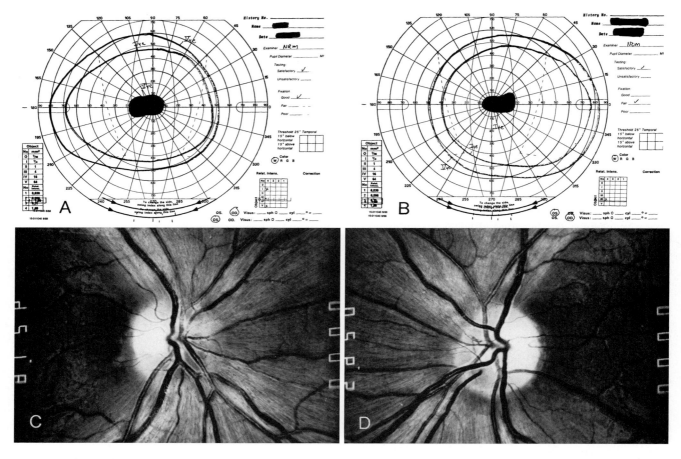

Figure 10.4.   Visual fields and appearance of ocular fundi in a patient with Cuban epidemic optic neuropathy. The patient was a 23-year-old Cuban man who developed progressive loss of vision in both eyes associated with a peripheral neuropathy in 1993. Examination revealed visual acuity of 20/200 OU. Visual fields performed by kinetic perimetry reveal a cecocentral scotoma in the field of both the left *(A)* and right *(B)* eyes. Photographs of the right *(C)* and left *(D)* optic fundi show temporal pallor of the optic discs associated with marked loss of the retinal nerve fiber layer in the papillomacular bundle.

intestinal disease, or gastrointestinal surgery accounts for only a few cases.

Pernicious anemia is by far the most common condition in which vitamin B_{12} deficiency and its complications are encountered. This presumably autoimmune disorder results from impaired absorption of the vitamin from the ileum, because the patient lacks the intrinsic factor elaborated by the parietal cells of the gastric mucosa. Pernicious anemia is most often found in, but is not limited to, middle-aged and elderly Caucasians of northern European extraction. The anemia is megaloblastic. It develops slowly and can be severe. Unless treatment is instituted early, most patients with pernicious anemia develop neurologic manifestations. The pathologic substrate is a white matter lesion that affects both myelin and axons initially in the posterior columns of the upper thoracic and lower cervical portions of the spinal cord (''subacute combined degeneration''). The process subsequently affects other white matter tracts and other levels of the spinal cord. Paresthesias and weakness in the extremities are heralding symptoms. With time, vibration sense is lost,

and the patient develops spasticity, with hyperactive knee and ankle jerks and Babinski reflexes. Dementia may also develop.

Deficiency of vitamin B_{12}, whether from inadequate diet or interference with absorption, can cause an optic neuropathy. Lesions in the optic nerves and optic chiasm have been demonstrated in some postmortem examinations of patients with pernicious anemia (64,65). There are also primate models of the disease (66–68). Severe optic nerve degeneration is found in experimental vitamin B_{12} deficiency in monkeys even before there is anemia or a spinal cord lesion (68). In light of this finding, it is not surprising that in humans, an optic neuropathy may be the first symptom of pernicious anemia and may precede the hematologic disturbance. Indeed, abnormal visual evoked responses can be recorded in patients with pernicious anemia who have no visual symptoms, suggesting that there may also be subclinical damage to the visual pathway in this disease (12).

The optic neuropathy that results from vitamin B_{12} deficiency resembles the other nutritional optic neuropathies

(69–73). The visual loss is symmetric, painless, and progressive. Central and centrocecal scotomas are the rule, and the optic disc appears normal in the early stages of the condition. Unless optic atrophy becomes well established, one can expect recovery of vision with intramuscular injections of hydroxocobalamin. The optic neuropathy of pernicious anemia, unlike the other deficiency optic neuropathies, does not usually respond to an improved diet.

Since the optic neuropathy of vitamin B_{12} deficiency is essentially indistinguishable from many other toxic and nutritional deficiency optic neuropathies, can present before there is anemia or myelopathy, and requires parenteral treatment, it is important to obtain a serum vitamin B_{12} level in all cases of unexplained bilateral optic neuropathy.

OTHER VITAMIN DEFICIENCIES

The association of visual loss with beriberi, known for centuries, focused attention on vitamin B_1 deficiency as a cause of nutritional optic neuropathy. This vitamin has received more attention in this regard than any other nutrient and, despite contrary evidence summarized in the following paragraphs, many authorities still consider thiamine (vitamin B_1) deficiency an important factor in the causation of nutritional deficiency optic neuropathy (74).

The role of thiamine deficiency in patients with nutritional deficiency optic neuropathy is controversial. Some studies of thiamine deprivation in rats have shown that an optic neuropathy may occur. However, the results of these experiments are not conclusive, since the animals may have suffered other deficiencies, and few animals were affected. When chronic thiamine deficiency was produced in human volunteers, their vision did not suffer (75,76). The prisoner-of-war studies present strong evidence against a primary role for thiamine deficiency in nutritional optic neuropathy. One study showed that vision loss developed just as the incidence of beriberi was declining. In fact, beriberi was as prevalent among prisoners of war with normal vision as it was among those who had loss of vision. Finally, among civilians in a Japanese prison camp, nutritional optic neuropathy could not be cured with injections of thiamine, and some prisoners developed visual loss while being treated with thiamine for beriberi.

The disorder consequent to thiamine depletion is Wernicke's encephalopathy. There is an excellent primate model of this disorder, and in this model there are no pathologic changes in the optic nerves (77,78). Indeed, loss of vision is uncommon among patients with Wernicke's disease (79,80). These observations cast further doubt on a role for thiamine deficiency in human nutritional optic neuropathy.

The role of pyridoxine, niacin, folic acid, and riboflavin deficiencies in causing an optic neuropathy was reviewed in an earlier edition of this book. As with thiamine, these vitamins are apt to be depleted in patients who are generally malnourished, but there is no definitive evidence indicating that such deficiencies play a primary etiological role in nutritional optic neuropathy. For example, low folate levels have been documented in the red blood cells and, occasionally, the serum of patients with nutritional optic neuropathy and some malnourished patients with optic neuropathy recover when treated with folic acid supplements (1,81,82). As discussed above, however, this does not prove that the folate deficiency caused the loss of vision or that the folic acid supplements affected the recovery.

Despite the lack of definitive evidence, it remains possible that there are some patients who develop an optic neuropathy consequent to dietary deficiency of thiamine, folate, and these other vitamins. It thus makes sense to enrich the diet of patients with loss of vision and evidence of poor nutrition with all of the vitamins in which they might be deficient.

TROPICAL OPTIC NEUROPATHY

There are optic neuropathies endemic to tropical regions for which a nutritional etiology has been invoked. An early report by Strachan from Jamaica appeared in 1897 (83). The clinical features of his patients resemble in some ways those of the epidemic cases described above. There was numbness and cramps in the hands and feet. The visual loss was bilateral and was sometimes accompanied by hearing loss. However, other features were unusual. Muscle wasting often developed. The pain was so severe that patients were kept awake. A dermatopathy was a constant finding. In any case, Strachan (83) made no claim for a nutritional etiology. When the disorder was subsequently reevaluated by others, they concluded that this was not a nutritional disease (84,85). Despite that, some authors use ''Strachan's syndrome'' to designate nutritional optic neuropathy. The eponym is inappropriate.

It should be noted that there is an otherwise unexplained bilateral optic neuropathy, called ''West Indian Amblyopia'' in black expatriates from the West Indies. Examples of this condition have been reported from Great Britain and the United States (86,87). The history is typically that of bilateral, painless progressive visual decline in a well-nourished adult. The visual field defects tend to be central or centrocecal, but annular scotomas and peripheral constriction have been reported. Optic atrophy develops. Deafness is also present in some of the patients. No treatment, including various vitamin regimens, is effective in reversing either the visual or the nonvisual manifestations of the disorder. Although a toxic basis (''bush tea'') has been postulated, there is no good evidence for either a toxic or nutritional etiology.

A disorder similar to Strachan's syndrome has been described in Nigerians (88,89). It differs from the West Indian cases (and the epidemic and sporadic nutritional optic neuropathies) in that the majority of patients have constricted visual fields and that total blindness can occur. Poor diet is said to be the common denominator in the African cases, but investigators have also suggested that exogenous cyanide from an excess of cassava in the diet is an etiologic factor. However, the manner in which cassava is prepared in this population would probably make for minimal exposure to cyanide (90). The evidence that cyanide plays a role in causing any optic neuropathy is tenuous at best and is discussed further in the section on tobacco optic neuropathy. The endemic tropical neuropathy in Nigeria might result from nutritional deficiency, but this has not been proved.

SPECIFIC TOXIC OPTIC NEUROPATHIES

No discussion of the toxic optic neuropathies can be considered complete without reference to the encyclopedic and authoritative text originated by Grant and subsequently coauthored by Schuman (91). The reader who wishes to pursue the subject of the toxic optic neuropathies in greater detail than is provided in this chapter is well advised to consult Grant and Schuman's ''Toxicology of the Eye.''

Table 10.1 lists substances that are suggested or presumed to be toxic to the human optic nerve. It also contains pertinent references so that the reader can decide whether the association of ingestion of, or exposure to a particular substance and the subsequent visual loss, is fortuitous or cause and effect. Several of the agents are of academic interest only, since they are no longer in use.

A recurrent dilemma in patients who develop loss of vision or a clear-cut optic neuropathy is deciding whether the disease or the treatment is responsible for the visual loss. In some cases, it is impossible to decide. In addition, the suspected toxin may not be the only agent to which the patient has been exposed, further confounding the issue of causation.

Several toxic-induced optic neuropathies are discussed below in detail.

METHANOL

Methanol ingestion is the most widely recognized cause of a toxic optic neuropathy, and methanol toxic neuropathy is also the best characterized pathogenetically and clinically. Unlike some of the intoxicants mentioned in this chapter, which are medications and therefore apt in time to be supplanted, methanol is likely to remain a permanent threat. Hence, it deserves special attention in this chapter. However, it must be noted that methanol intoxication is not an ideal paradigm for the toxic neuropathies. The combination of acute onset, life-threatening systemic symptoms, and severe irreversible visual loss is atypical.

Cases are encountered in both epidemic and sporadic form. The victim almost always has consumed the poison accidentally because it was mistaken for, substituted for, or added to, ethyl alcohol whose taste and smell it closely resembles. Although blindness can result from drinking an ounce or less of pure methanol, the toxic effect is ameliorated if it is ingested together with ethyl alcohol.

There is a well-studied primate model of methanol intoxication (92–94). In this model, there is disc swelling, but the lesion is retrobulbar. The evidence from human postmortem examinations also favors a retrobulbar locus (95–97). The early lesion is demyelinating (96); the later lesion is necrotic (97).

There is extensive literature on the clinical findings in methanol intoxication in humans (98–104). Initially, the patient has nausea and vomiting, but these symptoms may seem so insignificant that the physician falsely concludes that the patient has not been seriously intoxicated. After 18–48 hours, however, the patient begins to experience respiratory distress, headache, and visual loss. Abdominal pain, generalized weakness, confusion, and drowsiness are commonly present at this stage. Coma and death from respiratory failure may follow. Metabolic acidosis is one of the hallmarks of methanol intoxication, and it is consequent to the accumulation of formate (105). The severity of the acidosis is a rough guide to the severity of the intoxication but the visual complications are not consequent to the acidosis per se.

Methanol intoxication can reduce vision to any level, including total irrevocable blindness. Central and centrocecal scotomas predominate in cases of partial visual loss. The optic disc is often hyperemic, with blurred margins in the acute stage, and there may be some edema of the peripapillary retina. The reactions of the pupils to light are reduced in cases of severe, but not complete loss of vision; however, when the patient is blind, the pupils are dilated and nonreactive to light. Grant and Schuman (91) considered the lack of a pupillary reaction to light as signifying a poor prognosis. Patients may regain vision, usually within a week but occasionally later. In some cases, vision fails again weeks after first improving. The optic discs gradually become pale, and there is often cupping of the optic disc that may be indistinguishable from that in glaucoma. There may also be thinning of retinal arteries.

The diagnosis of methanol poisoning can be substantiated by demonstrating a serum methanol level of greater than 20 mg/dL. Other biochemical findings include a large anion gap, a high serum formate level, and a reduced serum bicarbonate level.

Treatment of methanol poisoning must be instituted promptly. In patients seen relatively early, who have ingested methanol but have not yet developed visual symptoms, there is the potential for preventing loss of vision, and even patients who have already lost vision may experience some degree of recovery if prompt treatment is instituted (106,107). Ethanol should be given, since it interferes with the metabolism of methanol. The metabolic acidosis responds to bicarbonate, and hemodialysis can help eliminate the toxin.

ETHYLENE GLYCOL

Ethylene glycol is the active ingredient in automobile antifreeze and may be consumed accidentally or in a suicide attempt. This poison deserves at least brief mention, since there is evidence that it is toxic to the optic nerve and because the metabolic consequences resemble those of methanol poisoning with which it could easily be confused (108).

As in methanol intoxication, the victim initially has nausea, vomiting, and abdominal pain. Stupor and coma follow, and there is cardiac failure within a few days. Unlike the situation in methanol intoxication, however, there is a high incidence of renal failure. The outcome can be fatal, or recovery can occur. Patients who survive may have permanent residual neurologic and ophthalmologic deficits.

Despite the metabolic similarities to methanol intoxication, the frequency of visual loss seems to be much lower in patients poisoned by ethylene glycol. Nevertheless, profound visual loss can occur, with dilated pupils that do not react to light. True papilledema, caused by cerebral edema,

Table 10.1
Substances Believed or Known to Cause Toxic Optic Neuropathy

Substance	References
Amantadine hydrochloride	223
Amiodarone	183–207
Amoproxan	224,225
Arsenicals	226
Aspidium (male fern)	227,228
Cafergot	229
Carbon disulfide	230–233
Carbon monoxide	234
Carbon tetrachloride	233,235–240
Catha edulis	241
Chlorambucil	242
Chloramphenicol	243–249
Chlorodinitrobenzene	250,251
Chlorpromazine	252
Chlorpropamide	253–255
Cisplatin	256–259
Clioquinol	152,155,158, 289–293
Clomiphene	260,261
Cobalt chloride	262
Cyclosporine	263–269
Dapsone	91
Desferrioxamine (desferoxamine; deferoxamine)	270–272
Dinitrobenzene	250,251
Dinitrochlorobenzene	250,251
Disulfiram	167–171,175, 273,274
Elcatonin (synthetic analog of calcitonin)	275
Emetine	276
Ergot	277
Ethambutol	109–119,122–151, 278–282
Ethchlorvynol	283,284
Ethylene glycol	285–287
5-Fluorouracil	288
Halogenated hydroxyquinolines	152,155,158, 289–293
Hexachlorophene	294,295
Infliximab	296,297
Interferon alpha	298–303
Iodoform	91
Iodoquinol	152,155,158, 289–293
Isoniazid	304–313
Lead	314–318
Methanol (methyl alcohol)	106,107,319,320
Methyl acetate	321,322
Methyl bromide	323
Octamoxin	324–329
Organic solvents	330
Penicillamine	120,331,332
Pheniprazine	333–335
Plasmocid	336,337
Quinine	338
Sildenafil	176–182
Streptomycin	339
Styrene (vinyl benzene)	340
Sulfonamides	341,342
Tacrolimus	343
Tamoxifen	344–347
Thallium	315,348–351
Tobacco	352,353
Toluene	354–359
Triethyltin	91
Trichloroethylene	360,361
Vincristine	362–366

may occur, or the optic discs can initially appear normal, only to become pale with time. Unlike the situation in methanol intoxication, patients with ethylene glycol intoxication may develop nystagmus and ophthalmoplegia.

One clue to the cause of the intoxication is the presence of oxalate crystals in the urine. The accumulation of glycolate causes a metabolic acidosis and a large anion gap. Treatment is essentially the same as the treatment of methanol intoxication. Bicarbonate is used to combat the acidosis; ethanol is administered to retard the metabolism of the ethylene glycol; and hemodialysis is employed to promote elimination of the poison.

ETHAMBUTOL

Of the drugs in wide use at the time this chapter was compiled, ethambutol is undoubtedly the one most often implicated in toxic optic neuropathy. The potential for visual impairment was recognized soon after this antituberculous agent was introduced (109). The original formulation was a racemic mixture. However, when it was discovered that the D-form was predominantly responsible for the therapeutic effect and the L-form for the toxicity, the L-form was withdrawn from the market.

There are good animal models of this disorder. Monkey experiments using the racemic mixture showed that ethambutol intoxication tended to first affect the optic chiasm (110,111). Studies in rats using the D-isomer showed that this was an axonal neuropathy and confirmed the special susceptibility of the optic chiasm (112). In rabbits, however, the lesion appeared in the optic nerves (113).

The biochemical basis of ethambutol toxicity has yet to be elucidated. Ethambutol's therapeutic effect is related to the metabolism of this drug to an agent that chelates metal-containing enzymes essential for bacterial replication. The chelation of copper or zinc containing enzymes within human mitochondria has been suggested as a mechanism for the optic neuropathy (114–116). Support for this mechanism includes the fact that reduced serum zinc levels are found in several toxic optic neuropathies (117) and patients with reduced plasma zinc levels maybe at increased risk for ethambutol toxic optic neuropathy (118,119). It is interesting in this regard that two other chelators–disulfiram (see later) and DL-penicillamine–have been implicated in toxic optic neuropathies (120,121).

Human ethambutol intoxication has been described in numerous publications (115,122–134). The occurrence of ocular toxicity is dose related; loss of vision most likely to occur in patients receiving 25 mg/kg/day or more. However, vision loss has been documented in approximately 1% of patients receiving the currently recommended therapeutic dose of 15–25 mg/kg/day (129,135,136). Visual loss rarely occurs before the patient has been receiving the drug for at least 2 months, with 7 months being the average. There is evidence that there is greater susceptibility to intoxication and more severe visual impairment in patients with renal tuberculosis, perhaps because ethambutol depends on the kidneys for excretion (125,137). Diabetes mellitus, liver damage, poor nutrition, as well as tobacco and alcohol use may be additional risk factors for ethambutol optic neuropathy (138–140).

Some authors claim that dyschromatopsia is the earliest symptom of the toxic optic neuropathy produced by ethambutol, with blue-yellow color changes being the most common (141). In any case, the loss of vision is bilaterally symmetric and begins insidiously. Reduced visual acuity with a central scotoma is the rule (134,142,143). However, patients may also present with peripheral visual field constriction and sparing of the central vision (135) or bitemporal defects (143,144). An initially normal optic nerve appearance may be followed by the development of optic nerve atrophy.

In some patients, the vision slowly improves over several months if ethambutol therapy is discontinued (129,143). However, the visual loss that results from ethambutol optic neuropathy is not necessarily reversible. Kumar et al. (133) described a series of seven consecutive patients with severe visual loss caused by ethambutol toxicity. Only 3 of the 7 patients (42.2%) achieved a visual recovery of better than 20/200 after an average follow-up of 8.3 ± 2.1 months after stopping the drug. There were no predisposing risk factors to contribute toward a poor prognosis. Kumar et al. (133) suggested that in light of their findings, ethambutol should not be used in patients with tuberculosis. Other investigators have documented that despite discontinuation of ethambutol at the onset of visual symptoms, only 40–50% of patients have improvement of vision and most patients with improved vision still sustain permanent visual deficits (122, 133,140,143,145).

It is important for the clinician to be aware that there are reports of patients who develop rapid onset, severe, bilateral, permanent visual loss despite treatment with a low therapeutic dose of ethambutol (130,133,143,146). In this regard, Chatterjee et al. (146) described a 26-year-old man who had "hazy vision" 3 days after starting treatment with ethambutol at a low dose of 15 mg/kg. Despite discontinuation of the drug 3 days later (6 days after starting treatment), he developed permanent "total blindness" OU.

Beyond stopping the drug, there is no specific therapy for ethambutol optic neuropathy. Recommendations regarding the appropriate screening strategy are controversial (122,136,139,147). Patients should be instructed to discontinue ethambutol immediately at the onset of any visual symptoms. Ethambutol is relatively contraindicated in patients who are unlikely to notice or describe visual symptoms such as adults with communication problems or poor baseline vision from unrelated causes and children. Most investigators agree that patients should have a baseline (pretreatment) ophthalmologic examination that includes assessment of visual acuity, color vision, and visual fields, and that this examination should be repeated at the onset of any visual symptoms. These parameters are often monitored periodically (every 1–3 months) during the treatment of asymptomatic patients (147). However, there is no consensus regarding the specific visual tests and testing intervals appropriate for monitoring asymptomatic patients during treatment (147). Some investigators suggest monitoring asymptomatic patients with more detailed visual testing such as contrast sensitivity (148), Farnsworth-Munsell 100 hue testing (119,149),

and visual evoked potentials (133,150,151) to detect the earliest evidence of a toxic effect on the optic nerves. Regardless of the screening strategy used, there is a small risk of permanent visual loss in patients treated with this drug.

HALOGENATED HYDROXYQUINOLINES

The halogenated hydroxyquinolines are amebacidal drugs. One of these (iodochlorhydroxyquin) was promoted in some parts of the world for preventing or treating traveler's diarrhea and chronic diarrheas. In that setting, it caused a syndrome of optic neuropathy, myelopathy, and peripheral neuropathy (SMON). This is ironic, since there is no evidence that the halogenated hydroxyquinolines actually prevent traveler's diarrhea. The impact on public health was significant, with over 10,000 cases documented in Japan between 1956 and 1970. SMON virtually disappeared in Japan when the use of these drugs was stopped.

Japanese investigators were the first to call attention to the problem, but the disorder was not limited to geographic or ethnic boundaries (152–157). The neurotoxicity of the halogenated hydroxyquinolines is dose related (158). Patients with gastrointestinal disease, who constitute a high proportion of those taking these drugs, were especially vulnerable.

Symptoms can appear as early as five days after beginning treatment. Initially, there is abdominal discomfort that is followed by paresthesias and dysesthesias in the legs. This may progress to paraparesis or paraplegia. One quarter of the patients suffer visual impairment in one form or another. Dyschromatopsia is an early symptom and occasionally is the only deficit; however, central acuity is usually affected, and about 5% of these patients become effectively blind.

Children with acrodermatitis enteropathica, a rare hereditary disease in which there is malabsorption of zinc, appear to have a low threshold for loss of vision from halogenated hydroxyquinolines (159). Interestingly, they often experience the visual loss without developing the other neurologic deficits (160–165).

DISULFIRAM

Disulfiram is a drug with a role, albeit a small one, in the treatment of chronic alcoholism. Disulfiram interferes with the metabolism of acetaldehyde, a metabolic product of ethanol. The concurrent ingestion of alcohol and disulfiram causes uncomfortable symptoms, including flushing, nausea, and vomiting as a result of the accumulation of acetaldehyde.

Disulfiram can cause an optic neuropathy, and since the optic neuropathy can occur in patients who have remained abstemious, alcohol toxicity presumably does not play a role in such cases. The mechanism of this toxicity is unknown, but disulfiram, like several other optic nerve toxins, is a chelating agent (117,166).

The symptoms and signs in patients with toxic optic neuropathy caused by disulfiram are quite typical of those of other toxic and nutritional optic neuropathies (167–175). The visual loss is subacute or chronic, affecting both eyes symmetrically. Pain is not a feature. The visual field defects are central or centrocecal. The optic discs are usually initially normal in appearance, but they can become pale late in the course. Some of the victims also develop a sensorimotor peripheral neuropathy. The prognosis for complete recovery is good if the disulfiram therapy is discontinued.

SILDENAFIL

Sildenafil citrate (Viagra, Pfizer Pharmaceuticals, New York, NY) is a phosphodiesterase type 5 inhibitor that is prescribed for erectile dysfunction (176). This drug facilitates erections by augmenting nitric oxide induced vasodilation in the corpus cavernosum. Systemic side effects are related to drug induced systemic vasodilation and include headache, flushing, and systemic hypotension. Severe systemic hypotension may occur when sildenafil is ingested with other nitrate medications. The most common ocular side effect is a transient alteration of color perception that presumably occurs from sildenafil's weak inhibitory effect on phosphodiesterase type 6, a phototransduction enzyme present in the retinal photoreceptor outer segments (176).

Pomeranz et al. recently described five patients who had nonarteritic anterior ischemic optic neuropathy (NAION) within minutes to hours after ingesting a therapeutic dose of sildenafil (177–179). These patients had symptoms and signs typical of NAION including acute visual loss, altitudinal visual fields deficits, a relative afferent pupillary defect, and disc edema. Visual deficits did not improve and the disc edema resolved to disc pallor. Although four of these patients did not have vasculopathic risk factors for NAION, they all had the classic small cupless "disc at risk" associated with this entity. Two other patients with sildenafil associated NAION have been described (180,181).

The association of sildenafil and NAION may be secondary to vascular effects induced by this drug. Nitric oxide induced vasodilation may precipitate NAION by interfering with vascular autoregulation at the optic nerve head or by inducing systemic hypotension (177). Alternatively, the drug may be directly toxic to the optic nerve as excessive nitric oxide has been postulated to damage retinal ganglion cell axons (182). Finally, the association may be coincidental as patients with vascular disease are at risk for erectile dysfunction and NAION. However, as noted above, most of these patients did not have known vasculopathy and the NAION occurred minutes to hours after ingestion of sildenafil.

It is important to specifically ask about sildenafil use in patients who present with NAION as they often do not volunteer this information. Until this association is better delineated, there is no screening strategy to determine which patients are at risk for NAION from sildenafil. However, Pomeranz recommends that a history of NAION should probably be a contraindication for sildenafil use (177).

Finally, patients contemplating treatment with this drug should be informed of the possible side effect of permanent visual loss.

AMIODARONE

Amiodarone is a benzofuran derivative that is primarily used to treat atrial or ventricular tachyarrhythmias that are unresponsive to other antiarrhythmic agents (183). Amioda-

rone's therapeutic mechanism of action is related to its ability to prolong the duration of action potentials and the refractory period in cardiac-conducting tissues. The most common ocular side effect is the formation of verticillate, pigmented, corneal epithelial deposits that eventually occur in most patients (70–100%) treated with the drug. The amount of corneal epithelial deposits observed in a given patient, as well as the incidence of these deposits in a group of patients, is related to the dose of the drug and the duration of treatment. With discontinuation of the drug, the deposits resolve over several months as amiodarone has a long half-life of up to 100 days. Other ocular side effects from amiodarone include anterior subcapsular lens opacities, multiple chalazia, and keratitis sicca. Fortunately, these ocular side effects rarely cause significant visual impairment and do not constitute a reason for discontinuing the drug (183).

Amiodarone is associated with an optic neuropathy that has many characteristics similar to nonarteritic anterior ischemic optic neuropathy. Gittinger and Asdourian (184) reported this association in two patients treated with therapeutic doses of amiodarone. They described a 45-year-old man who had unilateral, hemorrhagic disc edema noted on a routine examination 8 months after starting treatment with amiodarone. He was asymptomatic and had normal visual acuity, color vision, and visual fields. His disc edema resolved 1 month later despite continued treatment with the drug. The other patient was a 61-year-old man who complained of hazy vision in his right eye two months after starting treatment with amiodarone. He had a visual acuity of 20/25 OU, a right relative afferent pupillary defect and hemorrhagic disc edema in the right eye. Several days later, he developed hemorrhagic disc edema in the left eye. Three months later, he still had bilateral, hemorrhagic disc edema and his dosage of amiodarone was reduced. Five months after his visual loss, he had a visual acuity of 20/20 OU, an inferior arcuate defect in the right visual field, disc edema OD, and resolution of his disc edema OS.

Feiner et al. (185) subsequently described 13 patients who developed an optic neuropathy during treatment with amiodarone. The amiodarone dosage ranged from 200 to 600 mg/day and the time interval between initiation of amiodarone therapy and the manifestation of optic neuropathy ranged from 1–72 months. Three patients had no visual symptoms and disc edema was noted on a routine examination. The remaining 10 patients complained of blurry or decreased vision and presented with visual acuities ranging from 20/20 to 20/400. Nine patients had visual field deficits including arcuate scotomas, altitudinal deficits, centrocecal scotomas, enlarged blind spot, and visual field constriction. Among the 13 patients, 12 had disc edema and 5 had bilateral ocular involvement. Only 3 patients had recovery of vision after amiodarone was discontinued and 3 patients had a final visual acuity of 20/100 or worse.

Several other investigators have described patients that developed an optic neuropathy while being treated with amiodarone (186–197). In 1997, a 50-year-old man who became legally blind from a bilateral optic neuropathy that developed 6 weeks after the initiation of amiodarone therapy was awarded a $20 million judgment in a lawsuit against the pharmaceutical company that sells this drug (198).

The nature of the association of optic neuropathy and amiodarone treatment is controversial. Many of the patients described in the above reports developed an optic neuropathy that is indistinguishable from nonarteritic anterior ischemic optic neuropathy. Feiner et al. (185) noted that the 1.79% incidence of optic neuropathy among patients treated with amiodarone at the Mayo Clinic was significantly higher than the 0.3% incidence of ischemic optic neuropathy in the general population 50 years of age or older in Olmsted County, Minnesota. However, patients treated with amiodarone often have severe vascular disease and probably have a higher risk of developing anterior ischemic optic neuropathy compared with the general population.

Macaluso et al. (199) reviewed data from 73 patients who developed an optic neuropathy while taking amiodarone. They proposed several features that distinguish amiodarone-associated optic neuropathy from typical nonarteritic anterior ischemic optic neuropathy. Patients with amiodarone-induced optic neuropathy tend to have insidious bilateral visual loss and protracted, bilateral simultaneous disc edema that resolves several months after the drug is discontinued. In contrast, patients with typical nonarteritic anterior ischemic optic neuropathy tend to have acute unilateral visual loss and disc edema that resolves several weeks after visual loss. Despite these distinctions, there is certainly overlap in the clinical spectrum of these two entities and some patients reported in the literature as having optic neuropathy from amiodarone likely had typical nonarteritic anterior ischemic optic neuropathy.

The mechanism of amiodarone-induced optic neuropathy may be related to the fact that amiodarone binds phospholipids within lysosomes and forms a complex that is not degradable by phospholipase enzymes (183,200). The amiodarone-phospholipid complex accumulates within lysosomes and forms cytoplasmic lamellar inclusions. These lamellar inclusions have been observed in the cytoplasm of many tissues including corneal epithelial, stromal, and endothelial cells; lens epithelium; conjunctival epithelium; extraocular muscle fibers; scleral cells; uvea; blood vessel endothelial cells; retinal ganglion cells; retinal pigment epithelium; and optic nerve axons. Indeed, these inclusions are likely responsible for the corneal and lens deposits noted above.

The accumulation of these inclusions in Schwann cells has been implicated as a cause of the peripheral neuropathy that develops in some patients treated with amiodarone (201,202). Optic nerve axon inclusions have been observed by electron microscopy and may be related to the optic nerve dysfunction and disc edema that occur in association with amiodarone (200).

Several investigators have described a pseudotumor cerebri syndrome in patients treated with amiodarone (203–207). In these patients, amiodarone presumably causes disc edema by raising intracranial pressure.

The available data are insufficient to make firm recommendations regarding a screening protocol for patients treated with amiodarone. Macaluso et al. (199) obtained a baseline examination on all patients prior to starting amiodarone treatment and repeated this examination every 6 months during treatment. Any patient with visual symptoms during treatment should be promptly evaluated. Amiodarone may be a life-saving treatment and the occurrence of an optic neuropathy is therefore not an absolute contraindication to further treatment. However, in patients who have an optic neuropathy while on amiodarone, discontinuation of amiodarone and treatment with an alternative drug should be considered.

TOBACCO

Controversy concerning the mechanism, nature, nosology, semiology and existence of a toxic optic neuropathy caused by tobacco has been debated for many years (208). For much of this time, the designation "tobacco-alcohol amblyopia" has obfuscated these issues (209). It is our opinion that although tobacco probably can cause or contribute to a toxic optic neuropathy, alcohol is not a primary or contributing factor, and the two do not exert any toxic effect in concert. If ever a medical term deserved to be expunged, it is "tobacco-alcohol amblyopia."

The frequency with which tobacco optic neuropathy is encountered varies from time to time and place to place. This remarkable variability may reflect nothing more than the lack of good criteria for proving the diagnosis. In the mid-nineteenth century in Scotland, chronic cases were allegedly seen every day at one eye infirmary (210). One hundred years later, physicians at the Mayo Clinic were not even seeing one case a year (211), and investigators in Australia had also not seen a single case (26). One author essentially denied the existence of tobacco amblyopia (7). In 1977, most authorities agreed that this was a disease whose incidence was declining; an apparent paradox, since the consumption of tobacco products actually *increased* during the same period (212,213). A shift away from pipe and cigar smoking (which carries a higher risk) to cigarette smoking (which carries a lower risk) might explain the paradox.

In any case, convincing cases of tobacco amblyopia are still encountered (214). The field investigation of Cuban patients with epidemic optic neuropathy appears to provide further validation of a role for tobacco in optic nerve disease (49).

The mechanism by which tobacco damages the optic nerves has not been determined. One possibility relates to concurrent malnutrition. The Cuban experience suggests that tobacco may be a secondary factor in patients predisposed to an optic neuropathy by malnutrition. Schepens (215) made a pertinent observation about this relationship. He had rarely seen tobacco "amblyopia" in Belgium prior to World War II. However, during the Nazi occupation of Belgium, when there was widespread malnutrition, the incidence of the disease increased dramatically.

Vitamin B_{12} deficiency may also play a role in some cases of tobacco optic neuropathy as reported by Foulds et al. (216). Impaired vitamin B_{12} absorption was found in 40% of their patients, and there was overt pernicious anemia in 20%. Tobacco itself may actually interfere with the absorption of the vitamin (217). In most cases of tobacco optic neuropathy, however, there is no defect in vitamin B_{12} metabolism, and blood levels of the vitamin are within normal limits.

Cyanide is present in tobacco smoke, and this has led to a suspicion that tobacco optic neuropathy is a limited form of cyanide poisoning (218,219). The rationale for this theory was reviewed by Foulds and Pettigrew (212). In that review, they concluded that there is a defect in sulfur metabolism and of cyanide detoxification in patients with visual loss associated with smoking tobacco. The cyanide theory was reviewed again by Freeman (220).

Attempts to produce a cyanide optic neuropathy in large primates have failed on numerous occasions (212). Chronic cyanide injections caused an optic neuropathy in rats, but the characteristics were not those of human tobacco optic neuropathy (221). The onset was sudden. More importantly, the optic neuropathy only occurred when extensive brain lesions were already present. The role of cyanide in tobacco optic neuropathy has yet to be proved. As with nutritional deficiency optic neuropathy, it seems likely that the etiology of tobacco optic neuropathy in many cases is multifactorial.

Tobacco optic neuropathy is found mostly in middle-aged or elderly individuals. It is overwhelmingly a disease of men, perhaps because the victims are overwhelmingly pipe and cigar smokers. Why cigarette smokers should be less vulnerable is unknown. The disorder is painless and characterized by slowly progressive, bilateral dyschromatopsia and visual loss. The characteristic visual field defect is a centrocecal scotoma. The optic discs initially appear normal, with pallor being a late feature.

Patients with tobacco optic neuropathy slowly improve if they stop smoking, or in some cases, if they are treated with injections of hydroxocobalamin (222).

REFERENCES

1. Knox DL, Chen MF, Guilarte TR, et al. Nutritional amblyopia. Retina 1982;2: 288–293.
2. Dreyfuss PM. Blood transketolase levels in tobacco alcohol amblyopia. Arch Ophthalmol 1965;74:617–620.
3. Harrington DO. Amblyopia due to tobacco, alcohol and nutritional deficiency. Am J Ophthalmol 1962;53:967–972.
4. Carroll FD. Nutritional retrobulbar neuritis. Am J Ophthalmol 1947;30:172–176.
5. Victor M, Mancall EL, Dreyfuss PM. Deficiency amblyopia in the alcoholic patient. Arch Ophthalmol 1960;64:1–33.
6. Victor M. Tobacco amblyopia, cyanide poisoning and vitamin B12 deficiency: A critique of current concepts. In Smith JL, ed. Neuro-Ophthalmolgy Symposium of the University of Miami. Vol 5. Hallandale FL, Huffman, 1970:33–48.
7. Potts AM. Tobacco amblyopia. Surv Ophthalmol 1973;17:313–339.
8. Plant GT, Perry VH. The anatomical basis of the caecocentral scotoma. Brain 1990;113:1441–1457.
9. Carroll FD. Nutritional amblyopia. Arch Ophthalmol 1966;76:406–411.
10. Frisén L. Fundus changes in acute nutritional amblyopia. Arch Ophthalmol 1983; 101:577–579.
11. Ikeda H, Tremain KE, Sanders MD. Neurophysiological investigation in optic nerve disease: Combined assessment of the visual evoked response and electroretinogram. Br J Ophthalmol 1978;62:227–239.
12. Troncoso J, Mancall EL, Schatz NJ. Visual evoked potentials in pernicious anemia. Arch Neurol 1979;36:168–169.
13. Kupersmith MJ, Weiss PA, Carr RE. The visual evoked potential in tobacco alcohol and nutritional amblyopia. Am J Ophthalmol 1983;95:307–314.
14. Klien BA, Krill AE. Fundus flavimaculatus: Clinical, functional and histopathological observations. Am J Ophthalmol 1967;64:3–23.
15. Irvine AR, Wergland FL. Stargardt's hereditary progressive macular degeneration. Br J Ophthalmol 1972;56:817–826.
16. Fishman GA. Fundus flavimaculatus: A clinical classification. Arch Ophthalmol 1976;94:2061–2067.
17. Hadden OB, Gass JDM. Fundus flavimaculatus and Stargardt's disease. Am J Ophthalmol 1976;82:527–539.
18. Bresnick GH, Smith VC, Pokorney J. Autosomal dominantly inherited macular dystrophy with preferential short wavelength sensitive cone involvement. Am J Ophthalmol 1989;108:265–276.
19. Miyake Y, Ichikawa K, Shiose Y, et al. Hereditary macular dystrophy without visible fundus abnormality. Am J Ophthalmol 1989;108:292–299.
20. Matthews GP, Sandberg MA, Berson EL. Foveal cone electroretinograms in patients with central visual loss of unexplained etiology. Arch Ophthalmol 1992; 110:1568–1570.
21. Scott JA, Egan RA. Prevalence of organic neuro-ophthalmologic disease in patients with functional vision loss. Am J Ophthalmol 2003;135:670–675.
22. Eliott D, Traboulsi EI, Maumenee IH. Visual prognosis in autosomal dominant optic atrophy (Kjer type). Am J Ophthalmol 1993;115:360–367.
23. Newman NJ, Lott MT, Wallace DC. The clinical characteristics of pedigrees of Leber's hereditary optic neuropathy with the 11778 mutation. Am J Ophthalmol 1991;111:750–762.
24. Cullom ME, Heher KL, Miller NR, et al. Leber's hereditary optic neuropathy masquerading as tobacco alcohol amblyopia. Arch Ophthalmol 1993;111: 1482–1485.
25. Borruat FX, Hirt L, Regli F. Neuropathie optique alcoolo tabagique: Un piège diagnositique de la neuropathie optique de Leber. Rev Neurol 1994;150: 799–801.
26. Mackey D, Howell N. Tobacco amblyopia. Am J Ophthalmol 1994;117: 817–818.
27. Onishi K, Nakamura M, Sekiya Y, et al. Two cases of Leber's hereditary optic neuropathy simulating malnutritional optic neuropathy. Folia Ophthalmol Jpn 1994;45:891–894.
28. Glaser JS. Neuro-Ophthalmology, Ed 2. Philadelphia, JB Lippincott, 1990:156.
29. Nettleship E. Central amblyopia as an early symptom in tumour of the chiasma. Trans Ophthalmol Soc UK 1897;17:277–299.
30. Henderson WR. The pituitary adenomata: A follow up study of the surgical results in 338 cases (Dr. Harvey Cushing's series). Br J Surg 1939;26:811–879.
31. Hirsh O, Hamlin H. Fate of visual field and optic discs in pituitary tumors. Am J Ophthalmol 1954;37:880–883.
32. Sugita K, Sato O, Hirota T, et al. Scotomatous defects in the central visual fields in pituitary adenomas. Neurochirurgia 1975;18:155–162.
33. Trobe JD, Glaser JS. Quantitative perimetry in compressive optic neuropathy and optic neuritis. Arch Ophthalmol 1978;96:1210–1216.
34. Gutman I, Behrens M, Odel J. Bilateral central and centrocaecal scotomata due to mass lesions. Br J Ophthalmol 1984;68:336–342.
35. Page NGR, Sanders MD. Bilateral central scotomas due to intracranial tumour. Br J Ophthalmol 1984;68:449–457.
36. Spector RT, Smith JL, Parker JC. Cecocentral scotomas in gliomatosis cerebri. J Clin Neuroophthalmol 1984;4:229–238.
37. Bynke H. Pituitary adenomas with ocular manifestations: Incidence of cases and clinical findings 1946–1984. Neuroophthalmology 1984;6:303–311.
38. Beam AD. Amblyopia due to dietary deficiency: Report of eight cases. Arch Ophthalmol 1946;36:113–119.
39. Bloom SM, Merz EH, Taylor WW. Nutritional amblyopia in American prisoners of war liberated from the Japanese. Am J Ophthalmol 1946;29:1248–1257.
40. Hobbs HE. Ocular disturbances associated with malnutrition. Trans Ophthalmol Soc UK 1946;66:116–122.
41. Livingston PC. Ocular disturbances associated with malnutrition. Trans. Ophthalmol Soc UK 1946;66:19–44.
42. Ridley H. Ocular disturbances associated with malnutrition. Trans Ophthalmol Soc UK 1946;66:45–71.
43. Smith DA. Ocular disturbances in malnutrition. Trans Ophthalmol Soc UK 1946; 66:111–116.
44. Dekking HM. Tropical nutritional amblyopia ("camp eyes"). Ophthalmologica 1947;113:65–92.
45. Denny Brown D. Neurological conditions resulting from prolonged and severe dietary restriction. Medicine 1947;26:41–113.
46. Hirano M, Cleary JM, Stewart AM, et al. Mitochondria DNA mutations in an outbreak of optic neuropathy in Cuba. Neurology 1994;44:843–845.
47. Roman GC. An epidemic in Cuba of optic neuropathy, sensorineural deafness, peripheral sensory neuropathy, and dorsolateral myeloneuropathy. J Neurol Sci 1994;127:11–28.
48. Sadun AA, Martone JF, Muci Mendoza R, et al. Epidemic optic neuropathy in Cuba: Eye findings. Arch Ophthalmol 1994;112:691–699.
49. The Cuba Neuropathy Field Investigation Team. Epidemic optic neuropathy in Cuba: Clinical characterization and risk factors. N Engl J Med 1995;333: 1176–1182.
50. Thomas PK, Plant GT, Baxter P, et al. An epidemic of optic neuropathy and painful sensory neuropathy in Cuba: Clinical aspects. J Neurol 1995;242: 629–638.
51. Lessell S. Nutritional amblyopia. J Neuroophthalmol 1998;18:106–111.
52. Fisher CM. Residual neuropathological changes in Canadians held prisoners of war by the Japanese (Strachan's disease). Can Serv Med J 1955;11:157–199.
53. Smiddy WE, Green WR. Nutritional amblyopia: Histopathologic study with retrospective clinical correlation. Graefe's Arch Ophthalmol 1987;225:321–324.
54. Cuban National Operative Group on Epidemic Neuropathy: Epidemic neuropathy in Cuba. Cuban Ministry of Health, Havana, Cuba, July 30, 1993.

55. Lincoff NS, Odel JG, Hirano M. ''Outbreak'' of optic and peripheral neuropathy in Cuba? JAMA 1993;270:511–518.
56. Llanos G, Asher D, Brown P, et al. Epidemic neuropathy in Cuba. Epidemiol Bull 1993;14:1–4.
57. Centers for Disease Control. Epidemic neuropathy: Cuba, 1991–1994. MMWR 1994;43:183–192.
58. Roman GC. Epidemic optic neuropathy in Cuba: A plea to end the United States economic embargo on a humanitarian basis. Neurology 1994;44:1784–1786.
59. Newman NJ. Optic neuropathy. Neurology 1996;46:315–322.
60. Tucker K, Hedges TR. Food shortages and an epidemic of optic and peripheral neuropathy in Cuba. Nutritional Reviews 1993;51:349–357.
61. Mojon, DS, Kaufmann P, Odel JG et al. Clinical course of a cohort in the Cuban epidemic optic and peripheral neuropathy. Neurology 1997;48:19–22.
62. Milea D. Blindness in a strict vegan. N Engl J Med 2000;342:897–898.
63. Bjorkenheim B. Optic neuropathy caused by vitamin B12 deficiency in carriers of the fish tapeworm, Diphyllobothrium latum. Lancet 1966;1:688.
64. Bickel H. Funikulare Myelitis mit bulbaren und polyneuritischen Symptomen. Arch Psychiatr 1914;53:1106–1117.
65. Adams RD, Kubik CS. Subacute combined degeneration of the brain in pernicious anemia. N Engl J Med 1944;231:1–9.
66. Hind VMD. Degeneration in the peripheral visual pathway of vitamin B12 deficient monkeys. Trans Ophthalmol Soc UK 1970;90:839–846.
67. Hind VMD. The histology of vitamin B12 deficiency optic neuropathy in monkeys. In Cant JS, ed. The Optic Nerve. London, Henry Kimpton, 1972:257–269.
68. Agamanolis DP, Chester EM, Victor M, et al. Neuropathology of experimental vitamin B12 deficiency in monkeys. Neurology 1976;26:905–914.
69. Cohen H. Optic atrophy as the presenting sign in pernicious anemia. Lancet 1936;2:1202–1203.
70. Turner JAA. Optic atrophy associated with pernicious anemia. Brain 1940;63:225–236.
71. Hyland HH, Sharp VJH. Optic nerve degeneration in pernicious anemia. Can Med Assoc J 1952;67:660–665.
72. Hamilton HE, Ellis PP, Sheets RF. Visual impairment due to optic neuropathy in pernicious anemia. Blood 1959;14:378–385.
73. Lerman S, Feldmahn AL. Centrocecal scotoma as the presenting sign in pernicious anemia. Arch Ophthalmol 1961;65:381–385.
74. Burde RM, Savino PJ, Trobe JD. Clinical Decisions in Neuro Ophthalmology. Ed 2. St Louis, CV Mosby, 1985:46.
75. Williams RD, Nason HL, Wilder RM, et al. Observations on induced thiamine deficiency in man. Arch Intern Med 1940;66:785–799.
76. Williams RD, Nason HL, Power MH, et al. Induced thiamine (vitamin B1) deficiency in man. Arch Intern Med 1943;71:38–53.
77. Witt ED, Goldman Rakic PS. Intermittent thiamine deficiency in the rhesus monkey. I. Progression of neurological signs and neuroanatomical lesions. Ann Neurol 1983;13:376–395.
78. Cogan DG, Witt ED, Goldman Rakic PS. Ocular signs in thiamine deficient monkeys and in Wernicke's disease in humans. Arch Ophthalmol 1985;103:1212–1220.
79. De Wardener HE, Lennox B. Cerebral beri beri (Wernicke's encephalopathy): Review of 52 cases in Singapore prisoner of war hospital. Lancet 1947;1:11–17.
80. Cogan DG, Victor M. Ocular signs of Wernicke's disease. Arch Ophthalmol 1954;51:204–211.
81. Hsu CT, Miller NR, Wray ML. Optic neuropathy from folic acid deficiency without alcohol abuse. Ophthalmologica 2002;216:65–67.
82. Golnik KC, Schaible ER. Folate responsive optic neuropathy. J Clin Neuroophthalmol 1994;14:163–169.
83. Strachan H. On a form of multiple neuritis prevalent in the West Indies. Practitioner 1897;59:477–484.
84. Scott HH. An investigation into an acute outbreak of ''central neuritis.'' Ann Trop Med Parasitol 1918;12:109–196.
85. Montgomery RD, Cruickshank EK, Robertson WB, et al. Clinical and pathological observations on Jamaican neuropathy. Brain 1964;87:425–462.
86. Crews SJ. Bilateral amblyopia in West Indians. Trans Ophthalmol Soc UK 1963;83:653–667.
87. MacKenzie AD, Phillips CI. West Indian amblyopia. Brain 1968;91:249–260.
88. Osuntokun BO. An ataxic neuropathy in Nigeria: A clinical, biochemical and electrophysiological study. Brain 1968;91:215–248.
89. Osuntokun BO, Osuntokun O. Tropical amblyopia in Nigerians. Am J Ophthalmol 1971;72:708–716.
90. Tuboku Metzger AF. Diet and neuropathy. Br Med J 1969;4:239.
91. Grant WM, Schuman JS. Toxicology of the Eye. Ed 4. Springfield IL, Charles C Thomas, 1993.
92. Baumbach GL, Cancilla PA, Martin Amat G, et al. Methyl alcohol poisoning. IV. Alterations of the morphological findings of the retina and optic nerve. Arch Ophthalmol 1977;95:1859–1865.
93. Hayreh MS, Hayreh SS, Baumbach GL, et al. Methyl alcohol poisoning. III. Ocular toxicity. Arch Ophthalmol 1977;95:1851–1858.
94. Martin Amat G, Tephly TR, McMartin KE, et al. Methyl alcohol poisoning. II. Development of a model for ocular toxicity in methyl alcohol poisoning using the rhesus monkey. Arch Ophthalmol 1977;95:1847–1850.
95. McLean DR, Jacobs H, Mielke BW. Methanol poisoning: A clinical and pathological study. Ann Neurol 1980;8:161–167.
96. Sharpe JA, Hostovsky M, Bilbao JM, et al. Methanol optic neuropathy: A histopathological study. Neurology 1982;32:1093–1100.
97. Naeser P. Optic nerve involvement in a case of methanol poisoning. Br J Ophthalmol 1988;72:778–781.
98. Ziegler SL. The ocular menace of wood alcohol poisoning. Br J Ophthalmol 1921;5:365–373.
99. Roe O. Clinical investigation of methyl alcohol poisoning with special reference to the pathogenesis and treatment of amblyopia. Acta Med Scand 1943;113:558.
100. Jacobson BM, Russell HK, Grimm JJ, et al. Acute methyl alcohol poisoning: Report of 18 cases. US Naval Med Bull 1945;44:1099–1106.
101. Benton CD, Calhoun FP. The ocular effects of methyl alcohol poisoning. Trans Am Acad Ophthalmol Otolaryngol 1952;56:875–885.
102. Bennett IL, Cary FH, Mitchell GL Jr, et al. Acute methyl alcohol poisoning: A review based on experiences in an outbreak of 323 cases. Medicine 1953;32:431–463.
103. Kane RL. A methanol poisoning outbreak in Kentucky. Arch Environ Health 1968;17:119–129.
104. Dethlefs R, Naraqi S. Ocular manifestations and complications of acute methyl alcohol intoxication. Med J Aust 1978;2:483–485.
105. McMartin KE, Amber JJ, Tephly TR. Methanol poisoning in human subjects: Role for formic acid accumulation in the metabolic acidosis. Am J Med 1980;68:414–418.
106. Greiner JV, Pillai S, Limaye SR, et al. Sterno induced methanol toxicity and visual recovery after prompt dialysis. Arch Ophthalmol 1989;107:643.
107. Stelmach MZ, O'Day J. Partly reversible visual failure with methanol toxicity. Aust NZ J Ophthalmol 1992;20:57–64.
108. Jacobsen D, McMartin KE. Methanol and ethylene glycol poisonings: Mechanism of toxicity, clinical course, diagnosis and treatment. Med Toxicol 1986;1:309–334.
109. Carr RE, Henkind P. Ocular manifestations of ethambutol. Arch Ophthalmol 1962;67:566–571.
110. Schmidt IG. Central nervous system effects of ethambutol in monkeys. Ann NY Acad Sci 1966;135:759–774.
111. Schmidt IG, Schmidt LH. Studies of the neurotoxicity of ethambutol and its racemate for the rhesus monkey. J Neuropath Exp Neurol 1966;25:40–67.
112. Lessell S. Histopathology of experimental ethambutol intoxication. Invest Ophthalmol 1976;15:765–769.
113. Matsuoka Y, Mukyama M, Sobue I. Histopathological study of experimental ethambutol neuropathy. Clin Neurol 1972;12:453–459.
114. Kozak SF, Inderlied CB, Hsu HY, et al. The role of copper on Ethambutol's antimicrobial action and implications for Ethambutol-induced optic neuropathy. Diagn Microbiol Infect Dis 1998;30:83–87.
115. Lessell S. Toxic and deficiency optic neuropathies. In Glaser JS, Smith JL, eds. Neuro-Ophthalmology. Vol 7. St Louis, CV Mosby, 1973:21–37.
116. Leopold IH. Zinc deficiency and visual impairment. Am J Ophthalmol 1978;85:871–875.
117. Saraux H, Bechetoille A, Nou B, et al. La baisse du taux du zinc serique dans certaines névrites optiques toxique. Ann Ocul 1975;208:29–31.
118. Delacoux E, Moreau Y, Godefroy A, Evstigneef T. Prevention of ocular toxicity of ethambutol: Study of zincaemia and chromatic analysis. J Fr Ophtalmol 1978;1:191–196.
119. DePalma P, Franco F, Bragliani G, et al. The incidence of optic neuropathy in 84 patients treated with Ethambutol. Metab Pediatr Syst Ophthalmol 1989;2:80–82.
120. Tu J, Blackwell RQ, Lee P. DL-Penicillamine as a cause of optic axial neuritis. JAMA 1963;185:83–86.
121. Goldstein NP, Hollenhorst RW, Randall RV, Gross JB. Possible relationship of optic neuritis, Wilson's disease, and DL penicillamine therapy. JAMA 1966;196:734–735.
122. Citron K. Ethambutol: A review with special reference to ocular toxicity. Tubercle 1969;50(Suppl):32–36.
123. Leibold JE. Drugs having a toxic effect on the optic nerve. Int Ophthalmol Clin 1971;11:137–157.
124. Toth LC, Hermans G, Berthelon S. Névrite optique et l'ethambutol. Bull Soc Belge Opthtalmol 1973;165:382–394.
125. Bronte Stewart J, Pettigrew AR, Foulds WS. Toxic optic neuropathy and its experimental production. Trans Ophthalmol Soc UK 1976;96:355–358.
126. Yoshikawa T, Nagami P. Adverse drug interactions in TB therapy: Risks and recommendations. Geriatrics 1982;37:61–68.
127. Skjødt K, Fledelius HC. Ocular ethambutol toxicity in Denmark 1977–1981. Dansk Ugeskr Laeg 1985;147:1683–1686.
128. Fledelius HC, Petrera JE, Skjødt K, et al. Ocular ethambutol toxicity. Acta Ophthalmol 1987;65:251–255.
129. Kahana LM. Toxic ocular effects of ethambutol. Can Med Assoc J 1987;137:212–216.
130. Smith JL. Should ethambutol be barred? J Clin Neuroophthalmol 1987;7:84–86.
131. Kahana LM. Ethambutol and the eye. Lancet 1988;2:627.
132. Rahman M, Nizam R. Ethambutol toxic neuroretinopathy in Bangladesh. Pakistan J Ophthalmol 1989;5:37–40.

133. Kumar A, Sandramouli S, Verma L, et al. Ocular ethambutol toxicity: Is it reversible? J Clin Neuroophthalmol 1993;13:15–17.

134. Choi SY, Hwang JM. Optic neuropathy associated with Ethambutol in Koreans. Korean J Ophthalmol 1997;11:106–110.

135. Barron GJ, Tepper L, Iovine G. Ocular toxicity from Ethambutol. Am J Ophthalmol 1974;77:256–260.

136. Citron KM, Thomas GO. Ocular toxicity from Ethambutol. Thorax 1986;41:737–739.

137. De Vita EG, Miao M, Sadun AA. Optic neuropathy in ethambutol treated renal tuberculosis. J Clin Neuroophthalmol 1987;7:77–83.

138. Murray FJ. U.S. Public Health Service experience with ethambutol. International Congress of Chemotherapy, Vienna 1967;6:339.

139. Alvarez KL, Krop LC. Ethambutol-induced ocular toxicity revisited. Ann Pharmaco 1993;27:102–103.

140. Chuenkongkaew W, Samsen P, Thanasombatsakul N. Ethambutol and optic neuropathy. J Med Assoc Thai 2003;86:622–625.

141. Polak BCP, Leys M, van Lith GHM. Blue yellow colour vision changes as early symptoms of ethambutol oculotoxicity. Ophthalmologica 1985;119:223–226.

142. Kumar A, Sandramouli S, Verma L, et al. Ocular Ethambutol toxicity: is it reversible? J Clin Neuroophthal 1993;13:15–17.

143. Tsai RK, Lee YH. Reversibility of Ethambutol optic neuropathy. J Ocul Pharmacol Ther 1997;13:473–477.

144. Asayama T. Two cases of bitemporal hemianopsia due to ethambutol. Jpn J Clin Ophthalmol 1969;23:1209–1212.

145. Woung LC, Jou JR, Liaw SL. Visual function in recovered Ethambutol optic neuropathy. J Ocul Pharmaco Ther 1995;11:411–419.

146. Chatterjee VKK, Buchanan DR, Friedmann AI, Green M. Ocular toxicity following Ethambutol in standard dosage. Br J Dis Chest 1986;80:288–290.

147. Cornblath WT, Clavert PC. Best catch from NANOSNET. II. Monitoring for Ethambutol Optic Nerve Toxicity. J Neuroophthal 2002;22:124–125.

148. Salmon JF, Carmichael TR, Welsh NH. Use of contrast sensitivity measurement in the detection of subclinical ethambutol toxic optic neuropathy. Br J Ophthalmol 1987;71:192–196.

149. Trusiewicz D. Farnsworth 100-Hue Test in diagnosis of Ethambutol-induced damage to optic nerve. Ophthalmologica 1975;171:425–431.

150. Yiannikas C, Walsh JC, McLeod JG. Visual evoked potentials in the detection of subclinical optic toxic effects secondary to Ethambutol. Arch Neurol 1983;40:645–648.

151. Srivastava AK, Goel UC, Bajaj S, et al. J Assoc Phy India 1997;45:847–849.

152. Kono R. Subacute myelo neuropathy: A new neurological disease in Japan. Jpn J Med Sci Biol 1971;24:197–216.

153. Sobue I, Ando K, Iida M, et al. Myeloneuropathy with abdominal disorders in Japan. Neurology 1971;21:168–173.

154. Tsubaki T, Honma Y, Hoshi M. Neurological syndrome associated with clioquinol. Lancet 1971;1:696–697.

155. Nakae K, Yamamoto S, Shigematsu K, et al. Relation between subacute myelo optic neuropathy (SMON) and clioquinol: Nationwide survey. Lancet 1973;1:171–173.

156. Toyokura Y, Takusu T. Clinical features of SMON. Jpn J Med Sci Biol 1978;28:87–100.

157. Baumgartner G, Gawel MJ, Kaeser HE, et al. Neurotoxicity of halogenated hydroxyquinolines: clinical analysis of cases reported outside Japan. J Neurol Neurosurg Psych 1979;42:1073–1083.

158. Oakley GP. The neurotoxicity of the halogenated hydroxyquinolines. JAMA 1973;225:395–397.

159. Etheridge JE, Stewart GT. Treating acrodermatitis enteropathica. Lancet 1966;1:261–262.

160. Berggren L, Hansson O. Treating acrodermatitis enteropathica. Lancet 1966;1:52.

161. Hache JC, Woillez M, Breuillard F, et al. La nevrite optique des iodo quinolines. Bull Soc Ophtalmol Fr 1973;73:501–503.

162. Idriss ZH, Der Kaloustian VM. Acrodermatitis enteropathica: Report of three new cases. Clin Pediatr 1973;12:393–395.

163. Reich H. Acrodermatitis enteropathica. Dtsch Med Wschr 1973;98:1673–1676.

164. Behrens M. Optic atrophy in children after diiodohydroxyquin therapy. JAMA 1974;228:693–694.

165. Garcia Perez A, Castro C, Franco A, et al. A case of optic atrophy possibly induced by quinoline in acrodermatitis enteropathica. Br J Derm 1974;90:453–455.

166. Goodman LS, Gilman A. The Pharmacological Basis of Therapeutics, Ed 5. New York, MacMillan, 1975:148.

167. Humblet M. Nevrite retrobulbaire chronique par Antabuse. Bull Soc Belge Ophtalmol 1953;104:297–301.

168. Pommier A, Reiss Bryon M. Névrites retrobulbaires au disulfirame. Bull Soc Ophtalmol Fr 1963;63:254–256.

169. Perdriel G, Chevaleraud J. A propos d'un nouveau cas de névrite optique due au disulfiram. Bull Soc Ophtalmol Fr 1966;66:159–165.

170. Saraux H, Biais B. Névrites optiques par le disulfirame. Ann Ocul 1970;203:769–774.

171. Norton AL, Walsh FB. Disulfiram induced optic neuritis. Trans Am Acad Ophthalmol Otolaryngol 1972;76:1263–1265.

172. Corydon L. Optic neuritis and polyneuropathy and disulfiram (antabuse) therapy. Ugeskr Laeg 1973;135:1470–1472.

173. Norton AL. Drug can cause optic neuritis in alcoholics. JAMA 1971;218:808.

174. Maugery J, Magnard P, Villon JC. Optic neuritis in the course of treatment with esperal. Bull Soc Ophtalmol Fr 1974;74:779–781.

175. Acheson JF, Howard RS. Reversible optic neuropathy associated with disulfiram. A clinical and electrophysiological report. Neuroophthalmology 1988;8:175–177.

176. Marmor MF, Kessler R. Sildenafil (Viagra) and ophthalmology. Surv Ophthalmol 1999;44:153–162.

177. Pomeranz HD, Smith KH, Hart WM, Egan RA. Sildenafil-associated nonarteritic anterior ischemic optic neuropathy. Ophthalmology 2002;09:584–587.

178. Egan R, Pomeranz H. Sildenafil (Viagra) associated anterior ischemic optic neuropathy. Arch Ophthalmol 2000;118:291–292.

179. Cunningham AV, Smith KH. Anterior ischemic optic neuropathy associated with Viagra. J Neuroophthalmol 2001;21:22–25.

180. Dheer S, Rekhi GS, Merlyn S. Sildenafil associated anterior ischaemic optic neuropathy. JAPI 2002;50:265.

181. Boshier A, Pambakian N, Shakir SAW. A case of nonarteritic ischemic optic neuropathy (NAION) in a male patient taking sildenafil. Intl J Clin Pharmaco Ther 2002;40:422–423.

182. Neufeld AH, Sawada A, Becker B. Inhibition of nitric oxide synthase 2 by aminoguanidine provides neuroprotection of retinal ganglion cells in a rat model of chronic glaucoma. Proc Natl Acad Sci USA 1999;96:9944–9948.

183. Mantyjarvi M, Tuppurainen K, Ikaheimo K. Ocular side effects of Amiodarone. Surv Ophthalmol 1998;42:360–366.

184. Gittinger JW Jr, Asdourian GK. Papillopathy caused by amiodarone. Arch Ophthalmol 1987;105:349–351.

185. Feiner LA, Younge BR, Kazmier FJ, et al. Optic neuropathy and amiodarone therapy. Mayo Clin Proc 1987;62:702–717.

186. Garrett SN, Kearney JJ, Schiffman JS. Amiodarone optic neuropathy. J Clin Neuroophthalmol 1988;8:105–110.

187. Nazarian SM, Jay WM. Bilateral optic neuropathy associated with amiodarone therapy. J Clin Neuroophthalmol 1988;8:25–28.

188. Dewachter A, Lievens H. Amiodarone and optic neuropathy. Bull Soc Belge Ophtalmol 1988;227:47–50.

189. Krieg P, Schipper I. Bilaterale Optikusneuropathie nach Amiodarone Therapie. Klin Monatsbl Augenheilkd 1992;200:128–132.

190. Belec L, Davila G, Bleibel JM, et al. Bilateral optic neuropathy during prolonged treatment with amiodarone. Ann Med Interne 1992;143:349–350.

191. Palimar P, Cota N. Bilateral anterior ischaemic optic neuropathy following amiodarone. Eye 1998;12:894–896.

192. Seemongal-Dass RR, Spencer SR. Bilateral optic neuropathy linked with amiodarone. Eye 1998;12:474–477.

193. Sreih AG, Schoenfeld MH, Marieb MA. Optic neuropathy following Amiodarone therapy. PACE 1999;22:1108–1110.

194. Eryilmaz T, Atilla H, Batioglu F, Gunalp I. Amiodarone-related optic neuropathy. Jpn J Ophthalmol 2000;44:565–568.

195. Leifert D, Hansen LL, Gerling J. Amiodaron-Optikusneuropathie: ein eigneständiges Krankheitsbild? Klin Monatsbl Augenheilkd 2000;217:171–177.

196. Speicher MA, Goldman MH, Chrousos GA. Amiodarone optic neuropathy without disc edema. J Neuroophthalmol 2000;20:171–172.

197. Nagra PK, Foroozan R, Savino PJ, et al. Amiodarone induced optic neuropathy. Br J Ophthalmol 2003;87:420–422.

198. Mindel JM. Editorial: Amiodarone and optic neuropathy: A medicolegal issue. Surv Ophthalmol 1998;42:358–359.

199. Macaluso DC, Shults WT, Fraunfelder FT. Features of amiodarone-induced optic neuropathy. Am J Ophthalmol 1999;127:610–612.

200. Mansour AM, Puklin JE, O'Grady R. Optic nerve ultrastructure following amiodarone therapy. J Clin Neuroophthalmol 1988;8:231–237.

201. Pellissier JF, Pouget J, Cros D, et al. Peripheral neuropathy induced by amiodarone chlorhydrate: A clinopathological study. J Neurol Sci 1984;63:251–266.

202. Jacobs JM, Costa-Jussa FR. The pathology of amiodarone neurotoxicity. II. Peripheral neuropathy in man. Brain 1985;108:753–769.

203. Lopez AC, Lopez AM, Jimenez SF, De Elvira MJR. Acute intracranial hypertension during amiodarone infusion. Crit Care Med 1985;13:688–689.

204. Van Zandijcke M, Dewachter A. Pseudotumor cerebri with amiodarone (letter to the editor). J Neurol Neurosurg Psychiatry 1986;49:1463–1464.

205. Fikkers BG, Bogousslavsky J, Regli F, Glasson S. Pseudotumour cerebri with amiodarone. J Neurol Neurosurg Psychiatry 1986;49:606.

206. Grogan WA, Narkun DM. Pseudotumour cerebri with amiodarone. J Neurol Neurosurg Psychiatry 1987;50:651.

207. Borruat FX, Regli F. Pseudotumor cerebri as a complication of amiodarone therapy. Am J Ophthalmol 1993;116:776–777.

208. Solberg Y, Rosner M, Belkin M. The association between cigarette smoking and ocular diseases. Surv Ophthalmol 1998;42:535–547.

209. Sedwick LA. The perils of Pauline: Visual loss in a tippler. Surv Ophthalmol 1991;35:454–462.

210. Mackenzie W. A Practical Treatise on Diseases of the Eye. London, Longman, 1830.

211. Samples JR, Younge BR. Tobacco alcohol amblyopia. J Clin Neuroophthamol 1981;1:213–218.
212. Foulds WS, Pettigrew AR. Tobacco alcohol amblyopia. In Brockhurst RJ, Boruchoff SA, Hutchinson BT et al., eds. Controversy in Ophthalmology. Philadelphia, WB Saunders, 1977:851–865.
213. Harrington DO. What is the etiology of alcohol and tobacco amblyopia? In Brockhurst RJ, Boruchoff SA, Hutchinson BT et al., eds. Controversy in Ophthalmology. Philadelphia, WB Saunders, 1977:866–872.
214. Rizzo JF, Lessell S. Tobacco amblyopia. Am J Ophthalmol 1993;116:84–87.
215. Schepens CL. Is tobacco amblyopia a deficiency disease? Trans Ophthalmol Soc UK 1946;66:309–331.
216. Foulds WS, Chisholm IA, Bronte Stewart JM, et al. Vitamin B12 absorption in tobacco amblyopia. Br J Ophthalmol 1969;53:393–397.
217. Watson Williams EJ, Bottomley AC, Ainley RG et al. Absorption of vitamin B12 in tobacco amblyopia. Br J Ophthalmol 1969;53:549–552.
218. Lehmann JB, Gundermann K. Neue untersuchungen über die bedeutung der Balusaure fur die giftifheit des Tabakrauchs. Archiv Hyg 1912;76:319.
219. Wokes F. Tobacco amblyopia. Lancet 1958;2:526–527.
220. Freeman AG. Optic neuropathy and chronic cyanide intoxication: A review. J Roy Soc Med 1988;81:103–106.
221. Lessell S. Experimental cyanide optic neuropathy. Arch Ophthalmol 1971;86:194–204.
222. Krumesiek J, Kruger C, Patzold U. Tobacco-alcohol amblyopia, neuro-ophthalmological findings and clinical course. Acta Neurol Scand 1985;72:180–187.
223. Pearlman JT, Kadish AH, Ramsey JC. Vision loss associated with amantadine hydrochloride use. JAMA 1977;237:1200.
224. Saraux H, Cavicchi L. Névrite optique par l'amoproxan. Bull Soc Ophtalmol Fr 1970;70:664–665.
225. Francois P, Woillez M, Guilbert M, et al. Une nouvelle étiologie de névrite optique toxique: l'Amoproxan. Bull Soc Ophtalmol Fr 1970;70:665–666.
226. Longley BJ, Clausen NM, Tatum AL. Experimental production of primary atrophy in monkeys by administration of organic arsenical compounds. J Pharmacol 1942;76:202–206.
227. Agnello F. Amaurosi tossica da felce maschio. Rass Ital Ottal 1939;8:210–221.
228. Rosen ES, Edgar JT, Smith JLS. Male fern retrobulbar neuropathy in cattle. Trans Ophthalmol Soc UK 1969;89:289–299.
229. Gupta DR, Strobos RJ. Bilateral papillitis associated with cafergot therapy. Neurology 1972;22:793–797.
230. Lewin L, Guillery H. Die Wirkungen von Arzneimitteln und Giften auf das Auge. Ed 2. Berlin, August Hirschwald, 1913.
231. Villard H. Les brulures chimiques de l'oeil. Arch Ophtalmol 1927;44:21–40, 93–111, 167–177, 222–223.
232. Vigliani EC. Clinical observations on carbon disulfide intoxication in Italy. Industr Med Surg 1950;19:240–242.
233. Teleky L. Gewerbliche Vergiftungen. Berlin, Springer, 1955.
234. Simmons IG, Good PA. Carbon monoxide poisoning causes optic neuropathy. Eye 1998;12:809–814.
235. Wirtschafter ZT. Toxic amblyopia and accompanying physiological disturbances in carbon tetrachloride intoxication. Am J Public Health 1933;23:1035–1038.
236. Gocher TEP. Carbon tetrachloride poisoning. Northwest Med 1944;43:228–230.
237. Gray I. Carbon tetrachloride poisoning: Report of 7 cases with 2 deaths. NY J Med 1947;47:2311–2315.
238. Smith AR. Optic atrophy following inhalation of carbon tetrachloride. Arch Industr Hyg 1950;1:348–351.
239. Franceschetti A, Rickli JH. Nevrite retrobulbaire apres intoxication aigue aux hydrocarbures chlores. Ophthalmologica 1952;123:255–260.
240. Lyle DJ, Zavon MR. Blindness in a fur worker. Occup Med 1961;3:478–479.
241. Roper JP. The presumed neurotoxic effects of Catha edulis: An exotic plant now available in the United Kingdom. Br J Ophthalmol 1986;70:779–781.
242. Yiannakis PH, Larner AJ. Visual failure and optic atrophy associated with chlorambucil therapy. Br Med J 1993;306:109.
243. Joy RT, Scalettar R, Sodee DB. Optic and peripheral neuritis. JAMA 1960;173:1731–1734.
244. Cocke JG. Chloramphenicol optic neuritis. Am J Dis Child 1967;114:424–426.
245. Harley RD, Huang NN, Macri CH, et al. Optic neuritis and optic atrophy following chloramphenicol in cystic fibrosis patients. Trans Am Acad Ophthalmol Otolaryngol 1970;74:1011–1031.
246. Cogan DG, Truman JT, Smith TR. Optic neuropathy, chloramphenicol, and infantile genetic agranulocytosis. Invest Ophthalmol 1973;12:534–537.
247. Charache S, Finkelstein D, Lietman PS, et al. Peripheral and optic neuritis in a patient with hemoglobin SC disease during treatment of Salmonella osteomyelitis with chloramphenicol. Johns Hopkins Med J 1977;140:121–124.
248. Godel V, Nemet P, Lazar M. Chloramphenicol optic neuropathy. Arch Ophthalmol 1980;98:1417–1421.
249. Spaide RF, Diamond G, D'Amico RA, et al. Ocular findings in cystic fibrosis. Am J Ophthalmol 1987;103:204–210.
250. Nieden A. Über amblyopia durch roburitvergiftung. Zbl Prakt Augenheilkd 1888;12:193.
251. Sollier P, Jousset X. Névrites nitro phenolees. Clin Ophtalmol 1917;22:78–87.
252. Rab SM, Alam MN, Sadequzzaman MD. Optic atrophy during chlorpromazine therapy. Br J Ophthalmol 1969;53:208–209.
253. Givner I. Centrocecal scotomas due to chlorpropamide. Arch Ophthalmol 1961;66:64.
254. George CW. Central scotomata due to chlorpropamide. Arch Ophthalmol 1963;69:773.
255. Wymore J, Carter JE. Chlorpropamide-induced optic neuropathy. Arch Intern Med 1982;142:381.
256. Shimamura Y, Chikama M, Tanimoto T, et al. Optic nerve degeneration caused by supraophthalmic carotid artery infusion with cisplatin and ACNU: Case report. J Neurosurg 1990;72:285–288.
257. Maiese K, Walker RW, Gargan R, et al. Intra arterial cisplain associated optic and otic toxicity. Arch Neurol 1992;49:83–86.
258. Mansfield SH, Castillo M. MR of cis platinum induced optic neuritis. AJNR 1994;15:1178–1180.
259. Sugimoto M, Yokokawa M, Hoshina M, et al. Two females with presumed cisplatin associated visual disturbance. Jpn J Ophthalmol 1996;47:901–903.
260. Basteau F, Gérini Jamain S. Neuropathie optique et citrate de clomiphène. Bull Soc Ophtalmol Fr 1991;91:9–12.
261. Lawton AW. Optic neuropathy associated with clomiphene citrate therapy. Fertil Steil 1994;61:390–391.
262. Licht A, Oliver M, Rachmilewitz EA. Optic atrophy following treatment with cobalt chloride in a patient with pancytopenia and hypercellular marrow. Isr J Med Sci 1972;8:61–66.
263. Avery R, Jabs DA, Wingard JR, et al. Optic disc edema after bone marrow transplantation: Possible role of cyclosporine toxicity. Ophthalmology 1991;98:1294–1301.
264. Coskuncan NM, Jabs DA, Dunn JP, et al. The eye in bone marrow transplantation. VI. Retinal complications. Arch Ophthalmol 1994;112:372–379.
265. Katz B. Disk edema subsequent to renal transplantation. Surv Ophthalmol 1997;41:315–320.
266. Porges Y, Bluman S, Fireman Z, et al. Cyclosporine-induced optic neuropathy, ophthalmoplegia, and nystagmus in a patient with Crohn disease. Am J Ophthalmol 1998;126:607–609.
267. Suh DW, Ruttum MS, Stuckenschneider BJ, et al. Ocular findings after bone marrow transplantation in a pediatric population. Ophthalmology 1999;106:1564–1570.
268. Kerty E, Vigander K, Flage T, et al. Ocular findings in allogeneic stem cell transplantation without total body irradiation. Ophthalmology 1999;106:1334–1338.
269. Saito J, Kami M, Taniguchi F, et al. Unilateral papilledema after bone marrow transplantation. Bone Marrow Transplant 1999;23:963–965.
270. Lakhanpal V, Schocket SS, Rouben J. Deferoxamine (Desferal) induced toxic retinal pigmentary degeneration and presumed optic neuropathy. Ophthalmology 1984;91:443–451.
271. Marciani MG, Stefani N, Stefanini F, et al. Visual function during long term desferrioxamine treatment. Lancet 1993;341:491.
272. Dennerlein JA, Lang GE, Stahnke K, et al. Okuläre Befunde bei Desferaltherapie. Ophthalmologe 1995;92:38–42.
273. Dupuy O, Flocard F, Vial C, et al. Disulfiram (Esperal) toxicity: Apropos of 3 original cases. Rev Med Interne 1995;16:67–72.
274. Guillaume S, Joachim M. Neuropathie optique par disulfirame (Antabuse): une observation. Bull Soc Belge Ophtal 1998;268:161–162.
275. Kimura H, Masai H, Kashii S. Optic neuropathy following elcatonin therapy. J Neuroophthalmol 1996;16:134–136.
276. Jacovides A. Troubles visuels à la suite d'injections fortes d'emetine. Arch Ophthalmol 1923;40:657–660.
277. Kravitz D. Neuro retinitis associated with symptoms of ergot poisoning. Arch Ophthalmol 1935;13:201–206.
278. Hullo A. Les névrites optiques toxiques a l'ethambutol: Une realite. Bull Soc Ophtalmol Fr 1987;87:1329–1333.
279. Hamard H. Ethambutol et nerf optique. Bull Soc Ophtalmol Fr 1989;89:1001–1003.
280. Nasemann J, Zrenner E, Riedel KG. Recovery after severe ethambutol intoxication: Psychophysical and electrophysiological correlations. Doc Ophthalmol 1989;71:279–292.
281. Sato T, Amemiya T, Iwasaki M. Color vision in ethambutol optic neuropathy: Using standard pseudoisochromatic plates. Folia Ophthalmol Jpn 1992;43:424–427.
282. Russo PA, Chaglasian MA. Toxic optic neuropathy associated with ethambutol: Implications for current therapy. J Am Optom Assoc 1994;65:332–338.
283. Haining WM, Beveridge GW. Toxic amblyopia in a patient receiving ethchlorvynol as a hypnotic. Br J Ophthalmol 1964;48:598–600.
284. Brown E, Meyer GG. Toxic amblyopia and peripheral neuropathy with ethchlorvynol abuse. Am J Psychiatr 1969;126:882–884.
285. Friedman EA, Greenberg JB, Merrill JP et al. Consequences of ethylene glycol poisoning. Am J Med 1962;32:891–902.
286. Ahmed MM. Ocular effects of antifreeze poisoning. Br J Ophthalmol 1971;55:854–855.
287. Berger JR, Ayyar DR. Neurological complications of ethylene glycol intoxication: Report of a case. Arch Neurol 1981;38:724–726.
288. Adams JW, Bofenkamp TM, Kobrin J, et al. Recurrent acute toxic optic neuropathy secondary to 5-FU. Cancer Treatm Rep 1984;68:565–566.
289. Kjaersgaard K. Amnesia after clioquinol. Lancet 1971;2:1086.
290. McEwen LM. Neuropathy after Clioquinol. Br Med J 1971;3:169–170.
291. Reich JA, Billson FA. Toxic optic neuritis: Clioquinol ingestion in a child. Med J Aust 1973;2:593–595.

292. Soffer M, Basdevant A, Sarragoussi JJ, et al. Oxyquinoline toxicity. Lancet 1983;1:709.
293. Rose FC, Gawel M. Clioquinol neurotoxicity: An overview. Acta Neurol Scand 1984;70(Suppl 100):137–145.
294. Goutieres F, Aicardi J. Accidental percutaneous hexachlorophene intoxication in children. Br Med J 1977;2:663–667.
295. Slamovits TL, Burde RM, Klingele TG. Bilateral optic atrophy caused by chronic oral ingestion and topical application of hexachlorophene. Am J Ophthalmol 1980;89:676–679.
296. Foroozan R, Buono LM, Sergott RC, Savino PJ. Retrobulbar optic neuritis associated with infliximab. Arch Ophthalmol 2002;120:985–987.
297. Ten Tusscher MP, Jacobs PJ, Busch MJ, et al. Bilateral anterior toxic optic neuropathy and the use of infliximab. BMJ 2003;326:579.
298. Manesis EK, Petrou C, Brouzas D, Hadziyannis S. Optic tract neuropathy complicating low-dose interferon treatment. J Hepatology 1994;21:474–477.
299. Tadokoro Y, Ohtsuki H, Okano M, et al. A case of disc edema during systemic interferon therapy. Folia Ophthalmol Jpn 1995;46:653–656.
300. Purvin VA. Anterior ischemic optic neuropathy secondary to interferon alfa. Arch Ophthalmol 1995;113:1041–1044.
301. Lohmann CP, Kroher G, Bogenrieder T, et al. Severe loss of vision during adjuvant interferon alfa 2b treatment for malignant melanoma. Lancet 1999;353:1326.
302. Gupta R, Singh S. Anterior ischemic optic neuropathy caused by interferon alpha therapy. Am J Med 2002;112:683–684.
303. Vardizer Y, Linhart Y, Loewenstein A, et al. Interferon-α-associated bilateral simultaneous ischemic optic neuropathy. J Neuroophthalmol 2003;23:256–259.
304. Sutton PH, Beattie PH. Optic atrophy after administration of Isoniazid with P.A.S. Lancet 1955;1:650–651.
305. Keeping JA, Searle CW. Optic neuritis following isoniazid therapy. Lancet 1955;269:278.
306. Dixon GJ, Roberts GBS, Tyrrell WF. The relationship of neuropathy to the treatment of tuberculosis with isoniazid. Scot Med J 1956;1:350.
307. Kass K, Mandel W, Cohen H, Dressler SH. Isoniazid as a cause of optic neuritis and atrophy. JAMA 1957;164:1740–1743.
308. Ahmad I, Clark LA Jr. Isoniazid hypersensitivity reaction involving the eyes. Diseases Chest 1967;52:112–113.
309. Hughes RAC, Mair WGP. Acute necrotic myelopathy with pulmonary tuberculosis. Brain 1977;100:223–238.
310. Karmon G, Savir H, Zevin D, et al. Bilateral optic neuropathy due to combined ethambutol and isoniazid treatment. Ann Ophthalmol 1979;11:1013–1017.
311. Kiyosawa M, Ishikawa S. A case of isoniazid induced optic neuropathy. Neuroophthalmology 1981;2:67–70.
312. Jimenez-Lucho VE, del Busto R, Odel J. Isoniazid and ethambutol as a cause of optic neuropathy. Eur J Respir Dis 1987;71:42–45.
313. Boulanouar A, Abdallah E, El Bakkali M, et al. Neuropathies optiques toxiques graves induites par l'isoniazide: A propos de trois cas. J Fr Ophtalmol 1995;18:183–187.
314. Loewe O. A case of transient lead amaurosis. Arch Ophthalmol 1906;35:164–171.
315. Carroll FD. Optic neuritis. Am J Ophthalmol 1952;35:75–82.
316. Baghdassarian SA. Optic neuropathy due to lead poisoning. Arch Ophthalmol 1968;80:721–723.
317. Tennekoon G, Aitchison CS, Frangia J, et al. Chronic lead intoxication: Effects on developing optic nerve. Ann Neurol 1979;5:558–564.
318. Cavalleri A, Trimarchi F, Gelmi C, et al. Effects of lead on the visual system of occupationally exposed subjects. Scan J Work Environ Health 1982;8(Suppl 1):148–151.
319. Sekkat A, Maillard P, Dupeyron G, et al. Neuropathies optiques au cours d'une intoxication aiguë par le méthanol. J Fr Ophtalmol 1982;5:797–804.
320. Ninomiya H, Asahara S, Yokota K, et al. A case of optic neuropathy due to thinner inhalation. Folia Jpn Ophthalmol 1990;41:640–644.
321. Lund A. Toxic amblyopia after inhalation of methyl acetate. Ugeskr Laeger 1944;106:308–311.
322. Ogawa Y, Takatsuki R, Uema T, et al. Acute optic neuropathy induced by thinner sniffing. Industrial Health 1988;26:239–244.
323. Chavez CT, Hepler RS, Straatsma BR. Methyl bromide optic atrophy. Am J Ophthalmol 1985;99:715–719.
324. Delay J, Deniker P, Ginestet D, et al. Essais preliminaires d'un nouvel inhibiteur de la monoamine oxidase, l'hydrazino 2 octane(D 1514) comme antidepresseur. Encephale 1962;51:517–530.
325. Sourdille MJ. Névrites optiques par inhibiteurs de la mono amine oxidase (I.M.A.O.). Bull Soc Ophtalmol Fr 1964;64:981–990.
326. Joseph E, Berkman N. Complications oculaires dues aux inhibiteurs de la mono-amine oxidase. Presse Med 1965;73:1627–1629.
327. Kalt M. Névrite optique bilaterale à debut brutal, survenue chez un suject atherosclereux, grand fumeur et intoxique par un inhibiteur de la monoamine oxidase (I.M.A.O.). Bull Soc Ophtalmol Fr 1965;65:194–199.
328. Paufique L, Charleux J, Aimard G, et al. Alerte aux I.M.A.O. Bull Soc Ophtalmol Fr 1966;66:560–562.
329. Ardouin M, Urvoy M, Raoul T, et al. Étude électrorétinographique d'un cas d'intoxication par les I.M.A.O. Bull Soc Ophtalmol Fr 1967;67:920–924.
330. Blain L, Mergler D. La dyschromatopsie chez des personnes exposées professionnellement aux solvants organiques. J Fr Ophtalmol 1986;9:127–133.
331. Klingele TG, Burde RM. Optic neuropathy associated with penicillamine therapy in a patient with rheumatoid arthritis. J Clin Neuroophthalmol 1984;4:75–78.
332. Lee AHS, Lawton NF. Penicillamine treatment of Wilson's disease and optic neuropathy. J Neurol Neurosurg Psychiatry 1991;54:746.
333. Frandsen E. Toxic amblyopia during antidepressant treatment with pheniprazine (Catran). Acta Psychiatr Scand 1962;38:1–14. (See also Abl Ges Ophthalmol 1963;89:18.)
334. Jones OW III. Toxic amblyopia caused by pheniprazine. Arch Ophthalmol 1961;66:29–36.
335. Simpson JA, Evans JI, Sanderson ID. Amblyopia due to pheniprazine. Br Med J 1963;1:331.
336. Aksalonowa T. Die einwirkung normaler und toxischer Plamoziddosen auf die netzhaut (nach klinischen und experimentellen ergebnissen). Vestn Oftalmol 1937;10:91–94. (Transl German in Zbl Ges Ophthalmol 1937;38:551.)
337. Aksalonowa T. Die wirkung von therapeuticshen und toxischen gaben von Plasmocid auf die netzhaut und den sehnerv. Vestn Oftalmol 1938;13:26–37. (Transl German in Zbl Ges Ophthalmol 1939;43:345.)
338. Francois J, De Rouck A, Cambie E. Retinal and optic evaluation in quinine poisoning. Ann Ophthalmol 1972;4:177–185.
339. Sykowski P. Streptomycin causing retrobulbar optic neuritis. Am J Ophthalmol 1951;34:1446.
340. Pratt Johnson JA. Retrobulbar neuritis following exposure to vinyl benzene (styrene). Can Med Assoc J 1964;90:975–977.
341. Bucy PC. Toxic optic neuritis resulting from sulfanilamide. JAMA 1937;109:1007–1008.
342. Taub RG, Hollenhorst RW. Sulfonamides as a cause of toxic amblyopia. Am J Ophthalmol 1955;40:486–490.
343. Brazis PW, Spivey JR, Bolling JP, et al. A case of bilateral optic neuropathy in a patient on tacrolimus (FK506) therapy after liver transplantation. Am J Ophthalmol 2000;129:536–538.
344. Pugesgaard T, Von Eyben FE. Bilateral optic neuritis evolved during tamoxifen treatment. Cancer 1986;58:383–386.
345. Noureddin BN, Seoud M, Bashshur Z, et al. Ocular toxicity in low-dose tamoxifen: a prospective study. Eye 1999;13:729–733.
346. Ashford AR, Donev I, Tiwari RP, et al. Reversible ocular toxicity related to tamoxifen therapy. Cancer 1988;61:33–35.
347. Therssen R, Jansen E, Leys A, et al. Screening for tamoxifen ocular toxicity: A prospective study. Eur J Ophthalmol 1995;5:230–234.
348. Mahoney W. Retrobulbar neuritis due to thallium poisoning from depilatory cream: Report of 3 cases. JAMA 1932;98:618–620.
349. Lillie WI, Parker HL. Retrobulbar neuritis due to thallium poisoning. JAMA 1932;98:1347–1349.
350. Manschot WA. Ophthalmic pathological findings in a case of thallium poisoning. Excerpta Med Int Congr Ser 160 (III Congr Europ Soc Ophthal) Abstr. No. 26, June 1968. (See also Ophthalmologica Addit Ad 1969;158:348–349.)
351. Tabandeh H, Crowston JG, Thompson GM. Ophthalmologic features of thallium poisoning. Am J Ophthalmol 1994;117:243–245.
352. Costagliola C, Rinaldi M, Giacoia A, et al. Red cell glutathione as a marker of tobacco smoke induced optic neuropathy. Exp Eye Res 1989;48:583–586.
353. Wang Y, Wu L, Wu DZ, et al. Visual functions and trace elements metabolism in tobacco toxic optic neuropathy. Eye Science 1992;8:131–137.
354. Hamilton AS, Nixon CE. Optic atrophy and multiple neuritis developed in the manufacture of explosives (Binitrotoluene). JAMA 1918;70:2004–2006.
355. Keane JR. Toluene optic neuropathy. Ann Neurol 1978;4:390.
356. Holló G, Varga M. Toluene and visual loss. Neurology 1992;42:266.
357. Okada M, Masaoka N, Hashimoto K, et al. Effect of stellate ganglion block in optic neuropathy caused by glue sniffing. Folia Ophthalmol Jpn 1992;43:1257–1262.
358. Nakamura Y, Nagamine Y, Ogido T, et al. A case of optic neuropathy caused by sniffing toluene. Folia Ophthalmol Jpn 1996;47:832–834.
359. Kiyokawa M, Mizota A, Takasoh M, et al. Pattern visual evoked cortical potentials in patients with toxic optic neuropathy caused by Toluene abuse. Jpn J Ophthalmol 1999;43:438–442.
360. Heuner W, Petzold E. Schwere vergiftungen an einem sauerstoffatmungsgerat (durch trichlorathylen?) Zentrabl Arbeitsschutz Prophyl 1952;2:4–11.
361. Tabacchi G, Corsico R, Gallenelli R. Neurite retrobulbare da sospetta intossicazione cronica da trichloroetilene. Ann Ottal 1966;92:787–792.
362. Norton SW, Stockman JA. Unilateral optic neuropathy following vincristine chemotherapy. J Ped Ophthal Strab 1979;16:190–193.
363. Shurin SB, Rekate HL, Annable W. Optic atrophy induced by vincristine. Pediatrics 1982;70:288–291.
364. Teichmann KD, Dabbagh N. Severe visual loss after a single dose of vincristine in a patient with a spinal cord astrocytoma. J Ocular Pharmacol 1988;4:117–121.
365. Munier F, Perentes E, Herbort CP, et al. Selective loss of optic nerve β tubulin in vincristine induced blindness. Am J Med 1992;93:232–233.
366. Munier F, Uffer S, Herbort CP, et al. Perte des cellules ganglionnaires de la rétine secondaire à la prise de vincristine. Klin Monatsbl Augenheilkd 1992;200:550–554.

CHAPTER 11

Hereditary Optic Neuropathies

Nancy J. Newman

MONOSYMPTOMATIC HEREDITARY OPTIC
   NEUROPATHIES
  Leber's Optic Neuropathy
  Dominant Optic Atrophy
  Congenital Recessive Optic Atrophy
  Apparent Sex-Linked Optic Atrophy
  Presumed Autosomal-Recessive Chiasmal Optic Neuropathy
HEREDITARY OPTIC ATROPHY WITH OTHER
   NEUROLOGIC OR SYSTEMIC SIGNS
  Autosomal-Dominant Progressive Optic Atrophy and Deafness
  Autosomal-Dominant Optic Atrophy, Deafness and
    Ophthalmoplegia
  Autosomal-Dominant Progressive Optic Atrophy with
    Progressive Hearing Loss and Ataxia (CAPOS Syndrome)
  Hereditary Optic Atrophy with Progressive Hearing Loss and
    Polyneuropathy
  Autosomal-Recessive Optic Atrophy with Progressive Hearing
    Loss, Spastic Quadriplegia, Mental Deterioration, and
    Death (Opticocochleodentate Degeneration)

Opticoacoustic Nerve Atrophy with Dementia
Progressive Optic Atrophy with Juvenile Diabetes Mellitus,
    Diabetes Insipidus, and Hearing Loss (DIDMOAD/Wolfram's
    Syndrome)
Progressive Encephalopathy with Edema, Hypsarrhythmia, and
    Optic Atrophy (PEHO Syndrome)
Complicated Hereditary Infantile Optic Atrophy (Behr's
    Syndrome)
OPTIC NEUROPATHY AS A MANIFESTATION OF
   HEREDITARY DEGENERATIVE OR DEVELOPMENTAL
   DISEASES
Hereditary Ataxias
Hereditary Polyneuropathies
Hereditary Spastic Paraplegias
Hereditary Muscular Dystrophies
Storage Diseases and Cerebral Degenerations of Childhood
Mitochondrial Disorders

The hereditary optic neuropathies comprise a group of disorders in which the cause of optic nerve dysfunction appears to be heritable, based on familial expression or genetic analysis (1,2). Clinical variability, both within and among families with the same disease, often makes recognition and classification difficult. Traditionally, classification has relied on the recognition of similar characteristics and similar patterns of transmission, but genetic analysis now permits diagnosis of the hereditary optic neuropathies in the absence of family history or in the setting of unusual clinical presentations. As a result, the clinical phenotypes of each disease are broader, and it is easier to recognize unusual cases.

The inherited optic neuropathies typically present as symmetric, bilateral, central visual loss. In many of these disorders, the papillomacular nerve fiber bundle is affected, with resultant central or cecocentral scotomas. The exact location of initial pathology along the ganglion cell and its axon and the pathophysiologic mechanisms of optic nerve injury remain unknown. Optic nerve damage is usually permanent

and, in many diseases, progressive. Once optic atrophy is observed, substantial nerve injury has already occurred.

In classifying the hereditary optic neuropathies, it is important to exclude the primary retinal degenerations that may masquerade as primary optic neuropathies because of the common finding of optic disc pallor. Retinal findings may be subtle, especially among the cone dystrophies, where optic nerve pallor may be an early finding (3–6). Heckenlively et al. (7) reported 20 patients with hereditary, progressive, cone-rod degeneration and temporal optic atrophy, telangiectasia of optic disc vessels, and little or no pigmentary retinal changes. There are several possible explanations for the presence of optic atrophy in patients with hereditary cone-rod degenerations. If the pathologic processes have their primary effect in the bipolar layer of the retina, then transsynaptic degeneration could occur in both directions. In addition, a disease process affecting the cones could secondarily affect the bipolar cells and tertiarily affect the ganglion cells. The possibility of a primary retinal process should be considered in patients with temporal optic atrophy even when the retina itself is not obviously abnormal. Retinal arterial attenuation and abnormal electroretinography should help distinguish these diseases from the primary optic neuropathies. However, optic nerve disease and retinal pathology may also coexist. Weleber and Miyake (8) reported two families with affected members in two generations who had optic atrophy, moderate visual loss beginning in the second or third decades, and negative electroretinograms (ERGs) (markedly reduced b-wave amplitudes). It was believed that the ERG findings alone could not account for the degree of central visual loss in this autosomal-dominant disorder. Among the multisystem disorders (see below), primary retinal degeneration with secondary optic disc pallor is common and may be difficult to distinguish from primary optic nerve damage. There may be coexistent pathology.

The customary classification of the inherited optic neuropathies is by pattern of transmission. The most common patterns of inheritance include autosomal dominant, autosomal recessive, and maternal (mitochondrial). The same genetic defect may not be responsible for all pedigrees with optic neuropathy inherited in a similar fashion. Similarly, different genetic defects may cause identical or similar phenotypes—some inherited in the same manner, others not. Alternatively, the same genetic defect may result in different clinical expression, although the pattern of inheritance should be consistent. To complicate matters further, single cases are often presumed or proven to be caused by inherited genetic

defects, making the pattern of familial transmission unavailable as an aid in classification.

In some of the hereditary optic neuropathies, optic nerve dysfunction is typically the only manifestation of the disease. In others, various neurologic and systemic abnormalities are regularly observed. Additionally, inherited diseases with primarily neurologic or systemic manifestations, such as the multisystem degenerations, can include optic atrophy. This chapter continues the fifth edition's classification of the hereditary optic neuropathies into three major groups: (a) those that occur primarily without associated neurologic or systemic signs; (b) those that frequently have associated neurologic or systemic signs; and (c) those in which the optic neuropathy is secondary in the overall disease process. The hereditary optic neuropathies reflect a number of different inheritance patterns and can be caused by defects in either the nuclear or mitochondrial genomes. As more specific genetic defects are discovered, our concept of the phenotypes of these disorders will likely change, as will our classification. More accurate definition of the underlying genetic abnormalities will aid in genetic counseling. Furthermore, identification of the gene defect, elucidation of the gene product and its normal function, and clarification of the abnormality caused by the mutation should improve our understanding of the pathophysiologic mechanisms of optic nerve dysfunction and allow for the development of directed therapies.

MONOSYMPTOMATIC HEREDITARY OPTIC NEUROPATHIES

LEBER'S OPTIC NEUROPATHY

In 1871, Leber (9) first described the disease that bears his name, although similar cases were reported 50 years earlier (e.g., von Graefe in 1858 [10]). Leber considered this entity an inflammatory neuritis, but others supported an abiotrophic origin (11,12). Numerous pedigrees of Leber's hereditary optic neuropathy (LHON) have since been reported from Europe, North America, South America, Australia, and Asia (13–31). Since the late 1980s, LHON has received notoriety as a maternally inherited disease linked to abnormalities in mitochondrial DNA (32–90a). Genetic analysis has broadened our view of what constitutes the clinical presentation of LHON.

Clinical Features

Clinical descriptions prior to the availability of molecular confirmation must be assessed with caution, because quite possibly the individuals, and even pedigrees, described were not true cases of LHON. When large, typical pedigrees are used, individuals with atypical features can be assumed to represent unusual but valid cases of LHON.

Despite multiple studies describing hundreds of patients with LHON worldwide, the actual prevalence and incidence of visual loss from this disorder have been only rarely and geographically selectively investigated. Among individuals in Northeast England, there was a minimal prevalence of visual loss from LHON of 3.22 per 100,000 individuals and a prevalence for harboring a primary LHON-associated mitochondrial DNA (mtDNA) mutation of 11.82 per 100,000

individuals (91,92). Mackey et al. (93–95) extensively reviewed LHON in Australia and concluded that the disease accounts for about 2% of cases of legal blindness in individuals under age 65 and for about 11% of all patients with bilateral optic neuropathy of uncertain etiology in that country.

Men are affected with visual loss more frequently than women. This male predominance ranges from 80–90% in most pedigrees reported from North America, Europe, and Australia (15–18,20,22–26,28,96–100). Earlier reports indicated a male predominance of only 60% in Japan, but subsequent studies with molecular confirmation of LHON revealed that more than 90% of Japanese patients were males (27). Earlier reports may have inadvertently included pedigrees with autosomal-dominant optic atrophy (Kjer's disease) as LHON patients. Approximately 20–60% of men at risk for LHON experience visual loss (15,17,22,23,93,94). Among women at risk, the occurrence rate ranges from 4% to 32% (15,17,22,23,93,94). Affected women are more likely to have affected children, especially daughters, than unaffected female carriers (15,101). Mackey reported that approximately 20% of male and 4% of female carriers in Australia lose vision (93,94). Mackey and Howell (102) noted that there has been a dramatic decline in the risk of visual loss among pedigrees with LHON in Australia and a definite decrease in penetrance over the past century.

The onset of visual loss typically occurs between the ages of 15 and 35 years, but otherwise classic LHON has been reported in many individuals both younger and older (13–17,19,20,22,24,26–28,97). The range of age at onset is

1–80 years (15,16,20,22,103–107), but inclusion of all these cases as true examples of LHON may not be accurate. Among those cases of molecularly confirmed LHON, the age range is 2–80 years. This age variability occurs even among members of the same pedigree. We have observed a pedigree in which a boy was affected at age 8 years, two other boys at age 15, a woman at age 60, and her brother at age 67.

Visual loss typically begins painlessly and centrally in one eye. Some patients complain of a sensation of mist or fog obscuring their vision, whereas others note mild central fading of colors. The second eye is usually affected weeks to months later. Reports of simultaneous onset are numerous (14,15,24,98) and likely reflect both instances of true bilateral coincidence and those in which initial visual loss in the first eye went unrecognized. Rarely, loss of vision in the second eye occurs after a prolonged interval (more than 12 years) (107–109). Even more infrequently, visual loss remains monocular (20,28,96,110–112). Nikoskelainen et al. (28) reported one patient with unilateral disease for a 16-year follow-up period and a few patients with entirely subclinical disease. In general, however, greater than 97% of patients will have second eye involvement within 1 year (24,26).

The onset of visual loss is usually not associated with other symptoms. Uhthoff's symptom (a transient worsening of vision with exercise or warming) may occur in patients with LHON, as it does in patients with other optic neuropathies (24,26,113–115). Other reported symptoms at the time of visual loss are usually minor and nonspecific, such as headache; eye discomfort; flashes of light, color, or both; limb paresthesias; and dizziness (14,15,24,26,114,115).

The duration of progression of visual loss in each eye also varies and may be difficult to document accurately. Usually the course is acute or subacute, with deterioration of visual function stabilizing after months (14,15,20,24,98,114,115). In one study of molecularly confirmed LHON, progression of visual loss in each eye ranged from "sudden and complete" to 2 years, with a mean of 3.7 months (24). Nikoskelainen et al. (28) described rare patients with slowly progressive visual loss, ultimately with a favorable visual outcome.

Visual acuities at the point of maximum visual loss range from no light perception to 20/20 (14–16,20,24,25,98). Most patients deteriorate to acuities worse than 20/200 (14–16, 20,24–26,28,111,114,115). Color vision is affected severely, often early in the course, but rarely before significant visual loss (20,21,28,115). The Farnsworth-Munsell 100-Hue test may be the earliest indicator of optic nerve dysfunction, but subtle abnormalities of color vision can be demonstrated in asymptomatic family members (20,21). Pupillary light responses may be relatively preserved when compared with the responses in patients with optic neuropathies from other causes (28,116–118), although others have not confirmed this finding (119,120). Visual field defects are typically central or cecocentral (15,20,24,25,28,98,111,114, 115). The scotomas may be relative during the early stages of visual loss but rapidly become large and absolute, measuring at least 25–30° in diameter. A breakthrough of the scotoma is not uncommon, and according to Traquair (121), such an expansion usually occurs in the upper nasal field. Apparently unaffected eyes may show subtle cecocentral scotomas only to red test objects or as mild depression on central automated perimetry. Field abnormalities mimicking the bitemporal configuration of chiasmal defects have also been reported (122,123). In a few of these cases, the defects have strictly respected the vertical meridian.

Even the earliest descriptions of this disease noted funduscopic abnormalities other than optic atrophy (9,124,125). Especially during the acute phase of visual loss, hyperemia of the optic nerve head, dilation and tortuosity of vessels, retinal and disc hemorrhages, macular edema, exudates, retinal striations, and obscuration of the disc margin were recognized in some cases (9,97,113,124–127). Bell (97) concluded that the appearance of the disc might vary from completely normal to that "indicative of an acute inflammatory reaction."

In 1973, Smith et al. (114) reported a triad of signs believed pathognomonic for LHON: circumpapillary telangiectatic microangiopathy, swelling of the nerve fiber layer around the disc (pseudoedema), and absence of leakage from the disc or papillary region on fluorescein angiography (distinguishing the LHON nerve head from truly edematous discs) (Fig. 11.1). Nikoskelainen et al. (28,128,129) observed these funduscopic changes in all of their symptomatic patients with LHON, in some of their "presymptomatic" cases, and in a significant proportion of asymptomatic maternal relatives. However, having abnormalities of the peripapillary nerve fiber layer does not necessarily predict visual loss. Furthermore, some patients with LHON never exhibit the characteristic ophthalmoscopic appearance, even if examined at the time of acute visual loss (24,26,27,130,131). In one review, 22 of 52 patients did not have any abnormal funduscopic findings (24). In another review, 36% of 33 patients examined within 3 months of visual loss did not have retinal microangiopathy (26). The "classic" LHON ophthalmoscopic appearance may be helpful in suggesting the diagnosis if recognized in patients or their maternal relatives, but its absence, even during the period of acute visual loss, does not exclude the diagnosis of LHON. As the disease progresses, the telangiectatic vessels disappear and the pseudoedema of the disc resolves. Perhaps because of the initial hyperemia, the optic discs of patients with LHON may not appear pale for some time. This feature, coupled with the relatively preserved pupillary responses and the lack of pain, has led to the misdiagnosis of nonorganic visual loss in some LHON patients (116,123). Eventually, however, optic atrophy with nerve fiber layer dropout most pronounced in the papillomacular bundle supervenes (Fig. 11.2). Nonglaucomatous cupping of the optic discs (132–134) or arteriolar attenuation (111) may also be seen in patients with symptomatic LHON. Reports of other ocular manifestations, such as a Stargardt's-like maculopathy or retinal "vasculitis," are extremely rare and may represent coincidental findings (135,136).

In most patients with LHON, visual loss remains profound and permanent. However, not uncommonly, recovery of even excellent central vision occurs years after visual deterioration (15,24–26,28,96,98,104,137–146). Spontaneous improvement to some degree was reported in 29% of patients in one study (138), 45% in another (15), and in a surprising 11 of 13 patients in one Canadian pedigree (98). The

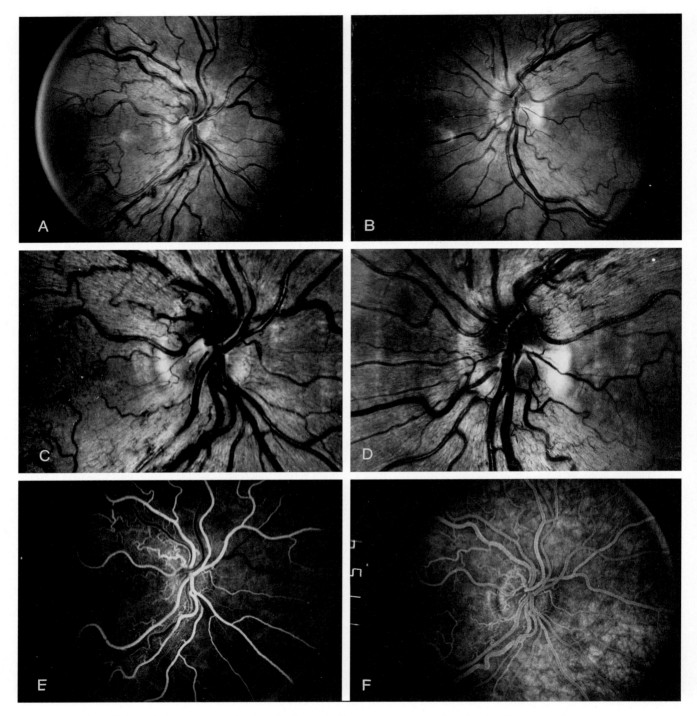

Figure 11.1.   Leber's optic neuropathy. *A and B,* Both optic discs in the acute phase of the disorder. Note hyperemic appearance of discs. Peripapillary telangiectatic vessels are present. *C and D,* Both optic discs photographed with red-free (540 nm) light. Note marked hyperemia of the discs with dilatation of small vessels both on the surface of the disc and in the peripapillary region. *E and F,* fluorescein angiogram in arteriovenous (*E*) and late (*F*) phases shows dilatation of right disc and peripapillary vessels but no leakage of fluorescein dye.

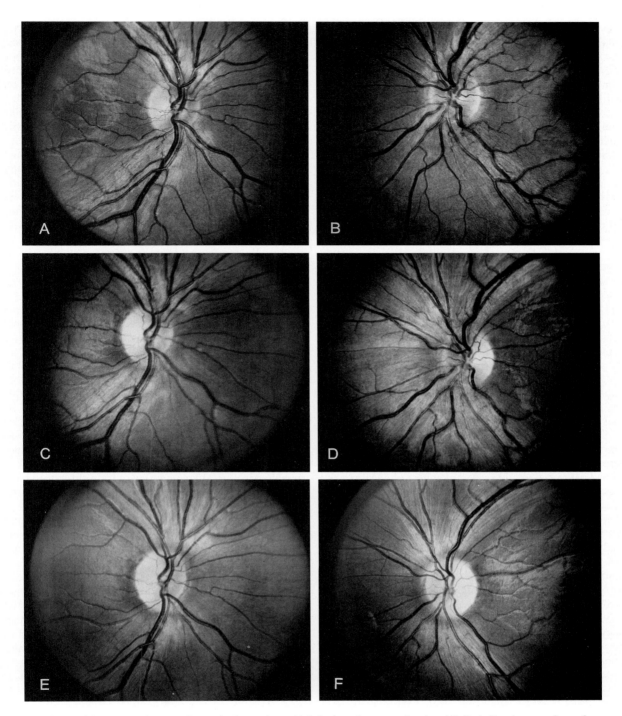

Figure 11.2. Progression to optic atrophy in a patient with Leber's optic neuropathy. *A and B,* Both discs in acute phase of the disease. Visual acuity is 20/100 in both eyes with large cecocentral scotomas. Telangiectatic vessels are evident adjacent to the inferior margin of both discs. The right disc is already pale temporally, and there is atrophy of the papillomacular nerve fiber layer. *C and D,* Two months after onset of visual loss, visual acuity is 5/200 in the right eye and 8/200 in the left eye. Both discs show moderate pallor, particularly temporally, with loss of nerve fiber layer that is especially evident in the papillomacular region. Previously seen telangiectatic vessels are disappearing. *E and F,* Six months after onset of visual loss, visual acuity has remained 5/200 in the right eye and 8/200 in the left eye. Both discs are pale, particularly temporally. The telangiectatic vessels have completely disappeared. One year after these photographs were obtained, the patient noted gradual, partial return of visual acuity in both eyes to 20/50.

recovery may occur gradually over 6 months to 1 year after initial visual loss or may suddenly occur up to 10 years after onset (140). It may take the form of a gradual clearing of central vision or be restricted to a few central degrees, resulting in a small island of vision within a large central scotoma. Visual field testing may be more sensitive to recovery than visual acuity testing, and the size of the central scotoma at the nadir may be one of the factors determining the extent to which visual function improves (145). Recovery is usually bilateral but may be unilateral. Patients whose vision improves most substantially appear to have a lower mean age at the time of initial visual loss (26,28,55,60,140,146). In the review by Riordan-Eva et al. (26) of 79 cases from 55 families, good visual outcome was strongly correlated with age at onset, all those with onset before 20 years having a final visual acuity better than 20/80. Furthermore, the particular mitochondrial DNA mutation also influences prognosis, with the 11778 mutation carrying the worst prognosis for vision and the 14484 mutation the best (see below). Recurrences of visual failure are rare among patients both with and without visual recovery (110,147–149).

Associated Findings

In most patients with LHON, visual dysfunction is the only significant manifestation of the disease. However, some pedigrees have members with associated cardiac conduction abnormalities (125,133,150–155a). Preexcitation syndromes, specifically Wolff-Parkinson-White and Lown-Ganong-Levine, were found in 14 of 163 individuals (9%) with LHON mutations among 10 Finnish families (151,153) and in 5 of 63 LHON patients (8%) among 35 Japanese pedigrees (154). Prolongation of the corrected QT interval was noted in the maternally related members of one molecularly confirmed LHON pedigree (133). Palpitations, syncope, and sudden death have been reported (9,23,151,152, 155,156), as have myocardial hypertrophy (155a) and isolated left ventricular abnormal trabeculation (155). Familial skeletal abnormalities may also occur in pedigrees with LHON (156–163).

Minor neurologic abnormalities, such as exaggerated or pathologic reflexes, mild cerebellar ataxia, tremor, movement disorders, myoclonus, seizures, muscle wasting, distal sensory neuropathy, auditory neuropathy, motor neuropathy, auditory neuropathy, and migraine, have been reported in patients with LHON (13,15,19,103,156,161,164–173a). Less commonly, pedigrees have been described in which multiple maternal members demonstrate the clinical features of LHON in addition to more severe neurologic abnormalities (156,157,159,174–190). We have termed these pedigrees "Leber's plus." The maternal members of a large Australian family demonstrated varied combinations of optic atrophy, movement disorders, spasticity, psychiatric disturbances, skeletal abnormalities, and acute infantile encephalopathic episodes (159). A Leber's-like optic neuropathy has been associated with dystonia and basal gangliar lesions in several pedigrees (178–184). Leigh-like encephalopathy, periaqueductal syndrome, and other brain stem involvement have also rarely been reported (187–189).

Disease clinically indistinguishable from multiple scle-

rosis may occur in families with LHON (19,26,111,157,161, 165,191–196). Harding et al. (197) reported molecularly confirmed 11778 pedigrees of LHON with individuals, especially females, exhibiting symptoms and signs of demyelinating disease combined with nonremitting visual loss typical of LHON. Cerebrospinal fluid and magnetic resonance (MR) imaging findings were characteristic of multiple sclerosis. Subsequent population surveys have not found the primary mutations associated with LHON to be overrepresented among multiple sclerosis patients (194,198). However, among multiple sclerosis patients selected specifically because of their prominent early optic neuropathy, the primary LHON mutations may be found more frequently (194). It is possible that this association between LHON and multiple sclerosis is no greater than the prevalence of the two diseases. An underlying LHON mutation, however, may worsen the prognosis of optic neuritis in patients with multiple sclerosis (196,198,199).

Ancillary Testing

Ancillary tests, aside from genetic analysis, are generally of limited usefulness in the evaluation of LHON. Fluorescein angiography is helpful in its illustration and confirmation of LHON funduscopic features and the lack of disc leakage (114,129). Electrocardiograms (ECGs) may reveal cardiac conduction abnormalities (114,151,155). Formal color testing with the D-15 panel and Farnsworth Munsell 100-Hue tests may reveal optic nerve dysfunction in LHON before any measurable visual loss has occurred (20,21,115). However, asymptomatic maternal relatives who demonstrate color defects and who do not go on to visual loss reduce the predictive value of these tests. Pattern-reversal visual evoked potentials (VEPs) may be absent or show prolonged latencies and decreased amplitudes, usually in eyes already afflicted with diminished acuity (20,21,23,24,200,201).

Brain stem auditory evoked potentials (BAEPs) were nonspecifically abnormal in 7 of 11 affected LHON patients in one study (202). A brief report from this same group suggested that VEPs and BAEPs may be abnormal in asymptomatic maternal relatives of LHON patients compared with control subjects (201). The standard flash ERG is typically normal (14,15,24,142,203), although occasional attenuation of the b-wave may be noted (26). Cerebrospinal fluid analysis is usually normal except in patients with a multiple sclerosis-like syndrome (24,26,197). Electroencephalograms are unremarkable (24).

Computed tomography (CT) scanning and MR imaging of the brain are typically normal in patients with LHON (24,204,205). Exceptions include patients with additional symptoms suggestive of multiple sclerosis and pedigrees with dystonia and basal gangliar lesions. One boy with LHON visual loss but no symptoms or signs suggestive of demyelinating disease was found to have extensive T2-hyperintense periventricular white matter changes (163). Two LHON patients were reported with distended optic nerve sheaths on orbital ultrasonography, CT scanning, and MR imaging (131,206). MR imaging of the optic nerves of symptomatic LHON patients typically reveals normal nerves in the acute phase of visual loss, often followed by high T2 signal in the intraorbital portions of the nerves after several months (26,204,205,207–209). Rarely, gadolinium enhancement and enlargement of the optic nerves and even chiasm are demonstrated during the acute phase of visual loss (210–212). Phosphorus-31 MR spectroscopy suggested impaired mitochondrial metabolism within limb muscle and the occipital lobes in several patients with LHON (213) as well as in unaffected carriers with the 11778 mutation (214).

Although morphologic abnormalities of mitochondria on skeletal muscle biopsy are rare in LHON (103,215,216), patients and carriers may exhibit abnormal lactate production with exercise (217). Sadun et al. (218) found an abundance of mitochondria and accumulation of mitochondrial debris in the extraocular muscles of one 11778 LHON patient, suggesting a compensatory increase in absolute numbers of mitochondria.

Pathology

In no case do we have optic nerve pathology from the early stages of the disease; hence, the location and nature of the initial injury remain uncertain. Kwittken and Barest (219) found atrophy of retinal ganglion cells and bilateral optic atrophy. The optic cup was shallow and filled with glial cells and connective tissue. There was symmetric destruction of the myelin sheaths in the papillomacular bundles. The lateral geniculate bodies were shriveled, and the optic radiations exhibited demyelination, suggesting transsynaptic degeneration.

Other authors have reported similar findings (156,175, 218,220–224). Kerrison et al. (225) noted marked atrophy of the nerve fiber and retinal ganglion cell layers and the optic nerves in a postmortem study of an 81-year-old affected woman from the large Australian family with "Leber's Plus" (159). Electron microscopy demonstrated retinal ganglion cell inclusions consisting of calcium circumscribed by a double membrane, suggesting intramitochondrial calcification. Histopathologic and morphometric analysis was performed on optic nerves from three other LHON patients, again years remote from the time of acute visual loss (222,223). Findings consisted of severe generalized depletion of optic nerve fibers (95–99% reduction), with sparing of only peripheral clusters of fibers, primarily those of larger diameter. There was fibrocytic scarring, scattered "degeneration dust," and evidence of minimal inflammation. These authors proposed a selective loss of the ganglion cell P-cell population (222,223).

Inheritance and Genetics

All pedigrees clinically designated as LHON have a maternal inheritance pattern (13,15,17,18,22,23). In maternal inheritance, all offspring of a woman carrying the trait will inherit the trait, but only the females can pass on the trait to the subsequent generation. Maternal transmission was elegantly demonstrated prior to genetic analysis by Nikoskelainen et al. (23) in four of their Finnish pedigrees with LHON. By using the classic funduscopic appearance as a marker of the disease in asymptomatic relatives, those investigators showed that every son or daughter of a female carrier inherited the LHON trait.

Both the father and the mother contribute to the nuclear portion of the zygote, but the mother's egg is virtually the sole provider of the zygote's cytoplasmic contents. The spermatozoon contributes only about 1% of that total (41,48, 226–228). Therefore, to explain maternal inheritance, a cytoplasmic determinant was sought. Initial theories included the transfer of a slow virus-like agent in the maternal ooplasm or transplacentally. Because the intracytoplasmic mitochondria are the only source of extranuclear DNA, mitochondrial inheritance was proposed as an explanation (229).

For more detailed reviews of mitochondrial genetics and diseases of mitochondrial DNA, the reader is referred to several comprehensive publications (33,41,48,,90a, 226–228,230–237). In brief, every cell contains several hundred intracytoplasmic mitochondria that generate the cellular energy necessary for normal cellular function and maintenance. Those cells in tissues particularly reliant on mitochondrial energy production, such as the central nervous system, will contain more mitochondria. Each mitochondrion contains 2–10 double-stranded circles of mtDNA. Each circle of mtDNA contains only 16,500 bases compared with the 3×10^9 bases contained within the nuclear genome. However, given that there are several mtDNAs in each mitochondrion and hundreds of mitochondria per cell, the mtDNA represents approximately 0.3% of the cell's total DNA. Its small size makes the mtDNA more accessible to study, and the entire gene sequence has been determined. Mitochondrial DNA codes for all the transfer RNAs and ribosomal RNAs required for intramitochondrial protein production, as well as for 13 proteins essential to the oxidative phosphorylation system. The majority of proteins crucial to normal oxidative phosphorylation function are encoded on nuclear genes, manufactured in the cytoplasm, and transported into the mitochondria. Hence, "mitochondrial disease" could result from genetic defects in either the nuclear or mitochondrial genomes. Over 100 mtDNA point mutations and countless mtDNA rearrangements have been proposed as etiologic factors in human disease (227,232,236). Expression of these diseases reflects complex genotypic–phenotypic interactions that likely involve nuclear modifying or susceptibility factors.

If a new mutation occurs in the mtDNA, there will be a period of coexistence of mutant and normal mtDNA within the same cell (heteroplasmy) (41,234,238). At each cell division, the mitochondrial genotype may drift toward pure normal or pure mutant or remain mixed (replicative segregation). The phenotype of the cell (and the tissue the cells comprise) depends on the proportional mixture of mtDNA genotypes and the intrinsic energy needs of the cell. The mutant phenotype may become apparent only when the amount of normal mtDNA can no longer provide sufficient mitochondrial function for cell and tissue maintenance (threshold effect). Because of the cytoplasmic location of mtDNA, mitochondrial diseases secondary to point mutations in the mtDNA follow a pattern of maternal inheritance.

In 1988, Wallace et al. (32) identified the first point mutation in mtDNA to be linked to an inherited disease. In multiple pedigrees with LHON, a single nucleotide substitution (adenine for guanine) was found at position 11778 in the mtDNA (Fig. 11.3). This region codes for subunit 4 (designated ND4) of complex I (NADH dehydrogenase) in the respiratory chain. The mutation at position 11778 changes an amino acid from arginine to histidine, likely a crucial substitution because arginine is found in this position in the ND4 protein in other species (evolutionarily conserved). Using polymerase chain reaction techniques, the ''Wallace mutation'' can be detected in any tissue sample that contains mitochondria, including whole blood, and even in archival preparations (239).

The Wallace mutation has been demonstrated in many racially divergent pedigrees with LHON, suggesting that the 11778 mutation has arisen independently on several occasions (24,26–29,31,32,34–37,39,40,42,48,51,52,55,72,101, 103,104,143,238,240). The 11778 mutation is not present in control subjects. Whereas 31–89% of European, North American, and Australian LHON pedigrees harbor the 11778 mutation (26,28,35,38–40,48,50–52,55,93,94,101, 143,241–244), greater than 90% of Japanese and Chinese LHON patients are 11778 positive (27,29,31,72,240).

Several other mutations have since been proposed as causal in LHON (Fig. 11.3). The majority are located within

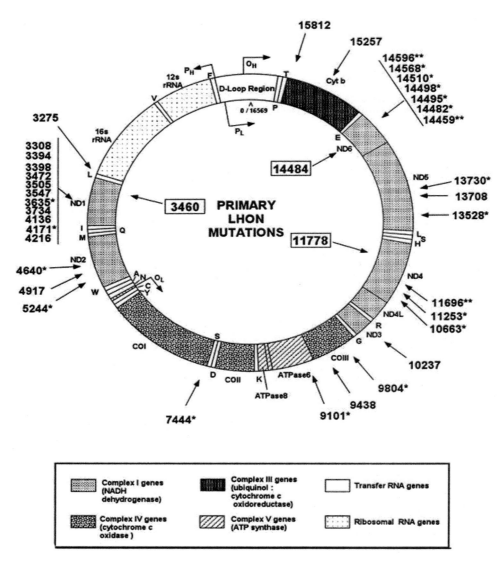

Figure 11.3. Mitochondrial genome showing the point mutations associated with Leber's hereditary optic neuropathy. The three primary mutations, accounting from more than 90% of cases, are shown inside the genome (*circle*), and the other mutations are shown outside the genome. Mutations noted with a single asterisk may be primary mutations, but they each account for only one or a few pedigrees worldwide. Mutations noted with two asterisks are primary mutations associated with Leber's optic neuropathy and dystonia. (Adapted from Newman NJ. From genotype to phenotype in Leber hereditary optic neuropathy: still more questions than answers. J Neuro-ophthalmol 2002;22:257–261.)

genes that also code for proteins representing complex 1, but most within subunits other than ND4. Huoponen et al. (45) and Howell et al. (43) identified a point mutation at mtDNA position 3460 within the gene coding for subunit 1 of complex I in nine independent families with LHON. This mutation has since been found in ethnically divergent pedigrees with LHON and accounts for 4–15% of LHON cases worldwide (28,29,43,47,50,54,63,64,72,93,94,101, 242–245). Johns et al. (53) discovered another mutation at position 14484 in the gene coding for the sixth subunit of complex I. The 14484 mutation accounts for 5–15% of LHON pedigrees worldwide (29,31,72,101), although it has a high prevalence (23 of 28 pedigrees) in French Canada (71). This high percentage of the 14484 mutation among French Canadian LHON patients is likely due to a founder effect, as further mtDNA haplotype analysis has confirmed the same maternal lineage (246).

The 11778, 3460, and 14484 mutations have been designated "primary" mutations for Leber's disease because they confer a genetic risk for LHON expression individually, change the coding for evolutionarily conserved amino acids in essential proteins, are found in multiple, different, ethnically divergent pedigrees, and are absent or rare among controls (64). Altogether, they probably account for more than 90% of LHON cases worldwide. Several other mtDNA mutations may be "primary," but they account individually for only a few pedigrees worldwide (see below) (Fig. 11.3). Other mtDNA point mutations have been associated with LHON (Fig. 11.3), but their pathogenetic significance remains less clear. They are considered "secondary" mutations because they are found with greater frequency among LHON patients than controls, but they may not in and of themselves confer a risk of blindness.

The other proposed mutations occur in other subunits of complex I (nucleotide positions 3308, 3394, 3398, 3472, 3505, 3547, 3635, 3734, 4136, 4171, and 4216 in ND1; 4640, 4917, and 5244 in ND2; 10237 in ND3; 10663 and 11253 in ND4; 13513, 13528, 13708, and 13730 in ND5; and 14482, 14495, 14498, 14510, and 14568 in ND6), in complex III (nucleotide positions 15257 and 15812 in the cytochrome b subunit), in complex IV (nucleotide position 7444 in cytochrome c oxidase subunit 1 and positions 9438 and 9804 in cytochrome c oxidase subunit 3), in complex V (nucleotide position 9101 in the ATPase 6 gene), and in the tRNA leucine 1 gene (46–49,53–59,62,64,66,67,69,70,74,76–80, 84–90a,247,248). They vary markedly in their prevalence, the degree of evolutionary conservation of the encoded amino acids altered, and their frequency among controls. Many of these mutations occur in combination with each other and the primary mutations and may simply define the mtDNA haplotypic background of the individual. Hence, caution must be used in assuming a primary causal significance for these mutations. Acknowledging this complexity, several of these other mtDNA mutations may indeed be causal ("primary") LHON mutations, specifically those at nucleotide positions 3635, 4171, 4640, 5244, 7444, 9101, 9804, 10663, 11253, 13528, 13730, 14482, 14495, 14498, 14510, and 14568. However, they in total represent less than 10% of all LHON pedigrees worldwide.

The pedigrees with LHON "plus" and severe neurologic abnormalities in multiple family members may be genetically distinct from those families with more typical, isolated Leber's-type visual loss. A few exceptions are worth noting, including spastic dystonia and basal ganglia lesions in at least two 11778 families and one 3460 family (103,168); a male 11778 patient with diabetes mellitus since age 2, seizures and visual loss at age 14, and unilateral sensorineural hearing loss at age 19 (167); one 3460 and one 11778 patient with asymptomatic periventricular brain lesions (163,168); a few patients with the primary LHON mutations and brain stem syndromes (187–189); one branch of a 11484-homoplasmic and 11778-heteroplasmic family with fatal infantile encephalopathy (190); and one remarkable 11778-positive pedigree with adult-onset multisystem degeneration with parkinsonism but no optic neuropathy (186). The maternal members of the Australian pedigree with optic neuropathies, movement disorders, spasticity, and acute encephalopathic episodes were found to carry the primary 14484 mutation as well as a mutation at mtDNA position 4160 (ND1) (44). Additionally, one branch of the family contained a second ND1 mutation (position 4136). Family members with both ND1 mutations failed to exhibit severe neurologic abnormalities, leading the authors to speculate that the second mutation acts as an intragenic suppressor mutation that ameliorates the expression of the disease.

Among the families with optic neuropathy and basal gangliar lesions (178–184), additional mtDNA primary mutations have been identified at nucleotide positions 14459 (178,249,250) and 14596 in the ND6 gene and nucleotide position 11696 in the ND4 gene (183). Other pedigrees with LHON and dystonia are as yet genetically unspecified. Of note, there is great variability among the maternally related family members harboring the 14459 mutation, with some individuals exhibiting optic neuropathy only, others dystonia only, and still others both (250). mtDNA mutations at nucleotide positions 13513 and 13045 in the ND5 gene usually cause findings typical of the mitochondrial encephalopathy with lactic acidosis and stroke-like episodes (MELAS) phenotype (73,251,251a). However, in rare patients with this mutation, LHON-like visual loss can occur in addition to MELAS symptoms.

Screening for LHON in a patient with visual loss from optic neuropathy should begin with the three primary mutations (248). In those primary mutation-negative patients in whom suspicion remains high, testing for the other mtDNA mutations associated with LHON is probably warranted, especially for those mutations deemed likely causal in a few previous pedigrees (Fig. 11.3). Alternatively, since the majority of these other mtDNA mutations reside in genes encoding subunits of complex I, complete sequencing of complex I, perhaps beginning with the so-called "hot spot" ND6 gene (80), might also be considered. Finally, sequencing the entire mitochondrial genome is possible, although labor intensive. This should be performed only in those cases of high suspicion and should be interpreted only by those versed in the complexities of mitochondrial genetics (70,236,252–254).

Determinants of Expression

Genetic analysis allows a broad view of what constitutes the clinical profile of LHON (2,56). Most striking is the number of patients without a family history of visual loss. Although there is undoubtedly a referral bias for the unusual cases, it is still remarkable that singleton cases constituted 57% of one series of molecularly confirmed LHON (24). In contrast, Mackey (93) reported only a small proportion of singleton cases in Australia, suggesting ascertainment difficulties or low penetrance in America. The use of high-resolution mtDNA haplotypes to aggregate multiple apparently unrelated pedigrees affected with LHON into single large maternal lineages descending from the same founder (246,255) may decrease the number of true singleton cases. Some of these singleton cases are women, some outside the typical age range for LHON, some without the classic ophthalmoscopic appearance (112,123). Clearly, the diagnosis of LHON should be considered in any case of unexplained bilateral optic neuropathy, regardless of age of onset, sex, family history, or funduscopic appearance.

Many questions remain unanswered regarding the determinants of phenotypic expression. For instance, does the specific mtDNA mutation dictate particular clinical features? Although those pedigrees with LHON "plus" demonstrate that certain mtDNA mutations may result in specific disease patterns of Leber's-like optic neuropathies with other neurologic abnormalities (84), few significant clinical differences have been demonstrated to date among LHON patients positive for the 11778 mutation, those with other mtDNA mutations, and those as yet genetically unspecified. One major exception is the difference in spontaneous recovery rates among patients with the 11778 mutation and those with the 14484 mutation. Among 136 patients with the 11778 mutation, only 5 (4%) reported spontaneous recovery (144), compared with 37–65% of 14484 patients (26,28,55,60, 244). Furthermore, the ultimate visual acuities in patients with the 14484 mutation are significantly better than those with the 11778 and 3460 mutations (26,244). Although Johns et al. (54) and Nikoskelainen et al. (28) reported a better visual prognosis among their 12 and 10 patients, respectively, with the 3460 mutation, other series have shown little difference between the 11778 and 3460 mutations (26,93,94,243,244). Cardiac conduction abnormalities occur in 11778 pedigrees (24,133,154,155a), but the 3460 mutation appears to have the highest association with the preexcitation syndromes in Finland (45,151,153).

Except for rare examples of de novo occurrence of a primary LHON mutation (256), a mtDNA mutation will be present in all maternally related family members of patients with LHON, even though many will never become symptomatic. Hence, whereas the presence of a mtDNA mutation may be necessary for phenotypic expression, it may not be sufficient. Does heteroplasmy among individuals in a pedigree play a role in phenotypic expression? Heteroplasmy for the primary LHON mutations has been demonstrated in several affected and unaffected individuals (24,39,43,84, 104,143,238,257–266). Within pedigrees, the proportion of mutant mtDNA in subsequent generations is largely determined by random genetic drift (265,266). Among individuals, the degree of heteroplasmy in blood generally correlates with the risk of visual loss. Additionally, mothers with 80% or less mutant mtDNA in blood are less likely to have clinically affected sons than mothers who are homoplasmic mutant (265). However, once a person becomes symptomatic, there does not appear to be any clinical difference in disease expression (260). Meiotic segregation can result in major differences in the proportion of mtDNA among siblings, potentially predisposing some individuals to visual loss. However, in most large reviews of molecularly confirmed LHON patients, heteroplasmy is documented in the blood of a minority of affected individuals (24,84,101). Although most of the probands themselves were homoplasmic for the mutation, it is possible that their unaffected relatives were heteroplasmic, helping to explain the pattern of expression.

Different proportions of mutant and normal mtDNA may also exist within the various tissues of the same heteroplasmic individual (238). The degree of tissue heteroplasmy might help to explain the variable phenotypes seen in patients whose mitochondrial genotypes measured in blood alone appear similar (41,238,267), since the amount of mutant mtDNA in the optic nerves of individuals at risk may differ. Howell et al. (268) performed postmortem genetic analysis on the optic nerve and retina of an affected LHON patient who was heteroplasmic in blood and found the ocular tissues to be essentially homoplasmic. Leukocyte mtDNA may be a "lagging indicator" of the mutational burden in other, more pathologically affected tissues, with a high proportion of mutated mtDNA in blood correlating with a high proportion of mutated mtDNA in other tissues (269).

Other genetic factors besides the specific mtDNA mutation and the presence and degree of heteroplasmy may play a role in expression. Although some investigators have claimed that multiple LHON-associated mtDNA mutations may be necessary for visual loss, this has not been corroborated in several studies (26,28,244,270). Indeed, case reports of unaffected individuals who even harbor two primary mutations (190,271) make this claim improbable. These rare pedigrees with two primary mutations exhibit no exceptional presentation of visual loss, including penetrance, the role of heteroplasmy, timing, severity, and even eventual recovery. Similarly, although the underlying mtDNA haplotype may influence the presence, penetrance, or expression of an mtDNA point mutation (272–277), this is unlikely to be the major factor in phenotypic expression. Nuclear-encoded factors modifying mtDNA expression, mtDNA products, or mitochondrial metabolism may influence phenotypic expression of LHON (278–281). The male predominance of visual loss in LHON may be explained by a modifying factor on the X chromosome (101,282,283). Most studies have not confirmed X-linkage in this disease (284–291), but the X-linked hypothesis may still be viable (84,101). The apolipoprotein E (APOE) gene is not a visual loss susceptibility gene in LHON (292).

Tissue energy utilization and reserve in an individual may also determine the timing and extent of visual loss. Mitochondrial energy production decreases with age (293), and the timing of visual loss in patients at risk for LHON may reflect the threshold at which already reduced mitochondrial function deteriorates to a critical level. Immunologic factors have also been proposed, especially to explain the association of LHON with multiple sclerosis (196,197,284). However, no association has been demonstrated between LHON and any HLA-DR genotype, suggesting that the HLA-DR locus is not a major genetic determinant for the development of visual loss (294).

Environmental factors may also play a role. Both the internal and external environment of the organism must be considered. Systemic illnesses, nutritional deficiencies, trauma, medications, or toxins that stress or directly or indirectly inhibit mitochondrial metabolism have been suggested to initiate or increase phenotypic expression of the disease (60,295–304). Widespread nutritional deficiency in Cuba did not appear to increase the expression of LHON in one large 11778-positive pedigree (305). Similarly, although some case and pedigree reports suggest a possible role for tobacco and excessive alcohol use as precipitants of visual loss (30a,65,148,170,296,298,306,307,307a), other studies, including one late case-control study of sibships (308), failed to confirm this. Other agents known to be toxic to the optic nerve, such as ethambutol (303,309), or to mitochondrial function, such as antiretroviral therapy (300–302), may have a heightened toxicity in patients with the LHON mutations and already compromised mitochondrial function. The evidence linking an abnormality of cyanide metabolism to patients with LHON and acute visual loss is inconclusive (203,310–313).

If the same clinical phenotype of LHON can arise from different mutations found in different subunits of complex I, and possibly even other complexes, most likely the phenotype is not the result of a specific enzyme defect. Indeed, theories on the pathogenesis of LHON must reconcile how multiple different mtDNA mutations located in different genes encoding different proteins result in an essentially identical clinical phenotype that is expressed only in the optic nerve, suddenly and bilaterally (248,252,314,315).

Theories on the pathogenesis of LHON usually begin at oxidative phosphorylation and the generation of ATP. After all, the three primary LHON mutations are found in genes that code for protein subunits of complex I of the respiratory chain. However, even demonstration of a definite deficiency of complex I activity and/or ATP synthesis as measured by enzyme assay has proved problematic (43,79,103,267,314, 316–324), especially with the 11778 mutation, the most common and severe mutation in terms of visual prognosis. Yen et al. (325,326) have shown probable compensatory increases in the absolute amount of mtDNA and in the level of complex II activity (a complex encoded entirely by nuclear genes) in patients with the 11778 mutation. However, although the central nervous system is very reliant on mitochondrial ATP, studies of the bioenergetics of vision do not indicate that ganglion cell function is markedly dependent upon mitochondrial energy production (314). Indeed, it is the photoreceptor layer of the retina rather than the retinal ganglion cell layer that is richest in enzymes for oxidative metabolism (314). This has led some to speculate that the pathogenesis in LHON is not via direct effects on oxidative

phosphorylation, but rather via more indirect mechanisms. Complex I is the site of NADH reoxidation, and it may be that maintenance of the proper NAD/NADH redox balance is particularly important for normal maintenance and function of the ganglion cells or their axons, especially for axonal transport (314,327). Transporter defects involving channels and pumps particularly reliant on mitochondrial ATP production could have specific tissue effects (252). Others propose free radical damage as crucial in LHON pathogenesis (315,328–331). Inhibition of the respiratory chain causes increased generation of free radicals, and the respiratory chain in turn may be inhibited by oxidative damage. This self-amplifying cycle of oxidative damage and respiratory chain dysfunction could cause direct or indirect damage to vulnerable tissues such as the ganglion cell or its axon. The different mtDNA mutations may cause different amounts of free radical production at the level of complex I, and this increased production of reactive oxygen species may occur particularly in a neuronal cell environment (294,328,332).

Even less clear are the subsequent mechanisms by which respiratory chain dysfunction or free radical production result in irreversible damage to the ganglion cells and their axons. Mitochondria play a major role in the induction of apoptosis (333). The collapse of the mitochondrial transmembrane potential and opening of the so-called permeability transition pore leads to the release of proapoptotic proteins, including cytochrome c, and resultant cell death (315,334,335). Many physiologic and pathologic stimuli can directly trigger opening of the mitochondrial transition pore. It is also probable that multiple consequences of mitochondrial dysfunction, including collapse of the transmembrane potential, uncoupling of the respiratory chain, hyperproduction of superoxide anions, disruption of mitochondrial biogenesis, outflow of matrix calcium and glutathione, and release of soluble intermembrane proteins, can indirectly activate apoptosis or necrosis (334). Alternatively, excitotoxic death can be initiated directly by reduced mitochondrial energy production, which leads to activation of the NMDA-type glutamate receptors (315). Additionally, free radicals are a key component in some excitotoxicity pathways and may also trigger apoptotic cell death directly.

Various mechanisms have been proposed on how any of these theorized pathophysiologic processes result in selective damage to the optic nerve, but supportive evidence is scarce. Based on the abnormal appearance of the papillary and peripapillary vasculature in many LHON patients, a primary vascular process with subsequent ischemia has been proposed (28). However, these vascular changes are likely secondary, especially given the intact vascular endothelium as demonstrated by the lack of fluorescein leakage, and the absence of these fundus findings in many patients. A mechanical mechanism has also been suggested in which the severe angle turn that the optic nerve axons need to make in the prelaminar area results in a "chokepoint" region where there is impaired or labile axoplasmic transport (314). Small-caliber, constantly firing P-cells may be particularly vulnerable (223). Histochemical studies of the optic nerve in animals have shown a high degree of mitochondrial respiratory activity within this unmyelinated, prelaminar portion of the optic nerve, suggesting a particularly high requirement for mitochondrial function in this region (336–338). Of great interest in this regard is the recent identification of the causative gene in autosomal dominant optic atrophy (see below) as a nuclear-encoded protein destined for the mitochondria and important in the formation and maintenance of the mitochondrial network (339). Similarly, a recent genetically induced mouse model of complex I deficiency shows the histopathologic features of optic nerve degeneration and demyelination (332,340). The retinal ganglion cell and its axon appear particularly vulnerable to defects in mitochondrial function (90a,248).

Treatment

In light of the possibility for spontaneous recovery in some patients with Leber's disease, any anecdotal reports of treatment efficacy must be considered with caution. Attempts to treat or prevent the acute phase of visual loss with systemic steroids, hydroxycobalamin (341), or cyanide antagonists have in general proved ineffective (111,114,115, 203,313). Reports from Japan advocated craniotomy with lysis of chiasmal arachnoid adhesions in patients with LHON, with 80% of more than 120 patients reporting visual improvement (16,342). Although the data are impressive, it is difficult to support a surgical therapy logistically removed from the site of ocular neurovascular changes. Optic nerve sheath decompression after progressive visual loss in two patients resulted in no improvement (131,206).

Some manifestations of other mitochondrial diseases, specifically the mitochondrial cytopathies, may respond to therapies designed to increase mitochondrial energy production (235,236,343–354). Most of the agents used are naturally occurring cofactors involved in mitochondrial metabolism, while others have antioxidant capabilities. Therapies tried include coenzyme Q_{10}, idebenone, L-carnitine, succinate, dichloroacetate, vitamin K_1, vitamin K_3, vitamin C, thiamine, vitamin B_2, and vitamin E. Mashima et al. (351) reported on 28 LHON patients, 14 of whom were treated with idebenone (a quinol that stimulates ATP formation) combined with vitamin B_2 and vitamin C. There was no significant difference in the number of eyes with visual recovery, although the authors claimed that the treatment seemed to speed recovery when it occurred. Topical agents deemed neuroprotective or antiapoptotic for ganglion cells could be administered directly to the eye (355). It remains to be seen whether any of these agents alone or in combination will prove consistently useful in the treatment of acute visual loss in LHON, in the prevention of second eye involvement, or in the prophylactic therapy of asymptomatic family members at risk.

A promising form of gene therapy known as allotypic expression may play a future role in the therapy of LHON and other mitochondrial diseases (356). In this approach, a nuclear-encoded version of a gene normally encoded by mtDNA (in this case, the ND4 gene containing nucleotide position 11778) is made synthetically, is inserted via an adeno-associated viral vector, and codes for a protein expressed in the cytoplasm that is then imported into the mitochondria. This protein increased the survival of cybrids harboring the 11778 mutation threefold and restored ATP synthesis to a level indistinguishable from that in cybrids containing normal mtDNA. The relative accessibility of the eye and its ganglion cells may provide the ideal setting in which to test this nuclear solution of a mitochondrial problem (357).

Nonspecific recommendations to avoid agents that might stress mitochondrial energy production have no proven benefit in LHON but are certainly reasonable. We advise our patients at risk for LHON to avoid tobacco use, excessive alcohol intake, and environmental toxins. An ECG should be obtained and any cardiac abnormalities treated accordingly. Considering the degree of visual acuity loss, it is remarkable that van Senus (15) reported that 82% of patients were gainfully employed despite their visual handicap. Low vision assessment may be helpful, especially because much of the useful peripheral vision may remain intact. Finally, the importance of genetic counseling in this disease should not be underestimated (358a).

DOMINANT OPTIC ATROPHY

Autosomal dominant optic atrophy, type Kjer (McKusick no. 165500, gene symbol OPA1) (359), is believed to be the most common of the hereditary optic neuropathies. The estimated disease prevalence is 1:50,000, or as high as 1:10,000 in Denmark (360,361).

Clinical Features

In addition to the cases described by Kjer (362,363), numerous other studies have established the clinical profile of patients with dominantly inherited optic atrophy (361,364–375). It is generally agreed that dominant optic atrophy (DOA) is an abiotrophy with usual onset in the first decade of life; however, no congenital case has been documented at birth or shortly thereafter. Kjer (362,363) noted that many of his patients were ignorant of the familial nature of their disease and, in fact, did not realize that they, themselves, had visual dysfunction. No individual in the series by Kline and Glaser (367) could identify a precise onset of reduced acuity. In Hoyt's series (368), the majority of affected patients dated the onset of visual symptoms between 4 and 6 years of age, although a few severely affected individuals were noted to have a visual disturbance, primarily because of nystagmus, prior to beginning schooling. Smith (365) reviewed the literature up to 1972 on this subject and collected 554 clear-cut cases, of whom 442 were actually examined. He emphasized that of this large group, only 15 patients (2.2%) were actually observed to have optic atrophy before age 10. Similarly, Johnston et al. (366) reported visual symptoms before the age of 10 years in only 58% of their 47 affected individuals. Three of the patients (12.5%) examined by Kline and Glaser (367), seven of Hoyt's (368) patients (22.6%), and five of the patients reported by Elliott et al. (370) (25%) were unaware of visual difficulties and were discovered to have optic atrophy as a direct consequence of examination of other affected family members. These phenomena attest to the usually imperceptible onset in childhood, often mild degree of visual dysfunction, absence of night blindness, and absence of acute or subacute progression.

Kjer (362,373) emphasized that visual acuity was usually reduced to the same mild extent in both eyes. Visual acuity remained between 20/20 and 20/60 throughout life in 40% of his cases, with severe visual loss (20/200 to 20/600) occurring in only 15%. None of the 200 patients examined by Kjer (362) had visual acuity reduced to hand motion or light perception levels. His findings are in accordance with the cases collected by Smith (365), who found that 37% had visual acuity of 20/60 or better, 46% had visual acuity between 20/60 and 20/200, and only 17% had visual acuity below 20/200. Other studies support this wide range of visual acuities from 20/20 to light perception (367,368,370–374). In an analysis of 87 affected patients from 21 molecularly confirmed families with DOA (373), the mean visual acuity was 20/120. In all studies, a few patients have been found with striking asymmetry between the acuities of the two eyes, and there is considerable interfamilial and intrafamilial variation in acuities (373,376,377).

Kjer (362,363) was able to obtain follow-up data in 98 patients, 75 of whom were observed for at least 5 years. Some progression occurred in about 50% of the patients. In addition, in Kjer's (363) series, no patients younger than 15 years of age had visual acuity below 20/200, but 10% of patients 15 to 44 years of age and 25% of patients 45 years and older had vision below 20/200. In a study of 20 patients with a mean follow-up of 16 years (370), visual acuity remained stable in both eyes of 13 patients (65%), decreased in one eye in 3 patients (15%), and decreased in both eyes in 4 patients (20%). There was no correlation between the rate of visual loss and initial visual acuity or individual pedigrees. Votruba et al. (373) documented deterioration of visual acuity with age in one third of their 21 families. These figures, as well as data from other reports (361,371, 378–380) suggest a mild, slow, insidious progression of visual dysfunction in some patients. The observation that some families have a marked decline in visual acuity with age while others do not has important implications for counseling (373). Grutzner (381) commented that rapid deterioration of vision may occur even after years of stable visual function, and Kjer et al. (361) also documented such rapid deterioration in a few patients. Spontaneous recovery of vision is not a feature of this disorder.

In the patients studied by Kjer (362,363), there was often an inability to perceive blue colors. Some studies (367, 368,382–384) subsequently demonstrated that tritanopia is the characteristic color vision defect in patients with DOA (385,386), particularly when patients are tested with the Farnsworth-Munsell 100-Hue test (367,368,387,388). However, other studies suggest that a generalized dyschromatopsia, with both blue-yellow and red-green defects, is even more common than an isolated tritanopia (370, 373,389). This mixed color defect accounted for more than 80% of the color deficits documented in a large study of 21 pedigrees (373).

Visual fields in patients with DOA characteristically show central, paracentral, or cecocentral scotomas. Often the defects are best delineated using red test objects, and in patients with acuities of 20/50 or better, static perimetry is necessary to identify the defects. The peripheral fields are usually normal in these patients; however, using chromatic testing with blue and red objects, there appears to be a characteristic inversion of the peripheral field, with the field being more contracted to blue isopters than red (390). Smith (365) collected 22 cases of "bitemporal hemianopia" detected with colored test objects, and Manchester and Calhoun (391) also reported this phenomenon. In the large study performed by Votruba et al. (373), 66% of the visual field defects in 50 affected patients were predominantly in the superotemporal visual fields. This pattern of visual field involvement has been demonstrated using a variety of techniques of field testing, and fixation has been monitored with scanning laser ophthalmoscopy (373), suggesting that these superobitemporal defects are not an artifact of the testing procedures or of eccentric fixation.

The optic atrophy in patients with dominantly inherited optic neuropathy may be subtle (363), may be temporal only (365,382), or may involve the entire optic disc (363,379) (Fig. 11. 4). Kline and Glaser (367) found the most characteristic change was a translucent pallor with absence of fine superficial capillaries of the temporal aspect of the disc, with a triangular excavation of the temporal portion of the disc. In the Votruba et al. analysis (373), wedge-shaped temporal pallor of the disc was documented in 44% of 172 eyes, total atrophy in another 44%, and subtle diffuse pallor in 12%. Other ophthalmoscopic findings reported in these patients included peripapillary atrophy, absent foveal reflex, mild macular pigmentary changes, arterial attenuation, and nonglaucomatous cupping with absence of a healthy neuroretinal rim and shallow saucerization of the cup (365,367,370, 392,393). Fournier et al. (394) emphasized several clinical features that help distinguish patients with DOA from those with normal tension glaucoma, including early age of onset, preferential loss of central vision, sparing of the peripheral fields, pallor of the remaining neuroretinal rim, and a family history of unexplained visual loss or optic atrophy. Sandvig (395) reported three families with autosomal-dominantly inherited excavated cupping and slowly progressive glaucomatous visual field defects but normal intraocular pressures. Visual loss was noted in the third and fourth decades and typically progressed to severe dysfunction. These families with dominant pseudoglaucoma are probably genetically distinct from the more common simple form of DOA.

Electrophysiologic studies have been performed in several patients with DOA (367,373,377,388). Visual evoked responses in affected individuals characteristically show diminished amplitudes and prolonged latencies, the latter usually less profound than in demyelinating disease (373, 377,388,396). Pattern ERGs show a reduced N95 component, in keeping with primary ganglion cell dysfunction (373). The extreme clinical variability among subjects with DOA suggests that on occasion combined clinical and functional evaluation, with computerized perimetry, tests of contrast sensitivity, and electrophysiologic testing, may be necessary to diagnose the most subtle cases (377).

Although there are dominantly inherited syndromes of

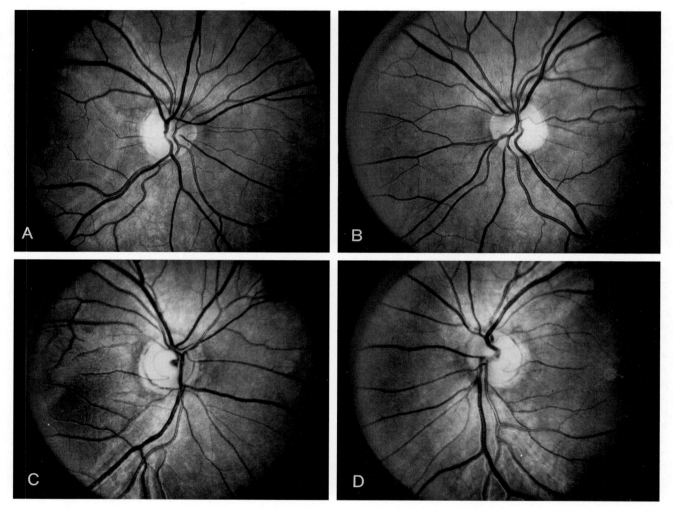

Figure 11.4. Dominant optic atrophy. *A and B,* Right and left optic discs in a patient with 20/40 visual acuity in both eyes, a tritanopic color vision defect, and bilateral, small central scotomas. Note minimal temporal pallor. *C and D,* Right and left discs of the above patient's father. Visual acuity is 20/100 in the right eye and 20/80 in the left eye, with severe dyschromatopsia and bilateral central scotomas. The pallor is extensive and is primarily temporal in a wedge shape.

optic atrophy associated with neurologic dysfunction, most of the patients with the syndrome of autosomal-dominant optic atrophy have no additional neurologic deficits. Nystagmus in some patients likely reflects early visual deprivation rather than central neurologic involvement. Kjer (362,363) found mental abnormalities in 10% of his cases, but this feature was not confirmed in subsequent studies. A mother and a daughter with bilateral optic atrophy with onset in infancy also had unilateral facial palsy (397). Eight of 31 patients described by Hoyt (368) had neural hearing loss, clustering in three of six families. Only one patient was aware of any hearing difficulties. More severe hearing loss associated with familial optic atrophy may or may not be a genetically distinct syndrome (see later).

Pathology/Pathophysiology

Johnston et al. (366) performed a histologic examination of the eyes and optic nerves of a 56-year-old woman from a family with a typical pedigree of autosomal-dominant hereditary optic atrophy. The patient had a long history of bilaterally reduced vision (20/100 in both eyes), bilateral central scotomas, and temporal pallor of both discs. In both eyes, there was diffuse atrophy of the retinal ganglion cell layer associated with diffuse atrophy and loss of myelin within the optic nerves. Johnston et al. (366) suggested, as did Kjer (362,363), that DOA is a primary degeneration of retinal ganglion cells. Electrophysiologic studies confirm loss of ganglion cell function predominantly from the central retina, but not the exclusive result of either parvocellular or magnocellular cell loss (373).

One study of a large pedigree of German descent suggested linkage of the gene responsible for DOA with the Kidd blood group antigen, subsequently localized to chromosome 18q12 (374,398). Further study of this family refined the chromosomal locus to a 3-centimorgan region at 18q12.2–12.3 (374). This family is clinically similar to the other pedigrees of DOA, including its intrafamilial variation, although the median visual acuity was somewhat better at 20/40.

Most of the other pedigrees with DOA, including several from Denmark, the United Kingdom, Germany, France, Cuba, Japan, and the United States, have genetic homogeneity in their linkage to the telomeric portion of the long arm of chromosome 3 (3q28–29) (339,360,361,399–403). Between 30–90% of these families have been found to harbor over 60 different missense and nonsense mutations, deletions, and insertions in a gene within this region that has been designated the OPA1 gene (339,401–406). Identification of those mutations requires sequencing of the OPA1 gene, a process currently available only on a research basis. The product of the OPA1 gene is targeted to the mitochondria and appears to exert its function in mitochondrial biogenesis and stabilization of mitochondrial membrane integrity (339,401,402). Downregulation of the OPA1 leads to fragmentation of the mitochondrial network and dissipation of the mitochondrial membrane potential, with cytochrome c release and caspase-dependent apoptosis (407). These findings demonstrate the crucial role of mitochondria in retinal ganglion cell pathophysiology (90a,339). Linkage analysis of patients with normal tension glaucoma has shown an association with polymorphisms of the OPA1 gene (408–410). Interestingly, there is a mutant strain of mice with dominantly inherited optic atrophy with variable expressivity (411). The mutation in these mice is located on the mouse chromosome 16, which is homologous to the human chromosome 3. There is currently no known treatment for DOA.

CONGENITAL RECESSIVE OPTIC ATROPHY

This form of optic atrophy is present at birth or develops at an early age and is usually discovered before the patient is 3 or 4 years old. It was described by Waardenburg (412) and others as having an autosomal-recessive transmission (413). According to Kjer (392), there is often consanguinity between parents. The clinical picture is that of visual acuity so severely affected that the patient may be completely blind with searching nystagmus. The visual fields, when they can be tested, show variable constriction, and there are often paracentral scotomas (414–416). The optic discs are completely atrophic and often deeply cupped.

Francois (417) remarked on the difficulty in separating this entity from infantile tapetoretinal degeneration in patients with both disc pallor and vascular narrowing. However, in primary optic atrophy, the ERG is normal or supranormal, whereas with the tapetoretinal degenerations, it is abolished. This form of optic atrophy is stationary and unassociated with other symptoms or signs of systemic or neurologic disease. It is, in our experience, rare, and its very existence as a distinct identity has been questioned (418).

APPARENT SEX-LINKED OPTIC ATROPHY

In 1975, Went et al. (419) reported a three-generation family with eight individuals with optic atrophy, all male and all related via the maternal lineage. The onset of visual loss was in early childhood, never acutely, with very slow progression. Visual acuities ranged from 20/50 to 20/1200. Visual evoked potentials showed prolonged latencies, and an ERG of the proband showed no abnormalities (420). One of the affected males had neurologic abnormalities, including ataxia, tremor, absent ankle jerks, and mental retardation. Subtle neurologic abnormalities were noted in the other males with optic atrophy, including absent ankle jerks, plantar responses, mild tremor, and gait disturbances (421). One branch of the pedigree had Huntington's disease, presumably coincidentally. This family has subsequently been found to show close linkage to the Xp11.4–11.2 region of the X chromosome and not to harbor any of the common primary mtDNA mutations associated with LHON (420,422). Another family described by Lysen and Oliver (423) demonstrated transmission from an affected grandfather to his grandson through an unaffected daughter, thereby strengthening the argument for sex-linked transmission. However, the documentation of optic atrophy was uncertain, and some affected individuals apparently had evidence of chorioretinitis.

PRESUMED AUTOSOMAL-RECESSIVE CHIASMAL OPTIC NEUROPATHY

In 1999, Pomerantz and Lessell (424) described a unique family in which all three siblings of one generation had incidentally noted bitemporal visual field defects and optic nerve pallor with retention of excellent visual acuity and no other neurologic or systemic symptoms or signs. Tests for the primary mtDNA mutations associated with LHON were negative. Of note, two maternal uncles had died in their early teens form a neurologic disease characterized initially by stuttering and loss of balance, progressing to bed confinement and aphasia. Examinations of the parents and children of the siblings were normal. The authors proposed an autosomal-recessively inherited chiasmal optic neuropathy, but a mitochondrial disorder is also possible.

HEREDITARY OPTIC ATROPHY WITH OTHER NEUROLOGIC OR SYSTEMIC SIGNS

AUTOSOMAL-DOMINANT PROGRESSIVE OPTIC ATROPHY AND DEAFNESS

In 1974, Konigsmark et al. (425) described six individuals in four generations who had congenital severe deafness and progressive midlife visual failure. Kollarits et al. (426) subsequently described a second family with the same syndrome. In all of the cases, there were no systemic or neurologic abnormalities except for congenital sensorineural hearing loss. The hearing loss in these pedigrees was severe at birth, with none of the reported patients having developed speech. Hearing evaluation in several of the affected individuals revealed that they could hear amplified speech so that they might have developed adequate speech if they had been provided amplification in early childhood and training in oral as well as in manual language. Subtle visual dysfunction was present at an early age, as demonstrated by the 9-year-old son of the proposita in the family examined by Konigsmark et al. (425), who had dyschromatopsia by the Farns-worth-Munsell 100-Hue test and bilateral optic pallor, worse temporally, despite visual acuity of 20/15 and bilaterally full fields. Most of the patients had normal acuity until at least 24 years of age.

Since 1979, several pedigrees with presumed autosomal-dominant optic atrophy and hearing loss have been described (368,427–434). There is great inter- and intrafamilial variability in the age of onset of the visual loss and the severity of the hearing loss. In most cases, visual loss remains better than 20/200. In one Turkish family, linkage analysis excluded the two known genes associated with autosomal dominant optic atrophy (see above) (434). It is unclear whether these pedigrees represent a phenotypic variant of DOA, a genetically distinct disorder, or a genetically heterogeneous group of disorders with a similar phenotype.

AUTOSOMAL-DOMINANT OPTIC ATROPHY, DEAFNESS AND OPHTHALMOPLEGIA

Treft et al. (434a) described a syndrome affecting 23 members of five generations of a Utah family characterized by optic atrophy, deafness, ptosis, ophthalmoplegia, dystaxia, and myopathy. The visual loss was first noted between the ages of 6 and 19 years, with an average age of onset of 11 years. Visual loss was occasionally sudden in onset but always progressive to the 20/30 to 20/400 range. Electroretinograms were abnormal, although retinal pigmentary changes were absent, suggesting the combination of a primary retinal degeneration and a primary optic neuropathy. Hearing loss was sensorineural and progressive, with onset in the first or second decades. Ophthalmoplegia, dystaxia, and myopathy occurred in midlife. One muscle biopsy showed ragged red fibers. Male-to-male transmission confirmed autosomal-dominant inheritance. An unrelated family from Belgium was reported with a similar phenotype (434b). Both these families have recently been genetically confirmed to carry the R445H mutation in the OPA1 gene (434c), previously reported in a single Japanese patient with optic atrophy (434d) and a single French woman with optic atrophy and deafness (434e). Other OPA1 mutations in this region (the GTPase domain) have been associated with monosymptomatic autosomal-dominant optic atrophy (Kjer's disease) (404,405; see above). These findings underscore the importance of mitochondrial dysfunction, whether the result of nuclear or mitochondrial DNA defects, as a final common pathway for many forms of syndromic and nonsyndromic optic atrophy.

AUTOSOMAL-DOMINANT PROGRESSIVE OPTIC ATROPHY WITH PROGRESSIVE HEARING LOSS AND ATAXIA (CAPOS SYNDROME)

In this syndrome, described by Sylvester (435) in 1958, a father and his six children were found to have bilateral optic atrophy and hearing loss, associated with ataxia and limb weakness. The onset of visual loss in these patients was between 2.5 and 9 years of age. The hearing loss was only moderate and, like the optic atrophy, was slowly progressive. The ataxia in these patients primarily affected the legs, with weakness and muscle wasting mainly affecting the shoulder girdle and hands. The relationship of this syndrome to Friedreich's ataxia was discussed in detail by Sylvester (435).

Nicolaides et al. (436) described three family members with a relapsing, early-onset cerebellar ataxia, progressive optic atrophy, and sensorineural hearing loss, with areflexia but no peripheral neuropathy and pes cavus deformity. The authors suggested autosomal-dominant or maternal mitochondrial inheritance and proposed the acronym CAPOS (cerebellar ataxia, areflexia, pes cavus, optic atrophy, and sensorineural deafness).

HEREDITARY OPTIC ATROPHY WITH PROGRESSIVE HEARING LOSS AND POLYNEUROPATHY

Rosenberg and Chutorian (437) reported the occurrence of progressive optic atrophy, sensorineural deafness, and polyneuropathy in three men belonging to two generations of a single family, two brothers and their nephew. The two brothers were 32 and 29 years-old and the nephew was 3.5 years-old when examined. All patients had poor hearing since childhood, with progression to virtually complete deafness. In the two older patients, gait disturbance began between 5 and 10 years of age, and the child had an awkward gait, absent deep tendon reflexes, and a partial Gowers' sign. One brother had visual acuity of 20/100 bilaterally with full visual fields and bilateral optic atrophy, temporal more than nasal. The other brother had visual acuity of 20/400 in both eyes with constricted fields and bilateral optic atrophy. The nephew had a normal ophthalmoscopic examination. All three individuals had abnormally slow nerve conduction velocities. The two brothers had gastrocnemius muscle biopsies showing severe neurogenic atrophy, whereas their nephew had a normal muscle biopsy but a sural nerve biopsy showing demyelination with axonal preservation. A similar family was reported by Iwashita et al. (438), consisting of a 25-year-old man and his 15-year-old sister. Both patients had bilateral optic atrophy, although the affected man had visual acuity of 20/100 in each eye while his sister had visual acuity of 20/20. Neurogenic hearing loss was present in both individuals; however, unlike the patients described by Rosenberg and Chutorian (437), nerve conduction velocities were normal in both patients, as were muscle biopsies. A sural nerve biopsy in the affected male showed mild demyelination. Subsequently, Hagemoser et al. (439) reported two families with autosomal-dominant optic atrophy in the first decade of life, followed by the development of hearing loss and peripheral neuropathy. These authors differentiated these families from those of Rosenberg and Chiturian (437) and Iwashita et al. (438) by the severity and early onset of the optic atrophy and by the mode of inheritance. Hagemoser et al. (439) suggested that the Rosenberg and Chiturian (437) pedigree represents an X-linked disorder and the Iwashita et al. (438) family an autosomal-recessive disorder. These disorders can be included in the spectrum of hereditary polyneuropathies that includes Charcot-Marie-Tooth disease (440–442; see following).

AUTOSOMAL-RECESSIVE OPTIC ATROPHY WITH PROGRESSIVE HEARING LOSS, SPASTIC QUADRIPLEGIA, MENTAL DETERIORATION, AND DEATH (OPTICOCOCHLEODENTATE DEGENERATION)

An autosomal-recessive syndrome characterized by severe optic atrophy with onset of visual loss in infancy, progressive hearing loss resulting in severe deafness, and progressive spastic quadriplegia beginning in infancy with progressive mental deterioration and death in childhood has been described by several authors (443–448). The common denominator in all these patients is a selective, systematized degeneration of the optic, cochlear, dentate, and medial lemniscal systems. The basal ganglia are unaffected in this condition. The diagnosis is made clinically because there are no pathognomonic histochemical, cytochemical, or electron microscopic characteristics found on brain biopsy (446).

OPTICOACOUSTIC NERVE ATROPHY WITH DEMENTIA

Jensen (449) described a 3-year-old boy and his two maternal uncles with a syndrome characterized by severe sensorineural hearing loss with onset in infancy, followed by progressive optic atrophy in the second or third decades and progressive dementia in adulthood. Subsequent autopsy studies (450,451) revealed generalized degeneration of the central nervous system with extensive calcification. Diffuse wasting of skeletal muscles was also found. An X-linked recessive inheritance was proposed, but mitochondrial inheritance may be as likely.

PROGRESSIVE OPTIC ATROPHY WITH JUVENILE DIABETES MELLITUS, DIABETES INSIPIDUS, AND HEARING LOSS (DIDMOAD/WOLFRAM'S SYNDROME)

In 1938, Wolfram (452) described a family in which four of eight siblings had diabetes mellitus and bilateral optic atrophy. Three of the four affected siblings subsequently developed neurosensory hearing loss and two developed neurogenic bladder. DeLawter (453) later reported a patient with diabetes mellitus and optic atrophy in whom diabetes insipidus was subsequently diagnosed. Since these initial reports, about 300 cases have been recorded, with a prevalence of 1 in 770,000 in the United Kingdom (454–471). The hallmark of all these cases is the association of juvenile diabetes mellitus and progressive visual loss with optic atrophy, almost always associated with diabetes insipidus, neurosensory hearing loss, or both (hence the acronym DIDMOAD for diabetes insipidus, diabetes mellitus, optic atrophy, and deafness). The progression and development of this syndrome are variable. Symptoms and signs of diabetes mellitus usually occur within the first or second decade of life and usually precede the development of optic atrophy. In several cases, however, visual loss with optic atrophy was the first sign of the syndrome. In the early stages, visual acuity may be normal despite mild dyschromatopsia and optic atrophy. In later stages, visual loss becomes severe,

usually worse than 20/200, suggesting progression (457, 468). Visual fields show both generalized constriction and central scotomas. Optic atrophy is uniformly severe, and there may be mild to moderate cupping of the disc.

The onset of hearing loss and of diabetes insipidus in this syndrome is equally variable. Both begin in the first or second decade of life and may be severe. Atonia of the efferent urinary tract is present in 46–58% of patients and is associated with recurrent urinary tract infections and even fatal complications (459,466). Other systemic and neurologic abnormalities include ataxia, axial rigidity, seizures, startle myoclonus, tremor, gastrointestinal dysmotility, vestibular malfunction, central apnea, neurogenic upper airway collapse, ptosis, cataracts, pigmentary retinopathy, iritis, lacrimal hyposecretion, tonic pupil, ophthalmoplegia, convergence insufficiency, vertical gaze palsy, mental retardation, psychiatric abnormalities, nystagmus, short stature, primary gonadal atrophy, other endocrine abnormalities, anosmia, megaloblastic and sideroblastic anemia, abnormal electroretinography, and elevated cerebrospinal fluid protein levels (457,466,467,470–472). Psychiatric disorders are also seen at an increased frequency among heterozygous carriers (473). Pathology and neuroimaging in some patients reveal widespread atrophic changes and suggest a diffuse neurodegenerative disorder, with particular involvement of the midbrain and pons (467,471,474). Median age at death is 30 years, most commonly due to central respiratory failure with brain stem atrophy (466,475).

Many of the associated abnormalities reported in Wolfram's syndrome are commonly encountered in patients with presumed mitochondrial diseases, especially patients with the chronic progressive external ophthalmoplegia syndromes (83,230). This has led to speculation that patients with Wolfram's syndrome may have a unifying pathogenesis in underlying mitochondrial dysfunction (167,476–480). Abnormalities of mitochondrial function can result from nuclear or mitochondrial DNA defects because both genomes code for proteins essential for normal mitochondrial function. Barrientos et al. (480) described a girl with diabetes mellitus at age 8, optic atrophy by age 11, bladder atony, diabetes insipidus, and ultimately sensorineural hearing loss. The patient was found to have a heteroplasmic mitochondrial DNA deletion, and the identical deletion was noted in lesser proportions in her asymptomatic sister, mother, and father. The presence of this deletion in both parents prompted the authors to propose that a defect in a nuclear gene was acting at the mitochondrial level to cause the disease. Most cases of Wolfram's have been classified as sporadic or recessively inherited, the latter usually concluded from sibling expression (which we now know could also occur from maternal transmission). Furthermore, some nuclear genetic defects can cause rearrangements of mitochondrial DNA, presumably if the altered gene codes for proteins involved in mtDNA regulation. Other investigators have not found mtDNA defects or evidence of mitochondrial dysfunction among patients with Wolfram's syndrome (466,467,477, 481). HLA typing reveals an association with the HLA-DR2 antigen in some patients, suggesting an influence of HLA on susceptibility to the disease (482,483). Using linkage analysis in 11 families, Polymeropoulos et al. (484) proposed localization of the Wolfram's gene to the short arm of chromosome 4. This locus was refined to chromosome 4p16.1 and accounts for many but not all DIDMOAD pedigrees (485,486). The gene responsible at this locus has been designated WFS1, in which multiple point mutations and deletions have been identified (486–488). Some of these mutations were subsequently found to be a common cause of inherited isolated low-frequency hearing loss (489). In one report, the locus on chromosome 4p16 was proposed as a predisposing factor for the formation of multiple mtDNA deletions (490). DIDMOAD patients were also found to concentrate on two major mtDNA haplotypes that are also overrepresented among LHON patients (273). A phenotypic variant of Wolfram's syndrome with peptic ulcer disease and bleeding secondary to a platelet aggregation defect, but without diabetes insipidus, was noted in four consanguineous Jordanian families and linked to a second locus (WFS2) on chromosome 4q22–24 (470,491). The Wolfram's phenotype may be nonspecific and reflect a wide variety of underlying genetic defects in either the nuclear or mitochondrial genomes. When the syndrome is accompanied by anemia, treatment with thiamine may ameliorate the anemia and decrease the insulin requirement (492).

PROGRESSIVE ENCEPHALOPATHY WITH EDEMA, HYPSARRHYTHMIA, AND OPTIC ATROPHY (PEHO SYNDROME)

Salonen et al. (493) described 14 patients from 11 families with a progressive encephalopathy with onset in the first 6 months of life, followed by severe hypotonia, convulsions with hypsarrhythmia, profound mental deterioration, hyperreflexia, transient or persistent facial and body edema, and optic atrophy (494). Optic atrophy is usually noted by the first or second year of life, and nystagmus is common. Microcephaly and brain atrophy develop, especially in the cerebellar and brain stem areas (495–498). A metabolic defect has yet to be determined, although elevations of nitric oxide have been noted (497), and an autosomal-recessive mode of inheritance is likely. This could be considered a form of Behr's syndrome, which probably represents a heterogeneous group of disorders (see below).

COMPLICATED HEREDITARY INFANTILE OPTIC ATROPHY (BEHR'S SYNDROME)

In 1909, Behr (499) described a syndrome of heredofamilial optic atrophy beginning in early childhood and associated with variable pyramidal tract signs, ataxia, mental retardation, urinary incontinence, and pes cavus. The syndrome has been reported in both sexes (380,413,500) and is believed to be autosomal-recessively inherited. Visual loss usually manifests before age 10 years, is moderate to severe, and is frequently accompanied by nystagmus. In most cases, the abnormalities do not progress after childhood. In one case of Behr's syndrome, MR imaging demonstrated diffuse symmetric white matter abnormalities (501). Horoupian et al. (502) reported two sisters with Behr's syndrome, one of whom came to autopsy. Findings included moderate atrophy of the optic nerves and optic tracts with extensive degeneration of the lateral geniculate nuclei and with mild attenuation of the visual radiations, but with normal striate cortex. Two other patients with Behr's syndrome were also autopsied, but in one patient the findings were overshadowed by an intracerebral hemorrhage (503) and in the other by necrotizing encephalopathy (504). Monaco et al. (505) reported a patient with Behr's syndrome associated with epilepsy, as well as slow motor nerve conduction velocities, a low testosterone level, and an amino acid imbalance in both plasma and cerebrospinal fluid.

In several Iraqi-Jewish pedigrees of Behr's syndrome, 3-methylglutaconic aciduria was identified, leading to mapping of the gene (designated OPA3) to chromosome 19q13.2–13.3 (506–512). These patients had infantile optic atrophy and an early-onset extrapyramidal movement disorder dominated by chorea. Approximately half of the patients developed spastic paraparesis by the second decade. The majority of affected individuals were female. In propionic acidemia, a rare autosomal recessive disorder, chronic metabolic decompensation occurs with paroxysmal ketoacidosis, failure to thrive, and mild developmental delay (512a). As a result of improved clinical intervention, survival has lengthened into adolescence. Male gender and age are associated with bilateral, progressive optic neuropathy (512a).

Korn-Lubetzki et al. (513) described a consanguineous Israeli-Jewish-Iraqi family with four of nine siblings (all males) affected within the first decade of life by a syndrome of optic atrophy, dystonia, and striatal atrophy on imaging, but with no identified causative metabolic or genetic defects. Clinical findings in other patients with Behr's syndrome may be similar to those in cases of hereditary ataxia; in fact, Francois (514) suggested that Behr's syndrome may be a transitional form between simple heredofamilial optic atrophy and the hereditary ataxias. Behr's syndrome is likely heterogeneous, reflecting different etiologic and genetic factors (515).

OPTIC NEUROPATHY AS A MANIFESTATION OF HEREDITARY DEGENERATIVE OR DEVELOPMENTAL DISEASES

HEREDITARY ATAXIAS

The inherited ataxias represent a group of chronic progressive neurodegenerative conditions involving the cerebellum and its connections (516,517). The most common classification of the hereditary ataxias is by pattern of inheritance: autosomal dominant (most common), autosomal recessive,

X-linked, and maternal (mitochondrial). Advances in biochemical and genetic analysis reveal a wide variability of clinical signs and neuropathology, even within families, and the overlap of clinical and pathologic phenotypes in disorders now known to be caused by different genetic defects makes diagnostic classification by phenotype often inaccurate (516,518–520). A genomic classification by chromosomal location is available for many of these disorders, and the abnormal gene products involved are under investigation. Optic atrophy is not uncommon among individuals with the hereditary ataxias (521,522).

The prototype of all forms of progressive ataxia was first described by Friedreich (523) in 1863. The onset of the disease is usually between the ages of 8 and 15 years, almost always before age 25 (524–528). The disorder is marked by degeneration of the large sensory neurons concerned with position sense and the afferent spinocerebellar tracts, causing a sensory ataxia. Characteristic clinical features include progressive ataxia of gait and clumsiness in walking and using the hands, dysarthria, loss of joint position and vibratory sensation, absent lower extremity tendon reflexes, and extensor plantar responses. Common findings include scoliosis, foot deformity, diabetes mellitus, and cardiac involvement. Other manifestations include pes cavus, distal wasting, deafness, nystagmus, eye movement abnormalities consistent with abnormal cerebellar function, and optic atrophy. The course is relentlessly progressive, with most patients unable to walk within 15 years of onset, and death from infectious or cardiac causes usually in the fourth or fifth decades. A later-onset, more slowly progressive form has been described (526,529).

Friedreich's ataxia is inherited in an autosomal-recessive manner, and the gene defect has been localized to the proximal long arm of the 9th chromosome (9q13–21) (526,530,531). The vast majority of cases are homozygous for an intronic, unstable, GAA trinucleotide expansion (532) in a gene designated FRDA/X25 that codes for a protein known as frataxin (516,533). Frataxin is a mitochondrial protein that appears to regulate iron levels in the mitochondria. Its absence leads to mitochondrial iron overload and overproduction of reactive oxygen species and cell death (534,534a). Optic atrophy is present in many cases of Friedreich's ataxia, although severe visual loss is uncommon. Bell and Carmichael (535) found optic disc pallor in 15 of 57 cases (26%), whereas Sjögren (536) noted optic atrophy in only 12% of his cases. In the Quebec cooperative study, Andermann et al. (537) found reduced visual acuity and optic atrophy in 4 of 13 cases (30%), and Geoffroy et al. (538), reviewing previous studies, reported a 50% prevalence of optic atrophy. Despite these figures, Heck (539) found no evidence of optic atrophy in members of a large family with this disease. Carroll et al. (540) performed clinical and electrophysiologic examinations on 22 patients with Friedreich's ataxia and found that although no patient had visual acuity below 20/80, the majority of the patients had either clinical or electrophysiologic evidence of visual sensory dysfunction. Livingstone et al. (541) examined 21 patients with Friedreich's ataxia and found that two thirds of the patients had some degree of visual impairment and abnormal visual evoked responses. These investigators found no correlation between the presence and severity of visual involvement and the age or duration of other neurologic symptoms. Wenzel et al. (542) found pathologic results on visual evoked responses in 25 of 45 patients (55%). Among series of genetically confirmed patients with Friedreich's ataxia, Müller-Felber et al. (543) found abnormal visual

evoked responses in 50% of patients, Durr et al. (544) found "reduced" visual acuity in 13% of 140 patients, and Montermini et al. (545) reported optic atrophy in 21% of 109 patients. It is unclear whether the variability in optic atrophy relates to the duration of the disease or the underlying genetic abnormality. Givre et al. (546) reported a 15-year-old boy with genetically confirmed Friedreich's ataxia with subacute bilateral optic neuropathies followed by partial spontaneous recovery, similar to the pattern of visual involvement seen in some patients with LHON.

Other autosomal-recessive ataxias less common than Friedreich's ataxia include ataxia telangiectasia, ataxia with vitamin E deficiency, abetalipoproteinemia, Refsum's disease, spastic ataxia, infantile-onset spinocerebellar ataxia, and ataxia with oculomotor apraxia (527). A condition resembling Friedreich's ataxia associated with decreased vitamin E levels has been localized to chromosome 8 (547) and also includes some patients with optic atrophy. Vitamin E supplementation of these patients may be efficacious early in the course of the disease. Early-onset autosomal-recessive spinocerebellar ataxia with hearing loss and optic atrophy shows linkage at 6p21–23 (548), congenital cerebellar ataxia with mental retardation, optic atrophy, and skin abnormalities (CAMOS) links at 15q24–26 (549), and pontocerebellar hypoplasia with progressive microcephaly (and optic atrophy) (CLAM) links to 7q11–21 (549a). In 1993, Arts et al. (550) described what they believed to be a unique clinical syndrome in a five-generation Dutch family. Transmission of the disease was X-linked recessive. Affected family members demonstrated optic atrophy, ataxia, deafness, flaccid tetraplegia, and areflexia. The course was generally progressive to death. No specific biochemical, immunologic, or genetic defects were identified, although pathologic examination showed almost complete absence of myelin in the posterior columns.

The most common of the hereditary ataxias are inherited in an autosomal-dominant pattern. The majority of these are now designated by the term **spinocerebellar ataxia** (SCA), reflecting their predominant pathology in the spinal cord and the cerebellar pathways (516,519,520,551–553). A wide range of clinical and pathologic findings can be seen within and among pedigrees. Although originally classified by clinical descriptions within specific families (554), they are now defined by the genetic loci and specific mutations in these families. Indeed, the same phenotype can be caused by a multitude of different gene defects. These diseases are inherited in an autosomal-dominant fashion, although sporadic cases can occur.

As of 2003, there were at least 23 different genetic loci for SCAs (SCA 1 to SCA 22) (552,553, personal communication, George Wilmot, MD, 2003). The combination of SCA1 (chromosome 6p), SCA 2 (chromosome 12q), SCA 3 (chromosome 14q and allelic with Machado-Joseph disease), SCA 6 (chromosome 19p), and SCA 7 (chromosome 3p) represents approximately 80% of the autosomal dominant ataxias (516). Many of the SCAs are caused by mutations involving the expansion of a CAG trinucleotide repeat in the protein coding sequences of specific genes, resulting in a series of glutamines. As with other diseases that involve abnormal repeats, the expanded regions can become larger with each successive generation, resulting in a younger age of onset in each generation (anticipation). Anticipation is seen particularly when the disease is inherited from the father.

Clinically, the SCAs are characterized by signs and symptoms attributable to cerebellar degeneration and sometimes other neurologic dysfunction secondary to neuronal loss. Loss of vision is usually mild but may be a prominent symptom, occurring in association with constricted visual fields and diffuse optic atrophy (522,554–556). However, it is not clear in some cases whether the primary process is retinal with secondary optic atrophy or primary optic nerve. Livingstone et al. (541) examined 17 patients with hereditary cerebellar or spastic ataxia, both clinically and electrophysiologically. They found visual sensory abnormalities in only three of the patients (17.6%), of whom only one had evidence of optic atrophy. Koeppen et al. (557) similarly found evidence of optic atrophy in 3 of 17 cases of adult-onset hereditary ataxia. In an autopsy study of one patient with temporal pallor of the discs in life, Staal et al. (558) found the eyes to be normal, including the ganglion cells. The retrobulbar portions of both optic nerves were atrophic and completely demyelinated, with severe axonal degeneration, but the prechiasmatic parts of the nerves were normal. Triau et al. (559) described a three-generation family with six members affected with progressive ataxia and blindness. The proband initially had optic atrophy but subsequently developed generalized chorioretinal degeneration. Pathologic examination showed demyelination and gliosis of the optic nerves and chiasm and gliosis of the retrochiasmal pathways back to the striate cortex. Hammond and Wilder (560) demonstrated abnormal VEPs in two patients with adult-onset spinocerebellar atrophy and no optic disc pallor.

Detailed analysis of the prevalence of optic atrophy among the different genotypes now associated with the spinocerebellar syndromes has not been performed. Prior to genetic analysis, Harding (554) categorized the autosomal-dominant cerebellar ataxias (ADCAs) into four types, with only the first type having individuals with primary optic atrophy (approximately 30% of cases). We now know that ADCA type I encompasses multiple genetic loci, including those pedigrees now classified genetically as SCA1, SCA2, SCA3, and probably SCA4 and SCA5. Initial studies suggest that patients with the SCA2 genotype do not exhibit optic atrophy (561), whereas SCA3 patients may have optic atrophy, especially if their ataxia is severe (562,563). In a study of six patients from three families of molecularly confirmed SCA 1, Abe et al. (556) found a gradual decrease in visual acuity and color vision, progressive contraction of visual fields, severely decreased corneal endothelial density, mild attenuation of oscillatory potentials on ERG, and optic atrophy with large cupping. Similarly, three patients from one molecularly confirmed SCA 1 family had optic atrophy (564). SCA 7 is essentially the only SCA associated with pigmentary retinal degeneration (565–567).

As of 2003, genetic testing was commercially available for SCA1, 2, 3, 6, 7, 8, 10, 12, and 17 and detatorubropallidoluysian atrophy (DRPLA) (516). Each test is specific for that SCA. Some spinocerebellar syndromes may result from mutations in mtDNA (568,569), including the point mutation at position 8993 (570) that is also associated with Leigh's syndrome (see later). There are currently no specific therapeutic options for the spinocerebellar syndromes.

Melberg et al. (571) described an autosomal dominant Swedish pedigree with five patients affected with cerebellar ataxia and sensorineural deafness, four of whom also had narcolepsy. Optic atrophy, other neurologic abnormalities, and psychiatric symptoms developed with increasing disease duration. Other inconsistent findings were diabetes mellitus and hypertrophic cardiomyopathy. A normal-sized SCA 1 repeat was observed and mitochondrial dysfunction was suggested.

Lundberg et al. (572) described a family with 29 members, of whom 15 had an autosomal-dominantly inherited syndrome of optic atrophy, ataxia, pyramidal tract signs, and absent Achilles reflex. Optic atrophy was present in seven of the family members and appeared to have begun during early life. In some instances, atrophy was severe and associated with nystagmus. Pes cavus was present even more often than optic atrophy and was severely disabling. In one third of the cases, there was a mild sensory disturbance in the lower limbs, with Achilles reflexes being absent in all cases. An autopsy performed in one patient revealed diffuse atrophy of both optic nerves, the optic chiasm, the optic tracts, and the lateral geniculate bodies. The posterior columns of the spinal cord were narrow and pale, and the inferior olives were firm and gray. The cerebellar cortex was mildly atrophic and most Purkinje cells were missing. Extensive demyelination was present in the anterior visual sensory system and both inferior olives, whereas the posterior columns were partially demyelinated. This family appears to have a transitional syndrome with features of both the predominantly spinal and the predominantly cerebellar hereditary ataxias. A similar family was described by Young (573).

HEREDITARY POLYNEUROPATHIES

In 1886, Charcot and Marie (574), as well as Tooth (575), collected 39 cases from personal observations and reports in the literature of a heredofamilial disorder characterized by progressive muscular weakness and atrophy that began during the first two decades of life. Subsequent classifications of **Charcot-Marie-Tooth disease** (CMT) have been by clinical syndrome, histopathology, and pattern of inheritance and, later, by genetic defect and affected gene products (576–578). This group of hereditary polyneuropathies accounts for 90% of all hereditary neuropathies, with the prevalence in the United States being about 40 per 100,000. Most forms of CMT begin between the ages of 2 and 15 years. The first signs are usually pes cavus, foot deformities, or scoliosis. There is slowly progressive weakness and wasting, first of the feet and legs and then of the hands. Motor symptoms predominate over sensory abnormalities. The most common form of CMT is type 1, a demyelinating neuropathy with autosomal-dominant inheritance, mapped most commonly to the short arm of chromosome 17 (17p11.2) (type 1A), although a few pedigrees with this phenotype are linked to the long arm of chromosome 1 (type 1B) (579–581). CMT type 2 is clinically similar, but nerve conductions are of normal velocity, suggesting the process is neuronal rather than demyelinating. Type 2 can be inherited in an autosomal-dominant fashion (linked to the short arm of chromosome 1) or autosomal-recessively (linked to the long arm of chromosome 8). Type 3 is the most severe form. When type 3 is inherited in an autosomal-dominant pattern, the linkage is to the same region on chromosome 1 associated with type 1B; when it is autosomal recessive, the linkage is to the same region on chromosome 17 associated with type 1A. There are also X-linked forms of CMT, both X-linked dominant (linked to defects on the long arm) and X-linked recessive (linked to regions on either the long arm or the short arm). As of 2002, causative mutations for the hereditary peripheral neuropathies had been identified in 17 different genes (577).

In 1889, Vizioli (582) reported progressive bilateral blindness and optic atrophy in a 59-year-old man and his 26-year-old son, both of whom had evidence of CMT. Since this initial report, numerous patients with CMT and optic atrophy have been reported (415,583–589). Alajouanine et al. (585) reported demyelination of the optic nerves in a postmortem study of a 65-year-old CMT patient in whom blindness and optic atrophy developed 40–50 years after the onset of his disease. Electrophysiologic testing reveals subclinical optic neuropathy in a high proportion of CMT patients (586,590–593). Tackmann and Radu (590) found abnormalities of VEPs in seven eyes of five patients with no clinical signs of optic nerve involvement. Burki (591) described the ocular findings in nine patients with CMT. Although only three patients complained of visual problems and all nine patients had normal visual acuity in both eyes, combined VEP and contrast sensitivity testing revealed evidence of optic neuropathy in one or both eyes of seven patients. Bird and Griep (592) performed VEPs on 25 patients with CMT and demonstrated abnormalities in 4 patients (16%), including the only patient with clinical optic atrophy. Carroll et al. (586) performed VEPs on 15 visually asymptomatic CMT patients and found definite abnormalities in 5 and possible abnormalities in another 3. Taking into account both electrophysiologic and clinical data, 73% of patients showed some afferent visual pathway dysfunction. Similarly, Gadoth et al. (593) reported prolongation of VEPs in 43.7% of 16 patients with CMT and clinically normal optic nerves.

Pedigrees specifically designated CMT type 6 show a regular association of CMT and optic atrophy (588,589,589a). Indeed, optic atrophy and neuropathy have been described in families that show autosomal-dominant, autosomal-recessive, and X-linked recessive inheritance. This type of CMT is as yet genetically unspecified and may prove genetically heterogeneous (588,589a).

We have already commented on the cases reported by Rosenberg and Chutorian (437) and their similarity to the hereditary ataxias as well as to CMT. Other cases have been reported (594,595) that also appear to link CMT to the hereditary ataxias, particularly Friedreich's ataxia.

Familial dysautonomia (Riley-Day syndrome) is an autosomal-recessive disease that almost exclusively affects Ashkenazi Jews (596). Abnormalities of the peripheral nervous system cause the clinical manifestations of sensory and autonomic dysfunction. The gene responsible has been identified on chromosome 9q31–33 (597). Optic atrophy has been demonstrated in patients with familial dysautonomia, usually after the first decade of life (598–600). Diamond et al. (599) found optic nerve pallor in all of their 12 patients, and 79% of eyes had abnormal VEPs. Older patients had more severe deficits than younger patients, suggesting progression. In some cases of familial dysautonomia, optic atrophy may go unrecognized because coincident corneal scarring prevents adequate fundus examination. However, in most cases, early mortality from the disease probably precludes the later development of large myelinated fiber deterioration and optic atrophy (598). Nevertheless, in those who survive beyond early childhood, optic atrophy is an important sign of central nervous system dysfunction in this disorder.

HEREDITARY SPASTIC PARAPLEGIAS

The hereditary spastic paraplegias (Strumpell-Lorrain disease) are autosomal-dominant disorders characterized by progressive spasticity of the lower limbs and pathologic reflexes with degeneration or demyelination of the corticospinal system and, to a lesser extent, of the posterior cord and the spinocerebellar system (601,602). Several loci have been identified, the most frequent of which is that linked to chromosome 2p22, followed by that linked to chromosome 14q11–21 (601). Optic neuropathy and dyschromatopsia with visual acuities ranging from 20/20 to 20/200 have been reported in a few patients with Strumpell-Lorrain disease (601,602).

Dillmann et al. (603) described two siblings with infantile spastic paraplegia and motor and sensory axonal polyneuropathy who developed progressive visual loss secondary to optic neuropathy in adolescence. The relationship to the hereditary motor and sensory neuropathy types 5 and 6 are discussed. Miyama et al. (604) described an 8-year-old girl with progressive infantile spastic paraplegia and severe developmental delay who developed peripheral neuropathy and optic atrophy at age 5 years.

HEREDITARY MUSCULAR DYSTROPHIES

Myotonic dystrophy, a relatively common autosomal dominant disorder with a prevalence of 1 in 20,000, is characterized by progressive myopathy, cataracts, cardiomyopathy with conduction defects, and diabetes mellitus (516,605,606). Other classic findings include frontal balding, bifacial weakness, ptosis, and cognitive and psychiatric dysfunction. Less common ophthalmologic manifestations can include ocular hypotonia, external ophthalmoplegia, pigmentary retinopathy, and optic atrophy (607). Most patients with myotonic dystrophy have an expansion of an unstable CTG repeat in a protein kinase gene on chromosome 19q13.3, although variants of the disease are genetically heterogeneous (516).

STORAGE DISEASES AND CEREBRAL DEGENERATIONS OF CHILDHOOD

About 100 inherited metabolic diseases with ocular manifestations have been described (608,609; see Chapter 46).

Among these, the lysosomal storage disorders are monogenic inborn errors of metabolism with heterogeneous pathophysiology and clinical manifestations (610–612). They represent more than 40 disorders, each of which is caused by the deficiency of a lysosomal enzyme or other protein. The stored material is usually a complex lipid or saccharide, and the nervous system is commonly affected. The inheritance pattern in these diseases is almost always recessive, usually autosomal recessive, but occasionally X-linked.

Of the inborn lysosomal disorders with ocular manifestations, the major diseases that include optic neuropathy are the mucopolysaccharidoses (MPS) and the lipidoses (613–618). Optic atrophy may occur in patients with MPS IH (Hurler), MPS IS (Scheie), MPS IHS (Hurler-Scheie), MPS IIA and IIB (Hunter), MPS IIIA and IIIB (Sanfilippo), MPS IV (Morquio), and MPS VI (Maroteaux-Lamy). In many cases, atrophy is caused by hydrocephalus that presumably occurs from meningeal mucopolysaccharide deposition, leading to delayed cerebrospinal fluid absorption (359,615,619–621). Meningeal or scleral mucopolysaccharide accumulation may also cause local compression of the optic nerve, resulting in disc swelling, optic atrophy, or both. In other cases, however, optic atrophy occurs in association with the deposition of mucopolysaccharides within glial cells of the optic nerve (622). Among the lipidoses, optic atrophy occurs in infantile and juvenile GM_1-gangliosidoses (GM_1-1 and GM_1-2), the GM_2-gangliosidoses (Tay-Sachs disease, Sandhoff disease, and late infantile, juvenile, and adult GM_2-gangliosidoses), and the infantile form of Niemann-Pick disease. Although reported in the neuronal ceroid lipofuscinoses, optic atrophy is most frequently a secondary feature of the severe retinal degeneration.

Other storage diseases in which optic atrophy figures prominently include the hereditary leukodystrophies, including the infantile and juvenile forms of Krabbe's disease, the Austin variant of sulfatidosis (mucosulfatidosis), and the infantile, juvenile, and adult forms of metachromatic leukodystrophy.

Metachromatic leukodystrophy (MLD) is an autosomal-recessive, degenerative disorder of central and peripheral myelin, secondary to arylsulfatase A deficiency. The genetic defect is localized to the long arm of chromosome 22. Optic atrophy occurs in up to 50% of cases, especially in the juvenile and adult forms (623–626). Pathology reveals diffuse ganglion cell loss with accumulation of cerebroside sulfate in optic nerve glial cells, with storage of metachromatic complex lipids in the retinal ganglion cells and optic nerves but not in the outer retinal layers (623,625,627–629).

Pathologic findings similar to those found in MLD are seen in the optic nerves of patients with Krabbe's disease and optic atrophy (630–633). In the storage diseases that are associated with optic atrophy, the atrophy appears to result from abnormal myelin metabolism, with secondary accumulation of abnormal storage materials within the optic nerve (631). Enlarged optic nerves with numerous globoid cells have been demonstrated on pathology and on neuroimaging (634,635). Krabbe's disease usually occurs in infancy, although a few cases with juvenile and even adult onset have been reported (636,637), some presenting with optic atrophy

and visual loss. Krabbe's disease is an autosomal recessive disease of both central and peripheral myelin, linked to chromosome 14, that results from a deficiency of galactocerebrosidase.

Adrenoleukodystrophy is an X-chromosome-linked recessive disorder characterized by primary atrophy of the adrenal glands, with or without Addison's disease and low plasma cortisol levels, and a severe degeneration of white matter in the central nervous system with blindness (638). Symptoms of behavioral changes signal the onset of the disease at the end of the first decade of life, followed by relentlessly progressive dementia, pyramidal tract dysfunction, and visual loss, with optic atrophy and demyelination of the entire visual pathway. Hence, visual loss may be of both anterior and retrochiasmal origin, although there appears to be an early predilection for the more posterior cerebral white matter (639,640). Wray et al. (641) reported the visual system findings in a 10-year-old boy with adrenoleukodystrophy and vision of light perception bilaterally with pale discs. These investigators found extensive demyelination throughout the visual sensory pathways. Within the optic nerve, some cells, thought by Wray et al. (641) to be either oligodendrocytes or macrophages, contained lipid-filled vacuoles, presumably myelin breakdown products. Similar findings were reported by others (642–644). The basic defect is accumulation of very long chain fatty acids secondary to a defective enzyme within the peroxisomes, subcellular organelles that contain enzymes necessary for normal cellular function (645). The defective gene in adrenoleukodystrophy is located at the distal end of the long arm of the X chromosome. Variants of adrenoleukodystrophy include adrenomyeloneuropathy, a clinically similar disorder except for later onset and slower progression, and a syndrome similar to adrenomyeloneuropathy seen in 15% of women heterozygous for the gene. Kaplan et al. (646) studied the visual system in 59 men with adrenomyeloneuropathy with VEPs, MR imaging, and clinical examination. They found that 63% of patients had involvement of the visual pathways from the optic nerves to the occipital cortex, presumably on the basis of primary demyelination. Interestingly, only five of the patients had visual complaints.

Zellweger syndrome (cerebrohepatorenal syndrome) is another peroxisomal disorder associated with optic atrophy (643,645,647,648). In this autosomal-recessive disease, there is dysfunction of multiple peroxisomal enzymes, with severe manifestations at birth, including floppiness, dysmorphic facial characteristics, cirrhosis, genital anomalies, skeletal anomalies, pigmentary retinopathy, and optic atrophy.

Another leukodystrophy, Pelizaeus-Merzbacher disease, is an X-linked recessive syndrome, and perhaps in some cases autosomal recessive, that is likely genetically heterogeneous (617,649–651). Symptoms are present either at birth or within the first year of life. They include nystagmus, head tremor, ataxia, spasticity, graying of the optic discs or optic atrophy, and ultimately seizures, microcephaly, athetoid movements, and failure to thrive. There is a frequent association with pes cavus and scoliosis. The course is progressive for several years, followed by slowing and some degree of stability. Pathologic examination reveals severe patchy absence of myelin in the central but not the peripheral nervous system, suggesting that this is a disorder of oligodendrocytes rather than Schwann cells. The disease has been linked to a gene on the long arm of the X chromosome (Xq22) that codes for myelin proteolipid protein and proteins involved in oligodendrocyte maturation (651–653). Pallor of the optic discs occurs in some patients with Pelizaeus-Merzbacher disease, although it is usually not severe, and visual acuity may not be significantly reduced. Rahn et al. (654) reported severe reduction in ganglion cells, thinning of the retinal nerve fiber layer, and widespread demyelination with loss of axon cylinders in the optic nerve of a patient with Pelizaeus-Merzbacher disease.

Infantile neuroaxonal dystrophy (INAD) is an autosomal-recessive, progressive neurologic disease characterized by severe, progressive motor disturbance; arrested mental development; and blindness with optic atrophy, beginning within the first year of life. Seizures and myoclonus may be severe, and most patients succumb within the first decade of life (655). Histopathologically, patients with this disorder have eosinophilic spheroids in the central, peripheral, and autonomic nervous systems; cerebellar degeneration; and degeneration of various neuronal, myelin, and glial elements (656–661). Optic atrophy is described in 40% of cases by age 3 years (660,661). Similar pathologic findings occur in Hallervorden-Spatz disease (pantothenate kinase-associated neurodegeneration), an autosomal-recessive disorder that is of later onset and is more insidiously progressive (662). The clinical syndrome is dominated by motor findings, both extrapyramidal and pyramidal. Patients with Hallervorden-Spatz disease will also have spheroids, but this pathology preferentially occurs in the basal ganglia (663). The brown discoloration of the globus pallidus, caused by iron-containing pigment deposition, serves to distinguish this disease. MR imaging reveals T2 hypointensities in the globus pallidus, the so-called eye of the tiger sign (664), and increased uptake of the iron isotope ^{59}Fe in the basal ganglia occurs. Visual loss, if present, may reflect retinal degeneration or primary optic atrophy (665–667), and the syndrome may even present initially with isolated optic atrophy (666). The responsible gene has been designated PANK2 on chromosome 20 (662), although the syndrome may be genetically heterogeneous.

Menkes syndrome (kinky hair disease) is an X-linked recessive disorder with maldistribution of body copper (668) and resultant cerebral copper deficiency. This degenerative disorder of gray matter manifests in the neonatal period with progressive psychomotor retardation, spasticity, seizures, and colorless, friable hair. Retinal abnormalities are not uncommon (669,670), and optic atrophy can also occur (671,672).

Canavan's disease (*N*-acetylaspartic aciduria) is an autosomal-recessive cerebral degeneration that occurs during the first year of life and is characterized by megalencephaly, poor head control, severe floppiness, spasticity, lack of psychomotor development, and optic atrophy (617,673). Neuroimaging shows increased lucency of the white matter, poor demarcation of gray and white matter, and eventually severe brain atrophy (674). Pathology is notable for "sponginess,"

with extensive demyelination from intramyelinic vacuolation and large abnormal mitochondria. Deficiency of aspartoacylase in skin fibroblasts is diagnostic of the disease. The abnormal gene is localized to the short arm of chromosome 17 (675–677).

Another cause of macrocephaly, Alexander disease, is believed to be a disorder primarily of the astrocytes, although marked cerebral demyelination with frontal predominance is characteristic of both the infantile and juvenile forms (678). Despite the severe demyelination, optic atrophy is not characteristic of this disease, the optic radiations are classically spared, and VEPs are usually normal (679). Nevertheless, patients with an adult-onset form of the disease have been reported with optic disc pallor and homonymous hemianopia (680). The majority of childhood cases of Alexander disease harbor mutations in the gene for glial fibrillary acidic protein (GFAP) (681).

Cockayne syndrome is an autosomal-recessive multisystem disease with both developmental anomalies and progressive degenerative changes (682). It is characterized clinically by severe dwarfism, failure to thrive, facial dysmorphisms (including enophthalmos), skin changes, and neurologic deterioration, with mental retardation and spasticity. Vision is usually impaired as a result of corneal opacities, cataracts, retinal degeneration, and optic atrophy (683,684). The disease is probably genetically heterogeneous and in some cases is related to dysfunctional RNA and DNA repair mechanisms, with mutations in several developmental genes (685–688). Cerebro-oculo-facio-skeletal syndrome (COFS) is a progressive disorder similar to Cockayne syndrome resulting in optic atrophy, brain atrophy, calcification, cataracts, microcornea, joint contractures, and growth retardation (688,689). COFS also results from mutations in several of the same DNA-repair genes mutated in Cockayne syndrome (688,690).

The Smith-Lemli-Opitz syndrome (691) is an autosomal-recessive disorder characterized by microcephaly, ambiguous male genitalia, anteverted nostrils, broad maxillary ridges, syndactyly of the second and third toes, failure to thrive, and death occurring in early childhood. It is a disorder of cholesterol biosynthesis caused by multiple different mutations in the DHCR7 gene on chromosome 11q13 (692,693). Ophthalmologic manifestations include blepharoptosis, strabismus, cataracts, optic atrophy, and optic nerve hypoplasia (694,695). Atchaneeyasakul et al. (695) reported the ocular histopathology in a case of the Smith-Lemli-Opitz syndrome. These investigators found, in addition to congenital bilateral cataracts, extensive loss of peripheral retinal axons with bilateral optic atrophy.

Allgrove or "4 A" syndrome is a rare autosomal recessive condition with alacrima, achalasia, autonomic disturbance, and ACTH insensitivity (696,697). The syndrome usually presents during the first decade of life with dysphagia or severe hypoglycemic or hypotensive attacks, related to adrenal insufficiency. There are often accompanying signs of multisystem neurologic disease, including pupil and cranial nerve abnormalities, frequent optic atrophy, autonomic neuropathy, upper and lower motor neuron signs, ataxia, and intellectual impairment. The disorder is caused by mutations in the AAAS gene on chromosome 12q13 (696,697).

Congential disorders of glycosylation (CDG) are autosomal-recessive multisystem disorders in which several different underlying enzymatic deficiencies have been identified (698). A 17-month-old girl with CDG-x (unknown enzymatic defect) had typical psychomotor retardation and truncal hypotonia, with additional dystonic hand movements and optic atrophy with nystagmus and strabismus (698).

The combination of growth retardation, alopecia, pseudoanodontia, and optic atrophy (GAPO syndrome) is likely inherited in an autosomal-recessive fashion (699–701). It may be the result of either ectodermal dysplasia or accumulation of extracellular connective tissue matrix (702). Despite the acronym, optic atrophy is not a constant finding in GAPO syndrome (701). The oculocerebrocutaneous syndrome (Delleman syndrome) is a rare and sporadic disorder characterized by congenital abnormalities of the eye, skin, and central nervous system, rarely with optic atrophy (703).

Heide (704), and later Al Gazali et al. (705), reported sibships with osteogenesis imperfecta, infantile blindness, optic atrophy, retinal abnormalities, severe developmental delay, growth retardation, paraplegia, abnormal electroencephalograms, and generalized atrophy on brain CT. This syndrome has overlapping features with the osteoporosis–pseudoglioma syndrome. Chitayat et al. (706) reported the association of skeletal dysplasia (dysosteosclerosis), intracerebral calcifications, hearing impairment, mental retardation, and optic atrophy. The optic atrophy appeared to be primary and not from compression of the optic nerves within the optic canals. Ohtagaki et al. (707) described a 15-year-old boy with epilepsy, optic atrophy, intracranial calcifications, and metaphyseal dysplasia.

Dumic et al. (708) reported two brothers with mental deficiency, short stature, microcephaly, alopecia, follicular ichthyosis, multiple skeletal anomalies, and recurrent respiratory infections, one of whom had optic atrophy. Al-Gazali (709) described an inbred Arab family with two children affected with mental retardation, iris coloboma, optic atrophy, nystagmus, and a distinctive narrow facial appearance, consistent with a previously undescribed autosomal-recessive syndrome.

Two male cousins with consanguineous parents were born with short stature, microcephaly, hypertelorism, ptosis, absent ear lobes, high-arched palates, abnormal EEG, severe mental retardation, and optic atrophy (710). This may represent an as yet undefined syndrome. Megarbane et al. (711) reported a large inbred Lebanese pedigree with autosomal-recessive congenital spastic ataxia, microcephaly, optic atrophy, short stature, speech defect, abnormal skin vessels, cerebellar atrophy, and severe mental retardation. None of the affected children had a metabolic abnormality or evidence of a respiratory chain complex defect. The same group described four children of both sexes from a highly inbred family with hypotonia, spastic diplegia, microcephaly, microphthalmia, congenital cataract, optic atrophy, ptosis, kyphoscoliosis, short stature, severe mental retardation, and cerebral malformations (712). A similar pedigree was previously reported by Warburg et al. (713) and termed the "micro syndrome."

Optic atrophy may also be a manifestation of quantitative chromosomal abnormalities. Bitoun et al. (714) described a 12-year-old girl with microcephaly, mild mental retardation, facial dysmorphism, and optic atrophy with 20/100 vision. Karyotyping revealed variegated mosaicism indicative of chromosomal instability. Two female siblings of a consanguineous Iranian family were found to have spastic paraplegia, optic atrophy with poor vision, microcephaly, and normal cognitive development (715). Karyotype analysis showed a normal female constitution in one and a male constitution (46,XY) in the other, leading the authors to conclude that the syndrome probably represents a new autosomal recessive trait of pleiotropic effects, including XY sex reversal.

Children with cerebral palsy have a higher prevalence of ocular defects than normal children. Black (716) found optic atrophy in 10.3% of 117 children with cerebral palsy. The etiology for the atrophy in these patients was not explained, nor were the clinical characteristics of the patients elaborated.

MITOCHONDRIAL DISORDERS

The prototype for a mitochondrial abnormality resulting in optic nerve dysfunction is, of course, LHON, with its classically isolated optic nerve involvement and its causal relationship to mtDNA point mutations (see above). Additionally, Kjer's DOA likely results from perturbations of mitochondrial function secondary to abnormalities in a nuclear gene whose product is destined for the mitochondria. Other multisystem hereditary disorders with prominent optic nerve involvement, such as Wolfram's syndrome, may also prove to have a final common pathway in mitochondrial dysfunction. Indeed, this apparent selective vulnerability of the ganglion cell or its axon to both hereditary and acquired mitochondrial abnormalities suggests a possible common pathophysiology for these disorders (90a,717). Given this relative selective involvement of the optic nerve in these disorders, however, it is somewhat surprising that other mitochondrial disorders do not regularly manifest optic neuropathies. Other presumed mitochondrial disorders of both nuclear and mitochondrial genomic origins may manifest optic atrophy, but often only as a secondary clinical feature that is variably present (82,83,230).

The subacute necrotizing encephalomyelopathy of Leigh (718) is a degenerative syndrome that may result from multiple different biochemical defects that all impair cerebral oxidative metabolism (232,719–727). The disorder may be inherited in an autosomal-recessive, X-linked, or maternal pattern, depending on the genetic defect. The onset of symptoms is typically between the ages of 2 months and 6 years; symptoms consist of progressive deterioration of brain stem functions, ataxia, seizures, peripheral neuropathy, intellectual deterioration, impaired hearing, and poor vision. Visual loss may be secondary to optic atrophy or retinal degeneration. In infants, the onset of the syndrome is insidious, with initial symptoms including failure to thrive, generalized weakness, and hypotonia. Three patients with a familial, adult form of Leigh's disease reported by Kalimo et al. (728) presented with bilateral visual loss, dyschromatopsia, central scotomas, and optic atrophy before developing other neurologic symptoms and signs. These patients were initially thought to represent examples of Leber's optic neuropathy (729).

Typical pathologic alterations in Leigh's syndrome consist of spongy necrotizing degeneration of the neuropil, capillary and glial proliferation, and loss of myelin with relative sparing of neurons. The most commonly affected areas are the tegmentum of the brain stem, the optic nerves, basal ganglia, substantia nigra, tectum of the midbrain, cerebellar cortex, dentate nucleus, and inferior olives (728,730,731). A predisposition for the periaqueductal and periventricular regions of the midbrain, pons, and medulla mimics the findings in Wernicke's encephalopathy, but Wernicke's affects the lower brain stem less frequently, and Leigh's syndrome tends to spare the hypothalamus and mammillary bodies. MR imaging demonstrates the distinctive pathologic localization, and MR proton spectroscopy may reveal pathologic lactate production (732).

In reviews of the pathologic ocular findings in patients with Leigh's syndrome, many of the cases have optic nerves with extensive atrophy with varying degrees of demyelination (504,733–736). Ultrastructural changes include distended mitochondria in all ocular tissues, particularly in the retinal pigment epithelium, nonpigmented ciliary epithelium, and corneal endothelium (735).

Enzyme defects associated with Leigh's syndrome include abnormalities of cytochrome c oxidase, the pyruvate dehydrogenase complex, biotinidase, and the NADH dehydrogenase complex (723,727). The syndrome of Leigh is likely a nonspecific phenotypic response to certain abnormalities of mitochondrial energy production. Most genetic defects that result in Leigh's syndrome probably occur in nuclear genes encoding proteins essential to mitochondrial oxidative phosphorylation, especially those genes involved in cytochrome c oxidase assembly (727). Approximately one third of Leigh's syndrome cases have been associated with a point mutation in the mtDNA at position 8993 (either T to G or T to C) within the gene for ATPase 6 (570,722,723, 737,738). This same genetic defect can cause the Leigh's phenotype, a syndrome of neuropathy, ataxia, and retinitis pigmentosa (NARP), or mild pigmentary degeneration of the retina and migraines (739,740). Visual loss may be caused by retinal or optic nerve degeneration. Another mtDNA point mutation that may be a relatively common cause of Leigh's syndrome occurs at position 13513 in the ND5 gene (251a,741). Interestingly, this same mutation has presented with phenotypes classic for mitochondrial encephalopathy with lactic acidosis and stroke-like episodes (MELAS) and even LHON (73). Another ND5 mutation at position 13084 is associated with a Leigh-MELAS overlap syndrome, with one family member exhibiting optic atrophy (741a). The Leigh's phenotype also occurs rarely in patients with mtDNA mutations that usually manifest with other phenotypes (723,726,742): at position 8344 (a mutation usually associated with the phenotype of myoclonic epilepsy with

ragged red fibers [MERRF]); at position 3243 (a mutation classically associated with MELAS); at position 14459 (a mutation usually associated with LHON or LHON plus dystonia); and with mtDNA deletions (typically a cause of chronic progressive ophthalmoplegia [CPEO] and pigmentary retinopathy).

Other presumed mitochondrial disorders of nuclear and mitochondrial genomic origins may manifest optic atrophy as a variable manifestation of their phenotype (82,83,230). Examples include cases of MERRF, MELAS, and chronic progressive external ophthalmoplegia, both with and without the full Kearns-Sayre phenotype (73,251,743–752).

Taylor et al. (753) described a 42-year-old man with progressive epilepsy, stroke-like episodes, cognitive decline, and bilateral optic atrophy, in whom a muscle biopsy revealed a defect in complex I activity and a novel heteroplasmic mtDNA ND3 gene mutation at position 10191. A point mutation in the mtDNA cytochrome b gene at position 14849 was presumed responsible for septo-optic dysplasia (with small, pale optic discs), retinitis pigmentosa, exercise intolerance, hypertrophic cardiomyopathy, and rhabdomyolysis in one male patient (754). Two brothers experienced profound irreversible visual loss over 2 months, associated with a metabolic disorder characterized by transient episodes of ataxia and paresis with slight elevation of blood and cerebrospinal fluid lactate; a defect in complex I activity was demonstrated (755). Taylor et al. (756) reported two sisters who presented with a late-onset neurodegenerative disease characterized by optic atrophy, encephalopathy, and ataxia. The optic neuropathy was notable for relatively well-preserved visual acuity (20/20–20/60), significant peripheral visual field constriction, and optic atrophy with cupping. Mitochondrial analysis revealed a partial deficiency of complex II, a complex entirely encoded by the nuclear genome. The other, more constant, phenotypic characteristics of all of these mitochondrial disorders distinguish them from diseases such as Leber's optic neuropathy, in which visual loss from optic nerve dysfunction is the primary, and most often only, manifestation of the disorder.

REFERENCES

1. Johns DR, Newman NJ. Hereditary optic neuropathies. Semin Ophthalmol 1995; 10:203–213.
2. Biousse V, Newman NJ. Hereditary optic neuropathies. Ophthalmol Clin North Am 2001;14:547–568.
3. Krill AE, Deutman AF. Dominant macular degenerations: The cone degenerations. Am J Ophthalmol 1972;73:352–369.
4. Krill AE, Deutman AF, Fishman M. The cone degenerations. Doc Ophthalmol 1973;35:1–80.
5. Zervas JP, Smith JL. Neuro-ophthalmic presentation of cone dysfunction syndromes in the adult. J Clin Neuroophthalmol 1987;7:202–218.
6. Newman NJ. Optic disc pallor: A false localizing sign. Surv Ophthalmol 1993; 37:273–282.
7. Heckenlively JR, Martin DA, Rosales TO. Telangiectasia and optic atrophy in cone-rod degenerations. Arch Ophthalmol 1981;99:1983–1991.
8. Weleber RG, Miyake Y. Familial optic atrophy with negative electroretinograms. Arch Ophthalmol 1992;110:640–645.
9. Leber T. Über hereditare und congenitalangelegte sehnervenleiden. Albrecht von Graefes Archiv fuer Ophthalmol 1871;17:249–291.
10. von Graefe A. Ein ungewohnlicher fall von hereditare amaurose. Archiv Fuer Ophthalmol 1858;4:266–268.
11. Gowers WR. A lecture on abiotrophy. Lancet 1902;1:1003–1021.
12. Collins ET. Hereditary ocular degenerations. Int Cong Ophthalmol Washington 1922;103–138.
13. Lundsgaard R. Leber's disease: A genealogic, genetic and clinical study of 101

cases of retrobulbar optic neuritis in 20 Danish families. Acta Ophthalmol 1944; 21(Suppl):300–306.

14. Asseman R. La maladie de Leber. Etude clinique et génétique á propos de 86 cas examinés. Thèse, Universitaire de Lille, 1958.

15. Van Senus AHC. Leber's disease in the Netherlands. Doc Ophthalmol 1963; 17:1–163.

16. Imachi J. Neuro-surgical treatment of Leber's optic atrophy and its pathogenetic relationship to arachnoiditis. In Brunette JR, Barbeau A, eds. Progress in Ophthalmology (Proceedings of the Second International Congress of Neuro-Genetics and Neuro-Ophthalmology). Vol 2. Amsterdam, Excerpta Medica, 1967: 121.

17. Seedorff T. Leber's disease. Acta Ophthalmol 1968;46:4–25.

18. Yamanaka H. The mode of inheritance of Leber's disease. Nippon Ganka Gakkai Zasshi 1971;75:1930–1936.

19. De Weerdt CJ, Went LN. Neurological studies in families with Leber's optic atrophy. Acta Neurol Scand 1971;47:541–554.

20. Carroll WM, Mastaglia FL. Leber's optic neuropathy. A clinical and visual evoked potential study of affected and asymptomatic members of a six-generation family. Brain 1979;102:559–580.

21. Livingstone IR, Mastaglia FL, Howe JW, et al. Leber's optic neuropathy: Clinical and visual evoked response studies in asymptomatic and symptomatic members of a 4-generation family. Br J Ophthalmol 1980;64:751–757.

22. Seedorff T. The inheritance of Leber's disease. A genealogical follow-up study. Acta Ophthalmol 1985;63:135–145.

23. Nikoskelainen EK, Savontaus ML, Wanne OP, et al. Leber's hereditary optic neuroretinopathy, a maternally inherited disease. A genealogic study in four pedigrees. Arch Ophthalmol 1987;105:665–671.

24. Newman NJ, Lott MT, Wallace DC. The clinical characteristics of pedigrees of Leber's hereditary optic neuropathy with the 11778 mutation. Am J Ophthalmol 1991;111:750–762.

25. Mackey D, Buttery RG. Leber hereditary optic neuropathy in Australia. Aust N Z J Ophthalmol 1992;20:177–184.

26. Riordan-Eva P, Sanders MD, Govan GG, et al. The clinical features of Leber's hereditary optic neuropathy defined by the presence of a pathogenic mitochondrial DNA mutation. Brain 1995;118:319–337.

27. Hotta Y, Fujiki K, Hayakawa M, et al. Clinical features of Japanese Leber's hereditary optic neuropathy with 11778 mutation of mitochondrial DNA. Jpn J Ophthalmol 1995;39:96–108.

28. Nikoskelainen EK, Huoponen K, Juvonen V, et al. Ophthalmologic findings in Leber hereditary optic neuropathy, with special reference to mtDNA mutations. Ophthalmology 1996;103:504–514.

29. Yamada K, Oguchi Y, Hotta Y, et al. Multicenter study on the frequency of three primary mutations of mitochondrial DNA in Japanese pedigrees with Leber's hereditary optic neuropathy: comparison with American and British counterparts. Neuroophthalmology 1999;22:187–193.

30. Sadun AA, Carelli V, Salomao SR, et al. A very large Brazilian pedigree with 11778 Leber's hereditary optic neuropathy. Trans Am Ophthalmol Soc 2002; 100:169–180.

30a. Sadun AA, Carelli V, Salomao SR, et al. Extensive investigation of a large Brazilian pedigree with 11778/haplogroup J Leber hereditary optic neuropathy. Am J Ophthalmol 2003;136:231–238.

31. Yen M-Y, Wang A-G, Chang W-L, et al. Leber's hereditary optic neuropathy—the spectrum of mitochondrial DNA mutations in Chinese patients. Jpn J Ophthalmol 2002;46:45–51.

32. Wallace DC, Singh G, Lott MT, et al. Mitochondrial DNA mutation associated with Leber's hereditary optic neuropathy. Science 1988;242:1427–1430.

33. Harding AE. The mitochondrial genome: Breaking the magic circle. N Engl J Med 1989;320:1341–1343.

34. Singh G, Lott MT, Wallace DC. A mitochondrial DNA mutation as a cause of Leber's hereditary optic neuropathy. N Engl J Med 1989;320:1300–1305.

35. Vilkki J, Savontaus ML, Nikoskelainen EK. Genetic heterogeneity in Leber hereditary optic neuroretinopathy revealed by mitochondrial DNA polymorphism. Am J Hum Genet 1989;45:206–211.

36. Yoneda M, Tsuji S, Yamauchi T, et al. Mitochondrial DNA mutation in a family with Leber's hereditary optic neuropathy. Lancet 1989;1:1076–1077.

37. Johns DR. Improved molecular-genetic diagnosis of Leber's hereditary optic neuropathy. N Engl J Med 1990;323:1488–1489.

38. Johns DR. The molecular genetics of Leber's hereditary optic neuropathy. Arch Ophthalmol 1990;108:1405–1407.

39. Bolhuis PA, Bleeker-Wagemakers EM, Ponne NJ, et al. Rapid shift in genotype of human mitochondrial DNA in a family with Leber's hereditary optic neuropathy. Biochem Biophys Res Commun 1990;170:994–997.

40. Morris, MA. Mitochondrial mutations in neuro-ophthalmological diseases. A review. J Clin Neuroophthalmol 1990;10:159–166.

41. Newman NJ, Wallace DC. Mitochondria and Leber's hereditary optic neuropathy. Am J Ophthalmol 1990;109:726–730.

42. Stone EM, Coppinger JM, Kardon RH, et al. Mae III positively detects the mitochondrial mutation associated with type I Leber's hereditary optic neuropathy. Arch Ophthalmol 1990;108:1417–1420.

43. Howell N, Bindoff LA, McCullough DA, et al. Leber hereditary optic neuropathy: Identification of the same mitochondrial ND1 mutation in six pedigrees. Am J Hum Genet 1991;49:939–950.

44. Howell N, Kubacka I, Xu M, et al. Leber hereditary optic neuropathy: Involvement of the mitochondrial ND1 gene and evidence for an intragenic suppressor mutation. Am J Hum Genet 1991;48:935–942.

45. Huoponen K, Vilkki J, Aula P, et al. A new mtDNA mutation associated with Leber hereditary optic neuroretinopathy. Am J Hum Genet 1991;48:1147–1153.

46. Johns DR, Berman J. Alternative, simultaneous complex I mitochondrial DNA mutations in Leber's hereditary optic neuropathy. Biochem Biophys Res Commun 1991;174:1324–1330.

47. Johns DR, Neufeld MJ. Cytochrome b mutations in Leber hereditary optic neuropathy. Biochem Biophys Res Commun 1991;181:1358–1364.

48. Brown MD, Voljavec AS, Lott MT, et al. Leber's hereditary optic neuropathy: a model for mitochondrial neurodegenerative diseases. FASEB J 1992;6: 2791–2799.

49. Brown MD, Voljavec AS, Lott MT, et al. Mitochondrial DNA complex I and III mutations associated with Leber's hereditary optic neuropathy. Genet 1992; 130:163–173.

50. Johns DR. Mitochondrial ND-1 mutation in Leber hereditary optic neuropathy. Am J Hum Genet 1992;50:872–874.

51. Labalette P, Hache JC, Hemery B, et al. Diagnosis of Leber's hereditary optic neuropathy without neurological abnormalities. Lancet 1992;340:368.

52. Poulton J, Deadman ME, Bronte-Stewart J, et al. Analysis of mitochondrial DNA in Leber's hereditary optic neuropathy. J Med Genet 1991;28:765–770.

53. Johns DR, Neufeld MJ, Park RD. An ND-6 mitochondrial DNA mutation associated with Leber hereditary optic neuropathy. Biochem Biophys Res Commun 1992;187:1551–1557.

54. Johns DR, Smith KH, Miller NR. Leber's hereditary optic neuropathy: Clinical manifestations of the 3460 mutation. Arch Ophthalmol 1992;110:1577–1581.

55. Mackey D, Howell N. A variant of Leber hereditary optic neuropathy characterized by recovery of vision and by an unusual mitochondrial genetic etiology. Am J Hum Genet 1992;51:1218–1228.

56. Newman NJ. Leber's hereditary optic neuropathy: New genetic considerations. Arch Neurol 1993;50:540–548.

57. Howell N, Kubacka I, Halvorson S, et al. Leber's hereditary optic neuropathy: the etiologic role of a mutation in the mitochondrial cytochrome b gene [letter]. Genetics 1993;133:133–136.

58. Howell N, Halvorson S, Burns J, et al. When does bilateral optic atrophy become Leber hereditary optic neuropathy? [letter] Am J Hum Genet 1993;53:959–963.

59. Johns DR, Neufeld MJ. Cytochrome c oxidase mutations in Leber hereditary optic neuropathy. Biochem Biophys Res Commun 1993;196:810–815.

60. Johns DR, Heher KL, Miller NR, et al. Leber's hereditary optic neuropathy: Clinical manifestations of the 14484 mutation. Arch Ophthalmol 1993;111: 495–498.

61. Johns DR, Smith KH, Savino PJ, et al. Leber's hereditary optic neuropathy: Clinical manifestations of the 15257 mutation. Ophthalmology 1993;100: 981–986.

62. Lamminen T, Majander A, Juvonen V, et al. A mitochondrial mutation at nt9101 in the ATP synthase 6 gene associated with deficient oxidative phosphorylation in a family with Leber hereditary optic neuroretinopathy. Am J Hum Genet 1995;56:1238–1240.

63. Howell N, Kubacka I, Halvorson S, et al. Phylogenetic analysis of the mitochondrial genomes from Leber's hereditary optic neuropathy pedigrees. Genetics 1995;140:285–302.

64. Brown MD, Torroni A, Reckord CL, et al. Phylogenetic analysis of caucasian 11778-positive and 11778-negative Leber's hereditary optic neuropathy patients indicates multiple independent occurrences of the common primary mitochondrial DNA mutations. Hum Mutat 1995;6:311–325.

65. Riordan-Eva P, Harding AE. Leber's hereditary optic neuropathy: The clinical relevance of different mitochondrial DNA mutations. J Med Genet 1995;32: 81–87.

66. Leo-Kottler B, Christ-Adler M, Baumann B, et al. Leber's hereditary optic neuropathy: Clinical and molecular genetic results obtained in a family with a new point mutation at nucleotide position 14498 in the ND6 gene. German J Ophthalmol 1996;5:233–240.

67. Mackey DA, Oostra R-J, Rosenberg T, et al. Primary pathogenic mtDNA mutations in multigeneration pedigrees with Leber hereditary optic neuropathy [letter]. Am J Hum Genet 1996;59:481–485.

68. Kerrison JB, Newman NJ. Clinical spectrum of Leber's hereditary optic neuropathy. Clin Neurosci 1997;4:295–301.

69. Wissinger B, Besch D, Baumann B, et al. Mutation analysis of the ND6 gene in patients with Lebers hereditary optic neuropathy. Biochem Biophys Res Comm 1997;234:511–515.

70. Howell N, Bogolin C, Jamieson R, et al. mtDNA mutations that cause optic neuropathy: how do we know? Am J Hum Genet 1998;62:196–202.

71. Macmillan C, Kirkman T, Fu K, et al. Pedigree analysis of French Canadian families with T14484C Leber's hereditary optic neuropathy. Neurology 1998; 50:417–422.

72. Mashima Y, Yamada K, Wakakura M, et al. Spectrum of pathogenic mitochondrial DNA mutations and clinical features in Japanese families with Leber's hereditary optic neuropathy. Curr Eye Res 1998;17:403–408.

73. Pulkes T, Eunson L, Patterson V, et al. The mitochondrial DNA G13513A transition in ND5 is associated with a LHON/MELAS overlap syndrome and may be a frequent cause of MELAS. Ann Neurol 1999;46:916–919.

74. Besch D, Leo-Kottler B, Zrenner E, et al. Leber's hereditary optic neuropathy: Clinical and molecular genetic findings in a patient with a new mutation in the ND6 gene. Graefes Arch Clin Exp Ophthalmol 1999;237:745–752.

75. Thieme H, Wissinger B, Jandeck C, et al. A pedigree of Leber's hereditary optic neuropathy with visual loss in childhood primarily in girls. Graefes Arch Clin Exp Ophthalmol 1999;237:714–719.

76. Batandier C, Picard A, Tessier N, et al. Identification of a novel T398A mutation in the ND5 subunit of the mitochondrial complex I and of three novel mtDNA polymorphisms in two patients presenting ocular symptoms. Hum Mutat 2000; 16:532.

77. Garcia-Lazano JR, Aguilera I, Bautista J, et al. A new mitochondrial DNA mutation in the tRNA leucine 1 gene (C3275A) in a patient with Leber's hereditary optic neuropathy. Hum Mutat 2000;15:120–212.

78. Isashiki Y, Ohba N, Izumo S, et al. Optic neuropathy and cerebellar ataxia associated with a rare missense variation (A14510G) of mitochondrial DNA. Br J Ophthalmol 2001;85:1009–1010.

79. Brown MD, Zhadanov S, Allen JC, et al. Novel mtDNA mutations and oxidative phosphorylation dysfunction in Russian LHON families. Hum Genet 2001;109: 33–39.

80. Chinnery PF, Brown DT, Andrews RM, et al. The mitochondrial ND6 gene is a hot spot for mutations that cause Leber's hereditary optic neuropathy. Brain 2001;124:209–218.

81. Huoponen, K. Leber hereditary optic neuropathy: Clinical and molecular genetic findings. Neurogenetics 2001;3:119–125.

82. Biousse V, Newman NJ. Neuro-ophthalmology of mitochondrial disorders. Sem Neurol 2001;21:275–291.

83. Biousse V, Newman NJ. Neuro-ophthalmology of mitochondrial disorders. Curr Opin Neurol 2003;16:35–43.

84. Man PYW, Turnbull DM, Chinnery PF. Leber hereditary optic neuropathy. J Med Genet 2002;39:162–169.

85. Luberichs J, Leo-Kottler B, Besch D, et al. A mutational hot spot in the mitochondrial ND6 gene in patients with Leber's hereditary optic neuropathy. Graefes Arch Clin Exp Ophthalmol 2002;240:96–100.

86. Kim JY, Hwang J-M, Park SS. Mitochondrial DNA C4171A/ND1 is a novel primary causative mutation of Leber's hereditary optic neuropathy with a good prognosis. Ann Neurol 2002;51:630–634.

87. Valentino ML, Avoni P, Barboni P, et al. Mitochondrial DNA nucleotide changes C14482G and C14482A in the ND6 gene are pathogenic for Leber's hereditary optic neuropathy. Ann Neurol 2002;51:774–778.

88. Fauser S, Leo-Kottler B, Besch D. Confirmation of the 14568 mutation in the mitochondrial ND6 gene as causative in Leber's hereditary optic neuropathy. Ophthalmic Genet 2002;23:191–197.

89. Leo-Kottler B, Luberichs J, Besch D, et al. Leber's hereditary optic neuropathy: Clinical and molecular genetic results in a patient with a point mutation at np T11253C (isoleucine to threonine) in the ND4 gene and spontaneous recovery. Graefes Arch Clin Exp Ophthalmol 2002;240:758–764.

90. Horvath J, Horvath R, Karcagi V, et al. Sequence analysis of Hungarian LHON patients not carrying the common primary mutation. J Inherit Metab Dis 2002; 25:323–324.

90a. Carelli V, Ross-Cisneros FN, Sadun AA. Mitochondrial dysfunction as a cause of optic neuropathies. Prog Retin Eye Res 2004;23:53–89.

91. Chinnery PF, Johnson MA, Wardell TM, et al. The epidemiology of pathogenic mitochondrial DNA mutations. Ann Neurol 2000;48:188–193.

92. Man PYW, Griffiths PG, Brown DT. The epidemiology of Leber hereditary optic neuropathy in the north east of England. Am J Hum Genet 2003;72:333–339.

93. Mackey DA. Epidemiology of Leber's hereditary optic neuropathy in Australia. Clin Neurosci 1994;2:162–164.

94. Mackey DA. Three subgroups of patients from the United Kingdom with Leber hereditary optic neuropathy. Eye 1994;8:431–436.

95. Chan C, Mackey DA, Byrne E. Sporadic Leber hereditary optic neuropathy in Australia and New Zealand. Aust N Z J Ophthalmol 1996;24:7–14.

96. Nettleship E. On some hereditary diseases of the eye. The Bowman Lecture Trans Ophthalmol Soc UK 1909;29 (Appendix VI):LVI–CXCII.

97. Bell J. Hereditary optic atrophy (Leber's disease). In Pearson K, ed. The treasury of human inheritance. Vol 2, Part 4. London, Cambridge University Press, 1931.

98. Bird A, McEachern D. Leber's hereditary optic atrophy in a Canadian family. Can Med Assoc J 1949;61:376–383.

99. Mackey DA. Misconceptions about Leber hereditary optic neuropathy. Med J Aust 1994;160:763–766.

100. Black GCM, Craig IW, Oostra RJ, et al. Leber's hereditary optic neuropathy: Implications of the sex ratio for linkage studies in families with the 3460 ND1 mutation. Eye 1995;9:513–516.

101. Harding AE, Sweeney MG, Govan GG, et al. Pedigree analysis in Leber hereditary optic neuropathy families with a pathogenic mtDNA mutation. Am J Hum Genet 1995;57:77–86.

102. Mackey D, Howell N. Tobacco amblyopia [letter]. Am J Ophthalmol 1994;117: 817–818.

103. Larsson NG, Andersen O, Holme E, et al. Leber's hereditary optic neuropathy and complex I deficiency in muscle. Ann Neurol 1991;30:701–708.

104. Zhu DP, Economou EP, Antonarakis SE. Mitochondrial DNA mutation and heteroplasmy in type I Leber hereditary optic neuropathy. Am J Med Genet 1992;42:173–179.

105. Oostra RJ, Tijmes NT, Cobben JM, et al. On the many faces of Leber hereditary optic neuropathy. Clin Genet 1997;51:388–393.

106. Ajax ET, Kardon R. Late-onset Leber's hereditary optic neuropathy. J Neuroophthalmol 1998;18:30–31.

107. Brenner L, Bynke G, Bynke H. Leber's hereditary optic neuropathy: A report of two unusual cases. Neuroophthalmology 1999;22:239–244.

108. Mathieu J. Contribution á l'étude de la neurite optique rétrobulbaire héréditaire. Thèse de Paris 1901; No 117, pp 51.

109. Taylor J, Holmes GM. Two families, with several members in each suffering from optic atrophy. Trans Ophthalmol Soc UK 1913;33:95–115.

110. Guzman E. Über hereditaire familiare sehnervenatrophie. Wien Klin Wochenschr 1913;26:139–141.

111. Nikoskelainen E, Hoyt WF, Nummelin K. Ophthalmoscopic findings in Leber's hereditary optic neuropathy. II. The fundus findings in the affected family members. Arch Ophthalmol 1983;101:1059–1068.

112. Dandekar SS, Graham EM, Plant GT. Ladies with Leber's hereditary optic neuropathy: an atypical disease. Eur J Ophthalmol 2002;12:537–541.

113. Norris WF. Hereditary atrophy of the optic nerves. Trans Am Ophthalmol Soc 1884;3:622–678.

114. Smith JL, Hoyt WF, Susac JO. Ocular fundus in acute Leber optic neuropathy. Arch Ophthalmol 1973;90:349–354.

115. Nikoskelainen E, Sogg RL, Rosenthal AR, et al. The early phase in Leber hereditary optic atrophy. Arch Ophthalmol 1977;95:969–978.

116. Wakakura M, Yokoe J. Evidence for preserved direct pupillary light response in Leber's hereditary optic neuropathy. Br J Ophthalmol 1995;79:442–446.

117. Nakamura M, Sekiya Y, Yamamoto M. Preservation of photic blink reflex in Leber's hereditary optic neuropathy. Invest Ophthalmol Vis Sci 1996;37: 2736–2743.

118. Bremner FD, Shallo-Hoffmann J, Riordan-Eva P, et al. Comparing pupil function with visual function in patients with Leber's hereditary optic neuropathy. Invest Ophthalmol Vis Sci 1999;40:2528–2534.

119. Jacobson DM, Stone EM, Miller NR, et al. Relative afferent papillary defects in patients with Leber hereditary optic neuropathy and unilateral visual loss. Am J Ophthalmol 1998;126:291–295.

120. Ludtke H, Kriegbaum C, Leo-Kottler B, et al. Pupillary light reflexes in patients with Leber's hereditary optic neuropathy. Graefes Arch Clin Exp Ophthalmol 1999;237:207–211.

121. Traquair HM. An Introduction to Clinical Perimetry. 5th ed. St Louis, CV Mosby, 1946:183–186.

122. Raaf JE, Bair HL. Leber's disease: Report of four cases in one family. Am J Ophthalmol 1938;21:384–389.

123. Weiner NC, Newman NJ, Lessell S, et al. Atypical Leber's hereditary optic neuropathy with molecular confirmation. Arch Neurol 1993;50:470–473.

124. Lauber H. Eine Fall con familiarer retrobulbarer Neuritis. Wien Klin Wochenschr 1902;15:1264–1265.

125. Van Heuven GJ. Die Diagnose der hereditaren Leberschen Sehnerven-atrophie. Klin Monatsbl Augenheilkd 1924;73:252–253.

126. Batten RD. Two cases of hereditary optic atrophy in a family with recovery with one case. Trans Ophthalmol Soc UK 1909;29:144–150.

127. Rossazza C, Degiovanni E, Larmande AM, et al. L'oedème papillaire et la maladie de Leber. Bull Soc Ophthalmol Fr 1973;73:595–597.

128. Nikoskelainen E, Hoyt WF, Nummelin K. Ophthalmoscopic findings in Leber's hereditary optic neuropathy. I. Fundus findings in asymptomatic family members. Arch Ophthalmol 1982;100:1597–1602.

129. Nikoskelainen E, Hoyt WF, Nummelin K, et al. Fundus findings in hereditary optic neuroretinopathy: III. Fluorescein angiographic studies. Arch Ophthalmol 1984;102:981–989.

130. Lopez PF, Smith JL. Leber's optic neuropathy. New observations. J Clin Neuroophthalmol 1986;6:144–152.

131. Smith JL, Tse DT, Byrne SF, et al. Optic nerve sheath distention in Leber's optic neuropathy and the significance of the ''Wallace mutation.'' J Clin Neuroophthalmol 1990;10:231–238.

132. Trobe JD, Glaser JS, Cassady JC. Optic atrophy. Differential diagnosis by fundus observation alone. Arch Ophthalmol 1980;98:1040–1045.

133. Ortiz RG, Newman NJ, Manoukian S, et al. Optic disk cupping and electrocardiographic abnormalities in an American pedigree with Leber's hereditary optic neuropathy. Am J Ophthalmol 1992;113:561–566.

134. Mashima Y, Kimura I, Yamamoto Y, et al. Optic disc excavation in the atrophic stage of Leber's hereditary optic neuropathy: Comparison with normal-tension glaucoma. Graefes Arch Clin Exp Ophthalmol 2003;241:75–80.

135. Yen M-Y, Wei Y-H, Liu J-H. Stargardt's type maculopathy in a patient with 11778 Leber's optic neuropathy. J Neuroophthalmol 1996;16:120–123.

136. Mann ES, Handler SP, Chung SM. Leber's hereditary optic neuropathy masquerading as retinal vasculitis. Arch Ophthalmol 2000;118:1587–1589.

137. Nettleship E. A case of family optic neuritis (Leber's disease) in which perfect recovery of sight took place. Trans Ophthalmol Soc UK 1903;23:108–112.

138. Holloway TB. Leber's disease. Arch Ophthalmol 1933;9:789–800.
139. Constantine EF. Leber's disease with recovery. Arch Ophthalmol 1955;53: 608–609.
140. Brunette JR, Bernier G. Study of a family of Leber's optic atrophy with recuperation. In Brunette JR, Barbeau A, eds. Progress in Neuro-Ophthalmology. Amsterdam, Excerpta Medica, 1969:91–97.
141. Saraux H, Biais B. Les formes spontanément curables de la névrite optique de leber. Bull Soc Ophthalmol Fr 1969;69:139–143.
142. Lessell S, Gise RL, Krohel GB. Bilateral optic neuropathy with remission in young men. Variation on a theme by Leber? Arch Neurol 1983;40:2–6.
143. Holt IJ, Miller DH, Harding AE. Genetic heterogeneity and mitochondrial DNA heteroplasmy in Leber's hereditary optic neuropathy. J Med Genet 1989;26: 739–743.
144. Stone EM, Newman NJ, Miller NR, et al. Visual recovery in patients with Leber's hereditary optic neuropathy and the 11778 mutation. J Clin Neuroophthalmol 1992;12:10–14.
145. Nakamura M, Yamamoto M. Variable pattern of visual recovery of Leber's hereditary optic neuropathy. Br J Ophthalmol 2000;84:534–535.
146. Mashima Y, Sato EA, Ohde H, et al. Macular nerve fibers temporal to fovea may have a greater potential to recover function in patients with Leber's hereditary optic neuropathy. Jpn J Ophthalmol 2002;46:660–667.
147. Bruyn GW, Went LN. A sex linked heredo-degenerative neurological disorder, associated with Leber's optic atrophy: Part 1. Clinical studies. J Neurol Sci 1964;1:59–80.
148. Chuman H, Nao-I N, Chuman T, et al. Atypical Leber's hereditary optic neuropathy: A case with five different episodes of visual disturbance. Neuroophthalmology 1999;22:195–198.
149. Newman-Toker DE, Horton JC, Lessell S. Recurrent visual loss in Leber hereditary optic neuropathy. Arch Ophthalmol 2003;121:288–291.
150. Rose FC, Bowden AN, Bowden PMA. The heart in Leber's optic atrophy. Br J Ophthalmol 1970;4:388–393.
151. Nikoskelainen E, Wanne O, Dahl M. Pre-excitation syndrome and Leber's hereditary optic neuroretinopathy. Lancet 1985;1:696.
152. Bower SPC, Hawley I, Mackey DA. Cardiac arrhythmia and Leber's hereditary optic neuropathy. Lancet 1992;339:1427–1428.
153. Nikoskelainen EK, Savontaus ML, Huoponen J, et al. Pre-excitation syndrome in Leber's hereditary optic neuropathy. Lancet 1994;344:857–858.
154. Mashima Y, Kigasawa K, Hasegawa H, et al. High incidence of pre-excitation syndrome in Japanese families with Leber's hereditary optic neuropathy. Clin Genet 1996;50:535–537.
155. Finsterer J, Stollberger C, Kopsa W, et al. Wolff-Parkinson-White syndrome and isolated left ventricular abnormal trabeculation as a manifestation of Leber's hereditary optic neuropathy. Can J Cardiol 2001;17:464–466.
155a. Sorajja P, Sweeney MG, Chalmers R, et al. Cardiac abnormalities in patients with Leber's hereditary optic neuropathy. Heart 2004;89:791–792.
156. Wilson J. Leber's hereditary optic atrophy: Some clinical and etiological considerations. Brain 1963;86:347–362.
157. Ferguson FR, Critchley M. Leber's optic atrophy and its relationship to the heredo-familial ataxias. J Neurol Psychopathol 1928;9:120–132.
158. Merritt HH. Hereditary optic atrophy (Leber's disease). Arch Neurol Psychiatr 1930;24:775–781.
159. Wallace DC. A new manifestation of Leber's disease and a new explanation for the agency responsible for its unusual pattern of inheritance. Brain 1970;93: 121–132.
160. Hodess AB, Harter DH. Leber's optic atrophy associated with spondyloepiphyseal dysplasia. Neurology 1974;24:1082–1085.
161. Nikoskelainen EK, Marttila RJ, Huoponen K, et al. Leber's "plus": neurological abnormalities in patients with Leber's hereditary optic neuropathy. J Neurol Neurosurg Psychiatry 1995;59:160–164.
162. Howell N, Kubacka I, McDonough B, et al. mtDNA analysis of Leber hereditary optic neuropathy associated with spondyloepiphyseal dysplasia. Am J Med Genet 2001;100:219–222.
163. Lev D, Yanoov-Sharav M, Watemberg N, et al. White matter abnormalities in Leber's hereditary optic neuropathy due to the 3460 mitochondrial DNA mutation. Eur J Paediatr Neurol 2002;6:121–123.
164. Ford FR. Diseases of the Nervous System in Infancy, Childhood and Adolescence. 5th ed. Springfield, IL, Charles C Thomas, 1966:291–293.
165. Palan A, Stehouwer A, Went LN. Studies on Leber's optic neuropathy III. Doc Ophthalmol 1989;71:77–87.
166. Prentice A, Engel WK. Leber's hereditary optic neuropathy associated with peripheral neuropathy and corticospinal tract signs: A kindred with unusual neurological manifestations. Ann Neurol 1992;32:252.
167. Pilz D, Quarrell OWJ, Jones EW. Mitochondrial mutation commonly associated with Leber's hereditary optic neuropathy observed in a patient with Wolfram syndrome (DIDMOAD). J Med Genet 1994;31:328–330.
168. Meire FM, Van Coster R, Cochaux P, et al. Neurological disorders in members of families with Leber's hereditary optic neuropathy (LHON) caused by different mitochondrial mutations. Ophthalmic Genet 1995;16:119–126.
169. Funakawa I, Kato H, Terao A, et al. Cerebellar ataxia in patients with Leber's hereditary optic neuropathy. J Neurol 1995;242:75–77.
170. Chalmers RM, Harding AE. A case-control study of Leber's hereditary optic neuropathy. Brain 1996;119:1481–1486.
171. Murakami T, Mita S, Tokunaga M, et al. Hereditary cerebellar ataxia with Leber's hereditary optic neuropathy mitochondrial DNA 11778 mutation. J Neurol Sci 1996;42:111–113.
172. Carelli V, Valentino ML, Liguori R, et al. Leber's hereditary optic neuropathy (LHON/11778) with myoclonus: Report of two cases. J Neurol Neurosurg Psychiatry 2001;71:813–816.
173. Cupini LM, Massa R, Floris R, et al. Migraine-like disorder segregating with mtDNA 14484 Leber hereditary optic neuropathy mutation. Neurology 2003; 60:717–720.
173a. Ćeranić B, Luxon LM. Progressive auditory neuropathy in patients with Leber's hereditary optic neuropathy. J Neurol Neurosurg Psychiatry 2004;75:626–630.
174. Bereday M, Cobb S. Relation of hereditary optic atrophy (Leber) to other familial degenerative diseases of the central nervous system. Arch Ophthalmol 1952;48: 669–680.
175. Adams JH, Blackwood W, Wilson J. Further clinical pathological observations on Leber's optic atrophy. Brain 1966;89:15–26.
176. McLeod JG, Low PA, Morgan JA. Charcot-Marie-Tooth disease with Leber optic atrophy. Neurology 1978;28:179–184.
177. McCluskey DJ, O'Conner PS, Sheehy JT. Leber's optic neuropathy and Charcot-Marie-Tooth disease. Report of a case. J Clin Neuroophthalmol 1986;6:76–81.
178. Novotny EJ, Singh G, Wallace DC. Leber's disease and dystonia. A mitochondrial disease. Neurology 1986;36:1053–1060.
179. Wallace DC, Singh G, Hopkins LC. Maternally inherited diseases of man. In Quagliariello E, Slater EC, Palmier F, et al., eds. Achievements and Perspectives of Mitochondrial Research. Vol 2. Amsterdam, Elsevier Science, 1986:427–436.
180. Marsden DC, Lang AE, Quinn NP, et al. Familial dystonia and visual failure with striatal CT lucencies. J Neurol Neurosurg Psychiatry 1986;49:500–509.
181. Bruyn GW, Vielvoye GJ, Went LN. Hereditary spastic dystonia: A new mitochondrial encephalopathy? Putaminal necrosis as a diagnostic sign. J Neurol Sci 1991;103:195–202.
182. Leuzzi V, Bertini E, De Negri AM, et al. Bilateral striatal necrosis, dystonia and optic atrophy in two siblings. J Neurol Neurosurg Psychiatry 1992;55:16–19.
183. De Vries DD, Went LN, Bruyn GW, et al. Genetic and biochemical impairment of mitochondrial complex I activity in a family with Leber hereditary optic neuropathy and hereditary spastic dystonia. Am J Hum Genet 1996;58:703–711.
184. Hanemann CO, Hefter H, Schlaug G, et al. Characterization of basal ganglia dysfunction in Leber "plus" disease. J Neurol 1996;243:297–200.
185. Murata M, Nakagawa M, Takahashi S. Optic atrophy associated with mitochondrial DNA 11778 mutation and epilepsy in a 4-year-old female. Folia Ophthalmol Jpn 1996;47:835–837.
186. Simon DK, Pulst SM, Sutton JP, et al. Familial multisystem degeneration with parkinsonism associated with the 11778 mitochondrial DNA mutation. Neurology 1999;53:1787–1793.
187. Riggs JE, Ellis BD, Hogg JP, et al. Acute periaqueductal syndrome associated with the G11778A mitochondrial DNA mutation. Neurology 2001;56:570–571.
188. Sadler M, Wiles CM, Stoodley N, et al. Ondine's curse in a woman with Leber's hereditary optic neuropathy. J Neurol Neurosurg Psychiatry 2002;73:347–348.
189. Funalot B, Reynier P, Vighetto A, et al. Leigh-like encephalopathy complicating Leber's hereditary optic neuropathy. Ann Neurol 2002;52:374–377.
190. Howell N, Miller NR, Mackey DA, et al. Lightning strikes twice: Leber hereditary optic neuropathy families with two pathogenic mtDNA mutations. J Neuroophthalmol 2002;22:262–269.
191. Lees F, MacDonald AME, Aldren Turner JW. Leber's disease with symptoms resembling disseminated sclerosis. J Neurol Neurosurg Psychiatr 1964;27: 415–421.
192. Flanigan KM, Johns DR. Association of the 11778 mitochondrial DNA mutation and demyelinating disease. Neurology 1993;43:2720–2722.
193. Paulus W, Straube A, Bauer W, et al. Central nervous system involvement in Leber's optic neuropathy. J Neurol 1993;240:251–253.
194. Kellar-Wood H, Robertson N, Govan GG, et al. Leber's hereditary optic neuropathy mitochondrial DNA mutations in multiple sclerosis. Ann Neurol 1994;36: 109–112.
195. Olsen NK, Hansen AW, Norby S, et al. Leber's hereditary optic neuropathy associated with a disorder indistinguishable from multiple sclerosis in a male harbouring the mitochondrial DNA 11778 mutation. Acta Neurol Scand 1995; 91:326–329.
196. Bhatti MT, Newman NJ. A multiple sclerosis-like illness in a man harboring the mtDNA 14484 mutation. J Neuroophthalmol 1999;19:28–33.
197. Harding AE, Sweeney MG, Miller DH, et al. Occurrence of a multiple sclerosis-like illness in women who have a Leber's hereditary optic neuropathy mitochondrial DNA mutation. Brain 1992;115:979–989.
198. Leuzzi V, Carducci C, Lanza M, et al. LHON mutations in Italian patients affected by multiple sclerosis. Acta Neurol Scand 1997;96:145–148.
199. Wakakura M, Mogi A, Ichibe Y, et al. Leber's hereditary optic neuropathy triggered by optic neuritis. Neuroophthalmology 1996;16:337–341.
200. Dorfman LF, Nikoskelainen E, Rosenthal AR, et al. Visual evoked potentials in Leber's hereditary optic neuropathy. Ann Neurol 1977;1:565–568.
201. Mondelli M, Rossi A, Scarpini C, et al. Leber's optic atrophy: VEP and BAEP changes in 16 asymptomatic subjects. Acta Neurol Scand 1991;84:366.

202. Mondelli M, Rossi A, Scarpini C, et al. BAEP changes in Leber's hereditary optic atrophy: Further confirmation of multisystem involvement. Acta Neurol Scand 1990;81:349–353.

203. Berninger TA, von Meyer L, Siess E, et al. Leber's hereditary optic atrophy: Further evidence for a defect of cyanide metabolism? Br J Ophthalmol 1989; 73:314–316.

204. Kermode AG, Moseley IF, Kendall BE, et al. Magnetic resonance imaging in Leber's optic neuropathy. J Neurol Neurosurg Psychiatry 1989;52:671–674.

205. Dotti MT, Caputo N, Signorini E, et al. Magnetic resonance imaging findings in Leber's hereditary optic neuropathy. Eur Neurol 1992;32:17–19.

206. Wilson DR, Kline LB. Leber's hereditary optic neuropathy with bilateral distended optic nerve sheaths. J Clin Neuroophthalmol 1992;12:73–74.

207. Mashima Y, Oshitari K, Imamura Y, et al. Orbital high-resolution magnetic resonance imaging with fast spin echo in the acute stage of Leber's hereditary optic neuropathy. J Neurol Neurosurg Psychiatry 1998;64:124–127.

208. Inglese M, Rovaris M, Bianchi S, et al. Magnetic resonance imaging, magnetization transfer imaging, and diffusion weighted imaging correlates of optic nerve, brain, and cervical cord damage in Leber's hereditary optic neuropathy. J Neurol Neurosurg Psychiatry 2001;70:444–449.

209. Batioglu F, Atilla H, Eryilmaz T. Chiasmal high signal on magnetic resonance imaging in the atrophic phase of Leber hereditary optic neuropathy. J Neuroophthalmol 2003;23:28–30.

210. Vaphiades MS, Newman NJ. Optic nerve enhancement on orbital magnetic resonance imaging in Leber's hereditary optic neuropathy. J Neuroophthalmol 1999; 19:238–239.

211. Vaphiades MS, Phillips PH, Turbin RE. Optic nerve and chiasmal enhancement in Leber hereditary optic neuropathy. J Neuroophthalmol 2003;23:104–105.

212. Phillips PH, Vaphiades M, Glasier CM, et al. Chiasmal enlargement and optic nerve enhancement on magnetic resonance imaging in Leber hereditary optic neuropathy. Arch Ophthalmol 2003;121:577–579.

213. Cortelli P, Montagna P, Avoni P, et al. Leber's hereditary optic neuropathy: Genetic, biochemical, and phosphorus magnetic resonance spectroscopy study in an Italian family. Neurology 1991;41:1211–1215.

214. Barbiroli B, Montagna P, Cortelli P, et al. Defective brain and muscle energy metabolism shown by in vivo ^{31}P magnetic resonance spectroscopy in nonaffected carriers of 11778 mtDNA mutation. Neurology 1995;45:1364–1369.

215. Nikoskelainen E, Hassinen IE, Paljarvi L, et al. Leber's hereditary optic neuroretinopathy: A mitochondrial disease? Lancet 1984;2:1474.

216. Nikoskelainen E, Asola M, Kalimo H, et al. Benzodiazepine sensitivity in Leber's hereditary optic neuroretinopathy. Lancet 1992;340:1223–1224.

217. Montagna P, Plazzi G, Cortelli P, et al. Abnormal lactate after effort in healthy carriers of Leber's hereditary optic neuropathy. J Neurol Neurosurg Psychiatry 1995;58:640–641.

218. Sadun AA, Kashima Y, Wurdeman AE, et al. Morphological findings in the visual system in a case of Leber's hereditary optic neuropathy. Clin Neurosci 1994;2:165–172.

219. Kwittken J, Barest HD. The neuropathology of hereditary optic atrophy (Leber's disease). The first complete anatomic study. Am J Pathol 1958;34:185–207.

220. Oud JSF, Henneman IP, Brugge RJ, et al. La maladie de Leber: Etude anatomique de deux cas dans une fratrie. J Neurol Sci 1968;6:401–417.

221. Dao J, Wurdeman AE, Sherman J, et al. The retinal ganglion cell and its axon in Leber's hereditary optic atrophy. Invest Ophthalmol Vis Sci 1994;35:1788.

222. Saadati HG, Hsu HY, Heller KB, et al. A histopathologic and morphometric differentiation of nerves in optic nerve hypoplasia and Leber hereditary optic neuropathy. Arch Ophthalmol 1998;116:911–916.

223. Sadun AA, Win P, Ross-Cisneros F, et al. Leber's hereditary optic neuropathy differentially affects smaller axons in the optic nerve. Trans Am Ophthalmol Soc 2000;98:1–13.

224. Sadun AA, Carelli V, Bose S, et al. First application of extremely high-resolution magnetic resonance imaging to study microscopic features of normal and LHON human optic nerve. Ophthalmology 2002;109:1085–1091.

225. Kerrison JB, Howell N, Miller NR, et al. Leber hereditary optic neuropathy: Electron microscopy and molecular genetic analysis of a case. Ophthalmology 1995;102:1509–1516.

226. Wallace DC. Mitochondrial DNA mutations and neuromuscular disease. Trends Genet 1989;5:9–13.

227. DiMauro S, Schon EA. Mitochondrial respiratory-chain diseases. N Engl J Med 2003;348:2656–2668.

228. Wallace DC. Mitochondrial diseases in man and mouse. Science 1999;283: 1482–1488.

229. Fine PEM. Mitochondrial inheritance and disease. Lancet 1978;2:659–661.

230. Newman NJ. Mitochondrial disease and the eye. Ophthalmol Clin North Am 1992;5:405–424.

231. Brown MD, Wallace DC. Molecular basis of mitochondrial DNA disease. J Bioenerg Biomembr 1994;26:273–289.

232. Chinnery PF, Schon EA. Mitochondria. J Neurol Neurosurg Psychiatry 2003; 74:1188–1199.

233. Johns DR. Mitochondrial DNA and disease. N Engl J Med 1995;333:638–644.

234. Zeviani M, Tiranti V, Piantadosi C. Mitochondrial disorders. Medicine 1998; 77:59–72.

235. Leonard JV, Schapira AHV. Mitochondrial respiratory chain disorders I: Mitochondrial DNA defects. Lancet 2000;355:299–304.

236. DiMauro S. Lessons from mitochondrial DNA mutations. Cell Devel Biol 2001; 9:397–405.

237. Wallace DC. Mouse models for mitochondrial disease. Am J Med Genet 2001; 106:71–93.

238. Lott MT, Voljavec AS, Wallace DC. Variable genotype of Leber's hereditary optic neuropathy patients. Am J Ophthalmol 1990;109:625–631.

239. Mitani I, Miyazaki S, Hayashi T, et al. Detection of mitochondrial DNA nucleotide 11778 point mutation of Leber hereditary optic neuropathy from archival stained histopathological preparations. Acta Ophthalmol Scand 1998;76:14–19.

240. Nakamura M, Ara F, Yamada M, et al. High frequency of mitochondrial ND4 gene mutation in Japanese pedigrees with Leber hereditary optic neuropathy. Jpn J Ophthalmol 1992;36:56–61.

241. Howell N, McCullough D. An example of Leber hereditary optic neuropathy not involving a mutation in the mitochondrial ND4 gene. Am J Hum Genet 1990;47:629–634.

242. Brown MD, Wallace DC. Spectrum of mitochondrial DNA mutations in Leber's hereditary optic neuropathy. Clin Neurosci 1994;2:138–145.

243. Obermaier-Kusser B, Lorenz B, Schubring S, et al. Features of mtDNA mutation patterns in european pedigrees and sporadic cases with Leber hereditary optic neuropathy. Am J Hum Genet 1994;55:1063–1066.

244. Oostra RJ, Bolhuis PA, Wijburg FA, et al. Leber's hereditary optic neuropathy. Correlations between mitochondrial genotype and visual outcome. J Med Genet 1994;31:280–286.

245. Nikoskelainen E. Leber hereditary optic neuropathy. Curr Opinion Ophthalmol 1991;2:531–537.

246. Macmillan C, Johns TA, Fu K, et al. Predominance of the T14484C mutation in French-Canadian families with Leber hereditary optic neuropathy is due to a founder effect. Am J Hum Genet 2000;66:332–335.

247. Wakakura M, Hayashi E, Toyo-oka Y, et al. Bilateral optic neuropathy with mitochondrial DNA 9804 mutation detected by non-isotopic single-strand conformational polymorphism. Neuroophthalmology 1998;19:7–12.

248. Newman NJ. From genotype to phenotype in Leber hereditary optic neuropathy: Still more questions than answers. J Neuroophthalmol 2002;22:257–261.

249. Jun AS, Brown MD, Wallace DC. A mitochondrial DNA mutation at nucleotide pair 14459 of the NADH dehydrogenase subunit 6 gene associated with maternally inherited Leber hereditary optic neuropathy and dystonia. Proc Natl Acad Sci USA 1994;91:6206–6210.

250. Shoffner JM, Brown MD, Stugard C, et al. Leber's hereditary optic neuropathy plus dystonia is caused by a mitochondrial DNA point mutation. Ann Neurol 1995;38:163–169.

251. Liolitsa D, Rahman S, Benton S, et al. Is the mitochondrial complex I ND5 gene a hot-spot for MELAS causing mutations? Ann Neurol 2003;53:128–132.

251a. Kirby DM, Boneh A, Chow CW, et al. Low mutant load of mitochondrial DNA G13513A mutation can cause Leigh's disease. Ann Neurol 2003;54:473–478.

252. Schon EA, Bonilla E, DiMauro S. Mitochondrial DNA mutations and pathogenesis. J Bioenergetics Biomembranes 1997;29: 131–149.

253. Howell N. Human mitochondrial diseases: Answering questions and questioning answers. Intl Rev Cytol 1999;186:49–116.

254. Chinnery PF, Howell N, Richard M, et al. Mitochondrial DNA analysis: Polymorphisms and pathogenicity. J Med Genet 1999;36:505–510.

255. Carelli V, Rengo C, Scozzari R, et al. mtDNA haplotypes allow genealogical aggregation of apparently unrelated LHON pedigrees. Neurology 2003; 60(Suppl):A3.

256. Biousse V, Brown MD, Newman NJ, et al. De novo 14484 mitochondrial DNA mutation in monozygotic twins discordant for Leber's hereditary optic neuropathy. Neurology 1997;49:1136–1138.

257. Vilkki J, Savontaus ML, Nikoskelainen EK. Segregation of mitochondrial genomes in a heteroplasmic lineage with Leber hereditary optic neuroretinopathy. Am J Hum Genet 1990;47:95–100.

258. Cormier V, Rötig A, Geny C, et al. mtDNA heteroplasmy in Leber hereditary optic neuroretinopathy. Am J Hum Genet 1991;48:813–814.

259. Howell N, McCullough D, Bodis-Wollner I. Molecular genetic analysis of a sporadic case of Leber hereditary optic neuropathy. Am J Hum Genet 1992;50: 443–446.

260. Smith KH, Johns DR, Heher KL, et al. Heteroplasmy in Leber's hereditary optic neuropathy. Arch Ophthalmol 1993;111:1486–1490.

261. Ghosh SS, Fahy E, Bodis-Wollner I, et al. Longitudinal study of a heteroplasmic 3460 Leber hereditary optic neuropathy family by multiplexed primer-extension analysis and nucleotide sequencing. Am J Hum Genet 1996;58:325–334.

262. Black GCM, Morten K, Laborde A, et al. Leber's hereditary optic neuropathy: Heteroplasmy is likely to be significant in the expression of LHON in families with the 3460 ND1 mutation. Br J Ophthalmol 1996;80:915–917.

263. Tanaka A, Kiyosawa M, Mashima Y, et al. A family with Leber's hereditary optic neuropathy with mitochondrial DNA heteroplasmy related to disease expression. J Neuroophthalmol 1998;18:81–83.

264. Jacobi FK, Leo-Kottler B, Mittelviethaus K, et al. Segregation patterns and heteroplasmy prevalence in Leber's hereditary optic neuropathy. Invest Ophthalmol Vis Sci 2001;42:1208–1214.

265. Chinnery PF, Andrews RM, Turnbull DM, et al. Leber hereditary optic neuropa-

thy: Does heteroplasmy influence the inheritance and expression of the G11778A mitochondrial DNA mutation? Am J Med Genet 2001;98:235–243.

266. Puomila A, Viitanen T, Savontaus M-L, et al. Segregation of the ND4/11778 and the ND1/3460 mutations in four heteroplasmic LHON families. J Neurol Sci 2002;205:41–45.

267. Carelli V, Ghelli A, Ratta M, et al. Leber's hereditary optic neuropathy: Biochemical effect of 11778/ND4 and 3460/ND1 mutations and correlation with the mitochondrial genotype. Neurology 1997;48:1623–1632.

268. Howell N, Xu M, Halvorson S, et al. A heteroplasmic LHON family: Tissue distribution and transmission of the 11778 mutation. Am J Hum Genet 1994; 55:203–206.

269. Juvonen V, Nikoskelainen E, Lamminen T, et al. Tissue distribution of the ND4/ 11778 mutation in heteroplasmic lineages with Leber hereditary optic neuropathy. Hum Mutat 1997;9:412–417.

270. Lodi R, Montagna P, Cortelli P, et al. 'Secondary' 4216/ND1 and 13708/ND5 Leber's hereditary optic neuropathy mitochondrial DNA mutations do not further impair in vivo mitochondrial oxidative metabolism when associated with the 11778/ND4 mitochondrial DNA mutation. Brain 2000;123:1896–1902.

271. Brown MD, Allen JC, VanStavern GP, et al. Clinical, genetic, and biochemical characterization of a Leber hereditary optic neuropathy family containing both the 11778 and 14484 primary mutations. Am J Med Genet 2001;104:331–338.

272. Brown MD, Sun F, Wallace DC. Clustering of Caucasian Leber hereditary optic neuropathy patients containing the 11778 or 14484 mutations on an mtDNA lineage. Am J Hum Genet 1997;60:381–387.

273. Hofmann S, Bezold R, Jaksch M, et al. Wolfram (DIDMOAD) syndrome and Leber hereditary optic neuropathy (LHON) are associated with distinct mitochondrial DNA haplotypes. Genomics 1997;39:8–18.

274. Torroni A, Petrozzi M, D'Urbano L, et al. Haplotype and phylogenetic analyses suggest that one European-specific mtDNA background plays a role in the expression of Leber hereditary optic neuropathy by increasing the penetrance of the primary mutations 11778 and 14484. Am J Hum Genet 1997;60:1107–1121.

275. Brown MD, Starikovskaya E, Derbeneva O, et al. The role of mtDNA background in disease expression: A new primary LHON mutation associated with Western Eurasian haplogroup J. Hum Genet 2002;110:130–138.

276. Carelli V, Vergani L, Bernazzi B, et al. Respiratory function in cybrid cell lines carrying European mtDNA haplogroups: Implications for Leber's hereditary optic neuropathy. Biochimica Biophysica Acta 2002;1588:7–14.

277. Sudoyo H, Suryadi H, Lertrit P, et al. Asian-specific mtDNA backgrounds associated with the primary G11778A mutation of Leber's hereditary optic neuropathy. J Hum Genet 2002;47:594–604.

278. Cock HR, Tabrizi SJ, Cooper JM, et al. The influence of nuclear background on the biochemical expression of 3460 Leber's hereditary optic neuropathy. Ann Neurol 1998;44:187–193.

279. Lodi R, Carelli V, Cortelli P, et al. Phosphorus MR spectroscopy shows a tissue specific in vivo distribution of biochemical expression of the G3460A mutation in Leber's hereditary optic neuropathy. J Neurol Neurosurg Psychiatry 2002; 72:805–807.

280. Carelli V, Wang K, Valentino ML, et al. Segregation analysis of a large LHON pedigree is consistent with the existence of a nuclear modifying gene. Neurology 2003;60(Suppl):A4.

281. Sangiori S, Farne S, Valentino ML, et al. MnSOD Ala9 Val polymorphism may be relevant as nuclear modifier of LHON mitochondrial DNA pathogenic mutations. Neurology 2003;60(Suppl):A4.

282. Vilkki J, Ott J, Savontaus ML, et al. Optic atrophy in Leber hereditary optic neuroretinopathy is probably determined by an X-chromosomal gene closely linked to DXS7. Am J Hum Genet 1991;48:486–491.

283. Bu X, Rotter JI. X-linked and mitochondrial gene control of Leber hereditary optic neuropathy (LHON): evidence from segregation analysis for dependence on X-inactivation. Clin Res 1991;39:96A.

284. Sweeney MG, Davis MB, Lashwood A, et al. Evidence against an X-linked locus close to DXS7 determining visual loss susceptibility in British and Italian families with Leber hereditary optic neuropathy. Am J Hum Genet 1992;51: 741–748.

285. Carvalho MRS, Muller B, Rotzer E, et al. Leber's hereditary optic neuroretinopathy and the X-chromosomal susceptibility factor: No linkage to DXS7. Hum Hered 1992;42:316–320.

286. Chalmers RM, Davis MB, Sweeney MG, et al. Evidence against an X-linked visual loss susceptibility locus in Leber hereditary optic neuropathy. Am J Hum Genet 1996;59:103–108.

287. Oostra RJ, Kemp S, Bolhuis PA, et al. No evidence for ''skewed'' inactivation of the X-chromosome as cause of Leber's hereditary optic neuropathy in female carriers. Hum Genet 1996;97:500–505.

288. Pegoraro E, Carelli V, Zeviani M, et al. X-inactivation patterns in female Leber's hereditary optic neuropathy patients do not support a strong X-linked determinant. Am J Med Genet 1996;61:356–362.

289. Juvonen V, Vikki J, Aula P, et al. Reevaluation of the linkage of an optic atrophy susceptibility gene to X-chromosomal markes in Finnish families with Leber hereditary optic neuroretinopathy. (LHON) [letter]. Am J Hum Genet 1993;53: 289–292.

290. Handoko HY, Wirapati PJ, Sudoyo HA, et al. Meiotic breakpoint mapping of a proposed X linked visual loss susceptibility locus in Leber's hereditary optic neuropathy. J Med Genet 1998;35:668–671.

291. Man PYW, Brown DT, Wehnert MS, et al. NDUFA-1 is not a nuclear modifier gene in Leber hereditary optic neuropathy. Neurology 2002;58:1861–1862.

292. Man PY, Morris CM, Zeviani M, et al. The role of APOE in the phenotypic expression of Leber hereditary optic neuropathy. J Med Genet 2003;40:e41.

293. Trounce I, Byrne E, Marzuki S. Decline in skeletal muscle mitochondrial respiratory chain function: Possible factor in ageing. Lancet 1989;1:637–639.

294. Govan GG, Smith PR, Kellar-Wood H, et al. HLA class II genotypes in Leber's hereditary optic neuropathy. J Neuro Sci 1994;126:193–196.

295. DuBois LG, Feldon SE. Evidence for a metabolic trigger for Leber's hereditary optic neuropathy. A case report. J Clin Neuroophthalmol 1992;12:15–16.

296. Johns DR, Smith KH, Miller NR, et al. Identical twins who are discordant for Leber's hereditary optic neuropathy. Arch Ophthalmol 1993;111:1491–1494.

297. Lam BL. Identical twins no longer discordant for Leber's hereditary optic neuropathy. Arch Ophthalmol 1998;116:956–957.

298. Cullom ME, Heher KL, Miller NR, et al. Leber's hereditary optic neuropathy masquerading as tobacco-alcohol amblyopia. Arch Ophthalmol 1993;111: 1482–1485.

299. Redmill B, Mutamba A, Tandon M. Leber's hereditary optic neuropathy following trauma. Eye 2001;15:544–547.

300. Luzhansky JZ, Pierce AB, Hoy JF, et al. Leber's hereditary optic neuropathy in the setting of nucleoside analogue toxicity. AIDS 2001;15:1588–1589.

301. Shaikh S, Ta C, Basham AA, et al. Leber hereditary optic neuropathy associated with antiretroviral therapy for human immunodeficiency virus infection. Am J Ophthalmol 2001;131:143–145.

302. Warner JE, Ries KM. Optic neuropathy in a patient with AIDS. J Neuroophthalmol 2001;21:92–94.

303. DeMarinis M. Optic neuropathy after treatment with anti-tuberculous drugs in a subject with Leber's hereditary optic neuropathy mutation. J Neurol 2001;248: 818–819.

304. Warner RB, Lee AG. Leber hereditary optic neuropathy associated with use of ephedra alkaloids. Am J Ophthalmol 2002;134:918–920.

305. Newman NJ, Torroni A, Brown MD, et al. Epidemic neuropathy in Cuba not associated with mitochondrial DNA mutations found in Leber's hereditary optic neuropathy patients. Am J Ophthalmol 1994;118:158–168.

306. Isashiki Y, Tabata Y, Kamimura K, et al. Genotypes of aldehyde dehydrogenase and alcohol dehydrogenase polymorphisms in patients with Leber's hereditary optic neuropathy. Jpn J Human Genet 1997;42:187–191.

307. Tsao K, Aitken PA, Johns DR. Smoking as an aetiological factor in a pedigree with Leber's hereditary optic neuropathy. Br J Ophthalmol 1999;83:577–581.

307a. Sadun F, De Negri AM, Carelli V, et al. Ophthalmologic findings in a large pedigree of 11778/haplogroup J Leber optic neuropathy. Am J Ophthalmol 2004;137:271–277.

308. Kerrison JB, Miller NR, Hsu F-C, et al. A case-control study of tobacco and alcohol consumption in Leber hereditary optic neuropathy. Am J Ophthalmol 2000;130:803–812.

309. Dotti MT, Plewnia K, Cardaioli E, et al. A case of ethambutol-induced optic neuropathy harbouring the primary mitochondrial LHON mutation at nt 11778. J Neurol 1998;245:302–303.

310. Wilson J. Skeletal manifestations in Leber's optic atrophy: A possible disorder of cyanide metabolism. Ann Phys Med 1965;44:91–95.

311. Wilson J, Linnell JC, Matthews DM. Plasma-cobalamins in neuro-ophthalmological diseases. Lancet 1971;1:259–261.

312. Cagianut B, Schnebli HP, Rhyner K, et al. Decreased thiosulfate sulfur transferase (rhodanese) in Leber's hereditary optic atrophy. Klin Wochenschr 1984;62: 850–854.

313. Nikoskelainen E. New aspects of the genetic, etiologic, and clinical puzzle of Leber's disease. Neurology 1984;34:1482–1484.

314. Howell N. Leber hereditary optic neuropathy: Respiratory chain dysfunction and degeneration of the optic nerve. Vision Res 1998;38:1495–1504.

315. Schapira AH. Mitochondrial disorders: An overview. J Bioenergetics Biomembranes 1997;29:105–107.

316. Majander A, Huoponen K, Savontaus ML, et al. Electron transfer properties of NADH: Ubiquinone reductase in the ND1/3460 and the ND4/11778 mutations of the Leber hereditary optic neuroretinopathy (LHON). FEBS Lett 1991;292: 289–292.

317. Toscano A, Harding AE, Gellera C, et al. Complex I multiple mitochondrial DNA mutations and biochemical deficiency in Leber's hereditary optic neuropathy. Neurology 1992;42(Suppl 3):266.

318. Smith PR, Cooper JM, Govan GG, et al. Platelet mitochondrial function in Leber's hereditary optic neuropathy. J Neurol Sci 1994;122:80–83.

319. Oostra RJ, Van Galen MJM, Bolhuis PA, et al. The mitochondrial DNA mutation ND*14,484C associated with Leber hereditary optic neuropathy, leads to deficiency of complex I of the respiratory chain. Biochem Biophys Res Commun 1995;215:1001–1005.

320. Hofhaus G, Johns DR, Hurko O, et al. Respiration and growth defects in transmitochondrial cell lines carrying 11778 mutation associated with Leber's hereditary optic neuropathy. J Biol Chem 1996;271:13155–13161.

321. Ghelli A, Degli Esposti M, Carelli V, et al. Changes in mitochondrial complex

I activity and coenzyme Q binding site in Leber's hereditary optic neuropathy (LHON). Molec Aspects Med 1997;18(suppl):S263–S267.

322. Yen M-Y, Lee J-F, Liu J-H, et al. Energy charge is not decreased in lymphocytes of patients with Leber's hereditary optic neuropathy with the 11778 mutation. J Neuroophthalmol 1998;18:84–85.

323. Carelli V, Ghelli A, Bucchi L, et al. Biochemical features of mtDNA 14484 (ND6/M64V) point mutation associated with Leber's hereditary optic neuropathy. Ann Neurol 1999;45:320–328.

324. Malik S, Sudoyo H, Marzuki S. Microphotometric analysis of NADH-tetrazolium reductase deficiency in fibroblasts of patients with Leber optic neuropathy. J Inherit Metab Dis 2000;23:730–744.

325. Yen M-Y, Lee H-C, Liu J-H, Compensatory elevation of complex II activity in Leber's hereditary optic neuropathy. Br J Ophthalmol 1996;80:78–81.

326. Yen M-Y, Chen C-S, Wang A-G, et al. Increase of mitochondrial DNA in blood cells of patients with Leber's hereditary optic neuropathy with 11778 mutation. Br J Ophthalmol 2002;86:1027–1030.

327. Levin LA, Schalow K. Differential susceptibility of retinal ganglion cells to redox modulation: A possible link to mitochondrial optic neuropathy [abstract]. Invest Ophthalmol Vis Sci 1998;39:S808.

328. Klivenyi P, Karg E, Rozsa C, et al. α-Tocopherol/lipid ratio in blood is decreased in patients with Leber's hereditary optic neuropathy and asymptomatic carriers of the 11778 mtDNA mutation. J Neurol Neurosurg Psychiatry 2001;70:359–362.

329. Kirkinezos IG, Moraes CT. Reactive oxygen species and mitochondrial diseases. Semin Cell Devel Biol 2001;12:449–457.

330. Wong A, Cavelier L, Collins-Schramm HE, et al. Differentiation-specific effects of LHON mutations introduced into neuronal NT2 cells. Hum Mol Genet 2002;11:431–438.

331. Qi X, Lewin AS, Hauswirth WW, et al. Oxygen toxicity induced by complex I deficiency is rescued with AAV mediated gene transfer of human SOD2. Neurology 2003;60(Suppl 1):A26.

332. Qi X, Lewin AS, Hauswirth WW, et al. Optic neuropathy induced by reductions in mitochondrial superoxide dismutase. Invest Ophthalmol Vis Sci 2003;44:1088–1096.

333. Danielson SR, Wong A, Carelli V, et al. Cells bearing mutations causing Leber's hereditary optic neuropathy are sensitized to fas-induced apoptosis. J Biol Chem 2002;277:5810–5815.

334. Zamzami N, Hirsch T, Dallaporta B, et al. Mitochondrial implication in accidental and programmed cell death: Apoptosis and necrosis. J Bioenergetics Biomembranes 1997;29:185–193.

335. Ghelli A, Zanna C, Porcelli AM, et al. Leber's hereditary optic neuropathy (LHON) pathogenic mutations induce mitochondrial-dependent apoptotic death in transmitochondrial cells incubated with galactose medium. J Biol Chem 2003;278:4145–4150.

336. Lessell S, Horovitz B. Histochemical study of enzymes of optic nerve of monkey and rat. Am J Ophthalmol 1972;74:118–126.

337. Andrews RM, Griffiths PG, Johnson MA, et al. Histochemical localization of mitochondrial enzyme activity in human optic nerve and retina. Br J Ophthalmol 1999;83:231–235.

338. Bristow EA, Griffiths PG, Andrews RM, et al. The distribution of mitochondrial activity in relation to optic nerve structure. Arch Ophthalmol 2002;120:791–796.

339. Delettre C, Lenaers G, Pelloquin L, et al. OPA1 (Kjer type) dominant optic atrophy: a novel mitochondrial disease. Mol Genet Metab 2002;75:97–107.

340. Qi X, Lewin AS, Hauswirth WW, et al. Suppression of complex I gene expression induces optic neuropathy. Ann Neurol 2003;53:198–205.

341. Foulds WS, Cant JS, Chisholm IA, et al. Ocular manifestations of the mucopolysaccharidoses. Ophthalmologica 1974;169:345–361.

342. Imachi J, Nishizaki K. The patients of Leber's optic atrophy should be treated neuro-surgically. Nippon Ganka Kiyo Jpn 1970;21:209–217.

343. Bresolin N, Bet L, Binda A, et al. Clinical and biochemical correlations in mitochondrial myopathies treated with coenzyme Q10. Neurology 1988;38:892–399.

344. Shoffner JM, Voljavec AS, Costigan DA, et al. Chronic external ophthalmoplegia and ptosis (CEOP): Improved retinal cone function with ascorbate, phylloquinone, and coenzyme Q10. Neurology 1989;39(Suppl):404.

345. Shoffner JM, Lott MT, Voljavec AS, et al. Spontaneous Kearns-Sayre/chronic external ophthalmoplegia plus syndrome associated with a mitochondrial DNA deletion: A slip-replication model and metabolic therapy. Proc Natl Acad Sci USA 1989;86:7952–7956.

346. Bresolin N, Doriguzzi C, Ponzetto C, et al. Ubidecarenone in the treatment of mitochondrial myopathies: A multi-center double-blind trial. J Neurol Sci 1990;100:70–78.

347. Mashima Y, Hiida Y, Oguchi Y. Remission of Leber's hereditary optic neuropathy with idebenone. Lancet 1992;340:368–369.

348. Cortelli P, Montagna P, Pierangeli G, et al. Clinical and brain bioenergetics improvement with idebenone in a patient with Leber's hereditary optic neuropathy: A clinical and P-MRS study. J Neurol Sci 1997;148:25–31.

349. Carelli V, Barboni P, Zacchini A, et al. Leber's hereditary optic neuropathy (LHON) with 14484/ND6 mutation in a North African patient. J Neurol Sci 1998;160:183–188.

350. Chinnery PF, Turnbull DM. Mitochondrial DNA and disease. Lancet 1999;354(1S):17–21.

351. Mashima Y, Kigasawa K, Wakakura M, et al. Do idebenon and vitamin therapy shorten the time to achieve visual recover in Leber hereditary optic neuropathy? J Neuroophthalmol 2000;20:166–170.

352. DiMauro S, Hirano M, Schon EA. Mitochondrial encephalomyopathies: Therapeutic approaches. Neurol Sci 2000;21:S901–S908.

353. Huang C-C, Kuo H-C, Chu C-C, et al. Rapid visual recovery after coenzyme Q10 treatment of Leber hereditary optic neuropathy. J Neuroophthalmol 2002;22:66.

354. Geromel V, Darin N, Chretien D, et al. Coenzyme Q(10) and idebenone in the therapy of respiratory chain diseases: Rationale and comparative benefits. Mol Genet Metab 2002;77:21.

355. Yoles E, Wheeler LA, Schwartz M. Alpha-2-adenoreceptor agonists are neuroprotective in a rat model of optic nerve degeneration. Invest Ophthalmol Vis Sci 1999;40:65–73.

356. Guy J, Qi X, Pallotti F, et al. Rescue of a mitochondrial deficiency causing Leber hereditary optic neuropathy. Ann Neurol 2002;52:534–542.

357. Larsson NG. Leber's hereditary optic neuropathy: A nuclear solution of a mitochondrial problem. Ann Neurol 2002;52:529–530.

358. Huoponen K, Puomila A, Savontaus M-L, et al. Genetic counseling in Leber hereditary optic neuropathy (LHON). Acta Ophthalmol Scand 2002;80:38–43.

358a. Thorburn DR, Dahl H-HM. Mitochondrial Disorders: genetics, counseling, prenatal diagnosis and reproductive options. A J Med Genet (Semin Med Genet) 2001;106:102–114.

359. McKusick VA. Mendelian Inheritance in Man: A Catalog of Human Genes and Genetic Disorders. 12th ed. Baltimore, The Johns Hopkins University Press, 1998.

360. Eiberg H, Kjer B, Kjer P, et al. Dominant optic atrophy (OPA1) mapped to chromosome 3q region. I. Linkage analysis. Hum Molec Genet 1994;3:977–980.

361. Kjer B, Eiberg H, Kjer P, et al. Dominant optic atrophy mapped to chromosome 3q region. II. Clinical and epidemiological aspects. Acta Ophthal Scand 1996;74:3–7.

362. Kjer, P. Hereditary infantile optic atrophy with dominant transmission (preliminary report). Dan Med Bull 1956;3:135–141.

363. Kjer P. Infantile optic atrophy with dominant mode of inheritance. A clinical and genetic study of 19 Danish families. Acta Ophthalmol 1959;164(suppl. 54):1–147.

364. Caldwell JBH, Howard RO, Riggs LA. Dominant juvenile optic atrophy: A study of two families and review of the hereditary disease in childhood. Arch Ophthalmol 1971;85:133–147.

365. Smith DP. Diagnostic criteria in dominantly inherited juvenile optic atrophy: A report of three new families. Am J Optom Physiol Opt 1972;49:183–200.

366. Johnston PB, Gaster RN, Smith VC, et al. A clinicopathologic study of autosomal dominant optic atrophy. Am J Ophthalmol 1979;88:868–875.

367. Kline LB, Glaser JS. Dominant optic atrophy: The clinical profile. Arch Ophthalmol 1979;97:1680–1686.

368. Hoyt CS. Autosomal dominant optic atrophy: A spectrum of disability. Ophthalmology 1980;87:245–251.

369. Neetens A, Rubbens MC. Dominant juvenile optic atrophy. Ophthalm Paediatr Genet 1985;5:79–83.

370. Elliott D, Traboulsi EI, Maumenee IH. Visual prognosis in autosomal dominant optic atrophy (Kjer type). Am J Ophthalmol 1993;115:360–367.

371. Brown J Jr, Fingert J, Taylor CM, et al. Clinical and genetic analysis of a family affected with dominant optic atrophy (OPA1). Arch Ophthalmol 1997;115:95–99.

372. Johnston RL, Burdon MA, Spalton DJ, et al. Dominant optic atrophy, Kjer type. Arch Ophthalmol 1997;115:100–103.

373. Votruba M, Fitzke FW, Holder GE, et al. Clinical features in affected individuals from 21 pedigrees with dominant optic atrophy. Arch Ophthalmol 1998;116:351–358.

374. Kerrison JB, Arnould VJ, Ferraz Sallum JM, et al. Genetic heterogeneity of dominant optic atrophy, Kjer type. Arch Ophthalmol 1999;117:805–810.

375. Johnston RL, Seller MJ, Behnam JT, et al. Dominant optic atrophy. Refining the clinical diagnostic criteria in light of genetic linkage studies. Ophthalmology 1999;106:123–128.

376. Kok-van Alphen CC. Four families with the dominant infantile form of optic nerve atrophy. Acta Ophthalmol 1970;48:905–916.

377. Del Porto G, Vingolo EM, Steindl K, et al. Clinical heterogeneity of dominant optic atrophy: the contribution of visual function investigations to diagnosis. Graefes Arch Clin Exp Ophthalmol 1994;32:717–727.

378. Scott JG. Hereditary optic atrophy with dominant transmission and early onset. Br J Ophthalmol 1941;25:461–479.

379. Lodberg CV, Lund A. Hereditary optic atrophy with dominant transmission: Three Danish families. Acta Ophthalmol 1950;28:437–468.

380. Francois J. Les atrophies optiques héréditaires. J Genet Hum 1976;24:183–200.

381. Grutzner P. Uber diagnose und funktionsstorungen bei der infantilen, dominant venerbten opticus-atrophie. Ber Dtsch Ophthalmol Ges 1963;65:268–277.

382. Smith DP. The assessment of acquired dyschromatopsia and clinical investigation of the acquired tritan defect in dominantly inherited juvenile atrophy. Am J Optom Physiol Opt 1972;49:574–588.

383. Smith DP, Cole BL, Isaacs I. Congenital tritanopia without neuroretinal disease. Invest Ophthalmol 1973;12:608–617.

384. Ohba N, Imamura PM, Tanino T. Colour vision in a pedigree with autosomal dominant optic atrophy. Mod Probl Ophthalmol 1976;17:315–319.

385. Jaeger W, Grutzner P. Le alterazioni del senso cromatico nelle degenerazioni famigliari maculari e nelle atrofie ottiche eraditarie. Bol d'Ocul 1966;45: 783–810.

386. Krill AE, Smith VC, Pokorny J. Similarities between congenital tritan defects and dominant optic-nerve atrophy: Coincidence or identity? J Optom Soc Am 1970;60:1132–1139.

387. Jaeger W. Hereditary optic atrophies in childhood. J Genet Hum 1966;15: 312–321.

388. Harding GFA, Crews SJ, Pitts SM. Psychophysical and visual evoked potential findings in hereditary optic atrophy. Trans Ophthalmol Soc UK 1979;99:96–102.

389. Mantyjarvi MI, Nerdrum J, Tuppurainen K. Color vision in dominant optic atrophy. J Clin Neuroophthalmol 1992;12:98–103.

390. Miller NR. In Discussion of paper by Hoyt. Ophthalmology 1980;87:250–251.

391. Manchester PT, Calhoun FP Jr. Dominant hereditary optic atrophy with bitemporal field defects. Arch Ophthalmol 1958;60:479–484.

392. Kjer P. Hereditary optic atrophies. The 1st Annual Hearst Lecture, presented at the 18th Annual Frederick C. Cordes Eye Society Meeting, University of California, San Francisco, April 23, 1966.

393. Votruba M, Thiselton D, Battacharya SS. Optic disc morphology of patients with OPA1 autosomal dominant optic atrophy. Br J Ophthalmol 2003;87:48–53.

394. Fournier AV, Damji KF, Epstein DL, et al. Disc excavation in dominant optic atrophy. Differentiation from normal tension glaucoma. Ophthalmology 2001; 108:1595–1602.

395. Sandvig K. Pseudoglaucoma of autosomal dominant inheritance. A report on three families. Acta Ophthalmol 1961;39:33–43.

396. Berninger TA, Jaeger W, Krastel M. Electrophysiology and colour perimetry in dominant infantile optic atrophy. Br J Ophthalmol 1991;75:49–53.

397. Thomson AP, Neugebauer M, Fryer A. Autosomal dominant optic atrophy with unilateral facial palsy: A new hereditary condition? J Med Genet 1999;36: 251–252.

398. Kivlin JD, Lovrien EW, Bishop DT, et al. Linkage analysis in dominant optic atrophy. Am J Hum Genet 1983;35:1190–1195.

399. Lunkes A, Hartung AU, Magarino C, et al. Refinement of the OPAI gene locus on chromosome 3q28–q29 to a region of 2–8 cM, in one Cuban pedigree with autosomal dominant optic atrophy type Kjer. Am J Hum Genet 1995;57: 968–970.

400. Jonasdottir A, Eiberg H, Kjer B, et al. Refinement of the dominant optic atrophy locus (OPA1) to a 1.4-cM interval on chromosome 3q28–3q29, within a 3-Mb YAC contig. Hum Genet 1997;99:115–120.

401. Delettre C, Lenaers G, Griffoin J-M, et al. Nuclear gene OPA1, encoding a mitochondrial dynamin-related protein, is mutated in dominant optic atrophy. Nature Genet 2000;26:207–210.

402. Alexander C, Votruba M, Pesch UEA, et al. OPA1, encoding a dynamin-related GTPase, is mutated in autosomal dominant optic atrophy linked to chromosome 3q28. Nature Genet 2000;26:211–215.

403. Shimizu S, Mori N, Kishi M, et al. A novel mutation in the OPA1Gene in a Japanese patient with optic atrophy. Am J Ophthalmol 2003;135:256–257.

404. Pesch UE, Leo-Kottler B, Mayer S, et al. OPA1 mutations in patients with autosomal dominant optic atrophy and evidence for semi-dominant inheritance. Hum Mol Genet 2001;10:1359–1368.

405. Toomes C, Marchbank NJ, Mackey DA, et al. Spectrum, frequency and penetrance of OPA1 mutations in dominant optic atrophy. Hum Mol Genet 2001; 10:1369–1378.

406. Marchbank NJ, Craig JE, Leek JP, et al. Deletion of the OPA1 gene in a dominant optic atrophy family: Evidence that haploinsufficiency is the cause of disease. J Med Genet 2002;39:e47.

407. Olichon A, Baricault L, Gas N, et al. Loss of OPA1 perturbates the mitochondrial inner membrane structure and integrity, leading to cytochrome c release and apoptosis. J Biol Chem 2003;278:7743–7746.

408. Aung T, Ocaka L, Ebenezer ND, et al. A major marker for normal tension glaucoma: Association with polymorphisms in the OPA1 gene. Hum Genet 2002; 110:52–56.

409. Buono LM, Foroozan R, Sergott RC, et al. Is normal tension glaucoma actually an unrecognized hereditary optic neuropathy? New evidence from genetic analysis. Curr Opin Ophthalmol 2002;13:362–370.

410. Aung T, Okada K, Poinoosawmy D, et al. The phenotype of normal tension glaucoma patients with and without OPA1 polymorphisms. Br J Ophthalmol 2003;87:49–152.

411. Rice DS, Williams RW, Ward-Bailey P, et al. Mapping the Bst mutation on mouse chromosome 16: A model for human optic atrophy. Mamm Genome 1995;6:546–548.

412. Waardenburg PJ. Different types of hereditary optic atrophy. Acta Genet Statist Med 1957;7:287–290.

413. Francois J. Mode d'hérédité des hérédo-dégénérescences du nerf optique. J Genet Hum 1966;15:147–220.

414. Norrie G. Causes of blindness in children. Acta Ophthalmol 1927;5:357–386.

415. Walsh FB, Ford FR. Central scotomas: Their importance in topical diagnosis. Arch Ophthalmol 1940;40:500–534.

416. Cordes FC. Optic atrophy in infancy, childhood and adolescence. Am J Ophthalmol 1952;35:1272–1284.

417. Francois J. Hereditary in Ophthalmology. St Louis, CV Mosby, 1961:508–509.

418. Moller H. Recessively inherited, simple optic atrophy: Does it exist? Ophthalm Paediatr Genet 1992;13:31–32.

419. Went LN, De Vries-De Mol EC, Voklker-Dieben HJ. A family with apparently sex-linked optic atrophy. J Med Genet 1975;12:94–98.

420. Assink JJM, Tijmes NT, ten Brink JB, et al. A gene for X-linked optic atrophy is closely linked to the Xp11.4-Xp11.2 region of the X chromosome. Am J Hum Genet 1997;61:934–939.

421. Volker-Dieben HJ, Van Lith GHM, Went LN, et al. A family with sex-linked optic atrophy (ophthalmological and neurological aspects). Doc Ophthalmol 1974;37:307–326.

422. Dimitratos SD, Stathakis DG, Nelson CA, et al. The location of human CASK at Xp11.4 identifies this gene as a candidate for X-linked optic atrophy. Genomics 1998;51:308–309.

423. Lysen JC, Oliver AP. Four generations of blindness. Bulletin of the Dight Institute 1947;5:20–25.

424. Pomeranz HD, Lessell S. A hereditary chiasmal optic neuropathy. Arch Ophthalmol 1999;117:128–131.

425. Konigsmark BW, Knox DL, Hussels IE, et al. Dominant congenital deafness and progressive optic nerve atrophy: Occurrence in four generations of a family. Arch Ophthalmol 1974;91:99–103.

426. Kollarits CR, Pinheiro ML, Swann ER, et al The autosomal dominant syndrome of progressive optic atrophy and congenital deafness. Am J Ophthalmol 1979; 87:789–792.

427. Gernet H. Hereditäre Opticus-atrophie in Kombination mit Taubheit. Berl Dtsch Ophthalmol Ges 1963;65:545–547.

428. Michal S, Ptasinska-Urbanska M, Mitkiewicz-Bochenek W. Atrophie optique hérédo-familiale dominante associée á la surdi-mutité. Ann Oculist 1968;201: 431–435.

429. Deutman AF, Baarsma GA. Optic atrophy and deaf-mutism, dominantly inherited. Doc Ophthalmol Proc Series 1977;17:145–154.

430. Grehn F, Kommerell G, Ropers H-H, et al. Dominant optic atrophy with sensorineural hearing loss. Ophthalm Paediatr Genet 1982;1:77–88.

431. Mets MB, Mhoon E. Probable autosomal dominant optic atrophy with hearing loss. Ophthalm Paediatr Genet 1985;5:85–89.

432. Ide K, Sugiura T, Miyazawa H. A pair of male siblings with dominant progressive optic atrophy and hearing loss. Rinsho Ganka (Jpn J Clin Ophthalmol) 1990;44:1739–1743.

433. Amemiya T, Honda A. A family with optic atrophy and congenital hearing loss. Ophthalm Genet 1994;15:87–93.

434. Ozden S, Duzcan F, Wollnik B, et al. Progressive autosomal dominant optic atrophy and sensorineural hearing loss in a Turkish family. Ophthalm Genet 2002;23:29–36.

434a. Treft RL, Sanborn GE, Carey J, et al. Dominant optic atrophy, deafness, ptosis, ophthalmoplegia, dystaxia, and myopathy. A new syndrome. Ophthalmology 1984;91:908–915.

434b. Meire F, DeLaey JJ, deBie S, et al. Dominant optic nerve atrophy with progressive hearing loss and chronic progrssive external ophthalmoplegia (CPEO). Ophthalmic Paediatr Genet 1985;5:91–97.

434c. Payne M, Yang Z, Katz BJ, et al. Dominant optic atrophy, sensorineural hearing loss, ptosis, and ophthalmoplegia: A syndrome caused by a missense mutation in OPA1. Am J Ophthalmol (in press).

434d. Shimizu S, Mori N, Kishi M, et al. A novel mutation in the OPA1 gene in a Japanese patient with optic atrophy. Am J Ophthalmol 2003;135:256–257.

434e. Amati-Bonneau P, Odent S, Derrien C, et al. The association of autosomal dominant optic atrophy and moderate deafness may be due to the R445H mutation in the OPA1 gene. Am J Ophthalmol 2003;136:1170–1171.

435. Sylvester PE. Some unusual findings in a family with Friedreich's ataxia. Arch Dis Child 1958;33:217–221.

436. Nicolaides P, Appleton RE, Fryer A. Cerebellar ataxia, areflexia, pes cavus, optic atrophy, and sensorineural hearing loss (CAPOS): A new syndrome. J Med Genet 1996;33:419–421.

437. Rosenberg RN, Chutorian A. Familial opticoacoustic nerve degeneration and polyneuropathy. Neurology 1967;17:827–832.

438. Iwashita H, Inoue N, Araki S, et al. Optic atrophy, neural deafness, and distal neurogenic amyotrophy: Report of a family with two affected siblings. Arch Neurol 1970;22:357–364.

439. Hagemoser J, Weinstein J, Bresnick G, et al. Optic atrophy, hearing loss, and peripheral neuropathy. Am J Med Genet 1989;33:61–65.

440. Pauli RM. Sensorineural deafness and peripheral neuropathy [letter]. Clin Genet 1984;26:383–384.

441. Sugano M, Hirayama K, Saito T, et al. Optic atrophy, sensorineural hearing loss and polyneuropathy: A case of sporadic Rosenberg-Chutorian syndrome. Fukushima J Med Sci 1992;38:57–65.

442. Saito T, Nishioka M, Ogino M, et al. A case of hereditary color and sensory neuropathy type I with optic atrophy, neural deafness and pyramidal trace signs. Clin Neurol 1993;33:519–524.

443. Nyssen R, van Bogaert L. La dégénérescence systématisée optico-cochléodentelée. Rev Neurol 1934;62:321–345.

444. Meyer JE. Uber eine kombinierte systemerkrankung in Klein, Mittel- und Endhirn (degenerescence systematisee optico-cochleo-dentelee). Arch Psychiatr Nervenkr 1949;182:731–758.

445. Levy M de L. Au sujet de deux cas de maladie heredo-degenerative du systeme nerveux. Rev Port Pediatr 1951;14:313–318.

446. Müller J, Zeman W. Dégénérescence systématisée optico-cochléo-dentelée. Acta Neuropathol 1965;5:26–39.

447. Ferrer I, Campistol J, Tobena L, et al. Dégénérescence systématisée optico-cochléo-dentelée. J Neurol 1987;234:416–420.

448. Larnaout A, Ben Hamida M, Hentati F. A clinicopathological observation of Nyssen-van Bogaert syndrome with second motor neuron degeration: Two distinct clinical entities. Acta Neurol Scand 1998;98:452–457.

449. Jensen PKA. Nerve deafness, optic nerve atrophy, and dementia: A new X-linked recessive syndrome? Am J Med Genet 1981;9:55–60.

450. Jensen PKA, Reske-Nielsen E, Hein-Sorensen O, et al. The syndrome of optico-acoustic nerve atrophy with dementia. Am J Med Genet 1987;28:517–518.

451. Jensen PKA, Reske-Nielsen E, Hein-Sorensen O. The syndrome of opticoacoustic nerve atrophy with dementia: A new X-linked recessive syndrome with extensive calcifications of the central nervous system [abstract]. Clin Genet 1989;35:222–223.

452. Wolfram DJ. Diabetes mellitus and simple optic atrophy among siblings. Mayo Clin Proc 1938;13:715–717.

453. DeLawter DE. Coexistence of diabetes insipidus and diabetes mellitus. Med Ann DC 1949;18:398–400.

454. Saraux H, Lestradet H, Biais B. La névrite optique du jeune diabétique. Ann d'Ocul 1972;205:35–42.

455. Marquardt JL, Loriaux DL. Diabetes mellitus and optic atrophy: With associated findings of diabetes insipidus and neurosensory hearing loss in two siblings. Arch Intern Med 1974;134:32–37.

456. Gunn T, Bortolussi R, Little JM, et al. Juvenile diabetes mellitus, optic atrophy, sensory nerve deafness, and diabetes insipidus: A syndrome. J Pediatr 1976;89:565–570.

457. Lessell S, Rosman NP. Juvenile diabetes mellitus and optic atrophy. Arch Neurol 1977;34:759–765.

458. Richardson JE, Hamilton W. Diabetes insipidus, diabetes mellitus, optic atrophy, and deafness: Three cases of DIDMOAD syndrome. Arch Dis Child 1978;52:796–798.

459. Dreyer M, Rudiger HW, Bujara K, et al. The syndrome of diabetes insipidus, diabetes mellitus optic atrophy, deafness, and other abnormalities (DIDMOAD syndrome). Two affected sibs and a short review of the literature (98 cases). Klin Wochenschr 1982;60:471–475.

460. Najjar SS, Saikaly MG, Zaytoun GM, et al. Association of diabetes insipidus, diabetes mellitus, optic atrophy, and deafness. The Wolfram or DIDMOAD syndrome. Arch Dis Child 1985;60:823–828.

461. Mtanda AT, Cruysberg JRM, Pinckers AJLG. Optic atrophy in Wolfram syndrome. Ophthalm Paediatr Genet 1986;7:159–165.

462. Bernhard C, Grange JD. Le syndrome de Wolfram ou DIDMOAD syndrome. Bull Soc Ophtalmol France 1987;87:651–653.

463. Van den Bergh L, Zeyen T, Verhelst J, et al. Wolfram syndrome: A clinical study of two cases. Doc Ophthalmol 1993;84:119–126.

464. Bitoun P. Wolfram syndrome. A report of four cases and review of the literature. Ophthalm Genet 1994;15:77–85.

465. Seynaeve H, Vermeiren A, Leys A, et al. Four cases of Wolfram syndrome: Ophthalmologic findings and complications. Bull Soc Belge Ophtalmol 1994;252:75–80.

466. Barrett TG, Bundley SE, Macleod AF. Neurodegeneration and diabetes: UK nationwide study of Wolfram (DIDMOAD) syndrome. Lancet 1995;346:1458–1463.

467. Scolding NJ, Kellar-Wood HF, Shaw C, et al. Wolfram syndrome: Hereditary diabetes mellitus with brainstem and optic atrophy. Ann Neurol 1996;9:352–360.

468. Barrett TG, Bundey SE, Fielder AR, et al. Optic atrophy in Wolfram (DIDMOAD) syndrome. Eye 1997;11:882–888.

469. Barrett TG, Bundey SE. Wolfram (DIDMOAD) syndrome. J Med Genet 1997;34:838–841.

470. Al-Till M, Jarrah NS, Ajlouni KM. Ophthalmologic findings in fifteen patients with Wolfram syndrome. Eur J Ophthalmol 2002;12:84–88.

471. Simsek E, Simsek T, Tekgul S, et al. Wolfram (DIDMOAD) syndrome: A multidisciplinary clinical study in nine Turkish patients and review of the literature. Acta Paediatr 2003;92:55–61.

472. Castro FJ, Barrio J, Perena MF, et al. Uncommon ophthalmologic findings associated with Wolfram syndrome. Acta Ophthalmol Scand 2000;78:118–119.

473. Swift RG, Perkins DO, Chase CL, et al. Psychiatric disorders in 36 families with Wolfram syndrome. Am J Psychiatry 1991;148:775–779.

474. Rando TA, Horton JC, Layzer RB. Wolfram syndrome: Evidence of a diffuse neurodegenerative disease by magnetic resonance imaging. Neurology 1992;42:1220–1224.

475. Kinsley BT, Dumont RH, Swift M, et al. Morbidity and mortality in the Wolfram syndrome. Diabetes Care 1995;18:1566–1570.

476. Bundey S, Pulton K, Whitwell H, et al. Mitochondrial abnormalities in the DIDMOAD syndrome. J Inherited Metab Dis 1992;15:315–319.

477. Van den Ouweland JMW, Bruining GJ, Lindhout D, et al. Mutations in mitochondrial tRNA genes: Non-linkage with syndromes of Wolfram and chronic progressive external ophthalmoplegia. Nucleic Acids Res 1992;20:679–682.

478. Bu X, Rotter JI. Wolfram syndrome: A mitochrondrial-mediated disorder? Lancet 1993;342:598–600.

479. Rötig A, Cormier V, Chatelain P, et al. Deletion of mitochondrial DNA in a case of early-onset diabetes mellitus, optic atrophy, and deafness (Wolfram syndrome, MIM 222300). J Clin Invest 1993;91:1095–1098.

480. Barrientos A, Casademont J, Saiz A, et al. Autosomal recessive Wolfram syndrome associated with an 8.5-kb mtDNA single deletion. Am J Hum Genet 1996;58:963–970.

481. Jackson MJ, Bindoff LA, Weber K, et al. Biochemical and molecular studies of mitochondrial function in diabetes insipidus, diabetes mellitus, optic atrophy, and deafness. Diabetes Care 1994;17:728–733.

482. Mattina T, Li Volti S, Palmeri P, et al. Wolfram's syndrome and HLA. Ophthalm Paediatr Genet 1988;9:25–28.

483. Vendrell J, Ercilla G, Faundez A, et al. Analysis of the contribution of the HLA system to the inheritance in the Wolfram syndrome. Diabetes Res Clin Pract 1994;22:175–180.

484. Polymeropoulos MH, Swift RG, Swift M. Linkage of the gene for Wolfram syndrome to markers on the short arm of chromosome 4. Nature Genet 1994;8:95.

485. Collier DA, Barrett TG, Curtis D, et al. Linkage of Wolfram syndrome to chromosome 4p16.1 and evidence for heterogeneity. Am J Hum Genet 1996;59:855–863.

486. Van Den Ouweland JM, Cryns K, Pennings RJ, et al. Molecular characterization of WFS1 in patients with Wolfram syndrome. J Mol Diagn 2003;5:88–95.

487. Khanim F, Kirk J, Latif F, et al. WFS1/wolframin mutations, Wolfram syndrome, and associated diseases. Hum Mutat 2001;17:357–367.

488. Domenech E, Gomez-Zaera M, Nunes V. WFS1 mutations in Spanish patients with diabetes mellitus and deafness. Eur J Hum Genet 2002;10:421–426.

489. Cryns K, Pfister M, Pennings RJ, et al. Mutations in the WFS1 gene that cause low-frequency sensorineural hearing loss are small non-inactivating mutations. Hum Genet 2002;110:389–394.

490. Barrientos A, Volpini V, Casademont J, et al. A nuclear defect in the 4p16 region predisposes to multiple mitochondrial DNA deletions in families with Wolfram syndrome. J Clin Invest 1996;97:1570–1576.

491. Ajlouni K, Jarrah N, El-Khateeb M, et al. Wolfram syndrome: Identification of a phenotypic and genotypic variant from Jordan. Am J Med Genet 2002;115:61–65.

492. Borgna-Pignatti C, Marradi P, Pinelli L, et al. Thiamine-responsive anemia in DIDMOAD syndrome. J Pediatr 1989;114:405–410.

493. Salonen R, Somer M, Haltia M, et al. Progressive encephalopathy with edema hypsarrhythmia, and optic atrophy (PEHO syndrome). Clin Genet 1991;39:287–293.

494. Somer M, Sainio K. Epilepsy and the electroencephalogram in progressive encephalopathy with edema, hypsarrhythmia, and optic atrophy (the PEHO syndrome). Epilepsia 1993;34:727–731.

495. Haltia M, Somer M. Infantile cerebello-optic atrophy. Acta Neuropathol 1993;85:241–247.

496. Somer M, Salonen O, Pihko H, et al. PEHO syndrome (progressive encephalopathy with edema, hypsarrhythmia, and optic atrophy): Neuroradiologic findings. Am J Neuroradiol 1993;14:861–867.

497. Riikonen R. The PEHO syndrome. Brain Dev 2001;23:765–769.

498. Vanhatalo S, Somer M, Barth PG. Dutch patients with progressive encephalopathy with edema, hypsarrhythmia, and optic atrophy (PEHO) syndrome. Neuropediatrics 2002;33:100–104.

499. Behr C. Die komplizierte, hereditar-familare optikusatrophie des kindesalters: ein bisher nicht beschriebener symptomkomplex. Klin Montasbl Augenheilkd 1909;47:138–160.

500. Pizzato MR, Pascual-Castroviejo I. Behr syndrome. A report of seven cases. Rev Neurol 2001;32:721–724.

501. Marzan KA, Barron TF. MRI abnormalities in Behr syndrome. Pediatr Neurol 1994;10:247–248.

502. Horoupian DS, Zucker DK, Moshe S, et al. Behr syndrome: A clinicopathologic report. Neurology 1979;29:323–327.

503. van Leeuwen M, van Bogaert L. Sur l'atrophie optique hérédo-familiale compliquée (Behr), forme de passage de l'atrophie de Leber aux hérédoataxies. Monatsschr Psychiatr Neurol 1942;105:314–350.

504. Dunn HG, Dolman CL. Necrotizing encephalomyelopathy: Report of a case with manifestations resembling Behr's syndrome. Eur Neurol 1972;7:34–55.

505. Monaco F, Pirisi A, Sechi GP, et al. Complicated optic atrophy (Behr's disease) associated with epilepsy and amino acid imbalance. Eur Neurol 1979;18:101–105.

506. Costeff H, Gadoth N, Apter N, et al. A familial syndrome of infantile optic atrophy, movement disorder, and spastic paraplegia. Neurology 1989;39:595–597.

507. Sheffer RN, Zlotogora J, Elpeleg ON, et al. Behr's syndrome and 3-methylglutaconic aciduria. Am J Ophthalmol 1992;114:494–497.

508. Costeff H, Elpeleg O, Apter N, et al. 3-methylglutaconic aciduria in "optic atrophy plus." Ann Neurol 1993;33:103–104.

509. Elpeleg ON, Costeff H, Joseph A, et al. 3-methyglutaconic aciduria in the Iraqi-Jewish ''optic atrophy plus'' (Costeff) syndrome. Dev Med Child Neurol 1994; 36:167–172.

510. Nystuen A, Costeff H, Bonné-Tamir B, et al. A syndrome involving optic atrophy demonstrates linkage disequilibrium with the CTG repeat in the 3′ untranslated region of the myotonic dystrophy protein kinse gene. Invest Ophthalmol Vis Sci 1997;38:S387.

511. Anikster Y, Kleta R, Shaag A, et al. Type III 3-methylglutaconic aciduria (optic atrophy plus syndrome, or Costeff optic atrophy syndrome): Identification of the OPA3 gene and its founder mutation in Iraqi Jews. Am J Hum Genet 2001; 69:1218–1224.

512. Kleta R, Skovby F, Christensen E, et al. 3-Methylglutaconic aciduria type III in a non-Iraqi-Jewish kindred: Clinical and molecular findings. Mol Genet Metab 2002;73:201–206.

512a. Ianchulev T, Kolin T, Moseley K, et al. Optic nerve atrophy in propionic acidemia. Ophthalmology 2003;110:1850–1854.

513. Korn-Lubetzki I, Blumenfeld A, Gomori JM, et al. Progressive dystonia with optic atrophy in a Jewish-Iraqi family. J Neurol Sci 1997;151:57–63.

514. Francois J. Hereditary degeneration of the optic nerve (hereditary optic atrophy). Intl Ophthalmol Clin 1968;8:999–1054.

515. Thomas PK, Workman JM, Thage O. Behr's syndrome. A family exhibiting pseudodominant inheritance. J Neurol Sci 1984;64:137–148.

516. Lynch DR, Farmer J. Practical approaches to neurogenetic disease. J Neuroophthalmol 2002;22:297–304.

517. Paulson H, Ammache Z. Ataxia and hereditary disorders. Neurol Clin 2001;19: 759–782.

518. Hamida MB, Attia-Romdhane N, Triki CH, et al. Analyse clinique et genetique de 188 familles d'heredo-degenerescence spino-cerebelleuse. Maladies de Friedreich et heredo-ataxies de P. marie. Rev Neurol (Paris) 1991;12:798–808.

519. Rosenberg RN. Autosomal dominant cerebellar phenotypes. The genotype has settled the issue. Neurology 1995;45:1–5.

520. Rosenberg RN. The genetic basis of ataxia. Clinical Neurosci 1995;3:1–4.

521. van Bogaert L. Hereditary optic atrophy as a manifestation of the heredoataxias. In Sorsby A, ed. Modern Trends in Ophthalmology. London, Butterworth & Co, 1948:317–331.

522. Schut JW. Hereditary ataxia: Clinical study through six generations. Arch Neurol Psychiatr 1950;63:535–568.

523. Friedreich N. Ueber degenerative atrophie der spinalen hinterstrange. Virchows Arch Pathol Anat 1863;26:391–419, 433–459; 27:1–26.

524. Harding AE. Friedreich's ataxia; a clinical and genetic study of 90 families with analysis of early diagnostic criteria and intrafamilial clustering of clinical features. Brain 1981;104:589–620.

525. Bressman SB. Inherited and acquired ataxias. In Rowland LP, ed. Merritt's Textbook of Neurology. 9th ed. Baltimore, Williams & Wilkins, 1995:686–694.

526. Johnson WG. Friedreich ataxia. Clin Neurosci 1995;3:33–38.

527. DiDonato S, Gellera C, Mariotti C. The complex clinical and genetic classification of inherited ataxias. II. Autosomal recessive ataxias. Neurol Sci 2001;22: 219–228.

528. Pilch J, Jamroz E, Marszal E. Friedreich's ataxia. J Child Neurol 2002;17: 315–319.

529. Lhatoo SD, Rao DG, Kane NM, et al. Very late onset Friedreich's ataxia presenting as spastic tetraparesis without ataxia or neuropathy. Neurology 2001;56: 1776–1777.

530. Chamberlain S, Shaw J, Wallis J, et al. Genetic homogeneity at the Friedreich's ataxia locus on chromosome 9. Am J Hum Genet 1989;44:518–521.

531. Hanauer A, Cherry M, Fujita R, et al. The Friedreich ataxia gene is assigned to chromosome 9q13-q21 by mapping of tightly linked markers and shows linkage disequilibrium with D9S15. Am J Hum Genet 1990;46:133–137.

532. Montermini L, Molto MD, Zara F, et al. Friedreich ataxia: Autosomal recessive disease caused by an intronic GAA triplet repeat expansion. Neurology 1996.

533. Campuzano V, Montermini L, Lutz Y, et al. Frataxin is reduced in Friedreich ataxia patients and is associated with mitochondrial membranes. Hum Mol Genet 1997;6:1771–1780.

534. Wilson RB, Lynch DR, Farmer JM, et al. Increased serum transferrin receptor concentrations in Friedreich ataxia. Ann Neurol 2000;47:659–661.

534a. Alldredge CD, Schlieve CR, Miller NR, et al. Pathophysiology of the optic neuropathy associated with Friedreich ataxia. Arch Ophthalmol 2003;121: 1582–1585.

535. Bell J, Carmichael EA. Hereditary ataxia and spastic paraplegia. In Fisher RA, ed. Treasury of Human Inheritance. Vol 4. London, Cambridge University Press, 1939:141–281.

536. Sjögren T. Klinische und erbbiologsiche untersuchungen uber die heredoataxien. Acta Psychiatr Scand Suppl 1943;27:1–97.

537. Andermann E, Remillard GM, Goyer C, et al. Genetic and family studies in Friedreich's ataxia. Can J Neurol Sci 1976;3:287–301.

538. Geoffroy GH, Barbeau A, Breton G, et al. Clinical description roentgenologic evaluation of patients with Friedreich's ataxia. Can J Neurol Sci 1976;3: 279–286.

539. Heck AF. A study of neural and extraneural findings in a large family with Friedreich's ataxia. J Neurol Sci 1964;1:226–255.

540. Carroll WM, Kriss A, Baraitser M, et al. The incidence and nature of visual pathway involvement in Friedreich's ataxia: A clinical and visual evoked potential study of 22 patients. Brain 1980;103:413–434.

541. Livingstone IR, Mastaglia FL, Edis R, et al. Visual involvement in Friedreich's ataxia and hereditary spastic ataxia: A clinical and visual evoked response study. Arch Neurol 1981;38:75–79.

542. Wenzel W, Camacho L, Claus D, et al. Visually evoked potentials in Friedreich's ataxia. Adv Neurol 1982;32:131–139.

543. Müller-Felber W, Rossmanith T, Spes C, et al. The clinical spectrum of Friedreich's ataxia in German families showing linkage to the FRDA locus on chromosome 9. Clin Invest 1993;71:109–114.

544. Durr A, Cossee M, Agid Y, et al. Clinical and genetic abnormalities in patients with Friedreich's ataxia. N Engl J Med 1996;335:1169–1175.

545. Montermini L, Richter A, Morgan K, et al. Phenotypic variability in Friedreich ataxia: Role of the associated GAA triplet repeat expansion. Ann Neurol 1997; 41:675–682.

546. Givre SJ, Wall M, Kardon RH. Visual loss and recovery in a patient with Friedreich ataxia. J Neuroophthalmology 2000;20:229–233.

547. Belal S, Hentati F, Hamida CB, et al. Friedreich's ataxia, vitamin E responsive type. The chromosome 8 locus. Clin Neurosci 1995;3:39–42.

548. Bomont P, Watanabe M, Gershoni-Barush R, et al. Homozygosity mapping of spinocerebellar ataxia with cerebellar atrophy and peripheral neuropathy to 9q33–34, and with hearing impairment and optic atrophy to 6p21–23. Eur J Hum Genet 2000;8:986–990.

549. Delague V, Bareil C, Bouvagnet P, et al. A new autosomal recessive non-progressive congenital cerebellar ataxia associated with mental retardation, optic atrophy, and skin abnormalities (CAMOS) maps to chromosome 15q24-q26 in a large consanguineous Lebanese Druze family. Neurogenetics 2002;4:23–27.

549a. Rajab A, Mochida GH, Hill A, et al. A novel form of pontocerebellar hypoplasia maps to chromosome 7q11–21. Neurology 2003;60:1664–1667.

550. Arts WFM, Loonen MCB, Sengers RCA, et al. X-linked ataxia, weakness, deafness, and loss of vision in early childhood with a fatal course. Ann Neurol 1993; 33:535–539.

551. Gilman S. The spinocerebellar ataxias. Clin Neuropharmacol 2000;23:296–303.

552. Subramony SH, Filla A. Autosomal dominant spinocerebellar ataxias and infinitum? Neurology 2001;56:287–289.

553. Tan EK, Ashizawa T. Genetic testing in spinocerebellar ataxias: Defining a clinical role. Arch Neurol 2001;58:191–195.

554. Harding AE. The clinical features and classification of late onset autosomal dominant cerebellar ataxias: A study of 11 families, including descendants of the ''Drew family of Walworth.'' Brain 1982;105:1–28.

555. Brown S. On hereditary ataxy, with a series of 21 cases. Brain 1892;15:250–282.

556. Abe T, Abe K, Aoki M, et al. Ocular changes in patients with spinocerebellar degeneration and repeated trinucleotide expansion of spinocerebellar ataxia type 1 gene. Arch Ophthalmol 1997;115:231–236.

557. Koeppen AH, Hans MB, Shepherd DI, et al. Adult-onset hereditary ataxia in Scotland. Arch Neurol 1977;34:611–618.

558. Staal A, Stefanko SZ, Busch HFM, et al. Autonomic nerve calcification and peripheral neuropathy in olivopontocerebellar atrophy. J Neurol Sci 1981;51: 383–394.

559. Triau E, Dom R, Ververken D, et al. Dominant olivopontocerebellar degeneration and optic pathway atrophy: A family report. Clin Neuropathol 1982;1: 67–72.

560. Hammond EJ, Wilder BJ. Evoked potentials in olivopontocerebellar atrophy. Arch Neurol 1983;40:366–369.

561. Durr A, Brice A, Lepage-Lezin A, et al. Autosomal dominant cerebellar ataxia type I linked to chromosome 12q (SCA2: spinocerebellar ataxia type 2). Clin Neurosci 1995;3:12–16.

562. Junck L, Fink JK. Machado-Joseph disease and SCA3: The genotype meets the phenotypes. Neurology 1996;46:4–8.

563. Higgins JJ, Nee LE, Vasconcelos O, et al. Mutations in American families with spinocerebellar ataxia (SCA) type 3: SCA3 is allelic to Machado-Joseph disease. Neurology 1996;46:208–213.

564. Illarioshkin SN, Slominsky PA, Ovchinnikov IV, et al. Spinocerebellar ataxia type 1 in Russia. J Neurol 1996;243:506–510.

565. Benomar A, Krols L, Stevanin G, et al. The gene for autosomal dominant cerebellar ataxia with pigmentary macular dystrophy maps to chromosome 3p12–21.1. Nature Genet 1995;10:84–88.

566. Gouw LG, Kaplan CD, Haines JH, et al. Retinal degeneration characterizes a spinocerebellar ataxia mapping to chromosome 3p. Nature Genet 1995;10: 89–93.

567. Ptacek LJ. Autosomal dominant spinocerebellar atrophy with retinal degeneration. Clin Neurosci 1995;3:28–32.

568. Shoffner JM, Kaufman A, Kootz D, et al. Oxidative phosphorylation diseases and cerebellar ataxia. Clin Neurosci 1995;3:43–53.

569. Lamperti C, Naini A, Hirano M, et al. Cerebellar ataxia and coenzyme Q10 deficiency. Neurology 2003;60:1206–1208.

570. Holt IJ, Harding AE, Petty RKH, et al. A new mitochondrial disease associated with mitochondrial DNA heteroplasmy. Am J Hum Genet 1990;46:428–483.

571. Melberg A, Hetta J, Dahl N, et al. Autosomal dominant cerebellar ataxia deafness and narcolepsy. J Neurol Sci 1995;134:119–129.

572. Lundberg PO, Wranne I, Brun A. Family with optic atrophy and neurological symptoms. Acta Neurol Scand 1967;43:87–105.

573. Young CA. Friedreich's ataxia showing transitional symptoms of Marie's disease (familial spinocerebellar ataxia). Trans Am Ophthalmol Soc 1934;32: 626–638.

574. Charcot JM, Marie P. Sur une forme particulière d'atrophie musculaire progressive souvent familiale. Rev Med Liege 1886;6:97–138.

575. Tooth HH. The Peroneal Type of Progressive Muscular Atrophy. Thesis for the Degree of M.D. University of Cambridge, London, HK Lewis, 1886.

576. Lovelace RE, Rowland LP. Hereditary neuropathies. In Rowland LP, ed. Merritt's Textbook of Neurology. 9th ed. Baltimore, Williams & Wilkins, 1995: 651–657.

577. Kuhlenbaumer G, Young P, Hunermund G, et al. Clinical features and molecular genetics of hereditary peripheral neuropathies. J Neurol 2002;249:1629–1650.

578. Pareyson D. Diagnosis of hereditary neuropathies in adult patients. J Neurol 2003;250:148–160.

579. Ionasescu VV, Ionasescu R, Searby C. Screening of dominantly inherited Charcot-Marie-Tooth neuropathies. Muscle Nerve 1993;16:1232–1238.

580. Suter L, Welcher AA, Snipes GJ. Progress in the molecular understanding of hereditary peripheral neuropathies reveals new insights into the biology of the peripheral nervous system. Trends Neurosci 1993;16:50–56.

581. Wise CA, Garcia CA, Davis SN, et al. Molecular analyses of unrelated Charcot-Marie-Tooth (CMT) disease suggests a high frequency of the CMTIA duplication. Am J Hum Genet 1993;53:853–863.

582. Vizioli F. Dell'atrofia muscolare progressiva nevrotica. Boll R Accad Med-Chir (Napoli), Aug–Sept, 1889.

583. Herishanu Y. Bilateral optic atrophy in Charcot-Marie's muscular atrophy. Confin Neurol 1969;31:383–387.

584. Hoyt WF. Charcot-Marie-Tooth disease with primary optic atrophy. Arch Ophthalmol 1960;64:925–928.

585. Alajouanine T, Castaigne P, Cambier J, et al. Maladie de Charcot-Marie: Etude anatomo-clinique d'une observation suivie pendant 65 ans. Presse Med 1967; 75:2745–2750.

586. Carroll WM, Jones SJ, Halliday AM. Visual evoked potential abnormalities in Charcot-Marie-Tooth disease and comparison with Friedreich's ataxia. J Neurol Sci 1983;61:123–133.

587. Ippel EF, Wittebol-Post D, Jennekens FG, et al. Genetic heterogeneity of hereditary motor and sensory neuropathy type VI. J Child Neurol 1995;10:459–463.

588. Chalmers RM, Bird AC, Harding AE. Autosomal dominant optic atrophy with asymptomatic peripheral neuropathy. J Neurol Neurosurg Psychiatry 1996;60: 195–196.

589. Chalmers RM, Riordan-Eva P, Wood NW. Autosomal recessive inheritance of hereditary motor and sensory neuropathy with optic atrophy. J Neurol Neurosurg Psychiatry 1997;62:385–387.

589a. Voo, I, Allf BE, Udar N, et al. Hereditary motor and sensory neuropathy type VI with optic atrophy. Am J Ophthalmol 2003;136:670–677.

590. Tackmann W, Radu EW. Pattern shift visual evoked potentials in Charcot-Marie-Tooth disease, HMSN type 1. J Neurol 1980;224:71–74.

591. Burki E. Ophthalmologische befunde be der neuralen muskelatrophie: Charcot-Marie-Tooth, HMSN type 1. Klin Monatsbl Augenheilkd 1981;179:94–96.

592. Bird TD, Griep E. Pattern reversal visual evoked potentials. Studies in Charcot-Marie-Tooth hereditary neuropathy. Arch Neurol 1981;38:739–741.

593. Gadoth N, Gordon CR, Bleich N, et al. Three modality evoked potentials in Charcot-Marie-Tooth Disease (HMSN-1). Brain Dev 1991;13:91–94.

594. van Bogaert L, Moreau M. Combinaison de l'amyotrophie de Charcot-Marie-Tooth et de la maladie de Friedreich chez plusieurs membres d'une famille. Encéphale 1939–1940;34:312–320.

595. Ross AT. Combination of Friedreich's ataxia and Charcot-Marie-Tooth atrophy in each of two brothers. J Nerv Ment Dis 1952;95:680–686.

596. Riley CM, Day R, Greeley D, et al. Central autonomic dysfunction with defective lacrimation. Report of five cases. Pediatrics 1949;3:468.

597. Slaugenhaupt SA, Blemenfeld A, Gill SP, et al. Tissue-specific expression of a splicing mutation in the IKBKAP gene causes familial dysautonomia. Am J Hum Genet 2001;68:598–605.

598. Rizzo JF (III), Lessell S, Liebman SD. Optic atrophy in familial dysautonomia. Am J Ophthalmol 1986;102:463–467.

599. Diamond GA, D'Amico RA, Axelrod FB. Optic nerve dysfunction in familial dysautonomia. Am J Ophthalmol 1987;104:645–648.

600. Groom M, Kay MD, Corrent GF. Optic neuropathy in familial dysautonomia. J Neuroophthalmology 1997;17:101–102.

601. Fink JK. The hereditary spastic paraplegias. Nine genes and counting. Arch Neurol 2003;60:1045–1049.

602. Makhoul J, Cordonnier M, Van Nechel C. Optic neuropathy in Strumpell-Lorrain disease: Presentation of a clinical case and literature review. Bull Soc Belge Ophtalmol 2002;286:9–14.

603. Dillmann U, Heide G, Dietz B, et al. Hereditary motor and sensory neuropathy with spastic paraplegia and optic atrophy: Report on a family. J Neurol 1997; 244:562–565.

604. Miyama S, Arimoto K, Kimiya S, et al. Complicated hereditary spastic paraplegia with peripheral neuropathy, optic atrophy and mental retardation. Neuropediatrics 2000;31:214–217.

605. Meola G. Clinical and genetic heterogeneity in myotonic dystrophies. Muscle Nerve 2000;23:1789–1799.

606. Lieberman AP, Fischbeck KH. Triplet repeat expansion in neuromuscular disease. Muscle Nerve 2000;23:843–850.

607. Gamez J, Montane D, Martorell L, et al. Bilateral optic nerve atrophy in myotonic dystrophy. Am J Ophthalmol 2001;131:398–400.

608. Kenyon KR. Lysosomal disorders affecting the ocular anterior segment. In Nicholson DH, ed. Ocular Pathology Update. New York, Masson, 1980:1–22.

609. Kolodny EH, Cable WJL. Inborn errors of metabolism. Ann Neurol 1982;11: 221–232.

610. Maire I. Is genotype determination useful in predicting the clinical phenotype in lysosomal storage diseases? J Inherit Metab Dis 2001;24(Suppl 2):57–61.

611. Desnick RJ, Schuchman EH. Enzyme replacement and enhancement therapies: Lessons from lysosomal disorders. Nat Rev Genet 2002;3:954–966.

612. Cabrera-Salazar MA, Novelli E, Barranger JA. Gene therapy for the lysosomal storage disorders. Curr Opin Mol Ther 2002;4:349–358.

613. Francois J. Ocular manifestations of the mucopolysaccharidoses. Ophthalmologica 1974;169:345–361.

614. Francois J. Ocular manifestations of inborn errors of carbohydrate and lipid metabolism. Bibl Ophthalmol 1975;84:1–175.

615. Kenyon KR. Ocular manifestations and pathology of systemic mucopolysaccharidoses. Birth Defects 1976;XII:133–153.

616. Johnson WG. Lysosomal diseases and other storage diseases. In Rowland LP, ed. Merritt's Textbook of Neurology. 9th ed. Baltimore, Williams & Wilkins, 1995:547–571.

617. Rapin I, Traeger E. Cerebral degenerations of childhood. In Rowland LP, ed. Merritt's Textbook of Neurology. 9th ed. Baltmore, Williams & Wilkins, 1995: 597–603.

618. Rapin I, Traeger E. Differential diagnosis. In Rowland LP, ed. Merritt's Textbook of Neurology. 9th ed. Baltimore, Williams & Wilkins, 1995:605–614.

619. McKusick VA, Kaplan D, Wise D, et al. The genetic mucopolysaccharidoses. Medicine 1965;44:445–483.

620. Goldberg MF, Scott CI, McKusick VA. Hydrocephalus and papilledema in the Maroteaux-Lamy syndrome (mucopolysaccharidosis type VI). Am J Ophthalmol 1970;69:969–975.

621. Collins MLZ, Traboulsi EI, Maumenee IH. Optic nerve head swelling and optic atrophy in the systemic mucopolysaccharidoses. Ophthalmology 1990;97: 1445–1449.

622. McDonnell JM, Green R, Maumenee IH. Ocular histopathology of systemic mucopolysaccharidosis, type II-A (Hunter syndrome, severe). Ophthalmology 1985;92:1772–1779.

623. Quigley HA, Green WR. Clinical and ultrastructural ocular histopathologic studies of adult-onset metachromatic leukodystrophy. Am J Ophthalmol 1976;82: 472–479.

624. Francois J. Ocular manifestations in demyelinating diseases. Adv Ophthalmol 1979;39:1–36.

625. Libert J, Van Hoof F, Toussaint D, et al. Ocular findings in metachromatic leukodystrophy: An electron microscopic and enzyme study in different clinical and genetic variants. Arch Ophthalmol 1979;97:1495–1504.

626. Baumann N, Masson M, Carreau V, et al. Adult forms of metachromatic leukodystrophy: Clinical and biochemical approach. Dev Neurosci 1991;13:211–215.

627. Cogan DG, Kuwabara T, Moser H. Metachromatic leucodystrophy. Ophthalmologica 1970;160:2–17.

628. Goebel HH, Argyrakis A. Adult metachromatic leukodystrophy. Am J Ophthalmol 1979;88:270–273.

629. Goebel HH, Busch-Hettwer H, Bohl J. Ultrastructural study of retina in late infantile metachromatic leukodystrophy. Ophthalm Res 1992;24:103–109.

630. Emery JM, Green WR, Huff DS. Krabbe's disease: Histopathology and ultrastructure of the eye. Am J Ophthalmol 1972;74:400–406.

631. Yunis EF, Lee RE. Further observations on the fine structure of globoid leukodystrophy. Hum Pathol 1972;3:371–388.

632. Harcourt B, Ashton N. Ultrastructure of the optic nerve in Krabbe's leucodystrophy. Br J Ophthalmol 1973;57:885–891.

633. Brownstein S, Mearher-Villemure K, Polomeno RC, et al. Optic nerve in globoid leukodystrophy (Krabbe's disease). Arch Ophthalmol 1978;96:864–870.

634. Hittmair K, Wimberger D, Wiesbauer P, et al. Early infantile form of Krabbe disease with optic hypertrophy: Serial MR examinations and autopsy correlation. Am J Neuroradiol 1994;15:1454–1458.

635. Jones BV, Barron TF, Towfighi J. Optic nerve enlargement in Krabbe's disease. Am J Neuroradiol 1999;20:1228–1231.

636. Baker RH, Trautmann JC, Younge BR, et al. Late juvenile-onset Krabbe's disease. Ophthalmology 1990;97:1176–1180.

637. Kolodny EH, Raghavan S, Krivit W. Late-onset Krabbe disease (globoid cell leukodystrophy): Clinical and biochemical features of 15 cases. Dev Neurosci 1991;13:232–239.

638. Blaw ME. Melanodermic type leukodystrophy (adrenoleukodystrophy). In Vinken PJ, Bruyn GW, eds. Handbook of Clinical Neurology. Vol 10. New York, American Elsevier, 1978:128–133.

639. Traboulsi EI, Maumenee IH. Ophthalmologic manifestations of X-linked childhood adrenoleukodystrophy. Ophthalmology 1987;94:47–52.

640. Jensen ME, Sawyer RW, Braun IF, et al. MR imaging appearance of childhood

adrenoleukodystrophy with auditory, visual, and motor pathway involvement. RadioGraphics 1990;10:53–66.

641. Wray SH, Cogan DG, Kuwabara T, et al. Adrenoleukodystrophy with disease of the eye and optic nerve. Am J Ophthalmol 1976;82:480–485.

642. Wilson WB. The visual system manifestations of adrenoleukodystrophy. Neuro-ophthalmology 1981;1:175–183.

643. Cohen SMZ, Brown III FR, Martyn L, et al. Ocular histopathologic and biochemical studies of the cerebrohepatorenal syndrome (Zellweger's syndrome) and its relationship to neonatal adrenoleukodystrophy. Am J Ophthalmol 1983;96:488–501.

644. Cohen SMZ, Green WR, De la Cruz ZC, et al. Ocular histopathologic studies of neonatal and childhood adrenoleukodystrophy. Am J Ophthalmol 1992;95:82–96.

645. Folz SJ, Trobe JD. The peroxisome and the eye. Surv Ophthalmol 1991;35:353–368.

646. Kaplan PW, Kruse B, Tusa RJ, et al. Visual system abnormalities in adrenomyeloneuropathy. Ann Neurol 1995;37:550–552.

647. Haddad R, Font RL, Friendly DS. Cerebro-hepato-renal syndrome of Zellweger. Ocular histopathologic findings. Arch Ophthalmol 1976;94:1927–1930.

648. Al-Essa M, Dhaunsi GS, Rashed M, et al. Zellweger syndrome in Saudi Arabia and its distinct features. Clin Pediatr 1999;38:77–86.

649. Saugier-Veber P, Munnich A, Bonneau D, et al. X-linked spastic paraplegia and Pelizaeus-Merzbacher disease are allelic disorders at the proteolipid protein locus. Nature Genet 1994;6:257–262.

650. Wang PJ, Young C, Lui HM. Neurophysiologic studies and MRI in Pelizaeus-Merzbacher disease: Comparison of classic and connatal forms. Pediatr Neurol 1995;12:47–53.

651. Koeppen AH, Robitaille Y. Pelizaeus-Merzbacher disease. J Neuropathol Exp Neurol 2002;61:747–759.

652. Doll R, Natowicz MR, Schiffmann R, et al. Molecular diagnostics for myelin proteolipid protein gene mutations in Pelizaeus-Merzbacher disease. Am J Hum Genet 1992;51:161–169.

653. Carango P, Funanage VL, Quirós RE, et al. Overexpression of DM20 messenger RNA in two brothers with Pelizaeus-Merzbacher disease. Ann Neurol 1995;38:610–617.

654. Rahn EK, Yanoff M, Tucker S. Neuro-ocular considerations in the Pelizaeus-Merzbacher syndrome: A clinicopathologic study. Am J Ophthalmol 1968;66:1143–1151.

655. Haberland C, Brunngraber EG, Witting LA. Infantile neuroaxonal dystrophy. Arch Neurol 1972;26:391–402.

656. Ellis WG, McCulloch JR, Yatsu F. Infantile neuroaxonal dystrophy: Ultrastructural and biochemical studies. Abstr Neurol 1969;19:304.

657. Herman MM, Huttenlocher PR, Bensch KG. Electron microscopic observations in infantile neuroaxonal dystrophy: Report of a cortical biopsy and review of the recent literature. Arch Neurol 1969;20:19–34.

658. Dorfman LF, Pedley TA, Tharp BR, et al. Juvenile neuroaxonal dystrophy: Clinical, electrophysiological, and neuropathological features. Ann Neurol 1978;3:419–428.

659. Goebel HH, Lehmann J. An ultrastructural study of the retina in human late infantile neuroaxonal dystrophy. Retina 1993;13:50–55.

660. Aicardi J, Castelein P. Infantile neuroaxonal dystrophy. Brain 1979;102:727–748.

661. Ferreira RC, Mierau GW, Bateman JB. Conjunctival biopsy in infantile neuroaxonal dystrophy. Am J Ophthalmol 1997;123:264–266.

662. Gordon N. Pantothenate kinase-associated neurodegeneration (Hallervorden-Spatz syndrome). Eur J Paediatr Neurol 2002;6:243–247.

663. Tripathi RC, Tripathi BJ, Bauserman SC, et al. Clinicopathologic correlation and pathogenesis of ocular and central nervous system manifestations in Hallervorden-Spatz syndrome. Acta Neuropathol 1992;83:113–119.

664. Porter-Grenn L, Silbergleit R, Mehta BA. Hallervorden-Spatz disease with bilateral involvement of globus pallidus and substantia nigra: MR demonstration. J Comput Assist Tomogr 1993;17:961–963.

665. Newell FW, Johnson RO III, Huttenlocher PR. Pigmentary degeneration of the retina in Hallervorden-Spatz syndrome. Am J Ophthalmol 1979;88:467–471.

666. Casteels I, Spileers W, Swinnen T, et al. Optic atrophy as the presenting sign in Hallervorden-Spatz syndrome. Neuropediatrics 1994;25:265–267.

667. Battistella PA, Midena E, Suppieg A, et al. Optic atrophy as the first symptom in Hallervorden-Spatz syndrome. Childs Nerv Syst 1998;14:135–138.

668. Menkes JH, Alter M, Steigleder GK, et al. A sex-linked recessive disorder with growth retardation, peculiar hair, and focal cerebral and cerebellar degeneration. Pediatrics 1962;29:764–779.

669. Taylor D. Ophthalmological features of some human hereditary disorders with demyelination. Bull Soc Belge Ophtalmol 1983;208:405–413.

670. Gasch AT, Caruso RC, Kaler SG, et al. Menkes' syndrome: Ophthalmic findings. Ophthalmology 2002;109:1477–1483.

671. Seelenfreund MH, Gartner S, Vinger PF. The ocular pathology of Menkes' disease. Arch Ophthalmol 1968;80:718–723.

672. Wray SH, Kuwabara T, Sanderson P. Menkes' kinky hair disease: A light and electron microscopic study of the eye. Invest Ophthalmol Vis Sci 1976;15:128–138.

673. Gascon GG, Ozand PT, Mahdi A, et al. Infantile CNS spongy degeneration—14 cases: Clinical update. Neurology 1990;40:1876–1882.

674. McAdams H, Geyer C, Done S, et al. CT and MR imaging of Canavan disease. Am J Neuroradiol 1990;11:397–399.

675. Bennett MJ, Gibson KM, Sherwood WG, et al. Reliable prenatal diagnosis of Canavan disease (aspartoacylase deficiency): Comparison of enzymatic and metabolite analysis. J Inher Metab Dis 1993;16:831–836.

676. Kaul R, Gao GP, Aloya M, et al. Canavan disease: Mutations among Jewish and non-Jewish patients. Am J Hum Genet 1994;55:34–41.

677. Gordon N. Canavan disease: A review of recent developments. Eur J Paediatr Neurol 2001;5:65–69.

678. Borrett D, Becker LE. Alexander disease: A disease of astrocytes. Brain 1985;108:367–385.

679. Ichiyama T, Hayaski T, Unita T. Two possible cases of Alexander disease. Multimodal evoked potentials and MRI. Brain Dev 1993;15:153–156.

680. Schwankhaus JD, Parisi JE, Gulledge WR, et al. Hereditary adult-onset Alexander's disease with palatal myoclonus, spastic paraparesis, and cerebellar ataxia. Neurology 1995;45:2266–2271.

681. Johnson AB. Alexander disease: A review and the gene. Int J Dev Neurosci 2002;20:391–394.

682. Cockayne EA. Dwarfism with retinal atrophy and deafness. Arch Dis Child 1946;21:52–54.

683. Levin PS, Green WR, Victor DI, et al. Histopathology of the eye in Cockayne syndrome. Arch Ophthalmol 1983;101:1093.

684. Traboulsi EI, De Becker I, Maumenee IH. Ocular findings in Cockayne syndrome. Am J Ophthalmol 1992;114:579–583.

685. Friedberg EC. Xeroderma pigmentosum, Cockayne syndrome, helicases and DNA repair. Cell 1992;128:1233–1237.

686. Nance MA, Berry SA. Cockayne syndrome: Review of 140 cases. Am J Med Genet 1992;42:68–84.

687. Troelstra C, van Gool A, de Wit J, et al. ERCC6, a member of a subfamily of putative helicases, is involved in Cockayne's syndrome and preferential repair of active genes. Cell 1992;71:939–953.

688. Bennett JL. Developmental neurogenetics and neuro-ophthalmology. J Neuro-ophthalmol 2002;22:286–296.

689. Pena SD, Shokeir MH. The cerebro-oculo-facio-skeletal (COFS) syndrome. Clin Genet 1974;5:285–293.

690. Graham JM Jr, Anyane-Yeboa K, Raams A, et al. Cerebro-oculo-facio-skeletal syndrome with nucleotide excision-repair defect and a mutated XPD gene, with prenatal diagnosis in a triplet pregnancy. Am J Hum Genet 2001;69:291–300.

691. Smith DW, Lemli L, Opitz JM. A newly recognized syndrome of multiple congenital anomalies. J Pediatr 1964;64:210–217.

692. Loeffler J, Utermann G, Witsch-Baumgartner M. Molecular prenatal diagnosis of Smith-Lemli-Opitz syndrome is reliable and efficient. Prenat Diagn 2002;22:827–830.

693. Herman GE. Disorders of cholesterol biosynthesis: Prototypic metabolic malformation syndromes. Hum Mol Genet 2003;12(Suppl 1):R75–88.

694. Kretzer FL, Hittner HM, Mehta RS. Ocular manifestations of the Smith-Lemli-Opitz syndrome. Arch Ophthalmol 1981;99:2000–2006.

695. Atchaneeyasakul LO, Linck LM, Connor WE, et al. Eye findings in 8 children and a spontaneously aborted fetus with RSH/Smith-Lemli-Opitz syndrome. Am J Med Genet 1998;80:501–505.

696. Houlden H, Smith S, DeCarvalho M, et al. Clinical and genetic characterization of families with triple A (Allgrove) syndrome. Brain 2002;125:2681–2690.

697. Kimber J, McLean BN, Prevett M, et al. Allgrove or 4 ''A'' syndrome: An autosomal recessive syndrome causing multisystem neurological disease. J Neurol Neurosurg Psychiatry 2003;74:654–657.

698. Prietsch V, Peters V, Hackler R, et al. A new case of CDG-x with stereotyped dystonic hand movements and optic atrophy. J Inherit Metab Dis 2002;25:126–130.

699. Moriya N, Mitsui T, Shibata T, et al. GAPO syndrome: Report on the first case in Japan. Am J Med Genet 1995;58:257–261.

700. Mullaney PB, Jacquemin C, Al-Rashed W, et al. Growth retardation, alopecia, pseudoanodontia, and optic atrophy (GAPO syndrome) with congenital glaucoma. Arch Ophthalmol 1997;115:940–941.

701. Ilker SS, Ozturk F, Kurt E, et al. Ophthalmic findings in GAPO syndrome. Jpn J Ophthalmol 1999;43:48–52.

702. Sandgren G. GAPO syndrome: A new case. Am J Med Genet 1995;58:87–90.

703. Tambe KA, Ambekar SV, Bafna PN. Delleman (oculocerebrocutaneous) syndrome: Few variations in a classical case. Eur J Paediatr Neurol 2003;7:77–80.

704. Heidi T. A syndrome of osteogenesis imperfecta, wormian bones, frontal bossing, brachytelephalangia, hyperextensible joints, congenital blindness and oligophrenia in three sibs. Klin Pediatr 1981;193:334–340.

705. Al Gazali LI, Sabrinathan K, Nair KGR. A syndrome of osteogenesis imperfecta, optic atrophy, retinopathy and severe developmental delay in two sibs of consanguinous parents. Clin Dysmorph 1994;3:55–62.

706. Chitayat D, Silver K, Azouz EM. Skeletal dysplasia, intracerebral calcifications, optic atrophy, hearing impairment, and mental retardation: Nosology of dysosteosclerosis. Am J Med Genet 1992;43:517–523.

707. Ohtagaki A, Hara T, Maegaki Y, et al. Intracranial calcifications, epilepsy, and

optic atrophy associated with metaphyseal dysplasia: A case report. Brain Dev 1997;19:414–417.

708. Dumic M, Cvitanovic M, Ille J, et al. Syndrome of short stature, mental deficiency, microcephaly, ectodermal dysplasia, and multiple skeletal anomalies. Am J Med Genet 2000;93:47–51.

709. Al-Gazali LI. Mental retardation, iris coloboma, optic atrophy and distinctive facial appearance in two sibs. Clin Dysmorphol 1998;7:201–203.

710. Megarbane A. Unknown diagnosis in two male cousins with facial abnormalities, optic atrophy, abnormal EEG, and severe psychomotor retardation. Am J Med Genet 2003;116A:381–384.

711. Megarbane A, Delague V, Ruchoux MM, et al. New autosomal recessive cerebellar ataxia disorder in a large inbred Lebanese family. Am J Med Genet 2001; 101:135–141.

712. Megarbane A, Choueiri R, Bleik J, et al. Microcephaly, microphthalmia, congenital cataract, optic atrophy, short stature, hypotonia, severe psychomotor retardation, and cerebral malformations: A second family with micro syndrome or a new syndrome. J Med Genet 1999;36:637–640.

713. Warburg M, Sjo O, Fledelius HC, et al. Autosomal recessive microcephaly, microcornea, cogenital cataract, mental retardation, optic atrophy, and hypogenitalism. Micro syndrome. Am J Dis Child 1993;147:1309–1312.

714. Bitoun P, Martin-Pont B, Tamboise E, et al. Optic atrophy, microcephaly, mental retardation and mosaic variegated aneuploidy: A human mitotic mutation. Ann Génét 1994;37:75–77.

715. Teebi AS, Miller S, Ostrer H, et al. Spastic paraplegia, optic atrophy, microcephaly with normal intelligence, and XY sex reversal: A new autosomal recessive syndrome? J Med Genet 1998;35:759–762.

716. Black PD. Ocular defects in children with cerebral palsy. Br Med J 1980;2: 487–488.

717. Carelli V, Ross-Cisneros FN, Sadun AA. Optic nerve degeneration and mitochondrial dysfunction: Genetic and acquired optic neuropathies. Neurochem Int 2002;40:573–584.

718. Leigh D. Subacute necrotizing encephalomyelopathy in an infant. J Neurol Neurosurg Psychiatr 1951;14:216–221.

719. Ugalde C, Triepels RH, Coenen MJH, et al. Impaired complex I assembly in a Leigh syndrome patient with a novel missense mutation in the ND6 gene. Ann Neurol 2003;54:665–669.

720. Van Coster RN, Lombes A, DeVivo DC, et al. Cytochrome c oxidase-associated Leigh syndrome: Phenotypic features and pathogenetic speculations. J Neurol Sci 1991;104:97–111.

721. DeVivo DC. The expanding clinical spectrum of mitochondrial diseases. Brain Dev 1993;15:1–21.

722. Santorelli FM, Shanske S, Macaya A, et al. The mutation at nt8993 of mitochondrial DNA is a common cause of Leigh's syndrome. Ann Neurol 1993;34: 827–834.

723. Rahman S, Blok RB, Dahl H-H M, et al. Leigh syndrome: Clinical features and biochemical and DNA abnormalities. Ann Neurol 1996;39:343–351.

724. DiMauro S, De Vivo DC. Genetic heterogeneity in Leigh syndrome. Ann Neurol 1996;40:5–7.

725. Morris AAM, Leonard JV, Brown GK, et al. Deficiency of respiratory chain complex I is a common cause of Leigh disease. Ann Neurol 1996;40:25–30.

726. Santorelli FM, Barmada MA, Pons R, et al. Leigh-type neuropathology in Pearson syndrome associated with impaired ATP production and a novel mtDNA deletion. Neurology 1996;47:1320–1323.

727. Shoubridge EA. Cytochrome c oxidase deficiency. Am J Med Genet 2001;106: 46–52.

728. Kalimo H, Lundberg PO, Olsson Y. Familial subacute necrotizing encephalomyelopathy of the adult form (adult Leigh syndrome). Ann Neurol 1979;6:200–206.

729. Enghoff E. Uber eine an Leber's opticusatrophie erinnernde heredodegenerative krankheit. Acta Med Scand 1963;173:83–90.

730. Jellinger K, Seitelberger F. Subacute necrotizing encephalomyelopathy (Leigh). Ergeb Inn Med Kinderheilkd 1970;29:155–219.

731. Friede RL. Developmental Neuropathology. New York, Springer-Verlag, 1975: 498–501.

732. Krageloh-Mann I, Grodd W, Niemann G, et al. Assessment and therapy monitoring of Leigh disease by MRI and proton spectroscopy. Pediatr Neurol 1992;8: 60–64.

733. Howard RO, Albert DM. Ocular manifestations of subacute necrotizing encephalomyelopathy (Leigh's disease). Am J Ophthalmol 1972;74:386–393.

734. Cavanagh JB, Harding BN. Pathogenic factors underlying the lesions in Leigh's disease. Tissue responses to cellular energy deprivation and their clinico-pathological consequences. Brain 1994;117:1357–1376.

735. Hayashi N, Geraghty MT, Green WR. Ocular histopathologic study of a patient with the T8993-G point mutation in Leigh's syndrome. Ophthalmology 2000; 107:1397–1402.

736. Carelli V, Sadun AA. Optic neuropathy in LHON and Leigh syndrome. Ophthalmology 2001;108:1172–1173.

737. Tatuch Y, Christodoulou J, Feigenbaum A, et al. Heteroplasmic mitochondrial DNA mutation (T to G) at 8993 can cause Leigh disease when the percentage of abnormal mtDNA is high. Am J Hum Genet 1992;50:852.

738. Tatuch Y, Pagon RA, Vlcek B, et al. The 8993 mtDNA mutation: Heteroplasmy and clinical presentation in three families. Eur J Hum Genet 1994;2:35–43.

739. Shoffner JM, Fernhoff PM, Krawiecki NS, et al. Subacute necrotizing encephalopathy: Oxidative phosphorylation defects and the ATPase 6 point mutation. Neurology 1992;42:2168–2174.

740. Ortiz RG, Newman NJ, Shoffner JM, et al. Variable retinal and neurologic manifestations in patients harboring the mitochondrial DNA 8993 mutation. Arch Ophthalmol 1993;111:1525–1530.

741. Chol M, Lebon S, Benit P, et al. The mitochondrial DNA G13513A MELAS mutation in the NADH dehydrogenase 5 gene is a frequent cause of Leigh-like syndrome with isolated complex I deficiency. J Med Genet 2003;40:188–191.

741a. Crimi M, Galbiati S, Moroni I, et al. A missense mutation in the mitochondrial ND5 gene associated with a Leigh-MELAS overlap syndrome. Neurology 2003; 60:1857–1861.

742. Kirby DM, Kahler SG, Freckmann ML, et al. Leigh disease caused by the mitochondrial DNA G14459A mutation in unrelated families. Ann Neurol 2000; 48:102–104.

743. Drachman DA. Ophthalmoplegia plus: The neurodegenerative disorders associated with progressive external ophthalmoplegia. Arch Neurol 1968;18:654.

744. Berenberg RA, Pellock JM, DiMauro S, et al. Lumping or splitting? ''Ophthalmoplegia-plus'' or Kearns-Sayre syndrome? Ann Neurol 1977;1:37–54.

745. Pavlakis SG, Phillips PD, DiMauro S, et al. Mitochondrial myopathy, encephalopathy, lactic acidosis, and stroke-like episodes: A distinctive clinical syndrome. Ann Neurol 1984;16:481.

746. Mullie MA, Harding AE, Petty RK, et al. The retinal manifestations of mitochondrial myopathy. Arch Ophthalmol 1985;103:1825.

747. Wallace DC, Zheng X, Lott MT, et al. Familial mitochondrial encephalomyopathy (MERRF): Genetic, pathophysiological, and biochemical characterization of a mitochondrial DNA disease. Cell 1988;55:601.

748. Pavlakis SG, Rowland LP, DeVivo DC, et al. Mitochondrial myopathies and encephalomyopathies. In Plum F, ed. Advances in Contemporary Neurology. Philadelphia, FA Davis Co, 1989:95–133.

749. Fabrizi GM, Tiranti V, Mariotti C, et al. Sequence analysis of mitochondrial DNA in a new maternally inherited encephalomyopathy. J Neurol 1995;242: 490–496.

750. Hwang JM, Park HW, Kim SJ. Optic neuropathy associated with mitochondrial tRNA [Leu(UUR)] A3243G mutation. Ophthalm Genet 1997;18:101–105.

751. Das CP, Prabhakar S, Sehgal S. Mitochondrial cytopathy, encephalomyopathy, lactic acidosis, stroke like episodes with optic atrophy: A rare association. J Assoc Phys India 1999;47:639–641.

752. Sakuta R, Honzawa S, Murakami N, et al. Atypical MELAS associated with mitochondrial tRNA (Lys) gene A8296G mutation. Pediatr Neurol 2002;27: 397–400.

753. Taylor RW, Singh-Kler R, Hayes CM, et al. Progressive mitochondrial disease resulting from a novel missense mutation in the mitochondrial DNA ND3 gene. Ann Neurol 2001;50:104–107.

754. Schuelke M, Krude H, Finckh B. Septo-optic dysplasia associated with a new mitochondrial cytochrome b mutation. Ann Neurol 2002;51:388–392.

755. Cahill M, Monavari A, Naughten E, et al. Two cases of hereditary optic atrophy associated with an enzymatic defect of the respiratory chain. Metab Pediatr Syst Ophthalmol 1996;19–20:27–29.

756. Taylor RW, Birch-Machin MA, Schaefer J, et al. Deficiency of complex II of the mitochondrial respiratory chain in late-onset optic atrophy and ataxia. Ann Neurol 1996;39:224–232.

CHAPTER 12

Topical Diagnosis of Chiasmal and Retrochiasmal Disorders

Leonard A. Levin

TOPICAL DIAGNOSIS OF OPTIC CHIASMAL LESIONS

The optic chiasm is one of the most important structures in neuro-ophthalmologic diagnosis. The arrangement of visual fibers in the chiasm accounts for the characteristic visual field defects caused by such diverse lesions as tumor, inflammation, demyelination, ischemia, and infiltration. In addition, damage to neurologic and vascular structures adjacent to the chiasm produces typical additional symptoms. Thus, accurate diagnosis depends on having knowledge of both the neuro-ophthalmologic and non–neuro-ophthalmologic manifestations of chiasmal lesions. Two early papers are of fundamental importance: Adler et al. (1) described early field changes in chiasmal lesions, and Gartner (2) outlined ocular pathology in the chiasmal syndrome. A paper of historical interest describes a case of chiasmal compression from the 16th century (3).

VISUAL FIELD DEFECTS

Although there are many variations in the visual field defects caused by damage to the optic chiasm, the essential feature is some type of bitemporal defect, the hallmark of damage to fibers that cross within the chiasm. The bitemporal defects may be superior, inferior, or complete, as well as peripheral, central, or both. Bitemporal field defects are also called heteronymous field defects, a term that distinguishes them from homonymous field defects.

Visual field defects caused by lesions of the optic chiasm are often classified according to the general site of the damage. In many cases this is an oversimplification, since many lesions that arise in the region of the chiasm affect not only the entire chiasm but the intracranial optic nerves as well. Nevertheless, it is reasonable to use this approach because it helps determine the precise management of the lesion and predict the visual outcome following treatment. This chapter classifies visual field defects produced by lesions that damage the optic chiasm as a result of damage at one of three locations: (*a*) the anterior angle of the chiasm, (*b*) the body of the chiasm, or (*c*) the posterior angle of the chiasm. A small number of lesions may damage nerve fibers at the lateral aspects of the chiasm.

Lesions that Damage the Distal Portion of One Optic Nerve at the Anterior Angle of the Optic Chiasm

Traquair (4) pointed out that it is at the anterior angle of the optic chiasm that the "junction" scotoma occurs because of the separation of nasal crossed and temporal uncrossed fibers. When a small lesion damages only the crossing fibers of the ipsilateral eye, the field defect is monocular and temporal and has a midline hemianopic character that extends to the periphery of the field. When only the macular crossed fibers from one eye are damaged, the resultant field defect is still monocular and temporal but is scotomatous and located in the paracentral region. If there is extensive damage to the visual fibers in an optic nerve, an extensive field defect or total blindness develops in the ipsilateral eye. In such cases, but also in less severe cases, the crossed ventral fibers that originate from ganglion cells inferior and nasal to the fovea of the contralateral eye may also be damaged, producing a defect in the superior temporal field of the contralateral eye (Fig. 12.1).

This contralateral field defect, which occurs in an eye without other evidence of visual dysfunction, may be overlooked when kinetic perimetry is performed unless the superior temporal region of the ''normal'' eye is carefully tested by the examiner, but it is almost always detected when automated static perimetry is used (Fig. 12.1). Bird (5) detailed the findings in eight patients with the anterior chiasmal syndrome. In each case, a central scotoma was present in the visual field of the eye on the side of the lesion, and there was temporal field loss in the contralateral eye. In five cases, the contralateral field loss was in the superior temporal field only, and in two of these five cases, the peripheral field was normal by kinetic perimetry, with the defect being scotomatous and detectable only in the paracentral upper temporal field with small test objects. In the remaining three patients, the contralateral field loss was in the paracentral temporal region, without preferential loss above or below the horizontal meridian.

The mechanism by which the fibers from the contralateral eye are damaged was ascribed to their anterior extension

into the affected ipsilateral optic nerve to form the structure called Wilbrand's knee (6,7) (see Chapters 1 and 4). Horton (8) suggested that this eponymous structure is more likely an artifact that develops during atrophy of the ipsilateral optic nerve. Against this are findings of superior temporal visual field defects in patients with acute avulsion injuries of the anterior chiasm (9,10). Whatever the mechanism, the importance of identifying the usually asymptomatic field defect cannot be sufficiently stressed, because it is at this point that the examiner can make an absolute diagnosis of an anterior optic chiasmal (distal optic nerve) syndrome, at a stage at which treatment of the underlying lesion is most likely to result in improvement in visual function.

Lesions that Damage the Body of the Optic Chiasm

Lesions that damage the body of the optic chiasm characteristically produce a bitemporal defect that may be quadrantic or hemianopic and that may be peripheral, central, or a combination of both, with or without so-called splitting of the macula (Fig. 12.2). In most cases, visual acuity is normal. In some patients, however, visual acuity is diminished, even though no field defect other than a bitemporal hemianopia is present (11). When the lesion compresses the chiasm from below, such as occurs with a pituitary adenoma, the field defects follow a stereotyped pattern (12). When the peripheral fibers are principally affected, the field defects usually begin in the outer upper quadrants of both eyes (Fig. 12.3). In the field of the right eye, the defect usually progresses in a clockwise direction and in the left eye in a counterclockwise direction (13).

The field defects may be unequal in the two eyes: one

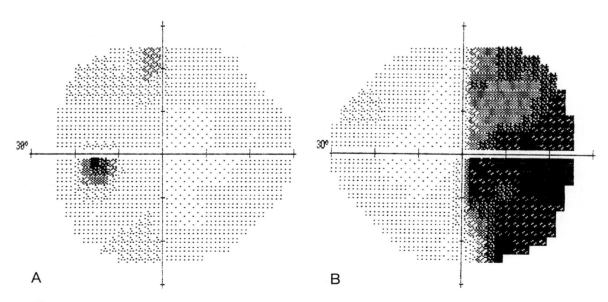

Figure 12.1. Syndrome of the distal optic nerve (anterior chiasmal syndrome). The patient was a 24-year-old woman with decreased vision in the right eye. Visual acuity was 20/25 OD and 20/20 OS. *A,* There was a small superior temporal defect in the visual field of the left eye on static perimetry, using a Humphrey 24-2 Threshold Test. This defect was not detected with kinetic perimetry. *B,* There was a dense temporal hemianopic defect in the visual field of the symptomatic right eye. The patient had a pituitary adenoma.

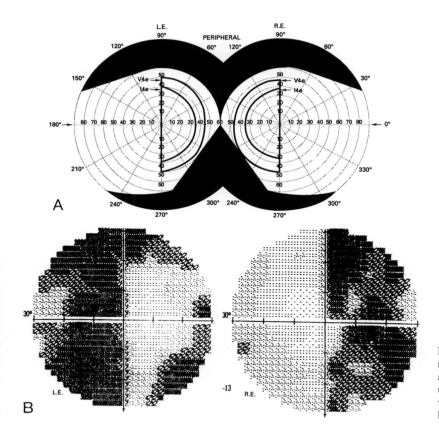

Figure 12.2. Optic chiasmal syndrome. *A*, Kinetic perimetry in a patient with a large pituitary adenoma reveals a complete bitemporal hemianopia. *B*, Static perimetry, using a Humphrey 24-2 Threshold Test, in another patient with a pituitary adenoma, reveals an incomplete bitemporal hemianopia.

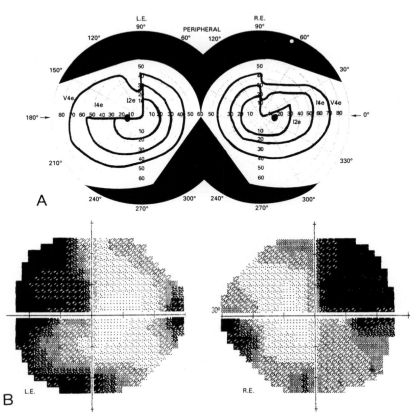

Figure 12.3. Bilateral superior temporal defects in patients with a pituitary adenoma. *A*, Kinetic perimetry in one patient demonstrates defects that are restricted to the superior temporal quadrants of the visual fields of both eyes (a bitemporal superior quadrantanopia). *B*, Static perimetry, using a Humphrey 24-2 Threshold Test, in another patient with a pituitary adenoma demonstrates bitemporal hemianopic defects that are much denser superiorly.

eye may become almost or completely blind, whereas the defect in the field of the other eye remains mild. In the charting of visual field defects resulting from pituitary adenomas and other compressive lesions, scotomas in the peripheral parts of the visual fields are usually dense and are not likely to be overlooked, although small relative paracentral scotomas are frequently missed when kinetic perimetry alone is performed. Automated perimetry can help in detecting some of the earliest signs of chiasmal compression, such as a subtle depression respecting the vertical meridian, detected by comparing pairs of thresholds across the meridian (14).

Pituitary adenomas are not, of course, the only lesions that can produce bitemporal field defects that are denser below. Suprasellar but infrachiasmal lesions, such as tuber-

culum sellae and medial sphenoid ridge meningiomas, craniopharyngiomas, and aneurysms, can also produce such defects. The field defects caused by such lesions are indistinguishable from those caused by pituitary adenomas.

Various suprasellar and suprachiasmal compressive lesions, such as tuberculum sellae meningiomas (15), craniopharyngiomas (16,17), aneurysms (18–21), and dolichoectatic anterior cerebral arteries, may damage the superior fibers of the optic chiasm, as may infiltrating lesions, such as germinomas (22–24), benign and malignant gliomas (25), and cavernous angiomas (26). The defects in the visual fields in such cases are still bitemporal but are located in the inferior rather than the superior fields of both eyes (Fig. 12.4). In addition, papilledema, which is quite unusual in patients

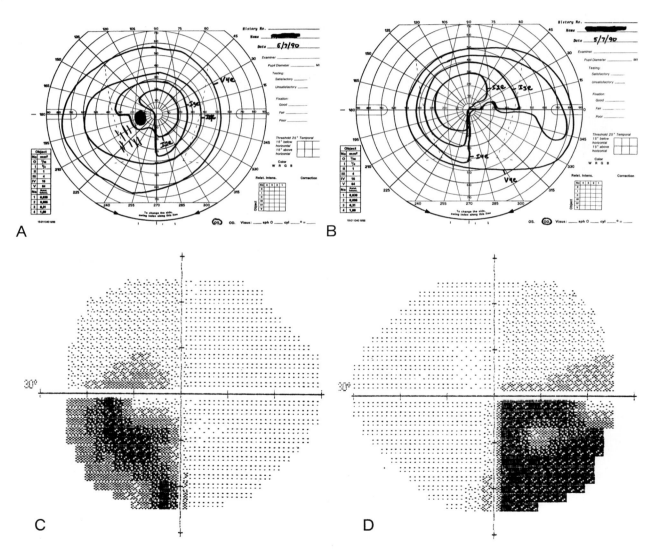

Figure 12.4. Bilateral inferior temporal field defects in a 32-year-old man with a suprasellar mass. Kinetic perimetry reveals inferior temporal quadrantic defects in the visual fields of the left (A) and right (B) eyes. The defects are scotomatous. Static perimetry, using a Humphrey 24-2 Threshold Test, in the same patient confirms the inferior temporal quadrantic nature of the defects. C, Visual field of left eye. D, Visual field of right eye. The patient underwent a craniotomy and was found to have a suprasellar suprachiasmatic germinoma.

with suprasellar, infrachiasmal lesions, is somewhat more common in suprachiasmal lesions because such lesions can extend into and occlude the third ventricle. Infiltrating tumors, such as gliomas and germinomas, as well as inflammatory and demyelinating lesions that affect the optic chiasm, may produce bitemporal field defects (Fig. 12.5), but such lesions may also produce other types of field defects, such as arcuate defects and nonspecific reduction in sensitivity, that do not necessarily correlate with the location, size, or extent of the lesion.

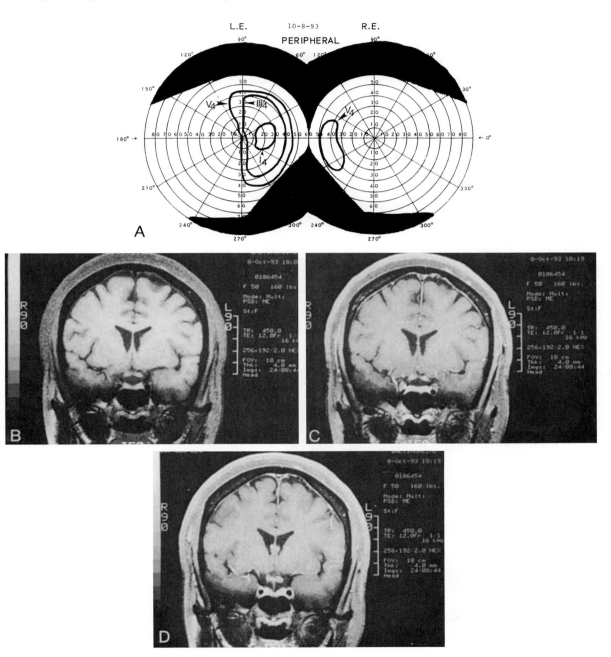

Figure 12.5. Optic chiasmal syndrome in multiple sclerosis. The patient was a 50-year-old woman with a previous history of transient lower extremity weakness who developed progressive loss of vision in both eyes. The patient reported that her vision would worsen considerably whenever she took a steam bath. Visual acuity was counting fingers at 3 feet OD and 20/100 OS. Color vision was diminished in both eyes, and there was a right relative afferent pupillary defect. *A,* Kinetic perimetry at presentation shows a complete temporal hemianopia in the field of vision of the left eye and only a small nasal island in the field of vision of the right eye. *B,* Unenhanced T1-weighted coronal magnetic resonace image shows an apparently normal optic chiasm. *C* and *D,* T1-weighted coronal magnetic resonance images after intravenous injection of contrast show enhancement of the intracranial portions of the optic nerves (*C*) and the optic chiasm (*D*). *(Figure continues.)*

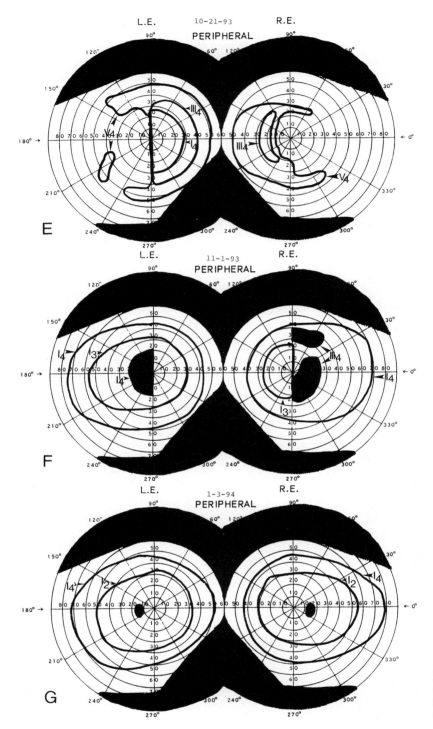

Figure 12.5. Continued. *E–G*, Kinetic perimetry after treatment with intravenous corticosteroids shows progressive improvement in visual fields over the subsequent 10 weeks. (Courtesy of Dr. John B. Kerrison.)

Although most compressive and infiltrative or inflammatory lesions that damage the body of the chiasm produce defects that are incomplete and that usually have a relative component, it is not uncommon for a tumor to produce a complete bitemporal hemianopia (Fig. 12.6). Successful de-

compression of the chiasm in such cases not infrequently results in improvement in the visual field, an outcome that might not have been expected from the severity of the visual field defect, and which can occur within days of surgery (27).

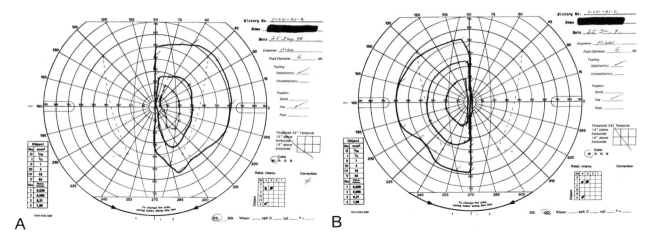

Figure 12.6. Complete bitemporal hemianopia in a 53-year-old woman from Bermuda who developed severe headache, nausea, and vomiting. She then noted difficulty reading. *A*, The visual field of the left eye shows a complete temporal hemianopia. *B*, The visual field of the right eye shows a complete temporal hemianopia. Magnetic resonance imaging revealed a large pituitary adenoma.

Lesions that Damage the Posterior Angle of the Optic Chiasm

Lesions that damage the posterior aspect of the optic chiasm produce characteristic defects in the visual fields, typically bitemporal hemianopic scotomas (28) (Fig. 12.7). Such defects may be mistaken for cecocentral scotomas and attributed to a toxic, metabolic, or even hereditary process rather than to a tumor; however, true bitemporal hemianopic scotomas are almost always associated with normal visual acuity and color perception, whereas cecocentral scotomas are invariably associated with reduced visual acuity and dyschromatopsia.

Traquair (4) wrote that a lesion that affects the posterior portion of the optic chiasm may be sufficiently focal that it damages only the crossed nasal fibers from the opposite retina, producing a monocular temporal field defect, or only the uncrossed temporal fibers from the ipsilateral eye, producing a monocular nasal field defect. In fact, this is uncommon, and most organic monocular nasal or temporal hemianopic field defects are caused by lesions affecting the optic nerve rather than the optic chiasm.

Lesions located toward the posterior aspect of the optic chiasm may damage one of the optic tracts, producing a homonymous field defect that is combined with whatever field defect has occurred from damage to the optic chiasm.

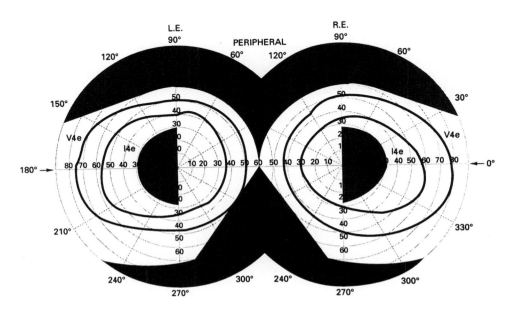

Figure 12.7. Bitemporal hemianopic scotomas in a patient with a pituitary adenoma. Such field defects result from damage to macular fibers in the posterior portion of the optic chiasm.

Bitemporal homonymous scotomas are particularly important in localizing a lesion, or at least the effects of such a lesion, to the posterior aspect of the optic chiasm. Lesions that produce such defects may be more difficult to treat successfully and are more likely to cause permanent residual field defects after surgical therapy or radiotherapy.

Lesions that Damage the Lateral Aspects of the Optic Chiasm

The lateral aspect of the optic chiasm occasionally is damaged by various tumors and, according to some authors, by pressure from the supraclinoid portion of sclerotic internal carotid arteries. When such damage occurs, both the uncrossed temporal fibers from the ipsilateral eye and crossed nasal fibers from the contralateral eye are affected, producing a contralateral homonymous hemianopic defect that cannot be differentiated from that produced by damage to the ipsilateral optic tract (29,30). Although a binasal hemianopia may rarely originate from pressure or other influences affecting the lateral aspects of the optic nerves, it probably never originates from damage to the lateral aspects of the optic chiasm.

Visual Field Defects Caused by Lesions that Damage the Optic Chiasm After Initially Damaging the Optic Nerve or Optic Tract

If there is extension of a lesion from the optic nerve or optic tract to the optic chiasm, the blind eye is usually on the side of the lesion. For example, if a patient with a blind right eye exhibits a defect in the temporal field of the left eye, the lesion obviously is on the right. Similarly, if there has been a left homonymous hemianopia from a right optic tract lesion and if there is extension of the lesion to affect the optic chiasm, blindness (or an extensive field defect) develops in the right eye. Conversely, if a lesion of the optic chiasm that has produced a bitemporal hemianopia extends to the right optic nerve, it will eventually produce loss of vision of the right eye. Similarly, if a chiasmal lesion extends into the right optic tract, there is again loss of vision of the right eye. In other words, if there is extension from an optic nerve or optic tract to the optic chiasm, the blind eye is on the side of the lesion, whereas when there is extension of a lesion from the optic chiasm to the optic nerve or to the optic tract, the blind eye is on the side of extension of the lesion. In such cases, it may be impossible to determine the nature and extent of the pathologic process from an examination of visual sensory function, and particularly visual fields, alone. Rather, it is the history of visual loss and its progression that provides an explanation of the visual findings.

ETIOLOGIES OF THE OPTIC CHIASMAL SYNDROME

Damage to the optic chiasm can occur from the direct or indirect effects of a variety of lesions. Bitemporal field defects are usually caused by damage to the optic chiasm from a cerebral mass lesion (31,32). In Rosen's (33) series, for example, tumors accounted for 80% of the cases of bitem-

poral field defects. The most common causes of an optic chiasmal syndrome are pituitary adenomas, suprasellar meningiomas, craniopharyngiomas, gliomas, and aneurysms originating from the internal carotid artery (34–38). Chiasmitis (39), particularly related to multiple sclerosis, sarcoi-

Table 12.1
Unusual Causes of Optic Chiasmal Syndromes

Cause	References
Aneurysm of basilar artery	21
Arachnoid cyst	43,44
Arteriovenous malformations (AVMs)	45–47
Brucellosis	48
Cavernous angioma	26,47,49–55
Chondroma	56
Choristoma	57
Choroid plexus papilloma	58
Cysticercosis	59–62
Demyelinating disease	63–69
Dolichoectatic sclerotic intracranial internal carotid arteries	70,71
Ectopic cerebellum	72
Ependymoma	73
Ethchlorvynol (Placidyl) abuse	66
Fibrous dysplasia	43
Ganglioglioma	74–77
Germinoma	24,78–80
Glioblastoma multiforme	81
Granular cell tumor of neurohypophysis	82,83
Inflammation (presumed) from Epstein-Barr viral infection	84
Ischemia from small vessel occlusive disease	85–87
Langerhans cell histiocytosis	43,88–90
Lymphoma	91,92
Malignant melanoma	93
Medulloblastoma	94
Metastatic carcinoma	95–97
Multiple myeloma	98
Nasopharyngeal carcinoma	43
Optochiasmatic arachnoiditis	99–101
Pachymeningitis associated with rheumatoid arthritis	102
Paraganglioma	103
Pituitary abscess	104
Plasmacytoma	98
Pneumatocele	105
Rathke's cleft cyst	106–111
Sarcoid granuloma	112,113
Sarcoid occurring in a pituitary adenoma	114
Septum pellucidum cyst	115
Sinus histiocytosis with lymphadenopathy	116
Sphenoid sinus mucocele	117
Syphilitic gumma	43
Toxoplasmosis	67
Tuberculoma	101,118,119
Varicella-zoster virus	120
Varix	121
Vasculitis	67,69
Venous angioma	122,123
Vitamin B_{12} deficiency	69
Whipple's disease	124

dosis (40), or systemic lupus erythematosus (41,42), is not uncommon. Other unusual causes of an optic chiasmal syndrome are listed in Table 12.1.

During pregnancy, preexisting intrasellar and suprasellar tumors, most commonly pituitary adenomas, may become symptomatic (125,126). In most cases, visual symptoms regress after delivery or abortion. In addition, the pituitary gland itself enlarges during the third trimester of pregnancy and may become sufficiently enlarged so that it compresses the chiasm, producing visual manifestations (127). In such cases, visual symptoms resolve spontaneously following delivery. Another cause of an optic chiasmal syndrome that occurs most often during or shortly after pregnancy is lymphocytic adenohypophysitis, an autoimmune disorder of unknown etiology (128–131), which can rarely cause pituitary apoplexy (132).

Extension of the subarachnoid space into the sella turcica through a deficient diaphragma sellae results in the empty sella syndrome (133). A primary empty sella syndrome occurs spontaneously and may be associated with an arachnoid cyst. It is rarely associated with significant visual acuity loss or visual field defects (134); however, a secondary empty sella syndrome follows surgery or radiation therapy in the sellar region. Patients in whom this syndrome develops may develop a true chiasmal syndrome, characterized by bitemporal field loss with and without a reduction in visual acuity and an acquired dyschromatopsia (135,136).

Occasionally the chiasm fails to develop, a syndrome called achiasmia or the non-decussating retinal-fugal fiber syndrome (137,138). In this syndrome the nasal retinal fibers do not decussate, resulting in routing of the fibers corresponding to the temporal visual field to the ipsilateral visual cortex (139). However, the visual fields are full (137), presumably as a result of cortical reorganization (139). These patients may have congenital nystagmus with or without seesaw nystagmus (138).

A complete bitemporal hemianopia can be produced by trauma to the optic chiasm (140–148) (Fig. 12.8). This can occur as a result of indirect injury (149), similar to that seen in indirect traumatic optic neuropathy (see Chapter 9), avulsion from globe traction (9,10), direct injury from a foreign body (e.g., chopsticks [150]), or sellar fracture (145). The most likely pathologic mechanisms in traumatic optic chiasmal syndrome are contusion necrosis (151) or avulsion (9). The syndrome of traumatic optic neuropathy is discussed in more detail in Chapter 9.

Clinical cases are occasionally observed in which bitemporal field defects occur not from a tumor compressing the chiasm but from a posterior fossa lesion that has caused increased intracranial pressure and consequent compression of the chiasm by an enlarged third ventricle. Most of these cases are also associated with papilledema. Wilbrand and Saenger (152) first observed a case of cerebellar tumor with associated hydrocephalus in which there was primary optic atrophy and bitemporal hemianopic scotomas. Cushing (153) and Sinclair and Dott (154) subsequently reported similar cases. Wagener and Cusick (155) initially suggested that dilation of the optic recess in the anterior extremity of the third ventricle may press directly upon the optic chiasm, producing a typical bitemporal defect. Hughes (156) noted that if the chiasm is in normal position, situated over the diaphragma sellae and projecting backward over the dorsum sellae, or is postfixed, overlying and behind the dorsum sellae, the third ventricle may tend to enlarge against its posterior aspect and spread over its superior surface. As a result, a bilateral depression of the inferior temporal central field occurs. On the other hand, if the chiasm is prefixed, overlying the diaphragma sellae or resting in the sulcus chiasmatis, the ventricle will tend to exert its pressure effects against the posterior inferior aspect of the chiasm and may even appear from beneath the chiasm between both optic nerves, pushing the nerves laterally. In such cases, bilateral central scotomas, bilateral nasal and arcuate defects, or even bilateral superior hemianopic scotomas could develop.

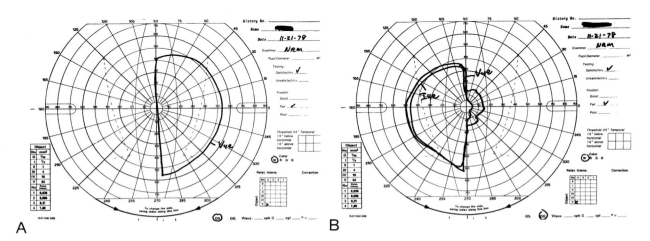

Figure 12.8. Complete bitemporal hemianopia in a 24-year-old man who was severely injured in a motor vehicle accident. Neuroimaging revealed no evidence of an intracranial mass lesion. Visual acuity was 20/20 OU. *A*, The visual field of the left eye shows a complete temporal hemianopia. *B*, The visual field of the right eye shows a complete temporal hemianopia except for about 15° of macular sparing. The field defects did not improve over a 5-year follow-up period.

Optic chiasmal syndromes can be iatrogenic. Most often, this occurs after attempted removal of a lesion compressing or infiltrating the chiasm. Chiasmal damage most often occurs during surgery to remove a suprasellar meningioma or craniopharyngioma and least often after surgery to remove a pituitary adenoma or to clip an intracranial aneurysm. A catheter placed in the lateral ventricle for hydrocephalus can migrate into the third ventricle and cause a bitemporal field defect (157,158). A chiasmal syndrome can also occur from exuberant packing of the sphenoid sinus with fat following transsphenoidal resection of a pituitary adenoma (159,160). In such cases, the fat is forced superiorly and compresses the inferior aspects of the optic nerves and optic chiasm. There is often immediate improvement after emergency removal of the fat. Similarly, a pneumatocele can result arising from the adjacent sphenoid sinus after surgery, for example if the patient sneezes (105,161). As mentioned above, the chiasm can prolapse into an empty sella (162), presumably as a consequence of traction from postoperative scar tissue.

Another cause of iatrogenic chiasm dysfunction is from radiation (163–166). This phenomenon appears to be related to a high dosage given over a short period of time. Radiation necrosis of the optic nerves and chiasm may begin months to several years after radiation. This syndrome is discussed in the section on radiation optic neuropathy (see Chapter 7). Finally, use of dopamine agonists for the treatment of prolactin-secreting pituitary adenomas can result in prolapse of the chiasm into the pituitary fossa (167–169). This syndrome is best treated by reducing the dosage of the dopamine agonist.

The noted neuro-ophthalmologist Simmons Lessell once remarked, "Someday, someone will report a meatball" compressing the optic chiasm, a prediction that reflects the enormous variety of lesions that can produce a chiasmal syndrome, including one that could result from eating an undercooked meatball (59). More important than the specific pathology of the lesion is the ability of the examiner to make the correct clinical diagnosis of an optic chiasmal syndrome at the earliest opportunity, so that confirmation by neuroimaging can be performed in a timely fashion and effective management initiated before permanent visual loss occurs.

MASQUERADERS OF THE OPTIC CHIASMAL SYNDROME

Manchester and Calhoun (170) reported bitemporal visual field defects in five patients with dominant hereditary optic atrophy. These and similar patients more likely had cecocentral scotomas, diagnosed by the crossing of the vertical midline and association with more severely reduced visual acuity than would be expected from the field defect alone. Similarly, cecocentral scotomas from toxic, metabolic, or other hereditary optic neuropathies can be confused with bitemporal hemianopias (171). Patients with nasal fundus ectasia may also have temporal field defects, which can be confused with the optic chiasmal syndrome. These pseudotemporal field defects can be distinguished by their failure to respect the vertical meridian and their diminution when minus refractive lenses are used in the perimeter. Since it is not un-

common for the pituitary gland to be physiologically convex (172), it behooves the clinician to search for other causes of bitemporal defects when the chiasm is radiographically normal and the visual field defects are atypical.

PATHOPHYSIOLOGY OF THE OPTIC CHIASMAL SYNDROME

The mechanism by which the chiasm is compressed from below was studied by Hedges (173), who used normal, adult, fresh necropsy material. He removed the pituitary gland and inserted the balloon tip of a Foley catheter into the sella turcica and then expanded it. As the balloon expanded and the optic chiasm was elevated, the crossing fibers were first affected, initially the lower nasal and later the upper nasal. The uncrossed upper temporal fibers were put "on stretch," whereas the lower temporal fibers, subserving the upper nasal visual field, were relatively unaffected. Hedges concluded that the results of this experiment explained the relative sparing of the upper nasal visual field in even advanced optic chiasmal syndromes. However, Harrington (174) disagreed with this theory and believed that the explanation for relative sparing of the superior nasal visual field in patients with severe damage to the optic chiasm was related in some way to the blood supply of the chiasm, although he gave no definitive evidence to support this contention.

Support for an ischemic mechanism was provided by Schneider et al. (175), who reported two patients with visual acuity and field loss thought to be secondary to infarction of the chiasmal and prechiasmal regions, associated with a chiasmal glioma in one case and a pituitary adenoma in the second case. Although many authors support the concept that ischemia is the primary explanation for the visual acuity and visual field loss that accompanies mass lesions that compress the optic nerves and chiasm, the role of axonal transport and its disruption from compression has yet to be examined in detail. Clearly if there is resolution of visual loss after relief of compression (27,176), permanent axonal loss cannot have occurred, absent axonal regeneration. Instead, conduction block, demyelination, and loss of axonal transport are more probable causes of decreased vision as a result of chiasmal or optic nerve compression. Finally, patients receiving radiation to the region of the optic chiasm may develop progressive acuity and field loss caused by radiation necrosis. The mechanism of radiation chiasmal damage probably reflects damage to endothelial cells, similar to the situation in radiation optic neuropathy (177).

NEURO-OPHTHALMOLOGIC SYMPTOMS ASSOCIATED WITH OPTIC CHIASMAL SYNDROMES

The most common complaints of patients with lesions that damage the optic chiasm are progressive loss of central acuity and dimming of the visual field, particularly in its temporal portion. In addition, bitemporal field defects, whether complete or scotomatous, may produce two other types of visual symptoms (178,179). One type consists of a disturbance of depth perception, and patients with this symptom complain of difficulties with such tasks as threading

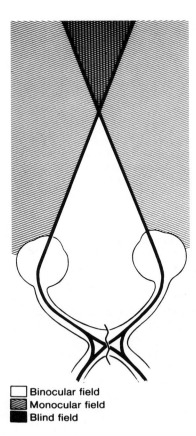

☐ Binocular field
▨ Monocular field
■ Blind field

Figure 12.9. The blind triangular area of the binocular visual field that occurs just beyond fixation in patients with a complete bitemporal hemianopia. Such patients have intact binocular vision in the triangular area up to fixation and intact monocular vision temporal and anterior to the triangular blind region. (Redrawn from Kirkham TH. The ocular symptomatology of pituitary tumors. Proc R Soc Med 1972;65:517–518.)

needles, sewing, and using precision tools. In such patients, convergence results in crossing of the two blind temporal hemifields. This produces a completely blind triangular area of field with its apex at fixation (Fig. 12.9). The image of an object posterior to fixation falls on blind nasal retinas and thus disappears. Testing for stereopsis can also be helpful in the clinical testing of patients with suspected chiasmal disorders (180).

Patients with bitemporal field defects may also experience diplopia or difficulty reading caused by a horizontal or vertical deviation of images unassociated with an ocular motor nerve paresis (179,181–184). Kirkham (179) called this phenomenon the "hemifield slide phenomenon." Such patients have difficulty reading because of doubling or loss of printed letters or words. The problems encountered by these patients result from loss of the normal partial overlap of the temporal field of one eye and the nasal visual field of the contralateral eye. This overlap normally permits fusion of images and helps to stabilize ocular alignment in patients with vertical or horizontal phorias. Because their remaining nasal visual fields represent only the temporal projection from each eye, patients with bitemporal hemianopia do not have a physio-

logic linkage between the two remaining hemifields. In such patients, a preexisting minor phoria becomes a tropia, and the consequent vertical or horizontal separation or overlap of the two heteronymous hemifields causes intermittent sensory difficulties (Fig. 12.10). A similar result may be seen in patients with heteronymous altitudinal field defects (185) (see Chapter 4).

Patients with lesions that damage the optic chiasm as well as one or more of the ocular motor nerves in the subarachnoid space or within the cavernous sinus on one or both sides may experience diplopia. The diplopia may be painless or painful depending on whether the trigeminal nerve is also affected. In some cases, individual oculomotor, trochlear, or abducens nerve pareses occur in association with a visual field defect that indicates optic chiasmal dysfunction. In other cases, multiple unilateral or bilateral ocular motor nerve pareses occur. Strabismus associated with evidence of single or multiple ocular motor nerve pareses in a patient with a bitemporal field defect suggests a process extrinsic to the chiasm rather than an infiltrative intrinsic lesion, unless there has been pituitary apoplexy that caused rapid chiasmal expansion.

Occasionally, patients with mass lesions compressing the chiasm complain of photophobia (186,187). This occurs via an unknown mechanism, distinct from thalamic dazzle

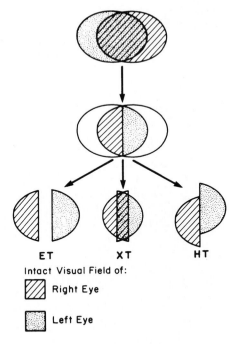

ET   XT   HT

Intact Visual Field of:

▨ Right Eye

▦ Left Eye

Figure 12.10. The hemifield slide phenomenon experienced by patients with bitemporal hemianopias. Patients with a preexisting exophoria or intermittent exotropia will have overlapping of the intact nasal fields, whereas patients with a preexisting esophoria or intermittent esotropia will have separation of the nasal hemifields, causing a blind area in the center of the field. Patients with preexisting hyperdeviations will complain of vertical separation of images crossing the vertical meridian. (Redrawn from Kirkham TH. The ocular symptomatology of pituitary tumors. Proc R Soc Med 1972;65:517–518.)

(188,189). Patients may also have decreased contrast sensitivity in the temporal hemifield, testing of which may be used for early detection of chiasmal compression (190).

NEURO-OPHTHALMOLOGIC SIGNS ASSOCIATED WITH OPTIC CHIASMAL SYNDROMES

Patients with chiasmal syndromes may or may not have ophthalmoscopically apparent nerve fiber layer or optic atrophy when first examined. However, when atrophy is present in patients with bitemporal hemianopia, its pattern is quite specific, appearing as a band across the disc (i.e., "band atrophy"). The reason for this is that degeneration occurs in fibers from peripheral and macular retinal ganglion cells located nasal to the fovea. Axons from peripheral retinal ganglion cells located nasal to both the disc and fovea course directly to the nasal aspect of the disc. Fibers from retinal ganglion cells located between the disc and fovea make up a small portion of the superior and inferior arcuate bundles, along with a larger number of fibers from peripheral temporal retinal ganglion cells. Finally, fibers from nasal macular retinal ganglion cells course directly to the temporal disc. Thus, when there is atrophy of nasal fibers, the normal striations of the nerve fiber layer are lost both nasal to the disc and in the papillomacular region. In addition, nerve fiber bundle slits or defects can be observed in the superior and

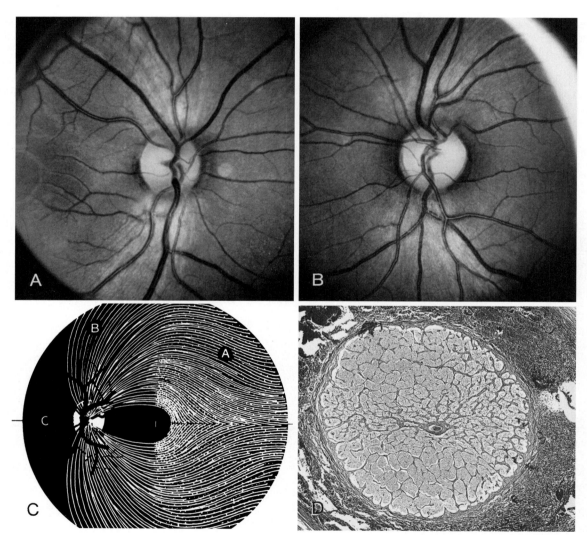

Figure 12.11.   Optic chiasmal syndrome. *A and B,* Both right and left optic discs show "band" atrophy with corresponding loss of nerve fibers from ganglion cells located nasal to the fovea. *C,* Diagram of nerve fiber loss in patients with temporal hemianopia. Regions marked A, B, and C denote areas of nerve fiber layer preservation, partial loss, and complete loss, respectively. *D,* Transverse section of orbital optic nerve in a patient with a temporal hemianopia shows "band" or "bowtie" pattern of atrophy with relative sparing of the superior and inferior portions of the nerve. (*C,* From Hoyt WF, Kommerell G. Der Fundus oculi bei Homonyer Hemianopia. Klin Monatsbl Augenheilkd 1973;162:456–464. *D,* From Unsöld R, Hoyt WF. Band atrophy of the optic nerve. Arch Ophthalmol 1980;98:1637–1638.)

inferior arcuate bundles. The optic disc shows corresponding atrophy at its nasal and temporal regions with relative sparing of the superior and inferior portions, where the majority of spared temporal fibers (subserving nasal field) enter (Fig. 12.11). Thus, the optic atrophy occupies a more or less horizontal band across the disc, wider nasally than temporally (191).

It is perhaps clinically more useful when atrophy is *absent* in patients with chiasmal (or optic nerve) compression than when it is present. Whereas patients with significant nerve fiber bundle defects and optic atrophy occasionally have impressive return of both acuity and field when successful decompression is obtained, patients with normal-appearing fundi frequently have complete return of visual function with successful decompression. It is crucial that decompression be carried out as soon as possible in these patients.

Papilledema is frequently associated with suprachiasmal tumors but rarely with intrasellar tumors. It is more commonly seen as a result of pre- and postchiasmal tumors.

The loss of retinal ganglion cells associated with damage to their axons from chiasmal compression (192) can be detected electrophysiologically with the pattern electroretinogram (193,194). Because retinal ganglion cell loss is irreversible, the presence of an abnormal-pattern electroretinogram presages a worse prognosis (194).

Most patients with lesions that affect the optic chiasm have no disturbances of ocular alignment or motility. Nevertheless, as mentioned above, when the ocular motor nerves are also damaged in the subarachnoid space or within the cavernous sinus, patients will have a strabismus with the characteristics of an oculomotor nerve paresis, trochlear nerve paresis, abducens nerve paresis, or a combination of these (Fig. 12.12). When the ocular motor nerves are damaged within the cavernous sinus, there may also be evidence of a trigeminal sensory (but not motor) neuropathy. In addition, if the oculosympathetic fibers are damaged, frequently with concurrent abducens nerve damage, there will be a postganglionic Horner's syndrome characterized by ipsilateral ptosis and a smaller but normally reactive pupil. When both the oculomotor nerve and oculosympathetic fibers are affected, the clinical picture will be one of an oculomotor nerve paresis with a small pupil that will be normally reactive if the paresis is pupil-sparing or poorly or nonreactive if the oculomotor nerve paresis has damaged pupillomotor fibers.

Not all patients with optic chiasmal lesions who develop strabismus do so because of damage to one or more ocular motor nerves. In some cases, as noted above, there is decompensation of a preexisting phoria caused by loss of the normal nasotemporal visual field overlap in patients with a complete or scotomatous bitemporal field defect (hemifield slide). This results in a manifest comitant strabismus, which may be vertical or horizontal.

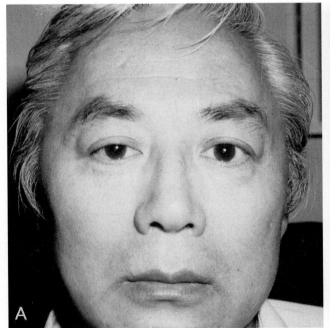
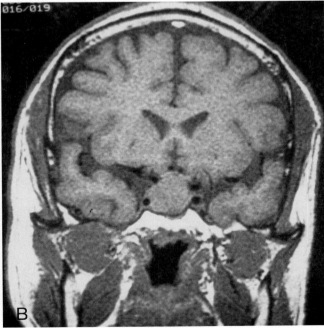

Figure 12.12. Partial oculomotor nerve paresis in a patient with a pituitary adenoma. The patient was referred to the Neuro-Ophthalmology Unit of the Johns Hopkins Hospital by an internist who thought he had a Horner's syndrome. Visual acuity was 20/20 OU. The pupils were isocoric and normally reactive. *A,* There is a moderate right ptosis. The patient also had mild limitation of upgaze in the right eye, and he developed a right hypotropia of about 4 prism-diopters on upgaze. A diagnosis of a partial right oculomotor nerve paresis was made, and magnetic resonance imaging was obtained. *B,* Noncontrast T1-weighted coronal magnetic resonance image reveals a sellar mass with suprasellar extension and invasion of both cavernous sinuses. The lesion was found to be a pituitary adenoma.

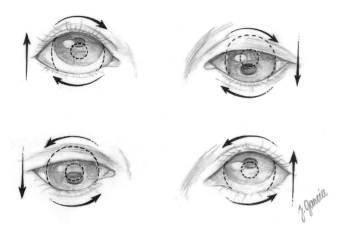

Figure 12.13. Seesaw nystagmus. As the right eye elevates, it also intorts. At the same time, the left eye depresses and extorts. The right eye then depresses and extorts, as the left eye elevates and intorts.

The unusual phenomenon of seesaw nystagmus may occur in patients with tumors of the diencephalon and chiasmal regions (195–198). This condition is characterized by synchronous alternating elevation and intorsion of one eye and depression and extorsion of the opposite eye (Fig. 12.13). The cause of seesaw nystagmus is unknown, but it may be related to damage to structures near the interstitial nucleus of Cajal, but not the nucleus itself (199–201). Rarely, seesaw nystagmus occurs in the absence of a brain stem or diencephalic lesion (202), for instance in congenital absence of the chiasm (203).

Lesions causing a chiasmal syndrome may arise from or extend to the hypothalamus. Such patients may develop dia-

betes insipidus and hypothalamic hypopituitarism; prepubertal children may also suffer both growth retardation and delayed sexual development; and young children and infants may have severe failure to thrive.

"CHIASMAL SYNDROME" OF CUSHING

In 1930, Cushing described the importance of optic atrophy and bitemporal field defects in adults as indicative of tumor when the sella turcica seemed normal in the plain lateral skull x-ray (153). This syndrome is most often produced by suprasellar meningiomas, aneurysms, and craniopharyngiomas. This notable contribution was once of great value in eliminating, or at least reducing, misdiagnosis of sinusitis and retrobulbar optic neuritis as common causes for slowly progressive bilateral loss of vision. Optic atrophy in such cases may be very slight, or the optic discs may remain normal in appearance for months despite pronounced loss of vision and extensive defects in the visual fields. The bitemporal field defects in some cases are extremely mild and detected only by careful kinetic perimetry or automated static perimetry. Finally, the normalcy of the sella turcica may only be relative. Since Cushing (153) described this syndrome, there have been substantial advances in neuroimaging. With the almost universal availability of computed tomography (CT) scanning and magnetic resonance (MR) imaging, most patients with progressive visual loss no longer undergo plain skull x-rays. Cushing's syndrome of the chiasm is thus more important for its historical significance than for its place in current neuro-ophthalmologic diagnosis. Nevertheless, there are still some areas in the world in which skull radiographs are used as the sole or initial step in assessing patients with an optic chiasmal syndrome. In such cases, the triad that represents Cushing's syndrome remains a useful clinical entity.

TOPICAL DIAGNOSIS OF RETROCHIASMAL VISUAL FIELD DEFECTS

With few exceptions, unilateral lesions of the visual sensory pathway posterior to the optic chiasm—affecting the optic tract, lateral geniculate body, optic radiation, or striate cortex—produce homonymous visual field defects without loss of visual acuity. When such defects are complete, they do not, in themselves, permit localization. In such instances, the clinician must rely on other symptoms and signs of neurologic disease or on neuroimaging to define both the area of damage and the etiology of the lesion (204). Nevertheless, some general comments about retrochiasmal field defects are worth noting before launching into a comprehensive discussion of the clinical syndromes associated with specific regions of the retrochiasmal visual sensory system.

Homonymous defects in the visual fields characteristically develop slowly if they are caused by intracranial tumors and rapidly when they originate from vascular processes such as hemorrhage or infarction. This applies wherever the lesion may be situated.

In the instance of homonymous hemianopia arising from cerebral tumor, a paper by Bender and Kanzer (205) is valuable. They noted progression of the field defects from the periphery of the field to its center in homonymous hemiano-

pias caused by brain tumors (206–208). When the cerebral tumor is removed or the visual system is decompressed, improvement first occurs in the central region and continues toward the periphery. Bender and Kanzer (205) also observed that defects for colored objects invariably appeared before disturbances for either form or for black-and-white objects. This observation may constitute another valid reason for including colored stimuli or objects in examination of visual fields. This should be done not only when testing for evidence of optic nerve disease but also when testing for chiasmal and retrochiasmal lesions, particularly when no defect has been found using standard kinetic perimetry with either white light or white test objects. Static perimetry seems to be as sensitive as manual testing using colored objects (especially red) for detecting subtle visual field defects (see Chapter 2).

The onset of homonymous hemianopias arising as the result of vascular lesions is sudden. Such defects include complete homonymous quadrantanopias and hemianopias, incomplete homonymous quadrantanopias and hemianopias with varying degrees of congruity, and homonymous paracentral scotomas. When and if improvement occurs, the central field resolves first, and such improvement may be followed by gradual enlargement of the peripheral fields if they have been affected.

Younge (209) described midline tilting between seeing and nonseeing areas in the perimetric evaluation of homonymous hemianopic field defects. A deviation from the absolute vertical meridian is often found when careful perimetry is performed in such patients. Stone et al. (210,211) and others (212–214) found that in nonhuman primates, a certain percentage of retinal ganglion cells nasal to the vertical midline bisecting the fovea have axons that do not cross at the optic chiasm, and a certain percentage of ganglion cells temporal to the same vertical midline have axons that do cross in the chiasm. It is not surprising, then, that there is some variation from a perfectly vertical separation of seeing and nonseeing field. Such a variation is rarely more than a few degrees (see below).

In 1962 Smith reported on the causes of homonymous hemianopia in 100 patients (215). Forty-three patients had proven etiologies, with the location of the lesion being in the occipital lobe in 12 patients, parietal lobe in 17 patients, and temporal lobe in 14 patients. Fifty-seven patients had lesions in which the location was assumed on the basis of clinical evidence alone. Of these patients, 27 had lesions presumed to be in the occipital lobe, 16 had lesions presumed to be in the parietal lobe, and 10 had lesions presumed to be in the temporal lobe. In addition, three patients had lesions presumed to be in the optic tract, and one patient had a presumed lateral geniculate lesion. Thus, almost 40% of patients with homonymous hemianopias had proven or presumed occipital lobe lesions, whereas 33% had parietal lobe lesions and only 24% had temporal lobe lesions. Optic tract and lateral geniculate lesions were rare. Smith found only a 42% incidence of vascular etiology in his series, compared with a 38% incidence of intracranial tumor.

Trobe et al. (216) reviewed 104 cases of isolated homonymous hemianopia and found, as might be expected, that the vast majority (86%) were caused by vascular disease in the territory of the posterior cerebral artery. Another three patients were believed to have suffered infarctions in the territory of the middle cerebral artery, bringing the total percentage of isolated homonymous hemianopias thought to be caused by infarction to 89%. These findings are similar to those of Shubova (217), although only 21 of the 104 cases reported by Trobe et al. (216) had etiologies proven angiographically or histologically, and the study was performed before the availability of modern neuroimaging. The 12 cases not caused by vascular lesions included occipital porencephaly, neoplasm, multiple sclerosis, and abscess. Interestingly, two thirds of the patients were between the ages of 50 and 70 years, and all five patients with isolated homonymous hemianopias under age 30 had nonvascular causes for their field defects. Older patients with isolated homonymous hemianopia apparently have an exceedingly high probability of vascular lesions, whereas younger patients may have either congenital or acquired nonvascular etiologies.

In 1986, Fujino et al. (218) retrospectively reviewed the location and causes of homonymous hemianopia in 140 patients. Patients were between the ages of 9 and 86 years,

with the greatest number in the sixth decade. The visual field defects were not necessarily isolated, and the location and properties of the underlying lesions were confirmed by surgery or CT scanning in about half the cases. Fifty-one percent of patients had occipital lobe pathology, 29% had lesions of the optic radiation, and 21% had lesions in the region of the optic tract and lateral geniculate. Vascular causes, including infarction, hemorrhage, and arteriovenous malformations, were responsible for 71% of cases and mass lesions, including tumors and abscesses, for another 19%. Other etiologies included trauma, inflammation, degeneration, and presumed demyelinating disease. Molia et al. (219) reported the development of homonymous hemianopic field defects in two children with intracranial shunts. In both cases the field defect was caused by displacement of the shunt catheter.

Given the preceding, it should be self-evident that neuroimaging (preferably MR imaging) should be the first diagnostic procedure used to determine the location and etiology of a homonymous hemianopia, following a complete history and examination.

Special consideration is given here to a syndrome originally emphasized by Hoyt et al. (220) and later by Bajandas et al. (221): homonymous hemioptic (hemianopic) hypoplasia. In this disorder, patients with cerebral hemiatrophy, presumably from fetal vascular insufficiency or trauma, suffer from mental retardation, a seizure disorder, congenital hemiplegia, and an ipsilateral complete homonymous hemianopia. Such patients have classic hemianopic ophthalmoscopic findings in the ocular fundi, with the eye ipsilateral to the hemispheric defect showing a slightly small optic disc with mild temporal pallor and impressive loss of the nerve fibers subserving ganglion cells temporal to the fovea. The superior and inferior arcuate bundles in such eyes are thus poorly visible. In the eye contralateral to the hemispheric defect, the optic disc is often small and oval, with a horizontal band of atrophy and loss of nerve fibers from ganglion cells nasal to the fovea, as occurs in patients with bitemporal hemianopia from lesions of the optic chiasm. Whether the ophthalmoscopic and histologic changes observed in these patients occur from retrograde degeneration after embryonic damage to the optic tract or from transsynaptic degeneration after damage to the optic radiation or striate cortex is unknown; indeed, either mechanism may be responsible in individual cases (222). It would appear that in humans, clinically apparent transsynaptic damage to the visual system occurs almost exclusively with prenatal or perinatal brain damage, including brain injury with porencephaly, cerebral ischemia, congenital ganglioglioma, and vascular malformations associated with Sturge-Weber syndrome (222–226). Other congenital lesions, such as arteriovenous malformations of the retrogeniculate visual pathways, may indirectly damage the optic tract or lateral geniculate body either prenatally or postnatally from the progressive effects of abnormal deep venous drainage (222). Patients with such lesions have retrograde optic nerve degeneration, and they will show homonymous hemioptic hypoplasia if the insult occurs early enough in development.

Another interesting phenomenon that occurs in some patients with congenital homonymous hemianopia is the development of exotropia and anomalous retinal correspondence (227–229). It is thought that in these patients the exotropia is a compensatory mechanism, allowing for anomalous retinal correspondence and, consequently, "panoramic" viewing. This "panoramic" vision facilitates horizontal enlargement of the visual field, with a shift of the hemianopic border toward the side of the defect. Whether the phenomenon is truly compensatory or merely the coincidental occurrence of two common congenital abnormalities of the visual system remains unclear. However, surgical correction of the exotropia may run the risk of not only intractable paradoxical diplopia, but also possible horizontal constriction of the visual field (229).

TOPICAL DIAGNOSIS OF OPTIC TRACT LESIONS

Although lesions of the optic tracts are infrequently recognized, they are of great importance because they represent the first region beyond the optic chiasm where lesions produce a homonymous field defect (Fig. 12.14). Common causes are tumor, vascular processes, demyelinating disease, and trauma (Figs. 12.15 and 12.16). In his series of 100 consecutive homonymous hemianopias, Smith (215) found only 3 that he attributed to a lesion of the optic tract. His criteria were extreme incongruity, a negative optokinetic response, a Behr's pupil (inequality of the pupils with the larger pupil on the side of the hemianopia), and evidence of neurologic disease in neighboring structures. Fujino et al. (178) reported 16 patients with lesions referable to the optic tract among their 140 patients with homonymous hemianopia. The causes were vascular in five, tumor in four, and miscellaneous in seven. Savino et al. (230) examined 21 patients who were thought to have lesions of the optic tract. The etiologies were primarily tumors, although one patient had demyelinating disease and two patients had suffered trauma.

Patients with optic tract lesions often have specific findings that permit the recognition of the location of the lesion on clinical grounds. In 1967, Burde (231) theorized that all patients with a complete homonymous hemianopia caused by an isolated optic tract lesion should have a relative afferent defect in the eye with the temporal field loss (contralateral to the side of the lesion). He made this assumption based on three phenomena: (*a*) the nasal visual field is considerably smaller than the temporal field; (*b*) the pupillomotor fibers within the visual sensory pathway hemidecussate in the optic chiasm along with or as part of the visual axons; and (*c*) the pupillomotor fibers are present within the optic tract for most of its extent. Bell and Thompson (232) subsequently confirmed Burde's (231) theory when they examined four patients with optic tract lesions. Each patient had normal visual acuity in both eyes, a complete homonymous hemianopia, and "band" atrophy in the eye on the side of the hemianopia (contralateral to the lesion). Color vision as tested with the Hardy-Rand-Rittler pseudoisochromatic plates was normal, and a Pulfrich test gave normal responses in all patients. However, all patients had an overt relative afferent pupillary defect in the eye on the side of the hemianopia (with the temporal field loss). Bell and Thompson (232) believed that the most likely etiology for this finding is that the temporal field is 60–70% larger than the nasal field, thus creating a disparity with respect to light input from the two eyes to the mesencephalic pupillary center. However, more recent evidence suggests that the relative afferent pupillary defect associated with an optic tract lesion is due to crossing of some fibers from the temporal retina destined for the pretectal nuclei, and subserving the pupillary light reflex (233).

O'Connor et al. (234) produced a relative afferent pupillary defect in two monkeys by experimental lesioning of the contralateral optic tract under direct visualization. Their results corroborated the clinical evidence of a relative afferent pupillary defect in patients with lesions of the contralateral optic tract producing complete homonymous hemianopia without evidence of optic neuropathy. A relative afferent pupillary defect was also present at some stage in 8 of 10 patients with optic tract syndromes reported by Newman and Miller (235).

Unilateral optic tract lesions, like other unilateral retrochiasmal lesions, do not cause loss of visual acuity. Such visual loss occurs from the effects of the lesion on one or both optic nerves. It is for this reason that when reduced visual acuity is present in a patient with a lesion in the region of the optic tract, it (and the associated relative afferent pupillary defect) is more often on the side of the lesion, as a result of accompanying optic nerve disease. On the other hand, in patients with pure optic tract lesions that do not damage either optic nerve or parts of the optic chiasm, a complete or nearly complete homonymous hemianopia is always associated with an obvious relative afferent pupillary defect on the side *opposite* the lesion. Such patients have normal visual acuity and color vision, and they have no sensation of reduced light brightness in the eye with the afferent pupillary defect.

Another pupillary phenomenon that is sometimes associated with lesions of the optic tract is pupillary hemiakinesia (hemianopic pupillary reaction or Wernicke's pupil). Because the pupillary afferents are present in this section of the visual system, when light is projected onto the "blind" retinal elements (subserving the nasal visual field in the ipsilateral eye and the temporal visual field in the contralateral eye), either no pupillary reaction occurs, or the reaction is markedly reduced. However, when light is projected onto the intact retinal elements (subserving the temporal visual field in the ipsilateral eye and the nasal visual field in the contralateral eye), a normal pupillary reaction is observed. Savino et al. (230) found this abnormality in only one of their patients and concluded that it is not helpful in diagnosing this syndrome; however, most of the patients in this study had lesions that extended to one or both optic nerves.

Patients with a complete or nearly complete homonymous hemianopia from an optic tract lesion eventually develop a characteristic pattern of optic atrophy (230,235). There is a wedge or "band" of horizontal pallor of the optic disc in the eye contralateral to the lesion (i.e., the eye with temporal field loss). This pattern of optic nerve atrophy is associated with atrophy of retinal nerve fibers originating from retinal ganglion cells nasal to the fovea and is identical with that

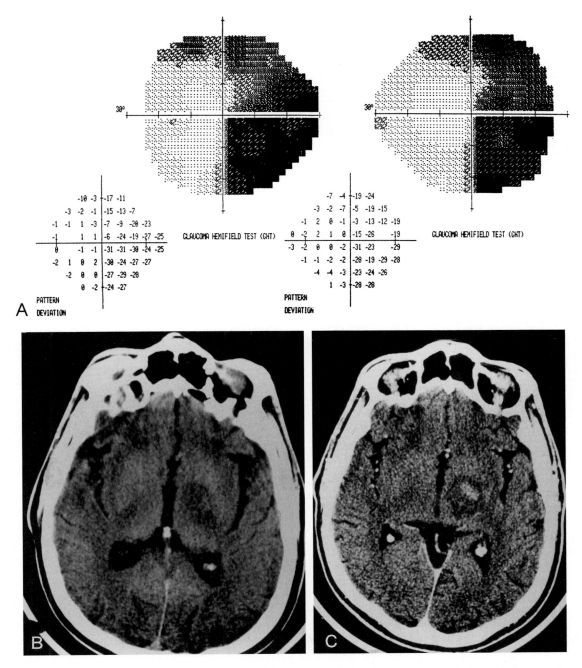

Figure 12.14. A 65-year-old man developed headache, sleepiness, personality changes, memory difficulties, right hemiparesis, and difficulty seeing to the right. *A,* Visual fields revealed an incongruent right homonymous hemianopia. Computed tomography scans before (*B*) and after (*C*) the administration of intravenous contrast revealed an enhancing lesion with surrounding edema in the region of the left optic tract, diagnosed ultimately as lymphoma.

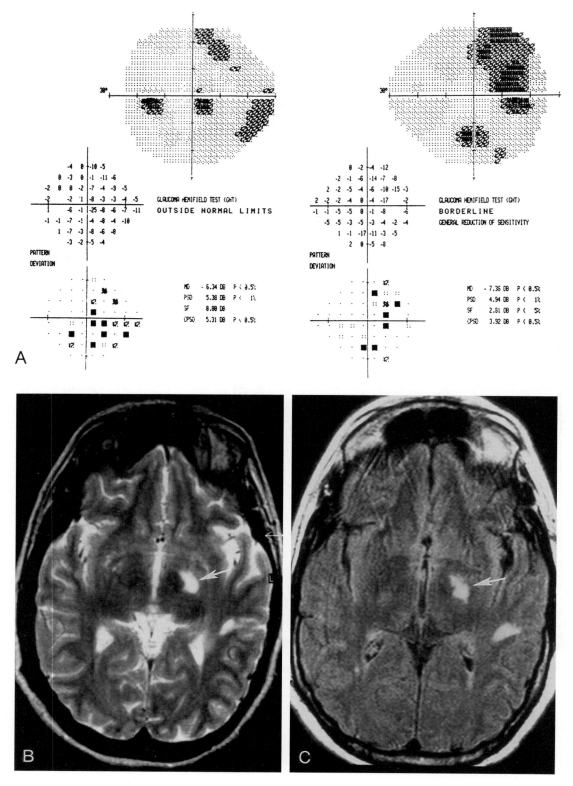

Figure 12.15. A 40-year-old man noted a "black spot" in front of both eyes that gradually worsened over 2 weeks. *A,* Visual acuities were normal, but there was a trace right relative afferent pupillary defect, and visual fields showed a highly incongruous right homonymous defect. *B and C,* Magnetic resonance imaging (*B,* T2-weighted; *C,* FLAIR) revealed multiple white matter lesions consistent with demyelinating disease, including a large plaque in the left optic tract (*arrows*).

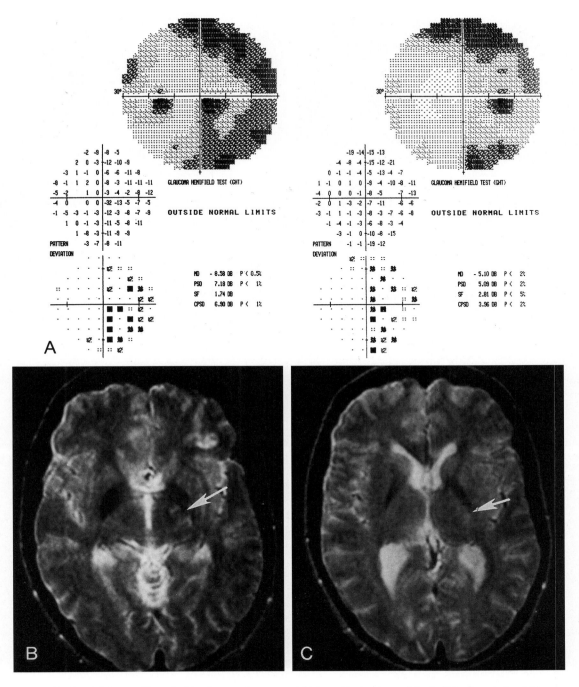

Figure 12.16. A 35-year-old man had head trauma in a motor vehicle accident and complained of blurriness in the right eye. *A,* Examination was notable for 20/20 vision in both eyes, a right relative afferent pupillary defect, pallor of the optic discs, and an incongruous right homonymous hemianopia. *B and C,* Magnetic resonance imaging revealed a subtle lesion in the left optic tract (*arrows*), presumably posttraumatic.

seen in both eyes of patients with bitemporal field loss from chiasmal syndromes (see above). At the same time, there is generalized pallor of the optic disc in the eye on the side of the lesion, and this is associated with severe loss of nerve fiber layer details in the superior and inferior arcuate regions that represent the majority of fibers subserving the nasal visual field and originating from retinal ganglion cells temporal to the fovea (Fig. 12.17).

Not all patients with optic tract lesions have complete homonymous hemianopias. Many have incomplete hemia-

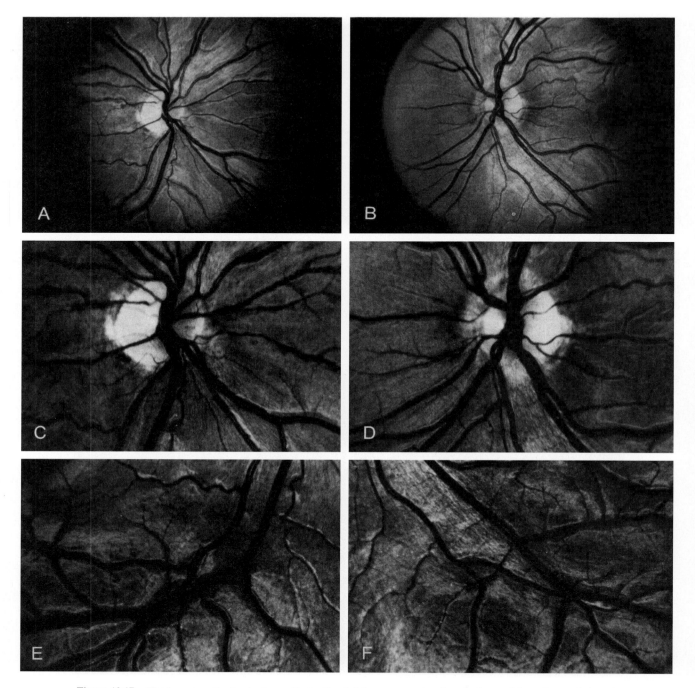

Figure 12.17. Hemianopic optic atrophy in a patient with a left homonymous hemianopia from a right optic tract lesion. *A,* The right optic disc has a somewhat diffuse temporal atrophy from loss of nerve fibers from ganglion cells temporal to the fovea. *B,* The left optic disc shows band atrophy from loss of nerve fibers from ganglion cells nasal to the fovea. *C and D,* Red-free (540 nm) photographs showing atrophy of right and left optic discs. Note band pattern of atrophy of the left disc. *E,* Inferior temporal peripapillary retina of right eye showing relative absence of visible arcuate bundle. *F,* Inferior temporal peripapillary retina of left eye showing relative preservation of arcuate bundle.

nopias or quadrantanopias, which as a rule are quite incongruous and may even be scotomatous (Fig. 12.18). Indeed, the optic tract is one of only two locations in the postchiasmal pathway in which homonymous scotomas can occur; the occipital lobe is the other.

Patients with optic tract lesions may have clinical manifestations in addition to homonymous visual field defects. Lesions that damage the optic tract may also damage adjacent neural structures, producing a variety of neurologic deficits (Fig. 12.19). Bender and Bodis-Wollner (236) examined 12 patients with optic tract lesions. Seven of the patients had disorders of mentation, and several had hypothalamic symptoms and signs. Eleven of the 21 patients studied by Savino et al. (230) had neurologic manifestations in addition to a homonymous visual field defect, as did 5 of the 10 patients evaluated by Newman and Miller (235).

In summary, a diagnosis of optic tract syndrome can be made in the setting of a highly incongruous homonymous hemianopia, with or without associated bilateral nerve fiber layer or optic atrophy, particularly when there is a relative afferent pupillary defect on the side opposite the lesion, despite normal visual acuity and color vision. In other words, a relative afferent pupillary defect in the eye on the side of a complete homonymous hemianopia in a patient with normal visual acuity and color vision in both eyes indicates a lesion of the optic tract (232,235). Unilateral lesions of the optic tract (or lateral geniculate body) that are associated with diminished visual acuity almost certainly produce the diminished acuity through damage to one or both optic nerves or the optic chiasm (11).

TOPICAL DIAGNOSIS OF LESIONS OF THE LATERAL GENICULATE BODY

Lesions affecting the lateral geniculate body (LGB; also lateral geniculate nucleus [LGN]) are less commonly diagnosed than those of the optic tract. At the beginning of the 20th century, it was accepted that incongruity of homonymous field defects is most pronounced with lesions near the junction of the optic chiasm and tract and diminishes progressively with more posterior lesions (237). This diagnostic perimetric axiom was attributed to a gradual alignment in the optic tract of the crossed and uncrossed visual axons from corresponding retinal areas. However, this theory was challenged by several clinicoanatomic case studies (238–240) and two clinical reports (241,242) suggesting that lesions of the lateral geniculate body produce significantly incongruous homonymous field defects. Gunderson and Hoyt (243) subsequently reported quantitative perimetric studies in two patients with lesions of the lateral geniculate body. One patient had a progressive hemianopia that began as an incongruous, relative wedge-shaped homonymous defect and ultimately resulted in a complete homonymous hemianopia with splitting of the macula. At autopsy, the patient had a diffuse pilocytic astrocytoma in the right temporal lobe, thalamus, and brain stem that completely replaced the right LGB. The second patient had a small arteriovenous malformation localized to the LGB. Hoyt (244) later described these two patients and two others in a more extensive discussion of perimetric findings in patients with lesions of the LGB. The most striking perimetric feature in these pa-

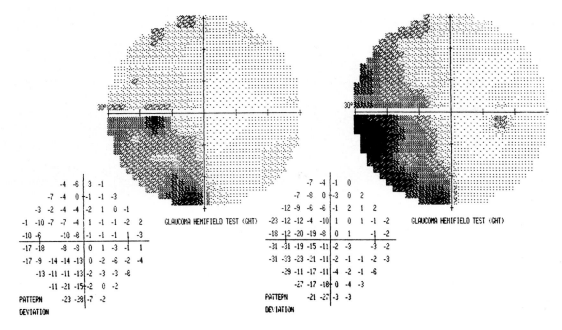

Figure 12.18. A 48-year-old woman with a history of migraines with left-sided visual aura had a typical aura without headache and without resolution of her visual symptoms. On examination, she had normal visual acuity, a left relative afferent pupillary defect, mild optic disc pallor in both eyes, and an incongruent left homonymous hemianopia. Magnetic resonance imaging revealed infarction in the region of the posterior right optic tract and lateral geniculate.

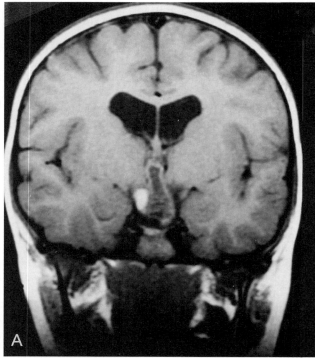

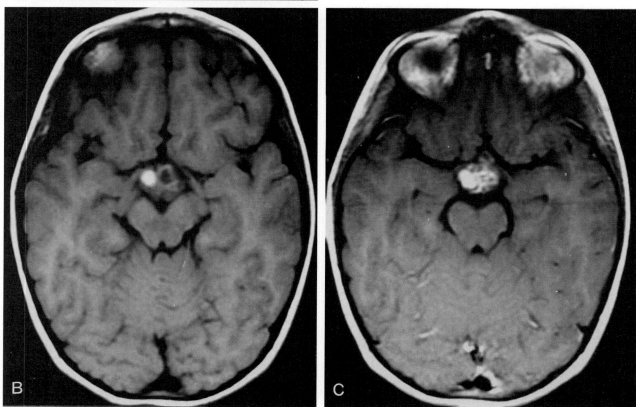

Figure 12.19. A 7-year-old girl presented with precocious puberty and was found to have a suprasellar mass with hydrocephalus. *A,* Coronal T1-weighted magnetic resonance image without gadolinium. *B,* Axial T1-weighted magnetic resonance image without gadolinium. *C,* Axial T1-weighted magnetic resonance image with gadolinium. *(Figure continues.)*

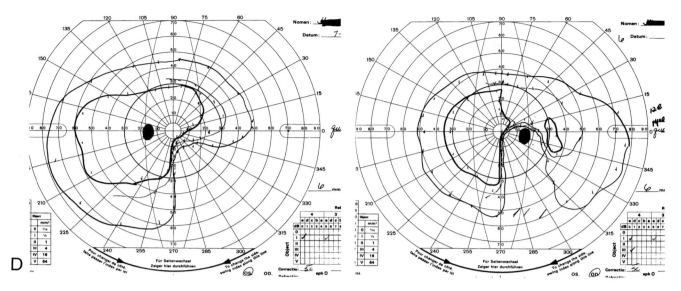

Figure 12.19. Continued. *D,* Examination revealed incongruous right inferior homonymous hemianopic defects consistent with damage to the left optic tract. Biopsy showed findings diagnostic of craniopharyngioma.

tients was the extensive incongruity of their visual field defects (Fig. 12.20).

It was mentioned in Chapter 1 that the dorsal region of the LGB subserves macular function, that the lateral aspect of the LGB subserves the superior visual field, and that the medial aspect subserves the inferior field. Case 1 of Hoyt (244) initially had incongruous, homonymous, wedge-shaped paracentral scotomas thought to be from damage to the dorsal crest of the LGB. Case 2 had an incongruous homonymous hemianopia, worse superiorly, which Hoyt thought was caused by extensive damage to the lateral aspect

of the LGB. It resulted in complete loss of the superior homonymous field, with minimal damage to the medial aspect, causing an incongruous loss of the inferior homonymous field. Case 4 had an incongruous, inferior homonymous hemianopia thought by Hoyt to indicate extensive damage to the medial aspect of the LGB. In addition, Hoyt emphasized the importance of hemianopic optic atrophy as an indication of irreversible damage to retrochiasmal visual fibers proximal to the visual radiations.

Frisén et al. (245,246) identified two specific patterns of relatively congruous homonymous field defects with sector

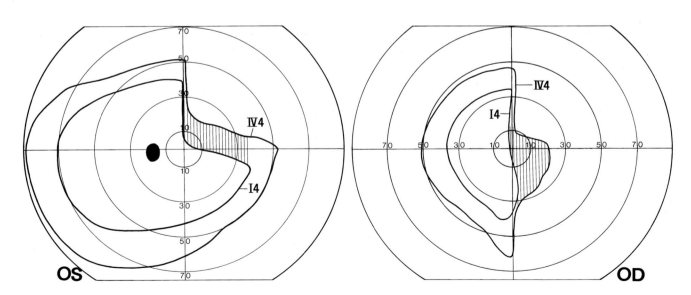

Figure 12.20. Incomplete, extremely incongruous, homonymous hemianopia in a patient with a lesion of the left lateral geniculate body. (Redrawn from Gunderson CH, Hoyt WF. Geniculate hemianopia: Incongruous homonymous field defects in two patients with partial lesions of the lateral geniculate nucleus. J Neurol Neurosurg Psychiatr 1971;34:1–6.)

optic atrophy, which they attributed to focal disease of the LGB caused by infarction in the territory of two specific arteries. Frisén et al. (245) described two patients with sector optic atrophy and homonymous, horizontal sectoranopia. One patient had a small arteriovenous malformation in the region of the LGB, whereas the second had a presumed infarction of the LGB. These authors believed that this specific pattern of field loss is indicative of ischemia or other damage in the territory of the lateral choroidal artery that supplies a portion of the LGB. They emphasized that the concept of an incongruous hemianopia as a hallmark of LGB damage is not necessarily correct. In addition, they argued, although the intricate retinotopic organization of the LGB may result in the production of relative defects, incongruous defects, and even (theoretically) monocular defects, vascular lesions are more likely to respect specific anatomic boundaries within the LGB and thus produce homonymous sector defects that are, in fact, quite congruous, with abruptly sloping borders (Fig. 12.21A and B).

In a second paper, Frisén (246) identified a syndrome characterized by loss of upper and lower homonymous sectors in the visual field that followed ligation of the distal portion of the anterior choroidal artery in a patient with a meningioma of the velum interpositum (Fig. 12.21C and D). In this patient, a CT scan showed a low-density region in the region of the LGB, thought to be compatible with an infarction. Frisén thus postulated that this "quadruple sectoranopia" syndrome was caused by ischemia or other damage to the portion of the LGB supplied by the anterior choroidal artery. Helgason et al. (247) reported a case similar to that of Frisén (246) and agreed that the field defects were caused by damage to the portion of the LGB supplied by the distal anterior choroidal artery. Both papers also emphasized the importance of focal nerve fiber layer atrophy with corresponding sector optic atrophy in establishing the diagnosis of a lesion of the LGB.

It seems clear that although incongruous homonymous field defects may arise from lesions in both the optic tract and LGB, lesions of the LGB may also produce fairly congruous defects (248,249). Indeed, Shacklett et al. (250) reported two patients with lesions of the LGB, both of whom had homonymous horizontal sectoranopias. One patient with a small arteriovenous malformation had an exquisitely congruous field defect. The other patient, who had a low-grade astrocytoma, had an incongruous field defect. The authors postulated that the arteriovenous malformation in the LGB of their first patient produced the highly congruous visual field defect by causing an infarction in the region of the LGB normally supplied by the lateral choroidal artery. The incongruous defect in the second patient was thought to be caused by infiltration of the portion of the LGB supplied by the lateral choroidal artery.

Although vascular lesions of the LGB tend to produce congruous homonymous field defects rather than incongruous ones, not all homonymous field defects caused by such lesions are congruous. Borruat and Maeder (251) described a patient with an incongruous left homonymous sectoranopia following head trauma. MR imaging revealed a hypointense lesion in the right LGB. The authors thought it

most likely that the lesion was an infarct in the territory of the right lateral choroidal artery, probably caused by shearing forces from the trauma.

Rarely, bilateral damage to the LGBs causes complete blindness (239,252). Most cases have resulted from vascular disease: syphilitic arteritis in the case reported by Mackenzie et al. (239) and coagulative ischemic necrosis, possibly associated with methanol ingestion, in the case reported by Merren (252). Donahue et al. (253) described a 37-year-old woman with central pontine myelinolysis and relatively congruous visual field defects in both halves of the visual field in an hourglass pattern (Fig. 12.22). The visual field defects resembled those described by Frisén (246) in patients with anterior choroidal artery infarction, but there was no evidence to suggest infarction in this case, leading the authors to postulate a preferential cellular susceptibility to myelinolysis among those cells supplied by this artery. Greenfield et al. (254) reported a 28-year-old woman who developed left homonymous wedge-shaped defects consistent with a lesion of the dorsal aspect of the right LGB and an incongruous right homonymous hemianopia after an episode of gastroenteritis. MR imaging revealed lesions of both LGBs and the left optic tract.

The specificity of homonymous sectoranopic visual field defects for lesions of the LGB is challenged by neuroimaging studies that reveal retrogeniculate lesions in some cases (255–259). Carter et al. (255), for example, reported three patients with homonymous horizontal sectoranopias consistent with the field defects caused by LGB lesions. CT scanning, however, revealed lesions of the optic radiation in all three cases: a presumed low-grade astrocytoma of the posterior temporal lobe in one patient, a large parietotemporal hemorrhage from an arteriovenous malformation in the second patient, and a posttraumatic hematoma in the temporal lobe in the third patient. Grossman et al. (258) reported similar visual field defects in a patient with an infarction in the occipital lobe.

Although three of the patients that Hoyt (244) described had no associated neurologic signs in addition to their visual field defects, patients with lesions of the LGB may also have neurologic symptoms and signs consistent with damage to the ipsilateral thalamus, the pyramidal tract, or both (247). As evidence of damage to the thalamus, there may be gross impairment of sensation on the side of the body opposite to the lesion, or there may be a complaint of pain of central origin that is referred to the opposite side of the body. Damage to the pyramidal tract causes weakness of the side of the body contralateral to the lesion.

Because the pupillomotor fibers leave the optic tract to ascend in the superior brachium, the pupillary reactions in patients with LGB lesions are normal unless the lesion also damages the optic tract or the brachium of the superior colliculus. As in lesions of the optic radiation, there is neither a contralateral relative afferent pupillary defect nor a hemianopic pupillary phenomenon. On the other hand, the visual axons from retinal ganglion cells first synapse in the LGB. Thus, sectoral or hemianopic atrophy of the retinal nerve fiber layer and optic disc occurs in patients with lesions of the LGB. Such defects, when associated with acquired

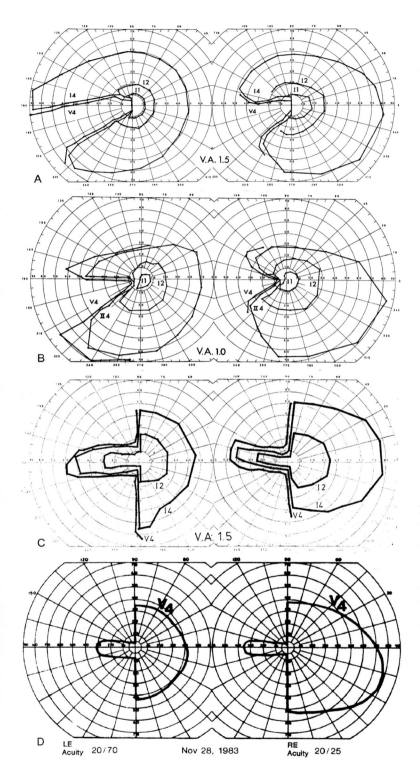

Figure 12.21. Visual field defects in patients with lesions of the lateral geniculate body (LGB). Homonymous horizontal sectoranopia from damage to the LGB in the territory of the lateral choroidal artery in a patient with a small arteriovenous malformation (*A*) and in a patient with presumed thrombosis of the lateral choroidal artery (*B*). Note the relative congruity of the field defect in both cases. Quadruple sectoranopia from damage to the LGB in the territory of the distal anterior choroidal artery in a patient with occlusion of the distal anterior choroidal artery (*C*) and in a patient with occlusion of the distal choroidal artery (*D*). (*A and B,* From Frisén L, Holmegaard L, Rosencrantz M. Sectorial optic atrophy and homonymous, horizontal sectoranopia: A lateral choroidal artery syndrome? J Neurol Neurosurg Psychiatr 1978;41:374–380. *C,* From Frisén L. Quadruple sectoranopia and sectorial optic atrophy: A syndrome of the distal anterior choroidal artery. J Neurol Neurosurg Psychiatry 1979;42:590–594. *D,* From Helgason C, Caplan LR, Goodwin J, et al. Anterior choroidal artery-territory infarction. Report of cases and review. Arch Neurol 1986;43:681–686.)

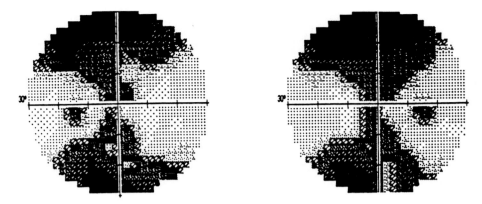

Figure 12.22. A 37-year-old woman suffered central pontine myelinolysis and complained of bilateral visual loss. Visual acuity was 20/25 OD and 20/30 OS, and automated static perimetry demonstrated fairly congruous defects having an hourglass configuration, with near-total depression superior and inferior to fixation. The visual field defects were similar to those reported after anterior choroidal artery infarction, prompting the authors to propose that the cells supplied by the anterior choroidal artery in the lateral geniculate might be particularly susceptible to metabolic insult, such as rapid changes in serum sodium level. (From Donahue SP, Kardon RH, Thompson HS. Hourglass-shaped visual fields as a sign of bilateral lateral geniculate myelinolysis. Am J Ophthalmol 1995;119:378–380.)

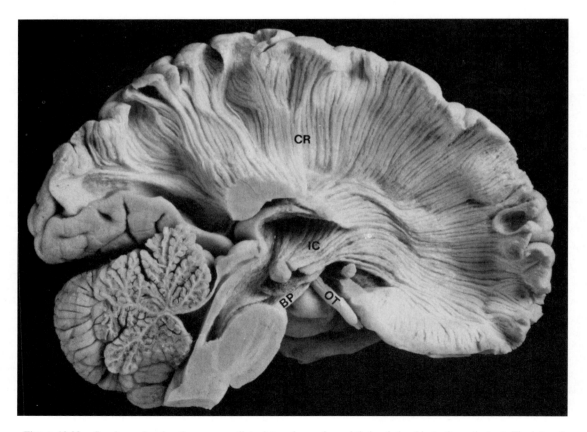

Figure 12.23. Specimen showing the corona radiata, internal capsule, and their relationship to the optic tract. The internal capsule and corona radiata have been exposed by removal of the corpus callosum, caudate nucleus, and diencephalon. The fibers of the basis pedunculi pass adjacent to the optic tract. CR, corona radiata; IC, internal capsule; BP, basis pedunculi; OT, optic tract. (From Ghuhbegovic N, Williams TH. The Human Brain. A Photographic Guide. Hagerstown, MD, Harper & Row, 1980.)

homonymous field defects, whether congruous or incongruous, must be taken as evidence of optic tract or lateral geniculate damage in all cases.

TOPICAL DIAGNOSIS OF LESIONS OF THE OPTIC RADIATION

Lesions of the Internal Capsule

Efferent projection fibers from and afferent projection fibers to the cerebral cortex traverse the subcortical white matter, where they form a radiating mass of fibers, the corona radiata, which converges toward the brain stem (Fig. 12.23). In the rostral brain stem, the fibers form a broad but compact fiber band, the internal capsule, that is bordered medially by the thalamus and caudate nucleus and laterally by the lenticular nucleus (260). The afferent fibers make up the thalamocortical radiation in the internal capsule. The efferent fiber bundles include (*a*) the corticospinal and corticobulbar tracts; (*b*) the frontopontine tract from the prefrontal and precentral regions of the cerebral cortex; (*c*) the temporoparietopontine tract from the temporal and parietal lobes; and (*d*) the optic radiation, which begins in the lateral geniculate body and occupies only a small region of the capsule, since it does not proceed to the brain stem. The internal capsule is thus composed of all fibers, afferent and efferent, that go to, or come from, the cerebral cortex.

Because of the curvature of fibers in the internal capsule, this structure has a broad, V-shaped appearance pointed medially when viewed in axial sections (Fig. 12.24). The anterior limb partially separates two structures of the basal ganglia, the head of the caudate nucleus and the lenticular nucleus (Figs. 12.24 and 12.25). The apex of the V, or genu, separates the head of the caudate nucleus and the thalamus. The posterior limb separates the thalamus and the lenticular nucleus (Fig. 12.24). The most posterior component of the internal capsule is the optic radiation. Interruption of the optic radiation is characterized by a contralateral homonymous hemianopic visual field defect.

The internal capsule receives the bulk of its blood supply from the lenticulostriate and lenticulo-optic branches of the middle cerebral artery. In addition, the anterior limb of the capsule is supplied by a branch of the anterior cerebral artery (Heubner's artery) (247).

A variety of clinical syndromes arise from lesions of the internal capsule. Obstruction of Heubner's artery causes paralysis of the face, tongue, and arm on the opposite side of the body; if the lesion is on the left, there is also motor dysphasia. The paralysis of the face spares the frontalis and orbicularis oculi in many instances, but occasionally during early stages there is transient lowering of the eyebrow and inability to completely close the eyelids. The sparing is related to the bilateral cortical innervation of these muscles. The muscles of deglutition and mastication and the larynx are similarly innervated.

If a lesion is extensive and affects the posterior limb of the capsule, there is a complete hemiplegia and hemianesthesia contralateral to the lesion. If there is damage to the posterior portion of the capsule, there is contralateral hemianesthesia and an homonymous hemianopia.

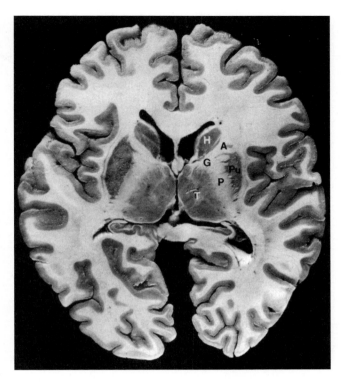

Figure 12.24. Horizontal section through the cerebral hemispheres at the level of the thalamus, showing the relationship of the portions of the internal capsule to the surrounding structures. A, anterior limb of the internal capsule; G, genu of the internal capsule; P, posterior limb of the internal capsule; H, head of the caudate nucleus; Pu, putamen; T, thalamic nuclei. (From Ghuhbegovic N, Williams TH. The Human Brain. A Photographic Guide. Hagerstown, MD, Harper & Row, 1980.)

Ocular findings in lesions of the internal capsule may be summarized as follows: (*a*) transient deviation of the eyes to the side of the lesion in many instances; (*b*) weakness of the frontalis and orbicularis oculi on the hemiplegic side in a minority of cases; (*c*) homonymous hemianopia in cases in which there is extensive damage to the posterior portion of the capsule.

The homonymous hemianopia that is associated with lesions of the internal capsule is often complete, but there is usually some degree of clearing with time. Only rarely does complete resolution or no resolution of the hemianopia occur.

Lesions of the Temporal Lobe

Unlike lesions of the internal capsule, which are frequently vascular, temporal lobe lesions are often neoplastic or infectious (i.e., abscess), and it is not until the occipital cortex is reached that vascular lesions again predominate. The disposition of the visual fibers in the temporal lobe is controversial. One has only to compare the report by Falconer and Wilson (261), whose 50 temporal lobectomy patients all had completely congruous hemianopic defects, denser above, with that of Van Buren and Baldwin (262), who found significant incongruity in their 41 temporal lobectomy

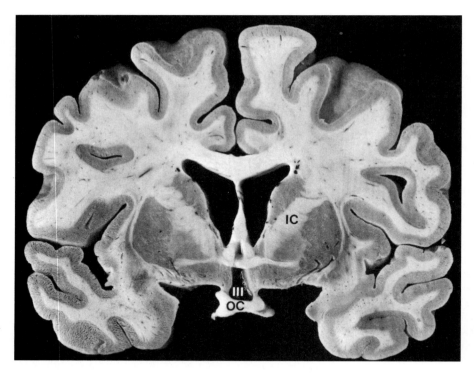

Figure 12.25. Coronal section through the cerebral hemispheres showing the relationship of the optic chiasm, third ventricle and internal capsule. OC, optic chiasm; III, 3rd ventricle; IC, internal capsule. (From Ghuhbegovic N, Williams TH. The Human Brain. A Photographic Guide. Hagerstown, MD, Harper & Row, 1980.)

patients with hemianopic defects, to realize that the issue is far from settled. Nevertheless, a few general comments can be made regarding the nature of homonymous defects seen with lesions of the temporal lobe.

If the temporal lobe is damaged or sectioned far enough posteriorly, the patient will have a homonymous visual field defect. In virtually all cases, the homonymous defect is incomplete and either is confined to the superior quadrants or is denser above, reflecting the anatomy of Meyer's loop, which courses anteriorly in the temporal lobe around the temporal horn of the lateral ventricle and consists entirely of axons subserving the superior visual fields of the two eyes (see Chapter 1). In many cases the homonymous defect is enough to interfere with everyday activities, particularly driving (263,264). On the other hand, the anterior temporal lobe may be damaged without producing any visual field defect. The amount of temporal lobe that may be removed without a resulting field defect is controversial. Penfield (265) reported 51 patients who underwent temporal lobectomy for temporal lobe epilepsy and wrote, ''When the line of removal is less than 6 cm posterior to the tip, it is apt to result in no postoperative visual field defect.'' Marino and Rasmussen (266) found that 17 of 50 patients who underwent temporal lobectomies had no detectable field defect, even though some of these patients had resections between 3.0 and 8.5 cm as measured both along the base of the middle fossa and along the sylvian fissure. On the other hand, Falconer and Wilson (261) found visual field defects when the line of removal was as little as 4.5 cm posterior to the tip of the temporal lobe. Removal of as little as 2 cm of anterior temporal lobe can result in a visual field defect detected by automated perimetry (267), and automated perimetry detects

abnormalities in almost all patients after temporal lobe resection (268). Attempts to prevent visual field defects from temporal lobe epilepsy surgery by doing amygdalohippocampectomy have not been successful (269).

The issue of how much temporal lobe can be removed or damaged without producing a homonymous visual field defect is complicated by several factors. First, most studies used kinetic rather than static perimetry. It is possible that some of the patients who had no evidence of a field defect by kinetic perimetry would have shown a defect if they had been tested with static perimetry, as in the study by Krolak-Salmon et al. (267). Second, when temporal lobectomy is performed for mass lesions, the lesion itself may influence the anatomy of the visual fibers within the temporal lobe. Even in studies that limit patient inclusion to epilepsy patients with mesial temporal sclerosis, thereby excluding patients with a major structural distortion of the optic radiation, the extent of resection often varies. The approach will depend on the results of electroencephalography, MR imaging, electrocorticography, and functional cortical mapping and the particular vascular anatomy of the patient's temporal lobe (270). In addition, there may be considerable individual variability in the spatial distribution of optic radiation fibers within the temporal lobe (270–272). Finally, infarction in the distribution of the anterior choroidal artery from surgical manipulation and resultant vasospasm may complicate temporal lobectomy in some cases (247,273), causing more extensive visual field defects from damage to the optic tract or the LGB.

Several patients in the series reported by Marino and Rasmussen (266) had defects following excisions 3.0–4.0 cm posterior to the temporal tip. However, it would appear that up to 4.0 cm of anterior temporal lobe can be removed in most patients without interrupting the visual fibers enough to produce a visual field defect. Once the temporal lobe is sectioned 4 cm or more posterior to its tip, most patients will develop a homonymous field defect. Bjork and Kugelberg (274) examined 26 patients who underwent temporal lobectomy for temporal lobe epilepsy unassociated with tumor. All patients had sections made 4.0–6.5 cm from the temporal tip, and all patients had homonymous superior quadrantic defects, although none of the patients was aware of the defect until the examination. Other investigators also report homonymous visual field defects after temporal lobectomies made 4–8 cm from the temporal tip in 74% (51/69) (275), 59% (13/22) (271), 69% (27/39) (276), and 52% (17/33) (270) of patients.

According to Van Buren and Baldwin (262), other characteristics of these field defects are (*a*) they do not affect visual acuity; (*b*) they do not alter the size of the blind spot; (*c*) they have sloping inferior margins; (*d*) they may cross the horizontal midline; (*e*) they may be either congruous or incongruous but when incongruous, the larger defect is often in the visual field of the eye on the side of the lesion (Fig. 12.26). In addition, the peripheral field, including the monocular crescent, is never spared in these field defects. Although Falconer and Wilson (261) concluded that excisions of varying magnitude between 4.5 and 8.0 cm produce homonymous defects, usually of the superior field, these investigators found that most of the defects were congruous and that there was no significant difference in the severity of the field defects that were produced when lesions were made between 4.5 and 6.0 cm from the tip and those that were produced after lesions made 6.0–8.0 cm from the tip. Marino and Rasmussen (266) noted incongruity in 79% of their patients with homonymous field defects after temporal lobectomy. Sixteen of these 26 patients exhibited the greater de-

fect in the visual field of the eye on the side of the lesion, whereas 10 patients exhibited the greater defect in the visual field of the eye contralateral to the lesion. Other investigators performed studies indicating that the gross dimensions of a temporal lobe resection generally correlate poorly with the presence, extent, and congruity of the resultant visual field defects (270,271,275,276). For example, although Jensen and Seedorff (275) found a higher frequency of extensive visual field defects after right-sided resections, Tecoma et al. (270) found no such effect of the side of the operation. Jensen and Seedorff (275) and Babb et al. (271) found a high degree of incongruity in the visual field defects among their patients and confirmed the finding of Marino and Rasmussen (266) and others of a consistently greater defect in the field of the eye on the side of the lobectomy; however, Tecoma et al. (270) reported more uniform visual fields with no consistent laterality, a finding that reflects the experience of many clinicians. These authors hypothesized that this variability in the congruity of the visual field defects after temporal lobectomy may reflect the individual reorganization within fiber bundles. The reorganization occurs in the optic radiation as the precise retinotopic organization of the LGB with its six monocular layers in vertical register becomes binocular at the visual cortex.

Although there seems to be no correlation between the amount of posterior section in temporal lobectomy and the severity of the visual field defect when sectioning is performed between 4 and 8 cm posterior to the temporal tip, most authors agree that sections beyond 8 cm tend to produce a complete homonymous hemianopia (261,262). Even this issue is controversial, however. In the study performed by Marino and Rasmussen (266), four patients with excisions of 7.5–8.0 cm as measured along the base of the middle fossa had no visual field defects, and none of the 11 patients with such excisions had a complete homonymous hemia-

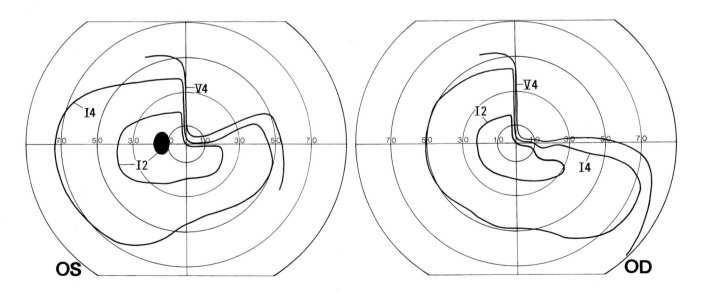

Figure 12.26. Homonymous quadrantanopia in a patient with a glioblastoma of the left temporal lobe. The defects are primarily superior and moderately incongruous. The greater defect is on the side opposite the lesion.

nopia. A rule of thumb (for which there are always exceptions) is that most patients in whom a temporal lobectomy is performed that extends at least 4 cm posterior to the temporal tip will have some degree of homonymous field defect denser superiorly than inferiorly, and patients in whom a lobectomy extends posteriorly beyond 8 cm should be expected to have a postoperative homonymous field defect that is complete or nearly so.

Penfield et al. (277) described splitting of the macula as the result of excision of the posterior portion of the temporal lobe; however, most series report a tendency for macular sparing in patients with partial or complete quadrantic defects. Marino and Rasmussen (266) found macular splitting primarily in patients whose field defects extended into the lower quadrants. When the field defect was confined to the superior quadrants, the macular field in these quadrants tended to be spared.

The visual field defects associated with temporal lobe lesions are summarized as follows:

1. A homonymous wedge-shaped defect in the upper visual fields, often called a ''pie-in-the-sky'' defect to emphasize its superior location and wedge shape, almost always indicates damage to the optic radiation in the temporal lobe (Fig. 12.26).
2. A superior homonymous quadrantic defect suggests damage to the inferior fibers of the optic tract, the optic radiation in the temporal lobe, or the inferior occipital cortex (Fig. 12.27). When the defect is congruous, an occipital lobe location is most likely, but the lesion may still be in the temporal lobe. When the defect is incongruous, the lesion is either in the optic tract or the temporal lobe, but not in the occipital lobe.

Horton and Hoyt (278) suggested that lesions of the occipital cortex, especially if they affect areas V2 and V3 of extrastriate cortex, are more likely to produce a sharply defined horizontal border to the quadrantanopia than are lesions of the optic radiation, which often produce incongruous defects with sloping borders. However, exquisite respect of the horizontal meridian can certainly occur with lesions in the optic radiation, including the temporal lobe (Fig. 12.28). Many but not all field defects associated with temporal lobe lesions are incongruous. The incongruity, when present, is not as severe as that seen with optic tract and some lateral geniculate lesions, and the more extensive defect is usually but not always in the eye on the side of the lesion (Fig. 12.26).

Nonvisual manifestations of lesions of the temporal lobe are described in detail in Chapter 28. Briefly, if there is a mass lesion of the temporal lobe, headache is common. Bilateral lesions of the transverse gyri of Heschl can cause cortical deafness, usually associated with aphasia, and unilateral lesions may cause a disturbance of hearing and sound discrimination contralateral to the lesion (279,280). If the lesion is in the dominant temporal lobe, the patient may have difficulty memorizing a series of spoken words, whereas if the lesion is in the nondominant temporal lobe, the patient may exhibit various forms of auditory agnosia (281). Auditory hallucinations or illusions may occur with lesions of

either temporal lobe. Severe disturbances of language can result from lesions in the dominant, usually left, temporal lobe. Disturbances of memory are common.

Tumors of the temporal lobe frequently cause seizures. Seizures of the temporal lobe often manifest as transient changes in emotions, mood, and behavior that are associated with motor automatisms: so-called complex partial seizures or psychomotor epilepsy. If the lesion is situated anteriorly and affects the uncinate gyrus, either directly or through pressure, so-called uncinate fits occur. These are characterized by an aura of unusual taste or smell, followed by abnormal motor activity of the mouth and lips, during which the patient is not in contact with his or her surroundings. There may be auditory or formed visual hallucinations.

Lesions of the Parietal Lobe

Lesions in the parietal lobe may produce ocular symptoms of diagnostic value. Homonymous hemianopia affecting primarily the lower fields is caused by damage to the optic radiation in the superior parietal lobe (Fig. 12.29). Such defects are usually more congruous than those produced by lesions of the temporal lobe (Fig. 12.30). Because the entire optic radiation passes through the parietal lobe, large lesions may produce complete homonymous hemianopia with macular splitting. Unawareness of the field defects characterizes many parietal lobe lesions in both the dominant and nondominant hemispheres (282,283), although this phenomenon is not limited to such lesions. Traquair (284) stated that before the appearance of other symptoms, there may be a disturbance of fixation reflexes sufficient to interfere with reading ability. This disturbance is sometimes manifest during visual field testing, during which the examiner notes that despite his or her best efforts, the patient cannot maintain central fixation. This often causes frustration on the part of the patient and exasperation on the part of the examiner or technician performing the field testing.

The anatomy of the optic radiation has been most extensively studied in the cat (285). Investigators noted a continuous sheet of fibers with no separation of fibers into those ultimately projecting to the superior and inferior visual cortices. Horton and Hoyt (278) argued that this lack of anatomic separation makes it unlikely that a lesion of the optic radiation could cause a visual field defect that strictly respects the horizontal meridian. Indeed, most field defects in patients with lesions of the optic radiation in the parietal lobe have sloping borders that do not precisely respect the horizontal (262). Exceptions occur, however, especially when the causative lesion is in the posterior optic radiation where the fascicles approach the calcarine cortex (Fig. 12.31). Borruat et al. (286) reported the case of a 45-year-old woman with probable multiple sclerosis and a congruous inferior homonymous quadrantanopia bordering the horizontal meridian secondary to a small white matter lesion in the contralateral trigone area (Fig. 12.32).

Neuro-ophthalmologic features suggesting a lesion in the parietal lobe include an incomplete and relatively congruous (or mildly incongruous) homonymous hemianopia that is denser below than above, conjugate movements of the eyes

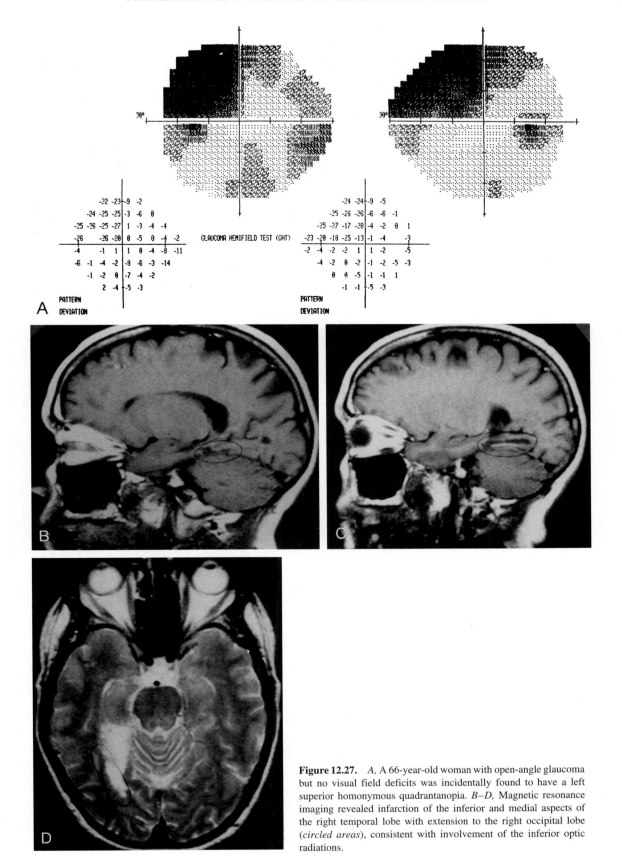

Figure 12.27. *A,* A 66-year-old woman with open-angle glaucoma but no visual field deficits was incidentally found to have a left superior homonymous quadrantanopia. *B–D,* Magnetic resonance imaging revealed infarction of the inferior and medial aspects of the right temporal lobe with extension to the right occipital lobe (*circled areas*), consistent with involvement of the inferior optic radiations.

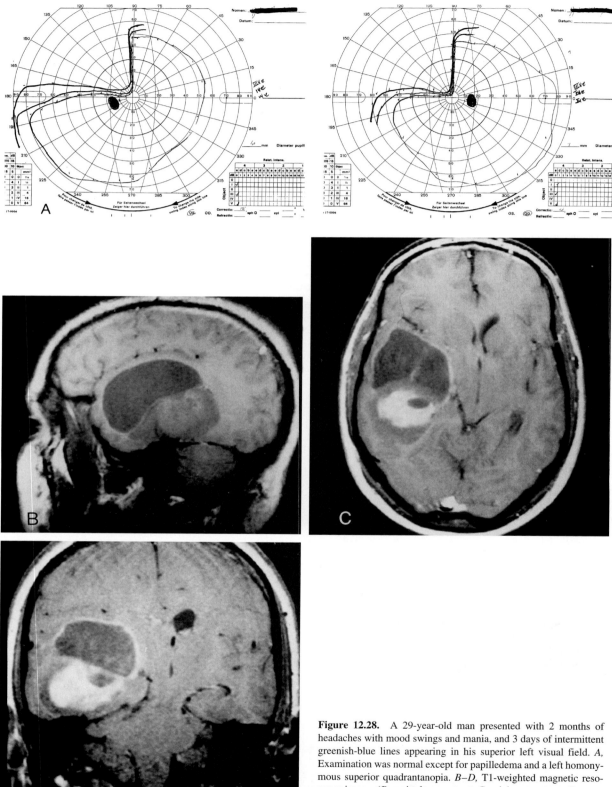

Figure 12.28. A 29-year-old man presented with 2 months of headaches with mood swings and mania, and 3 days of intermittent greenish-blue lines appearing in his superior left visual field. *A,* Examination was normal except for papilledema and a left homonymous superior quadrantanopia. *B–D,* T1-weighted magnetic resonance images (*B,* sagittal precontrast; *C,* axial postcontrast; *D,* coronal postcontrast) showed an inhomogenously enhancing cystic mass in the right temporal lobe. Biopsy was diagnostic of glioblastoma multiforme.

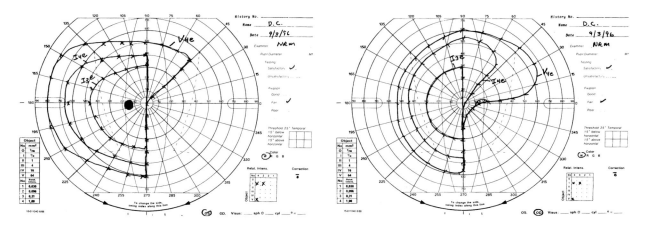

Figure 12.29. Incomplete mildly incongruous homonymous hemianopia in a patient with a left parietal lobe glioblastoma. The field defect in both eyes is denser inferiorly. The mild incongruity associated with the inferior nature of the defects is typical of damage to the optic radiations in the parietal lobe.

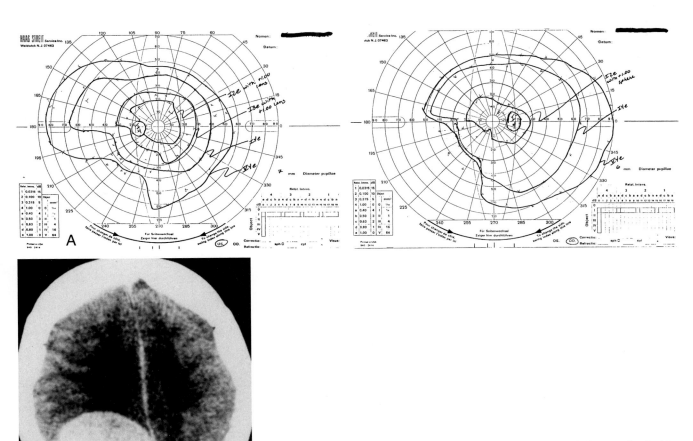

Figure 12.30. A 37-year-old woman complained of intermittent headaches associated with visual hallucinations of "a swirling black circle in the left eye." *A,* Examination was normal except for left homonymous inferior quadrantic visual field defects. *B,* Computed tomography scan after the administration of intravenous contrast revealed a large, dural-based homogenously enhancing right parietal lobe tumor with little mass effect, confirmed at surgery to be a meningioma.

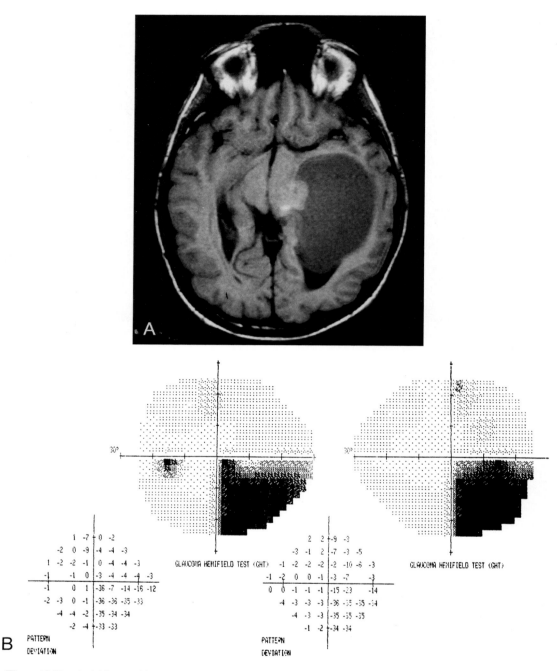

Figure 12.31. *A*, A 17-year-old man had a complex partial seizure and was found to have a left temporal lobe cystic fibrillary astrocytoma. The tumor was partially resected and then irradiated. *B*, Follow-up 6 years later showed a right inferior homonymous quadrantanopia. *(Figure continues.)*

to the side opposite the lesion on forced lid closure (Cogan's sign), and an abnormal optokinetic response. The abnormal optokinetic response consists of defective slow and fast phases when targets are moved toward the side of the lesion, a maneuver that necessitates pursuit movements to that side and saccades to the opposite side (287). The basis for such a response is discussed in Chapter 17. Other types of visual

disturbances caused by lesions in the parietal lobe include visual neglect, visual agnosia, and difficulties with word recognition (see Chapters 28 and 40 for more detailed discussion). As noted above, patients with parietal lobe lesions and homonymous visual field defects are often unaware of their visual deficits. This phenomenon is more likely to be observed when the underlying abnormality is in the nondomi-

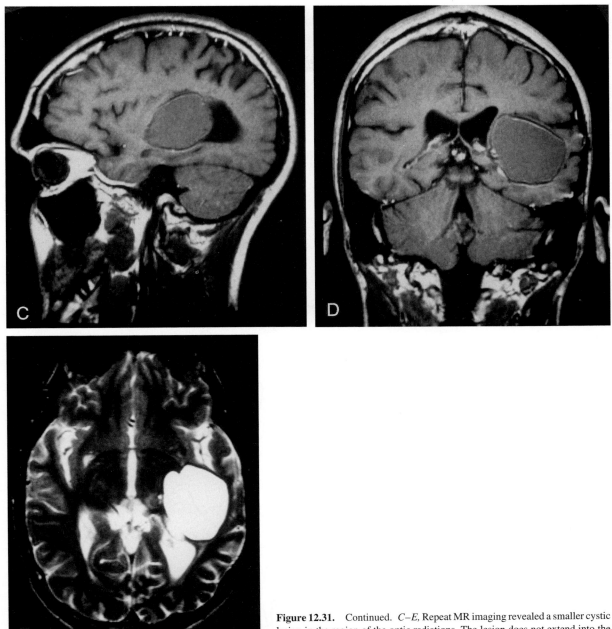

Figure 12.31. Continued. *C–E,* Repeat MR imaging revealed a smaller cystic lesion in the region of the optic radiations. The lesion does not extend into the occipital lobe.

nant cerebral hemisphere (usually the right parietal lobe), but it can also be observed in patients with dominant parietal lobe lesions. In other patients, the primary visual pathways may be unaffected or minimally affected, but the patient neglects the contralateral visual field (see Chapter 13).

Parietal lobe lesions cause other symptoms and signs. The parietal lobe is the principal sensory area of the cerebral cortex, and the postcentral gyrus is particularly important. The patient may complain of numbness, but more commonly there are more complex problems of sensory integration, as demonstrated on tests of tactile discrimination, position sense, stereognosis, and visual-spatial coordination (288). Irritative lesions of the postcentral gyrus cause sensory Jacksonian seizures that begin contralateral to the lesion at the part of the body corresponding to the excitation focus. Tingling or numbness spreads to adjacent parts of the body according to the order of their representation in the cortex (Jacksonian march). Lesions in the dominant parietal lobe can cause aphasia (usually fluent), apraxia, agnosia, acalculia, and agraphia. A lesion in the dominant parietal lobe affecting the angular gyrus may produce Gerstmann's syndrome (finger agnosia, right–left disorientation, agraphia,

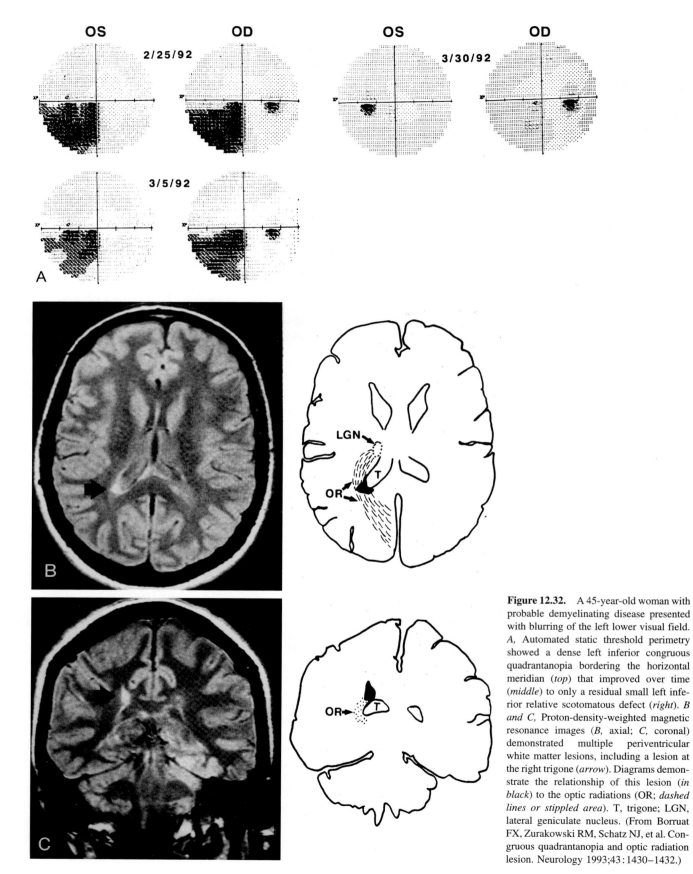

Figure 12.32. A 45-year-old woman with probable demyelinating disease presented with blurring of the left lower visual field. *A,* Automated static threshold perimetry showed a dense left inferior congruous quadrantanopia bordering the horizontal meridian (*top*) that improved over time (*middle*) to only a residual small left inferior relative scotomatous defect (*right*). *B and C,* Proton-density-weighted magnetic resonance images (*B,* axial; *C,* coronal) demonstrated multiple periventricular white matter lesions, including a lesion at the right trigone (*arrow*). Diagrams demonstrate the relationship of this lesion (*in black*) to the optic radiations (OR; *dashed lines or stippled area*). T, trigone; LGN, lateral geniculate nucleus. (From Borruat FX, Zurakowski RM, Schatz NJ, et al. Congruous quadrantanopia and optic radiation lesion. Neurology 1993;43:1430–1432.)

and acalculia) in association with a right homonymous hemianopia (289,290). Lesions in the nondominant parietal lobe may cause impaired constructional ability, dyscalculia, and, most commonly, inattention or neglect (291,292). Indeed, left spatial neglect after right hemisphere lesions may accentuate the left hemianopia, hemianesthesia, and hemiplegia and contribute to poor recovery (293).

LESIONS OF THE OCCIPITAL LOBE AND VISUAL CORTEX

In many cases the most posterior visual radiation and visual cortex are affected together. Most lesions in the occipital lobe are vascular or traumatic in origin, with tumor, abscess, demyelination, and toxic disorders of white matter occurring less frequently. Cole, a neurologist, has written a first-person account of his experience as a patient with an occipital stroke, which includes some of the symptomatology described below (294).

Because of the close anatomic relationship of fibers from corresponding portions of the two retinas, lesions of the occipital lobe cause defects that are not only overwhelmingly homonymous but also increasingly congruous the more posteriorly situated the lesion (295–299). Automated static perimetry may inaccurately portray homonymous visual fields as incongruous, compared to Goldmann or tangent screen perimetry (300).

Unilateral Lesions of the Posterior Occipital Lobe

Defects seen with these lesions are exclusively homonymous. With lesions of the tip of the occipital lobe (occipital pole), the field defects are always central homonymous scotomas that are exquisitely congruous (257,296,298,299) (Fig. 12.33). After a detailed examination of three patients with homonymous visual field defects produced by well-circumscribed lesions in the occipital lobe, Horton and Hoyt (298) estimated that the central 10° of the visual field are represented by at least 50–60% of the posterior striate cortex and that the central 30° is represented by about 80% of the cortex (Figs. 12.34 and 12.35). These findings were corroborated by McFadzean et al. (299). Instead of using lesions for mapping, it is possible to use functional MR imaging to detect those areas of the cortex activated by visual stimuli, and thus to produce a retinotopic map noninvasively (301). Wong and Sharpe used functional MR imaging to map the retinal representation on the occipital lobe and found that the central 15% of vision occupied only 37% of the cortex (302). Probably the most accurate method for determining cortical magnification (i.e., the degree by which areas of central retina are processed by magnified areas of visual cortex) is the use of angioscotoma mapping (303,304). Adams and Horton (305) used this mapping technique in squirrel monkeys and found that the central 16° of visual field is represented by approximately 70% of cortex. Similar cortical magnification of the central visual field is seen in the extrastriate areas V2 and V3 (306). The detailed anatomy of the visual cortex is discussed in Chapter 1.

Lesions located more anteriorly may produce primarily central field defects that break out into the periphery (Fig. 12.36). Impressive congruity is a feature of such field defects (257,307,308). The phenomenon of sparing of the macula is often seen in such cases (see below).

An unusual visual field defect is homonymous hemianopia associated with sparing of the horizontal or vertical meridian. This results from sparing from injury of the corresponding cortical representation of the meridian, with the vertical meridian represented at the lips of the calcarine fissure and the horizontal meridian represented at the base of the fissure (309,310).

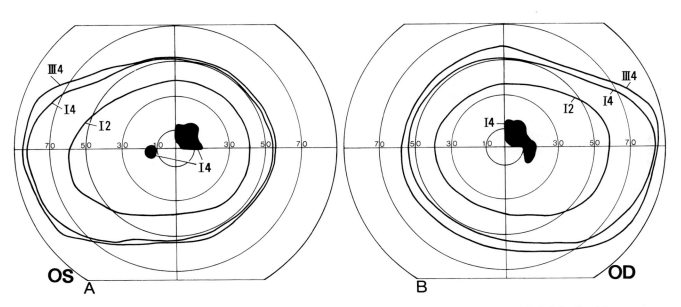

Figure 12.33.   Exquisitely congruous homonymous hemianopic scotomas in a patient with an infarct of the inferior lip of the left calcarine cortex. Note the few degrees of macular sparing.

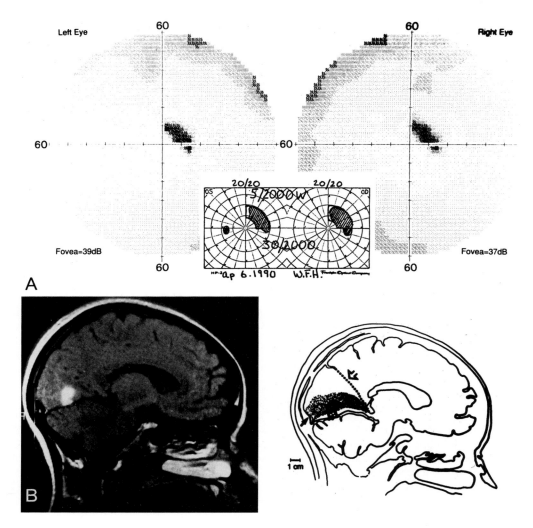

Figure 12.34. A 30-year-old woman reported several episodes of flashing colored lights in her right upper quadrant of vision. *A,* Merged 30-2 and 60-2 full-threshold visual field tests using a Humphrey Field Analyzer. A homonymous, congruous scotoma was present in the right upper quadrant. In the *inset,* the visual fields are mapped at the tangent screen. The scotoma extended from 6° to 18°. *B,* Parasagittal magnetic resonance image of the left occipital lobe. The lesion (*cross-hatched area on the right*) is within the visual cortex (*stippled area on the right*). The calcarine sulcus (*solid arrow*) and the parieto-occipital sulcus (*open arrow*) are marked by *dots.* On biopsy, the lesion was a presumed tuberculoma. (From Horton JC, Hoyt WF. The representation of the visual field in human striate cortex. Arch Ophthalmol 1991;109:816–824.)

Both Allen and Carman (311) and Barkan and Boyle (312) reported a syndrome in which an otherwise healthy patient develops the sudden onset of an isolated homonymous paracentral scotoma associated with normal visual acuity and no ophthalmoscopic abnormalities. Clinically, such a lesion must occur as the result of a vascular event in the posterior occipital cortex; however, in both cases, the homonymous scotomas were incongruous. The explanation for this apparent clinical–anatomic discrepancy is unclear.

Unilateral Lesions of the Anterior Occipital Lobe

Because the temporal field in each eye is larger than the nasal field, the fibers subserving that portion of the peripheral temporal field that has no nasal correlate must be un-

paired throughout the postchiasmal portion of the visual sensory pathway. Damage to these unpaired peripheral fibers produces a monocular defect in the extreme temporal visual field. This field defect is crescentic and its widest extent is in the horizontal meridian, where it extends from 60° out to approximately 90°. Because of its peculiar shape, a defect in this region has been termed a temporal crescent or half-moon syndrome (Figs. 12.35C, 12.37, and 12.38). Brouwer and Zeeman (313) demonstrated that after destruction of the peripheral nasal retina there was degeneration of a bundle of fibers localized in the median portion of the optic nerve, which continued into the optic chiasm to the median portion of the optic tract and spread ventrally into the lateral geniculate body. Wilbrand (6) confirmed that this bundle contained

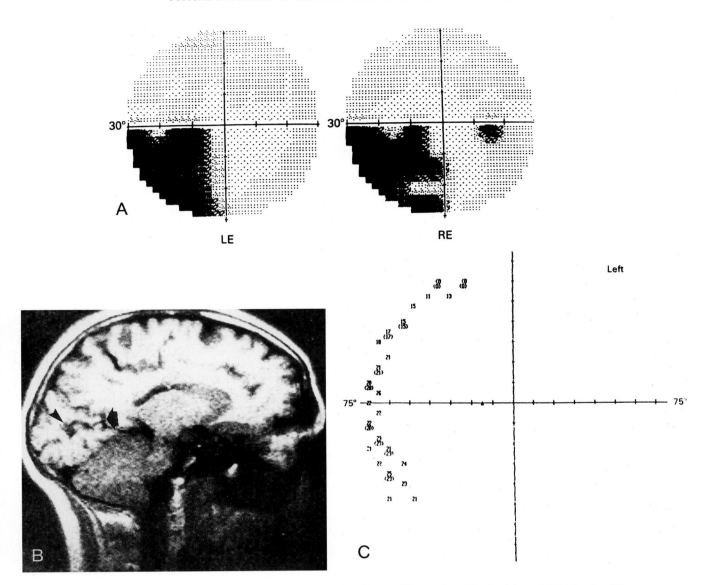

Figure 12.35. Humphrey visual fields (30-2 program) (*A*) in a 40-year-old man who suffered a right occipital infarction (*B*) involving the superior bank of the calcarine cortex (*arrowhead*). The infarction spared the posterior striate cortex as well as the anterior striate cortex at the junction of the parieto-occipital and calcarine fissures (*arrow*). *C,* The visual fields showed sparing of central fixation within 6° as well as sparing of the left monocular temporal crescent. (From McFadzean R, Brosnahan D, Hadley D, et al. Representation of the visual field in the occipital striate cortex. Br J Ophthalmol 1994;78:185–190.)

only crossed fibers. In 1929, Förster (quoted by Walsh [314]) produced the sensation of light in the extreme temporal periphery of one eye by electrically stimulating the most anterior portion of the striate cortex. Polyak (315) confirmed these findings and postulated that the most anterior portion of the striate cortex harbored the projected monocular temporal crescent of the contralateral eye. Ask-Upmark (316) and Kronfeld (317) performed further studies in patients in whom the temporal crescent was selectively spared or damaged. They agreed that lesions of the posterior striate cortex tended to spare the temporal crescent, whereas lesions of the anterior striate cortex could selectively produce a defect in

it or eliminate it entirely. Spence and Fulton (318) extirpated the entire left occipital lobe in a chimpanzee and later resected part of the right occipital lobe. They subsequently observed that the animal had vision only in the temporal periphery of the left eye. Postmortem examination of the brain disclosed that only the anterior portion of the right striate cortex was intact, confirming the conclusions reached by Polyak (315), Ask-Upmark (316), and Kronfeld (317).

According to Bender and Strauss (208), the unpaired nasal fibers corresponding to the extreme temporal peripheral visual field come together in the most anterior portion of the striate cortex, with the fibers for the inferior portion of the

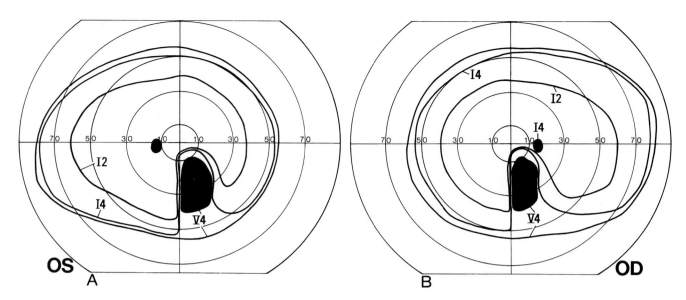

Figure 12.36. Inferior homonymous hemianopic scotomas that break out to the periphery in a patient with an infarct of the left superior occipital cortex.

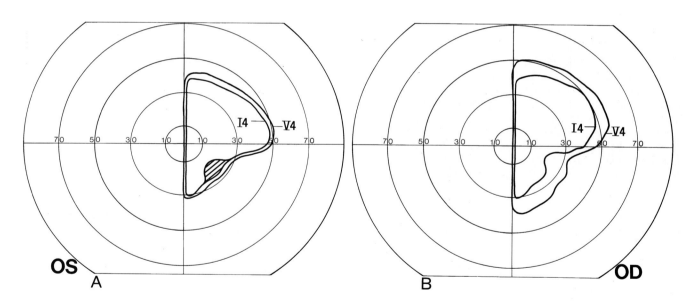

Figure 12.37. Visual field defects in a 22-year-old woman who suffered bilateral occipital lobe infarctions. There is a complete left homonymous hemianopia and an incomplete right inferior homonymous quadrantanopia. The temporal crescent is absent from the right visual field.

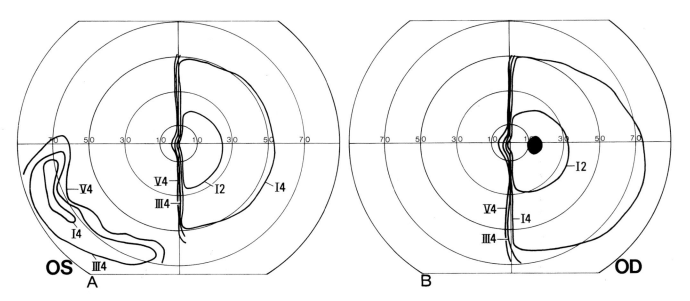

Figure 12.38. Visual field defects in a 56-year-old woman with a right occipital lobe infarction. There is a left homonymous hemianopia with sparing of the inferior portion of the left temporal crescent.

crescent terminating above the calcarine fissure and the fibers for the superior portion of the crescent terminating below the fissure.

Bender and Strauss (208) found that in 100 patients with verified cerebral tumor affecting the posterior optic radiation, there was a unilateral temporal crescentic defect in the visual field of 10 patients. The recognition of such a defect has value in the early diagnosis of a lesion of the posterior optic radiation or anterior visual cortex. Theoretically, a lesion anywhere in the postchiasmal visual pathway, from the optic tract to the occipital lobe (and particularly the dorsal LGB), could produce a monocular field defect in the temporal periphery (244); however, in practice, only lesions in the posterior optic radiation or anterior visual cortex produce such selective damage.

Both upper and lower temporal crescents may be scotomatous in the field of one eye, or only the upper or lower temporal crescent may be affected. Frequently, such a field defect is followed later by the development of an homonymous hemianopia (316). Bender and Strauss (208) fairly often found an unpaired crescentic relative scotoma medial to the peripheral absolute scotoma, indicating to them that the optic radiation has a lamellar arrangement.

Just as the temporal crescent may be affected by lesions destroying the most anterior occipital lobe, it may likewise be spared when the remainder of the temporal visual field is affected in an homonymous hemianopia (284,314,319,320) (Figs. 12.35 and 12.38). Such sparing seems to occur exclusively in patients with occipital lobe lesions that spare the anterior aspect of the visual cortex (208).

Two important facts should be kept in mind when considering the temporal crescent syndrome. First, monocular peripheral temporal visual field defects are probably caused most often by retinal lesions, not by intracranial ones. Thus, the nasal retinal periphery should be carefully examined ophthalmoscopically in such cases. Second, because these defects begin approximately 60° from fixation, central field testing (i.e., that performed using a tangent screen or most automated static perimetry programs) gives normal results and will not detect such defects (321,322) (Fig. 12.39).

Bilateral Effects of Unilateral Occipital Lobe Lesions

Although patients with unilateral lesions of the occipital lobe typically have visual deficits totally restricted to the contralateral field, area V1 and adjacent extrastriate areas often function or fail in concert. Pathologic lesions of the occipital lobe thus may disrupt not only area V1 but also adjacent underlying white matter and extrastriate cortex. Such damage may alter interhemispheric connections along their presplenial course and even disturb visual cortical–subcortical connections. Nonetheless, there is excellent evidence that there are regions of cortex ipsilateral to the field defect that process visual information (323,324). Rarely, cortical plasticity in the setting of congenital cerebral lesions can lead to developmental reorganization of the visual processing areas so that the visual field is represented ipsilaterally (325). There is also indirect evidence for reorganization of projections to extrastriate visual processing areas after injury to V1 (326).

For example, in a study by Bender and Teuber (327,328), dark adaptation was delayed in the apparently normal field. Rizzo and Robin (329) studied the vision of 12 patients with unilateral lesions of the visual cortex. All patients had homonymous defects in the contralateral visual fields, as expected, and all had visual acuity of 20/30 or better in both eyes. The first experiment performed by Rizzo and Robin (329) tested the subjects' ability to respond to transient sig-

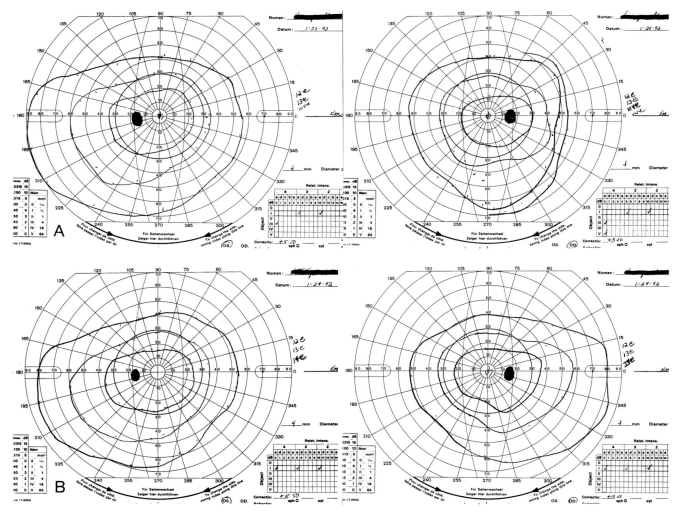

Figure 12.39. Migrainous loss of the temporal crescent. *A,* A 31-year-old woman with a history of migraine without aura had the sudden onset of a bright light in the temporal field of vision of the right eye, followed by loss of vision in this same region, and subsequent headache. The field deficit persisted for a few days and then resolved. *B,* Visual fields performed 5 days later were full in both eyes. Magnetic resonance imaging performed at the time of the initial deficit was completely normal.

nals presented at unpredictable temporal intervals and spatial locations among many spatially random and identical distracter elements. The results showed that compared with controls, the lesion group had a significantly reduced sensitivity to signal and increased response times in both hemifields. In a second experiment, Rizzo and Robin (329) tested the useful field of view in two of the patients under conditions of differing attention demand. Both patients showed bilateral constriction, consistent with the results of the first experiment. Rizzo and Robin suggested that one possible explanation for the bilateral effects of unilateral occipital lobe lesions is damage to interhemispheric connections along their presplenial course, affecting the synthesis of visual information from both hemifields. The disturbances are task-dependent and seem to result from a global reduction in visual attention capacity.

Subsequent experiments by Battelli et al. (329a) showed ipsilateral effects of right parietal lobe lesions on motion detection and suggested that some of these effects could be mediated by specific alterations in attention circuits. Although these disturbances are subtle compared with the homonymous visual field defects that occur in patients with unilateral occipital lobe lesions, they may be responsible for various unexplained complaints of reduced performance in tasks with high visual information-processing demands such as reading and driving.

Macular Sparing

When a portion of the central field of each eye in homonymous hemianopia is preserved as a result of deviation of the vertical meridian between the functioning and nonfunctioning halves of the visual fields, there is said to be "sparing of the macula" or "macular sparing." In a majority of such cases, visual acuity is normal, with the zone of preserved visual field ranging from 1° or 2° in width to almost 10° (Fig. 12.40). Another type of field in which there is sparing is the "overshot" field (284). In such a visual field, the sparing is not central alone but extends along the entire vertical meridian. A complete discussion of this phenomenon appears in the paper by Safran et al. (330).

Deviation of the vertical meridian accounting for macular sparing is a much-debated phenomenon. Although it is usually seen in patients with retrogeniculate (usually occipital) lesions, the absence of sparing does not imply that the lesion is pregeniculate or noncortical. The etiology of macular spar-

ing is controversial. Some authors consider it an artifact of testing. Others believe it is a real phenomenon related to the representation of a small portion of each macula in each occipital lobe. Finally, some authors believe that macular sparing results from incomplete damage of the visual pathways or occipital lobe. This section addresses each of these theories in turn.

What has been represented as wide sparing may often be shown in reality to be much narrower when ocular fixation is carefully controlled. Hence, imprecisely charted fields tend to show a wider sparing than actually exists. In many cases of homonymous hemianopia with sparing, it is possible to prove a shift in fixation by charting the blind spot in the single field in which it can be performed. Another method

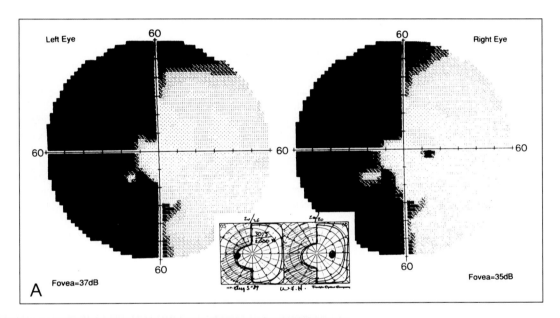

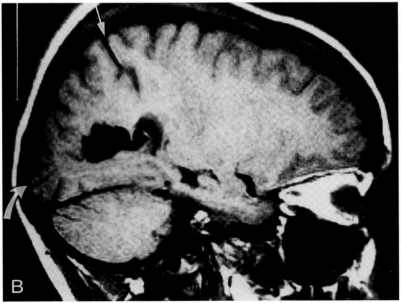

Figure 12.40. A 28-year-old woman suffered a persistent visual field defect after an unusually severe migraine attack. *A*, Full-threshold 60° visual fields using a Humphrey Field Analyzer show the central 15° of the left hemifield is intact. In the *inset*, the visual fields mapped at the tangent screen show that the field defect bisects the blind spot representation of the left eye. *B*, T1-weighted parasagittal magnetic resonance image through the right occipital lobe shows an arteriovenous malformation involving the anterior portion of the right calcarine cortex. The posterior margin of the lesion is situated 31 mm from the occipital tip, marking the approximate location of the representation of the left eye's blind spot. The calcarine (*curved arrow*) and parieto-occipital (*straight arrow*) sulci are indicated. (From Horton JC, Hoyt WF. The representation of the visual field in human striate cortex. Arch Ophthalmol 1991;109:816–824.)

is performing a tangent screen examination using three or more identical stimuli slowly brought horizontally from the defective hemifield toward the vertical meridian. One stimulus moves toward fixation, as the others simultaneously move inward to points 10–15° above and below fixation. With genuine macular sparing, the central stimulus is perceived before those above and below it. If there is defective fixation and shifting of the entire hemifield, however, all targets are simultaneously perceived.

It is impossible to obtain absolutely stable fixation, and physiologic movements of the fixing eye so slight that they cannot be detected by ordinary means probably account for 1–2° of deviation of the vertical meridian about the central area. Verhoeff (331) emphasized the importance of the optic fixation reflexes in cases of macular sparing. He suggested that loss of integration between the seeing field and the blind field in the conscious visual cortical area in use might result in eccentric fixation. As a result of fixation slippage, the original macular field would be split but would appear to be spared during field testing. Sugishita et al. (332) used fundus perimetry combined with fundus image analysis in two subjects with left occipital lesions and "macular sparing." Two of the four eyes tested showed eccentric fixation, and miniature eye movements to the blind hemifield were observed in 4–10% of the trials. Using microperimetry and a scanning laser ophthalmoscope, Bischoff et al. (333) also demonstrated rapid fixation shifts in their patients with "macular sparing" of 1–5°. These authors concluded that this typical macular sparing may be a functional adaptation of the ocular motor system to enhance the central visual field toward the blind hemifield.

In 1928 Lenz (334) proposed that a small fiber tract subserving the macular region branched from the optic tract through the corpus callosum to the opposite visual cortex, providing representation of the macula in both occipital lobes. The presence of bilateral representation of the macula was further suggested by Penfield et al. (277), who studied five patients after radical extirpation of the occipital lobe. In two instances, the posterior portion of the lobe was excised. In both, there was complete homonymous hemianopia with splitting of the macula. In two other cases, a large portion of the lobe was removed, and it was thought that the entire calcarine cortex was included. Nevertheless, following surgery, the patient had an homonymous hemianopia with macular sparing and retention of normal visual acuity. The fifth and most interesting case studied by Penfield et al. (277) was one in which there was complete destruction of the calcarine cortex of one side. This pathologic process resulted in homonymous hemianopia with sparing. When the diseased occipital lobe was extirpated, the line of resection was so far forward that it was adjacent to the splenium of the corpus callosum. Subsequent to the resection there were further field changes in that the vertical meridian failed to deviate about the point of fixation. Thus, "sparing of the macula" was converted into "splitting of the macula." Ohki et al. (335) described a case that was the reverse of Penfield's fifth case. The patient was a 62-year-old man who experienced a left parieto-occipital hemorrhage. When first examined, the patient had a right homonymous hemianopia with

macular splitting. As the hemorrhage resolved, the patient developed macular sparing, initially of 5° and then of 10°.

From a study of reported cases of occipital lobectomy and five cases studied personally, Dubois-Poulsen et al. (336) also supported the concept of macular representation in both occipital lobes as an explanation for macular sparing. These researchers endorsed a theory that had first been proposed by Morax (337), who suggested that in the foveal region of the retina there is a small vertical band of ganglion cells, some of which have crossed and others uncrossed fibers. Gramberg-Danielsen (338) supported this thesis in a thorough review of the problem of macular sparing. He emphasized the inexact nature of the vertical border between the two hemifields and called attention to a functional vertical overlap of the two sides of the visual field in the form of a narrow band that is widest near the fovea. At the retinal level, ganglion cells and their dendritic processes overlap and intertwine without any morphologic suggestion of the functional vertical separation of the two halves of the retina, corresponding to the temporal and nasal halves of the visual field. Halstead et al. (339) carefully studied the visual fields of two patients who underwent complete occipital lobectomy and found "splitting" in one case and "sparing" in the other. From a study of occipital lobectomy cases, Huber (340) (who subsequently declared macular sparing to be an artifact [333,341]) also confirmed the phenomenon of macular sparing, favoring the theory of bilateral foveal representation probably explained at the level of the retina.

Cowey (342) found occasional anomalous receptive fields for cells in the squirrel monkey's cortical fovea. All of his animals had previously had an occipital lobectomy. Recording from a microelectrode in a single cortical unit in the foveal area of the monkey' intact occipital lobe, he was able to evoke responses from the parafoveal area of the "blind" visual field. He recognized the similarity of his experimental finding to the clinical observation of macular sparing following occipital lobectomy in man.

It is clear from histochemical studies that, to some extent, a small portion of each macula probably has representation in each occipital lobe. As noted in Chapter 1, there is a small area of nasotemporal overlap on either side of the vertical meridian in which some axons from ganglion cells temporal to the fovea cross within the chiasm, whereas some axons from ganglion cells nasal to the fovea remain uncrossed (210,211,213,214,343). In the monkey, the nasotemporal overlap is smallest (about 1° of visual angle) near the fovea and increases at least twofold in more peripheral retina (213,214). Scanning laser ophthalmoscopy has demonstrated this zone of nasotemporal overlap in humans that extends into the blind hemifield, with a slightly concave shape (344).

Despite the presence of a nasotemporal overlap that exists in nonhuman primates and presumably in humans as well, the mere presence of an overlap does not necessarily have major visual consequences. Sugishita et al. (332) concluded that dual macular representation, if it exists in humans, must be less than 0.4° wide, and Brysbaert (345) also questioned the clinical significance of bilateral macular representation. Of more importance, however, is that a ganglion cell located on one side of the fovea does not necessarily receive input from a photoreceptor located on the same side. The much larger width of the cone pedicle compared with the foveal cone soma creates a packing problem that is only partly resolved by lateral displacement of cone pedicles and via the nerve fiber layer of Henle. This lateral shift could theoretically connect photoreceptors on one side of the vertical meridian to seemingly distant ganglion cells on the opposite side (266). Such an anatomic relationship would have no visual consequences, because it is the position of the photoreceptor and not the ganglion cell body that determines the location of visual input to the brain. The anatomic inexactness of the vertical demarcation can be observed clinically by visual field testing (289).

Nonetheless, the most likely cause of true macular sparing in clinical practice is incomplete damage to the visual pathways, particularly the occipital lobe. Wilbrand (347) suggested that macular sparing was the result of residual intact areas of the visual pathways. McAuley and Russell (308) noted an association between macular sparing and retained portions of the most posterior portion of the occipital cortex (Fig. 12.41). These observations are supported by the work of Horton and Hoyt (298), who demonstrated the extremely high cortical magnification of the macular representation (Fig. 12.40). The unique dual blood supply of the occipital cortex from the posterior cerebral and middle cerebral arteries (see Chapters 1 and 39) provides a mechanism for this partial damage. In patients with homonymous hemianopia and substantial macular sparing, not only is the location of the lesion almost always the occipital lobe, but also the pathogenesis is likely posterior cerebral artery infarction. In these cases, the most common cause for macular sparing is retention of some functioning posterior occipital cortex. In other cases, macular sparing may reflect fixation artifact or bilateral representation. Together, the consequences of these theories can explain the great variability in macular sparing seen in retrochiasmal disease.

Bilateral Occipital Lobe Lesions

Bilateral lesions of the occipital lobes may occur simultaneously or consecutively. Because such lesions are neurologically asymptomatic except with respect to the visual system, patients with unilateral lesions that have caused a homonymous field defect may not be aware of the defect until their attention is called to it (e.g., during a routine ocular examination or after a motor vehicle accident) or until they experience a similar event on the opposite side.

Förster first described a patient with a well-documented, partial, bilateral homonymous hemianopia in 1890 (348). The patient initially sustained a right homonymous hemianopia followed by a left homonymous hemianopia with sparing of central vision. Numerous case reports subsequently documented this condition and its many causes (349–358).

Bilateral homonymous hemianopia may appear simultaneously. In a majority of these cases, there is initially complete visual loss; however, this total blindness is usually transient, lasting from minutes to days (359,360). Nepple et al. (356) reviewed the findings in 15 patients with bilateral homonymous hemianopia. All patients had similarly shaped visual field defects on corresponding sides of the vertical midline for each eye, symmetric (and usually normal) visual acuity, normal pupils and fundi, and normal ocular motility unless there was a coexisting brain stem lesion. The majority

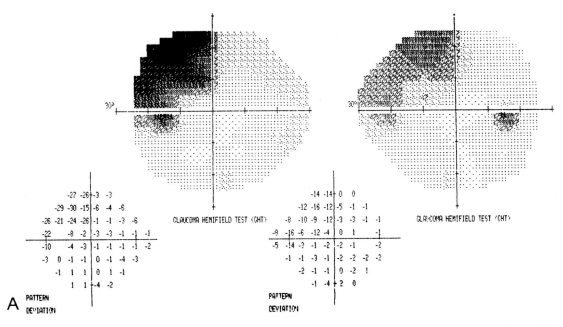

Figure 12.41. A 52-year-old man with coronary artery disease and thrombocytopenia purpura noticed trouble seeing to the left side with his left eye. *A,* Examination was normal except for visual fields, which showed an incongruous left homonymous quadrantic defect, denser in the left eye. *(Figure continues.)*

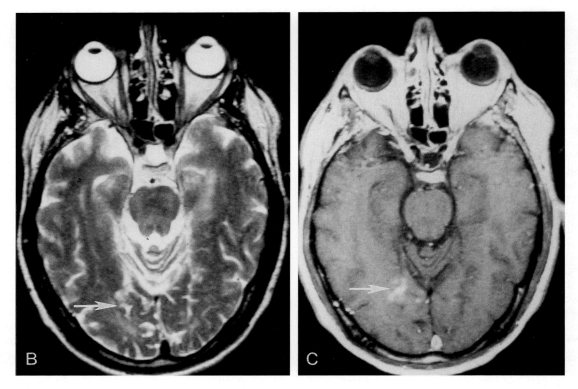

Figure 12.41. Continued. *B and C,* Magnetic resonance images (*B,* T2-weighted; *C,* T1-weighted after gadolinium) showed a curvilinear enhancing lesion in the medial, anterior, right occipital lobe consistent with infarction (*arrows*).

of patients had bilateral posterior cerebral artery insufficiency caused by arteriosclerosis (40%), uncal herniation from subdural hematoma (20%), or migraine (13%). Most of these patients had a history suggestive of simultaneous bilateral occurrence. Brain tumor did not occur in this series; conversely, in 849 patients with visual field defects and brain

tumors reviewed by Schaublin (361), there were no patients with bilateral homonymous hemianopias.

Bilateral homonymous hemianopia may also occur from consecutive events, invariably vascular (Fig. 12.42). This is a much more common phenomenon than is bilateral simultaneous homonymous hemianopia. In such cases, the patient

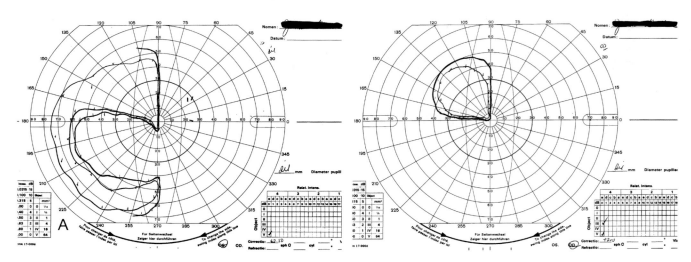

Figure 12.42. *A,* Bilateral homonymous hemianopic defects secondary to bilateral posterior cerebral artery infarction. Note the dense right homonymous hemianopia combined with a left inferior homonymous quadrantanopia with sparing of the left temporal crescent. *(Figure continues.)*

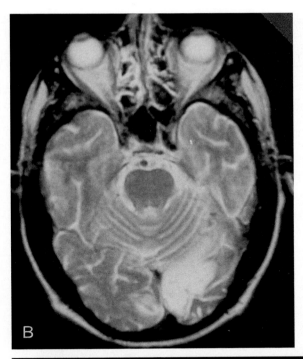

Figure 12.42. Continued. *B–D*, T2-weighted magnetic resonance images demonstrated bilateral posterior cerebral artery infarctions, worse on the left than the right, and extending less inferiorly and less anteriorly on the right.

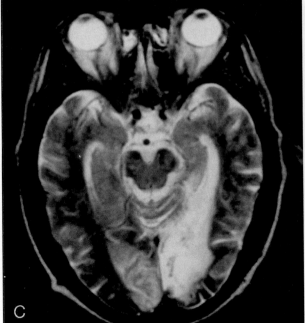

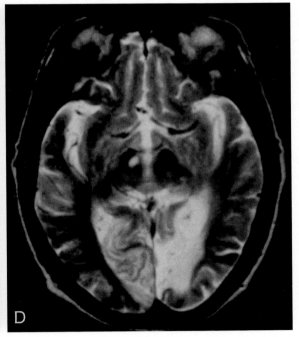

experiences an acute homonymous hemianopia with retention of normal vision with or without sparing of the macula. At a later time, varying from weeks to years, the patient develops a sudden homonymous hemianopia on the opposite side, again with or without macular sparing. After this second event, the patient is either blind or retains only a small central field around the point of fixation, similar to that seen in simultaneous cases.

The syndrome of bilateral nonsimultaneous homonymous

hemianopia from infarction of both occipital lobes is most frequently observed in elderly atherosclerotic individuals and may be associated with hypertensive crisis. In some instances, there are premonitory visual disturbances such as flashing lights or visual hallucinations. Because the vascular supply to association areas of the visual cortex may be interrupted, there may also be visual agnosia and other disturbances of higher cortical function.

Bilateral vascular lesions of the occipital lobes produce

bilateral homonymous lesions that are characteristic and vary only in their extent. They may be complete or scotomatous, and they may or may not be accompanied by macular sparing. Bender and Furlow (362,363), for instance, described "central scotomas" produced by bilateral lesions of the occipital lobes. Such defects are, in reality, bilateral homonymous scotomas that may be detected by careful field testing along the vertical midline (364) (Fig. 12.43A and B). Occasionally, such scotomas have enough central sparing to produce "ring" scotomas. One such patient had complete blindness transiently following a tractor accident. When vi-

sion returned, the patient noted that although he could see clearly in the exact center of his field, the paracentral area was blurred. Visual field testing demonstrated bilateral, congruous, homonymous scotomas with macular sparing (Fig. 12.43C and D).

Bilateral occipital lobe disease, whether from infarction, tumor, or trauma, may result in various degrees of bilateral homonymous hemianopia (Fig. 12.44). There may be complete (cortical or cerebral) blindness. The hemianopia may be complete on one side and incomplete (and congruous) on the other, or there may be a hemianopia on one side and a

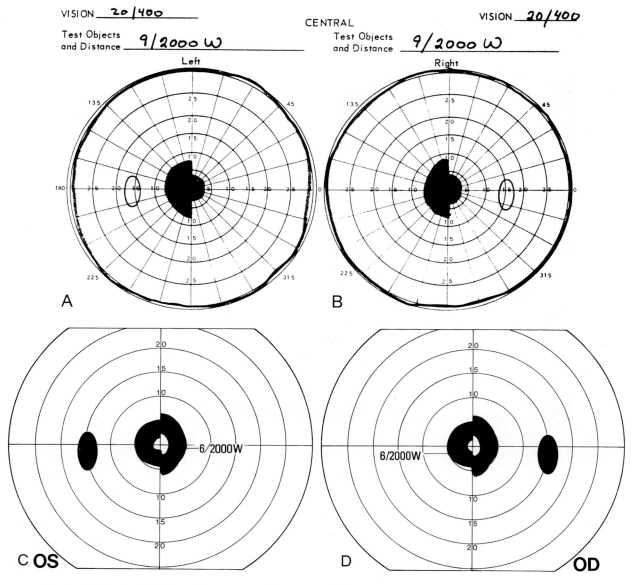

Figure 12.43. *A and B,* Bilateral homonymous hemianopic scotomas in a patient with bilateral nonsimultaneous occipital lobe strokes. *C and D,* Note vertical step that differentiates these defects from a true central scotoma with macular sparing in a patient who suffered trauma to the occipital region. The tractor on which he was riding overturned, pinning him underneath for several minutes. Initially, he was completely blind, but vision returned within several minutes. He subsequently realized that he had a "ring" of blurred vision around fixation. Note that the homonymous scotomas respect the vertical midline.

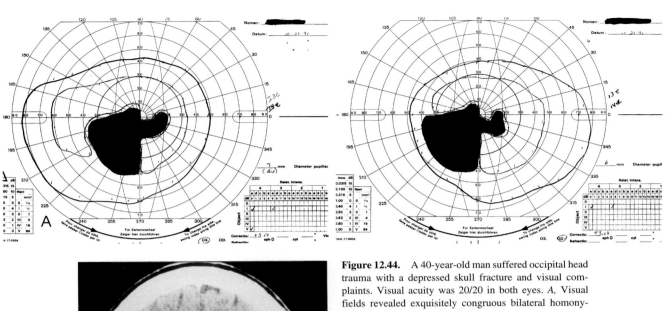

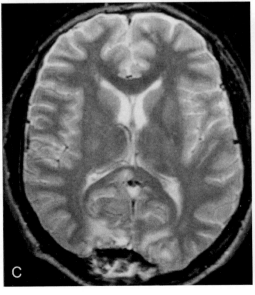

Figure 12.44. A 40-year-old man suffered occipital head trauma with a depressed skull fracture and visual complaints. Visual acuity was 20/20 in both eyes. *A,* Visual fields revealed exquisitely congruous bilateral homonymous scotomas, larger on the left than the right. A computed tomography scan (*B*) revealed a right occipital pole lesion, but magnetic resonance images (*C and D*) confirmed bilateral occipital pole involvement.

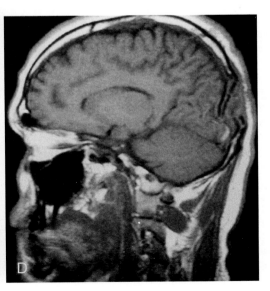

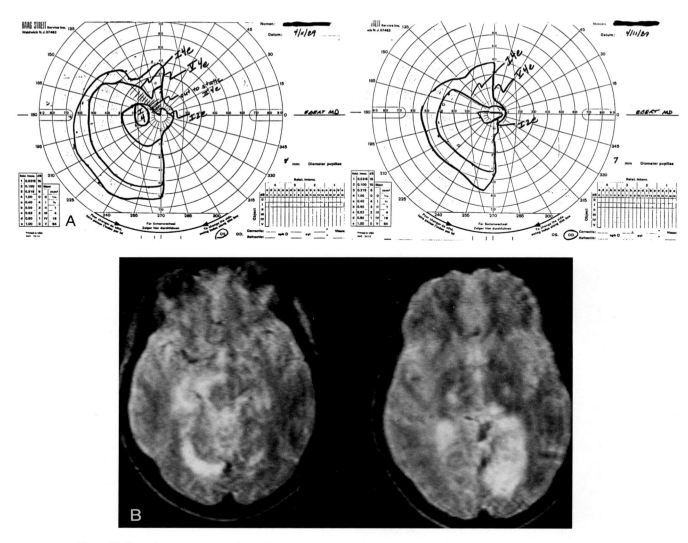

Figure 12.45. After strenuous exercise, a 33-year-old man suffered intermittent confusion, gait disturbances, and right facial weakness, followed by permanent left hemiparesis and difficulties with vision. *A,* Visual fields revealed a right homonymous hemianopia with macular sparing and a left superior homonymous quadrantanopia. *B,* Magnetic resonance imaging revealed the corresponding infarctions in the occipital lobes bilaterally. Note the involvement of the inferior occipital lobe on the right and the entire calcarine cortex on the left, with sparing of the most posterior pole. The patient also had cerebellar and brain stem infarctions, all secondary to artery-to-artery emboli from a vertebral artery dissection.

quadrantanopia on the other (307,365) (Figs. 12.42 and 12.45). In some instances, there may be a bilateral homonymous hemianopia with bilateral macular sparing of a different degree on each side. The remaining visual field thus appears to be severely constricted, and such patients may be thought to have bilateral optic nerve or retinal disease or may even be thought to have nonorganic visual field loss. As with bilateral homonymous hemianopic scotomas, however, careful testing along the vertical midline will establish the bilateral nature of the field defect and its correct origin (Fig. 12.46).

Crossed quadrant hemianopia results when patients develop bilateral quadrantic defects, either simultaneously or more commonly consecutively, that affect the superior oc-

cipital lobe above the calcarine fissure on one side and the inferior occipital lobe below the fissure on the other side. Such defects are sometimes called checkerboard fields and are infrequent (Fig. 12.47). Felix (366) described a case and reviewed the literature up to 1926, which included only two other cases. In the case reported by Felix and in one other case, this field defect followed a simultaneous bilateral homonymous hemianopia, although a case described by Groenouw (quoted by Felix [366]) occurred after two separate vascular events occurring 10 months apart.

Although bilateral altitudinal field defects are usually caused by bilateral anterior optic nerve disease (e.g., glaucoma or nonarteritic anterior ischemic optic neuropathy), they can also be caused by bilateral occipital lobe disease

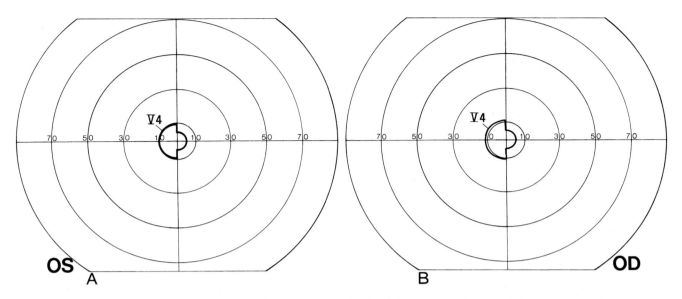

Figure 12.46. Bilateral homonymous hemianopias with macular sparing in a patient with severe cerebrovascular occlusive disease. The patient initially presented with 20/20 vision in both eyes but with "tubular" fields. The macular sparing respects the vertical midline.

(e.g., from trauma, infarction, hemorrhage, and rarely tumors). Such lesions were studied extensively by Holmes and Lister (375) and were subsequently described in more detail by Holmes (367), who observed that bullet wounds interrupting both occipital lobes were usually fatal if the lower portions were damaged because death occurred from intracranial bleeding as a result of laceration of the dural sinuses in the region of the torcular herophili. When the upper portions of the visual cortex or posterior radiations were damaged, however, the patient often survived, and the resultant field defects in such cases were altitudinal, with loss of the entire inferior field of both eyes.

Money and Nelson (1943) described field defects similar to those reported by Holmes (367), and Wortham et al. (368) reported bilateral inferior hemianopia occurring during or immediately following thoracoplasty. The defect was

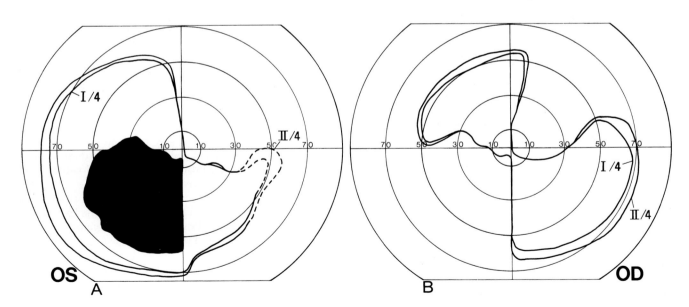

Figure 12.47. Crossed quadrant (checkerboard) hemianopia. These field defects occurred suddenly in a 70-year-old woman with basilar artery disease. Note the quadrantic defects in the right upper field and the left lower field with the narrow congruous isthmus near fixation. Also note the sparing of the left temporal crescent and the incongruity of the field defects along the upper vertical meridian and the right horizontal meridian. (Courtesy of University of California Hospital, San Francisco.)

thought to have resulted from anoxia, and slight improvement occurred over the next several months' observation. Newman et al. (369) described two cases of bilateral altitudinal hemianopia, one inferior and one superior, secondary to occipital infarctions that were demonstrated by CT scanning, and a similar case was confirmed both on neuroimaging and pathology by Vanroose et al. (370). Other cases secondary to occipital infarction or hemorrhage occur, occasionally in the setting of cardiac surgery or hypoxia (308,353,368, 371–376).

Based on the preceding, it can be understood why superior altitudinal defects from occipital lobe trauma are less common than inferior altitudinal defects. An example of the former, occurring in a patient where a bullet passed from right to left through the inferior portions of both occipital lobes but missing the dural sinuses, is depicted in Figure 12.48. On the other hand, both superior (Fig. 12.49) and inferior bilateral altitudinal defects can occur with vascular disease affecting the occipital lobes. When the lesion is far posterior, the field defect remains altitudinal but is central and scotomatous (Fig. 12.50). Spalding (296) confirmed the impressive congruity of these small field defects.

Cortical (Cerebral) Blindness

Cortical blindness and cerebral blindness are considered in the same section because in many instances it is impossible to differentiate between them on clinical grounds. The term "cortical blindness" indicates loss of vision in both eyes from damage to the striate cortex. "Cerebral blindness" is a more general term indicating blindness from damage to any portion of both visual pathways posterior to the lateral geniculate bodies. Thus, cortical blindness is a subset of cerebral blindness. Patients with cerebral blindness may have other neurologic deficits, including hemiplegia, sensory disorders, aphasia, and disorientation. Because of the similarity in the visual system symptomatology between these two conditions, for the sake of simplicity the term "cortical blindness" will be used in this section.

The essential features of cortical blindness as outlined by Marquis (377) are (a) complete loss of all visual sensation, including all appreciation of light and dark; (b) loss of reflex lid closure to bright illumination and to threatening gestures; (c) retention of the reflex constriction of the pupils to illumination and to convergence movements (the near-response); (d) integrity of the normal structure of the retinas as verified with the ophthalmoscope; (e) retention of full extraocular movements of the eyes, unless there is also damage to ocular motor structures. Many neuro-ophthalmologists use the term "cortical blindness" not only where the visual acuity is light perception or no light perception but also with any level of visual acuity, as long as the visual acuity is equal in the two eyes (assuming the anterior visual pathways are normal).

Hypoxia or ischemia of the occipital lobes is the most common etiologic factor producing cortical blindness. Such damage is necessarily bilateral. Most commonly, an infarction in the posterior cerebral artery territory is initially unrecognized, but this previously silent hemianopia contributes to complete cortical blindness when a contralateral lesion

occurs (378,379). The most common mechanism for the infarction is cerebral embolism from either the heart or the more proximal vessels of the vertebrobasilar system (380,381) (Fig. 12.51). Prolonged hypotension can cause cortical blindness from bilateral watershed infarctions at the parieto-occipital junction. Courville (382), among others, recognized that hypoxia causes laminar cortical necrosis and that the visual, premotor, and parietal areas are particularly apt to be damaged by this process. Courville (382) expressed the opinion that these areas seemingly had a higher oxygen requirement. Lindenberg (383) emphasized that the affected areas represent the border zones of cerebral circulation.

Cortical blindness is observed under many circumstances other than infarction, including trauma, neoplasm, malignant hypertension, toxemia of pregnancy, diseases of white matter (e.g., Schilder's disease, adrenoleukodystrophy, Pelizaeus-Merzbacher disease, metachromatic leukodystrophy, progressive multifocal leukoencephalopathy), Creutzfeldt-Jakob disease, mitochondrial encephalopathy lactic acidosis and stroke-like episodes (MELAS), cerebral angiography, ventriculography, blood transfusions, uremia, acute intermittent porphyria, syphilis, infectious and neoplastic meningitis, bacterial endocarditis, subacute sclerosing panencephalitis, hepatic encephalopathy, sudden elevation or reduction in intracranial pressure, cardiac arrest, hypoglycemia, correction of hyponatremia, epilepsy, electroshock, and after exposure to carbon monoxide, nitrous oxide, ethanol, licorice, methamphetamine, mercury, lead, cis-platinum, cyclosporin A, tacrolimus (FK506), methotrexate, vincristine, vindesine, and interferon (379,384–418). The mechanism of injury underlying the cortical blindness caused by these events or substances is not always known, but vascular insufficiency plays a role in many of them.

In certain situations, cortical blindness is transient. This is particularly true in patients who experience transient vascular insufficiency in the vertebrobasilar system, in hypertensive syndromes following restoration of normal blood pressure, after removal of many of the toxic agents listed above, and after trauma (417,419–421). Children are more likely to experience recovery from cortical blindness than adults, regardless of the underlying cause. Barnet et al. (419) studied six children who developed transient cortical blindness after respiratory or cardiac arrest, head trauma, or meningitis. In all cases, visual acuity returned to some extent in 1–10 weeks. Greenblatt (422) emphasized three clinical patterns of transient cortical blindness following head trauma:

1. Juvenile (up to age 8 years). These patients experience blindness of short duration (hours), accompanied by somnolence, irritability, and vomiting, with an excellent prognosis for full recovery.
2. Adolescent (late childhood through teenage years). These patients have blindness that does not develop immediately after the trauma but occurs several minutes later. The blindness lasts minutes to hours, is usually unaccompanied by other neurologic or systemic deficits, and also tends to resolve completely.
3. Adult. These patients have immediate blindness, a

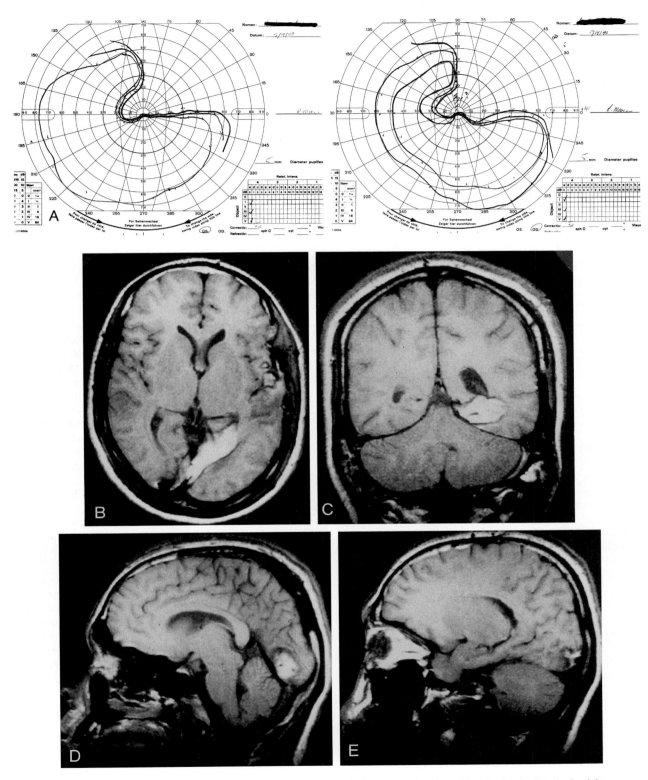

Figure 12.48. A 24-year-old man suffered a gunshot wound to the left temporal region with exit of the bullet via the right occipital pole. Visual acuity was 20/20 in both eyes, but there was cerebral dyschromatopsia and prosopagnosia. *A,* Visual fields showed a right superior homonymous quadrantanopia (probably resulting from damage to the left inferior radiations at the temporal–occipital lobe junction) and a left superior homonymous quadrantic scotoma (probably from damage to the right inferior occipital pole). *B–E,* Magnetic resonance images showed the hematoma created by the bullet track.

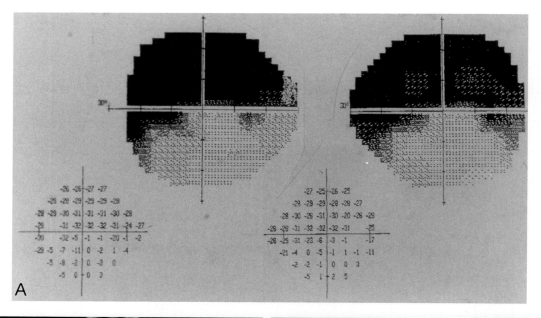

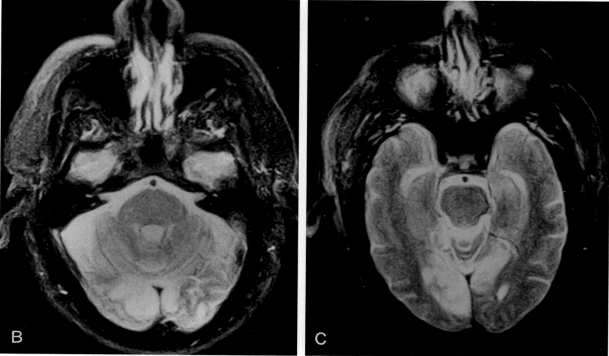

Figure 12.49.   A 71-year-old man had acute onset of complete visual loss, followed by clearing inferiorly. *A,* Examination was normal except for visual fields that showed bilateral superior altitudinal visual field defects (bilateral superior homonymous quadrantanopias). *B–F,* T2-weighted magnetic resonance images (*B–D,* axial views; *E and F,* sagittal views to the right and left of midline, respectively) demonstrated bilateral posterior cerebral artery infarctions involving primarily the inferior occipital lobes. *(Figure continues.)*

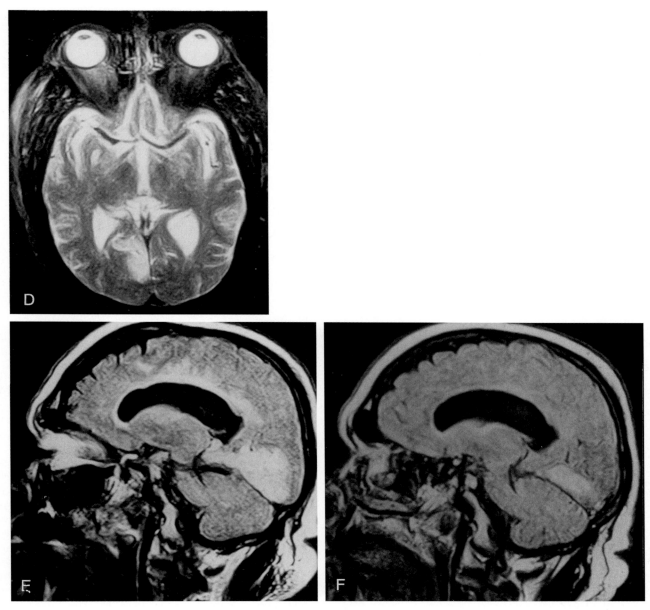

Figure 12.49. Continued.

protracted course with other neurologic defects, and a variable visual outcome.

Postictal cortical blindness is not uncommon (395, 423,424), and ictal cortical blindness as a manifestation of occipital seizures may occur (409,425–429). Ashby and Stephenson (430) analyzed 11 cases of blindness after seizures and concluded that there is a form of amaurosis that occurs in young children and infants that is postictal and is caused by depression of the visual centers. The seizures that accompany such blindness are usually violent and may be associated with aphasia and paresis of hemiplegic distribution. The hemiplegia may be permanent, although the visual loss is generally transient. Joseph and Louis (429) reviewed

the literature concerning seizure-induced bilateral blindness and divided affected patients into three groups. Fifteen patients, all under 12 years of age, had a long succession of seizures or status epilepticus. They developed blindness that was permanent or that lasted many months. Ten patients, seven of whom were between the ages of 10 and 20 years, had bilateral occipital seizures with blindness corresponding to atypical spike and wave activity. The blindness lasted less than 30 minutes in all cases. Finally, 18 patients had a focal seizure originating in or adjacent to an occipital lobe, with ictal spread to involve both occipital lobes. In these patients, blindness occurred either ictally or postictally. Because focal lesions may be responsible for ictal amaurosis, MR imaging

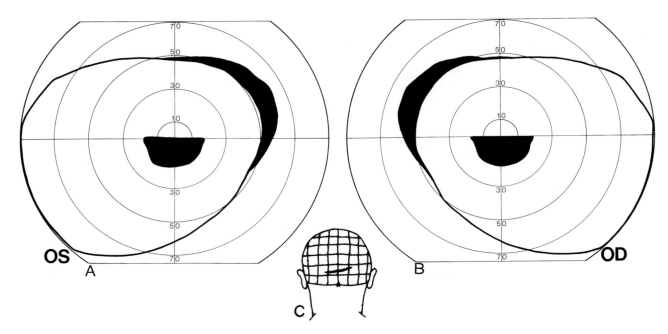

Figure 12.50. Occipital injury (shell fragment). Bilateral inferior hemianopic quadrantic scotomas, according to Holmes. (From Traquair HM. An Introduction to Clinical Perimetry, 3rd edition. St Louis, CV Mosby, 1940.)

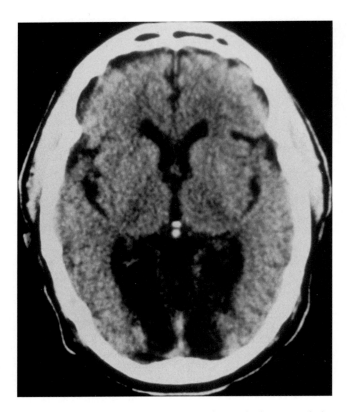

Figure 12.51. Bilateral simultaneous posterior cerebral artery occlusion secondary to embolic infarction from a cardiac arrhythmia. The patient was initially cortically blind with no light perception vision. Over the course of a few weeks he had 20/30 vision in each eye because of 5° of macular sparing.

should be performed in all cases (409). Complete recovery from ictal or postictal blindness can occur even though the blindness lasts for several days.

Visual-Evoked Responses in Cortical Blindness

The relationship between cortical blindness and the visual-evoked response (VER) is unclear. One of the earliest human studies on this subject was performed by Kooi and Sharbrough (431). Their patient had suffered head trauma and was initially blind with no evoked responses to light stimuli. Subsequently, both visual acuity and VERs underwent gradual and parallel improvement. This promising correlation was corroborated by other investigators (432–434). However, Spehlmann et al. (435) reported persistence of the VER to light in a blind patient who had extensive bilateral destruction of cortical visual areas and their association areas. Similarly, Celesia et al. (436) and Hess et al. (437) demonstrated normal VERs in both complete and incomplete cortical blindness. Aldrich et al. (379) found abnormal pattern and flash VERs in 15 of 19 patients with cortical blindness, but there was no correlation with the severity of visual loss or with visual outcome. Indeed, all four patients with normal VERs during blindness had poor visual outcomes, and three patients with good outcomes had no initial responses to pattern-reversal VERs. These investigators found that electroencephalography was a more helpful diagnostic indicator: the presence of a posterior dominant alpha rhythm responsive to eye opening appears to be incompatible with complete or incomplete cortical blindness. Hence, it would appear that at least in adults, VERs are not useful in establishing either the diagnosis or prognosis in patients with cortical blindness (379,438).

The usefulness of VERs in children with cortical visual dysfunction is controversial. Barnet et al. (419) reported two children who showed well-formed VERs shortly after the onset of their acute disease, even though they were completely blind. Bodis-Wollner et al. (439) described normal VERs to both flash and alternating grating patterns in a blind child in whom CT scanning showed destruction of the cerebral cortex corresponding to areas 18 and 19 bilaterally with preservation of primary visual cortex (area 17). Frank and Torres (440) recorded VERs to brief light flashes from occipital regions in a group of 30 cortically blind children aged 4 months to 15 years. These investigators compared their results with those obtained from 31 children of similar age range who had similar central nervous system diseases but no evidence of blindness. Only one patient with cortical blindness showed no response, and the presence of abnormal responses was not incompatible with normal vision. Mellor and Fielder (441) reported that poor or even absent VERs in infancy did not always indicate a poor prognosis, and Hoyt (442) showed a similar lack of correlation. Other authors also noted poor correlation of VERs and visual function in children with bilateral cerebral abnormalities, especially those with associated neurologic deficits (443–445), and it is not uncommon to see patients free of clinical neurologic or visual deficits who have incidentally discovered abnormal VERs.

Nevertheless, some investigators argue that the VER is indeed helpful in establishing both diagnosis and prognosis in children with cortical visual dysfunction. In a study of six children with cortical blindness after either bacterial meningitis or head trauma, Duchowny et al. (446) found that changes in short-latency VER components correlate with visual ability, whereas changes in longer-latency VER components correlate with the level of psychomotor function. Kupersmith and Nelson (447) reported that the presence of a VER wave, whether normal or abnormal, indicated the future development of vision. Lambert et al. (448) and Bencivenga et al. (449) also reported some correlation of the VER response to cerebral visual function. McCulloch and Taylor (450) argued that flash VERs are an excellent indicator of visual recovery for those children who have acute-onset cortical blindness and no preexisting neurologic disorder. In this subset of patients, many with presumed hypoxia, those with abnormal VERs had permanent visual impairment or blindness, and all but one patient with absent VERs remained blind (451,452). The variable results from previous studies may reflect the many different underlying etiologies of cortical blindness in children and the many other associated neurologic factors that might contribute to poor recovery.

Optokinetic Nystagmus in Cortical Blindness

Optokinetic nystagmus (OKN), the slow component of which is generally considered a conscious pursuit movement, is often used to distinguish patients with true blindness from those with nonorganic blindness. Most investigators agree that OKN is absent in patients with total cortical blindness (385,453–455). In fact, Brindley et al. (455) repeatedly

examined a patient with total cortical blindness over a 3.5-year period and could never elicit OKN.

Ter Braak (456) separated OKN into two types: passive and active. According to this investigator, passive OKN is produced by the movement of the majority of contrasts in the visual field and may still be present after ablation of the visual cortex, whereas active OKN depends on the movement of specific objects in the visual field and thus requires "vision" for its production. Using these definitions, Ter Braak et al. (457) examined a 71-year-old man with long-standing cortical blindness and found passive OKN in one direction. Subsequent necropsy revealed almost total destruction of both striate cortices and degeneration of both LGBs.

Despite these observations, the presence of OKN in an individual complaining of complete blindness or perception of light only is almost always evidence of nonorganic visual loss (see also Chapter 21).

Cortical Blindness with Denial of Blindness (Anton's Syndrome)

Patients with cortical blindness are often unaware of their deficit. This denial of blindness, a type of anosognosia, is called Anton's syndrome (458). The syndrome also occurs in patients with blindness from causes other than occipital lobe disease, including cataracts, retinopathies, or optic atrophy (459). The explanation for Anton's syndrome is unclear. Lessell (459) reviewed the various theories and concluded that each explains some of the cases. Geschwind (quoted by Lessell [459]) suggested that patients with denial commonly have an alteration in emotional reactivity. Such patients have emotions that are described as coarse and shallow and may predispose them to deny their blindness. Lessell also stated that "psychiatric" denial may occur as an accentuation of a common response to illness. In patients with Korsakoff's syndrome, denial of blindness may represent a memory disorder. Such patients cannot remember from minute to minute that they truly are blind. Finally, it is probable that in many patients with cortical blindness, there are lesions in various areas of the brain responsible for recognition and interpretation of visual images. In such patients, denial of blindness is caused not by the lesion in the primary visual pathway but by a lesion in another region of the brain.

Other Visual Features of Occipital Lobe Damage

Bender and Teuber (327) made noteworthy observations based on their study of 140 individuals who suffered penetrating head wounds in World War II. It was their belief that when macular function is spared, there is either an incomplete homonymous hemianopia or development of a pseudofovea. They also noted that when an incomplete homonymous field defect is produced by an occipital lobe lesion, there are often disturbances in the area of the homonymous visual fields that seem spared when "ordinary" methods of perimetry are performed. For instance, critical flicker fusion frequency falls in field areas adjacent to the scotoma and to a lesser degree in field areas far distant from the scotoma.

Dark adaptation is delayed in the apparently normal field. Luminous objects can be discerned within the scotomatous field when patients are placed in total darkness. Finally, when simple figures are presented to the patient so that part of the figure is in the area of scotoma and part in the seeing field, the entire figure is seen (completion phenomenon) (460). There are several different explanations for these observations. First, the methods of perimetry used in the 1940s were clearly less sensitive than automated static perimetry. It thus is likely that many of the patients studied by Bender and Teuber (327) actually had larger field defects than were detected by what was then "routine" perimetry. Second, it is likely that the observation of luminous objects in blind areas of the field represented artifacts of testing, since it is clear that some "luminous" objects have a larger area of stimulation of the retina than might normally be assumed. In addition, minor movements of the eyes during testing that might not be detected in total darkness with the equipment available to Bender and Teuber (327) may have moved the luminous target into the seeing field adjacent to the blind field.

Some patients with homonymous hemianopia, especially those with a vascular occlusion in the occipital lobe, report phosphenes in the blind visual field, particularly early in the course of their disorder (461–464) (see also the section on visual hallucinations in Chapter 13). Among 96 patients with homonymous hemianopia or quadrantanopia, most of vascular origin, Kolmel (463) noted that 14 had experienced colored patterns in their blind hemifield, typically red, green, blue, and yellow. Many of the visual field defects in these patients resolved substantially, suggesting that the phosphenes may be viewed as a prognostically favorable symptom. Of 32 patients with ischemic infarction of the retrochiasmal pathways studied prospectively by Vaphiades et al. (464), positive spontaneous visual phenomena in the blind hemifield were present in 13 patients (41%). Classifying these positive visual phenomena as photopsias, phosphenes, palinopsia, or visual hallucinations had no value in localizing the site of the lesion. However, there was a significant difference in the severity of associated neurologic deficits between hemianopic patients with and without these positive visual phenomena; specifically, larger lesions destroying anteriorly located visual association areas precluded the development of these positive phenomena. The authors proposed that visual association areas bordering damaged primary cortex were the source of these visual symptoms when they were released from normal inhibitory inputs from primary visual cortex.

An unusual visual phenomenon associated with unilateral or bilateral occipital lesions is cerebral diplopia or polyopia, in which two or more images are perceived monocularly (465,466). Cerebral polyopia may be due to reorganization of one or more of the multiple representations of the visual field in the visual cortex (466). Unlike monocular polyopia from irregularities of the ocular refractive media, cerebral polyopia does not improve with pinhole. This entity is discussed further in Chapter 13.

Lesions of the Striate Cortex Without Defects in the Visual Field

It is generally assumed that any lesion of the striate cortex produces a defect in the field of vision, but there are cases on record that suggest that this assumption may be incorrect. Teuber (467) stated that he had records on an extraordinary case of a 1-year-old child who sustained an accidental gunshot wound through the right parietal lobe. The bullet remained in the right calcarine area, where it could still be shown radiologically 30 years later. Teuber et al. could not demonstrate any evidence of a field defect, even though they used refined tests of flicker fusion and light thresholds. Weiskrantz (468) stressed that it is conceivable that an injury of the striate cortex must produce a critical minimum amount of damage before it produces any demonstrable scotoma. Evidence supporting this has been contributed by N. R. Miller, who searched in vain for tiny scotomas produced by stereotactically implanted depth electrodes (0.5 mm in diameter) that were inserted directly into and through the macular area of the occipital pole and the occipital portion of the optic radiations. It is unlikely that standard white-on-white automated perimetry can identify visual field defects associated with these small injuries, although it is possible that static color field testing could identify such defects. Similarly, stereotactic pallidotomy, a procedure used to treat patients with Parkinson's disease, requires precise positioning before the electrode is activated. The positioning includes placement of the electrode in the ipsilateral optic tract, the cells of which are then identified by recording from the electrode (468a). The electrode is then pulled back out of the optic tract into the globus pallidus, where a lesion is then made. It is difficult to identify visual field defects in the majority of patients in whom stereotactic pallidotomy is performed, regardless of whether the testing is performed using kinetic or static automated perimetry.

Weiskrantz and Cowey (469) contributed neurophysiologic evidence to support the aforementioned observations and conclusions. They showed that quantitative lesions in the macular cortex of the monkey produce a smaller drop in visual acuity than would be predicted from equivalent lesions of the macula. They suggested that the discrepancy between retinal and cortical effects is probably best explained in terms of lateral interaction of neuronal elements at the retinal level, the geniculate level, or both. An alternative explanation is that the visual cortex has a higher relative magnification factor for the foveal representation than is accounted for by the concentration of retinal ganglion cells in the macula (305).

Lesions of the Extrastrate Cortex with Defects in the Visual Field

As noted in Chapter 1, the striate cortex (V1, or Brodmann area 17) is the primary visual cortex and the principal recipient of output from the LGB. Surrounding the striate cortex within the occipital lobe are two visual association areas, Brodmann areas 18 and 19, also called the extrastriate visual cortex. Studies from primate electrophysiologic and pathway tracing methods indicate that areas 18 and 19 together represent at least five distinct cortical areas devoted to visual processing (278,470–472). These visual areas are designated V2, V3, V3a, V4, and V5 in the monkey, and corresponding regions are present in the human occipital cortex (472). Functional MR imaging has recently been able to demonstrate multiple visual areas in the human, each with their own retinotopic mapping (473,474). Regions V2 and V3 are the major recipient areas for projections from both the magnocellular and parvocellular systems in V1, the primary striate cortex. However, V1 also directly projects to areas V4 and V5, bypassing V2 (475). The sizes of V1 and V2 are highly correlated, but not V1 and V3 (306).

Feinsod et al. (476) suggested that a lesion in the extrastriate cortex alone might cause defects in the visual field. Others reported superior visual field defects from damage to the "nonvisual" lingual and fusiform gyri (373,477). Polyak (478) reported a case in which paracentral quadrantic scotomas were caused by an infarction primarily located in a region corresponding to the ventral portion of areas V2 and V3. Horton and Hoyt (278) reported two patients with homonymous quadrantic defects caused by tumors, one in the cuneus of the occipital lobe and the other in the upper peristriate cortex (Figs. 12.52 and 12.53). These investigators proposed not only that a lesion of V2/V3 may be sufficient to create a visual field defect, but also that such lesions are the principal cause of quadrantic defects that strictly respect the horizontal meridian. This hypothesis has been supported by functional MR imaging studies demonstrating selective loss of activation of extrastriate cortex areas in a patient with an upper right homonymous quadrantic defect (479).

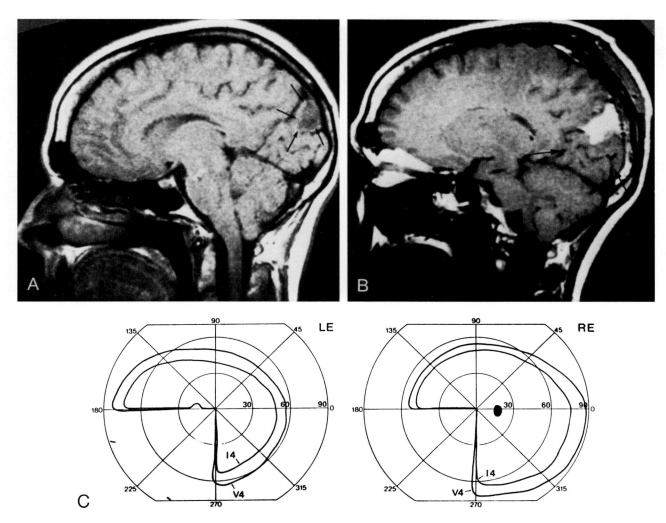

Figure 12.52. A 39-year-old woman had experienced multicolored visual hallucinations in her left lower quadrant since childhood. *A,* Magnetic resonance imaging revealed a lesion within the cuneus of the right occipital lobe that on en bloc resection was found to be a grade I astrocytoma. *B,* Postoperative magnetic resonance image revealed the area of resection. *C,* Postoperative visual fields demonstrated a left inferior homonymous quadrantanopia with precise respect of the horizontal and vertical meridians. The patient could detect gross hand motion within the quadrantic defect. (From Horton JC, Hoyt WF. Quadrantic visual field defects. A hallmark of lesions in extrastriate [V2/V3] cortex. Brain 1991;114:1703–1718.)

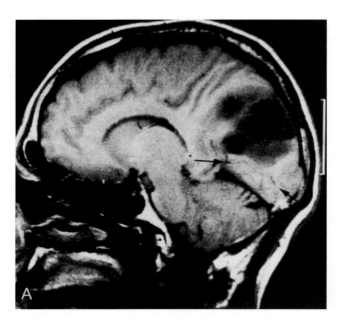

Figure 12.53. A 40-year-old man experienced increasing episodes of flashing lights in the left lower quadrant of vision and was found to have a large tumor of the right parieto-occipital cortex. *A,* On magnetic resonance imaging the calcarine sulcus (*between arrows*) and the occipital pole are preserved. *B,* After resection of the mass, he had a left lower quadrantanopia precisely bordering the horizontal meridian with sparing of the central 10°. (From Horton JC, Hoyt WF. Quadrantic visual field defects. A hallmark of lesions in extrastriate [V2/V3] cortex. Brain 1991;114:1703–1718.)

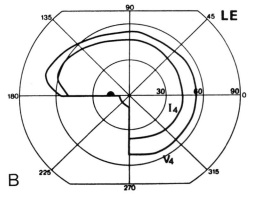
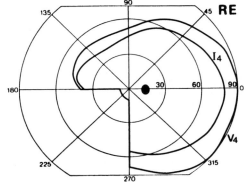

Cortical Visual Loss with Normal Neuroimaging

William F. Hoyt has suggested that the essence of neuro-ophthalmology is diagnosis in the presence of normal neuroimaging. A not uncommon example occurs when there is unilateral or bilateral homonymous hemianopia in the presence of normal MR imaging. Brazis et al. (480) reviewed several causes of this phenomenon, including the Heidenhain variant of Creutzfeldt-Jakob disease (481,482), variant Alzheimer dementia (483,484), nonketotic hypoglycemia, and ischemia without infarction. Many of these disorders can be detected with positron emission tomography scanning or functional MR imaging, which is sensitive to the effects of neural activity on blood oxygenation levels (485). Another etiology for visual loss without abnormalities on conventional MR imaging is occipital lobe seizures, which can disrupt visual perception not only during the ictus but also postictally (486) and even permanently (487).

Dissociation of Visual Perception

The chapter that follows (Chapter 13) discusses the topographic diagnosis of disorders of visual processing more dis-

tal to the primary visual cortex. Because many of these disorders result from lesions in the extrastriate cortex of the occipital lobes, it is worth mentioning a few of the more prominent syndromes in this chapter. As suggested by studies in monkeys, the human visual cortex is highly specialized with respect to specific functions (472). For instance, there are distinct areas of the cortex that subserve color vision. These can be identified either by studying patients with known lesions or by functional MR imaging mapping of activation of cortex after appropriate stimulation. One area in the lingual and fusiform gyri of the prestriate cortex corresponds to area V4 in the monkey and is responsible for color (472,488,489). Other areas adjacent to V3 can be identified by functional MR imaging as containing retinotopic maps for color (473). Lesions in any of these regions may spare the visual field but produce acquired dyschromatopsia in the contralateral hemifield (477,490,491). The disturbance of color vision in such cases may be permanent, especially if there are bilateral lesions. Conversely, transient achromatopsia may reflect temporary ischemia in this region, a phenomenon that may occur in migrainous aura (492).

The area of functional specialization for visual motion is

localized to the temporoparieto-occipital junction, a region corresponding to area V5 in the monkey (472,493,494). Lesions in this region, especially when bilateral, may cause a selective deficit in the perception of visual movement without a visual field defect and without impairment of nonvisual movement perception (i.e., movement perceived by acoustic or tactile stimulation) (495,496). A similar loss of motion detection, but in a single direction at a time, can be reproduced by electrical stimulation of the posterior temporal lobe (497).

In some patients, damage to an occipital lobe can cause a complete homonymous hemianopia to nonmoving objects, with retention of the ability to detect moving objects within the blind hemifield: static–kinetic dissociation, also called the Riddoch phenomenon. In 1917 Riddoch (498) noted that some wounded soldiers with complete homonymous hemianopia developed or retained the ability to perceive small moving objects in the affected hemifield. Riddoch divided his cases into three groups: those who perceived motion only on the affected side; those who perceived both moving and stationary objects but to a different degree; and those with no dissociation between moving and stationary objects. Static–kinetic dissociation may have prognostic significance since it usually means that some degree of recovery can be expected. Such a phenomenon has been observed not only after occipital trauma but also after removal of tumor, cortical blindness from cardiac arrest, and occipital apoplexy in patients with occipital arteriovenous malformations (see also (499)). Preservation of the human correlate of area V5 may be required for intact visual motion processing, perhaps via extrageniculostriate pathways (500) (see below).

Static–kinetic dissociation is not a purely pathologic phenomenon, nor is it limited to the striate cortex. In fact, all normal individuals perceive moving objects better than static objects of the same size, shape, and luminance. If objects are sufficiently small or dull, they will be perceived only during kinetic perimetry and not during static perimetry. Safran and Glaser (501) demonstrated variable degrees of physiologic dissociation of kinetic and static stimuli in 7 of 15 normal subjects. Interestingly, the dissociation occurred for achromatic target perception but not for chromatic perception of red. Safran and Glaser attributed this physiologic dissociation to a successive lateral summation of images, as previously noted by Greve (502). Spatial summation is more pronounced for rods than for cones, and this may explain the lack of dissociation of static and kinetic targets when hue recognition is required. Selective excitation of movement-dependent channels appears to be required for perception of movement (503). In addition, pathologic static–kinetic dissociation occurs in patients with nonoccipital lobe lesions. Zappia et al. (504) reported two patients, one with a lesion in the optic tract and one with a lesion of the optic chiasm. Both patients showed a dissociation between perception of static and kinetic objects in their affected hemifields. In addition, Safran and Glaser (501) studied 11 patients with compression of the anterior visual pathways and found some degree of static–kinetic dissociation in the defective field of all of them.

The Riddoch phenomenon of static–kinetic dissociation is one form of a general category of visual phenomena designated as ''blindsight'' (468,505–510). In a classic experiment, Mohler and Wurtz (511) removed the occipital lobe in trained monkeys. The monkeys appeared to be blind in the appropriate hemifield for several weeks but then began to make appropriate saccades into the previously blind hemifield. Mohler and Wurtz then extirpated the superior colliculi in the monkeys, who then became permanently blind in the hemifield. In another set of monkeys, Mohler and Wurtz first removed the superior colliculi. The monkeys showed some mild and transient difficulty with saccadic eye movements but no evidence of visual loss. The monkeys were then subjected to unilateral occipital lobe excision, following which they became permanently blind in the contralateral hemifield of both eyes. These experiments indicated that nonhuman primates have a subcortical vision sensory system that likely involves connections between the retina and the superior colliculus in addition to the retinogeniculo-occipital pathway for normal visual function. A similar subcortical pathway may exist in humans. Indeed, some patients with extensive damage to the occipital lobes appear to retain a rudimentary form of vision involving the perception of visual stimuli other than just moving objects. Most patients are not consciously aware of this ability to look, point, detect, and discriminate without truly ''seeing.'' In many cases blindsight is likely a result of islands of preserved area 17, as demonstrated by positron emission tomography, single photon-emission computed tomography, and image stabilization perimetry (512,513). Celesia et al. (512) argued that the sparing of portions of primary visual cortex, combined with probable scatter of light into the intact visual field during testing (514), accounts for blindsight in humans. However, other investigators contend that blindsight is a genuine phenomenon that reflects nonstriate visual pathways (see Cowey and Stoerig [508] for review), which can occur in the absence of functioning area 17 (515). In humans, examples of pathways invoked as an explanation for blindsight are a retinocollicular projection that reaches extrastriate cortical visual areas via the pulvinar nucleus (516) and a direct geniculo-extrastriate cortical projection (508). Interestingly, there appears to be an increase in the sensitivity of blindsight in a given individual over time, suggesting that training of visual function may have rehabilitative implications.

Another way in which visual perceptions may be dissociated is in the syndrome of unilateral inattention or neglect. Patients with this defect may appear to have normal visual function if tested in routine fashion, since they can correctly perceive objects in each hemifield with either eye. However, when two test objects are presented in the right and left hemifields of each eye simultaneously, the patient perceives only the test object in the hemifield ipsilateral to the lesion. This phenomenon, called visual extinction, can occur following damage to the parietal or occipitoparietal cortex as well as to the frontal lobe and thalamus. It can be demonstrated not only in patients with partial hemianopic defects on the same side but also in patients with previously recovered hemianopias or no documented visual field defects. Unilateral neglect can result from lesions in several different regions of the brain. This finding reflects the complex integrated network that exists for the modulation of directed attention within extrapersonal space (291). Functional MR imaging can demonstrate activation of visual cortex without activation of more distal cortical processing areas, demonstrating an anatomic basis for extinction (517).

Nonvisual Symptoms and Signs of Occipital Lobe Disease

As might be expected, vascular lesions of the occipital lobe are usually asymptomatic, except with regard to the visual system. Many patients with occipital infarctions experience acute pain of the head, brow, or eye ipsilateral to the lesion. This presumably reflects the dual trigeminal innervation of the posterior dural structures and the periorbital region (518). Patients with homonymous hemianopia may also complain of disturbances of equilibrium, particularly a feeling that their body is swaying toward the side of the hemianopia. Rondot et al. (519) called this phenomenon "visual ataxia" and proposed that the postural defect reflects unopposed tonic input of vision from the intact hemifield rather than any true vestibular impairment or neglect.

If a homonymous hemianopia is unrecognized by the patient, the first signs of its presence may be the functional consequence of hemifield blindness. Most clinicians have never seen the "door sign" (520), in which a patient with homonymous hemianopia acquires a linear wound in the forehead ipsilateral to the field defect from inadvertently striking the head on a door frame. However, it is not unusual to see patients with homonymous hemianopia that was discovered after a motor vehicle accident in which little or no injury was sustained to account for the field defect or the infarct in the occipital lobe (subsequently detected by neuroimaging) that clearly predated the accident.

If the posterior cerebral artery is occluded proximally, patients with an infarct in the occipital lobe may also have hemiplegia from damage to the posterior internal capsule or cerebral peduncle, language dysfunction from damage to posterior parietal structures, or symptoms reflecting damage to the ipsilateral thalamus (380,521). In addition, because the condition is ordinarily seen in patients with severe atherosclerosis, there may be other evidence of vertebrobasilar insufficiency, including ocular motor abnormalities referable to the rostral brain stem. Patients who develop a bilateral homonymous hemianopia in this setting may be more severely impaired than patients with blindness from bilateral retinal or optic nerve disease and may be difficult to rehabilitate (see below).

Tumors of the occipital lobe may cause nonvisual manifestations by virtue of their mass effect. Parkinson and Craig (522) examined the signs and symptoms of 50 patients with verified tumors limited to the occipital lobe. Headache was the most common symptom, occurring in 45 patients (90%). Other symptoms and signs included nausea and vomiting (46%), ataxia (30%), hallucinations that were usually unformed (24%), seizures (18%), and mental changes (16%). Most of the signs and symptoms noted by Parkinson and Craig are nonlocalizing and related to increased intracranial pressure. Ataxia and other cerebellar signs are usually re-

lated to direct downward pressure on the cerebellum by the tumor.

TREATMENT AND REHABILITATION FOR HOMONYMOUS HEMIANOPIA

Spontaneous recovery of homonymous visual field defects occurs in no more than 20% of patients within the first several months after brain injury (523–525). Thus, despite a certain amount of plasticity even in the adult cerebral cortex (526,527), patients with visual field defects have a consistently poor rehabilitation outcome (528–530). The exact anatomic location of the lesion causing the homonymous hemianopia does not appear to affect the functional outcome (531); however, the greater the number of associated neurologic deficits, the more difficult the rehabilitation and the poorer the functional performance (532). Contributing further to the poor functional improvement is the advanced age of most of these patients, a factor associated even in normal individuals with progressive cognitive, sensory, and motor deficits (533). Finally, the presence of neglect, especially in patients with nondominant hemisphere lesions, also interferes with the rehabilitation process.

Several techniques may assist in the treatment and rehabilitation of patients with homonymous hemianopia (534). A mirror attachment can be used to project the mirror image of the blind field into the seeing half-field (535). The mirror is attached to the nasal side of the spectacle frame behind the lens. Burns et al. (536) found that three of six patients learned to make some use of the device. For many patients, however, such mirrors do not prove satisfactory because the patient has to turn the head toward the mirror, because the mirror produces a scotoma that blocks a portion of the seeing field, and because spatial disorientation is common. Images seen in the mirror are reversed and projected to the opposite side of the midline (537), causing confusion. Mirrors on prongs fixed to a frame are available, but they are usually discarded by the patient because of the cosmetic appearance of such devices. Mintz (538) devised a small adjustable mirror that is mounted on a clip placed over the spectacle frames on the nasal side. Waiss and Cohen (539) suggested the use of a temporal mirror coating on the back surface of spectacles.

Smith (540) advocated the use of Fresnel press-on prisms in patients with a homonymous hemianopia. The prism is placed on the outside half of the lens ipsilateral to the hemianopia with the base oriented toward that side (i.e., for a patient with a left homonymous hemianopia, a 30-diopter prism was placed base-out on the left half of the left lens). Perlin and Dziadul (537) advocated placing 20 prism-diopter Fresnel prisms in front of both eyes, allowing for a 5° movement of the eyes before they encounter the prism edge (see also [541]). Prism power and placement are then modified, depending on patient adaptation. The goal is to increase the patient's scanning skills over time. Rossi et al. (542) randomly assigned 39 patients with stroke and homonymous hemianopia or unilateral visual neglect to treatment with 15 prism-diopter plastic press-on Fresnel prisms or to no treatment. Although the prism-treated group later performed significantly better than controls on visual perception tests, there was no difference in activities-of-daily-living function.

Pameijer (543) noted the extent of reading problems in patients with hemianopia. Patients with right hemianopias cannot see which letters or words follow those that they have already deciphered. Patients with left hemianopias may read without difficulty until they come to the end of the line. In attempting to return to the beginning of the next line, they move into their blind hemifield and lose their place, often beginning again on an unrelated line. Pameijer developed a "reading screen" for patients with a left homonymous hemianopia. This device is a black screen with an adjustable opening that the author claims helps patients find the beginning of each line. The same benefit can be achieved with a ruler or other straightedge positioned under each line of text. With respect to patients with right homonymous hemianopias, Pameijer recommended an "inversion telescope" that enables patients to read from right to left rather than left to right. For patients with bilateral homonymous hemianopias with macular sparing and restricted central fields (and also for patients with restricted fields from retinitis pigmentosa or glaucoma), Holm (464) recommended a reversed Galilean- or Keppler-type telescope that could be mounted in a regular spectacle frame.

Another strategy that may help rehabilitate patients with homonymous hemianopia is systematic training of saccadic eye movements and ocular scanning techniques (525,529, 545–548). Many hemianopic patients exhibit a restricted field of ocular motor visual exploration (547), and practice with spatially organized visual searching can improve functional outcome for these patients. Kerkhoff et al. (529) trained their hemianopic patients to perform large saccades into the blind field and to search their entire field in various patterns reflecting different search strategies, both in the laboratory and during activities of daily living. These investigators demonstrated training-related visual field improvement in 12 of 22 patients (54%) (mean increase, 6.7°; range, 2–24°), sustained improvement in functional ability as demonstrated by functional measurements in the laboratory and by subjective assessment, and return to part-time work in 20 of 22 patients (91%). Patients with visual neglect were not included in this study. Nelles et al. trained 221 hemianopic patients under either fixing or scanning conditions and found greater improvement in detection rates and reaction time with the latter (549).

Another proposed approach to patients with neurogenic visual field loss, including those with homonymous hemianopia, is to use training techniques which purportedly achieve actual restoration of visual field, presumably on the basis of neuroplasticity (550–552). Kasten et al. (550) achieved an average of 5 degree enlargement of the visual field with daily in-home training using a specialized computer device. Subjective improvement in visual function was reported by 72% of the patients, compared with 17% of the control group (550). Others have suggested that the mechanism of this improvement is increased saccadic movements into the blind hemifield (553), but debate is still ongoing.

Many patients do not have significant improvement with the devices or strategies described above, partly because of their physiologic and optical limitations and partly because of other perceptual, sensory, and motor difficulties associated with the disease process that damaged the retrochiasmal visual system. In many cases the most useful approach for reading is the use of a ruler placed under each line or having the patient turn the material 90° and reading vertically in the intact hemifield.

REFERENCES

1. Adler FH, Austin G, Grant FC. Localizing value of visual fields in patients with early chiasmal lesions. Arch Ophthalmol 1948;40:579–600.
2. Gartner S. Ocular pathology in the chiasmal syndrome. Am J Ophthalmol 1951;34:593–596.
3. Kivela T, Pelkonen R, Oja M, Heiskanen O. Diabetes insipidus and blindness caused by a suprasellar tumor: Pieter Pauw's observations from the 16th century. JAMA 1998;279:48–50.
4. Traquair HM. An Introduction to Clinical Perimetry. 6th ed. London, Kimpton, 1949.
5. Bird AC. Field loss due to lesions at the anterior angle of the chiasm. Proc R Soc Med 1972;65:519–521.
6. Wilbrand H. Schema des verlaus des Sehnervenfasern durch das Chiasma. Z Augenheilkd 1926;59:135–144.
7. Breen LA, Quaglieri FC, Schochet SS, Jr. Neuro-anatomical feature photo. J Clin Neuroophthalmol 1983;3:283–284.
8. Horton JC. Wilbrand's knee of the primate optic chiasm is an artefact of monocular enucleation. Trans Am Ophthalmol Soc 1997;95:579–609.
9. Arkin MS, Rubin PA, Bilyk JR, Buchbinder B. Anterior chiasmal optic nerve avulsion. Am J Neuroradiol 1996;17:1777–1781.
10. Parmar B, Edmunds B, Plant G. Traumatic enucleation with chiasmal damage: Magnetic resonance image findings and response to steroids. Br J Ophthalmol 2002;86:1317–1318.
11. Frisén L. The neurology of visual acuity. Brain 1980;103:639–670.
12. Hollenhorst RW, Younge BR. Ocular manifestations produced by adenomas of the pituitary gland: Analysis of 1,000 cases. In Kohler PO, Ross GT, eds. Diagnosis and Treatment of Pituitary Tumors. New York, Elsevier, 1973:53–64.
13. Cushing H, Walker CB. Distortions of the visual fields in cases of brain tumor. Brain 1915;37:341–400.
14. Fujimoto N, Saeki N, Miyauchi O, Adachi-Usami E. Criteria for early detection of temporal hemianopia in asymptomatic pituitary tumor. Eye 2002;16:731–738.
15. Gregorius FK, Hepler RS, Stern WE. Loss and recovery of vision with suprasellar meningiomas. J Neurosurg 1975;42:69–75.
16. Svolos D. Craniopharyngiomas: A study based on 108 verified cases. Acta Chir Scand 1969;403(Suppl):1–44.
17. Bartlett JR. Craniopharyngiomas: A summary of 85 cases. J Neurol Neurosurg Psychiatry 1971;34:37–41.
18. Berson E, Freeman M, Gay A. Visual field defects in giant suprasellar aneurysms of the internal carotid artery. Arch Ophthalmol 1966;76:52–58.
19. Cullen AF, Haining WM, Crombie AL. Cerebral aneurysms presenting with visual field defects. Br J Ophthalmol 1966;50:251–256.
20. Bird AC, Nolan B, Gargano FP, et al. Unruptured aneurysm of the supraclinoid carotid artery: A treatable cause of blindness. Neurology 1970;20:445–454.
21. Rush JA, Balis GA, Drake CG. Bitemporal hemianopsia in basilar artery aneurysm. J Clin Neuroophthalmol 1981;1:129–133.
22. Kageyama N. Ectopic pinealoma in the region of the optic chiasm. J Neurosurg 1971;35:755–759.
23. Camins MB, Mount LA. Primary suprasellar atypical teratoma. Brain 1974;97:447–456.
24. Isayama Y, Takahashi T, Inoue M. Ocular findings of suprasellar germinoma: Long-term follow-up after radiotherapy. Neuroophthalmology 1980;1:53–61.
25. Glaser JS, Hoyt WF, Corbett J. Visual morbidity with chiasmal glioma: Long-term studies of visual fields in untreated and treated cases. Arch Ophthalmol 1971;85:3–12.
26. Warner JEA, Rizzo JF 3rd, Brown EW, et al. Recurrent chiasmal apoplexy due to cavernous malformation. J Neuroophthalmol 1996;16:99–106.
27. Jakobsson KE, Petruson B, Lindblom B. Dynamics of visual improvement following chiasmal decompression. Quantitative pre- and postoperative observations. Acta Ophthalmol Scand 2002;80:512–516.
28. Larmande A, Larmande P. L'atteinte du genou posterieur du chiasma. Rev Otoneuroophtalmol 1977;49:1–2.
29. Enoksson P. Perimetry in neuro-ophthalmological diagnosis. Acta Ophthalmol 1965;82(Suppl):1–54.
30. Hoyt WF. Correlative functional anatomy of the optic chiasm, 1969. Clin Neurosurg 1970;17:189–208.
31. Huber A. Chiasmal syndrome. Klin Monatsbl Augenheilkd 1977;170:266–278.
32. Wybar K. Chiasmal compression. Proc R Soc Med 1977;70:307–317.
33. Rosen L. Contribution a l'étude des hemianopsies. Symptomatology et étiologie

de 97 cas examinés á la clinique ophtalmologique de bale entre 1925 et 1940. Confin Neurol 1941;4:271–293.

34. Arseni C, Ghitescu M, Cristescu A, et al. Intrasellar aneurysms simulating hypophyseal tumors. Eur Neurol 1970;3:321–329.

35. Huber A. Eye Signs and Symptoms in Brain Tumors. 3rd ed. St Louis, CV Mosby, 1976.

36. Quencer RM. Visual loss and bitemporal hemianopsia. J Clin Neuroophthalmol 1981;1:231–235.

37. Krauss HR, Slamovits TL, Sibony PA, et al. Carotid artery aneurysm simulating pituitary adenoma. J Clin Neuroophthalmol 1982;2:169–174.

38. Herold S, et al. Augensymptome bei Hypophysenadenomen, Kraniopharyngeomen und Meningeomen der vorderen und mittleren Schädelgrube. Klin Monatsbl Augenheilkd 1984;185:495–504.

39. Newman NJ, Lessell S, Winterkorn JM. Optic chiasmal neuritis. Neurology 1991;41:1203–1210.

40. Frohman LP, Guirgis M, Turbin RE, Bielory L. Sarcoidosis of the anterior visual pathway: 24 new cases. J Neuroophthalmol 2003;23:190–197.

41. Siatkowski RM, Scott IU, Verm AM, et al. Optic neuropathy and chiasmopathy in the diagnosis of systemic lupus erythematosus. J Neuroophthalmol 2001;21:193–198.

42. Frohman LP, Frieman BJ, Wolansky L. Reversible blindness resulting from optic chiasmitis secondary to systemic lupus erythematosus. J Neuroophthalmol 2001;21:18–21.

43. Weyand RD, Rucker CW. Unusual lesions involving the optic chiasm. Mayo Clin Proc 1952;27:505–511.

44. Segall HD, Hassan G, Ling SM, et al. Suprasellar cysts associated with isosexual precocious puberty. Radiology 1974;111:607–616.

45. Sibony PA, Lessell S, Wray S. Chiasmal syndrome caused by arteriovenous malformations. Arch Ophthalmol 1982;100:438–442.

46. Hopen G, Smith JL, Hoff JT, et al. The Wyburn-Mason syndrome: Concomitant chiasmal and fundus vascular malformations. J Clin Neuroophthalmol 1983;3:53–62.

47. Lavin PJM, McCrary JA, III, Roessmann U, et al. Chiasmal apoplexy: Hemorrhage from a cryptic vascular malformation in the optic chiasm. Neurology 1984;34:1007–1011.

48. Ciftci E, Erden I, Akyar S. Brucellosis of the pituitary region: MRI. Neuroradiology 1998;40:383–386.

49. Manz HJ, Klein LH, Fermaglich J, et al. Cavernous hemangiomas of optic chiasm, optic nerves and right optic tract. Virchows Arch (Pathol Anat) 1979;383:225–231.

50. Maitland CG, Abiko S, Hoyt WF, et al. Chiasmal apoplexy: Report of four cases. J Neurosurg 1982;56:118–122.

51. Castel JP, Delorge-Kerdiles C, Rivel J. Angiome caverneux du chiasma optique. Neurochirurgie 1989;35:252–256.

52. Corboy JR, Galetta SL. Familial cavernous angiomas manifesting with an acute chiasmal syndrome. Am J Ophthalmol 1989;108:245–250.

53. Hassler W, Zentner J, Wilhelm H. Cavernous angiomas of the anterior visual pathways. J Clin Neuroophthalmol 1989;9:160–164.

54. Regli L, DeTribolet N, Regli F, et al. Chiasmal apoplexy: Haemorrhage from a cavernous malformation in the optic chiasm. J Neurol Neurosurg Psychiatry 1989;52:1095–1099.

55. Hwang JF, Yau CW, Huang JK, et al. Apoplectic optochiasmal syndrome due to intrinsic cavernous hemangioma: Case report. J Clin Neuroophthalmol 1993;13:232–236.

56. Aoki H, Mori K, Tajima A, Maeda M. Sellar chondroma: Case report. Neurol Med Chir (Tokyo) 1999;39:870–874.

57. Kazim M, Kennerdell JS, Maroon J, et al. Choristoma of the optic nerve and chiasm. Arch Ophthalmol 1992;110:236–238.

58. Kimura M, Takayasu M, Suzuki Y, et al. Primary choroid plexus papilloma located in the suprasellar region: Case report. Neurosurgery 1992;31:563–566.

59. Chang GY, Keane JR. Visual loss in cysticercosis: Analysis of 23 patients. Neurology 2001;57:545–548.

60. Reddy DR, Reddy PS, Murthi DK, Reddy CS. A case of large suprasellar cysticercus cyst with bitemporal hemianopia. Neurol India 1973;21:44–45.

61. Rafael H, Gòmez-Llata S. Intrasellar cysticercosis: Case report. J Neurosurg 1985;63:975–976.

62. Del BOH, Guevara J, Sotelo J. Intrasellar cysticercosis. J Neurosurg 1988;69:58–60.

63. Endelmann L. Zwei Fälle plötzlich entstandener bitemporaler Hemianopsie mit unaufgeklärter Ätiologie. (Frühsymptom von multipler Sklerose). Z Augenheilkd 1932;78:234–242.

64. Sacks JG, Melen O. Bitemporal visual field defects in presumed multiple sclerosis. JAMA 1975;234:69–72.

65. Spector RH, Glaser JS, Schatz NJ. Demyelinative chiasmal lesions. Arch Neurol 1980;37:757–762.

66. Reynolds WD, Smith JL, McCrary JA III. Chiasmal optic neuritis. J Clin Neuroophthalmol 1982;2:93–101.

67. Kupersmith M, Frohman L, Warren F, et al. Diagnosis and treatment of unusual disorders of the chiasm. Ann Neurol 1986;20:140.

68. Newman NJ, Lessell S, Winterkorn JMS. Optic chiasmal neuritis. Neurology 1991;41:1203–1210.

69. Wilhelm H, Grodd W, Schiefer U, et al. Uncommon chiasmal lesions: Demyelinating disease, vasculitis, and cobalamin deficiency. German J Ophthalmol 1993;2:234–240.

70. Matsuo K, Kobayashi S, Sugita K. Bitemporal hemianopia associated with sclerosis of the intracranial internal carotid arteries. J Neurosurg 1980;53:566–569.

71. Hinshaw DB Jr, Jordan KR, Hasson AN, et al. CT cisternography of dolichoectatic arterial compression of the optic chiasm. Am J Neuroradiol 1985;6:837–839.

72. Chang AH, Kaufmann WE, Brat DJ. Ectopic cerebellum presenting as a suprasellar mass in infancy: implications for cerebellar development. Pediatr Dev Pathol 2001;4:89–93.

73. O'Connor PS, Smith JL. Chiasmal ependymoma. Ann Ophthalmol 1979;11:1424–1428.

74. Lowes M, Bojsen-Moller M, Vorre P, et al. An evaluation of gliomas of the anterior visual pathways: A 10–year survey. Acta Neurochir 1978;43:201–216.

75. Chilton J, Caughron MR, Kepes JJ. Ganglioglioma of the optic chiasm: Case report and reivew of the literature. Neurosurgery 1990;26:1042–1045.

76. Liu GT, Galetta SL, Rorke LB, et al. Gangliogliomas involving the optic chiasm. Neurology 1996;46:1669–1673.

77. Shuangshoti S, Kirsch E, Bannan P, Fabian VA. Ganglioglioma of the optic chiasm: Case report and review of the literature. Am J Neuroradiol 2000;21:1486–1489.

78. Isayama Y, Takahashi T, Inoue M, et al. Clinicopathological findings in the chiasmal region: Suprasellar germinoma. Jpn J Ophthalmol 1979;23:140–155.

79. Van Dalen JTW, Speelman HJD, De Waard RCB, et al. Chiasmal syndrome and Parinaud syndrome in a patient with a primary suprasellar germinoma. Neuroophthalmology 1983;3:225–233.

80. Chavy B, Rossazza C, Jan M, et al. Le germinome des voies optiques (a propos d'un cas). Bull Soc Ophtalmol Fr 1988;88:145–148.

81. Aroichane M, Miller NR, Eggenberger ER. Glioblastoma multiforme masquerading as pseudotumor cerebri: Case report. J Clin Neuroophthalmol 1993;13:105–112.

82. Waller RR, Riley FC, Sundt TM. A rare cause of the chiasmal syndrome. Arch Ophthalmol 1972;88:269–272.

83. Ji CH, Teng MMH, Chang T. Granular cell tumour of the neurohypophysis. Neuroradiology 1995;37:451–452.

84. Purvin V, Herr GJ, De MW. Chiasmal neuritis as a complication of Epstein-Barr virus infection. Arch Neurol 1988;45:458–460.

85. Hilton GF, Hoyt WF. An arteriosclerotic chiasmal syndrome. JAMA 1966;196:1018–1020.

86. Lee KF, Schatz NJ. Ischemic chiasmal syndrome. Acta Radiol 1975;347(Suppl):131–148.

87. Ahmadi J, Keane JR, McCormick GS, et al. Ischemic chiasmal syndrome and hypopituitarism associated with progressive cerebrovascular occlusive disease. Am J Neuroradiol 1984;5:367–372.

88. Smolik EA, Devecerski M, Nelson JS, et al. Histiocytosis X in the optic chiasm of an adult with hypopituitarism. J Neurosurg 1968;29:290–295.

89. Goodman RH, Post KD, Molitch ME, et al. Eosinophilic granuloma mimicking a pituitary tumor. Neurosurgery 1979;5:723–725.

90. Job OM, Schatz NJ, Glaser JS. Visual loss with Langerhans cell histiocytosis: Multifocal central nervous system involvement. J Neuroophthalmol 1999;19:49–53.

91. Zaman AG, Graham EM, Sanders MD. Anterior visual system involvement in non-Hodgkin's lymphoma. Br J Ophthalmol 1993;77:184–187.

92. Lee AG, Tang RA, Roberts D, Schiffman JS, Osborne A. Primary central nervous system lymphoma involving the optic chiasm in AIDS. J Neuroophthalmol 2001;21:95–98.

93. Hirst LW, Miller NR, Udvarhelyi GB. Metastatic malignant melanoma causing chiasmal syndrome. Neuroophthalmology 1983;3:21–27.

94. Teixeira F, Penagos P, Lozano D, et al. Medulloblastoma presenting as blindness of rapid evolution: A case report. J Clin Neuroophthalmol 1991;11:250–253.

95. Cohen MM, Lessell S. Chiasmal syndrome due to metastasis. Arch Neurol 1979;36:565–567.

96. Duvall J, Cullen JF. Metastatic disease in the pituitary: Clinical features. Trans Ophthalmol Soc UK 1982;102:481–486.

97. Baeesa SS, Benoit BG. Solitary metastasis of breast carcinoma in the optic chiasm. Br J Neurosurg 1999;13:319–321.

98. Poon MC, Prchal JT, Murad TM, et al. Multiple myeloma masquerading as chromophobe adenoma. Cancer 1979;43:1513–1516.

99. Bruetsch WL. Etiology of optochiasmatic arachnoiditis. Arch Neurol Psychiatry 1948;59:215–228.

100. Coyle JT. Chiasmatic arachnoiditis. Am J Ophthalmol 1969;68:345–349.

101. Iraci G, Giordano R, Fiore DL, et al. Tuberculosis and the anterior optic pathways. Neuroophthalmology 1984;4:111–127.

102. Weinstein GW, Powell SR, Thrush WP. Chiasmal neuropathy secondary to rheumatoid pachmeningitis. Am J Ophthalmol 1987;104:439–440.

103. Salame K, Ouaknine GE, Yossipov J, Rochkind S. Paraganglioma of the pituitary fossa: diagnosis and management. J Neurooncol 2001;54:49–52.

104. Har-El G, Swanson RM, Kent RH. Unusual presentation of a pituitary abscess. Surg Neurol 1996;45:351–353.

105. Lee AG, Van Gilder JC, White ML. Progressive visual loss because of a suprasel-

lar pneumatocele after trans-sphenoidal resection of a pituitary adenoma. J Neuroophthalmol 2003;23:142–144.

106. Iraci G, Giordano R, Gerosa M, et al. Ocular involvement in recurrent cyst of Rathke's cleft: Case report. Ann Ophthalmol 1979;11:94–98.

107. Lefkowitz DM, Quencer RM. Bitemporal hemianopsia. J Clin Neuroophthalmol 1984;4:209–212.

108. Voelker JL, Campbell RL, Muller J. Clinical, radiologic, and pathological features of symptomatic Rathke's cleft cysts. J Neurosurg 1991;74:535–544.

109. Fischer EG, DeGirolami U, Suojanen JN. Reversible visual deficit following debulking of a Rathke's cleft cyst: A tethered chiasm? J Neurosurg 1994;81:459–462.

110. Oka H, Kawano N, Suwa T, et al. Radiological study of symptomatic Rathke's cleft cysts. Neurosurgery 1994;35:632–637.

111. Rao GP, Blyth CPJ, Jeffreys RV. Ophthalmic manifestations of Rathke's cleft cysts. Am J Ophthalmol 1995;119:86–91.

112. Walsh TJ, Smith JL. Sarcoidosis and suprasellar mass. In Smith JL, ed. Neuro-Ophthalmology Symposium, Vol 4. St Louis, CV Mosby, 1968:167–177.

113. Decker RE, Mardayat M, Marc J, et al. Neurosarcoidosis with computerized tomographic visualization and transsphenoidal excision of a supra- and intrasellar granuloma: Case report. J Neurosurg 1979;50:814–886.

114. Rubin MR, Bruce JN, Khandji AG, Freda PU. Sarcoidosis within a pituitary adenoma. Pituitary 2001;4:195–202.

115. Kansu T, Bertan V. Fifth ventricle with bitemporal hemianopia. J Neurosurg 1980;52:276–278.

116. Bhattacharjee MB, Wroe SJ, Harding BN, et al. Sinus histiocytosis with massive lymphadenopathy: Isolated suprasellar involvement. J Neurol Neurosurg Psychiatry 1992;55:156–158.

117. Goodwin JA, Glaser JS. Chiasmal syndrome in sphenoid sinus mucocele. Ann Neurol 1978;4:440–444.

118. Hubault D, Brasseur G, Charlin JF, et al. Tuberculome de la region opto-chiasmatique: A propos de 2 observations. Bull Soc Ophtalmol Fr 1988;88:141–144.

119. Domingues FS, de Souza JM, Chagas H, et al. Pituitary tuberculoma: An unusual lesion of sellar region. Pituitary 2002;5:149–153.

120. Greven CM, Singh T, Stanton CA, Martin TJ. Optic chiasm, optic nerve, and retinal involvement secondary to varicella-zoster virus. Arch Ophthalmol 2001;119:608–610.

121. Mirabel S, Lindblom B, Halbach VV, et al. Giant suprasellar varix: An unusual cause of chiasmal compression. J Clin Neuroophthalmol 1991;11:268–272.

122. Fermaglich J, Kattah J, Manz H. Venous angioma of the optic chiasm. Ann Neurol 1978;4:470–471.

123. Carter JE, Wymore J, Ansbacher L, et al. Sudden visual loss and a chiasmal syndrome due to in intrachiasmatic vascular malformation. J Clin Neuroophthalmol 1982;2:163–167.

124. Kremer S, Besson G, Bonaz B, et al. Diffuse lesions in the CNS revealed by MR imaging in a case of Whipple disease. Am J Neuroradiol 2001;22:493–495.

125. Enoksson P, Lundberg N, Sjostedt S, et al. Influence of pregnancy on visual fields in suprasellar tumours. Acta Psychiatr Neurol Scand 1961;36:524–538.

126. Falconer MA, Stafford-Bell MA. Visual failure from pituitary and paraseller tumours occurring with favorable outcome in pregnant women. J Neurol Neurosurg Psychiatry 1975;38:919–921.

127. Elias Z, Powers SK, Grimson BS, et al. Chiasmal syndrome caused by pituitary-sellar disproportion. Surg Neurol 1987;28:395–400.

128. Asa SL, Bilbao JM, Kovacs K, et al. Lymphocytic hypophysitis of pregnancy resulting in hypopituitarism: A distinct clinicopathologic entity. Ann Intern Med 1981;95:166–171.

129. Baskin DS, Townsend JJ, Wilson CB. Lymphocytic adenohypophysitis of pregnancy simulating a pituitary adenoma: A distinct pathological entity. Report of two cases. J Neurosurg 1982;56:148–153.

130. Levine SN, Benzel EC, Fowler MR, et al. Lymphocytic adenohypophysitis: Clinical, radiological, and magnetic resonance imaging characterization. Neurosurgery 1988;22:937–941.

131. Stelmach M, O'Day J. Rapid change in visual fields associated with suprasellar lymphocytic hypophysitis. J Clin Neuroophthalmol 1991;11:19–24.

132. Dan NG, Feiner RI, Houang MT, Turner JJ. Pituitary apoplexy in association with lymphocytic hypophysitis. J Clin Neurosci 2002;9:577–580.

133. Kaufman B. The empty sella turcica: A manifestation of the intrasellar subarachnoid space. Radiology 1969;90:931–941.

134. Pollock SC, Bromberg BS. Visual loss in a patient with primary empty sella. Arch Ophthalmol 1987;105:487–488.

135. Neelon FA, Goree J, Lebovitz H. The primary empty sella: Clinical and radiographic characteristics and endocrine function. Medicine 1973;52:73–92.

136. Berke JP, Buxton LF, Kokmen E. The "empty" sella. Neurology 1975;25:1137–1143.

137. Apkarian P, Bour LJ, Barth PG, et al. Non-decussating retinal-fugal fibre syndrome. An inborn achiasmatic malformation associated with visuotopic misrouting, visual evoked potential ipsilateral asymmetry and nystagmus. Brain 1995;118(Pt 5):1195–1216.

138. Jansonius NM, van der Vliet TM, Cornelissen FW, et al. A girl without a chiasm: Electrophysiologic and MRI evidence for the absence of crossing optic nerve fibers in a girl with a congenital nystagmus. J Neuroophthalmol 2001;21:26–29.

139. Victor JD, Apkarian P, Hirsch J, et al. Visual function and brain organization in non-decussating retinal-fugal fibre syndrome. Cereb Cortex 2000;10:2–22.

140. Traquair HM, Dott NM, Russell WR. Traumatic lesions of the optic chiasma. Brain 1935;58:398–411.

141. Fisher NF, Jampolsky A, Scott AB. Traumatic bitemporal hemianopia. I. Diagnosis of macular splitting. Am J Ophthalmol 1968;65:237–242.

142. Obenchain TG, Killeffer FA, Stern WE. Indirect injury to the optic nerves and chiasm with closed head injury. Bull Los Angeles Neurol Soc 1972;37:13–20.

143. Tibbs PA, Brooks WH. Traumatic bitemporal hemianopia: Case report. J Trauma 1979;19:129–131.

144. Savino PJ, Glaser JS, Schatz NJ. Traumatic chiasmal syndrome. Neurology 1980;30:963–970.

145. Resneck JD, Lederman IR. Traumatic chiasmal syndrome associated with pneumocephalus and sellar fracture. Am J Ophthalmol 1981;92:233–237.

146. Neetens A. Traumatic bi-temporal hemianopia. Neuroophthalmology 1992;12:375–383.

147. Tang RA, Kramer LA, Schiffman J, et al. Chiasmal trauma: Clinical and imaging considerations. Surv Ophthalmol 1994;38:381–383.

148. Hassan A, Crompton JL, Sandhu A. Traumatic chiasmal syndrome: A series of 19 patients. Clin Experiment Ophthalmol 2002;30:273–280.

149. Atipo-Tsiba PW, Borruat FX. Traumatic dysfunction of the optic chiasm. Klin Monatsbl Augenheilkd 2003;220:138–141.

150. Matsumoto S, Hasuo K, Mizushima A, et al. Intracranial penetrating injuries via the optic canal. Am J Neuroradiol 1998;19:1163–1165.

151. Walsh FB. Indirect trauma to the optic nerves and chiasm. Invest Ophthalmol 1966;5:433–449.

152. Wilbrand H, Saenger A. Die neurologie des Auges. Wiesbaden, JB Bergman, 1915.

153. Cushing H. The chiasmal syndrome of primary optic atrophy and bitemporal field defects in adults with a normal sella turcica. Arch Ophthalmol 1930;3:505–551; 704–735.

154. Sinclair AH, Dott NM. Hydrocephalus simulating tumour in the production of chiasmal and other parahypophyseal lesions. Trans Ophthalmol Soc UK 1931;51:232–246.

155. Wagener HP, Cusick PL. Chiasmal syndromes produced by lesions in the posterior fossa. Arch Ophthalmol 1937;18:887–891.

156. Hughes EBC. Some observations on the visual fields in hydrocephalus. J Neurol Neurosurg Psychiatry 1945;9:30–39.

157. Coppeto JR, Gahm NG. Bitemporal hemianopic scotoma: A complication of intraventricular catheter. Surg Neurol 1977;8:361–362.

158. Slavin ML, Rosenthal AD. Chiasmal compression caused by a catheter in the suprasellar cistern. Am J Ophthalmol 1988;105:560–561.

159. McHenry JG, Spoor TC. Chiasmal compression from fat packing after transsphenoidal resection of intrasellar tumor in two patients. Am J Ophthalmol 1993;116:253.

160. Slavin ML, Lam BL, Decker RE, et al. Chiasmal compression from fat packing after transsphenoidal resection of intrasellar tumor in two patients. Am J Ophthalmol 1993;115:368–371.

161. Iplikcioglu AC, Bek S, Bikmaz K, Basocak K. Tension pneumocyst after transsphenoidal surgery for Rathke's cleft cyst: Case report. Neurosurgery 2003;52:960–963.

162. Czech T, Wolfsberger S, Reitner A, Gorzer H. Delayed visual deterioration after surgery for pituitary adenoma. Acta Neurochir (Wien) 1999;141:45–51.

163. Schatz NJ, Lichtenstein S, Corbett JJ. Delayed radiation necrosis of the optic nerves and chiasm. In Glaser JS, Smith JL, eds. Neuro-Ophthalmology. St Louis, CV Mosby, 1975:131–139.

164. Hammer HM. Optic chiasmal radionecrosis. Trans Ophthalmol Soc UK 1983;103(Pt 2):208–211.

165. Lessell S. Magnetic resonance imaging signs may antedate visual loss in chiasmal radiation injury. Arch Ophthalmol 2003;121:287–288.

166. Stafford SL, Pollock BE, Leavitt JA, et al. A study on the radiation tolerance of the optic nerves and chiasm after stereotactic radiosurgery. Int J Radiat Oncol Biol Phys 2003;55:1177–1181.

167. Jones SE, James RA, Hall K, Kendall-Taylor P. Optic chiasmal herniation: An underrecognized complication of dopamine agonist therapy for macroprolactinoma. Clin Endocrinol (Oxf) 2000;53:529–534.

168. Lohmann T, Trantakis C, Biesold M, et al. Minor tumour shrinkage in nonfunctioning pituitary adenomas by long-term treatment with the dopamine agonist cabergoline. Pituitary 2001;4:173–178.

169. Chuman H, Cornblath WT, Trobe JD, Gebarski SS. Delayed visual loss following pergolide treatment of a prolactinoma. J Neuroophthalmol 2002;22:102–106.

170. Manchester PT, Calhoun FP. Dominant hereditary optic atrophy with bitemporal field defects. Arch Ophthalmol 1958;60:479–484.

171. Danesh-Meyer H, Kubis KC, Wolf MA. Chiasmopathy? Surv Ophthalmol 2000;44:329–335.

172. Chanson P, Daujat F, Young J, et al. Normal pituitary hypertrophy as a frequent cause of pituitary incidentaloma: A follow-up study. J Clin Endocrinol Metab 2001;86:3009–3015.

173. Hedges TR. Preservation of the upper nasal field in the chiasmal syndrome: An anatomic explanation. Trans Am Ophthalmol Soc 1969;67:131–141.

174. Harrington DO. Discussion section following article by Hedges. Trans Am Ophthalmol Soc 1969;67:139–141.

175. Schneider RC, Kriss FC, Falls HF. Prechiasmal infarction associated with intrachiasmal and suprasellar tumors. J Neurosurg 1970;32:197–208.

176. Stark KL, Kaufman B, Lee BC, et al. Visual recovery after a year of craniopharyngioma-related amaurosis: Report of a nine-year-old child and a review of pathophysiologic mechanisms. J AAPOS 1999;3:366–371.

177. Levin LA, Gragoudas ES, Lessell S. Endothelial cell loss in irradiated optic nerves. Ophthalmology 2000;107:370–374.

178. Nachtigaller H, Hoyt WF. Storungen des seheindruckes bei bitemporaler hemianopsie und verschiebung der sehachsen. Klin Monatsbl Augenheilkd 1970;156:821–836.

179. Kirkham TH. The ocular symptomatology of pituitary tumours. Proc R Soc Med 1972;65:517–518.

180. Hirai T, Ito Y, Arai M, et al. Loss of stereopsis with optic chiasmal lesions and stereoscopic tests as a differential test. Ophthalmology 2002;109:1692–1702.

181. Kubie LS, Beckmann JW. Diplopia without extra-ocular palsies, caused by heteronymous defects in the visual fields associated with defective macular vision. Brain 1929;52:317–333.

182. Bardram MT. Oculomotor pareses and non-paretic diplopia in pituitary adenomata. Acta Ophthalmol 1949;27:225.

183. Chamlin M, Davidoff LM, Feiring EH. Ophthalmologic changes produced by pituitary tumors. Am J Ophthalmol 1955;40:353–368.

184. Elkington SG. Pituitary adenoma: Preoperative symptomatology in a series of 260 patients. Br J Ophthalmol 1968;52:322–328.

185. Borchert MS, Lessell S, Hoyt WF. Hemifield slide diplopia from altitudinal visual field defects. J Neuroophthalmol 1996;16:107–109.

186. Kawasaki A, Purvin VA. Photophobia as the presenting visual symptom of chiasmal compression. J Neuroophthalmol 2002;22:3–8.

187. Trobe JD. Photophobia in anterior visual pathway disease. J Neuroophthalmol 2002;22:1–2.

188. Du Pasquier RA, Genoud D, Safran AB, Landis T. Monocular central dazzle after thalamic infarcts. J Neuroophthalmol 2000;20:97–99.

189. Cummings JL, Gittinger JW, Jr. Central dazzle. A thalamic syndrome? Arch Neurol 1981;38:372–374.

190. Porciatti V, Ciavarella P, Ghiggi MR, et al. Losses of hemifield contrast sensitivity in patients with pituitary adenoma and normal visual acuity and visual field. Clin Neurophysiol 1999;110:876–886.

191. Unsöld R, Hoyt WF. Band atrophy of the optic nerve. Arch Ophthalmol 1980;98:1637–1638.

192. Kupfer C. Retinal ganglion cell degeneration following chiasmal lesions in man. Arch Ophthalmol 1963;70:256–260.

193. Ruther K, Ehlich P, Philipp A, et al. Prognostic value of the pattern electroretinogram in cases of tumors affecting the optic pathway. Graefes Arch Clin Exp Ophthalmol 1998;236:259–263.

194. Parmar DN, Sofat A, Bowman R, et al. Visual prognostic value of the pattern electroretinogram in chiasmal compression. Br J Ophthalmol 2000;84:1024–1026.

195. Kinder RSL, Howard GM. See-saw nystagmus. Am J Dis Child 1963;106:331–332.

196. Drachman DA. See-saw nystagmus. J Neurol Neurosurg Psychiatry 1966;29:356–361.

197. Fein JM, Williams RDB. See-saw nystagmus. J Neurol Neurosurg Psychiatry 1969;32:202–207.

198. Williams IM, Dickinson P, Ramsay RJ, et al. See-saw nystagmus. Aust NZ J Ophthalmol 1982;10:19–25.

199. Kanter DS, Ruff RL, Leigh RJ, Modic M. See-saw nystagmus and brainstem infarction: MRI findings. Neuroophthalmology 1987;7:279–283.

200. Halmagyi GM, Aw ST, Dehaene I, et al. Jerk-waveform see-saw nystagmus due to unilateral meso-diencephalic lesion. Brain 1994;117(Pt 4):789–803.

201. Rambold H, Helmchen C, Buttner U. Unilateral muscimol inactivations of the interstitial nucleus of Cajal in the alert rhesus monkey do not elicit seesaw nystagmus. Neurosci Lett 1999;272:75–78.

202. Epstein JA, Moster ML, Spiritos M. Seesaw nystagmus following whole brain irradiation and intrathecal methotrexate. J Neuroophthalmol 2001;21:264–265.

203. Apkarian P, Bour LJ. See-saw nystagmus and congenital nystagmus identified in the non-decussating retinal-fugal fiber syndrome. Strabismus 2001;9:143–163.

204. Huber A. Homonymous hemianopia. Neuroophthalmology 1992;12:351–366.

205. Bender MB, Kanzer MM. Dynamics of homonymous hemianopsias and preservation of central vision. Brain 1939;62:404–421.

206. Cushing H. Distortions of the visual fields in cases of brain tumor. The field defects produced by temporal lobe lesions. Trans Am Neurol Assoc 1921:374–423; Brain 1922;44:341–396.

207. Globus JH, Silverstone SM. Arch Ophthalmol 1935;14:325–386.

208. Bender MB, Strauss I. Defects in visual field of one eye only in patients with a lesion of optic radiation. Arch Ophthalmol 1937;17:765–787.

209. Younge BR. Midline tilting between seeing and nonseeing areas in hemianopia. Mayo Clin Proc 1976;51:562–568.

210. Stone J. The naso-temporal division of the cat's retina. J Comp Neurol 1966;126:585–600.

211. Stone J, Leicester J, Sherman SM. The naso-temporal division of the monkey's retina. J Comp Neurol 1973;150:333–348.

212. Bunt AH, Minckler DS, Johnson GW. Demonstration of bilateral projection of the central retina of the monkey with horseradish peroxidase neuronography. J Comp Neurol 1977;171:619–630.

213. Bunt AH, Minckler DS. Displaced ganglion cells in the retina of the monkey. Invest Ophthalmol Vis Sci 1977;16:95–96.

214. Bunt AH, Minckler DS. Foveal sparing: New anatomical evidence for bilateral representation of the central retina. Arch Ophthalmol 1977;95:1445–1447.

215. Smith JL. Homonymous hemianopia: A review of one hundred cases. Am J Ophthalmol 1962;54:616–622.

216. Trobe JD, Lorber ML, Schlezinger NS. Isolated homonymous hemianopia. Arch Ophthalmol 1973;89:377–381.

217. Shubova TB. Homonymous hemianopia in vascular diseases. Zh Nevropatol Psikhiatr 1963;63:511–521.

218. Fujino T, Kigazawa K, Yamada R. Homonymous hemianopia. A retrospective study of 140 cases. Neuroophthalmology 1986;6:17–21.

219. Molia L, Winterkorn JMS, Schneider SJ. Hemianopic visual field defects in children with intracranial shunts: Report of two cases. Neurosurgery 1996;39:599–603.

220. Hoyt WF, Rios-Montenegro EN, Behrens MM, et al. Homonymous hemioptic hypoplasia. Fundoscopic features in standard and red-free illumination in three patients with congenital hemiplegia. Br J Ophthalmol 1972;56:537–545.

221. Bajandas FJ, McBeath JB, Smith JL. Congenital homonymous hemianopia. Am J Ophthalmol 1976;82:498–500.

222. Kupersmith MJ, Vargas M, Hoyt WF, et al. Optic tract atrophy with cerebral arteriovenous malformations. Direct and transsynaptic degeneration. Neurology 1994;44:80–83.

223. Beatty RM, Sadun AA, Smith LEH, et al. Direct demonstration of transsynaptic degeneration in the human visual system: A comparison of retrograde and anterograde changes. J Neurol Neurosurg Psychiatry 1982;45:143–146.

224. Hoyt WF. Congenital occipital hemianopia. Neuroophthalmol Jpn 1985;2:252–260.

225. Fletcher WA, Hoyt WF, Narahara MH. Congenital quadrantanopia with occipital lobe ganglioglioma. Neurology 1988;38:1892–1894.

226. Ragge NK, Barkovich AJ, Hoyt WF, et al. Isolated congenital hemianopsia caused by prenatal injury to the optic radiation. Arch Neurol 1991;48:1088–1091.

227. Herzau V, Bleher I, Joos-Kratsch E. Infantile exotropia with homonymous hemianopia: a rare contraindication for strabismus surgery. Arch Ophthalmol 1988;226:148–149.

228. Gote H, Gregersen E, Rindziuski E. Exotropia and panoramic vision compensating for an occult homonymous hemianopia: a case report. Binocular Vision Eye Muscle Surg 1993;8:129–132.

229. Levy Y, Turetz J, Krakowski D, et al. Development of compensating exotropia with anomalous retinal correspondence after early infancy in congenital homonymous hemianopia. J Pediatr Ophthalmol Strabismus 1995;32:236–238.

230. Savino PJ, Paris M, Schatz NJ, et al. Optic tract syndrome: A review of 21 patients. Arch Ophthalmol 1978;96:656–663.

231. Burde RM. The pupil. Intl Ophthalmol Clin 1967;7:839–855.

232. Bell RA, Thompson HS. Relative afferent pupillary defect in optic tract hemianopias. Am J Ophthalmol 1978;85:538–540.

233. Schmid R, Wilhelm B, Wilhelm H. Naso-temporal asymmetry and contraction anisocoria in the pupillomotor system. Graefes Arch Clin Exp Ophthalmol 2000;238:123–128.

234. O'Connor PS, Kasdon D, Tredici TJ, et al. The Marcus Gunn pupil in experimental optic tract lesions. Ophthalmology 1982;89:160–164.

235. Newman SA, Miller NR. Optic tract syndrome. Arch Ophthalmol 1983;101:1241–1250.

236. Bender MB, Bodis-Wollner I. Visual dysfunctions in optic tract lesions. Ann Neurol 1978;3:187–193.

237. Kearns TP, Rucker CW. Clinics in perimetry No. 3: Incongruous homonymous hemianopsia. Am J Ophthalmol 1959;47:317–321.

238. Henschen SE. Über localisation innerhalb des ausseren knieganglions. Neurol Centralbl 1898;17:194–199.

239. Mackenzie I, Meighan S, Pollock EN. On the projection of the retinal quadrants on the lateral geniculate bodies, and the relationship of the quadrants to the optic radiations. Trans Ophthalmol Soc UK 1933;53:142–169.

240. Balado M, Malbran J, Franke E. Incongruencia hemianopsica derecha por lesion primivita del cuerpo geniculado externo izquierdo (isopteras internas). Arch Argentinos Neurologia 1934;11:143–151.

241. Smith JL, Nashold BS Jr, Kreshon MJ. Ocular signs after sterotactic lesions in the pallidum and thalamus. Arch Ophthalmol 1961;65:532–535.

242. Fite JD. Temporal lobe epilepsy: Association with homonymous hemianopsia. Arch Ophthalmol 1967;77:71–75.

243. Gunderson CH, Hoyt WF. Geniculate hemianopia: Incongruous homonymous field defects in two patients with partial lesions of the lateral geniculate nucleus. J Neurol Neurosurg Psychiatry 1971;34:1–6.

244. Hoyt WF. Geniculate hemianopias: Incongruous visual defects from partial involvement of the lateral geniculate nucleus. Proc Aust Assoc Neurol 1975;12:7–16.

245. Frisén L, Holmegaard L, Rosencrantz M. Sectorial optic atrophy and homonymous, horizontal sectoranopia: A lateral choroidal artery syndrome? J Neurol Neurosurg Psychiatry 1978;41:374–380.

246. Frisén L. Quadruple sectoranopia and sectorial optic atrophy: A syndrome of the distal anterior choroidal artery. J Neurol Neurosurg Psychiatr 1979;42:590–594.

247. Helgason C, Caplan LR, Goodwin J, et al. Anterior choroidal artery-territory infarction. Report of cases and review. Arch Neurol 1986;43:681–686.

248. Nakahashi K, Takeuchi H, Sekiya Y, et al. A case of hemorrhage in the lateral geniculate body, presenting a horizontal sectoranopia. Neuroophthalmol Jpn 1988;5:313–318.

249. Luco C, Hoppe A, Schweitzer M, et al. Visual field defects in vascular lesions of the lateral geniculate body. J Neurol Neurosurg Psychiatry 1992;55:12–15.

250. Shacklett DE, O'Connor PS, Dorwart RH, et al. Congruous and incongruous sectoral visual field defects with lesions of the lateral geniculate nucleus. Am J Ophthalmol 1984;98:283–290.

251. Borruat FX, Maeder P. Sectoranopia after head trauma: Evidence of lateral geniculate body lesion on MRI. Neurology 1995;45:590–592.

252. Merren MD. Bilateral lateral geniculate body necrosis as a cause of amblyopia. Neurology 1972;22:263–268.

253. Donahue SP, Kardon RH, Thompson HS. Hourglass-shaped visual fields as a sign of bilateral lateral geniculate myelinolysis. Am J Ophthalmol 1995;119:378–380.

254. Greenfield DS, Siatkowski RM, Schatz NJ, et al. Bilateral lateral geniculitis associated with severe diarrhea. Am J Ophthalmol 1996;122:280–281.

255. Carter JE, O'Connor P, Shacklett D, et al. Lesions of the optic radiations mimicking lateral geniculate nucleus visual field defects. J Neurol Neurosurg Psychiatry 1985;48:982–988.

256. Sato Y, Matusda S, Igarashi Y, et al. Horizontal homonymous sectoranopia due to a more proximal lesion than the lateral geniculate body: A report of four cases. Neuroophthalmology 1986;6:407–416.

257. Kolmel HW. Homonymous paracentral scotomas. J Neurol 1987;235:22–25.

258. Grossman M, Galatta SL, Nichols CW, et al. Horizontal homonymous sectorial field defect after ischemic infarction of the occipital cortex. Am J Ophthalmol 1990;109:234–236.

259. Grochowicki M, Vighetto A. Homonymous horizontal sectoranopia: report of four cases. Br J Ophthalmol 1991;75:624–628.

260. Bing R, Haymaker W. Compendium of Regional Diagnosis in Lesions of the Brain and Spinal Cord. 11th ed. St Louis, CV Mosby, 1940.

261. Falconer MA, Wilson JL. Visual field changes following anterior temporal lobectomy: Their significance in relation to ''Meyer's loop'' of the optic radiation. Brain 1958;81:114.

262. Van Buren JM, Baldwin M. The architecture of the optic radiation in the temporal lobe of man. Brain 1958;81:15–40.

263. Manji H, Plant GT. Epilepsy surgery, visual fields, and driving: A study of the visual field criteria for driving in patients after temporal lobe epilepsy surgery with a comparison of Goldmann and Esterman perimetry. J Neurol Neurosurg Psychiatry 2000;68:80–82.

264. Pathak-Ray V, Ray A, Walters R, Hatfield R. Detection of visual field defects in patients after anterior temporal lobectomy for mesial temporal sclerosis-establishing eligibility to drive. Eye 2002;16:744–748.

265. Penfield W. Temporal lobe epilepsy. Br J Surg 1954;41:337–343.

266. Marino R Jr, Rasmussen T. Visual field changes after temporal lobectomy in man. Neurology 1968;18:825–835.

267. Krolak-Salmon P, Guenot M, Tiliket C, et al. Anatomy of optic nerve radiations as assessed by static perimetry and MRI after tailored temporal lobectomy. Br J Ophthalmol 2000;84:884–889.

268. Hughes TS, Abou-Khalil B, Lavin PJ, et al. Visual field defects after temporal lobe resection: a prospective quantitative analysis. Neurology 1999;53:167–172.

269. Egan RA, Shults WT, So N, et al. Visual field deficits in conventional anterior temporal lobectomy versus amygdalohippocampectomy. Neurology 2000;55:1818–1822.

270. Tecoma ES, Laxer KD, Barbaro NM, et al. Frequency and characteristics of visual field deficits after surgery for mesial temporal sclerosis. Neurology 1993;43:1235–1238.

271. Babb TL, Wilson CL, Crandall PH. Asymmetry and ventral course of the human geniculostriate pathway as determined by hippocampal visual evoked potentials and subsequent visual field defects after temporal lobectomy. Exp Brain Res 1982;47:317–328.

272. Ebeling U, Reulen HJ. Neurosurgical topography of the optic radiation in the temporal lobe. Acta Neurochir (Wien) 1988;92:29–36.

273. Anderson DR, Trobe JD, Hood TW, et al. Optic tract injury after anterior temporal lobectomy. Ophthalmology 1989;96:1065–1070.

274. Bjork A, Kugelberg E. Visual field defects after temporal lobectomy. Acta Ophthalmol 1957;35:210–216.

275. Jensen I, Seedorff HH. Temporal lobe epilepsy and neuroophthalmology. Ophthalmological findings in 74 temporal lobe resected patients. Acta Ophthalmol 1976;54:827–841.

276. Katz A, Awad IA, Kong AK, et al. Extent of resection in temporal lobectomy for epilepsy. II. Memory changes and neurologic complications. Epilepsia 1989;30:763–771.

277. Penfield W, Evans JP, Macmillian JA. Visual pathway in man: With particular reference to macular representation. Arch Neurol Psychiatry 1935;33:816–834.

278. Horton JC, Hoyt WF. Quadrantic visual field defects. A hallmark of lesions in extrastriate (V2/V3) Cortex. Brain 1991;114:1703–1718.

279. Brain W. Diseases of the Nervous System. London, Oxford University Press, 1933.

280. Rubens AB. Agnosia. In Heilman KM, Valenstein E, eds. Clinical Neuropsychology. New York, Oxford University Press, 1979:233–267.

281. Kleist K. Gehirnpathologische und lokalisatorische Ergebnisse uber Horstorungen, Gerauschtaubheiten und Amusien. Monatsschr Psychiatr Neurol 1928;68:853–860.

282. Warrington BK Jr. The completion of visual forms across hemianopic field defects. J Neurol Neurosurg Psychiatry 1962;25:208–217.

283. Pahwa JM. Homonymous hemianopias from lesions of parietotemporal lobes. Mediscope 1963;5:543–547.

284. Traquair HM. An Introduction to Clinical Perimetry. 3rd ed. St Louis, CV Mosby, 1940.

285. Nelson SB, LeVay S. Topographic organization of the optic radiation of the cat. J Comp Neurol 1985;240:322–330.

286. Borruat FX, Siatkowski RM, Schatz NJ, et al. Congruous quadrantanopia and optic radiation lesion. Neurology 1993;43:1430–1432.

287. Baloh RW, Yee RD, Honrubia V. Optokinetic nystagmus and parietal lobe lesions. Ann Neurol 1980;7:269–276.

288. Sathian K. Tactile perception. In Beaumont JG, Kenealy P, Rogers M, eds. Blackwell Dictionary of Neuropsychology. Oxford, Blackwell, 1996:717–725.

289. Gerstmann J. Some notes on the Gerstmann syndrome. Neurology 1957;7:866–869.

290. Heimburger RF, Demeyer W, Reitan RM. Implications of Gerstmann's syndrome. J Neurol Neurosurg Psychiatry 1964;27:52–57.

291. Mesulam MM. A cortical network for directed attention and unilateral neglect. Ann Neurol 1981;10:309–325.

292. Heilman KM, Bowers D, Valenstein E, et al. The right hemisphere: Neuropsychological functions. J Neurosurg 1986;64:693–704.

293. Sterzi R, Bottini G, Celani MG, et al. Hemianopia, hemianaesthesia, and hemiplegia after right and left hemisphere damage. A hemispheric difference. J Neurol Neurosurg Psychiatry 1993;56:308–310.

294. Cole M. When the left brain is not right the right brain may be left: Report of personal experience of occipital hemianopia. J Neurol Neurosurg Psychiatry 1999;67:169–173.

295. Holmes G, Lister WT. Disturbances of vision from cerebral lesions with special reference to the cortical representation of the macula. Brain 1916;39:34–73.

296. Spalding JMK. Wounds of the visual pathway: Part II. The striate cortex. J Neurol Neurosurg Psychiatry 1952;15:169–183.

297. Spector RH, Glaser JS, David NJ, et al. Occipital lobe infarctions: Perimetry and computed tomography. Neurology 1981;31:1098–1106.

298. Horton JC, Hoyt WF. The representation of the visual field in human striate cortex. Arch Ophthalmol 1991;109:816–824.

299. McFadzean R, Brosnahan D, Hadley D, Mutlukan E. Representation of the visual field in the occipital striate cortex. Br J Ophthalmol 1994;78:185–190.

300. Wong AM, Sharpe JA. A comparison of tangent screen, Goldmann, and Humphrey perimetry in the detection and localization of occipital lesions. Ophthalmology 2000;107:527–544.

301. Sereno MI, Dale AM, Reppas JB, et al. Borders of multiple visual areas in humans revealed by functional magnetic resonance imaging. Science 1995;268(5212):889–893.

302. Wong AM, Sharpe JA. Representation of the visual field in the human occipital cortex: A magnetic resonance imaging and perimetric correlation. Arch Ophthalmol 1999;117:208–217.

303. Horton JC, Adams DL. The cortical representation of shadows cast by retinal blood vessels. Trans Am Ophthalmol Soc 2000;98:33–39.

304. Adams DL, Horton JC. Shadows cast by retinal blood vessels mapped in primary visual cortex. Science 2002;298(5593):572–576.

305. Adams DL, Horton JC. A precise retinotopic map of primate striate cortex generated from the representation of angioscotomas. J Neurosci 2003;23:3771–3789.

306. Dougherty RF, Koch VM, Brewer AA, et al. Visual field representations and locations of visual areas V1/2/3 in human visual cortex. J Vis 2003;3:586–598.

307. Koerner F, Teuber HL. Visual field defects after missile injuries in the geniculo-striate pathway in man. Exp Brain Res 1973;18:88–113.

308. McAuley DL, Russell RW. Correlation of CAT scan and visual field defects in vascular lesions of the posterior visual pathways. J Neurol Neurosurg Psychiatry 1979;42:298–311.

309. Galetta SL, Grossman RI. The representation of the horizontal meridian in the primary visual cortex. J Neuroophthalmol 2000;20:89–91.

310. Gray LG, Galetta SL, Schatz NJ. Vertical and horizontal meridian sparing in occipital lobe homonymous hemianopias. Neurology 1998;50:1170–1173.

311. Allen TD, Carman HF Jr. Homonymous hemianopic paracentral scotoma. Arch Ophthalmol 1938;20:846–849.

312. Barkan O, Boyle SF. Paracentral homonymous hemianopic scotoma. Arch Ophthalmol 1935;14:957–959.

313. Brouwer B, Zeeman WPC. The projection of the retina in the primary optic neuron of monkeys. Brain 1926;49:1–35.

314. Walsh TJ. Temporal crescent or half-moon syndrome. Ann Ophthalmol 1974; 6:501–505.
315. Polyak S. The Main Afferent Systems of the Cerebral Cortex in Primates. Berkeley, University of California Press, 1932.
316. Ask-Upmark E. On the cortical projection of the temporal half-moon of the visual field. Acta Ophthalmol 1932;10:271–290.
317. Kronfeld T. The temporal half-moon. Trans Am Ophthalmol Soc 1932;30: 431–456.
318. Spence KW, Fulton JF. The effects of occipital lobectomy on vision in the chimpanzee. Brain 1936;59:34–50.
319. Benton S, Levy I, Swash M. Vision in the temporal crescent in occipital infarction. Brain 1980;103:83–97.
320. Ceccaldi M, Brouchon M, Pelletier J, et al. Hemianopsia with preservation of temporal crescent and occipital infarction. Rev Neurol (French) 1993;149: 423–425.
321. Landau K, Wichmann W, Valavanis A. The missing temporal crescent. Am J Ophthalmol 1995;119:345–349.
322. Lepore FE. The preserved temporal crescent: the clinical implications of an "endangered" finding. Neurology 2001;57:1918–1921.
323. Tootell RB, Mendola JD, Hadjikhani NK, et al. The representation of the ipsilateral visual field in human cerebral cortex. Proc Natl Acad Sci USA 1998;95: 818–824.
324. Rossion B, de Gelder B, Pourtois G, et al. Early extrastriate activity without primary visual cortex in humans. Neurosci Lett 2000;279:25–28.
325. Kong CK, Wong LY, Yuen MK. Visual field plasticity in a female with right occipital cortical dysplasia. Pediatr Neurol 2000;23:256–260.
326. Baseler HA, Morland AB, Wandell BA. Topographic organization of human visual areas in the absence of input from primary cortex. J Neurosci 1999;19: 2619–2627.
327. Bender MB, Teuber HL. Spatial organization in visual perception after brain injury. Arch Neurol Psychiatr 1948;59:39–64.
328. Bender MB, Teuber HL. Spatial organization in visual perception after brain injury. Arch Neurol Psychiatr 1947;58:721.
329. Rizzo M, Robin DA. Bilateral effects of unilateral visual cortex lesions in human. Brain 1996;119:951–963.
329a. Battelli L, Cavanagh P, Thornton IM. Perception of biological motion in parietal patients. Neuropsychologia 2003;41:1808–1816.
330. Safran AB, Babel J, Werner A. Aspects campimetriques des lesions occipitales. J Fr Ophtalmol 1978;1:9–20.
331. Verhoeff FH. A new answer to the question of macular sparing. Arch Ophthalmol 1943;30:421–425.
332. Sugishita M, Hemmi I, Sakuma I, et al. The problem of macular sparing after unilateral occipital lesions. J Neurol 1993;241:1–9.
333. Bischoff P, Lang J, Huber A. Macular sparing as a perimetric artifact. Am J Ophthalmol 1995;119:72–80.
334. Lenz G. Der jetzige stand der Lehre von der Makulaaussparung. Klin Monatsbl Augenheilkd 1928;80:398–399.
335. Ohki K, Kase M, Yokoi M, et al. Transition from macular splitting to macular sparing in right homonymous hemianopia complicating a left occipitoparietal hemorrhage. Neuroophthalmology 1994;14:265–269.
336. Dubois-Poulsen A, Magis C, et al. Les consequences visuelles de la lobectomie occipital chez l'homme. Ann Oculist 1952;185:305–347.
337. Morax V. Discussion des hypotheses faites sur les connexions corticales des faisceaux maculaires. Ann Oculist 1919;156:103–107.
338. Gramberg-Danielsen B. Die doppelversorgung der macula. Graefe Arch Ophthalmol 1959;160:534–539.
339. Halstead WC, Walker EA, Bucy PC. Sparing and nonsparing of "macular" vision associated with occipital lobectomy in man. Arch Ophthalmol 1940;24: 948–962.
340. Huber A. Homonymous hemianopia after occipital lobectomy. Am J Ophthalmol 1962;54:623–629.
341. Huber A, Bischoff P, Lang J. Macular sparing: A perimetric artifact? In 10th Meeting of the International Neuro-Ophthalmology Society, June 5–9, 1994. Freiburg, Germany.
342. Cowey A. Projection of the retina onto striate and prestriate cortex in the squirrel monkey: Saimiri sciureus. J Neurophysiol 1964;27:366–393.
343. Leventhal AG, Ault SJ, Vitek DJ. The nasotemporal division in primate retina: the neural bases of macular sparing and splitting. Science 1988;240:66–67.
344. Reinhard J, Trauzettel-Klosinski S. Nasotemporal overlap of retinal ganglion cells in humans: a functional study. Invest Ophthalmol Vis Sci 2003;44: 1568–1572.
345. Brysbaert M. Interhemispheric transfer and the processing of foveally presented stimuli. Behav Brain Res 1994;64:151–161.
346. Schein SJ. Anatomy of macaque fovea and spatial densities of neurons in foveal representation. J Comp Neurol 1988;269:479–505.
347. Wilbrand H. Über die makulare Aussparung. Z Augenheilkd 1926;58:261–268.
348. Förster O. Uber rindenblindheit. Graefe Arch Ophthalmol 1890;36:94–108.
349. Biemond A. La projection des quadrants retiniens dans la radiation optique, etudiee dans un cas d'hemianopsie bilaterale. Folia Psychiatr Neurol Neurochir Neerl 1950;53:159–164.

350. Hoff H, Seitelberger F. Zur klinik und pathologie der doppelseitigen okzipitalen herderkrankungen. Wien Klin Wochenschr 1951;63:621–623.
351. Reese FH. Bilateral homonymous hemianopsia. Am J Ophthalmol 1954;38: 44–57.
352. Kearns TP, Wagner HP, Millikan CH. Bilateral homonymous hemianopsia. Arch Ophthalmol 1955;53:560–565.
353. Symonds C, MacKenzie I. Loss of vision from cerebral infarction. Brain 1957; 80:415–455.
354. Frontera AT. Bilateral homonymous hemianopsia with preservation of central vision. Mt Sinai J Med NY 1974;41:480–485.
355. Godtfredsen E. Bilateral homonymous hemianopia. Acta Ophthalmol 1975; 125(Suppl):20–21.
356. Nepple EW, Appen RE, Sackett JF. Bilateral homonymous hemianopia. Am J Ophthalmol 1978;86:536–543.
357. Drummond JW, Hall DL, Steen WH Jr. Bilateral homonymous hemianopia with hyponatremia. Ann Ophthalmol 1980;12:875–878.
358. Tanaka R, Miyasaka Y, Yada K, et al. Bilateral homonymous hemianopsia due to tentorial herniation, with sparing of central vision: Case report. Neurosurgery 1992;31:787–791.
359. Sachs T. Ungewohnliche formen hemianopischer gesichtsstorung. Wien Klin Wochenschr 1888;22:453–456.
360. Lloyd WI. Hemianopsia. Ophthalmol Rec 1917;26:491–515.
361. Schaublin A. Horizontal hemianopias. Confin Neurol 1967;29:327–337.
362. Bender MB, Furlow LT. Phenomenon of visual extinction in homonymous fields and psychologic principles involved. Arch Neurol Psychiatr 1945;53:29–33.
363. Bender MB, Furlow LT. Visual disturbances produced by bilateral lesions of the occipital lobes with central scotomas. Arch Neurol Psychiatr 1945;53:165–170.
364. Halpern JI, Sedler RR. Traumatic bilateral homonymous hemianopic scotomas. Ann Ophthalmol 1980;12:1022–1026.
365. Kaul SN, Du BGH, Kendall BE, et al. Relationship between visual field defect and arterial occlusion in the posterior cerebral circulation. J Neurol Neurosurg Psychiatr 1974;37:1022–1030.
366. Felix CH. Crossed quadrant hemianopsia. Br J Ophthalmol 1926;10:191–195.
367. Holmes G. Disturbances of vision by cerebral lesions. Br J Ophthalmol 1918; 2:353–384.
368. Wortham E, Levin G, Wick HW. Altitudinal anopsia following thoracoplasty. Arch Ophthalmol 1952;47:248–249.
369. Newman RP, Kinkel WR, Jacobs L. Altitudinal hemianopia caused by occipital infarctions. Arch Neurol 1984;41:413–418.
370. Vanroose E, Marchau M, Dehaene I, et al. Altitudinal hemianopia; a clinical and anatomical entity or a mere coincidence? Case report and review of literature. Acta Neurol Belg 1990;90:254–264.
371. Heller-Bettinger I, Kepes JK, Preskorn SH, et al. Bilateral altitudinal anopia caused by infarction of the calcarine cortex. Neurology 1976;26:1176–1179.
372. Camarda R, Bonavita V. Inferior cortical altitudinal hemianopia: Report of a case. Ital J Neurol Sci 1982;4:365–370.
373. Bogousslavsky J, Miklossy J, Deruaz JP, et al. Lingual and fusiform gyri in visual processing: A clinico-pathologic study of superior altitudinal hemianopia. J Neurol Neurosurg Psychiatr 1987;50:607–614.
374. Howard R, Trend P, Ross RRW. Clinical features of ischemia in cerebral arterial border zones after periods of reduced cerebral blood flow. Arch Neurol 1987; 44:934–940.
375. Lakhanpal A, Selhorst JB. Bilateral altitudinal visual fields. Ann Ophthalmol 1990;22:112–117.
376. Kerkhoff G. Displacement of the egocentric visual midline in altitudinal postchiasmatic scotomata. Neuropsychologia 1993;31:261–265.
377. Marquis DG. Effects of removal of visual cortex in mammals with observations on the retention of light discrimination in dogs. In: Williams & Wilkins, Baltimore; 1934:558.
378. Bogousslavsky J, Regli F, Van MG. Unilateral occipital infarction: Evaluation of the risk of developing bilateral loss of vision. J Neurol Neurosurg Psychiatr 1983;46:78–80.
379. Aldrich MS, Alessi AG, Beck RW, et al. Cortical blindness: Etiology, diagnosis, and prognosis. Ann Neurol 1987;21:149–158.
380. Fisher CM. The posterior cerebral artery syndrome. Can J Neurol Sci 1986;13: 232–239.
381. Pessin MS, Lathi ES, Cohen MB, et al. Clinical features and mechanism of occipital infarction. Ann Neurol 1987;21:290–299.
382. Courville C. Cerebral Anoxia. Los Angeles, San Lucas Press, 1953.
383. Lindenberg R. Compression of brain arteries as pathogenic factor for tissue necrosis and their areas of predilection. J Neuropathol Exp Neurol 1955;14: 223–243.
384. Magitot A, Hartmann E. La cecite corticale. Bull Soc Ophtalmol Fr 1926: 427–572.
385. Magitot A, Hartmann E. La cecite corticale. Rev Otoneuroroculo 1927;5:81–114.
386. Bergman PS. Cerebral blindness. Arch Neurol Psychiatr 1957;78:568–584.
387. Hoyt WF, Walsh FB. Cortical blindness with partial recovery following acute cerebral anoxia from cardiac arrest. Arch Ophthalmol 1958;60:1061–1069.
388. Lai CW, Hung T, Lin WSJ. Blindness of cerebral origin in acute intermittent porphyria. Arch Neurol 1977;34:310–312.
389. Margolis LH, Shaywitz BA, Rothman SA. Cortical blindness associated with

occipital atrophy: A complication of *H. influenzae* meningitis. Dev Med Child Neurol 1978;20:490–496.

390. Moel DI, Kwun YA. Cortical blindness as a complication of hemodialysis. J Pediatr 1978;93:890–894.

391. Beal MF, Chapman PH. Cortical blindness and homonymous hemianopia in the postpartum period. JAMA 1980;244:2085–2087.

392. Dobbins KR, Saul RF. Transient visual loss after licorice ingestion. J Neuroophthalmol 2000;20:38–41.

393. Keane JR. Blindness following tentorial herniation. Ann Neurol 1980;8:186–190.

394. Mukamel M, Weitz R, Nissenkorn I, et al. Acute cortical blindness associated with hypoglycemia. J Pediatr 1981;98:583–585.

395. Sadeh M, Goldhammer Y, Kuritsky A. Postictal blindness in adults. J Neurol Neurosurg Psychiatry 1983;46:566–569.

396. Sedwick LA, Klingele TG, Burde RM, et al. Schilder's disease. Total cerebral blindness due to acute demyelination. Arch Neurol 1986;43:85–87.

397. Eldridge PR, Punt JA. Transient traumatic cortical blindness in children. Lancet 1988;1:815–816.

398. Wilson SE, et al. Cyclosporin A-induced reversible cortical blindness. J Clin Neuroophthalmol 1988;8:215–220.

399. Heran F, Defer G, Brugieres P, et al. Cortical blindness during chemotherapy: Clinical, CT, and MR correlations. J Comput Assist Tomog 1990;14:262–266.

400. Kabra SK, Bagga A, Shankar V. Subacute sclerosing panencephalitis presenting as cortical blindness. Trop Doct 1992;22:94–95.

401. Lawrence-Friedl D, Bauer KM. Bilateral cortical blindness: An unusual presentation of bacterial endocarditis. Ann Emerg Med 1992;21:1502–1504.

402. Merimsky O, Loewenstein A, Chaitchik S. Cortical blindness: A catastrophic side effect of vincristine. Anticancer Drugs 1992;3:371–373.

403. Merimsky O, Nisipeanu P, Loewenstein A. Interferon-related cortical blindness. Cancer Chemother Pharmacol 1992;29:329–330.

404. Williamson PD, Thadani VM, Darcey TM, et al. Occipital lobe epilepsy: Clinical characteristics, seizure spread patterns, and results of surgery. Ann Neurol 1992;31:3–13.

405. Shutter LA, Green JP, Newman NJ, et al. Cortical blindness and white matter lesions in a patient receiving FK506 after liver transplantation. Neurology 1993;43:2417–2418.

406. Davis LE, Kornfeld M, Mooney HS, et al. Methylmercury poisoning: Long-term clinical, radiological, toxicological, and pathological studies of an affected family. Ann Neurol 1994;35:680–688.

407. Good WV, Jan JE, DeSa L, et al. Cortical visual impairment in children. Surv Ophthalmol 1994;38:351–364.

408. Cunningham FG, Fernandez CO, Hernandez C. Blindness associates with pre-eclampsia and eclampsia. Am J Obstet Gynecol 1995;172:1291–1298.

409. Gilliam F, Wyllie E. Ictal amaurosis: MRI, EEG, and clinical features. Neurology 1995;45:1619–1621.

410. Gospe SM Jr. Transient cortical blindness in an infant exposed to methamphetamine. Ann Emerg Med 1995;26:380–382.

411. Hagerty C, Licho R, Recht L. Cortical blindness after correction of symptomatic hyponatremia: Dynamic cerebral dysfunction visualized using serial SPECT scanning. J Nucl Med 1995;36:1272–1274.

412. Jackson A, Stewart G, Wood A, et al. Transient global amnesia and cortical blindness after vertebral angiography, further evidence for the role of arterial spasm. Am J Neuroradiol 1995;16:955–959.

413. Kupferschmidt H, Bont A, Schnorf H, et al. Transient cortical blindness and bioccipital brain lesions in two patients with acute intermittent porphyria. Ann Intern Med 1995;123:598–600.

414. Memon M, et al. Reversible cyclosporine-induced cortical blindness in allogeneic bone marrow transplant recipients. Bone Marrow Transplantation 1995;15:283–286.

415. Knower MT, Pethke SD, Valentine VG. Reversible cortical blindness after lung transplantation. South Med J 2003;96:606–612.

416. Vargas ME, Kupersmith MJ, Savino PJ, et al. Homonymous field defect as the first manifestation of Creutzfeldt-Jakob disease. Am J Ophthalmol 1995;119:497–504.

417. Hinchey J, Chaves C, Appignani B, et al. A reversible posterior leukoencephalopathy syndrome. N Engl J Med 1996;334:494–500.

418. Ammar T, Auwzinger G, Michaelides M. Cortical blindness and hepatic encephalopathy. Acta Ophthalmol Scand 2003;81:402–404.

419. Barnet AB, Manson JI, Wilner E. Acute cerebral blindness in childhood. Neurology 1970;20:1147–1156.

420. Dennis MS, Bamford JM, Sandercock PAG, et al. Lone bilateral blindness: A transient ischaemic attack. Lancet 1989;1:185–188.

421. Gleeson AP, Beattie TF. Post-traumatic transient cortical blindess in children: A report of four cases and a review of the literature. J Accid Emerg Med 1994;11:250–252.

422. Greenblatt SH. Posttraumatic transient cerebral blindness: Association with migraine and seizure diatheses. JAMA 1973;225:1073–1076.

423. Pritchard E. Case of amaurosis following violent convulsions. Proc R Soc Med 1918;11:1–2.

424. Mecca M. Reperti oculari nell'epilessia essenziale con particolare reguardo allo spasmo vasale. Ann Ottal 1938;66:457–469.

425. Jaffe SJ, Roach ES. Transient cortical blindness with occipital lobe epilepsy. J Clin Neuroophthalmol 1988;8:221–224.

426. Aldrich MS, Vanderzant CW, Alessi AG, et al. Ictal cortical blindness with permanent visual loss. Epilepsia 1989;30:116–120.

427. Roos KL, Tuite PJ, Below ME, et al. Reversible cortical blindness (Anton's syndrome) associated with bilateral occipital EEG abnormalities. Clin EEG 1990;21:104–109.

428. Lance JW, Smee RI. Partial seizures with visual disturbance treated by radiotherapy of cavernous hemangioma. Ann Neurol 1989;26:782–785.

429. Joseph JM, Louis S. Transient ictal cortical blindness during middle age. A case report and review of the literature. J Neuroophthalmology 1995;15:39–42.

430. Ashby H, Stephenson S. Acute amaurosis following infantile convulsions. Rep Soc Study Dis Child 1903;3:197–209.

431. Kooi KA, Sharbrough FW. Electrophysiological findings in cortical blindness. EEG Clin Neurophysiol 1966;20:260–263.

432. Crighel E, Botex MI. Photic evoked potentials in man in lesions of the occipital lobes. Brain 1966;89:311–316.

433. Chisholm IH. Cortical blindness in cranial arteritis. Br J Ophthalmol 1975;59:332–333.

434. Medina JL, Chokroverty S, Rubino FA. Syndrome of agitated delirium and visual impairment: A manifestation of medial temporo-occipital infarction. J Neurol Neurosurg Psychiatry 1977;40:861–864.

435. Spehlmann R, Gross RA, Ho SU, et al. Visual evoked potentials and postmodern findings in a case of cortical blindness. Ann Neurol 1977;2:531–534.

436. Celesia GG, Archer CR, Kuroiwa Y, et al. Visual function of the extrageniculocalcarine system in man: Relationship to cortical blindness. Arch Neurol 1980;37:704–706.

437. Hess CW, Meienberg O, Ludin HP. Visual evoked potentials in acute occipital blindness: diagnostic and prognostic value. J Neurol 1982;227:193–200.

438. Kuroiwa Y, Celesia GG. Visual evoked potentials with hemifield pattern stimulation: their use in the diagnosis of retrochiasmatic lesions. Arch Neurol 1981;38:86–90.

439. Bodis-Wollner I, Atkin A, Raab E, et al. Visual association cortex and vision in man: Pattern-evoked occipital potentials in a blind boy. Science 1977;198:629–630.

440. Frank Y, Torres F. Visual evoked potentials in the evaluation of "cortical blindness" in children. Ann Neurol 1979;6:126–129.

441. Mellor DH, Fielder AR. Dissociated visual development. Electrodiagnostic studies in infants who are "slow to see." Dev Med Child Neurol 1980;22:327.

442. Hoyt CF. Cortical blindness in infancy. Trans New Orleans Acad Ophthalmol 1986:235.

443. Wong VCN. Cortical blindness in children: A study of etiology and prognosis. Pediatr Neurol 1991;7:178–185.

444. Frank Y, Kurtzberg D, Kreuzer JA, et al. Flash and pattern-reversal visual evoked potential abnormalities in infants and children with cerebral blindness. Dev Med Child Neurol 1992;34:305–315.

445. Granet DB, Hertle RW, Quinn GE, et al. The visual-evoked response in infants with central visual impairment. Am J Ophthalmol 1993;116:437–443.

446. Duchowny MS, Weiss IP, Majlessi H, et al. Visual evoked responses in childhood cortical blindness after head trauma and meningitis: A longitudinal study of six cases. Neurology 1974;24:933–940.

447. Kupersmith MJ, Nelson JI. Preserved visual-evoked potential in infancy cortical blindness. Relationship to blindness. Neuroophthalmology 1986;6:85–94.

448. Lambert SR, Kriss A, Taylor D. Delayed visual maturation. Ophthalmology 1989;96:524.

449. Bencivenga R, Wong PKH, Woo S, et al. Quantitative VEP analysis in children with cortical visual impairment. Brain Topogr 1989;1:193–198.

450. McCulloch DL, Taylor MJ. Cortical blindness in children: Utility of flash VEPs. Pediatr Neurol 1992;8:156.

451. McCulloch DL, Taylor MJ, Whyte HE. Visual evoked potentials and visual prognosis following perinatal asphyxia. Arch Ophthalmol 1991;109:229–233.

452. Taylor MJ, McCulloch DL. Prognostic value of VEPs in young children with acute onset cortical blindness. Pediatr Neurol 1991;7:111–115.

453. Velzeboer CMJ. Bilateral cortical hemianopia and optokinetic nystagmus. Ophthalmologica 1952;123:187–188.

454. Morax PV. La cecite corticale. In Alajouanine T, ed. Les Grandes Activities du Lobe Occipital. Paris, Masson, 1960:217.

455. Brindley GS, Gautier-Smith PC, Lewin W. Cortical blindness and the functions of the nongeniculate fibres of the optic tracts. J Neurol Neurosurg Psychiatry 1969;32:259–264.

456. Ter Braak JWG. Untersuchungen über optokinetischen Nystagmus. Arch Neerl Physiol 1936;21:309–376.

457. Ter Braak JWG, Schenk VWD, van Vliet AGM. Visual reactions in a case of long-lasting cortical blindness. J Neurol Neurosurg Psychiatry 1971;34:140–147.

458. Anton G. Über die selbstwahrnehmung der herderkrankungen des gehirns durch den kranken bei rindenblindheitund Rindentaubheit. Arch Psychiatr Nervenkr 1899;32:86–127.

459. Lessell S. Higher disorders of visual function: Negative phenomena. In Glaser JS, Smith JL, eds. Neuro-Ophthalmology. St Louis, CV Mosby, 1975:3–4.

460. Ramachandran VS, Gregory RL. Perceptual filling in of artificially induced scotomas in human vision. Nature 1991;350:699–702.
461. Horrax G, Putnam T. Distortions of the visual fields in cases of brain tumour. The field defects and hallucinations produced by tumours of the occipital lobe. Brain 1932;55:499–523.
462. Lance JW. Simple formed hallucinations confined to the area of a specific visual field defect. Brain 1976;99:719–734.
463. Kolmel HW. Coloured patterns in hemianopic fields. Brain 1984;107:155–167.
464. Vaphiades MS, Celesia GG, Brigell MG. Positive spontaneous visual phenomena limited to the hemianopic field in lesions of central visual pathways. Neurology 1996;47:408–417.
465. Jones MR, Waggoner R, Hoyt WF. Cerebral polyopia with extrastriate quadrantanopia: Report of a case with magnetic resonance documentation of V2/V3 cortical infarction. J Neuroophthalmol 1999;19:1–6.
466. Cornblath WT, Butter CM, Barnes LL, Hasselbach MM. Spatial characteristics of cerebral polyopia: A case study. Vision Res 1998;38:3965–3978.
467. Teuber HL. Neuere beobachtungen über sehstrahlung und sehrinde. In Jung R, Kornhuber H, eds. The Visual System: Neurophysiology and Psychophysics: Symposium Freiburg, 1960. Berlin-Gottingen-Heidelberg, Springer-Verlag, 1961:264.
468. Weiskrantz L. Encephalization and the scotoma. Unpublished manuscript, Psychology Laboratory, Cambridge University, 1958.
468a.Biousse V, Newman NJ, Carroll C, et al. Visual fields in patients with posterior GPi pallidotomy. Neurology 1998;50:258–265.
469. Weiskrantz L, Cowey A. Comparison of the effects of striate cortex and retinal lesions on visual acuity in the monkey. Science 1967;155:104–106.
470. Zeki SM. Functional specialization in the visual cortex of the rhesus monkey. Nature London 1978;274:423–428.
471. Van Essen DC, Maunsell JHR. Hierarchical organization and functional streams in the visual cortex. Trends Neurosci 1983;6:370–375.
472. Zeki S, Watson JDG, Lueck CJ, et al. A direct demonstration of functional specialization in human visual cortex. J Neurosci 1991;11:641–649.
473. Wade AR, Brewer AA, Rieger JW, Wandell BA. Functional measurements of human ventral occipital cortex: Retinotopy and colour. Philos Trans R Soc Lond B Biol Sci 2002;357(1424):963–973.
474. Morland AB, Baseler HA, Hoffmann MB, et al. Abnormal retinotopic representations in human visual cortex revealed by fMRI. Acta Psychol (Amst) 2001; 107(1–3):229–247.
475. Nakamura H, Gattass R, Desimone R, et al. The modular organization of projections from areas V1 and V2 to areas V4 and TEO in macaques. J Neurosci 1993;13:3681–3691.
476. Feinsod M, Hoyt WF, Wilson WB. Suprastriate hemianopia. Lancet 1974;1: 1225–1226.
477. Damasio A, Yamada T, Damasio H, et al. Central achromatopsia: Behavioral, anatomic, and physiologic aspects. Neurology 1980;30:1064–1071.
478. Polyak S. The Vertebrate Visual System. Chicago, University of Chicago Press, 1957.
479. Slotnick SD, Moo LR. Retinotopic mapping reveals extrastriate cortical basis of homonymous quadrantanopia. Neuroreport 2003;14:1209–1213.
480. Brazis PW, Lee AG, Graff-Radford N, et al. Homonymous visual field defects in patients without corresponding structural lesions on neuroimaging. J Neuroophthalmol 2000;20:92–96.
481. Kropp S, Schulz-Schaeffer WJ, Finkenstaedt M, et al. The Heidenhain variant of Creutzfeldt-Jakob disease. Arch Neurol 1999;56:55–61.
482. Jacobs DA, Lesser RL, Mourelatos Z, et al. The Heidenhain variant of Creutzfeldt-Jakob disease: Clinical, pathologic, and neuroimaging findings. J Neuroophthalmol 2001;21:99–102.
483. Delamont RS, Harrison J, Field M, Boyle RS. Posterior cortical atrophy. Clin Exp Neurol 1989;26:225–227.
484. Benson DF, Davis RJ, Snyder BD. Posterior cortical atrophy. Arch Neurol 1988; 45:789–793.
485. Lee YJ, Chung TS, Soo Yoon Y, et al. The role of functional MR imaging in patients with ischemia in the visual cortex. Am J Neuroradiol 2001;22: 1043–1049.
486. Spatt J, Mamoli B. Ictal visual hallucinations and postictal hemianopia with anosognosia. Seizure 2000;9:502–504.
487. Valli G, Zago S, Cappellari A, Bersano A. Transitory and permanent visual field defects induced by occipital lobe seizures. Ital J Neurol Sci 1999;20:321–325.
488. Lueck CJ, Zeki S, Friston KJ, et al. The colour centre in the cerebral cortex of man. Nature 1989;340:386–389.
489. Zeki S, Bartels A. The clinical and functional measurement of cortical (in)activity in the visual brain, with special reference to the two subdivisions (V4 and V4 alpha) of the human colour centre. Philos Trans R Soc Lond B Biol Sci 1999;354(1387):1371–1382.
490. Green GJ, Lessell S. Acquired cerebral dyschromatopsia. Arch Ophthalmol 1977;95:121–128.
491. Rizzo M, Nawrot M, Blake R, et al. A human visual disorder resembling area V4 dysfunction in the monkey. Neurology 1992;42:1175–1180.
492. Lawden MC, Cleland PG. Achromatopsia in the aura of migraine. J Neurol Neurosurg Psychiatry 1993;56:708–709.
493. Probst T, Plendl H, Paulus W, et al. Identification of the visual motion area (area V5) in the human brain by dipole source analysis. Exp Brain Res 1993; 93:345–351.
494. Watson JDG, Myers R, Frackowiak RSJ, et al. Area V5 of the human brain: Evidence from a combined study using positron emission tomography and magnetic resonance imaging. Cerebral Cortex 1993;3:79–94.
495. Zihl J, von Cramon D, Mai N, et al. Disturbance of movement vision after bilateral posterior brain damage. Brain 1991;114:2235–2252.
496. Plant GT, Laxer KD, Barbaro NM, et al. Impaired visual motion perception in the contralateral hemifield following unilateral posterior cerebral lesions in humans. Brain 1993;116:1303–1335.
497. Blanke O, Landis T, Safran AB, Seeck M. Direction-specific motion blindness induced by focal stimulation of human extrastriate cortex. Eur J Neurosci 2002; 15:2043–2048.
498. Riddoch G. Dissociation in visual perceptions due to occipital injuries, with especial references to appreciation of movement. Brain 1917;40:15–57.
499. Troost BT, Newton TH. Occipital lobe arteriovenous malformations. Arch Ophthalmol 1975;93:250–256.
500. Mestre DR, Brouchon M, Ceccaldi M, et al. Perception of optical flow in cortical blindness: A case report. Neuropsychologia 1992;30:783–795.
501. Safran AB, Glaser JS. Statokinetic dissociation in lesions of the anterior visual pathways. Arch Ophthalmol 1980;98:291–295.
502. Greve EL. Single and multiple stimulus static perimetry in glaucoma: The two phases of visual field examination. Doc Ophthalmol 1973;36:1–355.
503. Tolhurst DJ. Separate channels for the analysis of the shape and movement of a moving visual stimulus. J Physiol 1973;231:385–402.
504. Zappia RJ, Enoch JM, Stamper R, et al. The Riddoch phenomenon revealed in non-occipital lobe lesions. Br J Ophthalmol 1971;55:416–420.
505. Perenin MT, Jeannerod M. Visual function within the hemianopic field following early cerebral hemidecortication in man. I. Spatial localization. Neuropsychologia 1978;16:1–13.
506. Rafal R, Smith J, Krantz J, et al. Extrageniculate vision in hemianopic humans: saccade inhibition by signals in the blind field. Science 1990;250:118–120.
507. Corbetta M, Marzi CA, Tassinari G, et al. Effectiveness of different task paradigms in revealing blindsight. Brain 1990;113:603–616.
508. Cowey A, Stoerig P. The neurobiology of blindsight. Trends Neurosci 1991;14: 140–145.
509. Weiskrantz L, Barbur JL, Sahraie A. Parameters affecting conscious versus unconscious visual discrimination with damage to the visaul cortex (V1). Proc Natl Acad Sci USA 1995;92:6122–6126.
510. Scharli H, Harman AM, Hogben JH. Residual vision in a subject with damaged visual cortex. J Cogn Neurosci 1999;11:502–510.
511. Mohler CW, Wurtz RH. Role of striate cortex and superior colliculus in visual guidance of saccadic eye movements in monkeys. J Neurophysiol 1977;40: 74–94.
512. Celesia GG, Bushnell D, Toleikis SC, et al. Cortical blindness and residual vision: Is the ''second'' visual system in humans capable of more than rudimentary visual perception? Neurology 1991;41:862–869.
513. Fendrich R, Wessinger CM, Gazzaniga MS. Residual vision in a scotoma: Implications for blindsight. Science 1992;258:1489–1491.
514. Campion J, Latto R, Smith YM. Is blindsight an effect of scattered light, spared cortex and near-threshold vision? Behav Brain Sci 1983;6:423–486.
515. Kleiser R, Wittsack J, Niedeggen M, Goebel R, Stoerig P. Is V1 necessary for conscious vision in areas of relative cortical blindness? Neuroimage 2001;13: 654–661.
516. Bittar RG, Ptito M, Faubert J, et al. Activation of the remaining hemisphere following stimulation of the blind hemifield in hemispherectomized subjects. Neuroimage 1999;10(3 Pt 1):339–346.
517. Rees G, Wojciulik E, Clarke K, et al. Neural correlates of conscious and unconscious vision in parietal extinction. Neurocase 2002;8:387–393.
518. Knox DL, Cogan DG. Eye pain and homonymous hemianopia. Am J Ophthalmol 1962;54:1091–1093.
519. Rondot P, Odier F, Valade D. Postural disturbances due to homonymous hemianopic visual ataxia. Brain 1992;115:179–188.
520. de Letona JML. Homonymous hemianopia and the ''door sign.'' Postgrad Med J 1992;68:301.
521. Milandre L, Brosset C, Botti G, et al. A study of 82 cerebral infarctions in the area of posterior cerebral arteries. Rev Neurol 1994;150:133–141.
522. Parkinson D, Craig W. Tumours of the brain, occipital lobe; their signs and symptoms. Can Med Assoc J 1951;64:111–113.
523. Zihl J, von Cramon D. Restitution of visual function in patients with cerebral blindness. J Neurol Neurosurg Psychiatry 1979;42:312–322.
524. Zihl J, von Cramon D. Visual field recovery from scotoma in patients with postgeniculate damage. Brain 1985;108:439–469.
525. Kerkhoff G, MunBinger U, Haaf E, et al. Rehabilitation of homonymous scotomata in patients with postgeniculate damage of the visual system: Saccadic compensation training. Restorative Neurol Neurosci 1992;4:245–254.
526. Safran AB, Landis T. Plasticity in the adult visual cortex. Implications for the diagnosis of visual field defects and visual rehabilitation. Curr Opin Ophthalmol 1996;7:53–64.
527. Safran AB, Landis T. From cortical plasticity to unawareness of visual field defects. J Neuroophthalmol 1999;19:84–88.

528. Balliet R, Blood KMT, Bach-y-Rita P. Visual field rehabilitation in the cortically blind? J Neurol Neurosurg Psychiatry 1985;48:1113–1124.

529. Kerkhoff G, MunBinger U, Meier EK. Neurovisual rehabilitation in cerebral blindness. Arch Neurol 1994;51:474–481.

530. Kerkhoff G. Restorative and compensatory therapy approaches in cerebral blindness: A review. Restor Neurol Neurosci 1999;15(2,3):255–271.

531. Dromerick AW, Reding MJ. Functional outcome for patients with hemiparesis, hemihypesthesia, and hemianopsia. Does lesion location matter? Stroke 1995; 26:2023–2026.

532. Nepomuceno CS, Hamilton S, Kelly PA, et al. The triad of left hemiplegia, hemihypesthesia, and homonymous hemianopsia: Implications for rehabilitation. South Med J 1994;87:905–908.

533. Szlyk JP, Brigell MI, Seiple W. Effects of age and hemianopic visual field loss on driving. Optometry Vis Sci 1993;70:1031–1037.

534. Pambakian AL, Kennard C. Can visual function be restored in patients with homonymous hemianopia? J Neurol Neurosurg Psychiatry 1997;81:324–328.

535. Bell E. A mirror for patients with hemianopia. JAMA 1949;140:1024.

536. Burns TA, Hanley WJ, Pietri JF, et al. Spectacles for hemianopia. Am J Ophthalmol 1952;35:1489–1492.

537. Perlin RR, Dziadul J. Fresnel prisms for field enhancement of patients with constricted or hemianopic visual fields. J Am Optom Assoc 1991;62:58–64.

538. Mintz MJ. A mirror for hemianopia. Am J Ophthalmol 1979;88:766–767.

539. Waiss B, Cohen JM. The utilization of a temporal mirror coating on the back surface of the lens as a field enhancement device. J Am Optom Assoc 1992; 63:576–580.

540. Smith JL. New pearls checklist. J Clin Neuroophthalmol 1981;1:78.

541. Gottlieb D, Freeman P, Williams M. Clinical research and statistical analysis of a visual field awareness system. J Am Optom Assoc 1992;63:518–188.

542. Rossi PW, Kheyfets S, Reding MJ. Fresnel prisms improve visual perception in stroke patients with homonymous hemianopia or unilateral visual neglect. Neurology 1990;40:1597–1599.

543. Pameijer JK. Reading problems in hemianopia. Ophthalmologica 1970;160: 322–325.

544. Holm OC. A simple method for widening restricted visual fields. Arch Ophthalmol 1970;84:611–612.

545. Schoepf D, Zangemeister WH. Correlation of ocular motor reading strategies to the status of adaptation in patients with hemianopic visual field defects. Ann NY Acad Sci 1993;682:404–408.

546. Zangemeister WH, Oechesner U, Freksa C. Short-term adaptation of eye movements in patients with visual hemifield defects indicates high level control of human scanpath. Optom Vis Sci 1995;72:467–477.

547. Zihl J. Visual scanning behavior in patients with homonymous hemianopia. Neuropsychologia 1995;33:287–303.

548. Zihl J. Eye movement patterns in hemianopic dyslexia. Brain 1995;118: 891–912.

549. Nelles G, Esser J, Eckstein A, Tiede A, et al. Compensatory visual field training for patients with hemianopia after stroke. Neurosci Lett 2001;306:189–192.

550. Kasten E, Wuse S, Behrens-Baumann W, et al. Computer-based training for the treatment of partial blindness. Nature Med 1998;4:1083–1087.

551. Kasten E, Poggel DA, Sabel BA. Computer-based training of stimulus detection improves color and simple pattern recognition in the defective field of hemianopic subjects. J Cogn Neurosci 2000;12:1001–1012.

552. Sabel BA, Kasten E. Restoration of vision by training of residual functions. Curr Opin Ophthalmol 2000;11:430–436.

553. Reinhard J, Schreiber A, Schiefer U, et al. Does visual restitution training change absolute homonymous visual field defects? A fundus-controlled study. Br J Ophthalmol (in press).

CHAPTER 13

Central Disorders of Visual Function

Matthew Rizzo and Jason Barton

This chapter addresses aspects of behavior disorders caused by damage to the visual cortex and white matter connections. These conditions are often referred to as "central disorders of vision," "cerebral disorders of vision," or "higher disorders of vision." The understanding of these disorders continues to improve with the development of new techniques for measuring visual dysfunction, imaging the behaving brain, rehabilitating visual dysfunction in patients with brain damage, and even creating visual sensations in the blind with prostheses to stimulate visual cortex. Insights into how the brain processes visual signals have altered the classic conceptualization of cerebral visual disorders, even

raising questions about the nature of the visual loss produced by damage to primary visual cortex.

Vision was once thought to be primarily a serial (or hierarchic) process in which visual signals were altered or enhanced at successive way stations from retina to brain until an image of the physical world somehow emerged at the level of conscious experience. The idea of serial processing of visual information was supported in the 1960s by the work of Hubel and Weisel (1), who interpreted data from experiments using microelectrode recordings in the visual cortex of cat and monkey in terms of serial connections among different functional modules called simple columns, complex columns, and hypercolumns. It subsequently became clear that serial processing is only one of several mechanisms used by the brain to process visual signals.

The primate visual system also uses parallel processing, beginning in the retina. Different types of retinal ganglion cells are specialized to transduce different types of physical signals and give rise to different channels (see Chapter 1). There is cross-talk among these channels at several levels from the retina to the cortex, and there also are feed-forward and feedback connections between early and late stages of the visual sensory system. Instead of just serial processing, visual functions are explained in terms of multiple interactions among specialized brain regions in the same hemisphere and across the corpus callosum. Felleman and van Essen (2) catalogued at least 30 functional representations of the visual fields in the cortex of the monkey, with over a hundred interconnections (see Chapter 1). How this model corresponds with the human arrangement is unclear, although homologies can be postulated, at least to the level of early prestriate cortex. Central disorders of vision thus can be interpreted as a consequence of disturbing the processing in different sectors or pathways in such a network.

SEGREGATION OF VISUAL INPUTS

For a historical perspective on the understanding of human vision, the interested reader is referred to several classic older references (3–14) and the previous edition of this text.

The functional segregation of visual inputs in the primate visual system is now well documented (see Chapter 1). Retinal information is communicated to cortical neurons through a set of pathways that appear specialized to convey a particular class of visual information. For example, the parvocellular or P-pathway, named for its connections to simian striate cortex (area V1) via parvocellular layers 3–6 of the lateral geniculate nucleus (LGN), is characterized by color opponency and slow-conducting axons that convey sustained signals (15,16). This pathway, which corresponds to a psychophysical sustained channel (17), has stronger projections to secondary areas such as V4 and inferior temporal (IT) cortex, located in the inferior occipital lobe and adjacent temporo-occipital regions (2). These regions, along the ventral or temporal cortical pathway (the "what" pathway), are presumed to play a role in the perception of color, luminance, stereopsis, and pattern recognition. In contrast, the magnocellular or M-pathway is characterized by large, fast-conducting axons that convey information about more transient visual signals. This pathway connects to areas in visual association cortex, including the middle temporal (MT) and medial superior temporal (MST) areas. These regions, located along the dorsal or parietal cortical pathway (the "where" pathway), are thought to analyze the spatial location and movement of objects in the panorama (Fig. 13.1). Recent

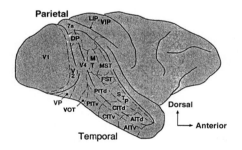

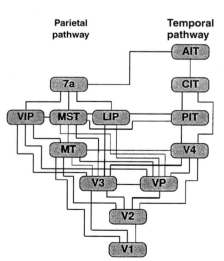

Figure 13.1. Parallel pathways for visual function in the cerebral cortex of the nonhuman primate. Borders between visual areas are indicated by *fine dashed lines.* The superior temporal sulcus has been opened to show areas that are normally out of sight. The medial hemisphere is not shown. The *lower panel* shows a flow diagram from area V1 (primary visual cortex) to the parietal pathway, which includes area MT, and the temporal pathway, which includes area V4. The visual information encoded by neurons varies greatly among these different areas. The human brain is likely to respect a similar organization. 7a, Brodmann's area 7a; AIT, anterior inferotemporal area (d, dorsal subdivision; v, ventral subdivision); CIT, central inferotemporal area (d, dorsal subdivision; v, ventral subdivision); DP, dorsal parietal area; FST, fundus of the superior temporal area; LIP, lateral intraparietal area; MST, medial superior temporal area; MT, middle temporal area; PIT, posterior inferotemporal area (d, dorsal subdivision; v, ventral subdivision); STP, superior temporal polysensory area; V1, visual area 1 (striate cortex); V2, visual area 2; V4, visual area 4; VIP, ventral intraparietal area; VOT, ventral occipitotemporal area; VP, ventral posterior area. (From Maunsell JH. The brain's visual world: Representation of visual targets in cerebral cortex. Science 1995; 270:764–768.)

research has identified a koniocellular or K-channel of retinal information that is distinct from the M- and P-channels; less is known about its central inputs, but it might be important for color (18,19).

The notion of two separate visual systems is a useful and fruitful paradigm in the macaque animal model (20), and it is also applicable to human vision. Analyses of data from a large number of patients with focal lesions of the visual cortex and its connections, as defined by computed tomographic (CT) scanning and magnetic resonance (MR) imaging, support the general concept of separate dorsal and ventral processing pathways as a framework for interpreting human clinical disorders (21). For example, damage in the inferior visual cortex, in the occipital lobe and adjoining temporal regions, impairs pattern recognition and learning, producing agnosia for objects and faces (prosopagnosia) or inability to read despite previous literacy (alexia). It can also reduce color perception in the contralateral field—cerebral achromatopsia (22–24). By contrast, damage in the superior visual cortex, in the occipital lobe and its adjacent parietal cortex, produces disorders of spatial-temporal analysis (i.e., inability to judge location, distance, orientation, size, or motion of objects), as well as marked disturbances of visually guided eye and hand control. Bálint's (25) syndrome is a striking example.

Although the dorsal visual cortex and the ventral visual cortex are associated with different, behaviorally separable functions, there is growing evidence that these two major divisions also have overlapping functions. For example, damage to the dorsal visual pathway is capable of impairing the recognition of shape defined by either motion or static texture cues (26), even though mechanisms for the processing of shape from static texture cues would be expected to depend on ventral pathways. Such findings suggest either a redundant representation of visual function within the two major visual pathways or interactions between the two pathways.

The patterns of dissociation of visual function observed with lesions of the dorsal and ventral visual association cortex further suggest that each of these major divisions has functional subdivisions. For instance, the dorsolateral visual association cortex may separately process several different types of motion, including first-order, second-order, and attention-generated apparent motion (27,28). Similarly, there may also be separate processing of shape-from-color as opposed to color sensation in the ventral pathways (29). There also appears to be significant separation for determining the distance of objects as opposed to their direction with respect to visually guided reaching (30,31), for pointing to as opposed to grasping of visual objects (32), and for perception of visual objects versus action upon them (33).

Explaining visual phenomena in human subjects on the basis of a neural substrate requires caution. There is a natural tendency to formalize the relationship of perceptual states to physiologic states (34). Blake (35) emphasized that as we learn more about the neural organization of the visual system, it becomes increasingly tempting to assign particular visual functions to particular stages. This issue can be addressed by using proper tests in a precise manner, such that the characteristics of the input stimulus are precisely defined (by mathematical techniques and physical measurements) and the perceptual and behavioral outputs are properly recorded (36). In this way, we can make inferences on the intervening stages of vision in normal healthy observers (37), and these strategies can also be applied in patients with focal brain lesions to obtain information on the anatomic constraints for different processing stages (35). Lesions of the visual cortex produce relative dissociations of function, such as color versus motion, that reveal the independence of certain perceptual properties. Thus, we are able to examine how certain types of information are condensed or dispersed, and which stages of visual processing precede others (35). This can contribute to a flow diagram of perceptual processing with potential cross-referencing with human neuroanatomy at the level of MR imaging analyses. Unique evidence from human lesion studies of vision can also be complemented by functional imaging (38–44) and by anatomic studies (45,46).

Behavior studies in patients with brain damage provide much of the critical data that underlie our understanding of vision. It is therefore important to understand the perspective and limitations of these studies, including the nature of the information they provide and the factors that affect their interpretation. Some patients with brain lesions can make sophisticated judgments on a wide variety of psychophysical procedures and can say what they see, allowing comparisons of their behavior with descriptions of their actual visual experience, thus motivating further inquiries (47). Other patients, however, cannot describe their perceptual experience because of an acquired damage in language processing areas of the left hemisphere, or because they may not be aware of their perceptual defect and therefore do not report it, a condition known as anosognosia (48–50). Alternatively, patients with cerebral lesions may have evidence of residual visual perception, even though they deny the existence of such perception (51,52), a phenomenon particularly well illustrated by "blindsight" (53–56).

BLINDSIGHT AND RESIDUAL VISION

Patients with visual loss due to lesions of the striate cortex or optic radiations may have some remnant visual function in their "blind" field. Some of these patients, including the often-studied patient G.Y. (Fig. 13.2), retain some awareness of visual stimuli and hence have residual vision (57–59), implying a severe field defect that is relative, not absolute. Others deny awareness of stimuli, even though they perform better than chance when asked to indicate or guess at some property of the stimulus: these are said to possess blindsight (53,60–63). Whether residual vision differs in pathophysiology from blindsight is unclear. For one, perceptual awareness varies along a spectrum: patients may retain a vague awareness of the presence of a stimulus, particularly of rapid onset or offset, but not of its particular features, which they can nonetheless discriminate or act upon (64). Also, stimulus parameters can be manipulated so that a patient shows resid-

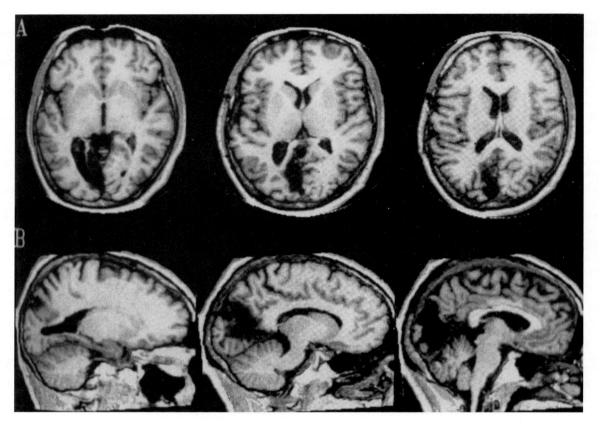

Figure 13.2. Magnetic resonance imaging of the lesion of patient G.Y., with residual vision. Axial (*A*) and sagittal (*B*) images of the left hemisphere, both T1-weighted, showing destruction of medial occipital cortex and the underlying optic radiation, from a lesion suffered at age 7 in a car accident. (From Barbur JL, Watson JD, Frackowiak RS, et al. Conscious visual perception without V1. Brain 1993;116 [Pt 6]:1293–1302.)

ual vision under some conditions and blindsight under others (65,66). Similar stimulus manipulations can degrade awareness and generate blindsight-like performance in normal subjects (67–69).

Philosophers have become interested in blindsight as a window into understanding vision and perceptual consciousness (70,71). Blindsight also fuels debates about the anatomic substrate of consciousness. In both monkey and human studies, some investigators conclude that conscious visual perception requires striate cortex (72–74), at odds with claims that hemispherectomized patients can retain awareness in the blind hemifield (75). Yet others have concluded that the decreased visual awareness in G.Y. reflects a defect in attention rather than vision, similar to syndromes of neglect and simultaneous extinction (64).

VARIETIES OF BLINDSIGHT PHENOMENA

Localization of Targets

Given expectations that the spatial functions of the superior colliculus would be most likely to persist after cerebral lesions, the first demonstration of blindsight asked whether patients could direct saccades to target locations within hemianopic fields (76). There was a weak correlation of saccadic size and target position, mainly for a limited range of paracentral locations, as also noted in subsequent reports too (60,77,78) (Fig. 13.3). In some cases, localization occurred in regions that later recovered on perimetry (53). Also, several studies have failed to find saccadic localization in the absence of awareness (79–81). Targets in blind hemifields also have been localized by hand reaching and pointing. In some studies manual localization is weak and variable, sometimes only in patients with residual vision (59,82,83), but there are other reports of nearly normal manual localization (64,78).

Motion

Many have speculated that target localization is easier with moving or oscillating rather than stationary targets (57,76,78,83), a claim supported by some reports (84,85) but not another (75). This is reminiscent of Riddoch's phenomenon (14), in which movement is appreciated before static targets in recovering hemianopic defects (14). Regarding perception of motion attributes, patient G.Y. could discriminate the speed and direction of rapid bright spots (57,59,86). With larger stimuli such as optokinetic gratings, some patients can discriminate motion direction (87), and a

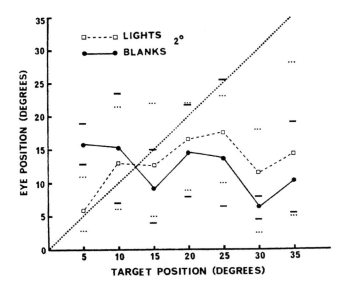

Figure 13.3. Saccadic localization in hemianopia (patient D.B.). Mean horizontal eye position plotted against target position, for trials with lights (n = 5 at each point) and control trials with no lights (in which case the meaning of target position is unclear from the study). *Bars* indicate range of values for each measure. Much of the correlation appears to rely upon the results for the 5-degree target. *Dotted line* shows position of ideal saccadic accuracy. (From Weiskrantz L, Warrington EK, Sanders MD, et al. Visual capacity in the hemianopic field following a restricted occipital ablation. Brain 1974;97:709–728.)

few experience an illusion of self-motion (88). One patient with bilateral lesions was said to differentiate between expanding and contracting patterns of optic flow, but his answers suggested that scatter into his remaining island of vision could not be excluded (89). Some of the reports of motion detection may actually represent information secondarily derived from spatial position or the detection of flicker rather than true motion perception. Studies using random dot stimuli that minimize such positional information and equilibrate flicker found no residual motion perception in 13 patients, including G.Y. (90,91).

Motion information might also guide eye movements. Recovery of optokinetic responses was reported in one patient with cortical blindness (92) but not in two others (83,93) nor in three hemianopic patients (87). Pursuit and saccadic responses to motion were not found in patients with medial occipital lesions sparing the lateral human motion area (80).

Form, Color, and Contrast

An early report claimed that patient D.B. could normally discriminate large X and O stimuli, perhaps through orientation perception (53,78). However, form discrimination was not found in seven other patients (59,77,89) nor orientation discrimination in two others, including G.Y. (94,95). Thus, these patients cannot use verbal responses to indicate residual form perception. Despite this, G.Y. and two other patients could arrange the orientation, shape, and size of their grasp correctly when they reached for objects in their blind

field (64,94,96). This may be consistent with evidence for a dissociation between pathways for object recognition and action (97).

While early studies found no evidence of chromatic perception (59,78), later studies showed detection of colored targets by 6 of 10 patients (98) and evidence of color-opponent interactions in the spectral sensitivity curves in three others (99). Studies of G.Y.'s residual vision showed that he could discriminate the motion of equiluminant colored spots (100) and was aware of hue, although these latter responses seem to represent an average from the entire blind hemifield (101). G.Y. could match and discriminate the color and motion of stimuli but could not compare the brightness of stimuli between his blind and seeing fields (86). The authors suggested that the impairment in perceiving the brightness dimension of color space was the critical factor causing his degraded awareness in the blind hemifield.

Studies of temporal and spatial contrast sensitivity have yielded mixed results, even when done on the same patient G.Y. (102–104). The investigators argued that stimulus parameters such as size and duration are critical.

Interactions between Blind and Normal Hemifields

Traditional blindsight methods are awkward in that they ask a patient to respond to something he or she cannot see. However, a number of innovative studies have circumvented this by examining how responses to visible stimuli might be modified by stimuli in the blind field.

Spatial summation occurs when two simultaneous stimuli generate faster responses than a single stimulus; temporal summation is the decrease in reaction time when a stimulus is preceded by another that provides a temporal prompt. Evidence for summation between seeing and blind fields has been inconsistent and found in only a minority of subjects (82,105,106), including G.Y. (107). The opposite, a distraction effect, in which targets in the blind field slow down response times to stimuli in the seeing field, has been shown for saccades but not manual reaction times (108). This finding could not be replicated in another study of six hemianopic patients (109), although it was found in a report on hemianopic monkeys (110). "Inhibition of return" is a normal phenomenon in which a stimulus delays the detection of a target appearing in the same location a short time later. Taking advantage of the fact that the effect is coded for position in external space rather than retinal position, one study of a hemianopic patient showed that a light flashed at a spot in the blind field delayed responses to a later target in the same spatial (not retinotopic) location, after a saccade had placed that location in the seeing field (111). From monkey physiology, the authors argued that this was mediated by the superior colliculus.

Evidence for form and letter perception using traditional methods has been mixed. One study of two patients showed that word perception in blindsight could be shown not by traditional methods but by an indirect strategy in which the choice of meaning of an ambiguous word (e.g., LIGHT) in the seeing field was influenced by a word in the blind field (e.g., DARK versus HEAVY) (64). Completion effects have been reported for form perception. Three patients could dis-

Stimulus conditions (s)

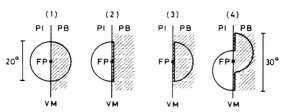

Figure 13.4. An experiment of figure completion in blindsight. With circular stimuli of radius 10 degrees centered between their seeing and blind hemifields (*shaded area*), subjects had to draw what they saw in the top row, with examples shown in the bottom row. Despite hemianopia, subjects perceived the whole circle as complete and different from the half-circle but did not tend to complete the half-displaced circle on the right. However, all subjects had macular sparing hemianopia and so would have perceived some of the right half of the stimuli, allowing a distinction between circles and half-circles. The placement of the half-displaced circle is such that the left half-circle is lower than that of the left sides of the other stimuli, affording another clue. PI, perimetrically intact area; PB, perimetrically blind area; VM, vertical meridian; FP, fixation point. (From Torjussen T. Visual processing in cortically blind hemifields. Neuropsychologia 1978; 16:15–21.)

criminate circles from semicircles when the critical half was in the hemianopic field, but the macular sparing of their hemianopia complicates the interpretation of this result (112) (Fig. 13.4). More recently two patients had completion effects with awareness for afterimages that were symmetric across the midline or with illusory contours such as the Kanisza triangle, despite the fact that they had no awareness or ability with stimuli restricted to the blind field (64). On a related note, the width of G.Y.'s grasp varied with object size only when the left-most part of the object fell in his seeing hemifield (96). Yet another study used an interference task with a stimulus flanked by distractors either different from or identical to the stimulus. Reaction times to seen letters and colors were prolonged by differing flankers

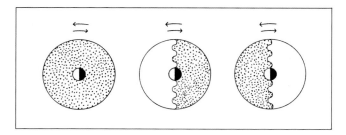

Figure 13.5. Display used to examine tilt induced by rotating motion. The dotted background rotates either clockwise or counterclockwise (*arrows*), while the patient rotates the black-and-white disc in the center to align the line marking the border between black and white with his or her perceived sense of vertical. The half-dotted backgrounds are used to examine hemifield responses. Although the curving boundaries exclude local cues to the true vertical, cues are still available from the overall configuration. (From Pizzamiglio L, Antonucci G, Francia A. Response of the cortically blind hemifields to a moving visual scene. Cortex 1984;20:89–99.)

placed in the blind field in a patient with an occipital lesion, but not in another with a lesion of the thalamus and optic radiations (113).

One study examined whether rotating motion in a blind field could tilt the patient's sense of the vertical (114). Stimulation of both fields induced more tilt in judgments of the vertical than stimulating the seeing hemifield alone, and some tilt was also induced by stimulating the blind hemifield. However, inadvertent cues to the true vertical were likely present in their half-field stimuli (Fig. 13.5). Another study tested whether perception of optic flow in a noise-filled pattern within the intact hemifield could be enhanced by optic flow in the blind hemifield: this could be shown in two patients with very limited damage to striate cortex (106) (Fig. 13.6). These subjects could not accurately guess the direction of motion when there was no stimulus in the intact field.

Pupillary Responses

The pupillary light reflex is preserved in cerebral lesions, since the afferent pathway leaves the optic tract to synapse in the pretectal nuclei of the midbrain. This light reflex primarily responds to overall luminance. However, responses to gratings and isoluminant colors also occur. While there is evidence that pupillary responses are modulated by cortical activity, it is unclear whether cortex is critical for responses to stimuli lacking a net flux in luminance (115). Nevertheless, pupillary responses to such stimuli in the blind hemifield have been shown in G.Y., with or without awareness (116,117). In another study, color stimuli caused afterimages that evoked pupillary responses in normal subjects; in the blind hemifield of two patients, including G.Y., there were "after" pupillary responses without any conscious afterimage (115).

Affective (Fear) Responses to Unseen Stimuli

Studies in normal subjects suggest that there may be a direct pathway between the pulvinar and the amygdala mediating emotional reactions to frightening stimuli, even when those stimuli are not consciously recognized (118). Studies of G.Y. suggest that he could process fearful and angry faces in his blind hemifield (119), and this may correlate with activity in his amygdala (120). Another study of a cortically blind patient showed that associating a neutral visual stimulus with a painful shock caused the development of startle reflexes to that stimulus, indicating that the subject could learn a fear reaction to an object that was not consciously perceived (121).

BLINDSIGHT AND HEMIDECORTICATION

Patients lacking a cerebral hemisphere are of obvious interest in the debate over the role of extrastriate cortex in blindsight functions. Visual localization studies in blindsight (76) were motivated by the hypothesis that the superior colliculus could mediate this function in the absence of striate cortex. Indeed, some have found that hemidecorticate infants will look toward their blind field when a target is presented

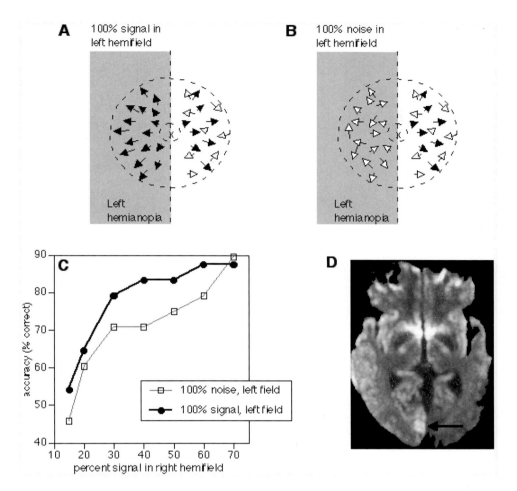

Figure 13.6. Interactions between blind and seeing hemifields in motion perception. Subjects with a discrete occipital lesion (*arrow* in *D*) are shown displays with optic flow patterns: expanding or contracting patterns of moving dots that give the impression of moving forward or backward in space. In their good hemifield they see a mixture of random noise motion and signal dots that have this motion. The ratio of this mixture is varied to give a range of performance in accuracy. The subject must guess whether they are moving forward or backward from these dots. At the same time, in the blind left hemifield, there is either a strong 100% signal pattern (*A*) or a meaningless 100% noise pattern (*B*). *C,* Accuracy of responses for different mixtures of signal and noise in the seeing hemifield. At all levels of signal/noise ratio, accuracy on the task performed with the stimuli in the good hemifield is enhanced when the blind hemifield contains a strong 100% motion signal.

there (122), and adults with such lesions have some residual manual localization of blind field targets (75,84), as well as a surprising awareness of these targets. Beyond localization, discrimination of motion and speed, but not direction, was reported in three patients, but the results could be explained by response bias (75). Some elementary form perception was reported in 3 of 10 patients (84,123). A "spatial summation" effect, in which normal subjects respond faster to two simultaneous flashes of light than to one, was found in two of four patients, even when one of the twin flashes was in the blind hemifield (124). A functional MR imaging (fMRI) study of these same patients suggested that blindsight may not be mediated solely by the superior colliculus, but also by activity in the ipsilateral V5 area (125). Similar ipsilateral extrastriate activity was found in a positron emission tomography (PET) study of another patient (126).

The validity of these findings is in question. Several recent studies have shown that the residual vision in hemispherectomized patients can be attributed to light scatter (127–130), despite the fact that some of the same authors have argued elsewhere for blindsight retinotectal function in hemispherectomized monkeys (131). Another study of two patients found that residual vision with preserved awareness was present in only a thin 3° strip near the vertical meridian, due to scatter or possibly receptive fields overlapping from one hemiretina to the other (132): no true blindsight was found.

ARTIFACT AND BLINDSIGHT

The importance of blindsight lies in the potential insights it provides about the anatomy of vision and conscious experience. However, such conclusions depend critically on the exclusion of more trivial explanations of blindsight-like performance. At least four issues need to be considered in evaluating any blindsight report:

1. A stimulus directed at a blind hemifield is actually stimulating the other (seeing) hemifield because of poor fixation. Inadvertent shifts of fixation can occur, especially if stimuli are not randomly located and last more than 150 ms, providing enough time for a saccade to be made. Eye position monitors can help but may be falsely reassuring (Fig. 13.7). Many techniques, such as electro-oculograms or infrared devices, reference eye position to the head, not to space. Because of this, a combined movement of the head and eyes can shift gaze into the blind field without being detected by the monitor. Thus, these head-referenced techniques are inadequate without rigorous head stabilization (133). A space-referenced system, such as the magnetic search coil technique, is better.
2. A stimulus directed at a blind hemifield is inadvertently stimulating the seeing hemifield because of light scatter.

Many early studies claimed that blindsight performance required very bright targets on a dark background. This is precisely the circumstance when light scatter is most problematic. Indeed, numerous studies have shown that light scatter can mimic or explain blindsight (80,127–129,134). Controlling for scatter is difficult and must take into account two potential sources of scatter, that on the screen and that within the eye. Physical measures of scatter on the screen are inadequate, as the eye is more sensitive than electronic equipment (80). As a physiologic control some have tried to show that similar blindsight performance could not be obtained with stimuli projected onto the normal blind spot (53). One strategy that can potentially control for both screen and intraocular scatter is to use patients with pregeniculate lesions as controls (76,77,84). Similarly, those who believe that extrastriate cortex is essential for blindsight also use control patients with thalamic lesions (113) or hemispherectomies (87,129). Flooding of the seeing field with light has also been used to minimize scatter.

3. The blind hemifield is not completely blind. Careful per-

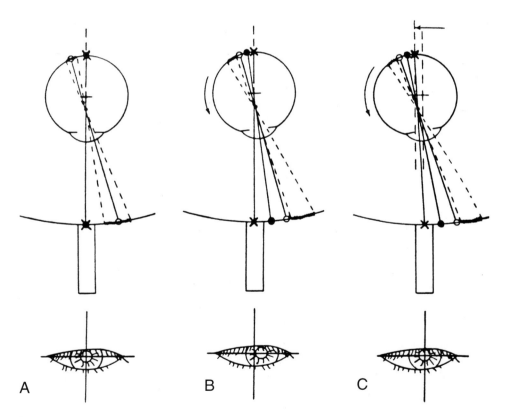

Figure 13.7. Problems with eye-head stabilization in perimetry. *A*, The subject fixates accurately on the fixation spot *X*, while a peripheral target (*white circle*) falls within the boundary of his left scotoma (*dashed lines*). The eye appears centered in the perimetric eye position monitor, as shown below. *B*, The subject fixates off to the left (*black circle*), rather than at the fixation spot X, and the target no longer falls within the scotoma. Thus, it is now visible. This off-fixation is detected by the eye position monitor below. *C*, If, however, the head is also shifted slightly laterally to the right (*straight arrows*), the eye appears to be centered in the monitor, although the patient is fixating off-center. This strategy could be used by patients who appear to have improving field defects. (From Balliet R, Blood KM, Bach-y-Rita P. Visual field rehabilitation in the cortically blind? J Neurol Neurosurg Psychiatry 1985;48:1113–1124.)

imetry may reveal surviving islands of vision that account for the residual perception (135–138). The demonstration that patients with optic neuropathy can exhibit blindsight-like abilities is also consistent with the suggestion that blindsight is based on residual function in the normal geniculostriate pathway (139). Some claim to exclude this hypothesis of surviving striate activation by means of fMRI (140). However, fMRI detects only small percentage changes in MRI signal even with strong stimulation, and its analysis uses arbitrary statistical thresholds to indicate activation. Its methodology is not designed for or capable of excluding weak residual activation in cortex.

4. Blindsight may simply represent a criterion shift. Subjects may reply more conservatively in detection tasks than when asked to choose between alternatives (134). Indeed, normal subjects show criterion shift with very brief stimuli (67,68,134), although this was not replicated recently (69,141). Signal detection analysis has been used to answer this criticism by calculating a measure of true sensitivity independent of the response criterion (98, 142,143). In G.Y., these have shown that shifts in criterion may explain some of his test results with motion perception but not his blindsight performance with static targets (144).

EXPLANATIONS OF BLINDSIGHT

Once these objections are met, one can turn to consideration of the anatomic origins of blindsight. The most common explanation invokes alternative visual pathways. A purely subcortical pathway from retina to superior colliculus may explain a function like spatial localization (76,132). It is claimed that better blindsight in the temporal than nasal hemifield of patients is a signature of collicular mediation (108,145). Other functions like pattern or motion detection may require extrastriate cortex, through a relay involving the superior colliculus and pulvinar. Since the colliculus lacks responses to color opponency, chromatic blindsight (98, 99,101,113,125,140) may indicate yet another relay, perhaps direct projections to extrastriate cortex from surviving lateral geniculate neurons (56) (Fig. 13.8).

The monkey evidence most strongly supports the retino-tecto-pulvinar relay to extrastriate regions, particularly those involved in motion perception. Lesions of V1 do not abolish responses in V5 (146–148) or V3A (149) unless accompanied by lesions of the superior colliculus (146,150). On the other hand, there is no evidence yet of remnant neuronal responses in regions of the monkey's ventral stream (149–151), at odds with the demonstrations of residual color and form perception in humans and in some monkeys (152). Stabilization of an early direct projection from LGN to V5, which normally regresses with development, may occur in infant cats with striate lesions (153), but evidence of this has not been found in infant monkeys (154).

Physiologic techniques in humans have also provided some support. In normal subjects, evoked potentials (155) and some transcranial magnetic stimulation studies (156) but not others (157) suggest that visual motion signals may arrive in V5 before and independent of V1. PET scans (58), magnetoencephalography (158), and evoked responses (159) have shown residual activation of V5 by rapid but not slow-

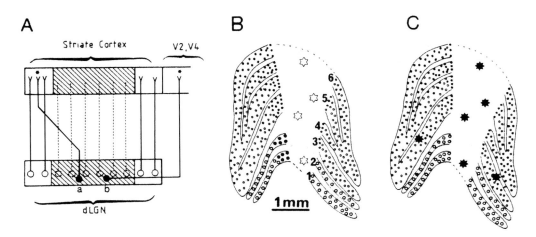

Figure 13.8. A geniculo-extrastriate hypothesis for blindsight. *A*, Neurons in the dorsal lateral geniculate nucleus (dLGN) normally project point to point to striate cortex, maintaining a strict topography. However, some neurons (black cell bodies) may project anomalously, either to neighboring striate areas (neuron a) or to extrastriate areas, such as areas V2 and V4 (neuron b), and either could survive after a restricted striate lesion (*shaded area*). These hypotheses were tested in a monkey with a long-standing partial striate lesion. *B*, After injection of the retrograde marker horseradish peroxidase (HRP) into adjacent striate cortex, label is present in appropriate parvocellular and magnocellular areas (*black dots*) adjacent to the region of the dLGN corresponding to the striate lesion but not in the scattered remnant neurons within the degenerated region (*white stars*). *C*, After injection of HRP into area V4, label is present not only in these remnants but also in scattered neurons throughout the dLGN, indicating the presence of a direct geniculo-extrastriate pathway. (From Cowey A, Stoerig P. The neurobiology of blindsight. Trends Neurosci 1991;14:140–145.)

moving stimuli in the blind hemifield in G.Y. In one of three patients with hemispherectomies, fMRI reportedly showed that moving stimuli activated V5 and V3A but not V1 in the remaining ipsilateral hemisphere (125). An intriguing fMRI study of G.Y. that varied stimuli to obtain responses with and without awareness showed that residual vision was associated with activation of extrastriate visual areas and dorsolateral prefrontal cortex, and blindsight was associated with activation in superior colliculus and medial prefrontal cortex (65).

One of the most important observations that any theory of blindsight must explain is its variability. Not all hemianopic patients have blindsight or residual vision; in fact, recent large studies, representing 46 patients in total, suggest that it is rare (90,136,137). One important variable may be how much the lesion extends beyond striate cortex to the optic radiations and extrastriate cortex. The pattern of extrastriate damage may also determine the type of blindsight found (53,160). However, correlations between abilities and lesion anatomy have proven elusive (79,80,90,105,161). A requirement for very focal striate damage is also difficult to distinguish from a need for partial striate damage (106), leading us back to a potential artifactual explanation.

Another important variable may be the timing of the lesion. Blindsight may require neural plasticity. If so, age at onset, time since lesion, and possibly training may be important—of note, G.Y. sustained his lesion at age 8 and has had extensive practice over many years (61). Infants or children may be more likely to develop blindsight or residual vision in both nonhuman primates (162) and man (59, 84,153), though not all studies find that age matters (123).

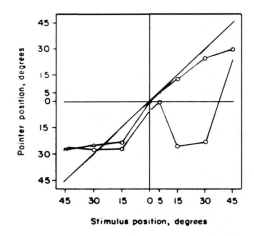

Figure 13.9. Learning of blindsight pointing. Median pointer position versus target position in the first trial block (*circles*) and after 205 trials (*diamonds*). The patient had bilateral occipital lesions and bilateral hemianopia, leaving only a small spared hemicentral island of vision from 0 to 9 degrees in the right field. The patient locates targets in his right hemifield better with training. The *diagonal solid line* shows position of perfect accuracy. (From Bridgeman B, Staggs D. Plasticity in human blindsight. Vision Res 1982;22:1199–1203.)

Though some deny that training helps (59,133), others claim that practice improves blindsight saccadic or manual localization (85,161,163–165) (Fig. 13.9). There are even claims that training may expand visual fields (166,167), a finding in need of verification.

CEREBRAL ACHROMATOPSIA

SYMPTOMS, ANATOMY, AND PATHOLOGY

Deficits in color perception after cerebral lesions have been described for over a hundred years (6,168–172). Achromatopsic patients are always symptomatic, complaining that the world appears in shades of gray, like a black-and-white movie (24,172–174). Some also feel that the world appears less bright (24) or has a "dirty gray" tinge (175). Less frequently, patients note abnormal color to their vision. Some find the world tinged with a hue, as if peering through a colored filter (171). Others see illusions of the residual colors perceived spreading beyond the boundaries of the objects from which they emanate, a type of visual perseveration (172). These positive color phenomena may occur transiently as the syndrome evolves after the acute lesion. For achromatopsic patients, daily activities that use color discrimination are impaired, such as distinguishing coins, stamps, or traffic lights; a good account of the experience of an achromatopsic artist exists (176).

Achromatopsia is seldom an isolated finding. Most commonly it forms one component of a tetrad that includes superior quadrantanopia, prosopagnosia, and topographagnosia. Superior quadrantanopia is almost always present, either bilaterally or unilaterally with complete hemianopia in the other hemifield, as the ventral occipitotemporal lesion that causes achromatopsia frequently extends into either the inferior calcarine cortex or the inferior optic radiation. Similarly, only a few cases without prosopagnosia have been reported (177). Topographagnosia is usually revealed by the patient becoming lost in familiar surroundings (172,178–180).

Other types of visual object agnosia can also occur (178,179). Achromatopsic patients with right homonymous hemianopias may have alexia without agraphia (172,177). If the lesions extend into more ventral temporal lobes bilaterally, there may also be associated amnesia (172,178). Experimental testing has revealed in some patients a problem with detecting stimuli with low salience (181), which has also been described in monkeys with V4 lesions and is thought to indicate inefficient attentional allocation in form processing.

Achromatopsia is caused by lesions of the lingual and fusiform gyri, in the ventromedial aspect of the occipital lobe (6,22), as confirmed by modern imaging (24,175,177, 179,180,182). Lesions of the middle third of the lingual gyrus or the white matter behind the posterior tip of the lateral ventricle are said to be critical (24,183). Bilateral lesions are necessary for complete achromatopsia (Fig. 13.10); unilateral right or left occipital lesions may produce a contralateral hemiachromatopsia.

Since achromatopsia requires bilateral occipital lesions, it is most often due to cerebrovascular disease. Bilateral se-

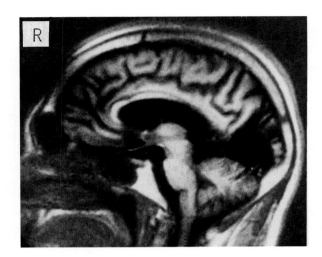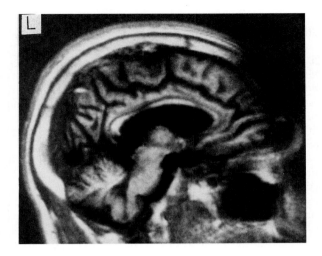

Figure 13.10. Magnetic resonance imaging in a patient with cerebral dyschromatopsia. Nonenhanced sagittal T1-weighted images show bilateral lesions in the visual cortices. The lesion of the right hemisphere (R) is responsible for the left homonymous hemianopia. The lesion of the left hemisphere (L) is located below the calcarine fissure in the inferior visual association cortex in regions thought to process color. (From Rizzo M, Nawrot M, Blake R, et al. A human visual disorder resembling area V4 dysfunction in the monkey. Neurology 1992;42:1175–1180.)

quential or simultaneous infarctions in the territories of both posterior cerebral arteries are not uncommon, given their shared origin from the basilar artery; multiple infarcts can also occur with coagulopathies (184). With occipital strokes, achromatopsia may be the initial symptom, or an initial cortical blindness may resolve into achromatopsia. Other bilateral lesions causing achromatopsia include herpes simplex encephalitis (179), cerebral metastases (177), repeated focal seizures (185), focal dementia (186), and even migraine aura, causing a transient achromatopsia (187). Subcortical temporo-occipital white matter damage (188) caused a reversible dyschromatopsia in one patient with carbon monoxide poisoning, a condition that usually causes an apperceptive agnosia with relative sparing of color perception (22).

Achromatopsia in the contralateral hemifield alone (hemiachromatopsia) can follow unilateral lesions in either the right or left occipital lobes. In contrast to complete achromatopsia, patients are typically asymptomatic until the defect is demonstrated on a visual examination (189,190), with one exception (175). Likewise, patients with complete achromatopsia after sequential bilateral lesions presumably have hemiachromatopsia after their first lesion but do not complain until their second lesion renders them achromatopsic in both hemifields (177,182). Hemiachromatopsia is usually associated with a superior quadrantanopia (175, 189,190); therefore, the color defect is demonstrable only in the remaining inferior quadrant. The preserved color vision in the ipsilateral hemifield allows normal or near-normal performance on centrally viewed tests of color vision such as pseudo-isochromatic plates and color-sorting tasks. Rather, the examiner must ask the patient to name or sort colors presented in the peripheral visual field. The incidence of hemiachromatopsia is probably underestimated, given its asymptomatic nature and the failure of routine clinical color tests to detect its presence.

Two rare cases with quadrantic field defects for color have also been described (191). However, as these quadrantic color defects evolved from more typical quadrantic defects for white lights, which in turn had evolved from initial hemianopias, it is not clear if these were true chromatic defects or subtle relative scotomata, particularly as color detection rather than color discrimination was tested. Nevertheless, the quadrantic retinotopic representation of the human V4 area on functional imaging (192) suggests that a very discrete lesion could theoretically create such a defect.

TESTING ACHROMATOPSIC PATIENTS

Color naming is not an adequate test for cerebral dyschromatopsia, since residual color perception may allow an approximate categorization of colors despite inability to make fine judgments about hue and saturation (Fig. 13.11); on the other hand, patients with color anomia may have intact color perception. Achromatopsia may be detected with pseudo-isochromatic plates, but some patients can achieve normal scores, especially if the plates are shown at a distance sufficient to obscure the resolution of the individual dots (172,179,180,193).

Color sorting or matching tests provide the best evidence of impaired color perception. Typical sorting tests include the Farnsworth-Munsell 100-Hue Test (Fig. 13.12), and the shorter items of Farnsworth D-15 (Fig. 13.13) and the Lanthony New Color Test, which test hue discrimination, and the Sahlgren Saturation Test, which measures saturation discrimination (194). Patients with cerebral achromatopsia are impaired on both hue and saturation tests (179,180,195). The abnormality affects all hue perceptions diffusely, unlike that of congenital color blindness, although the magnitude of the defect along red–green and blue–yellow axes may vary relatively (24). The degree of achromatopsia can vary be-

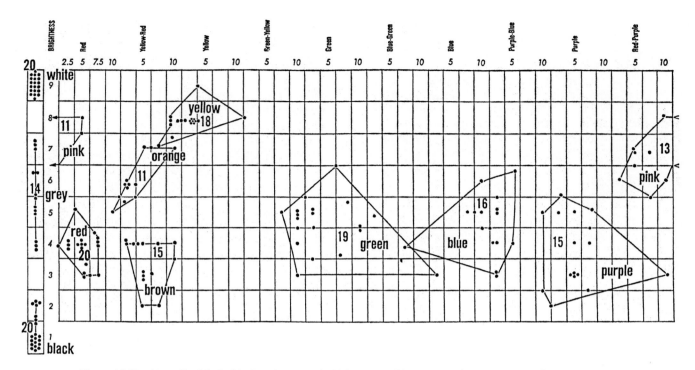

Figure 13.11. Normalized foci of basic color names in 20 languages. The numbers along the borders of the chart refer to the Munsell system of color notation. The numbers in the body of the chart refer to the number of languages in the sample of 20 that encode the corresponding color category. (From Berlin B, Kay P. Basic Color Terms; Their Universality and Evolution. Berkeley, University of California Press, 1969.)

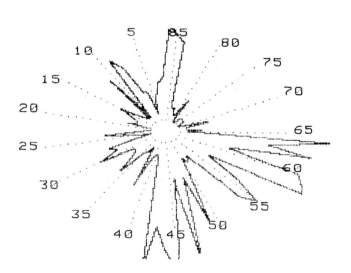

Figure 13.12. Results of Farnsworth-Munsell 100-Hue Test in the same subject as in Figure 13.10. The results are abnormal. The error score of 492 derived a major component from rack 3, which tests blue–green discrimination.

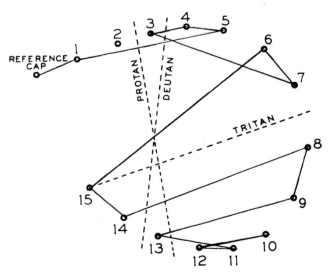

Figure 13.13. Plot of the Farnsworth D-15 test results in the same patient with cerebral dyschromatopsia discussed in Figures 13.10 and 13.12. The results are abnormal, showing an axis consistent with a tritan (blue–yellow) defect.

tween patients from complete to partial defects. Functional imaging studies suggest that this may depend on the extent of damage to not just one but a number of color-processing regions in occipitotemporal cortex (196).

In contrast, perception of brightness, the third (achromatic) dimension, tends to be normal (24,180,195). Because of this, care is required with matching tests to ensure that there are no inadvertent clues from differences in brightness, which these patients can perceive. Matching tests that use reflected colors are particularly vulnerable to this contamination. Colors should either vary randomly in brightness or have equal brightness (isoluminance), which requires attention to the illumination being used.

Since most patients view these tests with the fovea, patients with hemiachromatopsia often score normally (24). Clinical color-matching tasks can be used in the peripheral field but are cumbersome and require monitoring of eye movements.

NORMAL COLOR PERCEPTION

The perceptions of light by normal human observers can be characterized using a three-dimensional "color space." The three axes of this space are an achromatic dimension and two chromatic axes, which can be related to the activity of the three retinal cones. Relative differences in the activity of the three retinal cones give rise to chromatic differences. Thus, along the deutan chromatic axis, the activity of the S-cone (maximally sensitive for *S*hort wavelength light) remains constant, but the activity of the M-cone (*M*edium wavelength) changes with respect to that of the L-cone (*L*ong wavelength). Along the tritan axis, the ratio of M-cone to L-cone activity remains constant, but S-cone activity varies relative to the sum of M- and L-cone activity. Variations along these two chromatic dimensions cause differences in hue, which is related to the perceived dominant wavelength (i.e., red, yellow, blue), and differences in saturation, which is related to the purity of the spectral composition, with paler, less saturated shades representing greater mixture of white light with the dominant hue (e.g., pink, rose, red). Differences in brightness ("luminance" for light sources, "reflectance" for objects that reflect light) occur when light changes along the third dimension, the achromatic axis. Along this axis, the activity of all three cones changes together, such that the ratio of one cone's activity relative to another remains constant. Conventional color diagrams such as the CIE (Committee Internationale de l'Eclairage) chart depict the colors within a plane of the two chromatic dimensions, while omitting brightness. The CIE chart is a roughly polar diagram with hue represented by the angle of the vector from the central point representing white (equal mixture of all hues) and saturation represented by the vector length.

No single cone is able to distinguish the wavelength of the light it receives. This is because the firing rate of a cone is determined by both the intensity and the spectral composition of light. Increased firing may indicate either a more intense light or a change to a wavelength to which the cone is more sensitive. Wavelength selectivity requires a comparison between the responses of cones with maximal sensitivi-

ties in different regions of the light spectrum: this opponent process first occurs in retinal ganglion cells, where one comparison is between M-cone and L-cone activity and another is between S-cone and combined M- and L-cone activity. Hence these aspects of retinal physiology account for both trichromacy, due to the existence of the three different cones, and also for the two axes of wavelength opponency, due to comparisons occurring at the level of the retinal ganglion cells.

Wavelength perception is not the same as color perception, however. Color is a property of the appearance of surfaces and is not inherent in objects (197). Since most objects we see are not light sources themselves but are surfaces that reflect light, the wavelengths that they transmit to our eyes are determined by both the reflectant properties of the object and the illuminating light in the scene (198). When the illuminant changes, so too does the wavelength composition that reaches our eye from the object. Nevertheless, the perceived colors of objects are remarkably stable under different lighting conditions, a phenomenon known as "color constancy." Therefore, wavelength composition alone cannot determine perceived color (199). Rather, it is the relative proportion of received light at each wavelength reflected by the object that determines color. To determine proportion one needs to know the spectral composition of the illuminating light source, but this information is often not directly available.

To some degree, color constancy may be possible for simple stimuli by using low-level processes such as chromatic adaptation, local cone ratios (200), and the color opponency of retinal ganglion receptive fields. However, for complex scenes, the nervous system attempts an indirect estimate of the illumination. This may involve averaging the spectral luminance across large regions of the scene, deducing what kind of lighting is present, and then "discounting the illuminant" from the wavelengths reflected by a given object (199,201). This generates color as a stable property of objects, over a fairly wide range of natural illumination.

COLOR CONSTANCY AND ACHROMATOPSIA

A defect in color constancy should result in color percepts that vary with changes in illumination. Patients with achromatopsia have a more severe deficit in that they lack any color percept at all. Testing such patients for constancy of something they do not perceive is paradoxical; however, this can be done on dyschromatopsic patients, who have some residual hue sensitivity. One such patient was reported to have impaired color constancy (202). Three patients, two of whom had transient symptoms of achromatopsia, and all with subtle color-matching problems at the time of testing, had abnormal shifts of color matches when lighting was changed (203). Despite possessing some local color constancy based upon cone contrasts, one patient had impaired constancy for complex scenes, indicating abnormal global constancy mechanisms (200). Another shifted his color naming to black with increasing background luminance (204); this indicated that his naming depended heavily on relative luminance, representing a failure of "lightness" (rather than hue) constancy. All of these reports included patients with some dyschromatopsia and bilateral lingual and fusiform gyral lesions, except for one unilateral case (203). However, a report of a large series of 27 patients found 5 subjects with impaired color constancy on matching tasks, all asymptomatic, who did not have dyschromatopsia, and who had right or left lateral parietotemporal lesions (205). The authors argued that this was evidence of a larger network of cortical regions beyond the lingual/fusiform region that participated in generating color constancy.

TRICHROMACY, COLOR OPPONENCY, AND IMAGERY IN ACHROMATOPSIA

Not all color perception is lost in achromatopsia. Several methods have established that some aspects of color processing derived from the function of the cones and retinal ganglion cells of the parvocellular pathway can still be discerned in achromatopsic patients. Thus, both trichromacy and color opponency have been shown in photopic spectral sensitivity curves (179,202,206) and evoked potential or psychophysical measures of chromatic contrast sensitivity (206,207). Likewise, performance with anomaloscope testing can resemble an anomalous trichromat rather than a monochromat, despite the personal experience of the world in monochromatic "shades of gray" (182). On the other hand, some impairment in spectral sensitivity curves occurs in some patients, suggesting that there is some extrastriate contribution to chromatic contrast (208).

There is much evidence that achromatopsics can use color-opponent signals to locate chromatic boundaries, even though they cannot perceive the colors that determine those boundaries. In other words, these patients can detect a difference between colors, although they do not know what the colors are and cannot order them correctly by hue. This may account for the ability of some patients to read pseudo-isochromatic plates when they are placed far enough away that the individual dots on the plates are not resolvable (29, 179,180). Similarly, achromatopsics can detect the movement of chromatic stimuli (209,210), even performing at normal levels with suprathreshold chromatic contrast (208). Thus, wavelength variation is still perceived, even if color is not.

Also of interest in achromatopsia is the status of color imagery. This requires careful study, as some stereotyped color associations can be derived from verbal associations (e.g., yellow banana) without requiring visual imagery. There is good evidence that at least two patients with complete achromatopsia have normal imagery for colors (211–213). This contrasts with other patients who can match hues correctly but cannot imagine them or associate colors correctly with objects (214). This double dissociation may be explained by a separate "image buffer" that can be disconnected from either perceptual input about color or color memories (211).

PARALLELS WITH NONHUMAN PRIMATES

Zeki (170) first described color-selective neurons in area V4 of monkey. Wavelength selectivity has since been shown in other regions of macaque extrastriate cortex, including V2 (215,216) and inferotemporal cortex (217,218). Nevertheless, most attention has been focused on the role of V4 in color perception. Several studies suggest that area V4 in monkeys may be the site at which color constancy is generated. Zeki (219) reported that both V1 and V4 contained neurons with wavelength-selective responses, but only V4 had cells with responses that did not vary with the illumination and hence were specific for color rather than wavelength. Schein and Desimone (220) described a possible mechanism by which the illuminant could be discounted: they found that responses of V4 cells to wavelengths in the classical receptive field were suppressed by similar wavelengths in a large surrounding region that could even extend into the ipsilateral hemifield. One lesion study has shown that color constancy is impaired by lesions of V4 (221).

Does achromatopsia result from damage to a human homolog of area V4? This point remains contentious (222). Although defects in color constancy can be demonstrated in at least some achromatopsic patients, these subjects also suffer from a more severe defect of hue discrimination (24,195). In monkeys, lesions of V4 impair hue discrimination only mildly, if at all (221,223–227). Lesions of more anterior areas TE and TEO in inferotemporal cortex do impair hue discrimination, but to a less severe degree than in human achromatopsia (228). Rather, severe and permanent deficits in chromatic discrimination with spared achromatic vision appear to require extensive bilateral lesions of inferotemporal cortex (229). Along with the demonstrations on fMRI of multiple color-processing regions in human occipitotemporal cortex, this suggests that a severe achromatopsic defect may require damage to or disconnection of several components of a color-processing network rather than just a lesion of the human V4 homolog (192,222,225).

FUNCTIONAL IMAGING

A variety of brain-mapping studies support the existence of an extrastriate region specialized for color perception. PET first demonstrated color-selective responses in the lingual and fusiform gyri (42,230). Selective attention to the color of a stimulus increased blood flow in the lingual and fusiform gyri (39). fMRI has shown increased signal with colored stimuli and also during a color after-effect in the posterior fusiform gyri (231). Visual evoked potentials using depth and surface electrodes in epileptic patients have shown that stimuli of changing colors were associated with peaks at 200 to 300 ms in the lateral lingual gyrus and posterior fusiform gyrus (232). Also, stimulating at these sites specifically caused alterations in color perception in some patients (232).

There is considerable controversy over the homology between monkey V4 and the human color area in the posterior fusiform gyri (192,233). Studies have identified two regions in the fusiform gyri. One area adjacent to the V3 area may contain separate topographic maps for the upper and lower contralateral quadrants (234). This may be the human homolog of V4, which in monkey has both a dorsal and ventral component representing the lower and upper fields separately. However, adjacent and more anterior to this region is a second area that contains a nonretinotopic hemifield representation with even stronger color-specific responses. This has been variably named V8 (235) or V4 alpha (236). Experiments suggest that both V4 and V4 alpha are involved in the "ratio-taking" operations that are important in generating color constancy, without which the stable experience of color could not occur (236).

Thus, these studies suggest that color processing is not computed in a single area but in a cortical network. Studies of more complex tasks besides passive viewing of colors have also shown the involvement of additional cortical regions. Active color-sorting tasks are associated with signal changes not only in the fusiform gyri but also in more anterior fusiform areas and the collateral sulci (237). The naming of colors associated with perceived objects activates the fusiform gyrus just ventral to the area activated by color perception (238). Studies of color discrimination have shown activity in the precuneus, superior parietal parahippocampal, superior and lateral occipital gyri, as well as the lingual gyri (239,240). Perception of forms defined by color activates many areas, including the fusiform and lateral occipital gyri bilaterally, left precuneus, intraparietal sulcus, and inferior temporal gyrus (240).

PRESERVED COLOR VISION

Occasionally color discrimination is preserved in patients with other visual perceptual defects, most notably form agnosia (241–244). One of these cases provided evidence for impaired brightness discrimination with relatively preserved hue discrimination (244): in other words, the converse defect in color space to that of achromatopsic patients. A common feature of these reports is carbon monoxide poisoning. Zeki (22) hypothesized that this may reflect a differential toxic or hypoxic vulnerability of the color and form pathways in cortex, although whether this occurs in striate or prestriate cortex is unknown. None of these cases provided anatomic detail; however, a follow-up report of Adler's case with CT and MR imaging many years later showed only occipital atrophy without a focal lesion (245).

COLOR ANOMIA AND AGNOSIA

Some patients cannot recognize or name colors even though they can perceive them. Thus, while patients with achromatopsia cannot discriminate hue and saturation, though some can name some colors, those with color anomia and color agnosia can discriminate colors accurately but not name them. Such patients may not be aware of their deficits. Relevant to this type of defect, PET studies identified regions in the posterior inferior ventral temporal lobe (just anterior to that activated by color perception), parieto-occipital junc-

tion, and left lingual gyrus that were activated by color names (238,246).

Color anomia may occur as part of a more general anomia in aphasic patients or as an isolated entity. Several types of specific color anomia have been described, all occurring with left occipital lesions and often an associated right homonymous hemianopia, rather than the upper quadrant defects of achromatopsia. Apart from the disconnection variety, color-naming deficits are only rarely reported in the literature; however, it is probable that they are also underdiagnosed, as well as being unusual, deficits.

When it accompanies pure alexia and right homonomous hemianopia, color anomia may be part of an interhemispheric visual-verbal disconnection (214,247–249). Disruption of callosal connections in the splenium between the intact right striate cortex and the left angular gyrus prevents accurately perceived colors in the remaining left hemifield from gaining access to language processors. Thus, these subjects cannot read words or name colors that they see accurately in the left hemifield. On the other hand, some but not all of these subjects can name visual objects. Preservation of object naming has given rise to hypotheses that, unlike colors, objects can activate not only visual but also somesthetic representations of object shape, and that these more anterior representations could be transferred to the left hemisphere through more anterior corpus callosum (248). This remains to be proven.

In color dysphasia, another type of color anomia, patients cannot name not only visible colors but also the colors of familiar objects they see or imagine, tasks that patients with the disconnection anomia can do well (249). This defect is attributed to loss of an internal lexicon of colors, and indeed many have other dysphasic features. Most have left angular gyrus lesions, with associated alexia and agraphia, right hemifield defects, and Gerstmann's syndrome.

A third type of problem with color naming has been considered a short-term color amnesia. This patient could not name seen colors but could point accurately to colors named by the examiner. Verbal memory for color names was normal, but visual short-term memory for colors was impaired (250).

Color agnosia is also unusual (251–253). These patients can sort and match colors, and some can even name colors they see. However, they cannot name the colors for either visually presented or verbally named objects, cannot color line drawings of objects correctly, and cannot learn paired associations between seen objects and seen colors (a visual–visual task). Associated defects include pure alexia, object anomia, and poor performance on imagery tests for other object properties, although in at least one case the color agnosia was a relatively isolated defect (253). Most of these subjects had left occipitotemporal lesions, some with a right hemianopia, suggesting a left hemispheric dominance for semantic color knowledge.

PROSOPAGNOSIA AND RELATED DISTURBANCES OF OBJECT RECOGNITION

Prosopagnosia is the impaired ability to recognize familiar faces or to learn facial identity (254). While cases were described in the middle of the 19th century (255,256), detailed

study of prosopagnosia spans only the past 50 years. Early reports attributed prosopagnosia to a combination of generalized cognitive and visual disturbances (257,258). Indeed, impaired face recognition is still studied as one facet of more generalized problems of perception, cognition, and memory, as in macular degeneration (259), Alzheimer's disease (260–262), Huntington's disease (263), and Parkinson's disease (264,265), for example. However, as a diagnostic term, prosopagnosia should be reserved for patients with selective deficits in face recognition: that is, where the problem recognizing faces is disproportionately severe compared to other visual or cognitive dysfunction. This definition is a relative one, since many patients with prosopagnosia do have some mild object agnosia, complex visual disturbances, or abnormal nonverbal memory. The selectivity of this definition reflects the modern consensus that prosopagnosia is a specific functional disorder or family of disorders with specific neuroanatomic bases, as proposed decades ago (254,266).

CLINICAL ASPECTS OF PROSOPAGNOSIA

Patients with prosopagnosia cannot recognize most faces as familiar; rather, to identify people they rely mainly on voices or nonfacial visual cues, such as gait or mannerisms. On occasion they may use distinct face-related cues such as an unusual pair of glasses, a hairstyle, or a scar, cues that bypass the need to recognize the actual face. At other times the context of an encounter can prompt their recognition: they may recognize a physician in the hospital but not on the street (267–269). This may have a parallel in the laboratory phenomenon of ''provoked overt recognition'' (270). Here, when shown faces of people from a related category (e.g., sharing the same occupation), some patients with prosopagnosia can name the faces once they grasp the nature of the relationship. Another variation in recognition ability occurs in patients with the unusual anterograde form of prosopagnosia. Patients with this condition cannot learn to recognize new faces after the onset of their lesion, but their recognition of faces encountered before their lesion occurred is intact (51,271).

Most patients with prosopagnosia are aware of their perceptual problem and its attendant social difficulties, except for some cases with childhood onset (268,272,273). Some patients find their disability quite distressing and are severely dysphoric.

Identity is only one type of information present in faces. Gaze direction, emotional expression, age, and sex can also be determined. Some patients with prosopagnosia have a more extensive defect that also impairs these other facial functions (268,272,274,275), while others appear to make these judgments normally (276–280). Whether these functions are ever entirely preserved in prosopagnosia is a matter of debate, as some argue that these patients may use alternative feature cues (such as wrinkles for age) that normal subjects do not rely upon (272). However, evidence from functional imaging and monkey studies suggests that areas that encode facial identity and facial social signals may be separate, providing support for hypotheses that these functions are dissociable in brain-damaged patients.

Objective demonstration of impaired face recognition usually involves a battery of photographs of public persons, as in the Famous Faces Test (281). Ideally such a test should include unfamiliar faces as distractors (282), and the patient should be asked to provide names or biographical data belonging to the faces to exclude guessing. Failure should be contrasted with intact recognition of famous voices. Interpretation of results must take into account the cultural and social background of the patient to determine which faces should be familiar to him or her. If this is a problem, photographs of friends or relatives may be substituted.

The Faces subtest of the Warrington Recognition Memory Test (283) is a good test for short-term learning and retention of facial identity. This test shows subjects 50 faces and then asks them to identify the same faces later, when they are presented mixed with 50 other anonymous faces. The advantage of the Warrington test is that it dispenses with the issue of prior familiarity.

The Benton Face Recognition Test (BFRT) (284) shows subjects an unknown face and asks them to find the matching face in an array below. This matching test does not tap into the issue of familiarity and hence does not establish a diagnosis of prosopagnosia. However, failure to match faces suggests a degree of impaired face perception. The relevance of difficulties on this test to prosopagnosia is complicated by the fact that some patients are impaired on the BFRT and yet are not prosopagnosic (285).

There is no known treatment for prosopagnosia. One patient reportedly learned new faces when asked to rate faces for a personality trait or remember semantic data about them, but not when he focused on visual aspects of faces, but this benefit did not translate to recognition of other views of the same faces (286). Otherwise, patients may benefit socially from learning to use nonfacial and nonvisual cues more effectively in identifying people.

THE SPECIFICITY OF THE PROSOPAGNOSIC DEFECT

Can the prosopagnosic defect be truly specific for faces only? This point is of great relevance to debates about high-level visual processing, particularly as to whether its organization is highly modular for different stimuli (287,288). Most patients with prosopagnosia can identify objects at some basic level or category, unlike patients with severe generalized visual agnosia. However, some cannot identify subtypes (''subordinate categories'') such as types of cars, food, or coins, or specific individuals (''exemplars'') such as buildings, handwriting, or personal clothing (273,289–291). On the other hand, other patients reportedly can identify personal belongings (292), individual animals (276,293), specific places (276,279), cars (276,294), flowers (279), vegetables (294), and different eyeglasses (295). Thus, in some patients the defect appears to be highly specific for faces, in support of a modular account. However, a recent review with detailed measures of reaction time and signal detection parameters in two patients with prosopagnosia has argued that deficits in non-face processing are present even when accuracy rates suggest otherwise (296).

By the modular account, patients with prosopagnosia vary in the specificity of their recognition defect because of the variable extent of their lesion: the more other modules are damaged, the more difficulty with recognizing other object classes. However, assessments of specificity must take into account other factors that determine how easily subjects perform recognition tasks. First and foremost is premorbid perceptual expertise (297). Some normal subjects can expertly perceive subtle variations to determine the specific year of a single model of car, while others can barely distinguish cars from vans. To become expert, subjects must not only have frequent exposure to objects but also have an interest in discriminating between them. Thus, while our social interactions and motivations converge to make us all face experts, only some of us are car experts, even though we all see cars daily. Hence it is a challenge to determine what level of subordinate categorization to expect for nonfacial objects, based on a prosopagnosic patient's premorbid capability. Should one be able to tell the difference between a hawk and an eagle (class: birds of prey), or a buteo and an accipiter (class: hawks)?

A second potential source of variation in object recognition skills is that the types of perceptual processes needed with certain object categories may differ from those needed with other objects. For example, the rigid linear structures of man-made objects like houses and cars differ from the more randomly irregular curved surfaces of natural structures like faces, vegetables, and animals. Does the ability to distinguish one house from another hinge upon the same perceptual processes as the ability to distinguish between faces? This distinction may be reflected in reports of visual agnosias where the recognition of man-made objects is dissociated from the recognition of natural objects.

THE FUNCTIONAL DEFICIT IN PROSOPAGNOSIA

In cognitive models, a complex task such as face recognition is often depicted as a series of stages. The Bruce and Young model is typical (298). Visual processing generates a face percept. This percept is matched to "face recognition units," a memory store of previously encountered faces. A successful match activates person-identity nodes that contain names and biographical data, nodes that can also be accessed through other perceptual routes, such as voice or gait analysis.

This basic structure can be elaborated. Low-level visual processing may generate data for higher-level visual processing in at least two different streams. One analyzes the short- and long-term temporal variations in face structure that reveal expression and aging; the other ignores these temporal variations in favor of the more stable structural characteristics of faces that reveal identity. Top-down information flow is also present in the system. For example, matching of the face percept to face recognition units may be enhanced by top-down semantic activation from person-identity nodes, as when the subject knows the name of the person or his or her contextual category (actor, family, workmate).

In such a complex process, defective performance can theoretically arise at any one of several levels. In patients with extensive natural lesions, damage may not be restricted to a single level, although a certain type of dysfunction may predominate. Nevertheless, one can conceive of prosopagnosia as constituting two broad classes, one in which there is a failure to form a sufficiently accurate facial percept ("apperceptive prosopagnosia"), and one in which there is an inability to match an accurate percept to facial memories ("associative prosopagnosia") (299,300). More fine-grain delineations of disconnections between various elements of the process are also possible (269).

APPERCEPTIVE PROSOPAGNOSIA

In apperceptive prosopagnosia, patients cannot form an accurate picture of the face before them. In the past, this diagnosis has usually relied upon indirect deductions from performance on other visual tests not involving faces (299,300). These include overlapping figures, silhouettes, Gestalt completion tests (269,279,301), and global texture or moiré patterns (302). However, it is far from proven that the mechanisms probed by such tests are truly related to normal face recognition. Somewhat closer is the use of unfamiliar face-matching tests like the BFRT. Failure to match faces seen in different views or lighting may indicate a problem in extracting relevant facial structure. Though more logically appealing, this argument is problematic because the BFRT can also be failed by patients without prosopagnosia (285,303,304). This raises the possibility that performance on the BFRT depends upon facial information irrelevant to face recognition. (Although it seems counterintuitive that subjects would identify unfamiliar faces using criteria they do not apply to familiar faces, there is evidence that different strategies may indeed be used. For example, the internal facial features appear to play a greater role in recognizing familiar faces than in identifying unfamiliar ones (305,306).) Alternatively, prosopagnosia may require additional defects besides those that lead to poor BFRT performance.

The specific nature of the processing deficit in apperceptive prosopagnosia remains somewhat elusive. Data from normal subjects suggest two main hypotheses about the mechanisms of normal face perception. The holistic hypothesis argues that the elements of a face are integrated and processed as a complete whole, not subject to part decomposition (307–309). The configurational hypothesis argues that face recognition is a geometric problem in which the precise spatial relations between features encode the unique three-dimensional structure of a given face (310–312). This concept derives support from studies showing that IT cells in monkeys are selective for faces that differ in these internal spatial relations (313,314).

These two different hypotheses are not mutually exclusive. There are data that some patients with prosopagnosia are deficient in the perception of whole object structure, seeing only individual elements and relying on a feature-by-feature strategy in face perception (277,301). Recent studies show that many prosopagnosic patients with occipitotemporal lesions are markedly impaired in perceiving the configuration of facial features (315–317) (Fig. 13.14). Further work is needed to clarify which hypothesis best captures the nature of the prosopagnosic deficit.

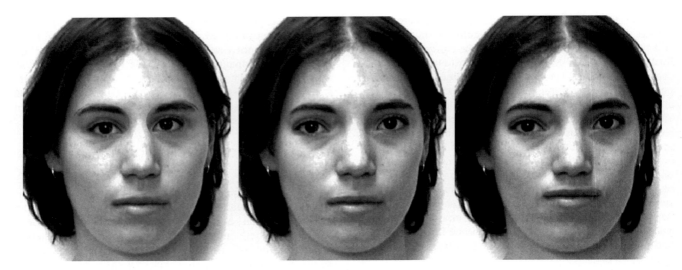

Figure 13.14. Stimuli used to test perception of facial configuration. The precise location of features within a face may be an important aspect of facial geometry that is relevant to identifying faces. Patients with lesions of the fusiform face area are impaired in perceiving faces that have been altered by moving the eyes closer (*left*) or the mouth higher (*right*), compared with the unaltered base face (*center*). (From Joubert S, Felician O, Barbeau E, et al. Impaired configurational processing in a case of progressive prosopagnosia associated with predominant right temporal lobe atrophy. Brain 2003;126:2537–2550.)

ASSOCIATIVE PROSOPAGNOSIA

An associative defect implies failure of perceptual data to gain access to memory stores (face-recognition units) (51,299,300). In some cases this may be because of a disconnection between facial percepts and the face-recognition units (269). In others the facial memories may be lost. The diagnosis of associative prosopagnosia has traditionally been indirect, based on demonstration of intact face perception, as from normal performance on the BFRT. However, as has been pointed out (318), a normal BFRT score does not prove normal face perception, as prosopagnosic patients who achieve such scores invariably take a long time to do the test, suggesting that they are using abnormal perceptual strategies.

A more direct probe of the status of facial memories is imagery (269). Batteries of questions can test whether subjects can recall details about the appearance of well-known faces, when they are not actually viewing those faces. While more posterior occipitotemporal lesions are associated with only mildly impaired face imagery, anterior temporal lesions are associated with severe loss, suggesting that facial memory stores are lost in these patients (319).

PEOPLE-SPECIFIC AMNESIA

The last element in the cognitive model of face processing is the person-identity node, containing biographic information about individuals. Because these biographic data can be accessed from several routes, this leads not to prosopagnosia, in which patients can still recognize people from other sensory cues, but to a people-specific amnesia, in which no cues can prompt recollection of other people, while other types of memories remain intact. This has been described with right temporal pole lesions (279,320,321). This localization

is consistent with functional imaging studies showing that name and face recognition both activate the anterior middle temporal gyrus and temporal pole (322,323). A disconnection between intact face memories and person-identity nodes was proposed in a patient with an unusual left hemispheric lesion who recognized faces as familiar, although he could provide names or biographical details only to the spoken name, not to faces (324).

COVERT FACIAL RECOGNITION

One of the intriguing observations in prosopagnosic patients is that a range of physiologic and behavioral techniques can show that these patients retain some unconscious "covert recognition" of these faces (325,326). Investigators have shown two main effects: covert familiarity, or distinguishing known from unknown faces, and covert semantic knowledge, or retained information about name, occupation, and other facts associated with a face.

Covert effects have been shown with physiologic measurements. Electrodermal skin conductance has shown larger responses with familiar than unfamiliar faces (51), or when names are paired correctly with faces (327,328). In one patient visual evoked potentials were used to study the P300 effect, in which the P300 wave is larger when an infrequent event is detected within a set of stimuli (329). Using familiar and unfamiliar faces, researchers showed that when familiar faces were infrequent they were associated with a large central P300 wave, indicating that faces were being categorized by familiarity.

Most commonly used are behavioral methods, including both direct and indirect techniques. Direct techniques force the subject to engage in a task involving face identity. When shown two faces and asked which face belongs to a certain name, several patients have been able to perform better than chance, even though they were not able to indicate which face was famous when they were not given the name (282,330,331). Numerous studies have shown that prosopagnosic patients are quicker to learn to associate a name with a famous face when the name is the correct one for that face (276,330–332). When scanning faces, the eye movements of two prosopagnosic patients showed a greater concentration on internal features when faces were familiar, just as occurs with normal subjects (52).

Indirect techniques ask the subject to perform some task not directly related to facial identity, and observe whether performance is influenced by the identity of a face shown with the task. Normal subjects are quicker at judging whether two facial pictures are from the same person when the face is familiar, and this difference depends on internal facial features: a similar difference in reaction time and reliance on inner features was shown in one patient (333). Matching the old and young faces of individuals across a 30-year gap was easier with famous faces for another patient (278). Another example is a "facial interference" paradigm, in which a subject classifies a famous name by occupation while a face is shown simultaneously (333). If the face belongs to someone with the alternative occupation, reaction times are normally slowed (the interference), and this was also found in one prosopagnosic patient (333). A similar phenomenon is "face priming," which measures the effects on name classification of a preceding (not simultaneous) face: here a face related to the name speeds up reaction times, as was found in the same prosopagnosic patient (334).

Not all prosopagnosic patients have covert recognition (272,273,277,335). Reasons why some have it and others not are unclear. Conjectures upon this point tend to reflect conflicting views on the origins of covert recognition. One concept proposes that it is generated by an alternate, "dissociated" route to normal face processing, through dorsal occipitoparietal cortex or amygdala (336). Proponents of a dissociated route often posit that to support covert function, face perception must be intact. Hence, the claim is that covert recognition is associated with associative prosopagnosia, in which accurate facial percepts cannot be matched to facial memory stores because of either disconnection or their loss, rather than apperceptive prosopagnosia, in which the facial percept is degraded (335,337). Another explanation is that covert function reflects residual processing within the surviving remnants of the normal face-processing network, a hypothesis that has been successfully modeled with computer simulations (338–340). In this model, the likelihood and strength of covert recognition would be inversely related to the degree of damage across the network (319).

Against the claim that covert recognition is absent in apperceptive prosopagnosia is the demonstration that several patients with impaired configural perception from unilateral right hemisphere lesions had good covert ability (319,341). Evidence for the network hypothesis comes from recent demonstrations that behavioral indices of covert recognition are correlated with the degree of residual overt familiarity in prosopagnosia (282). In this series of patients, impaired covert function was found mainly in two groups: those with bilateral occipitotemporal lesions causing apperceptive defects, and those with childhood-onset prosopagnosia. Early-onset prosopagnosia may be particularly problematic for covert recognition, as it may preclude the formation of facial memories needed to support it. Indeed, several of the previous cases without covert recognition had onset in childhood (272,273).

ASSOCIATED CLINICAL FINDINGS

Prosopagnosia is frequently associated with three other clinical findings. First is a field defect, commonly a left or bilateral upper quadrantanopia but sometimes a left homonymous hemianopia (52,269,342,343). Second is achromatopsia or hemiachromatopsia, particularly in those with lesions of the fusiform gyri. Last is topographagnosia, or getting lost in familiar surroundings (344). The latter may be related to a failure to recognize landmarks, as functional imaging studies suggest that there is a region specialized for building recognition adjacent to the fusiform face area (345). These three findings are not invariably associated, but with prosopagnosia they form a loosely associated quartet, likely reflecting the extent of damage among neighboring structures in the medial occipital lobe.

Some patients also have evidence of a mild visual object agnosia (272,273), though less severe than their prosopagnosia. Those with more anterior temporal damage can have visual or verbal memory disturbances (328,346). Other occasional deficits include simultanagnosia (276,333), palinopsia, visual hallucinations, constructional difficulties, and left hemineglect (269,346).

ANATOMY OF FACE PROCESSING AND PROSOPAGNOSIA

It is useful to place the anatomic data concerning prosopagnosia in the context of information from nonhuman primates and normal human functional imaging.

In monkeys, face-selective neuronal responses have been found in two main regions of cortex (Fig. 13.15). First is the inferotemporal cortex (IT) (313,347,348). This includes areas of the lower bank of the superior temporal sulcus (STS), such as areas TEa and TEm (349). Second is the upper bank of the STS (313,350), mainly in a multimodal area designated the superior temporal polymodal area (STPa) (351) or area TPO (349). Other areas with face-selective responses are located in the basal accessory nucleus of the amygdala (352), the ventral striatum, and the inferior prefrontal cortex (353). Face-sensitive neurons are a minority of cells in all these areas, ranging from 10% to 20% (349,354).

The face-selective cells in the STS have been studied the most (350,354). They do not respond to simple edges, bars, or complex nonfacial stimuli. All of the internal facial features contribute to the face-selective response, and the proper spatial arrangement of these features is crucial. It is debatable whether STS cells play a critical role in identifying faces, though. Most STS neurons respond vigorously to all faces (350). Only about 10% of cells in the fundus have selective responses to different faces (354), but, on the other

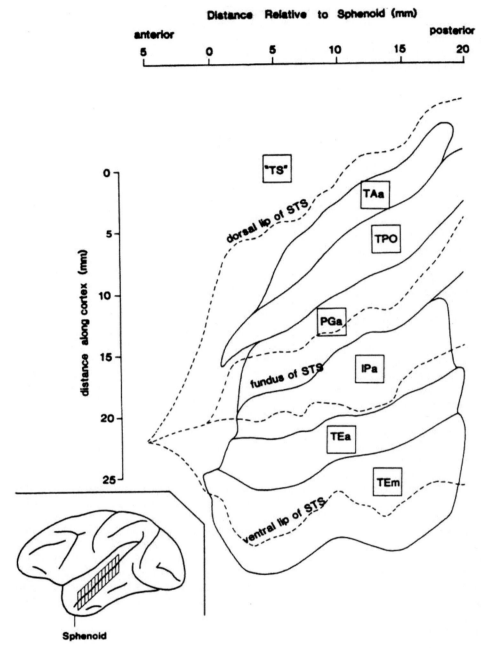

Figure 13.15. Face-processing areas in the monkey. *Bottom left diagram* is the lateral view of the cerebral hemisphere, with the superior temporal sulcus (STS) shaded. *Large diagram* is the unfolded STS. Areas TEa and TEm form part of IT, inferior temporal cortex, and area TPO is part of the dorsal STS. (From Leonard CM, Rolls ET, Wilson FA, et al. Neurons in the amygdala of the monkey with responses selective for faces. Behav Brain Res 1985;15:159–176.)

hand, there are reports claiming that 77% differentiate between faces to a degree, with a discriminative ability similar to human observers (355). Perhaps the most important evidence is that bilateral resections of the floor and banks of the STS only mildly affect object and face discrimination and do not impair judgments of facial familiarity (356). Rather, they impair the perception of important facial social signals, such as expression and direction of gaze (275).

IT neurons distinguish between faces that vary in the distances between internal features (313,314), and cooling of

IT profoundly impairs this type of perceptual judgment (357). The relevance of this to face recognition comes from observations that normal humans use internal features more than external ones to recognize familiar faces (306), and prosopagnosic patients can be severely impaired on perceiving the precise arrangement of internal features (315). IT neurons are also more sensitive to face orientation (358) than STS cells are (350,354), which is consistent with the fact that face recognition is disproportionately degraded by turning faces upside-down (the "inversion effect") (359).

While more data are needed, particularly on the effects of IT resection on face recognition, these results suggest that face processing differs in STS and IT (360,361). IT may play a greater role in facial identification, whereas the chief function of STS face cells may be the perception of socially relevant cues, such as gaze direction. In support, STS face cells also show sensitivity to head orientation and body posture, other cues to the direction of another animal's attention when the eyes are not visible (360).

Functional imaging has expanded our knowledge of the human anatomy of face processing. Early PET experiments (362) found that face identification activated the fusiform gyri and anterior temporal lobes bilaterally and the right parahippocampal gyrus, whereas object recognition activated the left occipitotemporal cortex. Another PET experiment confirmed bilateral activation of the fusiform gyri during a face-matching task (363,364). Recording from electrodes implanted in epileptic patients found significant potentials to faces but not cars, butterflies, or scrambled faces in the fusiform and inferior temporal gyri bilaterally (365) (Fig. 13.16). Stimulation of these regions impaired the naming of familiar faces.

fMRI studies (366) also support localization to the fusiform gyri, with a predominance of right-sided activity in some studies (367,368), although others found right, left, or symmetric activity in individuals, with no overall group asymmetry (369) (Fig. 13.17). The region on the right has been named the fusiform face area (FFA). In addition to this region, face-related activity occurs in the posterior STS and in an inferior occipital area (368,370,371). The latter is adjacent to both the fusiform and posterior STS and may be a perceptual input stage to both regions (366). As predicted from the monkey data (360), attention to direction of gaze

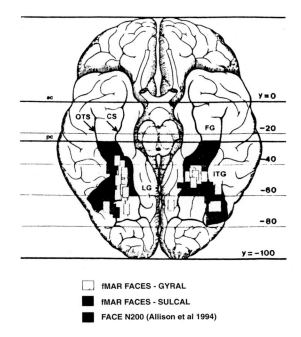

fMAR FACES - GYRAL

fMAR FACES - SULCAL

FACE N200 (Allison et al 1994)

Figure 13.17. Activation with fMRI during face perception. Schematic representation of voxels with increased intensity on MRI during perception of faces, superimposed on a view of the inferior brain surface. *Squares* show areas activated within sulci and upon gyral surfaces. For comparison, the areas activated in the evoked potential study shown in Figure 13.16 are superimposed in black. cs, collateral sulcus; fg, fusiform gyrus; itg, inferior temporal gyrus; lg, lingual gyrus; ots, occipitotemporal sulcus. (From Puce A, Allison T, Gore JC, et al. Face-sensitive regions in human extrastriate cortex studied by functional MRI. J Neurophysiol 1995;74:1192–1199.)

enhances the activity in the STS locus, whereas attention to identity enhances activity in the fusiform gyri (371). This has suggested a processing model with at least three modules: (*a*) an early perceptual stage in the inferior occipital area, which feeds into both (*b*) a fusiform area (IT homolog) for perception of identity and (*c*) an STS region for perception of dynamic facial aspects such as expression and gaze. This task segregation between IT (FFA) and STS (lateral occipitotemporal cortex) may be more relative than absolute, however (372).

In addition to localization, fMRI has been used to contribute to the debate about the face-specificity of the mechanisms involved in face identification (287,288). Faces and buildings activate separate adjacent structures in the fusiform gyrus (373), consistent with high stimulus-specificity of a face-processing module. The data on animals versus faces (two natural categories of objects) is mixed, however (374,375). Also, one study showed that stimuli such as cars and birds activated the fusiform face area if the subject was expert at their recognition (376). According to these authors, face recognition may be merely the most dramatic aspect of a type of perception that processes subtle differences in the shape of highly similar exemplars that belong to the same class of object.

In most cases, prosopagnosia is caused by lesions in the

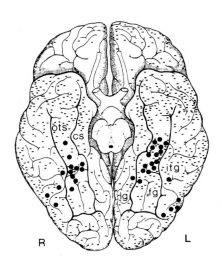

Figure 13.16. Evoked potentials during face perception. Summary of locations from which a surface-negative potential (N200) was recorded (*block dots*), and areas where it was not found (*dashes*), superimposed on a drawing of the inferior surface of the brain. cs, collateral sulcus; fg, fusiform gyrus; itg, inferior temporal gyrus; lg, lingual gyrus; ots, occipitotemporal sulcus. (From Allison T, Ginter H, McCarthy G, et al. Face recognition in human extrastriate cortex. J Neurophysiol 1994;71:821–825.)

medial occipitotemporal lobes (Figs. 13.18 and 13.19). The classic lesion is bilateral damage to the lingual and fusiform gyri of the medial occipitotemporal cortex (291,377) (Figs. 13.20 and 13.21). These relatively posterior lesions often involve the region identified on fMRI as the FFA (315). The importance of the bilateral nature of the lesions in this group is underscored by the report of a patient with sequential lesions, first on the right and then on the left, who became prosopagnosic only after the second lesion (378).

However, two other important categories of lesions can be encountered in prosopagnosia. First, there is a significant body of evidence that in some patients a unilateral right occipitotemporal lesion is sufficient to cause prosopagnosia (269,277,332,346,379,380) (Figs. 13.22 and 13.23). Such lesions may also affect the FFA (315). Second is the association of prosopagnosia with more anterior temporal lesions (279,381) (Fig. 13.24).

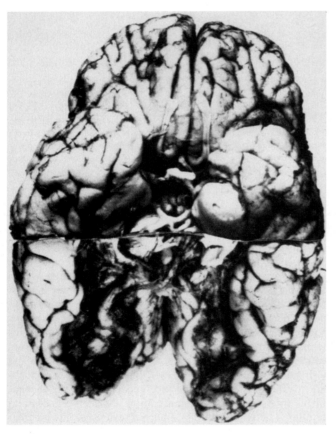

Figure 13.18. Pathology of prosopagnosia. The patient was a 59-year-old man who 2 years earlier had had sudden onset of cortical blindness that partially resolved, leaving bilaterally constricted visual fields, worse on the left and superiorly. The patient also had prosopagnosia, cerebral achromatopsia, and memory deficits. Basal view of the brain shows destruction of the occipital pole, pericalcarine tissues, caudal hippocampal gyrus, and entire fusiform gyrus of the right hemisphere. In the left hemisphere, there is some damage to the pericalcarine areas and the most caudal part of the hippocampal gyrus, with destruction of all the fusiform and most of the lingual gyri. (From Cohn R, Neumann MA, Wood DH. Prosopagnosia: a clinicopathological study. Ann Neurol 1977;1:177–182.)

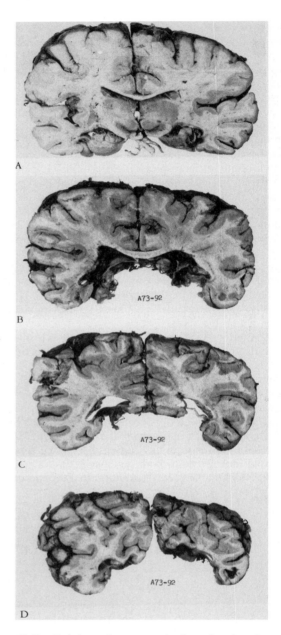

Figure 13.19. Pathology of prosopagnosia. Coronal sections through the brain of the same patient described in Figure 13.18. *A*, At the level of the thalamus. *B*, At the level of the fimbria. *C*, At the retrosplenial level. *D*, 2.5 cm caudal to *C*. As noted in the previous figure, the brain shows destruction of the occipital pole, pericalcarine tissues, caudal hippocampal gyrus, and entire fusiform gyrus of the right hemisphere. In the left hemisphere, there is some damage to the pericalcarine areas and the most caudal part of the hippocampal gyrus, with destruction of all the fusiform and most of the lingual gyri. (From Cohn R, Neumann MA, Wood DH. Prosopagnosia: a clinicopathological study. Ann Neurol 1977;1:177–182.)

How these three different patterns of lesions differ in the type of prosopagnosia they cause is not settled. One hypothesis is that unilateral right occipitotemporal lesions cause an apperceptive defect, whereas bilateral, more anterior tem-

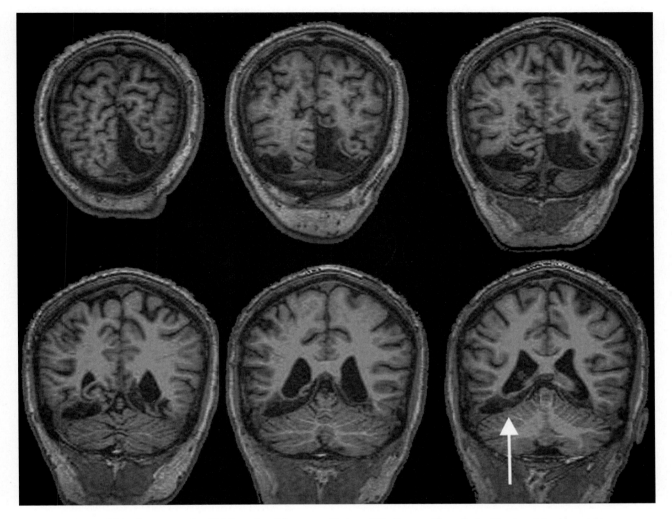

Figure 13.20. Prosopagnosia with bilateral occipitotemporal lesions. This 41-year-old man had suffered a subdural hematoma in a car accident 20 years earlier. He had been cortically blind for a few weeks. He now has right hemianopia, some mild object agnosia, and partial dyschromatopsia, as well as prosopagnosia.

poral lesions cause an associative one (299). While one study found paradoxically that an apperceptive patient who could not match faces had more anterior temporal lesions than one with intact matching ability (382), the results with a recent series of prosopagnosic patients are consistent with this hypothesis (315,319). Bilateral or unilateral occipitotemporal lesions that include the right fusiform face area impaired perceptual encoding of facial configuration but only mildly affected facial imagery, whereas anterior temporal lesions tended to eliminate facial memories, as accessed by imagery tests, but had much less effect on perceptual encoding of facial configuration. What remains to be determined is how unilateral occipitotemporal lesions differ from bilateral ones.

The most common causes of prosopagnosia are posterior cerebral artery infarctions, head trauma, and viral encephalitis (269,291,315), partly because of the potential of these lesions to cause bilateral damage. Tumors, hematomas, abscesses, and surgical resections are less frequent, but are

common causes in patients with unilateral lesions (300, 346,383). Progressive forms occur with focal temporal atrophy (279,317,384). It has been reported as a transient manifestation of migraine (385).

There is increasing interest in a developmental form of prosopagnosia also. The acquisition of face recognition depends on not only prenatal factors but also postnatal development in early childhood (268,272,273,386,387). Hence, developmental prosopagnosia covers both.

Because acquisition of adult-level face expertise may require experience in early childhood, defects with onset at or before this period are considered developmental prosopagnosia (268,272,273,316,386,387). This term covers patients with lesions acquired in early childhood and congenital cases, which in turn can be due to either prenatal insults or an inherited defect, which may be an autosomal-dominant trait. These patients often have associated deficits in judging social information from faces, and some have social develop-

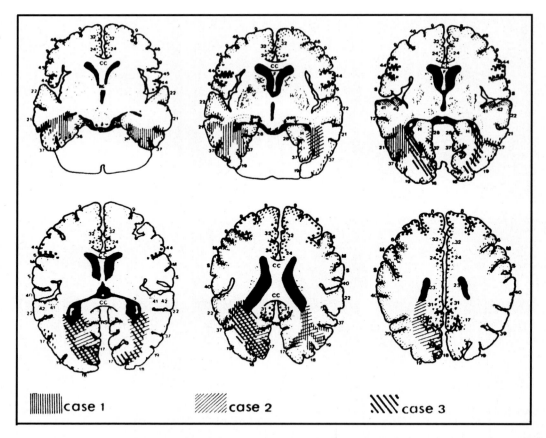

Figure 13.21.   Location of bilateral lesions in three patients with prosopagnosia. Axial template drawings with *shaded areas* representing the lesions of three patients with prosopagnosia. Bilateral damage, greater on the left than the right, is present in all three. (From Damasio AR, Damasio H, Van Hoesen GW. Prosopagnosia: anatomic basis and behavioral mechanisms. Neurology 1982;32:331–341.)

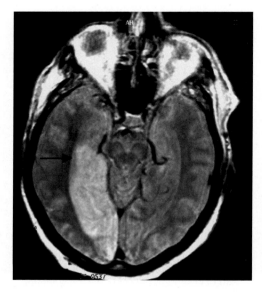

Figure 13.22.   Prosopagnosia with unilateral right occipitotemporal lesion. This 59-year-old man had had a right posterior cerebral arterial infarct 10 months earlier, involving the approximate level of the fusiform face area as well as, more posteriorly, the lateral occipital area, both of which are activated by faces in fMRI experiments. He has a left hemianopia as well.

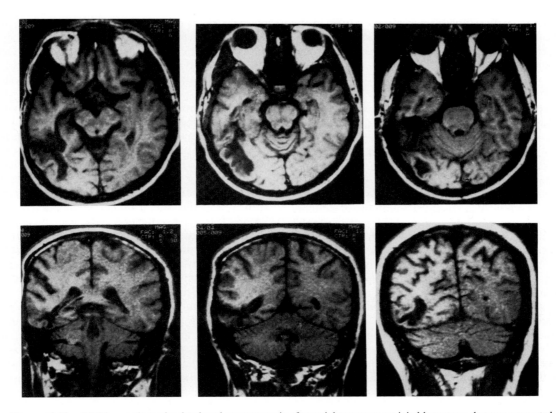

Figure 13.23. MRI in a patient who developed prosopagnosia after a right temporo-occipital hematoma that was evacuated 1 year previously. Axial T1-weighted images are shown in the *top row* and coronal T1-weighted images in the *bottom row*. The images all show only a unilateral right temporo-occipital hypointense area with no mass effect. No lesions are seen in the left hemisphere. (From Michel F, Poncet M, Signoret JL. Les lesions responsables de la prosopagnosie sont-elles toujours bilaterales? Rev Neurol 1989;145:764–770.)

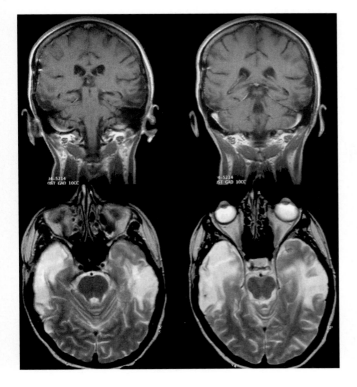

Figure 13.24. Prosopagnosia with bilateral anterior temporal lesions. This 33-year-old woman had a closed head injury and surgical resection of one temporal lobe 10 years earlier. She has full visual fields and no topographagnosia or color deficit. She performs well on tests of face perception but poorly on tests of face imagery, suggesting she has lost access to facial memory stores.

mental disorders such as Asperger syndrome (268). In the congenital cases, neuroimaging tends not to show the cortical lesions seen in adult-onset prosopagnosia, but sometimes there are more subtle anomalies.

OTHER DISORDERS OF FACE PERCEPTION

The use of unfamiliar face-matching tests has generated some interesting data on hemispheric processing of stimuli. One of the interesting observations has been that deficits in unfamiliar face matching can occur in subjects without prosopagnosia (303,304). This too tends to be associated with right hemispheric lesions. Since some prosopagnosic patients can match unfamiliar faces, though with some effort and increased test time, this raises the possibility of a double dissociation. However, a later study of 34 patients found that most subjects were impaired with both familiar face recognition and unfamiliar face matching (388). Also, in the two patients with preserved accuracy scores on one test but not the other, the reaction times were prolonged on the test with the normal accuracy score. The authors concluded that the processes for familiar and unfamiliar face identity were not independent.

A less-studied limb of the face-processing model is the analysis of dynamic facial information, such as gaze, expression, and age. Monkey and functional imaging data would suggest that these are more likely to be associated with damage to the lateral occipitotemporal region. There are few data to confirm or refute this at present. An older study did find that judgment of facial age could be impaired by right hemispheric lesions, but no detailed neuroanatomic data were provided (389). Another study showed that while defects in analyzing facial expression were usually associated with

other problems of identity recognition and face matching, a selective defect for facial expression alone occurred with left hemispheric lesions (388). Clearly the literature needs a more detailed exploration of relatively selective defects of dynamic facial interpretation, along with good neuroimaging.

Some patients mistake strangers for people known to them (390,391). Some persist in the belief of the mistaken identity, despite evidence to the contrary, and hence have some of the delusional quality of Capgras syndrome. As with prosopagnosia, false recognition of unfamiliar faces has been described mainly with right-sided lesions. Unlike prosopagnosia, the lesions are usually large middle cerebral artery strokes, affecting lateral frontal, temporal, and parietal cortex (390,391). Nevertheless, some patients appear to have associated prosopagnosia on testing, although they deny problems in recognizing people (391). In these cases, the fault may lie with either impaired perceptual input to face-recognition units or poor discriminative function of partial damaged face-recognition units (392).

False recognition without prosopagnosia has also been described (390,392). Most have right prefrontal damage, which may impair self-monitoring and decision making, leading to hasty mistaken judgments of facial similarity based on partial or fragmentary data, and failure to reject incorrect matches (392). These deficits in decision making and self-monitoring should be evident in other perceptual decisions, but evidence for this has not yet been gathered. Frontal lesions may also be responsible for the failure of some patients with the prosopagnosic variant of false recognition to recognize their impairment and to persist in their mistaken delusions.

ACQUIRED ALEXIA

Acquired alexia is the inability to read in previously literate individuals despite adequate visual acuity. The severity of the reading disorder and the pattern of accompanying neurologic defects vary depending on the location and extent of the underlying brain lesions. Reading is a complex behavior involving form perception, spatial attention, ocular fixation, scanning saccadic eye movements, and linguistic processing. Not surprisingly, many types of cerebral or visual dysfunction can disrupt the reading process; while other clinical signs may accompany the alexia, impaired reading is sometimes the chief or the only complaint. The severity of reading difficulty can range from a mild defect with slow reading and occasional errors, which requires comparison with normal controls matched for educational level (393), to a complete inability to read even numbers and letters. Analysis of the severity and type of reading errors can help differentiate between the various forms of reading disorders and their causes. Acquired alexia and milder forms of acquired reading disturbance must be distinguished from "dyslexia," a developmental defect that results in much less severe reading difficulties characterized by slow reading, letter or word reversals, and other inefficiencies. The label "dyslexia" has also been applied in acquired reading disturbance where the reading defect is incomplete (analogous to the use

of the term "dyschromatopsia" in cases of incomplete color vision loss).

Dejerine (394) first described a patient with alexia and agraphia but no other linguistic or visual defect, caused by a lesion of the left angular gyrus (Fig. 13.25). In 1892 he described a case of alexia without agraphia (pure alexia, or word blindness) with incomplete right homonymous hemianopia, due to a lesion of the left fusiform and lingual gyri (Fig. 13.26). This patient developed agraphia after a second infarct of the left angular gyrus, corroborating the findings of the previous case. Dejerine deduced that the left angular gyrus stored the visual representation of words needed for reading and writing. Furthermore, disconnecting the visual inputs of both hemispheres from the left angular gyrus could disrupt reading but leave writing intact. These early concepts have survived in modern disconnectionist theories of pure alexia (395), and his localization is consistent with the data from neuroimaging (396).

PURE ALEXIA (WORD BLINDNESS, OR ALEXIA WITHOUT AGRAPHIA)

Signs and Symptoms

The key feature of pure alexia is a dramatic dissociation between the ability to read and normal writing performance:

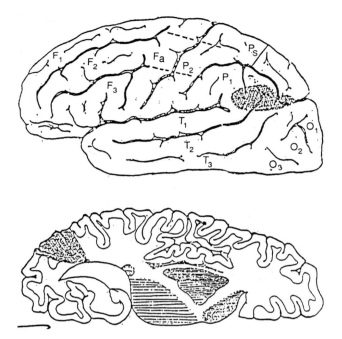

Figure 13.25. Location of the lesion causing alexia with agraphia. Drawings made by Déjérine of the case he reported in 1891 (see text for details). *Top,* Lateral surface of the left hemisphere. *Bottom,* Axial section of the same hemisphere. The drawings show a lesion (*shaded area*) of the left angular gyrus. (From Black SE, Behrmann M. Localization in alexia. In: Kertesz A, ed. Localization and Neuroimaging in Neuropsychology. San Diego, Academic Press, 1994:331–376.)

road signs, and map symbols (398,399), let alone words. At the mild end, patients have slow reading with occasional errors, diagnosable only by comparison with controls of similar educational level (393). These patients decipher words one letter at a time (letter-by-letter reading, or spelling dyslexia). The characteristic sign is the word-length effect, in that the time needed to read a word increases with the number of letters in the word (400,401).

In Japanese, which has two different writing systems, *kana* (phonetically based) and *kanji* (nonphonetic, ideographic form), there can be impaired reading of *kanji* but not *kana* (402) or vice versa (403). Dissociations in bilingual patients can also occur, with the more recently acquired language less affected (404), perhaps in keeping with hypotheses of right hemisphere involvement in new language acquisition. In patients with long-standing blindness, alexia for Braille can be caused by occipital lesions in the absence of somatosensory deficits (405).

Associated signs with pure alexia are common (396). There is often a right visual field defect, usually complete homonymous hemianopia but sometimes only a superior quadrantanopia, in which case there may also be a right hemiachromatopsia. Pure alexia cannot be attributed to right hemianopia, however, as pure alexia can occur without hemianopia (406–410), and many patients with right macula-splitting hemianopia do not have pure alexia. While any associated dyschromatopsia is restricted to the right hemifield, naming of colors in the left hemifield may be abnormal (248,396). Naming problems also extend to other visual objects and photographs frequently. Anomia is not necessarily restricted to the visual modality but can include objects perceived by touch, implying some nonvisual language disturbance (411). Verbal memory deficits and visual agnosia can occur (396,411). Some authors describe a disconnection optic ataxia in which the dominant right hand has difficulty with purposeful movements to objects in the nondominant left visual field (396).

such patients can write fluently and spontaneously, but having done so cannot read what they have just written. The severity of this defect can vary. At the severe end, patients with global alexia (397) cannot read numbers, letters, and other abstract symbols, such as musical notation for pitch,

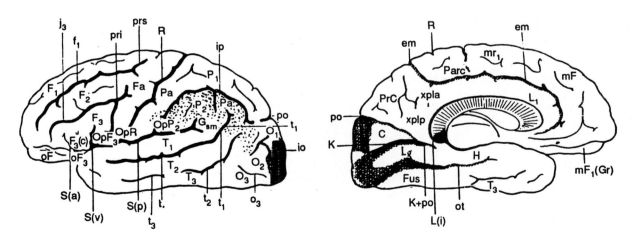

Figure 13.26. Location of the lesion causing alexia without agraphia (pure alexia). Drawing made by Déjérine of the case he reported in 1892 (see text for details). Drawing of the lateral and medial surface of the left hemisphere. *Dark shading* shows the first lesion, affecting the cuneus (C), lingual (TO2), and fusiform (TO1) gyri. (From Black SE, Behrmann M. Localization in alexia. In: Kertesz A, ed. Localization and Neuroimaging in Neuropsychology. San Diego, Academic Press, 1994:331–376.)

Covert Reading

Several studies have shown covert reading ability in patients with pure alexia. Some patients could indicate whether a string of letters formed a word (lexical decision task). This ability varied with linguistic features such as the frequency of the word in daily usage, the amount of visual imagery evoked by the word, and the grammatical category of the word, with better performance with nouns (401,412,413). The ability to distinguish words from non-words may use a mechanism separate from the laborious letter-by-letter strategy used to read words: the time required to make lexical decisions in one letter-by-letter reader was much less than the time needed to identify words and did not show the word-length effect characteristic of the latter (414). Other examples of covert determination of lexical status include one patient who could indicate which part of a long string of letters formed a word and point to a written word named by the examiner, even though she could not read it aloud (415). The ability to identify rapidly presented letters was better when the letters were part of words than if they were parts of random letter strings (word superiority effect) in one patient

(400) but not in another (416). The key distinctions between those with and without "covert" lexical classification ability remain to be elucidated.

Covert comprehension of word meaning has been reported also. Some patients could accurately categorize words semantically (i.e., indicating which are animals, foods, etc.) (401), though others could not (416). Words could be matched to objects or their pictures by some patients (412,417) but not others (418). Whether these demonstrations constitute "unconscious" covert ability has been challenged. One subject could not only make semantic matches but also was aware of the accuracy of her performance, showing preserved "metaknowledge" (417). Presence of metaknowledge may point to partial degradation of information rather than dissociations between conscious and nonconscious processes. Bub and Arguin (414) found that unlike covert lexical decisions, semantic categorizations took longer and also showed the word-length effect, suggesting that they were accomplished by the same mechanism that was used for explicit identification of words. They too concluded that semantic categorization may be due to partially decoded letter information allowing forced-choice responses

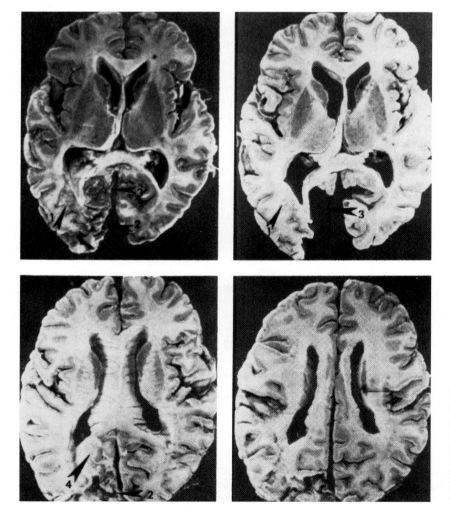

Figure 13.27. Pathology of pure alexia. Four axial sections through the brain of a 68-year-old man with pure alexia (alexia without agraphia), right homonymous hemianopia, color anomia, and optic ataxia. The infarction involves the left medial temporo-occipital lobe (*arrows 2 and 3*) and periventricular white matter (*arrow 1*), and also the forceps major (*arrow 4*). (From Damasio AR, Damasio H. The anatomic basis of pure alexia. Neurology 1983;33:1573–1583.)

if not verbal report, rather than covert knowledge. However, their findings contrast with the report by Coslett et al. (401) of a patient who could rapidly achieve both lexical decisions and semantic categorizations, suggesting that both types of covert processing used a "whole-word" identification strategy rather than the letter-by-letter technique for explicit reading. These authors attributed covert reading ability to right hemispheric language processing.

Anatomy, Pathology, and Mechanisms of Pure Alexia

Lesions causing pure alexia are almost always in the left hemisphere, most commonly in the medial and inferior occipitotemporal region (396,397) (Figs. 13.27 and 13.28). Most are due to infarction within the vascular territory of the left posterior cerebral artery. Other causes include primary and metastatic tumors (406,407,419), arteriovenous malformations (414,420), hemorrhage (408), herpes simplex encephalitis (410), multiple sclerosis (421), and posterior cortical atrophy (399,422).

One popular explanation of pure alexia is a disconnection of visual information from linguistic processing centers (395,423). Visual information from the right hemifield is either absent, in cases with right hemianopia, or interrupted in its course through left extrastriate centers to the "reading center" in the left angular gyrus. Callosal pathways transmitting visual information from visual association cortex of the right hemisphere to homologous regions in the left hemisphere are interrupted by a lesion in the splenium, forceps major, or periventricular white matter surrounding the occip-

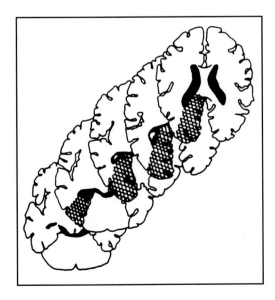

Figure 13.28. Location of lesions causing pure alexia, right homonymous hemianopia, and color dysnomia. Template drawings of axial computed tomographic images, combined from five patients, show lesions affecting the left medial and lateral occipital lobes, medial temporo-occipital lobe and paraventricular white matter, and forceps major, sometimes extending into the splenium proper. (From Damasio AR, Damasio H. The anatomic basis of pure alexia. Neurology 1983;33:1573–1583.)

ital horn of the lateral ventricle (396,424) (Fig. 13.29). Thus, words in the left hemifield also cannot access the left angular gyrus; similarly, other visual information is isolated, causing the associated anomia for colors and objects. Visuolinguistic disconnection may also result from the combined effects of bilateral occipital lesions in patients with bilateral field defects, without splenial damage (425).

Cases of pure alexia without hemianopia have been found with lesions of the white matter underlying the angular gyrus: such "subangular" lesions presumably disconnect the input from both hemispheres to the angular gyrus very distally (406–408,410). Some of these reports conclude that the right hemispheric callosal fibers travel in the white matter ventral to the occipital horn (407,408). Binder and Mohr (397) speculated that some callosal fibers travel dorsal to the occipital horn, and that these are preserved in letter-by-letter or spelling alexia, which they consider a partial form, but are destroyed in global alexia, which they consider the complete form.

Other non-disconnectionist interpretations of pure alexia exist. Some propose that it is a type of simultanagnosia (318). However, tests for simultanagnosia in some patients have been negative (418), although the adequacy of these tests has been disputed (318). Others have argued that letter-by-letter readers cannot access the visual word form, and that pure alexia may be a specific visual agnosia (418,426). The alexic deficit is magnified with script rather than print and with briefly shown words, maneuvers that stress identification of the word as a whole (418). Their use of a letter-by-letter strategy in reading and their need for more time with longer words point to an inability to grasp words as a whole and may represent residual visual processing in the right hemisphere (426). Such a visual agnosia may not be specific for words, but alexia may be its most troublesome manifestation. Apperceptive defects (302,427), simultanagnostic-like defects (418,428–430), and associative defects (431,432) have been proposed. A patient with pure alexia had difficulty in perceiving complex textures, a problem with local pattern analysis that may be relevant to word perception (302). Others have shown that alexia can be associated with subtle disturbances in visual recognition of nonverbal items (427). This agnosia may be restricted to the visual domain: when tested on imagery of letters and words, a patient was able to do much better when allowed to trace letters manually than when he was asked to manipulate visual images of letters mentally (433).

Some indirect support for the agnosia argument also comes from pathologic reports inconsistent with disconnection. One patient had a lesion of the left fusiform and lingual gyrus but no splenial degeneration, which should have occurred if callosal fibers had been affected (434). Another without hemianopia had a lesion in the left lateral occipito-temporal cortex, too ventral to interrupt fibers to the angular gyrus (435). Alexia in the setting of cortical dementia is presumably more likely to be agnosic than disconnective in nature (430).

While some cases of pure alexia may be a visual agnosia from left extrastriate damage, at least some cases do represent a true visual–verbal disconnection. The best evidence

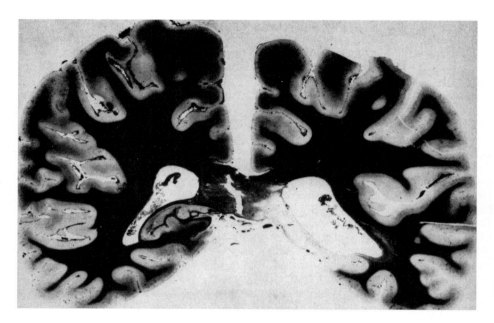

Figure 13.29. The splenium of the corpus callosum in pure alexia (alexia without agraphia). Coronal section through the brain of a 58-year-old man with pure alexia, a right homonymous hemianopia, color anomia, and memory deficits shows infarction and degeneration of the splenium, with associated destruction of the left hippocampus. (From Geschwind N, Fusillo M. Color-naming defects in association with alexia. Arch Neurol 1966;15:137–146.)

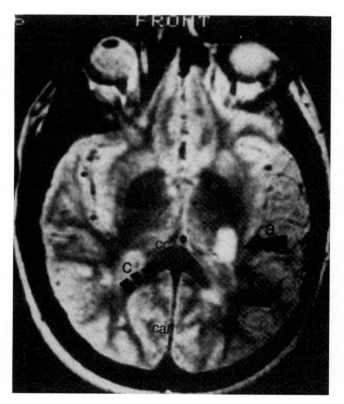

Figure 13.30. Neuroimaging in pure alexia (alexia without agraphia) caused by nonoccipital lesions. Axial magnetic resonance image in a patient with a right homonymous hemianopia, color anomia, and pure alexia shows an infarct of the left posterolateral thalamus affecting the lateral geniculate nucleus (*a*) and an infarct of the lateral aspect of the splenium of the corpus callosum (*b*). Both infarcts are in the distribution of the left posterior cerebral artery. An *arrow* (*c*) shows the direction of input from the intact right occipital lobe through the corpus callosum toward the left angular gyrus. cc, corpus callosum; cal, calcarine cortex. (From Stommel EW, Friedman RJ, Reeves AG. Alexia without agraphia associated with spleniogeniculate infarction. Neurology 1991;41:587–588.)

for disconnection comes from cases of pure alexia with atypical lesions. Pure alexia can occur with the combination of a splenial lesion and a left geniculate nuclear lesion causing right hemianopia (436,437) (Fig. 13.30); there is no damage to striate or extrastriate cortex in such patients. These cases demonstrate that disconnection is sufficient to cause pure alexia. In that light, any claim that an associated visual agnosia or simultanagnosia is responsible for pure alexia in a given patient must prove either that no such disconnection exists in that patient or that the case has features distinct from the pure alexia caused by verified disconnection above.

Prognosis and treatment depend on the underlying pathology as well as the severity of dyslexia. Global alexia can resolve into a spelling dyslexia (424). Interest in rehabilitation of reading in alexic patients is high, with many imaginative strategies currently evolving. These include altering text to highlight the spacing between words or phrases (438,439), enhancing oral articulation during reading (440), repetitive oral reading of text (438), attempts to enhance implicit or covert processing of whole words (439), and finger tracing of letters in patients presumed to have a disconnection syndrome (439,441). The success of these approaches in improving both speed and accuracy requires further evaluation

and will likely require tailoring to the specific reading defect in a given patient.

OTHER DISCONNECTION ALEXIAS

The disconnection hypothesis (395,423) involves two deafferentations of the left angular gyrus: the disconnection of right hemisphere vision and the disconnection or destruction of left hemisphere vision. Each of these has been described in isolation, as hemialexias. In left hemialexia, reading is impaired in the left hemifield only because of isolated damage to the posterior corpus callosum or callosal fibers elsewhere (442,443). This disconnection was visualized recently in one patient with a combination of fMRI and diffusion tensor imaging (443). Right hemialexia has been reported with a lesion of the left medial and ventral occipital lobe that spared other visual functions in the right field (444) (Fig. 13.31).

Left hemiparalexia is a rare syndrome attributed to splenial damage (445). The reading pattern is similar to that in neglect dyslexia, in that substitution and omission errors occur for the first letter of words. However, these patients do not have evidence of hemineglect, and while patients with

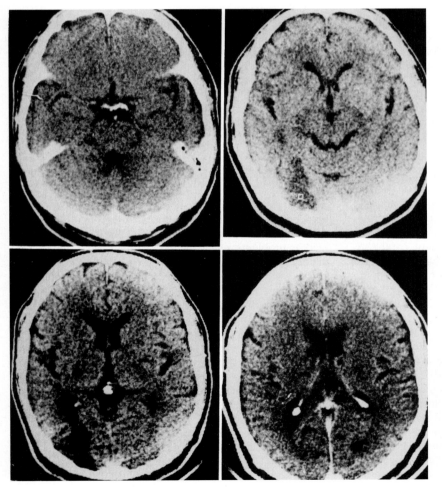

Figure 13.31. Neuroimaging in right hemialexia. Four axial computed tomographic images from a 54-year-old man with a stroke affecting the left medial and inferior occipital lobe, sparing striate cortex, and the forceps major. Although he did not have a homonymous field defect, he could not read letters, words, digits, or arithmetic symbols in his right homonymous hemifield. (From Castro-Caldas A, Salgado V. Right hemifield alexia without hemianopia. Arch Neurol 1984;41:84–87.)

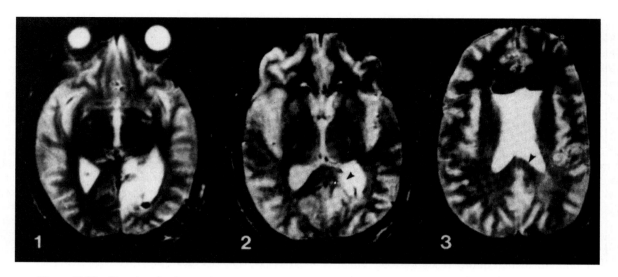

Figure 13.32. Neuroimaging in a patient with left hemiparalexia. *1–3*, Axial T2-weighted magnetic resonance images at three successive levels from a 40-year-old woman who underwent embolization of a left medial parieto-occipital arteriovenous malformation. After the procedure, she had a right homonymous hemianopia, left unilateral tactile dysnomia, and alien hand syndrome on the left. During reading, she missed the letters on the left side of words, even though she had an intact left homonymous hemifield and no left hemineglect. The images show changes consistent with infarction in the left ventral-caudal splenium (*arrowhead,* level 2) and medial occipital lobe (levels 1 and 2), with sparing of the rostral splenium (*arrowhead,* level 3). (From Binder JR, Lazar RM, Tatemichi TK, et al. Left hemiparalexia. Neurology 1992;42:562–569.)

neglect dyslexia often have right hemispheric lesions with left hemianopia, several of the patients reported (445) had left occipital lesions with right hemianopia (Fig. 13.32). There can be other signs of callosal disconnection, such as inability to name objects felt by the nondominant (left) hand, left-hand agraphia, and inability to duplicate the unseen movements of one hand by the other. All the patients reported by Binder et al. (445) had undergone surgery for arteriovenous malformations.

ALEXIA WITH AGRAPHIA

A combination of impaired reading and writing with relatively intact oral and auditory language function constitutes alexia with agraphia. This is associated with lesions of the left angular gyrus (394,423,446), although lesions of the adjacent temporoparietal junction have also been implicated (447). Little is known about this unusual disorder. In keeping with the parietal location, alexia with agraphia may be accompanied by acalculia, right–left disorientation, and finger agnosia, the other elements of Gerstmann's syndrome.

Another form of alexia and agraphia is described as an accompaniment of Broca's aphasia (nonfluent aphasia), which is due to lesions of the dominant (left) frontal lobe. While the difficulty these patients have with reading aloud and writing can be attributed to their difficulty with all forms of expressive language output, their comprehension of written material is also impaired, in contrast to relatively preserved comprehension of auditory language (448,449). In contrast with the letter-by-letter reading in pure alexia, these patients are better at occasionally grasping a whole word, while unable to name the letters of the word; thus, it is some-

times termed literal alexia or "letter blindness." These patients also have impaired comprehension of syntactic structure, just as their speech output often demonstrates a greater impairment of syntax, known as agrammatism. The underlying mechanism is unknown: gaze paresis and difficulty in maintaining verbal sequences have been proposed but not proven (449). It may be that this frontal alexia is a form of deep dyslexia, a type of central dyslexia (393).

DYSLEXIA SECONDARY TO ABNORMAL VISION, ATTENTION, OR EYE MOVEMENTS

Some patients with visual field defects have reading problems despite normal or near-normal visual acuity. Patients with complete homonymous hemianopia may complain of reading problems, hence the term hemianopic dyslexia. This mainly occurs when the central 5 degrees are affected (450). Overall reading speed is more prolonged for patients with right hemianopia than for those with left hemianopia (450,451). With languages written from left to right, patients with left hemianopia have trouble finding the beginning of lines, since the left margin disappears into the field defect as they scan rightwards (452,453) (Fig. 13.33). Marking their place with an L-shaped ruler can reduce this frustration. Right hemianopia prolongs reading times, with increased fixations and reduced amplitude of reading saccades to the right (451–453) (Fig. 13.33). Smaller type and learning to read obliquely with the page turned nearly 90 degrees may help. Reading performance can improve with time as both types of patients learn adaptive strategies (450).

Complete bitemporal hemianopia from damage to the optic chiasm can cause hemifield slide (see Chapter 12).

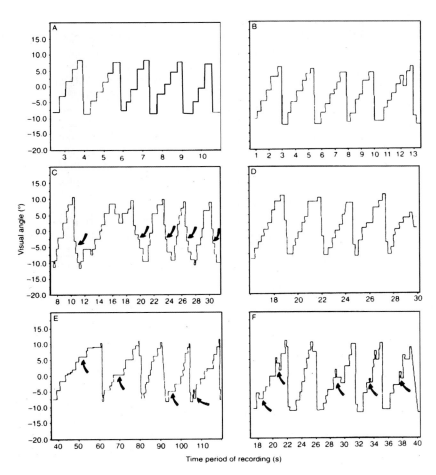

Figure 13.33. Eye movements during reading in normal subjects (*A* and *B*) and in patients with left homonymous and right homonymous hemianopia with either 1-degree (*C* and *E*) or 5-degrees sparing of the macula (*D* and *F*). Horizontal eye positions (on the *y* axis) are shown over time (on the *x* axis) as subjects read lines of a paragraph (positive visual angle is horizontal eye position to the right). *A* and *B*, Traces from normal subjects. *C* and *D*, Traces from patients with left homonymous hemianopia and either 1 degree (*C*) or 5 degrees (*D*) of macular sparing. Note the interruptions of the return sweeps to the beginning of the next line in *C* (*curved arrows*). *E* and *F*, Traces from patients with right homonymous hemianopia and either 1 degree (*E*) or 5 degrees (*F*) of macular sparing. *Curved arrows* in these patients indicate prolonged fixations and regressive leftward movements during line scanning. (From Zihl J. Eye movement patterns in hemianopic dyslexia. Brain 1995;118[Pt 4]: 891–912.)

With only nasal hemifields, there is no region of the visual field that has binocular representation, leading to difficulty keeping the eyes positionally registered with respect to each other and a breakdown of binocular alignment (454). The eyes wander slightly, causing episodic horizontal tropias, with transient diplopia or disappearance of objects along the vertical meridian, and episodic vertical tropias, with a vertical step in objects crossing the vertical meridian. Thus, when reading, letters may disappear or duplicate and lines of words may be confused as they cross from one hemifield into the other.

Disturbances of attention can cause a number of "peripheral dyslexias" (393). Simultanagnosia, in which perception of single items is adequate but perception of several objects simultaneously is impaired, has been implicated in attentional dyslexia (428,429). Patients read single words normally but not several words together; similarly, they identify single letters but not the letters in a word. Their reading may show literal migration errors, in which a letter from one word is substituted at the same place in another (e.g., LONG TURN becomes TONG TURN), and letters of similar appearance are more likely to be confused (e.g., G for C, rather than K for C) (429). Attentional dyslexia has been reported with lesions in the left temporo-occipital junction (429) and the left parietal lobe (428). Its diagnosis rests upon the difference between reading of single versus multiple words, and

the presence of simultanagnosia for other visual items besides words.

Left hemineglect is an attentional deficit that causes neglect dyslexia, manifest by left-sided reading errors (455). This can occur for the whole text, so that the patient misses the left side of a line or page. With individual words, the patient may make omissions (FLAME becomes LAME), additions (ACT becomes TACT), or substitutions (TONE becomes BONE) at the beginning. These defects are specific for left hemispace rather than word beginnings, as such errors do not occur for vertically printed words (455). Many patients with left hemineglect have left hemianopia as well, and the underlying lesion is often in the right parietal lobe, although right frontal and subcortical lesions can also cause neglect. Recognizing that mistakes are restricted to the left side of words or text leads to the diagnosis; associated hemineglect for nonverbal material is usually present, but neglect dyslexia dissociated from other manifestations of hemineglect can occur (456).

Abnormalities of ocular fixation and scanning saccades may impair reading. Most cortical lesions are single and unilateral and tend to cause fairly subtle saccadic abnormalities, if any; however, bilateral frontal or parietal lesions can cause an acquired ocular apraxia, in which the ability to make voluntary saccades to targets is disrupted (11,25,457,

458). As a result, the scanning of a scene is abnormal in these patients (457,458) and reading is consequently impaired (11,25,459,460). While the saccadic abnormality has been blamed for the dyslexia by some (459), simultanagnosia may contribute to the saccadic abnormality with biparietal lesions, and the reading disturbance may be attentional dyslexia. More severe and enduring saccadic and fixation dysfunction occurs with brain stem pathology. Reading difficulties from such lesions have not been well studied, but it has been reported, for example, that progressive supranuclear palsy causes difficulty reading, attributed to the disruption of fixation by square wave jerks and the disruption of scanning by hypometric and slow saccades (461).

CENTRAL DYSLEXIAS

Further types of more subtle acquired dyslexic deficits have been described. Many of these occur in association with other aphasic features and so might be classified as aphasic alexias; however, they occasionally occur as isolated dyslexias also (462). These reading defects are sometimes labeled central dyslexias, as they reflect dysfunction of central reading processes rather than "peripheral" attentional or visual processes. Central dyslexias are formulated in terms of reading models derived from cognitive neuropsychology (393). One of the main concepts involved is that of parallel information processing in reading. The perception of visual features and the abstraction of letter identity are followed by at least two distinct modes of processing. One route is a "direct" phonologic process, in which the units of a letter string are converted into units of sound (grapheme–phoneme correspondence), using the generic pronunciation rules of a given language. These components are then assembled into the pronounced whole word, found in an internal dictionary of word sounds (phonologic lexicon) and linked to information about word meaning in a semantic lexicon. Another route is an "indirect" lexical one, in which the whole word is perceived and identified in an internal dictionary of written words (orthographic lexicon): when the correct word form is activated, a corresponding entry in the semantic lexicon is also activated, leading in turn to access to the phonologic lexicon and the pronunciation of the word. A possible third "rule-based" phonologic route for pronunciation of non-words and unfamiliar words is postulated but controversial (463,464). The anatomic correlates of these different lexical and phonologic reading routes are still uncertain.

Surface dyslexia occurs with disruption of the indirect lexical reading process. Word recognition is critical for pronunciation of words with irregular spelling (e.g., compare LOSE with HOSE). Lacking the ability to access an internal semantic dictionary, patients with surface dyslexia are dependent on the grapheme-phoneme rules that usually apply but that fail with irregularly spelled words. Thus, these patients are revealed by their correct reading of regular words and overregularizing mispronunciations of irregular words (465), just as children might do with unfamiliar words. The best anatomic data on surface dyslexia points to lesions of the posterior superior and middle temporal gyri of the left

hemisphere (466). Surface dyslexia has also been reported in patients with Alzheimer's disease (467,468).

The converse of surface dyslexia is phonologic dyslexia (462–464,469). In the absence of access to grapheme–phoneme correspondence rules for pronunciation, these patients can pronounce only words that already have entries in their internal semantic dictionary. Thus, real words are easily pronounced, whether regular or irregular in spelling, but the reading of non- or pseudo-words (e.g., FRINE) is severely impaired. Their reliance on whole-word processing rather than component or letter processing is revealed by good performance in reading handwriting, contrasted with inability to read words printed backwards (462). Friedman (464) argues that there may be a second form of phonologic dyslexia in which it is not the direct route but the phonologic lexicon itself that is impaired, causing impaired repetition of heard pseudo-words as well as misreading of written pseudo-words. The responsible lesion for phonologic dyslexia is not well defined (393). In one patient an associated right inferior quadrantanopia was present (462), in contrast to the superior quadrantanopsias that accompany pure alexia (396).

Deep dyslexia resembles phonologic dyslexia in the inability to pronounce non-words because of damage to the phonologic route (470). However, patients with deep dyslexia also make semantic paralexic errors with familiar words, characteristically substituting words with a similar meaning for the correct one (e.g., JET for PLANE). Errors are more likely with function words (e.g., and, whether) than with verbs or nouns, and with abstract than with concrete words. Thus, it is argued that deep dyslexia may represent damage to both the direct and indirect reading routes (464). Extensive damage to the left hemisphere is associated with deep dyslexia, and it has been suggested that deep dyslexia represents the remnant reading ability of the right hemisphere (471).

FUNCTIONAL IMAGING OF READING

Only a few functional neuroimaging studies of visual language processing have been published, with conflicting results. Interestingly, activation of the left angular gyrus has not been found, with the possible exception of one study that found spread from the left posterior temporal lobe into the inferior parietal lobe (472). Petersen et al. (473) had subjects first passively view words, read words aloud, then describe uses for the objects represented by the words, a task that requires semantic processing. Striate and lateral temporal extrastriate areas were activated by viewing of a word, reading aloud recruited motor and articulation areas, and the semantic association task activated a left lateral inferofrontal area (474). A later study (475) found activation of the lateral extrastriate areas not only with words and pseudo-words but also with complex letter-like forms (false fonts), suggesting that this was related to processing of complex visual features and not specific for words. Words and pseudo-words, but not the letter-like forms, activated a left medial extrastriate area, which was attributed to activation of visual word forms. Similar preference for alphabetic characters over checkboards has been found in the left medial occipitotemporal sulcus, a region named the ''visual word form area'' (426). While Howard et al. (476) confirmed striate and lateral extrastriate activation with false fonts, they found that reading words activated the left posterior middle temporal gyrus, which they suggested was the location of the visual lexicon.

DISORDERS OF MOTION PERCEPTION (AKINETOPSIA)

Akinetopsia (cerebral akinetopsia) is the term used to describe complete loss of movement perception from an acquired cerebral lesion. Unlike cerebral achromatopsia, which was described in the late 1800s (see above), akinetopsia was not reported until the 1980s, after the discovery of motion-selective extrastriate regions in monkeys suggested that damage to homologous areas in humans might produce a defect in motion perception. Although akinetopsia requires bilateral cerebral lesions, subtler and generally asymptomatic disturbances of motion perception can occur with unilateral cerebral lesions.

Motion perception can play many roles in vision (477). One is the perception of moving objects in the environment. Because objects usually occupy only a small part of the visual field, their perception is facilitated by comparing their motion with that of the background. Object motion guides limb-reaching movements and smooth pursuit eye movements, and it influences saccadic accuracy. In addition to object motion, information about self-motion can be obtained from motion perception. As the observer moves or turns the head or eyes, the image of the entire visual environment moves in the opposite direction. Thus, motion of large portions of the visual field usually implies self-motion rather than motion of an external object. This large-field motion generates optokinetic responses that complement the vestibulo-ocular reflex in stabilizing sight during head motion or self-motion. Information about object identity is also available from visual motion. For example, the difference in motion between a figure and its background reveals two-dimensional shape, and the pattern of velocity gradients within a moving object encodes its three-dimensional form.

There are few clinical tests of motion perception. Smooth pursuit and optokinetic nystagmus can be observed and measured, but only indirect conclusions about the underlying state of motion perception can be made from these. More definitive tests of motion perception, such as animated displays of moving dots (random-dot kinematogram) or moving gratings can be designed to probe discrimination of motion direction, motion speed, the presence of a motion boundary, and forms defined by motion, but these are still experimental tools and are not widely used in the clinical setting.

SYMPTOMS AND SIGNS

Two cases of cerebral akinetopsia have been well described. Patient L.M. was first reported by Zihl et al. in 1983 (47) and subsequently was the subject of numerous reports (26,103,478–481). L.M. had no sensation of motion in depth or of rapid motion (47). When observing objects that were said to be moving rapidly, she noted that they appeared to ''jump'' rather than move (478).

On testing, her predictions of target trajectories were impaired at faster speeds, as was smooth pursuit, although her eyes could pursue a moving tactile target (47). Her perception of differences in temporal frequency or speed of gratings also was impaired (103). The minimum and maximum displacements needed by L.M. to distinguish motion direction were abnormal (103). During testing with random-dot kinematograms, small amounts of random motion (noise) or even stationary dots degraded her performance (26,482). Her use of motion cues for other tasks was also impaired. In a search task, she could not restrict her attention to moving targets, although she could focus her attention on objects of certain shapes or colors, implying an inability to apply a ''motion filter'' to visual scenes. Her use of motion clues to identify both three- and two-dimensional shapes was abnormal, especially when the image contained background noise (26).

Despite the above deficits, L.M. was able to perform a number of motion tasks well. She could distinguish moving from stationary stimuli (47), although her reaction times were slow (478). Contrast sensitivity testing showed that her detection of moving gratings was only mildly affected (103). She could discriminate motion direction for small spots (478) and for random-dot kinematograms that contained very little background noise (26,482).

The other patient, A.F., had somewhat similar deficits (483,484). His ability to discriminate differences in speed was severely impaired, and discrimination of direction in random-dot kinematograms with background noise was abnormal. His smooth pursuit appeared impaired, although it was not quantified. As with L.M., A.F. could not use relative speed differences to perceive two-dimensional forms, but in contrast to L.M., A.F. could use motion cues to discern three-dimensional forms. He also recognized shapes from biologic motion (485).

A.F. had a left incomplete homonymous hemianopia with some sparing in the superior quadrant. He was poor at recognizing objects in noncanonical (unusual) views (486) and in incomplete outline drawings. Tests of spatial vision, such as hyperacuity, line orientation, line bisection, and spatial location, gave abnormal results, as did tests of stereopsis. L.M.'s perception of form was abnormal, and she had an impaired ability to use cues from texture, dynamic stereopsis, or static density to determine form (26).

In L.M., Snellen visual acuity, critical flicker fusion, stereopsis using the Titmus test, color discrimination using the Farnsworth-Munsell 100-Hue Test, perimetry using static, dynamic, color, form, and flicker targets, object/word recognition, and saccadic accuracy were all normal (47). Further testing showed normal results on Lanthony gray luminance discrimination, distance perception, subjective vertical/horizontal, line bisection, line orientation, position matching, matching of object or facial parts, and face recognition (478). Similarly, A.F. had normal contrast sensitivity for static and moving gratings, normal shape discrimination, normal facial and object recognition, normal color discrimination (Farns-

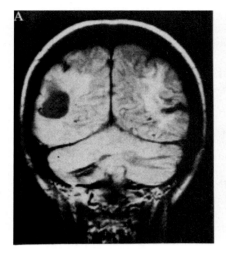

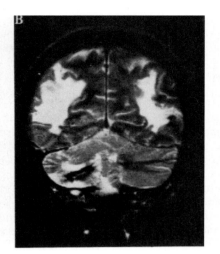

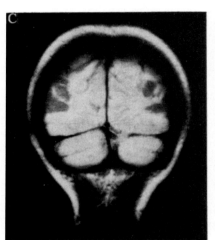

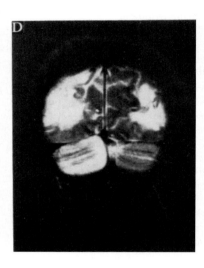

Figure 13.34. Conventional coronal magnetic resonance images through the occipital lobes in patient L.M., who developed bilateral temporo-occipital lesions from sagittal sinus thrombosis with resultant cerebral akinetopsia. *A*, T1-weighted image through midoccipital region shows hypointense areas, right greater than left, consistent with infarcts, surrounded by mild hyperintense areas consistent with edema. *B*, T2-weighted image at same location, showing large hyperintense areas with minimal mass effect on both sides. Note similar areas in cerebellum, primarily in right hemisphere and in the midline. *C*, T1-weighted image through posterior occipital lobes shows persistent bilateral hypointense areas with surrounding minimal hyperintensity. *D*, T2-weighted image at same location shows large areas of hyperintensity in both occipital lobes. (From Zihl J, von Cramon D, Mai N, et al. Disturbance of movement vision after bilateral posterior brain damage. Further evidence and follow-up observations. Brain 1991;114[Pt 5]:2235–2252.)

worth-Munsell 100-Hue Test), and normal color-naming ability.

L.M. had suffered sagittal sinus thrombosis, resulting in bilateral cerebral infarction involving the lateral aspects of Brodmann areas 18, 19, and 39 (lateral occipital, middle temporal, and angular gyri) (42) (Fig. 13.34). Shipp et al. (481) performed PET scanning on the patient, which showed that visual motion induced activation in the medial cuneus bilaterally (probably equivalent to monkey upper V3), the left fusiform gyrus (possibly the border between lower V3 and V4), and the superior temporal lobe (area 7), but not in area V5 (42,43).

A.F. had experienced an acute hypertensive hemorrhage and also had bilateral lesions in the lateral temporo-occipital regions (483,484).

MOTION PERCEPTION DEFICITS WITH UNILATERAL CEREBRAL LESIONS

Unilateral lesions of extrastriate cortex cause more subtle abnormalities of motion perception than cerebral akinetopsia. There are reports of contralateral hemifield defects for speed discrimination (487,488) (Fig. 13.35), for detection of boundaries between regions with different motion (484), and for discrimination of direction from backgrounds of motion noise (489). As in L.M. and A.F., motion detection and contrast thresholds for motion direction are normal in patients with these deficits (487,488), and lesions are located in lateral temporo-occipital cortex or the inferior parietal lobule, but only on one side of the brain. Hemiakinetopsia may not be commonly detected because of masking of the motion-perception deficits by a homonymous hemianopia caused by damage to the optic radiations or striate cortex.

Abnormalities in central motion perception also occur with unilateral lesions. Vaina (490) reported that patients with right temporo-occipital lesions could not identify two-dimensional structures from motion cues, whereas patients with right parieto-occipital lesions could not discriminate velocity or detect three-dimensional form-from-motion. Regan et al. (491) reported similar defects in detecting or recognizing two-dimensional form-from-motion in patients with both right- and left-sided lesions in the lateral temporo-occipital region (Fig. 13.36). Nawrot et al. (492) found ab-

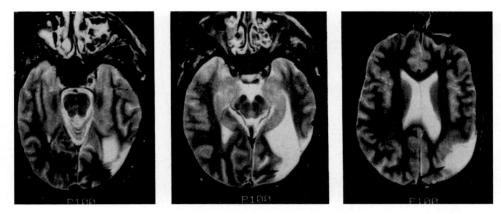

Figure 13.35. Neuroimaging in a patient with impaired contralateral hemifield motion perception. The patient had undergone resection of a seizure focus in the left parieto-occipital region. Following surgery, he had a deficit for speed discrimination in the contralateral (right) homonymous hemifield. T2-weighted axial magnetic resonance images show the extent of the left parieto-occipital lesion. (From Plant GT, Laxer KD, Barbaro NM, et al. Impaired visual motion perception in the contralateral hemifield following unilateral posterior cerebral lesions in humans. Brain 1993;116[Pt 6]:1303–1335.)

normal direction discrimination in seven subjects with right hemisphere lesions. Five had lesions in the temporoparietooccipital area, but two patients had lesions in other locations. In one patient, the lesion was in the ventromedial occipital region; the other patient had an insular lesion. Impaired direction discrimination for motion toward the side of the lesion was reported by Barton et al. (489) in patients with lesions of the lateral temporo-occipital area (Fig. 13.37). There is also some evidence that lesions of the cerebellum adversely affect the perception of motion (493).

The patients described above suggest that human lateral

temporo-occipital cortex participates in a variety of complex motion tasks, including speed discrimination, motion integration over a display to discern average direction and three-dimensional structure, and separation of regions with different motion to discern two-dimensional structure. Elementary spatial and temporal aspects of motion perception and simpler tasks such as detection of motion and discrimination of direction in the absence of noise are not impaired, however. Hence, motion perception is not completely abolished but is impaired in its more interpretative functions; the more elementary motion signals are processed at other cortical

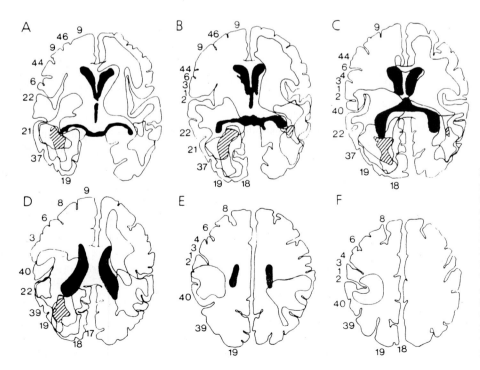

Figure 13.36. Impaired central perception of motion-defined form. Axial template drawings from computed tomographic scans showing the outlines of the lesions of seven patients who had abnormal speed thresholds for recognizing letters whose boundaries were defined by differences in motion from the background. Ventricles are *black,* and *hatched areas* indicate overlap between three or more patients. *Numbers* indicate Brodmann areas of the right hemisphere. (From Regan D, Giaschi D, Sharpe JA, et al. Visual processing of motion-defined form: selective failure in patients with parieto-temporal lesions. J Neurosci 1992;12:2198–2210.)

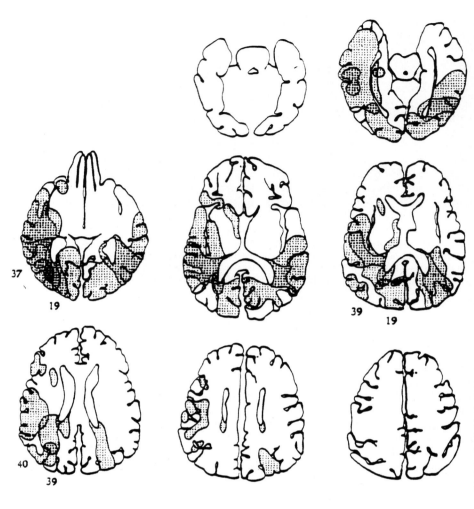

Figure 13.37.   Abnormal central motion direction discrimination. Axial template drawings from computed tomographic or magnetic resonance scans, showing lesions (*stippled areas*) of six patients with abnormal signal-to-noise thresholds for the discrimination of motion direction in foveally presented displays. In most, the defect affected motion primarily toward the side of the lesion. *Numbers* indicate Brodmann areas. Areas of denser stippling indicate greater overlap, with the highest density at the junction of Brodmann areas 19 and 37. (From Barton JJ, Sharpe JA, Raymond JE. Retinotopic and directional defects in motion discrimination in humans with cerebral lesions. Ann Neurol 1995;37:665–675.)

sites, probably at a lower level. The role of lateral temporo-occipital cortex may be to use elementary motion signals to derive a higher-order representation of motion, much as a color region may use elementary striate wavelength responses to derive a higher-order perception of color (22). It is for this reason that the destruction of lateral temporo-occipital cortex does not leave a patient completely motion-blind. Furthermore, other types of motion perception that do not depend upon derivation of local velocity signals, such as ''attention-based'' (or long-range) motion perception, may have a separate neuroanatomic substrate than that involved in akinetopsia. Thus, parietal rather than occipitotemporal lesions disrupt attention-based motion perception but do not affect functioning on the motion tests described above (28). These deficits in attention-based motion perception correlate more with dysfunction in transient attentional processes than defects in motion perception (494).

PHYSIOLOGY OF MOTION PERCEPTION IN NONHUMAN PRIMATES

Several areas in the primate brain respond to visual motion. The best-known is the middle temporal area. MT neu-

rons are selective for both direction and speed (495–499) but not for shape or color (497,500,501). MT has two major projections: to MST and to the ventral intraparietal area (VIP) (501–503). The ventral and dorsal regions of MST may be functionally distinct. Ventral MST responds best to the relative motion of small objects, whereas dorsal MST responds best when visual motion occurs over large portions of the visual field (307). Dorsal MST neurons also respond to large complex motion patterns, such as expanding or contracting radial patterns, and rotating or spiraling motion, which suggests a role in analyzing self-motion (504–510). VIP has not been extensively investigated, but it is known to have cells that are sensitive to moving stimuli (511).

The anterior superior temporal polysensory area contains form-selective and motion-selective cells (351,512). Some of these cells are selective for complex body movements such as hand actions, gait, and head movement (351,513), and these cells may integrate visual input from both cortical streams. A potential polysensory function of STP may be to determine motion relative to the observer by using both visual motion signals from an object and somatosensory, visual, or vestibular information about self-motion (514). Regions in the ventral pathway also have motion responses. Form-selective neurons in the inferotemporal cortex respond to their preferred stimulus regardless of whether the form is defined by luminance, texture, or motion information (515,516).

As there are already direction-selective neurons in V1, several studies have attempted to determine how MT contributes to motion perception. Experiments using transparent motion (517–519) and moving plaids (520,521) show that some MT neurons reduce motion noise by averaging motion vectors over large regions to derive a judgment of common global motion, and that this averaging function is restricted to the motion in the same depth plane, so that perception of moving natural transparent surfaces is not impaired (522). In contrast, V1 neurons respond whenever a motion stimulus in their preferred direction is present, without regard for the presence of other moving stimuli.

Motion can also be separated into first- and second-order types. First-order motion involves displacement of object boundaries that differ in luminance from the background, whereas second-order motion is movement of objects distinguished by cues other than luminance, such as texture and stereo disparity. Most MT cells respond to both first- and second-order motion, suggesting that MT functions as a general motion detector (523,524).

Another possible role for MT is the analysis of relative motion. The direction-selective responses of some MT neurons are inhibited by motion in a similar direction in the surrounding visual field (525–527). This surround inhibition may play a role in figure-ground discrimination, perceptual constancy, and motion cues to depth perception. It may also aid in accurate judgment of object trajectory during eye movements, by comparing object motion to the movement of the background across the retina as the eye moves. These neurons may also play a key role in perception of three-dimensional shape using motion cues (528).

Lesion and stimulation studies may elucidate the role of cortical areas in motion perception. MT or MST lesions cause pursuit and saccades to targets in the contralateral visual field to underestimate speed (529–532). Such lesions also cause deficient motion perception in the contralateral hemifield, as determined with the random-dot kinematogram (533). Schiller (227) also found mild to moderate contralateral impairments in motion detection, direction discrimination, and speed discrimination in monkeys with MT or MST lesions, although these defects were less severe than those from lesions of the LGN, suggesting that other cortical areas contribute to motion processing. Although large bilateral lesions of MT and MST create enduring impairments in a variety of motion tasks (534,535), some recovery after complete lesions of MT and MST does occur and presumably is mediated by other cortical areas (536).

Lesions of either monkey MT/MST (535) or IT (537) impair perception of motion-defined form, implying that both ventral and dorsal streams participate in perceiving form-from-motion. Schiller (227) found that lesions of either V4 or MT alone produced only mild defects in perceiving form-from-motion, but lesions of both together caused a moderate defect.

Microstimulation in MT affects the direction decisions of monkeys viewing a random-dot kinematogram (538–540). Small currents bias the decision in the preferred direction of the stimulated neurons, whereas large currents impair discrimination, presumably from motion noise as current spreads into adjacent neuronal columns.

Psychophysical and physiologic performance have been assessed simultaneously in monkeys viewing moving displays. ''Neurometric'' thresholds based on MT and MST neuronal firing rates for single neurons are similar to the psychophysical performance of the monkey for direction discrimination (537,541,542). Thus, the perceptual performance in monkeys may be supported by a surprisingly small number of MT or MST neurons. In fact, one study found that the perceptual decisions of monkeys could be simulated by the performance of as few as 100 weakly correlated neurons (543).

FUNCTIONAL IMAGING AND OTHER TECHNIQUES

PET scanning studies during motion perception show activation in the lateral occipital gyri, at the junction of Brodmann's areas 19 and 37 (39,42,544). This motion-selective area is most consistently related to the conjunction of the anterior limb of the inferior temporal sulcus with the lateral occipital sulcus (43). Other areas activated during motion perception include V1, V2 (43,545,546), and the dorsal cuneus, which may correspond to V3 (43,546) (Fig. 13.38). Viewing of optic flow increases blood flow in the dorsal cuneus, superior parietal lobe, and fusiform gyrus (547). More complex biologic motions similar to those that elicit responses in monkey area STP were studied by Bonda et al. (548). Goal-directed hand actions activated left hemispheric intraparietal sulcus and caudal superior temporal sulcus, which the investigators considered to be related to syndromes of apraxia with left hemisphere lesions. Expressive body movements activated right superior temporal sulcus, possibly corresponding to monkey area STP, and the amygdala, which is involved in perceiving emotional and social signals (271).

Studies with fMRI show motion-selective responses in the lateral temporo-occipital cortex as well as in V2 and the superior and inferior parietal lobules (549,550). Signal changes in lateral temporo-occipital cortex also correlate with motion after-effects (551). Both motion perception and pursuit-related signals are present in lateral temporo-occipital cortex, suggesting that a possible human homolog of MST is also located here (552).

Visual evoked potential dipoles revealed motion responses in the occipito-temporo-parietal region in a study performed by Probst et al. (553). These results have not been corroborated.

Magnetic stimulation can be used to create temporary dysfunction within specific cortical areas. Stimulation over lateral temporo-occipital cortex impairs motion direction discrimination but not form discrimination in the contralateral hemifield and, to a lesser degree, in the ipsilateral hemifield (156,157,554).

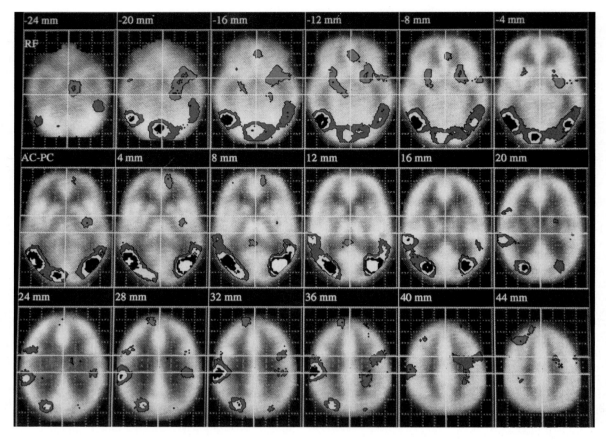

Figure 13.38. Positron emission tomographic study of motion perception. Areas with changing regional cerebral blood flow during motion perception, averaged over all normal subjects. Results are shown in axial section, with *numbers* indicating distance from a line joining the anterior and posterior commissures (negative values are inferior). Pixels indicate changes in blood flow, with black and white pixels indicating areas with highly significant increases in blood flow. Several areas of activation are seen, including the lateral temporo-occipital cortex. (From Dupont P, Orban GA, De Bruyn B, et al. Many areas in the human brain respond to visual motion. J Neurophysiol 1994;72:1420–1424.)

BÁLINT'S SYNDROME AND RELATED VISUOSPATIAL DISORDERS

In 1909, Bálint (25) described a triad of visual defects in a man with bilateral hemispheric lesions. Foremost was an inability to perceive together at any one time the several items of a visual scene, which Bálint interpreted as a "spatial disorder of attention." Holmes (11) used the term "visual disorientation" to describe a similar deficit, whereas Wolpert (555) coined the term "simultanagnosia," the "inability to interpret the totality of a picture scene despite preservation of ability to apprehend individual portions of the whole." Bálint's patient was also unable to move the eyes voluntarily to objects of interest despite unrestricted eye rotations. Bálint (25) called this "psychic paralysis of gaze," although other authors subsequently used such terms as "spasm of fixation" (556) and "acquired ocular apraxia" (557). Finally, Bálint's patient showed "optic ataxia," a defect of hand movements under visual guidance despite normal limb strength and position sense. Among the many reported causes of so-called Bálint's syndrome are cerebrovascular disease (especially watershed infarctions, as in Bálint's orig-

inal case) (Fig. 13.39) (49,558,559), tumor, trauma, prion diseases such as Jakob-Creutzfeldt disease, infection by human immunodeficiency virus (HIV) type 1 (560), and degenerative conditions such as Alzheimer's disease (561, 562).

Wolpert's (555) definition of simultanagnosia can be operationalized as an inability to report all the items and relationships in a complex visual display, despite unrestricted head and eye movements. A suitable screening tool is the Cookie Theft Picture from the Boston Diagnostic Aphasia Examination (563) or any similar picture containing a balance of information among the four quadrants (Fig. 13.40). The patient's report can be correlated with a checklist of the items in the picture. Exclusion criteria should include aphasia severe enough to impair the verbal descriptions of a display, so as to avoid confusing a defect of language with one of visual perception. It is also crucial to exclude or at least be aware of defective visual acuity or visual fields. For example, objects may seem to vanish into a central scotoma,

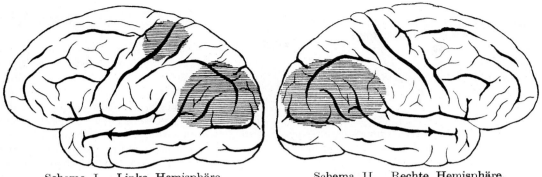

Schema I.   Linke Hemisphäre.   Schema II.   Rechte Hemisphäre.

Figure 13.39. Drawing of the locations of the major lesions in the case described by Bálint in 1909, as pictured on lateral views of the hemispheres. The views are idealized and do not convey the full extent of the pathology. The surface of the brain was actually atrophic. Not seen in this view are several lesions of potential importance to the patient's behavior presentation. These included lesions of the posterior white matter in which optic radiations travel on both sides, and of the pulvinar, a critical structure for visuospatial integration in primates. (From Bálint R. Seelenlahmung des "Schauens," optische Ataxie, röumliche Storung der Aufmerksamkeit. Monatschr Psychiatr Neurol 1909;25:51–181.)

paracentral scotoma, or hemianopia, causing complaints that mimic simultanagnosia. Extensive peripheral scotomata (564) or marked constriction of the visual fields, such as occurs in patients with retinitis pigmentosa or chronic atrophic papilledema, may hinder visual search and "simultaneous perception," despite unrestricted viewing, thus also producing an incoherent report.

Interestingly, the term "simultanagnosia" has little to do with the visual disorders now understood by the term "agnosia" (565). As noted above, patients with agnosia cannot recognize previously familiar objects or persons (49). Some patients diagnosed with "Bálint's syndrome" also may not recognize objects and faces (although Bálint's patient could). However, this is caused by their profound perceptual impair-

ments, as described under the old term "apperceptive agnosia" (566). This differs from true (associative) agnosia, in which relatively normal percepts are stripped of their meanings (567; see above).

The terms "ocular apraxia" (from the Greek word meaning "not acting") and "optic ataxia" (from the Greek word *ataktos,* meaning "disorderly") are also not helpful in conveying the underlying mechanisms in cases such as that described by Bálint (25), and some original investigators were even confused by the terminology and definitions (457,568). Also, acquired ocular apraxia must be distinguished from congenital ocular motor apraxia, a childhood disorder in which head thrusts occur with voluntary refixation despite a full range of reflexive saccades (557,569; see Chapter 19).

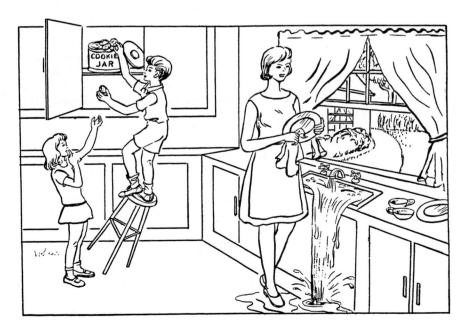

Figure 13.40. The Cookie Theft Picture from the Boston Diagnostic Aphasia Examination. This picture contains a balance of information among the four quadrants. The patient is asked to describe the events depicted in the picture.

According to Benton (570), a critical appraisal of a syndrome should include definition, behavior, anatomy, mechanism, and theory. Using these guidelines, Bálint's syndrome may not exist as a sufficiently autonomous complex. Affected patients often have a number of other devastating defects in behavior, such as hemineglect (571), and the triad of components in Bálint's syndrome are not as closely bound as might be expected. Moreover, individual components of the syndrome appear to represent broad categories comprising other, more specific defects. Furthermore, Bálint's syndrome does not appear to have the specific neuroanatomic significance attached to it by Bálint (25) (i.e., bilateral damage to the angular gyri), and it is not clear that the components of Bálint's triad have any special status compared with other defects associated with lesions in a similar location. Conversely, "Bálint's syndrome" occurs with bifrontal lesions (572), and a similar disorder was described by Ogren et al. (573) associated with lesions of the pulvinar. Simultanagnosia occurs in patients with bilateral lesions of the superior (dorsal) portions of both occipital lobes in Brodmann's areas 18 and 19 (565,574). Bilateral lesions of Brodmann's areas 6 and 8 (the frontal eye fields) may cause defective voluntary saccades, visual search, and scanning, compatible with ocular apraxia. Optic ataxia is associated with a wide variety of lesions in Brodmann's areas 5, 7, 19, 39, and 37, and a profound reaching disturbance was even reported with a relatively mesial right temporo-occipital lesion (575).

The wide variety of perceptual phenomena reported in cases such as Bálint's (including "vanishing" objects, tilted vision, metamorphopsia, palinopsia, and of the "positive" phenomena described below) are not likely to represent the behavioral expression of a single underlying neurophysiologic mechanism. Rather, Bálint's syndrome may include a combination of deficits resulting from lesions of the dorsolateral visual association cortices, which include the putative human area MT complex and its projections to the parieto-occipital cortex. Damage to these areas and to the cortices surrounding the angular gyrus and parietal insular cortex can disturb multiple aspects of spatial and temporal processing, including the perception of visual motion (47), structure from motion and dynamic stereopsis, the perception of egomotion, and coordination of visual (eye-centered) and vestibular (gravity-centered) coordinate systems that orient us in the physical world. Bilateral lower quadrantanopias may co-occur (11) from damage to the primary visual cortex lining the dorsal banks of the calcarine fissure (human area V1), thus adding to a patient's overall problem.

PSYCHOANATOMICAL SUBSTRATES IN BÁLINT'S SYNDROME

Twenty-four reports of "simultanagnosia/Bálint's syndrome," compiled by the Oxford University Press (576), provide an overview of key theoretical issues, lesion localization, underlying pathology, and standardized assessment techniques employed. A diversity of deficits, lesions, vision assessment, and opinions is clearly evident in these articles.

Rizzo and Vecera (577) reviewed psychoanatomic substrates of Bálint's syndrome and emphasized the role of deficits of visual short-term memory (working memory) and attention. James (578) defined attention in its modern sense as an ability that enhances our performance on behavioral tasks by focusing the mind on one item and withdrawing from other competing items. The report by Bálint (25) provided preliminary evidence of a neural substrate of attention. The lesions in his patient produced an attentional reduction in the visual fields manifested by failure to detect objects in the periphery (more so on the left). Indeed, reductions in the useful field of vision that are not caused by a visual field defect of luminance or form are now well described in elderly or demented patients (579,580; discussion following). This effective field reduction is associated with difficulty functioning in a complex visual environment, such as encountered while driving a motor vehicle (581,582).

Standard perimetry tasks (such as Goldmann and Humphrey perimetry) minimize attention demands to gain maximal estimates of sensory ability, leading to overestimates of functional ability in elderly or brain-damaged individuals engaging in real-world tasks that demand peripheral vision (581,583). Reduction in the useful field of view (UFOV), the visual area from which information can be acquired without moving the eyes or head, correlates with increased vehicle crash risk (579,582). UFOV task performance depends on speed of processing, divided attention, and selective attention. The efficiency with which we can extract information from a cluttered scene begins to deteriorate by age 20 years (584).

Patients described as having Bálint's syndrome may have impaired control over the focus of visual attention. Executive functions control our allocation of attention between competing sources of information (585,586). Focused attention helps consolidate information temporarily stored in working memory, the process that allows us to store representations for brief times until they can be attended to. Without focused attention, traces of retinal images in working memory fade without being consciously perceived or remembered (inattentional amnesia). We can be unaware of marked changes in an object or a scene (change blindness). The very act of perceiving one item in a rapid series of images briefly inhibits ability to perceive another image (the attentional blink).

Change blindness (CB) is a form of blindness that can occur despite normal vision and is the inability to detect critical changes in a scene due to a brief visual disruption. The disruptions can include saccades, flickers, blinks, camera cuts (587), or gradual image changes (588). CB probably depends on spatial attention and visual working memory (589). CB occurs when working memory is occupied by other information, is more likely when working memory capacity or duration is impaired (e.g., due to aging, drugs or fatigue, or neurologic disease (590,591)), and can help explain perceptual problems in patients like Bálint's.

The attentional blink (AB) is another type of blindness that can occur even in people with normal vision. When we identify a visual object, our ability to perceive a second object is impaired for several hundred milliseconds (because visual working memory is still occupied by the first object when the second arrives). This period, known as the AB, is not due to an eye blink and can be measured in a laboratory setting using a rapid serial visual presentation (RSVP) of visual targets (often a sequence of letters) on a computer monitor. The AB can increase pathologically due to reduced temporal processing speed and working memory in patients with a variety of brain lesions (592).

Navigating through the world, which was difficult for Bálint's patient, requires "executive attention" to switch the focus of attention between critical tasks such as tracking the terrain, monitoring the locations of nearby obstacles, finding landmarks, and perceiving the trajector of self-motion while walking (593). This involves switching attention between disparate spatial locations, local and global object details, and different visual tasks and is thought to rely on mechanisms in prefrontal areas (594).

PERCEPTION OF VISUAL OBJECT STRUCTURE, MOTION, AND DEPTH

In addition to the visual attention and working memory impairments described above, the lesions in Bálint's syndrome produce various defects in perception of visual object structure, motion, and depth. Information on object structure and depth is so important for interacting with objects and obstacles that our brains employ multiple cues (595). These cues include accommodation, convergence, binocular disparity, motion parallax, texture accretion/deletion, convergence of parallels, position relative to horizon, relative size, familiar size, texture gradients, edge interpretation, shading and shadows, and aerial perspective (596). Understanding the relationships among these redundant cues is an active research topic.

Perception of structure-from-motion (SFM) or kinetic depth is a real-world use of motion perception that may fail in patients with visual cortex lesions due to stroke (597) or early Alzheimer's disease (598). SFM deficits in drivers with brain lesions are associated with increased relative risk for safety errors and car crashes in driving simulation scenarios (599). Recovery of depth from motion relies on relative movements of retinal images. For motion parallax, relative movement of objects is produced by moving the head along the interaural axis. Impairments of motion parallax may be a factor in vehicle crashes in drivers with cerebral impairments or drug intoxication, who must make quick judgments with inaccurate perceptual information regarding the location of surrounding obstacles (600).

Displacement of images across the retina during self-motion (ego-motion) produces optic flow patterns that can specify the trajectory of self-motion with high accuracy (601–603). Perception of heading from optical flow patterns can decline due to aging and drugs such as marijuana (THC) and Ecstasy (MDMA), presumably due to chronic effects on cholinergic receptors (with THC) and serotoninergic/5HT-2 receptors (with MDMA) (604). Processing of visual motion cues also may be impaired in patients taking antidepressants such as nefazodone (Serzone®) that block serotonin reuptake (605).

Detecting and acting to avoid impending collision events requires information on self-motion and approaching ob-

jects. Objects on collision paths with us maintain a fixed location in the field of view, while "safe" objects will translate to the left or right side. Time-to-contact (TTC) is estimated from the expanding retinal image of the approaching object. Older drivers are less accurate than younger drivers at telling whether an approaching object in the environment will crash into them (606,607). Performance is worse for longer TTC conditions, possibly due to a greater difficulty in detecting the motion of small images in the field of view (608).

NAVIGATION

Navigating a route relies on visual perception, attention, spatial abilities, and memory. Topographic disorientation (TD) is a term that has been used to describe patients who have navigation problems despite normal or near-normal visual sensory abilities (609,610). Patients with TD may have lesions in inferotemporal regions, posterior parahippocampal regions, and hippocampus, especially in the right hemisphere. Causes of TD include stroke, trauma, and neurodegenerative diseases, including Alzheimer's disease (611). Associated problems include visual agnosia and other memory-related disturbances.

One form of navigation difficulty, "topographagnosia," is associated with prosopagnosia and achromatopsia (272,273,277,279,327,346,383). In these patients, the problem is an inability to identify familiar landmarks and buildings, "landmark agnosia" (612). This form occurs with right ventral temporo-occipital lesions (344,613). The origins of landmark agnosia are debated. Some propose that it reflects a selective multimodal memory disturbance rather than a strictly visual problem (344). However, functional imaging also suggests that buildings and places activate a specific region in occipitotemporal cortex, the "hippocampal place area," which is adjacent to the fusiform face area (614). Lesions of this region could create an agnosia specific for landmarks, and the frequent association with prosopagnosia may reflect the proximity of face and place processing in cortex.

In a second form, the spatial processing needed to describe, follow, or memorize routes is disrupted, usually by right parietotemporal lesions (613,615). It has been suggested that the key deficit with such lesions is an "egocentric disorientation," in which subjects cannot represent the location of objects and buildings with respect to themselves (609).

A third, related form is a "heading disorientation," in which there is a failure in representing direction with respect to cues in the external environment, rather than in reference to the subject. This has been associated with posterior cingulate lesions (616). This may have also been the case with a rare patient with a left parahippocampal and retrosplenial lesion who had defective route-finding associated with alexia and other severe visual amnestic deficits (617).

Parahippocampal lesions have also been implicated in an "anterograde topographagnosia," in which new routes cannot be learned though old routes are still known (618).

Aspects of complex disorders of visual processing associated with navigation impairments can be tested with the Trail Making Test, Benton Visual Retention Test, and Complex Figure Test (619,620). Lanca et al. (621) provided testing details in a recent review.

DISORDERS OF VISUALLY GUIDED REACHING AND GRASPING

Reaching and grasping external objects is a fundamental activity that demands the coordination of several different nervous system functions (622,623). To accomplish this task, the brain transforms a target's visual coordinates to body-centered space, plans a hand path and trajectory (the sequence of hand position and velocity to target), and computes multiple joint torques, especially about the shoulder and elbow. It also specifies the necessary limb segment orientations from among many possibilities, activates appropriate muscle groups, and inhibits others to meet those specifications. The sensory feedback, frames of reference, and neural mechanisms used to solve these complex motor control problems are active research topics (624–628).

Reaching can be separated into two different phases. In the transport phase of reaching, the hand is moved toward an object whose position is determined by vision or memory. In the acquisition phase, grasp formation depends on somatosensory and visual information on the limb and target (629), familiarity with the target, and, perhaps, predetermined motor programs. These two phases mature at different rates, may be controlled independently before becoming coordinated (630–632), and can be dissociated by focal brain lesions (633–635). Posterior parietal damage may affect neurons coding eye position in the head and stimulus location on the retina that, together with neurons in motor and premotor cortex, permit hand movements to visual targets in a body-centered coordinate system (628). The schema

proposed by Soechting and Flanders (626,636,637) takes origin at the shoulder, is closely related to the representation of object position and motion, and should depend on the visual cortex and its connections to other sensory and motor maps (638–640).

The observations of Bálint (25) on what he called optic ataxia sparked interest in the neural basis of visually guided reaching and grasping. In this condition, patients reportedly reach as if blind toward targets they nevertheless can see and describe (Fig. 13.41). Limb strength and position sense are normal; however, there is severe visual sensory loss and poor visuospatial perception, and patients may even appear demented because of their extensive bilateral lesions, as in the original case reported by Bálint (25) (discussed earlier). Inability to reach and grasp targets in these cases is often multifactorial, including V1-type visual field defects, defective visual attention, and inability to locate targets with the eyes. Another possibility is abnormal sensorimotor transformation, an inability to transform the visual coordinates of external objects to appropriate limb coordinates for generating accurate reaches.

The patient described by Bálint (25) had left hemineglect caused by extensive damage to the right inferior and superior parietal lobules. Lesions in these locations are likely to produce visuomotor difficulty in reaches conducted with the left hand to both visual fields (hand effects) and with both hands to the left visual fields (field effects) (634,641). Thus,

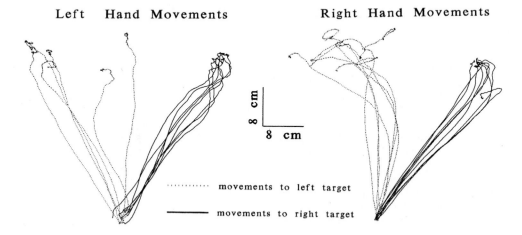

Figure 13.41. The paths of abnormal hand movements under visual guidance in a case of optic ataxia. The patient is viewed from above as he reaches for highly visible targets located at arm's length to the left and right of body midline. The recordings rely on an optoelectronic technique to transduce the position of an infrared light-emitting diode target fastened to the dorsum of each index fingertip. Multiple reaches are shown with the left hand and right hand. All movements begin from the same midline position just anterior to the patient. Head movement is unrestricted. The results show that trajectories of the hand movement are highly variable. The end positions of the movements are quite inaccurate, especially to the left target. The patient's hand movements actually improved for reaches to self-bound targets (body parts) and for reaches to remembered targets in the absence of vision (the latter conditions are not shown here). The patient also had simultanagnosia. (From Rizzo M. "Balint's syndrome" and associated visuospatial disorders. Baillieres Clin Neurol 1993;2:415–437.)

although Bálint (25) emphasized that his patient had trouble locating visual targets with the right hand, there is reason to suspect that left-hand control also was impaired. Observations on the reaching behavior in patients with focal circumscribed lesions of visual cortex can help clarify these issues (e.g., 79,567,575). Patterns of recovery in optic ataxia were reported by Goodale et al. (635). Anatomic substrates for visually guided reaching and lesions that affect underlying sensorimotor transformations were recently reported by Darling et al. (642,643).

POSITIVE VISUAL PHENOMENA

Most often cerebral lesions affect vision by creating deficits, or ''negative phenomena.'' On occasion, they may also create ''positive phenomena,'' when false visual images are seen by the patient. These false visual images can be classified as visual perseverations, hallucinations, and distortions (dysmetropia).

VISUAL PERSEVERATION

The persistence, recurrence, or duplication of a visual image is a rare complaint in patients with cerebral lesions. Several varieties exist, including palinopsia, polyopia, and illusory visual spread. Palinopsia (or paliopsia) is the perseveration of a visual image in time (644). Whereas the content of visual hallucinations is often imagery created de novo, or sometimes from the distant past (experiential hallucinations), the palinopsic illusion contains elements of a more recently viewed scene, or even one that is still being viewed. Nevertheless, the difference is not always distinct, and patients can have both perseverative and hallucinatory phenomena concurrently (644,645). Cerebral diplopia or polyopia is the perseveration of a visual image in space, when two or more copies of a seen object are perceived simultaneously (646–649).

Another spatial perseveration is ''illusory visual spread,'' in which the contents or surface appearance of an object spread beyond the spatial boundaries of the object (644). Thus, wallpaper patterns spread beyond the surface of the wall, and cloth patterns spread from a shirt to the wearer's face (644). In the experience of some (650), this is invariably associated with visual field defects, and it is suggested that the basis of this perseveration is analogous to the ''filling in'' process that minimizes the perceptual disruption at the physiologic blind spot.

Both spatial and temporal perseveration can occur in the same patient, as in palinopsic polyopia (647,651). Some patients report that as an object moves they see multiple copies of the object in its trail: though this may be considered an example of cerebral polyopia, it is clearly a form of palinopsia also. As yet another possible combination, Bender et al. (645) argued that since palinopsic images were often larger than the original images in their experience, this represented an illusory visual spread frequently concomitant with palinopsia; however, Critchley (644) thought that this combination was the exception rather than the rule.

Palinopsia

It is suggested that there are at least two forms of abnormal persistence of a visual image in time, an immediate and a delayed type. With the immediate type of palinopsia, an image persists after the disappearance of the actual scene, usually fading after a period of several minutes. This type of palinopsia bears some similarity to the normal phenomenon of an afterimage experienced after prolonged viewing of a bright object. Detailed studies of some patients have concluded that the differences between normal afterimages and such palinopsic images are primarily quantitative (651), although others disagree (645). With the delayed type of palinopsia, an image of a previously seen object reappears after an interval of minutes to hours, sometimes repeatedly for days or even weeks (651). Some patients have both immediate and delayed types of palinopsia (651).

The perseverated image can assume almost any location in the visual field. It may persist in the same retinal location as the original image, which is usually at the fovea, and thus move as the eyes move, much as a normal afterimage does (652). Sometimes the image is translocated into a coexistent visual field defect (644), and indeed this can be a transient feature in the evolution of cerebral homonymous field defects (645). Sometimes the image is multiplied across otherwise intact visual fields (647) (Fig. 13.42). On rare occasions, the location of palinopsic images is contextually specific, as when patients report that after viewing a face on television, everyone else in the room has the same face as the person on television, or that the sign over one shop reappears on the boards over other shops (644,647,653) (Fig. 13.43). While some of these cases may represent a complex form of palinopsic polyopia, others may also be consistent with a constant foveal or perifoveal perseverative image that manifests itself repeatedly when the context is appropriate.

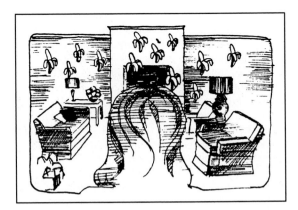

Figure 13.42. Palinopsia. Illustration of visual images experienced by a 71-year-old woman with complaints of seeing multiple objects. In this case, she had just peeled a banana and now saw multiple vivid images of the banana projected over the wall. She realized that they were only images and were not real. (From Michel EM, Troost BT. Palinopsia: cerebral localization with computed tomography. Neurology 1980;30:887–889.)

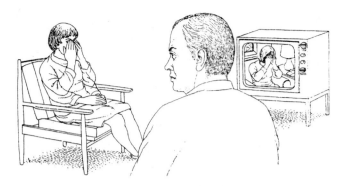

Figure 13.43. Palinopsia. The patient experienced the illusory image of hands rubbing across his wife's face after seeing an actress rubbing her own face on television. (From Bender M, Feldman M, Sobin A. Palinopsia. Brain 1968;91:321–338.)

A wide range of other symptoms can accompany palinopsia. An associated homonymous visual field defect is virtually always present, with reports of both upper (651,653) quadrantanopias. There may be other spatial illusions, such as metamorphopsia, macropsia, and micropsia (267,644,645, 651). Less frequently, "ventral stream" deficits have been reported, such as topographagnosia, prosopagnosia, and achromatopsia (346,645). Cummings et al. (652) reported an unusual patient with perseveration in both visual and somatosensory modalities, and another patient with a left temporoparietal tumor had both auditory and visual palinopsia (654).

The prognosis for visual perseveration is not clear. Bender et al. (645) considered palinopsia to be a rare transient phase in either the resolution or progression of a visual field defect, which usually lasted from days to months. However, other cases of palinopsia have persisted for months and years (651,652,655,656). Anticonvulsant medication such as carbamazepine may help some patients (655,657) but not others (652).

The pathophysiologic mechanism of palinopsia is still unclear. Four main hypotheses have been advanced (645): a pathologic exaggeration of the normal afterimage, a seizure disorder, hallucinations, and psychogenic origin.

Kinsbourne and Warrington (651) found many features in two patients that suggested that their (immediate-type) palinopsia represented an exaggeration of the normal afterimage. The vividness of the palinopsic image correlated with the intensity and duration of the initial stimulus. When the palinopsic image was visualized against a light background, it appeared as a negative (complementary color) afterimage. After monocular viewing of an object, the palinopsic image appeared binocularly. Lastly, the afterimage moved in the same direction as active eye movements but in the opposite direction when the eyes were moved passively. However, not all cases of immediate palinopsia exhibit these features; the color of palinopsic images does not depend strongly on the colors of the original stimulus, for one (645,656).

The hypothesis that palinopsia is a manifestation of epilepsy is supported mainly by circumstantial evidence. Several patients in early reports had other features that suggested seizures, such as episodic loss of consciousness, tongue biting, and confusion (644,645). More recently, epileptiform abnormalities on EEG and a good response to anticonvulsants have been reported in some patients with the immediate type of palinopsia (267,655,658), and in one patient with a delayed form (659), although improvement with anticonvulsants does not prove ictal origin.

The third hypothesis is that palinopsia may be a nonictal hallucinatory state. Some patients have both palinopsia and coexistent nonpalinopsic visual hallucinations. Also, the location of perseverative images within visual field defects is reminiscent of the release hallucinations of the Charles Bonnet syndrome. Furthermore, drugs that induce hallucinations can cause palinopsic illusions as well (651). Cummings et al. (652) suggested that delayed palinopsia with hemianopia was a release hallucination, whereas immediate palinopsia was more likely due to a seizure, especially when there was no accompanying visual field defect. The mechanistic value of this distinction has not yet been validated.

Psychogenic palinopsia was considered by Critchley (644), who postulated that palinopsic reports may be a confabulatory response to other visual dysfunction. Palinopsia may also occur without visual dysfunction in a psychiatric context, where it may be associated with other perseverative and misidentification delusions like Capgras syndrome (the belief that familiar people have been replaced by duplicates) (660).

Drug-induced palinopsia must first be considered. Intoxication with hallucinogens such as mescaline, LSD, and Ecstasy (MDMA) can cause palinopsia, sometimes permanently (661,662). Isolated reports have asserted that palinopsia and other visual illusions may occur with prescribed medication, such as clomiphene (663), interleukin-2 (664), trazodone (665), nefazodone (666), mitrazapine (667), or withdrawal from paroxetine (668). Second, it can occur with metabolic states such as nonketotic hyperglycemia (669). Third, palinopsia can occur in psychiatric conditions such as schizophrenia (660,670) and psychotic depression (671), but it is always accompanied by other signs of mental illness.

Once intoxication and metabolic and psychiatric conditions are excluded, however, visual perseveration suggests the possibility of a cerebral lesion. As always, a variety of lesions are possible, including brain abscess (672), tuberculoma (673), and hemorrhage (674). However, there are several cases of perseverative phenomena with other visual damage. Palinopsia has been reported in two patients with optic neuritis, one with Leber's hereditary optic neuropathy and one after photocoagulation for diabetic maculopathy (675,676). A survey of 50 patients with severe visual loss from ocular lesions found that in addition to release hallucinations, one or two had palinopsia, polyopia, or illusory visual spread (650). Also, some patients with palinopsia have apparently normal neurologic and ophthalmologic function and no history of drug use (676).

The localizing value of palinopsia is not clear. Bender et al. (645) found a predominance of right parieto-occipital lesions, although they acknowledged that left hemispheric lesions may have been underrepresented because of aphasia. Critchley (644) documented right, left, and bilateral lesions. While others have also found parietal pathology (674,677), there are also reports of medial occipital and occipitotemporal lesions in some cases with CT and autopsy specimens (647,653,673,678). In two cases, no lesion was found with neuroimaging (656,679), although in one the patient was eventually found to have Creutzfeldt-Jakob disease.

Cerebral Polyopia

Cerebral polyopia or diplopia is much less frequently described than palinopsia. It occurs with monocular viewing, distinguishing it from diplopia due to tropic misalignment of the eyes. As a cause of monocular polyopia, it must be distinguished from polyopia due to abnormalities of the refractive media, which often have specific treatments (680–682). However, unlike refractive polyopia, it does not resolve with viewing through a pinhole, and it is present with either eye viewing alone. In some patients cerebral polyopia occurs only in certain gaze positions, causing confusion with tropic diplopia until its monocular nature is realized (646). The number of images seen can range up to over a hundred, in one unique case of "entomopia" (649). Associated signs in Bender's series included frequent visual field defects, difficulties with visually guided reaching (optic ataxia), achromatopsia, object agnosia, fluctuations in the visual image, and abnormal visual afterimages. However, the diplopia in Meadows' (648) case was associated only with a small homonymous inferior left scotoma. The patient described by Lopez et al. (649) had no signs at all, although his symptoms were very brief, lasting only minutes, and a transient associated defect may have escaped detection. A recent review suggests that apart from such highly atypical cases, coexistent hemifield defects are the rule (683).

Among Bender's (646) wartime cases, cerebral polyopia often occurred as a transient phase in the recovery from cortical blindness due to occipital missile wounds. In two cases recovery followed a progression from cortical blindness to cerebral polyopia, then cerebral diplopia. Other causes in the older literature include encephalitis, multiple sclerosis, and tumors (646). A more recent patient had an infarct in peristriate cortex (683).

The origins of this rare symptom are obscure. It may be that polyopia is merely a variant of palinopsia, with perseverated and real images coexisting in time (683). Bender (646) suggested an analogy with the monocular diplopia that sometimes develops in strabismic patients who have both a true and a false macula, along with a disorder of unstable fixation that would cause the retinal image to shift over these falsely localizing regions. Gottlieb (684) also noted a correlation of polyopia with eye movements into the hemianopic field, but both Meadows (648) and Lopez (649) have contested the necessity of the abnormal fixation or eye movements.

VISUAL HALLUCINATIONS

Hallucinations are perceptions without external stimulation of the relevant sensory organ. Individuals vary in the degree of insight they possess—that is, whether they recognize these experiences as being "not real." Some propose the term "pseudohallucinations" for experiences with preserved insight. However, insight can fluctuate over time in an individual (sometimes it is gained only after attempted interaction with the phantom) and can vary within a group with a common pathology. Also there is no proof that insight has any pathogenetic significance, other than that it may correlate with the degree of associated cognitive or psychiatric impairment. Therefore, the term "hallucinations" is probably best used for all such experiences, regardless of insight.

Hallucinations are also sometimes divided into simple and complex forms. Simple hallucinations consist of brief flashes of points of light, colored lines, shapes, or patterns (phosphenes) (685–687) (Figs. 13.44 and 13.45). Complex hallucinations contain recognizable objects and figures (688), such as scenes of humans and animals moving (689–692), with a potential for bizarre, dreamlike imagery of considerable detail and clarity, including dragons, angels, and miniature policemen (693,694). There is considerable debate over the value of the simple/complex dichotomy in terms of its diagnostic and localizing value.

In the differential diagnosis of hallucinations, one of the chief considerations is whether there is any associated mental or cognitive dysfunction. When this is present, hallucinations can be associated with other conditions, the three most important being intoxication, psychiatric illness, and cogni-

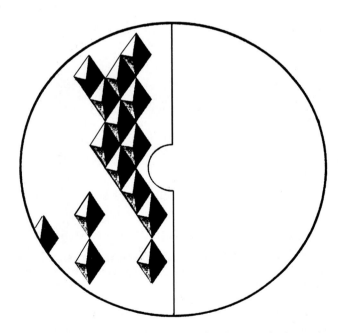

Figure 13.44. Appearance of simple hallucinations. Drawing by a patient with simple hallucinations in the left homonymous hemifield shows a pattern of pyramids adjacent to one another. The sides of each pyramid were colored red, yellow, green, or blue. The hallucinations gradually subsided, coincident with the development of a left homonymous hemianopia. Neuroimaging revealed changes consistent with an infarct in the right occipital lobe. (From Kölmel HW. Colored patterns in hemianopic fields. Brain 1984; 107:155–167.)

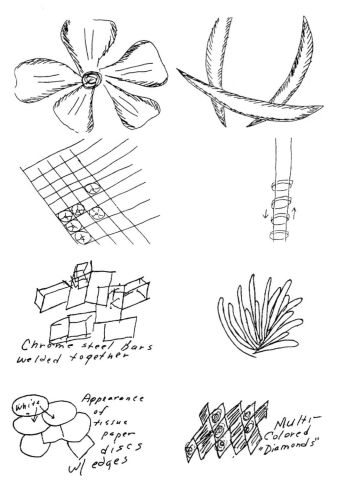

Figure 13.45. Appearance of both simple and complex hallucinations. Drawing by a patient with occipital lobe damage showing his most frequent hallucinations. Some are complex (*top*); others are simple (*middle and bottom*). (From Anderson SW, Rizzo M. Hallucinations following occipital lobe damage: the pathological activation of visual representations. J Clin Exp Neuropsychol 1994;16:651–663.)

tive dysfunction associated with neurodegenerative conditions.

Hallucinations with Altered Mental States

Drugs and intoxicants are particularly important cause of hallucinations. These include bupropion (695), baclofen withdrawal (696), dopaminergic agonists (697,698), ganciclovir (699), vincristine (700), and serotonin reuptake inhibitors such as fluoxetine and sertraline (701). With illicit drugs, hallucinations can occur for several months after use, sometimes recurring years later in relation to use of alcohol or medication (702). A transcranial magnetic stimulation study has shown that subjects with hallucinations related to Ecstasy (MDMA) use have hyperexcitable occipital cortex, probably related to alterations in serotonin levels (703).

Hallucinations also occur in psychiatric disorders, although visual hallucinations are usually accompanied by hallucinations in other sensory modalities (especially auditory) and by other signs of mental illness.

Hallucinations with Cognitive Dysfunction

Hallucinations are not rare in patients with dementia (704) or confusional states secondary to metabolic insults, including alcohol withdrawal, where they form the predominant type of hallucination (705). Among patients with Alzheimer's disease, hallucinations may be more common in patients with poor refraction or cataracts (706), and are correlated with atrophy of the occipital lobe (707). Other risk factors for hallucinations in Alzheimer's disease include not only greater cognitive deficits and accelerated rate of decline but also associated parkinsonism (708).

Of note, hallucinations are one of the defining criteria for diffuse Lewy body dementia, along with parkinsonism, dementia, and fluctuating levels of arousal. They occur in over 90% of patients with this condition, compared to 25% of patients with Alzheimer's (709). In diffuse Lewy body disease their incidence appears to correlate with the density of Lewy bodies in inferior temporal cortex (710).

Hallucinations also occur in about 25% of patients with Parkinson's disease (711). These are almost exclusively visual and almost always complex (712). While in some cases these can be caused by medications, it appears increasingly likely that they are a manifestation of the underlying disease process (712,713). A number of studies have shown that risk factors for hallucinations in this disease are longer duration and greater severity of the disease, depression and sleep disturbances, and some cognitive impairment (712–715). Many factors may contribute to the pathogenesis of hallucinations in Parkinson's disease. REM-sleep anomalies have been described, raising analogies with the hallucinatory experience in narcolepsy (716,717) and implicating cholinergic and serotonergic pathways in the brain stem (688). Impaired visual function may play a role, as some studies have shown that hallucinations are associated with worse visual acuity (713), defective visual memory (715), and poor performance on object-recognition tasks (718). Cognitive problems are more common and may contribute through a general degradation in information processing or a disruption in the ability of subjects to monitor reality and the origins of internal experience (715,718).

Treatment of hallucinations in neurodegenerative disorders involves consideration first of drugs that might be exacerbating the problem. A visual examination should determine whether there are any correctible causes of visual decline, such as cataracts or inadequate refraction (719). Better refraction can improve hallucinations in Alzheimer's disease (706). Last, medications could be used. In Parkinson's disease, there has been some success with cholinesterase inhibitors, such as rivastigmine (720), and with agents that treat REM-sleep disorders, such as clonazepam (717).

"Release Hallucinations" (Charles Bonnet Syndrome)

Visual loss of any origin can result in visual hallucinations (721). These are called "release hallucinations" because it is thought that they arise or are "released" in visual cortex through the absence of incoming sensory impulses. Release visual hallucinations are associated with central or peripheral visual field defects, which are usually binocular. Estimates of their prevalence vary, from 15% among patients with retinal disease (722) to 57% of patients with a variety of causes of visual loss (692).

The true incidence is underestimated because of the reluctance of patients to mention hallucinations for fear of being labeled "crazy": 73% of patients in one series had never mentioned the hallucinations to a physician (694). In fact, patients with release hallucinations are mentally lucid; most are aware that the visions are not real, and in general they are not distressed by them (694). Notable is the absence of other sensory hallucinations, although there are some exceptions.

Release hallucinations can be either simple or complex. Simple stimuli can include flashes or highly intense colors, termed "hyperchromatopsia" by some (650). Sometimes the vision is a recognizable image from the patient's past, such as a deceased relative (689,691,694,723). There are even reports of hallucinations of the self. Lepore (692) estimated that simple hallucinations are at least twice as common as complex ones. Even complex hallucinations may not be unusual, though, as several series have suggested an incidence of 10–30% for complex hallucinations in visual loss (692,693,724,725). Some authors reserve the term "Charles Bonnet syndrome" for the association of visual loss with complex formed hallucinations (693,725). However, some patients have simple hallucinations initially that evolve into complex ones (689,691,726). A similar progression in visual hallucinatory content is reported in normal people subject to sensory deprivation (727). Since the type of release hallucination also does not correlate with the site of visual loss (689), the distinction between complex and simple release hallucinations lacks diagnostic value.

Some of these visual hallucinations have perseverative features. A recent survey coined several terms for these (650). Among patients with ocular causes of severe visual loss, 37% had tessellopsia, in which the hallucinations had a fine repetitive geometric pattern, and 14% had dendropsia, in which a repetitive branching motif is seen.

There must be other contributing factors besides visual loss in the development of release hallucinations, since they do not develop in all patients with visual loss: of 505 patients with visual loss, only 60 (12%) met one study's criteria for complex release hallucinations (694). Age is one possibility. In the review by Schultz and Melzack (693), 80% of patients with hallucinations were over 60 years old, and the mean age at onset in the study by Teunisse et al. (694) was 72 years. This may simply represent the demographics of bilateral visual loss, however, and even subjects as young as 6 years can have release hallucinations (693,728,729). Social isolation is another potential factor, thought to act by accentuating the sensory deprivation of visual loss (730). The prospective study of Teunisse et al. (725) found a trend toward hallucinatory patients living alone or being widowed. The dictum that release hallucinations occur in patients with normal mental state has been questioned, as Cole (730) found that cognitive impairment was a feature in 9 of his

13 patients. On the other hand, Schultz and Melzack (731) found no evidence of cognitive dysfunction or depression in 14 patients on a psychological test battery, suggesting that cognitive decline is not a necessary factor. Hallucinations in some cases have been potentiated by drugs, such as estrogen (732).

Hallucinations often begin close to the time of visual loss. Most often they follow the onset of visual loss by several days or weeks, but this delay can be even longer (690,691). When the disease causing visual loss is ocular and occurs first in one eye and then in the other, it is often not until the second eye loses vision that hallucinations develop (690,726). Among patients undergoing photocoagulation for macular degeneration, hallucinations occur in about 60%, usually a few days after the procedure (426). Hallucinations may also occur simultaneous to the onset of visual loss, so that in some cases it is the complaint of visual hallucinations that leads to the discovery of a visual field defect. Rarely it has been possible to show that hallucinations actually preceded hemianopia by a few days (685). Among four patients with visual loss from giant cell arteritis, hallucinations were reported to begin 1–10 days before visual loss, and to disappear within a few weeks (733).

The hallucinations can be brief, with each episode lasting a few seconds or minutes, or they can be virtually continuous (693). Frequency varies from several per day to twice a year (694). They tend to occur in the evening and night, under poor lighting, and during periods of inactivity or solitude (694). The time during which patients suffer from continuous or recurrent hallucinations may be limited in some cases, lasting from a few days to a few months, but they often persist for long periods, sometimes years or decades (690,691,694). In Kölmel's series (724), the mean duration of complex hallucinations was 11.5 days. Kölmel (685) also felt that the occurrence of colored patterns in hemianopia indicated transient damage to the optic radiations rather than a permanent striate lesion, and that they were a good prognostic sign for the recovery of hemianopia.

Release hallucination do not bother many patients, and some subjects are reported to even enjoy them (693,694). Most patients have insight that the hallucinations are not real, although this can fluctuate and may be achieved only after an attempt to interact with the hallucinations (721). For these, treatment of the visual disturbance is not indicated, beyond reassurance concerning the significance of the hallucinations. However, a few patients may find them annoying, although only 6 of 60 patients studied by Teunisse et al. (694) were sufficiently troubled to consider pharmacotherapy. Unfortunately, there is no agreement on effective treatment. Anticonvulsant drugs have improved the hallucinations in some cases (691,734,735) but not others (690,691). Carbamazepine is probably the treatment of choice (736). Mixed results have occurred with haloperidol (726,730). There are isolated reports of benefit with tiapride (737), neuroleptics such as risperidone (738) and melperone (736), and gabapentin (739). Moving socially isolated patients into a more stimulating environment may lessen the hallucinations (730).

Any type of binocular visual loss can lead to release hallucinations (690). The most common damage in Lepore's (692) series of 104 patients was cerebral, mostly infarctions. Cataracts were most frequent among ocular causes of visual loss. In another series of 60 patients, macular degeneration and diabetic retinopathy were most common (694). Others have also reported retinal disease (726) and pathology of the optic nerves and chiasm (689). It is generally agreed that no other pathology besides the disorder causing visual loss is required for release visual hallucinations; that is, they are not a direct manifestation of an underlying cerebral lesion, but a physiologic reaction to loss of vision. However, if so it then remains to be determined why all subjects with binocular visual loss do not have hallucinations. As well as the factors mentioned above such as age, social isolation, and possibly subtle cognitive impairment, there is one report of increased incidence of posterior periventricular white matter lesions on MRI in patients with hallucinations from ocular disease (740), an interesting finding in need of verification.

In most reported series, there is some degree of bilateral visual loss in almost all patients (689,690). However, the need for binocular pathology has been questioned (692). Also, occasional patients have no or minimal demonstrable visual loss and yet have similar visual hallucinations (690,692,730). "Release" hallucinations can occur in normal subjects in sensory deprivation experiments (727), and it is possible that some subjects with hallucinations but without binocular visual loss suffer a similar deprivation in conditions of social isolation, especially since their hallucinations can resolve with a change in surroundings (730).

Schultz and Melzack (693) summarized the various theories about visual release hallucinations. When there has been intracranial pathology, hallucinations have sometimes been attributed to visual seizures (691); however, Cogan (690) distinguished release hallucinations from seizures by their longer duration and variable, nonstereotyped content, as well as association with visual loss rather than secondary motor or sensory epileptic events (693). By analogy with epilepsy, earlier reports of visual hallucinations with optic nerve pathology hypothesized a seizure-like "irritation" of the optic nerve (689). With visual loss due to media opacities such as cataracts, another hypothesis was that hallucinations were entoptic phenomena, being the subject's interpretation of the image of retinal blood vessels, the retinal ganglion network, and other ocular structures cast upon the retina. The entoptic theory is clearly untenable in patients with enucleations and hallucinations. Most today believe that all release hallucinations have a similar origin, within the brain rather than in the eye. In the brain, visual experience is represented by patterns of coordinated impulses within the vast neural network within visual cortex. These patterns are generated by sensory stimuli and represent the current experience of the individual; however, it is proposed that the brain has an inherent capacity to generate these neural patterns spontaneously, and will in fact do so during sensory deprivation from either imposed isolation (727) or pathologic denervation (693). These spontaneous neural patterns then correspond to hallucinations. For simple stimuli, it has even been proposed that the types of geometric patterns spontaneously

generated may reflect the underlying anatomy of the "stripes" in V2 cortex (741).

A similar explanation has been invoked for the phantom limb phenomenon after amputation, and presumably also underlies other release phenomena such as musical hallucinations in cases of deafness (742). Supporting evidence for the analogy with sensory deprivation includes the fact that these hallucinations tend to occur when patients are alone or inactive, in the evening or night, when the lighting is poor (694). More recently, single photon emission computed tomography (SPECT) and functional imaging have been used to demonstrate that release hallucinations are associated with hyperperfusion and increased metabolism or activity in extrastriate visual areas and thalamus (743–746).

Visual Seizures

Only about 5% of epileptic patients have visual seizures (747). These occur exclusively in patients with occipital or temporal lesions (748). When they do occur, they can be confused with migraine and release hallucinations. Indeed, much of the confusion around the localizing value of the visual content of hallucinations stems from failure to distinguish between release hallucinations and visual seizures. Conclusions that "the complexity of the hallucinations has no localizing value" originated in a discussion of release hallucinations with optic nerve disease (689). Clearly, the content of release hallucinations is highly variable and independent of the site of pathology: rather, it is the associated field defect that has localizing value in this setting. However, the same conclusion may not be valid for visual seizures (690). Older human stimulation experiments (749) found that simple unformed flashes of light and colors resulted from electrical activity in striate cortex, whereas stimulation of visual association cortex in areas 19 and temporal regions resulted in complex formed images. A similar distinction probably holds for epileptic visual hallucinations, though there are discrepancies in the literature. Patients with occipital lesions are more likely to have "elementary hallucinations," meaning simple geometric forms like squares, circles, zigzag lines, or unformed flashes or lights (748, 750,751) (Fig. 13.46), although there are some exceptional cases with complex hallucinations (751,752) (Figs. 13.47 and 13.48). In such cases, spread of ictal activity into extrastriate cortex is likely responsible for the complex character of the hallucinations (751,753). Seizures originating in occipitotemporal or anterior temporal structures are more likely to be associated with "complex hallucinations," such as objects, words, or animals (754), but these can also have elementary hallucinations (748). Whether the elementary characteristics are due to intrinsic visual properties of certain regions of the temporal lobe or to spread of ictal activity to the occipital lobe is not clear. Overall, a study of 20 patients concluded that elementary hallucinations could occur with either temporal or occipital foci, but that complex hallucinations were far more likely to indicate a temporal origin of seizures (748).

The distinction between visual seizures and release hallucinations can be difficult in patients with cerebral lesions.

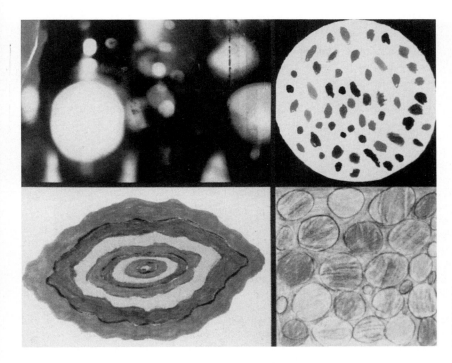

Figure 13.46. Visual illusions of occipital lobe epilepsy as perceived by four different patients. (From Panayiotopoulos CP. Elementary visual hallucinations in migraine and epilepsy. J Neurol Neurosurg Psychiatry 1994;57:1371–1374.)

Cogan (690) believed that release hallucinations were continuous and nonstereotyped in their content, whereas visual seizures were brief episodes with the same vision in all seizures. However, Schultz and Melzack (693) questioned this distinction, pointing out that release hallucinations can be episodic rather than continuous, and that their content can also be repetitive. They suggest that the association with other ictal phenomena or a visual field defect is more helpful. Accompanying head or eye deviation (usually but not always contralateral) and rapid blinking are common accompani-

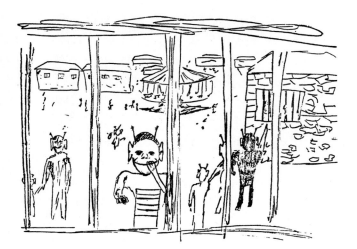

Figure 13.47. Appearance of complex visual hallucination caused by a right-sided occipital lobe cavernous hemangioma. (From Lance JW, Smee RI. Partial seizures with visual disturbance treated by radiotherapy of cavernous hemangioma. Ann Neurol 1989;26:782–785.)

ments of occipital seizures (751). Other features that also strongly support ictal origin are signs of more distant spread of seizure activity, such as confusion, dysphasia, tonic-clonic limb movements, and the automatisms of complex partial seizures. However, homonymous field defects indicate only the possibility of release hallucinations, since lesions that cause epilepsy may also cause visual field defects. In some cases, it has been felt that complex hallucinations in hemianopia might represent a combination of ictal and release phenomena (724). The diagnostic uncertainty may be resolved by seizure monitoring, although the routine scalp EEG leads often do not localize the occipital focus accurately (751,753). Suspicion of such a focus usually requires intracranial electrodes for confirmation (751).

Visual seizures are treated with the same anticonvulsants used for other focal seizures. Carbamazepine appears quite effective (747).

Although a variety of pathology in visual cortex may be associated with visual seizures, one syndrome requiring emphasis is "benign childhood epilepsy with occipital spike-waves" (755). This is an idiopathic epilepsy syndrome that begins between ages 5 and 9 and ceases spontaneously in the teenage years. Seizures are characterized by blindness and/or hallucinations of both simple and formed types and may progress to motor or partial complex seizures. Some children develop nausea and headache following the visual seizure, leading to an erroneous diagnosis of migraine. The diagnosis is established by occipital spike waves occurring during eye closure on EEG.

Migrainous Hallucinations

A variety of visual phenomena can occur in migraine (756). In classic migraine, the visual phenomena precede the

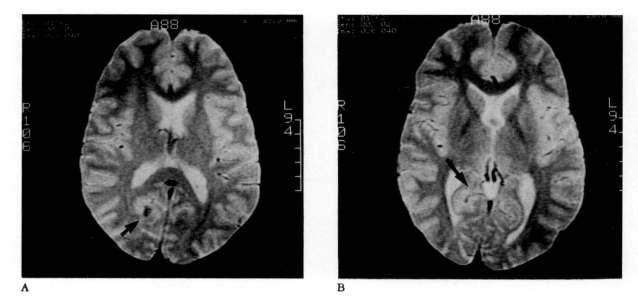

Figure 13.48. Neuroimaging appearance of the lesion causing the hallucination seen in Figure 13.47. *A*, T2-weighted MR image, axial view, shows small circumscribed hypointense lesion (*arrow*) consistent with a cavernous angioma in the right occipital lobe. *B*, Adjacent T2-weighted axial MR image shows small vessel adjacent to the region of the lesion (*arrow*). (From Lance JW, Smee RI. Partial seizures with visual disturbance treated by radiotherapy of cavernous hemangioma. Ann Neurol 1989;26:782–785.)

headache, whereas in migraine equivalent the visual phenomena occur without a subsequent headache. Photopsic images are most common, described as spots, wavy lines, or a shimmering like heat waves over a road on a hot day (757). The ''scintillating scotoma'' is a blind region surrounded by a margin of sparkling lights, which often slowly enlarges over the time of its presence. In some individuals the sparkling margin can be discerned as a zigzag pattern of lines oriented at 60° to each other (758), usually in one hemifield, and on the leading edge of a C-shaped scotoma (Fig. 13.49). This is the ''fortification spectrum'' or ''teichopsia'' (*teichos* being Greek for town wall), based on the resemblance of the zigzag margin to the ground plan of town fortifications in Europe (758) (Fig. 13.50). There may be several sets of zigzag lines in parallel, often shimmering or oscillating in brightness (759). They may be black and white (750) or vividly colored (758,759). These zigzag lines begin near central vision and expand toward the periphery with increasing speed over a period of about 20 minutes, with both the speed and the size of the lines increasing with retinal eccentricity (Fig. 13.49). The relation of speed and size to eccentricity is predicted by the cortical magnification factor, which is a measure of the area of visual field represented in a given amount of striate cortex as a function of retinal eccentricity (758,760). This suggests that these migrainous hallucinations are generated by a wave of neuronal excitation spreading from posterior to anterior striate cortex at a constant speed, leaving a transient neuronal depression that causes the temporary scotoma in its wake (759). It is also hypothesized that the zigzag nature of the lines reflects the sensitivity to line orientation of striate cortex and the pattern

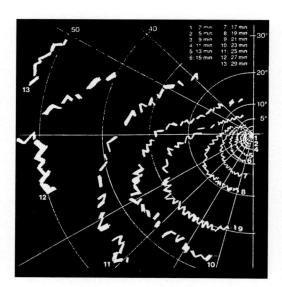

Figure 13.49. Photographic negative of a migraine phosphene protocol. The scintillating phosphene was progressing through the lower quadrant and part of the upper quadrant of the left visual hemifield. Thirteen drawings were made between 2 and 29 minutes after the phosphene first appeared near the center of the visual field. To evaluate the distance between the phosphene and the center of the visual field, several radii were drawn across the protocol. The angular distance from the fovea center, computed in degrees of visual angle, is indicated by *circles*. Circles and radii were added to the sheet after the observations were made. Observation distance = 34 cm. (From Grüsser OJ. Migraine phosphenes and the retino-cortical magnification factor. Vision Res 1995;35:1125–1134.)

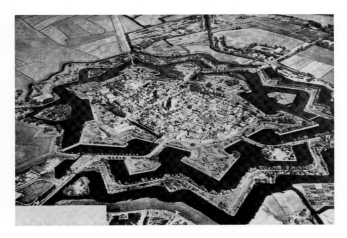

Figure 13.50. Aerial view of Naarden, a city with typical fortifications from which the concept of "fortification scotomas" originated. Note the jagged appearance of the walls and moats round the city. (From Plant GT. The fortification spectra of migraine. Br Med J [Clin Res Ed] 1986; 293:1613–1617.)

of inhibitory interconnections within and between striate columns (759,760).

Distinguishing migraine from epilepsy is an important problem for hallucinations, especially as visual seizures rarely progress to other clearly ictal symptoms (747). Both migraine and visual seizures can feature abnormal hallucinations followed by headache and vomiting (747,761). It has been suggested that the two disorders can be distinguished by their visual content, with black and white zigzag lines in migrainous hallucinations and colored circular patterns in ictal hallucinations (750,762). However, migraine-like hallucinations have been described with occipital seizures from cysticercosis (763). Other important distinguishing features are that seizures are briefer, usually lasting a few seconds or minutes, spread more rapidly than migrainous hallucinations, and always occur in the same hemifield (747). Episodes are also more frequent for visual seizures than migraine. Accompanying eyelid fluttering or eye deviation would also suggest seizure rather than migraine.

Other Hallucinatory States

Hallucinations with midbrain lesions were first described by Lhermitte (764), with coining of the term "peduncular hallucinations" and its first pathologic verification by van Bogaert (765). They are still considered rare. Their nature has many similarities to complex release hallucinations with visual loss, as described above. They can be continuous (766,767) or episodic (768,769), with detailed formed imagery such as flying birds, dogs, roaring lions (768), crawling snakes, gangsters with knife wounds (767), and men herding cattle (770), for example. These hallucinations are not stereotyped, varying from one episode to the next. As with release hallucinations, in some cases with thalamic rather than midbrain infarcts the hallucinations are from events in the patient's past (774). Patients often have insight that they are not real (766,768,771), but some do not possess

this (774) and may even interact with the hallucinations (772). Similar hallucinations have been described for sounds (773); some patients have multimodality hallucinations, involving vision, touch, sound, and even the sense of body posture (767,768).

Unlike release hallucinations with visual loss, peduncular hallucinations are almost invariably associated with inversion of the sleep–wake cycle, with diurnal somnolence and nocturnal insomnia (764,766,767,770,774). Other associated signs from damage to adjacent structures in the midbrain include unilateral or bilateral third nerve palsy (764, 766,770), hemiparkinsonism (769), hemiparesis (766), and gait ataxia (764,772). Many patients have had pre-existing visual loss (766,772), prompting some to speculate that this may be a contributing factor. However, there are other patients with relatively intact vision also (768,771).

Since the original pathologic description by van Bogaert (765), there have been reports with neuroimaging demonstrating unilateral or bilateral infarction of the peduncles with this condition (766,769). A detailed pathologic study showed bilateral infarction of the substantia nigra pars reticulata (768). The correlation of neuronal activity in this structure with REM-sleep stages and its connections to the pedunculopontine nucleus suggested an anatomic correlate to the disturbed sleep–wake cycle thought to underlie both the hallucinations and the associated inversion of the sleep–wake pattern in these patients. Others have postulated damage to the reticular formation and the ascending reticular activating system with similar consequences (772). There are also a few cases with similar hallucinations from lesions restricted to the paramedian thalamus, which may affect the thalamic reticular nucleus (772,774,775).

The most frequently described etiology is infarction (766,768,769,772), with peduncular hallucinosis included as one of the top-of-the-basilar syndromes (776). It has also been described as a vascular complication of angiography (771) and transiently after microvascular decompressive surgery for trigeminal neuralgia (767). There are two cases with extrinsic midbrain compression by tumors, a craniopharyngioma (777) and a medulloblastoma (770). In cases with infarction, the hallucinations can persist indefinitely (768), though the episodes may become shorter (774) or disappear (772). Hallucinations have resolved after relief of extrinsic tumor compression (770,777).

Miller Fisher has described a number of patients with hallucinations only with eye closure (778,779). In two cases the visual hallucinations were attributed to drug toxicity, due to atropine and probably lidocaine given for local anesthesia; in the other the hallucinations occurred during a respiratory infection with high fever. Parallels were drawn with hypnagogic hallucinations, and Fisher hypothesized a disturbance in sleep–wake cycle mechanisms. While these may be thought rare, we recently encountered two similar cases of visual hallucinations with eye closure occurring in the postoperative period after major surgery.

Local retinal dysfunction can cause hallucinations. These are being increasingly recognized as a common but transient side effect of photodynamic therapy for macular degeneration, for example, often developing several days after the procedure (426).

VISUAL DISTORTIONS (DYSMETROPSIA)

Illusions about the spatial aspect of visual stimuli include three main categories: micropsia, the illusion that objects are smaller than in reality; macropsia, the illusion that objects are larger than in reality; and metamorphopsia, the illusion that objects are distorted. Of these, micropsia is probably the most common and has the largest variety of possible etiologies.

Micropsia

Etiologically, several types of micropsia exist. Convergence-accommodative micropsia is a normal and long-recognized phenomenon in which an object at a set distance appears smaller when the observer focuses at near rather than far, although there has been no change in the retinal angle covered by the object and no change in its spatial relations to the surround. Investigations of this induced micropsia at near (or alternatively, macropsia at far) conclude that vergence rather than accommodation is responsible (780–782). Convergence micropsia may play a role in preserving size constancy at small distances (781). Its origins remain unclear, although there are older suggestions that the size of visual receptive fields is modified by the act of convergence (783). It is unusual for accommodative micropsia to be a source of complaint.

Psychogenic micropsia has also been reported among psychiatric patients, where it has been subject to psychoanalytic interpretations, with subjects literally trying to "distance" themselves from environments fraught with conflict (784–786).

Retinal micropsia occurs in conditions where the distance between photoreceptors is increased. The micropsia usually occurs in foveal vision, secondary to macular edema. There may be associated metamorphopsia if the edema and receptor separation is irregular. Visual acuity is also reduced due to photoreceptor separation, and it has been found that grating acuity correlates with psychophysical measures of micropsia (787). Causes of macular edema and micropsia include central serous retinopathy, severe papilledema (787), and retinal detachment (788). A prior history of macular detachment for at least 10 days was noted in a small sample by Sjostrand and Anderson (788), with the development of cystoid macular edema in some patients. In others, the micropsia was thought to indicate subclinical macular edema. The condition may resolve or may persist for years. While it has been suggested that retraction with scarring may cause micropsia to change into a more permanent macropsia, other studies show that micropsia from separation of photoreceptors can be long-standing (788). Retinal micropsia is often monocular but can be binocular, depending on the type of ocular pathology. Matching techniques that demand relative size judgments in relation to the normal eye have been developed and can serve as a useful monitor of disease progression (787,788).

Cerebral micropsia is rare. In contrast to retinal micropsia,

it is binocular. Unusual variants include hemimicropsia in the contralateral hemifield (789,790). One unusual case had hemimicropsia only for faces (791). Given the small number of cases, the localization value of cerebral micropsia is uncertain. Occipitotemporal lesions have been reported, with either medial (791,792) or lateral (790) involvement.

A recent survey of over 3,000 adolescent students revealed that complaints of episodic micropsia or macropsia were not rare, occurring in 9% (793). Some occurred in the hypnagogic state or during fever, and there was a correlation with a history of migraine. This possible migrainous micropsia, which we would presume to be a variant of cerebral micropsia, is reminiscent of an earlier description of micropsia occurring during migraine (794) (Fig. 13.51).

Macropsia

Macropsia is much less frequently described than micropsia. Retinal macropsia can occur in the late scarring stage of macular edema. It has been reported as a side effect of zolpidem use (795). Wilson (794) had a case of cerebral macropsia occurring during seizures. Cerebral hemimacropsia has also been reported with a left occipital tumor (796) and with a right occipital infarct (797). Both macropsia and micropsia occurred in a large sample of students surveyed (793).

Metamorphopsia

Peripheral causes of metamorphopsia are probably more common than cerebral metamorphopsia. Most often this occurs as a result of retinal pathology. Most often this is related to macular edema, and it may coexist with micropsia as a result (788), but disorders that cause traction on the retina may also distort the retinal map, such as an epiretinal membrane (798). Amemiya et al. (799) suggested a correlation with the segmental buckling procedure. As with retinal micropsia, the metamorphopsia from ocular disease is monocular; if due to binocular disease, it is unlikely that the distor-

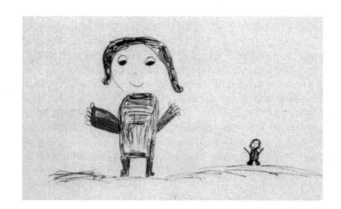

Figure 13.51. Drawing of cerebral micropsia by a child with migraine. The child stated that during some of her attacks, other children (*right*) appeared unusually small to her (*left*). (From Hachinski VC, Porchawka J, Steele JC. Visual symptoms in the migraine syndrome. Neurology 1973; 23:570–579.)

tions will be identical in the two eyes. Psychophysical tests of hyperacuity that require the alignment of dots or comparison of dot spacing in a dot bisection task have been developed to quantitate metamorphopsia in these conditions (800).

Cerebral metamorphopsia has been described with seizures (267,801,802). One patient had a right parietal glioma (267), and another was a boy with a right parietal arteriovenous malformation, whose metamorphopsia was limited to faces (802). It has also occurred with posterior cerebral infarction (803), once as a transient stage in the development of cortical blindness (804). The lesions with infarcts have been medial, however, with one lesion said to involve only the left cingulate gyrus and retrosplenial area (803). There is also one report of metamorphopsia due to brain stem lesions (805).

VISUAL LOSS IN AGING AND DEMENTIA

Many adults experience a decline in their ability to function effectively and independently in later life. Such a decline is multifactorial and includes impairment of vision from common eye conditions, such as age-related macular degeneration, glaucoma, and cataract. For instance, cataract can cause yellowing of the lens, producing a relative tritanopia; glaucoma causes visual field defects; and macular degeneration impairs central visual acuity and spatial contrast sensitivity and may also be associated with visual hallucinations, as described above. The risk of cerebrovascular disease increases with age, and ischemia with infarction causes the majority of visual impairments described earlier in this chapter.

Another cause of visual dysfunction in aging persons is dementia. Alzheimer's disease is the most common cause of dementia in the elderly, and the number of persons with this condition is projected to increase sharply by the middle of the 21st century. Alzheimer's disease often impairs recognition and visuospatial processing, and visual dysfunction can be the dominant early manifestation in a visual variant of the disease known as posterior cortical atrophy (576). In these patients, visuospatial dysfunction can be so marked as to suggest Bálint's syndrome (806). Impairment of motion perception (807) and visual recognition (260,562) also occurs in patients with Alzheimer's disease. Visual complaints may also be the earliest manifestation of Jakob-Creutzfeldt disease (808). However, visual abilities also decline as a function of normal aging of the nervous system in the absence of any diagnosable eye or brain disease. This important factor is often ignored in the interpretation of visual dysfunction.

Aging of the nervous system affects information processing at several levels, from the coding and storage of sensory inputs to the retrieval and modification of that stored information (809). There may also be a reduction in the powers of attention. Attention is needed to allocate a finite set of cognitive resources to a barrage of external and internal stimuli. Deterioration at one or more of these levels reduces the speed of processing and overall performance on a wide variety of everyday tasks ranging from walking and dialing a telephone to highly visual tasks such as driving, reading, or searching for a familiar face in a crowd.

Aging can also affect the temporal resolution of the visual system (810,811). Older adults require longer delays between successive stimuli before both are seen as separate percepts (812). Related changes also occur in critical flicker fusion (813,814), visual masking (815,816), and afterimages (817). In short, the aging nervous system appears to recover more slowly from the effects of visual stimulation, compatible with an overall slowing in processing time.

Aging also impairs inductive reasoning, spatial orientation, verbal memory, and perceptual speed (818). Such decline generally does not occur before age 60 and is not meaningful until age 80. After this, most abilities (except verbal and fund of knowledge) decline by about one standard deviation, mostly from slower processing speed (818–821). These reductions in the function of normally aging brain tissues add to the complications and symptoms in patients who have cerebral disturbances of vision from destructive lesions and also impair the ability of such patients to recover.

Slowing of neuronal processing speed can hinder function at each level of information processing in the central nervous system (822) and provides an adequate explanation for the cognitive decline with advancing age (823,824) that causes difficulties in a range of tasks from simple memory to complex reasoning and spatial abilities (819,825–828). These effects increase with the complexity of the task (824, 829,830). Fortunately, various strategies can be learned to mitigate the effects of slowed processing speed on the day-to-day functioning of elderly adults. For example, older typists can compensate for reduced speed of processing by planning and reading further ahead in the text (821,831), and older chess players with worse recall can plan their moves further ahead (832,833). External memory aids are also useful compensatory devices for such patients (834).

Many of the tests commonly employed to test the vision of older subjects do not measure age-related decline. For example, older adults can experience a reduction in the useful field of view (UFOV) because of reduced processing speed. Standard visual field testing using such instruments as the Goldmann perimeter for kinetic perimetry and the Humphrey field analyzer for static perimetry will fail to detect such deficits because they ignore speed of processing and intentionally minimize the role of attention to gain maximum estimates of sensory ability (835). This approach is effective for gauging retina or optic nerve function or for plotting a bitemporal or homonymous visual field defect, but it may overestimate the visual capacity in the elderly or in brain-damaged patients (836). The UFOV, defined as the visual area within what targets can be perceived without moving the eye in the head, can be markedly impaired in such persons under conditions of increased attention load (582). Practically speaking, the UFOV can be assessed using a commercially available instrument, the Visual Attention Analyzer Model 3000 (Visual Resources, Inc, Bowling

Green, KY). The results can be interpreted literally as a shrinkage of the visual fields, or may reflect a general loss of efficiency throughout the visual fields (584). More severe levels of UFOV impairment have been correlated with an unacceptable crash risk in older drivers in state crash records (582) and with a greatly increased relative risk of crashes in collision avoidance scenarios tested in high-fidelity driving simulations (599).

TESTS OF HIGHER VISUAL FUNCTION

Chapter 2 contains detailed descriptions of the standard vision tests used by ophthalmologists, neurologists, and neuro-ophthalmologists to measure patients' visual abilities and track deficits (621). However, as indicated above, standard vision and screening tools generally do not provide a measure of higher-order visual functions, nor are they meant to do so. Tranel (837) and Anderson and Rizzo (838) reviewed the assessment of high-order visual functions, including the proper selection and interpretation of tests and the categories of available tests. Basic categories of higher visual function tests included tests of (*a*) reading (e.g., the reading subtest of the Wide Range Achievement Test, the Chapman-Cook Speed of Reading Test); (*b*) visual recognition (the recognition of famous faces, Boston Naming Test, Visual Naming Test from the Multilingual Aphasia Examination); (*c*) mental imagery (the Hooper Visual Organization Test); (*d*) visual perception (Facial Recognition Test and Judgment of Line Orientation); (*e*) visual attention (Cookie Theft Picture, line bisection task); (*f*) visuoconstruction (drawing to dictation and copy, writing to dictation copy and spontaneously, 3-D Block Construction Test); and (*g*) visual memory (the Benton Visual Retention Test). Some of these tests are described next.

The Rey-Osterreith Complex Figure Test (CFT) requires subjects to copy a complex geometric figure. An extensive scoring system is provided. The CFT provides a reliable index of visuoconstructional ability independent of memory function (Fig. 13.52).

The Benton Visual Retention Test—Revised (BVRT) requires a subject to reproduce, by drawing, several line drawings depicting geometric designs (839). Typically, the subject is shown each plate for 10 seconds. The plate is then withdrawn and the subject is asked to reproduce the figure on a piece of white paper (Fig. 13.53). The BVRT is sensitive to visual memory, perception, and visuoconstructional impairments. It is well standardized and takes only about 10 minutes to administer in most subjects.

The Hooper Visual Organization Test (840) requires the subject to identify 30 different items (e.g., room, shoe, fish, scissors) from cut-up, rearranged line drawings of those items (Fig. 13.54). This test is memory-dependent in that it depends on the history of exposure to the items represented in the test.

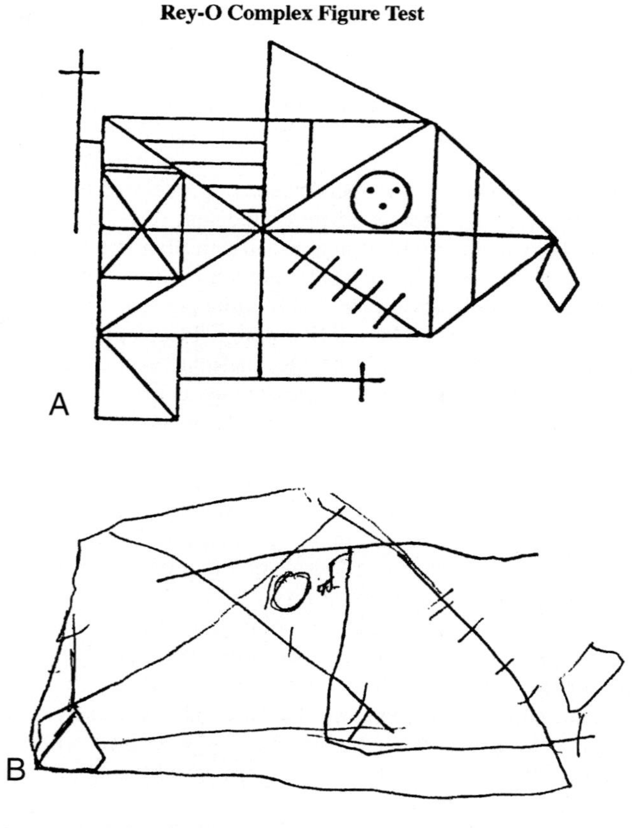

Rey-O Complex Figure Test

Figure 13.52. Tests of higher visual function. *A*, The Rey-Osterreith Complex Figure. *B*, Defective copy of this figure by a 74-year-old woman with Alzheimer's disease.

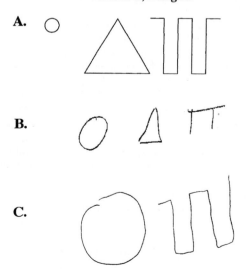

Benton Visual Retention Test
Form C, Design 5

Figure 13.53. Tests of higher visual function. *A*, Plate (design 5) from the Benton Visual Retention Test (BVRT). *B*, Defective reproduction by a patient with Alzheimer's disease. *C*, Omission of one of the left figures in a patient with a right hemisphere lesion causing left hemineglect.

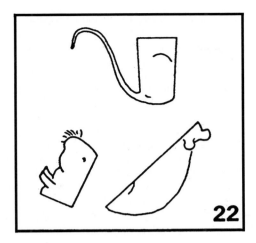

Figure 13.54. Tests of higher visual function. A plate (number 22/30) from the Hooper Visual Organization Test (HVOT). The patient is required to identify each of the 30 items on the plate from their cut-up, rearranged line drawings. This test is memory-dependent in that it depends on the history of exposure of the patient to the items on the plate.

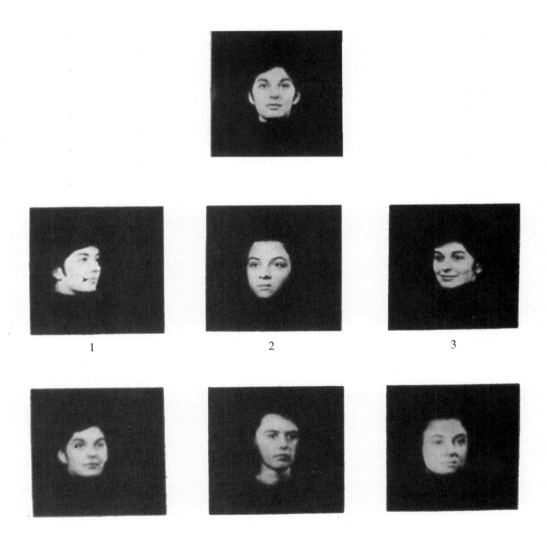

Figure 13.55. An item from the Benton Facial Recognition Test. This test measures visuoperceptual capacity. The subject is asked to choose which three of six face pictures below match the unfamiliar face pictured above. (Courtesy of Arthur Benton.)

Mooney's Closure Faces Test (841–843) is a "closure test" that provides information similar to that provided by the Hoopes Visual Organization Test. The patient is presented with 44 black-and-white, incomplete cartoons of faces and asked to judge the age and sex of the faces depicted. Performance on this test is memory-dependent, but recognition of previously familiar faces or famous faces is not required.

The Cookie Theft Picture (563) is a black-and-white line drawing of a complex picture from the Boston Diagnostic Aphasia Examination. It was designed with a balance of information among the four quadrants and tells a story. The subject is asked to view the picture and to report what he or she sees. Scoring is qualitative and depends on the report of the major items in the display (Fig. 13.40).

The Block Design subtest from the WAIS-R provides a very reliable measure of nonverbal intellectual capacity. It is highly correlated with performance IQ (844). It can be administered in a few minutes and is easily scored. In older populations, normative information is more robust for this subtest than for several other tests from the WAIS-R.

The Facial Recognition Test (845) measures visual perceptual capacity. The subject is asked to match unfamiliar faces under different lighting conditions and viewing angles or to match a face in one booklet with one of several faces in another booklet (Fig. 13.55). This is not a face-recognition test per se because the patient is being asked not to recognize

faces from memory but to match similar, although unfamiliar, faces. Thus, a patient can have severe prosopagnosia and still make the appropriate visual perceptive discriminations to pass this test (see above).

In the Judgment of Line Orientation Test, the patient must select, from an array of 11 line segments radiating from a semicircle, those segments that lie at the same angle as two target line segments. Performance on this test depends on visual perceptual discrimination and visuospatial judgment.

The findings from the tests described above can help provide a signature of the visuoperceptive impairments in a patient. For example, patients with right hemispheric dysfunction may perform poorly on the Judgment of Line Orientation, BVRT, and Block Design tasks. However, a patient's results cannot be properly interpreted without also having a clear idea of basic visual functions (such as spatial acuity and contrast sensitivity, visual fields, color perception, and motion perception) and intellectual capacities (such as verbal and performance IQ). More exhaustive reviews of neuropsychological tests, including tests of visual cognition, are available in the large compendia by Spreen and Strauss (846) and Lezak (620).

Acknowledgments

This work was supported by NIA AG 17177 and NIH PONS 19632 (M.R.), and NIMH MH 069898 and the Canada Research Chair program (J.B.).

GLOSSARY OF CEREBRAL VISUAL DEFICITS

Agnosia (also known as associative agnosia): The inability to recognize previously familiar objects despite adequate perception. Objects are effectively stripped of their meanings.

Alexia without agraphia (also known as pure alexia or acquired dyslexia): The acquired inability to read in previously literate subjects. Should not be confused with developmental dyslexia.

Anosognosia: Failure to recognize one's own impairment (see Anton's syndrome)

Anton's syndrome: The denial of cerebral blindness

Apperceptive agnosia: Failure to identify previously familiar objects due to impaired perception

Bálint's syndrome. Simultanagnosia, ocular apraxia, and optic ataxia

Blindsight: Residual vision in the fields of a putative striate scotoma; later redefined more broadly by Weiskrantz as a "visual capacity in a field defect in the absence of acknowledged awareness"

Central (paracentral) scotoma: A visual field defect at (or near) the fixation point

Cerebral achromatopsia (also known as central achromatopsia): An uncommon defect of color perception caused by damage to the visual cortex and connections. The term "achromatopsia" implies complete color loss. The term "dyschromatopsia" should be used when there is some sparing of color sensation.

Cerebral akinetopsia: Defective processing of visual motion cues due to cerebral lesions. The ability to perceive motion

direction, shape from motion, and other "higher-order" motion processes may be impaired.

Color agnosia: Inability to identify colors despite preserved ability to discriminate among colors

Color anomia: Inability to name colors despite adequate color perception and recognition

"Cortical blindness" (cerebral blindness): Inability to see following bilateral lesions of visual cortex and optic radiations. Affected patients generally have considerable damage that extends well beyond V1.

"Foveal sparing": A homonymous hemianopia in which the few degrees of vision near fixation are preserved

"Foveal splitting": A homonymous hemianopia that includes the entire foveal representation on the affected side

Hemianopia (or hemianopsia, or homonymous hemianopia): A visual field defect that occupies both the upper and lower visual portions of the same hemifield of both eyes

Keyhole vision (cerebral tunnel vision): Homonymous hemianopias may be bilateral (double homonymous hemianopia), leading to a severe loss of peripheral vision; if there is foveal sparing, a tunnel or keyhole of vision around fixation remains.

Metamorphopsia: The distortion of visual images due to a carnival mirror-like effect

Monocular temporal crescent: The peripheral-most sector of the visual fields of the eye represented in the depths of the contralateral calcarine fissure

Ocular apraxia (also called "psychic paralysis of gaze" and "spasm of fixation"): Inability to move the eyes to objects of interest despite unrestricted ocular rotations

Optic ataxia: A defect of hand movements under visual guidance despite adequate limb strength, position sense, and coordination

Palinopsia: Persistence of visual afterimages of an object despite looking away

Prosopagnosia: Inability to recognize previously familiar faces or to learn new faces despite adequate perception. This is a restricted form of (associative) agnosia.

Quadrantanopia: A visual field defect that is restricted to the upper or lower quadrant of a hemifield. A lesion below the calcarine fissure results in an upper (superior) quadrantanopia; a lesion above it causes a lower (inferior) quadrantanopia.

Scotoma (skotos, Greek for "darkness"): Scotomata are operationally defined by the inability to report the presence of targets of specific size and luminance in various portions of the visual field.

Simultanagnosia: This is often equated with Bálint's "spatial disorder of attention." According to Wolpert, an "inability to interpret the totality of a picture scene despite preservation of ability to apprehend individual portions of the whole."

REFERENCES

1. Hubel DH, Wiesel TN. Receptive fields and functional architecture of monkey striate cortex. J Physiol 1968;195:215–243.
2. Felleman DJ, Van Essen DC. Distributed hierarchical processing in the primate cerebral cortex. Cereb Cortex 1991;1:1–47.
3. Holmes G. The organization of the visual cortex in man. Proc R Soc Lond B Biol Sci 1945;132:348–361.
4. Polyak SL. The Vertebrate Visual System. Chicago, University of Chicago Press, 1957.
5. Ferrier D. The Functions of the Brain. London, Smith, Elder, 1876.
6. Verrey D. Hemiachromatopsie driote absolue. Arch Ophtalmol 1888;8:289–301.
7. Ewens GFW. A theory of cortical visual representation. Brain 1893;16:475–491.
8. Munk H. Ueber die Functionen der Grosshirnrinde; gesammelte Mittheilungen aus den Jahren 1877–80. Berlin, Hirschwald, 1881.
9. Schafer EA. On the functions of the temporal and occipital lobes: a reply to Dr. Ferrier. Brain 1888;11:145–165.
10. Inouye T. Die Sehstörungen bei Schussverletzungen der kortikalen Sehsphäre nach Beobachtungen an Verwundeten der letzten japanischen Kriege. Leipzig, W. Engelmann, 1909.
11. Holmes G. Disturbances of visual orientation. Br J Ophthalmol 1918;6:449–468.
12. Brodmann K. Vergleichende Lokalisationslehre der Grosshirnrinde in ihren Prinzipien dargestellt auf Grund des Zellenbaues. Leipzig, Barth, 1909.
13. Holmes G. Disturbances of vision by cerebral lesions. Br J Ophthalmol 1918;6:352–384.
14. Riddoch G. Dissociation of visual perceptions due to occipital injuries, with especial reference to appreciation of movement. Br J Med Psychol 1917;6:15–57.
15. Livingstone MS, Hubel DH. Psychophysical evidence for separate channels for the perception of form, color, movement, and depth. J Neurosci 1987;7:3416–3468.
16. Schiller PH, Logothetis NK, Charles ER. Role of the color-opponent and broadband channels in vision. Vis Neurosci 1990;5:321–346.
17. Kulikowski JJ, Tolhurst DJ. Psychophysical evidence for sustained and transient detectors in human vision. J Physiol 1973;232:149–162.
18. Troscianko T, Davidoff J, Humphreys G, et al. Human color discrimination based on a non-parvocellular pathway. Curr Biol 1996;6:200–210.
19. Hendry SH, Reid RC. The koniocellular pathway in primate vision. Annu Rev Neurosci 2000;23:127–153.
20. Ungerleider LG, Mishkin M. Two cortical visual systems. In: Ingle D, Goodale MA, Mansfield RJW, eds. Analysis of Visual Behavior. Cambridge, MA, MIT Press, 1982:549–586.
21. Rizzo M. The role of striate cortex: evidence from human lesion studies. In: Peters A, Rockland KS, eds. Cerebral Cortex. New York, London, Plenum Press, 1994:505–540.
22. Zeki S. A century of cerebral achromatopsia. Brain 1990;113(Pt 6):1721–1777.
23. Plant GT. Disorders of color vision in diseases of the nervous system. In: Foster DH, Cronly-Dillon J, eds. Inherited and Acquired Colour Vision Deficiencies:

Fundamental Aspects and Clinical Studies. Boca Raton, CRC Press, 1991:173–198.
24. Rizzo M, Smith V, Pokorny J, et al. Color perception profiles in central achromatopsia. Neurology 1993;43:995–1001.
25. Bálint R. Seelenlahmung des "Schauens," optische Ataxie, röumliche Storung der Aufmerksamkeit. Monatschr Psychiatr Neurol 1909;25:51–181.
26. Rizzo M, Nawrot M, Zihl J. Motion and shape perception in cerebral akinetopsia. Brain 1995;118(Pt 5):1105–1127.
27. Lu ZL, Sperling G. Attention-generated apparent motion. Nature 1995;377:237–239.
28. Batelli L, Cavanagh P, Intriligator J, et al. Unilateral right parietal brain damage leads to bilateral deficit for high-level motion. Neuron 2001;32:985–995.
29. Heywood CA, Cowey A, Newcombe F. On the role of parvocellular (P) and magnocellular (M) pathways in cerebral achromatopsia. Brain 1994;117(Pt 2):245–254.
30. Darling W, Butler A, Rizzo M. Increased sensorimotor transformation errors in a patient with inferior parietal lobe damage. Social Neuroscience Abstracts 1995;21:415.
31. Rizzo M, Darling W, Damasio H. Disorders of reaching with lesions of the posterior cerebral hemisphere. Abstr Soc Neurosci 1995;21:269.
32. Jeannerod M, Decety J, Michel F. Impairment of grasping movements following a bilateral posterior parietal lesion. Neuropsychologia 1994;32:369–380.
33. Goodale MA, Meenan JP, Bulthoff HH, et al. Separate neural pathways for the visual analysis of object shape in perception and prehension. Curr Biol 1994;4:604–610.
34. Teller DY. Linking propositions. Vision Res 1984;24:1233–1246.
35. Blake R. Psychoanatomical strategies for studying human visual perception. In: Papathomas TV, ed. Early Vision and Beyond. Cambridge, MA, MIT Press, 1995:17–25.
36. Nawrot M, Shannon E, Rizzo M. Measuring visual function. Curr Opin Ophthalmol 1993;4:30–37.
37. Julesz B. Foundations of Cyclopean Perception. Chicago, University of Chicago Press, 1971.
38. Fox PT, Mintun MA, Raichle ME, et al. Mapping human visual cortex with positron emission tomography. Nature 1986;323:806–809.
39. Corbetta M, Miezin FM, Dobmeyer S, et al. Selective and divided attention during visual discriminations of shape, color, and speed: functional anatomy by positron emission tomography. J Neurosci 1991;11:2383–2402.
40. Haxby JV, Grady CL, Horwitz B, et al. Dissociation of object and spatial visual processing pathways in human extrastriate cortex. Proc Natl Acad Sci USA 1991;88:1621–1625.
41. Grady CL, Haxby JV, Horwitz B, et al. Dissociation of object and spatial vision in human extrastriate cortex: age-related changes in activation of regional cerebral blood flow measured with [^{15}O] water and positron emission tomography. J Cogn Neurosci 1991;4:23–34.
42. Zeki S, Watson JD, Lueck CJ, et al. A direct demonstration of functional specialization in human visual cortex. J Neurosci 1991;11:641–649.
43. Watson JD, Myers R, Frackowiak RS, et al. Area V5 of the human brain: evidence from a combined study using positron emission tomography and magnetic resonance imaging. Cereb Cortex 1993;3:79–94.
44. Orban GA, Dupont P, De Bruyn B, et al. A motion area in human visual cortex. Proc Natl Acad Sci USA 1995;92:993–997.
45. Clarke S, Miklossy J. Occipital cortex in man: organization of callosal connections, related myelo- and cytoarchitecture, and putative boundaries of functional visual areas. J Comp Neurol 1990;298:188–214.
46. Tootell RB, Taylor JB. Anatomical evidence for MT and additional cortical visual areas in humans. Cereb Cortex 1995;5:39–55.
47. Zihl J, von Cramon D, Mai N. Selective disturbance of movement vision after bilateral brain damage. Brain 1983;106(Pt 2):313–340.
48. Anton F. Ueber die Selbstwharneh mungen der Herder Krankungen des Gehirns durch den Kranken bei Rinderblindheit und Rindentaubheit. Arch Psychiatr 1899;32:86–127.
49. Damasio AR. Disorders of complex visual processing: agnosias, achromatopsia, Bálint's syndrome, and related difficulties of orientation and construction. In: Mesulam M-M, ed. Principles of Behavioral Neurology. Philadelphia, FA Davis, 1985:259–288.
50. Damasio AR. Prosopagnosia. Trends Neurosci 1985;8:132–135.
51. Tranel D, Damasio AR. Knowledge without awareness: an autonomic index of facial recognition by prosopagnosics. Science 1985;228:1453–1454.
52. Rizzo M, Hurtig R, Damasio AR. The role of scanpaths in facial recognition and learning. Ann Neurol 1987;22:41–45.
53. Weiskrantz L. Residual vision in a scotoma. A follow-up study of 'form' discrimination. Brain 1987;110(Pt 1):77–92.
54. Weiskrantz L. Blindsight: a case study and implications. Oxford, New York, Clarendon Press, Oxford University Press, 1986.
55. Weiskrantz L. The Ferrier Lecture, 1989. Outlooks for blindsight: explicit methodologies for implicit processes. Proc R Soc Lond B Biol Sci 1990;239:247–278.
56. Cowey A, Stoerig P. The neurobiology of blindsight. Trends Neurosci 1991;14:140–145.
57. Barbur JL, Ruddock KH, Waterfield VA. Human visual responses in the absence of the geniculo-calcarine projection. Brain 1980;103:905–928.

58. Barbur JL, Watson JD, Frackowiak RS, et al. Conscious visual perception without V1. Brain 1993;116(Pt 6):1293–1302.
59. Blythe IM, Kennard C, Ruddock KH. Residual vision in patients with retrogeniculate lesions of the visual pathways. Brain 1987;110(Pt 4):887–905.
60. Sanders MD, Warrington EK, Marshall J, et al. ''Blindsight'': Vision in a field defect. Lancet 1974;1:707–708.
61. Stoerig P, Cowey A. Blindsight in man and monkey. Brain 1997;120:535–559.
62. Zeki S, Ffytche DH. The Riddoch syndrome: insights into the neurobiology of conscious vision. Brain 1998;121:25–45.
63. Weiskrantz L. Blindsight: a case study and implications. Oxford, Oxford University Press, 1998.
64. Marcel AJ. Blindsight and shape perception: deficit of visual consciousness or of visual function? Brain 1998;121:1565–1588.
65. Sahraie A, Weiskrantz L, Barbur J, et al. Pattern of neuronal activity associated with conscious and unconscious processing of visual signals. Proc Natl Acad Sci USA 1997;94:9406–9411.
66. Weiskrantz L, Barbur JL, Sahraie A. Parameters affecting conscious versus unconscious visual discrimination with damage to the visual cortex (V1). Proc Natl Acad Sci USA 1995;92:6122–6126.
67. Kolb FC, Braun J. Blindsight in normal observers. Nature 1995;377:336–338.
68. Meeres SL, Graves RE. Localization of unseen visual stimuli by humans with normal vision. Neuropsychologia 1990;28:1231–1237.
69. Morgan MJ, Mason AJS, Solomon JA. Blindsight in normal subjects? Nature 1997;385:401–402.
70. Tapp TD. Blindsight in hindsight. Consciousnesss Cogn 1997;6:67–74.
71. Natsoulas T. Blindsight and consciousness. Am J Psychol 1997;110:1–33.
72. Merigan WH, Nealey TA, Maunsell JHR. Visual effects of lesions of cortical area V2 in macaques. J Neurosci 1993;13:3180.
73. Celesia GG, Bushnell D, Toleikis SC, et al. Cortical blindness and residual vision: is the ''second'' visual system in humans capable of more than rudimentary visual perception? Neurology 1991;41:862–869.
74. Cowey A, Stoerig P. Visual detection in monkeys with blindsight. Neuropsychologia 1997;35:929–939.
75. Ptito A, Lepore F, Ptito M, et al. Target detection and movement discrimination in the blind field of hemispherectomized patients. Brain 1991;114(Pt 1B):497–512.
76. Pöppel E, Held R, Frost D. Residual visual function after brain wounds involving the central visual pathways in man. Nature 1973;243:295–296.
77. Perenin M, Jeannerod M. Residual vision in cortically blind hemifields. Neuropsychologia 1975;13:1–7.
78. Weiskrantz L, Warrington EK, Sanders MD, et al. Visual capacity in the hemianopic field following a restricted occipital ablation. Brain 1974;97:709–728.
79. Blythe IM, Bromley JM, Kennard C, et al. Visual discrimination of target displacement remains after damage to the striate cortex in humans. Nature 1986;320:619–621.
80. Barton JJ, Sharpe JA. Smooth pursuit and saccades to moving targets in blind hemifields. A comparison of medial occipital, lateral occipital and optic radiation lesions. Brain 1997;120:681–699.
81. Meienberg O, Zangemeister WH, Rosenberg M, et al. Saccadic eye movement strategies in patients with homonymous hemianopia. Ann Neurol 1981;9:537–544.
82. Corbetta M, Marzi CA, Tassinari G, et al. Effectiveness of different task paradigms in revealing blindsight. Brain 1990;113(Pt 3):603–616.
83. Perenin MT, Ruel J, Hecaen H. Residual visual capacities in a case of cortical blindness. Cortex 1980;16:605–612.
84. Perenin M, Jeannerod M. Visual function within the hemianopic field following early cerebral hemidecortication in man: I. Spatial localization. Neuropsychologia 1978;16:1–13.
85. Bridgeman B, Staggs D. Plasticity in human blindsight. Vision Res 1982;22:1199–1203.
86. Morland AB, Jones SR, Finlay AL, et al. Visual perception of motion, luminance and color in a human hemianope. Brain 1999;122:1183–1198.
87. Perenin MT. Discrimination of motion direction in perimetrically blind fields. Neuroreport 1991;2:397–400.
88. Heide W, Koenig E, Dichgans J. Optokinetic nystagmus, self-motion sensation and their aftereffects in patients with occipit-parietal lesions. Clin Vis Sci 1990;5:145–156.
89. Mestre DR, Brouchon M, Ceccaldi M, et al. Perception of optical flow in cortical blindness: a case report. Neuropsychologia 1992;30:783–795.
90. Barton JJ, Sharpe JA. Motion direction discrimination in blind hemifields. Ann Neurol 1997;41:255–264.
91. Azzopardi P, Cowey A. Motion discrimination in cortically blind patients. Brain 2001;124:30–46.
92. ter Braak JWG, Schenk VWD, van Vliet AGM. Visual reactions in a case of long-lasting cortical blindness. J Neurol Neurosurg Psychiatry 1971;34:140–147.
93. Verhagen W, Huygen P, Mulleners W. Lack of optokinetic nystagmus and visual motion perception in acquired cortical blindness. Neuro-Ophthalmology 1997;17:211–218.
94. Perenin MT, Rossetti Y. Grasping without form discrimination in a hemianopic field. Neuroreport 1996;7:793–797.
95. Morland A, Ogilvie J, Ruddock K, et al. Orientation discrimination is impaired in the absence of the striate cortical contribution to human vision. Proc Roy Soc Lond B Biol Sci 1996;263:633–640.
96. Jackson SR. Pathological perceptual completion in hemianopia extends to the control of reach-to-grasp movements. Neuroreport 1999;10:2461–2466.
97. Milner A, Goodale M. The Visual Brain in Action. Oxford, Oxford University Press, 1995.
98. Stoerig P. Chromaticity and achromaticity. Evidence for a functional differentiation in visual field defects. Brain 1987;110(Pt 4):869–886.
99. Stoerig P, Cowey A. Increment-threshold spectral sensitivity in blindsight. Evidence for color opponency. Brain 1991;114(Pt 3):1487–1512.
100. Guo K, Benson PJ, Blakemore C. Residual motion discrimination using color information without primary visual cortex. Neuroreport 1998;9:2103–2107.
101. Morland AB, Ruddock KH. Retinotopic organisation of cortical mechanisms responsive to color: evidence from patient studies. Acta Psychol 1997;97:7–24.
102. Barbur JL, Harlow AJ, Weiskrantz L. Spatial and temporal response properties of residual vision in a case of hemianopia. Philos Trans R Soc Lond B Biol Sci 1994;343:157–166.
103. Hess RF, Pointer JS. Spatial and temporal contrast sensitivity in hemianopia. A comparative study of the sighted and blind hemifields. Brain 1989;112(Pt 4):871–894.
104. Weiskrantz L, Harlow A, Barbur JL. Factors affecting visual sensitivity in a hemianopic subject. Brain 1991;114:2269–2282.
105. Marzi CA, Tassinari G, Aglioti S, et al. Spatial summation across the vertical meridian in hemianopics: a test of blindsight. Neuropsychologia 1986;24:749–758.
106. Intriligator JM, Xie R, Barton JJ. Blindsight modulation of motion perception. J Cogn Neurosci 2002;14:1174–1183.
107. Ward R, Jackson SR. Visual attention in blindsight: sensitivity in the blind field increased by targets in the sighted field. Neuroreport 2002;13:301–304.
108. Rafal R, Smith J, Krantz J, et al. Extrageniculate vision in hemianopic humans: saccade inhibition by signals in the blind field. Science 1990;250:118–121.
109. Walker R, Mannan S, Maurer D, et al. The oculomotor distractor effect in normal and hemianopic vision. Proc R Soc Lond B Biol Sci 2000;267:431–438.
110. Cowey A, Stoerig P, Le Mare C. Effects of unseen stimuli on reaction times to seen stimuli in monkeys with blindsight. Consciousness Cogn 1998;7:312–323.
111. Danziger S, Fendrich R, Rafal RD. Inhibitory tagging of locations in the blind field of hemianopic patients. Conscious Cogn 1997;6:291–307.
112. Torjussen T. Visual processing in cortically blind hemifields. Neuropsychologia 1978;16:15–21.
113. Danckert J, Maruff P, Kinsella G, et al. Investigating form and color perception in blindsight using an interference task. Neuroreport 1998;9:2919–2925.
114. Pizzamiglio L, Antonucci G, Francia A. Response of the cortically blind hemifields to a moving visual scene. Cortex 1984;20:89–99.
115. Barbur JL, Weiskrantz L, Harlow JA. The unseen color aftereffect of an unseen stimulus: insight from blindsight into mechanisms of color afterimages. Proc Natl Acad Sci USA 1999;96:11637–11641.
116. Weiskrantz L, Cowey A, Le Mare C. Learning from the pupil: a spatial visual channel in the absence of V1 in monkey and human. Brain 1998;121:1065–1072.
117. Weiskrantz L, Cowey A, Barbur JL. Differential pupillary constriction and awareness in the absence of striate cortex. Brain 1999;122:1533–1538.
118. Morris JS, Ohman A, Dolan RJ. A subcortical pathway to the right amygdala mediating ''unseen'' fear. Proc Natl Acad Sci USA 1999;96:1680–1685.
119. de Gelder B, Vroomen J, Pourtois G, et al. Non-conscious recognition of affect in the absence of striate cortex. Neuroreport 1999;10:3759–3763.
120. Morris JS, DeGelder B, Weiskrantz L, et al. Differential extrageniculostriate and amygdala responses to presentation of emotional faces in a cortically blind field. Brain 2001;124:1241–1252.
121. Hamm AO, Weike AI, Schupp HT, et al. Affective blindsight: intact fear conditioning to a visual cue in a cortically blind patient. Brain 2003;126:267–275.
122. Braddick O, Atkinson J, Hood B, et al. Possible blindsight in infants lacking one cerebral hemisphere. Nature 1992;360:461–463.
123. Ptito A, Lassonde M, Lepore F, et al. Visual discrimination in hemispherectomized patients. Neuropsychologia 1987;25:869–879.
124. Tomaiuolo F, Ptito M, Marzi CA, et al. Blindsight in hemispherectomized patients as revealed by spatial summation across the vertical meridian. Brain 1997;120:795–803.
125. Bittar RG, Ptito M, Faubert J, et al. Activation of the remaining hemisphere following stimulation of the blind hemifield in hemispherectomized subjects. Neuroimage 1999;10:339–346.
126. Ptito M, Johannnsen P, Faubert J, et al. Activation of human extrageniculostriate pathways after damage to area V1. Neuroimage 1999;9:97–107.
127. Stoerig P, Faubert J, Ptito M, et al. No blindsight following hemidecortication in human subjects? Neuroreport 1996;7:1990–1994.

128. Faubert J, Diaconu V, Ptito M, et al. Residual vision in the blind field of hemidecorticated humans predicted by a diffusion scatter model and selective spectral absorption of the human eye. Vision Res 1999;39:149–157.

129. King S, Azzopardi P, Cowey A, et al. The role of light scatter in the residual visual sensitivity of patients with complete cerebral hemispherectomy. Vis Neurosci 1996;13:1–13.

130. Faubert J, Diaconu V. From visual consciousness to spectral absorption in the human retina. Prog Brain Res 2001;134:399–409.

131. Ptito M, Herbin M, Boire D, et al. Neural bases of residual vision in hemicorticectomized monkeys. Prog Brain Res 1996;112:385–404.

132. Wessinger CM, Fendrich R, Gazzaniga MS, et al. Extrageniculostriate vision in humans: investigations with hemispherectomy patients. Prog Brain Res 1996; 112:405–413.

133. Balliet R, Blood KM, Bach-y-Rita P. Visual field rehabilitation in the cortically blind? J Neurol Neurosurg Psychiatry 1985;48:1113–1124.

134. Campion J, Latto R, Smith Y. Is blindsight an effect of scattered light, spared cortex, and near-threshold vision? Behav Brain Sci 1983;6:423–486.

135. Fendrich R, Wessinger CM, Gazzaniga MS. Residual vision in a scotoma: implications for blindsight. Science 1992;258:1489–1491.

136. Kasten E, Wuest S, Sabel B. Residual vision in transition zones in patients with cerebral blindness. J Clin Exp Neuropsychol 1998;20:581–598.

137. Scharli H, Harman A, Hogben J. Blindsight in subjects with homonymous visual field defects. J Cogn Neurosci 1999;11:52–66.

138. Scharli H, Harman AM, Hogben JH. Residual vision in a subject with damaged visual cortex. J Cogn Neurosci 1999;11:502–510.

139. Wust S, Kasten E, Sabel BA. Blindsight after optic nerve injury indicates functionality of spared fibers. J Cogn Neurosci 2002;14:243–253.

140. Stoerig P, Kleinschmidt A, Frahm J. No visual responses in denervated V1: high-resolution functional magnetic resonance imaging of a blindsight patient. Neuroreport 1998;9:21–25.

141. Robichaud L, Stelmach LB. Inducing blindsight in normal observers. Psychon Bull Rev 2003;10:206–209.

142. Azzopardi P, Cowey A. Is blindsight like normal, near-threshold vision? Proc Natl Acad Sci USA 1997;94:14190–14194.

143. Stoerig P, Hubner M, Poppel E. Signal detection analysis of residual vision in a field defect due to a post-geniculate lesion. Neuropsychologia 1985;23: 589–599.

144. Azzopardi P, Cowey A. Blindsight and visual awareness. Conscious Cogn 1998; 7:292–311.

145. Dodds C, Machado L, Rafal R, et al. A temporal/nasal asymmetry for blindsight in a localisation task: evidence for extrageniculate mediation. Neuroreport 2002; 13:655–658.

146. Rodman HR, Gross CG, Albright TD. Afferent basis of visual response properties in area MT of the macaque. I. Effects of striate cortex removal. J Neurosci 1989;9:2033–2050.

147. Girard P, Salin PA, Bullier J. Response selectivity of neurons in area MT of the macaque monkey during reversible inactivation of area V1. J Neurophysiol 1992;67:1437–1446.

148. Rosa MG, Tweedale R, Elston GN. Visual responses of neurons in the middle temporal area of new world monkeys after lesions of striate cortex. J Neurosci 2000;20:5552–5563.

149. Girard P, Salin PA, Bullier J. Visual activity in areas V3a and V3 during reversible inactivation of area V1 in the macaque monkey. J Neurophysiol 1991;66: 1493–1503.

150. Gross CG. Contribution of striate cortex and the superior colliculus to visual function in area MT, the superior temporal polysensory area and the inferior temporal cortex. Neuropsychologia 1991;29:497–515.

151. Girard P, Bullier J. Visual activity in area V2 during reversible inactivation of area 17 in the macaque monkey. J Neurophysiol 1989;62:1287–1302.

152. Cowey A, Stoerig P. Spectral sensitivity in hemianopic macaque monkeys. Eur J Neurosci 1999;11:2114–2120.

153. Payne BR, Lomber SG, Macneil MA, et al. Evidence for greater sight in blindsight following damage of primary visual cortex early in life. Neuropsychologia 1996;34:741–774.

154. Sorenson KM, Rodman HR. A transient geniculo-extrastriate pathway in macaques? Implications for 'blindsight.' Neuroreport 1999;10:3295–3299.

155. Ffytche DH, Guy CN, Zeki S. The parallel visual motion inputs into areas V1 and V5 of human cerebral cortex. Brain 1995;118(Pt 6):1375–1394.

156. Beckers G, Zeki S. The consequences of inactivating areas V1 and V5 on visual motion perception. Brain 1995;118(Pt 1):49–60.

157. Hotson J, Braun D, Herzberg W, et al. Transcranial magnetic stimulation of extrastriate cortex degrades human motion direction discrimination. Vision Res 1994;34:2115–2123.

158. Holliday IE, Anderson SJ, Harding GF. Magnetoencephalographic evidence for non-geniculostriate visual input to human cortical area V5. Neuropsychologia 1997;35:1139–1146.

159. Ffytche DH, Guy CN, Zeki S. Motion specific responses from a blind hemifield. Brain 1996;119:1971–1982.

160. Weiskrantz L. Outlooks for blindsight: explicit methodologies for implicit processes. Proc R Soc Lond B 1990;239:247–278.

161. Magnussen S, Mathiesen T. Detection of moving and stationary gratings in the absence of striate cortex. Neuropsychologia 1989;27:725–728.

162. Moore T, Rodman H, Repp A, et al. Greater residual vision in monkeys after striate damage in infancy. J Neurophysiol 1996;76:3928–3933.

163. Zihl J. ''Blindsight'': improvement of visually guided eye movements by systematic practice in patients with cerebral blindness. Neuropsychologia 1980;18: 71–77.

164. Zihl J, Werth R. Contributions to the study of ''blindsight''—I. Can stray light account for saccadic localization in patients with postgeniculate field defects? Neuropsychologia 1984;22:1–11.

165. Zihl J, Werth R. Contributions to the study of ''blindsight''—II. The role of specific practice for saccadic localization in patients with postgeniculate visual field defects. Neuropsychologia 1984;22:13–22.

166. Zihl J, von Cramon D. Restitution of visual function in patients with cerebral blindness. J Neurol Neurosurg Psychiatry 1979;42:312–322.

167. Zihl J. Recovery of visual functions in patients with cerebral blindness. Effect of specific practice with saccadic localization. Exp Brain Res 1981;44:159–169.

168. Swanzy HR. Case of hemiachromatopsia. Trans Ophthalmol Soc UK 1883;3: 185–189.

169. MacKay G, Dunlop JC. The cerebral lesions in a case of complete acquired color-blindness. Scott Med Surg J 1899;5:503.

170. Zeki S. Color coding in rhesus monkey prestriate cortex. Brain Res 1973;53: 422–427.

171. Critchley M. Acquired anomalies of color perception of central origin. Brain 1965;88:711–724.

172. Meadows JC. Disturbed perception of colors associated with localized cerebral lesions. Brain 1974;97:615–632.

173. MacKay G, Dunlop JC. The cerebral lesions in a case of complete acquired color-blindness. Scot Med Surg J 1899;5:503–512.

174. Pallis C. Impaired identification of faces and places with agnosia for colors. Report of a case due to cerebral embolism. J Neurol Neurosurg Psychiatry 1955; 18:218–224.

175. Damasio A, Yamada T, Damasio H, et al. Central achromatopsia: behavioral, anatomic, and physiologic aspects. Neurology 1980;30:1064–1071.

176. Sacks O. The case of the color-blind painter. In: Knopf AA, ed. An Anthropologist on Mars. New York, 1995.

177. Green GJ, Lessell S. Acquired cerebral dyschromatopsia. Arch Ophthalmol 1977;95:121–128.

178. Ogden JA. Visual object agnosia, prosopagnosia, achromatopsia, loss of visual imagery, and autobiographical amnesia following recovery from cortical blindness: case M.H. Neuropsychologia 1993;31:571–589.

179. Heywood CA, Cowey A, Newcombe F. Chromatic discrimination in a cortically color-blind observer. Eur J Neurosci 1991;3:802–812.

180. Victor JD, Maiese K, Shapley R, et al. Acquired central dyschromatopsia: analysis of a case with preservation of color discrimination. Clin Vis Sci 1989;4: 183–196.

181. Mendola J, Corkin S. Visual discrimination and attention after bilateral temporal-lobe lesions: a case study. Neuropsychologia 1999;37:91–102.

182. Pearlman AL, Birch J, Meadows JC. Cerebral color blindness: an acquired defect in hue discrimination. Ann Neurol 1979;5:253–261.

183. Damasio H, Frank R. Three-dimensional in vivo mapping of brain lesions in humans. Arch Neurol 1992;49:137–143.

184. Orrell RW, James-Galton M, Stevens JM, et al. Cerebral achromatopsia as a presentation of Trousseau's syndrome. Postgrad Med J 1995;71:44–46.

185. Aldrich MS, Vanderzant CW, Alessi AG, et al. Ictal cortical blindness with permanent visual loss. Epilepsia 1989;30:116–120.

186. Freedman L, Costa L. Pure alexia and right hemiachromatopsia in posterior dementia. J Neurol Neurosurg Psychiatry 1992;55:500–502.

187. Lawden MC, Cleland PG. Achromatopsia in the aura of migraine. J Neurol Neurosurg Psychiatry 1993;56:708–709.

188. Fine R, Parker G. Disturbance of central vision after carbon monoxide poisoning. Aust NZ J Ophthalmol 1996;24:137–141.

189. Albert ML, Reches A, Silverberg R. Hemianopic color blindness. J Neurol Neurosurg Psychiatry 1975;38:546–549.

190. Paulson HL, Galetta SL, Grossman M, et al. Hemiachromatopsia of unilateral occipitotemporal infarcts. Am J Ophthalmol 1994;118:518–523.

191. Kölmel HW. Pure homonymous hemiachromatopsia. Findings with neuro-ophthalmologic examination and imaging procedures. Eur Arch Psychiatry Neurol Sci 1988;237:237–243.

192. Wandell B, Wade A. Functional imaging of the visual pathways. Neurol Clin 2003;21:417–444.

193. Ichikawa K, Ichikawa H, Tanabe S. Detection of acquired color vision defects by standard pseudoisochromatic plates, part 2. Doc Ophthalmol Proc Ser 1987; 46:133–140.

194. Frisèn L, Kalm P. Sahlgren's saturation test for detecting and grading acquired dyschromatopsia. Am J Ophthalmol 1981;92:252.

195. Heywood CA, Wilson B, Cowey A. A case study of cortical color "blindness" with relatively intact achromatic discrimination. J Neurol Neurosurg Psychiatry 1987;50:22–29.

196. Beauchamp M, Haxby J, Rosen A, et al. A functional MRI case study of acquired cerebral dyschromatopsia. Neuropsychologia 2000;38:1170–1179.

197. Wyszecki G, Stiles WS. Color Science: Concepts and Methods, Quantitative Data and Formulae, 2nd ed. New York, Wiley, 1982.

198. Boynton RM. Human Color Vision, special limited ed. Washington, DC, Optical Society of America, 1992.

199. Land EH. Recent advances in Retinex theory. Vision Res 1986;26:7–21.

200. Hurlbert AC, Bramwell DI, Heywood C, et al. Discrimination of cone contrast changes as evidence for color constancy in cerebral achromatopsia. Exp Brain Res 1998;123:136–144.

201. Land E, Hubel D, Livingstone M, et al. Color-generating interactions across the corpus callosum. Nature 1983;303:616–618.

202. Kennard C, Lawden M, Morland AB, et al. Color identification and color constancy are impaired in a patient with incomplete achromatopsia associated with prestriate cortical lesions. Proc R Soc Lond B Biol Sci 1995;260:169–175.

203. Clarke S, Walsh V, Schoppig A, et al. Color constancy impairments in patients with lesions of the prestriate cortex. Exp Brain Res 1998;123:154–158.

204. D'Zmura MD, Knoblauch K, Henaff M-A, et al. Dependence of color on context in a case of cortical color vision deficiency. Vision Research 1998;38: 3455–3459.

205. Rüttiger L, Braun DI, Gegenfurtner KR, et al. Selective color constancy deficits after circumscribed unilateral brain lesions. J Neurosci 1999;19:3094–3106.

206. Heywood CA, Nicholas JJ, Cowey A. Behavioural and electrophysiological chromatic and achromatic contrast sensitivity in an achromatopsic patient. J Neurol Neurosurg Psychiatry 1996;60:638–643.

207. Adachi-Usami E, Tsukamoto M, Shimada Y. Color vision and color pattern evoked cortical potentials in a patient with acquired cerebral dyschromatopsia. Doc Ophthalmol 1997;90:259–269.

208. Cavanagh P, Hénaff M-A, Michel F, et al. Complete sparing of high-contrast color input to motion perception in cortical color blindness. Nature Neurosci 1998;1:242–247.

209. Heywood CA, Kentridge RW, Cowey A. Form and motion from color in cerebral achromatopsia. Exp Brain Res 1998;123:145–153.

210. Cole G, Heywood C, Kentridge R, et al. Attentional capture by color and motion in cerebral achromatopsia. Neuropsychologia 2003;41:1837–1846.

211. Shuren J, Brott T, Shefft B, et al. Preserved color imagery in an achromatopsic. Neuropsychologia 1996;34:485–489.

212. Bartolomeo P, Bachoud-Levi AC, Denes G. Preserved imagery for colors in a patient with cerebral achromatopsia. Cortex 1997;33:369–378.

213. Bartolomeo P, Bachoud-Levi AC, De Gelder B, et al. Multiple-domain dissociation between impaired visual perception and preserved mental imagery in a patient with bilateral extrastriate lesions. Neuropsychologia 1998;36:239–249.

214. de Vreese LP. Two systems for color-naming defects: verbal disconnection vs. color imagery disorder. Neuropsychologia 1991;29:1–18.

215. Hubel DH, Livingstone MS. Segregation of form, color, and stereopsis in primate area 18. J Neurosci 1987;7:3378–3415.

216. Leavitt J, Kiper D, Movshon J. Receptive fields and functional architecture of macaque V2. J Neurophysiol 1994;71:2517–2542.

217. Komatsu H, Ideura Y, Kaji S, et al. Color selectivity of neurons in the inferior temporal cortex of the awake macaque monkey. J Neurosci 1992;12:408–424.

218. Komatsu H, Ideura Y. Relationships between color, shape, and pattern selectivities of neurons in the inferior temporal cortex of the monkey. J Neurophysiol 1993;70:677–694.

219. Zeki S. Color coding in the cerebral cortex: the responses of wavelength-selective and color-coded cells in monkey visual cortex to changes in wavelength composition. Neuroscience 1983;9:767–781.

220. Schein SJ, Desimone R. Spectral properties of V4 neurons in the macaque. J Neurosci 1990;10:3369–3389.

221. Wild HM, Butler SR, Carden D, et al. Primate cortical area V4 important for color constancy but not wavelength discrimination. Nature 1985:133–135.

222. Merigan W. Human V4? Curr Biol 1993;3:226–229.

223. Dean P. Visual cortex ablation and thresholds for successively presented stimuli in rhesus monkeys: II. Hue. Exp Brain Res 1979;35:69–83.

224. Heywood CA, Cowey A. On the role of cortical area V4 in the discrimination of hue and pattern in macaque monkeys. J Neurosci 1987;7:2601–2617.

225. Heywood CA, Gadotti A, Cowey A. Cortical area V4 and its role in the perception of color. J Neurosci 1992;12:4056–4065.

226. Walsh V, Kulikowski JJ, Butler SR, et al. The effects of lesions of area V4 on the visual abilities of macaques: color categorization. Behav Brain Res 1992; 52:81–89.

227. Schiller PH. The effects of V4 and middle temporal (MT) area lesions on visual performance in the rhesus monkey. Vis Neurosci 1993;10:717–746.

228. Cowey A, Heywood C, Irving-Bell L. The regional cortical basis of achromatopsia: a study on macaque monkeys and an achromatopsic patient. Eur J Neurosci 2001;14:1555–1566.

229. Heywood CA, Gaffan D, Cowey A. Cerebral achromatopsia in monkeys. Eur J Neurosci 1995;7:1064–1073.

230. Lueck C, Zeki S, Friston K, et al. The color centre in the cerebral cortex of man. Nature 1989;340:386–389.

231. Sakai K, Watanabe E, Onodera Y, et al. Functional mapping of the human color center with echo-planar magnetic resonance imaging. Proc R Soc Lond B Biol Sci 1995;261:89–98.

232. Allison T, Begleiter A, McCarthy G, et al. Electrophysiological studies of color processing in human visual cortex. Electroencephalogr Clin Neurophysiol 1993; 88:343–355.

233. Heywood C, Kentridge R. Achromatopsia, color vision and cortex. Neurol Clin 2003;21:483–500.

234. Wade A. Functional measurements of human ventral occipital cortex: retinotopy and color. Philos Trans R Soc (B) (London) 2002;357:963–973.

235. Hadjikhani N, Liu AK, Dale AM, et al. Retinotopy and color sensitivity in human visual cortical area V8. Nat Neurosci 1998;1:235–241.

236. Bartels A, Zeki S. The architecture of the color centre in the human visual brain: new results and a review. Eur J Neurosci 2000;12:172–193.

237. Beauchamp M, Haxby J, Jennings J, et al. An fMRI version of the Farnsworth-Munsell 100-Hue test reveals multiple color-selective areas in human ventral occipitotemporal cortex. Cereb Cortex 1999;9:257–263.

238. Martin A, Haxby JV, Lalonde FM, et al. Discrete cortical regions associated with knowledge of color and knowledge of action. Science 1995;270:102–105.

239. Gulyás B, Roland P. Cortical fields participating in form and color discrimination in the human brain. Neuroreport 1991;2:585–588.

240. Gulyás B, Heywood C, Popplewell D, et al. Visual form discrimination from color or motion cues: functional anatomy by positron emission tomography. Proc Natl Acad Sci USA 1994;91:9965–9969.

241. Wechsler I. Partial cortical blindness with preservation of color vision. Arch Ophthalmol 1933;9:957–965.

242. Adler A. Course and outcome of visual agnosia. J Nerv Ment Dis 1950;111: 41–51.

243. Benson DF, Greenberg JP. Visual form agnosia. A specific defect in visual discrimination. Arch Neurol 1969;20:82–89.

244. Milner AD, Heywood CA. A disorder of lightness discrimination in a case of visual form agnosia. Cortex 1989;25:489–494.

245. Sparr SA, Jay M, Drislane FW, et al. A historic case of visual agnosia revisited after 40 years. Brain 1991;114(Pt 2):789–800.

246. Paulesu E, Harrison J, Baron-Cohen S, et al. The physiology of colored hearing: a PET activation study of color-word synaesthesia. Brain 1995;118:661–676.

247. Holmes G. Pure word blindness. Folia Psychiatr Neurol Neurochir Neerl 1950; 53:279–288.

248. Geschwind N, Fusillo M. Color-naming defects in association with alexia. Arch Neurol 1966;15:137–146.

249. Oxbury J, Oxbury SM, Humphrey N. Varieties of color anomia. Brain 1969; 92:847–860.

250. Davidoff JB, Ostergaard AL. Color anomia resulting from weakened short-term color memory. A case study. Brain 1984;107(Pt 2):415–431.

251. Kinsbourne M, Warrington EK. Observations on color agnosia. J Neurol Neurosurg Psychiatry 1964;27:296–299.

252. Luzzatti C, Davidoff J. Impaired retrieval of object-color knowledge with preserved color naming. Neuropsychologia 1994;32:933–950.

253. Miceli G, Fouch E, Capasso R, et al. The dissociation of color from form and function knowledge. Nat Neurosci 2001;4:662–667.

254. Bodamer J. Prosopagnosie. Arch Psychiatr Nervenkr 1947;179:6–54.

255. Benton A. Facial recognition 1990. Cortex 1990;26:491–499.

256. Della Sala S, Young AW. Quaglino's 1867 case of prosopagnosia. Cortex 2003; 39:533–540.

257. Bay E. Disturbances of visual perception and their examination. Brain 1953;76: 515–550.

258. Cohn R, Neumann MA, Wood DH. Prosopagnosia: a clinicopathological study. Ann Neurol 1977;1:177–182.

259. Tejeria L, Harper RA, Artes PH, et al. Face recognition in age related macular degeneration: perceived disability, measured disability, and performance with a bioptic device. Br J Ophthalmol 2002;86:1019–1026.

260. Mendez MF, Martin RJ, Smyth KA, et al. Disturbances of person identification in Alzheimer's disease. A retrospective study. J Nerv Ment Dis 1992;180:94–96.

261. Roudier M, Marcie P, Grancher A-S, et al. Discrimination of facial identity and of emotions in Alzheimer's disease. J Neurol Sci 1998;154:151–158.

262. Cronin-Coulomb A, Cronin-Coulomb M, Dunne T, et al. Facial frequency manipulation normalizes face discrimination in AD. Neurology 2000;54: 2316–2318.

263. Janati A. Kluver-Bucy syndrome in Huntington's chorea. J Nerv Ment Dis 1985; 173:632–635.

264. Dewick HC, Hanley JR, Davies AD, et al. Perception and memory for faces in Parkinson's disease. Neuropsychologia 1991;29:785–802.

265. Cousins R, Hanley JR, Davies AD, et al. Understanding memory for faces in

Parkinson's disease: the role of configural processing. Neuropsychologia 2000; 38:837–847.

266. Hoff H, Potzl O. Über eine optisch-agnostische Störung des 'Physiognomie—Gedachtnißes' (Bezeihungen zur Rückbildung ein Wortblindheit. Z Gesamte Neurol Pyschiatr 1937;159:367–395.

267. Young WB, Heros DO, Ehrenberg BL, et al. Metamorphopsia and palinopsia. Association with periodic lateralized epileptiform discharges in a patient with malignant astrocytoma. Arch Neurol 1989;46:820–822.

268. Kracke I. Developmental prosopagnosia in Asperger syndrome: presentation and discussion of an individual case. Dev Med Child Neurol 1994;36:873–886.

269. Takahashi N, Kawamura M, Hirayama K, et al. Prosopagnosia: a clinical and anatomical study of four patients. Cortex 1995;31:317–329.

270. Morrison D, Bruce V, Burton A. Understanding provoked overt recognition in prosopagnosia. Visual Cognition 2001;8:47–65.

271. Young AW, Aggleton JP, Hellawell DJ, et al. Face processing impairments after amygdalotomy. Brain 1995;118(Pt 1):15–24.

272. Young AW, Ellis HD. Childhood prosopagnosia. Brain Cogn 1989;9:16–47.

273. de Haan EH, Campbell R. A fifteen-year follow-up of a case of developmental prosopagnosia. Cortex 1991;27:489–509.

274. de Haan EH, Young AW, Newcombe F. Covert and overt recognition in prosopagnosia. Brain 1991;114:2575–2591.

275. Campbell R, Heywood CA, Cowey A, et al. Sensitivity to eye gaze in prosopagnosic patients and monkeys with superior temporal sulcus ablation. Neuropsychologia 1990;28:1123–1142.

276. Bruyer R, Laterre C, Seron X, et al. A case of prosopagnosia with some preserved covert remembrance of familiar faces. Brain Cogn 1983;2:257–284.

277. Sergent J, Villemure JG. Prosopagnosia in a right hemispherectomized patient. Brain 1989;112(Pt 4):975–995.

278. Sergent J, Poncet M. From covert to overt recognition of faces in a prosopagnosic patient. Brain 1990;113(Pt 4):989–1004.

279. Evans JJ, Heggs AJ, Antoun N, et al. Progressive prosopagnosia associated with selective right temporal lobe atrophy. A new syndrome? Brain 1995;118:1–13.

280. Tranel D, Damasio AR, Damasio H. Intact recognition of facial expression, gender, and age in patients with impaired recognition of face identity. Neurology 1988;38:690–696.

281. Albert M, Butters N, Levin J. Temporal gradients in retrograde amnesia of patients with alcoholic Korsakoff's disease. Arch Neurol 1979;36:211–216.

282. Barton JJ, Cherkasova M, O'Connor M. Covert recognition in acquired and developmental prosopagnosia. Neurology 2001;57:1161–1168.

283. Warrington E. Warrington Recognition Memory Test. Los Angeles, Western Psychological Services, 1984.

284. Benton A, van Allen M. Prosopagnosia and facial discrimination. J Neurol Sci 1972;15:167–172.

285. Parry F, Young A, Saul J, et al. Dissociable face processing impairments after brain injury. J Clin Exp Neuropsychol 1991;13:545–558.

286. Polster M, Rapcsak S. Representations in learning new faces: evidence from prosopagnosia. J Int Neuropsychol Soc 1996;2:240–248.

287. Kanwisher N. Domain specificity in face perception. Nat Neurosci 2000;3: 759–763.

288. Tarr MJ, Gauthier I. FFA: a flexible fusiform area for subordinate-level visual processing automatized by expertise. Nat Neurosci 2000;3:764–769.

289. Lhermitte F, Chain F, Escourolle R, et al. Étude anatomo-clinique d'un cas de prosopagnosie. Revue Neurologique 1972;126:329–346.

290. Whiteley AM, Warrington EK. Prosopagnosia: a clinical, psychological, and anatomical study of three patients. J Neurol Neurosurg Psychiatry 1977;40: 395–403.

291. Damasio AR, Damasio H, Van Hoesen GW. Prosopagnosia: anatomic basis and behavioral mechanisms. Neurology 1982;32:331–341.

292. de Renzi E. Current issues in prosopagnosia. In: Ellis HD, Jeeves MA, Newcome F, et al, eds. Aspects of Face Processing. Dordecht, The Netherlands, Martinus Nijhoff, 1986.

293. McNeil JE, Warrington EK. Prosopagnosia: a face-specific disorder. Q J Exp Psychol A 1993;46:1–10.

294. Henke K, Schweinberger S, Grigo A, et al. Specificity of face recognition: recognition of exemplars of non-face objects in prosopagnosia. Cortex 1998;34: 289–296.

295. Farah MJ, Levinson KL, Klein KL. Face perception and within-category discrimination in prosopagnosia. Neuropsychologia 1995;33:661–674.

296. Gauthier I, Behrmann M, Tarr MJ. Can face recognition really be dissociated from object recognition? J Cogn Neurosci 1999;11:349–370.

297. Diamond R, Carey S. Why faces are and are not special: an effect of expertise. J Exp Psychol Gen 1986;115:107–117.

298. Bruce V, Young A. Understanding face recognition. Br J Psychol 1986;77(Pt 3):305–327.

299. Damasio AR, Tranel D, Damasio H. Face agnosia and the neural substrates of memory. Annu Rev Neurosci 1990;13:89–109.

300. de Renzi E, Faglioni P, Grossi D, et al. Apperceptive and associative forms of prosopagnosia. Cortex 1991;27:213–221.

301. Levine DN, Calvanio R. Prosopagnosia: a defect in visual configural processing. Brain Cogn 1989;10:149–170.

302. Rentschler I, Treutwein B, Landis T. Dissociation of local and global processing in visual agnosia. Vision Res 1994;34:963–971.

303. de Renzi E, Faglioni P, Spinnler H. The performance of patients with unilateral brain damage on face recognition tasks. Cortex 1968;4:17–43.

304. Carlesimo G, Caltagirone C. Components in the visual processing of known and unknown faces. J Clin Exp Neuropsychol 1995;17:691–705.

305. Ellis H, Shepherd J, Davies G. Identification of familiar and unfamiliar faces from internal and external features: source implications for theories of face recognition. Perception 1979;8:431–439.

306. Young A, Hay D, McWeeney K, et al. Matching familiar and unfamiliar faces on internal and external features. Perception 1985;14:737–746.

307. Tanaka JW, Farah MJ. Parts and wholes in face recognition. Q J Exp Psychol A 1993;46:225–245.

308. Tanaka J, Sengco J. Features and their configuration in face recognition. Memory and Cognition 1997;25:583–592.

309. Farah M, Tanaka J, Drain H. What causes the face inversion effect? J Exp Psychol: Human Percept Performance 1995;21:628–634.

310. Rhodes G. Looking at faces: first-order and second-order features as determinants of facial appearance. Perception 1988;17:43–63.

311. Leder H, Bruce V. When inverted faces are recognized: the role of configural information in face recognition. Quarterly J Exp Psychol 2000;53A:513–536.

312. Barton J, Keenan J, Bass T. Discrimination of spatial relations and features in faces: effects of inversion and viewing duration. Br J Psychol 2001;92:527–549.

313. Yamane S, Kaji S, Kawano K. What facial features activate face neurons in the inferotemporal cortex of the monkey? Exp Brain Res 1988;73:209–214.

314. Young M, Yamane S. Sparse population coding of faces in the inferotemporal cortex. Science 1992;256:1327–1331.

315. Barton JJ, Press DZ, Keenan JP, et al. Lesions of the fusiform face area impair perception of facial configuration in prosopagnosia. Neurology 2002;58:71–78.

316. Barton JJ, Cherkasova MV, Press DZ, et al. Developmental prosopagnosia: a study of three patients. Brain Cogn 2003;51:12–30.

317. Joubert S, Felician O, Barbeau E, et al. Impaired configurational processing in a case of progressive prosopagnosia associated with predominant right temporal lobe atrophy. Brain 2003;126:2537–2550.

318. Farah MJ. Visual agnosia: disorders of object recognition and what they tell us about normal vision. Cambridge, MA, MIT Press, 1990.

319. Barton JJ, Cherkasova M. Face imagery and its relation to perception and covert recognition in prosopagnosia. Neurology 2003;61:220–225.

320. Ellis AW, Young AW, Critchley EM. Loss of memory for people following temporal lobe damage. Brain 1989;112(Pt 6):1469–1483.

321. Hanley J, Young AW, Pearson NA. Defective recognition of familiar people. Cognitive Neuropsychol 1989;6:179–210.

322. Gorno-Tempini M, Price C, Josephs O, et al. The neural systems sustaining face and proper name processing. Brain 1998;121:2103–2118.

323. Leveroni C, Seidenberg M, Mayer A, et al. Neural systems underlying the recognition of familiar and newly learned faces. J Neurosci 2000;20:878–886.

324. Verstichel P, Chia L. [Difficulties in face identification after lesion in the left hemisphere]. Rev Neurol (Paris) 1999;155:937–943.

325. Bruyer R. Covert face recognition in prosopagnosia: a review. Brain Cogn 1991; 15:223–235.

326. Young A. Covert recognition. In: Farah M, Ratcliff G, eds. The Neuropsychology of High-Level Vision. Hillsdale, Lawrence Erlbaum Associates, 1994: 331–358.

327. Bauer RM. Autonomic recognition of names and faces in prosopagnosia: a neuropsychological application of the Guilty Knowledge Test. Neuropsychologia 1984;22:457–469.

328. Bauer RM, Verfaellie M. Electrodermal discrimination of familiar but not unfamiliar faces in prosopagnosia. Brain Cogn 1988;8:240–252.

329. Renault B, Signoret JL, Debruille B, et al. Brain potentials reveal covert facial recognition in prosopagnosia. Neuropsychologia 1989;27:905–912.

330. McNeil JE, Warrington EK. Prosopagnosia: a reclassification. Q J Exp Psychol A 1991;43:267–287.

331. Sergent J, Signoret J-L. Implicit access to knowledge derived from unrecognized faces. Cerebral Cortex 1992;2:389–400.

332. Schweinberger SR, Klos T, Sommer W. Covert face recognition in prosopagnosia: a dissociable function? Cortex 1995;31:517–529.

333. de Haan EH, Young AW, Newcombe F. Face recognition without awareness. Cognitive Neuropsychol 1987;4:385–415.

334. Young A, Hellawell D, de Haan E. Cross-domain semantic priming in normal subjects and a prosopagnosic patient. Quart J Exp Psychol 1988;40A:561–580.

335. Newcombe F, Young AW, De Haan EH. Prosopagnosia and object agnosia without covert recognition. Neuropsychologia 1989;27:179–191.

336. Tranel D, Damasio H, Damasio A. Double dissociation between overt and covert face recognition. J Cognitive Neurosci 1995;7:425–432.

337. Schweinberger SR, Burton AM. Covert recognition and the neural system for face processing. Cortex 2003;39:9–30.

338. Farah MJ, O'Reilly RC, Vecera SP. Dissociated overt and covert recognition as an emergent property of a lesioned neural network. Psychol Rev 1993;100: 571–588.

339. Young A, Burton A. Simulating face recognition: implications for modelling cognition. Cognitive Neuropsychol 1999;16:1–48.

340. O'Reilly R, Farah M. Simulation and explanation in neuropsychology and beyond. Cognitive Neuropsychol 1999;16:49–72.

341. Stasheff SF, Barton JJ. Deficits in cortical visual function. Ophthalmol Clin North Am 2001;14:217–242.

342. Levine DN, Warach J, Farah M. Two visual systems in mental imagery: dissociation of ''what'' and ''where'' in imagery disorders due to bilateral posterior cerebral lesions. Neurology 1985;35:1010–1018.

343. Barton J, Cherkasova M, Press D, et al. Perceptual function in prosopagnosia. Perception 2004 (in press).

344. McCarthy R, Evans J, Hodges J. Topographic amnesia: spatial memory disorder, perceptual dysfunction, or category specific semantic memory impairment? J Neurol Neurosurg Psychiatry 1996;60:318–325.

345. O'Craven KM, Kanwisher N. Mental imagery of faces and places activates corresponding stimulus-specific brain regions. J Cogn Neurosci 2000;12: 1013–1023.

346. Landis T, Cummings JL, Christen L, et al. Are unilateral right posterior cerebral lesions sufficient to cause prosopagnosia? Clinical and radiological findings in six additional patients. Cortex 1986;22:243–252.

347. Gross CG, Rocha-Miranda CE, Bender DB. Visual properties of neurons in inferotemporal cortex of the Macaque. J Neurophysiol 1972;35:96–111.

348. Hasselmo M, Rolls E, Baylis G, et al. Object centered encoding by face-selective neurons in the cortex of the superior temporal sulcus of the monkey. Exp Brain Res 1989;75:417–429.

349. Baylis GC, Rolls ET, Leonard CM. Functional subdivisions of the temporal lobe neocortex. J Neurosci 1987;7:330–342.

350. Desimone R, Albright TD, Gross CG, et al. Stimulus-selective properties of inferior temporal neurons in the macaque. J Neurosci 1984;4:2051–2062.

351. Bruce C, Desimone R, Gross CG. Visual properties of neurons in a polysensory area in superior temporal sulcus of the macaque. J Neurophysiol 1981;46: 369–384.

352. Leonard CM, Rolls ET, Wilson FA, et al. Neurons in the amygdala of the monkey with responses selective for faces. Behav Brain Res 1985;15:159–176.

353. ó Scalaidhe S, Wilson F, Goldman-Rakic P. Areal segregation of face-processing neurons in prefrontal cortex. Science 1997;278:1135–1138.

354. Perrett DI, Rolls ET, Caan W. Visual neurones responsive to faces in the monkey temporal cortex. Exp Brain Res 1982;47:329–342.

355. Baylis GC, Rolls ET, Leonard CM. Selectivity between faces in the responses of a population of neurons in the cortex in the superior temporal sulcus of the monkey. Brain Res 1985;342:91–102.

356. Heywood CA, Cowey A. The role of the 'face-cell' area in the discrimination and recognition of faces by monkeys. Philos Trans R Soc Lond B Biol Sci 1992; 335:31–38.

357. Horel JA. Retrieval of a face discrimination during suppression of monkey temporal cortex with cold. Neuropsychologia 1993;31:1067–1077.

358. Tanaka K, Saito H, Fukada Y, et al. Coding visual images of objects in the inferotemporal cortex of the macaque monkey. J Neurophysiol 1991;66: 170–189.

359. Valentine T. Upside-down faces: a review of the effect of inversion upon face recognition. Br J Psychol 1988;79:471–491.

360. Perrett DI, Hietanen JK, Oram MW, et al. Organization and functions of cells responsive to faces in the temporal cortex. Philos Trans R Soc Lond B Biol Sci 1992;335:23–30.

361. Gauthier I, Logothetis N. Is face recognition not so unique after all? Cognitive Neuropsychol 2000;17:125–142.

362. Sergent J, Ohta S, MacDonald B. Functional neuroanatomy of face and object processing. A positron emission tomography study. Brain 1992;115(Pt 1):15–36.

363. Haxby JV, Horwitz B, Ungerleider LG, et al. The functional organization of human extrastriate cortex: a PET-rCBF study of selective attention to faces and locations. J Neurosci 1994;14:6336–6353.

364. Grady CL, Maisog JM, Horwitz B, et al. Age-related changes in cortical blood flow activation during visual processing of faces and location. J Neurosci 1994; 14:1450–1462.

365. Allison T, Ginter H, McCarthy G, et al. Face recognition in human extrastriate cortex. J Neurophysiol 1994;71:821–825.

366. Haxby J, Hoffman E, Gobbini M. The distributed human neural system for face perception. Trends Cogn Sci 2000;4:223–233.

367. McCarthy G, Puce A, Gore J, et al. Face-specific processing in the human fusiform gyrus. J Cogn Neurosci 1997;9:605–610.

368. Kanwisher N, McDermott J, Chun M. The fusiform face area: a module in human extrastriate cortex specialized for face perception. J Neurosci 1997;17: 4302–4311.

369. Puce A, Allison T, Gore JC, et al. Face-sensitive regions in human extrastriate cortex studied by functional MRI. J Neurophysiol 1995;74:1192–1199.

370. Haxby J, Ungerleider L, Clark V, et al. The effect of face inversion on activity in human neural systems. Neuron 1999;22:189–199.

371. Hoffman E, Haxby J. Distinct representations of eye gaze and identity in the distributed human neural system for face perception. Nature Neurosci 2000;3: 80–84.

372. Haxby JV, Gobbini MI, Furey ML, et al. Distributed and overlapping representations of faces and objects in ventral temporal cortex. Science 2001;293: 2425–2430.

373. Epstein R, Harris A, Stanley D, et al. The parahippocampal place area: recognition, navigation, or encoding? Neuron 1999;23:115–125.

374. Kanwisher N, Stanley D, Harris A. The fusiform face area is selective for faces not animals. Neuroreport 1999;10:183–187.

375. Chao L, Martin A, Haxby J. Are face-responsive regions selective only for faces? Neuroreport 1999;10:2945–2950.

376. Gauthier I, Skudlarski P, Gore JC, et al. Expertise for cars and birds recruits brain areas involved in face recognition. Nat Neurosci 2000;3:191–197.

377. Meadows JC. The anatomical basis of prosopagnosia. J Neurol Neurosurg Psychiatry 1974;37:489–501.

378. Ettlin TM, Beckson M, Benson DF, et al. Prosopagnosia: a bihemispheric disorder. Cortex 1992;28:129–134.

379. de Renzi E. Prosopagnosia in two patients with CT scan evidence of damage confined to the right hemisphere. Neuropsychologia 1986;24:385–389.

380. Michel F, Perenin MT, Sieroff E. Prosopagnosie sans hémianopsie après lésion unilatérale occipito-temporale droite. Revue Neurologique 1986;142:545–549.

381. Barton JJ, Zhao J, Keenan JP. Perception of global facial geometry in the inversion effect and prosopagnosia. Neuropsychologia 2003;41:1703–1711.

382. Clarke S, Lindemann A, Maeder P, et al. Face recognition and postero-inferior hemispheric lesions. Neuropsychologia 1997;35:1555–1563.

383. Malone DR, Morris HH, Kay MC, et al. Prosopagnosia: a double dissociation between the recognition of familiar and unfamiliar faces. J Neurol Neurosurg Psychiatry 1982;45:820–822.

384. Tyrell P, Warrington E, Frackowiak R, et al. Progressive degeneration of the right temporal lobe studied with positron emission tomography. J Neurol Neurosurg Psychiatry 1990;53:1048–1050.

385. Martins IP, Cunha e Sa M. Loss of topographic memory and prosopagnosia during migraine aura. Cephalalgia 1999;19:841–843.

386. McConachie HR. Developmental prosopagnosia. A single case report. Cortex 1976;12:76–82.

387. Ariel R, Sadeh M. Congenital visual agnosia and prosopagnosia in a child: a case report. Cortex 1996;32:221–240.

388. Young AW, Newcombe F, de Haan EH, et al. Face perception after brain injury. Selective impairments affecting identity and expression. Brain 1993;116(Pt 4): 941–959.

389. de Renzi E, Bonacini MG, Faglioni P. Right posterior brain-damaged patients are poor at assessing the age of a face. Neuropsychologia 1989;27:839–848.

390. Young A, Flude B, Hay D, et al. Impaired discrimination of familiar from unfamiliar faces. Cortex 1993;29:65–75.

391. Rapcsak S, Polster M, Comer J, et al. False recognition and misidentification of faces following right hemisphere damage. Cortex 1994;30:565–583.

392. Rapcsak S, Polster M, Glisky M, et al. False recognition of unfamiliar faces following right hemisphere damage: neuropsychological and anatomical observations. Cortex 1996;32:593–611.

393. Black SE, Behrmann M. Localization in alexia. In: Kertesz A, ed. Localization and Neuroimaging in Neuropsychology. San Diego, Academic Press, 1994: 331–376.

394. Dejerine J. Sur un cas de cecite verbale avec agraphie, suive d'autopsie. Comptes Rendus Societé du Biologie 1891;43:197–201.

395. Geschwind N. Disconnexion syndromes in animals and man. I. Brain 1965;88: 237–294.

396. Damasio AR, Damasio H. The anatomic basis of pure alexia. Neurology 1983; 33:1573–1583.

397. Binder JR, Mohr JP. The topography of callosal reading pathways. A case-control analysis. Brain 1992;115(Pt 6):1807–1826.

398. Horikoshi T, Asari Y, Watanabe A, et al. Music alexia in a patient with mild pure alexia: disturbed visual perception of non-verbal meaningful figures. Cortex 1997;33:187–194.

399. Beversdorf D, Heilman K. Progressive ventral posterior cortical degeneration presenting as alexia for music and words. Neurology 1998;50:657–659.

400. Bub DN, Black S, Howell J. Word recognition and orthographic context effects in a letter-by-letter reader. Brain Lang 1989;36:357–376.

401. Coslett HB, Saffran EM, Greenbaum S, et al. Reading in pure alexia. The effect of strategy. Brain 1993;116(Pt 1):21–37.

402. Jibiki I, Yamaguchi N. The Gogi (word-meaning) syndrome with impaired kanji processing: alexia with agraphia. Brain Lang 1993;45:61–69.

403. Sakurai Y, Ichikawa Y, Mannen T. Pure alexia from a posterior occipital lesion. Neurology 2001;56:778–781.

404. Ohno T, Takeda K, Kato S, et al. Pure alexia in a Japanese-English bilingual: dissociation between the two languages. J Neurol 2002;249:105–107.

405. Hamilton R, Keenan J, Catala M, et al. Alexia for Braille following bilateral occipital stroke in an early blind woman. Neuroreport 2000;11:237–240.

406. Greenblatt SH. Alexia without agraphia or hemianopsia. Anatomical analysis of an autopsied case. Brain 1973;96:307–316.

407. Vincent FM, Sadowsky CH, Saunders RL, et al. Alexia without agraphia, hemianopia, or color-naming defect: a disconnection syndrome. Neurology 1977;27:689–691.

408. Henderson VW, Friedman RB, Teng EL, et al. Left hemisphere pathways in reading: inferences from pure alexia without hemianopia. Neurology 1985;35:962–968.

409. Iragui VJ, Kritchevsky M. Alexia without agraphia or hemianopia in parietal infarction. J Neurol Neurosurg Psychiatry 1991;54:841–842.

410. Erdem S, Kansu T. Alexia without either agraphia or hemianopia in temporal lobe lesion due to herpes simplex encephalitis. J Neuroophthalmol 1995;15:102–104.

411. de Renzi E, Zambolin A, Crisi G. The pattern of neuropsychological impairment associated with left posterior cerebral artery infarcts. Brain 1987;110(Pt 5):1099–1116.

412. Albert ML, Yamadori A, Gardner H, et al. Comprehension in alexia. Brain 1973;96:317–328.

413. Coslett HB, Saffran EM. Evidence for preserved reading in 'pure alexia.' Brain 1989;112(Pt 2):327–359.

414. Bub DN, Arguin M. Visual word activation in pure alexia. Brain Lang 1995;49:77–103.

415. Caplan LR, Hedley-Whyte T. Cuing and memory dysfunction in alexia without agraphia. A case report. Brain 1974;97:251–262.

416. Behrmann M, Black SE, Bub D. The evolution of pure alexia: a longitudinal study of recovery. Brain Lang 1990;39:405–427.

417. Feinberg TE, Dyckes-Berke D, Miner CR, et al. Knowledge, implicit knowledge and meta knowledge in visual agnosia and pure alexia. Brain 1995;118(Pt 3):789–800.

418. Warrington EK, Shallice T. Word-form dyslexia. Brain 1980;103:99–112.

419. Uitti RJ, Donat JR, Romanchuk K. Pure alexia without hemianopia. Arch Neurol 1984;41:1130.

420. Ajax ET. Dyslexia without agraphia. Prognostic considerations. Arch Neurol 1967;17:645–652.

421. Jonsdóttir M, Magnússon T, Kjartansson O. Pure alexia and word-meaning deafness in a patient with multiple sclerosis. Arch Neurol 1998;55:1473–1474.

422. Freedman L, Selchen DH, Black SE, et al. Posterior cortical dementia with alexia: neurobehavioural, MRI, and PET findings. J Neurol Neurosurg Psychiatry 1991;54:443–448.

423. Dejerine J. Contributions a l'étude anatomopathologique et clinique des differentes varietes de cecite verbale. Memoires de la Societé Biologique 1892;44:61–90.

424. Lanzinger S, Weder B, Oettli R, et al. Neuroimaging findings in a patient recovering from global alexia to spelling dyslexia. J Neuroimaging 1999;9:48–51.

425. Lepore F. Visual deficits in alexia without agraphia. Neuro-Ophthalmology 1998;19:1–6.

426. Cohen SY, Bulik A, Tadayoni R, et al. Visual hallucinations and Charles Bonnet syndrome after photodynamic therapy for age related macular degeneration. Br J Ophthalmol 2003;87:977–979.

427. Behrmann M, Nelson J, Sekuler A. Visual complexity in letter-by-letter reading: ''pure'' alexia is not pure. Neuropsychologia 1998;36:1115–1132.

428. Shallice T, Warrington EK. The possible role of selective attention in acquired dyslexia. Neuropsychologia 1977;15:31–41.

429. Levine DN, Calvanio R. A study of the visual defect in verbal alexia-simultanagnosia. Brain 1978;101:65–81.

430. Mendez M, Cherrier M. The evolution of alexia and simultanagnosia in posterior cortical atrophy. Neuropsychiatry Neuropsychol Behav Neurol 1998;11:76–82.

431. Vaina L, Grzywacz N, Kikinis R. Segregation of computations underlying perception of motion discontinuity and coherence. Neuroreport 1994;5:2289–2294.

432. Chanoine V, Ferreira C, Demonet J, et al. Optic aphasia with pure alexia: a mild form of visual associative agnosia? A case study. Cortex 1998;34:437–448.

433. Bartolomeo P, Bachoud-Levi A, Chokron S, et al. Visually- and motor-based knowledge of letters: evidence from a pure alexic patient. Neuropsychologia 2002;40:1363–1371.

434. Beversdorf D, Ratcliffe N, Rhodes C, et al. Pure alexia: clinical-pathologic evidence for a lateralized visual language association cortex. Clin Neuropathol 1997;16:328–331.

435. Benito-León J, Sanchez-Suarez C, Diaz-Guzman J, et al. Pure alexia could not be a disconnection syndrome. Neurology 1997;49:305–306.

436. Silver FL, Chawluk JB, Bosley TM, et al. Resolving metabolic abnormalities in a case of pure alexia. Neurology 1988;38:730–735.

437. Stommel EW, Friedman RJ, Reeves AG. Alexia without agraphia associated with spleniogeniculate infarction. Neurology 1991;41:587–588.

438. Beeson P, Insalaco D. Acquired alexia: lessons from successful treatment. J Int Neuropsychol Soc 1998;4:621–635.

439. Maher L, Clayton M, Barrett A, et al. Rehabilitation of a case of pure alexia: exploiting residual reading abilities. J Int Neuropsychol Soc 1998;4:636–647.

440. Conway T, Heilman P, Rothi L, et al. Treatment of a case of phonological alexia with agraphia using the Auditory Discrimination in Depth (ADD) program. J Int Neuropsychol Soc 1998;4:608–620.

441. Nitzberg Lott S, Friedman R. Can treatment for pure alexia improve letter-by-letter reading speed without sacrificing accuracy? Brain Lang 1999;67:188–201.

442. Gazzaniga MS, Freedman H. Observations on visual processes after posterior callosal section. Neurology 1973;23:1126–1130.

443. Molko N, Cohen L, Mangin J, et al. Visualizing the neural bases of a disconnection syndrome with diffusion tensor imaging. J Cogn Neurosci 2002;14:629–636.

444. Castro-Caldas A, Salgado V. Right hemifield alexia without hemianopia. Arch Neurol 1984;41:84–87.

445. Binder JR, Lazar RM, Tatemichi TK, et al. Left hemiparalexia. Neurology 1992;42:562–569.

446. Benson DF. Alexia. In: Vinken PJ, Bruyn GW, Klawans HL, eds. Handbook of Clinical Neurology, rev. ser. Amsterdam, New York, Elsevier, 1985:433–455.

447. Kawahata N, Nagata K, Shishido F. Alexia with agraphia due to the left posterior inferior temporal lobe lesion—neuropsychological analysis and its pathogenetic mechanisms. Brain Lang 1988;33:296–310.

448. Benson DF, Brown J, Tomlinson EB. Varieties of alexia. Word and letter blindness. Neurology 1971;21:951–957.

449. Benson DF. The third alexia. Arch Neurol 1977;34:327–331.

450. Trauzettel-Klosinski S, Reinhard J. The vertical field border in hemianopia and its significance for fixation and reading. Invest Ophthalmol Vis Sci 1998;39:2177–2186.

451. de Luca M, Spinelli D, Zoccolotti P. Eye movement patterns in reading as a function of visual field defects and contrast sensitivity loss. Cortex 1996;32:491–502.

452. Zihl J. Eye movement patterns in hemianopic dyslexia. Brain 1995;118(Pt 4):891–912.

453. Trauzettel-Klosinski S, Brendler K. Eye movements in reading with hemianopic field defects: the significance of clinical parameters. Graefe's Arch Clin Exp Ophthalmol 1998;236:91–102.

454. Kirkham TH. The ocular symptomatology of pituitary tumours. Proc R Soc Med 1972;65:517–518.

455. Behrmann M, Moscovitch M, Black SE, et al. Perceptual and conceptual mechanisms in neglect dyslexia. Two contrasting case studies. Brain 1990;113(Pt 4):1163–1183.

456. Patterson KE, Wilson B. A ROSE is a ROSE or a NOSE: a deficit in initial letter identification. Cognitive Neuropsychol 1990;7:447–477.

457. Luria AR, Pravdina-Vinarskaya EN, Yarbus AL. Disturbances of ocular movement in a case of simultanagnosia. Brain 1962;86.

458. Rizzo M. 'Balint's syndrome' and associated visuospatial disorders. Baillieres Clin Neurol 1993;2:415–437.

459. Pierrot-Deseilligny C, Gray F, Brunet P. Infarcts of both inferior parietal lobules with impairment of visually guided eye movements, peripheral visual inattention and optic ataxia. Brain 1986;109(Pt 1):81–97.

460. Husain M, Stein J. Rezso Bálint and his most celebrated case. Arch Neurol 1988;45:89–93.

461. Friedman DI, Jankovic J, McCrary JA 3rd. Neuro-ophthalmic findings in progressive supranuclear palsy. J Clin Neuroophthalmol 1992;12:104–109.

462. Beauvois MF, Derouesne J. Phonological alexia: three dissociations. J Neurol Neurosurg Psychiatry 1979;42:1115–1124.

463. Funnell E. Phonological processes in reading: new evidence from acquired dyslexia. Br J Psychol 1983;74:159–180.

464. Friedman RB. Two types of phonological alexia. Cortex 1995;31:397–403.

465. Shallice T, Warrington EK, McCarthy R. Reading without semantics. Q J Exp Psychol A 1983;35A:111–138.

466. Patterson KE, Morton J. From orthograph to phonology: an attempt at an old interpretation. In: Patterson K, Marshall JC, Coltheart M, eds. Surface Dyslexia: Neuropsychological and Cognitive Studies of Phonological Reading. London, Hillsdale, NJ, Lawrence Erlbaum Associates, 1985:335–359.

467. Cummings JL, Houlihan JP, Hill MA. The pattern of reading deterioration in dementia of the Alzheimer type: observations and implications. Brain Lang 1986;29:315–323.

468. Friedman RB, Ferguson S, Robinson S, et al. Dissociation of mechanisms of reading in Alzheimer's disease. Brain Lang 1992;43:400–413.

469. Friedman RB, Kohn SE. Impaired activation of the phonological lexicon: effects upon oral reading. Brain Lang 1990;38:278–297.

470. Coltheart M, Patterson K, Marshall JC. Deep Dyslexia. London, Boston, Routledge & Kegan Paul, 1980.

471. Coltheart M. Deep dyslexia, a review of the syndrome. In: Coltheart M, Patterson K, Marshall JC, eds. Deep Dyslexia. London, Boston, Routledge & Kegan Paul, 1980:22–47.

472. Price CJ, Wise RJ, Watson JD, et al. Brain activity during reading. The effects of exposure duration and task. Brain 1994;117(Pt 6):1255–1269.

473. Petersen SE, Fox PT, Posner MI, et al. Positron emission tomographic studies of the cortical anatomy of single-word processing. Nature 1988;331:585–589.

474. Posner MI, Petersen SE, Fox PT, et al. Localization of cognitive operations in the human brain. Science 1988;240:1627–1631.

475. Petersen SE, Fox PT, Snyder AZ, et al. Activation of extrastriate and frontal cortical areas by visual words and word-like stimuli. Science 1990;249: 1041–1044.

476. Howard D, Patterson K, Wise R, et al. The cortical localization of the lexicons. Positron emission tomography evidence. Brain 1992;115(Pt 6):1769–1782.

477. Nakayama K. Biological image motion processing: a review. Vision Res 1985; 25:625–660.

478. Zihl J, von Cramon D, Mai N, et al. Disturbance of movement vision after bilateral posterior brain damage. Further evidence and follow-up observations. Brain 1991;114(Pt 5):2235–2252.

479. MacLeod DI, Chen B, Crognale M. Spatial organization of sensitivity regulation in rod vision. Vision Res 1989;29:965–978.

480. Baker CL, Jr., Hess RF, Zihl J. Residual motion perception in a "motion-blind" patient, assessed with limited-lifetime random dot stimuli. J Neurosci 1991;11: 454–461.

481. Shipp S, de Jong BM, Zihl J, et al. The brain activity related to residual motion vision in a patient with bilateral lesions of V5. Brain 1994;117(Pt 4):1023–1038.

482. Baker CJ, Hess R, Zihl J. Residual motion perception in a "motion-blind" patient, assessed with limited-lifetime random dot stimuli. J Neurosci 1991;11: 454–461.

483. Vaina LM, Lemay M, Bienfang DC, et al. Intact "biological motion" and "structure from motion" perception in a patient with impaired motion mechanisms: a case study. Vis Neurosci 1990;5:353–369.

484. Vaina LM. Functional segregation of color and motion processing in the human visual cortex: clinical evidence. Cereb Cortex 1994;4:555–572.

485. Johansson T, Fahlgren H. Alexia without agraphia: lateral and medial infarction of left occipital lobe. Neurology 1979;29:390–393.

486. Warrington EK, Taylor AM. The contribution of the right parietal lobe to object recognition. Cortex 1973;9:152–164.

487. Plant GT, Laxer KD, Barbaro NM, et al. Impaired visual motion perception in the contralateral hemifield following unilateral posterior cerebral lesions in humans. Brain 1993;116(Pt 6):1303–1335.

488. Greenlee MW, Lang HJ, Mergner T, et al. Visual short-term memory of stimulus velocity in patients with unilateral posterior brain damage. J Neurosci 1995;15: 2287–2300.

489. Barton JJ, Sharpe JA, Raymond JE. Retinotopic and directional defects in motion discrimination in humans with cerebral lesions. Ann Neurol 1995;37:665–675.

490. Vaina LM. Selective impairment of visual motion interpretation following lesions of the right occipito-parietal area in humans. Biol Cybern 1989;61: 347–359.

491. Regan D, Giaschi D, Sharpe JA, et al. Visual processing of motion-defined form: selective failure in patients with parietotemporal lesions. J Neurosci 1992;12: 2198–2210.

492. Nawrot M, Rizzo M, Damasio H. Motion perception in humans with focal cerebral lesions [abstract]. Invest Ophthalmol Vis Sci 1993;34(Suppl):1231.

493. Nawrot M, Rizzo M. Motion perception deficits from midline cerebellar lesions in human. Vision Res 1995;35:723–731.

494. Batelli L, Cavanagh P, Martini P, et al. Bilateral deficits of transient visual attention in right parietal patients. Brain 2003;126:2164–2174.

495. Dubner R, Zeki SM. Response properties and receptive fields of cells in an anatomically defined region of the superior temporal sulcus in the monkey. Brain Res 1971;35:528–532.

496. Maunsell JH, Van Essen DC. Functional properties of neurons in middle temporal visual area of the macaque monkey. I. Selectivity for stimulus direction, speed, and orientation. J Neurophysiol 1983;49:1127–1147.

497. Albright TD. Direction and orientation selectivity of neurons in visual area MT of the macaque. J Neurophysiol 1984;52:1106–1130.

498. Felleman DJ, Kaas JH. Receptive-field properties of neurons in middle temporal visual area (MT) of owl monkeys. J Neurophysiol 1984;52:488–513.

499. Lagae L, Raiguel S, Orban GA. Speed and direction selectivity of macaque middle temporal neurons. J Neurophysiol 1993;69:19–39.

500. van Essen DC, Maunsell JH, Bixby JL. The middle temporal visual area in the macaque: myeloarchitecture, connections, functional properties and topographic organization. J Comp Neurol 1981;199:293–326.

501. Maunsell JH, Van Essen DC. Functional properties of neurons in middle temporal visual area of the macaque monkey. II. Binocular interactions and sensitivity to binocular disparity. J Neurophysiol 1983;49:1148–1167.

502. Ungerleider LG, Desimone R. Cortical connections of visual area MT in the macaque. J Comp Neurol 1986;248:190–222.

503. Boussaoud D, Ungerleider LG, Desimone R. Pathways for motion analysis: cortical connections of the medial superior temporal and fundus of the superior temporal visual areas in the macaque. J Comp Neurol 1990;296:462–495.

504. Tanaka K, Saito H. Analysis of motion of the visual field by direction, expansion/contraction, and rotation cells clustered in the dorsal part of the medial superior temporal area of the macaque monkey. J Neurophysiol 1989;62:626–641.

505. Tanaka K, Fukada Y, Saito HA. Underlying mechanisms of the response specificity of expansion/contraction and rotation cells in the dorsal part of the medial superior temporal area of the macaque monkey. J Neurophysiol 1989;62: 642–656.

506. Duffy CJ, Wurtz RH. Sensitivity of MST neurons to optic flow stimuli. I. A continuum of response selectivity to large-field stimuli. J Neurophysiol 1991; 65:1329–1345.

507. Duffy CJ, Wurtz RH. Sensitivity of MST neurons to optic flow stimuli. II. Mechanisms of response selectivity revealed by small-field stimuli. J Neurophysiol 1991;65:1346–1359.

508. Graziano MS, Andersen RA, Snowden RJ. Tuning of MST neurons to spiral motions. J Neurosci 1994;14:54–67.

509. Duffy CJ, Wurtz RH. Response of monkey MST neurons to optic flow stimuli with shifted centers of motion. J Neurosci 1995;15:5192–5208.

510. Geesaman BJ, Andersen RA. The analysis of complex motion patterns by form/cue invariant MSTd neurons. J Neurosci 1996;16:4716–4732.

511. Colby CL, Duhamel JR, Goldberg ME. Ventral intraparietal area of the macaque: anatomic location and visual response properties. J Neurophysiol 1993;69: 902–914.

512. Oram MW, Perrett DI, Hietanen JK. Directional tuning of motion-sensitive cells in the anterior superior temporal polysensory area of the macaque. Exp Brain Res 1993;97:274–294.

513. Perrett DI, Smith PA, Potter DD, et al. Visual cells in the temporal cortex sensitive to face view and gaze direction. Proc R Soc Lond B Biol Sci 1985; 223:293–317.

514. Hietanen JK, Perrett DI. Motion sensitive cells in the macaque superior temporal polysensory area: response discrimination between self-generated and externally generated pattern motion. Behav Brain Res 1996;76:155–167.

515. Sáry G, Vogels R, Orban GA. Cue-invariant shape selectivity of macaque inferior temporal neurons. Science 1993;260:995–997.

516. Sáry G, Vogels R, Kovacs G, et al. Responses of monkey inferior temporal neurons to luminance-, motion-, and texture-defined gratings. J Neurophysiol 1995;73:1341–1354.

517. Snowden RJ, Treue S, Erickson RG, et al. The response of area MT and V1 neurons to transparent motion. J Neurosci 1991;11:2768–2785.

518. Qian N, Andersen RA. Transparent motion perception as detection of unbalanced motion signals. II. Physiology. J Neurosci 1994;14:7367–7380.

519. Qian N, Andersen RA, Adelson EH. Transparent motion perception as detection of unbalanced motion signals. I. Psychophysics. J Neurosci 1994;14:7357–7366.

520. Pasternak T, Schumer RA, Gizzi MS, et al. Abolition of visual cortical direction selectivity affects visual behavior in cats. Exp Brain Res 1985;61:214–217.

521. Rodman HR, Albright TD. Single-unit analysis of pattern-motion selective properties in the middle temporal visual area (MT). Exp Brain Res 1989;75:53–64.

522. Bradley DC, Qian N, Andersen RA. Integration of motion and stereopsis in middle temporal cortical area of macaques. Nature 1995;373:609–611.

523. Albright TD. Form-cue invariant motion processing in primate visual cortex. Science 1992;255:1141–1143.

524. Olavarria JF, DeYoe EA, Knierim JJ, et al. Neural responses to visual texture patterns in middle temporal area of the macaque monkey. J Neurophysiol 1992; 68:164–181.

525. Allman J, Miezin F, McGuinness E. Direction- and velocity-specific responses from beyond the classical receptive field in the middle temporal visual area (MT). Perception 1985;14:105–126.

526. Tanaka K, Hikosaka K, Saito H, et al. Analysis of local and wide-field movements in the superior temporal visual areas of the macaque monkey. J Neurosci 1986;6:134–144.

527. Born RT, Tootell RB. Segregation of global and local motion processing in primate middle temporal visual area. Nature 1992;357:497–499.

528. Buracas GT, Albright TD. Contribution of area MT to perception of three-dimensional shape: a computational study. Vision Res 1996;36:869–887.

529. Dürsteler MR, Wurtz RH. Pursuit and optokinetic deficits following chemical lesions of cortical areas MT and MST. J Neurophysiol 1988;60:940–965.

530. Dursteler MR, Wurtz RH, Newsome WT. Directional pursuit deficits following lesions of the foveal representation within the superior temporal sulcus of the macaque monkey. J Neurophysiol 1987;57:1262–1287.

531. Newsome WT, Wurtz RH, Dursteler MR, et al. Deficits in visual motion processing following ibotenic acid lesions of the middle temporal visual area of the macaque monkey. J Neurosci 1985;5:825–840.

532. Schiller PH, Lee K. The role of the primate extrastriate area V4 in vision. Science 1991;251:1251–1253.

533. Newsome WT, Pare EB. A selective impairment of motion perception following lesions of the middle temporal visual area (MT). J Neurosci 1988;8:2201–2211.

534. Cowey A, Marcar VL. The effect of removing superior temporal cortical motion areas in the macaque monkey: I. Motion discrimination using simple Dots. Eur J Neurosci 1992;4:1219–1227.

535. Marcar VL, Cowey A. The effect of removing superior temporal cortical motion

areas in the macaque monkey: II. Motion discrimination using random dot displays. Eur J Neurosci 1992;4:1228–1238.

536. Yamasaki DS, Wurtz RH. Recovery of function after lesions in the superior temporal sulcus in the monkey. J Neurophysiol 1991;66:651–673.

537. Britten KH, Newsome WT, Saunders RC. Effects of inferotemporal cortex lesions on form-from-motion discrimination in monkeys. Exp Brain Res 1992;88: 292–302.

538. Salzman C, Britten KH, Newsome WT. Cortical microstimulation influences perceptual judgements of motion direction. Nature 1990;346:174–177.

539. Salzman CD, Murasugi CM, Britten KH, et al. Microstimulation in visual area MT: effects on direction discrimination performance. J Neurosci 1992;12: 2331–2355.

540. Murasugi CM, Salzman CD, Newsome WT. Microstimulation in visual area MT: effects of varying pulse amplitude and frequency. J Neurosci 1993;13: 1719–1729.

541. Newsome WT, Britten KH, Movshon JA. Neuronal correlates of a perceptual decision. Nature 1989;341:52–54.

542. Celebrini S, Newsome WT. Microstimulation of extrastriate area MST influences performance on a direction discrimination task. J Neurophysiol 1995;73: 437–448.

543. Shadlen MN, Britten KH, Newsome WT, et al. A computational analysis of the relationship between neuronal and behavioral responses to visual motion. J Neurosci 1996;16:1486–1510.

544. Fox PT, Miezin FM, Allman JM, et al. Retinotopic organization of human visual cortex mapped with positron-emission tomography. J Neurosci 1987;7:913–922.

545. Zeki S, Watson JD, Frackowiak RS. Going beyond the information given: the relation of illusory visual motion to brain activity. Proc R Soc Lond B Biol Sci 1993;252:215–222.

546. Dupont P, Orban GA, De Bruyn B, et al. Many areas in the human brain respond to visual motion. J Neurophysiol 1994;72:1420–1424.

547. de Jong B, Shipp S, Skidmore B, et al. The cerebral activity related to the visual perception of forward motion in depth. Brain 1994;117:1039–1054.

548. Bonda E, Petrides M, Ostry D, et al. Specific involvement of human parietal systems and the amygdala in the perception of biological motion. J Neurosci 1996;16:3737–3744.

549. McCarthy G, Spicer M, Adrignolo A, et al. Brain activation associated with visual motion studied by functional magnetic resonance imaging in humans. Hum Brain Mapp 1994;2:234–243.

550. Tootell RB, Reppas JB, Kwong KK, et al. Functional analysis of human MT and related visual cortical areas using magnetic resonance imaging. J Neurosci 1995;15:3215–3230.

551. Tootell RB, Reppas JB, Dale AM, et al. Visual motion aftereffect in human cortical area MT revealed by functional magnetic resonance imaging. Nature 1995;375:139–141.

552. Barton JJ, Simpson T, Kiriakopoulos E, et al. Functional MRI of lateral occipito-temporal cortex during pursuit and motion perception. Ann Neurol 1996;40: 387–398.

553. Probst T, Plendl H, Paulus W, et al. Identification of the visual motion area (area V5) in the human brain by dipole source analysis. Exp Brain Res 1993; 93:345–351.

554. Beckers G, Homberg V. Cerebral visual motion blindness: transitory akinetopsia induced by transcranial magnetic stimulation of human area V5. Proc R Soc Lond B Biol Sci 1992;249:173–178.

555. Wolpert T. Die Simultanagnosie. Z Gesamte Neurol Pyschiatr 1924;93:397–415.

556. Johnston JL, Sharpe JA, Morrow MJ. Spasm of fixation: a quantitative study. J Neurol Sci 1992;107:166–171.

557. Cogan DG. Congenital ocular motor apraxia. Can J Ophthalmol 1966;1: 253–260.

558. Montero J, Pena J, Genis D, et al. Balint's syndrome. Report of four cases with watershed parieto-occipital lesions from vertebrobasilar ischemia or systemic hypotension. Acta Neurol Belg 1982;82:270–280.

559. Hijdra A, Meerwaldt JD. Balint's syndrome in a man with border-zone infarcts caused by atrial fibrillation. Clin Neurol Neurosurg 1984;86:51–54.

560. Schnider A, Landis T, Regard M. Balint's syndrome in subacute HIV encephalitis. J Neurol Neurosurg Psychiatry 1991;54:822–825.

561. Hof PR, Bouras C, Constantinidis J, et al. Selective disconnection of specific visual association pathways in cases of Alzheimer's disease presenting with Balint's syndrome. J Neuropathol Exp Neurol 1990;49:168–184.

562. Mendez MF, Mendez MA, Martin R, et al. Complex visual disturbances in Alzheimer's disease. Neurology 1990;40:439–443.

563. Goodglass H, Kaplan E. The Assessment of Aphasia and Related Disorders, 2nd ed. Philadelphia, Lea & Febiger, 1983.

564. Luria AR. Disorders of "simultaneous perception" in a case of bilateral occipito-parietal brain injury. Brain 1959;82:437–449.

565. Rizzo M, Robin DA. Simultanagnosia: a defect of sustained attention yields insights on visual information processing. Neurology 1990;40:447–455.

566. Lissauer H. Ein fall von Seelenblindheit nebst einem Beitrag zur Theorie derselben. Arch Psychiatr Nervenkr 1890;21:22–70.

567. Teuber HL. Alteration of perception and memory in man. In: Weiskrantz L, ed. Analysis of Behavioral Change. New York, Harper & Row, 1968.

568. Hécaen H, de Ajuriaguerra J. Bálint's syndrome (psychic paralysis of visual fixation) and its minor forms. Brain 1954;77:373–400.

569. Leigh RJ, Zee DS. The Neurology of Eye Movements, 2nd ed., rev. and enl ed. Philadelphia, FA Davis, 1991.

570. Benton AL. Gerstmann's syndrome. Arch Neurol 1992;49:445–447.

571. Rizzo M, Hurtig R. Visual search in hemineglect: what stirs idle eyes? Clin Vis Sci 1992;7:39–52.

572. Hausser CO, Robert F, Giard N. Balint's syndrome. Can J Neurol Sci 1980;7: 157–161.

573. Ogren MP, Mateer CA, Wyler AR. Alterations in visually related eye movements following left pulvinar damage in man. Neuropsychologia 1984;22:187–196.

574. Rizzo M, Hurtig R. Looking but not seeing: attention, perception, and eye movements in simultanagnosia. Neurology 1987;37:1642–1648.

575. Rizzo M, Rotella D, Darling W. Troubled reaching after right occipito-temporal damage. Neuropsychologia 1992;30:711–722.

576. Baylis G, Driver J, Baylis L, et al. Reading of letters and words in a patient with Balint's syndrome. Neurocase: case studies in neuropsychology, neuropsychiatry, and behavioural neurology. Oxford, Oxford University Press, 1995: 331–343.

577. Rizzo M, Vecera SP. Psychoanatomical substrates of Balint's syndrome. J Neurol Neurosurg Psychiatry 2002;72:162–178.

578. James W. The Principles of Psychology. New York, H Holt, 1890.

579. Ball KK, Beard BL, Roenker DL, et al. Age and visual search: expanding the useful field of view. J Opt Soc Am A 1988;5:2210–2219.

580. Ball KK, Roenker DL, Bruni JR. Developmental changes in attention and visual search throughout adulthood. In: Enns JTE, ed. The Development of Attention: Research and Theory. Advances in Psychology. North Holland, Elsevier Science Publishers, 1990;489–507.

581. Owsley C, Ball K, Sloane ME, et al. Visual/cognitive correlates of vehicle accidents in older drivers. Psychology Aging 1991;6:403–415.

582. Ball K, Owsley C, Sloane ME, et al. Visual attention problems as a predictor of vehicle crashes in older drivers. Invest Ophthalmol Vis Sci 1993;34:3110–3123.

583. Rizzo M, Robin DA. Bilateral effects of unilateral visual cortex lesions in human. Brain 1996;119(Pt 3):951–963.

584. Sekuler AB, Bennett PJ, Mamelak M. Effects of aging on the useful field of view. Exp Aging Res 2000;26:103–120.

585. Shallice T. Specific impairments of planning. Phil Trans R Soc B 1982;298: 199–209.

586. Baddeley A, Logie R, Bressi S, et al. Dementia and working memory. Q J Exp Psychol A 1986;38:603–618.

587. O'Regan JK, et al. Change-blindness as a result of "mudsplashes." Nature 1999; 398:34.

588. Simons DL, Franconeri SL, Reimer RL. Change blindness in the absence of visual disruption. Perception 2000;29:1143–1154.

589. Pani JR. Cognitive description and change blindness. Vis Cog 2000;7:107–126.

590. Batchelder S, Rizzo M, Vanderleest R, et al. Traffic Scene-Related Change Blindness in Older Drivers. Park City, UT, 2003.

591. Kellison I, Rizzo M, Vecera S, et al. Blindness to Context-Relevant Visual Change in Advancing Age. Society for Neurosciences, San Francisco, 2003.

592. Rizzo M, Akutsu H, Dawson J. Increased attentional blink after focal cerebral lesions. Neurology 2001;57:795–800.

593. Rizzo M. Safe and unsafe driving. In: Rizzo M, Eslinger PJ, eds. Principles and Practice of Behavioral Neurology and Neuropsychology. Philadelphia, WB Saunders, 2003:197–222.

594. Vecera SP, Rizzo M. Higher disorders of spatial vision and attention. In: Barton JJS, ed. Vision and the Brain. Neurologic Clinics of North America. Philadelphia, WB Saunders, 2003.

595. Kaufman L. Sight and Mind: An Introduction to Visual Perception. New York, Oxford University Press.

596. Palmer SE. Common region: a new principle of perceptual grouping. Cognit Psychol 1992;24:436–447.

597. Rizzo M, Nawrot M, Zihl J. Perception of structure-from-motion and non-motion cues in 'central akinetopsia.' Invest Ophthal Vis Sci 1995;34:1231.

598. Rizzo M, Nawrot M. Perception of movement and shape in Alzheimer's disease. Brain 1998;121:2259–2270.

599. Rizzo M, Reinach S, McGehee D, et al. Simulated car crashes and crash predictors in drivers with Alzheimer disease. Arch Neurol 1997;54:545–551.

600. Nawrot M. Depth perception in driving: alcohol intoxication, eye movement changes, and the disruption of motion parallax. First International Driving Symposium on Human Factors in Driver Assessment, Training and Vehicle Design. Aspen, CO, 2001:76–80.

601. Gibson JJ. The Ecological Approach to Visual Perception. Boston, Houghton Mifflin, 1979.

602. Warren WHJ, Blackwell AW, Morris MW. Age differences in perceiving the direction of self-motion from optical flow. J Gerontol 1989:147–153.

603. Warren WHJ, Mestre DR, Morris MW. Perception of circular heading from optical flow. J Exp Psychol Hum Percept Perform 1991;17:28–43.

604. Rizzo M, Lamers CTJ, Skaar N, et al. Perception of Heading in Abstinent MDMA and THC Users. Vision Sciences 3rd Annual Meeting, Sarasota FL, May 10, 2003.

605. Horton JC, Trobe JD. Akinetopsia from nefazodone toxicity. Am J Ophthalmol 1999;128:530–531.

606. Andersen GJ, Cisneros J, Atchley P, et al. Speed, size, and edge-rate information for the detection of collision events. J Exp Psychol: Hum Percept Perform 1999; 25:256–269.

607. Andersen GJ, Cisneros J, Saidpour A, et al. Age-related differences in collision detection during deceleration. Psychol Aging 2000;15:241–252.

608. Andersen GJ, Saidpour A, Enriquez A. Detection of Collision Events by Older and Younger Drivers. First International Driving Symposium on Human Factors in Driver Assessment, Training and Vehicle Design. Aspen CO, 2001:225–257.

609. Aguirre GK, D'Esposito M. Topographical disorientation: a synthesis and taxonomy. Brain 1999;122 (Pt 9):1613–1628.

610. Barrash J, Damasio H, Adolphs R, et al. The neuroanatomical correlates of route learning impairment. Neuropsychologia 2000;38:820–836.

611. Uc EY, Rizzo M, Qian S, et al. Driver route-following and safety errors in early Alzheimer's disease (in submission).

612. Takahashi N, Kawamura M. Pure topographical disorientation: the anatomical basis of landmark agnosia. Cortex 2002;38:717–725.

613. Pai M. Topographic disorientation: two cases. J Formos Med Assoc 1997;96: 660–663.

614. Kanwisher N. Faces and places: of central (and peripheral) interest. Nat Neurosci 2001;4:455–456.

615. de Renzi E, Faglioni P, Villa P. Topographical amnesia. J Neurol Neurosurg Psychiatry 1977;40:498–505.

616. Takahashi N, Kawamura M, Shiota J, et al. Pure topographic disorientation due to right retrosplenial lesion. Neurology 1997;49:464–469.

617. Sato K, Sakajiri K, Komai K, et al. A patient with amnesic syndrome with defective route finding due to left posterior cerebral artery territory infarction. No To Shinkei 1998;50:69–73.

618. Habib M, Sirigu A. Pure topographical disorientation: a definition and anatomical basis. Cortex 1987;23:73–85.

619. Rizzo M, et al. Principles and Practice of Behavioral Neurology and Neuropsychology. Philadelphia, Elsevier/WB Saunders, 2003:1200.

620. Lezak MD. Neuropsychological Assessment, 3rd ed. New York, Oxford University Press, 1995.

621. Lanca M, Jerskey BA, O'Connor MG. Neuropsychologic assessment of visual disorders. Vision and the Brain. Neurol Clin North Am 2003;21:363–386.

622. Georgopoulos AP. On reaching. Annu Rev Neurosci 1986;9:147–170.

623. Georgopoulos AP. Higher-order motor control. Annu Rev Neurosci 1991;14: 361–377.

624. Caminiti R, Johnson PB. Internal representations of movement in the cerebral cortex as revealed by the analysis of reaching. Cereb Cortex 1992;2:269–276.

625. Kalaska JF, Crammond DJ, Caminiti R, et al. Internal representations of movement in the cerebral cortex: cerebral cortical mechanisms of reaching movements. Science 1992;255:1517–1523.

626. Soechting JF, Flanders M. Moving in three-dimensional space: frames of reference, vectors, and coordinate systems. Annu Rev Neurosci 1992;15:167–191.

627. Darling WG, Miller GF. Transformations between visual and kinesthetic coordinate systems in reaches to remembered object locations and orientations. Exp Brain Res 1993;93:534–547.

628. Jeannerod M, Arbib MA, Rizzolatti G, et al. Grasping objects: the cortical mechanisms of visuomotor transformation. Trends Neurosci 1995;18:314–320.

629. Jeannerod M. The timing of natural prehension movements. J Mot Behav 1984; 16:235–254.

630. White BL, Castle P, Held R. Observations on the development of visually-directed reaching. Child Dev 1964;35:349–364.

631. Twitchell T. Reflex mechanisms and the development of prehension. In: Connolly K, ed. Mechanisms of Motor Skill Development. London, New York, Academic Press, 1970.

632. DiFranco D, Muir DW, Dodwell PC. Reaching in very young infants. Perception 1978;7:385–392.

633. Fisk JD, Goodale MA. The effects of unilateral brain damage on visually guided reaching: hemispheric differences in the nature of the deficit. Exp Brain Res 1988;72:425–435.

634. Jeannerod M. The Neural and Behavioral Organization of Goal-Directed Movements. New York, Oxford University Press, 1988.

635. Goodale M, Milner A, Jakobson L, et al. A neurological dissociation between perceiving objects and grasping them. Nature 1991;349:154–156.

636. Soechting JF, Flanders M. Sensorimotor representations for pointing to targets in three-dimensional space. J Neurophysiol 1989;62:582–594.

637. Soechting JF, Flanders M. Errors in pointing are due to approximations in sensorimotor transformations. J Neurophysiol 1989;62:595–608.

638. Mountcastle VB, Lynch JC, Georgopoulos A, et al. Posterior parietal association cortex of the monkey: command functions for operations within extrapersonal space. J Neurophysiol 1975;38:871–908.

639. Taira M, Mine S, Georgopoulos AP, et al. Parietal cortex neurons of the monkey related to the visual guidance of hand movement. Exp Brain Res 1990;83:29–36.

640. Ghez C, Gordon J, Ghilardi MF. Impairments of reaching movements in patients without proprioception: II. Effects of visual information on accuracy. J Neurophysiol 1995;73:361–372.

641. Perenin MT, Vighetto A. Optic ataxia: a specific disruption in visuomotor mechanisms. I. Different aspects of the deficit in reaching for objects. Brain 1988; 111(Pt 3):643–674.

642. Darling WG, Pizzimenti MA, Rizzo M. Unilateral posterior parietal lobe lesions affect representation of visual space. Vision Res 2003;43:1675–1688.

643. Darling WG, Bartelt R, Rizzo M. Unilateral posterior parietal lobe lesions disrupt kinaesthetic representation of forearm orientation. J Neurol Neurosurg Psychiatry 2004;75:428–435.

644. Critchley M. Types of visual perseveration: "paliopsia" and "illusory visual spread." Brain 1951;74:267–299.

645. Bender M, Feldman M, Sobin A. Palinopsia. Brain 1968;91:321–338.

646. Bender MB. Polyopia and monocular diplopia of cerebral origin. Arch Neurol Psychiatry 1945;54:323–338.

647. Michel EM, Troost BT. Palinopsia: cerebral localization with computed tomography. Neurology 1980;30:887–889.

648. Meadows JC. Observations on a case of monocular diplopia of cerebral origin. J Neurol Sci 1973;18:249–253.

649. Lopez JR, Adornato BT, Hoyt WF. 'Entomopia': a remarkable case of cerebral polyopia. Neurology 1993;43:2145–2146.

650. ffytche DH, Howard RJ. The perceptual consequences of visual loss: 'positive' pathologies of vision. Brain 1999;122:1247–1260.

651. Kinsbourne M, Warrington EK. A study of visual perseveration. J Neurol Neurosurg Psychiatry 1963;26:468–475.

652. Cummings JL, Syndulko K, Goldberg Z, et al. Palinopsia reconsidered. Neurology 1982;32:444–447.

653. Meadows JC, Munro SS. Palinopsia. J Neurol Neurosurg Psychiatry 1977;40: 5–8.

654. Auzou P, Parain D, Ozsancak C, et al. [EEG recordings during episodes of palinacousis and palinopsia]. Rev Neurol (Paris) 1997;153:687–689.

655. Swash M. Visual perseveration in temporal lobe epilepsy. J Neurol Neurosurg Psychiatry 1979;42:569–571.

656. Blythe IM, Bromley JM, Ruddock KH, et al. A study of systematic visual perseveration involving central mechanisms. Brain 1986;109(Pt 4):661–675.

657. Silva JA, Tekell JL, Penny G, et al. Resolution of palinopsia with carbamazepine. J Clin Psychiatry 1997;58:30.

658. Muller T, Buttner T, Kuhn W, et al. Palinopsia as sensory epileptic phenomenon. Acta Neurol Scand 1995;91:433–436.

659. Lefebre C, Kolmel HW. Palinopsia as an epileptic phenomenon. Eur Neurol 1989;29:323–327.

660. Joseph AB. Cotard's syndrome in a patient with coexistent Capgras' syndrome, syndrome of subjective doubles, and palinopsia. J Clin Psychiatry 1986;47: 605–606.

661. Kawasaki A, Purvin V. Persistent palinopsia following ingestion of lysergic acid diethylamide (LSD). Arch Ophthalmol 1996;114:47–50.

662. McGuire PK, Cope H, Fahy TA. Diversity of psychopathology associated with use of 3,4-methylenedioxymethamphetamine ('Ecstasy'). Br J Psychiatry 1994; 165:391–395.

663. Purvin VA. Visual disturbance secondary to clomiphene citrate. Arch Ophthalmol 1995;113:482–484.

664. Friedman DI, Hu EH, Sadun AA. Neuro-ophthalmic complications of interleukin 2 therapy. Arch Ophthalmol 1991;109:1679–1680.

665. Hughes MS, Lessell S. Trazodone-induced palinopsia. Arch Ophthalmol 1990; 108:399–400.

666. Faber RA, Benzick JM. Nafazodone-induced palinopsia. J Clin Psychopharmacol 2000;20:275–276.

667. Ihde-Scholl T, Jefferson JW. Mitrazapine-associated palinopsia. J Clin Psychiatry 2001;62:373.

668. Terao T. Palinopsia and paroxetine withdrawal. J Clin Psychiatry 2002;63:368.

669. Johnson SF, Loge RV. Palinopsia due to nonketotic hyperglycemia. West J Med 1988;148:331–332.

670. Marneros A, Korner J. Chronic palinopsia in schizophrenia. Psychopathology 1993;26:236–239.

671. Gates TJ, Stagno SJ, Gulledge AD. Palinopsia posing as a psychotic depression. Br J Psychiatry 1988;153:391–393.

672. Arnold RW, Janis B, Wellman S, et al. Palinopsia with bacterial brain abscess and Noonan syndrome. Alaska Med 1999;41:3–7.

673. Werring DJ, Marsden CD. Visual hallucinations and palinopsia due to an occipital lobe tuberculoma. J Neurol Neurosurg Psychiatry 1999;66:684.

674. Hayashi R, Shimizu S, Watanabe R, et al. Palinopsia and perilesional hyperperfusion following subcortical hemorrhage. Acta Neurol Scand 2002;105:228–231.

675. Jacome DE. Palinopsia and bitemporal visual extinction on fixation. Ann Ophthalmol 1985;17:251–257.

676. Pomeranz HD, Lessell S. Palinopsia and polyopia in the absence of drugs or cerebral disease. Neurology 2000;54:855–859.

677. Cleland PG, Saunders M, Rosser R. An unusual case of visual perseveration. J Neurol Neurosurg Psychiatry 1981;44:262–263.

678. Lazaro RP. Palinopsia: rare but ominous symptom of cerebral dysfunction. Neurosurgery 1983;13:310–313.

679. Purvin V, Bonnin J, Goodman J. Palinopsia as a presenting manifestation of Creutzfeldt-Jakob disease. J Clin Neuroophthalmol 1989;9:242–248.

680. Hirst LW, Miller NR, Johnson RT. Monocular polyopia. Arch Neurol 1983;40:756–757.

681. Crews J, Gordon A, Nowakowski R. Management of monocular polyopia using an artificial iris contact lens. J Am Optom Assoc 1988;59:140–142.

682. Basuk WL, Zisman M, Waring GO III, et al. Complications of hexagonal keratotomy. Am J Ophthalmol 1994;117:37–49.

683. Jones MR, Waggoner R, Hoyt WF. Cerebral polyopia with extrastriate quadrantanopia: report of a case with magnetic resonance documentation of V2/V3 cortical infarction. J Neuroophthalmol 1999;19:1–6.

684. Gottlieb D. The unidirectionality of cerebral polyopia. J Clin Neuroophthalmol 1992;12:257–262.

685. Kölmel HW. Colored patterns in hemianopic fields. Brain 1984;107:155–167.

686. Plant GT. A centrally generated colored phosphene. Clin Vis Sci 1986;1:161–172.

687. Anderson SW, Rizzo M. Hallucinations following occipital lobe damage: the pathological activation of visual representations. J Clin Exp Neuropsychol 1994;16:651–663.

688. Manford M, Andermann F. Complex visual hallucinations. Clinical and neurobiological insights. Brain 1998;121:1819–1840.

689. Weinberger L, Grant F. Visual hallucinations and their neuro-optical correlates. Arch Ophthalmol 1940;23:166–199.

690. Cogan DG. Visual hallucinations as release phenomena. Albrecht Von Graefes Arch Klin Exp Ophthalmol 1973;188:139–150.

691. Lance JW. Simple formed hallucinations confined to the area of a specific visual field defect. Brain 1976;99:719–734.

692. Lepore FE. Spontaneous visual phenomena with visual loss: 104 patients with lesions of retinal and neural afferent pathways. Neurology 1990;40:444–447.

693. Schultz G, Melzack R. The Charles Bonnet syndrome: 'phantom visual images.' Perception 1991;20:809–825.

694. Teunisse RJ, Cruysberg JR, Hoefnagels WH, et al. Visual hallucinations in psychologically normal people: Charles Bonnet's syndrome. Lancet 1996;347:794–797.

695. Ames D, Wirshing WC, Szuba MP. Organic mental disorders associated with bupropion in three patients. J Clin Psychiatry 1992;53:53–55.

696. Rivas DA, Chancellor MB, Hill K, et al. Neurological manifestations of baclofen withdrawal. J Urol 1993;150:1903–1905.

697. Lera G, Vaamonde J, Rodriguez M, et al. Cabergoline in Parkinson's disease: long-term follow-up. Neurology 1993;43:2587–2590.

698. Zoldan J, Friedberg G, Livneh M, et al. Psychosis in advanced Parkinson's disease: treatment with ondansetron, a 5-HT3 receptor antagonist. Neurology 1995;45:1305–1308.

699. Chen JL, Brocavich JM, Lin AY. Psychiatric disturbances associated with ganciclovir therapy. Ann Pharmacother 1992;26:193–195.

700. Gosh K, Sivakumaran M, Murphy P, et al. Visual hallucinations following treatment with vincristine. Clin Lab Hematol 1994;16:355–357.

701. Bourgeois JA, Thomas D, Johansen T, et al. Visual hallucinations associated with fluoxetine and sertraline. J Clin Psychopharmacol 1998;18:482–483.

702. Gaillard MC, Borruat FX. Persisting visual hallucinations and illusions in previously drug-addicted patients. Klin Monatsbl Augenheilkd 2003;220:176–178.

703. Oliveri M, Calvo G. Increased visual cortical excitability in Ecstasy users: a transcranial magnetic stimulation study. J Neurol Neurosurg Psychiatry 2003;74:1136–1138.

704. Lerner AJ, Koss E, Patterson MB, et al. Concomitants of visual hallucinations in Alzheimer's disease. Neurology 1994;44:523–527.

705. Platz WE, Oberlaender FA, Seidel ML. The phenomenology of perceptual hallucinations in alcohol-induced delirium tremens. Psychopathology 1995;28:247–255.

706. Chapman FM, Dickinson J, McKeith I, et al. Association among visual hallucinations, visual acuity, and specific eye pathologies in Alzheimer's disease: treatment implications. Am J Psychiatry 1999;156:1983–1985.

707. Holroyd S, Shepherd ML, Downs JH, et al. Occipital atrophy is associated with visual hallucinations in Alzheimer's disease. J Neuropsychiatry Clin Neurosci 2000;12:25–28.

708. Paulsen J, Salmon D, Thal L, et al. Incidence of and risk factors for hallucinations and delusions in patients with probable AD. Neurology 2000;54:1965–1971.

709. Ballard C, McKeith I, Harrison R, et al. A detailed phenomenological comparison of complex visual hallucinations in dementia with Lewy bodies and Alzheimer's disease. Int Psychogeriatr 1997;9:381–388.

710. Harding AJ, Broe GA, Halliday GM. Visual hallucinations in Lewy body disease relate to Lewy bodies in the temporal lobe. Brain 2002;125:391–403.

711. Barnes LL, Nelson JK, Reuter-Lorenz PA. Object-based attention and object working memory: overlapping processes revealed by selective interference effects in humans. Prog Brain Res 2001;134:471–481.

712. Sanchez-Ramos JR, Ortoll R, Paulson GW. Visual hallucinations associated with Parkinson disease. Arch Neurol 1996;53:1265–1268.

713. Holroyd S, Currie I, Wooten G. Prospective study of hallucinations and delusions in Parkinson's disease. J Neurol Neurosurg Psychiatry 2001;70:734–738.

714. Klein C, Kompf D, Pulkowski U, et al. A study of visual hallucinations in patients with Parkinson's disease. J Neurol 1997;244:371–377.

715. Barnes J, David AS. Visual hallucinations in Parkinson's disease: a review and phenomenological survey. J Neurol Neurosurg Psychiatry 2001;70:727–733.

716. Arnulf I, Bonnet A-M, Damier P, et al. Hallucinations, REM sleep, and Parkinson's disease. Neurology 2000;55:281–288.

717. Nomura T, Inoue Y, Mitani H, et al. Visual hallucinations as REM sleep behavior disorders in patients with Parkinson's disease. Mov Disord 2003;18:812–817.

718. Barnes J, Boubert L, Harris J, et al. Reality monitoring and visual hallucinations in Parkinson's disease. Neuropsychologia 2003;41:565–574.

719. Lepore FE. Visual loss as a causative factor in visual hallucinations associated with Parkinson disease. Arch Neurol 1997;54:799.

720. Bullock R, Cameron A. Rivastigmine for the treatment of dementia and visual hallucinations associated with Parkinson's disease: a case series. Curr Med Res Opin 2002;18:258–264.

721. Menon GJ, Rahman I, Menon SJ, et al. Complex visual hallucinations in the visually impaired: the Charles Bonnet Syndrome. Surv Ophthalmol 2003;48:58–72.

722. Scott IU, Schein OD, Feuer WJ, et al. Visual hallucinations in patients with retinal disease. Am J Ophthalmol 2001;131:590–598.

723. Adair DK, Keshavan MS. The Charles Bonnet syndrome and grief reaction. Am J Psychiatry 1988;145:895–896.

724. Kölmel HW. Complex visual hallucinations in the hemianopic field. J Neurol Neurosurg Psychiatry 1985;48:29–38.

725. Teunisse RJ, Cruysberg JR, Verbeek A, et al. The Charles Bonnet syndrome: a large prospective study in The Netherlands. A study of the prevalence of the Charles Bonnet syndrome and associated factors in 500 patients attending the University Department of Ophthalmology at Nijmegen. Br J Psychiatry 1995;166:254–257.

726. Siatkowski RM, Zimmer B, Rosenberg PR. The Charles Bonnet syndrome. Visual perceptive dysfunction in sensory deprivation. J Clin Neuroophthalmol 1990;10:215–218.

727. Heron W. The pathology of boredom. Sci Am 1957:196.

728. Schwartz TL, Vahgei L. Charles Bonnet syndrome in children. J Aapos 1998;2:310–313.

729. Mewasingh LD, Kornreich C, Christiaens F, et al. Pediatric phantom vision (Charles Bonnet) syndrome. Pediatr Neurol 2002;26:143–145.

730. Cole MG. Charles Bonnet hallucinations: a case series. Can J Psychiatry 1992;37:267–270.

731. Schultz G, Melzack R. Visual hallucinations and mental state. A study of 14 Charles Bonnet syndrome hallucinators. J Nerv Ment Dis 1993;181:639–643.

732. Fernandes LH, Scassellati-Sforzolini B, Spaide RF. Estrogen and visual hallucinations in a patient with Charles Bonnet syndrome. Am J Ophthalmol 2000;129:407.

733. Nesher G, Nesher R, Rozenman Y, et al. Visual hallucinations in giant cell arteritis: association with visual loss. J Rheumatol 2001;28:2046–2048.

734. Bhatia MS, Khastgir U, Malik SC. Charles Bonnet syndrome. Br J Psychiatry 1992;161:409–410.

735. Hori H, Terao T, Shiraishi Y, et al. Treatment of Charles Bonnet syndrome with valproate. Int Clin Psychopharmacol 2000;15:117–119.

736. Batra A, Bartels M, Wormstall H. Therapeutic options in Charles Bonnet syndrome. Acta Psychiatr Scand 1997;96:129–133.

737. Badino R, Trucco M, Caja A, et al. Release hallucinations and tiapride. Ital J Neurol Sci 1994;15:183–187.

738. Maeda K, Shirayama Y, Nukina S, et al. Charles Bonnet syndrome with visual hallucinations of childhood experience: successful treatment of 1 patient with risperidone. J Clin Psychiatry 2003;64:1131–1132.

739. Paulig M, Mentrup H. Charles Bonnet's syndrome: complete remission of complex visual hallucinations treated by gabapentin. J Neurol Neurosurg Psychiatry 2001;70:813–814.

740. Shedlack KJ, McDonald WM, Laskowitz DT, et al. Geniculocalcarine hyperintensities on brain magnetic resonance imaging associated with visual hallucinations in the elderly. Psychiatry Res 1994;54:283–293.

741. Burke W. The neural basis of Charles Bonnet hallucinations: a hypothesis. J Neurol Neurosurg Psychiatry 2002;73:535–541.

742. Fisman M. Musical hallucinations: report of two unusual cases [comment]. Can J Psychiatry 1991;36:609–611.

743. Ffytche DH, Howard RJ, Brammer MJ, et al. The anatomy of conscious vision: an fMRI study of visual hallucinations. Nat Neurosci 1998;1:738–742.

744. Wunderlich G, Suchan B, Volkmann J, et al. Visual hallucinations in recovery from cortical blindness: imaging correlates. Arch Neurol 2000;57:561–565.
745. Adachi N, Watanabe T, Matsuda H, et al. Hyperperfusion in the lateral temporal cortex, the striatum and the thalamus during complex visual hallucinations: single photon emission computed tomography findings in patients with Charles Bonnet syndrome. Psychiatry Clin Neurosci 2000;54:157–162.
746. Assadi M, Baseman S, Hyman D. Tc-SPECT scan in a patient with occipital lobe infarction and complex visual hallucinations. J Neurosci Nurs 2003;35:175–177.
747. Panayiotopoulos CP. Elementary visual hallucinations, blindness, and headache in idiopathic occipital epilepsy: differentiation from migraine. J Neurol Neurosurg Psychiatry 1999;66:536–540.
748. Bien C, Benninger F, Urbach H, et al. Localizing value of epileptic visual auras. Brain 2000;123:244–253.
749. Penfield W, Perot P. The brain's record of auditory and visual experience. Brain 1963;86:595–596.
750. Panayiotopoulos CP. Elementary visual hallucinations in migraine and epilepsy. J Neurol Neurosurg Psychiatry 1994;57:1371–1374.
751. Williamson PD, Thadani VM, Darcey TM, et al. Occipital lobe epilepsy: clinical characteristics, seizure spread patterns, and results of surgery. Ann Neurol 1992;31:3–13.
752. Lance JW, Smee RI. Partial seizures with visual disturbance treated by radiotherapy of cavernous hemangioma. Ann Neurol 1989;26:782–785.
753. Sveinbjornsdottir S, Duncan JS. Parietal and occipital lobe epilepsy: a review. Epilepsia 1993;34:493–521.
754. Rousseaux M, Debrock D, Cabaret M, et al. Visual hallucinations with written words in a case of left parietotemporal lesion. J Neurol Neurosurg Psychiatry 1994;57:1268–1271.
755. Gastaut H. A new type of epilepsy: benign partial epilepsy of childhood with occipital spike-waves. Clin Electroencephalogr 1982;13:13–22.
756. Hupp SL, Kline LB, Corbett JJ. Visual disturbances of migraine. Surv Ophthalmol 1989;33:221–236.
757. Lance JW, Anthony M. Some clinical aspects of migraine. A prospective survey of 500 patients. Arch Neurol 1966;15:356–361.
758. Plant GT. The fortification spectra of migraine. Br Med J (Clin Res Ed) 1986;293:1613–1617.
759. Richards W. The fortification illusions of migraines. Sci Am 1971;224:88–96.
760. Grüsser OJ. Migraine phosphenes and the retino-cortical magnification factor. Vision Res 1995;35:1125–1134.
761. Walker MC, Smith SJ, Sisodiya SM, et al. Case of simple partial status epilepticus in occipital lobe epilepsy misdiagnosed as migraine: clinical, electrophysiological, and magnetic resonance imaging characteristics. Epilepsia 1995;36:1233–1236.
762. Schulze-Bonhage A. [Differential diagnosis of visual aura in migraine and epilepsy]. Klin Monatsbl Augenheilkd 2001;218:595–602.
763. Sharma K, Wahi J, Phadke RV, et al. Migraine-like visual hallucinations in occipital lesions of cysticercosis. J Neuroophthalmol 2002;22:82–87.
764. Lhermitte J. Syndrome de la calotte du pedoncle cerebral: les troubles psychosensoriels dans les lesions du mescephale. Rev Neurol 1922;38:1359–1365.
765. van Bogaert L. L'hallucinose pedonculaire. Rev Neurol 1927;43:608–617.
766. Geller TJ, Bellur SN. Peduncular hallucinosis: magnetic resonance imaging confirmation of mesencephalic infarction during life. Ann Neurol 1987;21:602–604.
767. Tsukamoto H, Matsushima T, Fujiwara S, et al. Peduncular hallucinosis following microvascular decompression for trigeminal neuralgia: case report. Surg Neurol 1993;40:31–34.
768. McKee AC, Levine DN, Kowall NW, et al. Peduncular hallucinosis associated with isolated infarction of the substantia nigra pars reticulata. Ann Neurol 1990;27:500–504.
769. de la Fuente Fernandez R, Lopez J, Rey del Corral P, et al. Peduncular hallucinosis and right hemiparkinsonism caused by left mesencephalic infarction. J Neurol Neurosurg Psychiatry 1994;57:870.
770. Nadvi SS, van Dellen JR. Transient peduncular hallucinations secondary to brain stem compression by a medulloblastoma. Surg Neurol 1994;41:250–252.
771. Rozanski J. Peduncular hallucinosis following vertebral angiography. Neurology 1952;2:341–349.
772. Feinberg WM, Rapcsak SZ. 'Peduncular hallucinosis' following paramedian thalamic infarction. Neurology 1989;39:1535–1536.
773. Cascino GD, Adams RD. Brainstem auditory hallucinations. Neurology 1986;36:1042–1047.
774. Noda S, Mizoguchi M, Yamamoto A. Thalamic experiential hallucinosis. J Neurol Neurosurg Psychiatry 1993;56:1224–1226.
775. Serra Catafau J, Rubio F, Peres Serra J. Peduncular hallucinosis associated with posterior thalamic infarction. J Neurol 1992;239:89–90.
776. Caplan LR. "Top of the basilar" syndrome. Neurology 1980;30:72–79.
777. Dunn DW, Weisberg LA, Nadell J. Peduncular hallucinations caused by brainstem compression. Neurology 1983;33:1360–1361.
778. Fisher CM. Visual hallucinations and racing thoughts on eye closure after minor surgery. Arch Neurol 1991;48:1091–1092.
779. Fisher CM. Visual hallucinations on eye closure associated with atropine toxicity. A neurological analysis and comparison with other visual hallucinations. Can J Neurol Sci 1991;18:18–27.
780. Heinemann EG, Tulving E, Nachmias J. The effect of oculomotor adjustments on apparent size. Am J Psychol 1959;72:32–45.
781. Alexander KR. On the nature of accommodative micropsia. Am J Optom Physiol Opt 1975;52:79–84.
782. Hollins M. Does accommodative micropsia exist? Am J Psychol 1976;89:443–454.
783. Richards W. Apparent modifiability of receptive fields during accommodation and convergence and a model for size constancy. Neuropsychologia 1967;5:63–72.
784. Myers WA. Micropsia and testicular retractions. Psychoanal Q 1977;46:580–604.
785. Schneck JM. Micropsia. Psychosomatics 1969;10:249–251.
786. Schneck JM. Psychogenic micropsia and a spontaneous hypnotic auditory equivalent. Am J Clin Hypn 1986;29:53–58.
787. Frisen L, Frisen M. Micropsia and visual acuity in macular edema. A study of the neuro-retinal basis of visual acuity. Albrecht Von Graefes Arch Klin Exp Ophthalmol 1979;210:69–77.
788. Sjostrand J, Anderson C. Micropsia and metamorphopsia in the re-attached macula following retinal detachment. Acta Ophthalmol (Copenh) 1986;64:425–432.
789. Thiébaut F, Matavulj N. Hémi-micropsie relative homonyme driote en quadrant inférieur. Rev Otoneuroophtalmol 1949;21:245–246.
790. Cohen L, Gray F, Meyrignac C, et al. Selective deficit of visual size perception: two cases of hemimicropsia. J Neurol Neurosurg Psychiatry 1994;57:73–78.
791. Ebata S, Ogawa M, Tanaka Y, et al. Apparent reduction in the size of one side of the face associated with a small retrosplenial haemorrhage. J Neurol Neurosurg Psychiatry 1991;54:68–70.
792. Touge T, Takeuchi H, Yamada A, et al. [A case of posterior cerebral artery territory infarction with micropsia as the chief complaint]. Rinsho Shinkeigaku 1990;30:894–897.
793. Abe K, Oda N, Araki R, et al. Macropsia, micropsia, and episodic illusions in Japanese adolescents. J Am Acad Child Adolesc Psychiatry 1989;28:493–496.
794. Wilson SAK. Dysmetropsia and its pathogenesis. Trans Ophthalmol Soc U K 1916;36:412–444.
795. Iruela L, Ibanez-Rojo V, Baca E. Zolpidem-induced macropsia in anorexic woman. Lancet 1993;342:443–444.
796. Brégeat P, Klein M, Thiébaut F, et al. Hémi-macropsia homonyme droite et tumeur occipitale gauche. Rev Otoneuroophtalmol 1949;21:245–246.
797. Ardila A, Botero M, Gomez J. Palinopsia and visual allesthesia. Int J Neurosci 1987;32:775–782.
798. Enoch JM, Schwartz A, Chang D, et al. Aniseikonia, metamorphopsia and perceived entoptic pattern: some effects of a macular epiretinal membrane, and the subsequent spontaneous separation of the membrane. Ophthalmic Physiol Opt 1995;15:339–343.
799. Amemiya T, Lida Y, Yoshida H. Subjective and objective ocular disturbances in reattached retina after surgery for retinal detachment, with special reference to visual acuity and metamorphopsia. Ophthalmologica 1983;186:25–30.
800. Enoch JM, Baraldi P, Lakshminarayanan V, et al. Measurement of metamorphopsia in the presence of ocular media opacities. Am J Optom Physiol Opt 1988;65:349–353.
801. Ida Y, Kotorii T, Nakazawa Y. A case of epilepsy with ictal metamorphopsia. Folia Psychiatr Neurol Jpn 1980;34:395–396.
802. Nass R, Sinha S, Solomon G. Epileptic facial metamorphopsia. Brain Dev 1985;7:50–52.
803. Imai N, Nohira O, Miyata K, et al. A case of metamorphopsia caused by a very localized spotty infarct. Rinsho Shinkeigaku 1995;35:302–305.
804. Brau RH, Lameiro J, Llaguno AV, et al. Metamorphopsia and permanent cortical blindness after a posterior fossa tumor. Neurosurgery 1986;19:263–266.
805. Krizek GO. Metamorphopsias caused by pontine and peduncular lesions. Am J Psychiatry 1985;142:999.
806. Jackson GR, Owsley C. Visual dysfunction, neurodegenerative diseases, and aging. Neurol Clin 2003;21:709–728.
807. Graff-Radford NR, Bolling JP, Earnest F, et al. Simultanagnosia as the initial sign of degenerative dementia. Mayo Clin Proc 1993;68:955–964.
808. Gilmore GC, Wenk HE, Naylor LA, et al. Motion perception and Alzheimer's disease. J Gerontol 1994;49:P52–57.
809. Rizzo M, Corbett JJ, Thompson H, et al. Spatial contrast sensitivity in facial recognition. Neurology 1986;36:1254–1256.
810. Ball K, Vance D, Edwards J, et al. Aging and the brain. In: Rizzo M, Eslinger PJ, eds. Principles and Practice of Behavioral Neurology and Neuropsychology. Philadelphia, Saunders, 2004:795–809.
811. Sekuler R, Kline D, Dismukes K, et al. Some research needs in aging and visual perception. Vision Res 1983;23:213–216.
812. Botwinick J. Aging and Behavior: A Comprehensive Integration of Research Findings, 3rd ed. New York, Springer, 1984.
813. Kline DW, Orme-Rogers C. Examination of stimulus persistence as the basis

for superior visual identification performance among older adults. J Gerontol 1978;33:76–81.

814. Brozek J, Keys A. Changes in flicker-fusion frequency with age. J Consult Clin Psychol 1945;9:87–90.

815. Coppinger NW. The relationship between critical flicker frequency and chronological age for varying levels of stimulus brightness. J Gerontol 1955;10:48–52.

816. Kline DW, Birren JE. Age differences in backward dichoptic masking. Exp Aging Res 1975;1:17–25.

817. Kline DW, Szafran J. Age differences in backward monoptic visual noise masking. J Gerontol 1975;30:307–311.

818. Kline DW, Nestor S. Persistence of complementary afterimages as a function of adult age and exposure duration. Exp Aging Res 1977;3:191–201.

819. Schaie KW. The course of adult intellectual development. Am Psychol 1994; 49:304–313.

820. Schaie KW. Perceptual speed in adulthood: cross-sectional and longitudinal studies. Psychol Aging 1989;4:443–453.

821. Salthouse TA. Speed and knowledge as determinants of adult age differences in verbal tasks. J Gerontol 1993;48:P29–P36.

822. Salthouse TA. Effects of age and skill in typing. J Exp Psychol Gen 1984;113: 345–371.

823. Birren JE. Translations in gerontology—from lab to life. Psychophysiology and the speed of response. Am Psychol 1974;29:808–815.

824. Welford A. Motor performance. In: Birren JE, Schaie KW, eds. Handbook of the Psychology of Aging. New York, Van Nostrand Reinhold, 1977:450–496.

825. Salthouse TA. Speed of behavior and its implications for cognition. In: Birren JE, Schaie KW, eds. Handbook of the Psychology of Aging, 2nd ed. New York, Van Nostrand Reinhold, 1985:400–426.

826. Salthouse TA, Kausler DH, Saults J. Utilization of path-analytic procedures to investigate the role of processing resources in cognitive aging. Psychol Aging 1988;3:158–166.

827. Hertzog C. Influences of cognitive slowing on age differences in intelligence. Dev Psychol 1989;25:636–651.

828. Salthouse TA, Mitchell DR. Effects of age and naturally occurring experience on spatial visualization performance. Dev Psychol 1990;26:845–854.

829. Salthouse TA. Mediation of adult age differences in cognition by reductions in working memory and speed of processing. Psychol Sci 1991;2:179–183.

830. Cerella J, Poon LW, Williams DM. Age and the complexity hypothesis. In: Poon LW, ed. Aging in the 1980s: Psychological Issues. Washington, DC, American Psychological Association, 1980:332–340.

831. Cerella J. Age-related decline in extrafoveal letter perception. J Gerontol 1985; 40:727–736.

832. Bosman EA. Age-related differences in the motoric aspects of transcription typing skill. Psychol Aging 1993;8:87–102.

833. Charness N. Search in chess: Age and skill differences. J Exp Psychol Hum Percept Perform 1981;7:467–476.

834. Charness N, Krampe R, Mayr U. Coaching in entrepreneurial domains: Chess. Annual Meeting of the American Educational Research Association, San Francisco, 1995.

835. Loewen ER, Shaw RJ, Craik FI. Age differences in components of metamemory. Exp Aging Res 1990;16:43–48.

836. Ball K, Owsley C, Beard B. Clinical visual perimetry underestimates peripheral field problems in older adults. Clin Vis Sci 1990;5:113–125.

837. Tranel D. Assessment of higher-order visual function. Curr Opin Ophthalmol 1994;5:29–37.

838. Anderson SW, Rizzo M. Recovery and rehabilitation of visual cortical dysfunction. Neurorehabilitation 1995;5:129–140.

839. Benton AL, Van Allen MW. Visuoperceptual, visuospatial, and visuoconstructive disorders. In: Heilman KM, Valenstein E, eds. Clinical Neuropsychology, 2nd ed. New York, Oxford University Press, 1985:161–186.

840. Hooper HE. The Hooper Visual Organization Test Manual. Los Angeles, Western Psychological Services, 1958.

841. Mooney C, Ferguson G. A new closure test. Can J Psychol 1951;5:129–133.

842. Lansdell H. Relation of extent of temporal removals to closure and visuomotor factors. Percept Mot Skills 1970;31:491–498.

843. Newcombe F. Selective deficits after focal cerebral injury. In: Dimond SJ, Beaumont JG, eds. Hemisphere Function in the Human Brain. New York, Wiley, 1974:311–334.

844. Wechsler D. WAIS-R: Manual: Wechsler Adult Intelligence Scale–Revised. New York, Harcourt Brace Jovanovich, Psychological Corp, 1981.

845. Benton AL. Contributions to Neuropsychological Assessment: A Clinical Manual. New York, Oxford University Press, 1983.

846. Spreen O, Strauss E. A Compendium of Neuropsychological Tests: Administration, Norms, and Commentary. New York, Oxford University Press, 1991.

SECTION II:
The Autonomic Nervous System

Neil R. Miller, section editor

The autonomic nervous system provides innervation to the pupil, ciliary body, and lacrimal gland, all of which can be adversely affected by a variety of ocular, orbital, and neurologic disorders. This section contains three chapters. The first deals with the anatomy and physiology of the autonomic nervous system. The second chapter describes the techniques used to examine pupillary function, accommodation, and lacrimation. The final chapter describes disorders of pupillary function, accommodation, and lacrimation of neuro-ophthalmologic importance.

CHAPTER 14

Anatomy and Physiology of the Autonomic Nervous System

Randy Kardon

GENERAL ORGANIZATION OF THE AUTONOMIC NERVOUS SYSTEM

Body functions that are regulated independently of voluntary activity using reflex mechanisms involving afferent nerve input, efferent nerve output, and central integrating nerve pathways are part of the autonomic nervous system (1). Although the activity of this system is essentially autonomous, at higher levels of the central nervous system (CNS) voluntary modulation is still possible. As early as 1875, Hughlings Jackson offered clinical, physiologic, and experimental evidence to show that the autonomic nervous system, like the somatic nervous system, is integrated at all levels of nervous activity and that autonomic and somatic activities are closely correlated. Segmental autonomic reflexes are coordinated in the spinal cord, but regulation of functions such as respiration, blood pressure, swallowing, and pupillary movement requires suprasegmental integration higher in the brain stem. The autonomic subsystems in the brain stem are, in turn, influenced by more complicated integrating systems in the hypothalamus. Finally, certain cortical areas, particularly the frontal cortex, govern many of the activities of

the hypothalamus (2). Thus, coordination and integration of somatic and autonomic activities from the highest level of neurologic activity in cortex down to the spinal cord and peripheral nervous system (PNS) are used to attain fundamental adjustments of the organism to its environment.

Viewed broadly, the autonomic system ensures self-preservation of the organism by making continuous automatic adjustments so as to maintain homeostasis in the face of major and minor environmental changes. Sympathetic and parasympathetic elements in this system act in a balanced fashion to maintain homeostasis in bodily dynamics such as respiration, circulation, body temperature, and heart rate. At one extreme, sympathetic activity mobilizes mechanisms of the body to meet conditions of stress: the vessels of the skin and viscera constrict, and blood is shunted into dilated vessels of the skeletal muscles; the heart rate increases; respiration deepens; gastrointestinal activity ceases; skin is moistened with perspiration; hairs stiffen; and the pupils dilate. At the other extreme, parasympathetic activity has an opposite function, that of conservation and restoration of bodily resources: the heart is slowed, intestinal activity is increased, and the pupils constrict (3,4).

In addition to direct neural control of homeostatic functions, an autonomic neuroendocrine system is intimately linked to the same activities. For example, sympathetic nerve fibers stimulate the adrenal glands to liberate adrenaline to act on sympathetic effector organs in a manner homologous to their direct stimulation by sympathetic nerves. Similarly, the posterior lobe of the pituitary gland is stimulated by parasympathetic pathways from the hypothalamus to produce circulating hormones that participate in the homeostatic control of the organism's internal environment.

Neuro-ophthalmologic focus on the autonomic nervous system is concerned primarily with the control of the intrinsic muscles of the eye (the iris sphincter and dilator muscles and ciliary accommodative apparatus), lacrimation, and cerebral and orbital blood flow. In this chapter, we describe the basic anatomy, physiology, and pharmacology of the system as it pertains to the field of neuro-ophthalmology. A complete discussion of the autonomic nervous system is beyond the scope of this work; however, several excellent texts and monographs are available to the interested reader (5–13).

In the broadest sense, the autonomic nervous system covered in this chapter includes cortical and subcortical regions (including the hypothalamus), parts of the brain stem and spinal cord, and the peripheral sympathetic and parasympathetic nerves and ganglia.

CENTRAL LEVELS OF AUTONOMIC REGULATION

Limbic System

The term "limbic system" was applied by MacLean (14) to several areas within the CNS influencing autonomic function and emotional behavior (15) through direct connections with the hypothalamus. The limbic cortex consists of an arcuate band of cortex that includes the cingulate and parahippocampal gyri and the orbitofrontal and pyriform areas (Fig. 14.1). The concept of a greater limbic "system" was proposed to unite the limbic cortex and those structures with primary connections: the olfactory system, the preoptic area, the septum, the amygdala, the hypothalamus, and adjacent areas of neocortex (14,16–21).

From our standpoint, it is sufficient to be aware that stimulation of the limbic cortex produces visceral effects, such as vasomotor changes and gastrointestinal activity, as well as somatic and autonomic reactions that typify excitement and rage. Removal causes changes in behavior associated with a loss of emotional expression. Stimulation of the hippocampus elicits involuntary movements, rage reactions, sexual activity, and general hyperexcitability. Stimulation of the amygdala produces a mixture of parasympathetic and sympathetic reactions, including changes in respiration, blood pressure, and heart rate; pupillary constriction and dilation; and defecation or micturition. Ablation of the amygdala produces placidity. Stimulation in the septal region affects blood pressure, whereas injury to the septum reduces susceptibility to fear and anxiety. Thus, the regions of the CNS that are

collectively known as the limbic system exert some degree of central control over the autonomic system by modulating the more direct influence of the hypothalamus.

Cerebellum

The cerebellum is involved to some degree in the control of the autonomic nervous system (22,23). Stimulation of both anterior and posterior lobes produces changes in blood pressure and heart rate. Pupillary constriction and dilation also occur when portions of the cerebellum are stimulated, and accommodation can also be modulated by the cerebellum. Chemical stimulation of the posterior lobe of the cerebellum by local application of glutamate augments both sympathetic and parasympathetic tonic discharges (9). Therefore, although the full significance of cerebellar autonomic representation is not yet completely appreciated, it should be recognized that the cerebellum is capable of modulating different aspects of autonomic nervous system function.

Hypothalamus

Anatomy

The hypothalamus is the primary area of the brain concerned with the integration of autonomic functions. It forms the anterior inferior wall of the third ventricle and is located posterior and superior to the optic chiasm, and its superior border is the hypothalamic sulcus (Fig. 14.2). As noted previously, autonomic function is influenced from many regions of the brain, including parts of the cerebral cortex and thalamus, the hippocampus, the entorhinal area, the basal ganglia, the reticular formation, and the cerebellum. Generally, these influences appear to be mediated through involvement of the hypothalamus, which receives direct or indirect connections from most of these regions. Although the anatomic border of the hypothalamus is somewhat ill defined, the hypothalamus contains several cell clusters or nuclei (Fig 14.3).

The anterior group of nuclei includes the supraoptic and paraventricular nuclei, which differ in size and structure based on whether the brain is from a male or female (24,25). The supraoptic nucleus is believed to have parasympathetic function (26) and is located just superior and lateral to the optic chiasm, connecting to the pars intermedia and pars posterior of the hypophysis by the supraopticohypophyseal tract (Fig. 14.4). The paraventricular nucleus lies immediately beneath the anterior third ventricle. It undergoes atrophy after destruction of the nucleus of the vagus nerve or removal of the superior cervical ganglion.

The middle group of nuclei includes the tuberal nuclei, situated just posterior to the supraoptic nucleus within and near the surface of the tuber cinereum, and the ventromedial, dorsomedial, and lateral hypothalamic nuclei, located above the tuberal nuclei. The tuberal nuclei contain small multipolar cells, whereas the cells of the ventromedial, dorsomedial, and lateral hypothalamic nuclei are somewhat larger.

The posterior group of nuclei includes the nuclei of the mammillary body and the posterior hypothalamic nucleus.

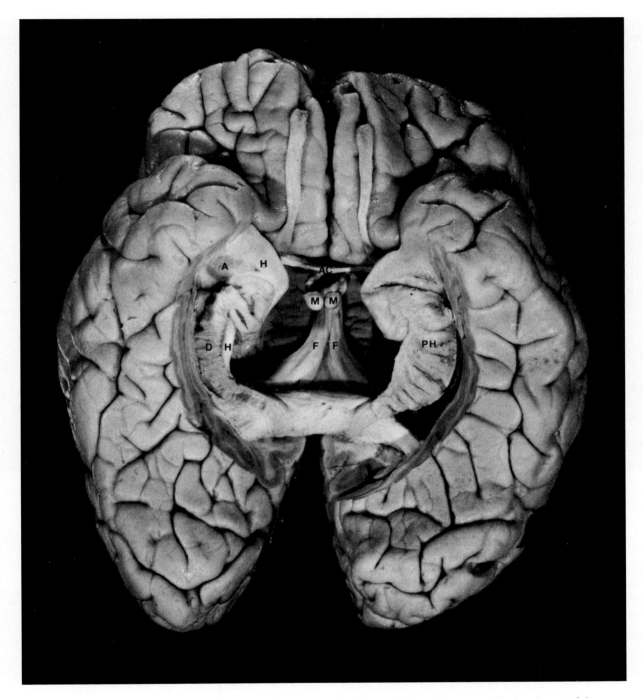

Figure 14.1. Components of the limbic system seen from below. The cerebellum, brain stem, thalami, and most of the basal ganglia have been removed. A, amygdaloid nuclear complex; AC, anterior commissure; D, dentate gyrus; F, fornix; H, hippocampus; M, mammillary body; PH, parahippocampal gyrus. (From Ghuhbegovic N, Williams TH. The Human Brain: A Photographic Guide. Hagerstown, MD, Harper & Row, 1980.)

The mammillary bodies are located in the interpeduncular space and are composed of two nuclear masses, the medial and lateral mammillary nuclei. Each mammillary body forms the posterior termination of the ipsilateral fornix and is also connected directly with the ipsilateral anterior nucleus of the thalamus. The posterior hypothalamic nucleus lies above and just rostral to the mammillary bodies. It is composed of large cells scattered among numerous smaller cells.

The hypothalamus also contains smaller nuclei, including the suprachiasmatic nucleus, located close to the midline

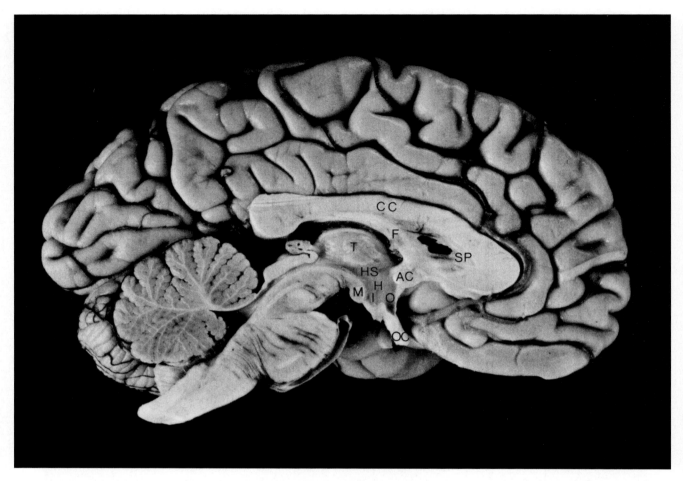

Figure 14.2. Hypothalamus and related structures. AC, anterior commissure; CC, corpus callosum; F, fornix; H, hypothalamus; HS, hypothalamic sulcus; I, infundibular recess; M, mammillary body; OC, optic chiasm; O, optic recess; SP, septum pellucidum; T, thalamus. (From Ghuhbegovic N, Williams TH. The Human Brain: A Photographic Guide. Hagerstown, MD, Harper & Row, 1980.)

above the optic chiasm, and the arcuate nucleus, a group of small cells located in the most ventral part of the third ventricle near the infundibular recess and extending into the medial eminence.

Neuromediators

Many different neuromediators are produced in various sites in the hypothalamic region, including angiotensin II, delta sleep-inducing peptide, dynorphin, enkephalin, endorphin, growth hormone release-inhibiting hormone (GHRIH, somatostatin), growth hormone-releasing factor (GHRF, somatocrinin), prolactin-releasing factor (PRF), prolactin-inhibiting factor (PIF), gonadotropin-releasing hormone (GnRH), corticotropin-releasing factor (CRF), thyrotropin-releasing hormone (TRH), vasopressin (antidiuretic hormone [ADH]), oxytocin, neurotensin, cholecystokinin, vasoactive intestinal peptide (VIP), substance P, glycine, glutamate, aspartate, gamma-aminobutyric acid (GABA), histamine, serotonin, adrenalin, noradrenaline, dopamine, and acetylcholine (27).

Fiber Connections

Knowledge of the hypothalamic connections to the brain and spinal cord is derived from comparative studies using anterograde and retrograde tracers in animals and from the study of normal and pathologic human material (28). These connections include afferent and efferent nerve fiber connections, as well as humoral connections to the hypophysis via a venous portal system (Figs. 14.5 and 14.6).

Afferent nerve pathways to the hypothalamus originate from ascending visceral sensory input, somatic sensory systems of the visual and olfactory systems, and numerous tracts from the brain stem, limbic structures, and neocortex. The hippocampal formation sends fibers directly to the hypothalamus, primarily via the fornix to the mammillary bodies (Figs. 14.2 and 14.5). Other hypothalamic afferents from cortical or subcortical structures include those from the cingulate gyrus, the piriform cortex, and the amygdala (10,12). Afferent projections to the hypothalamus from the spinal cord and brain stem also exist (29–31). Efferent nerve path-

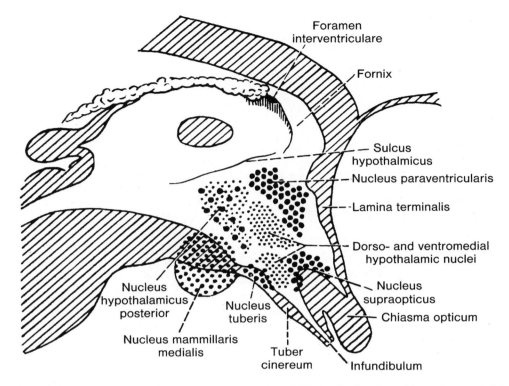

Figure 14.3.   Diagram of the ventricular surface of the human hypothalamus, showing the position and extent of the major hypothalamic nuclei. (From Brodal A. Neurological Anatomy. New York, Oxford University Press, 1981.)

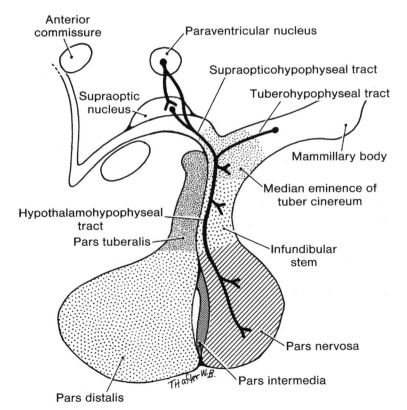

Figure 14.4.   Drawing of the hypophysis (pituitary gland) showing the origin and distribution of the hypothalamo-hypophyseal tract. (Redrawn from Crosby EC, Humphrey T, Lauer EW. Correlative Anatomy of the Nervous System. New York, Macmillan, 1962.)

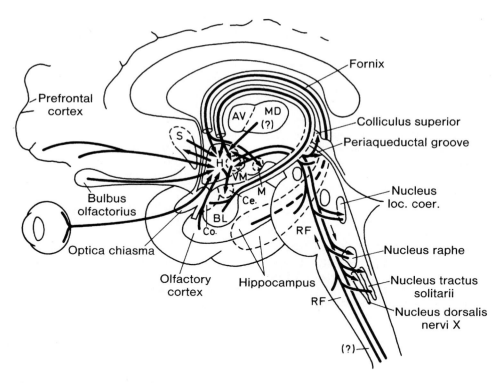

Figure 14.5. Diagram of the main afferent and efferent connections of the hypothalamus. The connections of the mammillary body and the hypothalamohypophyseal projections are not included. AV, anterior ventral thalamic nucleus; BL, basolateral amygdaloid nucleus; Ce, central amygdaloid nucleus; Co, cortical amygdaloid nucleus; H, hypothalamus; M, mammillary body; MD, dorsomedial thalamic nucleus; RF, reticular formation; S, septum pellucidum; VM, ventromedial hypothalamic nucleus. (From Brodal A. Neurological Anatomy. New York, Oxford University Press, 1981.)

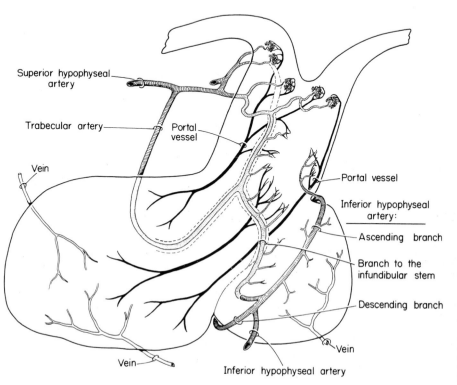

Figure 14.6. The blood supply of the pituitary gland. The major arteries that supply the gland are the superior, middle, and inferior hypophyseal arteries, all of which are branches of the internal carotid artery. The arteries that supply the median eminence and the superior portion of the pituitary stalk terminate in a host of capillary tufts and loops. In humans, blood is collected from this capillary plexus into several large trunks that carry it downward, chiefly on the anterosuperior surface of the pituitary stalk, to become continuous with sinusoids in the pars distalis. These trunks are called the hypophyseal portal system. (From Crosby EC, Humphrey T, Lauer WE. Correlative Anatomy of the Nervous System. New York, Macmillan, 1962.)

ways from the hypothalamus project reciprocally to these same sites, providing feedback control over brain stem, spinal cord, and peripheral autonomic nervous function (32–34). In addition, the hypothalamus influences the body's endocrine system via important connections with the anterior and posterior lobes of the pituitary gland. Fibers that pass from the supraoptic and paraventricular nuclei of the hypothalamus to the hypophysis make up the supraopticohypophyseal tract (35–38). Besides abundant nerve connections from the hypothalamus to the posterior lobe of the hypophysis, there is a vascular link between the hypophyseal stalk and the anterior lobe—the hypophyseal portal system—that brings the anterior lobe under control of the hypothalamus (Fig. 14.6). Some hypothalamic neurons sense various chemical constituents and the temperature of the blood directly, whereas other neurosecretory neurons produce and release hormones that act on the anterior pituitary and on various organ systems. Thus, neural and endocrine links to and from the hypothalamus combine to exert control over almost all autonomic functions.

From a neuro-ophthalmologic standpoint, the sensory input from the visual system to the hypothalamus has clinical significance. Autoradiographic studies demonstrate definite retinohypothalamic projections in various mammals (39–42), including humans (43). These projections, which are both crossed and uncrossed from the retina of each eye, were found to terminate in the midline hypothalamic suprachiasmatic nucleus, and degenerate following retinal lesions (40,41).

The function of retinohypothalamic afferents is concerned with photoneuroendocrine reflexes and photoperiodic functions, termed circadian cycles. The suprachiasmatic nucleus is the major center controlling circadian rhythms (44), and sensory input concerning the daily light cycle is essential for this function. There is strong evidence supporting a relationship between exposure to light and gonadal function in certain birds and mammals. Likewise, there are widely quoted anecdotes that connect the increase in springtime light in the Arctic with heightened sexual activity in the native Inuit people (ovulation is supposedly infrequent during the long winter nights). Zacharias and Wurtman (45) studied normal subjects who had been functionally blind since infancy and found that the onset of puberty was earlier in both boys and girls. In children who had no perception of light in either eye, the onset of puberty was even earlier. The authors suggested that this neuroendocrinologic phenomenon in blind children could be caused by altered retinohypothalamic stimulation.

The existence of a functional retinohypothalamic pathway in humans also comes from the work of Czeisler et al. (46), who evaluated the input of light to the circadian pacemaker by testing the ability of bright light to decrease plasma melatonin concentrations in 11 blind patients with no conscious perception of light and in six normal subjects. These investigators found that plasma melatonin concentrations decreased during exposure to bright light in three sightless patients by about 70% and in all six normal subjects by about 66%. When two of these blind patients were tested with their eyes covered during exposure to light, plasma melatonin did not

decrease. The three blind patients reported no difficulty sleeping, and they maintained apparent circadian conditioning to the 24-hour day. Plasma melatonin concentrations did not decrease during exposure to bright light in seven of the remaining blind patients; in the eighth, plasma melatonin was undetectable. These eight patients reported a history of insomnia, and in four of them, the circadian temperature rhythm was not conditioned to the 24-hour day. On the basis of these findings, Czeisler et al. concluded that the visual subsystem that mediates the light-induced suppression of melatonin secretion remains functionally intact in some sightless patients, probably via a retinohypothalamic pathway.

The fascinating story of the retinohypothalamic pathway was unraveled even further with the discovery of melanopsin-containing ganglion cells in the retina that are photosensitive, independent of rod and cone input (48–52,52a). These ganglion cells mediate the pupillary light reflex to the midbrain and also form projections to the suprachiasmatic nucleus in the hypothalamus. The discovery of this unique class of retinal neuron that is capable of modulating the circadian cycle may also explain why some patients blind from photoreceptor disease may still be capable of melatonin modulation by light, whereas other patients blind from optic nerve disease may lose this function. This topic is covered in greater detail later in this chapter in the section devoted to the anatomy of the pupil light reflex pathway.

Function

The hypothalamus is the coordinating center for the autonomic system complex. It mediates a vast number of autonomic mechanisms that adapt the body to its environment and control its reproductive activity, emotional behavior, and endocrine secretion (53). The complexity of hypothalamic function reflects the intricacy of its anatomy. The posterior part of the hypothalamus seems essential for functions associated with increases in sympathetic activity. Stimulation of the posterior hypothalamus induces vasoconstriction, heat production, increased metabolism, and pupillary dilation. The anterior part of the hypothalamus appears to be devoted to activity mediated by the parasympathetic system. Brooks and Koizumi (54) reviewed the role of the hypothalamus in the control of the endocrine system through the pituitary gland, reproduction, thirst and the control of water balance, control of body weight (hunger and satiation), temperature regulation, reactions to stress, control of emotional reactions, sleep and arousal, and control of somatic reactions.

Vasopressin and oxytocin, once thought to be produced and released by the posterior pituitary gland, are now known to be formed in the neurosecretory cells of the supraoptic and paraventricular hypothalamic nuclei (38,55,56). They reach the pituitary by axon transport along the fibers of the supraopticohypophyseal tract and then pass through the fenestrated capillaries within the pituitary into the bloodstream (57). Neurons in the supraoptic and paraventricular nuclei also contain other biologically active substances, including metenkephalin, cholecystokinin, glucagon, dynorphin, angiotensin, and CRF (58).

The hypothalamic influence on the anterior lobe of the pituitary gland involves nerve fibers from the tuberal region of the pituitary gland and the hypophyseal portal vascular system. The nerve fibers can be traced only to the median eminence and infundibular stem of the pituitary and are known collectively as the tuberohypophyseal or the tuberoinfundibular tract (Fig. 14.4) (38,59,60). Although the fibers are thin, secretory granules are found in their axons. Various releasing substances (GHRF, CRF, TRH, GnRH, PRF) and inhibiting substances (GHRIH, PIF) are manufactured in regions of the hypothalamus (Fig. 14.7). These substances are transported by the fibers of the tuberoinfundibular tract to the median eminence and infundibulum, where they are released into the portal vascular system that provides essentially all of the blood supply to the anterior lobe of the pituitary gland (60–64). Thus, the hypothalamus is intimately involved in the synthesis and transmission of factors that either stimulate or inhibit the secretion of hormones by the anterior pituitary (65).

Sexual behavior and reproduction are directed by the hypothalamus and hypophysis and are different in males and females. Estrogens and androgens influence the behavior of animals indirectly through their action on the hypothalamus. The tuberal region of the hypothalamus maintains basal levels of the gonadotrophic hormones, but the preoptic area is essential for the cyclic changes that induce ovulation (66,67). Radioactive-labeled estrogens accumulate in highest concentrations in the anterior hypothalamus, but they also accumulate in the amygdaloid complex.

A number of studies indicate that the supraoptic and paraventricular nuclei are specifically responsible for the maintenance of water balance by controlling the rate of vasopressin secretion. Destruction of these areas results in diabetes insipidus—an excessive loss of water via the kidneys (68). Although the hypothalamus is obviously important in regulating water intake, it is only part of a much more extensive system concerned with consumption of both food and water (69).

Certain regions of the hypothalamus appear to control aspects of food intake. Medially placed hypothalamic lesions may result in hyperphagia and obesity (70–72), indicating a medial satiety center, whereas lateral lesions often produce aphagia and consequent emaciation, indicating a lateral feeding center (72–76). Detailed neural models have been proposed to explain more fully homeostatic feeding behavior and may be more accurate (77,78).

The hypothalamus plays a major role in the regulation of body temperature. The anterolateral part of the hypothalamus appears to control the mechanism of heat loss, whereas the posterolateral part contains an area that regulates heat production. For example, some cells in the hypothalamus are sensitive to heating or cooling of the blood. These cells, which are found only in the anterolateral hypothalamus, appear to act as thermoreceptors, and it is this region of the hypothalamus that appears to act as the principal "thermostat" of the body, activating the posterior area when increased heat production is required. Catecholamines (adrenaline, noradrenaline, and dopamine) lower body temperature when injected into the anterior hypothalamic area, and serotonin increases body temperature. Thus, it is hypothesized that when a rise in body temperature is required, specific cells in the anterior hypothalamus release serotonin, which then triggers the specific pathways that induce heat production. When body cooling is needed, another group of cells in the same region release a catecholamine that activates the appropriate pathways promoting heat loss (79,80).

The response to stress occurs in two phases, short and prolonged, and the hypothalamus is involved in both. Initially, acute stressful stimuli of short duration evoke a strong sympathoadrenal discharge. Stored catecholamines are released and produce characteristic cardiovascular and metabolic reactions that may restore, or at least maintain, an acceptable degree of normality. Severe or prolonged stress is counteracted by additional reactions, including the release of corticosteroids from the adrenal cortex. These severe, persistent stress stimuli act on the hypothalamus either directly or via afferent neurons to promote secretion of CRF and the subsequent release of ACTH. Lesions of the hypothalamus interfering with the secretion of CRF result in an impaired resistance to infection and injury (81).

Von Economo (82) found that lesions to the posterior hy-

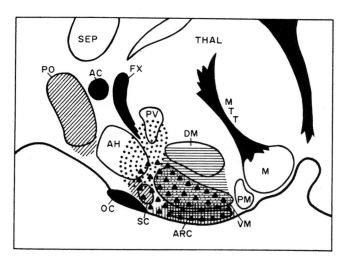

Corticotropin-releasing factor

Follicle-stimulating hormone-releasing factor

Luteinizing hormone-releasing factor

Growth hormone-releasing factor

Thyrotropin-releasing factor

Prolactin-inhibiting factor

Figure 14.7. Diagram of sagittal section through the hypothalamus showing the areas that have been implicated in the elaboration of some major releasing and inhibiting factors. AC, anterior commissure; AH, anterior hypothalamic area; ARC, arcuate nucleus; DM, dorsomedial nucleus; FX, fornix; M, mammillary body; MTT, mammillothalamic tract; OC, optic chiasm; PM, premammillary nucleus; PO, preoptic area; PV, paraventricular nucleus; SC, suprachiasmatic nucleus; SEP, septal nuclear complex; THAL, thalamus; VM, ventromedial nucleus. (From Brodal A. Neurological Anatomy. New York, Oxford University Press, 1981.)

pothalamus and rostral mesencephalon were usually associated with hypersomnia, whereas lesions in the anterior hypothalamus often resulted in insomnia. Subsequent investigators (83,84) confirmed the important role of the anterior hypothalamus and neighboring regions in the induction of sleep. Several studies also show that histamine-containing neurons in the posterior hypothalamus, including the tuberomammillary nucleus, are involved with the mechanism of arousal (85–87). These hypothalamic areas clearly play a role in the modulation of sleep but are highly influenced by afferents from the forebrain and brain stem and, therefore, do not function as the only "control center" for wakefulness.

The hypothalamus functions in modulating cardiovascular and digestive activities. For example, hypothalamic influences on the cardiovascular system can be demonstrated by stimulation of the posterior lateral hypothalamus, causing an increase in blood pressure and heart rate, whereas stimulation of the anterior hypothalamic regions causes vasodilation and lowering of blood pressure (88). Hypothalamic influences on digestion can be demonstrated by stimulation of the anterior hypothalamus, producing an increase in secretion and peristalsis in the stomach and intestines. If the posterior part of the hypothalamus is stimulated, these activities are depressed, coinciding with a general increase in sympathetic-induced behavior.

The hypothalamus plays a role not only in the control of visceral and endocrine function but also in the regulation of somatic activity. An intact hypothalamus helps to integrate reflex motor activity. In the absence of the hypothalamus, walking, running, and righting reflexes are imperfectly displayed and coordinated (54).

Of neuro-ophthalmologic interest is the influence of the hypothalamus on the intrinsic muscles of the eye, the position of the lids mediated by sympathetically innervated smooth muscle, the secretion of tears, the vasomotor system, and intraocular pressure. These are discussed later in this chapter.

Brain Stem

Preganglionic autonomic nerves, which originate in the visceral efferent columns of the brain stem, exit along various cranial nerves to connect with visceral, glandular, and vascular structures, as well as smooth muscles. The cell bodies of the brain stem preganglionic autonomic nerves form subnuclei of the oculomotor (3rd), facial (7th), glossopharyngeal (9th), vagus (10th), and spinal accessory (11th) cranial nerves and are concerned with pupillary, lacrimal, salivary, cardiovascular, respiratory, alimentary, and other visceral activities.

Apart from the autonomic neurons that make up the visceral efferent nuclei, there is also an autonomic representation of cell bodies in the gray matter of the reticular formation of the medulla, which modulate critical respiratory and cardiovascular functions. An inspiratory area lies in the ventral part of the medullary reticular formation adjacent to the inferior olive, whereas an expiratory area is located dorsal and slightly cephalic. Pneumotaxic centers are located near the midline in the ventral and rostral part of the tegmentum

of the pons and are connected to the respiratory areas by descending fibers (89). Many cardiovascular reflexes depend upon an intact medulla (90). The clustering of these essential functions in such a small area within the medulla explains the occasional catastrophic loss of neurologic function from small lesions. The "centers" that control and coordinate life-dependent functions are actually neural networks that are scattered over a region of brain stem and are not strictly localized to any single anatomic nuclear group.

PERIPHERAL AUTONOMIC NERVOUS SYSTEM

The peripheral component of the autonomic nervous system provides innervation to viscera, glands, blood vessels, and smooth (nonstriated) muscle, forming the visceral portion of the nervous system. Peripheral autonomic nerves also gather impulses from peripheral receptors whose input is used to modulate signals in the brain stem and spinal cord prior to the initiation of effector responses. The receptors and afferent fibers that transmit impulses to autonomic neurons within the spinal cord and brain stem are elements of the visceral sensory system. The efferent autonomic nerves belong to the visceral motor system.

Anatomy of the Peripheral Autonomic Nervous System

There are two major subdivisions of the efferent autonomic system, sympathetic and parasympathetic (91). Although both sympathetic and parasympathetic efferent nerves have cell bodies within the neural axis, there is always a synapse between the cell of origin and the cell of termination, and the ganglia where these synapses occur are always located outside the CNS. Both the sympathetic and parasympathetic efferent systems therefore contain two types of fibers: the preganglionic fiber, with its cell of origin in the CNS, either in the visceral efferent nuclei of cranial nerves (i.e., parasympathetic) or in the lateral gray columns of the spinal cord (i.e., sympathetic), and the postganglionic fiber, with its cell of origin in one of the ganglia outside of the CNS. In general, preganglionic fibers are finely myelinated, whereas postganglionic fibers are unmyelinated.

There are several morphologic and anatomic differences between the sympathetic and parasympathetic systems. The preganglionic efferent neurons of the sympathetic system receive input from the hypothalamus and have their cell bodies in the lower cervical, thoracic, and first two lumbar segments of the spinal cord, whereas the preganglionic fibers of the parasympathetic system have cell bodies located in specific regions of the brain stem and in the second, third, and fourth sacral segments of the spinal cord.

Another morphologic difference between the sympathetic and parasympathetic systems involves the location of the postganglionic cell bodies. In the sympathetic system, postganglionic cell bodies are found in the ganglia of the sympathetic trunk and, therefore, are almost always adjacent to the spinal cord. In contrast to the sympathetic system, cell bodies of postganglionic parasympathetic neurons are positioned farther from the CNS, either within or on the walls of the organ they supply or in ganglia close to the structure innervated.

There are three types of sympathetic ganglia, named according to their location. The three types are: (a) paravertebral—pairs of ganglia arranged in two chains close to each side of the vertebral column (e.g., superior, middle, and inferior cervical ganglia; 10 or 11 thoracic ganglia; 4 lumbar ganglia; and 2 to 6 sacral ganglia); (b) prevertebral—the celiac, mesenteric, and hypogastric ganglia lying in the abdominal cavity; and (c) terminal—several ganglia lying on or near the bladder and rectum.

The superior cervical ganglion, a structure of major interest to neuro-ophthalmologists because of its role in the anatomy of the oculosympathetic fibers to the pupil and to the upper and lower eyelids, is the largest of the cervical chain. It is located adjacent to the second and third cervical vertebrae, just behind the internal carotid artery. It gives off lateral, medial, and anterior branches and is the origin of the internal carotid nerve. The anterior branches of the superior cervical ganglion generate a plexus along the common and external carotid arteries. Within the neck, the external carotid plexus supplies various exocrine glands of the face and neck, including the sweat glands of the face; however, sweat glands within a small area of skin just above the brow usually are supplied by branches from the internal carotid nerve. Therefore, a specific pattern of sudomotor loss on the face may sometimes help to localize a lesion. The internal carotid nerve ascends behind the internal carotid artery and enters the carotid canal, where it forms a plexus surrounding the intracranial portion of the carotid artery, and finally along the ophthalmic artery to enter the orbit.

In the parasympathetic system, the preganglionic fibers originate within the CNS at the level of the midbrain (Edinger-Westphal nucleus), the medulla, and the second, third, and fourth sacral segments of the spinal cord. In the midbrain, parasympathetic preganglionic cell bodies give rise to axons that travel peripherally with axons of the oculomotor nerves and pass with the inferior division of the oculomotor nerve to synapse with the ciliary ganglion. Postganglionic parasympathetic fibers exit the ciliary ganglion as short ciliary nerves to innervate the muscles of the ciliary body and the sphincter pupillae muscle of the iris (27). In the medulla, myelinated preganglionic fibers travel with the facial, glossopharyngeal, vagus, and spinal accessory cranial nerves to synapse in the parasympathetic ganglia of the head: the pterygopalatine, submandibular, and otic ganglia. Neurons and synapses situated in these ganglia are exclusively efferent and parasympathetic, although afferent fibers and postganglionic sympathetic fibers do pass through the ganglia without interruption. Postganglionic parasympathetic efferents from these ganglia transmit the bulbar outflow to the lacrimal glands, salivary glands, and mucous membranes of the nose, mouth, and pharynx. In the sacrum, the preganglionic parasympathetic cell bodies lie in the second, third, and fourth sacral segments of the spinal cord. From this region, the preganglionic fibers exit the spinal cord with the sacral nerves and pass to ganglia located in or near the distal portion of the large intestine, the rectum, the bladder, and the organs of reproduction (10,12,92).

Of specific interest to neuro-ophthalmologists, the parasympathetic preganglionic lacrimal secretomotor efferents arise from the superior salivatory nucleus and travel with the facial nerve along the nervus intermedius and then via the greater superficial petrosal nerve through the pterygoid canal to synapse in the pterygopalatine (sphenopalatine) ganglion. The postganglionic course is somewhat variable, with some evidence suggesting that the postganglionic fibers travel via the zygomatic nerve to the lacrimal gland (Fig. 14.8) and via ganglionic branches to the nasal and palatal glands. The vagus nerve distributes large numbers of preganglionic fibers to the lungs, bronchi, heart, stomach, and small intestine, and to part of the large intestine. As noted previously, its ganglia are located close to, or embedded in, the visceral structures innervated, and the postganglionic fibers are very short.

Finally, the relationship between the number of preganglionic to postganglionic autonomic nerve fibers seems to differ among the sympathetic and parasympathetic divisions. In the sympathetic division, each sympathetic preganglionic neuron synapses with a large number of postganglionic neurons, and the postganglionic fibers ramify widely. In one study of the human superior cervical ganglion, Ebbesson (93) found a pre- to postganglionic fiber ratio of 1 to 196. In contrast, in the parasympathetic division, each parasympathetic preganglionic neuron typically synapses with one postganglionic neuron, and the distribution of its terminal arbors is much more limited. The anatomic arrangement of these two systems suggests that, physiologically, the sympathetic system is involved predominantly with diffuse reactions affecting the entire organism, whereas the parasympathetic system produces more restricted, localized effects. However, the sympathetic system is also capable of producing localized discrete effects to different organs in response to specific stimuli. For example, postganglionic sympathetic neurons may be activated independently or in concert depending on the stimulus and include the following: vasoconstrictor fibers to blood vessels supplying organs, vasodilatory fibers to skeletal muscle, secretomotor fibers to sweat glands, motor fibers to the erector pili muscles of skin, fibers to the pulmonary airways causing dilation of the bronchi and bronchioles, and fibers producing pupillary dilation. They can also alter glandular secretion and inhibit muscle contraction in the alimentary tract.

Physiology of the Peripheral Autonomic Nervous System

Many organs innervated by the autonomic nervous system receive fibers from both the sympathetic and parasympathetic divisions. Among these organs are the pupil, ciliary body, heart, bronchi, stomach, intestines, salivary glands, sex organs, and bladder. Other organs receive innervation from only one division of the autonomic system, such as the sweat glands, the piloerector muscles in the skin, the smooth muscles of the eyelid (Müller's muscle), the spleen, the arterioles, and probably the uterus.

When an organ receives both sympathetic and parasympathetic innervation, the effects produced by the two subsys-

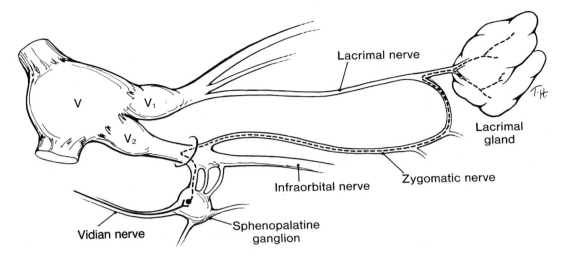

Figure 14.8. Diagram showing the postganglionic parasympathetic pathway for lacrimal secretion. The cell bodies of the postganglionic fibers originate in the sphenopalatine (pterygopalatine) ganglion, where they synapse with axons from the greater superficial petrosal nerve. The postganglionic fibers then leave the ganglion, join the maxillary nerve, and enter the zygomatic branch of the nerve. The fibers next enter the lacrimal nerve, a branch of the ophthalmic nerve, via anastomotic channels between the zygomatic and lacrimal nerves. The fibers ultimately enter the lacrimal gland within the lacrimal nerve. (Redrawn from Ruskell GL. The distribution of autonomic post-ganglionic nerve fibres to the lacrimal gland in monkeys. J Anat 1971; 109:229–242.)

tems are usually antagonistic. Heart rate, for example, is accelerated by stimulation of the sympathetic division and slowed by stimulation of the parasympathetic division. The tone of the small intestine increases with parasympathetic stimulation (along the vagus nerve) and decreases with sympathetic stimulation (4). The iris sphincter muscle contracts, causing pupil constriction with parasympathetic stimulation, whereas the iris dilator muscle dilates the pupil with sympathetic stimulation. Similarly, the ciliary muscle contracts with parasympathetic stimulation, causing active accommodation at near, whereas sympathetic stimulation inhibits accommodation. On the other hand, actions of the two divisions are not always antagonistic; they may actually summate. Salivary glands secrete profusely in response to stimulation of the parasympathetic division, but sympathetic stimulation also produces secretion from these glands. Thus, both systems participate in the intricate regulation of visceral functions, ensuring a proper balance in the action of various organs.

Pharmacology of the Autonomic Nervous System

Chemical Transmission of Autonomic Impulses

Both sympathetic and parasympathetic preganglionic fibers release acetylcholine (94). For both of these subsystems, the neural action potential originating in an autonomic neuron in the CNS is conducted along a myelinated nerve fiber to the presynaptic terminal, where it causes the release of acetylcholine from stores within the nerve ending. The acetylcholine crosses the narrow synaptic gap and combines with receptors located on the cell body of the postsynaptic (postganglionic) neuron, producing a localized depolariza-

tion called the "excitatory postsynaptic potential." This potential in turn initiates an action potential in the postganglionic neuron. Once its action is completed, acetylcholine is promptly hydrolyzed by acetylcholinesterase.

Acetylcholine is also the transmitter substance released by parasympathetic postganglionic fibers at the neuroeffector junction (94), whereas with few exceptions sympathetic postganglionic neurons typically release the catecholamine norepinephrine at the neuroeffector junction. Norepinephrine, bound loosely to adenosine triphosphate (ATP), is stored in the cytoplasmic granules of the nerve ending and is released from these concentrated stores when the nerve is stimulated. The action of norepinephrine on the effector cell is quickly terminated by reuptake of all available free norepinephrine into the cytoplasm of the presynaptic nerve ending. Norepinephrine is also broken down and inactivated by two relatively slow-acting enzymes: catechol-O-methyltransferase (COMT) and monoamine oxidase (MAO). The norepinephrine that is recovered by the nerve ending is retained, concentrated, and stored in the granules, or it is metabolized by intraneuronal monoamine oxidases.

The terms "adrenergic" and "cholinergic" were first used by Dale (95) to describe substances with sympathomimetic and parasympathomimetic properties, respectively. For many years, the idea of sympathetic adrenergic and parasympathetic cholinergic systems, operating antagonistically to control visceral function, has been accepted; however, there are many exceptions to this general concept. For example, the postganglionic fibers to the sweat glands are anatomically part of the sympathetic system, but they are cholinergic. Also, as noted above, acetylcholine is the neurotransmitter for both sympathetic and parasympathetic preganglionic fibers. In addition, some autonomic nerves are nonadrenergic and noncholinergic (NANC nerves). Such nerves, called ''purinergic'' by Burnstock (96), use ATP as their neurotransmitter. Nitric oxide (NO) and related substances also appear to mediate transmission from some autonomic nerves to smooth muscle (97,98), and many other substances that modulate neural activity in adjacent cells, including various peptides, are present in autonomic nerves (96).

Most autonomic nerves release more than one transmitter substance, a phenomenon called cotransmission. The principal cotransmitters in most sympathetic nerves are noradrenaline, ATP, and neuropeptide Y (NPY). In parasympathetic nerves, the principal transmitters are acetylcholine and VIP, although a minority of nerves use ATP, NO, or both. Another concept is that of neuromodulation, a term that refers to the effects that certain locally released agents have on neurotransmission. These effects are produced either by varying the amount of transmitter released from the presynaptic terminal or by acting on the postsynaptic neuron so that its response to the neurotransmitter is altered. A variety of interactions between cotransmitters and neuromodulators that influence neurotransmission have been described. In contrast to striated muscle, not all smooth muscle cells are activated directly by neurotransmitter released from terminal branches of the autonomic fibers. Instead, entire smooth muscle bundles can be stimulated via low-resistance pathways between the individual smooth muscle cells. The electric coupling between adjacent cells takes place at gap junctions that transmit and spread nerve impulses within the muscle bundle (99,100).

Denervation Supersensitivity

Destruction and degeneration of preganglionic or postganglionic autonomic axons is followed by greatly increased sensitivity of the deafferented autonomic effectors to their specific transmitter substances and to pharmaceutical compounds that mimic those transmitters. This supersensitivity of the denervated effector cell usually appears within 1 or 2 days after a parasympathetic nerve is sectioned. For sympathetic nerves, supersensitivity can be demonstrated within a few days and is fully developed within 1–2 weeks. In both the parasympathetic and sympathetic systems, the supersensitivity slowly declines if the efferent axons regenerate.

Regeneration of Autonomic Fibers

It once was thought that if a nerve was interrupted by injury or disease, no recovery could take place until new fibers grew out from the central stump. Murray and Thompson (101) showed, however, that when a nerve fiber is damaged and degenerates, adjacent normal fibers are stimulated to give off tiny side branches or sprouts. The stimulus for this growth is unknown but may be some humoral agent released from the degenerating fiber. In any event, the surface of adjacent normal fibers becomes locally disorganized, and tiny axonal strands develop on their surface and grow toward the degenerating fibers. These strands penetrate the fiber sheath and grow into the neural tubes of adjacent degenerated fibers, where they make contact with the adventitial or Schwann cells that presumably guide them toward the effector organ. Normal undamaged fibers thus actively contribute to the recovery of function (102).

The process of sprouting is very rapid. The new branches are visible by light microscopy within 4 or 5 days after the nerve axons are sectioned (101) and within 24 hours of the injury using electron microscopy (103). The sprouts continue to enlarge for at least 1–2 months (101).

Collateral nerve sprouting is particularly vigorous in the autonomic nervous system. Fibers from nearby nerves containing the same neurotransmitter, but often entirely unrelated in function, may send sprouts into the damaged nerve, and the impulses that these new collaterals carry may cause inappropriate activation of the end organ. Throughout this book, many clinical phenomena are described that are best explained by just this sort of uncontrolled sprouting of collaterals among the regenerating fibers. These include the pseudo-Argyll Robertson phenomenon with misdirection of regenerating oculomotor fibers, the light-near dissociation of the tonic pupil, gustatory sweating, crocodile tears, and postherpetic pain.

THE PUPIL LIGHT AND NEAR REFLEXES AND THEIR RELATIONSHIP TO THE AUTONOMIC NERVOUS SYSTEM

The major function of the pupil is to aid in optimizing retinal illumination to maximize visual perception. In dim light, dilation of the pupil provides an immediate means for maximizing the number of photons reaching the retina, which supplements the dark-adaptive mechanisms of retinal-gain control. Under bright light, pupil constriction can reduce retinal illumination by up to 1.5 log units. Although this reduction in retinal illumination is only a portion of the 12-log unit range of light sensitivity of the retina (104), it provides an important and immediate contribution to early light adaptation. Patients with a fixed immobile pupil are usually very symptomatic under conditions of changing illumination, emphasizing the important role of the pupil in optimizing visual perception over a wide range of lighting conditions of the environment.

In addition to its role in regulating the amount of light energy entering the eye, the iris can improve image quality on the retina by constricting, thus increasing the depth of focus of the eye's optical system (105) and reducing the degree of chromatic and spherical aberration (106,107). There is a limit to this beneficial effect, however, because constriction beyond a certain diameter results in image degradation secondary to increased diffraction (108). Because of the forward convexity of the anterior lens surface, the pupillary plane of the iris is farther forward in the eye than the iris root, and the iris plane thus forms the sides of a truncated cone. The magnification produced by the cornea causes the iris to appear one-eighth larger (and the pupil wider) than it actually is. Nevertheless, differences in corneal refractive power among eyes contribute only a minor degree to the difference between actual and apparent pupil size (109).

In this section, the anatomy and physiology of the normal pupil will be presented, including the afferent, efferent, and supranuclear pathways involved in the regulation of pupil size. The reader interested in pursuing these subjects in more detail is advised to consult the excellent book by Loewenfeld (109).

THE AFFERENT ARC OF THE PUPIL LIGHT REFLEX

The neuronal integration of the pupillary light reflex begins in the retina with the photoreceptors that pass information to the retinal ganglion cells by way of synapses with bipolar cells (110,111). For many years, it was assumed that only the photoreceptors contributed to the pupillary light reflex (109). It is now clear that other retinal elements—particularly certain ganglion cells—also play a role.

Rod and Cone Contribution to the Pupillary Light Reflex

The extent and nature of the contribution of rod and cone input to the pupillary light reflex was confusing for many years, because the responses measured were highly dependent upon the conditions of retinal adaptation, characteristics of the light stimulus (e.g., intensity, wavelength, and size), location of the portion of the retina that was stimulated, and sensitivity of the recording apparatus used to detect threshold pupil movements. Once sensitive infrared recording devices for precise measurement of small pupil movements and carefully controlled stimulus conditions were used, it became clear that both rods and cones contribute to the pupillary light reflex.

The relative contribution of the rods and cones depends on the conditions under which the pupil responses are measured. The same rods and cones that process light input for visual perception modify the pupillary response; there are no separate photoreceptors for vision and for the pupil. Thus, almost all modifications of stimulus conditions that produce a difference in visual perception also produce a comparable change in pupillary responsiveness. These modifications include changes in retinal adaptation, wavelength of light, stimulus duration, and stimulus light intensity. In fact, in almost every way in which responses are measured, the pupillary responses to light parallel those of visual perception. For example, the wavelength sensitivity profile of pupil threshold as the color of light is changed from blue to red exactly parallels the same wavelength sensitivity of visual perception. The shift in sensitivity is also the same as the eye is changed from a condition of light adaptation to dark adaptation (Purkinje shift), providing further evidence that the same photoreceptors are used for both pupillary responses and vision. In fact, patients with various abnormalities of either rods or cones can be shown to have the same deficits in color vision or lack of appropriate sensitivity change during dark adaptation when the results of visual threshold are compared with pupillary threshold to light stimuli (112).

Under conditions of dark adaptation, low-intensity light stimuli that are below the level of cone threshold produce small-amplitude pupil reactions that are only contributed to by rods. The recorded pupillary waveform movements caused by rod input under stimulus conditions of dark adaptation are indistinguishable in shape from those produced by dim stimuli under conditions of photopic light adaptation, where cone input is the primary source of signal to the pupillary motor center. Under dark adaptation, the threshold pupillary response also favors a blue wavelength, as would be expected for a rod-dominated response. In fact, under these conditions, there is a worsening of pupil threshold sensitivity at the fovea, causing a scotoma at the center of the visual field where rods are lacking. This is observed when the threshold for pupil contraction is observed using low-intensity lights below the level of cone threshold. As the intensity of light stimulus is increased above the cone threshold, pupil contractions can be recorded at the fovea, as the cone contribution comes into play. Under these stimulus conditions, both rods and cones contribute to the pupil response, a condition called "rod intrusion" (109). If a background light is used to adapt the eye to a photopic, relatively light-adapted state, the rod contribution is suppressed, and cones then provide the primary contribution to the pupillary light reflex.

Another important difference between the cone and rod contribution to the pupillary light reflex relates to the concept of pupillary threshold sensitivity versus pupillary amplitude of response. As stated above, under conditions of dark adaptation, the rods are far more sensitive than cones. The amount of light it takes to elicit a small, threshold pupillary response is over 2 log units less than what it would take to elicit a threshold pupil response from cone activation. Above the level of threshold, however, the amplitude of pupil contraction has a much greater valence from cone contribution compared with that of the rods. Therefore, although the rods are more sensitive in terms of the amount of light it takes to elicit a threshold pupil response in the dark-adapted state, the amount of pupil contraction produced at light levels above threshold for each photoreceptor type is greater for cones.

With focal light stimuli given at suprathreshold intensity levels, the amplitude of the pupillary light reflex has a large cone contribution for reasons stated above and is greater in amplitude at the center of the visual field and falls off in the peripheral field as shown by pupil perimetry. The density distribution of rods and cones (and bipolar cells) accounts for only one aspect of the pupillomotor response across the visual field.

Retinal Ganglion Cell Contributions to the Pupillary Light Reflex

Contributions from Ganglion Cells in General

Rods and cones relay the light signal to the retinal ganglion cells via synapses with bipolar cells (110,111). The ganglion cell distribution within the retina and receptive field properties thus provide the primary basis for the degree of pupillary response from light stimuli at different visual field locations.

The ganglion cells that serve the pupillomotor afferent input are densest in the central retina. The ganglion cells in the central area also have more of a one-to-one relationship with photoreceptor and bipolar cells, in contrast to those in the peripheral retina, where many more photoreceptors and bipolar cells map to one ganglion cell. Therefore, it is the central density of ganglion cells, their approximate one-to-one mapping with photoreceptors and bipolar cells, and their receptive field properties that account for the greater amplitude of pupillary response to stimuli in the central visual field.

The retinal ganglion cells, the first neurons in the chain to give rise to action potentials (the photoreceptors and bipolar cells give rise to generator potentials), are made up of different classes of neurons based on morphology, physiology, and projections. Although it appears that the pupillary and visual systems share the same photoreceptor input (and presumably bipolar cell input), the situation is more complicated for ganglion cell input. It appears that melanopsin-containing ganglion cells primarily serve the classical midbrain pupillary light reflex and circadian centers of the hypothalamus (discussed later). Other ganglion cells, which primarily serve visual perception via their synapses with the lateral geniculate nucleus (LGN) and the visual cortex, may also modulate the pupil light reflex under certain conditions of light stimulus. Over the years, many anatomic and physiologic studies have been performed in an attempt to classify retinal ganglion cells based on the size of their cell body, their dendritic field, their axon diameter, and their firing properties. This information has been collected in a number of species, most notably the cat and monkey, and with labeling techniques, the projections of the cell axons to the LGN and midbrain have been studied. Loewenfeld (109) summarized the properties of the major classes of ganglion cells in the retina and their projections. Based on these studies, it appears that in primates there are three main types of ganglion cells in the retina: α, β, and γ cells.

Two classes of ganglion cells—the α and β cells—have properties different from the γ cells. The α cells constitute 1–2% of the cells in the central retina and 10% in the periphery. They are densest in the parafoveal region and have the largest cell body size, which increases further in the peripheral retina. The axons of these cells are thick and have a corresponding fast conduction speed. Their receptive fields are large and have a phasic discharge. These cells respond to fast-moving stimuli, and they discharge in a transient fashion. The α cell axons project to the LGN, but almost 50% have attenuated branches that also project to the midbrain in areas such as the superior colliculus.

The β cells are the most numerous of all the ganglion cell classes, representing 50–60% of the total ganglion cell population. Like the γ cells, they are densest in the central retina. They have medium-sized cell bodies and axons, and they possess small-sized receptive fields. These ganglion cells fire tonically and are most responsive to contrast of small areas, such as fine-grating stimuli. They discriminate detail within the central field. The β cells also project primar-

ily to the LGN, but some of their axons have collateral branches that project to the tectum and pretectum.

The major contribution to the pretectal olivary neurons in the midbrain serving the classic pupillary light reflex pathway comes from the γ cells, which now appear to have been identified as the melanopsin-containing ganglion cells. These cells may also play a role in other visually evoked reflexes (such as circadian rhythm), because they also project to the superior colliculus and to the accessory optic system. The γ cells have small cell bodies and thin, slowly conducting axons, with large-sized receptive fields. They respond primarily to incremental changes in light intensity and are relatively insensitive to movement. These cells project almost exclusively to the midbrain and not to the LGN. They are densest in the central retina (posterior pole of the eye) and are less dense in the periphery. This accounts in large part for the central field weighting of pupillary response.

The proportion of γ ganglion cells that serves the pupillary light reflex is not known; the answer awaits specific labeling studies in primates. Such studies are technically difficult to perform, because the retrograde label must be microinjected into the specific pretectal olivary area where light-responding neurons can be identified using electric recordings. Even then, the label reaching the retinal ganglion cells is only weakly visible, and these neurons, once identified in flat mount preparations, must be individually injected using a micropipette containing a more visible dye that fills each cell body, dendrites, and axon (P.D.R. Gamlin, personal communication). At present, it is not known how many retinal ganglion cells project directly to the pretectal midbrain neurons serving the pupillary light reflex, but their number must be relatively small (on the order of 1%) in proportion to the total number of ganglion cells.

In summary, it would appear that the γ cells are primarily light-sensitive neurons with melanopsin that are activated by either rod or cone input but that also can be activated directly by light. These cells subserve the midbrain pupillary light reflex. The α cells are primarily movement-sensitive and provide afferent information for control of eye movements and foveation of peripherally moving targets. The β cells are mainly sensitive to high-contrast detail and probably provide the visual cortex with spatial frequency and orientation information used to interpret form. In view of evidence for cortical mediation of the pupillary movement to perimetric stimuli and isoluminant complex stimuli (gratings and randomly modulated patterns of varying spatial frequency), it is possible that other ganglion cells besides the γ type play a role in mediating the pupil response to other, nontraditional types of stimuli (113–121).

Contributions from Melanopsin-Containing Photoreceptive Ganglion Cells

In addition to the rods and cones, another retinal cell can modulate pupil size. Genetically altered mice that completely lack functional rods and cones nevertheless show a rather robust pupil light reflex (46–52). These mice possess a specific ganglion cell that contains melanopsin, a protein that is itself photosensitive, with a broad spectral peak centering on about 490 nm. Melanopsin-containing ganglion cells project to the suprachiasmatic nucleus in the hypothalamus and also to the pretectal nucleus (the site of the first midbrain interneuron synapse for the pupil light reflex pathway). Elegant electrophysiologic recordings coupled with the study of response properties of these ganglion cells have revealed that the cells provide the midbrain pathway for the pupil light reflex and also provide light sensing information for the diurnal regulating areas of the hypothalamus that modulate the circadian rhythm (46–52,52a). Thus, although as noted above the melanopsin-containing ganglion cells receive rod and cone input to the pupil light reflex, they also are capable of transduction of light directly, without photoreceptor input. This helps explain why some patients blind from photoreceptor loss continue to exhibit a circadian rhythm, whereas others blind from optic nerve lesions (and thus loss of melanopsin-ganglion cell input) lack a circadian rhythm.

With the discovery of a melanopsin-containing ganglion cell that is capable of direct activation by light in addition to photoreceptor input, a number of clinical observations may be unraveled in the near future. For example, input of this neuron to the pupil light reflex that can occur without photoreceptor input can help explain why some patients with extensive photoreceptor damage may still exhibit an intact pupil light reflex. This could also explain why such patients still maintain a circadian cycle. It may also explain other clinical examples that support the concept that separate ganglion cells exist for visual perception and the pupillary light reflex. These include cases of complete noncerebral monocular or binocular blindness in which the pupillary reaction to light persists, cases of recovered optic neuritis in which visual function has apparently returned to normal but the pupillary light reflex has not, and instances in which pupillomotor activity returns to normal before visual function in cases of amaurosis (122). Although the correlation between visual field loss and pupillary reactivity is sufficiently strong to be clinically useful (123), the correlation is not strong enough in optic nerve disease (124–126) to allow one to feel confident that the same ganglion cells serve both the visual and pupillomotor systems. Our own work comparing visual perimetry with pupil perimetry (Fig. 14.9) reveals many examples where the two types of perimetry correlate beautifully (e.g., anterior ischemic optic neuropathy) and other cases of optic nerve damage where large differences

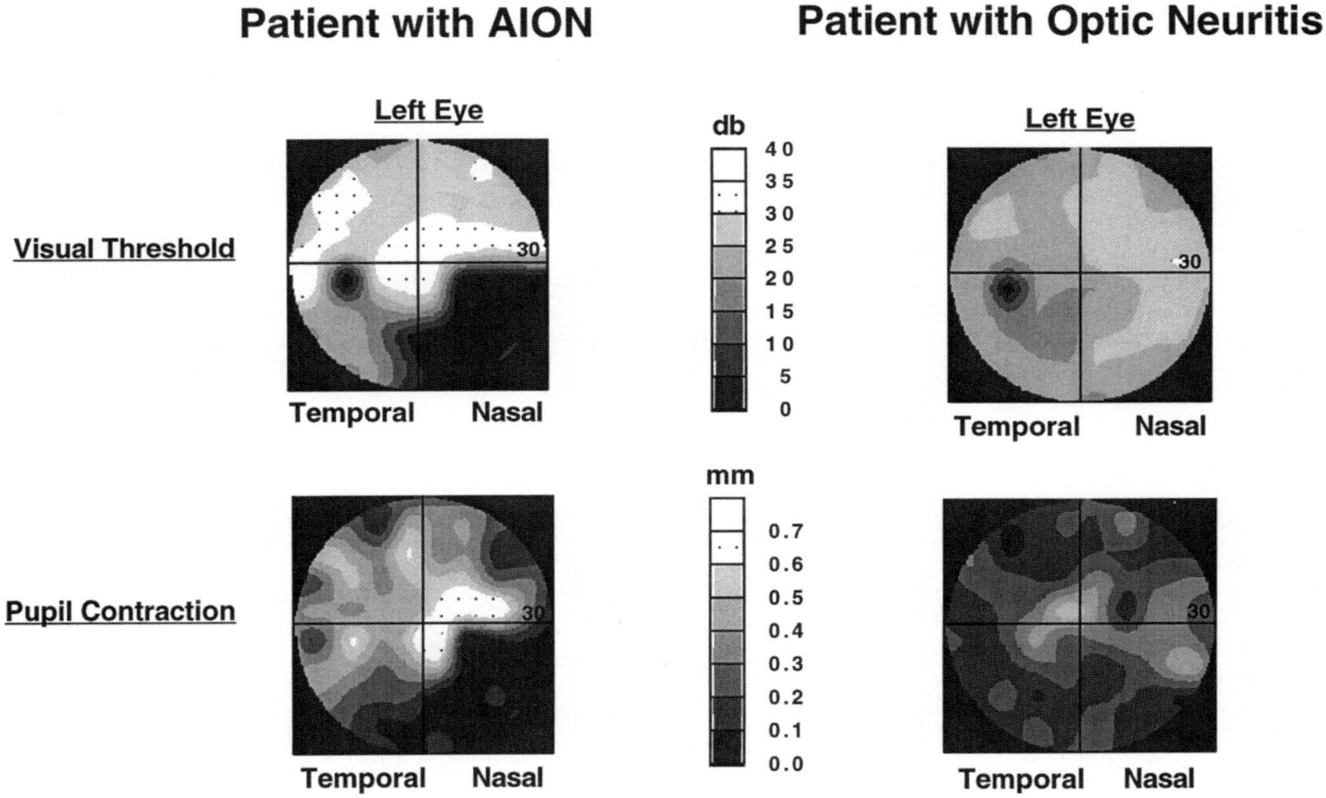

Figure 14.9. Clinical examples of the correlation between visual light sense perimetry and pupil perimetry in patients with optic nerve damage from anterior ischemic optic neuropathy (*left*) and acute optic neuritis (*right*). In the patient with anterior ischemic optic neuropathy there is good correlation between the areas of visual field loss (*top left*) and those with loss of pupillomotor sensitivity (*bottom left*). However, in the patient with acute optic neuritis there is much more damage to the "pupil field" (*bottom right*), showing poor correlation between the visual and pupillary systems.

exist between visual perimetry and pupil perimetry (e.g., optic neuritis and glaucoma) (127,128). Clinical examples such as this indicate that there may be differences between the ganglion cell integration of the pupillary response to light and the visual perception of light, and that separate ganglion cells and fibers may exist for each system, with different susceptibilities to optic nerve damage. It is also possible that some ganglion cells subserve each function independently, whereas others are shared by the visual and pupillary systems.

THE INTER-NEURON OF THE PUPIL LIGHT REFLEX

The axons of the ganglion cells travel intracranially within the optic nerve, optic chiasm, and optic tract. Just before these axons reach the LGN, some of them (or some of their branches) leave the optic tract (primarily the γ cell type) to reach the pretectal olivary nucleus in the mesencephalon via the brachium of the superior colliculus (129). As mentioned above, a small contribution of bifurcating fibers from the α and β ganglion cell axons also travel within the brachium.

As depicted in Figure 14.10, the ganglion cell axons from the nasal retina (temporal field) of the right eye cross at the chiasm and distribute to the contralateral (left) pretectal (olivary) nucleus. The ganglion cell axons from the temporal retina (nasal field) of the left eye remain on the same side and join the axons from the nasal retina of the right eye

(mapping to the same homonymous field) in the left optic tract to distribute to the left pretectal olivary nucleus. In this way, ganglion cell axons serving homonymous portions of the visual field distribute to the same pretectal nucleus. In other words, the axons serving right homonymous visual field space distribute to the left pretectal olivary nucleus, and the axons serving left homonymous visual field space distribute to the right pretectal olivary nucleus. At each pretectal olivary nucleus, a great deal of convergence occurs, with many ganglion cell axons forming connections with a relatively small number of dendritic processes of pretectal olivary neurons. Once the pupillary light signal is integrated at the level of the pretectal olivary nucleus, the signal is distributed in humans approximately equally to the right and left Edinger-Westphal nuclei, which in turn produce a right and left pupil contraction of similar amplitude.

The hemifield organization of the pupillary light reflex and the resulting degree of decussation in the chiasm and in the pretectum is specific to different species. In lower animals with little binocularity, such as the rabbit, almost all of the visual and pupillary input decussates in the chiasm from one eye to the opposite side. The pretectal decussation back to the opposite side is almost complete, thus producing a direct pupil response only in the eye being stimulated. In the cat, there is some binocularity, and there are more uncrossed fibers in the chiasm and pretectum, producing

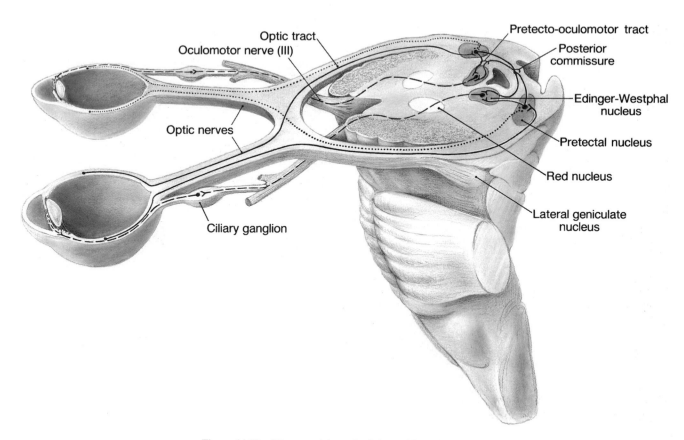

Figure 14.10.   Diagram of the path of the pupillary light reflex.

an incomplete consensual pupil response. In primates with significant binocularity, the uncrossed component of visual and pupillary input is even greater in both the chiasm and the pretectum, producing an almost equal direct and consensual pupil contraction when light is shined in only one eye (Fig. 14.11).

Proof of a hemifield organization and hemidecussation of pupillomotor fibers at the chiasm in humans comes from sagittal sectioning of the chiasm, which does not abolish either the direct or consensual reaction to light of either eye (130). Similarly, in nonhuman primates and in humans, destruction of an optic tract has only a small, subclinical effect on the symmetry of the direct and consensual reaction of either pupil to light but instead produces a relative afferent pupillary defect in the eye opposite the side of the lesion (131,132). This is because the intact temporal field of the eye on the same side of the tract lesion provides greater pupillomotor input (per unit area of retina stimulated) compared with the intact nasal field of the eye on the opposite side of the tract lesion. In addition, our own studies demonstrate absence of pupillary responses when hemifield stimuli are placed in the blind homonymous hemifields in patients with optic tract lesions. Thus, both experimental and clinical evidence supports the concept that the hemifield organization of visual and pupillomotor afferent fibers in humans is similar.

Ganglion cell fibers destined for the pretectal region of the mesencephalon leave the optic tracts before reaching the LGN. This anatomic feature is demonstrated by intact pupillary light responses in experimental animals following extirpation of the LGN. These pupillary fibers enter the mesencephalon via the brachium of the superior colliculus. Cutting the brachium to the superior colliculus on each side abolishes the light reflexes, whereas stimulation of the bra-

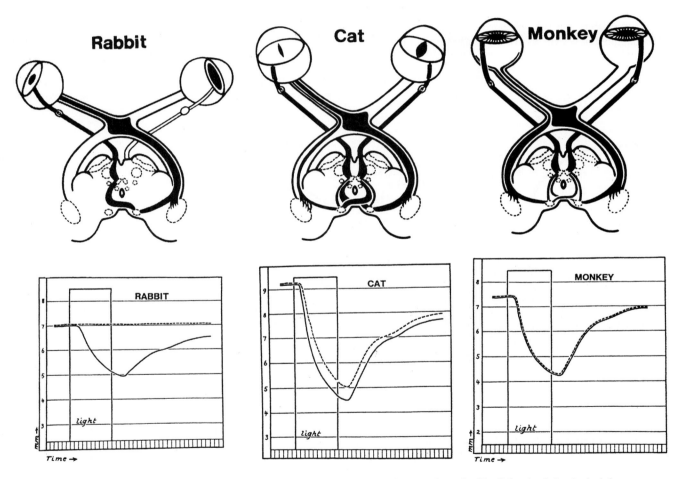

Figure 14.11. Chiasmal and pretectal decussations in rabbit, cat, and monkey as determined by light stimulation in the left eye. The proportion between crossed and uncrossed fibers in the central pretectal decussation of the light reflex arc parallels that between crossed and uncrossed chiasmal fibers. As a consequence, rabbits, with few uncrossed fibers in either decussation, have no consensual light reflex (*interrupted line*); cats, with many more crossed than uncrossed fibers in both decussations, have imperfect consensual reactions; and primates, with almost symmetric fiber distribution in the central pretectal decussation, have symmetric direct and consensual reactions. In no species is the consensual response larger than the direct one. (From Loewenfeld IE. Mechanisms of reflex dilatation of the pupil: historical review and experimental analysis. Surv Ophthalmol 1958;12:185–448.)

chium produces pupillary constriction (133). In humans with unilateral lesions of the brachium of the superior colliculus or of the pretectal olivary nucleus itself, pupillary responses to corresponding hemifield light stimuli are reduced even though visual field responses are normal (134,135). These rare lesions are often referred to as having a "tectal relative afferent pupil defect" with normal visual fields. This is in contrast to optic tract lesions, in which both visual and pupillary responses are reduced or absent when light is shined in the affected hemifield. These clinical cases provide further evidence for segregation of the pupillary and visual systems and also provide additional evidence for a hemifield organization of the pupillary light reflex pathway.

It once was assumed that pupillomotor fibers entered the superior colliculus, but this seems improbable because electric stimulation of that surface does not produce constriction of the pupil, and its removal does not impair the light reflex (136,137). Furthermore, Ranson and Magoun (138) obtained pupillary constriction by stimulation in the pretectal region and showed that bilateral destruction of the pretectal area abolished the light reflex under their conditions of light stimulus and observation. It is thus clear that the fibers that separate from the optic tract and enter the brachium of the superior colliculus synapse in the pretectal region of the mesencephalon (Fig. 14.10).

The pretectal region of the mesencephalon is located at the level of the posterior commissure, just rostral to the superior colliculus. Although this region is quite small, and there are considerable anatomic differences among species, various investigators have proposed separation of the pretectum into several subnuclei. The names given to these subnuclei are the nucleus of the optic tract, the sublentiform nucleus, the nucleus of the pretectal area, the pretectal olivary nucleus, the posterior nucleus, and the principal pretectal nucleus (138–143) (Fig. 14.12). Several of these subnuclei have been implicated as the sites of termination of afferent pupillomotor fibers from the retina, including the sublentiform nucleus, nucleus of the optic tract, nucleus of the pretectal area, and pretectal olivary nucleus (143–147). Of these subnuclei, the pretectal olivary nucleus is the region that most investigators favor as the primary site for the integration of the pupillary light reflex.

Kourouyan and Horton (148) injected tritiated proline unilaterally into the vitreous of monkeys and followed the distribution of anterograde transport of the tracer into the midbrain. They found label almost exclusively in the pretectal olivary nucleus on both sides of the midline. The tracer was also transported anterograde across the next synapse, labeling the lateral visceral cell columns of the Edinger-Westphal nucleus, further solidifying the pretectal olivary nucleus as

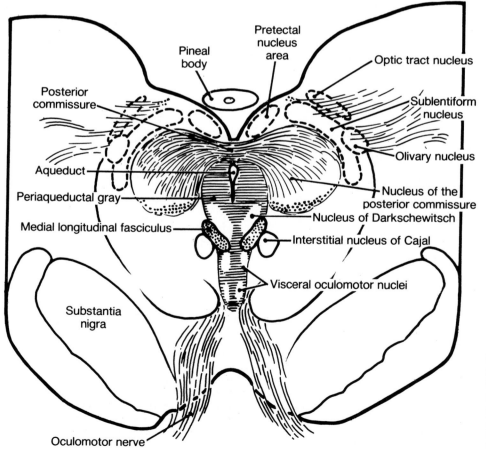

Figure 14.12. Drawing of the major pretectal nuclei and their relationship to the visceral and anterior median oculomotor nuclei. (From Carpenter MB, Pierson RJ. Pretectal region and the pupillary light reflex: an anatomical analysis in the monkey. J Comp Neurol 1973; 149:271–300.)

the integrating site of the pupillary light reflex. Fibers to the visceral cells of the Edinger-Westphal nucleus also were traced from the pretectal olivary nuclei by Carpenter and Pierson (141), whereas Benevento et al. (143) and Burde (149) traced fibers to the visceral nuclei from both ipsilateral and contralateral olivary and sublentiform pretectal nuclei.

Clarke and Gamlin (150) also labeled the pretectal olivary nucleus following tracer injections (WGA-HRP) into the retina. Furthermore, they recorded from units in the pretectal olivary nucleus that fired in response to retinal light stimuli (discussed later). In addition, a stimulus current given at the pretectal recording site produced pupillary constriction. These results provide overwhelming evidence that the pretectal olivary nucleus is the mesencephalic relay station for the pupillary light reflex (151).

The pretectal olivary nucleus in primates consists primarily of neuronal cell bodies located in the periphery of the nucleus in the shell surrounding the central neuropil (148,150). The integration and convergence of retinal impulses probably occurs in the central neuropil of the nucleus.

The firing properties of the neurons within the pretectal olivary nucleus and their relationship to stimulus luminance and pupil response were elucidated for monkeys studied in the awake state by Gamlin et al. (152). In response to a 5-second stimulus, these neurons respond with a phasic burst of action potentials at high frequency, followed by a transient sustained volley of action potentials at a lower frequency. Of the 16 separate neurons studied by these investigators, all had very linear increases in the sustained component of discharge frequency as the log stimulus intensity was increased linearly, and this corresponded to linear changes in pupil diameter. However, the slope of the response relationship between firing rate and log luminance was not the same for every neuron; some had a greater gain (steeper slope of the line) than others. In fact, in some cases where stimulus intensity was very low, an individual pretectal neuron could show an increase in firing frequency without any change in pupil size, demonstrating that the amount of neuronal increase in firing necessary to produce a measurable change in pupil diameter may be a summation of input from a number of pretectal neurons, especially at low-light levels of stimulation. It is not known whether the gain of individual pretectal neurons or the summation properties of many neurons firing in unison is regulated by higher supranuclear inputs. Perhaps the modulation of this firing rate and summation properties produce hippus, the random fluctuations of the pupil that are often observed under continual retinal illumination (discussed later). It is also of interest that Reiner et al. (153) reported specific neuropeptides within the pretectal nucleus that act as neuromodulators in other areas of the brain. The role of these neuropeptides in modulation of the pretectal response and the origin of these peptidergic nerve endings has not yet been completely elucidated.

The pretectal neurons possess temporal summation properties different from neurons involved in visual perception. The intensity-dependent time delay in the pupillary light reflex is longer than that which occurs at other synapses. For every log unit reduction in light intensity, the latency of the pupillary contraction may be prolonged by another 30–45 milliseconds. For this long delay in timing to occur, the pretectal neuron must be capable of summating input over a relatively long period of time before having to "start over." Therefore, the pupillary light reflex may be an indicator of damage to the retina or optic nerve by showing both a decrease in amplitude of pupil contraction and a prolongation of the latency time (Fig. 14.13).

Hess (154) thought that almost all pupillary responses to light were restricted to stimulation of an area of the retina 3 mm in diameter and centered at the macula. However, it is

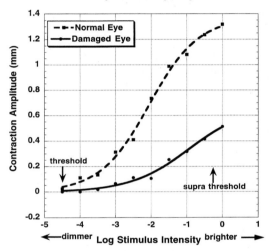

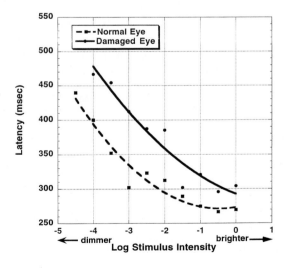

Figure 14.13. Example of pupil contraction amplitude as a function of stimulus luminance (*top*) and latency time as a function of stimulus luminance (*bottom*) in an eye with optic neuropathy and in the normal fellow eye. The response function of pupil contraction in the top graph shows more effects of damage at the brighter stimulus intensity range, whereas the latency time is more prolonged in the damaged eye at the dimmer light intensity range.

clear from studies using sensitive pupil-recording techniques and from clinical observations that stimulation of the retinal periphery can also produce constriction of the pupil and that lesions of the peripheral retina can produce an afferent pupillary defect (125,126) and corresponding decreases in the pupil contraction to small focal stimuli (127,128). There appear to be two major classes of pretectal neurons, based on their firing properties to stimuli presented in different locations within the visual field. One type of pretectal neuron responds with greater frequency to stimuli located toward the center of the visual field, and it responds with reduced frequency to stimuli at the periphery of its receptive field. This type of pretectal neuron has a foveal, center-weighted receptive field. The second type of pretectal neuron has a flatter response to stimuli placed in different locations within the visual field. Its discharge frequency does not change substantially regardless of the location of the light stimulus. Despite these experiments, it still is not clear how the topographic distribution of ganglion cells throughout the retina is distributed to these populations of pretectal neurons and how the simultaneous firing of these neurons is integrated within the Edinger-Westphal nucleus.

EXCITATORY INFLUENCES OF VISUAL CORTEX ON THE PUPIL LIGHT AND NEAR REFLEXES

In addition to the classic midbrain afferent pathway to the pupillomotor center, a second important excitatory influence on the pupillary constrictor neurons in the visceral nuclei of the oculomotor complex arrives via centrifugal pathways from the occipital cortex. These excitatory pathways almost certainly follow the same general route to the midbrain as the occipital motor pathways to somatic components of the oculomotor complex. Some of these centrifugal fibers appear to modulate pupil constriction to near stimuli and are distributed in a more ventrolaterally location in the upper midbrain compared with the light reflex pathways, as evidenced by their relative invulnerability to midline lesions in the region of the tectum or posterior commissure. Indeed, the supranuclear pathways for pupillary constriction associated with voluntary or involuntary effort to look at a near object are unaffected by many pretectal lesions that interrupt the pupillary light reflexes, producing a dissociation between the amplitude of the light and near reflexes—light-near pupillary dissociation.

Physiologic connections have been demonstrated between areas in the occipital lobes (areas 18 and 19 of Brodmann) and pupillary constrictor neurons; Barris (155), working with cats, found that stimulation of the occipital cortex produced constriction of the pupils as part of a near reaction. When these cortical areas were destroyed, degenerated fibers could be followed into the superior colliculus and the pretectal region. Jampel (156) confirmed these findings in nonhuman primates and found that stimulation of additional areas of the cortex resulted in pupillary constriction together with convergence and accommodation. In addition, tracer studies using tritiated leucine injected into cerebral cortex in primates reveal specific connections to various pretectal nuclei, including the olivary nucleus (157). Such anatomic connec-

tions point toward cortical modulation of pathways for both the pupillary constriction to near and the light reflex.

With regard to the possible modulation of the pupil light reflex by visual cortex, numerous investigators have demonstrated pupillary hemiakinesia or hemihypokinesia in response to focal light stimuli placed in the blind hemifield in patients with suprageniculate lesions (i.e, posterior to the LGN) (115,117,127,128,158–164). Studies using pupil perimetry show homonymous pupil field deficits that correspond to the borders of the visual field defects in patients with isolated occipital lesions (Fig. 14.14), anatomically confirmed by magnetic resonance (MR) imaging. Many of these patients were tested when the lesion was acute (within 1 week of onset), making transsynaptic degeneration unlikely. Thus, there may also be a significant, direct connection between the occipital cortex and the pretectal or Edinger-Westphal region of the mesencephalon. That such a connection between the occipital cortex and ocular motor brain stem centers does in fact exist is also suggested by studies of the role of the superior colliculus in the mediation of visually guided behavior in the cat (165), monkey (166), and human (167).

If the cortical injury occurs early in life, the phenomenon might result from transsynaptic degeneration across the LGN. Although Miller and Newman (168) found no clinical evidence of transsynaptic degeneration in an 86-year-old woman evaluated 57 years after suffering a cerebrovascular accident that resulted in a complete left homonymous hemianopia, Beatty et al. (169) used a paraphenylenediamine staining technique to demonstrate such degeneration in a patient who died at 86 years of age, 40 years after a craniotomy for removal of a right parieto-occipital arteriovenous malformation that left him with a complete left homonymous hemianopia.

INHIBITORY INFLUENCES ON THE PUPIL

Role of the Dark Reaction in Causing Pupil Dilation

When a light-adapted eye is suddenly exposed to a short period of darkness, the pupils dilate after a short latency period of about 300–400 milliseconds. This dilation still occurs, although it is slightly diminished, after the sympathetic innervation to the dilator muscle is interrupted. Thus, it must be partly caused by inhibitory impulses that affect the Edinger-Westphal nucleus. Because darkness is a positive stimulus for the photopic retina and evokes an "off-response" in the electroretinogram, it is reasonable to assume that this "off-stimulus" produces inhibitory impulses that are relayed to the mesencephalon, where they act on neurons concerned with pupillary constriction (170).

Cortical and Hypothalamic Inhibition of Pupillary Constriction

It is clear that the varying size of the normal pupil under different circumstances is primarily an expression of a varying tonic influence by the parasympathetic system and that the sympathetic system plays a supporting role. It is believed that in the awake subject, impulses travel via corticothalamo-hypothalamic pathways or corticolimbic pathways to inhibit

Occipital Lobe Infarct

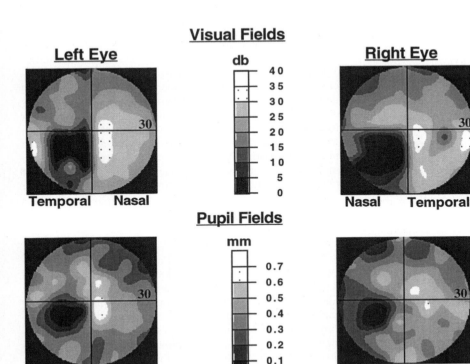

Figure 14.14. Example of a corresponding loss of pupil response in the same area of homonymous visual field loss in a patient with an acute, isolated occipital infarct. This result provides strong evidence for a cortical pupil light reflex pathway. Pupil perimetry was performed with 1.7° light stimuli given as a 6° grid pattern over the 30° visual field (same locations as in the visual perimetry). Grey scale of pupil field corresponds to amplitude of pupil contraction in each area of the visual field.

the mesencephalic parasympathetic outflow. Electric stimulation of the diencephalon or the cortex of sympathectomized cats and monkeys causes pupillary dilation and abolishes the light reflex (170). In addition, cortical stimulation of the sensorimotor areas of the brain and of the frontal lobes produces dilation of the pupil. We have found that transcranial magnetic stimulation placed over the occipital cortex in humans does not cause pupil dilation, but it does inhibit the pupil constriction elicited by a light stimulus given to the retina at the same time. This finding provides additional evidence for a modulating role of cerebral cortex on the pupillary light reflex. Fatigue and drowsiness in humans and in animals result in loss of this normal inhibition of the pupillary light reflex. During sleep, the pupils are small but retain their reaction to light. This miosis is a release phenomenon; that is, the central sympathetic inhibitory influences on the visceral oculomotor nuclei that originate in the cortex, the hypothalamus, and the reticular activating system are diminished during sleep. Conversely, stimulation of regions in the hypothalamus may provoke a burst of impulses that cause mydriasis, often with eyelid elevation and a rise in blood pressure (171–175).

Brain Stem and Spinal Cord Inhibition of Pupillary Constriction

The mydriasis that occurs with arousal or painful stimuli is reduced but not eliminated by sympathectomy (176,177)

and is present even in a decerebrate, sympathectomized preparation. Inhibition of a pupillary constriction "center" in the midbrain contributes to this reflex dilation (178,179). Thus, the dilation appears to depend in part on inhibition of neurons in the Edinger-Westphal nucleus. These pathways are located superficially in the anterolateral funiculus along with the descending sympathetic pupillodilator pathways (180). In the cat, the pathways extended from the dorsal root entry zone to the insertion of the dentate ligament. In the primate, they are located somewhat more anteriorly. Loewy et al. (181) identified two ascending pathways in the brain stem that produced pupillary dilation when stimulated, even if both sympathetic trunks were sectioned, and Kerr (182) traced some of these fibers from the spinal cord to the visceral oculomotor nuclei. Many of these inhibitory fibers are located in the periaqueductal gray area on their way to the visceral neurons of the Edinger-Westphal nucleus. Thus, it seems reasonably certain that ascending spinoreticular pathways produce direct inhibition of the motor neurons for pupillary constriction. Pharmacologic evaluation of inhibition of the Edinger-Westphal nucleus using microcannulae indicates that central adrenergic $\alpha2$ receptors play an important role (183,184). This work is also important because it provides an understanding of how centrally acting drugs that affect the sympathetic nervous sytem (e.g., antihypertensives such as clonidine) can affect pupil size.

THE EFFERENT ARC OF THE PUPIL LIGHT REFLEX

Midbrain Parasympathetic Outflow Pathway

All neural impulses that reach the sphincter of the pupil travel via a preganglionic parasympathetic pathway from the rostral midbrain to the ciliary ganglion in the orbit and then to the iris sphincter muscle via a postganglionic pathway within the short ciliary nerves (Fig. 14.15).

Visceral Oculomotor Nuclei

The visceral nuclei of the oculomotor nucleus, the nuclei that are believed to contain cell bodies of preganglionic, parasympathetic neurons that project to the ciliary ganglion and synapse with neurons that eventually produce both pupillary constriction and accommodation, are located in the dorsal midbrain. These consist of the Edinger-Westphal nuclei (185,186) (also called the dorsal visceral cell columns), the anterior median nuclei (187,188), and the nucleus of Perlia (187). The Edinger-Westphal nuclei are located dorsomedial to the somatic nuclei of the oculomotor nuclear complex (Fig. 14.16). Akert et al. (189) indicated that the origin of all parasympathetic neurons projecting to the ciliary ganglion in the monkey is limited to the Edinger-Westphal nucleus, but projections also arise from the ipsilateral half of the anterior median nucleus (145,149,190,191). In addition, Burde and Loewy (191) found that cell bodies in Perlia's nucleus also send axons that project to (or through) the ciliary ganglion in macaque monkeys.

Kourouyan and Horton (148) used unilateral injections of radioactively labeled proline into the vitreous of six monkeys to identify which neurons in the oculomotor nerve complex in the midbrain were involved in the pupil light reflex. After allowing sufficient time for the label to be transported to the midbrain (7–10 days), the authors localized the label to the pretectal olivary nucleus on each side of the midbrain (the site of the first synapse) and to the paired lateral visceral cell columns dorsal to the oculomotor nerve complex. These experiments provided strong evidence that the lateral visceral cell columns probably are the cells involved in the pupillary light reflex. To avoid confusion over nomenclature, these authors recommended that only neurons subserving pupillary constriction should be called the Edinger-Westphal nucleus. Jampel and Mindel (192) performed microelectrode studies in macaque monkeys and found that cells in the visceral nuclei that were concerned with pupillary constriction were located ventrally and somewhat caudally to those concerned with ciliary body constriction and accommodation. This finding suggested that the anterior median nuclei are the primary neurons involved in producing accommodation. According to Szentágothai (193), the number of preganglionic fibers from visceral cells of the oculomotor complex is about five times that of the postganglionic fibers that arise from the ciliary ganglion.

Pupillary Fibers in the Oculomotor Nerve

The determination of the position of the pupillomotor fibers in the oculomotor nerve is based on both anatomic and function studies. Within the brain stem, the pupillomotor fibers are located in the oculomotor fasciculus rostral to fibers originating from the other oculomotor subnuclei, consistent with the rostral location of the Edinger-Westphal nucleus (194) (Fig. 14.17). Sunderland and Hughes (195) found that between the brain stem and the middle of the cavernous sinus in humans, the pupillary fibers were concentrated at and around the superior surface of the nerve. In the anterior cavernous sinus and in the orbit, pupillary fibers were usually distributed among the somatic fibers of the inferior division of the oculomotor nerve.

Kerr and Hollowell (196) studied the location of the pupil-

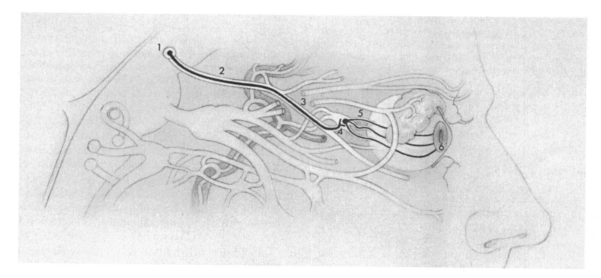

Figure 14.15. Parasympathetic pathway to the iris and ciliary body. 1, Edinger-Westphal and anterior median nuclei of the dorsal mesencephalon; 2, oculomotor nerve; 3, branch to the inferior oblique muscle; 4, motor root of the ciliary ganglion; 5, short ciliary nerves; 6, iris sphincter and ciliary muscle. (Chart prepared by Dr. H.S. Thompson and drawn by J. Esperson.)

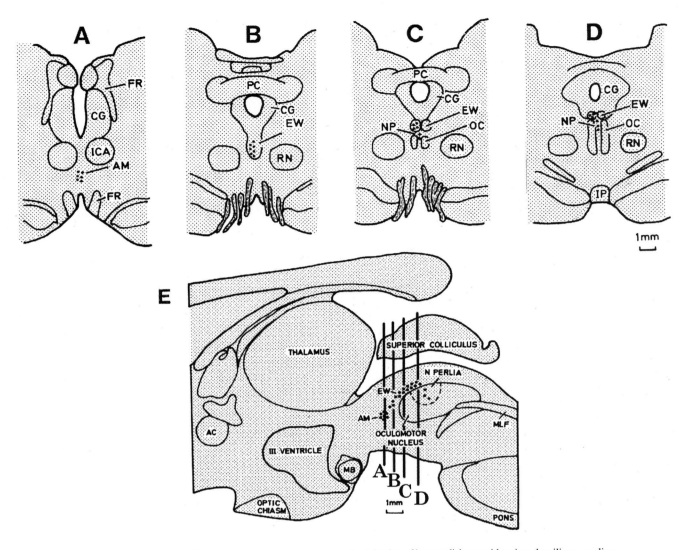

Figure 14.16. Visceral cells of the oculomotor nucleus, labeled by injection of horseradish peroxidase into the ciliary ganglion. The sagittal diagram *E* shows the levels of brain stem cross-sections *A* to *D*, where the tracer was found. The sections are arranged in rostral caudal order. AC, anterior commissure; AM, anteromedian nucleus; CG, central grey; EW, Edinger-Westphal nucleus; FR, fasciculus retroflexus; ICA, interstitial nucleus of Cajal; IP, interpeduncular nucleus; MB, mammillary body; MLF, medial longitudinal fasciculus; NP, nucleus of Perlia; PC, posterior commissure; OC, oculomotor nucleus; RN, red nucleus. (Redrawn from Burde RM, Loewy AD. Central origin of oculomotor parasympathetic neurons in the monkey. Brain Res 1980;198:434–439.)

lomotor fibers in the oculomotor nerve of humans and nonhuman primates. Although the results were much clearer in the nonhuman primates than in human specimens, these investigators confirmed the observations of Sunderland and Hughes (195) (Fig. 14.18). They found that the pupillomotor fibers are concentrated on the medial superior aspect of the oculomotor nerve as it leaves the brain stem and that they gradually move medially and slightly inferiorly as they run forward toward the cavernous sinus. This conveniently explains the propensity for pupil involvement by aneurysms of the posterior communicating artery that often compress

the medial and superior portion of the oculomotor nerve in the subarachnoid space. The preganglionic pupillomotor fibers occupy a very superficial location on the oculomotor nerve, with most lying immediately beneath the epineurium. Indirect evidence that the pupillomotor fibers occupy a superficial location in the subarachnoid portion of the oculomotor nerve also comes from histopathologic observations in diabetic patients with pupil-sparing oculomotor nerve palsies (197–199). In all cases in which the subarachnoid portion of the nerve is affected, the lesion is centrally located, sparing peripheral fibers.

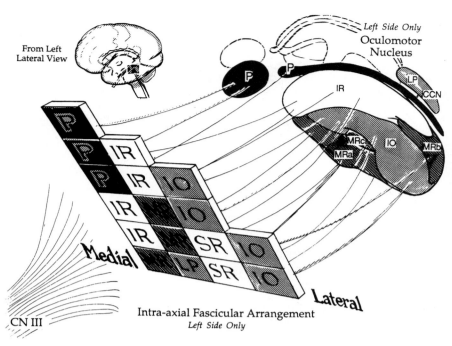

Figure 14.17. Schematic drawing of position of fibers in fascicle of human oculomotor nerve. Fibers destined for pupillary sphincter (P) occupy a rostral and medial position in the fascicle. CCN, central caudal nucleus; CN III, oculomotor nerve; IO, inferior oblique; IR, inferior rectus; LP, levator palpebrae superioris; MR, medial rectus; MRa, medial rectus subnucleus a; MRb, medial rectus subnucleus b; MRc, medial rectus subnucleus c; SR, superior rectus. (From Ksiazek S, Slamovits TL, Rosen CE, et al. Fascicular arrangement in oculomotor paresis. Am J Ophthalmol 1994;118:97–103.)

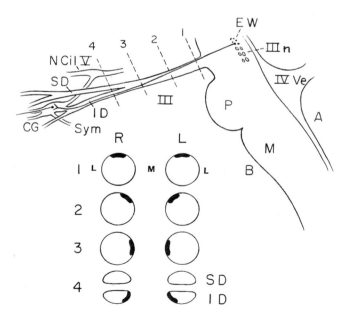

Figure 14.18. Course of preganglionic autonomic nerve fibers from the brain stem to the ciliary ganglion. A sagittal reconstruction of the brain stem with the course of the oculomotor nerve is shown at top. The corresponding locations of the preganglionic autonomic fibers for pupilloconstriction and accommodation within the right (R) and left (L) oculomotor nerves are shown in black in coronal sections through slices at 1 (emergence from the brain stem), 2 (midpoint in the subarachnoid space), 3 (at the point where the third nerve enters the dura), and 4 (in the anterior cavernous sinus where the fibers have entered the anatomic inferior division of the third nerve). The autonomic fibers are located superiorly as the oculomotor nerve exits the brain stem and then come to lie more medially as the oculomotor nerve passes toward the orbit. A, dorsal and B, ventral side of brain stem. P, pons; M, medulla; EW, Edinger-Westphal nucleus; IIIn, somatic portion of third nerve nucleus; III, third nerve; ID, inferior division of third nerve; SD, superior division of third nerve; NCilV, nasociliary branch of fifth nerve; CG, ciliary ganglion; Sym, sympathetic route; m, medial; l, lateral. (From Kerr FWL, Hollowell OW. Location of pupillomotor and accommodation fibres in the oculomotor nerve: experimental observations on paralytic mydriasis. J Neurol Neurosurg Psychiatry 1964;27:473.)

Ciliary Ganglion and Short Ciliary Nerves

The ciliary ganglion contains the postganglionic neurons that innervate the iris sphincter and the ciliary body. It is the site of the synapse with the preganglionic parasympathetic fibers. The ganglion is a small, irregular structure measuring 2 mm in the horizontal direction and about 1 mm in the vertical direction. It is located in the loose fatty tissue about 1 cm anterior to the medial end of the superior orbital fissure and the annulus of Zinn, and 1.5–2 cm behind the globe (Figs. 14.19 and 14.20). It lies on the temporal side of the ophthalmic artery between the optic nerve and the lateral rectus muscle in close association with the inferior division of the oculomotor nerve. Although Sinnreich and Nathan

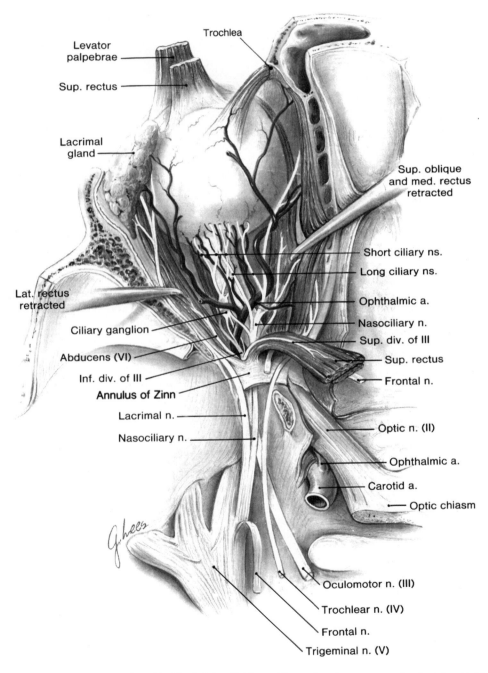

Figure 14.19. Superior view of the orbit. The inferior division of the oculomotor nerve supplies branches to the ciliary ganglion, which in turn gives off numerous short posterior ciliary nerves. (Redrawn from Wolff E. Anatomy of the Eye and Orbit. 6th ed. Philadelphia, WB Saunders, 1968.)

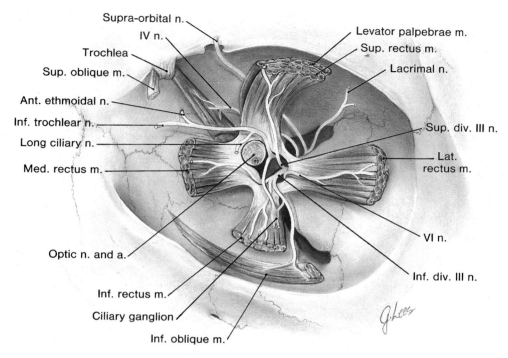

Figure 14.20. View of the posterior orbit showing the relationship of the optic nerve to the ocular motor nerves and extraocular muscles. Note the location of the ciliary ganglion. (Redrawn from Wolff E. Anatomy of the Eye and Orbit. 6th ed. Philadelphia, WB Saunders, 1971.)

(200) examined 30 orbits and found the location of the ganglia to be quite constant, other investigators (201,202) have found that the size, shape, and location of the human ciliary ganglion are extremely variable. The arterial branches supplying blood to the ganglion most frequently originate from the posterior lateral ciliary artery (supplying the anterior half of the ganglion) and from the lateral muscular arterial trunk (entering the ganglion from its lateral side) (202).

Most investigators agree that a majority, if not all, of the cell bodies in the ganglion are parasympathetic. Of considerable significance is the finding by Warwick (190) that only a small percentage of these cell bodies give rise to axons that supply the iris sphincter (3%), whereas a much larger percentage reaches the ciliary muscle (94%). This finding is consistent with the relative muscle mass of the iris sphincter and the ciliary muscle. Thus, over 90% of the mesencephalic parasympathetic outflow is concerned with accommodation and not with pupillary constriction.

In humans, there are 8–20 short ciliary nerves that leave the ciliary ganglion in two or three bundles and carry three types of fibers: (*a*) postganglionic, parasympathetic fibers to the iris sphincter and ciliary muscle; (*b*) postganglionic, sympathetic vasomotor fibers that originate in the superior cervical ganglion; and (*c*) afferent, sensory fibers of the trigeminal nerve. The short ciliary nerves are very tortuous and are intertwined with the posterior ciliary arteries. Most of these nerves pierce the sclera at the posterior pole of the globe temporal to the optic nerve. After the nerves enter the eye, they run anteriorly, first in the sclera and then in a

plexus in the suprachoroidal space (between the choroid and sclera) to innervate the anterior structures of the eye (200).

Sympathetic Outflow Pathway

The final common path of active dilator impulses extends from the hypothalamus to the iris. This path consists of a long three-neuron arc: (*a*) from the hypothalamus through the brain stem to the lateral cervical cord; (*b*) back out from the spinal cord to the cervical sympathetic chain and superior cervical ganglion in the neck; and (*c*) along the course of the internal carotid artery through the base of the skull and into the orbit and iris.

Hypothalamus

Karplus and Kreidl (171) and many subsequent investigators observed that maximum pupillary dilation could be induced by electric stimulation in the hypothalamus (172,175). This reaction can still be produced some weeks after the cortex is ablated. Thus, the efferent pathway destined for the pupillary dilator either originates in, or has a cell station in, the hypothalamus. Destruction of these hypothalamic centers, which are located mainly in the posterolateral region of the hypothalamus, results in miosis, ptosis, and reduction of pupillary reflex dilation.

Brain Stem and Spinal Cord Sympathetic Pathways

As noted above, the descending sympathetic pathways arise from the posterolateral region of the hypothalamus.

There may be a partial crossing in the decussation of Forel, but the fibers are largely uncrossed below that point. As these fibers run caudally, they come to occupy a lateral position in the brain stem. The pathway probably contains one or more synapses in the pontine and mesencephalic tegmentums, although some of the fibers descend directly, without synapse, to the "ciliospinal center of Budge and Waller" in the spinal cord (203–205). Within the spinal cord, the fibers are located superficially in the anterolateral columns (180).

The fibers descend within the substance of the spinal cord to the cervicothoracic region, where they pass medially to synapse with the preganglionic neurons of the peripheral sympathetic pathway at C8 to T2. Apparently, descending vasomotor and pupillomotor fibers are in juxtaposition until they leave the intermediolateral cell column, because stimulation of the cervical cord in the intermediolateral cell column causes both pupillary dilation and associated vasopressor responses, whereas the pupillomotor fibers can be stimulated separately as they approach the ventral (motor) root.

Preganglionic Sympathetic Fibers

The preganglionic sympathetic fibers pass via the ventral root to the paravertebral sympathetic chain as the white rami communicants (206). They then proceed without synapsing through the first thoracic or stellate ganglion close to the pleura at the apex of the lung. The fibers travel mainly in the anterior loop of the ansa subclavia (of Vieussens) and continue through the inferior and middle cervical ganglia to terminate in the superior cervical ganglion.

Superior Cervical Ganglion

This is the largest of the sympathetic ganglia and is often 2–3 cm long. It is located below the base of the skull between the internal jugular vein and the internal carotid artery and constitutes a fusion of the sympathetic ganglia associated with the first three or four cervical segments to which it sends gray rami. Histologically, the human superior cervical ganglion is composed of three different kinds of neural structures. There are cholinergic preganglionic sympathetic nerve terminals, adrenergic postganglionic cell bodies, and catecholamine-containing chromaffin cells, all in close proximity (207). In addition, Kondo and Fujiwara (208) described large, granule-containing cells in the human superior cervical ganglion that they believed to be a special type of postganglionic aminergic neuron. By far the most common type of nerve endings present are the cholinergic, preganglionic sympathetic nerve terminals.

Postganglionic fibers exit from the superior cervical ganglion in great numbers. Wolf (209) found that the ratio between preganglionic and postganglionic fibers in the cat varied from 1:11 to 1:17. These postganglionic fibers leave the superior cervical ganglion as two main sets of branches: (*a*) communicating branches composed of gray rami to the first four cervical segments and communicating branches to the glossopharyngeal, vagus, and hypoglossal nerves; and (*b*) branches to the pharynx, the heart, and the sympathetic effectors in the head via the internal and external carotid plexus (Fig. 14.21). The close anatomic relationship between the superior cervical ganglion and the lower cranial nerves explains the frequent simultaneous involvement of the cervical sympathetic trunk (producing a Horner syndrome) and the lower cranial nerves in cases of trauma, tumors, and infections at the base of the skull and in the retroparotid space.

Postganglionic Sympathetic Pathway

The postganglionic oculosympathetic fibers leave the superior cervical ganglion as a fairly thick bundle from its cephalic pole and accompany the internal carotid artery into the skull. These fibers form a plexus, first on the lateral surface of, and then surrounding, the artery. At the time of a carotid dissection, expansion of the arterial wall stretches this plexus, resulting in facial pain and a Horner syndrome. Almost immediately after joining the internal carotid artery, most of the sweat fibers (and piloerector fibers) to the face exit from the carotid plexus by following the external carotid artery to their effector organs in the skin (Fig. 14.21). The remainder of the carotid plexus extends upward through the carotid canal and the foramen lacerum to the region of the gasserian ganglion and cavernous sinus.

As the internal carotid plexus enters the skull, it gives off fibers that join the tympanic branch of the glossopharyngeal nerve to form the tympanic plexus on the promontory of the middle ear. These fibers are designated collectively as the caroticotympanic nerves and are located within the mucous membrane as well as in bony grooves of the promontory. After passing through the tympanic plexus, the sympathetic fibers rejoin the internal carotid plexus, at which point the plexus enters the skull with the internal carotid artery through the carotid canal, after which it is in close relation to the trigeminal ganglion. Within the carotid canal, some fibers leave the internal carotid plexus to form the deep petrosal nerve that joins the greater superficial petrosal nerve to form the vidian nerve. This nerve courses through the pterygoid or vidian canal and then joins the sphenopalatine ganglion. It carries visceral efferent fibers of the facial nerve, some of which supply the lacrimal gland.

The remainder of the sympathetic fibers continue through the carotid canal into the cavernous sinus. Within the sinus, the oculosympathetic fibers, the largest component of the sympathetic plexus, fuse with the abducens nerve for a short distance before separating and joining the ophthalmic nerve (210,211) (Fig. 14.22). Most, if not all, of the pupillary sympathetic fibers join the ophthalmic division of the trigeminal nerve and enter the orbit with the nasociliary nerve (Figs. 14.19 and 14.22). The remainder of the sympathetic plexus distributes some of its fibers to the ocular motor nerves within the cavernous sinus. It then exits the sinus with the internal carotid artery, at which point some of its branches are distributed along the ophthalmic artery and along the anterior cerebral, middle cerebral, and anterior choroidal arteries.

Postganglionic fibers of the sympathetic pathway include: (*a*) vasomotor fibers to the orbit; (*b*) oculosympathetic fibers to the intrinsic muscles of the eye; (*c*) fibers to the branched

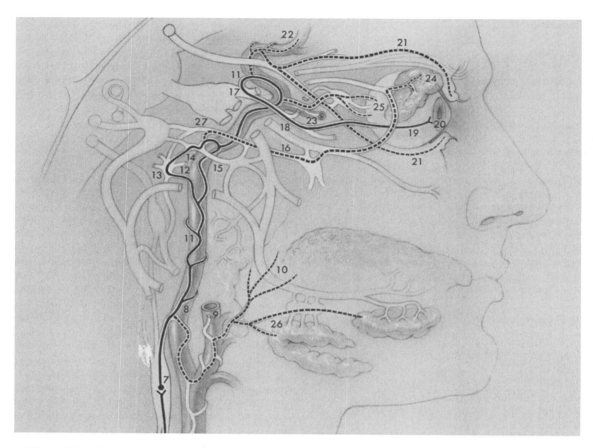

Figure 14.21. Sympathetic pathways to the face and eye. The *solid line* indicates the pathway of the pupillary dilator fibers, while the *dashed lines* show some of the other sympathetic pathways to the orbit and face. 7, superior cervical ganglion; 8, internal carotid artery; 9, external carotid artery; 10, sudomotor fibers to face; 11, carotid plexus; 12, caroticotympanic nerve; 13, tympanic plexus; 14, deep petrosal nerve; 15, lesser superficial petrosal nerve; 16, sympathetic contribution to vidian nerve; 17, ophthalmic division of the trigeminal nerve; 18, nasociliary nerve; 19, long ciliary nerve; 20, ciliary muscle and iris dilator muscle; 21, probable pathway of sympathetic contribution to retractor muscles of the eyelids; 22, vasomotor and some sudomotor fibers; 23, ophthalmic artery; 24, lacrimal gland; 25, short ciliary nerves; 26, sympathetic contribution to salivary glands; 27, greater superficial petrosal nerve. (Chart prepared by Dr. H.S. Thompson and drawn by J. Esperson.)

melanocytes of the uveal tract; (*d*) fibers to the extrinsic ocular muscles; (*e*) fibers to the smooth muscle of Müller; (*f*) fibers to the lacrimal gland; and (*g*) possibly fibers to the pigment layer of the retina (212).

Despite the apparent variability of peripheral sympathetic pathways, it seems certain that the fibers that innervate the pupillary dilator muscle enter the orbit with the nasociliary nerve, bypass the ciliary ganglion, and reach the eye as the long ciliary nerves (203,213) (Figs. 14.19 and 14.21). As noted above, other sympathetic fibers do pass through the ciliary ganglion but do not synapse there. They apparently serve a vasomotor function for the eye (201,214). Thus, sympathetic fibers are present in both the long and short ciliary nerves that enter the eye. The short and long ciliary nerves begin to cross each other as they pass forward between choroid and sclera, and by the time they have reached the iris root, they have all blended together to form a rich plexus from which the iris muscles, ciliary muscle, and vessel walls are supplied. Despite this appearance, Dr. H. Stanley

Thompson believes that the nerves of the iris maintain a segmental organization, specific with regard to their ultimate destinations to muscle bundles. Trauma to the nerves from heat during retinal or trabecular meshwork laser photocoagulation treatment or from cryotherapy may damage the short ciliary nerves. This may result in a tonic pupil with loss of the light reflex.

Peptidergic Innervation to the Iris

In addition to the autonomic nerves supplying the iris, sensory innervation is provided by the ophthalmic division of the trigeminal nerve (215,216). These sensory nerves may play an additional role in modulating pupil size. Every anterior segment surgeon knows that mechanical and chemical irritation of the eye can cause a strong miotic response that is noncholinergic and fails to reverse with autonomically acting drugs. In rabbits and cats, the response seems to be caused by the release of substance P or closely related pep-

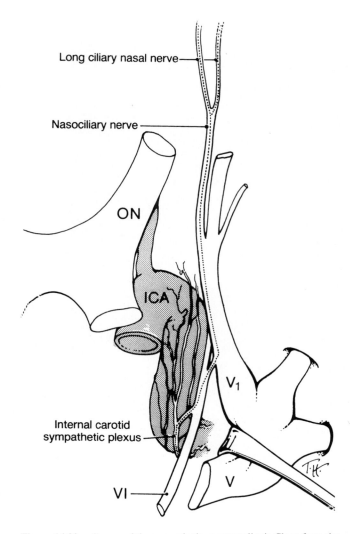

Figure 14.22. Course of the sympathetic, postganglionic fibers from the internal carotid plexus. They join briefly with the abducens nerve (VI) before entering the orbit with the nasociliary nerve, a branch of the ophthalmic division (V1) of the trigeminal nerve. After reaching the nasociliary nerve, the sympathetic fibers reach the iris dilator muscle as the long ciliary nerves. ICA, internal carotid artery; ON, optic nerve. (Modified from Solnitzky O. Horner's syndrome: its diagnostic significance. Georgetown Univ Med Cent Bull 1961;14:204–222.)

tides from the sensory nerve endings, but in monkeys and humans, substance P has little or no miotic effect. Almegaärd et al. (217) reported that cholecystokinin (in nanomolar amounts) caused contraction of isolated iris sphincter from monkeys and humans. Intracameral injections in monkeys caused miosis that was not prevented by tetrodotoxin or indomethacin, indicating that the miosis was not caused by stimulation of nerve endings or release of prostaglandins, but by direct action on sphincter receptors. The cholecystokinin antagonist lorglumide caused competitive inhibition of the response.

THE IRIS MUSCLES

The iris can be divided into four main parts from anterior to posterior: (*a*) the anterior border layer; (*b*) the stroma and sphincter muscle; (*c*) the anterior epithelium and dilator muscle; and (*d*) the posterior pigmented epithelium (Fig. 14.23). Light and electron microscopic, histochemical, and angiographic techniques have been used to elucidate the features of these structures (218–220). The color of the iris is determined by its mesodermal and ectodermal components. In Caucasians, the stroma is relatively free of pigment at birth. The stroma absorbs the long wavelengths of light, allowing the shorter (blue) wavelengths to pass through to the pigmented epithelium where they are reflected back, causing the iris to appear blue. If the stroma is dense and contains numerous, heavily pigmented melanosomes, the delicate lacework of iris vessels is hidden by the pigment, and the surface of the iris looks brown and velvety.

Iris Sphincter Muscle

The sphincter muscle is a ribbon-like, meridionally oriented band that measures 0.75–0.80 mm in diameter and 0.10–0.17 mm in thickness (Figs. 14.23 and 14.24). The sphincter muscle cells are spindle-shaped and are oriented parallel to the pupil margin. At the pupil margin, the muscle edge is separated from the pigment epithelium by a narrow band of collagen. Posteriorly, it is bound firmly to a dense layer of connective tissue that continues to the dilator muscle. This collagen layer contains arterioles, capillaries, and both sensory and motor nerves. The iris sphincter can be visualized in different states of contraction using infrared transillumination, in which case it appears as a darkened circumferential band adjacent to the pupil. During contraction, the sphincter becomes denser and thicker (Fig. 14.25).

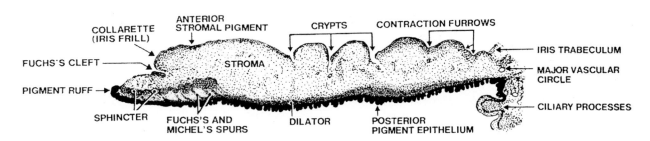

Figure 14.23. Schematic of the iris structure in sagittal cross-section. (From Loewenfeld IE. The Pupil: Anatomy, Physiology, and Clinical Applications. Ames, IA, Iowa State University Press, and Detroit, MI, Wayne State University Press, 1993:6.)

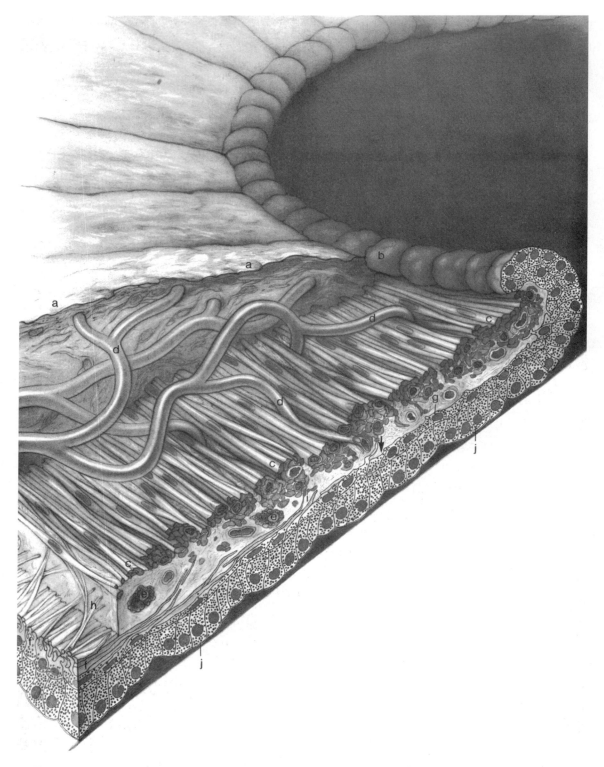

Figure 14.24. Schematic drawing of the pupillary portion of the iris showing the major layers. a, Anterior border layer; b, pigment ruff at the pupillary margin; c, sphincter muscle; d, vascular arcades within the anterior border layer and iris stroma; e, clump cells; f, dilator muscle; g, anterior epithelium anterior to termination of the dilator muscle (*arrow*); h and i, spur-like extensions from the dilator muscle that blend anteriorly with the sphincter muscle; j, posterior pigmented iris epithelium. (From Hogan MJ, Alvarado JA, Weddell JE. Histology of the Human Eye: An Atlas and Textbook. Philadelphia, WB Saunders, 1971.)

Normal Iris Sphincter Contraction

infrared transillumination   slit lamp front illumination

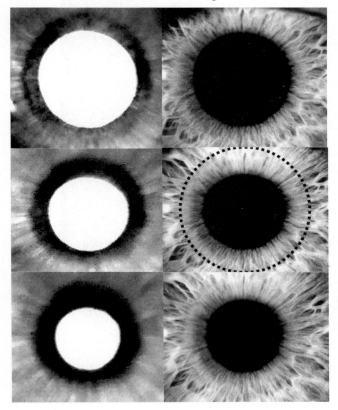

Figure 14.25. Changes in the iris sphincter during pupil contraction. The iris sphincter can be visualized in the human eye using infrared transillumination of the iris. The sphincter muscle has at least 20 segments, each innervated in series by separate branches of the parasympathetic postganglionic nerve. As the sphincter muscle shortens during contraction (*series on the left*), it transilluminates less, appearing as a denser darker band as the pupil becomes smaller. On the left is the same normal iris viewed with frontal illumination. The sphincter can often be distinguished within the iris stroma (*border outlined by broken circle*). (From Kardon RH, Corbett JJ, Thompson HS. Ophthalmology 1988;105:313–321.)

The sphincter muscle bundles are composed of small groups of five to eight muscle cells. The fibers of these cells are closely spaced and are in contact with each other by means of tight junctions and gap junctional complexes between the plasma membranes of adjacent cells. As with other smooth muscles, nerves do not enter these tight groups of muscle cells but lie close to their periphery. Because of this arrangement, it is believed that each muscle group functions as a unit. Apparently only one cell is innervated, and the junctional complexes spread the depolarizing current to the other cells of the group.

The Dilator Muscle–Anterior Iris Epithelial Layer

This layer measures about 12.5 microns in thickness and contains myoepithelial cells that have a muscular basal por-

tion that projects into the iris stroma and an epithelial apical portion adjacent to the posterior epithelial layer of the iris (Figs. 14.23 and 14.24). The muscular portions of the cells are oriented in a radial direction from the iris root toward the pupillary border and form three to five layers of dilator muscle. The myoepithelial processes are spindle-shaped and contain numerous myofilaments, although myofilaments are also present in the epithelial portion of the cells. Tight junctions and gap junctions similar to those described in the sphincter muscle are commonly found between the dilator muscle fibers. When the dilator contracts, it draws the iris up into folds and dilates the pupil. Interestingly, it would appear that during adrenergic mydriasis, the dilator muscle is the only part of the iris that is not thrown into folds (221–223) (Fig. 14.26).

Vascular Supply to the Iris Muscles

The iris has a rich supply of radially arranged vessels that arise from the greater or major arterial circle near the anterior part of the ciliary body and enter the iris between the ciliary crypts. They anastomose in an arteriovenous circle, the lesser or minor arterial circle, near the collarette. The major arterial circle is discontinuous and derives its blood supply partly from the nasal and temporal long posterior ciliary arteries that originate from the ophthalmic artery and the anterior ciliary arteries (109) (Fig 14.27). The anterior ciliary arteries are branches of the muscular arteries that also originate from the ophthalmic artery and reach the globe with the four rectus muscles and enter it from perforating branches. The relative contribution of each of the vessels to the iris varies among individuals, but the temporal iris seems the most susceptible to ischemia, particularly when multiple muscles are disinserted from the globe during strabismus or retinal reattachment surgery. The capillaries of the iris are formed by a single layer of unfenestrated endothelium with a rather thick basement membrane. These vessels are relatively impermeable to small molecules under normal conditions because of tight junctions between endothelial cells. In inflammatory conditions causing iritis, the tight junctions become incompetent, and permeability increases (109). The blood vessels of the iris have a serpentine course that allows them to accommodate to the changes in the length of the iris during dilation and constriction.

Nerve Supply to the Iris Muscles

The iris muscles, like other many other autonomic effector organs, are reciprocally innervated by both sympathetic and parasympathetic fibers. Immunohistochemistry and electron microscopy of nerve terminals in the iris reveal adrenergic terminals innervating the iris sphincter that are thought to arise from branches of adrenergic sympathetic nerves supplying the dilator muscle and cholinergic nerves innervating the dilator muscle that are thought to arise from branches of the cholinergic parasympathetic nerves supplying the sphincter (109). It is suspected that the adrenergic terminals innervating the sphincter inhibit that muscle during active dilation and that cholinergic terminals within the dilator are inhibitory during parasympathetic constriction of the sphinc-

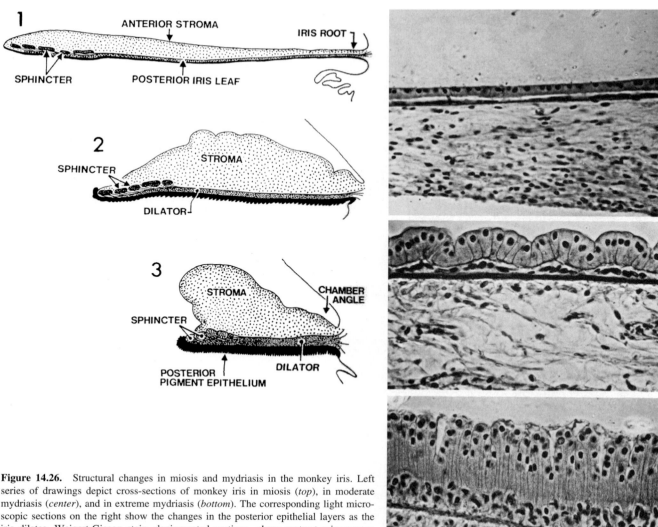

Figure 14.26. Structural changes in miosis and mydriasis in the monkey iris. Left series of drawings depict cross-sections of monkey iris in miosis (*top*), in moderate mydriasis (*center*), and in extreme mydriasis (*bottom*). The corresponding light microscopic sections on the right show the changes in the posterior epithelial layers as the iris dilates. Weigert-Gieson stain, depigmented sections, phase-contrast microscopy. (Drawings from Loewenfeld IE. The Pupil: Anatomy, Physiology, and Clinical Applications. Ames, IA, Iowa State University Press, and Detroit, MI, Wayne State University Press, 1993:6. Light micrographs from van Alphen GWHM. The structural changes in miosis and mydriasis of the monkey eye. Arch Ophthalmol 1963;69:802–814.)

ter (225–231) (Table 14.1). In other words, cholinergic excitatory nerves to the sphincter cause it to contract, but at the same time, branches to the dilator are inhibitory and cause it to relax, thus enhancing the miosis. On the other hand, mydriasis consists of adrenergic excitatory input to the dilator, causing it to contract. At the same time, not only is the central, cholinergic output to the sphincter inhibited, but also inhibitory branches of adrenergic nerves to the sphincter are activated, resulting in brisk dilation of the pupil.

One clinical correlate of the adrenergic inhibition of the sphincter is that a Horner pupil dilates very slowly. In some cases, interruption of the sympathetic nerves may cause a deficit not only in dilator activation, but also in sphincter inhibition. Also interesting are the effects of topical timolol (0.5%), as studied in humans with pupillography by Johnson et al. (232). These investigators found that this drug causes

a significant decrease in the amplitude of pupil redilation after a light stimulus, possibly by producing a β-adrenergic blockade of the inhibitory fibers to the sphincter, keeping the sphincter from relaxing properly and thus slowing dilation.

It is likely that with thoughtful selection of receptor-specific agonists and antagonists and continuous recording of the behavior of both pupils to dark and light stimuli, the pharmacology of the human iris can be better understood. In the meantime, it should be considered that every time a dilating drop is used, it is probable that one of the iris muscles is being stimulated and its antagonist is being inhibited.

INTEGRATED ACTIVITIES THAT INFLUENCE PUPIL SIZE AND MOVEMENT

Pupillary reflexes appear in the 5th month of development and are active by the 6th month. In infancy, the pupil is

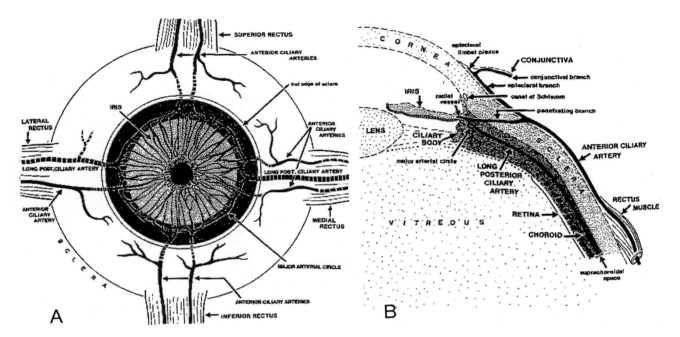

Figure 14.27. Pattern of blood supply of the iris and of other structures of the anterior ocular segment, as seen from frontal (*A*) and sagittal view (*B*). (*A*, From Loewenfeld IE. The Pupil: Anatomy, Physiology, and Clinical Applications. Ames, IA, Iowa State University Press, and Detroit, MI, Wayne State University Press, 1993:48. *B*, Modified after Marsh RJ, Ford SM. Blood flow in the anterior segment of the eye. Trans Ophthalmol Soc UK 1980;100:388–397 and after Hayreh SS, Scott W. Fluorescein iris angiography. Arch Ophthalmol 1978;96:1390–1400.)

small; however, during the first 6 months of life, the pupil begins to widen, and in adolescence it attains its widest diameter. This increase in size may be related to an incompletely developed iris sympathetic system at birth (233,234) and growth of the anterior segment of the eye during these years (235). From 20 to 60 years of age, the pupil steadily becomes smaller (236–240) (Fig. 14.28). Korczyn et al. (241) performed pharmacologic studies that suggested that although the iris dilator muscle does not lose its sensitivity to norepinephrine with age, sympathetic tone decreases with age. These investigators postulated that the decrease in sympathetic tone that occurs in persons over 60 years of age results from either degeneration or functional inactivity of the postganglionic neurons. In addition to a decrease in peripheral sympathetic tone, there is also probably a decrease in the amount of central inhibition of the Edinger-Westphal nucleus that contributes to the pupil becoming smaller with age (109). Both in infancy and in old age, pupillary responses to light and near stimuli appear to be less active than in adolescence and adult life.

Influence of Pupil Size on Pupillary Movements

That the size of the pupil can influence the dynamics of pupillary movements was shown by several investigators, although there is some discrepancy among their findings. Loewenfeld and Newsome (242) used infrared pupillographic techniques to demonstrate that the pupil has a linear range of movement within which both contractions to light and dilations to darkness move freely. Beyond this range, the movements decrease abruptly in both extent and velocity. This reduction in function occurs at a particular pupil diameter that is specific for an individual eye, regardless of the intensity of the stimulus or the pupil size at the beginning of stimulation. The limits of linearity vary slightly among normal persons but not between a person's two eyes. Loewenfeld and Newsome (242) used various pharmacologic agents to prove that linearities of dilation and constriction movements were, to a large extent, dependent on mechanical rather than pharmacologic factors.

Semmlow et al. (243) also studied variations in pupillary responsiveness with pupil size. These investigators were unable to confirm a linear range and a nonlinear range separated by a distinct "breakpoint," as suggested by Loewenfeld and Newsome (242). Instead, their data demonstrated

Table 14.1
Summary of Peripheral Cholinergic and Adrenergic Receptor Studies on the Iris Sphincter and Dilator Suggesting Reciprocal Innervation

	Iris Sphincter Muscle		Iris Dilator Muscle	
Receptor	Action	Result	Action	Result
Cholinergic	Excites	Miosis	Relaxes	Miosis
Adrenergic α1	Excites	Miosis	?	?
Adrenergic α2	Relaxes	Mydriasis	Excites	Mydriasis
Adrenergic β1	Relaxes	Mydriasis	Relaxes	?

Some of these actions may not cause any significant effect on static pupil size but may influence the rate of pupil constriction or dilation.

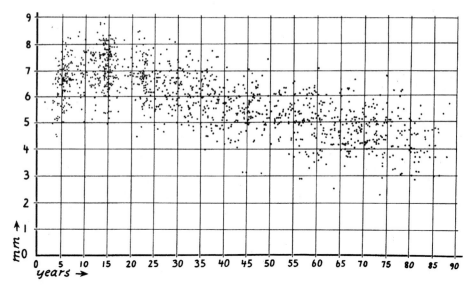

Figure 14.28. Age curve of pupil diameter among 1,263 normal subjects. Pupil diameters were measured from infrared flash photographs taken after 3 minutes in darkness. For each subject the average pupil diameters (right pupil diameter + left pupil diameter/ 2) were plotted as ordinate (mm) against age as the abscissa. The average line through this scatter plot indicates that the pupil size initially increases from infancy to early teens, then gradually declines as a function of age. (From Loewenfeld IE. Pupillary changes related to age. In Thompson HS, Daroff R, Frisén L, et al, eds. Topics in Neuro-Ophthalmology. Baltimore, Williams & Wilkins, 1979:124–150.)

a nonlinear process that was active in both constriction and dilation throughout the entire pupillomotor range, although it became most apparent at the extremes of pupil size. Nevertheless, Semmlow et al. (243) found that for pupil sizes between 3.5 and 6.0 mm, an assumption of ''approximate linearity'' is justified. According to these investigators, this relationship between pupillary size and response also occurs during the near response and is attributable to length-tension characteristics of the iris sphincter muscle.

To summarize, structural properties of the iris stroma vary among different persons and can limit pupil excursions in response to light or near. If the degree of pupil constriction is used as an indicator of light input, the pupil size range over which such measurements of contraction amplitude are made need to be considered. Obviously, a pupil that starts is 3.5 mm at rest will not contract to the same extent as one that is 5.0 mm, even when the same light stimulus is presented to the retina.

Pupil Size and Intraocular Pressure

Intraocular pressure exerts an influence on the size of the pupil (244–246). Elevation of the intraocular pressure in humans causes mydriasis, apparently through its effects on the iris sphincter muscle and not the neuromuscular junction (247). Part, but not all, of this effect is related to iris ischemia (248). Iris dilator function seems to be relatively resistant to the effects of increased intraocular pressure.

Benign (Simple, Central, ''Physiologic'') Anisocoria

Most normal persons have equal pupils. Nevertheless, pupillary inequality can be present in persons with normal pupillary constriction to light and normal dilation in darkness (249–251). This ''benign'' anisocoria is said to be present in about 20% of normal persons (249–254), but this figure is open to question, primarily because most studies use inadequate population samples, uncontrolled experimental con-

ditions, and/or lack of objective records of measurement. In addition, the true size of the pupil may be distorted by the cornea by 9–12%, depending upon pupil size (255). Nevertheless, Loewenfeld (239) examined 1,780 normal subjects using infrared flash photography (256) and found pupillary inequality with normal pupillary reflexes in 850 (48%). She emphasized that because pupillary inequality of less than 0.3 mm was very common and difficult to observe clinically, only inequality greater than 0.3 mm should be called ''anisocoria.'' Using this criterion, about 200 subjects (11%) in her study had clinically observable, benign anisocoria. Spencer and Czarnecki (257) found a similar prevalence of anisocoria (16%) in a study of 100 patients admitted to an intensive care stroke unit over a 1-year period.

Loewenfeld (239) believed that asymmetries of supranuclear inhibitory control of the dorsal mesencephalic visceral nuclei are responsible for this type of anisocoria and called it simple, central anisocoria, which always decreased in light. Simple anisocoria has no clinical significance with respect to visual function, but it is important that this type of anisocoria be recognized and differentiated from the acquired anisocoria that occurs in the setting of direct ocular trauma or damage to either the parasympathetic or sympathetic innervation of the iris, so that such patients are not subjected to unwarranted diagnostic studies. In such instances, the anisocoria may be benign, but the evaluation may not! Often, a preexisting anisocoria can be detected in previous photographs of the individual being examined, particularly if some type of magnification is used. This subject is discussed in more detail in Chapter 15.

Anisocoria in Lateral Gaze: Tournay's Phenomenon

In 1907, Gianelli noted that when some normal persons look in extreme lateral gaze, the pupil of the abducting eye becomes larger than the pupil of the opposite adducting eye, which becomes smaller (258) (Fig. 14.29). He hypothesized that this phenomenon resulted from mechanical traction

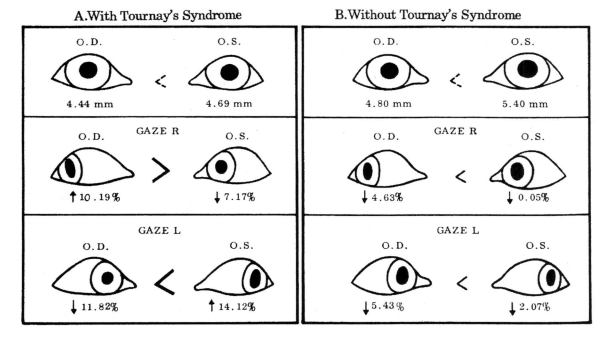

Figure 14.29. Percent changes in pupillary diameter during lateral gaze (Tournay's phenomenon). *A*, Changes in pupil size of a patient with bilateral Tournay's phenomenon. The pupil of the abducting eye dilates and the pupil of the adducting eye constricts. *B*, Pupil appearance in a patient without Tournay's phenomenon. The patient demonstrates slight pupillary constriction in both eyes on gaze to the right and left. Top frame is gaze straight ahead, middle frame is gaze to right, and lower frame is gaze to left. O.D., right eye; O.S., left eye; down-arrow, pupillary contraction; up-arrow, pupillary dilation. (From Loewenfeld IE, Friedlander RP, McKinnon PFM. Pupillary inequality associated with lateral gaze [Tournay's phenomenon]. Am J Ophthalmol 1974;78:449–469.)

caused by movement of the globe that stimulated the long ciliary nerves in abduction and the short ciliary nerves in adduction. Although this paper was largely ignored, Tournay (259) subsequently made similar, independent observations, emphasizing the dilation of the pupil ipsilateral to the direction of gaze. Although Tournay later discovered Gianelli's manuscript and credited him with the initial observation of this phenomenon (260), anisocoria that develops on extreme lateral gaze is called "Tournay's phenomenon." Some investigators (261,262) suggested that this phenomenon occurs in almost all normal persons; however, Sharpe and Glaser (263) studied 25 normal subjects and 5 patients with Duane's retraction syndrome by direct observation, photography, and infrared electronic pupillography and were unable to demonstrate anisocoria in lateral gaze in any of the subjects. Loewenfeld et al. (264) examined 150 normal subjects using infrared flash photography and concluded that Tournay's phenomenon occurs in normal subjects, but that its prevalence is low and its extent small (less than 10% of subjects showed a change in anisocoria greater than 0.3 mm). Loewenfeld (109) suggested that Tournay's phenomenon may result from "straying" of impulses that were meant for the medial rectus subnucleus to the nearby Edinger-Westphal nucleus. This would cause slight constriction of the pupil when the eye adducts and relative dilation of the pupil when the medial rectus subnucleus is inhibited (during abduction). Whatever the explanation, it is reasonable to conclude that

Tournay's phenomenon is relatively uncommon and has little or no clinical significance.

Hippus: Physiologic Pupillary Unrest

When observed in ordinary room illumination, the pupils of a young, healthy person are in almost constant motion (265). When the eyes are exposed to long-lasting light stimulation, both pupils constrict, then partially redilate, and begin to oscillate (111). In dim light, the pupils become large and the rate of oscillation is slow; however, with increasing light intensity, the mean diameter of the pupils becomes smaller and the rate of oscillation increases (maximally about 2 per second). These movements are synchronous in the two eyes and appear to continue indefinitely. This physiologic pupillary unrest, also called hippus, is present in all normal persons and is not triggered by accommodation (266). It is reduced or absent when the afferent or efferent path of the light reflex is impaired or in the presence of spastic miosis. Some investigators believe that physiologic pupillary unrest modulates the excitability of cells throughout the visual pathway by constantly changing the exposure of the retina to light (267); however, others emphasize that such a function of pupillary instability cannot be of major importance to the visual process because patients with fixed pupils have no impairment of visual function (268).

Physiologic pupillary unrest should not be confused with

two similar but unrelated phenomena: oscillatory pupillary movements that occur with reduced alertness (269) and edge-light induced pupillary oscillations.

That oscillatory movements of the pupil occur with changing states of wakefulness is not surprising. The iris is always under the influence of the labile, dynamic equilibrium of sympathetic and parasympathetic innervation, both of which are active in varying degrees. Specific excitatory and inhibitory reflexes are superimposed on this constantly wandering baseline of activity that influences the extent and shape of the reflex response. The same stimulus may, therefore, elicit an extensive reflex at one moment and none the next, depending on the state of alertness of the individual. Thus, these "fatigue waves" increase when a normal person is drowsy or very sleepy (269) and are suppressed by mental activity (270).

As far as edge-light induced pupillary oscillations are concerned, the pupil can be made to oscillate vigorously in a dark room by placing the narrow beam of the slit lamp across the pupillary margin of the iris (see Chapter 15). This is clearly the result of the photomotor reflex turning itself off and on. This phenomenon is unrelated to physiologic pupillary unrest, because the induced oscillations cease when the light is presented in "Maxwellian view," so that the constricting iris does not cut into the beam of light (271). Furthermore, when the iris of one eye is pharmacologically immobilized, stimulation of this eye no longer induces pupillary oscillations; however, the normal, physiologic unrest continues in the consensually reacting, untreated eye (111).

Although the term "hippus" is used to describe physiologic pupillary unrest, it is also used in numerous contradictory ways, including: (a) to describe "fatigue waves" related to the level of individual alertness (268–270); (b) to describe pathologic pupillary unrest (272–275); (c) to describe the pupillary changes that accompany Cheyne-Stokes respiration (276); and (d) to describe all pupillary unrest, whether physiologic or pathologic. The term "hippus" should be used synonymously with "physiologic pupillary unrest" because the phenomenon appears to have no clinical significance in most patients.

NORMAL PUPILLARY REFLEXES

Reaction to Light

When light is shined in either eye, both pupils constrict. The constriction in the ipsilateral eye is called the direct reaction to light and that in the contralateral eye is called the consensual reaction to light. For practical purposes, with unilateral light (as well as electric) stimulation, the direct and consensual reactions are of equal magnitude, provided that there is no lesion in the parasympathetic or sympathetic pathways (277,278).

Alternating Contraction Anisocoria

In 1954, Lowenstein described a phenomenon that he called "alternating contraction anisocoria" in which the direct pupillary constriction of the illuminated eye exceeded

the consensual constriction of the contralateral pupil (Fig. 14.30). This light-induced anisocoria was said to be "alternating" because it depended on which eye was stimulated. Smith and coworkers (279,280) studied 72 normal subjects using television pupillometry and found that the direct light reaction exceeded the consensual reaction in 61 of the subjects (84.7%). The degree of anisocoria was extremely small, with a mean value of 0.075 mm. It occurred in the presence and absence of previous dark adaptation and increased proportionally with reflex amplitude as the intensity of the stimulating light was raised. In addition, this light-induced anisocoria showed a high degree of repeatability in 20 subjects who were tested on two occasions, 1 year apart. Smith et al. (280) found three patterns of "contraction anisocoria" in their subjects. In the bilateral form, the amplitude of the direct pupillary response was always greater than that of the consensual reflex, no matter which eye was stimulated. In one form of unilateral contraction anisocoria, stimulation of only one side gave a greater direct response, whereas stimulation of the other side resulted in equal pupillary responses. In the second form of unilateral contraction anisocoria, the pupillary response of one side always exceeded that of the other side whether the response was direct or consensual, similar to an efferent pupillary defect. Dr. I.E. Loewenfeld was unable to confirm the presence of this second form of unilateral contraction anisocoria. She believed that in normal persons, the consensual light response is always slightly less than the direct response, even though this difference usually is not clinically evident.

Studies by several groups using temporal and nasal hemifield light stimuli indicate that contraction anisocoria may

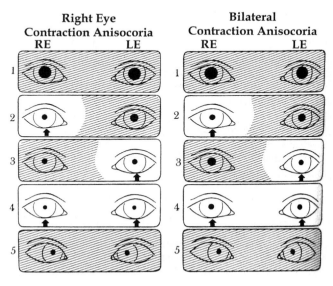

Figure 14.30. Consensual deficit (contraction anisocoria) unilateral versus bilateral. In frame 1, the eyes are in darkness, with equal pupils. In frames 2 and 3, one eye is stimulated by light (as indicated), and in frame 4, both eyes are exposed to light. The patient looks far away, except in frame 5, in which the near vision reaction is shown. RE, right eye; LE, left eye. (From Loewenfeld IE. The Pupil. Ames, Iowa State and Wayne State University Press, 1993.)

be related to the degree of crossed versus uncrossed pupillary light reflex fibers at both the chiasmal and pretectal decussations (109,281–283)—that is, when asymmetries of input and output of the light signal exist both at the chiasm and the pretectal olivary nucleus, respectively. At the pretectal level in some persons, there may be a greater crossed than uncrossed distribution of the light reflex to the recipient Edinger-Westphal nucleus, resulting in unequal contractions of the right and left pupil to a light stimulus. This would become apparent on full-field stimulation of the eye contralateral to the pretectal nucleus with the greater crossed output if there were also greater retinal input to this pretectal nucleus from the eye being stimulated. In other words, if the nasal retina (temporal visual field) provided greater input to the contralateral pretectal nucleus via its decussation at the chiasm compared with the uncrossed input from the temporal retina (nasal field) to the ipsilateral pretectal nucleus, full-field stimulation of this eye would then favor more input to the contralateral pretectal nucleus. If distribution of output from this nucleus was also unequal, favoring crossed output to the opposite Edinger-Westphal nucleus, the result would be a pupillary response favoring the pupil of the eye being stimulated; that is, the direct response would be greater than the consensual pupil response.

Contraction anisocoria may have clinical significance only in unilateral cases, where clinical observation of the direct pupil response during the swinging flashlight test may give the erroneous impression of a relative afferent pupillary defect, when in reality only contraction anisocoria is present. Based on our studies of pupillographic recordings of both pupils in normal subjects and in patients with organic causes of relative afferent pupillary defects who also happen to have unilateral contraction anisocoria, this condition may result in as much as a 0.3 log unit ''pseudo'' relative afferent pupillary defect. However, in most persons, there is no clinical relevance of this condition, and as far as clinical observation is concerned, in normal persons the direct and consensual pupillary light responses are almost always equal.

Effect of Age on the Pupillary Light reflex

Both in infancy and old age, the pupillary light reflex is less active than in adolescence and middle age. In addition, increasing age is associated not only with a decrease in resting pupillary size (239,240,284) but also with a reduction in maximum constriction velocity and an increased time to both maximum constriction velocity and reflex peak (284). Loewenfeld (240) evaluated pupillary reactivity to both short (0.8 sec) and long (3 sec) flashes of light in normal persons of all ages and found that for long flashes, the amplitude of the reaction and the resting pupillary diameter in darkness are related. This relation is linear in older persons, and there is little individual scatter; that is, the smaller the pupil, the smaller the amplitude of the light reaction. With decreasing age, there is increasing scatter, although the basic relationship remains the same. In addition, for a given pupil size in darkness, the light reactions of persons 40–60 years of age are more extensive than those of children or young adults with pupils of the same size. In persons over 60 years of age, for a given pupil diameter in darkness, the pupillary light reactions show slightly less amplitude than those of younger subjects. In contrast to the findings with long flashes of light, the pupillary reactions to short flashes are relatively insensitive to age-related changes in pupillary size (109).

The mechanism of these age-related changes is unknown. Iris degeneration could be responsible, but there are several reasons why this does not appear to be the case. First, age-related iris degeneration seldom begins before the age of 40, whereas the decline in pupil size and reactivity is already apparent at the beginning of the third decade of life and continues linearly until it levels off in later decades. Second, the light reactions of most normal persons remain brisk well into the sixth decade and often beyond. They appear to be limited in amplitude only by a smaller resting pupil size. Third, as already mentioned, for a given resting pupillary diameter in darkness, the pupillary reactions in middle-aged persons are even more extensive than those in the young. Finally, pupils of elderly persons usually react extensively to both adrenergic and cholinergic pharmacologic agents (240,285–287). Thus, in persons over about 60 years of age, structural changes in the iris tissues cannot be the primary reason for the age-related decline in pupillary size and function, although such changes probably contribute to the decreased pupil motility.

Decreased sympathetic tone could be responsible for decreased pupillary size and reactivity with advancing age. Korcyzn et al. (241) found that although the mydriasis produced by topical hydroxyamphetamine (Paredrine) did not decrease with increasing age, the mydriasis produced by topical cocaine did. Nevertheless, the decrease in size with age is much greater than can be explained solely on the basis of sympathetic paresis, there are no other signs of sympathetic paresis in otherwise normal persons, and the small pupils of elderly persons usually dilate well to atropinic agents. Thus, the miosis and decreased reactivity that occur with increasing age must occur from cholinergic impulses. Loewenfeld (240) believed that reduced central inhibition is responsible for the age-related changes in pupillary size and reactivity that occur in most normal persons. She emphasized that the pupillary changes that appear with increasing age are similar to those that occur with fatigue, except that they are irreversible.

Role of the Pupillary Light Reflex

The pupillary light reflex has several roles. One is to set the pupils at a size that is optimal for visual acuity (288,289). In addition, the reflex appears to reduce light adaptation in order to prepare the eyes in advance for the return to dim lighting (290,291).

Latent Period of the Pupillary Light Reflex

The latent period of the light reflex is relatively long, as is to be expected in a reflex with a smooth-muscle effector. With a bright light, the latent period is about 0.2 second. As the stimulus is dimmed, the latent period is prolonged until it approaches 0.5 second (292–294). Although the increase in latency is mainly linear, the overall curve of normal pupillary latency with decreasing stimulus intensity is somewhat nonlinear in response to brighter light stimuli (Fig. 14.13). This results in a latency period that is about 30–40 msec per log unit attenuation of light stimulus when given in the mesopic and low photopic-intensity range. However, over a brighter range of light stimuli, the latency period may only be delayed 10–15 msec per log unit attenuation.

Effect of Stimulus Intensity on the Pupillary Light Reflex

Within a critical period of 100 msec, the pupillary effectiveness of light intensity and duration are interchangeable. When a dark-adapted eye is exposed to light flashes of short duration, the pupillary threshold is very low. Using appropriate recording techniques, small but distinct pupillary reactions usually can be obtained well within the first log unit of stimulus luminance above a subject's scotopic visual threshold. When the intensity of the light is increased over a

range of about 3 log units, the pupillary constrictions become more extensive and constant. Throughout this low-intensity range of luminance, the responses are, however, typically shallow; that is, the constriction is preceded by a long latent period, and it is slow, small, and of short duration (Fig. 14.31). When the light intensity is increased, the pupillary reactions begin to increase markedly in amplitude, speed of movement, and duration of constriction until maximal values are reached at about 7–9 log units above the scotopic visual threshold. This sudden increase in effectiveness of the light stimuli occurs because the cone threshold has been exceeded, and cones produce much greater pupil contractions (111, 295,296). Very powerful light flashes fail to add further to the amplitude and speed, and they do not reduce the latent period of the reactions, but they greatly prolong the constriction. After such stimuli, the pupils may remain in spastic miosis for several seconds.

Spectral Sensitivity of the Pupillary Light Reflex

The pupillomotor effectiveness of a colored light stimulus is related to its apparent brightness. For each color, the threshold for pupillary reactions is almost as low as the corresponding visual threshold. This is true for all areas of the retina and in the dark-adapted as well as the light-adapted eye. In other words, the Purkinje shift exists for the pupil as well as for visual sensation (Fig. 14.32). This phenomenon provides further evidence that pupillary and visual function share the same photoreceptors (discussed previously). As described previously, melanopsin-containing retinal ganglion cells are capable of direct photic activation and provide the afferent input to the midbrain pathway of the pupil light reflex. These photosensitive neurons have a broad spectral sensitivity that is centered on approximately 490 nm.

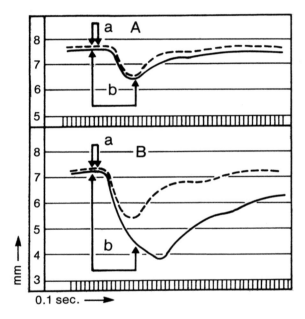

Figure 14.31. Reflexes to short and longer light stimuli at low and high levels of stimulus intensity. Pupillary diameter is recorded as the ordinate (mm) against time as the abscissa (0.1-second units). The *dashed lines* show the pupillary responses to 0.1-second light flashes (*double arrows in a*); the *solid lines*, those to 1.0-second stimuli (*double arrows in b*). In *A* (first line), dim light was used, about 3 log units above the subject's scotopic visual threshold. The reactions to short (*a*) and long (*b*) light flashes were similar. Both showed a long latent period, low peak speed, small extent, and short duration typical for low-intensity reactions. In *B* (second line), the light intensity was increased to about 9 log units above the visual threshold of the subject. The long bright light stimulus (*b*) caused the pupillary constriction to continue for a longer time and thus to become more extensive than the reflex elicited by the short bright light flash (*a*), even though latent period and peak speed of the two reactions were alike. Compared with the low-intensity reflexes of line A, the latent period was shortened and the constriction speed increased. (From Lowenstein O, Loewenfeld IE. Scotopic and photopic thresholds of the pupillary light reflex in normal man. Am J Ophthalmol 1959;48:87–98.)

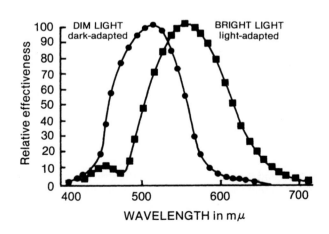

Figure 14.32. Purkinje shift in pupillary spectral sensitivity. The two curves were constructed from photographic records of pupil size obtained after 15 minutes of adaptation to darkness or light of different wavelengths (equal energy stimuli, with a tungsten light source and Hilger wavelength spectrometer). (From Loewenfeld IE. Recent Developments in Vision Research. Publ No 1272. Washington, DC, National Academy of Sciences, National Research Council, 1966.)

Pupillomotor Sensitivity of the Retina

The retinal periphery is far less efficient than the fovea in producing extensive pupillary constriction, and if the amplitude of the light reaction were used as a measure of retinal sensitivity, the pupillomotor sensitivity of the fovea would seem to be far greater than that of the periphery. However, when light stimuli of low intensity are presented, the periphery of the retina has a much lower pupillomotor threshold and is thus much more sensitive than the fovea, although the light reactions produced by stimulating the periphery are of low amplitude. The pupillary sensitivity of the retina is thus remarkably similar to the visual sensitivity (Fig. 14.33). In fact, visual acuity can be measured using pupil responses to checkerboard stimuli with a fair degree of accuracy (113,117,119). In addition, as is the case with vision, the threshold for pupillary reaction is elevated in a similar way

by bleaching and by real backgrounds (297–305), and this depression of sensitivity can be quantified by the construction of the equivalent background of the bleach that is used to describe psychophysical results (104,306).

In view of the many kinds of functional parallelism between pupillary responses and both objective and subjective visual sensory phenomena, it can safely be assumed that they use the same retinal photoreceptors. As noted above, the photosensitive melanopsin-containing retinal ganglion cells, which also can be activated by rod and cone input, appear to subserve the pupil light reflex and input to diurnal centers in the hypothalamus. It is also possible that a small number of ganglion cells serve both functions, with the impulses reaching their separate destinations by collateral branching in the final third of the optic tract, and the fibers affecting pupillary function descending into the mesencephalon to synapse in the pretectal nuclei.

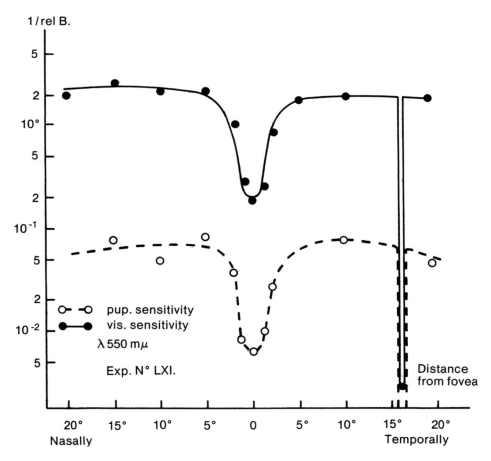

Figure 14.33. Pupillomotor and visual sensitivity to green light in the fovea and in the retinal periphery for the dark-adapted eye. Log relative effectiveness of 0.25-second test flashes in a 2° area is represented by the ordinate. A tungsten light with a rotating shutter and interference filter was used. Retinal positions are indicated on the abscissa. The visual thresholds (*solid line*) are parallel, with the pupil about 1.5 log units less sensitive than visual perception. In this experiment, the pupillary reactions were detected by visual observation with an infrared-sensitive image converter. When the pupillary reactions are recorded graphically and when larger testing areas are used, the pupillary threshold is closer to the visual threshold. Note the central depression for green light, shown in the pupillary reactions as well as for the visual threshold, and the lack of sensitivity at the blind spot. (From Loewenfeld IE. Recent Developments in Vision Research. Publ No 1272. Washington, DC, National Academy of Sciences, National Research Council, 1966.)

Modification of the Pupillary Light Reflex by Emotion and Fatigue

Fatigue and emotional excitement are so much a part of everyday life, and their modifying influence upon pupillary diameter and reactions is so profound, that their effects must be understood and constantly kept in mind when considering the pupillary reaction to light. The light response is dependent on a person's level of consciousness. When a normal person is alert, the central synapse of the pupillomotor reflex arc in the Edinger-Westphal nucleus is subject to central inhibitory influences. At the same time, hypothalamic discharges are produced by sensory or emotional stimuli provided by the environment or by spontaneous thoughts or emotions. These impulses travel via the brain stem, cervical cord, and peripheral sympathetic chain to the dilator muscle of the iris. As the subject drifts toward sleep, his or her cerebral and diencephalic centers cease to function in an orderly sequence. Central inhibition of the visceral oculomotor nuclei decreases, sympathetic activity is gradually lost, and the consequent relative preponderance of parasympathetic outflow results in miosis. At the moment of spontaneous or reactive awakening, sympathetic activity returns, and this, combined with supranuclear inhibition of the iris sphincter, results in pupillary dilation.

Thus, under the influence of the mechanisms described above, the pupil in healthy, alert persons is relatively large, with only a slight amount of physiologic pupillary unrest. As the subject becomes tired, the pupils gradually become smaller, and oscillatory fatigue waves become apparent. At the moment immediately preceding sleep, the pupils are quite small, but a psychosensory stimulus such as a sudden sound will restore the waking condition and redilate them (307). Pupillary light reflexes thus are superimposed upon a constantly shifting equilibrium of autonomic innervation of the iris that can be modified further by humoral adrenergic mechanisms (214) and influenced by the mechanical limitations of the iris (Fig. 14.34).

Binocular Interactions of the Pupillary Light Reflex

The extent of binocular interaction that exists in normal individuals has been the subject of much experimentation and controversy and appears to depend to some extent on the phenomena studied and the way the study is conducted. Although most investigations dealing with binocular interaction have been concerned with sensory phenomena, some have dealt with the pupillary reaction to light. Bárány and Halldén (308) reported that pupillary responses to light stimuli tended to be inhibited or abolished during suppression phases of binocular (retinal) rivalry; however, Lowe and Ogle (309) were unable to confirm these results. Simons and Ogle (310) performed carefully controlled experiments using infrared electronic pupillography and showed that the light threshold for pupillary constriction by foveal stimulation in one eye is essentially independent of the light adaptation level of the other eye. This finding suggests that there is no interocular influence as far as pupillary thresholds are concerned.

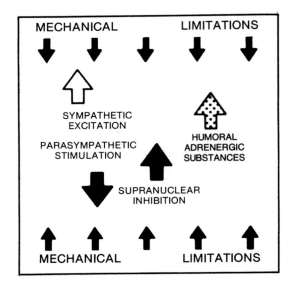

Figure 14.34. Mechanisms affecting pupillary size and reactivity. Parasympathetic innervation causes active pupillary constriction (*black arrow*); its central nervous inhibition causes incomplete, passive dilation of the pupil (*cross-hatched arrow*). Sympathetic excitation dilates the pupil rapidly and completely (*white arrow*). Adrenergic substances, entering the blood under the influence of central nervous mechanisms elicited by strong sensory or emotional stimulation, may reinforce and prolong pupillary dilation (*dotted arrow*). Finally, the limits of mechanical capacity of the iris muscles may modify the movements when extremes of mydriasis or miosis are approached (*small black arrows*). (From Loewenfeld IE. Recent Developments in Vision Research. Publ No 1272. Washington, DC, National Academy of Sciences, National Research Council, 1966.)

Conditioning of the Pupillary Light Reflex

Attempts to evoke experimentally the light response by conditioning the photomotor pupillary system to another stimulus have produced conflicting results. In such experiments, there are many possible sources of error, especially in the absence of continuous recording of the pupillary reactions. Some claims of successful conditioning of pupillary responses apparently resulted from confusion with unrecognized physiologic pupillary unrest and with the miosis of fatigue. In our opinion, the most careful investigators have been unable to demonstrate any conditioning of the light reflex (311,312).

Pupillary Light Reflex as a Servomechanism

The pupillary light response is mediated by fairly well-defined neuroanatomic processes and has a stimulus that can be quantitatively controlled in a laboratory environment. In addition, it is possible to obtain continuous recordings of pupil movement. Thus, the pupillary response system is particularly amenable to mathematically oriented studies (313). Stark and Sherman (314) initially constructed a system based on feedback control, and an analysis of the stochastic properties of light-induced pupillary movement led Stanten and Stark (315) to develop an overall system model, the components of which are related, at least grossly, to anatomic structure. Using this model, several investigators (243,316) defined the relationship between motor neuron activity and pupil size, and Terdiman et al. (317) described information transfer through the entire system (318). These papers as well as a summary of this work by Stark in Chapter 12 of Loewenfeld's book (109) are recommended to those interested in this approach to pupillary responses.

Pupillary Reaction to Darkness

The pupillary response to darkness is elicited by a short interval of darkness after an eye has been adapted to light. This dilation is bilateral and follows a latent period that is somewhat longer (about 300 msec) than that preceding pupillary constriction to light. The time course of the pupillary dark response does not change with age (319). This dilation may result from more than a simple cessation of the constriction to light. There may be active inhibition of the visceral oculomotor nuclei because of an ''off'' discharge in the retina as described above in the section on retinomesencephalic inhibition associated with the dark reaction (320). A disruption of the pupillary reaction to darkness may be responsible for the ''paradoxic'' pupillary response—constriction of the pupils in darkness —that is observed in patients with various retinal diseases.

Pupillary Reflex to Near and the Near Response

As fixation is shifted from a far to a near object, the eyes converge, the lenses accommodate, and both pupils constrict. This triad of ocular motor, accommodative, and pupillary activity is called the near response. Despite many contentions in the literature claiming that the pupillary constriction that occurs during the near response is exclusively dependent on either convergence or accommodation, clinical and experimental data indicate that any of the three functions can be selectively abolished or elicited without affecting the others (156). For example, convergence or accommodation may be eliminated selectively with prisms or lenses (321–323) and pupillary constriction alone can be blocked by weak, parasympatholytic substances without noticeable cycloplegia. In addition, isolated pupillary constriction, accommodation of the lens, and contraction of the medial rectus muscle can each be separately produced by electric stimulation of different parts of the cerebral cortex, oculomotor nucleus, or oculomotor nerve (156,192,324,325). Finally, clinical cases of isolated impairment or loss of pupillary constriction, accommodation, or convergence are not uncommon. These experimental and clinical observations confirm that the impulses that cause accommodation, convergence, and pupillary constriction arise from different cell groups within the oculomotor nucleus and travel via separate fibers to their effector muscles. Accommodation, convergence, and pupillary constriction are associated movements and are not tied to one another in the manner usually referred to by the term ''reflex.'' They are controlled, synchronized, and associated by supranuclear connections, but they are not caused by one another.

The miosis of the near response and the pupillary constriction to light have a single final common efferent pathway from the Edinger-Westphal nucleus to the iris sphincter via the ciliary ganglion. They differ mainly in the supranuclear pathways that are elicited by light and near that both converge on the Edinger-Westphal nucleus. Langley and Anderson (326), after careful exposure of a cat's orbit, painted the ciliary ganglion with nicotine and succeeded in blocking all pupillary response obtained by stimulating the oculomotor nerve, whereas stimulation of the short ciliary nerves remained effective. This experiment provided convincing physiologic evidence that there is a single final common pathway for pupillary constriction with a synapse at the ciliary ganglion.

It should be remembered that the pupillary constriction that is part of the near response is subject to the same central inhibitory and sympathetic antagonistic influences as is pupillary constriction to light. For example, the constriction associated with a near vision effort may be blocked by a simultaneous, psychosensory dilation.

Schäfer and Weale (327) studied the influence of age on the pupillary near response. These investigators found that aging results in a reduction of pupillary diameter as well as a reduction in the amplitude of pupillary constriction during the near response. Studies by these investigators and by Roth (328) also indicate an effect of retinal illumination on pupillary constriction during the near response. It appears that the pupillary near response is directly related in magnitude to the existing level of illuminance and that it functions in accord with other adaptive mechanisms that alter the overall sensitivity of the eye.

There appears to be no interocular modification of the pupillary response to near. Jagerman (329) found that when one pupil was dilated (but not cyclopleged) and forced to fixate a near target, there was no change in the degree of pupillary constriction that occurred in the opposite (unmedicated) eye. However, Jagerman (329) measured pupillary size using a mirror and a gauge with black semicircles of various diameters rather than by infrared pupillography.

The pupillary near reflex can be evaluated in terms of a servomechanism, just like the pupillary light reflex (315). Using this method, Semmlow and Stark (330) found that the dynamics of iris movement in the pupillary near response provide a relatively linear input to the iris motor system. Responses of the iris to step-like changes in target distance show two major nonlinearities: a range-dependent response gain that decreases as pupil size decreases and a direction dependence in which constriction is faster than dilation.

As a diagnostic tool for the physician, the pupillary near response is less reliable than the light reflex because of its subjective features. When pupillary constriction is poor or absent during near viewing, it is difficult to be certain that the patient has made a satisfactory effort to obtain clear near vision. For practical purposes, the reaction is important diagnostically only when it is more extensive than the constriction to light, as occurs in many cases of the dorsal midbrain syndrome or in patients with Argyll Robertson or tonic pupils.

Reflexes Following Eyelid Closure

Pupillary movements that occur after spontaneous blinking or voluntary blinking or as a reaction to corneal stimulation may be collectively called the "pupillary lid-closure reflexes." Considering the many conditions that produce eyelid closure, it is not surprising that the associated pupillary movements vary. When eyelid closure is spontaneous or voluntary, the pupillary reaction consists of a short constriction followed by redilation. When eyelid closure is elicited by a corneal or equivalent trigeminal sensory stimulus, the pupil dilates, and quite often this immediate reaction is followed by secondary blinks that produce pupillary constriction.

In any given eyelid-closure reaction, pupillary constriction or dilation is dependent on: (a) the intensity of the illumination present in the environment; (b) the duration of eyelid closure; and (c) the presence of any associated psychosensory stimulus. When observed in light, for example, long intentional closing of the eyes produces the dilation phase of the darkness reflex, whereas short intentional or reflex blinks dilate the pupils when accompanied by emotional overlay and constrict them in the absence of such psychosensory stimuli.

The cause of the pupillary movements with eyelid closure becomes clear when it is observed that spontaneous or voluntary eyelid closure in darkness fails to produce any pupillary reaction, and eyelid closure from corneal stimulation causes the usual pupillary dilation. Thus, the constriction on reexposure to light results from an increase in retinal sensitivity during the brief interval of darkness.

Reflex Dilation

In darkness, the pupils of normal, alert subjects are usually large and relatively steady. When the same persons are tired, relatively slow and irregular waves of pupillary contraction and dilation accompany the waves of drowsiness and arousal. As noted above, when someone is drifting off to sleep, there is miosis. This is the extreme example of the observation that arousal or any increase in alertness produces a reflex pupillary dilation. In waking animals or humans, any sensory or emotional stimulation causes the pupils to dilate. The mechanisms of this dilation are somewhat controversial (109,214), but two neural mechanisms appear to be involved, one active and one passive. The active component results from contraction of the radially arranged fibers of the dilator muscle via the cervical sympathetic pathway, and the passive component results from relaxation of the sphincter muscle caused by inhibition of the visceral oculomotor nuclei. These pupillary responses to sensory stimuli are part of a generalized arousal reaction that affects the entire body.

The active sympathetic discharges are the chief cause of rapid and extensive pupillary reflex dilation seen in conscious animals. In anesthetized animals, the active sympathetic component of pupillary dilation is abolished, and the pupils are dilated by inhibition of the sphincter nuclei alone. These inhibitory impulses converge upon the oculomotor nucleus from cortex, thalamus, and hypothalamus and from connections running in the diffuse reticular formation. The resulting pupillary dilation is slower and less extensive than reflex dilation in the conscious animal elicited by direct stimulation of the cervical sympathetic chain.

Confirmation of these mechanisms was provided by the electrophysiologic work of Bonvallet and Zbrozyna (331). These investigators stimulated the pontomesencephalic reticular formation of the cat while monitoring the activity of the short ciliary nerves in the retrobulbar space and in the sympathetic chain in the neck. They showed inhibition of the parasympathetic outflow occurring simultaneously with excitation of the cervical sympathetic chain. They also demonstrated that anesthesia eliminated the sympathetic outflow.

Humoral mechanisms can also influence pupillary dilation. Adrenergic substances reaching the dilator muscle via the blood cause it to contract, even when the sympathetic pathway and the oculomotor nerve have been cut. Norepinephrine, presumably released from the heart and great vessels, reaches the eye in 2–5 seconds and dilates the pupil. Adrenal catecholamines are released in sufficient quantity to affect the eye only after severe, stressful stimulation. Because the adrenaline is released into veins, it does not reach the eye until 12–15 seconds after the stimulus, and in the supersensitive, sympathectomized animal, the pupil may remain dilated for several minutes. In humans, pupillary dilation can result from any sensory, psychological, or emotional stimulus, and after spontaneous or voluntary motor activity; however, humoral mechanisms rarely produce pupillary changes except under conditions of catastrophic stress or following the development of denervation supersensitivity.

Psychosensory reflex dilation of the pupil may take many forms and may be produced in many ways. For the ciliospinal reflex, the neck is pinched; for the cochleopupillary reflex, a tuning fork is placed near the ear; and for the vestibulopupillary reflex, one labyrinth is stimulated. In "Flatau's neck mydriasis," the neck is flexed, whereas "Redlich's phenomenon" is produced by a vigorous and sustained muscular activity. In "Meyer's iliac phenomenon," pressure on McBurney's point produces pupillary dilation.

In addition to the reflexes described above, psychosensory activity is responsible for the pupillary abnormalities once thought to be characteristic of schizophrenic and neurotic patients (332,333) and also explains the ability of some persons to dilate both pupils voluntarily.

ACCOMMODATION AND THE AUTONOMIC NERVOUS SYSTEM

As noted above, when normal persons shift fixation from far objects to near objects, the near response occurs. During this response, both eyes converge, pupillary constriction occurs, and a change also occurs in the optical system of the eye. This optical change, termed accommodation, is controlled by an elaborate sensorimotor mechanism that monitors the clarity of the image focused upon the retina. The peripheral motor effector for this mechanism is the muscle of the ciliary body. This smooth muscle is activated primarily by the mesencephalic, parasympathetic outflow but is also influenced by cervical sympathetic outflow as well. The ciliary body containing the ciliary muscle encircles the anterior, inner surface of the eye as a girdle (Fig. 14.35). It conforms externally to the curvature of the overlying sclera

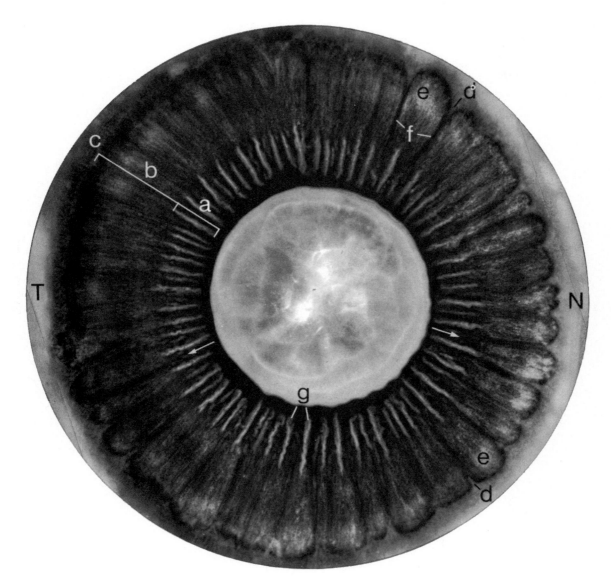

Figure 14.35. The inner surface of the ciliary body and lens. The nasal side of the eye is at N and the temporal is at T. a, pars plicata; b, pars plana; c, ora serrata; d, dentate processes; e, pars plana bays; f, striae of the dentate processes; g, ciliary processes; arrows, valleys of the pars plicata. (From Straatsma BR, Foos RY, Spencer LM. The New Orleans Academy of Ophthalmology: Symposium on Retina and Retinal Surgery. St Louis, CV Mosby, 1969.)

and has a triangular shape in cross-section (Fig. 14.36), with the base of the triangle facing the anterior chamber and the apex directed posteriorly toward the retina. Anteriorly, the ciliary body is continuous with the iris, whereas posteriorly, it is continuous with the rest of the uveal tract and with the overlying peripheral retina at the ora serrata. The external surface of the ciliary body lies adjacent to the sclera, being separated from it by the suprachoroidal space. The internal surface faces the vitreous. The ciliary body contains three layers: (a) unpigmented ciliary epithelium; (b) pigmented ciliary epithelium; and (c) the ciliary muscle, which controls accommodation (Figs. 14.36–14.38). The ciliary muscle consists of meridional, radial, and circular muscle fiber ori-

entations (Fig. 14.38). Rohen (334) suggested that the whole muscle is interconnected, with the muscle bundles forming a three-dimensional reticulum consisting of muscle cells that show considerable interweaving from layer to layer.

PATHWAYS FOR ACCOMMODATION

Parasympathetic Pathway for Accommodation

Bender and Weinstein (335) succeeded in producing ciliary muscle contraction without pupillary constriction by stimulating the caudal portion of the parasympathetic nucleus in the midbrain of the monkey. Jampel and Mindel (192) passed an electrode stereotaxically in a rostrocaudal

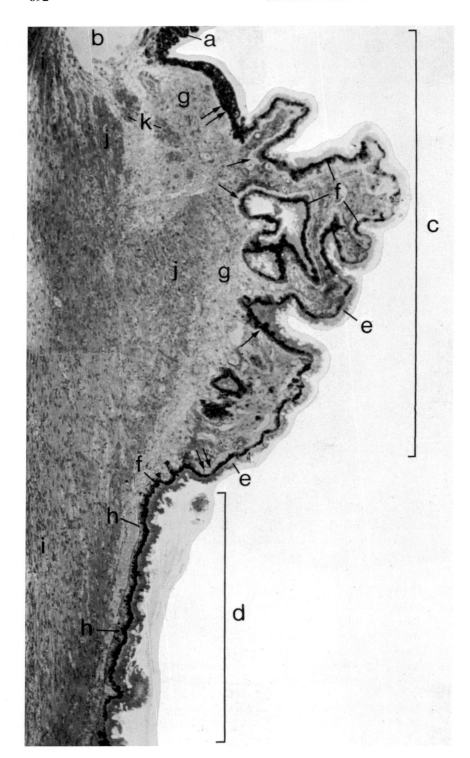

Figure 14.36. Light micrograph of a meridional section through a normal, human ciliary body. a, iris root; b, anterior chamber angle; c, pars plicata; d, pars plana; e, unpigmented ciliary epithelium; f, pigmented ciliary epithelium; g, connective tissue of the ciliary body stroma; h, elastic lamina that is part of Bruch's membrane; i, j, and k, longitudinal, radial, and circular portions of the ciliary muscle respectively. *Single arrows* and *double arrows* mark the extent of basement membrane-like material that forms the innermost boundary of the ciliary body stroma and separates it from the ciliary epithelium. (From Hogan MJ, Alvarado JA, Weddell JE. Histology of the Human Eye: An Atlas and Textbook. Philadelphia, WB Saunders, 1971.)

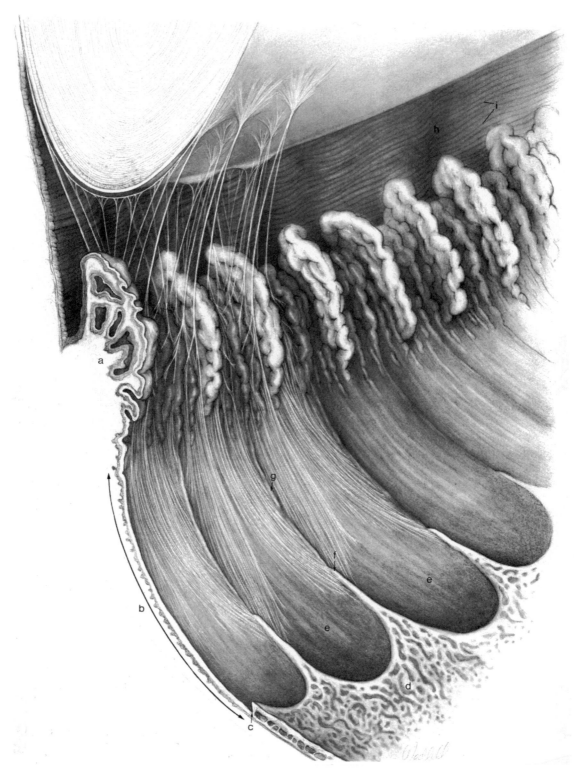

Figure 14.37. Drawing of the inner aspect of the ciliary body to show the pars plicata (*a*) and the pars plana (*b*). c, ora serrata; d, peripheral retina showing cystoid degeneration; e, oral bays; f, dentate processes; g, striae of the dentate processes; h, radial furrows of iris; i, circular furrows of iris. Note the origin of the zonular fibers from the pars plana and the insertion of the fibers onto the lens capsule. (From Hogan MJ, Alvarado JA, Weddell JE. Histology of the Human Eye: An Atlas and Textbook. Philadelphia, WB Saunders, 1971.)

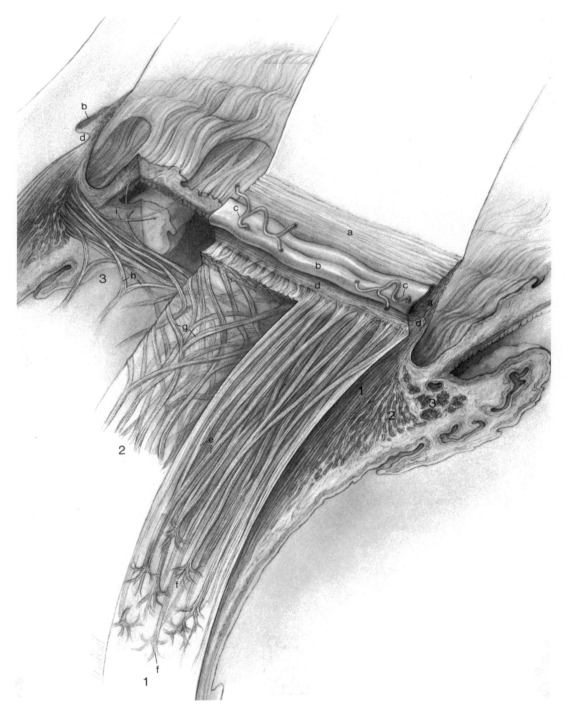

Figure 14.38. Drawing of the ciliary body showing the ciliary muscle and its components. The cornea and sclera have been dissected away, but the trabecular meshwork (a), Schlemm's canal (b), two external collecting veins (c), and the scleral spur (d) remain. The three components of the ciliary muscle are shown separately, viewed from the outside and sectioned meridionally. *Section 1* shows the longitudinal ciliary muscle; in *section 2*, the longitudinal muscle has been dissected away to show the radial ciliary muscle; and in *section 3*, only the innermost circular ciliary muscle is shown. The longitudinal muscle forms long V-shaped trellises (e) that terminate in the epichoroidal stars (f). The arms of the V-shaped bundles formed by the radial muscle meet at wide angles (g) and terminate in the ciliary processes. The V-shaped bundles of the circular muscle originate at such distant points in the ciliary tendon that their arms meet at a very wide angle (h). The iridic portion of this muscle (i) is shown joining the circular muscle cells. (From Hogan MJ, Alvarado JA, Weddell JE. Histology of the Human Eye: An Atlas and Textbook. Philadelphia, WB Saunders, 1971.)

direction through the small-cell component of the primate Edinger-Westphal nucleus and observed first a forward displacement of the iris diaphragm (i.e., accommodation) without constriction of the pupil. At a more caudal level, stimulation produced pupillary constriction without evidence of accommodation.

Studies in alert behaving rhesus monkeys have greatly clarified the details of the parasympathetic outflow to the ciliary muscle. Gamlin et al. (336–338) studied single-cell activity in the Edinger-Westphal nucleus during various near-viewing tasks. During normal viewing, accommodation and vergence are so closely matched that it is difficult to determine whether cellular activity is related to accommodation or to vergence. By carefully designing stimuli that created specific vergence and accommodative demands, these investigators were able to differentiate various cell types that responded primarily to accommodation (+A cells), to vergence (+V cells), or to both accommodation and vergence (+V + A cells).

Nearly all Edinger-Westphal cells that respond to pure accommodative stimuli can be antidromically stimulated from the ipsilateral oculomotor nerve and thus are considered to be preganglionic neurons innervating the ciliary muscle (336,337). These cells have a distinct pattern of activity unlike other cells in the vicinity of the oculomotor nucleus that respond to vergence stimuli, accommodative stimuli, or both. They are characterized by a low spontaneous firing rate in the dark or at optical infinity (mean 11.5 Hz) and a modest increase that is linearly related to the amplitude of the accommodative response. On the other hand, cells in the Edinger-Westphal nucleus that respond to near targets but cannot be antidromically stimulated through the oculomotor nerve are never purely accommodative (i.e., +A cells); they respond to either vergence stimuli (+V cells) or to both vergence and accommodative stimuli (+V + A cells). Their spontaneous firing rates and their overall sensitivity to accommodative stimuli are much higher than purely accommodative cells. The two cell types that cannot be antidromically stimulated are collectively designated as ''near-response'' neurons and are presumed not to innervate the ciliary muscle, although a nonsynapsing pathway cannot be ruled out for the +V + A cells. Gamlin et al. (337) suggest that these non-preganglionic neurons project efference copies of near-response activity to the spinal cord, cerebellum, or precerebellar structures, as has been suggested from other studies in both cats and primates (339,340). Alternatively, these Edinger-Westphal neurons may be premotor in nature and may project either directly or indirectly to preganglionic Edinger-Westphal neurons or to medial rectus motoneurons.

The predominant view of the innervation of the iris sphincter muscle and ciliary body is that preganglionic parasympathetic fibers from the mesencephalon synapse in the ciliary ganglion and that postganglionic fibers innervate the iris sphincter muscle and ciliary body. En route to the ciliary ganglion, these fibers travel superficially as part of the oculomotor nerve and occupy a topographic location adjacent to the pupillomotor fibers. Surgical removal of the short ciliary nerves in macaque monkeys produces chromatolysis in 97% of the cells in the ciliary ganglion, whereas iridectomy alone

causes 3% of these cells to become chromatolytic (190). These results highlight the fact that the vast majority of ciliary ganglion neurons innervate the ciliary body, whereas the minority provides innervation to the iris sphincter.

Effect of the Ciliary Muscle on Accommodation

The ciliary muscle, through its zonular attachments to the lens, produces distinct changes in its structure, which brings about changes in accommodation. The physical changes of accommodation were described in some detail by Adler (341) and consist of the following:

1. The anterior pole of the lens moves forward and the anterior chamber is narrowed.
2. The anterior surface of the lens becomes more convex.
3. The posterior surface of the lens becomes more convex, but the posterior pole remains fixed.
4. The anteroposterior diameter of the lens is increased.
5. The anterior surface of the lens assumes a hyperbolic curve; that is, the center of the lens surface becomes more convex while the periphery becomes flatter.
6. The diameter of the lens is narrowed.
7. During maximum accommodation, the lens sinks in the direction of gravity about 0.25–0.3 mm.

The means by which the ciliary muscle accomplishes its control of lens curvature has been the subject of lively debate for hundreds of years. There are two major theories: the relaxation theory and the tension theory (342). In 1855, Helmholtz (343) popularized the theory that the lens possesses elasticity, and believed that changes in the shape of the lens were brought about by an interplay between zonular tension generated by the ciliary body and lens tension generated from internal elastic properties. For example, increases in zonular tension would pull on the lens, resulting in a shortening of its anterior-posterior axis with an increase in equatorial diameter, thus making its surface flatter and less curved. When the pull of the zonules is relaxed, the internal elastic properties of the lens would allow the equatorial diameter of the lens to diminish, and the lens would get thicker in the middle, with both anterior and posterior surfaces becoming more curved. Henderson (344) accepted the principles enunciated by Helmholtz (343) but proposed that instead of the elasticity of the lens being balanced by the elasticity of the choroid, as Helmholtz believed, it is balanced by the tone of the ciliary muscle. The relaxation theory of accommodation, in which focusing at near results in relaxation of zonular tension and thickening of the lens, is supported by both clinical and experimental studies (345–348) as well as mathematical modeling (349).

Tscherning (350) proposed a diametrically opposite theory to the relaxation hypothesis. He visualized the zonular fibers becoming taut during accommodation, and he thought that this accounted for pressure upon the peripheral portions of the lens and for bulging of the central portion anteriorly. He later modified this view but continued to believe that the zonular fibers did not relax but became tighter during accommodation. He accepted the idea that the vitreous pressing upon the posterior surface of the lens accounted for anterior bulging of the portion of the lens not covered by iris. The tension theory of accommodation is not supported by clinical observations as is the relaxation theory but is based upon conclusions drawn from anatomic studies.

Most authors favor the relaxation theory of accommodation, but some remain unconvinced (351).

Sympathetic and Parasympathetic Control of the Ciliary Muscle

In 1860, Henke proposed that the circular and longitudinal fibers of the ciliary muscle have opposing actions in accommodation, known as reciprocal innervation. Working with animal eyes, Morat and Doyon (352) postulated that the parasympathetic nervous system was responsible for accommodation during the near response, whereas the sympathetic nervous system was responsible for relaxing accommodation through inhibition of the ciliary body muscle. Henderson (344) believed that the sympathetic system, at least in the monkey, was excitatory to longitudinal and radial fibers of the ciliary muscle and inhibitory to the circular fibers, and the parasympathetic system acted in the opposite manner. Cogan (353) suggested that the sympathetic system functions in adapting the eye for relatively distant objects and tends to oppose the parasympathetic system that functions in adapting the eye for near objects. He observed that following sympathectomy, there was greater accommodation amplitude, whereas after sympathetic stimulation, there was reduced accommodation in patients in whom one eye had adrenergic supersensitivity brought about by previous unilateral section of the cervical sympathetic trunk. Further evidence for sympathetic modulation of accommodation was demonstrated in enucleated cat eyes, where a change in shape of the ciliary body could be observed after application of adrenergic drugs (354) or when the long ciliary nerves were electrically stimulated (355).

Fenton and Hunter (356) reported on the histologic examination of the eyes of two patients with long-standing complete oculomotor palsy. Both eyes showed selective loss of the circular portion of the ciliary muscle, whereas the longitudinal and radial portions of the muscle remained intact. These findings lent support to the concept of a dual nerve supply to the ciliary muscle, with sympathetic innervation to the longitudinal and radial portions and parasympathetic innervation to the circular portion.

Hurwitz et al. (357,358) found that parasympathetic inhibition was the most potent mechanism in antagonizing accommodation in primates. Stimulation of α-adrenergic receptors produced no significant antagonistic response, whereas stimulation of β receptors depressed accommodation but did not abolish it. Gimpel et al. (359) measured the effect of topical 2.5% phenylephrine on amplitude of accommodation in 160 young adults. Although there was a statistically significant mean reduction of 11.7% after treatment, responses varied widely from a 30% increase to a 60% decrease.

Supranuclear Control of Accommodation

Jampel (360) contributed valuable experimental confirmation that the cerebral cortex participates in accommodative mechanisms. He recorded accommodative changes in the primate eye by using a retinoscope during faradic stimulation in overlapping areas of the preoccipital (peristriate) cortex. Accommodation was usually obtained in both eyes by unilateral cortical stimulation. It was always accompanied by convergence and often by pupillary constriction. Jampel (360) proposed that all three elements of the near response—accommodation, convergence, and pupillary constriction—are synthesized in the cerebral cortex and then are modified at a functionally lower level, in the pretectum and tectum of the midbrain, where they are influenced by less malleable systems, including the light reflex, afferent input from the extraocular muscles, and vestibular, postural, and cerebellar modulatory impulses (361,362). Ultimately, the impulses are projected onto the cell bodies of the neurons of the final common pathway that are located in the oculomotor nucleus and are transmitted separately to their effector organs.

Other studies suggest that cortical control of accommodation originates in the lateral suprasylvian (LS) area (363–364). This cortical area surrounds the middle suprasylvian area in the cat. Descending projections from accommodation-related neurons in this cortical area terminate mainly in the rostral portion of the superior colliculus (363). The accommodation-related areas of the superior colliculus also receive retinal afferents from the macular area and project to the pretectum. It is possible that the retino-collicular connections are part of an open-loop control system that is responsible for the initial phase of the accommodative response and that the LS-collicular-tectal system is responsible for fine-tuning the accommodative response using cortical control (366).

Other supranuclear mechanisms must influence accommodation. Hypothalamic pathways exist to inhibit activity in the ciliary neurons of the Edinger-Westphal nucleus in the same way that such pathways inhibit the pupillary constrictor neurons. Central sympathetic activity must also modify the function of the ciliary body. Although clinical evidence suggests that this is the case, systematic experimental investigations of these autonomic influences on ciliary activity have not been pursued with the vigor that has been applied to the problems of pupillomotor control.

CHARACTERISTICS OF ACCOMMODATION

Thus far, we have discussed the process of accommodation in terms of a motor system acting upon an effector organ, the ciliary muscle. We now consider this motor mechanism in terms of its integrated role in the process of vision.

Accommodation is controlled by visual sensory inputs and cerebral inputs that drive and monitor the motor output system. We will examine the control mechanism of accommodation in terms of the performance characteristics of the system.

Stimuli to Accommodate

During normal binocular viewing, the adjustment of the accommodative mechanism for different distances is produced by a voluntary convergence mechanism and retinal blur that evoke binocular fusion reflexes (367–371). In addition, the normal process of accommodation is greatly facilitated by voluntary efforts initiated by the awareness that the object of regard is nearby (367).

Small scanning movements of the eye represent another major factor in the ability of the eye to respond correctly to a change in the position of an accommodative target. Normal persons, when made to fix steadily on a target, cannot respond with a correct accommodative adjustment as the target is moved toward or away from them in monochromatic light. They can respond correctly to a change in the stimulus distance only when ocular scanning movements are permitted (372). It is believed that this scanning permits detection of the direction of the retinal defocus by means of the signal afforded by directional sensitivity of the cones (the Stiles-Crawford effect). Chromatic aberration is thought to be another cue for evoking accommodation (373,374), as is the amount of ambient light in the environment (375–377).

Time Characteristics of Accommodation

The reaction time of accommodation to rapid changes in the distance of a fixated object is relatively slow. The change in accommodation begins after a time delay of 0.36 second ($\pm$0.09 second) (379). Once the response starts, it continues in the proper direction in a more or less smooth manner until it levels off at the new accommodative level. This process can be made less exact and less smooth if the target differs only in focus but not in size. Interestingly, the total reaction time for far-to-near focus is about 20 msec longer than the reaction time from near to far.

Relation Between Pupil Size and Accommodation

As the size of the pupil diminishes, the speed and amount of pupillary constriction to either light or near stimulation also diminishes (380–383). In addition, as pupil size is reduced, the amplitude of accommodation generated at different target distances up to a distance of 1 meter is diminished (384). Very little accommodation is generated at target distances of greater than 1 meter, regardless of pupil size (385–392).

Stability of Accommodation

When normal individuals fixate on a target that is moving gradually toward or away from them, accommodation does not change in a gradual, steady manner (393). On the contrary, the accommodative response contains definite irregular fluctuations. It may not track the target accurately, and it may even make large errors in the opposite direction. Even when a target is stationary, there is instability of accommodation. When an eye fixates steadily upon an object inside optical infinity, the refractive power varies constantly over a small range. Whiteside (394) measured fluctuations as large as 0.25 diopters, whereas Campbell and Westheimer (395) recorded fluctuations as great as 0.4 diopters and noted that the fluctuations ceased when homatropine was instilled in the eye and when the subject fixated at optical infinity. The frequency characteristics of the fluctuations appeared to be most evident around 0–0.5 cycle/sec and 2 cycles/sec.

Stark and Takahashi (368) suggested that the high-frequency component (HFC) did not have a physiologic role but was a "consequence of important nonlinear characteristics of the accommodative servomechanism." Other studies show that the peak activity of the high-frequency component of fluctuations in accommodation (1.0–2.5 Hz) correlates closely with the arterial pulse and probably reflects intraocular tremor created by intraocular blood flow (396). The HFC is therefore unlikely to reflect a purposeful adaptive response of the accommodative system. The low-frequency component (LFC), on the other hand, increases in conditions that decrease depth of focus, including increased pupil size (397,398), decreased target luminance (398,399), increased target proximity (398,400), and decreased target contrast (337,398,401). The HFC is relatively impervious to changes in pupil size or these stimulus characteristics.

Based on early evidence, Alpern (402) first proposed that accommodative oscillations play an important role in "fine-tuning" the accommodative response. The continuous fluctuations may provide information on image quality via negative feedback. However, although the accommodative system operates relatively slowly in relation to other motor systems, only the HFC fluctuations are fast enough to provide useful information to the accommodative mechanism within its dynamic velocity range. The precise role of accommodative fluctuations is therefore not entirely clear. Whether these oscillations are similar in any way to the oscillation of the globe during steady fixation or to the oscillations of the pupil (i.e., hippus) during conditions of steady fixation and illumination is also unclear. Alternatively, the HFC and the LFC may not play functional roles in human accommodation; rather, the LFC may be a vestigial remnant of more slowly adaptive systems in nonmammalian vertebrates, and the HFC may be simply a consequence of ocular pulsations.

Feedback Control of Accommodation

Campbell and Westheimer (395) tested the response of the accommodative control system to momentary optic defocusing. These investigators found that the system continuously monitors the state of focus and that accommodative responses may be halted and modified according to changing stimulus conditions. Troelstra et al. (403) analyzed the initial directional tracking in three subjects. In this experiment, the investigators attempted to eliminate all extraneous clues, such as apparent vertical and horizontal target movement, size change, blur asymmetry, and illumination differences, as well as the possibility of learning the patterns of stimulus presentation. In one of their subjects, the initial direction of change in accommodation was in error about 50% of the time. Two other subjects made correct initial changes of accommodation in 100% of the trials. These two subjects apparently used subtle perceptual clues afforded by the imperfect test situation. Troelstra et al. concluded that the accommodative system can operate effectively as an "even-error servosystem" in which the retinal blur evokes movement in the system as a trial-and-error function.

Interocular Effects on Accommodation

Jagerman (404) studied eight normal subjects in whom he dilated one pupil or cyclopleged one eye and measured the amount of miosis and accommodation in the unmedicated eye when the medicated eye was forced to fixate an accommodative target. He found that dilation alone produced no change in the normal miotic or accommodative responses in the opposite eye, but when an eye under cycloplegia was forced to fixate a near object, "excessive" miosis and accommodation were noted in the opposite (unmedicated) eye.

Relation Between Accommodation and Convergence

During normal binocular viewing, accommodation and convergence operate in unison. The basic stimuli for the binocular adjustment for near vision are: (a) change in the vergence of the light reaching the two foveas and (b) temporal disparity of the two images relative to the two foveas.

The relationship between accommodation and the resulting vergence eye movement may differ depending on whether the fixing or non-fixing eye's movement is monitored. According to most investigators, accommodative vergence is a monocular phenomenon; that is, if one eye is covered and the viewing eye changes fixation from a far to a near target along its line of sight, the covered eye rotates inward (405–409). Although Kenyon et al. (410) used precise infrared photoelectric eye movement recordings to show the presence of movement in the viewing, as well as the nonviewing, eye during accommodation, the total vergence amplitude in the viewing eye was only about 12% that measured in the covered eye. According to Kenyon et al. (410), a fixation-holding mechanism exists that produces a general attenuation of both vergence and some saccadic movements in the viewing eye, enabling retention of the target on the fovea.

Accommodation is induced by convergence as an unconditioned reflex. The relationship of accommodation and convergence is not absolute or fixed, but under normal conditions a unit change in one is accompanied by a unit change in the other. A definite range of accommodation is possible at each position of convergence. Similarly, convergence can vary slightly relative to a fixed state of accommodation. The change in convergence produced by a change in accommodation is termed "accommodative convergence," whereas the change in accommodation produced by a change in convergence is termed "convergent accommodation" (411,412) (see also Chapter 15).

In subjects up to the age of 24 years, convergence-evoked accommodation is equal to the convergence, but beyond that age it gradually diminishes. The diminution of convergent accommodation with age probably is caused by progressive sclerosis of the lens and presbyopia, producing a reduced response to a given innervation and contraction of the ciliary muscle rather than a change in the relative innervations of the two functions (412). Although some investigators explain the relation between convergence stimulus and accommodation on the basis of an afferent feedback loop from the muscle spindles in the medial rectus to the Edinger-Westphal nucleus, others consider the association of convergence and accommodation to be a function of higher nervous activity, namely a function of the cerebral cortex (see previous section on supranuclear innervation of accommodation) (360).

Changes in Accommodation with Age

Some components of both static and dynamic accommodation change with age, whereas others remain constant throughout life (413,414). Specifically, both the speed and the amplitude of accommodation are greatest in the young and gradually decrease until about age 60 years, by which time most normal persons have no ability to perform tonic accommodation. On the other hand, as normal persons age, they show an increase in their subjective depth of focus, possibly from an increased tolerance to defocus related to the gradual onset of presbyopia. Other components of accommodation, including objective depth of focus and the peak velocity/amplitude relationship, remain stable, indicating absence of age effects on the neurologic control of reflex accommodation.

Accommodation in Infants

When examined under cycloplegia, infants tend to be hypermetropic. Attempts at dynamic retinoscopy in the newborn indicate that infants can focus their eyes at only one particular distance, roughly 19 cm (415). Apparently, the normal infant cannot adjust the focus of its eyes to changes in the distance of the object of regard during the 1st month of life. Images of targets nearer or farther away are said to be proportionally blurred. During the first few postnatal months, the range of accommodation increases and is said to approximate adult performance by the 4th month. Because the normal newborn infant is functionally decorticate, it seems reasonable to assume that a lack of inhibition of the Edinger-Westphal and anterior median nuclei would result in parasympathetic overactivity in the eye during the first weeks of life, which may help to explain why the point of focus is relatively close to the eyes during infancy.

Calculation of Accommodation with Age

The amplitude of accommodation diminishes gradually with age. The amount of accommodation remaining at any given age may be approximated using the "Rule of 4's:"

$$\text{Amount of accommodation} = 4^2 - \text{age}/4$$

Thus, for an 8-year-old, the dioptric power of the eye can be increased about 14 diopters by the contraction of the ciliary muscle and the consequent changes in the lens. By 20 years of age, this decreases to 11 diopters. For a 30-year-old, it decreases to 9 diopters, and by 50 years of age, it is about 3 diopters. A 60-year-old normal person has almost no accommodation.

Presbyopia

When the near point has become so far removed that an individual can no longer read fine print, he or she is said to be presbyopic. Presbyopia commences normally from about 35–50 years of age, usually somewhat earlier in women than in men. The principal symptom of presbyopia is inability to read small print. Initially, patients may complain that they are aware of a finite time that it takes them to focus on a near object after viewing at a distance. Often, inability to read is at first present only after prolonged use of the eyes or when the illumination is poor. It also may become evident during an unassociated illness or after surgery. Uncorrected presbyopia may be responsible for headaches, nonspecific eye pain, and chronic ocular irritation. Such symptoms occur only after prolonged use of the eyes and are actually relatively rare.

Presbyopia is a physiologic process that many investigators once thought was caused by increasing sclerosis or hardening of the lens nucleus (416). Clinical experience with lenses dislocated by trauma or removed during cataract surgery appeared to confirm this theory because the usual age-related cataract is discus-shaped, its shape being maintained by the firm lens substance (417). In addition, some investigators found normal or even supernormal ciliary muscle function in prepresbyopic and presbyopic subjects with diminished or absent accommodation (417–422), and in vitro studies of isolated ciliary muscle from rhesus monkeys show no loss of contractility with age (423).

Despite the attractiveness of progressive nuclear sclerosis as the cause of presbyopia, this does not seem to be the case. Numerous investigators have found that with increasing age, there is progressive sclerosis of the ciliary muscle (343,345). When the sclerotic muscle fails to relax the zonular fibers, presbyopia commences. In direct support of the contention that sclerosis of the ciliary muscle, rather than sclerosis of the lens, is responsible for presbyopia, there are many patients in whom presbyopia seems to develop within a few days or weeks. It is difficult to explain such sudden onset of presbyopia on the basis of lens changes, but it seems rational that a muscle functions only as long as its contraction produces the result for which it was intended.

Weale (425) agreed with the ciliary body theory of presbyopia but offered an alternative explanation for the progressive ineffectiveness of the ciliary muscle with age. He suggested that the effectiveness of the muscle is decreased by the constant approximation of the lens equator to the ciliary body. The cause of the proximity is, of course, the consequence of steady growth of both the lens and the ciliary body.

Observations using an animal model of presbyopia in rhesus monkeys show promise of resolving the controversy surrounding presbyopia. When expressed as a percentage of life span, the rate of decline of accommodation in the rhesus monkey closely parallels that in humans (426), supporting the use of this animal as a model for human presbyopia. As noted above, Neider et al. (350) performed slit-lamp and gonioscopic videography in iridectomized rhesus monkeys with stimulating electrodes implanted in the Edinger-Westphal nucleus. These techniques permitted real-time observations of movements of the ciliary body, lens, and zonules. The findings suggest that neither of the two previous theories about presbyopia is correct. During centrally induced accommodation in nonpresbyopic monkeys, Neider et al. observed that: (a) the lens became axially thicker; (b) the ciliary ring narrowed; and (c) at high levels of accommodation, the zonular fibers slackened and even folded, and the lens moved downward. In older presbyopic animals, these investigators noted an age-related decline in sphericization of the lens

induced by maximum stimulation of the Edinger-Westphal nucleus, with preservation of the circumlenticular space, as would be predicted by the classic theory of age-related loss of lenticular elasticity. However, there was a parallel decline in the centripetal excursion of the ciliary processes (i.e., a reduced response of the configurational response of the ciliary muscle to maximal stimulation of the Edinger-Westphal nucleus).

There are several possible explanations for the age-related loss of ciliary muscle responsiveness that produces presbyopia. Light and electron microscopic studies demonstrate only modest morphologic changes and suggest that reduced muscle contractility is not at fault (427). There is no age-related decline in ciliary muscle muscarinic receptor concentration or affinity, nor is there loss of choline acetyltransferase or acetylcholinesterase activity (428). As noted above, in vitro studies of isolated ciliary muscle from rhesus monkeys show no loss of contractility with age (423). It also seems unlikely that the aging zonule becomes rigid enough to ''splint'' the ciliary muscle. Thus, the best hypothesis, consistent with all available evidence, is that presbyopia is attributable primarily to deterioration of the elastic components of the ciliary body and choroids (350). Indeed, such deterioration has been demonstrated histologically (429).

METHODS OF MEASURING ACCOMMODATION

The principal difficulties encountered in the clinical quantitation of accommodation are the subjective nature of the end points and the number of variables that must be controlled if meaningful information is to be obtained.

The accommodative amplitude of an eye is visually estimated by bringing fine print toward it and recording the distance at which the print blurs. However, when the near point of accommodation is measured in this manner, the end point (blurring of the print) is often indistinct because the patient is required to make a judgment of the quality of the image. Egan (430) suggested the use of a cross cylinder in front of the eye with a series of horizontal and vertical lines to replace the fine print. Suddenly seeing the vertical lines blur while the horizontal lines remain sharp should result in an accurate and reproducible near point of accommodation. However, fine print may well represent a better accommodative stimulus than nonspecific lines.

Placing minus lenses in front of the eye is a second method of measuring accommodative power. Minus spheres of gradually increasing power are added to the distance correction until the patient reports a blurred image of a distant accommodative target. The amount of minus sphere that can be overcome by the subject's active focusing is a measure of the accommodative amplitude. If the test is performed at near ($\frac{1}{3}$ meter) with fine print, 3 diopters is added to the result.

Very accurate determinations of accommodative range and amplitude are possible with special instruments such as the high-speed infrared optometer devised by Campbell and Robson (431) and the laser optometer designed by Hennessy and Leibowitz (432).

ANATOMY AND PHYSIOLOGY OF NORMAL LACRIMAL FUNCTION

ANATOMY OF TEAR SECRETION BY THE LACRIMAL GLANDS

The lacrimal gland is situated in the superior lateral corner of the orbit, immediately behind the orbital rim within the lacrimal fossa of the frontal bone (Fig. 14.39). Inferiorly, it is in contact with the globe. Anteriorly, it is divided into an upper (orbital) and lower (palpebral) lobe by the lateral horn of the levator aponeurosis. The upper or superior lobe is bean-shaped, with its medial extremity lying on the levator and its lateral extremity lying on the lateral rectus muscle. The lower or inferior lobe, about half the size of the superior lobe, is situated underneath the levator aponeurosis and connects to the lateral superior conjunctival fornix by a series of excretory ducts. These ducts, about 12 in number, open into the conjunctival sac 4–5 mm above the upper border of the tarsus.

The lacrimal gland is a typical tubuloalveolar exocrine gland composed of small lobules made up of many fine tubules. Each tubule is composed of a layer of cylindrical cells lining the lumen and a layer of flat basal cells lying on a basement membrane. The basal cells are myoepithelial and contractile. The cylindrical cells contain granular cytoplasmic inclusions that histochemically differentiate these cells by their role in tear secretion. The collecting channels are initially intralobular, but later become extralobular, and finally empty into fine ducts. These ducts are lined with a double layer of epithelium. The ultrastructure of the human lacrimal gland has been described by several investigators (433–435).

The fluid produced within the acini of the primary lacrimal gland and secreted by the gland contains water, electrolytes, and protein. The concentrations of these components are then modified by cells of the duct system (436). Parasympathetic and sympathetic nerves innervate the acinar cells, duct cells, and blood vessels of the gland. The parasympathetic nerves contain acetylcholine and VIP. Norepinephrine is contained in the sympathetic nerves, whereas the sensory nerves contain substance P and possibly calcitonin gene-related peptide (CGRP).

Aqueous tear secretion occurs not only from the primary lacrimal gland but also from the accessory lacrimal glands of Krause and Wolfring. These small glands are similar in structure to the main lacrimal gland but are much smaller. The glands of Krause are located in the upper fornix; the glands of Wolfring are situated further down on the eyelid, above the tarsus (Fig. 14.39). It has generally been accepted

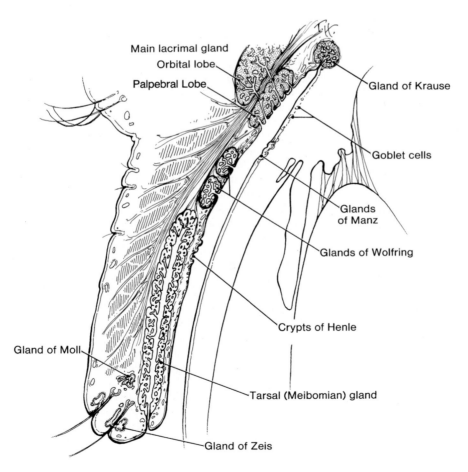

Figure 14.39. Partial schematic representation of secretory tear system. Note locations of primary and accessory lacrimal glands. (Redrawn from Jones LT, Reeh MJ, Wirtschafter JD. Manual of Ophthalmic Anatomy. Rochester, MN, American Academy of Ophthalmology and Otolaryngology, 1970.)

that the main lacrimal gland, having an efferent, parasympathetic innervation, functions primarily during reflex tear secretion, whereas the accessory lacrimal glands provide nonreflex, basal tear secretion (437–441) (see also Chapter 15).

Afferent stimuli causing discharge of the brain stem lacrimal secretory neurons arise from peripheral sensory nerve endings, usually from the trigeminal nerve, but occasionally from the retina. There are two neural pathways by which impulses from the lacrimal nucleus eventually reach the lacrimal gland to induce tear secretion. The parasympathetic pathway is primarily responsible for the gross production of reflex and continuous tears, but the role of the sympathetic system remains controversial.

PARASYMPATHETIC PATHWAY FOR LACRIMATION

The cell bodies of the preganglionic neurons responsible for parasympathetic lacrimal secretion are located in the lacrimal nucleus within the tegmental portion of the pons in a small area dorsal to the superior salivary nucleus (442). After traversing the facial nucleus, the preganglionic axons join the sensory root of the seventh nerve (the nervus intermedius) that emerges from the lateral portion of the pons between the facial and auditory nerves (Figs. 14.40). The ner-

vus intermedius passes through the cistern of the pontine angle and then joins with the rest of the facial nerve, occupying an anterior superior position within the combined nerve as it courses laterally (443) (Fig. 14.41). The surgical anatomy of the nervus intermedius is important because it can be injured during the resection of vestibular schwannomas and other procedures in this area. Symptoms of such injuries include crocodile tears (the gustolacrimal reflex), reduced or absent tear production, and taste abnormalities. These symptoms reflect the sensory and parasympathetic components of the nervus intermedius (444).

After joining the nervus intermedius, the facial nerve enters the internal auditory meatus within the petrous pyramid of the temporal bone (445–448). From here, the meatal segments of the facial nerve enter the labyrinthine segment of the facial canal, having pierced the meninges. After coursing above the vestibule of the inner ear and laterally 2.5–6 mm, the facial nerve trunk turns posteriorly at the geniculate ganglion (Fig. 14.42). The parasympathetic fibers destined for the lacrimal gland pass through the ganglion without synapsing and then separate anteriorly at the apex of the ganglion to become the greater superficial petrosal nerve (Figs. 14.42 and 14.43). The close relationship of the origin of the greater superficial petrosal nerve to the apex of the geniculate gan-

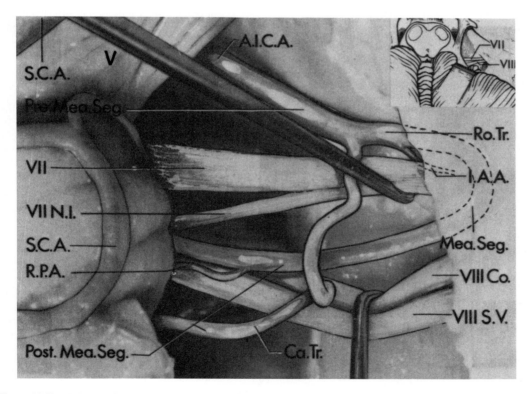

Figure 14.40. Relationships between nervus intermedius, facial nerve trunk, vestibulocochlear nerve trunk, and the superior cerebellar and anterior inferior cerebellar arteries. Nervus intermedius (VII N.I.) exits from the brain stem between the facial nerve trunk (VII) and the cochlear (VIII Co.) and superior vestibular (VIII S.V.) nerve trunks. Note relationships of the rostral (Ro. Tr.) and caudal (Ca. Tr.) trunks of the anterior inferior cerebellar artery (A.I.C.A) to the facial-vestibulocochlear nerve complex. V, trigeminal nerve; S.C.A., superior cerebellar artery; R.P.A., recurrent perforating artery; I.A.A., internal auditory artery; Mea. Seg., meatal segment. (From Martin RG, Grant JL, Peace D, et al. Microsurgical relationships of the anterior inferior cerebellar artery and the facial-vestibulocochlear nerve complex. Neurosurgery 1980;6:483–507.)

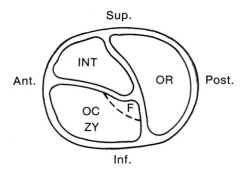

Figure 14.41. Location of the nervus intermedius within the facial nerve trunk just before it reaches the geniculate ganglion. The nervus intermedius (INT) occupies an anterior, superior position in the segment and makes up about 25% of the volume of the nerve at this point. Other branches of the facial nerve include F, frontal; OC, ocular; OR, oral; and ZY, zygomatic. (From Podvinec M, Pfaltz CR. Studies on the anatomy of the facial nerve. Acta Otolaryngol 1976;81:173–177.)

glion can be problematic, as this is the area where most of the facial sensory ganglion cell bodies are located. Thus, a geniculate ganglionectomy performed for facial neuralgia may include a section of the nervus intermedius to achieve a more complete deafferentation. Such a procedure may produce a severe decrease in tear secretion (449).

The greater superficial petrosal nerve, containing the para-

sympathetic fibers for tear secretion, emerges from the temporal bone in the floor of the middle cranial fossa (Fig. 14.43). The nerve then passes beneath the dura of the middle fossa under the gasserian ganglion in Meckel's cave. It enters the vidian canal at the anterior end of the foramen lacerum (Figs. 14.43 and 14.44), joining the deep petrosal nerve from the carotid sympathetic plexus to form the vidian nerve (450) (Fig. 14.44). The vidian nerve passes through the vidian canal directly to the sphenopalatine ganglion, where preganglionic lacrimal axons synapse with postganglionic secretomotor neurons (Figs. 14.8 and 14.44).

The sphenopalatine ganglion is a small structure measuring about 3 mm along its longest diameter. It is situated deep in the upper part of the pterygopalatine fossa, close to the sphenopalatine foramen and immediately below the maxillary nerve that has exited via the foramen rotundum (Figs. 14.8 and 14.44). The pterygopalatine fossa is directly posterior to the maxillary sinus antrum, from which it can be entered surgically or invaded by tumor or infection.

Secretory postganglionic neurons leave the sphenopalatine ganglion and immediately enter the adjacent maxillary division of the trigeminal nerve and travel into the inferior orbital fissure with its zygomatic branch (Figs. 14.8 and 14.44). These nerves run in the lateral wall of the orbit, reaching the lacrimal gland through an anastomosis between the zygomaticotemporal branch of this division and the lacrimal nerve, the latter being a branch of the ophthalmic divi-

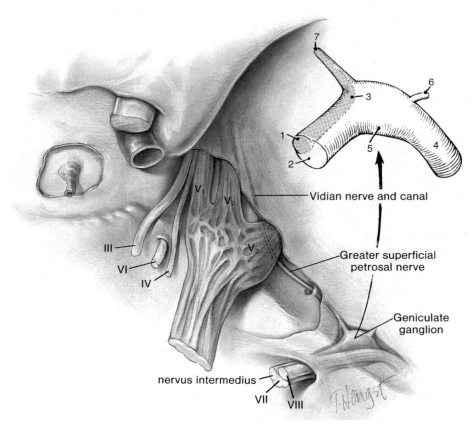

Figure 14.42. Drawing showing the relationship of the nervus intermedius to the facial-vestibulocochlear nerve complex as it enters the cerebrospinal fluid-filled internal acoustic meatus, the location of the geniculate ganglion within the labyrinthine segment of the facial (fallopian) canal, and the location of the greater superficial petrosal nerve within its canal as it courses up the petrous pyramid toward the vidian canal. Inset shows the anatomic relationship of the nervus intermedius (1) and the geniculate ganglion (5) to the facial nerve (2–4) in more detail. 2, first part of facial nerve; 3, genu of facial nerve; 4, second part of facial nerve; 6, lesser superficial petrosal nerve; 7, greater superficial petrosal nerve.

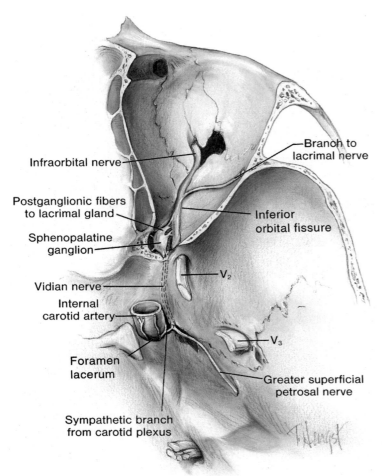

Infraorbital nerve

Postganglionic fibers
to lacrimal gland

Sphenopalatine
ganglion

Vidian nerve

Internal
carotid artery

Foramen
lacerum

Sympathetic branch
from carotid plexus

Branch to
lacrimal nerve

Inferior
orbital fissure

V₂

V₃

Greater superficial
petrosal nerve

Figure 14.43. Emergence of the greater superficial petrosal nerve from the temporal bone in the floor of the middle fossa, viewed from above. The greater superficial petrosal nerve joins with sympathetic fibers (the deep petrosal nerve) to form the vidian nerve. Note anatomic relationships of the inferior orbital fissure, sphenopalatine ganglion in the pterygopalatine fossa, and the maxillary nerve (V2) behind the posterior wall of the orbit and maxillary antrum. V3, mandibular nerve.

sion of the trigeminal nerve. The fibers terminate in the gland between the cells and around the ducts. The autonomic fibers of the lacrimal gland surround the acini but do not penetrate into the glandular cells (451–453). The terminal axons of most of the autonomic fibers to the lacrimal gland contain vesicle-filled varicosities that contain a cholinergic substance and are thought to be parasympathetic in nature. These parasympathetic nerves to the lacrimal gland also produce VIP and induce lacrimation by stimulating a cyclic adenosine monophosphate (cAMP)-dependent signal transduction pathway.

Some portions of the parasympathetic afferent pathway to the lacrimal gland can be evaluated by neuroimaging. In general, MR imaging is superior to computed tomographic (CT) scanning in imaging this pathway; however, CT scanning is more useful in imaging certain portions of the pathway. The lacrimal nucleus cannot be selectively imaged with any study. The nervus intermedius usually is too thin and too closely related to the main trunk of the facial nerve and the vestibulocochlear nerve complex to be imaged separately; however, the water-rich sleeve of cerebrospinal fluid in the internal auditory canal is easily demonstrated and provides an outline for the nerves it contains, including the

meatal segment of the facial nerve. The portion of the facial nerve within the cerebellopontine angle cistern and internal auditory canal is not normally enhanced after intravenous injection of gadolinium-DTPA (454); however, the intracanalicular portion of the facial nerve and the geniculate ganglion can be enhanced in pathologic settings because they have a fairly vascular perineurium. The facial canal can also be imaged by CT scanning (455), which is particularly helpful in the evaluation of fractures and other lesions of the tympanic and more distal portions of the facial canal (455). The portions of the parasympathetic pathway for lacrimation at and distal to the sphenopalatine ganglion may be imaged with CT scanning as a result of the natural contrast supplied by fat both within the pterygopalatine fossa and in the orbit and is complementary to MR imaging of these regions.

SYMPATHETIC PATHWAY FOR LACRIMATION

As discussed earlier in this chapter, preganglionic sympathetic fibers leave the lateral column of the spinal cord, travel along the cervical sympathetic chain, and synapse in the superior cervical ganglion. The postganglionic fibers join the carotid plexus, enter the base of the skull, and pass to

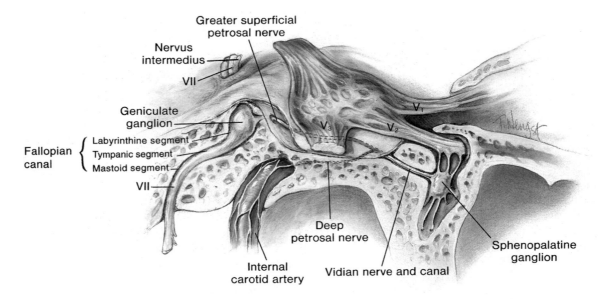

Figure 14.44. Vertical section through the axis of the petrous pyramid of the temporal bone showing the location of the geniculate ganglion and the course of the greater superficial petrosal nerve from the geniculate ganglion to the sphenopalatine ganglion. Some sympathetic fibers leave the internal carotid artery at the foramen lacerum to form the deep petrosal nerve. This nerve joins with the greater superficial petrosal nerve to form the vidian nerve. Also note the connections between the sphenopalatine ganglion and the maxillary nerve trunk (V2). V1, ophthalmic nerve; V3, mandibular nerve.

the lacrimal gland by multiple routes. One recognized route goes to the vidian nerve via the deep petrosal nerve (Fig. 14.44). These fibers pass through the sphenopalatine ganglion, join the zygomaticotemporal nerve, and then pass into the lacrimal gland with the parasympathetic motor fibers. Other sympathetic fibers reach the lacrimal gland via the carotid plexus, the ophthalmic division of the trigeminal nerve, and the lacrimal nerve. Still others may reach the gland via the cavernous sinus neural plexus, the ophthalmic artery, and the lacrimal artery.

Sympathetic nerves play a role in normal continuous tear secretion in humans (456) and in many animals (457–459), but the mechanism by which they do so is unclear (436,460). In addition, some investigators believe that sympathetic fibers to the lacrimal gland serve more of a vasomotor than a secretory function, as they are sparse in lacrimal glands of human (451,453,461,462).

SUPRANUCLEAR PATHWAYS MEDIATING TEAR SECRETION

The cerebral structures and pathways supporting emotional tearing include cortical, limbic, and hypothalamic systems that discharge through descending hypothalamotegmental pathways to the parasympathetic lacrimal nuclei of the pons. Experimental study of these systems is limited by the fact that psychic tearing is a function unique to humans. Pfuhl (463) suggested that psychic lacrimation results from stimulation of the frontal cortical fields responsible for eye motion (the second frontal convolution). In cats, direct projections were demonstrated to the superior salivatory nucleus

from the amygdala, a region in the anterior temporal lobe that is involved in emotional regulation. It is noteworthy that these projections did not pass through hypothalamic synapses, suggesting that lacrimation can be directly affected by the cerebral cortex. Takeuchi et al. (464) and Botelho et al. (457) stated that psychogenic tears may be decreased or increased by lesions of the frontal cortex, basal ganglia, or hypothalamus. Mizukawa et al. (465) reported that stimulation of the ventromedial hypothalamic nucleus of the rabbit causes lacrimation.

NORMAL TEAR FILM

The term ''tears'' refers to fluid that exists as a precorneal film and in the conjunctival sac. The volume of tear fluid is about 5–10 μL (466). Tears are produced by the lacrimal gland, the accessory lacrimal glands, and the goblet cells of the conjunctiva. Normal secretion of tears is about 1–2 μ>L/min (466,467). Except for those tears that evaporate, the tear fluid drains through the lacrimal puncta and canaliculi to the lacrimal sac, which then communicates with the nasal cavity.

Tears have a physically and chemically complex structure that interfaces between the ocular surface and the environment (468). The tear film is about 30–40 μm thick and is composed of three layers: (*a*) a thick inner mucous layer containing mucins, electrolytes, water, immunoglobulin (Ig) A, and several enzymes; (*b*) a thinner aqueous middle layer that contains proteins, including several antibacterial enzymes; and (*c*) a very thin outer lipid layer. A detailed description of the composition of the tear film and the lacrimal secretory system can be found in the volume edited by Sullivan (469) and in Chapter 15 of this text.

TYPES OF TEAR SECRETION

Four different types of lacrimation can be identified in humans: (*a*) continuous tearing, produced constantly for protection and maintenance of a healthy corneal epithelium and a perfectly smooth and transparent corneal refractive surface; (*b*) reflex tearing, stimulated by exposure of the free nerve endings in the eye, nose, and face to light, cold, wind, foreign bodies, or irritating gases and liquids; (*c*) induced tearing, which often develops as an allergically or chemically mediated response to local irritants or by direct nonsynaptic parasympathomimetic action of some drugs on the cAMP-dependent signal transduction pathways in the secretory cells of the lacrimal glands (Fig. 14.45); and (*d*) psychogenic tearing or tears of emotion, which are unique to humans. Young infants cry without shedding tears during the first days of life, and infants born prematurely may not shed tears for weeks. This delayed capacity for psychogenic weeping suggests that the connections within the CNS that indirectly innervate the lacrimal system are not fully developed in most newborns (470).

REGULATION OF TEAR SECRETION

Jones (439) hypothesized that tear secretion could be clinically separated into two types: basal secretion, which originated from the accessory lacrimal glands and occurred independent of stimulation, and reflex secretion, which originated from the main lacrimal gland and occurred only in response to neural stimulation. He believed that the tears that were produced after administration of topical anesthesia were caused by basal secretion. Regardless of the clinical advantages of this classification, this study may have led to the false impression that the role of the nervous system in the regulation of tear production is limited to parasympathetic neural stimulation of the main lacrimal gland. Proof that even basal tear production is neurologically regulated is that basal tearing is essentially eliminated in humans by the injection of lidocaine anesthetic into the sphenopalatine ganglion (471).

Indeed, the formation of all three layers of the tear film is regulated, and much of this regulation is neurally controlled (470a), involving either classic innervation via synaptic connections or atypical, nonsynaptic modulation from the release of neurotransmitters into the biosphere of cells, such as

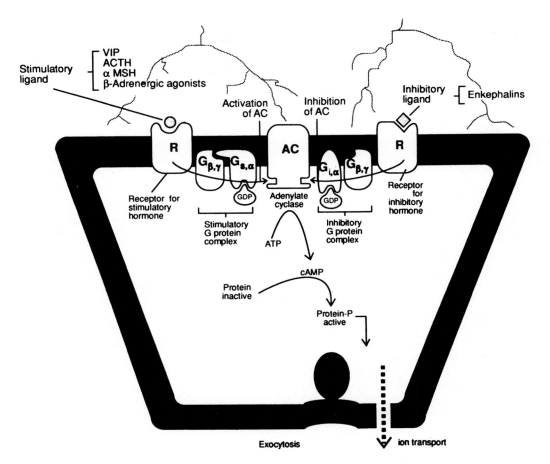

Figure 14.45. Schematic of the cAMP-dependent signal transduction pathway used to stimulate or inhibit main lacrimal gland electrolyte, water, and protein secretion. (From Dartt DA. Regulation of tear secretion. Adv Exp Med Biol 1994;350:1–9.)

the conjunctival goblet cells (436) (Fig. 14.46). For example, wounding of the corneal epithelium is followed by increased mucous secretion from conjunctival goblet cells. Secretion from goblet cells is also increased following the topical application of a number of neurotransmitters, including VIP, serotonin, epinephrine, dopamine, and phenylephrine. Thus, parasympathetic, serotoninergic, dopaminergic, and sympathetic nerves may all be involved in reflex secretion from conjunctival goblet cells (472).

Although sympathetic and parasympathetic nerves are present in the meibomian glands within the upper and lower eyelids, these nerves probably do not regulate the production of the lipid layer of tears (473). This is because the oily

secretion of these glands is produced by holocrine secretion, in which entire cells, including their stored lipids, are released. Lipid layer secretion is believed regulated primarily hormonally, with modulatory neural influences possible. Facial nerve and orbicularis oculi muscle function may play a role in both meibomian gland excretion and the maintenance of the lipid layer of tears by maintaining normal pressure on the excretory ducts (473).

The aqueous layer of the tear film most likely includes water derived not only from the main and accessory lacrimal glands but also from the corneal, and possibly the conjunctival, epithelium. Three classic neurologic pathways that stimulate secretion from the main lacrimal gland have been iden-

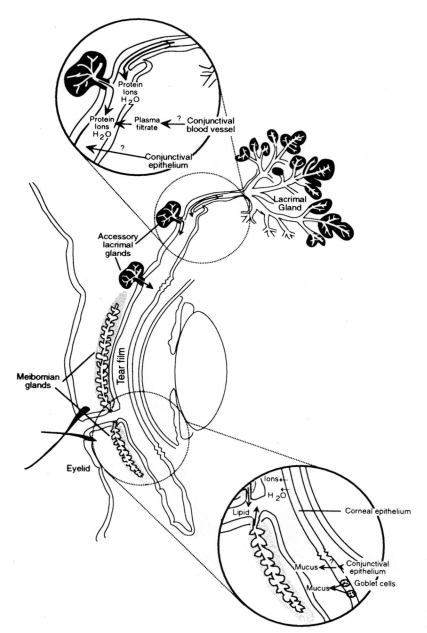

Figure 14.46. Schematic of the orbital glands and ocular epithelia that secrete the different layers of the tear film. (From Dartt DA. Physiology of tear production. In: Lemp MA, Marquardt R, eds. The Dry Eye: A Comprehensive Guide. Berlin: Springer-Verlag, 1992.)

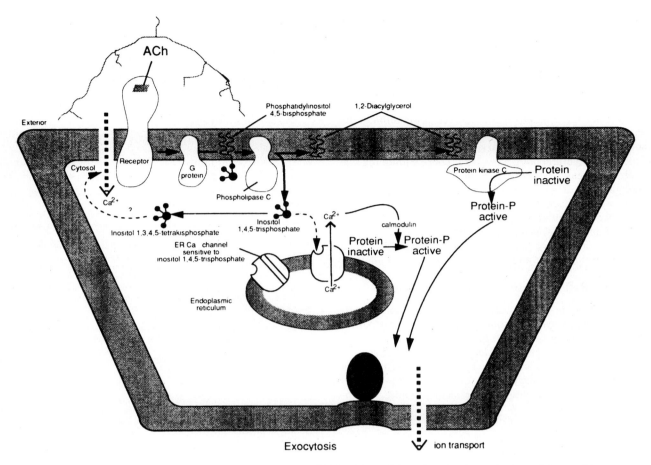

Figure 14.47. Schematic of 1,4,5 inositol triphosphate/Ca^{2+}/diacylglycerol-dependent signal transduction pathway used to stimulate main lacrimal gland electrolyte, water, and protein secretion. (From Dartt DA. Regulation of tear secretion. Adv Exp Med Biol 1994;350:1–9.)

tified: (*a*) the muscarinic cholinergic (Fig. 14.47); (*b*) the α1-adrenergic; and (*c*) the peptidergic (Fig. 14.45).

Acetylcholine acts on the main lacrimal gland via a classic synaptic pathway in which it stimulates a muscarinic receptor and a G protein, leading to a rise of intracellular calcium concentration and the activation of Ca^{2+}/calmodulin protein kinases that phosphorylate specific proteins to activate ion channels in the apical and basilateral membranes. There follows electrolyte, water, and protein secretion and, thus, the production of the primary fluid (Fig 14.47). The pathway just described is known as the 1,4,5-inositol triphosphate/Ca^{2+}/diacylglycerol-dependent signal transduction pathway and is unique to the main lacrimal gland.

The pathway and the mechanism by which α1-adrenergic agonists stimulate lacrimal secretion are unknown. The main lacrimal gland has a neurally controlled cAMP-dependent signal transduction pathway that can either stimulate or inhibit water, electrolyte, and protein secretion. A number of neurotransmitters and neuropeptides, including β-adrenergic agonists, VIP, dopamine, serotonin, and dibutyryl cAMP, all stimulate this cAMP-dependent signal transduction pathway

that phosphorylates protein kinases. The phosphorylated kinases, in turn, cause electrolyte and water secretion from the cytosol. Lacrimal secretion stimulated in this manner can be inhibited by the proenkephalin family of peptides acting through G proteins (Fig. 14.45).

Tears do not originate solely from the main lacrimal gland. Structures to support neurally regulated secretion have also been identified in the accessory lacrimal glands located within the eyelids. Parasympathetic axons with large, dense core vesicles and sympathetic axons with small, dense core vesicles appear to stimulate the cAMP-dependent signal transduction pathway for secretion of water and electrolytes by the accessory lacrimal glands in a manner similar to that for the main lacrimal gland (474). These nerves use a number of hormones, neuromodulators, and β-adrenergic agonists to accomplish this process (Fig. 14.45).

Commonly employed pharmacologic therapies also affect tear secretion. For example, the diuretic hydrochlorothiazide depresses basal tear secretion (475). Even the corneal epithelium contributes cytosolic water by secretion into the aqueous layer of the tear film following stimulation by classic neurotransmitters and neuropeptides, including β-adrenergic agonists, dopamine, serotonin, and dibutyryl cAMP, similar to the membrane system in the lacrimal gland cells.

REFLEXES ASSOCIATED WITH LACRIMATION

Trigeminal-Lacrimal Reflexes

Most reflex lacrimation originates from stimulation of the first division of the trigeminal nerve. The stimulus, if slight, may produce only ipsilateral lacrimation, but beyond a certain point it will affect both eyes (341). These stimuli include all painful diseases of the eye, corneal foreign bodies, and corneal irritants. Many nonocular sources of trigeminal stimulation produce lacrimation. These include tickling of the nasal mucous membrane, painful teeth, and painful sinus disease. Trigeminal-lacrimal reflexes may operate through brain stem connections between the descending spinal tract of the trigeminal nerve and the superior salivatory nucleus.

Other Reflexes Associated with Lacrimation

That bright light causes lacrimation is common knowledge, but the pathways that produce this reflex remain poorly understood. Strong gustatory stimuli may also cause lacrimation. Presumably, the gustatory-lacrimal reflex operates between the gustatory nuclei and the salivary nuclei (including the lacrimal nuclei) in the brain stem. Lacrimation can also be a part of the complicated synkineses of yawning, coughing, and vomiting.

REFERENCES

1. Langley JN, Dickinson WL. On the local paralysis of the peripheral ganglia and on the connection of different classes of nerve fibres with them. Proc R Soc Lond (Biol) 1889;46:423–431.
2. Kaada BR. Somato motor, autonomic and electrocorticographic responses to electrical stimulation of rhinencephalic and other structures in primates, cat and dog. Study of responses from limbic, subcallosal, orbito insular, piriform and temporal cortex, hippocampus, fornix, and amygdala. Acta Physiol Scand 1951; 24 (Suppl 83):1–285.
3. Cannon WB, Rosenblueth A. The sensitization of a sympathetic ganglion by preganglionic denervation. Am J Physiol 1936;16:408–413.
4. MacDonald IA. The sympathetic nervous system and its influence on metabolic function. In: Bannister R, Mathias CJ. Autonomic Failure: A Textbook of Clinical Disorders of the Autonomic Nervous System. Oxford, Oxford Medical Publishers, 1992:197–211 .
5. Pick J. The Autonomic Nervous System. Philadelphia, JB Lippincott, 1970.
6. Burn JH. The Autonomic Nervous System, 5th ed. Oxford, Blackwell Scientific Publications, 1975.
7. Appenzeller O. The Autonomic Nervous System. An Introduction to Basic and Clinical Concepts, 2nd ed. New York, Elsevier, 1976.
8. Gabella G. Structure of the Autonomic Nervous System. New York, John Wiley & Sons, 1976.
9. Koizumi K, Suda I. Induced modulation in autonomic efferent neuron activity. Am J Physiol 1963;205:738.
10. Brodal A. Neurological Anatomy in Relation to Clinical Medicine, 3rd ed. Oxford, Oxford University Press, 1981.
11. Hockman CH. Essentials of Autonomic Function. Springfield, IL, Charles C Thomas, 1987.
12. Parent A. Carpenter's Human Neuroanatomy, 9th ed. Baltimore, Williams & Wilkins, 1996.
13. Yates BJ, Miller AD. Vestibular Autonomic Regulation. Boca Raton, FL, CRC Publishing, 1996.
14. MacLean PD. Some psychiatric implications of physiological studies on frontotemporal portions of limbic system (visceral brain). Electroencephalogr Clin Neurophysiol 1952;4:407–418.
15. Papez JW. A proposed mechanism of emotion. Arch Neurol Psychiatry 1937; 38:725–743.
16. Adey WR, Tokizane T, eds. Structure and function of the limbic system. Prog Brain Res 1967;27:1–475.
17. Hockman CC. Limbic System Mechanics and Autonomic Function. Springfield, IL, Charles C Thomas, 1972.
18. DiCara LV, ed. Limbic and Autonomic Systems Research. New York, Plenum Press, 1974.
19. Isaacson RL. The Limbic System. New York, Plenum Press, 1974.
20. Hall E. The anatomy of the limbic system. In: Mogenson GJ, Calaresu FR, eds. Neural Integration of Physiological Mechanisms and Behavior. Toronto, University of Toronto Press, 1975:68–94.
21. MacLean PD. The Triune Brain in Evolution. New York, Plenum Press, 1989.
22. Dow R, Morruzzi G. Physiology and Pathology of the Cerebellum. Minneapolis, University of Minnesota Press, 1958.
23. Snider RS. Some cerebellar influences on autonomic function. In: Hockman CH, ed. Limbic System Mechanism and Autonomic Function. Springfield, IL, Charles C Thomas, 1972:87.
24. Gorski RA, Gordon JH, Shryne JE, et al. Evidence for a morphalogical sex difference within the medial preoptic area of the rat brain. Brain Res 1978;148: 333–346.
25. Braak H, Braak E. The hypothalamus of the human adult: chiasmatic region. Anat Embryol 1987;175:315–330.
26. Morton A. A quantitative analysis of the normal neuron population of the hypothalamic magnocellular nuclei in man and of their projections to the neurohypophysis. J Comp Neurol 1969;136:143–158.
27. Williams PL, Bannister R. Gray's Anatomy, 38th British ed. London, Churchill Livingstone, 1995.
28. Ingram WR. Nuclear organization and chief connections of the primate hypothalamus. Proc Assoc Res Nerv Ment Dis 1940;20:195–244.
29. Cowan WM, Guillery RW, Powell TPS. The origin of the mammillary peduncle and the hypothalamic connexions from the midbrain. J Anat 1964;98:345–363.
30. Cross BA, Silver IA. Electrophysiological studies on the hypothalamus. Br Med Bull 1966;22:254–258.
31. Palkovits MC, Léránth C, Záborszky L, et al. Electron microscopic evidence of direct neuronal connections from the lower brainstem to the median eminence. Brain Res 1977;136:339–344.
32. Saper CB, Loewy AD, Swanson LW, et al. Direct hypothalamo autonomic connections. Brain Res 1976;117:305–312.
33. Hancock MB. Cells of origin of hypothalamo spinal projections in the cat. Neurosci Lett 1976;3:179–184.
34. Hosoya Y, Matsushita M. Identification and distribution of the spinal and hypophyseal projection neurons in the paraventricular nucleus of the rat. A light and electron microscopic study with the horseradish peroxidase method. Exp Brain Res 1979;35:315–331.
35. Morton A. The time course of retrograde neuron loss in the hypothalamic magnocellular nuclei in man. Brain 1970;93:329–336.
36. Daniel PM, Prichard ML. Studies on the hypothalamus and the pituitary gland. Acta Endocrinol (Copenh) 1975;201 (Suppl 80):1–216.
37. Sherlock DA, Field PM, Raisman G. Retrograde transport of horseradish peroxidase in the magnocellular neurosecretory system of the rat. Brain Res 1975;88: 403–414.
38. Saper CB. Hypothalamus. In: Paxinos G, ed. The Human Nervous System. New York, Academic Press, 1990:389–713.
39. O'Steen WK, Vaughan GM. Radioactivity in the optic pathway and hypothalamus of the rat after intraocular injection of tritiated 5-hydroxytryptophan. Brain Res 1968;8:209–212.
40. Hendrickson AE, Wagoner N, Cowan WM. An autoradiographic and electron microscopic study of retino hypothalamic connections. Z Zellforsch Mikrosk Anat 1972;135:1–26.
41. Moore RY, Lenn NJ. A retinohypothalamic projection in the rat. J Comp Neurol 1972;146:1–14.
42. Moore RY. Retinohypothalamic projection in mammals. A comparative study. Brain Res 1973;49:403–409.
43. Sadun AA, Schaechter JD, Smith LEH. A retinohypothalamic pathway in man: light mediation of circadian rhythms. Brain Res 1984;302:371–377.
44. Moore RY. The organization of the human circadian timing system. Prog Brain Res 1992;93:99–115.
45. Zacharias L, Wurtman RJ. Blindness. Its relation to age of menarche. Science 1964;144:1154–1155.
46. Czeisler CA, Shanahan TL, Klerman EB, et al. Suppression of melatonin secretion in some blind patients by exposure to bright light. N Engl J Med 1995;332: 6–11.
47. Menaker M. Circadian photoreception. Science 2003;299:213–214.
48. Lucas RJ, Hattar S, Takao M, et al. Diminished pupillary light reflex at high irradiance in melanopsin-knockout mice. Science 2003;299:245–247.
49. Ruby NF, Brennan TJ, Xie X, et al. Role of melanopsin in circadian responses to light. Science 2002;298:2211–2213.
50. Hattar S, Liao HW, Takao M, et al. Melanopsin-containing retinal ganglion cells: architecture, projections, and intrinsic photosensitivity. Science 2002;295: 1065–1070.
51. Berson DM, Dunn FA, Takao M. Phototransduction by retinal ganglion cells that set the circadian clock. Science 2002;295:1070–1073.
52. Freedman MS, Lucas RJ, Soni B, et al. Regulation of mammalian circadian

behavior by non-rod, non-cone, ocular photoreceptors. Science 1999;284: 502–504.

52a. Sollars PJ, Smeraski CA, Kaufman JD et al. Melanopsin and non-melanopsin expressing retinal ganglion cells innervate the hypothalamic suprachlasmatic nucleus. Vis Neurosci 2003; 20:601–610.

53. Ganong WF. Review of Medical Physiology, 2nd ed. Los Altos, Lange Medical Publications, 1965.

54. Brooks CM, Koizumi K. The hypothalamus and control of integrative processes. In: Mountcastle VB, ed. Medical Physiology, Vol 1. St Louis, CV Mosby, 1980: 923–947.

55. Bodian D. Cytological aspects of neurosecretion in opossum neurohypophysis. Bull Johns Hopkins Hosp 1963;113:57–93.

56. Kupfermann I. Hypothalamus and limbic system: peptidergic neurons, homeostasis, and emotional behavior. In: Kandel ER, Schwartz JH, Jessell TM, eds. Principles of Neural Science. New York, Elsevier, 1991:735–749.

57. Scheithauer BW, Horvath E, Kovacs K. Ultrastructure of the neurohypophysis. Microsc Res Tech 1992;20:177–186.

58. Pelletier G, Désy L, Coté J, et al. Immunocytochemical localization of corticotropin releasing factor like immunoreactivity in the human hypothalamus. Neurosci Lett 1983;41:259–263.

59. Szentágothai J, Flerkó Mess B, Halász B. Hypothalamic Control of the Anterior Pituitary, 2nd ed. Budapest, Akadémiai Kiakó, 1968.

60. Haymaker W. Hypothalamo pituitary neural pathways and the circulatory system of the pituitary. In: Haymaker W, Anderson E, Nauta WJH, eds. The Hypothalamus. Springfield, IL, Charles C Thomas, 1969:219–250.

61. Popa GT, Fielding U. A portal circulation from the pituitary to the hypothalamic region. J Anat 1930;65:88–91.

62. Porter JC, Jones JC. Effect of plasma from hypophyseal portal vessel blood on adrenal ascorbic acid. Endocrinology 1956;58:62–67.

63. Bernardis LL. Localization of neuroendocrine functions within the hypothalamus. Can J Neurol Sci 1974;1:29–39.

64. Reichlin S, Baldessarini RJ, Martin JB, eds. The Hypothalamus. New York, Raven Press, 1978.

65. Harris GW, George R. Neurohumoral control of the adenohypophysis and regulation of the secretion of TSH, ACTH, and growth hormone. In: Haymaker W, Anderson E, Nauta WJH, eds. The Hypothalamus. Springfield, IL, Charles C Thomas, 1969:326–388.

66. Sawyer CH. Nervous control of ovulation. In: Lloyd CW, ed. Endocrinology of Reproduction. New York, Academic Press, 1959:1–18.

67. Everett JW. Central neural control of reproductive functions of the adenohypophysis. Physiol Rev 1964;44:373–431.

68. Andersson B. Polydipsia, antidiuresis and milk ejection caused by hypothalamic stimulation. In: Heller H, ed. Neurohypophysis. London, Butterworths, 1957: 131–140.

69. Fitzsimons JT. The hypothalamus and drinking. Br Med Bull 1966;22:232–237.

70. Hetherington AW, Ranson SW. Hypothalamic lesions and adiposity in the rat. Anat Rec 1940;78:149–172.

71. Stevenson JAF. Effects of hypothalamic lesions on water and energy metabolism in the rat. Recent Prog Horm Res 1949;4:363–394.

72. Stevenson JAF. Neural control of food and water intake. In: Haymaker W, Anderson E, Nauta WJH, eds. The Hypothalamus. Springfield, IL, Charles C Thomas, 1969:524–621.

73. Anand BK, Brobeck JR. Hypothalamic control of food intake in rats and cats. Yale J Biol Med 1951;24:123–140.

74. Fitzsimons JT. Thirst. Physiol Rev 1972;52:468–561.

75. Grossman SP. Role of the hypothalamus in the regulation of food and water intake. Psychol Rev 1975;82:200–224.

76. Novin D, Wyriecka W, Bray GA. Hunger: Basic Mechanisms and Clinical Applications. New York, Raven Press, 1976.

77. Leibowitz SF. Brain catecholaminergic mechanisms for control of hunger. In: Novin D, Wyriecka W, Bray GA, eds. Hunger: Brain Mechanisms and Clinical Implications. New York, Raven Press, 1976:1–18.

78. Brownstein MJ, Mezey E. Multiple chemical messengers in hypothalamic magnocellular neurons. Prog Brain Res 1986;68:161–168.

79. Myers RD. Temperature regulation. Neurochemical systems in the hypothalamus. In: Haymaker W, Anderson E, Nauta WJH, eds. The Hypothalamus. Springfield, IL, Charles C Thomas, 1969:506–523.

80. Hensel H. Neural processes in thermoregulation. Physiol Rev 1973;53: 948–1017.

81. Selye H. Homeostasis and the reactions to stress. A discussion of Walter B Cannon's contributions. In: Brooks CM, Koizumi K, Pinkston JO, eds. The Life and Contributions of Walter Bradford Cannon. Albany, State University of New York Press, 1975:89.

82. von Economo C. Die Encephalitis Lethargica ihre Nachkrankheiten und ihre Behandlung. Berlin, Urban & Schwarzenberg, 1929.

83. Clemente CD, Sterman MB. Cortical synchronization and sleep patterns in acute restrained and chronic behaving cats induced by basal forebrain stimulations. Electroencephalogr Clin Neurophysiol (Suppl) 1963;24:172–187.

84. Hernández Peón R, Chávez Ibarra G. Sleep induced by electrical or chemical stimulation of the forebrain. Electroencephalogr Clin Neurophysiol (Suppl) 1963;24:188–198.

85. Lin JS, Sakai K, Jouvet M. Evidence for histaminergic arousal mechanisms in the hypothalamus of cat. Neuropharmacology 1988;27:111–122.

86. Lin JS, Sakai K, Vannier Mercier G, et al. A critical role of the posterior hypothalamus in the mechanisms of wakefulness determined by microinjection of muscimol in freely moving cats. Brain Res 1989;479:225–240.

87. Sakai K, Yoshimoto Y, Luppi PH, et al. Lower brainstem afferents to the cat posterior hypothalamus. A double labelling study. Brain Res Bull 1990;24: 437–455.

88. Calaresu FR, Faiers AA, Mogenson GJ. Central neural regulation of heart and blood vessels in mammals. Neurobiology 1975;5:1–35.

89. Pitts RF, Magoun HW, Ranson SW. Localization of the medullary respiratory centers in the cat. Am J Physiol 1939;126:673–688.

90. Ranson SW, Billingsley PR. Vasomotor reactions from stimulation of the floor of the fourth ventricle. Am J Physiol 1916;41:85–90.

91. Langley JN. The Autonomic Nervous System. Cambridge, England, W Heffer and Sons, Ltd, 1921.

92. Crosby EC, Humphrey T, Lauer EW. Correlative Anatomy of the Nervous System. New York, Macmillan, 1962.

93. Ebbesson SOE. Quantitative studies of superior cervical sympathetic ganglia in a variety of primates including man. II. Neuronal packing density. J Morphol 1968;124:181–186.

94. Nieuwenhuys R. Chemoarchitecture of the Brain. Berlin, Springer Verlag, 1985.

95. Dale HH. Chemical transmission of the effects of nerve impulses. Br Med J 1934;1:834.

96. Burnstock G. Purinergic nerves. Pharmacol Rev 1972;24:509–581.

97. Bredt DS, Hwang PM, Snyder SH. Localization of nitric oxide synthase indicating a neural role for nitric oxide. Nature 1990;347:768–770.

98. Rand MJ. Nitrergic transmission. Nitric oxide as a mediator of nonadrenergic, noncholinergic neuroeffector transmission. Clin Exp Pharmacol Physiol 1992; 19:147–169.

99. Hillarp NA. The construction and functional organization of the autonomic innervation apparatus. Acta Physiol Scand 1959;46(Suppl 157):1–38.

100. Burnstock G. Autonomic neuromuscular junctions: current developments and future directions. J Anat 1986;146:1–30.

101. Murray JG, Thompson JW. The occurrence and function of collateral sprouting in the sympathetic nervous system of the cat. J Physiol (Lond) 1957;135: 133–162.

102. Murray JG. The consequences of injury and disease of nervous tissue: recent advances in knowledge. J R Coll Surg Edinb 1959;4:199–217.

103. Causey G, Hoffman H. Axon sprouting in partially deneurotized nerves. Brain 1955;78:661–668.

104. Rushton WAW. Visual adaptation: the Ferrier lecture. Proc R Soc Biol (Lond) 1965;162:20–46.

105. Campbell FW. The depth of field of the human eye. Optica Acta 1957;4: 157–164.

106. Westheimer G. Pupil size and visual resolution. Vision Res 1964;4:39–45.

107. Campbell FW, Green DG. Optical and retinal factors affecting visual resolution. J Physiol 1965;181:576–593.

108. Charman WN, Jenning JAM, Whitefoot H. The refraction of the eye in relation to spherical aberration and pupil size. Vision Res 1978;17:737–738.

109. Loewenfeld IE. The Pupil: Anatomy, Physiology, and Clinical Applications. Ames, Iowa, Iowa State University Press; Detroit, MI, Wayne State University Press, 1993.

110. Schweitzer NMJ. Threshold measurements on the light reflex of the pupil in the dark-adapted eye. Doc Ophthalmol 1956;10:1–78.

111. Loewenfeld IE. Pupillary movements associated with light and near vision: an experimental review of the literature. In: Whitcomb M, ed. Recent Developments in Vision Research. Publication No. 1272. Washington, DC, National Academy of Sciences, National Research Council, 1966:17–105.

112. ten Doesschate J, Alpern M. Response of the pupil to steady state retinal illlumination: contribution by cones. Science 1965;149:989–991.

113. Slooter J, Van Norren D. Visual acuity measured with pupil responses to checkerboard stimuli. Invest Ophthalmol Visual Sci 1980;19:105–108.

114. Ukai K. Spatial pattern as a stimulus to the pupillary system. J Opt Soc Am 1985;2:1094–1100.

115. Barbur JL, Forsyth PM. Can the pupil response be used as a measure of visual input associated with the geniculo-striate pathway? Clin Vision Sci 1986;1: 107–111.

116. Barbur JL, Thomson WD. Pupil response as an objective measure of visual acuity. Ophthal Physiol Opt 1987;7:425–429.

117. Barbur JL, Keenleyside MS, Thomson WD. Investigation of central visual processing by means of pupillometry. In: Kulikowski JJ, Dickinson CM, Murray IJ, eds. Seeing Color and Contour. Oxford, Pergamon Press, 1989:431–451.

118. Barbur JL, Harlow AJ, Sahraie A. Pupillary responses to stimulus structure, colour, and movement. Ophthal Physiol Opt 1992;12:137–141.

119. Cocker KD, Moseley MJ. Visual acuity and the pupil grating response. Clin Vision Sci 1992;7:143–146.

120. Young RSL, Han B, Wu P. Transient and sustained components of the pupillary responses evoked by luminance and color. Vision Res 1993;33:437–446.

121. Young RSL, Kennish J. Transient and sustained components of the pupil response evoked by achromatic spatial patterns. Vision Res 1993;33:2239–2252.

122. Duke-Elder S, Scott GI. System of Ophthalmology. Vol 12. London, Henry Kimpton, 1971:656.
123. Thompson HS, Montague P, Cox TA, et al. The relationship between visual acuity, pupillary defect, and visual field loss. Am J Ophthalmol 1982;93: 681–688.
124. Brown RH, Zillis JD, Lynch MG, et al. The afferent pupillary defect in asymmetric glaucoma. Arch Ophthalmol 1987;105:1540–1543.
125. Johnson LN, Hill RA, Bartholomew MJ. Correlation of afferent pupillary defect with visual field loss on automated perimetry. Ophthalmology 1988;95: 1649–1655.
126. Kardon RH, Haupert C, Thompson HS. The relationship between static perimetry and the relative afferent pupillary defect. Am J Ophthalmol 1993;115:351–356.
127. Kardon RH, Kirkali PA, Thompson HS. Automated pupil perimetry. Ophthalmology 1991;98:485–495.
128. Kardon RH. Pupil perimetry. Current Opin Ophthalmol 1992;3:565–570.
129. Bowling DB, Michael CR. Projection patterns of single physiologically characterized optic tract fibers in the cat. Nature 1980;286:899–902.
130. Parsons JH. The physiology of pupil reactions. Trans Ophthalmol Soc UK 1924; 44:1–11.
131. O'Connor PS, Kasdon D, Tredici TJ, et al. The Marcus Gunn pupil in experimental optic tract lesions. Ophthalmology 1982;89:160–164.
132. Newman SA, Miller NR. The optic tract syndrome: neuro-ophthalmologic considerations. Arch Ophthalmol 1983;101:1241–1250.
133. Karplus JP, Kreidl A. Ueber die bahn des pupillarreflexes (die reflectorische pupillenstarre). Pflugers Archiv Ges Physiol Menschen Tiere 1913;149: 115–155.
134. Ellis CJK. Afferent pupillary defect in pineal region tumour. J Neurol Neurosurg Psychiatry 1984;47:739–741.
135. Eliott D, Cunningham ET Jr, Miller NR. Fourth nerve paresis and ipsilateral relative afferent pupillary defect without visual sensory disturbance: a sign of contralateral dorsal midbrain disease. J Clin Neuroophthalmol 1991;11: 169–172.
136. Levinsohn G. Beitrag zur physiologie des pupillenreflexes. Albrecht von Graefes Arch Ophthalmol 1904;59:191–220.
137. Levinsohn G. Beitrag zur physiologie des pupillenreflexes. Albrecht von Graefes Arch Ophthalmol 1904;59:436–458.
138. Ranson SW, Magoun HW. The central path of the pupillo-constrictor reflex in response to light. Arch Neurol Psychiatr 1933;30:1193–1204.
139. Carpenter MB, Peter P. Accessory oculomotor nuclei in the monkey. J Hirnforsch 1970;12:405–418.
140. Scalia F. The termination of retinal axons in the pretectal region of mammals. J Comp Neurol 1972;145:223–257.
141. Carpenter MB, Pierson RJ. Pretectal region and the pupillary light reflex: an anatomical analysis in the monkey. J Comp Neurol 1973;149:271–300.
142. Kanaseki T, Sprague JM. Anatomical organization of pretectal nuclei and tectal laminae in the cat. J Comp Neurol 1974;158:319–338.
143. Benevento LA, Rezak M, Santos-Anderson R. An autoradiographic study of the projections of the pretectum in the rhesus monkey (Macaca mulatta): evidence for sensorimotor links to the thalamus and oculomotor nuclei. Brain Res 1977; 127:197–218.
144. Hendrickson A, Wilson ME, Toyne MJ. The distribution of optic nerve fibers in Macaca mulatta. Brain Res 1970;23:425–427.
145. Pierson R, Carpenter MB. Anatomical analysis of pupillary reflex pathways in the rhesus monkey. J Comp Neurol 1974;158:121–144.
146. Tigges J, O'Steen WK. Termination of retinofugal fibers in squirrel monkey: a reinvestigation using autoradiographic methods. Brain Res 1974;79:489–495.
147. Brodal A. Neurological Anatomy in Relation to Clinical Medicine. 3rd ed. New York, Oxford University Press, 1981.
148. Kourouyan HD, Horton JC. Transneuronal retinal input to the primate Edinger-Westphal nucleus. J Comp Neurol 1997;380:1–13.
149. Burde RM. The visceral nuclei of the oculomotor complex. Trans Am Ophthalmol Soc 1983;81:532–548.
150. Clarke RJ, Gamlin PDR. The role of the pretectum in the pupillary light reflex. In: Robbins J, ed. Basic and Clinical Perspectives in Vision Research. New York, Plenum Press, 1995.
151. Gamlin PDR, Clarke RJ. The pupillary light reflex pathway of the primate. J Am Optom Assoc 1995;66:415–418.
152. Gamlin PDR, Zhang H, Clarke RJ. Luminance neurons in the pretectal olivary nucleus mediate the pupillary light reflex in the rhesus monkey. Exp Brain Res 1995;106:177–180.
153. Reiner A, Williams J, Gamlin PDR. Characterization of neuropeptides, calcium binding proteins and glutamate receptors found in the olivary pretectal nucleus of the Rhesus monkey. Invest Ophthalmol Vis Sci 1995;36:S292.
154. Hess C. Untersuchungen über die ausdehnung des pupillomotorisch wirksamen bezirkes der netzhaut und über die pupillomotoischen aufnahmeorgane. Arch Augenheilkd 1907;58:182–205.
155. Barris RW. A pupillo-constrictor area in the cerebral cortex of the cat and its relationship to the pretectal area. J Comp Neurol 1936;63:353–368.
156. Jampel RS. Representation of the near-response on the cerebral cortex of the macaque. Am J Ophthalmol 1959;48:573–582.
157. Lui F, Gregory KM, Blanks HI, et al. Projections from visual areas of the cerebral

cortex to pretectal nuclear complex, terminal accessory optic nuclei, and superior colliculus in macaque monkey. J Comp Neurol 1995;363:439–460.
158. Frydrychowicz G, Harms H. Ergebnisse pupillomotorischer untersuchungen bei gesunden und kranken. Verh Dtsch Ophthalmol Ges 1940;53:71–80.
159. Harms H. Hemianopische pupillenstarre. Klin Monatsbl Augenheilkd 1951;118: 133–147.
160. Harms H. Möglichkeiten und grenzen der pupillometrischen perimetrie. Klin Monatsbl Augenheilkd 1956;129:518–534.
161. Cibis GW, Campos EC, Aulhorn E. Pupillary hemiakinesia in suprageniculate lesions. Arch Ophthalmol 1975;93:1322–1327.
162. Hamann KU, Hellner K, Müller-Jensen A, et al. Videopupillographic and VER investigations in patients with congenital and acquired lesions of the optic radiation. Ophthalmologica 1979;178:348–356.
163. Hamann KU, Hellner KA, Jensen W. The dynamics and latency of the pupillary response in cases of homonymous hemianopia. Neuroophthalmology 1981;2: 23–33.
164. Kardon RH. Pupil perimetry. In: Tusa RJ, Neuman SA, eds. Neuro-Ophthalmological Disorders. New York, Marcel Dekker Inc, 1995.
165. Sprague JM. Interaction of cortex and superior colliculus in mediation of visually guided behavior in the cat. Science 1966;153:1544–1547.
166. Mohler CW, Wurtz RH. Role of striate cortex and superior colliculus in visual guidance of saccadic eye movements in monkeys. J Neurophysiol 1977;40: 74–94.
167. Zihl J, von Cramon D. Perimetric testing of superior colliculus function in man: a case study. Nervenarzt 1978;49:488–491.
168. Miller NR, Newman SA. Transsynaptic degeneration. Arch Ophthalmol 1981; 99:1654.
169. Beatty RM, Sadun AA, Smith LEH, et al. Direct demonstration of transsynaptic degeneration in the human visual system: a comparison of retrograde and anterograde changes. J Neurol Neurosurg Psychiatry 1982;45:143–146.
170. Lowenstein O, Loewenfeld IE. The pupil. In: Davson H, ed. The Eye, Vol 3. New York, Academic Press, 1962:231–267.
171. Karplus JP, Kreidl A. Gehirn und sympathicus. I. Mitteilung zwischenhirnbasis und halssympathicus. Arch Anat Physiol 1909;129:138–144.
172. Sano K, Mayanagi Y, Sekino H, et al. Results of stimulation and destruction of the posterior hypothalamus in man. J Neurosurg 1970;33:689–707.
173. Balasubramaniam V, Kanaka TS, Ramanujam PB, et al. Electrophysiological studies during sedative neurosurgery. Neurology (Madras) 1972;20 (Suppl 2): 175–178.
174. Schvarcz JR, Driollet R, Rios E, et al. Stereotactic hypothalamotomy for behavior disorders. J Neurol Neurosurg Psychiatry 1972;35:356–359.
175. Kalyanaraman S. Some observations during stimulation of the human hypothalamus. Confin Neurol 1975;37:189–192.
176. Bechterew A. Über den verlauf der die pupille verengernden nervenfasern im gehirn und über die localisation eines centrums für die iris und contraction der augenmuskeln. Pflugers Archiv Ges Physiol Menschen Tiere 1883;31:60–87.
177. Kuntz A, Richins CA. Reflex pupillodilator mechanisms: an experimental analysis. J Neurophysiol 1946;9:1–7.
178. McSwiney BA, Suffolk SF. Segmental distribution of certain visceral afferent neurones of the pupillodilator reflex in the cat. J Physiol (Lond) 1938;98: 104–116.
179. Ury B, Gellhorn E. Role of sympathetic system in reflex dilatation of pupil. J Neurophysiol 1939;2:268–275.
180. Kerr FWL, Brown JA. Pupillomotor pathways in the spinal cord. Arch Neurol 1964;10:262–270.
181. Loewy AD, Araujo JC, Kerr FWL. Pupillodilator pathways in the brain stem of the cat: anatomical and electrophysiological identification of a central autonomic pathway. Brain Res 1973;60:65–91.
182. Kerr FWL. The ventral spinothalamic tract and other ascending systems of the ventral funiculus of the cord. J Comp Neurol 1975;159:335–356.
183. Koss MC. Pupillary dilation as an index of central nervous system alpha-2 adrenoceptor activation. J Pharmacol Methods 1986;15:1–19.
184. Christensen HD, Koss MC, Gherezghiher T. Synaptic organization in the oculomotor nucleus. Ann NY Acad Sci 1986;473:382–399.
185. Edinger L. Über den verlauf der centralen hirnnervenbahnen mit demonstration von präparaten. Neurol Zentralbl 1985;4:309.
186. Westphal C. Über einen fall von chronischer progressive lähmung des augenmuskeln (ophthalmoplegia externa) nebst beschreibung von ganglienzellengruppen im bereich des oculomotoriuskerns. Arch Psychiatr Nervenkr 1887;98:846.
187. Perlia R. Die anatomie des oculomotoriuscentrums deim menschen. Albrecht von Graefes Arch Ophthalmol 1889;35:287–304.
188. Olszewski J, Baxter D. Cytoarchitecture of the Human Brainstem. Philadelphia, Lippincott, 1954.
189. Akert K, Glicksman MA, Lang W, et al. The Edinger-Westphal nucleus in the monkey: a retrograde tracer study. Brain Res 1980;184:491–498.
190. Warwick R. The ocular parasympathetic nerve supply and its mesencephalic sources. J Anat 1954;88:71–93.
191. Burde RM, Loewy AD. Central origin of oculomotor parasympathetic neurons in the monkey. Brain Res 1980;198:434–439.
192. Jampel RS, Mindel J. The nucleus for accommodation in the midbrain of the macaque. Invest Ophthalmol 1967;6:40–50.

193. Szentágothai J. Die zentrale leitungsbahn des lichtreflexes der pupillen. Arch Psychiatr 1942;115:136–156.
194. Ksiazek SM, Slamovits TL, Rosen CE, et al. Fascicular arrangement in partial oculomotor paresis. Am J Ophthalmol 1994;118:97–103.
195. Sunderland S, Hughes ESR. The pupillo-constrictor pathway and the nerves to the ocular muscles in man. Brain 1946;69:301–309.
196. Kerr FWL, Hollowell OW. Location of pupillomotor and accommodation fibres in the oculomotor nerve: experimental observations on paralytic mydriasis. J Neurol Neurosurg Psychiatry 1964;27:473–481.
197. Dreyfus PM, Hakim S, Adams RD. Diabetic ophthalmoplegia: report of case, with postmortem study and comments on vascular supply of human oculomotor nerve. Arch Neurol Psychiatr 1957;77:337–349.
198. Asbury AK, Aldredge H, Hershberg R, et al. Oculomotor palsy in diabetes mellitus: a clinico-pathological study. Brain 1970;93:555–566.
199. Weber RB, Daroff RB, Mackey EA. Pathology of oculomotor nerve palsy in diabetics. Neurology 1970;20:835–838.
200. Sinnreich Z, Nathan H. The ciliary ganglion in man. Anat Anz 1981;150:287–297.
201. Grimes P, von Sallmann L. Comparative anatomy of the ciliary nerves. Arch Ophthalmol 1960;64:81–91.
202. Eliskova M. Blood vessels of the ciliary ganglion in man. Br J Ophthalmol 1973;57:766–772.
203. Budge J, Waller A. Recherches sur le système nerveaux: action de la partie cervicale du nerf grand sympathique et d'une portion de la moelle épinière sur la dilation de la pupille. C R Acad Sci (Paris) 1851;33:370–374.
204. Budge J, Waller A. Prix de physiologie expérimentale de l'année 1852. C R Acad Sci (Paris), 1852.
205. Carmel PW. Sympathetic deficits following thalamotomy. Arch Neurol 1968;18:378–387.
206. Palumbo LT. A new concept of the sympathetic pathways to the eye. Ann Ophthalmol 1976;8:947–954.
207. Matus AI. Ultrastructure of the superior cervical ganglion fixed with zinc iodide and osmium tetroxide. Brain Res 1970;17:195–203.
208. Kondo H, Fujiwara S. Granule-containing cells in the human superior cervical ganglion. Acta Anat 1979;103:192–199.
209. Wolff GA Jr. The ratio of preganglionic neurons to postganglionic neurons in the visceral nervous system. J Comp Neurol 1941;75:235–243.
210. Johnston JA, Parkinson D. Intracranial sympathetic pathways associated with the sixth cranial nerve. J Neurosurg 1974;39:236–243.
211. Parkinson D, Johnston J, Chaudhuri A. Sympathetic connections to the fifth and sixth cranial nerve. Anat Rec 1978;191:221–226.
212. Duke-Elder S. System of Ophthalmology. Vol 2. St Louis, CV Mosby, 1961.
213. Solnitzky O. Horner's syndrome: its diagnostic significance. Georgetown Univ Med Cent Bull 1961;14:204–222.
214. Loewenfeld IE. Mechanisms of reflex dilatation of the pupil: historical review and experimental analysis. Doc Ophthalmol 1958;12:185–448.
215. Saari M, Kiviniemi P, Johansson G, et al. Wallerian degeneration of the myelinated nerves of cat iris after denervation of the ophthalmic division of the trigeminal nerve: an electron microscopic study. Exp Eye Res 1973;17:281–287.
216. Huhtala A. Origin of myelinated nerves in the rat iris. Exp Eye Res 1976;22:259–265.
217. Almegraàd B, Stjernschantz J, Bill A. Cholecystokinin contracts isolated human and monkey iris sphincters: a study with CCK receptor antagonists. Eur J Pharmacol 1992;211:183–187.
218. Hogan MJ, Alvarado JA, Weddell JE. Histology of the Human Eye: An Atlas and Textbook. Philadelphia, Saunders, 1971:202–256.
219. Manuelli G, Carella G, Ghisolfi A. Ultrastructure, histoenzymologie et microangiotectonique de l'iris humain. Arch Ophthalmol 1972;32:633–652.
220. Fine BS, Yanoff M. Ocular Histology: A Text and Atlas. 2nd ed. New York, Harper and Row, 1979:197–214.
221. Salzmann M. The iris. In: The Anatomy and Physiology of the Human Eyeball in the Normal State [translated by Brown EVL]. Chicago, Chicago University Press, 1912.
222. van Alphen GW. The structural changes in miosis and mydriasis of the monkey eye. Arch Ophthalmol 1963;69:802–814.
223. van Alphen GW. Scanning electron microscopy of the monkey eye in miosis and mydriasis. Exp Eye Res 1979;29:511–526.
224. Newsome DA, Loewenfeld IE. Iris mechanics. II. Influence of pupil size on details of iris structure. Am J Ophthalmol 1971;71:553–573.
225. Schaeppi U, Koella WP. Innervation of the cat iris dilator. Am J Physiol 1964;207:1411–1416.
226. Ehinger B, Falck B, Persson H. Function of cholinergic nerve fibres in the cat. Acta Physiol Scand 1968;72:139–147.
227. Yoshitomi T, Ito Y. Double reciprocal innervations in dog iris sphincter and dilator muscles. Invest Ophthalmol Vis Sci 1986;27:83–121.
228. Narita S, Watanabe M. Response of isolated rat iris dilator to adrenergic and cholinergic agents and electrical stimulation. Life Sci 1982;30:1211–1218.
229. Suzuki R, Oso T, Kobayashi S. Cholinergic response in the bovine iris dilator muscle. Invest Ophthalmol Vis Sci 1983;24:760–765.
230. Yoshitomi T, Ito Y, Inomata H. Adrenergic excitatory and cholinergic inhibitory innervations in the human iris dilator. Exp Eye Res 1985;40:453–459.
231. Nomura T, Smelser GK. The identification of adrenergic and cholinergic nerve endings in the trabecular meshwork. Invest Ophthalmol 1974;13:525–532.
232. Johnson SH, Brubaker RF, Trautmann JC. Absence of an effect of timolol on the pupil. Invest Ophthalmol Vis Sci 1978;17:924–926.
233. Lind NA, Shinebourne E. Studies on the development of the autonomic innervation of the human iris. Br J Pharmacol 1972;38:462P.
234. Laor N, Korczyn AD, Nemet P. Sympathetic pupillary activity in infants. Pediatrics 1977;59:195–198.
235. Romano PE. Pupillary size in infants. Pediatrics 1977;60:762.
236. Kadlecová V, Peleska M. The effect of vegetative pupillary tone and iridic tissue on the pupillary diameter in aging. Cesk Oftalmol 1957;13:283–293.
237. Kadlecová V, Peleska M. The infrascopical study of the effect of cocaine on the pupil and its dependence on age. Cesk Oftalmol 1958;14:168–173.
238. Kadlecová V, Peleska M, Vasko A. Dependence on age of the diameter of the pupil in dark. Nature 1958;182:1520–1521.
239. Loewenfeld IE. "Simple, central" anisocoria: a common condition, seldom recognized. Trans Am Acad Ophthalmol Otolaryngol 1977;83:832–839.
240. Loewenfeld IE. Pupillary changes related to age. In: Thompson HS, Daroff R, Frisén L, et al, eds. Topics in Neuro-Ophthalmology. Baltimore, Williams & Wilkins, 1979:124–150.
241. Korczyn AD, Laor N, Nemet P. Sympathetic pupillary tone in old age. Arch Ophthalmol 1976;94:1905–1906.
242. Loewenfeld IE, Newsome DA. Iris mechanics. I. Influence of pupil size on dynamics of pupillary movements. Am J Ophthalmol 1971;71:347–362.
243. Semmlow J, Hansmann D, Stark L. Variation in pupillomotor responsiveness with mean pupil size. Vision Res 1975;15:85–90.
244. Tyner G, Scheie H. Mechanism of the miotic resistant pupil with increased intraocular pressure. Arch Ophthalmol 1953;50:572–579.
245. Jaeger EA, Weeks SD, Duane TD. Pupillary responses during ophthalmodynamometry. Arch Ophthalmol 1963;70:453–455.
246. Charles ST, Hamasaki DI. The effect of intraocular pressure on the pupil size. Arch Ophthalmol 1970;83:729–733.
247. Rutkowski PC, Thompson HS. Mydriasis and increased intraocular pressure. I. Pupillographic studies. Arch Ophthalmol 1972;87:21–24.
248. Rutkowski PC, Thompson HS. Mydriasis and increased intraocular presssure. II. Iris fluorescein studies. Arch Ophthalmol 1972;87:25–29.
249. French H. Index of Differential Diagnosis. 4th ed. New York, William Wood & Co, 1928.
250. Fuchs E. Diseases of the Eye. 10th ed. New York, JB Lippincott, 1932.
251. Meyer BC. Incidence of anisocoria and difference in size of palpebral fissures in five hundred normal subjects. Arch Neurol Psychiatr 1947;57:464–468.
252. Glaser JS. Neuro-ophthalmology. Hagerstown, MD, Harper and Row, 1978:174.
253. Lam BL, Thompson HS, Walls RC. Effect of light on the prevalence of simple anisocoria. Ophthalmology 1996;103:790–793.
254. Lam BL, Thompson HS, Corbett JJ. The prevalence of simple anisocoria. Am J Ophthalmol 1987;104:69–73.
255. Parker JA. Distortion of pupil size by the cornea. Can J Ophthalmol 1973;8:474–475.
256. Loewenfeld IE, Rosskothen HD. Infrared pupil camera: a new method for mass screening and clinical use. Am J Ophthalmol 1974;78:304–313.
257. Spencer JA, Czarnecki JSC. The pupil in stroke. Can J Ophthalmol 1983;18:226–227.
258. Gianelli A. Sulle modificazioni del diametro pupillare nei movimenti de lateralità dei bulbi oculari. Richerche Psichiatr Neurol Antropol Filosof IV S 1907;8:433.
259. Tournay A. Le lois d'isocorie et de l'anisocorie normales. Bull Acad Méd Paris 1917;3:680.
260. Tournay A. Sur l'anisocorie normale dans le regard latéral extrême. Arch Ophthalmol 1927;44:574–576.
261. Chenet L, Noyer A. Étude sur la réaction de Tournay. Arch Ophthalmol 1921;38:336.
262. Behr C. Die lehre von den pupillenbewegungen. In: von Graefe A, Saemisch T, eds. Handbuch der Gesammten Augenheilkunde. 3rd ed, Vol 2. Leipzig, W Engelmann, 1924:54.
263. Sharpe JA, Glaser JS. Tournay's phenomenon: a reappraisal of anisocoria in lateral gaze. Am J Ophthalmol 1974;77:250–255.
264. Loewenfeld IE, Friedlander RP, McKinnon PFM. Pupillary inequality associated with lateral gaze (Tournay's phenomenon). Am J Ophthalmol 1974;78:449–469.
265. Norrie G. Kleine beiträge. II. Oscillatio pupillae. Cent Augenheilkd 1888;12:232.
266. Hunter JD, Milton JG, Lüdtke H, et al. Spontaneous fluctuations in pupil size are not triggered by lens accommodation. Vision Res 2000;40:567–573.
267. Fernández-Guardiola A, Harmony T, Roldán E. Modulation of visual input by pupillary mechanisms. Electroencephalogr Clin Neurophysiol 1964;16:259–268.
268. Thompson HS, Franceschetti AT, Thompson PM. Hippus: semantic and historic considerations of the word. Am J Ophthalmol 1971;71:1116–1120.
269. Wilhelm H, Lüdtke H, Wilhelm B. Pupillographic sleepiness testing in hypersomniacs and normals. Graefes Arch Clin Exp Ophthalmol 1998;236:725–729.
270. Bouma H, Baghuis LCJ. Hippus of the pupil: periods of slow oscillations of unknown origin. Vision Res 1971;11:1345–1351.

271. Stark L, Baker F. Stability and oscillations in a neurological servomechanism. J Neurophysiol 1959;22:156–164.

272. Davson H. The Physiology of the Eye. London, Churchill, 1949:237.

273. Duke-Elder S. System of Ophthalmology. Vol 7. London, Henry Kimpton, 1962: 330

274. Sollberger A. Biological Rhythm Research. Amsterdam, Elsevier, 1965.

275. Walsh FB, Hoyt WF. Clinical Neuro-Ophthalmology. 3rd ed, Vol 1. Baltimore, Williams & Wilkins, 1969:482.

276. Sullivan KN, Manfredi F, Behnke RH. Hippus in Cheyne-Stokes respiration: observations in three patients with rhythmic respiratory and pupillary changes. Arch Intern Med 1968;112:116–121.

277. Ellis CJK. The pupillary light reflex in normal subjects. Br J Ophthalmol 1981; 65:754–759.

278. Tanino T, Kurihara K. Electrically evoked direct and consensual reflexes of the pupil. Jpn J Ophthalmol 1982;26:462–467.

279. Smith SA, Smith SE. Light-induced anisocoria in man. J Physiol (Lond) 1979; 293:58P.

280. Smith SA, Ellis CJK, Smith SE. Inequality of the direct and consensual light reflexes in normal subjects. Br J Ophthalmol 1979;63:523–527.

281. Smith SA, Smith SE. Contraction anisocoria. Nasal versus temporal illumination. Br J Ophthalmol 1980;64:933.

282. Lowenstein O. Alternating contraction anisocoria. Arch Neurol Psychiatr 1954; 72:742–757.

283. Cox TA, Drewes CP. Contraction anisocoria resulting from half-field illumination. Am J Ophthalmol 1984;97:577–582.

284. Bourne PR, Smith SA, Smith SE. Dynamics of the light reflex and the influence of age on the human pupil measured by television pupillometry. J Physiol (Lond) 1979;293:1P.

285. Lange F. Über die pupillomotorik im alter. Klin Monatsbl Augenheilkd 1954; 124:76–81.

286. Kadlecová V, Peleska M. The pupillary diameter in light and dark in various age categories. Cesk Oftalmol 1957;13:278–283.

287. Borthne A, Davanger M. Mydriatics and age. Acta Ophthalmol 1971;49: 380–387.

288. Campbell FW, Gregory AH. Effect of size of pupil on visual acuity. Nature 1960;187:1121–1123.

289. Hawkes CH, Stow B. Pupil size and the pattern-evoked visual response. J Neurol Neurosurg Psychiatry 1981;44:90–91.

290. Barlow HB. Dark and light adaptation: Psychophysics. In: Handbook of Sensory Physiology. Vol 7. New York, Springer, 1972.

291. Campbell FW, Woodhouse JM. The role of the pupil light reflex in dark adaptation. J Physiol (Lond) 1975;245:111P–112P.

292. Lowenstein O, Kawabata H, Loewenfeld IE. The pupil as an indicator of retinal activity. Am J Ophthalmol 1964;57:569–596.

293. Lee RE, Cohen HG, Boynton RM. Latency variation in human pupil contraction due to stimulus luminance and/or adaptation level. J Optom Soc Am 1969;59: 97–103.

294. Cibis GW, Campos EC, Aulhorn E. Pupillomotor latent period. Vision Res 1977; 17:737–738.

295. Lowenstein O, Loewenfeld IE. Scotopic and photopic thresholds of the pupillary light reflex in normal man. Am J Ophthalmol 1959;48:87–98.

296. Kadlecová V. The pupillomotorial adaptation of the eye. Ophthalmologica 1960; 140:379–387.

297. Alpern M, Benson DJ. Directional sensitivity of the pupillomotor photoreceptors. Am J Optom Physiol Opt 1953;30:569–580.

298. Alpern M, Kitai S, Isaacson JD. The dark-adaptation process of the pupillomotor photoreceptors. Am J Optom Physiol Opt 1959;48:583–593.

299. Schweitzer NMJ, Bouman MA. Differential threshold measurements on the light reflex of the human pupil. Arch Ophthalmol 1958;59:541–550.

300. Alexandridis E, Dodt E. Pupillenlichtreflexe und pupillenweite einer stäbchenmonochromatin. Albrecht von Graefes Arch Ophthalmol 1967;173:153–161.

301. Schubert E, Thoss F. Der einfluss verschiedener adaptation auf die schwelle sowie auf die reizstärkeabhängigkeit von latenzzeit und amplitude am konsensuellen pupillenreflex des menschen. Pflugers Archiv Ges Physiol Menschen Tiere 1967;294:541–550.

302. Webster JG. Pupillary light reflex: development of teaching models. IEEE Trans Biomed Eng BME 1971;18:187–194.

303. Webster JG, Cohen GH, Boynton RM. Optimizing the use of the criterion response for the pupil light reflex. J Optom Soc Am 1968;58:419–424.

304. Alexandridis E, Koeppe ER. Dis spektrale empfindlichkeit der für den pupillenlichtreflex verantwortlich photoreceptoren beim menschen. Albrecht von Graefes Arch Ophthalmol 1969;177:136–151.

305. Ohba N, Alpern M. Adaptation of the pupil light reflex. Vision Res 1972;12: 953–967.

306. Stiles WS, Crawford BH. Equivalent adaptation levels in localized retinal areas. Rep Disc Vision Phys Soc (Lond) 1932;3:194–211.

307. Lowenstein O, Feinberg R, Loewenfeld IE. Pupillary movements during acute and chronic fatigue: a new test for the objective evaluation of tiredness. Invest Ophthalmol 1963;2:138–157.

308. Bárány EH, Halldén U. Phasic inhibition of the light reflex of the pupil during retinal rivalry. J Neurophysiol 1948;11:25–30.

309. Lowe SW, Ogle KN. Dynamics of the pupil during binocular rivalry. Arch Ophthalmol 1966;75:395–403.

310. Simons SJ, Ogle KN. Pupillary response to momentary light stimulation to eyes unequally adapted to light. Am J Ophthalmol 1967;63:35–45.

311. Young FA. Studies of pupillary conditioning. J Exp Psychol 1958;55:97–109.

312. Morone G, Citroni M. Über die möglichkeit, den photomotorischen reflex der pupille hervorzurufen. Ophthalmologica 1962;143:423–430.

313. Stark L. The pupil as a paradigm example of a neurological control system: mathematical approaches in biology. In: Loewenfeld IE, ed. The Pupil: Anatomy, Physiology, and Clinical Applications. Detroit, Wayne State University Press, 1984.

314. Stark L, Sherman PM. A servoanalytic study of consensual pupil reflex to light. J Neurophysiol 1957;20:17–26.

315. Stanten F, Stark L. A statistical analysis of pupil noise. IEEE Trans Biomed Eng BME 1966;13:140–152.

316. Smith JD, Masek GA, Ichinose LY, et al. Single neuron activity in the pupillary system. Brain Res 1970;24:219–234.

317. Terdiman J, Smith JD, Stark L. Dynamic analysis of the pupil with light and electrical stimulation. IEEE Trans Systems Man Cybernetics SMC 1971;1: 239–251.

318. Usui S, Stark L. Sensory and motor mechanisms interact to control amplitude of pupil noise. Vision Res 1978;18:505–507.

319. Kollarits CR, Kollarits FJ, Schuette WH, et al. The pupil dark response in normal volunteers. Curr Eye Res 1983;2:255–259.

320. Lowenstein O, Givner I. Pupillary reflex to darkness. Arch Ophthalmol 1943; 30:603–609.

321. Donders FC. On the anomalies of accommodation and refraction of the eye. New Sydenham Soc (Lond) 1864;22:573–583.

322. Marg E, Morgan MW Jr. The pupillary near reflex: the relation of pupillary diameter to accommodation and the various components of convergence. Am J Optom Physiol Opt 1949;26:183–198.

323. Alpern M, Mason GL, Jardinico RE. Vergence and accommodation. V. Pupil size changes associated with changes in accommodative vergence. Am J Ophthalmol 1961;52:762–767.

324. Hensen V, Völckers C. Über den ursprung der accommodationsnerven nebst bermerkungen über die function der wurzeln des nervus oculomotorius: physioilglsche untersuchung. Albrecht von Graefes Arch Ophthalmol 1878;24:1–26.

325. Bender MB, Weinstein EA. Functional representation in the oculomotor and trochlear nuclei. Arch Neurol Psychiatr 1943;49:98–106.

326. Langley JN, Anderson HK. The action of nicotine on the ciliary ganglion and the endings of the third cranial nerve. J Physiol (Lond) 1892;13:460–468.

327. Schäfer WD, Weale RA. The influence of age and retinal illumination on the pupillary near reflex. Vision Res 1970;10:179–191.

328. Roth N. Effect of reduced retinal illuminance on the pupillary near reflex. Vision Res 1969;9:1259–1266.

329. Jagerman LS. Hering's law applied to the near reflex. Am J Ophthalmol 1970; 70:579–582.

330. Semmlow J, Stark L. Pupil movements to light and accommodative stimulation: a comparative study. Vision Res 1973:13:1087–1100.

331. Bonvallet MS, Zbrozyna A. Les commandes réticulaires du systeème autonome et en particulier de l'innervation sympathique et parasympathique de la pupille. Arch Ital Biol 1963;101:174–207.

332. Westphal A. Über bisher nicht beschriebene pupillenerscheinungen in katatonischen stupor mit krankendemonstration. Allg Z Psychiatr 1907;64:694–701.

333. Westphal A. Über ein im katatonischen stupor beobachtestes pupillenphaenomen sowie bemerkungen über die pupillenstarre bei hysterie. Dtsch Med Wochenschr 1907;33:1080–1085.

334. Rohen J. Das auge und seine hilfsorgene. In: Möllendorf WV. Handbuch der Mikroskopischen Anatomie den Menschen. Berlin, Erganz, 1964.

335. Bender MB, Weinstein EA. Functional representation in the oculomotor and trochlear nuclei. Arch Neurol Psychiatr 1953;49:98–106.

336. Zhang Y, Mays LE, Gamlin PDR. Characteristics of near-response cells projecting to the oculomotor nucleus. J Neurophysiol 1992;67:944–960.

337. Gamlin PD, Zhang Y, Clendaniel RA, et al. Behavior of identified Edinger-Westphal neurons during ocular accommodation. J Neurophysiol 1994;72: 2368–2382.

338. Gamlin PD, Clarke RJ. Single-unit activity in the primate nucleus reticularis tegmenti pontis related to vergence and ocular accommodation. J Neurophysiol 1995;73:2115–2119.

339. Burde RM, Parelman JJ, Luskin M. Lack of unity of Edinger-Westphal nucleus projections to the ciliary ganglion and spinal cord: a double-labeling approach. Brain Res 1982;249:379–382.

340. Roste GK, Dietrichs E. Cerebellar cortical and nuclear afferents from the Edinger-Westphal nucleus in the cat. Anat Embryol 1988;178:59–65.

341. Adler FH. Physiology of the Eye. 10th ed. St Louis, CV Mosby, 2002.

342. Fincham EF. The mechanism of accommodation. Br J Ophthalmol Suppl 1937; 8:5–80.

343. Helmholtz H. Über die akkommodation des auges. Albrecht von Graefes Arch Ophthalmol 1855;1:2.

344. Henderson T. Anatomy and physiology of accommodation in mammalia. Trans Ophthalmol Soc UK 1926;46:280–308.

345. Adler-Grinberg D. Questioning our classical understanding of accommodation and presbyopia. Am J Optom Physiol Optics 1986;63:571–580.

346. Neider MW, Crawford K, Kaufman PL, et al. In vivo videography of the rhesus monkey accommodative apparatus. Age-related loss of ciliary muscle response to central stimulation. Arch Ophthalmol 1990;108:69–74.

347. Glasser A, Kaufman PL. The mechanism of accommodation in primates. Ophthalmology 1999;106:863–872.

348. Ludwig K, Wegscheider E, Hoops JP, et al. In vivo imaging of the human zonular apparatus with high-resolution ultrasound biomicroscopy. Graefes Arch Clin Exp Ophthalmol 1999;237:361–371.

349. Burd HJ, Judge SJ, Flavell MJ. Mechanics of accommodation of the human eye. Vision Res 1999;39:1591–1595.

350. Tscherning M. Étude sur le mécanisme de l'accommodation. Arch Phys 1894; 1:1.

351. Schachar RA, Black TD, Kash RL, et al. The mechanism of accommodation and presbyopia in the primate. Ann Ophthalmol 1995;27:58–67.

352. Morat JP, Doyon M. Le grand sympathique, nerf de l'accommodation pour la vision des objets eloingés. Ann Oculist 1891;106:28–30.

353. Cogan DG. Accommodation and the autonomic nervous system. Arch Ophthalmol 1937;18:739–766.

354. Meesmann A. Experimentelle untersuchungen über die antagonistische innervation der ciliarmuskelatur. Albrecht von Graefes Arch Ophthalmol 1952;152: 335–356.

355. Melton CE, Purnell EW, Brecher GA. The effect of sympathetic nerve impulses on the ciliary muscle. Am J Ophthalmol 1955;40:155–162.

356. Fenton RH, Hunter WS. Histopathologic findings in eyes with paralysis of the oculomotor (third) nerve. Arch Ophthalmol 1965;73:224–228.

357. Hurwitz BS, Davidowitz J, Chin NB, et al. The effects of the sympathetic nervous system on accommodation: I. Beta sympathetic nervous system. Arch Ophthalmol 1972;87:668–674.

358. Hurwitz BS, Davidowitz J, Pachter BR, et al. The effects of the sympathetic nervous system on accommodation: II. Alpha sympathetic nervous system. Arch Ophthalmol 1972;87:675–678.

359. Gimpel G, Doughty MJ, Lyle WM. Large sample study of the effects of phenylephrine 2.5% eyedrops on the amplitude of accommodation in man. Ophthal Physiol Opt 1994;14:123–128.

360. Jampel RS. Representation of the near-response on the cerebral cortex of the macaque. Am J Ophthalmol 1959;48:573–582.

361. Clark BR, Randle RJ, Stewart JD. Vestibular ocular accommodation reflex in man. Aviat Space Environ Med 1975;46:1336–1339.

362. Hosoba M, Bando T, Tsukahara N. The cerebellar control of accommodation of the eye in the cat. Brain Res 1978;153:495–505.

363. Bando T, Yamamoto N, Tsukahara N. Cortical neurons related to lens accommodation in posterior lateral suprasylvian area in cats. J Neurophysiol 1984;52: 879–891.

364. Sawa M, Maekawa H, Ohtsuka K. Cortical area related to lens accommodation in cat. Jpn J Ophthalmol 1992;36:371–379.

365. Maekawa H, Ohtsuka K. Afferent and efferent connections of the cortical accommodation area in the cat. Neurosci Res 1993;17:315–323.

366. Sawa M, Ohtsuka K. Lens accommodation evoked by micro-stimulation of the superior colliculus in the cat. Vision Res 1994;34:975–981.

367. Ciuffreda KJ, Kruger PB. Dynamics of human voluntary accommodation. Am J Optom Physiol Optics 1988;65:365–370.

368. Stark L, Takahashi Y. Absence of an odd-error signal mechanism in human accommodation. IEEE Trans Biomed Eng 1965;12:138–146.

369. Phillips S, Stark L. Blur: a sufficient accommodative stimulus. Doc Ophthalmol 1977;43:65–89.

370. Charman WN, Tucker J. Dependence of accommodation response on the spatial frequency spectrum of the observed object. Vision Res 1977;17:129–139.

371. Charman WN, Tucker J. Accommodation and color. J Optom Soc Am 1978; 68:459–471.

372. Fincham EF. The accommodation reflex and its stimulus. Br J Ophthalmol 1951; 35:381–393.

373. Charman WN, Tucker J. Accommodation as a function of object form. Am J Optom Physiol Opt 1978;55:84–92.

374. Kruger PB, Pola J. Stimuli for accommodation: blur, chromatic aberration and size. Vision Res 1986;26:957–971.

375. Knoll HA. A brief history of "nocturnal myopia" and related phenomena. Am J Ophthalmol 1952;29:69–81.

376. Campbell FW. The minimum quantity of light required to elicit the accommodation reflex in man. J Physiol (Lond) 1954;123:357–366.

377. Alpern M, Larson BF. Vergence and accommodation: IV. Effect of luminance quantity on the AC/A. Am J Ophthalmol 1960;49:1140–1149.

378. Whiteside TCD. Accommodation of the human eye in a bright and empty visual field. J Physiol (Lond) 1952;118:65P.

379. Campbell FW, Westheimer G. Dynamics of accommodation responses of the human eye. J Physiol (Lond) 1960;151:285–295.

380. Schäfer WD, Weale RA. The influence of age and retinal illuminance on the pupillary near reflex. Vision Res 1970;10:179–191.

381. Semmlow J, Stark L. Pupil movements to light and accommodative stimulation: a comparative study. Vision Res 1973;13:1087–1100.

382. Bourne PR, Smith SA, Smith SE. Dynamics of the light reflex and the influence of age on the human pupil measured by television pupillometry. J Physiol (Lond) 1979;293:1P.

383. Ward PA, Charman WN. Effect of pupil size on steady state accommodation. Vision Res 1985;25:1317–1326.

384. Hennessey RT, Iida T, Shiina K, et al. The effect of pupil size on accommodation. Vision Res 1976;16:587–589.

385. Schober HAW. Über die akkommodationsruhelage. Optik 1954;11:282–290.

386. Morgan MW. A new theory for the control of accommodation. Am J Optom Physiol Opt 1946;23:99–110.

387. Otero JM. Influence of the state of accommodation on the visual performance of the human eye. J Optom Soc Am 1951;41:942–948.

388. Morgan MW. The resting state of accommodation. Am J Optom Physiol Opt 1957;34:347–353.

389. Helmholtz HW. Physiological Optics. Vol. 1. New York, Dover Publications, 1962:136–137.

390. Brown JL. The structure of the visual system. In: Graham CH, ed. Vision and Visual Perception. New York, John Wiley & Sons, 1965.

391. Ogle K. Optics. 2nd ed. Springfield, IL, Charles C Thomas, 1968.

392. Borish IM. Clinical Refraction. New York, Professional Press, 1970.

393. Westheimer G. Eye movement responses to a horizontally moving visual stimulus. Arch Ophthalmol 1954;52:932–941.

394. Whiteside TCD. The Problems of Vision in Flight at High Altitude. London, Butterworths, 1957.

395. Campbell FW, Westheimer G. Factors influencing accommodation responses of the human eye. J Opt Soc Am 1959;49:568–571.

396. Winn B, Gilmartin B. Current perspectives on microfluctuations of accommodation. Ophthal Physiol Opt 1992;12:252–256.

397. Gray LS, Winn B, Gilmartin B. Accommodation microfluctuations and pupil diameter. Vision Res 1993;33:2082–2090.

398. Heron G, Schor C. The fluctuations of accommodation and ageing. Ophthal Physiol Opt 1995;15:445–449.

399. Gray LS, Winn B, Gilmartin B. Effect of target luminance on microfluctuations of accommodation. Ophthal Physiol Opt 1993;13:258–265.

400. Kotulak JC, Schor CM. Temporal variations in accommodation during steady state conditions. J Opt Soc Am 1986;A3:223–227.

401. Charman WN. The retinal image in the human eye. In: Osborne N, Chader G, eds. Progress in Retinal Research. Vol 2. Oxford, UK, Pergamon, 1983:1–50.

402. Alpern M. Variability of accommodation during steady fixation at various levels of illuminance. J Opt Soc Am 1958;48:193–197.

403. Troelstra A, Zuber BL, Miller D, et al. Accommodative tracking: a trial-and-error function. Vision Res 1964;4:585–594.

404. Jagerman LS. Hering's law applied to the near reflex. Am J Ophthalmol 1970; 70:579–582.

405. Müller J. Elements of Physiology [translated by Baly W]. London, Taylor & Walton, 1826:1147–1148.

406. Alpern M, Ellen P. A quantitative analysis of the horizontal movements of the eyes in the experiment of Johannes Müller: I. Methods and results. Am J Ophthalmol 1956;42:289–303.

407. Hermann JS, Samson CR. Critical detection of the accommodative convergence to accommodation ratio by photosensor-oculography. Arch Ophthalmol 1967; 78:424–430.

408. Keller EL, Robinson DA. Abducens unit behavior in the monkey during vergence movements. Vision Res 1972;12:369–382.

409. Pickwell LD. Variation in ocular motor dominance. Br J Physiol Optics 1972; 27:115–119.

410. Kenyon RV, Ciuffreda KJ, Stark L. Binocular eye movements during accommodative vergence. Vision Res 1978;18:545–555.

411. Christoferson KW, Ogle KN. Effect of homatropine on the accommodation-convergence association. Arch Ophthalmol 1956;55:779–791.

412. Fincham EF, Walton J. The reciprocal actions of accommodation and convergence. J Physiol (Lond) 1957;137:488–508.

413. Mordi JA, Ciuffreda KJ. Static aspects of accommodation: age and presbyopia. Vision Res 1998;38:1643–1653.

414. Mordi JA, Ciuffreda KJ. Dynamic aspects of accommodation: age and presbyopia. Vision Res 2004;44:591–601.

415. Haynes H, White BL, Held R. Visual accommodation in human infants. Science 1965;148:528–530.

416. Gullstrand A. Appendices to Part I. In Helmholtz's Treatise on Physiological Optics, 1909. New York, Dover Publications, 1962.

417. Moses RA. Accommodation. In: Moses RA, ed. Adler's Physiology of the Eye Editor, 7th ed. St Louis, CV Mosby, 1981:304–325.

418. Saladin JJ, Stark L. Presbyopia: new evidence from impedance cyclography supporting the Hess-Gullstrand theory. Vision Res 1975;15:537–541.

419. Swegmark G, Olsson T. Impedance cyclography: a new method for accommodation recording. Acta Ophthalmol 1968;46:946–948.

420. Swegmark G. Studies with impedance cyclography on human ocular accommodation at different ages. Acta Ophthalmol 1969;46:1186–1206.

421. Saladin JJ, Usui S, Stark L. Impedance cyclography as an indication of ciliary muscle contraction. Am J Optom Physiol Opt 1974;51:613–625.

422. Fisher RF. The force of contraction of the human ciliary muscle during accommodation. J Physiol (Lond) 1977;270:51–74.

423. Poyer JF, Kaufman PL, Flugel C. Age does not affect contractile responses of the isolated rhesus monkey ciliary muscle to muscarinic agonists. Curr Eye Res 1993;12:413–422.

424. Duane A. Are the current theories of accommodation correct? Am J Ophthalmol 1925;8:196–202.

425. Weale RA. New light on old eyes. Nature 1963;198:944–946.

426. Bito LZ, DeRousseau CJ, Kaufman PL, et al. Age-dependent loss of accommodative amplitude in rhesus monkeys: an animal model for presbyopia. Invest Ophthalmol Vis Sci 1982;23:23–31.

427. Lutjen-Drecoll E, Tamm E, Kaufman PL. Age-related in rhesus monkey ciliary muscle by light and electron microscopy. Exp Eye Res 1988;47:885–889.

428. True-Gabelt B, Polansky JR, Kaufman PL. Ciliary muscle muscarinic receptors, ChAT and AChE in young and old rhesus monkeys. Inv Ophthalmol Vis Sci (ARVO suppl) 1987;28:65.

429. Miranda OC, Bito LZ, Kaufman PL. Ocular aging and presbyopia: comparison of the aging of iridial and ciliary muscles. Invest Ophthalmol Vis Sci (ARVO suppl) 1988;29:76.

430. Egan JA. A new test for accommodation. Am J Ophthalmol 1954;37:429–430.

431. Campbell FW, Robson JG. A high-speed infrared optometer. J Opt Soc Am 1959;49:268–272.

432. Hennessy RT, Leibowitz HW. Laser optometer incorporating the Badal principle. Behav Res Methods Instrum 1972;4:237–239.

433. Egeberg J, Jensen OA. The ultrastructure of the acini of the human lacrimal gland. Acta Ophthalmol 1969;47:400–410.

434. Orzalesi N, Riva A, Test F. Fine structure of human lacrimal gland: I. The normal gland. J Submicrosc Cytol 1971;3:282.

435. Sullivan DA, Wickham LA, Rocha EM, et al. Influence of gender, sex steroid hormones, and the hypothalamic-pituitary axis on the structure and function of the lacrimal gland. Adv Exp Med Biol 1998;438:11–42.

436. Dartt DA. Regulation of tear secretion. Adv Exp Med Biol 1994;350:1–9.

437. Axenfeld T. Die exstirpation der palpebralen tränendrüse. Klin Monatsbl Augenheilkd 1911;49:345–351.

438. Amdur J. Excision of palpebral lacrimal gland for epiphora. Arch Ophthalmol 1964;71:71–72.

439. Jones LT. The lacrimal secretory system and its treatment. Am J Ophthalmol 1966;62:47–60.

440. Newell FW. Ophthalmology. St. Louis, CV Mosby, 1969.

441. Maitchouk DY, Beuerman RW, Ohta T, et al. Tear production after unilateral removal of the main lacrimal gland in squirrel monkeys. Arch Ophthalmol 2000;118:246–252.

442. Crosby EC, Humphrey T, Lauer EW. Correlative Anatomy of the Nervous System. New York, Macmillan, 1962.

443. Podvinec M, Pfaltz CR. Studies on the anatomy of the facial nerve. Acta Otolaryngol 1976;81:173–177.

444. Irving RM, Viani L, Hardy DG, et al. Nervus intermedius function after vestibular schwannoma removal: clinical features and pathophysiological mechanisms. Laryngoscope 1995;105:809–813.

445. Anson BJ, Donaldson JA, Warpeha RL, et al. Surgical anatomy of the facial nerve. Arch Otolaryngol 1973;97:201–213.

446. Kudo H, Nori S. Topography of the facial nerve in the human temporal bone. Acta Anat 1974;90:467–480.

447. Proctor B, Nager GT. The facial canal: normal anatomy, variations and anomalies. Ann Otol Rhinol Laryngol 1982;91:33–61.

448. May M. The Facial Nerve. New York, Thieme Inc, 1986.

449. Rupa V, Weider DJ, Glasner S, et al. Geniculate ganglion: anatomic study with surgical implications. Am J Otol 1992;13:470–473.

450. Duke-Elder S, Wybar KC. The anatomy of the visual system. In: Duke-Elder S, ed. System of Ophthalmology. Vol 2. St Louis, CV Mosby, 1961.

451. Tsukahara S, Tanishima T. Histochemical and electron-microscopical study in the autonomic nerve distribution of human lacrimal gland. Acta Soc Ophthalmol Jpn 1973;77:712–718.

452. Kato Y. Distribution of the nerve fibers in the human lacrimal gland. Acta Soc Ophthalmol Jpn 1957;61:2264–2287.

453. Kato Y. Histochemical observation of the human lacrimal gland. Acta Soc Ophthalmol Jpn 1958;62:175–184.

454. Gebarski SS, Telian SA, Niparko JK. Enhancement along the normal facial nerve in the facial canal: MR imaging and anatomic correlation. Radiology 1992;183:391–394.

455. Weiglein AH, Andenhuber W, Jaske R, et al. Imaging of the facial canal by means of multiplanar angulated 2-D-high-resolution CT-reconstruction. Surg Radiol Anat 1994;16:423–427.

456. Whitwell J. Role of the sympathetic in lacrimal secretion. Br J Ophthalmol 1961;45:439–445.

457. Botelho SY, Hisada M, Fuenmayor N. Functional innervation of the lacrimal gland in the cat: origin of secretomotor fibers in the lacrimal nerve. Arch Ophthalmol 1966;76:581–588.

458. Tangkrisanavinont V. Stimulation of lacrimal secretion by sympathetic nerve impulses in the rabbit. Life Sci 1984;34:2365–2371.

459. Araie N. Neurophysiological mechanisms of reflex lacrimation. Nippon Seirigaku Zasshi 1984;46:191–204.

460. Gromada J, Jorgensen TD, Dissing S. The release of intracellar $Ca2+$ in lacrimal acinar cells by alpha-, beta-adrenergic and muscarinic cholinergic stimulation: the roles of inositol triphosphate and cyclic ADP-ribose. Pflugers Arch 1995;429:751–761.

461. Ehinger B. Adrenergic nerves to the eye and to related structures in man and in the cynomolgus monkey. Invest Ophthalmol 1966;5:42–52.

462. Ruskell GL. The fine structure of nerve terminations in the lacrimal glands of monkeys. J Anat 1968;103:65–76.

463. Pfuhl W. Warum weinen wir bei Kummer, Schmerz und Rührung? Med Wochenschr 1953;7:547–549.

464. Takeuchi Y, Fukui Y, Ichiyama M, et al. Direct amygdaloid projections to the superior salivatory nucleus: a light and electron microscopic study in the cat. Brain Res Bull 1991;27:85–92.

465. Mizukawa T, Takagi Y, Kamada K, et al. Study on lacrimal function. Tokushima J Exp Med 1954;1:67–72.

466. Mishima S, Gasset A, Klyce SD Jr, et al. Determination of tear volume and tear flow. Invest Ophthalmol 1966;5:264–276.

467. Sorensen T, Taagehoj K, Jensen F. Tear flow in normal human eyes: determination by means of radioisotope and gamma camera. Acta Ophthalmol 1979;57:564–580.

468. Van Haeringen NJ. Clinical biochemistry of tears. Surv Ophthalmol 1981;26:84–96.

469. Sullivan DE, ed. Lacrimal Gland, Tear Film, and Dry Eye Syndromes: Basic Science and Clinical Relevance. Advances in Experimental Medicine and Biology Series, Vol 350. New York, Plenum Press, 1994.

470. Allerhand J, Karilitz S, Penbharkkul S, et al. Electrophoresis and immunoelectrophoresis of neonatal tears. J Pediatr 1963;62:85–92.

470a. Dartt DA. Dysfunctional neural regulation of lacrimal gland secretion and its role in the pathogenesis of dry eye syndromes. Ocular Surface 2004;2:76–91.

471. Slade SG, Lindberg JV, Immediata AR. Control of lacrimal secretion after sphenopalatine ganglion block. Ophthalmic Plast Reconstr Surg 1986;2:65–70.

472. Kessler TL, Dartt DA. Neural stimulation of conjuctival goblet cell mucous secretion in rats. Adv Exp Med Biol 1994;350:393–398.

473. Korb DR, Baron DF, Herman JP, et al. Tear film lipid layer thickness as a function of blinking. Cornea 1994;13:354–359.

474. Seifer P, Spitznas M. Demonstration of nerve fibers in human accessory lacrimal glands. Graefes Arch Clin Exp Ophthalmol 1994;232:107–114.

475. Bergmann MT, Newman BL, Johnson NC Jr. The effect of a diuretic (hydrochlorothiazide) on tear production in humans. Am J Ophthalmol 1985;99:473–475.

CHAPTER 15

Principles and Techniques of Examination of the Pupils, Accommodation, and Lacrimation

Kathleen B. Digre

ASSESSMENT OF PUPILLARY SIZE, SHAPE, AND
   FUNCTION
   History
   Examination
   Pharmacologic Testing

ASSESSMENT OF ACCOMMODATION, CONVERGENCE, AND
   THE NEAR RESPONSE
   History
   Examination
ASSESSMENT OF LACRIMATION
   History
   Examination

ASSESSMENT OF PUPILLARY SIZE, SHAPE, AND FUNCTION

As is the case with any assessment in neuro-ophthalmology, assessment of the pupils requires a meticulous history and a rigorous examination. This is followed in some instances by pharmacologic testing of the pupil using a variety of topical agents. The reader interested in a more extensive discussion of this topic should read the excellent book by Loewenfeld (1).

HISTORY

Patients with disturbances of pupillary size or shape often are unaware that any abnormality is present. More often, their spouse, a friend, or a physician brings the abnormality to their attention. The disturbance may appear suddenly, or it may develop gradually over time. It may be present at all times, or it may be episodic. Some pupillary abnormalities may be present for years and are only detected when someone looks at the iris.

In obtaining a history from a patient with a disturbance in pupillary size or shape, particularly anisocoria, dating the onset of the abnormality may be important. The easiest and most reliable method is to view a driver's license, credit card, or a similar identification card with the patient's photograph on it which the patient is likely to have available at the time of the evaluation. The examination of family album photographs that have been taken over time (sometimes jokingly called "family album tomography" or "FAT scanning") can be performed with the naked eye or with a magnifying lens and may save both time and money in attempting to determine the date of onset of a pupillary disturbance.

Symptoms that may be elicited in any patient with disturbances of pupillary size and shape include light sensitivity or photophobia, difficulty focusing when going from dark to light or light to dark, and blurring of vision. The blurred vision is typically a nonspecific and poorly defined complaint. If one pupil is large, the blurring may be present when the patient enters brightly lighted environments, and if one pupil is abnormally small, images of objects observed with that eye may appear slightly dimmer than those observed with the opposite eye.

The past medical history also may be helpful in assessing the significance of a disturbance in pupillary size or shape. A history of previous infections (e.g., herpes zoster), trauma, surgery (e.g., in the neck or upper chest; cataract extraction), or chronic illnesses such as diabetes or migraine may suggest the etiology of the pupillary disturbance (2). The patient's occupation also may be important. A farmer or gardener may be exposed to plants or pesticides that can produce pupillary dilation or constriction by topical contamination.

A physician, nurse, or other health professional may work with or have access to topical dilating or constricting substances that may produce changes in pupillary size by design or chance. Medication history also is important because opiates cause constricted pupils (3) and anticholinergic medications, including atropinic substances used in inhalants for asthmatics, may cause pupillary dilation (4).

EXAMINATION

Simple inspection of the anterior segment at the slit-lamp biomicroscope is helpful in determining whether or not there is a pupillary abnormality. For example, examination of the cornea may reveal an abrasion or injury that could affect the pupillary size, whereas examination of the anterior chamber may reveal inflammation that explains a small pupil in the setting of ciliary spasm. It may also be important to perform gonioscopy to assess the anterior chamber angle in a patient with a dilated pupil, particularly when there is a history of pain or redness in the eye (5). Assessment of the iris should include not only inspection of the integrity of the sphincter muscle but also transillumination to determine if there is evidence of iris damage from previous ocular trauma. To retroilluminate the iris, the slit-lamp beam is directed obliquely through the pupil. A normal iris will not show defects, but an abnormality such as atrophy will show reflected light back to the observer. In addition, by placing a wide beam at an angle to the iris and turning the light off and on, the light reflex can be assessed for segmental defects, such as those that occur in eyes with tonic pupils or aberrant regeneration of the oculomotor nerve. One can even draw a diagram showing clock hours of denervation; the diagram can then be used to follow the patient's status. Transillumination of the iris and ciliary body under infrared lighting

conditions has been shown to be helpful to find other defects (6).

Pupil measurements can be performed in several ways. A simple handheld pupil gauge can be used to determine pupil size in both light and darkness. Pupil gauges may be circular or linear. They consist of a series of solid or open circles or half-circles with diameters that increase by 0.2 mm in steps (Fig. 15.1). They can be held next to the eye to estimate the size of the pupil. Other calipers and scales to measure pupillary size are also available (7).

An accurate method of measuring pupillary size and comparing pupils before and after pharmacologic testing is with a handheld pupil camera. With this device, the pupils can be photographed in various illuminations, although not in darkness (8).

Infrared video pupillometry is perhaps the most accurate method of assessing the size of the pupil (9). An infrared video pupillometer permits observation of the pupils not only in lighted conditions but also in total darkness. Furthermore, the iris sphincter can even be transilluminated to show the denervated and reinnervated portions (10). Some computer programs associated with these pupillometers allow the examiner to measure not only the diameter and area of the pupil but also the latency and velocity of the pupillary response to both light and near stimulation (11).

During the clinical evaluation of the pupils, it is helpful to determine the answers to several certain questions. For example, because the diameter of the pupil typically decreases with age (12) (Fig. 15.2), the examiner should determine if the pupillary size is appropriate for the patient's age. Other important questions to answer include the following:

Are the pupils equal in size? If not, is the difference greater in darkness or in the light?

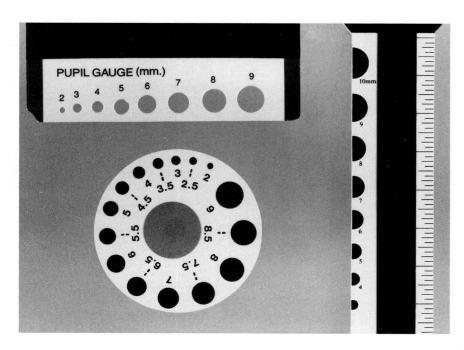

Figure 15.1. Pupil gauges. The best gauges measure in 0.1-mm steps.

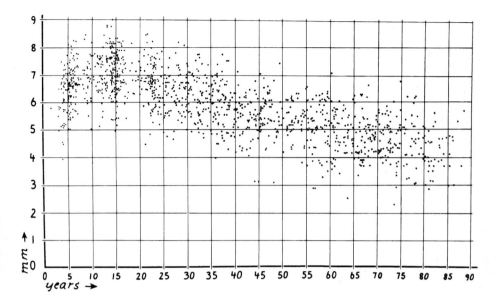

Figure 15.2. Graph showing relationship of age to pupil size in normal individuals. Note that, in general, pupillary size decreases with age. (From Loewenfeld IE. Pupillary changes related to age. In: Thompson HS, ed. Topics in Neuro-ophthalmology. Baltimore: Williams & Wilkins, 1979:124–150).

Do the pupils constrict to light equally and with the same velocity?

Do they redilate equally and with the same velocity?

Is the pupillary reaction to light stimulation equal to the pupillary reaction to near stimulation?

Is there reflex dilation to psychosensory stimulation?

Is there a relative afferent pupillary defect?

Assessing Pupillary Size

The diameter of both pupils should be estimated or measured in light, using either normal room light or a handheld transilluminator or other light source. The diameter of the pupils then should be assessed in darkness, using the dimmest room light in which the examiner can still see the edge of the pupil (13). Finally, the pupillary size should be assessed during near stimulation using an accommodative target to achieve maximum constriction of the pupils. The measurements of the two pupils in light and darkness also should be compared to determine if there is **anisocoria**: a difference of at least 0.4 mm between the two pupils. A substantial percentage of the normal population has clinically detectable anisocoria of 0.4 mm or more, with the percentage increasing with increasing age (14). Whereas 20% of the general population aged 17 years and under have so-called physiologic anisocoria, the prevalence rises to 33% in otherwise normal persons over 60 years of age (15). In addition, anisocoria may be produced by damage to the iris sphincter or dilator muscles or to their nerve supply. The amount of anisocoria may be affected by illumination. For instance, a greater degree of anisocoria is present in darkness than in light in patients with physiologic anisocoria or Horner syndrome (13,16). Anisocoria also can also be affected by the degree of accommodation, by patient fatigue, and by sympathetic drive (e.g., anxiety) (13,16,17).

Recent advances in refractive surgery have made measurement of pupillary diameters in darkness clinically important to reduce the risk of nocturnal halos due to the improper calculation of pupillary size in darkness. Numerous pupillographic devices are available commercially to measure pupillary sizes in darkness (18).

Testing the Direct Pupillary Reaction to Light

When testing the reaction of a pupil to light shined in the eye—**the direct pupillary light reaction**—it is important to have a dimly lit room that is quiet so as to reduce or eliminate emotional effects on the pupil (19). Furthermore, one must be certain that the patient is fixating on a distance target to eliminate any effect of accommodation on pupillary size. The examiner must be certain that the patient is not attempting to close the eyelids during the test, because this produces a variable degree of pupillary constriction.

A relatively bright light source should always be used to illuminate the pupil and produce pupillary constriction, because increased stimulus intensity is associated with an increased light reflex amplitude and a maximum rate of constriction and redilation (20,21). If the light source is too bright, however, a prolonged contraction lasting several seconds ("spastic miosis") will occur and make determination of the normal light reflex difficult or impossible (22). In general, a fully charged transilluminator or an indirect ophthalmoscope with maximum brightness is the optimum light source. In addition, it is helpful to use a dim secondary light source to provide oblique illumination of the pupil in some cases, because this technique increases visualization of darkly pigmented irides (Fig. 15.3).

The light source should be shined straight into the eye for a few seconds and then moved downward away from the eye to eliminate the stimulation. The pupil response should be assessed during this maneuver, which should be repeated several times. The normal response to a bright light is a contraction called **pupillary capture** (23) (also called the

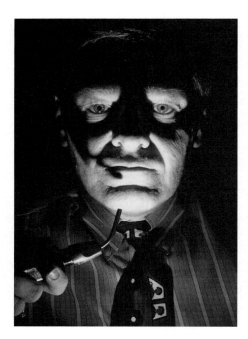

Figure 15.3. Indirect lighting to view pupils in darkness is helpful in viewing dilation.

phasic response). An abnormal response is **pupillary escape**, in which the pupil initially constricts and then slowly redilates and returns to its original size. Pupillary escape most often occurs on the side of a diseased optic nerve or retina, particularly in patients with a central field defect, although it also occurs in patients with lesions of the contralateral optic tract, in patients with lesions of the brachium conjunctivum, and in normal persons tested with a low-intensity light source (24,25) (see also Chapter 16).

The initial size of the pupil is important in assessing both pupillary capture and pupillary escape; a larger pupil is more likely to show pupillary escape, whereas a smaller pupil is more likely to show pupillary capture (26–28).

The latency and speed with which a pupil constricts to light and redilates after light stimulation can be assessed using pupillography. This technique reveals that normal persons have pupillary wave forms with latency of 0.20–0.28 seconds and duration of contraction of 0.45 seconds (29). There is a modest interindividual difference in latency in normal subjects (between 8.3–35 milliseconds) (30). The use of pupillography to record wave forms of pupillary constriction and dilation is generally limited to pupillary research laboratories.

Testing the Consensual Response to Light

When light is shined in one eye, the contralateral pupil should constrict. This is the **consensual light response**. The consensual response to light is best assessed using a light source for illumination of the pupil of one eye and a dimmer light source that can be held obliquely to the side of the contralateral eye to be observed. The consensual pupillary response should be approximately equal in both velocity and extent to the direct response, because the pupillary decussation in the midbrain is about 50% to each eye. In fact, the consensual reaction to light in normal humans is slightly less than the direct reaction, producing about 0.1 mm or less of what has been called **alternating contraction anisocoria** (22,31). Contraction anisocoria is difficult to see without using pupillography.

Testing the Near Response

The near response, a co-movement of the near triad that also includes accommodation and convergence (discussed later), should be tested in a room with light that is adequate for the patient to fixate an accommodative target. A nonaccommodative target, such as a pencil, pen, or the patient's own thumb may not be a sufficient stimulus to produce a normal near response, even in a normal person, and these targets should be avoided (except in a patient who is blind, in which case one must stimulate the pupillary near response using proprioception from one of the patient's own fingers or thumb). Similarly, the near response should not be induced by having the patient look at a bright light stimulus, because the light itself may produce pupillary constriction. The examiner should attempt to test the pupillary near response several times to give the patient practice. One can document the light and near response with photographs or pupillometry (Fig. 15.4).

If a patient is unable to cooperate for a near effort, some authors advocate using the **lid closure reflex**, in which the patient attempts to squeeze the eyes shut while the physician tries to open them (22). This maneuver typically causes the pupils to constrict.

Assessment of Pupillary Dilation

Dilation of the pupils occurs in a variety of settings. Most often, the pupils dilate after they have constricted to light or near stimulation. In patients with certain retinal and, less often, optic nerve disease, they may actually dilate when light is shined in one eye, or the pupils may constrict to darkness (paradoxical pupillary responses) (32,33). Reflex pupillary dilation can be elicited by sudden noise or by pinching the back of the neck (the ciliospinal reflex).

When assessing pupillary dilation, the examiner should look specifically for **dilation lag** (34). This phenomenon is present when there is more anisocoria 5 seconds after pupillary constriction to light than there is 15 seconds after pupillary constriction (35). Dilation lag typically occurs in patients with a defect in the sympathetic innervation of the pupil (i.e., a Horner pupil).

Dilation lag usually is easy to detect. One method is simply to observe both pupils simultaneously in very dim light after a bright room light has been turned off. Normal pupils return to their widest size within 12–15 seconds, with most of the dilation occurring in the first 5 seconds. Pupils that show dilation lag may take up to 25 seconds to return to maximal size in darkness, with most of the dilation occurring about 10–12 seconds after the light goes out. A second way to determine if dilation lag is present is to take flash photo-

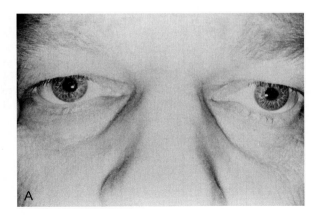

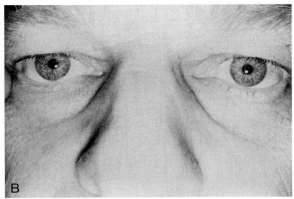

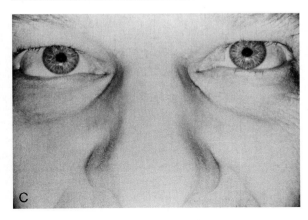

Figure 15.4. A handheld camera documents size of the pupils in light and darkness in a normal subject. *A,* In room light without any other stimulation. *B,* In room light during stimulation with a bright light. *C,* In room light during stimulation with an accommodative target. Note associated convergence.

graphs at 5 and 15 seconds after the lights are turned off. If there is a difference in anisocoria of greater than 0.4 mm at 5 seconds minus the anisocoria at 15 seconds, a Horner syndrome is present (35).

Infrared videography beautifully demonstrates dilation lag because even the most darkly pigmented iris will appear bright with this technique (36). Using infrared videography, some investigators have found that re-dilation lag is the most

sensitive diagnostic test to detect either unilateral or bilateral Horner syndrome (37).

Testing for Light-Near Dissociation

Dissociation between the pupillary response to light stimulation and the pupillary response to near stimulation—**light-near dissociation**—occurs in patients with a variety of disorders, including blindness (from optic nerve or retinal damage), neurosyphilis, oculomotor nerve paresis with aberrant regeneration, tonic pupil (e.g., Adie pupil), hydrocephalus, pineal region tumors, and intrinsic mesencephalic disease (see Chapter 16). In almost all cases, **the pupillary reaction to light is impaired, whereas the pupillary response to near is normal or near normal**. Thus, the potential for light-near dissociation should be considered in any patient with an impaired pupillary light reaction.

Although there are rare intracranial lesions that can produce a light-near pupillary dissociation in which the reaction to light is normal and the reaction to near is abnormal, the vast majority of cases of this type of light-near dissociation are caused by lack of effort on the part of the patient during attempted near stimulation.

Testing for a Relative Afferent Pupillary Defect

When a patient has an optic neuropathy in one eye or an asymmetric bilateral optic neuropathy, covering one eye and then the other reveals that the pupil of the normal eye constricts when it is uncovered and the abnormal eye is covered, whereas the pupil of the abnormal eye dilates when it is uncovered and the pupil of the normal eye is covered. (Fig. 15.5). This is known as the ''Marcus Gunn'' or ''Gunn'' phenomenon, and the abnormal pupil is often called a **Marcus Gunn pupil**. In fact, a better term for this phenomenon is ''relative afferent pupillary defect,'' because this term, usually abbreviated as **RAPD**, describes the nature of the pupillary abnormality rather than being an eponym.

The concept of an RAPD is not new. In 1884, Hirschberg described a young woman with retrobulbar neuritis in whom he diagnosed an organic visual loss because of reduced pupillary light reactions when the affected eye was stimulated (38). In addition, he noted that the consensual pupillary reaction in the affected eye was better than the direct reaction. Gunn stated that he was able to differentiate retrobulbar optic neuritis from non-organic loss of vision by the difference in pupillary reactions to prolonged exposure to light and recommended comparing the behavior of the two pupils when one was stimulated directly or consensually for a continued period. He emphasized that the pupil on the side of an eye with optic nerve dysfunction dilated spontaneously after initial constriction if the pupil continued to be exposed to light, whereas the pupil in an eye with non-organic visual loss tended to remain fairly constricted as long as the light was on (39,40). Kestenbaum subsequently popularized the concept of the RAPD and credited Gunn with its discovery (41). The phenomenon described by Kestenbaum and attributed to Gunn thus became known as ''Gunn'' pupil. Kestenbaum also modified the test by covering each eye individ-

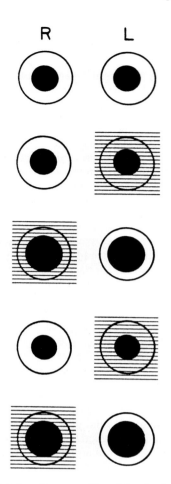

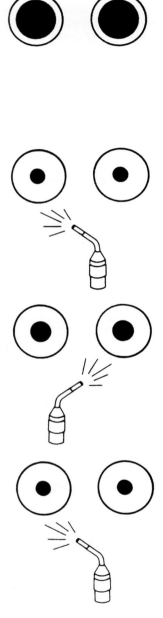

Figure 15.5. Relative afferent pupillary defect in the left eye demonstrated by the alternate cover test as described by Kestenbaum. The left pupil dilates (as does the right) when the left eye is uncovered and the right eye is covered. (From Thompson HS. Pupillary signs in the ophthalmologic diagnosis of optic nerve disease. Trans Ophthalmol Soc UK 1976; 96:377–381.)

Figure 15.6. Relative afferent pupillary defect in the left eye demonstrated using the swinging flashlight test. The pupils constrict when the light is shined directly into the right eye; however, when the flashlight is swung back to the left eye, both pupils dilate. (From Thompson HS. Pupillary signs in the ophthalmologic diagnosis of optic nerve disease. Trans Ophthalmol Soc UK 1976;96:377–381.)

ually and measuring the size of each pupil. Indeed, he was one of the first investigators to quantify the RAPD (41).

Levatin substituted an alternating flashlight for the alternating cover test (42) (Fig. 15.6). His theory was that the differences in pupillary response to light would be accentuated if, instead of simply covering one eye and then the other in a lighted room, the patient focused on a distant target in a darkened room, and a pocket flashlight was swung back and forth multiple times to bring out the best response. Levatin et al. subsequently reported on the use of this **swinging flashlight test** to screen patients with possible optic neuropathies and emphasized that the sign was not always obvious (43). In fact, in 1998, Enyedi et al. compared the efficacy of the swinging flashlight test with that of the Gunn test for detecting an RAPD and found the former to be more sensitive (44).

Indeed, the swinging flashlight test is probably the most valuable clinical test of optic nerve dysfunction available to

the general physician because it can detect dysfunction of the prechiasmal (and, in fact, pregeniculate) afferent visual sensory system in the absence of any ophthalmoscopic evidence of such a dysfunction.

Thompson and colleagues (45–47) described the method

for performing the swinging flashlight test and emphasized several important points, a few of which are repeated here:

First, a bright handlight and a darkened room are essential. The more contrast there is between the light beam and the darkened room, the greater will be the amplitude of the pupillary movement, and the easier it will be to see a small RAPD. It is possible, however, to use too much light. In such cases, a bright afterimage is produced that may keep the pupils small for several seconds, thus obscuring the pupillary dilation in the abnormal eye (48).

Second, the patient must fixate on a distant target during the test. This prevents the miosis that occurs during the near response, making the assessment of pupillary constriction difficulty if not impossible.

Third, in patients with ocular misalignment (i.e., strabismus or displacement of the globe by an orbital or intracranial process), care must be taken to shine the light along the visual axis. Shining the light directly into one eye and obliquely into the other may produce an RAPD.

Fourth, the light should cross from one eye to the other fairly rapidly but should remain on each eye for 3–5 seconds to allow pupillary stabilization.

Thus, there really are two parts of the pupillary response that must be observed during the swinging flashlight test: the initial pupillary constriction response, and the pupillary escape that is observed for 2–5 seconds after the light is shined into the eye. Most examiners vary the rate at which they move the light from eye to eye, and there is often an optimum ''swing rate'' that brings out an RAPD that varies among patients. Some authors recommend moving the light from one pupil to the other before the latter can escape from the consensual response to bring out an RAPD (49); however, **the light should never be left longer on one eye than on the other** as this might tend to create an RAPD in the eye with the longer light exposure, because the longer the light is kept on the eye, the more pupillary dilation occurs as the eye adapts to the light. In addition, if the retina becomes bleached in one eye and not in the other, a small RAPD will be produced. Special care must be taken to keep retina bleach equal, especially when measuring with neutral density filters greater than 1.2 log units in density (50) (see later).

Finally, the swinging flashlight test can be performed as long as there are two pupils, even when one pupil is nonreactive and dilated or constricted from neurologic disease, iris trauma, or topical drugs. Recall that as the light is shifted from the normal to the abnormal eye, the total pupillomotor input is reduced. Thus, the efferent stimulus for pupillary constriction is reduced in **both eyes** so that both pupils dilate. In performing the swinging flashlight test, one tends to observe only the pupil that is being illuminated; however, **the opposite pupil is responding in an identical fashion**. Thus, if one pupil is mechanically or pharmacologically nonreactive, the examiner can simply perform a swinging flashlight test observing only the reactive pupil. If the abnormal eye is the eye with a fixed pupil, then the pupil of the normal eye will constrict briskly when light is shined directly in it and will dilate when the light is shined in the opposite eye. If the abnormal eye is the eye with the reactive pupil, the pupil will constrict when light is shined in the opposite eye and dilate when the light is shined directly in it. This is extremely helpful in attempting to determine if a patient with an oculomotor nerve paresis or traumatic iridoplegia also has an optic neuropathy or retinal dysfunction (22).

The swinging flashlight test can be refined further in patients in whom a unilateral optic neuropathy is suspected but who do not seem to have an RAPD when a standard swinging flashlight test is performed. In such patients, the use of a neutral density filter with a transmission of 0.3

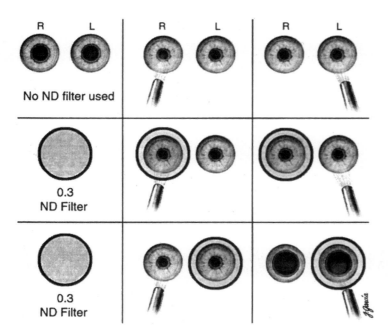

Figure 15.7. The use of neutral density filters to bring out a relative afferent pupillary defect (RAPD). *Above,* The patient has decreased vision in the left eye, but a swinging flashlight test fails to demonstrate a convincing RAPD in the left eye. *Middle,* A 0.3 log unit neutral density filter is placed over the right eye, and a swinging flashlight test is performed. No relative afferent pupillary defect is induced. *Bottom,* The filter is then place over the left eye, and the test is repeated. There is now a left relative afferent in the left eye, when the filter is placed in front of the right eye and the swinging flashlight test is performed, the reduced brightness in the right eye will tend to balance the reduced brightness in the left eye (from the optic neuropathy), and no RAPD will be seen. However, placing the filter in front of the left eye while performing the swinging flashlight test further reduces the light input in the left eye and further increases the difference in light input between the two eyes. Thus, there is now an obvious RAPD during the test.

logarithmic units often permits the detection of the defect (51) (Fig. 15.7). The test is performed as follows. The filter is first placed over one eye, and the swinging flashlight test is performed. The filter is then placed over the opposite eye, and the swinging flashlight is repeated. If there is truly no defect in the afferent system in either eye, placing the filter over either eye will simply induce a slight but symmetric RAPD in the eye covered by the filter from reduction in the amount of light entering the system through that eye. On the other hand, if one eye already has a mild RAPD, placement of the filter over that eye will further reduce the amount of light entering the system through that eye, thus increasing the previously inapparent or subtle defect and causing it to become obvious, whereas placement of the filter over the opposite (normal) eye will simply balance the RAPD in the opposite eye, and there will be no significant asymmetry in pupillary responses to light.

One can also quantify the RAPD using graded neutral density filters that are calibrated in percent transmittance (52). After determining that an RAPD is present, the examiner balances the defect by adding successive neutral density filters in 0.3 logarithmic steps over the **normal eye** while performing the swinging flashlight test, until the defect disappears (Fig. 15.8). The most useful neutral density filters are those ranging in transmission from 80% (0.1 log unit) to 1% (2.0 log units). Separate filters can be used individually or in combination in front of the eye (Fig. 15.9).

When using neutral density filters to quantify an RAPD, the examiner should make a decision about the presence of absence of the RAPD within 2–3 swings after the filter is placed in front of the normal eye. If more swings are needed, he or she must rebleach the retina of the covered eye and resume measuring. The neutral density filters should be held near the nose, so that stray light does not affect the measurement. Filters more than 1.2 log units in density are so dark that it is hard to see the pupil through them, even when light is shined on the eye. The examiner thus may need to peek around the filter to make a judgment. To reach the endpoint of the test, the examiner should overshoot the endpoint; i.e., produce an RAPD in the normal (covered) eye. The examiner should then rebleach the retina of that eye and perform the swinging flashlight test with another filter at the next lower amount. Several ''rules of thumb'' in measuring the RAPD for various conditions are found in Table 15.1.

Although some authors (53) have used a grading scale for the RAPD based on the initial pupillary constriction and how quickly the pupil redilates (e.g., Grade I: weak initial constriction followed by greater redilation; Grade II: a slight ''stall'' in movement, followed by a definite dilation; Grade III: immediate pupillary dilation [i.e., pupillary escape]; Grade IV: pupillary dilation during prolonged illumination of the contralateral eye for 6 seconds, followed by constriction; Grade V: immediate pupillary dilation and no signs of constriction), these systems are subject to inter-observer errors and are affected by pupillary size; e.g., the small pupil may not show a detectable initial constriction.

There is some correlation between the severity of an RAPD and the size of a peripheral field defect in the eye

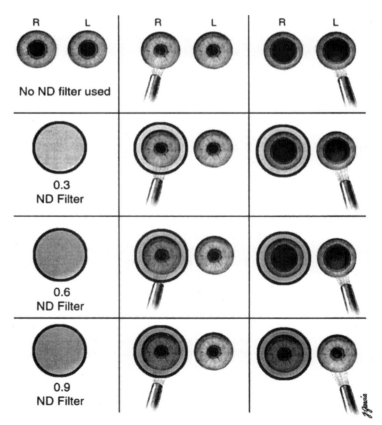

Figure 15.8. Quantification of the relative afferent pupillary defect (RAPD) using neutral density filters and the swinging flashlight test. Neutral density filters of increasing density are placed in front of the normal eye in a patient with a contralateral RAPD, and a swinging flashlight test is performed until the RAPD disappears. In this case, the RAPD is balanced with a 0.9 log unit filter.

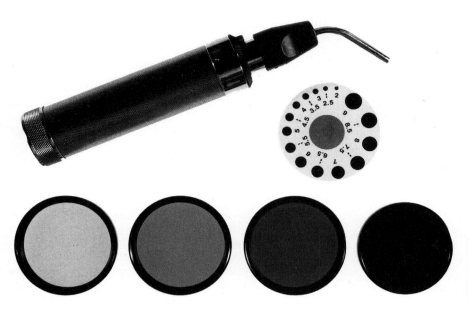

Figure 15.9. The equipment needed to quantify or bring out a relative afferent pupillary defect includes a bright handheld light source, a pupil gauge, and a set of photographic neutral density filters in 0.3, 0.6, 0.9, and 1.2 steps.

Table 15.1
Expected Relative Afferent Pupillary Defect in Various Settings

Condition	Expected RAPD	Comment	References
Optic nerve	0.3–3 log units	If no RAPD, either no optic neuropathy or bilateral disease	22,143
Chiasm	Only if asymmetric		
Optic tract	0.4–0.6 log units in the eye with the temporal visual field defect (contralateral to the tract lesion)	From asymmetry of the pupillomotor fibers (more crossed fibers than uncrossed)	144–146
Pretectal lesion	Contralateral RAPD without associated loss of visual acuity, color vision, or visual field		147
Visual field defect	RAPD correlates with severity of visual field loss		55
Central visual field defects	Greater pupillary escape		148
Peripheral visual field defects	Greater sustained pupillary response		25
Amblyopia	<0.5 log unit	If >1.0 log unit, look for other explanation	22,149
Anisocoria	0.1 log unit for every 1 mm difference; <3 mm of anisocoria induces RAPD that may be difficult to measure	Must assess in light	150
Macular disease	If visual acuity >20/200, RAPD of ≤0.5 log units	Even worst macular disease causes RAPD of <1.0 log unit	22,151
Central serous choridopathy	<0.3 log units		152
Central retinal vein occlusion	Ischemic: 0.9–1.2 log units; Nonischemic: <0.6 log units		153
Retinal hemorrhage	Small: none; large: major intraocular can produce RAPD of ≤1.2 log units	Depends on amount of light blocked	154
Retinal detachment	1 quadrant: 0.3 log units; 2 quadrants: 0.6 log units; macula: 0.9 log units. Total: 2 log units		46,155,156
Retinitis pigmentosa	≤0.3 log units		157
Cataract	≤0.3 in opposite eye but only if cataract very dense	From upregulation of photoreceptors in eye with cataract	158,159
Patching; dark adaptation	≤1.5 log units in nonoccluded eye	Maximum RAPD in 30 minutes; reverses in 10 minutes	160,161
Glaucoma	Usually none unless unilateral or markedly asymmetric	Corresponds with remaining neuroretinal rim	162,163
Refractive error	None		164
Nonorganic visual loss	None		22,39

RAPD, relative afferent pupillary defect.

detected by kinetic perimetry (54). There is less convincing evidence of a correlation between the pupillary response and a central field defect in the eye detected by static perimetry (55).

Tests other than the swinging flashlight test can be used to detect a relative afferent pupillary defect. Kestenbaum proposed a test that is loosely based on the Gunn phenomenon, in which the patient fixes in the distance with one eye, while the other eye is occluded by the palm of the hand (56). The examiner holds a handlight with fresh batteries 1 inch from the uncovered eye for 5 seconds to allow the pupils to stabilize. The size of the uncovered pupil is then measured with a pupil gauge to the nearest 0.25 mm. The size of the opposite pupil is then measured in the same fashion, and the difference between the two eyes is determined after correcting for any initial anisocoria. This result is called ''Kestenbaum's number.''

Jiang and Thompson measured the RAPD in a group of patients using the swinging flashlight test with neutral density filters (57). They compared the results with the results of the Kestenbaum test and found a distinct relationship between the severity of the RAPD measured with neutral density filters and Kestenbaum's number (r = 0.86). The major problem with the Kestenbaum test includes the need for two intact iris sphincters and the problem of miosis of the elderly and hippus in the young (57).

A highly sensitive way to detect an RAPD is by using pupillography (58,59). Pupillary reactions that occur during stimulation of an eye with a damaged retina or optic nerve have a prolonged latent period and a shortened duration and diminished amplitude of constriction. These parameters can be evaluated by pupillography. For example, inflammatory diseases of the optic nerve and optic atrophy are associated with significant prolongation of the latent period, ischemic optic neuropathy produces a lesser prolongation, and acute papilledema does not affect latency at all (60). Furthermore, portable pupillography units can detect and measure large RAPDs quickly, even in a clinical setting (61), and such devices can be linked to computerized systems to test the visual field (62,63).

Tests used to detect an RAPD, particularly the swinging flashlight test, are sensitive tests for optic nerve dysfunction; however, they represent only one type of test used to determine whether or not a patient has an optic neuropathy and, if so, the degree of severity of the optic nerve dysfunction.

Other tests of optic nerve function are reviewed in Chapter 4 of this text.

Other Clinical Tests of Pupillary Function

The swinging flashlight test provides only relative information regarding the visual sensory system of the two eyes, because the pupillary light response of one eye is compared with that of the other eye. In order to assess the pupillary light reflex of each eye separately, however, one can evaluate the number of pupillary oscillations that occur over a fixed amount of time or determine the time it takes for a pupil to oscillate a specific number of times when stimulated by light (64–66). In this test, a thin beam of light (0.5 mm wide) is placed horizontally across the inferior aspect of the pupillary margin (Fig. 15.10). The light induces pupillary constriction that moves the light out of the pupil. The pupil then redilates until the beam is once again at the edge of the pupillary margin, whereupon the pupil again constricts, creating a cycle. A set number of cycles (usually 10, 20, or 30) are then timed by a stopwatch to the nearest 0.1 second, and the time of the cycle—the **edge-light pupil cycle time**—is calculated as msec/cycle. Alternatively, the number of cycles that occur during a fixed period of time, usually 1 minute, are counted. In both cases, the results are compared with results from normal control subjects. For instance, normal pupils generally cycle at a rate of 900 msec/cycle.

Unfortunately, the edge-light pupil cycle time is not a particularly sensitive indicator of optic nerve disease compared with the swinging flashlight test or visual evoked potentials. In addition, it may be difficult or impossible to induce regular oscillations in some patients and, as with other tests of pupillary constriction, the edge-light pupil cycle time is affected by the efferent arm of the pupillary light reflex (e.g., oculomotor nerve function). Nevertheless, it is a potentially useful initial diagnostic test in one-eyed patients or in patients with presumed bilateral symmetric retinal or optic nerve disease (67,68).

Pupil Cycle Induction Test

The **pupil cycle induction test** is a variation of the edge-light pupil cycle time (69). It is used to assess the difficulty in producing regular and sustained light-induced pupillary oscillations. In this test, a beam with a thickness of 0.45 mm or less is placed horizontally at the lower edge of the pupil-

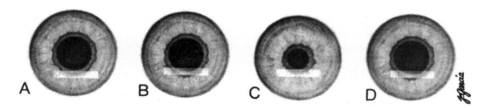

Figure 15.10. Testing the edge-light pupil cycle time. The pupil can be induced to cycle at the slit lamp by placing a horizontally oriented slit beam on the lower pupil margin. The beam is then moved slightly upward, inducing pupillary constriction that moves the light out of the pupil. The pupil then redilates until the beam is once again at the edge of the pupillary margin, whereupon the pupil again constricts, creating a cycle.

Table 15.2
Pharmacologic Testing in Diagnosing Common Pupil Conditions

Agent	Setting/Purpose	Dose	Time	Lighting	Measure	End Point	Caution
Testing for denervation supersensitivity							
Dilute pilocarpine (165–167)	Dilated, poorly reactive or nonreactive pupil to distinguish tonic pupil from 3rd nerve palsy pupil or pharmacologic blockade	0.0625–0.1% (168)	30 min	Dim light or darkness	Change in pupil diameter	>0.5 mm difference between two eyes *or* the larger abnormal pupil becomes the smaller pupil	Limited usefulness-bilateral Adie pupil; normals can react variably to medication; cannot reliably distinguish between 3rd nerve palsy and tonic pupil (167)
Testing for Pharmacologic Blockade							
Pilocarpine	Dilated, fixed pupil to distinguish pharmacologic blockade from tonic pupil or 3rd nerve palsy pupil	2%	40 min	darkness	Change in pupil diameter	Pupil that is pharmacologically blockaded should not constrict at all or should constrict minimally	Other causes of dilated pupil may prevent constriction; e.g., traumatic or post-herpetic iridoplegia; angle-closure glaucoma; fixed pupil after cataract surgery (154)
Testing for Horner Syndrome							
Cocaine (169)	Anisocoria with normal pupillary reactions to light to determine if sympathetic defect present	2–10%	40–60 min	Light	Larger pupil dilates; smaller pupil either dilates poorly or not at all	>0.8 mm inequality is positive; <0.3 negative	If the affected pupil dilates >2 mm to cocaine, be wary (170); keep patient alert because sleep may give a false-negative test; always assess test result in dark
Hydroxyamphetamine (and Tyramine) (171)	In proven Horner syndrome to differentiate between first/second order and third order Horner syndrome	5%	50–60 min	Light	Dilation of Horner pupil indicates first or second order Horner syndrome; dilation of normal pupil but not of Horner pupil indicates third-order syndrome	>1 mm change in anisocoria **OR** a change of anisocoria (difference in pre to post-anisocoria) of >0.5 mm suggests post-ganglionic (171); increased size of smaller pupil over normal pupil suggests preganglionic defect (154)	Should not be performed on same day as cocaine test; some authors suggest waiting 3 days; not always accurate in congenital Horner syndrome because of trans-synaptic degeneration (154)
Apraclonidine (172,173)	Anisocoria with normally reactive pupils; to determine if sympathetic defect present	0.5–1%	60 min	Light	Dilation of the smaller pupil (reversal of anisocoria)	Dilation of smaller pupil with reversal of anisocoria (normal pupils never dilate >0.5 mm)	Helpful when cocaine not available, but does *not* differentiate pre- and postganglionic Horner syndromes
Phenylephrine 2.5%	To confirm a Horner syndrome and to exclude a small immovable pupil causing a positive test	2.5%	30–60 min	Light	Pupillary size after treatment	The Horner pupil should dilate as well as or more than other pupil	A normal pupil will also dilate

lary margin in much the same way as in testing the edge-light pupil cycle time. The pupils of almost all eyes with normal optic nerves can generally be induced to cycle at regular intervals, whereas the pupils of almost all eyes with optic nerve disease show altered responses, such as complete failure to cycle or prolonged pauses in the cycle. We have found the results of testing edge-light pupil cycle time and pupil cycle induction difficult to interpret, not particularly reproducible, and less sensitive than the results of a simple swinging flashlight test. We thus use these tests only when assessing monocular patients.

PHARMACOLOGIC TESTING

A few cautionary comments should be made regarding the interpretation of pupillary responses to topically instilled drugs.

First, the test variables must be carefully controlled whenever possible, both before and after pharmacologic testing. This means that the ambient lighting should be optimal for the test performed, the patient must fixate in the distance for at least 1 minute to minimize miosis and relax the pupil, and the patient should be alert throughout the test, because the psychic state of the individual can influence pupillary size (e.g., the pupils tend to be miotic in persons who are tired or listless and mydriatic in patients who are upset or anxious) (70).

Second, the pupil sizes must be measured as accurately as possible. The CU-5 camera manufactured by the Polaroid Company allows the direct measurement of pupillary size; however, one can simply paste or tape a ruler on the patient's brow and then use any camera to obtain photographs from which accurate measurements can be made. Pupillometers also provide accurate measurements but are not well suited to most clinical practices.

Third, it is ideal, whenever possible, to use the presumably normal pupil as an internal control. For instance, if a judgment is to be made about the dilation or constriction of one of the pupils in response to a drop of some topical agent, such as 0.1% pilocarpine, 10% cocaine, or 5% hydroxyam-phetamine (see Chapter 16), the drug should be placed in **both eyes** so that the responses of the two eyes can be compared. When the condition is bilateral, no such comparisons are possible, but an attempt should be made to make certain that the observed response is indeed caused by the instilled drug. In such cases, the drug may be placed in one eye only so that the responses of the medicated and unmedicated eyes can be compared. Occasionally, in patients with presumed bilateral pupillary abnormalities, we and others (22) place drops in both of the patient's eyes and also in one of our own, to serve as a type of external control.

Finally, the drug should always be placed in the eye of concern **first** and then placed in the contralateral eye so that if there is no response in the presumably abnormal eye, one cannot blame squeezing or tearing as the cause.

Problems can occur when performing pharmacologic testing of the pupil using topical drugs. The drug may be outdated and thus more or less potent. The patient may develop sufficient tearing that the strength of the drug is altered by dilution, or it is washed out of the inferior conjunctival sac before it can be absorbed. The patient may squeeze the eyes tightly during instillation of the drug, thus preventing a sufficient amount of drug from being placed in the inferior conjunctival sac. Penetration of the drug through the cornea may be altered, especially if other topical medications have been used; e.g., anesthetics for testing of intraocular pressure, or if the integrity of the corneal epithelium has been altered by manipulation of the cornea during tonometry or testing of corneal sensation. One must also consider individual variations in the action of the drug on patients of different ages or with different colored irides.

Determining the results of pupillary testing can also be difficult depending on the initial size of the pupil. Differences in pupillary diameter or area can have profound results on the ultimate outcome in pharmacologic testing (Table 15.2).

Finally, it is important to remember why a particular test is being performed in the first place (Table 15.2). The correct drug must be used and placed in the eyes in the proper fashion.

ASSESSMENT OF ACCOMMODATION, CONVERGENCE, AND THE NEAR RESPONSE

Most visual problems associated with accommodation occur because accommodation is too great, too little, or too slow. Disturbances of the other two components of the near response—convergence and pupillary miosis—also can be of importance if they are too active or if they have reduced activity.

HISTORY

The symptoms of patients with disturbances of accommodation tend to be nonspecific but some aspects of the history may be important. Patients with accommodative insufficiency, for instance, usually complain of blurred vision at near but not in the distance. Patients with the most common problem with accommodation—**presbyopia**—may report that the farther away they hold an object, the better they can see it. Some patients with accommodative insufficiency report monocular diplopia; others complain of discomfort during attempted reading, a noticeable delay in focusing when changing fixation from a distant to a near or a near to a distant object, or a combination of these symptoms. Some patients report headache, light intolerance, and other asthenopic symptoms (71). Frequently, presbyopia and other accommodative insufficient states can be precipitated with medications having anticholinergic effects.

Accommodative excess or spasm is typically associated with clear vision at near and poor distance vision. Objects may look larger or smaller (macropsia or micropsia) than normal in this setting. In addition, patients with accommodative excess or spasm often complain of brow ache (72). When convergence also is affected, other symptoms may be present. For example, convergence excess often is associated with diplopia in the distance, blurring of vision, oscillopsia, and/or pain; whereas convergence insufficiency most often is associated with trouble reading, diplopia at near, blurred vision that clears when either eye is covered, and pain or discomfort during near tasks.

In patients with **spasm of the near reflex**, symptoms are related to dysfunction of all three components. Such patients have accommodative spasm (up to 8–10 diopters), extreme miosis, an esotropia in primary position, and apparent but inconsistent bilateral limitation of abduction. These patients tend to complain of blurred or dim vision, binocular horizontal diplopia at both distance and near, temple or diffuse headache, pain in the eyes, and even trouble walking (73,74). Spasm of the near reflex is discussed in detail in Chapter 16 of this text.

EXAMINATION

Accommodation is the ability of the lens to change its refractive power in order to keep the image of an object clear on the retina. The primary stimulus for accommodation is blurring (75), and most tests of accommodation depend on producing or eliminating blur. There are, however, stimuli for accommodation other than blur, including chromatic aberration and perceived nearness (76), and these can also be used to test accommodation.

General Principles Related to the Components of the Near Triad

Accommodation is part of a complex triad that maintains clear near vision and is called the **near response** or the **near reflex**. Even though the components of the near response—accommodation, convergence, and pupillary miosis—normally work together during near viewing, each component can be tested separately. For example, one can weaken the stimulus to accommodation with plus lenses or strengthen the stimulus to accommodation with weak minus lenses without stimulating convergence or miosis. One can use weak base-out prisms to stimulate convergence without changing accommodation. Under certain conditions, one can test accommodation without inducing pupillary constriction (77). In addition, even in presbyopia in which accommodation fails, convergence and miosis continue. Furthermore, if one paralyzes accommodation with drugs, convergence remains intact. **Relative accommodation** is the term used to describe the amount of accommodation that is unrelated to convergence; **relative convergence** describes the amount of convergence unrelated to accommodation (78).

Depth of focus is slightly different from accommodation. It is the distance for any given accommodative state that an object can be viewed without a change in acuity or generation of blur. Depth of focus is more dependent on pupillary size and amount of illumination than is accommodation. For example, accommodation is not significantly affected by miosis and bright illumination; however, in patients with small pupils and bright illumination, the depth of focus is increased. Thus, a patient over 60 years of age will have very little, if any, accommodation; however, if one compares two patients, one with large pupils and the other with small pupils, the patient with the smaller pupils will have an increased

depth of focus, and this increased depth of focus may be mistaken for accommodation. Many traditional tests of accommodation thus may overestimate the amount or range of accommodation in a patient because the tests cannot distinguish true accommodation from combined accommodation and depth of focus (79).

Accommodation

There are actually three aspects of accommodation: the near point of accommodation, the accommodative amplitude, and the range of accommodation. The **near point of accommodation** (NPA) is the point closest to the eye at which a target is sharply focused on the retina. The **accommodative amplitude** is the power of the lens that permits such clear vision. This power is measured in units called diopters (D) and is calculated by dividing the NPA in centimeters into 100. The accommodative amplitude is thus simply the reciprocal of the NPA (e.g., a patient with an NPA of 25 cm has an accommodative amplitude of 100/25 = 4 D). The **range of accommodation** is the distance between the furthest point an object of a certain size is in clear sight and the nearest point at which the eye can maintain that clear vision.

Convergence

Convergence is a vergence adduction movement that increases the visual angle to permit single binocular vision during near viewing. Convergence can be voluntary but need not be; i.e., no stimulus need be present to elicit it. It is also reflexive and a co-movement in the near response. Accommodation and convergence are related; a unit change in one normally causes a unit change in the other (80).

Convergence may be separated into four subtypes: (a) tonic convergence; (b) accommodative convergence; (c) fusional convergence; and (d) voluntary convergence.

The eyes normally tend to diverge. Keeping the eyes straight thus requires increased tone in the medial rectus muscles. This tone is **tonic convergence** (81).

Accommodative convergence is the amount of convergence elicited for a given amount of accommodation. The relationship between accommodation and convergence is usually expressed as the ratio of accommodative convergence in prism diopters (PD) to accommodation in diopters: the AC/A ratio. Because accommodation decreases with age, the AC/A ratio increases with age (72,82). Just as convergence can be stimulated by accommodation, so accommodation can be stimulated by convergence. The ratio of convergence accommodation in diopters to convergence in PD is called the CA/C ratio.

Fusional convergence is convergence that is stimulated not by changes in accommodation but by disparate retinal images (81). It is thought to be used to "fine tune" normal convergence. Pupillary constriction can occur with fusional vergence, but the amplitude of this form of convergence is not as great as that of accommodative convergence.

Voluntary convergence is measured by determining the near point of convergence (NPC)—the nearest point to which the eye can converge. It is closer to the eyes than the near point of accommodation and, in general, does not deteriorate with age as does the NPA. The NPC usually is 10 cm or less.

Miosis

The pupil constricts when changing fixation from distance to near. This movement can occur in darkness, is slower than the light reflex, and is maintained as long as the near reaction is maintained. Miosis improves the range through which an object is seen clearly without any change in accommodation; i.e., the depth of field (see above). The miotic response to the near effort is directly dependent on that effort. Normal persons usually need a visible target to view to reach maximal pupillary miosis and accompanying accommodation. This miotic response also can be inadvertently stimulated by forceful eyelid closure (83). In patients with presbyopia, pupil size continues to decrease even when accommodation has reached its maximum. This probably occurs because aging changes limit alterations in the lens or ciliary muscles, whereas the pupillary sphincter is still functional and responsive to stimulation (84). On the other hand, artificially induced miosis (e.g., pharmacologic) reduces the amplitude of accommodation (85).

In testing accommodation and the near vision response, the above relationships must be remembered. Furthermore, one must remember that accommodation is never measured or tested in an absolute sense, but rather in response to how it changes under certain testing conditions (86).

Testing Techniques

The techniques one uses to determine the range and amplitude of accommodation, degree of convergence, etc. depend in part on the setting and the questions to be answered.

Accommodation

The principal handicaps in the clinical application of adequate tests of accommodation are the subjective nature of the end points and the number of variables that must be controlled. The first step in any testing of components of accommodation or the near triad, is to perform an adequate refraction for both distance and near viewing. For children and some adults, a cycloplegic refraction with an agent such as cyclopentolate (Cyclogyl) is needed to prevent the patient from accommodating and thus increasing the degree of myopia requiring correction during the refraction (87,88). Indeed, this "pseudomyopia" may be the first clue to accommodative spasm. Conversely, excellent distant vision and poor near vision may indicate accommodative insufficiency or presbyopia.

The NPA is most easily measured clinically using a scale device such as the Prince, Krimsky, or Berens rules (89–91). These instruments are simply rulers with markings in both centimeters and diopters on which there is a small sliding chart containing Snellen letters (Fig. 15.11). The technique of testing accommodation with them is called the "push-up method" (92) and is performed as follows.

Wearing an optimum distance refraction and with the op-posite eye occluded, the patient fixes on small (usually 5 point) type on a card that is attached to the rule and that can be slid forward and backward. The size of the type is important, because the smallest type will evoke the strongest accommodative response (93). The zero point of the rule should be 11–14 mm in front of the cornea. This corresponds to the approximate position of the spectacle correction. The card is moved from a distance to the closest point at which the patient can see the print before it starts to blur. This is the NPA and, as noted above, is expressed in centimeters. The maneuver is repeated several times until the test gives reproducible results.

Once the NPA is determined, the accommodative amplitude in diopters, as indicated above, is calculated by dividing 100 by the NPA in centimeters. Using the push-up method, Duane (94) developed age-related normative data for the accommodative amplitude that are still in use today (Fig. 15.12).

Although the push-up method of determining the NPA and the accommodation amplitude has the disadvantage of overestimating accommodation, it is the most widely used method, the quickest in clinical practice, and the most popular. When interpreting the results of testing of accommodation using the push-up method, the examiner must be sure that the patient fully cooperated with the testing. Nevertheless, if, on repeated testing, the NPA (and thus the accommodative amplitude) is consistently out of the range considered to be normal for age, the results should be considered truly abnormal (94).

Adequate room lighting obviously must be available when testing accommodation, and it usually is recommended that the light be directed over the right shoulder when testing the right eye and over the left shoulder when testing the left eye. Indeed, illumination is a critical factor in performing the test. By increasing illumination from 1 to 25 foot-candles, the accommodative range can be increased by 28% in non-presbyopes and by 73% in presbyopes (95).

The range of accommodation can be tested in a fashion similar to that used to test the accommodative amplitude. The patient is instructed to indicate when the object blurs at near (the near point or NPA) and when it blurs in the distance (the far point). The range of accommodation is then calculated by determining the far point and near point in diopters (i.e., dividing each of the distances in centimeters into 100) and by subtracting the far point from the near point. For an emmetrope, the range of accommodation corresponds to the accommodative amplitude because the far point is at infinity. For a myope whose near point is 10 cm and whose far point is 50 cm **in front** of the eye, the range of accommodation is $100/10 - 100/50 = 10 - 2 = 8$ D. For a hyperope with a near point of 10 cm and a far point of 25 cm **behind** the eye, the range of accommodation is $100/10 - (-100/25) = 10 - (-4) = 10 + 4 = 14$ D. If the patient is too presbyopic or myopic to do the test, corrective lenses should be used. One must then adjust the results to reflect the correction. If a minus lens has been used, the diopter power of the lens is added to the result; if a plus lens has been used, the diopter power is subtracted.

The push-up method of measuring the NPA and the ac-

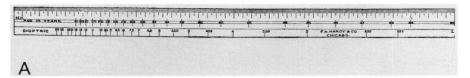

A

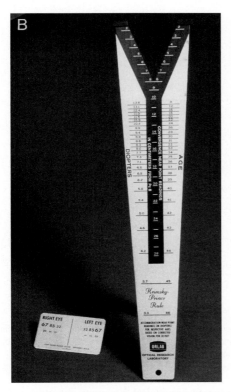

B

Figure 15.11. Photographs of accommodative rules. *A,* The Prince Rule. *B,* The Krimsky-Prince Rule. *C,* The Berens Rule. (*A,* From Wood CA. The American Encyclopedia and Dictionary of Ophthalmology. Chicago, Cleveland Press, 1919: 10961. *B,* Photo courtesy Paul Montague, CRP.)

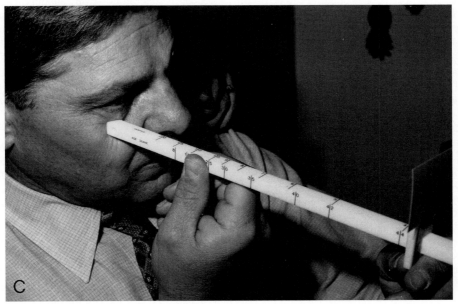

C

Numerical Values of Limits for Each Age

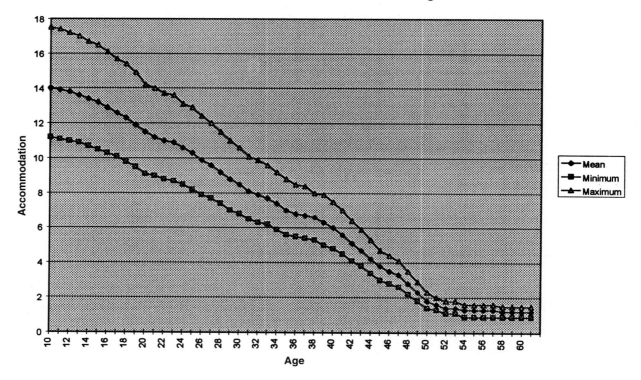

Figure 15.12.   The relationship between accommodation and age. Note the relatively linear decrease in accommodation with age until about age 52, when almost all accommodation has been lost. (Graph data from Duane A. The accommodation and Donders curve and the need of revising our ideas regarding them. JAMA 1909;52:1992–1996.)

commodative amplitude is not the only one that can be used. A second method is the **method of the spheres**. In this test, the patient fixates on a reading target at 40 cm, and accommodation is stimulated by progressively adding minus (i.e., concave) lenses until the print blurs. Accommodation is then relaxed by adding stronger plus (i.e., convex) lenses until the print again blurs. The sum of the lenses is the measure of the accommodative amplitude. For example, if a patient accepts up to a −4.0 D sphere before print blurs and then accepts the addition of +2.50 D sphere before print again blurs, the total accommodative amplitude is 4.0 D + 2.5 D = 6.50 D (72). Like the push-up method for determining the NPA and the accommodative amplitude, the method of the spheres depends on patient cooperation.

The most objective method of measuring accommodation is the use of refractometers (96,97). Most of these machines use increasingly minus lenses to stimulate accommodation and measure the accommodative response. Alternatively, one can stimulate accommodation not with lenses but pharmacologically by using a topical agent muscarinic agonist like pilocarpine and measure the response using a refractometer (98).

Convergence

Like accommodation, there is a near point of convergence (NPC), a convergence amplitude, and a range of conver-

gence. In general, however, the only measurement of importance is the NPC. This measurement usually is determined by having the patient fixate on an accommodative target held 33 cm from the eyes. The target then is moved toward the nose, with the patient being instructed to try to keep the target in focus. The end-point of the test is when the patient reports horizontal diplopia. The distance at which this occurs is then measured with a millimeter ruler placed alongside the patient's nose.

The NPC also can be determined by placing a red glass over one eye and moving a light forward until the patient experiences diplopia (99) or, more objectively, by performing the above test and noting the distance from the nose at which one of the inward turning eyes is observed to turn suddenly outward. In normal persons, the NPC is usually between 5–10 cm (100). An NPC greater than 30 cm indicates convergence insufficiency.

Yet another way to determine if convergence is normal is to perform a cover-uncover test (see Chapter 18) while the patient is reading. This is helpful only if the patient has full versions and no previous strabismus.

In addition to determining the NPC, it may be useful to determine if a patient's convergence is sufficient for the amount of accommodation; i.e., the AC/A ratio. There are two different methods for measuring the AC/A ratio.

The **gradient method** determines the AC/A ratio by the

change in deviation in prism diopters (PD) that occurs when a lens of a specific power is placed over both eyes to stimulate or relax accommodation (101). An accommodative target must be used, and the working distance is held constant. Plus or minus lenses are used to vary the accommodative requirement, and the difference between the ocular alignment with and without the lens, divided by the power of the lens, is the AC/A ratio. For example, a patient's ocular alignment is measured with the patient viewing the accommodative target at a specific distance such as 33 cm, and the patient is found to have an esophoria of 2 PD. A -1.00 D spherical lens is placed over each eye, and ocular alignment is again measured with the patient viewing the same target at the same distance. The patient is now found to have an esophoria of 6 PD. The difference between the ocular alignment with and without the lens, divided by the power of the lens, is the AC/A ratio and is $6 - 2/1 = 4/1 = 4$. This means that when 1 diopter of accommodation was stimulated in this patient by placing a -1.00 D spherical lens in front of the eyes, the patient's convergence, measured at the same distance from the eyes, increased from 2 to 6 PD. In another patient, a $+3.00$ sphere might be used to reduce accommodation, and a change in deviation from an exotropia of 4 PD to an exotropia of 10 PD might be noted. The AC/A ratio then would be $10 - 4/3 = 6/3 = 2$.

The second method for determining the AC/A ratio is the **heterophoria method**. This method uses the distance-near relationship to determine the AC/A ratio. Instead of measuring ocular alignment at near with and without a specific power lens, ocular alignment is measured at distance and near, and the difference in alignment in PD between distance and near viewing is divided by the fixation distance used for near viewing as expressed in diopters. Normal persons should have the same ocular alignment when viewing both distant and near objects. If a patient is more exotropic or less esotropic at near compared with distance, this indicates less convergence, or a low AC/A ratio; if the patient is more esotropic or less exotropic at near compared with distance, this indicates a high AC/A ratio. For example, if a patient has an exophoria of 5 PD at distance and an esophoria of 4 PD at 33 cm, the AC/A ratio is $5 - (-4)/3 = 9/3 = 3$.

The normal AC/A ratio is between 3 and 6, regardless of the method of testing that is used (72). It should be noted, however, that the AC/A ratio varies from person to person and from day to day or hour to hour in a given individual depending on that person's level of fatigue or alertness. In addition, the AC/A ratio rises sharply after the age of 40 as accommodation begins to be lost but convergence remains stable (102). Nevertheless, values above 6 usually indicate an excess of convergence per unit of accommodation, whereas values below 3 suggest convergence insufficiency. An elevated AC/A ratio in a cooperative child is a risk factor for the rapid onset of myopia (103).

Testing convergence accommodation; i.e., the CA/A ratio, requires that the patient experience no blur during the test. This can be accomplished by the use of a pin hole device (104), performing the test in dim illumination (105), or using a Gaussian target (106). In this test, accommodation is measured as convergence is produced using progressively stronger base-out prisms. Unlike accommodation, convergence does not decline significantly with age (102). Thus, just as the AC/A ratio increases with age, the CA/C ratio decreases with age (102,105).

ASSESSMENT OF LACRIMATION

The most anterior optical surface of the eye, the **tear film**, is also one of the greatest optical powers of the eye, and a deficient tear film thus is one of the most common causes of fluctuating blurred vision in clinical practice. In fact, optical aberrations caused by an early break-up of the tear film have been shown objectively to diminish image quality (107).

The tear film is a trilaminar structure consisting of a superficial lipid layer, an aqueous middle component that accounts for over 90% of the film, and a mucin component in the innermost layer. In order to discern a problem of the tear secretion, one must attempt to determine if only one layer is affected or all the layers are affected.

The main function of the lipid layer is to retard evaporation of the tear film. Removal of this layer causes a 19-fold increase in evaporation (108,109).

The aqueous layer, being the thickest component of the tear film, contributes the most to its volume, and most of the tests that measure the quantity of the tear film test this layer. The aqueous layer of the tear film is produced by both the primary lacrimal gland located in the lacrimal fossa in the superior lateral orbit and the accessory lacrimal glands of Krause and Wolfring that are similar in structure to the main lacrimal gland but are much smaller in size. The glands of Krause are located in the upper fornix, whereas the glands of Wolfring are situated further down on the eyelid, above the tarsus. The relative importance of the main and accessory lacrimal glands in the maintenance of normal tear secretion is somewhat controversial. It generally is accepted that the main lacrimal gland, having an efferent parasympathetic innervation, functions primarily during **reflex** tear secretion, whereas the accessory lacrimal glands provide **basal** tear secretion (110,110a).

The mucin layer is a biphasic layer that allows the aqueous component to adhere to the hydrophobic cornea epithelium. This layer thus helps to maintain the integrity of the aqueous component of tears and the quality of the tear film. Abnormalities in this layer (and also in the oil layer) can create tear film disturbances despite good aqueous tear production. The mucin layer is produced by goblet cells located in the conjunctiva.

The normal basal tear volume is 5–9 μL, and the normal flow rate averages 0.5 to 2.2 μL/min (111). In general, neither basal tear volume nor flow changes with increasing age, but reflex tearing decreases with age (112).

The main disturbances of lacrimation relate to excess or insufficient tear production and to obstruction of the normal passage of tears through the lacrimal drainage apparatus. Thus, the assessment of patients with difficulties should be oriented to an evaluation of tear production and drainage.

HISTORY

Excessive drying of the eyes occurs in several settings, including reduced production, increased evaporation, and excessive drainage of tears. **Epiphora**—excessive tearing—also occurs under several different circumstances, including increased production of tears, an obstructed lacrimal drainage system, or excessive dryness of the eyes caused by a deficiency of normal basal tearing from hypofunction of the glands of Krause and Wolfring. In this last setting, the excess tearing is reflexive in nature and results from stimulation of the primary lacrimal gland in response to dryness and irritation of the cornea. Indeed, epiphora and irritation from dry eyes is one of the most common ocular problems in the United States (113) and the world (114).

The causes of dry eyes initially may be suspected from the results of a validated short questionnaire developed by Schein et al. (115) (Table 15.3). This questionnaire consists of six major questions. Even though these questions do not significantly correlate with tests of reduced tear function (e.g., lower Schirmer scores or abnormalities on Rose Bengal testing; see below), the questions nevertheless seem to be able to identify patients likely to have dry eyes.

Like dryness of the eyes, epiphora may cause blurred vision that is present during both distance and near viewing. Patients with epiphora should be asked about recent trauma to the eyelids or nose and about previous surgery in this area. They also should be queried about any symptoms or signs of recent infections or inflammations.

EXAMINATION

The examination of a patient with a disturbance of lacrimation is directed toward three main abnormalities: decreased tear production, increased tear production, and partial or complete obstruction of the lacrimal drainage apparatus.

Lid function is critical to spreading the tear film and should be assessed in any patient suspected of having an abnormality of tear function. Disturbances of eyelid structure and function can be detected both by simple external examination and by slit-lamp biomicroscopy. Slit-lamp examination can also detect punctate staining of the inferior cornea related to dry eyes, exposure (lagophthalmos), or a lid abnormality (112).

Table 15.3
Questions to Ask to Diagnose Dry Eyes

1. Do your eyes ever feel dry?
2. Do you ever have a gritty or sandy sensation in your eyes?
3. Do your eyes ever have a burning sensation?
4. Are your eyes ever red?
5. Do you notice much crusting on your lashes?
6. Do your eyes ever get stuck shut in the morning?

(From Schein OD, Hochberg MC, Munoz B, et al. Dry eye and dry mouth in the elderly: A population-based assessment. Arch Intern Med 1999;159:1359–1363; and Brewitt H, Sistani F. Dry eye disease: The scale of the problem. Surv Ophthalmol 2001;45[Suppl 2]:S199-S202.)

Tests of the tear film may be separated into those that test a particular part of the tear film or a particular function of the tears, those that measure the amount of tear secretion, and those that detect obstruction of tear drainage (115a).

The lipid layer can be studied using optical interference patterns, matching the color interference with known color controls. This method is used mainly for research purposes; however, lipid layer thickness measurements were strongly correlated with an assessment of fluorescein break-up time and the Schirmer 1 test in a series of patients evaluated by Isreb and colleagues (116) (see later). Thus, it would appear that a deficiency of the lipid layer of the tear film can be associated with clinical tests of tear film production and function.

An examination of the aqueous layer should begin with an assessment of the tear meniscus, which should be observed for evidence of protein precipitates and debris. A normal tear meniscus is about 1 mm; less than 0.3 mm is abnormal (117). At the same time, the relation of the tear meniscus to the lower eyelid can be assessed. The eyelids and lashes should be observed for evidence of entropion, ectropion, and stray lashes, and for the position and integrity of the lower lacrimal punctum, because such abnormalities may cause disturbances that simulate those caused by abnormal tear production.

Specific tests of the mucin layer of the tears include a conjunctival biopsy to determine if goblet cells are present and, if so, in what number. A qualitative test for mucin also can be performed. In this test, a cotton strip (3 mm × 10 mm) is placed in the inferior cul de sac of an unanesthetized eye for 5 minutes. The strip is then placed on a glass slide and stained with the periodic acid-Schiff (PAS) stain. If the stain is positive, mucin is present (112).

Impression cytology also can be used to determine if goblet cells are present and in what numbers. In this simple technique, cellulose acetate filter strips are placed on the conjunctival epithelium and then transferred to a glass slide where they are stained with hematoxylin and PAS. This procedure can be used to diagnose not only dry-eye conditions but also vitamin A deficiencies (118).

Other qualities of the tear film can be tested individually. For example, the tear film contains various proteins including albumin, immunoglobulins, and lysozyme (119). Lysozyme, an enzyme that lyses bacterial walls and is reduced in dry-eye syndromes, can be detected using the lysozyme lysis test. This test is said to be more reliable and sensitive than the Schirmer test (discussed later); however, the lysozyme lysis test requires gels, broth cultures, and measurements after incubating tear-soaked filter papers in the gel for 24 hours, whereas the Schirmer test requires only a strip of filter paper and a topical anesthetic. Other assays, such as an assay for tear lactoferrin (120), also may be useful in diagnosing such conditions as keratoconjunctivitis sicca (121). The osmolarity of the tear film can be measured. An increasing osmolarity may be diagnostic of keratoconjunctivitis sicca (122).

In patients with symptoms suggesting insufficient tear production, the most common tests performed are nonspecific tests of tear secretion. The sensitivity and specificity

Table 15.4
Sensitivity and Specificity of Tests for Tear Production

Test Name	Basis of Test	Reference Values	Sensitivity	Specificity
NIBUT	Noninvasive test of tear stability	<10 seconds suggests unstable tear film	82%	86%
Rose Bengal	Assess ocular surface damage	<3 sec, <1 sec	95%, 92%	96%, 86%
Schirmer 1	Assess reflex tear flow	≤5.5 mm, ≤3 mm, ≤5 mm, ≤10 mm	85%, 10%, 25%, 79%	83%, 100%, 90%, 97%
Schirmer 2	Assess reflex tear flow			
Phenol red thread	Assess tear volume	<6–10 mm	Unknown	Unknown

NIBUT, noninvasive tear breakup timen.
(Adapted from Mainstone JC, Bruce AS, Golding TR. Tear meniscus measurement in the diagnosis of dry eye. Curr Eye Res 1996;15:653–661; and from Versura P, Cellini M, Torreggiani V, et al. Dryness symptoms, diagnostic protocol and therapeutic management: a report on 1200 patients. Ophthalmic Res 2001;33:221–227.)

of these tests vary greatly (Table 15.4), depending on the specific test used and the reference criteria for normal values.

Judging the height of the tear meniscus may predict the amount of tear production and secretion as may assessment of radius of curvature, height, width, and cross-sectional area; however, there is little correlation between the results of this technique and the results of more objective tests of tear production (e.g., the Schirmer test) unless quantitative measurements of the meniscus are made (123).

The **noninvasive tear film break-up time** test is perhaps the simplest test used to determine the adequacy of the tear film (124). In this test, the examiner touches the conjunctiva of an unanesthetized eye with a fluorescein strip or places a small drop of fluorescein on the cornea of the eye. The fluorescein stains the mucin layer of the tear film and spreads across the cornea, which is then assessed using the cobalt blue filter of the slit lamp. The patient is asked to blink once, then look straight ahead without blinking. A normal test is characterized by the persistence of the fluorescein over the cornea for 10 seconds or longer. A break up and disappearance of the fluorescein in less than 10 seconds is abnormal and indicates an abnormality in one of the layers of the tear film (125). This simple test has relatively good sensitivity (82%) and specificity (86%) for adequacy of the tear film (126).

Another test of tear function is the **Rose Bengal test**. In this test, the eye is first anesthetized with a 5% solution of proparacaine, and a small drop of a 1% solution of Rose Bengal is placed either directly on the cornea or just superior to it. This solution stains dead and degenerating cells. Normal patients should have little if any staining of the conjunctiva and cornea, whereas patients with a dry eye or a poor mucin layer will have mild to severe staining of both (112). Some authors have found that Rose Bengal staining in non-exposure zones of the bulbar conjunctiva characterize tear deficiencies caused by an abnormality of the lipid layer and help to differentiate it from dry-eye syndromes caused by a deficiency of the aqueous component of the tear film (127).

As noted above, tear secretion may be classified as basal, reflex, or total. Tests of tear secretion can be separated into those that test basal tear production (i.e., from the glands of Krause and Wolfring) and those that test reflex tear production (i.e., from the primary lacrimal gland).

The **Schirmer test** was first described in 1903 (128) and remains a simple and practical clinical test of tear secretion

(125). Total tear secretion usually is tested first, because no anesthetic drop is applied to the eye in this test, often called the Schirmer 1 test. In this test, the patient sits in a dimly lit, quiet room. After drying the inferior conjunctival fornices on both sides with a cotton-tipped applicator or the edge of a tissue, the examiner places a strip of special absorbent filter paper in the lower conjunctival sac on both sides, with care being taken to keep the strip from touching the cornea by placing it either medially or laterally (Fig. 15.13). The strips are stabilized by folding the indented end over the lid margin. The patient is then advised to look straight ahead or slightly upward for 5 minutes, during which time he or she can blink normally. After 5 minutes, the strip is removed, and the amount of wetting is measured from the folded end. Because the eyes have not been anesthetized, the irritation from the filter paper produces wetting of the filter paper from both basal tear secretion and reflex secretion.

A variant of the Schirmer 1 test can be performed by anesthetizing the eyes with a topical drug such as proparacaine 0.5%. Topical cocaine should not be used as an anesthetic, because it irritates the cornea and inflames the eye. Once the eye has been anesthetized, the paper strips are placed as indicated above, and the nasal mucosa is stimulated using a cotton-tipped applicator or a tissue or piece of cotton that has been soaked with benzene or a similar trigeminal stimulant (129). This test provides a more consistent means of stimulating reflex tear secretion (in addition to the basal secretion that occurs). Regardless of the technique used, normal persons have a total tear secretion (e.g., wetting of the filter paper) of 10–30 mm in 5 minutes (112).

Basal tear secretion is determined using the Schirmer 2 test. In this test, a topical anesthetic is placed in the inferior conjunctival sac of both eyes. After a minute or so, the examiner uses a small piece of cotton or filter paper to dry the inferior fornices as in the Schirmer 1 test and its variant described above. The paper strips are then placed in the manner of the Schirmer 1 test, and the patient is given instructions identical with those given for the Schirmer 1 test. After 5 minutes, the strips are removed, and the amount of wetting is measured. The wetting in this test should represent only the basal tear secretion, because the topical anesthetic should prevent stimulation of the main lacrimal gland. In addition, by subtracting the amount of basal tear secretion obtained from the Schirmer 2 test from the total secretion

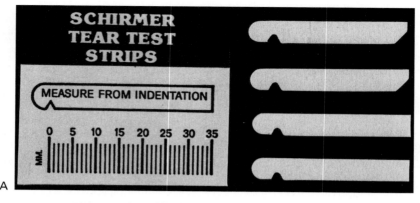

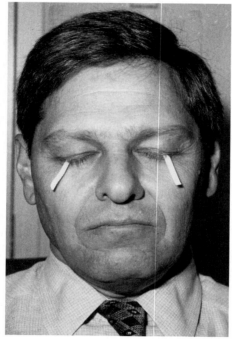

Figure 15.13. *A,* Schirmer filter strips and measuring scale on packet of strips. *B,* Patient with Schirmer strips properly placed laterally in inferior fornix of both eyes.

measured in the Schirmer 1 test or its variant, one should obtain the amount of reflex tearing (see later, however).

The **phenol red thread test** also assesses tear volume and deficient aqueous. It uses a cotton thread that has been soaked with phenol red. This substance is actually yellow but is sensitive to the pH of tears and will change from yellow to red when soaked with tears. One end of the thread is placed in the inferior conjunctival sac with the other end hanging over the edge of the lid, and the length of thread that has changed color is measured after 15 seconds. A change of color from yellow to red of less than 6 mm is diagnostic of dry eyes (125).

All of the tests of tear secretion described above have their proponents and detractors. Korb surveyed practitioners as to their preferred diagnostic method for the determination of dry-eye syndrome (130). Besides a complete history and use of the dry-eye questionnaire developed by Schein et al. described above (115), most practitioners used the fluores-

cein tear film break-up time or Rose Bengal test as their first test. In fact, a study that compared the Schirmer 1 and 2 tests, the Rose Bengal test, the tear film break-up time test, and the assay for lactoferrin level in patients with Sjögren syndrome reported that the best balance between sensitivity and specificity was achieved by performing both a Rose Bengal test and a Schirmer 1 test (131).

Fluorophotometric methods can be used to measure both tear volume and flow. These techniques are not clinically applicable, however, and are best used as research tools (132). Corneal sensitivity testing does not correlate with dry eyes (133).

Patients who have epiphora, particularly those in whom the epiphora is unilateral, should be evaluated not only for excess or reduced tear production but also for possible blockage of the tear drainage system. The punctae should be examined to see if they are patent, and the examiner should gently press on the lacrimal sac to see if there is regurgitation of contents through the punctae, indicating a block at the naso-lacrimal duct.

The patency of the drainage system can be assessed using the **fluorescein dye disappearance test**. The test is performed by instillation of one drop of 2% fluorescein dye into the inferior conjunctival sac of both eyes. The conjunctival sacs of the two eyes are then assessed after 5 minutes for any difference between the two eyes of residual fluorescein in the sac and on the sclera, as indicated by a difference in color intensity (134). A slightly more quantitative version of this test is to instill the dye in both inferior conjunctival sacs and to place a small cotton pledget, cotton-tipped applicator, or strip of Schirmer filter paper in the nose on each side just beneath the inferior turbinate (135,136). The pledgets, applicators, or strips are removed 1–5 minutes later and examined to see if they are stained with dye that should have passed through the lacrimal punctae into the lacrimal canaliculi and then to the lacrimal sac, eventually exiting the lacrimal duct just below the inferior turbinate. If no dye is present, a **secondary dye test** can be performed by flushing the lacrimal system with clear saline checking the fluid emanating from the nose for fluorescein staining (135). If there still is no dye, the nasolacrimal apparatus can be probed. If, after probing, dye is present at the inferior turbinate, incomplete blockage exists, and the lacrimal pump is functioning. If, however, there is clear fluid at the inferior turbinate, a non-functioning pump exists, and a complete block is present (112,129).

In addition to the tests described above, lacrimal scintillography has been used to test lacrimal flow. This technique uses technetium-99 combined with specific scanning techniques, allowing abnormal secretion and abnormal tear flow patterns to be identified (137). The procedure is useful for research but is impractical for the daily assessment of patients in the clinic. Finally, taste tests in which a specific substance, such as saccharin or Chloromycetin, is placed in the inferior conjunctival sac, can be used to determine if there is an intact lacrimal drainage system; however, these tests give results that are not reproducible and that have not been standardized (112).

Dacryocystography is a radiologic evaluation of the lacrimal drainage system in which contrast is placed into the lower fornix on the side of the presumed obstruction, and radiographs, computed tomographic scans, magnetic resonance images, or angiographic images are obtained to determine if and where the contrast material hangs up, thus localizing the obstruction (138). This test may be helpful in selected patients, particularly those in whom a structural lesion is suspected.

Just as in testing for dry eyes, sometimes a combination of testing is necessary for the evaluation of patients with epiphora (139). The physician involved with such patients should be aware of the tests that can be performed as well as their relative sensitivities and specificities.

ACKNOWLEDGMENTS   This work was supported in part by a grant from Research to Prevent Blindness, Inc., New York, NY, to the Department of Ophthalmology, University of Utah.

REFERENCES

1. Loewenfeld I. The Pupil. Boston, Butterworth-Heinemann, 1999.
2. Jacobson DM. Benign episodic unilateral mydriasis. Ophthalmology 1995;102: 1623–1627.
3. Murray RB, Adler MW, Korczyn AD. The pupillary effects of opioids. Life Science 1983;33:495–509.
4. Weir REP, Whitehead DEJ, Zaid FH, et al. Pupil Blown by a Puffer. Lancet 2004;363:1853.
5. Bienfang DC. Neuro-ophthalmology of the pupil and accommodation. In Albert DM, Jakobiec FA, eds. Principles and Practice of Ophthalmology. Philadelphia, WB Saunders, 1994:2470–2482.
6. Kardon RH, Corbett JJ, Thompson HS. Segmental denervation and reinnervation of the iris sphincter as shown by infrared videographic transillumination. Ophthalmology 1998;105:313–321.
7. Loewenfeld IE. The Pupil. Boston, Butterworth, 1999:833–839.
8. Czarnecki JSC, Pilley SFJ, Thompson HS. The analysis of anisocoria. Can J Ophthalmol 1979;14:297–302.
9. Wachler BSB, Krueger RR. Agreement and repeatability of infrared pupillometry and the comparison method. Ophthalmology 1999;106;319–323.
10. Kardon RH, Corbett JJ, Thompson HS. Segmental denervation and reinnervation of the iris sphincter as shown by infrared videographic transillumination. Ophthalmology 1998;105:313–321.
11. Loewenfeld IE. The Pupil. Boston, Butterworth, 1999:869–894.
12. Loewenfeld IE. Pupillary changes related to age. In Thompson HS, ed. Topics in Neuro-Ophthalmology. Baltimore, Williams & Wilkins, 1979:124–150.
13. Ettinger ER, Wyatt HJ, London R. Anisocoria: Variation and clinical observation with different conditions of illumination and accommodation. Invest Ophthalmol Vis Sci 1991;32:501–509.
14. Thompson HS. The pupil and accommodation. In Lessell S, van Dalen JTW, eds. Neuro-Ophthalmology. Amsterdam, Excerpta Medica, 1980:226–240.
15. Lam BL, Thompson HS, Corbett JJ. The prevalence of simple anisocoria. Am J Ophthalmol 1987;104:69–73.
16. Rosenberg ML. Physiological anisocoria: A manifestation of physiologic asymmetry of sympathetic tone. Invest Ophthalmol Vis Sci 1988;29(Suppl):79.
17. Cheng MMP, Catalano RA. Fatigue-induced familial anisocoria. Am J Ophthalmol 1990;109:480–481.
18. Wilhelm H, Wilhelm B. Clinical applications of pupillography. J Neuroophthalmol 2003;23:42–49.
19. Lowenstein O, Loewenfeld IE. Influence of retinal adaptation upon the pupillary reflex to light in normal man. II. Effect of adaptation to dim illumination upon pupillary reflexes elicited by bright light. Am J Ophthalmol 1961;51:644–654.
20. Lowenstein O, Loewenfeld IE. Influence of retinal adaptation upon the pupillary reflex to light in normal man. I. Effect of adaptation to bright light on pupillary threshold. Am J Ophthalmol 1959;48:536–549.
21. Ellis CJK. The pupillary light reflex in normal subjects. Br J Ophthalmol 1981; 65:754–759.
22. Thompson HS. The pupil. In Hart WM, ed. Adler's Physiology of the Eye. Ed 9. St Louis, Mosby Year Book, 1992:412–441.
23. Sun F, Stark L. Pupillary escape intensified by large pupillary size. Vision Res 1983;23:611–615.
24. Thompson HS. Afferent pupillary defects: Pupillary findings associated with defects of the afferent arm of the pupillary light reflex arc. Am J Ophthalmol 1966;62:860–873.
25. Bergamin O, Kardon RH. Greater pupillary escape differentiates central from peripheral visual field loss. Ophthalmology 2002;109:771–780.
26. Semmlow J, Stark L. Pupil movements to light and accommodative stimulation: A comparative study. Vision Res 1973;13:1087–1100.
27. Loewenfeld IE, Newsome DA. Iris mechanics. I. Influence of pupil size on dynamics of pupillary movements. Am J Ophthalmol 1971;71:347–362.
28. Sun F, Tauchi P, Stark L. Dynamic pupillary response controlled by pupil size effect. Exp Neurol 1983;82:313–324.
29. Lowenstein O, Friedman ED. Pupillographic studies. Arch Ophthalmol 1942; 27:969–993.
30. Bergamin O, Kardon RH. Latency of the pupil light reflex: sample rate, stimulus intensity and variation in normal subjects. Invest Ophthalmol Vis Sci 2003;44: 2597–2605.
31. Lowenstein O. Alternating contraction anisocoria. Arch Neurol Psychiatr 1954; 72:742–757.
32. Price MJ, Thompson HS, Judisch GF, et al. Pupillary constriction to darkness. Br J Ophthalmol 1985;69:205–211.
33. Frank JW, Kushner BJ, France TD. Paradoxical pupillary phenomena. Arch Ophthalmol 1988;106:1564–1566.
34. Riley FC, Moyer NJ. Experimental Horner's syndrome: a pupillographic evaluation of guanethidine-induced adrenergic blockade in humans. Am J Ophthalmol 1970;69:442–447.
35. Pilley SFJ, Thompson HS. Pupillary "dilation lag" in Horner's syndrome. Br J Ophthalmol 1975;59:731–735.
36. Alward WL, Munden PM, Verdick RE, et al. Use of infrared videography to detect and record iris transillumination defects. Arch Ophthalmol 1990;108: 748–750.

37. Smith SA, Smith SE. Bilateral Horner's syndrome: detection and occurrence. J Neurol Neurosurg Psychiatry 1999;66:48–51.
38. Hirschberg J. Neuritis retrobulbaris. Zentralbl Prakt Augenheilkd 1884;8:185–186.
39. Gunn RM. Functional or hysterical amblyopia. Ophthal Rev 1902;21:271–280.
40. Gunn RM. Discussion on retro-ocular neuritis. Lancet 1904;4:412.
41. Kestenbaum A. Clinical Methods of Neuro-Ophthalmological Examination. New York, Grune & Stratton, 1946:288–291.
42. Levatin P. Pupillary escape in disease of the retina or optic nerve. Arch Ophthalmol 1959;62:768–779.
43. Levatin P, Prasloski PF, Collen MF. The swinging flashlight test in multiphasic screening for eye disease. Can J Ophthalmol 1973;8:356–359.
44. Enyedi LB, Dev S, Cox TA. A comparison of the Marcus Gunn and alternating light tests for afferent papillary defects. Ophthalmology 1998;105:871–873.
45. Thompson HS. Pupillary signs in the diagnosis of optic nerve disease. Trans Ophthalmol Soc UK 1976;96:377–381.
46. Thompson HS. Putting a number on the relative afferent pupillary defect. In Thompson HS, Daroff R, Frisén L, et al., eds. Topics in Neuro-Ophthalmology. Baltimore, Williams & Wilkins, 1979:157–158.
47. Thompson HS, Corbett JJ, Cox TA. How to measure the relative afferent pupillary defect. Surv Ophthalmol 1981;26:39–42.
48. Borchert M, Sadun AA. Bright light stimuli as a mask of relative afferent pupillary defect. Am J Ophthalmol 1988;106:98–99.
49. Kawasaki A, Moore P, Kardon RH. Variability of the relative afferent pupillary defect. Am J Ophthalmol 1995;120:622–633.
50. Thompson HS, Jiang MQ. Letter to the Editor. Ophthalmology 1987;94:1360–1362.
51. Thompson HS. 12th Pupil Colloquium. Am J Ophthalmol 1981;92:435–436.
52. Fineberg E, Thompson HS. Quantitation of the afferent pupillary defect. In Smith JL, ed. Neuro-Ophthalmology Focus 1980. New York, Masson, 1979:25–30.
53. Bell RA, Waggoner PM, Boyd WM, et al. Clinical grading of relative afferent pupillary defects. Arch Ophthalmol 1993;111:938–942.
54. Thompson HS, Montague P, Cox TA, et al. The relationship between visual acuity, pupillary defect, and visual field loss. Am J Ophthalmol 1982;93:681–688.
55. Kardon RH, Hauper CL, Thompson HS. The relationship between static perimetry and the relative afferent pupillary defect. Am J Ophthalmol 1993;115:351–356.
56. Kestenbaum A. Clinical Methods of Neuro-Ophthalmological Examination. Ed 2. New York, Grune & Stratton, 1961:420–456.
57. Jiang MQ, Thompson HS, Lam BL. Kestenbaum's number as an indicator of pupillomotor input asymmetry. Am J Ophthalmol 1989;107:528–530.
58. Lowenstein O, Loewenfeld IE. Electronic pupillography: A new instrument and some clinical applications. Arch Ophthalmol 1958;59:352–363.
59. Kawasaki A, Moore P, Kardon RH. Long-term fluctuation of relative afferent pupillary defect in subjects with normal visual function. Am J Ophthalmol 1996;122:875–882.
60. Alexandridis E, Argyropoulos TR, Krastel H. The latent period of the pupil light reflex in lesions of the optic nerve. Ophthalmologica 1981;182:211–217.
61. Volpe NJ, Plotkin EES, Maguire MG, et al. Portable pupillography of the swinging flashlight test to detect afferent papillary defects. Ophthalmology 2000;107:1913–1922.
62. Kardon RH, Kirkali PA, Thompson HS. Automated pupil perimetry. Pupil field mapping in patients and normal subjects. Ophthalmology 1991;98:485–495.
63. Kardon RH. Pupil perimetry. Curr Opin Ophthalmol 1992;3:565–570.
64. Stern HJ. A simple method for the early diagnosis of abnormality of the pupillary reaction. Br J Ophthalmol 1944;28:275–276.
65. Miller SD, Thompson HS. Edge-light pupil cycle time. Br J Ophthalmol 1978;62:495–500.
66. Miller SD, Thompson HS. Pupil cycle time in optic neuritis. Am J Ophthalmol 1978;85:635–642.
67. Weinstein JM, Van Gilder JC, Thompson HS. Pupil cycle time in optic nerve compression. Am J Ophthalmol 1980;89:263–267.
68. Milton JG, Longtin A, Kirkham TH, et al. Irregular pupil cycling as a characteristic abnormality in patients with demyelinative optic neuropathy. Am J Ophthalmol 1988;105:402–407.
69. Safran AB, Walser A, Roth A, et al. Pupil cycle induction test: A way of evaluating the pupillary light reflex. Ophthalmologica 1981;183:205–213.
70. Lowenstein O, Loewenfeld IE. The pupil. In Davson H, ed. The Eye. Vol. 3. New York, Academy Press, 1969:255–337.
71. Duke-Elder WS. System of Ophthalmology. St Louis, CV Mosby, 1970:476–479,
72. Michaels DD. Visual Optics and Refraction, St Louis, CV Mosby, 1985.
73. Cogan DG, Freese CG. Spasm of the near reflex. Arch Ophthalmol 1955;54:752–759.
74. Goldstein JH, Schneekloth BB. Spasm of the near reflex: A spectrum of anomalies. Surv Ophthalmol 1996;40:269–278.
75. Kruger PB, Pola J. Stimuli for accommodation: Blur, chromatic aberration and size. Vision Res 1986;26:957–971.
76. Kotulak JC, Morse SE. The effect of perceived distance on accommodation under binocular steady-state conditions. Vision Res 1995;35:791–795.
77. Stakenburg M. Accommodation without pupillary constriction. Vision Res 1991;31:267–273.
78. Duke-Elder WS. Text-Book of Ophthalmology. St Louis, CV Mosby, 1949:4415–4450.
79. Glasser A, Kaufman PL. Accommodation and presbyopia. In Kaufman PL, Alm A, eds. Adler's Physiology of the Eye, Ed 10. St Louis, CV Mosby, 2003:197–233,
80. Schor CM. A dynamic model of cross coupling between accommodation and convergence: Simulations of step and frequency responses. Optom Vis Sci 1992;69:258–269.
81. Von Noorden G. Binocular Vision and Ocular Motility, Ed 4. St Louis, CV Mosby, 1990:85–100.
82. Bruce AS, Atchison DA, Bhoola H. Accommodation-convergence relationships and age. Invest Ophthalmol Vis Sci 1995;36:406–413.
83. Loewenfeld IE. The Pupil. Boston, Butterworth, 1999:317.
84. Alpern M. Testing distance effect on phoria measurement at various accommodation levels. Arch Ophthalmol 1955;54:906–915.
85. Hennessy RT, Iida T, Shiina K, et al. The effect of pupil size on accommodation. Vision Res 1975;16:587–589.
86. Miller RJ. Pitfalls in the conception, manipulation and measurement of visual accommodations. Hum Factors 1990;32:27–44.
87. Egashira SM, Kish LL, Twelker JD, et al. Comparison of cyclopentolate versus tropicamide cycloplegia in children. Optom Vis Sci 1993;70:1019–1026.
88. Mutti D, Zadnick K, Egashira S, et al. The effect of cycloplegia on measurement of the ocular components. Invest Ophthalmol Vis Sci 1994;35:515–527.
89. Prince AE. A combined age and refraction scale. Arch Ophthalmol 1897;16:24–27.
90. Krimsky E. A modified Prince rule. Am J Ophthalmol 1960;49:827–829.
91. Berens C, Sells SB. Experimental studies on fatigue of accommodation. Am J Ophthalmol 1950;33:47–58.
92. Duane A. Studies in monocular and binocular accommodation with their clinical applications. Am J Ophthalmol 1922;5:865–877.
93. Atchison DA, Capper EJ, McCabe KL. Critical subjective measurement of amplitude of accommodation. Optom Vis Sci 1994;71:699–706.
94. Duane A. The accommodation and Donders curve and the need of revising our ideas regarding them. JAMA 1909;52:1992–1996.
95. Ferree CE, Rand G. Intensity of light in relation to the examination of the eye. Br J Ophthalmol 1936;20:331–346.
96. Schaeffel F. Wilhelm H, Zrenner E. Inter-individual variability in the dynamics of natural accommodation in humans: relation to age and refractive errors. J Physiol 1993;461:301–320.
97. Mathews S. Scleral expansion surgery does not restore accommodation in human presbyopia. Ophthalmology 1999;106:873–877.
98. Wold JE, Ju A, Chen S, Glasser A. Subjective and objective measurement of human accommodative amplitude. J Cataract Refract Surg 2003;29:1878–1888.
99. Mazow ML, France TD, Finkleman S, et al. Acute accommodative and convergence insufficiency. Trans Am Ophthalmol Soc 1989;87:158–173.
100. Von Noorden GK. Binocular Vision and Ocular Motility. St Louis, CV Mosby, 1990.
101. Morgan MW. A comparison of clinical methods of measuring accommodative convergence. Am J Optom 1950;102:385–396.
102. Heron G, Charman WN, Schor CM. Age changes in the interactions between the accommodation and vergence systems. Optom Vis Sci 2001;78:754–762.
103. Mutti DO, Jones LA, Moeschberger ML, et al. AC/A ratio, age, and refractive error in children. Invest Ophthalmol Vis Sci 2000;41:2469–2478.
104. Fincham EF. The proportion of ciliary muscular force required for accommodation. J Physiol 1955;128:99–113.
105. Wick B, Currie D. Convergence accommodation: Laboratory and clinical evaluation. Optom Vis Sci 1991;68:226–231.
106. Tsuetaki TK, Schor CM. Clinical method for measuring adaptation of tonic accommodation and vergence accommodation. Am J Optom Physiol Optom 1987;64:437–439.
107. Tutt R, Bradley A, Begley C, et al. Optical and visual impact of tear break-up in human eyes. Invest Ophthalmol Vis Sci 2000;41:4117–4123.
108. McCulley JP, Shine WE. The lipid layer: The outer surface of the ocular surface tear film. Biosci Rep 2001;21:407–418.
109. McCulley JP, Shine W. A compositional based model for the tear film lipid layer. Trans Am Ophthalmol Soc 1997;95:79–88.
110. Rolando M, Zierhut M. The ocular surface and tear film and their dysfunction in dry eye disease. Surv Ophthalmol 2001;45(Suppl 2):S203–S210.
110a. Dartt DA. Dysfunctional neural regulation of lacrimal gland secretion and its role in pathogenesis of dry eye syndromes. Ocular Surface 2004;2:76–91.
111. Mishima S, Gasset A, Klyce SD, et al. Determination of tear volume and tear flow. Invest Ophthalmol 1966;5:264–276.
112. Doughman DJ. Clinical tests. Int Ophthalmol Clin 1973;13:199–217.
113. Schaumberg DA, Sullivan DA, Buring JE, et al. Prevalence of dry eye syndrome among US women. Am J Ophthalmol 2003;136:318–326.
114. Chia EM, Mitchell P, Rochtchina E, et al. Prevalence and associations of dry eye syndrome in an older population: The Blue Mountains Eye Study. Clin Exp Ophthalmol 2003;31:229–232.

115. Schein OD, Hochberg MC, Munoz B, et al. Dry eye and dry mouth in the elderly: A population based assessment. Arch Intern Med 1999;159:1359–1363.

115a. Dogru M. Tsubota K. New insights into the diagnosis and treatment of dry eye. Ocular Surface 2004;2:59–75.

116. Isreb MA, Greiner JV, Korb DR, et al. Correlation of lipid layer thickness measurements with fluorescein tear film break-up time and Schirmer's test. Eye 2003;17:79–83.

117. Nichols KK, Nichols JJ, Lynn Mitchell G. The relation between tear film tests in patients with dry eye disease. Ophthalmic Physiol Opt 2003;23:553–560.

118. Newman NJ, Capone A, Leeper HF, et al. Clinical and subclinical findings with retinal deficiency. Ophthalmology 1994;101:1077–1083.

119. Mircheff AK. Lacrimal fluid and electrolyte secretion: A review. Exp Eye Res 1989;8:607–617.

120. McCollum CJ, Foulks GN, Bodner B, et al. Rapid assay of lactoferrin in keratoconjunctivitis sicca. Cornea 1994;13:505–508.

121. Da Dalt S, Moncada A, Priori R, et al. The lactoferrin tear test in the diagnosis of Sjögren's syndrome. Eur J Ophthalmol 1996;6:284–286.

122. Lemp MA. Recent developments in dry eye management. Ophthalmology 1987; 94:1299–1304.

123. Mainstone JC, Bruce AS, Golding TR. Tear meniscus measurement in the diagnosis of dry eye. Curr Eye Res 1996;15:653–661.

124. Norn MS. Desiccation of the precorneal tear film. I. Corneal wetting time. Acta Ophthalmol 1969;47:856–880.

125. Bron AJ. Diagnosis of dry eye. Surv Ophthalmol 2001;45(Suppl 2):S221–S226.

126. Mengher LS, Pandher KS, Bron AJ. Non-invasive tear film break-up time: Sensitivity and specificity. Acta Ophthalmol 1986;64:441–444.

127. Lee SH, Tseng SCG. Rose Bengal staining and cytologic characteristics associated with lipid tear deficiency. Am J Ophthalmol 1997;124:736–750.

128. Schirmer O. Studien zur physiologie und pathologie der tränenabsonderung und tränenabfuhr. Albrecht von Graefes Arch Ophthalmol 1903;56:197–291.

129. Jones LT. Anatomy of the tear system. Int Opthalmol Clin 1973;13:3–22.

130. Korb DR. Survey of preferred tests for diagnosis of the tear film and dry eye. Cornea 2000;19:483–486.

131. Vitali C, Moutsopoulos HM, Bombardieri S. The European Community Study Group on diagnostic criteria for Sjogren's syndrome: Sensitivity and specificity for ocular and oral involvement in Sjogren's syndrome. Ann Rheum Dis 1994; 53:637–647.

132. Afonso AA, Monroy D, Stern ME, et al. Correlation of tear fluorescein clearance and Schirmer test scores with ocular irritation symptoms. Ophthalmology 1999; 106:803–810.

133. Bjerrum KB. Test and symptoms in keratoconjunctivitis sicca and their correlation. Acta Ophthalmol Scand 1996;74:436–441.

134. Zappia RJ, Milder B. Lacrimal drainage function. 2. The fluorescein dye disappearance test. Am J Ophthalmol 1972;74:160–162.

135. Zappia RJ, Milder B. Lacrimal drainage function. 1. The Jones fluorescein test. Am J Ophthalmol 1972;74:154–159.

136. Toprak AB, Erkin EF, Kayikcioglu O, et al. Fluorescein dye disappearance test in patients with different degrees of epiphora. Eur J Ophthalmol 2002;12: 359–365.

137. Hurwitz JJ, Victor WH. The role of sophisticated radiological testing in the assessment and management of epiphora. Ophthalmology 1985;92:407–413.

138. Rubin PA, Bilyk JR, Shore JW, et al. Magnetic resonance imaging of the lacrimal drainage system. Ophthalmology 1994;101:235–243.

139. Guzek JP, Ching AS, Hoang TA, et al. Clinical and radiologic lacrimal testing in patients with epiphora. Ophthalmology 1997;104:1875–1881.

140. Loewenfeld IE. Pupillary changes related to age. In Thompson HS, ed. Topics in Neuro-Ophthalmology. Baltimore: Williams & Wilkins, 1979:124–150.

141. Bitsios P, Prettyman R, Szabadi E. Changes in autonomic function with age: A study of pupillary kinetics in healthy young and old people. Age and Aging 1996;25:432–438.

142. Thompson HS. Pupillary signs in the ophthalmologic diagnosis of optic nerve disease. Trans Ophthalmol Soc UK 1976;96:377–381.

143. Cox TA, Thompson HS, Corbett JJ. Relative afferent pupillary defects in optic neuritis. Am J Ophthalmol 1981;92:685–690.

144. Bell RA, Thompson HS. Optic tract lesions and relative afferent pupillary defect. In Thompson HS, ed. Topics in Neuro-Ophthalmology. Baltimore, Williams & Wilkins, 1979:164–168.

145. Newman SA, Miller NR. The optic tract syndrome: Neuro-ophthalmologic considerations. Arch Ophthalmol 1983;101:1241–1250.

146. Schmid R, Wilhelm B, Wilhelm H. Naso-temporal asymmetry and contraction anisocoria in pupillomotor system. Graefes Arch Clin Exp Ophthalmol 2000; 238:123–128.

147. Forman S, Behrens MM, Odel JG, et al. Relative afferent pupillary defect with normal visual function. Arch Ophthalmol 1990;108:1074.

149. Portnoy JZA, Thompson HS, Lennarson L, et al. Pupillary defects in amblyopia. Am J Ophthalmol 1983;96:609–614.

150. Lam BL, Thompson HS. An anisocoria produces a small relative afferent papillary defect in the eye with the smaller pupil. J Neuroophthalmol 1999;19: 153–159.

151. Newsmen DA, Milton RC, Gass JDM. Afferent pupillary defect in macular degeneration. Am J Ophthalmol 1981;92:396–402.

152. Han DP, Thompson HS, Folk JC. Differentiation between recently resolved optic neuritis and central serous retinopathy. Arch Ophthalmol 1985;103:394–396.

153. Servais GE, Thompson HS, Hayreh SS. Relative afferent pupillary defect in central retinal vein occlusion. Ophthalmology 1986;93:301–303.

154. Kardon R. The pupil. In Kaufman P, Alm A, eds. Adler's Physiology of the Eye. Ed 10. St Louis, CV Mosby, 2003:713–743.

155. Folk JC, Thompson HS, Farmer SG, et al. Relative afferent pupillary defects in eyes with retinal detachment. Ophthalmic Surg 1987;18:757–759.

156. Bovino JA, Burton TC. Measurement of the relative afferent pupillary defect in retinal detachment. Am J Ophthalmol 1980;90:19–21.

157. Jiang MQ, Thompson HS. Pupillary defects in retinitis pigmentosa. Am J Ophthalmol 1985;99:607–608.

158. Sadun AA, Bassi CJ, Lessell S. Why cataracts do not produce afferent pupillary defects. Am J Ophthalmol 1990;110:712–714.

159. Lam BL, Thompson HS. A unilateral cataract produces a relative afferent pupillary defect in the contralateral eye. Ophthalmology 1990;97:334–338.

160. Lam BL, Thompson HS. Relative afferent pupillary defect induced by patching. Am J Ophthalmol 1989;107:305–306.

161. DuBois LG, Sadun AA. Occlusion-induced contralateral afferent pupillary defect. Am J Ophthalmol 1989;107:306–307.

162. Kohn AN, Moss AP, Podos SM. Relative afferent pupillary defects in glaucoma without characteristic field loss. Arch Ophthalmol 1979;77:294–296.

163. Jonas JB, Zach FM, Naumann GO. Quantitative pupillometry of relative afferent defects in glaucoma. Arch Ophthalmol 1990;108:479–480.

164. Quigley HA, Addicks EM, Green WR. Optic nerve damage in human glaucoma. Arch Ophthalmol 1982;100:135–146.

165. Thompson HS. Adie's syndrome: some new observations. Trans Am Ophthalmol Soc 1977;75:587–626.

166. Drummond PD. The effect of light intensity and dose of dilute pilocarpine eye drops on pupillary constriction in healthy subjects. Am J Ophthalmol 1991;112: 195–199.

167. Jacobson DM, Olson KA. Influence of pupil size, anisocoria, and ambient light on pilocarpine miosis. Ophthalmology 1993;100:275–280.

168. Leavitt JA, Wayman LL, Hodge DO, et al. Pupillary response to four concentrations of pilocarpine in normal subjects: Application to testing for Adie tonic pupil. Am J Ophthalmol 2002;133:333–336.

169. Kardon RH, Denison CE, Brown CK, et al. Critical evaluation of the cocaine test in the diagnosis of Horner's syndrome. Arch Ophthalmol 1990;108:384–387.

170. Wilhelm H. Neuro-ophthalmology of papillary function: Practical guidelines. J Neurol 1998;373–583.

171. Cremer SA, Thompson HS, Digre KB, et al. Hydroxyamphetamine mydriasis in Horner's syndrome. Am J Ophthalmol 1990;110:71–76.

172. Morales J, Brown SM, Abdul-Rahim AS, et al. Ocular effects of apraclonidine in Horner syndrome. Arch Ophthalmol 2000;118:951–954.

173. Brown SM, Aouchiche R, Freedman KA. The utility of 0.5% apraclonidine in the diagnosis of Horner syndrome. Arch Ophthalmol 2003;121:1201–1203.

174. Brewitt H, Sistani F. Dry eye disease: the scale of the problem. Surv Ophthalmol 2001;45(Suppl 2):S199–S202.

175. Versura P, Cellini M, Torreggiani V, et al. Dryness symptoms, diagnostic protocol and therapeutic management: Report on 1,200 patients. Ophthalmic Res 2001;33:221–227.

CHAPTER 16

Disorders of Pupillary Function, Accommodation, and Lacrimation

Aki Kawasaki

In this chapter I describe various disorders that produce dysfunction of the autonomic nervous system as it pertains to the eye and orbit, including congenital and acquired disorders of pupillary function, accommodation, and lacrimation. Although many of these disorders are isolated phenomena that affect only a single structure, others are systemic disorders that involve various other organs in the body.

DISORDERS OF THE PUPIL

The value of observation of pupillary size and motility in the evaluation of patients with neurologic disease cannot be overemphasized. In many patients with visual loss, an abnormal pupillary response is the only objective sign of organic visual dysfunction. In patients with diplopia, an impaired pupil can signal the presence of an acute or enlarging intracranial mass. An adequate clinical examination of the pupils requires little time and can be meaningful when approached with a sound understanding of the principles of pupillary innervation and function. In most cases, one needs only a hand light with a bright, even beam, a device for measuring pupillary size (preferably in half-millimeter steps), a few pharmacologic agents, and an examination room that permits easy control of the background illumination.

This section commences with an overview of congenital and acquired diseases of the iris that affect pupil size, shape, and reactivity because these structural defects may be the cause of "abnormal pupils" and often are easy to diagnose at the slit lamp. Furthermore, if a preexisting structural iris defect is present, it may confound interpretation of the neurologic evaluation of pupillary function; at the very least, it should be kept in consideration during such evaluation.

STRUCTURAL DEFECTS OF THE IRIS

Congenital Defects

Aniridia

Aniridia is a rare congenital abnormality in which the iris is partially hypoplastic or completely absent (1,2) (Fig. 16.1*A*). Patients with aniridia initially may be thought to have fixed, dilated pupils until a more careful examination is performed. In almost all cases, histologic or gonioscopic

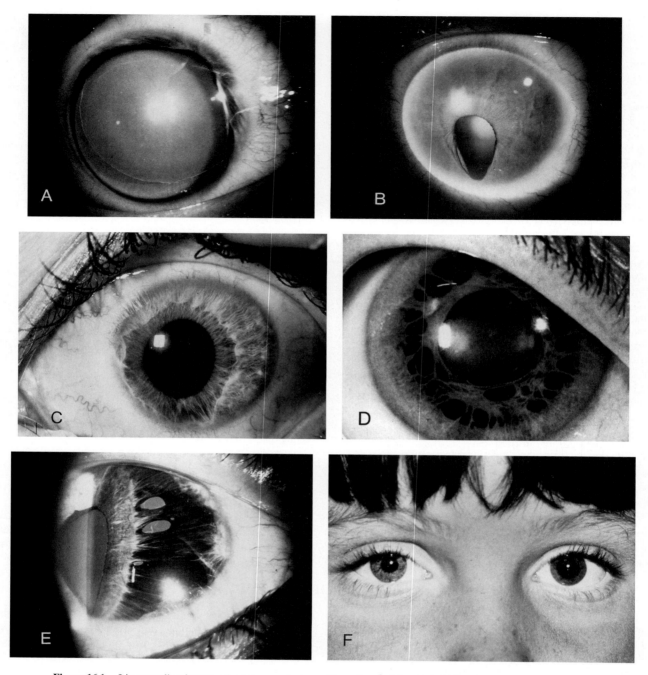

Figure 16.1. Iris anomalies that may simulate neurologic pupillary abnormalities. *A,* Aniridia. Note associated upward lens dislocation. *B,* Typical iris coloboma. *C,* Acquired corectopia in iridocorneal–endothelial adhesion syndrome. *D,* Persistent pupillary membrane. *E,* Pseudopolycoria from iridocorneal–endothelial adhesion syndrome. *F,* Heterochromia iridis in a patient with congenital Horner syndrome. The lighter iris is in the eye with Horner syndrome. (*A* and *B,* Courtesy of Dr. Irene H. Maumenee. *C,* Courtesy of Dr. Harry A. Quigley. *D,* From Gutman ED, Goldberg MF. Persistent pupillary membrane and other ocular abnormalities. Arch Ophthalmol 1976;94:156–157. *E,* Courtesy of Dr. Harry A. Quigley.)

examination reveals small remnants of iris tissue. The iris is only minimally developed, and the iris musculature usually is hypoplastic. Patients with aniridia often have photophobia, poor visual acuity, and other ocular defects, including glaucoma, cataracts, ectopia lentis, corneal opacification, ciliary body hypoplasia, optic nerve hypoplasia, foveal hypoplasia, strabismus, and nystagmus (3). The condition usually is bilateral, and two thirds of cases are inherited in autosomal-dominant fashion (4).

The gene defect resulting in aniridia is a nonsense or frameshift mutation in the large PAX6 gene on chromosome 11p13 (3). The PAX6 gene is a master regulator gene, critical in the development of the eye and central nervous tissues. Mutations of this gene are associated with other ocular abnormalities, such as anterior segment defects and foveal hypoplasia, in addition to aniridia. Mutations can be sporadic or inherited; in most cases, loss of one allele (heterozygous PAX6 mutation) is sufficient to result in ocular structural defects. Detection of a PAX6 mutation necessitates genetic counseling.

Systemic abnormalities found in patients with aniridia are many and varied. They include polydactyly, oligophrenia, cranial dysostosis, malformations of the extremities and external ears, hydrocephalus, and mental retardation (2). The most important association, however, is with the childhood cancer, Wilms' tumor. Aniridia occurs in 1 in 73 patients with Wilms' tumor, compared with a frequency of 1 in 50,000–100,000 in the general population (1). The reason for this high association is the close proximity of the aniridia gene to the gene for Wilms' tumor (WT1) (5). The association of Wilms' tumor, aniridia, genitourinary anomalies, and mental retardation is known as WAGR syndrome and is due to a contiguous defect on chromosome 11p13 that encompasses both the PAX6 and the WT1 genes. Although spontaneous deletions can occur simultaneously in both genes, the detection of an intragenic PAX6 mutation in a patient with sporadic aniridia can eliminate the need for routine kidney ultrasounds (3).

Coloboma of the Iris

A coloboma is a notch, hole, or fissure in any of the ocular structures (cornea, iris, ciliary body, zonules, choroids, retina, and optic disc) due to defective embryogenesis. Affected eyes are frequently microphthalmic. The term "typical" coloboma specifically refers to one caused by defective closure of the fetal fissure. Typical colobomata occur in the inferonasal quadrant and are the most common type (Fig. 16.1*B*). According to Pagon, only iris colobomata that are "typical" are associated with chorioretinal or optic disc colobomas (6). "Atypical" colobomata may result from (*a*) interference with embryonic growth of the neuroepithelial layers; (*b*) mechanical blockage of the advancing neuroectoderm by mesodermal elements present at the edge of the optic cup; and (*c*) occlusion of vessels within the embryonic iris tissue, with subsequent iris atrophy. When an atypical iris coloboma does not extend to the pupillary margin, it produces pseudopolycoria, a defect in the iris that has the clinical appearance of an accessory pupil.

A "complete" iris coloboma extends the full thickness of the iris and typically produces an oval-shaped or keyhole-shaped pupil, whereas an "incomplete" iris coloboma is a partial-thickness defect best seen as a wedge-shaped transillumination defect of the iris (7). An isolated coloboma in a microphthalmic eye has an established autosomal-dominant inheritance pattern, but penetrance is incomplete. A few pedigrees supporting an autosomal-recessive or X-linked–recessive inheritance pattern have been reported. Nevertheless, regardless of the type, location, and completeness of a colobomatous defect, patients with a coloboma should undergo an evaluation to determine whether it truly is an isolated finding or part of a multisystem disorder.

One well-known congenital multisystem syndrome with heterogeneous etiologies is the CHARGE association (coloboma, heart defects, atresia of the choanae, retardation of growth and development, genital hypoplasia, and ear anomalies or hearing loss) (6). Patients with the phenotypic CHARGE association can be given a more specific diagnosis if an etiologic basis is found, such as a teratogenic agent (retinoic acid) or a gene defect (partial tetrasomy of chromosome 22, the cat-eye syndrome) (8).

Cat-eye syndrome is one clinical phenotype resulting from a genomic disorder of 22q11. Specifically, there is a partial tetrasomy (four copies) of this region of chromosome 22. Patients commonly have ocular colobomata, anal atresia, and preauricular skin tags. Other anomalies include heart defects (particularly total anomalous pulmonary venous return), renal malformations, craniofacial anomalies, genital anomalies, and mental retardation (9).

Square Pupils

Square pupils are thought to represent incomplete aniridia. White and Fulton observed, in homozygous twins whose mother showed the same defect, large, irregular, roughly quadrilateral pupils that responded to constricting stimuli only in certain quadrants (10). Similar pupils were observed in a mother and daughter with incomplete aniridia and cataracts (11).

Elliptic Pupils

Elliptic pupils occasionally occur. In strong illumination, such pupils take on the form of elliptical slits (12,13).

Scalloped Pupils

Irregular, cup-shaped indentations in the pupillary margins have been described as a congenital anomaly in large pupils that otherwise react normally to light and near stimuli (14). Scalloped pupils probably are more commonly an acquired disorder, particularly in familial amyloidosis (15,16). The pupil also may develop a scalloped appearance after trauma to the sphincter muscle, causing multiple tears, segmental sphincter atrophy, or both. A scalloped pupil can occur after uveitis that is complicated by the development of posterior synechiae (adhesions between the iris and lens).

Peninsula Pupils

Bosanquet and Johnson reported 40 patients from Newfoundland and Labrador with an unusual form of partial iris sphincter atrophy that resulted in an oval pupil (17). The condition, called peninsula pupils, was bilateral in most cases. The anomaly was confined to the iris, and there were no associated systemic disorders. Most of the affected individuals were male, and all had blue irides. Three of the patients believed that their pupils had been large and oval since birth. This pupillary anomaly may be an inherited trait peculiar to the Newfoundland-Labrador region.

Ectopic (Misplaced) Pupils

Misplaced or ectopic pupils (corectopia, ectopia pupillae) are observed frequently. Isolated ectopic pupils may be inherited as either a dominant or a recessive trait. The condition usually is usually bilateral and symmetric (18). Although the pupils may be displaced in any direction, they often are up and out from the center of the cornea. Such displacement of the pupils is frequently associated with ectopia lentis, congenital glaucoma, microcornea, ocular coloboma, and high myopia (19). Ectopic pupils also occur in some patients with albinism and some patients with Axenfeld-Rieger anomaly. In addition, three families were reported in which affected members had ectopic pupils, ptosis, and ophthalmoplegia (20–22).

Although acquired corectopia may occur in patients with severe midbrain damage, the clinical setting and the variability of the acquired defect usually allow the physician to distinguish easily between the congenital and acquired forms (23–25). Similarly, the corectopia that occurs during the course of purely ocular disorders such as the iridocorneal–endothelial (ICE) adhesion syndromes and posterior polymorphous corneal dystrophy should be differentiated easily from congenital and neurologic corectopia by the clinical setting and the associated ocular signs (Fig. 16.1C).

Persistent Pupillary Membrane Remnants

Persistent pupillary membrane remnants are vestiges of the embryonic pupillary membrane that can appear as threadlike bands running across the pupillary space and attaching to the lesser circle of the iris (26,27) (Fig. 16.1D). Occasionally, such remnants are attached to the lens and may be associated with an anterior capsular cataract. Persistence of the entire membrane can block visual input, but most cases are visually insignificant. Excision of the membrane has been performed in young patients who are at risk for amblyopia and in others with visual impairment during pupillary constriction (e.g., in bright sunlight) (28).

Polycoria and Pseudopolycoria

In true polycoria, the extra pupil or pupils are equipped with a sphincter muscle that contracts on exposure to light (29). This is an extremely rare condition. Most additional pupils are actually just holes in the iris without a separate sphincter muscle. This pseudopolycoria may be a congenital disorder, such as an iris coloboma or persistent pupillary membrane, or it may be part of one of several syndromes characterized by mesodermal dysgenesis (30). A distinctive feature of pseudopolycoria is passive constriction, distortion, or even occlusion of the accessory pupil when the true pupil is dilated (31). More commonly, pseudopolycoria occurs as an acquired disorder from direct iris trauma including surgery, photocoagulation, ischemia, or glaucoma or as part of a degenerative process such as the ICE syndrome (Fig. 16.1E).

Congenital Miosis

Congenital miosis usually is bilateral and characterized by extremely small pupils that react slightly to light stimuli and dilate poorly after instillation of sympathomimetic agents (32,33). The anomaly appears to result from congenital absence of the iris dilator muscle. Additionally, the iris sphincter muscle may be contracted excessively because of the lack of counterpull normally supplied by the dilator muscle. Congenital miosis may occur sporadically or may be inherited. Most of the inherited cases are transmitted as an autosomal-dominant trait, although pedigrees with autosomal-recessive inheritance have been reported (34,35).

Congenital miosis may be an isolated phenomenon, or it may be associated with other ocular abnormalities, including microcornea, iris atrophy, myopia, and anterior chamber angle deformities (32). In addition, congenital miosis can occur in patients with systemic disorders. Patients with congenital miosis also may have albinism, the congenital rubella syndrome, the oculocerebrorenal syndrome of Lowe, Marfan syndrome, or multiple skeletal anomalies (33,36–39). Congenital miosis was noted in four members of a family with hereditary spastic ataxia, and it is one of the main features in Stormorken syndrome, a dominantly inherited metabolic disorder also characterized by bleeding tendency, thrombocytopathia, muscular weakness, postexertional muscle spasms, ichthyosis, asplenia, dyslexia, and headache (40).

Congenital Mydriasis

Congenital mydriasis may be similar to or identical with the condition described above as square pupils. This condition may be difficult to distinguish from aniridia unless a careful ocular examination is performed. Caccamise and Townes described a 73-year-old woman with bilaterally large, round pupils that were present from birth (41). The condition appeared to have been inherited as an autosomal-dominant trait, although all other affected family members were female. Both pupils constricted to topical 4% pilocarpine solution, suggesting an intact iris sphincter muscle, and both pupils dilated rapidly to topical 10% phenylephrine solution, indicating an intact iris dilator muscle. However, neither pupil reacted to a potent topical cholinesterase inhibitor, suggesting an abnormality of acetylcholine production at the parasympathetic neuromuscular junction.

Magnetic resonance (MR) imaging has shown an enlarged fourth ventricle and atrophy of the cerebellar vermis in one case report of congenital mydriasis (42). In another patient with bilateral congenital mydriasis and absent accommodation, the pupils did not react to light, lid closure, or administration of topical 1% pilocarpine solution; however, both pupils dilated further after topical administration of 2.5% phenylephrine (43). A patient with the Waardenburg syndrome who had a unilateral, congenitally fixed, dilated pupil has been reported (44). Pharmacologic studies in this patient suggested the possibility of congenital agenesis of the iris sphincter muscle.

Congenital Abnormalities of Iris Color

The color of the iris depends on the pigment in the iris stroma. In albinism, there is failure of mesodermal and ectodermal pigmentation. Consequently, the iris has a transparent, grayish-red color and transilluminates readily.

In a number of congenital and acquired conditions, the iris of one eye differs in color from the iris of the other eye. In other instances, one iris is entirely normal, and a part of the iris in the opposite eye has a different color than the rest of the iris surrounding it (iris bicolor). These abnormalities, collectively called heterochromia iridis, may occur (*a*) as an isolated congenital anomaly; (*b*) in association with other ocular abnormalities, such as iris or optic disc coloboma; (*c*) in association with systemic congenital abnormalities, as in patients with the Waardenburg syndrome, congenital Horner syndrome, or incontinentia pigmenti; or (*d*) from an acquired ocular condition (45) (Fig. 16.1*F*). When iris heterochromia is part of a pathologic condition, it is necessary to determine which iris is abnormal. For example, the darker iris is abnormal in patients with a diffuse iris and ciliary body melanoma and in siderosis from an intraocular foreign body or vitreous hemorrhage. The lighter iris is pathologic in congenital Horner syndrome, in Fuchs heterochromic iridocyclitis, and after iris atrophy following a unilateral iritis or acute glaucoma.

Acquired Defects

Inflammation

Iritis or iridocyclitis in its acute stages produces swelling of the iris, miosis, and slight reddening of the circumcorneal tissues. The miosis of iritis results from the release of a neurohumor, substance P, that produces miosis through interaction with a specific receptor in the iris sphincter muscle (46).

In patients with intraocular inflammation, dilation of the pupil with mydriatics may be difficult because of adhesions between the iris and the lens (posterior synechiae). These adhesions in chronic iritis may distort the shape of the pupil. They also may fix the pupil in a dilated position. Occasionally, the adhesions are not evident until the pupil is further dilated by a mydriatic. Such adhesions and black pigment on the lens suggest iritis, active or inactive. True neurogenic, paralytic mydriasis may occur as part of certain inflammatory disorders that affect the eye and orbit, such as herpes zoster.

Ischemia

Ischemia of the anterior segment of the globe may be acute or chronic. Both types can produce iridoplegia. Transient

dilation of the pupil may occur during an episode of monocular amaurosis associated with carotid occlusive disease, migraine, or Raynaud disease. This unilateral pupillary change is not caused by the blindness but by the hypoxic process that affects the entire eye, including the iris sphincter. Emboli that enter the central retinal artery frequently involve other branches of the ophthalmic artery, particularly the posterior ciliary arteries. If venous outflow from the globe is briefly impaired, the retina may shut down temporarily without producing an ipsilateral mydriasis. If the whole globe is ischemic (as in angle-closure glaucoma), iris ischemia will relax the iris sphincter and dilate the pupil (47).

Chronic ischemia of the anterior segment of the globe results in neovascularization of the chamber angle and the surface of the iris (rubeosis iridis), producing iris atrophy, ectropion of the pigment layer at the pupillary margin (ectropion uveae), glaucoma, and immobility of the iris. This type of chronic ischemia of the anterior segment may result from severe occlusive disease in the carotid system or the aortic arch. It also may be produced by microvascular disease or drug toxicity (e.g., quinine).

Severe, generalized atherosclerosis may result in vascular insufficiency of both irides, producing oval pupils from bitemporal palsy of the pupillary sphincters (48). Such patients have no evidence of iris atrophy or synechiae. Conversely, local iris ischemia was postulated to cause focal temporal atrophy of the iris and a nonreactive pupil in a patient with advanced keratoconus (49).

Tumor

Very few tumors affect the iris, but those that do can cause irregularity of the iris border, anisocoria, and an abnormally reactive pupil. Leiomyoma, malignant melanoma, and lymphoma can all present in this fashion.

Trauma

Spastic miosis is a constant and immediate result of trauma to the globe and occurs immediately after blunt trauma to the cornea. A similar spastic miosis follows perforating injury to the eye. The constriction of the pupil is profound but usually transient and often followed by iridoplegia. Transient spasm of accommodation often occurs in this setting and lasts 1–2 hours.

Dilation of the pupil frequently occurs after concussion of the globe and often is followed by paralysis of accommodation after the initial intense miosis has resolved. Because both the iris sphincter and dilator muscles are involved, the term "traumatic mydriasis" is misleading, as it suggests injury to the sphincter alone. The functions of the iris and ciliary muscle usually are affected together, but occasionally one is impaired without the other. The clinical picture is that of a moderately dilated pupil with both the direct and consensual reactions to light and near stimuli being diminished or absent. The deformity may resolve in a few weeks, but it usually is permanent. This abnormality may have several causes. The frequent absence of detectable pathologic change suggests that the effect may occur from injury of the fine nerves of the ciliary plexus. These may be damaged or

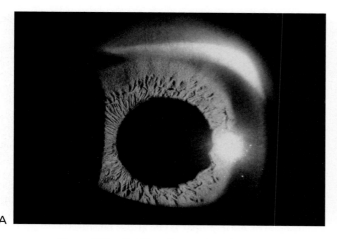

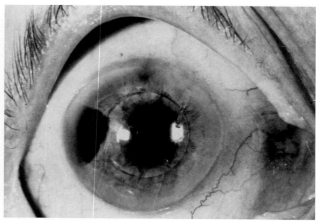

A   B

Figure 16.2. Pupillary changes after direct iris trauma. *A*, Tears in the iris sphincter causing pupillary dilation. *B*, Iris dialysis producing pseudopolycoria. (Courtesy of Dr. Walter J. Stark.)

torn by the tissue distortion caused by a pressure wave initiated by the impact. In other cases, contusion necrosis directly produces a lesion in the iris and ciliary body. Finally, as noted above, tears in the iris or rupture of the iris sphincter may be identified using slit-lamp biomicroscopy with transillumination (Fig. 16.2*A*), and a traumatic, peripheral iridodialysis may be present, with resultant distortion of the normally round pupil (Fig. 16.2*B*).

Traumatic iridoplegia in the unconscious patient with multiple head injuries may pose a difficult diagnostic problem. If it cannot be established beyond question that the iridoplegia is the result of direct ocular or orbital damage, it must be assumed that the patient has a tentorial herniation from subdural or epidural hematoma.

Acute Angle-Closure Glaucoma

An acute attack of angle-closure glaucoma usually presents no problem in diagnosis, but occasionally the pain is minimal or nonexistent. Redness of the eye is common. The pupil is usually mid-dilated and fixed (Fig. 16.3), but it may be oval. If the acute rise in intraocular pressure abates in an hour or two, the patient may never complain about the pain but instead may seek medical attention for iridoplegia. If the physician fails to notice the shallow anterior chamber or measure the intraocular pressure, he or she may be unable to explain the iridoplegia or may mistakenly attribute it to an oculomotor nerve lesion (11).

The dilated pupil that is associated with acute glaucoma initially occurs because there is maximum contact between the iris and the lens when the pupil is in a mid-dilated position. Thus, most angle-closure attacks occur when the pupil is mid-dilated (e.g., in darkness), and tonic pupil has been reported as a possible risk for angle closure (50). The iris becomes trapped in this position as intraocular pressure rises. Eventually, the increased pressure results in iris ischemia so that even when the pressure is reduced, the iris no longer functions properly and remains in the mid-dilated position.

Atrophy

Iris atrophy may be caused by inflammation, ischemia, or trauma (Fig. 16.4). It may be circumscribed or diffuse and may involve the anterior border layer, the stroma and sphincter muscle, the anterior epithelium and dilator muscle, the posterior pigmented epithelium, or a combination of these structures. Patients with unilateral iris atrophy that involves the dilator muscle often develop anisocoria, with the smaller pupil on the side of the atrophy. Patients in whom iris atrophy involves the sphincter muscle develop anisocoria with the larger pupil on the side of the atrophy.

Feibel and Perlmutter reported that patients with the pig-

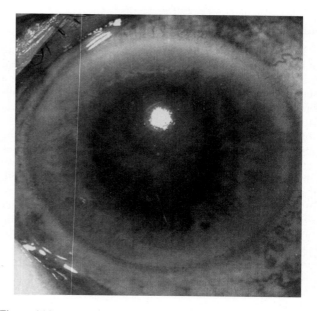

Figure 16.3. Appearance of the eye during an attack of acute angle-closure glaucoma. The pupil is fixed and asymmetrically dilated. Note the opaque, thickened cornea and dilation of the conjunctival vessels.

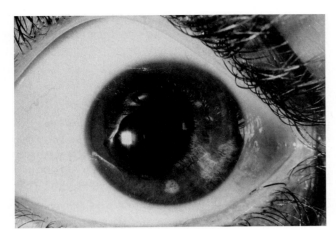

Figure 16.4. Iris atrophy following several attacks of herpes zoster ophthalmicus. (Courtesy of Dr. David L. Knox.)

ment dispersion syndrome and anisocoria had greater transillumination defects of the iris on the side of the larger pupil (51). Histologic studies of affected irides in patients with this syndrome show both atrophic and hypertrophic focal changes in the dilator muscle. The etiology of the anisocoria in these patients remains unclear; in some cases, it stems from an unrelated, coexisting condition such as a tonic pupil, Horner syndrome, or physiologic anisocoria. In others, the anisocoria may be a result of structural change or irritative stimulation of the iris due to pigment dispersion (51–53).

With age, the iris may become gray and of a more uniform color. Its stroma becomes thin, and the sphincter appears as a gray-brown ring. Stromal fibers may be partly torn and may float in the anterior chamber (iridoschisis). Typical of the aged iris are changes on the edge of the pupil, which becomes thin and loses its pigment so that it resembles a fine lacework. Another characteristic finding easily seen by slit-lamp biomicroscopy in elderly persons is the deposition of hyaline about the pupillary margin (54). Histologic examination of excised iris tissue in such cases shows deposition of hyaline in the iris stroma and in the muscles of the iris that also are atrophic.

Postoperative Mydriasis

In 1963, Urrets-Zavalia described several patients who suffered an irreversible mydriasis and pupillary immobility after an otherwise uncomplicated keratoplasty for keratoconus (55). In the typical case, a patient with keratoconus and a normally reacting pupil undergoes an uncomplicated penetrating keratoplasty, following which the pupil dilates and will not react to miotics of any type or strength. The cause of this dilation is unknown, but certain patients may be predisposed to develop this disorder because of preexisting hypoplasia of the iris stroma (56). In patients who develop microperforations in Descemet's membrane during deep lamellar keratoplasty, a fixed and dilated pupil can occur after the air/gas injection into the anterior chamber (57). The mechanism here is speculated to be induced pupil block

causing an acute rise of intraocular pressure and secondary iris ischemia.

Postoperative mydriasis occasionally occurs after an otherwise uneventful cataract extraction with placement of an intraocular lens (58,59). It sometimes is called an "atonic pupil." This condition presumably occurs from direct damage to the iris sphincter muscle during surgery.

Surgical or laser-induced damage to the short ciliary nerves or ciliary ganglion can produce a postoperative tonic pupil. Affected patients show a mild mydriasis with anisocoria that is less than 1.0 mm. The most common setting is after excimer laser photorefractive keratectomy. The mechanism may be a medication effect of topical steroids on a susceptible cornea. The mydriasis seems to improve with time in these cases (60).

AFFERENT ABNORMALITIES

Relative Afferent Pupillary Defect

The relative afferent pupillary defect (RAPD) is one of the most important objective signs of dysfunction in the afferent visual pathway. The methods of RAPD detection and quantification were reviewed in Chapter 15. In this section, we discuss the various conditions that should be considered when one finds an RAPD.

Optic Nerve Disorders

Most patients with a unilateral or asymmetric bilateral optic neuropathy, regardless of the cause, have an RAPD (61). In general, the magnitude of an RAPD correlates with the extent of central visual field loss (62–64). The correlation is higher with compressive and ischemic optic neuropathies than with demyelinating optic neuritis (62,65). Patients with acute optic neuritis have a substantial RAPD (1.0–3.0 log units) (66). After recovery, even when there are no remaining visual complaints, there often is a small RAPD (0.3–0.6 log units) still present in the affected eye. In optic nerve compression, the RAPD can be used as an additional test to monitor progression or recovery of optic nerve damage. Patients with glaucoma have an RAPD when the cupping and field loss is unilateral or asymmetric (67,68). Likewise, patients with optic disc drusen have an RAPD when there is functional asymmetry of vision between the two eyes (68).

Initial studies of patients with visual loss from Leber hereditary optic neuropathy (LHON) found that their pupil responses were not significantly different from those of normal persons and suggested that this visual–pupil dissociation was a characteristic finding of this optic neuropathy (69). Subsequent studies of patients with LHON, including those with clinical or electrophysiologic evidence of uniocular involvement, have demonstrated a pupil response deficit consistent with the visual deficit (70,71). Bremner et al. quantified the focal pupil and visual sensitivity at various points within the visual scotoma of patients with LHON (72). A pupil deficit was detected at all test locations, but it was smaller than the corresponding visual deficit (about 7.5 dB difference; i.e., a relative pupil sparing). The authors hypothesized that there may be a lower susceptibility of pupil fibers to damage in LHON.

The RAPD appears to have some prognostic value in traumatic optic neuropathy. In 19 patients with indirect traumatic optic neuropathy treated acutely with similar megadoses of methylprednisolone, patients who had an initial RAPD less than 2.1 log units improved to visual acuity of 20/30 or better. Patients with an initial RAPD larger than 2.1 log units showed little improvement of vision (73).

Retinal Disease

Diseases of the retina are uncommon causes of an RAPD. Most of the pupillomotor input derives from the central retina, so in a suspected retinopathy, the presence of a RAPD usually indicates macular involvement (see Table 15.1). In macular visual loss with visual acuity of 20/200 or better, the RAPD usually is 0.5 log units or less. A RAPD greater than 1.0 log units with a lesion confined to the macula is unusual (74,75). Kerrison et al. demonstrated that in monkeys with controlled laser destruction of the macula, approximately 25–50% loss of ganglion cells was needed to produce a 0.6 log-unit RAPD (76). Central serous maculopathy produces very little RAPD, usually 0.3 log units or less. When the subretinal fluid disappears, so does the RAPD (77). An RAPD can occur in a patient with a retinal detachment (78). In this setting, each quadrant of a fresh, bullous detachment produces about 0.3 log of RAPD, and when the macula detaches, the RAPD increases by about another 0.7 log units (79).

An RAPD can be used to help separate nonischemic from ischemic central retinal vein occlusion (CRVO). Servais et al. studied 120 patients with a unilateral CRVO and found that 90% of nonischemic CRVOs had an RAPD of 0.3 log units or less, and none had an RAPD larger than 0.9 log units (80). In contrast, in 33 patients with ischemic CRVO, 91% had an RAPD of 1.2 log units or more, and none had an RAPD smaller than 0.6 log units. In eyes that initially were nonischemic, a significant increase in the RAPD was an early indicator of ischemic conversion, even when the fundus appeared relatively unchanged.

Induced RAPD from Asymmetric Retinal Adaptation

An eye that is occluded by a ptotic lid or eye patch becomes increasingly dark-adapted during the first 30 minutes of occlusion. This can produce up to 1.5 log units of a false RAPD in the unpatched eye (81,82). Therefore, assessment of an RAPD in a patient wearing an eye patch should not be performed immediately after patch removal because of underlying asymmetry of retinal light sensitivity between the two eyes. This is particularly important to remember in patients with traumatic optic neuropathy (a real RAPD in the patched eye may be overlooked) and in patients with nonorganic visual loss (an RAPD may mistakenly be attributed to the opposite eye). After 10–15 minutes in room light with both eyes open, retinal sensitivity equalizes, and any RAPD detected should be considered valid.

An anisocoria of 2 mm or more, especially if one pupil is very small, can produce a clinically significant difference in the amount of light entering the retina. A general rule put forth is 0.1 log unit RAPD on the side of the smaller pupil for every 1 mm of anisocoria (83).

Amblyopia

A small RAPD, generally less than 0.5 log units, often can be seen in an amblyopic eye. The magnitude of the RAPD does not correlate well with the visual acuity (84,85), nor does it predict the effect of occlusion therapy (86). That such pupillomotor asymmetry is not always observed suggests that it may be seen only in patients who do not take up fixation in the amblyopic eye, even though a bright light is effectively blocking the good eye.

Local Anesthesia and RAPD

A transient RAPD typically is seen following local anesthesia in the orbit. In one study, the method of anesthetic delivery (peribulbar versus retrobulbar versus sub-Tenon) did not affect the degree of induced RAPD or its recovery time (87).

Media Opacities

Dense intraocular hemorrhage that mechanically blocks light from reaching the retina can produce an RAPD that resolves as the hemorrhage clears (88). In contrast, a dense unilateral cataract does not produce an RAPD in the affected eye. Instead, a very small RAPD occasionally is found in the opposite eye. This may be partly because of the dark-adapted retina behind the cataract and partly because the incoming light is scattered by the opaque lens, allowing more light to hit the macular area directly (89–92). DuBois and Sadun also suggested that retinal sensitivity may be upregulated slowly behind a cataract by a neurogenic mechanism that is unrelated to routine receptor photochemistry (81).

Optic Tract Disorders

A complete or nearly complete lesion of the optic tract produces a contralateral homonymous hemianopia and a small to moderate RAPD (0.3–1.6 log units) in the contralateral eye (i.e., the eye with the temporal field loss) (93–95). Assuming an asymmetric distribution of crossed and uncrossed pupillomotor fibers in each optic tract similar to that of visual fibers, the contralateral side of the RAPD found in optic tract (and midbrain tectal) lesions can be understood. However, the large range and magnitude of tract RAPDs is not explained by the percentage of decussating pupillomotor input and may be related instead to individual differences in the pupillomotor sensitivity of the temporal and nasal retina. Additionally, an asymmetric distribution of efferent impulses from each pretectal nucleus to the Edinger-Westphal nuclei would produce an efferent deficit in the eye contralateral to the lesion (i.e., the eye with the afferent deficit). This relative efferent deficit, which is most evident when comparing only the direct pupil response between the two eyes in a patient with an optic tract (or tectal) lesion, can lead to overestimation of the RAPD. Cox and Drewes suggested that this efferent part of the asymmetry can be avoided by watching one eye only and comparing its direct and consensual responses (96). This makes the examination more difficult, but it is necessary in some clinical settings.

Pretectal Nucleus

A unilateral lesion in the pretectal nucleus or in the brachium of the superior colliculus from an arteriovenous malformation, infarct, tumor, or other lesion will damage the afferent pupillomotor fibers that derive from the ipsilateral optic tract. This can produce a contralateral RAPD without any visual field defect (97,98). The tectal RAPD occasionally is associated with an ipsilateral or contralateral trochlear nerve paresis if the lesion affects the ipsilateral trochlear nerve nucleus, the predecussation portion of the ipsilateral trochlear nerve fascicle, or the postdecussation portion of the contralateral trochlear nerve fascicle (99,100).

Geniculate and Retrogeniculate Lesions

Lesions that involve the lateral geniculate nucleus or the proximal portion of the retrogeniculate pathway may be associated with a contralateral RAPD if there is also involvement of the adjacent intercalated (pretectal) neurons in the dorsal midbrain that serve as the link between the afferent visual pathway (optic tract) and the efferent pupillomotor centers (Edinger-Westphal nuclei). These are, then, essentially the same as tectal RAPDs (101). Congenital postgeniculate lesions causing homonymous hemianopia also have a contralateral RAPD, presumably from transsynaptic degeneration of the optic tract ipsilateral to the lesion (102).

Nonorganic Visual Loss

Neither nonorganic loss of visual acuity nor nonorganic constriction of the visual field in one eye ever produces an RAPD (103). This obviously is of great clinical importance. Although Kosmorsky et al. (104) reported five patients with neurogenic monocular temporal visual field defects who did not have an RAPD, the vast majority of patients with monocular neurogenic loss of the visual field do have one in the eye with visual loss. We have no explanation for the findings of Kosmorsky et al.

RAPD in Normal Eyes

Some normal subjects show a small RAPD, clinically and pupillographically, in the absence of any detectable pathologic disease (105,106). The RAPD in such cases usually is 0.3 log units or less and variable in degree. It also may vary from side to side. The RAPD in normal subjects was hypothesized as representing, in part, a real but "normal" degree of asymmetry in interocular retinal sensitivity as well as the degree of uncertainty inherent in quantifying a fluctuating, biologic process (i.e., the pupil light reflex). Thus, the presence of a very small RAPD in a healthy subject with no visual or neurologic complaints or deficits probably is of no significance. It also is possible that some normal patients, especially those with a small but persistent RAPD on the same side, harbor underlying pathology (i.e., an early compressive lesion of the optic nerve, subclinical optic neuritis)

(11). Whether further investigation is warranted for such patients should be individualized based on the clinical setting.

Wernicke Pupil

When the optic chiasm is bisected sagittally, the nasal halves of each retina become insensitive to light so that there is not only a bitemporal hemianopia but also a bitemporal pupillary hemiakinesia; that is, light falling on the nasal retina of either eye will fail to produce a pupillary constriction. Clinical demonstration of this sign with a flashlight is difficult because of intraocular scatter: when light strikes the retina in one quadrant, it tends to be spread evenly, and the beam from a flashlight directed upon the blind hemiretina thus spills onto the seeing half, causing pupillary constriction. Thus, if a very bright but small beam of light such as that produced by a slit lamp is shined on the nonseeing hemiretina of a patient with damage to the optic chiasm or optic tract and then is shined on the seeing hemiretina, it is possible to see that the pupil reacts better when the light shines on the seeing hemiretina than when it shines on the nonseeing retina. However, for practical purposes, the results of this test when performed at the bedside are often inconclusive and unreliable, and this has disappointed several generations of ophthalmologists and neurologists since Wernicke popularized the test in 1883.

Poorly Reacting Pupils from Midbrain Disease

Fixed dilated pupils and pupils that react poorly to both light and near stimuli may be produced by damage to the visceral oculomotor nuclei and their efferent fiber tracts. The precise location of such lesions is almost impossible to determine unless there is associated evidence of ocular motor nerve dysfunction. Other midbrain lesions damage the afferent input to the Edinger-Westphal nuclei or cause combined afferent and efferent damage. Seybold et al. described a variety of pupillary abnormalities in patients with tumors in the pineal region (107). With a bright light stimulus, four patients had impairment of both light and near reactions, two patients had markedly impaired light reactions and relatively intact responses to near stimuli (classic light–near dissociation), and two patients had relatively intact light reactions but impaired responses to near stimuli (inverse Argyll Robertson pupils). With a dim light stimulus, five patients had impairment of reactions to both light and near stimuli and three patients had impaired light reactions but relatively intact reactions to near stimuli. In addition, four of the patients had an asymmetric sympathetic reflex dilation. It seems that various combinations of defects involving the pupil light reflex, the pupil near response, and accommodation can occur with lesions of the rostral midbrain.

Bilateral complete internal ophthalmoplegia, when caused by damage to the rostral oculomotor nuclear complex, rarely occurs in isolation. Lesions that produce these changes must be located in the periaqueductal gray matter near the rostral end of the aqueduct. Vascular, inflammatory, neoplastic, and demyelinating diseases that affect this area almost always produce associated signs, including nuclear ophthalmoplegia, paralysis of vertical gaze, loss of convergence, exotropia, ptosis, and other defects of ocular movement.

Paradoxical Reaction of the Pupils to Light and Darkness

Barricks et al. described three unrelated boys, 2, 6, and 10 years of age, with congenital stationary night blindness, myopia, and abnormal electroretinograms, who showed a "paradoxical" pupillary constriction in darkness (108). In a lighted room, all three patients had moderately dilated pupils; however, when the room lights were extinguished, the patients' pupils briskly constricted and then slowly redilated. Subsequent investigators confirmed this observation and reported similar paradoxical pupillary responses in children and adults with congenital achromatopsia, blue-cone monochromatism, and Leber congenital amaurosis (109,110). In addition, such responses occasionally occur in patients with optic disc hypoplasia, dominant optic atrophy, and bilateral optic neuritis. Flynn et al. suggested that the pupillary responses seen in these patients occur not from abnormalities in the central nervous system (CNS) but from selective delays in afferent signals from the retinal photoreceptors to the pupillomotor center (111).

EFFERENT ABNORMALITIES: ANISOCORIA

The presence of anisocoria usually indicates a structural defect of one or both irides or a neural defect of the efferent pupillomotor pathways innervating the iris muscles in one or both eyes. A careful slit-lamp examination to assess the health and integrity of the iris stroma and muscles is an important step in the evaluation of anisocoria. If the irides are intact, then an innervation problem is suspected. As most efferent disturbances causing anisocoria are unilateral, two simple maneuvers are helpful in determining whether it is the sympathetic or parasympathetic innervation to the eye that is dysfunctional: (1) checking the pupillary light reflex and (2) measuring the anisocoria in darkness and in bright light.

When the larger pupil has an obviously impaired reaction to light stimulation, it is likely the cause of the anisocoria. One can presume the problem lies somewhere along the parasympathetic pathway to the sphincter muscle. Common etiologies include an acute tonic pupil, oculomotor nerve palsy, or pharmacologic blockade. If both pupils have a good light reflex and the degree of anisocoria decreases in bright light (i.e., anisocoria is greater in darkness), then there is either a deficit of sympathetic innervation to the dilator muscle in the eye with the smaller pupil (as in Horner syndrome)

ANISOCORIA

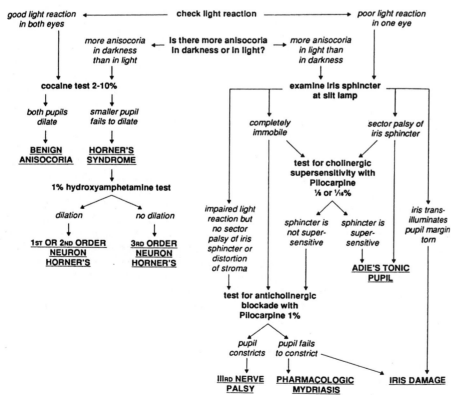

Figure 16.5. Steps that assist the evaluation of anisocoria.

or a physiologic anisocoria. The evaluation of anisocoria is described in the following sections and outlined in Figure 16.5

Anisocoria Greater in Darkness

Physiologic (Benign) Anisocoria

Inequality of pupil size becomes clinically observable when the difference between pupils is about 3 mm. In dim light or darkness, almost 20% of the normal population has an anisocoria of 0.4 mm or more at the moment of examination. In room light, this number drops to about 10% (112–114). This form of anisocoria is known by several names, including physiologic anisocoria, simple central anisocoria, essential anisocoria, and benign anisocoria. It is typically 0.6 mm or less; a difference in size of 1.0 or more is rare (114–116) (Fig. 16.6). The degree of pupillary inequality in physiologic anisocoria may change from day to day or even from hour to hour, however. The anisocoria usually diminishes slightly in bright light, perhaps because the smaller pupil reaches the zone of mechanical resistance first, giving the larger pupil a chance to make up the size difference (117).

Physiologic anisocoria is not caused by damage to the peripheral nerves that innervate the sphincter and dilator muscles of the iris. The pupillary reactions to light and darkness are normal. Instead, it is presumed to occur because the supranuclear inhibition of the parasympathetic pupilloconstrictor nuclei in the midbrain is not balanced with any more precision than is necessary for clear, binocular vision. It is unrelated to refractive error. Occasionally, a reversal of physiologic anisocoria is seen, a phenomenon termed ''seesaw anisocoria'' (112,116).

When physiologic anisocoria is suspected, reviewing old photographs, such as a driver's license or especially a family album, can be a valuable diagnostic tool (Fig. 16.7). In the latter case, the anisocoria usually can be traced back to infancy or early childhood.

Horner Syndrome

When the sympathetic innervation to the eye is interrupted, the retractor muscles in the eyelids are weakened, allowing the upper lid to droop and the lower lid to rise. The dilator muscle of the iris also is weakened, allowing the pupil to become smaller, and vasomotor and sudomotor control of parts of the face may be lost. This combination of ptosis, miosis, and anhidrosis is called **Horner syndrome** (Fig 16.8)

HISTORICAL BACKGROUND

In 1869, Johann Friedrich Horner, a Swiss ophthalmologist, published a short case report in which he emphasized that eyelid ptosis could be caused by a lesion as far away from the eye as the neck by denervating the sympathetically innervated muscle in the upper lid that had recently been described by H. Müller. Although he was not the first to report the clinical condition, his meticulous and scientifically substantiated account of the clinical effects of cervical sympathetic paralysis has firmly attached his name to this syndrome (118). In the French literature, this condition is called the Claude Bernard-Horner syndrome to honor the work of Claude Bernard in 1852 on the physiology of the sympathetic nerves.

Although Horner and Bernard generally are credited with identifying the clinical signs of oculosympathetic paresis, these signs were first produced experimentally in the dog by François Pourfour du Petit in 1727. Pourfour du Petit was never recognized for these contributions; however, Pourfour du Petit syndrome is the term used for the combination of

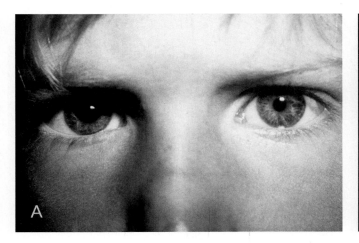
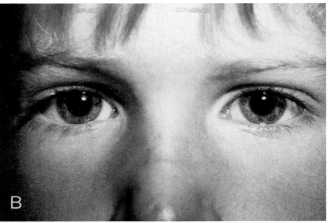

Figure 16.6. Physiologic (benign) anisocoria. The patient was a 5-year-old boy whose parents noted that the right pupil was larger than the other. The anisocoria was more obvious in dark than in light, and both pupils reacted normally to light stimulation. *A*, Appearance of the patient. Note anisocoria with right pupil larger than left. *B*, 45 minutes after instillation of a 10% solution of cocaine into both inferior conjunctival sacs, both pupils are dilated, indicating that anisocoria is not caused by sympathetic denervation.

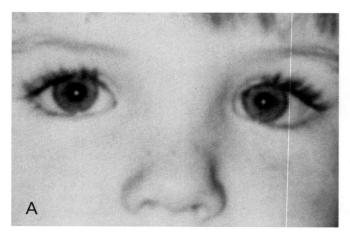

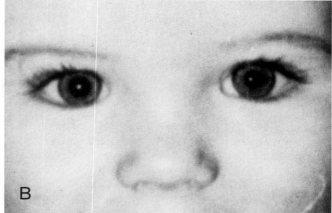

Figure 16.7. Value of old photographs in the assessment of anisocoria. *A*, This 3-year-old boy was noted by his parents to have intermittent anisocoria, with the right pupil larger than the left. The anisocoria was greater in darkness than in light, and both pupils reacted normally to light stimulation. *B*, Photograph of patient at age 7 months shows obvious anisocoria.

signs caused by sympathetic stimulation (i.e., lid retraction, mydriasis, and conjunctival blanching). This eponym is remarkable because Pourfour du Petit never actually stimulated the sympathetic nerve in his experimental animals (119).

CLINICAL CHARACTERISTICS

Ptosis. The affected eye often looks small or sunken in patients with Horner syndrome. The upper eyelid is slightly drooped because of paralysis of the sympathetically innervated smooth muscle (Müller muscle) that contributes to the position of the opened upper eyelid. This ptosis sometimes is so slight and variable that it escapes attention. In one study, ptosis was frankly absent in 12% of patients (120). Similar smooth muscle fibers in the lower eyelid also lose their nerve supply in Horner syndrome; thus, the lower lid

usually is slightly elevated, producing an "upside-down ptosis," further narrowing of the palpebral fissure, and an apparent enophthalmos. That the enophthalmos is apparent rather than real has been confirmed by several studies (119,121,122).

Pupillary Signs. *Miosis.* The palsy of the iris dilator muscle in Horner syndrome allows unantagonized action of the iris sphincter, producing a smaller pupil. However, in some patients in the setting of intense emotional excitement, the pupil on the side of the sympathetic lesion becomes larger than the normal pupil. Likewise, if the dilator muscle is stimulated directly (e.g., after an adrenergic eye drop is used), the pupil will dilate widely. This "paradoxical pupillary dilation" is caused by denervation supersensitivity of the dilator muscle to circulating and topical adrenergic substances.

Topical apraclonidine is an alpha-adrenergic receptor ago-

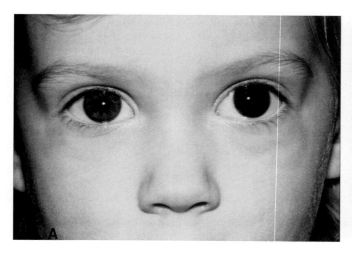

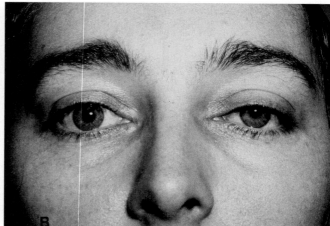

Figure 16.8. Horner syndrome in two patients. *A*, Congenital right Horner syndrome. Note associated heterochromia iridis and minimal ptosis. *B*, Left Horner syndrome after neck trauma.

nist that has little or no effect on a normal pupil but can dilate a Horner pupil due to denervation supersensitivity of the alpha-1 receptors on the iris dilator muscle. Thus, reversal of anisocoria following topical instillation of apraclonidine has been seen in patients with unilateral Horner syndrome (123,124).

Anisocoria.   Any anisocoria, when caused by weakness of a single iris muscle, increases in the direction of action of that muscle. With a unilateral oculosympathetic defect, the weakness of the dilator muscle in the affected eye (and resultant anisocoria) is most apparent in darkness. Conversely, the anisocoria almost disappears in light because the normal action of both sphincters (oculoparasympathetic activity) constricts the pupils to almost equal sizes. In regular room light, the degree of anisocoria in Horner syndrome is rather small, on the order of 1.0 mm or less, and can be overlooked or mistakenly attributed to simple anisocoria (125). Furthermore, when a patient is fatigued or drowsy, the size of the pupils and the degree of anisocoria diminish as the hypothalamic sympathetic outflow to both eyes subsides and uninhibited parasympathetic outflow augments. Some patients with Horner syndrome have anisocoria measuring up to 2.5 mm; such a large anisocoria is not seen with benign anisocoria. The actual amount of anisocoria in Horner syndrome thus varies with (*a*) the resting size of the pupils; (*b*) the completeness of the injury; (*c*) the alertness of the patient; (*d*) the extent of reinnervation of the dilator muscle; (*e*) the brightness of the examiner's light or the ambient light in the room; (*f*) the degree of denervation supersensitivity; (*g*) the fixation of the patient at distance or near; and (*h*) the concentration of circulating adrenergic substances in the blood.

Dilation Lag.   Paresis of the iris dilator muscle results in a smaller resting pupil size (miosis) and also in impaired pupillary movement during dilation, called dilation lag. Dilation lag can be seen clinically by illuminating the patient's

eyes tangentially from below with a hand-held flashlight, and then abruptly turning the room lights out. The normal pupil will immediately dilate, but several seconds will elapse before the Horner pupil begins to dilate. The dilation dynamics of a normal pupil compared with a Horner pupil have been well documented using continuous recording pupillography (119). Immediately following a bright light flash, both pupils are strongly constricted. In the first second of darkness, both pupils synchronously enlarge a small degree, presumably from acute inhibition of parasympathetic impulses. In the next few seconds, the normal pupil, stimulated by an active burst of sympathetic discharges, rapidly dilates, whereas the Horner pupil, denervated of sympathetic impulses, hardly moves. This results in an increasing anisocoria during in the first 5 seconds or so of darkness. Thereafter, the Horner pupil slowly dilates from decreasing parasympathetic tone and catches up in size to the normal pupil. Thus, if both pupils are observed simultaneously for 15–20 seconds after turning off the room light, one sees an initial increase in the degree of anisocoria, followed by decreasing anisocoria (Fig. 16.9).

A psychosensory stimulus such as a sudden noise will cause a normal pupil to dilate. When looking for dilation lag in darkness, interjection of a sudden loud noise just as the lights go out tends to augment the initial increase in anisocoria when a unilateral oculosympathetic defect is present. One can also pinch the patient's neck (the ciliospinal reflex), press over McBurney's point (Meyer's iliac sign), or flex the patient's neck (Flatau's neck mydriasis) to bring this out (126).

There remains controversy about which aspect of pupillary reflex dilation in darkness best identifies the impaired dilation dynamics of a Horner syndrome. Several methods of detecting dilation lag have been proposed. Taking Polaroid photographs 5 seconds after the lights go out and again after 15 seconds of darkness is a simple and readily available

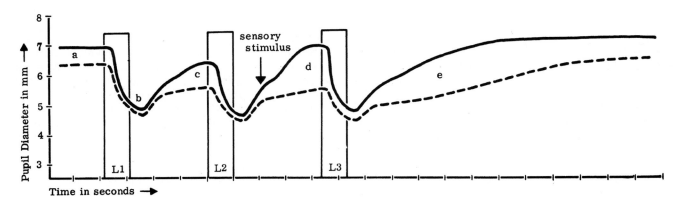

Figure 16.9. Pupillogram of a patient with a left Horner syndrome (*solid line* is a normal pupil; *broken line* is a Horner pupil). Point a is the resting size of both pupils (and anisocoria) in darkness. Following a 1-second pulse of light, the pupils are maximally constricted at b. As the pupils redilate in the darkness, increasing anisocoria seen in c is due to the relative inactivity of the Horner pupil. Addition of a sensory stimulus after the pulse of light further enhances the asymmetric dilation dynamics (d) between the normal pupil and the Horner pupil. In e, the dilation of both pupils is observed over a longer period of time. After the initial increase in anisocoria, there is a gradual decreasing of the anisocoria as the slowly dilating Horner pupil eventually recovers its baseline size in darkness.

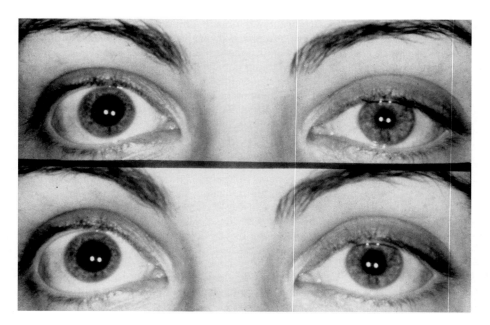

Figure 16.10. Dilation lag in a patient with a left Horner syndrome, observed using regular flash color photos. *Top,* Photo taken 5 seconds after the room lights were turned off. *Bottom,* Photo taken after 15 seconds of darkness. The right pupil is already maximally dilated within 5 seconds of turning the room lights off, but the left pupil still has not dilated maximally after 15 seconds of darkness.

means to assess for dilation lag. Patients with Horner syndrome show more anisocoria in the 5-second photograph than in the 15-second photograph, emphasizing that the absence of continued dilation after 5 seconds in darkness (i.e., demonstration of decreasing anisocoria in the later phase of dilation) is a defining characteristic of an oculosympathetic defect (127,128) (Fig. 16.10). Videography with infrared illumination is one of the best ways to show this phenomenon (129). Others have reported that a single measurement of anisocoria taken within the first 5 seconds of darkness (i.e., assessment of the increase in anisocoria in the early phase of dilation) is adequate for identifying dilation lag. One study reported that 0.6 mm or more at 4 seconds was 82% sensitive for diagnosing a unilateral Horner syndrome (130) Using a binocular infrared video pupillometer with continuous recording of pupil diameters, Smith and Smith found that after a light flash, a delay in the time needed to recover three quarters of the baseline pupil size had a 70% sensitivity and 95% specificity of detecting unilateral Horner syndrome (131). This definition of dilation lag based on a measure of time, instead of the degree of anisocoria, is particularly useful for detecting bilateral Horner syndrome.

Hypochromia Iridis. Depigmentation of the ipsilateral iris is a typical feature of congenital Horner syndrome and occasionally is seen in patients with a long-standing, acquired Horner syndrome (132). It is never seen in patients with an acute or recently acquired Horner syndrome.

Anhidrosis. Characteristic vasomotor and sudomotor changes of the facial skin can occur on the affected side in some patients with Horner syndrome. Immediately following sympathetic denervation, the temperature of the skin rises on the side of the lesion because of loss of vasomotor control and consequent dilation of blood vessels. Additionally, there may be facial flushing, conjunctival hyperemia, epiphora, and nasal stuffiness in the acute stage.

Some time after the injury, the skin of the ipsilateral face

and neck may have a lower temperature and may be paler than that of the normal side. This occurs from supersensitivity of the denervated blood vessels to circulating adrenergic substances, with resultant vasoconstriction.

The distribution of the loss of sweating (anhidrosis) and flushing depends on the location of sympathetic lesion. For example, in lesions of the preganglionic neuron, the entire side of the head, the face, and the neck down to the clavicle usually are involved, whereas in postganglionic lesions, anhidrosis is limited to a patch on the forehead and the medial side of the nose. In a warm environment, the skin on the affected side will feel dry, whereas the skin on the normal side will be so damp that a smooth object, such as a plastic bar, will not slide easily on the skin but will stick. Because most persons live and work in temperature-controlled spaces, patients with Horner syndrome rarely complain of disturbances of sweating or asymmetric facial flushing.

Paradoxic unilateral sweating with flushing of the face, neck, and sometimes the shoulder and arm can be a late development in patients with a surgically induced Horner syndrome following cervical sympathectomy (133) or a cervical injury. Apparently, some axons in the vagus nerve normally pass into the superior cervical ganglion. These parasympathetic axons can establish, by collateral sprouting, anomalous vagal connections with postganglionic sympathetic neurons to the head and neck. Affected patients may experience bizarre sudomotor and pilomotor (gooseflesh) activity and vasomotor flushing geared reflexively to certain functions of the vagus nerve. The patterns of anomalous sweating vary but often involve the central portions of the face and forehead (119).

Accommodation. Most reports describe an increase in accommodative amplitude on the side of a Horner syndrome (119). It would appear that an intact sympathetic innervation of the ciliary muscle helps that muscle loosen and tighten the zonules with alacrity. This is a minor effect and is clinically insignificant.

DIAGNOSIS

Not all patients with unilateral ptosis and ipsilateral miosis have Horner syndrome (134). The prevalence of simple anisocoria in the normal population is about 20%. A ptosis from any cause, such as dehiscence of the levator insertion, eyelid inflammation, or myasthenia gravis, may occur coincidentally on the side of the smaller pupil in a patient who also happens to have simple anisocoria, resulting in a "pseudo-Horner syndrome."

The most widely used confirmatory test for the diagnosis of Horner syndrome is the cocaine eyedrop test (135). In 1884, Koller first described using a 2% cocaine solution as a topical ocular anesthetic, at which time it was noted that this substance also dilated the pupil. It was subsequently noted that cocaine also widened the palpebral fissure and blanched the conjunctiva of a normal eye—the same combination of signs that was known to occur when the cervical sympathetic nerve was stimulated. Shortly thereafter, Uhthoff suggested that cocaine be used as a clinical test of the sympathetic integrity to the eye (119).

Cocaine blocks the reuptake of the norepinephrine that is released continuously from sympathetic nerve endings at the neuromuscular synapse, allowing norepinephrine to accumulate at the receptors of the effector cells. In a normal eye, a 2–10% solution of cocaine causes dilation of the pupil. One study noted a mean pupil dilation of 2.14 mm (range, 0.6–4.0 mm) in normal eyes in response to a 5% cocaine solution (125). A lesion anywhere along the three-neuron sympathetic pathway that impairs neural impulses will interrupt the normal spontaneous release of norepinephrine from presynaptic nerve endings. Thus, cocaine has no significant mydriatic effect on a sympathetically denervated iris.

Rarely, a normal pupil will fail to dilate after topical application of 2% cocaine, perhaps because the oculosympathetic nerves of a few lethargic individuals do not release enough norepinephrine for 2% cocaine to have an effect, or because some heavily pigmented irides bind the drug so that it does not reach the dilator muscle (11). Whatever the reason, a 10% solution most often is used to test for a Horner pupil (Fig. 16.11). The first drop stings briefly, then the anesthetic effect takes effect and a second drop can be placed about 1 minute later. Peak effect is attained in 40–60 minutes. There are no apparent psychoactive effects from a 10% solution of cocaine, but metabolites of the drug can be found in the urine in 100% of patients after 24 hours, in 50% at 36 hours, and in 2% after 48 hours (136,137). The odds of an anisocoria being caused by an oculosympathetic palsy increase with the amount of post-cocaine anisocoria, regardless of the amount of baseline anisocoria. For clinical purposes, a post-cocaine anisocoria of 0.8 mm measured in standard room light is sufficient to diagnose a Horner syndrome (138). However, if the smaller (suspected Horner) pupil dilates more than 2 mm, even if the post-cocaine anisocoria is greater than 0.8 mm, a Horner syndrome is unlikely (125).

Some patients with very dark irides simply do not dilate well to cocaine. If the normal pupil has not dilated by 2 mm or more at 40–60 minutes after cocaine instillation, the differential effect of cocaine on a sympathetically denervated iris may not be evident. Apparent inaction of cocaine also can result from an overly bright room and patient drowsiness, both of which promote pupillary constriction.

LOCALIZATION

Localization of the site of injury of a Horner syndrome often can be determined from associated signs and symptoms and can be helpful in the appropriate evaluation of these patients.

Central Horner Syndrome. The central sympathetic pathway has components in the brain, brain stem, and spinal cord. Experimental data suggest that this central sympathetic pathway has cerebral cortical representation and is polysyn-

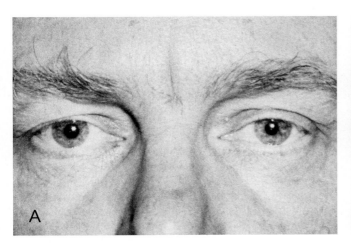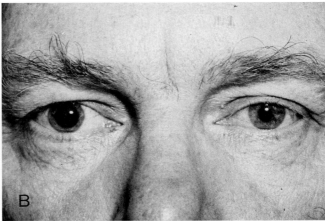

Figure 16.11. Response of normal pupil and a Horner pupil to cocaine. *A,* A 55-year-old man with left Horner syndrome associated with Raeder paratrigeminal neuralgia. *B,* 45 minutes after conjunctival instillation of two drops of a 10% cocaine solution in each eye, the right pupil is dilated, whereas the left pupil remains unchanged (small).

aptic (139). A patient with Horner syndrome after a transient ischemic episode showed only a lesion in the ipsilateral insular cortex (140). From the posterolateral hypothalamus, sympathetic fibers pass through the lateral brain stem and extend to the ciliospinal center of Budge in the intermediolateral gray column of the spinal cord at C8–T1. A central Horner syndrome caused by damage to any of these structures is ipsilateral to the lesion and almost always unilateral. A lesion in this neuron often produces a hemihypohidrosis of the entire body. Lesions of the hypothalamus such as tumor or hemorrhage can cause an ipsilateral Horner syndrome (141,142) with contralateral hemiparesis, contralateral hypesthesia, or both. Patients with a central Horner syndrome caused by a lesion of the thalamus also show a contralateral hemiparesis that often is ataxic (143). Contralateral hypesthesia, vertical gaze paresis, and dysphasia are other associated findings.

The occurrence of a unilateral Horner syndrome and a contralateral trochlear nerve paresis indicates a lesion of the dorsal mesencephalon. The lesion injures either the trochlear nucleus on the side of the Horner syndrome or the ipsilateral fascicle (140,144–146).

Although a Horner syndrome associated with an ipsilateral abducens nerve paresis is most often caused by a lesion in the cavernous sinus (see below), this combination of signs also may occur in patients with pontine lesions (147). In such cases, the Horner syndrome is central rather than postganglionic.

The classical brain stem syndrome characterized in part by a central Horner syndrome is Wallenberg syndrome, also called the lateral medullary syndrome. The typical findings of Wallenberg syndrome are ipsilateral impairment of pain and temperature sensation over the face, Horner syndrome, limb ataxia, and a bulbar disturbance causing dysarthria and dysphagia. Contralaterally, pain and temperature sensation is impaired over the trunk and limbs. The symptoms of Wallenberg syndrome include vertigo and a variety of unusual sensations of body and environmental tilt, often so bizarre as to suggest a psychogenic origin (148,149). Patients may report the whole room tilted on its side or even upside down; with their eyes closed, they may feel themselves to be tilted. Lateropulsion, a compelling sensation of being pulled toward the side of the lesion, is often a prominent complaint and also is evident in the ocular motor findings (150,151). If the patient is asked to fixate straight ahead and then gently close the lids, the eyes deviate conjugately toward the side of the lesion. This is reflected by the corrective saccades that the patient must make on eye opening to reacquire the target. Lateropulsion may even appear with a blink. Wallenberg syndrome is most commonly caused by thrombotic occlusion of the ipsilateral vertebral artery, although isolated posterior inferior cerebellar artery disease is occasionally seen (152). In a series of 130 patients with lateral medullary infarction, the pathogenesis was large vessel infarction in 50%, arterial dissection in 15%, small vessel infarction in 13%, and cardiac embolism in 5% (153). Demyelinating disease of the medulla has also been reported in a case of Wallenberg syndrome (154).

Although most patients with a central neuron Horner syn-

drome have other neurologic deficits, occasional patients with cervical spondylosis present only with a Horner syndrome and perhaps some neck pain. An isolated central Horner syndrome also can occur from a brain stem syrinx (155).

Lesions of the spinal cord (lower cervical or upper thoracic area) can cause a central Horner syndrome. In most cases there are other neurologic deficits, although in some patients the Horner syndrome is the only neurologic abnormality. Spinal cord lesions that may cause a central Horner syndrome include trauma (most common), inflammatory or infectious myelitis, vascular malformation, demyelination, syrinx, syringomyelia, neoplasms, and infarction. What appears to be an alternating Horner syndrome (i.e., alternating oculosympathetic deficit) can be seen in patients with cervical cord lesions and in some patients with systemic dysautonomias (156–159). Other patients have attacks of autonomic hyperreflexia that excite the ciliospinal center of Budge on the affected side (the C8–T1 intermediolateral gray column may, in fact, be supersensitive as a result of its disconnection). This excess firing of sympathetic impulses (oculosympathetic spasm) dilates the pupils, lifts the eyelid, blanches the conjunctiva, and increases sweating of the face (160). When the oculosympathetic spasm occurs unilaterally and intermittently on the side of an underlying Horner syndrome, the anisocoria appears to reverse; this mechanism may account for some cases of alternating Horner syndrome (161).

Preganglionic (Second-Order Neuron) Horner Syndrome. The preganglionic (second-order) neuron exits from the ciliospinal center of Budge and passes across the pulmonary apex. It then turns upward, passes through the stellate ganglion, and goes up the carotid sheath to the superior cervical ganglion, near the bifurcation of the common carotid artery.

In one large series, malignancy was the cause of about 25% of cases of preganglionic Horner syndrome (162). The most common tumors, not surprisingly, were lung and breast cancer, but Horner syndrome was not an early sign of either of these tumors. Indeed, by the time the Horner syndrome had appeared, the tumor already was known to be present.

Apical lung lesions that spread locally at the superior thoracic outlet cause symptoms of ipsilateral shoulder pain (the most common initial symptom) and pain and paresthesia along the medial arm, forearm, and fourth and fifth digits (the distribution of the C8 and T1 nerve roots) as well as a preganglionic Horner syndrome and weakness/atrophy of the hand muscles. This combination of signs is called the Pancoast syndrome. The majority of lesions causing Pancoast syndrome are carcinomas of the lung (163). Other tumors and infectious processes, including tuberculosis, bacterial pneumonias, and fungal infection, have been reported. A patient with a preganglionic Horner syndrome and ipsilateral shoulder pain should be investigated thoroughly for neoplastic involvement of the pulmonary apex, the pleural lining, and the brachial plexus.

Tumors that spread behind the carotid sheath at the C6 level may produce a preganglionic Horner syndrome associated with paralysis of the phrenic, vagus, and recurrent laryngeal nerves: the Rowland Payne syndrome (164). Just 3 inches lower, at the thoracic outlet, these nerves are more widely separated and less likely to be involved together. Thus, if a patient is newly hoarse and has a preganglionic Horner syndrome, a chest radiograph may be warranted to see whether the hemidiaphragm ipsilateral to the Horner syndrome is elevated.

Nonpulmonary tumors that produce a preganglionic Horner syndrome include sympathetic chain or intercostal nerve schwannoma, paravertebral primitive neuroectodermal tumor, vagal paraganglioma, mediastinal tumors or cysts, and thyroid carcinoma. Injury to the brachial plexus or spinal roots, pneumothorax, fracture of the first rib, or neck hematoma should be considered in patients whose preganglionic Horner syndrome follows neck or shoulder trauma.

The preganglionic neuron is the most common site of injury for an iatrogenic Horner syndrome. The varied anesthetic, radiologic, and surgical procedures that can produce the condition include coronary artery bypass surgery, lung or mediastinal surgery, carotid endarterectomy, insertion of a pacemaker, epidural anesthesia, interpleural placement of chest tubes, internal jugular catheterization, and stenting of the internal carotid artery (165–170).

Despite advances in neuroimaging and other diagnostic tests, many cases of preganglionic Horner syndrome have no explanation. In one series, about 28% of cases of preganglionic Horner syndrome were of unknown etiology (125).

Postganglionic (Third-Order Neuron) Horner Syndrome. The postganglionic (third-order) sympathetic neuron to the iris dilator muscle begins in the superior cervical ganglion and travels in the wall of the internal carotid artery, where it is called the carotid sympathetic plexus or sometimes the carotid sympathetic nerve. The latter may be a more appropriate term, as the majority of sympathetic fibers ascend as a single bundle. Within the cavernous sinus, the sympathetic fibers leave the internal carotid artery, join briefly with the abducens nerve, and then leave it to join the ophthalmic division of the trigeminal nerve, entering the orbit with its nasociliary branch (171,172). The sympathetic fibers in the nasociliary nerve divide into the two long ciliary nerves that travel with the lateral and medial suprachoroidal vascular bundles to reach the anterior segment of the eye and innervate the iris dilator muscle.

Most lesions that damage the postganglionic sympathetic neuron are vascular lesions that produce headache or ipsilateral facial pain as well and often are lumped under the clinical description of a ''painful postganglionic Horner syndrome.'' Responsible lesions may be extracranial, affecting postganglionic sympathetics in the neck, or intracranial, affecting the sympathetics at the base of the skull, in the carotid canal and middle ear, or in the region of the cavernous sinus. It is unusual for an orbital lesion to produce an isolated Horner syndrome.

Lesions of or along the internal carotid artery are a common cause of a painful postganglionic Horner syndrome, the most common being a traumatic or spontaneous dissection of the cervical internal carotid artery. In 146 such patients, a Horner syndrome was the most common ocular finding (44%) (173). In half of these cases, the Horner syndrome was the initial and sole manifestation of the carotid artery dissection. In the other half, an associated ocular or cerebral ischemic event occurred within a mean of 7 days of the Horner syndrome, emphasizing the need for early recognition and diagnosis of this cause of Horner syndrome. Carotid dissections are discussed in Chapter 40.

Pathologic conditions of the internal carotid artery other than dissection that are associated with a Horner syndrome include aneurysms, severe atherosclerosis, acute thrombosis, fibromuscular dysplasia, and arteritis (174). Mass lesions in the neck that can compress the carotid sympathetic neuron include tumors, inflammatory masses, enlarged lymph nodes, and even an ectatic jugular vein (175,176).

In the deep retroparotid space and around the jugular foramen, oculosympathetic fibers are in close proximity with several lower cranial nerves. Lesions in this area of the neck, usually trauma, tumors, and masses, can result in a Horner syndrome associated with ipsilateral paralysis of the tongue, soft palate, pharynx, and larynx. Such lesions may cause dysphagia, dysphonia, and hoarseness. The ipsilateral posterior pharynx may be hypesthetic. This combination of paralysis of the cervical sympathetics and the last four cranial nerves (the glossopharyngeal, vagus, accessory, and hypoglossal nerves) is called Villaret syndrome (177).

The superior cervical ganglion lies about 1.5 cm behind the palatine tonsil and thus can be damaged by iatrogenic or traumatic penetrating intraoral injury. Tonsillectomy, intraoral surgery, peritonsillar injections, and accidental punctures through the soft palate are some of the etiologies that have been reported to cause a postganglionic Horner syndrome from damage to the superior cervical ganglion (178,179).

Lesions at the skull base can cause a postganglionic Horner syndrome. A middle fossa mass encroaching on Meckel's cave and on the internal carotid artery at the foramen lacerum can produce a postganglionic Horner syndrome associated with trigeminal pain or sensory loss. A basal skull fracture involving the petrous bone can damage the postganglionic sympathetic fibers within the carotid canal, producing a postganglionic Horner syndrome associated with an ipsilateral abduction deficit, facial palsy, and/or sensorineural hearing loss (abducens, facial, and vestibulocochlear cranial nerves) (180).

Any lesion in the cavernous sinus may produce a postganglionic Horner syndrome. In many cases, there is associated ipsilateral ophthalmoparesis caused by involvement of one or more ocular motor nerves as well as pain or dysesthesia of the ipsilateral face caused by trigeminal nerve dysfunction. The occurrence of an abducens palsy and a postganglionic Horner syndrome (Parkinson sign) without other neurologic signs should raise suspicion of a cavernous sinus lesion (181–183). When a Horner syndrome and oculomotor nerve palsy occur together, there is combined sympathetic and parasympathetic dysfunction of the iris muscles. In such cases, the anisocoria is minimal or absent despite the impaired light reaction of the affected pupil, and pharmacologic testing may be the only means to detect an underlying sympathetic paresis (184).

Cluster headaches are severe lancinating unilateral headaches that usually occur in middle-aged men. The headaches often are nocturnal, last 30–120 minutes, and are accompanied by ipsilateral tearing, nasal stuffiness, conjunctival injection, and ptosis (signs of acute oculosympathetic palsy). A postganglionic Horner syndrome occurs in 5–22% of patients with cluster headache (185,186). Otherwise, no other neurologic deficits are present. Cluster headache is thought to be a vasospastic process affecting the carotid arterial system. Raeder paratrigeminal neuralgia is an eponym used for a painful postganglionic Horner syndrome characterized by a persistent ipsilateral trigeminal neuralgia and/or trigeminal nerve dysfunction. It is the trigeminal nerve involvement (pain or sensory change) that is distinctive and warrants investigation for a lesion in the middle cranial fossa medial to the trigeminal ganglion (185–187).

The hydroxyamphetamine test can be used to assist the differentiation between a postganglionic and a preganglionic or central Horner syndrome (188–190) (Fig. 16.12). Hydroxyamphetamine releases stored norepinephrine from the postganglionic adrenergic nerve endings, producing variable mydriasis in normal subjects (191). A lesion of the postganglionic neuron results in loss of terminal nerve endings

and their stores of norepinephrine; thus, hydroxyamphetamine has no mydriatic effect. With lesions of the preganglionic or central neuron, the postganglionic nerve endings, though nonfunctioning, remain structurally intact. Thus, the pupil dilates fully and may even become larger than the opposite pupil from upregulation of the postsynaptic receptors on the dilator muscle. A postganglionic Horner pupil occasionally dilates in response to topical hydroxyamphetamine (false-negative result) when patients are tested within the first week of sympathetic injury before the stores of norepinephrine at the presynaptic nerve endings have been depleted (192). Hydroxyamphetamine hydrobromide 1% (Paredrine) is commonly used in the United States but is difficult to obtain or unavailable in other countries. Both tyramine hydrochloride 5% and hydroxymethylamphetamine (Pholedrine) have a mode of action similar to that of hydroxyamphetamine and serve equally well as agents for a localizing pharmacologic test (193,194).

A smaller pupil that fails to dilate to both cocaine and hydroxyamphetamine most likely has a lesion of the post-

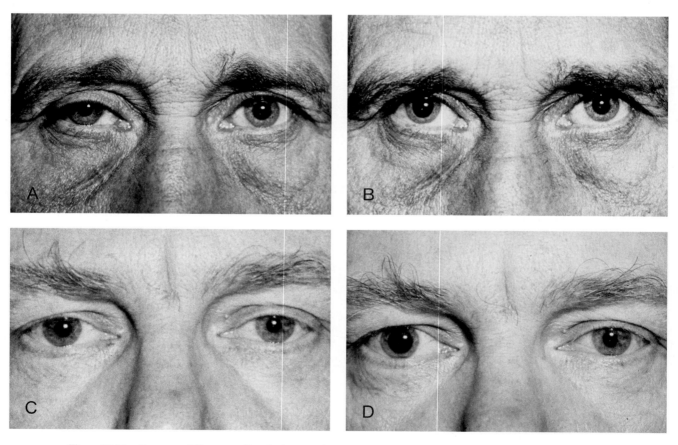

Figure 16.12.   Response of Horner pupils to hydroxyamphetamine. *A,* Right Horner syndrome in a 45-year-old man with an apical lung tumor. *B,* 45 minutes after conjunctival instillation of 2 drops of 1% hydroxyamphetamine solution (Paredrine) in each eye, both pupils are dilated, indicating an intact postganglionic neuron (i.e., a preganglionic Horner syndrome). *C,* Left Horner syndrome associated with cluster headaches in a 55-year-old man. *D,* 45 minutes after conjunctival instillation of two drops of 1% hydroxyamphetamine solution in each eye, only the right (normal) pupil is dilated. The left pupil is unchanged, indicating damage to the postganglionic neuron (i.e., a postganglionic Horner syndrome).

ganglionic sympathetic neuron. Such a pupil should dilate to a weak, direct-acting topical adrenergic drug, such as a 1% solution of phenylephrine hydrochloride or a 2% solution of epinephrine due to adrenergic denervation supersensitivity of the iris dilator muscle. Indeed, such a pupil not only will dilate but also will become larger than the opposite normal pupil. Denervation supersensitivity of the iris to adrenergic drugs apparently does not occur immediately after damage to the postganglionic sympathetic nerve but may take as long as 17 days to develop (195). Occasionally, this test is used to differentiate a mechanically restricted pupil (e.g., iris damage) from a postganglionic Horner pupil because the restricted pupil fails to dilate to direct-acting adrenergic agents.

ACQUIRED HORNER SYNDROME IN CHILDREN

Horner syndrome in childhood (under age 18 years) may be congenital (42%), postoperative (42%), or truly acquired (15%) (196). It is this last group that often results from an underlying neoplasm or serious neurologic disease. For example, neuroblastoma is responsible for up to 20% of such cases (197). Other reported etiologies include spinal cord tumors, brachial plexus trauma, intrathoracic aneurysm, embryonal cell carcinoma, rhabdomyosarcoma, thrombosis of the internal carotid artery, and brain stem vascular malformations (196,198). Thus, an acquired Horner syndrome in a child with no prior surgical history, even if the finding is isolated, warrants immediate further investigation. This is particularly important for neuroblastoma because younger age (less than 1 year) is strongly correlated with better outcome.

CONGENITAL HORNER SYNDROME

Patients with a congenital Horner syndrome have ptosis, miosis, facial anhidrosis, and hypochromia of the affected iris (119,199). Even a child with very blue eyes usually has a paler iris on the affected side from impaired development of iris melanophores, causing hypochromia of the iris stroma. This occurs whether the lesion is preganglionic or postganglionic because of anterograde transsynaptic dysgenesis (200). Children with naturally curly hair and a congenital Horner syndrome have straight hair on the side of the Horner syndrome (201). The reason for this abnormality is unclear, but it probably relates to lack of sympathetic innervation to the hair shafts on the affected side of the head.

Parents of an infant with congenital Horner syndrome sometimes report that the baby develops a hemifacial flush when nursing or crying. The flushed side probably is the normally innervated side that appears dramatically reddish when seen against the opposite side with pallor from impaired facial vasodilation and perhaps overactive vasoconstriction as well. In other words, hemifacial flushing in infants is likely to be opposite the side of a congenital Horner syndrome (202,203). Sometimes, a cycloplegic refraction unexpectedly answers the question by producing an atropinic

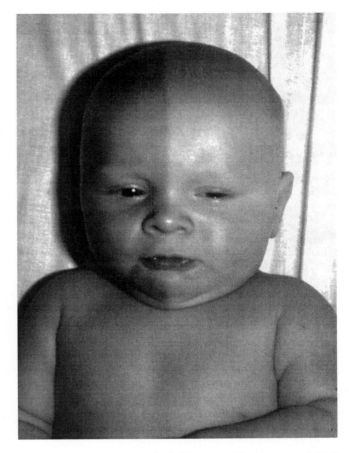

Figure 16.13. Lack of atropinic flushing in a child with a congenital left Horner syndrome. The atropinic flush is present only on the side of the face opposite the Horner syndrome.

flush. This reaction occurs only when there is an intact sympathetic innervation to the skin (Fig. 16.13).

Some patients with congenital Horner syndrome have clinical evidence that indicates a preganglionic lesion (e.g., facial anhidrosis, evidence of a brachial plexus injury, history of thoracic surgery), but pharmacologic localization with hydroxyamphetamine indicates a postganglionic lesion. Possible explanations include an embryopathy directly involving the superior cervical ganglion, damage to the vascular supply of the superior cervical ganglion, and transsynaptic dysgenesis of the superior cervical ganglion following a defect located more proximally in the sympathetic pathway (200,204).

Birth trauma probably is the most common etiology of congenital Horner syndrome (196). Use of forceps, history of shoulder dystocia, and fetal rotation can lead to injury of the sympathetic plexus along its course in the neck or near the thoracic outlet. Associated upper extremity weakness is indicative of concomitant damage to the ipsilateral brachial plexus (200) (Fig. 16.14). Neuroblastoma was found in one of 31 congenital cases (''congenital'' being defined as a Horner syndrome detected before 4 weeks of age) (196). Even if the definition of ''congenital'' is extended to include

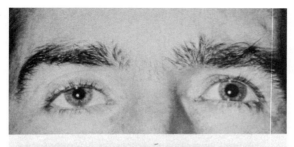

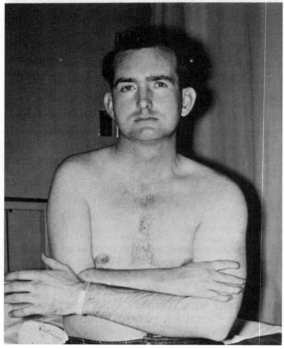

Figure 16.14. Horner syndrome (*top*) associated with injury of the right brachial plexus at birth. Note the underdeveloped right arm and forearm (*bottom*).

cases of Horner syndrome detected within the first year of life, the incidence of neuroblastoma is low, less than 10% (200,205). Other etiologies include congenital tumors, postviral complication, iatrogenic Horner syndrome, and abnormalities of the internal carotid artery such as fibromuscular dysplasia and congenital agenesis (206–209).

Many cases of congenital Horner syndrome are idiopathic, even after initial work-up and long-term follow-up. George et al. reported that no etiology was found in 16 of 23 (70%) infants who were found to have a Horner syndrome in the first year of life. In young infants with an isolated Horner syndrome and no history of birth trauma, a congenital basis may be suspected. Careful general examination and a urine test for catecholamines, with regular follow-up thereafter, constitutes the minimum evaluation (205). For infants in whom the onset of Horner syndrome is firmly established after the first 4 weeks of life (i.e., an acquired process), immediate and thorough imaging is recommended.

Pharmacologic Stimulation of the Iris Sphincter

Almost all cases of acute pharmacologically induced anisocoria are caused by parasympathetic blockade of the iris sphincter muscle, resulting in a fixed and dilated pupil. In such cases, the anisocoria is greater in light than darkness. However, in rare instances, a pharmacologic agent produces anisocoria by stimulating the parasympathetic system, thus producing a fixed miotic pupil in which the anisocoria is greater in darkness. In such cases, a 1% solution of tropicamide typically fails to dilate the pharmacologically constricted pupil. Anisocoria caused by parasympathetic stimulation can occur after handling of a pet's flea collar (210,211) that contains an anticholinesterase pesticide or a garden insecticide that contains parathion, a synthetic organophosphate ester.

Pharmacologic Inhibition of the Iris Dilator

Brimonidine tartrate is an alpha-2-adrenergic agonist that presumably decreases iris dilator action by its effect at the presynaptic alpha-2 inhibitory receptors of postganglionic sympathetic neurons. The resultant pupillary miosis is more apparent in darkness than in light (212).

Anisocoria Greater in Light

Damage to the Preganglionic Parasympathetic Outflow to the Iris Sphincter

The efferent pupillomotor pathway for pupillary constriction to light and near stimulation begins in the mesencephalon with the visceral oculomotor (Edinger-Westphal) nuclei and continues via the oculomotor nerve to the ciliary ganglion. The postganglionic impulses are carried through the short ciliary nerves to reach the iris sphincter (see Chapter 14). Because accommodative impulses begin in the same midbrain nuclei as pupilloconstrictor impulses and follow the same peripheral course to the eye, accommodative paralysis frequently accompanies pupillary paralysis in lesions of the efferent parasympathetic pathway to the iris sphincter. This combination of iridoplegia and cycloplegia was called internal ophthalmoplegia by Hutchinson to distinguish it from the external ophthalmoplegia that occurs when the extraocular muscles are paralyzed in the setting of normal pupillary responses.

Lesions anywhere along the two-neuron parasympathetic pathway to the intraocular muscles cause mydriasis at rest and impaired reflex constriction that ranges from mildly sluggish light reactions to complete pupillary unreactivity. Damage to the preganglionic portion of this pathway to the iris sphincter is caused by lesions involving the parasympathetic midbrain nuclei and the oculomotor nerve.

The Edinger-Westphal Nuclei

When there is isolated damage to the Edinger-Westphal nuclei, bilateral pupillary abnormalities are the rule. Most lesions in this region that produce pupillary abnormalities also affect other parts of the oculomotor nucleus, causing ptosis, ophthalmoparesis, or both.

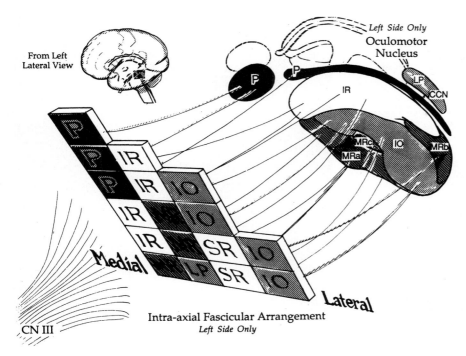

Figure 16.15. Position of the pupillomotor fibers in the fascicle of the human oculomotor nerve. The fibers destined to innervate the iris sphincter muscle (P) are located rostral and medial to the fibers that innervate the extraocular muscles and the levator palpebrae superioris (LP). IO, inferior oblique; IR, inferior rectus; MR, medial rectus; SR, superior rectus; MRa, MRb, and MRc, subnuclei serving medial rectus function in the oculomotor nuclear complex; CCN, central caudal nucleus. (From Ksiazek SM, Slamovits TL, Rosen CE, et al. Fascicular arrangement in partial oculomotor paresis. Am J Ophthalmol 1994;118:97–103.)

Pupillomotor Fascicle of the Oculomotor Nerve

Because the fibers emerging from the Edinger-Westphal nucleus are among the most rostral of the oculomotor fascicles in the midbrain tegmentum, it is possible for a lesion to selectively damage the parasympathetic fibers (213) (Fig. 16.15). Indeed, a unilateral fixed and dilated pupil or bilateral internal ophthalmoplegia may be the sole clinical manifestation of a fascicular oculomotor nerve palsy due to a rostral midbrain lesion (214,215). The fascicular oculomotor nerve can be damaged by a variety of processes, including ischemia, hemorrhage, inflammation, and infiltration. Such processes often involve other structures in the rostral mesencephalon, leading to an oculomotor palsy associated with other neurologic signs such as contralateral hemiparesis or tremor. These well-recognized syndromes are considered in Chapter 20.

Pupillomotor Fibers in the Subarachnoid Portion of the Oculomotor Nerve

As the separate fascicles of the oculomotor nerve exit the mesencephalon, they merge to form one oculomotor nerve trunk in the interpeduncular fossa. The oculomotor nerve passes between the posterior cerebral and superior cerebellar arteries and courses anteriorly to the cavernous sinus. In this part of the oculomotor nerve pathway, the pupillary fibers are superficially located and migrate from a superior medial position to the inferior part of the nerve (216). The location of the pupil fibers makes them particularly susceptible to infectious injury from basal meningitis and direct compression from aneurysms, tumors, and uncal herniation. Basal meningitis (bacterial, fungal, tuberculosis) can produce uni-lateral or bilateral poorly reactive pupils with complete or relative sparing of the extraocular muscles (217,218). In addition, hemosiderin deposits along the superficial surfaces of the cranial nerves from recurrent blood in the cerebrospinal fluid (CSF) can cause pupillary dysfunction and hearing loss in patients with superficial siderosis (219).

An expanding aneurysm is always a feared potential cause of a large and poorly reactive pupil. However, aneurysms at the junction of the internal carotid artery and the posterior communicating artery that compress the oculomotor nerve nearly always produce some extraocular muscle or eyelid dysfunction, even if such involvement is subtly or variably present, in addition to the pupil impairment. In the oft-quoted case of Payne and Adamkiewicz, a 35-year-old woman developed an acute unilateral internal ophthalmoplegia as the "principal feature" of a posterior communicating artery aneurysm (220). It was, however, not the sole manifestation of her aneurysm: she had noticed slight drooping of her eyelid 6 months previously. At the time her pupil became dilated, a "slight" and inconstant ptosis was noted. A preexisting strabismus made difficult the possible detection of any subtle extraocular muscle dysfunction. It appears that a dilated and poorly reactive pupil in isolation is rarely due to an aneurysm, and in the case where it is, it is more likely due to an aneurysm of the tip of the basilar artery than an aneurysm of the internal carotid artery (221,222).

Occasionally, intrinsic lesions of the oculomotor nerve in the subarachnoid space produce only an internal ophthalmoplegia. In two cases of an oculomotor nerve schwannoma in the interpeduncular fossa, an isolated dilated pupil and reduced accommodation were the sole manifestations of the tumor for 1 year or longer, before ptosis and external ophthalmoplegia appeared (223,224).

Cavernous Portion of the Oculomotor Nerve

The pupillomotor fibers are located inferiorly and superficially in the portion of the oculomotor nerve located within the cavernous sinus. Any lesion of the cavernous sinus can potentially compress and damage the oculomotor nerve and the pupil fibers. When oculosympathetic fibers in the cavernous sinus are damaged as well, the pupil light reflex may be sluggish, but there may not be an apparent change in the resting pupil size (i.e., there may be no anisocoria) (184).

Damage to the Ciliary Ganglion and Short Ciliary Nerves: The Tonic Pupil

Any injury to the ciliary ganglion or the short ciliary nerves in the retrobulbar space or in the intraocular, suprachoroidal space will cause internal ophthalmoplegia. Within a few days, cholinergic supersensitivity may develop. These findings are due to denervation of the iris sphincter and ciliary muscle. In some cases, denervation is the only pathologic process; when permanent, it results in unilateral paralysis of accommodation and a dilated pupil that reacts poorly to light and near stimulation but constricts well to weak topical pilocarpine. In others, denervation is followed by subsequent reinnervation (both appropriate and aberrant) of the iris muscles that results in recovery of accommodation, a pupillary response to near stimuli that is unusually strong and tonic, and redilation after constriction to near stimuli that is delayed and slow. These are the characteristic features of a tonic pupil (Fig. 16.16). Tonic pupils are generally divided into three categories: local, neuropathic, and Adie syndrome (225,226).

LOCAL TONIC PUPILS

This type of tonic pupil, typically unilateral, is due to orbital or systemic lesions that affect the ciliary ganglion or short ciliary nerves in isolation. Disorders that have been reported to cause this type of ''local'' tonic pupil include herpes zoster, chickenpox, measles, diphtheria, syphilis (both congenital and acquired), Lyme disease, sarcoidosis, scarlet fever, pertussis, smallpox, influenza, sinusitis, Vogt-Koyanagi-Harada syndrome, rheumatoid arthritis, polyarteritis nodosa, giant cell arteritis, migraine, lymphomatoid granulomatosis, viral hepatitis, choroiditis, primary and metastatic choroidal and orbital tumors, blunt injury to the globe, intraocular siderosis from foreign body, and penetrating orbital injury (227–237). In some of these cases, the tonic pupil may have occurred as happenstance. In others, ancillary testing such as MR imaging or orbital color Doppler imaging have demonstrated clear abnormalities at the ciliary ganglion, suggesting local injury related to the primary systemic disease process (238,239).

Various ocular or orbital surgical procedures, including retinal reattachment surgery, inferior oblique muscle surgery, orbital surgery, optic nerve sheath fenestration, retinal photocoagulation, argon laser trabeculoplasty, transconjunctival cryotherapy, transscleral diathermy, retrobulbar injections of alcohol, and even inferior dental blocks, can cause denervation injury (iridoplegia and cycloplegia) and a ''local'' tonic pupil (240–247).

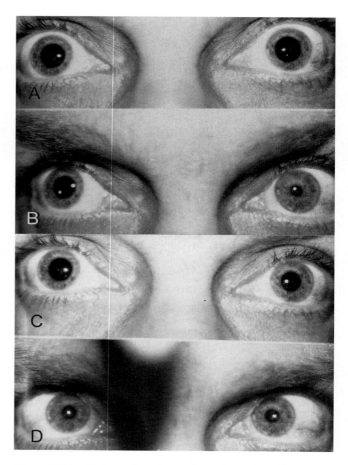

Figure 16.16. Tonic pupil syndrome. About 4 months earlier, this 38-year-old man noted that his right pupil was larger than his left pupil. *A*, In the dark looking in the distance, both pupils are dilated and relatively equal in size. *B*, In bright light, the right pupil does not constrict, whereas the left pupil constricts normally, producing a marked anisocoria. *C*, In room light looking in the distance, there is a moderate anisocoria. *D*, During near viewing, however, both pupils constrict. The right pupil constricted much more slowly than the left and redilated slowly.

NEUROPATHIC TONIC PUPILS

This type of tonic pupil, usually with bilateral involvement, represents one manifestation of a widespread, peripheral, and autonomic neuropathy that also involves the ciliary ganglion, the short ciliary nerves, or both (248). In some cases, there is evidence of both a sympathetic and a parasympathetic disturbance. These include syphilis, chronic alcoholism, diabetes mellitus, amyloidosis, systemic lupus erythematosus, Sjögren syndrome, some of the spinocerebellar degenerations, hereditary motor-sensory neuropathy (Charcot-Marie-Tooth disease), Landry-Guillain-Barré syndrome, and the Miller Fisher syndrome (249–254). Dysautonomias associated with tonic pupils are subacute autonomic neuropathy, Shy-Drager syndrome, and Ross syndrome. Tonic pupils can occur from the distant effects of cancer, occurring either as an isolated phenomenon or as part of a more extensive paraneoplastic autonomic polyneuropathy (255,256).

They also may develop in patients with trichloroethylene intoxication (257).

ADIE (HOLMES-ADIE) TONIC PUPIL SYNDROME

Adie syndrome is an uncommon, idiopathic condition that may develop in otherwise healthy persons and in patients with unrelated conditions. It nearly always occurs as a sporadic entity, although it has been described in three sisters and in twins (258,259). Such reports are simply too rare to suggest any hereditary origin. Adie syndrome is rare before age 15 years (260,261). In a child, secondary causes of a tonic pupil should be ruled out first, and then attention should be directed to management of the anisometropia to avoid amblyopia (262).

Most patients with Adie syndrome are 20–50 years of age. Although the syndrome occurs in both sexes, there is a clear predilection for women (about 70% of cases). Adie syndrome is unilateral in about 80% of cases. When the condition is bilateral, the onset occasionally is simultaneous but usually occurs in separate episodes months or even years apart (263).

Historical Background. William Adie's name most often is associated with the syndrome of tonic pupil and benign areflexia, but he was not the first to describe the syndrome or its features. The earliest description of a tonically reacting pupil was by Piltz, who mentioned the occurrence of a bilateral, tonic light reflex in patients with general paresis (264). Gordon Holmes published a series of 19 cases and reviewed the previous literature on the subject just before the publications of his student William Adie (265). In the United Kingdom, therefore, this condition is called the Holmes-Adie syndrome.

Clinical Characteristics. *Symptoms.* Around 80% of patients with Adie syndrome have visual complaints, usually related to the iridoplegia. These include photophobia and difficulty with dark adaptation (266). Symptoms related to ciliary muscle dysfunction are blurred near vision and brow ache or headache with near work. Over time, the dilated pupil becomes smaller and accommodation improves; however, some patients continue to have difficulty focusing. Such patients can see clearly at rest for both distance and near; however, they experience visual blur when shifting fixation from near to distance (tonicity of accommodation). This is particularly troublesome if the unaffected eye has poor vision from other causes.

If, some years later, the other eye also develops a tonic pupil, the condition seems to produce far fewer symptoms and may even pass unnoticed. This is in part because both eyes are now affected and because the patient has become presbyopic in the interim; therefore, less accommodative difference is induced between the two eyes.

Although patients with Adie syndrome not uncommonly have abnormal tests of autonomic function, they are relatively asymptomatic. Symptoms may include chronic cough, abnormal sweating, or postural dizziness (267,268).

Sectoral Palsy of the Iris Sphincter. As mentioned above, the pathophysiology of an Adie pupil is acute denervation followed by appropriate and inappropriate reinnervation of the ciliary body and iris sphincter. The clinical findings depend in part on the stage of evolution in which the pupil is examined. Acutely following a denervation injury, there is an internal ophthalmoplegia. The pupil is markedly dilated and appears unresponsive to light or near stimulation. At this stage, it often is confused with a pharmacologically induced mydriasis and cycloplegia. However, a careful slit-lamp examination using a bright light usually reveals segmental contractions of the iris sphincter (Fig. 16.16). These segmental contractions to bright light represent remaining areas of normally innervated iris sphincter. Under the slit lamp, the iris segments that contract are seen to tighten and bunch up like a purse-string bag being closed. Conversely, in denervated segments, the iris stroma appears thin and flat. The adjacent pupillary ruff is meager, and the radius of curvature of the pupil margin is flatter. These denervated segments do not contract to a bright light, but the radial markings of the stroma in these denervated segments show a "streaming" movement that is caused by mechanical pull from normally contracting segments. These findings are characteristic of sectoral palsy of the iris sphincter (Fig. 16.17). Sectoral palsy of the iris sphincter is a critical diagnostic observation, present in about 90% of Adie pupils. In these cases, the amount of sphincter palsy (estimated in clock-hour segments around the pupil margin) is 70% or more, so detection requires attentive observation of each clock-hour segment (269). Sectoral palsy is not seen with pharmacologic anticholinergic blockade, which paralyzes 100% of the sphincter. About 10% of Adie pupils also have no segmental contraction to bright light (100% sphincter palsy), at least not acutely.

The "vermiform movements" of the iris in Adie syndrome probably represent spontaneous pupillary unrest, or hippus, in normally innervated segments of the sphincter and are essentially the same as segmental contractions of the iris. In a rare patient with Adie tonic pupil in one eye, the ciliary muscle in the other eye suddenly shows evidence of dysfunction, even though the pupillary light and near reactions appear normal (272). This probably is a limited form of Adie syndrome.

Accommodative Paresis. In most patients with Adie syndrome, the acute accommodative paresis is moderate to severe because of ciliary muscle denervation and paralysis. Accommodation gradually improves over several months as injured axons begin to regenerate and reinnervate the ciliary muscle. Most of the recovery occurs in the first 2 years after the acute injury.

Aberrant Reinnervation of the Iris Sphincter. In the acute stage, both the pupil light reflex and pupillary constriction to near effort are equally and severely impaired. After several weeks or months, the near response of the pupil begins to increase in amplitude while the light response remains severely impaired (light–near dissociation). However, the pupil movement now is distinctly different than normal. The pupil constriction to a near effort is strong, slow, and sustained (tonic near response). In addition, the redilation movement after cessation of near effort is equally slow and sustained, delaying visual refocus by several seconds (tonicity of accommodation). These findings are caused by aber-

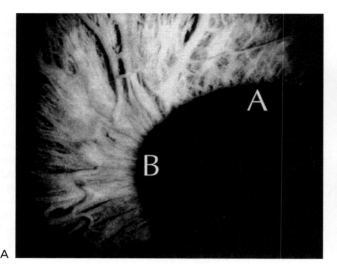

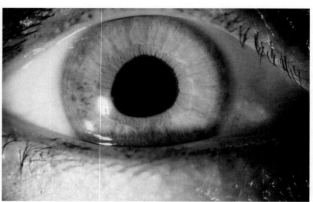

A   B

Figure 16.17.   Segmental palsy of the iris sphincter in Adie tonic pupil syndrome. *A,* One part of the iris sphincter is denervated and does not react to light. Another segment (*B*) of the iris sphincter constricts to light in this irregularly shaped Adie tonic pupil. *B,* In another case, the area of iris sphincter between 12 and 4 o'clock demonstrates intact pupillary ruff and puckering of the iris stroma consistent with active contraction in this segment, but most of the remainder of the iris sphincter is denervated. The pupillary ruff is mostly absent, the iris stroma is less dense, and the radius of pupil curvature is flatter in this area, particularly between 5 and 7 o'clock and between 8 and 12 o'clock (sectoral palsy). (Courtesy of Dr. F-X Borruat.)

rant reinnervation of the iris sphincter by regenerating accommodative fibers.

Warwick and others showed that the pupillomotor fibers to the iris sphincter constitute about 3% of the total number of postganglionic neurons that leave the ciliary ganglion, whereas the remaining 97% of neurons innervate the ciliary muscle (271). Thus, when the ciliary ganglion is injured, there is a numerically greater chance of survival of cells serving accommodation compared with those serving pupil constriction. In 1967, Loewenfeld and Thompson suggested that the fibers of these surviving cells, originally destined for the ciliary muscle, resprouted randomly, with some of the fibers reaching and reinnervating their appropriate target, the ciliary muscle (272). This explained the recovery of accommodation over time. Other resprouting fibers, however, mistakenly reinnervated the iris sphincter. Thus, pupil constriction also recovered, but only as a misdirection synkinesis. When the patient made a near effort, the accommodative impulses stimulated both ciliary muscle and iris sphincter activity (Fig. 16.18). The long latency and slow, prolonged contraction of the iris sphincter were thought to be related to its inappropriate reinnervation and its cholinergic supersensitivity (272,273).

The light reflex of a tonic pupil remains impaired. Furthermore, in about one third of patients, more segments of sphincter become increasingly impaired over time, suggesting that the degenerative changes in the ciliary ganglion are progressive. Besides being less numerous in quantity, perhaps pupillary fibers have an inherently greater susceptibility to the primary insult that causes these degenerative changes. In any event, it is clear that the pupillary light–near dissociation of a tonic pupil results from impairment of the light reflex with restoration of the near reflex and not from sparing

of near reflex fibers, as occurs in some dorsal midbrain lesions.

Decreased Corneal Sensation.   Purcell et al. used the Cochet-Bonnet aesthesiometer to demonstrate a regional decrease in corneal sensation in 10 of 11 patients with unilateral Adie syndrome (acute and chronic), consistent with the theory that the lesion in Adie syndrome is located in the ciliary ganglion or short ciliary nerves (275). Interestingly, the areas with reduced sensation did not correlate to the extent or distribution of the iris sphincter denervation.

Absent Muscle Stretch Reflexes.   Deep-tendon hyporeflexia or areflexia can be demonstrated in almost 90% of patients with Adie syndrome. As is the case with the pupil light reflex, there can be progressive loss of reflex activity over time. The reflexes of the upper extremities are abnormal almost as often as the reflexes of the lower extremities (226).

Electrophysiologic studies suggest that the cause of areflexia is loss of large-diameter afferent fibers or impairment in their synaptic connections to motor neurons (275–277). Histopathologic studies in patients with Adie syndrome have demonstrated moderate degeneration of both axons and myelin sheaths in the fasciculus gracilis and fasciculus cuneatus (278,279). The dorsal and ventral roots appeared normal, as did the remaining spinal cord. There appears to be a degeneration of cell bodies in the dorsal root ganglia similar to that which occurs in the ciliary ganglion (280).

Cholinergic Denervation Supersensitivity.   In 1940, Adler and Scheie reported that the tonic pupil of patients with Adie syndrome constricted intensely to 2.5% methacholine chloride (due to cholinergic supersensitivity), whereas normal pupils did not (281) (Fig. 16.19). Later studies demonstrated large interindividual variability of pupil responses such that it was subsequently dropped as a test for tonic

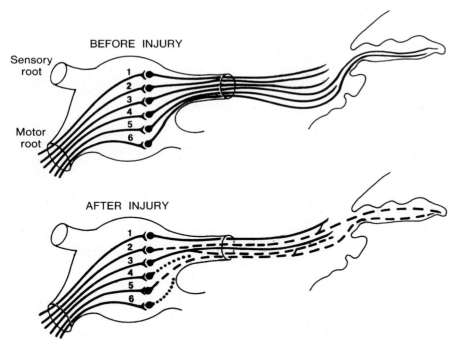

Figure 16.18. Misregeneration theory as it pertains to the findings in the tonic pupil syndrome. *Top,* Before injury, most of the fibers in the ciliary ganglion are destined for the ciliary muscle to produce accommodation. *Bottom,* Following injury, it is more likely that a regenerating postganglionic fiber will be one for accommodation; however, many of these fibers send branches or collaterals to the iris, producing pupillary constriction during attempted accommodation-convergence. In this drawing, postganglionic fiber 1, for accommodation, has not been injured; fibers 2 and 5, also accommodative, have regenerated, sending sprouts to both the ciliary muscle and the iris sphincter; fiber 3, for pupillary constriction, has sent a sprout to the ciliary muscle via the remaining nerve sheath of fiber 4, which has been damaged; fiber 6, for pupillary constriction, has been destroyed and has not regenerated. Thus, accommodation and pupillary constriction will occur primarily on attempted accommodation-convergence.

pupils (282). Instead, dilute pilocarpine (0.1% or less) has become the most popular pharmacologic agent for demonstrating cholinergic denervation supersensitivity of the iris sphincter (283,284). A 0.1% pilocarpine solution can be prepared in a syringe from 1 part commercially available 1% pilocarpine and 9 parts normal saline, although bacteriostatic water also can be used and may have less constricting effect on a normal iris sphincter (285). The criterion for diagnosing cholinergic supersensitivity has been proposed as either (*a*) the affected pupil constricts 0.5 mm more than the unaffected pupil under dim ambient lighting or (*b*) the suspected pupil that is larger than the normal pupil before instillation of

pilocarpine becomes the smaller pupil after instillation of pilocarpine (286). Cholinergic supersensitivity develops quickly, usually within days after injury. About 80% of tonic pupils demonstrate cholinergic supersensitivity; the test result is influenced by intersubject variability, differential corneal penetration, mechanical influence of the iris stroma (how small the pupil is at baseline), and the state of reinnervation.

As preganglionic injury can also produce end-organ supersensitivity, oculomotor nerve palsy can also cause a "positive" pilocarpine test. Furthermore, the degree of cholinergic supersensitivity is about the same in patients with

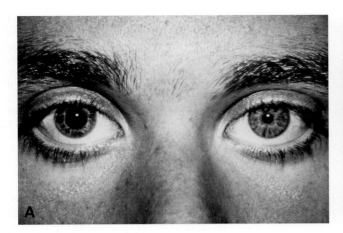
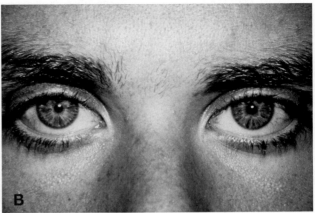

Figure 16.19. *A,* A right tonic pupil in a 36-year-old woman. *B,* 45 minutes after conjunctival instillation of two drops of 0.1% pilocarpine solution in each eye, the right pupil is constricted and nonreactive. The left pupil remains unchanged and normally reactive.

oculomotor nerve palsies and patients with Adie pupils (287).

Ciliary muscle supersensitivity also can be established by measuring the near point of accommodation before and after instillation of dilute pilocarpine, but only if the patient is under age 45 years and has normal accommodation in the normal eye.

Long-Term Features and Prognosis. Several features of Adie syndrome change over time. Accommodation recovers significantly over a year or two. The size of the tonic pupil decreases by 2–3 mm or more over several years (Fig. 16.20). In some patients, it can become the smaller pupil, even in room light, and bilateral cases of chronic Adie pupils can be mistaken for Argyll Robertson pupils (288). The explanation for the progressive miosis in Adie syndrome was proposed by Kardon et al., who used infrared transillumination to evaluate the distribution of segmental iris sphincter reactivity under various stimulus conditions (289). In darkness, reinnervated segments of the sphincter appeared "denser" under transillumination compared with normal pupils and became even denser with near effort (i.e., during active contraction). This finding suggested that in darkness, a tonic pupil has a constant volley of low-level impulses from accommodative neurons that keeps reinnervated segments of iris sphincter in a greater state of contraction compared with a normally innervated sphincter that receives no parasympathetic impulses in darkness. In addition, the number and extent of reinnervated segments appear to increase with time. Both of these phenomena probably contribute to the decreasing size of a tonic pupil (Fig. 16.21). Additionally, the active reinnervation process apparently prevents development of iris atrophy, a feature not typically found in chronic Adie syndrome.

Kardon et al. also demonstrated that the degree of cholin-

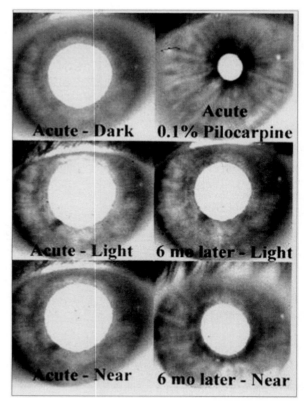

Figure 16.21. Six infrared transillumination views of the same iris in a patient with an acute Adie pupil affecting all but one of the segments. The middle and lower photographs on the right are from the same eye 6 months later. The photographs of the left side show that there is only one small segment (the dense area at the pupil border at the 7 o'clock position) that still contracts appropriately to light and near. This example was chosen because all the rest of the iris sphincter has been denervated so that the changes in density of the remaining, normally reacting segment can be discerned in darkness, in light and at near. In the "acute-dark" photograph (*top left*), the area of the 7 o'clock position cannot be seen but becomes dense in response to light stimulation (*middle left*, "acute-light") and in response to near stimulation (*bottom left*, "acute-near"). The change in the sphincter also is shown in response to low-concentration pilocarpine (*top right*). All of the denervated segments show an increase in density after 0.1% pilocarpine, except for the one segment that normally is innervated and, therefore, presumably not supersensitive, which appears translucent at the 7:30 position (*top right*, "acute 0.1% pilocarpine"). This same patient was examined 6 months later (*right side, middle and bottom photographs*), and the results show a light–near dissociation with an increase in density on near response. The pupil is slightly smaller in light than in the acute state because of some sustained firing of accommodative fibers that have started to reinnervate the sphincter areas. (From Kardon RH, Corbett JJ, Thompson HS. Segmental denervation and reinnervation of the iris sphincter as shown by infrared videographic transillumination. Ophthalmology 1998;105:313–321.)

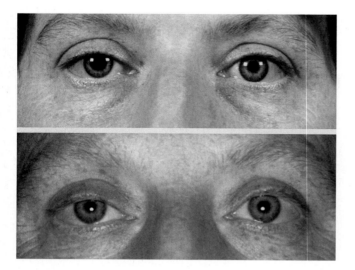

Figure 16.20. Changes in size of an Adie tonic pupil over time. *Top,* Appearance of an acute right-sided Adie pupil in a 33-year-old woman. *Bottom,* Appearance of the same patient 10 years later. The right pupil has become smaller in resting size so that in ambient lighting, there is no apparent anisocoria. (Courtesy of Dr. F-X Borruat.)

ergic sensitivity decreases as reinnervation increases (289). Denervated segments that are unreactive to light and near stimulation show an intense increase in density following dilute pilocarpine. However, as these segments are reinnervated and become reactive to near effort, they become less reactive to the pilocarpine.

The light reaction of the Adie pupil generally does not recover. Like the muscle-stretch reflexes, it deteriorates further with passing years in most patients.

Patients with unilateral Adie syndrome tend to develop a tonic pupil in the opposite eye with time. This occurs in about 4% of cases per year (263). Overall, this is a benign condition; however, in some patients with shallow anterior chamber angles, an acute tonic pupil can precipitate an attack of angle-closure glaucoma (50,290).

TREATMENT

Weak solutions of eserine or pilocarpine can be used to constrict a tonic pupil for relief of photophobia and for cosmetic purposes (reduction of anisocoria, especially in patients with light-colored irides) (291,292). Most patients do not need this treatment for very long because within a year or two, the tonic pupil becomes smaller in size and in dim light, and it soon is the smaller of the two pupils (293). For symptoms related to abnormal accommodation, a bifocal add usually suffices, even if it is not yet needed by the unaffected eye.

Damage to the Iris Sphincter

Tears in the iris sphincter or the iris base may occur from blunt trauma to the eye. Such damage may produce a nonreactive or poorly reactive irregularly dilated pupil that may be mistaken for the dilated pupil of an oculomotor nerve palsy, particularly if the patient is lethargic or comatose from the injury. In most cases, careful examination of the dilated pupil with a hand light reveals subtle irregularities in its normally smooth contour, and the iris tears or dialysis are easily observed using a standard or portable slit lamp (Fig. 16.2).

Pharmacologic Blockade with Parasympatholytic Agents

A fixed dilated pupil can be caused by topical administration of one of several parasympatholytic agents, many of which are described in the section on drug effects. It suffices here to emphasize that such agents block the action of acetylcholine on the iris sphincter and ciliary muscles, that they produce both mydriasis and cycloplegia, and that the mydriasis produced by such drugs is extreme, usually more than 8 mm. It is necessary to differentiate a pupil that is pharmacologically dilated from one that is neurologically dilated. Thompson et al. suggested using a 0.5–1% solution of pilocarpine for this task (294). A pupil that is dilated from pharmacologic blockade of the sphincter will be unchanged or poorly constricted by a topical solution of pilocarpine strong enough to constrict the opposite pupil (Fig. 16.22), whereas a tonic pupil that constricts to weak solutions of pilocarpine because of denervation supersensitivity should certainly constrict to 0.5–1% pilocarpine. A pupil that is dilated from oculomotor nerve dysfunction also will constrict well after instillation of pilocarpine.

Pharmacologic Stimulation of the Iris Dilator

Topical cocaine placed in the nose for medical or other reasons can back up the lacrimal duct into the conjunctival sac. Most eye-whitening drops that contain sympathomimetic components are too weak to dilate the pupil, but if the cornea is abraded (e.g., by a contact lens) enough of the oxymetazoline or the phenylephrine in the solution may get into the aqueous humor to dilate the pupil. In addition, mists containing adrenergic or anticholinergic drugs for bronchodilation may escape around the edge of the facemask and condense in the conjunctival sac, inadvertently causing unilateral pupillary dilation.

Anisocoria Due to Sympathetic Hyperactivity

Sympathetic hyperactivity occurs in a number of settings, usually as an episodic phenomenon. In several of these settings, the pupils are affected, and in cases of unilateral or asymmetric oculosympathetic hyperactivity, there may be an anisocoria.

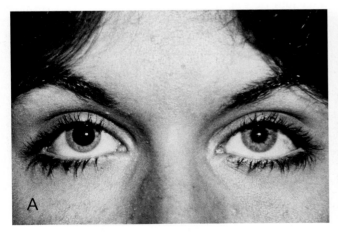
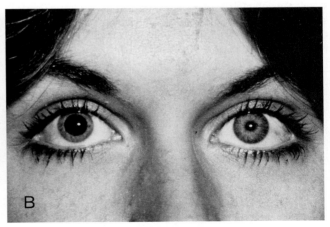

Figure 16.22. Pharmacologically dilated pupil. *A*, Fixed, dilated right pupil in an 18-year-old woman complaining of headache and blurred vision. *B*, 45 minutes after conjunctival instillation of two drops of 1% pilocarpine in each eye, the right pupil is unchanged, whereas the left pupil is markedly constricted. The patient subsequently admitted having placed topical scopolamine in the right eye.

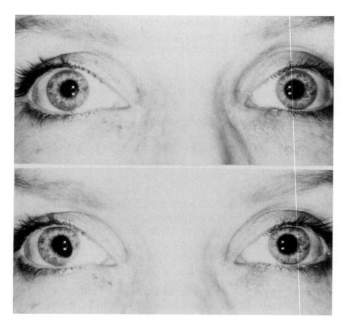

Figure 16.23. Tadpole pupil. *Top*, Before the episode, the pupils are normal in size and shape. *Bottom*, During the episode, the right pupil develops an eccentric shape, with the 5 o'clock portion of the pupil being displaced outward. (From Thompson HS, Zackon DH, Czarnecki JSC. Tadpole-shaped pupils caused by segmental spasm of the iris dilator muscle. Am J Ophthalmol 1983;96:467–477.)

Tadpole-Shaped Pupils

An occasional patient reports that the pupil of one eye becomes distorted for a minute or two. In most cases, the eye feels "funny" and the vision in the eye becomes slightly blurred. Looking in the mirror reveals that the pupil is pulled in one direction like the tail of a tadpole, hence the term "tadpole pupil" (Fig. 16.23). Often patients describe the direction of the tadpole tail to be different on different occasions. This phenomenon usually occurs many times a day for several weeks, spontaneously remits, and then recurs several months later. Eventually, the condition abates and does not recur (295).

The etiology of tadpole pupils is unclear. Presence of an intact pupil light reflex suggests dilator spasms rather than sphincter paresis. In a review of 26 cases, Thompson et al. noted that 11 patients (42%) also had a partial postganglionic Horner syndrome on the affected side (295). The authors postulated that repeated bursts of sympathetic impulses asymmetrically pulled one segment of the iris toward the limbus and that this repeated irritation eventually could have caused loss of fibers and the Horner syndrome. Thus, testing for Horner syndrome is recommended for patients who give a history of episodic tadpole-shaped pupils (296), even if there is no anisocoria at the time of the examination.

Another mechanism may be responsible for tadpole pupils in the setting of a congenital Horner syndrome. Tang reported the case of a young man with a hypoplastic right internal carotid artery and ipsilateral congenital Horner syndrome who experienced exercise-induced pupillary distortion of the right pupil (297). The same segment of the iris always dilated after strenuous exercise, and it was the same area that failed to dilate with hydroxyamphetamine. In this case, the tadpole pupil presumably resulted from local supersensitivity of a denervated segment of the iris dilator muscle, occurring at moments when the level of circulating catecholamines was increased.

Aberrant regeneration causing segmental spasm of the iris dilator

An iris dilator–deglutition synkinesis resulting in episodic segmental dilator contraction was described in a young boy with Horner syndrome and paresis of the glossopharyngeal, vagus, and hypoglossal nerves (Villaret-like syndrome) following resection of a neuroblastoma in his right upper neck during infancy (298). Later, he had focal dilator spasms of his right pupil that resulted in an elliptical pupil (Fig. 16.24) and were associated with swallowing. Presumably, this dilator–deglutition synkinesis was caused by aberrant vagal nerve sprouts that made an inappropriate synaptic connection at the superior cervical ganglion.

Pourfour du Petit Syndrome

This syndrome is the clinical opposite of Horner syndrome. It represents oculosympathetic overactivity instead of underactivity and usually is caused by lesions along the

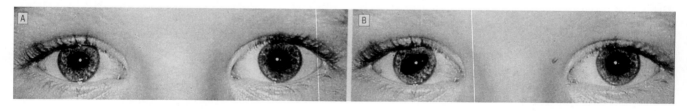

Figure 16.24. Iris dilator–deglutition synkinesis causing segmental iris dilator muscle contraction in 10-year-old boy with a long-standing right Horner syndrome. *A*, The child has a right Horner syndrome that had been present since removal of a cervical neuroblastoma when he was 6 days old. At age 2 years, his parents first noted that while he was drinking, his right pupil would become transiently distorted in shape. *B*, Appearance of the pupils during the act of swallowing. There is segmental dilation of the right pupil at the 1 o'clock and 7 o'clock positions, causing a distorted pupil. The dilation occurs only when the child is swallowing. (From Boehme BI, Graef MH. Acquired segmental iris dilator muscle synkinesis due to deglutition. Arch Ophthalmol 1998;116:248–249.)

cervical sympathetic chain. The clinical signs are unilateral mydriasis, lid retraction, apparent exophthalmos, and conjunctival blanching, all of which may be episodic or constant. The phenomenon is rare and has been described after trauma, brachial plexus anesthetic block or other injury, and parotidectomy and in patients with tumors of the pleural lining or mediastinum (299,300). The oculosympathetic hyperactivity sometimes precedes the development of a Horner syndrome. Presumably, the lesion first irritates the sympathetic fibers and later damages them.

Sympathetic Hyperactivity and Spinal Cord Lesions

Autonomic hyperreflexia is a phenomenon seen in quadriplegic patients who have experienced severe spinal cord injury. It usually appears weeks to months after the acute injury and results from absent cerebral control of the spinal sympathetic neurons that leads to paroxysms of sympathetic hyperactivity that either occur spontaneously or are triggered by nonspecific stimuli below the level of cord injury (301). Occasionally, the oculosympathetic pathway is affected unilaterally or a patient undergoes a local anesthetic procedure that blocks sympathetic activity on one side, making evident the eye findings of autonomic hyperreflexia as episodes of unilateral mydriasis, blurry vision, and lid retraction on the unanesthetized side (302,303). In other patients, passive arm or leg stretching or limb movement can induce a transient asymmetric mydriasis. This may represent a localized form of autonomic hyperreflexia (oculosympathetic spasm) that occurs in response to proprioceptive impulses that ascend to reach the damaged area of the spinal cord (160).

Oculosympathetic hyperactivity has been reported after a relatively minor cord injury. Saito and Nakazawa described a young man who sustained a whiplash injury in a car accident and shortly thereafter developed episodes of unilateral mydriasis (304). The episodes lasted several hours to a few days and occurred once or twice a week. The patient had no other neurologic deficits. Radiographic studies revealed slight narrowing of the disc space at the C5–C6 level. Pharmacologic testing suggested that the mydriasis was caused by episodic sympathetic irritation.

An "alternating Horner syndrome" has been reported in patients with lower cervical and upper thoracic cord lesions and in some patients with primary dysautonomia, such as the Shy-Drager syndrome (see below). Some authors believe that it results from a transient oculosympathetic deficit that changes sides at intervals of 2 hours or 2 weeks (157,158,305); however, Moniz and Czarnecki studied pharmacologically two patients with this phenomenon and concluded that the clinical findings also could be explained by a unilateral lesion that causes alternating oculosympathetic hypofunction and hyperfunction (161).

Other Anisocorias

Anisocoria in Lateral Gaze: The Tournay Phenomenon

In 1907, Gianelli noted that when some normal persons look in extreme lateral gaze, the pupil on that side becomes larger and the pupil on the opposite side becomes smaller (306). Gianelli hypothesized that this phenomenon resulted from mechanical traction caused by movement of the globe that stimulated the long ciliary nerves in abduction and the short ciliary nerves in adduction. Tournay independently made similar observations, emphasizing the dilation of the pupil ipsilateral to the direction of gaze, and later recognized Gianelli as the first to observe this phenomenon (307,308). Nonetheless, an anisocoria that develops on extreme lateral gaze is called the Tournay's phenomenon. Sharpe and Glaser studied 25 normal subjects and 5 patients with Duane retraction syndrome by direct observation, photography, and infrared electronic pupillography (309) and could not demonstrate anisocoria in lateral gaze in any of the subjects (309). Loewenfeld et al. examined 150 normal subjects using infrared flash photography and concluded that the Tournay phenomenon does exist but that its prevalence is low and its extent small (e.g., less than 10% of subjects showed a change in anisocoria greater than 0.3 mm) (310). Loewenfeld postulated that the Tournay phenomenon results from "straying" of impulses that were meant for the medial rectus subnucleus to the nearby Edinger-Westphal nucleus (119). This would cause slight constriction of the pupil when the eye adducts and relative dilation of the pupil when the medial rectus subnucleus is inhibited during abduction. Whatever the explanation, it is reasonable to conclude that the Tournay phenomenon is relatively uncommon and has little or no clinical significance.

Anisocoria During Migraine Headache

The best-known association of an anisocoria and vascular headache is the cluster headache syndrome mentioned previously. This section deals with those occasional patients who report having one dilated pupil or unequal-sized pupils only during a classic or common migraine headache attack. The induced anisocoria generally is rather small but ranges from 0.3 mm to 2.5 mm (Fig. 16.25) (311–313).

The mechanism of anisocoria during migraine is not fully established. A study that found diminished velocity and amplitude of the pupil light reflex in 10 migraineurs (312) implicates parasympathetic dysfunction as one possibility. In such cases, the abnormal pupil is the larger one, and other evidence for oculoparasympathetic hypofunction should exist. The series by Woods et al. supports this hypothesis in that it showed reduced light responses in five of seven patients examined during their migraine and reduced accommodation in two others (311). One patient had a history of ophthalmoplegic migraines since childhood that evolved into an isolated unilateral mydriasis accompanying her migraine headaches as an adult. Such a limited form of ophthalmoplegic migraine must be rare (314,315). Another etiologic site of oculoparasympathetic dysfunction that has been described with migraine is the ciliary ganglion (316,317). Presumably, migrainous vasospasm can cause local and reversible ischemia of the ciliary ganglion and could also account for the findings described by Woods et al. (311).

Although parasympathetic hypofunction may be the most common cause of unilateral dilation during a migraine attack, it is not the only possible mechanism. An episodic unilateral sympathetic hyperactivity or spasm accompanying

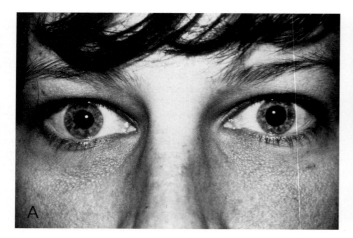
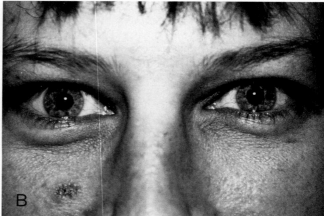

Figure 16.25. Intermittent unilateral pupillary dilation in a young woman during severe migraine headache. *A*, During the migraine attack, the left pupil is dilated and poorly reactive. Accommodation is normal, however, suggesting that the dilation is caused by sympathetic hyperactivity rather than parasympathetic hypoactivity. *B*, Between attacks, the pupils are isocoric.

the attack might cause a similar process. In such a case, the patient would experience no loss of accommodation in the affected eye. We have seen such patients and believe that this mechanism is not uncommon.

Yet another hypothesis for anisocoria during migraine is sympathetic hypofunction. In some migraineurs, pharmacologic pupillary testing has suggested that a bilateral postganglionic oculosympathetic deficit occurs during the headache attack, and in those migraineurs who develop a clinically apparent but transient anisocoria, there is asymmetry of their sympathetic dysfunction (313).

Finally, it is possible that some cases of anisocoria during migraine represent an exaggeration of an underlying benign physiologic anisocoria. At any rate, a transient and isolated anisocoria that is associated temporally with migraine headache attacks and recurs periodically in stereotypic fashion in an otherwise healthy person appears to be a fairly benign syndrome. This clinical picture has not been reported with intracranial aneurysm, midbrain tumor, seizures, or arterial dissection (316).

Sarkies reported that intermittent angle-closure glaucoma can produce a clinical picture similar to the episodic mydriasis that occurs in association with a migraine attack (47). Thus, it is important to consider that entity in patients who experience intermittent episodes of unilateral mydriasis with periocular or retrobulbar pain, especially if there is an associated redness of the eye and blurred vision.

Benign Episodic Mydriasis

Benign episodic mydriasis is the term used to describe recurrent episodes of unilateral mydriasis that are not associated with a concurrent headache or migraine (Fig. 16.26). This condition probably is a variant of the transient mydriasis that occurs during migraine headaches and that is described above. Indeed, about half the patients with benign episodic mydriasis have a history of migraines (318,319).

Benign episodic mydriasis typically occurs and recurs in

the same eye. There are no associated neurologic deficits. The duration of mydriasis averages 12 hours, but the range is wide (10 minutes to 7 days). In Jacobson's series, 11 of 24 patients were examined during an episode (319). In these patients, the anisocoria ranged from 1 to 3 mm. Associated symptoms included blur (62%), orbital pain (21%), and red eye (17%). Five patients had a normal pupil light reflex with normal vision, four patients had decreased accommodative function, and one patient demonstrated cholinergic supersensitivity.

Because a small but significant percentage of patients with benign episodic mydriasis experience simultaneous ipsilateral blurred vision, orbital pain, red eye, or a combination of these manifestations, intermittent angle-closure glaucoma must be eliminated as a possibility in patients in whom such a diagnosis is considered (47).

Differentiation Between Causes of Anisocoria

From a practical standpoint, anisocoria that is more evident in darkness than in light indicates that the parasympathetic pathway that constricts the pupils and the iris sphincter muscles are intact (i.e., both eyes have a normal pupil light reflex). The problem thus lies with asymmetric sympathetic activity and dilation in darkness. Most cases represent either simple anisocoria or a Horner syndrome. These two entities are differentiated using 10% cocaine. If the cocaine test indicates that the patient has a Horner syndrome, a hydroxyamphetamine test is performed on another occasion at least 24 hours later to differentiate a central or preganglionic Horner syndrome from a postganglionic Horner syndrome. Once the Horner syndrome is diagnosed and localized, appropriate evaluation for the etiology is required (320).

Anisocoria that is more evident in light than in darkness indicates a defect of the parasympathetic system or the iris sphincter muscle. Thus, the faulty pupil has a poor light reflex. The iris should be examined using a slit-lamp biomicroscope to determine whether there is a sphincter tear or

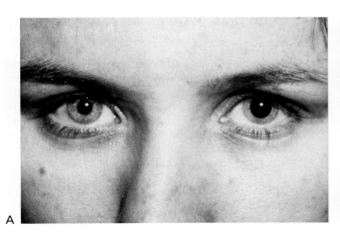
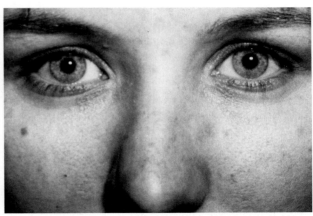

A   B

Figure 16.26. Intermittent unilateral pupillary dilation unassociated with migraine. This operating room nurse was noted to have a dilated left pupil while she was assisting at surgery. She had no headache at the time, nor did she have any visual symptoms other than a vague sense of blurred vision. *A*, During the episode, the left pupil is markedly dilated. Visual acuity at this time was 20/20 OU at both distance and near. The right pupil constricted normally to light stimulation; the left pupil constricted minimally under the same conditions. *B*, 2 hours later, the pupils are isocoric. Both pupils now reacted normally to light stimulation.

other iris damage. If there is no evidence of iris damage, clinical examination usually bears out a diagnosis of oculomotor nerve palsy or tonic pupil. In uncertain cases, a 0.1% solution of pilocarpine can be used to test for denervation supersensitivity. If neither pupil constricts, a 1% solution of pilocarpine can then be used to distinguish between a pharmacologically blocked pupil and a neurologically denervated pupil (321) (Fig. 16.5).

DISTURBANCES IN DISORDERS OF THE NEUROMUSCULAR JUNCTION

Myasthenia Gravis

Myasthenia gravis (MG) is an autoimmune disorder characterized by pathogenic antibodies against acetylcholine receptors at motor terminals. Clinically apparent weakness of the intraocular muscles is rare. Nonetheless, abnormalities of pupillary function and accommodation are occasionally reported in patients with MG. Two patients with anisocoria and sluggish pupil light reflexes that resolved following treatment with cholinesterase inhibitor have been described (322,323). Pupillary fatigue during prolonged light stimulation has also been noted in other patients (323,324). Yamazaki and Ishikawa used an open-loop stimulus and infrared video pupillography to record direct pupillary responses to light as well as their velocities and acceleration in seven patients with MG and in three healthy persons (325). Their results suggest that involvement of the iris sphincter is common in patients with MG. Lepore et al. reported abnormalities of pupil cycle time, but most of these patients were taking anticholinesterase agents, systemic corticosteroids, or both, which may have affected their pupillary movements (326). In addition, it is not clear whether the pupillary abnormalities observed were caused by direct involvement of the iris musculature, the neuromuscular junction, or central path-

ways of the pupillary light reflex. Bryant concluded that patients with severe MG tend to show significant interocular differences in pupil cycle times, with the degree of difference correlating with the severity of the illness (327).

It thus appears that some degree of pupillary dysfunction can occur from MG but that in the vast majority of patients, such pupillary dysfunction is not clinically significant and should not confuse the diagnosis; that is, MG should be considered in patients with an ocular motility disturbance and clinically normal pupil responses. On the other hand, patients with ocular motility disturbances and abnormally reactive pupils or anisocoria should first be considered to have a neurologic disorder, not myasthenia. MG is described in detail in Chapter 21.

Botulism

Botulinum toxin is produced by one of several strains of the organism *Clostridium botulinum*. The toxin blocks cholinergic neurotransmission at the neuromuscular junction and cholinergic autonomic synapses. Dilated, poorly reactive pupils and paralysis of accommodation are nearly universally present in patients with clinical botulism (328–331). Interestingly, the accommodation dysfunction often is more severely affected than the pupillary dysfunction. The reason is not clear. There are seven different strains of *C. botulinum*, A–F (including Cα and Cβ), with A, B, and E being of most clinical importance. In type E botulism, internal ophthalmoplegia and ptosis often are the initial neurologic manifestations of the disease, whereas in types A and B, systemic autonomic symptoms tend to occur simultaneously with the onset of ocular symptoms.

Common routes of infection are ingestion of contaminated canned goods or meats, wound infection (particularly in heroin addicts who use subcutaneous injections known as "skin popping"), and gastrointestinal colonization in infants. Botulism should be considered in any patient with symmetric, descending muscular weakness; blurred near vision; and poorly reactive pupils. The differential diagnosis and details of this disease are in Chapters 21 and 49.

Lambert-Eaton Myasthenic Syndrome

Lambert-Eaton syndrome is an immune-mediated disorder (primary or paraneoplastic) in which antibodies are directed against PQ-type voltage-gated calcium channels, resulting in inhibition of neurotransmitter release at cholinergic synapses. The pupil dysfunction is one feature of the cholinergic dysautonomia. One study reported that six of 50 (8%) patients with Lambert-Eaton myasthenic syndrome (LEMS) had sluggish pupil responses to light on clinical examination (332); however, another study using a more quantitative technique found abnormal pupil cycle times in 69% of eyes in seven patients with LEMS (333). Tonic pupils also have been reported in patients with LEMS. One of these patients showed some recovery of the light reaction following administration of 3,4-diaminopyridine and pyridostigmine (334,335).

DRUG EFFECTS

The iris is easy to see because it is suspended in a clear fluid behind a clear cornea. Thus, the actions of the sphincter and dilator muscles on the size of the pupil can be monitored easily. Parasympathetic and sympathetic neural impulses to the iris muscles can be modified by drugs at the synapses and at the effector sites, because it is at these locations that the transmission of the impulses depends on chemical mediators. Thus, the pupil can be and frequently is used as an indicator of drug action.

A few cautionary words should first be said about the interpretation of pupillary responses to topically instilled drugs. There are large interindividual differences in the responsiveness of the iris to drugs placed in the conjunctival sac, and this becomes most evident when weak concentrations are used. For example, a 0.25% solution of pilocarpine will produce a minimal constriction in some patients and a marked miosis in others. The general status of the patient can also influence the size of the pupils (336). If the patient becomes uncomfortable or anxious while waiting for the drug to act, both pupils may dilate. If the patient becomes drowsy, both pupils will constrict. Thus, if a judgment is to be made about the dilation or constriction of the pupil in response to a topical drug, one pupil should be used as a control whenever possible (119).

If only one eye is involved, the drug should be put in both eyes so that the response of the normal and abnormal eye can be compared. When the condition is bilateral, no such comparisons are possible, but an attempt should be made to make sure that the observed response is indeed caused by the instilled drug. Thus, if both eyes are involved, the drop should be put in one eye only so that the responses of the medicated and unmedicated eyes can be compared.

Drugs that Dilate the Pupils

Parasympatholytic (Anticholinergic) Drugs (Fig. 16.27)

Plants from the family Solanaceae occur naturally and contain belladonna alkaloids in various proportions. These plants include deadly nightshade (*Atropa belladonna*), black henbane (*Hyoscyamus niger*), jimson weed (*Datura stramonium*), "angel's trumpet" (*Datura suaveolens*), and morning glory. The word belladonna ("beautiful lady") was derived from the cosmetic use of these substances as mydriatics in 16th-century Venice. The mischief caused by the ubiquitous jimson weed is typical of this group of plants. Jimson weed has been used as a poison, has been taken as a hallucinogen, and has caused accidental illness and death. It also can cause a marked accidental mydriasis if it is inadvertently or purposefully applied to the conjunctiva of one or both eyes (337).

Other solanaceous plants like blue nightshade (*Solanum dulcamara*) and Jerusalem cherry are found in home gardens. They contain solanine, which has effects similar to the belladonna alkaloids. Inadvertent topical ocular application with the juice from the plant can produce a dilated nonreactive pupil that gradually returns to normal in 1–6 days (338–340).

Atropine and scopolamine block parasympathetic activity by competing with acetylcholine at the effector cells of the iris sphincter and ciliary muscle, thus preventing depolarization. Accidental mydriasis and anisocoria can be caused by topical absorption after ocular contact with these drugs in their natural form, but the most frequent ways the drug reaches the eye is by a finger from a scopolamine patch (used for vertigo, seasickness, or postoperative pain) to the conjunctival sac (341), by accidental topical adsorption of the inhalant used to treat asthma (341a) or by the deliberate instillation of the drug into one or both eyes by a person attempting to feign a neurologic disorder. After conjunctival instillation of 1% atropine, mydriasis begins within about 10 minutes and is complete in 35–45 minutes; cycloplegia is complete in about an hour. When concentrations of 2–4% atropine are used, the pupil may stay dilated for several days, but accommodation usually returns in 48 hours. Scopolamine (0.2%) causes mydriasis that lasts, in an uninflamed eye, for 2–5 days. This drug is a less effective cycloplegic than atropine.

A dilated, fixed pupil caused by pharmacologic blockade of the iris sphincter by atropine may be difficult to distinguish from a denervated iris sphincter. One clinically helpful feature is the presence of segmental contractions of the iris sphincter. Atropine weakens the sphincter equally at all segments because convective circulation of the aqueous humor distributes the drug to all parts of the sphincter (342). Thus, at the slit lamp, if there is still any segment of the sphincter that constricts to light, the pupil is not pharmacologically dilated, it is denervated. If the sphincter is diffusely paralyzed (i.e., no segmental contractions seen), then no distinction between a pharmacologically dilated pupil and a parasympathetically denervated one can be made. Preganglionic denervation of the iris sphincter (i.e., oculomotor nerve palsy) may not always be associated with ophthalmoplegia

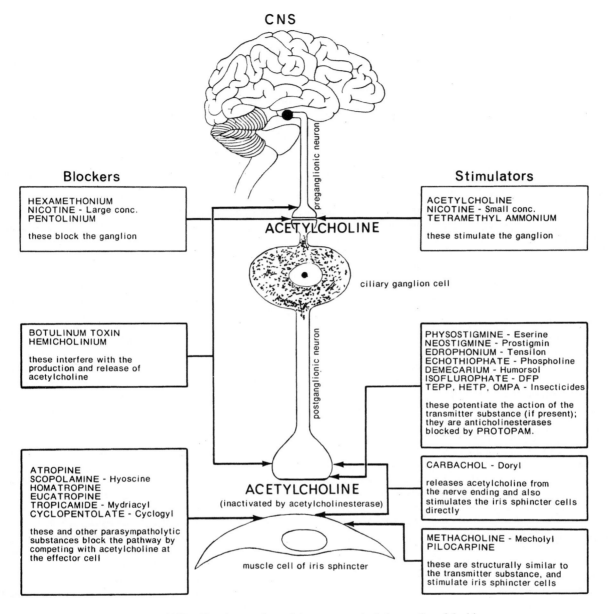

Figure 16.27.   The pharmacology of the parasympathetic innervation of the iris.

or ptosis. A minority (about 10%) of postganglionic iris sphincter denervations (i.e., tonic pupils) involve 100% of the muscle (255). As noted above, one can use pharmacologic testing to differentiate between a pharmacologically dilated pupil and a pupil that is parasympathetically denervated (one or two drops of a 0.5–1% solution of pilocarpine in both conjunctival sacs). This concentration of pilocarpine will not displace an anticholinergic drug from the receptors of the iris sphincter muscle, but it will produce a definite constriction of the other normal pupil, and it also will constrict a denervated pupil (from oculomotor nerve palsy or tonic pupil) (226). Even a partial response to 0.5–1% pilocarpine indicates pharmacologic blockade, because a dener-

vated pupil should constrict at least as well as the normal pupil and perhaps even more, if denervation supersensitivity is present.

Results of the pilocarpine test may be misleading in cases of trauma. A pupil that is dilated because of blunt ocular trauma tends to constrict poorly to pilocarpine, not because of pharmacologic manipulation but because the sphincter muscle itself has been damaged. Other observations suggesting related damage to the eye (e.g., tears of the pupillary margin, Vossius' ring, lenticular changes, choroidal rupture, scattered pigment on the anterior iris stroma) generally make it clear that the globe has been severely injured. Iron mydriasis, however, from an unsuspected intraocular iron foreign body, is mostly caused by toxic damage to the iris nerves rather than to the iris muscle, and these pupils constrict vigorously to pilocarpine like a denervated pupil (236,343).

Tropicamide (Mydriacyl) and cyclopentolate (Cyclogyl) are synthetic parasympatholytics with a relatively short duration of action (344). Tropicamide (1%) is an effective, short-acting mydriatic; its action peaks at 25 minutes and lasts 3–6 hours. The 1% drops produce little loss of accommodation, although mild cycloplegia may be detected between the 25th and 35th minutes after instillation. Compared with tropicamide, a 1% solution of cyclopentolate is a much more effective cycloplegic and perhaps a slightly less effective mydriatic, especially in dark eyes. Mydriasis and cycloplegia approach a maximum in about 30 minutes; accommodation takes about half a day to return, and the pupil still may not be working normally after more than 24 hours. To be completely confident of cycloplegia, second and third drops sometimes are used. In a child, especially a small blond child, enough cyclopentolate may be absorbed through the nasal mucosa after three drops in each eye to produce mild transient symptoms of toxicity, such as flushing of the skin and restlessness (345).

Because patients with Alzheimer dementia have abnormalities in the cholinergic pathways of the brain, it has been hypothesized that the cholinergic pathway to the eye may be defective as well. In 1994, Scinto et al. reported that patients with Alzheimer disease showed greater mydriasis to weak (0.01%) tropicamide (i.e., cholinergic supersensitivity) compared with normal controls (346). Some subsequent studies have confirmed these findings, whereas others have refuted them. As the debate continues, recent investigators have suggested that reducing the peak constriction amplitude is a more sensitive indicator of central cholinergic dysfunction compared with tropicamide-induced pupil dilation, and others have proposed that an even more dilute solution (0.005%) might lower false-positive rates (347,348). At present, there are no standardized guidelines for clinical use of weak tropicamide eyedrops as a diagnostic or differentiating test of Alzheimer dementia.

Botulinum toxin blocks the release of acetylcholine, and hemicholinium interferes with the synthesis of acetylcholine both at the preganglionic and at the postganglionic nerve endings, thus interrupting the parasympathetic pathway in two places. Topical gentamicin may produce a similar effect (349). The outflow of sympathetic impulses also is interrupted by systemic doses of these drugs, because the chemical mediator in sympathetic ganglia also is acetylcholine.

Lidocaine and similar anesthetic agents produce a dilated pupil following intraocular or intraorbital injection (350). In most cases, the anesthetic agent is injected to produce both anesthesia and akinesia for intraocular or strabismus surgery, and the dilation is expected. In other cases, however, the anesthetic is injected anteriorly but diffuses posteriorly. For example, Perlman and Conn described three patients who developed transient fixed dilated pupils after undergoing blepharoplasties using a local anesthetic consisting of a 50/50 mixture of 2% lidocaine with epinephrine 1:200,000 and 0.75% bupivacaine with epinephrine 1:200,000 (351). In most of these cases, the pupil returns to normal within 24

hours. Local anesthesia occasionally enters the orbit by other means. Unilateral mydriasis following dental surgery has been reported after inadvertent injection of lidocaine through the pterygopalatine fossa and inferior orbital fissure into the orbit (11).

Nebulized treatments for asthma containing anticholinergic drugs such as ipratropium bromide sometimes cause a unilateral or bilateral mydriasis when the eye is accidentally exposed to the aerosol from an incorrectly placed mask (352).

Sympathomimetic (Adrenergic) Drugs (Fig. 16.28)

Epinephrine (Adrenalin) stimulates the receptor sites of the dilator muscle cells directly. When applied to the conjunctiva, a 1:1,000 solution does not usually penetrate into the normal eye in sufficient quantity to have an obvious mydriatic effect. Indeed, even a solution of 1.25% epinephrine is insufficient to dilate most pupils of normal subjects (353). If, however, the receptors are supersensitive from previous denervation, or if the corneal epithelium is damaged, allowing more of the drug to get into the eye, these concentrations of epinephrine will dilate the pupil.

Phenylephrine (Neo-Synephrine) in a 10% solution has a powerful mydriatic effect. Its action is almost exclusively a direct α-stimulation of the effector cell. The pupil recovers in 8 hours and shows a "rebound miosis" that lasts several days. A 2.5% solution most often is used for mydriasis, in part because this rarely produces systemic hypertension, as does a 10% solution (354). Even weak solutions of phenylephrine may be sufficient to dilate a pupil, but pupils dilated with this drug should still react to light stimulation. Roberts described a patient thought to be comatose from alcohol and benzodiazepine (diazepam, lorazepam) overdose who developed a fixed dilated left pupil after nasotracheal intubation and gastric lavage (355). A diagnosis of possible cerebral herniation was made, and the patient was treated with intravenous mannitol, furosemide, and hyperventilation. A computed tomographic (CT) scan showed no abnormalities. The fixed dilated pupil returned to normal over 3–4 hours, and the patient's condition subsequently improved. It was suspected that the fixed dilated pupil was caused by inadvertent topical ocular contamination with phenylephrine nose spray (0.5%) that had been used in the left nostril in preparation for the endotracheal intubation; however, we would not expect a pupil dilated in this manner to be nonreactive to light stimulation.

Ephedrine acts chiefly by releasing endogenous norepinephrine from the nerve ending. It also has a definite direct stimulating effect on iris dilator muscle cells and can produce significant mydriasis, depending on the concentration used.

Tyramine hydrochloride (5%) and hydroxyamphetamine hydrobromide (1%) have an indirect adrenergic action on the pupillary dilator muscle, releasing norepinephrine from the stores in the postganglionic nerve endings. As far as is known, this is their only effective mechanism of action.

Cocaine (5–10%) is applied to the conjunctiva as a topical anesthetic, a mydriatic, and a test for Horner syndrome (see above). Its mydriatic effect is the result of an accumulation

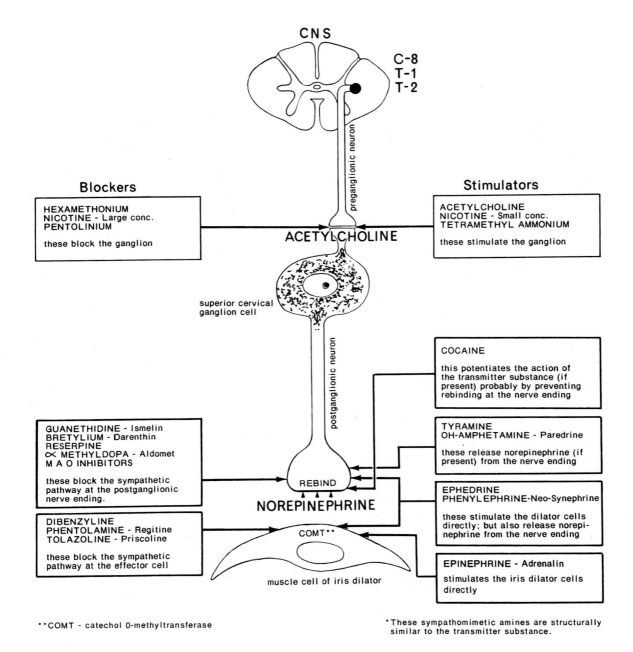

Figure 16.28.   The pharmacology of the sympathetic innervation of the iris.

of norepinephrine at the receptor sites of the dilator cells. The transmitter substance builds up at the neuroeffector junction because cocaine prevents the reuptake of the norepinephrine back into the cytoplasm of the nerve ending. Cocaine itself has no direct action on the effector cell, nor does it release norepinephrine from the nerve ending, and it does not retard the physiologic release of norepinephrine from the stores in the nerve ending. Its action is indirect in that it interferes with the mechanism for prompt disposition of the chemical mediator. In this respect, its action is analogous to that of the anticholinesterases at the cholinergic junction. The dura-

tion of cocaine mydriasis is quite variable. It may last more than 24 hours. Pupils that dilate from cocaine do not show rebound miosis as the effect of the drug dissipates.

Tetrahydrozoline hydrochloride, pheniramine maleate, and chlorpheniramine maleate are sympathomimetic agents often used in topical ocular decongestants. Instillation of eye drops containing these substances may produce mydriasis, particularly when the drops contain more than one of the drugs (356).

Ibopamine is an ester of N-methyl-dopamine that is nonselectively active on DA1 and DA2 dopaminergic receptors

ectopia, an upward, inward movement of the pupils in a comatose patient with mesencephalic disease (23). Such pupillary abnormalities presumably are caused by incomplete damage to the parasympathetic pupillary fibers in the mesencephalon. Midbrain corectopia is not limited to patients in coma, however (24).

Lesions of the tegmental portion of the pons may interrupt descending sympathetic pathways and produce bilaterally small pupils. In many cases, especially those with pontine hemorrhage, the pupils are pinpoint, presumably from a combination of sympathetic interruption and parasympathetic disinhibition. Despite the size of such pupils, a pupil light reflex usually is present and can be observed with the aid of magnification within several hours after the onset of the primary intracranial event (398).

The pupillary fibers within the peripheral oculomotor nerve are particularly susceptible when uncal herniation compresses the nerve against the posterior cerebral artery or the edge of the cerebellar tentorium (399). In these instances, pupil dilation may precede other signs of ocular motor nerve paralysis, and such patients may present with fixed, dilated or fixed, oval pupils (25,400).

The nature of pupillary dysfunction in a comatose patient often reflects the level and degree of brain stem dysfunction. This is particularly true when brain stem dysfunction is produced by an expanding supratentorial lesion. Such lesions accounted for 20% of patients initially diagnosed as ''coma'' in the series reported by Plum and Posner (395). Supratentorial lesions produce neurologic dysfunction by two mechanisms: primary cerebral damage and secondary brain stem dysfunction from displacement, tissue compression, swelling, and vascular stasis. Of the two processes, secondary brain stem dysfunction is the more threatening to life. It usually presents as one of two main patterns. Most patients develop signs of bilateral diencephalic impairment: the central syndrome or rostral-caudal deterioration. In this syndrome, pupillary, ocular motor, and respiratory signs develop that indicate that diencephalic, mesencephalic, pontine, and, finally, medullary function are being lost in an orderly rostral to caudal fashion. Other patients develop signs of uncal herniation with oculomotor nerve and lateral mesencephalic compression (uncal herniation syndrome). The following discussion is obtained from the excellent monograph ''The Diagnosis of Stupor and Coma'' by Plum and Posner (395).

Central Syndrome of Rostral-Caudal Deterioration

The first evidence that a supratentorial mass is beginning to impair the diencephalon usually is a change in alertness or behavior. Initially, patients with such lesions find it difficult to concentrate and tend to lose the orderly details of recent events. Some patients become agitated, whereas others become increasingly drowsy. Respiration in the early diencephalic stage of the central syndrome is commonly interrupted by deep sighs, yawns, and occasional pauses. Many patients have periodic breathing of the Cheyne-Stokes type, particularly as they become increasingly somnolent. The pupils are small (1–3 mm) but maintain a small and brisk

reaction to light stimulation unless there is concomitant compression of one or both oculomotor nerves. Some patients show conjugate or slightly divergent roving eye movements and have an inconsistent response to oculocephalic testing (doll's head maneuver). More frequently, the eyes are conjugate and stable at rest, responding briskly to oculocephalic testing. In such patients, caloric testing using cold water evokes a full, conjugate, slow tonic movement toward the irrigated side with impairment or absence of the fast component of the response. Early diencephalic dysfunction in such patients is suggested by the development of bilateral signs of corticospinal or extrapyramidal dysfunction. A few patients develop diabetes insipidus, reflecting severe downward traction on the pituitary stalk and the median eminence of the hypothalamus.

The clinical importance of the diencephalic stage of the central stage of rostral-caudal deterioration caused by a supratentorial mass lesion is that it warns that a potentially reversible lesion is about to become irreversible by progressively encroaching on the brain at or below the level of the tentorium. Once signs of mesencephalic dysfunction appear, however, it becomes increasingly likely that the patient has suffered a brain stem infarction, rather than reversible compression and hypoxia, and the outlook for neurologic recovery is poor.

As mesencephalic and upper pontine damage ensues, abnormally wide fluctuations of body temperature are common. Respirations gradually change from the Cheyne-Stokes type to a sustained tachypnea. The initially small pupils dilate and become fixed in midposition. It is unclear whether this dilation is caused by interruption of the afferent light reflex pathway, damage to the dorsal visceral nuclei of the oculomotor nerve complex, or both. In this stage, the pupils no longer dilate to psychosensory stimuli. Oculocephalic testing often fails to elicit appropriate eye movements, and even caloric testing may fail to produce normal tonic movements toward the irrigated side. Motor dysfunction progresses from decorticate to bilateral extensor rigidity in response to noxious stimuli. Of the adult patients examined by Plum and Posner (1980), none with a supratentorial lesion recovered full neurologic function once mesencephalic signs were fully developed. The prognosis for recovery is often better in children.

After the mesencephalic/upper pons stage, ischemia continues to progress caudally down the brain stem. Hyperventilation resolves, giving rise to a fairly regular breathing pattern with a shallow depth and rapid rate (20–40 per minute). The pupils remain in midposition and do not respond to light stimulation. Oculocephalic testing elicits no ocular movements, and the extremities become increasingly flaccid.

The medullary stage is terminal. Respiration slows and often becomes irregular in rate and depth; it is interrupted by deep sighs or gasps. The pulse is variable, and the blood pressure drops. The eyes are immobile and no longer respond to caloric or oculocephalic stimulation. The pupils may dilate widely during this stage (terminal mydriasis). In the absence of an intact sympathetic outflow pathway, the mydriasis may be caused by hypoxia of the neurons of the Edinger-Westphal nucleus that had previously been deafferented. Alternatively, it may be caused by an agonal release of adrenergic substances into the blood in response to hypoxia, thus causing the pupil to dilate. Both mechanisms may occur simultaneously.

The size and reactivity of the pupils should never, by themselves, be used as an indication of irreversible coma and brain death. In the first place, some comatose patients whose mid-dilated pupils are thought to be unreactive to light when examined with a hand-held penlight can be shown to react when assessed with infrared pupillometry (401). In addition, even widely dilated, fixed pupils can be observed in comatose patients who eventually recover neurologic function. For example, Cleveland reported the complete neurologic recovery of a 14-year-old boy who suffered a cardiac arrest lasting 3 hours (402). During the entire resuscitation episode, the patient's pupils were widely dilated and fixed. Gauger also emphasized that the observation of widely dilated, nonreactive pupils during the period of resuscitation after a cardiac or respiratory arrest does not, in itself, signify irreversible brain injury (403). Conversely, some patients with irreversible coma develop nonreactive small or pinpoint pupils (404,405). The reason for the small size of the pupils in some of these patients is previous use of miotic agents to treat glaucoma.

Uncal Herniation Syndrome

Patients with the syndrome of uncal herniation have asymmetric pupillary changes in the early phases of coma. During the early third nerve stage, signs of oculomotor nerve dysfunction may occur with almost any level of altered consciousness, from slight drowsiness to complete unconsciousness. The earliest consistent sign is unilateral dilation of one pupil that initially is sluggishly reactive to light but soon becomes widely dilated (6–9 mm) and nonreactive to light stimulation. This pupillary disturbance may last for several hours before neurologic signs other than an altered state of consciousness appear (406).

Traditional teaching held that if a supratentorial mass lesion such as acute hemorrhage causes altered consciousness and an acutely dilated pupil, the dilated pupil indicates the side of the lesion. The iridoplegia occurs from uncal descent and compression of the superolateral aspect of the ipsilateral oculomotor nerve. Occasionally, however, the dilated pupil is contralateral to the lesion, a finding called a "false-localizing" pupil (407,408). This phenomenon occurs from shift of the midline away from the lesion, with compression either of the contralateral oculomotor nerve or the contralateral side of the mesencephalon against the lateral tentorial edge. The localizing value of this pupil sign is far less important in this era of modern neuroimaging, but it remains useful in understanding the sequence of events during uncal herniation. In any event, during this early phase, respiration may be normal, extraocular movements and oculocephalic responses may be unimpaired, and motor abnormalities may reflect only a supratentorial process. Nevertheless, once other signs of herniation or brain stem compression appear, deterioration may proceed rapidly, with the patient becoming comatose within a few hours.

Once the pupil is fully dilated, ophthalmoplegia related to oculomotor nerve dysfunction soon follows. In this late third nerve stage, the patient usually becomes deeply stuporous, then comatose. Oculocephalic testing initially shows evidence of ocular motor impairment, with eventual disappearance of all responses. As the opposite cerebral peduncle becomes compressed against the contralateral tentorial edge, hemiplegia develops ipsilateral to the expanding supratentorial lesion (409). The signs of mesencephalic damage continue to develop. The pupil opposite the one that originally dilated may become fixed and widely dilated or assume a midposition (410,411). Eventually, both pupils become dilated and nonreactive to light stimulation. Most patients at this stage show sustained hyperpnea, impaired or absent oculocephalic and caloric responses, and bilateral decerebrate rigidity. From this stage, progression of the uncal syndrome is clinically indistinguishable from that of the central syndrome.

Coma from Metabolic Disease

In patients in deep coma, the state of the pupils may become the single most important criterion that clinically distinguishes between metabolic and structural disease. Pupillary pathways are relatively resistant to metabolic insults. Thus, the presence of preserved pupil light reflexes despite concomitant respiratory depression, caloric unresponsiveness, decerebrate rigidity, or motor flaccidity suggests metabolic coma. Conversely, if asphyxia, drug ingestion, or preexisting pupillary disease can be eliminated as a cause of coma, the absence of pupillary light reflexes in a comatose patient strongly implicates a structural lesion rather than a metabolic process.

In a study of 115 patients presenting to the emergency department with coma (mean Glasgow Coma Scale score of 4) from a variety of structural and metabolic etiologies (cardiopulmonary arrest excluded), both loss of the pupil light reflex and anisocoria were found to be independent predictors of underlying structural pathology (412). Loss of the light reflex had greater sensitivity (83%) for predicting a structural lesion, whereas the presence of anisocoria was less sensitive (39%) but very specific (96%) for a structural lesion. Structural causes of coma included intracerebral hemorrhage, subarachnoid hemorrhage, acute infarction, subdural and epidural hematoma, brain contusion, and tumor. In the same series, 16 of 69 patients (23%) with coma of metabolic origin demonstrated loss of the pupil light reflex; half of these patients were comatose from drug overdose (412).

Normal pupil shape, size, and reactivity are highly indicative of intact midbrain function. In one series of 162 patients with severe head injury, pupillary dysfunction was the feature that correlated best with brain stem ischemia from damage to perforating vessels from the basilar artery (413).

Cheyne-Stokes Respiration

Cheyne-Stokes respiration (CSR) is a pattern of periodic breathing in which phases of hyperpnea regularly alternate with apnea. The breathing waxes from breath to breath in a smooth crescendo and then, once a peak is reached, wanes in an equally smooth decrescendo. CSR implies bilateral dysfunction of neurologic structures usually lying deep in the cerebral hemispheres or diencephalon, but rarely as low as the upper pons (414).

During CSR, the size of the pupils fluctuates. The pupils dilate in the hyperpneic phase unless there is a concomitant sympathetic nerve paralysis, and they constrict during the apneic phase unless there is a concomitant oculomotor nerve paralysis (415). The cyclic breathing and pupillary movement also are associated with cyclic changes in the level of consciousness. During the apneic phase, the patient slips into a deeper coma; in the hyperpneic phase, the patient may become agitated. In humans, the mydriasis of the hyperpneic phase is almost, but not entirely, blocked by topical sympatholytic drugs (e.g., 5% guanethidine) and does not occur when there is an associated or unrelated Horner syndrome. This suggests that neural activity, mediated by the peripheral sympathetic pathway to the eye, plays an important role in the dilation. This suggests, in turn, that the mechanism of the mydriasis of the agitated phase of CSR may be similar to that of reflex pupillary dilation and related to the intermittent partial arousal of a semicomatose patient.

DISORDERS OF ACCOMMODATION

Abnormalities of accommodation usually are acquired and occur most frequently as part of the normal aging process (presbyopia). However, disturbances of accommodation also may occur in otherwise healthy persons, in persons with generalized systemic and neurologic disorders, and in persons with lesions that produce a focal interruption of the parasympathetic (and rarely the sympathetic) innervation of the ciliary body. Also, accommodative function can be voluntarily disrupted.

ACCOMMODATION INSUFFICIENCY AND PARALYSIS

Congenital and Hereditary Accommodation Insufficiency and Paralysis

Congenital defects are a rare cause of isolated accommodation insufficiency. The ciliary body is defective in a number of congenital ocular anomalies, but in most cases vision is so defective that an inability to accommodate is never noted by either the patient or the physician. Aniridia and choroidal coloboma cause obvious defects of the ciliary body. Ciliary aplasia can occur in well-formed eyes in which the iris is intact and reacts normally to light.

Sédan and Roux described three brothers who could see normally for distance without glasses but required +4.00 spherical lenses for reading (416). None of the children had pupillary constriction during near viewing, although their other ocular functions were normal. The children's retinoscopic findings were not reported, but neither atropine nor physostigmine influenced the state of their accommodation. Aplasia of the ciliary body was the presumed congenital defect. In another family of 10 affected members, an accommodative defect was present in infancy and thereafter nonprogressive by history (417). Pharmacologic assessment with various topical agents suggested a difficulty with either the ciliary musculature or the lens of the affected eyes.

Congenital absence of accommodation has been noted in combination with congenital mydriasis. In three such cases, patent ductus arteriosus was an associated anomaly (43). Defective accommodation was noted in 21 of 78 (27%) dyslexic children, suggesting an association between the two disorders (418).

Acquired Accommodation Paresis

Isolated Accommodation Insufficiency

Accommodation insufficiency refers to an accommodative ability that measures below the minimum for the age of the patient. Most clinicians use the near point of accommodation as their diagnostic criterion for accommodation insufficiency (accommodative amplitude that is 2 diopters or more below the age-appropriate minimum). Isolated accommodation insufficiency occurring in otherwise healthy eyes can be divided into two groups: (a) static insufficiency and (b) dynamic insufficiency (419).

Static accommodation insufficiency is an inadequate response of either the lens or the ciliary muscle, despite normal ciliary body innervation and neural function. It usually occurs gradually from changes occurring in either the lens or the ciliary body. The most common cause of isolated static insufficiency is presbyopia. In some patients, however, there is sudden loss of accommodation that does not recover. Treatment consists of appropriate spectacle correction.

Dynamic accommodation insufficiency occurs in patients who have inadequate parasympathetic impulses required to stimulate the ciliary musculature but have normal pupil size and reactivity. Such patients usually are asthenopic persons who become ill, often hospitalized, with some unrelated condition. Dynamic accommodation insufficiency also may occur in otherwise healthy young individuals, particularly in children with nonspecific viral illnesses (420,421). The transient loss of accommodation that can occur just before or after childbirth may be another example of this phenomenon (422). Raskind listed various systemic disorders associated with an acquired accommodation insufficiency (423). In all these cases, it is likely that the accommodation insufficiency represents a nonspecific manifestation of the systemic disorder.

The symptoms of dynamic accommodation insufficiency are asthenopia, tiring of the eyes sometimes associated with brow ache, irritation and burning of the eyes, blurred vision particularly for near work, inability to concentrate, and photophobia. As a general rule, symptoms resolve and accommodation recovers following treatment of the underlying illness and restitution of the patient's former state of health. If accommodation insufficiency remains, the prescription of convex (plus) lenses is indicated, regardless of the patient's age. In patients with an associated convergence insufficiency, convergence exercises or base-out prisms added to the near correction may be of benefit.

Accommodation Insufficiency Associated with Primary Ocular Disease

Iridocyclitis may cause profound dysfunction of the ciliary body. In the acute stage, there may be ciliary spasm and loss of accommodation. In the chronic stage, atrophy of the ciliary body results in accommodation insufficiency. The more severe the uveitis, the more commonly mydriasis and cycloplegia (internal ophthalmoplegia) are associated with it. In addition, viruses such as herpes zoster may produce a uveitis associated with a ciliary ganglionitis, resulting in a tonic pupil syndrome.

Glaucoma in children or young adults causes accommodation insufficiency from secondary atrophy of the ciliary body. The drugs used in the management of glaucoma affect the ciliary body as well as the iris. In patients who still are able to accommodate, miotic drugs frequently produce ciliary spasm with symptoms of blurred vision.

Metastases to the suprachoroidal space may produce cycloplegia and pupillary dilation from damage to the ciliary neural plexus. Lymphoma and carcinoma of the breast, lung, or colon are the most common tumors that produce this condition.

Internal ophthalmoplegia associated with contusion of the globe was discussed in the section above on the pupil. In most cases, when accommodation is paralyzed, the pupil is dilated and fixed. Recovery of accommodation is common, but full recovery of pupillary function is less likely. On rare occasions, the pupil is spared or recovers fully but the ciliary muscle remains paralyzed. Patients who ''accidentally'' notice the inability to accommodate in one eye should be questioned specifically for previous trauma to that eye (11).

Immediately following a concussion injury to the globe, the pupil is small and accommodation is spastic. Subsequently, the pupil dilates and the ciliary muscle becomes paretic. Accommodation usually returns in 1–2 months. The traumatic etiology of the accommodation paresis may be suspected by slit-lamp biomicroscopic observation of tears in the iris sphincter, tears at the root of the iris, or recession of the angle of the anterior chamber with posterior displacement of the ciliary attachment. There also may be associated ocular hypotension or glaucoma. Following trauma to the globe, rupture of zonular fibers with partial subluxation of the lens also may produce loss of accommodation.

Iatrogenic trauma to the eye, such as that which occurs during retinal reattachment surgery, cryotherapy, or panretinal photocoagulation, may injure the ciliary nerves, producing accommodation paresis and mydriasis (424–426). Laser applications at or anterior to the equator and long exposure times are important factors in the development of accommodation paresis following photocoagulation (427). Optic nerve sheath fenestration performed from the lateral approach can damage the short ciliary nerves that penetrate the temporal sclera, causing a postoperative tonic pupil (245). Sector palsy of the iris sphincter has been reported after argon laser trabeculoplasty (244). Transient internal ophthalmoplegia also can result from local anesthesia injected into the lids or gums that inadvertently enters into the orbit (see also the section above on Local Tonic Pupils).

Accommodation Insufficiency Associated with Neuromuscular Disorders

Some diseases produce myopathic changes in the smooth muscle fibers of the ciliary body, but isolated ocular involvement of this type is rare.

Myasthenia gravis may cause defective accommodation (428,429). Manson and Stern studied patients with MG and patients with unexplained accommodation disturbances (430). All patients were questioned about diplopia, ptosis, and the effects of sustained reading or close work upon their vision. Binocular and uniocular accommodation amplitudes were measured. Of nine patients with MG (six with generalized and three with ocular disease), eight had abnormal fatigue of visual accommodation. The accommodation defect improved rapidly after an intravenous injection of edrophonium hydrochloride (Tensilon).

Botulism nearly always causes an acute accommodation paralysis. The toxins produced by *C. botulinum* interfere with the release of acetylcholine at the neuromuscular junction and in the cholinergic autonomic nervous system. Although several different subtypes of toxin exist and routes of human infection can vary (food-borne, wound, gastrointestinal tract colonization in infants), clinical manifestations are similar. These include progressive descending skeletal muscle weakness, ocular motor palsies, bulbar paralysis, and cardiovascular lability (431). Food-borne botulism produces prominent gastrointestinal symptoms as well.

Almost 90% of patients with botulism of any type complain of blurred vision. Paralysis of accommodation and impairment of the pupillary light reflex are common and early signs of botulism, often appearing suddenly about the 4th or 5th day of the illness. Accommodation is usually more severely affected than pupil function, for unclear reasons (Fig. 16.31). In some cases, accommodative failure is the initial and sole sign of nervous system involvement. In a series of nine patients with food-borne botulism, all patients examined acutely had marked or complete accommodative loss but full mydriasis was present in only one patient, and another patient had sluggish pupillary reactions (328). Recognition of the clinical syndrome of botulism is critical, as respiratory failure can result in mortality rates up to 20% (431).

Tetanus can produce accommodation paralysis. In most cases, the accommodation paralysis occurs in the setting of generalized ophthalmoparesis; however, one patient described had normal eye movements and normally reactive pupils to light stimulation (432).

Myotonic dystrophy frequently produces degenerative changes in the lens, the region of the ora serrata, and the anterior chamber angle. It also may be associated with ocular hypotension. It is reasonable to assume that the ciliary muscle also is affected, because other smooth muscle dysfunction occurs in such patients (433).

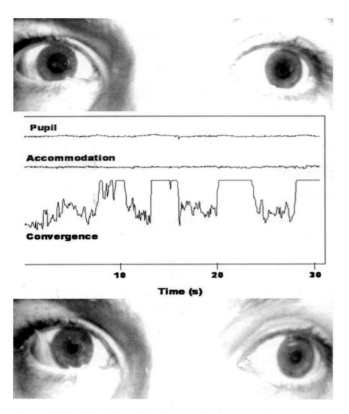

Figure 16.31. The effect of botulism on the elements of the near reflex. The patient was a 33-year-old man with acute food-borne botulism. His symptoms were 4 days of blurred vision, abdominal pain, nausea, and sweating. *Top,* The patient's pupils are large and unreactive to light. *Middle,* Simultaneous recordings of pupil size, accommodation, and convergence to near effort confirm complete paralysis of pupil responsiveness and accommodation, whereas convergence is intact. *Bottom,* Both pupils constrict following instillation of 0.1% pilocarpine. (Courtesy of Dr. Helmut Wilhelm.)

Accommodation Insufficiency Associated with Focal or Generalized Neurologic Disease

Accommodation paresis may be caused by both focal and generalized neurologic disorders that interrupt the innervation of the ciliary body. Supranuclear lesions can influence the signal inputs to the parasympathetic midbrain nuclei for accommodation, resulting in paresis or even paralysis of accommodation. Such lesions include damage to the cerebral cortex, rostral midbrain, superior colliculus, and possibly the cerebellum (434,435). In these cases, convergence insufficiency usually accompanies the accommodation insufficiency because of cross-coupling between these two systems.

Acute infectious or epidemic encephalitis as well as postinfectious acute disseminated encephalomyelitis (ADEM) such as that which is associated with or follows measles, chickenpox, or other viral infections can cause accommodative paralysis (436). Typically, patients have loss of the near triad (convergence palsy, absence of pupillary near response, failure of accommodation) and normal pupil responses to light. Histopathologic examination in fatal cases shows diffuse perivenous white-matter lesions throughout the cerebral hemispheres and brain stem.

An acute focal lesion of the hemispheres may cause acute bilateral accommodation insufficiency. Specifically, this has been reported with an acute ischemic stroke in the territory of the left middle cerebral artery and an acute hematoma in the left pariteo-occipital region (437,438). The issue is whether the accommodation insufficiency is related to a direct effect of these lesions on supranuclear pathways for accommodation or is a nonspecific sequela of a significant focal cerebral lesion. If the former, it remains to be determined whether a lesion in either hemisphere can cause accommodation insufficiency or just a lesion in the left hemisphere.

Acute problems with near vision resulting from an abnormality of accommodation can be one of the earliest symptoms of pressure on the dorsal mesencephalon such as from obstructive hydrocephalus or a pineal tumor. These complaints may appear weeks before the pupil light reaction or ocular motility becomes clinically abnormal. Particularly in previously healthy children and young adults who suddenly lose accommodation, a careful evaluation should be undertaken to exclude lesions in the area of the rostral dorsal midbrain, including the superior colliculus (439,440). Some of these patients also demonstrate a sudden increase of myopia (pseudomyopia) related to accommodation spasm with blurring of distant vision.

Wilson disease is an hereditary disorder of copper metabolism characterized by progressive degeneration of the CNS associated with hepatic cirrhosis. The neurologic syndrome frequently includes rigidity, difficulty speaking and swallowing, and a characteristic tremor of the wrists and shoulders. Ocular findings include a peripheral corneal ring of copper deposition involving Descemet's membrane (Kayser-Fleischer ring), copper pigment under the lens capsule, and various ocular motor disturbances, including jerky oscillations of the eyes, involuntary upgaze, paresis of upgaze, and slowed saccadic movements. Paresis of accommodation is common (441,442), but the location of the lesion responsible for the accommodation paresis is controversial. Some investigators favor a supranuclear lesion (441,443), whereas others postulate a lesion in the region of the oculomotor nucleus that serves the near response (442).

In contrast to the aforementioned supranuclear lesions that result in bilateral paralysis of accommodation with sparing of the pupil light reflex, lesions of the peripheral oculoparasympathetic pathway typically result in unilateral paralysis of accommodation and paralysis of the pupillary light reflex in the same eye. This is because the peripheral impulses for pupil constriction and accommodation originate in the same visceral (Edinger-Westphal) nuclei and follow the same peripheral pathway to the eye. Thus, the patient with an acute lesion in the peripheral pathway subserving accommodation will more likely seek medical consultation for the associated mydriasis than the blurred near vision. The evaluation of such an anisocoria was outlined in an earlier section of this chapter. Common types of injury along this oculoparasympathetic pathway are infection, ischemia, and compression, resulting in an oculomotor nerve palsy or a tonic pupil syndrome.

Primary and secondary aberrant reinnervation of the oculomotor nerve also can involve the ciliary muscle. Herzau and Foerster described three young patients who had increased myopia during attempted adduction of the affected eye, presumably from aberrant reinnervation (444).

An isolated accommodation paralysis—accommodation paralysis without mydriasis—theoretically can be caused by a lesion of the ciliary ganglion or short ciliary nerves. We are unaware of any well-documented cases of this phenomenon.

Accommodation Insufficiency Associated with Systemic Disease

Children and adults may develop transient accommodation paresis following various systemic illnesses. In such cases, the accommodation paresis often appears to occur as an indirect complication of the systemic disorder rather than from direct damage to the ciliary body or its innervation. There are, however, certain systemic diseases that produce accommodation insufficiency through direct effects on the ciliary body and lens or on their innervation.

In patients with diphtheria, accommodative paralysis usually is bilateral and occurs during or after the 3rd week following the onset of infection. Recovery is the rule but may take several years (445). Because of regular vaccination, the infection from *Corynebacteria diphtheriae* is now rare in most developed countries. Accommodation paralysis has been reported following injection of diphtheria antitoxin. The mechanism of diphtheritic accommodation palsy appears to be related to toxin-induced segmental demyelination of peripheral nerves with preservation of axons (446).

Loss of accommodation may occur in patients with diabetes mellitus from several mechanisms (447). For example, accommodation paresis may develop in young patients with previously uncontrolled diabetes who have just begun treatment. Hyperopia and accommodation weakness develop concurrently within a few days after the patient's blood glucose has been lowered and then gradually return to normal over 2–6 weeks. The mechanisms for the refractive and accommodative changes in diabetes are poorly understood. Sorbitol accumulates in the lens during periods of hyperglycemia, causing it to swell, and the lens appears responsible for the shifts in refraction because these shifts do not occur in aphakic or pseudophakic eyes. The same mechanism may account for accommodation paresis, because lens resiliency probably is decreased from the swelling. Persistent loss of accommodation can occur in patients with both controlled and uncontrolled diabetes mellitus from damage to the parasympathetic innervation to the eye. In this setting, accommodation paresis and mydriasis are due to denervation injury rather than to effects on the lens. Thus, either metabolic or neurologic mechanisms can be responsible for reduced accommodation in patients with this disease.

Lieppman described 12 professional divers who had visual complaints after decompression sickness (448). All of the divers had evidence of severe accommodation and convergence insufficiency that was thought to be caused by a "central" lesion. These findings were reproduced in two rhesus monkeys experimentally subjected to similar hyperbaric conditions.

Accommodation Insufficiency Associated with Trauma to the Head and Neck

Theoretically, any cerebral injury could impair the highly complex neurophysiologic system involved in the coordination of the near response. Similarly, abnormal input from the upper posterior cervical roots or contusion to the side of the cervical cord could disturb transmission in the ascending spinotegmental and spinomesencephalic pathways that influence parasympathetic outflow from the Edinger-Westphal median nuclei. Symptoms of difficulty with focusing at near and at far, commonly associated with headache and pains about the eyes, are common complaints in patients who have suffered cerebral concussion or craniocervical extension injuries (449). These vague and ill-defined complaints are most prominent during the first weeks or months after injury. The prevalence of accommodation dysfunction in patients with head or neck trauma is not exactly defined and may be influenced in part by the average age of patients studied, as older patients likely have presbyopia prior to trauma.

In a series of 161 patients with head injury (average age 29 years), Kowal found that 16% had poor accommodation, 19% had over-accommodation (pseudomyopia), and 14% had convergence insufficiency (450). In about half of these patients, near vision complaints improved or resolved within the first year after their injury. Similarly, among 39 patients with whiplash or indirect injury to the neck, Burke et al. found decreased accommodation and convergence in nine (23%), six of whom were symptomatic (451). Five of these six patients recovered accommodation after 9 months.

Tests of accommodation depend upon an earnest, volitional effort by a motivated patient. Thus, patients who have cortical deficits, loss of concentration, poor comprehension, excessive somnolence, or pain often perform poorly on accommodative tests. Other patients attempting to gain material or psychological compensation may intentionally perform poorly on these tests (452). The persistence of symptoms for many months or even years is most common in patients who are seeking compensation for their injury through litigation.

Accommodation Insufficiency and Paralysis from Pharmacologic Agents

Most topical pharmacologic agents that produce pupillary mydriasis also produce cycloplegia, including atropine, scopolamine, homatropine, eucatropine, tropicamide, cyclopentolate, and oxyphenonium. Various investigators have compared the duration and effectiveness of cycloplegia produced by these agents when used as ocular solutions (453,454). None of these agents causes persistent paralysis of accommodation after discontinuation, although there may be some confusion when loss of accommodation occurs after treatment of a severe viral uveitis (e.g., herpes zoster, varicella) with a cycloplegic agent. In such cases, the accommodation paralysis occurs from the effects of the virus on the ciliary ganglion and not from the cycloplegic drug.

When cycloplegic agents or related substances are incorporated in medications that are taken internally or applied to the skin as ointments or plasters, there may be sufficient absorption to produce paresis of accommodation. In such cases, the accommodation deficit is partial and recovery begins shortly after the medication is discontinued.

Accommodation Paralysis for Distance: Sympathetic Paralysis

Lesions of the cervical sympathetic outflow may produce a defect that prevents the patient from accommodating fully from near to far, but most reports describe an increase in accommodative amplitude on the side of the Horner syndrome (455). Cogan described an ipsilateral increase in near accommodation in five patients with Horner syndrome and noted an apparent paresis of accommodation in one patient (456).

ACCOMMODATION SPASM AND SPASM OF THE NEAR REFLEX

General Considerations

Accommodation spasm is due to excessive activity of the ciliary muscle that results in an abnormally close point of focus. Clinically, there is an apparent or increased myopia that disappears following cycloplegia (pseudomyopia). Accommodation spasm typically affects both eyes, but unilateral cases have been reported (457). It can occur in isolation as pseudomyopia or in association with convergence spasm and excessive pupillary miosis in varying combinations and degrees, all of which probably represent the spectrum of clinical presentations of spasm of the near reflex (458).

Symptoms of isolated accommodation spasm are blurry vision, especially at distance, fluctuating vision, asthenopia, eyestrain, poor concentration, brow ache, and headaches. The diagnostic finding is a greater myopia on manifest refraction compared with cycloplegic refraction, the difference ranging from 1 to 10 diopters. Additionally, the patient will not accept the majority of the cycloplegic refraction, preferring instead the greater myopic correction for visual improvement.

In addition to the symptoms of accommodation spasm, patients with spasm of the near reflex who have convergence spasm also complain of a horizontal diplopia that often is variable in nature. Because of the diplopia and apparent esotropia, such patients initially may be mistaken as having a unilateral or bilateral abducens nerve palsy or ocular myasthenia and undergo extensive neurologic and neuroimaging investigations (428,459). Spasm of the near reflex should be suspected in a patient with an apparent unilateral or bilateral limitation of abduction that is associated with severe bilateral miosis (459,460). The diagnosis is confirmed by demonstrating that the miosis resolves as soon as either eye is occluded with a hand-held occluder or patch (461). Additionally, the apparent abduction weakness present on horizontal gaze testing with both eyes open will disappear when the opposite

eye is patched (monocular ductions testing) or when the oculocephalic maneuver is performed. Refraction with and without cycloplegia will establish the presence of pseudomyopia as well.

Accommodation Spasm Unassociated with Organic Disease

Most cases of accommodation spasm (usually as part of spasm of the near reflex) appear to be nonorganic, being triggered by an underlying emotional disturbance or occurring as part of malingering. In such cases, spasm of the near reflex typically occurs as intermittent attacks lasting several minutes (462,463). The degree of accommodation spasm and convergence spasm in such patients is variable; however, miosis is always present and impressive (Fig. 16.32). However, many young persons, when undergoing a noncycloplegic refraction, can accept increasing degrees of overcorrecting concave (minus) lenses. When these same patients undergo a cycloplegic refraction, they are found to be emmetropic or at least significantly less myopic than they appeared to be when not cyclopleged. However, unlike patients with accommodation spasm who prefer the greater myopic correction, these otherwise healthy young persons prefer their cycloplegic refraction for best-corrected visual acuity.

The management of most patients with nonorganic spasm of the near reflex begins with simple reassurance that they have no irreversible visual or neurologic disorder. In other instances, referral for psychiatric counseling is appropriate. Symptomatic relief may be necessary with a cycloplegic agent and bifocal spectacles or reading glasses. Glasses with an opaque inner third of the lens to occlude vision when the eyes are esotropic have been proposed for the convergence spasm (464). Nonorganic spasm of the near reflex also is discussed in Chapter 27.

Accommodation Spasm Associated with Organic Disease

Accommodative spasm has been reported, mostly as single case occurrences, in association with various organic diseases and CNS lesions. These include neurosyphilis, ocular inflammation, Raeder paratrigeminal neuralgia syndrome, cyclic oculomotor palsy, congenital ocular motor apraxia, congenital horizontal gaze palsy, pineal tumor, Chiari malformation, pituitary tumor, metabolic encephalopathy, vestibulopathy, Wernicke-Korsakoff syndrome, epilepsy, cerebellar lesions, and acute stroke (465–471).

Several investigators have reported spasm of the near reflex in patients with MG (472,473). Romano and Stark described a 26-year-old man who developed isolated pseudomyopia as a presenting sign of ocular MG (428). The pseudomyopia was thought to have occurred from ''substitute convergence'' that the patient used to compensate for bilateral medial rectus weakness rather than from true accommodation spasm.

Isolated accommodation spasm and spasm of the near reflex appear to be increasingly recognized as a consequence of head injury (450,474–477). In one series, accommodation

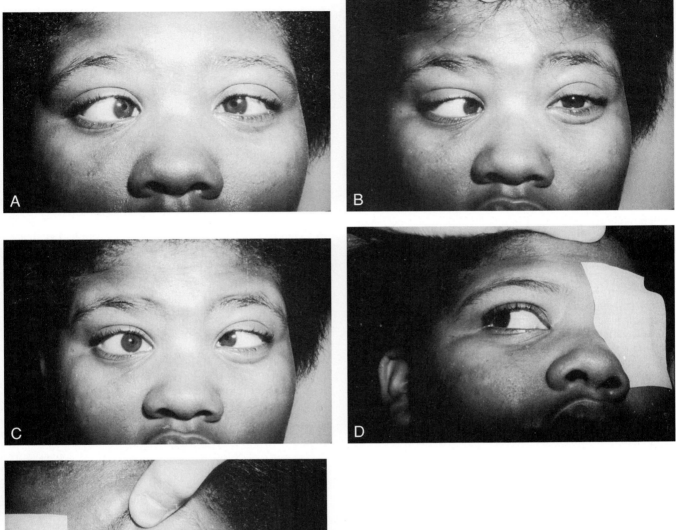

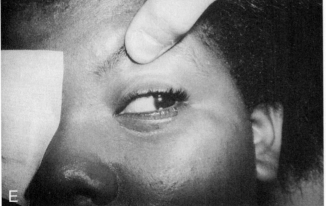

Figure 16.32. Spasm of the near reflex in an otherwise healthy 15-year-old female. *A,* In primary position, the eyes are esotropic and the pupils are constricted. *B,* On attempted right gaze, the right eye does not abduct and both pupils become even smaller. *C,* On attempted left gaze, the left eye does not abduct and both pupils become smaller. *D,* With the left eye patched, the right eye abducts fully on oculocephalic testing and the pupil dilates. *E,* With the right eye patched, the left eye abducts fully on oculocephalic testing and the pupil dilates.

spasm was found in 19% of patients following closed head injury (450). Chan and Trobe reported six patients who recovered from severe brain injury (i.e., comatose more than 1 week, increased intracranial pressure, brain stem deficits) and complained of reduced distance vision (474). Isolated pseudomyopia was found in all six patients, and full manifest correction alleviated the visual blur. Posttraumatic accommodation spasm may be a persistent condition, lasting up to 9 years after head trauma (474,476,478).

DRUG EFFECTS ON ACCOMMODATION

Most of the cholinergic agents mentioned in the earlier section of this chapter concerning pharmacologically induced miosis also produce an increase in accommodation and, occasionally, accommodation spasm. Pilocarpine, physostigmine, and the organophosphate esters produce the most

accommodation, whereas the effect of aceclidine on accommodation is minimal (478).

DISORDERS OF LACRIMATION

Disorders that disrupt the neural control of lacrimation include cerebral diseases and trigeminal nerve lesions as well as lesions along the parasympathetic secretomotor pathway from pons to lacrimal gland. The disorders of lacrimation produced by these lesions generally can be divided into three types: reduced tearing (hypolacrimation), excessive tearing (hyperlacrimation), and inappropriate tearing.

HYPOLACRIMATION

Lesions of the Trigeminal Nerve

The majority of afferent inputs for reflex lacrimation are carried via the ophthalmic division of the trigeminal nerve. Significant hypolacrimation can result from deafferentation of the tear reflex on one side, such as occurs in severe trigeminal neuropathy. However, lesions that damage the trigeminal nerve at the pontine angle, petrous tip, or Meckel's cave often simultaneously damage the nearby parasympathetic lacrimal fibers (either the nervus intermedius or the greater superficial petrosal nerve). In these cases, trigeminal nerve-related reduction of tears represents combined dysfunction in the afferent and efferent limbs of the tear reflex.

Brain Stem Lesions

It might be assumed that any lesion of the brain stem that involves the facial nucleus automatically produces decreased tearing and loss of taste because of the proximity of the structures conveying these modalities. In fact, abnormalities of tear secretion seldom are recognized in patients with lesions of the brain stem. Two patients with Moebius syndrome had bilateral congenital sensorineural deafness and facial motor palsy with intact lacrimation and taste sensation, demonstrating that lesions in this area of the pons can spare both taste and tearing as these functions are anatomically separate from the motor function (479).

Crosby and DeJonge called attention to an acquired brain stem syndrome with unilateral involvement of the superior salivary nucleus (480). One of the small vessels supplying the area near the fourth ventricle at the level of the superior salivary nucleus is prone to develop thrombosis. The vascular accident that develops when this vessel becomes occluded is characterized by a peripheral facial motor palsy, ipsilateral dry eye, and reduced salivary flow from the submaxillary gland. The rostral end of the vestibular nucleus lies in the immediate vicinity, and these patients usually have vertical or torsional nystagmus. The pathways and neurons concerned with lateral gaze also may be affected, causing an ipsilateral palsy of horizontal gaze.

Lesions Affecting the Nervus Intermedius

A peripheral facial palsy associated with ipsilateral loss of reflex tearing suggests a more proximal site of damage along the facial nerve pathway, either at the cerebellopontine

angle or in the petrous bone. The secretomotor fibers for lacrimation and salivation exit the brain stem in the nervus intermedius. This nerve is sandwiched between the motor trunk of the facial nerve and the vestibulocochlear nerve as they traverse the cerebellopontine angle and the internal auditory meatus. Lesions in this area, usually tumors, can produce loss of hearing, vestibular dysfunction, facial palsy, decreased salivation, altered taste sensation, and a dry eye on the affected side.

Pulec and House found that 10 of 15 patients with vestibular schwannomas had demonstrable but asymptomatic deficiency of tearing on the side of the lesion (481). Because this sign often is present before any overt clinical evidence of the lesion, such as facial palsy or corneal hypesthesia, careful testing of reflex tearing in such patients may aid in initial diagnosis. Dysfunction of the nervus intermedius also occurs after surgical resection of vestibular schwannomas. In a series of 257 patients who had surgical removal of these tumors, 72% reported significant ipsilateral dry eye (loss or significant reduction of tears) postoperatively compared with 4% preoperatively (482). In addition, crocodile tears (see below) and abnormal taste were reported postoperatively in 44% and 48% of patients, respectively, compared with 2% and 6% preoperatively.

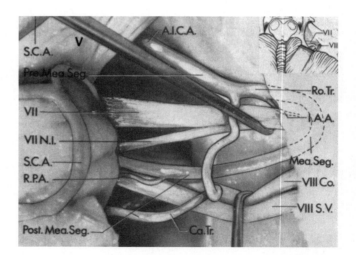

Figure 16.33. Relationships between nervus intermedius, facial nerve trunk, vestibulocochlear nerve trunk, and the superior cerebellar and anterior inferior cerebellar arteries. Nervus intermedius (VII N.I.) exits from the brain stem between the facial nerve trunk (VII) and the cochlear (VIII Co.) and superior vestibular (VIII S.V.) nerve trunks. Note the relationships of the rostral (Ro. Tr.) and caudal (Ca. Tr.) trunks of the anterior inferior cerebellar artery (A.I.C.A) to the facial-vestibulocochlear nerve complex. V, trigeminal nerve; S.C.A., superior cerebellar artery; R.P.A., recurrent perforating artery; I.A.A., internal auditory artery; Mea, Seg., meatal segment. (From Martin RG, Grant JL, Peace D, et al. Microsurgical relationships of the anterior inferior cerebellar artery and the facial-vestibulocochlear nerve complex. Neurosurgery 1980;6:483–507.)

At the end of the internal acoustic meatus, the motor trunk of the facial nerve and the nervus intermedius enter the facial canal that houses the geniculate ganglion (Fig. 16.33). Patients with injury to the facial nerve in the facial canal proximal to or at the geniculate ganglion do not have hearing loss; in fact, they may complain of hyperacusis from loss of the normal damping action of the stapedius muscle. Idiopathic and viral inflammation within the facial canal, skull base fractures, infection of the geniculate ganglion (e.g.,

herpes zoster, syphilis), and otitis media are common causes of facial nerve injury at this site.

Lesions Affecting the Greater Superficial Petrosal Nerve

Any lesion that involves the floor of the middle cranial fossa in the neighborhood of the gasserian ganglion may injure the lacrimal fibers in the greater superficial petrosal nerve (Figs. 16.34 and 16.35). The resulting deficiency of

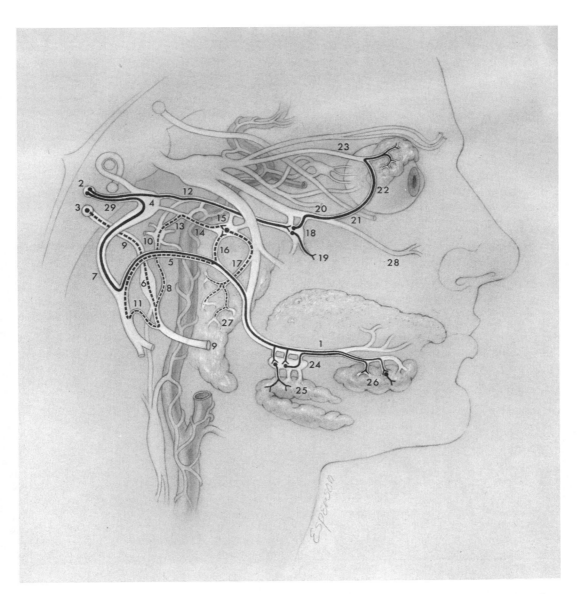

Figure 16.34.   Secretomotor pathways for lacrimation and salivation: The efferent visceromotor (parasympathetic) outflow. 1, lingual nerve; 2, superior salivatory and lacrimal nucleus; 3, inferior salivatory nucleus; 4, geniculate ganglion of the seventh nerve; 5, chorda tympani; 6, petrosal ganglion; 7, facial nerve; 8, tympanic nerve; 9, glossopharyngeal nerve; 10, tympanic plexus; 11, anastomotic branch (cranial nerves 9 to 7); 12, greater superficial petrosal nerve; 13, deep petrosal nerve; 14, lesser superficial petrosal nerve; 15, otic ganglion; 16, anastomotic branch; 17, auriculotemporal nerve; 18, sphenopalatine ganglion; 19, branches to nasal mucosa and palatine glands; 20, maxillary division of trigeminal nerve; 21, zygomatic nerve; 22, zygomaticolacrimal anastomosis; 23, lacrimal nerve; 24, submaxillary ganglion; 25, submaxillary gland; 26, sublingual gland; 27, parotid gland; 28, infraorbital nerve; 29, nervus intermedius.

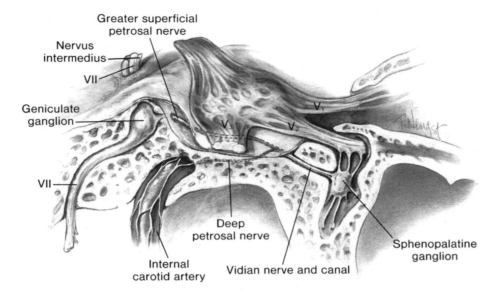

Figure 16.35. Vertical section through the axis of the petrous pyramid of the temporal bone showing the location of the geniculate ganglion and the course of the greater superficial petrosal nerve from the geniculate ganglion to the sphenopalatine ganglion. Some sympathetic fibers leave the internal carotid artery at the foramen lacerum to form the deep petrosal nerve. This nerve joins with the greater superficial petrosal nerve to form the vidian nerve. Note the connections between the sphenopalatine ganglion and the maxillary nerve trunk (V_2). V_1, ophthalmic nerve; V_3, mandibular nerve.

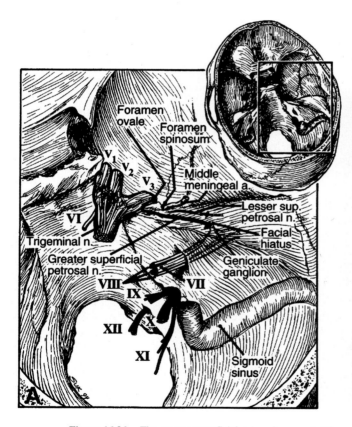

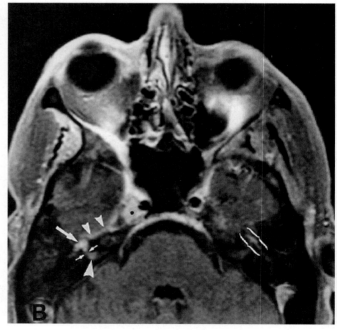

Figure 16.36. The greater superficial petrosal nerve. *A,* Diagram of the proximal facial nerve, including the takeoff of the greater superficial petrosal nerve (GSPN). *B,* Axial contrast-enhanced T1-weighted magnetic resonance image with fat suppression at the level of Meckel's cave and the temporal bone in a patient with perineural spread of adenoid cystic carcinoma along the right GSPN. Note tumor in the right cavernous sinus and anterior aspect of Meckel's cave (*black dot*). The GSPN courses directly beneath this area. Note the enhancement of the GSPN (*small arrowheads*). The geniculate region enhances brightly and is grossly enlarged (*large arrow*). The labyrinthine and distal intracanalicular segments of the facial nerve also show enhancement (*small arrows and large arrowhead,* respectively); these two segments of the facial nerve normally do not enhance. On the left side, the geniculate ganglion is of normal size (and enhances normally), and only the proximal GSPN and the proximal tympanic segment of the facial nerve enhance (*brackets*). (From Ginsberg LE, De Monte F, Gillenwater AM. Greater superficial petrosal nerve: Anatomy and MR findings in perineural tumor spread. AJNR Am J Neuroradiol 1996;17:389–393.)

tears on the affected side rarely is noted unless the patient has an associated palsy of the trigeminal or facial nerve and develops signs of keratitis from drying and exposure of the cornea. Acquired lesions that may damage the greater superficial petrosal nerve include nasopharyngeal tumors, meningeal sarcomas, facial nerve schwannomas, perineural tumor infiltration, inflammations of the gasserian ganglion (e.g., herpes zoster), petrositis, sphenoid sinus disease, aneurysms of the petrous portion of the internal carotid artery, fractures through the middle fossa, alcohol injections, and extradural operations for trigeminal neuralgia (483) (Fig. 16.36).

The finding of impaired tear secretion on the side of an acquired palsy of the abducens nerve is of great localizing value because it indicates a lesion (usually extradural) in the middle cranial fossa. Thus, patients with "isolated" abducens nerve palsies should undergo careful testing of reflex tear function in addition to other tests of facial and trigeminal nerve function. Most patients with a combination of an abducens nerve palsy and ipsilateral decreased reflex tearing have nasopharyngeal tumors.

Lesions Affecting the Sphenopalatine Ganglion

Lesions of the sphenopalatine ganglion (also called the pterygopalatine ganglion) frequently cause pain and hypesthesia in the cheek (the area supplied by the maxillary division of the trigeminal nerve) in addition to decreased tearing and dryness of the nasal mucosa on the same side. Thus, the combination of dry eye and cheek pain or numbness on the same side should prompt investigation for a lesion, usually a malignant tumor, in the pterygopalatine fossa (Fig. 16.37). Similarly, a patient with a known tumor or infection of the maxillary (or sphenoid) sinus who develops unilateral reduction of tear secretion should be suspected to have extension of the process beyond the confines of the sinus.

Lesions of the Zygomaticotemporal Nerve

Damage to the zygomaticotemporal nerve produces postganglionic denervation of the lacrimal gland. Such damage usually occurs from facial trauma involving the posterior lateral orbital wall. Occasionally, tumors in this area, particularly metastatic carcinoma, will damage these fibers, resulting in a reduction of reflex tearing.

HYPERLACRIMATION

Reflex hypersecretion can result from excessive afferent triggers of the tear reflex arc or from overstimulation of the efferent parasympathetic fibers.

Supranuclear Lesions

The tear reflex normally can be elicited by a strong emotion such as sadness. This is called psychogenic tearing or crying. In cerebral diseases that significantly damage the frontal lobes, basal forebrain, thalami, or especially the posterior ventral hypothalamus, unexpected and excessive spells of crying (pathologic crying) can occur (484). Pharmacologic studies suggest dysfunction of the serotoninergic system as the cause of this syndrome, which may be treated

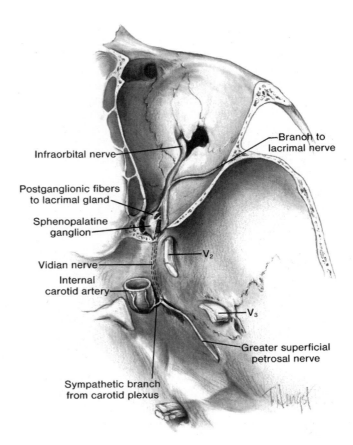

Figure 16.37. Anatomic relations of the sphenopalatine ganglion, the vidian nerve, and the maxillary nerve behind the posterior wall of the orbit and maxillary antrum, viewed from above.

with serotonin reuptake inhibitors (485). The main characteristics of pathologic crying are an absence of voluntary control and a lack of corresponding mood, such as intense sadness or grief. Pathologic crying and pathologic laughing, often termed emotional incontinence, frequently are associated with diverse neurologic and psychiatric findings. Emotional incontinence associated with dysphagia and dysarthria make up the syndrome of pseudobulbar palsy that may be seen in patients with parkinsonism, various age-related dementias, amyotrophic lateral sclerosis, giant-cell arteritis, hypothalamic tumors, and encephalitis.

Excessive lacrimation also can be associated with the photophobia caused by meningitis or encephalitis. Intermittent spells of excessive tearing were the first indication of recurrence of a craniopharyngioma in a 14-year-old boy (222). The lesion was suprasellar in location and compressed hypothalamic structures in the floor of the third ventricle.

SUNCT Syndrome

SUNCT syndrome (short-lasting unilateral neuralgiform headache attacks with conjunctival injection and tearing) is characterized by moderately severe, strictly unilateral attacks of burning or stabbing pain confined to the orbital and periorbital area associated with excessive lacrimation. The attacks are typically 10–120 seconds in duration, with symptomatic periods lasting days to months. Ipsilateral hyperlacrimation and conjunctival injection are considered essential to the diagnosis, and rhinorrhea and vasomotor signs such as forehead sweating also can occur in patients with this condition. Although certain clinical features suggest a similarity to trigeminal neuralgia or cluster headaches, the pathophysiology of SUNCT remains unknown. Hyperactivity in the thalamus and hypothalamus has been noted using functional MR imaging.

Sphenopalatine Neuralgia

Sphenopalatine neuralgia, also called Sluder neuralgia, is a syndrome of nasal pain accompanied by ipsilateral hyperlacrimation, rhinorrhea, salivation, photophobia, and hemifacial redness. Anesthesia or ablation of the sphenopalatine ganglion abolishes the symptoms (487). Initially thought to be an idiopathic inflammation of the sphenopalatine ganglion, this condition more likely is a neurovascular headache syndrome (488).

INAPPROPRIATE LACRIMATION

Commonly known as crocodile tears (Bogorad syndrome), the gustolacrimal reflex results from an anomalous lacrimal gland innervation that causes profuse and inappropriate tearing in response to stimulation of the taste buds. Most commonly, crocodile tears develop unilaterally in the eye on the side of a facial palsy. However, crocodile tears should not be confused with the watery eye of an acute facial palsy that is due to excess pooling and impaired drainage of tears from loss of normal orbicularis oculis action (blinking). Before discussing the congenital and acquired gustolacrimal reflexes, we will review some of the afferent pathways responsible for transmission of gustatory stimuli and the adjacent efferent pathways to the salivary glands.

Anatomy of the Afferent and Efferent Pathways Involved in the Gustolacrimal Reflex

Anatomy of the Afferent Gustatory Pathways

The taste buds of the tongue are the receptors for gustatory sensation. These afferent impulses are carried by the facial nerve (mediating taste from the anterior two thirds of the tongue) and the glossopharyngeal nerve (mediating taste from the posterior third of the tongue). The gustatory afferent fibers for the anterior two thirds of the tongue pass centripetally with the lingual branch of the mandibular nerve, split off under the base of the skull in the chorda tympani, and in this nerve pass through the petrotympanic fissure, the middle ear, and a special canal in the posterior wall of the tympanic cavity to the facial canal, then upward with the trunk of the facial nerve to the geniculate ganglion, where the cell bodies of these bipolar sensory neurons are located

(Fig. 16.38). In the geniculate ganglion, the gustatory fibers continue centrally in the nervus intermedius. Upon entering the pons, they turn caudally as the tractus solitarius and finally synapse in the rostral end of the nucleus solitarius. Gustatory afferents from the posterior third of the tongue travel via the glossopharyngeal nerve to the brain stem and also synapse in the nucleus solitarius.

Anatomy of the Secretomotor (Parasympathetic) Nerves to the Salivary Glands

Preganglionic salivary neurons arise in two different nuclei in the brain stem and follow two separate pathways to their respective parasympathetic ganglia and end organs. Salivary neurons of the superior salivary nucleus leave the lower pons with the lacrimal fibers as the nervus intermedius, pass through the geniculate ganglion without synapsing, proceed down the facial nerve, and leave the facial canal with the chorda tympani. With this nerve, they join the lingual nerve and pass to the submandibular ganglion and the diffuse sublingual ganglia, where they synapse with the postganglionic neurons that innervate the submandibular and sublingual salivary glands.

Salivary neurons of the inferior salivary nucleus leave the medulla with the fibers of the glossopharyngeal nerve and pass through the jugular foramen with the vagus and spinal accessory nerves. These salivary fibers pass through the petrous ganglion of the glossopharyngeal nerve without synapsing, branch off at the base of the skull, and ascend as the tympanic nerve (of Jacobson) to the tympanic cavity through a small canal in the undersurface of the petrous portion of the temporal bone on the jugular fossa. Within the tympanic cavity, the tympanic nerve divides into branches that form the tympanic plexus and are contained in grooves on the surface of the promontory. It is in this location that an anastomosing branch from the tympanic plexus joins the greater superficial petrosal nerve through a foramen in the roof of the tympanic cavity. The secretory fibers leave the tympanic cavity, course through the anterior surface of the petrous bone, enter the middle fossa as the lesser superficial petrosal nerve, and leave through a foramen in the base of the middle fossa (or through the foramen ovale) to end in the otic ganglion, where they synapse with neurons that supply the parotid gland as the auriculotemporal nerve.

The otic ganglion lies at the base of the skull medial to the mandibular nerve and inferior to the foramen ovale. It has a sensory root from the fibers of the glossopharyngeal and facial nerves via the lesser superficial petrosal nerve, a motor root from the nerve to the internal pterygoid muscle, and a sympathetic root from the carotid sympathetic plexus. The otic ganglion gives origin to three communicating nerves: (a) the nerve to the pterygoid canal; (b) a twig to the chorda tympani; and (c) the auriculotemporal nerve. In addition, two motor branches supply the tensor tympani and the tensor veli palatini.

General Considerations Concerning the Gustolacrimal Reflex

The syndrome of unilateral lacrimation associated with eating and drinking was described initially by Oppenheim

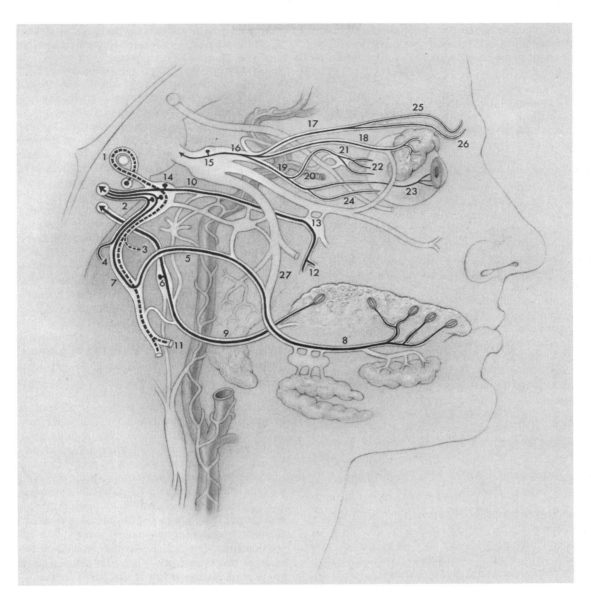

Figure 16.38. Sensory pathways for lacrimal and salivary reflexes. Afferent components of the trigeminal, facial, and glosso-pharyngeal nerves (*solid lines*). The motor outflow to the facial muscles is indicated as a *dashed line*. 1, motor root of facial nerve; 2, nervus intermedius; 3, motor nerve to stapedius muscle; 4, sensory fibers from eardrum and external auditory canal; 5, chorda tympani; 6, petrosal ganglion; 7, facial nerve; 8, lingual nerve; 9, glossopharyngeal nerve; 10, greater superficial petrosal nerve; 11, motor branches to face; 12, sensory fibers from soft palate and tonsillar region; 13, sphenopalatine ganglion; 14, geniculate ganglion; 15, gasserian ganglion; 16, ophthalmic division of the trigeminal nerve; 17, frontal nerve; 18, lacrimal nerve; 19, nasociliary nerve; 20, sensory root of ciliary ganglion; 21, ciliary ganglion; 22, short ciliary nerves; 23, long ciliary nerve; 24, infratrochlear nerve; 25, supraorbital nerve; 26, supratrochlear nerve; 27, mandibular nerve.

and later in more detail by Bogorad, who called it the syndrome of crocodile tears (489,490). The term appears to have derived from the notion that the crocodile "will weep over a man's head after he has devoured the body and then eat up the head too" (491). Bing applied the term "gustolachrymal reflex," a more appropriate designation (492). This reflex may not be as rare as believed (493). In most patients, the symptom of tearing during eating or drinking is little more

than an inconvenience and medical advice is not sought. In some, however, the tearing is so profuse that they must hold a handkerchief to their cheek to absorb the flow of tears.

Types of Gustolacrimal Reflexes

It is possible to differentiate at least three separate types of gustolacrimal reflexes. A congenital variety often is associated with congenital paralysis of abduction. One acquired variety has its onset either in the initial stage of a facial palsy or without clinical evidence of facial palsy. The second acquired—and most common—variety develops after a peripheral facial palsy.

Congenital Gustolacrimal Reflex

Lutman described three patients with a congenital gustolacrimal reflex, two of whom also had congenital paralysis of abduction (494). One of these two patients had a unilateral gustolacrimal reflex and an ipsilateral abduction weakness; the other patient had bilateral gustolacrimal reflexes and bilateral paralysis of abduction. Other authors have described congenital cases in which mastication (chewing and sucking motions) seemed to provide more powerful stimuli for lacrimation than did gustatory stimuli alone (495). It has been speculated that the etiology of the congenital gustolacrimal reflex is related to abnormal differentiation of the lacrimal and the salivary nuclei in the pons associated with a supranuclear or nuclear abnormality of the abducens nerve (495,496).

In support of a central developmental origin of the congenital gustolacrimal reflex is the occurrence of the reflex in some patients with the Duane retraction syndrome, a syndrome known to result from defective development of the abducens nucleus and anomalous reinnervation of the lateral rectus muscle (497–499; also see Chapter 20). An alternative mechanism may be peripheral facial nerve and abducens nerve palsy due to birth trauma with subsequent anomalous reinnervation of the former (11).

Acquired Gustolacrimal Reflex with Onset in the Early Stage of Facial Palsy

Kaminsky reported a patient with onset of the gustolacrimal reflex 3 weeks after the appearance of a facial palsy (500), whereas Christoffel reported another with onset at the time the facial palsy began (501). Bauer reported a 15-year-old girl in whom an acquired gustolacrimal reflex was the presenting symptom of an ipsilateral vestibular schwannoma (502). On examination, the patient also had slight facial weakness, moderate corneal hypalgesia, and subtotal hearing loss. Following surgery to remove the tumor, her facial palsy was complete, but the gustolacrimal symptoms had disappeared.

Chorobski argued that crocodile tears occurring simultaneously with or shortly after the appearance of a facial palsy cannot be explained by misdirection of regenerating fibers (491). He proposed that such cases are best explained by compression, demyelination, and cross-stimulation of neural impulses between the afferent fibers for taste and the secretomotor fibers for lacrimation within the nervus intermedius (i.e., ephaptic transmission between the autonomic fibers of the proximal seventh cranial nerve). This theory of ephaptic transmission also may be particularly attractive for patients in whom the gustolacrimal reflex resolves either spontaneously or after decompression of the proximal portion of the facial nerve (491).

Acquired Gustolacrimal Reflex Following Facial Palsy or Sectioning of the Greater Superficial Petrosal Nerve

The most common type of gustolacrimal reflex develops weeks or months after a total facial palsy from a lesion in the proximal portion of the nerve. The syndrome may follow skull fracture, herpes zoster oticus, or idiopathic facial palsy (Bell's palsy) with reduction in reflex tearing and unilateral loss of taste in the anterior two thirds of the tongue (503). The accepted mechanism in these cases is misdirection of secretomotor salivary fibers into the pathway of the secretomotor lacrimal fibers at the level of the greater superficial petrosal nerve.

Initially, it was thought that this condition developed when preganglionic salivary fibers in the nervus intermedius mistakenly passed into the greater superficial petrosal nerve with the lacrimal fibers. However, in 1949, Boyer and Gardner reported the syndrome of crocodile tears following surgical section of the greater superficial petrosal nerve where it exits from the petrous bone (504). Their findings indicated that salivary fibers could not have established lacrimal innervation via the greater superficial petrosal nerve. On the other hand, they found that sectioning of the glossopharyngeal nerve relieved crocodile tears in two of their patients, suggesting that this nerve was crucial to the development of the condition.

In 1963, Golding-Wood reported additional cases of the gustolacrimal reflex following proximal sectioning of the greater superficial petrosal nerve (505). He proposed that collateral axonal sprouting occurs from the glossopharyngeal preganglionic salivary nerves, where the tympanic branch joins the greater superficial petrosal nerve (493), and that these misdirected salivary branches aberrantly reinnervate the sphenopalatine ganglion and thus stimulate the lacrimal gland. These collateral axons are the aberrant sprouts of intact salivary fibers that have their normal pathway destined to the otic ganglion and the parotid gland. This theory would explain how salivary axons could circumvent a proximally sectioned greater superficial petrosal nerve and still connect into the pathway of the lacrimal gland.

In support of his theory, Golding-Wood demonstrated in his patients that electrical stimulation of the glossopharyngeal nerve exposed surgically within the tympanic cavity reproduced the patients' tearing phenomenon (505). Subsequent anesthetic block of the glossopharyngeal nerve at the jugular foramen stopped the reflex lacrimation. In three other patients, surgical section of the glossopharyngeal nerve within the inner ear was performed with immediate and lasting cure of the abnormal lacrimation.

Transtympanic resection of the tympanic branch of the glossopharyngeal nerve has remained a highly successful surgical treatment of crocodile tears. Other treatment options, including anticholinergic drugs, intraorbital injections to destroy the sphenopalatine ganglion, and subtotal resection of the lacrimal gland, have had variable success rates. Botulinum toxin type A was introduced as an alternative treatment for crocodile tears in 1998 (506,507). Due to its high efficacy in relieving symptoms with minimal complications, especially when the transconjunctival approach to the lacrimal gland is used (508), this may be the optimal treatment.

DRUG EFFECTS ON LACRIMATION

Lacrimation may be altered by the effects of topical and systemic agents on the main lacrimal gland, its nerve supply, or the accessory lacrimal glands. Some drugs, including methacholine and pilocarpine, induce tearing by direct parasympathomimetic action on the secretory cells of the lacrimal gland (see Chapter 14). Topical drug effects must be differentiated from tearing produced through corneal irritation, local allergic reaction, and so forth. The number of agents that reduce tear secretion is small; they include psychotropic drugs and practolol (509,510).

GENERALIZED DISTURBANCES OF AUTONOMIC FUNCTION

''Dysautonomia'' is a term used to describe any congenital or acquired anomaly in the autonomic nervous system that adversely affects health. This can result in a variety of clinical symptoms, ranging from transient episodes of hypotension to tonic pupil syndrome to progressive neurodegenerative disease. It is not the intention of this chapter to provide a detailed description on the numerous dysautonomic syndromes; however, a few comments will be made on the disorders in which ocular findings are early or prominent signs.

ROSS SYNDROME

In 1958, Ross described a 32-year-old man with Adie syndrome who had become progressively anhidrotic over 12 years (511). Ross syndrome is the eponym now given to the triad of tonic pupils, absent muscle-stretch reflexes, and progressive segmental impairment of sweating. Some patients have a compensatory hyperhidrosis in the early stages of the disease. In the late stage, most patients have generalized anhidrosis.

Histopathologic studies in patients with this condition demonstrate that severe degeneration and loss of cholinergic sudomotor neurons and fibers account for the clinical anhidrosis (512–514). The tonic pupils observed in the Ross syndrome can be unilateral or bilateral and show the same clinical characteristics as an idiopathic tonic pupil.

The combination of idiopathic tonic pupils and areflexia without anhidrosis is known as the Adie (or Holmes-Adie) syndrome (see above). In fact, many patients with Adie syndrome show abnormal sweating patterns when they are formally tested, thus creating confusion in the clinical distinction between Adie syndrome and Ross syndrome (267, 268,515,516). Furthermore, findings of other autonomic deficits such as orthostatic hypotension, abnormalities of cardiovascular reflexes, and chronic cough suggest more widespread autonomic involvement than previously thought in both Adie syndrome and Ross syndrome (267,268,516,517). Shin et al. speculated that Adie syndrome and Ross syndrome (as well as another condition called the harlequin syndrome) may represent a spectrum of clinical manifestations of disorders of neural crest derivatives that include the parasympathetic ganglia, sympathetic ganglia, and dorsal root ganglia (518).

Other studies provide clinical evidence of sympathetic nervous system dysfunction in Ross syndrome. An oculosympathetic defect (Horner syndrome), usually postganglionic, on the side of the facial anhidrosis occurs in some patients with Ross syndrome (518–520). Mild postganglionic sympathetic denervation of the heart also has been demonstrated in some patients (517). Another study showed electrophysiologic evidence of impairment of tactile, temperature, and pain sensation as well as the histopathologic finding of moderately decreased vasomotor and sensory nerve fibers in the epidermis of three patients with Ross syndrome, suggesting progressive degeneration in sensory myelinated and unmyelinated fiber populations in addition to the progressive loss of cholinergic sudomotor fibers (514).

Despite reports of more widespread autonomic and sensory degenerative changes in Ross syndrome, it is the benign and slowly progressive course that distinguishes it from other dysautonomic syndromes (see below).

FAMILIAL DYSAUTONOMIA

Riley-Day syndrome, also called familial dysautonomia, is a rare disorder found almost exclusively in persons of Ashkenazi Jewish descent. The responsible gene maps to chromosome 9q31–33 and is inherited in autosomal-recessive fashion (521). The diagnosis is suspected from clinical signs of generalized autonomic instability such as abnormal sweating, loss of vasomotor control, labile hypertension, episodic fever, and attacks of vomiting. Relative pain insensitivity and a peripheral sensory neuropathy are other features. Two ocular findings are present in all patients: absence or marked insufficiency of tears and corneal anesthesia. Diagnosis is based on five clinical signs: (a) lack of flare following intradermal histamine injection; (b) absence of fungiform papillae on the tongue; (c) pupillary miosis to dilute muscarinic agents such as pilocarpine (cholinergic denervation supersensitivity); (d) severe hypolacrimation; and (e) absent muscle-stretch reflexes (522,523).

Patients with familial dysautonomia produce an insufficient quantity of tears when crying, an important diagnostic feature of the disease at all ages other than in infancy (because the normal infant does not produce tears in any significant quantity before the 6th–8th week after birth). Reflex lacrimation in response to irritants such as the odor of onions, scratching of the middle turbinate, or filter paper in the conjunctival sac also is deficient (524). Yet these same patients produce a copious flow of tears after a parenteral dose of methacholine, suggesting parasympathetic denervation supersensitivity of the lacrimal gland. Histologically, the lacrimal glands appear to be normal (525).

Topical parasympathomimetic agents administered in low concentration produce miosis in patients with familial dysautonomia. The cholinergic supersensitivity of the pupils most often results from parasympathetic denervation, as occurs in other tonic pupil syndromes (526,527); however, the authors of one study proposed increased drug penetration across damaged corneal epithelium as another explanation for the strong miotic effect of dilute pilocarpine in their 10 patients with familial dysautonomia who had normal pupil responses to light and near with infrared pupillography (528).

Ocular findings other than markedly diminished tear secretion, corneal anesthesia, and pupillary dysfunction include corneal ulceration and/or keratopathy, exodeviation, anisometropia, myopia, optic atrophy, anisocoria, ptosis, and tortuosity of retinal vasculature (527,529,530).

Consistent histopathologic lesions have not been identified in familial dysautonomia. Pearson et al. (531,532) described several similar pathologic features in two patients with familial dysautonomia: (a) marked reduction in sympathetic postganglionic neurons and their peripheral axons; (b) marked reduction in sensory dorsal root ganglia and small myelinated and nonmyelinated axons in peripheral nerves; (c) variable reduction in sensory axons and neurons thought to be parasympathetic in nature in the submucosa of the tongue; and (d) variable reduction of mucosal papillae and taste buds. These pathologic findings, although not substantiated completely by others, fit well with biochemical findings in patients with familial dysautonomia that implicate a disturbed catecholamine metabolism (533). On the other hand, Mittag et al. (534) found evidence of a deficiency or absence of choline acetyltransferase enzyme in the cholinergic nerve terminals of a patient with familial dysautonomia. Although a cholinergic defect could affect both the sympathetic and parasympathetic nervous systems through its effect at the ganglion level, it cannot explain the sensory defects in patients with familial dysautonomia.

SHY-DRAGER SYNDROME

Shy-Drager syndrome is a subtype of multiple system atrophy (MSA), one of the three idiopathic neurodegenerative syndromes (onset usually after age 50 years) that primarily affect the autonomic nervous system. The other two are pure autonomic failure, in which impairment of the autonomic nervous system (orthostasis, bladder dysfunction, sexual impotence) occurs without other neurologic features, and Parkinson disease, in which autonomic impairment occurs with an extrapyramidal movement disorder. In MSA, autonomic impairment occurs with an extrapyramidal movement disorder, a cerebellar movement disorder, or both (535). Patients with MSA are said to have ''Shy-Drager syndrome'' when their symptoms and signs are primarily those related to autonomic failure.

Despite the criteria described above, making the clinical distinction among MSA, Parkinson disease, and pure autonomic failure can be difficult. For example, some patients in the early stages of MSA show only autonomic deficits, and others develop only motor deficits that are strikingly similar to those that occur in patients with Parkinson disease. Certain diagnostic tests may aid in the early differentiation of these disorders, particularly functional tests of myocardial sympathetic function, such as myocardial scintigraphy using [123]I (536,537). Patients with Parkinson disease show signifi-

cantly decreased isotope uptake compared with patients with MSA, consistent with other studies indicating that postganglionic sympathetic cardiac denervation occurs in patients with Parkinson disease and pure autonomic failure but not in patients with MSA.

Histopathologic findings described in patients with MSA are inclusion bodies in the oligodendrocytes and neurons in the CNS and intact normal postganglionic sympathetic neurons, further supporting the theory that the degenerative process of MSA is limited to the autonomic neurons in the CNS (538,539).

MR imaging in 29 patients with MSA (subclassified into the syndromes of Shy-Drager, olivopontocerebellar atrophy, and striatonigral degeneration) included high signal in the basis pontis and middle cerebellar peduncles on T2-weighted images consistent with atrophy, signal abnormalities in the putamen, and cerebral atrophy predominantly involving the frontal and parietal lobes (540). These features were commonly present in all patients, regardless of their clinical presentation.

Common ocular signs in patients with Shy-Drager syndrome include anisocoria, iris atrophy, convergence insufficiency, and nystagmus. Other patients have evidence of significant ocular sympathetic and parasympathetic insufficiency, including alternating Horner syndrome, cholinergic sensitivity, decreased lacrimation, and corneal hypesthesia (541,542).

AUTOIMMUNE AUTONOMIC NEUROPATHY

Idiopathic (Primary) Autonomic Neuropathy

Two forms of primary or idiopathic autonomic neuropathy once were classified by the temporal profile of symptomatic autonomic nervous system dysfunction they produced: (a) subacute autonomic neuropathy (also called acute pandysautonomia), having an acute or subacute onset; and (b) pure autonomic failure, having a gradual onset and slow progression of symptoms (see the section above on Multiple System Atrophy). Subsequent studies indicate that these two forms of idiopathic autonomic neuropathy are, in fact, two pathogenetically different diseases. Idiopathic subacute autonomic neuropathy is an immune-mediated disorder that often follows a viral or systemic illness, progresses over several days to weeks, and then tends to improve spontaneously or after treatment with immunomodulatory drugs, whereas pure autonomic failure is an idiopathic, progressive, degenerative disorder (543).

Idiopathic subacute autonomic neuropathy is characterized by findings of autonomic dysfunction, including orthostatic hypotension with a fixed cardiac rate, decreased salivation and lacrimation, impaired pupil reactions, anhidrosis, atony of the bladder, gastroparesis, severe constipation, impotence, and abnormal flushing of the skin (544,545).

The pupillary disturbances that occur in idiopathic subacute autonomic neuropathy are seen early in the course of the disease. They include mydriasis, poor or absent constriction to light and near stimuli, and irregularity of the pupillary margin (546,547). Pharmacologic testing of the pupils in such patients is consistent with both parasympathetic and sympathetic postganglionic denervation, with denervation supersensitivity of both the iris sphincter and iris dilator muscles (548,549).

Patients with pure autonomic failure generally have less prominent pupillary dysfunction, sicca symptoms, and gastrointestinal dysmotility compared with patients with subacute autonomic neuropathy.

Paraneoplastic Autonomic Neuropathy

Paraneoplastic autonomic neuropathy is clinically indistinguishable from idiopathic subacute autonomic neuropathy (543,550). It occurs in about 30% of patients with cancer who have anti-Hu antibodies, and of these, more than half have a clinical and temporal profile similar to subacute autonomic neuropathy (551).

Autoimmune Autonomic Neuropathy

Not only do idiopathic subacute autonomic neuropathy and paraneoplastic autonomic neuropathy have identical clinical findings, they appear to have a similar autoimmune basis. Patients with both disorders test positive for ganglionic nicotinic acetylcholine receptor autoantibodies, as opposed to patients with pure autonomic failure and MSA, who have no evidence of these antibodies (543). Thus, idiopathic subacute optic neuropathy and paraneoplastic autonomic neuropathy are now considered to be forms of a new category of autonomic optic neuropathy called autoimmune autonomic optic neuropathy (AAN). The diagnosis of AAN thus is given to any patient with symptoms of autonomic dysfunction who has positive serum titers of ganglionic acetylcholine receptor antibodies (552). In a study of 18 patients with autoimmune autonomic neuropathy, the mean age was 61.4 years, with a female predominance (544). High titers of ganglionic acetylcholine receptor antibody were associated with symptoms of severe cholinergic dysautonomia such as sicca, upper gastrointestinal dysfunction, large pupils with impaired light and near reactions, and neurogenic bladder. Impaired pupillary function was the clinical feature that most reliably predicted seropositivity; conversely, low antibody titers correlated with mild cholinergic neuropathy. It appears that these receptor antibodies have a pathophysiologic role in the development and severity of clinical symptoms, but the full clinical spectrum of AAN remains to be determined. Thus, if a previously healthy person develops acute or subacute symptoms of autonomic dysfunction, and especially if there is involvement of the pupils, serologic testing for ganglionic acetylcholine receptor antibodies as well as cancer-related antibodies is crucial for both diagnosis and therapy (544).

MILLER FISHER SYNDROME

Miller Fisher syndrome (MFS) is considered a variant of Guillain-Barré syndrome (acute idiopathic polyneuritis). The majority (80–100%) of patients with MFS are positive for anti-GQ1b IgG antibodies. Some patients also show clinical and/or imaging evidence of CNS involvement. Pupillary abnormalities are rather common, being present in 21 of 50

(42%) patients in one study (553). Bilateral mydriasis, poor or no light reaction, anisocoria, and reduced accommodation are typical findings (439,554–556) and indicate primary oculoparasympathetic dysfunction. The results from one patient whose pupils were studied pharmacologically in the acute and recovery stages of MFS suggested that the pupillary involvement was caused by involvement of both the sympathetic and parasympathetic nervous systems (557). MFS is discussed in more detail in Chapter 61.

REFERENCES

1. Shaw MW, Falls HG, Neel JV. Congenital aniridia. Am J Hum Genet 1960;12: 389–415.
2. Flanagan JC, DiGeorge AM. Sporadic aniridia and Wilms' tumor. Am J Ophthalmol 1969;67:558–561.
3. Vincent M-C, Pujo A-L, Olivier D, et al. Screening for PAX6 gene mutations is consistent with haploinsufficiency as the main mechanism leading to various ocular defects. Eur J Hum Genet 2002;11:163–169.
4. Waardenburg PJ, Franceschetti A, Klein D. Genetics and Ophthalmology. Assen, The Netherlands, R. Van Gorcum, 1961.
5. Muto R, Yamamori S, Ohashi H, et al. Prediction by FISH analysis of the occurrence of Wilms tumor in aniridia patients. Am J Med Genet 2002;108: 285–289.
6. Pagon RA. Ocular coloboma. Surv Ophthalmol 1981;25:223–236.
7. Onwochei B, Simon JW, Bateman JB, et al. Ocular colobomata. Surv Ophthalmol 2000;45:175–194.
8. Russell-Eggitt IM, Blake KD, Wyse RKH. The eye in the CHARGE association. Br J Ophthalmol 1990;74:421–426.
9. Berends MJ, Tan-Sindhunata G, Leegte B, et al. Phenotypic variability of cat-eye syndrome. Genet Counsel 2001;12:23–34.
10. White BV, Fulton MN. A rare pupillary defect. J Hered 1937;28:177–179.
11. Thompson HS, Miller NR. Disorders of pupillary function, accommodation and lacrimation. In Miller NR, Newman NJ. Walsh and Hoyt's Clinical Neuro-Ophthalmology. 5th ed, Vol 1. Baltimore, Williams &Wilkins, 1998:961–1040.
12. de Schweinitz GE. Diseases of the Eye. 10th ed. Philadelphia, WB Saunders, 1924.
13. Von Noorden GK, Baller RS. The chamber angle in slit-pupil. Arch Ophthalmol 1963;70:598–602.
14. Lindberg JG. Beiträge zurklinischen bilde der angeborenen sog: ''Kerben am pupillarande'' und zu ihrer entwicklungsgeschichtlichen erklärung. Klin Monatsbl Augenheilkd 1920;65:723–733.
15. Andrade C. A peculiar form of peripheral neuropathy: Familial atypical generalized amyloidosis with special involvement of peripheral nerves. Brain 1952;75: 408–427.
16. Lessell S, Wolf PA, Benson MD, et al. Scalloped pupils in familial amyloidosis. N Engl J Med 1975;293:914–915.
17. Bosanquet RC, Johnson GJ. Peninsula pupil: Anomaly unique to Newfoundland and Labrador? Arch Ophthalmol 1981;99:1824–1826.
18. Gangadharan M, Menon G. Bilaterally symmetrical isolated corectopia: A case report. Jpn J Ophthalmol 1986;30:266–268.
19. Byles DB, Nischal KK, Cheng H. Ectopia lentis et pupillae. A hypothesis revisited. Ophthalmology 1998;105:1331–1336.
20. Li TM. Congenital total bilateral ophthalmoplegia. Am J Ophthalmol 1923;6: 816–821.
21. Salleras A, de Zarate JCL. Recessive sex-linked inheritance of external ophthalmoplegia and myopia coincident with other dysplasias. Br J Ophthalmol 1950; 18:213–255.
22. McPherson E, Robertson C, Cammarano A, et al. Dominantly inherited ptosis, strabismus and ectopic pupils. Clin Genet 1976;10:21–26.
23. Selhorst JB, Hoyt WF, Feinsod M, et al. Midbrain corectopia. Arch Neurol 1976;33:193–195.
24. Bril V, Sharpe JA, Ashby P. Midbrain asterixis. Ann Neurol 1979;6:362–364.
25. Fisher CM. Oval pupils. Arch Neurol 1980;37:502–503.
26. Merin S, Crawford JS, Cardarelli J. Hyperplastic persistent pupillary membrane. Am J Ophthalmol 1971;78:717–719.
27. Gutmann ED, Goldberg MF. Persistent pupillary membrane and other ocular abnormalities. Arch Ophthalmol 1976;94:156–157.
28. Pandey SK, Ram J, Werner L et al. Pupillary abnormality. Br J Ophthalmol 2000;84:554.
29. Jaffe NS, Knie P. True polycoria. Am J Ophthalmol 1952;35:253–255.
30. Waring GO III, Rodrigues MM, Laibson PR. Anterior chamber cleavage syndrome: A stepladder classification. Surv Ophthalmol 1975;20:3–27.
31. Hofeldt GT, Simon JW. Polycoria, miosis, and amblyopia. J AAPOS 2002;6: 328–329.
32. Veirs ER, Brown W. Congenital miosis associated with a narrow angle of the anterior chamber and abnormally placed iris tissue. Arch Ophthalmol 1961;65: 59–60.

33. Harms WA. Congential eye defects. J Kansas Med Soc 1977;78:497–502.
34. Holth S, Berner S. Congenital miosis or pinhole pupils owing to developmental faults of the dilator muscle. Br J Ophthalmol 1923;7:401–419.
35. Van Lint A. Congenital miosis. Bull Soc Belge Ophtalmol 1940;79:24–25.
36. Agoston I, Grof P. La miose congénitale et l'albinisme. Ophthalmologica 1968; 155:399–408.
37. Ramsey MS, Fine BS, Shields JA, et al. The Marfan syndrome. Am J Ophthalmol 1973;76:102–116.
38. Kissel P, Cordier J, Raspiller A, et al. Microcorie, manifestation ophtalmologique rare des malformations associées oculo-vertebro-acromeliques. Otoneuroophtalmol 1973;45:241–245.
39. Dick DJ, Newman PK, Cleland PG. Hereditary spastic ataxia with congenital miosis: Four cases in one family. Br J Ophthalmol 1983;67:97–101.
40. Sjaastad O, Aasly J, Stormorken H, et al. A new hereditary synrome with a bleeding tendency, extreme miosis, spasms, dyslexia, thrombocytopathia, etc: Pupillometric, evaporimetric, and ophthalmological observations. Acta Ophthalmol 1992;70:713–720.
41. Caccamise WC, Townes PL. Bilateral congenital mydriasis. Am J Ophthalmol 1976;81:515–517.
42. Richardson P, Schulenburg WE. Bilateral congenital mydriasis. Br J Ophthalmol 1992;76:632–633.
43. Gräf MH, Jungherr A. Congenital mydriasis, failure of accommodation, and patent ductus arteriosus. Arch Ophthalmol 2002;120:509–510.
44. Laor N, Korczyn AD. Waardenburg syndrome with a fixed dilated pupil. Br J Ophthalmol 1978;62:491–494.
45. Drews RC. Heterochromia iridum with coloboma of the optic disc. Arch Ophthalmol 1973;90:437.
46. Cohen S, Dusman E, Blumberg S, et al. In vitro contraction of the pupillary sphincter by substance P and its stable analogs. Invest Ophthalmol Vis Sci 1981; 20:717–721.
47. Sarkies NJC, Sanders MD, Gautier-Smith PC. Episodic unilateral mydriasis and migraine. Am J Ophthalmol 1985;99:217–218.
48. Safran AB, Janin Y, Roth A. Bitemporal palsy of the pupillary sphincters: A sign of diffuse circulatory insufficiency. J Clin Neuroophthalmol 1983;3:185–189.
49. Baumann J, Insler MS. Pupillary abnormalities in keratoconus. Ann Ophthalmol 1985;17:766–767.
50. Kawana K, Okamoto F, Nose H, et al. A case of angle closure glaucoma caused by plateau iris and Adie's pupil. Am J Ophthalmol 2003;135:717–718.
51. Feibel RM, Perlmutter JC. Anisocoria in the pigmentary dispersion syndrome. Am J Ophthalmol 1990;110:657–660.
52. Krebs DB, Colquhoun J, Ritch R, et al. Asymmetric pigment dispersion syndrome in a patient with unilateral Horner's syndrome. Am J Ophthalmol 1989; 108:737–738.
53. Murthy S, Hawksworth N. Asymmetric pigment dispersion in a patient with the unilateral Adie pupil. Am J Ophthalmol 2001;132:410–411.
54. Larsson S, Osterlind G. Studies on the cause of senile miosis and rigidity of the pupil. Acta Ophthalmol 1944;21:1–25.
55. Urrets-Zavalia A Jr. Fixed, diated pupil, iris atrophy and secondary glaucoma: Distinct clinical entity following penetrating keratoplasty in keratoconus. Am J Ophthalmol 1963;56:257–265.
56. Bertelsen TI, Seim V. The cause of irreversible mydriasis following keratoplasty in keratoconus: A preliminary report. Ophthalm Surg 1974;5:56–58.
57. Maurino V, Allan BDS, Stevens JD et al. Fixed dilated pupil (Urrets-Zavalia syndrome) after air/gas injection after deep lamellar keratoplasty for keratoconus. Am J Ophthalmol 2002;133:266–268.
58. Lam BL, Beck RW, Hall D, et al. Atonic pupil after cataract surgery. Ophthalmology 1989;96:589–590.
59. Halpern BL, Pavilack MA, Gallagher SP. The incidence of atonic pupil following cataract surgery. Arch Ophthalmol 1995;113:448–450.
60. Geerling G, Neppert B, Wirbelauer C, et al. Relative mydriasis after photorefractive keratectomy. J Refract Surg 2000;16:69–74.
61. Miyazawa H. Relative afferent pupillary defect in several types of optic neuropathy. Acta Soc Ophthalmol Jpn 1988;92:2103–2109.
62. Kardon R, Haupert C, Thompson HS. The relationship between static perimetry and the relative afferent pupillary defect. Am J Ophthalmol 1993;115:351–356.
63. Johnson L, Hill R, Bartholomew M. Correlation of afferent pupillary defect with visual field loss on automated perimetry. Ophthalmology 1988;95:1649–1653.
64. Thompson HS, Montague P, Cox TA, et al. The relationship between visual acuity, pupillary defect, and visual field loss. Am J Ophthalmol 1982;93: 681–688.
65. Bobak SP, Goodwin JA, Guevara RA, et al. Predictors of visual acuity and the relative afferent pupillary defect in optic neuropathy. Doc Ophthalmol 1999;97: 81–95.
66. Cox TA, Thompson HS, Corbett JJ. Relative afferent pupillary defects in optic neuritis. Am J Ophthalmol 1981;92:685–690.
67. Brown RH, Zilis JD, Lynch MG, et al. The afferent pupillary defect in asymmetric glaucoma. Arch Ophthalmol 1987;105:1540–1543.
68. Girkin CA. Evaluation of the pupillary light response as an objective measure of visual function. Ophthalmol Clin North Am 2003;16:143–153.
69. Wakakura M, Yokoe J. Evidence for preserved direct pupillary light response in Leber's hereditary optic neuropathy. Br J Ophthalmol 1995;79:442–446.
70. Jacobson DM, Stone EM, Miller NR, et al. Relative afferent pupillary defects in patients with Leber's hereditary optic neuropathy and unilateral visual loss. Am J Ophthalmol 1998;126:291–295.
71. Ludtke H, Kreigbaum C, Leo-Kottler B, et al. Pupillary light reflexes in patients with Leber's hereditary optic neuropathy. Graefes Arch Clin Exp Ophthalmol 1999;237:207–211.
72. Bremner FD, Shallo-Hoffman J, Riordan-Eva P, et al. Comparing pupil function with visual function in patients with Leber's hereditary optic neuropathy. Invest Ophthalmol Vis Sci 1999;40:2528–2534.
73. Alford MA, Nerad JA, Carter KD. Predictive value of the initial quantified relative afferent pupillary defect in 19 consecutive patients with traumatic optic neuropathy. Ophthal Plast Reconstr Surg 2001;17:323–327.
74. Newsome DA, Milton RC, Gass JDM. Afferent pupillary defect in macular degeneration. Am J Ophthalmol 1981;92:396–402.
75. Thompson H, Watzke R, Weinstein J. Pupillary dysfunction in macular disease. Trans Am Ophthalmol Soc 1980;78:311–317.
76. Kerrison JB, Buchanan K, Rosenberg ML, et al. Quantification of optic nerve axon loss associated with a relative afferent pupillary defect in the monkey. Arch Ophthalmol 2001;119:1333–1341.
77. Folk JC, Thompson HS, Han D, et al. Visual function abnormalities in central serous retinopathy. Arch Ophthalmol 1984;102:1299–1302.
78. Bovino JA, Burton TC. Measurement of the relative afferent pupillary defect in retinal detachment. Am J Ophthalmol 1980;90:19–21.
79. Folk JC, Thompson HS, Farmer SG, et al. Relative afferent pupillary defect in eyes with retinal detachment. Ophthalm Surg 1987;18:757–759.
80. Servais GE, Thompson HS, Hayreh SS. Relative afferent pupillary defect in central retinal vein occlusion. Ophthalmology 1986;93:301–303.
81. DuBois LG, Sadun AA. Occlusion-induced contralateral afferent pupillary defect. Am J Ophthalmol 1989;107:306–307.
82. Lam BL, Thompson HS. Relative afferent pupillary defect induced by patching (the other eye). Am J Ophthalmol 1989;107:305–306.
83. Lam BL, Thompson HS. An anisocoria produces a small relative afferent pupillary defect in the eye with the smaller pupil. J Neuroophthalmol 1999;19: 153–159.
84. Portnoy JZ, Thompson HS, Lennarson L, et al. Pupillary defects in amblyopia. Am J Ophthalmol 1983;96:609–614.
85. Kase M, Nagata R, Yoshida A, et al. Pupillary light reflex in amblyopia. Invest Ophthalmol Vis Sci 1984;25:467–471.
86. Firth AY. Pupillary responses in amblyopia. Br J Ophthalmol 1990;74:676–680.
87. Ramsay AS, Ray-Chaudhuri N, Dayan M, et al. Quantification of relative afferent pupillary defects induced by posterior sub-Tenon's, peribulbar, and retrobulbar anaesthetics. Br J Ophthalmol 2001;85:1445–1446.
88. Striph GG, Halperin LS, Stevens JL, et al. Afferent pupillary defect caused by hyphema. Am J Ophthalmol 1988;106:352.
89. Bullock JD. Relative afferent pupillary defect in the "better" eye. J Clin Neuroophthalmol 1990;10:45–51.
90. Sadun AA, Libondi T. Transmission of light through cataracts. Am J Ophthalmol 1990;110:710–712.
91. Sadun AA, Bassi CJ, Lessell S. Why cataracts do not produce afferent pupillary defects. Am J Ophthalmol 1990;110:712–714.
92. Lam BL, Thompson HS. A unilateral cataract produces a relative afferent pupil defect in the contralateral eye. Ophthalmology 1990;97:334–337.
93. Bell RA, Thompson HS. Relative afferent pupillary defect in optic tract hemianopias. Am J Ophthalmol 1978;85:538–540.
94. Loewenfeld IE. Pupils in optic tract lesions. J Clin Neuroophthalmol 1983;3: 221–222.
95. Newman SA, Miller NR. The optic tract syndrome: Neuro-ophthalmologic considerations. Arch Ophthalmol 1983;101:1241–1250.
96. Cox TA, Drewes CP. Contraction anisocoria resulting from half-field illumination. Am J Ophthalmol 1984;97:577–582.
97. Ellis CJK. Afferent pupillary defect in pineal region tumour. J Neurol Neurosurg Psychiatry 1984;47:739–741.
98. Forman S, Behrens MM, Odel J, et al. Relative afferent pupillary defect with normal visual function. Arch Ophthalmol 1990;108:1074–1075.
99. Eliott D, Cunningham ET Jr, Miller NR. Fourth nerve paresis and ipsilateral relative afferent pupillary defect without visual sensory disturbance: A sign of contralateral dorsal midbrain disease. J Clin Neuroophthalmol 1991;11: 169–171.
100. King JT Jr, Galetta SL, Flamm ES. Relative afferent pupillary defect with normal vision in a glial brainstem tumor. Neurology 1991;41:945–946.
101. Wilhelm H, Wilhelm B, Petersen D, et al. Relative afferent pupillary defects in patients with geniculate and retrogeniculate lesions. Neuro-ophthalmology 1996; 16:219–224.
102. Tychsen L, Hoyt WF. Relative afferent pupillary defect in congenital occipital hemianopia. Am J Ophthalmol 1985;100:345–346.
103. Thompson H. Functional visual loss. Am J Ophthalmol 1985;100:209–213.
104. Kosmorsky GS, Tomsak RL, Diskin DK. Absence of the relative afferent pupillary defect with monocular temporal visual field loss. J Clin Neuroophthalmol 1992;12:181–191.
105. Kawasaki A, Moore P, Kardon RH. Long-term fluctuation of relative afferent

pupillary defect in subjects with normal visual function. Am J Ophthalmol 1996; 122:875–882.

106. Kawasaki A, Moore P, Kardon RH. Variability of the relative afferent pupillary defect. Am J Ophthalmol 1995;120:622–633.

107. Seybold ME, Yoss RE, Hollenhorst RW, et al. Pupillary abnormalities associated with tumors of the pineal region. Neurology 1971;21:232–237.

108. Barricks ME, Flynn JT, Kushner BJ. Paradoxical pupillary responses in congenital stationary night blindness. Arch Ophthalmol 1977;95:1800–1804.

109. Frank JW, Kushner BJ, France TD. Paradoxical pupillary phenomena: A review of patients with pupillary constriction to darkness. Arch Ophthalmol 1988;106: 1564–1566.

110. Sobol WM, Kimura AE, Kardon RH, et al. Pupillary constriction to darkness in a patient with blue-cone monochromatism. J Clin Neuroophthalmol 1991;11: 53–54.

111. Flynn JT, Kazarian E, Barricks M. Paradoxical pupil in congenital achromatopsia. Intl Ophthalmol 1981;3:91–96.

112. Loewenfeld IE. "Simple, central" anisocoria: A common condition, seldom recognized. Trans Am Acad Ophthalmol Otolaryngol 1977;83:832–839.

113. Lam BL, Thompson HS, Corbett JJ. The prevalence of simple anisocoria. Am J Ophthalmol 1987;104:69–73.

114. Lam BL, Thompson HS, Walls R. Effect of light on the prevalence of simple anisocoria. Ophthalmology 1996;103:790–793.

115. Safran AB, Petrovic D, Roth A, et al. Les limites de l'anisocorie physiologique. Bull Mem Soc Fr Ophtalmol 1984;95:268–271.

116. Brodsky MC, Sharp GB, Fritz KJ, et al. Idiopathic alternating anisocoria. Am J Ophthalmol 1992;114:509–510.

117. Loewenfeld I, Newsome D. Iris mechanics, part I and part II. Am J Ophthalmol 1971;71:347–362 (Part I) (Part II, Newsome and Loewenfeld) 553–573.

118. Thompson H. Johann Friedrich Horner (1831–1886). Am J Ophthalmol 1986; 102:792–795.

119. Loewenfeld I. The Pupil: Anatomy, Physiology and Clinical Applications. Ames, IA and Detroit, MI: Iowa State University Press in collaboration with Wayne State University Press, 1993.

120. Maloney WF, Younge BR, Moyer NJ. Evaluation of the causes and accuracy of pharmacologic localization in Horner's syndrome. Am J Ophthalmol 1980; 90:394–402.

121. Van der Wiel HL, Van Gijn J. No enophthalmos in Horner's syndrome. J Neurol Neurosurg Psychiatry 1987;50:498.

122. Nielsen PJ. Upside-down ptosis in patients with Horner's syndrome. Acta Ophthalmol 1983;61:952–957.

123. Morales J, Brown SM, Abdul-Rahim AS, et al. Ocular effects of apraclonidine in Horner syndrome. Arch Ophthalmol 2000;118:951–954.

124. Brown SM, Aouchiche R, Freedman KA. The utility of 0.5% apraclonidine in the diagnosis of Horner syndrome. Arch Ophthalmol 2003;121:1201–1203.

125. Wilhelm H, Ochsner H, Kopyziok E, et al. Horner's syndrome: A retrospective analysis of 90 cases and recommendations for clinical handling. German J Ophthalmol 1992;1:96–102.

126. Flatau E. Le phénomène nuquo-mydriatique. Rev Neurol 1921;37:1200–1205.

127. Pilley S, Thompson H. Pupillary "dilatation lag" in Horner's syndrome. Br J Ophthalmol 1975;59:731–735.

128. Van der Wiel HL, Van Gijn J. Horner's syndrome: Criteria for oculo-sympathetic denervation. J Neurol Sci 1982;56:293–298.

129. Verdick R, Thompson HS. Infrared videography of the eyes. J Ophthalm Photogr 1991;13:19–21.

130. Krzizok T, Gräf M, Kraus S. Foto- und videografische Messung des Dilatationsdefizits zur Differentialdiagnose des Horner-Syndroms. Ophthalmologe 1995; 92:125–131.

131. Smith SA, Smith SE. Bilateral Horner's syndrome: Detection and occurrence. J Neurol Neurosurg Psychiatry 1999;66:48–51.

132. Diesenhouse MC, Palay DA, Newman NJ, et al. Acquired heterochromia with Horner syndrome in two adults. Ophthalmology 1992;99:1815–1817.

133. Romano A, Kurchin A, Rudich R, et al. Ocular manifestations after upper dorsal sympathectomy. Ann Ophthalmol 1979;11:1083–1086.

134. Thompson B, Corbett J, Kline L, et al. Pseudo-Horner's syndrome. Arch Neurol 1982;108:111.

135. Thompson HS. Diagnosing Horner's syndrome. Trans Am Acad Ophthalmol Otolaryngol 1977;83:840–842.

136. Bralliar B, Skarf B, Owens J. Ophthalmic use of cocaine and the urine test for bezoyl ecgonine. N Engl J Med 1989;320:1757–1758.

137. Jacobson DM, Berg R, Grinstead GF, Kruse JR. Duration of positive urine for cocaine metabolite after ophthalmic administration: Implications for testing patients with suspected Horner's syndrome using ophthalmic cocaine. Am J Ophthalmol 2001;131:742–747.

138. Kardon RH, Denison CE, Brown CK, et al. Critical evaluation of the cocaine test in the diagnosis of Horner's syndrome. Arch Ophthalmol 1990;108:384–387.

139. Amonoo-Kuofi HS. Horner's syndrome revisited: with an update of the central pathway. Clin Anat 1999;12:345–361.

140. Nagy AN, Hayman LA, Diaz-Marchan PJ, et al. Horner's syndrome due to first-order neuron lesions of the oculosympathetic pathway. AJR Am J Roentgenol 1997;169:581–584.

141. Stone WM, de Toledo J, Romanul FCA. Horner's syndrome due to hypothalamic

infarction: Clinical, radiologic and pathologic correlations. Arch Neurol 1986;43:199–200.

142. Austin CP, Lessell S. Horner's syndrome from hypothalamic infarction. Arch Neurol 1991;48:332–334.

143. Rosetti AO, Reichhart MD, Bogousslavsky J. Central Horner's syndrome with contralateral ataxic hemiparesis: a diencephalic alternate syndrome. Neurology 2003;61:334–338.

144. Coppeto JR. Superior oblique paresis and contralateral Horner's syndrome. Ann Ophthalmol 1983;15:681–683.

145. Guy JR, Day AL, Mickle JP, et al. Contralateral trochlear nerve paresis and ipsilateral Horner's syndrome. Am J Ophthalmol 1989;107:73–76.

146. Müri RM, Baumgartner RW. Horner's syndrome and contralateral trochlear nerve palsy. Neuroophthalmology 1995;15:161–163.

147. Kellen RI, Burde RM, Hodges FJ 3rd, et al. Central bilateral sixth nerve palsy associated with a unilateral preganglionic Horner's syndrome. J Clin Neuroophthalmol 1988;8:179–184.

148. Hornsten G. Wallenberg's syndrome. I. General symptomatology, with special reference to visual disturbances and imbalance. Acta Neurol Scand 1974;50: 434–446.

149. Tiliket C, Ventre J, Vighetto A, et al. Room tilt illusion: A central otolith dysfunction. Arch Neurol 1996;53:1259–1264.

150. Hornsten G. Wallenberg's syndrome. II. Oculomotor and oculostatic disturbances. Acta Neurol Scand 1974;50:447–468.

151. Baloh RW, Yee RD, Honrubia V. Eye movements in patients with Wallenberg's syndrome. Ann NY Acad Sci 1981;374:600–613.

152. Fisher CM, Tapia J. Lateral medullary infarction extending to the lower pons. J Neurol Neurosurg Psychiatry 1987;50:620–624.

153. Kim JS. Pure lateral medullary infarction: Clinical-radiological correlation of 130 acute, consecutive patients. Brain 2003;126:1864–1872.

154. Smith DB, Demasters BKK. Demyelinative disease presenting as Wallenberg's syndrome: Report of a patient. Stroke 1981;12:877–878.

155. Pomerantz H. Isolated Horner syndrome and syrinx of the cervical spinal cord. Am J Ophthalmol 2002;133:702–704.

156. Kramer W, van der Does de Willebois JJM. Occlusion of the anterior spinal artery in the cervical cord with sympathetic spasm of the pupil on finger movement. Folia Psychiatr Neurol 1959;62:458–464.

157. Furukawa T, Toyokura Y. Alternating Horner syndrome. Arch Neurol 1974;30: 311–313.

158. Ottomo M, Heimburger RF. Alternating Horner's syndrome and hyperhidrosis due to dural adhesions following cervical spinal cord injury. J Neurosurg 1980; 53:97–100.

159. Tan E, Kansu T, Saygi S, et al. Alternating Horner's syndrome: A case report and review of the literature. Neuroophthalmology 1990;10:19–22.

160. Kline LB, McCluer SM, Bonikowski FP. Oculopathic spasm with cervical spinal cord injury. Arch Neurol 1984;41:61–64.

161. Moniz E, Czarnecki J. The alternating Horner's syndrome: Is it or isn't it? Am J Ophthalmol 1980;90:577.

162. Thompson H, Maxner C, Corbett J. Horner's syndrome due to damage to the preganglionic neuron of the oculosympathetic pathway: In Huber A, ed. Sympathicus und Auge. Stuttgart: Ferdinand Enke, 1990:99–104.

163. Arcasoy SM, Jett JR. Superior pulmonary sulcus tumors and Pancoast's syndrome. N Engl J Med 1997;337:1370–1376.

164. Vaghadia H, Spittle M. Newly recognized syndrome in the neck. J R Soc Med 1983;76:799.

165. Gedde SJ, Clark FJ, Johns JA, et al. Horner's syndrome as a complication of pacemaker insertion. Am J Ophthalmol 1991;112:97–99.

166. Barbut D, Gold JP, Heinemann MH, et al. Horner's syndrome after coronary artery bypass surgery. Neurology 1996;19:181–184.

167. Schachner SM, Reynolds AC. Horner syndrome during lumbar epidural analgesia for obstetrics. Obstet Gynecol 1982;59:31S.

168. Jeret JS, Mazurek AA. Acute postpartum Horner's syndrome due to epidural anesthesia. Arch Ophthalmol 1995;113:560.

169. Davis P, Watson D. Horner's syndrome and vocal cord paralysis as a complication of percutaneous internal jugular vein catheterisation in adults. Anaesthesia 1982;37:587–588.

170. Gasch AT. Horner's syndrome secondary to chest tube placement. Ann Ophthalmol 1996;28:235–239.

171. Parkinson D, Johnston J, Chaudhuri A. Sympathetic connections of the fifth and sixth cranial nerves. Anat Rec 1978;191:221–226.

172. Parkinson D. Further observations on the sympathetic pathways to the pupil. Anat Rec 1988;220:108–109.

173. Biousse V, Touboul P-J, D'Anglejan-Chatillon J, et al. Ophthalmologic manifestations of internal carotid artery dissection. Am J Ophthalmol 1998;126: 565–577.

174. Monteiro MLR, Coppeto JR. Horner's syndrome associated with carotid artery atherosclerosis. Am J Ophthalmol 1988;105:93–94.

175. Cengiz K, Aykin A, Diren B. Intrathoracic goiter with hyperthyroidism, tracheal compression, superior vena cava syndrome and Horner's syndrome. Chest 1990; 87:1005–1006.

176. Inci S, Bertan V, Kansu T, et al. Horner's syndrome due to jugular venous ectasia. Childs Nerv Syst 1995;11:533–535.

177. Boon P, de Reuck J, van de Velde E. Villaret's syndrome due to thrombosis of the jugular vein. Clin Neurol Neurosurg 1990;92:337–341.
178. Keane JR. Oculosympathetic paresis: Analysis of 100 hospitalized patients. Arch Neurol 1979;36:13–16.
179. Liu GT, Deskin RW, Bienfang DC. Horner's syndrome caused by intra-oral trauma. J Clin Neuroophthalmol 1992;12:110–115.
180. Worthington JP, Snape L. Horner's syndrome secondary to a basilar skull fracture after maxillofacial trauma. J Oral Maxillofac Surg 1998;56:996–1000.
181. Striph GG, Burde RM. Abducens nerve palsy and Horner's syndrome revisited. J Clin Neuroophthalmol 1988;8:13–17.
182. Smith EF, Santamarina L, Wolintz AH. Herpes zoster ophthalmicus as a cause of Horner syndrome. J Clin Neuroophthalmol 1993;13:250–253.
183. Myles WM, Maxner CE. Localizing value of concurrent sixth nerve paresis and postganglionic Horner's syndrome. Can J Ophthalmol 1994;29:39–42.
184. Trobe JD, Glaser JS, Post JD. Meningiomas and aneurysms of the cavernous sinus. Arch Ophthalmol 1978;96:457–467.
185. Riley FC, Moyer NJ. Oculosympathetic paresis associated with cluster headaches. Am J Ophthalmol 1971;72:763–768.
186. Grimson BS, Thompson HS. Raeder's syndrome: A clinical review. Surv Ophthalmol 1980;24:199–210.
187. Goadsby PJ. Raeder's syndrome: Paratrigeminal paralysis of the oculopupillary sympathetic system. J Neurol Neurosurg Psychiatry 2002;72:297–299.
188. Thompson HS, Mensher JH. Adrenergic mydriasis in Horner's syndrome: Hydroxyamphetamine test for diagnosis of postganglionic defects. Am J Ophthalmol 1971;72:472–480.
189. Thompson HS, Mensher JH. Hydroxyamphetamine test in Horner's syndrome. Am J Ophthalmol 1975;79:523–526.
190. Cremer SA, Thompson HS, Digre KB, et al. Hydroxyamphetamine mydriasis in Horner's syndrome. Am J Ophthalmol 1990;110:71–76.
191. Cremer SA, Thompson HS, Digre KB, et al. Hydroxyamphetamine mydriasis in normal subjects. Am J Ophthalmol 1990;110:66–70.
192. Donahue SP, Lavin PJM, Digre K. False-negative hydroxyamphetamine (Paredrine) test in acute Horner's syndrome. Am J Ophthalmol 1996;122:900–901.
193. Wilhelm H, Schäffer E. Pholedrin zur Lokalisation des Horner-Syndroms. Klin Monatsbl Augenheilkd 1994;204:169–175.
194. Bates AT, Chamberlain S, Champion M, et al. Pholedrine: A substitute for hydroxyamphetamine as a diagnostic eyedrop test in Horner syndrome. J Neurol Neurosurg Psychiatry 1995;58:215–217.
195. Oono S, Inoue T. Development of supersensitivity of the pupil in Horner's syndrome: Case report. Neuroophthalmology 1991;11:241–245.
196. Jeffrey AR, Ellis FJ, Repka MX, et al. Pediatric Horner syndrome. JAAPOS 1998;2:159–167.
197. Woodruff G, Buncic JR, Morin JD. Horner's syndrome in children. J Pediatr Ophthalmol Strabis 1988;25:40–44.
198. Sauer C, Levinsohn MW. Horner's syndrome in childhood. Neurology 1976;26:216–220.
199. Hyodo T, Kase M, Shintomi Y. Two cases of congenital Horner's syndrome. Folia Ophthalmol Jpn 1983;34:387–390.
200. Weinstein JM, Zweifel TJ, Thompson HS. Congenital Horner's syndrome. Arch Ophthalmol 1980;98:1074–1078.
201. Shewmon DA. Unilateral straight hair in congenital Horner syndrome due to stellate ganglion tumor. Ann Neurol 1983;13:345–346.
202. Kuramoto Y, Sasaki Y, Tagami H, et al. Congenital Horner's syndrome. Arch Dermatol 1989;125:1145–1146.
203. Saito H. Congenital Horner's syndrome with unilateral facial flushing. J Neurol Neurosurg Psychiatry 1990;53:85–86.
204. Sears ML, Kier EL, Chavis RM. Horner's syndrome caused by occlusion of the vascular supply to sympathetic ganglia. Am J Ophthalmol 1974;77:717–724.
205. George NDL, Gonzalez G, Hoyt CS. Does Horner's syndrome in infancy require investigation? Br J Ophthalmol 1998;82:51–54.
206. Sayed AK, Miller BA, Lack EE, et al. Heterochromia iridis and Horner's syndrome due to paravertebral neurilemmoma. J Surg Oncol 1983;22:15–16.
207. Borzyskowski M, Harris RF, Jones RW. The congenital varicella syndrome. Eur J Pediatr 1981;137:335–338.
208. Bayatpour M, Logan J, Perry HP, et al. Horner's syndrome due to congenital cytomegalovirus infection. South Med J 1982;75:220–221.
209. Reader AL 3rd, Massey EW. Fibromuscular dysplasia of the carotid artery: A cause of congenital Horner's syndrome? Ann Ophthalmol 1980;12:326–330.
210. Ellenberg DJ, Spector LD, Lee A. Flea collar pupil. Ann Emerg Med 1994;21:1170.
211. Flach AJ, Donahue ME. Pet flea and tick collar-induced anisocoria. Arch Ophthalmol 1994;112:586.
212. McDonald JE, El-Mpatassem AM, Decker BB. Effect of brimonidine tartrate ophthalmic solution 0.2% on pupil size in normal eyes under different luminance conditions. J Cataract Refract Surg 2001;27:560–564.
213. Ksiazek SM, Slamovits TL, Rosen CE, et al. Fascicular arrangement in partial oculomotor paresis. Am J Ophthalmol 1994;118:97–103.
214. Shuaib A, Israelian G, Lee MA. Mesencephalic hemorrhage and unilateral pupillary deficit. J Clin Neuroophthalmol 1989;9:47–49.
215. Hashimoto M, Ohtsuka K. Bilateral internal ophthalmoplegia as a feature of

oculomotor fascicular syndrome disclosed by magnetic resonance imaging. Am J Ophthalmol 1998;125:121–123.
216. Kerr FWL, Hollowell OW. Location of pupillomotor and accommodation fibers in the oculomotor nerve: Experimental observation on paralytic mydriasis. J Neurol Neurosurg Psychiatry 1964;27:473–481.
217. Lesser RL, Simon RM, Leon H, et al. Cryptococcal meningitis and internal ophthalmoplegia. Am J Ophthalmol 1979;87:682–687.
218. McGravey AR. A dilated unreactive pupil in acute bacterial meningitis: Oculomotor nerve inflammation versus herniation. Pediatr Emerg Care 1989;5:187–188.
219. Pelak VS, Galetta SL, Grossman RI, et al. Evidence for preganglionic pupillary involvement in superficial siderosis. Neurology 1999;53:1130–1132.
220. Payne JW, Adamkiewicz J Jr. Unilateral internal ophthalmoplegia with intracranial aneurysm: Report of a case. Am J Ophthalmol 1969;68:349–352.
221. Bartleson JD, Trautmann JC, Sundt TM Jr. Minimal oculomotor nerve palsy secondary to unruptured intracranial aneurysm. Arch Neurol 1986;43:1015–1020.
222. Walsh FB, Hoyt WF. Clinical Neuro-Ophthalmology. 3rd ed, Vol 1. Baltimore, Williams & Wilkins, 1969:494.
223. Kaye-Wilson LG, Gibson R, Bell JE, et al. Oculomotor nerve neurinoma: Early detection by magnetic resonance imaging. Neuroophthalmology 1994;14:37–41.
224. Wilhelm H, Klier R, Tóth B, et al. Oculomotor nerve paresis starting a isolated internal ophthalmoplegia. Neuroophthalmology 1995;15:211–215.
225. Thompson HS. Adie's syndrome. Some new observations. Trans Am Ophthalmol Soc 1977;75:587–626.
226. Thompson HS. A classification of "tonic pupils." In Thompson HS, Daroff R, Frisén L, et al, eds. Topics in Neuro-Ophthalmology. Baltimore, Williams & Wilkins, 1979.
227. Rogers JW. Internal ophthalmoplegia following chickenpox. Arch Ophthalmol 1964;71:617–618.
228. Levy NS, Kramer SG, de Barros T. Pupillary and accommodative abnormalities in the Vogt-Koyanagi-Harada syndrome. Am J Ophthalmol 1970;69:582–588.
229. Victor DI, Green WR, Stark WJ, et al. A non-permanent tonic pupil in rheumatoid arteritis. Can J Neurol Sci 1977;4:209–212.
230. Sen DK. Isolated pupillary paralysis in a case of herpes zoster. J Pediatr Ophthalmol Strabis 1979;16:33–34.
231. Sundaram MBM. Pupillary abnormalities in congenital neurosyphilis. Can J Neurol Sci 1985;12:134–135.
232. Haider S. Tonic pupil in lymphomatoid granulomatosis. J Clin Neuroophthalmol 1993;13:38–39.
233. Brooks-Kayal AR, Liu GT, Menacker SJ, et al. Tonic pupil and orbital glial-neural hamartoma in infancy. Am J Ophthalmol 1995;119:809–811.
234. Massey EW. Pupillary dysautonomia and migraine: Is Adie's pupil caused by migraine? Headache 1981;21:143–146.
235. Currie J, Lessell S. Tonic pupil with giant cell arteritis. Br J Ophthalmol 1984;68:135–138.
236. Monteiro MLR, Coppeto JR, Milani J. Iron mydriasis: Pupillary paresis from an occult intraocular foreign body. J Clin Neuroophthalmol 1993;13:254–257.
237. Bennett JL, Pelak VA, Mourelatos Z, et al. Acute sensorimotor polyneuropathy with tonic pupils and an abduction deficit: An unusual presentation of polyarteritis nodosa. Surv Ophthalmol 1999;43:341–344.
238. Bowie EM, Givre SJ. Tonic pupil and sarcoidosis. Am J Ophthalmol 2003;135:417–419.
239. Foroozan R, Buono LM, Savino PJ, et al. Tonic pupils from giant cell arteritis. Br J Ophthalmol 2003;87:510–512.
240. Newsome DA, Einaugler RB. Tonic pupil following retinal detachment surgery. Arch Ophthalmol 1971;86:233–234.
241. Bajart AM, Robb RM. Internal ophthalmoplegia following inferior oblique myectomy: A report of three cases. Ophthalmology 1979;86:1401–1406.
242. Lobes LA Jr, Bourgon P. Pupillary abnormalities induced by argon laser photocoagulation. Ophthalmology 1985;92:234–236.
243. Stromberg BV, Knibbe M. Anisocoria following reduction of bilateral orbital floor fractures. Ann Plast Surg 1988;21:486–488.
244. Pfeiffer N, Kommerell G. Sector palsy of the sphincter pupillae muscle after argon laser trabeculoplasty. Am J Ophthalmol 1991;111:511–512.
245. Corbett JJ, Nerad JA, Tse D, et al. Results of optic nerve sheath fenestration for pseudotumor cerebri: the lateral orbitotomy approach. Arch Ophthalmol 1988;106:1391–1397.
246. O'Connor M, Eustace P. Tonic pupil and lateral rectus palsy following dental anaesthesia. Neuroophthalmology 1983;3:205–208.
247. Patel JI, Jenkins L, Benjamin L, et al. Dilated pupils and loss of accommodation following diode panretinal photocoagulation with sub-tenon local anaesthetic in four cases. Eye 2002;16:628–632.
248. Miller RG, Nielsen SL, Sumner AJ. Hereditary sensory neuropathy and tonic pupils. Neurology 1976;26:931–935.
249. Williams D, Brust JCM, Abrams G, et al. Landry-Guillain-Barré syndrome with abnormal pupils and normal eye movements: A case report. Neurology 1979;29:1033–1036.
250. Fukushima M, Kawashima S, Hirokawa H, et al. A case of spinocerebellar degeneration associated with bilateral tonic pupil and downbeat nystagmus: An electrophysiological investigation. Folia Ophthalmol Jpn 1985;36:1117–1121.

251. Fletcher WA, Sharpe JA. Tonic pupils in neurosyphilis. Neurology 1986;36: 188–192.
252. Straub RH, Jeron A, Kerp L. The pupillary light reflex: Prevalence of pupillary autonomic neuropathy in diabetics using age-dependent and age-independent pupillary parameters. Ophthalmologica 1992;204:143–148.
253. Keltner JL, Swisher CN, Gay AJ, et al. Myotonic pupils in Charcot-Marie-Tooth disease: Successful relief of symptoms with 0.025% pilocarpine. Arch Ophthalmol 1975;93:1141–1148.
254. Hoyle C, Ewing DJ, Parker AC. Acute autonomic neuropathy in association with systemic lupus erythematosus. Ann Rheum Dis 1985;44:420–424.
255. Maitland CG, Scherokman BJ, Schiffman J, et al. Paraneoplastic tonic pupils. J Clin Neuroophthalmol 1985;5:99–104.
256. Bruno MK, Winterkorn JMS, Edgar MA, et al. Unilateral Adie pupil as sole ophthalmic sign of anti-Hu paraneoplastic syndrome. J Neuroophthalmol 2000; 20:248–249.
257. Feldman RG, Lessell S, Travers PH, et al. Neuro-ophthalmologic and neuropsychological effects of trichloroethylene intoxication: 18-year follow-up. Neurology 1984;34(Suppl 1):242.
258. Dressler M. Familiäres vorkommen von Adieschem syndrom mit hippus. Klin Wochenschr 1937;16:1013–1017.
259. Hough WH. Adie's syndrome in twins: A preliminary report. Med Ann DC 1941;10:137–140.
260. Dutton GN, Paul R. Adie syndrome in a child: Case report. J Pediatr Ophthalmol Strabis 1992;29:126.
261. Phillips PH, Newman NJ. Tonic pupil in a child. J Pediatr Ophthalmol Strabis 1996;33:331–332.
262. Firth AY. Adie syndrome: Evidence for refractive error and accommodative asymmetry as the cause of amblyopia. Am J Ophthalmol 1999;128:118–119.
263. Thompson HS, Bell RA, Bourgon P. The natural history of Adie's syndrome. In Thompson HS, Daroff R, Frisén L et al, eds. Topics in Neuro-Ophthalmology. Baltimore, Williams & Wilkins, 1979:96–99.
264. Piltz J. Experimentell erzeugter reziproker wechsel der pupillendifferenz bei progressiver paralyse. Neurol Zentralbl 1900;19:434–441.
265. Holmes G. Partial iridoplegia with symptoms of other diseases of the nervous system. Trans Ophthalmol Soc UK 1931;51:209–228.
266. Bell RA, Thompson HS. The symptoms of Adie's syndrome. In Thompson HS, Daroff R, Frisén L, eds. Topics in Neuro-Ophthalmology. Baltimore, Williams & Wilkins, 1979:99–104.
267. Jacobson DM, Hiner BC. Asymptomatic autonomic and sweat dysfunction in patients with Adie's syndrome. J Neuroophthalmol 1998;18:143–147.
268. Kimber J, Mitchell D, Mathias CJ. Chronic cough in the Holmes-Adie syndrome: Association in five cases with autonomic dysfunction. J Neurol Neurosurg Psychiatry 1998;65:583–586.
269. Thompson HS. Segmental palsy of the iris sphincter in Adie's syndrome. Arch Ophthalmol 1978;96:1615–1620.
270. Bell RA, Thompson HS. Ciliary muscle dysfunction in Adie's syndrome. Arch Ophthalmol 1978;96:638–642.
271. Warwick R. The ocular parasympathetic nerve supply and its mesencephalic sources. J Anat 1954;88:71–93.
272. Loewenfeld IE, Thompson HS. The tonic pupil: A reevaluation. Am J Ophthalmol 1967;63:46–87.
273. Loewenfeld IE, Thompson HS. Mechanism of tonic pupil. Ann Neurol 1981; 10:275–276.
274. Purcell JJ Jr, Krachmer JH, Thompson HS. Corneal sensation in Adie's syndrome. Am J Ophthalmol 1977;84:496–500.
275. Abbruzzese G, Abbruzzese M, Favale E, et al. Tonic vibration reflex in Holmes-Adie syndrome: An electrophysiological study. J Neurol Neurosurg Psychiatry 1979;42:943–947.
276. Pavesi G, Macaluso GM, Medici D, et al. On the cause of hyporeflexia in the Holmes-Adie syndrome. Electromyogr Clin Neurophysiol 1994;34:111–115.
277. Miyasaki JM, Ashby P, Sharpe JA, et al. On the cause of hyporeflexia in the Holmes-Adie syndrome. Neurology 1988;38:262–265.
278. Ulrich J. Morphological basis of Adie's syndrome. Eur Neurol 1980;19:390–395.
279. Selhorst JB, Madge G, Ghatak N. The neuropathology of the Holmes-Adie syndrome. Ann Neurol 1984;16:138.
280. Harriman DGF, Garland H. The pathology of Adie's syndrome. Brain 1968;91: 401–418.
281. Adler FH, Scheie HG. The site of disturbance in tonic pupils. Trans Am Ophthalmol Soc 1940;38:183–192.
282. Loewenfeld IE, Oono S. The iris as a pharmacologic indicator: The supposed instability of Mecholyl. Eye Ear Nose Throat Monthly 1966;45:69–77.
283. Leavitt JA, Wayman LL, Hodge DO, et al. Pupillary response to four concentrations of pilocarpine in normal subjects: Application to testing for Adie tonic pupil. Am J Ophthalmol 2003;133:333–336.
284. Younge BR, Buski ZJ. Tonic pupil: A simple screening test. Can J Ophthalmol 1976;11:295–299.
285. Slavin ML, Rosenberg RA. Dilute pilocarpine solutions in Adie's syndrome. Ann Ophthalmol Glaucoma 1994;26:205–206.
286. Jacobson DM, Olson KA. Influence on pupil size, anisocoria, and ambient light on pilocarpine miosis: Implications for supersensitivity testing. Ophthalmology 1993;100:275–280.
287. Jacobson DM, Vierkant RA. Comparison of cholinergic supersensitivity in third nerve palsy and Adie's syndrome. J Neuroophthalmol 1998;18:171–175.
288. Rosenberg ML. Miotic Adie's pupils. J Clin Neuroophthalmol 1989;9:43–45.
289. Kardon RH, Corbett JJ, Thompson HS. Segmental denervation and reinnervation of the iris sphincter as shown by infrared videographic transillumination. Ophthalmology 1998;105:313–321.
290. Leibovitch I, Kurtz S, Almog Y. Adie's tonic pupil-induced angle-closure glaucoma. Ophthalmologica 2002;216:71–72.
291. Flach AJ, Dolan BJ. The therapy of Adie's syndrome with dilute pilocarpine hydrochloride solutions. J Ocular Pharmacol 1985;1:353–362.
292. Wirtschafter JD, Herman WK. Low concentration eserine therapy for the tonic pupil (Adie) syndrome. Ophthalmology 1980;87:1037–1043.
293. Ishida O, Utsumi T, Sugasawa J, et al. Long-term follow-up study on the tonic pupil. Folia Ophthalmol Jpn 1993;44:1162–1167.
294. Thompson HS, Newsome DA, Loewenfeld IE. The fixed dilated pupil: Sudden iridoplegia or mydriatic drops? A simple diagnostic test. Arch Ophthalmol 1971; 86:21–27.
295. Thompson HS, Zackon DH, Czarnecki JSC. Tadpole-shaped pupils caused by segmental spasm of the iris dilator muscle. Am J Ophthalmol 1983;96:467–477.
296. Balaggan KS, Hugkulstone CE, Bremner FD. Episodic segmental iris dilator muscle spasm. The tadpole-shaped pupil. Arch Ophthalmol 2003;121:744–745.
297. Tang RA. Unilateral pupillary distortion: A case report. J Clin Neuroophthalmol 1985;5:105–108.
298. Boehme BI, Graef MH. Acquired segmental iris dilator muscle synkinesis due to deglutition. Arch Ophthalmol 1998;116:248–249.
299. Byrne P, Clough C. A case of Pourfour du Petit syndrome following parotidectomy. J Neurol Neurosurg Psychiatry 1990;53:1014.
300. Teeple E, Ferrer E, Ghia J, et al. Pourfour du Petit syndrome: Hypersympathetic dysfunctional state following a direct non-penetrating injury to the cervical sympathetic chain and brachial plexus. Anaesthesiology 1981;55:591–592.
301. Mathias CJ. Autonomic disorders and their recognition. N Engl J Med 1997; 336:721–724.
302. Wayne EM, Vukov JG. Eye findings in autonomic hyperreflexia. Ann Ophthalmol 1977;9:41–42.
303. Saper CB, DeMarchena O. Somatosympathetic reflex unilateral sweating and pupillary dilatation in a paraplegic man. Ann Neurol 1986;19:389–390.
304. Saito H, Nakazawa S. Episodic unilateral mydriasis after neck trauma. Neuro-ophthalmology 1990;10:209–216.
305. Hopf H. Intermittent Horner's syndrome on alternate sides: A hint for locating spinal lesions. J Neurol 1980;224:155.
306. Gianelli A. Sulle modificazioni del diametro pupillare nei movimenti de lateralità dei bulbi oculari. Richerche Psichiatr Neurol Antropol Filosof IV S 1907;8:433.
307. Tournay A. Le lois d'isocorie et de l'anisocorie normales et pathologiques. Bull Acad Méd Paris 1917;3:680.
308. Tournay A. Sur l'anisocorie normale dans le regard latéral extrème. Arch Ophthalmol 1927;44:574–576.
309. Sharpe JA, Glaser JS. Tournay's phenomenon: A reappraisal of anisocoria in lateral gaze. Am J Ophthalmol 1974;77:250–255.
310. Loewenfeld IE, Friedlander RP, McKinnon PFM. Pupillary inequality associated with lateral gaze (Tournay's phenomenon). Am J Ophthalmol 1974;78:449–469.
311. Woods D, O'Connor PS, Fleming R. Episodic unilateral mydriasis and migraine. Am J Ophthalmol 1984;98:229–234.
312. Mylius V, Braune HJ, Schepelmann K. Dysfunction of the pupillary light reflex following migraine headache. Clin Auton Res 2003;13:16–21.
313. DeMarinis M, Assenza S, Carletto F. Oculosympathetic alternations in migraine patients. Cephalalgia 1998;18:77–84.
314. van Pelt W, Andermann F. On the early onset of ophthalmoplegic migraine. Am J Dis Child 1964;107:628–631.
315. Edelson RN, Levy DE. Transient benign unilateral pupillary dilation in young adults. Arch Neurol 1974;31:12–14.
316. Evans RW, Jacobson DM. Transient anisocoria in a migraineur. Headache 2003; 43:416–418.
317. Purvin VA. Adie's tonic pupil secondary to migraine. J Neuroophthalmol 1995; 15:43–44.
318. Hallett M, Cogan DG. Episodic unilateral mydriasis in otherwise normal patients. Arch Ophthalmol 1970;84:130–136.
319. Jacobson DM. Benign episodic unilateral mydriasis: Clinical characteristics. Ophthalmology 1995;102:1623–1627.
320. Digre KB, Smoker WR, Johnston P, et al. Selective MR imaging approach for evaluation of patients with Horner's syndrome. AJNR Am J Neuroradiol 1992; 13:223–227.
321. Thompson HS, Pilley SFJ. Unequal pupils: A flow chart for sorting out the anisocorias. Surv Ophthalmol 1976;21:45–48.
322. Baptista AG, Souza HS. Pupillary abnormalities in myasthenia gravis: Report of a case. Neurology 1961;11:210–213.
323. Herishanu Y, Lavy S. Internal "ophthalmoplegia" in myasthenia gravis. Ophthalmologica 1971;163:302–305.
324. Dutton GN, Garson JA, Richardson RB. Pupillary fatigue in myasthenia gravis. Trans Ophthalmol Soc UK 1982;102:510–513.
325. Yamazaki A, Ishikawa S. Abnormal pupillary responses in myasthenia gravis: A pupillographic study. Br J Ophthalmol 1976;60:575–580.

326. Lepore FE, Sanborn GE, Slevin JT. Pupillary dysfunction in myasthenia gravis. Ann Neurol 1979;6:29–33.

327. Bryant RC. Asymmetrical pupillary slowing and degree of severity in myasthenia gravis. Ann Neurol 1980;7:288–289.

328. König H, Gassman HB, Jenzer G. Ocular involvement in benign botulism B. Am J Ophthalmol 1975;80:430–432.

329. Miller NR, Moses H. Ocular involvement in wound botulism. Arch Ophthalmol 1977;95:1788–1789.

330. Terranova W, Palumbo J, Breman JG. Ocular findings in botulism type B. JAMA 1979;241:475–477.

331. Friedman DI, Fortanasce VN, Sadun AA. Tonic pupils as a result of botulism. Am J Ophthalmol 1990;109:236–237.

332. O'Neill JH, Murray NM, Newsom-Davis J. The Lambert-Eaton myasthenic syndrome. A review of 50 cases. Brain 1988;111:577–596.

333. Clark CV, Newsom-Davis J, Sanders MD. Ocular autonomic nerve function in Lambert-Eaton myasthenic syndrome. Eye 1990;4:473–481.

334. Wirtz PW, de Keizer RJW, de Visser M, et al. Tonic pupils in Lambert-Eaton myasthenic syndrome. Muscle Nerve 2001;24:444–445.

335. Rubenstein AE, Horowitz SH, Bender AN. Cholinergic dysautonomia and Eaton-Lambert syndrome. Neurology 1979;29:720–723.

336. McLaren JW, Erie JC, Brubaker RF. Computerized analysis of pupillograms in studies of alertness. Invest Ophthalmol Vis Sci 1992;33:671–676.

337. Simmons FH. Jimson weed mydriasis in farmers. Am J Ophthalmol 1957;44:109–110.

338. Voltz R, Hohlfeld R, Liebler M, et al. Gardener's mydriasis. Lancet 1992;339:752.

339. Rubinfeld RS, Currie JN. Accidental mydriasis from blue nightshade "lipstick." J Clin Neuroophthalmol 1987;7:34–37.

340. Reader AL 3rd. Mydriasis from *Datura wrightii*. Am J Ophthalmol 1977;84:263–264.

341. Rubin MM, Sadoff RS, Cozzi GM. Unilateral mydriasis caused by transdermal scopolamine. Oral Surg Oral Med Oral Pathol 1990;70:569–570.

341a. Weir REP, Whitehead DEJ, Zaid FH, et al. Pupil blown by a puffer. Lancet 2004;363:1853.

342. Wyatt H. Ocular pharmacokinetics and convectional flow: Evidence from spatio-temporal analysis of mydriasis. J Ocular Pharmacol Ther 1996;12:441–459.

343. Monteiro MLR, Coppeto JR, Milani J. Iron mydriasis: Pupillary paresis from an occult intraocular foreign body. J Clin Neuroophthalmol 1993;13:254–257.

344. Dillon JR, Tyhurst CW, Yolton RL. The mydriatic effect of tropicamide on light and dark irides. J Am Optom Assoc 1977;48:653–658.

345. Praeger DL, Miller SN. Toxic effects of cyclopentolate (Cyclogyl): Report of a case. Am J Ophthalmol 1964;58:1060–1061.

346. Scinto LF, Daffner KR, Dressler D, et al. A potential noninvasive neurobiological test for Alzheimer's disease. Science 1994;266:1051–1054.

347. Iijima A, Haida M, Ishikawa N, et al. Re-evaluation of tropicamide in the pupillary response test for Alzheimer's disease. Neurobiol Aging 2003;24:789–796.

348. Granholm E, Morris S, Galasko D, et al. Tropicamide effects on pupil size and pupillary light reflexes in Alzheimer's and Parkinson's disease. Intl J Psychophysiol 2003;47:95–115.

349. Awan KJ. Mydriasis and conjunctival paresthesia from local gentamicin. Am J Ophthalmol 1985;15:723–724.

350. Lee JJ, Moster MR, Henderer JD, et al. Pupil dilation with intracameral 1% lidocaine during glaucoma filtering surgery. Am J Ophthalmol 2003;136:201–203.

351. Perlman JP, Conn H. Transient internal ophthalmoplegia during blepharoplasty: A report of three cases. Ophthalmic Plast Reconstr Surg 1991;7:141–143.

352. Cabana MD, Johnson H, Lee CK, et al. Transient anisocoria secondary to nebulized ipratropium bromide. Clin Pediatr 1998;37:445–447.

353. Atsumi K, Sobue G, Ariki G, et al. Autonomic nerve function in spino-cerebellar degeneration. Folia Ophthalmol Jpn 1991;42:1875–1881.

354. Duffin RM, Pettit TH, Straatsma BR. 2.5% vs. 10% phenylephrine in maintaining mydriasis during cataract surgery. Arch Ophthalmol 1983;101:1903–1906.

355. Roberts JR. Pseudo cerebral herniation due to phenylephrine nasal spray. N Engl J Med 1989;320:1757.

356. Gelmi C, Ceccuzzi R. Mydriatic effects of ocular decongestants studied by pupillography. Ophthalmologica 1994;208:243–246.

357. Marchini G, Babighian S, Tosi R, et al. Comparative study of the effects of 2% ibopamine, 10% phenylephrine and 1% tropicamide on the anterior segment. Invest Ophthalmol Vis Sci 2003;44:281–289.

358. Hendrix LE, Dion JE, Jensen ME, et al. Papaverine-induced mydriasis. AJNR Am J Neuroradiol 1994;15:716–718.

359. Taylor P. Agents acting at the neuromuscular junction ant autonomic ganglia. In Gilman AG, Rall TW, Nies AS, et al, eds. The Pharmacological Basis of Therapeutics. New York, Pergamon, 1990:166–186.

360. Lowenstein O, Loewenfeld IE. Effect of physostigmine and pilocarpine on iris sphincter of normal man. Arch Ophthalmol 1953;50:311–318.

361. Babikian PV, Thompson HS. Arecoline miosis. Am J Ophthalmol 1984;98:514–515.

362. Schuman JS, Horwitz B, Choplin NT, et al. A 1-year study of brimonidine twice daily in glaucoma and ocular hypertension. A controlled, randomized,

363. Mitchell AA, Lovejoy FH Jr, Goldman P. Drug ingestions associated with miosis in comatose children. J Pediatr 1976;89:303–305.

364. Robertson DA. Four cases of spinal miosis; with remarks on the action of light on the pupil. Edinburgh Med J 1869;15:487–493.

365. Robertson DA. On an interesting series of eye symptoms in a case of spinal disease with remarks on the action of belladonna on the iris, etc. Edinburgh Med J 1869;14:696–708.

366. Loewenfeld IE. The Argyll Robertson pupil, 1869–1969: A critical survey of the literature. Surv Ophthalmol 1969;14:199–299.

367. Lanigan-O'Keeffe FM. Return to normal of Argyll Robertson pupils after treatment. Br Med J 1977;2:1191–1192.

368. Sears ML. The cause of the Argyll Robertson pupil. Am J Ophthalmol 1971;72:488–489.

369. Dahlström A, Fuxe K, Hillarp NA, et al. Adrenergic mechanisms in the pupillary light-reflex path. Acta Physiol Scand 1964;62:119–124.

370. Ichinohe N, Shoumura K. Marked miosis caused by deafferenting the oculomotor nuclear complex in the cat. Auton Neurosci 2001;94:42–45.

371. Lowenstein O. Miosis in Argyll Robertson syndrome and related pupillary disorders. Arch Ophthalmol 1956;55:356–370.

372. Kirkham TH, Kline LB. Monocular elevator paresis, Argyll Robertson pupils and sarcoidosis. Can J Ophthalmol 1976;11:330–335.

373. Rogers TD, Mitchell JD, Smith MA, et al. Argyll Robertson pupil in multiple sclerosis: A case report. Neuroophthalmology 1985;5:223–225.

374. Koudstaal PJ, Vermeulen M, Wokke JHJ. Argyll Robertson pupils in lymphocytic meningoradiculitis (Bannwarth's syndrome). J Neurol Neurosurg Psychiatry 1987;50:363–365.

375. Averbuch-Heller L, von Maydell RD, Poonyathalang A, et al. "Inverse Argyll Robertson pupil" in botulism: Late central manifestation. Neuroophthalmology 1996;16:351–354.

376. Freeman JW, Cox TA, Batnitzky S, et al. Craniopharyngioma simulating bilateral internal ophthalmoplegia. Arch Neurol 1980;37:176–177.

377. Czarnecki JSC, Thompson HS. The iris sphincter in aberrant regeneration of the third nerve. Arch Ophthalmol 1978;96:1606–1610.

378. Lotufo DG, Smith JL, Hopen GR, et al. The pupil in congenital third nerve misdirection syndrome. J Clin Neuroophthalmol 1983;3:193–195.

379. Coppeto JR, Monteiro MLR, Young D. Tonic pupils following oculomotor nerve palsies. Ann Ophthalmol 1985;17:585–588.

380. Jammes JL. Fixed dilated pupils in petit mal attacks. Neuroophthalmology 1980;1:155–159.

381. Goh KYC, Conway EJ, DaRosso RC, et al. Sympathetic storms in a child with a midbrain glioma: a variant of diencephalic seizures. Pedriatr Neurol 1999;21:742–744.

382. Boeve BF, Wijdicks EFM, Benarroch EE, et al. Paroxysmal sympathetic storms ("diencephalic seizures") after severe diffuse axonal head injury. Mayo Clin Proc 1998;73:148–152.

383. Pant SS, Benton JW, Dodge PR. Unilateral pupillary dilatation during and immediately following seizures. Neurology 1966;16:837–840.

384. Lance JW. Pupillary dilatation and arm weakness as negative ictal phenomena. J Neurol Neurosurg Psychiatry 1995;58:261–262.

385. Masjuan J, Garcia-Segovia J, Baron M, et al. Ipsilateral mydriasis in focal occipitotemporal seizures. J Neurol Neurosurg Psychiatry 1997;63:810–811.

386. Zee DS, Griffin J, Price DL. Unilateral pupillary dilatation during adversive seizures. Arch Neurol 1974;30:403–405.

387. Gadoth N, Margalith D, Bechar M. Unilateral pupillary dilatation during focal seizures. J Neurol 1981;225:227–230.

388. Swartz BE, Delgado-Escueta AV, Maldonado HM. A stereoencephalographic study of ictal propagation producing anisocoria, auras of fear, and complex partial seizures of temporal lobe origin. J Epilepsy 1990;3:149–156.

389. Jampel RS. Convergence, divergence, pupillary reactions and accommodations of the eye from faradic stimulation of the macaque brain. J Comp Neurol 1960;115:371–399.

390. Hashida N, Shoumura K, Ichinohe N, et al. Anisocoria: A pupillary sign of hippocampal lesions: an experimental study in the cat by using neurotoxins. J Hirnforsch 1997;38:9–26.

391. Berreen JP, Vrabec MP, Penar PL. Intermittent pupillary dilatation associated with astrocytoma. Am J Ophthalmol 1990;109:237–239.

392. Lance JW, Smee RI. Partial seizures with visual disturbance treated by radiotherapy of cavernous hemangioma. Ann Neurol 1989;26:782–785.

393. Afifi AK, Corbett JJ, Thompson HS, et al. Seizure-induced miosis and ptosis: Association with temporal lobe magnetic resonance imaging abnormalities. J Child Neurol 1990;5:142–146.

394. Rosenberg ML, Jabbari B. Miosis and internal ophthalmoplegia as a manifestation of partial seizures. Neurology 1991;41:737–739.

395. Plum F, Posner JB. The Diagnosis of Stupor and Coma. 3rd ed. Philadelphia, FA Davis, 1980.

396. Crill WE. Horner's syndrome secondary to deep cerebral lesions. Neurology 1966;16:325.

397. Carmel PW. Sympathetic deficits following thalamotomy. Arch Neurol 1968;18:378–387.

multicenter clinical trial. Chronic Brimonidine Study Group. Ophthalmology 1997;115:847–852.

398. Fisher CM. Some neuro-ophthalmological observations. J Neurol Neurosurg Psychiatry 1967;30:383–392.
399. Sunderland S, Bradley KC. Disturbances of oculomotor function accompanying extradural haemorrhage. J Neurol Neurosurg Psychiatry 1953;16:35–46.
400. Marshall LF, Barba D, Toole BM, et al. The oval pupil: Clinical significance and relationship to intracranial hypertension. J Neurosurg 1983;58:566–568.
401. Larson MD, Muhiudeen I. Pupillometric analysis of the ''absent light reflex.'' Arch Neurol 1995;52:369–372.
402. Cleveland JC. Complete recovery after cardiac arrest for three hours. N Engl J Med 1971;284:334–335.
403. Gauger GE. What do ''fixed, dilated pupils'' mean? N Engl J Med 1971;284:1105.
404. Sims JK. Pupillary diameter in irreversible coma. N Engl J Med 1971;285:57.
405. Fogelholm R, Laru-Sompa R. Brain death and pinpoint pupils. J Neurol Neurosurg Psychiatry 1988;51:1002.
406. Chesnut RM, Gautille T, Blunt BA, et al. The localizing value of asymmetry in pupillary size in severe head injury: Relation to lesion type and location. Neurosurgery 1994;34:840–846.
407. Chen R, Sahjpaul R, Del Maestro RF, et al. Initial enlargement of the opposite pupil as a false localising sign in intraparenchymal frontal haemorrhage. J Neurol Neurosurg Psychiatry 1994;57:1126–1128.
408. Marshman LA, Polkey CE, Penney CC. Unilateral fixed dilation of the pupil as a false-localizing sign with intracranial hemorrhage: Case report and literature review. Neurosurgery 2001;49:1251–1255.
409. Kernohan JW, Woltman HW. Incisura of the crus due to contralateral brain tumor. Arch Neurol Psychiatr 1929;21:274–287.
410. Ropper AH, Cole D, Louis DN. Clinicopathologic correlation in a case of pupillary dilation from cerebral hemorrhage. Arch Neurol 1991;48:1166–1169.
411. Ropper AH. The opposite pupil in herniation. Neurology 1990;40:1707–1709.
412. Tokuda Y, Nakazato N, Stein GH. Pupillary evaluation for differential diagnosis of coma. Postgrad Med J 2003;79:49–51.
413. Ritter AM, Muizelaar JP, Barnes T, et al. Brain stem blood flow, pupillary response, and outcome in patients with severe head injuries. Neurosurgery 1999;44:941–948.
414. Cherniack NS, von Euler C, Homma I, et al. Experimentally induced Cheyne-Stokes breathing. Respir Physiol 1979;37:185–200.
415. Gonyea EF. The abnormal pupil in Cheyne-Stokes respiration. J Neurosurg 1990;72:810–812.
416. Sédan J, Roux A. Paralysie ou absence congénitale de l'accommodation chez trois frères. Bull Soc Ophtalmol Fr 1933;46:163–167.
417. Hibbert FG, Goldstein V, Oborne SM. Defective accommodation in members of one family with an account of an apparatus for recording electrical potential changes. Trans Ophthalmol Soc UK 1975;95:455–461.
418. Hammerberg E, Norn MS. Defective dissociation of accommodation and convergence in dyslectic children. Br Orthopt J 1974;31:96–98.
419. Duane A. Anomalies of accommodation clinically considered. Arch Ophthalmol 1916;45:124–136.
420. Törnqvist G. Paralysis of accommodation. Acta Ophthalmol 1971;49:702–706.
421. Chrousos GA, O'Neill JF, Lueth BD, et al. Accommodation deficiency in healthy young individuals. J Pediatr Ophthalmol Strabismus 1988;25:176–179.
422. Alpers BJ, Palmer HD. The cerebral and spinal complications occurring during pregnancy and the puerperium: A critical review and illustrative cases. J Nerv Ment Dis 1929;70:465–470.
423. Raskind RH. Problems at the reading distance. Am Orthopt J 1976;26:53–59.
424. Pruett RC. Internal ophthalmoplegia after panretinal therapy. Arch Ophthalmol 1979;97:2212.
425. Rogell GD. Internal ophthalmoplegia after Argon laser panretinal photocoagulation. Arch Ophthalmol 1979;97:904–905.
426. Lerner BC, Lakhanpal V, Schocket SS. Transient myopia and accommodative paresis following retinal cryotherapy and panretinal photocoagulation. Am J Ophthalmol 1984;97:704–708.
427. Dellaporta A. Laser application and accommodation paralysis. Arch Ophthalmol 1980;98:1133–1134.
428. Romano PE, Stark WJ. Pseudomyopia as a presenting sign in ocular myasthenia gravis. Am J Ophthalmol 1973;75:872–875.
429. Cooper J, Kruger P, Panariello GF. The pathognomonic pattern of accommodative fatigue in myasthenia gravis. Binoc Vis 1988;3:141–148.
430. Manson N, Stern G. Defects of near vision in myasthenia gravis. Lancet 1965;1:935–937.
431. Caya JG. Clostridium botulinum and the ophthalmologist: A review of botulism, including biological warfare ramifications of botulinum toxin. Surv Ophthalmol 2001;46:25–34.
432. Mohan K, Khandalavala B, Gupta A, et al. Accommodation failure following tetanus. J Clin Neuroophthalmol 1991;11:122–124.
433. Kohn NN, Faires JS, Rodman T. Unusual manifestations due to involvement of involuntary muscle in dystrophica myotonica. N Engl J Med 1964;271:1179–1183.
434. Gamlin PDR, Yoon K, Zhang H. The role of cerebro-ponto-cerebellar pathways in the control of vergence eye movements. Eye 1996;10:167–171.
435. Ohtsuka K, Nagasaka Y. Divergent axon collaterals from the rostral superior colliculus to the pretectal accommodation-related areas and the omnipause neuron area in the cat. J Comp Neurol 1999;413:68–76.
436. Noel LP, Watson AG. Internal ophthalmoplegia following chickenpox. Can J Ophthalmol 1976;11:267–269.
437. Ohtsuka K, Maekawa H, Takeda M, et al. Accommodation and convergence insufficiency with left middle cerebral artery occlusion. Am J Ophthalmol 1988;106:60–64.
438. Manor RS, Heilbronn YD, Sherf I, et al. Loss of accommodation produced by peristriate lesion in man? J Clin Neuroophthalmol 1988;8:19–23.
439. DeRespinis PA, Shen JJ, Wagner RS. Guillain-Barré syndrome presenting as a paralysis of accommodation. Arch Ophthalmol 1989;107:1282.
440. Ohtsuka K, Maeda S, Oguri N. Accommodation and convergence palsy caused by lesions in the bilateral rostral superior colliculus. Am J Ophthalmol 2002;133:425–427.
441. Klingele TG, Newman SA, Burde RM. Accommodation defect in Wilson's disease. Am J Ophthalmol 1980;90:22–24.
442. Curran RE, Hedges TR III, Boger WP III. Loss of accommodation and the near response in Wilson's disease. J Pediatr Ophthalmol Strabis 1982;19:157–160.
443. Goldberg MF, von Noorden GK. Ophthalmologic findings in Wilson's hepatolenticular degeneration wih emphasis on ocular motility. Arch Ophthalmol 1966;75:162–170.
443. Kohn NN, Faires JS, Rodman T. Unusual manifestations due to involvement of involuntary muscle in dystrophica myotonica. N Engl J Med 1964;271:1179–1183.
444. Herzau V, Foerster MH. Fehlinnervation nach okulomotoriusparalyse mit beteiligung des ziliarmuskels. Klin Monatsbl Augenheilkd 1976;169:61–65.
445. Stephenson RW. Paralysis of accommodation with recovery after 5 years. Br J Ophthalmol 1960;44:51.
446. Fisher CM, Adams RD. Diphtheritic polyneuritis: A pathological study. J Neuropathol Exp Neurol 1956;15:243–268.
447. Marmor MF. Transient accommodative paralysis and hyperopia in diabetes. Arch Ophthalmol 1973;89:419–421.
448. Lieppman ME. Accommodative and convergence insufficiency after decompression sickness. Arch Ophthalmol 1981;99:453–456.
449. Harrison RJ. Loss of fusional vergence with partial loss of accommodative convergence and accommodation following head injury. Binoc Vis 1987;2:93–100.
450. Kowal L. Ophthalmic manifestations of head injury. Aust NZ J Ophthalmol 1992;20:35–40.
451. Burke JP, Orton HP, West J, et al. Whiplash and its effect on the visual system. Graefes Arch Clin Exp Ophthalmol 1992;230:335–339.
452. Westcott V. Concerning accommodative asthenopia following head injury. Am J Ophthalmol 1936;19:385–391.
453. Milder B. Tropicamide as a cycloplegic agent. Arch Ophthalmol 1961;66:70–72.
454. Miranda MN. Residual accommodation: A comparison between between cyclopentolate 1% and a combination of cyclopentolate 1% and tropicamide 1%. Arch Ophthalmol 1972;87:515–517.
455. Giles CL, Henderson JW. Horner's syndrome. An analysis of 216 cases. Am J Ophthalmol 1958;46:289–296.
456. Cogan DG. Accommodation and the autonomic nervous system. Arch Ophthalmol 1937;18:739–766.
457. Rutstein RP, Marsh-Tootle W. Acquired unilateral visual loss attributed to an accommodative spasm. Optom Vis Sci 2001;78:492–495.
458. Goldstein JH, Schneekloth BB. Spasm of the near reflex: A spectrum of anomalies. Surv Ophthalmol 1996;40:269–278.
459. Griffin JF, Wray SH, Anderson DP. Misdiagnosis of spasm of the near reflex. Neurology 1976;26:1018–1020.
460. Troost BT, Troost EG. Functional paralysis of horizontal gaze. Neurology 1979;29:82–85.
461. Newman NJ, Lessell S. Pupillary dilatation with monocular occlusion as a sign of nonorganic oculomotor dysfunction. Am J Ophthalmol 1989;108:461–462.
462. Cogan DG, Freese CG. Spasm of the near reflex. Arch Ophthalmol 1955;54:752–759.
463. Keane JR. Neuro-ophthalmic signs and symptoms of hysteria. Neurology 1982;32:757–762.
464. Manor RS. Use of special glasses in treatment of spasm of near reflex. Ann Ophthalmol 1979;11:903–905.
465. Bielschowsky A. Lectures of motor anomalies of the eye: Paralysis of individual eye muscles. Arch Ophthalmol 1935;13:33–59.
466. Safran AB, Roth A, Gauthier G. Le syndrome des spasmes de convergence plus. Klin Monatsbl Augenheilkd 1982;180:471–473.
467. Dagi L, Chrousos GA, Cogan DC. Spasm of the near reflex associated with organic disease. Am J Ophthalmol 1987;103:582–585.
468. Moster ML, Hoenig EM. Spasm of the near reflex associated with metabolic encephalopathy. Neurology 1998;39:150.
469. Shahar E, Andraus J. Near reflex accommodation spasm: Unusual presentation of generalized photosensitive epilepsy. J Clin Neurosci 2002;9:605–607.
470. Kawasaki T, Kiyosawa M, Fujino T, et al. Slow accommodation release with a cerebellar lesion. Br J Ophthalmol 1993;77:678.
471. Raymond GL, Compton JL. Spasm of the near reflex associated with cerebrovascular accident. Austr NZ J Ophthalmol 1990;18:407–410.

472. Van Bogaert L. Sur des modalités exceptionnelles des crises oculogyres. J Neurol Psychiatr (Brussels) 1928;28:379.

473. Rabinovitch V, Vengrjenovsky G. Sur un cas de myasthénie progressive avec participation des muscles lisses de l'oeil. Arch Ophthalmol 1935;52:23–31.

474. Chan RVP, Trobe JD. Spasm of accommodation associated with closed head trauma. J Neuroophthalmol 2002;22:15–17.

475. Knapp C, Sachdev A, Gottlob I. Spasm of the near reflex associated with head injury. Strabismus 2002;10:1–4.

476. Monteiro MLR, Curi ALL, Pereira A, et al. Persistent accommodative spasm after severe head trauma. Br J Ophthalmol 2003;87:243–244.

477. Bohlmann BJ, France TD. Persistent accommodative spasm nine years after head trauma. J Clin Neuroophthalmol 1987;7:129–134.

478. Fechner PU, Teichmann KD, Weyrauch W. Accommodative effects of aceclidine in the treatment of glaucoma. Am J Ophthalmol 1975;79:104–106.

479. Jamal MN, Samara NS, Al-Lozi MT. Moebius' syndrome: A report of two cases. J Laryngol Otol 1988;102:350–352.

480. Crosby EC, DeJonge BR. Experimental and clinical studies of the central connections and central relations of the facial nerve. Ann Otolaryngol 1963;72:735–755.

481. Pulec JL, House WF. Facial nerve involvement and testing in acoustic neuromas. Arch Otolaryngol 1964;80:685–692.

482. Irving RM, Viani L, Hardy DG, et al. Nervus intermedius function after vestibular schwannoma removal: Clinical features and pathophysiological mechanisms. Laryngoscope 1995;105:809–813.

483. Ginsberg LE, De Monte F, Gillenwater AM. Greater superficial petrosal nerve: Anatomy and MR findings in perineural tumor spread. AJNR Am J Neuroradiol 1996;17:389–393.

484. Brown JW. Physiology and phylogenesis of emotional expression. Brain Res 1967;5:1–14.

485. Iannaccone S, Ferini-Strambi L. Pharmacologic treatment of emotional lability. Clin Neuropharmacol 1996;19:532–535.

486. Pareja JA, Caminero AB, Sjaastad O. SUNCT syndrome: Diagnosis and treatment. CNS Drugs 2002;16:373–383.

487. Day M. Sphenopalatine ganglion analgesia. Curr Rev Pain 1999;3:342–347.

488. Ahamed SH, Jones NS. What is Sluder's neuralgia? J Laryngol Otol 2003;117:437–443.

489. Oppenheim H. Lehrbuch der Kervenkrankheiten. Basel, S Karger, 1913.

490. Bogorad FA. Das syndrom der krokodilstränen. Vrach Delo 1928;11:1328.

491. Chorobski J. Syndrome of crocodile tears. Arch Neurol Psychiatr 1951;65:299–318.

492. Bing R. Lehrbuch der Nervenkrankheiten. 3rd ed. Munich, Urban and Achwarzenberg, 1924.

493. Axelsson A, Laage-Hellman JE. The gusto-lachrymal reflex: The syndrome of crocodile tears. Acta Otolaryngol 1962;54:239–254.

494. Lutman FC. Paroxysmal lacrimation when eating. Am J Ophthalmol 1947;30:1583–1585.

495. Jampel RS, Titone C. Congenital paradoxical gustatory-lacrimal reflex and lateral rectus paralysis: Case report. Arch Ophthalmol 1962;67:123–126.

496. Fabriani F. Lacrimation disorders in bulbopontine disorders. Riv Patol Nerv Ment 1954;75:731–743.

497. Biedner B, Geltman C, Rothkoff L. Bilateral Duane's retraction syndrome associated with crocodile tears. J Pediatr Ophthalmol Strabis 1979;16:113–114.

498. Ramsay J, Taylor D. Congenital crocodile tears: A key to the aetiology of Duane's syndrome. Br J Ophthalmol 1980;64:518–522.

499. Hotchkiss MG, Miller NR, Clark AW, et al. Bilateral Duane's retraction syndrome: A clinical-pathologic case report. Arch Ophthalmol 1980;98:870–874.

500. Kaminsky SD. Ueber das syndrom der krokodils-tränen. Dtsch Nervenheilkd 1929;110:151–160.

501. Christoffel H. Verhinderung von krokodilstränen durch monokel. Schweiz Med Wochenschr 1939;69:455.

502. Bauer M. Crocodile tears in a case of acoustic neurinoma. Pract Otorhinolaryngol 1964;26:22–28.

503. McCoy FJ, Goodman RC. The crocodile tear syndrome. J Plast Reconstr Surg 1979;63:58–62.

504. Boyer FC, Gardner WJ. Paroxysmal lacrimation (syndrome of crocodile tears) and its surgical treatment: Relation to auriculotemporal syndrome. Arch Neurol Psychiatr 1949;61:56–64.

505. Golding-Wood PH. Crocodile tears. Br Med J 1963;2:1518–1521.

506. Boroojerdi B, Ferbert A, Schwarz M, et al. Botulinum toxin treatment of synkinesia and hyperlacrimation after facial palsy. J Neurol Neurosurg Psychiatry 1998;65:111–114.

507. Riemann R, Pfennigsdorf S, Riemann E, et al. Successful treatment of crocodile tears by injection of botulinum toxin into the lacrimal gland: Case report. Ophthalmology 1999;106:2322–2324.

508. Montoya FJ, Riddell CE, Caesar R, et al. Treatment of gustatory hyperlacrimation (crocodile tears) with injection of botulinum toxin into the lacrimal gland. Eye 2002;16:705–709.

509. Saraux H, Martin P, Morax S, et al. Hyposecretion lacrymale et medicaments psychotropes. Ann Oculist 1976;209:193–197.

510. Felix RH, Ive FA, Dahl MGC. Cutaneous and ocular reactions to practolol. Br Med J 1974;4:321–324.

511. Ross AT. Progressive selective sudomotor denervation: A case with coexisting Adie's syndrome. Neurology 1958;8:809–817.

512. Bergmann I, Dauphin M, Naumann M, et al. Selective degeneration of sudomotor fibers in Ross syndrome and successful treatment of compensatory hyperhidrosis with botulinum toxin. Muscle Nerve 1998;21:1790–1793.

513. Sommer C, Lindenlaub T, Zillikens D et al. Selective loss of cholinergic sudomotor fibers causes anhidrosis in Ross syndrome. Ann Neurol 2002;52:247–250.

514. Peretti A, Nolano M, De Joanna G, et al. Is Ross syndrome a dysautonomic disorder only? An electrophysiologic and histologic study. Clin Neurophysiol 2003;114:7–16.

515. Johnson RH, McLellan DL, Love DR. Orthostatic hypotension and the Holmes-Adie syndrome. J Neurol Neurosurg Psychiatry 1971;34:562–570.

516. Bacon PJ, Smith SE. Cardiovascular and sweating dysfunction in patients with Holmes-Adie syndrome. J Neurol Neurosurg Psychiatry 1993;56:1096–1102.

517. Druschky K, Hilz M, Koelsch C, et al. Cardiac sympathetic denervation in Ross syndrome demonstrated by MIBG-SPECT. J Auton Nerv Syst 1999;76:184–187.

518. Shin RK, Galetta SL, Ting TY, et al. Ross syndrome plus. Beyond Horner, Holmes-Adie, and harlequin. Neurology 2000;55:1841–1846.

519. Wolfe GI, Galetta SL, Teener JW, et al. Site of autonomic dysfunction in a patient with Ross' syndrome and postganglionic Horner's syndrome. Neurology 1995;45:2094–2096.

520. Drummond PD, Edis RH. Loss of facial sweating and flushing in Holmes-Adie syndrome. Neurology 1990;40:847–849.

521. Eng CM, Slaugenhaupt SA, Blumenfeld A, et al. Prenatal diagnosis of familial dysautonomia by analysis of linked CA-repeat polymorphisms on chromosome 9q31–q33. Am J Med Genet 1995;59:349–353.

522. Brunt PW, McKusick VA. Familial dysautonomia: A report of genetic and clinical studies, with a review of the literature. Medicine 1970;49:343–374.

523. Francois J. The Riley-Day syndrome: Familial dysautonomy, central autonomic dysfunction. Ophthalmologica 1977;174:20–34.

524. Kroop IG. The production of tears in familial dysautonomia: Preliminary report. J Pediatr 1956;48:328–329.

525. Dunnington JH. Congenital alacrima in familial autonomic dysfunction. Arch Ophthalmol 1954;52:925–931.

526. Smith AA, Dancis J, Breinin G. Ocular responses to autonomic drugs in familial dysautonomia. Invest Ophthalmol 1965;72:358–361.

527. Goldberg MF, Payne JW, Brunt PW. Ophthalmologic studies of familial dysautonomia: The Riley-Day syndrome. Arch Ophthalmol 1968;80:732–743.

528. Korczyn AD, Rubenstein AE, Yahr MD, et al. The pupil in familial dysautonomia. Neurology 1981;31:628–629.

529. Rizzo JF 3rd, Lessell S, Liebman SD. Optic atrophy in familial dysautonomia. Am J Ophthalmol 1986;102:463–467.

530. Josiatis CA, Matisoff M. Familial dysautonomia in review: Diagnosis and treatment of ocular manifestations. Adv Exp Med Biol 2003;506:71–79.

531. Pearson J, Axelrod F, Dancis J. Current concepts of dysautonomia: Neuropathological defects. Ann NY Acad Sci 1974;22:288–300.

532. Pearson J, Budzilovich G, Finegold MJ. Sensory, motor and autonomic dysfunction: The nervous system in familial dysautonomia. Neurology 1971;21:486–493.

533. Weinshilboum RM, Axelrod J. Reduced plasma dopamine-β-hydroxylase activity in familial dysautonomia. N Engl J Med 1971;285:938–942.

534. Mittag TW, Mindel JW, Green JP. Choline acetyltransferase in familial dysautonomia. Ann NY Acad Sci 1974;22:301–306.

535. Consensus Committee of the American Autonomic Society and the American Academy of Neurology. Consensus statement on the definition of orthostatic hypotension, pure autonomic failure, and multiple system atrophy. Neurology 1996;46:1470.

536. Goldstein DS, Holmes C, Li S, et al. Cardiac sympathetic denervation in Parkinson disease. Ann Intern Med 2000;133:338–347.

537. Druschky A, Hilz MJ, Platsch G, et al. Differentiation of Parkinson's disease and multiple system atrophy in early disease stages by means of I-123-MIBG-SPECT. J Neurol Sci 2000;175:3–12.

538. Papp MI, Lantos PL. Accumulation of tubular structures in oligodendroglial and neuronal cells as the basic alteration in multiple-system atrophy. J Neurol Sci 1992;107:172–182.

539. Orimo S, Ozawa E, Oka T, et al. Different histopathology accounting for a decrease in myocardial MIBG uptake in PD and MSA. Neurology 2001;57:1140–1141.

540. Naka H, Ohshita T, Murata Y, et al. Characteristic MRI findings in multiple system atrophy: comparison of three subtypes. Neuroradiology 2002;44:204–209.

541. Rosen J, Brown SI. New ocular signs in Shy-Drager syndrome. Am J Ophthalmol 1974;78:1032–1033.

542. Nirankari VS, Khurana RK, Lakhanpal V. Ocular manifestations of the Shy-Drager syndrome. Ann Ophthalmol 1982;14:635–638.

543. Vernino S, Low PA, Fealey RD, et al. Autoantibodies to ganglionic acetylcholine receptors in autoimmune autonomic neuropathies. N Engl J Med 2000;343:847–855.

544. Klein C, Vernino S, Lennon VA, et al. The spectrum of autoimmune autonomic neuropathies. Ann Neurol 2003;53:752–758.

545. Low PA. Autonomic neuropathies. Curr Opin Neurol 1994;7:402–406.

546. Andersen O, Lindberg J, Modigh K, et al. Subacute dysautonomia with incomplete recovery. Acta Neurol Scand 1972;48:510–519.

547. Li S, Guo Y. Pandysautonomia: Clinicopathological report of 5 cases. Chin Med J 1995;108:829–834.

548. Yee RD, Trese M, Zee DS, et al. Ocular manifestations of acute pandysautonomia. Am J Ophthalmol 1976;81:740–744.

549. Okada F, Shintomi Y, Kase M. Pupillary symptoms in three patients with pandysautonomia. Neuroophthalmology 1988;8:87–93.

550. Winkler AS, Dean A, Hu M, et al. Phenotypic and neuropathologic heterogeneity of anti-Hu antibody-related paraneoplastic syndrome presenting with progressive dysautonomia: Report of 2 cases. Clin Auton Res 2001;11:115–118.

551. Camdessanche JP, Antoine JC, Honnorat J, et al. Paraneoplastic peripheral neuropathy associated with anti-Hu antibodies. A clinical and electrophysiological study of 20 patients. Brain 2002;125:166–175.

552. Lennon VA, Ermilov LG, Szurszewski JH, et al. Immunization with neuronal nicotinic acetylcholine receptor induces neurological autoimmune disease. J Clin Invest 2003;111:907–913.

553. Mori M, Kuwabara S, Fukutake T, et al. Clinical features and prognosis of Miller Fisher syndrome. Neurology 2001;56:1104–1106.

554. Elizan TS, Spire JP, Andiman RM, et al. Syndrome of acute idiopathic ophthalmoplegia with ataxia and areflexia. Neurology 1971;21:281–292.

555. Keane JR. Tonic pupils with acute ophthalmoplegic polyneuritis. Ann Neurol 1977;2:393–396.

556. Oomura M, Yamawaki T, Oe H, et al. Association of cardiomyopathy caused by autonomic nervous system impairment with the Miller Fisher syndrome. J Neurol Neurosurg Psychiatry 2003;74:689–690.

557. Okajima T, Imamura S, Kawasaki S, et al. Fisher's syndrome: A pharmacological study of the pupils. Ann Neurol 1977;2:63–65.

SECTION III:
The Ocular Motor System

Nancy J. Newman

The term "ocular motor system" refers to the entire somatic motor system that controls the position and movement of the eyes. This system includes the extraocular muscles, the cranial nerves and nuclei that innervate them, and the pathways in the cerebral hemispheres, cerebellum, and brainstem that coordinate and control ocular motility and alignment. The first of the seven chapters in this section

describes the anatomy and physiology of the ocular motor system. The second chapter is concerned with the techniques used to examine ocular motility and alignment. The remaining five chapters are devoted to various neurologic, neuromuscular, and myopathic disorders of neuro-ophthalmologic importance.

CHAPTER 17

Anatomy and Physiology of Ocular Motor Systems

James Sharpe and Agnes M.F. Wong

In this chapter we describe physiologic processes and anatomic bases for the control of eye movements. Many concepts in this chapter are based on information from anatomic and physiologic experiments on monkeys, and to a lesser extent on lower animals. Since the ocular motor behavior of the monkey is similar to that of man, it is valid to use information obtained from such experimental animals to understand the control of eye movements in humans. Quantitative methods of eye movement recording in normal human subjects and patients with brain lesions, together with high-resolution brain imaging, have advanced our knowledge considerably.

SIX EYE MOVEMENT SYSTEMS AND THEIR TWO GOALS

Eye movements are divided into different types called systems, each of which performs a specific, quantifiable function and has a distinctive anatomic substrate and physiologic organization. We can best understand the types of eye movements when we consider the major goals of the ocular motor systems (1). There are six systems: saccadic, smooth pursuit, fixation, vergence, vestibulo-ocular, and optokinetic. All six systems interact during visual tasks. They have two goals: attaining fixation with both eyes, and preventing slippage of images on the retina. The saccadic system uses fast eye movements to attain fixation of images that lie off the fovea, whereas the other systems generate slower smooth eye movements to maintain fixation and prevent image slip on the retina.

When an object of interest moves within the environment or when the head moves, there must be mechanisms to bring the image of the object on the fovea of each eye and keep it there. When an object moves horizontally, vertically, or obliquely in a frontal plane, both eyes must move simultaneously in the same direction. Binocular movements in the same direction are termed conjugate eye movements or versions. When an object moves toward or away from the viewer in a sagittal plane, the eyes must move in opposite directions. Binocular movements in opposite directions are termed disjunctive or vergence eye movements; they are achieved by the vergence system. More than a century ago, Hering and Helmholtz debated the neural basis of binocular coordination (2,3). Helmholtz believed that each eye is controlled independently and that binocular coordination is learned. Hering believed that both eyes are innervated by common command signals that yoke the movements of both eyes (Hering's law of equal innervation). For example, the right lateral rectus and left medial muscles are yoked agonists for rightward version; the left superior oblique and right inferior rectus muscles are yoked agonists for downward version to the right. Conjugate control remains a subject of debate (4,5), since anatomic, physiologic, and behavioral evidence indicates independent supranuclear innervation of motoneurons to each eye that are considered to be yoked (6–9).

We shall discuss the operations of the six systems and how they generate eye movements to achieve binocular fixation and prevent retinal image slip. First we consider the anatomy and functions of the peripheral ocular motor nerves and extraocular muscles.

EXTRAOCULAR MUSCLES

Each eyeball is rotated by six extraocular muscles: the medial rectus, lateral rectus, superior rectus, inferior rectus, superior oblique, and inferior oblique. These muscles, with the exception of the inferior oblique, take origin from a fibrotendinous ring at the orbital apex called the annulus of Zinn, which surrounds a central opening known as the oculomotor foramen. The oculomotor foramen encircles the optic foramen and the central part of the superior orbital fissure (Fig. 17.1). The optic nerve and the ophthalmic artery pass through the optic foramen, whereas the superior and inferior divisions of the oculomotor nerve, the abducens nerve, and the nasociliary branch of the trigeminal nerve pass through

the superior orbital fissure within the annulus of Zinn (10). The trochlear nerve and the frontal and lacrimal branches of the trigeminal nerve enter the orbit through the superior orbital fissure outside the annulus of Zinn.

The four rectus muscles pass anteriorly from the orbital apex, parallel to their respective orbital walls. Anterior to the equator, the muscles insert onto the sclera by tendinous expansions. The distance from the corneal limbus to the insertion of each rectus muscle gradually increases around the globe from the medial rectus (5.3 mm) to the inferior rectus (6.8 mm), lateral rectus (6.9 mm), and superior rectus (7.9 mm) (11). An imaginary line drawn through these muscle insertions is called the spiral of Tillaux (Fig. 17.2).

The superior oblique muscle runs forward for a short distance from its origin at the orbital apex before forming a long tendon that passes through the trochlea. The trochlea is a fibrous cartilaginous structure anchored in the trochlear fossa of the frontal bone, just inside the superior medial orbital rim (12). After passing through the trochlea, the superior oblique tendon turns obliquely backward and outward to attach to the upper sclera behind the equator and beneath the superior rectus (Fig. 17.3).

The inferior oblique is the only extraocular muscle that does not originate from the annulus of Zinn. It arises from the inferior nasal aspect of the orbit just inside the orbital rim and passes obliquely backward and outward to insert on the lower portion of the globe behind the equator. A more thorough discussion of the gross anatomy of the extraocular muscles can be found in other sources (10,13,14).

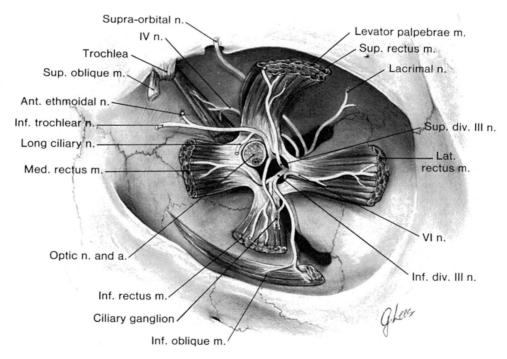

Figure 17.1. View of the posterior orbit showing the origins of the extraocular muscles and their relationships to the optic and ocular motor nerves. (Redrawn from Warwick R. Eugene Wolff's Anatomy of the Eye and Orbit. 7th ed. Philadelphia: WB Saunders, 1976.)

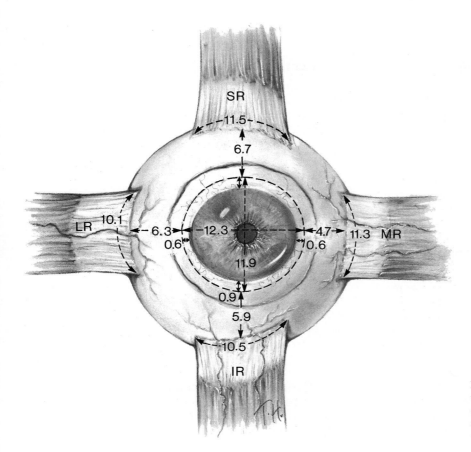

Figure 17.2. The anatomic relationships of rectus muscle insertions, cornea, and limbus (the spiral of Tillaux). (Redrawn from Apt L. An anatomical reevaluation of rectus muscle insertions. Trans Am Ophthalmol Soc 1980;78:365–375.)

The actions that the extraocular muscles exert on the globe are determined by the axis of rotation of the globe, the bony anatomy of the orbit, and the origin and insertion of the muscles. In addition, the orbital layer of each rectus muscle inserts onto a sleeve and ring of collagen in Tenon's fascia called ''pulleys'' (Figs. 17.4 and 17.5). The pulleys are linked to the orbital wall, adjacent extraocular muscles, and equatorial Tenon's fascia by sling-like bands that contain collagen, elastin, and richly innervated smooth muscles (15,16). Pulleys limit side-slip movement of the muscles during eye movements and act as the functional origin of the rectus muscles (15–18).

Extraocular Muscle Fiber Types

Extraocular muscles are composed of a variable number of fibers. The medial rectus has the largest muscle mass, while the inferior oblique has the smallest (19). Although they vary in overall structure such as length, mass, and tendon size, certain features are common to all extraocular muscles. Each muscle consists of muscle fibers with a diameter of 9–30 μm, which are smaller than those of muscles in other parts of the body. Each fiber is surrounded by a sarcolemma that covers a granular sarcoplasm in which individual myofibrils are apparent. Connective tissue surrounds individual muscle fibers (endomysium), groups of fibers (internal perimysium), and the muscles themselves (external peri-

mysium; epimysium). This connective tissue contains many elastic fibers, as well as blood vessels and nerves.

All human extraocular muscle fibers have the light and electron microscopic appearance of a typical striated muscle (20). Likewise, the mechanism of contraction of these fibers is identical to that of voluntary muscles in other parts of the body, with the exception of the multiply innervated fibers (discussed later). The similarities, however, end there, as the muscle fiber types composing the extraocular muscles are very much different from those in any other skeletal muscles (21,22). Each extraocular muscle exhibits two distinct layers: an outer *orbital layer* adjacent to the periorbita and orbital bone, and an inner *global layer* adjacent to the eye and the optic nerve (Figs. 17.6 and 17.7). While the global layer extends the full muscle length and inserts to the globe via a well-defined tendon, the orbital layer ends before the muscle becomes tendinous and inserts into the pulley of the muscle. Each layer contains fibers suited for either sustained contraction or brief rapid contraction.

Six types of fibers have been identified in the extraocular muscles (Table 17.1 and Fig. 17.6) (23–26). In the orbital layer, about 80% are singly innervated fibers. These fibers have an extremely high content of mitochondria and oxidative enzymes. They have fast-twitch capacity and are the most fatigue-resistant. They are the only fiber type that show long-term effects after the injection of botulinum toxin (27). The remaining 20% of orbital fibers are multiply innervated

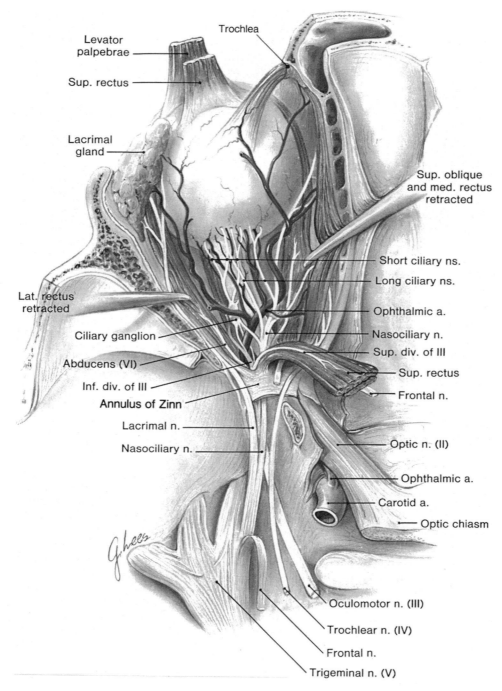

Figure 17.3.   View of the normal orbit from above, showing the relationships of the extraocular muscles, ocular motor nerves, and vessels. (Redrawn from Warwick R. Eugene Wolff's Anatomy of the Eye and Orbit. 7th ed. Philadelphia: WB Saunders, 1976.)

fibers. Unlike most mammalian skeletal muscles, the orbital layer multiply innervated fibers exhibit multiple nerve terminals distributed along their length. They have twitch capacity near the center of the fiber and nontwich activity proximal and distal to the endplate band (28).

In the global layer, about 33% are red singly innervated fibers, which are fast-twitch and highly fatigue-resistant. Another 33% are pale singly innervated fibers with fast-twitch properties but low fatigue resistance. Intermediate singly innervated fibers constitute about another 23% of fibers. They

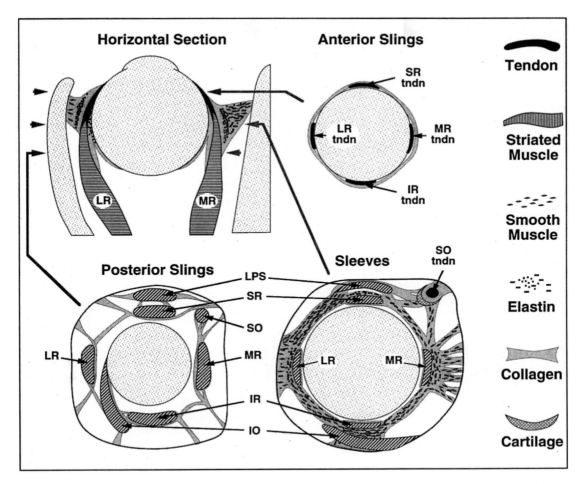

Figure 17.4. Structure of the orbital connective tissues, including the rectus muscle pulleys. IO, inferior oblique; IR, inferior rectus; LPS, levator palpebrae superioris; LR, lateral rectus; MR, medial rectus; SO, superior oblique; SR, superior rectus. The three coronal views are represented at the levels indicated by *arrow*s in horizontal section. (From Demer JL, Miller JM, Poukens V. Surgical implications of the rectus extraocular muscle pulleys. J Pediatr Ophthalmol Strabismus 1996;33:208–218.)

have fast-twitch properties and an intermediate level of fatigue resistance. The remaining 10% of global layer muscle fibers are multiply innervated fibers, with synaptic endplates along their entire length, as well as at the myotendinous junction, where palisade ending proprioceptors are found. The multiply innervated fibers are nontwitch, having tonic properties, with slow, graded, nonpropagated responses to neural or pharmacologic activation. The twitch and nontwitch muscle fibers are innervated by different types of motoneurons. Large motoneurons within the abducens, trochlear, and oculomotor nuclei innervate twitch, singly innervated fibers, whereas smaller motoneurons around the periphery of these nuclei innervate nontwitch, multiply innervated fibers (29).

It was suggested that different muscle fiber types may subserve different types of eye movements; slower or vestibularly induced eye movements were attributed to contraction of the slower tonic fibers, while rapid movements were attributed to contraction of the faster twitch fibers (30–32). However, more recent studies argue against this concept

(33–35). Using intraoperative electromyography, Scott and Collins (33) demonstrated that all muscle fiber types participate in all classes of eye movements. In addition, different fiber types are recruited at specific eye positions, regardless of the type of eye movements. Robinson (36) proposed that the functional arrangement of muscle fiber types is related to the threshold at which motor units are recruited. In saccades and quick phases of nystagmus, all motor units are recruited and burst synchronously. There is no differential in the recruitment order of different muscle fiber or motor unit types (36). However, after saccades, or in slow smooth eye movements, the recruitment of individual motoneurons into sustained discharge is dependent on eye position. Motor units containing orbital singly innervated fibers and global red singly innervated fibers are recruited first, well in the off-direction of muscle action (36). Those motor units containing multiply innervated fiber types are recruited next, probably near straight ahead position, where their fine increments of force would be of value for fixation (36). The in-

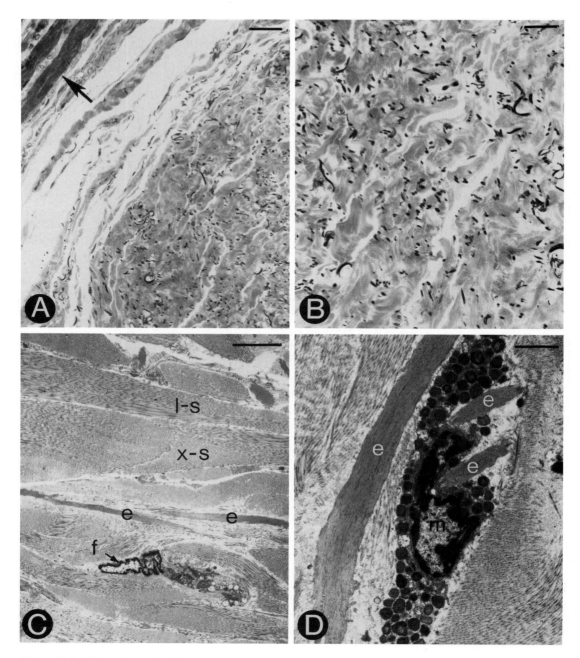

Figure 17.5. Photomicrographs of rectus muscle pulley structure. *A* and *B*, Light micrographs of dense connective tissue on the orbital side of a human medial rectus (*arrow*) pulley. Dense collagen matrix is intermixed with elastin filaments. *C* and *D*, Electron photomicrographs of rectus muscle pulleys. Collagen is arranged in bundles running at right angles to one another (x-s, bundles cut in cross-section; l-s, bundles cut in longitudinal section). Elastin filaments (e) are scattered individually in collagen matrix. (From Porter JD, Poukens D, Baker RS, et al. Structure function correlations in the human extraocular muscle pulleys. Invest Vis Sci 1996;37:468–472.)

creasingly faster but fatigable fibers are recruited last, at positions well into the on-direction of muscle action (36). Thus, although the global intermediate and global white singly innervated fiber types are transiently recruited during all on-direction saccades, they are recruited into continuous activity only in intermediate to extreme positions of gaze.

Another unique feature of the extraocular muscles is their rich nerve supply. Each motoneuron from the ocular motor nerves supplies very few muscle fibers compared with the ratio of motoneurons to muscle fibers in other striated muscles (37–39). Motor unit size is only about one muscle fiber per motoneuron in the global layer, and two to five muscle

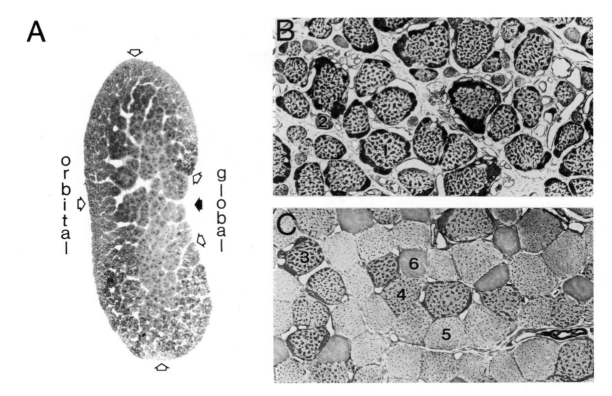

Figure 17.6. Light photomicrographs of Macaca monkey rectus muscle organization. *A,* Layered organization of typical rectus muscle; C-shaped orbital and central, global layers are indicated. *B,* Fiber types present in orbital muscle layer. Orbital singly innervated and multiply innervated fibers are present. *C,* Fiber types present in the global muscle layer. Global red, global intermediate, and global white singly innervated muscle fiber types and the global multiply innervated fiber type are indicated. (From Porter JD, Baker RS, Ragusa RJ, et al. Extraocular muscles: basic and clinical aspects of structure and function. Surv Ophthalmol 1995;39:451–484.)

fibers per motoneuron in the orbital layer of human rectus muscles (40). The low innervation ratio allows extraocular muscles to increase or decrease force in small amounts for the precise control of eye position.

Extraocular Muscle Proprioception

Human extraocular muscles contain neuromuscular spindles, Golgi tendon organs, and palisade endings (41–43).

Muscle spindles occur only in the orbital layer of muscles. Golgi tendon organs and palisade endings are found only in nontwich, multiply innervated fibers and only in the global layer. Palisade endings lie at myotendinous junctions and have the microscopic features of immature Golgi tendon organs (43). The function of muscle spindles and Golgi tendon organs is not settled. Muscle spindles are positioned to serve as feedback to any adjustment of the pulleys to which the orbital muscle layers attach. Ocular motoneurons do not par-

Table 17.1
Functional Properties of Extraocular Muscle Fiber Types

	Orbital		Global			
	SIF	MIF	Red SIF	Intermediate SIF	White SIF	MIF
% of layer	80	20	33	23	33	10
Contraction mode	Twitch	Mixed	Twitch	Twitch	Twitch	Nontwitch
Contraction speed	Fast	Fast/slow	Fast	Fast	Fast	Slow
Fatigue resistance	High	Variable	High	Intermediate	Low	High
Recruitment order	1st	3rd	2nd	5th	6th	4th

SIF, singly innervated fiber; MIF, multiply innervated fiber.
(Modified from Porter JD, Baker RS, Ragusa RJ, Brueckner JK. Extraocular muscles: basic and clinical aspects of structure and function. Surv Ophthalmol 1995;39:451–484.)

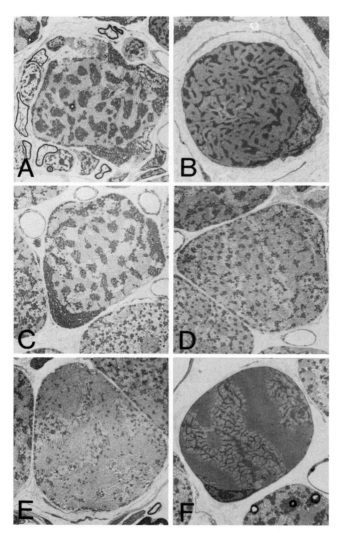

Figure 17.7. Electron photomicrographs of fiber types present in primate extraocular muscle. *A,* Orbital singly innervated. *B,* Orbital multiply innervated. *C,* Global red singly innervated. *D,* Global intermediate singly innervated. *E,* Global white singly innervated. *F,* Global multiply innervated.

ticipate in any stretch reflex. Palisade endings appear to be the primary proprioceptors (44,45). Extraocular muscle afferents project from these proprioceptors, via the ophthalmic branch of the trigeminal nerve and the gasserian ganglion, to the spinal trigeminal nucleus (46). Proprioceptive inputs may also project centrally via the ocular motor nerves (47). From the trigeminal nucleus, proprioceptive information is distributed widely to structures involved in ocular motor control, including the superior colliculus, vestibular nuclei, nucleus prepositus hypoglossi, cerebellum, and frontal eye fields. Proprioceptive information is also distributed to structures involved in visual processing, including the lateral geniculate body, pulvinar, and visual cortex.

Deafferentation of the eye muscles does not affect ocular motor control or visually mediated adaptation of eye movements in primates (48). Vision and efferent eye movement commands (efference copy, or nonretinal feedback, which we discuss later) provide sufficient information to the brain for accurate eye movement control, and this information is modified by visual feedback independently of proprioception (48). Although visual input and internal (nonretinal) feedback massively dominate any contribution of proprioception to the control of eye motion, extraocular proprioception has been implicated in various functions (49). It may specify visual direction (50–53), modulate visual processing (54), contribute to spatial localization (50,55), and participate in binocular functions (56), particularly during the critical period of development of the visual sensory system (57,58). Proprioception may also participate in the control of different oculomotor systems (56,59–65). Abnormalities in proprioception might contribute to fixation instabilities in congenital nystagmus (66) and to strabismus (56,67). For an in-depth discussion of extraocular muscle proprioception, see Donaldson's (49) excellent review.

LEVATOR PALPEBRAE SUPERIORIS

The levator palpebrae superioris arises as a short tendon that is blended with the underlying origin of the superior rectus from the undersurface of the lesser wing of the sphenoid bone, above and anterior to the optic foramen. The flat muscle belly passes forward below the orbital roof and just superior to the superior rectus until it is about 1 cm behind the orbital septum, where it ends in a membranous expansion or aponeurosis. The aponeurosis of the levator spreads out in a fan-shaped manner across the width of the eyelid, inserting primarily into the tarsal plate that separates the bundles of the orbicularis oculi muscle in the lower half of the eyelid. The lateral and medial extensions of the aponeurosis are its lateral and medial horns. The lateral horn is attached to the orbital tubercle and to the upper aspect of the lateral canthal ligament. The medial horn is attached to the medial canthal ligament (68).

Each levator palpebrae muscle contains the three singly innervated muscle fiber types found in the global layer of the extraocular muscles, and a true slow-twitch fiber type. The multiply innervated fiber type and the fatigue-resistant singly innervated type seen in the orbital layer of extraocular muscles are absent. The levator muscle is also more interspersed with fat and less sharply separated from adjacent connective tissue than are the fibers of the superior rectus.

The nerve supply to the levator muscle is via branches from the superior division of the oculomotor nerve (discussed later) that reach the muscle either by piercing the medial edge of the superior rectus or by winding around its medial border (Fig. 17.1). The vascular supply originates from the lateral muscular branch of the ophthalmic artery, the supraorbital artery, the lacrimal artery, and the posterior ethmoidal artery (69).

OCULAR MOTOR NUCLEI AND NERVES

Oculomotor Nucleus and Nerve

The oculomotor nerve (the third nerve) is the largest and most complex of the three ocular motor nerves. It contains somatic motor fibers that innervate the superior, inferior, and medial recti, the inferior oblique, and the levator palpebrae superioris. It also contains visceral (parasympathetic) motor fibers that innervate the ciliary and the iris sphincter muscles. In addition to somatic and visceral motor fibers, the oculomotor nerve carries fibers from the trigeminal nerve and the sympathetic plexus. In humans, the oculomotor nerve has about 15,000 axons (four times the number in the abducens nerve and seven times the number in the trochlear nerve), most of which are distributed to about 40,000 muscle fibers.

Oculomotor Nucleus

The oculomotor nucleus consists of an elongated mass of cells lying ventral to the periaqueductal gray matter of the mesencephalon. Its rostral extent is the posterior commissure, and its caudal extent is the trochlear nucleus near the pontomesencephalic junction (Figs. 17.8 and 17.9). Unlike the trochlear and abducens nuclei, the oculomotor nucleus has both midline unpaired and lateral paired portions. Contemporary neuroanatomic retrograde tracing techniques in monkeys reveal that the organization of the somatic components of the oculomotor nucleus (70–73) is more complex than that described by Warwick (74) (Fig. 17.10). The superior rectus is represented on the contralateral side of the medial portion of the oculomotor nucleus. Fibers from this subnucleus cross the midline and pass through the superior rectus subnucleus on the opposite side before turning ventrally to enter the fascicle of the oculomotor nerve (75). The inferior rectus motoneurons lie dorsally, primarily in the rostral portion of the ipsilateral nucleus. The medial rectus motoneurons lie in three separate subgroups in the ipsilateral oculomotor nucleus (70,71) (Fig. 17.11). Inferior oblique motoneurons are found ipsilaterally, between the ventral medial rectus subgroup and the inferior rectus representation.

The oculomotor nucleus also contains, in addition to motoneurons, many internuclear neurons that project to and from other nuclei concerned with ocular motor function. These internuclear neurons project primarily to the ipsilateral abducens nucleus, with a small population of neurons projecting to the contralateral abducens nucleus (76–79).

In addition to motoneurons and internuclear neurons, the oculomotor nucleus also contains preganglionic, parasympathetic neurons whose axons project to the ciliary ganglion and ultimately control pupillary constriction and accommodation. These cell bodies are located in the visceral nuclei of the oculomotor nucleus: the Edinger-Westphal nuclei, the anterior median nuclei, and, possibly, Perlia's nucleus (80). The caudal central nucleus is a single midline structure located in the caudal end of the oculomotor nucleus. It supplies both levator palpebrae superioris muscles.

Fascicular Portion of the Oculomotor Nerve

The fascicular portion of the oculomotor nerve, which lies within the substance of the brain stem, arises from the ventral side of the nucleus. These fibers descend ventrally and spread laterally as they pass through the red nucleus to partially penetrate the medial part of the cerebral peduncle (Fig. 17.12). The origin of these fibers from the rostral to the

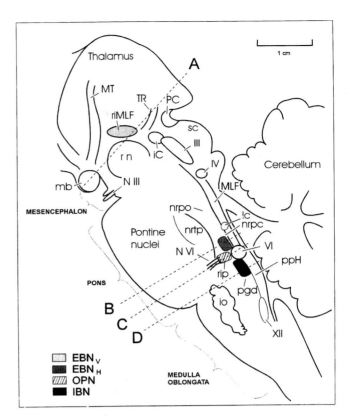

Figure 17.8. Sagittal view of a human brain stem showing the location of saccadic premotor neurons. *Shaded areas* mark the location of premotor saccadic neurons: excitatory short-lead burst neurons of the horizontal (EBN$_H$) system in the nrpc, and of the vertical (EBN$_V$) system in the riMLF; inhibitory short-lead burst neurons (IBN) in the pgd and omnipause neurons (OPN) in the rip. The broken lines A to D indicate the planes of the corresponding sections shown in Figure 17.9. III, oculomotor nucleus; IV, trochlear nucleus t; VI, abducens nucleus; XII, hypoglossal nucleus, iC, interstitial nucleus of Cajal; io, inferior olive; mb, mammillary body; MLF, medial longitudinal fasciculus; MT, mammillothalamic tract, N III, oculomotor nerve; NVI, abducens nerve; lc, locus ceruleus; nrpc, nucleus reticularis pontis caudalis; nrpo, nucleus reticular is pontis oralis; nrtp, nucleus reticularis tegmenti pontis; PC, posterior commissure; pgd, nucleus paragigantocellularis dorsalis; ppH, nucleus prepositus hypoglossi; PX, pyramidal decussation; riMLF, rostral interstitial nucleus of the MLF; rip, nucleus raphe interpositus; rn, red nucleus; sc, superior colliculus; TR, tractus retroflexus. (From Horn AKE, Büttner-Ennever JA, Büttner U. Saccadic premotor neurons in the brainstem: functional neuroanatomy and clinical implications. Neuroophthalmology 1996;16:229–240.)

caudal ends of the oculomotor nuclear columns explains their dispersion throughout the ventral mesencephalon. Although this arrangement may seem haphazard, it is clear that the fibers actually are arranged in a divisional pattern within the brain stem. Indeed, superior and inferior division oculomotor nerve pareses frequently occur in patients with intrinsic lesions of the mesencephalon (81–85). As the fibers emerge on both sides of the interpeduncular fossa, the fiber bundles immediately coalesce to form two large nerve trunks.

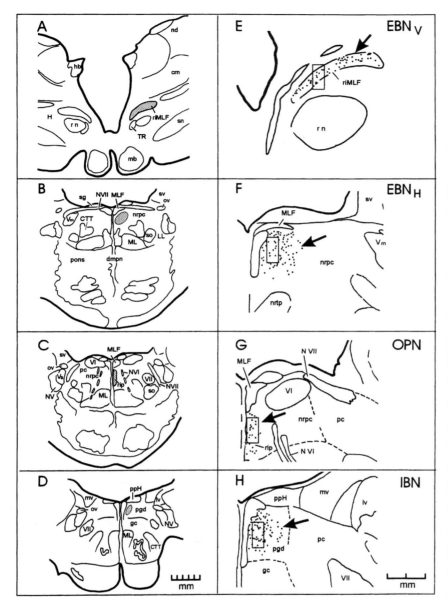

Figure 17.9. Transverse sections through the human brain stem at levels indicated in Figure 17.8, showing the localization of saccadic premotor neuron groups (*shaded areas*) from rostral to caudal through the riMLF (*A*), the nrpc (*B*), the rip (*C*), and the pgd (*D*). *E–H*, Magnification of the areas containing premotor saccadic neurons in *A* to *D*. Immunoreactive human neurons (only within the relevant areas) are indicated by dots. *E*, The riMLF contains vertical short-lead burst neurons (EBN$_V$) (*arrow*). The dorsal border of the riMLF is outlined by the thalamosubthalamic artery, which serves as a useful landmark. *F*, The area containing horizontal excitatory short-lead burst neurons (EBN$_H$) is confined to the medial part of the nrpc (*arrow*). *G*, The saccadic omnipause neurons (OPN) lie within the rip scattered at the midline (*arrow*). *H*, The horizontal inhibitory short-lead burst neurons (IBN) lie within the medial part of the pgd. cm, centromedian nucleus; CTT, central tegmental tract; dmpn, dorsomedial pontine nuclei; gc, gigantocellular nucleus; H, field H of Forel; hb, habenular nuclei; LL, lateral lemniscus; lv, lateral vestibular nucleus; mb, mammillary body; ML, medial lemniscus; MLF, medial longitudinal fasciculus; mv, medial vestibular nucleus; nd, dorsal thalamic nucleus; nrpc, nucleus reticularis pontis caudalis; nrtp, nucleus reticularis tegmenti pontis; NV, trigeminal nerve; NVI, abducens nerve; NVII, facial nerve; ov, nucleus ovalis, pc, parvocellular nucleus; pgd, nucleus paragigantocellularis dorsalis; ppH, nucleus prepositus hypoglossi; riMLF, rostral interstitial nucleus of the MLF; rip, nucleus raphe interpositus; rn, red nucleus; sn, substantia nigra; so, superior olive; sv, superior vestibular nucleus; TR, tractus retroflexus; Vm, motor trigeminal nucleus; Vs, sensory trigeminal nucleus; VI, abducens nucleus; VII, facial nucleus. (From Horn AKE, Büttner-Ennever JA, Büttner U. Saccadic premotor neurons in the brainstem: functional neuroanatomy and clinical implications. Neuroophthalmology 1996; 16:229–240.)

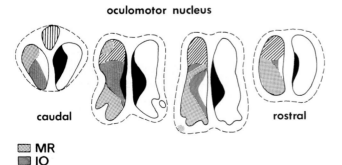

Figure 17.10. Oculomotor nucleus subgroups as determined by contemporary retrograde tracer techniques in Macaca monkey. (Courtesy of Jean A. Büttner Ennever.)

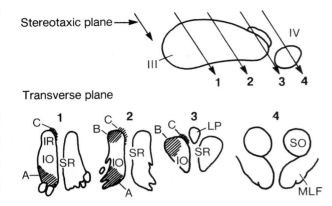

Figure 17. 11. Transverse sections of the oculomotor and trochlear nuclei showing multifocal labeling of motoneurons after injection of horseradish peroxidase into the ipsilateral medial rectus. Top of drawing shows lateral view of nuclei, with *arrows* indicating levels at which the transverse sections (below) were taken. Three separate subgroups (*A, B, C*) are labeled. Nonlabeled areas include the motoneurons that innervate the ipsilateral inferior oblique (IO), inferior rectus (IR), and superior rectus (SR) muscles; LP, motoneuron pool supplying both levator palpebrae superioris muscles; MLF, medial longitudinal fasciculus; SO, motoneuron pool supplying the ipsilateral superior oblique muscle. (Redrawn from Henn V, Büttner Ennever JA, Hepp K. The primate oculomotor system. I. Motoneurons. Hum Neurobiol 1982;1:77–85.)

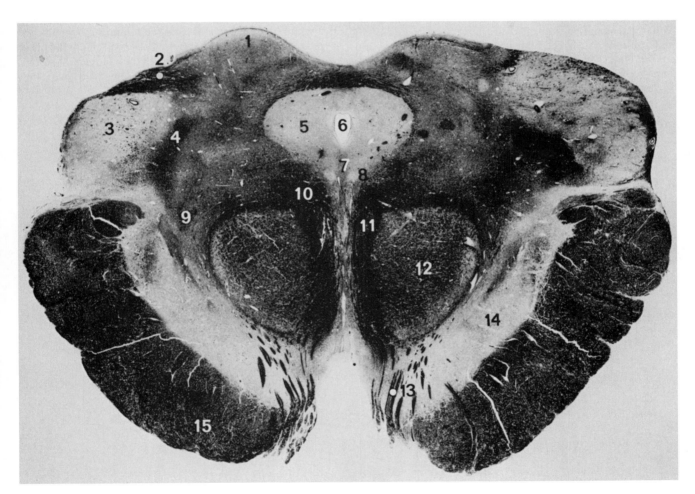

Figure 17.12. Section through rostral mesencephalon showing the oculomotor nuclei and the fasciculi of the oculomotor nerves. 1, superior colliculus; 2, brachium of the inferior colliculus; 3, medial geniculate nucleus; 4, spinal and trigeminal lemnisci; 5, central gray substance; 6, cerebral aqueduct; 7, visceral (parasympathetic) nuclei of the oculomotor nuclear complex; 8, motor nuclei of the oculomotor nuclear complex; 9, medial lemniscus; 10, central tegmental tract; 11, medial longitudinal fasciculus; 12, red nucleus; 13, fasciculus of the oculomotor nerve; 14, substantia nigra; 15, cerebral peduncle. (From Gluhbegovic N, Williams TH. The Human Brain: A Photographic Guide. Hagerstown, MD: Harper & Row, 1980.)

Oculomotor Nerve

Most of the axons in the oculomotor nerve are myelinated and have diameters that vary from 3 to 18 microns. These fibers may be classified as large (6–18 microns) and small (3–6 microns). The large-caliber axons originate from motoneurons and are destined for the extraocular muscles, whereas most of the smaller axons transmit parasympathetic impulses to the ciliary body and iris.

The oculomotor nerve emerges from the interpeduncular fossa at the ventral surface of the mesencephalon as a number of horizontally arranged bundles that immediately fuse into a single nerve trunk. The nerve, invested by pia, passes obliquely downward, forward, and laterally through the subarachnoid cistern at the level of the tentorial incisura and pierces the dura at the top of the clivus just lateral to the posterior clinoid process.

Shortly after leaving the mesencephalon, the nerve passes between two major branches of the basilar artery, the superior cerebellar artery and the posterior cerebral artery (Fig. 17.13). As it continues distally, the nerve is adjacent to the medial inferior surface of the posterior communicating artery for about 0.5 cm before it penetrates the dura to enter the cavernous sinus.

The oculomotor nerve is medial to, and slightly beneath, the ridge of the free edge of the tentorium cerebelli as it enters the cavernous sinus (86). This point is slightly lateral and anterior to the dorsum sellae and 2–7 mm posterior to the initial segment of the supraclinoid portion of the carotid artery.

Within the cavernous sinus, the oculomotor nerve is located just above the trochlear nerve, and both, along with the first (and sometimes the second) division of the trigeminal nerve, lie within the deep layer of the lateral wall of the sinus (Fig. 17.14). This deep layer is formed by the sheaths of these nerves, supplemented by a reticular membrane extending between the sheaths (87) (Fig. 17.15). Anteriorly in the cavernous sinus, the oculomotor nerve apparently receives sympathetic fibers from the carotid trunk; however, the anatomic features of this anastomosis are unclear.

The vascular supply of the oculomotor nerve in the subarachnoid space is via vascular twigs from the posterior cerebral artery, the superior cerebellar artery, and the tentorial and dorsal meningeal branches of the meningohypophyseal trunk of the internal carotid artery. In the cavernous sinus, the tentorial, dorsal meningeal, and inferior hypophyseal branches of the meningohypophyseal trunk supply the nerve along with branches from the ophthalmic artery (88–91).

As the oculomotor nerve leaves the cavernous sinus through the superior orbital fissure to enter the orbit, it is crossed superiorly by the trochlear and ophthalmic division

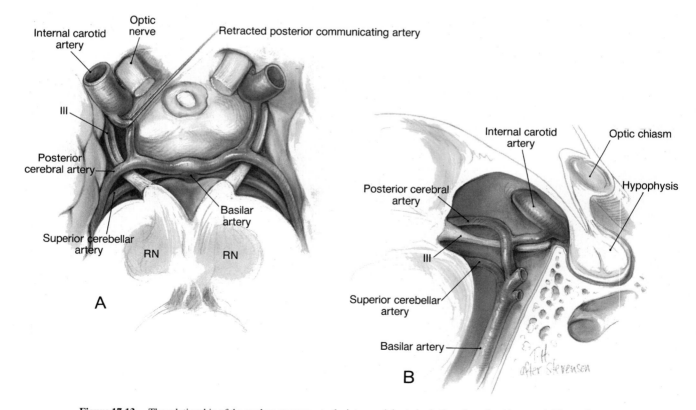

Figure 17.13. The relationship of the oculomotor nerve to the intracranial arteries in the subarachnoid space. *A,* The oculomotor nerves (III) are viewed from above. On the left, the posterior communicating artery has been retracted to show the groove that it may produce through its contact with the oculomotor nerve. RN, red nucleus. *B,* Lateral view of the left oculomotor nerve (III) showing its arterial relationships.

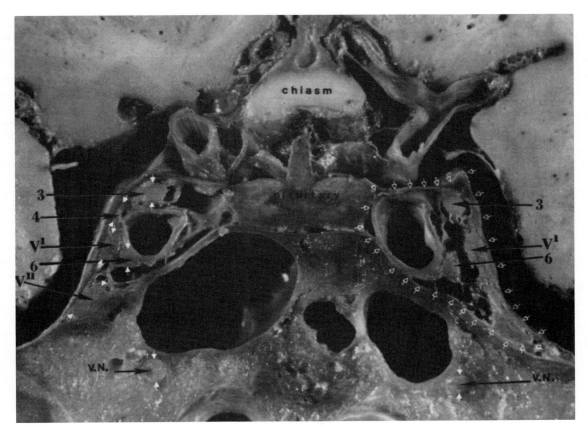

Figure 17.14. Transverse section through the optic chiasm, pituitary gland, and cavernous sinuses, showing the location of the ocular motor nerves. *White hollow arrow*s (right side of photograph) indicate the boundaries of the cavernous sinus. *White solid arrow*s (left side of photograph) outline boundaries of nerves. 3, oculomotor nerve; 4, trochlear nerve; VI, ophthalmic division of the trigeminal nerve; VII, mandibular division of the trigeminal nerve; 6, abducens nerve; VN, vidian nerve. (Courtesy of Dr. William F. Hoyt.)

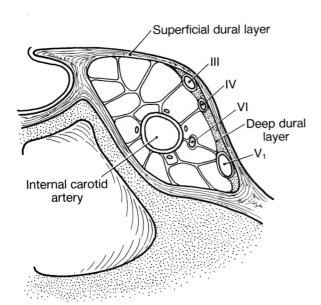

Figure 17.15. Diagram of the cavernous sinus showing that the lateral wall is composed of two layers: a superficial layer (sl) and a deep layer (dl). The deep layer is formed by the sheaths of the oculomotor (III), trochlear (IV), and ophthalmic (V1) nerves, with a reticular membrane between these sheaths. VI, abducens nerve. (Redrawn from Umansky F, Nathan H. The lateral wall of the cavernous sinus: with special reference to the nerves related to it. J Neurosurg 1982;56:228–234.)

of the trigeminal nerves. In this region, the oculomotor nerve divides into two discrete trunks, the superior and inferior divisions. Both divisions pass through the annulus of Zinn adjacent to the abducens nerve (92,93) (Fig. 17.1). The superior division, the smaller of the two, passes up and over the lateral aspect of the optic nerve, dividing into multiple small branches just anterior to the orbital apex. The branches run anteriorly for several millimeters before entering the substance of the superior rectus. The fibers that will supply the levator palpebrae superioris then coalesce briefly, forming a few bundles. These bundles pass along the lateral aspect of the superior rectus and reach the undersurface of the levator palpebrae superioris, at which point they penetrate the muscle.

The inferior division divides into multiple branches in the posterior orbit. These branches innervate the medial and inferior recti and then pass anteriorly beneath the optic nerve or through the inferior rectus itself to penetrate the inferior oblique. The nerve to the inferior oblique, after running along the lateral border of the inferior rectus, splays into several fascicles that penetrate the posterior lateral border of the inferior oblique where it is in contact with the lateral border of the inferior rectus (93). The inferior division also transmits parasympathetic axons to the ciliary ganglion as the motor root of the ganglion (Figs. 17.1 and 17.16).

The topographic arrangement of the fibers within the oculomotor nerve is unclear. Within the subarachnoid space,

pupilloconstrictor fibers appear to be located superficially in the superior portion of the nerve (94,95). There is strong clinical evidence to suggest that fibers in this portion of the oculomotor nerve are arranged in a ''superior'' and ''inferior'' division, but their precise topographic anatomy is not known. Within the cavernous sinus and orbit, the pupillary fibers are located in the inferior division of the nerve, but the position of the fibers going to specific extraocular muscles is unknown except for the major division of the oculomotor nerve into its superior and inferior divisions.

Morphopathologic and neurogenetic studies reveal that some developmental ocular motility disorders are a consequence of altered development of oculomotor motoneurons. Engle et al. (96) suggested that a syndrome previously thought to be an extraocular muscle disorder, congenital fibrosis of the extraocular muscles, may have its origin in oculomotor motoneurons. Individuals with an autosomal-dominant mutation linked to chromosome 12 exhibit congenital, bilateral ptosis, external ophthalmoplegia, and eyes fixed in down gaze. Morphopathologic analysis revealed absence of the superior division of the oculomotor nerve, absence of the caudal central subnucleus of the oculomotor nucleus (which innervates the levator palpebrae), apparent loss of superior rectus motoneurons, and severe levator palpebrae superioris and superior rectus muscle abnormalities (97). These data suggest that congenital fibrosis of the extraocular muscles results from a developmental abnormality in

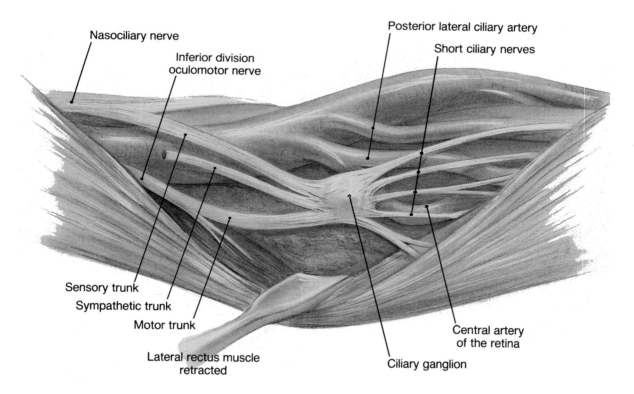

Figure 17.16.   The human ciliary ganglion and its relationship to the orbital arteries, viewed from the lateral aspect of the orbit. The lateral rectus has been retracted away from the ganglion and the optic nerve so that the nerves to and from the ganglion can be identified. (From Eliskóva M. Blood vessels of the ciliary ganglion in man. Br J Ophthalmol 1973;57:766–772.)

the ocular motor lower motor neuron system, much like that proposed for Duane's retraction syndrome (see Chapter 20).

Trochlear Nucleus and Nerve

The trochlear, or fourth, nerve is the smallest of the ocular motor nerves, containing only about 2,100 axons and innervating only the superior oblique muscle.

Trochlear Nucleus

The paired trochlear nuclei are located in the gray matter in the floor of the cerebral aqueduct just caudal to the oculomotor nuclear complex (Fig. 17.17). The trochlear nucleus lies within the dorsal and medial aspect of the medial longitudinal fasciculus (MLF) (98). Motoneurons of one trochlear nucleus innervate the superior oblique muscle of the contralateral eye, although a few (3%–5%) of them innervate the ipsilateral superior oblique muscle (72,99).

Fascicular Portion of the Trochlear Nerve

The axons that emerge from the nuclei initially pass laterally a short distance below the cerebral aqueduct, then curve dorsocaudally, and finally converge to decussate over the roof of the aqueduct in the anterior medullary velum (Fig. 17.18). Each fascicle exits from the dorsal surface of the brain stem on the opposite side (100). The trochlear nerve is the only cranial nerve that crosses and exits from the dorsal side of the brain stem. Thus, the axons from each nucleus innervate the contralateral superior oblique muscle. The decussation, however, is incomplete, with about 5% of the motoneurons passing through the ipsilateral trochlear nerve (72). Because of the dorsal location of the trochlear nuclei, the fascicles of the trochlear nerves are extremely short and are not related to neural structures other than the roof of the cerebral aqueduct. This explains the virtual impossibility of differentiating isolated trochlear nerve damage due to intrinsic brain stem disease from that arising from injury to the subarachnoid portion of the nerve.

Trochlear Nerve

The two trochlear nerves emerge on the dorsal surface of the brain stem just below the inferior colliculi and immediately pass forward around the mesencephalon between the posterior cerebral and superior cerebellar arteries. They then

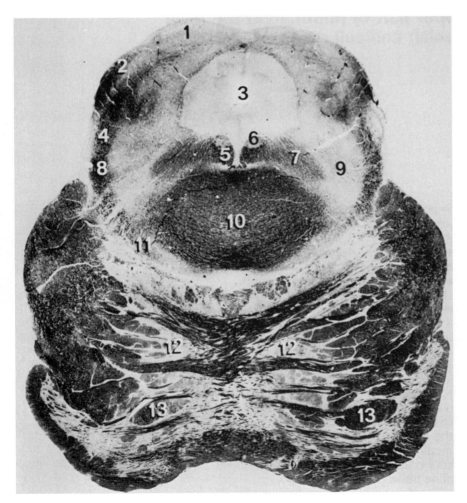

Figure 17.17. Section through the caudal mesencephalon at the level of the trochlear nucleus. *1*, inferior colliculus; *2*, brachium of the inferior colliculus; *3*, cerebral aqueduct; *4*, lateral lemniscus; *5*, medial longitudinal fasciculus; *6*, trochlear nucleus; *7*, central tegmental tract; *8*, spinal and trigeminal lemnisci; *9*, tegmental reticular formation; *10*, decussation of superior cerebellar peduncles; *11*, medial lemniscus; *12*, pontine nuclei and transverse fibers; *13*, corticospinal and corticonuclear fibers. (From Gluhbegovic N, Williams TH. The Human Brain: A Photographic Guide. Hagerstown, MD: Harper & Row, 1980.)

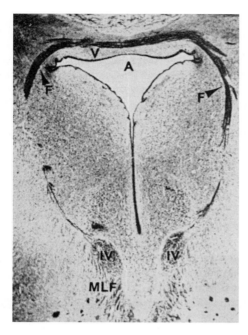

Figure 17.18. The decussation of the trochlear nerves. In this transverse section through the caudal mesencephalon, the trochlear nuclei (IV) can be seen just dorsal to the medial longitudinal fasciculus (MLF). The fascicles of the trochlear nerve (F) course dorsally around the cerebral aqueduct (A) and decussate in the anterior medullary velum (V) before emerging from the dorsal surface of the brainstem. (From Duke Elder S. System of Ophthalmology. Vol 3. London: Henry Kimpton, 1963:265.)

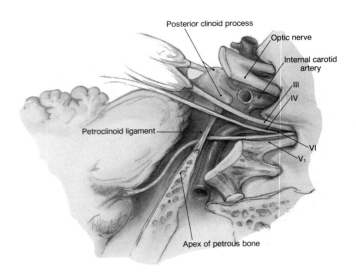

Figure 17.19. Dissection to illustrate the subarachnoid and intracavernous courses of the ocular motor nerves. Note the long subarachnoid course of the trochlear nerve as it proceeds around the brain stem compared with the shorter courses of the oculomotor and abducens nerves. The abducens nerve penetrates the dura at the base of the skull inferior to the points at which the oculomotor and trochlear nerves penetrate the dura.

course around the cerebral peduncles and pierce the dura to enter the cavernous sinus, where the attached and free borders of the tentorium cross one another (Fig. 17.19). This point is inferior and lateral to the point at which the oculomotor nerve enters the cavernous sinus.

Within the cavernous sinus, the trochlear nerve is adjacent and just inferior to the oculomotor nerve, lying in the deep layer of the lateral wall (Figs. 17.14 and 17.15). As the trochlear nerve leaves the cavernous sinus to pass through the superior orbital fissure, it crosses over the oculomotor nerve to lie superior to it. In this region, it receives filaments from the sympathetic plexus and perhaps from the ophthalmic division of the trigeminal nerve.

The trochlear nerve enters the orbit through the superior orbital fissure, outside the annulus of Zinn (Figs. 17.1 and 17.3). It runs anteriorly and medially beneath the superior periorbita to cross over the superior rectus as a single fascicle until just before it enters the superior oblique at its superior nasal aspect (93).

Abducens Nucleus and Nerve

The sixth (abducens) nerve is somewhat larger than the trochlear nerve, but it is only about one-third the size of the oculomotor nerve. It innervates the ipsilateral lateral rectus muscle.

Abducens Nucleus

Each abducens nucleus is located just beneath the floor of the fourth ventricle and lateral to the midline of the pons at the junction of the pons and the medulla (Fig. 17.20). A prominent band of fibers, the genu of the facial nerve, curves over its dorsal and lateral surface. Adjacent and medial to each nucleus is the MLF.

The abducens nucleus contains two neuron populations, the abducens motoneurons and the abducens internuclear neurons. The abducens motoneurons innervate the lateral rectus, while the abducens interneurons give rise to axons that ascend in the contralateral medial longitudinal fasciculus and participate in the internuclear neurons system that controls horizontal conjugate gaze.

Fascicular Portion of the Abducens Nerve

The fascicular portion of the abducens nerve courses ventrally, laterally, and caudally through the pons, passing medial to the superior olivary nucleus to emerge in a groove between the pons and medulla. During this passage, the fascicle is adjacent to the motor nucleus of the facial nerve and the facial nerve fascicle, the motor nucleus of the trigeminal nerve, the spinal tract of the trigeminal nerve (and its nucleus), the superior olivary nucleus, the central tegmental tract, and the corticospinal tract.

The vascular supply of the abducens nuclei and fascicles is via arteries arising from the basilar artery (101,102). These arterial branches can be separated into three groups by their length and the general regions of the brain stem that they serve: (a) the median or paramedian vessels; (b) the short circumferential (or short lateral) branches; and (c) the long circumferential (or long lateral) branches.

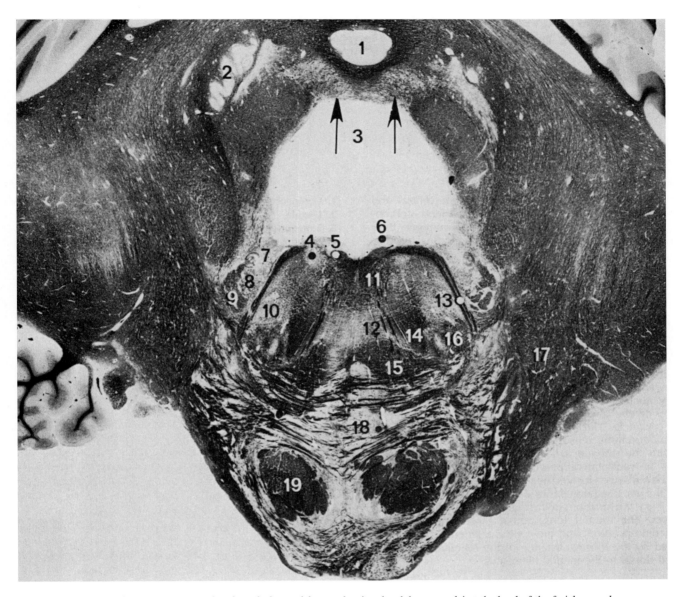

Figure 17.20. Transverse section through the caudal pons showing the abducens nuclei at the level of the facial genu. *1*, cerebellar vermis; *2*, dentate nucleus; *3*, fourth ventricle; *4*, abducens nucleus; *5*, genu of the facial nerve; *6*, facial colliculus; *7*, lateral vestibular nucleus; *8*, spinal nucleus of the trigeminal nerve; *9*, spinal tract of the trigeminal nerve; *10*, facial nucleus; *11*, medial longitudinal fasciculus; *12*, reticular formation; *13*, fasciculus of facial nerve; *14*, central tegmental tract; *15*, medial lemniscus and trapezoid body; *16*, spinal and trigeminal nuclei; *17*, middle cerebellar peduncle; *18*, pontine nuclei and transverse pontine fibers; *19*, pyramidal tract. The *arrow*s show the position of the cerebellar fastigial nuclei. (From Gluhbegovic N, Williams TH. The Human Brain: A Photographic Guide. Hagerstown, MD: Harper & Row, 1980.)

The median branches emerge from the undersurface of the basilar artery and penetrate the pons and medulla at regular intervals. Their course is straight or slightly curved. The circumferential branches encircle the brain stem, entering its substance laterally and superiorly (102,103).

The proximity of the fascicular portion of the abducens nerve to other important neural structures within the brain stem explains the tendency for lesions that produce abducens nerve paresis within the brain stem to cause other neurologic signs.

Abducens Nerve

The abducens nerve emerges from the brain stem between the pons and the medulla, lateral to the pyramidal prominence. The nerve then turns upward along the base of the pons lateral to the basilar artery (Fig. 17.19). The abducens nerve is usually a single trunk that passes between the pons and the anterior inferior cerebellar artery; however, it occasionally exists as two separate trunks (104–106). In one pattern, the abducens nerve originates as a single trunk but splits into two branches that enter the cavernous sinus separately; in a second pattern, the abducens nerve originates as two separate trunks that also enter the cavernous sinus separately (107).

Whether as one trunk or more, the abducens nerve ascends through the subarachnoid space along the face of the clivus and perforates the dura of the clivus about 1 cm below the crest of the petrous bone. It bends laterally around or passes through the inferior petrosal sinus and under the petroclinoid ligament (Grüber's ligament) to enter the cavernous sinus. Within the sinus, the abducens nerve courses anteriorly, bending laterally around the proximal portion of the cavernous carotid artery and running medially and parallel to the ophthalmic division of the trigeminal nerve (86). The abducens nerve is not located within the lateral wall of the cavernous sinus as are the oculomotor and trochlear nerves, but it lies within the body of the sinus instead (86,87) (Figs. 17.14 and 17.15). In addition, within the cavernous sinus, the abducens nerve is fused briefly with a branch of the carotid sympathetic chain, which then splits off and fuses with the ophthalmic division of the trigeminal nerve to enter the orbit with the nasociliary nerve (108–111). The abducens nerve occasionally divides into up to five rootlets that rejoin later to form a single nerve trunk before entering the orbit (86).

The abducens nerve enters the orbit through the superior orbital fissure within the annulus of Zinn adjacent to the lateral rectus (Fig. 17.1). In some individuals, a collagenous septum separates the abducens nerve and the lateral rectus from the other nerves at the orbital apex. In others, the nerve continues for a short distance under the muscle belly before it is separated from the rest of the orbital contents by a sheath along the undersurface of the muscle (93). As with the other ocular motor nerves, the abducens nerve ramifies posteriorly in the orbit, with the branches gradually entering the lateral rectus in a diffuse manner.

THREE DIMENSIONS OF EYE MOTION

The eyeball and the head undergo rotation with three degrees of freedom: rotation about the yaw axis is horizontal, about the pitch (interaural) axis is vertical, and about the roll (naso-occipital) axis is torsional. In theory, the eye could assume an infinite number of torsional positions for any gaze direction. However, during fixation, saccades, and smooth pursuit movements, eye rotation has only two degrees of freedom, with torsion being constrained. In other words, there is only one fixed torsional eye position for each combination of horizontal and vertical eye position. This constraint on torsion is mediated by neural innervation (112–114), by the mechanical properties of the orbital tissue (18,115–120), or a combination of both. Donders first described this phenomenon by observing the rotation of his own eye about the visual axis using afterimages (121). Listing quantitatively defined the amount of torsion for each gaze direction (122,123): any position of the eyeball can be reached from primary position by rotation about an axis that is perpendicular to the line of sight in primary position. The collection of these axes for all rotations that start from primary position constitutes Listing's plane. Donders' and Listing's observations have been heralded as "laws." Listing's law specifies the constraint on torsion expressed by Donders' law. One consequence of Listing's and Donders' laws is that motor efficiency is optimized. By ensuring that the eye stays near the center of its torsional range, the laws permit quick responses to unpredictable targets that may appear from any direction.

For the vestibulo-ocular and optokinetic reflexes, however, Listing's law is violated. This violation is determined by the innervation of extraocular muscles in the planes of the semicircular canals. Head movement about the roll axis elicits ocular torsion to prevent images from slipping on the retina (124,125). Similarly, rotation of retinal images around the roll axis elicits torsional optokinetic smooth eye movements (126). Vestibular and optokinetic movements are discussed later in the chapter. Here we emphasize that three-dimensional control of eye of movements is an important feature of ocular motor systems. For in-depth discussions of three-dimensional eye movements, see Hepp (123) and Wong (127).

PHASIC VELOCITY AND TONIC POSITION COMMANDS TO ORBITAL FORCES THAT DETERMINE OCULAR MOTILITY

Before discussing the central organization of the different ocular motor systems, it is useful to review the nature of the mechanical properties of the orbital tissues, since passive forces must be overcome to move the eyes and, once the eyes are in position, to hold them in place. The predominant orbital forces are elasticity and viscosity (128,129). The moment of inertia of the human eye is so small relative to other tissue forces that for practical purposes it can be ignored. Viscous forces are the major hindrance to movement of the globe within the orbit. For fast eye movements, therefore, a powerful phasic contraction of the extraocular muscles is necessary to overcome viscous drag. This high-frequency phasic discharge provides a "burst" of neural activity that stimulates muscle contraction. The very-high-frequency burst that is required to drive the eyes at saccadic speeds is called a pulse of innervation (128,130).

Once the eyes have been brought to a new position, they must be held there against orbital elastic forces that tend to rotate the globe toward the primary position. To prevent this centripetal drift, a sustained, tonic contraction of the extraocular muscles must follow the phasic contraction produced by the pulse of innervation. This sustained contraction is called a step of neural activity (Fig. 17.21). For each position of the eye there is a specific step discharge rate of agonist motor units and a reciprocally lower step discharge rate for their antagonist motor units. Thus, because of the viscous and elastic forces in the orbit, the ocular motor control signal for a saccadic eye movement is a pulse and a step of innerva-

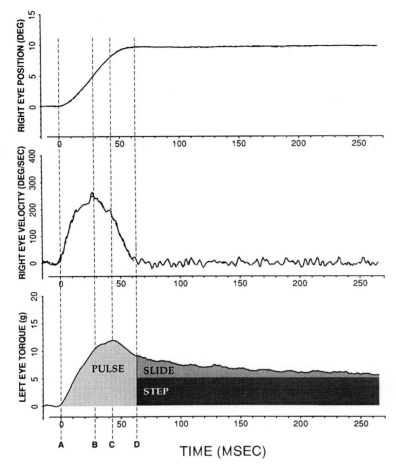

Figure 17.21. The pulse and step of force during and after a saccade. Position (*top*) and velocity (*center*) of the right eye during a rightward saccade and isometric torque developed in the left eye (*bottom*) are shown while it is prevented from moving. The pulse of torque ends with a gradual transition into a slide to the step of torque required to hold the eyes in about 10° of abduction. *A*, saccade onset; *B*, time of peak velocity; *C*, time of peak torque; *D*, end of saccade. (Adapted from Goldstein H, Reinecke R. Clinical applications of oculomotor plant models. In: AF Fuchs, T Brandt, U Büttner, D Zee, eds. Contemporary Ocular Motor and Vestibular Research: A Tribute to David A. Robinson. New York: Thieme Medical Publishers, 1994:10–17.)

tion (128,131). Both the pulse and the step must be of the correct amplitude and appropriately matched for the eyes to be moved rapidly from one position to another and held steady at the end of the movement. The pulse does not actually have an abrupt offset before the step change in the activity of eye muscles. Instead there is a gradual decline (called a slide) in muscle torque after the saccade lands the eye at a specified position in the orbit (128,132,133). This slide probably reflects a gradual transition from the high-frequency discharge of motoneurons during the pulse to a lower-frequency discharge for the step (134). The innervation for a saccade then consists of a pulse-slide-step (Fig. 17.21).

The saccadic pulse and step are eye velocity (phasic) and eye position (tonic) commands. Indeed, ocular motor neurons discharge in relation to both velocity and position for all types of eye movements. When the discharge occurs for low-velocity eye movements (i.e., smooth pursuit, or vestibular or optokinetic smooth eye movements), the phasic increase (a velocity command) is usually smaller than that required for saccades. The tonic firing rate is an eye position command. Phasic-tonic (velocity-position) commands are required for conjugate movements (versions) and vergence movements (135). Groups of neurons in the brain stem tegmentum provide the prenuclear velocity and position commands for the phasic and tonic changes in innervation required for eye movements of appropriate speed and amplitude.

CENTRAL ORGANIZATION OF THE OCULAR MOTOR SYSTEMS

SACCADIC SYSTEM

Saccades are the rapid eye movements that quickly redirect the eye such that an image of an object is brought to the fovea. Here we use the term "saccade" for all fast eye movements, including both voluntary and involuntary changes of fixation, the quick phases of vestibular and optokinetic nystagmus, and the rapid eye movements that occur during sleep (REM sleep) (136). The involuntary fast eye movements that make up one phase of jerk nystagmus are often termed quick phases rather than saccades, but vestibular and optokinetic nystagmus quick phases have amplitude–velocity relationships like voluntary and visually evoked saccades (137–141) (Figs. 17.22 and 17.23).

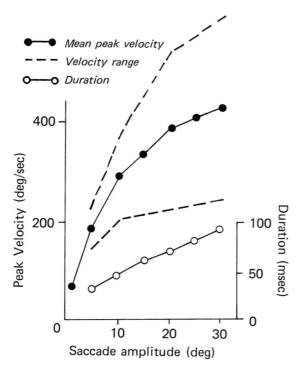

Figure 17.22. The relationship of saccadic amplitude to saccadic peak velocity and duration in normal individuals. Note the broad range of maximum and minimum peak velocity. (Redrawn from Zee DS, Robinson DA. In: Thompson HS, Daroff R, Frisén L, et al, eds. Topics in Neuro-Ophthalmology. Baltimore: Williams & Wilkins, 1979:266–285.)

Characteristics of Saccades

The visual stimulus for a saccade is usually an image of an object of interest seen in the visual periphery. The ocular motor system responds to the appearance of such a stimulus with a saccade of the appropriate amplitude after a latency period of several hundred milliseconds. Saccades can be identified by their velocities and durations (138,142–148).

Saccadic Speed

Saccades show a relatively invariant relationship between their peak velocity and their size: the larger the eye movement, the higher its top speed (Fig. 17.22). The values for most normal subjects fall within a relatively limited range (137,142,147). This amplitude–peak velocity relationship has been called the main sequence and can be used to identify saccades as such (143). In normal individuals, the peak velocity of saccades varies from 30 to 700 deg/sec, and their duration varies from 30 to 100 msec for movements from 0.5°–40° in amplitude (143,149,150). The peak velocity saturates for large-amplitude saccades. This relationship is the same for vertical and horizontal saccades and changes little with age (147,148).

Saccadic velocities cannot be voluntarily controlled, but they are reduced in association with mental fatigue or inattention and are higher when directed to unpredictable visual targets than when made to predictable targets or in darkness (137,150–152). The saccades of REM sleep are slower than saccades made while awake (153). Furthermore, REMs are not usually conjugate but are disjunctive or even monocular in horizontal or vertical directions. Binocular misalignment and disjunctive (even monocular) REMs during sleep

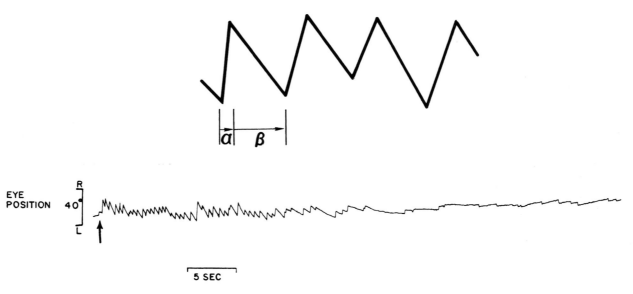

Figure 17.23. The vestibulo-ocular response to sustained rotation. Horizontal eye position is plotted against time. In the lower tracing, the *arrow* represents the beginning of rotation of the patient to the right side in darkness. Note that the nystagmus dies away after about 30–35 seconds. The nystagmus waveform is enlarged in the upper tracing. The nystagmus can be seen to consist of slow phases (β) opposite to the direction of head rotation that hold gaze steady and quick phases (α) that not only reset the eyes to prevent them from drifting to the side of the orbit but also move them in the direction of head rotation. After about 45 seconds of content speed rotation there is reversal of the direction of nystagmus.

provide evidence that separate left eye and right eye pathways generate saccades in each eye and control the position of each eye (6). Although saccadic velocities may be affected by the alertness of a subject, they are not reduced by neuromuscular fatigue (154,155).

For a typical saccade, the eye accelerates rapidly, reaching its peak velocity between one-third and one-half the way through the movement (Fig. 17.21). The eye then gently decelerates but usually stops relatively abruptly (150). Occasionally, even in normal individuals, the eye drifts for a few hundred milliseconds after the initial rapid portion of the horizontal saccade is finished. Such postsaccadic drift has been called a glissade (156,157) and may represent a mismatch between the sizes of the phasic (pulse) and tonic (step) innervation that produce saccades. They can be conjugate (version), correcting for undershoot of the target, or disjunctive (vergence), compensating for divergence during the saccade, or purely monocular. Normal human saccades typically have no postsaccadic drift in the abducting eye and some onward drift in the adducting eye (158). Glissades occur more frequently in fatigued individuals (157,159).

At the end of a saccade, the eye occasionally makes an immediate, oppositely directed, small saccade of about 0.25°–0.50° before coming to rest. This small saccade has been called a dynamic overshoot (160) The incidence of dynamic overshoot is idiosyncratic and is thought to be caused by a brief reversal of the central saccadic command, or by elastic restoring force in the eye muscle (158,161). Dynamic overshoot is most conspicuous after small saccades and often monocular, in the abducting eye. In fact, the microsaccades (about 0.20°) that occur during normal fixation often consist of a pair of to-and-fro saccades of almost equal size, with the latter saccade being a correction of dynamic overshoot, so that the eye ends up almost where it started.

Saccadic Latency (Initiation Time)

The interval between the appearance of a target of interest and the onset of a saccade is normally about 150–250 msec. The latency period increases somewhat with ageing (147,162) and varies according to target luminance and predictability (163). The introduction of a brief temporal "gap" of several hundred milliseconds between the disappearance of an initial fixation point and the presentation of a peripheral target leads to a general reduction in saccadic latency to about 100 ms; these short latency saccades are called express saccades (164–167). Conversely, if the original fixation target remains on while a saccade is made to a new target, the "overlap" target condition delays the saccade onset well over 200–250 msec. These gap and overlap conditions illustrate effects of fixation and attention on the timing of saccades to new visual targets.

Saccadic Accuracy

Small degrees of both conjugate and disconjugate saccadic dysmetria are normal: slight overshooting (hypermetria) tends to occur with small-amplitude saccades and slight undershooting (hypometria) is usual with larger-amplitude saccades (168). The degree of dysmetria is normally about

10% of the amplitude of the initial saccade (152) but is more prominent in older individuals (147,148,162) and with fatigue or inattention (159).

After a hypometric saccade is made, a corrective saccade occurs, after a latency of only 100–130 msec, considerably less than the normal saccadic reaction time. Such corrective movements can occur even when the target is extinguished before the initial saccade is completed. Therefore, a nonvisual or "extraretinal" signal can provide information about whether the first movement is accurate, so that a corrective saccade can be triggered if necessary. This nonvisual information is not proprioceptive (i.e., not using afferent signals from the extraocular muscles) but is based upon monitoring of efferent ocular motor commands, called efference copy or corollary discharge (48,169,170). Vision is certainly important, however, since both the probability and accuracy of a corrective saccade increase if visual information about retinal error (the distance of the image of an object from the fovea) is available at the end of the initial saccade (171). Undershoots appear to improve the efficiency of the saccadic system (172,173).

Although saccades can be made to imagined target locations in darkness, such saccades are inaccurate. For attempted saccades made in darkness between the remembered locations of two targets 5°–70° apart, the first attempts deviate by about 5° from the appropriate angle (174). With successive attempts, there is increasing deviation. In darkness, between saccades to eccentric positions in the orbit, the eyes drift slowly toward the midposition (175,176).

Processing of Visual Information for Saccades

During the period between the initial presentation of a visual target in the periphery and the subsequent saccade to that target, if a target suddenly jumps to a new position and then rapidly returns to its initial location before a saccade to the new position, subjects still make a complete saccade toward the new (transient) target location (177) (Fig. 17.24). Then, after a fairly constant interval of about 150–200 msec, subjects make a corrective saccade back to the original target position. The interval between saccades is relatively independent of the interval between the changes in target position. This suggested that (a) the saccadic system reacts to only one stimulus at a time, and (b) there is an obligatory refractory period following the end of a saccade during which a second saccade cannot be produced. This is in part the rationale for the characterization of saccades as "preprogrammed" (177): once initiated, they cannot be modified and thus run their course unaffected by either visual or nonvisual feedback. That behavior led to the "sampled data" system hypothesis that visual information is sampled to generate saccades (178,179). According to this hypothesis, when a decision is made to generate a saccade based on the retinal error (the distance between the peripheral retinal location of an image and the fovea), the size and direction of the required saccade are calculated and are irrevocable. A preprogrammed saccadic eye movement command is then generated based upon the visual information that was acquired during the initial visual sample. Once the saccade is com-

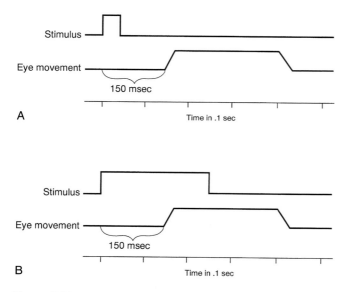

Figure 17.24. The apparent ''preprogrammed'' nature of saccadic eye movements. *A*, In response to a double target jump, there is a 150-msec latency period before the eye moves. The eye then moves to where the target was after its initial movement, stays in this location for a set period of time, and then moves back to the new (original) location of the target. *B*, Even when the target jumps to a new location and then moves back to its original location following the eye movement, the eye remains in its new position for the same amount of time as in *A* before moving back to the new (original) target position. (Redrawn from Westheimer G. Eye movement responses to a horizontally moving visual stimulus. Arch Ophthalmol 1954;52:932–941.)

pleted, the visual world is again sampled to determine whether another saccade is required to bring the image of the object of interest onto the fovea. If a retinal error still exists, the entire process is repeated.

Although this ''sampled data'' system hypothesis accounts for some aspects of the saccadic system, it can acquire and use visual information continuously up to about 70 msec before a saccade begins (180). This is about the time it takes visual information to traverse the retina and central visual pathways and reach brain stem ocular motor structures. In addition, under certain conditions, two saccades may occur back to back with virtually no intersaccadic interval (180). Thus, there is no obligatory refractory period between saccades. Rather, the central nervous system appears to be able to process information in parallel and to program more than one saccade at a time (181). Visual information can be acquired even during a saccade and influence the time of the occurrence, size, and direction of subsequent saccades. When a target is briefly flashed directly on the fovea during a saccade, a subsequent saccade can be produced that takes the eye to the actual location of the target even though no retinal error ever existed (since the target was flashed on the fovea) and the target is no longer visible (182). Thus, the saccadic system can calculate the position of the target relative to the head using a combination of knowledge of the position of the eye in the orbit during the saccade at the

instant the target was flashed and the retinal error (in this case, zero). The saccadic system can program movement in a head coordinate as well as a retinal coordinate scheme (182,183). Moreover, the amplitude of saccades can be adapted to increase or decrease by moving a target to a new position while the saccades are in flight. This adaptation requires several hundred intrasaccadic movements of a target and is a form of motor learning (184,185). Finally, saccade trajectories of patients with abnormally slow saccades can be modified when the target position is changed after the eye has already begun moving (186). Thus, normal saccades appear to be preprogrammed only because of their high velocities and brief durations. Once a saccade has begun, there is usually not enough time to process the new visual information required to modify the saccade before it has finished.

Vision During Saccades

Although the visual world is rapidly sweeping across the retina during a saccade, there is no sense of a blurred image. We do not seem to see during saccadic eye movements. However, there are instances where vision is quite clear during saccades. For example, when looking at the track from a fast-moving train, the sleepers become visible only when we make saccade opposite to the motion of the train, thereby stabilizing their image on the retina. Absence of blurring of images during saccades has been called saccadic omission (187) and is caused by two factors: saccadic suppression, consisting of elevation of the threshold for detecting light during a saccade (188,189), and visual masking, a process by which the presence of a stationary, highly contoured visual background before or after a saccade eliminates the perception of the blurred visual image during the saccade. Visual masking is independent of eye movements, since it also occurs if a pattern is briefly moved across a stationary retina at saccadic velocities (190–194).

Visual interactions reduce the response to visual stimulation of many neurons in the striate cortex (area V1) and the superficial layers of the superior colliculus of monkeys during saccades (195–197). Reduced sensitivity in the activity in the magnocellular visual pathway is a cellular correlate of saccadic omission (198). Many neurons in the middle temporal (MT), middle superior temporal cortical (MST), and lateral intraparietal (LIP) (199) areas of monkeys are selectively silenced during image motion induced by saccades, but they respond well to identical external image motion, when no saccades occur. In addition, some neurons in areas MT and MST reverse their preferred direction of motion sensitivity during saccades. Consequently, oppositely directed motion signals annul one another, and motion percepts are suppressed (200).

Constancy of spatial relations is also maintained during after saccades. Although the visual scene shifts with each saccade, we maintain our sense of straight ahead and piece together one view from many ''snapshots'' taken between saccades. This spatial constancy is probably accomplished by extraretinal signals of the eye movement commands (efference copy) to perceptual areas that register retinal input with motor commands (170,201). Efference copy may reduce visual sensitivity, making motion less visible, and expand receptive fields of neurons to enable a smooth shift of targets that flash into view at the onset of a saccade (199,202).

Neurophysiology and Neuroanatomy of Saccadic Eye Movements

Two classes of cells are essential components of the brain stem circuits that produce saccades: burst neurons and omnipause neurons. Burst neurons are divided into excitatory and inhibitory types. Excitatory burst neurons in turn are divided into short-lead burst neurons and long-lead burst neurons (short-lead burst neurons are sometimes called medium-lead burst neurons). The immediate premotor command for the saccadic pulse is generated by excitatory short-lead burst neurons that lie within the paramedian reticular formation in the pons (for horizontal saccades) (203) and in the paramedian mesencephalon (for vertical and torsional saccades) (204) (Fig. 17.8). They deliver high-frequency discharges, at rates up to 1,000 Hz, to motoneurons 8–15 msec before and during saccades but are silent during fixation and during pursuit, vestibular, and optokinetic smooth eye movements. Long-lead burst neurons discharge irregularly for up to 100 msec before a saccade burst, and some are thought to activate short-lead burst neurons. Long-lead burst neurons are located predominantly in the rostral paramedian pontine reticular formation (PPRF) and the midbrain reticular formation (205,206); they also show a burst of activity just before and during the saccade, and they may trigger saccades, encode their direction or size, or relay saccadic commands from the superior colliculus and other areas (207,208). Omnipause neurons show a reverse pattern of firing to short-lead burst neurons; they have a high tonic discharge rate (over 100 Hz), which is interrupted 10–12 msec before and during saccades in any direction (Figs. 17.9 and 17.25). Omnipause neurons exert a tonic inhibition during fixation and smooth eye movements on short-lead burst neurons, preventing them from firing. During a saccade omnipause neurons are inhibited, possibly by long-lead burst neurons in the rostral PPRF and superior colliculus. Inhibition of omnipause neurons releases short-lead burst neurons to activate motoneurons and dispatch a saccade (209) (Fig. 17.25). Inhibitory burst neurons are activated by the excitatory short-lead burst neurons at the same time as the omnipause cells cease firing (210). Omnipause cells serve as latch to release saccades and stop them. Inhibitory burst neurons inhibit the motoneurons to antagonist muscles just before and during the saccade. The discharge rate of motoneurons encodes saccadic velocity, and the discharge duration encodes saccade duration. Saccadic amplitude is consequently a function of both firing frequency and duration (211,212).

Brain Stem Generation of Horizontal Saccades

The PPRF receives bilateral projections from the frontal eye field (FEF), in the frontal cortex around the arcuate sulcus; the intermediate and deep layers of mainly the contralat-

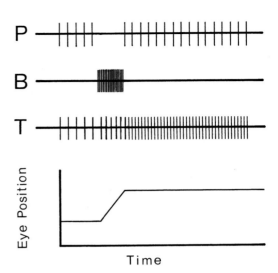

Figure 17.25. The relationship among the discharges of excitatory short lead burst cells (B), tonic cells (T), and omnipause pause cells (P) in the generation of a saccadic eye movement. Omnipause cells cease discharging just before the saccade, allowing the excitatory burst cells to generate a pulse of innervation with a rapidly increasing firing rate. During this period, the eye moves to its new position. The tonic firing rate increases during the saccade and at the end of the burst cell activity, tonic firing rate is appropriate to hold the eye in its new position. The rate remains constant as long as the eye is held in the new position of gaze. (Redrawn from Zee DS. In: Lessell S, van Dalen JTW. Neuro-Ophthalmology. Vol. 1. Amsterdam: Excerpta Medica, 1980:131–145.)

eral superior colliculus; and ipsilateral projections from brain stem structures, including the nucleus interstitialis of Cajal, nucleus of Darkschewitsch, and nucleus of the posterior commissure, the mesencephalic reticular formation, the vestibular nuclei, the nucleus prepositus hypoglossi, and the cerebellar fastigial nucleus (213–215).

Electric stimulation within the caudal PPRF generates ipsiversive saccades (216). Damage that is confined to short-lead burst neurons in the caudal PPRF causes slow ipsiversive saccades, having prolonged durations, reduced peak velocities, and normal or near-normal amplitudes (217,218). Paralysis of all ipsiversive conjugate eye movements was reported in earlier studies (219,220) and may have reflected damage to vestibular nucleus projections carrying eye position and smooth eye movement signals across the pons to the abducens nucleus (221). Large, bilateral, pontine lesions that include the midline may also produce a vertical saccadic paresis in addition to the horizontal defect (217,220,222). Thus, pontine structures also participate in the generation of vertical saccades.

Excitatory short-lead burst neurons in the caudal PPRF excite the lateral rectus motoneurons and internuclear neurons that lie within the abducens nucleus (134,209). These internuclear neurons are surrogate motoneurons for the medial rectus muscle. Their axons cross the midline and ascend within the MLF to excite medial rectus motoneurons in the contralateral oculomotor nucleus. Interruption of axons of these abducens nucleus internuclear neurons causes paresis of adduction in the eye on the side of a lesion in the MLF, the cardinal manifestation of internuclear ophthalmoplegia (see Chapter 19). About 80% of short-lead burst neurons in the caudal PPRF, which were once thought to encode conjugate velocity commands for saccades, actually encode monocular movements of either abduction or adduction (7). This behavior is contrary to Hering's law. Moreover, most abducens motor neurons, which innervate the lateral rectus muscle, fire with both ipsilateral and contralateral eye movements (5,7).

Inhibitory burst neurons for horizontal saccades are located just caudal and ventral to the abducens nucleus in the reticular formation of the rostral medulla (Fig. 17.9) and send their axons across the midline to the motoneurons and internuclear neurons in the contralateral abducens nucleus (210,223). Inhibitory burst neurons act to suppress activity of the contralateral (antagonist) abducens nucleus during ipsiversive saccades. Saccades in one direction are driven by yoked agonist muscles in the two eyes. Normal trajectories of saccades require reciprocal inhibition of yoked antagonist muscles. Inhibitory burst neurons provide this reciprocal pulse of inhibition. A pulse-step of excitation in agonist motoneurons is accompanied by a pulse-step of reduced firing rate in antagonist motoneurons.

In humans, excitatory short-lead burst neurons lie in the nucleus reticularis pontis caudalis, and inhibitory burst neurons are the medial part of the nucleus paragigantocellularis dorsalis (Figs. 17.8 and 17.9) (203). Omnipause neurons reside in the nucleus raphe interpositus (rip) in the midline of the caudal pons, between the excitatory burst neurons rostrally and the inhibitory burst neurons caudally, at the level of the abducens nuclei (Fig. 17.9) (224,225).

Brain Stem Generation of Vertical and Torsional Saccades

Vertical saccades are generated by excitatory short-lead burst neurons in the rostral interstitial nucleus of the MLF (riMLF) (Figs. 17.8 and 17.9). Those for upward and downward saccades are intermingled in this nucleus (204, 226–228), although in cats upward burst neurons are concentrated in its caudal part and downward burst neurons are more rostral (229). In squirrel monkeys, short-lead burst neurons with upward on directions descend directly in the MLF bilaterally to the superior rectus and inferior oblique subnuclei of the oculomotor nucleus with axon collaterals crossing within the oculomotor nucleus. They supply the superior rectus and inferior oblique muscles of both eyes (230,231) (Fig. 17.26). They also give collateral axons to the interstitial nucleus of Cajal (INC), which integrates the pulse delivered to it from the riMLF into a step and transmits it to motoneurons (neural integration of the pulse is discussed below). riMLF short-lead burst neurons for downward saccades project directly to the inferior rectus subnucleus of the oculomotor nucleus and to the trochlear nucleus, on the same side, and send collaterals to the ipsilateral INC (230,231) (Fig. 17.26). Inferior rectus motoneurons innervate the muscle of

the ipsilateral eye and superior oblique motoneurons innervate the muscle of the contralateral eye. Thus, these riMLF burst neurons on one side excite downward movements of both eyes and dysconjugate torsion, greater in the contralateral eye, with the upper poles rolling toward the ipsilateral side. One short-lead burst cell in one riMLF sends axons to motoneurons of yoked pairs of muscles: By this dual projection pattern, short-lead burst neurons can each drive vertical motoneuron pools of both eyes during conjugate vertical rapid eye movements (Fig. 17.26); these data support Hering's law (4,232).

The omnipause neurons located in the caudal pons cease firing to generate vertical and torsional saccades as well as horizontal saccades (Fig. 17.9). Inhibitory burst neurons for vertical and torsional saccades reside within the riMLF (230,231,233,234).

Unilateral lesions of the riMLF abolish torsional saccades toward the side of damage and induce torsional nystagmus and tonic torsional deviation, with the upper poles of the eyes beating and rotated toward the opposite side, in monkeys (235,236) and humans (237,238). Unilateral lesions of the INC cause tonic torsion to the opposite side, like the effect of riMLF lesions. INC lesions also produce torsional nystagmus, but the nystagmus fast phases are directed toward the side of the lesion, unlike the effect of riMLF lesions (239). Unilateral INC lesions also cause the ocular tilt reaction, as we discuss later in this chapter. While the deficits after a riMLF lesion result from an imbalance of the saccade generator, a vestibular imbalance probably causes the deficits after an INC lesion (239,240).

Effects of discrete lesions on vertical gaze in monkeys and humans are largely consistent with information that is emerging from single neuron studies. Lesions in structures within the mesencephalon, namely the riMLF, the posterior commissure, and the INC, create vertical saccadic palsies (241–245). The mixture of neurons with up-and-down presaccadic activity in the riMLF and INC indicates that selective palsies of upward and downward conjugate eye movements are not produced by discrete lesions within these small nuclei, but rather by lesions that disrupt projections from the nuclei to the oculomotor and trochlear nuclei. Such lesions are bilateral, or unilateral and so close to the midline that they involve axons that cross the midline within commissural fiber tracts. Since excitatory burst neurons with upward on-direction project bilaterally to oculomotor nucleus neurons, whereas neurons with downward on-directions project ipsilaterally to motoneurons of the oculomotor and trochlear nuclei (230,231), isolated lesions of the riMLF are more likely to selectively impair downward saccades (245). Either unilateral or bilateral pretectal lesion near the posterior commissure may destroy projections from both riMLF and the INC, selectively abolishing upward saccades.

The nucleus of the posterior commissure also contains upward short-lead burst neurons that project across the commissure (230). The nucleus of the posterior commissure projects to the contralateral nucleus of the posterior commissure, riMLF, and INC and intralaminar nucleus of the thalamus. Lesions of the posterior commissure paralyze upward

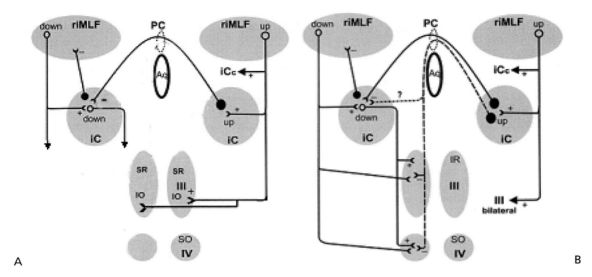

Figure 17.26. Midbrain pathways for the generation of vertical saccades. Downward acting neurons are shown on the left side and upward acting neurons on the right side of *A* and *B*. *A*, Projections to superior rectus (SR) and inferior oblique (IO) motoneurons for upward saccades. *B*, Projections to inferior rectus (IR) and superior oblique (SO) motoneurons for downward saccades. *Open circles* indicate excitatory neurons and *filled circles* indicate inhibitory neurons. The riMLF provides only excitatory projections to motoneurons in the oculomotor (III) and trochlear nuclei (IV), and presumably to premotor down-burst-tonic neurons in the iC, which themselves excite SO motoneurons of the same side. Further, the motoneurons receive an inhibitory GABA-ergic input from the contralateral iC. These inhibitory neurons could be activated by premotor up-burst neurons in the riMLF, thereby inhibiting the SO and IR motoneurons during upward saccades. It is not clear whether inhibitory projection via the posterior commissure (PC) is mediated via collaterals from premotor burst-tonic neurons in the contralateral interstitial nucleus of Cajal (iC) (question mark) or by separate projections. It is possible that inhibitory neurons in the iC may include non-premotor saccade-related up- and down-burst neurons in the iC (question mark, left side). Down-burst neurons project back to the ipsilateral riMLF, and there is some evidence that saccade-related up-burst neurons project to the contralateral iC (iCc). Aq, aqueduct of Sylvius. (Adapted from Horn AK, Helmchen C, Wahle P. GABA-ergic neurons in the rostral mesencephalon of the macaque monkey that control vertical eye movements. Ann NY Acad Sci 2003;1004:19–28.)

saccades in monkeys and humans (241,243,246) as part of the pretectal syndrome (see Chapter 19); anatomic or electrophysiologic evidence that nucleus of the posterior commissure fibers transmitting commands for upward saccades traverse this prominent structure is scanty (230,247). Discrete posterior commissure lesions in squirrel monkeys produce postsaccadic drifts, velocity reduction, and phase advance of the vestibulo-ocular reflex (VOR). Posterior commissure fibers are necessary for conveying the output of the vertical neural integrator to vertical oculomotor neurons (247).

As noted above, bilateral PPRF lesions that include the midline may also produce a vertical saccadic paresis in addition to a bidirectional horizontal saccadic palsy (217, 220,222). The PPRF contains excitatory burst neurons with on-directions for oblique saccades having either upward or downward vectors (207,248). Signals from these oblique burst neurons on each side of the PPRF might sum to cancel horizontal vectors in opposite directions, and transmit velocity commands for upward or downward saccades to the riMLF neurons on each side. Damage to either the oblique burst neurons in the PPRF or pause neurons in the rip (249) might cause paresis of vertical saccades. Direct projections from the FEF in the cerebral hemispheres to the riMLF have been demonstrated (250). The relative importance of ascend-

ing signals from the PPRF and descending signals from the superior colliculus (SC) and cerebral hemispheres to the riMLF seems uncertain.

Neural Integration of the Saccadic Pulse

The pulse-step of innervation that drives ocular motoneurons during saccades (Fig. 17.21) is generated by premotor neurons in the brain stem tegmentum. Short-lead burst neurons deliver the pulse, an eye velocity command, to motoneurons. The saccadic step, an eye position command, is created from the pulse by a neural network that integrates, in the mathematical sense, conjugate eye velocity commands into the appropriate position-coded information (step) for the ocular motoneurons. This neural integrator is reflected in the activity of neurons located within the INC and vestibular nucleus for vertical and torsional movements (251–254) and in the medial vestibular nucleus (MVN) and adjacent nucleus prepositus hypoglossi (NPH) for horizontal movement (255–259). Burst-tonic neurons in the MVN and the NPH, which lies immediately medial to the MVN (Fig. 17.9), carry eye position and eye velocity signals during conjugate saccades and fixation as well as during disjunctive saccades and fixation. Burst-tonic neurons preferentially encode the position and the velocity of a single eye (9), contrary to expectations from Hering's law. These burst-tonic neurons shape the pulse-slide-step saccadic discharges of abducens nucleus neurons to which they project.

The velocity-to-position neural integrator is not perfect. In darkness, after an eccentric saccade, the eyes drift back toward orbital midposition at a rate that is determined by elastic restoring forces in the orbit relative to the opposite force generated by the tonic step of muscle discharge (257). The centripetal drift occurs because the integrator discharges. It is said to be "leaky." Drift rate declines exponentially and can be expressed by a time constant; after one time constant, the eye velocity declines to 37% of its initial value and after three time constants, eye movements have nearly stopped. The time constant of centripetal eye drift in darkness is 20–70 seconds (174,260). The time constant of orbital restoring forces that return the eye toward midposition is about 200 msec. Thus, even in darkness, the neural integrator greatly prolongs the mechanically determined centripetal drift of the eyes. In the light, visual feedback prevents the integrator from leaking. This eye position holding depends on the integrity of the flocculus, the ventral paraflocculus, or both (261). The activity of the horizontal neural integrator is distributed among the NPH, the vestibular nucleus, and the flocculus. Damage to the NPH and MVN or flocculus causes gaze-evoked nystagmus with centripetal decelerating slow phases (255,259,262). Destruction of the NPH alone does not eliminate the integrator; rather, the time constant of centripetal drift decreases to 10% of its normal values but remains 10 times longer than that attributable to the mechanics of the orbit (257).

Because the eye moves in three dimensions and the order of movements is independent, the integral of angular eye velocity does not yield angular eye position in three dimensions. Therefore, the neural integrator does not process eye velocity signals alone. Instead, eye position signals must be fed back and multiplied by eye velocity signals before they are integrated to transform eye velocity into appropriate eye position commands (263). Velocity-to-position transformation is used by all eye movement systems, as we discuss later in this chapter.

Feedback Control of Saccades

Precisely how the central nervous system controls the intensity and duration of the saccadic burst is unknown. Studies of patients with slow saccades have led to the hypothesis that saccades may be generated by a mechanism that drives the eyes to a specific orbital position (186). Through a "feedback loop" that allows continuous comparison of the actual (based on monitoring of internal ocular motor commands—efference copy) and the desired (based on visual information regarding target position) eye position, the burst neurons could be driven until the eye reaches the target (208,264,265). Further support for this type of mechanism comes from recordings of the activity of burst neurons during saccades (264), from the behavior of vestibular quick phases during high-velocity head rotations (266), and from the finding that certain drugs slow saccades but do not alter their accuracy (267).

Saccades are initiated by trigger signals from the cerebral hemispheres and superior colliculi that inhibit omnipause neurons. Inhibition of these omnipause cells releases the discharge of excitatory burst neurons and the duration of their firing determines the amplitude of saccades. A command signal of desired eye position (e.g., retinal target error), which is independent of the trigger signal, determines how long the burst cells fire (Fig. 17.27). Collaterals of short-lead burst neurons excite inhibitory burst neurons, which inhibit the omnipause cells and antagonist motoneurons during the saccade. The burst output provides an eye velocity command, which is also integrated to create a new eye position command (the step). The pulse is also believed to be integrated by another resettable integrator to provide a feedback signal of eye position, which inhibits the excitatory burst neurons (131,208,218,265,268). The eye velocity signal must also be multiplied by an eye position signal before being transformed by the neural integrator into an eye position command (263). Once the actual eye position matches the desired eye position, the burst cells cease firing, the omnipause cells resume their tonic activity, and the saccade stops.

Cerebral Control of Saccadic Eye Movements

Two major classes of saccades are generated by the cerebral hemispheres: (a) reflexive visually guided saccades in response to the sudden appearance of targets on the retina and (b) volitional saccades that are internally triggered toward a target. In actual behavior, both modes of saccade generation act in concert, as when a person decides to look at one of several suddenly appearing objects. Visually guided saccades are often elicited to a newly appearing target while a person is looking at a prior target. In the laboratory this is tested with a continually appearing target and a sudden peripheral target that the person is required to refixate; this

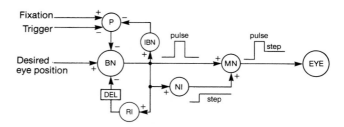

Figure 17.27. Model for generation of saccades. Fixation maintains activity of omnipause pause neurons (P) until a trigger signal inhibits them, releasing excitatory short-lead burst neurons (BN). BNs excite inhibitory burst neurons (IBN), which stop pause cell activity and also inhibit motor neurons of antagonist muscles. The burst neurons send a velocity command (the pulse) to motoneurons (MN) and to the neural integrator (NI), which creates a position command (the step) for the eye. Another integrator, resettable after each saccade (RI), creates a negative feedback signal of eye position, delivered after a delay (DEL), to BN. When actual eye position equals desired eye position, BNs cease firing, pause cells are disinhibited, and the saccade stops.

is called the overlap task. The refixation saccade requires disengagement of attention, shifting of attention from the fixation target to the new target, and the disengagement of fixation. If the original fixation target is extinguished for a gap of about 200 msec before the new target appears (a paradigm named the gap task), fixation is disengaged more rapidly and many "express" saccades are dispatched at very short latencies of about 100 msec (165,269).

Volitional saccades may themselves be of three categories: (*a*) predictive, when a target is expected at a location but has not yet appeared or when self-paced saccades are made between preselected targets; (*b*) memory guided, toward the remembered positions of targets on the retina (i.e., with visual memory) or toward the remembered position of gaze direction before the head is rotated (i.e., with vestibular input); and (*c*) saccades directed away from the position of a suddenly appearing target; the latter are called antisaccades since they direct the fovea away from a visual target (182,270,271). Attention and volitional effort are especially demanded when making antisaccades, since reflexive saccades to the visual target must be suppressed.

FRONTAL EYE FIELDS

Two structures, the FEF and the SC, appear to be critical for the generation of visually guided and volitional saccadic eye movements. Positron emission tomography (PET), func-

tional MRI (fMRI), and cortical stimulation indicate that the FEF in humans is located in the posterior part of the middle frontal gyrus and the adjacent precentral sulcus and gyrus (272–277) (Fig. 17.28). The FEF receives projections from several cortical areas, notably the lateral intraparietal area (LIP; also called the parietal eye field), supplementary eye field in the cingulate gyrus, prefrontal cortex, and superior temporal cortex as well as from the pulvinar and intralaminar nuclei of the thalamus. Cerebral metabolism increases in the FEF during fixation, self-paced saccades in darkness, reflexive visually guided saccades, memory-guided saccades in a delayed task after target disappearance, and antisaccades (270,274,278). Metabolic activity in the human FEF increases progressively from tasks requiring fixation, to paradigms that elicit reflexive saccades to visual targets, to paradigms for volitional saccades guided by memory or away from targets (274). This is consistent with the observation by Funahashi et al. (279) that FEF lesions in monkeys impair memory-guided saccades more than visually guided saccades. A population of neurons in the FEF discharge before and specifically in relation to visually guided saccades to seen or remembered targets (280). Lesions of the FEF produce deficits in generating saccades to briefly presented targets, in the production of saccades to two or more sequentially presented targets, and in the selection of simultaneously presented targets (281).

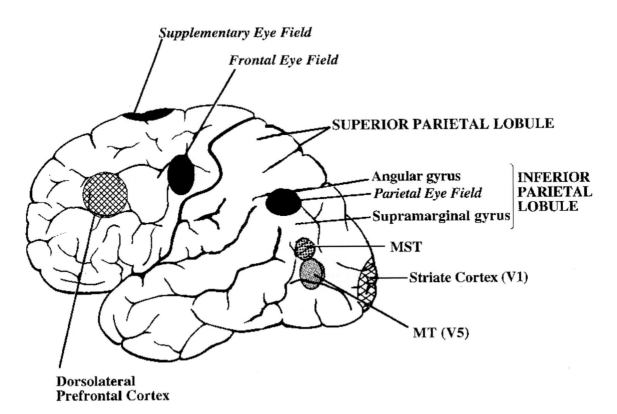

Figure 17.28. Probable locations of cortical areas involved in cerebral control of eye movements in humans. MT, middle temporal visual area; MST, medial superior temporal visual area. (Adapted from Leigh RJ, Zee DS. The Neurology of Eye Movements. Oxford, UK: Oxford University Press, 1999.)

Stimulation within the FEF produces contralateral saccades, usually with a vertical component. The size and direction of the saccade are determined by which region is stimulated; the organization is in retinal coordinates. Purely vertical saccades can be produced by simultaneously stimulating corresponding points in the FEF of both hemispheres, thus nullifying the horizontal components (282).

FEF neurons project caudally in the anterior limb of the internal capsule and reach the premotor structures of the brain stem by four pathways: fibers to the striatum (caudate nucleus and putamen); a dorsal, transthalamic pathway to thalamic nuclei; a ventral pedunculo-tegmental pathway; and an intermediate pathway (214,215). Projections are to the ipsilateral superior colliculus and to the rip of the caudal pons, and to the nucleus reticularis tegmenti pontis (NRTP) and riMLF (Fig. 17.9), and to the caudal PPRF on each side (213,250,283). Projections to the omnipause neurons in the nucleus rip probably trigger saccades, whereas projections to the NRTP may be important in transmitting saccade direction and amplitude information to burst neurons in the PPRF (214,215,283).

SUPERIOR COLLILCULUS

The paired superior and inferior colliculi appear as four small swellings or eminences that protrude from the tectum (i.e., the roof of the mesencephalon; Fig. 17.8). Although the SC is a brain stem structure, we discuss it here with cerebral cortical areas because of its close relationship to cerebral generation of saccades. Each SC has seven alternating layers of cells and fibers (284) that can be divided into two functional parts, superficial and deep. The superficial layers are primarily involved in visual sensory function. The SC receives visual input both from the retina directly via the optic tract and indirectly from the visual cortex. The deep layers of the SC are concerned with ocular motor function. Cortical afferents to the deep layers include the striate, prestriate, auditory, and somesthetic cortex, parietal and temporal cortical areas, prefrontal cortex, and FEF.

The SC receives two projections from the FEF: a direct one (285) and an indirect one via the caudate nucleus and the pars reticulata of the substantia nigra (SNpr) (286–290). The parietal eye field (area LIP) also projects to the SC (291). Intermediate layers of the SC contain saccade-related burst neurons, called T cells in monkeys because of their morphology. T cells discharge in relation to contraversive horizontal and vertical saccades. Saccadic eye movements of different sizes and directions are represented in an orderly topographic map across the intermediate and deep layers of the SC, where large saccades are encoded caudally and small saccades rostrally. T neurons for downward saccades are lateral, neurons for upward saccades are medial, neurons for large horizontal saccades are caudal, and those for small horizontal saccades are rostral in the SC (292,293). Thus, the SC contains a retinotopically organized motor map in which each site is thought to encode a specific saccade vector.

Three types of SC cells participate in generating saccades:

burst T neurons, buildup neurons, and fixation neurons. Fixation neurons in the rostral pole of the SC keep the buildup neurons silent and the eyes still until a new target appears and activates the buildup cell population, which discharges as a rostrally spreading wave, or moving hill, to inhibit fixation cells (294,295). Buildup cells (also referred to as prelude cells) were thought to activate saccades through their trajectories; however, this spreading wave theory is challenged by the finding that buildup activity would arrive at the fixation zone much too late to terminate saccades at the appropriate time (296). Instead, buildup neurons may help to trigger saccades by inhibiting the collicular fixation cells, which excite omnipause neurons in the midline of the pons. The colliculus projects to omnipause neurons (297). The rostral SC fixation cells excite them monosynaptically to maintain fixation. Cells in the caudal and rostral SC inhibit the pontine omnipause neurons disynaptically (298) (Fig. 17.29). The inhibitory interneurons may be located close to the omnipause neurons in the rip, or in the NRTP (298). Short-lead

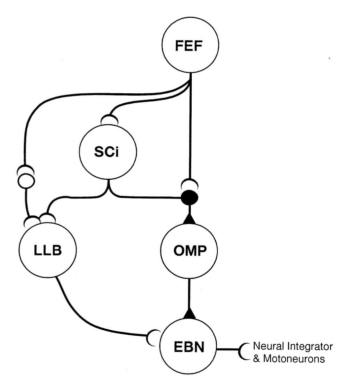

Figure 17.29. Frontal eye field projections to brain stem showing hypothetical connections for triggering saccades. Frontal eye field (FEF) neurons turn off omnipause neurons (OMP) by exciting inhibitory interneurons. Signals from FEF or the SC determine saccade amplitude and direction. This spatial command is translated into a temporal code, the duration of EBN cell discharge. EBN cells are called short-lead burst neurons in the text. Filled synapses are inhibitory. SCi, intermediate layer of superior colliculus; LLB, long-lead burst neuron; EBN, medium-lead excitatory burst neuron. (Adapted from Segraves MA. Activity of monkey frontal eye field neurons projecting to oculomotor regions of the pons. J Neurophysiol 1992; 68:1967–1985.)

and long-lead burst neurons in the PPRF receive excitatory projections from the SC (205,206,299,300). SC fixation neurons and pontine omnipause neurons are inhibited to dispatch saccades, and burst T neurons are proposed to activate short-lead excitatory burst neurons in the PPRF to drive them to their targets (Fig. 17.29).

Damage to either the FEF or the SC alone produces relatively subtle ocular motor defects. A unilateral FEF lesion in humans causes increased latency and reduced amplitude of initial visually triggered random, predictable saccades, and memory-guided saccades contralateral to the lesion or in both directions (301,302). Patients with large chronic frontal lobe lesions on one side involving prefrontal cortex (area 46) show another defect in higher-level control of saccadic eye movement. When a visual stimulus is presented in their contralateral visual field and they are instructed to make saccades away from it (antisaccades), they cannot suppress an unwanted saccades toward that stimulus (303,304). However, according to Rivaud et al. (302), lesions more restricted to the human FEF do not impair the ability to make antisaccades and suppress reflexive saccades. FEF ablation in monkeys does not eliminate express saccades, whereas SC ablation does (305). The FEF may participate in the unlocking of fixation required to dispatch saccades (302,306), but it is not critical for this function.

Inactivation of the FEF in one hemisphere does not eliminate the generation of contralateral saccades. After intracarotid injection of sodium amobarbital to suspend function of one cerebral hemisphere, patients can produce both ipsilateral and contralateral saccades similar to those produced before injection (307). In addition, voluntary saccades are preserved while visually guided saccades show only prolonged latency and mild slowing in both horizontal directions after chronic hemidecortication (308,309). These findings indicate that other structures, namely the intact cerebral hemisphere and the SC, can generate saccades even when the FEF and parietal lobe are inactivated, and demonstrate that the inability to perform contralateral saccades after an acute hemispheric lesion is not caused solely by inactivation of the frontal lobe.

In monkeys, bilateral ablation of the FEF causes a transient decrease in frequency and amplitude of saccadic eye movements (305,310,311). Bilateral removal of the SC causes only a slight increase in saccadic latency and a decrease in saccade amplitude (312,313). Such monkeys also show enhanced fixation with decreased distractibility. When viewing a central target, they are less likely to glance at a distracting stimulus presented in the visual periphery. However, lesions restricted to the rostral pole of the SC impair fixation and increase the frequency of express saccades by disinhibiting the rest of the intermediate layer (314).

In marked contrast to the above findings, sequential bilateral ablations or cooling of both SCs as well as both FEFs, with either structure being removed before the other, produces a marked paralysis of visually guided saccades and spontaneous saccades in all directions (310,311). The ocular motor range for saccades is limited to only 5°–10° away from central fixation. Stimulation of the occipital or parietal lobe will evoke saccades only if either the FEF or SC remains intact. The FEF and SC appear to be parallel gatekeepers of cerebral control of saccadic eye movements.

Thus, there are two parallel pathways through which saccades may be triggered: one through the FEF and the other through the SC. Lesions of either pathway alone produce only mild defects, while lesions of both cause profound, permanent saccadic defects. As noted above, ablation of the SC alone eliminates express saccades, perhaps being activated more directly by visual afferents to the SC (305,310).

SUPPLEMENTARY EYE FIELD

The anterior part of the supplementary motor area in the upper part of the paracentral sulcus of the dorsomedial frontal cortex is also called the supplementary eye field (SEF) (Fig. 17.28) since it contains neurons that discharge before volitional and visually guided saccades and stimulation there elicits saccades. The pre-SEF located just anterior to the SEF also participates in saccade control (315–317). Unlike the effect of FEF or SC stimulation, where contralateral saccades of specific amplitude are evoked irrespective of initial eye position, stimulation of SEF elicits saccades toward a specific region of the orbit. In other words, the FEF and the SC elicits saccades in retinotopic space, whereas the SEF elicits saccades in craniotopic space, which is synonymous with eye position in the orbit (317). Neurons in the SEF fire individually in relation to retinal goals (315), but populations of SEF neurons extract craniotopic information from them (316). The anterior part of the SEF encodes saccade termination zones in the contralateral hemirange of the orbit, and the posterior SEF encodes saccades that finish straight ahead or in the ipsilateral hemirange. Furthermore, the lateral SEF encodes for saccades terminating in the upper orbit, while the medial SEF encodes saccades ending in the lower orbit. Continuing stimulation of the SEF regions maintains fixation in specific fixation regions of the orbit and inhibits visually evoked saccades.

The SEF has anatomic connections to the parietal eye field (PEF) in the LIP area, the FEF, and the SC (318). Ablation of the FEF has a negligible effect on saccades evoked by stimulation of the ipsilateral SEF, and ablation of the SC merely increases their latency and reduces their amplitude but does not eliminate them (319). The SEF is thought to mediate saccades to specific orbital positions by projections to the SC and mesencephalic reticular formation and perhaps the NRTP (320,321). The SEF's role in fixation might be effected by its excitation of the fixation cells of the rostral SC (294,295,314), since ablation of the SC eliminates the inhibition of saccades that occurs during SEF stimulation while the eyes are positioned in specific fixation regions (319).

Effects of lesions and transcortical magnetic stimulation study in humans suggest that the SEF participates in learning, planning, and triggering of memory-guided sequences of saccades (322,323). PET shows that the SEF and adjacent cingulate gyrus are active during volitional saccades, be they self-paced, or antisaccades, or memory-guided to previous visual targets, but this region is not active during reflexive saccades to visual targets (272–274,278). It seems that the SEF plays a predominant role in directing voluntary sequences of saccades to positions relative to the head and maintaining fixation there. The SEF is more involved in the learning of new tasks than is the FEF. Also, with continued training on behavioral tasks, the responsivity of the SEF drops. Accordingly, the SEF is more involved in learning operations, whereas the FEF is more specialized for the execution of saccades (281). The SEF is primarily involved in the process of planning, decoding, and updating new saccade sequences, whereas the FEF plays a major role in determining the direction of forthcoming saccades (324).

DORSOLATERAL PREFRONTAL CORTEX

Neurons in the dorsolateral prefrontal cortex (Fig. 17.28) in Brodmann areas 46 and 9 (Fig. 17.30), located anterior to the FEF, are active in visuospatial memory coding and when making antisaccades and suppressing reflexive saccades (279). They project to the FEF, SEF, and SC and receive input from the posterior parietal cortex. Lesions to this area impair the ability to make antisaccades and suppress unwanted reflexive saccades to visual targets in humans (304) and impair memory-guided saccade sequences in humans and monkeys (279,322). PET in humans indicates that the dorsolateral prefrontal cortex is not activated during voluntary self-paced saccades in darkness (325), although it is activated during memory-guided saccades to a single target

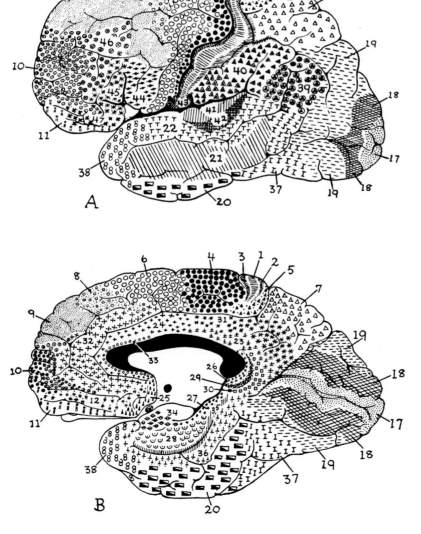

Figure 17.30. Cytoarchitectural map of the human cortex showing Brodmann areas. *A*, Convex surface. *B*, Medial surface. The cortical areas of greatest importance with respect to ocular motor activity are areas *6*, *8*, *19*, *37*, *39*, *40*, and *46*. (From Strong OS, Elwyn A. Human Neuroanatomy. 3rd ed. Baltimore: Williams & Wilkins, 1953.)

(274,278). During antisaccades, the most demanding type of volitional saccade, the dorsolateral prefrontal cortex, FEF, and SEF are preferentially activated (274). Functional imaging indicates metabolic activity in a cortical location during a task relative to fixation, darkness, or another eye movement task, whereas the lesion location identified with a behavioral deficit signifies a critical cerebral area (including subcortical white matter connections), without prompt compensation by other cerebral areas that have redundant functions. The dorsolateral prefrontal cortex contributes mainly to the advanced planning of environmental scanning using memory of target location.

PARIETAL CORTEX

Stimulation of the LIP area, in the intraparietal sulcus of the inferior parietal lobule of monkeys, elicits saccades, and lesions to it delay reflexive saccades to visual targets (326,327). The LIP area is designated as the PEF (328,329) (Fig. 17.28). Neurons in this area discharge in relation to visually guided saccades but are independent of visual stimulation since they also discharge during memory-guided and learned saccade tasks (330,331). The PEF receives projections from the FEF, and PEF neurons project to the FEF and SC (332) While destruction of either the PEF or the FEF produces subtle saccadic defects of visually guided saccades in monkeys, combined bilateral ablation of the PEF and ablation of one FEF, or bilateral ablation of the FEF and ablation of one PEF, produces paralysis of visually guided saccades for several days, followed by some recovery to profound delay and hypometria of saccades (333). The recovery may be mediated by the SEF, or superior temporal polysensory area (334), and their projections to the SC and other brain stem structures.

Area 7a of the monkey posterior parietal cortex in the inferior parietal lobule also contain neurons that discharge in relationship to saccades (335–337). These cells, however, are more tightly linked to directed visual attention than to any specific type of motor behavior, since they also discharge with limb movements as well as when the animal is simply required to pay attention to—but not saccade to—a peripheral target (338). The superior parietal lobule (Fig. 17.28) is also concerned with attention shifting as a prelude to saccades (337,339,340).

Functional imaging has revealed that the human posterior parietal cortex is activated during visually guided reflexive saccades, volitional saccades to remembered visual targets, and antisaccades (273,278,341). The homolog of the simian LIP area is uncertain but possibly includes the angular and supramarginal gyri (Brodmann areas 39 and 40) (329) (Figs. 17.28 and 17.30); lesions of the posterior parietal cortex involving this region delay visually guided saccades in the gap and overlap tasks, but more so in the overlap task (304,342). Right-sided lesions impair visually guided saccades more than left-sided lesions, as is the case with other visuospatial functions. Thus, the PEF of the posterior parietal cortex participates in visually guided reflexive saccades, and it might participate in disengaging fixation. The PEF has a signal that describes a saccade target and maintains the memory of a saccade plan, which is probably derived from the FEF and dorsolateral prefrontal cortex. The PEF renders the goal of the saccade to a salient location for attentional processes and possibly to provide targets for future saccades. The PEF contains a salience map that uses the saccade signal to provide information that updates visual representation to compensate for an eye movement, thus maintaining a spatially accurate vector map of the visual world despite a moving eye (343).

The MST and the foveal region of the MT area of monkeys and its human homolog, area V5, which participate in motion perception and smooth pursuit generation (discussed below), also provide information to generate saccades to moving targets. Lesions to these areas cause retinotopic defects so that saccades to a target moving in the contralateral visual field are inaccurate in all directions (344–347). Projections from striate cortex (area V1) to V5, and from V1 to the lateral intraparietal area make up part of the dorsal, magnocellular pathway for processing motion, attention, and visuomotor interaction (348) that is concerned with generating saccades to visual targets.

BASAL GANGLIA

The caudate nucleus receives input from the FEF and projects to the SNpr, which in turn projects to the intermediate layer of the SC. Caudate neurons discharge before contralateral memory-guided and visually evoked saccades (349–351). Output from the FEF is routed through the caudate, with the caudonigral circuit disinhibiting the SC. The caudate inhibits the SNpr and the SNpr inhibits the SC, both inhibitory synapses being GABA-ergic. SNpr neurons are tonically active during fixation and they pause, disinhibiting SC burst neurons that fire before and during saccades to visual and remembered targets (287–290,352,353). Thus, the FEF has a powerful two-pronged excitatory effect on the SC, one direct and the other through the caudate and SNpr. The ventral part of the subthalamic nucleus sends excitatory signals to the SNpr and might act to suppress unwanted eye movements, and recover fixation after saccades by indirectly inhibiting burst cells in the SC (354).

Functional imaging indicates that the putamen and globus pallidus as well as the thalamus are metabolically activated with voluntary self-paced saccades and memorized sequences of saccades in darkness, but not with visually guided saccades (273,274). Volitional saccades may utilize a basal ganglia-thalamo-cortical circuit, involving putamen to globus pallidus to thalamus to the FEF and SMA. This circuit is analogous to the striatal, thalamic, and cortical pathways described for face, arm, and leg movements, but it is distinct from the caudo-nigral collicular circuit responsible for triggering and suppressing both voluntary and visually guided saccades (349,352,353). Patients with bilateral lesions of the putamen and globus pallidus have inaccurate or delayed internally triggered voluntary saccades but normal externally triggered saccades to visual targets (355).

THALAMUS

The intramedullary nucleus of the thalamus contains long-lead burst neurons that discharge before mainly contraversive self-initiated and visually triggered saccades in monkeys. They might provide relevant cortical areas with information on gaze behavior, or to relay command from cortex to the deep layers of the SC or other brain stem neurons. Pause neurons and visual fixation neurons are also found in this thalamic region (356,357). The central thalamus may fetch eye movement-related activity of the cortex, signal that a target response is imminent, and capture control from other interfering commands (356,357). Lesions of the intramedullary lamina could contribute to the syndrome of thalamic neglect (356,357). Patterns of saccadic responses in the pregeniculate complex of the monkey thalamus suggest its role as a relay between the parietal cortex and brain stem ocular motor pathways, such as the SC and pretectal nucleus of the optic tract (358).

CENTRAL MIDBRAIN RETICULAR FORMATION

An important relay for projections to and from the SC may be the nucleus subcuneiformis, a structure that lies lateral to the oculomotor nucleus in the central mesencephalic reticular formation (320,359). Microstimulation in the central mesencephalic reticular formation elicits contralaterally directed saccades; recordings from the nucleus indicate that its neurons discharge in relation to visually guided contralateral saccades, and lesions of it impair the generation of contralateral visually guided saccades but not vestibularly induced quick phases. Neurons of the central mesencephalic reticular formation receive collaterals from SC axons in the predorsal bundle descending to the PPRF and receive ascending from the PPRF. They project dorsally to the SC as well as caudally to the NRTP and rip. However, inactivation of the central mesencephalic reticular formation results in hypermetria of contraversive and upward saccades and reduced latency for initiation of contraversive saccades (360). Fixation is also destabilized by large square-wave jerks. The hypermetria supports the idea that the central mesencephalic reticular formation participates in the feedback control of saccade accuracy. Reduction in contraversive saccade latency and development of square-wave jerks after central mesencephalic reticular formation inactivation support its role in saccade triggering (360). The central mesencephalic reticular formation may also participate in extracting the horizontal vector from oblique saccade signals from the SC and relaying feedback of eye displacement from excitatory burst neurons in the PPRF to T burst and buildup cells in the SC (361).

Another region of the midbrain reticular formation, just lateral to the INC (the peri-INC midbrain reticular formation), contains long-lead burst neurons that play a role in generating vertical saccades Inactivation of this region produces hypometria and slowing of upward and downward saccades. The vertical saccade hypometria may indicate that the peri-INC midbrain reticular formation provides long-lead burst activity to the short-lead burst neurons in the riMLF and also activates omnipause neurons (362).

On the basis of his pioneering lesion and stimulation studies in the brain stem tegmentum of monkeys, Bender (220)

concluded that there is a decussation of an ocular motor pathway occurring in the midbrain reticular formation between the levels of the oculomotor and trochlear nuclei. Structures above this ocular motor decussation in the midbrain reticular formation govern contraversive gaze, and structures below it generate ipsiversive gaze. The anatomic and physiologic basis for this decussation remains uncertain, but it may comprise the predorsal bundle from the SC, which crosses the midline ventral to the oculomotor nucleus in the decussation of Meynert and descends in the contralateral tegmentum to the PPRF.

Cerebellar Regulation of Saccades

Through its connections to the vestibular nuclei and to the reticular formation by way of the deep cerebellar nuclei, the cerebellum participates in three major ocular motor functions: (a) regulation of saccadic amplitude and repair of saccadic dysmetria; (b) stabilization of images upon the retina by regulating smooth pursuit; and (c) regulation of the duration of vestibulo-ocular responses and recalibrating them when visual or vestibular input is altered. Some details of cerebellar functions will be discussed in the following sections on the smooth pursuit, vergence, and vestibulo-ocular systems. Here we describe cerebellar control of saccadic accuracy.

Lobules VI and VII of dorsal cerebellar vermis (also called the ocular motor vermis), the underlying fastigial nuclei, and the flocculus are important for saccadic eye movement control (261,363,364) (Fig. 17.31). Functional imaging reveals increased activity in the human vermis during saccades to predictable targets, self-paced and memorized sequences of saccades in darkness (273,365). Purkinje cells in lobules VI and VII discharge in relation to saccades, including nystagmus quick phases (366–369), and electric stimulation of the dorsal cerebellar vermis in alert monkeys evokes conjugate saccades with an horizontal ipsiversive component (370). Stimulation of lobule V produces saccades that range from upward to horizontal, while stimulation of lobules VI and VII produce saccades that range from horizontal to downward. Saccadic direction is apparently encoded by anatomic location in the cerebellum, as it is in the FEF and SC. Unlike saccades evoked by stimulation of these latter structures, however, saccades evoked by cerebellar stimulation are graded in amplitude as a function of stimulus intensity. The amplitude of the saccade also depends upon the initial position of the eye in the orbit, and the end of the saccade tends to be at the same point in the orbit regardless of the starting position (370,371). Such saccades are made in craniotopic coordinates and are said to be ''goal-directed'' since they take the eye to the same orbital position.

Complete cerebellectomy in monkeys creates persistent saccadic dysmetria without abnormalities in velocity or latency (372). In this setting, all saccades overshoot, although the degree of overshoot is greatest for centripetally directed movements. The saccadic abnormality in such monkeys consists of both pulse size dysmetria and pulse-step match dysmetria. The size of the saccadic pulse is usually too large,

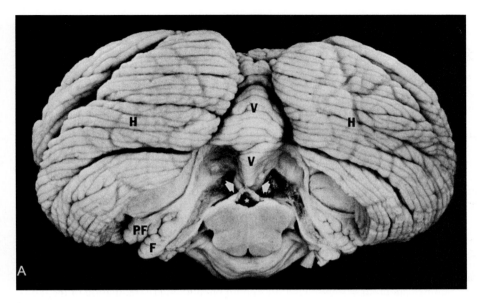

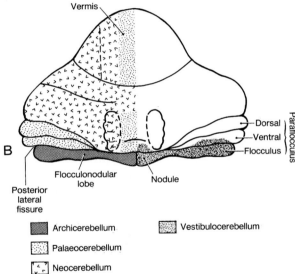

Figure 17.31. The human cerebellum. *A,* Anterior inferior view shows the cerebellar hemispheres (H), vermis (V), flocculus (F), and paraflocculus (PF). *White arrowheads,* nodulus; *asterisk,* fourth ventricle. *B,* Subdivisions of the human cerebellum. The left half of the drawing shows the three main subdivisions: the archicerebellum, the flocculonodular lobe; the paleocerebellum, the anterior vermis, the pyramis, the uvula, and the paraflocculus; and the neocerebellum. The right half of the diagram shows the structures of the vestibulocerebellum, the flocculonodular lobe, and the dorsal and ventral paraflocculi. (*A,* From Ghuhbegovic N, Williams TH. The Human Brain: A Photographic Guide. Hagerstown, MD, Harper & Row, 1980. *B,* After Brodal A. Neurological Anatomy in Relation to Clinical Medicine. 3rd ed. New York: Oxford University Press, 1981.)

creating saccadic overshoot (pulse size dysmetria). At the end of the rapid, pulse portion of the saccade, the eye drifts on for a few hundred milliseconds toward the final eye position, as a glissade (pulse-step match dysmetria). The dysmetria is a feature of damage to the ocular motor vermis (363), and the postsaccadic drift reflects damage to the flocculus and ventral paraflocculus (261) (Fig. 17.31). In this chapter, both the flocculus and the paraflocculus are often referred to as the flocculus.

In contrast to total cerebellectomy, ablation of only the dorsal cerebellar vermis and the underlying fastigial nuclei creates saccadic pulse size dysmetria in monkeys but no postsaccadic drift (372). Experimental lesions of the dorsal vermis create a saccadic dysmetria in which centripetal saccades overshoot the target (hypermetric dysmetria) while centrifugal saccades undershoot the target (hypometric dys-

metria) (363,373), a pattern that is recognized in patients with cerebellar disease. Acutely, ablation of the ocular motor vermis increases saccade latency and reduces their speed, but these deficits recover while hypometria persists (363). The cerebellum can adjust saccade amplitude and saccade dynamics independently. On the other hand, ablation of the cerebellar flocculus creates pulse-step match dysmetria with postsaccadic drift but no pulse size dysmetria (261,374). The two components of saccadic dysmetria caused by total cerebellectomy are thus related to ablation of two different regions of the cerebellum. The dorsal cerebellar vermis and underlying fastigial nuclei control of saccadic pulse size, while the flocculus is responsible for appropriately matching the saccadic pulse and step.

The caudal part of the fastigial nucleus (Figs. 17.20 and 17.32) is termed the fastigial ocular motor region (FOR). It

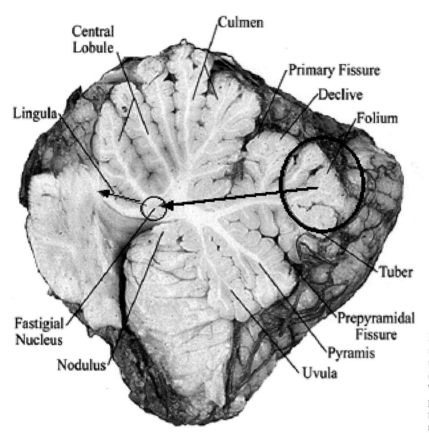

Figure 17.32. Sagittal view of human cerebellum showing the ocular motor vermis, comprising parts of the declive, folium, and tuber (*large oval*), projecting (*large arrow*) to the fastigial nucleus (*small circle*). The fastigial nucleus projects (*small arrow*) to the opposite side of the brain stem tegmentum. (Adapted from Leigh RJ, Zee DS. The Neurology of Eye Movements. Oxford: Oxford University Press, 1999.)

receives inhibitory input from Purkinje cells in dorsal vermis lobules VI and VII, which receive mossy fiber input from brain stem nuclei. The FOR also receives projections from the dorsolateral pontine nucleus (DLPN), dorsomedial pontine nucleus, NRTP, pontine raphe, paramedian nucleus reticularis pontis caudalis, NPH (Fig. 17.8), subnucleus b of the medial accessory olivary nucleus, vestibular nucleus (375,376), and inferior olivary nucleus (377). Neurons in the caudal fastigial nucleus project through the opposite fastigial nucleus, and then over the contralateral superior cerebellar peduncle in the hook bundle of Russell within the uncinate fasciculus, to the contralateral SC and brain stem tegmentum. Their axons terminate in the region of cells in the pons that generate saccades, namely the excitatory and inhibitory burst neurons, and omnipause neurons (376,378). Neurons in the FOR are responsible for accelerating contraversive saccades and decelerating ipsiversive saccades (364, 379,380). Neurons in one FOR fire at the end of ipsiversive saccades, but neurons in the opposite FOR fire at their beginning. Chemical inactivation of the FOR on both sides makes all saccades hypermetric, indicating that they influence the saccade burst generator in the brain stem to make saccades more consistent and accurate. Chemical inactivation of the FOR neurons on one side makes ipsiversive saccades hypermetric and contraversive saccades hypometric (381,382).

Unilateral FOR lesions in patients have bilateral effects, since neurons from the contralateral FOR pass though it.

Lateropulsion of saccades is a form of dysmetria consisting of overshooting of horizontal saccades in one direction, undershooting in the other, and oblique misdirection of vertical saccades (Fig. 17.33). Lateropulsion occurs toward the side of lateral medullary infarcts, a phenomenon we call ipsipulsion to specify the direction of dysmetria relative to the side of the lesion (383). Ipsipulsion consists of overshoot of ipsiversive saccades, undershoot of contraversive saccades, and ipsiversive deviation of vertical saccades (383–387). Lateropulsion occurring contralateral to lesions of the superior cerebellar peduncle and uncinate fasciculus is named contrapulsion, which is the combination of overshoot of contraversive saccades, undershoot of ipsiversive saccades, and contraversive deviation of vertical saccades (388,389) (Fig. 17.33). Ipsipulsion might arise from damage to climbing fiber projections from the opposite-side inferior olivary nucleus through the inferior cerebellar peduncle to the cortex of the dorsal vermis; climbing fiber damage increases Purkinje cell activity and in turn inhibits the ipsilateral fastigial nucleus (390). If the damage occurs before decussation of olivocerebellar projections, contrapulsion results (389). Contrapulsion of saccades from cerebellar outflow damage can be explained by disruption of the uncinate

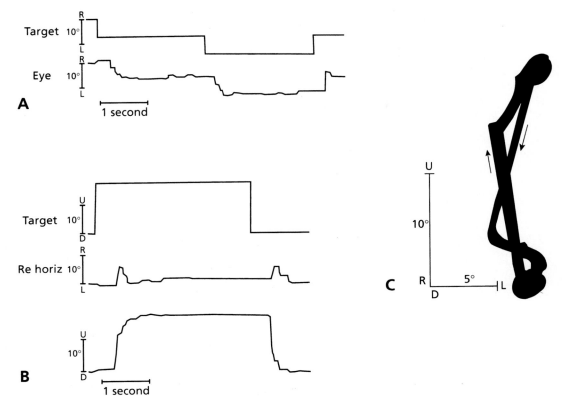

Figure 17.33. Unidirectional saccadic dysmetria (contrapulsion of saccades) from an infarct involving the left superior cerebellar peduncle and uncinate fasciculus. *A,* Rightward saccades are hypermetric and leftward saccades are hypometric. *B,* Vertical saccades (*lower trace*) are accompanied by rightward saccades (*middle trace*). *C,* Rightward pulsion of vertical saccades. *Arrows* beside misdirected oblique saccades indicate their direction. R, right; L, left; U, up; D, down. (Redrawn from Ranalli PJ, Sharpe JA. Ann Neurol 1986;20:311–316.)

fasciculus, from the contralateral fastigial nucleus, as it passes around the superior cerebellar peduncle (Fig. 17.34) (388,391).

Adaptive Control of Saccade Amplitude

Saccadic adaptation is a process by which errors in the saccadic amplitude, induced by errors in target position or weakness of extraocular muscles, can be corrected (392,393). It exemplifies motor learning (394). Errors in saccadic amplitude can result from brain, peripheral nerve, or muscle diseases, and aging. Another function of rapid saccadic adaptation is to overcome reduction in saccade amplitude caused by fatigue (395). Saccadic dysmetria can be simulated by changing the position of a visual target during saccades, forcing the subject to make a corrective saccade after every target jump. After many such trials, subjects unknowingly adjust the amplitude of their saccades to land closer to the new target position (392,396). Saccadic adaptation is specific to the direction or amplitude of the target movement so that a change induced in saccade size in one direction and amplitude is not induced for saccades to other directions and amplitudes. Furthermore, saccadic adaptation is specific to the stimulus for saccade, whether visually guided saccades or memory-guided saccades, with little transfer of adaptation among different stimulus conditions (392,397–399).

The ocular motor vermis (lobules VI and VII) and the FOR participate in saccadic adaptation (400–402). Ablation of lobules VI and VII in monkeys impairs saccadic adaptation (395). Functional imaging in humans shows increased activity in the ocular motor vermis while they learn to change the amplitude of their saccades (403).

The mechanism of adaptation could have its origin in a signal from a group of saccade-related Purkinje cells in lobules VI and VII that give a precise account of the timing when a saccade ends. The duration of burst responses in these cells changes with saccadic amplitude (404). Saccadic adaptation could be the consequences of changing time representation in pulse duration of the neural signal in the cerebellum (405). Studies in rhesus monkeys during saccadic adaptation to extraocular muscle weakness (402) or to changes in target position (406) reported two mechanisms for saccadic adaptation: an earlier burst for ipsiversive saccades in the FOR when saccade size is decreasing, and a change in spike number when saccade size is increasing (402) or decreasing (406).

Adaptation is shown by patients who develop a unilateral

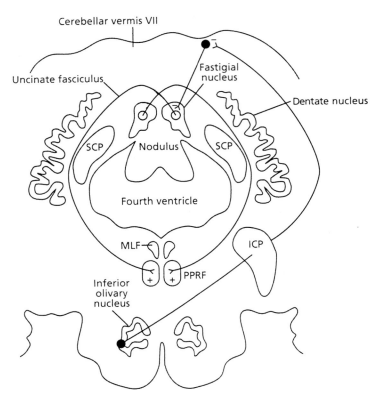

Figure 17.34. Schema of projections from the inferior olivary nuclei (IO) through the inferior cerebellar peduncle (ICP) to lobule VII of cerebellar cortex where Purkinje cells inhibit the fastigial nucleus (FN). The caudal part of the FN probably excites the contralateral paramedian pontine reticular formation (PPRF) via its projections in the uncinate fasciculus. A lesion in the left ICP increases Purkinje cell activity, leading to decreased firing of the ipsilateral FN and decreased activation of the contralateral (right) PPRF; this causes ipsipulsion of saccades. A lesion of the left uncinate fasciculus (from the right FN) decreases activity in the ipsilateral (left) PPRF, causing contrapulsion of saccades. SP, superior cerebellar peduncle. (From Sharpe JA, Morrow MJ, Newman NJ, et al. Disturbances of ocular motility. Continuum 1995;1:41–92.

peripheral ocular motor nerve palsy but for various reasons habitually fixate with their paretic eye (407,408). Such individuals modify their saccadic innervation to compensate for both the saccadic undershoot and the postsaccadic drift created by the palsy. If the patient is forced (by patching the paretic eye) to use the nonparetic eye for viewing, saccadic innervation will, within a few days, revert to a pattern satisfying the visual needs of the nonparetic, viewing eye.

After surgically induced ocular muscle weakness, monkeys can adjust the size of the saccadic pulse and suppress postsaccadic drift (372). Removal of only the dorsal cerebellar vermis and underlying fastigial nuclei abolishes the ability of the monkey to modify the size of the saccadic pulse, while preserving the ability to suppress postsaccadic drift. Thus, the dorsal cerebellar vermis and the fastigial nuclei (Fig. 17.20) are important for adjustments of the saccadic pulse amplitude but not for appropriately matching the size of the saccadic step to that of the pulse to prevent postsaccadic drift. This adaptive matching of the saccadic pulse and step is controlled by the flocculus (374). Flocculectomized monkeys cannot appropriately adjust the saccadic step to eliminate postsaccadic drift.

SMOOTH PURSUIT SYSTEM

Characteristics of Smooth Pursuit Eye Movements

Smooth pursuit stabilizes the image of an object on or near the fovea during slow movement of the object or of the body. Smooth pursuit is needed to hold the eye on a stationary target during locomotion. When one views a target located off to one side during locomotion, smooth pursuit holds its image at the fovea, despite relative motion of the background. The pursuit system ensures optimal visual acuity for relative motion of a small visual target by reducing the speed of target image movement over the retina; this movement is called retinal slip and it is measured as retinal velocity error, the difference between target velocity and smooth eye movement velocity. Attention and the intent to pursue are required to sustain smooth tracking with a target image on the central retina. In that sense smooth pursuit is voluntary, but in another context it is reflexive since a percept of retinal image motion is required. Very few individuals can make conjugate smooth eye movements in darkness without an externally derived sensory percept of target motion. The speed of retinal images that can be tolerated for clear vision depends on the spatial frequency of the image. Image motion exceeding 5°–6° per second reduces visual acuity for the higher spatial frequencies of high-contrast letters (409,410).

Under normal conditions, retinal slip is detected by the visual system and provides the necessary stimulus for pursuit, a velocity error (411,412). Under special circumstances, however, a stationary target located away from the fovea, a position error, may also act as a pursuit stimulus (413,414). Patients with diminished central vision can also generate smooth pursuit movements by using their central scotoma as a target, by using peripheral retinal slip as a stimulus, or by using both mechanisms (415).

Image motion on the retina is not the only stimulus capable of eliciting smooth pursuit movements. Some subjects can smoothly track their own outstretched finger when it is moving in front of them in darkness. Both knowledge of the motor command to the limb (efference) and its proprioceptive input (afference) are probably being used to generate these pursuit eye movements (416–418). Certain patients with acquired blindness can also pursue in this manner (419). Very few individuals, however, can generate smooth eye movements voluntarily, without any external perception of movement (see reference (420) for exception). Conversely, the perception of movement itself (for example, induced by pursuing the imaginary center of a rolling wheel when only two points on its rim are visible) is an adequate stimulus even when no actual image motion has occurred in the direction of the eye movement (411,421). Therefore, in addition to using information from the retina, the brain can generate smooth pursuit eye movements by using information about target motion from other sensory systems, by monitoring motor commands, or by higher-level perceptual representations of target movement in space (422).

The latency for initiation of smooth pursuit movements is 100 to 130 msec (423,424). When a gap with no target precedes a pursuit target, the shortest latencies are recorded; this phenomenon has been termed express smooth pursuit (425–427). Pursuit initiation consists of smooth eye acceleration. By using step-ramp targets, in which a stimulus spot steps quickly to one area of retina, then moves at a constant velocity, Rashbass (428) showed that this initial pursuit eye movement is in the direction of target velocity, rather than target position (Fig. 17.35). Because of processing delays, the initial 100- to 130-msec interval of pursuit acceleration is as an open-loop condition, without feedback, while the pursuit system is responding only to target motion that took place before the eyes started to move.

For the first 20–40 msec, pursuit initiation responds only to target direction (412,423,429). After 40 msec, smooth eye acceleration increases while target stimuli remain off the fovea (423,430). During the 100- to 130-msec open-loop period, smooth eye acceleration reduces retinal slip, closing the negative visual feedback loop. Smooth eye velocity must then be maintained close to target velocity, although retinal slip speeds are a fraction of target speed (410). If pursuit acted upon retinal slip information alone, smooth eye velocity would fall as it approached target velocity, creating instability in the system. This implies that extraretinal signals are used to drive pursuit at steady state, called pursuit maintenance.

Eye motion feedback is a source of extraretinal input. The brain adds a signal representing eye velocity to retinal slip input to construct a representation of target velocity in space to drive smooth pursuit (Fig. 17.36). Extraretinal feedback of eye velocity, an efference copy (or corollary discharge), accounts for sustained smooth pursuit (412,431). Eye veloc-

SMOOTH PURSUIT EYE MOVEMENTS

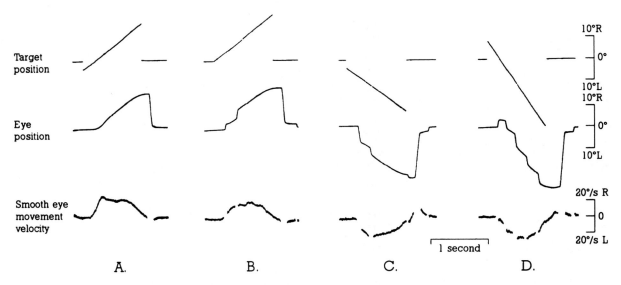

Figure 17.35. Recordings of pursuit responses to step-ramp stimuli, showing pursuit initiation in a normal subject. *A,* The step and ramp are in opposite directions and the eye accelerates toward the ramp after a latency of 110 msec and a saccade to the step of target position is canceled. The ramp moves toward the fovea at 20°/sec. The initial foveal position is at the primary position (0°). *D,* With the step and ramp again in opposite directions but at a ramp speed of 40°/sec, the step elicits a saccade followed by low-velocity pursuit in the direction of the ramp and a series of catch-up saccades and smooth pursuit movements to foveate the target. Ramps at 20°/sec away from the fovea (*B* and *C*) elicit slower pursuit than the 20° ramp toward the fovea (*A*). (From Morrow MJ, Sharpe JA. Smooth pursuit initiation in young and elderly subjects. Vision Res 1993; 33:203–210.)

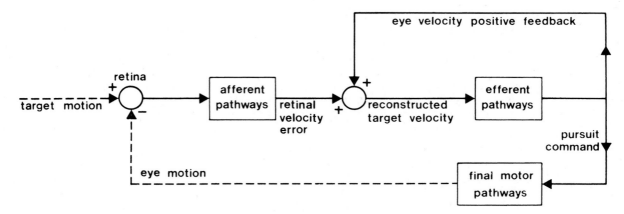

Figure 17.36. A model of the smooth pursuit system. A negative feedback loop provides a retinal image slip signal (retinal velocity error, being target velocity minus eye velocity) to drive smooth pursuit. Maintenance of stable pursuit requires an internal positive feedback loop that uses a copy of the eye velocity signal. The copy is "efference copy" or "corollary discharge." When this eye velocity signal is added to the retinal velocity error, a signal of target velocity in the environment is reconstructed. When retinal velocity error is reduced to zero by effective smooth pursuit, the positive feedback loop sustains the smooth eye motion at the speed of the target. (From Lisberger SG, Morris EJ, Tychsen L. Visual motion processing and sensory-motor integration for smooth pursuit eye movements. Annu Rev Neurosci 1987;10:97–129.)

ity feedback becomes available to cortical visual motion processing areas in monkeys 50–100 msec after pursuit is initiated (432). Neural mechanisms that anticipate target trajectory also provide an extraretinal input that enhances smooth pursuit maintenance (412,429).

Targets can usually be followed accurately (with eye velocity approximating target velocity) provided that the target velocity is less than about 50° per second and, for periodic targets such as sine waves, the frequency of oscillation is less than about 1 Hz. Ongoing smooth pursuit also shows very small oscillations of the smooth eye movements, called ringing (431,433). As the retinal image of a stimulus slips off the fovea, catch-up saccades are dispatched toward the target to reposition its image near the fovea. Saccadic rather than smooth pursuit is a sign that the system has reached its velocity or acceleration saturation. The efficacy of smooth pursuit is usually measured by its gain, the speed of smooth eye movement divided by target speed. Ideal gain is 1.0. When gain falls much below unity, catch-up saccades are required to foveate the target, and pursuit is said to be saccadic rather than smooth. Some human subjects can attain smooth pursuit eye speeds of up to 150° per second for sinusoidal target motion (429) and 100° per second for constant-velocity motion (434). However, even the highest pursuit eye speeds fall well below peak speeds of saccades (137,154) or the vestibulo-ocular reflex (266). Since it is not due to ocular motor constraints, smooth pursuit velocity must saturate because of limits of sensory motion processing, or the conversion of sensory inputs to motor commands. Normal elderly persons have smooth pursuit gains below unity at much lower target velocities and accelerations than younger persons (435–437).

Smooth pursuit is also limited by eye acceleration. Humans can attain smooth pursuit accelerations of about $1,200°/sec^2$, although smooth pursuit becomes considerably less effective as target acceleration exceeds $200°/sec^2$. Increases in target acceleration best explain decreases in pursuit eye velocity as target frequency rises (429). Initial pursuit responses are faster for accelerating targets (430). Inputs of retinal image acceleration as well as retinal image velocity drive smooth pursuit (412).

Smooth pursuit eye movements follow the trajectory of predictable targets more faithfully than unpredictable targets (429,438). Processing delays of the pursuit system should cause phase lag of the eyes behind a target, but smooth pursuit of predictable targets can often be maintained with no phase lag, or even a small phase lead. This phase matching during pursuit maintenance is probably achieved by an internal positive feedback of the eye velocity command (412) (Fig. 17.36). Furthermore, pursuit may continue in the anticipated trajectory of a target after the target has been blanked or stabilized on the fovea or has changed its path (439,440). Subjects can anticipate target motion and initiate predictive eye acceleration before the target moves, even when target motion is unpredictable (440), but they cannot maintain smooth pursuit at the speed of unpredictable target motion.

Neurophysiology of Pursuit Eye Movements

Cerebral Initiation and Maintenance of Smooth Pursuit

Visual processing is divided into two parallel but anatomically and functionally interconnected pathways. One, the magnocellular (M) pathway, is concerned with motion and spatial analysis; the other, the parvocellular (P), is concerned with form and color perception (441–443). Within the cerebral hemisphere of monkeys, the M pathway is dorsal to the P pathway, and they are designated as the dorsal and ventral streams. The dorsal occipito-temporal-parietal stream conveys information about location and motion (the "where pathway''), whereas the more ventral occipito-temporal stream conveys color, form, and pattern information (the ''what pathway''). The M visual channel in monkeys projects to striate cortex (area V1), then to cortical areas V2 and V3, and MT (middle temporal, area V5), then adjacent area MST (medial superior temporal, area V5a), and then posterior parietal cortex.

Functional imaging and magnetoencephalography of the human brain show cortical areas in addition to the ascending limb of the inferior temporal sulcus (the homolog of MT/V5) that are activated by moving patterns (444–447). The ascending limb of the inferior temporal sulcus is considered to include satellites of MT and has been referred to as hMT/V5 + . Other cortical areas that also respond to moving in preference to stationary patterns are lingual cortex, lateral occipital sulcus (area LOS/KO), dorsolateral-posterior-occipitoparietal cortex (hV3A), anterior-dorsal-intraparietal sulcus (DIPSA), postcentral sulcus, and a small area in the precentral cortex, being perhaps the FEF (444,448); these areas are activated to different amounts in individual subjects, but not at all in some subjects. Only hMT/V5 + is significantly activated in practically every brain (444). The contributions, if any, of the other areas to motion processing, perception, and behavior are uncertain. Lesion as well as fMRI evidence points to the junction of Brodmann areas 19 and 39 as the homolog of simian MT/MST in humans (344,347,432,449–452).

Humans and monkeys with unilateral striate cortex or optic radiation lesions cannot pursue a target confined to the contralateral visual hemifield (453–455). Patients are also unable to discriminate motion direction or to perceive motion in the affected hemifield (456), but there is controversy about the existence of residual vision after destruction of area V1 (457,458) (see also Chapter 13). Monkeys with bilateral striate ablation eventually recover substantial smooth pursuit, implying adaptive use of extrastriate visual motion inputs after cortical blindness (262), but humans with cortical blindness cannot pursue visual targets.

AREA V5: MIDDLE TEMPORAL AND MEDIAL SUPERIOR TEMPORAL CORTEX

Neurons in the foveal part of simian area MT (V5) and dorsal and lateral area MST discharge during smooth pursuit (459,460) (Fig. 17.37). Their receptive fields include the fovea but do not respect the vertical meridian and extend far into the ipsilateral visual field. Every V5 neuron receives input from both eyes (461). Discharge that occurs during pursuit of a target isolated in darkness can be either a response to the residual retinal slip velocity or an extraretinal signal of eye velocity. Cells in the foveal region of area MT respond only to retinal slip, whereas the lateral and dorsal area MST contain cells that respond even in the absence of retinal image motion, indicating an extraretinal input (432). The foveal MT and lateral MST provide retinal slip information for pursuit, and the dorsal and lateral MST receive either a corollary motor discharge or proprioceptive information regarding eye motion (432,462), which is required for pursuit maintenance (412).

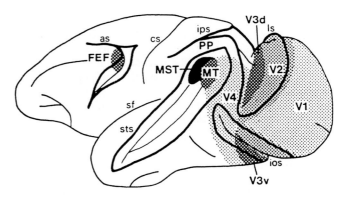

Figure 17.37. Left cerebral hemisphere of rhesus monkey showing area important in visual motion analysis and smooth ocular pursuit. The lateral part of the middle temporal (MT) area containing foveal receptive fields and the lateral part of the medial superior temporal area (MST) participate in generating ipsiversive pursuit by conveying visual signals to the pursuit system. VI, striate cortex; V2–V4, prestriate cortical areas; PP, posterior parietal cortex; FEF, frontal eye field. Sulci are opened to reveal the arcuate sulcus (AS), inferior occipital sulcus (IOS), lunate sulcus (LS), and superior temporal sulcus (STS). SF, sylvian fissure; CS, central sulcus, IPS, intraparietal sulcus. (From Tusa RJ, Ungerleider LG. Fiber pathways of cortical areas mediating smooth pursuit eye movements in monkeys. Ann Neurol 1988;23:174–183.)

Lesions in areas MST and MT cause two types of pursuit defect: retinotopic and directional. Retinotopic pursuit defects consist of lower smooth pursuit speed and inaccurate saccades in the contralateral area of the visual field subserved by the damaged area; the defects are for pursuit and saccades in all directions. Directional pursuit defects consist of lowered smooth pursuit speed toward the side of the damaged area, in response to a target presented anywhere in either hemifield; saccades are not affected (344,345). Both area MT and area MST have retinotopic maps of the contralateral visual field. Damage to neurons responding to visual motion in a specific area of visual field causes defective smooth pursuit initiation to targets moving in that region (450). Retinotopic deficits result from damage to any portion of area MST (345), or to the extrafoveal representation within area MT (432); receptive fields are larger in MST, and retinotopic deficits resulting from MST damage cover a larger portion of visual field. During smooth pursuit, but not while the eyes are still, electrical stimulation within either the foveal MT or lateral MST alone causes ipsiversive smooth eye movements to accelerate (463). Directional pursuit deficits are caused by lesions in only the foveal region of MT or the lateral region of MST (345).

The ipsiversive smooth pursuit defect is not explained by directional motion sensitivity of the MT and MST, because all directions of motion are represented in the preferences of their neurons (464,465) and because there is no defect in generating ipsiversive saccades to moving targets after MST or foveal MT lesions. Instead, the directional smooth pursuit bias lies in the projection patterns of the population of MST neurons to brain stem structures (466,467). Paresis of ipsiversive smooth pursuit corresponds to the ipsiversive bias in the preferred directions of output neurons from MST to the brain stem (467). A specific selection of cortical neurons from areas MT and MST forms the projection to the nucleus of the optic tract (NOT) and dorsal terminal nucleus of the accessory optic system (AOS), and this subpopulation has the same directional bias as their brain stem target neurons (467). Ipsiversive pursuit defects also result from lesions at subcortical levels of the pursuit pathway, as we discuss below.

HUMAN HOMOLOGS OF AREA V5

Patients with lesions at the junction of Brodmann areas 19, 37, and 39 (Fig. 17.30) and subcortical white matter have retinotopic defects of pursuit initiation and directional defects of pursuit initiation and maintenance (346,347,449, 468). Retinotopic defects are far less commonly detected than directional defects, unless of course the optic radiation or striate cortex is damaged. This area (Fig. 17.30) is homologous to simian MT and MST (Fig. 17.37); a zone within this cortical region of humans has the same distinctive myelination pattern as simian MT (469). Furthermore, functional imaging in normal human subjects shows increased activity in this region during smooth pursuit (452). Damage in this area, at the lateral junction of the parietal, temporal, and occipital lobes (Fig. 17.28), can account for impairment of ipsiversive pursuit or optokinetic nystagmus (OKN) slow phases after posterior cerebral lobe lesions (470–475, 476,449,477).

Despite this lateralization of directional pursuit pathways, each hemisphere contributes to smooth pursuit in both horizontal directions. After hemidecortication, monkeys have severe impairment of ipsiversive pursuit, but contraversive pursuit is also impaired for high-speed targets (478). Similarly, patients with unilateral focal lesions exhibit reduction of contraversive pursuit velocity, but less reduction than of ipsiversive pursuit (347,449,477). Contraversive smooth pursuit recovers in monkeys 6–8 months after hemispheric damage (478). Humans who have had hemidecortication a decade earlier do not have impaired contraversive pursuit (308), but patients with smaller areas of unilateral damage that spare V5 may have symmetrically reduced pursuit gain in both horizontal directions (347,449,479,480).

In both humans and monkeys, hemidecortication or large focal hemispheric lesions cause abnormally high contraversive pursuit velocities toward slow targets, with gains above unity (308,449,478,481). Ipsiversive pursuit requires catch-up saccades and contraversive pursuit requires back-up saccades to foveate a target. The marked asymmetries of horizontal smooth pursuit, with high contraversive and low ipsiversive gain, in patients with large cerebral lesions is associated with slow ocular drift away from the damaged side. Corrective saccades toward the side of damage create a low-amplitude nystagmus called pursuit paretic nystagmus (308,482). Pursuit paretic nystagmus may be caused by imbalanced smooth pursuit or optokinetic drive to brain stem neurons that generate horizontal smooth eye movements. A cortical bias of smooth pursuit direction might also explain

the occurrence of latent nystagmus that accompanies strabismus (461) (see also Chapter 23).

Lesions of the posterior limb of the internal capsule also lower the speed of ipsiversive smooth pursuit (449,480). Projections from V5, at the junction of occipito-temporal cortex, are conveyed through the internal sagittal stratum to the internal capsule, then to the basis pontis (483). The internal sagittal stratum lies medial to the optic radiation. Damage to striate cortex, the optic radiation, or the posterior part of the internal sagittal stratum does not cause directional impairment of smooth pursuit but does cause retinotopic loss of pursuit in the affected hemifield (455,471). Ipsiversive smooth pursuit defects from extrastriate cortical lesions are often associated with optic radiation or V1 damage that causes contralateral homonymous hemianopia, but the ipsiversive pursuit impairment is independent of the visual field defect (449,455,471).

Despite interruption of the optic radiation or area V1, visual information is delivered from the seeing hemisphere to the damaged hemisphere across the splenium of the corpus callosum. Reduced ipsiversive smooth pursuit gain in patients with normal visual fields results from involvement of cortical area V5 or its projections to the basal pontine nuclei, or alternatively from damage to subcortical white matter that disconnects V5 from visual motion information received from areas V1 of both cerebral hemispheres (347,449,480).

ANATOMIC CONNECTIONS OF AREAS MT AND MST

In addition to direct inputs from areas V1, V2, and V3, area MT also has reciprocal direct subcortical connections with the pulvinar. Area MT projects to areas MST, ventral intraparietal area (VIP), floor of the superior temporal sulcus, FEF, ventral bank of the intraparietal sulcus of posterior parietal cortex, and through the forceps major of the corpus callosum to the contralateral MT, MST, and V4. Subcortical projections are to the lateral pontine nucleus (LPN) and DLPN, striatum, thalamic nuclei (pulvinar, lateral geniculate nucleus, reticular nucleus), NOT, dorsal terminal nucleus, and SC (467,483–490).

Inputs to area MST originate within areas V2, V3a, MT, PO, V4, and dorsal prelunate cortex; within V1, only the representation of peripheral retina projects to MST. Cortical projections from MST are to the posterior parietal cortex, inferotemporal cortex, FEF, and contralateral MST (466, 483,489,491–493). The rich cortical connections of MT and MST engage other cerebral areas in generating pursuit.

POSTERIOR PARIETAL CORTEX

Cortical neuronal responses during smooth pursuit were first demonstrated in area 7a (or PG) in the inferior parietal lobule of the posterior parietal cortex (494,495), although some of the visual tracking neurons reported in area 7a (496–498) are actually in the dorsal MST. Among cells in area 7a that are active during looking, some discharge only when the target is a novel stimulus (494). Area 7a contains (*a*) visual fixation neurons that discharge during stationary fixation or smooth pursuit of an object, (*b*) visual tracking neurons with directionally selective responses during pursuit but no responses during stationary fixation, and (c) neurons that discharge during combined eye and hand tracking.

The discharge of fixation neurons and visual tracking neurons in area 7a depends upon the motivational content of the target; unless the target is of interest to the monkey (e.g. food), pursuit responses cease (495). Saccadic, visual fixation, and visual tracking neurons all respond to visual stimuli independently of eye motion and lack responses in the absence of visual stimuli (336). Their sensory responses are enhanced if the stimulus is the target for a movement, indicating that activity in area 7a is related to visual attention rather than to a command function. A subset of visual tracking cells do retain responses to a target moving in the dark (true pursuit cells) (496). Half of true pursuit cells have directionally selective visual responses in the direction opposite to their preferred pursuit direction, and in all of these cells the discharge during pursuit with a visible background is greater than that during pursuit in darkness, suggesting a synergistic convergence of signals from extraretinal pursuit activity (efference copy) and background retinal image motion. These "anti-directional" cells are thought to be involved in perception of relative motion (496). The other true pursuit neurons have similar directional preferences for both pursuit and visual motion. These "iso-directional" cells may represent a converging point for retinal velocity error and eye velocity. This could serve to create an efferent motor signal for pursuit or to signal the trajectory of an object in space, relative to the head rather than the retina. True pursuit neurons have ipsidirectional preferences (497,499).

Many neurons have no response to vestibular stimulation in the dark but respond similarly during pursuit of a moving target with the head fixed, and during passive head movement with a head-fixed target, so that the vestibulo-ocular reflex is canceled (497); these cells appeared to encode pursuit and head motion similar to gaze Purkinje cells of the flocculus. Other neurons increase their firing during head motion in the dark to the same side as the preferred direction for pursuit, whereas some neurons have opposite pursuit and vestibular responses. Vestibular and smooth pursuit information converges upon these cells, and many receive a smooth pursuit signal for head fixed or for combined eye and head tracking (497).

Evidence for a role of the parietal lobe in generating smooth pursuit has been based on clinical observations of patients, made before the era of computed tomography (CT) or MRI, of saccadic pursuit toward the side of posterior cerebral hemispheric lesions (500–502). Modern imaging indicates that unidirectional impairment of smooth pursuit and motion perception correlates better with more ventral damage at the temporo-occipital junction (347,449,455,480, 503). Nevertheless, Lynch and McLaren (333) found that bilateral lesions of the parietal and superior temporal cortex in monkeys create enduring pursuit deficits, and direction-specific pursuit-related responses are found in neurons of areas 7a and LIP (the parietal eye field) (504,505).

VISUAL ATTENTION AND THE PARIETAL LOBES

In addition to visual motion information, the pursuit system requires attention on a target of interest. Pursuit is a voluntary function. Distracted subjects do not pursue smoothly. Areas MT and MST in monkeys project to several cortical areas known to be involved in visual attention, including area 7a, and the VIP area (486). Functional imaging shows increased activity in both the parietal (506,507) and rostral temporal lobes of humans during smooth pursuit (508); these areas correspond to simian posterior parietal cortex and superior temporal polysensory area, a region in the floor and bank of the anterior superior temporal sulcus, receiving converging input from components of the ventral and dorsal streams of visual processing. Both the inferior and superior parietal lobules are probably concerned with attentive eye movements (339,340,495).

Some patients with hemineglect due to acute nondominant parietal lobe lesions are transiently unable to make smooth pursuit eye movements that cross the orbital midline away from the side of damage (473,509). Contralateral pursuit in these patients seems to be impaired in a craniotopic (head-centered) frame of reference. However, inattention to the left visual field after acute right-sided parietal lobe lesions or the frequently associated hemianopia (which causes retinotopic loss of smooth pursuit) might be misinterpreted as a directional palsy of smooth pursuit to the left (510). Lawden et al. (511) studied the smooth pursuit of a foveal target against structured backgrounds and in darkness in patients with unilateral cerebral lesions overlapping in the anterior inferior portion of Brodmann area 40 of the parietal lobe and in frontal white matter. The structured background significantly decreased pursuit gain in patients with either right or left hemispheric lesions. Some patients had a significant smooth pursuit asymmetry when measured either in darkness or with the structured background; however, a few patients had significant pursuit asymmetry in darkness but not with the background, and others had pursuit asymmetry with the background but not in darkness. Most patients had ipsiversive impairment of pursuit, but several patients with pursuit asymmetry had a contraversive defect. Those investigators (511) also hypothesized that hemineglect or hemianopia was responsible for contraversive pursuit defects. Those studies did not test eye movements in different orbital positions, making it difficult to distinguish craniotopic from retinotopic deficits, since the head-centered and eye-centered frames of reference are the same when the eyes are near the orbital midline (512).

Morrow (512) has demonstrated craniotopic defects of smooth pursuit speed and saccade amplitude in the hemirange contralateral to the orbital midline in patients with frontal or parietal lobe lesions. The craniotopic defects did not correlate with contralateral neglect and occurred with either right- or left-sided lesions. The patients also had lowered ipsiversive pursuit gains. Acutely, hemidecorticate monkeys also have defects of both pursuit and saccades in the contralateral orbital hemirange, in addition to persisting ipsiversive pursuit defects, but the larger lesions are accompanied by neglect of contralateral space (309,478).

These varieties of impaired pursuit lead to the classification of four categories of defective smooth pursuit caused by cerebral hemispheric damage (513):

Ipsiversive: Pursuit gain is lowered toward the side of lesions. Contralateral smooth pursuit velocities may be normal, high, or low (but greater than ipsiversive smooth eye movement velocities).

Omnidirectional: Gain is reduced for targets in both hemifields in all directions, without asymmetry.

Retinotopic: Pursuit gain is lowered in all directions in the contralateral visual hemifield.

Craniotopic: Gain is reduced in all directions in the hemirange contralateral to the orbital midline, after recent unilateral hemispheric lesions.

FRONTAL EYE FIELDS AND SMOOTH PURSUIT

Neurons with pursuit responses are also found in the FEF, in the fundus of the arcuate sulcus of monkeys (514,515). These cells have excitatory responses to pursuit movements in their preferred direction but minimal activity during saccades and stationary fixation. Some cells have weaker responses to visual motion, but since responses begin well before the onset of pursuit, responses cannot be attributed to retinal slip of the background, corollary eye movement discharge, or sensitivity to orbital eye position. Directional tuning is broad, without preponderance of ipsidirectional preferences. The early response of these cells suggests that they contribute to pursuit initiation. Microstimulation of this part of the FEF elicits ipsiversive pursuit when the eyes are still in the dark, during fixation, and during ongoing pursuit (514–516).

Unilateral lesions of the pursuit region of the monkey FEF cause ipsiversive or omnidirectional pursuit defects (514,517,518). Bilateral FEF lesions lower pursuit speed in all directions in monkeys but do not eliminate smooth pursuit (518,519). However, optokinetic smooth eye movements evoked by large field stimulation remain normal (520). Sparing of large field tracking responses suggests that the FEF pursuit zone has a retinotopic organization, receiving input from neurons in the posterior cortex that detect predominantly retinal motion close to the fovea, and subserve pursuit. The ipsiversive bias of the FEF pursuit zone might reflect direction preferences of its neuronal projections to the brain stem, as identified for the output neurons from MST (466,467). The FEF is anatomically positioned to participate in smooth pursuit; it receives ipsilateral input from MT and MST (486) and projects to the ipsilateral DLPN and NRTP (214,215,318).

Functional imaging shows increased activity in the human FEF during smooth pursuit (506). Patients with frontal lobe lesions that involve the FEF have directional defects of smooth pursuit toward the side of damage (302,449,521) or bidirectional defects (477,521). Step-ramp presentation of targets reveals no retinotopic pursuit defects, but saccades to contralaterally moving ramps are hypometric (521).

OTHER CEREBRAL REGIONS AND SMOOTH PURSUIT

Microstimulation of the simian SEF evokes smooth eye motion (522), specifically accelerating the initiation but not the maintenance of pursuit (523). Neurons in the SEF respond in relation to the initiation of smooth pursuit (524). In humans, lesions involving the SEF and dorsolateral prefrontal cortex might lower ipsiversive pursuit gain (477,521), but lesions to the SEF are reported to delay the reversal of pursuit direction in response to periodic target motion without reduction in smooth pursuit gain (468). Pursuit responses are recorded in the VIP (525). In the hierarchy of regions, the VIP is similar to the MST, since it too receives a heavy projection from the MT. Lesions involving the corpus striatum are reported to cause errors in the phase between target and smooth eye motion, attributed to impaired target prediction (479), but patients with diffuse or focal cortical lesions do not show phase lag of smooth pursuit behind predictably moving targets (449,521,526,527).

Recovery of Smooth Pursuit

After focal MT and MST lesions, monkeys recover directional and retinotopic pursuit within 1–2 weeks (344,451,528). Complete eradication of areas MT and MST together severely prolongs recovery, and it is incomplete after 7 months. Area VIP and the FEF may mediate the recovery after MST lesions. Pursuit defects from lesions outside the superior temporal sulcus also recover. Partial recovery of pursuit defects after bilateral FEF ablations occurs over 6 weeks and may be mediated by MT and MST or the SEF (519). Substantial recovery also occurs over weeks to months following unilateral FEF ablations in monkeys (514,517).

Patients studied weeks to months after hemispheric damage demonstrate that pursuit defects endure beyond the acute lesion stage (346,347,449,455,503,511,521). Focal lesions or even total hemidecortication do not eliminate ipsiversive pursuit. Persistence of ipsiversive pursuit palsy for some 30 years after a temporal-parietal cyst (449), and for at least a decade after hemidecortication (308,478), testifies to limited adaptation by redundant subcortical pathways in the damaged hemisphere or the other, intact, hemispheric cortex.

Pursuit Control from Cerebrum to Cerebellum

Neurons in areas MST and MT and the FEF project to the DLPN located in the dorsal part of the basal pons (483,529–531). DLPN neurons have many properties in common with MT and MST neurons, and lesions in the DLPN in monkeys produce ipsidirectional deficits of the initiation and maintenance of pursuit (532). Motor commands do not originate in the DLPN, since stimulation there produces only smooth eye acceleration when the eyes are already engaged in smooth tracking; DLPN neurons carry visual and nonvisual, probably efference copy, signals. The dorsomedial pontine nucleus and the rostral part of the nearby NRTP also participate in smooth pursuit (533). Microstimulation in the rostral part of one NRTP elicits predominantly upward smooth eye movements, perhaps because it receives input from both FEFs and their horizontal components cancel (215,534). Stimulation of FEF or NRTP evokes smooth eye movements during fixation or in the dark, unlike the effects of stimulating in DLPN or MT and MST, which produces pursuit movement only when pursuit is ongoing. Unilateral paramedian chemical lesions in the NRTP severely impair upward pursuit and to a lesser degree horizontal pursuit (535). NRTP is a component of a corticoponto-cerebellar circuit from the pursuit area of FEF and projects to the cerebellum. This FEF-NRTP-cerebellum pathway parallels the MT and MST-DLPN-cerebellum pathway in regulating smooth-pursuit eye movements (535).

The DLPN and NRTP project mossy fibers through the contralateral middle cerebellar peduncle to cortex of the flocculus and vermis lobules VI, VII (the ocular motor vermis), and IX (the uvula) and send collaterals to the deep cerebellar nuclei (536,537). Their neurons discharge during pursuit, and lesions in them impair pursuit (532,533,535,538). Ipsiversive smooth pursuit deficits occur in patients with unilateral damage in the basis pontis (539–541), possibly by involving connections of the DLPN or NRTP. The NOT and dorsal terminal nucleus of the AOS receive projection neurons from areas MT and MST (467). The NOT is also engaged during pursuit. Electrolytic lesions of NOT in monkeys reduce ipsiversive pursuit gains to below 0.5, with partial recovery after about 2 weeks. Vertical pursuit is not affected by unilateral or bilateral NOT lesions. Rostral lesions of NOT in and around the pretectal olivary nucleus, which interrupt cortical input through the brachium of the SC, impair smooth pursuit, OKN, and optokinetic after-nystagmus (OKAN). Cortical pathways through rostral NOT play an important role in maintenance of ipsiversive ocular pursuit (542). OKN is discussed later in this chapter. Directionally selective cells in the monkey NOT provide input to the pursuit system through efferent projections: through the NRTP to the cerebellum, as well as to the optokinetic system through projections to the inferior olive (543).

Cerebellum and Smooth Pursuit

The cerebellum is crucial for smooth pursuit. Cerebellectomy abolishes it and stimulation of cerebellar cortex produces smooth eye motion, signifying excitation of pathways responsible for generating the motor commands for smooth pursuit (370,544,545). Flocculectomy in monkeys lowers the speed of smooth pursuit (261) Unilateral lesions of the ventral paraflocculus alone impair smooth pursuit in all horizontal directions, whereas bilateral lesions of the flocculus alone do not impair smooth pursuit in any direction (546).

Neurons in the flocculus and dorsal vermis modulate their firing during smooth pursuit eye movements (547–552). Purkinje cells in the flocculus and ventral paraflocculus (also inclusively referred to as the flocculus in this chapter) encode gaze velocity and acceleration during tracking with the eyes or with the head and eyes; they do not discharge during fixation of a stationary target while the head is moved, since during this activity gaze does not change, even though the eyes move in the orbit at the same speed as the opposed head movement. They are called gaze velocity Purkinje cells (553,554). Neurons of posterior vermis lobules VI and VII also encode gaze velocity (the sum of eye velocity and head velocity) and target velocity in space (the sum of gaze velocity and retinal image velocity) using inputs of eye, retinal image, and head velocities (549,550).

Lesions of the vermis at lobules VI and VII of monkeys cause a small decrease in steady pursuit gain during triangular-wave tracking and a decrease in peak eye acceleration of initial pursuit. In a pursuit adaptation paradigm, where targets change velocity during ongoing pursuit, normal animals can adaptively adjust eye their eye acceleration to match the new target velocity. Following lesions in the oculomotor vermis, this adaptive capability is impaired (555). The ocular motor vermis plays a role in smooth pursuit and its adaptive control.

Smooth pursuit function is lateralized in the cerebellum. Hemicerebellectomy in monkeys lowers ipsiversive pursuit velocities more than contraversive velocities (544). Floccular Purkinje cells discharge with ipsiversive pursuit more than contraversive pursuit (552,553), or more with downward-contraversive pursuit (552). Stimulation of the simian cerebellar cortex produces predominantly ipsiversive smooth eye movements (370). In humans, unilateral lesions of the cerebellar hemisphere, apparently sparing the vermis and fastigial nucleus, have been reported to reduce the gain of ipsiversive initial pursuit and to mildly reduce the gain of maintained pursuit in both horizontal directions (556).

The fastigial nucleus (Fig. 17.20) receives inhibitory projections from the ocular motor vermis (Fig. 17.34), and many neurons in the caudal part of the fastigial nucleus discharge in relation to initial acceleration and maintenance of smooth pursuit, especially when it is contraversive and downward (557). Chemical inhibition of its caudal part impairs contraversive pursuit acceleration or increases ipsiversive acceleration. However, pursuit maintenance is affected only slightly in all directions. Bilateral inactivation of this FOR leaves pursuit acceleration intact and produces moderate decreases in pursuit speed (558). The role of the FOR may be to add a supplementary signal to other pursuit circuits. Nonetheless, patients with lesions involving the fastigial nuclei on both sides are reported to have saccadic hypermetria but well-preserved smooth pursuit (559).

Brain Stem Generation of Smooth Pursuit

Floccular gaze velocity Purkinje cells inhibit floccular target neurons (FTNs) in the ipsilateral medial vestibular nucleus (560,561). Purkinje cells of the flocculus project caudally and medially between the middle cerebellar peduncle and the flocculus, over the caudal surface of the middle cerebellar peduncle, then over the dorsal surface of the cochlear nuclei, and then caudally along the lateral surface of the inferior cerebellar peduncle (the restiform body) to pass over its dorsal surface in the cerebellopontine angle, and they terminate exclusively in the ipsilateral vestibular nuclei. Some project medially into the y-group. Others continue rostrally and medially to terminate in the superior vestibular nucleus. Many axons stream caudal and ventral to the y-group to form a compact tract (the angular bundle of Löwy) adjacent to the lateral angle of the fourth ventricle and dorsal to the MVN, and terminate in the rostral part of the MVN and the ventrolateral vestibular nucleus (562).

FTNs inhibit neurons in the ipsilateral abducens nucleus, and they discharge during contraversive smooth pursuit

(560,561). Cells identified as smooth pursuit or eye-head neurons in the MVN are probably FTNs (563–565). FTNs are considered to be the major premotor input to motoneurons during pursuit (560,564,566). Position-vestibular-pause (PVP) cells are other second-order neurons in the MVN that also discharge during contraversive pursuit, but PVP cells act by exciting the contralateral abducens nucleus (561). They are called PVP neurons because they have firing rates proportional to eye position and vestibular eye velocity, and they pause during saccades. The source of pursuit information to PVP cells is uncertain (566,567). Thus, the flocculus or ventral paraflocculus participates in ipsiversive pursuit by inhibiting ipsilateral FTNs, and both FTN and PVP cells are active during contraversive pursuit.

The fastigial nucleus also projects to the vestibular nucleus, to the reticular formation near the abducens nucleus, and to the DLPN (378,568), but it is unclear how smooth pursuit neurons in the caudal fastigial nucleus gain access to the smooth pursuit machinery in the brain stem, and whether floccular and fastigial signals merge at common brain stem structure (558).

Smooth pursuit and saccadic eye movements share some brain stem pathways. The midline cells in the pons called omnipause neurons, which keep excitatory burst neurons for saccades under constant inhibition during fixation and stop firing during saccades, reduce their firing rate during smooth pursuit. Electrical microstimulation of the omnipause neurons decelerates the eyes during smooth pursuit. Omnipause neurons provide inhibition to control the time course of pursuit. The same inhibitory cells control both saccades and smooth pursuit (569). Another type of cell in the PPRF, near the omnipause neurons, discharges in bursts during saccades in a preferred direction, and they discharge in a sustained fashion at a lower frequency for the duration of pursuit in the same preferred direction. These saccade-pursuit neurons may participate in the eye-velocity modulation of omnipause cell discharge (570).

The smooth and saccadic eye movement subregions of the FEF both send direct projections to the ipsilateral riMLF, suggesting a possible role of the riMLF in smooth pursuit eye movements and providing further evidence for interaction between the saccadic and pursuit systems at the brain stem level (250).

Direct connections from the vestibular nuclei to ocular motor nuclei may complete the principal horizontal pursuit circuit in the brain stem. The excitatory circuit from the cerebral cortex to the ipsilateral pontine nuclei, then to the contralateral cerebellar vermis and flocculus, next to the vestibular nucleus, and finally from the vestibular nucleus to the abducens nucleus generates horizontal smooth pursuit by exciting lateral rectus motoneurons and medial rectus internuclear neurons in the contralateral abducens nucleus and inhibiting them in the ipsilateral abducens nucleus. This pathway constitutes a double decussation of the horizontal pursuit pathway (571). The first decussation is the pontocerebellar projections through the contralateral middle cerebellar peduncle to the vermis and flocculus. The second decussation is from second-order vestibular neurons in the MVN to the contralateral abducens nucleus (571) (Fig. 17.38).

In contrast to the impairment of ipsiversive pursuit that results from lesions at sites more upstream in the pursuit pathway, lesions in the medulla oblongata often lower the speed of contraversive pursuit more than ipsiversive pursuit (385,571,572). Damage to projections from vestibular nuclei to the abducens nucleus or damage to the inferior cerebellar peduncle interrupting olivary climbing fibers to the cerebellar cortex may explain the contraversive pursuit defect. Loss of climbing fiber input would increase the activity of ipsi-

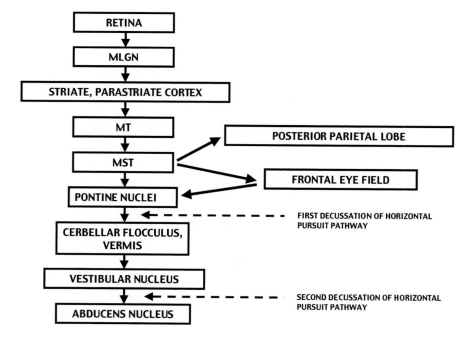

Figure 17.38. Flow of visual motion and motor signals that generate smooth pursuit. *Dashed lines* indicate double decussation of pathway for horizontal pursuit. A double decussation for the horizontal pursuit pathway makes it effectively ipsilateral, so that unilateral lesions cause ipsiversive pursuit defects. MLGN, magnocellular lateral geniculate nucleus; MT, middle temporal visual area; MST, medial temporal area. (Adapted from Morrow MJ, Sharpe JA. Smooth pursuit eye movements. In: Sharpe JA, Barber HO, eds. The Vestibulo-Ocular Reflex and Vertigo. New York: Raven, 1993:141–162.)

lateral Purkinje cells (382). Consequently, the ipsilateral fastigial nucleus would be inhibited, therefore impairing contraversive smooth pursuit (382).

Other brain stem structures also participate in pursuit. The NPH together with the adjacent MVN (Fig. 17.9) performs integration, in the mathematical sense, for conjugate horizontal eye movements by transforming eye velocity signals to eye position signals (255,256,258). A pre-emphasis force is required to accelerate the eyes to a constant velocity during pursuit (573). Integration transforms an acceleration command to a constant velocity command for maintained pursuit, and also transforms a velocity command to a position command for sustained eccentric eye position holding after pursuit stops. Damage in both the MVN and NPH sharply limits the rapid rise of the velocity of the slow phases of optokinetic nystagmus, which are thought to be accomplished by pursuit, but inactivation of the NPH alone has little effect on pursuit (258).

Lesions in the PPRF were thought to paralyze all conjugate eye movements toward the side of damage, including smooth pursuit (216,219,574). Destruction of fibers passing near this region, rather than destruction of neuronal cell bodies, may account for this ipsiversive pursuit paralysis. Injections of the excitotoxin kainic acid, which damages cell bodies but not axons, into the PPRF slows only ipsiversive saccades. Thus, a lesion confined to the burst neurons in the PPRF leaves a full range of smooth eye movements (217,221). In fact, the amplitude range of saccades is also normal after chemical inactivation of excitatory burst neurons (218), indicating that the inactivation spares the eye position internal (nonvisual) feedback circuit that drives the eyes until they reach their target (264,265).

Vertical smooth pursuit channels in the brain stem are distinct from those that control horizontal pursuit. Cells in the rostral part of the vestibular nucleus send vertical pursuit signals to ocular motoneurons via the MLF (575) (Figs. 17.8 and 17.9). The y-group of the vestibular nucleus, located at junction of the brain stem and cerebellum and the adjacent dentate nucleus, has neurons that fire for upward pursuit, and stimulation in this area produces smooth upward eye movements (576). Thus, the MLF and probably the superior cerebellar peduncle in monkeys carry signals used for vertical pursuit (575,577–579). Patients with MLF damage have only mildly impaired vertical smooth pursuit (580), suggesting that pathways outside the MLF carry much of the vertical smooth pursuit command signal in humans. Vertical smooth pursuit is selectively impaired by damage in the midbrain. Lesions in the pretectum degrade upward pursuit (574, 581,582). Both upward and downward smooth pursuit are limited in range or reduced in gain by damage in the ventral tegmentum of the midbrain, involving the INC and probably commissural projections ventral as well as dorsal to the aqueduct of Sylvius (244,582). INC neurons in animals modulate their firing during vertical pursuit (583,584), and pursuit-related neurons in the FEF project to the riMLF (250). Burst neurons in the INC may be a site of convergence of both vertical saccadic and smooth pursuit signals, or they might provide input to the eye velocity to eye position integrator for vertical motion (584).

VERGENCE SYSTEM

Vergence eye movements permit stereopsis and prevent diplopia. By moving the eyes in opposite horizontal directions, the vergence system maintains the image of an object on the fovea of each eye, whether the object is located far away or nearby and whether it is moving toward or away from the viewer. Fixation of a near object induces not only convergence but also accommodation of the lenses and constriction of the pupils, as described in Chapters 14 and 15; these three responses constitute the near reaction (585). Two major types of vergence stimuli may be distinguished: retinal blur and retinal disparity. Retinal blur refers to a loss of image sharpness, while retinal disparity is the separation of images of a single object such that they fall on noncorresponding parts of the retina (586). Retinal blur elicits accommodative vergence and retinal disparity elicits fusional vergence. In most natural circumstances, both stimuli combine to produce appropriate vergence eye movements; however, accommodative and fusional vergence can be tested separately under experimental conditions (587–590). Voluntary control of convergence without visual stimuli, and, to a minor degree, of divergence, is variable among individuals.

Accommodative vergence can be elicited by covering one eye and changing the distance of the fixation target seen by the other eye (the Müller paradigm) (585,587,588). If the fixation target is accurately aligned with the visual axis of the viewing eye, that eye moves only slightly, but the covered eye moves nasally, and its movement reflects the accommodative-induced vergence. When a vergence command is sent to both eyes, the command to the viewing eye may be canceled by an opposing pursuit command, keeping the viewing eye on target (591). The Müller paradigm elicits a small abducting saccade in the viewing eye that is followed by a vergence adduction back to the target (592).

Fusional vergence alone can be elicited by placing a prism in front of one eye during binocular fixation of a stationary target. This induces retinal disparity without changing the distance of the target. There is thus no need for a change in accommodation.

Characteristics of Vergence Eye Movements

Vergence movements are slow, often lasting as long as 1 second when the stimulus is an abrupt change in target distance. The latency of a vergence movement is about 200 msec for retinal blur stimuli and about 80 to 160 msec for retinal disparity stimuli (593). The waveform is typically that of an exponential function, with a time constant of 150–200 msec, reflecting the viscous and elastic properties of the orbit (594). For constant velocity targets or target steps, the trajectory is one of increasing velocity for convergent movements and decreasing velocity for divergent movements. Peak velocities for convergence are higher than for divergence. Premotor commands for conjugate eye movements (versions) and vergence eye movements are generated independently. However, under natural viewing conditions when targets move tangentially as well as in depth, combined vergence and versional movements are required, and the speed of vergence increases to decrease the delay in bringing the target image to both foveae. Most vergence eye movements are accompanied by disconjugate saccades, and saccades speed up vergence. Combined saccade–vergence eye movements often induce miniature conjugate saccadic oscillations of about 0.3° at 20 to 30 Hz (595,596).

Moreover, vergence occurs during horizontal and vertical saccades to pure versional targets, altering the trajectory of saccades and making them transiently disconjugate (597–599). The eyes diverge then converge during horizontal saccades, coming to alignment 30–100 msec after the saccades stop. During upward saccades there is often an initial divergence, and during downward saccades, an initial convergence.

Visual sensitivity is markedly reduced during vergence eye movements (600). Thus, visual suppression occurs not only for saccades (as discussed above) but also for vergence eye movements.

Neurophysiology of Vergence Eye Movements

The stimulus for fusional vergence is a position error—the presence of the image of an object on noncorresponding parts of the two retinas (601). A vergence command is then generated until this retinal disparity is reduced to the small degree necessary for stereopsis. This may be considered a negative feedback control system. Important interactions occur between vergence and accommodation, resulting in convergence-evoked accommodation and accommodation-evoked convergence. They are expressed in the ratio of accommodative-linked convergence to accommodation (AC/A) and by the ratio of convergence-linked accommodation to convergence (CA/C) (585,602).

Brain Stem Mechanisms

Although vergence movements are mediated by the same ocular motoneurons that subserve versional movements of the saccadic, smooth pursuit, vestibulo-ocular, and optokinetic systems (134,603–605), the sensitivity of individual neurons differs depending on whether eye position is changed by a vergence or by a versional movement (606). Some motoneurons in the abducens and oculomotor nuclei play a more important role than others in either vergence or conjugate movements (606). The medial rectus muscle of macaque monkeys is innervated by three separate subgroups of motoneurons in the ipsilateral oculomotor nucleus (607,608) (Fig. 17.11). Neurons in all three of these locations receive inputs from the contralateral abducens nucleus via the MLF. The cells in the dorsomedial part of the nucleus are smaller than the cells in the other two areas and are preferentially labeled when tracer substances are injected in the outer orbital layer of the medial rectus muscle, believed to contain primarily "tonic" fibers. These cells might be a subpopulation of medial rectus motoneurons that are principally concerned with vergence movements, but this speculation is contrary to electrophysiologic evidence that all motoneurons are in a final common pathway and participate in all classes of eye movements (212,603).

Three sets of neurons in the midbrain reticular formation discharge only in relation to convergence or divergence

movements: vergence burst, vergence tonic, and vergence burst-tonic cells (609–611). These cells are intermixed in the reticular formation 1–2 mm dorsal and dorsolateral to the oculomotor nucleus. Vergence tonic cells discharge in relation to the angle of convergence and carry eye position commands for medial and lateral rectus motoneurons. Vergence burst neurons have higher-frequency discharge before and during vergence and transmit eye velocity commands for motoneurons (135). Burst neurons for either convergence or divergence are present. Vergence burst-tonic cells combine the velocity and position commands. The inputs to these neurons are uncertain. The similarities of burst and tonic activities of vergence neurons to those neurons that generate saccades (discussed above) and the interactions of vergence movements with saccades suggest that pause cells and a vergence velocity-to-position neural integrator are also elements of the vergence system (599). However, omnipause neurons in the rip do not inhibit vergence. Although saccades made during both convergence and divergence are significantly slower than conjugate saccades, modulation of omnipause neurons is not responsible for the slower saccades during vergence movements (612).

Convergence cells project to medial rectus subdivisions of the ipsilateral oculomotor nucleus, providing medial rectus motoneurons with their convergence signal, but divergence cells are not found to project to either oculomotor nucleus (613). Abducens motoneurons decrease their firing rate during convergence, but their vergence inputs are unknown. Internuclear neurons in the abducens nucleus, which project through the MLF to excite medial rectus motoneurons in the contralateral oculomotor nucleus, activate the medial rectus muscle during conjugate eye movements, but they carry an inappropriate direction signal for vergence; they decrease their activity during convergence (610,614). Internuclear neurons in the oculomotor nucleus lie along the lateral border of the medial rectus motoneuron subdivisions in the monkey (607). These oculomotor internuclear neurons excite contralateral abducens motoneurons and are probably involved in the coordination of horizontal conjugate movements, but they carry the wrong direction signal for convergence (615). The MLF does, however, carry signals related to vergence, and lidocaine-induced internuclear ophthalmoplegia in monkeys increases the amount of convergence evoked by accommodation, suggesting that the MLF transmits information that inhibits convergence (616). The internuclear neurons of the oculomotor nucleus (607) increase their activity during both version and convergence, and they may inhibit convergence by exciting lateral rectus motoneurons (615). Other neurons in the vicinity of the abducens nucleus that display activity similar to the midbrain vergence cells are possible candidates for the source of convergence signals, by inhibiting lateral rectus motoneurons (617).

Cerebral Control of Vergence Eye Movements

Frontal cortex immediately anterior to the saccade-related FEF in monkeys is involved in vergence and accommodation (618), and neurons of the pursuit region of the FEF modulate strongly during both frontal pursuit and vergence tracking

(619). Neurons in the striate cortex of the monkey respond to retinal disparity and also indicate the distance of the image ahead or behind the actual fixation point (620). Neurons with identical properties are found in area MT of macaque monkeys (464) (Fig. 17.37). Cells in area MST that are sensitive to retinal image motion play an active role in the generation of vergence eye movements at short latencies (621). Neurons in the posterior parietal lobe of monkeys are activated during visual tracking of objects moving in the sagittal plane (496,622). Lateral intraparietal area neurons that discharge before saccades also respond preferentially to far or distant targets when the depth of the target is cued by either binocular image disparity or its accommodative demand (623).

Cerebellar Control of Vergence Eye Movements

The cerebellum also regulates vergence eye movements. Total cerebellectomy in monkeys causes a transient paralysis of convergence (544,545). The NRTP contains neurons that discharge in relation to elements of the near reaction, including vergence (624,625) (Fig. 17.8). The NRTP projects to the ocular motor vermis (537) and the nucleus interpositus in monkeys (corresponding to the emboliform and globose cerebellar nuclei in humans) and receives input from the FEF. The posterior interpositus nucleus contains neurons that are active during convergence, divergence, and accommodation (626). Cerebral cortex, the NRTP, and the interpositus form part of a cerebro-ponto-cerebellar pathway modulating or controlling vergence and ocular accommodation (625).

The monkey flocculus contains neurons that discharge in relationship to the angle of vergence eye position (627). They might participate in the necessary modulation of the amplitude of the vestibulo-ocular reflex for changes in target distance; VOR amplitude and speed increase when a near target is viewed (628,629), as we discuss below with otolith-ocular reflexes. Stimulation of the flocculus can cause movements in one eye only (630). Nonetheless, monkeys with lesions of the flocculus retain the ability to make adaptive changes in vergence and their AC/A ratio (631).

Patients with Arnold-Chiari malformation or cerebellar degeneration can have an esotropia consisting of a convergence bias (or a divergence weakness) with full abduction of each eye (632–634). In rabbits the flocculus has inhibitory projections to the medial rectus muscle but not to the lateral rectus motoneurons (635); if this is the case in humans, it provides a possible mechanism for the esotropia sometimes associated with cerebellar disease.

FIXATION SYSTEM

Although the eyes may appear to an examiner to be still during steady viewing, fixation actually consists of three distinct types of miniature movements that are not detected by visual inspection of the eyes: microsaccades, microtremor, and microdrift. They occur in horizontal, vertical and torsional directions (636,637). Microsaccades usually have amplitudes of less than 26 minutes of arc (average about 6 minutes; there are 60 arc-minutes in 1°). By ophthal-

moscopy, the examiner can detect saccades as small as about 10 minutes of arc. Microsaccades occur at a mean frequency of approximately 120 per minute. Although it has been suggested that microsaccades prevent images from fading on the retina (638,639), vision remains clear when they are voluntarily suppressed. Normal individuals can voluntarily reduce the rate of microsaccades (640). When they are asked to suppress them, saccade rate is reduced to about 30 per minute. Microsaccades stop during finely guided visual motor tasks such as threading a needle or sighting a rifle. Microsaccades have no known visual function (641,642), but they may reflect shifting of visual attention away from a fixated object (643,644). Some investigators (645) maintain that microsaccades refresh images to prevent the fading that occurs when the eyes are immobile (646).

Microtremor consists of a continuous high-frequency buzz of eye motion underlying both miniature saccades and microdrift. Microtremor has spectral peaks at lower (up to 25 Hz) and higher (60–90 Hz) frequencies and is coherent between the eyes. It therefore has, at least in part, a central origin (647). Microtremor could reflect the synchronous discharge of ocular motor units. The average amplitude of microtremor is much less than 1 minute of arc, usually 5 to 30 arc-seconds (60 arc-seconds are equal to one arc-minute).

The eyes also drift smoothly at rates less than 20 minutes of arc per second and amplitudes of about 2 to 5 arc-minutes. This microdrift is considered to be necessary to prevent fading of a stable image (636). During eccentric gaze over about 40°, drift becomes directed toward the orbital midposition at rates over 30 arc-minutes per second, and fixation of a target is restored by centrifugal saccades; this pattern of drift and fast eye movements creates end-point nystagmus (175,176). Microdrift rates increase considerably when no target is visible, implying the operation of a fixation mechanism when an object is viewed.

Normal persons have small conjugate horizontal saccades that intrude upon fixation. These saccadic intrusions are larger than microsaccades and are called square wave jerks (648). They have amplitudes over about 0.5°. Each intrusive saccade is followed after an interval of about 200 msec by a horizontal corrective saccade, back to the fixation position. They normally occur less than 10 times per minute (648,649). More frequent square wave jerks can accompany focal or diffuse cerebral, brain stem, or cerebellar disease, and they are larger in amplitude and more frequent in cerebellar conditions (650).

The concept of visual fixation as an active process, not merely the absence of visible eye movements, was emphasized by Holmes (651) and has been supported by modern observations. Fixation of a stationary target is distinct from smooth pursuit. Pursuit of a slowly moving target is characterized by small oscillations of eye velocity (1°–2° per second at 3–4 Hz), called ringing. Time delays in the closed-loop pursuit system account for ringing. Ringing is absent during fixation, indicating that fixation is not equivalent to ''pursuit at zero velocity'' and that smooth pursuit is ''switched off'' (431,433). Visual enhancement of the VOR may also be a function of the fixation system (652,653). Furthermore, a rare variant of congenital nystagmus occurs during pursuit, but not during fixation (654). Cerebral lesions can cause spasm of fixation, a defect in initiating saccades when a target is viewed that improves when no target is present for fixation (651,655).

Neurophysiologic Basis of Fixation

Several cerebral areas participate in visual fixation. Fixation-related activity is recorded in neurons in the posterior parietal areas LIP and 7a (504) and in areas MT and MST of the superior temporal sulcus of monkeys (505,656). The neuronal discharge is determined by eye position in the orbit and subserves an internal representation of the external space in a non-retinotopic frame of reference (504). The discharge of fixation neurons and visual tracking neurons in area 7 depends upon the motivational content of the target; unless the target is of interest to the monkey, responses cease (327,495). Visual fixation neurons, like saccadic and visual tracking neurons in area 7, respond to visual stimuli independently of eye motion and lack responses in the absence of visual stimuli. Their sensory responses are enhanced if the stimulus is the target for a movement, indicating that the fixation activity in area 7 is related to visual attention (336).

Stimulation of the SEF in the dorsomedial frontal cortex of the monkey maintains fixation in specific fixation regions of the orbit and inhibits visually evoked saccades (317). Neuronal recordings in the SEF show activity related to saccadic eye movement or visual fixation or both. This activity depends upon the position of a fixation target in a topographic distribution: neurons in the rostral SEF are more active with the eyes to the contralateral position, while those in the caudal part are more active with eyes to the ipsilateral position; also, cells in the medial part of the area have higher activity with a downward fixation position, whereas those in the lateral part have higher activity with an upward fixation position. This distribution of units is in agreement with the map of termination zones of saccadic eye movements evoked by electrical stimulation of the same area (316), but there is conflicting evidence on this point (315). The SEF role in fixation might be effected by its excitation of the fixation cells of the rostral SC (294,295,314), since ablation of the SC eliminates the inhibition of saccades that occurs during SEF stimulation while the eyes are positioned in specific fixation regions (281,319). Dorsolateral prefrontal cortex (Brodmann area 46) contains neurons that have increased activity during fixation and neurons that appear to suppress unwanted saccades (279,657–659).

Steady fixation raises the threshold for eliciting saccades by stimulation of the FEF or the SC of the monkey (183,660). In monkeys many FEF neurons with presaccadic activity actually increase their discharge in response to the disappearance of a fixation target (306). This ''fixation disengagement discharge'' is an element of switching off fixation.

Functional imaging reveals that fixation increases activity in several regions of human cerebral cortex (278,340,661). Area 17 at the occipital pole and up to 2.5 cm of adjacent lateral occipital lobe surface (Brodmann area 18) and ventrolateral occipito-temporal cortex (areas 19 and 37) are activated by a foveal target light subtending less than 20 minutes of arc (278). The ventromedial frontal lobe including the anterior cingulate gyrus is activated predominantly in the dominant hemisphere when compared to activation by saccade tasks. Fixation also activates the dominant ventrolateral frontal lobe, including areas Brodmann areas 8, 9, 10, 45, and 46 (278) (Fig. 17.30). A concordant finding is that some patients with medial or ventrolateral frontal lobe lesions cannot maintain central fixation when competing peripheral stimuli are presented (662). Brodmann areas 10, 11, and 32 of the orbitofrontal cortex appear to be engaged in fixation by processing limbic motivational or memory input to frontal and parietal lobe ocular motor areas, since PET shows activation of the orbitofrontal region specifically during fixation in comparison with saccades to remembered target locations, or during attention to details of the fixation stimulus (278,340). The human FEF is also activated during fixation, but regional cerebral blood flow increases progressively from a fixation task to tasks evoking reflexive saccades to targets, to tasks requiring antisaccades or volitional saccades guided by memory (274), and as mentioned above, the FEF is probably involved in disengaging fixation.

Among brain stem structures, neurons in the SNpr are tonically active during fixation and inhibit burst neurons in the SC that fire in relation to saccades made to visual and remembered targets; SNpr neurons pause before and during saccades, disinhibiting the SC burst neurons (288,290). As discussed previously in the chapter, fixation neurons in the rostral pole of the SC keep presaccadic buildup neurons in the caudal SC silent, and the eyes remain fixated, until a new target appears and activates the buildup neurons. The buildup cells in turn inhibit the fixation neurons and excite burst neurons in a more dorsal sublayer of the SC (294,295,314). SC burst neurons project to omnipause neurons in the rip (224,297) (Figs. 17.8, 17.9, and 17.29). The fixation cells of the SC might activate omnipause neurons that sustain fixation by tonically inhibiting presaccadic short-lead burst neurons in the PPRF and riMLF, and preventing them from firing.

VESTIBULO-OCULAR SYSTEM

During normal behavior, it is natural to use a combination of eye and head movements, whether to voluntarily acquire or track a target of interest or to reflexively stabilize gaze in response to a passive body movement. Even foveate animals that have acquired a high degree of independent control over their eyes and head commonly use both eye and head movements together. This cooperation between eye and head movement is reflected in the anatomic and physiologic similarities between the head and ocular motor control systems. When the head moves, peripheral labyrinthine and cervical proprioceptors reflexes, inducing vestibulo-ocular (head-eye), cervico-ocular (neck-eye), and vestibulo-collic (head-neck) reflexes, are stimulated to stabilize gaze. We have described cervico-ocular and vestibulo-collic reflexes, combined eye and head saccades, and combined eye and head pursuit in a prior edition of this book (663), and readers may consult that and other works (565,664–673) for further information on eye–head coordination. Here we discuss the vestibulo-ocular reflex.

Vestibulo-Ocular Reflex

When the head moves, VOR eye movements are generated in the opposite direction to maintain the direction of viewing and to prevent retinal image slip. Side-to-side, fore-and-aft, or up-and-down head movement activates the translational VOR, and roll of the head around the interaural axis elicits the torsional VOR. Translation and static roll with respect to the gravitational vector are detected by the otolith receptors in the maculae of the utricle and saccule. Head rotation about its yaw (earth-vertical), pitch (interaural), or roll (naso-occipital) axes elicits the angular VOR, detected by the cupulae in the semicircular canals.

The VOR stabilizes gaze (eye position in space) during head motion so that images can be held steady on the retina. It produces an eye movement in the orbit that is equal and opposite to the head movement, so that the sum of eye position in the orbit and head position in space—the eye position in space—is held constant (Fig. 17.39). The VOR thereby maintains the line of sight despite any head motion, be it translational or rotational. The angular VOR detects acceleration of the head in the plane of the semicircular canals. The head acceleration stimulus is integrated by the mechanical property of the semicircular canals (Fig. 17.40) so that the signal carried in the vestibular nerve is proportional to head velocity (674). The VOR functions well for brief, high-frequency head movements; however, because of the mechanical characteristics of the semicircular canals, the peripheral vestibular apparatus cannot accurately estimate head velocity during sustained-velocity or low-frequency head rotation. Thus, during a constant-velocity rotation in the dark, after the inertia of the endolymph is overcome and it is moving with the canal, the cupula returns to its initial position, the peripheral vestibular signal fades away, and vestibular nystagmus (as well as the sensation of rotation) slowly disappears (Fig. 17.23). During rotation in the light, the optokinetic system (discussed below) compensates for this low-frequency limitation in function of the angular VOR.

To maintain clear vision, the angular VOR responds promptly with a latency of 7 to 10 msec (652,675–677), well below that of ocular following responses, which exceed 70 msec in humans (678,679). The ratio of the output of the reflex (smooth eye movement speed in one direction) to the

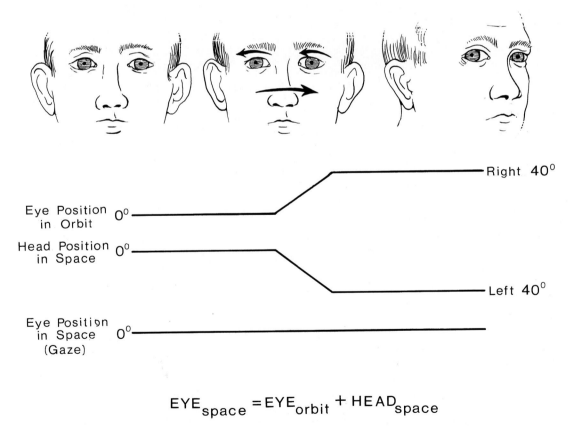

$$EYE_{space} = EYE_{orbit} + HEAD_{space}$$

Figure 17.39. The function of the vestibulo-ocular reflex. When the head is rapidly turned to one side, the eyes move a corresponding amount in the orbit toward the opposite side. Because the movements of head and eyes are equal and opposite, the position of the eyes in space (gaze position) remains unchanged. (Redrawn from Leigh RJ, Zee DS. The Neurology of Eye Movement. Philadelphia: FA Davis, 1991.)

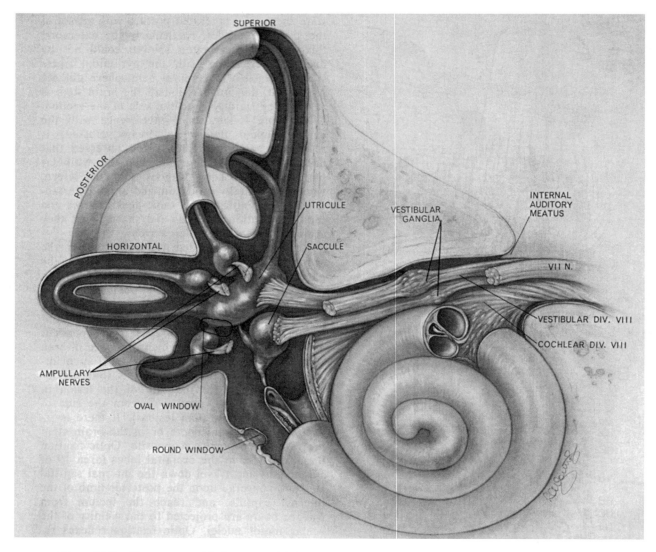

Figure 17.40.   The structures of the inner ear and their sensory nerves. The right labyrinth and cochlea are viewed from the anterior aspect. Note the three semicircular canals, with their bony and membranous components. At one end of each of the canals are enlargements, the ampullae, connected to which are the ampullary nerves, branches of the vestibular nerve. The ampullary nerves conduct impulses centrally from each of the semicircular canals and affect the ocular muscles by specific connections to the vestibular nuclei and premotor structures in the brainstem. At the other end of the semicircular canals are the utricle and saccule, attached to which are other branches of the vestibular nerve. Note the position of the superior and inferior parts of the vestibular ganglion within the internal auditory meatus. (Drawing by Lynn Young, University of California School of Medicine, San Francisco.)

input of the reflex (head speed in the opposite direction) is its gain. VOR gain must approximate 1.0 to prevent slippage of retinal images. The eyes and head must also be 180° out of phase; this phase difference is called zero, by convention. VOR phase lead or lag must be absent for clear vision. If the gain is too much above or below its ideal value of unity, a target image remains off the fovea, although it may be transiently stable on the retina. If there is a phase lead of the eyes before the head or a phase lag behind it, the target image is never stationary on the retina. Abnormal gain or

phase of the reflex causes visual blur and oscillopsia. The VOR gain varies with the frequency of head motion and is less dependent on head velocity; its gain begins to decline only if head velocities exceed 350°/sec (266). The eyes have a phase lead before the head at very low frequencies of head motion (under 0.2 Hz) and a phase lag behind the head at very high frequencies (over 3 Hz), but phase differences remain about zero during most natural head motion. During passive head rotation in darkness (without optokinetic or pursuit influences), angular VOR gain is below unity under

1 Hz, is near 1.0 from 1–2 Hz, decreases somewhat between 2–8 Hz, then increases continuously from 8 Hz to about 1.3 at 20 Hz; it has been recorded as high as 3.0 at 70 Hz (676,680–682). However, during natural passive head motions while running or walking, or during self-generated head oscillation, predominant frequencies are under 5–6 Hz. Head velocities do not exceed 100°/sec during walking and running, but gaze velocity rises up to about 9°/sec and visual acuity declines (683,684). Active head-shaking can attain head velocities over 780°/sec (683,684). Normal persons see illusionary movement of the world (oscillopsia) during rapid self-generated head shaking.

Translational VOR and Tilt-Roll Otolith-Ocular Reflexes

The otolith system contributes to the VOR when the head moves linearly in the earth-horizontal plane, or tilts relative to gravity, or moves up and down. Otolith-ocular responses can be considered a subsystem of the vestibulo-ocular system. They elicit the translational VOR and the static torsional VOR. The semicircular canals also generate angular torsional VOR responses, as well as the horizontal and vertical angular VOR. Otolith-ocular responses are divided into two categories: translational responses and tilt responses. Translational otolith-ocular responses are generated by up-down (bob), anterior-posterior (surge), and lateral (heave) movements of the head. They elicit vertical or horizontal eye movements whose amplitude depends on the angle of vergence and the direction of gaze (685,686). They generate short-latency compensatory eye movements and provide gaze stabilization during fast translatory head movements when visual mechanisms are insufficient. Tilt otolith-ocular responses are evoked by movement of the labyrinths during head motion around the roll (naso-occipital) axis or the pitch (inter-aural) axis, producing torsional or vertical eye movements, respectively. In contrast to translational VOR responses, tilt otolith-ocular responses occur when the head undergoes static changes with respect to gravity—in positions of roll or pitch, both being angular head movements. The translational VOR is measured by its sensitivity, rather than by gain, as for the angular VOR arising from the canals or from the otolith receptors during tilt (gain is the ratio of angular eye movement to angular head movement), since linear movement of the head produces angular rotation of the eyes, and the two movements are in different reference frames. Sensitivity is typically stipulated by the ratio, rotation of the eyes in degrees per head translation in centimeters.

The translational VOR functions well at high frequencies (above 1 Hz, being optimal near 4 Hz), where smooth pursuit does not function. Both the angular VOR and translation VOR operate with high-pass characteristics relative to a head velocity input, although the cutoff frequency of the angular VOR (less than 0.1 Hz) is far below that of the translational (approximately 1 Hz), and both perform well at high frequencies that exceed the capabilities of smooth pursuit (687). Smooth pursuit supplements the VOR at frequencies below 1–2 Hz. The translational VOR has a latency of about 20

msec (688), being much shorter than visual following reflexes but twice as long as the latency of the angular VOR. At low frequencies of head translation, only very distant targets can be stabilized by the translational VOR alone, but smooth pursuit can compensate to stabilize images on the retina. Even at high acceleration, lateral head movement (heave) is not fully compensatory. Only about 40% of the vestibular eye position and 60% of the eye velocity required for image stabilization is achieved during high-acceleration heaves (688,689). The low vestibular response is supplemented by vestibular catch-up saccades during the head heave, in the same direction as the vestibular smooth eye movements. Despite the smooth eye movements and vestibular catch-up saccades during the heave, at the end of the head movement only about 70% of the heave is compensated by eye rotation, and foveating saccades are required after the VOR stops.

During head rotation about its earth-vertical (yaw) axis, the translational VOR is activated together with the angular VOR, because the eyes and labyrinths are positioned off the center of head and neck rotation. The linear translation of the eyes varies inversely with the viewing distance. For example, when shaking the head side-to side (''no''), viewing an object 10 cm from the eyes requires eye movements approximately twice as large as those while viewing an object 30 cm away, to stabilize its image on the fovea. The gain of the angular VOR and the sensitivity of the translational VOR depend on the intended viewing distance (628,629,686, 690). In monkeys, augmentation in VOR sensitivity occurs 50–200 msec *before* the intended convergence of the eyes (691).

In addition to their responses to linear acceleration during head translation and to static head orientation with respect to gravity, otolith-ocular detectors respond to angular motion involving a dynamic reorientation of the head relative to gravity. Otolith-borne head angular velocity signals contribute to the VOR during both constant-velocity rotations and very-low-frequency sinusoidal oscillations (692,693).

The macula of the utricle (Fig. 17.40) lies in the horizontal plane and is positioned to sense fore-and-aft and lateral head translations, or tilts of the head around its naso-occipital roll axis. The macula of the saccule is orientated vertically to sense up-and-down and fore-and-aft translations, as well as tilts of the head. The otolith receptors of both the saccule and utricle (Fig. 17.40) can probably respond to translations or tilts in all directions (694), but the saccules are thought to detect predominantly accelerations along the gravity vector, and otolith-induced vertical eye movements during vertical linear accelerations are attributed to the saccules.

Otolith-ocular reflexes also operate during constant-velocity head rotation when the axis of rotation is directed off-vertical, against the pull of gravity, in contrast to the canal-mediated angular VOR, which fades away. In lateral-eyed animals like rabbits the otolithic VOR supplements the poor low-frequency response of the angular VOR. Otolith-ocular reflexes modulate the angular VOR when the head assumes different positions in the gravitational field.

During roll of the head, the eyes undergo torsion in the opposite direction, representing dynamic counter-roll, which is mediated by the vertical semicircular canals. The dynamic counter-roll is counteracted by torsional quick phases in the same direction as the head roll. If the head is kept tilted after it rolls, there is a residual static counter-roll of about 10%–25% of the amplitude of the head roll. Static counter-roll is an utricular otolith reflex to the pull of gravity; this static reflex response is so small that the upper and lower poles of the eyes appear to be nearly aligned with the sagittal plane of the head in any position of head roll (695).

Experimental stimulation of the utricular nerve in the cat produces elevation of the ipsilateral eye, depression of the contralateral eye, and torsion of both eyes, with their upper poles rolling contralaterally (696,697). A similar reaction occurs with stimulation of the INC of monkeys, but the lower eye is on the side of INC stimulation and the head tilts and the eyes roll toward the side of stimulation (698). This triad of binocular torsion, head tilt, and vertical strabismus is called the ocular tilt reaction. It has been attributed to a central imbalance of utricular input to the INC and finally to the oculomotor and trochlear nuclei (699,700). Evidence from lesions in patients indicates that excitatory projections from one utricle to the ipsilateral vestibular nuclei decussate in the tegmentum of the mid-pons while ascending to the contralateral INC (701,702).

In animals with laterally placed eyes, rolling the head about the naso-occipital axis results in disjunctive vertical rather than conjugate torsional eye movements: when the animal's head rolls to the right, the right eye goes up and the left eye down, maintaining alignment of the eyes with the earth's horizontal meridian (703). The vertical divergence occurring during roll is stimulated by the vertical semicircular canals and the maintained position is mediated by the otoliths. The vertical divergence of the ocular tilt reaction in humans and animals with frontally placed eyes is a skew deviation. In humans, clockwise head rotation (from the subject's reference—toward the right shoulder) is accompanied by counter-rolling, combined with slight upward movement of the right eye and downward movement of the left eye in the orbits. This reflexive vertical divergence of the optical axes is compensatory to downward translation of the right eye and upward translation of the left eye relative to the earth-horizontal plane, due to the head roll (704). Counterclockwise head roll (from the subject's reference—toward the left shoulder) causes torsion with vertical translation of the eyes, in the opposite directions to clockwise head roll. The reflex causes the intorting eye to move upward and the extorting eye to move downward, compensating for opposed vertical translation of the eyes. The magnitude of vertical divergence is about 5° for head roll at 0.4 Hz. This physiologic dynamic skew deviation in humans is attributed to activation of the vertical semicircular canals (705,706).

Central otolith-ocular projections are less well known than those concerned with the angular VOR. Horizontal utricular evoked responses are brought about by excitatory projections to the ipsilateral abducens nucleus neurons and internuclear neurons to the opposite medial rectus subnucleus (Fig. 17.41). These effects are opposite in direction to the

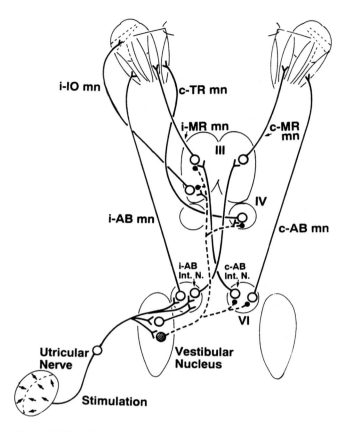

Figure 17.41. Connections from the utricle to extraocular muscles in the cat. AB, abducens; IO, inferior oblique; TR trochlear; MR, medial rectus; i, ipsilateral to stimulation; c, contralateral. *Solid lines* indicate short-latency circuits and *dashed lines* indicate long-latency circuits. *Lines ending in open angles* show excitatory projection and *lines ending in filled circles* show inhibitory projection. The hatched cell body denotes populations of excitatory or inhibitory neurons, as depicted by their terminations. (From Uchino Y, Sasaki M, Sato H, et al. Utriculoocular reflex arc of the cat. J Neurophysiol 1996;76:1896–1903.)

effects of stimulating the nerve from the horizontal semicircular canal. Polysynaptic pathways from the utricle in cats excite contralateral trochlear motoneurons to contract the ipsilateral superior oblique muscle, and they inhibit ipsilateral inferior oblique motoneurons (697). Stimulating different parts of the utricular macula evokes upward, downward, or lateral eye movements (694,707). As mentioned above, stimulation of one utricular nerve results in vertical ocular divergence and contralateral ocular torsion (696); the ipsilateral eye deviates up, the contralateral eye deviates down, and the upper poles of both eyes rotate to the opposite side. Saccular nerve stimulation excites or inhibits superior rectus, inferior rectus, superior oblique, and inferior oblique motoneurons at polysynaptic latencies but does not influence lateral or medial rectus motoneurons (708). Saccular innervation to motoneurons with vertical and torsional actions is indirect, through the lateral vestibular nucleus and the y-group of the vestibular nuclei (709).The y-group comprises small clusters of dorsolateral accessory vestibular nuclei located dorsal to the restiform body (inferior cerebellar peduncle) and ventral to the dentate nucleus. They participate in the generation of vertical smooth eye movements (576,710).

Angular VOR

Three neuron arcs underlie each semicircular canal extraocular muscle reflex (Fig. 17.42). Central connections of the angular VOR pathways follow three general features:

1. Each semicircular canal activates two extraocular muscles in its own plane, one muscle in each eye.
2. Excitatory projections are contralateral, whereas inhibitory projections are ipsilateral. This inhibition is achieved by inhibitory postsynaptic potentials on motoneurons. Disfacilitation of the paired reciprocal canal in the opposite labyrinth also achieves inhibition. The right anterior canal is reciprocally paired with the left posterior canal, the right posterior canal with the left anterior canal, and the right lateral canal with the left lateral canal (Fig. 17.40). For example, when the head rotates in yaw to the right side, the ampullary nerve of the right lateral canal is excited and the ampullary nerve of the left lateral canal is disfacilitated.
3. Anterior canal projections are partly conveyed to vertically acting motoneurons through the cerebellum via the brachium conjunctivum (superior cerebellar peduncle),

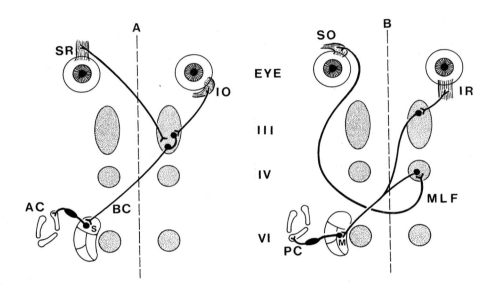

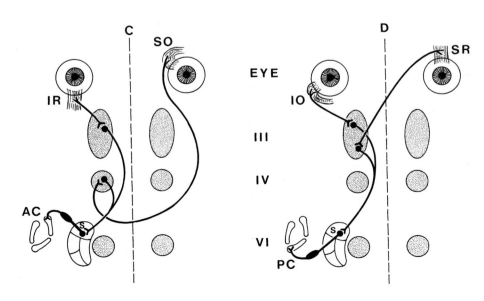

Figure 17.42. Direct vertical vestibulo-ocular projections from the vertical semicircular canals. *A* and *B*, Excitatory connections. *C* and *D*, Inhibitory connections. *A*, Excitatory afferents from the anterior semicircular canals (AC) synapse in the superior vestibular nucleus (S), and their signals are relayed via the brachium conjunctivum (BC) to ocular motor subnuclei that drive the ipsilateral superior rectus (SR) and contralateral inferior oblique (IO) muscles. *B*, Excitatory afferents from the posterior semicircular canals (PC) synapse in the medial vestibular nucleus (M), and their signals are relayed via the contralateral medial longitudinal fasciculus (MLF) to the ocular motor subnuclei that drive the ipsilateral superior oblique (SO) and contralateral inferior rectus (IR) muscles. *C*, Inhibitory afferents from the anterior semicircular canals. *D*, Inhibitory afferents from the posterior semicircular canals. (Redrawn from Ghelarducci B, Highstein SM, Ito M. In: Baker R, Berthoz A, eds. Control of Gaze by Brain Stem Neurons. New York: Elsevier/North-Holland, 1977:167–175.)

whereas posterior and horizontal canal projections ascend in the brain stem tegmentum to motoneurons.

HORIZONTAL ANGULAR VOR

Stimulation of a horizontal canal by ipsilateral head acceleration results in the deviation of both eyes away from the side of the canal. The semicircular canals on each side work in a reciprocal push–pull fashion. When the head rotates to the right, the right horizontal canal's ampullary nerve is stimulated by deflection of its cupula and the left horizontal canal's nerve is disfacilitated by deflection of its cupula. The horizontal VOR is served by a direct excitatory projection from the horizontal (lateral) semicircular canal to the medial vestibular nucleus that synapses on second-order PVP neurons. A direct excitatory pathway from PVP cells of the horizontal VOR projects to the contralateral abducens nucleus (Fig. 17.43). As described above, the contralateral abducens nucleus contains both motoneurons to the lateral rectus muscle and internuclear neurons that project in the contralateral MLF to medial rectus motor neurons (711). These abducens nucleus internuclear neurons are thought to be the most important VOR pathway to the medial rectus muscle and constitute the third neuron in a four-neuron reflex; they also transmit saccadic and pursuit eye movement signals to medial rectus motoneurons (577,578). Another pathway of PVP cell axons passes through the ipsilateral abducens nucleus without synapse and ascends to the ipsilateral medial rectus subnucleus through the ascending tract of Deiters, which lies just lateral to the MLF (711–714) (Fig. 17.43). These simple reflex arcs consisting of three or four neurons are called the direct VOR (Figs. 17.42 and 17.43). The direct VOR transmits head velocity commands from the vestibular nerve to the ocular motoneurons to ensure that eye velocity matches head velocity.

The indirect VOR refers to processed signals of head velocity that have undergone alteration by adaptation, or velocity storage, or integration to eye position commands. These processes are reviewed below. In monkeys, head velocity signals, which represent the eye velocity commands of the direct pathway, and eye position signals of the indirect pathway share PVP cells in the vestibular nucleus and their axons in the MLF (577,578). The terms indirect and direct VOR denote physiologic operations that have both distinct and shared anatomic circuits between second-order vestibular neurons and ocular motoneurons.

VERTICAL AND TORSIONAL ANGULAR VOR

The ampullary nerve from the anterior semicircular canal on one side excites the ipsilateral superior rectus muscle and the contralateral inferior oblique muscle, resulting in elevation and contralateral torsion of both eyes. The ampullary nerve from one posterior canal excites the ipsilateral superior oblique muscle and the contralateral inferior rectus muscle (Fig. 17.42); thus, one posterior canal activates depression and contralateral torsion of both eyes, the movement vectors being different in each eye and dependent on the position of the eye in the orbit (715,716). When an anterior canal is stimulated by head acceleration in its plane, the posterior canal in the opposite labyrinth is disfacilitated (inhibited) by that same head acceleration. Stimulation of both anterior canals by downward head acceleration activates the upward angular VOR. Stimulation of both posterior canals by upward head acceleration activates the downward angular VOR (Fig. 17.44). Stimulation of the anterior and posterior canals on one side by ipsilateral head roll activates the torsional angular VOR so that the upper poles of the eyes roll toward the contralateral shoulder.

Axons from the ampullae of the vertical canals on one side synapse in the ipsilateral superior medial and ventrolateral vestibular nuclei (717). Their excitatory projections cross the midline to innervate the contralateral inferior oblique and inferior rectus motoneurons and the ipsilateral superior rectus and superior oblique motoneurons (635,717). The motoneurons innervating those four vertically and torsionally acting muscles are all located on the same side of the brain stem (Fig. 17.42).

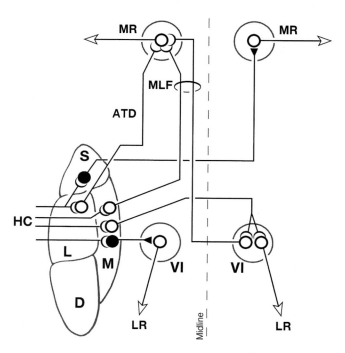

Figure 17.43. The direct horizontal VOR pathway from horizontal semicircular canal (HC) to medial rectus (MR) subnucleus of the oculomotor nucleus and to the abducens nucleus (VI). Excitatory second-order vestibular neurons project to the MR through the medial longitudinal fasciculus (MLF) and the ascending tract of Deiters (ATD). Axons of the ATD actually course through the abducens nucleus without synapse (not shown). The abducens nucleus contains motoneurons of the lateral rectus muscle (LR) and internuclear neurons that project through the opposite MLF to the MR subnucleus. *Open symbols* indicate excitatory neurons and *filled symbols* indicate inhibitory neurons. Inhibition of internuclear neurons in the ipsilateral abducens nucleus is not illustrated. S, superior; L, lateral; M, medial; and D, descending vestibular nuclei. LR, lateral rectus muscles. (From Sharpe JA, Johnston JL. The vestibulo-ocular reflex: clinical, anatomic and physiologic correlates. In: Sharpe JA, Barber HO, eds. The Vestibulo-ocular Reflex and Vertigo. New York: Raven, 1993:15–39.)

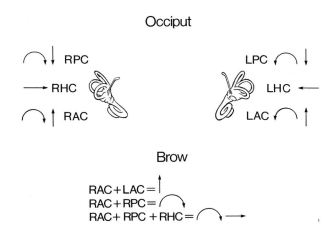

Occiput

RPC   LPC

RHC   LHC

RAC   LAC

Brow

RAC+LAC =
RAC+RPC =
RAC+ RPC + RHC =

Figure 17.44. Summary of the ocular motor effects of stimulating individual semicircular canals and combinations of canals. Stimulation of the right posterior canal (RPC) produces depression of both eyes, combined with intorsion of the right eye and extorsion of the left eye. Stimulation of the right horizontal canal (RHC) produces leftward movement of both eyes. Stimulation of the right anterior canal (RAC) produces elevation of both eyes, combined with intorsion of the right eye and extorsion of the left eye. Similar ocular changes occur with stimulation of the left semicircular canals (LPC, left posterior canal; LHC, left horizontal canal; LAC, left anterior canal). When the right and left anterior canals are stimulated simultaneously, intorsion of the right eye and extorsion of the left eye produced by stimulation of the right anterior canal are counteracted by extorsion of the right eye and intorsion of the left eye produced by stimulation of the left anterior canal. With all torsional movements neutralized, the only observed eye movement is elevation of both eyes. Similarly, stimulation of the right anterior and posterior canals produces only torsional eye movements. (Redrawn from Leigh RJ, Zee DS. The Neurology of Eye Movement. Philadelphia: FA Davis, 1991.)

Anterior canal excitation is relayed through second-order neurons of the vestibular nucleus through the brachium conjunctivum, the MLF (Fig. 17.42), and a ventral tegmental pathway (not shown in Fig. 17.42) to the contralateral inferior oblique and superior rectus motoneurons (579,718,719). Reciprocal inhibition of anterior canal signals is transmitted by superior vestibular nucleus neurons that ascend in the ipsilateral reticular formation and MLF to the ipsilateral trochlear nucleus and inferior rectus subnucleus (720,721). Posterior canal excitatory signals are transmitted by neurons in the rostral part of the medial vestibular nucleus through the contralateral MLF to the trochlear nucleus and inferior rectus subnucleus (722). The trochlear nucleus innervates the superior oblique muscle of the opposite eye and the inferior rectus subnucleus innervates the ipsilateral eye. Thus, one posterior canal activates the superior oblique muscle of the ipsilateral eye and the inferior rectus muscle of the contralateral eye. Reciprocal inhibition to antagonist muscles is conveyed by the superior and rostral part of the medial vestibular nucleus via the ipsilateral reticular formation and MLF to the ipsilateral superior rectus and inferior oblique subnuclei (718,721,723). The ipsilateral superior rectus subnucleus innervates the contralateral superior rectus muscle, as described above.

The y-group of accessory vestibular nuclei participates in the generation of vertical smooth eye movements (579,724). The y-nuclei receive input from second-order neurons in the superior and medial vestibular nuclei that receive primary afferents from the anterior and posterior canals (724). The flocculus (562) and the posterior part of cerebral cortical areas 7 or caudal part of the superior bank of superior temporal sulcus (725) also project to the y-group. It projects to the oculomotor nucleus (726,727). Neurons with activity related to vertical head velocity and eye velocity are recorded in the y-group, indicating its role in vertical gaze. It sends excitatory projections to superior rectus and inferior oblique motoneurons (576,710). The y-group cells are activated during visual following and during suppression of the VOR (produced by rotation of the head and an optokinetic drum in the same direction). Their response is in phase with eye velocity during visual following and in phase with head velocity during suppression of the VOR. However, during the VOR in darkness, y-cells exhibit only slight modulation, suggesting that visual following and vestibular signals on y-cells are mainly involved in vertical visual–vestibular interaction (710). The flocculus plays a role in the eye velocity-to-position integrator of the vertical VOR (252).

Velocity to Position Integration and the VOR

Ocular motoneurons discharge at rates in proportion to eye position and to eye velocity. The signals carried by primary vestibular afferents encode head velocity and provide an eye velocity command to motor neurons to move the eyes at an appropriate speed and overcome orbital viscous forces. To maintain eccentric eye position against the elastic restoring forces in eye muscles that cause the eyes to drift toward the orbital midposition, a tonic level of muscle firing is achieved by an eye position command to motoneurons. The same neural network within the brain stem that we discussed in the section on the saccadic system also integrates, in the mathematical sense, eye velocity signals for the VOR to create eye position commands and transforms the vestibular velocity information into the appropriate tonic firing rate (131,263). Velocity-to-position integration also regulates the phase of the VOR. Defective integration creates a phase lead of the eyes before the head. A neural integrator is also required to generate position-coded information for other conjugate eye movement systems, pursuit and optokinetic, and all of these systems share a common integrator. Thus, an eye position command is created from, and added to, an eye velocity command for delivery to motoneurons. The neural integrator for horizontal eye movements is located in the MVN and the NPH, which lies just medial to it (255,256). The neural integrator for vertical and torsional eye movements is located in the INC of the rostral midbrain and the vestibular nucleus (251–254).

Commissures between these neural integrator structures on each side of the brain stem are important in transforming velocity to position commands for horizontal and vertical movements. Neural integration for horizontal eye motion may be brought about by inhibitory connections between the MVN and NPH on each side of the brain stem that pass through the vestibular commissure (728). MVN neurons that project to the contralateral abducens nucleus give collateral axons to the contralateral MVN and NPH. Mutual inhibition creates positive feedback loops that allow MVN and NPH neurons to perseverate (integrate) eye velocity commands, thereby creating eye position commands. Transection of the vestibular commissure at the level of the abducens nuclei damages the horizontal velocity to position integrator while preserving the peak velocity response of the VOR (729). For vertical eye movements, INC neurons projecting to the oculomotor nucleus and trochlear nuclei pass through the posterior commissure (730). Small lesions in the posterior commissure of monkeys cause defective eccentric gaze holding, decrease the low-frequency vertical VOR gain, and cause a phase lead in the vertical VOR—all being effects of damage to the velocity-to-position integrator of vertical eye motion (247).

Cells in the paramedian tracts in the midline of the pontine and medullary tegmentum also participate in vertical eye movements (731,732). They receive projections from the INC (730), and anterior semicircular canals, after synaptic relay from the vestibular nucleus (717,732). The pontine paramedian tract cells lie within the MLF and dorsal to the omnipause neurons of the rip. Their neurons discharge as burst-tonic units with activity related to vertical eye position (732). Their efferents project along the midline, then pass laterally to follow the ventral external arcuate fibers around the surface of the medulla into the restiform body (731) to terminate in the flocculus and ventral paraflocculus. In cats, lesions of paramedian tract cells, just rostral to the level of the abducens nucleus, cause gaze-evoked vertical nystagmus and primary position upbeat nystagmus with decelerating slow phases (732), indicating their role in eye velocity-to-position integration.

Velocity Storage for the VOR

Central vestibular mechanisms perform another operation on the peripheral vestibular signal. They extend the range of performance (bandwidth) over which the VOR reliably signals head velocity to ocular motoneurons. This process, called velocity storage, is used by the VOR to make it effective during low-frequency head motion (733–735). The semicircular canals are effective at transferring higher-frequency head motion so that eye velocities match head velocity, but they are ineffective at very low head frequencies, below about 0.02 Hz, and the vestibular response dies away after constant-velocity rotation for several seconds (Fig. 17.23). For example, during constant-velocity head motion, the cupula gradually returns toward the neutral position with a time constant of about 5–7 seconds, and the firing rate of first-order vestibular neurons, which varies as the angle of deviation of the cupula, incorrectly informs the brain that the head is moving at progressively lower velocities. Velocity storage boosts the time constant to about 20 seconds.

Velocity storage is responsible for postrotatory nystagmus, which appears after prolonged rotation stops (736) (Fig. 17.45). The postrotatory nystagmus reflects the discharge of velocity storage. During a constant-velocity rotation, after

the original nystagmus dies out, a reversal phase of nystagmus may develop with slow phases in the opposite direction—that is, in the same direction as head rotation (Fig. 17.23). Visual fixation normally stops postrotatory vestibular nystagmus by shortening the time constant of velocity storage, a process called dumping. The vestibular signal is dumped when it conflicts with visual information from the retina, or with gravitational information from the utricles. Tilting of the head laterally or in pitch attenuates postrotatory nystagmus by activating otolithic receptors, which are responsible for dumping velocity storage. The nodulus (Fig. 17.31) and uvula (Fig. 17.32) are necessary for dumping by head tilts, since stimulation of this part of the cerebellum reduces the time constant of horizontal postrotatory nystagmus (737) and ablation of it prevents dumping (738). Nodular lesions in monkeys cause periodic alternating nystagmus in darkness by increasing the activity within the velocity storage mechanism (738). Patients with posterior vermis lesions involving the nodulus and uvula cannot decrease the vestibular response from the semicircular canals when the head is tilted (739).

The velocity storage mechanism is located in the superior and medial vestibular nuclei (255,740). The transformed vestibular signal is reflected in the discharge of secondary vestibular neurons within the vestibular nuclei, since they show a time constant of decay that is comparable to the behaviorally measured nystagmus response, not to the signals carried on primary vestibular afferents (741). The velocity storage mechanism uses the peripheral labyrinthine signal, and by the process of integration, in the mathematical sense, increases the response duration of the VOR three-fold—that is, the time constant of decay of vestibular nystagmus is prolonged to about 20 seconds, three times longer than the signal actually delivered from the semicircular canals. This velocity storage integrator is used by both the vestibulo-ocular and the optokinetic systems. The otolith-ocular reflexes described earlier are also important in charging the velocity storage mechanism of the canal-based reflex, in all planes (742). The velocity storage integrator is distinctive from the velocity-to-position integrator that each eye movement system employs to transform eye velocity commands to position commands.

Microstimulation in parts of the superior and medial vestibular nuclei, but not the NPH, of monkeys induces nystagmus with characteristics that indicate activation of velocity storage (740). Midsagittal section of the medulla caudal to the level of the abducens nuclei abolishes velocity storage in monkeys (743). The time constant of the horizontal and vertical VOR is reduced to that of the semicircular canal signal conveyed to the vestibular nuclei. The storage mechanism appears to depend on crossing commissural fibers between the MVN on each side. Commissural section does not alter the gain of the reflex (the ratio of eye velocity to head velocity) or its adaptation to visual input induced by magnifying or reducing lenses (discussed later). The velocity-to-position integrator is not altered, since saccades and eccentric gaze holding remain intact (743). Midline lesions of the rostral medulla may abolish velocity storage by disrupting

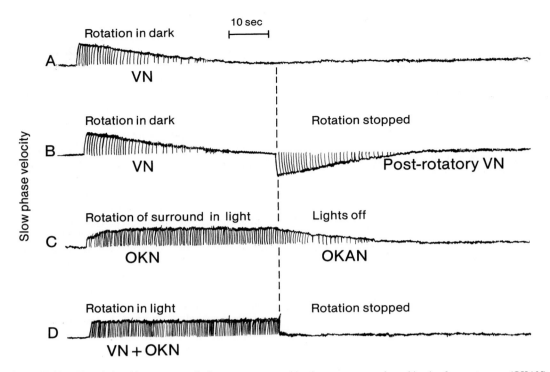

Figure 17.45. The relationship among vestibular nystagmus, optokinetic nystagmus, and optokinetic after-nystagmus (OKAN) in the rhesus monkey. *A,* When the animal is rotated in the dark at 60°/sec, vestibular nystagmus (VN) occurs that dies away over about 60 seconds as the cupula returns to its original position. *B,* If, after vestibular nystagmus has died away, rotation is suddenly stopped, a postrotatory vestibular nystagmus (postrotatory VN) begins with slow phases in the opposite direction. *C,* When the surround is rotated around the monkey while it is immobile and the lights are on, optokinetic nystagmus (OKN) develops. Note the rapid onset of slow phases (rapid-rise OKN) followed by a slow-rise in OKN slow-phase velocity over about 10 seconds to a steady maximum velocity. The combination of rapid and slow rise is typical of primates. In humans the rapid rise in the slow-phase velocity of OKN obscures the slow rise that is evident in animals, and humans exhibit only rapid-rise OKN. If the lights are suddenly turned off, the nystagmus does not stop immediately but gradually fades away as OKAN. *D,* When the monkey is rotated in light, the nystagmus is a sum of VN and OKN. The summed slow-phase velocities rapidly attain a maximum that prevents slippage of retinal images, and the nystagmus does not fade away as it does with vestibular stimulation alone (*A*). For the first 40–60 seconds, a combination of VN and OKN prevents retinal image slip. Then OKN sustains retinal image stability after VN has decayed. When the rotation is suddenly stopped, the postrotatory VN is balanced by OKAN in the opposite direction, and no nystagmus occurs. The upward or downward spikes in each recording are nystagmus quick-phase velocities. (Redrawn from Cohen B, Matsuo V, Raphan T. J Physiol [Lond] 1977;270:321–344.)

crossing axons of type I secondary vestibular neurons from the MVN (which are excited by ipsilateral head motion) or crossing axons of type II secondary vestibular neurons (which are inhibited by ipsilateral head motion) (743). As noted above, section of the vestibular commissure in the caudal pons between the abducens nuclei damages the velocity-to-position integrator for horizontal motion; this more rostral damage to commissure fibers also impairs velocity storage (729).

Visual–Vestibular Interaction and Voluntary Control of the VOR

VISUAL ENHANCEMENT OF THE VOR

In darkness the VOR functions suboptimally, with a gain below 1 during passive head movement at frequencies below 1 Hz. However, during self-generated active head movement in darkness, VOR gain is near unity at frequencies from 0.25–2 Hz (437). Enhancement by preprogrammed eye movements can account for higher VOR gain during active head motion in darkness, and an efference copy of head motor commands contributes to the higher gains of compensatory smooth eye movements. When a target is viewed, vision enhances VOR gain to unity, providing stability of retinal images even at lower frequencies (744,745). This visually enhanced VOR is sometimes abbreviated as the VVOR. As head velocity increases, the velocity of opposed smooth eye movements increases to keep retinal image speed below 5°–6°/sec to maintain high visual acuity (746).

Visual enhancement is a function of the optokinetic system at very low frequencies, and at usual frequencies, below 1 to 2 Hz, smooth pursuit is considered to be responsible for gain enhancement. Nonetheless, when the head starts to move, visual enhancement of vestibular smooth eye movement speed can occur within the latent period before initiation of smooth pursuit or optokinetic tracking (652,747). Furthermore, small oscillations of eye velocity that occur during smooth pursuit (called ringing) do not occur during the VVOR (653), and enhancement occurs at head movement frequencies as high as 2.8 Hz (746) where pursuit is limited or absent. Another mechanism, perhaps the fixation system, may also enhance the VOR (652,653).

VISUAL CANCELLATION OF THE VOR

During smooth tracking of an object that moves in the same direction as the head, the VOR must be canceled; otherwise the VOR would move the eyes opposite to the direction of intended gaze. Cancellation can be achieved by the smooth pursuit system. Visual cancellation shares properties with smooth pursuit and smooth pursuit is sufficient to cancel the VOR. However, other mechanisms are also available to cancel the VOR during passive and head movement and during active eye-head tracking. Some patients show impaired cancellation and spared smooth pursuit, or vice versa (580,745,748,749). Readers may consult our previous discussion (663) of mechanisms of VOR cancellation and the roles of fixation and pursuit for further information.

VOLUNTARY ENHANCEMENT AND CANCELLATION OF THE VOR

In addition to visual-vestibular interactions described above, the VOR can be partially enhanced or canceled by voluntary, nonvisual, mechanisms. Normal individuals can voluntarily change the gain of the VOR when they attempt to fixate imaginary targets during rotation in darkness (687,750). Fixation of an imaginary stationary target increases the gain, while fixation of an imaginary target moving with the head decreases the gain. Voluntary control of the reflex is less robust than visual control.

The cerebral hemispheres exert some governance of the VOR since VOR imbalance in darkness occurs in patients with focal cerebral lesions (751) and in monkeys and humans after hemidecortication (482,752,753). Unilateral ablation of area 7 in the posterior parietal cortex in monkeys causes imbalance of the VOR for 2–4 weeks; ipsiversive VOR gain is decreased (754). Area 7 or the caudal end of the superior bank of the superior temporal sulcus projects to the MVN and NPH and the y-group of vestibular nuclei (725). The human cerebrum is crucial for smooth pursuit and optokinetic responses that modify the VOR during visual vestibular interactions. Cerebral hemidecortication impairs ipsiversive smooth pursuit, voluntary and visual enhancement of the ipsiversive VOR, and voluntary and visual cancellation of the contraversive VOR (482).

Motor Learning and Memory: Adaptive Plasticity in the VOR

Adaptive changes in the VOR occur in response to certain visual stimuli. The VOR is a feed-forward, open-loop control system. In other words, the labyrinthine receptors, which provide the input of the reflex, receive no information about eye movements, the output of the reflex. Visual feedback could guide smooth eye movements with a latency of about 100 msec but that is too long and visual following responses are too slow to maintain image stability at the speed of most head movements. In contrast, other eye movement systems are closed-loop, negative-feedback systems; that is, the retinal receptors receive feedback about eye motion and change the input to the system. In the absence of rapid feedback, the VOR must undergo continuous calibration by short-term and long-term adaptations to correct any errors induced by visual or vestibular changes. Those errors are sensed by vision and the visual input recalibrates the VOR by a process of motor learning.

For example, wearing magnifying glasses causes the angular VOR gain and the translational VOR sensitivity to increase (755–758). The retinal image slip caused by magnifying or miniaturizing spectacles increases or decreases the amplitude of the eye movement relative to the amplitude of the head movement. This recalibration has a course of many hours but starts within 15 minutes (756). A nearsighted person who consistently wears minus lenses in glasses for myopia has a lower VOR gain (in light and when measured in darkness) than an emmetropic person, and a farsighted (hyperopic) person who wears plus lenses has a higher gain (759). Individuals who wear contact lenses have no changes in gain since there is no rotational magnification or reduction of retinal image displacement. Both visual and vestibular inputs are necessary for motor learning. The VOR does not recalibrate during head turns in the dark or during retinal image motion with the head stationary. The adapted changes are retained if either visual or vestibular input is withheld. This is memory in the VOR. In the early stages of adaptation, the VOR changes that develop may be rapidly reversed in the absence of continuous visual stimulation; however, the changes that occur after 1 or 2 weeks of altered visual input persist for some time in the absence of vestibular activity or continued visual stimulation (760). These more persistent changes are called plastic and are considered important in the repair of altered visual input to the VOR or damage to the reflex arc by ageing or disease.

Normal human subjects who wear reversing prisms see a laterally inverted world, right to left, and head turns cause the observed environment to move in the same direction as the head turn itself. In such individuals, adaptive changes in the VOR apparently occur almost immediately after they begin to wear the prisms. After only 1 hour of wearing vision-reversal prisms, normal individuals have a 50% adaptation of gain (761). VOR phase also shifts, and after wearing such prisms for 1 or 2 weeks, they actually reverse their VOR. Head rotations are associated with smooth eye movements in the same direction (760,762,763). Thus, the gain and phase of the VOR are altered to stabilize images on the retina during head movements. Even the relationship between the axis of head rotation and the axis of compensatory eye movements can be changed by coupling retinal image motion in one plane to head rotation in another (764). The three pairs of semicircular canals are not perfectly aligned with the pulling directions of the six extraocular muscles. Therefore, for head movement in one plane, the VOR depends upon central neural mechanisms that couple the canals to the muscles with the appropriate gains to generate a response that rotates each around the correct axis. A consequence of these neural connections is a cross-axis adaptive capability when head rotation is around one axis and visual motion or eye movement responses are about another axis (764). Monocular VOR adaptation occurs in three dimensions in response to unilateral peripheral ocular motor nerve palsies. The gain of the antagonists of weak muscles is adjusted to make the VOR of the affected eye symmetrical in the directions of action of the weak and intact muscles (8) (765–767). Asymmetrical retinal slip drives the adaptation to the palsy.

An indirect VOR pathway mediates motor learning and memory in the VOR in response to retinal slip. The cerebellum is a crucial structure for motor learning (394,768). The ventral paraflocculus (Fig. 17.31) appears to be most important in motor learning, since lesions of the ventral paraflocculus alone degrade VOR adaptation, as well as smooth pursuit and visual cancellation of the VOR in monkeys (546). The floccular complex probably uses visual input, from mossy fibers, to detect retinal image slip, and then its gaze velocity Purkinje cells relay that information to the vestibular nucleus (769). Inactivation of the flocculus in cats by stimulating climbing fibers from the olivary nucleus prevents optically induced changes in VOR gain (770), but it does not change previously adapted changes in gain. However, damage to the flocculus of monkeys reverses VOR adaptation (771,772). The sites of learning and memory must be at points of convergence of visual and vestibular inputs, where visual–vestibular mismatch, in the form of retinal image slip, can recalibrate the VOR. This convergence occurs in the flocculus and ventral paraflocculus and in the vestibular nucleus, which actually serves as the deep cerebellar nucleus for the flocculus

Two sites of motor learning and memory in the VOR are probable: one in the brain stem at vestibular afferent synapses onto FTNs in the medial vestibular nucleus or in the membranes of FTNs themselves; the other in the cerebellum at gaze velocity Purkinje cells of the flocculus and paraflocculus (546), which receive both visual information and vestibular information (773) (Fig. 17.46). FTNs are inhibited by gaze velocity Purkinje cells and receive excitatory input from first- or second-order vestibular neurons (560). Differences between vestibular nerve and floccular inputs to FTNs could cause them to increase or decrease the modifiable VOR gain (Fig. 17.46) (773). In addition to modifying their head velocity sensitivity during VOR adaptation, Purkinje cells in the flocculus change their eye velocity sensitivity and eye position sensitivity to effect modification in the neural integrator of the indirect VOR pathway (774). Adaptation must involve the velocity-to-position integrator so that smooth eye movements have appropriate gain and phase at both low and high frequencies of head motion (774). Long-term depression at synapses of parallel fibers onto Purkinje cells is one signature of motor learning. Transgenic knockout mice lacking a protein kinase required for long-term depression at Purkinje cells exhibit impaired adaptation of the VOR (775). For a thorough analysis of behavioral, cellular, and molecular mechanisms of VOR learning and memory, readers may consult a review by Broussard and Kassardjian (776).

THE OPTOKINETIC SYSTEM

Characteristics of Optokinetic Movements

The optokinetic system is the helpmate of the angular VOR. Optokinetic smooth eye movements are necessary to sustain compensatory eye speed at the same speed as the head during prolonged rotations, after the VOR fades away (Fig. 17.45A). It has been emphasized above that the angular VOR responds best to brief, high-frequency changes in head position. During a constant-velocity head rotation in darkness, the cupula returns to its normal position and the compensatory eye movements that are stimulated by the VOR cease. During rotation in the light, therefore, there must be a backup optokinetic mechanism to ensure adequate image

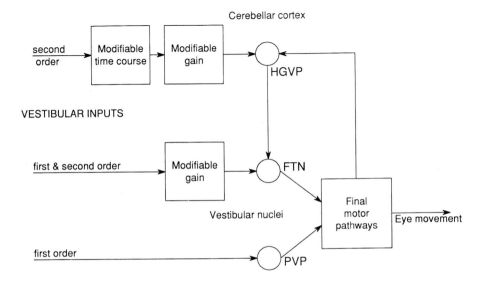

Figure 17.46. Hypothesis for motor learning in the VOR. *Circles* indicate sites of signal convergence (summing junctions). Horizontal gaze velocity Purkinje (HGVP) neurons in the flocculus inhibit floccular target neurons (FTN) in the vestibular nucleus. Position-vestibular-pause neurons (PVP) transmit the direct unmodifiable VOR. A positive feedback loop from HVP to FTN to final motor pathways sustains memory. *Large boxes* indicate other transformations. (From Lisberger SG. Neural basis for motor learning in the vestibuloocular reflex of primates. III. Computation and behavioral analysis of the sites of learning. J Neurophysiol 1994;72:974–998.)

stabilization during very-low-frequency head motion. The optokinetic system aids the VOR to keep the eyes still in space during low-frequency head motion by moving them at the same speed as the head. The optokinetic image stabilizing system also uses the vestibular nuclei to generate slow phases of nystagmus. Smooth pursuit is induced with both voluntary assent and sensory stimulation by small objects whose images are guided to the foveal or parafoveal retina, but optokinetic slow phases are induced reflexively by large scenes that stimulate large areas of the retina.

In the rather artificial situation when a normal human subject sits with the head still inside a large, patterned, revolving drum that fills the visual field, the optokinetic system generates smooth eye movements to reduce slip of the retinal images; the slow smooth eye movements are opposed by fast eye movements creating a nystagmus, the slow phases of which are in the direction of the revolving drum. This is optokinetic nystagmus (OKN). Full-field image motion also causes an illusionary sensation of self-rotation (called circularvection) in the direction opposite to the drum rotation. When the lights are turned off, there is also an optokinetic after-nystagmus (OKAN) that has the same direction as the prior OKN (Fig. 17.45C). Thus, during the more natural situation—rotation of the head in the light—OKN can supplant the fading vestibular responses by producing compensatory eye movements that have been stimulated by retinal signals rather than labyrinthine signals. When head rotation ceases, OKAN acts to nullify the inappropriate postrotatory vestibular nystagmus that would be expected to occur from the change in angular head velocity to zero (Fig. 17.45D). Thus, OKN and OKAN help ensure clear, stable vision and an appropriate perception of motion both during and after head rotation. OKAN and the opposed postrotatory nystagmus are both produced by the velocity storage mechanism (734) discussed previously.

Smooth pursuit and OKN are often activated simultaneously in naturally occurring situations. Nevertheless, antagonistic stimulations of pursuit and OKN occur during pursuit of a small object against a stationary visual scene. A stationary background or a background moving in the same direction as a horizontally moving target improves pursuit. In contrast, a background moving in the direction opposite to that of the target impairs pursuit, and pursuit suppresses optokinetic following (777–779). Smooth pursuit may have evolved, in part, to suppress reflexive optokinetic following. The optokinetic system is sensitive to relative depth cues such as motion parallax and disparity, which segregate an object of regard from other elements in the scene. Complex optic flow patterns (e.g., those experienced by the moving observer who looks a little off to one side of his direction of heading) are dealt with by the smooth pursuit system, which spatially filters visual motion inputs so as to exclude all but the motion of the object of interest (779).

Speed limitations of OKN slow phases are similar to those of smooth pursuit; both have smooth eye speeds that peak at 80°–90°/sec (434,780). OKN responses are divided into two classes based on their time courses:

1. *Slow-rise OKN* causes a gradual initial increase of smooth eye movement speed (Fig. 17.45C) and a slow decrease

of speed beginning when the visual scene disappears; this gradual fall produces OKAN and is recorded only in darkness. The slow rise of OKN slow-phase velocity accompanies charging of the same velocity storage mechanism used by the VOR. OKAN accompanies discharging of velocity storage.

2. *Rapid-rise OKN* causes a quick initial jump in smooth eye movement speed at target onset and a proportionate, quick drop in speed at target offset. The rapid rise in slow-phase eye speed might be produced by smooth pursuit, not by the optokinetic system.

Since foveate animals also have the smooth pursuit system for visually tracking a small moving object, the ocular motor response elicited in such animals by larger stimuli probably reflects a combination of pursuit and optokinetic tracking. The rapid-rise component occludes the slow-rise component in normal humans. Small handheld drums or tapes that are used in clinics to test OKN do not elicit the illusion of circularvection, and OKAN does not follow the nystagmus elicited by small OKN stimuli; this OKN is generated by the smooth pursuit and optokinetic systems, but activation of genuine OKN is ensured by the illusion of circularvection and the presence of OKAN in darkness, as achieved by full visual field stimulation.

Afoveate animals like rabbits have only slow-rise OKN. Their responses are symmetrical to the right and left during binocular viewing, but monocular stimulation in these animals produces asymmetric OKN; slow phases are faster for targets moving in the temporal-to-nasal direction than those moving in the nasal-to-temporal direction. Healthy human infants (781), patients with central scotomas or amblyopia (782–784), and patients with bilateral, and occasionally unilateral, parieto-occipital lesions (476,785) may show temporal-nasal asymmetries of OKN, when viewing with only one eye. These characteristics of slow-rise OKN that appear in infants and patients with scotomas or cerebral damage indicate that the slow-rise optokinetic system exists in humans. In contrast, humans and animals with both rapid-rise and slow-rise OKN have symmetrical slow phases to monocular OKN (782). The cerebral cortical rapid-rise, presumed smooth pursuit, component of OKN in foveate animals produces equal nasal-to-temporal slow phase responses, canceling out the temporal-to-nasal bias evident during stimulation of one eye in afoveate species.

Monkeys have both rapid-rise and slow-rise components of OKN (Fig. 17.45), but human OKN responses have predominantly rapid-rise responses. Human OKAN is not as prominent as in monkeys or lower animals (735,780,786). OKAN in darkness has been used as a measure of the ''pure'' action of the optokinetic system since it is not obscured by pursuit or ocular following responses to head translation (discussed below). OKN in the torsional plane is not well developed in humans and torsional slow-phase velocities do not exceed 8°/sec (527,787); torsional OKAN is typically absent and if present exhibits only a few beats (527). Human vertical OKN is robust and has a higher slow phase/stimulus gain for upward stimulus movement (138), and vertical OKAN upward slow phases are faster than downward slow phases (788). In humans, smooth pursuit or short latency following responses presumably play an important role in maintaining steady gaze during and after head movement.

The rapid-rise component of OKN might be generated by the smooth pursuit system, since pursuit deficits in monkeys correlate with defective rapid-rise OKN (733) and patients with impaired pursuit from cerebellar (789) or parieto-occipital (470,476) damage can exhibit poor rapid-rise OKN and the emergence of slow buildup of OKN slow-phase velocities. However, other ocular following responses that are normally activated by head translation may be responsible for the rapid rise in slow-phase velocities (779).

Ocular Following Responses to Head Translation

Just as the optokinetic smooth eye movements supplement the angular VOR during head rotation, another visual following mechanism supplements the translational VOR during head translation. Miles et al. (678,779,790) identified this tracking response and determined that it is distinct from smooth pursuit of a small target and distinct from the optokinetic response to full visual field image motion. It responds best to movement of large objects subtending about 40° of the visual field, and its response is enhanced when the background visual scene moves in the opposite direction. Miles (779) contended that this tracking mechanism is engaged by movement of the observer as he or she views the foreground moving against the distant background.

As an example, consider viewing the world from a moving train, when nearby objects appear to rush by in a blur while the distant scene remains clear. The observer's perception of visual motion is determined by the angular velocity of the object relative to himself or herself and the angular velocity varies inversely with viewing distance; that is, the relative angular velocity is greater for nearby objects than for distant ones. Little tracking is required to stabilize distant objects on the retina, but if the moving observer inspects foreground objects and tracks them, the distant background is swept across the retina. The resulting opposed movement of foreground and background is the optimal stimulus for the ocular following response that stabilizes the foreground images on the retina (779).

This ocular following mechanism has a very short latency of just over 50 msec in monkeys and as low as 70 msec in humans (679,791,792), in contrast to the 100- to 130-msec delay in initiating pursuit of a small target (423,424). Unlike OKN, there is no after-nystagmus subsequent to this ocular following response and therefore no charging of the velocity storage mechanism. Like smooth pursuit but unlike OKN, ocular following responses are sensitive to high-acceleration and high-velocity targets. Miles (779) has proposed that the ocular following mechanism corresponds to the early-rise component of OKN and that it uses the cerebral to pontocerebellar circuit described below. Since it subserves ocular stabilization during translational otolith-ocular responses, it may also share brain stem pathways that convey information from the otolith receptors.

To summarize, the ocular following response is a third mechanism for conjugate ocular tracking. It differs from both the smooth pursuit and slow-rise optokinetic tracking mechanisms. It acts to prevent slippage of retinal images during translation of the head or during movement of large areas of the visual field when the head is still. We regard this ocular following mechanism as an optokinetic subsystem that supplements the otolith-ocular vestibular subsystem.

Neurophysiology of Optokinetic Movements

The optokinetic system has been divided into two functional pathways: an indirect subcortical pathway involving the accessory optic pathway in the brain stem, and a direct transcortical one involving the cerebral hemispheres, cerebellum, and brain stem. The indirect pathway subserves the slow-rise component of OKN and the direct pathway corresponds to the rapid-rise component (733,793). The terms ''direct'' and ''indirect'' are functional designations and do not specify anatomic connections of a direct or indirect nature (793). Indeed, the slow-rise (indirect) OKN pathway is anatomically more ''direct'' than the transcortical rapid-rise (direct) OKN pathway of primates.

Subcortical Optokinetic Pathway

The slow-rise element of OKN in afoveate animals is attributed to subcortical mechanisms. Subcortical OKN pathways may also operate independently of cerebral cortical pathways in nonhuman primates, but in humans cortical pathways overlie and dominate them. Projections from the retina cross in the optic chiasm and project to the contralateral nucleus of the optic tract (NOT) in the midbrain pretectum and mediate the slow-rise component of horizontal OKN in afoveate animals and probably in nonhuman primates (793,794). The lateral terminal nucleus of the AOS receives input from the contralateral retina and participates in vertical OKN in non-primate mammals (793). Although the role of the AOS in vertical OKN of primates is undefined, the simian NOT is a pivotal visual relay in generating horizontal OKN. The NOT projects to the vestibular nuclei, the NPH, and the dorsal cap of the inferior olivary nuclei, which is the major source of climbing fiber input to the flocculus (543,794,795).

Neurons in the vestibular nuclei that respond to head acceleration in one direction also respond to optokinetic stimulation in the opposite direction, but they have little or no eye position sensitivity and do not project directly to ocular motoneurons (794,796). Microstimulation of the primate superior and medial vestibular nuclei, but not the NPH, activates velocity storage for both OKN and the VOR (740). The storage mechanism for OKN requires eighth-nerve input since bilateral labyrinthectomy abolishes OKAN (797). Visual fixation normally stops OKAN and postrotatory vestibular nystagmus by shortening the time constant of velocity storage, a process discussed earlier in this chapter called dumping. The nodulus and uvula are necessary for dumping (738).

Cerebral Cortical Participation in the Optokinetic Pathway

Cortical circuits are superimposed on the phylogenetically older brain stem OKN pathways. Bilateral striate cortex ablation in monkeys abolishes the initial rapid rise of OKN slow phases and causes a temporal-to-nasal bias of monocular OKN but does not alter OKAN duration (262). Humans with blindness from bilateral occipital lesions do not have any optokinetic responses unless some striate and extrastriate visual cortex is spared (798,799); however, patients with bilateral incomplete occipital lobe damage are reported to have nasal/temporal asymmetry of OKN during monocular stimulation and slow buildup of OKN slow-phase speed, like monkeys after bilateral occipital lobectomy and like animals without foveas (785,799). Combined unilateral lesions in prestriate cortex and the inferior parietal lobule of monkeys impair ipsilateral OKN slow-phase responses (333). These lesions may involve area MST and MT, since damage to this region slows the slow phases of rapid-rise and slow-rise OKN, toward the side of the lesion (345). The defects last only 2 weeks, indicating that other areas compensate for damage to this cortical region.

Defective generation of OKN has long been a well-recognized clinical sign of cerebral hemispheric lesions involving the parietal, posterior temporal, and prestriate lateral occipital cortex or their descending projections (474,475,800,801). The defective OKN is evident when targets move toward the side of cerebral damage. A clinical convention is to name the direction of OKN according to the direction of the fast phases, but defective OKN consists of lowered slow-phase speeds and altered frequency of the opposed fast phases. When the OKN defect caused by cerebral lesions is elicited with small handheld striped tapes or drums, it corresponds to lowering of ipsiversive smooth pursuit velocity. Slow buildup of OKN elicited by full-field stimulation has been reported in patients with parietal lobe lesions and attributed to loss of the rapid-rise component with sparing of the slow-rise component (470). However, OKAN and circularvection may also be impaired in patients with parieto-occipital lesions (476), implying damage to the slow-rise component as well.

If one cerebral hemisphere is deprived of visual input by section of the ipsilateral optic tract, or by midline section of the optic chiasm and occlusion of the ipsilateral eye in monkeys, optokinetic nystagmus remains normal in all directions. However, if the corpus callosum is then sectioned, OKN is defective when visual targets move toward the "blind" hemisphere (802). This affirms that the hemianopia from involvement of the optic radiation, which is often associated with parieto-temporal lobe lesions, is *not* responsible for the impairment of ipsiversive smooth eye movements (449,471,574), and that visual information is delivered from the seeing hemisphere to the blind hemisphere across the corpus callosum, despite interruption of the classic optic pathway in the optic radiation. Asymmetry of OKN (or smooth pursuit) in patients who do not have hemianopia might result from involvement of cortical area V5 or its projections to the basal pontine nuclei, or from damage to subcortical white matter that disconnects V5 from visual information relayed from area V1 of both cerebral hemispheres (308,455,474).

Neurons in temporal lobe area MST exhibit optokinetic responses. These neurons also respond during pursuit in the dark, with most neurons exhibiting the same directional pref-

erence for pursuit as for optokinetic stimuli (497,498). MST neurons also discharge in relation to short-latency ocular following responses (803). These are the eye movements generated by sudden motion of large portions of the visual scene and distinguished from OKN by their optimal stimulation by motion over a large (40°) central region with reversed visual motion in the far periphery (678,790). As reviewed above, short latency ocular following responses are thought to play a role in stabilizing gaze on large nearby objects during head translation, and possibly in generating the rapid initial rise in smooth eye movement velocity that makes up the early component of OKN (678,790). Responses in MST precede ocular following responses and neuronal latencies correlate with eye movement latencies (803). MST provides visual input to the DLPN for ocular following responses (803). In addition, most MST neurons with ocular following responses also have genuine smooth pursuit responses with similar directional preferences for both, and some also discharge during full-field OKN. In summary, there is mounting evidence in primates that these motion-processing areas of the cerebral cortex are engaged in three types of smooth tracking: the slow-rise and rapid-rise components of OKN, short latency ocular following responses, and smooth pursuit. Either short-latency ocular following responses (779) or smooth pursuit may produce the rapid-rise component of OKN.

Ablation of the pursuit zone of the FEF impairs smooth pursuit but spares OKN and OKAN. It also leaves the rapid rise of OKN slow phases intact (520), providing evidence that smooth pursuit is not the source of the early component of OKN. This dissociation of pursuit and OKN illustrates that distinction between the nature of the targets that activate the two systems is critical; pursuit of large field stimulation is normal, but pursuit of a small target is degraded. If neural elements that mediate ocular tracking have a retinotopic organization, those with weighting toward the fovea could process smooth pursuit, whereas those representing all or most of the retina could process optokinetic tracking.

Cortical visual areas can generate OKN by way of projections to the NOT and dorsal terminal nucleus of the AOS (466,530,543), where neurons have features of binocular responses, sensitivity to small spots, and directional preference, all bestowed by the cerebral cortex. Lesions of the NOT in monkeys cause a deficit in ipsiversive pursuit and decrease the rapid and slow-rise components of OKN slow-phase velocity and affect OKAN (542). Since lesions that affect ocular pursuit have similar effects on ipsilateral OKN, processing for these two functions is closely linked in NOT, as it is elsewhere. The NOT provides direction-sensitive input to the pursuit system through efferent projections: to the NRTP, as well as to the optokinetic system through projections to the inferior olive (543).

The DLPN of the basal pons also receives projections from area MST of extrastriate cortex, as described above in our discussion of smooth pursuit. Lesions to simian DLPN impair ipsiversive pursuit, the rapid rise in OKN and ocular following responses, but spare slow-rise OKN and OKAN (532). The DLPN projects to the cerebellar flocculus and vermis, areas known to participate in smooth eye movement control. Removal of the monkey flocculus and paraflocculus reduces the rapid rise in slow-phase speed of OKN and causes ultimate slow phases to saturate at subnormal speed, but does not impair OKAN (261). Thus, the primate cerebellum participates in rapid-rise but not slow-rise OKN. The anatomic circuits from the cerebellum to the brain stem for the rapid-rise OKN component are presumed to be the same as for smooth pursuit. In foveate animals, which have developed robust pursuit systems, all smooth tracking mechanisms (smooth pursuit, and optokinetic and short latency ocular following responses) share some cerebral, cerebellar, and brain stem pathways.

SUMMARY OF EYE MOVEMENT CONTROL

In this chapter, we have described roles that the peripheral nerves and muscles and regions of the cerebral hemispheres, brain stem, and cerebellum play in the two goals of ocular motor systems, attaining binocular fixation and preventing retinal image slip. In this final section, we summarize some of this information and provide a brief outline of central nervous system control of ocular motility.

SACCADES

Saccades function to move the fovea rapidly to a target located on the peripheral retina. Phasic high-frequency discharges of ocular motoneurons provide a pulse of innervation, an eye velocity command, to extraocular muscles that drive the eyes against the viscous resistance of orbital tissue. Tonic discharge of motoneurons provides a step of innervation, an eye position command, to the muscles that maintains eye position against elastic restoring forces of the muscles and their tendons and orbital soft tissue. Other eye movement systems also use phasic velocity commands to overcome orbital viscous forces and tonic step commands to prevent the eyes from gliding back to the midposition of the orbit. For each eye position, there is a level of tonic contraction in agonist muscles and a reciprocal level of lesser tonic contraction in their antagonist muscles.

The cerebral hemispheres dispatch trigger signals to omnipause neurons in the brain stem to start saccades and signals of desired saccade amplitude and direction, or of final eye position, that determine the durations and directions of saccades. Cerebral control of saccades involves the parietal eye fields (PEF) and the frontal eye fields (FEF). The PEF processes signals for visually guided saccades and transmits them to the ipsilateral superior colliculus (SC) and to the FEF. The FEF is involved in dispatching volitional and visually guided saccades, but either the FEF or the PEF can assume these functions through parallel pathways from both the PEF and FEF to the SC and brain stem presaccadic structures. Output from the FEF is also routed through the caudate nucleus, which projects to the nucleus substantia nigra pars reticulata (SNpr). The SNpr projects to the SC. The caudate inhibits the SNpr and the SNpr inhibits the SC. SNpr neurons discharge during fixation and they pause, thereby disinhibiting SC burst neurons that fire before and during voluntary and visually evoked saccades. Thus, the FEF has a powerful two-pronged excitatory effect on the SC, one direct and the other through the caudate and SNpr.

Together, the FEF and SC form an obligatory route for saccadic commands originating in the cerebrum, since ablation of both the SC and FEF, but not of either alone, causes severe deficits in the generation of saccadic eye movements. The FEF and SC project to the contralateral paramedian reticular formation of the pons (PPRF) and the mesencephalon in the region of the rostral interstitial nucleus of the medial longitudinal fasciculus (riMLF). Each FEF or SC generates contralateral horizontal saccades, while vertical saccades require simultaneous activity in both FEFs or both SCs.

The final premotor circuits for saccades are located within the paramedian reticular formations of the pons and mesencephalon. Short-lead burst neurons in the PPRF discharge at high frequencies just before and during horizontal saccades. These cells project to the abducens nucleus to generate horizontal saccades. Inhibitory burst neurons in the medulla provide reciprocal inhibition to the contralateral abducens nucleus. Short-lead excitatory burst neurons in the riMLF project to the ocular motoneurons to generate vertical and torsional saccades. The activity of both horizontal and vertical burst neurons is inhibited by the omnipause cells that lie in the midline of the caudal pons. These pause cells cease discharging before and during every saccade.

For horizontal saccades and the other types of conjugate eye movements (pursuit, vestibular, and optokinetic), abducens motoneurons innervate the lateral rectus muscle and internuclear neurons in the abducens nucleus, project via the contralateral medial longitudinal fasciculus (MLF) to the medial rectus divisions of the oculomotor nucleus. For vertical saccades, commands from the riMLF are transmitted to the oculomotor and trochlear nuclei.

SMOOTH PURSUIT

Smooth pursuit eye movements serve to maintain the image of a small object on or near the fovea if the object or the head moves slowly. Areas V5 (MT) and V5a (MST) at the junction of temporal-occipital cortex are important structures in the cortical control of smooth pursuit. Lesions in this region lower the speed of ipsiversive smooth pursuit; they also lower the speed of pursuit of a slowly moving target and the accuracy of saccades in all directions in the contralateral visual field. FEF lesions also cause ipsiversive smooth pursuit defects. Projections from V5 and V5a are to nuclei in the ipsilateral basal pons that, in turn, project to the dorsal cerebellar vermis and the flocculus. Each flocculus controls pursuit by inhibiting neurons in the vestibular nucleus. Second-order vestibular neurons share smooth pursuit and vestibulo-ocular reflex signals and deliver them to motoneurons.

VERGENCE

Vergence eye movements permit stereopsis and prevent diplopia by moving the eyes in opposite horizontal directions. The vergence system maintains the image of an object on the fovea of each eye whether the object is located far away or nearby, and whether it is moving toward or away from the viewer. Posterior temporal, prestriate, and dorsal prefrontal cortex of monkeys are involved in vergence. Neurons in the parietal lobe of monkeys are activated during visual tracking of objects moving in the sagittal plane. Three types of vergence cells (vergence burst, vergence tonic, and vergence burst-tonic cells) are intermixed in the midbrain reticular formation dorsal to the oculomotor nucleus. These neurons process supranuclear convergence and divergence commands that are delivered to medial rectus and lateral rectus motoneurons.

FIXATION

Visual fixation consists of three types of miniature movements: microdrift, microsaccades, and microtremor. Attentive fixation controls slow drift and suppresses microsaccades. Several cerebral areas are engaged in fixation. Area 7 of the parietal lobe is active in attending to the target. The supplementary eye field (SEF) participates in maintaining fixation with the eyes in specific regions of the orbit and inhibiting visually evoked saccades. The lateral prefrontal cortex contains neurons that have increased activity during fixation and neurons that appear to suppress unwanted saccades in monkeys. The FEF participates in disengaging fixation.

Neurons in the SNpr are tonically active during fixation and inhibit presaccadic burst neurons in the SC. The SNpr functions as a gatekeeper for saccadic commands from the cerebral hemispheres to the brain stem and prevents unwanted saccades to extraneous targets. Fixation neurons in the rostral pole of the SC keep presaccadic neurons in the caudal SC silent, while the eyes remain fixated, until a new target appears and activates presaccadic buildup neurons, which inhibit the fixation neurons. The SC projects to omnipause neurons in the midline of the pontine tegmentum. The fixation cells of the SC activate omnipause neurons that sustain fixation by tonically inhibiting presaccadic burst neurons in the PPRF and riMLF.

VESTIBULO-OCULAR REFLEX

The vestibulo-ocular reflex (VOR) prevents slippage of retinal images by moving the eyes at the same speed as the head as it accelerates in the opposite direction. The angular VOR is activated by the semicircular canals as the head rotates. The translational VOR operates when the head moves in the horizontal plane or frontal plane or up and down; it is activated by otolith receptors, which also generate the tilt VOR when the head rotates relative to gravity. Head acceleration signals are integrated by mechanical properties of the semicircular canals so that the vestibular nerve transmits head velocity signals to the vestibular nucleus. Second-order neurons in the vestibular nuclei take several routes. For the horizontal VOR, axons of second-order neurons in the medial vestibular nucleus transmit velocity commands to the abducens nucleus where they synapse on lateral rectus motoneurons, and abducens internuclear neurons that project through the MLF to the medial rectus subdivisions of the

oculomotor nucleus. The horizontal VOR is also served by another direct excitatory projection from the horizontal semicircular canal to second-order neurons in the medial vestibular nucleus. Their axons pass through the ipsilateral abducens nucleus without synapse and ascend to the ipsilateral medial rectus subnucleus through the ascending tract of Deiters, which lies just lateral to the MLF. Second-order vestibular neurons in the medial and superior vestibular nuclei transmit vertical and torsional smooth eye movement signals through the MLF and the brachium conjunctivum to the oculomotor and trochlear nuclei.

To maintain eccentric eye position against elastic restoring forces in eye muscles that cause the eyes to drift toward the orbital midposition, a tonic level of muscle contraction is achieved by an eye position command to motoneurons. Eye velocity position signals are obtained from eye velocity signals by neural integration. A neural integrator is also required to generate position-coded information for other conjugate eye movement systems: saccadic, pursuit, and optokinetic. The velocity-to-position neural integrator for horizontal eye movements is located in the medial vestibular nucleus and the adjacent nucleus prepositus hypoglossi. The neural integrator for vertical and torsional eye movements is located in the interstitial nucleus of Cajal of the rostral midbrain and the vestibular nucleus.

Vision also interacts with the VOR to enhance it during low-frequency head motion. Visual enhancement is required to raise the ratio of eye speed to head speed (VOR gain) to near unity to stabilize images of the stationary environment on the retina. During pursuit of an object with combined eye and head movements, vision cancels the VOR; otherwise the VOR would drive the eyes in the direction opposite to head pursuit, away from the pursued object.

OPTOKINETIC MOVEMENTS

Optokinetic smooth eye movements sustain compensatory eye speed at the same speed as the head during low-frequency or prolonged rotations. The VOR responds best to brief, higher-frequency changes in head position. The optokinetic system is the helpmate of the angular VOR in keeping the eyes still in space during low-frequency head motion. Optokinetic slow phases are induced reflexively by large scenes that stimulate much of the retina, whereas smooth pursuit is usually induced by a small moving object with its image located near the fovea. Optokinetic responses are naturally evoked during head motion with the environment stable but also occur with the head still and the visual scene in motion. Sequential slow phases and opposed quick phases represent optokinetic nystagmus (OKN).

Another visual tracking mechanism supplements the translational VOR, just as the optokinetic system supplements the angular VOR. This short latency ocular following response is distinct from smooth pursuit of foveal targets and from the optokinetic response to full visual field image motion. The ocular following response is best to movement of large objects subtending about 40° of the visual field and is enhanced when the background visual scene moves in the opposite direction.

Cerebral areas V5 and V5A neurons discharge in relation to short-latency ocular following responses and smooth pursuit, and some also discharge during full-field OKN. This motion processing area of cerebral cortex participates in all three conjugate tracking mechanisms: OKN, short-latency ocular following responses, and smooth pursuit. OKN also uses pathways in the brain stem in common with smooth pursuit. A subcortical pathway involving the AOS in the brain stem subserves OKN in afoveate animals. Cortical circuits for the optokinetic system of primates are superimposed on this phylogenetically older brain stem pathway and share its connections.

REFERENCES

1. Robinson DA. The purpose of eye movements. Invest Ophthalmol Vis Sci 1978; 17:835–837.
2. Hering E. The theory of binocular vision (Die Lehre vom Binokularen Sehen). New York (original Leipzig): Plenum (original Wilhelm Englemann), 1977 (original 1868).
3. Helmholz JA. A Treatise on Physiological Optics. New York, Dover, 1910.
4. Moschovakis AK. Are laws that govern behavior embedded in the structure of the CNS? The case of Hering's law. Vision Res 1995;35:3207–3216.
5. King WM, Zhou W. Neural basis of disjunctive eye movements. Ann NY Acad Sci 2002;956:272–283.
6. Zhou W, King WM. Binocular eye movements not coordinated during REM sleep. Exp Brain Res 1997;117:153–160.
7. Zhou W, King WM. Premotor commands encode monocular eye movements. Nature 1998;393:692–695.
8. Sharpe JA, Tweed D, Wong AM. Adaptations and deficits in the vestibulo-ocular reflex after peripheral ocular motor palsies. Ann NY Acad Sci 2003; 1004:111–121.
9. Sylvestre PA, Choi JT, Cullen KE. Discharge dynamics of oculomotor neural integrator neurons during conjugate and disjunctive saccades and fixation. J Neurophysiol 2003;90:739–754.
10. Burde RM, Feldon SE. The extraocular muscles. In: Hart WM, ed. Adler's physiology of the eye. 9th ed. St Louis: CV Mosby, 1992:101–134.
11. Helveston EM, Merriam WW, Ellis FD, et al. The trochlea: a study of the anatomy and physiology. Ophthalmology 1982;89:124–133.
12. Patuhet G. Traite d'Anatomie Humaine. Paris, Masson et Cie, 1951:281.
13. Warwick R. In: Eugene Wolff's Anatomy of the Eye and Orbit. 7th ed. Philadelphia, WB Saunders, 1976:303–305.
14. Spencer RF, McNeer KW. The periphery: extraocular muscles and motor neurones. In: Carpenter RHS, ed. Eye Movements. Boca Raton, CRC Press, 1991: 175–199.
15. Demer JL, Miller JM, Poukens V, et al. Evidence for fibromuscular pulleys of the recti extraocular muscles. Invest Ophthalmol Vis Sci 1995;36:1125–1136.
16. Porter JD, Poukens V, Baker RS, et al. Structure function correlations in the human medial rectus extraocular muscle pulleys. Invest Ophthalmol Vis Sci 1996;37:468–472.
17. Demer JL, Poukens V, Miller JM, Micevych P. Innervation of extraocular pulley smooth muscle in monkeys and humans. Invest Ophthalmol Vis Sci 1997;38: 1774–1785.
18. Demer JL, Oh SY, Poukens V. Evidence of active control of rectus extraocular muscle pulleys. Invest Ophthalmol Vis Sci 2000;41:1280–1290.
19. Peachey L. The structure of the extraocular muscle fibers of mammals. In: Bach-y-Rita P, Collins CC, Hyde JE, eds. The Control of Eye Movements. New York, Academic Press, 1971:47–66.
20. Huxley HE. The mechanism of muscular contraction. Sci Am 1965;213:18–27.
21. Porter JD, Baker RS, Ragusa RJ, et al. Extraocular muscles: basic and clinical aspects of structure and function. Surv Ophthalmol 1995;39:451–484.
22. Porter JD, Baker RS. Muscles of a different 'color': the unusual properties of the extraocular muscles may predispose or protect them in neurogenic and myogenic disease. Neurology 1996;46:30–37.
23. Spencer RF, McNeer KW. Morphology of the extraocular muscles in relation to the clinical manifestations of strabismus. In: Lennerstrand G, von Noorden GK, Campos EC, eds. Strabismus and Amblyopia. New York, Plenum Press, 1988:37–45.
24. Spencer RF, Porter JD. Structural organization of the extraocular muscles. In: Büttner-Ennever JA, ed. Neuroanatomy of the Oculomotor System. Amsterdam, Elsevier, 1988:33–79.
25. Spencer RF, McNeer KW. The periphery: Extraocular muscles and motoneurons. In: Cronly-Dillon JR, ed. Vision and Visual Function. London, MacMillan, 1991: 175–199.
26. Porter JD, Baker RS, Ragusa RJ, Brueckner JK. Extraocular muscles: basic and clinical aspects of structure and function. Surv Ophthalmol 1995;39:451–484.
27. Spencer RF, McNeer KW. Botulinum paralysis of adult monkey extraocular muscle: Structural alterations in the orbital, singly innervated muscle fibers. Arch Ophthalmol 1987;105:1703–1711.
28. Jacoby J, Chiarandini DJ, Stefani E. Electrical properties and innervation of fibers in the orbital layer of rat extraocular muscles. J Neurophysiol 1989;61: 116–125.
29. Buttner-Ennever JA, Horn AKE, Scherberger H, D'Ascanio P. Motoneurons of twitch and nontwitch extraocular muscle fibers in the abducens, trochlear, and oculomotor nuclei of monkeys. J Comp Neurol 2001;438:318–335.
30. Verhoeff FH. Problems concerning convergence. Trans Am Acad Ophthalmol Otolaryngol 1947;52:15–19.
31. Alpern M, Wolter JR. The relation of horizontal saccadic and vergence movements. Arch Ophthalmol 1956;56:685–690.
32. Jampel RS. Multiple motor systems in the extraocular muscles of man. Invest Ophthalmol 1967;6:288–293.
33. Scott AB, Collins CC. Division of labor in human extraocular muscles. Arch Ophthalmol 1973;90:319–322.
34. Collins CC. The human ocular system. In: Lennerstrand G, Bach-y-Rita P, eds. Basic Mechanisms of Ocular Motility and Their Clinical Implications. New York, Pergamon, 1975:145–180.
35. Barmack NH. Laminar organization of the extraocular muscles of the rabbit. Exp Neurol 1978;59:304–321.
36. Robinson DA. The functional behavior of the peripheral ocular motor apparatus: a review. In: Kommerell G, ed. Disorders of Ocular Motility. Munich, Bergman Verlag, 1978:43–61.
37. Adler FH. Physiology of the Eye. 4th ed. St Louis, CV Mosby, 1965:400.
38. Bach-y-Rita P. Neurophysiology of eye movements. In: Bach-y-Rita P, Hyde JE, eds. The Control of Eye Movements. New York, Academic Press, 1971: 7–46.
39. Alvarado JA, van Horn C. Muscle cell types of the cat inferior oblique. In: Lennerstrand G, Bach-y-Rita P, eds. Basic Mechanisms of Ocular Motility and Their Clinical Implication. Oxford, UK, Pergamon, 1975:15–43.
40. Lam H, Poukens V, Oh SY, et al. Laminar analysis of motor unit size in human rectus extraocular muscles. Soc Neurosci Abstr 2002;7:857.
41. Ruskell GL. The fine structure of human extraocular muscle spindles and their potential proprioceptive capacity. J Anat 1989;167:199–214.
42. Lukas JR, Aigner M, Blumer R, et al. Number and distribution of neuromuscular spindles in human extraocular muscles. Invest Ophthalmol Vis Sci 1994;35: 4317–4327.
43. Buttner-Ennever JA, Eberhorn A, Horn AK. Motor and sensory innervation of extraocular eye muscles. Ann NY Acad Sci 2003;1004:40–49.
44. Richmond FJR, Johnston WSW, Baker RS, Steinbach MJ. Palisade endings in human extraocular muscles. Invest Ophthalmol Vis Sci 1984;25:471–476.
45. Steinbach MJ. Proprioceptive knowledge of eye position. Vision Res 1987;27: 1737–1744.
46. Porter JD. Brainstem terminations of extraocular muscle primary afferent neurons in the monkey. J Comp Neurol 1986;247:133–143.
47. Gentle A, Ruskell G. Pathway of the primary afferent nerve fibers serving proprioception in monkey extraocular muscles. Ophthalmic Physiol Opt 1997;17: 225–231.
48. Lewis RF, Zee DS, Hayman MR, et al. Oculomotor function in the rhesus monkey after deafferentation of the extraocular muscles. Exp Brain Res 2001; 141:349–358.
49. Donaldson IM. The functions of the proprioceptors of the eye muscles. Phil Trans R Soc Lond B 2000;355:1685–1754.
50. Steinbach MJ, Smith DR. Spatial localization after strabismus surgery: evidence for inflow. Science 1981;213:1407–1409.
51. Gauthier GM, Nommay D, Vercher JL. The role of ocular muscle proprioception in visual localization of targets. Science 1990;249:58–61.
52. Gauthier GM, Nommay D, Vercher JL. Ocular muscle proprioception and visual localization of targets in man. Brain 1990;113:1857–1871.
53. Bridgeman B, Stark L. Ocular proprioception and efference copy in registering visual direction. Vision Res 1991;31:1903–1913.
54. Lal R, Friedlander MJ. Effect of passive eye movement on retinogeniculate transmission in the cat. J Neurophysiol 1990;63:523–538.
55. Steinbach MJ, Kirshner EL, Arstikaitis MJ. Recession vs marginal myotomy surgery for strabismus: effects on spatial localization. Invest Ophthalmol Vis Sci 1987;28:1870–1872.
56. Lewis RF, Zee DS, Gaymard BM, Guthrie BL. Extraocular muscle proprioception functions in the control of ocular alignment and eye movement conjugacy. J Neurophysiol 1994;72:1028–1031.
57. Trotter Y, Celebrini S, Beaux JC, Grandjean B. Neuronal stereoscopic processing following extraocular proprioception deafferentation. Neuroreport 1990;1: 187–190.
58. O'Keefe LP, Berkley MA. Binocular immobilization induced by paralysis of the extraocular muscles of one eye: evidence for an interocular proprioceptive mechanism. J Neurophysiol 1991;66:2022–2033.
59. Knox PC, Donaldson IM. Afferent signals from the extraocular muscles of the

pigeon modify the electromyogram of these muscles during the vestibulo-ocular reflex. Proc R Soc London 1991;B246:243–250.

60. Gauthier GM, Vercher J-L. Ocular motor proprioception and ocular motor control. In: Jami L, Pierrot-Deseilligny E, Zytnicki D, eds. Muscle Afferents and Spinal Control of Movement. Oxford, UK, Pergamon, 1992:277–285.

61. Knox PC, Donaldson IM. Afferent signals from the extraocular muscles of the pigeon modify the vestibulo-ocular reflex. Proc R Soc London 1993;B253:77–82.

62. Allin F, Velay JL, Bouquerel A. Shift in saccadic direction induced in humans by proprioceptive manipulation: a comparison between memory-guided and visually guided saccades. Exp Brain Res 1996;110:473–481.

63. Fahy FL, Donaldson IM. Extraocular muscle proprioception and the vestibulo-ocular reflex (VOR) in the pigeon. J Physiol 1996;495:149P.

64. Lewis RF, Zee DS, Goldstein HP, Guthrie BL. Proprioceptive and retinal afference modify postsaccadic ocular drift. J Neurophysiol 1999;82:551–563.

65. Donaldson IM, Knox PC. Afferent signals from the extraocular muscles affect the gain of the horizontal vestibulo-ocular reflex in the alert pigeon. Vision Res 2000;40:1001–1011.

66. Optican LM, Zee DS. A hypothetical explanation of congenital nystagmus. Bio Cybernet 1984;50:119–134.

67. Corsi M, Sodi A, Salvi G, Faussone-Pellegrini MS. Morphological study of extraocular muscle proprioceptor alterations in congenital strabismus. Ophthalmologica 1990;200:154–163.

68. Warwick R. In: Eugene Wolff's Anatomy of the Eye and Orbit. 7th ed. Philadelphia, WB Saunders, 1976:266.

69. George JL. La vascularisation artérielle du muscle releveur de la paupiäre supérieure. J Fr Ophtalmol 1984;7:143–149.

70. Büttner Ennever JA, Akert K. Medial rectus subgroups of the oculomotor nucleus and their abducens internuclear input in the monkey. J Comp Neurol 1981;197:17–27.

71. Spencer RF, Porter JD. Innervation and structure of extraocular muscles in the monkey in comparison to those of the cat. J Comp Neurol 1981;198:649 665.

72. Porter JD, Guthrie BL, Sparks DL. Innervation of monkey extraocular muscles: localization of sensory and motor neurons by retrograde transport of horseradish peroxidase. J Comp Neurol 1983;218:208–219.

73. Porter JD, Burns LA, May PJ. Morphological substrate for eyelid movements: innervation and structure of primate levator palpebrae superioris and orbicularis oculi muscles. J Comp Neurol 1989;287:64–81.

74. Warwick R. Representation of the extra ocular muscles in the oculomotor nuclei of the monkey. J Comp Neurol 1953;98:449–503.

75. Bienfang DC. Crossing axons in the third nerve nucleus. Invest Ophthalmol 1975;12:927–931.

76. Maciewicz RJ, Kaneko CRS, Highstein SM, et al. Morphophysiological identification of interneurons in the oculomotor nucleus that project to the abducens nucleus in the cat. Brain Res 1975;96:60–65.

77. Maciewicz RJ, Spencer R. Oculomotor and abducens internuclear pathways in the cat. In: Baker R, Berthoz A, eds. Control of Gaze by Brain Stem Neurons. Amsterdam, Elsevier/North Holland, 1977:99–108.

78. Maciewicz RJ, Romagnano MA, Baker R, et al. Two projections of the oculomotor internuclear neurons. Anat Rec 1977;187:642.

79. Maciewicz RJ, Phipps BS. The oculomotor internuclear pathway: a double retrograde labeling study. Brain Res 1983;262:1–8.

80. Burde RM, Loewy AD. Central origin of oculomotor parasympathetic neurons in the monkey. Brain Res 1980;198:434–439.

81. Ksiazek SM, Repka MX, Maguire A, et al. Divisional oculomotor nerve paresis caused by intrinsic brainstem disease. Ann Neurol 1989;26:714–718.

82. Hriso E, Masdeu JC, Miller A. Monocular elevation weakness and ptosis: an oculomotor fascicular syndrome? J Clin Neuroophthalmol 1991;11:111–113.

83. Eggenberger ER, Miller NR, Hoffman PN, et al. Mesencephalic ependymal cyst causing an inferior division paresis of the oculomotor nerve: case report. Neurology 1993;43:2419–2420.

84. Zak R, Slamovits T, Burde R. Oculomotor brainstem anatomy: nuclei to fasciculus. J Neurooncol 1994;18:241–248.

85. Schwartz TH, Lycette CA, Yoon SS, et al. Clinicoradiologic evidence for oculomotor fascicular anatomy. J Neurol Neurosurg Psychiatry 1995;59:338.

86. Harris FS, Rhoton ALJ. Anatomy of the cavernous sinus: a microsurgical study. J Neurosurg 1976;45:169–180.

87. Umansky F, Nathan H. The lateral wall of the cavernous sinus: with special reference to the nerves related to it. J Neurosurg 1982;56:228–234.

88. Parkinson D. Collateral circulation of cavernous carotid artery. Anat Can J Surg 1964;7:251–268.

89. Parkinson D. A surgical approach to the cavernous portion of the carotid artery: anatomical studies and case report. J Neurosurg 1965;23:474–483.

90. Asbury AK, Aldredge H, Hershberg R, et al. Oculomotor palsy in diabetes mellitus: a clinico-pathological study. Brain 1970;93:555–566.

91. Nadeau SE, Trobe JD. Pupil sparing in oculomotor palsy: a brief review. Ann Neurol 1983;13:143–148.

92. Miller NR, Kiel SM, Green WR, et al. Unilateral Duane's retraction syndrome (type 1). Arch Ophthalmol 1982;100:1468–1472.

93. Sacks JG. Peripheral innervation of extraocular muscles. Am J Ophthalmol 1983;95:520–527.

94. Sunderland S, Hughes ESR. The pupillo-constrictor pathway and the nerves to the ocular muscles in man. Brain 1946;69:301–309.

95. Kerr FWL, Hollowell OW. Location of pupilomotor and accommodation fibers in the oculomotor nerve: experimental observations on paralytic mydriasis. J Neurol Neurosurg Psychiatry 1964;27:473–481.

96. Engle E, Kunkel L, Specht L, et al. Mapping a gene for congenital fibrosis of the extraocular muscles to the centromeric region of chromosome. Nat Genet 1994;127:69–73.

97. Engle EC, Gumnerov BC, McKeown CA, et al. Oculomotor nerve and muscle abnormalities in congenital fibrosis of the extraocular muscles. Ann Neurol 1997;41:314–325.

98. Olszewski J, Baxter D. Cytoarchitecture of the human brain stem. Basel, Karger, 1954.

99. Miyazaki S. Bilateral innervation of the superior oblique muscle by the trochlear nucleus. Brain Res 1985;348:52–56.

100. Barton NB, Clark RG. Neuro-anatomical feature photo. J Clin Neuroophthalmol 1982;2:143–144.

101. Stopford JSB. The arteries of the pons and medulla oblongata. J Anat 1915;50:131–164.

102. Hassler O. Arterial pattern of human brainstem: Normal appearance and deformation in expanding supratentorial conditions. Neurology 1967;17:368–375.

103. Gillilan LA. Angioarchitecture of the human brainstem. Anat Rec 1955;121:299.

104. Testut L. Tratado de Anatomia Humana. Barcelona, Salvat y Cia, 1902.

105. Cushing H. Strangulation of the nervi abducentes by lateral branches of the basilar artery in cases of brain tumour: with an explanation of some obscure palsies on the basis of arterial constriction. Brain 1910;33:204–235.

106. Jain KK. Aberrant roots of the abducens nerve. J Neurosurg 1964;21:349–351.

107. Nathan H, Ouaknine G, Kosary IZ. The abducens nerve: anatomical variations in its course. J Neurosurg 1974;41:561–566.

108. Monro A. The Anatomy of the Human Bones and Nerves. Edinburgh, Hamilton & Balfour, 1746:363.

109. Johnston JA, Parkinson D. Intracranial sympathetic pathways associated with the sixth cranial nerve. J Neurosurg 1974;39:236–243.

110. Parkinson D, Johnston J, Chaudhuri A. Sympathetic connections of the fifth and sixth cranial nerves. Anat Rec 1978;191:221–226.

111. Parkinson D, et al. Horner syndrome and others. Surg Neurol 1979;11:221–223.

112. Tweed D, Vilis T. Geometric relations of eye position and velocity vectors during saccades. Vision Res 1990;30:111–127.

113. Crawford JD, Vilis T. How do motor systems deal with the problem of controlling three-dimensional rotations? J Motor Behavior 1995;27:89–99.

114. Straumann D, Zee DS, Solomon D, Kramer PD. Validity of Listing's law during fixations, saccades, smooth pursuit eye movements, and blinks. Exp Brain Res 1996;112:135–146.

115. Schnabolk C, Raphan T. Modeling three-dimensional velocity-to-position transformation in oculomotor control. J Neurophysiol 1994;71:623–638.

116. Demer JL, Miller JM, Poukens V, et al. Evidence for fibromuscular pulleys of the recti extraocular muscles. Invest Ophthalmol Vis Sci 1995;36:1125–1136.

117. Straumann D, Zee DS, Solomon D, et al. Transient torsion during and after saccades. Vision Res 1995;35:3321–3334.

118. Quaia C, Optican LM. Commutative saccadic generator is sufficient to control a 3-D ocular plant with pulleys. J Neurophysiol 1998;79:3197–3215.

119. Raphan T. Modeling control of eye orientation in three dimensions. I. Role of muscle pulleys in determining saccade trajectory. J Neurophysiol 1998;79:2653–2667.

120. Thurtell MJ, Kunin M, Raphan T. Role of muscle pulleys in producing eye position-dependence in the angular vestibuloocular reflex: a model-based study. J Neurophysiol 2000;84:639–650.

121. Donders FC. Beitrag zur Lehre von den Bewegungen des menschlichen Auges. Holland Beitr Anat Physiol Wiss 1848;1:104–384.

122. von Helmholtz H. Handbuch der Physiologischen Optik. 3rd ed. Hamburg, Voss, 1867.

123. Hepp K. On Listing's law. Commun Math Physics 1990;132:285–292.

124. Collewijn H, Van der Steen J, Ferman L, Jansen TC. Human ocular counterroll: assessment of static and dynamic properties from electromagnetic scleral coil recordings. Exp Brain Res 1985;59:185–196.

125. Crawford JD, Vilis T. Axes of eye rotation and Listing's law during rotations of the head. J Neurophysiol 1991;65:407–423.

126. Morrow MJ, Sharpe JA. The effects of head and trunk position on torsional vestibular and optokinetic eye movements in humans. Exp Brain Res 1993;95:144–150.

127. Wong AM. Listing's law: clinical significance and implications for ocular motor control. Surv Ophthalmol 2004 (in press).

128. Robinson DA. The mechanics of human saccadic eye movement. J Physiol 1964;174:245–264.

129. Robinson DA. Eye movement control in primates. Science 1968;161:1219–1224.

130. Robinson DA. Oculomotor unit behavior in the monkey. J Neurophysiol 1970;33:393–404.

131. Robinson DA. Oculomotor control signal. In: Lennerstrand G, Bach-y-Rita P,

eds. Basic mechanisms of ocular motility and their clinical implications. Oxford: Pergamon Press, 1975:337–374.

132. Miller JM, Robins D. Extraocular muscle forces in alert monkey. Vision Res 1992;32:1099–1113.

133. Goldstein H, Reinecke R. Clinical applications of ocular motor plant models. In: Fuchs AF, Brandt T, Büttner U, Zee D, eds. Contemporary ocular motor and vestibular research: a tribute to David A. Robinson. Thieme Medical Publishers: New York, 1994:10–17.

134. Sylvestre PA, Cullen KE. Quantitative analysis of abducens neuron discharge dynamics during saccadic and slow eye movements. J Neurophysiol 1999;82: 2612–2632.

135. Gamlin PDR, Mays LE. Dynamic properties of medial rectus motoneurons during vergence eye movements. J Neurophysiol 1992;67:64–74.

136. Jacobs L, Feldman M, Bender MB. Eye movements during sleep: I. The pattern in the normal human. Arch Neurol 1971;25:151–159.

137. Sharpe JA, Troost BT, Dell'Osso LF, Daroff RB. Comparative velocities of different types of fast eye movements in man. Invest Ophthalmol 1975;14: 689–692.

138. Garbutt S, Han Y, Kumar AN, et al. Vertical optokinetic nystagmus and saccades in normal human subjects. Invest Ophthalmol Vis Sci 2003;44:3833–3841.

139. Curthoys IS. Generation of the quick phase of horizontal vestibular nystagmus. Exp Brain Res 2002;143:397–405.

140. Melvill Jones G. Predominance of anti-compensatory oculomotor response during rapid head rotation. Aerospace Med 1964;35:965–968.

141. Lau CY, Honrubia V, Baloh RW. The Pattern of Eye Movement Trajectories During Physiological Nystagmus in Humans. London, Academic Press, 1978.

142. Boghen D, Troost BT, Daroff RB, et al. Velocity characteristics of normal human saccades. Invest Ophthalmol 1974;13:619–623.

143. Bahill AT, Clark MR, Stark L. The main sequence: a tool for studying human eye movements. Math Biosci 1975;24:191–204.

144. Baloh RW, Sills AW, Kumley WE, Honrubia V. Quantitative measurement of saccade amplitude, duration and velocity. Neurology 1975;25:1065–1070.

145. Abel LA, Troost BT, Dell'Osso LF. The effects of age on normal saccadic characteristics and their variability. Vision Res 1983;23:33–37.

146. Bahill AT, Brockenbrough A, Troost BT. Variability and development of a normative data base for saccadic eye movements. Invest Ophthalmol Vis Sci 1981;21:116–125.

147. Sharpe JA, Zackon DH. Senescent saccades: effects of aging on their accuracy, latency and velocity. Acta Otolaryngol 1987;104:422–428.

148. Huaman A, Sharpe JA. Vertical saccades in senescence. Invest Ophthalmol Vis Sci 1993;34:2588–2595.

149. Smeets JB, Hooge IT. Nature of variability in saccades. J Neurophysiol 2003; 90:12–20.

150. Smit AC, Van Gisbergen J, Cools AR. A parametric analysis of human saccades in different experimental paradigms. Vision Res 1987;27:1745–1762.

151. Fletcher WA, Sharpe JA. Saccadic eye movement dysfunction in Alzheimer's disease. Ann Neurol 1986;20:464–471.

152. Becker W, Fuchs AF. Further properties of the human saccadic system: eye movements and correction saccades with and without visual fixation points. Vision Res 1969;9:1247–1258.

153. Fukuda T, Wakakura M, Ishikawa S. Comparative study of eye movements in the alert state and rapid eye movement in sleep. Neuroophthalmology 1981;1: 253–260.

154. Fuchs AF, Binder MD. Fatigue resistance of human extraocular muscles. J Neurophysiol 1983;49:28–34.

155. Barton JJ, Huaman AG, Sharpe JA. Effects of edrophonium on saccadic velocity in normal subjects and myasthenic and nonmyasthenic ocular palsies. Ann Neurol 1994;36:585–594.

156. Weber RB, Daroff RB. Corrective movements following refixation saccades: type and control system analysis. Vision Res 1972;12:467–475.

157. Bahill AT, Hsu FK, Stark L. Glissadic overshoots are due to pulse width errors. Arch Neurol 1978;35:138–142.

158. Kapoula Z, Optican LM, Robinson DA. Visually induced plasticity of postsaccadic ocular drift in normal humans. J Neurophysiol 1989;61:879–891.

159. Bahill AT, Stark L. Overlapping saccades and glissades are produced by fatigue in the saccadic eye movement system. Exp Neurol 1975;48:95–106.

160. Bahill AT, Clark MR, Stark L. Dynamic overshoot in saccadic eye movements is caused by neurological control signed reversals. Exp Neurol 1975;48:107–122.

161. Enderle JD. Neural control of saccades. Progr Brain Res 2002;140:21–49.

162. Warabi T, Kase M, Kato T. Effect of aging on the accuracy of visually guided saccadic eye movement. Ann Neurol 1984;16:449–454.

163. Findlay JM. Spatial and temporal factors in the predictive generation of saccadic eye movements. Vision Res 1981;21:347–354.

164. Isa T, Kobayashi Y. Switching between cortical and subcortical sensorimotor pathways. Progr Brain Res 2004;143:299–305.

165. Fisher B, Ramsperger E. Human express saccades, extremely short reaction times of goal directed eye movements. Exp Brain Res 1984;57:191–195.

166. Fisher B, Ramsberger E. Human express saccades, effects of randomization and daily practice. Exp Brain Res 1986;64:569–578.

167. Kalesnykas RP, Hallett PE. The differentiation of visually guided and anticipatory saccades in gap and overlap paradigms. Exp Brain Res 1987;68:115–121.

168. Weber RB, Daroff RB. The metrics of horizontal saccadic eye movements in normal humans. Vision Res 1971;11:921–928.

169. Grusser OJ. On the history of the ideas of efference copy and reafference. Clio Med 1995;33:35–55.

170. Bridgeman B. A review of the role of efference copy in sensory and oculomotor control systems. Ann Biomed Engineer 1995;23:409–422.

171. Prablanc C, Masse D, Echallier JF. Error-correcting mechanisms in large saccades. Vision Res 1978;18:557–560.

172. Henson DB. Corrective saccades: effects of altering visual feedback. Vision Res 1978;18:63–67.

173. Optican LM. Saccadic dysmetria. In: Lennerstrand G, Zee D, Keller EL, eds. Functional basis of ocular motility disorders. Oxford: Pergamon Press, 1982: 291–302.

174. Becker W, Klein HM. Accuracy of saccadic eye movements and maintenance of eccentric eye positions in the dark. Vision Res 1973;13:1021–1034.

175. Eizenman M, Cheng P, Sharpe JA, et al. End-point nystagmus and ocular drift: an experimental and theoretical study. Vision Res 1990;30:863–877.

176. Sharpe JA, Cheng P, Eizenman M. End-point nystagmus in the vertical plane. In: Fuchs AF, Brandt T, Buettner U, Zee DS, eds. Contemporary Ocular Motor and Vestibular Research: A Tribute to David A. Robinson. New York, Thieme Medical Publishers, 1994:348–350.

177. Westheimer G. Eye movement responses to a horizontally moving visual stimulus. Arch Ophthalmol 1954;52:932–941.

178. Young LR, Stark L. A sampled data model for eye tracking movements. Q Progr Res Lab Electr MIT 1962;66:370–383.

179. Young LR, Stark L. Variable feedback experiments testing a sampled data model for eye tracking movements. IEEE Trans Hum Factors Electron HFE 1963;4: 38.

180. Becker W, Jürgens R. An analysis of the saccadic system by means of double step stimuli. Vision Res 1979;19:967–983.

181. Robinson DA. Models of the saccadic eye movement control system. Kybernetik 1973;14:71–83.

182. Hallett PE, Lightstone AD. Saccadic eye movements to flashed targets. Vision Res 1976;16:107–114.

183. Sparks DL, Mays LE. Spatial localization of saccade targets. I. Compensation for stimulation-induced perturbations in eye position. J Neurophysiol 1983;49: 45–63.

184. Deubel H. Separate adaptive mechanisms for the control of reactive and volitional saccadic eye movements. Vision Res 1995;35:3529–3540.

185. Straube A, Fuchs AF, Usher S, Robinson FR. Characteristics of saccadic gain adaptation in rhesus macaques. J Neurophysiol 1997;77:874–895.

186. Zee DS, Optican LM, Cook JD, et al. Slow saccades in spinocerebellar degeneration. Arch Neurol 1976;33:243–251.

187. Campbell FW, Wurtz RH. Saccadic omission: why we do not see a grey out during saccadic eye movement. Vision Res 1978;18:1297–1303.

188. Diamond MR, Ross J, Morrone MC. Extraretinal control of saccadic suppression. J Neurosci 2000;20:3349–3455.

189. Matin E. Saccadic suppression: a review and an analysis. Psychol Bull 1974; 81:899–917.

190. MacKay DM. Elevation of visual threshold by displacement of retinal image. Nature 1970;225:90–92.

191. MacKay DM. Interocular transfer of suppression effects of retinal image displacement. Nature 1970;225:872–873.

192. Mitrani L, Mateeff S, Yakimoff N. Is saccadic suppression really saccadic? Vision Res 1971;11:1157–1161.

193. Rolls ET, Tovee MJ. Processing speed in the cerebral cortex and the neurophysiology of visual masking. Proc R Soc London Series B Biol Sci 1994;257:9–15.

194. Macknik SL, Livingstone MS. Neuronal correlates of visibility and invisibility in the primate visual system. Nature Neurosci 1998;1:144–149.

195. Judge SJ, Wurtz RH, Richmond BJ. Vision during saccadic eye movements: I. Visual interactions in striate cortex. J Neurophysiol 1980;43:1133–1155.

196. Richmond BJ, Wurtz RH. Vision during saccadic eye movements. II. A corollary discharge to monkey superior colliculus. J Neurophysiol 1980;43:1156–1167.

197. Wurtz RH, Richmond BJ, Judge SJ. Vision during saccadic eye movements: III. Visual interactions in monkey superior colliculus. J Neurophysiol 1980;43: 1168–1181.

198. Burr DC, Morrone MC, Ross J. Selective suppression of the magnocellular visual pathway during saccadic eye movements. Nature 1994;371:511–513.

199. Kusunoki M, Goldberg ME. The time course of perisaccadic receptive field shifts in the lateral intraparietal area of the monkey. J Neurophysiol 2003;89: 31519–1527.

200. Thiele A, Henning P, Kubischik M, et al. Neural mechanisms of saccadic suppression. Science 2002;295:2460–2462.

201. Ilg UJ, Bridgeman B, Hoffmann KP. An influence of mechanical disturbance on oculomotor behaviour. Vision Res 1989;29:545–551.

202. Ross J, Morrone MC, Goldberg ME, et al. Changes in visual perception at the time of saccades. Trends Neurosci 2001;24:113–121.

203. Horn AKE, Büttner-Ennever JA, Suzuki Y, et al. Histological identification of premotor neurons for horizontal saccades in monkey and man by parvalbumin immunostaining. J Comp Neurol 1995;359:350–363.

204. Horn AK, Buttner-Ennever JA. Premotor neurons for vertical eye movements

in the rostral mesencephalon of monkey and human: histologic identification by parvalbumin immunostaining. J Comp Neurol 1998;392:413–427.

205. Scudder CA, Moschovakis AK, Karabelas AB, et al. Anatomy and physiology of saccadic long-lead burst neurons recorded in the alert squirrel monkey. I. Descending projections from the mesencephalon. J Neurophysiol 1996;76:332–352.

206. Scudder CA, Moschovakis AK, Karabelas AB, et al. Anatomy and physiology of saccadic long-lead burst neurons recorded in the alert squirrel monkey. II. Pontine neurons. J Neurophysiol 1996;76:353–370.

207. Hepp K, Henn V. Neuronal activity preceding rapid eye movements in the brain stem of the alert monkey. Progr Brain Res 1979;50:645–652.

208. Scudder CA, Kaneko CS, Fuchs AF, et al. The brainstem burst generator for saccadic eye movements: a modern synthesis. Exp Brain Res 2002;142:439–462.

209. Moschovakis AK, Highstein SM. The anatomy and physiology of primate neurons that control rapid eye movements. Ann Rev Neurosci 1994;17:465–488.

210. Strassman A, Highstein SM, McCrea RA. Anatomy and physiology of saccadic burst neurons in the alert squirrel monkey. II. Inhibitory burst neurons. J Comp Neurol 1986;249:358–380.

211. Keller EL. Participation of the medial pontine reticular formation in eye movement generation in monkey. J Neurophysiol 1974;37:316–332.

212. Robinson DA. The control of eye movements. In: Brooks VB, ed. Handbook of physiology, vol 2, part 2. Bethesda, MD: American Physiology Society, 1981:1275–1320.

213. Schnyder H, Reisine H, Hepp K, et al. Frontal eye field projection to the paramedian pontine reticular formation traced with wheat germ agglutinin in the monkey. Brain Res 1985;329:151–160.

214. Stanton GB, Goldberg ME, Bruce CJ. Frontal eye field efferents in the macaque monkey. J Comp Neurol 1988;27:473–506.

215. Stanton GB, Goldberg ME, Bruce CJ. Frontal eye field efferents in the macaque monkey: II Topography of terminal fields in midbrain and pons. J Comp Neurol 1988;27:493–506.

216. Cohen B, Komatsuzaki A. Eye movements induced by stimulation of the pontine reticular formation: evidence for integration in oculomotor pathways. Exp Neurol 1972;36:101–117.

217. Henn V, Lang W, Hepp K, et al. Experimental gaze palsies in monkeys and their relation to human pathology. Brain 1984;107:619–636.

218. Barton EJ, Nelson JS, Gandhi NJ, et al. Effects of partial lidocaine inactivation of the paramedian pontine reticular formation on saccades of macaques. J Neurophysiol 2003;90:372–386.

219. Goebel HH, Komatsuzaki A, Bender MB, et al. Lesions of the pontine tegmentum and conjugate gaze paralysis. Arch Neurol 1971;24:431–440.

220. Bender M. Brain control of conjugate horizontal and vertical eye movements. Brain 1980;103:23–69.

221. Johnston JL, Sharpe JA. Sparing of the horizontal vestibulo-ocular reflex with lesions of the paramedian pontine reticular formation. Neurology 1989;39:876.

222. Lang W, Henn V, Hepp K. Gaze palsies offer selective pontine lesions in monkeys. In: Roncoux A, Crommelinck M, eds. Physiological and pathological aspects of eye movements. The Hague: Dr. W Junk Publishers, 1982:209–218.

223. Hikosaka O, Igusa Y, Nakao S, et al. Direct inhibitory synaptic linkage of pontomedullary reticular burst neurons with abducens motoneurons in the cat. Exp Brain Res 1978;33:337–352.

224. Büttner-Ennever JA, Cohen B, Pause M, et al. Raphe nucleus of the pons containing omnipause neurons of the oculomotor system in the monkey and its homologue in man. J Comp Neurol 1988;267:307–321.

225. Horn AKE, Büttner-Ennever JA, Wahle P, et al. Neurotransmitter profile of saccadic omnipause neurons in nucleus raphe interpositus. J Neurosci 1994;14:2032–2046.

226. Buttner U, Buttner-Ennever JA, Henn V. Vertical eye movement related unit activity in the rostral mesencephalic reticular formation of the alert monkey. Brain Res 1977;130:239–252.

227. Buttner-Ennever JA, Buttner U. A cell group associated with vertical eye movements in the rostral mesencephalic reticular formation of the monkey. Brain Res 1978;151:31–47.

228. Shiraishi Y, Nakao S. Differential locations in the midbrain of distinct groups of vertical eye movement-related neurones in cat: their projections and direct connections with oculomotor neurones. Acta Physiol Scand 1995;154:151–163.

229. Wang SF, Spencer RF. Spatial organization of premotor neurons related to vertical upward and downward saccadic eye movements in the rostral interstitial nucleus of the medial longitudinal fasciculus (riMLF) in the cat. J Comp Neurol 1996;366:163–180.

230. Moschovakis AK, Scudder CA, Highstein SM. Structure of the primate oculomotor burst generator. I. Medium-lead burst neurons with upward on-directions. J Neurophysiol 1991;65:203–217.

231. Moschovakis AK, Scudder CA, Highstein SM. Structure of the primate oculomotor burst generator. II. Medium-lead burst neurons with downward on-directions. J Neurophysiol 1991;65:218–229.

232. Moschovakis AK, Scudder CA, Highstein SM. A structural basis for Hering's law: projections to extraocular motoneurons. Science 1990;248:1118–1119.

233. Crossland WJ, Hu XJ, Rafols JA. Morphological study of the rostral interstitial nucleus of the medial longitudinal fasciculus in the monkey, *Macaca mulatta*, by Nissl, Golgi and computer reconstruction and rotation methods. J Comp Neurol 1994;347:47–63.

234. Spencer RF, Wang SF. Immunohistochemical localization of neurotransmitters utilized by neurons in the rostral interstitial nucleus of the medial longitudinal fasciculus (riMLF) that project to the oculomotor and trochlear nuclei in the cat. J Comp Neurol 1996;366:134–148.

235. Vilis T, Hepp K, Schwarz U, et al. On the generation of vertical and torsional rapid eye movements in the monkey. Exp Brain Res 1989;77:1–11.

236. Suzuki Y, Büttner-Ennever JA, Straumann D, et al. Deficits in torsional and vertical rapid eye movements and shift of Listing's plane after uni- and bilateral lesions of the rostral interstitial nucleus of the medial longitudinal fasciculus (riMLF). Exp Brain Res 1995;106:215–232.

237. Leigh RJ, Seidman SH, Grant MH, et al. Loss of ipsidirectional quick phases of torsional nystagmus with a unilateral midbrain lesion. J Vestibular Research 1993;3:115–121.

238. Helmchen C, Glasauer S, Bartl K, et al. Contralesionally beating torsional nystagmus in a unilateral rostral midbrain lesion. Neurology 1996;47:482–486.

239. Helmchen C, Rambold H, Fuhry L, et al. Deficits in vertical and torsional eye movements after uni- and bilateral muscimol inactivation of the interstitial nucleus of Cajal of the alert monkey. Exp Brain Res 1998;119:436–452.

240. Buttner U, Buttner-Ennever JA, Rambold H, et al. The contribution of midbrain circuits in the control of gaze. Ann NY Acad Sci 2002;956:99–110.

241. Pasik P, Pasik T, Bender MB. The pretectal syndrome in monkeys: I. Disturbances of gaze and body posture. Brain 1969;92:521–534.

242. Kömpf D, Pasik T, Pasik P, et al. Downward gaze in monkeys: stimulation and lesion studies. Brain 1979;102:527–558.

243. Büttner-Ennever JA, Büttner U, Cohen B, et al. Vertical gaze paralysis and the rostral interstitial nucleus of the medial longitudinal fasciculus. Brain 1982;105:125–149.

244. Ranalli PJ, Sharpe JA, Fletcher WA. Palsy of upward and downward saccadic, pursuit and vestibular movements with a unilateral midbrain lesion: pathophysiologic correlations. Neurology 1988;38:114–122.

245. Bhidayasiri R, Plant GT, Leigh RJ. A hypothetical scheme for the brainstem control of vertical gaze. Neurology 2000;54:1985–1993.

246. Keane DR, Jr. Pretectal syndrome with metastatic malignant melanoma to the posterior commissure. Am J Ophthalmol 1976;82:910–914.

247. Partsalis AM, Highstein SM, Moschovakis AK. Lesions of the posterior commissure disable the vertical neural integrator of the primate oculomotor system. J Neurophysiol 1994;71:2582–2585.

248. Hepp K, Henn V. Spatio-temporal recoding of rapid eye movement signals in the monkey paramedian pontine reticular formation (PPRF). Exp Brain Res 1983;52:105–120.

249. Kaneko CR. Effect of ibotenic acid lesions of the omnipause neurons on saccadic eye movements in rhesus macaques. J Neurophysiol 1996;75:2229–2242.

250. Yan YJ, Cui DM, Lynch JC. Overlap of saccadic and pursuit eye movement systems in the brain stem reticular formation. J Neurophysiol 2001;86:3056–3060.

251. Fukushima K. The interstitial nucleus of Cajal in the midbrain reticular formation and vertical eye movements. Neurosci Res 1991;10:151–187.

252. Fukushima K, Kaneko CR. Vestibular integrators in the oculomotor system. Neurosci Res 1995;22:249–258.

253. Crawford JD, Cadera W, Vilis T. Generation of torsional and vertical eye position signals by the interstitial nucleus of Cajal. Science 1991;252:1551–1553.

254. Crawford JD. The oculomotor neural integrator uses a behaviour-related coordinate system. J Neurosci 1994;14:6911–6923.

255. Cannon SC, Robinson DA. Loss of the neural integrator of the oculomotor system from brainstem lesions in monkeys. J Neurophysiol 1987;57:1383–1409.

256. Cheron G, Godaux E. Disabling the oculomotor neural integrator by kainic acid injections of the prepositus-vestibular complex of the cat. J Physiol 1987;394:267–290.

257. Kaneko CR. Eye movement deficits after ibotenic acid lesions of the nucleus prepositus hypoglossi in monkeys. I. Saccades and fixation. J Neurophysiol 1997;78:1753–1768.

258. Kaneko CR. Eye movement deficits following ibotenic acid lesions of the nucleus prepositus hypoglossi in monkeys. II. Pursuit, vestibular, and optokinetic responses. J Neurophysiol 1999;81:668–681.

259. Arnold DB, Robinson DA, Leigh RJ. Nystagmus induced by pharmacological inactivation of the brainstem ocular motor integrator in monkey. Vision Res 1999;39:4286–4295.

260. Hess K, Reisine H, Dürsteler M. Normal eye drift and saccadic drift correction in darkness. Neuroophthalmology 1985;5:247–252.

261. Zee DS, Yamazaki A, Butler PH, et al. Effects of ablation of flocculus and paraflocculus on eye movements in primate. J Neurophysiol 1981;46:878–899.

262. Zee DS, Tusa RJ, Herdman SJ, et al. Effects of occipital lobectomy upon eye movements in primate. J Neurophysiol 1987;58:883–907.

263. Tweed D, Vilis T. Implications of rotational kinematics for the oculomotor system in three dimensions. J Neurophysiol 1987;58:832–849.

264. Van Gisbergen JAM, Robinson DA, Gielen S. A quantitative analysis of the generation of saccadic eye movements by burst neurons. J Neurophysiol 1981;45:417–442.

265. Scudder CA. A new local feedback model of the saccadic burst generator. J Neurophysiol 1988;59:1455–1475.
266. Pulaski PD, Zee DS, Robinson DA. The behavior of the vestibulo-ocular reflex at high velocities of head rotation. Brain Res 1981;222:159–165.
267. Jürgens R, Becker W, Kornhuber HH. Natural and drug-induced variations of velocity and duration of human saccadic eye movements: evidence for a control of the neural pulse generator by local feedback. Biol Cybern 1981;39:87–96.
268. Ashe J, Hain TC, Zee DS, et al. Microsaccadic flutter. Brain 1991;114:461–472.
269. Fisher B, Weber H, Biscaldi M, et al. Separate populations of visually guided saccades in humans: reaction times and amplitudes. Exp Brain Res 1993;92:528–541.
270. Kristjansson A, Chen Y, Nakayama K. Less attention is more in the preparation of antisaccades, but not prosaccades. Nature Neurosci 2001;4:1037–1042.
271. Olk B, Kingstone A. Why are antisaccades slower than prosaccades? A novel finding using a new paradigm. Neuroreport 2003;14:151–155.
272. Fox PT, Fox JM, Raichle ME, et al. The role of the cerebral cortex in the generation of voluntary saccades. J Neurophysiol 1985;54:348–369.
273. Petit L, Orssaud C, Tzourio N, et al. PET study of voluntary saccadic eye movements in humans: basal ganglia-thalamocortical system and cingulate cortex involvement. J Neurophysiol 1993;69:1009–1017.
274. Sweeney JA, Mintun MA, Kwee S, et al. Positron emission tomography study of voluntary saccadic eye movements and spatial working memory. J Neurophysiol 1996;75:454–468.
275. DeSouza JF, Menon RS, Everling S. Preparatory set associated with pro-saccades and anti-saccades in humans investigated with event-related FMRI. J Neurophysiol 2003;89:1016–1023.
276. Cornelissen FW, Kimmig H, Schira M, et al. Event-related fMRI responses in the human frontal eye fields in a randomized pro- and antisaccade task. Exp Brain Res 2002;145:270–274.
277. Godoy J, Luders H, Dinner DS, et al. Versive eye movements elicited by cortical stimulation of the human brain. Neurology 1990;40:296–299.
278. Anderson TJ, Jenkins IH, Brooks DJ, et al. Cortical control of saccades and fixation in man. A PET study. Brain 1994;117:1073–1084.
279. Funahashi S, Bruce CJ, Goldman-Rakic PS. Dorsolateral prefrontal lesions and oculomotor delayed response performance: evidence for mneumonic ''scotomas.'' J Neurosci 1993;13:1479–1497.
280. Goldberg ME, Bushnell MC. Behavioral enhancement of visual responses in monkey cerebral cortex: II. Modulation in frontal eye fields specifically related to saccades. J Neurophysiol 1981;46:773–787.
281. Tehovnik EJ, Sommer MA, Chou IH, et al. Eye fields in the frontal lobes of primates. Brain Res Rev 2000;32:413–418.
282. Robinson DA, Fuchs AF. Eye movements evoked by stimulation of frontal eye fields. J Neurophysiol 1969;32:637–648.
283. Seagraves MA. Activity of monkey frontal eye field neurons projecting to oculomotor regions of the pons. J Neurophysiol 1992;68:1967–1985.
284. Kanaseki T, Sprague JM. Anatomical organization of pretectal nuclei and tectal laminae in the cat. J Comp Neurol 1974;158:319–338.
285. Helminski JO, Segraves MA. Macaque frontal eye field input to saccade-related neurons in the superior colliculus. J Neurophysiol 2003;90:1046–1062.
286. Jayaraman A, Batton RR, Carpenter MB. Nigrotectal projection in the monkey: an autoradiographic study. Brain Res 1977;135:147–152.
287. Hikosaka O, Wurtz RH. Visual and oculomotor functions of monkey substantia nigra pars reticulata: I. Relation of visual and auditory responses to saccades. J Neurophysiol 1983;49:1230–1253.
288. Hikosaka O, Wurtz RH. Visual and oculomotor functions of monkey substantia nigra pars reticulata: II. Visual responses related to fixation of gaze. J Neurophysiol 1983;49:1254–1267.
289. Hikosaka O, Wurtz RH. Visual and oculomotor functions of monkey substantia nigra pars reticulata: III. Memory contingent visual and saccade responses. J Neurophysiol 1983;49:1268–1284.
290. Hikosaka O, Wurtz RH. Visual and oculomotor functions of monkey substantia nigra pars reticulata: IV. Relation of substantia nigra to superior colliculus. J Neurophysiol 1983;49:1285–1301.
291. Gaymard B, Lynch J, Plone CJ, et al. The parieto-collicular pathway: anatomical location and contribution to saccade generation. Eur J Neurosci 2003;17:1518–1526.
292. Sparks DL, Hartwich-Young R. The Deep Layers of the Superior Colliculus. Amsterdam, Elsevier, 1989.
293. Sparks DL. The brainstem control of saccadic eye movements. Nature Rev Neurosci 2002;3:952–964.
294. Munoz DP, Wurtz RH. Saccade-related activity in monkey superior colliculus. I. Characteristics of burst and buildup cells. J Neurophysiol 1995;73:2313–2333.
295. Munoz DP, Wurtz RH. Saccade-related activity in monkey superior colliculus. II. Spread of activity during saccades. J Neurophysiol 1995;73:2334–2348.
296. Soetedjo R, Kaneko CR, Fuchs AF. Evidence against a moving hill in the superior colliculus during saccadic eye movements in the monkey. J Neurophysiol 2002;87:2778–2789.
297. King WM, Precht W, Dieringer N. Afferent and efferent connections of cat omnipause neurons. Exp Brain Res 1980;38:395–403.
298. Yoshida K, et al. Disynaptic inhibition of omnipause neurons following electrical stimulation of the superior colliculus in alert cats. J Neurophysiol 2001;85:2639–2642.
299. Raybourn MS, Keller EL. Cooliculoreticular organization in primate oculomotor system. J Neurophysiol 1977;40:861–878.
300. May PJ, Porter JD. The laminar distribution of macaque tectobulbar and tectospinal neurons. Vis Neurosci 1992;8:257–276.
301. Sharpe JA. Adaptation to frontal lobe lesions. In: Keller EL, Zee D, eds. Adaptive processes in visual and oculomotor systems. Oxford: Pergamon Press, 1986:239–246.
302. Rivaud S, Muri RM, Gaymard B, et al. Eye movement disorders after frontal eye field lesions in humans. Exp Brain Res 1994;102:110–120.
303. Guitton D, Buchtel HA, Douglas RM. Frontal lobe lesions in man cause difficulties in suppressing reflexive glances and generating goal-directed saccades. Exp Brain Res 1985;58:455–472.
304. Pierrot-Deseilligny C, Rivaus S, Gaymard B, et al. Cortical control of reflexive visually guided saccades in man. Brain 1991;114:1473–1485.
305. Schiller PH, Sandell JH, Maunsell JHR. The effect of frontal eye field and superior colliculus lesions on saccadic latencies in the rhesus monkey. J Neurophysiol 1987;57:1033–1049.
306. Dias EC, Bruce CJ. Physioloigcal correlate of fixation disengagement in the primate's frontal eye field. J Neurophysiol 1994;72:2532–2537.
307. Lesser RP, Dinner DS, Leigh RJ, et al. Acute inactivation of the frontal eye fields does not eliminate the generation of contralateral saccades. Neurology 1984;34(Suppl 1):95.
308. Sharpe JA, Lo AW, Rabinovitch HE. Control of the saccadic and smooth pursuit systems after cerebral hemidecortication. Brain 1979;102:387–403.
309. Tusa RJ, Zee DS, Herdmann SJ. Effects of on unilateral cerebral cortical lesions on ocular motor behavior in monkeys. Saccades and quick phases. J Neurophysiol 1986;56:1509–1625.
310. Schiller PH, True SD, Conway JL. Deficits in eye movements following frontal eye field and superior colliculus ablations. J Neurophysiol 1980;44:1175–1189.
311. Keating EG, Gooley SG. Saccadic disorders caused by cooling the superior colliculus or frontal eye field, or from combined lesions of both structures. Brain Res 1988;438:247–255.
312. Wurtz RH, Albano JE. Visual-motor function of the primate superior colliculus. Annu Rev Neurosci 1980;3:189–226.
313. Albano JE, Mishkin M, Westbrook LE, et al. Visuomotor deficits following ablation of monkey superior colliculus. J Neurophysiol 1982;48:388–351.
314. Munoz DP, Wurtz RH. Role of the rostral superior colliculus in active fixation and execution of express saccades. J Neurophysiol 1992;67:1000–1002.
315. Russo GS, Bruce CJ. Neurons in the supplementary eye field of rhesus monkeys code visual targets and saccadic eye movements in an oculocentric coordinate system. J Neurophysiol 1996;76:825–848.
316. Lee K, Tehovnik EJ. Topographic distribution of fixation-related units in the dorsomedial frontal cortex of the rhesus monkey. Eur J Neurosci 1995;7:1005–1011.
317. Tehovnik EJ, Lee K. The dorsomedial frontal cortex of the rhesus monkey: topographic representation of saccades evoked by electrical stimulation. Exp Brain Res 1993;96:430–442.
318. Shook BL, Schlag-Ray M, Schlag J. Primate supplementary eye field: I. Comparative aspects of mesencephalic and pontine connections. J Comp Neurol 1990;301:618–642.
319. Tehovnik EJ, Lee K, Schiller PH. Stimulation-evoked saccades from the dorsomedial frontal cortex of the rhesus monkey following lesions of the frontal eye fields and superior colliculus. Exp Brain Res 1994;98:179–190.
320. Cohen B, Waitzman DM, Buttner-Ennever JA, et al. Horizontal saccades and the central midbrain reticular formation. Progress Brain Res 1986;64:243–256.
321. Crandall WF, Keller EL. Visual and oculomotor signal in the nucleus reticularis tegmenti pontis. J Neurophysiol 1985;54:1326–1345.
322. Pierrot-Deseilligny C, Israel I, Berthoz A, et al. Role of the different frontal lobe areas in the control of the horizontal component of memory-guided saccades in man. Exp Brain Res 1993;95:166–171.
323. Muri RM, Rivaud S, Vermersch AI, et al. Effects of transcranial magnetic stimulation over the region of the supplementary motor area during sequences of memory-guided saccades. Exp Brain Res 1995;104:163–166.
324. Isoda M, Tanji J. Contrasting neuronal activity in the supplementary and frontal eye fields during temporal organization of multiple saccades. J Neurophysiol 2003;90:3054–3065.
325. Petit L, Orssaud C, Tsourio N, et al. Functional anatomy of a prelearned sequence of horizontal saccades in human. J Neurosci 1996;16:3714–3716.
326. Keating EG, Gooley SG, Pratt SE, et al. Removing the superior colliculus silences eye movements normally evoked from stimulation of the parietal and occipital eye fields. Brain Res 1983;269:145–148.
327. Lynch JC, McLaren JW. Deficits of visual attention and saccadic eye movements after lesions of parietooccipital cortex in monkeys. J Neurophysiol 1989;61:74–90.
328. Andersen RA, Brotchie PR, Mazzoni P. Evidence for the lateral intraparietal area as the parietal eye field. Curr Opinion Neurobiol 1992;2:840–846.
329. Muri RM, Iba-Zizen MT, Derosier C, et al. Location of the human posterior eye field with functional magnetic resonance imaging. J Neurol Neurosurg Psychiatry 1996;60:445–448.

330. Barash S, Bracewell RM, Fogassi L, et al. Saccade related activity in the lateral inintraparietal area I; Temporal properties; comparison with area 7a. J Neurophysiol 1991;66:1095–2108.

331. Colby CL, Duhamel J-R, Goldberg ME. Visual, presaccadic and cognitive activation of single neurons in monkey lateral intraparietal area. J Neurophysiol 1996;76:2841–2852.

332. Stanton GB, Bruce CJ, Goldberg ME. Topography of projections to posterior cortical areas from the macaque frontal eye fields. J Comp Neurol 1995;353:291–305.

333. Lynch JC, McLaren JW. The Contribution of Parieto-Occipital Association Cortex to the Control of Slow Eye Movements. Oxford, UK, Pergamon, 1982.

334. O Scalaidhe SP, Albright TD, Rodman HR, et al. Effects of superior temporal polysensory area lesions on eye movements in the macaque monkey. J Neurophysiol 1995;73:1–19.

335. Mountcastle VB, Lynch JC, Georgopoulos A, et al. Posterior parietal association cortex of monkey: command functions for operations within extrapersonal space. J Neurophysiol 1975;38:871–908.

336. Robinson DL, Goldberg ME, Stanton GB. Parietal association cortex in the primate: sensory mechanisms and behavioral modulations. J Neurophysiol 1978;41:910–932.

337. Yin TCT, Mountcastle VB. Mechanisms of neural integration in the parietal lobe for visual attention. Fed Proc 1978;37:2251–2257.

338. Bushnell MC, Goldberg ME, Robinson DL. Behavioral enhancement of visual responses in monkey cerebral cortex: I. Modulation in posterior parietal cortex related to selective visual attention. J Neurophysiol 1981;46:755–772.

339. Posner MI, Walker JA, Fredrich FJ, et al. Effect of parietal injury on covert orientating of attention. J Neurosci 1984;4:1863–1874.

340. Corbetta M, Miezen FM, Shulman GI, et al. A PET study of visuospatial attention. J Neurosci 1993;13:1202–1226.

341. Tobler PN, Felblinger J, Burki M, et al. Functional organisation of the saccadic reference system processing extraretinal signals in humans. Vision Res 2001;41:1351–1358.

342. Walker R, Findlay JM, Young AW, et al. Disengaging neglect and hemianopia. Neuropsychologia 1991;29:1019–1027.

343. Bisley JW, Goldberg ME. The role of the parietal cortex in the neural processing of saccadic eye movements. Adv Neurol 2003;93:141–157.

344. Dürsteler MR, Wurtz RH, Newsome WT. Directional pursuit deficits following lesions of the foveal representation within the superior temporal sulcus of the macaque monkey. J Neurophysiol 1987;57:1262–1287.

345. Dürsteler MR, Wurtz RH. Pursuit and optokinetic deficits following chemical lesions of cortical areas MT and MST. J Neurophysiol 1988;60:940–965.

346. Thurston SE, Leigh RJ, Crawford T, et al. Two distinct deficits of visual tracking caused by unilateral lesions of cerebral cortex in humans. Ann Neurol 1988;23:266–273.

347. Morrow MJ, Sharpe JA. Retinotopic and directional deficits of smooth pursuit initiation after posterior cerebral hemispheric lesions. Neurology 1993;43:595–603.

348. Van Essen DC. Functional Organization of Primate Visual Cortex. New York, Plenum Press, 1985.

349. Hikosaka O, Sakamoto M, Usui S. Functional properties of monkey caudate nucleus. I. Activities related to saccadic eye movements. J Neurophysiol 1989;61:780–798.

350. Hikosaka O, Imai H, Sagawa M. Saccadic eye movements in parkinsonism. Basel, Switzerland, Japan Scientific Society Press and S Kaerger, 1992.

351. Hikosaka O, Sakamoto M, Miyashita N. Effects of caudate nucleus stimulation on substantia nigra cell activity in monkey. Exp Brain Res 1993;95:457–472.

352. Hikosaka O, Wurtz RH. Modification of saccadic eye movements by GABA related substances. I. Effect of muscimol and bicuculline in monkey superior colliculus. J Neurophysiol 1985;53:266–291.

353. Hikosaka O, Wurtz RH. Modification of saccadic eye movements by GABA-related substances. I. Effect of muscimol in monkey substantia nigra pars reticula. J Neurophysiol 1985;53:292–308.

354. Matsumura M, Kojima J, Gardiner TW, et al. Visual and oculomotor functions of monkey subthalamic nucleus. J Neurophysiol 1992;67:1615–1632.

355. Vermersch A-I, Muri RM, Rivaud S, et al. Saccade disturbances after bilateral lentiform nucleus lesions in humans. J Neurol Neurosurg Psychiatry 1996;60:179–184.

356. Schlag-Ray M, Schlag J. Visuomotor functions of the central thalamus in monkey. I. Unit activity related to spontaneous eye movements. J Neurophysiol 1984;51:1149–1174.

357. Schlag J, Schlag-Ray M. Visuomotor functions of the central thalamus in monkey. II. Unit activity related to visual events, targeting, and fixation. J Neurophysiol 1984;51:1175–1195.

358. Livingston CA, Fedder SR. Visual-ocular motor activity in the macaque pregeniculate complex. J Neurophysiol 2003;90:226–244.

359. Cohen B, Matsuo V, Fraden J, et al. Horizontal saccades elicited by stimulation of the central mesencephalic reticular formation. Exp Brain Res 1985;57:605–616.

360. Waitzman DM, Silakov VL, DePalma-Bowles S, et al. Effects of reversible inactivation of the primate mesencephalic reticular formation. I. Hypermetric goal-directed saccades. J Neurophysiol 2000;83:2260–2284.

361. Waitzman DM, Sikalov VL, Cohen B. Central mesencephalic reticular formation (cMRF) neurons discharging before and during eye movements. J Neurophysiol 1996;75:1546–1572.

362. Waitzman DM, Silakov VL, DePalma-Bowles S, et al. Effects of reversible inactivation of the primate mesencephalic reticular formation. II. Hypometric vertical saccades. J Neurophysiol 2000;83:2285–2299.

363. Takagi M, Zee DS, Tamargo RJ. Effects of lesions of the oculomotor vermis on eye movements in primate: saccades. J Neurophysiol 1998;80:1911–1931.

364. Kleine JF, Guan Y, Buttner U. Saccade-related neurons in the primate fastigial nucleus: what do they encode? J Neurophysiol 2003;90:3137–3154.

365. Hayakawa Y, Nakajima T, Takagi M, et al. Human cerebellar activation in relation to saccadic eye movements: a functional magnetic resonance imaging study. Ophthalmologica 2002;216:399–405.

366. Kase M, Miller DC, Noda H. Discharges of Purkinje cells and mossy fibers in the cerebellar vermis of the monkey during saccadic eye movements and fixation. J Physiol 1980;300:539–555.

367. McElligott JG, Keller EL. Neuronal Discharge in the Posterior Cerebellum: Its Relationship to Saccadic Eye Movement Generation. Oxford, UK, Pergamon, 1982.

368. Ohtsuka K, Noda H. Discharge properties of Purkinje cells in the oculomotor vermis during visually guided saccades in the macaque monkey. J Neurophysiol 1995;74:1828–1840.

369. Helmchen C, Büttner U. Saccade-related Purkinje cell activity in the oculomotor vermis spontaneous eye movements in light and darkness. Exp Brain Res 1995;103:198–208.

370. Ron S, Robinson DA. Eye movements evoked by cerebellar stimulation in the alert monkey. J Neurophysiol 1973;36:1004–1022.

371. McElligott JG, Keller EL. Cerebellar vermis involvement in monkey saccadic eye movements: Microstimulation. Exp Neurol 1984;86:543–558.

372. Optican LM, Robinson DA. Cerebellar-dependent adaptive control of the primate saccadic system. J Neurophysiol 1980;44:1058–1076.

373. Ritchie L. Effects of cerebellar lesions on saccadic eye movements. J Neurophysiol 1976;39:1246–1256.

374. Optican LM, Zee DS, Miles FA. Floccular lesions abolish adaptive control of post-saccadic ocular drift in primates. Exp Brain Res 1986;64:596–598.

375. Gonzalo-Ruiz A, Leichnetz GR. Afferents of the caudal fastifial nucleus in a New World monkey (Cebus apella). Exp Brain Res 1990;80:600–608.

376. Noda KH, Sugita S, Ikeda Y. Afferents and efferent connections of the oculomotor region of the fastigial nucleus of macaque monkeys. J Comp Neurol 1990;302:330–348.

377. Ikeda Y, Noda H, Sugita S. Olivocerebellar and cerebelloolivary connections of the oculomotor region of the fastigial nucleus in the macaque monkey. J Comp Neurol 1989;284:463–488.

378. Batton RR, Jayaraman A, Ruggiero D, et al. Fastigial efferent projections in a monkey: an autoradiographic study. J Comp Neurol 1977;174:281–306.

379. Fuchs AF, Robinson FR, Straube A. Role of the caudal fastigial nucleus in saccade generation. I. Neuronal discharge patterns. J Neurophysiol 1993;70:1723–1740.

380. Fuchs AF, Robinson FR, Straube A. Preliminary Observations on the Role of the Caudal Fastigial Nucleus in the Generation of Smooth-Pursuit Eye Movements. New York, Thieme Medical Publishers, 1994.

381. Robinson FR, Straube A, Fuchs AF. Role of the caudal fastigial nucleus in saccade generation. II. Effects of Muscimol inactivation. J Neurophysiol 1993;70:1741–1758.

382. Straube A, Helmchen C, Robinson F, et al. Saccadic dysmetria is similar in patients with a lateral medullary lesion and in monkeys with a lesion of the deep cerebellar nucleus. J Vestibular Res 1994;4:327–333.

383. Morrow MJ, Sharpe JA. Torsional nystagmus in the lateral medullary syndrome. Ann Neurol 1988;24:390–398.

384. Kommerell G, Hoyt WF. Lateropulsion of saccadic eye movements. Electroculographic studies in a patient with Wallenberg's syndrome. Arch Neurol 1973;28:313–318.

385. Waespe W, Wichmann W. Oculomotor disturbances during visual-vestibular interaction in Wallenberg's lateral medullary syndrome. Brain 1990;113:821–846.

386. Waespe W, Baumgartner R. Enduring dysmetria and impaired gain adaptivity of saccadic eye movements in Wallenberg's lateral medullary syndrome. Brain 1992;115:1125–1146.

387. Solomon D, Galetta SL, Liu GT. Possible mechanisms for horizontal gaze deviation and lateropulsion in the lateral medullary syndrome. J Neuroophthalmol 1995;51:26–30.

388. Ranalli PJ, Sharpe JA. Contrapulsion of saccades and ipsilateral ataxia: a unilateral disorder of the rostral cerebellum. Ann Neurol 1986;20:311–316.

389. Tilikete C, Hermier M, Pelisson D, et al. Saccadic lateropulsion and upbeat nystagmus: disorders of caudal medulla. Ann Neurol 2002;53:658–662.

390. Helmchen C, Straube A, Büttner U. Saccadic lateropulsion in Wallenberg's syndrome may be caused by a functional lesion of the fastigial nucleus. J Neurol 1994;241:421–426.

391. Sharpe JA, Morrow MJ, Newman NJ, et al. Continuum, Neuro-ophthalmology. Baltimore, Lippincott Williams & Wilkins, 1995.

392. Deubel H. Separate adaptive mechanisms for the control of reactive and volitional saccadic eye movements. Vision Res 1995;35:3529–3540.
393. Scudder CA, Batourina EY, Tunder GS. Comparison of two methods of producing adaptation of saccade size and implications for the site of plasticity. J Neurophysiol 1998;79:704–715.
394. Raymond JL. Learning in the oculomotor system: from molecules to behavior. Curr Opin Neurobiol 1998;8:770–776.
395. Barash S, Melikyan A, Sivakov A, et al. Saccadic dysmetria and adaptation after lesions of the cerebellar cortex. J Neurosci 1999;19:10931–10939.
396. Albano JE, King WM. Rapid adaptation of saccadic amplitude in humans and monkeys. Invest Ophthalmol Vis Sci 1989;30:1883–1893.
397. Chaturvedi V, van Gisbergen JA. Specificity of saccadic adaptation in three-dimensional space. Vision Res 1997;37:1367–1382.
398. Shelhamer M, Clendaniel R. Sensory, motor, and combined contexts for context-specific adaptation of saccade gain in humans. Neurosci Lett 2002;332:200–204.
399. Shelhamer M, Clendaniel RA. Context-specific adaptation of saccade gain. Exp Brain Res 2002;146:441–450.
400. Robinson FR, Fuchs AF, Noto CT. Cerebellar influences on saccade plasticity. Ann NY Acad Sci 2002;956:155–163.
401. Robinson FR, Fuchs AF. The role of the cerebellum in voluntary eye movements. Ann Rev Neurosci 2001;24:981–1004.
402. Scudder CA, McGee DM. Adaptive modification of saccade size produces correlated changes in the discharges of fastigial nucleus neurons. J Neurophysiol 2003;90:1011–1026.
403. Desmurget M, Pelisson D, Urquizar C, et al. Functional anatomy of saccadic adaptation in humans. Nature Neurosci 1998;1:524–528.
404. Thier P, Dicke PW, Haas R, et al. Encoding of movement time by populations of cerebellar Purkinje cells. Nature 2000;405:72–76.
405. Thier P, Dicke PW, Haas R, et al. The role of the oculomotor vermis in the control of saccadic eye movements. Ann NY Acad Sci 2002;978:50–62.
406. Inaba N, Iwamoto Y, Yoshida K. Changes in cerebellar fastigial burst activity related to saccadic gain adaptation in the monkey. Neurosci Res 2003;46:359–368.
407. Kommerell G, Olivier D, Theopold H. Adaptive programming of phasic and tonic components in saccadic eye movements: investigations in patients with abducens palsy. Invest Ophthalmol 1976;15:657–660.
408. Abel LA, Schmidt D, Dell'Osso LF, et al. Saccadic system plasticity in humans. Ann Neurol 1978;4:313–318.
409. Burr DC, Ross J. Contrast sensitivity at high velocities. Vision Res 1982;22:479–484.
410. Murphy BJ. Pattern thresholds for moving and stationary gratings during smooth eye movements. Vision Res 1978;18:521–530.
411. Steinbach MJ. Pursuing the perceptual rather than the retinal stimulus. Vision Res 1976;16:1371–1376.
412. Lisberger SG, Morris EJ, Tychsen L. Visual motion processing and sensory-motor integration for smooth pursuit eye movements. Ann Rev Neurosci 1987;10:97–129.
413. Pola J, Wyatt HJ. Target position and velocity: the stimuli for smooth pursuit eye movements. Vision Res 1980;20:523–534.
414. Segraves MA, Goldberg ME. Effect of stimulus position and velocity upon the maintenance of smooth pursuit eye velocity. Vision Res 1994;34:2477–2482.
415. Gresty M, Halmagyi M. Following eye movements in the absence of central vision. Acta Otolaryngologica 1979;87:477–483.
416. Steinbach MJ. Eye tracking of self-moved objects: the role of efference. J Exp Psychol 1969;82:366–376.
417. Gauthier GM, Hofferer JM. Eye tracking of self-moved targets in the absence of vision. Exp Brain Res 1976;26:121–139.
418. Mather JA, Lackner JR. The influence of efferent, proprioceptive, and timing factors on the accuracy of eye-hand tracking. Exp Brain Res 1981;43:406–412.
419. Leigh RJ, Zee DS. Eye movements of the blind. Invest Ophthalmol Vis Sci 1980;19:328–331.
420. Heywood S. Voluntary control of smooth eye movements and their velocity. Nature 1972;238:408–410.
421. Yasui S, Young LR. Perceived visual motion as effective stimulus to pursuit eye movement system. Science 1975;190:906–908.
422. Mack A, Fendrich R, Wong E. Is perceived motion a stimulus for smooth pursuit? Vision Res 1982;22:77–88.
423. Carl JR, Gellman RS. Human smooth pursuit: stimulus-dependent responses. J Neurophysiol 1987:1446–1463.
424. Morrow MJ, Sharpe JA. Smooth pursuit initiation in young and elderly subjects. Vision Res 1993;33:203–210.
425. Merrison AFA, Carpenter RHS. ''Express'' smooth pursuit. Vision Res 1995;35:1459–1462.
426. Krauzlis RJ, Miles FA. Release of fixation for pursuit and fixation and saccades in humans: evidence for shared inputs acting on different neural substrates. J Neurophysiol 1996;76:2822–2833.
427. Krauzlis RJ, Miles FA. Decreases in the latencies of smooth pusuit and saccadic eye movements produced by the gap paradigm in monkeys. Vision Res 1996;36:1973–1985.
428. Rashbass C. The relationship between saccadic and smooth tracking eye movements. J Physiol 1961;159:326–338.
429. Lisberger SG, Evinger C, Johanson GW, et al. Relation between eye acceleration and retinal image velocity during foveal smooth pursuit in man and monkey. J Neurophysiol 1981;46:229–249.
430. Tychsen L, Liesberger SG. Visual motion processing for the initiation of smooth-pursuit eye movements in humans. J Neurophysiol 1986;56:953–968.
431. Robinson DA, Gordon JL, Gordon SE. A model of the smooth pursuit eye movement system. Biol Cybernetics 1986;55:43–57.
432. Newsome WT, Wurtz RH, Komatsu H. Relation of cortical areas MT and MST to pursuit eye movements. III. Differentiation of retinal from extraretinal inputs. J Neurophysiol 1988;60:604–620.
433. Luebke AE, Robinson A. Transition dynamics between pursuit and fixation suggest different mechanisms. Vision Res 1988;28:941–946.
434. Meyer CH, Lasker AG, Robinson DA. The upper limit of human smooth pursuit velocity. Vision Res 1985;25:561–563.
435. Sharpe JA, Sylvester TO. Effect of aging on horizontal smooth pursuit. Invest Ophthalmol Vis Sci 1978;17:465–468.
436. Zackon DH, Sharpe JA. Smooth pursuit in senescence: effects of target acceleration and velocity. Acta Otolaryngol 1987;104:290–297.
437. Kim JS, Sharpe JA. The vertical vestibulo-ocular reflex, and its interaction with vision during active head motion: effects of aging. J Vestib Res 2001;11:13.
438. McKinley PA, Peterson BW. Voluntary modulation of the vestibuloocular reflex in humans and its relation to smooth pursuit. Exp Brain Res 1985;60:454–464.
439. Becker W, Fuchs AF. Prediction in the oculomotor system: smooth pursuit during transient disappearance of a visual target. Exp Brain Res 1985;57:562–575.
440. Kowler E, Steinman RM. The effect of expectations on slow oculomotor control. III. Guessing unpredictable target displacements. Vision Res 1981;21:191–203.
441. Livingstone MS, Hubel DH. Psychophysical evidence for separate channels for the perception of form, color, movement, and depth. J Neurosci 1987;7:3416–3468.
442. Livingstone MS, Hubel DH. Segregation of form, color, movement and depth: anatomy, physiology and perception. Science 1988;240:740–749.
443. DeYoe EA, Van Essen DC. Concurrent processing streams in monkey visual cortex. Trends Neurosci 1988;11:219–226.
444. Sunaert S, Van Hecke P, Marchal G, et al. Motion-responsive regions of the human brain. Exp Brain Res 1999;127:355–370.
445. Nakamura H, Kashii S, Nagamine T, et al. Human V5 demonstrated by magneto-encephalography using random dot kinematograms of different coherence levels. Neurosci Res 2003;46:423–433.
446. Schoenfeld MA, Woldorff M, Duzel E, et al. Form-from-motion: MEG evidence for time course and processing sequence. J Cogn Neurosci 2003;15:157–172.
447. Ahlfors SP, Simpson GV, Dale AM, et al. Spatiotemporal activity of a cortical network for processing visual motion revealed by MEG and fMRI. J. Neurophysiol 1999;82:2545–2555.
448. Ferber S, Humphrey GK, Vilis T. The lateral occipital complex subserves the perceptual persistence of motion-defined groupings. Cerebral Cortex 2003;13:716–721.
449. Morrow MJ, Sharpe JA. Cerebral hemispheric localization of smooth pursuit asymmetry. Neurology 1990;40:284–292.
450. Newsome WT, Wurtz RH, Dürsteler MR, et al. Deficits in visual motion processing following ibotenic acid lesions of the middle temporal visual area of the macaque monkey. J Neurosci 1985;5:825–840.
451. Newsome WT, Paré EB. A selective impairment of motion perception following lesions of the middle temporal visual area (MT). J Neurosci 1988;8:2201–2211.
452. Barton JJS, Simpson T, Kirakopolos E, et al. Functional MRI of lateral occipito-temporal cortex during pursuit and motion perception. Ann Neurol 1996;40:387–398.
453. Segraves MA, Goldberg ME, Deng S-Y, et al. The role of striate cortex in the guidance of eye movements in the monkey. J Neurosci 1987;7:3040–3058.
454. Barton JJS, Sharpe JA, Raymond JE. Retinotopic and directional deficits in motion discrimination in humans with cerebral lesions. Ann Neurol 1995;37:665–675.
455. Barton JJS, Sharpe JA. Smooth pursuit and saccades to moving targets in blind hemifields. A comparison of medial occipital, lateral occipital and optic radiation lesions. Brain 1997;120:681–689.
456. Barton JJS, Sharpe JA. Motion direction discrimination in blind hemifields. Ann Neurol 1997;41:255–264.
457. Ffytche D, Guy CN, Zeki S. Motion specific responses from a blind hemifield. Brain 1996;119:1971–1982.
458. Weiskrantz L. Roots of blindsight. Progress Brain Res 2004;144:229–241.
459. Komatsu H, Wurtz RH. Relation of cortical areas MT and MST to pursuit eye movements. I. Localization and visual properties of neurons. J Neurophysiol 1988;60:580–603.
460. Erickson RG, Dow BM. Foveal tracking cells in the superior temporal sulcus of the macaque monkey. Exp Brain Res 1989;78:113–131.
461. Kiorpes L, Walton PJ, O'Keefe LP, et al. Effects of early-onset artificial strabismus on pursuit eye movements and on neuronal responses in area MT of macaque monkeys. J Neurosci 1996;16:6537–6553.
462. Thier P, Erickson RG. Responses of visual-tracking neurons from cortical area MST-l to visual, eye and head motion. European J Neurosci 1992;4:539–553.
463. Komatsu H, Wurtz RH. Modulation of pursuit eye movements by stimulation of cortical areas MT and MST. J Neurophysiol 1989;62:31–47.

464. Maunsell JHR, Van Essen DC. Functional properties of neurons in middle temporal area of the macaque monkey: II. Binocular interactions and sensitivity to binocular disparity. J Neurophysiol 1983;49:1148–1167.

465. Tanaka K, Hikosaka H, Saito H, et al. Analysis of local and wide-field movement in the superior temporal visual areas of the macaque monkey. J Neurosci 1986; 6:134–144.

466. Hoffmann K-P, Distler C, Ilg U. Callosal and superior temporal sulcus contributions to receptive field properties in the macaque monkey's nucleus of the optic tract and dorsal terminal nucleus of the accessory optic tract. J Comp Neurol 1992;321:150–162.

467. Hoffmann K, Bremmer F, Thiele A, et al. Directional asymmetry of neurons in cortical areas MT and MST projecting to the NOT-DTN in macaques. J Neurophysiol 2002;87:2113–2123.

468. Heide W, Kurzidim K, Kompf D. Deficits of smooth pursuit eye movements after frontal and parietal lesions. Brain 1996;119:1951–1969.

469. Clarke S, Miklossy J. Occipital cortex in man: organization of callosal connections, related myelo- and cutoarchitecture, and putative boundaries of functional visual areas. J Comp Neurol 1990;298:188–214.

470. Baloh RW, Yee RD, Honrubia V. Optokinetic nystagmus and parietal lobe lesions. Ann Neurol 1980;7:269–276.

471. Sharpe JA, Deck JHN. Destruction of the internal sagittal stratum and normal smooth pursuit. Ann Neurol 1978;4:473–476.

472. Leigh RJ, Tusa RJ. Disturbance of smooth pursuit caused by infarction of occipitoparietal cortex. Ann Neurol 1985;17:185–187.

473. Bogousslavsky J, Regli F. Pursuit gaze defects in acute and chronic unilateral parieto-occipital lesions. Eur Neurol 1986;25:10–18.

474. Kömpf D. The signifcance of optokinetic nystagmus asymmetry in hemispheric lesions. Neuroophthalmology 1986;6:61–64.

475. Kjallman L, Frisén L. The cerebral ocular pursuit pathways. A clinicoradiological study of small-field optokinetic nystagmus. J Clin Neuroophthalmol 1986;6:209–214.

476. Heide W, Koenig E, Dichgans J. Optokinetic nystagmus, self-motion sensation and their after effects in patients with occipito-parietal lesions. Clin Vis Sci 1990;5:145–156.

477. Lekwuwa GU, Barnes GR. Cerebral control of eye movements. I. The relationship between cerebral lesions and smooth pursuit deficits. Brain 1996;119: 473–490.

478. Tusa RJ, Zee DS, Herdmann SJ. Recovery of Oculomotor Function in Monkeys with Large Unilateral Cortical Lesions. Oxford, UK, Pergamon, 1986.

479. Lekwuwa GU, Barnes GR. Cerebral control of eye movements. II. Timing of anticipatory eye movements, predictive pursuit and phase errors in focal cerebral lesions. Brain 1996;119:491–505.

480. Barton JJS, Sharpe JA. Directional defects in pursuit and motion perception in humans with unilateral cerebral lesions. Brain 1996;119:1535–1550.

481. Barton JJS, Sharpe JA. Ocular tracking of step-ramp targets by patients with unilateral cerebral lesions. Brain 1998;121:1165–1183.

482. Sharpe JA, Lo AW. Voluntary and visual control of the vestibuloocular reflex after cerebral hemidecortication. Ann Neurol 1981;10:164–172.

483. Tusa RJ, Ungerleider LG. Fiber pathways of cortical areas mediating smooth pursuit eye movements in monkeys. Ann Neurol 1988;23:174–183.

484. Desimone R, Ungerleider LG. Multiple visual areas in the caudal superior temporal sulcus of the macaque. J Comp Neurol 1986;248:164–189.

485. Ungerleider LG, Desimone R. Cortical connections of visual area MT in the macaque. J Comp Neurol 1986;248:190–222.

486. Boussaoud D, Ungerleider LG, Desimone R. Pathways for motion analysis: cortical connections of the medial superior temporal and fundus of the superior temporal visual areas in the macaque. J Comp Neurol 1990;206:462–495.

487. Morel A, Bullier J. Anatomical segregation of two cortical visual pathways in the macaque monkey. Vis Neurosci 1990;4:555–578.

488. Cusick CG, Scripter JL, Darensbourg JG, et al. Chemoarchitectonic subdivisions of the visual pulvinar in monkeys and their connectional relations with the middle temporal and rostral dorsolateral visual areas, MT and DLr. J Comp Neurol 1993;336:1–30.

489. Schall JD, Morel A, King DJ, Bullier J. Topography of visual cortex connections with frontal eye field in macaque: convergence and segregation of processing streams. J Neurosci 1995;15:4464–4487.

490. Lock TM, Baizer JS, Bender DB. Distribution of corticotectal cells in macaque. Exp Brain Res 2003;151:455–470.

491. Baizer JS, Ungerleider LG, Desimone R. Organization of visual inputs to the inferior temporal and posterior parietal cortex in macaques. J Neurosci 1991; 11:168–190.

492. Boussaoud D, Desimone R, Ungerleider LG. Subcortical connections of visual areas MST and FST in macaques. Vis Neurosci 1992;9:291–302.

493. Steele GE, Weller RE, Cusick CG. Cortical connections of the caudal subdivision of the dorsolateral area (V4) in monkeys. J Comp Neurol 1991;306:495–520.

494. Hyvärinen J, Poranen A. Function of the parietal associative area 7 as revealed from cellular discharges in alert monkeys. Brain 1974;97:673–692.

495. Lynch JC, Mountcastle VB, Talbot WH, et al. Parietal lobe mechanisms for directed visual attention. J Neurophysiol 1977;40:362–389.

496. Sakata H, Shibutani H, Kawano K. Functional properties of visual tracking neurons in posterior parietal cortex of the monkey. J Neurophysiol 1983;49: 1364–1380.

497. Kawano K, Sasaki M, Yamashita M. Response properties of neurons in posterior parietal cortex of monkey during visual-vestibular stimulation: I. Visual tracking neurons. J Neurophysiol 1984;51:340–351.

498. Kawano K, Sasaki M. Response properties of neurons in posterior parietal cortex of monkey during visual-vestibular stimulation: II. Optokinetic neurons. J Neurophysiol 1984;51:352–360.

499. Erickson RG, Thier P. A neuronal correlate of spatial stability during periods of self-induced visual motion. Exp Brain Res 1991;86:608–616.

500. German WJ, Fox JC. Observations following unilateral lobectomies. Association for Research and Nervous and Mental Disease 1934;13:378–434.

501. Cogan DG. Neurology of the Ocular Muscles. Springfield, IL, Charles C Thomas, 1948.

502. Cogan DG. Ophthalmic manifestations of bilateral non-occipital cerebral lesions. Br J Ophthalmol 1965;49:281–297.

503. Leigh RJ. The Cortical Control of Ocular Pursuit Movements. Paris, Revue Neurologique, 1989;145:605–620.

504. Bremmer F, Distler C, Hoffmann KP. Eye position effects in monkey cortex. II. Pursuit- and fixation-related activity in posterior parietal areas LIP and 7A. J Neurophysiol 1997;772:962–977.

505. Bremmer F, Ilg UJ, Thiele A, et al. Eye position effects in monkey cortex. I. Visual and pursuit-related activity in extrastriate areas MT and MST. J Neurophysiol 1997;77:944–961.

506. Petit L, Haxby JV. Functional anatomy of pursuit eye movements in humans as revealed by fMRI. J Neurophysiol 1999;82:463–471.

507. Berman RA, Colby CL, Genovese CR, et al. Cortical networks subserving pursuit and saccadic eye movements in humans: an FMRI study. Human Brain Mapping 1999;8:209–225.

508. Colby CL, Zeffiro T. Cortical activation in humans during visual and oculomotor processing measured by positron emission tomography (PET). Soc Neurosci Abstr 1990;16:621.

509. Reeves AG, Perret J, Jenkyn LR, et al. Pursuit gaze and the occipitoparietal region: a case report. Arch Neurol 1984;41:83–84.

510. Sharpe JA. Pursuit gaze and the occipito-parietal region: comment. Survey Ophthalmol 1985;29:453–454.

511. Lawden MC, Bagelmann H, Crawford TJ, et al. An effect of structured backgrounds on smooth pursuit eye movements in patients with cerebral lesions. Brain 1995;118:37–48.

512. Morrow MJ. Craniotopic defects of smooth pursuit and saccadic eye movement. Neurology 1996;46:514–521.

513. Sharpe JA, Morrow MJ. Cerebral hemispheric smooth pursuit disorders. Neuroophthalmology 1991;11:87–98.

514. MacAvoy MG, Gottlieb GP, Bruce CJ. Smooth-pursuit eye movement representation in the primate frontal eye field. Cerebral Cortex 1991;1:95–102.

515. Gottlieb JP, MacAvoy MG, Bruce CJ. Neural responses related to smooth-pursuit eye movements and their correspondence with electrically elicited smooth eye movements in the primate frontal eye field. J Neurophysiol 1994;72: 1634–1653.

516. Gottlieb JP, Bruce CJ, MacAvoy MG. Smooth eye movements elicited by microstimulation in the primate frontal eye field. J Neurophysiol 1993;69:786–799.

517. Keating EG. Frontal eye field lesions impair predictive and visually-guided pursuit eye movements. Exp Brain Res 1991;86:311–323.

518. Keating EG. Lesions of the frontal eye field impair pursuit eye movements, but preserve the predictions driving them. Behav Brain Res 1993;53:91–104.

519. Lynch JC. Frontal eye field lesions in monkeys disrupt visual pursuit. Exp Brain Res 1987;68:437–441.

520. Keating EG, Pierre A, Chopra S. Ablation of the pursuit area in the frontal cortex of the primate degrades foveal but not optokinetic smooth eye movements. J Neurophysiol 1996;76:637–641.

521. Morrow MJ, Sharpe JA. Deficits of smooth-pursuit eye movement after unilateral frontal lobe lesions. Ann Neurol 1995;37:443–451.

522. Tian JR, Lynch JC. Slow and saccadic eye movements evoked by microstimulation in the supplementary eye field of the cebus monkey. J Neurophysiol 1995; 74:2204–2210.

523. Missal M, Heinen SJ. Facilitation of smooth pursuit initiation by electrical stimulation in the supplementary eye fields. J Neurophysiol 2001;86:2413–2425.

524. Heinen SJ. Single neuron activity in the dorsomedial frontal cortex during smooth pursuit eye movements. Exp Brain Res 1995;104:357–361.

525. Colby CL, Duhamel J-R, Goldberg ME. Ventral intraparietal area of the macaque: Anatomic location and visual response properties. J Neurophysiol 1993; 69:902–914.

526. Fletcher WA, Sharpe JA. Smooth pursuit dysfunction in Alzheimer's disease. Neurology 1988;38:272–277.

527. Morrow MJ, Sharpe JA. The effects of head and trunk position on torsional vestibular and optokinetic eye movements in humans. Exp Brain Res 1993;95: 144–150.

528. Yamasaki DS, Wurtz RH. Recovery of function after lesions in the superior temporal sulcus in the monkey. J Neurophysiol 1991;66:651–673.

529. Leichnetz GR. Inferior frontal eye field projections to the pursuit-related dorso-

lateral pontine nucleus and middle temporal area (MT) in the monkey. Vis Neurosci 1989;3:171–180.

530. Distler C, Mustari MJ, Hoffmann KP. Cortical projections to the nucleus of the optic tract and dorsal terminal nucleus and to the dorsolateral pontine nucleus in macaques: a dual retrograde tracing study. J Comp Neurol 2002;444:144–158.

531. Giolli RA, Gregory KM, Suzuki D, et al. Cortical and subcortical afferents to the nucleus reticularis tegmenti pontis and basal pontine nuclei in the macaque monkey. Vis Neurosci 2001;18:725–740.

532. May JG, Keller EL, Suzuki DA. Smooth-pursuit eye movement deficits with chemical lesions in the dorsolateral pontine nucleus of the monkey. J Neurophysiol 1988;59:952–975.

533. Suzuki DA, Yamada T, Yee RD. Smooth-pursuit eye-movement–related neuronal activity in macaque nucleus reticularis tegmenti pontis. J Neurophysiol 2003;89:2146–2158.

534. Yamada T, Suzuki DA, Yee RD. Smooth pursuit-like eye movements evoked by microstimulation in macaque nucleus reticularis tegmenti pontis. J Neurophysiol 1996;76:3313–3324.

535. Suzuki DA, Yamada T, Hoedema R, et al. Smooth-pursuit eye-movement deficits with chemical lesions in macaque nucleus reticularis tegmenti pontis. J Neurophysiol 1999;82:1178–1186.

536. Langer T, Fuchs AF, Scudder CA, et al. Afferents to the flocculus of the cerebellum in the rhesus macaque as revealed by retrograde transport of horseradish peroxidase. J Comp Neurol 1985;235:1–25.

537. Thielert CD, Thier P. Patterns of projections from the pontine nuclei and the nucleus reticularis tegmenti pontis to the posterior vermis in the rhesus monkey: a study using retrograde tracers. J Comp Neurol 1993;337:113–26.

538. Keller EL, Heinen SJ. Generation of smooth-pursuit eye movements: neuronal mechanisms and pathways. Neurosci Res 1991;11:79–107.

539. Kato I, Watanabe J, Nakamura T, Harada K, et al. Mapping of brainstem lesions by the combined use of tests of visually induced eye movements. Brain 1990; 113:921–935.

540. Their P, Bachor A, Faiss J, et al. Selective impairment of smooth-pursuit eye movements due to an ischemic lesion of the basal pons. Ann Neurol 1991;29: 443–448.

541. Gaymard B, Pierrot-Desseilligny C, Rivaud S, et al. Smooth pursuit eye movement deficits after pontine nuclei lesions in humans. J Neurol Neurosurg Psychiatry 1993;56:799–807.

542. Yakushin SB, Gizzi M, Reisine H, et al. Functions of the nucleus of the optic tract (NOT). II. Control of ocular pursuit. Exp Brain Res 2000;131:433–437.

543. Ilg UJ, Hoffmann KP. Responses of monkey nucleus of the optic tract neurons during pursuit and fixation. Neurosci Res 1991;12:101–110.

544. Westheimer G, Blair SM. Oculomotor defects in cerebellectomized monkeys. Invest Ophthalmol 1973;12:618–621.

545. Westheimer G, Blair SM. Functional organization of primate oculomotor system revealed by cerebellectomy. Exp Brain Res 1974;21:463–472.

546. Rambold H, Churchland A, Selig Y, Jasmin L, et al. Partial ablations of the flocculus and ventral paraflocculus in monkeys cause linked deficits in smooth pursuit eye movements and adaptive modification of the VOR. J Neurophysiol 2002;87:912–924.

547. Noda H, Suzuki DA. Processing of eye movement signals in the flocculus of the monkey. J Physiol 1979;294:349–364.

548. Noda H, Suzuki DA. The role of the flocculus of the monkey in fixation and smooth pursuit eye movements. J Physiol 1979;294:335–348.

549. Suzuki DA, Keller EL. The role of the posterior vermis of monkey cerebellum in smooth-pursuit eye movement control. I. Eye and head movement-related activity. J Neurophysiol 1988;59:1–18.

550. Suzuki DA, Keller EL. The role of the posterior vermis of monkey cerebellum in smooth-pursuit eye movement control. II. Target velocity-related Purkinje cell activity. J Neurophysiol 1988;59:19–40.

551. Sato H, Noda H. Posterior vermal Purkinje cells in macaques responding during saccades, smooth pursuit, chair rotation and/or optokinetic stimulation. Neurosci Res 1992;12:583–595.

552. Krauzlis RJ, Lisberger SG. Directional organization of eye movement and visual signals in the floccular lobe of the monkey cerebellum. Exp Brain Res 1996; 109:289–302.

553. Lisberger SG, Fuchs AF. Role of primate flocculus during rapid behavioral modification of vestibulo-ocular reflex: I. Purkinje cell activity during visually guided horizontal smooth pursuit eye movements and passive head rotation. J Neurophysiol 1978;41:733–763.

554. Krauzlis R, Lisberger SG. Visual motion commands for pursuit eye movements in the cerebellum. Science 1991;253:568–571.

555. Takagi M, Zee DS, Tamargo RJ. Effects of lesions of the oculomotor cerebellar vermis on eye movements in primate: smooth pursuit. J Neurophysiol 2000;83: 2047–2062.

556. Straube A, Scheuerer W, Eggert T. Unilateral cerebellar lesions affect initiation of ipsilateral smooth pursuit eye movements in humans. Ann Neurol 1997;42: 891–898.

557. Fuchs AF, Robinson FR, Straube A. Participation of the caudal fastigial nucleus in smooth-pursuit eye movements. I. Neuronal activity. J Neurophysiol 1994; 72:2714–2718.

558. Robinson FR, Straube A, Fuchs AF. Participation of caudal fastigial nucleus in

smooth pursuit eye movements. II. Effects of muscimol inactivation. J Neurophysiol 1997;78:848–859.

559. Buttner U, Straube A, Spuler A. Saccadic dysmetria and ''intact'' smooth pursuit eye movements after bilateral deep cerebellar nuclei lesions. J Neurol Neurosurg Psychiatry 1994;57:832–834.

560. Lisberger SG, Pavelko TA, Broussard DM. Responses during eye movements of brainstem neurons that receive monosynaptic inhibition from the flocculus and ventral paraflocculus in monkeys. J Neurophysiol 1994;72:909–927.

561. Broussard DM, de Charms RC, Lisberger SG. Input from the ipsilateral and contralateral vestibular apparatus to behaviorally-characterized abducens neurons in rhesus monkeys. J Neurophysiol 1995;74:2445–2459.

562. Langer T, Fuchs AF, Chubb MC, et al. Floccular efferents in the rhesus macaque as revealed by autoradiography and horseradish peroxidase. J Comp Neurol 1985;235:26–37.

563. Cullen KE, McCrea RA. Firing behaviour of brain stem neurons during voluntary cancellation of the horizontal vestibuloocular reflex I. Secondary vestibular neurons. J Neurophysiol 1993;70:828–843.

564. Cullen KE, McCrea RA. Firing behaviour of brain stem neurons during voluntary cancellation of the horizontal vestibuloocular reflex. II. Eye movement related neurons. J Neurophysiol 1993;70:844–856.

565. Roy JE, Cullen KE. Brain stem pursuit pathways: dissociating visual, vestibular, and proprioceptive inputs during combined eye-head gaze tracking. J Neurophysiol 2003;90:271–290.

566. Scudder CA, Fuchs AF. Physiological and behavioural identification of vestibular nucleus neurons mediating the horizontal vestibuloocular reflex in trained rhesus monkeys. J Neurophysiol 1992;68:244–264.

567. McFarland JL, Fuch AF. Discharge patterns of the nucleus prepositus hypoglossi and adjacent medial vestibular nucleus during horizontal eye movement in behaving macaques. J Neurophysiol 1992;68:319–332.

568. Yamada J, Noda H. Afferent and efferent connections of the oculomotor cerebellar vermis in the macaque monkey. J Comp Neurol 1987;265:224–241.

569. Missal M, et al. Common inhibitory mechanism for saccades and smooth-pursuit eye movements. J Neurophysiol 2002;88:1880–1892.

570. Keller EL, Missal M. Shared brainstem pathways for saccades and smooth-pursuit eye movements. Ann NY Acad Sci 2003;1004:29–39.

571. Johnston JL, Sharpe JA, Morrow MJ. Paresis of contralateral smooth pursuit and normal vestibular smooth eye movements after unilateral brainstem lesions. Ann Neurol 1992;31:495–502.

572. Baloh RW, Yee RD, Honrubia V. Eye movements in patients with Wallenberg's syndrome. Ann NY Acad Sci 1981;374:600–613.

573. Robinson DA. The mechanics of human smooth pursuit eye movement. J Physiol 1965;180:569–591.

574. Daroff RB, Hoyt WF. Supranuclear disorders of ocular control systems in man. In: Bach-y-Rita P, Collins CC, Hyde J, eds. The control of eye movements. New York: Academic Press, 1971:117–235.

575. Tomlinson RD, Robinson DA. Signals in vestibular nucleus mediating vertical eye movements in the monkey. J Neurophysiol 1984;51:1121–1136.

576. Chubb MC, Fuchs AF. Contribution of y-group of vestibular nuclei and dentate nucleus of cerebellum to generation of vertical smooth eye movements. J Neurophysiol 1982;48:75–99.

577. King WM, Lisberger SG, Fuchs AF. Response of fibers in medial longitudinal fasciculus (MLF) of alert monkeys during horizontal and vertical conjugate eye movements evoked by vestibular or visual stimuli. J Neurophysiol 1976;39: 1135–1149.

578. Pola J, Robinson DA. Oculomotor signals in medial longitudinal fasciculus of the monkey. J Neurophysiol 1978;41:245–259.

579. Carpenter MB, Cowie RJ. Connections and oculomotor projections of the superior vestibular nucleus and cell group 'y'. Brain Res 1985;336:265–287.

580. Ranalli PJ, Sharpe JA. Vertical vestibulo-ocular reflex, smooth pursuit, and eye-head tracking dysfunction in internuclear ophthalmoplegia. Brain 1988;111: 1299–1317.

581. Baloh RW, Furman JM, Yee RD. Dorsal midbrain syndrome: clinical and oculographic findings. Neurology 1985;35:54–60.

582. Sharpe JA, Kim JS. Midbrain disorders of vertical gaze: a quantitative re-evaluation. Ann NY Acad Sci 2002;956:143–154.

583. King WM, Fuchs AF, Magnin M. Vertical eye movement-related responses of neurons in midfrain near interstitial nucleus of Cajal. J Neurophysiol 1981;46: 549–562.

584. Missal M, de Brouwer S, Lefevre P, et al. Activity of mesencephalic vertical burst neurons during saccades and smooth pursuit. J Neurophysiol 2000;83: 2080–2092.

585. Semmlow JL. Oculomotor responses to near stimuli: the near triad. In: Zuber B, ed. Models of oculomotor behavior and control. Boca Raton, FL: CRC Press, 1981:161–191.

586. Westheimer G, Mitchell AM. Eye movement responses to convergent stimuli. Arch Ophthalmol 1956;55:848–856.

587. Semmlow JL, Hung GK. Accommodative and fusional components of fixation disparity. Invest Ophthalmol Vis Sci 1979;18:1082–1086.

588. Semmlow JL, Venkiteswaran N. Dynamic accommodative vergence components in binocular vision. Vision Res 1976;16:403–410.

589. Semmlow JL, Wetzel P. Dynamic contributions of the components of binocular vergence. J Optical Soc Am 1979;69:639–645.

590. Hung GK, Semmlow JL, Ciuffreda KJ. Identification of accommodative vergence contribution to the near response using response variance. Invest Ophthalmol Vis Sci 1983;24:772–777.

591. Kenyon RV, Ciuffreda KJ, Stark L. Binocular eye movements during accommodative vergence. Vision Res 1978;18:545–565.

592. Ramat S, Das VE, Somers JT, et al. Tests of two hypotheses to account for different-sized saccades during disjunctive gaze shifts. Exp Brain Res 1999;129:450–510.

593. Busettini C., Fitzgibbon E, Miles F. Short-latency disparity vergence in humans. J Neurophysiol 2001;85:1129–1152.

594. Robinson DA. The mechanics of human vergence eye movement. J Pediatr Ophthalmol 1966;3:31–37.

595. Ramat S, Somers JT, Das VE, et al. Conjugate ocular oscillations during shifts of the direction and depth of visual fixation. Invest Ophthalmol Vis Sci 1999;40:1681–1686.

596. Bhidayasiri R, Somers JT, Kim JI, et al. Ocular oscillations induced by shifts of the direction and depth of visual fixation. Ann Neurol 2001;49:24–28.

597. Collewijn H, Erkelens CJ, Stinman RM. Voluntary binocular gaze-shifts in the plane of regard: dynamics of version and vergence. Vision Res 1985;35:3335–3358.

598. Erkelens CJ, Stinman RM, Collewijn H. Ocular vergence under natural conditions. II. Gaze-shifts between real targets differing in distance and directions. Proc R Soc Lond Biol Sci 1989;236:441–465.

599. Zee DS, Fitzgibbon EJ, Optican LM. Saccade-vergence interactions in humans. J Neurophysiol 1992;68:1624–1641.

600. Manning KA, Riggs LA. Vergence eye movements and visual suppression. Vision Res 1984;24:521–526.

601. Rashbass C, Westheimer G. Disjunctive eye movements. J Physiol 1961;159:339–360.

602. Fincham EF, Walton J. The reciprocal actions of accommodation and convergence. J Physiol 1957;137:488–508.

603. Keller EL, Robinson DA. Abducens unit behavior in the monkey during vergence eye movements. Vision Res 1972;12:369–382.

604. Keller EL. Accommodative vergence in the alert monkey. Motor unit analysis. Vision Res 1973;13:1565–1575.

605. Robinson DA, Keller EL. The behavior of eye movement motoneurons in the alert monkey. Bibliotheca Ophthalmologica: Supplementa Ophthalmologica 1972;82:7–16.

606. Mays LE, Porter JD. Neural control of vergence movements: Activity of abducens and oculomotor neurons. J Neurophysiol 1984;52:743–761.

607. Büttner-Ennever JA, Akert K. Medial rectus subgroups of the oculomotor nucleus and their abducens internuclear input in the monkey. J Comp Neurol 1981;197:17–27.

608. Porter JD, Guthrie BL, Sparks DL. Innervation of monkey extraocular muscles: localization of sensory and motor neurons by retrograde transport of horseradish peroxidase. J Comp Neurol 1983;218:208–219.

609. Mays LE. Neural control of vergence eye movements: convergence and divergence neurons in the midbrain. J Neurophysiol 1984;51:1091–1108.

610. Mays LE, Porter JD, Gamlin PDR, et al. Neural control of vergence eye movements: neurons encoding vergence velocity. J Neurophysiol 1986;56:1007–1021.

611. Judge S, Cumming BG. Neurons in the monkey midbrain with activity related to vergence eye movement and accommodation. J Neurophysiol 1986;555:915–930.

612. Busettini C, Mays LE. Pontine omnipause activity during conjugate and disconjugate eye movements in macaques. J Neurophysiol 2003;90:3838–3853.

613. Zhang Y, Mays LE, Gamlin PDR. Characterisitics of near response cells projecting to oculomotor nucleus. J Neurophysiol 1992;67:944–960.

614. Gamlin PDR, Gnadt JW, Mays LE. Abducens internuclear neurons carrying inappropriate signal for ocular convergence. J Neurophysiol 1989;62:70–81.

615. Clendaniel RA, Mays LE. Characteristics of antidromically identified oculomotor internuclear neurons during vergence and versional eye movements. J Neurophysiol 1994;71:1111–1127.

616. Gamlin PDR, Gnadt JW, Mays LE. Lidocaine-induced unilateral internuclear ophthalmoplegia: effects on convergence and conjugate eye movements. J Neurophysiol 1989;62:82–95.

617. Gnadt JW, Gamblin PDR, Mays LE, et al. Vergence-related cells near the abducens nuclei. Soc Neurosci Abstr 1988;14:612.

618. Gamlin PD, Yoon K. An area for vergence eye movement in primate frontal cortex. Nature 2000;407:1003–1007.

619. Fukushima K, Yamanobe T, Shinmei Y, et al. Coding of smooth eye movements in three-dimensional space by frontal cortex. Nature 2002;419:157–162.

620. Poggio GF, Gonzalez F, Krause F. Stereoscopic mechanisms in monkey visual cortex binocular correlation and disparity selectivity. J Neurosci 1988;8:4531–4550.

621. Takemura A, Inoue Y, Kawano K, at al. Single-unit activity in cortical area MST associated with disparity-vergence eye movements: evidence for population coding. J Neurophysiol 2001;85:2245–2266.

622. Motter BC, Mountcastle VB. The functional properties of the light-sensitive neurons of the posterior parietal cortex studied in waking monkeys: foveal sparing and opponent vector organization. J Neurosci 1981;1:326.

623. Gnadt JW, Mays LE. Neurons in monkey parietal area LIP are tuned for eye-movements in three-dimensional space. J Neurophysiol 1995;73:280–297.

624. Gamlin PD, Clarke RJ. Single-unit activity in the primate nucleus reticularis tegmenti pontis related to vergence and ocular accommodation. J Neurophysiol 1995;17:2115–2119.

625. Gamlin PD, Yoon K, Zhang H. The role of the cerebro-ponto-cerebellar pathways in the control of vergence eye movements. Eye 1996;10:167–171.

626. Zhang H, Gamlin PD. Neurons in the posterior interposed nucleus of the cerebellum related to vergence and accommodation. I. Steady-state characteristics. J Neurophysiol 1998;79:1255–1269.

627. Miles FA, Fuller JH, Braitman DJ, Dow BM. Long-term adaptive changes in primate vestibulo-ocular reflex: III. Electrophysiological observations in flocculus of normal monkeys. J Neurophysiol 1980;43:1437–1476.

628. Virre E, Tweed D, Milner K, et al. A re-examination of the gain of the vestibulo-ocular reflex. J Neurophysiol 1986;56:439–450.

629. Snyder LH, King WM. Effect of viewing distance and location of the axis of head rotation on the monkey's vestibuloocular reflex I. Eye movement responses. J Neurophysiol 1992;67:861–874.

630. Balaban CD, Watanabe E. Functional representation of eye movement in the flocculus of monkeys (Macaca fuscata). Neurosci Lett 1984;49:199–205.

631. Judge SJ. Optically-induced changes in tonic vergence and AC/A ratio in normal monkeys and monkeys with lesions of the flocculus and ventral paraflocculus. Exp Brain Res 1987;66:1–9.

632. Akman S, Dayanir V, Sanac A, et al. Acquired esotropia as presenting sign of cranial-cervical junction anomalies. Neuroophthalmology 1995;15:311–314.

633. Lewis AR, Kline LB, Sharpe JA. Acquired esotropia due to Arnold-Chiari I malformation. J Neuroophthalmol 1996;16:49–54.

634. Versino M, Hurko O, Zee DS. Disorders of binocular control of eye movements in patients with cerebellar dysfunction. Brain 1996;119:1933–1950.

635. Ito M, Nisimaru N, Yamamoto M. Pathways for the vestibulo-ocular reflex excitation arising from semicircular canals of rabbits. Exp Brain Res 1976;24:257–271.

636. Steinman RM, Haddad GM, Skavenski AA, et al. Miniature eye movements. Science 1973;181:810–819.

637. Ferman L, Collewijn H, Jansen TC, et al. Human gaze stability in the horizontal, vertical and torsional direction during horizontal head movements, evaluated with three-dimensional sclero induction coil technique. Vision Res 1987;27:811–828.

638. Ditchburn RW. The function of small saccades. Vision Res 1980;20:271–272.

639. Martinez-Conde S, Macknik SL, Hubel DH. Microsaccadic eye movements and firing of single cells in the striate cortex of macaque monkeys. Nature Neurosci 2000;3:251–258.

640. Winterson BJ, Collewijn H. Microsaccades during finely guided visuomotor tasks. Vision Res 1976;16:1387–1390.

641. Kowler E, Steinman RM. Small saccades serve no useful purpose [reply to a letter]. Vision Res 1980;20:273–276.

642. Hamstra SJ, Sinha T, Hallett PE. The joint contributions of saccades and ocular drift to repeated ocular fixations. Vision Res 2001;41:1709–1721.

643. Hafed ZM, Clark JJ. Microsaccades as an overt measure of covert attention shifts. Vision Res 2002;42:2533–2545.

644. Engbert R, Kliegl R. Microsaccades uncover the orientation of covert attention. Vision Res 2003;43:1035–1045.

645. Martinez-Conde S, Macknik SL, Hubel DH, et al. Microsaccadic eye movements and firing of single cells in the striate cortex of macaque monkeys. Nature Neurosci 2000;3:251–258.

646. Ditchburn RW, Ginsborg BL. Vision with a stabilized retinal image. Nature 1952;170:36–37.

647. Spauschus A, Marsden J, Halliday DM, et al. The origin of ocular microtremor in man. Exp Brain Res 1999;126:4556–4562.

648. Herishanu YO, Sharpe JA. Normal square wave jerks. Invest Ophthalmol Vis Sci 1981;20:268–272.

649. Shaffer DM, Krisky CM, Sweeney JA. Frequency and metrics of square-wave jerks: Influences of task-demand characteristics. Invest Ophthalmol Vis Sci 2003;44:1082–1087.

650. Sharpe JA, Herishanu YO, White OB. Cerebral square wave jerks. Neurology 1982;321:57–62.

651. Holmes G. Spasm of fixation. Trans Ophthalmol Soc UK 1930;50:253–262.

652. Johnston JL, Sharpe JA. The initial vestibulo-ocular reflex and its visual enhancement and cancellation in humans. Exp Brain Res 1994;99:302–308.

653. Leigh RJ, Huebner WP, Gordon JL. Supplementation of the human vestibulo-ocular reflex by visual fixation and smooth pursuit. J Vestib Res 1994;4:347–353.

654. Kelly BJ, Rosenberg ML, Zee DS, et al. Unilateral pursuit-induced congenital nystagmus. Neurology 1989;39:414–416.

655. Johnston JL, Sharpe JA, Morrow MJ. Spasm of fixation: a quantitative study. J Neurol Sci 1992;107:166–171.

656. Bair W, O'Keefe LP. The influence of fixational eye movements on the response of neurons in area MT of the macaque. Vis Neurosci 1998;15:779–786.

657. Suzuki H, Azuma M. Prefrontal neuronal activitiy during gazing at a light spot in the monkey. Brain Res 1977;126:497–508.

658. Funahashi S, Bruce CJ, Goldman-Rakic PS. Visuospatial coding in primate prefrontal neurons revealed by oculomotor paradigms. J Neurophysiol 1990;63: 813–831.

659. Funahashi S, Chaffe MV, Goldman-Rakic PS. Prefrontal neuronal activity in rhesus monkeys performing a delayed anti-saccade task. Nature 1993;365: 753–758.

660. Goldberg ME, Bushnell MC, Bruce CJ. The effect of attentive fixation of eye movements evoked by electrical stimulation of the frontal eye fields. Exp Brain Res 1986;61:579–584.

661. Gusnard DA, Raichle ME, Raichle ME. Searching for a baseline: functional imaging and the resting human brain. Nature Rev Neurosci 2001;2:685–694.

662. Paus T, Kalina M, Patockova L, et al. Medial versus lateral frontal lobe lesions and differential impairment of central-gaze fixation maintenance in man. Brain 1991;114:2051–2067.

663. Sharpe JA. Neural control of ocular motor systems. In: Miller NR, Newman NJ, eds. Walsh and Hoyt's Clinical Neuro-ophthalmology. Baltimore, Lippincott Williams & Wilkins, 1998:1101–1167.

664. Leigh RJ, Zee DS. The Neurology of Eye Movements. Oxford, Oxford University Press, 1999.

665. Bronstein AM, Hood JD. The cervico-ocular reflex in normal subjects and patients with absent vestibular function. Brain Res 1986;373:399–408.

666. Jurgens R, Mergner T. Interaction between cervico-ocular and vestibulo-ocular reflexes in normal adults. Exp Brain Res 1989;77:381–390.

667. Sawyer RNJ, Thurston SE, Becker KR, et al. The cervico-ocular reflex of normal human subjects in response to transient and sinusoidal trunk rotations. J Vestib Res 1994;4:245–249.

668. Kasai T, Zee DS. Eye-head coordination in labyrinthine-defective human beings. Brain Res 1978;144:123–141.

669. Keshner EA, Peterson BW. Mechanisms controlling human head stabilization. I. Head-neck dynamics during random rotations in the horizontal plane. J Neurophysiol 1995;73:2293–2301.

670. Keshner EA, Cromwell RL, Peterson BW. Mechanisms controlling human head stabilization. II. Head-neck characteristics during random rotations in the vertical plane. J Neurophysiol 1995;73:2302–2312.

671. Cullen KE, Roy JE, Sylvestre PA. Signal processing by vestibular nuclei neurons is dependent on the current behavioral goal. Ann NY Acad Sci 2001;942: 345–346.

672. Roy JE, Cullen KE. Vestibuloocular reflex signal modulation during voluntary and passive head movements. J Neurophysiol 2002;87:2337–2357.

673. Tomlinson RD. Combined eye-head gaze shifts in the primate. III: Contributions to the accuracy of gaze saccades. J Neurophysiol 1990;64:1873–1891.

674. Wilson VJ, Melvill Jones G. Mammalian Vestibular Physiology. New York, Plenum, 1979.

675. Maas EF, Huebner WP, Seidman SH, et al., Leigh RJ. Behaviour of human horizontal vestibulo-ocular reflex in response to high acceleration stimuli. Brain Res 1989;499:153–156.

676. Tabak S, Collewijn H. Human vestibulo-ocular responses to rapid, helmet-driven head movements. Exp Brain Res 1994;102:367–378.

677. Collewijn H, Smeets JB. Early components of the human vestibulo-ocular response to head rotation: latency and gain. J Neurophysiol 2000;84:376–389.

678. Miles FA, Kawano K. Visual stabilization of the eyes. Trends Neurosci 1987; 10:153–158.

679. Gellman RS, Carl JR, Miles FA. Short latency ocular following responses in man. Vis Neurosci 1990;5:107–122.

680. Stott JRR. The vertical vestibulo-ocular reflex and ocular resonance. Vision Res 1984;24:949–960.

681. Gauthier GB, Piron JP, Roll JP, et al. High-frequency vestibulo-ocular reflex activation through forced head rotation. Aviation Space Environmental Med 1984;55:1–7.

682. Vercher JL, Gauthier GM, Marchetti E, et al. Origin of eye movements induced by high-frequency rotation of the head. Aviation Space Environmental Med 1984;55:1046–1050.

683. Grossman GE, Leigh RJ, Abel LA, et al. Frequency and velocity of rotational head pertubations during locomotion. Exp Brain Res 1988;70:470–476.

684. Grossman GE, Leigh RJ, Bruce EN, et al. Performance of the human vestibulo-ocular reflex during locomotion. J Neurophysiol 1989;62:264–272.

685. Paige GD. The influence of target distance on eye movement responses during vertical linear motion. Exp Brain Res 1989;77:585–593.

686. Paige GD, Tomko DL. Eye movement responses to linear head motion in the squirrel monkey I: Basic characteristics. J Neurophysiol 1991;65:1170–1182.

687. Paige GD, Telford L, Seidman SH, et al. Human vestibuloocular reflex and its interactions with vision and fixation distance during linear and angular head movement. J Neurophysiol 1998;80:2391–2404.

688. Ramat S, Zee DS, Shelhamer MJ. Ocular motor responses to abrupt interaural head translation in normal humans. J Neurophysiol 2003;90:887–902.

689. Tian JR, Crane BT, Demer JL. Vestibular catch-up saccades augmenting the human transient heave linear vestibulo-ocular reflex. Exp Brain Res 2003;151: 435–445.

690. Vilis T. Interactions between the angular and translational components of the vestibulo-ocular reflex. In: Sharpe JA, Barber HO, eds. New York, Raven Press, 1993:117–124.

691. Snyder LH, Lawrence DM, King WM. Changes in vestibulo-ocular reflex (VOR) anticipate changes in vergence angle in monkey. Vision Res 1992;32:569–575.

692. Angelaki DE, Hess BJ. Three-dimensional organization of otolith-ocular reflexes in rhesus monkeys. I. Linear acceleration responses during off-vertical axis rotation. J Neurophysiol 1996;75:2405–2424.

693. Angelaki DE, Hess BJ. Three-dimensional organization of otolith-ocular reflexes in rhesus monkeys. II. Inertial detection of angular velocity. J Neurophysiol 1996;75:2425–2440.

694. Curthoys IS. Eye movements produced by utricular and saccular stimulation. Aviation Space Environmental Med 1987;58(Suppl):A192–A197.

695. Collewijn H, Van der Steen J, Ferman L, et al. Human ocular counter roll: assessment of static and dynamic properties from electromagnetic scleral coil recordings. Exp Brain Res 1985;59:185–196.

696. Suzuki JI, Tokumasu K, Goto K. Eye movements from single utricular nerve stimulation in the cat. Acta Otolaryngol 1969;68:350–362.

697. Uchino Y, Sasaki M, Sato H, et al. Utriculoocular reflex arc of the cat. J Neurophysiol 1996;76:1896–1903.

698. Westheimer G, Blair SM. The ocular tilt reaction: a brainstem oculomotor routine. Invest Ophthalmol 1975;14:833–839.

699. Rabinovitch HE, Sharpe JA, Silvester TO. The ocular tilt reaction. Arch Ophthalmol 1977;95:1395–1398.

700. Halmagyi JM, Brant TH, Dieterich M, et al. Tonic contraversive ocular tilt reaction due to unilateral meso-diencephalic lesion. Neurology 1990;40: 1503–1509.

701. Zackon DH, Sharpe JA. The ocular tilt reaction and skew deviation. In: Sharpe JA, Barber HO, eds. The vestibulo-ocular reflex and vertigo. New York, Raven Press, 1993:129–140.

702. Brandt T, Dieterich M. Skew deviation with ocular torsion: a vestibular brainstem sign of topographic diagnostic value. Ann Neurol 1993;33:528–534.

703. Van der Steen J, Collewijn H. Ocular stability in the horizontal, frontal and sagittal planes in the rabbit. Exp Brain Res 1984;56:263–274.

704. Harris L, Beykirch K, Fetter M. The visual consequences of deviations in the orientation of the axis of rotation of the human vestibulo-ocular reflex. Vision Res 2001;41:3271–3281.

705. Jauregui-Renaud K, Faldon M, Clarke A, et al. Skew deviation of the eyes in normal human subjects induced by semicircular canal stimulation. Neurosci Lett 1996;205:135–137.

706. Jauregui-Renaud K, Faldon ME, Gresty M, et al. Horizontal ocular vergence and the three-dimensional response to whole-body roll motion. Exp Brain Res 2001;136:79–82.

707. Fluur E, Mellström A. Utricular stimulation and oculomotor reactions. Laryngoscope 1970;80:1701–1712.

708. Isu N, Graf W, Sato H, et al. Sacculo-ocular reflex connectivity in cats. Exp Brain Res 2000;131:262–268.

709. Hwang JC, Poon WF. An electrophysiological study of the sacculo-ocular pathways in cats. Jpn J Physiol 1981;25:241–251.

710. Partsalis AM, Zhang Y, Highstein SM. Dorsal Y group in the squirrel monkey. I. Neuronal responses during rapid and long-term modifications of the vertical VOR. J Neurophysiol 1995;73:615–631.

711. McCrea RA, Strassman A, May E, et al. Anatomical and physiological characteristics of vestibular neurons mediating the horizontal vestibulo-ocular reflex of the squirrel monkey. J Comp Neurol 1987;264:547–570.

712. Reisine H, Strassman A, Highstein SM. Eye position and head velocity signals are conveyed to medial rectus motoneurons in the alert cat by the ascending tract of Deiters. Brain Res 1981;211:153–157.

713. Chen-Huang C, McCrea RA. Viewing distance related sensory processing in the ascending tract of deiters vestibulo-ocular reflex pathway. J Vestib Res 1998; 8:175–184.

714. Nguyen L, Baker R, Spencer RF. Abducens internuclear and ascending tract of Deiters inputs to medial rectus motoneurons in the cat oculomotor nucleus: synaptic organization. J Comp Neurol 1999;405:141–159.

715. Cohen B, Suzuki I. Eye movements induced by ampullary nerve stimulation. Am J Physiol 1963;204:347–351.

716. Cohen B. The Vestibulo-ocular Reflex Arc. New York, Springer-Verlag, 1974.

717. McCrea RA, Stassman A, Highstein SM. Anatomical and physiological characteristics of vestibular neurons mediating the vertical vestibulo-ocular reflexes of the squirrel monkey. J Comp Neurol 1987;264:571–594.

718. Uchino Y, Suzuki S. Axon collaterals to the extraocular motoneuron pools of inhibitory vestibuloocular neurons activated from the anterior, posterior and horizontal semicircular canals in the cat. Neurosci Lett 1983;37:129–135.

719. Hirai N, Uchino Y. Superior vestibular nucleus neurones related to the excitatory vestibulo-ocular reflex of anterior canal origin and their ascending course in the cat. Neurosci Res 1984;1:73–79.

720. Graf W, Ezure K. Morphology of vertical canal related second-order vestibular neurons in the cat. Exp Brain Res 1986;63:35–48.

721. Uchino Y, Hirari N, Watanabe S. Vestibulo-ocular reflex from the posterior canal nerve to extraocular motoneurons in the cat. Exp Brain Res 1978;32: 377–388.

722. Graf W, McCrea RA, Baker R. Morphology of posterior canal related secondary vestibular neurons in rabbit and cat. Exp Brain Res 1983;52:125–138.

723. Tokumasu K, Goto K, Cohen B. Eye movements from vestibular nuclei stimulation in monkeys. Ann Otol Rhinol Laryngol 1969;78:1105–1119.

724. Blazquez P, Partsalis A, Gerrits NM, et al. Input of anterior and posterior semicircular canal interneurons encoding head-velocity to the dorsal Y group of the vestibular nuclei. J Neurophysiol 2000;83:2891–2904.

725. Ventre J, Faugier-Grimaud S. Projections of the temporo-parietal cortex on vestibular complex in the macaque monkey (Macaca fascicularis). Exp Brain Res 1988;72:653–658.

726. Steiger HJ, Buttner-Ennever JA. Oculomotor nucleus afferents in the monkey demonstrated with horseradish peroxidase. Brain Res 1979;160:1–15.

727. Gonzalo-Ruiz A, Leichnetz GR, Smith DJ. Origin of cerebellar projections to the region of the oculomotor complex, medial pontine reticular formation, and superior colliculus in New World monkeys: a retrograde horseradish peroxidase study. J Comp Neurol 1988;268:508–526.

728. Galiana HL, Outerbrege JS. A bilateral model for central neural pathways in vestibuloocular reflex. J Neurophysiol 1984;51:210–241.

729. Anastasio TJ, Robinson DA. Failure of the oculomotor neural integrator from a discrete midline lesion between the abducens nuclei in the monkey. Neurosci Lett 1991;127:82–86.

730. Kokkoroyannis T, Scudder CA, Balaban CD, et al. Anatomy and physiology of the primate interstitial nucleus of Cajal: I. Efferent projections. J Neurophysiol 1996;75:725–739.

731. Buttner-Ennever JA, Horn AK. Pathways from cell groups of the paramedian tracts to the floccular region. Ann NY Acad Sci 1996;781:532–540.

732. Nakamagoe K, Iwamoto Y, Yoshida K. Evidence for brainstem structures participating in oculomotor integration. Science 2000;288:857–859.

733. Cohen B, Matsuo V, Raphan T. Quantitative analysis of the velocity characteristics of optokinetic nystagmus and optokinetic after-nystagmus. J Physiol 1977; 270:321–344.

734. Raphan T, Matsuo V, Cohen B. Velocity storage in the vestibulo-ocular reflex arc (VOR). Exp Brain Res 1979;35:229–248.

735. Cohen B, Henn V, Raphan T, et al. Velocity storage, nystagmus and visual-vestibular interactions in humans. Ann NY Acad Sci 1981;374:421–433.

736. Schrader V, Koenig E, Dichgans J. The effect of lateral head tilt on horizontal postrotatory nystagmus I and II and the Purkinje effect. Acta Otolaryngol 1985; 100:98–105.

737. Solomon D, Cohen B. Stimulation of the nodulus and uvula discharges velocity storage in the vestibulo-ocular reflex. Exp Brain Res 1994;102:57–68.

738. Waespe W, Cohen B, Raphan T. Dynamic modification of the vestibulo-ocular reflex by the nodulus and uvula. Science 1985;228:199–202.

739. Hain TC, Zee DS, Maria BL. Tilt suppression of vestibulo-ocular reflex in patients with cerebellar lesions. Acta Otolaryngol 1988;105:13–20.

740. Yokota J-I, Reisine H, Cohen B. Nystagmus induced by electrical stimulation of the vestibular and prepositus hypoglossi nuclei in the monkey: evidence for the site of induction of velocity storage. Exp Brain Res 1992;92:123–138.

741. Buttner UW, Büttner U, Henn V. Transfer characteristics of neurons in vestibular nuclei of the alert monkey. J Neurophysiol 1978;41:1614–1628.

742. Dizio P, Lackner JR. Influence of gravitational force level on vestibular and visual velocity storage in yaw and pitch. Vision Res 1992;32:111–120.

743. Katz E, Vianney de Jong JMB, Buettner-Ennever J, et al. Effects of midline section on velocity storage and the vestibulo-ocular reflex. Exp Brain Res 1991; 87:505–520.

744. Barnes GR. Visual-vestibular interaction in the control of head and eye movement: the role of visual feedback and predictive mechanisms. Progress Neurobiol 1993;41:435–472.

745. Sharpe JA, Goldberg HJ, Lo AW, et al. Visual-vestibular interaction in multiple sclerosis. Neurology 1981;31:427–433.

746. Das VE, Leigh RJ, Thomas CW, et al. Modulation of high-frequency vestibulo-ocular reflex during visual tracking in humans. J Neurophysiol 1995;74: 624–632.

747. Lisberger SG. Visual tracking in monkeys: evidence for short-latency suppression of the vestibuloocular reflex. J Neurophysiol 1990;63:676–688.

748. Halmagyi GM, Gresty MA. Clinical signs of visual-vestibular interaction. J Neurol Neurosurg Psychiatry 1979;42:934–939.

749. Chambers BR, Gresty MA. The relationship between disordered pursuit and vestibulo-ocular reflex suppression. J Neurol Neurosurg Psychiatry 1983;46: 61–66.

750. Barr CC, Schultheis LW, Robinson DA. Voluntary, non-visual control of the human vestibulo-ocular reflex. Acta Otolaryngol 1976;81:365–375.

751. Carmichael EA, Dix MR, Hallpike CS, et al. Some further observations upon the effect of unilateral cerebral lesions on caloric and rotational nystagmus. Brain 1961;84:571–584.

752. Pasik P, Pasik T, Bender MB. Oculomotor function following cerebral hemidecortication in the monkey: a study with special reference to optokinetic and vestibular nystagmus. Arch Neurol 1960;3:298–305.

753. Estanol B, Romero R, Saenz de Viteri M, et al. Oculomotor and oculovestibular functions in a hemispherectomy patient. Arch Neurol 1980;37:365–368.

754. Ventre J, Faugier-Grimaud S. Effects of posterior parietal lesions (area 7) on VOR in monkeys. Exp Brain Res 1986;62:654–658.

755. Gauthier GM, Robinson DA. Adaptation of the human vestibuloocular reflex to magnifying lenses. Brain Res 1975;92:331–335.

756. Demer JL, Porter FI, Goldberg J, et al. Adaptation to telescopic spectacles: vestibulo-ocular reflex plasticity. Invest Ophthalmol Vis Sci 1989;30:159–170.

757. Paige GD, Sargent EW. Visually-induced adaptive plasticity in the human vestibulo-ocular reflex. Exp Brain Res 1991;84:25–34.

758. Crane B, Demer JL. Effect of adaptation to telescopic spectacles on the initial human horizontal vestibuloocular reflex. J Neurophysiol 2000;83:38–49.

759. Cannon SC, Leigh RJ, Zee DA, et al. The effect of rotational magnification of corrective spectacles on the quantitative evaulation of the VOR. Acta Otolaryngol 1985;100:81–88.

760. Melvill Jones G. Plasticity in the adult vestibulo-ocular reflex arc. Phil Trans R Soc Lond Biol Sci 1977;278:319–314.

761. Yagi T, Shimizu M, Sekine S, Kamio T. New neurotological test for detecting cerebellar dysfunction: vestibulo-ocular reflex changes with horizontal vision-reversal prisms. Ann Otol Rhinol Laryngol 1981;90:276–280.

762. Gonshor A, Melvill Jones G. Changes of human vestibulo-ocular response induced by vision-reversal during head rotation. J Physiol 1973;234:102P–103P.

763. Melvill Jones G, Gonshor A. Oculomotor response to rapid head oscillation (0.5–5.0 Hz) after prolonged adaptation to vision-reversal: ''simple'' and ''complex'' effects. Exp Brain Res 1982;45:45–58.

764. Trillenberg P, Shelhamer M, Roberts DC, et al. Cross-axis adaptation of torsional components in the yaw-axis vestibulo-ocular reflex. Exp Brain Res 2003;148: 158–165.

765. Wong AM, Tweed D, Sharpe JA. The vestibulo-ocular reflex in fourth nerve palsy: deficits and adaptation. Vision Res 2002;42:2205–2218.

766. Wong AMF, Sharpe JA. Adaptations and deficits in the vestibulo-ocular reflex after third nerve palsy. Arch Ophthalmol 2002;120:360–368.

767. Wong AMF, Tweed D, Sharpe JA. Adaptations and deficits in the vestibulo-ocular reflex after sixth nerve palsy. Invest Ophthalmol Vis Sci 2002;43:99–111.

768. Lisberger SG, Miles FA, Zee DS. Signals used to compute errors in monkey vestibuloocular reflex: possible role of flocculus. J Neurophysiol 1984;52: 1140–1153.

769. Watanabe E. Neuronal events correlated with long-term adaptation of the horizontal vestibulo-ocular reflex in the primate flocculus. Brain Res 1984;297: 169–174.

770. Luebke AE, Robinson DA. Gain changes of the cat's vestibulo-ocular reflex after flocculus deactivation. Exp Brain Res 1994;98:379–390.

771. Partsalis AM, Zhang Y, Highstein SM. Dorsal Y group in the squirrel monkey. II. Contribution of the cerebellar flocculus to neuronal responses in normal and adapted animals. J Neurophysiol 1995;73:632–650.

772. Nagao S, Kitazawa H. Effects of reversible shutdown of the monkey flocculus on the retention of adaptation of the horizontal vestibulo-ocular reflex. Neurosci Lett 2003;118:563–570.

773. Lisberger SG. Neural basis for motor learning in the vestibuloocular reflex of primates. III Computation and behavioural analysis of the sites of learning. J Neurophysiol 1994;72:974–998.

774. Blazquez PM, Hirata Y, Heiney SA, et al. Cerebellar signatures of vestibulo-ocular reflex motor learning. J Neurosci 2003;2330:9741–9742.

775. Feil R, Hartmann J, Luo C, et al. Impairment of LTD and cerebellar learning by Purkinje cell-specific ablation of cGMP-dependent protein kinase. J Cell Biol 2003;163:295–302.

776. Broussard DM, Kassardjian CD. Learning in a simple motor system. Learn Memory 2004;11:127–146.

777. Yee RD, Daniels SA, Jones OW, et al. Effects of an optokinetic background on pursuit eye movements. Invest Ophthalmol Vis Sci 1983;24:1115–1122.

778. Collewijn H, Tamminga EP. Human smooth and saccadic eye movements during voluntary pursuit of different target motions on different backgrounds. J Physiol 1984;351:217–250.

779. Miles FA. The sensing of rotational and translational optic flow by the primate optokinetic system. Rev Oculomot Res 1993;5:393–403.

780. Fletcher WA, Hain TC, Zee DS. Optokinetic nystagmus and afternystagmus in human beings: Relationship to nonlinear processing of information about retinal slip. Exp Brain Res 1990;81:46–52.

781. Schor CM, Narayan V, Westall C. Postnatal development of optokinetic after nystagmus in human infants. Vision Res 1983;23:1643–1647.

782. Westall CA, Schor CM. Asymmetries of optikinetic nystagmus in amblyopia: the effect of selected retinal stimulation. Vision Res 1985;25:1431–1438.

783. Van Die G, Collewijn H. Control of human optokinetic nystagmus by the central and peripheral retina: effects of partial visual field masking, scotopic vision and central retinal scotomata. Brain Res 1986;383:185–194.

784. Shawkat F, Harris CM, Taylor DS, et al. The optokinetic response differences between congenital profound and nonprofound unilateral visual deprivation. Ophthalmology 1995;102:1615–1622.

785. Mehdorn E. Naso-temporal asymmetry of the optokinetic nystagmus after bilateral occipital infarction in man. In: Lennerstrand G, Zee D, Keller EL, eds. Functional basis of ocular motility disorders. Oxford: Pergamon Press, 1982: 321–324.

786. Baloh RW, Yee RD, Honrubia V. Clinical Abnormalities of Optokinetic Nystagmus. Oxford, UK, Pergamon, 1982.

787. Suzuki Y, Shinmei Y, Nara H, et al. Effects of a fixation target on torsional optokinetic nystagmus. Invest Ophthalmol Vis Sci 2000;41:2954–2959.

788. Bohmer A, Baloh RW. Vertical optokinetic nystagmus and optokinetic afternystagmus in humans. J Vestib Res 1990–1991;1:309–315.

789. Baloh RW, Yee RD, Honrubia V. Late cortical cerebellar atrophy: clinical and oculographic features. Brain 1986;109:159–180.

790. Miles FA, Kawano K, Optican LM. Short-latency ocular following responses of monkey. I. Dependence on temporal spatial properties of the visual input. J Neurophysiol 1986;56:1321–1354.

791. Miles FA. Short-latency visual stabilization mechanisms that help to compensate for translational disturbances of gaze. Ann NY Acad Sci 1999;871:260–271.

792. Masson GS, Yang DS, et al. Reversed short-latency ocular following. Vision Res 2002;42:2081–2087.

793. Precht W. Anatomical and functional organization of optikinetic pathways. In: Lennerstrand G, Zee D, Keller EL, eds. Functional basis of ocular motility disorders. Oxford: Pergamon Press, 1982:291–302.

794. Fuchs AF, Mustari MJ. The optokinetic response in primates and its possible neuronal substrate. Rev Oculomot Res 1993;5:343–369.

795. Maekawa K, Takeda T. Origin of descending afferents to the rostral part of dorsal cap of inferior olive which transfers contralateral optic activities to the flocculus: a horseradish peroxidase study. Brain Res 1979;172:393–405.

796. Waespe W, Henn V. Gaze stabilization in the primate. The interaction of the vestibuloocular reflex optokinetic nystagmus and smooth pursuit. Rev Physiol Biochem Pharmacol 1987;106:33–125.

797. Zee DS, Yee RD, Robinson DA. Optokinetic responses in labyrinthine-defect of human beings. Brain Res 1976;113:423–428.

798. Brindley GS, Gautier-Smith PC, Lewin W. Cortical blindness and the functions of the nongeniculate fibres of the optic tracts. J Neurol Neurosurg Psychiatry 1969;32:259–264.

799. Ter Braak JWG, Schenk VWD, Van Vliet AGM. Visual reactions in a case of long-lasting cortical blindness. J Neurol Neurosurg Psychiatry 1971;34:140–147.

800. Fox C, Holmes G. Optic nystagmus and its value in the localization of cerebral lesions. Brain 1926;39:333–371.

801. Fox C. Disorders of optic nystagmus due to cerebral tumors. Arch Neurol Psychiatry 1932;28:1007–1029.

802. Pasik T, Pasik P. Optokinetic nystagmus: an unlearned response altered by sectioning of chiasma and corpus callosum in monkeys. Nature 1964;203:609–611.

803. Kawano K, Shidara M, Watanabe Y, et al. Neuroactivity in cortical area MST of alert monkeys during ocular following responses. J Neurophysiol 1994;71:2305–2324.

Principles and Techniques of the Examination of Ocular Motility and Alignment

Mark S. Borchert

In the previous chapter, we discussed the anatomy and physiology of the major intracranial and extracranial structures that control eye movements. In this chapter, we discuss normal and abnormal monocular and binocular eye movements as they pertain to the techniques used in the examina-tion of patients with disorders of ocular motility. The reader in further pursuit of the subjects considered in this chapter should consult the books by Nelson and Catalano (1), Leigh and Zee (2), and von Noorden (3).

HISTORY

A careful history should always precede a complete exam-ination of the ocular motor system. Patients with ocular motor disorders may complain of a number of visual difficul-ties, including diplopia, visual confusion, blurred vision, and the vestibular symptoms of vertigo, oscillopsia, or tilt.

DIPLOPIA

Since misalignment of the visual axes causes the image of an object of interest to fall on noncorresponding parts of the two retinas, usually the fovea of one eye and the extrafo-veal retina of the other eye, a sensory phenomenon occurs that is usually interpreted as *diplopia*, the visualization of an object in two different spatial locations. Depending on the nature of the misalignment, the diplopia may be horizontal, vertical, torsional, or a combination of these.

Diplopia that results from ocular misalignment disappears with either eye closed: it is a binocular phenomenon. Binocu-lar diplopia is almost never caused by intraocular disease, although Burgess et al. reported a series of patients who developed binocular diplopia from the presence of a subreti-nal neovascular membrane in one eye (4). The pathophysiol-ogy of binocular diplopia with uniocular disease is unclear, but it may represent the establishment of rivalry between central and peripheral fusion mechanisms.

Diplopia that persists with one eye closed, *monocular di-plopia*, is rarely caused by neurologic disease. In almost all cases, it is produced by local ocular phenomena, including uncorrected astigmatism or other refractive errors, corneal and iris abnormalities, cataract, and macular disease (5–10). Most patients with this type of monocular diplopia will rec-ognize a difference in the intensity of the two images they see. One image will be fairly clear, but the second image will be perceived as "fuzzy" and may be described as a "ghost image" that overlaps the clear image.

Rare cases of monocular diplopia and polyopia are occasionally reported in patients with central nervous system disease (11–15). Patients with "cerebral polyopia" usually do not complain of overlapping images and generally see each image with equal clarity. In addition, the monocular diplopia in these patients is always seen with both eyes (i.e., with either eye covered). Such patients usually have lesions in the parieto-occipital region. The mechanism of cerebral diplopia-polyopia is unknown. Bender postulated that an instability of fixation from occipital disease could produce rapid ocular excursions with consequent stimulation of retinal areas or "competing maculae" (11). Other evidence suggesting a role for the occipital lobe in the pathogenesis of cerebral diplopia or polyopia came from the work of Brindley and Lewin, who stimulated different sites in the visual cortex of a patient who was blind from glaucoma (16). The patient reported seeing two, three, or multiple points of light.

Monocular diplopia is occasionally described by patients after surgery to correct congenital strabismus (3,17). In such patients, it is believed that a portion of the extrafoveal retina in the previously deviated eye has been used as a "fovea" for many years. Once the true foveae of the two eyes are aligned, there is apparently a sensory conflict in the previously deviated eye between the true fovea and the portion of the retina that previously corresponded to the fovea of the opposite eye. Such patients may complain of monocular diplopia or binocular triplopia. These symptoms usually disappear with time.

Monocular diplopia may be a complaint of individuals with no evidence of ocular or cerebral disease. Such patients should not undergo extensive neurologic or neuroimaging evaluations.

Thus, in any patient complaining of "diplopia," one should first determine if it is binocular or monocular. If the diplopia is monocular and the patient is otherwise healthy, the examiner may concentrate on ocular, rather than neurologic or myopathic, disorders that affect ocular alignment. In patients with binocular diplopia, the eyes are presumably misaligned, and the examiner should ascertain whether the diplopia is horizontal, vertical, or so forth; if it is better or worse in any particular direction of gaze; if it is different when viewing at distance or near; and if it is affected by head posture.

VISUAL CONFUSION

In patients with misalignment of the visual axes, the maculae of the two eyes are simultaneously viewing two different objects or areas. Occasionally, both macular images may be interpreted as existing at the same point in space. This sensory phenomenon is called *visual confusion*. Patients with visual confusion complain that the images of objects of interest are superimposed on inappropriate backgrounds.

BLURRED VISION

Misalignment of the visual axes does not always produce diplopia or visual confusion. In some patients, the images of an object seen by noncorresponding parts of the retina are so close together that the patient does not recognize diplopia but instead complains that the vision is blurred when both eyes are open. Similarly, some patients interpret visual confusion not as image superimposition but as simple "blurred vision." Blurred vision that exists only with both eyes viewing is quite common in the early stages of an ocular motor nerve paresis. In such patients, the blurred vision clears completely if either eye is closed.

Blurred vision that resolves with one but not either eye closed usually suggests a primary visual sensory disturbance. Blurred vision that does not resolve with either eye closed also usually occurs from visual sensory disease but may also occur in some patients with disorders of saccades (e.g., saccadic oscillations such as ocular flutter; see Chapter 23) and in patients with impaired pursuit leading to disordered tracking.

VESTIBULAR SYMPTOMS: VERTIGO, OSCILLOPSIA, AND TILT

Patients with disorders that affect the vestibular system may complain of disequilibrium or unsteadiness, symptoms that reflect imbalance of vestibular tone. A common complaint of patients with vestibular imbalance is *vertigo*, the illusory sensation of motion of self or of the environment. Vertigo usually reflects a mismatch between vestibular, visual, and somatosensory inputs concerning the position or motion of one's body in space (see Chapter 17) (18). Although it is helpful to question patients with vertigo as to the direction of their vertiginous illusions, they are often uncertain because their vestibular sense indicates head rotation in one direction, whereas their eye movements (the slow phases of vestibular nystagmus) are producing visual image movements that connote rotation of the head in the opposite direction. It is best to evaluate the vestibular sense alone by asking the patient about the perceived direction of self-rotation with the eyes closed, thus eliminating conflicting visual stimuli.

Oscillopsia is an illusory to-and-fro movement of the environment that may be horizontal, vertical, torsional, or a combination of these directions. It is usually caused by an instability of fixation from mechanical or neurologic disorders (19–21). When oscillopsia is produced or accentuated by head movement, it is usually of vestibular origin. Oscillopsia is rarely present when ocular motor dysfunction is congenital.

A third group of vestibular symptoms include the perception of *tilts*—static rotations of the perceived world or the body. These complaints usually reflect a disturbance of the otolith organs, from either peripheral or central causes (see also Wallenberg's syndrome in Chapter 19) (22). When dealing with such patients, as with patients who complain of vertigo, the examiner should ask about the perception of the positions of the body with the eyes closed, to eliminate conflicting visual stimuli.

EXAMINATION

The examination of the ocular motor system generally consists of the assessment of (*a*) fixation and gaze-holding ability, (*b*) range of monocular and binocular eye movements, (*c*) ocular alignment, and (*d*) performance of versions (saccades, pursuit). In addition, depending upon the findings of the basic examination, it may be appropriate to test the vestibulo-ocular and optokinetic reflexes and to attempt mechanically to move the eyes using forced duction testing.

FIXATION AND GAZE-HOLDING ABILITY

Principles

In an awake individual, the eyes are never absolutely still. Fixation is interrupted by three distinctive types of miniature eye movements: (*a*) microsaccades, with an average amplitude of about 6 minutes of arc and a mean frequency of about 2 per second; (*b*) continuous microdrift at rates of less than 20 minutes of arc/second; and (*c*) microtremor, consisting of high frequency (40–60 Hz) oscillations of 5–30 seconds of arc (23–25). Square wave jerks—spontaneous, horizontal saccades of about 0.5°, followed about 200 msec later by a corrective saccade and occurring at a rate of less than 9 per minute—can also be observed during fixation in normal individuals. Herishanu and Sharpe suggested that in normal individuals, square wave jerks are sporadically enlarged microsaccades (26). St. Cyr and Fender (27) postulated that the spontaneous eye movements that occur during fixation correct minor fixation errors, whereas Ditchburn (28) believed that such movements may prevent images from fading on the retina. Kowler and Steinman, however, stated that these small saccades serve no useful purpose, since vision remains clear when they are voluntarily suppressed (29).

When no efforts are being made toward ocular fixation or accommodation, the eyes are said to be in a ''physiologic'' position of rest. With total ophthalmoplegia, there is usually a slight divergence of the visual axes, and this position usually also occurs during sleep, deep anesthesia, and death (30–35).

Technique

In patients complaining of intermittent diplopia, visual confusion, or strabismus, tests of sensory fusion (e.g., stereoacuity) and fixation should be performed before the eyes are dissociated by tests of monocular visual function (e.g., visual acuity, color vision, visual fields).

The initial part of the ocular motor examination should consist of a careful study of fixation (36). The patient should be instructed to focus on a distant target, and the eyes should be observed carefully. Asking the patient to describe the target can control attention. If strabismus is present, any preference for fixation with one eye should be noted. Constant or intermittent monocular and binocular eye movements, whether conjugate or dissociated, should be noted. Subtle degrees of abnormal fixation can often be easily detected during the ophthalmoscopic examination (37). The

types of fixation abnormalities that may be observed are described in Chapters 19 and 23.

RANGE OF EYE MOVEMENTS

Principles

To discuss eye movements, it is necessary to have a frame of reference against which any movement may be quantified. Accordingly, the primary position of the eyes has been arbitrarily designated as that position from which all other ocular movements are initiated or measured (38,39).

It was once assumed that all ocular motions occurred around a fixed point in the orbit called the center of rotation. It has been shown, however, that there is no fixed center of rotation that does not move when the globe rotates and that the globe translates during every eye movement (40–41). Thus, horizontal movements rotate the center of the globe in a semicircle in the plane of eye rotation, called the *space centroid*. Nevertheless, for practical purposes, the globe can be considered to rotate around a fixed point that lays 13.5 mm posterior to the corneal apex and 1.6 mm nasal to the geometric center of the globe.

All movements of the globe around the hypothetical center of rotation can be analyzed in terms of a coordinate system with three axes perpendicular to each other and intersecting at the center of rotation (Fig. 18.1). These three axes, described by Fick in 1854, are called the *x*, *y*, and *z* axes of Fick (42). The *y* axis is equivalent to the visual axis; the *z* axis is vertical (around which the eye rotates horizontally); and the *x* axis is horizontal (around which the eye rotates vertically). These axes are stable with respect to a frontal plane, fixed in the skull, that corresponds roughly with the equatorial plane of the eye when it is directed straight ahead (Listing's plane) (43).

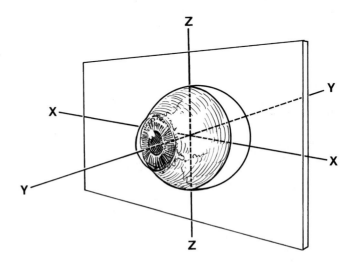

Figure 18.1. The axes of rotation of the eye. The *y* axis corresponds to the line of sight when the eye is in the primary position, looking straight ahead.

Rotations of both eyes (relative to one another) in the same direction are called *versions*. Rotations in opposite directions are called *vergences*. Only *convergence* (movement of the eyes toward one another) in the horizontal plane is volitionally significant. *Divergence* amplitudes (movement of the eyes away from one another) are small in normal individuals.

Rotations of either eye alone without attention to the movements of the other eye are called *ductions*. Horizontal rotation (rotation around the z axis of Fick) is termed *adduction* if the anterior pole of the eye is rotated nasally (i.e., inward, medially) and *abduction* if the anterior pole of the eye is rotated temporally (i.e., outward, laterally). Vertical rotation (around the x axis) is called *elevation* (or sursumduction) if the anterior pole of the eye rotates upward and *depression* (or deorsumduction) if it rotates downward.

Rotation during ductions or versions around either the horizontal or vertical axis places the eye in a secondary position of gaze. In achieving this position, there is no rotation of the globe around the y axis (i.e., there is no torsion).

The oblique positions of gaze are called tertiary positions. They are achieved by a simultaneous rotation around the horizontal and vertical axes, a movement that can be considered to occur around an oblique axis lying in Listing's plane. When an eye moves obliquely out of primary position, the vertical axis of the globe tilts with respect to the x and z axes of Fick; however, this tilt is considered "false torsion" since it does not represent a true rotation around the y axis but rather an apparent movement with respect to the planar coordinate system. For an excellent video demonstration of this phenomenon and its effect on visual perception, see *www.med.uwo.ca/physpharm/courses/llconsequencesweb/*. The amount of false torsion associated with any particular oblique position of gaze is constant, regardless of how the eye reaches that position (Donders' law) (44). Tertiary positions of gaze are thus positions of gaze associated with false torsion.

True ocular torsion is defined by the direction of the rotation around the y axis of Fick (i.e., the visual axis) relative to the nose. If the 12 o'clock region of the limbus rotates toward the nose, the movement is called *intorsion* (incycloduction; incyclotorsion). If the same area rotates away from the nose, the movement is called *extorsion* (excycloduction; excyclotorsion).

True ocular torsion occurs only minimally during voluntary versions. Volitional head tilts are preceded by a brief torsion movement of the eye in the direction of the anticipated head tilt that disappears by the time the head reaches its desired position (45). Thereafter torsion in the opposite direction occurs to compensate for the head tilt (46). In this setting, the torsion movements are called *countertorsion* or *counterrolling*. Countertorsion has two components, dynamic and static. Dynamic countertorsion occurs during head tilt and reflects the semicircular canal-induced torsional vestibulo-ocular reflex (VOR) (47,48). Static countertorsion persists at a given angle of any head tilt, but the amount of rotation is minor compared with that which occurs from dynamic countertorsion (49–51). Static countertorsion reflects a tonic otolith-ocular reflex (52,53). Each utricle influ-

ences both eyes in both directions but primarily controls tilt to the contralateral side (54–56). In addition, abnormalities in static countertorsion that are found in patients with intracranial compressive lesions have been found to correspond in part to the extent to which they impinge on the utricular nerve and brain stem (56).

The entire concept of static countertorsion was challenged by Jampel, who believed that the anatomy of the oblique muscle tendon insertions prevents such torsion movements from occurring (57–61). Numerous other investigators using sophisticated magnetic search coil techniques subsequently confirmed that static countertorsion does exist (62,63).

Most investigators find that static countertorsion represents only about 10% of the total amount of torsion associated with any large head tilt (64–66). Dynamic and static torsion apparently work only within a small range to attempt to keep the sensory vertical raphes of each retina perpendicular to the horizon (67). It is suggested that countertorsion is a primitive compensatory adaptation of lateral-eyed animals to head movements in the roll plane (68). With evolution of the eyes to the frontal plane (to promote stereopsis) and development of upright posture, this movement is merely vestigial.

True torsion does occur as a normal component of voluntary convergence. Both eyes extort, and the extorsion is greater in downward convergence than in upward convergence (69). This may be a phylogenetically recent adaptation in frontal-eyed animals to prevent distortions in pitch stereopsis of vertical lines caused by false intorsion during downward convergence (68). (It is during downward gaze that accurate pitch stereopsis is most important for walking and reading.)

To discuss the independent action of any individual extraocular muscle or any pair of extraocular muscles is strictly a hypothetical convenience. In any actual rotation of the globe, all six muscles are affected and act as a single muscle unit with a single axis of rotation at any given moment (70). The complete muscle unit can produce an infinite variety of rotations consistent with Listing's and Donders' laws that, together, state that when the line of fixation passes from the primary to any other position, the angle of false torsion is the same as if the eye had arrived at this position by turning around a fixed axis perpendicular to the initial and final positions of the line of fixation. Listing's law has been modified to allow temporal rotation of Listing's plane to account for the necessary torsion during convergence (71). Nevertheless, some studies show that Listing's and Donders' laws are not precisely followed in that some true torsion does develop during eccentric gaze (72–74).

Demer et al. have shed light on the anatomic correlates of an extraocular muscle pulley system surrounding the globe roughly parallel to Listing's plane that anchors the functional origins of the muscles relative to one another and largely explains how Listing's and Donders' laws are obeyed (75–77). They have shown histologic and magnetic resonance imaging (MRI) evidence of orbital fibrous connective tissues that create this pulley system, allowing the extraocular muscles to function commutatively.

Within the concept of a single muscle unit, it nevertheless

seems acceptable to discuss the action of the extraocular muscles in the setting of individual antagonist pairs. Boeder emphasized that the two horizontal rectus muscles have only the primary action of either adduction (for the medial rectus) or abduction (for the lateral rectus) (70). The primary action of the two vertical rectus muscles is vertical eye movement (elevation for the superior rectus and depression for the inferior rectus), with both muscles additionally having secondary actions of adduction and torsion (intorsion for the superior rectus and extorsion for the inferior rectus). According to Boeder, torsion is the primary action of the two oblique muscles, with the superior oblique producing intorsion and the inferior oblique producing extorsion. The secondary actions of these muscles are abduction and vertical movement (depression for the superior oblique; elevation for the inferior oblique). For the oblique muscles, the secondary vertical actions are at least as great as the primary torsion effects.

Normal eye movements are binocular. Such movements are called *versions* if the movements of the two eyes are in the same direction. For practical purposes, the extraocular muscles of each eye work in pairs during such movements, with one muscle contracting (the *agonist*) and the other muscle relaxing (the *antagonist*). The three agonist–antagonist muscle pairs for each eye are the medial and lateral rectus muscles, the superior and inferior rectus muscles, and the superior and inferior oblique muscles. From experimentally produced ocular motor palsies, Sherrington proposed that whenever an agonist muscle receives a neural impulse to contract, an equivalent inhibitory impulse is sent to the motor neurons supplying the antagonist muscle so that it will relax (78). This is called Sherrington's law of reciprocal innervation.

For the eyes to move together to produce a horizontal version, the lateral rectus of one eye and the medial rectus of the opposite eye must contract together. These muscles constitute a *yoke pair*. The other two yoke pairs are (*a*) the superior rectus muscle of one eye and the inferior oblique muscle of the other eye and (*b*) the superior oblique muscle of one eye and the inferior rectus muscle of the other eye. Implicit in the concept of a yoke pair is the premise that such muscles receive equal innervation so that the eyes move together. This is the simplest statement of Hering's law of motor correspondence (79).

Techniques

When testing the range of ocular movement, the examiner should ask the patient to follow a target through the full range of movement, including the cardinal (or diagnostic) positions of gaze. The eyes are tested individually with one eye covered (ductions) and together with both eyes open (versions). The normal range of movements is fairly stable throughout life for all directions except upgaze. Normal abduction is usually 50°; adduction, 50°; and depression, 45° (3). Upward gaze decreases somewhat with advancing age. Chamberlain examined 367 "normal" individuals ranging in age from 5 to 94 years of age (80). He found that there was a progressive decrease in upward rotation of the eyes from 40° in patients 5–14 years of age to only 16° in patients 85–94 years of age. Thus, limitation of upward gaze in an older individual may simply be age-related and not necessarily a new, pathologic process.

When the range of motion is limited, it is necessary to determine whether the limitation is mechanical and, if not, whether the disturbance is supranuclear or peripheral.

Several tests may be used to determine whether a mechanical restriction of ocular motion is present. Mechanical limitation of motion (such as that seen in patients with thyroid ophthalmopathy or orbital floor fracture with entrapment) can be inferred if intraocular pressure increases substantially when the patient attempts to look in the direction of gaze limitation (81–84). The intraocular pressure measurements are most easily performed using a Tonopen or a pneumatic tonometer, although any similar instrument may be used (83).

Mechanical limitation of motion can more reliably be detected with forced duction (or traction) testing. In such tests, an attempt is made to move the eye forcibly in the direction(s) of gaze limitation (Fig. 18.2). As described by Jaensch, this test is performed as follows (85). The cornea is anesthetized using several drops of a topical anesthetic such as proparacaine or tetracaine hydrochloride. The conjunctiva is further anesthetized by holding a cotton swab or cotton-tipped applicator soaked with 5–10% cocaine against it for about 30 seconds. The conjunctiva is then grasped with a fine-toothed forceps near the limbus on the side opposite

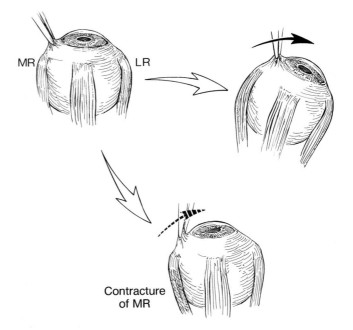

Figure 18.2. Forced duction testing. After the eye has been anesthetized with topical proparacaine and cocaine, the conjunctiva just posterior to the limbus is grasped with a fine-toothed forceps at a point opposite the direction of limitation. An attempt is then made to rotate the eye in the direction of limitation. If no mechanical limitation is present, the eye can be moved fully into the direction of limitation (*solid black arrow*). If mechanical limitation is present, the eye will resist attempts to rotate it into the field of limitation (*dashed black arrow*).

the direction in which the eye is to be moved. The patient is instructed to try to look in the direction of limitation, and an attempt is made to move the eye in that direction (i.e., opposite that in which mechanical restriction is suspected). If no resistance is encountered, the motility defect is not restrictive; however, if resistance is encountered, then mechanical restrictions exist (86–90). In some patients, particularly those who are cooperative and have substantial limitation of movement, the forced duction test can be performed simply by asking the patient to look in the direction of limitation and then attempting to move the eye by placing a cotton-tipped applicator stick against the eye on the opposite side just posterior to the limbus (91). Other investigators recommend using a suction device to perform and quantify forced duction testing (92–94).

Forced ductions can also be used to test restriction of the oblique muscles (95). For this test, the conjunctiva is grasped near the limbus at the 3 o'clock and 9 o'clock position with toothed forceps. Retropulsion of the globe is then applied, putting the oblique muscles on stretch. The eye is then moved from medially to laterally in an arc that follows the orbital rim while depressed (to test the inferior oblique muscle) or elevated (to test the superior oblique muscle). During this process, a distinct bump is encountered as the globe passes over the stretched oblique tendon or muscle. The resistance of this bump toward passage of the globe is an indication of the tightness of the muscle.

Often, particularly in children or when testing restriction of the oblique muscles, the forced duction test can be performed only under general anesthesia (Fig. 18.3). However, succinylcholine, which is often given to patients under general anesthesia, produces tonic contraction of the extraocular muscles, thereby altering the results of the forced duction test (96–98).

In addition to the forced duction test, mechanical determination of muscle force can be used to assess the function of apparently paretic muscles with contracture of their antagonists. An estimate of active muscle force present in patients with limitation of ocular motility can be made by stabilizing the anesthetized eye with a toothed forceps in a position near the limbus on the side of the limitation while the eye attempts to look into the field of the limitation (Fig. 18.4) (99,100). The presence of a tug on the forceps indicates that a contraction of the suspected paralytic muscle has occurred. The results of this "forced generation test" can even be quantified (101).

Nonrestrictive limitation of eye movements may occur from disease of supranuclear or infranuclear structures. Since the workup and management of the patient will vary considerably depending on the location of the lesion, supranuclear disorders must be distinguished from infranuclear disorders. From a practical standpoint, supranuclear disorders that cause abnormalities in the range of eye movements usually result from lesions of the cerebral hemispheres or the brain stem premotor structures. In such cases, stimulation of the vestibular apparatus can be used to assess the integrity of the peripheral ocular motor pathways either by oculocephalic testing (the doll's head maneuver) or by caloric testing (102–105).

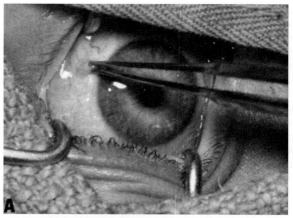

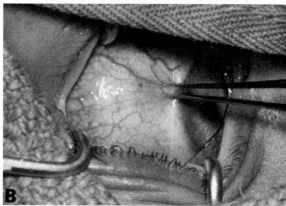

Figure 18.3. Forced duction testing in a patient under general anesthesia. *A,* The conjunctiva and episclera are grasped near the limbus with a fixation forceps. *B,* The eye is moved medially to test for mechanical restriction of adduction. The eye can be moved medially without difficulty. (From von Noorden G, Maumenee AE. Atlas of Strabismus. Ed 2. St Louis, CV Mosby, 1973:113.)

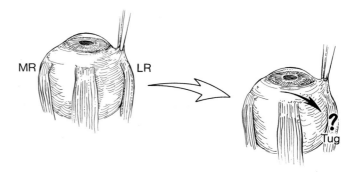

Figure 18.4. Estimation of active, generated muscle force. After the eye has been anesthetized with topical proparacaine and cocaine, the conjunctiva just posterior to the limbus is grasped with a fine-toothed forceps on the side of the limitation. The examiner then holds the eye while the patient attempts to look in the direction of limitation. If there is an intact nerve supply to the muscle that could move the eye into the field of limitation, the examiner will feel a tug on the forceps.

In the oculocephalic test, the awake patient is asked to fixate a target straight ahead while the head (or the entire body) is rotated from side to side and up and down. A normal response consists of a conjugate eye deviation in the direction away from head or body rotation such that the eyes remain stable with respect to space despite the head movement. Asking the patient to read a Snellen chart during head or body rotation can demonstrate the remarkable integrity of this VOR. In patients with intact vestibular systems, there is no degradation of visual acuity, even with rotations of up to 40°/sec (106). Patients with vestibular disease have a rapid decline in this dynamic visual acuity with head rotation.

To perform the oculocephalic test in comatose patients, the eyelids are simply held open and the rotational head movements are performed. Chu et al. modified this procedure for patients with severe neck rigidity or injuries that prevent neck flexion and extension (107). These investigators place such patients on a stretcher with wheels. The stretcher is then sharply pushed in the direction of either the patient's head or feet. This maneuver does not produce a rotational stimulus but is simply a linear or translational movement that may stimulate otolith-ocular reflexes (which are minimal) and visual tracking. In fact, it probably functions as a full-field pursuit test, and similar results can be obtained using a slowly moving "optokinetic" tape or drum. Although these tests may not give exact information regarding the VOR, they nevertheless provide important information regarding ocular motility that may be otherwise impossible to obtain.

In unconscious patients, oculocephalic testing may be the most useful method of assessing eye movements. The VOR is often intact in such patients, whereas saccadic and pursuit eye movements are absent. Thus, rapid horizontal rotation of the head results in deviation of the eyes away from the direction of the head turn. The eyes then make an exponential drift back to primary position if the head rotation is maintained. Though not saccadic, this recentration of the eyes may be quite rapid, occurring with a time constant of less than 0.5 seconds in the most severe vegetative states (105). Normal responses during oculocephalic testing indicate that the nuclear and infranuclear ocular motor structures are intact and capable of being stimulated by an intact vestibular system. This test can also be used in patients with functional (nonorganic) limitation of gaze to show that a full range of eye movement can be elicited despite apparent gaze restriction during testing of voluntary eye movements (108,109).

Another way to stimulate the vestibular system is by caloric irrigation (102–104,110–115). In this test, performed in the light with the patient in a supine position, the external auditory canal is first inspected to make certain that the tympanic membrane is intact. The patient's head is flexed 30°. This places the lateral (horizontal) semicircular canals in a nearly vertical position, allowing the thermal stimulus to induce maximal convection currents in the endolymph. Up to 200 cc of warm (44°C) or cold (30°C) water is infused into the external canal using a small tube fitted onto a syringe (116). In the awake patient, a normal response consists of conjugate nystagmus, with the slow phase toward the side of cold water irrigation (or away from the side of warm

water irrigation) and the fast phase away from the side of cold water irrigation (or toward the side of warm water irrigation). Temperature stimulation of the vestibular system causes a slow-phase movement followed by a quick refixation movement (saccade) resulting in nystagmus. If the induced nystagmus is consistently less when one ear is irrigated, regardless of the stimulus temperature, a peripheral vestibular disturbance is present on that side. If the nystagmus is consistently greater in one direction, regardless of which ear is stimulated, the patient has a directional preponderance of the vestibular system that may occur with central or peripheral vestibular lesions and is otherwise nonlocalizing (2).

The eye movements that occur during caloric irrigation can best be observed by placing Frenzel's spectacles on the patient (117). These spectacles eliminate patient fixation and provide magnification for the examiner; some models also provide illumination of the patient's eyes.

In practical terms, the caloric irrigation test is messy, uncomfortable for the awake patient, and usually useful only for detecting relatively gross asymmetry in vestibular function. Nevertheless, attempts have been made to quantify subtle vestibular dysfunction with this test. The duration of nystagmus after caloric irrigation seems to be a reproducible measure of vestibular function, and the slow-phase velocity of caloric stimulation nystagmus, as measured with electronystagmography, is a commonly used parameter for assessing vestibular function (118).

Itaya and Kitahara described an air caloric test that causes a continuous thermal change in the semicircular canals, thus avoiding the use of water (119). These inventors claimed that this test is more sensitive than water irrigation for detecting vestibular disorders.

In comatose patients with intact nuclear and infranuclear ocular motor structures and an intact vestibular system, a normal response is simply a tonic, conjugate ocular deviation toward the side of cold water irrigation and away from the side of warm water irrigation. There are no significant refixation movements, since all horizontal quick phases are generated by the paramedian pontine reticular formation (PPRF), which is not functioning in such patients. Absence of the VOR by either oculocephalic or caloric stimulation in comatose patients is consistently associated with poor outcome (120–122).

Caloric testing may be used to evaluate the integrity of vertical gaze by infusing warm or cold water simultaneously into both external auditory canals. A normal response in the awake individual is a conjugate jerk nystagmus with a slow phase that is upward when warm water is used and downward when cold water is used. A normal response in the comatose individual is a tonic, conjugate movement of the eyes upward (for warm water) or downward (for cold water). Although caloric testing is the best way to evaluate unilateral peripheral vestibular function, our experience with bilateral caloric irrigation suggests that it is of limited value in assessing the integrity of vertical gaze and that oculocephalic and rotation testing provides more accurate and reproducible results.

Caloric testing in patients with abolished vestibular function can occasionally induce nystagmus. This pseudocaloric nystagmus always beats away from the affected ear, regardless of whether cold or warm water is used for irrigation (123,124). It can thus be distinguished from caloric nystagmus that beats away from the irrigated ear when cold irrigation is used and toward the irrigated ear when warm irrigation is used. According to Becker et al., pseudocaloric nystagmus probably represents unmasking of a pre-existing vestibular nystagmus through tactile (caloric) stimulation (see Chapter 23) (124).

In some patients with paresis of upward gaze, Bell's phenomenon may be helpful in differentiating an infranuclear from a supranuclear lesion. Bell's phenomenon consists of outward and upward rolling of the eyes when forcible efforts are made to close the eyelids against resistance. It does not occur with blinks, and it is observed in only 50% of individuals during voluntary unrestrained lid closure (125). The presence of this movement in individuals who cannot voluntarily elevate their eyes usually indicates that brain stem pathways between the facial nerve nucleus and that portion of the oculomotor nucleus responsible for ocular elevation are intact, and thus that an upward gaze paresis is supranuclear in origin (126). However, an intact Bell's phenomenon may occur in patients with Guillain-Barré syndrome and was also demonstrated in a patient with complete ophthalmoplegia caused by myasthenia gravis (127,128). Absence of a Bell's phenomenon has less diagnostic usefulness, since about 10% of normal subjects do not have this fascio-ocular movement (129,130). A downward Bell's response is present in up to 8% of individuals (130).

OCULAR ALIGNMENT

Principles

When the eyes are not aligned on the same object, *strabismus* is present. The strabismus may be congenital or acquired and may be caused by central or peripheral dysfunction. In some individuals, particularly those with isolated congenital strabismus, the amount of ocular misalignment is unchanged regardless of the direction of gaze or of which eye is fixating the target. This type of strabismus is termed *comitant* or *concomitant*. On the other hand, when the amount of an ocular deviation changes in various directions of gaze, with either eye fixing, or both, the strabismus is said to be *incomitant* or *noncomitant*. Congenital comitant strabismus is occasionally associated with other neurologic dysfunction (131–134), and acquired comitant strabismus may rarely occur as a sign of intracranial disease (135–147). Most cases of acquired comitant strabismus appear in otherwise normal children and adults, as well as in persons with neurologic or systemic disease, from decompensation of a pre-existing phoria, or as a result of latent hypermetropia (3,148,149). Thus, most instances of neuropathic or myopathic strabismus are of the incomitant variety. The reasons for this incomitance are described in the next section.

Primary and Secondary Deviations

Any patient with a manifest deviation of one eye (heterotropia) will fixate a target with only one eye at a time. During viewing with one eye, the visual axis of the opposite (nonfixing) eye will be deviated a certain amount away from the target. Patients with a comitant strabismus have the same amount of deviation of the nonfixing eye regardless of the eye that is fixing or the field of gaze. Most patients with incomitant (and especially paralytic) strabismus tend to fix with the nonparetic eye if visual acuity is equal in the two eyes. In these patients, the deviation of the nonfixing eye is called the primary deviation. When such patients are forced to fix the same target with the paretic eye, the deviation that results, the secondary deviation, is always greater than the primary deviation (Fig. 18.5). The explanation for this phenomenon is related to the position of the eyes within the

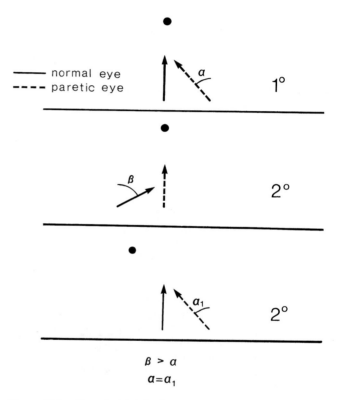

Figure 18.5. The principle of primary and secondary deviations. *Top,* When the normal eye fixes on a target directly ahead, the paretic eye deviates from the primary position by a certain amount (α). This is called the primary deviation. *Middle,* When the paretic eye fixes on a target in primary position, the normal eye also deviates from primary position by a certain amount (β), but this secondary deviation of the normal eye when the paretic eye is fixing is greater than the amount of deviation of the paretic eye when the normal eye is fixing ($\beta > \alpha$). *Bottom,* Although the common explanation of primary and secondary deviation is based on Hering's law of equal innervation to yoke muscles, Leigh and Zee (1991) suggested that the secondary deviation is greater than the primary deviation in paretic strabismus because when the paretic eye is fixing in primary position, it is forced further into its field of limitation. If the paretic eye were fixing on an object in the opposite direction, the deviation of the eye from primary position (α1) would be the same as if the normal eye were fixing on an object straight ahead ($\alpha = \alpha$1). Thus, although Hering's law is maintained, the explanation for primary and secondary deviations is based upon the position of the eyes within the orbit and not upon which eye is fixing.

orbits (2). When a single muscle is paretic, the deviation between the two eyes is proportional to the difference between the forces generated by the paretic muscle and its normal yoke muscle. Furthermore, the amount of force contributed by each muscle toward holding the eye in a specific orbital position increases as the eye is moved into the direction of action of that muscle. Under normal circumstances, this force, thus obeying Hering's law, is equal for yoke pairs of muscles. However, as the eyes move into the direction of action of the paretic muscle, the difference in forces generated by the normal and paretic yoke muscles increases, thus increasing the deviation between the two eyes. When this change in deviation is tested as a function of orbital position, it is actually found to be independent of which eye is fixing. Thus, when the paretic eye is fixating a target, it is held in an orbital position further in the direction of action of the paretic muscle than when the nonparetic eye is fixating the same target. This results in a secondary deviation that is greater than the primary deviation simply because of the change in eye position toward the direction of action of the paretic muscle when the paretic eye is forced to take up

fixation. The innervation to both muscles in the yoke pair is increased in that direction as predicted by Hering's law, and this increased innervation is more effective in the nonparetic muscle. However, the innervation is not increased any more than if the nonparetic eye is forced to take up fixation in eccentric gaze to achieve the same final orbital position.

Past-pointing and Disturbances of Egocentric Localization

Von Graefe first described anomalies of spatial localization that he referred to as *past-pointing* or *false orientation* in patients with paralytic strabismus (150). If a patient is asked to point at an object in the field of action of a paretic muscle while the paretic eye is fixating, the patient's finger will point beyond the object *toward* the field of action of the paretic muscle (Fig. 18.6). During this test, it is important that the hand be covered or that the patient point rapidly toward the object so as to avoid visual correction of the error of localization while the hand is still moving toward the object. Patients with accommodative esotropia exhibit a sim-

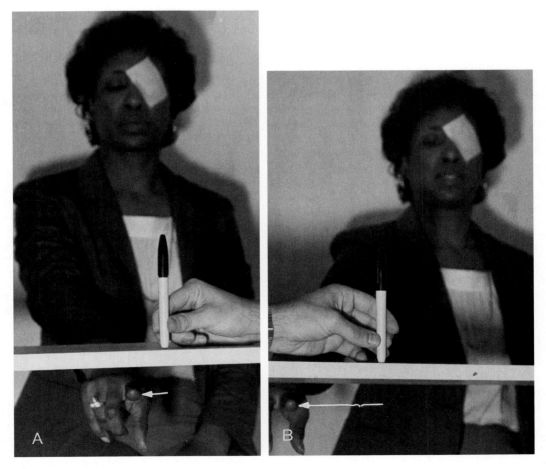

Figure 18.6. Past-pointing in a patient with a right sixth nerve paresis. *A,* In primary position, there is only a slight amount of past-pointing. *B,* In right gaze, however, the amount of past-pointing increases. The *white arrows* indicate the amount of past-pointing (the difference between the actual target location and the area in space to which the patient points).

ilar phenomenon while they have a manifest esotropia, pointing in the direction that the nonfixating eye is looking (151).

The explanation of past-pointing is controversial. One explanation is that the image of the target lies in an abnormal location relative to the fovea so that the patient incorrectly localizes the object into that field. This explanation, however, does not account for the past-pointing that is observed when the image of the target lies on the fovea of the paretic eye (152–154). Clearly nonvisual information about eye position is involved in spatial localization, and an argument has raged over the relative role of efferent command to the eye muscles versus proprioceptive afferent information from the eye muscles. In support of the efferent command theory, Helmholtz argued that past-pointing depends on the "intensity of the effort of will" that is sent to the paretic muscle (155). For a thorough description of the evidence for proprioceptive feedback from the muscles in spatial localization, see the review by Weir (156).

Head Turns and Tilts

Patients with strabismus commonly turn or tilt the head to minimize diplopia. Head turns are frequently associated with paresis of the horizontal extraocular muscles. Similarly, patients with vertical extraocular muscle paresis may carry their head flexed or extended. Most patients with such head turns adopt the particular posture to minimize or eliminate diplopia by moving the eyes away from the field of action of the paretic muscle; however, some patients adopt a head posture that actually increases the distance between the two images, allowing one of the images to be more easily ignored.

Head turns also occur in patients with congenital nystagmus. In such patients, keeping the eyes in an eccentric (null) position in the orbit by means of the head turn may result in reduction in the amplitude or frequency of the nystagmus.

Head tilts are most commonly observed with paresis of the oblique muscles, particularly the superior oblique. With an acquired superior oblique palsy, for example, the face is usually turned away from the paretic eye, the chin is down slightly, and the head is tilted toward the side opposite the paretic muscle. This permits fusion of images. Patients with congenital superior oblique palsy may adopt a similar head tilt or one in the opposite direction (i.e., toward the side of the paretic muscle) to more widely separate the images. Head tilts that occur from ocular causes often must be differentiated from nonocular torticollis.

Finally, some patients develop head turns that seem to be caused by central visual field defects and not by ocular misalignment (157). Such patients turn their heads toward the hemianopic field under both monocular and binocular conditions. The explanation for the head turn in these patients is unclear.

Techniques

Ocular alignment may be tested subjectively or objectively, depending on the circumstances under which the examination is performed and the physical and mental state of the patient.

Subjective Testing

When a patient is cooperative, subjective testing of diplopia reliably indicates the disparity between retinal images. The simplest subjective tests of ocular alignment use colored filters to dissociate the deviation and to emphasize and differentiate the images so that the patient and the observer can interpret them. A fixation light is used to provide the image. A red filter held over one eye suffices in most cases. However, the addition of a green filter over the opposite eye gives better results in children, in patients with a tendency to suppress or ignore one of the images, and in patients with a slight paresis and good fusion ability who can overcome their deviation. The use of complementary colored filters, one over each eye, produces maximum dissociation of images, since there is no part of the visible spectrum common to both eyes.

The red filter is always placed over the patient's right eye, and all questions posed to the patient relate to the relationship of the red image with respect to the white (or green) image. The patient is first asked if he or she sees one or two lights. If the patient sees two lights, he or she is then asked what color they are. After the appropriate answer, the patient is asked if the red light is to the right or left of the other light and if it is above or below the other light. The information thus received will be that the patient sees two lights, one red and one white or green, that they are crossed (each image is perceived on the side opposite the eye that is seeing it) or uncrossed (each image is perceived on the same side as the eye that is seeing it), and that the image relating to the right eye (red image) is higher or lower than the other image. The image of an object is always displaced in the *opposite* direction to the position of the eye (Fig. 18.7). Thus, if an eye is exotropic, the patient will have *crossed* diplopia,

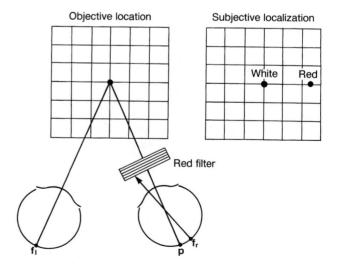

Figure 18.7. The principle of diplopia tests. A red filter is placed in front of the right eye, and the patient fixes a single light in the distance. If the eyes are misaligned, the light is imaged on the fovea of one eye (fl) and the nonfoveal retina (p) of the opposite eye. The patient thus sees two images, white and red, in different locations in space.

and (with a red filter over the right eye) the patient will see the red image to the *left* of the other image. Similarly, if the patient has an esotropia, the red image will be seen to the *right* of the other image (*uncrossed* diplopia). If the patient has a vertical deviation of the eyes, the eye that is higher will see the image of an object *below* that of the opposite eye.

Once the patient indicates that there is a clear separation of images when he or she is fixing on a light held straight ahead, the examiner can determine the area of maximum vertical separation, horizontal separation, or both, by having the patient look at a light held in the eight other cardinal positions of gaze (right, upper right, up, upper left, left, lower left, down, lower right).

In addition to the use of filters placed over one or both eyes, one can place a red Maddox rod over one eye and have the patient fixate on a white light (158). The "rod" is, in fact, a set of small half-cylinders aligned side by side in a frame in such a way that when the eye views a light through the cylinders, the image seen is that of a line perpendicular to the cylinder axis. Thus, if one views a white light with one eye covered by a red Maddox rod, the images will be those of a red line and a white light. The Maddox rod can be placed in such a manner as to produce a vertical, horizontal, or oblique line. Individuals who are orthophoric will see the line pass through the light. When the rod is oriented to produce the image of a vertical line, patients with a horizontal strabismus will see the line to the left or right of the light. When the rod is oriented so that a horizontal line image is produced, patients with a vertical strabismus will see the line above or below the light.

Torsional misalignment of the eyes (e.g., superior oblique palsy) can be tested with two Maddox rods, one over each eye (159). This is best performed using a trial lens frame. If both rods are oriented so as to produce a horizontal line image, an eye with torsional dysfunction will see the line as oblique rather than horizontal. The patient is then asked to rotate the rod until the line is perceived as horizontal. By this method, the amount of torsion can be measured and followed. Traditionally, one clear (or white) Maddox rod and one red Maddox rod are used for this test. However, Simons et al. showed that the subjective torsion more reliably localizes to the paretic eye if two red Maddox rods are used and if the room is dark during testing (160).

The precise methods of testing and documenting positions of gaze have been described in detail by numerous authors and are not discussed further in this chapter (2,3,161).

In addition to the tests described above, other subjective techniques may be used in which two test objects rather than one are presented to the patient in such a way that each object is viewed with only one eye (Fig. 18.8). The patient is then required to place the two objects in such a fashion that they appear to be superimposed. The objects appear superimposed only when their images fall on the fovea of each eye. Misalignment of the foveas results in the patient placing the objects in different locations in space. The eyes are differentiated and dissociated in various ways. Each eye may be presented with a different target, or complementary colors may be placed into the visual field, either directly or

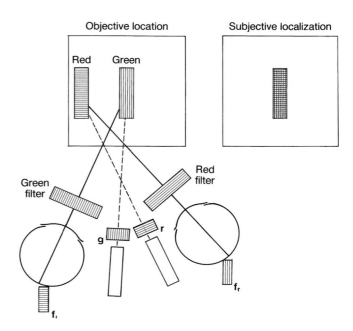

Figure 18.8. The principle of haploscopic tests. Red and green test objects are used, and the patient has a red filter placed in front of one eye and a green filter in front of the other eye.

by projection, with each eye being provided with a corresponding colored filter. These haploscopic tests include the use of a major amblyoscope and the Hess screen and Lancaster red-green tests (162,163).

In general, the Hess test uses a gray or black screen marked with a tangent scale on which red targets are projected or positioned where the tangent lines cross. A green target or light is superimposed subjectively on the red fixation target. Complementary red and green filters are worn to permit (and stimulate) binocular dissociation, thus revealing the ocular deviation in each position of fixation. The test is performed with the patient 0.5 meters from the screen.

The Lancaster test incorporates the same principles as the Hess screen but uses a two-dimensional grid rather than a tangent screen and is performed with the patient 1 or 2 meters from the grid.

Although the Hess and Lancaster tests use red and green colors to dissociate images, as in the more simple "red glass" test described above, they differ from that test in principle. In the red glass test, one white fixation light is used that can be seen by each eye through the red and green (if used) filters. In the Hess or Lancaster tests, instead of a white light, two different-colored test objects are used. These are projected red and green lines that can be perceived only by the fovea of the eye that is viewing through the corresponding colored filter. Thus, the eye that is viewing through the red filter (usually the right eye) sees only the red line, whereas the eye that is viewing through the green filter (usually the left eye) sees only the green line. Each fovea perceives the image from its respective target as being located straight ahead. This is macular-macular projection (confusion). The binocular dissociation produced in this manner is sufficient to reveal even a minimal and well-controlled heterophoria. The patient, wearing the red filter over the right eye, is asked to superimpose the green line on the red line as each fixation position on the screen or grid is illuminated consecutively. The nonfixing left eye is deviated behind the green filter, but the patient merely guides the flashlight so that the green line is positioned where the deviated eye is pointing. At this point, the patient sees the red and green lights superimposed. The examiner, however, can see the deviation of the green line from the red line and can plot the position of the green line onto a chart. The test is then repeated with the red and green filters reversed, so that the left eye now fixates the red line, and the field of the deviating right eye is plotted. Not only is this test helpful in assessing the degree of deviation of both comitant and noncomitant strabismus at any given time, but also it may be used in patients with paralytic strabismus to detect subtle changes in ocular alignment that occur over time. It thus may help in the planning and evaluation of therapy for such patients (164). In addition, subjective torsion of the eyes can be detected when the patient rotates one line at an oblique angle relative to the other line. We believe that this test is the best way to subjectively determine the degree of ocular torsion present in one or both eyes. The interested reader should consult von Noorden (3), Burde (39), and Zee et al. (164) for excellent descriptions of these tests.

Objective Testing

The simplest objective method of determining ocular alignment is the use of a hand light to cast a reflection on the corneal surfaces of both eyes in the cardinal positions of gaze. If the images from the two corneas appear centered, then the visual axes are often correctly aligned. If the light reflexes are not centered, one can either estimate the amount of misalignment based on the apparent amount of decentra-

tion of the light reflex (with the fixation light held 33 cm from the patient, 1 mm of decentration equals 7° of ocular deviation) (165), or prisms can be placed over either of the eyes until the light reflexes appear centered. Krimsky recommended that the prisms be placed over the nonfixing eye (166), but von Noorden considered this technique less precise and more difficult than placing prisms over the fixing eye (3), and we agree; however, if the nonfixing eye is so eccentric and limited in its excursion that centration of the light reflex is impossible or requires excessive prism over the fixing eye, holding the prism over the fixing eye results in a measurement of the deviation only in eccentric gaze. As noted above, this is essentially the same as measuring the secondary, rather than the primary, deviation.

A number of conditions other than a heterotropia may cause decentration of the corneal light reflex and must be considered to interpret tests correctly based on centration of the light reflex. The angle kappa is defined as the angle between the visual line (line connecting the point of fixation with the fovea) and the pupillary axis (line through the center of the pupil perpendicular to the cornea). The angle is measured at the center of the pupil. It is called positive when the light reflex is displaced nasally and negative when the light reflex is displaced temporally. A positive angle kappa may simulate an exodeviation (Fig. 18.9), and a negative angle kappa may simulate an esodeviation. Conversely, strabismus may be less apparent when a large angle kappa is associated with esotropia or a large negative angle is associated with exotropia. Other ocular abnormalities that produce decentration of the corneal light reflex include eccentric fixation and ectopic macula (e.g., in patients with retinopathy of prematurity or other retinal disease with macular traction).

The most precise objective methods of measuring ocular alignment are the cover tests (153,167,168). Although these tests require that the patient be able to fixate a target with either eye, they generally require less cooperation than do

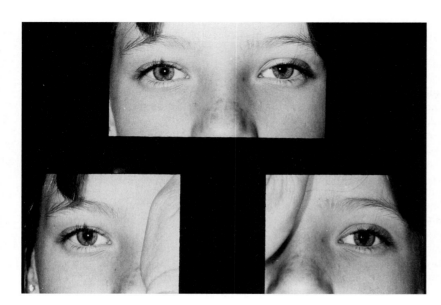

Figure 18.9. Positive angle kappa with the corneal light reflex test. With both eyes open (*top*), the eyes appear exotropic because the light reflection is decentered nasally in the left eye. The reflex remains centered in the right eye when the left eye is covered (*bottom left*). When the right eye is covered (*bottom right*), there is no shift of fixation, and the light reflection remains nasally displaced.

the subjective tests described above. The three types of cover tests used by most clinicians are the single cover test, the cover/uncover test, and the alternate cover (cross-cover) test.

In the single cover test, the patient fixates an accommodative target at 33 cm (near target) or 6 meters (distant target). An opaque occluder is placed in front of one eye, and the examiner observes the opposite eye to see whether it moves to take up fixation of the target (Fig. 18.10). If movement is observed, its direction and speed should be noted. The test is then repeated on the opposite eye. If the patient has a manifest ocular deviation (heterotropia), the previously nonfixing eye will be observed to change position to take up fixation when the fixing eye is covered. On the other hand, when the nonfixing eye is covered, no movement of the fixing eye will be observed (since it is already fixing on the target). This test is usually performed with the patient fixing in primary position and with the eyes in the other cardinal positions of gaze. In our experience, movements of as little as 1° can be easily observed.

In the cover/uncover test, the patient fixates on an accommodative target, and one eye is occluded. The behavior of that eye is then observed as the cover is removed (Fig. 18.10). The direction of any deviation and the speed and rate of recovery to binocular fixation are noted. If no movement of the uncovered eye is observed when the cover/uncover test is performed, an alternate cover test may be used to detect a latent deviation of the eyes (heterophoria). Instead of occluding one eye and then taking the occluder away, first one eye and then the other are alternately occluded. The cover should remain in front of each eye long enough to allow the patient to take up fixation with the uncovered eye. This test prevents fusion and dissociates the visual axes. Any movement of either uncovered eye suggests that although the eyes are straight during binocular viewing, loss of fusion (i.e., by the alternate occlusion of the two eyes) results in a deviation of whichever eye is covered (Fig. 18.11).

The importance of distinguishing between heterophorias and heterotropias cannot be overemphasized, since patients with heterophorias have binocular central fusion, whereas patients with heterotropias do not.

If either the cover/uncover or alternate cover test detects evidence of ocular misalignment, prisms can be used to neutralize the movement and thereby measure the deviation, whether it is a heterotropia or heterophoria. Prisms are placed in front of either eye such that the apex of the prism is oriented in the direction of the deviation, and the prism strength is altered until the deviation is no longer observed. The technique for measuring the amount of strabismus with ophthalmic prisms was beautifully described by Thompson and Guyton, and their manuscript should be reviewed by the physician or technician planning to perform such measurements (169).

When there is a vertical ocular deviation, it is often helpful to perform cover tests with the head tilted first toward one side and then toward the other (170,171). The patient is instructed to maintain fixation on a distant target, and the position of the eyes relative to each other is measured. The patient is then instructed to tilt the head to one side while maintaining fixation on the target, and the eyes are again

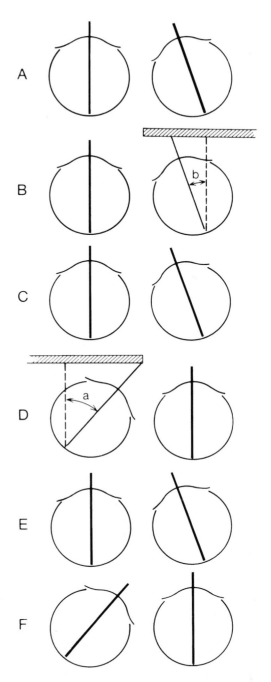

Figure 18.10. The single cover and cover/uncover tests. In both tests, one eye is covered at a time; however, in the single cover test, one eye is covered and the opposite eye is observed. In the cover/uncover test, one eye is covered and the behavior of that eye is observed when the cover is removed. *A,* Initially, with both eyes viewing, the left eye is fixating the target and the right eye is esotropic. When the right eye is covered (*B*), no movement of the left (uncovered) eye is observed, nor is any movement of the right eye observed when the cover is removed (*C*). *D,* When the left eye is covered, the right eye moves outward to take up fixation. The deviation of the normal eye under cover (the secondary deviation, a) is greater than that of the paretic eye under cover (primary deviation, b). When the cover is removed, either the left eye again takes up fixation (E) or the paretic right eye continues to fixate (F).

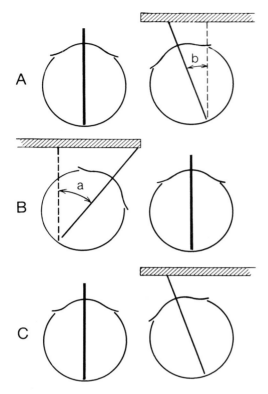

Figure 18.11. The alternate cover test. This test prevents fusional vergence and thus tests both phorias and tropias but does not differentiate between them. In this test, the cover is quickly moved from one eye to the other, and any movement of either eye is noted. In this example, there is an esodeviation.

examined to see whether one eye has moved higher than the other. Measurements are made with the head tilted to each side.

This test is useful primarily in the diagnosis of superior oblique palsy, since patients with this disorder consistently show a hypertropia of the damaged eye when the head is tilted toward the affected side (159). It has been suggested that the physiologic basis of this test lies in the fact that the vertical eye muscles are not driven in their usual yoked pairs when the head is tilted. Instead, the vestibular apparatus produces compensatory torsion of the eyes by co-innervation of the ipsilateral (to the side of the tilt) superior oblique and superior rectus muscles, producing intorsion, and of the contralateral inferior oblique and inferior rectus muscles, producing extorsion. When a patient with a trochlear nerve palsy tilts the head toward the affected side, intorsion of that eye should occur to keep the vertical meridian perpendicular to the horizon. As noted above, this intorsion is usually about 10° and is produced by the otolith-ocular reflex, resulting in synergistic contractions of the superior rectus and superior oblique muscles. If, however, the superior oblique muscle is paretic, its secondary actions, one of which is depression, are also impaired. The superior rectus muscle is therefore the only means by which the eye is intorted, and its main action, elevation of the eye, is unopposed. This mechanism

is contested by authors who find no relationship between the amount of hypertropia and the amount of countertorsion with the head tilt test (172).

The head tilt test is best used as part of a three-step diagnostic test first described by Haagedorn (173) and popularized by Parks (174) and Hardesty (175). This test is used to isolate the affected paretic muscle in concomitant or incomitant vertical deviations. It is useful only if the paresis is of a single cyclovertical muscle (176). The steps are as follows:

1. The presence of a vertical heterotropia is determined in primary position. Depending on the eye that is hypertropic, one of four muscles may be paretic: the ipsilateral inferior rectus, the ipsilateral superior oblique, the contralateral superior rectus, or the contralateral inferior oblique. Thus, if the patient has a right hypertropia, the muscles that may be paretic are the right superior oblique, the right inferior rectus, the left superior rectus, or the left inferior oblique.
2. Whether the hypertropia increases in right or left horizontal gaze is determined. This reduces the potential paretic muscles to two. Thus, in a patient with a right hypertropia, if the deviation increases in right gaze, the affected muscles can only be the right inferior rectus (which has its maximum vertical action when the eye is in an abducted position) or the left inferior oblique (which has its maximum vertical action when the eye is in an adducted position). If the deviation increases in left gaze, the affected muscles could be either the right superior oblique or the left superior rectus.
3. The differential diagnosis between the two muscles, one in each eye, that are potentially responsible for the vertical heterotropia, is now made using the head tilt test as described above. Thus, if the patient has a right hypertropia that increases in left gaze, an increase in the hypertropia when the head is tilted to the right side indicates a paretic superior oblique muscle.

Although we believe the three-step test is extremely useful in patients with presumed trochlear nerve palsies (159,177), we and others find that its reliability in the diagnosis of pareses of other vertical muscles is questionable (178). Furthermore, both restrictive ophthalmoplegia and myasthenia gravis can mimic superior oblique palsy using the three-step test (179).

A final objective method of determining ocular torsion is direct observation of the ocular fundus (180–182). The normal fovea is generally located about 7° below the center of the optic disc (range 0–16°) or along a horizontal line originating from a point between the middle and lower thirds of the optic disc (183). When an eye is extorted, the foveal reflex rotates below this plane, whereas intorsion results in upward rotation of the reflex (Fig. 18.12). The amount of torsion can be determined using a variety of ophthalmoscopic and photographic methods (180–186).

PERFORMANCE OF VERSIONS

Versions may be tested by examining the saccadic, pursuit, vestibular, and optokinetic systems.

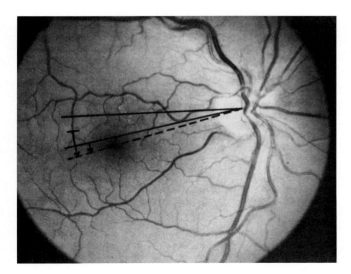

Figure 18.12. Torsion of the ocular fundus. Photograph of an extorted right fundus, direct view, with a *dashed line* drawn from the center of the optic disc through the fovea. The normal angular range of the fovea from the center of the disc is shown by the two *solid lines*. The amount of extorsion can be measured in degrees from the center of the normal range (*long arrow*) or from the limit of the normal range (*short arrow*). (Courtesy of Dr. David L Guyton.)

Clinical Examination of Saccades

Saccadic eye movements are examined clinically by instructing the patient to alternately fixate upon two targets, usually the examiner's finger and nose. Saccades in each direction can be examined in each field of gaze in both the horizontal and vertical planes. The examiner must determine whether the saccades are promptly initiated, of normal velocity, and accurate.

Saccadic latencies can be appreciated by noting the time it takes the patient to initiate the saccade. Abnormal voluntary saccadic velocities may be accentuated by using a drum or hand-held tape with repetitive patterns. Rotating the drum or passing the tape horizontally and vertically across the patient's visual field stimulates the optokinetic system to produce nystagmus (see Chapter 17). Abnormal saccadic velocities, particularly slowing, thus become more evident when the patient is forced to make multiple, repetitive saccades to refixate the passing targets. Altered saccadic velocities that occur in only one plane of movement can also be appreciated by using obliquely placed targets to stimulate oblique saccades. In such patients, the normal-velocity component of the saccade (e.g., the horizontal) will be completed before the other component (e.g., the vertical), so that the trajectory appears L-shaped.

Disorders of saccadic accuracy (e.g., saccadic dysmetria) can be inferred from the direction and size of corrective saccades that the patient must make to ultimately acquire the fixation target. Since saccades as small as $\frac{1}{2}°$ can be easily identified during clinical observation, minimal degrees of saccadic dysmetria can be easily appreciated during the clinical examination. Normal individuals may under-

shoot a target by a few degrees when refixations are large. Similarly, such individuals may overshoot a target during centripetal, and especially downward, saccades. This dysmetria is transient, gradually disappearing during repetitive refixations between the same targets.

When a saccadic abnormality is detected during the clinical examination, the examiner must attempt to localize the disturbance within the hierarchical organization of the saccadic eye movement system (see Chapters 17 and 19). The first step in localization is to establish whether the disease process affects reflexive saccades. Quick phases can be examined by spinning the patient in a swivel chair to elicit vestibular and optokinetic nystagmus. Next, an attempt should be made to determine whether saccades can be performed without visual targets or in response to auditory targets, by asking the patient to refixate under closed lids. The eye movements thus generated can be observed, palpated, and even heard (with a stethoscope applied to the lids).

During the evaluation of saccadic eye movements, it is often helpful to observe gaze changes when the patient makes a combined eye/head movement to see whether an accompanying head movement can facilitate the production of a saccade. This strategy is used by some patients with ocular motor apraxia (see Chapter 19). The effect of blinks should also be noted, since they may facilitate both the ability to initiate saccades and the subsequent saccadic velocity. Finally, asking the patient to repetitively refixate between two targets may reveal fatigue of saccadic eye movements.

Clinical Examination of Pursuit

Patients with isolated deficiency of smooth pursuit do not usually complain of visual symptoms, since they can track moving objects with a series of saccades. Only very demanding tracking tasks (e.g., playing tennis, handball, or baseball) may cause patients with impaired pursuit to report difficulties. The vision of normal subjects deteriorates during tracking of targets moving at high frequencies, however, so that even complaints of inability to track fast-moving objects may not signify a disorder of smooth pursuit (187).

To test the pursuit system, the patient should be asked to track a small target, such as a pencil tip held a meter or more from the eyes, with the head held still. The target should initially be moved at a low, uniform velocity. Pursuit movements that do not match the target velocity result in corrective saccades. If these are "catch-up" saccades, then the pursuit gain is low. If pursuit gain is too high, then "back-up" saccades are observed. Small children, uncooperative patients, or individuals thought to have nonorganic blindness may be tested with a slowly rotating large mirror held before their eyes.

Although hand-held drums or tapes with repetitive targets do not truly test the optokinetic system (see Chapter 17), they do stimulate pursuit and may be useful in the detection of pursuit asymmetries and other abnormalities of the pursuit system.

The VOR generates eye movements that compensate for angular displacement of the head and maintain the visual axes "on target." If one observes a slowly moving target by moving the head, so that the target remains stationary relative to the head, the eye movements generated by the VOR are inappropriate and must be suppressed. The ability of a patient to suppress (or cancel) the VOR can be evaluated by using a central fixation target that moves in the same direction and at the same velocity as the head (37,188). Patients often do this best by fixating on their thumbnail with their arm outstretched while being rotated in the examination chair. Those who have limb muscle weakness can be rotated in a wheelchair while fixating a target that rotates with the chair (189). When suppression of the VOR and pursuit are compared in normal human subjects, similar frequency response curves are obtained, leading to the hypothesis that suppression of the VOR depends directly on information derived from the smooth pursuit system (190,191). This hypothesis is supported by the clinical observation that patients with impaired smooth pursuit also have abnormal suppression of the VOR (192–194). The evaluation of VOR suppression is thus another way to test the integrity of the pursuit system. Deficits in VOR suppression, however, are nonlocalizing, since they may occur with either cerebral or cerebellar disease (195–197).

In some patients, it is difficult to test smooth pursuit because of spontaneous nystagmus; however, in some of these patients, the nystagmus is less prominent in a specific position of gaze (the null point; see Chapter 23). In these patients, cancellation of the VOR during head rotation can be tested with the eyes fixing on a target in this position. As with pursuit, the head rotation should be gentle at first. In patients with inadequate cancellation, the eyes are continually taken off target by the intact VOR, and corrective saccades therefore occur. An asymmetric deficit may imply a pursuit imbalance provided that the VOR is intact and symmetric: deficient cancellation of the VOR on rotation to one side corresponds to a low pursuit gain to that side. Furthermore, when there is a discrepancy between the performance of smooth pursuit and cancellation of the VOR (e.g., poor pursuit but good cancellation), one should suspect an inadequate or asymmetric VOR.

Clinical Examination of the Vestibular and Optokinetic Systems

We previously described the clinical methods used to test the vestibular system (oculocephalic and caloric testing), and we will not repeat them here. Although the optokinetic system can be tested in the laboratory (discussed later), the system cannot be tested as part of a routine clinical examination.

QUANTITATIVE ANALYSIS OF EYE MOVEMENTS

Voluntary Eye Movements

Most disturbances of ocular motility and alignment can be detected during a standard clinical examination; however, performing a quantitative analysis of eye movements may more accurately reveal subtle abnormalities of the pursuit, saccadic, optokinetic, and vestibulo-ocular systems. The most common methods used to record eye movements are

electro-oculography and infrared oculography (198–207). These techniques may be used to distinguish myopathic (restrictive) from neuropathic conditions that affect ocular motility and to determine the presence or absence of improvement of ocular motor function (208–212). The value of vertical saccadic velocity or amplitude determinations in adduction versus abduction to identify and monitor superior oblique muscle dysfunction remains controversial (213–215).

Although electro-oculography can yield reasonable recordings of horizontal eye movements, vertical measurements with this technique are affected by eyelid artifacts and nonlinearities (206). Changes in illumination and skin resistance also affect the readings with this method. Infrared oculography provides higher-resolution measurements of both horizontal and vertical eye movements, but over a limited range, especially vertically. In addition, the signal is lost when the eyes are closed. Finally, neither electro-oculography nor infrared oculography measures ocular torsion.

The magnetic field-search coil method, which uses coils embedded in a silicone rubber ring that adheres to the sclera by suction, overcomes most of the problems that limit both electro-oculography and infrared oculography (62,216). Further advances in this system using a digital microprocessor enable this technique to be used with great accuracy to measure virtually all types of normal and abnormal eye movements (206,207).

Vestibulo-Ocular Reflex

As explained above, the oculocephalic and caloric tests that are performed in patients with apparent limitation of eye movement primarily test the function of the semicircular canals of the vestibular system. More extensive testing is usually directed toward determining gain, phase, and balance. Rotation tests give more accurate and reproducible results than do caloric tests, although the mental state of the patient while in darkness may influence the results (217). The gain of the VOR may be obtained by measuring the peak eye velocity in response to a velocity step (e.g., sudden sustained rotation at 60°/sec) in darkness. This is usually done in vestibular laboratories equipped with servo-controlled chairs and eye monitoring equipment, although portable systems for this purpose are available (217,218).

Although the otolith organs respond to linear acceleration, tests of their function are rarely performed. Several investigators have suggested that muscle responses that occur less than 100 ms after release into free-fall are part of a normal startle reflex that originates in the otoliths (219–221). Using this theory, Halmagyi and Gresty developed a technique for measuring otolith integrity by recording eye blink reflexes that occur following sudden free-falls (222). Such testing may confirm the presence of otolith function in patients with impaired semicircular canal function or show impaired otolith function in patients with normal semicircular canal function.

Optokinetic System

The hand-held "optokinetic" drums or tapes that are used to elicit smooth movements primarily test the pursuit system.

True optokinetic testing requires a stimulus that fills the field of vision. A common technique is to have the patient sit inside a large, patterned optokinetic drum that is rotated around the patient. A true optokinetic stimulus induces a sensation of self-rotation (223). Another method of eliciting a true optokinetic response is rotation of an individual at a constant velocity in the light for over 1 minute. The sustained nystagmus that results is caused by purely visual stimuli (the vestibular response having died away); however, it is still difficult to separate its pursuit and optokinetic components.

REFERENCES

1. Nelson LB, Catalano RA. Atlas of Ocular Motility. Philadelphia: WB Saunders, 1989.
2. Leigh RJ, Zee DS. The Neurology of Eye Movements. Ed 3. Philadelphia: FA Davis, 1999.
3. von Noorden GK. Binocular Vision and Ocular Motility. Ed 5. St Louis: CV Mosby, 1996.
4. Burgess D, Roper-Hall G, Burde RM. Binocular diplopia associated with subretinal neovascular membranes. Arch Ophthalmol 1980;98:311–317.
5. Fincham EF. Monocular diplopia. Br J Ophthalmol 1963;47:705–712.
6. Ho PC, Elliott JH, O'Day DM. Multirefractile cataract. Invest Ophthalmol Vis Sci (Suppl) 1981;20:50.
7. Amos JF. Diagnosis and management of monocular diplopia. J Am Optom Assoc 1982;53:101–115.
8. Hirst LW, Miller NR, Johnson RT. Monocular polyopia. Arch Neurol 1983;40:756–757.
9. Coffeen P, Guyton DL. Monocular diplopia accompanying ordinary refractive errors. Am J Ophthalmol 1988;105:451–459.
10. Woods RL, Bradley A, Atchison DA. Monocular diplopia caused by ocular aberrations and hyperopic defocus. Vision Res 1996;36:3597–3606.
11. Bender MB. Polyopia and monocular diplopia of cerebral origin. Arch Neurol 1945;54:323–338.
12. Kinsbourne M, Warrington EK. A study of visual perseveration. J Neurol Neurosurg Psychiatr 1963;26:468–475.
13. Meadows JC. Observations on a case of monocular diplopia of cerebral origin. J Neurol Sci 1973;18:249–253.
14. Safran AB, Kline LB, Glaser JS, et al. Television-induced formed visual hallucinations and cerebral diplopia. Br J Ophthalmol 1981;65:707–711.
15. Kasmann B, Ruprecht KW. Eclamptogenic Gerstmann's syndrome in combination with cortical agnosia and cortical diplopia. Germ J Ophthalmol 1995;4:234–238.
16. Brindley GS, Lewin WS. The sensations produced by electrical stimulation of the visual cortex. J Physiol (Lond) 1968;196:479–493.
17. Cass EE. Monocular diplopia occurring in cases of squint. Br J Ophthalmol 1941;25:565–577.
18. Brandt T, Daroff RB. The multisensory physiological and pathological vertigo syndromes. Ann Neurol 1980;7:195–203.
19. Knight RT, St. John JN, Nakada T. Chewing oscillopsia: a case of voluntary visual illusions of movement. Arch Neurol 1984;41:95–96.
20. Bender MB. Oscillopsia. Arch Neurol 1965;13:204–213.
21. Gresty MA, Hess K, Leech J. Disorders of the vestibulo-ocular reflex producing oscillopsia and mechanisms compensating for loss of labyrinthine function. Brain 1977;100:693–716.
22. Ropper AH. Illusion of tilting of the visual environment: report of five cases. J Clin Neuroophthalmol 1983;3:147–151.
23. Steinman RM, Haddad GM, Skavenski AA, et al. Miniature eye movement: the pattern of saccades made by man during maintained fixation may be a refined but useless motor habit. Science 1973;181:810–819.
24. Winterson BJ, Collewijn H. Microsaccades during finely guided visuomotor tasks. Vis Res 1976;16:1387–1390.
25. Ciuffreda KJ, Kenyon RV, Stark L. Fixational eye movements in amblyopia and strabismus. J Am Optom Assoc 1979;50:1251.
26. Herishanu YO, Sharpe JA. Normal square wave jerks. Invest Ophthalmol Vis Sci 1981;20:268–272.
27. St Cyr GJ, Fender DH. The interplay of drifts and flicks in binocular fixation. Vision Res 1969;9:245–265.
28. Ditchburn RW. The function of small saccades. Vision Res 1980;20:271–272.
29. Kowler E, Steinman RM. Small saccades serve no useful purpose [reply to a letter]. Vision Res 1980;20:273–276.
30. Grut EH. A contribution to the pathogeny of concomitant squinting. Trans Ophthalmol Soc UK 1890;10:1–41.
31. Breinin GW. The position of rest during anesthesia and sleep. Arch Ophthalmol 1957;57:323–326.
32. Worth C, Chavasse B. Squint. 9th ed. London, Bailliere, Tindal, and Cox, 1959:714.
33. Abraham SV. The basic position of rest: convergence and divergence. J Pediatr Ophthalmol 1964;1:9–24.
34. Jacobs L, Feldman M, Bender MB. Eye movements during sleep: I. The pattern in the normal human. Arch Neurol 1971;25:151–159.
35. Duke-Elder S, Wybar KC. Ocular motility and strabismus. In: Duke-Elder S, ed. System of Ophthalmology. Vol 6. St Louis, CV Mosby, 1973:96.
36. Hayashi S. Studies of the fixation movements of the eye ball. Jpn J Ophthalmol 1960;4:234–247.
37. Zee DS. Ophthalmoscopy in examination of patients with vestibular disorders. Ann Neurol 1978;3:373–374.
38. Scobee RG. The Oculorotary Muscles. 2nd ed. St Louis, CV Mosby, 1952.
39. Burde RM. The extraocular muscles: anatomy, physiology, and pharmacology. In: Moses RA, ed. Adler's Physiology of the Eye. 7th ed. St Louis, CV Mosby, 1981.
40. Park R, Park G. The center of ocular rotation in the horizontal plane. Am J Physiol 1933;104:545–552.
41. Verrijp C. Movements of the eyes. In: Behrens C, ed. The Eye and Its Diseases. Philadelphia, WB Saunders, 1949.
42. Fick A. Die Bewegungen des menschlichen Augapfels. Henle und Pfeufer, Ztschr 4:101, 1854.
43. Listing JB. In: Ruete CG, ed. Lehrbuch der Ophthalmologie für Aerzte and Studierende. 2nd ed, Vol 1. Braunschweig, Friedr Vieweg & Sohn GmbH, 1855; 37ff.
44. Donders FC. Beitrag zur lehre von den bewegungen des menschlichen auges. Holländ Beitr Anat Physiol Wiss 1848;1:104, 384.
45. Tweed D, Haslwanter T, Fetter M. Optimizing gaze control in three dimensions. Science 1998;281:1363–1366.
46. Cohen B. The vestibulo-ocular reflex arc. In: Kornhuber HH, ed. Handbook of Sensory Physiology. Vol 6. Berlin, Springer-Verlag, 1974:477–540.
47. Leigh RJ, Brandt T. A re-evaluation of the vestibulo-ocular reflex: new ideas of its purpose, properties, neural substrate, and disorders. Neurology 1993;43:1288–1295.
48. Dieterich M, Brandt T. Vestibulo-ocular reflex. Curr Opin Neurol 1995;8:83–88.
49. Nelson JR, Cope D. The otoliths and the ocular countertorsion reflex. Arch Otolaryngol 1971;94:40–50.
50. Nelson JR, House WF. Ocular countertorsion as an indicator of otolith function: effects of unilateral vestibular lesions. Trans Am Acad Ophthalmol Otolaryngol 1971;75:1313–1321.
51. Woellner RC, Graybiel A. Counterrolling of the eyes and its dependence on the magnitude of gravitational or inertial force acting laterally on the body. J Appl Physiol 1959;14:632–634.
52. Uemura T, Cohen B. Effects of vestibular nuclei lesions on vestibulo-ocular reflexes and posture in monkeys. Acta Otolaryngol (Suppl) 1973;315:1–71.
53. Suzuki J, Cohen B, Bender MB. Compensatory eye movements induced by vertical semicircular canal stimulation. Exp Neurol 1964;9:137–160.
54. Diamond SG, Markham CH, Simpson NE, et al. Binocular counterrolling in humans during dynamic rotation. Acta Otolaryngol 1979;87:490–498.
55. Diamond SG, Markham CH. Binocular counterrolling in humans with unilateral labyrinthectomy and in normal controls. Ann NY Acad Sci 1981;374:69–79.
56. Diamond SG, Markham CH. Ocular counterrolling as an indicator of vestibular otolith function. Neurology 1983;33:1460–1469.
57. Jampel RS. The action of the superior oblique muscle. Arch Ophthalmol 1966; 75:535–544.
58. Jampel RS. The fundamental principle of the action of the oblique ocular muscles. Am J Ophthalmol 1970;69:623–638.
59. Jampel RS. Ocular torsion and the function of the vertical extraocular muscles. Am J Ophthalmol 1975;79:292–304.
60. Jampel RS. Ocular torsion and the law of the primary retinal meridians. In: Glaser JS, ed. Neuro-ophthalmology. Vol 10. St Louis, CV Mosby, 1980:201–216.
61. Jampel RS. Ocular torsion and the primary retinal meridians. Am J Ophthalmol 1981;91:14–24.
62. Collewijn H, Van der Steen J, Ferman L, et al. Human ocular counterroll: assessment of static and dynamic properties from electromagnetic scleral coil recordings. Exp Brain Res 1985;59:185–196.
63. Vogel R, Thümler R, von Baumgarten RJ. Ocular counterrolling. Some practical considerations of a new evaluation method for diagnostic purposes. Acta Otolaryngol (Stockh) 1986;102:457–462.
64. Krejcova H, Highstein S, Cohen B. Labyrinthine and extra-labyrinthine effects on ocular counter-rolling. Acta Otolaryngol 1971;72:165–171.
65. Linwong M, Herman SJ. Cycloduction of the eyes with head tilt. Arch Ophthalmol 1971;85:570–573.
66. Miller EF, Graybiel A. Effect of gravitoinertial force on ocular counter-rolling. J Appl Physiol 1971;35:697–700.
67. Horn G, Stechler G, Hill RM. Receptive fields of units in the visual cortex of the cat in the presence or absence of bodily tilt. Exp Brain Res 1972;15:113–132.
68. Brodsky MC. Do you really need your oblique muscles? Arch Ophthalmol 2002; 120:820–828.
69. Hering E. In: Bridgeman B, Stark L, eds. The Theory of Binocular Vision. New York, Plenum Press, 1977:129–145.
70. Boeder P. The cooperation of extraocular muscles. Am J Ophthalmol 1961;51:469–481.

71. Mok D, Ro A, Cadera W, Crawford JD, Vilis T. Rotation of Listing's plane during vergences. Vision Res 1992;32:2055–2064.
72. Ferman L, Collewijn H, Van den Berg AV. A direct test of Listing's law: I. Human ocular torsion measured in static tertiary positions. Vision Res 1987;27: 929–938.
73. Ferman L, Collewijn H, Van den Berg AV. A direct test of Listing's law: II. Human ocular torsion measured under dynamic conditions. Vision Res 1987; 27:939–951.
74. Tweed D, Vilis T. Geometric relations of eye position and velocity vectors during saccades. Vis Res 1990;30:111–127.
75. Demer JL, Miller JM, Poukens V, et al. Evidence for fibromuscular pulleys of the recti extraocular muscles. Invest Ophthalmol Vis Sci 1995;36:1125–1136.
76. Kono R, Poukens V, Demer JL. Quantitative analysis of the structure of the human extraocular muscle pulley system. Invest Ophthalmol Vis Sci 2002;43: 2923–2932.
77. Demer JL, Oh SY, Clarke RA, Poukens V. Evidence for a pulley of the inferior oblique muscle. Invest Ophthalmol Vis Sci 2003;44:3856–3865.
78. Sherrington CS. Experimental note on two movements of the eyes. J Physiol (Lond) 1894;17:27.
79. Hering E. Die Lehre von Binocularen Sehen. Leipzig. Wilhelm Engelmann, 1868.
80. Chamberlain W. Restriction in upward gaze with advancing age. Am J Ophthalmol 1971;71:341–346.
81. Zappia RJ, Winkelman JZ, Gay AJ. Intraocular pressure changes in normal subjects and the adhesive muscle syndrome. Am J Ophthalmol 1971;71: 880–883.
82. Helveston E. The clinical applications of passive ductions and generated muscle force. Ophthalmology 1979;86:30.
83. Saunders RA, Helveston EM, Ellis FD. Differential intraocular pressure in strabismus diagnosis. Ophthalmology 1981;87:59–70
84. Reader AL III. Normal variations of intraocular pressure on vertical gaze. Ophthalmology 1982;89:1084–1087.
85. Jaensch PA. Paresen der schrügen Heber. Albrecht von Graefes Arch Klin Exp Ophthalmol 1929;121:113–125.
86. Wolff J. The occurrence of retraction movements of the eyeball together with congenital defects in the external ocular muscles. Arch Ophthalmol 1900;29: 297–309.
87. Dunnington JH, Berke RN. Exophthalmos due to chronic orbital myositis. Arch Ophthalmol 1943;30:446–466.
88. Duane TD, Schatz HJ, Caputo AR. Pseudo-Duane's retraction syndrome. Trans Am Ophthalmol Soc 1976;74:121–132.
89. Goldstein JH, Sachs DB. Bilateral Duane's syndrome. J Pediatr Ophthalmol 1977;14:12–17.
90. Oei TH, Verhagen WIM, Horsten GPM. Forced duction test in clinical practice. Ophthalmologica 1983;186:87–90.
91. Smith JL. The office forced duction test. Ophthalmic Surg 1975;6:62–63.
92. Stephens KF, Reinecke RD. Quantitative forced duction. Trans Am Acad Ophthalmol Otolaryngol 1967;71:324–329.
93. Knox DL. Suction cup forced duction. Am J Ophthalmol 1974;77:762–763.
94. Miller FS III, Kalina RE. Suction cup for forced duction testing. Am J Ophthalmol 1984;97:390–391.
95. Guyton DL. Exaggerated traction test for the oblique muscles. Ophthalmology 1981;88:1035–1040.
96. Jampolsky A. Strabismus: surgical overcorrections. Highlights Ophthalmol 1965;8:78–79.
97. Katz RL, Eakins KE. Pharmacologic studies of extraocular muscles. Invest Ophthalmol 1967;6:261–268.
98. Smith RB. Succinylcholine and the forced duction test. Ophthalmic Surg 1974; 5:53–55.
99. Scott AB. Active force tests in lateral rectus paralysis. Arch Ophthalmol 1971; 85:397–404.
100. Scott AB. Extraocular muscle forces in strabismus. In: Bach-y-Rita P, Collins CC, Hyde JE, eds. The Control of Eye Movements. New York, Academic Press, 1971:327–342.
101. Scott AB, Collins CC, O'Meara DM. A forceps to measure strabismus forces. Arch Ophthalmol 1972;88:330–333.
102. Bender MB, Bergman PS, Nathanson M. Ocular movements on passive head turning and caloric stimulation in comatose patients. Trans Am Neurol Assoc 1955;80:184–185.
103. Nathanson M, Bergman PS, Anderson PJ. Significance of oculocephalic and caloric responses in the unconscious patient. Neurology 1957;7:829–832.
104. Fisher CM. Neurological examination of the comatose patient. Acta Neurol Scand 1969;45(Suppl 36):1–56.
105. Leigh RJ, Hanley DF, Munschauer FE III, et al. Eye movements induced by head rotation in unresponsive patients. Ann Neurol 1984;15:465–473.
106. Demer JL, Honrubia V, Baloh RW. Dynamic visual acuity: a test for oscillopsia and vestibulo-ocular reflex function. Am J Otol 1994;15:340–347.
107. Chu FC, Reingold D, Cogan DG. A maneuver to elicit vertical dolls' eye movements. Am J Ophthalmol 1979;87:724.
108. Griffin JF, Wray SH, Anderson DP. Misdiagnosis of spasm of the near reflex. Neurology 1976;26:1018–1020.
109. Troost BT, Troost EG. Functional paralysis of horizontal gaze. Neurology 1979; 29:82–85.
110. Klingon GH. Caloric stimulation in localization of brainstem lesions in the comatose patient. Arch Neurol 1952;68:233–235.
111. Vaernet K. Caloric vestibular reactions in transtentorial herniation of the brainstem. Neurology 1957;7:833–836.
112. Blegvard B. Caloric vestibular reactions in transtentorial herniation of the brainstem. Acta Psychiatr Neurol Scand 1962;30:187–196.
113. Rodriguez Barrios R, Mottinelli MD, Medoc J. The study of ocular motility in the comatose patient. J Neurol Sci 1966;3:183–206.
114. Johnkees LBW. The caloric test and its value in evaluation of the patient with vertigo. Otolaryngol Clin North Am 1973;6:73–93.
115. Eviatar A. A critical look at the "cold calorics." Arch Otolaryngol 1974;89: 361–365.
116. Plum F, Posner JB. The Diagnosis of Stupor and Coma. 3rd ed. Philadelphia, FA Davis, 1980.
117. Frenzel H. Spontan- und Provokations-nystagmus als Krankheitssymptom: Ein Leitfaden für seine Beobachtung, Aufzeichnung, und Formanalyse. Berlin, Springer-Verlag, 1955.
118. Luxon L. Comparison of assessment of caloric nystagmus by observation of suration and by electronystagmographic measurement of slow-phase velocity. Br J Audiol 1995;29:107–115.
119. Itaya T, Kitahara M. Air caloric test with continuous thermal change in patients with vestibular disorders. Acta Oto-Laryngol (Suppl) 1995;519:184–187.
120. Facco E, Zuccarello M, Pittoni G, et al. Early outcome prediction in severe head injury: Comparison between children and adults. Childs Nerv Sys 1986;2:67–71.
121. Kennedy CR, Duffy SW, Smith R, et al. Clinical predictors of outcome of encephalitis. Arch Dis Child 1987;62:1156–1162.
122. Müller-Jensen A, Neunzig HP, Emskotter T. Outcome prediction in comatose patients: signficance of reflex eye movement analysis. J Neurol Neurosurg Psychiatr 1987;50:389–392.
123. Griesen O. Pseudocaloric nystagmus. Acta Otolaryngol 1972;73:341–343.
124. Becker GD, Davis JL, Parell GJ. Pseudocaloric nystagmus. Arch Neurol 1978; 35:93–94.
125. Collewijn H, van der Steen J, Steinman RM. Human eye movements associated with blinks and prolonged eyelid closure. J Neurophysiol 1985;54:11–27.
126. Jampel RS, Haidt SJ. Bell's phenomenon and acute idiopathic polyneuritis. Am J Ophthalmol 1972;74:145–153.
127. Ropper AH. The CNS in Guillain-Barré syndrome. Arch Neurol 1983;40: 397–398.
128. Miller NR, Griffin J, Cornblath D, et al. Intact Bell's phenomenon in a patient with myasthenia gravis and upward gaze paresis. Arch Ophthalmol 1989;107: 1117.
129. Hall A. The origin and purposes of blinking. Br J Ophthalmol 1945;29:455–467.
130. Francis IC, Loughhead JA. Bell's phenomenon. A study of 508 patients. Austral J Ophthalmol 1984;12:15–21.
131. Guibor GP. Some eye defects seen in cerebral palsy, with some statistics. Am J Phys Med 1953;32:342–347.
132. Frandsen AD. Occurrence of squint. Acta Ophthalmol (Suppl) 1960;62:9–158.
133. Hiles DA, Wallar PH, McFarlane F. Current concepts in the management of strabismus in children with cerebral palsy. Ann Ophthalmol 1975;7:789–798.
134. Hoyt CS. Abnormalities of the vestibulo-ocular response in congenital esotropia. Am J Ophthalmol 1982;93:704–708.
135. Anderson WD, Lubow M. Astrocytoma of the corpus callosum presenting with acute comitant esotropia. Am J Ophthalmol 1970;69:594–598.
136. Wolter JR, Kindt GW, Waldman J. Concomitant exotropia: following Reye's syndrome. J Pediatr Ophthalmol 1975;12:162–164.
137. Goldstein JH, Wolintz AH, Stein SC. Concomitant strabismus as a sign of intracranial disease. Ann Ophthalmol 1983;15:53–55.
138. Bixenman WW, Laguna JF. Acquired esotropia as initial manifestation of Arnold-Chiari malformation. J Pediatr Ophthalmol Strabismus 1987;24:83–86.
139. Vollrath-Junger C, Lang J. Akuter Strabismus convergens bei erhöhtem Hirndruck. Klin Monatsbl Augenheilkd 1987;190:359–362.
140. Slavin ML. Transient comitant esotropia in a child with migraine. Am J Ophthalmol 1989;107:190–192.
141. Williams AS, Hoyt CS. Acute comitant esotropia in children with brain tumors. Arch Ophthalmol 1989;107:376–378.
142. Astle WF, Miller SJ. Acute comitant esotropia: a sign of intracranial disease. Can J Ophthalmol 1994;29:151–154.
143. Akman A, Dayanir V, Sanaç AS, et al. Acquired esotropia as presenting sign of cranio-cervical junction anomalies. Neuroophthalmology 1995;15:311–314.
144. Hoyt CS, Good WV. Acute onset concomitant esotropia: when is it a sign of serious neurological disease? Br J Ophthalmol 1995;79:498–501.
145. Lewis AR, Kline LB, Sharpe JA. Acquired esotropia due to Arnold-Chiari I malformation. J Neuroophthalmol 1996;16:49–54.
146. Macpherson H, De Becker I, MacNeill JR. Beware: armed and dangerous—acquired non-accommodative esotropia. Am Orthop J 1996;46:44–56.
147. Simon JW, Waldman JB, Couture KC. Cerebellar astrocytoma manifesting as isolated, comitant esotropia in childhood. Am J Ophthalmol 1996;121:584–586.
148. Hiatt RL, Boyer SL, Cope-Troupe C. Decompensated strabismus. Ann Ophthalmol 1979;11:1581–1588.

149. Legmann Simon A, Borchert M. Etiology and prognosis of acute, late-onset esotropia. Ophthalmology 1997;104:1348–1352.
150. von Graefe A. Beiträge zur physiologie und pathologie der schiefen augenmuskeln. Albrecht von Graefes Arch Klin Exp Ophthalmol 1854;1:1–81.
151. Weir CR, Cleary M, Parks S, Dutton GN. Spatial localization in esotropia: does extraretinal eye position information change? Invest Ophthalmol Vis Sci 2000; 41:3782–3786.
152. von Noorden GK, Awaya S, Romano PE. Past pointing in paralytic strabismus. Trans Am Ophthalmol Soc 1970;68:72–85.
153. von Noorden GK, Awaya S, Romano PE. Past pointing in paralytic strabismus. Am J Ophthalmol 1971;71:27–33.
154. Perenin MT, Jeannerod M, Prablanc C. Spatial localisation with paralysed eye muscles. Ophthalmologica 1977;175:206–214.
155. Helmholtz H. Treatise on Physiological Optics. Vol 3 [Southall JPC, translator]. New York, Dover Publications, 1962.
156. Weir CR. Spatial localization: does extraocular muscle proprioception play a role? Graefes Arch Clin Exp Ophthalmol 2000;238:868–873.
157. Paysse EA, Coates DK. Anomalous head posture with early-onset homonymous hemianopia. J AAPOS 1997;1:209–213.
158. Maddox EE. A new test for heterophoria. Ophthalmol Rev 1890;9:129–133.
159. Trobe JD. Cyclodeviation in acquired vertical strabismus. Arch Ophthalmol 1984;102:717–20.
160. Simons K, Arnoldi K, Brown MH. Color dissociation artifacts in double Maddox rod cyclodeviation testing. Ophthalmology 1994;101:1897–1901.
161. Roper-Hall G. Methods and theories of testing extraocular movements. Int Ophthalmol Clin 1978;18:1–18.
162. Hess WR. Ein einfaches messendes Verfahren zur Motilitätsprufung der Augen. Z Augenheilkd 1916;35:201–219.
163. Lancaster WB. Detecting, measuring, plotting and interpreting ocular deviations. Trans Sect Ophthalmol AMA, 1939;78–94.
164. Zee DS, Chu FC, Optican LM, et al. Graphic analysis of paralytic strabismus with the Lancaster red-green test. Am J Ophthalmol 1984;97:587–592.
165. Hirschberg J. Über die messung des schieldgrades und die dosierung der schieloperation. Zentrabl Prakt Augenheilkd 1885;8:325.
166. Krimsky E. The Management of Binocular Imbalance. Philadelphia, Lea & Febiger, 1948:175ff.
167. Kornder LD, Nursey JN, Pratt-Johnson JA, et al. Detection of manifest strabismus in young children: I. A prospective study. Am J Ophthalmol 1974;77: 207–210.
168. Kornder LD, Nursey JN, Pratt-Johnson JA, et al. Detection of manifest strabismus in young children: II. A retrospective study. Am J Ophthalmol 1974;77: 211–214.
169. Thompson JT, Guyton DL. Ophthalmic prisms: measurement errors and how to minimize them. Ophthalmology 1983;90:204–210.
170. Bielschowsky A. Lectures on Motor Anomalies of the Eyes. Hanover, Dartmouth Publications, 1940:88.
171. Urist MJ. Head tilt in vertical muscle paresis. Am J Ophthalmol 1970;69: 440–442.
172. Ohtsuki H, Kishimoto F, Kobashi R, et al. Motor adaptation in the Bielschowsky head-tilt test in cases of superior oblique palsy. Nippon Ganka Gakkai Zashi [Acta Soc Ophthalmol Jpn] 1992;96:1055–1060.
173. Haagedorn A. A new diagnostic motility scheme. Am J Ophthalmol 1942;25: 726–728.
174. Parks MM. Isolated cyclovertical muscle palsy. Arch Ophthalmol 1958;60: 1027–1035.
175. Hardesty HH. Diagnosis of paretic vertical rotators. Am J Ophthalmol 1963;56: 811–816.
176. Kushner BJ. Errors in the three-step test in the diagnosis of vertical strabismus. Ophthalmology 1989;96:127–132.
177. Sydnor CF, Seaber JH, Buckley EG. Traumatic superior oblique palsies. Ophthalmology 1982;89:134–138.
178. von Noorden GK, Hansell R. Clinical characteristics and treatment of isolated inferior rectus paralysis. Ophthalmology 1991;98:253–257.
179. Moster ML, Bosley TM, Slavin ML, et al. Thyroid ophthalmopathy presenting as superior oblique paresis. J Clin Neuroophthalmol 1992;12:94–97.
180. Guyton DL. Clinical assessment of ocular torsion. Am Orthopt J 1983;33:7–15.
181. Guyton DL, Weingarten P. Sensory torsion as the cause of primary oblique muscle overaction/underaction and A- and V-pattern strabismus. Binoc Vision Eye Muscle Qtrly 1994;9:209–236.
182. Guyton DL. Strabismus surgery decisions based on torsion findings. In: Long AD, ed. Anterior Segment and Strabismus Surgery. Amsterdam, Kugler, 1996: 129–137.
183. Madigan WP Jr, Katz NN. Ocular torsion: direct measurement with indirect ophthalmoscope and protractor. J Pediatr Ophthalmol Strabismus 1992;29: 171–174.
184. Morton GV, Lucchese N, Kushner BJ. The role of fundoscopy and fundus photography in strabismus diagnosis. Ophthalmology 1983;90:1186–1191.
185. Ruttum M, von Noorden GK. Adaptation to tilting of the environment in cyclotropia. Am J Ophthalmol 1983;96:229–237.
186. De Ancos E, Klainguti G. An objective measure of ocular torsion: a new indirect ophthalmoscopy lens. Klin Monatsbl Augenheilkd 1994;204:360–362.
187. Benson AJ, Barnes GR. Vision during angular oscillation: the dynamic interaction of visual and vestibular mechanisms. Aviat Space Environ Med 1978;49: 340–345.
188. Barnes GR, Benson AJ, Prior ARJ. Visual-vestibular interaction in the control of eye movement. Aviat Space Environ Med 1978;49:557–564.
189. Zee DS. Suppression of vestibular nystagmus. Ann Neurol 1977;1:207.
190. Chambers BR, Gresty MA. Effects of fixation and optokinetic stimulation on vestibulo-ocular reflex suppression. J Neurol Neurosurg Psychiatr 1982;45: 998–1004.
191. Barnes GR, Grealy MA. Predictive mechanisms of head-eye coordination and vestibulo-ocular reflex suppression in humans. J Vestib Res 1992;2:193–212.
192. Dichgans J. Optokinetic nystagmus as dependent on the retinal periphery via the vestibular nucleus. In: Baker R, Berthoz A, eds. Control of Gaze by Brain Stem Neurons. New York, Elsevier, 1977:261–267.
193. Halmagyi GM, Gresty MA. Clinical signs of visual-vestibular interaction. J Neurol Neurosurg Psychiatr 1979;42:934–939.
194. Buttner U, Grundei T. Gaze-evoked nystagmus and smooth pursuit deficits: their relationship studied in 52 patients. J Neurol 1995;242:384–389.
195. Waterson JA, Barnes GR, Grealy MA. A quantitative study of eye and head movements during smooth pursuit in patients with cerebellar disease. Brain 1992; 115:1343–1358.
196. Catz A, Ron S, Solzi P, Korczyn AD. Vestibulo-ocular reflex suppression following hemispheric stroke. Scand J Rehab Med 1993;25:149–152.
197. Fetter M, Klockgether T, Schulz JB, et al. Oculomotor abnormalities and MRI findings in idiopathic cerebellar ataxia. J Neurol 1994;241:234–241.
198. Baloh RW, Sills AW, Kumley WE, et al. Quantitative measurement of saccade amplitude, duration, and velocity. Neurology 1975;25:1065–1070.
199. Collewijn H, Van der Mark F, Jansen TC. Precise recording of human eye movements. Vision Res 1975;15:447–450.
200. Young LR, Sheena D. Survey of eye movement recording models. Behav Res Method Instrum 1975;7:397–429.
201. Baloh RW, Kumley WE, Sills AW, et al. Quantitative measurement of smooth pursuit eye movements. Ann Otolaryngol 1976;85:111–119.
202. Dell'Osso LF, Daroff RB. Eye movement characteristics and recording techniques. In: Glaser JS, ed. Neuro-ophthalmology. Hagerstown, Harper and Row, 1978:185–198.
203. Robinson DA. The control of eye movements. In: Brooks VB, ed. Handbook of Physiology. Vol 2. Bethesda, American Physiology Society, 1981:1275–1320.
204. Yee RD. Eye movement recording as a clinical tool. Ophthalmology 1983;90: 211–222.
205. Eizenman M, Frecker RC, Hallett PE. Precise non-contacting measurement of eye movements using the corneal reflex. Vis Res 1984;24:167–174.
206. Bechert K, Koenig E. A search coil system with automatic field stabilization, calibration, and geometric processing for eye movement recordings in humans. Neuroophthalmology 1996;16:163–170.
207. Koenig E, Westermann H, Jäger K, et al. A new multiaxis rotating chair for oculomotor and vestibular function testing in humans. Neuroophthalmology 1996;16:157–162.
208. Metz HS, Scott AB, O'Meara DM, et al. Ocular saccades in lateral rectus palsy. Arch Ophthalmol 1970;84:453–460.
209. Metz HS. III nerve palsy: I. Saccadic velocity studies. Ann Ophthalmol 1973; 5:526–528.
210. Metz HS, Scott WE, Madison E, et al. Saccadic velocity and active force studies in blowout fractures of the orbit. Am J Ophthalmol 1974;78:665–670.
211. Zee DS, Yee RD. Abnormal saccades in paralytic strabismus. Am J Ophthalmol 1977;83:112–114.
212. Metz HS. Saccades with limited downward gaze. Arch Ophthalmol 1980;98: 2204–2205.
213. Stathacopoulos RA, Yee RD, Bateman JB. Vertical saccades in superior oblique palsy. Inv Ophthalmol Vis Sci 1991;32:1938–1943.
214. Tian S, Lennerstrand G. Vertical saccadic velocity and force development in superior oblique palsy. Vis Res 1994;34:1785–1798.
215. Lewis RF, Zee DJ, Repka MX, et al. Regulation of static and dynamic ocular alignment in patients with trochlear nerve paresis. Vision Res 1995;35: 3255–3264.
216. Ferman L, Collewijn H, Jansen TC, et al. Human gaze stability in the horizontal, vertical and torsional direction during voluntary head movements, evaluated with a three-dimensional scleral induction coil. Vision Res 1987;27:811–828.
217. Saadat D, Oleary DP, Pulec JL, et al. Comparison of vestibular autorotation and caloric testing. Otolaryngol Head Neck Surg 1995;113:215–222.
218. Goebel JA, Hanson JM, Langhofer LR, et al. Head-shake vestibulo-ocular reflex testing: comparison of results with rotational chair testing. Otolaryngol Head Neck Surg 1995;112:203–209.
219. Greenwood R, Hopkins A. Muscle responses during sudden falls in man. J Physiol (Lond) 1976;254:507–518.
220. Greenwood R, Hopkins A. Landing from an unexpected fall and a voluntary step. Brain 1976;99:375–386.
221. Watt DGD. Responses of cats to sudden falls: an otolith-originating reflex assisting landing. J Neurophysiol 1976;39:257–265.
222. Halmagyi GM, Gresty MA. Eye blink reflexes to sudden free falls: a clinical test of otolith function. J Neurol Neurosurg Psychiatr 1983;46:844–847.
223. Dichgans J, Von Reutern GM, Rommelt U. Impaired suppression of vestibular nystagmus by fixation in cerebellar and noncerebellar patients. Arch Psychiatr Nervenkr 1978;226:183–199.

CHAPTER 19

Supranuclear and Internuclear Ocular Motility Disorders

David S. Zee and David Newman-Toker

In this chapter, we survey clinicopathologic correlations for supranuclear ocular motor disorders. The presentation follows the schema of the 1999 text by Leigh and Zee (1), and the material in this chapter is intended to complement that of Chapters 17 and 23. We emphasize an anatomic approach, although we also discuss certain metabolic, infectious, degenerative, and inflammatory diseases in which supranuclear and internuclear disorders of eye movements are prominent. Details about these conditions can be found in the appropriate chapters in other volumes of this text.

OCULAR MOTOR SYNDROMES CAUSED BY LESIONS IN THE MEDULLA

Many structures within the medulla are important in the control of eye movements: the vestibular nuclei, perihypoglossal nuclei, and inferior olive and its outflow pathway through the inferior cerebellar peduncle. The perihypoglossal nuclei consist of the nucleus prepositus hypoglossi (NPH), which lies in the floor of the fourth ventricle, the intercalatus nucleus, and ventrally the nucleus of Roller. These nuclei are interconnected with other ocular motor structures in the brain stem and cerebellum. The NPH and the adjacent medial vestibular nuclei (MVN) are critical for holding horizontal positions of gaze (the neural integrator) (2). These structures also participate in vertical gaze-holding, although more rostral structures, especially the interstitial nucleus of Cajal (INC), also contribute. With lesions in the paramedian structures of the medulla, nystagmus—commonly upbeat—is the most common finding (3). Upbeat nystagmus may also reflect involvement of a ventral tegmental pathway for the upward vestibulo-ocular reflex (VOR) producing a downward vestibular bias and a consequent upbeat nystagmus (4). Wernicke's disease commonly affects the region of NPH and MVN, which may account for the horizontal gaze-evoked nystagmus and spontaneous vertical nystagmus and loss of vestibular responses that occur with this disease.

Lesions of the inferior olivary nucleus or its connections may produce the oculopalatal myoclonus (oculopalatal tremor) syndrome (5,6). This condition usually develops weeks to months after a brain stem or cerebellar infarction, although it may also occur with degenerative conditions (7,8). The term *myoclonus* is misleading because the movements of affected muscles are to and fro and are approximately synchronized, typically at a rate of 2–4 cycles/sec. *Ocular palatal tremor* is the better term (6). The abnormal ocular movements consist of pendular oscillations that are often vertical but may have a horizontal or torsional component. Predominantly vertical oscillations are usually associated with symmetric bilateral palatal tremor. Mixed vertical and torsional movements, sometimes disconjugate and with a seesaw quality, are associated with unilateral or asymmetric palatal tremor (9,10). Occasionally, patients develop the eye oscillations without movements of the palate. Closing the eyes may bring out the vertical ocular oscillations (11). The nystagmus sometimes disappears with sleep, but the palatal movements usually persist. Occasionally, the oscillations resolve spontaneously. Gabapentin may partially ameliorate the eye oscillations (12).

The main pathologic finding with palatal tremor is hypertrophy of the inferior olivary nucleus, which is often seen on magnetic resonance (MR) imaging (13). The olivary nucleus contains enlarged, vacuolated neurons with expanded dendrites and enlarged astrocytes (Fig. 19.1). The hypertrophic

neurons and their dendrites contain increased acetylcholinesterase reaction product (14). Guillain and Mollaret (15) suggested that disruption of connections between the dentate and the contralateral olivary nucleus (which run via the red nucleus and central tegmental tract) causes this syndrome. Another hypothesis is that the ocular oscillations are caused by instability in circuits that include the projection from the inferior olive to the flocculus, which is thought to be important in the adaptive control of the VOR (10).

Occasionally, lesions are restricted to the vestibular nuclei. For example, vertigo may be the sole symptom of an exacerbation of multiple sclerosis (MS) (16,17) and of brain stem ischemia (18–21). Nystagmus caused by lesions in the vestibular nuclei may be purely horizontal, vertical, or torsional, or mixed. Moreover, nystagmus from a central vestibular lesion can mimic that caused by peripheral vestibular disease (22,23). Dolichoectasia of the basilar artery may produce a variety of combinations of central and peripheral vestibular syndromes (24,25). Microvascular compression of the vestibulocochlear nerve may produce paroxysmal vertigo (26,27). Brandt and Dieterich (28), Büttner et al. (29), and Dieterich (30) provide useful topographic schemes for localizing central vestibular syndromes and central vestibular nystagmus within the brain stem and cerebellum.

WALLENBERG'S SYNDROME (LATERAL MEDULLARY INFARCTION)

Lesions of the vestibular nuclei commonly affect neighboring structures, in particular the cerebellar peduncles and perihypoglossal nuclei. The best-recognized syndrome involving the vestibular nuclei is caused by a lateral medullary infarction (Wallenberg's syndrome) (Fig. 19.2). The typical findings of Wallenberg's syndrome are impairment of sensation of pain and temperature over the ipsilateral face, ipsilateral Horner's syndrome and limb ataxia, and dysarthria and dysphagia. Sensation of pain and temperature are impaired over the contralateral trunk and limbs. The ipsilateral facial nerve may also be affected if the infarct extends more

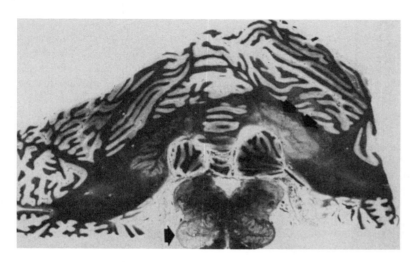

Figure 19.1. Pathology of palato-ocular myoclonus. A section through the cerebellum and medulla shows marked demyelination of the right dentate nucleus and restiform body (*double arrows*). The left inferior olive is hypertrophic and shows mild demyelination (*arrow*). (From Nathanson M. Palatal myoclonus: further clinical and pathophysiological observations. Arch Neurol Psychiatry 1956;75:285–296.)

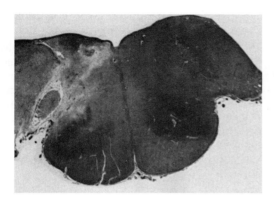

Figure 19.2. Wallenberg's syndrome. Transverse section through the medulla oblongata showing a unilateral infarction in its dorsolateral region. (From Ongerboer de Visser BW, Kuypers HGJM. Late blink reflex changes in lateral medullary lesions: an electrophysiological and neuroanatomical study of Wallenberg's syndrome. Brain 1978;101:285–294.)

rostrally (Fig. 19.3). Wallenberg's syndrome is most commonly caused by occlusion of the ipsilateral vertebral artery; occasionally, the posterior inferior cerebellar artery is selectively involved (31,32) (Fig. 19.4). Dissection of the vertebral artery (either spontaneous or traumatic, such as following chiropractic manipulation) may cause Wallenberg's syndrome (33). Rarely, demyelinating disease is the cause (34).

The symptoms of Wallenberg's syndrome include vertigo

and unusual sensations of body and environmental tilt, often so bizarre as to suggest a psychogenic origin (35,36). Patients may report that the whole room appears tilted on its side or even upside down; with their eyes closed, they may feel themselves to be tilted. Such symptoms are occasionally reported in patients without signs of lateral medullary infarction and may be caused by transient brain stem or cerebellar ischemia (37–40) and occasionally with lesions in the thalamus (41), cerebral hemispheres (42), or peripheral vestibular apparatus (43).

Lateropulsion, a compelling sensation of being pulled toward the side of the lesion, is often a prominent symptom in patients with Wallenberg's syndrome and is also reflected in the ocular motor system (44–46). If the patient is asked to fix straight ahead and then gently close the lids, the eyes deviate conjugately toward the side of the lesion. This is reflected in the corrective saccades that the patient must make on eye opening to reacquire the target. Lateropulsion may appear with a blink.

Saccadic eye movements are also affected by lateropulsion (Fig. 19.5) (44,46–49). Horizontal saccades directed toward the side of the lesion usually overshoot the target, and saccades directed away from the side of the lesion undershoot the target; this is referred to as *ipsipulsion* of saccades and should be differentiated from the *contrapulsion* of saccades that occurs with lesions in the superior cerebellar peduncle due, for example, to superior cerebellar artery occlusions (discussed later). Quick phases of nystagmus are similarly affected in Wallenberg's syndrome, so that sac-

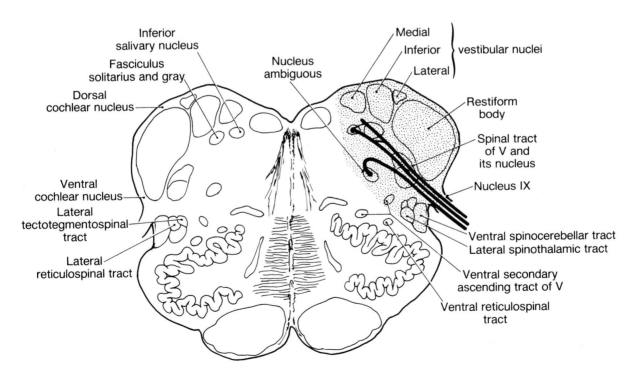

Figure 19.3. Medulla oblongata showing the specific neural structures (*shaded area*) that are commonly damaged in Wallenberg's syndrome.

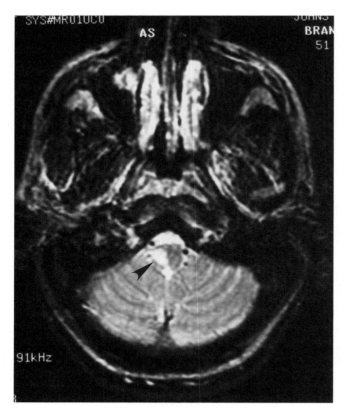

Figure 19.4. Neuroimaging of Wallenberg's syndrome. T2-weighted magnetic resonance image, axial view, in a 51-year-old man with Wallenberg's syndrome characterized in part by lateropulsion of saccades toward the right side, a skew deviation with the right eye being hypotropic, and the ocular tilt reaction, shows a hyperintense area (*arrowhead*) consistent with an infarct on the right side of the medulla.

phases) can also occur (54). The ocular tilt reaction (discussed later) commonly occurs in Wallenberg's syndrome (55), including a skew deviation with an ipsilateral hypotropia. The eyes counter-roll with the top poles rotated toward the side of the lesion, but unequally, so that there is also a cyclodeviation. The lower eye is usually more extorted. Some patients show ipsilateral head tilt (56). The skew deviation and head tilt arise from imbalance in pathways mediating otolith responses. The subjective sensations of tilt or inversion of the world probably also reflect involvement of central projections from the graviceptors—the utricle and saccule.

Smooth pursuit is usually impaired in Wallenberg's syndrome, particularly for tracking targets moving away from the side of the lesion (46). Caloric testing usually shows intact horizontal canal function. During both rotational and caloric testing, there is a directional preponderance of slow phases, usually toward the side of the lesion (45,46,57). Head nystagmus also occurs in some patients (44).

Many of the findings in Wallenberg's syndrome, including the bizarre visual disturbances and the skew deviation, may reflect imbalance of otolith influences caused by direct damage to the caudal aspects of the vestibular nuclei. Damage to the restiform body, which carries olivocerebellar projections, may also account for some of the ocular motor findings, especially the steady-state deviation of the eyes toward the side of the lesion and the ipsipulsion of saccades (47–49,58,59). Ipsipulsion of saccades, with deviation of the eyes to the side of the lesion, can be reproduced experimentally by lesions of the fastigial nucleus (60). This finding supports the hypothesis that in Wallenberg's syndrome, the interruption of climbing fiber input to the dorsal cerebellar vermis releases Purkinje cell inhibition upon the underlying fastigial nucleus, thus leading to the equivalent of a lesion in the fastigial nucleus (58). An analogous increase in Purkinje cell inhibition from the flocculus to the vestibular nucleus may also play a role in the nystagmus (slow phase toward the side of the lesion) seen in these patients.

SYNDROME OF THE ANTERIOR INFERIOR CEREBELLAR ARTERY

The anterior inferior cerebellar artery (AICA) supplies portions of the vestibular nuclei and the adjacent dorsolateral brain stem, and the inferior lateral cerebellum. The AICA is also the origin of the labyrinthine artery in most persons and also sends a twig to the cerebellar flocculus in the cerebellopontine angle. Consequently, ischemia in the distribution of the AICA may cause vertigo, vomiting, hearing loss, facial palsy, and ipsilateral limb ataxia, along with deficits in gaze-holding and pursuit as well as vestibular nystagmus (61–63) (Fig. 19.6). The ocular motor signs reflect a combination of involvement of the labyrinth, vestibular nuclei, and flocculus (discussed later) .

SKEW DEVIATION AND THE OCULAR TILT REACTION

Skew deviation is a vertical misalignment of the visual axes caused by a disturbance of prenuclear vestibular inputs

cades directed away from the side of the lesion are smaller than those toward the lesion. On attempting a purely vertical refixation, an oblique saccade directed toward the side of the lesion is produced. Corrective saccades then bring the eyes back to the target (50). Saccades made in total darkness also show lateropulsion, although in one report the patient was still able to make corrective saccades to the remembered location of a previously seen target (51). This finding implied that the central nervous system "knew" actual eye position. With time, vertical saccades may become more bizarre; S-shaped saccadic trajectories can appear a week or more after the onset of the illness and may reflect an adaptive strategy to correct the saccadic abnormality. *Torsipulsion,* inappropriate torsional saccades during attempted horizontal or vertical saccades, also may occur, sometimes in association with torsional nystagmus (52,53).

Spontaneous nystagmus in Wallenberg's syndrome, when present, is usually horizontal or mixed horizontal and torsional with a small vertical component (52). In primary position, the slow phase is directed toward the side of the lesion, although it may reverse direction in eccentric positions, suggesting that the gaze-holding mechanism is also impaired. Lid nystagmus (synkinetic lid twitches with horizontal quick

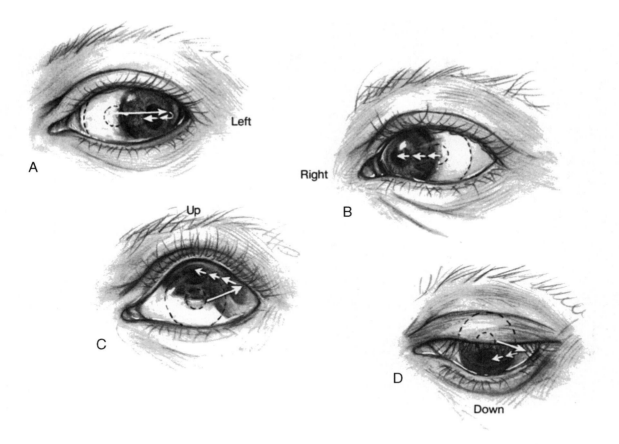

Figure 19.5. Lateropulsion of saccades in a patient with a left Wallenberg's syndrome. *A,* On attempted leftward gaze, the patient overshoots the target and must make a corrective saccade. *B,* On attempted rightward gaze, the patient makes a series of hypometric saccades. *C* and *D,* On attempted upward and downward gaze, the eyes move obliquely to the left and must make several refixation movements back to center. (Redrawn from Kommerell G, Hoyt WF. Lateropulsion of saccadic eye movements: electro-oculographic studies in a patient with Wallenberg's syndrome. Arch Neurol 1973;28:313–318.)

to the oculomotor nuclei. Torsional and horizontal deviations may be associated findings. The hypertropia may be the same (comitant) in all positions of gaze, or it may vary and even alternate (typically with an alternating abducting hypertropia—i.e., right hypertropia on right gaze, left hypertropia on left gaze) (64–67). When skew deviation is incomitant, it may mimic an isolated superior (68) or inferior (69) oblique palsy by the Bielschowsky three-step test. In such cases, however, it appears that the addition of a fourth step, assessment of ocular torsion in both eyes, may be able to distinguish skew deviation from isolated oblique weakness: with skew mimicking superior oblique palsy, the hypertropic eye is incyclotorted (rather than excyclotorted, as one would expect if the hypertropia were the result of superior oblique weakness) (68). By analogy, when skew mimics inferior oblique palsy, the hypotropic eye is excyclotorted (rather than incyclotorted, as one would expect if the hypotropia were the result of inferior oblique weakness) (69). It remains to be seen, however, whether the addition of this fourth step will reliably distinguish between superior oblique palsy and all forms of skew deviation, or whether some cases will simply be indistinguishable at the bedside.

In many patients, skew deviation is associated with ocular torsion and head tilt, the pathologic ocular tilt reaction (OTR), which may be tonic (sustained) (56) or paroxysmal (70,71). Such patients also show a deviation of the subjective vertical (72,73). The ocular torsion may be dissociated, producing a cyclodeviation (74). The OTR is usually attributed to an imbalance in otolith-ocular and otolith-collic reflexes that are part of a phylogenetically old righting response to a lateral tilt of the head (75). In patients with more rostral lesions, interruption of descending pathways involved with controlling head posture may also contribute to the head tilt of the OTR (75,76).

Skew deviation occurs with a variety of abnormalities in the vestibular periphery, brain stem, or cerebellum (66,77–83) and with raised intracranial pressure from supratentorial tumors or pseudotumor cerebri (84,85). In infants, a skew deviation may be the harbinger of a subsequent horizontal strabismus (86).

Why does skew deviation occur with lesions at so many sites within the posterior fossa? An imbalance in otolith pathways is the most likely cause (77). An imbalance of posterior semicircular canal inputs may also play a role (56,87), al-

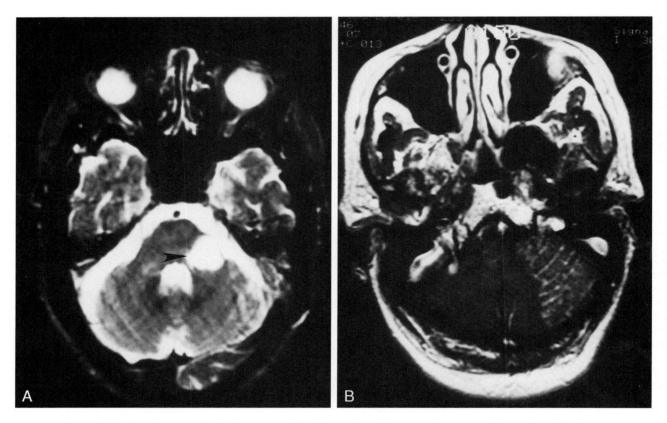

Figure 19.6. Neuroimaging of infarct in territory of the left anterior inferior cerebellar artery (AICA). *A*, T2-weighted axial magnetic resonance (MR) scan shows hyperintense area in the region of the left middle cerebellar peduncle (*arrowhead*). *B*, T1-weighted axial MR scan after intravenous injection of paramagnetic contrast material shows diffuse enhancement in the distal distribution of the AICA involving the left cerebellar hemisphere. The 69-year-old patient had, among other manifestations, left-beating gaze-evoked nystagmus.

though if that is the case nystagmus should also be present (88).

To understand skew deviation, it is helpful to consider physiologic aspects of otolith-ocular reflexes (75). In lateral-eyed animals, tilting the head laterally around the longitudinal (anterior-posterior) axis causes a disjunctive, vertical (skew) deviation (i.e., one eye goes up, the other down) that acts to hold the visual axis of each eye close to the horizontal. In human subjects, who are frontal-eyed, a static head tilt (ear to shoulder) causes sustained, largely conjugate counter-rolling of the eyes (ocular torsion) that is about 10% of the head roll (89–91), although the actual amount may be related to various factors, including the angle of vergence. Thus, the static ocular response does not compensate for the head tilt and is thought to be vestigial. There may also be a small amount of skewing in normal subjects during rotation of the head around its roll (anterior-posterior) axis (92). In contrast, peripheral or central lesions that disrupt otolith inputs often cause large amounts of skew deviation (e.g., 7°) and ocular torsion (e.g., 25°). Usually, any pathologic head tilt (ear to shoulder) is contralateral to the hypertropic eye, and the ocular torsion is such that the upper poles of the eyes rotate toward the lower ear. The contralateral head tilt may be a

compensatory response to the perceived tilt of the subjective visual vertical, although it may also reflect direct involvement of descending projections from the vestibular nuclei or the INC to cervical motoneurons (76).

Lesions of the vestibular organ or its nerve can cause both skew deviation and the OTR by producing an imbalance in utricle inputs (80,93). The ocular tilt reaction may also occur as a component of Tullio phenomenon, which is characterized by sound-induced vestibular symptoms (94–96). It occurs in patients with perilymph fistula either at the oval or round window, with other abnormal communications between the membranous labyrinth and the perilymph space, or with abnormalities of the ossicular chain and its connection with the membranous labyrinth. Dehiscence of the roof of the superior semicircular canal is another recently identified cause (96–98). The OTR is consistent with the effects of experimental stimulation of the otoliths (100) and the utricular nerve (101), which cause ipsilateral hypertropia and conjugate ocular counter-rolling (i.e., top pole of the eyes toward the contralateral ear).

The utricle projects predominantly to the ipsilateral lateral vestibular nucleus, whereas the saccule projects to the y-group of vestibular nuclei (101,102). Thus, lesions of the vestibular nuclei (e.g., as part of Wallenberg's lateral medullary syndrome) may also cause skew deviation with hypotropia on the side of the lesion (55). In addition, some patients show an ipsilateral head tilt and disconjugate ocular torsion. The latter is an excylotropia, with excyclodeviation of the ipsilateral, lower eye, but small or absent incyclodeviation of the contralateral, higher eye (52,103).

Skew deviation is encountered in patients with cerebellar lesions (66,67,104–106). Some of these patients show an alternating skew deviation that is characterized by a hyperdeviation of the abducting eye. This abnormality also may be analogous to a phylogenetically old, otolith-mediated, righting reflex present in lateral-eyed animals, which in this case is related to the ocular motor response that compensates for fore-and-aft motion (as opposed to lateral roll) of the head. Although the brain stem is likely also involved in some of these patients, skew deviation can occur in some patients who appear to have pure cerebellar disease. This suggests that just as the cerebellum governs the semicircular canal-ocular reflex, it also influences the otolith-ocular reflexes. Indeed, downbeat nystagmus, which is sometimes attributable to disease of the flocculus (discussed later), commonly coexists with this pattern of skew deviation that alternates with lateral gaze.

Utricular projections from the vestibular nuclei probably cross the midline and ascend in the medial longitudinal fasciculus (MLF). Therefore, unilateral internuclear ophthalmoplegia (INO) is often associated with a skew deviation, presumably because lesions of one MLF cause an imbalance of ascending otolith inputs. The INO is usually on the side of the hypertropic eye, likely reflecting that utricular projections are generally damaged in the MLF after crossing at the level of the mid-pons (i.e., a right MLF lesion damages utricular inputs from the left ear, leading to a right hypertropia similar conceptually to that seen with a left lateral medullary syndrome or right rostral midbrain syndrome) (107).

In the midbrain, otolith projections contact the oculomotor and trochlear nerve nuclei as well as the INC. Lesions in the mesencephalon, in or around the INC, thus may cause skew deviation (78,108,109) and the OTR (56,110). When the head tilt is sustained (tonic), it is contralateral to the side of the lesion; in addition, there is usually a hypertropia that is ipsilateral to the lesion and a conjugate cyclotorsion that is characterized by intorsion of the ipsilateral eye and extorsion of the contralateral eye (i.e., ocular counter-rolling away from the side of the mesencephalic lesion). Defects of vertical eye movements and oculomotor or trochlear nerve function are also common in this setting. Combined prenuclear and fascicular or nuclear lesions in the midbrain may create torsion of one eye and the OTR (111,112).

In patients with meso-diencephalic lesions, spontaneous ocular oscillations may also be present that suggest involvement of otolith inputs to the oculomotor system, such as seesaw nystagmus (113) or, more rarely, slowly alternating skew deviation (114–116). In the latter case, skew deviation slowly alternates or varies cyclically in magnitude over the course of a few minutes. The periodicity of the phenomenon (with each eye typically being hypertropic for about 30 seconds to a minute) is reminiscent of periodic alternating nystagmus, and the two phenomena can coexist (117).

In some patients, the skew deviation (with or without a head tilt) is not sustained but paroxysmal (70,71). In one patient with a clearly defined lesion close to the right INC, episodes of contralateral hypertropia and ipsilateral head tilt occurred, suggesting an irritative mechanism (71). This interpretation of the findings in paroxysmal skew deviation is supported by the results of electric stimulation near the INC in the monkey. This produces an ocular tilt reaction that consists of depression and extorsion of the ipsilateral eye and elevation and intorsion of the contralateral eye (118). With the head free to move, an ipsilateral head tilt also occurs (119). In human patients, stimulation in the region of the INC causes an ipsilateral OTR (120). Microvascular compression may also cause a paroxysmal skew deviation with torsional nystagmus (121). Skew deviation has also been reported as an epileptic phenomenon (122).

OCULAR MOTOR SYNDROMES CAUSED BY LESIONS IN THE CEREBELLUM

Clinicians are appropriately cautious in attributing eye movement abnormalities specifically to cerebellar dysfunction, because the brain stem is so frequently damaged in patients with lesions of the cerebellum. Likewise, brain stem lesions can produce a ''functional'' cerebellar lesion and corresponding cerebellar eye signs by virtue of a change in the climbing fiber activity projecting to cerebellar Purkinje cells, as occurs in Wallenberg's syndrome (discussed previously). Holmes (123) and Cogan (77), however, recognized specific cerebellar eye signs, and Daroff (124) listed more than 30 ''cerebellar eye signs'' in a compendium published in 1982. Recent clinical and experimental studies provide additional evidence that cerebellar lesions alone can cause specific ocular motor abnormalities (104,125,126). In essence, three principal syndromes can be identified: the syndrome of the dorsal vermis and underlying posterior fastigial nuclei, the syndrome of the flocculus and paraflocculus, and the syndrome of the nodulus and ventral uvula. The main features of each of these syndromes are summarized in Table 19.1.

LOCATION OF LESIONS AND THEIR MANIFESTATIONS

Experimental lesions of the dorsal vermis (lobules VI and VII) and of the underlying fastigial nuclei (called the fastigial oculomotor region) cause saccadic dysmetria, typically hypometria if the vermis alone is involved and hypermetria if the deep nuclei are affected (127). Pursuit, especially the initial acceleration of the eyes during tracking, is also affected by dorsal vermis lesions (128). Lesions of the deep nuclei can lead to macrosaccadic oscillations, an extreme degree of hypermetria. Lesions restricted to the dorsal vermis produce not only saccadic dysmetria but also impaired initiation of pursuit with a decrease in the acceleration of the eyes during tracking, and disturbances of eye alignment

Table 19.1
Localization of Cerebellar Eye Movement Abnormalities

Structure	Function	Disorder
Flocculus and paraflocculus	Retinal-image stabilization (smooth tracking with head still or free suppression of inappropriate vestibular nystagmus, holding positions of gaze, adaptive control of the VOR and pulse-step match)	Impaired smooth pursuit, VOR cancellation and fixation suppression of caloric nystagmus; gaze-evoked, rebound, centripetal and downbeat nystagmus; postsaccadic drift; inappropriate amplitude or direction of the VOR
Nodulus and ventral uvula	Control of low-frequency response of the VOR	Periodic alternating nystagmus, impaired tilt suppression of postrotatory nystagmus, positional nystagmus, impaired habituation of the VOR, increased duration of vestibular responses.
Dorsal vermis and posterior fastigial nucleus	Saccade accuracy, smooth-pursuit eye alignment	Saccadic dysmetria, impaired pursuit, esodeviations

VOR, vestibulo-ocular reflex.
(Zee DS, Walker MF. Cerebellar control of eye movements. In: Chalupa LM, Werner JS, eds. The Visual Neurosciences. Cambridge, MA: MIT Press, 2003:1485–1498.)

including the development of an esodeviation. The pattern of saccadic dysmetria that occurs in cerebellar disease, as well as whether corrective saccades occur, may also vary with the type of visual stimulus. Saccades to remembered targets are more dysmetric (129–131). In some cerebellar patients, only corrective saccades are dysmetric (132). Saccadic dysmetria may be present for externally triggered movements to a visual target but not for internally triggered saccades during scanning of a visual scene (133). Deficits of pursuit may also be produced by lesions of the dorsal vermis (130), as can defects in motion perception (134). Bilateral symmetric lesions of the deep nuclei do not lead to pursuit deficits during sustained tracking, although unilateral lesions lead to a contralateral deficit (135,136), probably because of an imbalance in eye acceleration signals.

Experimental lesions of the flocculus and paraflocculus cause gaze-evoked nystagmus, rebound nystagmus, and downbeat nystagmus. Such lesions also cause impaired smooth tracking (either with head still [smooth pursuit] or with head moving), postsaccadic drift, and loss of some adaptive capabilities, such as the ability to adjust the amplitude and direction of the VOR or the pulse-step (phasic-tonic) match for saccades. Unilateral lesions produce ipsilateral deficits in pursuit and gaze-holding (47,137,140). In patients with cerebellar disease, pursuit defects with the head still, defects in combined eye and head tracking, and gaze-holding deficits frequently occur together, reflecting their common substrate in the flocculus and vestibular nuclei (139). Quantitatively, however, pursuit with the head still is sometimes relatively more impaired (140,141). Patients with cerebellar disease may show timing errors during tracking of periodic targets (141), but there is some preservation of predictive capability (142). The ability to generate anticipatory smooth eye movements of high speed at the onset of tracking is also impaired in some cerebellar patients (143).

Experimental lesions of the nodulus lead to an increase in the duration of vestibular responses that predisposes the animal to the development of periodic alternating nystagmus (144). Other abnormalities of the ''velocity-storage mechanism'' also are present, including abnormally directed slow

phases of nystagmus during sustained rotations, a failure of tilt suppression of postrotatory nystagmus (145), loss of habituation (146) and positional nystagmus (147).

Syndromes of the dorsal vermis and fastigial nucleus, flocculus and paraflocculus, and nodulus are frequently encountered in patients with degenerative disorders that presumably affect only the cerebellum. In some instances, pathologic examination confirms disease restricted to the cerebellum (148). Similar findings occur in patients with focal structural lesions of the cerebellum.

FitzGibbon et al. (149) attributed another ocular motor sign to a focal cerebellar lesion. Patients with cavernous angiomas in the middle cerebellar peduncle show torsional nystagmus during vertical pursuit. The direction of the torsional nystagmus changes with the direction of the pursuit, with the eye velocity of the slow phase of the torsional nystagmus being directly proportional to the eye velocity of the slow phase of pursuit. This finding probably relates to the fact that smooth pursuit is organized in, and superimposed on, a phylogenetically old vertical ''labyrinthine-optokinetic'' coordinate system. Thus, for a pure vertical pursuit movement to occur, opposite torsional components must cancel (as is the case for pure vertical vestibular nystagmus). The middle cerebellar peduncle probably carries information to and from the cerebellum (perhaps between the flocculus and the nucleus reticularis tegmenti pontis in the pons) and contains vertical pursuit signals encoded with a torsional component (150).

Other signs that occur in patients with lesions restricted to the cerebellum cannot always be attributed to dysfunction of a particular part of the cerebellum. They include square-wave jerks (151,152), alternating skew deviation (67,104), cross-coupled VOR responses (inappropriately directed slow phases) (147,153,154), disconjugate (poorly yoked) saccades with disconjugate gaze-evoked nystagmus (104,126) and divergent nystagmus (155), centripetal nystagmus (156), primary position upbeating nystagmus (157), positional nystagmus (158), increased responsiveness of the cervico-ocular reflex (159), and impaired responses to linear translation (L-VOR) (154,160,161).

The cerebellum is also important in long-term adaptive functions that keep eye movements appropriate to the visual stimulus (162). Experimentally, it has been shown that control of VOR amplitude and direction, saccade amplitude, pursuit initiation, and phoria adaptation are all under cerebellar control. For example, adaptation of the gain of the VOR is impaired in patients with cerebellar lesions (163). This adaptive or "repair shop" function of the cerebellum probably accounts for both the enduring nature of the ocular motor deficits that accompany diffuse cerebellar lesions and, perhaps, the somewhat variable effects of cerebellar lesions. Thus, inherent, idiosyncratic abnormalities in brain stem or peripheral ocular motor mechanisms that are normally "repaired" by the cerebellum may reappear after cerebellar lesions. For example, some patients with cerebellar disease may not be able to adapt to a phoria induced by wearing prisms (164,165), and the same is true for monkeys with cerebellar vermis lesions (126). Children with cerebellar lesions often make better recoveries than adults (166). If cerebellar ablation is performed in neonatal monkeys, almost-complete recovery occurs, provided the deep cerebellar nuclei are left intact; if they are not, gaze-holding and smooth pursuit never fully recover (167).

ETIOLOGIES

There are many conditions that produce cerebellar eye signs. These include developmental anomalies, degenerative diseases, vascular diseases, and tumors.

Developmental Anomalies of the Hindbrain

The Arnold-Chiari malformation is an abnormality of the hindbrain involving the caudal cerebellum (including the vestibulocerebellum, flocculus, paraflocculus [tonsils], uvula, and nodulus) and the caudal medulla (168,169). In the type I malformation, the cerebellar tonsils are displaced caudally into the foramen magnum and the medulla is elongated. A meningomyelocele usually is not present. Such patients often develop symptoms in adult life. In the type II malformation, both the fourth ventricle and the inferior vermis extend below the foramen magnum; the brain stem and spinal cord are thin; and a lumbar meningomyelocele is usually present. Patients with type II malformation usually present in childhood, but in milder cases, the onset of symptoms is delayed until adulthood. Presenting symptoms of the Arnold-Chiari malformation include oscillopsia that is brought on or exacerbated by head movements, and dizziness, vertigo, cervical pain, and headaches, all of which can be brought on by Valsalva maneuvers. A variety of ocular motor abnormalities, and especially downbeat nystagmus (both spontaneous and positional), occur in patients with the Arnold-Chiari malformation (Table 19.2). Many of these signs are reproducible by vestibulocerebellar lesions in monkeys (170). Diagnosis is by MR imaging, with sagittal views of the craniocervical junction (Fig. 19.7). Patients often improve after suboccipital decompression, although it may take months for the eye movement abnormalities to diminish (171). A similar ocular motor syndrome can occur in patients

Table 19.2
Eye Signs in the Arnold-Chiari Malformation

Downbeat nystagmus (occasionally with a torsional component), worse on lateral gaze
Sidebeat nystagmus (primary position, unidirectional, horizontal nystagmus)
Periodic alternating nystagmus
Divergent nystagmus
Esotropia
Gaze-evoked nystagmus
Rebound nystagmus including torsional rebound
Impaired pursuit (and VOR cancellation)
Impaired OKN with slow build-up of eye velocity in response to a constant velocity stimulus
Convergence nystagmus
Divergence paralysis
Skew deviation accentuated or alternating on lateral gaze
Saccadic dysmetria
Internuclear ophthalmoplegia
Increased VOR gain
Shortened VOR time constant
Positional nystagmus

OKN, optokinetic nystagmus; VOR, vestibulo-ocular reflex.

with other lesions located at the craniocervical junction (172). The positional nystagmus of posterior fossa lesions (173–175) must be differentiated from the more common benign paroxysmal positional nystagmus of the labyrinth (147,158,176–181).

The Dandy-Walker syndrome consists of a malformation of the cerebellar vermis, a membranous cyst of the fourth

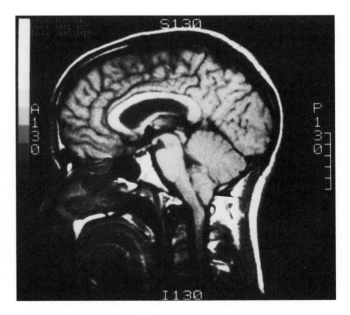

Figure 19.7. Neuroimaging of an Arnold-Chiari malformation. T1-weighted sagittal magnetic resonance image shows herniation of cerebellar tonsils below the foramen magnum (*arrowhead*). Note flattening of the brain stem in this region.

ventricle, and malformations of the cerebellar cortex and deep cerebellar nuclei. Patients with this condition often show a mild saccadic dysmetria, although some patients have normal eye movements (182). Ocular motor abnormalities, including nystagmus and strabismus, also occur in patients with agenesis of the vermis (183) or hypoplasia of the entire cerebellum (184). Other rare syndromes associated with anomalous cerebellar development include Coffin-Siris syndrome (developmental delay, hypotonia, cutaneous changes, and abnormalities of the roof of the fourth ventricle) (185) and Joubert's syndrome (a variable combination of episodic tachypnea, psychomotor retardation, retinal dystrophy, torsional nystagmus, skew deviation, ocular motor apraxia, agenesis of the cerebellar vermis, and fibrosis of the extraocular muscles) (186–188).

Degenerative Diseases

Many degenerative processes can affect the cerebellum or its connections and produce cerebellar eye signs. The hereditary ataxias show considerable variability in phenotypic expression. As a result, there have been difficulties with classification, a problem that is being partially resolved with the discovery of genetic markers and the realization that phenotype is influenced by both primary and modifier genes (189–195). Moreover, many of these conditions also affect brain stem structures. Thus, other, presumably noncerebellar, ocular motor signs may be present (e.g., slow saccades, prolonged saccadic latencies, decreased or absent vestibulo-ocular responses, and ophthalmoplegia). It remains to be proved whether eye movement abnormalities can be used to reliably detect extracerebellar involvement or early signs of disease in persons at risk for developing hereditary ataxias In general, patients with Friedreich's ataxia show a decrease of vestibulo-ocular responses and prominent square-wave jerks. Slow saccades point to brain stem involvement, as occurs with SCA2. In one form of a recessively inherited cerebellar degeneration with peripheral neuropathy and prominent square-wave jerks (saccadic intrusions) and saccadic dysmetria, the speed of large saccades was actually too fast (196). In general, the gross amount of atrophy of different parts of the cerebellum as shown by MR imaging does not correlate well with the severity of ocular motor dysfunction (197), although more sensitive imaging analysis techniques of individual lobules will likely reveal better clinical-anatomic correlations.

Paraneoplastic cerebellar degeneration is a rare remote effect of cancer, usually occurring with breast, ovarian, or small-cell lung cancer (198,199). The onset of symptoms is usually acute or subacute, with severe midline and appendicular ataxia, dysarthria, and downbeat nystagmus. Autopsies show a total loss of Purkinje cells. Such patients have lost the output from the cerebellar cortex, and the common finding of primary position downbeat nystagmus is compatible with the hypothesis that a preponderance of inhibitory projections of the cerebellum to the central connections of the superior semicircular canals can cause this nystagmus.

The episodic vertigo and ataxia syndromes, often responsive to acetazolamide, may be associated with prominent cerebellar eye signs, including downbeat nystagmus, and many are mapped to the same area of chromosome 19 in which hemiplegic migraine and SCA6 are mapped (200–202). Such syndromes may be associated with migraine, essential tremor, or myokymia; many are channelopathies (203,204).

Vascular Diseases

The cerebellum is supplied by three branches of the vertebrobasilar circulation: the posterior inferior cerebellar artery (PICA), the AICA, and the superior cerebellar artery (SCA). Occlusion of one or more of these vessels often produces brain stem infarction too, making precise clinicopathologic correlation difficult. Infarction in the distribution of the distal PICA may cause acute vertigo and nystagmus that often simulates an acute peripheral vestibular lesion (205). These symptoms probably reflect a central imbalance in horizontal VOR pathways created by asymmetric infarction of the vestibulocerebellum. The vestibulocerebellum also influences the gaze-holding networks within the vestibular nuclei, and patients with lesions in the vestibulocerebellum may have prominent gaze-evoked nystagmus that helps differentiate this cerebellar lesion from an acute peripheral vestibulopathy.

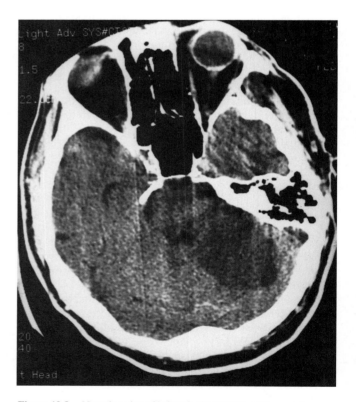

Figure 19.8. Neuroimaging of infarct in the territory of the superior cerebellar artery (SCA) in a 69-year-old man with hypertension. Computed tomographic scan shows a large hypodense area in the left cerebellar hemisphere corresponding to the distribution of the left SCA. The patient had a left horizontal gaze palsy from compression of the left side of the brain stem.

Infarction in the territory of the AICA, the branches of which often supply the flocculus, may cause vertigo, vomiting, hearing loss, facial palsy, and ipsilateral limb ataxia, along with gaze-holding and pursuit deficits as well as vestibular nystagmus (61–63,206) (Fig. 19.6). The ocular motor signs reflect a combination of involvement of the labyrinth, vestibular nuclei, and flocculus.

Infarction in the territory of the SCA causes ataxia, limb dysmetria, and vertigo (206,207) (Fig. 19.8). A characteristic abnormality is saccadic contrapulsion. Contralateral saccades overshoot and ipsilateral saccades undershoot the target. Attempted vertical saccades are oblique, with a horizontal component away from the side of the lesion (208–210). Thus, this saccadic disorder is the opposite of the saccadic ipsipulsion seen in Wallenberg's syndrome (discussed previously) and probably reflects interruption of outputs from the fastigial nucleus running in the uncinate fasciculus next to the superior cerebellar peduncle (121,211). Infarction restricted to the posterior-inferior vermis can selectively impair pursuit and optokinetic eye movements (212).

Mass Lesions

Cerebellar hemorrhage, tumors, infarcts, abscesses, cysts, and extra-axial hematomas may all cause cerebellar eye signs by direct damage to the cerebellar parenchyma. Cerebellar lesions, however, may also compress the brain stem and produce additional signs. Vertical or horizontal gaze disorders can occur, depending on whether the direction of compression is upward or directly forward, respectively. The oculomotor, trochlear, and abducens nerves may also be affected. Ocular motor dysfunction may also be caused by secondary obstructive hydrocephalus and increased intracranial pressure.

Medulloblastomas arising in the posterior medullary velum frequently produce or are associated with positional nystagmus. Involvement of the nodulus and uvula is presumably responsible for this finding (213) and may also account for the inability to suppress postrotational nystagmus by tilting the head (145,146). Tumors within the fourth ventricle may affect the cerebellar nuclei, vestibulocerebellum, and dorsal medulla. Upbeating nystagmus may occur in such cases.

Vestibular schwannomas may compress the cerebellar flocculus (which lies in the cerebellopontine angle) and produce eye signs of vestibulocerebellar lesions (214), including Brun's nystagmus, in which there is a coarse nystagmus beating to the side of the lesion (reflecting a gaze-holding deficit) and a fine nystagmus beating away from the side of the lesion (reflecting a vestibular imbalance). Head-shaking nystagmus may be present (215). MR imaging after intravenous injection of contrast is the most sensitive and specific method used to detect small lesions in this region. Acute cerebellar hemorrhage frequently causes nystagmus, gaze palsy (usually toward the side of the lesion), abducens nerve palsy, and skew deviation (216–218). These signs are, in part, caused by compression of the brain stem.

OCULAR MOTOR SYNDROMES CAUSED BY LESIONS OF THE PONS

LESIONS OF THE INTERNUCLEAR SYSTEM: INTERNUCLEAR OPHTHALMOPLEGIA

Among the fibers that make up the MLF, many carry a conjugate horizontal eye movement command from abducens internuclear neurons in the pons to the medial rectus subdivision of the contralateral oculomotor nuclear complex in the midbrain. Other fibers in the MLF carry signals for holding vertical eye position, for vertical smooth pursuit, and for the vertical VOR.

Manifestations

Lesions of the MLF produce INO (219,220) (Fig. 19.9). When the lesion is unilateral, the INO is characterized by weakness of adduction ipsilateral to the side of the lesion (Fig. 19.10). This weakness may vary from a complete loss of adduction beyond the midline to a mild decrease in the velocity or acceleration of adduction without any limitation in range of motion (Fig. 19.11). The fibers subserving horizontal gaze in the MLF each carry commands for all types of conjugate eye movements. Hence, vestibular slow phases, pursuit and optokinetic following, and saccades and quick phases of nystagmus are all affected by the MLF lesion. The weakness of adduction, however, may be more obvious for saccades because damaged axons, especially those that are demyelinated, show a greater defect for carrying high- rather than low-frequency impulses. This dissociation is reflected in a "pulse-step mismatch" that occurs because saccade speed (determined by the high-frequency "pulse" of innervation) is diminished out of proportion to the limitation in range of adduction (determined by the low-frequency "step" of innervation). An adduction lag is brought out clinically by asking the patient to make large-amplitude (which

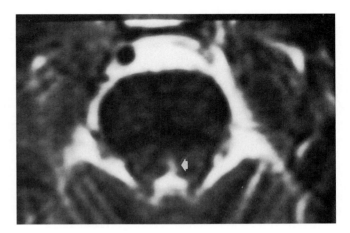

Figure 19.9. Neuroimaging in a patient with a left internuclear ophthalmoplegia. T2-weighted magnetic resonance image, axial view, shows a tiny area of hyperintensity consistent with an infarct in the region corresponding to the location of the left medial longitudinal fasciculus (*arrowhead*). The patient also had a skew deviation.

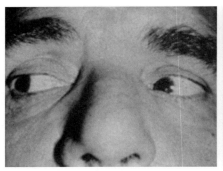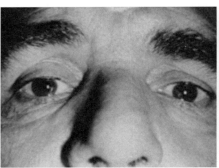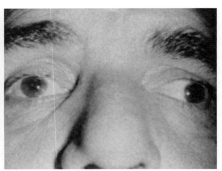

Figure 19.10. Unilateral, right internuclear ophthalmoplegia in a 32-year-old man with multiple sclerosis. Note complete lack of adduction in the right eye on attempted left horizontal gaze.

require the highest speeds) horizontal saccades back and forth across the midline or by using an "optokinetic" tape or drum with repetitive symbols to produce nystagmus that allows easy comparison of the movements of the two eyes (221). Quantitative recordings of eye movements in patients with MS show that the most sensitive sign of adduction weakness in INO is a decreased ratio either of peak eye velocity (222) or of peak acceleration (223) of the adducting saccades of the eye on the side of the lesion to the abducting saccades of the other eye (224).

When patients with INO are able to converge, despite absence of voluntary adduction, the lesion is located caudally with preservation of the medial rectus subdivision of the oculomotor nuclear complex (225). Patients with INO and intact convergence were said to have a posterior INO by Cogan (77). Although the presence of intact convergence is important in such cases, the absence of convergence in the setting of an INO (the "anterior" INO of Cogan) does not necessarily imply a rostral lesion involving the medial rectus nuclear subdivision. Some patients simply are not able to produce a strong convergence effort, and the vertical dis-

parity that occurs when a unilateral INO is associated with a skew deviation also may interfere with convergence effort.

In some patients with an INO, abducting saccades in the affected eye may also be slow or "fractionated" (226,227). This phenomenon may reflect impaired inhibition of the affected medial rectus, although Kommerell (228) was unable to find any evidence of impaired medial rectus inhibition in one patient with a unilateral INO in whom he performed electromyography. Slowing of abducting saccades tends to be more prominent in bilateral INO, probably because of damage to extra-MLF pathways running through the pontine tegmentum (229,230).

The second cardinal sign of an INO is nystagmus in the contralateral eye when it is abducted. This nystagmus consists of a centripetal (inward) drift, followed by a corrective saccade that may be hypermetric, hypometric, or orthometric. It is present in nearly all patients with INO (231). A number of mechanisms could account for the abduction nystagmus of INO (220) and may not be mutually exclusive. They include (*a*) an increase in convergence tone; (*b*) impaired inhibition of the medial rectus contralateral to the

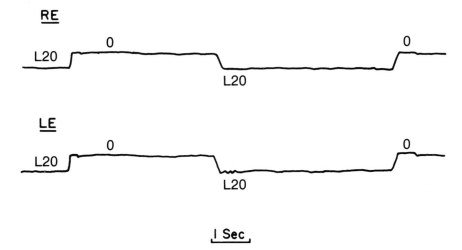

Figure 19.11. Ocular motor recording of a patient with a mild right internuclear ophthalmoplegia. On attempted left horizontal gaze, the velocity of the adducting right eye is less than the velocity of the abducting left eye, which overshoots the target and shows mild abducting nystagmus.

lesion (232); (*c*) interruption of descending internuclear fibers that project to the abducens nucleus (233); (*d*) a superimposed gaze-evoked nystagmus; and (*e*) adaptation to the contralateral medial rectus weakness (234–236). Because abduction nystagmus is not observed in acute experimental INO induced by injection of lidocaine into the MLF of monkeys (237), the cause of abduction nystagmus must relate either to lesions outside the MLF or to an adaptive response to the initial adduction weakness.

Patching experiments in patients with INO show that in many cases the abducting nystagmus diminishes if the patient is required to habitually view with the nonparetic eye (235,236). In these patients, the abducting nystagmus relates, at least in part, to a conjugate (because of Hering's law of equal innervation to the two eyes) adaptive change in innervation that acts to improve adduction of the paretic eye, but at the expense of a disturbance in abducting saccades of the contralateral eye. Abducting saccades overshoot the target and are followed by a centripetal drift (''pulse-step mismatch''), giving the appearance of an abducting nystagmus. Such nystagmus usually dies out after a beat or two, and the postsaccadic drift is brief. It would bring the eye to a stable eccentric position if it were not interrupted by corrective eccentric saccades.

The other common mechanism for abduction nystagmus is a dissociated gaze-evoked nystagmus that appears more prominent in the abducting eye because the adducting eye is weak. In contrast to the abducting nystagmus produced by adaptation, such gaze-evoked abduction nystagmus is more sustained, and the postsaccadic drift would bring the eye to the primary position if it were not interrupted by corrective eccentric saccades. Interruption of the paramedian tracts that run near the MLF and carry fibers to and from the flocculus may be responsible for the gaze-evoked nystagmus that is associated with INO (238).

Skew deviation commonly occurs with unilateral INO but rarely with bilateral INO. When skew deviation is associated with INO, the higher eye is usually on the side of the lesion (Fig. 19.12). It is usually easy to differentiate skew deviation of an INO from trochlear nerve palsy because of the adducting weakness and abducting nystagmus, but at times skew deviation and trochlear nerve palsy may be hard to separate (68). Skew deviation may reflect imbalance of otolith inputs that cross in the medulla and ascend in the MLF (discussed previously).

Dissociated vertical nystagmus (downbeat in the ipsilateral eye, torsional in the contralateral eye) may occur with an INO (239). This pattern of dissociated nystagmus reflects the fact that posterior semicircular canal pathways mediating excitation pass through the MLF, but some anterior semicircular canal pathways do not (240). Experimental INO produced by lidocaine blockade causes ipsilateral hypertropia and unilateral downbeating nystagmus (237). Patients with a unilateral INO may also have an ipsiversive torsional nystagmus (top poles of the eyes cyclorotate so as to beat toward the side of the lesion) (241,242). The torsional nystagmus is sometimes dissociated and is usually but not always associated with a skew deviation. It may relate to interruption of pathways between the vestibular nuclei and the INC. Some

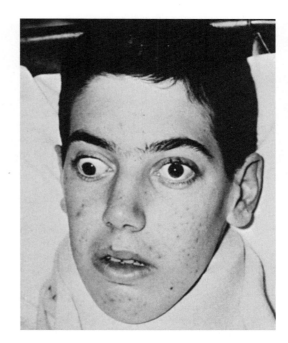

Figure 19.12. Skew deviation in a patient following an operation on the posterior fossa for a superiorly placed vermis tumor. The deviation persisted for 3 weeks.

patients with bilateral INO cannot fix steadily. In such patients, sporadic bursts of monocular abducting saccades may occur in each eye (243).

Patients with bilateral INO have bilateral adduction weakness and abducting nystagmus (Figs. 19.13 and 19.14). Such patients also have impaired vertical vestibular and pursuit eye movements and impaired vertical gaze-holding with gaze-evoked nystagmus on looking up or down (244–247).

Many patients with an INO have no visual symptoms, particularly when there is no limitation of adduction (231). In other cases, the presence of either limitation of adduction or skew deviation may cause diplopia that is horizontal, vertical, or oblique. Patients with INO occasionally complain of oscillopsia (248). Horizontal oscillopsia usually occurs from either the adduction lag or the abduction nystagmus, whereas vertical oscillopsia occurs during head movements and is caused by a deficient vertical VOR (249). In many patients, visual symptoms become less bothersome or resolve completely, either because of recovery of function of MLF axons or because of more central adaptive mechanisms.

Lesions that damage the MLF may also damage the abducens nucleus, fascicle, or both on either side of the brain stem. Lesions that damage the MLF on one side and the ipsilateral abducens nucleus produce the one-and-a-half syndrome (discussed later), whereas lesions that damage the ipsilateral abducens fascicle produce horizontal ophthalmoplegia in the ipsilateral eye from the combination of an INO and an abducens nerve palsy. Lesions that damage the MLF on one side and the paramedian pontine reticular for-

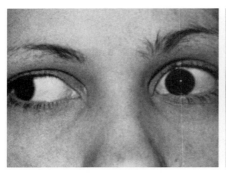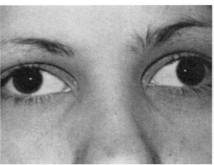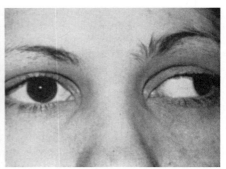

Figure 19.13.   Bilateral internuclear ophthalmoplegia in a young woman with multiple sclerosis. The pupils have been dilated with mydriatics.

mation (PPRF) or abducens nucleus on the opposite side produce a horizontal gaze palsy toward the side of the damaged PPRF or abducens nucleus. In such cases, the INO cannot be diagnosed because of the overriding horizontal gaze palsy. Damage to the MLF on one side and to the contralateral abducens nerve fascicle will produce abduction weakness of the contralateral eye combined with adduction weakness of the ipsilateral eye. In this setting, there will be a ''pseudo-horizontal gaze palsy'' on attempted horizontal gaze away from the side of the MLF lesion. The diagnosis may be suspected in a patient who appears to have a horizontal gaze palsy that is asymmetric, with one eye (usually the adducting eye) being more limited than the other.

As with patients having conjugate gaze palsy from damage to the abducens nucleus, patients with the one-and-a-half syndrome often have an associated facial nerve paralysis. This paralysis is ipsilateral to the horizontal gaze palsy and occurs from damage to the fascicle of the facial nerve as it loops around the abducens nucleus (discussed later).

Etiologies

Table 19.3 summarizes some causes of INO. In general, a unilateral INO is most commonly caused by ischemia, although there is often subtle involvement of the other side (Fig. 19.15). Bilateral INO is commonly caused by demyelination associated with MS, but even in MS, the INO may be quite asymmetric (250) (Fig. 19.16). Although MR imaging frequently shows a lesion in the MLF in patients with INO (250a) (Fig. 19.9), there are many exceptions (251,252). Thin cuts and sagittal T2-weighted imaging are sometimes required.

Posterior INO of Lutz

In 1923, Lutz (253) described a condition in which abduction (not adduction) was impaired with respect to saccades and pursuit but not with respect to vestibular stimulation. As noted above, Cogan (77) described an INO as one in which there was slowed or limited adduction of one eye,

BILATERAL INO

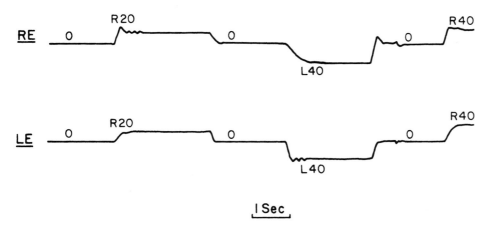

Figure 19.14. Ocular motor recording showing the saccadic velocities of a patient with bilateral internuclear ophthalmoplegia. On attempted right horizontal gaze, the velocity of the adducting left eye is less than the velocity of the abducting right eye. The right eye overshoots the target and shows abducting nystagmus. On attempted left horizontal gaze, the velocity of the adducting right eye is less than the velocity of the abducting left eye. The left eye overshoots the target and shows abducting nystagmus.

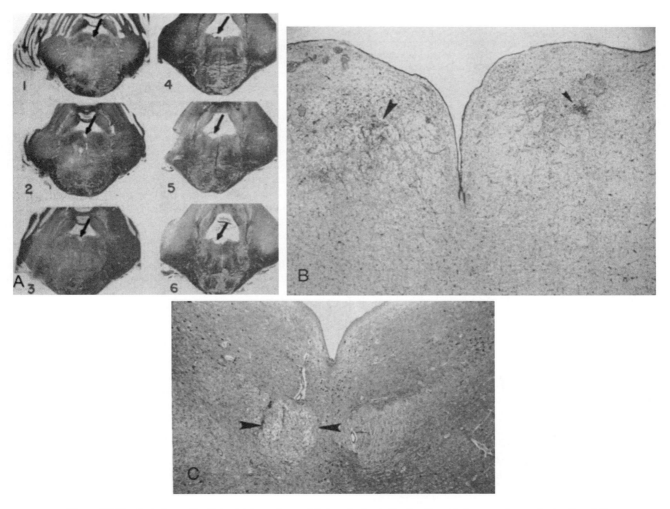

Figure 19.15. Pathology of unilateral internuclear ophthalmoplegia. *A,* Section through the pons in a patient with a left internuclear ophthalmoplegia shows a small infarction in the region of the left medial longitudinal fasciculus (*arrows*). Sections are numbered from rostral to caudal. *B,* Area from the infarct indicated by the *arrow* in *A* and the surrounding region. The *large arrowhead* points to the infarct involving the left medial longitudinal fasciculus. The *small arrowhead* points to a small infarct just lateral to the right medial longitudinal fasciculus. *C,* Section through the rostral pons in a patient with a left internuclear ophthalmoplegia. There is a septic infarction involving the left medial longitudinal fasciculus (*arrowheads*). Many axons of the left medial longitudinal fasciculus have been destroyed, but the right medial longitudinal fasciculus is entirely normal. (*A* and *B,* From Cogan DG, Kubik CS, Smith JL. Internuclear ophthalmoplegia: a review of 58 cases. Arch Ophthalmol 1950;44:783–796. *C,* From Ross AT, DeMyer WE. Isolated syndrome of the medial longitudinal fasciculus in man. Arch Neurol 1966;15:203–205.)

associated with overshoot of the abducting eye. Because this condition appeared to be the opposite of the INO that Lutz (253) had described, some authors began to refer to the eye movement abnormality observed by Lutz as the "posterior INO of Lutz" and the eye movement abnormality observed by Cogan (77) as the "anterior INO of Cogan." This resulted in confusing terminology because Cogan (77) had his own anterior and posterior types of INO that were based on whether convergence was present. In any event, the INO described by Cogan (77) is quite common, whereas the posterior INO of Lutz is rare (254–256).

The pathogenesis of the posterior INO of Lutz is difficult to understand because the abducens nucleus contains neurons that innervate both lateral and medial rectus muscles for all conjugate eye movements (219,257,258). Patients with abducens palsy thus may show nystagmus in the contralateral adducting eye, if the weak abducting eye is used preferentially for fixation (256). This nystagmus could reflect the same type of mechanisms (an adaptive response or a dissociated nystagmus) that accounts for the abducting nystagmus that develops in patients with typical INO.

Çelebisoy and Akyürekli (259) described a patient in whom a posterior INO of Lutz was mimicked by a rostral brain stem infarction that caused a horizontal gaze paresis

Table 19.3
Etiology of Internuclear Ophthalmoplegia

Multiple sclerosis (commonly bilateral [223]); postirradiation demyelination

Brain stem infarction (commonly unilateral), including complication of arteriography and hemorrhage (250)

Brain stem and fourth ventricular tumors

Arnold-Chiari malformation, and associated hydrocephalus and syringobulbia

Infection: bacterial, viral, and other forms of meningoencephalitis

Hydrocephalus, subdural hematoma, supratentorial arteriovenous malformation

Nutritional disorders: Wernicke's encephalopathy and pernicious anemia (864)

Metabolic disorders: hepatic encephalopathy

Drug intoxication: phenothiazines, tricyclic antidepressants, narcotics, propranolol, lithium, barbiturates, D-penicillamine, toluene

Cancer: due to carcinomatous infiltration or remote effect

Head trauma, and cervical hyperextension or manipulation

Degenerative conditions: progressive supranuclear palsy

Syphilis

Pseudo-internuclear ophthalmoplegia of myasthenia gravis and Fisher's syndrome

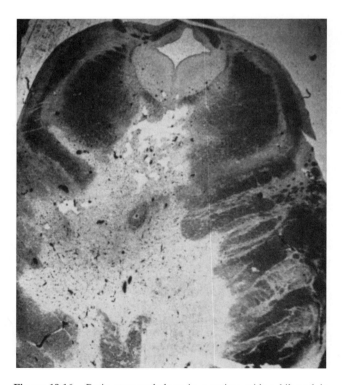

Figure 19.16. Brain stem pathology in a patient with a bilateral internuclear ophthalmoplegia and severe cerebrovascular and cardiovascular disease. Section at pontomesencephalic junction shows paramedian necrosis with areas of coalescing cavitation in the regions normally occupied by both medial longitudinal fasciculi. This lesion involves both sides of the midline. (From Gonyea EF. Bilateral internuclear ophthalmoplegia: association with occlusive cerebrovascular disease. Arch Neurol 1974; 31:168–173.)

to one side and a pseudo-abducens paresis on attempted gaze to the other side. The patient also had bilateral vertical gaze palsy and other evidence of midbrain dysfunction. The mechanisms of posterior INO using examples with more rostral brain stem lesions have been discussed (227). In other cases an infranuclear cause has been suggested (260).

LESIONS OF THE ABDUCENS NUCLEUS

Lesions of the abducens nucleus cause an ipsilateral palsy of horizontal conjugate gaze because the abducens nucleus contains two groups of neurons: abducens motoneurons that innervate the ipsilateral lateral rectus muscle, and abducens internuclear neurons that innervate the contralateral medial rectus motor neurons via the MLF. Vergence movements of the eyes are spared, however, so that adduction is possible with a near stimulus. Such a localized lesion can be produced experimentally (261), but it occurs rarely in humans (262–264) except in Möbius syndrome, a congenital brain stem anomaly with horizontal gaze disturbances, often with an associated facial palsy (265). This condition occurs in at least some cases from aplasia or hypoplasia of both abducens nuclei. More often, however, the abducens nucleus is affected in association with adjacent tegmental structures, particularly the genu of the facial nerve, the MLF, and the PPRF (229,266). Lesions restricted to the abducens nucleus can often be distinguished from those in the adjacent caudal PPRF (see also below), because only in the latter may pursuit and vestibular movements be spared, and only in the former may ipsilateral saccades in the contralateral field be spared by virtue of intact inhibition upon the contralateral abducens nucleus. Gaze-evoked nystagmus on contralateral gaze also occurs in patients with presumed abducens nucleus lesions (263). Possible mechanisms for the gaze-evoked nystagmus include damage to adjacent vestibular or NPH pathways that are involved in neural integration for gaze-holding, or damage to the paramedian cells and tracts that lie in part in the rostral abducens nucleus and have reciprocal connections with the cerebellar flocculus, a structure also involved in gaze-holding (238).

LESIONS OF THE PARAMEDIAN PONTINE RETICULAR FORMATION (PPRF)

The PPRF, which corresponds principally to medial portions of the nucleus reticularis pontis caudalis, contains burst neurons that are important in the generation of saccades, and the paramedian nucleus raphe interpositus contains pause neurons that inhibit burst neurons at all times except during saccades.

Destructive lesions of the PPRF, such as infarction and hemorrhage, tend to affect all cell groups, along with fibers of passage that convey pursuit and vestibular signals to the ipsilateral abducens nucleus. Unilateral destructive lesions cause an ipsilateral, conjugate, horizontal, gaze palsy (233,267,268). With acute lesions, the eyes may be deviated contralaterally. Nystagmus occurs when gaze is directed into the intact contralateral field of movement with quick phases directed away from the lesioned side; this is usually accentuated in darkness. Ipsilaterally directed saccades and quick phases are small and slow and do not carry the eye past the midline. The degree of slowing of saccades directed toward the lesioned side, when made in the intact field of gaze, probably depends on whether projections to inhibitory burst neurons, which project to the contralateral abducens nucleus, are damaged. Recall that excitatory saccadic inputs reach the abducens nucleus from the ipsilateral population of excitatory burst cells in the PPRF, whereas inhibitory saccadic inputs originate from contralateral inhibitory burst cells in the medulla. If the lesion is restricted to the ipsilateral abducens nucleus, saccades from the opposite field of gaze to the midline may be relatively rapid, because inhibition of the antagonist is intact. If the PPRF is extensively damaged, particularly in its more caudal part, inhibition is also affected so that saccades beginning from the field of gaze opposite to the lesioned side and moving to the midline are extremely slow. Rapid eye movements directed to the side opposite the lesion appear normal. Vertical saccades may be slightly slow, and an inappropriate horizontal component, directed away from the side of the lesion, may occur during attempted vertical saccades (269).

Smooth-pursuit movements and slow phases of optokinetic nystagmus may be preserved in both directions within the intact field of movement of a patient with a lesion of the PPRF, but they usually cannot bring the eyes across the midline. Sometimes horizontal pursuit is asymmetrically impaired, more so for contralateral target motion (270). This is in contrast to the effects of more basal lesions in the pons that impair ipsilateral or bilateral pursuit (271–273). Because of the confluence of pursuit pathways in the brain stem and its cerebellar connections, the direction of a pursuit deficit with a brain stem lesion is not reliable for determining the side of the lesion (274). In some patients with PPRF lesions, vestibular stimuli drive the eyes past the midline. Presumably, in such individuals, either the ipsilateral abducens nucleus or its direct vestibular input is intact, or the PPRF lesion is more rostral (269,275). With more restricted lesions, usually hemorrhages, both smooth pursuit and the VOR may be preserved, whereas saccades are absent or slow (276). Occasionally in such patients, vestibular stimuli can drive only the contralateral adducting eye and not the ipsilateral abducting eye into the ipsilateral field. This finding implies a lesion of one PPRF and the ipsilateral abducens nerve but sparing the abducens nucleus (277).

Bilateral lesions restricted to the PPRF are uncommon. Discrete infarction (278) or tumor (279) can cause a selective loss of saccades, leaving smooth pursuit and the VOR relatively preserved. Such a selective deficit implies loss or dysfunction of saccadic burst neurons but sparing of fibers of passage conveying smooth pursuit and the VOR. Experimental lesions of the PPRF in monkeys, using neurotoxins that spare fibers of passage, may cause a similar deficit (280). Patients with horizontal gaze palsies may substitute convergence for impaired conjugate adduction and then cross-fixate to extend their range of view (281). Furthermore, during the recovery phase from bilateral gaze palsies from vascular lesions, involuntary synkinetic divergence and convergence movements may appear with horizontal or vertical gaze (282,283). Bilateral pontine lesions may abolish all horizontal eye movements, but, particularly with chronic lesions such as tumors, reflexive eye movements may be spared.

Bilateral pontine lesions may impair vertical eye movements (284–286). Signals for vertical vestibular and smooth pursuit eye movements ascend in the MLF and other pathways through the pons; consequently, vestibular and pursuit eye movements can be impaired with pontine lesions. Abnormal (usually slow) vertical saccades occur in patients with discrete, bilateral pontine lesions (278,287–289) and in monkeys with bilateral neurotoxic lesions of the PPRF (280,290). Pause cells project rostrally to vertical burst neurons located in the midbrain. Pontine lesions, therefore, may lead to desynchronization of vertical (and horizontal) burst neuron discharge and consequently to slow vertical (and horizontal) saccades. Ocular flutter has been reported with a PPRF lesion (291).

COMBINED UNILATERAL CONJUGATE GAZE PALSY AND INTERNUCLEAR OPHTHALMOPLEGIA (ONE-AND-A-HALF SYNDROME)

Combined lesions of the abducens nucleus or PPRF and adjacent MLF on one side of the brain stem cause an ipsilateral horizontal gaze palsy and INO, so that the only preserved horizontal eye movement is abduction of the contralateral eye; hence the name *one-and-a-half syndrome* (Figs. 19.17–19.19) (18,229,282,292,293). Such patients may show an exotropia when attempting to look straight ahead; the eye opposite the side of the lesion is deviated outward. This misalignment of the eyes is thought to be caused by the unopposed drives of the intact pontine gaze center to the spared abducens nucleus and is called *paralytic pontine exotropia* (294). Many patients, however, have an esotropia or no deviation in primary position (as with many cases of INO), though it may be always present when fixation is eliminated (295). The spared abduction saccades of the contralateral eye are followed by centripetal drift, so that a nystagmus similar to that of the abducting eye in INO is present. Occasionally, the ipsilateral horizontal vestibular responses are preserved when voluntary gaze is abolished (275, 282,293), suggesting that the pontine lesion is more rostral in the PPRF or more discrete in the caudal PPRF (296), thus sparing the vestibular projections to the abducens nucleus. Although attempts at conjugate movements elicit no adduction, vergence movements may be preserved. Ocular bobbing may accompany the one-and-a-half syndrome (297).

The one-and-a-half syndrome may result from brain stem ischemia (298–302), MS (292), tumor (303,304), hemorrhage (305), trauma (306), and other miscellaneous causes, including HIV infection with tuberculosis, (302). Bilateral INO with associated abducens nerve palsy also may mimic the one-and-a-half syndrome, as can myasthenia gravis (299). A "one-and-a-half syndrome" has been described in which only adduction in one eye was spared (307). The patient had mucormycosis that caused an abducens nerve palsy from cavernous sinus infiltration on one side and a contralateral horizontal gaze palsy from simultaneous carotid artery occlusion.

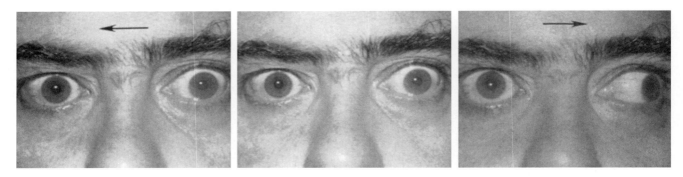

Figure 19.17. One-and-a-half syndrome in a 23-year-old man with multiple sclerosis. *Arrows* indicate direction of attempted gaze. All ocular motor signs cleared within 3 months after onset.

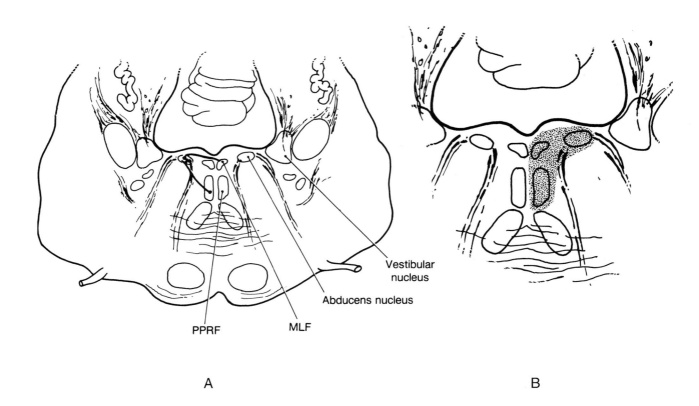

Figure 19.18. Location of lesions producing the one-and-a-half syndrome. *A*, The important structures involved in the production of horizontal gaze. MLF, medial longitudinal fasciculus; PPRF, paramedian pontine reticular formation. Neurons project from the PPRF to the abducens nucleus and neurons in the abducens nucleus are both motoneurons whose axons represent the abducens nerve and internuclear neurons whose axons ascend in the *contralateral* MLF. *B*, The areas that may be involved when a one-and-a-half syndrome is present. Involvement of either the abducens nucleus or the PPRF can cause the horizontal gaze palsy. Damage to the ipsilateral medial longitudinal fasciculus produces the internuclear ophthalmoplegia. (Modified from Sharpe JA, Rosenberg MA, Hoyt WF, et al. Paralytic pontine exotropia: a sign of acute unilateral pontine gaze palsy and internuclear ophthalmoplegia. Neurology 1974;24:1076–1081.)

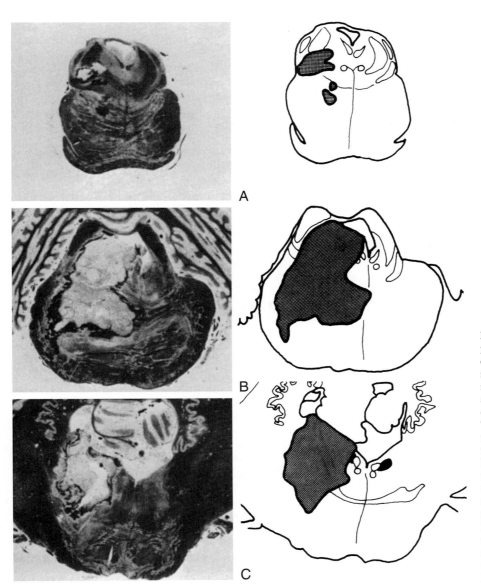

Figure 19.19. Brain stem findings in a 48-year-old hypertensive man with a recent myocardial infarction who developed a complete right horizontal gaze palsy and a complete right internuclear ophthalmoplegia (one-and-a-half syndrome). Sections through the pons demonstrate an extensive area of hemorrhage. The drawings on the *right* illustrate the relationship of the hemorrhage to the fourth ventricle, superior cerebellar peduncles, medial longitudinal fasciculi, medial tectospinal tracts, medial lemnisci, dentate nuclei (all outlined in *heavy black lines*), and the abducens nuclei (*black*). *A*, Rostral pons. *B*, Midpons. *C*, Caudal pons. (From Pierrot-Deseilligny C, Chain F, Serdaru M, et al. The "one-and-a-half" syndrome: electro-oculographic analyses of five cases with deductions about the physiological mechanisms of lateral gaze. Brain 1981;104:665–699.)

SLOW SACCADES FROM PONTINE LESIONS

Slow saccades are characteristic of many degenerative and metabolic diseases (Table 19.4). Horizontal saccades may be slowed in patients with spinocerebellar degenerations; vertical saccades are often relatively less affected in such patients. In diseases that principally affect the midbrain, such as progressive supranuclear palsy, vertical saccades are the first to become slow. In some patients with slow saccades, blinks of the eyelids may actually speed up the movements (308). The explanation for this phenomenon is uncertain, but it probably reflects the effects of blinks upon pause and burst neurons rather than a momentary deprivation of vision. Some patients with slow saccades can generate smooth-pursuit movements of up to about 20°/sec. It is difficult to distinguish a considerably slowed saccade from pursuit, however, so that whether pursuit function is truly intact in such pa-

tients is not established. Conversely, if the saccades are so slow that they cannot bring the eye to the moving target, then even if pursuit is intact, it may not appear so because the eye seems to lag the target. Vestibular stimulation elicits normal compensatory slow phases, but quick phases of nystagmus are slow and show approximately the same abnormal relationship between amplitude and peak velocity, as do voluntary saccades. Patients with SCA2 usually make saccades of normal amplitude despite their low velocity. Progressive supranuclear palsy, however, causes both slow and small horizontal saccades (discussed later). Patients with slow saccades may use a variety of strategies of combining eye and head movements to move their gaze more quickly to the target.

Slow horizontal saccades may be caused by disease of saccadic burst cells in the PPRF. Autopsy examinations of

Table 19.4
Etiology of Slow Saccades

Olivopontocerebellar atrophy and related spinocerebellar degenerations
Huntington's disease
Progressive supranuclear palsy
Parkinson's (advanced cases) and related diseases; Lytico-Bodig and
    Caribbean Parkinson's
Whipple's disease
Lipid storage diseases
Wilson's disease
Drug intoxication: anticonvulsants, benzodiazepines
Tetanus
In dementia: Alzheimer's disease (stimulus-dependent) and in association
    with AIDS
Lesions of the paramedian pontine reticular formation
Internuclear ophthalmoplegia
Peripheral nerve palsy, diseases affecting the neuromuscular junction and
    extraocular muscle, restrictive ophthalmopathy
Paraneoplastic syndromes

the brains of patients with SCA2 with slow saccades demonstrate a marked loss of neurons from the nucleus reticularis pontis caudalis and the adjacent raphe nuclei (309). Alternatively, slowing of saccades may reflect abnormal inputs to the paramedian reticular formation from the cerebral hemispheres, the superior colliculus, or the cerebellum. Lesions in the pause cell region also may produce slow saccades (290).

SACCADIC OSCILLATIONS FROM PONTINE LESIONS

Saccadic oscillations that lack an intersaccadic interval, such as opsoclonus and ocular flutter, probably result from pontine lesions in the pause cell region (310). A number of other mechanisms are possible, however. Macrosaccadic oscillations (an extreme form of saccadic dysmetria) also occur with pontine lesions (311), as can ocular flutter (291) (see Chapter 23).

OCULAR MOTOR SYNDROMES CAUSED BY LESIONS IN THE MESENCEPHALON

SITES AND MANIFESTATIONS OF LESIONS

Disturbances of vertical eye movements from midbrain lesions are usually caused by damage to one or more of three main structures: the posterior commissure, the rostral interstitial nucleus of the medial longitudinal fasciculus, or the INC (312).

Posterior Commissure

Lesions of the posterior commissure cause a syndrome characterized by loss of upward gaze and other associated findings (Table 19.5 and Figs. 19.20 and 19.21). The condi-

Table 19.5
Features of the Syndrome of the Posterior Commissure (aka Dorsal Midbrain Syndrome)

Limitation of upward eye movements (Parinaud's syndrome)
    Saccades
    Smooth pursuit
    Vestibulo-ocular reflex
    Bell's phenomenon
Lid retraction (Collier's sign); occasionally ptosis
Disturbances of downward eye movements
    Downward gaze preference ("setting sun" sign)
    Downbeating nystagmus
    Downward saccades and smooth pursuit may be impaired, but vestibular
        movements are relatively preserved.
Disturbances of vergence eye movements
    Convergence-retraction nystagmus (Koerber-Salus-Elschnig syndrome)
    Paralysis of convergence
    Spasm of convergence
    Paralysis of divergence
    "A" or "V" pattern exotropia
    Pseudo-abducens palsy
Fixation instability (square-wave jerks)
Skew deviation
Pupillary abnormalities (light–near dissociation)

tion is known by a variety of names: Parinaud's syndrome, Koerber-Salus-Elschnig syndrome, pretectal syndrome, dorsal midbrain syndrome, and the sylvian aqueduct syndrome (313,314). Unilateral midbrain lesions can also create the same ocular motor syndrome, possibly by interrupting the afferent and efferent connections of the posterior commissure, or possibly by disturbing supranuclear inputs from the nucleus of the posterior commissure directly to the midbrain oculomotor nuclei (discussed later). Although paralysis of upward gaze in this syndrome has, in the past, been ascribed to destruction of the superior colliculi, this is not the case. Experimental lesions restricted to the superior colliculus in nonhuman primates produce no limitation of upward gaze (315). Furthermore, the selective upgaze paralysis seen in this syndrome cannot be explained on the basis of different crossing patterns of premotor burst neurons originating in the riMLF (downward premotor neurons are uncrossed to the third and fourth cranial nerve nuclei, while upward premotor neurons are both uncrossed and crossed), since none of these neurons appear to cross via the posterior commissure (312,316). Although sparse data are available, damage to premotor neurons in the nucleus of the posterior commissure that selectively subserve upward eye movements (or their axons, which appear to traverse the posterior commissure to arrive at their oculomotor targets) may be involved in the genesis of the selective loss of upward eye movements in the syndrome of the posterior commissure (317).

The vertical gaze deficit caused by lesions of the posterior commissure usually affects all types of eye movements, although the VOR and Bell's phenomenon are sometimes spared. Below the horizontal meridian, vertical saccades can be made but are usually slow. Acutely, the eyes may be tonically deviated downward (setting-sun sign); this finding is prominent in premature infants with intraventricular hemorrhage (318). Transient downward deviation of the eyes occasionally occurs in healthy neonates, but in such cases, the eyes can be easily driven above the horizontal meridian

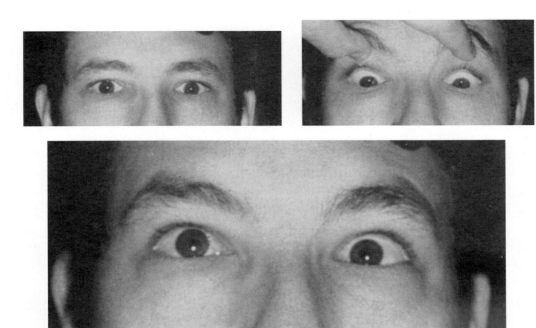

Figure 19.20. Appearance of a patient with Parinaud's dorsal midbrain syndrome. *Above left,* The eyes are straight in primary position. Note bilateral upper eyelid retraction. *Above right,* Downward gaze is normal. *Below center,* There is marked limitation of upward gaze bilaterally, worse on the left, producing a right hypertropia. (From Bajandas FJ, Aptman M, Stevens S. The sylvian aqueduct syndrome as a sign of thalamic vascular malformation. In: Smith JL, ed. Neuro-Ophthalmology Focus 1980. New York: Masson, 1979:401–406.)

by the vertical doll's head maneuver (86). Tonic upward deviation of the eyes occurs in some patients with midbrain lesions (319). Oculogyric crises may also occur in patients with midbrain lesions and are discussed below. Episodic (paroxysmal) tonic up-gaze may also occur in otherwise normal infants, in patients with other neurologic deficits, including ataxia, as a familial dominantly inherited disorder, and, occasionally, with structural lesions in the midbrain (320–327).

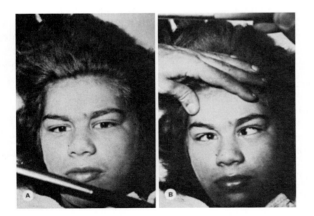

Figure 19.21. Dorsal midbrain syndrome. *A,* Gaze straight ahead. *B,* On attempted upward gaze, the patient develops convergence-retraction nystagmus.

The dorsal midbrain syndrome is also characterized by disturbances of horizontal eye movements. In some patients convergence is paralyzed, whereas in others it is excessive and causes convergence spasm. During horizontal saccades, the abducting eye may move more slowly than its adducting fellow. This finding is called *pseudo-abducens palsy* (313) and may reflect an excess of convergence tone (328). It may be responsible for an early symptom of evolving posterior commissure lesions—reading difficulty caused by a transient inability to find, and to focus both eyes on, the beginning of the next line when a horizontal saccade is made.

Convergence-retraction nystagmus is another sign often evident in patients with disease affecting the dorsal midbrain (329,330) (Fig. 19.22). Experimental lesions suggest that this eye movement disturbance results from damage to the posterior commissure (331). Originally thought to be a saccadic disorder consisting of asynchronous, opposed saccades, recent quantitative measures suggest that the adducting movements are abnormal convergence movements (332).

Abnormalities of the eyelids occur in patients with dorsal midbrain lesions. The most common is eyelid retraction (Collier's tucked lid sign), but ptosis occasionally occurs. In some patients, the abnormalities of the lids may be more prominent than those of the eye movements (333,334).

Pupillary reactions are also commonly affected in patients with lesions in the region of the posterior commissure. The pupils are usually large and react better to an accommodative stimulus than to light (i.e., light-near dissociation).

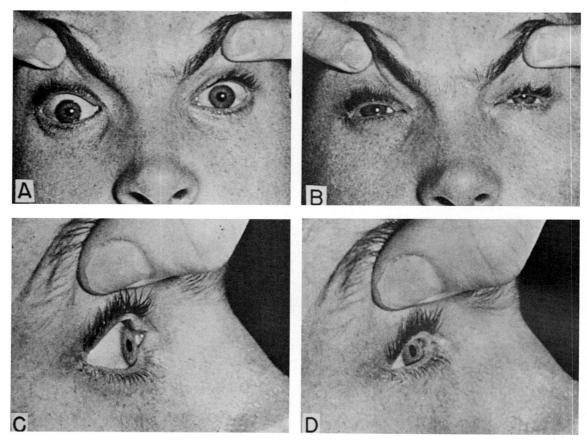

Figure 19.22.   Dorsal midbrain syndrome. *A*, Position of eyes in primary position. *B*, Retraction on attempted upward gaze. *C*, Lateral view of right eye when the patient is looking straight ahead. *D*, On attempted upward gaze, obvious retraction of the globe occurs. (From Lyle DJ, Mayfield FH. Retraction nystagmus: a case report. Am J Ophthalmol 1954;37:177–182.)

Many disease processes can affect the region of the posterior commissure (Table 19.6 and Figs. 19.23–19.25). Pineal tumors (335,336) produce the dorsal midbrain syndrome either by direct pressure on the posterior commissure or by causing obstructive hydrocephalus. Hydrocephalus may pro-

duce this syndrome by enlarging the aqueduct and third ventricle or the suprapineal recess, thus stretching or compressing the posterior commissure (337,338). Shunt dysfunction may produce Parinaud's syndrome before dilation of the ventricles is apparent on neuroimaging or measures of intra-

Table 19.6
Etiology of Disorders of Vertical Gaze

Tumor: Classically, pineal germinoma or teratoma in an adolescent male; also pineocytoma, pineoblastoma, glioma, metastasis
Hydrocephalus: Usually aqueductal stenosis leading to dilatation of the third ventricle and aqueduct or enlargement of the suprapineal recess with pressure on the posterior commissure
Vascular: Midbrain or thalamic hemorrhage or infarction
Metabolic: Lipid storage disease: Niemann-Pick variants
Drug-induced
Degenerative: Progressive supranuclear palsy, cortical basal degeneration, Lytico-Bodig diffuse Lewy body disease; miscellaneous degenerations
Miscellaneous: Multiple sclerosis, Whipple's disease, hypoxia, encephalitis, syphilis, aneurysm, neurosurgical procedure, mesencephalic clefts, tuberculoma, trauma, benign transient form of childhood

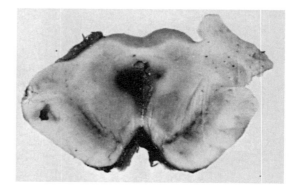

Figure 19.23.   Pathology of dorsal midbrain syndrome. Contusion hemorrhages are present in the region of the oculomotor nucleus and posterior commissure after a fall that resulted in an impact to the right side of the vertex. (Courtesy of Dr. Richard Lindenberg.)

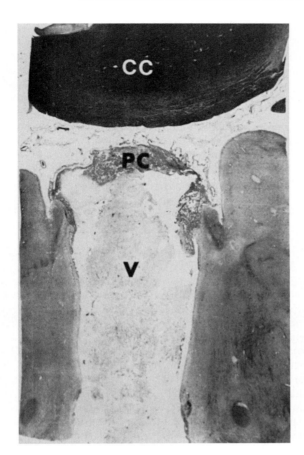

Figure 19.24. Metastatic malignant melanoma causing a dorsal mid-brain syndrome. Horizontal section through the inferior third ventricle (V) shows replacement of posterior commissure (PC) by metastatic melanoma. CC, corpus callosum. (From Keane JR, Davis RL. Pretectal syndrome with metastatic melanoma to the posterior commissure. Am J Ophthalmol 1976;82:910–914.)

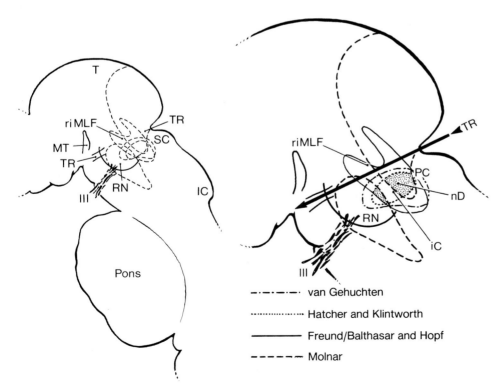

van Gehuchten
Hatcher and Klintworth
Freund/Balthasar and Hopf
Molnar

Figure 19.25. Locations of lesions producing isolated paralysis of upward gaze. *Left,* Four lesions giving rise to upward gaze paralysis have been superimposed on a sagittal section of the human brain stem. The enlargement of the lesions on the *right* shows that the common areas involved (*stippled regions*) include the interstitial nucleus of Cajal (iC), the nucleus of Darkschewitsch (nD), and fibers of the posterior commissure (PC). IC, inferior colliculus; MT, mammillothalamic tract; riMLF, rostral interstitial nucleus of the medial longitudinal fasciculus; RN, red nucleus; SC, superior colliculus; T, thalamus; TR, tractus retroflexus; III, oculomotor nerve. (Redrawn from Büttner-Ennever JA, Büttner U, Cohen B, et al. Vertical gaze paralysis and the rostral interstitial nucleus of the medial longitudinal fasciculus. Brain 1982;105:125–149.)

cranial pressure are consistently high (339). An intermittent Parinaud's syndrome dependent on head position was described in a patient with a posterior fossa subdural hematoma (340).

Rostral Interstitial Nucleus of the Medial Longitudinal Fasciculus

The rostral interstitial nucleus of the medial longitudinal fasciculus (riMLF), which lies in the prerubral fields of the mesencephalon, contains the burst neurons that generate vertical and torsional saccades (analogous to the PPRF in the pons for horizontal saccades). The riMLF lies dorsomedial to the rostral half of the red nucleus, medial to the fields of Forel, lateral to the periventricular gray and the nucleus of Darkschewitsch, and immediately rostral to the INC. The riMLF projects to ipsilateral more than contralateral third and fourth nerve nuclei, the INC (important for vertical gaze-holding [discussed later]), and caudal targets, including the cell groups of paramedian tract, that relay ocular motor signals to the cerebellum. Although the right and left riMLF nuclei are interconnected, the projections are now believed to course ventral to the cerebral aqueduct rather than via the posterior commissure, as thought previously (312,316).

Given this information, it is not unexpected that bilateral experimental lesions of the riMLF abolish all vertical and torsional saccadic movements (341,342). However, unilateral experimental lesions of the riMLF produce slowed downward saccades, loss of ipsilesional torsional quick phases of the VOR, contralesional beating torsional nystagmus, and tonic contralesional ocular torsion (343). An anatomic explanation for these findings follows.

Burst neurons within the riMLF have mixed vertical and torsional vectors rather than subpopulations of neurons with either vertical or torsional vectors, echoing the anatomic structure of the vertical semicircular canals (presumably since the vestibulo-ocular system is the phylogenetically-older substrate underlying the saccadic system (344)). The net vector sum of various burst neurons firing may, however, lead to purely vertical or purely torsional saccadic eye movements. Burst neurons within the riMLF subserving upward-torsional saccades appear to be redundant (i.e., project to both ipsilateral and contralateral third and fourth nerve nuclei), while those subserving downward-torsional saccades are not (i.e., project to the ipsilateral third and fourth nerve nuclei only (312,316)). Each vertical-torsional saccade burst neuron sends axon collaterals to yoke muscle pairs that subserve the same pulling direction in each eye; specifically, these pairings are as follows: (a) *right* superior rectus and *left* inferior oblique (serving upward-leftward torsional saccades, innervated by individual burst neurons within *each* riMLF nucleus); (b) *left* superior rectus and *right* inferior oblique (serving upward-rightward torsional saccades, innervated by individual burst neurons within *each* riMLF nucleus); (c) *right* inferior rectus and *left* superior oblique (serving downward-rightward torsional saccades, innervated by individual burst neurons within the *right* riMLF nucleus only); and (d) *left* inferior rectus and *right* superior oblique (serving downward-leftward torsional saccades, innervated

by individual burst neurons within the *left* riMLF nucleus only).

Because infranuclear fibers innervating the superior oblique (fourth) and superior rectus (third) muscles are crossed projections, each riMLF burst neuron for downward saccades can control the movement of both eyes without sending axon collaterals across the midline. Thus, unilateral midbrain lesions in the riMLF can produce selective loss of downward saccades.

The same burst neurons that lack right–left asymmetry with respect to vertical saccades are "lateralized" with respect to "directionality" of torsional saccades; that is to say, all of the right riMLF vertical-torsional burst neurons drive saccades toward the right shoulder (top pole rotating to the right), and all of the left riMLF vertical-torsional burst neurons drive saccades toward the left shoulder. Thus, unilateral midbrain lesions in the riMLF can also produce selective loss of ipsilesional torsional saccades. The associated left–right asymmetry in tonic firing rates between the two riMLF nuclei may explain both the contralesional-beating torsional nystagmus (a sign of vertical VOR imbalance), and the tonic ocular torsion toward the contralesional side (a sign of otolith ocular imbalance).

Clinically, bilateral lesions of the riMLF are more common than unilateral lesions. They generally cause either loss of downward saccades or loss of all vertical saccades (345) (Figs. 19.26–19.28). Lesions of the riMLF are usually infarcts in the distribution of a small perforating vessel (the posterior thalamo-subthalamic paramedian artery) that arises between the bifurcation of the basilar artery and the origin of the posterior communicating artery (Fig. 19.28). This vessel may be paired or single (346,347); it supplies structures that include the riMLF, the rostromedial red nucleus, the adjacent subthalamus, the posterior inferior portion of the dorsomedial nucleus, and the parafascicular nucleus of the thalamus. Some investigators think that paralysis of downward saccades results from lateral lesions of both riMLFs, whereas medial bilateral lesions cause a total palsy of vertical saccades (Figs. 19.28–19.32) (348). Others (349), however, have observed that downward gaze paresis is more often associated with medial lesions than with lateral ones. Although vertical smooth pursuit and the VOR may be affected with lesions in this area, this probably reflects damage to nearby structures, such as the MLF and INC (350). Deleu et al. (351) reported a patient with a vertical one-and-a-half syndrome. The patient had loss of all downward movements and selective loss of upward movements in one eye. A vertical one-and-a-half syndrome in which there was impairment of all upward eye movements and a selective deficit of downward saccades in the eye on the side of the lesion has also been reported (352,353,354). Unilateral lesions of the midbrain can also produce combined complete up-gaze and down-gaze palsy, isolated up-gaze palsy, or monocular elevator palsy (353).

Clinically, unilateral lesions of the riMLF generally produce a down-gaze palsy, mainly affecting saccades or, more rarely, a complete vertical gaze palsy for all eye movement types (268,348,355,356). As seen with experimental lesions, unilateral lesions of the riMLF also produce a contralaterally

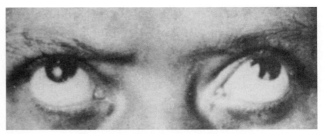

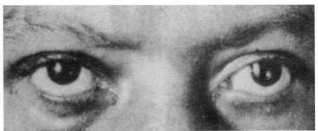

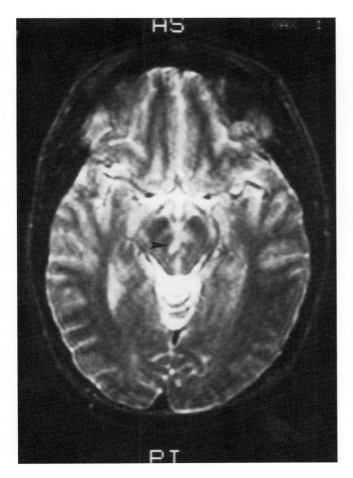

Figure 19.26. Neuroimaging of a lesion in a patient with bilateral conjugate vertical saccadic gaze palsy and cognitive dysfunction. T2-weighted axial magnetic resonance image shows a hyperintense midline lesion (*arrowhead*) affecting the region of the rostral interstitial nucleus of the medial longitudinal fasciculus.

Figure 19.27. Isolated paralysis of downward gaze in a 42-year-old alcoholic man. *Above,* Upward gaze is normal. *Below,* The patient cannot make voluntary downward eye movements. Bilateral simultaneous caloric stimulation with warm water induced downward nystagmus, but the excursion of the fast phases was truncated at the level of direct forward gaze. (From Jacobs L, Anderson PJ, Bender MB. The lesions producing paralysis of downward but not upward gaze. Arch Neurol 1973;28:319–323.)

Interstitial Nucleus of Cajal

The INC, which lies adjacent and caudal to the riMLF in the midbrain reticular formation, contains premotor neurons that subserve vertical gaze-holding (analogous to the perihypoglossal nucleus in the medulla for horizontal gaze) (312). The INC projects to contralateral (more than ipsilateral) third and fourth nerve nuclei, the riMLF (important for vertical and torsional saccades [discussed previously]), and caudal targets, including the cell groups of paramedian tract, which relay ocular motor signals to the cerebellum, as well as the ipsilateral vestibular and perihypoglossal nuclei (subserving horizontal gaze-holding), and the ipsilateral C1-C2 ventral horns (involved in eye–head coordination), among others (312,316,360). The right and left INC are interconnected via the posterior commissure.

Given this information, it is not surprising that bilateral experimental lesions of the INC severely impair both vertical and torsional gaze-holding and disrupt normal vertical and torsional VOR responses (361). Unilateral experimental lesions of the INC produce similar (though less profound) vertical and torsional gaze-holding deficits (vertical gaze-evoked nystagmus, and spontaneous, ipsilesional beating torsional nystagmus), along with tonic contralesional ocular torsion (362).

Lesions restricted to the INC are not well studied in humans, apparently because isolated lesions of INC are rare (due to frequent involvement of riMLF). Nevertheless, available evidence suggests that such lesions produce a clinical syndrome characterized by vertical gaze-evoked nystagmus, impaired vertical smooth pursuit, tonic torsional deviation

beating torsional nystagmus, a tonic torsional deviation to the contralateral side, and a deficit in generating ipsilaterally directed torsional quick phases (i.e., top pole rolling toward the side of the lesion) (357,358). As pointed out above, the selective impairment of downward saccades with unilateral riMLF lesions appears to result from a lack of redundancy in the premotor pathways for down-gaze—burst neurons subserving downward(-torsional) saccades project only to the ipsilateral third and fourth nerve nuclei, while those subserving upward(-torsional) saccades project both ipsilaterally and contralaterally (312,316). These apparent facts notwithstanding, Ranalli et al. (359) described a patient with a unilateral lesion of the riMLF (which partially involved the adjacent INC) that led to a loss of saccades above the primary position and slow and limited saccades below. Smooth pursuit and the VOR were also affected in the vertical plane, being restricted in range and reduced in gain. The anatomic underpinnings of this clinical picture remain uncertain.

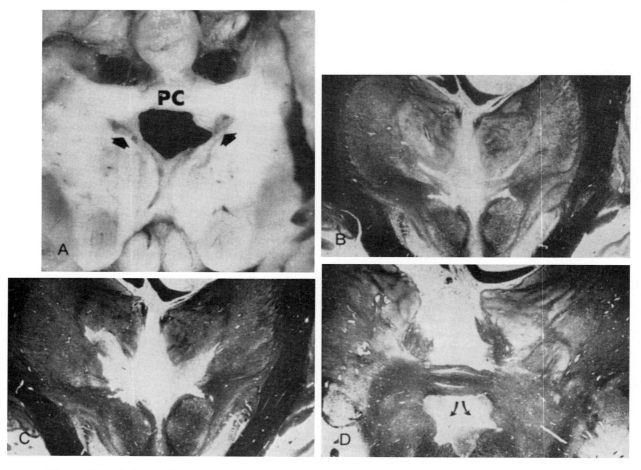

Figure 19.28. Pathology of isolated paralysis of downward gaze. *A*, In a 58-year-old man who died of septic shock and was noted to have selective paralysis of downward gaze, the cut surface of the rostral mesencephalon reveals bilateral cavitary infarcts (*arrows*). The posterior commissure (PC) is intact. *B* and *C*, In a 42-year-old man who suffered an infarction of the brain stem and was noted to have selective paralysis of downward gaze, sections through the rostral mesencephalon show zones of bilateral infarction and necrosis involving portions of the tractus retroflexus and red nuclei on both sides. Zones of necrosis also involve portions of the intralaminar, dorsomedial, lateral, and posteromedial thalamic nuclei. *D*, Section through the mesencephalon at the level of the posterior commissure shows bilateral zones of infarction (*arrows*) in the periaqueductal gray matter. The posterior commissure itself and other portions of the pretectal region of the mesencephalon are normal. (*A*, From Trojanowski JQ, Wray SH. Vertical gaze ophthalmoplegia: selective paralysis of downgaze. Neurology 1980;30:605–610. *B–D*, From Jacobs L, Anderson PJ, Bender MB. The lesions producing paralysis of downward but not upward gaze. Arch Neurol 1973;28:319–323.)

to the contralateral side, and torsional nystagmus (110,358,363). The torsional nystagmus has been variably reported as contralesional beating or ipsilesional beating (110,358). Recent studies suggest that the apparent confusion may stem from the comorbid presence of riMLF damage in those cases where contralesional-beating nystagmus is present (358). A jerk seesaw nystagmus may also occur in patients with lesions that damage the INC (364), although seesaw nystagmus has not been reproduced in the monkey with INC lesions (365). The INC may also contribute to dynamic properties of the VOR, especially its low-frequency behavior, by virtue of the effect on the vestibular velocity storage mechanism (366). Lesions in the midbrain produce a change in the phase of the VOR (367), and electric stimula-

tion of the INC in a human produced torsional nystagmus and the OTR (120).

Periaqueductal Gray Matter and Mesencephalic Reticular Formation

The effects of lesions localized to mesencephalic structures other than the posterior commissure, INC, and the riMLF are less clear. The periaqueductal gray matter of the mesencephalon contains neurons that stop discharging during saccades. A patient with bilateral lesions of the periaqueductal gray matter, caudal to the posterior commissure and ventral to the superior colliculus, showed a selective defect of down-gaze, with tonic upward deviation of the eyes (368).

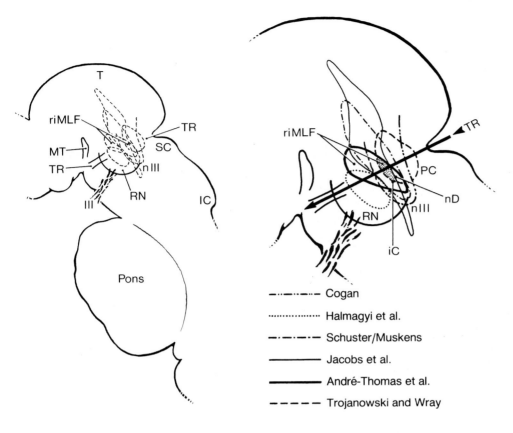

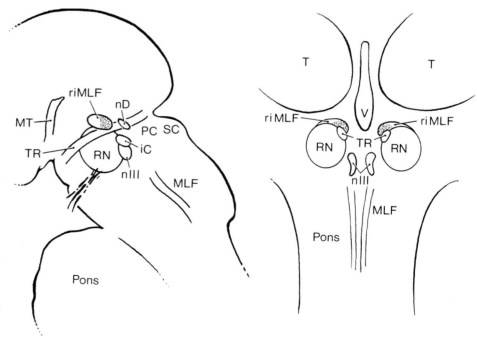

Figure 19.29. Locations of lesions producing isolated paralysis of downward gaze. *Left,* Sagittal section through the human brain stem on which the bilaterally destroyed areas in the six autopsied cases of isolated downward gaze paralysis are superimposed. *Right,* An enlargement of the lesions shows that the common area destroyed in these cases (*stippled region*) lies dorsal to the red nucleus at the level of the tractus retroflexus (TR)—that is, around the rostral interstitial nucleus of the medial longitudinal fasciculus (riMLF) and the nucleus of Darkschewitsch (nD). iC, interstitial nucleus of Cajal; IC, inferior colliculus; MT, mammillothalamic tract; PC, posterior commissure; RN, red nucleus; SC, superior colliculus; T, thalamus; III, oculomotor nerve; nIII, oculomotor nucleus. (Redrawn from Büttner-Ennever JA, Büttner U, Cohen B, et al. Vertical gaze paralysis and the rostral interstitial nucleus of the medial longitudinal fasciculus. Brain 1982;105:125–149.)

Figure 19.30. Smallest area critical for the selective mediation of downgaze (*stippled area*). *Left,* Sagittal view of the brain stem as seen from the midline. *Right,* Coronal view of the critical region as seen from a rostral approach. The involved region is rostral to the posterior commissure (PC) in a region that has been designated as the rostral interstitial nucleus of the medial longitudinal fasciculus (riMLF). iC, interstitial nucleus of Cajal; MLF, medial longitudinal fasciculus; MT, mammillothalamic tract; nD, nucleus of Darkschewitsch; nIII, oculomotor nucleus; RN, red nucleus; SC, superior colliculus; T, thalamus; TR, tractus retroflexus; V, third ventricle. (Redrawn from Pierrot-Deseilligny C, Chain F, Gray F, et al. Parinaud's syndrome: electro-oculographic analysis of six cases with deductions about vertical gaze organization in the premotor structures. Brain 1982;105:667–696.)

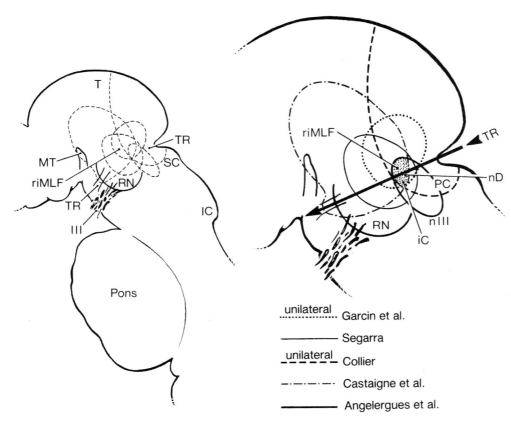

Figure 19.31. Locations of brain stem lesions that produce paralysis of both upward and downward gaze. *Left,* Five unilateral or bilateral lesions producing upward and downward gaze paralysis are superimposed on a sagittal section of the human brain. The enlargement on the *right* shows the common area involved (*stippled region*). This area includes parts of the rostral interstitial nucleus of the medial longitudinal fasciculus (riMLF), the interstitial nucleus of Cajal (iC), and the nucleus of Darkschewitsch (nD). IC, inferior colliculus; MT, mammillothalamic tract; PC, posterior commissure; RN, red nucleus; SC, superior colliculus; T, thalamus; TR, tractus retroflexus; III, oculomotor nerve; nIII, oculomotor nucleus. (Redrawn from Büttner-Ennever JA, Büttner U, Cohen B, et al. Vertical gaze paralysis and the rostral interstitial nucleus of the medial longitudinal fasciculus. Brain 1982; 105:125–149.)

Another reported lesion of the periaqueductal gray matter caused persistent up-gaze palsy (369). Thus, it seems that lesions of the periaqueductal gray matter of the midbrain may cause an imbalance of the vertical gaze-holding mechanism. Areas of the mesencephalic reticular formation outside of the riMLF and INC have also been implicated in control of saccades. Lesions there affect horizontal and vertical saccade accuracy; the pattern depends on the exact location within the mesencephalic reticular formation (370,371).

Other Sites and Manifestations

Unilateral, paramedian midbrain lesions sometimes cause impairment of ipsilateral, horizontal smooth pursuit by affecting the descending smooth-pursuit pathway; contralateral saccades may also be affected (372), but the horizontal VOR tends to be spared (Roth-Bielschowsky phenomenon) (313). Paramedian midbrain lesions often damage the oculomotor nerve nucleus, thereby producing a combination of nuclear and prenuclear deficits (372,373). Lesions that damage the oculomotor nucleus are characterized by bilateral elevator and eyelid weakness, because the superior rectus subnucleus is located contralaterally, and the levator subnucleus is located in the midline. Abnormal pupils are common in patients with such lesions. Occasionally, large midbrain lesions also cause complete loss of horizontal eye movements (374,375).

Rarely, midbrain lesions selectively impair the function of both elevator muscles (the superior rectus and inferior oblique muscles) of one eye. This double elevator palsy is thought to be supranuclear in origin, because in the primary position, the eyes are nearly straight, and only on looking upward does a vertical disconjugacy become evident (376). This condition occurs in patients with midbrain infarction and tumor; the lesion may be ipsilateral or contralateral (353,377,378). Rarely, it is congenital (379,380). Because the superior rectus is a stronger elevator than the inferior oblique, it is not always possible to be sure of inferior oblique weakness. If, however, the inferior oblique is weak in addition to the superior rectus, then a nuclear lesion is unlikely, because these two muscles are supplied by the ipsilateral and contralateral oculomotor subnuclei, respectively. More likely, prenuclear inputs to the oculomotor nuclei are impaired in such patients. The VOR is variably affected. Monocular elevator palsy may be associated with a contralateral down-gaze palsy (381). Occasionally monocular elevator palsy is caused by a lesion selectively involving the inferior oblique and superior rectus muscle fascicles of the oculomotor nerve as it exits the brain stem (382). In most instances, however, a monocular paresis of elevation results from causes other than midbrain disease, such as thyroid ophthalmopathy, blowout fracture of the orbit, myasthenia gravis, or restrictive ophthalmopathies. MR scanning of the orbit may be helpful in differentiating restrictive eye muscle diseases causing a similar clinical picture (383).

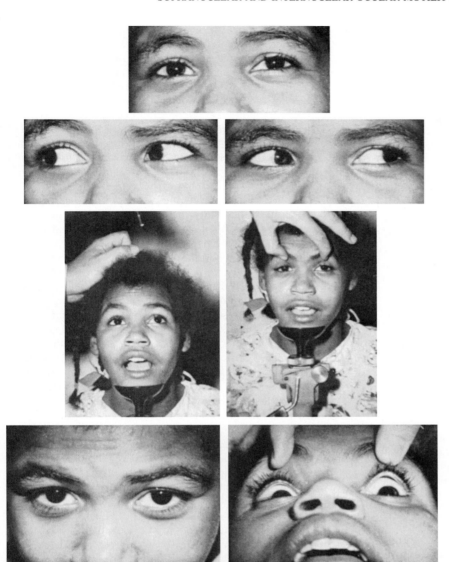

Figure 19.32. Supranuclear vertical ophthalmoplegia in a patient with a metabolic storage disease (DAF syndrome). *Top,* In primary position, the patient's eyes are straight. She is also able to make normal voluntary horizontal eye movements. *Center,* The patient cannot make voluntary upward or downward vertical eye movements. *Bottom,* On oculocephalic testing, full vertical ocular excursions are elicited. (From von Noorden GK, Maumenee AE. Atlas of Strabismus, 2nd ed. St Louis: CV Mosby, 1973:161.)

NEUROLOGIC DISORDERS THAT PRIMARILY AFFECT THE MESENCEPHALON

Two neurologic disorders produce profound disturbances of ocular motility, primarily because of their effects on cells in the mesencephalon: progressive supranuclear palsy and Whipple's disease.

Progressive Supranuclear Palsy

Progressive supranuclear palsy (PSP) is a degenerative disease of later life characterized by disturbances of tone and posture leading to falls, difficulties with swallowing and speech, and mental slowing (384–389). PSP is one of the tauopathies (385,390). Abnormal eye movements are usually present early in the course of the disease, but occasionally they are noted late or not at all (391). Although familial cases

of PSP occur and appear to be inherited in an autosomal-dominant fashion (392,393), the disease is usually sporadic.

The initial ocular motor deficit of PSP is usually impairment of vertical saccades and quick phases, either down or up (245). The saccades are at first slow and later also small, with eventual complete loss of voluntary vertical refixations. Vertical smooth pursuit is usually relatively preserved, and the VOR is intact until later in the disease, although a characteristic nuchal rigidity may make the vertical doll's head maneuver difficult to perform. A large-field visual stimulus often elicits much better visual tracking than does a small target (394). Bell's phenomenon is usually absent. There are many types of eyelid abnormalities in PSP, including blepharospasm, apraxia of eyelid closing or opening, lid retraction, and lid lag (395).

Horizontal eye movements also show characteristic abnormalities in patients with PSP, including impaired fixation with square-wave jerks, impaired pursuit, impaired vestibular cancellation, and saccades and quick phases that are small and eventually slow (396–398). In some patients, the abnormality of voluntary horizontal eye movements resembles an INO; however, vestibular stimulation may overcome the limitation of adduction in such cases (399). Convergence eye movements are commonly impaired in patients with PSP, and many patients have severe convergence insufficiency (400). Late in the disease, the ocular motor deficit may progress to a complete ophthalmoplegia.

Studies of eye movements in patients with PSP may also reflect the disturbances of attention that occur in this disorder. The latency (reaction time) of horizontal saccades in PSP is prolonged in some patients, but in others, saccadic latency (using a gap paradigm in which the fixation target goes out before the new peripheral target appears) is reduced so that patients show short-latency or express saccades (401–403). Patients with PSP also make errors with an antisaccade task in which they are required to look away from a presented target. Both the express saccades and errors on the antisaccade task suggest defects in frontal lobe function (401) and, although neuropathologic changes in the frontal lobe are mild in patients with PSP, positron emission tomographic (PET) scanning indicates profound frontal hypometabolism in such patients (404). Defects of visual attention are more prominent in the vertical than in the horizontal plane (405), and poor performance on visual search tasks may be related in part to loss of voluntary saccades and disruption of steady fixation by square-wave jerks (406).

PSP is a diffuse brain stem disorder, although cortical involvement also occurs (407). Both computed tomographic (CT) scanning and MR imaging show atrophy of the midbrain and dilation of the quadrigeminal cisterns, cerebral aqueduct, and third and fourth ventricles (408). There is a characteristic "hummingbird sign" due to the midbrain atrophy (409). Histologically, neuronal loss, neurofibrillary tangles, and gliosis principally affect the brain stem reticular formation and the ocular motor nuclei (384,410). The midbrain may bear the brunt of the early pathology, accounting for the relative vulnerability of vertical saccades (411). Thus, the slowing of vertical saccades probably results from dysfunction of burst neurons in the riMLF, whereas the neck stiffness, often with dorsiflexion, may be caused by damage to the INC, which contributes to the control of head movements (412). Abnormalities are also present in the nucleus raphe interpositus in the pons in which omnipause neurons, important for control of velocity and amplitude of both horizontal and vertical saccades, are located (413). Recent studies suggest that PSP likely causes the abnormal saccade velocity by virtue of its direct effect on premotor saccade burst neurons within the midbrain (414,415). Pathology within the substantia nigra pars reticulata may also play a role (416). Pursuit abnormalities may reflect damage to the deep pontine nuclei (417). The pedunculopontine nucleus is also specifically affected and may be associated with secondary damage to a number of other cortical and subcortical structures (407).

The differential diagnosis of PSP includes a similar syndrome caused by multiple infarcts that affect the basal ganglia, internal capsule, and midbrain (418–420). Hydrocephalus may also mimic PSP (421), as can Whipple's disease (422) and a delayed syndrome following aortic valve replacement (423). At the bedside, slowing of vertical saccades, the inability to suppress blinks to a bright light (a visual "glabellar sign"), the "applause sign" (persistent clapping after instructed to clap just three times), and tonic deviation of the eyes and head following sustained rotation of the body in a vestibular chair are helpful diagnostic findings (424).

PSP should be differentiated from cortical-basal ganglionic degeneration, which may affect vertical and horizontal gaze but which also causes focal dystonia, ideomotor apraxia, alien hand syndrome, myoclonus, and an asymmetric akinetic-rigid syndrome with late onset of gait or balance disturbances (402,403,425–429). A syndrome similar to PSP has been reported from Guadeloupe and has been attributed to exposure to mitochondrial complex 1 inhibitors such as quinolones, acetogenins, and rotenoids (430). It also is a tauopathy. The Parkinson-dementia complex of Guam (Lytico-Bodig variant) also resembles PSP (431,432). PSP should also be differentiated from Parkinson's disease (discussed later). Although upward gaze may be limited in PSP and in Parkinson's disease, impaired downward gaze, slow vertical saccades, abnormal horizontal saccades, and square-wave jerks are much more characteristic of PSP. Diffuse Lewy body disease may present a problem in differential diagnosis and mimic PSP (433) or Parkinson's disease (434). Other basal ganglia disorders that may mimic PSP include idiopathic striopallidodentate calcification (435), autosomal-dominant parkinsonism and dementia with pallidopontonigral degeneration (436), multisystem atrophy, and olivopontocerebellar atrophy (398). Some of the neurologic deficits of PSP, but generally not the eye movements, have been reported to improve modestly with methysergide therapy (437), tricyclic antidepressants (438), or dopamine agonists such as bromocriptine (388,439,440).

Whipple's Disease

Whipple's disease is a rare multisystem disorder characterized by weight loss, diarrhea, arthritis, lymphadenopathy, and fever that may involve and even be confined to the central nervous system (441,442). This disease can cause a defect of ocular motility that may mimic PSP (443). Initially, vertical saccades and quick phases are abnormal (444); eventually, all eye movements may be lost (445). A highly characteristic finding is pendular vergence oscillations and concurrent contractions of the masticatory muscles: oculomasticatory myorhythmia (446–448). The pendular vergence oscillations are always associated with vertical saccade palsy. Rhythmic palatal tremor may also be present (449). Rajput and Mchattie (450) described ophthalmoplegia with myorhythmia of the leg, but not of the eyes or jaw. Whipple's disease can be diagnosed using molecular analysis and can be treated with antibiotics (442).

OCULAR MOTOR SYNDROMES CAUSED BY LESIONS OF THE SUPERIOR COLLICULUS

Lesions restricted to the superior colliculi are rare in humans. One patient (297) underwent removal of a cavernous angioma from the right superior colliculus. Following surgery, he had persistently impaired upward gaze, implying pretectal damage, but a full range of horizontal eye movements. Systematic testing of horizontal saccades demonstrated a paucity of spontaneous refixations contralateral to the side of the lesion. Saccades to the left occurred after a

normal latency but were hypometric. These findings are similar to those seen after experimental ablation of the superior colliculi in monkeys (451). Pierrot-Deseilligny et al. (452) reported a patient who had a hematoma largely restricted to the right superior colliculus. The patient showed defects in latency and accuracy for contralateral saccades and increased numbers of inappropriate saccades during the anti-saccade task.

OCULAR MOTOR SYNDROMES CAUSED BY LESIONS OF THE THALAMUS

Thalamic lesions are characterized by disturbances of both horizontal and vertical gaze (453). Conjugate deviation of the eyes contralateral to the side of the lesion (also called wrong-way deviation) may occur with hemorrhage affecting the medial thalamus (Fig. 19.33) (18,454). The reason for this contraversive deviation is unclear. The descending pathways from the frontal eye fields to the pons have not yet crossed at this level, although the notion of a precise ocular motor decussation is less certain now than in the past. Damage to the descending pathway for smooth pursuit might lead to a paretic, contraversive deviation of the eyes (305). Nevertheless, a patient with a defect of smooth pursuit directed toward the side of a small hemorrhage in the posterior thalamus and adjacent internal capsule still showed an ipsiversive gaze preference (455). Another possibility is that wrong-way deviation may be an irritative phenomenon, because neurophysiologic studies show that saccade-related neurons in the intralaminar thalamic nuclei mainly discharge for contralateral saccades.

Forced downward deviation of the eyes, with convergence and miosis, is another common feature of thalamic hemorrhage; affected patients appear to peer at their noses (456,547). In autopsied cases, the hemorrhage usually extends into or compresses the midbrain. Hence, forced down-

ward deviation of the eyes may represent either an irritant effect of the hemorrhage on structures responsible for downward gaze or an imbalance created by an acute up-gaze palsy. Resolution of the downward deviation occurs after treatment of raised intracranial pressure; thus, traction on mesencephalic structures or hydrocephalus may cause this condition.

Esotropia, sometimes quite marked, occurs in patients with caudal thalamic lesions. Although it is usually associated with downward gaze deviation, it may occur as an isolated finding (458,459). The esotropia that occurs with thalamic lesions may reflect a disturbance of inputs to premotor vergence neurons in the midbrain (328). Combined lesions of the thalamus and midbrain may cause paresis of convergence (460).

Patients with posterolateral thalamic infarctions may have disturbances of the subjective visual vertical (either ipsilateral or contralateral) (72). The ocular tilt reaction is not present, however, unless the rostral midbrain is also damaged.

Infarction of the caudal thalamus caused by occlusion of the proximal portion of the posterior cerebral artery or its perforator branch, the posterior thalamosubthalamic paramedian artery, is reported to cause paralysis of downgaze. In fact, this deficit is probably caused not by damage to

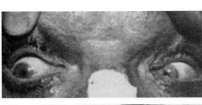
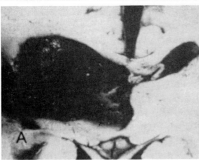
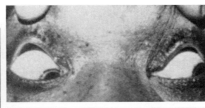
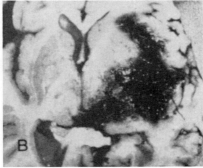

Figure 19.33. Contralateral (''wrong-side'') gaze deviation with supratentorial, thalamic-basal ganglia hemorrhage. *A, top,* The patient's eyes are deviated to the right. *Bottom,* Coronal section immediately posterior to the mammillary bodies shows a left intracerebral hemorrhage involving the thalamus, internal capsule, and basal ganglia. *B, top,* In another patient, the eyes are deviated down and left. *Bottom,* Horizontal section through the mid-diencephalon reveals a right intracerebral hemorrhage involving the pretectum, thalamus, posterior limb of the internal capsule, globus pallidus, and putamen. In both patients, the hemorrhage also involved the lateral midbrain tegmentum. (From Keane JR. Contralateral gaze deviation with supratentorial hemorrhage: three pathologically verified cases. Arch Neurol 1975;32:119–122.)

the thalamus but by damage to the adjacent riMLF or its immediate premotor inputs (461,462). Some patients have impairment of horizontal gaze, perhaps from interruption of descending pathways (463,464). Associated disturbances of arousal and short-term memory occur in some patients with thalamic lesions and may be caused by damage to specific thalamic nuclei (465,466). Experimentally, combined lesions of the superior colliculus and caudal thalamus in monkeys produce an enduring saccadic hypometria without corrective saccades (467), implying a role for these structures in generating efference copy signals (468–470).

Patients with central thalamic lesions show defects in double-step saccade paradigms (making successive accurate saccades after a target has quickly jumped twice to different locations), suggesting that information for saccades pro-grammed using extraretinal information about eye position must pass through the thalamus and possibly the internal medullary lamina (471). Lesions in the posterior parietal cortex and in the supplementary eye field in the frontal lobes create similar deficits in the double-step paradigm. Patients with thalamic lesions also show defects in saccade adaptation, likely reflecting interruption in pathways that carry information to and from the cerebellum (472).

Patients with lesions of the pulvinar develop difficulties in shifting attention and gaze into the contralateral hemifield, manifested by a paucity and prolonged latency of visually guided saccades (473,474). These results are consistent with some reported effects of pharmacologic and destructive lesions of the pulvinar in the monkey and indicate the importance of this thalamic nucleus in directing visual attention (475,476).

OCULAR MOTOR ABNORMALITIES AND DISEASES OF THE BASAL GANGLIA

PARKINSON'S DISEASE

Patients with Parkinson's disease may show a number of ocular motor findings (477). Steady fixation is often disrupted by square-wave jerks (478). Upward gaze is often moderately restricted (479), although this abnormality frequently is observed in normal, elderly persons (480). Convergence insufficiency is a common and often symptomatic disturbance (481,481a).

Saccades made reflexively to novel visual stimuli in Parkinson's disease are usually of relatively normal amplitude (426,428,482). In contrast, saccades in Parkinson's disease become hypometric in more complicated tasks such as when patients are asked to perform rapid, self-paced refixations between two stationary targets (478,482–486). During such a test, which relies on an internally generated, predictive strategy, intersaccadic intervals increase above values during unpredictable tracking to suddenly appearing targets (482,483). This effect is not, however, related simply to the persistence of the target light, because saccades made in anticipation of the appearance of a target light or to a remembered target location are also hypometric (482,487–491), and patients with Parkinson's disease have difficulty in generating sequences of memory-guided saccades to all types of stimuli (492,493). Despite this hypometria, patients can still shift their gaze, using a series of saccades, to the location of a target that is briefly flashed, indicating a retained ability to encode the location of objects in extrapersonal space (478,494). Saccadic latencies during nonpredictive tracking may be normal or mildly increased (478,485,495,496). Patients with Parkinson's disease often show defects in generating predictive saccades (495,497). Saccadic velocity may be normal or, particularly in advanced cases, mildly reduced (478,498). Patients with mild disease perform normally on the antisaccade task (499,500), but with advanced disease, errors increase, especially when patients are also taking anticholinergic drugs (501,502) Patients with Parkinson's disease have also been shown to be impaired in saccade search strategies that require use of "working memory" (503,504) although this may depend upon the difficulty of the task (505). Saccade adaptation may be affected in Parkinson's disease, implicating the basal ganglia in ocular motor learning (506).

Pallidotomy causes no improvement in ocular motor performance and may actually cause mild deficits in internally generated saccades and square-wave jerks (507,508). In contrast, stimulation of the subthalamic nucleus has been reported to improve saccade performance in Parkinson's patients (403).

Clinically, the saccadic initiation defect to command or to continuously visible targets appears to be more marked in the vertical plane. Upward saccades especially may be hypometric. In contrast, vertical saccades to randomly appearing visual targets are normal (496). If downward saccades are abnormal, or the velocity of vertical saccades in either direction is decreased, PSP is a more likely diagnosis than Parkinson's.

Combined movements of the eye and head may be abnormal in Parkinson's disease. Affected patients tend not to move their heads unless instructed to do so (509–511). During rapid eye-head gaze shifts, in response to either predictable or unpredictable step displacements of the target, patients show increased latency and slowing of head or eye movements (510).

Smooth-pursuit movements are usually impaired, although minimally so in mildly affected patients (497). During tracking of a target moving in a predictable, sinusoidal pattern, pursuit gain (eye velocity/target velocity) is decreased, leading to catch-up saccades (512). Because the catch-up saccades are hypometric, however, the cumulative tracking eye movement is less than that of the target, and this may be one mechanism for defective smooth tracking (497,513). Despite the impairment of smooth-pursuit gain, the phase relationship between eye and target movement during tracking of a periodic target is normal (495); this implies a normal predictive smooth tracking strategy (484). Cancellation of the VOR, by fixing upon an object moving with the head, is abnormal, however, so that during combined, active eye-head tracking, gain (gaze velocity/target velocity) is reduced (510).

Both caloric and low-frequency rotational vestibular responses, in darkness, may be hypoactive in patients with Parkinson's disease (514,515). At higher frequencies of head rotation, however, and particularly during visual fixation, the gain of the VOR is close to 1.0, which accounts for the lack of complaint of oscillopsia in such patients (515).

Patients with the syndrome of amyotrophic lateral sclerosis plus parkinsonism plus dementia (Lytico-Bodig syndrome), who live on the islands of the South Pacific Ocean, including Guam, may show more severe deficits than patients with idiopathic Parkinson's, including limitation of vertical gaze (432). Patients with diffuse Lewy body disease, Creutzfeldt-Jakob disease, multisystem atrophy (516), cortical-basal ganglion degeneration, Guadeloupean parkinsonism, and PSP must also be distinguished from those with idiopathic Parkinson's (402,424,426,428,430,433,517,518). Antisaccade testing is abnormal in cortical-basal ganglion degeneration (519) and in PSP (discussed previously). MR imaging may help in the differential diagnosis between Parkinson's and similar disorders (408,520).

Oculogyric crises, once encountered mainly in patients with postencephalitic parkinsonism, now occur primarily as a side effect of drugs, especially neuroleptic agents (521), although they may occur in other conditions such as reversible posterior leukoencephalopathy (522). A typical attack begins with feelings of fear or depression, which give rise to an obsessive fixation of a thought. The eyes typically deviate upward and sometimes laterally (Fig. 19.34); they rarely deviate downward. During the period of upward deviation, the movements of the eyes in the upper field of gaze appear nearly normal. Affected patients have great difficulty looking down, except when they combine a blink and downward saccade. Thus, the ocular disorder may reflect an imbalance of the vertical gaze-holding mechanism. Anticholinergic drugs promptly terminate both the thought disorder and the ocular deviation, a finding that suggests that the disorders of thought and eye movements are linked by a pharmacologic imbalance common to both (521). Oculogyric crises are distinct from the brief upward ocular deviations that occur in Tourette's syndrome (discussed later), in Rett's syndrome (523), and in most patients with tardive dyskinesia (524). In some patients with tardive dyskinesias, however, the upward eye deviations are longer-lasting and also are associated with the characteristic neuropsychological features of oculogyric crises (525), thus making the differentiation between the two entities difficult. Delayed oculogyric crises occurred in one patient after a focal striatocapsular infarction (526) and in another with bilateral lentiform lesions (527). Episodic brief spells of tonic upgaze occurred after bilateral lentiform lesions in a patient (528).

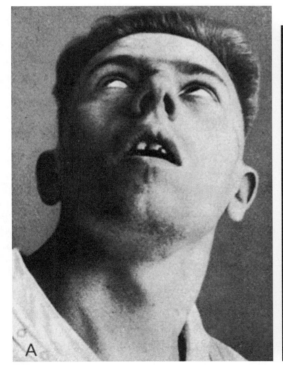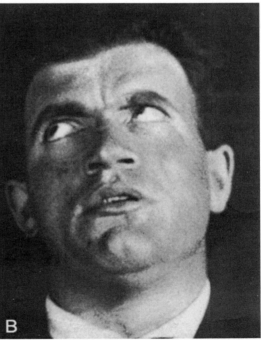

Figure 19.34. Oculogyric crisis in patients with postencephalitic parkinsonism. *A*, In a young man. Note hyperextension of neck, opening of the mouth, and conjugate deviation of the eyes up and to the right. *B*, In a middle-aged man. Again, the eyes are conjugately deviated up and to the right. (From Kyrieleis W. Die Augenveränderungen bei entzündlichen Erkrankungen des Zentralnervensystems. III. Die nichteitrigen entzündlichen Erkrankungen des Zentralnervensystems. A. Die nichteitrige epidemische Encephalitis [Encephalitis epidemica, lethargica]. In: Schieck F, Brückner A, eds. Kurzes Handbuch der Ophthalmologie, vol 6. Berlin: Julius Springer, 1931:712–738.)

In general, treatment of Parkinson's disease with L-dopa does not seem to improve the ocular motor deficits (479), except for saccadic accuracy (i.e., saccades become larger) (498,529). Occasionally, reversal of saccadic slowing occurs with treatment (530), and newly diagnosed patients with idiopathic disease may experience improved smooth pursuit after institution of dopaminergic therapy (529). In patients with parkinsonism caused by methyl-4-phenyl-1,2,3,6-tetrahydropyridine (MPTP) toxicity, saccadic latency is shortened and saccadic accuracy improved by dopaminergic agents (531). In addition, reflex blepharospasm is improved in these patients with treatment. These findings are similar to those in monkeys. When these animals are given MPTP, they develop increased latency and duration of saccades, decreased rate of spontaneous saccades, and inappropriate saccades, all of which are reversed by dopaminergic therapy (532,533). In patients with idiopathic disease who show pronounced drug-related fluctuations, there is disagreement as to whether smooth pursuit shows increase in gain during "on" periods (498,534,535). Although patients who are receiving L-dopa and who show dyskinetic movements of other body parts (536) are said to have unsteady gaze, particularly in darkness, this phenomenon usually is not evident clinically.

The dopaminergic pars compacta of the substantia nigra does not appear to contain neurons related to eye movement, whereas the pars reticulata does (537,538). In monkeys with MPTP-induced parkinsonism, the cerebral metabolic rate was reduced in the frontal eye field and paralamellar mediodorsal thalamus (539). It is possible that these metabolic changes are related to loss of projections from the dopamine-depleted substantia nigra.

HUNTINGTON'S DISEASE

Huntington's disease produces disturbances of voluntary gaze, particularly saccades (540–543). It is caused by a genetic defect of the IT15 gene (the "Huntington" gene) on chromosome 4, producing a CAG triplet repeat (544). Initiation of saccades in patients with Huntington's disease may be difficult. Such patients show prolonged latencies, especially when the saccade is to be made on command, in anticipation of a target moving in a predictable fashion, or in a self-paced fashion. An obligatory blink or head turn may be used to start the eye moving (545). Saccades may be slow in the horizontal or vertical plane; this deficit can often be detected early in the disease if eye movements are measured (89), but it may not be evident clinically until late in the course (541). Saccades may be slower in patients who become symptomatic at an earlier age, and such persons are more likely to have inherited the disease from their father (546). The slowing of vertical saccades in Huntington's disease probably does not occur in patients with chorea from nondegenerative conditions or tardive dyskinesia (547). Longitudinal studies of saccades can be used to quantify the progression of the disease (540,548).

Smooth pursuit may also be impaired with decreased gain in patients with Huntington's disease, but it often is relatively spared compared with saccades. By contrast, gaze-

holding and the VOR are preserved, though there may be a deficit in VOR adaptive capability (550). Late in the disease, rotational stimulation causes the eyes to tonically deviate with few or no quick phases.

Fixation is abnormal in some patients with Huntington's disease because of saccadic intrusions (541,551). This defect of steady fixation is particularly evident when the patient views a textured background (89). The paradoxical findings of difficulty in initiating voluntary saccades but with an excess of extraneous saccades during attempted fixation can be further elucidated using novel test stimuli. Such studies reveal an excessive distractibility in, for example, an antisaccade task (542). A second finding is that saccades to visual stimuli are made at normal latency, whereas those made to command are delayed. These findings may be related to the parallel pathways that control the various types of saccadic responses. On the one hand, disease affecting either the frontal lobes or the caudate nucleus, which inhibits the pars reticulata of the substantia nigra, may lead to difficulties in initiating voluntary saccades in tasks that require learned or predictive behavior (537,538). On the other hand, Huntington's also affects the pars reticulata of the substantia nigra (552). Because the pars reticulata of the substantia nigra inhibits the superior colliculus and therefore suppresses reflexive saccades to visual stimuli, one might expect excessive distractibility during attempted fixation. The slowing of saccades may reflect damage to saccadic burst neurons (553), but at least some pathologic evidence (554) suggests that disturbance of prenuclear inputs, such as the superior colliculus or frontal eye field, is responsible.

Despite the nearly ubiquitous finding of abnormal eye movements in patients with Huntington's, some persons with the disease who are evaluated before they become symptomatic show normal eye movements (89,555). Thus, routine testing of eye movements is not a reliable method for determining which offspring of affected patients will go on to develop the disease. Reveley et al. (556) reported some improvement in the eye movement abnormalities in patients with Huntington's who were treated with sulpiride.

Neuroacanthocytosis (557) must be distinguished from Huntington's disease (and PSP), but eye movement abnormalities do not seem to be an important feature of this disorder. Dentatorubropallidoluysian atrophy (558), also called the Haw River syndrome (559), is another CAG triplet repeat disease (B37, chromosome 12) that must be distinguished from Huntington's, although myoclonus and ataxia are more common in dentatorubropallidoluysian atrophy than in Huntington's.

OTHER DISEASES OF BASAL GANGLIA

A number of conditions other than Parkinson's and Huntington's that affect the basal ganglia cause abnormal eye movements. Hepatolenticular degeneration (Wilson's disease) and juvenile dystonic lipidosis (Niemann-Pick type 2s) are discussed below. Other conditions include caudate hemorrhage, which has been associated with ipsilateral gaze preference (560) and, rarely, Sydenham's chorea. Vermersch et al. (561) recorded saccadic eye movements in patients with bilateral lesions in the lentiform nucleus and found prominent abnormalities in saccades that required an internal representation of the target (remembered saccades, saccades to sequences, predictive saccades) but normal responses for visually guided saccades, including antisaccades (which are nonetheless triggered by a visual target). Lekwuwa et al. (562) suggested that defects in control of predictive pursuit eye movements are a feature of striatal damage.

Patients with Tourette's syndrome may show a variety of ocular abnormalities, including blepharospasm and eye tics that include involuntary gaze deviations (563,564), but saccades, fixation, and pursuit, when tested in conventional laboratory testing paradigms, show no abnormalities (565). The gaze deviations must be distinguished from benign eye movement tics, which children often outgrow (566,567). Quantitative testing of patients with Tourette's syndrome have shown various saccade abnormalities in "higher-level" tasks such as the antisaccade task and "go/no-go"

tasks, though there is considerable disagreement among these studies as to the exact deficits (568–573). A confounding factor in these studies is the presence or absence of associated attention-deficit/hyperactivity disorder (ADHD) (572,574,575).

Routine ocular motor functions are normal in most patients with essential blepharospasm (576). In some studies, however, abnormal saccade latencies are seen for both visually guided and memory-guided saccades (577,578), suggesting a possible basal ganglia localization. Patients with spasmodic torticollis may show abnormalities in vestibular function, including the torsional VOR (88,579). Patients with tardive dyskinesia may show increased saccade distractibility (580). Severely affected patients with Lesch-Nyhan syndrome (hypoxanthine-guanine phosphoribosyltransferase [HPRT] deficiency) show excessive distractibility, difficulty initiating saccades, and an oculomotor apraxia-like condition (581).

OCULAR MOTOR SYNDROMES CAUSED BY LESIONS IN THE CEREBRAL HEMISPHERES

Extensive reviews of the effects of cerebral hemisphere lesions on eye movements were done by Pierrot-Deseilligny (582) and Leigh and Kennard (583). One particular issue that must be considered in assessing abnormalities of eye movements in patients with lesions in the cerebral hemispheres is the sometimes confounding role of defects in directing visual attention and the associated neglect (584–587).

ACUTE LESIONS

Following an acute lesion of one cerebral hemisphere, the eyes usually deviate conjugately toward the side of the lesion (Prevost's or Vulpian's sign) (588) (Fig. 19.35). Gaze deviations are more common after large strokes involving predominantly the right postrolandic cortex (589,590) (Fig. 19.36). Visual hemineglect often accompanies such gaze deviations (590,591). Gaze deviation that occurs after a stroke usually resolves within a few days to a week; if gaze deviation persists, there may be a previous lesion in the contralateral frontal lobe (592). In general, for comparably sized lesions, ocular motor defects—both pursuit and saccades—are more profound when the lesion is in the nondominant hemisphere (593).

In the acute phase, patients may not voluntarily direct their eyes toward the side of the intact hemisphere, in part because of neglect. Shortly thereafter, however, vestibular stimulation usually produces a full range of horizontal movement (with the slow phase), in contrast to most gaze palsies associated with pontine lesions (313). When quick phases of caloric nystagmus directed away from the side of the lesion are absent, consciousness is usually impaired. Sometimes, in addition to ipsiversive deviation of the eyes, there is a small-amplitude nystagmus with ipsilateral quick phases. A similar finding occurs acutely after hemidecortication in the monkey (594). The slow phases of this nystagmus may reflect unopposed pursuit drives directed away from

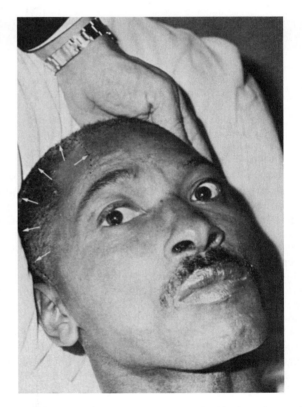

Figure 19.35. Persistent hemispheral (supranuclear) horizontal gaze palsy following severe frontal head trauma. Five weeks before this photograph was taken, the patient sustained a severe blow to the head, causing a depressed right frontal skull fracture. Operation disclosed extensive contusion and necrosis of the right frontal lobe (*arrows* indicate the site of the surgical incision). The patient had akinetic mutism and was hemiplegic on the right side. His eyes remained in right conjugate gaze at all times, but he could follow a very slowly moving target to the left.

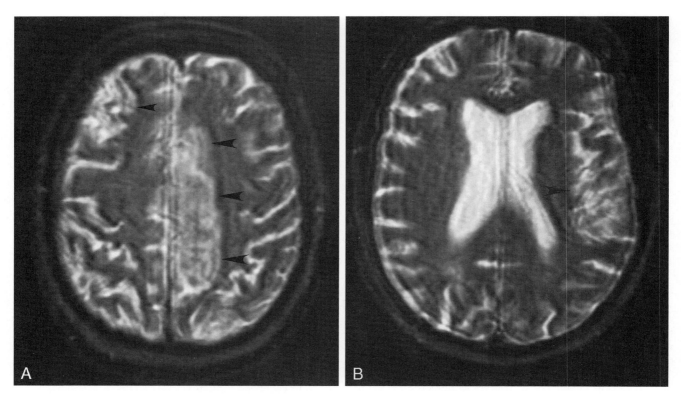

Figure 19.36.   Neuroimaging of an acute infarct in the territory of the left anterior cerebral and middle cerebral arteries. *A,* T2-weighted axial magnetic resonance image shows diffuse hyperintensity in the distribution of the left anterior cerebral artery (*large arrowheads*). Note the small area of hyperintensity in the right frontal region, consistent with an old infarct (*small arrowhead*). *B,* T2-weighted magnetic resonance image at a lower plane reveals an area of hyperintensity in the region of the left middle cerebral artery (*arrowhead*). The patient had a supranuclear conjugate gaze paresis to the left side and right hemineglect. He also had difficulty generating rightward saccades. The ocular motor signs were transient, as expected from a left-sided cerebral lesion.

the side of the lesion. Vertical saccades may be abnormal; they are dysmetric with an inappropriate horizontal component toward the side of the lesion (595). Because both hemispheres usually must be activated to elicit a purely vertical saccade, the loss of one hemisphere may cause such oblique saccades.

Following intracarotid injection of barbiturate (Wada test to determine cerebral dominance), a transient gaze preference may occur in association with hemiparesis; such a deviation occurs more commonly with right-sided injections, providing further evidence for the dominance of the right hemisphere in directing attention (596). During the period of hemiparesis of the Wada test, contralateral and ipsilateral saccades are still possible, with relatively minor slowing of the former. This persistence of voluntary saccades is probably related to the influence of posterior cerebral areas, which receive blood supply from the vertebrobasilar system and which project to the superior colliculus, independently of the frontal eye fields (597).

As noted above, acute cerebral hemisphere lesions are frequently associated with a conjugate deviation of the eyes (598) (Fig. 19.35). The deviation is usually ipsilateral to the side of the affected hemisphere and is more common with

right hemisphere lesions. In the right hemisphere, the lesions are located predominantly in the subcortical frontoparietal region and the internal capsule. In the left hemisphere, the lesions are usually larger, covering the entire frontotemporoparietal area. The larger the lesion, the more persistent the conjugate deviation. Quantitative recordings in such patients show that both the pursuit and the saccade deficits associated with conjugate deviation of the eyes are predominantly contralateral, but as the conjugate deviation resolves, an ipsilateral pursuit defect becomes more apparent (599). Craniotopic defects in saccades and especially pursuit may outlast the conjugate deviation, however, being greater in the field contralateral to the lesion (600). The initial conjugate deviation may reflect the effect on eye movements of cerebral hemisphere asymmetries in attention mechanisms (596), whereas the more enduring eye movement defects after the conjugate deviation resolves may reflect more specific defects in motor control mechanisms mediated by the hemispheres. Conjugate eye deviation is occasionally "wrongway" (i.e., contralateral to the side of the lesion) (601). The lesions are almost always hemorrhagic, most commonly in the thalamus. Affected patients usually have signs of rostral brain stem dysfunction and a shift of midline structures. Epileptic phenomena, impairment of ipsilateral pursuit pathways, and more caudal damage to descending pathways near the brain stem are evoked as explanations. In most cases, the last cause seems most plausible. Acute hemisphere lesions may cause epileptic seizures with contralateral deviation of the eyes or nystagmus, often with an associated head turn. The ocular motor manifestations of epilepsy are discussed below. Unilateral or bilateral ptosis may also occur with acute lesions in the cerebral hemispheres, usually in the nondominant hemisphere (311,602).

PERSISTENT DEFICITS CAUSED BY LARGE UNILATERAL LESIONS

Persistent ocular motor deficits caused by lesions such as hemidecortication for intractable seizures are summarized in Table 19.7. Although there may be no resting deviation of the eyes, forced eyelid closure may cause a contralateral spastic conjugate eye movement, the mechanism of which is not understood (Fig. 19.37) (603,604). This tonic deviation (Cogan's sign) differs from the tonic deviation associated with Wallenberg's syndrome, because in the former, active or attempted eyelid closure is necessary to cause the eyes to deviate, whereas in the latter, the deviation occurs even with eyes open in darkness. Cogan's sign occurs most frequently with parietotemporal lesions.

In primary position, a small-amplitude nystagmus may be present that is best seen during ophthalmoscopy. It is characterized by slow phases directed toward the side of the intact hemisphere and may represent an imbalance in smooth-pursuit tone (605). Horizontal pursuit gain (eye velocity/target velocity) is low for tracking of targets moving toward the side of the lesion for all stimulus velocities. For targets moving slowly toward the intact hemisphere, the eye

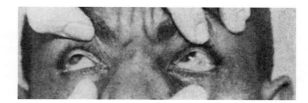

Figure 19.37. Conjugate lateral deviation of the eyes on forced closure of the eyelids in a patient with a tuberculoma of the left occipitoparietal region. (From Cogan DG. Neurologic significance of lateral conjugate deviation of the eyes on forced closure of the lids. Arch Ophthalmol 1948; 39;37–42.)

movements may be too fast (pursuit gain more than 1); for higher target velocities, pursuit gain toward the intact side is normal (605,606). This disturbance of smooth pursuit probably reflects loss of both posterior (occipital-parietal-temporal) and frontal influences.

A convenient way to demonstrate the asymmetry of smooth pursuit that occurs with large hemisphere lesions is with a hand-held optokinetic tape or drum (607). The response is decreased when the stripes are moved or the drum is rotated toward the side of the lesion. At the bedside, this optokinetic response is usually judged by the frequency and amplitude of quick phases, but because these quick-phase variables also depend on slow-phase velocity, a decreased response may reflect impaired slow-phase generation, impaired quick-phase generation, or a combination of the two.

Hemidecortication causes abnormalities of both contralateral and ipsilateral horizontal saccades (605,608). Saccades are usually slower than normal for refixations into and sometimes out of the hemianopic field. Saccadic latency is also prolonged in both directions (605). For small refixations, contralaterally directed saccades have greater latencies than ipsilateral saccades. Prolonged saccadic reaction time may reflect (*a*) defects in visual detection because of the hemianopia, (*b*) defects in directing visual attention, and (*c*) abnormal motor programming. Saccadic accuracy is impaired asymmetrically: most contralaterally directed saccades do not put the eye on target (608).

The horizontal VOR may be mildly asymmetric in hemidecorticate patients, with the gain (eye velocity/head velocity) being greater for compensatory eye movements directed away from the side of the lesion (609,610). More asymmetry appears when visual fixation and vestibular stimulation are combined (during rotation while fixating a stationary object), probably reflecting the ipsilateral smooth-pursuit deficit. The asymmetry is still present during head rotation if the patient imagines a stationary object (610).

FOCAL LESIONS

Ocular motor disturbances that occur from focal lesions of the cerebral hemispheres depend on a variety of factors, including the location and size of the lesion and whether the lesion is unilateral or bilateral.

Table 19.7
Persistent Effects of Large Unilateral Lesions of the Cerebral Hemispheres on Ocular Motor Function

Fixation: In darkness, eyes usually drift away from the side of the lesion. This may also be evident during fixation (on ophthalmoscopic exam) as nystagmus with quick phases toward the side of the lesion. Square-wave jerks.

Saccades: Slower saccades to both sides, especially contralaterally; latency longer for small saccades directed contralateral to the side of the lesion; inaccurate (hypometric and hypermetric) saccades into the "blind" hemifield.

Smooth pursuit: Reduced pursuit gain toward the side of the lesion; smooth-pursuit gain away from the side of the lesion may be increased for low-velocity targets.

Optokinetic: Reduced gain for stimuli directed toward the side of the lesion; impaired optokinetic after-nystagmus; may be relatively preserved compared with pursuit, with prolonged build-up of slow-phase velocity.

Vestibular: During sinusoidal rotation, VOR gain in darkness may be slightly asymmetric (greater for eye movements away from the side of the lesion); with attempted fixation of an imagined or real stationary target, the asymmetry is increased.

Forced eyelid closure: Eyes usually deviate conjugately away from the side of the lesion ("spasticity of conjugate gaze").

VOR, vestibulo-ocular reflex.

Occipital Lobe Lesions

A unilateral lesion of either occipital lobe causes a contralateral visual field defect and an ocular motor deficit (saccadic dysmetria) that reflects the patient's homonymous hemianopia. Saccades into the hemianopic visual field are dysmetric, usually hypometric, and similar patterns of saccades are seen with acoustic targets, implying some degree of common motor programming, perhaps influenced by associated defects in directing spatial attention (611). Characteristic patterns also occur in patients who have hemianopic dyslexia (612). Patients with hemianopia usually show a variety of compensatory strategies to increase saccadic accuracy (613), unless hemineglect is also present (614). These strategies include (a) a staircase of search saccades with backward, glissadic drifts; (b) a deliberate overshooting saccade to bring the target into the intact hemifield of vision; and (c) with predictable targets, saccades using memory of previous attempts. Such findings have been used to develop simple clinical tests for distinguishing homonymous hemianopias with and without neglect (615). Rapid gaze shifts achieved by combined movements of eye and head also show increased latency of head movements and development of compensatory strategies when looking to the hemianopic side (616). Smooth pursuit remains intact with unilateral lesions of the striate cortex, as long as the moving stimulus is presented to the intact hemifield (617). Optokinetic nystagmus elicited at the bedside is usually symmetric, unless subcortical pathways involved in smooth tracking are also affected (618; discussed later).

Bilateral occipital lesions cause cortical blindness. A patient with bilateral, congenital occipital lesions and little residual vision was reported to be able to make voluntary saccades but not smooth pursuit (619). Optokinetic responses are present in monkeys following bilateral occipital lobectomy (620), but this may not be the case in humans (621). Focal occipital seizures may cause either contralateral or ipsilateral deviation of the eyes and nystagmus (discussed later).

Parietal Lobe Lesions

Unilateral lesions of the parietal lobes, especially those involving the inferior parietal lobule and underlying deep white matter, cause abnormalities of ocular tracking of moving targets, including an asymmetry of smooth pursuit and of optokinetic nystagmus as tested at the bedside with handheld drums or tapes (607,622–625). Lesions at the temporoparieto-occipital junction probably affect secondary visual areas that are important for motion processing and for programming of smooth-pursuit eye movements (626). One such area is likely to be the human homologue of what in monkeys is called the middle temporal (MT) visual area.

Lesions of MT in monkeys impair the ability to estimate the speed of a moving target that is within the affected visual field, although stationary objects can be seen and accurately localized. The ocular motor consequences of this scotoma for motion or retinotopic defect are that saccades made to targets moving in the affected, contralateral hemifield are inaccurate and that the initiation of smooth pursuit is impaired (627). Such a behavior deficit occurs in patients with lesions affecting the temporoparieto-occipital cortex (625,628–631).

Lesions of adjacent cortex (including Brodmann areas 19 and 39), which probably correspond to the medial superior temporal (MST) visual area and underlying white matter, lead to a directional defect in smooth pursuit that is characterized by impaired tracking (reduced gain) for targets moving toward the side of the lesion, irrespective of the visual hemifield in which the target lies (628,632,633). Barton et al. (630) did not find a direct correlation between pursuit and motion detection deficits. Either could be present without the other, although unavoidable differences in the paradigms for eye movement and for motion perception precluded a strict one-to-one correspondence. Lawden et al. (634) showed that pursuit is also influenced by the presence of a stationary-structure background in patients with cerebral lesions. Lesions in the inferior parietal cortex (area 40) and in white matter containing frontoparietal connections were associated with a significant degradation in pursuit capability when patients had to track a small target moving on a structured background rather than a small target moving in darkness.

In some patients, pursuit gain away from the side of the parietal lobe lesion is also somewhat reduced, especially when the eyes move into the contralateral field of gaze. This phenomenon probably results from contralateral neglect (600,635) and may be associated with a paucity of exploratory eye movements in the contralateral field (636). In other patients, contralateral pursuit gain is increased (628,637). Subcortical, thalamic, and brain stem lesions may cause an ipsilateral defect from damage to involvement of the descending pathway for smooth pursuit (623,638,639). Full-field optokinetic stimulation is also impaired with experimental lesions of MST in monkeys (627). In human patients with parietal lesions, optokinetic nystagmus (OKN) is often impaired in response to stimuli moving toward the side of the lesion, although it may be relatively spared compared with foveal tracking (624,640). Optokinetic after-nystagmus (OKAN) and circularvection (the sensation of self-rotation) may also be impaired (625). In monkeys, acute lesions of the parietal lobe cause asymmetries of the VOR (641), but comparable studies in humans are lacking.

Unilateral lesions of the parietal lobe may affect saccadic initiation, causing an increase in saccadic latencies, either bilaterally (642) or only for saccades to contralateral targets (643,644). These changes are independent of any visual field defect. The latency defects are enhanced when the fixation target remains on and a new target appears in the periphery (the "overlap" task) and are diminished when the fixation target is extinguished before the presentation of the new target in the periphery (the "gap" task). Other deficits reported with unilateral parietal lesions include inaccuracy and hypometria of contralaterally directed visually guided saccades (645), mild saccadic slowing (646), and disturbances of predictive saccadic tracking (647). Memory-guided saccades are especially impaired, being both delayed and inaccurate (648,649). These changes in saccades are more prominent with right hemisphere lesions. The saccade defects associated with parietal lesions may be caused in part by difficulties in shifting attention from one position to another in extrapersonal space (650), but there are no strict correlations between attention and the ocular motor deficits (651–653). In a double-step paradigm in which subjects had to be able to use nonretinal, corollary discharge information about the saccade to the first target to compute the size and direction of the second saccade, patients with parietal lesions were not able to make the appropriate computation about the size and direction of the saccade (i.e., their spatial computation was impaired, implying a defect in using extraretinal signals of eye position) (645,654,655). In general, parietal lesions have relatively little effect on generation of more volitional internally guided saccades (i.e., when the target position is memorized or known) or on reflexive saccade inhibition (as in the antisaccade task) but seem more involved with triggering the superior colliculus directly to initiate reflexive saccades to the unexpected appearance of novel targets in the visual environment (656). Patients with parietal lesions also show defects in visual search tasks, though they may involve both the ipsilateral and contralateral visual fields (587,649,657,658). Selection of targets of interest among competing visual stimuli is also affected by experimental parietal lesions (659), and this finding may be related to parietal patients who show simultagnosia.

Bilateral parietal lobe lesions may cause acquired ocular motor apraxia, particularly if the lesions are large (discussed later). When smooth pursuit is possible, it is particularly limited with higher-acceleration target motion (660).

Temporal Lobe Lesions

The effects of temporal lobe lesions on eye movements are less well studied. In patients with posterior temporal lesions, fixation-suppression of caloric-induced nystagmus is said to be impaired when slow phases are directed away from the side of the lesion (661). This abnormality may reflect impairment of visual-motion or smooth-pursuit pathways rather than any effect on vestibular nystagmus per se. Patients with homonymous hemianopia and lesions affecting the temporal lobes may lack the sensation of self-rotation (circularvection) that normally occurs during full-field optokinetic stimulation, compared with patients who have a homonymous hemianopia from occipital lesions and who do experience circularvection (662). These findings support the localization of the vestibular cortex to the superior temporal gyrus and, perhaps, the adjacent parietal cortex (663–670). Patients with parietoinsular lesions may have tilts of the subjective visual vertical, usually contraversive (107). This is not associated with a skew deviation, although occasionally there is some monocular torsion. Patients with lesions in the same area may also have a defect in generating memory-guided saccades after a vestibular (rotational) stimulus (671). Finally, patients with lesions in the medial temporal lobe—the hippocampus—show marked impairment of generating sequences of saccades, whereas their spatial memory is intact (672).

Seizures emanating in the temporal lobes may cause a variety of vestibular sensations, although lesions in the frontal lobes may produce similar phenomenon. Although a mild feeling of dizziness is common with a variety of seizure types, a true sensation of rotation—tornado epilepsy—is a rare but well-described epileptic phenomenon (664, 673–679).

Frontal Lobe Lesions

Lesions of the frontal lobe, in both monkeys and humans, may produce an ipsilateral conjugate deviation of the eyes that resolves with time (313,680). Rarely, contralateral deviation occurs with acute frontal lesions (305), which may include just the frontal eye fields (681) or frontoparietal lesions (682). Enduring deficits after frontal lobe lesions include abnormalities of saccades and smooth pursuit (651). Three areas within the frontal lobes that play an important role in the control of eye movements are (*a*) the frontal eye fields; (*b*) the supplementary eye fields in the supplementary motor area; and (*c*) the prefrontal cortex, especially the dorsolateral portion (683).

Unilateral frontal eye field lesions lead to a slight increase in saccade latency to reflexively triggered saccades with a predominantly contralateral hypometria (684–687). Latencies are greatest in the overlap task (when the initial fixation target remains on, even after the peripheral target appears), suggesting a role for the frontal eye fields in disengagement from central fixation. Saccades may show a prolonged latency to predictable target jumps, particularly in patients with right-sided frontal lesions (684,688). There is also a bilateral deficit in latency and accuracy for saccades to a remembered visual target but not for remembered saccades after a vestibular (rotation) input (671). With attempted vertical saccades, a horizontal component directed toward the side of the lesion often causes an oblique movement (595). Mild slowing of contralateral saccades occurs in some patients (684). Deep, unilateral frontal lobe lesions cause increased latency for contralateral saccades (642). This deficit is probably caused by damage of efferent and afferent connections of the frontal eye fields.

Patients with unilateral frontal lesions show defects in the antisaccade task. This requires the subject to suppress a reflexive glance toward a peripheral visual target and, instead, look toward its mirror location in the contralateral visual field (689). Patients with unilateral frontal lobe lesions that involve the dorsolateral portion of the frontal cortex have difficulty in suppressing the reflexive glance, especially if the visual stimulus appears in the visual hemifield contralateral to the side of the lesion (690). Patients with lesions in the frontal eye fields alone do not have this problem, though they do have difficulty in generating the antisaccade when the target lies in the visual hemifield ipsilateral to the lesion (689,691). After lesions in the dorsolateral portion of the frontal cortex, there is also a deficit in both vestibular (rotation) and visually guided memory saccades (692) as well as deficits in generating predictive saccades (693) and in visual search (587,694). Taken together, the results of lesion studies suggest that the dorsolateral portion of the frontal cortex has an overall role in decisional processes related to suppressing unwanted saccades and facilitating saccades to known upcoming target locations. Lesion studies also suggest that the anterior cingulate cortex may also play a role in suppressing unwanted saccades (695). Lesions affecting the supplementary eye fields, especially in the left hemisphere, impair the ability of patients to make a remembered sequence of saccades (696,697). Likewise, patients with such lesions cannot make a memory-guided saccade to a visual target, but they can do so after a body rotation (692,698). Patients with lesions of the supplementary eye fields may also show abnormalities in changing the direction of saccades from a previously learned sequence (699).

Patients with unilateral frontal lobe lesions also show pursuit deficits (562,593,625,687,700,701). The frontal and supplementary eye fields and perhaps the dorsolateral portion of the prefrontal cortex play a role in this abnormality. Defects are in both initiation and maintenance (more so at higher target speeds and frequencies). If lesions are in the supplementary eye field, defects are ipsilateral; if lesions are in the frontal eye field, defects are bilateral but usually greater for ipsilateral tracking. Patients with lesions of the supplementary eye field may have delayed reversal with periodic constant-velocity stimuli, implying impaired anticipation of the target trajectory. Saccades to moving targets are also inaccurate in some of these patients. Patients with lesions affecting the frontal eye fields may also show craniotopic as well as directional (ipsilateral) defects in pursuit (600). Tracking in the field contralateral to the lesion is worse than in the ipsilateral field. Visual exploration deficits may also play a role in some of the eye movement deficits seen with frontal lesions (702).

Acute bilateral frontal or frontoparietal lesions may produce a striking disturbance of ocular motility that is called *acquired ocular motor apraxia*. It is characterized by loss of voluntary control of eye movements, both saccades and pursuit, with preservation of reflex movements, including the VOR and quick phases of nystagmus. There is also relative preservation of saccades made to visual targets, compared with internally guided saccades made on command, and preservation of saccades made with blinking or with head movements (703,704). Voluntary movements of the eyes are limited in the horizontal and usually also in the vertical plane. The defect of voluntary eye movements probably reflects disruption of descending pathways from both the frontal eye fields and the parietal cortex so that the superior colliculus and brain stem reticular formation are bereft of their supranuclear inputs. The behavior deficit is similar to that produced by combined, experimental lesions of the frontal eye fields and superior colliculus (705).

When a similar disorder of ocular motility, called "psychic paralysis of gaze," is associated with optic ataxia and disturbance of visual attention (simultanagnosia), the eponym Bálint's syndrome is used (703–706) (see Chapter 13). The main abnormalities are a defect in the visual guidance of saccades (increased latency and decreased accuracy) and inaccurate searching saccades. Voluntary saccades may be made with greater ease than those in response to visual targets, the converse of what one usually finds with more frontal lesions (707–709). Spontaneous blinking may be lost (710). In one patient, the visual scene faded during fixation and intentional blinking restored it (711). In Bálint's syn-

drome, the lesions are usually bilateral and located in the parietal or occipital lobes. The anatomic basis for this disturbance is not known, although it has been attributed to defects in the inhibitory control of the superior colliculus by the substantia nigra, pars reticulata (712). Spasm of fixation refers to a rare defect in generating voluntary eye movements when a fixation target is continuously present; it is alleviated when the central fixation target is removed (712).

OCULAR MOTOR APRAXIA

Ocular motor apraxia is characterized by an impaired ability to generate saccades on command (Fig. 19.38). Congenital ocular motor apraxia was first described by Cogan in 1965. An abnormality in eye movements may be recognized shortly after birth, when the child does not appear to fixate upon objects normally and may appear blind (713). Some children with congenital ocular motor apraxia are said to have a transient head and limb tremor in the first few days of life. Between ages 4 and 6 months, characteristic thrusting horizontal head movements develop, sometimes with prominent blinking or even rubbing of the eyelids, when the child attempts to change fixation. In children with poor head control, development of head thrusting may be delayed or absent. Almost all patients also show a defect in generating quick phases of nystagmus, which can usually be appreciated at the bedside by manual spinning of the patient, either when holding the child out at arm's length or by rotating the child on a swivel chair (if necessary sitting in an adult's lap). Despite difficulties in shifting horizontal gaze, vertical voluntary eye movements are normal.

Measurements of eye and head movements have further characterized congenital ocular motor apraxia (714–716). With the head immobilized, patients show both impaired initiation (increased latency) and decreased amplitude (hypometria) of voluntary saccades in response to either a simple verbal command to look left or right or in tracking a step displacement of a target. Saccades are also delayed during attempted refixations between auditory targets in complete darkness. Thus, abnormal visual-fixation reflexes cannot ex-

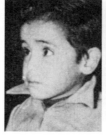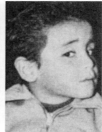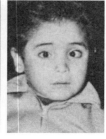

Figure 19.38. Congenital ocular motor apraxia. The patient was looking to the right (*left*) when he was told to glance at the camera. His head rapidly moved to the left, while the eyes remained deviated toward the right. As a result, the patient's head had to turn further to the left in order to permit fixation ahead (*center*). Once the patient was able to fixate on the camera, his head turned slowly back to the right until it was straight (*right*). (From Urrets-Zavalia A, Remonda C. Congenital ocular motor apraxia. Ophthalmologica 1957;134:157–167.)

plain the difficulty initiating saccades. Saccadic velocities are normal, however, and saccades or quick phases of nystagmus of large amplitude can occasionally be generated. These findings indicate that in these patients, the premotor brain stem burst neurons that generate saccadic eye movements are intact. In younger patients, however, the timing and amplitude (but not velocity) of quick phases of vestibular and optokinetic nystagmus may be impaired (i.e., the eyes intermittently deviate tonically in the direction of the slow phase because of a defect in the initiation of quick phases). Sometimes the saccade defects and head thrusts are asymmetric (717). Pursuit eye movements may also be of low gain, but the corrective saccades are usually promptly generated. The defects in congenital ocular motor apraxia are usually restricted to the horizontal plane, an important differential diagnostic point because most acquired cases of ocular motor apraxia also cause defects in the vertical plane.

The head thrusts made by patients with congenital ocular motor apraxia probably reflect one of several adaptive strategies to facilitate changes in gaze (714,718). Younger patients appear to use their intact VOR, which drives their eyes into an extreme contraversive position in the orbit. As the head continues to move past the target, the eyes are dragged along in space until they become aligned with the target. The head then rotates backward and the eyes maintain fixation as they are brought back to the primary position in the orbit by the VOR. In contrast, older patients appear to use the head movement alone to trigger the generation of a saccadic eye movement that cannot normally be made with the head still. This strategy may reflect the use of a phylogenetically old linkage between head and saccadic eye movements that occurs reflexively in afoveate animals such as the rabbit when they desire to redirect their center of visual attention.

The cause of congenital ocular motor apraxia is unknown. Cogan (719) suggested a delay in the normal development of the mechanisms by which we assume voluntary control over eye movements. Delayed psychomotor development (especially in learning to read and in speech), infantile hypotonia, strabismus, incoordination, torsional nystagmus, and clumsiness occur in some patients (720). Associated anomalies, especially agenesis of the corpus callosum and cerebellar dysplasia and hypoplasia (e.g., as part of Joubert's syndrome), are found in a number of patients with congenital ocular motor apraxia (721–724). Most likely, however, such anomalies are markers of abnormal development rather than being directly responsible for the eye movement disorder. Congenital ocular motor apraxia is occasionally familial and has been reported in monozygotic twins (725,726). Patients usually improve with age, with the head movements becoming less prominent as the patients are better able to direct their eyes voluntarily.

A variety of disorders that directly involve the brain stem mechanisms for generating saccades, including structural or degenerative processes within the pontine and mesencephalic reticular formations, are characterized by the development of a strategy of head thrusting or blinking to shift gaze that superficially resembles congenital ocular motor apraxia. These disorders usually can be differentiated from congenital ocular motor apraxia because all types of saccades and

quick phases (both horizontal and vertical) are typically affected, and because saccades may be slow. In the early stages of these diseases, however, the ocular motor apraxia may be indistinguishable from congenital ocular motor apraxia. Thus, patients with ataxia-telangiectasia (Louis-Bar syndrome, 11q22-23) and its variants (ataxia-oculomotor apraxia syndrome of Aicardi, types 1 and 2), Gaucher's disease (types 2 and 3,1q21-31), Niemann-Pick disease type 2s, Pelizaeus-Merzbacher disease, Cockayne's syndrome, Huntington's disease, hepatolenticular degeneration, vitamin E deficiency, some of the peroxisome disorders, Whipple's disease, and many other storage diseases and aminoacidurias may appear to have ocular motor apraxia (723,724,727–735) (Fig. 19.32).

A few features that can be used to distinguish some of these disorders from congenital ocular motor apraxia include the following:

1. In Pelizaeus-Merzbacher disease, pendular, elliptical nystagmus, upbeat nystagmus, saccade dysmetria, and other cerebellar signs (especially truncal titubation) are often present.
2. Patients with Niemann-Pick disease characteristically show a vertical and especially downgaze disturbance along with dysarthria, ataxia, cognitive dysfunction, and emotional changes. Such patients have so-called foam cells in the bone marrow. Rarely, a horizontal gaze disturbance dominates the picture. The typical vertical pattern of gaze disturbance in Niemann-Pick must be distinguished from the vertical gaze palsies associated with kernicterus, in which athetosis and hearing loss are commonly associated.
3. In Gaucher's disease, vertical gaze may be affected, but horizontal gaze disturbances are more common.
4. Tay-Sachs disease impairs vertical and, subsequently, horizontal eye movements.
5. Late-onset hexosaminidase deficiency also preferentially affects vertical gaze.
6. In Whipple's disease, supranuclear and especially vertical gaze palsy is frequent and may be associated with the convergence oscillations of "oculomasticatory myorhythmia."
7. In Joubert's syndrome, patients commonly have skew deviations that change with lateral gaze and also spontaneously alternate as to which eye is higher, along with seesaw and pendular nystagmus. Patients with Joubert's syndrome may also have pigmentary degeneration of the retina as well as breathing disturbances early in life.
8. In vitamin E deficiency (e.g., abetalipoproteinemia), a slow but full range of abduction and limited range but normal speed of adduction are characteristic.
9. Patients with ataxia-telangiectasia have other cerebellar eye signs and elevated levels of alpha-fetoprotein.
10. In childhood Huntington's disease, slowing of saccades is prominent, and rigidity may be more apparent than chorea.

The role of blinking in facilitating eye movements in patients with congenital ocular motor apraxia may be related to a natural synkinesis of blinking and saccade-generating or in some cases to lesions in the posterior fossa. Zee et al. (308) studied two patients who could make saccades of normal velocity and amplitude only in association with a simultaneous blink. In one patient, the initiation of saccades was also facilitated by blinks, much like patients with typical congenital ocular motor apraxia; however, both patients had other signs of cerebellar or brain stem dysfunction, suggesting a posterior fossa localization for blink facilitation of saccadic velocity and amplitude.

ABNORMAL EYE MOVEMENTS AND DEMENTIA

Patients with various dementing processes have abnormal eye movements, reflecting either disturbances in cerebral cortical structures or in other subcortical structures that may also be affected by that particular disease. Excessive errors on the antisaccade test (736–739), particularly when associated with a ''visual grasp reflex'' (741), are a useful indicator of an organic process when pseudodementia is a diagnostic consideration in a patient with a possible cognitive decline. Patients with Alzheimer's disease have excessive numbers of square-wave jerks and defects in saccade latency and, occasionally, accuracy and velocity (737,739,740). Alzheimer's patients show longer mean fixation durations and a reduced number of exploring saccades when viewing simple but not complex scenes, perhaps reflecting a motivation deficit. Impaired predictive tracking and excessive number of anticipatory saccades are a feature of Alzheimer's disease (737), as is difficulty generating saccades during reading (738). Eye movements may be used to monitor higher-level processes, such as ''curiosity,'' by looking at exploratory behavior (visual search and scan paths) while a subject views novel visual stimuli (587). This capability too appears to be diminished in Alzheimer's patients (742). Impairment of spatially directed attention may also be reflected in eye movement abnormalities (743), and a Bálint-like syndrome may develop (744). Pursuit abnormalities also occur in Alzheimer's patients (745,746).

Patients with Creutzfeldt-Jakob disease may show limitation of vertical gaze and slow vertical saccades (747,748) as well as two rare forms of nystagmus: periodic alternating nystagmus (748) and centripetal nystagmus (749). Overdoses of lithium or bismuth may lead to syndromes that mimic Creutzfeldt-Jakob disease (750,751). Cerebellar eye signs are typically found in another prion disorder: Gerstmann-Strüssler-Scheinker disease (752,753).

Patients infected with the human immunodeficiency virus (HIV) show a number of ocular motor abnormalities that usually reflect the effects of an opportunistic infection or coexistent neoplasia (754–758). However, HIV encephalopathy itself can cause disturbed ocular motility (759), including errors on the antisaccade task, increased fixation instability, increased latencies of horizontal and, especially, vertical saccades (760), acquired ocular motor apraxia (761), cerebellar and brain stem signs, including gaze-evoked and dissociated nystagmus (762,763), slow saccades (764), and decreased but especially asymmetric pursuit gain (760,765).

OCULAR MOTOR MANIFESTATIONS OF SEIZURES

Eye and head movements are common manifestations of epileptic seizures, and the wide representation of oculomotor and vestibular control within the cerebral cortex leads to a number of possible ways that seizures can affect eye movements themselves and visual or vestibular perceptions (670).

A variety of eye movements can occur with seizures, including horizontal or vertical gaze deviation, skew deviation, and spontaneous, retractory, periodic alternating or monocular nystagmus (122,766–776). Epileptic convergence nystagmus may occur with periodic lateralizing epileptiform discharges (777) and with burst-suppression patterns (778,779). The seizure focus may arise from any lobe, although the lesions usually are more posterior. Epileptic nystagmus can occur with typical absence seizures (780) and with infantile spasms (781).

Patients with epileptic foci affecting the temporoparieto-occipital cortex may show either ipsiversive or contraversive eye deviation and nystagmus (766,782–784). Seizures are usually accompanied by relatively fast cortical activity. Ipsiversive gaze deviation may be caused by a smooth-pursuit movement, with the quick phases of nystagmus being triggered by the eccentric eye position and ipsilateral drift of the eyes. Contraversive deviation may be initiated by saccades and the subsequent nystagmus from an impaired gaze-holding mechanism (deficient neural integrator). Furman et al. (678) described a patient with a temporoparietal seizure focus who showed no gaze deviation before the onset of nystagmus. Her attacks were accompanied by vertigo, suggesting involvement of the ''vestibular cortex'' of the superior temporal sulcus.

Overall, contraversive deviation of the eyes is more common than ipsiversive deviation during seizures. In cases with posterior foci (temporal, parietal, or occipital lobes), experimental studies suggest that eye movements may be mediated by projections via either the superior colliculus or the frontal eye fields (785). Thus, saccades may be generated by more than one of the descending parallel pathways. Frontal lobe foci are also reported to cause contraversive deviations unless they are bilateral, in which case vertical deviations also may occur (786). These results are consistent with stimulation studies in monkeys, in which unilateral stimulation of the frontal eye fields typically causes oblique saccades with a contralateral horizontal component; the direction of the vertical saccade depends upon a cortical map (787). Purely vertical movements require bilateral stimulation of the frontal eye fields. Because there are also neurons in the frontal eye fields that contribute to smooth pursuit, it is theoretically possible that frontal lobe foci could lead to an ipsiversive deviation.

Head turning is a common accompaniment of epileptic gaze deviation. In patients who are conscious during the seizure, a frontal focus is likely, and the initial direction of head turning is usually, but not invariably, contralateral to the seizure focus (788–790). A contralateral focus is also likely in a patient who shows marked, sustained, and unnatural lateral positioning of the head and eyes (789,790). In patients who are unconscious during the seizure, the focus may arise from any lobe, and head turning may be toward or away from the side of the lesion (788,791,792). As discussed above, seizures emanating in the superior temporal lobes may cause a variety of vestibular sensations (670), and occipital lobe seizures may produce oscillopsia (793). Rarely, seizures are precipitated by movements of the eyes, such as convergence (794) or sustained lateral deviation (795).

EYE MOVEMENTS IN STUPOR AND COMA

The ocular motor examination is especially useful for evaluating the unconscious patient, because both arousal and eye movements are controlled by neurons in the brain stem reticular formation. Comatose patients do not make eye movements that depend upon cortical visual processing. Voluntary saccades and smooth pursuit are in abeyance, and quick phases of nystagmus also may be absent. The ocular motor examination of the unconscious patient, therefore, consists of observing the resting position of the eyes, looking for any spontaneous movements, and reflexively inducing eye movements (796–798).

Gaze Deviations

Conjugate, horizontal deviation of the eyes is common in coma. When this is caused by lesions above the brain stem ocular motor decussation between the midbrain and pons, the eyes are usually directed toward the side of the lesion and away from the hemiparesis. A vestibular stimulus, however, usually drives the eyes across the midline. If the conjugate deviation is caused by a lesion below the ocular motor decussation, the eyes will be directed away from the side of the lesion and toward the hemiparesis. The latter is typically seen with pontine lesions, but also in some patients with thalamic (18) and rarely hemispheric disease above the thalamus (so-called wrong-way deviations) (305,682).

Intermittent deviations of the eyes and head are usually caused by seizure activity. At the onset of each attack, gaze is usually deviated contralateral to the side of the seizure focus and may be followed by nystagmus with contralaterally directed quick phases. Toward the end of the seizure, gaze drifts to an ipsilateral (paretic) position.

Tonic downward deviation of the eyes, often accompanied by convergence, occurs in patients with thalamic hemorrhage (453,456) and with lesions affecting the dorsal midbrain. It may be induced by unilateral caloric stimulation, after the initial horizontal deviation subsides, in patients with coma induced by sedative drugs (799). Forced downward deviation of the eyes can also be seen in patients with nonorganic (feigned) coma or seizures (800).

Tonic upward deviation of the eyes is uncommon in coma, but it may be seen after an hypoxic-ischemic insult, even when no pathologic lesions are found in the midbrain (801). Patients who survive after manifesting this ocular motor disturbance typically develop downbeating nystagmus, the upward drift of which is thought to be caused by loss of inhibition on the upward vertical VOR (802). Upward deviation of the eyes also occurs as a component of oculogyric crisis, which usually occurs as a side effect of certain drugs, especially neuroleptic agents (521). Tonic uninhibited elevation

of the lids (eyes-open coma) may also occur in unconscious patients and may be related to pontomesencephalic dysfunction (803).

Deviations of the visual axes in coma may be caused by skew deviation, by a phoria that is normally compensated for by fusional mechanisms, or by paralysis of the oculomotor, trochlear, or abducens nerves. Restrictive ophthalmopathy, particularly blowout fracture of the orbit, may be an additional mechanism in patients who have suffered facial trauma. The diagnosis of the cause of the deviation depends upon determining whether the range of movement of the eyes induced by head rotation or caloric stimulation (discussed later) is reduced in a pattern corresponding to specific muscle weakness. In addition, assessment of the pupils and other brain stem reflexes may help. Complete oculomotor nerve palsy causes pupillary dilation, ipsilateral ptosis, and deviation of the eye down and out. Pupillary involvement is an early sign of uncal herniation (797), and disturbances of eye movements usually follow (804). Vertical misalignment of the eyes is usually caused by skew deviation or trochlear nerve palsy, the latter being particularly common following head trauma. Bilateral abducens palsy occurs when increased intracranial pressure compromises the nerves as they bend over the petroclinoid ligament. Occasionally, skew deviation and INO occur in patients with metabolic encephalopathy or drug intoxication.

Spontaneous Eye Movements

Spontaneous eye movements that occur in unconscious patients may help establish the etiology of the coma. Slow conjugate or disconjugate roving eye movements are similar to the eye movements of light sleep but slower than the rapid eye movements (REM) of paradoxic or REM sleep. If a complete range can be shown, their presence indicates that brain stem gaze mechanisms are intact (796).

Other types of spontaneous eye movements consist of various forms of vertical to-and-fro movements, often called "bobbing." Typical ocular bobbing consists of intermittent, usually conjugate, rapid downward movement of the eyes followed by a slower return to the primary position (805,806). Reflex horizontal eye movements are usually absent. Ocular bobbing is a classic sign of intrinsic pontine lesions, usually hemorrhage, but it also occurs in patients with cerebellar lesions that compress the pons and in metabolic or toxic encephalopathy. Inverse bobbing also occurs in this setting. This eye movement abnormality, which is also called ocular dipping, is characterized by a slow downward movement, followed by a rapid return to midposition. Reverse bobbing consists of rapid deviation of the eyes upward and a slow return to the horizontal, whereas converse bobbing (also called reverse dipping) is characterized by a slow upward drift of the eyes that is followed by a rapid return to primary position. These variants of ocular bobbing are less reliable for localization than is straightforward ocular bobbing. Nevertheless, the occurrence in some patients of several different types of ocular bobbing during their illness suggests a common underlying pathophysiology (807–810). Because the pathways that mediate upward and downward eye movements differ anatomically and probably pharmacologically, it seems likely that these movements represent a varying imbalance of mechanisms for vertical gaze. Rarely, large-amplitude pendular vertical oscillations occur in the acute phase of a brain stem stroke (804).

Repetitive vertical eye movements, including variants of ocular bobbing, may contain convergent-divergent components. Such movements are usually caused by disease affecting the dorsal midbrain (109,808,812).

Monocular bobbing movements may occur as a synkinesis with jaw movement. Such movements are similar to those seen in the congenital condition called the Marcus Gunn jaw-winking phenomenon and primarily involve the neural pathways to the inferior rectus muscle (813).

Ping-pong gaze consists of slow, horizontal, conjugate deviations of the eyes that alternate every few seconds. In more alert patients, ping-pong gaze has been shown to be a series of small saccades that take the eyes back and forth from one extreme orbital position to the other (814,815). Although ping-pong gaze can occur in patients with posterior fossa hemorrhage (816), it is usually a sign of bilateral infarction of the cerebral hemispheres. In one reported case, no cerebral hemispheric lesions were noted, but bilateral lesions of the cerebral peduncles were present (817). Sometimes oscillations with a periodicity similar to that of ping-pong gaze can be induced transiently by a rapid head rotation in patients with bilateral hemisphere disease (818).

Rapid, small-amplitude, vertical eye movements may be the only manifestation of epileptic seizures in patients with coexistent brain stem injury (819). Rapid, monocular eye movements with horizontal, vertical, or torsional components that occur in patients with coma may also indicate brain stem dysfunction.

Identification of patients who are conscious but quadriplegic, the *locked-in syndrome* or de-efferented state, depends on identifying preserved voluntary vertical eye movements (797,820). The syndrome is typically caused by pontine infarction and is characterized in part by a variable loss of voluntary and reflex horizontal movements, such that eyelid or vertical eye movements may be the only means of communication during the acute illness. The locked-in syndrome also occurs with midbrain lesions, in which case ptosis and ophthalmoplegia may be present (821).

Reflex Eye Movements

Reflex eye movements may be elicited in unconscious patients either by head rotation (the doll's head or oculocephalic maneuver) or by caloric stimulation (798). Head rotation, with the patient supine, stimulates the labyrinthine semicircular canals, the otoliths, and neck muscle proprioceptors. However, unless there has been prior loss of vestibular function (e.g., from aminoglycoside toxicity), the contribution made by neck muscle proprioceptors to generating reflex eye movements (the cervico-ocular reflex) is insignificant (818). Furthermore, the otolith contribution is probably small compared with that of the labyrinthine semicircular canals. Finally, although visually mediated eye movements, such as fixation and smooth pursuit, can influence the eye movements produced by head rotation in normal, awake subjects, this is unlikely to be the case in unconscious patients. Therefore, eye rotations induced by head rotation in unconscious individuals principally result from the effects of the semicircular canals and their central connections (i.e., the VOR). The head should not be rotated in unconscious patients unless there is certainty that no neck injury or abnormality is present. Conventionally, high-frequency (1–2 Hz) quasi-sinusoidal rotations or position-step stimuli are applied; the latter consists of a sudden head turn to a new position. Both horizontal and vertical rotations should be performed. If small-amplitude head rotations are performed, the adequacy of the VOR can be estimated by observing the optic disc of one eye with an ophthalmoscope (344).

Caloric irrigation of the external auditory meatus causes convection currents of the vestibular endolymph that displace the cupula of a semicircular canal; thus, this procedure also tests the VOR. The canal stimulated depends on the orientation of the head (e.g., with the head elevated 30° from the supine position, the horizontal canals are principally stimulated). Before caloric stimulation, the physician should always check that the tympanic membrane is intact. Usually only about 5 cc of ice water need be introduced into the external auditory meatus, but large quantities (100 cc or more) may be necessary to induce a response in some comatose patients.

Caloric stimulation with ice water is sometimes a more effective stimulus than head rotation, in part because of the sustained nature of the stimulus and in part because of the arousing effect of the cold water. Combined cold caloric stimulation and head rotation may be the most effective stimulus in the deeply unconscious patient (796). This usually produces tonic deviation of the eyes toward the irrigated ear in patients with intact vestibular function.

In testing reflex eye movements in unresponsive patients, it is important to note (*a*) the magnitude of the response; (*b*) whether the ocular deviation is conjugate; (*c*) the dynamic response to position-step head rotations; and (*d*) the occurrence of any quick phases of nystagmus, particularly during caloric stimulation. Impaired abduction suggests abducens nerve palsy. Impaired adduction usually indicates either INO or oculomotor nerve palsy, although occasionally impaired adduction to vestibular stimulation is observed in patients with metabolic coma or drug intoxication. Vertical responses may be impaired with disease of the midbrain (822) or bilateral lesions of the MLF. Pontine lesions may abolish the reflex eye movements in the horizontal plane but spare the vertical responses. When reflex eye movements are present in an unresponsive patient, the brain stem is likely to be structurally intact. When reflex eye movements are abnormal or absent, the cause may be structural disease, profound metabolic coma, or drug intoxication (823). Intoxication with a variety of medications may lead to partial or total loss of reflexive eye movements. Metabolic disturbances can cause restriction of reflex eye movements, but usually only with profound coma (824). When used in combination with other clinical signs, reflex eye movements are useful in evaluating the prognosis of comatose patients (825,826).

If reflex eye movements are intact in an unconscious patient, the eyes are carried into a corner of the orbit when the head is rapidly rotated horizontally to a new position (position step stimulus). If the head is held stationary in its new position, the eyes may slowly drift back to the midline. This implies that the gaze-holding mechanism (neural integrator) is not functioning normally. Patients with more rapid centripetal drift may have more severe brain injury (818).

Quick phases of nystagmus are usually absent in acutely unconscious patients. Their presence, without a tonic deviation of the eyes, should raise the possibility of nonorganic (i.e., feigned) coma. In patients who are stuporous but uncooperative, caloric nystagmus may be a useful way of inducing eye movements that cannot be initiated voluntarily. For example, in a patient with a pineal tumor but no overt abnormalities during testing of voluntary eye movements,

Singh and Strobos (827) induced retraction nystagmus with caloric stimulation. Patients who survive coma but who are left in a persistent vegetative state, with severe damage of the cerebral hemispheres but preservation of the brain stem (828), regain nystagmus with caloric or rotational stimulation (818). Caloric nystagmus was present in patients with neocortical death and an isoelectric electroencephalogram (829).

Normal subjects have been studied during syncope (830). Subjects developed downbeat nystagmus and tonic upward deviation of the eyes. There was also an increased amplitude of the VOR in most of the subjects. These findings are most compatible with cerebellar hypoperfusion.

OCULAR MOTOR DYSFUNCTION AND MULTIPLE SCLEROSIS

MS causes a variety of ocular motor deficits; bilateral INO, cerebellar eye signs (including gaze-evoked nystagmus), and acquired pendular nystagmus are the most common (224,250,831–835) (see Chapter 60). Pendular or elliptical nystagmus is a frequent disabling manifestation of the disease (836,837). Measurement of eye movements may help establish the diagnosis of MS during early stages of the disease. Saccadic abnormalities may be more readily detected when targets are presented randomly so that neither their time of onset nor their location can be predicted. Large saccades (20° or more) are more likely to show changes in velocity than are small saccades (838). Because normal subjects show differences in the peak velocity of abducting and adducting saccades, it is worth developing a normative database for each of these. With these provisos, most patients with MS show saccadic abnormalities that include prolonged latency, inaccuracy, and decreased velocity. In particular, minor slowing of adducting saccades may indicate an INO that may not be evident with clinical testing (839).

Some patients with MS show saccadic oscillations (243,840–842). Smooth-pursuit gain may be decreased

(610,843,844), and impaired cancellation of the horizontal VOR may be present (610). Abnormalities of vertical gaze-holding, smooth pursuit, and eye-head tracking occur in patients with an INO (359). Other abnormalities in patients with MS include horizontal and vertical gaze palsies (845), gaze-evoked blepharoclonus (846), vertical nystagmus, saccadic pulsion (847), various vestibular abnormalities (832), and superior oblique myokymia.

Diagnosis of early MS depends on the demonstration of lesions disseminated throughout the nervous system. Subtle deficits of ocular motility can provide a sensitive method for identifying subclinical lesions, but there is a need for caution because these tests are not specific for MS (848). The clinician must compare the results of ocular motor studies with other clinical or laboratory findings before making a diagnosis (849).

A number of drugs, including gabapentin and memantine (an agent with NMDA blocking, AMPA receptor modulation, and dopaminergic action) may ameliorate the visually disabling pendular nystagmus commonly observed in MS (12,850).

OCULAR MOTOR MANIFESTATIONS OF SOME METABOLIC DISORDERS

Some babies who ultimately develop normally show transient ocular motor disturbances, including upward or downward deviation of the eyes (but with a full range of reflex vertical movement), intermittent opsoclonus, and skew deviation (86,320,851,852). The last may be associated with the eventual development of horizontal strabismus. In addition, premature babies may show reduced excursion of the adducting eye with caloric stimulation, suggesting an INO. In such infants, full deviation of both eyes usually occurs with rotational stimuli (853), although quick phases of nystagmus may be absent (854). The time constant of the VOR (as reflected in the duration of nystagmus to a sustained constant velocity stimulus) in newborns is low (typically 6 seconds) and does not attain adult values until the infant is about 2 months old (854). Thus, normal infants may have abnormal eye movements.

The lipid storage diseases are often characterized by gaze palsies. Tay-Sachs disease impairs vertical and, subsequently, horizontal eye movements. Adult-onset hexosamin-

idase deficiency also preferentially affects vertical gaze (855). Variants of Niemann-Pick disease that begin after the first year of life (e.g., the sea-blue histiocyte syndrome or juvenile dystonic lipidosis) are characterized by deficits of voluntary vertical eye movements, particularly saccades and smooth pursuit; vertical vestibular and horizontal eye movements are relatively preserved (856–859) (Fig. 19.32). Gaucher's disease is associated with a prominent deficit of horizontal gaze, and slow saccades may be a prominent finding in adults with this condition (860).

Wernicke's encephalopathy is characterized by the triad of ophthalmoplegia, mental confusion, and gait ataxia. It is caused by thiamine deficiency and is most commonly encountered in alcoholics. The ocular motor findings include weakness of abduction, gaze-evoked nystagmus and primary position vertical nystagmus, impaired vestibular responses to caloric and rotational stimulation, INO, the one-and-a-half syndrome, and horizontal and vertical gaze palsies that may progress to total ophthalmoplegia (861–866). The ophthalmoplegia is bilateral but may be asymmetric. Experimental thiamine deficiency in monkeys causes an orderly progression of ophthalmoplegia associated with well-circumscribed histopathologic changes (867). These changes consist of neuronal loss and gliosis in the oculomotor, trochlear, abducens, and vestibular nuclei. In humans, demyelination, vascular changes, and hemorrhage also may occur. In addition to the sites listed above, lesions are found in the paraventricular regions of the thalamus, hypothalamus, periaqueductal gray matter, superior vermis of the cerebellum, and dorsal motor nucleus of the vagus. Thus, gaze-evoked nystagmus and the impaired caloric responses can be attributed to vestibular nucleus involvement. The abduction weakness and INO may reflect damage to the abducens nerve and the MLF, respectively, whereas paralysis of horizontal gaze may be caused by damage to the PPRF or abducens nucleus.

The one-and-a-half syndrome indicates dysfunction of the MLF and either the abducens nucleus or the PPRF, and total ophthalmoplegia may be caused by damage to all of the ocular motor nerve nuclei. Most likely, affected areas of the brain contain neurons that use high amounts of glucose and, therefore, are particularly dependent upon thiamine, an important coenzyme in glucose metabolism (868). Administration of thiamine usually causes rapid improvement of the ocular motor signs, although complete recovery may take several weeks. Coexistent magnesium deficiency should also be treated. In patients with Wernicke's disease who go on to develop Korsakoff's syndrome, which is primarily characterized by a severe and enduring memory loss, ocular motor abnormalities may persist (869,870). The ocular motor abnormalities include slow and inaccurate saccades, impaired smooth pursuit, and gaze-evoked nystagmus. MR imaging shows a distinctive pattern of abnormality in Wernicke's disease, with T2 intensity in structures around the third and fourth ventricles and the aqueduct (871).

Leigh's syndrome is a fatal subacute necrotizing encephalopathy of infancy or childhood characterized by psychomotor retardation, seizures, and brain stem abnormalities, including eye movements. It is an inherited disorder caused either by abnormalities of mitochondrial deoxyribonucleic acid (DNA), in which case it is maternally inherited, or by a chromosomal abnormality, in which case it is transmitted as an autosomal-recessive disorder. Some cases show an underlying defect of pyruvate dehydrogenase (872); others reflect a mitochondrial cytopathy (873,874). Both the disturbances of ocular motility and the pathologic findings resemble those caused by experimental thiamine deficiency or Wernicke's encephalopathy (875,876). Halmagyi et al.

(113) reported seesaw nystagmus and the OTR in a patient with Leigh's disease.

Pelizaeus-Merzbacher disease is an X-linked recessive leukodystrophy (877) with severe cerebellar signs, including saccadic dysmetria. Some patients also show difficulty initiating saccades and pendular nystagmus (730,878).

Deficiency of vitamin E may cause a progressive neurologic condition characterized by areflexia, cerebellar ataxia, and loss of joint position sense. Ocular motor involvement includes progressive gaze restriction, sometimes with strabismus. Vitamin E deficiency is more common in children, in whom it may be caused by abetalipoproteinemia (Bassen-Kornzweig disease). It is also reported in adults who have bowel or liver diseases that interfere with fat absorption or as an inherited ataxia on chromosome 8q13, the site of the α-tocopherol transfer protein gene (879). Vitamin E deficiency is characterized by a dissociated ophthalmoplegia and by nystagmus in which adduction is fast but with a limited range and abduction is slow but with a full range (880). A posterior INO of Lutz (discussed previously) occurs in some patients (254,255). The combination of ocular motor findings in patients with vitamin E deficiency probably reflects a mixture of central and peripheral pathology.

Wilson's disease, hepatolenticular degeneration, is an inherited disorder of copper metabolism that is transmitted in an autosomal-recessive fashion. The defect is in a copper-transporting adenosine triphosphatase (ATPase) gene at q14.3 on chromosome 13. CT scanning in patients with this condition shows hypodense areas, and PET scanning indicates a decreased rate of glucose metabolism in the globus pallidus and putamen (881). The classic clinical picture is a prominent dysarthria, abnormal movements, psychiatric symptoms, and liver disease. Ocular motor disorders in hepatolenticular degeneration include a distractibility of gaze, with inability to voluntarily fix upon an object unless other competing visual stimuli are removed (e.g., fixation of a solitary light in an otherwise dark room) (882). Slow saccades were reported in one patient with this condition (883), and apraxia of eyelid opening can also occur (884).

Amyotrophic lateral sclerosis is associated with various eye-movement disorders, including nystagmus (885), saccade disturbances that suggest a frontal lobe disturbance (886–888), and impaired pursuit (889). Occasionally slow saccades are a feature (886). However, the existence of multisystem diseases in which motor neuron degeneration is just one neurologic feature makes specific clinical diagnoses difficult (890,891). Ocular motor abnormalities were reported in a single patient with Kugelberg-Welander disease (892).

EFFECTS OF DRUGS ON EYE MOVEMENTS

Many substances affect eye movements (Table 19.8). In some cases, the drug induces abnormalities of eye movements at therapeutic concentrations (e.g., anticonvulsants) (893). In other cases, abnormalities of eye movements develop only when concentrations of the drug in the central nervous system are inappropriately elevated. In still other cases, the eye-movement abnormalities are caused by substances not meant for internal use.

Patients with drug-induced abnormalities of eye movements most often complain of diplopia, caused by ocular misalignment, or oscillopsia, caused by spontaneous nystagmus or an inappropriate VOR (894). Many drugs have their effect on central vestibular and cerebellar connections and cause ataxia and gaze-evoked nystagmus (895).

Although all classes of eye movements may be affected by therapeutic doses of various drugs, smooth pursuit, eccentric

Table 19.8
Effect of Drugs on Eye Movements

Benzodiazepines: Reduced velocity and increased duration of saccades, impaired smooth pursuit, decreased gain and increased time constant of VOR, divergence paralysis

Tricyclic antidepressants: Internuclear ophthalmoplegia, partial or total gaze paresis, opsoclonus

Phenytoin: Impaired smooth pursuit and VOR suppression, gaze-evoked nystagmus, downbeat nystagmus, periodic alternating nystagmus, total gaze paresis, convergence spasm

Carbamazepine: Decreased velocity of saccades, impaired smooth pursuit, gaze-evoked nystagmus, oculogyric crisis, downbeat nystagmus, total gaze paresis

Phenobarbital and other barbiturates: Reduced peak saccadic velocity, gaze-evoked nystagmus, impaired smooth pursuit, impaired vergence, decreased VOR gain, perverted caloric responses, vertical nystagmus, partial or total gaze paresis

Phenothiazines: Oculogyric crisis, internuclear ophthalmoplegia

Lithium carbonate: Saccadic dysmetria, impaired smooth pursuit, gaze-evoked nystagmus, downbeat nystagmus, oculogyric crisis, internuclear ophthalmoplegia, total gaze paresis, opsoclonus

Amphetamines: Reduced saccade latency, increased accommodative convergence/accommodation ratio

Ethyl alcohol: Reduced peak velocity, increased latency, and hypometria of saccades, impaired smooth pursuit and VOR suppression, gaze-evoked nystagmus, positionally induced nystagmus, normal static VOR compensation, reversed compensation of vestibular lesions

Nicotine: Upbeat nystagmus, in darkness: Square-wave jerks, impaired horizontal and vertical pursuit

Methadone: Saccadic hypometria, impaired smooth pursuit

Baclofen: Reduced VOR time constant, total gaze paresis

β-Blockers: Diplopia, internuclear ophthalmoplegia

Chloral hydrate: Impaired smooth pursuit

Nitrous oxide: Reduced saccadic peak velocity, impaired smooth pursuit

VOR, vestibulo-ocular reflex.

gaze holding, and convergence are particularly susceptible. For example, diazepam, methadone, phenytoin, barbiturates, chloral hydrate, and alcohol all impair smooth-pursuit tracking. Some drugs have specific effects on ocular motility and thus provide insights into both the function of the ocular motor system and the mode of drug action. For example, diazepam reduces saccadic peak velocity but does not impair accuracy; methadone shows the converse effect. Diazepam reduces the gain of the VOR; in experimental animals the time constant is prolonged, but in humans it is reduced (896). In contrast, baclofen reduces the time constant of the VOR (897). Nicotine causes upbeat nystagmus (898–900). Alcohol affects eye movements by virtue of its effects on the density of endolymph and the cupula in the labyrinth as well as on more central structures (901–906).

At toxic levels, neuroactive drugs can impair all eye movements, particularly when consciousness is also impaired. Phenytoin may cause a complete ophthalmoplegia in awake patients, and therapeutic levels may cause ophthalmoplegia in patients in stupor (823). Phenytoin and diazepam can lead to opsoclonus (907). The tricyclic antidepressants may cause complete ophthalmoplegia or an INO in stuporous patients. Lithium causes a variety of abnormali-

ties, including fixation instability and downbeat nystagmus (908). In one patient who showed marked impairment of all types of horizontal eye movements and downbeat nystagmus prior to death, neuronal loss was mainly confined to the NPH and adjacent MVN (909). Thus, the pathophysiology was similar to that produced by experimental lesions of these nuclei in monkeys (910); that is, the neural integrator (gaze-holding network) was disrupted. The propensity of lithium to damage this area of the medulla is related to its proximity to the choroid plexus of the fourth ventricle and thus to elevated local concentrations of lithium (909). Cerebellar damage may also occur after lithium intoxication (911). Amiodarone can cause prominent cerebellar eye signs, including downbeat nystagmus (912).

In addition to drugs, certain toxins can cause abnormal eye movements. Some, such as chlordecone (913) and thallium (914), cause saccadic oscillations. Intoxication with hydrocarbons can cause a vestibulopathy (915,916), and exposure to trichloroethylene and other solvents may affect pursuit, suppression of the VOR, and saccades (917,918). Prolonged exposure to toluene, especially in glue-sniffing addiction, may lead to a variety of ocular motor disturbances, including pendular (919) and downbeat (920) nystagmus, saccadic oscillations (921–923), and INO (924). Tobacco has a number of ocular motor effects. It causes upbeat nystagmus (925,926), impaired pursuit (926), decreased saccade latency (927), and increased square-wave jerks during pursuit (928), although performance is normal on the antisaccade test (898,929,930). Cocaine can affect eye movements, with opsoclonus being the most dramatic abnormality (931).

Ototoxicity, especially that associated with administration of aminoglycosides, is an important cause of VOR loss (934). Intravenous gentamicin is most often responsible. Its toxicity may be insidious, occurring without hearing symptoms and even with normal blood levels and relatively short periods of administration (935). Some patients who develop ototoxicity may be genetically predisposed to its toxic side effects (936,937). Topical (intratympanic) gentamicin is used to purposefully ablate labyrinthine function as part of the treatment of intractable Ménière's syndrome but occasionally leads to unwanted labyrinthine loss when used to treat external ear infections (938). Cisplatin is probably not as vestibulotoxic as originally thought (939–941).

REFERENCES

1. Leigh RJ, Zee DS. The Neurology of Eye Movements. Philadelphia: FA Davis, 1999.
2. Arnold DB, Robinson DA, Leigh RJ. Nystagmus induced by pharmacological inactivation of the brainstem ocular motor integrator in monkey. Vision Res 1999;39:4286–4295.
3. Tilikete C, Hermier M, Pelisson D, Vighetto A. Saccadic lateropulsion and upbeat nystagmus: disorders of caudal medulla. Ann Neurol 2002;52:658–662.
4. Ranalli PJ, Sharpe JA. Upbeat nystagmus and the ventral tegmental pathway of the upward vestibulo-ocular reflex. Neurology 1988;38:1329–1330.
5. Guillain G. The syndrome of synchronous and rhythmic palato-pharyngo-laryngo-oculo-diaphragmatic myoclonus. Proc R Soc Med (UK) 1938;31:1031–1038.
6. Deuschl G, Toro C, Valls-Solé J, et al. Symptomatic and essential palatal tremor. 1. Clinical, physiological, and MRI analysis. Brain 1994;117:767–774.
7. Schwankhaus JD, Parisi JE, Gulledge WR, et al. Hereditary adult-onset Alexander's disease with palatal myoclonus, spastic paraparesis, and cerebellar ataxia. Neurology 1995;45:2266–2271.
8. Deuschl G, Wilms H. Palatal tremor: the clinical spectrum and physiology of a rhythmic movement disorder. Adv Neurol 2002;89:115–130.

9. Gresty MA, Ell JJ, Findley LJ. Acquired pendular nystagmus: its characteristics, localising value and pathophysiology. J Neurol Neurosurg Psychiatry 1982;45: 431–439.
10. Nakada T, Kwee IL. Oculopalatal myoclonus. Brain 1986;109:431–441.
11. Jacobs L, Bender MB. Palato-ocular synchrony during eyelid closure. Arch Neurol 1976;33:289–291.
12. Stahl JS, Rottach K, Averbuch-Heller L, et al. A pilot study of gabapentin as treatment for acquired nystagmus. Neuroophthalmology 1996;16:107–113.
13. Kulkarni PK, Muthane UB, Taly AB, et al. Palatal tremor, progressive multiple cranial nerve palsies, and cerebellar ataxia: a case report and review of literature of palatal tremors in neurodegenerative disease. Mov Disord 1999;14:689–693.
14. Koeppen AH, Barron KD, Dentinger MP. Olivary hypertrophy: histochemical demonstration of hydrolytic enzymes. Neurology 1980;30:471–480.
15. Guillain G, Mollaret P. Deux cas myoclonies synchrones et rhythmées vélo-pharyngo-laryngooculo-diaphragmatiques: le problème anatomique et physio-pathologique de ce syndrome. Rev Neurol (Paris) 1931;2:545–566.
16. Alpini D, Caputo D, Pugnetti L, et al. Vertigo and multiple sclerosis: aspects of differential diagnosis. Neurol Sci 2001;22:584–587.
17. Frohman EM, Kramer PD, Dewey RB, et al. Benign paroxysmal positioning vertigo in multiple sclerosis: diagnosis, pathophysiology and therapeutic techniques. Mult Scler 2003;9:250–255.
18. Fisher CM. Some neuro-ophthalmological observations. J Neurol Neurosurg Psychiatry 1967;30:383–392.
19. Gomez CR, Cruz-Flores S, Malkoff MD, et al. Isolated vertigo as a manifestation of vertebrobasilar ischemia. Neurology 1996;47:94–97.
20. Baloh RW. Vertebrobasilar insufficiency and stroke. Otolaryngol Head Neck Surg 1995;112:114–117.
21. Thömke F, Hopf HC. Pontine lesions mimicking acute peripheral vestibulopathy. J Neurol Neurosurg Psychiatry 1999;66:340–349.
22. Meienberg O, Rover J, Kommerell G. Prenuclear paresis of homolateral inferior rectus and contralateral superior oblique eye muscles. Arch Neurol 1978;35: 231–233.
23. Lawden MC, Bronstein AM, Kennard C. Repetitive paroxysmal nystagmus and vertigo. Neurology 1995;45:276–280.
24. Büttner U, Ott M, Helmchen C, et al. Bilateral loss of eighth nerve function as the only clinical sign of vertebrobasilar dolichoectasia. J Vestib Res 1995;5: 47–51.
25. Passero S, Nuti D. Auditory and vestibular findings in patients with vertebrobasilar dolichoectasia. Acta Neurol Scand 1996;93:50–55.
26. Brackmann DE, Kesser BW, Day JD. Microvascular decompression of the vestibulocochlear nerve for disabling positional vertigo: the House Ear Clinic experience. Otol Neurotol 2001;22:882–887.
27. Brandt T, Dieterich M. Vestibular paroxysmia (disabling positional vertigo). Neuroophthalmology 1994;14:359–369.
28. Brandt T, Dieterich M. Central vestibular syndromes in roll, pitch and yaw. Neuroophthalmology 1995;15:291–303.
29. Büttner U, Helmchen C, Büttner-Ennever JA. The localizing value of nystagmus in brainstem disorders. Neuroophthalmology 1995;15:283–290.
30. Dieterich M. The topographic diagnosis of acquired nystagmus in brainstem disorders. Strabismus 2002;10:137–145.
31. Fisher CM, Karnes WE, Kubik CS. Lateral medullary infarction: the pattern of vascular occlusion. J Neuropathol Exp Neurol 1961;20:323–378.
32. Fisher CM, Tapia J. Lateral medullary infarction extending to the lower pons. J Neurol Neurosurg Psychiatry 1987;50:620–624.
33. Menendez-Gonzalez M, Garcia C, Suarez E, et al. [Wallenberg's syndrome secondary to dissection of the vertebral artery caused by chiropractic manipulation]. Rev Neurol 2003;37:837–839.
34. Smith DB, Demasters BKK. Demyelinative disease presenting as Wallenberg's syndrome. Report of a patient. Stroke 1981;12:877–878.
35. Hornsten G. Wallenberg's syndrome. I. General symptomatology, with special reference to visual disturbances and imbalance. Acta Neurol Scand 1974;50: 434–446.
36. Tiliket C, Ventre J, Vighetto A, et al. Room tilt illusion: a central otolith dysfunction. Arch Neurol 1996;53:1259–1264.
37. Slavin ML, LoPinto RJ. Isolated environmental tilt associated with lateral medullary compression by dolichoectasia of the vertebral artery. J Clin Neuroophthalmol 1987;7:29–33.
38. Mehler MF. Complete visual inversion in vertebrobasilar ischaemic disease. J Neurol Neurosurg Psychiatry 1988;51:1236–1237.
39. Charles N, Froment C, Rode G, et al. Vertigo and upside down vision due to an infarct in the territory of the medial branch of the posterior inferior cerebellar artery caused by dissection of a vertebral artery. J Neurol Neurosurg Psychiatry 1992;55:188–189.
40. López L, Ochoa S, Mesropian H, et al. Acute transient upside-down inversion of vision with brainstem-cerebellar infarction. Neuroophthalmology 1995;15: 277–280.
41. Aldridge AJ, Kline LB, Girkin CA. Environmental tilt illusion as the only symptom of a thalamic astrocytoma. J Neuroophthalmol 2003;23:145–147.
42. Solms M, Kaplan-Solms K, Saling M, et al. Inverted vision after frontal lobe disease. Cortex 1988;24:499–509.
43. Malis DD, Guyot JP. Room tilt illusion as a manifestation of peripheral vestibular disorders. Ann Otol Rhinol Laryngol 2003;112:600–605.
44. Kommerell G, Hoyt WF. Lateropulsion of saccadic eye movements. Electrooculographic studies in a patient with Wallenberg's syndrome. Arch Neurol 1973;28:313–318.
45. Hornsten G. Wallenberg's syndrome. II. Oculomotor and oculostatic disturbances. Acta Neurol Scand 1974;50:447–468.
46. Baloh RW, Yee RD, Honrubia V. Eye movements in patients with Wallenberg's syndrome. Ann NY Acad Sci 1981;374:600–613.
47. Waespe W, Baumgartner R. Enduring dysmetria and impaired gain adaptivity of saccadic eye movements in Wallenberg's lateral medullary syndrome. Brain 1992;115:1125–1146.
48. Büttner U, Straube A. The effect of cerebellar midline lesions on eye movements. Neuroophthalmology 1995;15:75–82.
49. Solomon D, Galetta SL, Liu GT. Possible mechanisms for horizontal gaze deviation and lateropulsion in the lateral medullary syndrome. J Neuroophthalmol 1995;15:26–30.
50. Kirkham TH, Guitton D, Gans M. Task-dependent variations of ocular lateropulsion in Wallenberg's syndrome. Can J Neurol Sci 1981;8:21–22.
51. Ohtsuka K, Sawa M, Matsuda S, et al. Nonvisual eye position control in a patient with ocular lateropulsion. Ophthalmologica 1988;197:85–89.
52. Morrow MJ, Sharpe JA. Torsional nystagmus in the lateral medullary syndrome. Ann Neurol 1988;24:390–398.
53. Helmchen C, Glasauer S, Büttner U. Pathological torsional eye deviation during voluntary saccades: a violation of Listing's law. J Neurol Neurosurg Psychiatry 1997;62:253–260.
54. Daroff RB, Hoyt WF, Sanders MD, et al. Gaze-evoked eyelid and ocular nystagmus inhibited by the near reflex: unusual ocular motor phenomena in a lateral medullary syndrome. J Neurol Neurosurg Psychiatry 1968;31:362–367.
55. Dieterich M, Brandt T. Wallenberg's syndrome: lateropulsion, cyclorotation, and subjective visual vertical in thirty-six patients. Ann Neurol 1992;31:399–408.
56. Brandt T, Dieterich M. Pathological eye-head coordination in roll: tonic ocular tilt reaction in mesencephalic and medullary lesions. Brain 1987;110:649–666.
57. Estanol B, Lopez-Rios G. Neuro-otology of the lateral medullary infarct syndrome. Arch Neurol 1982;39:176–179.
58. Waespe W, Wichmann W. Oculomotor disturbances during visual-vestibular interaction in Wallenberg's lateral medullary syndrome verified by magnetic resonance imaging. Brain 1990;113:821–846.
59. Waespe W. Saccadic gain adaptivity in the two eyes in Wallenberg's lateral medullary syndrome. Neuroophthalmology 1995;15:193–201.
60. Robinson FR, Straube A, Fuch AF. Role of the caudal fastigial nucleus in saccade generation. II. Effects of muscimol inactivation. J Neurophysiol 1993;70: 1741–1758.
61. Grad A, Baloh RW. Vertigo of vascular origin. Clinical and electronystagmographic features in 84 cases. Arch Neurol 1989;46:281–284.
62. Oas J, Baloh RW. Vertigo and the anterior inferior cerebellar artery syndrome. Neurology 1992;42:2274–2279.
63. Lee H, Sohn SI, Jung DK, et al. Sudden deafness and anterior inferior cerebellar artery infarction. Stroke 2002;33:2807–2812.
64. Keane JR. Alternating skew deviation: 47 patients. Neurology 1985;35:725–728.
65. Rousseaux M, Petit H, Dubois F, et al. ''Laterally alternating'' skew deviation. Mechanism and significance. Neuroophthalmology 1985;5:277–280.
66. Moster ML, Schatz NJ, Savino PJ, et al. Alternating skew on lateral gaze (bilateral abducting hypertropia). Ann Neurol 1988;23:190–192.
67. Zee DS. Considerations on the mechanisms of alternating skew deviation in patients with cerebellar lesions. J Vest Res 1996;6:1–7.
68. Donahue SP, Lavin PJ, Hamed LM. Tonic ocular tilt reaction simulating a superior oblique palsy: diagnostic confusion with the 3-step test. Arch Ophthalmol 1999;117:347–352.
69. Donahue SP, Lavin PJ, Mohney B, Hamed L. Skew deviation and inferior oblique palsy. Am J Ophthalmol 2001;132:751–756.
70. Rabinovitch HE, Sharpe JA, Sylvester TO. The ocular tilt reaction. A paroxysmal dyskinesia associated with elliptical nystagmus. Arch Ophthalmol 1977;95: 1395–1398.
71. Hedges TR III, Hoyt WF. Ocular tilt reaction due to an upper brainstem lesion: paroxysmal skew deviation, torsion, and oscillation of the eyes with head tilt. Ann Neurol 1982;11:537–540.
72. Dieterich M, Brandt T. Ocular torsion and tilt of subjective visual vertical are sensitive brainstem signs. Ann Neurol 1993;33:292–299.
73. Brandt T, Dieterich M. Vestibular syndromes in the roll plane: topographic diagnosis from brain stem to cortex. Ann Neurol 1994;36:337–347.
74. Galetta SL, Liu GT, Raps EC, et al. Cyclodeviation in skew deviation. Am J Ophthalmol 1994;118:509–514.
75. Brodsky MC. Three dimensions of skew deviation. Br J Ophthalmol 2003;87: 1440–1441.
76. Brandt T, Dieterich M. Two types of ocular tilt reactions: the ''ascending'' pontomedullary VOR-OTR and the ''descending'' mesencephalic integrator-OTR. Neuroophthalmology 1998;19:83–92.
77. Cogan DG. Neurology of the Ocular Muscles, ed 2. Springfield, IL, Charles C Thomas, 1956.

78. Keane JR. Ocular skew deviation. Analysis of 100 cases. Arch Neurol 1975; 32:185–190.

79. Brandt T, Dieterich M. Skew deviation with ocular torsion: a vestibular sign of topographic diagnostic value. Ann Neurol 1993;33:528–534.

80. Riordan-Eva P, Harcourt JP, Faldon M, et al. Skew deviation following vestibular nerve surgery. Ann Neurol 1997;41:94–99.

81. Arbusow V, Dieterich M, Strupp M, et al. Herpes zoster neuritis involving superior and inferior parts of the vestibular nerve causes ocular tilt reaction. Neuroophthalmology 1998;19:17–22.

82. Verhulst E, Van Lammeren M, Dralands L. Diplopia from skew deviation in Ramsey-Hunt syndrome. A case report. Bull Soc Belge Ophtalmol 2000;27–32.

83. Tilikete C, Vighetto A. Internuclear ophthalmoplegia with skew deviation. Two cases with an isolated circumscribed lesion of the medial longitudinal fasciculus. Eur Neurol 2000;44:258–259.

84. Merikangas JR. Skew deviation in pseudotumor cerebri. Ann Neurol 1978;4:583.

85. Frohman LP, Kupersmith MJ. Reversible vertical ocular deviations associated with raised intracranial pressure. J Clin Neuroophthalmol 1985;5:158–163.

86. Hoyt CS, Mousel DK, Weber AA Transient supranuclear disturbances of gaze in healthy neonates. Am J Ophthalmol 1980;89:708–713.

87. Glasauer S, Dieterich M, Brandt T. Simulation of pathological ocular counterroll and skew-torsion by a 3-D mathematical model. Neuroreport 1999;10:1843–1848.

88. Averbuch-Heller L, Rottach KG, Zivotofsky AZ, et al. Torsional eye movements in patients with skew deviation and spasmodic torticollis: responses to static and dynamic head roll. Neurology 1997;48:506–514.

89. Collewijn H, Van der Steen J, Ferman L, et al. Human ocular counterroll: assessment of static and dynamic properties from electromagnetic scleral coil recordings. Exp Brain Res 1985;59:185–196.

90. Pansell T, Schworm HD, Ygge J. Torsional and vertical eye movements during head tilt dynamic characteristics. Invest Ophthalmol Vis Sci 2003;44:2986–2990.

91. Kushner BJ. Ocular torsion: rotations around the ''WHY'' axis. J AAPOS 2004;8:1–12.

92. Jauregui-Renaud K, Faldon M, Clarke AH, et al. Otolith and semicircular canal contributions to the human binocular response to roll oscillation. Acta Otolaryngol 1998;118:170–176.

93. Halmagyi GM, Gresty MA, Gibson WPR. Ocular tilt reaction with peripheral vestibular lesion. Ann Neurol 1979;6:80–83.

94. Deecke L, Mergner T, Plester D. Tullio phenomenon with torsion of the eyes and subjective tilt of the visual surround. Ann NY Acad Sci 1981;374:650–655.

95. Dieterich M, Brandt T, Fries W. Otolithic function in man. Results from a case of otolithic Tullio phenomenon. Brain 1989;112:1377–1392.

96. Minor LB, Solomon D, Zinreich JS, Zee DS. Sound- and/or pressure-induced vertigo due to bone dehiscence of the superior semicircular canal. Arch Otolaryngol Head Neck Surg 1998;124:249–258.

97. Minor LB. Labyrinthine fistulae: pathobiology and management. Curr Opin Otolaryngol Head Neck Surg 2003;11:340–346.

98. Baloh RW. Superior semicircular canal dehiscence syndrome: leaks and squeaks can make you dizzy. Neurology 2004;62:684–685.

99. Curthoys IS. Eye movements produced by utricular and saccular stimulation. Aviat Space Environ Med 1987;58(Suppl):A192–A197.

100. Suzuki JI, Tokumasu K, Goto K. Eye movements from single utricular nerve stimulation. Acta Otolaryngol (Stockh) 1969;68:350–362.

101. Gacek RR. Neuroanatomical correlates of vestibular function. Ann Otol Rhinol Laryngol 1980;89:2–5.

102. Uchino Y. Otolith and semicircular canal inputs to single vestibular neurons in cats. Biol Sci Space 2001;15:375–381.

103. Brandt T, Dieterich M. Different types of skew deviation. J Neurol Neurosurg Psychiatry 1991;54:549–550.

104. Versino M, Hurko O, Zee DS. Disorders of binocular control of eye movements in patients with cerebellar dysfunction. Brain 1996;119:1933–1950.

105. Mossman S, Halmagyi GM. Partial ocular tilt reaction due to unilateral cerebellar lesion. Neurology 1997;49:491–493.

106. Radtke A, Bronstein AM, Gresty MA, et al. Paroxysmal alternating skew deviation and nystagmus after partial destruction of the uvula. J Neurol Neurosurg Psychiatry 2001;70:790–793.

107. Brandt T, Dieterich M. Vestibular syndromes in the roll plane: topographic diagnosis from brainstem to cortex. Ann Neurol 1994;36:337–347.

108. Nashold BS Jr, Gills JP Jr. Ocular signs from brain stimulation and lesions. Arch Ophthalmol 1967;77:609–618.

109. Keane JR. Pretectal pseudobobbing. Five patients with ''V''-pattern convergence nystagmus. Arch Neurol 1985;42:592–594.

110. Halmagyi GM, Brandt T, Dieterich M, et al. Tonic contraversive ocular tilt reaction due to unilateral meso-diencephalic lesion. Neurology 1990;40:1503–1509.

111. Dieterich M, Brandt T. Ocular torsion and perceived vertical in oculomotor, trochlear and abducens palsies. Brain 1993;116:1095–1104.

112. Dichgans M, Dieterich M. Third nerve palsy with contralateral ocular torsion and binocular tilt of visual vertical, indicating a midbrain lesion. Neuroophthalmology 1995;15:315–320.

113. Halmagyi GM, Pamphlett R, Curthoys IS. Seesaw nystagmus and ocular tilt reaction due to adult Leigh's disease. Neuroophthalmology 1992;12:1–9.

114. Corbett JJ, Schatz NJ, Shults WT, et al. Slowly alternating skew deviation: description of a pretectal syndrome in three patients. Ann Neurol 1981;10:540–546.

115. Mitchell JM, Smith CL, Quencer RB. Periodic alternating skew deviation. J Clin Neuroophthalmol 1981;1:5–8.

116. Greenberg HS, DeWitt LD. Periodic nonalternating ocular skew deviation accompanied by head tilt and pathologic lid retraction. J Clin Neuroophthalmol 1983;3:181–184.

117. Lewis JM, Kline LB. Periodic alternating nystagmus associated with periodic alternating skew deviation. J Clin Neuroophthalmol 1983;13:115–117.

118. Westheimer G, Blair SM. The ocular tilt reaction. A brainstem oculomotor routine. Invest Ophthalmol 1975;14:833–839.

119. Westheimer G, Blair SM. Synkinese der Augenund Kopfbewegungen bei Hirnstammreizungen am Wachen Macaws-Affen. Exp Brain Res 1975;24:89–95.

120. Lueck CJ, Hamlyn P, Crawford TJ, et al. A case of ocular tilt reaction and torsional nystagmus due to direct stimulation of the midbrain in man. Brain 1991;114:2069–2079.

121. Straube A, Büttner U. Pathophysiology of saccadic contrapulsion in unilateral rostral cerebellar lesions. Neuroophthalmology 1994;14:3–7.

122. Galimberti CA, Versino M, Sartori I, et al. Epileptic skew deviation. Neurology 1988;50:1469–1472.

123. Holmes G. The symptoms of acute cerebellar injuries due to gunshot injuries. Brain 1917;40:461–535.

124. Daroff RB. Eye signs in humans with cerebellar dysfunction. In: Lennerstrand G, Zee DS, Keller EL, eds. Functional Basis of Ocular Motility Disorders. Oxford, UK, Pergamon, 1982:463–465.

125. Zee DS, Walker MF. Cerebellar control of eye movements. In: Chalupa LM, Werner JS, eds. The Visual Neurosciences. Cambridge, MA, MIT Press, 2003:1485–1498.

126. Takagi M, Tamargo R, Zee DS. Effects of lesions of the cerebellar oculomotor vermis on eye movements in primate: binocular control. Prog Brain Res 2003;142:19–33.

127. Takagi M, Zee DS, Tamargo R. Effects of lesions of the oculomotor vermis on eye movements in primate: saccades. J Neurophysiol 1998;80:1911–1930.

128. Takagi M, Zee DS, Tamargo R. Effects of lesions of the oculomotor cerebellar vermis on eye movements in primate: smooth pursuit. J Neurophysiol 2000;83:247–262.

129. Gaymard B, Rivaud S, Amarenco P, et al. Influence of visual information on cerebellar saccadic dysmetria. Ann Neurol 1994;35:108–112.

130. Kanayama R, Bronstein AM, Shallo-Hoffmann J, et al. Visually and memory guided saccades in a case of cerebellar saccadic dysmetria. J Neurol Neurosurg Psychiatry 1994;57:1081–1084.

131. Bronstein AM, Shallo-Hoffmann J, Kanayama R, et al. Corrective saccades in cerebellar dysmetria. Ann Neurol 1995;37:413–414.

132. Bötzel K, Rottach K, Büttner U. Normal and pathological saccadic dysmetria. Brain 993;116:337–353.

133. Straube A, Deubel H, Spuler A, et al. Differential effect of bilateral deep cerebellar nuclei lesion on externally and internally triggered saccades in humans. Neuroophthalmology 1995;15:67–74.

134. Nawrot M, Rizzo M. Motion perception deficits from midline cerebellar lesions in human. Vision Res 1995;35:723–731.

135. Kurzan R, Straube A, Büttner U. The effect of muscimol micro-injections into the fastigial nucleus on the optokinetic response and the vestibulo-ocular reflex in the alert monkey. Exp Brain Res 1993;94:252–260.

136. Büttner U, Straube A, Spuler A. Saccadic dysmetia and ''intact'' smooth-pursuit eye movements after bilateral deep cerebellar nuclei lesion. J Neurol Neurosurg Psychiatry 1994;57:832–834.

137. Westheimer G, Blair SM. Functional organization of primate oculomotor system revealed by cerebellectomy. Exp Brain Res 1974;21:463–472.

138. Rambold H, Churchland A, Selig Y, et al. Partial ablations of the flocculus and ventral paraflocculus in monkeys cause linked deficits in smooth pursuit eye movements and adaptive modification of the VOR. J Neurophysiol 2002;87:912–924.

139. Büttner U, Grundei T. Gaze-evoked nystagmus and smooth-pursuit deficits: their relationship studied in 52 patients. J Neurol 1995;242:384–389.

140. Grant MP, Leigh RJ, Seidman SH, et al. Comparison of predictable smooth ocular and combined eye-head tracking behaviour in patients with lesions affecting the brainstem and cerebellum. Brain 1992;115:1323–1342.

141. Waterston JA, Barnes GR, Grealy MA. A quantitative study of eye and head movements during smooth pursuit in patients with cerebellar disease. Brain 1992;115:1343–1358.

142. Lekwuwa GU, Barnes GR, Grealy MA. Effects of prediction on smooth-pursuit eye velocity gain in cerebellar patients and controls. In: Findlay JM, Walker R, Kentridge RW, eds. Eye Movement Research: Mechanisms, Processes, and Applications. Amsterdam, Elsevier, 1995:119–129.

143. Moschner C, Zangemeister WH, Demer JL. Anticipatory smooth eye movements of high velocity triggered by large target steps: normal performance and effect of cerebellar degeneration. Vision Res 1996;36:1341–1348.

144. Cohen B, John P, Yakushin SB, et al. The nodulus and uvula: source of cerebellar

control of spatial orientation of the angular vestibulo-ocular reflex. Ann NY Acad Sci 2002;978:28–45.

145. Hain TC, Zee DS, Maria BL. Tilt suppression of vestibulo-ocular reflex in patients with cerebellar lesions. Acta Otolaryngol (Stockh) 1988;105:13–20.

146. Wiest G, Deecke L, Trattnig S, Mueller C. Abolished tilt suppression of the vestibulo-ocular reflex caused by a selective uvulo-nodular lesion. Neurology 1999;52:417–419.

147. Walker MF, Steffen H, Zee DS Three-axis approaches to ocular motor control: a role for the cerebellum. In: Harris LR, Jenkin M, eds. Levels of Perception. New York, Springer-Verlag, 2002:399–413.

148. Zee DS. Cerebellar control of eye movements. In: Honrubia V, Brazier MAB, eds. Nystagmus and Vertigo: Clinical Approaches to the Patient with Dizziness. New York, Academic Press, 1982:241–249.

149. FitzGibbon E, Calvert P, Zee DS, et al. Torsional nystagmus during vertical smooth pursuit. J Neuroophthal 1996;16:79–90.

150. Angelaki DE, Dickman JD. Premotor neurons encode torsional eye velocity during smooth-pursuit eye movements. J Neurosci 2003;23:2971–2979.

151. Zee DS, Yee RD, Cogan DG, et al. Ocular motor abnormalities in hereditary cerebellar ataxia. Brain 1976;99:207–234.

152. Hotson JR. Cerebellar control of fixation eye movements. Neurology 1982;32:31–36.

153. Walker MF, Zee DS. Directional abnormalities of vestibular and optokinetic responses in cerebellar disease. Ann NY Acad Sci 1999;871:205–220.

154. Zee DS, Walker MF, Ramat S. The cerebellar contribution to eye movements based upon lesions: binocular, three-axis control and the translational vestibulo-ocular reflex. Ann NY Acad Sci 2002.

155. Yee RD, Baloh RW, Honrubia V, et al. Slow build-up of optokinetic nystagmus associated with downbeat nystagmus. Invest Ophthalmol Vis Sci 1979;18:622–629.

156. Leech J, Gresty M, Hess K, et al. Gaze failure, drifting eye movements, and centripetal nystagmus in cerebellar disease. Br J Ophthalmol 1977;61:774–781.

157. Daroff RB, Troost BT. Upbeat nystagmus. JAMA 973;225:312.

158. Bertholon P, Bronstein AM, Davies RA, et al. Positional down-beating nystagmus in 50 patients: cerebellar disorders and possible anterior semicircular canalithiasis. J Neurol Neurosurg Psychiatry 2002;72:366–372.

159. Bronstein AM, Hood JD. Cervical nystagmus due to loss of cerebellar inhibition on the cervicoocular reflex: a case report. J Neurol Neurosurg Psychiatry 1985;48:128–131.

160. Wiest G, Tian JR, Baloh RW, et al. Otolith function in cerebellar ataxia due to mutations in the calcium channel gene CACNA1A. Brain 2001;124:2407–2416.

161. Wiest G, Tian JR, Baloh RW, et al. Initiation of the linear vestibulo-ocular reflex in cerebellar dysfunction. Ann NY Acad Sci 2001;942:505–507.

162. Ito M. Mechanisms of motor learning in the cerebellum. Brain Res 2000;886:237–245.

163. Yagi T, Shimizu M, Sekine S, et al. New neurotological test for detecting cerebellar dysfunction. Vestibulo-ocular reflex changes with horizontal vision-reversal prisms. Ann Otorhinolaryngol 1981;90:276–280.

164. Milder DG, Reinecke RD. Phoria adaptation to prisms. A cerebellar–dependent response. Arch Neurol 1983;40:339–342.

165. Hain TC, Luebke A. Phoria adaptation in patients with cerebellar lesions. Invest Ophthalmol Vis Sci 1990;31:1394–1397.

166. Wania JH, Walsh FB. Absence of ocular signs with cerebellar ablation in an infant. Arch Ophthalmol 1959;61:655–656.

167. Eckmiller R, Westheimer G. Compensation of oculomotor deficits in monkeys with neonatal cerebellar ablations. Exp Brain Res 1983;49:315–326.

168. Cheng JS, Nash J, Meyer GA. Chiari type I malformation revisited: diagnosis and treatment. Neurologist 2002;8:357–362.

169. Schijman E. History, anatomic forms, and pathogenesis of Chiari I malformations. Childs Nerv Syst 2004;2–13.

170. Zee DS, Yamazaki A, Butler PH, et al. Effects of ablation of flocculus and paraflocculus on eye movements in primate. J Neurophysiol 1981;46:878–899.

171. Spooner JW, Baloh RW. Arnold-Chiari malformation. Improvement in eye movements after surgical treatment. Brain 1981;104:51–60.

172. Spillane JD, Pallis C, Jones AM. Developmental abnormalities in the region of the foramen magnum. Brain 1957;80:11–48.

173. Gregorius FK, Crandall PH, Baloh RW. Positional vertigo with cerebellar astrocytoma. Surg Neurol 1976;6:283–286.

174. Watson P, Barber HO, Deck J, et al. Positional vertigo and nystagmus of central origin. Can J Neurol Sci 1981;8:133–137.

175. Kattah JC, Kolsky MP, Luessenhop AJ. Positional vertigo and the cerebellar vermis. Neurology 1984;34:527–529.

176. Baloh RW, Honrubia V, Jacobson K. Benign positional vertigo: clinical and oculographic features in 240 cases. Neurology 1987;37:371–378.

177. Sakata E, Ohtsu K, Shimura H, et al. Positional nystagmus of benign paroxysmal type (BPPN) due to cerebellar vermis lesions. Pseudo–BPPN. Auris Masus Larynx (Tokyo) 1987;14:17–21.

178. Brandt T, Steddin S. Current view of the mechanism of benign paroxysmal positioning vertigo: cupulolithiasis or canalolithiasis. J Vestibular Res 1993;3:373–382.

179. Baloh RW, Yue Q, Jacobson BA, et al. Persistent direction-changing positional nystagmus: Another variant of benign positional nystagmus? Neurology 1995;45:1297–1301.

180. Strupp M, Brandt T, Steddin S. Horizontal canal benign paroxysmal positioning vertigo: reversible ipsilateral caloric hypoexcitability caused by canalolithiasis. Neurology 1995;45:2072–2076.

181. Nuti D, Vannucchi P, Pagnini P. Benign paroxysmal positional vertigo of the horizontal canal: a form of canalolithiasis with variable clinical features. J Vest Res 1996;6:173–184.

182. Leigh RJ, Mapstone T, Weymann C. Eye movements in children with the Dandy-Walker syndrome. Neuroophthalmology 1992;12:285–288.

183. Calogero JA. Vermian agenesis and unsegmented midbrain tectum. Case report. J Neurosurg 1977;47:605–608.

184. Sarnat HB, Alcala H. Human cerebellar hypoplasia: a syndrome of diverse causes. Arch Neurol 1980;37:300–305.

185. DeBassio WA, Kemper TL, Knoefel JE. Coffin-Siris syndrome. Neuropathologic findings. Arch Neurol 1985;42:350–353.

186. Lambert SR, Kriss A, Gresty M, et al. Joubert syndrome. Arch Ophthalmol 1989;107:709–713.

187. Boltshauser E. Joubert syndrome: more than lower cerebellar vermis hypoplasia, less than a complex brain malformation. Am J Med Genet 2002;109:332.

188. Lagier-Tourenne C, Boltshauser E, Breivik N, et al. Homozygosity mapping of a third Joubert syndrome locus to 6q23. J Med Genet 2004;41:273–277.

189. Margolis RL. The spinocerebellar ataxias: order emerges from chaos. Curr Neurol Neurosci Rep 2002;2:447–456.

190. Di Donato S, Gellera C, Mariotti C. The complex clinical and genetic classification of inherited ataxias. II. Autosomal recessive ataxias. Neurol Sci 2001;22:219–228.

191. Di Donato S. The complex clinical and genetic classification of inherited ataxias. I. Dominant ataxias. Ital J Neurol Sci 1998;19:335–343.

192. Rivaud-Pechoux S, Gaymard B, Canel G, et al. Eye movement abnormalities correlate with genotype in autosomal dominant cerebellar ataxia type 1. Ann Neurol 1998;43:297–302.

193. Buttner N, Geschwind D, Jen JC, et al. Oculomotor phenotypes in autosomal dominant ataxias. Arch Neurol 1998;55:1353–1357.

194. Durig JS, Jen JC, Demer JL. Ocular motility in genetically defined autosomal dominant cerebellar ataxia. Am J Ophthalmol 2002;133:718–721.

195. Schols l, Bauer P, Schmidt T, et al. Autosomal dominant cerebellar ataxias: clinical features, genetics, and pathogenesis. Lancet Neurol 2004;3:291–304.

196. Swartz BE, Li S, Bespalova I, et al. Pathogenesis of clinical signs in recessive ataxia with saccadic intrusions. Ann Neurol 2003;54:824–828.

197. Fetter M, Klockgether T, Schulz JB, et al. Oculomotor abnormalities and MRI findings in idiopathic cerebellar ataxia. J Neurol 1994;241:234–241.

198. Bataller L, Dalmau J. Paraneoplastic neurologic syndromes. Neurol Clin 2003;21:221–247.

199. Darnell RB, Posner JB. Paraneoplastic syndromes involving the nervous system. N Engl J Med 2003;349:1543–1554.

200. Jen J, Kim GW, Baloh RW. Clinical spectrum of episodic ataxia type 2. Neurology 2004;62:17–22.

201. Jen J. Familial episodic ataxias and related ion channel disorders. Curr Treat Options Neurol 2000;2:429–431.

202. Subramony SH, Schott K, Raike RS, et al. Novel CACNA1A mutation causes febrile episodic ataxia with interictal cerebellar deficits. Ann Neurol 2003;54:725–731.

203. Kullmann DM. The neuronal channelopathies. Brain 2002;125:1177–1195.

204. Pietrobon D. Calcium channels and channelopathies of the central nervous system. Mol Neurobiol 2002;25:31–50.

205. Lee H, Yi HA, Cho YW, Sohn CH, et al. Nodulus infarction mimicking acute peripheral vestibulopathy. Neurology 2003;60:1700–1702.

206. Amarenco P, Hauw J-J. Cerebellar infarction in the territory of the anterior and inferior cerebellar artery. A clinicopathological study of 20 cases. Brain 1990;113:139–155.

207. Kase CS, White JL, Joslyn JN, et al. Cerebellar infarction in the superior cerebellar artery distribution. Neurology 1985;35:705–711.

208. Ranalli PJ, Sharpe JA. Contrapulsion of saccades and ipsilateral ataxia: a unilateral disorder of the rostral cerebellum. Ann Neurol 1986;20:311–316.

209. Benjamin EE, Zimmerman CF, Troost BT. Lateropulsion and upbeat nystagmus are manifestations of central vestibular dysfunction. Arch Neurol 1986;43:962–964.

210. Uno A, Mukuno K, Sekiya H, et al. Lateropulsion in Wallenberg's syndrome and contrapulsion in the proximal type of the superior cerebellar artery syndrome. Neuroophthalmology 1989;9:75–80.

211. Waespe W, Müller-Meisser E. Directional reversal of saccadic dysmetria and gain adaptivity in a patient with a superior cerebellar artery infarction. Neuroophthalmology 1996;16:65–74.

212. Vahedi K, Rivaud S, Amarenco P, et al. Horizontal eye movement disorders after posterior vermis infarctions. J Neurol Neurosurg Psychiatry 1995;58:91–94.

213. Ekbom K, Horsten G, Johansson T. Posterior cranial fossa tumors. Headaches, oculostatic disorders and scintillation camera findings. Headache 1974;14:119–132.

214. Yamazaki A, Zee DS. Rebound nystagmus: EOG analysis of a case with a flocular tumor. Br J Ophthalmol 1979;63:782–786.

215. Humphriss RL, Baguley DM, Moffat DA. Head-shaking nystagmus in patients with a vestibular schwannoma. Clin Otolaryngol 2003;28:514–519.

216. Ott KH, Kase CS, Ojemann RG, et al. Cerebellar hemorrhage: diagnosis and treatment. Arch Neurol 1974;31:160–167.

217. Brennen RW, Bergland RM. Acute cerebellar hemorrhage. Analysis of clinical findings and outcome in 12 cases. Neurology 1977;27:527–532.

218. Dunne JW, Chakera T, Kermode S. Cerebellar haemorrhage: diagnosis and treatment: a study of 75 consecutive cases. Q J Med 1987;64:739–754.

219. Cogan DG. Internuclear ophthalmoplegia: typical and atypical. Arch Ophthalmol 1970;84:583–589.

220. Zee DS. Internuclear ophthalmoplegia: clinical and pathophysiological considerations. In: Büttner U, Brandt T, eds. Oculomotor Disorders in the Brain Stem. London, WB Saunders, 1992:455–470.

221. Smith JL, David NJ. Internuclear ophthalmoplegia: two new clinical signs. Neurology 1964;14:307–309.

222. Ventre J, Vighetto A, Bailly G, et al. Saccade metrics in multiple sclerosis: versional velocity disconjugacy as the best clue? J Neurol Sci 1991;102:144–149.

223. Flipse JP, Straathof CSM, Van der Steen J, et al. Binocular saccadic acceleration in multiple sclerosis. Neuroophthalmology 1996;16:43–46.

224. Frohman EM, Frohman TC, O'Suilleabhain P, et al. Quantitative oculographic characterisation of internuclear ophthalmoparesis in multiple sclerosis: the versional dysconjugacy index Z score. J Neurol Neurosurg Psychiatry 2002;73:51–55.

225. Kupfer C, Cogan DG. Unilateral internuclear ophthalmoplegia: a clinicopathological case report. Arch Ophthalmol 1966;75:484–489.

226. Feldon SE, Hoyt WF, Stark L. Disordered inhibition in internuclear ophthalmoplegia. Analysis of eye movement recordings with computer simulations. Brain 1980;103:113–137.

227. Thömke F, Hopf HC. Abduction paresis with rostral pontine and/or mesencephalic lesions: pseudoabducens palsy and its relation to the so-called posterior internuclear ophthalmoplegia of Lutz. BMC Neurol 2001;1:4.

228. Kommerell G. Unilateral internuclear ophthalmoplegia. The lack of inhibitory involvement in medial rectus muscle activity. Invest Ophthalmol Vis Sci 1981;21:592–599.

229. Bronstein AM, Rudge P, Gresty MA, et al. Abnormalities of horizontal gaze. Clinical, oculographic and magnetic resonance imaging findings. II. Gaze palsy and internuclear ophthalmoplegia. J Neurol Neurosurg Psychiatry 1990;53:200–207.

230. Thömke F, Hopf HC, Breen LA. Slowed abduction saccades in bilateral internuclear ophthalmoplegia. Neuroophthalmology 1992;12:241–246.

231. Crane TB, Yee RD, Baloh RW, et al. Analysis of characteristic eye movement abnormalities in internuclear ophthalmoplegia. Arch Ophthalmol 1983;101:206–210.

232. Pola J, Robinson DA. An explanation of eye movements seen in internuclear ophthalmoplegia. Arch Neurol 1976;33:447–452.

233. Pierrot-Deseilligny C, Chain F. L'ophtalmoplégie internucléaire. Rev Neurol (Paris) 1979;135:485–513.

234. Baloh RW, Yee RD, Honrubia V. Internuclear ophthalmoplegia. I. Saccades and dissociated nystagmus. Arch Neurol 1978;35:484–489.

235. Zee DS, Hain TC, Carl JR. Abduction nystagmus in internuclear ophthalmoplegia. Ann Neurol 1987;21:383–388.

236. Thömke F. Some observations on abduction nystagmus in internuclear ophthalmoplegia. Neuroophthalmology 1996;16:27–38.

237. Gamlin PDR, Gnadt JW, Mays LE. Lidocaine-induced unilateral internuclear ophthalmoplegia: effects on convergence and conjugate eye movements. J Neurophysiol 1989;62:82–95.

238. Büttner-Ennever JA, Horn AKE, Schmidtke K. Cell groups of the medial longitudinal fasciculus and paramedian tracts. Rev Neurol (Paris) 1989;145:533–539.

239. Nozaki S, Mukuno K, Ishikawa S. Internuclear ophthalmoplegia associated with ipsilateral downbeat nystagmus and contralateral incyclorotatory nystagmus. Ophthalmologica 1983;187:210–216.

240. Cremer PD, Migliaccio AA, Halmagyi GM, Curthoys IS. Vestibulo-ocular reflex pathways in internuclear ophthalmoplegia. Ann Neurol 1999;45:529–533.

241. Lin HY, Tsai RK. Internuclear ophthalmoplegia associated with transient torsional nystagmus. J Formos Med Assoc 2002;101:446–448.

242. Srivastava AK, Tripathi M, Gaikwad SB, et al. Internuclear ophthalmoplegia and torsional nystagmus: an MRI correlate. Neurol India 2003;51:271–272.

243. Herishanu YO, Sharpe JA. Saccadic intrusions in internuclear ophthalmoplegia. Ann Neurol 1983;14:67–72.

244. Evinger LC, Fuchs AF, Baker R. Bilateral lesions of the medial longitudinal fasciculus in monkeys: effects on the horizontal and vertical components of voluntary and vestibular induced eye movements. Exp Brain Res 1977;28:1–20.

245. Leigh RJ, Newman SA, King WM. Vertical gaze disorders. In: Lennerstrand G, Zee DS, Keller EL, eds. Functional Basis of Ocular Motility Disorders. Oxford, UK, Pergamon, 982:257–266.

246. Kirkham TH, Katsarkas A. An electrooculographic study of internuclear ophthalmoplegia. Ann Neurol 1977;2:385–392.

247. Guitton D, Kirkham T. Vertical oculomotor deficits following MLF lesions in man and monkey are similar. Soc Neurosci Abst 1978;4:163.

248. Gordon RM, Bender MB. Visual phenomena in lesions of the medial longitudinal fasciculus. Arch Neurol 1966;15:238–240.

249. Gresty MA, Hess K, Leech J. Disorders of the vestibulo-ocular reflex producing oscillopsia and mechanisms compensating for loss of labyrinthine function. Brain 1977;100:693–716.

250. Frohman EM, Solomon D, Zee DS. Nuclear, supranuclear and internuclear eye movement abnormalities in multiple sclerosis. Int J MS 1996;2:79–89.

250a. Kim JS. Internuclear ophthalmoplegia as an isolated or predominant symptom of brainstem infarction. Neurology 2004;62:1491–1496.

251. Mutschler V, Eber AM, Rumbach L, et al. Internuclear ophthalmoplegia in 14 patients. Clinical and topographic correlation using magnetic resonance imaging. Neuroophthalmology 1990;10:319–325.

252. Schmidt F, Kastrup A, Nagele T, et al. Isolated ischemic internuclear ophthalmoplegia: toward the resolution limits of DW-MRI. Eur J Neurol 2004;11:67–68.

253. Lutz A. Ueber die Bahnen der Blickwendung und deren Dissoziierung. Klin Monatsble Augenheilkd 1923;70:213–235.

254. Kommerell G. Internuclear ophthalmoplegia of abduction. Isolated impairment of phasic ocular motor activity in supranuclear lesions. Arch Ophthalmol 1975;93:531–534.

255. Cremer PD, Halmagyi GM. Eye movement disorders in a patient with liver disease. Neuroophthalmology 1996;16(Suppl):276.

256. Oliveri RL, Bono F, Quattrone A. Pontine lesion of the abducens fasciculus producing so-called posterior internuclear ophthalmoplegia. Eur Neurol 1997;37:67–69.

257. Bogousslavsky J, Regli F, Ostinelli B, et al. Paresis of lateral gaze alternating with so-called posterior internuclear ophthalmoplegia. A partial paramedian pontine reticular formation-abducens nucleus syndrome. J Neurol 1985;232:38–42.

258. Thömke F, Hopf HC, Krämer G. Internuclear ophthalmoplegia of abduction: clinical and electrophysiological data on the existence of an abduction paresis of prenuclear origin. J Neurol Neurosurg Psychiatry 1992;55:105–111.

259. Çelebisoy N, Akyürekli Ö. One-and-a-half syndrome, type II: a case with rostral brain stem infarction. Neuroophthalmology 1996;16:373–377.

260. Wiest G, Wanschitz J, Baumgartner C, et al. So-called posterior internuclear ophthalmoplegia due to a pontine glioma: a clinicopathological study. J Neurol 1999;246:412–415.

261. Carpenter MB, McMasters RE, Hanna GR. Disturbances of conjugate horizontal eye movements in the monkey. I. Physiological effects and anatomical degeneration resulting from lesions of the abducens nucleus and nerve. Arch Neurol 1963;8:231–247.

262. Hirose G, Furui K, Yoshioka A, et al. Unilateral conjugate gaze palsy due to a lesion of the abducens nucleus. J Clin Neuroophthalmol 1993;13:54–58.

263. Müri RM, Chermann JF, Cohen L, et al. Ocular motor consequences of damage to the abducens nucleus area in humans. J Neuroophthalmol 1996;16:191–195.

264. Miller NR, Biousse V, Hwang T, et al. Isolated acquired unilateral horizontal gaze paresis from a putative lesion of the abducens nucleus. J Neuroophthalmol 2002;22:204–207.

265. Amaya LG, Walker J, Taylor D. Möbius syndrome: a study and report of 18 cases. Binoc Vis Q 1990;5:119–132.

266. Bronstein AM, Morris J, Du Boulay G, et al. Abnormalities of horizontal gaze. Clinical, culographic and magnetic resonance imaging findings. I. Abducens palsy. J Neurol Neurosurg Psychiatry 1990;53:194–199.

267. Goebel HH, Komatsuzaki A, Bender MB, et al. Lesions of the pontine tegmentum and conjugate gaze paralysis. Arch Neurol 1971;24:431–440.

268. Pierrot-Deseilligny C, Chain F, Lhermitte F. Syndrome de la formation réticulaire pontine. Précisions physiopathologiques sur les anomalies des mouvements oculaires volontaires. Rev Neurol (Paris) 1982;138:517–532.

269. Johnston JL, Sharpe JA, Ranalli PJ, et al. Oblique misdirection and slowing of vertical saccades after unilateral lesions of the pontine tegmentum. Neurology 1993;43:2238–2244.

270. Johnston JL, Sharpe JA, Morrow MJ. Paresis of contralateral smooth pursuit and normal vestibular smooth eye movements after unilateral brainstem lesions. Ann Neurol 1992;31:495–502.

271. Thier P, Bachor A, Faiss J, et al. Selective impairment of smooth-pursuit eye movements due to an ischemic lesion of the basal pons. Ann Neurol 1991;29:443–448.

272. Gaymard B, Pierrot-Deseilligny C, Rivaud S, et al. Smooth-pursuit eye movement deficits after pontine nuclei lesions in humans. J Neurol Neurosurg Psychiatry 1993;56:799–807.

273. Deleu D, Michotte A, Ebinger G. Impairment of smooth pursuit in pontine lesions: functional topography based on MRI and neuropathologic findings. Acta Neurol Belg 1997;97:28–35.

274. Furman JMR, Hurtt MR, Hirsch WL. Asymmetrical ocular pursuit with posterior fossa tumors. Ann Neurol 1991;30:208–211.

275. Pierrot-Deseilligny C, Goasguen J. Isolated abducens nucleus damage due to histiocytosis X. Brain 1984;107:1019–1032.

276. Kommerell G, Henn V, Bach M, et al. Unilateral lesion of the paramedian pontine reticular formation. Loss of rapid eye movements with preservation of vestibulo-ocular reflex and pursuit. Neuroophthalmology 1987;7:93–98.

277. Monteiro MLR, Coppeto JR. Cryptic disseminated tuberculosis presenting as gaze palsy. J Clin Neuroophthalmol 1985;5:27–29.
278. Hanson MR, Hamid MA, Tomsak RL, et al. Selective saccadic palsy caused by pontine lesions: clinical, physiological, and pathological correlations. Ann Neurol 1986;20:209–217.
279. Nishida T, Tychsen L, Corbett JJ. Resolution of saccadic palsy after treatment of brain-stem metastasis. Arch Neurol 1986;43:1196–1197.
280. Henn V, Lang W, Hepp K, et al. Experimental gaze palsies in monkeys and their relation to human pathology. Brain 1984;107:619–636.
281. Beigi B, O'Keeffe M, Logan P, et al. Convergence substitution for paralysed horizontal gaze. Br J Ophthalmol 1995;79:229–232.
282. Bogousslavsky J, Regli F. Convergence and divergence synkinesis. A recovery pattern in benign pontine hematoma. Neuroophthalmology 1984;4:219–225.
283. Brusa G, Meneghini S, Piccardo A, et al. Regressive pattern of horizontal gaze palsy. Case report. Neuroophthalmology 1987;7:301–306.
284. Christoff N. A clinicopathologic study of vertical eye movements. Arch Neurol 1974;31:1–8.
285. Dominguez RO, Bronstein AM. Complete gaze palsy in pontine haemorrhage. J Neurol Neurosurg Psychiatry 1988;51:150–151.
286. Toyoda K, Hasegawa Y, Yonehara T, et al. Bilateral medial medullary infarction with oculomotor disorders. Stroke 1992;23:1657–1659.
287. Hennerici M, Fromm C. Isolated complete gaze palsy: an unusual ocular movement deficit probably due to a bilateral parapontine reticular formation (PPRF) lesion. Neuroophthalmology 1981;1:165–173.
288. Slavin ML. A clinicoradiographic correlation of bilateral horizontal gaze palsy with slowed vertical saccades and midline dorsal pontine lesion on magnetic resonance imaging. Am J Ophthalmol 1986;101:118–120.
289. Izaki A, Shimo-oku M, Suzuki A. Two cases of bilateral medial longitudinal fasciculus syndrome with vertical saccades of slow velocity. Neuroophthalmology 1996;16(suppl):289.
290. Kaneko CRS. Effect of ibotenic acid lesions of the omnipause neurons on saccadic eye movements in rhesus macaques. J Neurophysiol 1996;75:2229–2242.
291. Schon F, Hodgson TL, Mort D, Kennard C. Ocular flutter associated with a localized lesion in the paramedian pontine reticular formation. Ann Neurol 2001;50:413–416.
292. Wall M, Wray SH. The one-and-a-half syndrome: a unilateral disorder of the pontine tegmentum: a study of 20 cases and review of the literature. Neurology 1983;33:971–980.
293. Deleu D, Solheid C, Michotte A, et al. Dissociated ipsilateral horizontal gaze palsy in one-and-a-half syndrome: a clinicopathologic study. Neurology 1988;38:1278–1280.
294. Sharpe JA, Rosenberg MA, Hoyt WF, et al. Paralytic pontine exotropia: a sign of acute unilateral pontine gaze palsy and internuclear ophthalmoplegia. Neurology 1974;24:1076–1081.
295. Johkura H, Komiyama A, Kuroiwa Y. Eye deviation in patients with one-and-a-half syndrome. Eur Neurol 2000;44:210–215.
296. Johnston JL, Sharpe JA. Sparing of the vestibulo-ocular reflex with lesions of the paramedian pontine reticular formation. Neurology 1989;39:876.
297. Heywood S, Ratcliff G. Long-term oculomotor consequences of unilateral colliculectomy in man. In: Lennerstrand G, Bach-y-Rita P, eds. Basic Mechanisms of Ocular Motility and Their Clinical Implications. Oxford, Pergamon, 1975:561–564.
298. de Seze J, Lucas C, Leclerc X, et al. One-and-a-half syndrome in pontine infarcts: MRI correlates. Neuroradiology 1999;41:666–669.
299. Bandini F, Faga D, Simonetti S. Ocular myasthenia mimicking a one-and-a-half syndrome. J Neuroophthalmol 2001;21:210–211.
300. Kunavarapu C, Kesavan RB, Pevil-Ulysee M, Mohan SS. Systemic lupus erythematosus presenting as "one-and-a-half syndrome." J Rheumatol 2001;28:874–875.
301. Larner AJ, Rudge P. One-and-a-half syndrome resulting from spontaneous vertebral artery dissection. Int J Clin Pract 2002;56:480–481.
302. Minagar A, Schatz NJ, Glaser JS. Case report: one-and-a-half-syndrome and tuberculosis of the pons in a patient with AIDS. AIDS Patient Care STDS 2000;14:461–464.
303. Crisostomo EA. One-and-a-half syndrome in a patient with metastatic breast disease. J Clin Neuroophthalmol 1985;5:270–272.
304. Jackel RA, Gittinger JW Jr, Smith TW, et al. Metastatic adenocarcinoma presenting as a one-and-a-half syndrome. J Clin Neuroophthalmol 1986;6:116–119.
305. Sharpe JA, Bondar RL, Fletcher WA. Contralateral gaze deviation after frontal lobe haemorrhage. J Neurol Neurosurg Psychiatry 1985;48:86–88.
306. Smith MS, Buchsbaum HW, Masland WS. One and a half syndrome. Occurrence after trauma with computerized tomographic correlation. Arch Neurol 1980;37:251.
307. Carter JE, Rauch RA. One-and-a-half syndrome, type II. Arch Neurol 1994;51:87–89.
308. Zee DS, Chu FC, Leigh RJ, et al. Blink-saccade synkinesis. Neurology 1983;33:1233–1236.
309. Büttner-Enever JA, Wadia NH, Sakai H, et al. Neuroanatomy of oculomotor structures in olivo-pontocerebellar atrophy (OPCA) patients with slow saccades. J Neurol 1985;232(suppl):285.
310. Zee DS, Robinson DA. A hypothetical explanation of saccadic oscillations. Ann Neurol 1979;5:405–414.
311. Averbuch-Heller L, Kori AA, Rottach K, et al. Dysfunction of pontine omnipause neurons causes impaired fixation: macrosaccadic oscillations with a unilateral pontine lesion. Neuroophthalmology 1996;16:99–106.
312. Bhidayasiri R, Plant GT, Leigh RJ. A hypothetical scheme for the brainstem control of vertical gaze. Neurology 2000;54:1985–1993.
313. Daroff RR, Hoyt WE. Supranuclear disorders of ocular control systems in man: clinical, anatomical and physiological correlations, 1969. In: Bach-y-Rita P, Collins CC, Hyde JE, eds. The Control of Eye Movements. New York, Academic Press, 1971:175–235.
314. Keane JR. The pretectal syndrome: 206 patients. Neurology 1990;40:684–690.
315. Pasik T, Pasik P, Bender MB. The superior colliculi and eye movements: an experimental study in the monkey. Arch Neurol 1966;15:420–436.
316. Büttner U, Büttner-Enever JA, Rambold H, Helmchen C. The contribution of midbrain circuits in the control of gaze. Ann NY Acad Sci 2002;956:99–110.
317. Moschovakis AK, Scudder CA, Highstein SM. Structure of the primate oculomotor burst generator. I. Medium-lead burst neurons with upward on-directions. J Neurophysiol 1991;65:203–217.
318. Tamura EE, Hoyt CS. Oculomotor consequences of intraventricular hemorrhages in premature infants. Arch Ophthalmol 1987;105:533–535.
319. Barontini F, Simonetti C, Ferranini F, et al. Persistent upward eye deviation. Report of two cases. Neuroophthalmology 1983;3:217–224.
320. Ouvrier RA, Billson F. Benign paroxysmal tonic upgaze of childhood. J Child Neurol 1988;3:177–180.
321. Apak RA, Topcu M. A case of paroxysmal tonic upgaze of childhood with ataxia. Eur J Paediatr Neurol 1999;3:129–131.
322. Hayman M, Harvey AS, Hopkins IJ, et al. Paroxysmal tonic upgaze: a reappraisal of outcome. Ann Neurol 1998;43:514–520.
323. Lispi ML, Vigevano F. Benign paroxysmal tonic upgaze of childhood with ataxia. Epileptic Disord 2001;3:203–206.
324. Rouveyrol F, Stephan JL. Benign paroxysmal tonic upgaze of infancy: 2 additional cases. Arch Pediatr 2003;10:527–529.
325. Ruggieri VL, Yepez II, Fejerman N. [Benign paroxysmal tonic upward gaze syndrome]. Rev Neurol 1998;27:88–91.
326. Spalice A, Parisi P, Iannetti P. Paroxysmal tonic upgaze: physiopathological considerations in three additional cases. J Child Neurol 2000;15:15–18.
327. Verrotti A, Trotta D, Blasetti A, et al. Paroxysmal tonic upgaze of childhood: effect of age-of-onset on prognosis. Acta Paediatr 2001;90:1343–1345.
328. Pullicino P, Lincoff N, Truax BT. Abnormal vergence with upper brainstem infarcts: pseudoabducens palsy. Neurology 2000;55:352–358.
329. Ochs AL, Stark L, Hoyt WF, et al. Opposed adducting saccades in convergence-retraction nystagmus. A patient with sylvian aqueduct syndrome. Brain 1979;102:497–508.
330. Schnyder H, Bassetti C. Bilateral convergence nystagmus in unilateral dorsal midbrain stroke due to occlusion of the superior cerebellar artery. Neuroophthalmology 1996;16:59–63.
331. Pasik T, Pasik P, Bender MB. The pretectal syndrome in monkeys. II. Spontaneous and induced nystagmus, and ''lightning'' eye movements. Brain 1969;92:871–884.
332. Rambold H, Kompf D, Helmchen C. Convergence retraction nystagmus: a disorder of vergence? Ann Neurol 2001;50:677–681.
333. Galetta SL, Gray LG, Raps EC, et al. Pretectal eyelid retraction and lag. Ann Neurol 1993;33:554–557.
334. Saeki N, Yamaura A, Sunami K. Bilateral ptosis with pupil sparing because of a discrete midbrain lesion: magnetic resonance imaging evidence of topographic arrangement within the oculomotor nerve. J Neuroophthalmol 2000;20:130–134.
335. Wray SH. The neuro-ophthalmic and neurologic manifestations of pinealomas. In: Schmider HH, ed. Pineal Tumors. New York, Masson, 1977:21–59.
336. Baloh RW, Furman JM, Yee RD. Dorsal midbrain syndrome: clinical and oculographic findings. Neurology 1985;35:54–60.
337. Swash M. Periaqueductal dysfunction (the Sylvian aqueduct syndrome): a sign of hydrocephalus? J Neurol Neurosurg Psychiatry 1974;37:21–26.
338. Corbett JJ. Neuro-ophthalmologic complications of hydrocephalus and shunting procedures. Semin Neurol 1986;6:111–123.
339. Bleasel AF, Ell JJ, Johnston I. Pretectal syndrome and ventricular shunt dysfunction. Neuroophthalmology 1992;12:193–196.
340. Rismondo V, Borchert M. Position-dependent Parinaud's syndrome. Am J Ophthalmol 1992;114:107–108.
341. Kömpf D, Pasik T, Pasik P, et al. Downward gaze in monkeys. Stimulation and lesion studies. Brain 1979;102:527–558.
342. Henn V, Hepp K, Vilis T. Rapid eye movement generation in the primate. Physiology, pathophysiology, and clinical implications. Rev Neurol (Paris) 1989;145:540–545.
343. Suzuki Y, Buttner-Ennever JA, Straumann D, et al. Deficits in torsional and vertical rapid eye movements and shift of Listing's plane after uni- and bilateral lesions of the rostral interstitial nucleus of the medial longitudinal fasciculus. Exp Brain Res 1995;106:215–232.
344. Zee DS. The organization of the brainstem ocular motor subnuclei. Ann Neurol 1978;4:384–385.

345. Cogan DG, Chu FC, Bachman DM, et al. The DAF syndrome. Neuroophthalmology 1981;2:7–16.
346. Percheron C. Les artères du thalamus humain. II. Arteres et territoires thalamique paramedians de l'artère basilair communicante. Rev Neurol (Paris) 1976;132:309–324.
347. Castaigne P, Lhermitte F, Buge A, et al. Paramedian thalamic and midbrain infarcts: clinical and neuropathological study. Ann Neurol 1981;10:127–148.
348. Büttner-Ennever JA, Büttner U, Cohen B, et al. Vertical gaze paralysis and the rostral interstitial nucleus of the medial longitudinal fasciculus. Brain 1982;105:125–149.
349. Pierrot-Deseilligny C, Chain F, Gray F, et al. Parinaud's syndrome: electro-oculographic and anatomical analyses of six vascular cases with deductions about vertical gaze organization in the premotor structures. Brain 1982;105:667–696.
350. Dehaene I, Casselman JW, Van Zandijcke M. Selective paralysis of downward saccades. Cerebrovasc Dis 1994;4:377–378.
351. Deleu D, Buisseret T, Ebinger G. Vertical one-and-a-half syndrome: supranuclear downgaze paralysis with monocular elevation palsy. Arch Neurol 1989;46:1361–1363.
352. Bogousslavsky J, Regli F. Upgaze palsy and monocular paresis of downward gaze from ipsilateral thalamo-mesencephalic infarction: a vertical "one-and-a-half syndrome." J Neurol 1984;231:43–45.
353. Hommel M, Bogousslavsky J. The spectrum of vertical gaze palsy following unilateral brainstem stroke. Neurology 1991;41:1229–1234.
354. Sekine S, Utsumi H, Kaku H, et al. [A case presenting vertical one-and-a-half syndrome and seesaw nystagmus due to thalamomesencephalic infarction]. No To Shinkei 2003;55:699–703.
355. Ranalli PJ, Sharpe JA, Fletcher WA. Palsy of upward and downward saccadic, pursuit, and vestibular movements with a unilateral midbrain lesion: pathophysiologic correlations. Neurology 1988;38:114–122.
356. Green JP, Newman NJ, Winterkorn JS. Paralysis of downgaze in two patients with clinical-radiologic correlation. Arch Ophthalmol 1993;111:219–222.
357. Riordan-Eva P, Faldon M, Büttner-Ennever JA, et al. Abnormalities of torsional fast eye movements in unilateral rostral midbrain disease. Neurology 1996;47:201–207.
358. Helmchen C, Rambold H, Kempermann U, et al. Localizing value of torsional nystagmus in small midbrain lesions. Neurology 2002;59:1956–1964.
359. Ranalli PJ, Sharpe JA. Vertical vestibulo-ocular reflex, smooth-pursuit and eye-head tracking dysfunction in internuclear ophthalmoplegia. Brain 1988;111:1299–1317.
360. Kokkoroyannis T, Scudder CA, Balaban CD, et al. Anatomy and physiology of the primate interstitial nucleus of Cajal: Efferent projections. J Neurophysiol 1996;75:725–739.
361. Helmchen C, Rambold H, Fuhry L, Buttner U. Deficits in vertical and torsional eye movements after uni- and bilateral muscimol inactivation of the interstitial nucleus of Cajal of the alert monkey. Exp Brain Res 1998;119:436–452.
362. Helmchen C, Rambold H, Fuhry L, Buttner U. Deficits in vertical and torsional eye movements after uni- and bilateral muscimol inactivation of the interstitial nucleus of Cajal of the alert monkey. Exp Brain Res 1998;119:436–452.
363. Fukushima K. The interstitial nucleus of Cajal and its role in the control of movements of head and eyes. Prog Neurobiol 1987;29:107–192.
364. Halmagyi GM, Aw ST, Dehaene I, et al. Jerk-waveform seesaw nystagmus due to unilateral meso-diencephalic lesion. Brain 1994;117:775–788.
365. Rambold H, Helmchen C, Buttner U. Unilateral muscimol inactivations of the interstitial nucleus Cajal in the alert rhesus monkey do not elicit seesaw nystagmus. Neurosci Lett 1999;272:75–78.
366. Rambold H, Helmchen C, Buttner U. Vestibular influence on the binocular control of vertical-torsional nystagmus after lesions in the interstitial nucleus of Cajal. Neuroreport 2000;11:779–784.
367. Sharpe JA, Ranalli PJ. Vertical vestibulo-ocular reflex control after supranuclear midbrain damage. Acta Otolaryngol Suppl 1991;481:194–198.
368. Jacobs L, Heffner RR Jr, Newman RP. Selective paralysis of downward gaze caused by bilateral lesions of the mesencephalic periaqueductal gray matter. Neurology 1985;35:516–521.
369. Thames PB, Trobe JD, Ballinger WE. Gaze paralysis caused by lesion of the periaqueductal gray matter. Arch Neurol 1984;41:437–440.
370. Waitzman DM, Silakov VL, DePalma-Bowles S, Ayers AS. Effects of reversible inactivation of the primate mesencephalic reticular formation. II. Hypometric vertical saccades. J Neurophysiol 2000;83:2285–2299.
371. Waitzman DM, Silakov VL, DePalma-Bowles S, Ayers AS. Effects of reversible inactivation of the primate mesencephalic reticular formation. I. Hypermetric goal-directed saccades. J Neurophysiol 2000;83:2260–2284.
372. Zackon DH, Sharpe JA. Midbrain paresis of horizontal gaze. Ann Neurol 1984;16:495–504.
373. Reagan TJ, Trautmann JC. Combined nuclear and supranuclear defects in ocular motility. A clinicopathologic study. Arch Neurol 1978;35:133–137.
374. Ropper AH, Miller DC. Acute traumatic midbrain hemorrhage. Ann Neurol 1985;18:80–86.
375. Worthington JM, Halmagyi GM. Bilateral total ophthalmoplegia due to midbrain hematoma. Neurology 1996;47:1176–1177.
376. Jampel RS, Fells P. Monocular elevation paresis caused by a central nervous system lesion. Arch Ophthalmol 1968;80:45–57.
377. Lessell S, Wolf PA, Chronley D. Prolonged vertical nystagmus after pentobarbital sodium administration. Am J Ophthalmol 1975;80:151–152.
378. Ford CS, Schwartze GM, Weaver RG, et al. Monocular elevation paresis caused by an ipsilateral lesion. Neurology 1984;34:1264–1267.
379. Bell JA, Fielder AR, Viney S. Congenital double elevator palsy in identical twins. J Clin Neuroophthalmol 1990;10:32–34.
380. Ziffer AJ, Rosenbaum AL, Demer JL, et al. Congenital double elevator palsy: vertical saccadic velocity utilizing the scleral search coil technique. J Pediatr Ophthalmol Strabis 1992;29:142–149.
381. Wiest G, Baumgartner C, Schnider P, et al. Monocular elevation paresis and contralateral downgaze paresis from unilateral mesodiencephalic infarction. J Neurol Neurosurg Psychiatry 1996;60:579–581.
382. Gauntt CD, Kashii S, Nagata I. Monocular elevation paresis caused by an oculomotor fascicular impairment. J Neuroophthalmol 1995;15:11–14.
383. Cadera W, Bloom JN, Karlik S, Viirre E. A magnetic resonance imaging study of double elevator palsy. Can J Ophthalmol 1997;32:250–253.
384. Steele JC, Richardson JC, Olszewski J. Progressive supranuclear palsy: a heterogeneous degeneration involving the brain stem, basal ganglia and cerebellum with vertical gaze and pseudobulbar palsy, nuchal dystonia and dementia. Arch Neurol 1964;10:333–359.
385. Burn DJ, Lees AJ. Progressive supranuclear palsy: where are we now? Lancet 2002;1:359–369.
386. Nath U, Ben Shlomo Y, Thomson RG, et al. Clinical features and natural history of progressive supranuclear palsy: a clinical cohort study. Neurology 2003;60:910–916.
387. Goetz CG, Leurgans S, Lang AE, Litvan I. Progression of gait, speech and swallowing deficits in progressive supranuclear palsy. Neurology 2003;60:917–922.
388. Litvan I. Diagnosis and management of progressive supranuclear palsy. Semin Neurol 2001;21:41–48.
389. Morris HR, Gibb G, Katzenschlager R, et al. Pathological, clinical and genetic heterogeneity in progressive supranuclear palsy. Brain 2002;125:969–975.
390. Golbe LI. Progressive supranuclear palsy in the molecular age. Lancet 2000;356:870–871.
391. Riley DE, Fogt N, Leigh RJ. The syndrome of "pure akinesia" and its relationship to progressive supranuclear palsy. Neurology 1994;44:1025–1029.
392. de Yébenes JG, Sarasa JL, Daniel SE, et al. Familial progressive supranuclear palsy: description of a pedigree and review of the literature. Brain 1995;118:1095–1103.
393. Tetrud JW, Golbe LI, Forno LS, et al. Autopsy-proven progressive supranuclear palsy in two siblings. Neurology 1996;46:931–934.
394. Seemungal BM, Faldon M, Revesz T, et al. Influence of target size on vertical gaze palsy in a pathologically proven case of progressive supranuclear palsy. Mov Disord 2003;18:818–822.
395. Hamilton SR. Neuro-ophthalmology of movement disorders. Curr Opin Ophthalmol 2000;11:403–407.
396. Dix MR, Harrison MJG, Lewis PD. Progressive supranuclear palsy (the Steele-Richardson-Olszewski syndrome). A report of 9 cases with particular reference to the mechanism of the oculomotor disorder. J Neurol Sci 1971;13:237–256.
397. Troost BT, Daroff RB. The ocular motor defects in progressive supranuclear palsy. Ann Neurol 1977;2:397–403.
398. Rascol O, Hain TC, Brefel C, et al. Antivertigo medications and drug-induced vertigo. Drugs 1995;50:777–791.
399. Mastaglia FL, Grainger KMR. Internuclear ophthalmoplegia in progressive supranuclear palsy. J Neurol Sci 1975;25:303–308.
400. Kitthaweesin K, Riley DE, Leigh RJ. Vergence disorders in progressive supranuclear palsy. Ann NY Acad Sci 2002;956:504–507.
401. Pierrot-Deseilligny C, Rivaud S, Pillon B, et al. Lateral visually guided saccades in progressive supranuclear palsy. Brain 1989;112:471–487.
402. Pierrot-Deseilligny C, Rivaud-Pechoux S. [Contribution of oculomotor examination for the etiological diagnosis of parkinsonian syndromes]. Rev Neurol (Paris) 2003;159:3S75–3S81.
403. Rivaud-Pechoux S, Vermersch AI, Gaymard B, et al. Improvement of memory-guided saccades in parkinsonian patients by high-frequency subthalamic nucleus stimulation. J Neurol Neurosurg Psychiatry 2000;68:381–384.
404. Goffinet AM, De Volder AG, Gillian C, et al. Positron tomography demonstrates frontal lobe hypometabolism in progressive supranuclear palsy. Ann Neurol 1989;25:131–139.
405. Rafal RD, Posner MI, Friedman JH, et al. Orienting of visual attention in progressive supranuclear palsy. Brain 1988;111:267–280.
406. Fisk JD, Goodale MA, Burkhart G, et al. Progressive supranuclear palsy: the relationship between ocular motor dysfunction and psychological test performance. Neurology 1982;32:698–705.
407. Verny M, Duyckaerts C, Agid Y, et al. The significance of cortical pathology in progressive supranuclear palsy: clinico-pathological data in 10 cases. Brain 1996;119:1123–1136.
408. Yekhlef F, Ballan G, Macia F, et al. Routine MRI for the differential diagnosis of Parkinson's disease, MSA, PSP, and CBD. J Neural Transm 2003;110:151–169.

409. Kato N, Arai K, Hattori T. Study of the rostral midbrain atrophy in progressive supranuclear palsy. Neurol Sci 2003;210:57–60.

410. Kida M, Koo H, Grossniklaus HE, et al. Neuropathologic findings in progressive supranuclear palsy. J Clin Neuroophthalmol 1988;8:161–170.

411. Juncos JL, Hirsch EC, Malessa S, et al. Mesencephalic cholinergic nuclei in progressive supranuclear palsy. Neurology 1991;41:25–30.

412. Fukushima-Kudo J, Fukushima K, Tashiro K. Rigidity and dorsiflexion of the neck in progressive supranuclear palsy and the interstitial nucleus of Cajal. J Neurol Neurosurg Psychiatry 1987;50:1197–1203.

413. Revesz T, Sangha H, Daniel SE. The nucleus raphe interpositus in the Steele-Richardson-Olszewski syndrome (progressive supranuclear palsy). Brain 1996; 119:1137–1143.

414. Averbuch-Heller L, Gordon C, Zivotofsky A, et al. Small vertical saccades have normal speeds in progressive supranuclear palsy (PSP). Ann NY Acad Sci 2002; 956:434–437

415. Bhidayasiri R, Riley DE, Somers JT, et al. Pathophysiology slow vertical saccades in progressive supranuclear palsy. Neurology 2001;57:2070–2077.

416. Halliday GM, Hardman CD, Cordato NJ, et al. A role for the substantia nigra pars reticulata in the gaze palsy of progressive supranuclear palsy. Brain 2000; 123:724–732.

417. Malessa S, Gaymard B, Rivaud S, et al. Role of pontine nuclei damage in smooth-pursuit impairment of progressive supranuclear palsy: a clinical pathologic study. Neurology 1994;44:716–721.

418. Dubinsky RM, Jankovic J. Progressive supranuclear palsy and a multi-infarct state. Neurology 1987;37:570–576.

419. Moses Ill H, Zee D. Multi-infarct PSP. Neurology 1987;37:1819.

420. Josephs KA, Ishizawa T, Tsuboi Y, et al. A clinicopathological study of vascular progressive supranuclear palsy: a multi-infarct disorder presenting as progressive supranuclear palsy. Arch Neurol 2002;59:1597–1601.

421. Curran T, Lang AE. Parkinsonian syndromes associated with hydrocephalus: case reports, a review of the literature, and pathophysiological hypotheses. Mov Disord 1994;9:508–520.

422. Averbuch-Heller L, Paulson GW, Daroff RB, Leigh RJ. Whipple's disease mimicking progressive supranuclear palsy: the diagnostic value of eye movement recording. J Neurol Neurosurg Psychiatry 1999;66:532–535.

423. Mokri B, Ahlskog JE, Fulgham JR, Matsumoto JY. Syndrome resembling PSP after surgical repair of ascending aorta dissection or aneurysm. Neurology 2004; 62:971–973.

424. Kuniyoshi S, Riley DE, Zee DS, et al. Distinguishing progressive supranuclear palsy from other forms of Parkinson's disease: evaluation of new signs. Ann NY Acad Sci 2002;956:484–486.

425. Riley DE, Lang AE, Lewis A, et al. Cortical-basal ganglionic degeneration. Neurology 1990;40:1203–1212.

426. Vidailhet M, Rivaud S, Gouider-Khouja N, et al. Eye movements in parkinsonian syndromes. Ann Neurol 1994;35:420–426.

427. Bergeron C, Pollanen MS, Weyer L, et al. Unusual clinical presentations of cortical-basal ganglionic degeneration. Ann Neurol 1996;40:893–900.

428. Rottach K, Riley DE, DiScenna AO, et al. Dynamic properties of horizontal and vertical eye movements in parkinsonian syndromes. Ann Neurol 1996;39: 368–377.

429. Litvan I, Agid Y, Goetz C, et al. Accuracy of the clinical diagnosis of corticobasal degeneration: a clinicopathologic study. Neurology 1997;48:119–125.

430. Caparros-Lefebvre D, Sergeant N, Lees A, et al. Guadeloupean parkinsonism: a cluster of progressive supranuclear palsy-like tauopathy. Brain 2002;125: 801–811.

431. Lepore FE, Steele JC, Cox TA, et al. Supranuclear disturbances of ocular motility in Lytico-Bodig. Neurology 1988;38:1849–1853.

432. Steele JC, Caparros-Lefebvre D, Lees AJ, Sacks OW. Progressive supranuclear palsy and its relation to pacific foci of the parkinsonism-dementia complex and Guadeloupean parkinsonism. Parkinsonism Relat Disord 2002;9:39–54.

433. Brett FM, Henson C, Staunton H. Familial diffuse Lewy body disease, eye movement abnormalities, and distribution of pathology. Arch Neurol 2002;59: 464–467.

434. Louis ED, Klataka LA, Liu Y, et al. Comparison of extrapyramidal features in 31 pathologically confirmed cases of diffuse Lewy body disease and 34 pathologically confirmed cases of Parkinson's disease. Neruology 1997;48:376–380.

435. Saver JL, Liu GT, Charness ME. Idiopathic striopallidodentate calcification with prominent supranuclear abnormality of eye movement. J Neuroophthalmol 1994; 14:29–33.

436. Wszolek ZK, Pfeiffer RF, Bhatt MH, et al. Rapidly progressive autosomal dominant parkinsonism and dementia with pallido-ponto-nigral degeneration. Ann Neurol 1992;32:312–320.

437. Rafal RD, Grimm RJ. Progressive supranuclear palsy: functional analysis of the response to methysergide and antiparkinsonian agents. Neurology 1981;31: 1507–1518.

438. Newman GC. Treatment of progressive supranuclear palsy with tricyclic antidepressants. Neurology 1985;35:1189–1193.

439. Jackson JA, Jankovic J, Ford J. Progressive supranuclear palsy: clinical features and response to treatment in 16 patients. Ann Neurol 1983;13:273–278.

440. Golbe LI. Progressive supranuclear palsy. Curr Treat Options Neurol 2001;3: 473–477.

441. Knox DL, Green Wm R, Troncoso JC, et al. Cerebral ocular Whipple's disease: a 62-year odyssey from death to diagnosis. Neurology 1995;45:617–625.

442. Misbah SA, Aslam A, Costello C. Whipple's disease. Lancet 2004;363:654–656.

443. Averbuch-Heller L, Paulson GW, Daroff RB, Leigh RJ. Whipple's disease mimicking progressive supranuclear palsy: the diagnostic value of eye movement recording. J Neurol Neurosurg Psychiatry 1999;66:532–535.

444. Finelli PF, McEntee WJ, Lessell S, et al. Whipple's disease with predominantly neuroophthalmic manifestations. Ann Neurol 1977;1:247–252.

445. Knox DL, Bayless TM, Pittman FE. Neurologic disease in patients with treated Whipple's disease. Medicine 1976;55:467–476.

446. Schwartz MA, Selhorst JB, Ochs AL, et al. Oculomasticatory myorhythmia: a unique movement disorder occurring in Whipple's disease. Ann Neurol 1986; 20:677–683.

447. Grotta JC, Pettigrew LC, Schmidt WA, et al. Oculomasticatory myorhythmia. Ann Neurol 1987;22:395–396.

448. Simpson DA, Wishnow R, Gargulinski RB, et al. Oculofacial-skeletal myorhythmia in central nervous system Whipple's disease: additional case and review of the literature. Mov Disord 1995;10:195–200.

449. Quinn N. Rhythmic tremor of the palate and other cranial limb muscles, with cerebellar ataxia: consider Whipple's disease. Mov Disord 2001;16:787.

450. Rajput AJ, Mchattie JD. Ophthalmoplegia and leg myorhythmia in Whipple's disease. Mov Disord 1997;12:111–114.

451. Albano JE, Mishkin M, Westbrook LE, et al. Visuomotor deficits following ablation of monkey superior colliculus. J Neurophysiol 1982;48:338–350.

452. Pierrot-Deseilligny C, Rosa A, Masmoudi K, et al. Saccade deficits after a unilateral lesion affecting the superior colliculus. J Neurol Neurosurg Psychiatry 1991; 54:1106–1109.

453. Fisher A, Knezevic W. Ocular and ocular motor aspects of primary thalamic haemorrhage. Clin Exp Neurol 1985;21:129–139.

454. Keane JR. Contralateral gaze deviation with supratentorial hemorrhage: three pathologically verified cases. Arch Neurol 1975;32:119–122.

455. Brigell M, Babikian V, Goodwin JA. Hypometric saccades and low-gain pursuit resulting from a thalamic hemorrhage. Ann Neurol 1984;15:374–378.

456. Fisher CM. The pathologic and clinical aspects of thalamic hemorrhage. Trans Am Neurol Assoc 1959;84:56–59.

457. Choi KD, Jung DS, Kim JS. Specificity of "peering at the tip of the nose" for a diagnosis of thalamic hemorrhage. Arch Neurol 2004;61:417–422.

458. Gomez CR, Gomez SM, Selhorst JB. Acute thalamic esotropia. Neurology 1988; 38:1759–1762.

459. Hertle RW, Bienfang DC. Oculographic analysis of acute esotropia secondary to a thalamic hemorrhage. J Clin Neuroophthalmol 1990;10:21–26.

460. Lindner K, Hitzenberger P, Drlicek M, et al. Dissociated unilateral convergence paralysis in a patient with thalamotectal haemorrhage. J Neurol Neurosurg Psychiatry 1992;55:731–733.

461. Siatkowski RM, Schatz NJ, Sellitti TP, et al. Do thalamic lesions really cause vertical gaze palsies? J Clin Neuroophthalmol 1993;13:190–193.

462. Clark JM, Albert GW. Vertical gaze palsies from medial thalamic infarctions without midbrain involvement. Stroke 1995;26:1467–1470.

463. Biller J, Sand JJ, Corbett JJ, et al. Syndrome of the paramedian thalamic arteries: clinical and neuroimaging correlation. J Clin Neuroophthalmol 1985;5:217–223.

464. Lepore FE, Gulli V, Miller DC. Neuro-ophthalmological findings with neuropathological correlation in bilateral thalamic-mesencephalic infarction. J Clin Neuroophthalmol 1985;5:224–228.

465. Weisbrod M, Kölmel HW, Hättig H, et al. The significance of vertical gaze palsy in the paramedian thalamic artery syndrome. Neuroophthalmology 1992; 12:85–90.

466. Beversdorf DQ, Jenkyn LR, Petrowski III JT, et al. Vertical gaze paralysis and intermittent unresponsiveness in a patient with a thalamomesencephalic stroke. J Neuroophthalmol 1995;15:230–235.

467. Albano JE, Wurtz RH. Deficits in eye position following ablation of monkey superior colliculus, pretectum, and posterior-medial thalamus. J Neurophysiol 1982;48:318–337.

468. Gaymard B, Rivaud S, Pierrot-Deseilligny C. Impairment of extraretinal eye position signals after central thalamic lesions. Exp Brain Res 1994;102:1–9.

469. Sommer MA, Wurtz RH. What the brain stem tells the frontal cortex. I. Oculomotor signals sent from superior colliculus to frontal eye field via mediodorsal thalamus. J Neurophysiol 2004;91:1381–1402.

470. Sommer MA, Wurtz RH. What the brain stem tells the frontal cortex. II. Role of the SC-MD-FEF pathway in corollary discharge. J Neurophysiol 2004;91: 1403–1423.

471. Gaymard B, Rivaud S, Pierrot-Deseilligny C. Impairment of extraretinal eye position signals after central thalamic lesions. Exp Brain Res 1994;102:1–9.

472. Gaymard B, Rivaud-Pechoux S, Yelnik J, et al. Involvement of the cerebellar thalamus in human saccade adaptation. Eur J Neurosci 2001;14:554–560.

473. Zihl J, Von Cramon D. The contribution of the "second" visual system to directed visual attention in man. Brain 1979;102:835–856.

474. Ogren MP, Mateer CA, Wyler AR. Alterations in visually related eye movements following left pulvinar damage in man. Neuropsychologia 1984;22:187–196.

475. Vilkki J. Visual hemi-inattention after ventrolateral thalamotomy. Neuropsychologia 1984;22:399–408.

476. Bender DB, Baizer JS. Saccadic eye movements following kainic acid lesions of the pulvinar in monkeys. Exp Brain Res 1990;79:467–478.

477. Kennard C, Lueck CJ. Oculomotor abnormalities in diseases of the basal ganglia. Rev Neurol 1989;145:587–595.

478. White OB, Saint-Cyr JA, Tomlinson RD, et al. Ocular motor deficits in Parkinson's disease. II. Control of the saccadic and smooth-pursuit systems. Brain 1983;106:571–587.

479. Corin MS, Elizan TS, Bender MB. Oculomotor function in patients with Parkinson's disease. J Neurol Sci 1972;15:251–265.

480. Chamberlain W. Restriction in upward gaze with advancing age. Am J Ophthalmol 1971;71:341–346.

481. Repka MX, Claro MC, Loupe DN, et al. Ocular motility in Parkinson's disease. Pediatr Ophthalmol Strabis 1996;33:144–147.

481a. Biousse V, Skibell BC, Watts RL, et al. Ophthalmologic feature of Parkinson's disease. Neurology 2004;62:177–180.

482. Crawford T, Goodrich S, Henderson L, et al. Predictive responses in Parkinson's disease: manual keypresses and saccadic eye movements to regular stimulus events. J Neurol Neurosurg Psychiatry 1989;52:1033–1042.

483. DeJong JD, Melvill Jones G. Akinesia, hypokinesia, and bradykinesia in the oculomotor system of patients with Parkinson's disease. Exp Neurol 1971;32:58–68.

484. Melvill Jones C, DeJong JD. Dynamic characteristics of saccadic eye movements in Parkinson's disease. Exp Neurol 1971;31:17–31.

485. Teravainen H, Calne DB. Studies of parkinsonian movement: I. Programming and execution of eye movements. Acta Neurol Scand 1980;62:137–148.

486. Muller C, Wenger S, Fertl L, et al. Initiation of visual-guided random saccades and remembered saccades in parkinsonian patients with severe motor-fluctuations. J Neural Transm 1994;7:101–108.

487. Hikosaka O, Segawa M, Imai H. Voluntary saccadic eye movements. Application to analyze basal ganglion functions. In: Highlights in Neuro-Ophthalmology. Proceedings of Sixth Meeting of the International Neuroophthalmology Society (INOS). Amsterdam, Aeolus Press, 1987:133–138.

488. Lueck CJ, Tanyeri S, Crawford TJ, et al. Saccadic eye movements in Parkinson's disease. I. Delayed saccades. Quart J Exp Psychol 1992;45A:193–210.

489. Lueck CJ, Crawford TJ, Henderson L, et al. Saccadic eye movements in Parkinson's disease. II. Remembered saccades—towards a unified hypothesis? Q J Exp Psychol 1992;45A:211–233.

490. Kimmig H, Haussmann K, Mergner T, Lucking CH. What is pathological with gaze shift fragmentation in Parkinson's disease? J Neurol 2002;249:683–692.

491. Shaunak S, O'Sullivan E, Blunt S, et al. Remembered saccades with variable delay in Parkinson's disease. Mov Disord 1999;14:80–86.

492. Nakamura T, Bronstein AM, Lueck CJ, et al. Vestibular, cervical and visual remembered saccades in Parkinson's disease. Brain 1994;117:1423–1432.

493. Vermersch AI, Rivaud S, Vidailhet M, et al. Sequences of memory-guided saccades in Parkinson'sdisease. Ann Neurol 1994;35:487–490.

494. Crawford TJ, Henderson L, Kennard C. Abnormalities of nonvisually guided eye movements in Parkinson's disease. Brain 1989;112:1573–1586.

495. Bronstein AM, Kennard C. Predictive ocular motor control in Parkinson's disease. Brain 1985;108:925–940.

496. Tanyeri S, Lueck CJ, Crawford TJ, et al. Vertical and horizontal saccadic eye movements in Parkinson's disease. Neuroophthalmology 1989;9:165–177.

497. Waterston JA, Barnes GR, Grealy MA, et al. Abnormalities of smooth eye and head movement control in Parkinson's disease. Ann Neurol 1996;39:749–760.

498. Rascol O, Clanet M, Montastruc JL, et al. Abnormal ocular movements in Parkinson's disease. Evidence for involvement of dopaminergic systems. Brain 1989;112:1193–1214.

499. Lueck CJ, Tanyeri S, Crawford TJ, et al. Antisaccades and remembered saccades in Parkinson's disease. J Neurol Neurosurg Psychiatry 1990;53:284–288.

500. Fukushima J, Fukushima K, Miyasaka K, et al. Voluntary control of saccadic eye movement in patients with frontal cortical lesions and parkinsonian patients in comparison with that in schizophrenics. Biol Psychiatry 1994;36:21–30.

501. Briand KA, Strallow D, Hening W, et al. Control of voluntary and reflexive saccades in Parkinson's disease. Exp Brain Res 1999;129:38–48.

502. Vidailhet M, Rivaud S, Gouider-Khouja N, et al. Saccades and antisaccades in parkinsonian syndromes. Adv Neurol 1999;80:377–382.

503. Hodgson TL, Tiesman B, Owen AM, Kennard C. Abnormal gaze strategies during problem solving in Parkinson's disease. Neuropsychologia 2002;40:411–422.

504. Ketcham CJ, Hodgson TL, Kennard C, Stelmach GE. Memory-motor transformations are impaired in Parkinson's disease. Exp Brain Res 2003;149:30–39.

505. Shaunak S, O'Sullivan E, Blunt S, et al. Remembered saccades with variable delay in Parkinson's disease. Mov Disord 1999;14:80–86.

506. MacAskill MR, Anderson TJ, Jones RD. Saccadic adaptation in neurological disorders. Prog Brain Res 2002;140:417–431.

507. Averbuch-Heller L, Stahl JS, Hlavin ML, Leigh RJ. Square-wave jerks induced by pallidotomy in parkinsonian patients. Neurology 1999;52:185–188.

508. Blekher T, Siemers E, Abel LA, Yee RD. Eye movements in Parkinson's disease: before and after pallidotomy. Invest Ophthalmol Vis Sci 2000;41:2177–2183.

509. Kennard C, Zangemeister WH, Mellors S, et al. Eye-head coordination in Parkinson's disease. In: Lennerstrand G, Zee DS, Keller EL, et al. Functional Basis of Ocular Motility Disorders. Oxford, UK, Pergamon, 1982:517–520.

510. White OB, Saint-Cyr JA, Tomlinson RD, et al. Ocular motor deficits in Parkinson's disease. III. Coordination of eye and head movements. Brain 1988;111:115–129.

511. Baloh RW, Jacobson K, Honrubia V. Idiopathic bilateral vestibulopathy. Neurology 1989;39:272–275.

512. Lekwuwa GU, Barnes GR, Collins CJ, Limousin P. Progressive bradykinesia and hypokinesia of ocular pursuit in Parkinson's disease. J Neurol Neurosurg Psychiatry 1999;66:746–753.

513. Melvill Jones G, DeJong JD. Visual tracking of sinusoidal target movement in Parkinson's disease. In D.R.B. Aviation Medical Research Unit (Department of Physiology), Vol 5. McGill University, Montreal, 1974–1976:271–288.

514. Reichert WH, Doolittle J, McDowell FH. Vestibular dysfunction in Parkinson disease. Neurology 1982;32:1133–1138.

515. White OB, Saint-Cyr JA, Sharpe JA. Ocular motor deficits in Parkinson's disease. I. The horizontal vestibulo-ocular reflex and its regulation. Brain 1983;106:555–570.

516. Merchut MP, Brigell M. Olivopontocerebellar atrophy presenting with hemiparkinsonian ocular motor signs. J Clin Neuroophthalmol 1990;10:210–214.

517. Rinne JO, Lee MS, Thompson PD, et al. Corticobasal degeneration: a clinical study of 36 cases. Brain 1994;117:1183–1196.

518. Garbutt S, Harwood MR, Kumar AN, et al. Evaluating small eye movements in patients with saccadic palsies. Ann NY Acad Sci 2003;1004:337–346.

519. Jacobs DH, Adair JC, Heilman KM. Visual grasp in corticobasal degeneration. Ann Neurol 1994;36:679.

520. Eckert T, Sailer M, Kaufmann J, Schrader C, et al. Differentiation of idiopathic Parkinson's disease, multiple system atrophy, progressive supranuclear palsy, and healthy controls using magnetization transfer imaging. Neuroimage 2004;21:229–235.

521. Leigh RJ, Foley JM, Remler BF, et al. Oculogyric crisis: a syndrome of thought disorder and ocular deviation. Ann Neurol 1987;22:13–17.

522. Antunes NL, Small TN, George D, Boulad F, Lis E. Posterior leukoencephalopathy syndrome may not be reversible. Pediatr Neurol 1999;20:241–243.

523. FitzGerald P, Jankovic J. Tardive oculogyric crises. Neurology 1989;39:1434–1437.

524. FitzGerald PM, Jankovic J, Glaze DG, et al. Extrapyramidal involvement in Rett's syndrome. Neurology 1990;40:293–295.

525. Sachdev P. Tardive and chronically recurrent oculogyric crises. Mov Disord 1993;8:93–97.

526. Liu GT, Carrazana EJ, Macklis JD, et al. Delayed oculogyric crises associated with striatocapsular infarction. J Clin Neuroophthalmol 1991;11:198–201.

527. Shimpo T, Fuse S, Yoshizawa A. Retrocollis and oculogyric crisis in association with bilateral putaminal hemorrhages. Clin Neurol 1933;33:40–44.

528. Kim JS, Kim HK, Im JH, et al. Oculogyric crisis and abnormal magnetic resonance imaging signals in bilateral lentiform nuclei. Mov Disorders 1996;11:756–758.

529. Gibson JM, Pimlott R, Kennard C. Ocular motor and manual tracking in Parkinson's disease and the effect of treatment. J Neurol Neurosurg Psychiatry 1987;50:853–860.

530. Highstein SM, Cohen B, Mones R. Changes in saccadic eye movements of patients with Parkinson's disease before and after L-dopa. Trans Am Neurol Assoc 1969;94:277–279.

531. Hotson JR, Langston EB, Langston JW. Saccade responses to dopamine in human MPTP-induced parkinsonism. Ann Neurol 1986;20:456–463.

532. Brooks BA, Fuchs AR, Finocchio D. Saccadic eye movement deficits in the MPTP monkey model of Parkinson's disease. Brain Res 1986;383:404–407.

533. Schultz W, Romo R, Scarnati E, et al. Saccadic reaction times, eye–arm coordination and spontaneous eye movements in normal and MPTP–treated monkeys. Exp Brain Res 1989;78:253–267.

534. Gibson JM, Kennard C. Quantitative study of "on-off" fluctuations in the ocular motor system in Parkinson's disease. Adv Neurol 1986;45:329–333.

535. Sharpe JA, Fletcher WA, Lang AE, et al. Smooth pursuit during dose-related on-off fluctuations in Parkinson's disease. Neurology 1987;37:1389–1392.

536. Shimizu N, Cohen B, Bala SP, et al. Ocular dyskinesias in patients with Parkinson's disease treated with levodopa. Ann Neurol 1977;1:167–171.

537. Hikosaka O. Role of basal ganglia in saccades. Rev Neurol (Paris) 1989;145:580–586.

538. Hikosaka O, Wurtz RH. The basal ganglia. In: Wurtz RH, Goldberg ME, eds. The Neurobiology of Saccadic Eye Movements. Reviews of Oculomotor Research. Vol 3. Amsterdam, Elsevier, 1989:257–281.

539. Ho PC, Feman SS. Internuclear ophthalmoplegia in Fabry's disease. Ann Ophthalmol 1981;13:949–951.

540. Starr A. A disorder of rapid eye movements in Huntington's chorea. Brain 1967;90:545–567.

541. Leigh RJ, Newman SA, Folstein SE, et al. Abnormal ocular motor control in Huntington's disease. Neurology 1983;33:1268–1275.

542. Lasker AG, Zee DS, Hain TC, et al. Saccades in Huntington's disease: initiation defects and distractability. Neurology 1987;37:364–370.

543. Winograd-Gurvich CT, Georgiou-Karistianis N, et al. Hypometric primary saccades and increased variability in visually-guided saccades in Huntington's disease. Neuropsychologia 2003;41:1683–1692.

544. Schapira AH. Mitochondrial function in Huntington's disease: clues for pathogenesis and prospects for treatment. Ann Neurol 1997;41:141–142.

545. Zangemeister WN, Mueller Jensen A. The co-ordination of gaze movements in Huntington's disease. Neuroophthalmology 1985;5:193–206.

546. Lasker AG, Zee DS, Hain TC, et al. Saccades in Huntington's disease: slowing and dysmetria. Neurology 1988;38:427–431.

547. Hotson JR, Louis AA, Langston EB, et al. Vertical saccades in Huntington's disease and nondegenerative choreoathetoid disorders. Neuroophthalmology 1984;4:207–217.

548. Rubin AJ, King WM, Reinbold KA, et al. Quantitative longitudinal assessment of saccades in Huntington's disease. J Clin Neuroophthalmol 1993;13:59–66.

549. Garcia Ruiz PJ, Cenjor C, Ulmer E, et al. [Speed of ocular saccades in Huntington disease. Prospective study]. Neurologia 2001;16:70–73.

550. Fielding J, Georgiou-Karistianis N, Bradshaw J, et al. Impaired modulation of the vestibulo-ocular reflex in Huntington's disease. Mov Disord 2004;19:68–75.

551. Avanzini G, Girotti F, Caraceni T, et al. Oculomotor disorders in Huntington's chorea. J Neurol Neurosurg Psychiatry 1979;42:581–589.

552. Oyanagi K, Takeda S, Takahashi H, et al. A quantitative investigation of the substantia nigra in Huntington's disease. Ann Neurol 1989;26:13–19.

553. Koeppen AH. The nucleus pontis centralis caudalis in Huntington's disease. J Neurol Sci 1989;91:129–141.

554. Leigh RJ, Parhad IM, Clark AW, et al. Brainstem findings in Huntington's disease. Possible mechanisms for slow vertical saccades. J Neurol Sci 1985;71:247–256.

555. Rothlind JC, Brandt J, Zee D, et al. Verbal memory and oculomotor control are unimpaired in asymptomatic adults with the genetic marker for Huntington's disease. Arch Neurol 1993;50:799–802.

556. Reveley MA, Dursun SM, Andrews H. Improvement of abnormal saccadic eye movements in Huntington's disease by sulpiride: a case study. J Psychopharmacol 1994;8:262–265.

557. Rinne JO, Daniel SE, Scaravilli F, et al. The neuropathological features of neuroacanthocytosis. Mov Disord 1994;9:297–304.

558. Nielsen JE, Sorensen S, Hasholt L, et al. Dentatorubral-pallidoluysian atropy. Clinical features of a five-generation Danish family. Mov Disord 1996;11:533–541.

559. Burke JR, Wingfield MS, Lewis KE, et al. The Haw River syndrome: dentatorubropallidoluysian atrophy (DRPLA) in an African-American family. Nature Genet 1994;7:521–524.

560. Stein RW, Kase CS, Hier DB, et al. Caudate hemorrhage. Neurology 1984;34:1549–1554.

561. Vermersch AI, Müri RM, Rivaud S, et al. Saccade disturbances after bilateral lentiform nucleus lesions in humans. J Neurol Neurosurg Psychiatry 1996;60:179–184.

562. Lekwuwa GU, Barnes GR. Cerebral control of eye movements. II. Timing of anticipatory eye movements, predictive pursuit and phase errors in focal cerebral lesions. Brain 1996;119:491–505.

563. Frankel M, Cummings JL. Neuro-ophthalmic abnormalities in Tourette's syndrome: functional and anatomic implications. Neurology 1984;34:359–361.

564. Elston JS, Casgranje F, Lees AJ. The relationship between eye-winking tics, frequent eye-blinking and blepharospasm. J Neurol Neurosurg Psychiatry 1989;52:477–480.

565. Bollen EL, Roos RAC, Cohen AP, et al. Oculomotor control in Gilles de 1a Tourette syndrome. J Neurol Neurosurg Psychiatry 1988;51:1081–1083.

566. Binyon S, Prendergast M. Eye-movement tics in children. Dev Med Child Neurol 1991;33:343–355.

567. Shawkat F, Harris CM, Jacobs M, et al. Eye movement tics. Br J Ophthalmol 1992;76:697–699.

568. Dursun SM, Burke JG, Reveley MA. Antisaccade eye movement abnormalities in Tourette syndrome: evidence for cortico-striatal network dysfunction? J Psychopharmacol 2000;14:37–39.

569. Farber RH, Swerdlow NR, Clementz BA. Saccadic performance characteristics and the behavioural neurology of Tourette's syndrome. J Neurol Neurosurg Psychiatry 1999;66:305–312.

570. LeVasseur AL, Flanagan JR, Riopelle RJ, Munoz DP. Control of volitional and reflexive saccades in Tourette's syndrome. Brain 2001;124:2045–2058.

571. Munoz DP, Le Vasseur AL, Flanagan JR. Control of volitional and reflexive saccades in Tourette's syndrome. Prog Brain Res 2002;140:467–481.

572. Mostofsky SH, Lasker AG, Singer HS, et al. Oculomotor abnormalities in boys with Tourette syndrome with and without ADHD. J Am Acad Child Adolesc Psychiatry 2001;40:1464–1472.

573. Straube A, Mennicken J-B, Riedel M, et al. Saccades in Gilles de la Tourette's syndrome. Mov Disorders 1997;12:536–546.

574. Klein CH, Raschke A, Brandenbusch A. Development of pro- and antisaccades in children with attention-deficit hyperactivity disorder (ADHD) and healthy controls. Psychophysiology 2003;40:17–28.

575. Munoz DP, Armstrong IT, Hampton KA, Moore KD. Altered control of visual fixation and saccadic eye movements in attention-deficit hyperactivity disorder. J Neurophysiol 2003;90:503–514.

576. Demer JL, Holds JB, Hovis LA. Ocular movements in essential blepharospasm. Am J Ophthalmol 1990;110:674–682.

577. Aramideh M, Bour LJ, Koelman JHTM, et al. Abnormal eye movements in blepharospasm and involuntary levator palpebrae inhibition. Brain 1994;117:1457–1474.

578. Bollen E, Van Exel E, van der Velde EA, et al. Saccadic eye movements in idiopathic blepharospasm. Mov Disord 1996;11:678–682.

579. Stell R, Bronstein AM, Marsden CD. Vestibulo-ocular abnormalites in spasmodic torticollis before and after botulinum toxin injections. J Neurol Neurosurg Psychiatry 1989;52:57–62.

580. Thaker GK, Nguyen JA, Tamminga CA. Increased saccadic distractibility in tardive dyskinesia: functional evidence for subcortical GABA dysfunction. Biol Psychiatry 1989;25:49–59.

581. Jinnah HA, Lewis RF, Visser JE, et al. Ocular motor dysfunction in Lesch-Nyhan disease. Pediatr Neurol 2001;24:200–204.

582. Pierrot-Deseilligny C. Eye movement control by the cerebral cortex. Curr Opin Neurol. 2004;17:17–25.

583. Leigh RJ, Kennard C. Using saccades as a research tool in the clinical neurosciences. Brain 2004;127:460–477.

584. Mort DJ, Malhotra P, Mannan SK, Rorden C, et al. The anatomy of visual neglect. Brain 2003;126:1986–1997.

585. Gitelman DR. Attention and its disorders. Br Med Bull 2003;65:21–34.

586. Mapstone M, Weintraub S, Nowinski C, et al. Cerebral hemispheric specialization for spatial attention: spatial distribution of search-related eye fixations in the absence of neglect. Neuropsychologia 2003;41:1396–1409.

587. Mort DJ, Kennard C. Visual search and its disorders. Curr Opin Neurol 2003;16:51–57.

588. Goodwin JA, Kansu T. Vulpian's sign: conjugate eye deviation in acute cerebral hemisphere lesions. Neurology 1986;36:711–712 .

589. Tijssen CC. Horizontal conjugate eye deviation. A clinical and electrophysiological study. Doctoral thesis, Nijmegen University, The Netherlands, 1988.

590. Kömpf D, Gmeiner HJ. Gaze palsy and visual hemineglect in acute hemisphere lesions. Neuroophthalmology 1989;9:49–53.

591. Johnston CW. Eye movements in visual hemi-neglect. In: Johnston CW, Pirozzolo FJ, eds. Neuropsychology of Eye Movements. Hillsdale, NJ, Lawrence Earlbaum, 1988:235–263.

592. Steiner I, Melamed E. Conjugate eye deviation after acute hemispheric stroke: delayed recovery after previous contralateral frontal lobe damage. Ann Neurol 1984;16:509–511.

593. Lekwuwa GU, Barnes GR. Cerebral control of eye movements. I. The relationship between cerebral lesion sites and smooth-pursuit deficits. Brain 1996;119:473–490.

594. Tusa RJ, Zee DS, Nerdman SJ. Effect of unilateral cerebral cortical lesions on ocular motor behavior in monkeys: saccades and quick phases. J Neurophysiol 1986;56:1590–1625.

595. Fletcher WA, Gellman RS. Saccades in humans with lesions of frontal eye fields (FEF). Society for Neuroscience Abstracts 1989;15:1203.

596. Meador KJ, Loring DW, Lee GP, et al. Hemisphere asymmetry for eye gaze mechanisms. Brain 1989;112:103–111.

597. Lesser RP, Leigh RJ, Dinner DS, et al. Preservation of voluntary saccades after intracarotid injection of barbiturate. Neurology 1985;35:1108–1112.

598. Tijssen CC, Van Gisbergen JAM, Schulte BPM. Conjugate eye deviation: side, site, and size of the hemispheric lesion. Neurology 1991;41:846–850.

599. Tijssen CC, Van Gisbergen JAM. Conjugate eye deviation after hemispheric stroke: a contralateral saccadic palsy? Neuroophthalmology 1993;13:107–118.

600. Morrow MJ. Craniotopic defects of smooth-pursuit and saccadic eye movement. Neurology 1996;46:514–521.

601. Tijssen CC. Contralateral conjugate eye deviation in acute supratentorial lesions. Stroke 1994;25:1516–1519.

602. Blacker DJ, Wijdicks EF. Delayed complete bilateral ptosis associated with massive infarction of the right hemisphere. Mayo Clin Proc 2003;78:836–839.

603. Cogan DG. Neurologic significance of lateral conjugate deviation of the eyes on forced closure of the lids. Arch Ophthalmol 1948;39:37–42.

604. Sullivan HC, Kaminski HJ, Maas EF, et al. Lateral deviation of the eyes on forced lid closure in patients with cerebral lesions. Arch Neurol 1991;48:310–311.

605. Sharpe JA, Lo AW, Rabinovitch HE. Control of the saccadic and smooth-pursuit systems after cerebral hemidecortication. Brain 1979;102:387–403.

606. Troost BT, Daroff RB, Weber RB, et al. Hemispheric control of eye movements. II. Quantitative analysis of smooth pursuit in a hemispherectomy patient. Arch Neurol 1972;27:449–452.

607. Cogan DG, Loeb DR. Optokinetic response and intracranial lesions. Arch Neurol Psychiatry 1949;61:183–187.

608. Troost BT, Daroff RB, Weber RB, et al. Hemispheric control of eye movements. II. Quantitative analysis of smooth pursuit in a hemispherectomy patient. Arch Neurol 1972;27:449–452.

609. Estanol B, Romero R, de Viteri MS, et al. Oculomotor and oculovestibular functions in a hemispherectomy patient. Arch Neurol 1980;37:365–368.

610. Sharpe JA, Lo AW. Voluntary and visual control of the vestibuloocular reflex after cerebral hemidecortication. Ann Neurol 1981;10:164–172.

611. Traccis S, Puliga MV, Ruiu MC, et al. Unilateral occipital lesion causing hemianopia affects the acoustic saccadic programming. Neurology 1991;41:1633–1638.

612. Zihl J. Eye movement patterns in hemianopic dyslexia. Brain 1995;118: 891–912.

613. Meienberg O, Büttner-Ennever JA, Kraus-Ruppert R. Unilateral paralysis of conjugate gaze due to lesion of the abducens nucleus: clinico-pathological case report. Neuroophthalmology 1981;2:47–52.

614. Meienberg O, Harrer M, Wehren C. Oculographic diagnosis of hemineglect in patients with homonymous hemianopia. J Neurol 1986;233:97–101.

615. Meienberg O. Clinical examination of saccadic eye movements in hemianopia. Neurology 1983;11:1315.

616. Zangemeister WN, Meienenberg O, Stark L, et al. Eye-head coordination in homonymous hemianopia. J Neurol 1982;43:254.

617. Segraves MA, Goldberg ME, Deng SY, et al. The role of striate cortex in the guidance of eye movements in the monkey. J Neurosci 1987;7:3040–3058.

618. Kolmel HW, Nabel HJ. Optokinetic nystagmus in homonymous hemianopia due to a strictly occipital lesion. Eur Arch Psychiatry Neurol Sci 1989;99:202.

619. Rizzo M, Hurtig R. The effect of bilateral visual cortex lesions on the development of eye movements. Neurology 1989;6:413.

620. Zee DS, Tusa RJ, Herdman SJ, et al. Effects of occipital lobectomy upon eye movements in primate. J Neurophysiol 1987;58:883–907.

621. Brindley GS, Gautier-Smith PC, Lewin W. Cortical blindness and the functions of the nongeniculate fibers of the optic tracts. J Neurol Neurosurg Psychiatry 1969;9:264.

622. Fox JC, Holmes G. Optic nystagmus and its value in the localization of cerebral lesions. Brain 1926;3:371.

623. Kjallman L, Frisén L. The cerebral ocular pursuit pathways: a clinicoradiological study of small-field optokinetic nystagmus. J Clin Neuroophthalmol 1986;6: 209–217.

624. Heide W, Koenig E, Dichgans J. Optokinetic nystagmus, self-motion sensation and their after-effects in patients with occipitoparietal lesions. Clin Vis Sci 1990; 156:133–143.

625. Heide W, Kurzidim K, Kömpf D. Deficits of smooth-pursuit eye movements after frontal and parietal lesions. Brain 1996;119:1951–1969.

626. Morrow MJ, Sharpe JA. Retinoptic and directional deficits of smooth-pursuit initiation after posterior cerebral hemispheric lesions. Neurology 1993;43: 595–603.

627. Dursteler MR, Wurtz RH. Pursuit and optokinetic deficits following chemical lesions of cortical areas MT and MST. J Neurophysiol 1988;60:940–965.

628. Leigh RJ. The cortical control of ocular pursuit movements. Rev Neurol (Paris) 1989;5:612.

629. Barton JJS, Sharpe JA, Raymond JE. Retinoptic and directional defects in motion discrimination in humans with cerebral lesions. Ann Neurol 1995;5:675.

630. Barton JJS, Sharpe JA, Raymond JE. Directional defects in pursuit and motion perception in humans with unilateral cerebral lesions. Brain 1996;535:1550.

631. Barton JJS, Simpson T, Kiriakopoulos E, et al. Functional MRI of lateral occipitotemporal cortex during pursuit and motion perception. Ann Neurol 1996;7: 398.

632. Thurston SE, Leigh RJ, Crawford T, et al. Two distinct deficits of visual tracking caused by unilateral lesions of cerebral cortex in humans. Ann Neurol 1988;6: 266–273.

633. Morrow MJ, Sharpe JA. Smooth-pursuit initiation in humans with cerebral hemispheric lesions. Society for Neuroscience Abstracts 1989;14:612.

634. Lawden MC, Bagelmann H, Crawford TJ, et al. An effect of structured backgrounds on smooth-pursuit eye movements in patients with cerebral lesions. Brain 1995;118:37–48.

635. Bogousslavsky J, Regli F. Pursuit gaze defects in acute and chronic unilateral parieto-occipital lesions. Eur Neurol 1986;25:10–18.

636. Ghika J, Ghika-Schmid F, Bogousslavsky J. Parietal motor syndrome: a clinical description in 32 patients in the acute phase of pure parietal strokes studied prospectively. Clin Neurol Neurosurg 1998;100:271–282.

637. Morrow MJ, Sharpe JA. Cerebral hemispheric localization of smooth-pursuit asymmetry. Neurology 1990;40:284–292.

638. Kömpf D, Oppermann J. Vertical gaze palsy and thalamic dementia. Syndrome of the posterior thalamosubthalamic paramedian artery. Neuroophthalmology 1986;6:121–124.

639. Pierrot-Deseilligny C, Rivaud S, Samson Y, et al. Some instructive cases concerning the circuitry of ocular smooth pursuit in the brainstem. Neuroophthalmology 1989;9:31–42.

640. Baloh RW, Yee RD, Honrubia V. Optokinetic nystagmus and parietal lobe lesions. Ann Neurol 1980;7:269–276.

641. Ventre J, Faugier-Grimaud S. Effects of posterior parietal lesions (area 7) on VOR in monkeys. Exp Brain Res 1986;62:654–658.

642. Pierrot-Deseilligny C, Rivaud S, Penet C, et al. Latencies of visually guided saccades in unilateral hemispheric cerebral lesions. Ann Neurol 1987;21: 138–148.

643. Sundqvist A. Saccadic reaction-time in parietal-lobe dysfunction. Lancet 1979; 1:870.

644. Lynch JC, McLaren JW. Deficits of visual attention and saccadic eye movements after lesions of parieto-ocipital cortex in monkeys. J Neurophysiol 1989;61: 74–90.

645. Heide W, Blankenburg M, Zimmerman E, et al. Cortical control of double-step saccades: implications for spatial orientation. Ann Neurol 1995;38:739–748.

646. Bogousslavsky J. Impairment of visually evoked eye movements with a unilateral parieto-occipital lesion. J Neurol 1987;234:160–162.

647. Ron S, Schmid R, Orpaz D. Applying a model of saccadic prediction to patients' saccadic eye movements. Brain Behav Evol 1989;33:179–182.

648. Muri RM, Gaymard B, Rivaud S, et al. Hemispheric asymmetry in cortical control of memory-guided saccades. A transcranial magnetic stimulation study. Neuropsychologia 2000;38:1105–1111.

649. Shimozaki SS, Hayhoe MM, Zelinsky GJ, et al. Effect of parietal lobe lesions on saccade targeting and spatial memory in a naturalistic visual search task. Neuropsychologia 2003;41:1365–1386.

650. Posner MI, Walker JA, Friedrich FJ, et al. Effects of parietal injury on covert orienting of attention. J Neurosci 1984;4:1863–1874.

651. Pierrot-Deseilligny C. Saccades and smooth-pursuit impairment after cerebral hemispheric lesions. Eur Neurol 1994;34:121–134.

652. Walker R, Findlay JM. Saccadic eye movement programming in unilateral neglect. Neuropsychologia 1996;34:493–508.

653. Ferber S, Danckert J, Joanisse M, et al. Eye movements tell only half the story. Neurology 2003;60:1826–1829.

654. Duhamel J-R, Goldberg ME, Fitzgibbon EJ, et al. Saccadic dysmetria in a patient with a right frontoparietal lesion: the importance of corollary discharge for accurate spatial-behavior. Brain 1992;115:1387–1402.

655. Vuilleumier P, Schwartz S. Modulation of visual perception by eye gaze direction in patients with spatial neglect and extinction. Neuroreport 2001;12: 2101–2104.

656. Gaymard B, Lynch J, Ploner CJ, et al. The parieto-collicular pathway: anatomical location and contribution to saccade generation. Eur J Neurosci 2003;17: 1518–1526.

657. Zihl J, Hebel N. Patterns of oculomotor scanning in patients with unilateral posterior parietal or frontal lobe damage. Neuropsychologia 1997;35:893–906.

658. Niemeier M, Karnath HO. Exploratory saccades show no direction-specific deficit in neglect. Neurology 2000;54:515–518.

659. Wardak C, Olivier E, Duhamel JR. Saccadic target selection deficits after lateral intraparietal area inactivation in monkeys. J Neurosci 2002;22:9877–9884.

660. Leigh RJ, Tusa RJ. Disturbance of smooth pursuit caused by infarction of occipitoparietal cortex. Ann Neurol 1985;17:185–187.

661. Carmichael EA, Dix MR, Hall-Pike CS. Lesions of the cerebral hemispheres and their effects upon optokinetic and caloric nystagmus. Brain 1954;77:345–372.

662. Straube A, Brandt T. Importance of the visual and vestibular cortex for self-motion perception in man (circularvection). Hum Neurobiol 1987;6:211–218.

663. Bottini G, Karnath HO, Vallar G, et al. Cerebral representations for egocentric space: functional-anatomical evidence from caloric vestibular stimulation and neck vibration. Brain 2001;124:1182–1196.

664. Kluge M, Beyenburg S, Fernandez G, Elger CE. Epileptic vertigo: evidence for vestibular representation in human frontal cortex. Neurology 2000;55: 1906–1908.

665. Brandt T, Dieterich M. The vestibular cortex. Its locations, functions, and disorders. Ann NY Acad Sci 1999;871:293–312.

666. Bucher SF, Dieterich M, Wiesmann M, et al. Cerebral functional magnetic resonance imaging of vestibular, auditory, and nociceptive areas during galvanic stimulation. Ann Neurol 1998;44:120–125.

667. Dieterich M, Brandt T. Vestibular system: anatomy and functional magnetic resonance imaging. Neuroimaging Clin North Am 2001;11:263–273.

668. Dieterich M, Brandt T. Brain activation studies on visual-vestibular and ocular motor interaction. Curr Opin Neurol 2000;13:13–18.

669. Schneider D, Schneider L, Claussen CF, Kolchev C. Cortical representation of the vestibular system as evidenced by brain electrical activity mapping of vestibular late evoked potentials. Ear Nose Throat J 2001;80:251–260.

670. Kahane P, Hoffmann D, Minotti L, Berthoz A. Reappraisal of the human vestibular cortex by cortical electrical stimulation study. Ann Neurol 2003;54:615–624.

671. Israël I, Rivaud S, Gaymard B, et al. Cortical control of vestibular-guided saccades. Brain 1995;118:1169–1184.

672. Müri RM, Rivaud S, Timsit S, et al. Role of the medial temporal lobe in the control of memory-guided saccade. Exp Brain Res 1994;101:165–168.

673. Nielsen JM. Tornado epilepsy simulating Ménière's syndrome. Neurology 1959; 9:794–796.

674. Smith BN. Vestibular disturbances in epilepsy. Neurology 1960;10:465–469.

675. Barac B. Vertiginous epileptic attacks and so-called "vestibulogenic seizures." Epilepsia 1968;9:137–144.

676. Schneider RC, Calhoun HD, Crosby EC. Vertigo and rotational movement in cortical and subcortical lesions. J Neurol Sci 1968;6:493–516.

677. Kogeorgos J, Scott DF, Swash M. Epileptic dizziness. Br Med J 1981;282: 687–689.

678. Furman JMR, Crumrine PK, Reinmuth OM. Epileptic nystagmus. Ann Neurol 1990;27:686–688.

679. Wiest G, Zimprich F, Prayer D, et al. Vestibular processing in human paramedian precuneus as shown by electrical cortical stimulation. Neurology 2004;62: 473–475.

680. Latto R, Cowey A. Fixation changes after frontal eye-field lesions in monkey. Brain Res 1971;30:25–36.

681. Tanaka H, Arai M, Kubo J, Hirata K. Conjugate eye deviation with head version due to a cortical infarction of the frontal eye field. Stroke 2002;33:642–643.

682. Pessin MS, Adelman LS, Prager RJ, et al. "Wrong-way eyes" in supratentorial hemorrhage. Ann Neurol 1981;9:79–81.
683. Blanke O, Spinelli L, Thut G, et al. Location of the human frontal eye field as defined by electrical cortical stimulation: anatomical, functional and electrophysiological characteristics. Neuroreport 2000;11:1907–1913.
684. Sharpe JA. Adaptation to frontal lobe lesions. In: Keller EL, Zee DS, eds. Adaptive Processes in Visual and Oculomotor Systems. Oxford, Pergamon, 1986: 239–246.
685. Magel-Leiby S, Buchtel HA, Welch A. Cerebral control of directed visual attention and orienting saccades. Brain 1990;113:237–276.
686. Braun DI, Weber H, Mergner T, et al. Saccadic reaction times in patients with frontal and parietal lesions. Brain 1992;115:1359–1386.
687. Rivaud S, Muri RM, Gaymard B, et al. Eye movement disorders after frontal eye field lesions in humans. Exp Brain Res 1994;102:110–120.
688. Deng S-Y, Goldberg ME, Segraves MA, et al. The effect of unilateral ablation of the frontal eye fields on saccadic performance in the monkey. In: Keller EL, Zee DS, eds. Adaptive Processes in Visual and Oculomotor Systems. Oxford, Pergamon, 1986:201–208.
689. Guitton D, Buchtel HA, Douglas RM. Frontal lobe lesions in man cause difficulties in suppressing reflexive glances and in generating goal-directed saccades. Exp Brain Res 1985;58:455–472.
690. Pierrot-Deseilligny C, Rivaud S, Gaymard B, et al. Cortical control of reflexive visually-guided saccades. Brain 1991;114:1473–1485.
691. Machado L, Rafal RD. Control of fixation and saccades during an anti-saccade task: an investigation in humans with chronic lesions of oculomotor cortex. Neuropsychology 2004;18:115–123
692. Pierrot-Deseilligny C, Israël I, Berthoz A, et al. Role of the differential frontal lobe areas in the control of the horizontal component of memory-guided saccades in man. Exp Brain Res 1993;95:166–171.
693. Pierrot-Deseilligny C, Muri RM, et al. Decisional role of the dorsolateral prefrontal cortex in ocular motor behaviour. Brain 2003;126:1460–1473.
694. Iba M, Sawaguchi T. Involvement of the dorsolateral prefrontal cortex of monkeys in visuospatial target selection. J Neurophysiol 2003;89:587–599.
695. Milea D, Napolitano M, Dechy H, et al. Complete bilateral horizontal gaze paralysis disclosing multiple sclerosis. J Neurol Neurosurg Psychiatry 2001;70: 252–255.
696. Gaymard B, Pierrot-Deseilligny C, Rivaud S. Impairment of sequences of memory guided saccades after supplementary motor area lesions. Ann Neurol 1990; 28:622–626.
697. Lu X, Matsuzawa M, Hikosaka O. A neural correlate of oculomotor sequences in supplementary eye field. Neuron 2002;34:317–325.
698. Pierrot-Deseilligny C, Rivaud S, Gaymard B, et al. Cortical control of memory-guided saccades in man. Exp Brain Res 1991;83:607–617.
699. Husain M, Parton A, Hodgson TL, et al. Self-control during response conflict by human supplementary eye field. Nat Neurosci 2003;6:117–118.
700. Morrow MJ, Sharpe JA. Deficits of smooth-pursuit eye movement after unilateral frontal lobe lesions. Ann Neurol 1995;37:443–451
701. Fukushima K. Frontal cortical control of smooth-pursuit. Curr Opin Neurobiol 2003;13:647–654.
702. Moser A, Kömpf D. Unilateral visual exploration deficit in a frontal lobe lesion. Neuroophthalmology 1990;10:39–44.
703. Pierrot-Deseilligny C, Gautier JC, Loron P. Acquired ocular motor apraxia due to bilateral frontoparietal infarcts. Ann Neurol 1988;23:199–202.
704. Dehaene I, Lammens M. Paralysis of saccades and pursuit: clinicopathologic study. Neurology 1991;41:414–415.
705. Schiller PH, True SD, Conway JL. Deficits in eye movements following frontal eye-field and superior colliculus ablations. J Neurophysiol 1980;44:1175–1189.
706. Rizzo M. "Balint's syndrome" and associated visuospatial disorders. Baillieres Clin Neurol 1993;2:415–437.
707. Tsutsui J, Takeda J, Ichihashi S, et al. Ocular motor apraxia and lesions of the visual association area. Neuroophthalmology 1980;1:149–154.
708. Pierrot-Deseilligny C, Gray F, Brunet P. Infarcts of both inferior parietal lobules with impairment of visually guided eye movements, peripheral visual attention and optic ataxia. Brain 1986;109:81–97.
709. Pierrot-Deseilligny C. Controle cortical des saccades. Rev Neurol (Paris) 1989; 145:596–604.
710. Watson RT, Rapcsak SZ. Loss of spontaneous blinking in a patient with Balint's syndrome. Arch Neurol 1989;46:567–570.
711. Gottlieb D, Calvanio R, Levine DN. Reappearance of the visual percept after intentional blinking in a patient with Balint's syndrome. J Clin Neuroophthalmol 1991;11:62–65.
712. Johnston JL, Sharpe JA, Morrow MJ. Spasm of fixation: a quantitative study. J Neurol Sci 1992;107:166–171.
713. Gittinger JW Jr, Sokol S. The visual-evoked potential in the diagnosis of congenital ocular motor apraxia. Am J Ophthalmol 1982;93:700–703.
714. Zee DS, Yee RD, Singer HS. Congenital ocular motor apraxia. Brain 1977;100: 581–589.
715. Fielder AR, Gresty MA, Dodd KL, et al. Congenital ocular motor apraxia. Trans Ophthalmol Soc UK 1986;105:589–598.
716. Harris C, Shawkat F, Russell-Eggitt I, et al. Intermittent horizontal saccade failure ("ocular motor apraxia") in children. Br J Ophthalmol 1996;80:151–158.

717. Catalano RA, Calhoun JH, Reinecke RD, et al. Asymmetry in congenital ocular motor apraxia. Can J Ophthalmol 1988;23:318–321.
718. Eustace P, Beigi B, Bowell R, et al. Congenital ocular motor apraxia: an inability to unlock the vestibulo-ocular reflex. Neuroophthalmology 1994;14:167–174.
719. Cogan DG. Ophthalmic manifestations of bilateral non-occipital cerebral lesions. Br J Ophthalmol 1965;49:281–297.
720. Russo PA, Flynn MF, Veith J. Congenital ocular motor apraxia with torsional oscillations: a case report. Optom Vis Sci 1995;72:925–930.
721. Shawkat FS, Kingsley D, Kendall B, et al. Neuroradiological and eye movement correlates in children with intermittent saccade failure: "ocular motor apraxia." Neuropediatrics 1995;26:298–305.
722. Le BI, Moreira MC, Rivaud-Pechoux S, et al. Cerebellar ataxia with oculomotor apraxia type 1: clinical and genetic studies. Brain 2003;126:2761–2772.
723. Le B, Bouslam N, Rivaud-Pechoux S, et al. Frequency and phenotypic spectrum of ataxia with oculomotor apraxia 2: a clinical and genetic study in 18 patients. Brain 2004;127:759–767.
724. Tusa RJ, Hove MT. Ocular and oculomotor signs in Joubert syndrome. J Child Neurol 1999;14:621–627.
725. Prasad P, Nair S. Congenital ocular motor apraxia: sporadic and familial. J Neuroophthalmol 1994;14:102–104.
726. Gurer YK, Kukner S, Kunak B, et al. Congenital ocular motor apraxia in two siblings. Pediatr Neurol 1995;13:261–262.
727. Stell R, Bronstein AM, Plant GT, et al. Ataxia telangiectasia: a reappraisal of the ocular motor features and their value in the diagnosis of atypical cases. Mov Disord 1989;4:320–329.
728. Patterson MC, Horowitz M, Abel RB, et al. Isolated horizontal supranuclear gaze palsy as a marker of severe systemic involvement in Gaucher's disease. Neurology 1993;43:1993–1997.
729. Gascon GG, Abdo N, Sigut D, et al. Ataxia-oculomotor apraxia syndrome. J Child Neurol 1995;10:118–122.
730. Nezu A. Neurophysiological study in Pelizaeus-Merzbacher disease. Brain Dev 1995;17:175–181.
731. Aicardi J, Barbosa C, Andermann E, et al. Ataxia-ocular motor apraxia: a syndrome mimicking ataxia-telangiectasia. Ann Neurol 1988;24:497–502.
732. Farr AK, Shalev B, Crawford TO, et al. Ocular manifestations of ataxia-telangiectasia. Am J Ophthalmol 2002;134:891–896.
733. Lewis RF, Crawford TO. Slow target–directed eye movements in ataxia-telangiectasia. Invest Ophthalmol Vis Sci 2002;43:686–691.
734. Lewis RF. Ocular motor apraxia and ataxia-telangiectasia. Arch Neurol 2001; 58:1312.
735. Lewis RF, Lederman HM, Crawford TO. Ocular motor abnormalities in ataxia telangiectasia. Ann Neurol 1999;46:287–295.
736. Currie J, Ramsden B, McArthur C, et al. Validation of a clinical antisaccade eye movement test in the assessment of dementia. Arch Neurol 1991;48:644–648.
737. Abel LA, Unverzagt F, Yee RD. Effects of stimulus predictability and interstimulus gap on saccades in Alzheimer's disease. Dement Geriatr Cogn Disord 2002; 13:235–243.
738. Lueck KL, Mendez MF, Perryman KM. Eye movement abnormalities during reading in patients with Alzheimer disease. Neuropsychiatry Neuropsychol Behav Neurol 2000;13:77–82.
739. Schewe HJ, Uebelhack R, Vohs K. Abnormality in saccadic eye movement in dementia. Eur Psychiatry 1999;14:52–53.
740. Shafiq-Antonacci R, Maruff P, Masters C, Currie J. Spectrum of saccade system function in Alzheimer disease. Arch Neurol 2003;60:1272–1278.
741. Fletcher WA, Sharpe JA. Saccadic eye movement dysfunction in Alzheimer's disease. Ann Neurol 1986;20:464–471.
742. Daffner KR, Scinto LFM, Weintraub S, et al. Diminished curiosity in patients with probable Alzheimer's disease as measured by exploratory eye movements. Neurology 1992;42:320–328.
743. Scinto LFM, Daffner KR, Castro L, et al. Impairment of spatially directed attention in patients with probable Alzheimer's disease as measured by eye movements. Arch Neurol 1994;51:682–688.
744. Hof PR, Bouras C, Constantinidis J, et al. Balint's syndrome in Alzheimer disease: specific disruption of the occipito-parietal visual pathway. Brain Res 1989; 493:368–375.
745. Fletcher WA, Sharpe JA. Smooth-pursuit dysfunction in Alzheimer's disease. Neurology 1988;38:272–277.
746. Zaccara G, Gangemi PF, Muscas GC, et al. Smooth-pursuit eye movements: alterations in Alzheimer's disease. J Neurol Sci 1992;112:81–89.
747. Bertoni JM, Label LS, Sackelleres JC, et al. Supranuclear gaze palsy in familial Creutzfeldt-Jakob disease. Arch Neurol 1983;40:618–622.
748. Grant MP, Cohen M, Petersen RB, et al. Abnormal eye movements in Creutzfeldt-Jakob disease. Ann Neurol 1993;34:192–197.
749. Helmchen C, Büttner U. Centripetal nystagmus in a case of Creutzfeldt-Jacob disease. Neuroophthalmology 1985;15:187–192.
750. Smith SJM, Kocen RS. A Creutzfeldt-Jakob-like syndrome due to lithium toxicity. J Neurol Neurosurg Psychiatry 1988;51:120–123.
751. Gordon MF, Abrams RI, Rubin DB, et al. Bismuth subsalicylate toxicity as a cause of prolonged encephalopathy with myoclonus. Mov Disord 1995;10: 220–222.

752. Farlow MR, Yee RD, Dlouhy SR, et al. Gerstmann-Straussler-Scheinker disease. I. Extending the clinical spectrum. Neurology 1989;39:1446–1452.

753. Yee RD, Farlow MR, Suzuki DA, et al. Abnormal eye movements in Gerstmann-Sträussler-Scheinker disease. Arch Ophthalmol 1992;110:68–74.

754. Currie J, Benson E, Ramsden B, et al. Eye movement abnormalities as a predictor of the acquired immunodeficiency syndrome dementia complex. Arch Neurol 1988;9:953.

755. Hamed LM, Schatz NJ, Galetta SL. Brainstem ocular motility defects and AIDS. Am J Ophthalmol 1988;106:437–442.

756. Jabs DA, Green WR, Fox R, et al. Ocular manifestations of acquired immune deficiency syndrome. Ophthalmology 1989;92:1099.

757. Keane JR. Neuro-ophthalmologic signs in AIDS: 50 patients. Neurology 1991; 1:845.

758. Hedges TR III. Ophthalmoplegia associated with AIDS. Surv Ophthalmol 1994; 39:51.

759. Merril PT, Paige GD, Abrams RA, et al. Ocular motor abnormalities in human immunodeficiency virus infection. Ann Neurol 1991;30:130–138.

760. Johnston JL, Miller JD, Nath A. Ocular motor dysfunction in HIV-1-infected subjects: a quantitative oculographic analysis. Neurology 1996;1:457.

761. Brekelmans GJF, Tijssen CC. Acquired ocular motor apraxia in an AIDS patient with bilateral fronto-parietal lesions. Neuroophthalmology 1990;56.

762. Tagliati M, Simpson D, Morgello S, et al. Cerebellar degeneration associated with human immunodeficiency virus infection. Neurology 1998;4:251.

763. Pfister HW, Einhaupl KM, Büttner U, et al. Dissociated nystagmus as a common sign of ocular motor disorders in HIV-infected patients. Eur Neurol 1989;7:280.

764. Nguyen N, Rimmer S, Katz B. Slowed saccades in the acquired immunodeficiency syndrome. Am J Ophthalmol 1989;107:356–360.

765. Sweeney JA, Brew BJ, Keilp JG, et al. Pursuit eye movement dysfunction in HIV-1 seropositive individuals. J Psychiatr Neurosci 1991;16:247–252.

766. Thurston SE, Leigh RJ, Osorio L. Epileptic gaze deviation and nystagmus. Neurology 1985;35:1518–1521.

767. Kaplan PW, Tusa RJ. Neurophysiologic and clinical correlations of epileptic nystagmus. Neurology 1993;43:2508–2514.

768. Gire C, Somma-Mauvais H, Nicaise C, et al. Epileptic nystagmus: electroclinical study of a case. Epileptic Disord 2001;3:33–37.

769. Grant AC, Jain V, Bose S. Epileptic monocular nystagmus. Neurology 2002; 59:1438–1441.

770. Hughes JR, Fino JJ. Epileptic nystagmus and its possible relationship with PGO spikes. Clin Electroencephalogr 2003;34:32–38.

771. Kellinghaus C, Loddenkemper T, Luders HO. Epileptic monocular nystagmus. Neurology 2003;61:145–147.

772. Moster ML, Schnayder E. Epileptic periodic alternating nystagmus. J Neuroophthalmol 1998;18:292–293.

773. Goodfellow GW, Allison CL, Schiange DG. Unusual eye movements in a patient with complex partial seizure disorder. Optometry 2002;73:160–165.

774. Garcia-Pastor A, Lopez-Esteban P, Peraita-Adrados R. Epileptic nystagmus: a case study video-EEG correlation. Epileptic Disord 2002;4:23–28.

775. Bogacz J, Bogacz D, Bogacz A. Oculomotor phenomena in petit-mal. Clin Neurophysiol 2000;111:959–963.

776. Kent L, Blake A, Whitehouse W. Eyelid myoclonia with absences: phenomenology in children. Seizure 1998;7:193–199.

777. Young GB, Brown JD, Bolton CF, et al. Periodic lateralized epileptiform discharges (PLEDs) and nystagmus retractorius. Ann Neurol 1977;2:61–62.

778. Brenner RP, Carlow TJ. PLEDS and nystagmus retractorius. Ann Neurol 1979; 5:403.

779. Nelson KR, Brenner RP, Carlow TJ. Divergent-convergent eye movements and transient eyelid opening associated with an EEG burst-suppression pattern. J Clin Neuroophthalmol 1986;6:43–46.

780. Watanabe K, Negoro T, Matsumoto A, et al. Epileptic nystagmus associated with typical absence seizures. Epilepsia 1984;25:22–24.

781. Horita H, Hoashi E, Okuyama Y, et al. The studies of the attacks of abnormal eye movement in a case of infantile spasms. Folia Psychiatrica Neurol Jpn 1977; 31:393–402.

782. Rosenbaum DA, Siegel M, Rowan AJ. Contraversive seizures in occipital epilepsy: case report and review of the literature. Neurology 1986;36:281–284.

783. Tusa RJ, Kaplan PW, Main TC, et al. Ipsiversive eye deviation and epileptic nystagmus. Neurology 1990;40:662–665.

784. Stolz SE, Chatrian G, Spence AM. Epileptic nystagmus. Epilepsia 1991;32: 910–918.

785. Keating EG, Gooley SG. Disconnection of parietal and occipital access to the saccadic oculomotor system. Exp Brain Res 1988;70:385–398.

786. Kaplan PW, Lesser RP. Vertical and horizontal epileptic gaze deviation and nystagmus. Neurology 1989;39:1391–1393.

787. Bruce CJ, Goldberg ME, Bushnell MC, et al. Primate frontal eye fields. II. Physiological and anatomical correlates of electrically evoked eye movements. J Neurophysiol 1985;54:714–734.

788. Quesney LF. Seizures of frontal lobe origin. In: Pedley TA, Meldrum BS, eds. Recent Advances in Epilepsy, 3. Edinburgh, Churchill Livingstone, 1986: 81–110.

789. Wyllie E, Luders H, Morris HH, et al. The lateralizing significance of versive head and eye movements during epileptic seizures. Neurology 1986;36:606–611.

790. Wyllie E, Luders H, Morris HH, et al. Ipsilateral forced head and eye turning at the end of the generalized tonic-clonic phase of versive seizures. Neurology 1986;36:1212–1217.

791. Ochs R, Gloor P, Quesney F, et al. Does headturning during a seizure have lateralizing or localizing significance? Neurology 1984;34:884–890.

792. Gloor P, Quesney F, Ives J, et al. Significance of direction of head turning during seizures. Neurology 1987;37:1092.

793. Bender MB. Oscillopsia. Arch Neurol 1965;13:204–213.

794. Vignaendra V, Lim CL. Epileptic discharges triggered by eye convergence. Neurology 1978;28:589–591.

795. Shanzer S, April R, Atkin A. Seizures induced by eye deviation. Arch Neurol 1965;13:621–626.

796. Fisher CM. The neurological examination of the comatose patient. Acta Neurol Scand 1969;45(Suppl 36):1–56.

797. Plum F, Posner JB. Diagnosis of Stupor and Coma, 3rd ed. Philadelphia, FA Davis, 1980.

798. Buettner UW, Zee DS. Vestibular testing in comatose patients. Arch Neurol 1989;46:561–563.

799. Simon RP. Forced downward ocular deviation. Occurrence during oculovestibular testing in sedative drug-induced coma. Arch Neurol 1978;35:456–458.

800. Rosenberg ML. The eyes in hysterical states of unconsciousness. J Clin Neuroophthalmol 1982;2:259–260.

801. Keane JR. Sustained upgaze in coma. Ann Neurol 1981;9:409–412.

802. Nakada T, Kwee IL, Lee H. Sustained upgaze in coma. J Clin Neuroophthalmol 1984;4:35–37.

803. Keane JR. Spastic eyelids. Failure of levator inhibition in unconscious states. Arch Neurol 1975;32:695–698.

804. Keane JR. Acute vertical ocular myoclonus. Neurology 1986;36:86–89.

805. Fisher CM. Ocular bobbing. Arch Neurol 1964;11:543–546.

806. Mehler MF. The clinical spectrum of ocular bobbing and ocular dipping. J Neurol Neurosurg Psychiatry 1988;51:725–727.

807. Brusa A, Firpo MP, Massa S, et al. Typical and reverse bobbing: a case with localizing value. Eur Neurol 1984;23:151–155.

808. Rosenberg ML, Calvert PC. Ocular bobbing in association with other signs of midbrain dysfunction. Arch Neurol 1986;43:314.

809. Goldschmidt TJ, Wall M. Slow upward ocular bobbing. J Clin Neuroophthalmol 1987;7:241–243.

810. Titer EM, Laureno R. Inverse/reverse ocular bobbing. Ann Neurol 1988;23: 103–104.

811. Rosenberg ML, Calvert PC. Ocular bobbing in association with other signs of midbrain dysfunction. Arch Neurol 1986;43:314.

812. Noda S, Ide K, Umezaki M, et al. Repetitive divergence. Ann Neurol 1987;21: 109–110.

813. Oesterle CS, Faulkner WJ, Clay R, et al. Eye bobbing associated with jaw movement. Ophthalmology 1982;89:63–67.

814. Ishikawa H, Ishikawa S, Mukuno K. Short-cycle periodic (ping-pong) gaze. Neurology 1993;43:1067–1070.

815. Johkura K, Komiyama A, Tobita M, Hasegawa O. Saccadic ping-pong gaze. J Neuroophthalmol 1998;18:43–46.

816. Senelick RC. ''Ping-pong'' gaze. Periodic alternating gaze deviation. Neurology 1976;26:532–535.

817. Larmande P, Dongmo L, Limodin J, et al. Periodic alternating gaze: a case without any hemispheric lesion. Neurosurgery 1987;20:481–483.

818. Leigh RJ, Hanley DF, Munschauer FE III, et al. Eye movements induced by head rotation in unresponsive patients. Ann Neurol 1984;15:465–473.

819. Simon RP, Aminoff MJ. Electrographic status epilepticus in fatal anoxic coma. Ann Neurol 1986;20:351–355.

820. Larmande P, Henin D, Jan M, et al. Abnormal vertical eye movements in the locked-in syndrome. Ann Neurol 1982;11:100–102.

821. Meienberg O, Mumenthaler M, Karbowski K. Quadriparesis and nuclear oculomotor palsy with total bilateral ptosis mimicking coma. A mesencephalic ''locked-in syndrome''? Arch Neurol 1979;36:708–710.

822. Uematsu D, Suematsu M, Fukuuchi Y, et al. Midbrain locked-in state with oculomotor subnucleus lesion. J Neurol Neurosurg Psychiatry 1985;48:952–956.

823. Rosenberg M, Sharpe J, Hoyt WF. Absent vestibulo-ocular reflexes and acute supratentorial lesions. J Neurol Neurosurg Psychiatry 1975;38:6–10.

824. Hanid MA, Silk DBA, Williams R. Prognostic value of the oculovestibular reflex in fulminant hepatic failure. Br Med J 1978;1:1029.

825. Mueller-Jensen A, Neunzig HP, Emskotter T. Outcome prediction in comatose patients: significance of reflex eye movement analysis. J Neurol Neurosurg Psychiatry 1987;50:389–392.

826. Levy DE, Plum F. Outcome prediction in comatose patients: significance of reflex eye movement analysis. J Neurol Neurosurg Psychiatry 1988;51:318.

827. Singh BM, Strobos RJ. Retraction nystagmus elicited by bilateral simultaneous cold caloric stimulation. Ann Neurol 1980;8:79.

828. Dougherty JH, Rawlinson DG, Levy DE, et al. Hypoxic-ischemic brain injury and the vegetative state: clinical and neuropathologic correlation. Neurology 1981;31:991–997.

829. Nayyar M, Strobos RJ, Singh BM, et al. Caloric-induced nystagmus with isoelectric electroencephalogram. Ann Neurol 1987;21:98–100.

830. Lempert T, von Brevern M. The eye movements of syncope. Neurology 1996; 46:1086–1088.
831. Barnes D, McDonald WI. The ocular manifestations of multiple sclerosis: 2. Abnormalities of eye movements. J Neurol Neurosurg Psychiatry 1992;55: 863–888.
832. Frohman EM, Solomon D, Zee DS. Vestibular dysfunction and nystagmus in multiple sclerosis. Int J MS 1997;3:13–26.
833. Gnanaraj L, Rao VJ. Partial unilateral third nerve palsy and bilateral internuclear ophthalmoplegia: an unusual presentation of multiple sclerosis. Eye 2000;14(Pt 4):673–675.
834. Frohman EM, Zhang H, Kramer PD, et al. MRI characteristics of the MLF in MS patients with chronic internuclear ophthalmoparesis. Neurology 2001;57: 762–768.
835. Frohman EM, O'Suilleabhain P, Dewey RB Jr, et al. A new measure of dysconjugacy in INO: the first-pass amplitude. J Neurol Sci 2003;210:65–71.
836. Aschoff JC, Conrad B, Kornhuber HH. Acquired pendular nystagmus with oscillopsia in multiple sclerosis: a sign of cerebellar nuclei disease. J Neurol Neurosurg Psychiatry 1974;37:570–577.
837. Lopez LI, Bronstein AM, Gresty MA, et al. Clinical and MRI correlates in 27 patients with acquired nystagmus. Brain 1996;119:465–472.
838. Meienberg O, Muri R, Rabineau PA. Clinical and oculographic examinations of saccadic eye movements in the diagnosis of multiple sclerosis. Arch Neurol 1986;43:438–443.
839. Frohman TC, Frohman EM, O'Suilleabhain P, et al. Accuracy of clinical detection of INO in MS: corroboration with quantitative infrared oculography. Neurology 2003;61:848–850.
840. Gresty MA, Findley LJ, Wade P. Mechanism of rotatory eye movements in opsoclonus. Br J Ophthalmol 1980;64:923–925.
841. Francis DA, Heron JR. Ocular flutter in suspected multiple sclerosis: a presenting paroxysmal manifestation. Postgrad Med J 1985;61:333–334.
842. Ashe J, Hain TC, Zee DS, et al. Microsaccadic flutter. Brain 1991;114:461–472.
843. Solingen LD, Baloh RW, Myers L, et al. Subclinical eye movement disorders in patients with multiple sclerosis. Neurology 1977;27:614–619.
844. Reulen JPH, Sanders EACM, Hogenhuis LAM. Eye movement disorders in multiple sclerosis and optic neuritis. Brain 1983;106:121–140.
845. Milea D, Napolitano M, Dechy H, et al. Complete bilateral horizontal gaze paralysis disclosing multiple sclerosis. J Neurol Neurosurg Psychiatry 2001;70: 252–255.
846. Keane JR. Sustained upgaze in coma. Ann Neurol 1981;9:409–412.
847. Frohman EM, Solomon D, Zee DS. Vestibular dysfunction and nystagmus in multiple sclerosis. Int J MS 1997;3:13–26.
848. Downey DL, Stahl JS, Bhidayasiri R, et al. Saccadic and vestibular abnormalities in multiple sclerosis: sensitive clinical signs of brainstem and cerebellar involvement. Ann NY Acad Sci 2002;956:438–440.
849. Frohman EM, Goodin DS, Calabresi PA, et al. The utility of MRI in suspected MS: report of the Therapeutics and Technology Assessment Subcommittee of the American Academy of Neurology. Neurology 2003;61:602–611.
850. Starck M, Albrecht H, Pöllmann W, et al. Drug therapy for acquired pendular nystagmus in multiple sclerosis. J Neurol 1997;244:9–16.
851. Hoyt CS. Nystagmus and other abnormal ocular movements in children. Pediatr Clin North Am 1987;34:1415–1423.
852. Ahn JC, Hoyt WF, Hoyt CS. Tonic upgaze in infancy. A report of three cases. Arch Ophthalmol 1989;107:57–58.
853. Donat JFG, Donat JR, Lay KS. Changing response to caloric stimulation with gestational age in infants. Neurology 1980;30:776–778.
854. Weissman BM, DiScenna AO, Leigh RJ. Maturation of the vestibulo-ocular reflex in normal infants during the first 2 months of life. Neurology 1989;39: 534–538.
855. Harding AE, Young EP, Schon F. Adult onset supranuclear ophthalmoplegia, cerebellar ataxia, and neurogenic proximal muscle weakness in a brother and sister: another hexosaminidase. A deficiency syndrome. J Neurol Neurosurg Psychiatry 1987;50:687–690.
856. Neville BGR, Lake BD, Stephens R, et al. A neurovisceral storage disease with vertical supranuclear ophthalmoplegia, and its relationship to Niemann-Pick disease. Brain 1973;96:97–120.
857. Cogan DG, Chu FC, Reingold D, et al. Ocular motor signs in some metabolic diseases. Arch Ophthalmol 1981;99:1802–1808.
858. Shawkat FS, Carr L, West P, et al. Vertical saccade palsy: a presenting sign of Niemann-Pick type IIS. Eur J Neurol 1994;1:93–95.
859. Natowicz MR, Stoler JM, Prence EM, et al. Marked heterogeneity in Niemann-Pick disease, type C: clinical and ultrastructural findings. Clin Ped 1995; 190–197.
860. Vivian AJ, Harris CM, Kriss A, et al. Oculomotor signs in infantile Gaucher disease. Neuroophthalmology 1993;13:151–155.
861. Cogan DG, Victor M. Ocular signs of Wernicke's disease. Arch Ophthalmol 1954;51:204–211.
862. Ghez C. Vestibular paresis: a clinical feature of Wernicke's disease. J Neurol Neurosurg Psychiatry 1969;32:134–139.
863. Deramo VA, Jayamanne DG, Auerbach DB, Danesh-Meyer H. Acute bilateral ophthalmoplegia in a young woman. Surv Ophthalmol 2000;44:513–517.
864. Kumar PD, Nartsupha C, West BC. Unilateral internuclear ophthalmoplegia

and recovery with thiamine in Wernicke syndrome. Am J Med Sci 2000;320: 278–280.
865. Mulder AH, Raemaekers JM, Boerman RH, Mattijssen V. Downbeat nystagmus caused by thiamine deficiency: an unusual presentation of CNS localization of large cell anaplastic CD 30-positive non-Hodgkin's lymphoma. Ann Hematol 1999;78:105–107.
866. Sharma S, Sumich PM, Francis IC, et al. Wernicke's encephalopathy presenting with upbeating nystagmus. J Clin Neurosci 2002;9:476–478.
867. Cogan DG, Witt ED, Goldman-Rakic PS. Ocular signs in thiamine-deficient monkeys and in Wernicke's disease in humans. Arch Ophthalmol 1985;103: 1212–1220.
868. Witt ED, Goldman-Rakic PS. Intermittent thiamine deficiency in the rhesus monkey. I. Progression of neurological signs and neuro-anatomical lesions. Ann Neurol 1983;13:376–395.
869. Kenyon RV, Becker JT, Butters N, et al. Oculomotor function in Wernicke-Korsakoff syndrome. I. Saccadic eye movements. Int J Neurosci 1984;25:53–65.
870. Kenyon RV, Becker JT, Butters N. Oculomotor function in Wernicke-Korsakoff syndrome. II. Smooth-pursuit eye movements. Int J Neurosci 1984;25:67–69.
871. Ramulu P, Moghekar A, Chaudhry V, et al. Wernicke's encephalopathy. Neurology 2002;59:846.
872. Miranda AF, Ishii S, DiMauro S, et al. Cytochrome c oxidase deficiency in Leigh's syndrome: genetic evidence for a nuclear DNA-encoded mutation. Neurology 1989;39:697–702.
873. DiMauro S, Servidei S, Zeviani M, et al. Cytochrome c oxidase deficiency in Leigh syndrome. Ann Neurol 1987;22:498–506.
874. Adams PL, Lightowlers RN, Turnbull DM. Molecular analysis of cytochrome c oxidase deficiency in Leigh's syndrome. Ann Neurol 1997;41:268–270.
875. Howard RO, Albert DM. Ocular manifestations of subacute necrotizing encephalomyelopathy (Leigh's disease). Am J Ophthalmol 1972;74:386–393.
876. Dooling EC, Richardson EP Jr. Ophthalmoplegia and Ondine's curse. Arch Ophthalmol 1977;95:1790–1793.
877. Blanco-Barca MO, Eiris-Punal J, Soler-Regal C, Castro-Gago M. [Duplication of the PLP gene and the classical form of Pelizaeus-Merzbacher disease]. Rev Neurol 2003;37:436–438.
878. Trobe JD, Sharpe JA, Hirsh DK, et al. Nystagmus of Pelizaeus-Merzbacher disease: a magnetic search-coil study. Arch Neurol 1991;48:87–91.
879. Ouahchi K, Arita M, Kayden H, et al. Ataxia with isolated vitamin E deficiency is caused by mutations in the alpha-tocopherol transfer protein. Nature Genet 1995;9:141–145.
880. Yee RD, Cogan DC, Zee DS. Ophthalmoplegia and dissociated nystagmus in abetalipoproteinemia. Arch Ophthalmol 1976;94:571–575.
881. Hawkins RA, Mazziotta JC, Phelps ME. Wilson's disease studied with FDG and positron emission tomography. Neurology 1987;37:1707–1711.
882. Lennox G, Jones R. Gaze distractibility in Wilson's disease. Ann Neurol 1989; 25:415–417.
883. Kirkham TH, Kamin DF. Slow saccadic eye movements in Wilson's disease. J Neurol Neurosurg Psychiatry 1974;37:191–194.
884. Keane JR. Lid-opening apraxia in Wilson's disease. J Clin Neuroophthalmol 1988;8:31–33.
885. Kushner MJ, Parrish M, Burke A, et al. Nystagmus in motor neuron disease: clinicopathological study of two cases. Ann Neurol 1984;16:71–77.
886. Averbuch-Heller L, Helmchen C, Horn AK, et al. Slow vertical saccades in motor neuron disease: correlation of structure and function. Ann Neurol 1998; 44:641–648.
887. Evdokimidis I, Constantinidis TS, Gourtzelidis P, et al. Frontal lobe dysfunction in amyotrophic lateral sclerosis. J Neurol Sci 2002;195:25–33.
888. Vaphiades MS, Husain M, Juhasz K, Schmidley JW. Motor neuron disease presenting with slow saccades and dementia. ALS Other Motor Neuron Disord 2002;3:159–162.
889. Abel LA, Williams IM, Gibson KL, et al. Effects of stimulus velocity and acceleration on smooth pursuit in motor neuron disease. J Neurol 1995;242: 419–424.
890. Gizzi M, DiRocco A, Sivak M, et al. Ocular motor function in motor neuron disease. Neurology 1992;42:1037–1046.
891. Okuda B, Yamamoto T, Yamasaki M, et al. Motor neuron disease with slow eye movements and vertical gaze palsy. Acta Neurol Scand 1992;85:71–76.
892. Gruber H, Zeitlhofer J, Prager J, et al. Complex oculomotor dysfunctions in Kugelberg-Welander disease. Neuroophthalmology 1983;3:125–128.
893. Thurston SE, Leigh RJ, Abel LA, et al. Slow saccades and hypometria in anticonvulsant toxicity. Neurology 1984;34:1593–1596.
894. Remler BF, Leigh RJ, Osorio I, et al. The characteristics and mechanisms of visual disturbances associated with anticonvulsant therapy. Neurology 1990;40: 791–796.
895. Rascol O, Hain TC, Brefel C, et al. Antivertigo medications and drug-induced vertigo. Drugs 1995;50:777–791.
896. Padoan S, Korttila K, Magnusson M, et al. Effect of intravenous diazepam and thipental on voluntary saccades and pursuit eye movements. Acta Otolaryngol 1992;112:579–588.
897. Cohen B, Helwig D, Raphan T, et al. Baclofen and velocity storage: a model of the effects of the drugs on the vestibulo-ocular reflex in the monkey. J Physiol (Lond) 1987;393:703–725.

898. Pereira CB, Strupp M, Eggert T, et al. Nicotine-induced nystagmus: three-dimensional analysis and dependence on head position. Neurology 2000;55:1563–1566.
899. Pereira CB, Strupp M, Holzleitner T, Brandt T. Smoking and balance: correlation of nicotine-induced nystagmus and postural body sway. Neuroreport 2001;12:1223–1226.
900. Sibony PA, Evinger C, Manning K, et al. Nicotine and tobacco-induced nystagmus. Ann Neurol 1990;28:198.
901. Booker JL. End-position nystagmus as an indicator of ethanol intoxication. Sci Justice 2001;41:113–116.
902. Citek K, Ball B, Rutledge DA. Nystagmus testing in intoxicated individuals. Optometry 2003;74:695–710.
903. Crevits L. Effect of alcohol on saccades. Clin Experiment Ophthalmol 2002;30:450–451.
904. Fetter M, Haslwanter T, Bork M, Dichgans J. New insights into positional alcohol nystagmus using three-dimensional eye-movement analysis. Ann Neurol 1999;45:216–223.
905. Wegner AJ, Fahle M. Alcohol and visually guided saccades: gap effect and predictability of target location. Psychopharmacology (Berl) 1999;146:24–32.
906. Zingler VC, Strupp M, Krafczyk S, et al. Does alcohol cancel static vestibular compensation? Ann Neurol 2004;55:144–145.
907. Dehaene I, Van Vleymen B. Opsoclonus induced by phenytoin and diazepam. Ann Neurol 1987;21:216.
908. Flechtner K-M, Mackert A, Thies K, et al. Lithium effect on smooth-pursuit eye movements of healthy volunteers. Biol Psychiatr 1992;32:932–938.
909. Corbett JJ, Jacobson DM, Thompson HS, et al. Downbeating nystagmus and other ocular motor defects caused by lithium toxicity. Neurology 1989;39:481–487.
910. Cannon SC, Robinson DA. Loss of the neural integrator of the oculomotor system from brain stem lesions in monkey. J Neurophysiol 1987;5:1383–1409.
911. Schneider JA, Mirra SS. Neuropathologic correlate of persistent neurological deficit in lithium intoxication. Ann Neurol 1994;36:928–931.
912. Green JF, King DJ, Trimble KM. Antisaccade and smooth pursuit eye movements in healthy subjects receiving sertraline and lorazepam. J Psychopharmacol 2000;14:30–36.
913. Taylor JR, Selhorst JB, Houff SA, et al. Chlordecone intoxication in man. I. Clinical observations. Neurology 1978;28:626–630.
914. Maccario M, Seelinger D, Snyder R. Thallotoxicosis with coma and abnormal eye movements (opsoclonus): clinical and EEG correlations. Electroencephalogr Clin Neurophysiol 1975;38:98–99.
915. Hodgson MJ, Furman J, Ryan C, et al. Encephalopathy and vestibulopathy following short-term hydocarbon exposure. J Occup Med 1989;31:51–54.
916. Ödkvist LM, Möller C, Thuomas K. Otoneurologic disturbances caused by solvent polution. Otolarygol Head Neck Surg 1992;106:687–692.
917. Larsby B, Tham R, Eriksson B, et al. I. Effects of trichloroethylene on the human vestibulo-oculomotor system. Acta Orolaryngol (Stockh) 1986;101:193–199.
918. Moller C, Ödkvist LM, Thell J, et al. Otoneurological findings in psycho-organic syndrome caused by industrial solvent exposure. Acta Otolaryngol (Stockh) 1989;107:5–12.
919. Rosenberg NL, Kleinschmidt-DeMasters BJ, Davis KA, et al. Toluene abuse causes diffuse central nervous system white matter changes. Ann Neurol 1988;23:611–614.
920. Malm C, Lying-Tunell U. Cerebellar dysfunction related to toluene sniffing. Acta Neurol Scand 1980;62:188–190.
921. Lazar RB, Ho SU, Melen O, et al. Multifocal central nervous system damage caused by toluene abuse. Neurology 1983;33:1337–1340.
922. Maas EF, Ashe J, Spiegel PS, et al. Acquired pendular nystagmus in toluene addiction. Neurology 1991;41:282–285.
923. Morata TC, Nylén P, Johnson A, et al. Auditory and vestibular functions after single or combined exposure to toluene: a review. Arch Toxicol 1995;69:431–443.
924. Hunnewell J, Miller NR. Bilateral internuclear ophthalmoplegia and pendular nystagmus in a patient with chronic toluene toxicity from glue-sniffing. Neurology, 1997.
925. Sibony PA, Evinger C, Manning KA. Tobacco-induced primary-position upbeat nystagmus. Ann Neurol 1987;21:53–58.
926. Sibony PA, Evinger C, Manning KA. The effects of tobacco smoking on smooth-pursuit eye movements. Ann Neurol 1988;23:238–241.
927. Roos YBWEM, de Jongh FE, Crevits L. The effect of smoking on ocular saccadic latency time. Neuroophthalmology 1993;13:75–79.
928. Thaker GK, Ellsberry R, Moran M, et al. Tobacco smoking increases square-wave jerks during pursuit eye movements. Biol Psychiatry 1991;29:82–88.
929. Roos YBWEM, de Jongh FE, Crevits L. The effects of smoking on anti-saccades. Neuroophthalmology 1995;15:3–8.
930. Kim JI, Somers JT, Stahl JS, Bhidayasiri R, Leigh RJ. Vertical nystagmus in normal subjects: effects of head position, nicotine and scopolamine. J Vestib Res 2000;10:291–300.
931. Demer JL, Volkow ND, Ulrich I, et al. Eye movements in cocaine abusers. Psychiat Res 1989;29:123–136.
932. Scharf D. Opsoclonus-myoclonus following the intranasal usage of cocaine. J Neurol Neurosurg Psychiatry 1989;52:1447–1448.
933. Elkardoudi-Pijnenburg Y, Van Vliet AGM. Opsoclonus, a rare complication of cocaine misuse. J Neurol Neurosurg Psychiatry 1996;60:592.
934. Brandt T. Bilateral vestibulopathy revisited. Eur J Med Res 1996;1:361–368.
935. Halmagyi GM, Fattore CM, Curthoys IS, et al. Gentamicin vestibulotoxicity. Otolaryngol Head Neck Surg 1994;111:571–574.
936. Fishel-Ghodsian N, Prezant TR, Bu X, et al. Mitochondrial ribosomal RNA gene mutation in a patient with sporadic aminoglycoside ototoxicity. J Otolaryngol 1993;14:399–403.
937. Prezant TR, Agapian JV, Bohlman MC, et al. Mitochondrial ribosomal RNA mutation associated with both antibiotic-induced and nonsyndromic deafness. Nature Genet 1993;4:289–294.
938. Longridge NS. Topical gentamicin vestibular toxicity. J Otolaryngol 1994;23:444–446.
939. Kitsigianis G-A, O'Leary DP, Davis LL. Active head-movement analysis of cisplatin-induced vestibulotoxicity. Otolaryngol Head Neck Surg 1988;98:82–87.
940. Myers SF, Blakely BW, Schwan S. Is cis-platinum vestibulotoxic? Otolaryngol Head Neck Surg 1993;108:322–328.
941. Nakayama M, Riggs LC, Matz GJ. Quantitative study of vestibulotoxicity induced by gentamicin or cisplatin in the guinea pig. Laryngoscope 1996;106:162–167.

CHAPTER 20

Nuclear and Infranuclear Ocular Motility Disorders

Jane C. Sargent

Lesions of the oculomotor, trochlear, and abducens nerves may be located anywhere from the ocular motor nuclei to the termination of the nerves in the extraocular muscles in the orbit. Ocular motor nerve palsies present to the clinician in one of four ways: (*a*) as an isolated partial or complete nerve palsy without any other neurologic signs and without symptoms except those related to the palsy itself; (*b*) in association with symptoms such as pain or proptosis, but without any signs of neurologic or systemic disease; (*c*) in associa-tion with other ocular motor nerve palsies, but without any other neurologic signs; and (*d*) in association with other neurologic signs. Most large series that document the percentage of ocular motor nerve palsies caused by each pathologic condition ignore these modes of presentation and thus are of limited value to the clinician. For this reason, we discuss ocular motor nerve palsies in relation to their presentation, their known or presumed site of origin, and the lesions that cause them.

OCULOMOTOR (THIRD) NERVE PALSIES

CONGENITAL

Congenital oculomotor nerve palsies are rarer than ac-quired palsies, but they constitute nearly half of the oculomo-tor nerve pareses seen in children (1–11) (Fig. 20.1). Most cases are unilateral, but bilateral cases also occur (3,6,7,9, 12,13). As a general rule, patients with congenital oculomo-tor nerve palsy have no other neurologic or systemic abnor-malities, but there are many reports of associated problems such as additional cranial nerve dysfunction, developmental delay, asymmetric hypoplasia of the midbrain and corpus callosum, septo-optic dysplasia, and cerebral palsy (3,7,8, 14–16). Most cases are sporadic, although rare familial cases occur (2,13).

All affected patients have some degree of ptosis and ophthalmoparesis, and most have pupillary involvement (1,7,15). Usually the pupil is miotic rather than dilated, pre-sumably because of misdirected oculomotor nerve regenera-tion (17). It may be large at birth, becoming miotic at several months of age as other signs of aberrant regeneration appear (7,15,17) (discussed later). The pupil is sometimes spared (1,3,15).

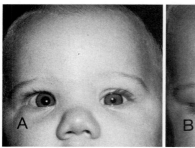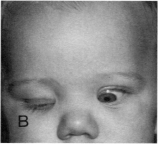

Figure 20.1. Congenital left oculomotor nerve palsy with aberrant regeneration in a child with a history of birth trauma. Note the miotic left pupil. *A*, In primary position, there is a left hypotropia. *B*, On attempted downward gaze, there is retraction of the left upper eyelid (pseudo-Graefe sign).

Usually there is some degree of amblyopia, which may be severe (5,7,15). However, visual acuity may be better in the paretic eye (2,5,7,15), especially if there is associated nystagmus, which will probably be less in the paretic eye. Some children learn to hold the ptotic lid open with a finger if that eye has the better acuity (15).

Congenital oculomotor palsy may be caused by absent or incomplete development of the nucleus or nerve (18–20) or damage to the nucleus or nerve (20), and it may be complete or incomplete. When the cause is birth injury, recovery may be rapid and complete, but more often it is incomplete, or aberrant regeneration develops (1,10). How birth injury causes oculomotor palsy is unclear.

Several congenital syndromes result from the failure of oculomotor axons to innervate their target muscles. Intact motor neurons from other oculomotor subnuclei or from the trochlear or abducens nuclei then send axons into the muscles, causing anomalous or paradoxic innervation patterns. If no innervation occurs, fibrosis of the muscles results (21). These syndromes include (*a*) congenital fibrosis of the extraocular muscles; (*b*) congenital adduction palsy with synergistic divergence; (*c*) vertical retraction syndrome; and (*d*) oculomotor nerve paresis with cyclic spasm. Duane's syndrome is a related condition discussed with the abducens nerve.

Congenital Fibrosis of the Extraocular Muscles

Congenital fibrosis of the extraocular muscles (CFEOM) (22) is the extreme form of absence of oculomotor innervation. It occurs in at least three genetic forms and is usually dominantly inherited (23,24). In the classic type, CFEOM1, there is nonprogressive bilateral restrictive ophthalmoplegia and ptosis. In the primary position, both eyes are infraducted with an inability to move above the horizontal midline. Each eye may be esotropic, exotropic, or midline. Forced ductions show restriction. There may be aberrant movements, but the pupils are usually normal. Muscles may be small on imaging (25). High astigmatism and unilateral amblyopia are common (23). CFEOM1 is dominantly inherited and maps to chromosome 12p. The superior division of the oculomotor nerve and its subnuclei are absent. The levator palpebrae

superioris and the superior rectus are fibrotic, but the other oculomotor muscles are not.(25)

CFEOM2 was described in three Saudi Arabian families and one Turkish family and is caused by maldevelopment of both the oculomotor and trochlear nerves. Affected patients have ptosis and bilateral fixed exotropia with or without hypertropia or hypotropia. CFEOM2 is recessively inherited and is caused by homozygous defects in the ARIX (PHOX2A) gene at chromosome 11q13. This gene is necessary for the development of oculomotor and trochlear alpha motor neurons and other adrenergic brain stem neurons in mice and zebrafish (23).

CFEOM3 is a dominantly inherited disorder characterized by congenital fibrosis of the extraocular muscles, with absence of vertical eye movements, preservation of horizontal movements, except for some cases with adduction deficit, and variable degrees of ptosis (23–26). It may be asymmetric. Mildly affected family members of the Canadian family described have only slight limitation of vertical gaze. All have superficial keratopathy, presumably related to their absent Bell's phenomenon. Computed tomography shows small extraocular muscles, especially the superior recti. In addition, three of the five patients scanned had ventricular asymmetry, and two patients had asymmetrically shaped globes (26). CFEOM3 maps to 16q24.2-q24.3 and appears to be autosomal dominant with incomplete penetrance (27). It probably results from maldevelopment of the oculomotor and trochlear nuclei by a mechanism different from that causing CFEOM1.

Congenital restrictive external ophthalmoplegia with gustatory epiphora has been reported in children exposed prenatally to isotretinoin (28) or thalidomide (29), and gustatory epiphora can occur even in Duane's syndrome (30). These conditions suggest that loss of brain stem neurons in the oculomotor nuclei can cause fibrosis of the extraocular muscles, and that loss of brain stem neurons can cause aberrant rewiring from nearby surviving nuclei.

Congenital Adduction Palsy with Synergistic Divergence

Patients with this syndrome have congenital unilateral paralysis of adduction associated with simultaneous bilateral abduction on attempted gaze into the field of action of the paretic medial rectus muscle (21,31–34) (Figs. 20.2 and 20.3). Most patients have no other neurologic abnormalities (35). Electromyography shows absent oculomotor nerve innervation of the affected medial rectus muscle, combined with innervation of the lateral rectus by an aberrant branch of the oculomotor nerve instead of the abducens nerve (36). Electro-oculographic findings are similar to those of patients with Duane's retraction syndrome, suggesting that anomalous innervation of the extraocular muscles is responsible (32,37,38). It may, indeed, be a variant of Duane's syndrome (39). Synergistic divergence sometimes occurs with the hereditary congenital fibrosis syndrome and the Marcus Gunn jaw-wink phenomenon, again suggesting aberrant rewiring (40).

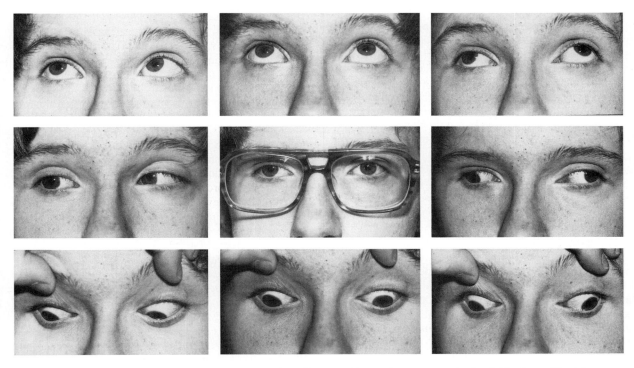

Figure 20.2. Congenital adduction palsy and synergistic divergence. Extraocular movements in nine fields of gaze. The right eye has the most marked lateral movement on attempted left lateral gaze, but also abducts on right lateral gaze. (From Wilcox LM Jr, Gittinger JW Jr, Breinin GM. Congenital adduction palsy and synergistic divergence. Am J Ophthalmol 1981;91:1–7.)

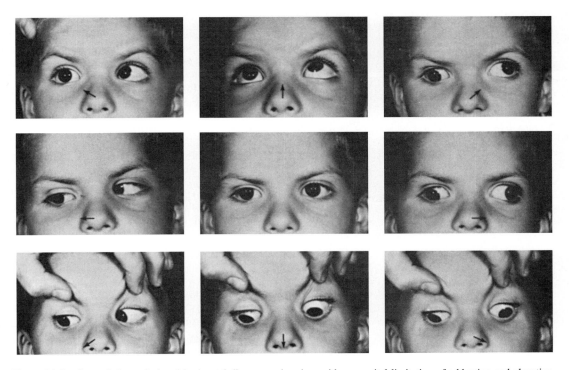

Figure 20.3. Synergistic vertical and horizontal divergence in a boy with congenital limitation of adduction and elevation of the right eye. On attempted left horizontal gaze (and to some extent on right horizontal gaze), the right eye abducts and shoots downward. Optokinetic stimuli and clockwise constant rotation in a Bárány chair caused divergent nystagmus. (Courtesy of Dr. Maurice Van Allen.)

Vertical Retraction Syndrome

In the vertical retraction syndrome, limitation of movement of the affected eye on attempted elevation or depression is associated with a retraction of the globe and narrowing of the palpebral fissure. There may be an associated esotropia or exotropia, more marked in the direction of the restricted vertical field of action. The superior rectus muscle is usually more affected than the inferior rectus muscle, so that the retraction may be evident only during attempted depression of the eyes. The condition may be unilateral (41–44), bilateral (45), and sporadic or familial (44,45). (Figs. 20.4–20.6). Electro-oculography and electromyography suggest anomalous oculomotor innervation of the vertical rectus muscles of the affected eye (42,44). Presumably this syndrome is another pattern of neuronal misdirection resulting from insufficient innervation of the eye muscles, like synergistic divergence and Duane's syndrome (23,44).

Oculomotor Paresis *with* Cyclic Spasms (Cyclic Oculomotor Paresis)

In 1884, Rampoldi (46) described the first case of what he described as an ''oculopalpebral imbalance.'' Since this time, numerous similar cases have been reported. The condi-

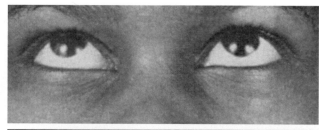
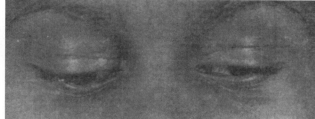
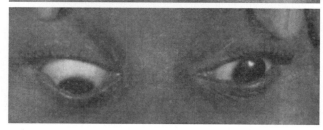

Figure 20.5. Vertical gaze in a patient with bilateral vertical retraction syndrome. *Top,* Minimal limitation of elevation bilaterally. *Middle,* Slight limitation of depression bilaterally, with left exotropia. The deviated left eye is slightly retracted. *Below,* The upper eyelids are elevated to show the position of the left eye on attempted downward gaze. Note exotropia, limitation of depression, and retraction. (From Khodadoust AA, von Noorden GK. Bilateral vertical retraction syndrome: A family study. Arch Ophthalmol 1967;78:606–612.)

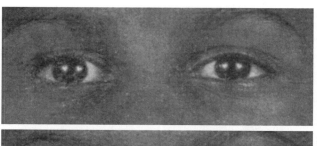
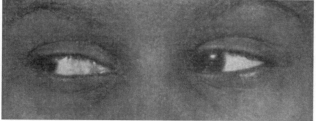
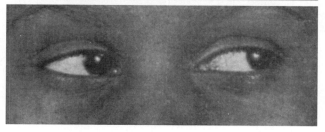

Figure 20.4. Normal horizontal gaze in a patient with bilateral vertical retraction syndrome. *Top,* Primary position. *Middle,* Normal versions of both eyes on attempted right lateral gaze. *Below,* Normal versions of both eyes on attempted left lateral gaze. (From Khodadoust AA, von Noorden GK. Bilateral vertical retraction syndrome: A family study. Arch Ophthalmol 1967;78:606–612.)

tion is usually unilateral and is in most cases present from birth (1,2,47–54). Typically there is an oculomotor nerve paresis with ptosis, mydriasis, reduced accommodation, and ophthalmoparesis (Fig. 20.7, *top* and *bottom left*). About every 2 minutes, the ptotic eyelid elevates, the globe begins to adduct, the pupil constricts, and accommodation increases (Fig. 20.7, *bottom right*). These spasms last 10–30 seconds and then give way again to the paretic phase.

The cycling is usually present when the oculomotor deficit is first discovered, but may develop months to years later. Once present, it usually persists unchanged throughout life, although occasionally it evolves into a static oculomotor deficit (55). The cycles continue even during sleep, although they do so at a reduced rate and amplitude, subsiding only during deep sleep. Most patients with unilateral cyclic oculomotor paresis have some degree of amblyopia in the affected eye.

In some patients, movements of the eyes influence the cycling. Adduction or accommodation-convergence efforts, or less commonly vertical gaze or forced eyelid closure, often increase the extent and duration of the spastic phase. Conversely, abduction efforts may shorten and reduce the spasms and accentuate or prolong the paretic phase.

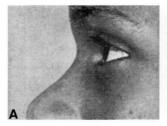
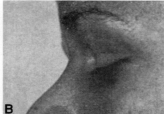
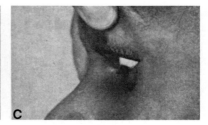

Figure 20.6. Lateral view of left eye in a patient with bilateral vertical retraction syndrome. *A*, Primary position. *B*, When looking down, there is almost complete pseudoptosis and enophthalmos of the fixating left eye. *C*, With the eyelid held open, retraction of the left eye during attempted downward gaze is clear. (From Khodadoust AA, von Noorden GK. Bilateral vertical retraction syndrome: A family study. Arch Ophthalmol 1967;78:606–612.)

Cyclic oculomotor paresis is occasionally associated with other pathologic conditions, including birth trauma and congenital infections (47). There are four current theories regarding the pathogenesis of cyclic oculomotor paresis. The first is that the primary lesion is in the oculomotor nerve, with secondary reorganization of synaptic input to the nuclear cells (47). The second is that a peripheral oculomotor nerve lesion is responsible, as suggested by electromyography and muscle pathology (49,56–59). This could be chronic compression from a blood vessel (59). The third theory is that there is aberrant third nerve regeneration with intermittent conduction block (49). Our own theory is that there is a relationship with ocular neuromyotonia (60).

Cyclic oculomotor paresis is usually but not always congenital (58,59,61,62). In one reported case (61), a brain stem glioma was associated. Neuroimaging is generally normal (62).

ACQUIRED

Acquired dysfunction of the oculomotor nerve is far more common than congenital dysfunction, being caused by nearly every pathologic process (63). The precise site of the responsible lesion is clear in some cases and speculative in others. Neuroimaging has made localization easier.

Lesions of the Oculomotor Nucleus

The oculomotor nerve supplies motor innervation to the superior rectus, inferior rectus, medial rectus, inferior oblique, and levator palpebrae superioris muscles and parasympathetic innervation by way of the ciliary ganglion to the pupillary constrictor and the ciliary muscles. Because of the anatomy of the oculomotor subnuclei, however, a pure oculomotor nuclear lesion produces a somewhat different clinical picture.

Damage to the oculomotor nucleus is not uncommon (63–83). When it occurs, it results in bilateral defects (84). Bilateral involvement is explained by the anatomy of the nucleus and its fibers (85,86). Both levator palpebrae superioris muscles are innervated by a single midline subnucleus located at the caudal end of the oculomotor nerve complex (Fig. 20.8). Symmetric bilateral ptosis that progresses rapidly to total ptosis, when neuropathic in origin, usually indi-

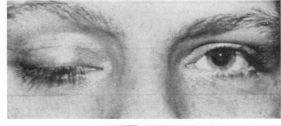

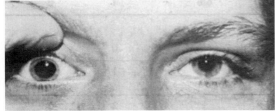
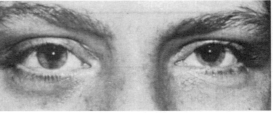

Figure 20.7. Right oculomotor paresis with cyclic spasm (cyclic oculomotor paresis) in a 21-year-old man. *Top,* Paretic phase with maximum ptosis. *Bottom left,* Paretic phase with eyelid held up to reveal markedly dilated right pupil. *Bottom right,* Spastic phase showing right eyelid in almost normal position and constricted right pupil. (From Fells P, Collin JRO. Cyclic oculomotor palsy. Trans Ophthalmol Soc UK 1979;99:192–196.)

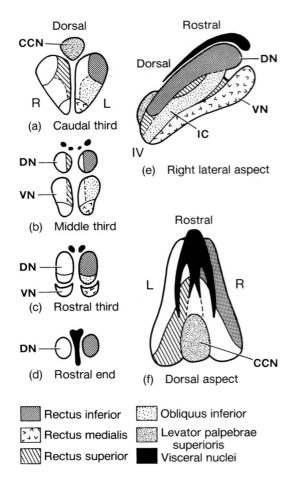

Figure 20.8. Warwick's schema of topographic organization within the oculomotor nucleus. Note the caudal dorsal midline position of caudal central nucleus (CCN), the motor pool for the levator palpebrae superioris. The motor pool of the superior rectus (*hashed area*) is contralateral to the extraocular muscle it innervates. The visceral (parasympathetic) nuclei are shown in black. DN, dorsal nucleus; IC, intermediate column; IV, region of the trochlear nucleus; VN, ventral nucleus. (From Warwick R. Representation of the extra-ocular muscles in the oculomotor nuclei of the monkey. J Comp Neurol 1953;98:449–504.)

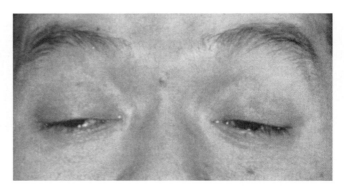

Figure 20.9. Isolated, bilateral ptosis in a patient with brain stem encephalitis and discrete inflammatory foci in the caudal mesencephalon. (From Conway VH, Rozdilsky B, Schneider RJ, et al. Isolated bilateral complete ptosis. Can J Ophthalmol 1983;18:37–40.)

cates a nuclear lesion with involvement of caudal midline structures (66,77,87–90) (Figs. 20.9–20.11). In some cases the ptosis is isolated, whereas in others there is associated ophthalmoplegia that may be significant or so minimal as to be overlooked (90). Alternatively, more rostral lesions of the oculomotor nuclear complex spare the central caudal nucleus, preserving levator function bilaterally (70,91,92).

A second anatomic feature of the oculomotor nuclear complex that results in bilateral ocular dysmotility is the innervation of the superior rectus muscle. This pathway is primarily crossed, with its fibers passing through, but not originating from, the subnucleus for superior rectus function ipsilateral to the affected eye. Thus, the subnucleus for superior rectus function on either side of the brain stem gives rise to fibers that pass through the contralateral superior rectus subnucleus without synapse and innervate the contralateral

superior rectus muscle. Lesions in this region cause not only ipsilateral weakness of the superior rectus, medial rectus, inferior rectus, inferior oblique, or a combination of these muscles, but also limitation of elevation in the contralateral eye from impairment of superior rectus function on that side (68–71,74–76,78,93–95). Such patients have bilateral limitation of upward gaze, usually worse on the contralateral side (96) (Figs. 20.12 and 20.13).

Nuclear lesions sometimes spare the pupil (97), but when the pupil is involved, it indicates dorsal, rostral damage. The subnuclei for pupillary constriction, the Edinger-Westphal nuclei, are dorsal and medial to the somatic subnuclei.

Incomplete oculomotor nerve pareses, occasionally restricted to a nerve supplying a single extraocular muscle, may be produced by focal lesions of the oculomotor nuclear complex. Nuclear lesions are frequently associated with supranuclear gaze palsies and other signs of midbrain damage.

Lesions of the oculomotor nucleus are most often caused by ischemia, usually from embolic or thrombotic occlusion of isolated perforating paramedian arterioles or the basilar artery occlusion ("top of the basilar" syndrome) (7,65,69, 72,76,98–106). Other etiologies include hemorrhage (106–108), tumor (70,77), inflammation (109), tuberculoma (110), Behçet's disease (111), cephalic tetanus (112), and brain stem compression (113) (Fig. 20.14).

Degenerative diseases can involve the ocular motor nuclei. Machado-Joseph disease is an autosomal-dominant spinocerebellar degeneration caused by an expanded CAG repeat on chromosome 14q32.1. It frequently causes ophthalmoplegia because of loss of neurons in the ocular motor nuclei. Nystagmus, optic atrophy, bulging eyes, lid retraction, supranuclear palsy, facial and lingual fasciculations, rigidity, and ataxia are often associated (114).

Amyotrophic lateral sclerosis (ALS) is not usually considered to cause ophthalmoplegia, and neither are other anterior horn cell diseases such as Kennedy's disease, spinal muscular atrophy (115–117), and poliomyelitis (118). Oculomotor neurons differ from other bulbar and spinal neurons in a number of ways (119). They have more excitatory glutamatergic inputs, different metabotropic glutamate receptors

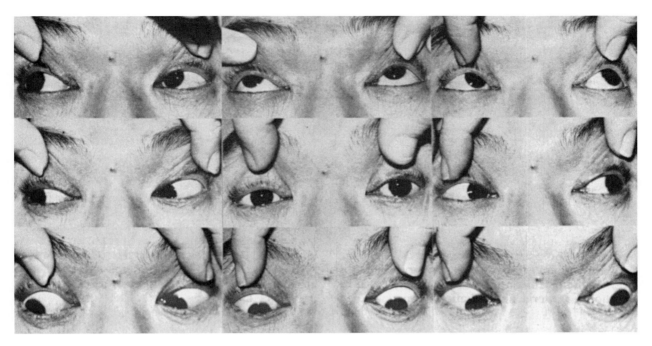

Figure 20.10. Ocular motility in the patient with isolated, bilateral ptosis from brain stem encephalitis seen in Figure 20.9. Note normal extraocular movements. (From Conway VH, Rozdilsky B, Schneider RJ, et al. Isolated bilateral complete ptosis. Can J Ophthalmol 1983;18:37–40.)

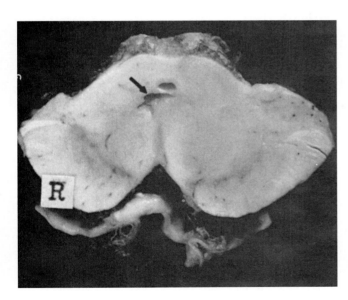

Figure 20.11. Pathophysiology of bilateral ptosis in a patient with an infarction in the oculomotor nucleus. A discrete lesion (*arrow*) is present in the caudal portion of the oculomotor nucleus just ventral to the cerebral aqueduct. (From Growdon JH, Winkler GF, Wray SH. Midbrain ptosis: A case with clinicopathologic correlation. Arch Neurol 1974;30:179–181.)

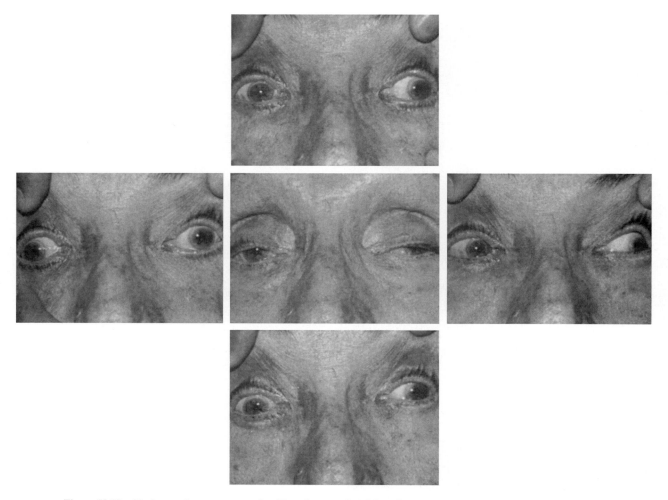

Figure 20.12. Nuclear oculomotor nerve palsy. There is a complete left oculomotor nerve palsy. In addition, however, there is bilateral ptosis and absence of elevation of the right eye. The right eye also has marked limitation of depression, suggesting that the lesion is not limited to the left oculomotor nerve nucleus but involves the right nucleus as well. Neither oculocephalic nor caloric stimulation produced any improvement in vertical gaze.

(120), a higher firing rate, different calcium binding proteins, fewer androgen receptors, and different trophic factors. In spite of this, rare ALS patients develop bilateral complete ophthalmoplegia (with normal pupillary responses) late in the course of the disease. Postmortem examination then discloses neuronal loss and gliosis in the ocular motor nuclei (121–127). Most ALS patients have relative preservation of neurons in the oculomotor and trochlear nuclei, but often there are subtle morphologic changes, worse in demented patients and those with ophthalmoplegia (125). The majority of eye movement abnormalities seen in ALS are supranuclear in origin (128–131).

Lesions just adjacent to the oculomotor nuclear complex may mimic damage to the nucleus itself. These can usually be distinguished from their nuclear and infranuclear counterparts by stimulation of the vestibular system using oculocephalic or caloric testing, or by eliciting Bell's phenomenon (132,133) (see Chapter 18). When this causes improvement in ocular motility, a supranuclear lesion is unquestionably present. If there is no improvement, either isolated infranuclear or (more commonly) a combination of infranuclear and nuclear damage may exist (68,134).

In some cases of the Miller Fisher variant of the Guillain-Barré syndrome (132,135), an antibody-mediated peripheral neuropathy, ophthalmoplegia occurs from damage to nuclear and adjacent structures in the brain stem, as demonstrated by neuroimaging, although in most cases the predominant pathology is in the cranial nerves themselves (136–139) (discussed later). In especially severe cases, the brain stem syndrome overlaps that of Bickerstaff's encephalitis (140), both in neuroimaging and in pathology (141).

Lesions of the Oculomotor Nerve Fascicle

Beyond the nucleus but still within the brain stem, fascicular lesions of the oculomotor nerves produce both complete and incomplete palsies identical to those caused by lesions outside the brain stem, and it is by their accompanying brain

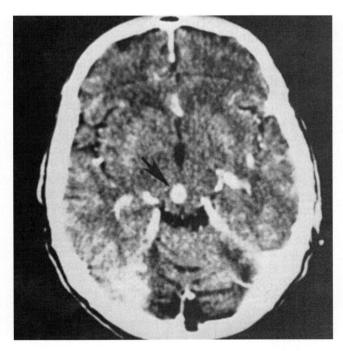

Figure 20.13. Computed tomographic scan in the patient seen in Figure 20.12. Note the enhancing lesion in the dorsal mesencephalon (*arrow*).

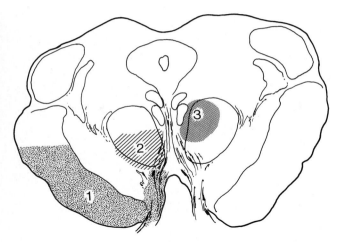

Figure 20.15. Diagram of a section through the mesencephalon showing regions in which the oculomotor nerve fascicle may be injured, causing specific neurologic syndromes. 1, Weber's syndrome; 2, Benedikt's syndrome; 3, Claude's syndrome.

stem signs and neuroimaging (142–144) that we can localize them. Sometimes there are no brain stem signs at all (145).

Fascicular oculomotor nerve palsy forms part of several classic midbrain syndromes. Nothnagel's syndrome is ipsilateral oculomotor nerve palsy and ipsilateral cerebellar ataxia from a lesion involving the oculomotor nerve fascicle and the brachium conjunctivum (146,147). (Nothnagel's

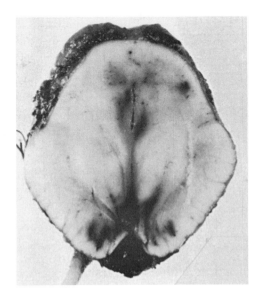

Figure 20.14. Hemorrhages in the mesencephalon in the region of the oculomotor nucleus after transtentorial herniation.

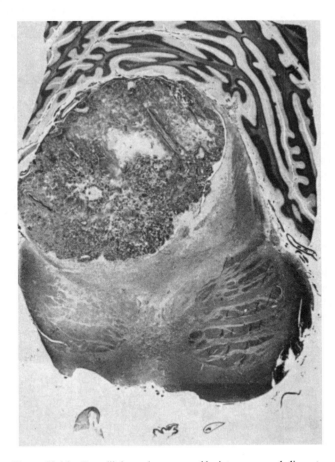

Figure 20.16. Benedikt's syndrome caused by intramesencephalic metastasis of a prostatic carcinoma. (From Loseke N, Retif J, Noterman J, et al. Inferior red nucleus syndrome [Benedikt's syndrome] due to a single intramesencephalic metastasis from a prostatic carcinoma: Case report. Acta Neurochir 1981;56:59–64.)

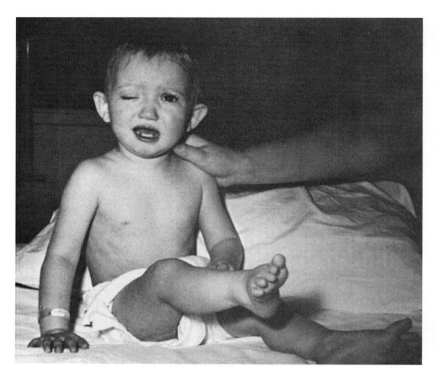

Figure 20.17. Weber's syndrome produced by a brain stem glioma infiltrating the mesencephalon. Note the oculomotor nerve palsy on the right and the hemiplegia on the left.

original patients had tumors of the quadrigeminal area, one described as the size of "a small apple," and a multitude of assorted signs) (147). The other syndromes are crossed (Fig. 20.15). Benedikt's syndrome is ipsilateral oculomotor nerve palsy with contralateral involuntary movements, which may be hemichorea, hemiathetosis, hemiballismus, or Parkinsonian tremor (147,148). These signs result from damage to the red nucleus, especially its dorsocaudal portion, through which the oculomotor fascicle passes (147,149) (Figs. 20.15 and 20.16). Weber's syndrome is ipsilateral oculomotor palsy with contralateral hemiplegia or hemiparesis, including the lower face and tongue, from damage to the oculomotor nerve fascicle and the cerebral peduncle (106,150,151) (Figs. 20.15, 20.17–20.19). Claude's syndrome is ipsilateral oculomotor nerve palsy with contralateral ataxia. It results from a lesion of the oculomotor nerve fascicle and usually the superior cerebellar peduncle just below and medial to the red nucleus (152), although the red nucleus itself is often involved as well (147,153,154). Slightly larger infarcts can cause combinations of these syndromes (151) (Fig. 20.20). The pontine, cerebellar, thalamic, and hemispheric strokes that frequently accompany midbrain infarction can cause associated horizontal and vertical gaze defects, internuclear ophthalmoplegia, dysarthria, ataxia, gait disturbance, hemiparesis, decreased level of consciousness, and visual field cuts (106,151).

Although the fascicular syndromes usually involve the pupil, this is not invariable (97,143–145,155–158), and pupil sparing may occur, as well as other incomplete oculomotor pareses (159). Pareses of just the superior division of the oculomotor nerve (levator palpebrae superioris and superior rectus weakness) or of just the inferior division (me-

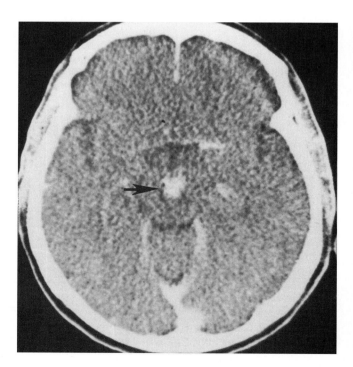

Figure 20.18. Computed tomogram in a patient with Weber's syndrome showing an enhancing lesion in the ventral mesencephalon (*arrow*). The lesion was thought to be a solitary metastasis from a breast carcinoma.

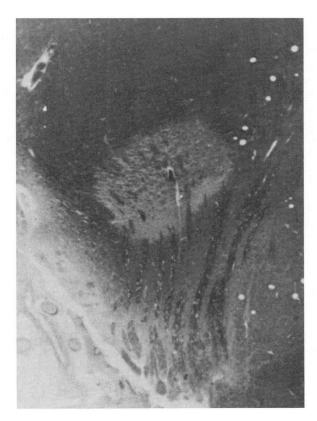

Figure 20.19. Demyelinating plaque in the mesencephalon damaging oculomotor fascicular fibers in the region of the cerebral peduncle. This lesion could produce Weber's syndrome.

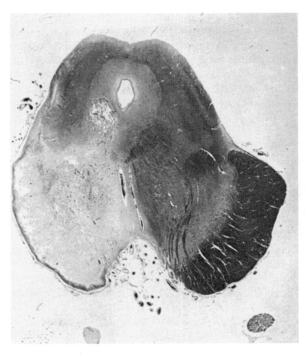

Figure 20.20. Histologic section through the mesencephalon of a patient who had a basilar artery occlusion. An infarct is present that involves the right oculomotor nerve nucleus and fascicle, the ipsilateral red nucleus, and the ipsilateral cerebral peduncle. The patient had a right oculomotor nerve palsy, a left rubral tremor, and a left hemiparesis. (Courtesy of Dr. Richard Lindenberg.)

dial rectus, inferior oblique, and inferior rectus weakness, with pupillary involvement) are most often caused by lesions in the superior orbital fissure or posterior orbit where the nerve is divided into its two main branches (see below), but fascicular lesions in the midbrain can produce them as well because of the organized anatomic arrangement of the fibers within the fascicle (160–164). Small fascicular lesions occasionally cause isolated weakness of one or two muscles (165–167).

The majority of midbrain syndromes are vascular in origin, are parts of more extensive strokes including the cerebellum, thalamus, pons, or cerebrum, and are caused by ischemia in the territory of the middle or upper basilar artery, less commonly by occlusion of perforating arterioles of the posterior cerebral artery. Paramedian arteriolar occlusions more commonly cause nuclear lesions, while more lateral ones cause fascicular lesions (104–106,151,154,164,168). Large-artery disease, lacunar disease, and cardioembolism are each frequent causes of midbrain infarction (151).

Fascicular oculomotor palsy also can be caused by hemorrhage (169,170), compression (70,149,166,171), trauma (82,172), inflammation (75,173–175), and demyelination (176–178). Because the fascicle contains central nervous system myelin, it can be involved in multiple sclerosis (MS), occasionally in isolation or even as the first MS clinical event. Oculomotor nerve palsy in this location may or may not involve the pupil. It may be painful and even associated with apoplectic headache, thus falsely suggesting a bleed from a posterior communicating artery aneurysm (177,179,180). Neuroimaging with high-quality magnetic resonance imaging (MRI) usually but not invariably shows the midbrain lesion, although some are missed (178,181). In one report, enhancement of the cisternal portion of the oculomotor nerve, not initially present, became evident 10 days after the appearance of a fascicular lesion from MS. While the authors discussed the possibility of an associated lesion of peripheral myelin, enhancement from Wallerian degeneration is a likelier explanation (181).

Lesions of the Oculomotor Nerve in the Subarachnoid Space

The most common site of an isolated acquired oculomotor paresis is in the subarachnoid space. The oculomotor nerve emerges from the cerebral peduncle of the midbrain into the interpeduncular fossa and runs forward and laterally in the subarachnoid space between the posterior cerebral and superior cerebellar arteries, beside the posterior communicating artery, and then penetrates the dura lateral to the posterior clinoid process and enters the cavernous sinus. The pupillary fibers are superficial and dorsal in the nerve. In rare patients, the nerve has an aberrant course (182).

A subarachnoid oculomotor palsy may be complete, incomplete, or progressive (183). Often it is isolated, without associated clinical findings. Usually there is some degree of accommodative paresis, but pupillary involvement is variable and depends primarily on the nature and location of the lesion. There may be (*a*) isolated pupillary involvement; (*b*) ophthalmoplegia with pupillary involvement; or (*c*) ophthalmoplegia with pupillary sparing.

Isolated Fixed, Dilated Pupil as the Sole Manifestation of Subarachnoid Oculomotor Nerve Palsy

The pupillary fibers run superficially and dorsally in the subarachnoid oculomotor nerve, so they are most vulnerable to compression from external masses such as aneurysms. Occasionally compressive lesions produce a dilated, fixed pupil without ophthalmoplegia, although this usually evolves in time into a more complete oculomotor palsy (184,185). There are numerous reports of isolated pupillary involvement from aneurysmal compression or aneurysmal subarachnoid hemorrhage, most commonly from a posterior communicating artery aneurysm (186–191). Usually there is severe headache as well, developing instantaneously in only 50% of the patients with aneurysmal subarachnoid hemorrhage and developing gradually within 1 to 5 minutes in another 19% (191). Frequently there are focal signs or symptoms or loss of consciousness (192). Most aneurysmal oculomotor nerve palsies involve the pupil but also have ophthalmoplegia (see below).

A third nerve palsy in the setting of a decreased level of consciousness is suspicious for transtentorial uncal herniation (193,194), a true surgical emergency, and ipsilateral pupillary enlargement often precedes the ophthalmoplegia. This pupillary dilation with a sluggish response to light may be the first clinical sign of increasing cerebral edema or of an expanding supratentorial mass such as an epidural,

subdural, or intracerebral hematoma (195,196). To supplement a century and a half of clinical observation, infrared pupillometry has documented pupillary changes during transtentorial uncal herniation. Several mechanisms have been implicated. Herniation of the hippocampal gyrus itself can press on the upper surface of the ipsilateral oculomotor nerve where the nerve passes over the ridge of the dura associated with the clival attachment of the free edge of the tentorium (197) (Fig. 20.21). Uncal herniation may push the mesencephalon laterally, pulling the compressed nerve more firmly into contact with the posterior clinoid process (198). The nerve may develop a deep groove (Kernohan's notch) where it is compressed upon the tentorial shelf between the free and the attached borders of the tentorium (199). The nerve may be displaced medially, causing its distal portion to ''kink'' over the clivus just posterior to the clinoid (195). Hemorrhage may develop within the compressed nerve (200). The basilar artery, which is tethered to the surface of the pons and midbrain by numerous short branches, moves downward with the herniating brain stem, further stretching both oculomotor nerves. The posterior cerebral arteries are therefore also drawn tightly down across the dorsal surface of the oculomotor nerves, where the pupillary fibers are concentrated, producing even more compression (201) (Fig. 20.22). The oculomotor complex may be shut down in the midbrain by decreased local blood flow, with or without direct brain stem compression (202).

With worsening herniation, contralateral hemiparesis and additional signs of impaired ipsilateral oculomotor nerve function appear. In addition to the previously mentioned ipsilateral pupillary dilation, weakness of eye muscles supervenes. The sequence of extraocular muscle involvement is not consistent, but ptosis and medial rectus muscle weakness are usually the most apparent and easily demonstrable signs in the obtunded or semicomatose patient.

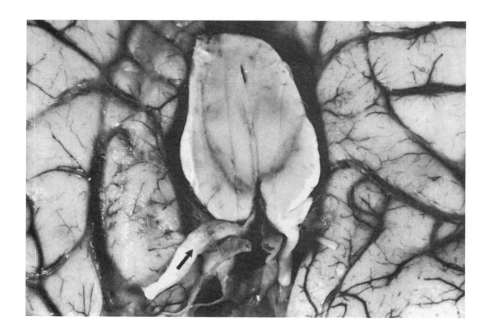

Figure 20.21. Compression of the oculomotor nerve (*arrow*) from a herniated hippocampal gyrus. (Courtesy of Dr. Richard Lindenberg.)

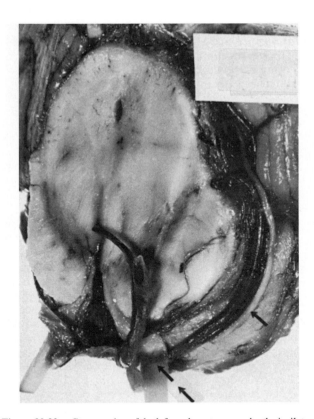

Figure 20.22. Compression of the left oculomotor nerve by the ipsilateral posterior cerebral artery in a case of transtentorial herniation. The artery has been reflected forward, exposing the site of compression (*double arrows*) on the nerve at its exit from the brain stem. The left superior cerebellar artery passes just beneath the oculomotor nerve and bends around the left side of the mesencephalon. Also note the location of the trochlear nerve (*single arrow*). (Courtesy of Dr. Richard Lindenberg.)

Variations on the typical pattern include "wrong side" (contralateral) pupillary dilation (203–205), "wrong side" (ipsilateral) hemiparesis from pressure of the tentorium on the contralateral displaced cerebral peduncle (204), early ipsilateral complete oculomotor nerve palsy with pupillary involvement (200,204,206), transiently oval pupils (207), and pupil-sparing oculomotor nerve palsy (171,208). Sometimes there are subtle abnormalities of the "normal" contralateral pupil. It may be midsize with a sluggish light reaction and may progress through a stage of mild miosis to dilation (209).

Postcompression recovery of oculomotor nerve function proceeds in the reverse order of the involvement. Following improvement in eye movement and resolution of ptosis, the pupil may remain slightly dilated and sluggishly reactive to light. We have found that the pupillary function is the least likely of all functions to return to normal.

Conditions other than aneurysms and herniation can produce a fixed, dilated pupil without immediate ophthalmoplegia. Head trauma can tear the oculomotor pupillary fibers in the medial part of the nerve as it leaves the brain stem (210). Other causes include tumors such as

schwannoma (211), arachnoid cyst of the interpeduncular cistern (212), basal meningitis (213–215), superficial siderosis (216), anti–GQ1-antibody syndrome (217), and a number of infections such as leprosy, herpes zoster, chickenpox, smallpox, measles, diphtheria, scarlet fever, pertussis, and influenza, although the site of injury in these cases is more likely the ciliary ganglion or the postganglionic parasympathetic fibers rather than the oculomotor nerve in the subarachnoid space. Truly isolated pupillary dilation from involvement of the subarachnoid portion of the oculomotor nerve is exceptionally rare. The occurrence of a widely dilated, nonreactive pupil in an otherwise healthy patient, even a patient complaining of headache, is far more likely to be caused by either ciliary ganglion involvement (i.e., a tonic pupil) or direct pharmacologic blockade, both of which can be diagnosed by pharmacologic testing (see Chapter 16).

Subarachnoid Oculomotor Nerve Palsy with Pupillary Involvement

The oculomotor nerve enters the subarachnoid space by exiting from the cerebral peduncle of the midbrain. Extra-axial mass lesions in this area may compress the peduncle as well as the nerve, causing Weber's syndrome (oculomotor palsy with contralateral hemiparesis or hemiplegia) and falsely suggesting an intrinsic midbrain lesion (218) (Fig. 20.23).

Intracranial aneurysms are the most common cause of isolated oculomotor nerve palsy with pupillary involvement (219,220), usually with pain in or around the eye (191,192,221), as mentioned above (Figs. 20.24–20.26). The symptomatic aneurysms most commonly arise from the junction of the internal carotid and posterior communicating arteries, where they are in close proximity to the oculomotor nerve, especially its pupillary fibers (222,223), but aneurysms located at the top of the basilar artery and aneurysms located at the junction of the basilar artery and superior cerebellar artery may produce a similar clinical picture (224–226). Bilateral oculomotor nerve palsies developed in one case from a ruptured anterior communicating artery aneurysm (227). Aneurysms may injure the oculomotor nerve by direct compression (228), from a small hemorrhage, or at the time of a major rupture (229). More than 90% of patients with major subarachnoid hemorrhage from rupture of a posterior communicating artery aneurysm had symptoms of oculomotor palsy prior to the rupture (194, 229–231). The oculomotor palsy is usually incomplete, at least at first (232). The earliest sign is a mild ptosis that may progress to a complete painful pupil-involving oculomotor palsy within hours to a few days, with the average interval from onset to maximum ophthalmoplegia being 3 days (183,233). In exceptional cases it may fluctuate in severity or be intermittent (234), or spontaneous resolution of the palsy may even occur without surgery. This does not rule out an aneurysm (235). Pupil-sparing oculomotor palsies are much less common from aneurysms but do occur (236) (see later).

Even with the use of the operating microscope, trauma to the oculomotor nerve during aneurysm surgery is common,

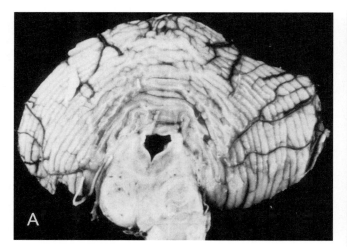

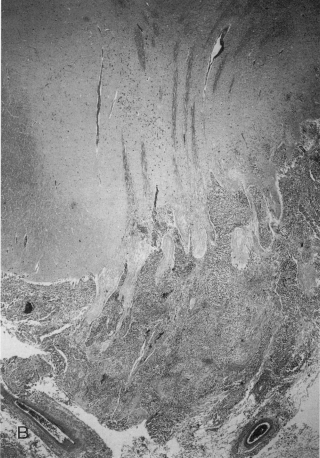

Figure 20.23. Leptomeningeal sarcoma that initially presented as an isolated oculomotor nerve palsy in a young boy who later developed a Weber's syndrome. *A*, Gross appearance showing tumor compressing and infiltrating the left ventral surface of the mesencephalon. *B*, Histopathologic section through the ventral mesencephalon showing infiltration and compression of the left cerebral peduncle by a tumor that is also destroying oculomotor nerve fibers as they exit from the brain stem.

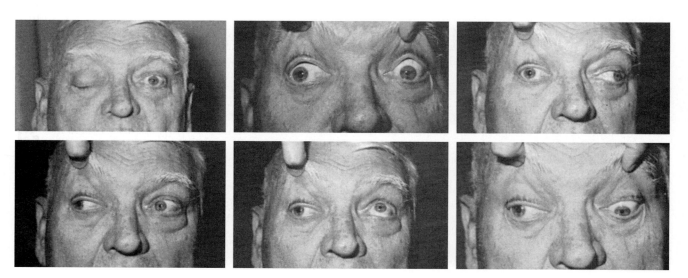

Figure 20.24. Complete right oculomotor nerve palsy with involvement of the pupil. The patient also complained of severe right-sided retroorbital pain.

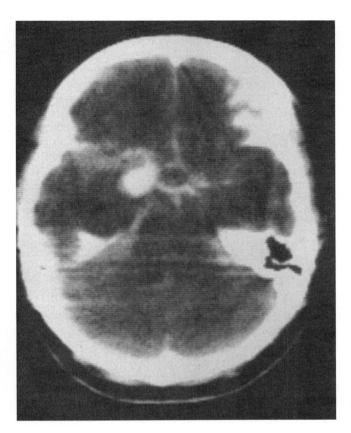

Figure 20.25. Computed tomographic scan shows a large aneurysm at the junction of the right internal carotid and right posterior communicating arteries in the patient in Figure 20.24.

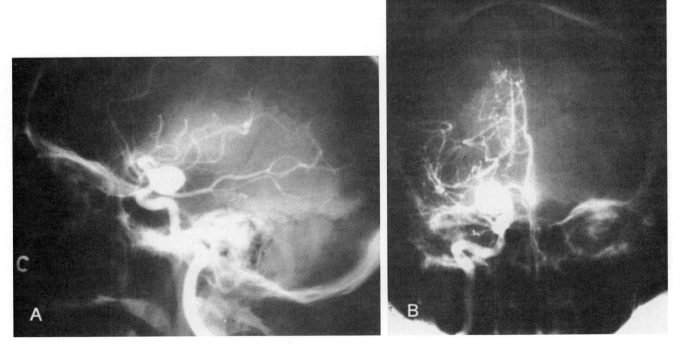

Figure 20.26. Selective right internal carotid arteriograms showing a large aneurysm at the junction of the right internal carotid and right posterior communicating arteries in the patient in Figure 20.24. *A*, Lateral view. *B*, Anteroposterior view.

either from manipulation of the nerve during surgery or from the aneurysm clip. The resulting weakness may be transient or permanent (237–240). Even without surgical complications, not all aneurysmal third nerve palsies recover (240). It remains to be seen whether there will be a better oculomotor outcome with endovascular treatment of saccular aneurysms (241,241a).

Tumors and other compressive lesions located in the subarachnoid space can stretch, infiltrate, or compress the oculomotor nerve. The patient may have no complaint until minor trauma produces enough damage in an already compromised nerve to cause ophthalmoparesis, ptosis, and mydriasis (242,243). A dolichoectatic basilar artery (157,244) or posterior cerebral artery (245,246) may compress the nerve painlessly, sometimes with intermittent ophthalmoplegia (245). Infiltrating lesions such as sarcoma (247), acute myeloid leukemia (248), Langerhans cell histiocytosis (i.e., eosinophilic granuloma) (249), glioma (250), and sarcoidosis (251) also sometimes cause oculomotor palsy.

Schwannomas of the subarachnoid portion of the oculomotor nerve produce progressive oculomotor paresis that usually becomes complete over months to years (252–254). In some cases, these tumors extend into the orbit, producing proptosis (255). Surgical treatment tends to worsen the oculomotor palsy (256). We examined a 31-year-old woman with neurofibromatosis type 1 who developed progressive bilateral complete oculomotor nerve pareses with pupillary involvement. MRI in this patient revealed bilateral interpeduncular lesions consistent with schwannomas (Fig. 20.27). Intrinsic lesions of the oculomotor nerve other than schwannomas, such as cavernous angiomas, can produce an acute or progressive oculomotor nerve paresis (257).

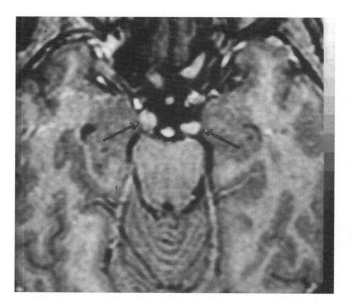

Figure 20.27. T1-weighted magnetic resonance image (axial view) in a 31-year-old-woman with progressive bilateral pupillary-involved oculomotor pareses and neurofibromatosis. There are bilateral enhancing lesions in the interpeduncular cistern (*arrows*) consistent with schwannomas of the oculomotor nerves.

When paralysis of the oculomotor nerve occurs in the setting of basilar meningitis, it is often bilateral and usually associated with other cranial nerve palsies (258–260) Nevertheless, meningitis, whether infectious, inflammatory, or neoplastic, occasionally produces isolated oculomotor nerve palsies, both with and without pupillary involvement (1,261,262).

The Miller Fisher syndrome is defined clinically as the triad of ophthalmoplegia, ataxia, and areflexia (132). While in some patients there is unquestionable brain stem involvement, perhaps causing nuclear and fascicular lesions of the oculomotor nerves (140,141), in most cases the lesion is in the peripheral nerves themselves (135). MRI studies bear this out (139,142). Usually there is bilateral involvement of the oculomotor, trochlear, and abducens nerves, with or without pupillary involvement, but partial and asymmetrical syndromes exist. About a third develop facial weakness, and a fifth develop generalized weakness. Most have proprioceptive sensory problems, as demonstrated by their inability to localize the thumb with their eyes closed (263). Areflexia develops by the end of the first week. If the paralysis is localized to the eye muscles and the face, the prognosis for full recovery is excellent, with or without treatment. With extensive paralysis, the outcome is less favorable. This is an acute immune axonal polyneuropathy, most commonly associated with *Campylobacter jejuni* infection, usually serotype 0-2 or 0-10, or less commonly with *Haemophilus influenzae* or infectious mononucleosis (264). About 80% of patients have an antibody to the GQ1b or GT1b ganglioside. There is molecular mimicry between lipopolysaccharides of *C. jejuni* and the human GQ1b ganglioside (265). Plasmapheresis has little effect on the ophthalmoplegia in the typical case (266). However, plasmapheresis and IVIg are useful in typical Guillain-Barré syndrome and are often helpful in Miller Fisher syndrome when the paralysis is more severe. Anti-GQ1b, anti-GT1a, and other ganglioside antibodies are sometimes found in typical Guillain-Barré syndrome as well, suggesting that there may be a clinical continuum of self-limited antibody-mediated syndromes from isolated internal ophthalmoplegia (217) through isolated incomplete oculomotor palsies such as an inferior division palsy (267), isolated oculomotor neuropathies such as an otherwise unexplained unilateral oculomotor nerve palsy (268), Miller Fisher syndrome, Guillain-Barré syndrome (269), to Bickerstaff's encephalitis (141,270). Chronic ophthalmoplegia can be associated with anti-GQ1b antibodies (271). Anti-GQ1b antibodies can be associated with a paraneoplastic syndrome of ophthalmoplegia and neuropathy (272). A chronic ataxic sensory neuropathy with ophthalmoplegia (CANOMAD syndrome) (273,274) is associated with anti-GD1b (disialosyl) antibodies.

While the ''vasculopathic'' diabetic painful oculomotor nerve palsy classically spares the pupil, the pupil may be involved 10–38% of the time (220,275). At least sometimes, the lesion is in the subarachnoid portion of the nerve (276).

Severe cranial trauma may produce oculomotor nerve palsy, both in isolation and in association with other cranial nerve palsies (210,277–280). Isolated involvement of the oculomotor nerve is usually caused by a frontal blow to a forward-moving head and in most patients is associated with skull fracture and concussion. Such fractures cause momentary displacement of bone fragments that may lacerate the nerve or impair its blood supply. Stretching, contusion, and avulsion are the major causes of the tissue damage (281,282). Cranial nerve avulsions are common in patients who die of closed head injuries. Obviously, such trauma may injure the oculomotor nerve fibers at any point from the mesencephalon to the orbit. If the subarachnoid portion of the oculomotor nerve is injured, variations in the size of the tentorial incisura may be important. A large tentorial opening may allow freer movement or rotation of the mesencephalon and adjacent structures at the instant of impact. Mild head injury rarely causes oculomotor nerve palsy (283), but when it does, it may signal the existence of an underlying mass lesion.

Elevated intracranial pressure very rarely injures the oculomotor nerve as it does the abducens nerve, and oculomotor palsy has developed in the settings of pseudotumor cerebri (284) and of chronic bilateral subdural hematomas (285).

Painful oculomotor nerve palsy with pupillary involvement may result from a posteriorly draining carotid–cavernous sinus fistula (286,287). The paresis may be complete or incomplete and the pupil spared or involved. These patients are usually older women. The fistula usually is of the spontaneous dural type, and the patient may be thought to have an aneurysm until angiography reveals the true etiology.

In the subarachnoid space, a lesion of the oculomotor nerve is most likely to produce an isolated palsy without other neurologic signs; thus, it is possible that the oculomotor nerve palsies with pupillary involvement that occur in association with various viral syndromes, perhaps immunologically mediated (see above), following immunization (288), and as part of a migraine syndrome (289), originate in the subarachnoid portion of the oculomotor nerve.

Subarachnoid Oculomotor Nerve Palsy with Pupillary Sparing

This syndrome occurs frequently in the form of the ''painful pupil-sparing diabetic third-nerve palsy,'' is clinically isolated, and is blamed on microvascular ischemia (Fig. 20.28). Considering how common it is, there are relatively few pathologic reports (290–293). It can occur in the midbrain from infarction or hemorrhage, often without being visible on MRI (97,143,144,155,170), or in the peripheral nerve in the subarachnoid space, cavernous sinus, or superior orbital fissure (291,294–297), apparently from an ischemic stroke of the nerve. Because the pupil fibers are peripheral in the nerve and may have a better blood supply than the rest of the nerve, they are relatively spared. The deep core of the subarachnoid oculomotor nerve has a scantier collateral blood supply than the interpeduncular or cavernous portions (185,290,298).

The degree of pupil sparing depends on when the pupil is examined and how much anisocoria has to be present to be counted. The degree of anisocoria, when present, is almost always 1 mm or less, and the pupil is reactive. In one study, 38% of affected patients had anisocoria, but in only two patients was it greater than 2 mm (299).

In one study of 55 patients with vasculopathic oculomotor paresis, in 55% eye muscle weakness was incomplete but diffusely involved all of the oculomotor muscles. Only 13% showed focal superior division weakness. Aneurysmal oculomotor paresis was more often focal (232).

Pain around the eye is very common and can be severe.

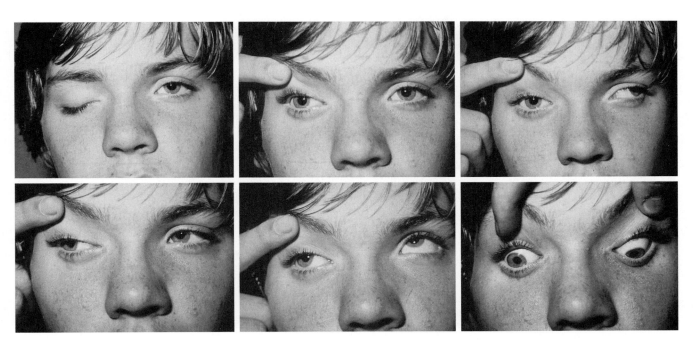

Figure 20.28. Pupil-sparing oculomotor nerve palsy in a patient with diabetes mellitus.

In animals, sensory fibers from the ophthalmic division of the trigeminal nerve join the first division of the oculomotor nerve within the lateral wall of the cavernous sinus and reach the spinal trigeminal nucleus (300,301). Both infarction and compression cause similar pain, and infarctions and aneurysms cannot be differentiated by the nature or severity of the pain. For that reason, patients with pupil-sparing oculomotor palsies deserve neuroimaging (302,303), and those with an anisocoria of 2 mm or more deserve angiography. Weakness typically worsens over a few to 10 days (304). Occasionally in diabetes, multiple cranial neuropathies appear simultaneously (305,306).

Identical painful ischemic palsies can occur without diabetes. Hypertension (275), atherosclerosis (142,219), migraine (276), systemic lupus erythematosus (307,308), temporal arteritis (309,310), use of sildenafil citrate (311), carotid–cavernous fistula (312), and dissection or occlusion of the carotid artery (313–315) are all rarely associated with the same clinical syndrome.

Ischemic oculomotor nerve palsies characteristically resolve within 4 to 16 weeks without treatment. Any not resolving in that time should be considered due to a mass such as an aneurysm or tumor (183). Resolution is almost always complete, and there is rarely (316–318) evidence of aberrant regeneration (Fig. 20.29).

While a pupil-sparing oculomotor palsy, with or without pain, is the hallmark of ischemia and a pupil-involving oculomotor palsy is the hallmark of compression, compressive lesions such as aneurysms do sometimes cause pupil-sparing oculomotor palsy. These tend to cause incomplete palsies (319). The compression can be from a posterior fossa tumor (320), temporal lobe astrocytoma putting pressure on the nerve or the brain stem (321), or subdural hematoma (208).

Other conditions occasionally associated with isolated, pupil-sparing oculomotor palsy include viral inflammations, monoclonal gammopathy (322), lymphoma, and leukemia.

Ophthalmoplegic migraine is a puzzling syndrome often beginning in childhood: prolonged attacks of migraine are sometimes followed by the development of an oculomotor palsy. Usually the child has a well-established migraine pattern before the first occurrence of ophthalmoplegia. While the headache may last hours, the ophthalmoplegia may last days to weeks, or after a number of attacks it may become permanent. It may or may not involve the pupil. Neuroimaging shows an area of enhancement or swelling (323) in the nerve in the interpeduncular fossa. Autopsy material typically shows a focal enlargement of the nerve, but the pathology is often confusing because of associated conditions that are probably not related (324). The possibility exists that ophthalmoplegic migraine is a recurrent focal demyelinating mononeuropathy related to the porous blood–nerve barrier where the nerve emerges from the brain stem (325–327) (Fig. 20.30). Another possibility is that it represents an intraneural occult vascular malformation (328). The abducens nerve or trochlear nerve can be involved instead. Aneurysms

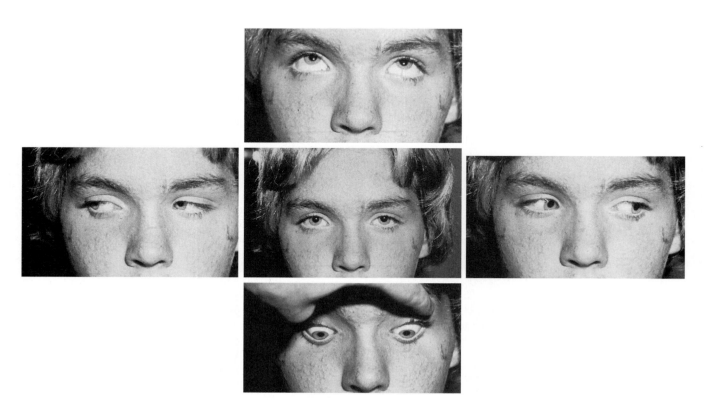

Figure 20.29.   Resolution of pupil-sparing oculomotor nerve palsy in the patient in Figure 20.28. Improvement began to occur about 3 weeks following onset of the palsy.

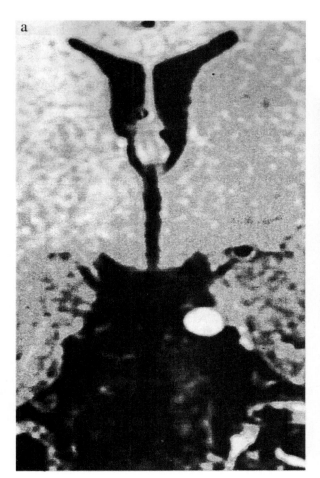
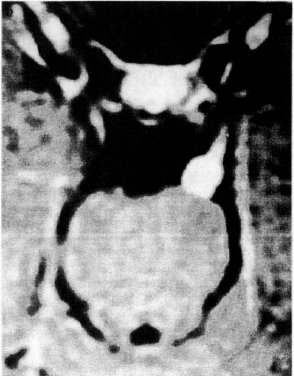

Figure 20.30. Magnetic resonance inaging showing enhancement of the intracisternal portion of the oculomotor nerve with gadolinium in a case of ophthalmoplegic migraine. *A,* Coronal image. *B,* Axial image. (From Lance JW, Zagami AS. Ophthalmoplegic migraine: A recurrent demyelinating neuropathy? Cephalalgia 2001;21:84–89.)

can cause this syndrome in older children or adults and need to be ruled out.

Subarachnoid Oculomotor Nerve Palsy From Involvement at or Near Its Entrance to the Cavernous Sinus

Like the trochlear and abducens nerves (see below), the oculomotor nerve is particularly vulnerable to stretch and contusion injuries where it is firmly attached to the dura adjacent to the posterior clinoid process, just posterior to the cavernous sinus (282) (Fig. 20.31). Frontal head trauma and aneurysms are common causes of injury at this site. In addition, oculomotor nerve dysfunction can be a complication of surgery in the parasellar region. The oculomotor nerve is damaged probably at this immediate precavernous site (239).

Lesions of the Oculomotor Nerve Within the Cavernous Sinus and Superior Orbital Fissure: The Sphenocavernous Syndrome

Lesions within the cavernous sinus or superior orbital fissure may produce isolated oculomotor nerve dysfunction but more often cause a unilateral cranial polyneuropathy. Because the cavernous sinus contains structures that continue through the superior orbital fissure, it is often impossible to determine clinically whether the lesion is confined to the sinus, is in the fissure, or involves both structures. The sphenocavernous syndrome, therefore, is characterized by paralysis or paresis of the oculomotor, trochlear, and abducens nerves, usually with involvement of the ophthalmic division (and in the cavernous sinus, the maxillary division) of the trigeminal nerve (329–331) (Fig. 20.32). It is usually due to a mass lesion (332). Patients often complain of severe periorbital or supraorbital pain because of trigeminal involvement. There may be numbness over the forehead or cheek. Often there is a Horner's syndrome, and there may be proptosis, edema of the eyelids, and chemosis of the conjunctiva. In patients with combined oculomotor paresis and Horner's syndrome, the pupil may be small or midposition and poorly reactive. This appearance is virtually pathognomonic of a cavernous sinus lesion (332).

Lesions commonly producing the sphenocavernous syndrome include aneurysms (333), meningiomas, pituitary tu-

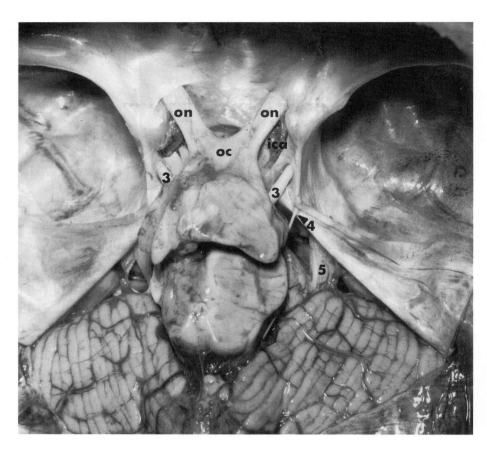

Figure 20.31. Base of the brain, showing position of the oculomotor (3) and trochlear (4) nerves as they penetrate the dura to enter the cavernous sinus. 5, trigeminal nerve; ica, internal carotid artery; oc, optic chiasm; on, optic nerve.

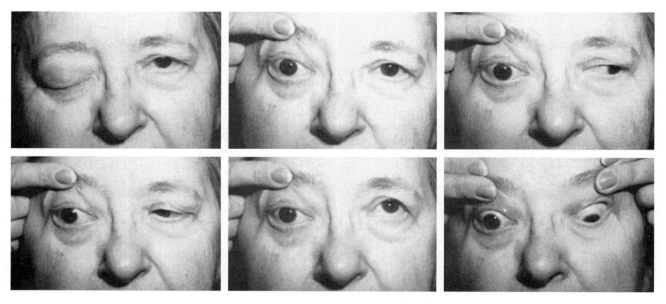

Figure 20.32. Patient with cavernous sinus syndrome from basal meningioma. The patient has right proptosis associated with a complete right oculomotor nerve palsy, a right abducens nerve paresis, and a right Horner's syndrome. The right pupil is slightly smaller than the left pupil.

mors, craniopharyngiomas, nasopharyngeal tumors, metastatic tumors, lymphoma, and infectious and inflammatory processes (332,334–342). Less common lesions include venous malformations of the cavernous sinus (343,344); schwannomas arising from the third, fourth, fifth, or sixth cranial nerve or from the intracavernous sympathetic nerves (345–349), rhabdomyosarcoma (350); sarcoid granuloma (351); and multiple myeloma with and without deposition of amyloid (352). Trigeminal schwannomas may be associated with pathologic laughter.

The Tolosa-Hunt syndrome (337,353) of painful ophthalmoplegia is caused by idiopathic granulomatous inflammation, anywhere from the orbit to the superior orbital fissure, cavernous sinus, or even intracranially. It is sometimes associated with Crohn's disease or systemic lupus erythematosus (354). Both pain and ophthalmoplegia improve rapidly and dramatically with systemic corticosteroids. Steroids are usually given for several months. In refractory cases, radiotherapy, cyclophosphamide, methotrexate, and cyclosporine have been tried (355). Unfortunately, steroids sometimes cause marked improvement in symptoms from tumors, aneurysms, and inflammatory disorders, so improvement is not helpful diagnostically (356). Biopsy of cavernous sinus lesions is difficult and dangerous. Careful follow-up and neuroimaging is therefore mandatory in cases of painful ophthalmoplegia, and MRI is the modality of choice, often requiring high-resolution multiplanar sequences and the use of gadolinium-based contrast agents (357). The signal intensity within the cavernous sinus of patients with Tolosa-Hunt syndrome is similar to that of orbital pseudotumor, meningioma, lymphoma, metastatic tumor, and sarcoidosis, and in some

cases there is sellar erosion (358) (Fig. 20.33). Careful follow-up is mandatory.

Septic thrombosis of the cavernous sinuses is an uncommon but life-threatening illness, with a mortality rate of 20–30% with antibiotic treatment and essentially 100% without treatment. The superior ophthalmic and cerebral veins and the pterygoid plexus veins are valveless and drain into the cavernous sinus, potentially bringing in bacteria and fungi from infections of the ethmoid and sphenoid sinuses and from the face, ear, nose, and teeth. Clinical signs include fever, proptosis, external ophthalmoplegia, sometimes with a large pupil from oculomotor nerve involvement, and sometimes with a Horner's syndrome and smaller pupil. Pain is significant. There may be decreased facial sensation in the first and second trigeminal divisions. The infection and thrombosis may become bilateral by spread through the circular sinus. Signs of impaired venous drainage from the orbit and face are common. If the lesion progresses, visual loss, meningitis, seizures, hemiparesis, and coma may develop. The most common organism implicated is *Staphylococcus aureus*. Other pathogens responsible are *Streptococcus* and gram-negative bacilli, anaerobes, and fungi (359).

Carotid–cavernous fistulas can produce typical cavernous sinus syndromes (286,335). Painful ophthalmoplegia occurs also in patients with syphilis, giant cell (temporal) arteritis, diabetes mellitus, rheumatoid arthritis, and systemic lupus erythematosus (332).

Isolated Oculomotor Nerve Involvement in the Cavernous Sinus

The same lesions that produce the cavernous sinus syndrome may also cause isolated oculomotor nerve dysfunc-

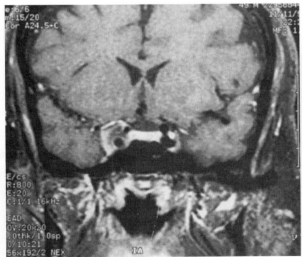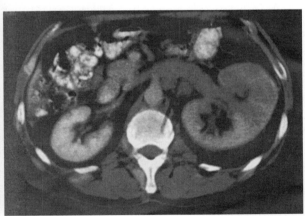

Figure 20.33. Neuroimaging in a patient with painful ophthalmoplegia. The patient was a 49-year-old man with right retrobulbar pain and generalized limitation of movement of the right eye. He was thought to have the Tolosa-Hunt syndrome and was treated with oral corticosteroids without improvement. The ophthalmoparesis progressed to a complete ophthalmoplegia associated with loss of vision in the eye. *A*, T1-weighted, coronal magnetic resonance image after intravenous injection of paramagnetic contrast material reveals enlargement of the right cavernous sinus. *B*, Computed tomography scan of the abdomen reveals a left renal mass. The patient was found to have a metastatic renal cell carcinoma. (From Mehelas TJ, Kosmorsky GS. Painful ophthalmoplegia syndrome secondary to metastatic renal cell carcinoma. J Neuroophthalmol 1996;16:289–290.)

tion, with and without pupillary involvement. In particular, extrinsic lesions, including pituitary adenomas (334), craniopharyngiomas, suprasellar aneurysms (332), and suprasellar meningiomas, can cause isolated oculomotor nerve dysfunction. Lesions that infiltrate the cavernous sinus, such as multiple myeloma, Tolosa-Hunt syndrome, metastatic carcinoma (142), and nasopharyngeal carcinoma (360), may also produce an oculomotor nerve palsy as the initial sign of the disease, as may intrinsic schwannomas of the oculomotor nerve (Figs. 20.34 and 20.35).

The ischemia that produces oculomotor nerve dysfunction in patients with diabetes mellitus is, at least in some instances, caused by a lesion in the intracavernous portion of the nerve (297). Pupil-sparing oculomotor nerve palsies may develop in patients with a persistent primitive trigeminal artery (361). In such cases, the palsy is thought to result from direct pressure on the cavernous portion of the oculomotor nerve by this congenital vessel that provides a connection between the infraclinoid internal carotid artery and the rostral basilar artery.

Lesions of the Oculomotor Nerve Within the Orbit

Orbital lesions that produce oculomotor nerve dysfunction usually produce other ocular motor dysfunction as well as visual loss and, in some cases, significant proptosis. The complete orbital apex syndrome is the association of lesions of the third, fourth, sixth, and ophthalmic division of the fifth cranial nerve, with optic neuropathy. Proptosis is common. While the orbital apex syndrome can usually be distinguished clinically from the more painful sphenocavernous syndrome, some lesions extend from the cavernous sinus

into the orbital apex. In addition, large intracranial mass lesions occasionally expand to such a degree that they compress the intracranial optic nerve and the subarachnoid or cavernous sinus portion of the oculomotor nerves, and also prevent adequate venous drainage from the orbit, resulting in a ''pseudo-orbital apex syndrome'' (157,362) (Fig. 20.36).

The oculomotor nerve enters the orbit as two separate divisions: the superior division, which innervates the levator palpebrae superioris and the superior rectus muscle, and the inferior division, which innervates the medial and inferior rectus muscles, the inferior oblique muscle, and the ciliary ganglion. An incomplete oculomotor nerve paresis in the distribution of either division is most often caused by a lesion in either the sphenocavernous region or the orbital apex. Because the oculomotor nerve has a divisional topographic arrangement beginning in the brain stem, divisional oculomotor nerve pareses occasionally result from lesions in the brain stem or subarachnoid space (Fig. 20.37).

Orbital lesions can interrupt the function of the entire oculomotor nerve, a division of the oculomotor nerve, or a branch to one or a few muscles. In addition, the globe may be displaced or the muscles infiltrated. It is hard to tell muscle dysfunction from nerve dysfunction. Myasthenia gravis can mimic oculomotor nerve dysfunction, although it does not involve the pupil. Orbital pseudotumor, like Tolosa-Hunt syndrome in the cavernous sinus, is a steroid-responsive granulomatous condition (see above) that can involve any or all of the ocular motor nerves in the orbit.

Partial or complete oculomotor nerve dysfunction also may occur following dental anesthesia (363,364). The most commonly accepted explanation is that the anesthetic solution is inadvertently injected into the inferior dental artery,

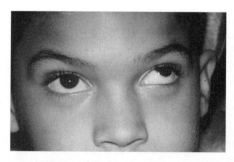

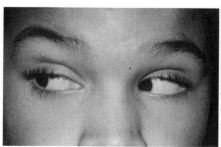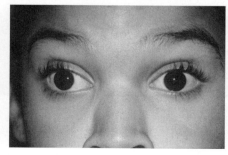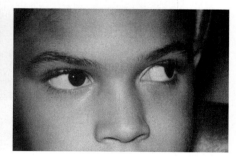

Figure 20.34. Appearance of a 10-year-old boy with a slowly progressive, pupil-involved right oculomotor nerve paresis. The patient has an exotropia in primary position (*center*), associated with marked limitation of elevation (*above*) and mild limitation of adduction (*right*) of the right eye. Abduction of the eye is normal (*left*), as is depression (not shown).

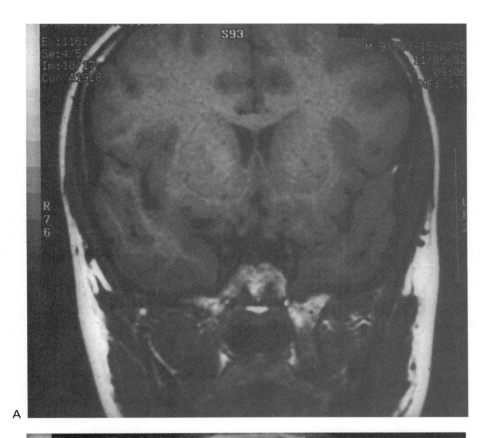

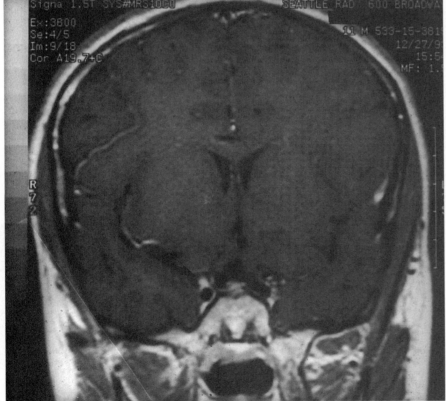

Figure 20.35. *A*, T1-weighted coronal image shows slight enlargement of the right oculomotor nerve within the cavernous sinus (*arrow*). *B*, After intravenous injection of paramagnetic contrast material, the enlarged nerve enhances (*arrow*). The appearance is consistent with a schwannoma of the cavernous portion of the oculomotor nerve.

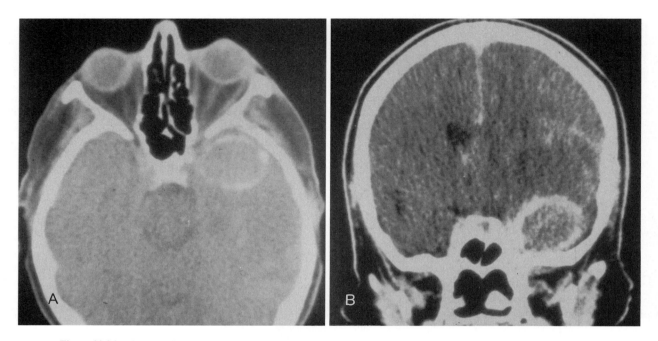

Figure 20.36. Computed tomographic scan showing a giant, partially thrombosed, intracranial aneurysm that was responsible for producing a pseudoorbital apex syndrome in a 69-year-old woman. Note the location of the aneurysm adjacent to the superior orbital fissure and optic canal. The patient had left proptosis, ophthalmoplegia, and optic neuropathy. *A,* Axial view. *B,* Coronal view.

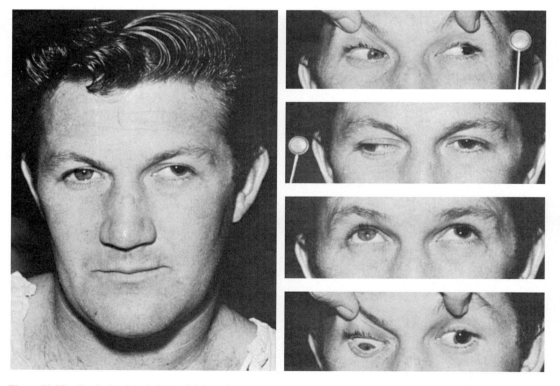

Figure 20.37. Paralysis of the inferior division of the left oculomotor nerve. The left levator palpebrae superioris muscle and the superior rectus muscle are not involved. This palsy occurred spontaneously and without pain. Neuroradiologic investigations, including cerebral arteriography, were normal. The palsy cleared almost completely (the pupil remained slightly dilated) within 6 weeks. The etiology was never determined.

which is immobile as it enters the inferior dental canal, or into the superior alveolar artery. In either instance, the solution then travels by retrograde flow into the maxillary artery. From the maxillary artery, the solution reaches the middle meningeal artery, the orbital branch of which forms a fairly constant anastomosis with the lacrimal branch of the ophthalmic artery. In some persons in whom the origin of the ophthalmic artery is absent or narrowed, this anastomosis dominates the arterial supply to the orbit (365).

Lesions of the Oculomotor Nerve of Uncertain or Variable Location

In both adults and children, the site of the lesion causing an isolated oculomotor palsy is often unclear (275,366). Many types of lesion can affect the nerve at several potential sites. For example, patients with diabetic or hypertensive oculomotor nerve pareses may have ischemic lesions of the brain stem or the subarachnoid or cavernous sinus portions of the nerve. The site of immunologic damage to the oculomotor nerve and its companion nerves is variable as well. Isolated weakness of the inferior oblique muscle can result from a fascicular lesion in the midbrain or a small lesion in the orbit (165) (Fig. 20.38). The ''double elevator palsy'' of the inferior oblique and superior rectus muscles is usually due to a supranuclear lesion in the pretectum but can occur also in the oculomotor fascicle or the orbit. A pretectal location is responsible if the Bell's phenomenon is preserved (367,368).

Recovery from Acquired Oculomotor Nerve Palsy

Oculomotor nerve paralysis, whether complete or incomplete, may have several outcomes. First, complete recovery may occur, sometimes in as little as a week or two. This suggests recovery from neurapraxia, without axonal loss.

With presumed nerve infarcts associated with diabetes, hypertension, or ophthalmoplegic migraine, recovery does not begin for a month or more but is usually complete within 3 months (369). This suggests a lesion of axons, with preservation of nerve connective tissue. With aneurysmal compression (240,370) or trauma, it can take up to 2 or 3 years to recover completely, suggesting more severe anatomic disruption of the nerve. If ptosis following trauma is going to recover completely, it usually does so within 6 months but occasionally takes as long as 2 years (371).

In some cases of oculomotor nerve palsy, the paralysis persists completely unchanged. These nerves have usually been transected by trauma or chronic compression or have been infiltrated by tumor. Sometimes recovery is only partial. This occurs especially after damage to the fascicular portion of the nerve. Partial recovery may be characterized by oculomotor nerve synkinesis, so-called ''aberrant regeneration'' (see below). Usually this synkinesis becomes apparent within 9 weeks after injury, but it has taken 3 to 6 months (371).

Acquired Oculomotor Synkinesis: Misdirection of Regenerating Fibers in the Oculomotor Nerve (Aberrant Regeneration)

General Considerations

There are several competing theories to explain the clinical findings of oculomotor nerve synkinesis. Peripheral motor and sensory nerves, including the autonomic nerves, can regenerate to some degree, and the degree of recovery is related to the severity of the lesion. If only the myelin is damaged, conduction block will result but axonal transport continues, the axon does not degenerate, and its muscle does not atrophy. Once the myelin has regenerated, nerve conduction recommences.

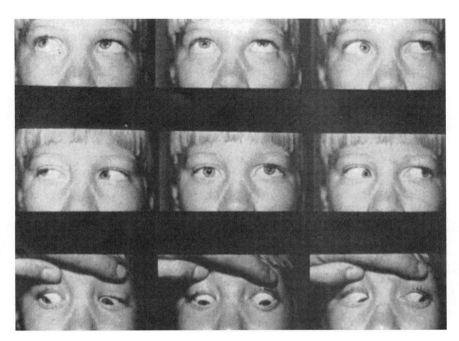

Figure 20.38. Isolated paresis of the right inferior oblique muscle in a healthy 11-year-old boy who had a history of a right hypotropia of several years' duration. (From Scott WE, Nankin SJ. Isolated inferior oblique paresis. Arch Ophthalmol 1977;5:1586–1593.)

If a nerve is crushed, interrupting axons but not the connective tissue tubes investing them, Wallerian degeneration takes place. The axon disintegrates distal to the lesion. Central chromatolysis appears in the nerve cell bodies, which then manufacture proteins and other molecules for axon repair and pump them down to the regenerating part of the axons. The axons grow slowly down their connective tissue tubes to reconnect with their targets, and only then does useful nerve conduction recommence. The anatomy of the nerve and its relationship to its target is basically unchanged. In cases where the nerve is lesioned very close to its cell body (and the oculomotor nerve is short, so this may be relevant), axonal degeneration may progress proximally as well, sometimes leading to loss of the cell body.

If the nerve is transected but the two ends are very near together, regeneration may be possible. Wallerian degeneration takes place. New axon sprouts fan out in all directions from the severed end of the proximal segment. Those that find the distal nerve segment will bridge the gap and grow down the connective tissue tubes. Often they are misdirected and grow down each other's tubes. This could result in an axon that previously innervated the superior rectus now innervating the medial rectus or the ciliary ganglion. This results in oculomotor nerve synkinesis. If the nerve is avulsed, or if it is transected with the two ends being far apart, the new axon sprouts will not be able to find connective tissue tubes, and reinnervation will not occur. In the brain stem, glia and signaling molecules form the scaffolding to direct nerve regeneration. Further evidence for regenerating nerve misdirection (described earlier) includes the findings after section and anastomosis of the oculomotor nerve in man (372,373).

Ephaptic transmission and central synaptic reorganization are two other mechanisms proposed to account for the synkinesis (374). It has been proposed that ephaptic activation of axons can occur centrally within a partially demyelinated lesion or peripherally at a compressed or severed segment of nerve. Lepore and Glaser (374) suggested that that this mechanism could account for the insidious transition from paresis to synkinesis that occurs in some patients. An ephapse develops where adjacent nerve fibers were injured (axo-axonal transmission). Similarly, they believed that the recovery from associated ocular movements to normal function argued strongly for transient "cross-talk" between adjacent axons rather than for misdirection of regenerating fibers (Figs. 20.39 and 20.40).

Another theory proposed by Lepore and Glaser is that major structural changes responsible for acquired oculomotor nerve synkinesis actually occur within the oculomotor subnuclei rather than in the peripheral axons. Chromatolysis that is initiated by axonal injury, in this theory, could induce structural, metabolic, and physiologic alterations in the nerve cell body and its connections. Thus, anomalous co-contraction might occur because after axon injury, central brain stem neurons at the level of the oculomotor subnuclei undergo synaptic reorganization. Animal studies show that after oculomotor nerve section and reapproximation, the contralateral oculomotor nucleus and ipsilateral abducens, trochlear, and trigeminal nuclei send intraaxial sprouts through the brain

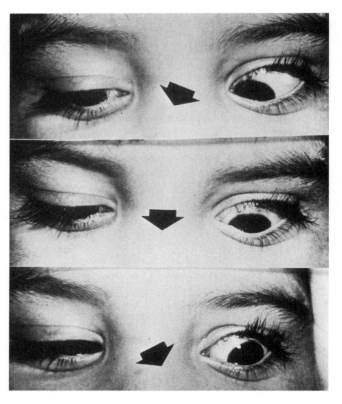

Figure 20.39. Pseudo-Graefe eyelid retraction in a 3-year-old boy 10 months following the development of a complete left oculomotor nerve palsy associated with a severe migraine episode. Ocular motility was otherwise normal. (From Lepore FE, Glaser JS. Misdirection revisited: A critical appraisal of acquired oculomotor nerve synkinesis. Arch Ophthalmol 1980; 98:2206–2209.)

stem down the previously injured nerve to the muscles, causing aberrant reinnervation. In addition, there is some central topographic reorganizing at the level of the nucleus (375–377).

In humans, acquired synkinesis has involved the opposite eyelid (378), the abducens nerve (379), the facial nerve (380), the trigeminal nerve (381), and the oculomotor nerve (382). It may be that damage to the third nerve (or to the fourth or sixth nerve) causes loss of the axon and cell body, followed by sprouting of nearby motor axons. These would be guided down the preexisting glial tracks in the brain stem out to the connective tissue tubes in the peripheral nerve and eventually connect to muscles and the ciliary ganglion. There would later be some degree of central reorganization of the nuclei involved. There might be ephaptic conduction as well, especially between peripheral nerve axons that had lost myelin. All these mechanisms are probably correct to some degree. While there is as yet no evidence that new oculomotor cell bodies can arise, there is also no evidence that they cannot. Neural plasticity is a powerful force.

Considerations Relating to the Oculomotor Nerve

Following injury to the oculomotor nerve at any point along its pathway from the brain stem to the orbit, a syn-

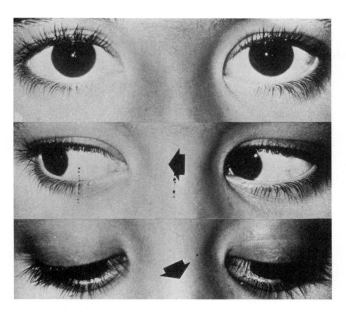

Figure 20.40. Disappearance of pseudo-Graefe sign seen in Figure 20.39. The eyelid retraction resolved within 3 months after it was first noted. Ocular motility and eyelid motility are normal. (From Lepore FE, Glaser JS. Misdirection revisited: A critical appraisal of acquired oculomotor nerve synkinesis. Arch Ophthalmol 1980;98:2206–2209.)

drome of oculomotor nerve synkinesis may occur. In adults, synkinesis first appears about 9 weeks after injury (371), whereas in infants with birth trauma, it first appears 1 to 6 weeks following birth. Oculomotor nerve synkinesis is thought to occur from misdirection of regenerated axons in the nerve or brain stem, ephaptic transmission, and/or nuclear reorganization (see above). If the nerve has been transected neurosurgically and reanastomosed or grafted, synkinesis has developed as expected. Thus, the levator palpebrae superioris may receive fibers that were originally destined for the medial rectus muscle, or fibers originally intended for the superior rectus muscle may reach the inferior oblique, inferior rectus, or medial rectus muscles. Finally, fibers originally destined for any of these muscles may reach the ciliary ganglion to synapse with the postganglionic parasympathetic fibers that innervate the iris sphincter muscle or the ciliary body.

The signs of aberrant regeneration of the oculomotor nerve are as follows: (*a*) horizontal gaze–eyelid synkinesis—elevation of the involved eyelid in attempted adduction of the eye; (*b*) pseudo-Graefe sign—retraction and elevation of the eyelid on attempted downward gaze (Fig. 20.41); (*c*) limitation of elevation and depression of the eye with occasional retraction of the globe on attempted vertical movement; (*d*) adduction of the involved eye on attempted elevation or depression; (*e*) pseudo-Argyll Robertson pupil—the involved pupil does not react, or reacts poorly and irregularly to light stimulation, but constricts on adduction during conjugate gaze; and (*f*) monocular vertical optokinetic responses—the normal eye responds normally, but the involved eye has suppressed vertical responses (383).

Partial involvement may occur. Rarely, the eyelid of the contralateral eye is involved, resulting in elevation on downgaze (378).

In most but not all cases of aberrant regeneration the pupil is involved, because motor axons (also cholinergic) have innervated the ciliary ganglion. The pupil constricts when the patient is asked to look in a direction requiring oculomotor nerve function (Figs. 20.42 and 20.43). In other cases, the pupil may appear to be permanently paralyzed in the mid-dilated position, but slit-lamp biomicroscopy shows slight movement that reflects aberrant reinnervation (384). In still other cases, particularly in patients with congenital oculomotor palsy with aberrant regeneration, the pupil may be quite miotic (17). Some of these pupils show further constriction on attempted ocular movement, whereas others do not appear to constrict further under any circumstances. Segmental iris contraction to light may occur (384,385). Because these pupils have a poor reaction to light but do constrict during adduction, their reactions simulate the light–near dissociation of the Argyll Robertson pupil, and they have been called "pseudo-Argyll Robertson pupils." Oculomotor synkinesis may be subtle and partial rather than blatant. The ciliary body may be anomalously reinnervated as well, with increased myopia and increased intraocular pressure on attempted adduction (386).

Secondary Oculomotor Nerve Synkinesis

This is oculomotor nerve synkinesis developing after an acquired or congenital oculomotor palsy, usually complete. The responsible lesion may be an aneurysm, trauma, compression, Guillain-Barré syndrome (387), ophthalmoplegic migraine, or almost anything, but the rule remains: aberrant regeneration is extremely rare (but never say never [316,388]) following a diabetic painful pupil-sparing oculomotor palsy or any other ischemic lesion. Its occurrence in this setting demands a work-up for an aneurysm or other missed lesion. Most cases of oculomotor nerve synkinesis are unilateral, but some are bilateral (387).

Primary Oculomotor Nerve Synkinesis

Less frequently, oculomotor nerve synkinesis occurs as a "primary" phenomenon, without a preexisting acute oculomotor nerve paresis. Patients with primary oculomotor nerve synkinesis usually harbor slow-growing lesions of the cavernous sinus, most commonly meningiomas or aneurysms, but schwannomas can be responsible as well (157,374,389, 390) (Fig. 20.44). Sometimes the responsible slow-growing mass lesion is not in the cavernous sinus. It might be an unruptured aneurysm at the junction of the internal carotid artery and the posterior communicating artery.

EVALUATION AND MANAGEMENT OF PATIENTS WITH ACQUIRED OCULOMOTOR NERVE PALSY

The evaluation of a patient with an acquired oculomotor nerve palsy depends on the associated symptoms and signs, the pattern of oculomotor nerve involvement, and the age of the patient. As should be clear from the preceding discus-

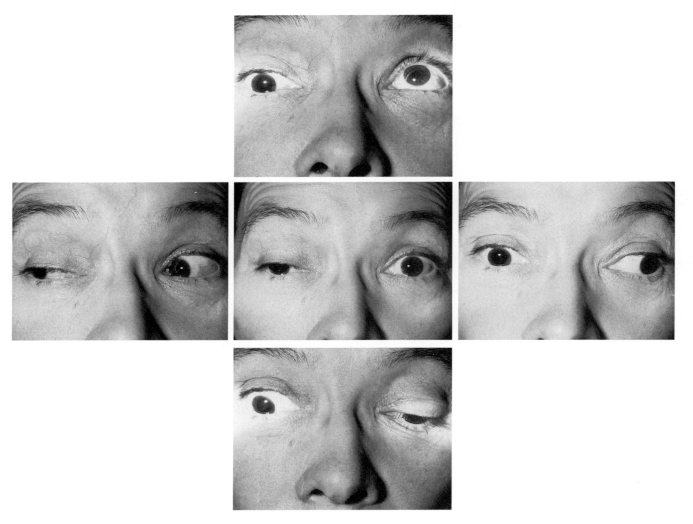

Figure 20.41.   Misdirected regeneration of the right oculomotor nerve following trauma (secondary aberrant regeneration). Note elevation of the right upper eyelid on attempted downward gaze and on attempted adduction of the right eye (pseudo-Graefe sign). Although the right pupil was markedly dilated and poorly reactive to light, it constricted slightly on attempted adduction of the eye.

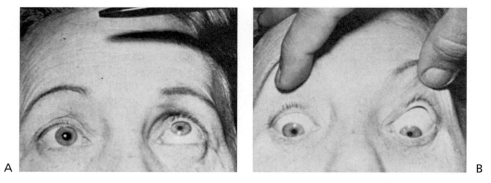

Figure 20.42.   Aberrant regeneration of the right oculomotor nerve with involvement of the pupil. *A*, During attempted elevation of the eyes, the right pupil remains mid-dilated. *B*, During depression of the eyes, the right pupil constricts.

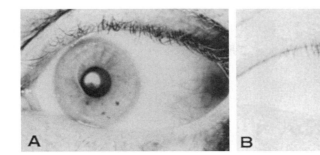

Figure 20.43. Aberrant regeneration of the pupillary sphincter associated with aberrant regeneration of the left oculomotor nerve. The pupil does not constrict significantly to a light stimulus. *A*, During attempted adduction of the left eye, the pupil constricts. *B*, When the left eye abducts, the pupil redilates.

sion, oculomotor nerve dysfunction may present in one of five ways:

1. With a dilated, nonreactive or poorly reactive pupil without ophthalmoplegia or ptosis. This is rare and usually occurs in a comatose or obtunded patient with an expanding supratentorial mass lesion. In the awake, alert patient with a widely dilated pupil, pharmacologic blockade or a tonic pupil is far more likely than a posterior cerebral aneurysm. Magnetic resonance angiography may still be needed to rule out an aneurysm.
2. With ophthalmoplegia, ptosis, and a dilated, poorly reactive or nonreactive pupil. This may be caused by any pathologic process at any point along the pathway of the oculomotor nerve. If the anisocoria is 2 mm or greater, ischemia is probably not the cause, and catheter angiography is appropriate (299,391) if MRI does not show a nonaneurysmal mass lesion. Magnetic resonance angiog-

raphy can detect more than 95% of aneurysms large enough to bleed (263,392), but conventional angiography remains the most sensitive test for detecting intracranial aneurysms and should be performed in any patient in whom this possibility is considered likely. Catheter angiography has a morbidity or mortality of 1–2% (393). Aneurysms are occasionally reported (394,395) in children in the first decade of life. In a young child with an acquired pupil-involved oculomotor nerve palsy, with negative noninvasive imaging, the decision to perform conventional angiography must be made on a case-by-case basis.

3. With ophthalmoplegia and ptosis, but without any pupillary involvement. Pupil-sparing oculomotor nerve palsies are most commonly caused by ischemia, but compression and inflammation may also produce them. An underlying ischemic or inflammatory process such as diabetes mellitus, giant cell arteritis, or systemic hypertension should

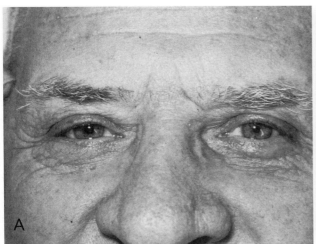
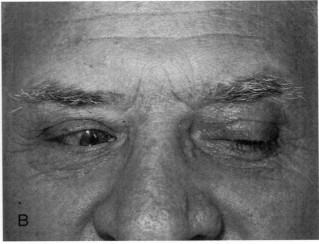

Figure 20.44. Primary aberrant regeneration in a 63-year-old man. The patient had never had an acute oculomotor nerve palsy but had begun to notice intermittent diplopia. He was found to have a large right intracavernous trigeminal schwannoma. *A*, The patient has a small, intermittent exotropia caused by right medial rectus weakness. There is also slight anisocoria with a larger pupil on the right. *B*, On attempted gaze downward and to the left, the patient develops right upper eyelid retraction (pseudo-Graefe sign).

be sought. Evaluation should include measurement of systemic blood pressure, serum glucose, and sedimentation rate. Aneurysms involve the pupil 96% of the time, and when they spare it, they tend to cause incomplete motor paresis (396). Some favor performing MRI and magnetic resonance angiography in a pupil-sparing complete oculomotor nerve palsy, while other expert clinicians choose observation, especially in the older patient with vascular risk factors. Certainly, if there is no improvement after 3 months, imaging needs to be performed to rule out a mass lesion. Whenever the pupils are normal, an ophthalmoplegia may represent the effects of myopathic or neuromuscular disease (e.g., myasthenia gravis) rather than a neuropathy.

4. With ophthalmoplegia, ptosis, and a small or midpositioned fixed pupil. Patients with this clinical picture usually have lesions in the cavernous sinus that have damaged not only the oculomotor nerve but also the oculosympathetic fibers.

5. With aberrant regeneration. Patients with primary aberrant regeneration have slow-growing mass lesions compressing or infiltrating the oculomotor nerve in the cavernous sinus or, less often, in the subarachnoid space.

After diagnosis and treatment of the responsible lesion, the degree of recovery determines the need for further treatment. Ischemic palsies usually begin to recover after a month and are completely recovered in 3 months. If not, imaging is required, because there is probably an underlying mass lesion. After aneurysm clipping or the removal of a compressive lesion, recovery usually takes 3 months but may take as long as 3 years (370). Ptosis is usually resolved in 6 months if it is going to resolve at all, but again it may take up to 2 years. Some oculomotor palsies recover partially or never recover at all.

Once it is clear that recovery will not be complete, the patient has several choices. In patients with partial recovery, various strabismus procedures may be of benefit in providing binocular single vision, at least in the primary position (397,398), and ptosis surgery may also be used to improve the position of the affected eyelid. Botulinum toxin injections of the lateral rectus may realign the eyes in mild cases, while waiting for improvement (399). Some patients seem content simply to patch the affected eye or are able to ignore the double image. An opaque contact lens provides a cosmetically acceptable means of alleviating diplopia in these patients. The surgical management of patients with complete oculomotor nerve palsy is more difficult. The goal is to regain fusion in primary position. Several different techniques are in use, probably because none produces consistently excellent results (397,398,400,401). Surgical reanastomosis of a severed oculomotor nerve has resulted in aberrant regeneration (372,373).

TROCHLEAR (FOURTH) NERVE PALSIES

Trochlear nerve palsy is the most common cause of acquired vertical strabismus in the general population. A nuclear or fascicular lesion causes partial or complete paralysis of the contralateral superior oblique muscle, usually associated over time with overaction of its antagonist, the ipsilateral inferior oblique muscle (Figs. 20.45 and 20.46). After issuing from the dorsum of the brain stem, the trochlear nerves cross almost immediately in the anterior medullary velum. Each nerve then runs in the subarachnoid space, through the cavernous sinus and superior orbital fissure, into the orbit, to the superior oblique muscle. Patients with a trochlear nerve palsy complain of vertical diplopia that is greatest in downgaze and gaze to the opposite side, because the superior oblique muscle is a depressor in adduction, when the muscle axis is parallel to the visual axis. The patients also have excyclotorsion when tested with double Maddox rods or Lancaster red-green glasses (402,403). The superior oblique muscle is an intorter, particularly when the eye is in abduction. The ability of the superior oblique muscle to intort the eye is particularly important when assessing superior oblique function in the presence of an oculomotor nerve palsy. The absence of intorsion when the patient attempts to depress the abducted eye indicates lack of superior oblique function as well.

Most patients with trochlear nerve palsy have compensatory torticollis (Fig. 20.47). They typically tilt the head to the side opposite the paralyzed superior oblique muscle to avoid torsional diplopia (404). This spontaneous ocular torticollis is absent in patients with poor vision in either eye and in patients with large vertical fusional amplitudes that allow them to fuse in all positions of gaze (405). Less commonly, patients with trochlear nerve palsy tilt their heads to the side of the palsy, presumably resulting in greater separation of images, thus allowing one of the images to be ignored.

Paralysis of the trochlear nerve is far less commonly recognized than paralysis of either the oculomotor or abducens nerves (219,275,406,407).

CONGENITAL

Congenital trochlear nerve palsy accounts for 29–67% of trochlear nerve palsies (408,409). The etiology is unknown. Aplasia of one trochlear nerve nucleus has been documented as part of a congenital nuclear aplasia syndrome or, together with aplasia of the abducens nerve, in a patient with the oculoauriculovertebral dysplasia–hemifacial microsomia syndrome (Goldenhar-Gorlin syndrome) (19,410). Most isolated trochlear nerve palsies are sporadic, but autosomal-dominant transmission occasionally occurs (411–413). Usually patients with congenital trochlear nerve palsy are neurologically normal. Some have other neurologic deficits, including cerebral palsy (414). Many have some degree of facial asymmetry (415–417). The patients usually develop large vertical fusion amplitudes and a head tilt, allowing them to avoid diplopia. There may be decompensation after a minor head injury or without any antecedent event (418). When these patients are evaluated, a review of old photo-

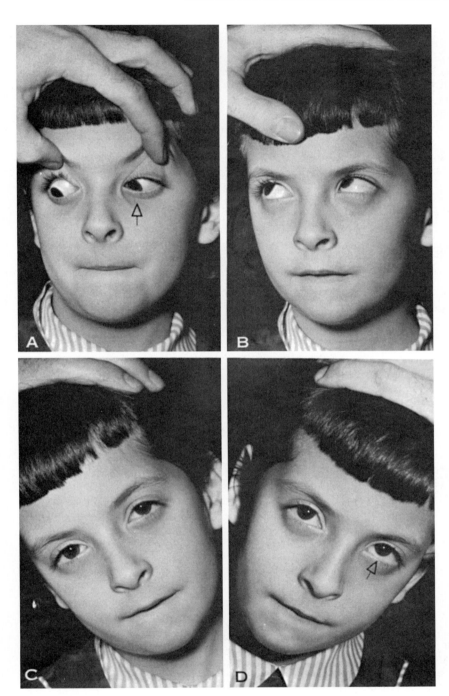

Figure 20.45. Left trochlear nerve palsy. *A*, Downward movement of the left eye (*arrow*) is limited in gaze down and right. *B*, Upward gaze to the right shows secondary overaction of the left inferior oblique muscle, the antagonist of the left superior oblique muscle. *C*, Head tilt to the right produces orthophoria and eliminates diplopia. *D*, Head tilt to the left results in upward deviation of the left eye (*arrow*). (Courtesy of Dr. R. D. Harley.)

graphs, such as a driver's license, may reveal a preexisting head tilt (419,420). In addition, direct measurement of vertical fusion amplitudes may establish the diagnosis. Normal persons have a vertical fusion range of only 3–6 prism diopters (421), whereas patients with congenital superior oblique paresis may have 10–25 prism diopters of vertical fusion amplitude.

Congenital superior oblique palsy may be bilateral. It may appear to be unilateral until corrected surgically, at which time the contralateral palsy becomes apparent (422–424). In most cases, however, careful measurements of both vertical and torsional deviation (including direct visualization of the ocular fundi to determine whether torsion is present) permit differentiation between unilateral and bilateral palsies.

ACQUIRED

When an etiology can be determined, blunt head trauma, usually a direct orbital, frontal, basal, or oblique cranial

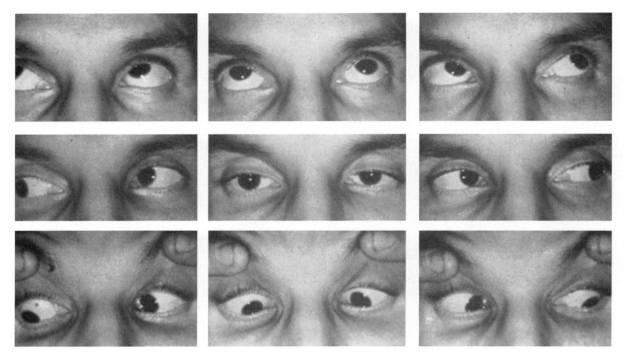

Figure 20.46. Bilateral trochlear nerve palsies in a 28-year-old man following a motorcycle accident. The patient suffered a severe blow to the vertex of his head. Note the patient's inability to depress either eye fully in adduction. There is bilateral overaction of both inferior oblique muscles. (Courtesy of Jacqueline Morris, C.O.)

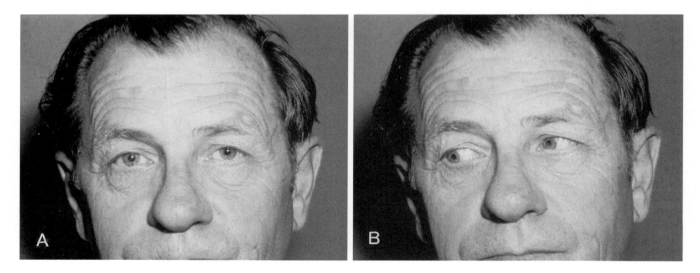

Figure 20.47. Head tilt in a patient with a left trochlear nerve palsy following head trauma. *A*, In primary position, the patient has a left hypertropia. (Note difference in position of the light reflexes on the two corneas.) *B*, On gaze right and down, there is underaction of the left superior oblique. *(Figure continues.)*

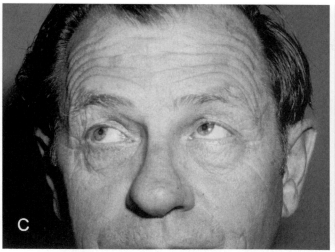
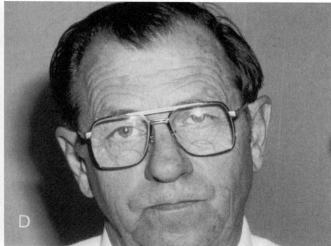

Figure 20.47. Continued. *C*, On gaze right and up, there is overaction of the left inferior oblique. *D*, The patient has adopted a head tilt toward the right shoulder (the side opposite the palsy) that allows him to fuse in primary position.

blow, is the most common cause of isolated, acquired, unilateral and bilateral trochlear nerve palsy in both adults and children (219,275,408,409,424–429). As with other ocular motor nerve palsies, almost any pathologic process can damage the trochlear nerve at any point from its nucleus to its termination in the orbit where it innervates the superior oblique muscle (430).

Lesions of the Trochlear Nerve Nucleus

Lesions of the brain stem that damage the trochlear nerve nucleus cannot be localized clinically unless there are neighborhood neurologic signs suggesting intrinsic mesencephalic damage (431) or positive neuroimaging. Even when brain stem signs are present, distinguishing nuclear from fascicular involvement is almost impossible. In addition, extrinsic lesions that compress the dorsal mesencephalon may injure the trochlear nerves as they emerge from the brain stem and at the same time damage the brain stem itself. Cells of the trochlear nucleus are often damaged by lesions of the tegmentum at the junction of the pons and mesencephalon, particularly contusion and hemorrhage caused by impact against the tentorial margin. MRI misses a number of these lesions. Lesions that can damage the trochlear nuclei include ischemia, medulloblastoma, astrocytoma, ependymoma, metastatic tumor, MS, hemorrhage, and vascular malformations (408,425,430,432–436) (Figs. 20.48–20.50). Conjugate or internuclear gaze defects can obscure a superior oblique palsy, which may be recognized only once the horizontal gaze difficulties resolve (437). We have seen both unilateral and bilateral superior oblique paresis associated with Parinaud's dorsal midbrain syndrome from pineal tumors, aqueductal stenosis, and hydrocephalus (438). Vertical diplopia in this setting is commonly caused by trochlear nerve dysfunction (420,439). We and others have also seen trochlear nerve palsy following neurosurgical procedures in the posterior fossa and following some brain stem strokes

(239). In some of these cases, the trochlear nuclei must have been affected. The trochlear nuclear motor neurons are sometimes involved in ALS (127), although usually subclinically. Herpes zoster occasionally causes a trochlear nerve palsy (440).

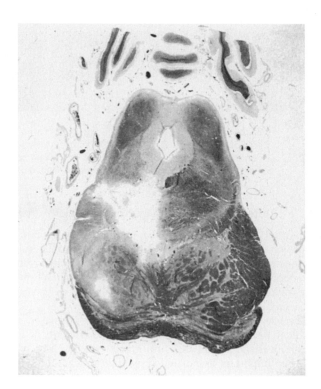

Figure 20.48. Histologic section through the caudal mesencephalon in a patient with a basilar artery occlusion showing an infarct involving the right trochlear nerve nucleus. (Courtesy of Dr. Richard Lindenberg.)

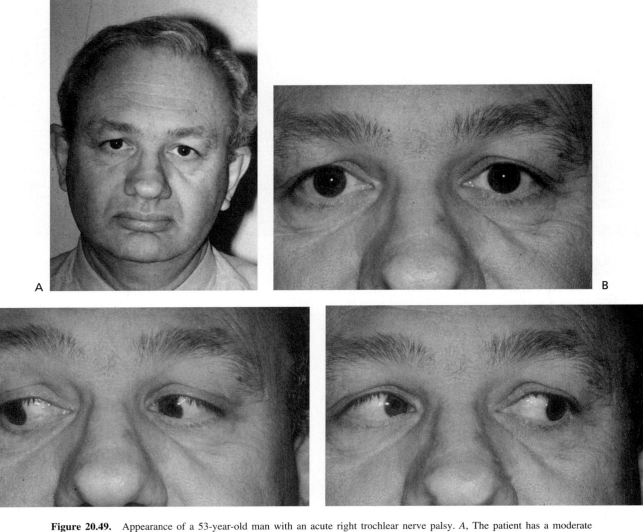

Figure 20.49. Appearance of a 53-year-old man with an acute right trochlear nerve palsy. *A*, The patient has a moderate head tilt toward the left shoulder. *B*, In primary position, there is a small right hypertropia. *C*, On gaze right and down, both eyes move normally. *D*, On gaze left and down, there is underaction of the right superior oblique muscle, with an increased right hypertropia. (Courtesy of Dr. Steven R. Hamilton.)

Lesions of the Trochlear Nerve Fascicle

Fascicular involvement of the trochlear nerves can be caused by the same processes that cause damage to the trochlear nuclei. These processes include compression, infiltration, demyelination, ischemia, hemorrhage, superficial siderosis, infection, and trauma (79,425,430,441–443) (Figs. 20.51 and 20.52).

Because of the dorsal location and short course of the trochlear fascicles, associated neurologic signs are of less help in localization than are neuroimaging studies. Nevertheless, two important associated signs that indicate a nuclear or fascicular lesion are Horner's syndrome and a relative afferent pupillary defect unassociated with evidence of an optic neuropathy or optic tract syndrome. The sympathetic pathways run through the dorsolateral tegmentum of the mesencephalon adjacent to the trochlear fascicles, so they may both be injured together, causing a trochlear paresis and contralateral Horner's syndrome (444–446). A relative afferent pupillary defect can be caused by damage to afferent pupillomotor fibers in the brachium of the superior colliculus, and a trochlear paresis can be caused by damage to either the nearby trochlear nucleus or the predecussation portion of the trochlear nerve fascicle (447,448) (Fig. 20.53).

Lesions of the Trochlear Nerve in the Subarachnoid Space

The trochlear nerve is particularly vulnerable to injury or compression as it emerges from the dorsal surface of the brain stem (79,407,425). Trauma in this location may avulse the rootlets of the emerging nerve (450), or there may be

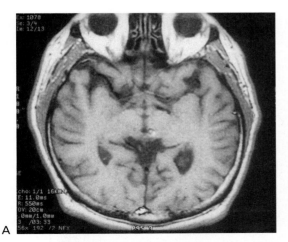

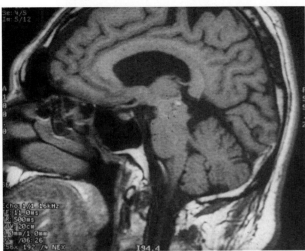

Figure 20.50. Magnetic resonance imaging performed on the patient in Figure 20.49. The study was performed when the patient did not recover in several months. T1-weighted axial (*A*) and sagittal (*B*) images show a small vascular malformation in the region of the left trochlear nucleus.

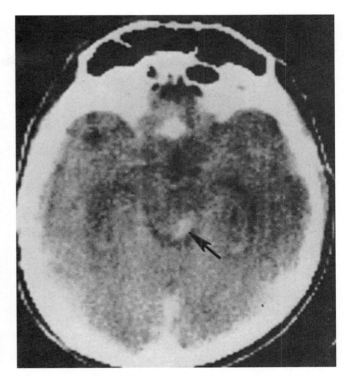

Figure 20.51. Computed tomographic scan showing hemorrhage within the mesencephalic tectum (*arrow*) in a 56-year-old man with hypertension and the sudden onset of headache associated with vertical and torsional diplopia. The patient had bilateral superior oblique palsies, probably caused by damage to the trochlear nerve fascicles in the anterior medullary velum of the mesencephalon. (From Wise J, Gomolin J, Goldberg LL. Bilateral superior oblique palsy: Diagnosis and treatment. Can J Ophthalmol 1983; 18:28–32.)

stretching or contusion injury with hemorrhage within the nerve or localized subarachnoid hemorrhage (449). Increased intracranial pressure can damage the nerve unilaterally or bilaterally (450,451).

As the trochlear nerve traverses the subarachnoid space, it is vulnerable to trauma. Often the site of damage is unclear. This is especially true when the palsy is accompanied by evidence of blunt trauma to the ipsilateral or contralateral orbit. There may be both a trochlear nerve palsy and an orbital blowout fracture (452), or the patient's appearance may suggest an orbital cause for the vertical diplopia when the real culprit is a trochlear palsy (453). Iatrogenic trauma is often subarachnoid in location (454).

Trauma that is insufficient to cause loss of consciousness may nevertheless cause a trochlear nerve palsy because of the extremely fragile nature of the nerve, its long subarachnoid course, and its propinquity to the tentorial edge (455,456). The oculomotor and abducens nerves are less sus-

ceptible. Ocular motor nerve palsies that occur after apparently trivial head trauma, including trochlear nerve palsy, may be associated with asymptomatic basal intracranial tumors that have stretched, thinned, or infiltrated the nerve, which nevertheless has continued to function. Some of these patients may have other neurologic findings on careful examination. Patients who develop cranial neuropathies from trivial trauma deserve careful neuroimaging (457).

The subarachnoid portion of the trochlear nerve is occasionally damaged by aneurysms of the superior cerebellar artery (458,459). Meningitis caused by syphilis, tuberculosis, Lyme disease, ehrlichiosis (460,461), and even aseptic meningitis can cause a trochlear nerve palsy. In addition, we and others have encountered cases of trochlear nerve palsy associated with tentorial meningioma, pinealoma, sphenoid sinusitis, encephalitis, migraine, Sjögren's syndrome, and arteriovenous malformations. In some cases, the palsy is the only neurologic sign of the underlying condition (425,462,463). Usually, however, there are other signs of focal or systemic neurologic disease.

Schwannomas, both solid and cystic, may cause trochlear nerve palsy by involvement of the nerve in the subarachnoid space or by brain stem compression, along with other signs

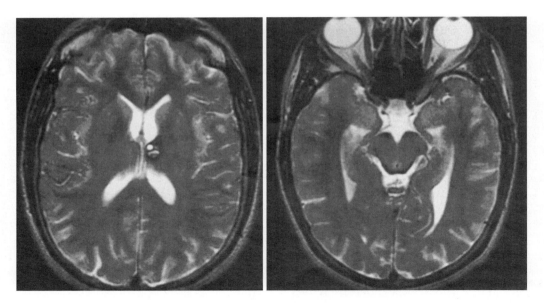

Figure 20.52. Neuroimaging of patient with an intermittent trochlear nerve palsy associated with superficial siderosis caused by recurrent hemorrhage from a small periventricular cavernous angioma. *A,* T2-weighted magnetic resonance image, axial view, shows a small, round, well-demarcated, left periventricular lesion with a mixed signal intensity, consistent with a cavernous angioma. *B,* T2-weighted axial magnetic resonance image at the level of the superior colliculi shows a rim of low signal intensity covering the dorsal surface of the mesencephalon. (From Hashimoto M, Hoyt WF. Superficial siderosis and episodic fourth nerve paresis: Report of a case with clinical and magnetic resonance imaging findings. J Neuroophthalmol 1996; 16:277–280.)

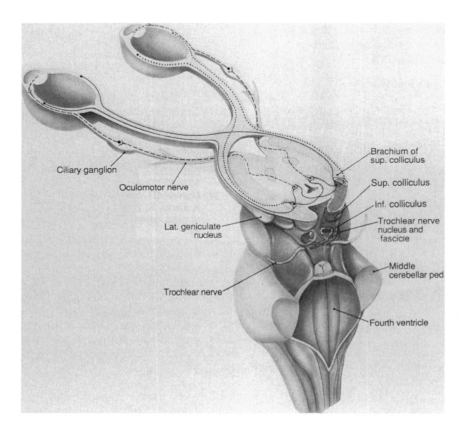

Figure 20.53. Presumed site of damage in a young woman who developed a left trochlear nerve paresis and was found to have a left relative afferent pupillary defect unassociated with any visual sensory deficit. The *shaded portion* indicates a lesion involving the brachium of the right superior colliculus and the right dorsal mesencephalon, including the right trochlear nucleus or the predecussation portion of the right trochlear nerve fascicle. The patient was found to have an anaplastic astrocytoma of the brain stem. (From Eliott D, Cunningham ET Jr, Miller NR. Fourth nerve paresis and ipsilateral relative afferent pupillary defect without visual sensory disturbance: A sign of contralateral dorsal midbrain disease. J Clin Neuroophthalmol 1991;11:169–171.)

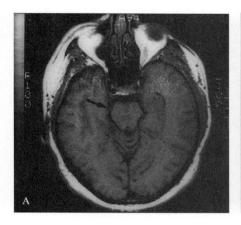
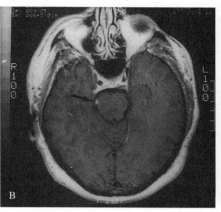
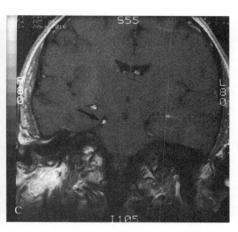

Figure 20.54. Neuroimaging in a 53-year-old man with vertical diplopia and a left head tilt. An examination revealed a right trochlear nerve paresis. Magnetic resonance imaging was performed when the patient's diplopia did not improve within several months. *A,* T1-weighted axial magnetic resonance image shows slight enlargement of the subarachnoid portion of the right trochlear nerve (*arrow*). *B,* T1-weighted axial magnetic resonance image in same plane after intravenous injection of paramagnetic contrast material shows enhancement of the trochlear nerve in this region (*arrow*). *C,* Enhanced T1-weighted coronal magnetic resonance image of the same area shows the location of the right trochlear nerve lesion just beneath the tentorium cerebelli (*arrow*). The signal characteristics of the lesion are most consistent with a schwannoma or meningioma of the trochlear nerve.

of brain stem dysfunction. In other cases, diplopia may be the only manifestation of the tumor (Fig. 20.54). Both trochlear and trigeminal schwannomas occasionally present with pathologic laughter (348,464–466). Intrinsic trochlear nerve lesions other than schwannomas can also produce a trochlear nerve palsy in this region. These include cavernous angiomas and arteriovenous malformations (257,467).

Patients with posteriorly draining dural carotid–cavernous sinus fistulas sometimes develop acute, painful ophthalmoplegia without conjunctival chemosis, dilation of conjunctival vessels, or proptosis. This can result in trochlear or abducens nerve paresis (468–471).

The association of trochlear nerve palsy with elevated intracranial pressure (ICP) is well documented. Trochlear nerve palsy occurs with obstructive hydrocephalus, shunt malfunction, and otitic hydrocephalus. Bilateral trochlear nerve paresis may be a localizing sign of involvement of the superior medullary velum by a dilated sylvian aqueduct or downward pressure from an enlarged third ventricle (438). Trochlear nerve palsy can rarely develop with decreased ICP, such as that following a lumbar puncture or the development of spontaneous intracranial hypotension (472,473).

Lesions of the Trochlear Nerve Within the Cavernous Sinus and Superior Orbital Fissure

Lesions that produce a cavernous sinus syndrome were discussed in an earlier section of this chapter. When they produce combined ocular motor nerve palsies, the trochlear nerve is often involved (332). It is unusual, however, to see an isolated trochlear nerve palsy in cavernous sinus disease, although ischemia (e.g., diabetes mellitus) may conceivably affect the nerve in this location. It is also possible that the isolated trochlear nerve palsy occurring in some patients

with trigeminal herpes zoster or geniculate herpes zoster originates in the cavernous sinus (474). Dural carotid–cavernous sinus fistula can cause a painful trochlear nerve palsy, even without the signs of a red eye and proptosis (471). Wegener's granulomatosis may involve the nerve in the cavernous sinus (475). The nerve may occasionally be compressed by a persistent primitive trigeminal artery. This occurs either in or right before the cavernous sinus (476).

Lesions of the Trochlear Nerve Within the Orbit

Trauma (including surgery) may damage the trochlear nerve in the orbit, but in many cases it is impossible to know whether the damage has occurred to the nerve, the trochlea, the superior oblique muscle or tendon, or several of these structures. A similar problem arises in assessing patients with orbital inflammation, ischemia, tumors, or vascular malformations that are associated with superior oblique dysfunction (436,477,478). The superior oblique paralysis that occurs in patients with Paget's disease and with hypertrophic arthritis may be caused by mechanical disruption of the superior oblique tendon within the trochlea and not by damage to the trochlear nerve itself.

We have already commented on the occurrence of oculomotor nerve palsy after dental anesthesia. The third and fourth nerves may be involved together (363).

Lesions of the Trochlear Nerve of Uncertain or Variable Location

Isolated, acquired paralysis of the superior oblique muscle without any systemic or neurologic signs or symptoms is not uncommon. Spontaneous recovery often occurs within 1 to 4 months. This is most likely inflammatory or ischemic in origin (369,479) and has been associated with diabetes, hypertension, HIV infection, progressive systemic sclerosis, and Churg-Strauss allergic granulomatous angiitis.

Anterior temporal lobectomy for treatment of epilepsy sometimes results in ipsilateral paresis of the superior oblique muscle. This usually resolves completely within 14 weeks. It might result from indirect traction on the subarachnoid portion of the trochlear nerve during surgery. We have seen three cases of transient trochlear nerve paresis following anterior temporal lobectomy. The paresis cleared completely in all of our patients within 3 months of the surgery (480,481).

Recovery from Acquired Trochlear Nerve Palsy

A trochlear nerve palsy may recover or not, or it may recover incompletely. Complete recovery is the rule after ischemia or most head injury, or after relief of compression from tumor or aneurysm (369). Incomplete recovery leaves the patient with mild but persistent vertical or torsional diplopia. Absence of recovery occurs primarily after mesencephalic injury or with transection of the trochlear nerve by trauma or compression.

DIFFERENTIAL DIAGNOSIS OF ACQUIRED TROCHLEAR NERVE PALSY: SKEW DEVIATION

Although trochlear nerve paresis is the most common cause of acquired vertical diplopia, other causes include ocular myopathies (e.g., dysthyroid eye disease), disorders of the neuromuscular junction (e.g., myasthenia gravis), and skew deviation (420). The ocular myopathies and disorders of the neuromuscular junction are described in Chapters 22 and 21, respectively. Skew deviation is discussed in Chapter 19, but we chose to discuss it in this chapter as well in order to contrast the findings with those seen in patients with trochlear nerve palsy.

Skew deviation is a vertical misalignment of the visual axis caused by defective supranuclear inputs. The hypertropia may be constant for all positions of gaze (comitant), or it may vary and may even alternate depending on the direction of gaze (420,482). Skew deviation may be transient, constant, or alternating. Both transient and periodic vertical divergence can occur in patients with basilar artery insufficiency or basilar artery migraine or as the first sign of a pontine astrocytoma (157,213,483). It can be caused by lesions in a number of brain stem locations, on either side, and is usually associated with other signs and symptoms of brain stem or cerebellar disease (420,482). Mild skew deviation may not be recognized as such and may be misdiagnosed as an incomplete palsy of a single vertically acting muscle. It may closely resemble a trochlear nerve palsy. The easiest way to differentiate between them is by using double Maddox rods or the Lancaster red-green test to find the associated unilateral cyclotorsional deviation of trochlear nerve palsy. Ophthalmoscopic examination or fundus photography can also be used to detect ocular torsion (407,420,484). These tests are described in Chapter 18. Unlike a trochlear nerve palsy, skew deviation is usually not associated with torsional diplopia or cyclodeviation, but there is an exception. The ocular tilt reaction is a skew deviation associated

with a head tilt and bilateral ocular torsion. This results from damage to the utricular pathway on its way from the utricle, synapsing in the vestibular nuclei, then crossing the midline and ascending in the medial longitudinal fasciculus (MLF) to the vertically acting oculomotor and trochlear nuclei. The hypertropia is contralateral to a utricular nerve lesion and ipsilateral to an MLF lesion. The bilaterality of the cyclotorsion can be seen by funduscopy or with double Maddox rods. Often there is an internuclear ophthalmoplegia as well.

EVALUATION AND MANAGEMENT OF TROCHLEAR NERVE PALSY

The three-step test is used to diagnose a trochlear nerve palsy. It is used to isolate the involved paretic muscle in concomitant or incomitant vertical deviations. It is useful only when the paresis involves a single cycloverted muscle (485–487). The steps are as follows:

1. A vertical heterotropia is determined in primary position. Depending on the eye that is hypertropic, one of four muscles may be paretic: the ipsilateral inferior rectus, the ipsilateral superior oblique, the contralateral superior rectus, or the contralateral inferior oblique. Thus, if the patient has a right hypertropia, the muscles that may be paretic are the right superior oblique, the right inferior rectus, the left superior rectus, or the left inferior oblique.
2. Whether the hypertropia increases in right or left horizontal gaze is determined. This reduces the potential paretic muscles to two. Thus, in a patient with a right hypertropia, if the deviation increases in right gaze, the affected muscles can only be the right inferior rectus (which has its maximum vertical action when the eye is in an abducted position) or the left inferior oblique (which has its maximum vertical action when the eye is in an adducted position). If the deviation increases in left gaze, the affected muscles would be either the right superior oblique or the left superior rectus.
3. The choice between the two muscles, one in each eye, that are potentially responsible for the vertical heterotropia is now made using the head tilt test. Thus, if the patient has a right hypertropia that increases in left gaze, an increase in the hypertropia when the head is tilted to the right side indicates a paretic right superior oblique muscle.

The three-step test is extremely useful in patients with trochlear nerve palsies, but its reliability in the diagnosis of pareses of other vertical muscles is less certain (403,488). In addition, both restrictive ophthalmoplegia and myasthenia gravis can mimic superior oblique palsy on the three-step test (489).

The easiest method of treating diplopia while awaiting resolution of a trochlear nerve palsy is occluding one eye with a patch or an opaque contact lens. In other patients, particularly those with mild vertical displacement, the use of a vertical press-on (Fresnel) prism may be of benefit (490), although some degree of diplopia in extremes of gaze is almost always present. In cases of acquired trochlear nerve palsy, no attempt at surgical correction should be considered until at least 8–12 months have elapsed without improvement in superior oblique function, unless the physician knows with certainty that the trochlear nerve has been severed (e.g., after intracranial surgery).

Botulinum toxin has been used in both acquired and decompensated congenital trochlear nerve paresis (491,492). The botulinum toxin is injected into the ipsilateral inferior oblique muscle. Care must be taken to avoid spread of the toxin to the adjacent inferior rectus muscle. We have not found this treatment particularly useful.

When a trochlear nerve palsy has been stable for 8–12 months, surgery may be considered, using any one of several operative procedures. These procedures are designed to (*a*) strengthen all or a portion of the superior oblique muscle; (*b*) weaken its antagonist, the ipsilateral inferior oblique muscle; or (*c*) weaken its yoke muscle, the contralateral inferior rectus muscle. The decision to use one or another of these procedures or to use several in combination depends upon the results of a careful orthoptic examination (404,493–495). Similar considerations apply to the treatment of bilateral trochlear nerve palsy (496). The results of surgery for both congenital and acquired trochlear nerve palsies are usually excellent.

ABDUCENS (SIXTH) NERVE PALSY AND NUCLEAR HORIZONTAL GAZE PARALYSIS

The abducens nerve is unique in that damage to its nucleus results not in ipsilateral abduction weakness but in horizontal gaze paralysis toward the side of the lesion. Beyond the nucleus, damage results in abduction weakness only, because of weakness of the ipsilateral lateral rectus muscle. In the section below, we examine these syndromes in detail (497).

CONGENITAL

Congenital absence of abduction as an isolated phenomenon is exceedingly rare but may occur from injury to the abducens nerve shortly before or during birth. In one study (498), abduction paresis was present in 35 of 6,360 newborns, and in all but one it disappeared by 6 weeks of age. Birth trauma was suspected. In another study of 6,886 neonates, 0.4% had abduction paresis, increasing progressively from 0% for deliveries by caesarean section to 0.1% for spontaneous vaginal delivery, 2.4% for forceps delivery, and 3.2% for vacuum extraction, again suggesting birth trauma as the cause (499).

Congenital paralysis of conjugate horizontal eye movements occurs more frequently than does unilateral or bilateral abduction weakness and may be sporadic (500,501) or familial (502). Convergence is usually preserved (Fig. 20.55). An autopsy on a child with isolated bilateral horizontal gaze palsy showed that the abducens nuclei were present but hypoplastic. Several nerve fibers extended from the nuclei into the pons for about one quarter of the normal distance. No abducens nerves could be identified grossly (503).

Congenital absence of abduction, either alone or as part of a horizontal gaze palsy, usually occurs with other neurologic or systemic anomalies. Patients with cerebral palsy seem to have an increased prevalence of congenital abducens paresis (414). In addition, congenital paralysis of both abduction and horizontal gaze occurs in patients with a variety of skeletal abnormalities. There is a recessive disorder of congenital horizontal gaze palsy with progressive scoliosis (504,505). The Athabascan brain stem dysgenesis syndrome is a recessive disorder with congenital horizontal gaze palsy, sensorineural deafness, central hypoventilation, and developmental delay (506). Klippel-Feil syndrome (fusion of several cervical vertebrae) can occur with congenital horizontal gaze palsy (507). This may represent a *forme fruste* of Wildervanck's cervico-oculo-acoustic syndrome: Duane's syndrome with the Klippel-Feil anomaly and deafness. A syndrome of congenital horizontal gaze paralysis and ear dysplasia is well described (508). Unilateral agenesis of the abducens nucleus and nerve (as well as the trochlear nucleus and nerve) was described in a patient with oculoauriculovertebral dysplasia–hemifacial microsomia (Goldenhar-Gorlin syndrome) (410). All of these syndromes, however, are rare. Far more common are congenital disturbances of horizontal

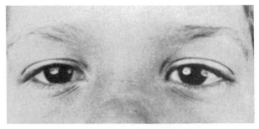
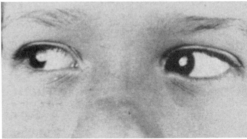
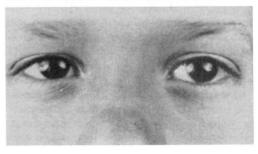

Figure 20.55. Congenital, isolated, unilateral horizontal gaze palsy in a 5-year-old boy. *Top,* In primary position, the patient's eyes are straight. *Middle,* Both eyes move fully to the right. *Bottom,* On attempted gaze to the left, neither eye moves more than a few degrees. (From Hoyt CS, Billson FA, Taylor H. Isolated unilateral gaze palsy. J Pediatr Ophthalmol 1977; 14:343–345.)

gaze associated with two conditions: Möbius syndrome and Duane's retraction syndrome.

Möbius Syndrome (Congenital Bulbar Paralysis)

This congenital syndrome was described at about the same time by Harlan, Chisholm, and Möbius (509–511). There is facial diplegia with absent abduction or absent horizontal gaze bilaterally. The face is devoid of expression, with the lips constantly open. The facial weakness may prevent adequate nursing. Some patients cannot close their eyes at all, while others close them incompletely. There may be excess lacrimation and epiphoria. In milder cases, there may be only an esotropia associated with unilateral or bilateral limitation of abduction, and some patients may even be able to converge (512). In most cases, however, the eyes are straight and do not move horizontally (Fig. 20.56). In a review of 61 cases of Möbius syndrome in the literature, bilateral abducens palsy was present in 43 cases, unilateral abducens palsy in 2 cases, and horizontal gaze palsy in the rest. Complete bilateral ophthalmoplegia was present in 15 and oculomotor palsy in 12 (513).

Associated congenital defects sometimes seen in Möbius syndrome include deafness, webbed fingers or toes, supernumerary digits, and even absence of the hands, feet, fingers, or toes. Poland syndrome (absence of the sternal head of the pectoralis major with or without symbrachydactyly) may be associated (514). Tongue weakness is often present (512, 513,515). Abnormalities of the lower cranial nerves, with speech and swallowing difficulties, were noted in all patients in one series (516). Disorders of respiratory control occur, such as continuous tachypnea (517). Many patients with Möbius syndrome have mental retardation or frank autism

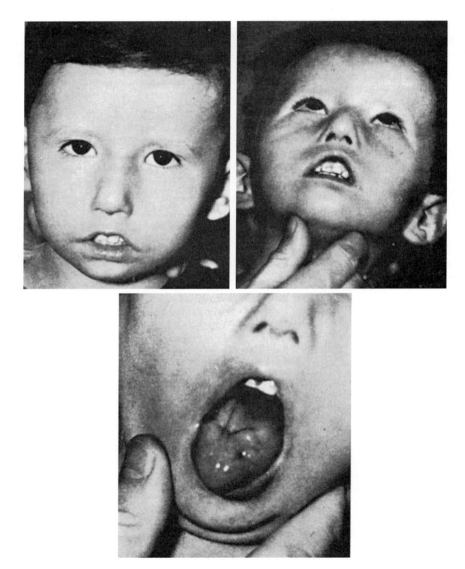

Figure 20.56. Möbius syndrome in a 3-year-old boy. The boy had spontaneous vertical eye movements but no horizontal eye movements. Note bilateral facial palsy and atrophy of the tongue.

(518). A Möbius-like facies can occur in facioscapulohumeral dystrophy and in infantile myotonic dystrophy, on the basis of myopathic weakness of the face (519).

Most cases of Möbius syndrome are sporadic, but at least three dominantly inherited types occur, at different loci (520–522). Penetrance is incomplete. These families do not have primary skeletal defects. The risk is reported to be no greater than 2% for another affected sibling in pedigrees in which the syndrome includes limb abnormalities (516).

Möbius syndrome was reported in one patient whose mother took the drug thalidomide during her pregnancy (523) and one whose mother took cocaine (524), but the most dramatic association is with misoprostol. Of 96 Brazilian children with Möbius syndrome, 47 had been exposed to misoprostol in the first trimester of gestation (525,526).

A woman suffered splenic rupture and hypotension while 8 weeks pregnant. The child was born with Möbius syndrome with bilateral sixth and seventh nerve palsies and abnormal brain stem evoked responses (527).

Pathologic findings commonly demonstrate focal brain stem necrosis with calcifications in the dorsal tectum at the junction of the midbrain and pons or in the pontine and medullary tegmentum, with mineralized foci of necrosis in brain stem nuclei. These appear to be prenatal encephalomalacic lesions (528–531). In other cases, there has been hypoplasia or atrophy of cranial nerve nuclei without signs of necrosis (528).

In most cases, Möbius syndrome is the result of a prenatal vascular insult to the brain stem. The fetal paramedian brain stem may be especially vulnerable to ischemia (531). The product of the mutated gene in one dominantly inherited form of Möbius syndrome is PLEXIN-D1, expressed in vascular endothelium and probably playing a role in embryonic vasculogenesis (532). Disruption of the fetal subclavian arterial supply at around 6 weeks of gestation causes the specific pattern of combinations of the Klippel-Feil, Poland, and Möbius anomalies (533). Severe maternal hypotension has been associated. Other vascular malformations may occur, such as transposition of the great vessels, suggesting an intrapartum insult during the 4th to 7th week (534). The high occurrence of autism with Möbius syndrome suggests that autism may be caused also by a prenatal brain stem event.

Duane's Retraction Syndrome (Stilling-Türk-Duane Syndrome)

Duane's retraction syndrome (DRS) is a predominantly congenital eye movement disorder characterized by marked limitation or absence of abduction, variable limitation of adduction, and palpebral fissure narrowing and globe retraction on attempted adduction (Figs. 20.57 and 20.58). Vertical ocular movements are often noted on adduction, most frequently in an upward direction (535). The condition was first described at the end of the 19th century (536–538). In 1906, Duane described 54 cases, summarized all findings, and offered theories on pathogenesis and treatment (539). After his original report, several large series were described (540–547).

All patients with DRS have abnormal horizontal eye movements (21,548). In most cases this is unilateral, but it is bilateral in 15–20% of affected patients (549). It is more common in females than males, except in China, where the sexes are equally affected (546). The left eye is more frequently affected than the right. In most patients, gaze is directed toward the side of the unaffected eye, sometimes with

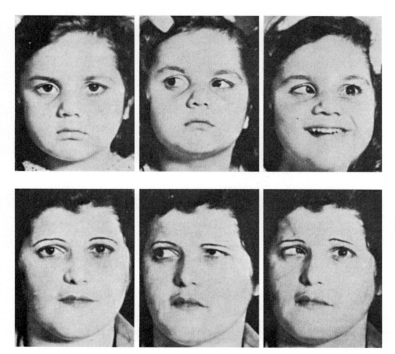

Figure 20.57. Unilateral left Duane's retraction syndrome in a young girl (*above*) and her mother (*below*). The syndrome was present in five members of three generations. (From Laughlin RC. Am J Ophthalmol 1937;20:396–398.)

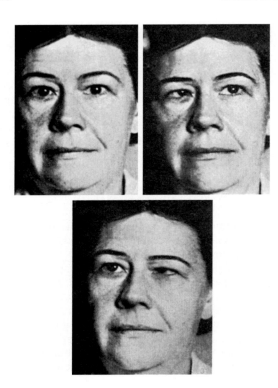

Figure 20.58.   Bilateral Duane's retraction syndrome. The patient has bilateral limitation of abduction. Note retraction of the adducting eye with associated narrowing of the lid fissure with gaze to either side.

a head turn toward the affected side to allow binocular single vision. Visual symptoms are conspicuous by their absence. Vision is almost always normal unless there is associated anisometropia. Thus, in the majority of cases, no treatment is necessary unless the patient has a marked head turn.

Early histologic studies demonstrated abnormalities of the lateral or medial rectus muscles and led investigators to conclude that DRS was a local myogenic phenomenon. It was generally believed that the cause of the abduction deficiency was fibrosis of the lateral rectus muscle, and that limitation of adduction was caused by a posterior insertion of the medial rectus muscle. Adhesions between the medial rectus muscle and the medial orbital wall were also reported (540). Subsequent electromyographic studies showed that DRS is a neurogenic disorder in which branches of the oculomotor nerve innervate the lateral rectus muscle (550–553) (Fig. 20.59) and that retraction of the globe, once thought to have a mechanical cause, is produced by a co-contraction of horizontal rectus muscles.

Huber distinguished three types of DRS based on electromyographic recordings and speculated on the pathophysiology of each type. Duane type I, the most common type, consists of limited or absent abduction with relatively normal adduction. The lateral rectus does not contract during attempted abduction; the medial and lateral recti co-contract during adduction, causing retraction of the globe. Usually the patient is orthotropic in the primary position. Duane type II consists of limited or absent adduction with relatively normal abduction. The lateral rectus contracts on abduction, but the lateral and medial recti co-contract during adduction, causing retraction of the globe and limitation of adduction. Duane type III consists of defective abduction and adduction both. The lateral and medial recti co-contract during both abduction and adduction, causing retraction and limitation of horizontal movements (552,554). Electromyography shows anomalous dual innervation of these muscles by the oculomotor and abducens nerves.

Until 1980, the only pathologic study performed on a patient with DRS showed no abducens nerve on the affected side. Histologically, the abducens nucleus was hypoplastic,

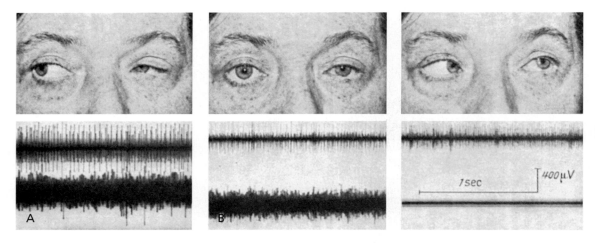

Figure 20.59.   Electromyogram in left Duane's retraction syndrome. Simultaneous recording from left lateral rectus (*A*) and medial rectus (*B*) muscles shows paradoxic innervation of the lateral rectus muscle during attempted adduction of the left eye. In fact, the lateral rectus muscle receives its maximal innervation during adduction and its minimal innervation during attempted abduction. The innervation pattern of the left medial rectus is normal. Note its inhibition during abduction of the eye. (From Huber A, Esslen E, Kloti R, et al. Zum problem des Duane syndromes. Albrecht von Graefes Arch Klin Exp Ophthalmol 1964; 167:169–191.)

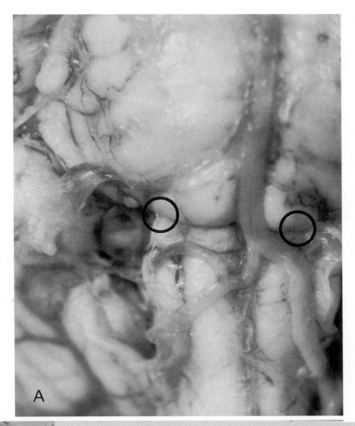

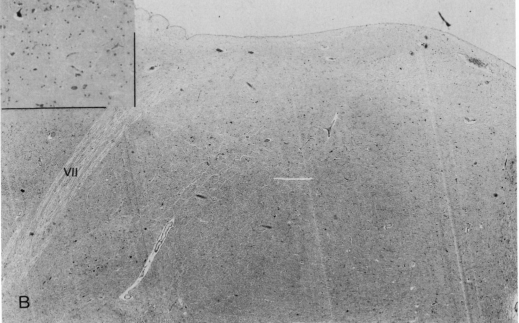

Figure 20.60. Pathology of bilateral Duane's retraction syndrome. *A*, View of ventral surface of brain stem in a patient with bilateral Duane's retraction syndrome who died of metastatic carcinoma shows no evidence of abducens nerves at the pontomedullary junction (*circles*). *B*, Histologic section through the pons reveals no evidence of motoneurons in the region of the abducens nucleus (see also *inset*). The facial nerve fascicle (VII) is intact and courses around the area normally occupied by the abducens nucleus. (From Hotchkiss MG, Miller NR, Clark AW, et al. Bilateral Duane's retraction syndrome: A clinical-pathologic case report. Arch Ophthalmol 1980;98:870–874.)

the lateral rectus muscle was fibrotic, and the medial rectus muscle was hypertrophic. The innervation of the lateral rectus muscle was not discussed, nor were the terminal branches of the oculomotor nerve followed (555). Subsequent autopsies on two patients with DRS showed that the abducens nuclei and nerves were absent bilaterally and that the lateral rectus muscles were partially innervated by branches from the inferior division of the oculomotor nerves (556,557) (Figs. 20.60 and 20.61). The lateral rectus muscles were fibrotic in areas lacking innervation but appeared relatively normal where innervated.

Miller et al. reported the complete pathologic findings in a 43-year-old woman with a left-sided DRS type I. The patient's eye movement disorder was verified clinically and electro-oculographically before her death from metastatic carcinoma. In this patient, the right side of the brain stem, the right cavernous sinus, and the right orbit were normal. The left abducens nucleus contained no cell bodies of abducens motoneurons, but in its rostral portion there were many small cell bodies believed by the investigators to be internuclear neurons for lateral gaze (Fig. 20.62). The left abducens nerve was absent, and the left lateral rectus muscle was innervated by branches from the inferior division of the oculomotor nerve (Fig. 20.63). The affected lateral rectus muscle was fibrotic in those areas that were not innervated (37).

MRI is now sensitive enough to show the absence of the abducens nerve in some cases (558,559). It thus seems clear that DRS is caused by agenesis of or damage to the abducens nerve in the brain stem, followed by anomalous innervation from the oculomotor nerve. This bears similarities to congenital fibrosis of the ocular muscles, acquired oculomotor synkinesis, the vertical retraction syndrome, and the synergistic divergence syndrome. Other misdirection syndromes such as the Marcus Gunn jaw-wink phenomenon and crocodile tears have been reported with DRS (24,548).

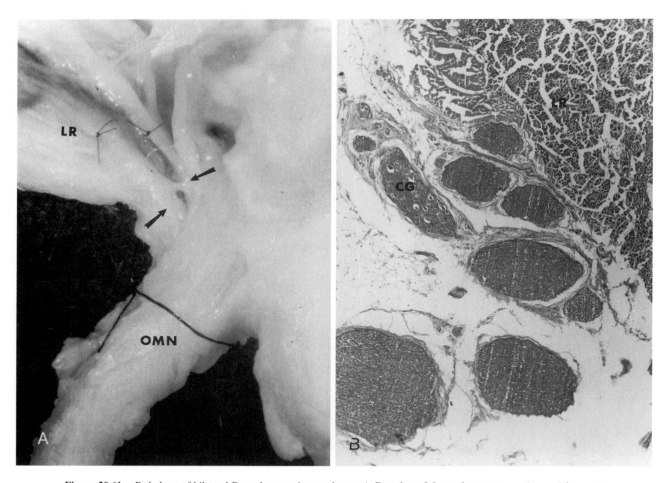

Figure 20.61. Pathology of bilateral Duane's retraction syndrome. *A*, Branches of the oculomotor nerve (*arrows*) innervate the lateral rectus muscle (LR). The large suture is tied around the oculomotor nerve (OMN), and the small sutures are tied around several branches of the nerve innervating the lateral rectus muscle. *B*, Histologic section through the posterior portion of the right orbit shows branches of the oculomotor nerve innervating the lateral rectus muscle (LR). The branches originate from the inferior division of the oculomotor nerve, as evidenced by their close association with the ciliary ganglion (CG). (From Hotchkiss MG, Miller NR, Clark AW, et al. Bilateral Duane's retraction syndrome: A clinical-pathologic case report. Arch Ophthalmol 1980;98:870–874.)

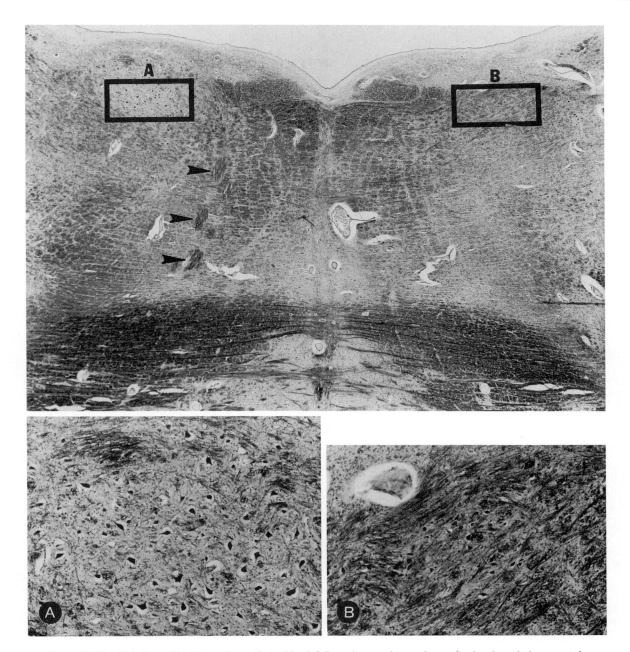

Figure 20.62. Pathology of brain stem in a patient with a left Duane's retraction syndrome. Section through the pons at the level of the rostral portion of the abducens nucleus. Right abducens nucleus is present (*box A, left side* of section), and portions of the fascicle of the abducens nerve can be identified (*arrowheads*). In the region normally occupied by the left abducens nucleus (*box B, right side* of section), only a few small cells are present. *Inset A,* Magnified view of right abducens nucleus shows that it is composed of large cell bodies typical of normal motoneurons. *Inset B,* Magnified view of area normally occupied by left abducens nucleus shows several small dark cells, possibly representing cell bodies of abducens internuclear neurons. No typical motoneurons are visible. (From Miller NR, Kiel SM, Green WR, et al. Unilateral Duane's retraction syndrome [type 1]. Arch Ophthalmol 1982;100:1468–1472.)

Thirty percent to 50% of patients with DRS have associated congenital defects involving ocular, skeletal, and neural structures (541,543,560–566). The differentiation of these frequently affected structures occurs between the 4th and 8th week of gestation, coincident with the development of the oculomotor nerves (567). This suggests a teratogenic event during the 2nd month of gestation as the cause of DRS.

Most cases of DRS are sporadic, but dominantly inherited familial unilateral and bilateral cases occur (538,545) and may constitute about 10% of observed cases (541). In two

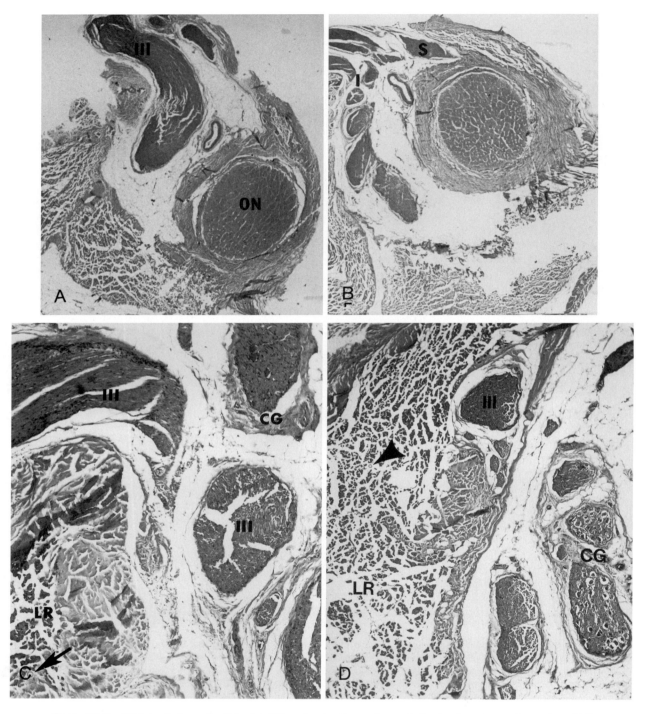

Figure 20.63. Orbital pathology of unilateral, left Duane's retraction syndrome. *A*, Section through posterior portion of left orbit shows oculomotor nerve (III) entering the orbit lateral and superior to the optic nerve (ON). *B*, In a section through the orbit slightly more anteriorly, the oculomotor nerve has split into a superior (S) and an inferior (I) division. The inferior division lies lateral to the optic nerve and adjacent to the lateral rectus muscle. *C*, Higher power of the section seen in *B* shows branches of the inferior division of the oculomotor nerve (III) adjacent to the lateral rectus muscle (LR). *Arrow* points to 10-0 suture used to mark the location of the lateral rectus muscle before processing. CG, ciliary ganglion. *D*, In a section taken further anteriorly through the left orbit, a branch of the oculomotor nerve (III) innervates the lateral rectus muscle (LR). The *arrowhead* points to the 10-0 suture used to mark the location of the lateral rectus muscle before processing. (From Miller NR, Kiel SM, Green WR, et al. Unilateral Duane's retraction syndrome [type 1]. Arch Ophthalmol 1982;100:1468–1472.)

different families, DRS has been associated with mutations at 2q31 and translocations at 8q (568,569).

Okihiro syndrome is an autosomal dominant condition characterized by radial ray malformations, such as absent thumbs, absent radii, and shortened humeri (or milder manifestations such as thenar muscle hypoplasia), deafness, and DRS. Okihiro syndrome is caused by a mutation of the human SALL4 gene on chromosome 20q13.13–q13.2 (570). DRS has occurred in children of mothers who have taken the drug thalidomide during pregnancy (571,572). Some of these children may have had the SALL4 mutation instead of thalidomide embryopathy.

Wildervanck's syndrome is the cervico-oculo-acoustic syndrome, consisting of the Klippel-Feil anomaly, deafness, and DRS (573). This is similar to some cases of Möbius syndrome.

DRS has been reported as an acquired syndrome in a few patients after damage to the abducens nerve, from pontine glioma, skull base meningioma, surgery for trigeminal rhizotomy, and after removal of an orbital cavernous hemangioma via a lateral orbitotomy (574–577). Presumably direct trauma to the abducens nerve was followed by aberrant regeneration. Pseudo-DRS can be caused by entrapment of the medial rectus muscle in an orbital blowout fracture or by a metastasis to the orbit causing mechanical limitation (578,579).

ACQUIRED

As with oculomotor and trochlear nerve palsies, many series report a variety of causes of abducens nerve palsy (219,220,275,580,581). These articles have the same limitations as those described with respect to other ocular motor nerve palsies. Nevertheless, certain specific syndromes do occur, depending on the location and nature of the lesion producing the palsy.

Lesions of the Abducens Nerve Nucleus

The abducens nucleus contains not only motor neurons that innervate the ipsilateral lateral rectus but also cell bodies of internuclear neurons that cross the midline and ascend in the contralateral MLF to synapse in the medial rectus subnucleus on that side (582,583). Thus, lesions that damage the abducens nucleus produce a conjugate gaze palsy to the ipsilateral side, and lesions of both abducens nuclei completely eliminate conjugate horizontal gaze (584–588). Neither unilateral nor bilateral isolated abduction weakness ever occurs from a lesion of the abducens nucleus. In most but not all cases in which the abducens nucleus is damaged, an ipsilateral peripheral facial nerve palsy is also present, because the facial nerve fascicle loops around the abducens nucleus before exiting from the brain stem.

Lesions of the abducens nucleus sometimes damage the ipsilateral MLF, producing the "one-and-a-half" syndrome. This consists of a horizontal gaze palsy combined with an internuclear ophthalmoplegia (INO) (213,262,589–594).

Electromyography of the lateral rectus muscle can determine the nature of an abduction defect in many cases. When

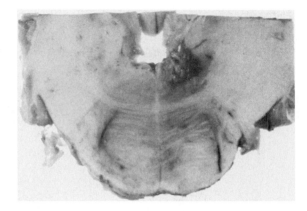

Figure 20.64. Pathology of a lesion producing an acquired right horizontal gaze palsy. Hemorrhage and softening are present in the lateral pontine tegmentum in the region of the right abducens nucleus. (Courtesy of Dr. Richard Lindenberg.)

normal electric activity is recorded from the resting lateral rectus muscle, significant nuclear involvement is excluded. Decreased electric activity, fibrillation potentials, or polyphasic potentials indicate nuclear or infranuclear involvement.

The abducens nuclei can be damaged unilaterally or bilaterally from brain stem ischemia (169,588,595–597) (Fig. 20.64), infiltration (598,599), trauma (600), inflammation (601), compression (602–605), or demyelination (606,607) (Figs. 20.65–20.67). Horizontal gaze palsies were present in several affected members of a family with pontine cavernous angiomas (608). We have seen similar cases. Herpes zoster can cause an abducens nerve palsy on the basis of brain stem inflammation and loss of nuclear cells, with or without long tract signs (609).

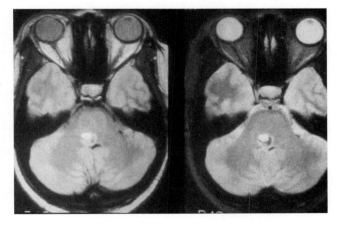

Figure 20.65. Magnetic resonance image in a 62-year-old woman with a slowly progressive right horizontal gaze paresis and ipsilateral facial weakness. Axial proton-density (*left*) and T2-weighted (*right*) images demonstrate a lesion in the region of the abducens nerve nucleus. An evaluation revealed breast carcinoma with evidence of systemic metastases, and the lesion was thought to be a metastasis.

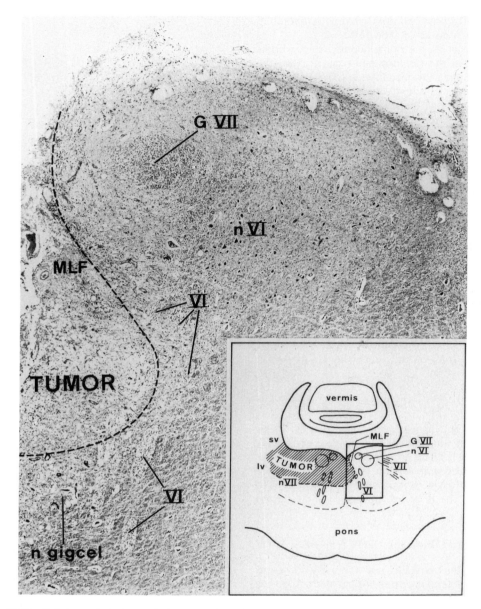

Figure 20.66. Pathology of a lesion producing an acquired, rightward horizontal gaze palsy. Transverse section through the pons at the level of the abducens nuclei shows an intact left abducens nucleus, while the right abducens nucleus is destroyed by an infiltrating tumor. Some damage across the midline involves both the medial longitudinal fasciculus and some fibers of the left abducens fascicle to a minor degree. The *inset* is a low-power drawing showing the area photographed (*rectangle*) and the extent of tumor. MLF, medial longitudinal fasciculus; VI, left abducens fascicle; n VI, left abducens nucleus; VII, fascicle of the left facial nerve; G VII, genu of the left facial nerve; n VII, region of the nucleus of the right facial nerve; n gigcel, nucleus gigantocellularis; lv, lateral vestibular nucleus; sv, superior vestibular nucleus. (From Meienberg O, Büttner-Ennever JA, Kraus-Ruppert R. Unilateral paralysis of conjugate gaze due to lesion of the abducens nucleus. Neuroophthalmology 1981; 2:47–52.)

Patients with the Wernicke-Korsakoff syndrome often develop paralysis of conjugate gaze, presumably from a metabolic insult to the abducens nuclei (610,611). Wernicke-Korsakoff syndrome can be seen after bariatric surgery, hyperemesis gravidarum, gamma hydroxybutyrate abuse, anorexia nervosa, peptic ulcer, acute pancreatitis, esophageal metastasis, carcinoma of the stomach or esophagus, and celiac disease, as well as alcoholism (612–615). Loss of nuclear motor neurons in ALS is discussed above in the oculomotor nerve section.

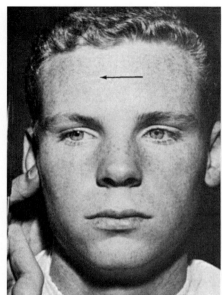 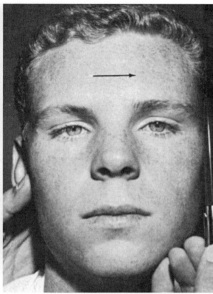

Figure 20.67. Acute bilateral paralysis of horizontal gaze in a 16-year-old boy with multiple sclerosis. Two weeks after this photograph was obtained, all neurologic signs had resolved.

Lesions of the Abducens Nerve Fascicle

When an abducens nerve palsy coexists with a gaze palsy to the same side from damage to both the abducens nucleus and the ipsilateral abducens nerve fascicle, the fascicular nerve element in the gaze palsy cannot be assessed unless there is a marked asymmetry between the two eyes, with the abducting eye being more limited in movement than the adducting eye (616). More commonly, fascicular involvement of the abducens nerve produces an isolated abduction weakness just like that of peripheral nerve involvement, without a gaze palsy, and the lesion may not be visible on MRI (105,178,617). Often fascicular lesions can be diagnosed by neighborhood pontine signs. There is much confusion and overlap in the eponymous syndromes, and what we now call them is often not what was originally described (618). In one study of 36 patients with isolated pontine strokes, not one patient fit into any of the "classical" eponymous alternating syndromes. Incomplete syndromes are common, and sometimes there is abducens nuclear involvement as well as fascicular involvement. Strokes of the cerebellum and multiple strokes in the posterior circulation territory are commonly associated with pontine strokes.

The pons can be divided into the basis pontis, which is ventral and medial and which contains the pyramidal tracts, the pontine nuclei, and their pontocerebellar fibers; and the pontine tegmentum, which is more lateral and dorsal and which contains the fifth, sixth, and seventh nerve nuclei, the superior salivatory nucleus, the nucleus of the tractus solitarius, the descending tract of V, the lateral lemniscus, the medial lemniscus, the sympathetic fibers, and the inferior cerebellar peduncle. A lesion in the basis pontis, usually a stroke involving paramedian arterioles from the basilar artery, causes the medial pontine syndrome or Millard-Gubler syndrome of ipsilateral sixth and seventh nerve fascicular

palsies with contralateral hemiplegia (Fig. 20.68). A lesion in the pontine tegmentum, usually a stroke involving the anterior inferior cerebellar artery, causes Foville's syndrome of ipsilateral sixth and seventh nerve palsy, fascicular or nuclear, with contralateral ataxia and contralateral sensory disturbance. Associated findings may include loss of taste from the anterior two thirds of the tongue, ipsilateral Horner's syndrome, ipsilateral analgesia of the face, ipsilateral peripheral deafness, contralateral ataxia, and contralateral loss of pain and temperature sensation on the body, usually from occlusion of the anterior inferior cerebellar artery (618–620) (Foville's original patient had an ipsilateral sixth and seventh nerve palsy and contralateral weakness; Millard's and Gubler's patients had seventh nerve weakness without sixth nerve involvement, associated with contralateral weakness). A lesion of the sixth nerve, sparing the seventh, with contralateral hemiparesis is the Raymond-Cestan syndrome. Larger strokes, trauma, and large hemorrhages can cause combinations of these syndromes.

Fascicular lesions may be due to ischemia, tumor, compression or infiltration, infection, or inflammation, with MS being the most common form of inflammation (178,580). *Listeria monocytogenes* meningoencephalitis has a tendency to cause brain stem lesions, and abducens nuclear or fascicular involvement can occur (621). Although the abducens nerve palsies that occur in association with diabetes mellitus are usually assumed to be peripheral, they can be caused by small pontine hemorrhages or ischemic lesions. As imaging improves, more "peripheral" abducens lesions are seen to be central (169,622). In one report, MRI showed a small, transient, enhancing lesion in the lower pons associated with ophthalmoplegic migraine and abducens palsy (623).

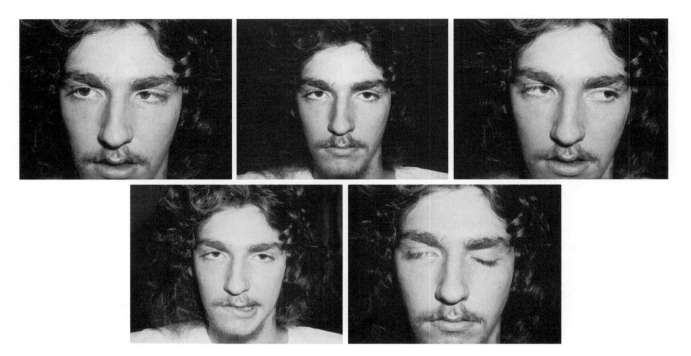

Figure 20.68. Millard-Gubler syndrome in a 23-year-old man with an intrapontine hemorrhage. The patient has a right abducens nerve paresis, a right peripheral facial nerve paresis, and a left (contralateral) hemiparesis.

Lesions of the Abducens Nerve in the Subarachnoid Space

Causes of abducens nerve damage in the subarachnoid space are many and varied and are similar to those of the oculomotor and trochlear nerves (see above) (Fig. 20.69). The long subarachnoid course of the abducens nerve is usually blamed for its frequent injury. However, the trochlear nerve is longer, yet trochlear nerve palsies are rarer. The abducens nerve has an eventful course, passing through many potentially hazardous areas. It lies along the ventral surface of the pons and is bound to it by the anterior inferior cerebellar artery. The nerve may therefore be compressed by this vessel, the posterior inferior cerebellar artery, or the basilar artery, particularly when they are either atherosclerotic or dolichoectatic (624). Dolichoectatic or atherosclerotic arteries can cause either single or multiple cranial neuropathies (624,625). Aneurysms of the vessels can also cause abducens palsy (225), usually in isolation and usually with severe headache.

After its exit from the pons, the abducens nerve passes almost vertically through the subarachnoid space to pierce the dura overlying the clivus, where it is held in place (see Chapter 17). It is vulnerable to stretch from descent of the brain stem associated with vertex blows, transtentorial herniation, Arnold-Chiari malformations, intracranial hypotension, and infratentorial masses. In these circumstances, it may be injured at its attachment at either the pons or the

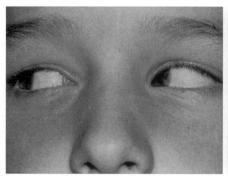
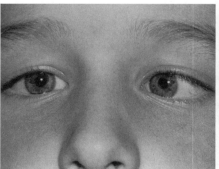
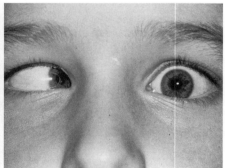

Figure 20.69. Left abducens nerve palsy in a 7-year-old boy with aseptic meningitis. It was assumed that the palsy was caused by damage to the abducens nerve in the subarachnoid space. The palsy cleared without treatment.

clivus. It may be traumatized directly, such as by neurosurgical mishap (239), or indirectly by blunt trauma such as closed head injury (580). Bilateral abducens palsy after blunt head trauma suggests that the forces involved were considerable and that there may be intracranial bleeding or other severe damage (626,627). Of particular interest is the development of abducens paralysis, either unilateral or bilateral and usually associated with lower cranial nerve palsies, during halo-pelvic traction (628). The pathophysiology appears to be distortion of the abducens nerve itself or ischemia from distortion of its nutrient blood vessels, during traction on the brain stem.

Meningitis, whether bacterial, neoplastic, spirochetal, or viral, often produces abducens nerve paralysis, sometimes bilateral (629–633). Patients with AIDS are particularly vulnerable to opportunistic organisms causing meningitis, including *Mycobacterium, Cryptococcus, Toxoplasma gondii, Cytomegalovirus,* and herpes simplex virus. Patients frequently exhibit abducens and other cranial nerve palsies in the course of meningitis (634–636). Idiopathic hypertrophic cranial pachymeningitis is chronic inflammatory thickening of the meninges (Fig. 20.70). It is sometimes associated with rheumatoid arthritis, syphilis, Tolosa-Hunt syndrome, Wegener's granulomatosis, Churg-Strauss syndrome, or sinus infection. When it involves the basal meninges, it can produce an abducens palsy, which is usually reversible with steroids if treated early (637–639).

Skull base tumors, benign and malignant, common and rare, may directly involve the subarachnoid portion of the abducens nerve by compression, stretching, or infiltration, and often an isolated abducens palsy is the first sign of the tumor (640–643). Early on, the paresis may be intermittent (644). Trigeminal schwannomas may present with abducens nerve signs without trigeminal signs (645). Acoustic neuromas may cause abducens palsy, but almost never as their first or sole manifestation. Similarly, although the abducens nerve may be damaged by exophytic spread of intrinsic pos-

terior fossa tumors such as glioma, medulloblastoma, or ependymoma, patients with these tumors almost always have other neurologic symptoms and signs.

Less common are intrinsic tumors of the nerve itself. As with the oculomotor and trochlear nerves, schwannomas and neurofibromas of the subarachnoid portion of the abducens nerve may produce an isolated abducens palsy (646–648). Cavernous angiomas and fibroblastic tumors of the nerve produce a similar clinical picture (649,650).

Changes in ICP, either increased or decreased, can cause unilateral or bilateral abducens palsy, which may be a false localizing sign (580,651). Unilateral (and occasionally bilateral) abducens palsy with headache sometimes develops after lumbar puncture, shunting for hydrocephalus, myelography, or spinal anesthesia, from loss of spinal fluid. The palsy may be delayed in onset up to 14 days and inevitably recovers, although it may take as long as 4 to 6 weeks to do so. After lumbar puncture with a 22-gauge needle, the incidence of abducens palsy has been reported to be 1 in 5,800, and after myelography, 1 in 500 (652–655).

Spontaneous intracranial hypotension may cause severe orthostatic headaches, meningeal enhancement with gadolinium, and abducens paresis (656,657). Meningeal biopsy in longstanding intracranial hypotension shows fibroblasts and thin-walled small vessels on the inner surface of the dura mater, without inflammation.

Abducens nerve paresis resulting from increased ICP probably occurs because the abducens nerve becomes compressed between the pons and the basilar artery or clivus or is stretched across the sharp edge of the petrous temporal bone (658,659). Similar mechanisms may operate when a low-pressure state develops after lumbar puncture, after cerebrospinal fluid shunting, or spontaneously. Although the possibility of a toxic process must be considered in patients who develop abducens paralysis following spinal anesthesia or myelography, it seems unlikely that chemical irritation would produce only unilateral isolated cranial nerve palsy.

Anteriorly draining dural carotid–cavernous sinus fistulas frequently cause an abducens palsy from compression or ischemia of the nerve in the cavernous sinus (see below). These fistulas are associated with chemosis, proptosis, and redness. Posterior-draining dural carotid–cavernous sinus fistulas may also produce an abducens palsy, without the orbital signs (468,660). The palsy may be bilateral, and there may be ocular motor nerve involvement from drainage into the inferior petrosal sinus.

Lesions of the Extradural Portion of the Abducens Nerve at the Petrous Apex

After the abducens nerve penetrates the dura overlying the clivus, it passes beneath the petroclinoid (Gruber's) ligament. Here it is adjacent to the mastoid air cells. In patients with severe mastoiditis, the inflammatory process may extend to the tip of the petrous bone, producing localized inflammation of the meninges in the epidural space and a classic syndrome: Gradenigo's syndrome of the petrous apex (661,662). The adjacent abducens nerve becomes inflamed and paretic. Because the Gasserian ganglion and facial nerve

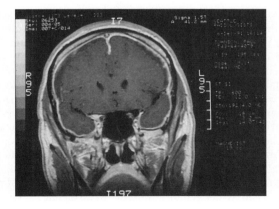

Figure 20.70. Neuroimaging in a 39-year-old man with a slowly progressive right abduction deficit associated with headache. Axial T1-weighted magnetic resonance image shows diffuse meningeal enhancement as well as inflammatory changes in the right cavernous sinus. Biopsy of the meninges established a diagnosis of idiopathic hypertrophic cranial pachymeningitis. The disease was arrested with cranial irradiation and immunotherapy.

are nearby, patients have severe pain on the ipsilateral side of the face and around the eye and may also develop facial paralysis. Occipital pain may be caused by irritation of the tentorial branch of the trigeminal nerve. Abducens paresis is sometimes delayed until 2 or 3 days after the onset of the pain. There may be photophobia, lacrimation, and decreased corneal sensation. Usually the inflammation is localized, but sometimes meningitis develops. Because of the prompt and almost universal use of antibiotics in children with known or presumed acute otitis media, the incidence of Gradenigo's syndrome has markedly declined.

Pathologic processes other than inflammation can involve the petrous apex and produce symptoms suggesting Gradenigo's syndrome. These include tumors (663,664) and aneurysms of the intrapetrosal segment of the internal carotid artery. Patients presenting with the petrous apex syndrome should be carefully evaluated with appropriate neuroimaging studies.

When lateral sinus thrombosis or phlebitis extends into the inferior petrosal sinus, the nerve may become paretic (665). A similar situation may occur when one jugular vein (particularly the larger right jugular) is ligated during radical neck dissection. Both of these conditions cause increased ICP.

The nerve may be injured in its petrous segment when the skull is fractured (627,666,667). A persistent primitive trigeminal artery may compress the nerve. Whether this takes place just outside or inside the cavernous sinus is unclear (668).

Lesions in the superior aspect of the sphenopalatine (pterygopalatine) fossa often present with the classic picture of abducens palsy, loss of tearing, irritation of the eye on the side of the paresis, and trigeminal sensory neuropathy in the distribution of the maxillary division of the trigeminal nerve. The lesion is usually a malignant tumor (e.g., nasopharyngeal carcinoma) that has extended through foramina at the base of the skull and has spread beneath the dura to damage the extradural portions of the abducens and trigeminal nerves.

Lesions of the Abducens Nerve in the Cavernous Sinus and Superior Orbital Fissure: The Sphenocavernous Syndrome

Lesions in the cavernous sinus and superior orbital fissure often involve more than one cranial nerve, but isolated palsies sometimes occur. Because most of the structures in the cavernous sinus continue out through the superior orbital fissure, it is difficult to differentiate between these areas clinically. The maxillary division of the trigeminal nerve leaves the cavernous sinus through the foramen rotundum and can be injured in the cavernous sinus but not in the superior orbital fissure. The abducens nerve may be damaged in the cavernous sinus, either alone or with other nerves, by a variety of pathologic processes (332).

The abducens nerve runs centrally within the sinus itself, while the oculomotor and trochlear nerves and the ophthalmic division of the trigeminal nerve run in its lateral wall. Intracavernous vascular lesions such as aneurysms therefore preferentially injure the abducens nerve (669–672), as do direct and dural carotid–cavernous fistulas (231,673,674), hemangiomas (675), and, rarely, internal carotid artery dissection (676). Tumors that infiltrate the cavernous sinus as well as those that compress the structures within it may produce isolated abducens palsy (677,678). These include meningioma (679), schwannoma (680), metastatic carcinoma (681,682), nasopharyngeal carcinoma (644), Burkitt's lymphoma (683,684), pituitary adenoma with and without apoplexy (334), craniopharyngioma (685), suprasellar germinoma (686), juvenile nasopharyngeal angiofibroma (687), osteogenic sarcoma (688), Rosai-Dorfman histiocytosis (689), teratoma (690), and multiple myeloma or plasmacytoma (691,692). Larger lesions may involve both cavernous sinuses and produce bilateral abducens nerve palsies.

Hypertension, diabetes mellitus, giant cell arteritis, systemic lupus erythematosus, and perhaps migraine cause ischemic abducens nerve lesions within the cavernous sinus, usually painful. These typically resolve within 3 months. Granulomatous processes such as tuberculosis, sarcoidosis, and the Tolosa-Hunt syndrome occur in the cavernous sinus and cause abducens palsy. Nongranulomatous inflammation such as bacterial and fungal sphenoid sinusitis occurs as well (693). Herpes zoster can cause abducens palsy in the same location.

Although isolated involvement of the abducens nerve in the cavernous sinus is not rare, it is far more common to have associated neurologic signs and symptoms, even if there are no other ocular motor nerve palsies (332). One of the more important of these intracavernous syndromes is the combination of isolated abducens paralysis and ipsilateral Horner's syndrome (157,694) (Fig. 20.71). Oculosympathetic fibers leave the internal carotid artery within the cavernous sinus and briefly join with the abducens nerve before separating off and fusing with the ophthalmic division of the trigeminal nerve (Fig. 20.72). Involvement of the segment of the abducens nerve that is carrying the oculosympathetic fibers results in this syndrome (695).

Lesions of the Abducens Nerve Within the Orbit

The abducens nerve has a very short course in the orbit, piercing the lateral rectus muscle only a few millimeters from the superior orbital fissure (696). For this reason, isolated orbital involvement is rare. Schwannomas can arise from nerves in the orbit, including the abducens nerve (697). Dental anesthesia can cause transient abduction weakness. There is controversy over whether the anesthetic is injected intraarterially into the inferior dental artery and then flows retrograde into the maxillary and middle meningeal arteries, or whether there is direct injection through the inferior orbital fissure (364,698). In the orbit, differentiation between neural and muscular involvement producing abduction weakness may not be possible. Occasionally the lateral rectus muscle is congenitally absent. Myasthenia gravis can easily mimic an abducens palsy.

Lesions of the Abducens Nerve of Uncertain or Variable Location

Spontaneously remitting isolated abducens nerve palsy is uncommon in the general population. In adults, there are

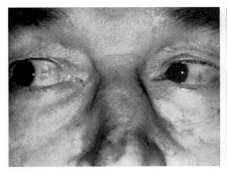
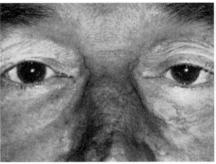
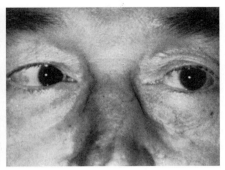

Figure 20.71. Left abducens nerve paresis associated with left Horner's syndrome in a patient with a probable meningioma of the left cavernous sinus. Note the mild left ptosis and miosis.

often vascular risk factors such as diabetes mellitus or hypertension, or a history of a recent viral syndrome (369). Spontaneous remission is even less common in children, where tumor is the most common cause of abducens palsy. Benign, remitting palsies do occur in children, however, and may even recur (699–705). The location of these lesions is unknown. The lesion in abducens palsy from ophthalmoplegic migraine is variable, either central (623) or peripheral, and it may be impossible in an individual case to decide which,

if the imaging is unrevealing (706). Immunologic damage to the abducens nerve can probably happen anywhere along its course (707).

A number of substances may produce an abducens nerve palsy, including arsenic, carbon tetrachloride, chloroquine, dichloracetylene, diphenylhydantoin, ethylene glycol, isoniazid, nitrofurans, piperazine, thalidomide, trichloroethylene, Orthoclone OKT3, and interferon α-2a. These intoxications are discussed in the final section of this chapter. In none

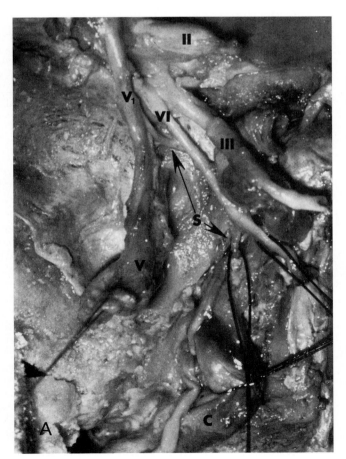

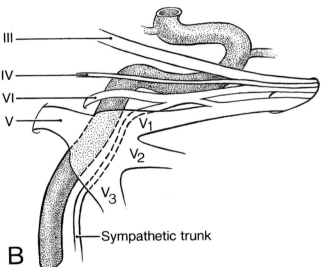

Figure 20.72. Oculosympathetic connections with the abducens nerve in the cavernous sinus. *A,* The sympathetic nerve (S) enters the cavernous sinus with the internal carotid artery (C). Within the sinus, it joins briefly (*short arrow*) with the abducens nerve (VI). It then separates from the nerve (*long arrow*) and joins with the ophthalmic branch (V1) of the trigeminal nerve (V). III, oculomotor nerve; II, optic nerve. *B,* Drawing of relationship of oculosympathetic fibers, abducens nerve, and trigeminal nerve. (*A,* From Parkinson D, Johnston J, Chaudhur A. Sympathetic connections to the fifth and sixth cranial nerves. Anat Rec 1978;191:221–226.)

of these cases is the precise mechanism of damage clearly understood.

Chronic, Isolated Abducens Nerve Paralysis

Truly isolated abducens nerve palsies (no other signs or symptoms) are usually caused by vascular, inflammatory, and compressive lesions. It is our experience and that of others that "benign" vascular or inflammatory abducens nerve palsies usually resolve within about 3 months. Any abducens palsy of unclear or presumed vascular origin that does not resolve or at least begin to improve within 3 months should be investigated fully (581). The most important issue in a patient with an abducens nerve palsy is whether or not the palsy is truly isolated. If other neurologic signs (e.g., trigeminal sensory neuropathy, facial paresis, hearing loss, Horner's syndrome) are present, the chance of a mass lesion is greater, and the patient should undergo an appropriate work-up without delay. If no other findings are present, and the patient is over 60 with vascular risk factors, it is safe to follow him or her clinically at regular intervals, although not necessarily wrong to obtain imaging studies (708).

The development of an abducens nerve palsy following minimal head trauma suggests the presence of a compressive lesion such as a tumor (709). Spontaneous recovery of an abducens nerve palsy may occur even with a skull base tumor or leukemia, perhaps from remyelination, axonal regeneration, resorption of hemorrhage in a tumor, recovery of blood flow, slippage of a nerve that had been stretched by the tumor, or immune responses to the tumor (644,710).

EVALUATION AND MANAGEMENT OF ABDUCENS NERVE PALSY

There is a tendency to assume that all patients with an esotropia and unilateral or bilateral abduction weakness have an abducens nerve paresis. The physician should first consider the possibility that the condition is myopathic (e.g., thyroid eye disease) or neuromuscular (e.g., myasthenia gravis). A careful history and examination directed at these possibilities may be sufficient to eliminate them. Alternatively, the physician may need to perform further studies, including orbital MRI, thyroid function studies, serum assay for anti-acetylcholine and MuSK antibodies, and repetitive nerve stimulation and single-fiber electromyography.

When an abducens palsy is likely, the evaluation depends on the medical history, associated signs and symptoms, and age of the patient. A thoughtful and thorough neurologic examination should determine whether there are any intraaxial or extraaxial signs, such as INO, gaze palsy, hemiparesis, ataxia, trigeminal sensory neuropathy, facial paresis, hearing loss, oculomotor or trochlear palsy, or Horner's syndrome, to try to determine the site and identity of the lesion. Redness, swelling, or proptosis of the affected eye suggests a spontaneous dural carotid–cavernous sinus fistula. Cavernous sinus thrombosis, particularly the aseptic variety, can produce a clinical picture similar to that seen in patients with carotid–cavernous sinus fistulas. Patients with septic cavernous sinus thrombosis nearly always have prominent systemic manifestations of sepsis.

If a patient with an apparent abducens nerve paresis has no other findings and has diabetes or underlying systemic vascular disease or is in the vasculopathic age group (i.e., over age 60), and if the onset of the palsy is sudden, he or she should be followed at regular intervals, with an interval history obtained and a complete examination performed each time. If during this time the patient develops other neurologic signs or the paresis worsens, a complete work-up, including neuroimaging or reimaging and an otolaryngologic evaluation, is necessary. If no improvement occurs in 3 months, the patient needs a complete reassessment (581). On the other hand, if the patient is under age 60 and has no risk factors for ischemic or inflammatory disease, we perform MRI with careful attention to the pathway of the abducens nerve from the brain stem to the orbit. A lumbar puncture, cerebral angiography, and otolaryngologic assessment may be indicated in some patients.

As with trochlear nerve paralysis, abducens nerve paralysis may or may not resolve, and the resolution may be complete or incomplete. Ischemic pareses almost always recover completely, usually within 2 to 4 months (369). Some degree of spontaneous recovery of traumatic abducens pareses occurs in 30–54% of cases and may take more than a year (711). Of 213 patients with isolated acquired abducens nerve paresis, 78% recovered spontaneously, with recovery beginning within 4 months of the onset of symptoms. Among the 35 patients who did not recover, serious pathology (e.g., tumor, stroke, aneurysm) was identified in 14, underscoring the importance of performing an evaluation in patients whose abducens nerve palsy does not recover within 3 to 6 months (581) (see above). Patients whose abducens nerve is transected during a neurosurgical procedure may recover function within 9 months if the nerve is reapproximated at the time of surgery (712).

Strabismus surgery should not be considered for an abducens nerve palsy until at least 10 to 12 months have passed without improvement, unless the abducens nerve is no longer in continuity (e.g., after neurosurgical transection without reapproximation). During this period, some patients prefer to occlude one eye with a patch or an opaque contact lens, whereas others may be able to ignore their diplopia. Patients under 8 years old should undergo alternate patching of the eyes to prevent amblyopia. Prisms are not usually very helpful, though exceptions occur. Botulinum toxin injections to the ipsilateral medial rectus muscle may be helpful. Surgery, when required, usually consists of either weakening of the ipsilateral medial rectus muscle combined with strengthening of the ipsilateral lateral rectus muscle or some type of vertical muscle transposition procedure (404,713,714), often combined with chemodenervation of the ipsilateral medial rectus muscle with botulinum toxin.

Chemodenervation of the antagonist medial rectus muscle with botulinum toxin can be used to treat patients with both acute and chronic abducens nerve palsy. Early use of botulinum toxin in acute abducens nerve palsy does not affect the eventual outcome of the condition (714). In chronic abducens nerve palsy, surgery is generally more beneficial than botulinum toxin (715). The decision to perform any procedure depends upon the etiology and severity of the abducens weakness as well as the results of forced duction and force-generation tests (716,717) (see Chapter 18).

DIVERGENCE WEAKNESS AND ITS RELATIONSHIP TO ABDUCENS NERVE PALSY

Despite the controversy about its cause, divergence weakness appears to be a well-defined entity. It was first described by Parinaud in 1883 and is diagnosed by Bielschowski's five criteria (718,719):

1. There is sudden uncrossed, horizontal diplopia at distance but not at near.
2. The angle of the esophoria or esotropia remains unchanged or may decrease on horizontal gaze to either side.
3. When an object is brought near to the patient, the two images approach each other and become fused when the object is at a distance of 25–40 cm from the patient.
4. Ductions are full.
5. Fusion divergence is reduced or absent.

Divergence weakness is distinguished from convergence spasm because patients with convergence spasm maintain an esotropia at near, have miotic pupils, have reduced distance visual acuity from induced myopia, and show normal fusional divergence. It is possible, however, that these conditions are on a clinical continuum (720).

A distinction is made between the syndromes of divergence insufficiency, in which an otherwise healthy patient suddenly develops comitant esotropia at distance with normal-appearing ductions, and divergence paralysis, in which the patient has associated neurologic disease. Divergence insufficiency is most frequently observed in adults, although it may occur at any age. Sometimes it is preceded by minor head trauma or mild nonspecific illness. It is usually self-limited. Base-out prisms are often helpful. In persistent cases, after an interval of 12 months, strabismus surgery can be performed (404,720–723).

Divergence paralysis has been associated with many conditions, including intracranial masses, trauma, medication effect, intracranial hemorrhage, inflammation, temporal arteritis, progressive supranuclear palsy, cerebellar degeneration, Miller Fisher syndrome, brain stem stroke, and syphilis (723–729). We see divergence paralysis most often in patients with MS and in patients with increased ICP from brain tumor or pseudotumor cerebri or Arnold-Chiari malformation.

The cause is controversial. Some observers believe the condition is merely bilateral abducens nerve palsies (724,730), and bolster the argument with recordings of saccadic velocities. Other investigators believe there is a divergence center in the brain stem, as yet not discovered, and point to brain stem recordings from the reticular formation of monkeys (718,731). In humans, upper brain stem infarcts at the level of the diencephalic–mesencephalic junction, just rostral to the oculomotor nucleus, can cause inappropriate convergence, but this is associated with upgaze palsy and convergence-retraction nystagmus (732). We agree with von

Noorden (404) that two findings in patients with divergence paralysis separate it from simple bilateral abducens nerve pareses. First, fusional divergence is markedly reduced or absent if measured from the fusion-free position at near and distance fixation. Second, the esotropia not only remains unchanged during horizontal gaze but may even decrease. We therefore consider divergence paralysis an entity separate from abducens nerve paresis.

Whatever the pathogenesis of divergence weakness, patients with this disorder should be assumed to have neurologic disease until proven otherwise and should undergo a detailed neurologic evaluation. Most patients with an underlying neurologic disorder will be identified clinically and should then be worked up accordingly. Those with a normal clinical examination are not likely to have a lesion on neuroimaging but certainly need careful sequential follow-up if it is not performed (720,733–735).

CYCLIC ESOTROPIA AND ITS RELATIONSHIP TO ABDUCENS NERVE PALSY

Cyclic, or alternate-day, esotropia is a rare condition characterized by a regularly recurring esotropia that may at first be mistaken for an unusual form of abducens paralysis. It usually appears in children 3 to 4 years old, but it occurs also in adults (736–739). Usually 24 hours of unilateral esotropia and diplopia alternates with 24 hours of orthophoria and fusion. It is unrelated to visual activity, accommodation, or interruption of fusion. On esotropic days, a constant deviation of 30–40 prism diopters is typical. Cyclic esotropia occurs without any abnormalities of eyelid or pupillary activity, suggesting that it is not caused by oculomotor nerve hyperactivity. Most cases occur with regular 48-hour cycles, although some recur every 3rd or 4th day (740). Although cyclic esotropia usually begins spontaneously, it may develop after strabismus surgery, after cataract extraction, after tumor removal, in association with retinal detachment, in patients with optic atrophy, after traumatic aphakia, and after acquired sixth nerve palsy (741–745). All of these conditions have the potential for interrupting binocularity. Eventually the esotropia may become constant.

The cause of cyclic esotropia is mysterious. Circadian rhythmicity occurs in a variety of physiologic parameters, including intraocular pressure, temperature, headache, and psychological states, but the usual period is 24 rather than 48 hours (746–748). Even circadian sneezing occurs (749). One patient had a phase shift after travel through six time zones (750). Among the suggested causes of cyclic esotropia are an abnormal hypothalamic "biologic clock," incomplete or unusual cerebral dominance, prior encephalitis, and trauma. Velocity–amplitude relationships and saccadic dynamics are normal in both eyes on both orthotropic and esotropic days (751). It therefore seems unlikely that cyclic esotropia is caused simply by either oculomotor nerve hyperactivity or abducens nerve hypoactivity. It may be that strabismus is interrupted by periodic intervals of fusion, rather than that normal function is interrupted by periodic intervals of strabismus, and that central adaption to a peripheral defect may be partly responsible for some forms of this phenomenon (751,752). An even rarer condition is cyclic vertical deviation, in which 24 hours of vertical strabismus with diplopia alternates with 24 hours of orthophoria.

The appropriate treatment for cyclic esotropia is surgery aimed at correcting the maximum ocular deviation. Patients usually obtain good results with straight eyes and central fusion. Once corrected, the cyclic pattern does not recur, and there is no overcorrection on previously straight days.

DIAGNOSIS OF INFRANUCLEAR OPHTHALMOPLEGIA

In patients with monocular ophthalmoplegia involving more than one ocular motor nerve, or in patients with bilateral ophthalmoplegia, several possibilities must be considered. Myopathies or disorders of the neuromuscular junction may be responsible, rather than the ocular motor nerves. These disorders are considered in Chapters 21 and 22. When the etiology is neurologic, the lesion may be anywhere from the brain stem to the orbit. Intrinsic brain stem lesions may produce mixtures of ocular motor nerve pareses on one or both sides combined with supranuclear disorders of gaze (753). Extrinsic masses adjacent to the brain stem (especially those that grow along the skull base) and lesions in or near the cavernous sinus, such as meningiomas and pituitary adenomas, are particularly prone to produce both unilateral and bilateral ocular motor polyneuropathies (685,754–758). Pathologic processes including ischemia, hemorrhage, inflammation, compression, infiltration, metabolic dysfunction, toxic reactions, trauma, and degeneration may each be responsible (305,754,759,760). In most cases, the clinical history and a careful examination, when combined with appropriate neuroimaging, systemic, and otolaryngologic studies, are sufficient to identify the site and nature of the disease process.

Acute complete bilateral ophthalmoplegia is usually from pituitary apoplexy, botulism, myasthenia gravis, Wernicke's encephalopathy, the Miller Fisher variant of the Guillain-Barré syndrome, brain stem stroke or hemorrhage, and less commonly from phenytoin overdose, amitriptyline overdose, meningitis, or bilateral involvement of the cavernous sinus by infection or masses (761,762).

Ocular motor nerve palsies may be familial and recurrent, often associated with facial paralysis (704,763–766). The inheritance pattern appears to be autosomal dominant. Usually the patients are over 40 years of age and healthy.

Recurrent cranial nerve palsies occur also in individuals without a family history (767–771). Some of these patients have an underlying systemic vasculopathy, most often diabetes mellitus. Others have no evidence of a systemic illness but have asymptomatic aseptic meningitis. Still others have no clinical or laboratory evidence of systemic or neurologic disease. In most cases, there is involvement of the ocular motor nerves followed or preceded by facial nerve paralysis. Some of these may represent partial expression of the Miller Fisher syndrome. The relationship of these palsies to the Tolosa-Hunt syndrome, particularly when they are associated with pain, is unclear.

Some generalized neuropathies can produce ophthalmoplegia. As the ocular motor nerves are short, ophthalmoplegia may occur late in the clinical syndrome, after involvement of the longer nerves. Refsum's disease, Friedreich's ataxia, Charcot-Marie-Tooth disease, chronic inflammatory demyelinating polyneuropathy, and the Guillain-Barré syndrome are occasionally complicated by ophthalmoplegia (772,773). CANOMAD (chronic ataxic neuropathy with ophthalmoplegia, M-protein, agglutination, and disialosyl antibodies) is a chronic generalized immunologically mediated neuropathy that usually causes ophthalmoplegia (274). Eosinophilia-myalgia syndrome, which is both a neuropathy and a myopathy, is sometimes severe enough to involve eye muscles, either because of nerve or direct muscle involvement. Mitochondrial diseases such as the various types of chronic progressive external ophthalmoplegia, the Kearns-Sayre syndrome, and MELAS (mitochondrial myopathy, encephalopathy, lactic acidosis, and stroke-like episodes) probably cause their ophthalmoplegia on a myopathic basis (774,775). However, there is evidence for peripheral neuronal loss as well in some cases of chronic progressive external ophthalmoplegia (CPEO), suggesting that the ophthalmoplegia may be multifactorial (776,777). The recessive syndrome of intestinal pseudo-obstruction with external ophthalmoplegia is a combination of a myopathy resembling facioscapulohumeral muscular dystrophy and a peripheral neuropathy that is both axonal and demyelinating (778). The ophthalmoplegia here may be multifactorial as well, but in our one case, the myopathy was much more prominent than the neuropathy. The ophthalmoplegia seen in Machado-Joseph disease, a spinocerebellar degeneration, is from loss of neurons in ocular motor nuclei (114).

HYPERACTIVITY OF THE OCULAR MOTOR NERVES

Several ocular motor syndromes are characterized by hyperactivity, rather than hypoactivity, of one or more of the ocular motor nerves. Two of these are ocular neuromyotonia and superior oblique myokymia. Both of these disorders are considered in Chapter 23 because of their relationship to nystagmus and other ocular oscillations. We consider them also in this chapter because they affect the ocular motor nerves.

OCULAR NEUROMYOTONIA

This is an acquired condition in which various eye muscles go into brief intermittent spasm, causing diplopia that comes and goes (779) (Fig. 20.73). Usually the muscles relate to one ocular motor nerve, but they may relate to more than one or be bilateral. Sometimes only one muscle, such as the levator palpebrae superioris, is involved. Occasionally the condition is self-limited (60,779–784). Most patients had undergone radiation therapy for brain tumors or pituitary tumors months to years before. The history of radiation is not always obvious. One 72-year-old man developed ocular neuromyotonia after having undergone myelography many years earlier using thorium dioxide (Thorotrast), a substance that is weakly radioactive and that remained in his subarachnoid space (785). Ocular neuromyotonia can develop without radiation injury in patients with Graves' dysthyroid orbitopathy, internal carotid aneurysm, compression of the oculomotor nerve by a dolichoectatic basilar artery, or months after cavernous sinus thrombosis from mucormycosis (786–789). It is unclear whether ocular neuromyotonia is related to the delayed myotonia of limb muscles that can follow radiation to the brachial plexus.

Low-dose carbamazepine and quinine have both been used to stop the spasms. One patient was able to stop spasms by suddenly directing her gaze in the opposite direction, abruptly stretching the overactive muscle (790). Another patient, who had had radiation for a pituitary tumor, experienced superior oblique neuromyotonia only after drinking alcohol. The condition was relieved by abstinence (781). The evaluation of patients with neuromyotonia, particularly those without a history of prior radiation therapy, should include MRI of the brain, with particular attention to the posterior fossa, and thyroid studies.

SUPERIOR OBLIQUE MYOKYMIA (SUPERIOR OBLIQUE MICROTREMOR)

Superior oblique myokymia (SOM) was first described by Duane in 1906, but clinicians became generally aware of the disorder following the description by Hoyt and Keane in 1970. Typical symptoms are monocular blurring of vision or tremulous sensations in the eye (791,792). Patients typically experience brief episodes of vertical or torsional diplopia, vertical or torsional oscillopsia, or both. Attacks usually last less than 10 seconds but may occur many times a day. The attacks may be spontaneous or be brought on by looking downward, by tilting the head toward the side of the affected eye, or by blinking. Most patients with SOM have no underlying disease, although cases have been reported following trochlear nerve palsy, after mild head trauma, in the setting of MS, after brain stem stroke, in a patient with a dural arteriovenous fistula, and in patients with cerebellar tumor (792–795). The eye movements of SOM are often difficult to appreciate on gross examination but are usually apparent with the ophthalmoscope or slit-lamp biomicroscope. They consist of spasms of cyclotorsional and vertical movements. Measurement of the movements of SOM using the magnetic search coil technique (795–797) reveal an initial intorsion and depression of the affected eye, followed by irregular oscillations of small amplitude. The frequency of these oscillations is variable. Some resemble jerk nystagmus, with frequencies of 2 to 6 Hz, but superimposed upon these oscillations are low-amplitude, irregular oscillations with frequencies ranging up to 50 Hz.

Electromyographic recordings from superior oblique muscles affected by SOM reveal some motor units that discharge either spontaneously or following contraction of the muscle. These units are abnormal, being of long duration

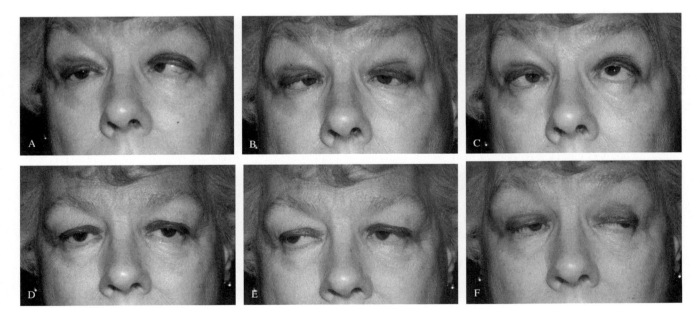

Figure 20.73. Ocular neuromyotonia. Appearance of a 62-year-old woman who had been treated with whole-brain radiation for a pituitary tumor 15 years prior to her presentation. The patient had paroxysmal spasms of adduction of the right eye, left eye (*A*), or both eyes (*B*), lasting several seconds. The pupils remained normal during the spasms, and there was no evidence of accommodation spasm, as might be expected if the patient were experiencing spasm of the near response. In addition, there was occasional spasm of elevation of the left eye (*C*). Between episodes of spasm, the eyes were straight (*D*) and horizontal gaze to the right (*E*) and left (*F*) was normal. The spasms initially responded to quinine (tonic water) but later required carbamazepine.

(greater than 2 msec) and increased amplitude, and they are polyphasic, with a spontaneous discharge rate of approximately 45 Hz. Spontaneous activity is absent only with large saccades in the ''off'' (upward) direction and is less affected by vestibular eye movements. Some firing units show an irregular discharge following muscle contraction before subsiding to a regular discharge of 35 Hz (792,798,799). Electromyography findings are similar to those of facial muscles with hemifacial spasm. The electromyogram suggests that the etiology of SOM is neuronal damage and subsequent regeneration. SOM is only occasionally preceded by an ipsilateral trochlear nerve palsy, but the possibility remains that mild chronic damage to the trochlear nerve could trigger regeneration (792,798,799). Vascular compression of the trochlear nerve by the posterior cerebral artery may be etiologic in some cases and may be disclosed by thin-slice MRI.

Microvascular decompression carries the risk of trochlear nerve palsy (244,800–802).

SOM spontaneously resolves in some patients (791); others tolerate it and do not need treatment. For those whose symptoms are distressing, both medical and surgical therapies are available. Individual patients may respond to a number of drugs, including carbamazepine, baclofen, gabapentin, and topically or systemically administered α-adrenergic blocking agents (791,803). Those who do not respond to drugs may benefit from extraocular muscle surgery (791,792). The procedure used by most surgeons is a superior oblique tenotomy combined with myectomy of the ipsilateral inferior oblique muscle, but nasal transposition of the anterior portion of the affected superior oblique tendon, thereby weakening cyclorotation, is also performed. The role of neurovascular compression has yet to be determined.

SYNKINESIS INVOLVING THE OCULAR MOTOR AND OTHER CRANIAL NERVES

A synkinesis (''moving together'') is a simultaneous movement or a coordinated set of movements of muscles supplied by different nerves or different branches of the same nerve. Normally occurring cranial synkineses are exemplified by sucking, chewing, conjugate eye movements, and Bell's phenomenon.

Abnormal cranial nerve synkineses occur most commonly in DRS (discussed earlier) and in the Marcus Gunn jaw-winking phenomenon (trigemino-ocular motor synkinesis) (see Chapter 24). Similar synkineses involving various facial and neck muscles and the extraocular muscles occur in rare

patients (804). One child had her ptotic lid elevate whenever she sat up, perhaps from a synkinesis between the levator and the neck muscles (805). One woman experienced diplopia every time she swallowed, because of intorsion and depression of one eye. She appears to have had a synkinesis between the superior oblique muscle and one of the muscles of deglutition (806). Some patients with the Marcus Gunn jaw-wink phenomenon have more extensive synkineses, with movements of both the eye and the lid related to jaw movement (807). The Marcus Gunn phenomenon and DRS may coexist (808).

NEUROPATHIC TOXICOLOGY OF THE OCULAR MOTOR SYSTEM

Exogenous agents sometimes cause peripheral ocular motor neuropathies. They can also cause supranuclear damage, extrapyramidal reactions, neuromuscular blockade, and myopathic damage.

Toxic ocular motor neuropathies are rare. They may be confined to a single nerve or involve some or all of the ocular motor nerves. They may be associated with other signs and symptoms, either neurologic or systemic. There are no characteristic features that clearly identify them as toxic; unless the patient is rechallenged with a drug or poison and develops the ophthalmoplegia again, diagnosis may have to be tentative.

In most cases of toxic ophthalmoplegia, the mechanism is unknown. In a few, there is an immunologic attack. Enzymatic processes may be blocked. Some patients have idiopathic reactions because of their own genetic makeup. Some reported cases may be pure coincidence.

Before the availability of penicillin, organic arsenicals were used extensively to treat syphilis. An abducens nerve paresis was observed in one patient with chronic arsenic poisoning (809).

A transient oculomotor nerve palsy developed in a 2.5-year-old child who consumed a large amount of aspirin and then developed convulsions and coma. We wonder whether this was a sign of herniation from cerebral edema (810).

Atorvastatin, a lipid-lowering agent, was associated in one

case with the development of ptosis and limitation of upgaze bilaterally, with ataxia and paresthesias. The patient had anti-AChR antibodies. The antibodies and the ophthalmoplegia disappeared within 10 weeks of discontinuing the drug. The product monographs for three other HMC-CoA reductase inhibitors (lovastatin, simvastatin, and fluvastatin) list ''impairment of ocular movement'' as an adverse effect (811).

A man industrially exposed to carbon tetrachloride, an organic cleaning solvent, developed bilateral abducens pareses associated with evidence of systemic toxicity (812).

Subtenon carboplatin has been use as chemotherapy for intraocular retinoblastoma. Ten consecutive patients developed restricted ocular motility as a result of fibrosis of orbital soft tissues. This does not appear to be specifically neurogenic. It may represent fibrotic change after fat necrosis (813).

Chloroquine diphosphate, a quinoline derivative, is sometimes used to treat malaria and a number of rheumatic disorders. A patient who had undergone long-term treatment with chloroquine developed bilateral abducens palsies (814).

Cocaine abuse has been implicated in several cases of myasthenia gravis. While the associated ophthalmoplegia is not caused by a nerve lesion, it is easy to confuse with one. One case was associated with pseudotonic pupils (815). A midbrain hematoma from smoking crack cocaine caused a bilateral INO (816). A small wound infection from cocaine injection caused ophthalmoplegia and descending weakness from botulism. A patient experienced diplopia from a tension orbital pneumocele, caused by nasal obstruction from cocaine abuse (817). Prenatal exposure to cocaine may have resulted in a case of Möbius syndrome (524).

A patient developed a reversible bilateral abducens nerve palsy and cerebellar dysfunction while being treated with high-dose cytosine arabinoside and mitoxantrone for acute myelogenous leukemia (818).

Dichloracetylene is known to cause trigeminal neuropathy. Two men exposed to monochloracetylene and dichloracetylene fumes developed trigeminal neuropathy, followed days later by herpes zoster of the lips. One of them developed transient trigeminal and abducens palsies, perhaps related to the herpes zoster (819).

Diphenylhydantoin was introduced as an anticonvulsant by Merritt and Putnam in 1938. Nystagmus and reversible generalized ophthalmoplegia occur with increasing dosages of diphenylhydantoin. We have seen patients with therapeutic levels of Dilantin referred for presumed abducens nerve paresis who actually had a decompensated esophoria. Patients may also exhibit divergence insufficiency. This breakdown of fusional ability is reversible (820,821).

Ecstasy (MDMA) abuse has been associated with one case of bilateral abducens nerve palsy (822).

Ethylene glycol (antifreeze) is usually drunk by mistake. It is oxidized in part to oxalic acid. Two men developed transient horizontal diplopia from bilateral abduction weakness during recovery from ethylene glycol poisoning. Interestingly, both patients could see clearly in primary position at near, suggesting that they may actually have had divergence paralysis rather than true abducens nerve palsies (823). A man developed left abducens paresis and bilateral optic disc swelling after drinking 3 or 4 ounces of ethylene glycol (40).

Gelsemium sempervirens, the yellow jasmine flower, yields a mixture of alkaloids used in the folk treatment of headache and neuralgias. Severe systemic reactions to the mixture are characterized by bradycardia, hypothermia, dysphagia, weakness, and ocular motor paralysis with diplopia and ptosis. Involvement of the abducens nerve is most common. In nonfatal cases, the ocular symptoms always disappear within several days (824).

Black tar heroin is injected subcutaneously or snorted. It has caused outbreaks of wound botulism with ophthalmoplegia (825).

A 13-year-old boy newly diagnosed with diabetes developed ophthalmoplegia and cerebral edema while receiving an insulin infusion of 0.1 units/kg/hr. One dose of intravenous mannitol reversed the cerebral edema. The ophthalmoplegia improved immediately and was completely gone in 2 weeks (826).

α-2a-Interferon is used in the treatment of hepatitis C. A woman developed a left abducens nerve paresis 3 days after beginning treatment with this drug. The abducens nerve paresis cleared within 6 weeks after treatment was stopped (827).

Isoniazid (INH) is used primarily to treat tuberculosis. Toxic reactions rarely occur when small doses are used (3 mg/kg/day), but they occur frequently with progressively larger doses. Optic neuropathy is the most dreaded complication. A patient who ingested 7,500 mg became comatose and developed a bilateral abducens nerve paresis (828).

Isotretinoin (Accutane, 13-*cis*-retinoic acid) is a vitamin A analog used for the treatment of cystic acne. Used during pregnancy, it is teratogenic. A child exposed in utero was born with congenital restrictive ophthalmoplegia, which may have been congenital ocular fibrosis syndrome, and gustatory epiphora, a misdirection syndrome involving the seventh cranial nerve. Both these conditions could have arisen because of loss of neurons in brain stem nuclei, around the 5th week of gestation. In addition, the child had stigmata of retinoic acid embryopathy (craniofacial and ear abnormalities, micrognathia, and a tall forehead) (829).

Systemic lead poisoning can cause a wide variety of visual and ocular disturbances and a peripheral neuropathy. Bilateral abducens nerve pareses occurred in 60% of a group of 75 soldiers who developed acute lead poisoning from eating chili powder contaminated with lead chromate (830). This may have resulted from increased ICP; however, cases of paralysis of the oculomotor and trochlear nerves have also been reported (824).

Prenatal exposure to misoprostol has been associated with Möbius syndrome (525,526).

The nitrofurans nitrofurantoin (Furadantin) and furaltadone are antibacterial agents that cause both cranial and generalized polyneuropathies. Toxicity is related to dosage and length of treatment. Impaired renal function hinders their excretion. The polyneuropathy is reversible if the drug is withdrawn, but recovery may be quite slow. Abducens nerve palsy appears together with other cranial nerve palsies and recovers in 2 weeks after the drug is withdrawn (831).

Orthoclone OKT3 is a monoclonal murine immunoglobulin G used to treat acute cellular rejection of allografted organs. It can cause increased ICP with optic disk swelling and bilateral abducens palsy (832).

Phenylbutazone is an anti-inflammatory agent previously widely used in the treatment of a number of conditions, including gout, rheumatoid arthritis, and bursitis. Two patients developed unilateral abducens nerve palsies within 3 weeks of beginning the drug. The palsies resolved in both patients after the drug was stopped (833).

Once used in the treatment of gout, piperazine citrate, a phenothiazine derivative, is employed as a base for medications used for parasitic diseases in humans and animals (e.g., ascariasis). In humans, overdosage produces diarrhea, urticaria, weakness, extrapyramidal tremor, and disturbed coordination and equilibrium. A 4-year-old child developed a unilateral abducens nerve paresis after he was given piperazine syrup for treatment of intestinal parasites. The paralysis recovered within several months but recurred 5 days after the drug was restarted (834).

A 50-year-old man with erectile dysfunction developed a pupil-sparing third nerve palsy 36 hours after the use of sildenafil citrate (Viagra) (835).

Ophthalmoplegia is a very common manifestation of envenomation by Russell's viper, the Sri Lankan krait, the Papuan taipan, and some other Asiatic snakes. If the patient does not die of respiratory paralysis, rhabdomyolysis, coagulopathy, or hemolysis, the ophthalmoplegia resolves in about 2 weeks (836,837).

Thalidomide, a nonbarbiturate hypnotic, is a teratogen, causing phocomelia and sporadic occurrences of facial, palatal, and abducens nerve palsies. Möbius syndrome was reported in a patient whose mother took the drug during her pregnancy (523,838).

Thallium, a heavy metal, is highly toxic, causing peripheral neuropathy, brain swelling, and visual system dysfunction. In a few cases, thallium has injured the ocular motor nerves, either a single nerve or multiple nerves. If ocular motility is affected, there is always a polyneuritis involving the extremities (839).

Trichloroethylene (Trichloroethene) is a nonflammable volatile liquid used as a solvent. Toxic exposure to the fumes causes cranial polyneuropathy. One patient had incomplete bilateral external ophthalmoplegia. Neuropathologic examination revealed pronounced degenerative changes of the brain stem nuclei, fascicles, and peripheral cranial nerves. Another had facial diplegia, trigeminal motor weakness, numbness, loss of taste on the anterior two thirds of the tongue, ptosis, and left abduction weakness (840).

The vinca alkaloids, vincristine and vinblastine, are derived from the periwinkle plant. They bind to tubulin, prevent microtubular formation, and arrest cells in metaphase. Vincristine is used intravenously as cancer chemotherapy. Abducens nerve palsy may occur as a complication of vincristine therapy, usually as part of a generalized axonal polyneuropathy (841–843).

REFERENCES

1. Miller N. Solitary oculomotor nerve palsy in childhood. Am J Ophthalmol 1977;83:106–111.
2. Victor DI. The diagnosis of congenital unilateral third-nerve palsy. Brain 1976;99:711–718.
3. Balkan R, Hoyt CS. Associated neurologic abnormalities in congenital third nerve palsies. Am J Ophthalmol 1984;97:315–319.
4. Keith CG. Oculomotor nerve palsy in childhood. Aust NZ Ophthalmol 1987;15:181–184.
5. Schumacher-Feero LA, Yoo KW, Soleri FM, et al. Third cranial nerve palsy in children. Am J Ophthalmol 1999;128:216–221.
6. Good WV, Barkovich AJ, Nickel BL, et al. Bilateral congenital oculomotor palsy in a child with brain anomalies. Am J Ophthalmol 1991;111:555–558.
7. Hamed LM. Associated neurologic and ophthalmologic findings in congenital oculomotor nerve palsy. Ophthalmology 1991;98:708–714.
8. Ing EB, Sullivan TJ, Clarke MP, et al. Oculomotor nerve palsies in children. J Pediatr Ophthalmol Strabis 1992;29:331–336.
9. Parmeggiani A, Posar A, Leonardi M, et al. Neurological impairment in congenital bilateral ptosis with ophthalmoplegia. Brain Dev 1992;14:107–109.
10. Patel CK, Taylor DS, Russell Eggitt IM, et al. Congenital third nerve palsy associated with mid-trimester amniocentesis. Br J Ophthalmol 1993;77:530–533.
11. Prats JM, Monson MJ, Zuazo E, et al. Congenital nuclear syndrome of the oculomotor nerve. Pediatr Neurol 1993;9:476–478.
12. Flanders M, Watters GB, Draper J, et al. Bilateral congenital third cranial nerve palsy. Can J Ophthalmol 1989;24:28–30.
13. Al-Gazali LI, Sztriha L, Punnose J, et al. Absent pituitary gland and hypoplasia of the cerebellar vermis associated with partial ophthalmoplegia and postaxial polydactyly: A variant of orofaciodigital syndrome VI or a new syndrome? J Med Genet 1999;36:161–166.
14. Papst W, Esslen E. Elektromyographischer beitrag zum Mobius syndrom. Klin Monatsbl Augenheilkd 1960;137.
15. Tsaloumas M, Willshaw H. Congenital oculomotor palsy: Associated neurological and ophthalmological findings. Eye 1997;11:500–503.
16. Sun CC, Kao LY. Unilateral congnital third cranial nerve palsy with central nervous system anomalies: Report of two cases. Chang Gung Med J 2000;23:776–781.
17. Lotufo DG, Smith JL, Hopen GR, et al. The pupil in congenital third nerve misdirection syndrome. J Clin Neuro Ophthalmol 1983;3:193–195.
18. Wilbrand HO, Saenger A, Die kongenitalen augenmuskellahmungen (kernplasie). In Neurologie des Auges. Munich, JF Bergmann Verlag, 1921:179–182.
19. Mellinger JF, Gomez MR, Agenesis of the cranial nerves. In Vinken PJ, Bruyn GW, eds. Handbook of Clinical Neurology. New York, Elsevier, 1977:395–414.
20. Norman MG. Unilateral encephalomalacia in cranial nerve nuclei in neonates: Report of two cases. Neurology 1974;24:424–427.
21. Freedman HL, Kushner BJ. Congenital ocular aberrant innervation: New concepts. J Pediatr Ophthalmol Strabis 1997;34:10–16.
22. Brown HW, Congenital structural muscle anomalies. In Allen JH, ed. Strabismus Ophthalmic Symposium. St Louis, Mosby, 1950:205–236.
23. Engle E. Applications of molecular genetics to the understanding of congenital ocular motility disorders. Ann NY Acad Sci 2002;956:55–63.
24. Engle E. The genetics of strabismus: Duane, Moebius, and fibrosis syndromes. In Traboulsi E, ed. Genetic Diseases of the Eye: A Textbook and Atlas. New York, Oxford University Press, 1998:477–512.
25. Engle E, Goumnerov B, McKeown CA, et al. Oculomotor nerve and muscle abnormalities in congenital fibrosis of the extraocular muscles. Ann Neurol 1997;41:314–325.
26. Gillies WE, Harris AJ, Brooks AM, et al. Congenital fibrosis of the vertically acting extraocular muscles. A new group of dominantly inherited ocular fibrosis with radiologic findings. Ophthalmology 1996;103:1517–1519.
27. Doherty EJ, Macy ME, Wang SM, et al. CFEOM3: A new extraocular congenital fibrosis syndrome that maps to 16q24.2-q24.3. Invest Ophthalmol Vis Sci 1999;40:1687–1694.
28. Guirgis MF, Wong AMF, Tychsen L. Congenital restrictive external ophthalmoplegia and gustatory epiphora associated with fetal isotretinoin toxicity. Arch Ophthalmol 2002;120:1094–1095.
29. Miller MT, Stromland K. Ocular motility in thalidomide embryopathy. J Pediatr Ophthalmol Strabis 1991;28:47–54.
30. Ramsay J, Taylor T. Congenital crocodile tears: A key to the aetiology of Duane's syndrome. Br J Ophthalmol 1980;64:518–522.
31. Burian HM, Cahill JE. Congenital paralysis of medial rectus muscle with unusual synergism of the horizontal muscles. Trans Am Ophthalmol Soc 1952;50:87–102.
32. Cruysberg JR, Mtanda AT, Duinkerke-Eerola KU, et al. Congenital adduction palsy and synergistic divergence: A clinical and electro-oculographic study. Br J Ophthalmol 1989;73:68–75.
33. Shivaram SM, Engle E, Petersen RA, et al. Congenital fibrosis syndromes. Int Ophthalmol Clin 2001;41:105–113.
34. Phillips PH. Strabismus surgery in the treatment of paralytic strabismus. Curr Opin Ophthalmol 2001;12:408–418.
35. Jimura T, Tagami Y, Isayama Y, et al. A case of synergistic divergence associated with Horner's syndrome. Folia Ophthalmol Jpn 1983;34:477–480.
36. Wilcox LMJ, Gittinger JWJ, Breinin GM. Congenital adduction palsy and synergistic divergence. Am J Ophthalmol 1981;91:1–7.
37. Miller NR, Kiel SM, Green WR, et al. Unilateral Duane's retraction syndrome (type 1). Arch Ophthalmol 1982;100:1468–1472.
38. Hotchkiss MG, Miller NR, Clark AWea. Bilateral Duane's retraction syndrome: A clinical pathologic case report. Arch Ophthalmol 1980;98:870–874.
39. Wagner RS, Caputo AR, Frohman LP. Congenital unilateral adduction deficit with simultaneous abduction. A variant of Duane's retraction syndrome. Ophthalmology 1987;94:1049–1053.
40. Brodsky M. Hereditary external ophthalmoplegia synergistic divergence, jaw winking, and oculocutaneous hypopigmentation: A congenital fibrosis syndrome caused by deficient innervation to ocular muscles. Ophthalmology 1998;105:717–725.
41. Scassellati-Sforzolini G. Una sindroma molto rare: Diffeto congenito monolaterale della elevazione con retrazione del globe. Riv Oto Neuro Oftalmol Cir Neurol Sud Am 1958;33:431–439.
42. Pruksacholawit K, Ishikawa S. Atypical vertical retraction syndrome: A case study. J Pediatr Ophthalmol 1976;13:215–220.
43. Kommerell G, Bach M. A new type of Duane's syndrome. Neuroophthalmology 1986;6:159–164.
44. Weinacht S, Huber A, Gottlob I. Vertical Duane's retraction syndrome. Am J Ophthalmol 1996;122:447–449.
45. Khodadoust AA, von Noorden GK. Bilateral vertical retraction syndrome: A family study. Arch Ophthalmol 1967;78:606–612.
46. Rampoldi R. Casuistica clinica. II. Singolarissimo caso squilibrio motorio oculopalpebrale. Ann Ottal 1884;12:463–469.
47. Loewenfeld IE, Thompson HS. Oculomotor paresis with cyclic spasms: A critical review of the literature and a new case. Surv Ophthalmol 1975;20:81–124.
48. Fells P, Collin JRO. Cyclic oculomotor palsy. Trans Ophthalmol Soc UK 1979;99:192–196.
49. Bateman DE, Saunders M. Cyclic oculomotor palsy: Description of a case and hypothesis of the mechanism. J Neurol Neurosurg Psychiatry 1983;46:451–453.
50. Parlato CJ, Nelson LB, Harley RD. Cyclic strabismus. Ann Ophthalmol 1983;15:1126–1129.
51. Frenkel REP, Brodsky MC, Spoor TC. Adult-onset cyclic esotropia and optic atrophy. J Clin Neuro Ophthalmol 1986;6:27–30.

52. Friedman DI, Wright KW, Sadun AA. Oculomotor palsy with cyclic spasms. Neurology 1989;39:1263–1264.

53. Barroso LH, Abreu SG, Finkel E, et al. Cyclic oculomotor paresis in Rio. J Clin Neuroophthalmol 1991;11:136.

54. Bielschowsky A. Über die okulomotoriouslähmung mit cyclischem wechsel von krampf und erschlaffungszuständen am gelähmten auge. Albrecht Von Graefes Archiv fur Klinische und Experimentelle Ophthalmologie 1929;121:659–685.

55. Petrovic A, Tschemolossow A. Zur frage der rhythmischen angiospasmem im gebiete der augenkerne. Klin Monatsbl Augenheilkd 1931;86:491–496.

56. Burde RM. Cyclic oculomotor paralysis: Discussion of a case presentation by J.O. Susac. In Smith JL, ed. Neuro-Ophthalmology. St Louis: CV Mosby, 1973: 139.

57. Salus R. Okulomotoriuslahmung mit abnormer zyklischer innervation der inneren este. Klin Monatsbl Augenheilkd 1912;50:66–80.

58. Troost BT, Noreika J. Acquired cyclic esotropia in an adult. Am J Ophthalmol 1981;91:8–13.

59. Kommerell G, Mehdorn E, Ketelsen UP, et al. Oculomotor palsy with cyclic spasms. Electromyographic and electron microscopic evidence of chronic peripheral neuronal involvement. Neuroophthalmology 1988;8:9–21.

60. Abdulla N, Eustace P. A case of ocular neuromyotonia with tonic pupil. J Neuroophthalmol 1999;19:125–127.

61. Stevens H. Cyclic oculomotor paralysis. Neurology 1965;15:556–559.

62. Yazici B, Unal M, Koksal M, et al. Oculomotor palsy with cyclic spasms: A case report. Orbit 2000;19:129–133.

63. Biousse V, Newman NJ. Third nerve palsies. Semin Neurol 2000;20:55–74.

64. Roper Hall G, Burde RM. Inferior rectus palsies as a manifestation of atypical third cranial nerve disease. Am J Orthop 1975;25:122–130.

65. Reagan TJ, Trautman JC. Combined nuclear and supranuclear defects in ocular motility: A clinicopathologic study. Arch Neurol 1978;35:133–137.

66. Meienberg O, Mumenthaler M, Karbowski K. Quadriparesis and nuclear oculomotor palsy with total bilateral ptosis mimicking coma: A mesencephalic "locked in syndrome"? Arch Neurol 1979;36:708–710.

67. Pierrot Deseilligny C, Schaison M, Bousser MG, et al. Syndrome nucléaire du nerf moteur oculaire commun: À propos de deux observations cliniques. Rev Neurol 1981;137:217–222.

68. Bogousslavsky J, Regli F. Nuclear and prenuclear syndromes of the oculomotor nerve. Neuroophthalmology 1983;3:211–216.

69. Biller J, Shapiro R, Evans LS, et al. Oculomotor nuclear complex infarction: Clinical and radiological correlation. Arch Neurol 1984;41:985–987.

70. Keane JR, Zaias B, Itabashi HH. Levator sparing oculomotor nerve palsy caused by a solitary midbrain metastasis. Arch Neurol 1984;41:210–212.

71. Kobayashi S, Mukuno K, Ishikawa S, et al. Oculomotor nerve nuclear complex syndrome: A case with clinicopathologic correlation. Presented at the Fifth Meeting of the International Neuro-Ophthalmology Society, 1984, Antwerp, Belgium.

72. Zackon DH, Sharpe JA. Midbrain paresis of horizontal gaze. Ann Neurol 1984; 16:495–504.

73. Traboulsi EI, Azar DT, Achram M, et al. Brain stem tuberculoma and isolated third nerve palsy. Neuroophthalmology 1985;5:43–45.

74. Kobayashi S, Mukuno K, Tazak Y, et al. Oculomotor nerve nuclear complex syndrome. A case with clinicopathologic correlation. Neuroophthalmology 1986;6:55–59.

75. Antworth MV, Beck RW. Third nerve palsy as a presenting sign of acquired immune deficiency syndrome. J Clin Neuroophthalmol 1987;7:125–128.

76. Kömpf D, Erbguth F, Kreiten K, et al. Bilateral third nerve palsy in basilar vertebral artery disease. Neuroophthalmology 1987;7:355–362.

77. Pusateri TJ, Sedvick LA, Margo CE. Isolated inferior rectus muscle palsy from a solitary metastasis to the oculomotor nucleus. Arch Ophthalmol 1987;105: 675–677.

78. Tognetti F, Godano U, Glassi E. Bilateral traumatic third nerve palsy. Surg Neurol 1988;29:120–124.

79. Meienberg O, Müri R. Nuclear and infranuclear disorders. Baillieres Clin Neurol 1992;1:417–434.

80. Hattori S, Utsunomiya K. Isolated oculomotor nerve palsy caused by mesencephalic hemorrhage. Rinsho Shinkeigaku 1994;34:1021–1025.

81. Roig C, Gironell A, Marti Vilalta JL, et al. Nuclear oculomotor nerve syndrome due to mesencephalic infraction or hemorrhage. Five cases and a review of literature. Neurologia 1994;9:224–232.

82. Guerrero AL, Onzain JI, Martin JA, et al. Isolated lesion of the Edinger Westphal nucleus in topographical relation with a posttraumatic mesencephalic hematoma. Rev Neurol 1996;24:982–984.

3. Tokuno T, Nakazawa K, Yoshida S, et al. Primary oculomotor nerve palsy due to head injury: Analysis of 10 cases. No Shinkei Geka [Neurol Surg] 1995;23: 497–501.

84. Getenet JC, Vighetto A, Nighoghossian N, et al. Isolated bilateral third nerve palsy caused by a mesencephalic hematoma. Neurology 1994;44:981.

85. Warwick R. Representation of extra-ocular muscles in oculomotor nucleus of the monkey. J Comp Neurol 1953;98:449–495.

86. Donzelli R, Marinkovic S, Brigante L, et al. The oculomotor nerve complex in humans. Microanatomy and clinical significance. Surg Radiol Anat 1998;20: 7–12.

87. Stevenson GC, Hoyt WF. Metastasis to midbrain from mammary carcinoma: Cause of bilateral ptosis and ophthalmoplegia. JAMA 1963;186:514–516.

88. Growdon JH, Winkler GF, Wray SH. Midbrain ptosis: A case with clinicopathologic correlation. Arch Neurol 1974;30:179–181.

89. Conway VH, Rozdilsky B, Schneider RJ, et al. Isolated bilateral complete ptosis. Can J Ophthalmol 1983;18:37–40.

90. Martin TJ, Corbett JJ, Babikian PV. Bilateral ptosis due to mesencephalic lesions with relative preservation of ocular motility. J Neuroophthalmol 1996;16: 258–263.

91. Elliott RL. Encephalitis with ophthalmoplegia. Confinia Neurologica 1969;31: 184–197.

92. Bryan JS, Mamed LM. Levator-sparing nuclear oculomotor palsy: Clinical and magnetic resonance imaging findings. J Clin Neuroophthalmol 1992;12:26–30.

93. Daroff RB. Ocular motor manifestations of brain stem and cerebellar dysfunction. In Neuro-Ophthalmology: Symposium of the University of Miami and the Bascom Palmer Eye Institute. Miami: Huffman Publishing Co, 1970.

94. Kaji R, Akiguchi I, Kameyama M, et al. Oculomotor nerve nucleus syndrome: Crossed innervation of the superior rectus muscle. Rinsho Shinkeigaku 1983; 23:242–246.

95. Bogousslavsky J, Regli F. Atteinte intra-axiale du nerf moteur oculaire commun dans les infarctus mesencephaliques. Rev Neurol 1984;140:263–270.

96. Saeki N, Yamaura A. Ocular signs due to an oculomotor intranuclear lesion: Palsy of adduction and contralateral eye elevation. J Clin Neurosci 2000;7: 153–154.

97. Fleet WS, Rapcsak SZ, Huntley WW, et al. Pupil sparing oculomotor palsy from midbrain hemorrhage. Ann Ophthalmol 1988;20:345–346.

98. Mehler MF. The neuroophthalmic spectrum of the rostral basilar artery syndrome. Arch Neurol 1988;45:966–971.

99. Kubic CS, Adams RD. Occlusion of the basilar artery: A clinical and pathological study. Brain 1946;69:73–121.

100. Anderson WW, R.M. J. Basilar artery disease: Clinical manifestations. Calif Med 1960;92:400–402.

101. Masucci EF. Bilateral ophthalmoplegia in basilar vertebral artery disease. Brain 1965;89:97–196.

102. Shutt HKR, David NJ, Smith JL. Complete bilateral III and IV nerve palsies due to basilar artery disease. In Smith JL, ed. Neuro-Ophthalmology. St Louis, Mosby, 1970:356–362.

103. Caplan LR. "Top of the basilar" syndrome. Neurology 1980;30:72–79.

104. Bogousslavsky J, Maeder P, Regli F, et al. Pure midbrain infarction: Clinical syndromes, MRI, and etiologic patterns. Neurology 1994;44:2032–2040.

105. Thömke F, Gutmann L, Stoeter P, et al. Cerebrovascular brain stem diseases with isolated cranial nerve palsies. Cerebrovascular Dis 2002;13:147–155.

106. Martin PJ, Chang HM, Wityk R, et al. Midbrain infarction: Associations and aetiologies in the New England Medical Center Posterior Circulation Registry. J Neurol Neurosurg Psychiatry 1998;64:392–395.

107. Caplan LR, Zervas NT. Survival with permanent midbrain dysfunction after surgical treatment of traumatic subdural hematoma: The clinical picture of a Duret hemorrhage? Ann Neurol 1977;1:587–589.

108. Pratt DV, Orengo-Nania S, Horowitz BL, et al. Magnetic resonance findings in a patient with nuclear oculomotor palsy. Arch Ophthalmol 1995;113:141–142.

109. Pou Serradell A, Pascual Calvet J, Roquer Gonzalez J. Atteinte bilatérale intra axiale du nerf moteur oculaire commun (III): Deux cas. Rev Neurol 1996;152: 744–747.

110. Dierssen G, Trigueros F, Sanz F, et al. Surgical treatment of a mesencephalic tuberculoma. J Neurosurg 1978;49:753–755.

111. Aydin MD, Aydin N. A neuro-Behçet's lesion in oculomotor nerve nucleus. Acta Neurol Scand 2003;108:139–141.

112. Park DM. Cranial nerve palsies in tetanus: Cephalic tetanus. J Neurol Neurosurg Psychiatry 1970;33:212–215.

113. Durward QJ, Barnett HJM, Barr HWK. Presentation and management of mesencephalic hematoma: Report of two cases. J Neurosurg 1982;56:123–127.

114. Jardim LB, Pereira ML, Silveira I, et al. Neurologic findings in Machado-Joseph disease: Relation with disease duration, subtypes, and (CAG)n. Arch Neurol 2001;58:899–904.

115. Gruber H, Zeitlhofer J, Prager J, et al. Complex oculomotor dysfunctions in Kugelberg Welander disease. Neuroophthalmology 1983;3:125–128.

116. Korinthenberg R, Sauer M, Ketelsen U-P, et al. Congenital axonal neuropathy caused by deletions in the spinal muscular atrophy region. Ann Neurol 1997; 42:364–368.

117. Aberfeld DC, Namba T. Progressive ophthalmoplegia in Kugelberg-Welander disease. Arch Neurol 1969;20:253–256.

118. Murray RG, Walsh FB. Ocular abnormalities in poliomyelitis and their pathogenesis. Can Med Assoc J 1954;70:141–147.

119. Kaminski HJ, Richmonds CR, Kusner LL, et al. Differential susceptibility of the ocular motor system to disease. Ann NY Acad Sci 2002;956:42–54.

120. Laslo P, Lipski J, Funk GD. Differential expression of group I metabotropic glutamate receptors in motoneurons at low and high risk for degeneration in ALS. Neuroreport 2001;12:1903–1908.

121. Van Bogaert L. Contribution à la connaissance des troubles oculaires et vestibulaires dans la S.L.A. Rev Otoneuroophtalmol 1925;3:263–274.

122. Lawyer TJ, Netsky MG. Amyotrophic lateral sclerosis (a clinicoanatomic study of fifty-three cases). Arch Neurol Psychiatr 1953;69:171–192.

123. Gizzi M, DiRocco A, Sivak M, et al. Ocular motor function in motor neuron disease. Neurology 1992;43:1037–1046.

124. Norris FH. ALS and eye movements. Neurology 1993;43:451.

125. Okamoto K, Hirai S, Amari M, et al. Oculomotor nuclear pathology in amyotrophic lateral sclerosis. Acta Neuropathologica 1993;85:458–462.

126. Okuda B. ALS and eye movements. Neurology 1993;43.

127. Harvey DG, Torack RM, Rosenbaum HE. Amyotrophic lateral sclerosis with ophthalmoplegia: A clinicopathologic study. Arch Neurol 1979;36:615–617.

128. Hayashi H, Kato T, Kawada A, et al. Amyotrophic lateral sclerosis: Oculomotor function in patients on respirators. Neurology 1987;37:1431.

129. Ohki M, Kanayama R, Nakamura T, et al. Ocular abnormalities in amyotrophic lateral sclerosis. Acta Otolaryngol Suppl 1994;511.

130. Shaunak S, Orrell RW, O'Sullivan E, et al. Oculomotor function in amyotrophic lateral sclerosis. Ann Neurol 1995;38:38–44.

131. Kori A, Averbuch Heller L, Büttner Ennever J, et al. Slow vertical saccades in motor neuron disease. Presented at the 29th Annual Frank Walsh Meeting of the North American Neuro-Ophthalmology Society, Baltimore, April 5–6, 1997.

132. Fisher CM. An unusual variant of acute idiopathic polyneuritis (syndrome of ophthalmoplegia, ataxia and areflexia). N Engl J Med 1956;255:57–65.

133. Jampel RS, Haidt SJ. Bell's phenomenon and acute idiopathic polyneuritis. Am J Ophthalmol 1972;74:145–153.

134. Bogousslavsky J, Regli F, Ghika J, et al. Internuclear ophthalmoplegia, prenuclear paresis of contralateral superior rectus, and bilateral ptosis. J Neurol 1984;230:197–203.

135. Mori M, Kuwabara S, Fukutake T. Clinical features and prognosis of Miller Fisher syndrome. Neurology 2001;56:1104–1106.

136. Carvalho M, Cordeiro E, Alves M, et al. The Miller Fisher syndrome. Review of the cases of the Santa Maria Hospita. Acta Med Port 1996;9:167–170.

137. Nagaoka U, Kato T, Kurita K, et al. Cranial nerve enhancement on three-dimensional MRI in Miller Fisher syndrome. Neurology 1996;47.

138. Yee RD, Zasorin N, Baloh RW, et al. Transient ophthalmoplegia and ataxia. In Frank B. Walsh Society, Cleveland, OH, 1984.

139. Garcia-Rivera CA, Rozen TD, Zhou D, et al. Miller Fisher syndrome: MRI findings. Neurology 2001;57:1755.

140. Bickerstaff ER. Mesencephalitis and rhombencephalitis. Br Med J 1951;2:77–81.

141. Odaka M, Yuki N, Yamada M, et al. Bickerstaff's encephalitis: Clinical features of 62 cases and a subgrooup associated with Guillain-Barré syndrome. Brain 2003;126:2279–2290.

142. Blake PY, Mark AS, Kattah Jea. MR of oculomotor nerve palsy. Am J Neuroradiol 1995;16:1665–1672.

143. Thömke F, Tettenborn B, Hopf HC. Third nerve palsy as the sole manifestation of midbrain ischemia. Neuroophthalmology 1995;15:327–335.

144. Breen LA, Hopf HC, Farris BK, et al. Pupil-sparing oculomotor nerve palsy due to midbrain infarction. Arch Neurol 1991;48:105–106.

145. Keane JR. Isolated brain stem third nerve palsy. Arch Neurol Psychiatr 1988;45:813–814.

146. Nothnagel H. Topische Diagnostik der Gehirnkrankheiten. Berlin, A. Hirschwald, 1879.

147. Liu GT, Crenner CW, Logigian EL, et al. Midbrain syndromes of Benedikt, Claude, and Nothnagel: Setting the record straight. Neurology 1992;42:1820–1822.

148. Benedikt M. Tremblement avec paralysie croisee du moteur oculaire commun. Bull Med 1889;3:547–548.

149. Loseke N, Retif J, Noterman J, et al. Inferior red nucleus syndrome (Benedikt's syndrome) due to a single intramesencephalic metastasis from a prostatic carcinoma: Case report. Acta Neurochirurgica 1981;56:59–64.

150. Weber HD. A contribution to the pathology of the crura cerebri. Med Chirurg Trans 1865;28:121–189.

151. Kumral E, Bayulkem G, Akyol A, et al. Mesencephalic and associated posterior circulation infarcts. Stroke 2002;33:2224–2231.

152. Seo SW, Heo JH, Lee KY, et al. Localization of Claude's syndrome. Neurology 2001;57:2304–2307.

153. Claude H. Syndrome pédonculaire de la région du noyau rouge. Rev Neurol 1912;1.

154. Duncan GW. Posterior cerebral artery stenosis with midbrain infarction. Stroke 1995;26:900–902.

155. Saeki N, Murai N, Sunami K. Midbrain tegmental lesions affecting or sparing the pupillary fibers. J Neurol Neurosurg Psychiatry 1996;61:401–406.

156. Boccardo M, Ruelle A, Banchero MA. Isolated oculomotor palsy caused by aneurysm of the basilar artery bifurcation. J Neurol Neurosurg Psychiatry 1986;233:61–62.

157. Miller N. Walsh and Hoyt's Clinical Neuro-Ophthalmology. Baltimore, Williams & Wilkins, 1985:652–784.

158. Koennecke H-C, Seyfert S. Mydriatic pupil as the presenting sign of common carotid artery dissection. Stroke 1998;29:2653–2655.

159. Thömke F, Gutmann L, Hopf HC. Comment on: Most diabetic third nerve palsies are peripheral. Neurology 1999;53:894–895.

160. Ksiazek SM, Slamovits TL, Rosen CE, et al. Fascicular arrangement in partial oculomotor paresis. Am J Ophthalmol 1994;118:97–103.

161. Schwartz TH, Lycette CA, Yoon SS, et al. Clinicoradiographic evidence for oculomotor fascicular anatomy. J Neurol Neurosurg Psychiatry 1995;59:338.

162. Guy JR, Savino PJ, Schatz NJ. Superior division paresis of the oculomotor nerve. Ophthalmology 1985;92:777–784.

163. Ksiazek SM, Repka MX, Maguire A, et al. Divisional oculomotor nerve paresis caused by intrinsic brain stem disease. Ann Neurol 1989;26:714–718.

164. Eggenberger ER, Miller NR, Hoffman PN, et al. Mesencephalic ependymal cyst causing an inferior divisional paresis of the oculomotor nerve: Case report. Neurology 1993;43:2419–2420.

165. Castro O, Johnson LN, Mamourian AC. Isolated inferior oblique paresis from brain stem infarction: Perspective on oculomotor fascicular organization in the ventral midbrain tegmentum. Arch Neurol 1990;47:235–237.

166. Gauntt CD, Kashii S, Nagata I. Monocular elevation paresis caused by an oculomotor fascicular impairment. J Neuroophthalmol 1995;15:11–14.

167. Sato K, Yoshikawa H, Takamori M. A case of partial fascicular oculomotor paresis. Rinsho Shinkeigaku [Clin Neurol] 1997;37:854–856.

168. Tatu L, Moulin T, Bogousslavsky J, et al. Arterial territories of human brain. In Bogousslavsky J, Caplan LR, eds. Stroke Syndromes. Cambridge, Cambridge University Press, 2001:371–404.

169. Fujioka T, Segawa F, Ogawa K. Ischemic and hemorrhagic brain stem lesions mimicking diabetic ophthalmoplegia. Clin Neurol Neurosurg 1995;97:167–171.

170. Hopf HC, Gutmann L. Diabetic 3rd nerve palsy: Evidence for a mesencephalic lesion. Neurology 1990;40.

171. Keane JR. Oculomotor palsy with pupillary sparing in subdural hematoma: Two cases with documented tentorial herniation. Mt Sinai J Med 1974;41:161–164.

172. Tokuno T, Kawakami Y, Yamamoto T. Isolated infranuclear oculomotor nerve palsy caused by traumatic midbrain hemorrhage: Case report. No Shinkei Geka [Neurol Surg] 1996;24:849–852.

173. Wilson WB, Sharpe JA, Deck JHN. Cerebral blindness and oculomotor nerve palsies in toxoplasmosis. Am J Ophthalmol 1980;89:714–718.

174. Kowalska B, Stankiewicz C, Lipowski P, et al. Ocular and orbital symptoms of Wegener's disease. Otolaryngol Polska 1997;51:169–175.

175. Shintani S, Tsuruoka S, Yamada M. Churg-Strauss syndrome associated with third nerve palsy and mononeuritis multiplex of the legs. Clin Neurol Neurosurg 1995;97:172–174.

176. Newman NJ, Lessell S. Isolated pupil-sparing third nerve palsy as the presenting sign of multiple sclerosis. Arch Neurol 1990;47:817–818.

177. Bentley PI, Kimber T, Schapira AHV. Painful third nerve palsy in MS. Neurology 2002;58:1532.

178. Thömke F, Lensch E, Ringel K, et al. Isolated cranial nerve palsies in multiple sclerosis. J Neurol Neurosurg Psychiatry 1997;63:682–685.

179. Galer BS, Lipton RB, Weinstein S, et al. Apoplectic headache and oculomotor nerve palsy: An unusual presentation of multiple sclerosis. Neurology 1990;40:1465–1466.

180. Clavelou P, Colamarino R, Plane C, et al. Paralysie due IIIe nerf cranien et céphalée brutale: Une étiologie inhabituelle. Bull Soc Ophtalmol Fr 1994;94:117–118.

181. Bhatti MT, Schmalfuss IM, Williams LS, et al. Peripheral third cranial nerve enhancement in multiple sclerosis. AJNR Am J Neuroradiol 2003;24:1390–1395.

182. Katayama M, Kawase T, Sato S, et al. Abnormal course of the oculomotor nerve on the clivus combined with a petroclival meningioma: Case report. Skull Base 2002;12:141–144.

183. Capo H, Warren F, Kupersmith MJ. Evolution of oculomotor nerve palsies. J Clin Neurol Ophthalmol 1992;12:21–25.

184. Sunderland S, Hughes ESR. The pupillo-constrictor pathway and the nerves to the ocular muscles in man. Brain 1946;69:301–309.

185. Kerr FWL, Hollowell OW. Location of pupillomotor and accommodation fibers in the oculomotor nerve: Experimental observations on paralytic mydriasis. J Neurol Neurosurg Psychiatry 1964;27:473–481.

186. Walsh FB, Hoyt WF, eds. Clinical Neuro-Ophthalmology. Baltimore, Williams & Wilkins, 1969:252.

187. Crompton JL, Moore CE. Painful third nerve palsy: How not to miss an intracranial aneurysm. Aust J Ophthalmol 1981;9:113–115.

188. Gale AN, Crockard HA. Transient unilateral mydriasis with basilar aneurysm. J Neurol Neurosurg Psychiatry 1982;45:565–566.

189. Biousse V, Newman NJ. Aneurysms and subarachnoid hemorrhage. Neurosurg Clin North Am 1999;10:631–651.

190. Pia HW, Fontana H. Aneurysms of the posterior cerebral artery. Acta Neurochirurgica 1977;39:13–35.

191. Linn FH, Rinkel GJE, Algra A, et al. Headache characteristics in subarachnoid haemorrhage and benign thunderclap headache. J Neurol Neurosurg Psychiatry 1998;65:791–793.

192. Linn FHH, Wijdicks EFM, van der Graaf Y, et al. Prospective study of sentinel headache in aneurysmal subarachnoid haemorrhage. Lancet 1994;344.

193. Liu GT. Coma. Neurosurg Clin North Am 1999;10:579–586.

194. Liu GT, Volpe NJ, Galetta SL. Neuro-Ophthalmology: Diagnosis and Management. Philadelphia, WB Saunders, 2001:531.

195. Ropper AH, Cole D, Louis DN. Clinicopathological correlation in a case of pupillary dilation from cerebral hemorrhage. Arch Neurol 1991;48:1166–1169.
196. Safran AB, Berney J. Les modifications pupillaires des hématomes sous duraux aigus. Arch Suisses Neurol Neurochir Psychiatr 1977;120:27–42.
197. Jefferson G. On the saccular aneurysms of the internal carotid artery in the cavernous sinus. Br J Surg 1938;26:267–302.
198. Hutchinson J. Four lectures on the compression of the brain. Clin Lect Rep London Hosp 1867;4:10–55.
199. Keefe WP, Rucker CW, Kernohan JW. Pathogenesis of paralysis of the third cranial nerve. Arch Ophthalmol 1960;63:585–592.
200. Weiner LP, Porro RS. Total third nerve paralysis: A case with hemorrhage in the oculomotor nerve in subdural hematoma. Neurology 1965;15:87–90.
201. Sunderland S. The tentorial notch and complications produced by herniations of the brain through that aperture. Br J Surg 1958;45:422–438.
202. Ritter AM, Muizelaar JP, Barnes TM, et al. Brain stem blood flow, pupillary response, and outcome in patients with severe head injuries. Neurosurgery 1999; 44:941–948.
203. Chen R, Sahjpaul R, Del Maestro RF. Initial enlargement of the opposite pupil as a false localizing sign in intraparenchymal frontal haemorrhage. J Neurol Neurosurg Psychiatry 1994;57:1126–1128.
204. Pevehouse BC, Bloom WH, McKissock W. Ophthalmic aspects of diagnosis and localization of subdural hematoma: An analysis of 389 cases and review of the literature. Neurology 1960;10:1037–1041.
205. Roberts M, Owens G, O'Rourke J. Third nerve paresis with contralateral subdural hematoma following cerebrospinal fluid loss. EENT Monthly 1971;50: 59–62.
206. Berger B, Frenkel M. Complete third nerve paralysis and decreasing vision secondary to subdural hematoma. Ann Ophthalmol 1979;11:1817–1819.
207. Fisher CM. Oval pupils. Arch Neurol Psychiatr 1980;37:502–503.
208. Kavieff RD, Miller JA, Klepach GL. Pupillary sparing oculomotor palsy from acute subdural hematoma. Ann Ophthalmol 1984;16:387–390.
209. Ropper AH. The opposite pupil in herniation. Neurology 1990;40:1707–1709.
210. Mariak Z, Mariak Z, Lewko J, et al. Pathogenesis of primary internal ophthalmoplegia after head injury. Eur J Ophthalmol 1995;5:56–58.
211. Wilhelm H, Klier R, Tóth B. Oculomotor paresis starting as isolated internal ophthalmoplegia. Neuroophthalmology 1995;15:211–215.
212. Cohn EM. Isolated third nerve palsy caused by an arachnoid cyst. Presented at the Fifth meeting of the International Neuro-Ophthalmology Society, Antwerp, Belgium, 1984.
213. Fisher CM. Some neuroophthalmological observations. J Neurol Neurosurg Psychiatry 1967;30:383–392.
214. Swaminathan TR, Kalyanaraman S, Narendran P. Ocular manifestations of central nervous system tuberculosis correlated with CT scan findings. In Henkind P, ed. ACTA: XXIV International Congress of Ophthalmology. Philadelphia: JB Lippincott, 1982:841–845.
215. Lesser RL, Simon RM, Leon H, et al. Cryptococcal meningitis and internal ophthalmoplegia. Am J Ophthalmol 1979;87:682–687.
216. Pelak VS, Galetta SL, Grossman RI, et al. Evidence for preganglionic pupillary involvement in superficial siderosis. Neurology 1999;53:1130–1132.
217. Radziwill AJ, Steck AJ, Borruat FX, et al. Isolated internal ophthalmoplegia associated with IgG anti-GQ1b antibody. Neurology 1998.
218. Waga S, Morikawa A, Sakakura M. Craniopharyngioma with midbrain involvement. Arch Neurol 1979;36:319–320.
219. Rucker CW. The causes of paralysis of the third, fourth, and sixth cranial nerves. Am J Ophthalmol 1966;61:1293–1298.
220. Richards BW, Jones FR, Younge BR. Causes and prognosis in 4,278 cases of paralysis of the oculomotor, trochlear, and abducens cranial nerves. Am J Ophthalmol 1992;113:489–496.
221. Berlit P. Isolated and combined pareses of cranial nerves III, IV and VI: A retrospective study of 412 patients. J Neurol Sci 1991;103:10–15.
222. Huige WM, Van Vliet AG, Bastiaensen LA. Early symptoms of subarachnoid haemorrhage due to aneurysms of the posterior communicating artery. Doc Ophthalmol 1988;70:251–256.
223. Soni SR. Aneurysms of the posterior communicating artery and oculomotor paresis. J Neurol Neurosurg Psychiatry 1974;37:475–484.
224. Trobe JD, Glaser JS, Quencer RC. Isolated oculomotor paralysis: The product of saccular and fusiform aneurysms of the basilar artery. Arch Ophthalmol 1978; 96:1236–1240.
225. McKinna AJ. Eye signs in 611 cases of posterior fossa aneurysms: Their diagnostic and prognostic value. Can J Ophthalmol 1983;18:3–6.
226. DiMario FJJ, Rorke LB. Transient oculomotor nerve paresis in congenital distal basilar artery aneurysm. Pediatr Neurol 1992;8:303–306.
227. Coyne TJ, Wallace MC. Bilateral third cranial nerve palsies in association with a ruptured anterior communicating artery aneurysm. Surg Neurol 1994;42:52–56.
228. Kanaka K, Matsumaru Y, Mashiko R, et al. Small unruptured cerebral aneurysms presenting with oculomotor nerve palsy. Neurosurgery 2003;52:553–557.
229. Locksley HB. Natural history of subarachnoid hemorrhage, intracranial aneurysm and arteriovenous malformations. J Neurosurg 1966;25:219–239.
230. Okawara S. Warning signs prior to rupture of an intracranial aneurysm. J Neurosurg 1973;38:575–580.
231. Kupersmith MJ. Neurovascular Neuro-Ophthalmology. Berlin, Springer-Verlag, 1993.
232. Sanders S, Kawasaki A, Purvin VA. Patterns of extraocular muscle weakness in vasculopathic pupil-sparing incomplete third nerve palsy. J Neuroophthalmol 2001;21:256–259.
233. Hamer J. Prognosis of oculomotor palsy in patients with aneurysms of the posterior communicating artery. Acta Neurochirurgica 1982;66:173–175.
234. Tummala R, Harrison A, Madison MT, et al. Pseudomyasthenia resulting from a posterior carotid artery wall aneurysm: A novel presentation: Case report. Neurosurgery 2001;49:1466–1469.
235. Foroozan R, Slamovits TL, Thomas L, et al. Spontaneous resolution of aneurysmal third nerve palsy. J Neuroophthalmol 2002;22:211–214.
236. Kissel JT, Burde RM, Klingele TG, et al. Pupil-sparing oculomotor palsies with internal carotid posterior communicating artery aneurysms. Ann Neurol 1983; 13:149–154.
237. Wakai S, Eguchi T, Asano T, et al. Oculomotor palsy caused by aneurysm clip: Report of two cases. Neurosurgery 1981;9:429–432.
238. Goto K, Imai H, Nakazato O, et al. Inferior branch palsy of the oculomotor nerve following clipping of basilar apex aneurysm. Clin Neurol 1993;33.
239. Yoss RE, Rucker CW, Miller RH. Neurosurgical complications affecting the oculomotor, trochlear, and abducent nerves. Neurology 1968;18:594–600.
240. Grayson MC, Soni SR, Spooner VA. Analysis of the recovery of third nerve function after direct surgical intervention for posterior communicating aneurysms. Br J Ophthalmol 1974;58:118–125.
241. Inamasu J, Nakamura Y, Saito R, et al. Early resolution of third nerve palsy following endovascular treatment of a posterior communicating artery aneurysm. J Neuroophthalmol 2002;22:12–14.
241a. Stiebel-Kalish H, Maimon S, Amsalem J, et al. Evolution of oculomotor nerve paresis after endovascular coiling of posterior communicating artery aneurysms: A neuro-ophthalmological perspective. Neurosurgery 2003;53:1268–1274.
242. Eyster EF, Hoyt WF, Wilson CB. Oculomotor palsy from minor head trauma: An initial sign of basal intracranial aneurysm. JAMA 1972;220:1083–1086.
243. Walter KA, Newman NJ, Lessell S. Oculomotor palsy from minor head trauma: Initial sign of intracranial aneurysm. Neurology 1994;44:148–150.
244. Hashimoto M, Ohtsuka K, Akiba H, et al. Vascular compression of the oculomotor nerve disclosed by thin-slice magnetic resonance imaging. Am J Ophthalmol 1998;125:881–882.
245. Hopkins EW, Poser CM. Posterior cerebral artery ectasia: An unusual cause of ophthalmoplegia. Arch Neurol 1973;29:279–281.
246. Scotti G. Internal carotid origin of a tortuous posterior cerebral artery: A cause of ophthalmoplegia. Arch Neurol 1974;31:273–275.
247. Miller NR. Isolated oculomotor nerve palsy in childhood from leptomeningeal polymorphic cell sarcoma. J Pediatr Ophthalmol 1976;13:211–214.
248. Haase R, Wiegand P, Hirsch W, et al. Unusual presentation of central nervous system relapse with oculomotor nerve palsy in a case of CD56-positive acute myeloid leukemia following allogenic stem cell transplantation. Pediatr Transplant 2002;6:260–265.
249. Hardenack M, Völker A, Schröder JM, et al. Primary eosinophilic granuloma of the oculomotor nerve: Case report. J Neurosurg 1994;81:784–787.
250. Reifenberger G, Bostrom J, Bettag M, et al. Primary glioblastoma multiforme of the oculomotor nerve. Case report. J Neurosurg 1997;86:739–741.
251. Ueyama H, Kumamoto T, Fukuda S, et al. Isolated third nerve palsy due to sarcoidosis. Sarcoidosis Vasc Diffuse Lung Dis 1997;14:169–170.
252. Leunda G, Vaquero J, Cabezudo J, et al. Schwannoma of the oculomotor nerves: Report of four cases. J Neurosurg 1982;57:563–565.
253. Celli P, Ferrante L, Acqui M, et al. Neurinoma of the third, fourth, and sixth cranial nerves: A survey and report of a new fourth nerve case. Surg Neurol 1992;38.
254. Niazi W, Boggan JE. Schwannoma of extraocular nerves: Survey of literature and case report of an isolated third nerve schwannoma. Skull Base Surg 1994; 4:219–226.
255. Shen WC, Yang DY, Ho WL, et al. Neurilemmoma of the oculomotor nerve presenting as an orbital mass: MR findings. Am J Neuroradiol 1993;14:1253.
256. Asaoka K, Sawamura Y, Murai H, et al. Schwannoma of the oculomotor nerve: A case report with consideration of the surgical treatment. Neurosurgery 1999; 45:630–634.
257. Matias-Guiu X, Alejo M, Sole T, et al. Cavernous angiomas of cranial nerves: Report of two cases. J Neurosurg 1990;73:620–622.
258. Freeman WR, Lerner CW, Mines JA, et al. A prospective study of the ophthalmologic findings in the acquired immune deficiency syndrome. Am J Ophthalmol 1984;97:133–142.
259. Beck RW, Janssen RS, Smiley L, et al. Melioidosis and bilateral third-nerve palsies. Neurology 1984;34:105–107.
260. Kay MC, McCrary JA. Multiple cranial nerve palsies in late metastasis of midline malignant reticulosis. Am J Ophthalmol 1979;88:1087–1090.
261. Keane JR. Intermittent third nerve palsy with cryptococcal meningitis. J Clin Neurol Ophthalmol 1993;13:124–126.
262. Newman NJ, Slamovits TL, Friedland S, et al. Neuro-ophthalmic manifestations of meningocerebral inflammation from the limited form of Wegener's granulomatosis. Am J Ophthalmol 1995;120:613–621.
263. Hirayama K, Fukutake T, Kawamura M. "Thumb localizing test" for detecting

a lesion in the posterior column-medial lemniscal system. J Neurol Sci 1999; 167:45–47.

264. Salazar A, Martinez H, Soltelo J, et al. Ophthalmoplegic polyneuropathy associated with infectious mononucleosis. Ann Neurol 1983;13:219–220.

265. Yuki N, Taki T, Takahashi T, et al. Molecular mimicry between GQ1b gangliosides and lipopolysaccharides of *Campylobacter jejuni* isolated from patients with Fisher's syndrome. Ann Neurol 1994;36.

266. Mori M, Kuwabara S, Fukutake T, et al. Plasmapheresis and Miller Fisher syndrome: Analysis of 50 consecutive cases. J Neurol Neurosurg Psychiatry 2002; 72:680.

267. Go T. Partial oculomotor nerve palsy associated with elevated anti-galactocerebroside and anti-GM1 antibodies. J Pediatr Ophthalmol Strabismus 2000;137: 425–426.

268. Ichikawa H, Kamiya Y, Susuki K, et al. Unilateral oculomotor nerve palsy associated with anti-GQ1b antibody. Neurology 2002;59:957–958.

269. Koga M. Anti-GT1a IgG in Guillain-Barré syndrome. J Neurol Neurosurg Psychiatry 2002;72:767–771.

270. Odaka M, Yuki N, Hirata K. Anti-GQ1b syndrome: Clinical and immunological range. J Neurol Neurosurg Psychiatry 2001;70:50–55.

271. Reddel SW, Barnett MH, Yan W. Chronic ophthalmoplegia with anti-GQIb antibody. Neurology 2000;54:1000.

272. Kloos L, Sillevis Smit P, Ang CW, et al. Paraneoplastic ophthalmoplegia and subacute axonal neuropathy associated with anti-GQ1b antibodies in a paitent with malignant melanoma. J Neurol Neurosurg Psychiatry 2003;74:507–509.

273. Susuki K, Yuki N, Hirata K. Features of sensory ataxic neuropathy associated with anti-GD1b IgM antibody. J Neuroimmunol 2001;112:181–187.

274. Willison HJ, O'Leary CP, Veitch J, et al. The clinical and laboratory features of chronic sensory ataxic neuropathy with anti-disialosyl IgM antibodies. Brain 2001;124:1968–1977.

275. Rush JA, Younge BR. Paralysis of cranial nerves III, IV, and VI: Cause and prognosis in 1000 cases. Arch Ophthalmol 1981;99:76–79.

276. Renowden SA, Harris KM, Hourihan MD. Isolated atraumatic third nerve palsy: Clinical features and imaging techniques. Br J Radiol 1993;66:1111–1117.

277. Mariak Z, Mariak Z, Proniewska-Skretek E, et al. Injuries of cranial nerves II-VII in 350 patients hospitalized due to closed head trauma. Klin Oczna 1995; 97:130–132.

278. Balcer L, Galetta SL, Bagley LJ, et al. Localization of traumatic oculomotor nerve palsy to the midbrain exit site by magnetic resonance imaging. Am J Ophthalmol 1996;122:437–439.

279. Keane JR. Neurologic eye signs following motorcycle accidents. Arch Neurosurg 1989;46:761–762.

280. Adam T, Schumacher M. Traumatic lesions of the optic, oculomotor, and abducens nerves: Computed tomographic findings. Neurosurg Rev 1988;11:231–237.

281. Mariak Z, Mariak Z, Rydzewska M. Injuries of cranial nerves II-VII from mortal closed head injuries. Klin Oczna 1995;97:133–135.

282. Memon MY, Paine KWE. Direct injury of the oculomotor nerve in craniocerebral trauma. J Neurosurg 1971;35:461–464.

283. Muthu P, Pritty P. Mild head injury with isolated third nerve palsy. Emerg Med J 2001;18:310–311.

284. McCammon A, Kaufman HH, Sears ES. Transient oculomotor paralysis in pseudotumor cerebri. Neurology 1981;31:182–184.

285. Phookan G, Cameron M. Bilateral chronic subdural haematoma: An unusual presentation with isolated oculomotor nerve palsy. J Neurol Neurosurg Psychiatry 1994;57:1146.

286. Acierno MD, Trobe JD, Cornblath WT, et al. Painful oculomotor palsy caused by posterior-draining dural carotid-cavernous fistulas. Arch Ophthalmol 1995; 113:1045–1049.

287. Miyachi S, Negoro M, Handa T, et al. Dural carotid cavernous sinus fistula presenting as isolated oculomotor nerve palsy. Surg Neurol 1993;39:105–109.

288. Chan CC, Sogg RL. Isolated oculomotor palsy after measles immunization. Am J Ophthalmol 1980;89:446–448.

289. Lincoff HA, Cogan DG. Unilateral headache and oculomotor paralysis not caused by aneurysm. Arch Ophthalmol 1957;57:181–189.

290. Dreyfus PM, Hakin S, Adams RD. Diabetic ophthalmoplegia. AMA Arch Neurol Psychiatry 1957;77.

291. Weber RB, Daroff RB, Mackey EA. Pathology of oculomotor nerve palsy in diabetics. Neurology 1970;20:835–838.

292. Usui Y, Mukoyama M, Hashizume M, et al. Diabetic ophthalmoplegia: A clinico-pathological study of the first case in Japan. Rinsho Shinkeigaku [Clin Neurol] 1989;29:442–449.

293. Smith BE, Dyck PJ. Subclinical histopathological changes in the oculomotor nerve in diabetes mellitus. Ann Neurol 1992;32:376–385.

294. Lenzi GL, Fieschi C. Superior orbital fissure syndrome: Review of 130 cases. Eur Neurol 1977;16:23–30.

295. Boghen D. Pupil-sparing oculomotor palsy. Ann Neurol 1983;14:698.

296. Keane JR, Ahmadi J. Most diabetic third nerve palsies are peripheral. Neurology 1998;51:1510.

297. Asbury AK, Aldredge H, Hershberg R, et al. Oculomotor palsy in diabetes mellitus: A clinical-pathological study. Brain 1970;93:555–566.

298. Cahill M, Bannigan J, Eustace P. Anatomy of the extraneural blood supply to the intracranial oculomotor nerve. Br J Ophthalmol 1996;80:177–181.

299. Jacobson DM. Pupil involvement in patients with diabetes-associated oculomotor nerve palsy. Arch Ophthalmol 1998;116:723–727.

300. Lanzino G, Andreoli A, Tognetti F, et al. Orbital pain and unruptured carotid posterior communicating artery aneurysms: The role of sensory fibers of the third cranial nerve. Acta Neurochirurgica 1993;120:7–11.

301. Bortolami R, D'Alessandro R, Manni E. The origin of pain in "ischemic-diabetic" third nerve palsy. Arch Neurol 1993;50:795.

302. Jacobson DM. Relative pupil-sparing third nerve palsy etiology and clinical variables predictive of a mass. Neurology 2001:6.

303. Cullom ME, Savino PJ, Sergott RC. Relative pupillary-sparing third nerve palsies: To arteriogram or not? J Clin Neuroophthalmol 1995;15:136–141.

304. Jacobson DM, Broste SK. Early progression of ophthalmoplegia in patients with ischemic oculomotor nerve palsies. Arch Ophthalmol 1995;113:1535–1537.

305. Sergott RC, Glaser JS, Berger LJ. Simultaneous, bilateral diabetic ophthalmoplegia. Report of two cases and discussion of differential diagnosis. Ophthalmology 1984;91:18–22.

306. Eshbaugh CG, Siatkowski RM, Smith JL, et al. Simultaneous, multiple cranial neuropathies in diabetes mellitus. J Neuroophthalmol 1995;15:219–224.

307. Keane JR. Eye movement abnormalities in systemic lupus erythematosus. Arch Neurol 1995;52:1145–1149.

308. Amris K, Lausen T. Oculomotor nerve paralysis in patients with rheumatic disease, possible causes and anatomical localization of the lesions. Ugeskr Laeger 1993;155:320–323.

309. Barton JJ, Corbett JJ. Neuro-ophthalmologic vascular emergencies in the elderly. Clin Geriatr Med 1991;7:525–548.

310. Davies GE, Shakir RA. Giant cell arteritis presenting as oculomotor nerve palsy with pupillary dilatation. Postgrad Med J 1994;70:298–299.

311. Donahue SP, Taylor RJ. Pupil-sparing third nerve palsy associated with sildenafil citrate (Viagra). Am J Ophthalmol 1998;126:476–477.

312. Ono Y, Umeda F, Nawata H, et al. A case of NIDDM associated with oculomotor palsy due to atypical carotid cavernous sinus fistula. Fukuoka Igaku Zasshi Fukuoka Acta Medica 1993;84:488–492.

313. Hegde VI, Coutinho CMA, Mitchell JD. Dissection of the intracranial internal carotid artery producing isolated oculomotor nerve palsy with sparing of pupil. Acta Neurol Scand 2002;105:330–332.

314. Schievink WI, Mokri B, Garrity JA. Ocular motor nerve palsies in spontaneous dissections of the cervical internal carotid artery. Neurology 1993;43: 1938–1941.

315. Ringel K, Schindler H, et al. Pupil-sparing oculomotor palsy as the only clinical sign of an internal carotid artery occlusion. Eur J Neurol 1999;6:378.

316. Barr D, Kupersmith M, Turbin R. Synkinesis following diabetic third nerve palsy. Arch Ophthalmol 2000;118:132–134.

317. Zorilla E, Kozak GP. Ophthalmoplegia in diabetes mellitus. Ann Intern Med 1967;67:968–976.

318. Sibony PA, Lessell S. Transient oculomotor synkinesis in temporal arteritis. Arch Neurol Psychiatr 1984;41:87–88.

319. Keane JR. Aneurysms and third nerve palsies. Ann Neurol 1983;14:696–697.

320. Winterkorn JM, Bruno M. Relative pupil-sparing oculomotor nerve palsy as the presenting sign of posteror fossa meningioma. J Neuroophthalmol 2001;21: 207–209.

321. So SC, Leiguarda RC, Hankinson J. Pupillary sparing in oculomotor palsy from temporal lobe astrocytoma: Report of two cases. Acta Neurol Latinoam 1976; 22:27–30.

322. Ruggles KH, Massey EW. Pupil-sparing oculomotor palsy with IgG monoclonal paraproteinemia. Ann Ophthalmol 1981;13:875–876.

323. Ramelli GP, Vella S, Lovblad K, et al. Swelling of the third nerve in a child with transient oculomotor paresis: A possible cause of ophthalmoplegic migraine. Neuropediatrics 2000;31:145–147.

324. Carlow TJ. Reply to "Oculomotor ophthalmoplegic migraine: What really causes it?" J Neuroophthalmol 2003;23:240–241.

325. Carlow TJ. Oculomotor ophthalmoplegic migraine: Is it really migraine? J Neuroophthalmol 2002;22:215–221.

326. Lance JW, Zagami AS. Ophthalmoplegic migraine: A recurrent demyelinating neuropathy? Cephalalgia 2001;21:84–89.

327. Durkan GP, Troost BT, Slamovits TL, et al. Recurrent painless oculomotor palsy in children. A variant of ophthalmoplegic migraine? Headache 1981;21:58–62.

328. Lee AG. Oculomotor ophthalmoplegic migraine: What really causes it? J Neuroophthalmol 2003;23:240.

329. Newman NJ. Third-, fourth-, and sixth-nerve palsies and the cavernous sinus. In Albert DM, Jakobiec FA, eds. Principles and Practice of Ophthalmology. Philadelphia, Saunders, 2000:3992–4028.

330. Bartholow R. Aneurysms of the arteries at the base of the brain: Their symptomatology, diagnosis, and treatment. Am J Med Sci 1872;64:373–386.

331. Lenzi GL, Fieschi C. Superior orbital fissure syndrome: Review of 130 cases. Eur Neurol 1977;16:23–30.

332. Keane JR. Cavernous sinus syndrome. Analysis of 151 cases. Arch Neurol 1996; 53:967–971.

333. Date I, Sugiu K, Ohmoto T. A giant thrombosed aneurysm of the petrous carotid artery presenting with cavernous sinus syndrome. Skull Base Surg 1999;9: 65–70.

334. Hollenhorst RW, Younge BR. Ocular manifestations produced by adenomas of

the pituitary gland: Analysis of 1000 cases. In Kohler PO, Ross GT, eds. Diagnosis and Treatment of Pituitary Tumors. New York, Elsevier, 1973:53–64.

335. De Keizer RJW. Spontaneous carotid cavernous fistulas. Neuroophthalmology 1981;2:35–46.

336. Hamada H, Endo S, Fukuda O, et al. Giant aneurysm in the cavernous sinus causing subarachnoid hemorrhage 13 years after detection: A case report. Surg Neurol 1996;45:143–146.

337. Montecucco C, Caporali R, Pacchetti C, et al. Is Tolosa Hunt syndrome a limited form of Wegener's granulomatosis? Report of two cases with antineutrophil cytoplasmic antibodies. Br J Rheumatol 1993;32:640–641.

338. Trobe JD, Glaser JS, Post JD. Meningiomas and aneurysms of the cavernous sinus: Neuroophthalmic features. Arch Ophthalmol 1978;96:457–467.

339. Unsöld R, Safran AB, Safran E, et al. Metastatic infiltration of nerves in the cavernous sinus. Arch Ophthalmol 1980;37:59–61.

340. Barr HWK, Blackwood W, Meadows SP. Intracavernous carotid aneurysms: A clinical-pathological report. Brain 1971;94:607–622.

341. Kim DK, Grieve J, Archer DJ. Meningiomas in the region of the cavernous sinus: A review of 21 patients. Br J Neurosurg 1996;10:439–444.

342. Dinubile MJ. Septic thrombosis of the cavernous sinus. Arch Neurol 1988;45:567–572.

343. Spiro FI, Myerson L. A venous malformation of the cavernous sinus. Br J Radiol 1976;49:92–94.

344. do Souto AA, Marcondes J, da Silva MR, et al. Sclerosing cavernous hemangioma in the cavernous sinus: Case report. Skull Base 2003;13:93–98.

345. Ture U, Seker A, Kurtkaya O, et al. Internal carotid plexus schwannoma of the cavernous sinus. Neurosurgery 2003;52:435–439.

346. Nakamura M, Carvalho GA, Samii M. Abducens nerve schwannoma: A case report and review of the literature. J Neuroophthalmol 2003;23:172.

347. Goel A, Muzumdar D. Trigeminal neurinomas. Neurosurg Quarterly 2003;13:162–178.

348. Veshchev I, Spektor S. Trochlear nerve neuroma manifested with intractable atypical facial pain: Case report. Neurosurgery 2002;50:889–892.

349. Kurokawa Y, Uede T, Honda O, et al. Successful removal of intracavernous neurinoma originating from the oculomotor nerve: A case report. Neurol Med Chir (Tokyo) 1992;32.

350. Aysun S, Topcu M, Gunay M, et al. Neurologic features as initial presentations of childhood malignancies. Pediatr Neurol 1994;10:40–43.

351. Quinones-Hinojosa A, Chang EF, Khan SA, et al. Isolated trigeminal nerve sarcoid granuloma mimicking trigeminal schwannoma: Case report. Neurosurgery 2003;52:700–705.

352. O'Brien TJ, McKelvie PA, Vrodos N. Bilateral trigeminal amyloidoma: An unusual case of trigeminal neuropathy with a review of the literature. Case report. J Neurosurg 1994;81:780–783.

353. Kline LB, Hoyt WF. The Tolosa-Hunt syndrome. J Neurol Neurosurg Psychiatry 2001;71:577–582.

354. Evans OB, Lexow SS. Painful ophthalmoplegia in systemic lupus erythematosus. Ann Neurol 1978;4:584–585.

355. Jacobs D, Galetta SL. Diagnosis and management of orbital pseudotumor. Curr Opinion Ophthalmol 2002;13:347–351.

356. Thomas JE, Yoss RE. The parasellar syndrome: Problems in determining etiology. Mayo Clin Proc 1970;45:617–623.

357. Hudgins PA. Imaging of the cavernous sinus. Techniques Neurosurg 2003;8:211–219.

358. Yousem DM, Atlas SW, Grossman RI, et al. MR imaging of Tolosa-Hunt syndrome. AJR Am J Roentgenol 1990;154:167–170.

359. Ebright JR, Pace MT, Niazi AF. Septic thrombosis of the cavernous sinuses. Arch Intern Med 2001;161:2671–2676.

360. Krisht AF, Kadri PAS, Raja A, et al. Pathology of the cavernous sinus. Techniques Neurosurg 2003;8:204–210.

361. Tibbs PA, Walsh JW, Minix MB. Persistent primitive trigeminal artery and ipsilateral acquired blepharoptosis. Arch Neurol 1981;38:323–324.

362. Acers TE. Pseudo-orbital apex syndrome. Am J Ophthalmol 1979;88:623–625.

363. Hyams SW. Oculomotor palsy following dental anesthesia. Arch Ophthalmol 1976;94.

364. Penarrocha-Diago M, Sanchis-Bielsa JM. Ophthalmologic complications after intraoral local anesthesia with articaine. Oral Surg Oral Med Oral Pathol Oral Radiol Endodontics 2000;921–924.

365. Hayreh SS, Dass R. The ophthalmic artery. I. Origin and intracranial and intracanalicular course. Br J Ophthalmol 1962;46:65–98.

366. Kodsi SR, Younge BR. Acquired oculomotor, trochlear and abducent cranial nerve palsies in pediatric patients. Am J Ophthalmol 1992;114:568–574.

367. Wiest G, Baumgartner C, Schnider P, et al. Monocular elevation paresis and contralateral downgaze paresis from unilateral mesodiencephalic infarction. J Neurol Neurosurg Psychiatry 1996;60.

368. White JW. Paralysis of the superior rectus and inferior oblique muscles of the same eye. Arch Ophthalmol 1942;27:366–371.

369. Kobashi R, Ohtsuki H, Hasebe S. Clinical studies of ocular motility disturbances: Part 2. Ischemic ocular motor nerve palsy risk factors. Jpn J Ophthalmol 1997;41.

370. Golnik KC, Miller NR. Late recovery of function after oculomotor nerve palsy. Am J Ophthalmol 1991;111:566–570.

371. Krohel GB. Blepharoptosis after traumatic third nerve palsies. Am J Ophthalmol 1979;88:598–601.

372. Iwabuchi T, Suzuki M, Nakaoka T, et al. Oculomotor nerve anastomosis. Neurosurgery 1982;10:490–491.

373. Mariniello G, Horvat A, Dolene VV. En bloc resection of an intracavernous oculomotor nerve schwannoma and grafting of the oculomotor nerve with sural nerve. Case report and review of the literature. J Neurosurg 1999;91:1045–1049.

374. Lepore FE, Glaser JS. Misdirection revisited: A critical appraisal of acquired oculomotor nerve synkinesis. Arch Ophthalmol 1980;98:2206–2209.

375. Pallini R, Fernandez E, Lauretti L, et al. Experimental repair of the oculomotor nerve: The anatomical paradigms of functional regeneration. J Neurosurg 1992;77:768–777.

376. Fernandez E, Di Rocco F, Lauretti L, et al. Reinnervation of extraocular muscles by facial-to-oculomotor nerve anastomosis in rats: Anatomic nuclear changes. Neurosurgery 2003;53:409–415.

377. Sibony PA, Evinger C, Lessell S. Retrograde horseradish peroxidase transport after oculomotor nerve injury. Invest Ophthalmol Vis Sci 1986;27:975–980.

378. Guy JR, Engle HM, Lesser AM. Acquired contralateral oculomotor synkinesis. Arch Neurol 1989;46:1021–1023.

379. Packer AJ, Bienfang DC. Aberrant reinnervation involving the oculomotor and abducens nerves. Ophthalmologica 1984;189:80–85.

380. Lemke C, Bably I. Synkinesis between facial nerve and oculomotor nerve. A case report. Anat Anz 1998;180:339–342.

381. Gotlob I, Jain S, Engle E. Elevation of one eye during tooth brushing. Am J Ophthalmol 2002;134:459–460.

382. Krzizok T, Graf M. Post-traumatic anomalous innervation of the lateral rectus muscle by trigeminal fibers. Klin Monatsbl Augenheilkd 1994;205.

383. Forster RK, Schatz NJ, Smith JL. A subtle eyelid sign in aberrant regeneration of the third nerve. Am J Ophthalmol 1969;67:696–698.

384. Behrens MM. Failure of the light reaction. Trans Am Acad Otolaryngol 1977;83:827–831.

385. Czarnecki JSC, Thompson HS. The iris sphincter in aberrant regeneration of the third nerve. Arch Ophthalmol 1978;96:1606–1610.

386. Herzau V, Foerster MH. Fehlinnervation nach okulomotoriusparalyse mit beteiligung des ziliarmuskels. Klin Monatsbl Augenheilkd 1976;169:61–65.

387. Georgiou T, McKibbin M, Doran RML. Bilateral third-nerve palsy with aberrant regeneration in Guillain-Barré syndrome. Eye 2003;17:254–256.

388. Weinstein EA, Dolger H. External ocular muscle palsies occurring in diabetes mellitus. Arch Psychiatry 1948;60:597–603.

389. Schatz NJ, Savino PJ, Corbett JJ. Primary aberrant oculomotor regeneration: A sign of intracavernous meningioma. Arch Neurol 1977;34:29–32.

390. Boghen D, Chartrand JP, Laflamme P, et al. Primary aberrant third nerve regeneration. Ann Neurol 1979;6:415–418.

391. Trobe JD. Managing oculomotor palsy. Arch Ophthalmol 1998;166:798.

392. Horikoshi T, Fukamachi A, Nishi H, et al. Detection of intracranial aneurysms by three-dimensional time-of-flight magnetic resonance angiography. Neuroradiology 1994;36:203–207.

393. Heiserman JE, Dean BL, Hodak JA, et al. Neurologic complications of cerebral angiography. AJNR Am J Neuroradiol 1994;15:1401–1407.

394. Branley MG, Wright KW, Borchert MS. Third nerve palsy due to cerebral artery aneurysm in a child. Aust NZ Ophthalmol 1992;20:137–140.

395. Wolin MJ, Saunders RA. Aneurysmal oculomotor nerve palsy in an 11-year-old boy. J Clin Neuroophthalmol 1992;17:178–180.

396. Trobe JD. Third nerve palsy and the pupil. Arch Ophthalmol 1988;106:601–602.

397. Noonan CP, O'Connor M. Surgical management of third nerve palsies. Br J Ophthalmol 1995;79.

398. Kushner BJ. Surgical treatment of paralysis of the inferior division of the oculomotor nerve. Arch Ophthalmol 1999;117:485–489.

399. Saad N, Lee J. The role of botulinum toxin in third nerve palsy. Aust NZ Ophthalmol 1992;20:121–127.

400. Saunders RA, Rogers GL. Superior oblique transposition for third nerve palsy. Ophthalmology 1982;89:310–316.

401. Sato M, Maeda M, Ohmura T, et al. Myectomy of lateral rectus muscle for third nerve palsy. Jpn J Ophthalmol 2000;44:555–558.

402. Lyle TK. Torsional diplopia due to cyclotropia and its surgical treatment. Trans Am Acad Ophthalmol Otolaryngol 1964;387–411.

403. Trobe JD. Cyclodeviation in acquired vertical strabismus. Arch Ophthalmol 1984;102:717–720.

404. von Noorden GK. Binocular Vision and Ocular Motility: Theory and Management of Strabismus. 5th ed. St Louis, CV Mosby, 1996.

405. Burian HM, Rowan PJ, Sullivan MS. Absence of spontaneous head tilt in superior oblique muscle palsy. Am J Ophthalmol 1975;79:972–977.

406. Tiffin PA, MacEwen CJ, Craig EA, et al. Acquired palsy of the oculomotor, trochlear and abducens nerves. Eye 1996;19:377–384.

407. Brazis PW. Palsies of the trochlear nerve: Diagnosis and location, recent concepts. Mayo Clin Proc 1993;68:501–509.

408. Younge BR, Sutula F. Analysis of trochlear nerve palsies: Diagnosis, etiology, and treatment. Mayo Clin Proc 1977;52:11–18.

409. Harley RD. Paralytic strabismus in children: Etiologic incidence and management of the third, fourth, and sixth nerve palsies. Ophthalmology 1980;86:24–43.

410. Aleksic S, Budzilovich G, Choy A, et al. Congenital ophthalmoplegia in oculo-

vertebral dysplasia-hemifacial microsomia (Goldenhaar-Gorlin syndrome): A clinicopathologic study and review of the literature. Neurology 1976;26: 638–644.

411. Botelho PJ, Giangiacomo JG. Autosomal-dominant inheritance of congenital superior oblique palsy. Ophthalmology 1996;103:1508–1511.

412. Astle WF, Rosenbaum AL. Familial congenital fourth cranial nerve palsy. Arch Ophthalmol 1985;103:532–535.

413. Bhola RM, Horne GV, Squirrell DM, et al. Autosomal dominant congenital superior oblique palsy. Eye 2001;15:479–484.

414. Erkkilä H, Lindberg L, Kallio AK. Strabismus in children with cerebral palsy. Acta Ophthalmol Scand 1996;74:636–638.

415. Lee JP. Paralytic and incomitant strabismus. Curr Opin Ophthalmol 1996;7: 19–23.

416. Paysee EA, Coats DK, Plager DA. Facial asymmetry and tendon laxity in superior oblique palsy. J Pediatr Ophthalmol Strabismus 1995;32:158–161.

417. Goodman CR, Chabner E, Guyton DL. Should early strabismus surgery be performed for ocular torticollis to prevent facial asymmetry? J Pediatr Ophthalmol Strabismus 1995;32:162–168.

418. Varrato J, Galetta S. Fourth nerve palsy unmasked by botulinum toxin therapy for cervical torticollis. Neurology 2000;55:896.

419. McHenry LCJ. Dr. Samuel Johnson's head tilt: A hitherto unrecognized example of IVth cranial nerve palsy. Neurology 1983;33:230.

420. Spector RH. Vertical diplopia. Surv Ophthalmol 1993;38:31–62.

421. Parks MM. Ocular Motility and Strabismus. Hagerstown, MD, Harper & Row, 1975.

422. Urist MJ. Bilateral superior oblique paralysis. Arch Ophthalmol 1953;49: 382–391.

423. Hermann JS. Masked bilateral superior oblique paresis. J Pediatr Ophthalmol Strabismus 1981;18:43–48.

424. Von Noorden GK, Murray E, Wong SY. Superior oblique paralysis. A review of 270 cases. Arch Ophthalmol 1986;104:1771–1776.

425. Keane JR. Fourth nerve palsy: Historical review and study of 215 inpatients. Neurology 1993;43:2439–2443.

426. Rucker CW. Paralysis of the third, fourth, and sixth cranial nerves. Am J Ophthalmol 1958;46:787–794.

427. Khawam E, Scott AB, Jampolsky A. Acquired superior oblique palsy: Diagnosis and management. Arch Ophthalmol 1967;77:761–768.

428. Rougier J, Girod M, Bongrand M. Etiology of and recovery from trochlear nerve paralysis: Apropos of 40 cases. Bull Soc Ophtalmol Fr 1973;73:739–744.

429. Bennett JL, Pelak VS. Palsies of the third, fourth, and sixth cranial nerves. Ophthalmol Clin North Am 2001;14:169–185.

430. Burger LJ, Kalvin NH, Smith JL. Acquired lesions of the fourth cranial nerve. Brain 1970;93:567–574.

431. Coppeto JR, Lessell S. Cryptogenic unilateral paralysis of the superior oblique muscle. Arch Ophthalmol 1978;96.

432. Krohel GB, Mansour AM, Petersen WL. Isolated trochlear nerve palsy secondary to a juvenile pilocytic astrocytoma. J Clin Neuroophthalmol 1982;1:119–123.

433. Chen CH, Hwang WJ, Tsai TT, et al. Midbrain hemorrhage presenting with trochlear nerve palsy. Zhonghua Yi Xue Za Zhi (Taipei) 2000;63:138–143.

434. Jacobson DM, Moster ML, Eggenberger ER, et al. Isolated trochlear nerve palsy in patients with multiple sclerosis. Neurology 1999;53:877.

435. Thomke F, Ringel K. Isolated superior oblique palsies with brain stem lesions. Neurology 1999;53:1126.

436. Wilcsek GA, Francis IC, Egan CA, et al. Superior oblique palsy in a patient with a history of perineural spread from a periorbital squamous cell carcinoma. J Neuroophthalmol 2000;20:240–241.

437. Vanooteghem P, Dehaene I, Van Zandycke M, et al. Combined trochlear nerve palsy and internuclear ophthalmoplegia. Arch Neurol 1992;49:108–109.

438. Guy JR, Friedman WF, Mickle JP. Bilateral trochlear nerve paresis in hydrocephalus. J Clin Neuroophthalmol 1989;9:105–111.

439. Cobbs WH, Schatz NJ, Savino PJ. Nontraumatic bilateral fourth nerve palsies: A dorsal midbrain sign. Ann Neurol 1980;8:107–108.

440. Grimson BS, Glaser JS. Isolated trochlear nerve palsies in herpes zoster ophthalmicus. Arch Ophthalmol 1978;96:1233–1235.

441. Orwitz JI, Galetta SL, Teener JW. Bilateral traochlear nerve palsy and downbeat nystagmus in a patient with cephalic tetanus. Neurology 1997;49:894–895.

442. Hashimoto M, Hoyt WF. Superficial siderosis and episodic fourth nerve paresis: Report of a case with clinical and magnetic resonance imaging findings. J Neuroophthalmol 1996;16:277–280.

443. Mielke C, Alexander MS, Anand N. Isolated bilateral trochlear nerve palsy as the first clinical sign of a metastatic bronchial carcinoma. Am J Ophthalmol 2001;132:593–594.

444. Coppeto JR. Superior oblique paresis and contralateral Horner's syndrome. Ann Ophthalmol 1983;15:681–683.

445. Müri RM, Baumgartner RW. Horner's syndrome and contralateral trochlear nerve palsy. Neuroophthalmology 1995;15.

446. Guy JR, Day AL, Mickle JP, et al. Contralateral trochlear nerve paresis and ipsilateral Horner's syndrome. Am J Ophthalmol 1989;107:73–76.

447. King JT, Galetta SL, Flamm ES. Relative afferent pupillary defect with normal vision in a glial brain stem tumor. Neurology 1991;41:945–946.

448. Eliott D, Cunningham ETJ, Miller NR. Fourth nerve paresis and ipsilateral rela-

tive afferent pupillary defect without visual sensory disturbance: A sign of contralateral dorsal midbrain disease. J Clin Neuroophthalmol 1991;11.

449. Hara N, Kan S, Simizu K. Localization of post-traumatic trochlear nerve palsy asociated with hemorrhage at the subarachnoid space by magnetic resonance imaging. Am J Ophthalmol 2001;132:443–445.

450. Heinze J. Cranial nerve avulsion and other neural injuries in road accidents. Med J Aust 1969;2:1246–1249.

451. Bechac G, Gigaud M, Mathis A. Une etiologie peu commune d'excyclophorie bilaterale avec pseudo-ectopie maculaire: La stenose de l'aqueduc. Bull Soc Ophtalmol Fr 1982;82:1030–1035.

452. Knapp P. Blowout fractures. In Symposium on Strabismus: Transactions of the New Orleans Academy of Ophthalmology. St Louis, CV Mosby, 1978:285–291.

453. Keane JR. Fourth nerve palsy opposite a black eye: Two patients simulating orbital blowout fractures. J Clin Neuroophthalmol 1981;1:209–211.

454. Grimson BS, Ross MJ, Tyson G. Return of function after intracranial suture of the trochlear nerve. J Neurosurg 1984;61:191–192.

455. Lepore FE. Disorders of ocular motility following head trauma. Arch Neurol 1995;52:924–926.

456. Hoya K, Kirino T. Traumatic trochlear nerve palsy following minor occipital impact: Four case reports. Neurol Med Chir (Tokyo) 2000;40:358–360.

457. Neetens A. Extraocular muscle palsy from minor head trauma: Initial sign of intracranial tumor. Neuroophthalmology 1983;3:43–48.

458. Agostinis C, Caverni L, Moschini Lea. Paralysis of fourth cranial nerve due to superior-cerebellar artery aneurysm. Neurology 1992;42:457–458.

459. Hall JK, Jacobs DA, Movsas T, et al. Fourth nerve palsy, homonymous hemianopia, and hemisensory deficit caused by a proximal posterior cerebral artery aneurysm. J Neuroophthalmol 2002;22:95–98.

460. Carter N, Miller NR. Fourth nerve palsy caused by *Ehrlichia chaffeensis*. J Neuroophthalmol 1997;17:47–50.

461. Muller D, Neubauer BA, Waltz S, et al. Neuroborreliosis and isolated trochlear palsy. Eur J Paediatr Neurol 1998;2:275–276.

462. Chu K, Kang DW, Song YW, et al. Trochlear nerve palsy in Sjögren's syndrome. J Neurol Sci 2000;177:157–159.

463. Kuhl V, Urban PP, Mayet WJ, et al. Isolated trochlear nerve palsy and repetitive Raynaud's phenomenon of the tongue in primary Sjögren's syndrome. J Neurol 1999;246:974–975.

464. Al-Mefty O, Ayoubi S, Gaber E. Trigeminal schwannomas: Removal of dumbbell-shaped tumors from the expanded Meckel cave and outcomes of cranial nerve function. J Neurosurg 2002;96:453–463.

465. Dolenc VV, Coscia S. Cystic trochlear nerve neurinoma. Br J Neurosurg 1996; 10:593–597.

466. Nadkarni TD, Goel A. Trochlear nerve neurinoma presenting as pathological laughter. Br J Neurosurg 1999;13:212–213.

467. Bassetti C, de Tribolet N, Deruaz JP, et al. Arteriovenous malformation of the trochlear nerve: A rare cause of acquired isolated fourth nerve palsy. Neuroophthalmology 1994;14:135–139.

468. Kosmorsky GS, Hanson MR, Tomsak RL. Carotid cavernous fistula presenting as painful ophthalmoplegia without external ocular signs. J Clin Neuro Ophthalmol 1988;8:131–135.

469. Sogg RL. Comment on "Isolated trochlear nerve palsy secondary to dural carotid cavernous sinus fistula" by Aki K. Selky and Valerie A. Purvin. J Neuroophthalmol 1996;16:69.

470. Selky AK, Purvin VA. Isolated trochlear nerve palsy secondary to dural carotid cavernous sinus fistula. J Neuroophthalmol 1994;14:52–54.

471. Tsai RK, Chen HY, Wang HZ. Painful fourth cranial nerve palsy caused by posteriorly-draining dural carotid-cavernous sinus fistula. J Formos Med Assoc 2000;99:730–732.

472. Follens I, Godts D, Evens PA, et al. Combined fourth and sixth cranial nerve palsy after lumbar puncture a rare complication. Bull Soc Belge Ophtalmol 2001; 281:29–33.

473. Brady-McCreery KM, Speidel S, Mussein MA, et al. Spontaneous intracranial hypotension with unique strabismus due to third and fourth cranial neuropathies. Binocular Vision Strabismus Quarterly 2002;17:43–48.

474. Keane JR. Delayed trochlear nerve palsy in a case of herpes zoster oticus. Arch Ophthalmol 1975;93:382–383.

475. Hermann M, Bobek-Billewicz B, Bullo B, et al. Wegener's granulomatosis with unusual cavernous sinus and sella turcica extension. Eur Radiol 1999;9: 1859–1861.

476. Wise BL, Palubinskas AJ. Persistent trigeminal artery (carotid basilar anastomosis). J Neurosurg 1964;21:199–206.

477. Muir J. Strabismic manifestations in Apert's syndrome. Am Orthopt J 1981;31: 60–64.

478. Bagolini B, Campos EC, Chiesi C. Plagiocephaly causing superior oblique deficiency and ocular torticollis: A new clinical entity. Arch Ophthalmol 1982;100: 1093–1096.

479. Moulignier A, Laloum L, Chauveau E, et al. HIV-1-related ischaemic trochlear nerve palsy. J Neurol 2003;250:108–109.

480. Cohen-Gadol AA, Leavitt JA, Lynch JJ, et al. Prospective analysis of diplopia after anterior temporal lobectomy for mesial temporal lobe sclerosis. J Neurosurg 2003;99:496–499.

481. Jacobson DM, Warner JJ, Ruggles KH. Transient trochlear nerve palsy following anterior temporal lobectomy for epilepsy. Neurology 1995;45:1465–1468.
482. Keane JR. Ocular skew deviation: Analysis of 100 cases. Arch Neurol 1975; 32:185–190.
483. Allerand CD. Paroxysmal skew deviation in association with a brain stem glioma: Report of an unusual case. Neurology 1962;12:520–523.
484. Beck RW, Smith CH. Neuroophthalmology: A Problem-Oriented Approach. Boston, Little, Brown and Company, 1988:1–33.
485. Hardesty HH. Diagnosis of paretic vertical rotators. Am J Ophthalmol 1963;56: 811–816.
486. Haagedorn A. A new diagnostic motility scheme. Am J Ophthalmol 1942;25: 726.
487. Kushner BJ. Errors in the three-step test in the diagnosis of vertical strabismus. Ophthalmology 1989;96:127–132.
488. von Noorden GK, Hansell R. Clinical characteristics and treatment of isolated inferior rectus paralysis. Ophthalmology 1991;98:253–257.
489. Moster ML, Bosley TM, Slavin ML. Thyroid ophthalmopathy presenting as superior oblique paresis. J Clin Neuroophthalmol 1992;12:94–97.
490. Bixenman WW. Vertical prisms: Why avoid them? Surv Ophthalmol 1984;29: 70–78.
491. Buonsanti JL, Rivera Sanchez-Covisa ME, Scarfone H, et al. Botulinum toxin chemodenervation of the inferior oblique muscle for chronic and acute IV nerve palsies: Results in 15 cases. Binocular Vision Strabismus Quarterly 1996;11: 119–124.
492. Garnham L, Lawson JM, O'Neill D, et al. Botulinum toxin in fourth nerve palsies. Aust NZ Ophthalmol 1997;25:31–35.
493. Kubatko Zielinska T, Krzystkowa KM, Madroszkiewicz A, et al. Principles and results of treatment in acquired paralysis. Klin Oczna 1995;97.
494. Gonzalez C, Cinciripini G. Anterior transposition of the inferior oblique in the treatment of unilateral superior oblique palsy. J Pediatr Ophthalmol Strabis 1995; 32:107–113.
495. Maruo T, Iwashige H, Akatsu S, et al. Superior oblique palsy: Results of surgery in 443 cases. Binocular Vision Strabismus Quarterly 1991;6:143.
496. Ohtsuki H, Hasebe H, Hanabusa K, et al. Intraoperative adjustable suture surgery for bilateral superior oblique palsy. Ophthalmology 1994;101:188–193.
497. Bajandas FJ. The six syndromes of the sixth nerve. In Smith JL, ed. Neuroophthalmology Update. New York, Masson, 1977:49–68.
498. Reisner SH, Perlman M, Ben Tovim N, et al. Transient lateral rectus muscle paresis in the newborn infant. J Pediatr 1971;78:461–465.
499. Galbraith RS. Incidence of neonatal sixth nerve palsy in relation to mode of delivery. Am J Obstet Gynecol 1994;170.
500. Hoyt CS, Billson FA, Taylor H. Isolated unilateral gaze palsy. J Pediatr Ophthalmol 1977;14.
501. Zweifach PH, Walton DS, Brown RH. Isolated congenital horizontal gaze paralysis: Occurrence of the near reflex and ocular retraction on attempted lateral gaze. Arch Ophthalmol 1969;81:345–350.
502. Francois J. Congenital ophthalmoplegias. In Brunette JR, Barbeau A, eds. Progress in Neuroophthalmology. Amsterdam, Excerpta Medica, 1969:387–421.
503. Phillips WH, Dirion JK, Graves GO. Congenital bilateral palsy of the abducens. Arch Ophthalmol 1932;8:355–364.
504. Jen J, Coulin CJ, Bosley TM, et al. Familial horizontal gaze palsy with progressive scoliosis maps to chromosome 11q23–25. Neurology 2002;59:432–435.
505. Sharpe JA, Silversides JL, Blair RDG. Familial paralysis of horizontal gaze: Associated with pendular nystagmus, progressive scoliosis, and facial contraction with myokymia. Neurology 1975;25:1035–1040.
506. Holve S, Friedman B, Hoyme HE, et al. Athabascan brain stem dysgenesis syndrome. Am J Med Genet 2003;120:169–173.
507. Witzel SH. Congenital paralysis of lateral gaze: Occurrence in a case of Klippel Feil syndrome. Am J Ophthalmol 1958;59:463–464.
508. Safran AB, Roth A, Haenggeli CA. Congenital horizontal gaze paralysis and ear dysplasia: A syndrome. Ophtalmologica 1983;187:157–160.
509. Möbius PJ. Über angeborene doppelseitige abducens facialis lähmung. Muench Med Wochenschr 1888;35:91–108.
510. Chisholm JJ. Congenital paralysis of the sixth and seventh pairs of cranial nerves in an adult. Arch Ophthalmol 1882;11:323–325.
511. Harlan GC. Congenital paralysis of both abducens and both facial nerves. Trans Am Ophthalmol Soc 1880;3:216–218.
512. Rodrigues Alves CA, Caldeira JAF. Moebius' syndrome: A case report with multiple congenital anomalies. J Pediatr Ophthalmol 1975;12:103–106.
513. Henderson JL. The congenital facial diplegia syndrome: Clinical features, pathology and aetiology. Brain 1939;62:381–403.
514. Kuklik M. Poland-Mobius syndrome and disruption spectrum affecting the face and extremities: A review paper and presentation of five cases. Acta Chir Plast 2000;42:95–103.
515. Verzijl HT, Van Der Zwaag B, Cruysberg JR, et al. Mobius syndrome redefined: A syndrome of rhombencephalic maldevelopment. Neurology 2003;61: 327–333.
516. Baraitser M. Genetics of Mobius syndrome. J Med Genet 1977;14:415–417.
517. Hamaguchi H, Hashimoto T, Mori K, et al. Continuous tachypnea verified by a polygraphic study. Neuropediatrics 1993;24:319–323.
518. Bandim JM, Ventura LO, Miller MT, et al. Autism and Mobius sequence: an exploratory study of children in northeastern Brazil. Arq Neuropsiquiatr 2003; 61:181–185.
519. Hanson PA, Rowland LP. Möbius syndrome and facioscapulohumeral muscular dystrophy. Arch Neurol 1971;24:31–39.
520. Kremer H, Kuyt LP, van den Helm B, et al. Localization of a gene for Moebius syndrome to chromosome 3q by linkage analysis in a Dutch family. Hum Molec Genet 1996;5:1367–1371.
521. Verzijl HTFM, van den Helm B, Veldman B, et al. A second gene for autosomal dominant Moenius syndrome is localized to chromosome 10q, in a Dutch family. Am J Hum Genet 1999;65:752–756.
522. Slee JJ, Smart RD, Viljoen DL, et al. Deletion of chromosome 13 in Moebius syndrome. J Med Genet 1991;28:413–414.
523. Elsahy N. Möbius syndrome associated with the mother taking thalidomide during gestation. Plast Reconstr Surg 1973;51:93–95.
524. Kankirawatana P, Tennison MB, D'Cruz O, et al. Mobius syndrome in infant exposed to cocaine in utero. Pediatr Neurol 1993;9:71–72.
525. Sanchez O, Guerra D. Moebius syndrome due to the use of misoprostol. Case report. Invest Clin 2003;44:147–153.
526. Pastuszak AL, Schuler L, Speck-Martins CE, et al. Use of misoprostol during pregnancy and Mobius' syndrome in infants. N Engl J Med 1998;338: 1881–1885.
527. Lipson AH, Gillerot Y, Tannenberg AE, et al. Two cases of maternal antenatal splenic rupture and hypotension associated with Moebius syndrome and cerebral palsy in offspring. Eur J Pediatr 1996;155:800–804.
528. Towfighi J, Marks K, Palmer E, et al. Mobius syndrome. Neuropathologic observations. Acta Neuropath (Berl) 1979;48:11–17.
529. D'Cruz OF, Swisher CN, Jaradeh S, et al. Mobius syndrome: Evidence for a vascular etiology. J Child Neurol 1993;8:260–265.
530. Thakkar N, O'Neil W, Duvally J, et al. Mobius syndrome due to brain stem tegmental necrosis. Arch Neurol 1977;34:124–126.
531. Leong S, Ashwell KW. Is there a zone of vascular vulnerability in the fetal brain stem? Neurotoxicol Teratol 1997;19:265–275.
532. Van Der Zwaag B, Hellemons AJ, Leenders WP, et al. PLEXIN-D1, a novel plexin family member, is expressed in vascular endothelium and the central nervous system during mouse embryogenesis. Dev Dyn 2002;225:336–343.
533. Issaivanan M, Virdi VS, Parmar VR. Subclavian artery supply disruption sequence: Klippel-Feil and Mobius anomalies. Indian J Pediatr 2002;69:441–442.
534. Raroque HGJ, Hershewe GL, Snyder RD. Mobius syndrome and transposition of the great vessels. Neurology 1988;38:1894–1895.
535. Oohira A, Masuzawa K. A case of congenital oblique retraction syndrome with upshoot in adduction. Strabismus 2002;10:39–44.
536. Bahr K. Vorstellung eines falles von eigenartiger muskelanomalie eines auges. Ber Dtsch Ophthalmol Ges 1896;25:334–336.
537. Stilling J. Untersuchungen Uber die Entstehung der Kurzsichtigkeit. Wiesbaden, JF Bergmar, 1887:13.
538. Türk S. Bemerkurgen zu einem falle von retraction des auges. Zentrabl Prakt Augenheilkd 1899;23:14–18.
539. Duane A. Congenital deficiency of abduction, associated with impairment of adduction, retraction movements, contraction of the palpebral fissure and oblique movements of the eye. Arch Ophthalmol 1905;34:133–159.
540. Gundersen T, Zeavin B. Observations on the retraction syndrome of Duane. Arch Ophthalmol 1956;55:576–580.
541. Kirkham TH. Inheritance of Duane's syndrome. B J Ophthalmol 1970;54.
542. Isenberg S, Urist MJ. Clinical observations in 101 consecutive patients with Duane's retraction syndrome. Am J Ophthalmol 1977;84:419–425.
543. Maruo T, Kubota N, Arimoto H, et al. Duane's syndrome. Jpn J Ophthalmol 1979;23:453–468.
544. Celic M, Dorn V. Zur diagnostik und behandlung des Stilling Türk Duane syndroms (klinische, elektromyographische und elektrookulographische untersuchungen). Klin Monatsbl Augenheilkd 1983;183:285–290.
545. Mehel E, Quere MA, Lavenant F, et al. Epidemiological and clinical aspects of Stilling Turk Duane syndrome. J Fr Ophtalmol 1996;19:533–542.
546. Zhang F. Clinical features of 201 cases with Duane's retraction syndrome. Chinese Med J 1997;110:789–791.
547. Gutowski NJ. Duane's syndrome. Eur J Neurol 2000;7:145–149.
548. DeRespinis PA, Caputo AR, Wagner RS, et al. Duane's retraction syndrome. Surv Ophthalmol 1993;38:257–288.
549. Zhang F. Clinical features of 31 cases with bilateral Duane's retraction syndrome. Chung-Hua Yen Ko Tsa Chih [Chinese J Ophthalmol] 1998;34:127–129.
550. Sato S. Electromyographic study on retraction syndrome. Jpn J Ophthalmol 1960;4:57–66.
551. Huber A, Esslen E, Kloti R, et al. Zum problem des Duane syndromes. Albrecht von Graefes Arch Klin Exp Ophthalmol 1964;167:169–191.
552. Huber A. Electrophysiology of the retraction syndromes. Br J Ophthalmol 1974; 58:293–300.
553. Strachan IM, Brown BH. Electromyography of extraocular muscles in Duane's syndrome. Br J Ophthalmol 1972;56:594–599.
554. Liu GT, Volpe NJ, Galetta SL. Neuroophthalmology: Diagnosis and Management. Philadelphia, WB Saunders, 2001:547–548.
555. Matteuci P. I difetti congeniti di abduzione con particolare riguardo alia patogenesi. Rass Ital Ottal 1946;15:345–380.

556. Hickey WF, Wagoner MD. Bilateral congenital absence of the abducens nerve. Virchows Arch Pathol Anat 1983;402:91–98.

557. Hotchkiss MG, Miller NR, Clark AW, et al. Bilateral Duane's retraction syndrome: A clinical pathologic case report. Arch Ophthalmol 1980;98:870–874.

558. Ozkurt H, Basak M, Oral Y, et al. Magnetic resonance imaging in Duane's retraction syndrome. J Pediatr Ophthalmol Strabismus 2003;40:19–22.

559. Parsa CF, Grant E, Dillon WP Jr, et al. Absence of the abducens nerve in Duane syndrome verified by magnetic resonance imaging. Am J Ophthalmol 1998;125: 399–401.

560. Imaizumi K. Wildervanck (cervico-oculo-acoustic) syndrome. Ryoikibetsu Shokogun Shirizu 2001;361–362.

561. Marshman WE, Schalit G, Jones RB, et al. Congenital anomalies in patients with Duane retraction syndrome and their relatives. J AAPOS 2000;4:106–109.

562. Zhang F. A clinical analysis of 25 cases with Duane's retraction syndrome combined with congenital crocodile tears. Chung-Hua Yen Ko Tsa Chih [Chinese J Ophthalmol] 2002;38:217–219.

563. Tillman O, Kaiser HJ, Killer HE. Pseudotumor cerebri in a patient with Goldenhar's and Duane's syndromes. Ophthalmologica 2002;216:296–299.

564. Becker K, Beales PL, Calver DM, et al. Okihiro syndrome and acro-renal-ocular syndrome: Clinical overlap, expansion of the phenotype, and absence of PAX2 mutations in two new families. J Med Genet 2002;39:68–71.

565. Aguirre-Aquino BI, Rogers DG, Traboulsi EI. A patient with de Morsier and Duane syndromes. J AAPOS 2000;4:243–245.

566. Haciyakupoglu G, Pelit AA, Altunbasak S, et al. Crocodile tears and Dandy-Walker syndrome in cervico-oculo-acoustic syndrome. J Pediatr Ophthalmol Strabismus 1999;36:301–303.

567. Cross HE, Pfaffenbach DD. Duane's retraction syndrome and associated congenital malformations. Am J Ophthalmol 1972;73:442–450.

568. Appukuttan B, Gillanders E, Juo SH, et al. Localization of a gene for Duane retraction syndrome to chromosome 2q31. Am J Hum Genet 1999;65: 1639–1646.

569. Pizzuti A, Calabrese G, Bozzali M, et al. A peptidase gene in chromosome 8q is disrupted by a balanced translocation in a Duane syndrome patient. Invest Ophthalmol Vis Sci 2002;43:3609–3612.

570. Kohlhase J, Heinrich M, Schubert L, et al. Okihiro syndrome is caused by SALL4 mutations. Hum Molec Genet 2002;11:2979–2987.

571. McBride WG. Thalidomide may be a mutagen. Br Med J 1994;308:1635–1636.

572. Cullen JF. Ocular and ocular muscle abnormalities in thalidomide children. Br Orthopt J 1967;24:2–14.

573. Brodsky MC, Fray KJ. Brain stem hypoplasia in the Wildervanck (cervico-oculo-acoustic) syndrome. Arch Ophthalmol 1998;116:383–385.

574. Otradovec J. Obraz Duanova retrack cniko smdru u nadoru ugozkoucho kmene. Cesk Oftalmol 1968;27:90–95.

575. Silverberg M, Demer J. Duane's syndrome with compressive denervation of the lateral rectus muscle. Am J Ophthalmol 2001;131:146–148.

576. Smith JL, Damast M. Acquired retraction syndrome after sixth nerve palsy. Br J Ophthalmol 1973;57:110–114.

577. Sood GC, Srinath BS, Krishnamurthy G. Acquired Duane's retraction syndrome following Kronlein's operation. EENT Monthly 1975;54:308–310.

578. Gittinger JW, Hughes JP, Suran EL. Medial orbital wall blowout fracture producing an acquired retraction syndrome. J Clin Neuroophthalmol 1986;6:153–156.

579. Kivlin JD, Lundergan MK. Acquired retraction syndrome associated with orbital metastasis. J Pediatr Ophthalmol Strabismus 1985;22:109–112.

580. Keane JR. Bilateral sixth nerve palsy: Analysis of 125 cases. Arch Neurol 1976; 33.

581. King AJ, Stacey E, Stephenson G, et al. Spontaneous recovery rates for unilateral sixth nerve palsies. Eye 1995;9:476–478.

582. Buttner-Ennever JA, Buttner U. Neuroanatomy of the ocular motor pathways. Baillieres Clin Neurol 1992;1:263–287.

583. Carpenter MB, Batton RR. Abducens internuclear neruons and their role in conjugate horizontal gaze. J Comp Neurol 1980;189:191–209.

584. Meienberg O, Büttner Ennever JA. Unilateral paralysis of conjugate gaze due to lesion of the abducens nucleus. Neuroophthalmology 1981;2:47–52.

585. Henn V, Büttner U. Disorders of horizontal gaze. In Lennerstrand G, Zee DS, Keller EL, eds Functional Basis of Ocular Motility Disorders. Oxford, Pergamon Press, 1982:239–245.

586. Miller NR, Biousse V, Hwang T, et al. Isolated acquired unilateral horizontal gaze paresis from a putative lesion of the abducens nucleus. J Neuroophthalmol 2002;22:204–207.

587. Muri RM, Chermann JF, Cohen L, et al. Ocular motor consequences of damage to the abducens nucleus area in humans. J Neuroophthalmol 1996;16:191–195.

588. Bennett AH, Savill T. A case of permanent conjugate deviation of the eyes and head, the result of a lesion limited to the sixth nerve nucleus; with remarks on associated lateral movements of the eyeballs, and rotation of the head and neck. Brain 1889;12:102–116.

589. Sharpe JA, Rosenberg MA, Hoyt WF, et al. Paralytic pontine exotropia: A sign of acute unilateral pontine gaze palsy and internuclear ophthalmoplegia. Neurology 1974;24.

590. Crevits L, de Reuck J, et al. Paralytic pontine exotropia in subarachnoid hemorrhage: A clinicopathological correlation. Clin Neurol Neurosurg 1975;78: 269–274.

591. Wall M, Wray SH. The one and a half syndrome: A unilateral disorder of the pontine tegmentum: A study of 20 cases and review of the literature. Neurology 1983;33:971–980.

592. Pierrot Deseilligny C, Chain F, Serdaru M, et al. The ''one and a half'' syndrome: Electrooculographic analyses of five cases with deductions about the physiological mechanisms of lateral gaze. Brain 1981;104:665–699.

593. Bronstein AM, Rudge P, Gresty MA, et al. Abnormalities of horizontal gaze: Clinical, oculographic and magnetic resonance imaging findings. II. Gaze palsy and internuclear ophthalmoplegia. J Neurol Neurosurg Psychiatry 1990;53: 200–207.

594. Deleu D, Solheid C, Michotte A, et al. Dissociated ipsilateral horizontal gaze palsy in one-and-a-half syndrome: A clinicopathologic study. Neurology 1988; 38:1278–1280.

595. Hamed LM, Silbiger J, Silbiger M, et al. MRA of vascular lesions causing neuro ophthalmic deficits. Surv Ophthalmol 1993;37:425–434.

596. Dehaene I, Dom R, Marchau M, et al. Locked-in syndrome with bilateral ptosis: Combination of bilateral horizontal pontine gaze paralysis and nuclear oculomotor nerve paralysis. J Neurol 1985;232:366–367.

597. Bogousslavsky J, Miklossy J, Regli F, et al. One-and-a-half syndrome in ischaemic locked-in state: A clinico-pathological study. J Neurol Neurosurg Psychiatry 1984;47:927–935.

598. Pierrot Deseilligny C, Goasguen J. Isolated abducens nucleus damage due to histiocytosis X. Brain 1984;107:1019–1032.

599. Derby BM, Guiang RL. Spectrum of symptomatic brain stem metastasis. J Neurol Neurosurg Psychiatry 1975;38:888–895.

600. Klingele TG, Schultz R, Murphy MG, et al. Pontine gaze paresis due to traumatic craniocervical hyperextension: Report of two cases. J Neurosurg 1980;53: 249–251.

601. Abad VC, Wolintz A. Bilateral horizontal gaze palsy. Ann Ophthalmol 1982; 14:1046–1048.

602. Sakata K, Yamamoto I. Tentorial meningioma: Surgical anatomy and approaches. No Shinkei Geka Neurol Surg 2000;28:1047–1056.

603. Meienberg O, Muri R. Nuclear and infranuclear disorders. Baillieres Clin Neurol 1992;1:417–434.

604. Tripathi M, Padma MV, Jain S, et al. Pontine hematoma and one and a half syndrome. J Assoc Physicians India 2000;48:450–451.

605. Azevedo Junior D. Pontine tegmentum hematoma: A case report with the ''one-and-a-half'' syndrome without pyramidal tract deficit. Arquiv Neuropiquiatria 1995;53:475–480.

606. Miller NR, Newman NJ, eds. Walsh & Hoyt's Clinical Neuroophthalmology. 5th ed, Vol 1. Baltimore, Williams & Wilkins.

607. Joseph R, Pullicino P, Goldberg CD, et al. Bilateral pontine gaze palsy. Nuclear magnetic resonance findings in presumed multiple sclerosis. Arch Neurol 1985; 42:93–94.

608. Bicknell JM, Carlow TJ, Dornfeld M, et al. Familial cavernous angiomas. Arch Neurol 1978;35:746–749.

609. Reshef E, Greengerg SB, Jancovic J. Herpes zoster ophthalmicus followed by contralateral hemiparesis: Report of two cases and review of literature. J Neurol Neurosurg Psychiatry 1985;48:122–127.

610. Cogan DG, Victor M. Ocular signs of Wernicke's disease. Arch Ophthalmol 1954;51:204–211.

611. Todd KG, Butterworth R. Mechanisms of selective neuronal cell death due to thiamine deficiency. Ann NY Acad Sci 1999;893:404–411.

612. Friedman J, Westlake R, Furman M. Grievous bodily harm: Gamma hydroxybutyrate abuse leading to a Wernicke-Korsakoff syndrome. Neurology 1996;46: 469–471.

613. Perkin GD, Murray-Lyon I. Neurology and the gastrointestinal system. J Neurol Neurosurg Psychiatry 1998;65:291–300.

614. Hermaszewski RA, Rigby S, Dalgleish AG. Coeliac disease presenting with cerebellar degeneration. Postgrad Med J 1991;67:1023–1024.

615. Cirignotta F, Manconi M, Mondini S, et al. Wernicke-Korsakoff encephalopathy and polyneuropathy after gastroplasty for morbid obesity: Report of a case. Arch Neurol 2000;57:1356–1359.

616. Mukuno K, Aoki S, Ishikawa S, et al. Abducens nucleus lesion in the spectrum of internuclear ophthalmoplegia. Presented at the Fifth Meeting of the International Neuro-Ophthalmology Society, 1984, Antwerp, Belgium.

617. Mastrianni JA, Galetta SL, Raps EC, et al. Isolated fascicular abducens nerve palsy and Lyme disease. J Neuroophthalmol 1994;14:2–5.

618. Silverman IE, Liu GT, Volpe NJ, et al. The crossed paralyses: The original brain stem syndromes of Millard Gubler, Foville, Weber, and Raymond Cestan. Arch Neurol 1995;52:635–638.

619. Foville A. Note sur une paralysie peu connue de certains muscle de l'oeil, et sa liaison avec quelques points de l'anatomie et la physiologie de la protuberance annulaire. Bull Soc Anat Paris 1858;33:373–405.

620. Balkan S, Zulkuf O. Clinical and biochemical neuroanatomy. In Bogousslavsky J, Fisher M, eds. Textbook of Neurology. Boston, Butterworth Heinemann, 1998: 32–34.

621. Mrowka M, Graf L-P, Odin P. MRI findings in mesenrhombencephalitis due to *Listeria monocytogenes*. J Neurol Neurosurg Psychiatry 2002;73:775.

622. Bronstein AM, Morris J, Du Boulay G, et al. Abnormalities of horizontal gaze: Clinical, oculographic and magnetic imaging findings. I. Abducens palsy. J Neurol Neurosurg Psychiatry 1990;53:194–199.

623. Lee TG, Choi W-S, Chung K-C. Ophthalmoplegic migraine with reversible enhancement of intraparenchymal abducens nerve on MRI. Headache 2002;42:140–141.

624. Ohtsuka K, Sone A, Igarashi Y, et al. Vascular compressive abducens nerve palsy disclosed by magnetic resonance imaging. Am J Ophthalmol 1996;122:416–419.

625. Durand JR, Samples JR. Dolichoectasia and cranial nerve palsies. J Clin Neuroophthalmol 1989;9:249–253.

626. Caldicott DGE, Wurm A, Edwards NA. The eyes have it: An uncommon but useful sign after serious craniocervical trauma. J Trauma 2002;53:1001–1005.

627. Ozveren MF, Uchida K, Erol FS. Isolated abducens paresis associated with incomplete Horner's syndrome caused by petrous apex fracture: Case report and anatomical study. Neurologia Medico-Chirurgica 2001;41:494–498.

628. Wilkins C, MacEwen GD. Cranial nerve injury from halo traction. Clin Orthop Rel Res 1977;126.

629. Kim L, Glantz MJ. Neoplastic meningitis. Current Treatment Options Oncol 2001;2:517–527.

630. Kindstrand E. Lyme borreliosis and cranial neuropathy. J Neurol Neurosurg Psychiatry 1995;242:658–663.

631. Olson ME, Chernik NL, Posner JB. Infiltration of the leptomeninges by systemic cancer: A clinical and pathological study. Arch Neurol 1974;30:122–137.

632. Bodur H, Erbay A, Akinci E, et al. Neurobrucellosis in an endemic area of brucellosis. Scand J Infect Dis 2003;35:94–97.

633. Hosoglu S, Geyik MF, Balik I, et al. Predictors of outcome in patients with tuberculous meningitis. Intl J Tuberculosis Lung Dis 2002;6:64–70.

634. Sacktor N. The epidemiology of human immunodeficiency virus-associated neurological disease in the era of highly active antiretroviral therapy. J Neurovirol 2002;8:115–121.

635. Mamidi A, DeSimone JA, Pomerantz RJ. Central nervous system infections in individuals with HIV-1 infection. J Neurovirol 2002;8:158–167.

636. Bensalem MK, Berger JR. HIV and the central nervous system. Comp Therapy 2002;28:23–33.

637. Tajima Y, Kishimoto R, Sudoh K, et al. Two cases of hypertrophic cranial pachymeningitis associated with infection in the external auditory canal and paranasal sinus. Rinsho Shinkeigaku [Clin Neurol] 2003;43:258–264.

638. Campisi P, Rappaport JM, Leblanc R. Idiopathic pachymeningitis: A nonspecific relapsing inflammatory intracranial lesion presenting as multiple cranial nerve palsies. J Otolaryngol 2002;31:329–332.

639. Marano E, D'Armiento FP, Scarano V, et al. Focal hypertrophic cranial pachymeningitis associated with temporal arteritis: A new case report. J Neurol 2003;250:98–100.

640. Harada T, Ohashi T, Ohki K, et al. Clival chordoma presenting as acute esotropia due to bilateral abducens palsy. Ophthalmologica 1997;211:109–111.

641. Balcer LJ. Neuro-ophthalmologic manifestations of Maffucci's syndrome and Ollier's disease. J Neuroophthalmol 1999;19:62–66.

642. Slavin ML. Metastatic malignant melanoma. J Clin Neuroophthalmol 1989;9:55–59.

643. Inoue R, Katayama S, Kusakabe T, et al. Cerebral gumma showing linear dural enhancement on magnetic resonance imaging: Case report. Neurologia Medico-Chirurgica 1995;35:813–817.

644. Volpe NJ, Lessell S. Remitting sixth nerve palsy in skull base tumors. Arch Ophthalmol 1994;111:1391–1395.

645. Del Priore LV, Miller NR. Trigeminal schwannoma as a cause of chronic, isolated sixth nerve palsy. Am J Ophthalmol 1989;108:726–729.

646. Okada Y, Shima T, Nishida M, et al. Large sixth nerve neuroma involving the prepontine region: Case report. Neurosurgery 1997;40:608–610.

647. Katz DM, reviewer. Nakamura M, Carvalho GA, Samii M. Abducens nerve schwannoma. A case report and review of the literature. J Neuroophthalmol 2003;23:172.

648. Char G, Charles CF, Moule NJ, et al. Syndrome of inappropriate antidiuretic hormone secretion in a patient with intrasellar neurofibroma of the sixth nerve. West Indian Med J 1991;40:143–146.

649. Nehls DG, Sonntag VK, Murphy AR, et al. Fibroblastic tumor of the abducens nerve. Case report. J Neurosurg 1985;62:296–299.

650. Ogata S, Shimazaki H, Aida S, et al. Giant intracranial granular-cell tumor arising from the abducens. Pathol Intl 2001;51:481–486.

651. Krishna R, Kosmorsky GS, Wright KW. Pseudotumor cerebri sine papilledema with unilateral sixth nerve palsy. J Neuroophthalmol 1998;18:53–55.

652. Insel TR, Kalin NH, Risch SC, et al. Abducens palsy after lumbar puncture. N Engl J Med 1980;303:703.

653. Kestenbaum A. Clinical Methods of the Neuro-Ophthalmologic Examination. New York, Grune & Stratton, 1961:287.

654. Thomke F, Mika-Gruttner A, Visbeck A, et al. The risk of abducens palsy after diagnostic lumbar puncture. Neurology 2000;54:768–769.

655. Bell HA, McIlwain GG, O'Neill D. Iatrogenic lateral rectus palsies: A series of five postmyelographic cases. J Neuroophthalmol 1994;14:205–209.

656. Kuhl V, Andreas J, Muller-Forell W, et al. [Spontaneous intracranial hypotension syndrome in cervicothorackc cerebrospinal fluid leak]. Nuklearmedizin 2000;39:N22–24.

657. Mokri B, Parisi JE, Scheithauer BW. Meningeal biopsy in intracranial hypotension: Meningeal enhancement on MRI. Neurology 1995;45:1801–1807.

658. Cushing H. Strangulation of the nerve abducentes by lateral branches of the basilar artery in cases of brain tumor: With an explanation of some obscure palsies of arterial constriction. Brain 1910;33:204–235.

659. Sachsenwegen R. Clinical localisation of oculomotor disturbances. In Vinken PJ, Bruyn GW, eds. Handbook of Clinical Neurology. New York, John Wiley & Sons, 1969.

660. Kurata A, Takano M, Tokiwa K, et al. Spontaneous carotid cavernous fistula presenting only with cranial nerve palsies. AJNR Am J Neuroradiol 1993;14:1097–1101.

661. Gradenigo G. A special syndrome of endocranial otitic complications (paralysis of the motor oculi externus of otitic origin). Ann Otol Rhinol Laryngol 1904;13:637.

662. DeGraaf J, Cats H, de Jager AEJ. Gradenigo's syndrome: A rare complication of otitis media. Clin Neurol Neurosurg 1988;90:237–239.

663. Alexander MP, Goodkin DE, Poser CM. Solitary plasmacytoma producing cranial neuropathy. Arch Neurol 1975;32:777–778.

664. Yamashita J, Asato R, Handa H, et al. Abducens nerve palsy as an initial symptom of trigeminal schwannoma. J Neurol Neurosurg Psychiatry 1977;40:1190–1197.

665. Symonds C. Discussion of cranial nerve palsies associated with otitis. Proc R Soc Med 1944;37:387.

666. Marconi F, Parenti G, Dobran M. Bilateral traumatic abducens nerve palsy. Case report. J Neurosurg Sci 1994;38:177–180.

667. Antoniades K, Karakasis D, Taskos N. Abducent palsy following transverse fracture of the middle cranial fossa. J Craniomaxillofac Surg 1993;21:172–174.

668. Harrison CR, Luttrell C. Persistent carotid basilar anastomosis. J Neurosurg 1953;10:205–219.

669. Nishio A, Nishijima Y, Komiyama M, et al. Primitive trigeminal artery variant aneurysm treated with Guglielmi detachable coils: Case report. Neurologia Medico-Chirurgica 2001;41:446–449.

670. Tsuboi K, Shibuya F, Yamada T, et al. Giant aneurysm at the junction of the left internal carotid and persistent primitive trigeminal arteries: Case report. Neurologia Medico-Chirurgica 1992;32:778–781.

671. Killer HE, Matzkin DC, Sternman D, et al. Intracavernous carotid aneurysm as a rare case of isolated sixth nerve palsy in an eight-year-old child. Neuroophthalmology 1993;13:147–150.

672. O'Connor PS, Glaser JS. Intracavernous aneurysms and isolated sixth nerve palsy. In Smith JL, ed. Neuro-Ophthalmology Focus. New York, Masson, 1981:155–159.

673. Lewis AI, Tomsick TA, Tew JM, Jr. Management of 100 consecutive direct carotid-cavernous fistulas: Results of treatment with detachable balloons [comment]. Neurosurgery 1995;36:239–245.

674. Brismar G, Brismar J. Spontaneous carotid-cavernous fistulas: Clinical symptomatology. Acta Ophthalmol 1976;54:542–552.

675. Zhou LF, Mao Y, Chen L. Diagnosis and surgical treatment of cavernous sinus hemangiomas: An experience of 20 cases. Surg Neurol 2003;60:31–37.

676. Lal V, Sawhney IM, Bansal SK, et al. Abducens nerve palsy due to spontaneous internal carotid artery dissection: A case report. Comput Med Imaging Graph 1994;18:381–383.

677. Sakalas R, Harbison JW, Vines FS, et al. Chronic sixth nerve palsy: An initial sign of basisphenoid tumors. Arch Ophthalmol 1975;93:186–190.

678. Eisenberg MB, Al-Mefty O, DeMonte F, et al. Benign nonmeningeal tumors of the cavernous sinus. Neurosurgery 1999;44:949–955.

679. Iwai Y, Yamanaka K, Ishiguro T. Gamma knife radiosurgery for the treatment of cavernous sinus meningiomas. Neurosurgery 2003;52:517–524.

680. Du R, Dhoot J, McDermott MW, et al. Cystic schwannoma of the anterior tentorial hiatus. Case report and review of the literature. Pediatr Neurosurg 2003;38:167–173.

681. Takami T, Ohata K, Tsuyuguchi N, et al. Cavernous sinus metastasis from thyroid papillary adenocarcinoma: A case report. J Clin Neurosci 2002;9:598–600.

682. Zorlu F, Yildiz F, Ertoy D, et al. Dermatofibrosarcoma protuberans metastasizing to cavernous sinuses and lungs: A case report. Jpn J Clin Oncol 2001;31:557–561.

683. Dufour H, Diaz A, Metellus P, et al. [Burkitt lymphoma of the cavernous sinus. Apropos of a case]. Neuro-Chirurgie 2001;47:564–567.

684. Arimoto H, Shirotani T, Nakau H, et al. Primary malignant lymphoma of the cavernous sinus: A case report. Neurologia Medico-Chirurgica 2000;40:275–279.

685. Bartlett JRJ. Craniopharyngiomas: A summary of 85 cases. J Neurol Neurosurg Psychiatry 1971;34:725–732.

686. Isayama Y, Takahashi T, Inoue M, et al. Clinicopathological findings in the chiasmal region: Suprasellar germinoma. Jpn J Ophthalmol 1979;23:140–155.

687. Dare AO, Gibbons KJ, Proulx GM, et al. Resection followed by radiosurgery for advanced juvenile nasopharyngeal angiofibroma: report of two cases. Neurosurgery 2003;52:1207–1211.

688. Reichenthal E, Cohen ML, Manor R, et al. Primary osteogenic sarcoma of the sellar region: Case report. J Neurosurg 1981;55:299–302.

689. Hadjipanayis CG, Bejjani G, Wiley C, et al. Intracranial Rosai-Dorfman disease treated with microsurgical resection and stereotactic radiosurgery. Case report. J Neurosurg 2003;98:165–168.

690. Becherer TA, Davis DG, Hodes JE, et al. Intracavernous teratoma in a school-aged child. Pediatr Neurosurg 1999;30:135–139.

691. O'Sullivan F, Elton JS, Rossor M. Solitary intracranial plasmacytoma presenting as lateral rectus palsy. Neuroophthalmology 1990;10:109–113.

692. Ampil FL, Borski TG, Nathan CA, et al. Cavernous sinus involvement by extramedullary plasmacytoma of the sphenoid sinus. An argument for the use of adjuvant chemotherapy. Leukemia Lymphoma 2002;43:2037–2040.

693. Nelson DA, Holloway WJ, Kara Eneff SC, et al. Neurological syndromes produced by sphenoid sinus abscess: With neuroradiologic review of pituitary abscess. Neurology 1967;17:981–987.

694. Abad JM, Alvarez F, Blazquez MG. An unrecognized neurological syndrome: Sixth nerve palsy and Horner's syndrome due to traumatic intracavernous aneurysm. Surg Neurol 1981;16:140–144.

695. Striph GG, Burde RM. Abducens nerve palsy and Horner's syndrome revisited. J Clin Neurol Ophthalmol 1988;8:13–17.

696. Sacks JG. Peripheral innervation of the extraocular muscles. Am J Ophthalmol 1983;95:520–527.

697. Rootman J, Goldberg C, Robertson W. Primary orbital schwannomas. Br J Ophthalmol 1982;66:194–204.

698. O'Connor M, Eustace P. Tonic pupil and lateral rectus palsy following dental anaesthesia. Neuroophthalmology 1983;3:205–208.

699. Cohen HA, Nussinovitch M, Ashkenazi A, et al. Benign abducens nerve palsy of childhood. Pediatr Neurol 1993;9:394–395.

700. Hedges TR. Idiopathic oculomotor paresis in childhood. Neuroophthalmology 1996;16:129–131.

701. Afifi AK, Bell WE, Bale JF, et al. Recurrent lateral rectus palsy in childhood. Pediatr Neurol 1990;6:315–318.

702. Afifi AK, Bell WE, Menezes AH. Etiology of lateral rectus palsy in infancy and childhood. J Child Neurol 1992;7:295–299.

703. Barnett AM. Benign recurrent abducens palsy in children. S Afr Med J 1972;46:1662–1663.

704. Golnik KC, Miller NR. Familial recurrent cranial nerve palsy. J Neurol Neurosurg Psychiatry 1992;55:976–977.

705. Lee MS, Galetta SL, Volpe NJ. Sixth nerve palsies in children. Pediatr Neurol 1999;20:49–52.

706. De Renzi E, Nichelli P. Ophthalmoplegic migraine with persistent abducens nerve palsy. Eur Neurol 1977;15:227–230.

707. Balcer LJ, Galetta SL, Salhany K, et al. Serum sickness and a sixth nerve palsy. In 29th annual Frank B. Walsh Meeting, 1997, Baltimore, MD.

708. Currie J, Lubin JH, Lessell S. Chronic isolated abducens paresis from tumors at the base of the brain. Arch Neurol 1983;40:226–229.

709. Depper MH, Truwit CL, Dreisbach JN, et al. Isolated abducens nerve palsy: MR imaging findings. AJR Am J Roentgenol 1993;160:837–841.

710. Wolfe GI. Spontaneous remission of papilledema and sixth nerve palsy in acute lymphoblastic leukemia. J Neuroophthalmol 1994;14:91–94.

711. Mutyala S, Holmes JM, Hodge DO, et al. Spontaneous recovery rate in traumatic sixth nerve palsy. Am J Ophthalmol 1996;122:898–899.

712. Sawamura Y, Ikeda J, Miyamachi K, et al. Full functional recovery after surgical repair of transected abducens nerve: Case report. Neurosurgery 1997;40:605–608.

713. Laby DM, Rosenbaum AL. Adjustable vertical rectus muscle transposition surgery. J Pediatr Ophthalmol Strabis 1994;31:75–78.

714. Lee DA, Dyer JA, O'Brien PC, et al. Surgical treatment of lateral rectus muscle paralysis. Am J Ophthalmol 1984;97:511–518.

715. Repka MX, Lam GC, Morrison NA. The efficacy of botulinum neurotoxin A for the treatment of complete and partially recovered chronic sixth nerve palsy. J Pediatr Ophthalmol Strabismus 1994;31:79–83.

716. Metz HS. The diagnosis and treatment of abduction deficiencies. Ann Ophthalmol 1976;8:683–693.

717. Metz HS, Mazow M. Botulinum toxin treatment of acute sixth and third nerve palsy. Graefes Arch Clin Exp Ophthalmol 1988;226:141–144.

718. Bielschowsky A. Lecture on Motor Anomalies of the Eyes. Hanover, NH, Dartmouth College Publications, 1943:152ff.

719. Parinaud H. Clinique nerveuse: Paralysie des mouvements associés des yeux. Arch Neurol (Paris) 1883;5:145–172.

720. Jacobson DMMD, Jacobson DM. Divergence insufficiency revisited: Natural history of idiopathic cases and neurologic associations relative to afferent pupillary defect with normal vision: a localizing sign of midbrain or brachium injury. 2000:1237–1241.

721. Bruce GM. Ocular divergence: Its physiology and pathology. Arch Ophthalmol 1935;13:639–660.

722. Burian HM, Anomalies of the convergence and divergence functions and their treatment. In Symposium on Strabismus. Transactions of the New Orleans Academy of Ophthalmology. St Louis, CV Mosby, 1971:223.

723. Krohel GB, Tobin DR, Hartnett ME, et al. Divergence paralysis. Am J Ophthalmol 1982;94:506–510.

724. Kirkham TH, Bird AC, Sanders MD. Divergence paralysis with raised intracranial pressure. Br J Ophthalmol 1972;56:776–782.

725. Savitsky N, Madonick MJ. Divergence paralysis associated with tumor of the brain. Arch Neurol Psychiatr 1946;55:232–235.

726. Savitsky N, Madonick MJ. Divergence paralysis and head trauma. Arch Neurol Psychiatr 1945;53:135–137.

727. Arai M, Fuji S. Divergence paralysis associated with the ingestion of diazepam. J Neurol 1990;237:45–46.

728. Friling R, Yassur Y, Merkin L, et al. Divergence paralysis versus bilateral sixth nerve palsy in an incomplete Miller Fisher syndrome. Neuroophthalmology 1993;13:215–217.

729. Alger EM. Paralysis of divergence. Trans Am Ophthalmol Soc 1916;14:665–677.

730. Jampolsky A. Ocular divergence mechanisms. Trans Am Ophthalmol Soc 1970;68:730–822.

731. Mays LE. Neural control of vergence eye movements: Convergence and divergence neurons in the midbrain. J Neurophysiol 1984;51:1091–1108.

732. Pullicino P, Lincoff N, Truax BT. Abnormal vergence with upper brain stem infarcts: Pseudoabducens palsy. Neurology 2000;55:352–358.

733. Wiggins RE, Baumgartner S. Diagnosis and management of divergence weakness in adults. Ophthalmology 1999;106:1353–1356.

734. Lepore FE. Divergence paresis: A nonlocalizing cause of diplopia. J Neuroophthalmol 1999;19:242–245.

735. Schanzer B, Bordaberry M. The child with divergence paresis. Surv Ophthalmol 1998;42:571–576.

736. Burian HM. Discussion. In Allen JH, ed. Strabismus Ophthalmic Symposium. St Louis, CV Mosby, 1958:488.

737. Bagheri AMD, Ahmadieh HMD, Repka MXMD. Acquired cyclic strabismus in an adult. J Pediatr Ophthalmol Strabismus 2002;39:310–312.

738. Tapiero B, Pedespan JM, Rougier MB, et al. Cyclic strabismus. Presentation of two new cases and critical review of the literature. J Fr Ophthalmol 1995;18:411–420.

739. Riordan Eva P, Vickers SF, McCarry B, et al. Cyclic strabismus without binocular function. J Pediatric Ophthalmol Strabismus 1993;30:106–108.

740. Costenbader FD, Mousel DK. Cyclic esotropia. Arch Ophthalmol 1964;71:180–181.

741. Hutcheson KA, Lambert SR. Cyclic esotropia after a traumatic sixth nerve palsy in a child. J AAPOS 1998;2:376–377.

742. Troost BT, Abel L, Noreika J, et al. Acquired cyclic esotropia in an adult. Am J Ophthalmol 1981;91:8–13.

743. Frenkel RE, Brodsky MC, Spoor TC. Adult-onset cyclic esotropia and optic atrophy. J Clinical Neuroophthalmol 1986;6:27–30.

744. Cole MD, Hay A, Eagling EM. Cyclic esotropia in a patient with unilateral traumatic aphakia: Case report. Br J Ophthalmol 1988;72:305–308.

745. Pillai P, Dhand UK. Cyclic esotropia with central nervous system disease: Report of two cases. J Pediatr Ophthalmol Strabismus 1987;24:237–241.

746. Roper Hall MJ, Yapp JMS. Alternate day squint. In The First International Congress of Orthoptics. St Louis, CV Mosby, 1968:262–271.

747. Richter CP. Clock mechanism esotropia in children: Alternate day squint. Johns Hopkins Med J 1968;122:218–223.

748. Caputo AR, Greenfield PS. Cyclic esotropia. Ann Ophthalmol 1978:775–778.

749. Grant AC. Circadian sneezing. Neurology 1994;44:369–375.

750. Metz HS, Bigelow C. Change in the cycle of circadian strabismus. Am J Ophthalmol 1995;120:124–125.

751. Troost BT, Abel L, Noreika J, et al. Acquired cyclic esotropia in an adult. Am J Ophthalmol 1981;91:8–13.

752. Gusek-Schneider GC, Uberall MA, Wenzel D. Intermittent esotropia as equivalent of absence in epilepsy. J Pediatr Ophthalmol Strabismus 2000;37:363–364.

753. Worthington JM, Halmagyi GM. Bilateral total ophthalmoplegia due to midbrain hematoma. Neurology 1996;46:1176–1177.

754. Agarwal P, Sharma K, Gupta RK, et al. Acute bilateral ophthalmoplegia secondary to metastatic prostate carcinoma. J Neuroophthalmol 1995;15:45–47.

755. Bills DC, Meyer FB, Laws ERJ. A retrospective analysis of pituitary apoplexy. Neurosurgery 1993;33:602–608.

756. Bonicki W, Kasperlik-Zaluska A, Koszewski W, et al. Pituitary apoplexy: Endocrine, surgical, and oncological emergency: Incidence, clinical course and treatment with reference to 799 cases of pituitary adenomas. Acta Neurochir (Wien) 1993;120:118–122.

757. McFadzean RM, Doyle D, Rampling R. Pituitary apoplexy and its effect on vision. Neurosurgery 1991;29:669–675.

758. Kennedy HB, Smith RJS. Eye signs in craniopharyngioma. Br J Ophthalmol 1975;59:689–695.

759. Mehelas TJ, Kosmorsky GS. Painful ophthalmoplegia syndrome secondary to metastatic renal cell carcinoma. J Neuroophthalmol 1996;16:289–290.

760. Spector RH, Fiandaca MS. The "sinister" Tolosa Hunt syndrome. Neurology 1986;36:198–203.

761. Liu GT, Volpe NJ, Galetta S. Neuroophthalmology: Diagnosis and Management. Philadelphia, WB Saunders, 2001:505.

762. Randeva HS. Classical pituitary apoplexy: Clinical features, management, and outcome. Clinical Endocrinology 1999;51:181–188.

763. Sangla I, Ceccaldi M, Poncet M. Recurrent idiopathic facial paralysis and other

cranial nerve involvement in 2 members of a family. Rev Neurol 1996;152: 291–293.

764. Currie S. Familial oculomotor palsy with Bell's palsy. Brain 1970;93:193–198.

765. Aldrich MS, Beck RW, Alers JW. Recurrent facial and ocular motor palsies. Neurology 1984;34 (Suppl.):165.

766. Aldrich MS, Beck RW, Albers JW. Familial recurrent Bell's palsy with ocular motor palsies. Neurology 1987;37:1369–1371.

767. Kansu T, Us Ö, Sarpel G, et al. Recurrent multiple cranial nerve palsies (Tolosa Hunt plus?). J Clin Neuro Ophthalmol 1983;3.

768. Boeri R, Caraceni T. Trois cas d'ophtalmoloplegie douloureuse benigne suivis de paralysie faciale. Rev Otoneuroophthalmol 1970;42:109–112.

769. Uncini A, Lugaresi A, Porrini AM, et al. Recurrent cranial nerve palsies, midbrain infarction and hydrocephalus due to megadolichobasilar artery. Ital J Neurol Sci 1991;11:489–492.

770. Symonds C. Recurrent multiple cranial nerve palsies. J Neurol Neurosurg Psychiatry 1958;21:95–99.

771. TakahashI A. Migrating disseminated multiple cranial neuropathy. Clin Neurol 1974;14:838–843.

772. Spector RH, Neuroophthalmologic manifestations of Charcot Marie Tooth disease and related disorders. In Smith JL, ed. Neuro-Ophthalmology Update. New York, Masson, 1977:329–335.

773. Arroyo JG, Horton JC. Acute, painful, pupil-involving third nerve palsy in chronic inflammatory demyelinating polyneuropathy. Neurology 1995;45: 845–846.

774. Biousse V, Newman NJ. Neuro-ophthalmology of mitochondrial diseases. Curr Opin Neurol 2003;16:35–43.

775. Chinnery PF, Schon EA. Mitochondria. J Neurol Neurosurg Psychiatry 2003; 74:1188–1199.

776. Schwartzman MJ, Mitsumoto H, Shields RWJ, et al. Neurogenic muscle weakness in chronic progressive external ophthalmoplegia (CPEO). Muscle Nerve 1990;13:1183–1184.

777. Drachman DA. Ophthalmoplegia plus: The neurodegenerative disorders associated with progressive external ophthalmoplegia. Arch Neurol 1968;18:654–674.

778. Ionasescu V. Oculogastrointestinal muscular dystrophy. Am J Med Genet 1983; 15:103–112.

779. Ricker K, Mertens HG. Okuläre neuromyotonie. Klin Monatsbl Augenheilkd 1970;156:837–842.

780. Shults WT, Hoyt WF, Behrens MM, et al. Ocular neuromyotonia: A clinical description of six patients. Arch Ophthalmol 1986;104:1028–1034.

781. Ezra E, Spalton D, Sanders MD, et al. Ocular neuromyotonia. Br J Ophthalmol 1996;80.

782. Yee RD, Purvin VA. Ocular neuromyotonia: Three case reports with eye movement recordings. J Neuroophthalmol 1998;18:1–8.

783. Morrow MJ, Kao GW, Arnold AC. Bilateral ocular neuromyotonia: Oculographic correlations. Neurology 1996;46:264–266.

784. Barroso LH, Hoyt WF. Episodic exotropia from lateral rectus neuromyotonia: Appearance and remission after radiation therapy for a thalamic glioma. J Pediatr Ophthalmol Strabismus 1993;30:56–67.

785. Yee RD, Nelson P, Azzarelli B. Cross your "I's" (eyes) and dot your "T's" (threes). Presented at the 25th Annual Meeting of the Frank B. Walsh Society, 1996, Salt Lake City, UT.

786. Chung SM, Lee AG, Holds JB, et al. Ocular neuromyotonia in Graves dysthyroid orbitopathy. Arch Ophthalmol 1997;115:365–370.

787. Harrison AR, Wirtschafter JD. Ocular neuromyotonia in a patient with cavernous sinus thrombosis secondary to mucormycosis. Am J Ophthalmol 1997;124: 122–123.

788. Chung SM, Lee AG, Holds JB, et al. Ocular neuromyotonia in Graves dysthyroid orbitopathy. Arch Ophthalmol 1997;115:365–370.

789. Tilikete C, Vial C, Nederlaender M, et al. Idiopathic ocular neuromyotonia: A neurovascular compression syndrome? J Neurol Neurosurg Psychiatry 2000;69: 642–644.

790. Safran AB, Magistris M. Terminating attacks of ocular neuromyotonia. J Neuroophthalmol 1998;18:47–48.

791. Miller NR. The clinical manifestations, natural history and results of treatment of superior oblique myokymia. Am Orthopt J 1996;46.

792. Hoyt WF, Keane JR. Superior oblique myokymia: Report and discussion on five cases of benign intermittent uniocular microtremor. Arch Ophthalmol 1970; 84:461–467.

793. Geis TC, Newman NJ, Dawson RC. Superior oblique myokymia associated with a dural arteriovenous fistula. J Neuroophthalmol 1996;16:41–43.

794. Susac JO, Smith JL, Schatz NJ. Superior oblique myokymia. Arch Neurol 1973; 29:432–434.

795. Thurston SE, Saul RF. Superior oblique myokymia. Quantitative description of the eye movement. Neurology 1991;41:1679–1681.

796. Morrow MJ, Sharpe JA, Ranalli PJ. Superior oblique myokymia associated with a posterior fossa tumor: Oculographic correlation with an idiopathic case. Neurology 1990;40.

797. Leigh RJ, Tomsak RL, Seidman SH, et al. Superior oblique myokymia. Quantitative characteristics of the eye movements in three patients. Arch Ophthalmol 1991;109:1710–1713.

798. Kommerell G, Schaubele G. Superior oblique myokymia: An electromyographical analysis. Trans Ophthalmol Soc UK 1980;100:504–506.

799. Komai K, Mimura O, Umaya J, et al. Neuro-ophthalmological evaluation of superior oblique myokymia. Neuroophthalmology 1992;12:135–140.

800. Scharwey K, Krzizok T, Samii M, et al. Remission of superior oblique myokymia after microvascular decompression. Ophthalmologica 2000;214:426–428.

801. Ehongo A, Abi FH, Neugroschl C, et al. [Superior oblique myokymia secondary to neurovascular compression]. Bulletin Societe Belge d'Ophtalmol 2003: 79–83.

802. Samii M, Rosahl SK, Carvalho GA. Microvascular decompression for superior oblique myokymia: first experience. Case report. J Neurosurg 1998;89.

803. Tomsak RL, Kosmorsky GS, Leigh RJ. Gabapentin attenuates superior oblique myokymia. Am J Ophthalmol 2002;133:721–723.

804. Schwartz GA. A note on an unusual facio-ocular synkinesis. Arch Neurol 1962; 6:358–365.

805. Hwang J-M, Yi KY, Kang G. Unilateral eyelid retraction induced by a change from supine to sitting position. Arch Ophthalmol 1996;114:1287.

806. McLeod AR, Glaser JS. Deglutition trochlear synkinesis. Arch Ophthalmol 1974;92:171–172.

807. Oesterle CS, Faulkner WJ, Clay R, et al. Eye bobbing associated with jaw movement. Ophthalmology 1982;89:63–67.

808. Agarwal LP, Dayal Y, Gupta AK. Marcus-Gunn phenomenon associated with Duane's retraction syndrome. Orient Arch Ophthalmol 1963;1:224–225.

809. Chhuttani PN, Chawla LS, Sharma TD. Arsenical neuropathy. Neurology 1967; 17:269–274.

810. Walsh FB, Hoyt WF. Clinical Neuro-Ophthalmology. Baltimore, Williams & Wilkins, 1969:2612.

811. Negvesky GJ, Kolsky MP, Laureno R. Reversible atorvastatin-associated external ophthalmoplegia, anti-acetylcholine receptor antibodies, and ataxia. Arch Ophthalmol 2000;118:427–428.

812. Lyle DJ, Zavon MR. Blindness in a fur worker. J Occup Med 1961;3:478–479.

813. Mulvihill A, Budning A, Jay V, et al. Ocular motility changes after subtenon carboplatin chemotherapy for retinoblastoma. Arch Ophthalmol 2003;121: 1120–1124.

814. Kalsbeek F. Bilateral paralysis of the abducent nerve as cause of diplopia after the use of chloroquine. Med Geneesk 1960;104:1414–1416.

815. Valmaggia C, Gottlob IM. Cocaine abuse, generalized myasthenia, complete external ophthalmoplegia, and pseudotonic pupil. Strabismus 2001;9:9–12.

816. Diaz-Calderon E, Del Brutto OH, Aguirre R, et al. Bilateral internuclear ophthalmoplegia after smoking ''crack'' cocaine. J Clin Neuroophthalmol 1991;11: 297–299.

817. Ayala C, Watkins L, Deschler D. Tension orbital pneumocele secondary to nasal obstruction from cocaine abuse: A case report. Otolaryngol Head Neck Surg 2002;127:572–574.

818. Ventura GJ, Keating MJ, Castellanos AM, et al. Reversible bilateral lateral rectus muscle palsy associated with high-dose cytosine arabinoside and mitoxantrone therapy. Cancer 1896;58:1633–1635.

819. Broser F, Henschler D, Hopf HC. Chlorierte acetylene als ursache einer irreparablen trigeminusstorung bei zwei patienten. Dtsch Z Nervenheilkd 1970;197: 163–170.

820. Horii K, Fujitake J, Tatsuoka Y, et al. A case of phenytoin intoxication induced by hypothyroidism. Rinsho Shinkeigaku [Clin Neurol] 1991;31:528–533.

821. Larsen JR, Larsen LS. Clinical features and management of poisoning due to phenytoin. Med Toxicol Adverse Drug Exp 1989;4:229–245.

822. Schroeder B, Brieden S. Bilateral sixth nerve palsy associated with MDMA ''ecstasy'' abuse. Am J Ophthalmol 2000;129:408–409.

823. Brekke A. To tilfelle av forgifning mid etylenglykol. Norsk Mag Laegevid 1930; 91:318–388.

824. Grant WM. Toxicology of the Eye. Springfield, IL, Charles C Thomas, 1986.

825. Spitters C, Moran J, Kruse D, et al. Wound botulism among black tar heroin users, Washington, 2003. JAMA 2003;290:1848.

826. Franklin B, Liu JK, Ginsberg-Fellner F. Cerebral edema and ophthalmoplegia reversed by mannitol in a new case of insulin-dependent diabetes mellitus. Pediatrics 1982;69:87–90.

827. Fukumoto Y, Shigemitsu T, Kajii N, et al. Abducens nerve paralysis during interferon-2a therapy in a case of chronic active hepatitis. Intern Med 1994;33: 637–640.

828. Van Oettingen WF. Poisoning: A Guide to Clinical Diagnosis and Treatment. 2d ed. Philadelphia, WB Saunders, 1958.

829. Guirgis MF, Wong AMF, Tychsen L. Congenital restrictive external ophthalmoplegia and gustatory epiphora associated with fetal isotretinoin toxicity. Arch Ophthalmol 2002;120:1094–1095.

830. Power JG, Barnes RM, Nash WN, et al. Lead poisoning in Gurkha soldiers in Hong Kong. Br Med J 1969;2:336–337.

831. Masaros MP, Seymour J, Sadjadpour K. Lateral rectus muscle palsy associated with nitrofurantoin (Macrodantin). Am J Ophthalmol 1982;94.

832. Strominger MB, Liu GT, Schatz NJ. Optic disk swelling and abducens palsies associated with OKT3. Am J Ophthalmol 1995;119:664–665.

833. Crismer R, Pirot G, Naome J, et al. A case of diplopia caused by phenylbutazone intoxication of the abducens nerve. Rev Med Liege 1965;20:549–550.

834. Rouher F, Cantat MA. Observation instructive d'une paralysie oculaire après absorption de piperazine. Bull Mem Soc Fr Ophtalmol 1962;75:460–466.

835. Donahue SP, Taylor RJ. Pupil-sparing third nerve palsy associated with sildenafil citrate (Viagra). Am J Ophthalmol 1998;126:476–477.

836. Seneviratne U, Dissanayake S. Neurological manifestations of snake bite in Sri Lanka. J Postgrad Med 2002;48:275–279.

837. Lalloo DG, Trevett AJ, Korinhona A, et al. Snake bites by the Papuan taipan (*Oxyuranus scutellatus canni*): Paralysis, hemostatic and electrocardiographic abnormalities, and effects of antivenom. Am J Tropical Med Hygiene 1995;52: 525–531.

838. d'Avignon M, Barr B. Ear abnormalities and cranial nerve palsies in thalidomide children. Arch Otolaryngol 1964;80:136–140.

839. Pentschew A, Intoxikationen: Handbuch der speziellen pathologischen ana tomie und histologie. In Lubarsch O, Henke F, Rossle R, eds. Erkrankungen des Zentralen Nervensystems. Berlin, Springer, 1958:1907–2502.

840. Buxton PH, Hayward M. Polyneuritis cranialis associated with industrial trichloroethylene poisoning. J Neurol Neurosurg Psychiatry 1967;30:511–518.

841. Sandler SG, Tobin W, Henderson ES. Vincristine-induced neuropathy: A clinical study of fifty leukemic patients. Neurology 1969;19:367–374.

842. Albert DM, Wong VG, Henderson ES. Ocular complications of vincristine therapy. Arch Ophthalmol 1967;78:709–713.

843. Verstappen CCP, Heimans JJ, Hoekman K, et al. Neurotoxic complications of chemotherapy in patients with cancer: Clinical signs and optimal management. Drugs 2003;63:1549–1563.

CHAPTER 21

Disorders of Neuromuscular Transmission

Preston C. Calvert

NORMAL NEUROMUSCULAR TRANSMISSION

To understand the pathophysiology of the defects in myasthenia gravis (MG) and other disorders that damage the neuromuscular junction (NMJ), it is necessary to have some knowledge of the basic events of neuromuscular transmission. The reader interested in pursuing the subject may wish to consult the reviews by Drachman or Vincent et al., as well as the monograph edited by Engel (1–3).

Acetylcholine (ACh), the natural transmitter, is synthesized chiefly in the motor nerve terminals and is stored in vesicles for subsequent release (4,5) (Fig. 21.1). Neurotransmission begins with the release of the contents of the vesicles by a process of exocytosis that occurs at specialized release sites (6,7). The probability of vesicular binding and release at these sites depends directly on calcium concentrations in nerve terminals. A change in this probability of release is the main pathophysiologic feature in the Lambert-Eaton myasthenic syndrome and botulism (see below). The vesicle release sites are located directly opposite the areas of highest concentration of ACh receptors on the postsynaptic membranes (8,9) (Fig. 21.2), thus minimizing the distance that the transmitter must travel to reach the receptor site. When ACh combines with its receptor, a transient increase of permeability to sodium and potassium ions occurs (10), resulting in membrane depolarization.

Quanta of ACh are normally released spontaneously, producing local endplate depolarizations of small amplitude called miniature endplate potentials (mepps) (11); a much greater amount of ACh (150–200 quanta) is released when a nerve impulse arrives at the motor nerve terminal, resulting in a larger depolarization, the endplate potential (12). The amplitude of the endplate potential is normally sufficient to trigger an action potential that is propagated along the muscle membrane. The muscle action potential, in turn, initiates the sequence of events that leads to muscle contraction. The entire process of neuromuscular transmission is rapid, on the order of a millisecond. It is terminated by the removal of ACh, in part by its diffusion away from the NMJ, but mostly by the action of acetylcholinesterase, which rapidly hydrolyzes ACh.

The ACh receptor (ACHR) is the target of the autoimmune response in most cases of acquired MG and the site of the genetic mutation in many congenital myasthenic syndromes (see below). The nicotinic AChR of skeletal muscle is a ligand-gated channel, composed of five subunits that are arranged around a central pore and span the muscle membrane (13–18). Each AChR molecule consists of two α-subunits and one each of β, δ, and either γ or ϵ. Each of the two α-subunits has an extracellular ACh bind-

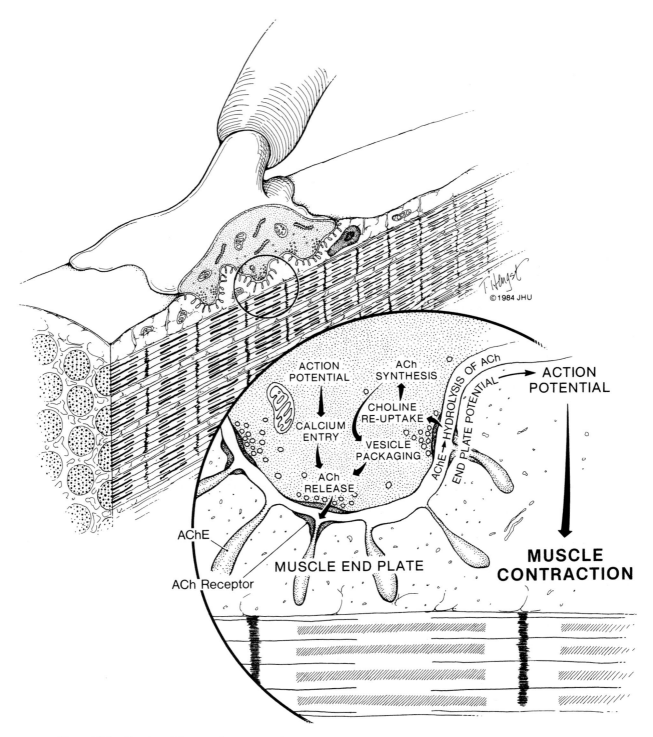

Figure 21.1. Drawing of the normal neuromuscular junction. Note the sites of acetylcholine (ACh) release, the location of acetylcholine receptors, and the location of acetylcholinesterase (AChE).

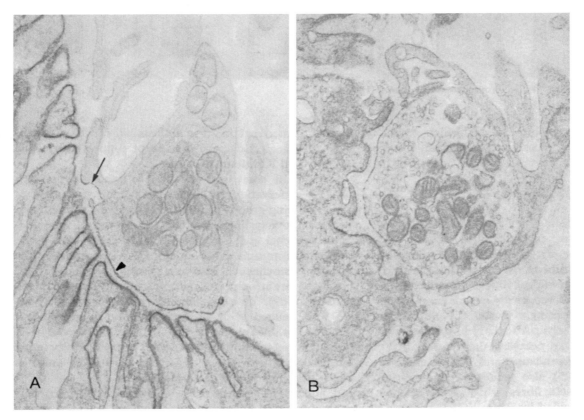

Figure 21.2. Skeletal muscle endplate regions. Acetylcholine receptor sites are stained by α-bungarotoxin conjugated to horseradish peroxidase, ×22,300. *A*, In normal muscle, the acetylcholine receptors are associated with terminal expansions and deep surfaces of the postsynaptic folds. The presynaptic membrane (*arrowhead*) and Schwann's cell membrane (*arrow*) facing the crest of the folds are lightly stained by leaching. *B*, In skeletal muscle from a patient with severe myasthenia gravis, the postsynaptic regions are abnormal with virtually no staining of acetylcholine receptor sites. (From Engel AG, Lindstrom JM, Lambert EH, et al. Ultrastructural localization of the acetylcholine receptor in myasthenia gravis and in its autoimmune model. Neurology 1977;27:307–315.)

ing site. The ion channel of the receptor is functionally closed in the resting state. It is opened when both α-subunit binding sites are occupied by the agonist, ACh. Blocking agents, such as α-bungarotoxin or curare, bind at or near the same site, preventing access to ACh. Acetylcholine receptors in muscle cells undergo active turnover by endocytosis and subsequent lysosomal degradation (19,20).

MYASTHENIA GRAVIS

MG is a disease characterized clinically by muscle weakness and fatigability, caused by a reduction in the number of available ACh receptors at NMJs. Receptor depletion is mediated by one or more antibodies directed against ACh receptors or other NMJ postsynaptic membrane constituents, resulting in impaired neuromuscular transmission.

MG is the most common disorder that affects the NMJ. The reader interested in pursuing this subject in more detail should consult the reviews by Drachman and Vincent, as well as the superb monograph edited by Engel (1–3).

ETIOLOGY AND PATHOGENESIS

The earliest clues that the ACh receptor was the molecular target in MG came from experimental autoimmune MG; immunization with purified ACh receptor faithfully reproduced in rabbits and rodents the immunologic and electrophysiologic features of the human disease (21–24). At about the same time, Fambrough et al. (25) demonstrated that myasthenic patients had less than one-third of the ACh receptors present in normal control subjects. This reduction in the number of available ACh receptors is usually caused by the actions of antibodies to those receptors (see below; Fig. 21.2). Such antibodies are found in the serum of 80–90% of patients with MG (26,27). In addition to increased degradation and decrease in ACh receptor number, receptor blockade may be caused by steric hindrance of the ligand ACh by binding of the antibody to a portion of the receptor molecule near the active site (28). Across patients, the serum anti-

ACh receptor antibody concentration does not correlate well with disease severity (26,29,30). There is recent evidence that genetic polymorphisms in the genes for the α and δ subunits of the ACh receptor may predispose certain individuals to develop MG (31–33). Despite the frequency of mutations in the ϵ subunit in congenital ACh receptor deficiency (discussed later), there is no apparent linkage between such mutations and the development of autoimmune MG (34). There is also no evidence for linkage of β or γ subunit polymorphisms with MG (33,35).

Some ''antibody-negative'' patients have mild or localized disease (e.g., ocular myasthenia) (36), whereas others have generalized, even severe disease. Acquired anti-ACh receptor antibody-negative MG is nonetheless autoimmune because it responds to immunotherapy and pheresis (37,38) and can be passively transferred (39). Recent studies of patients seronegative for anti-ACh receptor antibody have revealed additional IgG and non-IgG serum components that induce NMJ dysfunction by indirectly affecting the state or number of ACh receptors. An IgG antibody that binds to muscle specific kinase (MuSK) was found in some MG patients who lacked anti-ACh receptor antibodies (40). MuSK is a membrane-located tyrosine kinase that interacts during myotube development with agrin and RAPsyn to help determine the clustering and localization of erbB receptors in the membrane, which is important for the subsequent proper clustering and localization of ACh receptors in the NMJ postsynaptic membrane (41,42). Patients with anti-MuSK antibodies rarely also have anti-ACh receptor antibodies, supporting the concept that these patients form a distinct subclass of MG.

Anti-MuSK antibodies are found in about 6% of patients with MG; anti-ACh antibodies are found in about 85% of patients overall, with a lower rate of anti-ACh antibodies in purely ocular patients. The frequency of anti-MuSK antibodies in purely ocular MG patients is not yet established. The anti-MuSK–positive patients are much more likely to be women than those who are negative for both anti-ACh receptor and anti-MuSK antibody (43). There is reportedly a high incidence of dysphagia, dysarthria, and facial weakness in patients positive for anti-MuSK (43,44), and these patients have a high risk of respiratory crisis. Ophthalmoparesis was present in 95% of a small series of patients with anti-MuSK antibodies, similar to the percentage in those who are negative for both anti-ACh receptor and anti-MuSK antibody (43). The anti-MuSK antibody test is available commercially in North America.

There is still a subpopulation of patients who are seronegative for both anti-ACh receptor antibodies and anti-MuSK antibodies, estimated at about 9% of MG patients overall (42). These doubly seronegative patients show relatively mild, limb-predominant weakness with a low risk of respiratory crisis in series from MG clinics (42,43), or may have purely ocular disease. Additional, non-IgG serum factors that inhibit ACh receptor function have been detected in the serum of patients with seronegative MG. The molecular identity of these factors is as yet unknown, but preliminary evidence suggests they may include an IgM antibody (41,45).

EPIDEMIOLOGY

Autoimmune MG affects all races and ages, with an incidence of 4–5 per 100,000. There is a female predominance overall, but the sex predilection is age-dependent, with women predominating among younger patients and men among those who are older at diagnosis (46–48). The prevalence of MG has been increasing slowly in most epidemiologic studies over the past 50 years, in part due to improved treatment and reduced mortality of the disease (48,49). Patients with thymomas are more likely to be over 30 years old, with a mean age at diagnosis of 50 years in one large series, and about equally male and female (50).

SYMPTOMS AND SIGNS

The hallmark clinical feature of MG is variability in the strength of the affected muscles (18). Weakness varies from day to day and from hour to hour, typically increasing toward evening. Transient weakness is often associated with physical exertion. Affected muscles fatigue if contraction is maintained or repeated. This must be differentiated from the neurasthenic ''fatigue'' of tiredness or depression. The most commonly affected muscles, in descending frequency, are the levator palpebrae superioris, the extraocular muscles, and orbicularis oculi; the proximal limb muscles, especially the triceps brachii, deltoids, and iliopsoas; the muscles of facial expression, mastication, and speech; and the neck extensors.

The levator palpebrae superioris and extraocular muscles are initially affected in about 70% of cases, and these muscles are eventually affected in over 90% of patients (51–54). When weakness of these muscles is combined with weakness of the orbicularis oculi, the combination is highly suggestive of MG.

Ptosis and Other Signs of the Levator Palpebrae Superioris

Ptosis may occur as an isolated sign or in association with extraocular muscle involvement. It is characterized by its fluctuating nature and frequently shifts from one eye to the other (55,56). Ptosis is often initially unilateral but eventually almost always becomes bilateral. When signs are limited to one eye, despite obvious myasthenic features, it is essential to image the orbit and brain for a mass lesion. When ptosis is bilateral, it is usually asymmetric, but severe symmetric ptosis may occur, particularly in patients with severe ophthalmoplegia. The ptosis is frequently absent when the patient awakens, but it appears later in the day, becoming most pronounced in the evening. Repeated closure of the eyelids may make ptosis appear or may worsen it when it is initially minimal. Similarly, prolonged upward gaze will often result in gradual lowering of the eyelids (Fig. 21.3). The demonstration of fatigability of bilateral ptosis does not exclude a nonmyasthenic cause, such as dorsal midbrain compression by a mass lesion (57).

Gorelick et al. (58) emphasized the phenomenon of enhancement of ptosis in patients with MG. Such patients, who appear to have either unilateral or symmetric bilateral ptosis, will have worsening of ptosis on one side when the opposite

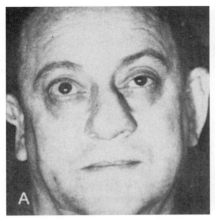
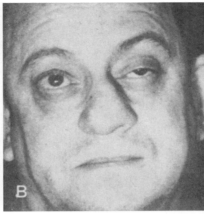
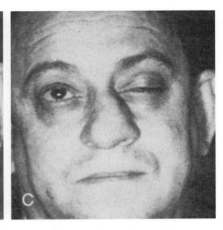

Figure 21.3. Increasing ptosis on maintained upward gaze in a patient with myasthenia gravis. *A–C* represent three frames from a movie showing progressive ptosis over a 3-minute period as the patient maintained fixation above the horizontal meridian. (From Cogan DG. Myasthenia gravis: A review of the disease and a description of lid twitch as a characteristic sign. Arch Ophthalmol 1965;74:217–221.)

eyelid is elevated and held in a fixed position (Fig. 21.4). The explanation of this "seesaw" phenomenon is Hering's law of equal innervation, which relates to the levator muscles as it does to the extraocular muscles (59). Manual eyelid elevation decreases the effort required for eyelid elevation ipsilaterally and thus results in relaxation of the contralateral levator palpebrae superioris and consequent worsening ptosis on that side. This is a corollary to the contralateral eyelid retraction that is often seen in patients with unilateral ptosis. Enhancement of ptosis is not pathognomonic for MG. It can be seen in patients with congenital ptosis and in patients with acquired ptosis from causes other than MG. Nevertheless, in a patient with an appropriate history, the observation of enhancement of ptosis is highly suggestive of MG.

Cogan (55) first emphasized the presence of an eyelid twitch response, Cogan's lid twitch, in patients with MG. When the patient's eyes are directed downward for 10–20 seconds and the patient is then instructed to make a vertical saccade back to primary position, the upper eyelid elevates and either slowly begins to droop or else twitches several times before settling into a stable position (Fig. 21.5). This eyelid twitch phenomenon is caused by the rapid recovery and easy fatigability of myasthenic muscle.

Transient, spontaneous eyelid retraction occurs in some patients with MG without evidence of thyroid dysfunction (60). This phenomenon, which usually occurs on return of the eyes from upward gaze to primary position, may be caused by post-tetanic facilitation of the levator palpebrae superioris.

Thus, four types of eyelid retraction may be observed in patients with MG. First, patients with unilateral ptosis may develop contralateral eyelid retraction as they attempt to elevate the ptotic eyelid. Second, patients with ptosis may develop brief eyelid retraction lasting only a few seconds following a saccade from downward gaze to primary position (Cogan's lid twitch). Third, patients may develop transient eyelid retraction lasting several seconds or minutes after star-

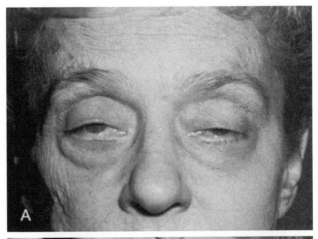
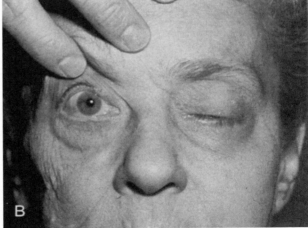

Figure 21.4. Enhanced ptosis in a 78-year-old woman with myasthenia gravis. *A,* The patient has bilateral ptosis. *B,* When the right eyelid is elevated, the patient develops increased (enhanced) ptosis on the opposite side.

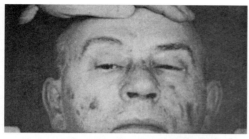

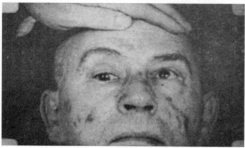

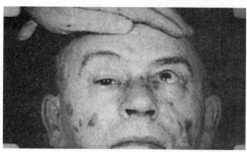

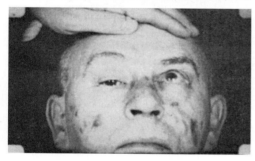

Figure 21.5. Cogan's eyelid twitch phenomenon in a patient with myasthenia gravis. The photograph is made from successive frames of a movie. As the patient looks upward, the left eyelid elevates fully while the right eyelid elevates only partially. The right eyelid then immediately becomes successively more ptotic. The entire process takes only a few seconds. In motion, this transient eyelid elevation gives the appearance of a twitch. (From Cogan DG. Myasthenia gravis: A review of the disease and a description of lid twitch as a characteristic sign. Arch Ophthalmol 1965; 74:217–221.)

ing straight ahead or looking upward for several minutes. Finally, there is an increased prevalence of thyroid eye disease among patients with MG (see later), and persistent bilateral eyelid retraction or unilateral eyelid retraction without contralateral ptosis in a patient with MG should suggest a diagnosis of coincident thyroid ophthalmopathy.

Ophthalmoparesis and Other Abnormalities of Eye Movement

Involvement of the extraocular muscles, like ptosis, is extremely common in patients with MG, although the reason for this is unknown (61,62). Possible explanations are that (*a*) minimal weakness of the extraocular muscles is likely to be symptomatic, in contrast to that in limb muscles; (*b*) extraocular muscles comprise 80% single-innervated twitch fibers, and such fibers, which have high nerve-firing frequencies, may be more sensitive to fatigue and reduction of the safety factor of transmission; (*c*) the graded, continuous depolarization of the postjunctional membrane of multiply innervated extraocular muscles means they have no safety factor, and this may make them especially sensitive to a loss of functional ACh receptors; and (*d*) the reduced expression of complement inhibitory proteins such as decay accelerating factor in the extraocular muscles compared to limb muscles may enhance complement-mediated injury of the NMJ after antibody deposition.

In most cases, disturbances of ocular motility and alignment are associated with ptosis; however, cases without clinical involvement of the levator muscles occur. There is no set pattern to extraocular muscle involvement. All degrees of ocular motor dysfunction, from apparent involvement of a single isolated muscle to complete external ophthalmoplegia, occur. Thus, the abnormalities may mimic ocular motor nerve palsies, internuclear ophthalmoplegia, or gaze palsies. Glaser (63) emphasized the frequent involvement of the medial rectus muscle. This involvement may produce either a variable, incomitant strabismus (64) or a clinical picture simulating unilateral or bilateral internuclear ophthalmoplegia with weakness of adduction of one eye and abducting nystagmus in the opposite eye (65) (Fig. 21.6). Downshoot of the adducting (66) or abducting (67) eye has been proposed to suggest MG as the cause of apparent unilateral or bilateral internuclear ophthalmoplegia. The wall-eyed bilateral internuclear ophthalmoplegia (WEBINO) pattern of ophthalmoparesis may also be simulated (68).

Individual muscles other than the medial rectus may also be selectively involved in patients with MG. Several investigators (69–71) reported patients who developed the sudden onset of an isolated inferior rectus paresis as the initial sign of MG, and Rush and Shafrin (72) reported a 39-year-old man whose initial presentation of MG was the sudden onset of superior oblique muscle weakness that mimicked a trochlear nerve palsy (Fig. 21.7). The involvement of multiple muscles innervated by the oculomotor nerve may mimic a pupil-sparing oculomotor nerve palsy (73) or a "double elevator palsy" (unilateral limitation of upward gaze) (74).

Many patients with MG present either with dysfunction of extraocular muscles in one eye that are innervated by more than one cranial nerve or with dysfunction of muscles in both eyes. As MG progresses, weakness of the extraocular muscles may simulate the progressive external ophthalmoplegia encountered in patients with mitochondrial myopathies (75,76). In severely affected patients, there may be complete external ophthalmoplegia. This is almost always associated with complete or almost complete ptosis.

The tendency for affected muscles, including the extraoc-

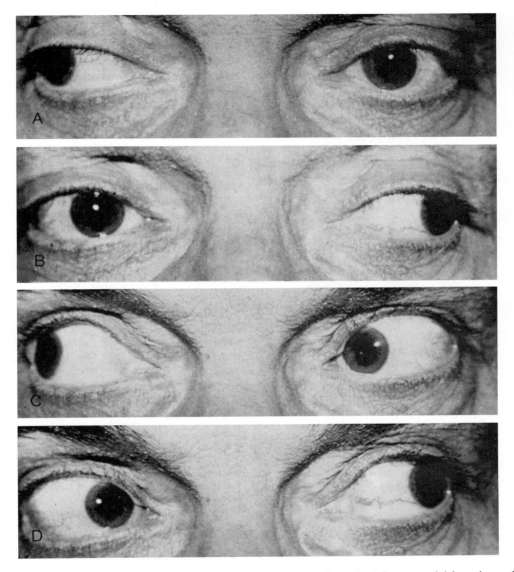

Figure 21.6. Pseudo-internuclear ophthalmoplegia in a patient with myasthenia gravis. *A*, On attempted rightward gaze, there is adduction lag of the left eye. Note bilateral ptosis. *B*, On attempted leftward gaze, there is adduction lag of the right eye. Following intravenous administration of edrophonium chloride (Tensilon), there is marked improvement of adduction of both the left eye (*C*) and the right eye (*D*). (From Glaser JS. Myasthenic pseudo-internuclear ophthalmoplegia. Arch Ophthalmol 1966;75:363–366.)

ular muscles, to fatigue may cause patients with a full range of eye movements to show fatigue on sustained eccentric gaze (Fig. 21.8) (77). Such patients show a "muscle paretic" fatigue that may be mistaken for a brain stem or cerebellar process.

Even in patients in whom the clinical examination does not reveal evidence of fatigue of eye muscles, recordings of eye movements may demonstrate a variety of ocular motor abnormalities (78). Metz et al. (79) found abnormally slow saccades in patients with MG, but most investigators emphasize relative preservation of saccadic velocity, at least in the initial stages of the saccade. In fact, most of the saccadic

abnormalities in patients with MG are related to saccadic accuracy and final saccadic velocity. Schmidt et al. (80–84) described four kinds of saccadic abnormalities in such patients: (*a*) hypermetric saccades; (*b*) hypometric saccades that begin with normal velocity but ultimately show a decrease in velocity (intrasaccadic fatigue) and undershoot the target; (*c*) small, jerking ("quiver") eye movements; and (*d*) gaze-evoked nystagmus. In addition, Baloh and Keesey (85) found that the velocity and amplitude of saccades decreased after repetitive refixations. Cogan et al. (86) also described preservation of saccadic eye movements in patients with MG and observed the characteristic twitch-like

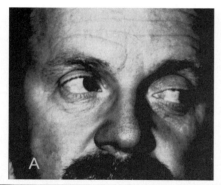

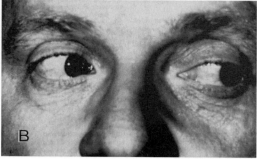

Figure 21.7. Pseudotrochlear nerve palsy in a patient with myasthenia gravis. *A,* Before intravenous injection of edrophonium chloride, the patient has mild left ptosis and a right hypertropia with overaction of the right inferior oblique muscle. *B,* Following intravenous injection of edrophonium, the ptosis has disappeared, as has the right inferior oblique overaction. (From Rush JA, Shafrin F. Ocular myasthenia presenting as superior oblique weakness. J Clin Neuroophthalmol 1982;2:125–127.)

or quiver movements of the eyes on attempted changes of gaze observed by other investigators (55,80–82,87,88). Even patients with severe myasthenic ophthalmoparesis may achieve initial saccadic velocities that are not significantly different from those in normal persons (89).

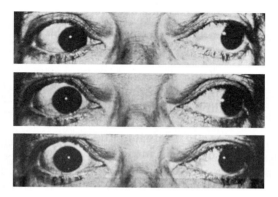

Figure 21.8. Myasthenic sustained gaze fatigue. *Top,* Initial eye movements in left gaze show minimal adduction limitation. *Middle and bottom,* As right medial rectus fatigue develops, the right eye drifts back toward primary position despite efforts to sustain left gaze. (From Osher RH, Glaser JS. Myasthenic sustained gaze fatigue. Am J Ophthalmol 1980; 89:443–445.)

Barton et al. (90) compared the duration and amplitude of voluntary saccades in a repetitive task in eight patients with MG with those in patients with nonmyasthenic palsies and control subjects. Saccades were of prolonged duration in both patient groups initially, but durations decreased in patients with MG after intravenous injection of edrophonium hydrochloride, whereas they increased in patients with nonmyasthenic palsies.

Several investigators (65,91–95) described fatigue of optokinetic quick phases producing a decreased amplitude of the movement that disappears after intravenous injection of edrophonium hydrochloride. This reversal of ocular motor fatigue is highly suggestive of MG, although it occasionally occurs in other myasthenic syndromes (96) (discussed later). In a detailed retrospective meta-analysis of prior reports of changes in optokinetic nystagmus by edrophonium administration in myasthenic and nonmyasthenic patients, using a detection theory analysis, Barton (97) showed little ability of the baseline pretreatment data to discriminate myasthenic ophthalmoparesis from other causes. However, the increase in amplitude of optokinetic nystagmus after edrophonium was found to be an almost ideal screening test for myasthenic fatigue, showing 97% sensitivity and specificity. Recent studies using quantitative magnetic search coil eye movement recording with an open-loop optokinetic paradigm also showed a transient improvement in optokinetic gain, fast-phase summed amplitude, and fast-phase velocity in myasthenic ophthalmoparesis during this testing paradigm after neostigmine administration (98,99). This effect was not seen in nonmyasthenic ophthalmoparesis or normal subjects. The use of an open-loop test paradigm was found to increase the sensitivity of this test without significant effect on specificity and did not require individual optimization of the stimulus for each patient.

Not all features of myasthenic eye movements can be ascribed solely to changes in peripheral mechanisms. Because the brain monitors the accuracy of saccades and makes appropriate innervation changes to optimize ocular motor performance, when MG causes paretic saccades, central adaptation is stimulated. Thus, patients with MG often show hypometric large saccades but hypermetric small saccades (81,82,89,100,101). Saccadic hypermetria occurs because the central nervous system has adaptively increased the size of the saccadic pulse in an attempt to overcome the myasthenic weakness. These central changes can be observed and recorded before and after an intravenous injection of edrophonium (Fig. 21.9). After injection, saccade size increases. Many saccades become too large, and occasionally an extreme degree of hypermetria produces continuous, to-and-fro saccadic movements about the target—macrosaccadic oscillations (102). These eye movement abnormalities occur because edrophonium has transiently removed the neuromuscular blockade, exposing the increased saccadic innervation.

The trajectories of saccades made by myasthenic patients are often characteristic of the disorder. For large refixations, the eye may begin rapidly but slow in midflight and slide up to the desired position. This phenomenon is caused by intrasaccadic fatigue of muscle fibers. These fibers cannot

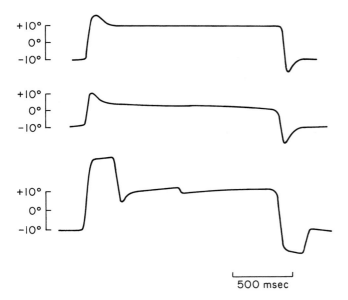

Figure 21.9. Saccadic eye movement abnormalities in myasthenia gravis and their alteration after intravenous injection of edrophonium chloride. *Top,* The saccades are mildly hypermetric in both directions, overshooting the target and drifting back. This occurs because of a discrepancy between the saccadic pulse and the step. *Middle,* After repetitive refixations, fatigue occurs: the saccadic pulse becomes smaller. *Bottom,* After intravenous injection of edrophonium, saccades become markedly hypermetric. (Redrawn from Yee RD, Cogan DG, Zee DS, et al. Rapid eye movements in myasthenia gravis. II. Electro-oculographic analysis. Arch Ophthalmol 1976; 94:1465–1472.)

sustain the vigorous muscle contraction required for the duration of the saccadic pulse. The step of innervation then carries the eye slowly to its final position. The peak velocity of such saccades may be normal, but the duration is prolonged. In fact, patients with little residual ocular motility may seem to make overly fast saccades within their limited range of motion. The peak velocity of these saccades is often greater than would be expected for the size of the saccade. Although central adaptive changes may be partly responsible, similar changes in other types of ocular muscle palsies do not produce super-fast saccades (103,104). A more likely explanation is that the fast-twitch fibers of the agonist muscle, fibers that are relatively inactive and rested during fixation, can begin the saccade with a normal pulse of activity, but fatigue develops rapidly, aborting the pulse. Because the tonic fibers may also become fatigued during the saccade, the eye stops and may even begin to drift backward. When the tonic fibers are completely fatigued, the step is absent. This creates a rapid drift backward—the quiver movement. Peak saccadic velocity may thus be higher than normal for the observed (but not the intended) saccade. Occasionally, a quiver-like movement may be followed by a slow continuation of the saccade. This occurs because a fatigued pulse is followed, after a brief period of electric silence, by either a renewed step from tonic fibers or another corrective saccadic pulse.

Nystagmus

Patients with MG may have involvement of one or both medial rectus muscles, producing a syndrome that mimics a unilateral or bilateral internuclear ophthalmoplegia with abduction nystagmus. Others develop upgaze paresis and convergence-retraction nystagmus that mimics a dorsal midbrain syndrome. However, isolated nystagmus as a sign of MG is rare. Bender (105) stated that myasthenic nystagmus may occur as a unilateral phenomenon without obvious paresis of eye movement. Finelli and Hoyt (106) observed bilateral, sustained, high-frequency abduction nystagmus in a patient with hyperthyroidism but no other clinical or electro-oculographic abnormalities of eye movement. Following intravenous administration of edrophonium, the nystagmus stopped, supporting a diagnosis of MG. Keane and Hoyt (107) observed spontaneous, conjugate, vertical nystagmus in a patient with MG. The nystagmus occurred several seconds after the patient looked upward and was characterized by an upward, slightly torsional fast phase with a rate of 2–3 Hz and a low amplitude. These investigators also noted dissociated horizontal nystagmus that was most marked in the abducting eye after the patient was given an intravenous injection of *d*-tubocurarine.

It seems clear that isolated abduction nystagmus and delayed nystagmus that occurs following a change in gaze may occur as presenting signs of MG. This nystagmus occurs because myasthenic fatigue limits the ability to hold the eye steady after a saccade. Depending on whether the pulse or the step is more affected, the resulting pulse–step mismatch causes a forward or backward postsaccadic drift. Thus, sustained eccentric gaze often brings out nystagmus with slow-phase waveforms that follow a linear or negative exponential time course. This type of nystagmus has been called muscle-paretic nystagmus (82) and probably occurs when the tonic fibers are fatigued. In this setting, the fast-twitch fibers are relatively spared because they discharge vigorously only during saccades or quick phases.

Orbicularis Oculi Involvement

Patients with MG often have involvement of the orbicularis oculi muscles that may not be apparent when ptosis or ophthalmoplegia predominates. The combination of ptosis, ocular motility disturbances, and weakness of the orbicularis oculi is found in only a few disorders, including MG, myotonic dystrophy, oculopharyngeal dystrophy, and mitochondrial myopathy. Of these, MG is the most common. Patients suspected of having MG should therefore have testing of orbicularis oculi strength by having the patient forcefully shut the eyes while the examiner manually attempts to open the eyelids against the forced lid closure. Osher and Griggs (108) described the ''peek'' sign of orbicularis fatigue in patients with MG. In such patients, upon gentle eyelid closure, the orbicularis oculi muscle contracts, initially achieving eyelid apposition; however, the orbicularis muscle rapidly fatigues and the palpebral fissure widens, thereby exposing the sclera. The patient thus appears to ''peek'' at the examiner. A similar phenomenon is probably responsible for ectropion of the lower eyelid that develops as the day progresses in some patients with MG.

Pupillary Function

Although most investigators report no pupillary abnormalities in patients with MG, Baptista and Souza (109) described a patient with generalized MG who had a larger pupil on the side of the more severe ophthalmoplegia. Both pupils showed sluggish responses to light, and both were constricted after injection of neostigmine. Herishanu and Lavy (110) reported a similar patient with ocular MG who had anisocoria and sluggishly reactive pupils that showed fatigue on prolonged light stimulation. Anticholinesterase therapy resulted in complete resolution of pupillary inequality and return of normal pupillary reflexes. Dutton et al. (111) also noted pupillary fatigue during constant light stimulation in eyes of patients with MG. Yamazaki and Ishikawa (112) used an open-loop stimulus and infrared video pupillography to record the velocity and acceleration of pupillary responses to light in seven patients with MG and in three normal subjects. The patients with MG showed reduced velocity and acceleration of pupillary constriction to both light and near stimuli, suggesting that the iris sphincter is commonly involved in MG. Lepore et al. (113) also reported pupillary dysfunction in patients with MG as indicated by abnormalities of pupil cycle times; however, most of these patients were taking anticholinesterase agents, systemic corticosteroids, or both, which may have affected their pupillary movements. In addition, it is not clear whether the pupillary abnormalities observed by Lepore et al. (113) were caused by direct involvement of the iris musculature, the NMJ, or central pathways of the pupillary light reflex. Bryant (114) concluded that patients with more severe MG tend to show significant interocular differences in pupil cycle times, with the degree of difference correlating with the severity of the illness.

The recent identification of a group of patients suffering from autoimmune autonomic neuropathy (AAN) who have antibodies directed against autonomic ganglion nicotinic ACh receptors is of potential relevance to these observations of pupillary abnormalities in patients with MG (115,116). Patients with AAN often show a poorly reactive pupillary light reflex. It is possible that some patients with MG have circulating antibodies that cross-react with the ACh receptors in the ciliary ganglia, leading to impairment of the pupillary light reflex and a partial overlap with the syndrome of AAN, as suggested in a recent study of seven patients with features of both MG and AAN (117).

It seems clear that some degree of pupillary dysfunction can occur in patients with MG; however, in most patients, this dysfunction is not clinically significant and should not confuse the diagnosis. In patients with nonspecific ocular motility disturbances and clinically normal pupillary responses, MG should be strongly considered in the differential diagnosis. Conversely, when ocular motor disturbances occur in the setting of a dilated, poorly reactive pupil, MG should not be considered a likely cause.

Accommodation

Rabinovitch and Vengrjenovsky (118) reported diminished accommodation in patients with MG, and several patients with MG examined by Bonnet (119) demonstrated progressive weakening of accommodation during prolonged convergence. Manson and Stern (120) studied patients with MG and patients with unexplained disturbances of accommodation. Of nine patients with MG, eight had excessive fatigue of accommodation that rapidly improved after an intravenous injection of edrophonium. In addition, 6 of 11 patients with isolated defects in accommodation responded favorably to anticholinesterase agents. Walsh and Hoyt (121) observed a patient with MG and reduced accommodation in whom an intramuscular injection of neostigmine enabled the person to discard 1.5 diopters of hyperopic correction. A patient with seronegative MG was reported to have both atonic bladder and accommodation paresis, indicating involvement of autonomic cholinergic receptors in more than one organ system (122). The patient reportedly had improvement of both problems after thymectomy and corticosteroid therapy, with recurrence of symptoms with tapering of the steroids. These observations of accommodation impairment and other autonomic involvement in patients with MG may be related to overlap of the specificity of the anti-ACh antibodies in MG with the autonomic ganglia nicotinic ACh receptors, and may provide additional evidence of an overlap syndrome with AAN (see above) (115,117).

Most patients with MG who experience difficulties with accommodation have accommodation fatigue with blurring of near vision. However, some have blurring of distant vision from "pseudomyopia" caused by spasm of convergence and accommodation (118,123).

Nonocular Features

In patients with generalized involvement of skeletal muscles, the facies may be characteristic, showing a generalized weakness of expression (Fig. 21.10). Weakness frequently affects the neck extensors (head "ptosis") and proximal limb muscles. When the muscles of expression, phonation, articulation, swallowing, and chewing are affected, there may be a characteristic facial "snarl," dysarthric speech, nasal regurgitation of liquids, and the need to prop the jaw closed. When the muscles of respiration or swallowing are involved, the term "myasthenic crisis" indicates the gravity of the disease. Rarely, MG presents with respiratory insufficiency alone. In some patients, the stapedius muscle is involved, resulting in hyperacusis or a decrease in the intensity of sound required to elicit an acoustic reflex (124). There is usually a history of fluctuation and fatigability (worse with repeated activity, improved by rest). In women, weakness may show a catamenial pattern of worsening in relation to the menstrual cycle (125). If the weakness occurs in a vague and variable pattern, it may be misinterpreted as having a psychogenic origin. Patients may complain of pain in weak muscles, especially in the neck and back and around the eyes, but this complaint may be attributable to the extra effort required to maintain posture and fusion. On physical examination, the findings are limited entirely to the lower

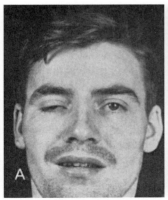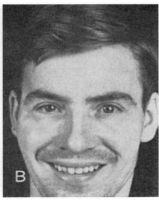

Figure 21.10. Clinical appearance of a patient with myasthenia gravis before and after intramuscular injection of neostigmine methylsulfate (Prostigmin). *A*, Prior to injection there is bilateral ptosis, more marked on the right side, as well as generalized weakness of the facial muscles. The patient had been asked to smile as widely as possible. *B*, Fifteen minutes after intramuscular injection of neostigmine, the patient's ptosis has disappeared and his facial musculature now appears to function normally. (From Mattis RD. Ocular manifestations of myasthenia gravis. Arch Ophthalmol 1941;26:969–982.)

motor unit, without loss of reflexes or altered sensation or coordination.

DIAGNOSTIC TESTING

The tests devised to diagnose MG include clinical tests, assays for circulating antibodies to components of the NMJ, pharmacologic tests, repetitive nerve stimulation, and single-fiber electromyography.

Clinical Tests

Two clinical tests may be helpful in supporting the diagnosis of MG: the sleep test and the ice test. They are particularly useful in elderly or ill patients for whom pharmacologic testing may be considered potentially dangerous.

Sleep Test

As noted earlier, many patients with MG state that when they awaken in the morning, they have little or no ptosis or diplopia, but that these manifestations appear or worsen during the day. Odel et al. (126) studied the effects of a 30-minute period of sleep or rest on 42 patients with edrophonium-positive MG and 26 patients with other causes of ptosis or ophthalmoparesis. After undergoing a complete ocular examination and external photographs, each patient was taken to a quiet, darkened room and instructed to close the eyes and try to sleep. Thirty minutes later, a physician awoke the patient and immediately photographed and measured the patient's palpebral fissures, ocular alignment, and ocular motility. These investigators found that most patients with MG showed marked improvement in ptosis, ocular motor dysfunction, or both immediately upon awakening from

sleep (Fig. 21.11). The improvement lasted 2–5 minutes, following which the ptosis and ophthalmoparesis recurred. Patients with ptosis and ophthalmoparesis caused by disorders other than MG showed no such improvement after sleep. Odel et al. (126) concluded that this sleep test was a safe, moderately sensitive, and specific way to confirm a presumptive diagnosis of MG.

Ice Test

The use of local cooling to eliminate ptosis in patients with possible MG is a rapid, simple, and inexpensive test with a high degree of specificity and sensitivity (127–129). The ice test is particularly useful in patients in whom the use of anticholinesterase agents is contraindicated by either cardiac status or age.

Local cooling from 35°C to 28°C reduces decrement, neuromuscular jitter, and weakness, and all of these effects are reversed on rewarming (130). Significant cooling of the superotemporal cul-de-sac and beneath the lateral rectus muscles has been measured with temperature probes after 5 minutes of local cooling of the orbit as in the ice test (131). Cooling the eyelids with an ice pack improved ptosis in 92% of patients with myasthenia but not in any of 24 control patients with ptosis attributable to oculomotor nerve palsy (15 patients), myopathy (5 patients), or congenital ptosis (4 patients) (127–129). These findings suggest that a positive response to the ice test may be diagnostic for MG. Recent investigators have studied the importance of cooling for the effectiveness of the ice test by comparing cooling to heating of the orbit and have found surprisingly little difference between these two interventions (132). Thus, it has been suggested that the part of the effect of the ice test may be to enforce levator palpebrae rest, although some authors report that adding ice to the same duration of brief rest produces a larger change in lid position (133).

The ice test is performed as follows. The size of the palpebral fissure is measured, photographed, or both. A surgical glove containing crushed ice or ice cubes is then applied to the more involved eyelid for 2 minutes, with the opposite lid serving as a control. After 2 minutes, the glove is removed, and the size of the palpebral fissure is immediately measured or photographed. The test is considered positive if the size of the palpebral fissure is greater after cooling than after the rest period; this difference is usually greater than 2 mm in patients with MG (129). The improvement in ptosis typically lasts less than 1 minute (127).

Specific Autoantibody Assays

A radioimmunoassay using human ACh receptor labeled with [125I] α-bungarotoxin to detect antireceptor antibodies is one of the standard diagnostic tests for MG (27,134). It is positive in about 85% of all patients with MG, in studies combining generalized disease and limited ocular disease. Although the presence of anti-ACh receptor antibodies is quite specific for MG, these antibodies are not detectable in about 15% of all patients subsequently proven to have MG and in no more than 50% of patients with weakness confined to the extraocular muscles (26,27,36). Some assays measure

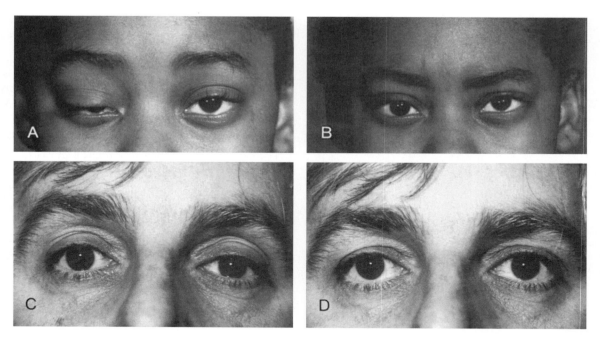

Figure 21.11. The sleep test for myasthenia gravis. *A*, A 10-year-old girl has right ptosis. Note use of the frontalis to help elevate the eyelid. *B*, After 30 minutes of sleep, the ptosis has resolved. The frontalis is no longer contracted. *C*, A 48-year-old man has bilateral symmetric ptosis. *D*, After 30 minutes of sleep, the ptosis has resolved. (From Odel JG, Winterkorn JMS, Behrens MM. The sleep test for myasthenia gravis: A safe alternative to Tensilon. J Clin Neuroophthalmol 1991;11:288–292.)

all antireceptor antibodies, sometimes referred to as binding antibodies; others specifically measure antibodies that produce blocking of the ACh binding site on the receptor or antibodies that accelerate degradation (modulation) of the ACh receptor (135,136). Antibodies that block the ACh binding site are unlikely to be the only positive antibody study because at least some assays for modulating antibodies may detect both blocking and modulating antibodies (136). Because of this overlap, and the fact that 8% of MG patients will have only either binding or modulating antibodies detected, the most productive sequence of testing is to perform the assay for binding anti-ACh antibodies, followed by an assay for modulating antibodies if the binding antibody assay is negative. Some additional patients with MG may have detectable antibodies only when tested in an assay that uses exclusively adult-type ACh receptors containing the ε-subunit, unlike the usual assay that uses muscle cells expressing fetal-type receptors. There is evidence that patients with ocular MG are more likely to produce this adult-type receptor selective antibody (137,138). False-positive results are rare but sometimes occur in patients with amyotrophic lateral sclerosis (139), mitochondrial myopathy (140), and possibly in patients with a history of general anesthesia with muscle paralysis (136). Anti-ACh receptor antibodies were reported in 8% of 50 patients with thyroid ophthalmopathy, who did not develop evidence of clinical MG over mean follow-up of 4.5 years (141).

As noted in the section above on clinical–pathophysiologic correlations, about 40–50% of patients who are seronegative for anti-ACh receptor antibodies, or about 6% of

MG patients overall, will be found to have anti-MuSK antibodies in an immunoprecipitation assay (42). Anti-MuSK antibodies are almost never seen in patients who have anti-ACh receptor antibodies, and vice versa. The usefulness of anti-MuSK antibodies in diagnosing patients with purely ocular manifestations is not yet clear, although many patients with anti-MuSK antibodies are reported to show ophthalmoparesis (43). The incidence of false-positive anti-MuSK antibodies is unknown but probably low.

Pharmacologic Tests

The abnormal fatigability of skeletal muscles may be evaluated by observing or quantifying their strength before and after the injection of anticholinesterase agents. Nearly any objectively quantifiable motor endpoint can be used, such as millimeters of ptosis at rest, timed fatigue of the lids on upgaze, vital capacity, timed swallow of 4 oz of water by straw (the "slurp test," especially useful in children), forward arm abduction time, or the cine-esophagram. Anticholinesterase pharmacologic testing has a sensitivity of about 50–75% in MG. Thus, when MG is strongly suspected, serologic testing is normal or inconclusive, and pharmacologic testing is negative or cannot be performed, patients should undergo more extensive electrophysiologic tests.

Edrophonium Test

Edrophonium (supplied as the chloride or bromide salt) is a rapidly acting and quickly hydrolyzed anticholinesterase (142). It competes with ACh for the enzyme acetylcholinesterase and thus allows prolonged and repetitive action of ACh at the synapse. It is commonly chosen because of the rapid onset (30 sec) and short duration (about 5 min) of its effect.

In patients with ptosis, edrophonium has particular value. An intravenous dose of up to 10 mg is usually used. Once the position of the eyelids is verified, a test dose of 1–2 mg of edrophonium is injected, and the patient is observed carefully for any idiosyncratic reaction (see below) or for improvement in ptosis. If definite improvement occurs, the test is considered positive and is terminated. If no such reactions occur within 30 seconds, additional 1- to 2-mg doses are administered at 30-second intervals, or a single 5-mg bolus can be administered, as the patient is observed (143,144). A positive response is elevation of one or both eyelids, sometimes accompanied by an improvement in facial expression, which lasts not just a few seconds but 2–5 minutes (Fig. 21.12). If no improvement in eyelid position occurs within about 3 minutes of achieving the maximal edrophonium dose, the test is negative. The mean dose required to achieve a diagnostic change in ptosis was 3.3 mg in one study (143). Occasionally, a paradoxical reaction (worsening of ptosis) occurs following administration of edrophonium. This should not be considered a positive response. Similarly, virtually all patients experience transient quivering of the eyelids, lacrimation, and salivation. These responses also do not constitute a positive test.

Edrophonium also may be used in patients without ptosis but with diplopia. Such patients may be tested by having them hold a red glass over one eye (or use red-green glasses), fixate a distant white light, and describe the relative positions of the two lights seen (red and white or green) (145). Edrophonium is then injected, and the patient is asked to describe any change in the position of the two lights. Another option is to use the Lancaster red-green test or the Hess screen to plot the position of the two eyes before and after the injection of edrophonium. This technique provides an extremely accurate determination of eye position (146,147). The alternate prism-cover test can also be used to document the effects of edrophonium on ocular motor balance (143,148), but this test may be better suited to the more prolonged effects of neostigmine (see below). When ocular deviations are used as the endpoint of the edrophonium test, the mean dose necessary to achieve a significant change was 2.6 mg in one recent study (143).

Edrophonium produces an increase in near exophorias of normal subjects and in vertical distance deviations of nonmyasthenic strabismus (148). These changes are clinically insignificant, however, and easily distinguished from the major changes in ocular motility and alignment that constitute a positive edrophonium test.

It is not sufficient simply to ask a patient if his or her diplopia resolves after injection of edrophonium, because patients with diplopia may have a change in ocular alignment without recognizing a corresponding change in diplopia. Thus, a patient with an objectively positive edrophonium

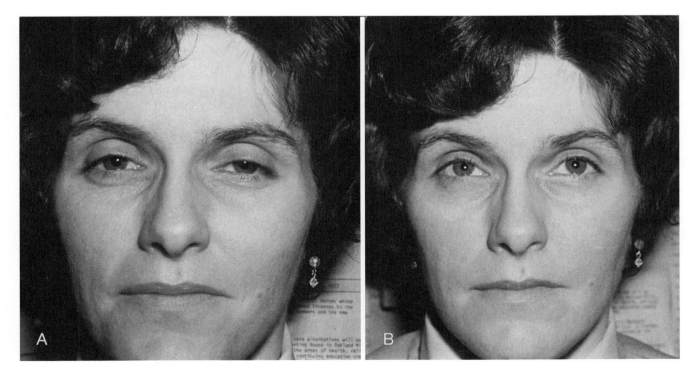

Figure 21.12. The edrophonium test for myasthenia gravis. The patient was a 27-year-old woman with ptosis and intermittent diplopia. *A*, Before injection of edrophonium, the patient has bilateral ptosis and weakness of facial musculature. *B*, One minute following an intravenous injection of 2 mg of edrophonium, the patient's ptosis has disappeared and her facial muscles appear to function more normally.

test may have no subjective awareness that his or her strabismus has improved unless the improvement is substantial.

When ocular motility is minimally affected, a careful study of eye movements before and after intravenous injection of edrophonium may be particularly helpful in diagnosis. Small changes in saccadic accuracy, particularly the development of saccadic hypermetria, suggest MG. Care must be taken, however, not to overinterpret tiny changes in saccade metrics so as to avoid false-positive diagnoses of MG from saccade interpretation; the effect must be obvious and reproducible to be relied upon. Saccadic fatigability during repetitive refixations or optokinetic nystagmus, which is reversed by edrophonium, is also a useful sign (81,85,91–95, 149–152). As described above, quantitative measurement of the amplitude of optokinetic nystagmus before and after edrophonium administration provides a very sensitive and specific test for myasthenic ophthalmoparesis (97).

Because edrophonium is a peripheral anticholinesterase agent, it allows ACh to accumulate briefly in ganglia, at parasympathetic nerve endings, and at NMJs in all types of muscle: cardiac, smooth, and striated. It is the transient excess of ACh at nicotinic synapses that produces a positive test in patients with MG, but this same excess also may produce muscarinic cholinergic side effects from a brief overstimulation of the parasympathetic nervous system. Although the original description of this test by Osserman and Kaplan (153) included no report of any complications, Van Dyk and Florence (154) accumulated a list of side effects by conducting a telephone survey of 25 neuro-ophthalmologists. Three instances of severe, untoward reactions were reported. A 50-year-old man became faint and then unresponsive about 1 minute after edrophonium was injected. His pupils dilated, and no radial or precordial pulse could be obtained. Cardiopulmonary resuscitation was begun, and the patient was revived without difficulty and without any permanent sequelae. A single case of bradycardia with symptomatic hypotension also was reported, as was a case of loss of consciousness and apnea. Ing et al. reported the results of a survey of 357 members of the North American Neuro-Ophthalmology Society about their experience with edrophonium testing (155). The 199 responders had performed at least 23,111 edrophonium tests and reported 37 serious reactions, an estimated rate of 0.16%. Most of these major adverse events involved syncope, convulsive syncope, or other manifestations of bradycardia. The respondents also reported respiratory failure, generalized seizure, severe vomiting, and transient ischemic attack as severe adverse reactions. A case of asystole has been reported after edrophonium administration in a patient with beta-blockade (156). In addition to these major reactions, less severe side effects of edrophonium testing include near-syncope, dizziness, and involuntary defecation. Although most side effects associated with the edrophonium test can probably be prevented by pretreating patients with an intramuscular injection of atropine sulfate, such reactions are rare. Accordingly, it is not necessary to pretreat with atropine, but it is prudent always to have the drug available during the test. In addition, great caution should be used in performing edrophonium (or neostigmine) tests in older patients, particularly those with

known cardiac disease. Instead, the clinician may depend on the results of other features of the presentation, or the results of an ice or sleep test (see above) to direct a further diagnostic evaluation. Should it be necessary to perform a edrophonium test in a patient with cardiac disease, the patient should always have an intravenous line in place and be hooked up to an electrocardiograph machine, in an environment with advanced cardiac life support immediately available.

A positive edrophonium test is usually, but not always, indicative of MG. No reliable quantitative estimates of the specificity of the test are available (157), but the specificity is believed to be fairly high. On rare occasions, patients with intracranial lesions producing pupil-sparing oculomotor nerve palsies and other ocular motor disorders may show transient improvement of their findings when tested with edrophonium. Intracranial disorders reported to produce a false-positive edrophonium response include brain stem glioma (158,159), pineal region tumor (160), parasellar tumor or aneurysm (161), and parasellar schwannoma (162). Some of these patients may have had both MG and an intracranial lesion. In others, however, there was no other evidence of MG, and the response to edrophonium was thought to be falsely positive. For this reason, it is advisable to perform neuroimaging in all patients with isolated, unilateral, pupil-sparing ophthalmoparesis and in selected patients with other ocular muscle pareses, even when the diagnosis of MG seems certain. Other neuromuscular disorders may produce a positive edrophonium test, including Lambert-Eaton myasthenic syndrome (163–165), botulism (166–169), some congenital myasthenic syndromes (170), snake envenomation by cobras (171) or death adders (172), Guillain-Barré syndrome (173), amyotrophic lateral sclerosis (174), and post-poliomyelitis syndrome (175).

A negative edrophonium test in no way rules out MG. The sensitivity of the test in patients with generalized MG has been estimated at 73–96% (143,157). In ocular MG, the sensitivity has been estimated at 60–95% (157). Most experienced neuro-ophthalmologists have seen patients in whom several edrophonium tests were unequivocally negative but who had other evidence of MG. Patients may have several negative edrophonium tests before a positive edrophonium test is observed. In patients suspected of having MG, a negative edrophonium test should be followed either by a neostigmine test or by other nonocular diagnostic tests (see later).

Neostigmine Test

Because of the transient nature of the ocular (and systemic) changes in muscle strength that occur following the administration of edrophonium, the neostigmine bromide test remains an exceptionally valuable method of diagnosing MG, particularly in patients with diplopia but without ptosis. The longer duration of the effects of this drug is sufficient to permit repeated testing of muscle strength and evaluation of ocular motility (176). In adults with obvious ptosis and ophthalmoparesis, it is appropriate to mix 0.6 mg of atropine sulfate with 0.5–1.5 mg of neostigmine in a 3-cc syringe and inject the mixture into one of the deltoid muscles. A change in ocular motility and ptosis is usually apparent within 15 minutes and is most obvious 30 minutes following the injection (Figs. 21.10 and 21.13). When there is only minor ophthalmoparesis, one option is to perform quantitative measurements of ocular motility before and after neostigmine injection (177). This procedure involves performing prism-cover testing in primary position at distance and near and in the cardinal positions of gaze. Another aspect of this test is to measure the extent of ductions for the cardinal positions of gaze. These measurements are repeated 30–45 minutes following the intramuscular injection of neostigmine. The extent of the difference between preinjection and postinjection measurements determines whether the test is positive or negative. This approach allowed correct diagnosis of 70% of patients studied (177). A recent study reported that 93.8% of patients with MG showed a diagnostic response to neostigmine, with similar sensitivity in patients with generalized and ocular MG (178). The specificity of the neostigmine test has apparently not been quantitatively studied.

The neostigmine test may be particularly helpful in the diagnosis of MG in children, in whom intravenous injection of edrophonium may be accompanied by crying and lack of cooperation, precluding any meaningful assessment of its effect (179). In such patients, neostigmine may be injected, and by the time the neostigmine takes effect, the child usually has stopped crying and can be observed and the eye movements measured if necessary. In children, the amount of neostigmine given is related to body weight and is 0.025–0.04 mg/kg, not exceeding a total dose of 1.5 mg (the adult dose). The dose of atropine in children is adjusted to 0.011 mg/kg, up to a maximum of 0.4 mg (180).

Adverse effects of neostigmine testing include bradycardia, syncope, near-syncope, and paradoxical tachycardia (especially at low doses). The combined muscarinic autonomic effects of neostigmine and atropine are often not completely balanced, and if neostigmine predominates, the patient may transiently experience increased salivation, tearing, borborygmi, and the urge to defecate or urinate. Atropine predominance produces dry mouth, tachycardia, and so forth. The

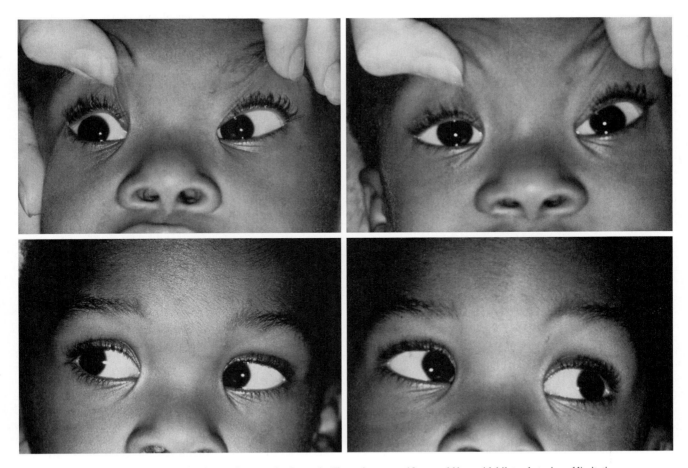

Figure 21.13. The neostigmine test for myasthenia gravis. The patient was a 10-year-old boy with bilateral ptosis and limitation of eye movements. *Top left,* The patient has moderate limitation of eye movement on attempted right horizontal gaze. His eyelids are being manually elevated because of his ptosis. *Top right,* There is almost no horizontal eye movement on attempted left lateral gaze. *Bottom,* Thirty minutes after intramuscular injection of neostigmine, the child's ptosis has resolved. Horizontal eye movements to the right (*bottom left*) and left (*bottom right*) are almost normal.

relative balance of these competing effects may change over time during the test period. In addition, fasciculations are almost always induced in normal subjects as well as myasthenic patients by the administration of neostigmine (181). Fasciculations are a useful marker of neostigmine pharmacologic effect and are not blocked by atropine.

As with edrophonium, a positive neostigmine test usually, but not always, indicates MG. Walsh and Hoyt (182) observed a positive response to neostigmine in one patient with multiple sclerosis, in another patient with a brain stem tumor, and in a third patient with congenital ptosis. In the patient with congenital ptosis, the eyelid elevated almost fully on one occasion following an intramuscular neostigmine injection, but subsequent injections had no effect. Isolated, nonreproducible positive neostigmine tests may thus occur in nonmyasthenic persons.

Electrophysiologic Tests

Repetitive nerve stimulation has long been used to diagnose MG. In recent years, however, single-fiber electromyography has been shown to be a much more sensitive and specific technique.

Repetitive Nerve Stimulation

The primary technique used by most clinical electrophysiologists in the diagnosis of MG consists of eliciting a decremental response between the first and fourth or fifth response to repetitive supramaximal motor nerve stimulation (Fig. 21.14). Supramaximal electric stimuli are delivered at a rate of 2–3 Hz to the appropriate nerves, and compound muscle action potentials are recorded from muscles. A decrement in amplitude of 10% or more is usually considered abnormal (183,184). The sensitivity of repetitive nerve stimulation in diagnosing generalized MG has been reported to vary from 51% to as much as 100%, depending on the technique used and the severity of myasthenia in sampled patients (145,185,186). Özdemir and Young (184) tested 80 selected

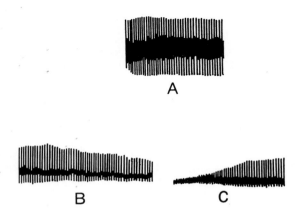

Figure 21.14. Drawing of the results of an electromyogram during repetitive nerve stimulation in a normal subject (*A*), in a patient with myasthenia gravis (*B*), and in a patient with the Lambert-Eaton myasthenic syndrome (*C*). Note the decremental response in myasthenia gravis and the facilitation response in the myasthenic syndrome.

patients with MG with this technique and were able to document the diagnosis in 95% of the patients, providing that several clinically weak muscles, including a proximal one such as the deltoid, were studied. Study of patients with more severe disease increases the likelihood of a positive test. The sensitivity of repetitive nerve stimulation in patients with ocular MG is much lower, 10–17% (186,187). The study of facial muscles such as orbicularis oculi (188) or nasalis (189) has been reported to produce an increased yield over extremity muscles, especially in patients with ocular MG. Technical factors in the performance of repetitive nerve stimulation may increase the likelihood of false-negative responses. These include the temperature in the extremity muscles (130,190,191) and the eyelid (130). Cessation of acetylcholinesterase-inhibiting medicines at least 12 hours before the test is important to maximize sensitivity (188,192). The specificity of repetitive nerve stimulation test has not been formally assessed. Decremental responses are not pathognomonic of MG, because low-level decrement may be seen in other disorders, including Lambert-Eaton myasthenic syndrome, amyotrophic lateral sclerosis (174), and polymyositis, as well as X-linked spinal and bulbar muscular atrophy (193). The relatively low sensitivity of the test implies that a normal test does not exclude MG.

Single-Fiber Electromyography

Endplate potentials in the postsynaptic membrane of the NMJ reach the threshold for triggering an action potential of the muscle fiber with random variability, and this results in a variable latency between a nerve stimulus and the action potential of the responding muscle fiber. The latencies of responses of fibers belonging to the same motor unit are therefore not quite synchronous. The variability between any fiber and a reference fiber from the same unit is called "jitter." When the safety factor for transmission is low, these latency variabilities (jitters) are increased. There are also more response failures ("blocking"), in which an action potential of the muscle fiber is not triggered by arrival of a nerve terminal action potential. Both blocking and jitter are worsened by exercising or heating the muscle. Jitter and blocking can be detected in human muscles using suitably selective electrodes, and the latencies can be studied statistically during either voluntary contraction (194) or indirect stimulation (195) in a technique called collectively single-fiber electromyography (single-fiber EMG). In patients undergoing evaluation for MG who are antibody-negative and in whom repetitive nerve stimulation is negative or equivocal, single-fiber EMG is an extremely useful diagnostic test. In a study of single-fiber EMG and repetitive nerve stimulation of the same muscles, Gilchrist et al. (196) found that a significant decrement of the response to repetitive nerve stimulation was never found without increased jitter and blocking in the same muscle, and concluded that these two test abnormalities result from the same physiologic phenomenon. On the basis of similar results, another interpretation of the physiology was proposed, based on the effects of the different rates of stimulation of the motor endplates in 3-Hz repetitive stimulation and voluntarily activated single-fiber EMG (197). The single-fiber EMG was more sensitive to the presence of the disordered NMJ function in each muscle.

An experienced electrophysiologist is required to perform single-fiber EMG and should perform the technique regularly to maintain the appropriate skills. Single-fiber EMG is a highly sensitive test. It is positive in 88–99% of all patients with MG (185,198,199). In generalized MG, the sensitivity of repetitive nerve stimulation is high, about that of anti-ACh receptor antibody, and the sensitivity of single-fiber EMG is highest (more than 95%) (198). Like the edrophonium and neostigmine tests, however, single-fiber EMG may be negative initially only to be positive several months later. Thus, a negative single-fiber EMG test in a muscle with normal strength is not absolute evidence that the patient does not have MG. However, if a clinically weak muscle has normal jitter at all endplates, the diagnosis of MG can be excluded (185,194,200).

In known ocular MG, defined by positive ACh receptor antibody or clinical response to acetylcholinesterase inhibitors, the sensitivity of repetitive nerve stimulation is low, even in facial muscles (187), whereas the sensitivity of single-fiber EMG is higher, especially in the frontalis or orbicularis oculi muscles, where it may be as high as 62–100% (187,201). In patients with suspected ocular MG but without positive antibodies or response to cholinesterase inhibitors, the rate of positive single-fiber EMG is lower, 21% in one series (187). In patients determined by clinical criteria to have ocular MG, the absence of abnormal single-fiber EMG in the extensor digitorum communis of the forearm was associated with a higher probability (82%) of continuing with restricted ocular disease without generalization, over a mean follow-up period of 55 months, than those with abnormal results (42%) (202). Single-fiber EMG in extraocular muscles is rarely performed clinically but has very high sensitivity for ocular MG (201).

Single-fiber EMG abnormalities are frequently seen in other disorders of neuromuscular transmission, including the Lambert-Eaton myasthenic syndrome, congenital myasthenic syndromes, and botulism. Increased jitter may have causes other than defective neuromuscular transmission, such as denervation of many causes (203), amyotrophic lateral sclerosis (204), mitochondrial cytopathy, and oculopharyngeal dystrophy (205), and the results are considered positive only in the context of normal fiber density and routine EMG.

Additional Tests

Because a thymic tumor is found in about 10% of patients with MG, the evaluation of a patient with suspected or proven MG should include imaging of the anterior mediastinum (206). Both computed tomography (CT) and magnetic resonance imaging (MRI) have greater sensitivity than plain radiographs, whose sensitivity is 58% for thymoma in patients with MG (207). Plain radiographs should no longer be used alone to detect thymoma in patients with MG. A recent study showed that helical CT of the chest with intravenous contrast in patients with MG had 88.5% sensitivity

for thymoma and 77% specificity (208). Other studies have placed the specificity of a normal nonhelical CT as high as 98.7% (207). The ability of chest CT to distinguish thymoma from benign thymic hyperplasia may be limited (209,210). Some patients with MG have no evidence of thymoma on initial chest CT but develop evidence of thymoma when repeat scanning is done at 1–2 years (208). CT features of a mass with lobulated or irregular contours, multiple foci of calcification, and areas of low attenuation suggest invasive thymoma (211). MRI with cardiac gated images is capable of detecting about the same percentage of thymomas in patients with MG (212). Dynamic MRI imaging with bolus contrast injection showed sensitivity of 79% and specificity of 84% for thymoma in a recent study (213). The longer scanning time and breathhold for chest MRI compared to helical CT may be a limitation in some patients by producing movement artifacts. MRI is useful in distinguishing invasive thymoma from noninvasive tumors due to its ability to show the relationships of the tumor to adjacent anatomic structures (208,210,214). In patients demonstrated to have a likely thymoma by CT scanning, MRI may provide evidence of invasion of adjacent tissues, which is useful for surgical planning and decisions about preoperative treatment such as radiotherapy or chemotherapy. A useful clinical approach would be to use chest CT scanning for detection of likely thymoma in patients with suspected or known MG, followed by chest MRI in those who show evidence of thymic enlargement or mass. Radionuclide imaging studies such as thallium-201 single photon emission computed tomography (215), indium-111-labeled octreotide imaging (216), and 2-fluoro-18-deoxyglucose positron emission tomography (217,218) have been shown to demonstrate the presence of thymomas reliably. The lack of detailed anatomic information in these radionuclide studies has limited their usefulness in the screening of patients with MG and the preoperative evaluation of patients with suspected thymoma. However, these studies may have value in evaluating patients with suspected recurrence of thymoma after resection.

Antibodies to striated muscle membrane and other components are known to be associated with the presence of thymoma (219) and are present in about 75% of MG patients with thymoma (220). The antigens involved in this reactivity to striated muscle sections have been determined to include the ryanodine receptor, a calcium ion release channel of the sarcoplasmic reticulum (221), and titin, a very large filamentous structural protein of the muscle fiber (222). A study of cortical thymoma tissue showed that it expresses ryanodine receptor and titin epitopes along with costimulatory molecules on thymoma antigen-presenting cells. This suggests that there is autosensitization to these epitopes in patients with thymoma, leading to production of the corresponding antibodies (223). A similar mechanism has been postulated to account for autosensitization to the ACh receptor in patients with thymoma. There is no evidence that these anti-ryanodine receptor or anti-titin antibodies are involved in the clinical pathogenesis of MG, even though there is some electrophysiologic evidence of a disruption of excitation–contraction coupling in affected muscles, and titin binding correlates somewhat with myopathic features in patients with MG (224). Ryanodine receptor antibodies are present in 70% of MG patients with thymoma, compared to only 14% of such patients without thymoma. Titin antibodies are present in 95% of MG patients with thymoma, contrasted to 34% of those patients without thymoma (220). Another study found titin antibodies in 94% of MG patients with thymoma but only in 3% of such patients without thymoma (225). The specificity of ryanodine receptor antibodies for the detection of thymoma in MG patients is 70%, and the specificity of titin antibodies for this purpose is only 39%, using the data of reference (220). Among MG patients without thymoma, those with onset of disease later than 60 years have a similar incidence of anti-titin antibodies as patients with thymoma (226). Taken together, the data suggest that these antibody tests, including the original anti-striated muscle antibody test, are not very useful for the detection or exclusion of thymoma when each is used alone, and even in combination add only limited additional information to the results of imaging.

A complete blood count, erythrocyte sedimentation rate, antinuclear antibody test, and thyroid function tests should be performed in all patients diagnosed with MG because of the increased prevalence of other autoimmune diseases in these patients. Any patient who may be a candidate for corticosteroid treatment should be screened for diabetes mellitus, and all patients should undergo a skin test for tuberculosis prior to institution of chronic immunosuppression.

DISORDERS ASSOCIATED WITH MYASTHENIA GRAVIS

Patients with MG have a higher prevalence of other autoimmune disorders than otherwise normal persons, about 14% in a Danish cohort (227) and 15% in a Dutch patient series (228). Disorders of the thyroid gland, including subclinical disease indicated by serum antibody studies, are more common in a myasthenic population than in a normal population. Such patients are as commonly hypothyroid as hyperthyroid (229–234). Millikan and Haines (235) found that the incidence of hyperthyroidism before, during, and after detectable MG is about 5%. If all thyroid disorders are considered, the prevalence may be as high as 9% in males and 18% in females (46,236). Many of these patients have dysthyroid symptoms that precede myasthenic symptoms by months or years. In other cases, dysthyroid symptoms may be subsiding when symptoms and signs of MG first appear, and vice versa. The linkage between them appears to be the genetic and other factors predisposing to autoimmunity (237). All diseases of the thyroid gland are overrepresented, including nontoxic goiter (46,238–240), spontaneous myxedema (241,242), Hashimoto's disease (47,243–247), Graves' disease, and thyroid carcinoma (248). A particularly difficult clinical issue relates to the infrequent coexistence of thyroid ophthalmopathy and ocular manifestations of MG (249). The mechanism of this association remains uncertain, but there may be an immunologic cross-reaction to shared epitopes of the target tissues in the orbital muscles (250,251). Thyroid ophthalmopathy has been reported to be present in about 60% of patients with Graves' disease, whether or not

MG is also known to be present (251). Anti-ACh receptor antibodies have been found in 8% of patients with thyroid ophthalmopathy, although none of these patients showed clinical signs of MG over median follow-up of 4.5 years (141). The incidence of clinical MG in patients with thyroid ophthalmopathy has been estimated to be less than 1% (252–254). On the other hand, the incidence of exophthalmos in patients with MG has been reported to be as high as 23% in a Japanese series, with thyrotropin inhibitory immunoglobulin present in 19% (255). In the case of coexistence of these two ocular motor disorders, the presence of exotropia has been suggested to be a myasthenic feature much more likely than a thyroid ophthalmopathy feature (256). When a patient with thyroid ophthalmopathy develops ptosis, orbicularis oculi weakness, exotropia, or new ocular deviations after a period of stability, the possibility of coexisting MG should always be considered. Similarly, if a patient with MG develops proptosis, lid retraction, hypotropia with infraorbital edema, chemosis, or superficial ocular irritation, the development of thyroid ophthalmopathy should be suspected. In treating such overlap patients, efforts must be made to delineate the contribution of each underlying ocular motor disorder to the patient's clinical status, and the appropriate therapy given specific to the effects of each disorder. The relative contribution of each disorder to the patient's problems may evolve over time. It has been well documented that the clinical features of MG tend to become milder and easier to control with acetylcholinesterase inhibitors when coexisting hyperthyroidism is effectively treated, although there are reported exceptions (257–259).

Other autoimmune disorders also occur more commonly in patients with MG than in the normal population. Rheumatoid arthritis and ankylosing spondylitis are common in patients with MG and their relatives (47,244,260–262). Aplastic anemia associated with a thymic tumor can occur in patients with MG (47,263), as can pure red cell aplasia (264) and pernicious anemia (265,266). Other immune-mediated disorders occasionally associated (individually and familially) with MG are systemic lupus erythematosus (47,262, 267–272), pemphigus vulgaris (269,273–275), ulcerative colitis (268,276), sarcoidosis (47,236,277), Sjögren's syndrome (236,244,278), type I diabetes mellitus (47,279), scleroderma (280,281), mixed connective tissue disease (282), dermatomyositis (283,284), polymyositis (285), stiff person syndrome (286), autoimmune neuromyotonia due to voltage-gated potassium channel antibodies (287), Lambert-Eaton myasthenic syndrome due to voltage-gated calcium channel antibodies (288), recurrent transverse myelitis (289), multiple sclerosis (290,291), idiopathic thrombocytopenia purpura (292), psoriasis (293), vitiligo (294), antiglomerular basement membrane glomerulonephritis (295), interstitial pneumonitis (296), primary ovarian failure (297–299), and autoimmune hepatitis (47,300). Primary adrenal insufficiency of the autoimmune type is another rare association (301,302).

Other associated disorders that may relate to immune system dysfunction in patients with MG include acrocyanosis, heterozygous C2 deficiency (303), autoimmune hemolytic anemia (304), nephritis (47,260), the reticuloses

(47,305–307), Satoyoshi's syndrome (308), herpes zoster, Kaposi's sarcoma (309), HTLV-1-associated myelopathy (310), alopecia totalis (311), autoimmune deafness (312), chronic graft-versus-host disease (313,314), antiphospholipid syndrome (315), anticardiolipin antibodies (316), MALT lymphoma (317), and lymphoid tumor of the orbit (318).

LOCALIZED OR OCULAR MYASTHENIA

Although 50–75% of patients with MG initially present with so-called "ocular MG," with only ptosis, diplopia, or both, 53–85% of these patients eventually develop other signs and symptoms of "clinically generalized MG," including proximal muscle weakness, difficulty with speech, and difficulty swallowing (53,143,319–325). Thus, only a remainder of 15–47% of patients whose manifestations remain localized to the eyelids and extraocular muscles continue to have ocular MG. The percentage of patients with only ocular manifestations at onset who go on to develop systemic manifestations within 2 years is 43–87% (202,319, 320,326,327). Grob (328) estimated from his well-analyzed, large experience that when the disease had remained localized for a year from onset, the likelihood of remaining localized was 84%. Age and sex are not reliable indicators of the risk of progression of disease. The presence of positive anti-ACh receptor antibodies may increase the risk of generalization (323). The absence of single-fiber EMG abnormalities in limb muscles has been associated with a reduced risk of progression to clinically generalized MG, but the presence of such abnormalities does not significantly increase the risk of generalization over the baseline likelihood (202).

Spontaneous remission of symptoms lasting variable durations may occur in ocular MG in about 20% of patients, usually during the first year of the disease (244,321,329). Remissions may be permanent, but relapses may occur after 1 or more years of remission and may cause progressive worsening of symptoms. Rollinson and Fenichel (330) described three patients with ocular MG with childhood onset who experienced complete and prolonged remissions lasting 4–14 years and then experienced recurrences of their ocular MG. One patient had a second spontaneous remission followed by another relapse. There is evidence from several retrospective studies that the administration of immunosuppressive treatment to patients with ocular MG can reduce the frequency of progression to clinical generalization (143,323–325,331,332) by 50–75%. The need for a controlled study of the effect of immunosuppressive treatment on the risk of generalization has been recognized (331,333).

TREATMENT

Most patients with MG can lead full and productive lives with proper therapy. Treatment includes cholinesterase inhibitors, thymectomy, immunosuppressive drugs, and, for selected patients with ocular manifestations, local therapy.

Cholinesterase Inhibitors

Anticholinesterase agents are the primary symptomatic therapy for patients with MG. These drugs prolong the action of ACh by slowing its degradation at the NMJ, thereby enhancing neuromuscular transmission. Although many patients experience some benefit from anticholinesterase agents, the response is often incomplete, particularly in patients with ocular manifestations, necessitating additional therapy (discussed later). Anticholinesterase drugs, unlike immunosuppressive regimens, do not alter the natural history or likelihood of progression of MG to generalized disease.

Mestinon (pyridostigmine bromide) is the most widely used anticholinesterase agent. Its onset of action occurs within 30 minutes and peaks at 1–2 hours. The usual starting dose is one tablet (60 mg) taken orally every 3–4 hours. Doses higher than 120 mg given five or six times daily are not often useful. A sustained-release anticholinesterase preparation, Mestinon Timespan 180 mg, is available, but because of its irregular absorption, it should be used only for night-time dosing in patients who have weakness during the night or upon awakening.

Anticholinesterases are safe, well-tolerated drugs, although they should be used with caution in patients with asthma or cardiac conduction defects. The most common side effects are diarrhea and abdominal cramping, which are dose-related and can be controlled with diphenoxylate or loperamide once or twice a day. It would appear that many physicians who treat patients with pyridostigmine are unaware of these side effects or their treatment; experienced clinicians frequently encounter patients who believe that they are "allergic" to pyridostigmine because they developed diarrhea or other gastrointestinal side effects during therapy, and their physicians discontinued the drug without attempting to treat these side effects. Other symptoms of cholinergic excess are tearing, sialorrhea, and fasciculations. Muscarinic symptoms such as tearing and increased salivation usually do not interfere with treatment and may respond to judicious use of selective muscarinic anticholinergic agents such as propantheline bromide, oxybutynin chloride, or hyoscyamine sulfate. Fasciculations are not reduced by muscarinic anticholinergic medications. Excessive anticholinesterase administration may cause increased weakness that is reversible after decreasing or discontinuing the drug.

Thymectomy

The data for the efficacy of thymectomy come from retrospective, uncontrolled experience, but a multicenter, randomized, controlled trial of thymectomy is being organized to address the many residual questions about this treatment (334,335). Thymectomy is usually recommended for patients with MG in two settings. First, patients with clinically generalized MG between puberty and 50 years of age may benefit from thymectomy (336). Thymectomy results in clinical improvement in about 85% of such patients, with drug-free remission in up to 35% and reduced medication requirements in up to 50% (337). The benefit from thymectomy is delayed, however, rarely occurring within 6 months and usually requiring 2–5 years for demonstrated efficacy (337–339). The surgery is more difficult in older patients, and such patients are less likely to improve after thymectomy. Because of involution, no significant thymic tissue remains beyond middle age. Second, thymectomy should be performed in any patient with a thymoma, regardless of age, because these tumors may spread locally and become invasive, even though they rarely metastasize. The use of thymectomy in patients with purely ocular disease is controversial and currently not often undertaken (340). The small, uncontrolled series of patients with ocular MG treated by thymectomy have usually included high numbers of patients also taking immunosuppressive medicines (323, 341–343), so evaluation of the effect of thymectomy in inducing remission is confounded. Similar problems produce difficulty in interpreting the results of thymectomy for prevention of generalization of ocular MG. A controlled trial of thymectomy in ocular MG, compared to immunosuppressive drug therapy, would be desirable. When both thymectomy and immunosuppressive medications are to be used to treat a patient with MG, thymectomy is usually performed before placing the patient on medication. This avoids poor wound healing as well as the potential increased risk of postoperative infection related to immunosuppression. If immunosuppressive therapy after thymectomy is indicated, it is generally begun 2–6 weeks postoperatively for prednisone or 1–2 weeks postoperatively for azathioprine.

A number of different approaches can be used to perform a thymectomy, including a median sternotomy and limited transcervical or transcervical endoscopic approaches (344). A trans-sternal approach is still preferred by most centers, however, because this permits dissection and removal of all thymus tissue, which can extend throughout the mediastinum from the diaphragm to the neck (345,346). This is particularly true in cases of thymoma, which can spread throughout the thoracic cavity. If thymomatous tissue cannot be completely excised, nonferromagnetic clips should be placed at the site of remaining tumor and postoperative radiotherapy administered.

The risks of surgery include injury to the phrenic or recurrent laryngeal nerves, atelectasis, pleural effusion, pneumonia, myasthenic crisis, intercurrent pulmonary embolism, impaired wound healing, and late sternal instability (347). Therefore, thymectomy should always be performed in an institution where this procedure is performed expertly and regularly, and where the staff is experienced in the anesthetic care and the pre- and postoperative management of MG.

Immunosuppressive Drugs

Immunosuppressive pharmacologic treatment intended to induce a clinical remission is desirable in most patients with MG, including patients with ocular MG. Options include several drugs that provide chronic immunosuppression: prednisone, azathioprine, cyclosporine, and mycophenolate mofetil. The choice among them is made by considering three factors: (a) how the toxicity profile fits the patient; (b) how quickly the patient must improve; and unfortunately (c) the patient's financial ability to afford long-term treatment.

Common errors in therapy include not immunosuppressing patients aggressively enough, not treating long enough, and treating without adequate management of side effects or infections. In such cases, the predictably poor outcomes may convince both the patient and his or her physician that a particular drug is either ineffective or too dangerous to continue when, in fact, this is not the case.

Before immunosuppression is begun, the patient's history of tuberculosis exposure should be obtained and a tuberculin skin test performed. Tuberculosis complicating immunosuppressive therapy of MG is not common, although detailed studies have not been published. Some studies are available that describe the risk of tuberculosis in patients who are immunosuppressed after organ transplantation (348–350). In that posttransplant setting, with intensive immunosuppression, the incidence of clinical tuberculosis is low. These considerations suggest that if the patient has a positive skin test reaction and is a recent tuberculin convertor or has had recent contact with an untreated patient with tuberculosis, empiric prophylaxis against tuberculosis might be given concurrent with immunosuppressive treatment. Another alternative in such a patient is to use other immunomodulatory therapies for MG, such as maintenance plasmapheresis or human immune globulin therapy, which might have a lower risk of reactivating tuberculosis. The risk of reactivation of tuberculosis in a tuberculin reactor of unknown duration, without recent exposure, is probably low, and the need for concurrent antituberculous treatment in that setting is unclear.

Corticosteroids

Long-term, alternate-day treatment with systemic corticosteroids has been the mainstay of MG therapy since the 1970s (351–355). Corticosteroids are indicated when MG symptoms are insufficiently controlled by anticholinesterase agents and are sufficiently disabling to the patient that the frequent side effects of these drugs are worth the risk. "Sufficient control" is best defined functionally for each individual patient. For example, some patients are willing to live with moderate generalized weakness or to patch one eye to eliminate diplopia, whereas for others, even mild ptosis or diplopia is intolerable. Corticosteroids can produce improvement in patients with all degrees of weakness, from diplopia to severe respiratory involvement. Diplopia, which is rarely corrected by anticholinesterase agents alone, usually responds well to steroid treatment. Older men with MG seem to respond particularly well to steroid therapy (356). Steroids may also improve overall results following removal of a thymoma, probably because of their lympholytic effects (357,358).

More than 80% of patients with MG can be expected to improve with steroid treatment alone (359,360). Improvement usually begins within 2–3 weeks after beginning treatment, although maximum benefit may not occur for up to 6 months or more.

Patients with moderate to severe generalized weakness or significant respiratory insufficiency or bulbar weakness are at risk of a transient steroid-induced exacerbation and should be admitted to the hospital for initiation of steroid therapy and observation. Nearly 50% of such patients have an exacerbation, which lasts days and occurs most commonly during the second 5 days of induction (360). This precaution generally is not necessary for patients with ocular MG. The cause of this initial steroid-induced deterioration is not clear. In patients with generalized MG, some authors prefer a gradually increasing schedule because larger initial doses may exacerbate weakness (351). In these patients with generalized MG, prednisone is begun at a dosage of 15–20 mg/day and is increased gradually by about 5 mg every 2 or 3 days until the patient reaches a satisfactory clinical response or reaches the level of 60 mg/day. There is little rationale for gradual introduction in patients with ocular MG, given the low risk of major transient worsening, and prednisone can be started at the total expected effective dosage of 40–60 mg/day. Prednisolone is chosen only if a problem in the hepatic metabolism of prednisone to prednisolone is known or suspected.

Once a patient receiving daily prednisone experiences a clinical response to the medication, the dosage is kept constant until the improvement levels off or 3 months, whichever comes first. The same total dose is then maintained but the dosage schedule is gradually changed to an alternate-day regimen. When the patient reaches a plateau of improvement on an alternate-day regimen, the total dosage is tapered gradually to seek the smallest effective dosage. The goal is not to eliminate all medication, because steroid treatment must be continued indefinitely in 64–90% of patients. In other words, the goal for most patients is not a drug-free remission but a stable, pharmacologically maintained remission, using the lowest dose of medication possible (228).

Some patients should be considered candidates for forms of immunotherapy other than systemic corticosteroids, such as azathioprine, cyclosporine, mycophenolate mofetil, or thymectomy if not already performed. These include patients who have an exacerbation when prednisone is slowly tapered, patients who fail to respond to prednisone, patients who require more than 40–50 mg/day of prednisone, and patients in whom the toxicity of prednisone exceeds its benefit.

Physicians must make their patients familiar with the unfortunately long list of side effects of chronic steroid therapy and of their potential seriousness. Of course, not every patient will develop every symptom, but most patients will have some side effects. Almost every patient will gain weight and develop part of the cushingoid habitus. Fortunately, many of the side effects can be minimized with alternate-day dosing and scrupulous attention to follow-up. Patients should undergo routine monitoring of weight, blood pressure, fasting blood glucose, and electrolytes. Much of the toxicity caused by prednisone can also be prevented by early intervention. For example, preventative treatment of osteoporosis, especially in postmenopausal women, includes exercise, calcium supplements (1,500 mg/day, monitoring 24-hour urinary calcium), vitamin D (400–800 IU/day, monitoring serum vitamin D levels), and replacement of gonadal hormones. Use of calcitonin or etidronate should be considered in patients who develop steroid osteopenia (detected by monitoring baseline and follow-up quantitative bone mineral densitometry) or fractures (361). Obesity, hypertension, and diabetes mellitus can be prevented or at least identified early

by monitoring caloric intake to prevent weight gain, restricting sodium intake, using potassium supplements as needed, and monitoring fasting serum glucose levels. Dyspepsia and possibly ulcers may be prevented by giving antacids (Tums and Rolaids double as calcium supplements), histamine receptor antagonists, or both in susceptible persons. Adrenal insufficiency can be prevented by supplementing maintenance steroid doses during acute periods of stress. Finally, the physician treating a patient with MG with systemic corticosteroids should use the smallest, single, alternate-day, effective dose possible.

Patients with MG being treated with chronic systemic steroids or other immunosuppressive agents are at risk for developing infections caused by opportunistic organisms, including certain bacteria, fungi, and viruses. In addition, such patients are at risk to develop lymphoma. In some cases, these secondary disorders are confused with an exacerbation of the patient's myasthenia.

Azathioprine (Imuran)

Because a completely intact immune response requires antigen processing and presentation (dependent in part on RNA synthesis) as well as proliferation and differentiation of immunocompetent cells (dependent on DNA and RNA synthesis), purine analog pro-drugs like azathioprine can interrupt the immune response at multiple sites (362). Azathioprine is metabolized to 6-mercaptopurine, which is then further metabolized to thioguanine moieties such as 6-methyl-mercaptopurine and others (363). The thioguanines are incorporated into replicating DNA molecules in rapidly dividing cells, such as those in the immune system, and prevent effective DNA replication. The effect is to reduce the proliferation of dividing T and B lymphocytes, as well as the production of cytotoxic T lymphocytes and plasma cells. There is also a reduction of the production of cytokines by active T lymphocytes (364). The accumulation of 6-mercaptopurine and other active metabolites may take many weeks after beginning a maintenance dose of azathioprine, contributing to the usually long delay of onset of the clinical effect on autoimmune diseases. A close relationship exists between azathioprine dosage and biologic effects on dividing cells, particularly lymphoid and erythroid cells. Leukopenia and macrocytosis occur predictably and are monitored as guides to azathioprine dosage (365). The drug is extensively oxidized and methylated in liver and red blood cells. Concurrent administration of allopurinol (for treatment of gout or hyperuricemia) can increase the toxicity of azathioprine by interfering with its metabolism by xanthine oxidase, an important degradative pathway. Therefore, the azathioprine dosage must be reduced by as much as 75% in patients who take allopurinol.

Azathioprine can be used effectively as initial therapy in MG as indicated in evidence from case series (323,365–367) as well as randomized, double-blind controlled trials (368,369). The manner in which azathioprine is most often used derives from its chief disadvantage, namely that beneficial effects may take 6 months or more to appear. It therefore tends to be used as additional therapy in patients whose MG is not adequately controlled after thymectomy and corticosteroid therapy (370,371). The combination affords the relatively rapid onset of immunosuppression produced by the steroids and allows tapering of corticosteroids once the azathioprine has had time to take effect. The addition of azathioprine also allows a reduction of steroid dosage in patients with otherwise well-controlled disease who experience unacceptable side effects of prednisone and in patients who require a chronic maintenance dosage of prednisone of more than 30 mg on alternate days.

Patients who are unable or unwilling to comply with close medical follow-up should never be treated with azathioprine. Approximately 10% of patients cannot tolerate azathioprine because of abnormal liver function, bone marrow depression, or an idiosyncratic reaction consisting of flu-like symptoms of fever and myalgia (372). The risk of myelosuppression may be correlated with the level of activity of one of the degradative enzymes for 6-mercaptopurine and subsequent active metabolites, thiopurine methyl-transferase (TPMT). Several studies have shown that common genetic polymorphisms that reduce TPMT activity may increase the risk of myelosuppression with azathioprine use (373,374). In the near future, measurement of TPMT activity may be useful prior to initiation of azathioprine therapy to predict the likelihood of myelosuppression and allow adjustment of the initial dosage (363). The issue of a small increased risk of malignancy in azathioprine-treated patients is unresolved. Experience with azathioprine in organ transplantation suggests an increased risk of malignancy, but many patients with MG or rheumatoid arthritis have been treated for years with the drug, and no increase in the incidence of malignancies has been seen in such patients (367,375,376).

The usual target dosage of azathioprine is 2–3 mg/kg/day. In obese patients, the optimal dosage depends on the total body weight, not on lean body weight. A test dosage of approximately 50 mg/day should be given for the first week. If this is well tolerated, the dosage should be gradually increased by 50 mg each week while the white blood cell (WBC) count, differential count, platelet count, and liver function tests are closely monitored. To establish the optimal dosage, several endpoints may be used. A total WBC count of 3,000–4,000/mm^3 is one safe endpoint. Azathioprine should be briefly discontinued if the WBC falls below 2,500/mm^3 or the absolute neutrophil count is less than 1,000/mm^3. It can then be reintroduced at a lower dosage. This measure cannot be used in patients receiving prednisone because of the steroid-induced leukocytosis. In that situation, a lymphocyte differential count percentage of 5–10% is an appropriate target. A rise in the red blood cell mean corpuscular volume to above 100 fl also provides a useful gauge of biologic activity and in MG usually correlates with clinical improvement (365). Macrocytosis does not require discontinuation of therapy.

An adequate therapeutic trial of azathioprine as sole therapy must last at least 1–2 years, because the lag to onset of effect may be 3 to 12 months, and maximum benefit may take 1–3 years. Although azathioprine is decidedly slow to act, it is well tolerated by most patients. Close monitoring for toxicity should continue indefinitely, and patients should be seen at least every 3 months after a stable, nontoxic dosage is reached. Although most patients with MG require life-long immunosuppression, as with prednisone, it is often worthwhile to attempt to taper azathioprine to establish a minimum effective dosage. A doubling of the anti-ACh receptor antibody titer (optimally in sera from two different dates measured in simultaneous assay) may predict clinical relapse (377). Based on European experience with the drug as sole therapy (378), we know that only a few patients with MG remain in remission after discontinuation of azathioprine (366,377); thus, continued close follow-up is necessary after therapy is stopped.

As with other immunosuppressive agents, azathioprine increases susceptibility to opportunistic infections, which should be treated promptly and vigorously. The hematologic toxicities discussed above (leukopenia, anemia, and thrombocytopenia) are all reversible upon reduction of the dosage of azathioprine. Hepatic toxicity with mild elevation of transaminases is common and responds to lowering the dosage. A rise in transaminase levels up to twofold is usually well tolerated by patients. Gastrointestinal discomfort, with nausea and anorexia, is usually mild and responds to the use of divided doses taken after meals. There are potential effects of azathioprine on the fertility of women, although an effect on male fertility is controversial (379). The drug should therefore be used with caution in all patients of childbearing age. Azathioprine should be discontinued several weeks prior to planned efforts at conception, and efforts should be made to avoid its use during pregnancy (380,381).

Cyclosporine

Cyclosporine is a cyclic polypeptide that inhibits the activation of helper/inducer (CD4+) T cells (382,383) and their production of the cytokine interleukin-2 (384,385) via a calcineurin-mediated mechanism, while relatively sparing suppressor (CD8+) T cells. Its therapeutic effect in MG is thus explained because the activation of B cells and production of anti-ACh receptor antibodies are T-cell–dependent. This relatively selective immunomodulatory action contrasts with the broad-spectrum effects of corticosteroids, azathioprine, and cyclophosphamide. Unlike cytotoxic immunosuppressants, cyclosporine does not cause generalized myelosuppression, thereby limiting the risk of opportunistic infections.

Cyclosporine reaches peak plasma concentrations within 3–4 hours after ingestion. The drug has a large volume of distribution and is sequestered in tissues. It is cleared from blood with a half-life of about 19 hours. Most of the drug is metabolized in the liver and excreted in the bile. This accounts for its ability to potentiate greatly the risk of necrotizing myopathy or myoglobinuria from lovastatin, a drug that also depends on biliary excretion. Because cytochrome P$_{450}$-mediated oxidation of the drug is extensive, hepatic dysfunction or concomitant administration of agents that affect the cytochrome P$_{450}$ system can cause dramatic changes in the elimination of cyclosporine.

Cyclosporine's independent mechanism of action produces an effect that is additive to that of corticosteroids, and because of evidence that the combination of cyclosporine with azathioprine and prednisone for suppression of organ rejection causes an increased risk of malignancies and infectious complications (386), most centers prefer to use only prednisone in combination with cyclosporine. Corticosteroids also have been noted to increase plasma cyclosporine levels.

Cyclosporine was the first drug shown to be effective primary immunotherapy for the treatment of MG in a prospective double-blinded, randomized, placebo-controlled trial (387,388). Improvement began at about 2 weeks, with maximum improvement by 4 months, correlating with a reduction in anti-ACh receptor antibody levels. Although the original trial was small and limited, experience with the drug in open trials for MG is also generally positive (389–391).

The efficacy of cyclosporine is similar to that of azathioprine (392), but it has the advantage of a more prompt effect, usually occurring within weeks (387,389,390,392–394). The rate of clinical response is 78–96%. For this reason, it is reasonable to consider using cyclosporine as a first-line immunosuppressive drug in patients with MG, because its immunomodulatory effects are more targeted than those of either systemic corticosteroids or azathioprine. It is also indicated in patients in whom treatment with corticosteroids or azathioprine has either failed or resulted in excessive toxicity. The general indications for use of the drug in MG are the same as for any immunosuppressant: the severity of the MG must not be functionally trivial, the expected benefit must outweigh the risks of toxicity, and the patient must be reliable. The cost of this drug is quite high, and this may be a factor discouraging its use in some patients.

The efficacy of cyclosporine relates to the lowest ("trough") plasma levels, whereas toxicity depends on peak concentrations. Therefore, the drug is given in a divided dosage schedule to minimize peak drug levels, initially at 2.5 mg/kg twice a day (5 mg/kg daily). There is no need to increase the drug dosage slowly. Because it is lipid-soluble and variably absorbed, cyclosporine should be taken with a fat-containing meal.

Although the dosage is eventually guided by clinical efficacy, it is initially adjusted by monitoring plasma cyclosporine levels and side effects. Plasma levels should be measured every 2 weeks until stable, and then approximately monthly. Trough levels are measured in the morning, 12–14 hours after the last dose. The reported levels depend on the method of assay; using the RIA with a specific monoclonal antibody, the trough level should be maintained between 100 and 200 ng/mL. The blood pressure, serum creatinine, and serum urea nitrogen are monitored, and the dosage of cyclosporine is decreased if the creatinine level rises more than 1.4 times above the baseline level.

Compared with corticosteroids, cyclosporine has less frequent serious chronic toxicity. The most worrisome side effects are nephrotoxicity and hypertension (388,393–395). It should therefore be used only with great caution in patients with preexisting uncontrolled hypertension or significant renal disease. There is an increased risk of nephrotoxicity in elderly patients. Nonsteroidal anti-inflammatory drugs that inhibit prostaglandin generation will potentiate cyclosporine nephrotoxicity. Other side effects include facial hirsutism, gastrointestinal disturbance, headache, tremor, convulsions, and rarely hepatotoxicity. These are related to drug level and are reversible with dosage reduction. Optic disc swelling may occur in patients taking cyclosporine. In some cases, the disc swelling is caused by increased intracranial pressure (396,397), whereas in other patients it represents a toxic anterior optic neuropathy that may have clinical similarity to anterior ischemic optic neuropathy (398,399). Other visual complications of cyclosporine include reversible cortical blindness and complex visual hallucinations (400–405). Hypertension usually responds either to dosage reduction or, if levels are appropriate, to weight reduction, salt restriction, an antihypertensive drug, or a combination of these therapies. As with other immunosuppressive agents, there is an increase in the long-term risk of malignancy. The increased incidence of skin cancer of various types in association with long-term use of cyclosporine is particularly well established (406). With close attention to management, however, cyclosporine can be used safely in nearly 90% of patients (407).

Mycophenolate Mofetil (CellCept)

Mycophenolate mofetil is a newer immunosuppressive agent that takes advantage of a biochemical difference between lymphocytes and all other body cells. Lymphocytes are unique in being dependent on de novo synthesis of purines for nucleic acids, because they are unable to use the purine salvage pathway. This allows selective inhibition of lymphocyte DNA replication and cell proliferation by mycophenolate mofetil, which acts to block inosine monophosphate dehydrogenase, a key enzyme in the de novo purine synthesis pathway. Mycophenolate mofetil also suppresses antibody secretion by B lymphocytes. Similar to cyclosporine, the selective nature of the effects of mycophenolate mofetil on the immune system makes myelosuppression infrequent. Mycophenolate mofetil is well absorbed after oral administration. Its absorption is not significantly affected by food. The half-life of the drug after an oral dose is about 18 hours. Mycophenolate mofetil is hydrolyzed to mycophenolate, which is the active metabolite. The drug is 97% protein-bound; its free concentration is increased by other protein-bound drugs, such as salicylates. The route of excretion is primarily by glucuronidation by glucuronyl transferase to mycophenolate glucuronide. The glucuronide is then excreted by the kidney, with 93% of a dose recovered in the urine and the remainder in the feces. Dosing must be adjusted for severe renal failure, but metabolism is less sensitive to hepatic disease. A number of other drug interactions exist and must be considered, including probenecid, magnesium- or aluminum-containing antacids, and cholestyramine resin.

Individual case reports initially indicated that mycophenolate mofetil could be beneficial for patients with MG (408,409). Small, uncontrolled open-label pilot studies seemed to confirm the benefit of mycophenolate mofetil in patients with MG (410–412). The patients in these pilot studies were generally already taking other immunosuppressive agents, most often prednisone and cyclosporine. Rates of improvement of 63–67% were reported. The time to improvement varied by study; Ciafaloni et al. (411) reported improvement in all responding patients by 2 months, and as early as 2 weeks; Chaudhry et al. (410) reported an onset of apparent benefit in responding patients averaging 5 months, with a range of 2–12 months. A subsequent, larger open-label study from the Duke group on 85 patients analyzed retrospectively showed clinical improvement in 73%. Many patients were able to reduce their doses of other immunosuppressives and pyridostigmine. The mean time to improvement for this larger study was about 8 weeks for subjective first improvement, 11 weeks for first objective improvement, and 27 weeks to maximal improvement (413). Severe side effects were uncommon, leading to discontinuation of the drug in about 6% of patients. Diarrhea was the most common significant side effect. A small randomized, placebo-controlled, double-blind trial was reported of mycophenolate mofetil in patients with MG (414). A strong trend existed toward greater improvement in the mycophenolate-treated patients, but due to the small numbers in the trial it did not reach significance. Larger randomized, controlled trials are needed. There are as yet no data specifically addressing the use of mycophenolate mofetil in patients with ocular MG, or as primary therapy. The likelihood of a relatively rapid onset of action and the paucity of side effects are factors that may favor the use of mycophenolate mofetil as primary immunomodulatory therapy in patients with ocular MG with sufficient disability to warrant such an approach. The relatively high cost of the drug may be a barrier to its use in some patients.

Mycophenolate mofetil is usually started at a full dosage of 1 g b.i.d., for a total dosage of 2 g daily. In children, the dosage is 600 mg/m^2 bid, up to the adult dosage of 1,000 mg bid. The dosage is maintained for at least 6 months to evaluate possible efficacy. Higher dosages of mycophenolate mofetil, up to 1.5 g b.i.d., are sometimes used in suppression of allograft rejection but have not been systematically studied in MG. The dosage of mycophenolate mofetil is maintained at the effective level. Some patients respond to dosages as low as 500 mg b.i.d., and it would be rational to try to lower the dosage to the lowest level that maintains the improvement after a period of stability.

The most frequent symptomatic side effect of mycophenolate mofetil is diarrhea. Up to 40% of patients receiving the drug for prevention of allograft rejection develop leukopenia or anemia, but this problem has not been seen frequently in the small series of patients treated for MG with the drug (410,411). This lower incidence of myelosuppression is also typical of the experience with this drug in the treatment of rheumatoid arthritis (415). When mycophenolate mofetil was used for prevention of allograft rejection in renal, cardiac, or liver transplant patients, it was associated with the development of hypertension, edema, headache, hyperglycemia, hypercholesterolemia, hypokalemia, hyperkalemia, diarrhea, gastrointestinal bleeding, cytomegalovirus infections, and skin rashes in a significant number of patients. With the exception of diarrhea, these problems were not reported in the small series of MG patients treated with this drug.

Short-Term Immunotherapies

Three forms of short-term immunotherapy are extremely useful in selected patients with severe, generalized MG: high-dose cyclophosphamide (416–421), plasmapheresis (plasma exchange) (422–425) and its newer variants (426,427), and intravenous injection of human immune globulin (HIG) (428–432). Such treatments are not usually used in the treatment of patients with ocular MG.

An Approach to Immunosuppressive Therapy of Myasthenia Gravis

There are as many specific approaches to the management of MG as there are neurologists involved actively in the care of these complex patients. There is clearly a great deal of ''art'' in this area, and several approaches work well for the patient when applied by a dedicated and experienced clinician. No approach will work well if haphazardly administered or when given to a noncompliant patient. One commonsense approach to the treatment of a patient presenting to the neuro-ophthalmologist with ocular MG is presented here. Of primary importance, the diagnosis must have been confirmed with sufficient confidence that therapy can be initiated, which is essential to avoid subjecting patients with other disorders to the risks and toxicity associated with the immunomodulatory agents used in MG therapy.

Patients with pure ocular MG showing minimal diplopia or ptosis can be managed by obtaining a chest CT or MRI to exclude thymoma, and then following them carefully while using prisms to correct diplopia. The patient must be carefully briefed regarding symptoms to monitor that should prompt a rapid return visit, and all patients with suspected but not proven MG should be seen in scheduled follow-up for a 24-month period to monitor any changes in the clinical pattern. The patient may try pyridostigmine (Mestinon) for temporary symptomatic relief of diplopia or ptosis, although experience is not encouraging that this drug can produce adequate and sufficiently consistent alignment of the eyes to relieve diplopia.

Patients with pure ocular MG with more severe diplopia or ptosis are unlikely to obtain sufficient relief from prism therapy or pyridostigmine, but these interventions can be tried for temporary symptomatic relief. In these patients, even when the clinical extent of their disease is purely ocular, immunosuppressive therapy is indicated. The advantages of this approach include the likely benefit to prevent progression to generalized MG, and relief of disability, usually with relatively mild adverse side effects. It is rarely appropriate to refer patients with pure ocular MG without evidence of thymoma for thymectomy. All patients who are to be started on long-term immunosuppressive medications should have a PPD placed in addition to their chest CT or MRI to exclude tuberculosis (unless BCG immunized). Only reliable and compliant patients can be safely treated with these medications, and the importance of careful follow-up and adherence to the medication and monitoring regimen must be stressed to the patient. For patients who are relatively young, with mild or no history of hypertension or renal disease, and for whom the cost of the drug does not represent a barrier, cyclosporine A should be considered as the primary treatment. This agent works rapidly and has relatively few bothersome symptomatic side effects. With careful monitoring as outlined in the discussion above, it is quite safe and can be given long term. Alternatively, mycophenolate mofetil may be considered for primary therapy, given its relatively rapid onset of action and generally mild side effects. The same cost considerations as exist for cyclosporine apply to the use of mycophenolate mofetil. If financial or medical issues preclude the use of mycophenolate mofetil or cyclosporine A but there are no severe prednisone contraindications, the patient may be started on prednisone (every day, tapered to every other day; see above discussion). To achieve steroid sparing and facilitate tapering, it is often appropriate to add azathioprine to prednisone. As tapering of prednisone proceeds after achieving maximal benefit, azathioprine may end up being a partial or complete substitute for prednisone therapy for long-term maintenance. Reasons to add azathioprine to prednisone include an inadequate response to prednisone alone or inability to taper prednisone below 30–40 mg qod, intolerable acute steroid side effects, or to minimize long-term steroid side effects. In patients who can not take mycophenolate mofetil or cyclosporine A and who have strong contraindications to prednisone or just do not want to take it, it is sometimes reasonable to use patching to control diplopia and start azathioprine as primary immunosuppressive therapy. The main drawback to azathioprine as primary therapy is its long delay to onset of effect, and the patient needs to be reminded of this frequently.

Each of the available immunotherapeutic options for MG has its advantages and disadvantages. Prednisone generally acts rapidly and is effective, but it has substantial side effects. Azathioprine is safe and moderately effective, with few side effects, but slow. Cyclosporine and mycophenolate mofetil are about equal to azathioprine in effectiveness and patient tolerability and are much more rapid in their effects, but they are expensive. The therapeutic armamentarium now available provides a broad spectrum of effective treatment modalities; however, more specific, long-lasting, and affordable treatments are still needed.

Local Treatment

Patients with ocular symptoms alone may not require systemic therapy. Ptosis, the single most frequent finding and complaint, may be reduced in many patients by placing a wire attachment on the top of one or both sides of a spectacle frame to keep the eyelids elevated. Almost invariably, patients develop irritation of the eyes from exposure because these "ptosis crutches" prevent normal blinking, but many patients nevertheless prefer this method of treatment. This is particularly true when the amount or type of medication required to relieve the ptosis has intolerable side effects. Ptosis surgery may be necessary in some patients with MG, particularly in patients refractory to appropriate medical therapy, thymectomy, or both, or in whom ptosis is the only (or predominant) finding (433–437). Success is sometimes short-lived, however, because myasthenic ptosis is variable and can recur. Some patients with intermittent diplopia may require no therapy, but most are sufficiently bothered that some type of treatment is usually necessary. In patients with diplopia along a relatively fixed plane, prisms can be used, particularly when there is a relatively comitant deviation. Some patients may be content to wear prisms that correct their diplopia only in primary position. Other patients may be forced to wear a patch over one eye. Rare patients improve with small doses of botulinum toxin A (438). Extraocular muscle surgery is rarely warranted in patients with MG and diplopia unless the strabismus has been stable for at least a year and no other treatment options are available (438–441).

PEDIATRIC MYASTHENIA GRAVIS

Autoimmune MG can occur at any age (442). One clinical challenge in "juvenile-onset" myasthenia is to distinguish antibody-mediated disease from gene mutations affecting NMJ ion channels (see below) (443). Juvenile-onset autoimmune MG differs little from adult-onset disease, except that it may improve with age (444). It responds to anticholinesterase agents and immunotherapy (443,445). Amblyopia may occur with extraocular muscle involvement and must be prevented by careful ophthalmologic follow-up (446). The optimal age for thymectomy and the choice of immunosuppressive agents in such young patients is controversial (443, 444,447).

CONGENITAL MYASTHENIC SYNDROMES

Once thought to be a single clinical and pathologic entity (261,448–452), congenital MG is now known to be a heterogeneous group of genetic neuromuscular transmission disorders (170,453–455). These conditions can be differentiated from acquired autoimmune MG on the basis of clinical, electromyographic, electrophysiologic, cytochemical, structural, and molecular genetic grounds. Many but not all cases present neonatally or in infancy with ptosis, fluctuating ophthalmoparesis, poor feeding, and respiratory difficulty. Symptoms may be episodic or may demonstrate fatigability that is worsened by crying, activity, or fever. Persistence of symptoms, rather than a transient monophasic course, distinguishes a congenital myasthenic syndrome from neonatal MG. Some syndromes may not even present until adoles-

cence or adulthood. Serum anti-ACh receptor antibodies are absent. In many cases, siblings or parents are affected, but a negative family history does not exclude autosomal-recessive inheritance. The edrophonium test, which relies on intact acetylcholinesterase and normal channel open times for its effect, is negative in many congenital myasthenic syndromes. Thus, a negative test does not exclude the diagnosis, and a positive test cannot distinguish any of the congenital myasthenic syndromes from autoimmune myasthenia. The diagnosis instead rests on the results of electrophysiologic testing and other key features.

Congenital myasthenic syndromes may be separated into those in which the defect is primarily presynaptic and those in which the defect is primarily postsynaptic. The major syndromes in which the defect is presynaptic are related to defects in ACh synthesis, mobilization, or release (456,457). Postsynaptic syndromes are mainly those caused by endplate acetylcholinesterase deficiency (458,459) and ACh receptor deficiency (454,460), as well as disorders of the ACh receptor kinetics, including the fast- and slow-channel syndromes (461). Nevertheless, almost any gene or process involved in neuromuscular transmission is a potential target for these rare genetic mutations (454).

PRESYNAPTIC CONGENITAL MYASTHENIC SYNDROMES

These disorders were previously called "familial infantile myasthenia" (462,463). In 1979, however, Hart et al. (464) described an autosomal-recessive congenital myasthenic disorder in two siblings. An 18-year-old boy and his 5-year-old sister had fluctuating ptosis since birth, feeding difficulties during infancy, easy fatigability on exertion, and episodic apnea following crying, vomiting, or febrile illnesses. Symptoms responded to neostigmine but not to prednisone and improved with age. No circulating anti-ACh receptor antibody was found in either child. Repetitive nerve stimulation in the older child showed decremental responses during 2-Hz stimulation after exercise. Subsequent cases were described by Mora et al. (456), who found that the size of synaptic vesicles was reduced in some patients. The defective step or steps in ACh synthesis are unknown but could involve choline reuptake, ACh assembly via choline acetyltransferase, or vesicle packaging (465). A related autosomal-recessive presynaptic syndrome marked by less episodic symptoms is associated with a paucity of synaptic vesicles and reduced quantal release (457).

POSTSYNAPTIC CONGENITAL MYASTHENIC SYNDROMES

Congenital Acetylcholinesterase Deficiency

In patients with a congenital deficiency of acetylcholinesterase, weakness, atrophy, fatigability, ptosis, and ophthalmoparesis are usually recognized in the first 2 years of life. Autosomal-recessive inheritance is the rule. In most patients, pupillary light responses are abnormally slow (453,459).

Engel et al. (458) first described this syndrome in a 14-year-old boy with lifelong ptosis and external ophthalmoparesis as well as bulbar, truncal, and proximal extremity weakness worsened by exertion (Fig. 21.15). The child showed no response to anticholinesterase drugs or guanidine and had minimal improvement with corticosteroid treatment. Subsequent reports have revealed variability of the occurrence of ophthalmoparesis in these patients (459).

EMG studies in these patients show decremental responses at 2-Hz stimulation, postactivation facilitation, and postactivation exhaustion. Microelectrode studies reveal prolonged delay of mepps. However, the most distinguishing electrophysiologic finding is a reduplicated compound muscle action potential (CMAP) response to single stimuli (466). This is caused by absent acetylcholinesterase activity, the action of which is normally the rate-limiting step for termina-tion of the action of ACh. In acetylcholinesterase deficiency, ACh can bind or rebind to more than one ACh receptor before diffusing from the synapse, prolonging the decay phase of the endplate potentials. The prolonged endplate potential can trigger more than one muscle fiber action potential because its amplitude remains above threshold. Alternatively, unhydrolyzed ACh can excite nerve terminals to fire to branch points, giving "double discharge" (466). The physiology is similar to that of organophosphate poisoning (467). Double discharges are also characteristic of the slow-channel syndrome (discussed later).

The genetic defect that produces endplate acetylcholinesterase deficiency has been determined (468). Muscle endplate acetylcholinesterase is made up of one to three tetramers of the acetylcholinesterase globular form attached to a triple helical collagen like tail called ColQ. This ColQ tail is essential for localization of the acetylcholinesterase tetramers to the postsynaptic membrane of the endplate. Several truncation and missense mutations of the ColQ gene result in the acetylcholinesterase deficiency phenotype (170,468). Unfortunately, no effective treatment for endplate acetylcholinesterase deficiency has been found, with no useful benefit from acetylcholinesterase inhibitors, 3,4-diaminopyridine, quinidine, ephedrine, pseudoephedrine, or prednisone (3).

Primary Acetylcholine Receptor Deficiency

Patients with autosomal-recessive congenital MG caused by reduced numbers of ACh receptors were described by Vincent et al. (454,460). These children may present with poor feeding and ptosis in the neonatal period. Milder phenotypes may have normal neonatal periods and show motor milestone delay beginning at a later time. Most eventually develop some degree of bilateral ptosis and ophthalmoparesis (3). More severely affected individuals had complete external ophthalmoplegia by 13 years of age. Limb and facial weakness were present. Repetitive stimulation of motor nerves at 3 Hz showed decremental muscle responses, and single-fiber EMG revealed jitter and blocking.

The genetic defect in congenital ACh receptor deficiency producing reduced numbers of receptor molecules is one of several recessive, loss-of-function mutations in the ACh receptor subunit genes. These may be premature termination defects or various missense mutations. The patient may be homozygous for the deficiency or heterozygous (3,170).

Unlike patients with acetylcholinesterase deficiency, patients with a deficiency of ACH receptors improve when treated with anticholinesterase-inhibiting agents such as pyridostigmine. There may be further improvement following the addition to the regimen of 3,4-diaminopyridine, which acts by blocking potassium channels in neuronal and muscle membranes. Potassium channel blockade produces prolonged action potential durations and may facilitate neuromuscular transmission by facilitating ACh release in response to each action potential arriving at the presynaptic nerve terminal (469). Engel reported that combination therapy with pyridostigmine and 3,4-diaminopyridine produced

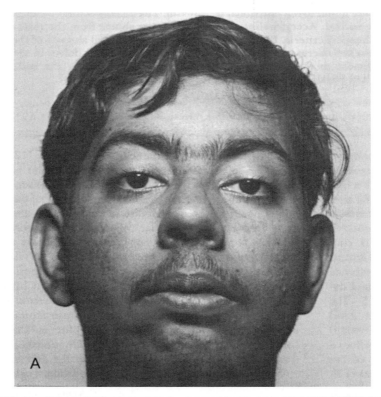

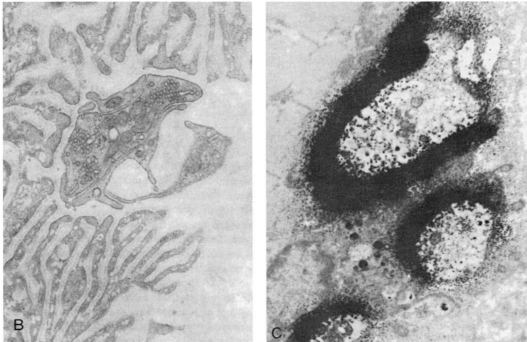

Figure 21.15. Congenital myasthenic syndrome caused by acetylcholinesterase deficiency. *A,* A 16-year-old boy with bilateral ptosis, facial and skeletal muscle weakness, reduced muscle bulk, and scoliosis. *B and C,* Electron cytochemical localization of acetylcholinesterase activity. *B,* Patient's endplate shows no reaction after incubation with α-bungarotoxin. *C,* Control endplate from a normal subject shows marked reaction after only 30 minutes of incubation. (From Engel AG, Lambert EH, Gomez MR. A new myasthenic syndrome with end-plate acetylcholinesterase deficiency, small nerve terminals, and reduced acetylcholine release. Ann Neurol 1977;1:315–330.)

improvement in ptosis and overall endurance but did little for ophthalmoparesis (3).

Primary Acetylcholine Receptor Kinetic Abnormality—Fast-Channel Syndrome

A group of congenital myasthenic patients show only mild reduction in the number of ACh receptor molecules but demonstrate a lowered binding affinity for acetylcholine, a shortened duration of the opening of the ACh receptor ion channel after ligand binding, or both (3). These patients are exceedingly rare, originating from only a few known kindreds. The three syndromes that have been described are called the low-affinity, fast-channel syndrome, the fast-channel syndrome due to a gating abnormality, and the mode-switching kinetics syndrome (3). Ptosis and ophthalmoparesis are common features of all three syndromes, with onset of these and other myasthenic symptoms and signs in early childhood.

Patients with fast-channel syndromes typically show a decremental response of the combined muscle action potential to repetitive stimulation at 3 Hz (3). Specific diagnosis of each syndrome requires specific electrophysiologic studies of the motor endplate, sometimes including patch clamp recordings.

The genetic defects in these fast-channel congenital myasthenic syndromes are recessive, loss-of-function, missense mutations in the α or ϵ subunits of the ACh receptor (470,471). The mutation causes a conformational change in the receptor subunit that alters the kinetics of channel opening or closing. Some mutations may be revealed only when another mutation in the ACh receptor genes is present that allows the phenotype to be expressed.

Treatment of the fast-channel syndromes is usually possible with acetylcholinesterase inhibitors such as pyridostigmine, combined with 3,4-diaminopyridine. Good clinical responses to this approach have been reported (3), and improvement in the pathologic electrophysiologic findings has been demonstrated in some patients.

Primary Acetylcholine Receptor Kinetic Abnormality—Slow-Channel Syndrome

Engel et al. (461,472) reported the first two families with slow-channel syndrome. The age of onset, rate of progression, severity, and pattern of weakness were highly variable (453). Apparent onset of clinical symptoms may be delayed to adult life, and symptoms may worsen intermittently. Skeletal muscle atrophy was common. Some patients had predominant involvement of cervical, scapular, and finger extensor muscles, the last of which may be a clinical distinguishing feature. Ophthalmoparesis and ptosis were often prominent. Predictably from this presentation, the diseases confused with this disorder include mitochondrial myopathy, myotonic dystrophy, congenital myopathy, spinal muscular atrophy, limb girdle dystrophy, Möbius syndrome, and peripheral neuropathies.

Like acetylcholinesterase deficiency, slow-channel syndrome is characterized by reduplicated CMAP responses to single stimuli. This phenomenon is ubiquitous in all muscles from birth onward, indicating a primary defect. Repetitive nerve stimulation shows decrement at low rates of stimulation.

Slow-channel syndrome is an example of calcium-mediated cellular excitotoxicity. Eleven mutations causing the syndrome have been described that result in single amino-acid substitutions in the α, β, and ϵ subunits of the ACh receptor at regions that are crucial to the gating kinetics of the ion pore (170,454,473). Prolonged channel openings result in abnormal ingress of Ca^{2+}, Mg^{2+}, Mn^{2+}, and ammonium into junctional folds and junctional sarcoplasm. The result of this open-channel cationic toxicity is not only a myasthenic syndrome but also a fixed, vacuolar myopathy (473).

Treatment with pyridostigmine, transmitter releasers such as guanidine, and prednisone is generally unsuccessful, although Gomez et al. (473) reported an exception. Quinidine has been shown to produce an improvement in the prolonged open duration of the pathologic ion channels in the slow-channel syndrome (474,475), with clinical improvement in some patients (476). Effective serum levels of quinidine were reported to be 0.7–2.5 μg/mL, which are at the low end of the usual therapeutic range for this potentially toxic drug.

ACQUIRED DISORDERS OF NEUROMUSCULAR TRANSMISSION OTHER THAN MYASTHENIA GRAVIS

As with congenital "myasthenic" syndromes, acquired disorders of neuromuscular transmission other than MG may be caused by presynaptic or postsynaptic abnormalities. In addition, some syndromes are characterized by both pre- and postsynaptic abnormalities. Most of the acquired disorders of neuromuscular transmission other than MG are caused by the effects of exogenous agents on the NMJ.

LAMBERT-EATON MYASTHENIC SYNDROME

A disorder resembling MG in patients with bronchogenic carcinoma was first described by Anderson et al. in 1953 (477), and subsequent investigators reported similar cases (478,479). Following these reports, Eaton, Lambert, Rooke, and coworkers studied the clinical and physiologic characteristics of this syndrome in 30 such cases and concluded that it was a syndrome distinct from MG (480–482).

Clinical Features

Lambert-Eaton myasthenic syndrome is characterized primarily by weakness but also by fatigability, hyporeflexia, and autonomic dysfunction. Weakness is proximal and more prominent in legs and truncal muscles than in arms. Ocular and bulbar muscles are sometimes affected but mildly so, in contrast to their prominent involvement in MG (discussed later). Weakness is more disabling than life-threatening because the disorder rarely produces respiratory failure. Therefore, Lambert-Eaton myasthenic syndrome is really part of the differential diagnosis of acquired myopathy in adults. It is not often confused with MG, although the two autoimmune disorders may coexist. Reflexes are reduced or absent, but muscle wasting is infrequent. Autonomic symptoms and signs include dry mouth, decreased sweating, erectile impotence, and loss of the pupillary light reflex (163,483).

Lambert-Eaton myasthenic syndrome is associated commonly as a paraneoplastic syndrome with small cell lung cancer and occasionally with non-Hodgkin's lymphoma, leukemia, and other malignancies (484). Paraneoplastic Lambert-Eaton myasthenic syndrome presents before (up to 6 years preceding) the discovery of the neoplasm in 86% of patients, with a median anticipation of 6 months (484). The vast majority of patients with paraneoplastic Lambert-Eaton syndrome will be found to have a tumor within 2 years of onset of neurologic symptoms (484,485). As in MG, sex and age affect case incidence. About two thirds of all cases are paraneoplastic (484). Men constitute 70% of the paraneoplastic cases. One-third of cases are primarily autoimmune and show an equal sex distribution. Taken together, these statistics account for the overall male predominance (M:F 1.6:1) in the disorder (484). Although most affected patients are adults, the disorder can also occur in children (486–488). The disorder can occur alone but develops in association with other autoimmune disorders (489) in up to 27% of the non-cancer-associated cases. The myasthenic syndrome may develop in patients with MG (see later), pernicious anemia (490), thyroid disease (491–493), systemic lupus erythematosus (484), vitiligo (493), celiac disease (494), type I diabetes mellitus (484), ulcerative colitis (484), Addison's disease (484), rheumatoid arthritis (484), or Sjögren's syndrome (495). There is a strong association between Lambert-Eaton syndrome and the presence of the HLA B8 marker overall, but especially in cases without underlying malignancy (496). In younger female patients with non-tumor Lambert-Eaton myasthenic syndrome, there is also an association with HLA DR3 and DQ2, both of which are in strong linkage disequilibrium with HLA B8 (497,498). Occasionally patients have features of both autoimmune MG and the myasthenic syndrome (499–504). Paraneoplastic Lambert-Eaton myasthenic syndrome may be associated with other paraneoplastic neurologic disorders, including cerebellar degeneration, sensorimotor polyneuropathy, sensory polyneuropathy, and limbic encephalitis (485, 505–507).

Pathophysiology

The neuromuscular transmission defect in Lambert-Eaton myasthenic syndrome is presynaptic. It is caused by impaired release of ACh at motor nerve terminals (508) because of antibodies directed against voltage-gated calcium channels in the motor nerve terminal and cholinergic autonomic nerve terminals (509,510), especially the P/Q form (485). These antibodies reduce the number of calcium channels and thus the probability of synaptosomal release of ACh at active zones (511). Small cell lung carcinomas enriched in voltage-gated calcium channels provide the shared antigenic stimulus in paraneoplastic Lambert-Eaton myasthenic syndrome. Close to 100% of patients with the myasthenic syndrome

associated with small cell lung carcinoma have antibodies to voltage-gated calcium channels. In patients with the Lambert-Eaton syndrome without underlying cancer, 85–90% have voltage-gated calcium channel antibodies (485). The antibodies are also seen rarely in the generalized hyperimmunoglobulinemic state associated with systemic lupus erythematosus or rheumatoid arthritis, and in less than 5% of MG patients (485). A small residual percentage of patients with clinical and electrophysiologic evidence of Lambert-Eaton myasthenic syndrome, usually without associated cancer, have no detectable antibodies to voltage-gated calcium channels. Purified IgG from these patients can induce a myasthenic syndrome when passively transferred to mice, indicating that there is a circulating antibody that is able to induce the myasthenic syndrome that is not detected by the assay for antibody to voltage-gated calcium channels (512,513). The specificity of this transferable antibody has not yet been determined.

Acetylcholine synthesis and mobilization are unimpaired in Lambert-Eaton myasthenic syndrome, and the amount of depolarization produced by single quanta is normal. The impaired ACh release results in compound endplate potentials that may be too small to trigger muscle action potentials. As a result, muscles fatigue and evoked compound muscle action potentials are low in amplitude. The normally increased mobilization of calcium that occurs in the nerve terminal immediately following exercise or electric activation of motor nerves at rates above 10 Hz transiently increases the release of ACh, the resultant endplate potential amplitude, and therefore muscle strength (508,514). This facilitation is the basis for the electrophysiologic diagnosis, but it is only occasionally evident on physical examination (as in ptotic eyelids on sustained upgaze). Repetitive nerve stimulation reveals decrement at 2 Hz but marked (40–1,000%) facilitation of the compound muscle action potential after brief exercise or 50-Hz stimulation (Fig. 21.14C) (481,515). Single-fiber EMG reveals increased jitter and blocking that improve as units fire at higher rates (502,516). As in MG, failure of neuromuscular transmission and weakness worsen when the temperature is raised (517,518).

Ocular Manifestations

In contrast to MG, ocular symptoms are less common in Lambert-Eaton syndrome, but ptosis and both clinical and subclinical ocular motor involvement do occur in these patients (96,484,519–523). Wirtz et al. reviewed 227 individual reported patient descriptions of Lambert-Eaton myasthenic syndrome from 155 papers (484). At some time during the course of the illness, 21% of the patients reported ptosis and 21% reported diplopia. Individual studies have reported ptosis during the illness in as high as 54% of patients (524). Tearing was impaired and caused dry eyes in 4% of patients reported overall, but one study showed deficient reflex tear secretion in 69% (525). Signs noted by examiners at some point during the illness included ptosis in 30%, indicating that ptosis was sometimes asymptomatic. An ocular motor disturbance was suggested to neurologic examiners by signs in 12%. While the occurrence of neuro-ophthalmologic symptoms and signs was actually relatively frequent at some point during the illness, these signs were rare as the presenting manifestations of Lambert-Eaton myasthenic syndrome, in strong contrast to the presentation of MG. A patient with weakness limited to the eyelids or extraocular muscles who is suspected of having an NMJ disorder is very unlikely to have Lambert-Eaton myasthenic syndrome (526).

Cruciger et al. (523) examined five patients with the Lambert-Eaton syndrome, all of whom complained of intermittent ptosis and three of whom complained of intermittent diplopia. These investigators observed ptosis in three of the patients. In addition, of three patients whose eye movements were measured before and after exercise, two had saccadic velocities that were normal before exercise but increased up to 40% after exercise. This finding is similar to that seen in peripheral muscles of such patients and demonstrated electromyographically as facilitation. Dell'Osso et al. (96) examined saccades in five patients with the Lambert-Eaton syndrome. All patients made saccades that were similar to those made by patients with MG in that the saccades were often hypometric or multiple and closely spaced. Two patients demonstrated both saccadic facilitation and positive edrophonium tests; however, all of the patients had slow or normal saccadic velocities rather than the "super-fast" velocities found in patients with MG (see above).

Fatigable ptosis after sustained upgaze is a clinically useful sign in MG. Paradoxical lid elevation after sustained upgaze may be a clinically useful sign in Lambert-Eaton syndrome (527,528). Brazis has also described enhancement of ptosis in the Lambert-Eaton syndrome by elevating the contralateral lid (528).

Abnormalities of pupillary responses are common in patients with Lambert-Eaton myasthenic syndrome (525). One study found impaired light responses of the pupils in 69% of Lambert-Eaton patients using the pupil cycle time, compared with 18% of a "control" group (525). This is not surprising in light of the incidence of significant autonomic involvement in the myasthenic syndrome, estimated to be as high 93% (529). Clinical abnormalities of pupillary responses that are apparent by bedside examination have been less frequently observed. Well-documented bilateral tonic pupils have been reported in the myasthenic syndrome (530). Impaired pupillary responses may improve transiently with administration of 3,4-diaminopyridine and pyridostigmine, even in the presence of a tonic pupil syndrome, suggesting that the poor pupil responses result from impaired cholinergic transmission at the ganglionic nicotinic synapses by a process similar to that operating at the NMJ (530). Evidence of denervation sensitivity of the sympathetic and parasympathetic iris musculature has been reported in two-thirds of patients with Lambert-Eaton syndrome (525). Bilateral adrenergic denervation sensitivity has been reported in a patient with Lambert-Eaton syndrome without associated cancer, possibly due to involvement of nicotinic cholinergic synapses in the superior cervical ganglion (531).

Therapy

In general, the Lambert-Eaton myasthenic syndrome responds to therapy somewhat less well than does MG. An individualized, combined approach to therapy includes treatment of any underlying cancer, pharmacotherapy of the neuromuscular transmission defect, and immunosuppression. Because the syndrome may precede the discovery of a tumor by several years, the evaluation should include not only an initial extensive search for underlying malignancy, including chest CT or MRI, but also frequent surveillance if the initial evaluation is negative. Partial but rarely complete remission may be achieved by removal or control of the underlying small cell cancer with surgery, radiation therapy, or chemotherapy (532,533). A more detailed discussion of pharmacologic therapy of Lambert-Eaton syndrome is beyond the scope of this text. Therapies include 3,4-diaminopyridine, anticholinesterase agents, immunosuppressants, and sometimes plasmapheresis or intravenous immunoglobulin.

NEUROMUSCULAR DISORDERS CAUSED BY DRUGS OR TOXINS

Substances that cause neuromuscular disturbances do so by affecting presynaptic mechanisms, postsynaptic mechanisms, or both. These substances are primarily drugs and toxins.

The common settings in which the effects of drugs appear are (a) in a patient at increased risk because of abnormally increased drug concentration; (b) as part of a drug-induced generalized immunologic disorder; (c) with delayed recovery of strength following general anesthesia during which neuromuscular blocking agents may have been used; and (d) unmasking or worsening of MG or the myasthenic syndrome (534). Drug-induced disturbances of neuromuscular transmission usually resemble naturally occurring MG, causing prominent ptosis and ophthalmoparesis as well as variable degrees of facial, bulbar, and extremity muscle weakness. Respiratory difficulties may occur early and are often severe. Treatment consists of discontinuing the offending agent and reversing the block with various agents, including calcium gluconate, potassium, and anticholinesterases (535,536).

Toxins that disturb neuromuscular transmission may be acquired from many sources, including bacteria, arthropods, and snakes. Treatment depends on the recognition of the specific toxin, the availability of antitoxin, and supportive therapy.

Drug-Induced Autoimmune Damage to the Neuromuscular Junction

A myasthenic syndrome may develop in patients receiving D-penicillamine for rheumatoid arthritis or Wilson's disease (537–549). The syndrome may consist of ocular symptoms and signs alone or may be associated with generalized muscle involvement (550). It mimics true MG not only in its clinical features but also in that affected patients have the same histocompatibility antigens and anti-ACh receptor antibodies (551–553). Such antibodies either block or increase the degradation of ACh receptors, just as they do in true MG (549). D-penicillamine thus has no direct neuromuscular blocking effect but produces a myasthenic syndrome in much the same way that MG occurs naturally. The onset averages 8 months after the onset of therapy, and the syndrome is unrelated to D-penicillamine dosage or cumulative dosage (540,550). When the drug is withdrawn, strength improves in a few weeks or months as antibody titers fall (549). Treatment with D-penicillamine is also associated with a systemic lupus erythematosus-like syndrome, Goodpasture's syndrome, thyroiditis, and polymyositis (537,550).

Drugs that Affect Neuromuscular Transmission Through Presynaptic and Postsynaptic Effects

A variety of drugs act at both pre- and postsynaptic sites of the NMJ to disturb neuromuscular transmission in humans (536,554–556). Such drugs can "unmask" subclinical MG or worsen known MG. It is rare for such drug effects to be clinically important in patients with normal neuromuscular transmission. Antibiotics, antihypertensives, and neuromuscular blockers in particular are cited based on experimental electrophysiologic data, and at times such drugs are listed as "contraindicated" in MG. This made more sense in an era before widespread availability of sophisticated respiratory monitoring and intensive care units. Several common drugs implicated as peripherally acting neuromuscular blockers, such as phenytoin (557–559), calcium channel blockers (560), and propranolol (561), can be used safely in vivo (562). Jonkers et al. (563) showed that there is no rapid deterioration of neuromuscular transmission in patients with moderately severe MG after intravenous injections with therapeutic doses of propranolol and verapamil. In antibiotic usage, a nonblocking agent should always be chosen if possi-

ble, but an effective aminoglycoside should never be routinely avoided in favor of a cephalosporin, for example, if the antibiotic sensitivities do not support that decision. In a severe infection, or when a myasthenic patient is already on a ventilator, the indicated antibiotic should be used despite its potential effects on neuromuscular transmission. Table 21.1 lists some of the drugs that interfere with the function of the NMJ.

Toxins that Damage Presynaptic Neuromuscular Transmission

Arthropod Envenomation

Envenomation by the female black widow spider (*Latrodectus mactans*) causes diffuse central and peripheral nervous system stimulation with vasoconstriction, hypertension, and autonomic hyperactivity (627). The effects on muscle and neuromuscular transmission begin 15–60 minutes after envenomation, with muscle cramps involving the trunk and extremities. The abdomen may become rigid, and pain may be extreme (628). Persistent ocular manifestations seem limited to a single report of Horner's syndrome proven by cocaine testing ipsilateral to a black widow spider bite on the hand several weeks prior (629). The mechanism producing the Horner's syndrome was unclear in this case, with the authors hypothesizing that an otherwise unrecognized internal carotid artery dissection might have occurred during

Table 21.1
Drugs that Interfere with the Function of the Neuromuscular Junction

Drug	Site of Action	References
Neuromuscular blocking agents (pancuronium, vecuronium, alcuronium)	Postsynaptic	555,564–566
Acetylcholinesterase inhibitors:		
Medications—pyridostigmine, neostigmine	Postsynaptic	142,567–569
Pesticides—organophosphates, carbamates		
Biowarfare agents—Sarin, VX		
Phenothiazines	Postsynaptic	570
Trimethaphan	Postsynaptic	571,572
D,L-Carnitine	Postsynaptic	555,573
Inhalational anesthetics (ether, ketamine, halothane)	Postsynaptic	574,575
Amphetamine	Presynaptic	576
Corticosteroids	Pre- and postsynaptic	360,577
Antiarrhythmics (procainamide, quinidine)	Pre- and postsynaptic	578–583
Antibiotics:		
Aminoglycosides (e.g., gentamicin)	Pre- and postsynaptic	556,584
Polymyxins (e.g., polymyxin B)		585,586
Penicillins (e.g., ampicillin)		587,588
Macrolides (e.g., erythromycin)		589–593
Tetracyclines (e.g., minocycline)		594,595
Quinolones (e.g., ciprofloxacin)		596–600
Monobasic amino acids (e.g., clindamycin)		601,602
Anticonvulsants (e.g., phenytoin)	Pre- and postsynaptic	558,603–605
Beta-adrenergic blocking agents	Pre- and postsynaptic	561,606,607
Chloroquine	Pre- and postsynaptic	608–614
Cis-platinum	Unknown	615
Lithium	Pre- and postsynaptic	616–619
Magnesium	Pre- and postsynaptic	620–622
Iodinated radiographic contrast agents	Unknown	623–626

the acute phase of muscular rigidity and severe pain, with arterial hypertension, leaving the patient with a new Horner's syndrome.

Black widow spider venom has a presynaptic site of action when tested in nerve–muscle preparations. The purified toxin (α-latrotoxin) increases the release of ACh quanta at vertebrate NMJs until the vesicles in the nerve terminal become depleted (630). The venom of the brown widow spider (*Latrodectus geometricus*) has similar properties but causes intermittent release of ACh (631).

Treatment is empiric, consisting of warming and calcium gluconate infusions to reduce muscle cramping. The administration of magnesium sulfate intravenously may help to reduce transmitter release (627), and atropine is sometimes helpful (632). Antivenom is available for *Latrodectus* envenomation and should be administered promptly whenever possible (628).

Paralysis may also occur in humans as a result of a salivary toxin elaborated by female ticks (633,634). *Dermacentor* (wood and dog ticks) and *Amblyomma* species are the most frequently involved in North America, although other genera are also possible causes elsewhere in the world, especially *Ixodes holocyclus* (635). In most cases, irritability precedes paralysis by 12–24 hours. Paralysis of the legs usually occurs first, often associated with pain, paresthesias, and numbness. In severe cases, paralysis of the upper extremities follows within 24 hours. Bulbar paralysis quickly follows, and death may occur from respiratory paralysis.

The paralysis that occurs in tick paralysis is usually bilateral, symmetric, and flaccid. Deep tendon and superficial reflexes disappear beginning at the ankles and extending upward to include the upper extremities. Hyperesthesia, anesthesia, or dysesthesia may be present. As bulbar paralysis develops, the lower cranial nerves are affected first. Cerebellar ataxia is frequently present. Myoclonic twitching and choreiform movements may occur (635).

Ocular signs occur late in the course of the disorder. The pupils dilate and do not react to either light or near stimulation (636). The extraocular muscles may become paralyzed, usually in association with the onset of facial paralysis (635). Photophobia may occur and is often severe.

Electrophysiologic studies of patients with tick paralysis reveal slowing of motor and sensory nerve conduction. Endplate potentials at NMJs from patients poisoned with toxin from North American ticks (*Dermacentor andersoni, Dermacentor variabilis*) are normal (637), but toxin from the Australian tick (*Ixodes holocyclus*) produces a temperature-dependent reduction in evoked release of transmitter, suggesting that presynaptic inhibition of ACh release may contribute to paralysis (638).

Patients with tick paralysis do not respond to anticholinesterase agents because the pathology is presynaptic. The treatment is to remove the offending tick immediately and to provide supportive measures, including assisted ventilation, until the intoxication phase subsides. The neurologic symptoms and signs usually resolve after the tick is removed, and the ultimate prognosis is therefore favorable. If the tick is not removed before bulbar signs have appeared, however, death may occur despite supportive measures (635).

Scorpion toxin increases ACh release at the NMJ secondarily by inducing repetitive potentials in nerve terminal membrane (639). This effect occurs by delaying the normal sodium channel inactivation that occurs during the action potential. Similar effects on voltage-gated sodium channels occur in muscle membrane (640). The scorpion sting results in serious visceral effects, but neuromuscular transmission is little affected. Nevertheless, some patients develop abnormal eye movements after being stung (641–643). The abnormal movements are generally involuntary, conjugate, slow, and roving, but occasionally they are dysconjugate. A primary position unsustained nystagmus may occur. Two children who were stung by a bark scorpion (*Centruroides sculpturatus*) had rapid, conjugate, multidirectional saccades resembling opsoclonus (643). Ptosis has been described after envenomation by *Parabathus transvaalicus* (644). Treatment of envenomations by *C. sculpturatus* and other neurotoxic scorpion species is with either species-specific antivenom or sedatives. Neurologic and systemic manifestations of the envenomation, including the abnormal eye movements, generally resolve within 1 hour after treatment with species-specific antivenom and within 24 hours when only symptomatic treatment is given.

A syndrome resembling ocular MG was reported in a patient within 24 hours of a wasp sting by Brumlik (645). The syndrome persisted for weeks and responded to anticholinesterase drugs and prednisone. Although bee, wasp, and hornet venoms can cause NMJ disturbances in other arthropods, the case reported by Brumlik was unusual because such disturbances are not a regular feature of human envenomation by these species. Singh et al. (646) reported a case of bilateral ptosis after a wasp sting that was apparently reversible.

Botulism

Botulism occurs in three forms: food-borne, wound, and infantile (647,648). The disease is produced by a polypeptide toxin elaborated by the organism *Clostridium botulinum* (630). It is the most potent poison known. A cholinergic synapse may be blocked by as few as 10 molecules of toxin. In food-borne botulism, symptoms begin about 8–36 hours after food containing the toxin is eaten. The toxin is intact because proper cooking that normally would denature the toxin has not been performed (649). In wound botulism, organisms contaminating wounds produce toxin that is absorbed systemically (650). Nearly all cases develop from extremity wounds that occur outside the home, which may include intravenous drug abuse. Symptoms begin 4–17 days after the injury, with an average incubation time of 7 days. Wounds that cause botulism may appear clinically uninfected; however, when the wound is carefully explored and cultured, the organism is usually found. In infantile botulism, organisms in the gastrointestinal tract produce toxin that is systemically absorbed (651–653).

At least eight types of botulinum toxin are characterized (A, B, Cα, Cβ, D, E, F, and G) (567). Types A and B are the most common causes of botulism in the United States (654–656), although type E should be suspected when seafood is eaten (657).

Botulinum toxins impair neuromuscular transmission presynaptically (658) by interfering with the exocytotic release of ACh vesicles after the stimulus-induced influx of calcium into the nerve terminal (630,659). Recovery eventually occurs when nerve fibers sprout, and new NMJs are established (660), but the process may take months to years. The clostridial neurotoxins are secreted as a 150-kD holotoxin that is cleaved during or shortly after secretion into a 100-kD heavy chain and a 50-kD light chain, which are joined by disulfide bonds and high-affinity noncovalent interactions. The heavy chain is responsible for the specific targeting of these toxins to the presynaptic membrane of cholinergic terminals and for the translocation of the catalytic light chain into the presynaptic cytosol.

The diagnosis of botulism depends on clinical, epidemiologic, and electrophysiologic findings and may be confirmed by the discovery of the toxin or the organism in food, stool, or a wound. Signs of infantile botulism are constipation, listlessness, poor suck, regurgitation, and generalized weakness. In children and adults, the symptoms of botulism include nausea, vomiting, blurred vision, dysphagia, and pooling of secretions in the mouth and pharynx, followed by generalized weakness mostly proximal in the upper extremities and diplopia (649). Examination of affected patients reveals facial, pharyngeal, and generalized proximal weakness but normal sensation. Urinary retention and hypoactive bowel sounds are frequently present (661).

Ophthalmologic findings include dilated pupils in 52%, poor pupillary light reaction in 59%, ptosis in 80%, nystagmus in 55%, diplopia in 59%, and examination evidence of ophthalmoparesis or ophthalmoplegia in 36% (662–667) (Fig. 21.16). Pupillary dilation may be the only clinical sign of botulism and must be sought (668). Paralysis of accommodation is reported in 59% of patients (666). Photophobia, probably related to mydriasis, is also reported frequently. The pupillary dilation may be persistent, with features of tonic pupils (669). Bilateral tonic pupils may be present acutely, and resolve over a period of weeks (670). Decreased lacrimation and subjective ocular dryness are frequently noted (666).

Hedges et al. (665) noted rapid quivering eye motions in two patients with botulism. These eye movements were observed during attempts to refixate laterally placed objects and occurred in association with ophthalmoparesis. Electrooculographic examination showed that the quivering motions were composed of multiple hypometric saccades, many of which had subnormal, variable velocities. Hedges et al. (665) postulated that by blocking ACh release at the NMJ (see below), botulinum toxin appears to limit the duration of the extraocular muscle response to the saccadic burst of innervation. Stahl et al. (169) used magnetic search coil recording to investigate a patient with food-borne botulism who had ophthalmoparesis and also found variable saccadic velocities, with saccadic hypometria, but no quiver movements. The static alignment of the eyes was exotropic, with severely limited ductions in all directions of gaze for each eye. Administration of intravenous edrophonium 10 mg partially relieved all aspects of the ocular motor abnormalities. Saccadic velocities were significantly improved for the dura-

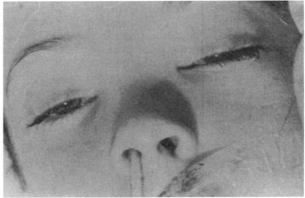

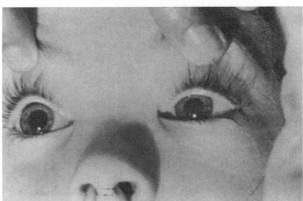

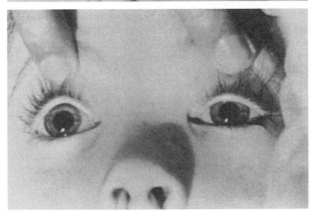

Figure 21.16. Clinical appearance of an 8-year-old girl who developed wound botulism after she fell from a horse and sustained a compound fracture of the humerus. Although the wound appeared clean, *Clostridium botulinum* was cultured from it. *Top,* The patient has severe bilateral ptosis. *Middle,* On attempted rightward gaze, there is marked limitation of movement of both eyes. Note dilated pupils. *Bottom,* On attempted leftward gaze, there is almost no movement of the eyes. The patient was quadriparetic but was awake and alert. She recovered completely within several months.

tion of the medication effect, and ocular ductions were also much improved. All abnormalities had resolved when the patient was retested 7 months later (169).

Electromyography can establish the diagnosis of botulism (671–673). The findings suggest a presynaptic disorder analogous to Lambert-Eaton myasthenic syndrome. Motor and sensory nerve conduction velocities are normal. The amplitude of the evoked muscle action potential is usually reduced. There may be no decrement at low rates of stimulation. Following exercise or at high stimulus frequencies, significant facilitation is present. Single-fiber EMG shows increased jitter and blocking. These abnormalities are less prominent at higher frequencies of innervation (674). Fibrillations in affected muscles may appear about 2 weeks after the disorder begins.

Botulism is treated with bivalent (A and B) or trivalent (A, B, and E) antitoxin, 20,000–40,000 units, two or three times per day, in addition to removal of stomach and intestinal contents (649) if ingestion was the likely route of entry. Early antitoxin treatment is important to maximize its effectiveness (675). Because most commercially available antitoxins are equine immunoglobulins, serious allergic reactions may develop during therapy. The CDC must be contacted to obtain the antitoxin in most areas of the United States. In patients with wound botulism, the most important treatment is to open and extensively débride the wound. Penicillin or another antibiotic should be given, with the choice of the antibiotic being based on sensitivies from wound culture. By contrast, treatment of patients with food-borne botulism with oral penicillin to destroy organisms in the gastrointestinal tract is of no benefit (653). Regardless of the apparent severity of the disease when the patient is first seen, full respiratory and nutritional support may be required.

Although guanidine may reverse the electrophysiologic defect and increase the amplitude of the muscle action potential in patients with botulism (672,673,676), it may not help such patients clinically (677,678). Similarly, 4-aminopyridine may also produce electrophysiologic improvement (679), but neither guanidine nor 4-aminopyridine seems to reverse respiratory depression. The efficacy of 3,4-diaminopyridine in the treatment of botulism is controversial, with individual case reports finding both improvement and no benefit in botulism of different serotypes (680–682). Patients with botulism do not respond well to treatment with anticholinesterase agents.

Tetanus

Like *Clostridium botulinum, Clostridium tetani* produces a neurotoxin that blocks the calcium-dependent release of ACh at NMJs (630), but this effect is overshadowed by its effects on the CNS. Tetanus is described in detail in Chapter 49.

Toxins that Damage Both Pre- and Postsynaptic Neuromuscular Transmission

Envenomation by poisonous snakes is an important problem around the world. Of the four largest families of poisonous snakes (*Elapidae,* cobras, coral snakes, mambas, kraits; *Hydrophiidae,* sea snakes; *Viperidae,* Old World vipers; and *Crotalidae,* rattlesnakes and related species), only the first two have venom with potent neuromuscular blocking properties (683,684). (The South American rattlesnake [*Crotalus*

durissus terrificus] is an exception.) The venom of the Papuan taipan snake (*Oxyuranus scutellatus canni*) contains a variety of toxins, including neurotoxins, a procoagulant, and a calcium channel blocking toxin. The effects of taipan snake venom are predominantly presynaptic.

In most cases of *Elapidae* envenomation, neuromuscular blocking activity of the venoms is a major cause of death and disability. Envenomation is followed in minutes to hours by signs of neuromuscular blockade resembling that caused by competitive neuromuscular blocking drugs. Patients initially develop bilateral ptosis, ophthalmoparesis, and dysphagia, followed by tongue, laryngeal, and pharyngeal weakness (685–688). Respiratory paralysis eventually occurs, leading to death if patients are not treated. Ophthalmoparesis and ptosis are frequent components, related to both pre- and postsynaptic effects on neuromuscular transmission (689). Sea snakes, members of *Hydrophiidae,* produce a neurotoxic venom that can also produce ptosis and ophthalmoplegia (690). Many of the symptoms show improvement with anticholinesterase agents (691), although antivenom administration and ventilatory and cardiocirculatory support are the mainstays of treatment.

REFERENCES

1. Drachman DB. Myasthenia gravis. N Engl J Med 1994;330:1797–1810.
2. Vincent A, Palace J, Hilton-Jones D. Myasthenia gravis. Lancet 2001;357:2122–2128.
3. Engel AG. Myasthenia Gravis and Myasthenic Disorders. New York, Oxford, 1999.
4. Hebb CO, Krnjevic K, Silver A. Acetylcholine and choline acetyltransferase in the diaphragm of the rat. J Physiol 1964;171:504–513.
5. Hubbard JI. Microphysiology of vertebrate neuromuscular transmission. Physiol Rev 1973;53:674–723.
6. Heuser JE, Reese TS. Evidence for recycling of synaptic vesicle membrane during transmitter release at the frog neuromuscular junction. J Cell Biol 1973;57:315–344.
7. Heuser JE, Reese TS, Landis DMD. Functional changes in frog neuromuscular junctions studied with freeze-fracture. J Neurocytol 1974;3:109–131.
8. Hubbard JI, Kwanbunbumpen S. Evidence for the vesicle hypothesis. J Physiol 1968;194:407–420.
9. Fertuck HC, Salpeter MM. Localization of acetylcholine receptor by ^{125}I-labeled alpha-bungarotoxin binding at mouse motor endplates. Proc Natl Acad Sci USA 1974;71:1376–1378.
10. Takeuchi A, Takeuchi N. On the permeability of end-plate membrane during the action of transmitter. J Physiol 1960;154:52–67.
11. Fatt P, Katz B. Spontaneous subthreshold activity at motor nerve endings. J Physiol 1952;117:109–128.
12. Katz B. The Release of Neural Transmitter Substances. Springfield, IL, Charles C Thomas, 1969.
13. Kistler J, Stroud R, Klymkowsky M, et al. Structure and function of an acetylcholine receptor. Biophys J 1982;37:371–383.
14. Ratnam M, LeNguyen D, Rivier J, et al. Transmembrane topography of the nicotinic acetylcholine receptor: Immunochemical tests contradict theoretical predictions based on hydrophobicity profile. Biochem 1986;25:2633–2643.
15. Kubalek E, Ralston S, Lindstrom J, et al. Location of subunits within the acetylcholine receptor by electron image analysis of tubular crystals from *Torpedo marmorata.* J Cell Biol 1987;105:9–18.
16. Stevens CF. Channel families in the brain. Nature 1987;328:198–199.
17. Changeux JP. Functional architecture and dynamics of the nicotinic acetylcholine receptor: An allosteric ligand-gated ion channel. In Fidia Research Foundation N.S. Award Lectures. New York, Raven Press, 1990:21–168.
18. Newsom-Davis J. Myasthenia gravis and the Miller Fisher variant of Guillain-Barré syndrome. Curr Opin Neurol 1997;10:18–21.
19. Berg DK, Hall ZW. Loss of alpha-bungarotoxin from junctional and extrajunctional acetylcholine receptors in rat diaphragm muscle in vivo and in organ culture. J Physiol 1975;252:771–789.
20. Devreotes PN, Fambrough DM. Acetylcholine receptor turnover in membranes of developing muscle fibers. J Cell Biol 1975;65:335–358.
21. Patrick J, Lindstrom J. Autoimmune response to acetylcholine receptor. Science 1973;180:871–872.
22. Lambert EH, Lindstrom JM, Lennon VA. End-plate potentials in experimental autoimmune myasthenia gravis in rats. Ann NY Acad Sci 1976;274:300–318.

23. Penn AS, Chang HW, Lovelace RE, et al. Antibodies to acetylcholine receptors in rabbits: Immunochemical and electrophysiological studies. Ann NY Acad Sci 1976;274:354–376.

24. Sanders DB, Schleifer LS, Eldefrawi ME, et al. An immunologically induced defect of neuromuscular transmission in rats and rabbits. Ann NY Acad Sci 1976;274:319–336.

25. Fambrough DM, Drachman DB, Satyamurti S. Neuromuscular junction in myasthenia gravis: Decreased acetylcholine receptors. Science 1973;182:293–295.

26. Lindstrom JM, Seybold ME, Lennon VA, et al. Antibody to acetylcholine receptor in myasthenia gravis. Prevalence, clinical correlates, and diagnostic value. Neurology 1976;26:1054–1059.

27. Vincent A, Newsom-Davis J. Acetylcholine receptor antibody as a diagnostic test for myasthenia gravis: results in 153 validated cases and 2967 diagnostic assays. J Neurol Neurosurg Psychiatry 1985;48:1246–1252.

28. Lennon VA, Lindstrom JM, Seybold ME. Experimental autoimmune myasthenia gravis: Cellular and humoral immune responses. Ann NY Acad Sci 1976;274:283–299.

29. Roses AD, Olanow CW, McAdams MW, Lane RJ. No direct correlation between serum antiacetylcholine receptor antibody levels and clinical state of individual patients with myasthenia gravis. Neurology 1981;31:220–224.

30. Drachman DB, Adams RN, Josifek LF, Self SG. Functional activities of autoantibodies to acetylcholine receptors and the clinical severity of myasthenia gravis. N Engl J Med 1982;307:769–775.

31. Garchon HJ, Djabiri F, Viard JP, et al. Involvement of human muscle acetylcholine receptor alpha-subunit gene (CHRNA) in susceptibility to myasthenia gravis. Proc Natl Acad Sci USA 1994;91:4668–4672.

32. Heckmann JM, Morrison KE, Emeryk-Szajewska B, et al. Human muscle acetylcholine receptor alpha-subunit gene (CHRNA1) association with autoimmune myasthenia gravis in black, mixed-ancestry and Caucasian subjects. J Autoimmun 1996;9:175–180.

33. Giraud M, Eymard B, Tranchant C, et al. Association of the gene encoding the delta-subunit of the muscle acetylcholine receptor (CHRND) with acquired autoimmune myasthenia gravis. Genes Immun 2004;5:80–83.

34. Bonifati DM, Willcox N, Vincent A, Beeson D. Lack of association between acetylcholine receptor epsilon polymorphisms and early onset myasthenia gravis. Muscle Nerve 2004;29:436–439.

35. Djabiri F, Gajdos P, Eymard B, et al. No evidence for an association of AChR beta-subunit gene (CHRNB1) with myasthenia gravis. J Neuroimmunol 1997;78(1–2):86–89.

36. Vincent A, Newsom-Davis J. Acetylcholine receptor antibody characteristics in myasthenia gravis. I. Patients with generalized myasthenia or disease restricted to ocular muscles. Clin Exp Immunol 1982;49:257–265.

37. Mossman S, Vincent A, Newsom-Davis J. Myasthenia gravis without acetylcholine-receptor antibody: A distinct disease entity. Lancet 1986;1:116–119.

38. Evoli A, Bartoccioni E, Batocchi AP, et al. Anti-AChR-negative myasthenia gravis: Clinical and immunological features. Clin Invest 1989;12:104–109.

39. Drachman DB, de Silva S, Ramsay D, Pestronk A. Humoral pathogenesis of myasthenia gravis. Ann NY Acad Sci 1987;505:90–105.

40. Hoch W, McConville J, Helms S, et al. Auto-antibodies to the receptor tyrosine kinase MuSK in patients with myasthenia gravis without acetylcholine receptor antibodies. Nat Med 2001;7:365–368.

41. Vincent A, McConville J, Farrugia ME, et al. Antibodies in myasthenia gravis and related disorders. Ann NY Acad Sci 2003;998:324–335.

42. Vincent A, Bowen J, Newsom-Davis J, McConville J. Seronegative generalised myasthenia gravis: clinical features, antibodies, and their targets. Lancet Neurol 2003;2:99–106.

43. Evoli A, Tonali PA, Padua L, et al. Clinical correlates with anti-MuSK antibodies in generalized seronegative myasthenia gravis. Brain 2003;126(Pt 10):2304–2311.

44. Scuderi F, Marino M, Colonna L, et al. Anti-p110 autoantibodies identify a subtype of "seronegative" myasthenia gravis with prominent oculobulbar involvement. Lab Invest 2002;82:1139–1146.

45. Yamamoto T, Vincent A, Ciulla TA, et al. Seronegative myasthenia gravis: A plasma factor inhibiting agonist-induced acetylcholine receptor function copurifies with IgM. Ann Neurol 1991;30:550–557.

46. Simpson JA. An evaluation of thymectomy in myasthenia gravis. Brain 1958;81:112–144.

47. Simpson JA. Myasthenia gravis: A new hypothesis. Scot Med J 1960;5:419–436.

48. Wirtz PW, Nijnuis MG, Sotodeh M, et al. The epidemiology of myasthenia gravis, Lambert-Eaton myasthenic syndrome and their associated tumours in the northern part of the province of South Holland. J Neurol 2003;250:698–701.

49. Phillips LH 2nd. The epidemiology of myasthenia gravis. Ann NY Acad Sci 2003;998:407–412.

50. Lopez-Cano M, Ponseti-Bosch JM, Espin-Basany E, et al. Clinical and pathologic predictors of outcome in thymoma-associated myasthenia gravis. Ann Thorac Surg 2003;76:1643–1649.

51. Mattis RD. Ocular manifestations of myasthenia gravis. Arch Ophthalmol 1941;26:969–982.

52. Osserman KE. Myasthenia Gravis. New York, Grune & Stratton, 1957.

53. Daroff RB. Ocular myasthenia: Diagnosis and therapy. In Glaser JS, ed. Neuro-Ophthalmology. St Louis, CV Mosby, 1980:62–71.

54. Oosterhuis HJ. The ocular signs and symptoms of myasthenia gravis. Doc Ophthalmol 1982;52(3–4):363–378.

55. Cogan DG. Myasthenia gravis: A review of the disease and a description of lid twitch as a characteristic sign. Arch Ophthalmol 1965;74:217–221.

56. Cogan DG, Chu FC. Ocular manifestations of myasthenia gravis. In Smith JL, ed. Neuro-Ophthalmology Focus 1982. New York, Masson, 1981:131–138.

57. Kao YF, Lan MY, Chou MS, Chen WH. Intracranial fatigable ptosis. J Neuroophthalmol 1999;19:257–259.

58. Gorelick PB, Rosenberg M, Pagano RJ. Enhanced ptosis in myasthenia gravis. Arch Neurol 1981;38:531.

59. Gay AJ, Salmon ML, Windsor CE. Hering's law, the levators, and their relationship in disease states. Arch Ophthalmol 1967;77:157–160.

60. Puklin JE, Sacks JG, Boshes B. Transient eyelid retraction in myasthenia gravis. J Neurol Neurosurg Psychiatry 1976;39:44–47.

61. Kaminski HJ, Maas E, Spiegel P, Ruff RL. Why are eye muscles frequently involved in myasthenia gravis? Neurology 1990;40:1663–1669.

62. Kaminski HJ, Richmonds CR, Kusner LL, Mitsumoto H. Differential susceptibility of the ocular motor system to disease. Ann NY Acad Sci 2002;956:42–54.

63. Glaser JS. Ocular manifestations in Symposium on Neuro-Ophthalmology. Transactions of the New Orleans Academy of Ophthalmology. St. Louis, CV Mosby, 1976:232–240.

64. Acers TE. Ocular myasthenia gravis mimicking pseudointernuclear ophthalmoplegia and variable esotropia. Am J Ophthalmol 1979;88(3 Pt 1):319–321.

65. Glaser JS. Myasthenic psuedo-internuclear ophthalmoplegia. Arch Ophthalmol 1966;75:363–366.

66. Jay WM, Nazarian SM, Underwood DW. Pseudo-internuclear ophthalmoplegia with downshoot in myasthenia gravis. J Clin Neuroophthalmol 1987;7:74–76.

67. Ito K, Mizutani J, Murofushi T, Mizuno M. Bilateral pseudo-internuclear ophthalmoplegia in myasthenia gravis. J Otorhinolaryngol Relat Spec 1997;59:122–126.

68. Fagundez Vargas MA, Andres Domingo ML, Calvo Arrabal MA. [The WEB-INO syndrome as presentation form of myasthenia gravis]. Arch Soc Esp Oftalmol 2000;75:485–488.

69. Cleary PE. Ocular manifestations of myasthenia gravis. Br Orthopt J 1973;30:38–51.

70. Spoor TC, Shippman S. Myasthenia gravis presenting as an isolated inferior rectus paresis. Ophthalmology 1979;86:2158–2160.

71. Van Dalen JTW, Van Mourek-Noordenbos AM. Isolated inferior rectus paresis: A report of six cases. Neuroophthalmology 1984;4:89–94.

72. Rush JA, Shafrin F. Ocular myasthenia presenting as superior oblique weakness. J Clin Neuroophthalmol 1982;2:125–127.

73. Osher RH. Myasthenic "oculomotor" palsy. Ann Ophthalmol 1979;11:31–34.

74. McCrary JA. Tensilon and the pseudo-double elevator palsy. In Smith JL, ed. Neuro-Ophthalmology Symposium of the University of Miami and the Bascom Palmer Eye Institute, 1970. Hallandale, FL, Huffman Publishing Co, 1970:119–122.

75. Brust JC, List TA, Catalano LW, Lovelace R. Ocular myasthenia gravis mimicking progressive external ophthalmoplegia. Rare case of myasthenia associated with peripheral neuropathy and spastic paraparesis. Neurology 1974;24:755–760.

76. Das JC, Chaudhuri Z, Bhomaj S, et al. Ocular myasthenia presenting as progressive external ophthalmoplegia. J Pediatr Ophthalmol Strabismus 2002;39:52–54.

77. Osher RH, Glaser JS. Myasthenic sustained gaze fatigue. Am J Ophthalmol 1980;89:443–445.

78. Spooner JW, Baloh RW. Eye movement fatigue in myasthenia gravis. Neurology 1979;29:29–33.

79. Metz HS, Scott AB, O'Meara DM. Saccadic eye movements in myasthenia gravis. Arch Ophthalmol 1972;88:9–11.

80. Schmidt D. Saccadic eye movements in myasthenic ocular muscle pareses. In Glaser JS, ed. Neuro-Ophthalmology. St Louis, CV Mosby, 1977:177–189.

81. Schmidt D, Dell'Osso LF, Abel LA, Daroff RB. Myasthenia gravis: Dynamic changes in saccadic waveform, gain, and velocity. Exp Neurol 1980;68:365–377.

82. Schmidt D, Dell'Osso LF, Abel LA, Daroff RB. Myasthenia gravis: Saccadic eye movement waveforms. Exp Neurol 1980;68:346–364.

83. Szmeja Z, et al. [The value of stapedius reflex examinations in patients with myasthenia gravis]. HNO 1978;26:198–200.

84. Lande S, Black J, Dolly JO, et al. Effects of botulinum neurotoxin and Lambert-Eaton myasthenic syndrome IgG at mouse nerve terminals. J Neural Transm Park Dis Dement Sect 1989;1:229–242.

85. Baloh RW, Keesey JC. Saccade fatigue and response to edrophonium for the diagnosis of myasthenia gravis. Ann NY Acad Sci 1976;274:631–641.

86. Cogan DG, Yee RD, Gittinger J. Rapid eye movements in myasthenia gravis. I. Clinical observations. Arch Ophthalmol 1976;94:1083–1085.

87. Yamazaki A, Ishikawa S. Eye movements. In Ishikawa S, ed. Neuro-Ophthalmology. Tokyo, Egaku Shoin, 1974.

88. Schmidt D. [Diagnosis of myasthenic eye signs. Clinical signs and electronystagmographical findings of saccadic eye movements]. Klin Monatsbl Augenheilkd 1975;167:651–664.

89. Yee RD, Cogan DG, Zee DS, et al. Rapid eye movements in myasthenia gravis. II. Electro-oculographic analysis. Arch Ophthalmol 1976;94:1465–1472.

90. Barton JJ, Sharpe JA. ''Saccadic jitter'' is a quantitative ocular sign in myasthenia gravis. Invest Ophthalmol Vis Sci 1995;36:1566–1572.

91. Blomberg LH, Persson T. A new test for myasthenia gravis. Preliminary report. Acta Neurol Scand Suppl 1965;13(pt 1):363–364.

92. Stella S. Optokinetic nystagmus in patients with ocular myasthenia. Invest Ophthalmol 1967;6:668–669.

93. Campbell MJ, Simpson E, Crombie AL, Walton JN. Ocular myasthenia: Evaluation of Tensilon tonography and electronystagmography as diagnostic tests. J Neurol Neurosurg Psychiatry 1970;33:639–646.

94. Spector RH, Daroff RB, Birkett JE. Demonstration of Tensilon responsiveness with infrared optokinetic nystagmography. In Glaser JS, Smith JL, eds. Neuro-Ophthalmology Symposium of the University of Miami and the Bascom Palmer Eye Institute, 1975. St Louis, CV Mosby, 1975:270–276.

95. Spector RH, Daroff RB, Birkett JE. Edrophonium infrared optokinetic nystagmography in the diagnosis of myasthenia gravis. Neurology 1975;25:317–321.

96. Dell'Osso LF, Ayyar DR, Daroff RB, Abel LA. Edrophonium test in Eaton-Lambert syndrome: Quantitative oculography. Neurology 1983;33:1157–1163.

97. Barton JJ. Quantitative ocular tests for myasthenia gravis: A comparative review with detection theory analysis. J Neurol Sci 1998;155:104–114.

98. Yang Q, Wei M, Sun F, et al. Open-loop and closed-loop optokinetic nystagmus (OKN) in myasthenia gravis and nonmyasthenic subjects. Exp Neurol 2000;166:166–172.

99. Tian J, Yang Q, Wei M, et al. Neostigmine-induced alterations in fast phase of optokinetic responses in myasthenic ocular palsies. J Neurol 2002;249:867–874.

100. Feldon SE, Hoyt WF, Stark L. Saccadic abnormalities in diseases of the peripheral nervous system. In Lennerstrand G, Zee DS, Keller EL, eds. Functional Basis of Ocular Motility Disorders. Oxford, Pergamon Press, 1982:545–548.

101. Feldon SE, Stark L, Lehman SL, Hoyt WF. Oculomotor effects of intermittent conduction block in myasthenia gravis and Guillain-Barré syndrome. An oculographic study with computer simulations. Arch Neurol 1982;39:497–503.

102. Komiyama A, Toda H, Johkura K. Edrophonium-induced macrosaccadic oscillations in myasthenia gravis. Ann Neurol 1999;45:522–525.

103. Abel LA, Schmidt D, Dell'Osso LF. Saccadic system plasticity in humans. Ann Neurol 1978;4:313–318.

104. Optican LM, Robinson DA. Cerebellar-dependent adaptive control of primate saccadic system. J Neurophysiol 1980;44:1058–1076.

105. Bender MB. Disorders of eye movements. In Vinken PH, Bruyn GW, eds. Handbook of Clinical Neurology. Amsterdam, North Holland Publishing Co, 1969:598.

106. Finelli PF, Hoyt WF. Myasthenic abduction mystagmus in a patient with hyperthyroidism. Neurology 1976;26(6 pt 1):589–590.

107. Keane JR, Hoyt WF. Myasthenic (vertical) nystagmus. Verification by edrophonium tonography. JAMA 1970;212:1209–1210.

108. Osher RH, Griggs RC. Orbicularis fatigue: The ''peek'' sign of myasthenia gravis. Arch Ophthalmol 1979;97:677–679.

109. Baptista AG, Silva ESH. Pupillary abnormalities in myasthenia gravis. Report of a case. Neuropsihijatrija 1961;11:210–213.

110. Herishanu Y, Lavy S. Internal ''ophthalmoplegia'' in myasthenia gravis. Ophthalmologica 1971;163:302–305.

111. Dutton GN, Garson JA, Richardson RB. Pupillary fatigue in myasthenia gravis. Trans Ophthalmol Soc UK 1982;102 (pt 4):510–513.

112. Yamazaki A, Ishikawa S. Abnormal pupillary responses in myasthenia gravis. A pupillographic study. Br J Ophthalmol 1976;60:575–580.

113. Lepore FE, Sanborn GE, Slevin JT. Pupillary dysfunction in myasthenia gravis. Ann Neurol 1979;6:29–33.

114. Bryant RC. Asymmetrical pupillary slowing and degree of severity in myasthenia gravis. Ann Neurol 1980;7:288–289.

115. Vernino S, Low PA, Fealey RD, et al. Autoantibodies to ganglionic acetylcholine receptors in autoimmune autonomic neuropathies. N Engl J Med 2000;343:847–855.

116. Sandroni P, Vernino S, Klein CM, et al. Idiopathic autonomic neuropathy: Comparison of cases seropositive and seronegative for ganglionic acetylcholine receptor antibody. Arch Neurol 2004;61:44–48.

117. Vernino S, Cheshire WP, Lennon VA. Myasthenia gravis with autoimmune autonomic neuropathy. Auton Neurosci 2001;88:187–192.

118. Rabinovitch V, Vengrjenovsky G. Sur un cas de myasthenie progressive avec participation des muscles lisses de l'oeil. Arch Ophthalmol 1935;52:23–31.

119. Bonnet M. [The ocular manifestations of primary diseases of striated muscle]. J Med Lyon 1965;46:867–891.

120. Manson N, Stern G. Defects of near vision in myasthenia gravis. Lancet 1965;62:935–937.

121. Walsh FB, Hoyt WF. Clinical Neuro-Ophthalmology. 3rd ed. Baltimore, Williams & Wilkins, 1969:1285.

122. Matsui M, Enoki M, Matsui Y, et al. Seronegative myasthenia gravis associated with atonic urinary bladder and accommodative insufficiency. J Neurol Sci 1995;133(1–2):197–199.

123. Van Bogaert L. Sur des modalites exceptionnelles des crises oculgyres. J Neurol Psychiatry 1928;28:379.

124. Morioka WT, Neff PA, Boisseranc TE, et al. Audiotympanometric findings in myasthenia gravis. Arch Otolaryngol 1976;102:211–213.

125. Leker RR, Karni A, Abramsky O. Exacerbation of myasthenia gravis during the menstrual period. J Neurol Sci 1998;156:107–111.

126. Odel JG, Winterkorn JM, Behrens MM. The sleep test for myasthenia gravis. A safe alternative to Tensilon. J Clin Neuroophthalmol 1991;11:288–292.

127. Saavedra J, Femminini R, Kochen S, deZarate JC. A cold test for myasthenia gravis. Neurology 1979;29:1075.

128. Sethi KD, Rivner MH, Swift TR. Ice pack test for myasthenia gravis. Neurology 1987;37:1383–1385.

129. Ertas M, Arac N, Kumral K, Tuncbay T. Ice test as a simple diagnostic aid for myasthenia gravis. Acta Neurol Scand 1994;89:227–229.

130. Borenstein S, Desmedt JE. Local cooling in myasthenia. Improvement of neuromuscular failure. Arch Neurol 1975;32:152–157.

131. Ellis FD, Hoyt CS, Ellis FJ, et al. Extraocular muscle responses to orbital cooling (ice test) for ocular myasthenia gravis diagnosis. J AAPOS 2000;4:271–281.

132. Movaghar M, Slavin ML. Effect of local heat versus ice on blepharoptosis resulting from ocular myasthenia. Ophthalmology 2000;107:2209–2214.

133. Kubis KC, Danesh-Meyer HV, Savino PJ, Sergott RC. The ice test versus the rest test in myasthenia gravis. Ophthalmology 2000;107:1995–1998.

134. Lindstrom J. An assay for antibodies to human acetylcholine receptor in serum from patients with myasthenia gravis. Clin Immunol Immunopathol 1977;7:36–43.

135. Kao I, Drachman DB. Myasthenic immunoglobulin accelerates acetylcholine receptor degradation. Science 1977;196:527–529.

136. Howard FM Jr, Lennon VA, Finley J, et al. Clinical correlations of antibodies that bind, block, or modulate human acetylcholine receptors in myasthenia gravis. Ann NY Acad Sci 1987;505:526–538.

137. Beeson D, Jacobson L, Newsom-Davis J, Vincent A. A transfected human muscle cell line expressing the adult subtype of the human muscle acetylcholine receptor for diagnostic assays in myasthenia gravis. Neurology 1996;47:1552–1555.

138. MacLennan C, Beeson D, Buijs AM, et al. Acetylcholine receptor expression in human extraocular muscles and their susceptibility to myasthenia gravis. Ann Neurol 1997;41:423–431.

139. Mittag TW, Caroscio J. False-positive immunoassay for acetylcholine receptor antibody in amyotrophic lateral sclerosis. N Engl J Med 1980;302:868.

140. Mitsikostas D, Manta P, Kalfakis N, et al. External ophthalmoplegia with ragged-red fibres and acetylcholine receptor antibodies. Funct Neurol 1995;10(4–5):209–215.

141. Jacobson DM. Acetylcholine receptor antibodies in patients with Graves' ophthalmopathy. J Neuroophthalmol 1995;15:166–170.

142. Koelle GB. Anticholinesterase agents. In Goodman LS, Gilman A, eds. Pharmacologic Basis of Therapeutics. 5th ed. New York, MacMillan, 1975:445–466.

143. Kupersmith MJ, Latkany R, Homel P. Development of generalized disease at 2 years in patients with ocular myasthenia gravis. Arch Neurol 2003;60:243–248.

144. Kupersmith MJ, Weinberg H, Frohman L, et al. Ocular myasthenia: diagnosis and treatment. In Lawton-Smith, Katz RS, eds. Neuroophthalmology Enters the Nineties. Hialeah, FL, Dutton Press, 1988:178–182.

145. Kelly JJ Jr, Daube JR, Lennon VA, et al. The laboratory diagnosis of mild myasthenia gravis. Ann Neurol 1982;12:238–242.

146. Retzlaff JA, Kearns TP, Howard FM Jr, Cronin ML. Lancaster red-green test in evaluation of edrophonium effect in myasthenia gravis. Am J Ophthalmol 1969;67:13–21.

147. Younge BR, Bartley GB. Lancaster test with Tensilon for myasthenia. Arch Neurol 1987;44:472–473.

148. Siatkowski RM, Shah L, Feuer WJ. The effect of edrophonium chloride on muscle balance in normal subjects and those with nonmyasthenic strabismus. J Neuroophthalmol 1997;17:7–11.

149. Breinin GM. Electromyography; a tool in ocular and neurologic diagnosis. I. Myasthenia gravis. AMA Arch Ophthalmol 1957;57:161–164.

150. Gil R, Lefevre JP. [Optokinetic nystagmus and the Tensilon test in myasthenia]. Rev Electroencephalogr Neurophysiol Clin 1983;13:88–95.

151. Barton JJ, Huaman AG, Sharpe JA. Effects of edrophonium on saccadic velocity in normal subjects and myasthenic and nonmyasthenic ocular palsies. Ann Neurol 1994;36:585–594.

152. Barton JJ, Jama A, Sharpe JA. Saccadic duration and intrasaccadic fatigue in myasthenic and nonmyasthenic ocular palsies. Neurology 1995;45:2065–2072.

153. Osserman KE, Kaplan LI. Rapid diagnostic test for myasthenia gravis: Increased muscle strength, without fasciculation after intravenous administration of edrophonium (Tensilon) chloride. JAMA 1952;150:265–269.

154. Van Dyk HJ, Florence L. The Tensilon test. A safe office procedure. Ophthalmology 1980;87:210–212.

155. Ing EB, Ing SY, Ing T, Ramocki JA. The complication rate of edrophonium testing for suspected myasthenia gravis. Can J Ophthalmol 2000;35:141–145.

156. Okun MS, Charriez CM, Bhatti MT, et al. Asystole induced by edrophonium following beta blockade. Neurology 2001;57:739.

157. Pascuzzi RM. The edrophonium test. Semin Neurol 2003;23:83–88.

158. Dirr LY, Donofrio PD, Patton JF, Troost BT. A false-positive edrophonium test in a patient with a brainstem glioma. Neurology 1989;39:865–867.

159. Ragge NK, Hoyt WF. Midbrain myasthenia: Fatigable ptosis, ''lid twitch'' sign, and ophthalmoparesis from a dorsal midbrain glioma. Neurology 1992;42:917–919.

160. Fierro B, Croce G, Filosto L, et al. Ocular pseudomyasthenia: report of a case with a pineal region tumor. Ital J Neurol Sci 1991;12:593–596.

161. Moorthy G, Behrens MM, Drachman DB, et al. Ocular pseudomyasthenia or ocular myasthenia ''plus'': A warning to clinicians. Neurology 1989;39:1150–1154.

162. Gupta M, Davis H, Rennie IG. Positive Tensilon test and intracranial tumor: A case report. Eur J Ophthalmol 2003;13:590–592.

163. Henriksson KG, Nilsson O, Rosen I, Schiller HH. Clinical, neurophysiological and morphological findings in Eaton Lambert syndrome. Acta Neurol Scand 1977;56:117–140.

164. Oh SJ, Cho HK. Edrophonium responsiveness not necessarily diagnostic of myasthenia gravis. Muscle Nerve 1990;13:187–191.

165. Nakashima I, Kikuchi A, Onodera J, et al. [A juvenile case of Lambert-Eaton myasthenic syndrome with severe emaciation]. Rinsho Shinkeigaku 1997;37:402–406.

166. Hughes JM, Blumenthal JR, Merson MH, et al. Clinical features of types A and B food-borne botulism. Ann Intern Med 1981;95:442–445.

167. Edell TA, Sullivan CP Jr, Osborn KM, et al. Wound botulism associated with a positive Tensilon test. West J Med 1983;139:218–219.

168. Rapoport S, Watkins PB. Descending paralysis resulting from occult wound botulism. Ann Neurol 1984;16:359–361.

169. Stahl JS, Averbuch-Heller L, Remler BF, Leigh RJ. Clinical evidence of extraocular muscle fiber-type specificity of botulinum toxin. Neurology 1998;51:1093–1099.

170. Engel AG, Ohno K, Sine SM. Congenital myasthenic syndromes: Recent advances. Arch Neurol 1999;56:163–167.

171. Watt G, Theakston RD, Hayes CG, et al. Positive response to edrophonium in patients with neurotoxic envenoming by cobras (*Naja naja philippinensis*). A placebo-controlled study. N Engl J Med 1986;315:1444–1448.

172. Hudson BJ. Positive response to edrophonium in death adder (*Acanthophis antarcticus*) envenomation. Aust NZ J Med 1988;18:792–794.

173. Diamond S, Schear HE, Leeds MF. Pseudo-internuclear oculomotor ophthalmoplegia secondary to Guillain-Barré polyneuronitis simulating myasthenia gravis in a air transport pilot. Aviat Space Environ Med 1975;46:204–207.

174. Mulder DW, Lambert EH, Eaton LM. Myasthenic syndrome in patients with amyotrophic lateral sclerosis. Neurology 1959;9:627–631.

175. Truffert A, Lalive PH, Janssens JP, et al. Endplate dysfunction causing respiratory failure in a patient with prior paralytic poliomyelitis. J Neurol Neurosurg Psychiatry 2003;74:370–372.

176. Viets HR, Schwab RS. Prostigmin in the diagnosis of myasthenia gravis. N Engl J Med 1935;213:1280–1283.

177. Miller NR, Morris JE, Maquire M. Combined use of neostigmine and ocular motility measurements in the diagnosis of myasthenia gravis. Arch Ophthalmol 1982;100:761–763.

178. Hsu SY, Tsai RK, Wang HZ, Su MY. A comparative study of ocular and generalized myasthenia gravis. Kaohsiung J Med Sci 2002;18:62–69.

179. Afifi AK, Bell WE. Tests for juvenile myasthenia gravis: Comparative diagnostic yield and prediction of outcome. J Child Neurol 1993;8:403–411.

180. Gunn VL, Nechyba C, eds. The Harriet Lane Handbook: A Manual for Pediatric House Officers. 16th ed. St Louis, CV Mosby, 2002.

181. Heijnsbroek GJ, van Gijn J. Neostigmine-induced fasciculations: A useful diagnostic test? Clin Neurol Neurosurg 1983;85:231–234.

182. Walsh FB, Hoyt WF. Clinical Neuro-Ophthalmology. 3rd ed. Baltimore, Williams & Wilkins, 1969:1287.

183. Özdemir C, Young RR. Electrical testing in myasthenia gravis. Ann NY Acad Sci 1971;183:287–302.

184. Özdemir C, Young RR. The results to be expected from electrical testing in the diagnosis of myasthenia gravis. Ann NY Acad Sci 1976;274:203–222.

185. Stalberg E. Clinical electrophysiology in myasthenia gravis. J Neurol Neurosurg Psychiatry 1980;43:622–633.

186. Literature review of the usefulness of repetitive nerve stimulation and single-fiber EMG in the electrodiagnostic evaluation of patients with suspected myasthenia gravis or Lambert-Eaton myasthenic syndrome. Muscle Nerve 2001;24:1239–1247.

187. Padua L, Stalberg E, LoMonaco M, et al. SFEMG in ocular myasthenia gravis diagnosis. Clin Neurophysiol 2000;111:1203–1207.

188. Oh SJ, Eslami N, Nishihira T, et al. Electrophysiological and clinical correlation in myasthenia gravis. Ann Neurol 1982;12:348–354.

189. Niks EH, Badrising UA, Verschuuren JJ, Van Dijk JG. Decremental response of the nasalis and hypothenar muscles in myasthenia gravis. Muscle Nerve 2003;28:236–238.

190. Borenstein S, Desmedt JE. Temperature and weather correlates of myasthenic fatigue. Lancet 1974;2:63–66.

191. Ricker K, Hertel G, Stodieck S. Influence of temperature on neuromuscular transmission in myasthenia gravis. J Neurol 1977;216:273–282.

192. Krarup C. Electrical and mechanical responses in the platysma and in the adductor pollicis muscle in normal subjects. J Neurol Neurosurg Psychiatry 1977;40:234–240.

193. Yamada M, Inaba A, Shiojiri T. X-linked spinal and bulbar muscular atrophy with myasthenic symptoms. J Neurol Sci 1997;146:183–185.

194. Stalberg E, Ekstedt J, Broman A. Neuromuscular transmission in myasthenia gravis studied with single-fibre electromyography. J Neurol Neurosurg Psychiatry 1974;37:540–547.

195. Schwartz MS, Stalberg E. Single-fibre electromyographic studies in myasthenia gravis with repetitive nerve stimulation. J Neurol Neurosurg Psychiatry 1975;38:678–682.

196. Gilchrist JM, Massey JM, Sanders DB. Single-fiber EMG and repetitive stimulation of the same muscle in myasthenia gravis. Muscle Nerve 1994;17:171–175.

197. Sonoo M, Uesugi H, Mochizuki A, et al. Single-fiber EMG and repetitive nerve stimulation of the same extensor digitorum communis muscle in myasthenia gravis. Clin Neurophysiol 2001;112:300–303.

198. Sanders DB. The electrodiagnosis of myasthenia gravis. Ann NY Acad Sci 1987;505:539–556.

199. Oh SJ, Kim DE, Kuruoglu R, et al. Diagnostic sensitivity of the laboratory tests in myasthenia gravis. Muscle Nerve 1992;15:720–724.

200. Stalberg E, Ekstedt J. Single-fibre EMG (clinical experience). Electroencephalogr Clin Neurophysiol 1971;30:259.

201. Rivero A, Crovetto L, Lopez L, et al. Single fiber electromyography of extraocular muscles: A sensitive method for the diagnosis of ocular myasthenia gravis. Muscle Nerve 1995;18:943–947.

202. Weinberg DH, Rizzo JF III, Hayes MT, et al. Ocular myasthenia gravis: Predictive value of single-fiber electromyography. Muscle Nerve 1999;22:1222–1227.

203. Stalberg E, Ekstedt J. Single-fiber EMG and microphysiology of the motor unit in normal and diseased human muscle. In Desmedt JE, ed. New Developments in Electromyography and Clinical Neurophysiology. Basel, S Karger, 1973:113–129.

204. Mercelis R. Abnormal single-fiber electromyography in patients not having myasthenia: Risk for diagnostic confusion? Ann NY Acad Sci 2003;998:509–511.

205. Ukachoke C, Ashby P, Basinski A, Sharpe JA. Usefulness of single-fiber EMG for distinguishing neuromuscular from other causes of ocular muscle weakness. Can J Neurol Sci 1994;21:125–128.

206. Kaye AD, Janssen R, Arger PH, et al. Mediastinal computed tomography in myasthenia gravis. J Comput Tomogr 1983;7:273–279.

207. Ellis K, Austin JH, Jaretzki A III. Radiologic detection of thymoma in patients with myasthenia gravis. AJR Am J Roentgenol 1988;151:873–881.

208. Pirronti T, Rinaldi P, Batocchi AP, et al. Thymic lesions and myasthenia gravis. Diagnosis based on mediastinal imaging and pathological findings. Acta Radiol 2002;43:380–384.

209. Nicolaou S, Muller NL, Li DK, Oger JJ. Thymus in myasthenia gravis: Comparison of CT and pathologic findings and clinical outcome after thymectomy. Radiology 1996;201:471–474.

210. Camera L, Brunetti A, Romano M, et al. Morphological imaging of thymic disorders. Ann Med 1999;31(Suppl 2):57–62.

211. Tomiyama N, Muller NL, Ellis SJ, et al. Invasive and noninvasive thymoma: Distinctive CT features. J Comput Assist Tomogr 2001;25:388–393.

212. Emskotter T, Trampe H, Lachenmayer L. [Magnetic resonance imaging in myasthenia gravis. An alternative to mediastinal computerized tomography?] Dtsch Med Wochenschr 1988;113:1508–1510.

213. Sakai S, Murayama S, Soeda H, et al. Differential diagnosis between thymoma and non-thymoma by dynamic MR imaging. Acta Radiol 2002;43:262–268.

214. Tregnaghi A, De Candia A, Calderone M, et al. [Imaging of the thymus gland in myasthenia gravis (computerized tomography and magnetic resonance)]. Radiol Med (Torino) 1995;90:404–409.

215. Higuchi T, Taki J, Kinuya S, et al. Thymic lesions in patients with myasthenia gravis: Characterization with thallium 201 scintigraphy. Radiology 2001;221:201–206.

216. Lastoria S, Vergara E, Palmieri G, et al. In vivo detection of malignant thymic masses by indium-111-DTPA-D-Phe1-octreotide scintigraphy. J Nucl Med 1998;39:634–639.

217. Liu RS, Yeh SH, Huang MH, et al. Use of fluorine-18 fluorodeoxyglucose positron emission tomography in the detection of thymoma: A preliminary report. Eur J Nucl Med 1995;22:1402–1407.

218. Kubota K, Yamada S, Kondo T, et al. PET imaging of primary mediastinal tumours. Br J Cancer 1996;73:882–886.

219. Aarli JA, Skeie GO, Mygland A, Gilhus NE. Muscle striation antibodies in myasthenia gravis. Diagnostic and functional significance. Ann NY Acad Sci 1998;841:505–515.

220. Romi F, Skeie GO, Aarli JA, Gilhus NE. Muscle autoantibodies in subgroups of myasthenia gravis patients. J Neurol 2000;247:369–375.

221. Skeie GO, Mygland A, Treves S, et al. Ryanodine receptor antibodies in myasthenia gravis: Epitope mapping and effect on calcium release in vitro. Muscle Nerve 2003;27:81–89.

222. Voltz RD, Albrich WC, Nagele A, et al. Paraneoplastic myasthenia gravis: Detection of anti-MGT30 (titin) antibodies predicts thymic epithelial tumor. Neurology 1997;49:1454–1457.

223. Romi F, Bo L, Skeie GO, et al. Titin and ryanodine receptor epitopes are expressed in cortical thymoma along with costimulatory molecules. J Neuroimmunol 2002;128(1–2):82–89.

224. Skeie GO, Romi F, Aarli JA, et al. Pathogenesis of myositis and myasthenia associated with titin and ryanodine receptor antibodies. Ann NY Acad Sci 2003;998:343–350.

225. Li YF, Zhang JB, Cui LY. Serum anti-titin antibody in patients with myasthenia gravis. Zhongguo Yi Xue Ke Xue Yuan Xue Bao 2003;25:725–727.
226. Buckley C, Newsom-Davis J, Willcox N, Vincent A. Do titin and cytokine antibodies in MG patients predict thymoma or thymoma recurrence? Neurology 2001;57:1579–1582.
227. Christensen PB, Jensen TS, Tsiropoulos I, et al. Associated autoimmune diseases in myasthenia gravis. A population-based study. Acta Neurol Scand 1995;91: 192–195.
228. Beekman R, Kuks JB, Oosterhuis HJ. Myasthenia gravis: Diagnosis and follow-up of 100 consecutive patients. J Neurol 1997;244:112–118.
229. Johns RJ, Knox DL, Walsh FB, Renken HJ. Involuntary eye movements in a patient with myasthenia and hyperthyroidism. Arch Ophthalmol 1962;67:35–41.
230. Drachman DB. Myasthenia gravis and the thyroid gland. N Engl J Med 1962; 266:330–333.
231. Simpson JA. The biochemistry of myasthenia gravis. In Kuhn E, ed. Progressive Muskeldystrophie, Myotonie, Myasthenie. Berlin, Springer Verlag, 1966: 339–349.
232. Gaelen LH, Levitan S. Myasthenia gravis and thyroid function. Arch Neurol 1968;18:107–110.
233. Schlezinger NS, Corin MS. Myasthenia gravis associated with hyperthyroidism in childhood. Neurology 1968;18:1217–1222.
234. Cohen JS. Optic neuropathy of Graves disease, hyperthyroidism, and ocular myasthenia gravis. Arch Ophthalmol 1973;90:131–132.
235. Millikan CH, Haines SF. The thyroid gland in relation to neuromuscular disease. AMA Arch Intern Med 1953;92:5–39.
236. Downes JM, Greenwood BM, Wray SH. Auto-immune aspects of myasthenia gravis. Q J Med 1966;35:85–105.
237. Behan PO. Immune disease and HLA associations with myasthenia gravis. J Neurol Neurosurg Psychiatry 1980;43:611–621.
238. Rowland LP, Hoefer PF, Aranow H Jr, Merritt HH. Fatalities in myasthenia gravis; a review of 39 cases with 26 autopsies. Neurology 1956;6:307–326.
239. Simpson JA. The correlations between myasthenia gravis and disorders of the thyroid gland. In Research in Muscular Dystrophy, Proceedings of the 4th Symposium, 1968. London, Pitman, 1968:31–41.
240. Bundey S, Doniach D, Soothill JF. Immunological studies in patients with juvenile-onset myasthenia gravis and in their relatives. Clin Exp Immunol 1972;11: 321–332.
241. Feinberg WD, Underdahl LO, Eaton LM. Myasthenia gravis and myxedema. Mayo Clin Proc 1957;32:299–305.
242. Sahay BM, Blendis LM, Greene R. Relation between myasthenia gravis and thyroid disease. Br Med J 1965;5437:762–765.
243. Simpson JA. Immunological disturbances in myasthenia gravis with a report of Hashimoto's disease developing after thymectomy. J Neurol Neurosurg Psychiatry 1964;27:485–492.
244. Simpson JA. Myasthenia gravis as an autoimmune disease: Clinical aspects. Ann NY Acad Sci 1966;135:506–516.
245. Becker KL, Titus JL, McConahey WM, Woolner LB. Morphologic evidence of thyroiditis in myasthenia gravis. JAMA 1964;187:994–996.
246. Daly JJ, Jackson E. Case of Hashimoto's disease with myasthenia gravis. Br Kuo J 1964;5385:748.
247. Osher RH, Smith JL. Ocular myasthenia gravis and Hashimoto's thyroiditis. Am J Ophthalmol 1975;79:1038–1043.
248. Donaldson JO, Grunnet ML, Thompson HG. Concurrence of myasthenia gravis, thymoma, and thyroid carcinoma. Arch Neurol 1980;40:122–124.
249. Raef H, Ladinsky M, Arem R. Concomitant euthyroid Graves' ophthalmopathy and isolated ocular myasthenia gravis. Postgrad Med J 1990;66:849–852.
250. Marino M, Ricciardi R, Pinchera A, et al. Mild clinical expression of myasthenia gravis associated with autoimmune thyroid diseases. J Clin Endocrinol Metab 1997;82:438–443.
251. Marino M, Barbesino G, Pinchera A, et al. Increased frequency of euthyroid ophthalmopathy in patients with Graves' disease associated with myasthenia gravis. Thyroid 2000;10:799–802.
252. Peacey SR, Belchetz PE. Graves' disease: Associated ocular myasthenia gravis and a thymic cyst. J R Soc Med 1993;86:297–298.
253. Bartley GB. The epidemiologic characteristics and clinical course of ophthalmopathy associated with autoimmune thyroid disease in Olmsted County, Minnesota. Trans Am Ophthalmol Soc 1994;92:477–588.
254. Bartley GB, Fatourechi V, Kadrmas EF, et al. Clinical features of Graves' ophthalmopathy in an incidence cohort. Am J Ophthalmol 1996;121:284–290.
255. Okada S, Saito E, Ogawa T, et al. Grades of exophthalmos and thyrotropin-binding inhibitory immunoglobulin in patients with myasthenia gravis. Eur Neurol 1995;35:99–103.
256. Vargas ME, Warren FA, Kupersmith MJ. Exotropia as a sign of myasthenia gravis in dysthyroid ophthalmopathy. Br J Ophthalmol 1993;77:822–823.
257. Ali AS, Akavaram NR. Neuromuscular disorders in thyrotoxicosis. Am Fam Physician 1980;22:97–102.
258. Ohno M, Hamada N, Yamakawa J, et al. Myasthenia gravis associated with Graves' disease in Japan. Jpn J Med 1987;26:2–6.
259. Teoh R, Chow CC, Kay R, et al. Response to control of hyperthyroidism in patients with myasthenia gravis and thyrotoxicosis. Br J Clin Pract 1990;44: 742–744.
260. Oosterhuis HJ. Studies in myasthenia gravis. 1. A clinical study of 180 patients. J Neurol Sci 1964;38:512–546.
261. Namba T, Grob D. Familial concurrence of myasthenia gravis and rheumatoid arthritis. Arch Intern Med 1970;125:1056–1058.
262. Goulon M, Estournet B, Tulliez M. Myasthenia gravis and associated diseases. Int J Neurol 1980;14:61–72.
263. Green RA, Booth CB. The development of myasthenia gravis after removal of thymoma. Am J Med 1958;25:293–302.
264. Bailey RO, Dunn HG, Rubin AM, Ritaccio AL. Myasthenia gravis with thymoma and pure red blood cell aplasia. Am J Clin Pathol 1988;89:687–693.
265. Simpson JA, Behan PO, Dick HM. Studies on the nature of autoimmunity in myasthenia gravis. Evidence for an immunodeficiency type. Ann NY Acad Sci 1976;274:382–389.
266. Green ST, Ng JP, Chan-Lam D. Insulin-dependent diabetes mellitus, myasthenia gravis, pernicious anaemia, autoimmune thyroiditis and autoimmune adrenalitis in a single patient. Scot Med J 1988;33:213–214.
267. Harvey AM, Shulman LE, Tumulty PA, et al. Systemic lupus erythematosus: Review of the literature and clinical analysis of 138 cases. Medicine (Balt) 1954; 33:291–437.
268. Alarc'on-Segovia D, Galbraith RF, Maldonado JE, Howard FM Jr. Systemic lupus erythematosus following thymectomy for myasthenia gravis. Report of two cases. Lancet 1963;186:662–665.
269. Wolf SM, Barrows HS. Myasthenia gravis and systemic lupus erythematosus. Arch Neurol 1966;14:254–258.
270. Branch CE Jr, Swift TR. Systemic lupus erythematosus, myasthenia gravis, and Ehlers-Danlos syndrome. Ann Neurol 1978;4:374–375.
271. Fujii Y, Miyoshi S, Kido T, et al. [Myasthenia gravis with systemic lupus erythematosus: Report of two cases and review of the literature]. Nippon Kyobu Geka Gakkai Zasshi 1983;31:106–111.
272. Park MJ, Kim YA, Lee SS, et al. Appearance of systemic lupus erythematosus in patients with myasthenia gravis following thymectomy: Two case reports. J Korean Med Sci 2004;19:134–136.
273. Beutner EH, Chorzelski TP, Hale WL, Hausmanowa-Petrusewicz I. Autoimmunity in concurrent myasthenia gravis and pemphigus erythematosus. JAMA 1968;203:845–849.
274. Hausmanowa-Petrusewicz I, Chorzelski T, Strugalska H. Three-year observation of a myasthenic syndrome concurrent with other autoimmune syndromes in a patient with thymoma. J Neurol Sci 1969;9:273–284.
275. Vetters JM, Saikia NK, Wood J, Simpson JA. Pemphigus vulgaris and myasthenia gravis. Br J Dermatol 1973;88:437–441.
276. Osserman KE, Kornfeld P, Cohen E, et al. Studies in myasthenia gravis; review of two hundred eighty-two cases at the Mount Sinai Hospital, New York City. AMA Arch Intern Med 1958;102:72–81.
277. Nishida H, Tanaka Y, Nakao N, et al. [A case of myasthenia gravis following sarcoidosis and Hashimoto's thyroiditis]. Rinsho Shinkeigaku 2000;40: 797–800.
278. Wolf SM, Rowland LP, Schotland DL, et al. Myasthenia as an autoimmune disease: Clinical aspects. Ann NY Acad Sci 1966;135:517–535.
279. Kuo CC, Chiu HC, Lin BJ. Myasthenia gravis and insulin-dependent diabetes mellitus in two adolescents. Zhonghua Min Guo Wei Sheng Wu Ji Mian Yi Xue Za Zhi 1989;22:31–37.
280. Bhalla R, Swedler WI, Lazarevic MB, et al. Myasthenia gravis and scleroderma. J Rheumatol 1993;20:1409–1410.
281. Wanchu A, Sud A, Bambery P. Linear scleroderma and autoimmune hemolytic anaemia. J Assoc Physicians India 2002;50:441–442.
282. Johansson EA, Niemi KM, Lassus A, Gripenberg M. Mixed connective tissue disease: A follow-up study of 12 patients with special reference to cold sensitivity and skin manifestations. Acta Derm Venereol 1981;61:225–231.
283. Vasilescu C, Bucur G, Petrovici A, Florescu A. Myasthenia in patients with dermatomyositis: clinical, electrophysiological and ultrastructural studies. J Neurol Sci 1978;38:129–144.
284. van de Warrenburg BP, Hengstman GJ, Vos PE, et al. Concomitant dermatomyositis and myasthenia gravis presenting with respiratory insufficiency. Muscle Nerve 2002;25:293–296.
285. Yamaguchi T, Sakurai Y, Mannen T, Shimizu J. Rapidly progressive polymyositis with elevated antiacetylcholine receptor antibody activity. Intern Med 2000; 39:1108–1110.
286. Aso Y, Sato A, Narimatsu M, et al. Stiff-man syndrome associated with antecedent myasthenia gravis and organ-specific autoimmunopathy. Intern Med 1997; 36:308–311.
287. Vincent A, Jacobson L, Plested P, et al. Antibodies affecting ion channel function in acquired neuromyotonia, in seropositive and seronegative myasthenia gravis, and in antibody-mediated arthrogryposis multiplex congenita. Ann NY Acad Sci 1998;841:482–496.
288. Oh SJ, Dwyer DS, Bradley RJ. Overlap myasthenic syndrome: Combined myasthenia gravis and Eaton-Lambert syndrome. Neurology 1987;37:1411–1414.
289. Lindsey JW, Albers GW, Steinman L. Recurrent transverse myelitis, myasthenia gravis, and autoantibodies. Ann Neurol 1992;32:407–409.
290. Shakir RA, Hussien JM, Trontelj JV. Myasthenia gravis and multiple sclerosis. J Neuroimmunol 1983;4:161–165.

291. Fryze W, Obiedzinski R, Klos M. [Coexistence of multiple sclerosis and myasthenia gravis]. Neurol Neurochir Pol 1991;25:259–262.

292. Ho SL, Shah M, Williams AC. Idiopathic thrombocytopenic purpura and autoimmune thyroiditis in a patient with myasthenia gravis. Muscle Nerve 1992;15:966–967.

293. Kwan SY, Lin JH, Su MS. Coexistence of epilepsy, myasthenia gravis and psoriasis vulgaris. Zhonghua Yi Xue Za Zhi (Taipei) 2000;63:153–157.

294. Topaktas S, Dener S, Kenis M, Dalkara T. Myasthenia gravis and vitiligo. Muscle Nerve 1993;16:566–567.

295. Drube S, Maurin N, Sieberth HG. Coincidence of myasthenia gravis and antiglomerular basement membrane glomerulonephritis: A combination of two antibody-mediated autoimmune diseases on day 15. Nephrol Dial Transplant 1997;12:1478–1480.

296. McFadden RG, Craig ID, Paterson NA. Interstitial pneumonitis in myasthenia gravis. Br J Dis Chest 1984;78:187–191.

297. Williamson HO, Phansey SA, Mathur S, et al. Myasthenia gravis, premature menopause, and thyroid autoimmunity. Am J Obstet Gynecol 1980;137:893–901.

298. Kuki S, Morgan RL, Tucci JR. Myasthenia gravis and premature ovarian failure. Arch Intern Med 1981;141:1230–1232.

299. Coulam CB. The prevalence of autoimmune disorders among patients with primary ovarian failure. Am J Reprod Immunol 1983;4:63–66.

300. Whittingham S, Mackay IR, Kiss ZS. An interplay of genetic and environmental factors in familial hepatitis and myasthenia gravis. Gut 1970;11:811–816.

301. Bosch EP, Reith PE, Granner DK. Myasthenia gravis and Schmidt syndrome. Neurology 1977;27:1179–1180.

302. Okada T, Kawamura T, Tamura T, et al. Myasthenia gravis associated with Addison's disease. Intern Med 1994;33:686–688.

303. Efthimiou J, D'Cruz D, Kaplan P, Isenberg D. Heterozygous C2 deficiency associated with angioedema, myasthenia gravis, and systemic lupus erythematosus. Ann Rheum Dis 1986;45:428–430.

304. Iwasaki Y, Kinoshita M. Ocular myasthenia gravis associated with autoimmune hemolytic anemia and Hashimoto's thyroiditis. Am J Ophthalmol 1989;107:90–91.

305. Alter NM, Osnato M. Myasthenia gravis with status lymphaticus and mutltiple thymic granulomas. Arch Neurol Psychiatr 1930;23:345–360.

306. Symmers D. Malignant tumors and tumor-like growths of the thymic region. Ann Surg 1932;95:544–572.

307. Cohen SM, Waxman S. Myasthenia gravis, chronic lymphocytic leukemia, and autoimmune hemolytic anemia. A spectrum of thymic abnormalities? Arch Intern Med 1967;120:717–720.

308. Satoh A, Tsujihata M, Yoshimura T, et al. Myasthenia gravis associated with Satoyoshi syndrome: Muscle cramps, alopecia, and diarrhea. Neurology 1983;33:1209–1211.

309. Bedrick JJ, Savino PJ, Schatz NJ. Conjunctival Kaposi's sarcoma in a patient with myasthenia gravis. Arch Ophthalmol 1981;99:1607–1609.

310. Fukui T, Sugita K, Ichikawa H, et al. Human T lymphotropic virus type I associated myelopathy and myasthenia gravis: A possible association? Eur Neurol 1994;34:158–161.

311. Noguchi Y, Fuchigami T, Morimoto S, Harada K. Myasthenia gravis with alopecia totalis. Acta Paediatr Jpn 1998;40:99–101.

312. Ammar-Khodja A. [Autoimmune deafness and myasthenia]. Rev Laryngol Otol Rhinol (Bord) 1991;112:161–163.

313. Nelson KR, McQuillen MP. Neurologic complications of graft-versus-host disease. Neurol Clin 1988;6:389–403.

314. Zaja F, Barillari G, Russo D, et al. Myasthenia gravis after allogeneic bone marrow transplantation. A case report and a review of the literature. Acta Neurol Scand 1997;96:256–259.

315. Watanabe H, Hakusui S, Yanagi T, et al. [A case of antiphospholipid syndrome associated with myasthenia gravis]. Rinsho Shinkeigaku 1997;37:641–644.

316. Colaco CB, Scadding GK, Lockhart S. Anti-cardiolipin antibodies in neurological disorders: Cross-reaction with anti-single stranded DNA activity. Clin Exp Immunol 1987;68:313–319.

317. Gabrielli GB, Codella O, Capra F, De Sandre G. Pulmonary mucosa-associated lymphoid tissue lymphoma and myasthenia gravis. A case report. Haematologica 1998;83:381–382.

318. Van de Mosselaer G, Van Deuren H, Dewolf-Peeters C, Missotten L. Pseudotumor orbitae and myasthenia gravis. A case report. Arch Ophthalmol 1980;98:1621–1622.

319. Bever CT Jr, Aquino AV, Penn AS, et al. Prognosis of ocular myasthenia. Ann Neurol 1983;14:516–519.

320. Grob D, Arsura EL, Brunner NG, Namba T. The course of myasthenia gravis and therapies affecting outcome. Ann NY Acad Sci 1987;505:472–499.

321. Oosterhuis HJ. The natural course of myasthenia gravis: A long-term follow-up study. J Neurol Neurosurg Psychiatry 1989;52:1121–1127.

322. Sommer N, Melms A, Weller M, Dichgans J. Ocular myasthenia gravis. A critical review of clinical and pathophysiological aspects. Doc Ophthalmol 1993;84:309–333.

323. Sommer N, Sigg B, Melms A, et al. Ocular myasthenia gravis: Response to long-term immunosuppressive treatment. J Neurol Neurosurg Psychiatry 1997;62:156–162.

324. Kupersmith MJ, Moster M, Bhuiyan S, et al. Beneficial effects of corticosteroids on ocular myasthenia gravis. Arch Neurol 1996;53:802–804.

325. Mee J, Paine M, Byrne E, et al. Immunotherapy of ocular myasthenia gravis reduces conversion to generalized myasthenia gravis. J Neuroophthalmol 2003;23:251–255.

326. Grob D. Course and management of myasthenia gravis. JAMA 1953;153:529–532.

327. Ferguson FR, Hutchinson EC, Liversedge LA. Myasthenia gravis; results of medical management. Lancet 1955;269:636–639.

328. Grob D. Natural history of myasthenia gravis. In Engel AG, ed. Myasthenia Gravis and Myasthenic Disorders. New York, Oxford, 1999:135.

329. Grob D, Brunner NG, Namba T. The natural course of myasthenia gravis and effect of therapeutic measures. Ann NY Acad Sci 1981;377:652–669.

330. Rollinson RD, Fenichel GM. Relapsing ocular myasthenia. Neurology 1981;31:325–326.

331. Kupersmith MJ. Does early immunotherapy reduce the conversion of ocular myasthenia gravis to generalized myasthenia gravis? J Neuroophthalmol 2003;23:249–250.

332. Monsul NT, Patwa HS, Knorr AM, et al. The effect of prednisone on the progression from ocular to generalized myasthenia gravis. J Neurol Sci 2004;217:131–133.

333. Kupersmith MJ. Does early treatment of ocular myasthenia gravis with prednisone reduce progression to generalized disease? J Neurol Sci 2004;217:123–124.

334. Gronseth GS, Barohn RJ. Practice parameter: Thymectomy for autoimmune myasthenia gravis (an evidence-based review): Report of the Quality Standards Subcommittee of the American Academy of Neurology. Neurology 2000;55:7–15.

335. Wolfe GI, Kaminski HJ, Jaretzki A III, et al. Development of a thymectomy trial in nonthymomatous myasthenia gravis patients receiving immunosuppressive therapy. Ann NY Acad Sci 2003;998:473–480.

336. Lanska DJ. Indications for thymectomy in myasthenia gravis. Neurology 1990;40:1828–1829.

337. Buckingham JM, Howard FM Jr, et al. The value of thymectomy in myasthenia gravis: A computer-assisted matched study. Ann Surg 1976;184:453–458.

338. Papatestas AE, Genkins G, Horowitz SH, Kornfeld P. Thymectomy in myasthenia gravis: Pathologic, clinical, and electrophysiologic correlations. Ann NY Acad Sci 1976;274:555–573.

339. Olanow CW, Wechsler AS, Sirotkin-Roses M, et al. Thymectomy as primary therapy in myasthenia gravis. Ann NY Acad Sci 1987;505:595–606.

340. Evoli A, Batocchi AP, Minisci C, et al. Therapeutic options in ocular myasthenia gravis. Neuromuscul Disord 2001;11:208–216.

341. Schumm F, Wietholter H, Fateh-Moghadam A, Dichgans J. Thymectomy in myasthenia with pure ocular symptoms. J Neurol Neurosurg Psychiatry 1985;48:332–337.

342. Evoli A, Batocchi AP, Provenzano C, et al. Thymectomy in the treatment of myasthenia gravis: report of 247 patients. J Neurol 1988;235:272–276.

343. Nakamura H, Taniguchi Y, Suzuki Y, et al. Delayed remission after thymectomy for myasthenia gravis of the purely ocular type. J Thorac Cardiovasc Surg 1996;112:371–375.

344. Shrager JB, Deeb ME, Mick R, et al. Transcervical thymectomy for myasthenia gravis achieves results comparable to thymectomy by sternotomy. Ann Thorac Surg 2002;74:320–327.

345. Younger DS, Jaretzki A, Penn AS, et al. Maximum thymectomy for myasthenia gravis. Ann NY Acad Sci 1987;505:832–835.

346. Jaretzki A, 3rd. Thymectomy for myasthenia gravis: Analysis of controversies, patient management. Neurology 2003;9:77–92.

347. Spath G, Brinkmann A, Huth C, Wietholter H. Complications and efficacy of transsternal thymectomy in myasthenia gravis. Thorac Cardiovasc Surg 1987;35:283–289.

348. Korner MM, Hirata N, Tenderich G, et al. Tuberculosis in heart transplant recipients. Chest 1997;111:365–369.

349. Lichtenstein IH, MacGregor RR. Mycobacterial infections in renal transplant recipients: Report of five cases and review of the literature. Rev Infect Dis 1983;5:216–226.

350. Meyers BR, Halpern M, Sheiner P, et al. Tuberculosis in liver transplant patients. Transplantation 1994;58:301–306.

351. Seybold ME, Drachman DB. Gradually increasing doses of prednisone in myasthenia gravis. Reducing the hazards of treatment. N Engl J Med 1974;290:81–84.

352. Brunner NG, Berger CL, Namba T, Grob D. Corticotropin and corticosteroids in generalized myasthenia gravis: Comparative studies and role in management. Ann NY Acad Sci 1976;274:577–595.

353. Howard FM Jr, Duane DD, Lambert EH, Daube JR. Alternate-day prednisone: Preliminary report of a double-blind controlled study. Ann NY Acad Sci 1976;274:596–607.

354. Sghirlanzoni A, Peluchetti D, Mantegazza R, et al. Myasthenia gravis: Prolonged treatment with steroids. Neurology 1984;34:170–174.

355. Jacobson ME. The rationale of alternate-day corticosteroid therapy. Postgrad Med 1971;49:181–186.

356. Engel WK. Myasthenia gravis, corticosteroids, anticholinesterases. Ann NY Acad Sci 1976;274:623–630.

357. Taylor R, Tandan R, Roberts J, et al. Disseminated thymoma and myasthenia gravis: Dramatic response to prednisone. Ann Neurol 1989;25:208–209.

358. Kodama K, Doi O, Higashiyama M, et al. Dramatic response of postthymomectomy myasthenia gravis with multiple lung nodules to corticosteroids. Ann Thorac Surg 1997;64:555–557.

359. Pascuzzi RM, Coslett HB, Johns TR. Long-term corticosteroid treatment of myasthenia gravis: Report of 116 patients. Ann Neurol 1984;15:291–298.

360. Johns TR. Long-term corticosteroid treatment of myasthenia gravis. Ann NY Acad Sci 1987;505:568–583.

361. Lane NE. An update on glucocorticoid-induced osteoporosis. Rheum Dis Clin North Am 2001;27:235–253.

362. Handschumacher RE. Immunosuppressive agents. In Gilman AG, Rall TW, Nies AS, et al., eds. Goodman and Gilman's The Pharmacological Basis of Therapeutics. 8th ed. New York, Pergamon, 1990:1264–1276.

363. Baker DE. Pharmacogenomics of azathioprine and 6-mercaptopurine in gastroenterologic therapy. Rev Gastroenterol Disord 2003;3:150–157.

364. Hildner K, Marker-Hermann E, Schlaak JF, et al. Azathioprine, mycophenolate mofetil, and methotrexate specifically modulate cytokine production by T cells. Ann NY Acad Sci 1998;859:204–207.

365. Witte AS, Cornblath DR, Parry GJ, et al. Azathioprine in the treatment of myasthenia gravis. Ann Neurol 1984;15:602–605.

366. Mertens HG, Hertel G, Reuther P, Ricker K. Effect of immunosuppressive drugs (azathioprine). Ann NY Acad Sci 1981;377:691–699.

367. Matell G. Immunosuppressive drugs: Azathioprine in the treatment of myasthenia gravis. Ann NY Acad Sci 1987;505:589–594.

368. Bromberg MB, Wald JJ, Forshew DA, et al. Randomized trial of azathioprine or prednisone for initial immunosuppressive treatment of myasthenia gravis. J Neurol Sci 1997;150:59–62.

369. Palace J, Newsom-Davis J, Lecky B. A randomized double-blind trial of prednisolone alone or with azathioprine in myasthenia gravis. Myasthenia Gravis Study Group. Neurology 1998;50:1778–1783.

370. Mantegazza R, Antozzi C, Peluchetti D, et al. Azathioprine as a single drug or in combination with steroids in the treatment of myasthenia gravis. J Neurol 1988;235:449–453.

371. Kuks JB, Djojoatmodjo S, Oosterhuis HJ. Azathioprine in myasthenia gravis: Observations in 41 patients and a review of literature. Neuromuscular Disord 1991;1:423–431.

372. Kissel JT, Levy RJ, Mendell JR, Griggs RC. Azathioprine toxicity in neuromuscular disease. Neurology 1986;36:35–39.

373. Dubinsky MC, Lamothe S, Yang HY, et al. Pharmacogenomics and metabolite measurement for 6-mercaptopurine therapy in inflammatory bowel disease. Gastroenterology 2000;118:705–713.

374. Campbell S, Kingstone K, Ghosh S. Relevance of thiopurine methyltransferase activity in inflammatory bowel disease patients maintained on low-dose azathioprine. Aliment Pharmacol Ther 2002;16:389–398.

375. Pirofsky B, Dawson PJ, Reid RH. Lack of oncogenicity with immunosuppressive therapy. Cancer 1980;45:2096–2101.

376. Whisnant JK, Pelkyelkey J. Rheumatoid arthritis: Treatment with azathioprine (Imuran): Clinical side effects and laboratory abnormalities. Ann Rheum Dis 1982;41:44–47.

377. Michels M, Hohlfeld R, Hartung HP, et al. Myasthenia gravis: Discontinuation of long-term azathioprine. Ann Neurol 1988;24:798.

378. Hohlfeld R, Toyka KV, Besinger UA, et al. Myasthenia gravis: Reactivation of clinical disease and of autoimmune factors after discontinuation of long-term azathioprine. Ann Neurol 1985;17:238–242.

379. Dejaco C, Mittermaier C, Reinisch W, et al. Azathioprine treatment and male fertility in inflammatory bowel disease. Gastroenterology 2001;121:1048–1053.

380. Janssen NM, Genta MS. The effects of immunosuppressive and anti-inflammatory medications on fertility, pregnancy, and lactation. Arch Intern Med 2000; 160:610–619.

381. Tendron A, Gouyon JB, Decramer S. In utero exposure to immunosuppressive drugs: Experimental and clinical studies. Pediatr Nephrol 2002;17:121–130.

382. Borel JF, Feurer C, Gubler HU, et al. Biological effect of cyclosporin A: A new antilymphocytes agent. Agents Actions Suppl 1976;6:468–475.

383. Kahn BD, Bach JF. Proceedings of the Second International Congress on Cyclosporine. Transplant Proc 1988;20:1–1131.

384. Elliott JF, Lin Y, Mizel SB, et al. Induction of interleukin 2 messenger RNA inhibited by cyclosporine A. Science 1984;226:1439–1441.

385. Kronke M, Leonard WJ, Depper JM, et al. Cyclosporine A inhibits T-cell growth factor gene expression at the level of mRNA transcription. Proc Natl Acad Sci USA 1984;81:5214–5218.

386. Salamon JR, Griffin PJA. Immunosuppression with a combination of cyclosporin, azathioprine, and prednisolone may be unsafe. Lancet 1985;2: 1066–1067.

387. Tindall RS, Rollins JA, Phillips JT, et al. Preliminary results of a double-blind, randomized, placebo-controlled trial of cyclosporine in myasthenia gravis. N Engl J Med 1987;316:719–724.

388. Tindall RS, Phillips JT, Rollins JA, et al. A clinical therapeutic trial of cyclosporine in myasthenia gravis. Ann NY Acad Sci 1993;681:539–551.

389. Goulon M, Elkharrat D, Lokiec F, Gajdos P. Results of a one-year open trial of cyclosporine in ten patients with severe myasthenia gravis. Transplant Proc 1988;20(3 Suppl 4):211–217.

390. Nyberg-Hansen R, Gjerstad L. Myasthenia gravis treated with ciclosporin. Acta Neurol Scand 1988;77:307–313.

391. Antonini G, Bove R, Filippini C, Millefiorini M. Results of an open trial of cyclosporine in a group of steroid-dependent myasthenic subjects. Clin Neurol Neurosurg 1990;92:317–321.

392. Schalke B, Kappos L, Dommasch D, et al. Cyclosporin A treatment of myasthenia gravis: Initial results of a double blind trial of cyclosporin A versus azathioprine. Ann NY Acad Sci 1988;505:872–875.

393. Bonifati DM, Angelini C. Long-term cyclosporine treatment in a group of severe myasthenia gravis patients. J Neurol 1997;244:542–547.

394. Ciafaloni E, Nikhar NK, Massey JM, Sanders DB. Retrospective analysis of the use of cyclosporine in myasthenia gravis. Neurology 2000;55:448–450.

395. Mihatsch MJ, Bach JF, Coovadia HM, et al. Cyclosporine-associated nephropathy in patients with autoimmune diseases. Klin Wochenschr 1988;66:43–47.

396. Cruz OA, Fogg SG, Roper-Hall G. Pseudotumor cerebri associated with cyclosporine use. Am J Ophthalmol 1996;122:436–437.

397. Katz B, Moster ML, Slavin ML. Disk edema subsequent to renal transplantation. Surv Ophthalmol 1997;41:315–320.

398. Avery R, Jabs DA, Wingard JR, et al. Optic disk edema after bone marrow transplantation: Possible role of cyclosporine toxicity. Ophthalmology 1991;98: 1294–1301.

399. Porges Y, Blumen S, Fireman Z, et al. Cyclosporine-induced optic neuropathy, ophthalmoplegia, and nystagmus in a patient with Crohn disease. Am J Ophthalmol 1998;126:607–609.

400. Noll R, Kulkarni R. Complex visual hallucinations and cyclosporine. Arch Neurol 1984;41:329–330.

401. Katirji MB. Visual hallucinations and cyclosporine. Transplantation 1987;43: 768–769.

402. Rubin AM, Kang H. Cerebral blindness and encephalopathy with cyclosporin A toxicity. Neurology 1987;37:1072–1076.

403. Steg RE, Garcia EG. Complex visual hallucinations and cyclosporine toxicity. Neurology 1991;41:1156.

404. Apaydin C, Gur B, Yakupoglu G, et al. Ocular and visual side effects of systemic cyclosporine. Ann Ophthalmol 1992;24:465–468.

405. Garg RK. Posterior leukoencephalopathy syndrome. Postgrad Med J 2001;77: 24–28.

406. Euvrard S, Kanitakis J, Claudy A. Skin cancers after organ transplantation. N Engl J Med 2003;348:1681–1691.

407. The Multiple Sclerosis Study Group. Efficacy and toxicity of cyclosporine in chronic progressive multiple sclerosis: A randomized, double-blinded, placebo-controlled clinical trial. Ann Neurol 1990;27:591–605.

408. Hauser RA, Malek AR, Rosen R. Successful treatment of a patient with severe refractory myasthenia gravis using mycophenolate mofetil. Neurology 1998;51: 912–913.

409. Meriggioli MN, Rowin J. Treatment of myasthenia gravis with mycophenolate mofetil: A case report. Muscle Nerve 2000;23:1287–1289.

410. Chaudhry V, Cornblath DR, Griffin JW, et al. Mycophenolate mofetil: A safe and promising immunosuppressant in neuromuscular diseases. Neurology 2001; 56:94–96.

411. Ciafaloni E, Massey JM, Tucker-Lipscomb B, Sanders DB. Mycophenolate mofetil for myasthenia gravis: An open-label pilot study. Neurology 2001;56: 97–99.

412. Mowzoon N, Sussman A, Bradley WG. Mycophenolate (CellCept) treatment of myasthenia gravis, chronic inflammatory polyneuropathy and inclusion body myositis. J Neurol Sci 2001;185:119–122.

413. Meriggioli MN, Ciafaloni E, Al-Hayk KA, et al. Mycophenolate mofetil for myasthenia gravis: An analysis of efficacy, safety, and tolerability. Neurology 2003;61:1438–1440.

414. Meriggioli MN, Rowin J, Richman JG, Leurgans S. Mycophenolate mofetil for myasthenia gravis: A double-blind, placebo-controlled pilot study. Ann NY Acad Sci 2003;998:494–499.

415. Goldblum R. Therapy of rheumatoid arthritis with mycophenolate mofetil. Clin Exp Rheumatol 1993;Suppl 8:S117–119.

416. Nouza K, Smat V. The favourable effect of cyclophosphamide in myasthenia gravis. Rev Fr Etud Clin Biol 1968;13:161–163.

417. Niakan E, Harati Y, Rolak LA. Immunosuppressive drug therapy in myasthenia gravis. Arch Neurol 1986;43:155–156.

418. Badurska B, Ryniewicz B, Strugalska H. Immunosuppressive treatment for juvenile myasthenia gravis. Eur J Pediatr 1992;151:215–217.

419. De Feo LG, Schottlender J, Martelli NA, Molfino NA. Use of intravenous pulsed cyclophosphamide in severe, generalized myasthenia gravis. Muscle Nerve 2002;26:31–36.

420. Drachman DB, Jones RJ, Brodsky RA. Treatment of refractory myasthenia: "Rebooting" with high-dose cyclophosphamide. Ann Neurol 2003;53:29–34.

421. Hirano M. Use of intravenous pulsed cyclophosphamide in severe, generalized myasthenia gravis. Curr Neurol Neurosci Rep 2003;3:55–56.

422. Pinching AJ, Peters DK. Remission of myasthenia gravis following plasma-exchange. Lancet 1976;2:1373–1376.

423. Dau PC, Lindstrom JM, Cassel CK, et al. Plasmapheresis and immunosuppressive drug therapy in myasthenia gravis. N Engl J Med 1977;297:1134–1140.

424. Keesey J, Buffkin D, Kebo D, Ho W, Herrmann C Jr. Plasma exchange alone as therapy for myasthenia gravis. Ann NY Acad Sci 1981;377:729–743.

425. Batocchi AP, Evoli A, Di Schino C, Tonali P. Therapeutic apheresis in myasthenia gravis. Ther Apher 2000;4:275–279.

426. Yeh JH, Chen WH, Chiu HC. Double filtration plasmapheresis in the treatment of myasthenic crisis: Analysis of prognostic factors and efficacy. Acta Neurol Scand 2001;104:78–82.

427. Takamori M, Maruta T. Immunoadsorption in myasthenia gravis based on specific ligands mimicking the immunogenic sites of the acetylcholine receptor. Ther Apher 2001;5:340–350.

428. Fateh-Moghadam A, Wick M, Besinger U, Geursen RG. High-dose intravenous gammaglobulin for myasthenia gravis. Lancet 1984;1:848–849.

429. Gajdos P, Chevret S, Clair B, et al. Plasma exchange and intravenous immunoglobulin in autoimmune myasthenia gravis. Ann NY Acad Sci 1998;841:720–726.

430. Dalakas MC. Intravenous immunoglobulin in the treatment of autoimmune neuromuscular diseases: present status and practical therapeutic guidelines. Muscle Nerve 1999;22:1479–1497.

431. Achiron A, Barak Y, Miron S, Sarova-Pinhas I. Immunoglobulin treatment in refractory myasthenia gravis. Muscle Nerve 2000;23:551–555.

432. Gajdos P, Chevret S, Toyka K. Intravenous immunoglobulin for myasthenia gravis. Cochrane Database Syst Rev 2003:CD002277.

433. Callahan A. Reconstructive Surgery of the Eyelids and Ocular Adnexa. Birmingham, AL, Aesculapius, 1966:114.

434. Iliff CE, Iliff WJ, Iliff NT. Oculoplastic Surgery. Philadelphia, WB Saunders, 1979:45.

435. Kapetansky DI. Surgical correction of blepharoptosis in myasthenia gravis. Am J Ophthalmol 1972;74:818–820.

436. Castronuovo S, Krohel GB, Kristan RW. Blepharoptosis in myasthenia gravis. Ann Ophthalmol 1983;15:751–754.

437. Bernardini FP, de Conciliis C, Devoto MH. Frontalis suspension sling using a silicone rod in patients affected by myogenic blepharoptosis. Orbit 2002;21:195–198.

438. Bentley CR, Dawson E, Lee JP. Active management in patients with ocular manifestations of myasthenia gravis. Eye 2001;15(Pt 1):18–22.

439. Acheson JF, Elston JS, Lee JP, Fells P. Extraocular muscle surgery in myasthenia gravis. Br J Ophthalmol 1991;75:232–235.

440. Ohtsuki H, Hasebe S, Okano M, Furuse T. Strabismus surgery in ocular myasthenia gravis. Ophthalmologica 1996;210:95–100.

441. Bhatti MT. Double trouble. Surv Ophthalmol 2003;48:347–355.

442. Evoli A, Batocchi AP, Bartoccioni E, et al. Juvenile myasthenia gravis with prepubertal onset. Neuromuscul Disord 1998;8:561–567.

443. Andrews PI. A treatment algorithm for autoimmune myasthenia gravis in childhood. Ann NY Acad Sci 1998;841:789–802.

444. Mullaney P, Vajsar J, Smith R, Buncic JR. The natural history and ophthalmic involvement in childhood myasthenia gravis at the Hospital for Sick Children. Ophthalmology 2000;107:504–510.

445. Lindner A, Schalke B, Toyka KV. Outcome in juvenile-onset myasthenia gravis: A retrospective study with long-term follow-up of 79 patients. J Neurol 1997;244:515–520.

446. Ellenhorn N, Lucchese N, Greenwald M. Juvenile myasthenia gravis and amblyopia. Am J Ophthalmol 1986;101:214–217.

447. Herrmann DN, Carney PR, Wald JJ. Juvenile myasthenia gravis: Treatment with immune globulin and thymectomy. Pediatr Neurol 1998;18:63–66.

448. Levin PM. Congenital myasthenia in siblings. Arch Neurol 1949;62:745–748.

449. Millichap JG, Dodge PR. Diagnosis and treatment of myasthenia gravis in infancy, childhood, and adolescence: A study of 51 patients. Neurology 1960;10:1007–1014.

450. Namba T, Brown SB, Grob D. Neonatal myasthenia gravis: Report of two cases and review of the literature. Pediatrics 1970;45:488–504.

451. Namba T, Brunner NG, Brown SB, et al. Familial myasthenia gravis. Report of 27 patients in 12 families and review of 164 patients in 73 families. Arch Neurol 1971;25:49–60.

452. Bundey S. A genetic study of infantile and juvenile myasthenia gravis. J Neurol Neurosurg Psychiatry 1972;35:41–51.

453. Engel AG. Congenital myasthenic syndromes. Neurol Clin 1994;12:401–437.

454. Vincent A, Newland C, Croxen R, Beeson D. Genes at the junction: Candidates for congenital myasthenic syndromes. Trends Neurosci 1997;20:15–22.

455. Kullmann DM, Hanna MG. Neurological disorders caused by inherited ion-channel mutations. Lancet Neurol 2002;1:157–166.

456. Mora M, Lambert EH, Engel AG. Synaptic vesicle abnormality in familial infantile myasthenia. Neurology 1987;37:206–214.

457. Walls TJ, Engel AG, Nagel AS, et al. Congenital myasthenic syndrome associated with paucity of synaptic vesicles and reduced quantal release. Ann NY Acad Sci 1993;681:461–468.

458. Engel AG, Lambert EH, Gomez MR. A new myasthenic syndrome with endplate acetylcholinesterase deficiency, small nerve terminals, and reduced acetylcholine release. Ann Neurol 1977;1:315–330.

459. Hutchinson DO, Walls TJ, Nakano S, et al. Congenital endplate acetylcholinesterase deficiency. Brain 1993;116:633–653.

460. Vincent A, Cull-Candy SG, Newsom-Davis J, et al. Congenital myasthenia: End-plate acetylcholine receptors and electrophysiology in five cases. Muscle Nerve 1981;4:306–318.

461. Engel AG, Lambert EH, Mulder DM, et al. A newly recognized congenital myasthenic syndrome attributed to a prolonged open time of the acetylcholine-induced ion channel. Ann Neurol 1982;11:553–569.

462. Greer M, Schotland M. Myasthenia gravis in the newborn. Pediatrics 1960;26:101–108.

463. Robertson WC, Chun RW, Kornguth SE. Familial infantile myasthenia. Arch Neurol 1980;37:117–119.

464. Hart ZH, Sahashi K, Lambert EH, et al. A congenital, familial myasthenic syndrome caused by a presynaptic defect of transmitter resynthesis or mobilization. Neurology 1979;29:556.

465. Engel AG. Morphologic and immunopathologic findings in myasthenia gravis and in congenital myasthenic syndromes. J Neurol Neurosurg Psychiatry 1980;43:577–589.

466. van Dijk JG, Lammers GJ, Wintzen AR, Molenaar PC. Repetitive CMAPs: Mechanisms of neural and synaptic genesis. Muscle Nerve 1996;19:1127–1133.

467. Maselli RA, Soliven BC. Analysis of the organophosphate-induced electromyographic response to repetitive nerve stimulation: Paradoxical response to edrophonium and D-tubocurarine. Muscle Nerve 1991;14:1182–1188.

468. Ohno K, Brengman J, Tsujino A, Engel AG. Human endplate acetylcholinesterase deficiency caused by mutations in the collagen-like tail subunit (ColQ) of the asymmetric enzyme. Proc Natl Acad Sci USA 1998;95:9654–9659.

469. Maddison P, Newsom-Davis J, Mills KR. Effect of 3,4-diaminopyridine on the time course of decay of compound muscle action potential augmentation in the Lambert-Eaton myasthenic syndrome. Muscle Nerve 1998;21:1196–1198.

470. Ohno K, Wang HL, Milone M, et al. Congenital myasthenic syndrome caused by decreased agonist binding affinity due to a mutation in the acetylcholine receptor epsilon subunit. Neuron 1996;17:157–170.

471. Milone M, Ohno K, Fukudome T, et al. Congenital myasthenic syndrome caused by novel loss-of-function mutations in the human AChR epsilon subunit gene. Ann NY Acad Sci 1998;841:184–188.

472. Engel AG, Lambert EH, Mulder DM, et al. Investigations of 3 cases of a newly recognized familial, congenital myasthenic syndrome. Trans Am Neurol Assoc 1979;104:8–11.

473. Gomez CM, Maselli R, Gammack J, et al. A beta-subunit mutation in the acetylcholine receptor channel gate causes severe slow-channel syndrome. Ann Neurol 1996;39:712–723.

474. Sieb JP, Tolksdorf K, Dengler R, Jerusalem F. An autosomal-recessive congenital myasthenic syndrome with tubular aggregates in a Libyan family. Neuromuscul Disord 1996;6:115–119.

475. Fukudome T, Ohno K, Brengman JM, Engel AG. AChR channel blockade by quinidine sulfate reduces channel open duration in the slow-channel congenital myasthenic syndrome. Ann NY Acad Sci 1998;841:199–202.

476. Harper CM, Engel AG. Quinidine sulfate therapy for the slow-channel congenital myasthenic syndrome. Ann Neurol 1998;43:480–484.

477. Anderson HJ, Churchill-Davidson HD, Richardson AT. Bronchial neoplasm with myasthenia. Lancet 1953;2:1291–1293.

478. Henson RA. Unusual manifestations of bronchial carcinoma. Proc R Soc Med 1953;46:859–861.

479. Borelli VM, Keen H. Bronchial neoplasm with myasthenia. Lancet 1954;1:315–316.

480. Lambert EH, Eaton LM, Rooke ED. Defect of neuromuscular conduction associated with malignant neoplasms. Am J Physiol 1956;187:612–613.

481. Eaton LM, Lambert EH. Electromyography and electric stimulation of nerves in diseases of motor unit; observations on myasthenic syndrome associated with malignant tumors. JAMA 1957;163:1117–1124.

482. Lambert EH, Kane C, Rowland LP, et al. Symposium on muscle disease. Arch Phys Med Rehabil 1965;46:Supp:146–159.

483. Rubenstein AE, Horowitz SH, Bender AN. Cholinergic dysautonomia and Eaton-Lambert syndrome. Neurology 1979;29:720–723.

484. Wirtz PW, Smallegange TM, Wintzen AR, Verschuuren JJ. Differences in clinical features between the Lambert-Eaton myasthenic syndrome with and without cancer: An analysis of 227 published cases. Clin Neurol Neurosurg 2002;104:359–363.

485. Sanders DB. Lambert-Eaton myasthenic syndrome: diagnosis and treatment. Ann NY Acad Sci 2003;998:500–508.

486. Shapira Y, Harel S, Russell A. Mitochondrial encephalomyopathies, a group of neuromuscular disorders with defects in oxidative metabolism. Israel J Med Sci 1984;13:161–164.

487. Chelmicka-Schorr E, Bernstein LP, Zurbrugg EB, Huttenlocher PR. Eaton-Lambert syndrome in a 9-year-old girl. Arch Neurol 1979;36:572–574.

488. Tsao CY, Mendell JR, Friemer ML, Kissel JT. Lambert-Eaton myasthenic syndrome in children. J Child Neurol 2002;17:74–76.

489. Kennedy WR, Jimenez-Pabon E. The myasthenic syndrome associated with small cell carcinoma of the lung (Eaton-Lambert syndrome). Neurology 1968;18:757–766.

490. Gutmann L, Crosby TW, Takamori M, Martin JD. The Eaton-Lambert syndrome and autoimmune disorders. Am J Med 1972;53:354–356.
491. Norris FH Jr. Neuromuscular transmission in thyroid disease. Ann Intern Med 1966;64:81–86.
492. Kissel P, Schmitt J, Duc M, et al. Myasthenia and thyrotoxicosis. In Walton JN, Canal N, Scarlato G, eds. Muscle Diseases. Amsterdam, Exerpta Medica, 1970.
493. Hoffman WH, Helman SW, Sekul E, et al. Lambert-Eaton myasthenic syndrome in a child with an autoimmune phenotype. Am J Med Genet 2003;119A:77–80.
494. Lang B, Pinto A, Giovannini F, et al. Pathogenic autoantibodies in the Lambert-Eaton myasthenic syndrome. Ann NY Acad Sci 2003;998:187–195.
495. Brown JW, Nelson JR, Hermann C Jr. Sjögren's syndrome with myopathic and myasthenic features. Bull Los Angeles Neurol Soc 1968;33:9–20.
496. Willcox N, Demaine AG, Newsom-Davis J, et al. Increased frequency of IgG heavy chain marker Glm and of HLA-B8 in Lambert-Eaton myasthenic syndrome with and without associated lung carcinoma. Hum Immunol 1985;14:29–36.
497. Parsons KT, Kwok WW, Gaur LK, Nepom GT. Increased frequency of HLA class II alleles DRB1*0301 and DQB1*0201 in Lambert-Eaton myasthenic syndrome without associated cancer. Hum Immunol 2000;61:828–833.
498. Wirtz PW, Roep BO, Schreuder GM, et al. HLA class I and II in Lambert-Eaton myasthenic syndrome without associated tumor. Hum Immunol 2001;62:809–813.
499. Brown JC, Johns RJ. Clinical and physiological studies of the effect of guanidine of patients with myasthenia gravis. Johns Hopkins Med J 1969;124:1–8.
500. Takamori M, Gutmann L. Intermittent defect of acetylcholine release in myasthenia gravis. Neurology 1971;21:47–54.
501. Dahl DS, Sato S. Unusual myasthenic state in a teen-age boy. Neurology 1974;24:897–901.
502. Schwartz MS, Stalberg E. Myasthenia gravis with features of the myasthenic syndrome. An investigation with electrophysiologic methods including single-fiber electromyography. Neurology 1975;25:80–84.
503. Katz JS, Wolfe GI, Bryan WW, et al. Acetylcholine receptor antibodies in the Lambert-Eaton myasthenic syndrome. Neurology 1998;50:470–475.
504. Leavitt JA. Myasthenia gravis with a paraneoplastic marker. J Neuroophthalmol 2000;20:102–105.
505. Kleopa KA, Teener JW, Scherer SS, et al. Chronic multiple paraneoplastic syndromes. Muscle Nerve 2000;23:1767–1772.
506. Vernino S, Lennon VA. New Purkinje cell antibody (PCA-2): Marker of lung cancer-related neurological autoimmunity. Ann Neurol 2000;47:297–305.
507. Hiasa Y, Kunishige M, Mitsui T, et al. Complicated paraneoplastic neurological syndromes: A report of two patients with small cell or non-small cell lung cancer. Clin Neurol Neurosurg 2003;106:47–49.
508. Lambert EH, Elmqvist D. Quantal components of end-plate potentials in the myasthenic syndrome. Ann NY Acad Sci 1971;183:183–199.
509. Lennon VA, Lambert EH. Autoantibodies bind solubilized calcium channel-omega-conotoxin complexes from small cell lung carcinoma: A diagnostic aid for Lambert-Eaton myasthenic syndrome. Mayo Clin Proc 1989;64:1498–1504.
510. Johnston I, Lang B, Leys K, Newsom-Davis J. Heterogeneity of calcium channel autoantibodies detected using a small-cell lung cancer line derived from a Lambert-Eaton myasthenic syndrome patient. Neurology 1994;44:334–338.
511. Nagel A, Engel AG, Lang B, et al. Lambert-Eaton myasthenic syndrome IgG depletes presynaptic membrane active zone particles by antigenic modulation. Ann Neurol 1988;24:552–558.
512. Nakao YK, Motomura M, Fukudome T, et al. Seronegative Lambert-Eaton myasthenic syndrome: Study of 110 Japanese patients. Neurology 2002;59:1773–1775.
513. Abicht A, Lochmuller H. What's in the serum of seronegative MG and LEMS? Neurology 2002;59:1672–1673.
514. Lambert EH. Defects of neuromuscular transmission in syndromes other than myasthenia gravis. Ann NY Acad Sci 1966;135:367–384.
515. Wise RP, Macdermot V. A myasthenic syndrome associated with bronchial carcinoma. J Neurol Neurosurg Psychiatry 1962;25:31–39.
516. Schwartz MS, Stalberg E. Myasthenic syndrome studied with single-fiber electromyography. Arch Neurol 1975;32:815–817.
517. Ward CD, Murray NM. Effect of temperature on neuromuscular transmission in the Eaton-Lambert syndrome. J Neurol Neurosurg Psychiatry 1979;42:247–249.
518. Swift TR, Sackellares JC, Harper KE. The effect of temperature on neuromuscular transmission in myasthenic syndrome. Electroencephalogr Clin Neurophysiol 1978;45:18P.
519. Hedges TR Jr. Ophthalmoplegia of myasthenia and bronchial neoplasm. Arch Ophthalmol 1963;70:333–334.
520. Elmqvist D, Lambert EH. Detailed analysis of neuromuscular transmission in a patient with the myasthenic syndrome sometimes associated with bronchogenic carcinoma. Mayo Clin Proc 1968;43:689–713.
521. Oh SJ. The Eaton-Lambert syndrome in ocular myasthenia gravis. Arch Neurol 1974;31:183–186.
522. Black JT. Neuromuscular diseases that affect the eye. Int Ophthalmol Clin 1978;18:83–121.
523. Cruciger MP, Brown B, Denys EH, et al. Clinical and subclinical oculomotor findings in the Eaton-Lambert syndrome. J Clin Neuroophthalmol 1983;3:19–22.
524. O'Neill JH, Murray NM, Newsom-Davis J. The Lambert-Eaton myasthenic syndrome. A review of 50 cases. Brain 1988;111(Pt 3):577–596.
525. Clark CV, Newsom-Davis J, Sanders MD. Ocular autonomic nerve function in Lambert-Eaton myasthenic syndrome. Eye 1990;4(Pt 3):473–481.
526. Wirtz PW, Sotodeh M, Nijnuis M, et al. Difference in distribution of muscle weakness between myasthenia gravis and the Lambert-Eaton myasthenic syndrome. J Neurol Neurosurg Psychiatry 2002;73:766–768.
527. Breen LA, Gutmann L, Brick JF, Riggs JR. Paradoxical lid elevation with sustained upgaze: A sign of Lambert-Eaton syndrome. Muscle Nerve 1991;14:863–866.
528. Brazis PW. Enhanced ptosis in Lambert-Eaton myasthenic syndrome. J Neuroophthalmol 1997;17:202–203.
529. O'Suilleabhain P, Low PA, Lennon VA. Autonomic dysfunction in the Lambert-Eaton myasthenic syndrome: Serologic and clinical correlates. Neurology 1998;50:88–93.
530. Wirtz PW, de Keizer RJ, de Visser M, et al. Tonic pupils in Lambert-Eaton myasthenic syndrome. Muscle Nerve 2001;24:444–445.
531. Kanzato N, Motomura M, Suehara M, Arimura K. Lambert-Eaton myasthenic syndrome with ophthalmoparesis and pseudoblepharospasm. Muscle Nerve 1999;22:1727–1730.
532. Jenkyn LR, Brooks PL, Forcier RJ, et al. Remission of the Lambert-Eaton syndrome and small cell anaplastic carcinoma of the lung induced by chemotherapy and radiotherapy. Cancer 1980;46:1123–1127.
533. Chalk CH, Murray NM, Newsom-Davis J, et al. Response of the Lambert-Eaton myasthenic syndrome to treatment of associated small-cell lung carcinoma. Neurology 1990;40:1552–1556.
534. Weisman SJ. Masked myasthenia gravis. JAMA 1949;141:917–918.
535. Critchley M, Herman KJ, Harrison M, et al. Value of exchangeable electrolyte measurement in the treatment of myasthenia gravis. J Neurol Neurosurg Psychiatry 1977;40:250–252.
536. Argov Z, Mastaglia FL. Drug therapy: Disorders of neuromuscular transmission caused by drugs. N Engl J Med 1979;301:409–413.
537. Bucknall RC, Dixon ASJ, Glick EN, et al. Myasthenia gravis associated with penicillamine treatment for rheumatoid arthritis. Br Med J 1975;1:600–602.
538. Cylonkowska A. Myasthenia syndrome during penicillamine treatment. Br Med J 1975;2:726.
539. Schmidt D, Kommerell G. [Ocular myasthenia caused by D-penicillamine]. Klin Monatsbl Augenheilkd 1976;168:409–413.
540. Gordon RA, Burnside JW. D-Penicillamine-induced myasthenia gravis in rheumatoid arthritis. Ann Intern Med 1977;87:578–579.
541. Francois J, Verbraeken H, Gabriel P, Wille C. [Myasthenic syndrome following oral treatment with penicillamine]. Bull Soc Belge Ophtalmol 1978;182:126–130.
542. Bucknall RC, Balint G, Dawkins RL. Myasthenia associated with D-penicillamine therapy in rheumatoid arthritis. Scand J Rheumatol Suppl 1979:91–93.
543. Froelich CJ, Hashimoto F, Searles RP, Bankhurst AD. D-penicillamine-induced myasthenia gravis in rheumatoid arthritis. J Rheumatol 1979;6:237–239.
544. Keesey J, Novom S. HLA antigens in penicillamine-induced myasthenia gravis. Neurology 1979;29:528–529.
545. Sundstrom WR, Schuna AA. Penicillamine-induced myasthenia gravis. Arthritis Rheum 1979;22:197–198.
546. Kimbrough RL, Mewis L, Stewart RH. D-penicillamine and the ocular myasthenic syndrome. Ann Ophthalmol 1981;13:1171–1172.
547. Fawcett PR, McLachlan SM, Nicholson LV, et al. D-Penicillamine-associated myasthenia gravis: immunological and electrophysiological studies. Muscle Nerve 1982;5:328–334.
548. Scadding G, Newsom-Davis J. D-pen-associated MG. Muscle Nerve 1983;6:170–171.
549. Kuncl RW, Pestronk A, Drachman DB, Rechthand E. The pathophysiology of penicillamine-induced myasthenia gravis. Ann Neurol 1986;20:740–744.
550. Liu GT, Bienfang DC. Penicillamine-induced ocular myasthenia gravis in rheumatoid arthritis. J Clin Neuroophthalmol 1990;10:201–205.
551. Masters CL, Dawkins RL, Zilko PJ, et al. Penicillamine-associated myasthenia gravis, antiacetylcholine receptor and antistriational antibodies. Am J Med 1977;63:689–694.
552. Russell AS, Lindstrom JM. Penicillamine-induced myasthenia gravis associated with antibodies to acetylcholine receptor. Neurology 1978;28:847–849.
553. Vincent A, Newsom-Davis J, Martin V. Anti-acetylcholine receptor antibodies in D-penicillamine-associated myasthenia gravis. Lancet 1978;1:1254.
554. Howard JF. Adverse drug interactions in disorders of neuromuscular transmission. J Neurol Orthop Med Surg 1991;12:26–34.
555. Barrons RW. Drug-induced neuromuscular blockade and myasthenia gravis. Pharmacotherapy 1997;17:1220–1232.
556. Wittbrodt ET. Drugs and myasthenia gravis. An update. Arch Intern Med 1997;157:399–408.
557. Norris FH, Colella JAB, McFarlin D. Effect of diphenylhydantoin on neuromuscular synapse. Neurology 1964;14:869–876.
558. Yaari Y, Pincus JH, Argov Z. Phenytoin and transmitter release at the neuromuscular junction of the frog. Brain Res 1979;160:479–487.

559. Milonas J, Kountouris D, Scheer E. [Myasthenic syndrome following long-term diphenylhydantoin therapy]. Nervenarzt 1983;54:437–438.
560. Lee SC, Ho ST. Acute effects of verapamil on neuromuscular transmission in patients with myasthenia gravis. Proc Natl Sci Counc Repub China B 1987;11:307–312.
561. Herishanu Y, Rosenberg P. Beta-blockers and myasthenia gravis [letter]. Ann Intern Med 1975;83:834–835.
562. Matell G, Bjelak S, Jonkers I, Pirskanen R, et al. Calcium channel and beta-receptor antagonists and agonists in MG. Ann NY Acad Sci 1998;841:785–788.
563. Jonkers I, Swerup C, Pirskanen R, et al. Acute effects of intravenous injection of beta-adrenoreceptor and calcium channel at antagonists and agonists in myasthenia gravis. Muscle Nerve 1996;19:959–965.
564. Tota G, Vagella A, Busoni P. Richerche sull'ipotonia oculare da alloferina durante anestesia generale. Ann Ottal 1967;93:171–179.
565. Eisenkraft JB, Sawhney RK, Papatestas AE. Vecuronium in the myasthenic patient. Anaesthesia 1986;41:666–667.
566. Eisenkraft JB, Book WJ, Mann SM, et al. Resistance to succinylcholine in myasthenia gravis: a dose-response study. Anesthesiology 1988;69:760–763.
567. Wadia RS, Chitra S, Amin RB, et al. Electrophysiological studies in acute organophosphate poisoning. J Neurol Neurosurg Psychiatry 1987;50:1442–1448.
568. Weinbroum AA, Rudick V, Paret G, et al. Anaesthesia and critical care considerations in nerve agent warfare trauma casualties. Resuscitation 2000;47:113–123.
569. White SM. Chemical and biological weapons. Implications for anaesthesia and intensive care. Br J Anaesth 2002;89:306–324.
570. McQuillen MP, Gross M, Johns RJ. Chlorpromazine-induced weakness in myasthenia gravis. Arch Neurol 1963;8:286–290.
571. Randall LO, Peterson WG, Lehmann G. The ganglionic blocking action of thiophanium derivatives. J Pharmacol Exp Ther 1949;97:48–57.
572. Dale RC, Schroeder ET. Respiratory paralysis during treatment of hypertension with trimethaphan camsylate. Arch Intern Med 1976;136:816–818.
573. Bazzato G, Mezzina C, Ciman M, Guarnieri G. Myasthenia-like syndrome associated with carnitine in patients on long-term haemodialysis. Lancet 1979;1:1041–1042.
574. Abel M, Eisenkraft JB. Anesthetic implications of myasthenia gravis. Mt Sinai J Med 2002;69(1–2):31–37.
575. Eisenkraft JB, Neustein SM, Cohen E. Anesthesia for thoracic surgery. In Barash PG, Cullen BF, Stoelting RK, eds. Clinical Anesthesia. 2nd ed. Philadelphia, JB Lippincott, 1992:977–979.
576. Nagorka AR, Bergeson PS. Infant methamphetamine toxicity posing as scorpion envenomation. Pediatr Emerg Care 1998;14:350–351.
577. Dengler R, Rudel R, Warelas J, Birnberger KL. Corticosteroids and neuromuscular transmission: Electrophysiological investigation of the effects of prednisolone on normal and anticholinesterase-treated neuromuscular junction. Pflugers Arch 1979;380:145–151.
578. Drachman DA, Skom JH. Procainamide: A hazard in myasthenia gravis. Arch Neurol 1965;13:316–320.
579. Lee DC, Kim YI, Liu HH, Johns TR. Presynaptic and postsynaptic actions of procainamide on neuromuscular transmission. Muscle Nerve 1983;6:442–447.
580. Godley PJ, Morton TA, Karboski JA, Tami JA. Procainamide-induced myasthenic crisis. Ther Drug Monit 1990;12:411–414.
581. Miller CD, Oleshansky MA, Gibson KF, Cantilena LR. Procainamide-induced myasthenia-like weakness and dysphagia. Ther Drug Monit 1993;15:251–254.
582. Kornfeld P, Horowitz SH, Genkins G, Papatestas AE. Myasthenia gravis unmasked by antiarrhythmic agents. Mt Sinai J Med 1976;43:10–14.
583. Stoffer SS, Chandler JH. Quinidine-induced exacerbation of myasthenia gravis in patient with Graves' disease. Arch Intern Med 1980;140:283–284.
584. L'Hommedieu C, Stough R, Brown L, et al. Potentiation of neuromuscular weakness in infant botulism by aminoglycosides. J Pediatr 1979;95:1065–1070.
585. Onishi A, Shida K, Kuroiwa Y. [Problems of antibiotic administration in myasthenia gravis]. Shinkei Kenkyu No Shimpo 1971;15:906–910.
586. McQuillen MP, Cantor HA, O'Rourke JR. Myasthenic syndrome associated with antibiotics. Trans Am Neurol Assoc 1967;92:163–167.
587. Rosenberger K. [Myasthenic reactions during penicillin therapy]. Med Welt 1978;29:976–978.
588. Argov Z, Brenner T, Abramsky O. Ampicillin may aggravate clinical and experimental myasthenia gravis. Arch Neurol 1986;43:255–256.
589. Nieman RB, Sharma K, Edelberg H, Caffe SE. Telithromycin and myasthenia gravis. Clin Infect Dis 2003;37:1579.
590. May EF, Calvert PC. Aggravation of myasthenia gravis by erythromycin. Ann Neurol 1990;28:577–579.
591. Absher JR, Bale JF Jr. Aggravation of myasthenia gravis by erythromycin. J Pediatr 1991;119(1 [Pt 1]):155–156.
592. Cadisch R, Streit E, Hartmann K. [Exacerbation of pseudoparalytic myasthenia gravis following azithromycin (Zithromax)]. Schweiz Med Wochenschr 1996;126:308–310.
593. Pijpers E, van Rijswijk RE, Takx-Kohlen B, Schrey G. A clarithromycin-induced myasthenic syndrome. Clin Infect Dis 1996;22:175–176.
594. Wullen F, Kast G, Bruck A. [On side-effects of tetracycline administration in myasthenic patients]. Dtsch Med Wochenschr 1967;92:667–669.
595. Gibbels E. [Further observations on side effects of intravenous administration of reverin in myasthenia gravis pseudoparalytica]. Dtsch Med Wochenschr 1967;92:1153–1154.
596. Vial T, Chauplannaz G, Brunel P, et al. [Exacerbation of myasthenia gravis by pefloxacin]. Rev Neurol (Paris) 1995;151:286–287.
597. Sieb JP. Fluoroquinolone antibiotics block neuromuscular transmission. Neurology 1998;50:804–807.
598. Moore B, Safani M, Keesey J. Possible exacerbation of myasthenia gravis by ciprofloxacin. Lancet 1988;1:882.
599. Mumford CJ, Ginsberg L. Ciprofloxacin and myasthenia gravis. Br Med J 1990;301:818.
600. Roquer J, Cano A, Seoane JL, Pou Serradell A. Myasthenia gravis and ciprofloxacin. Acta Neurol Scand 1996;94:419–420.
601. Singh YN, Marshall IG, Harvey AL. Depression of transmitter release and postjunctional sensitivity during neuromuscular block produced by antibiotics. Br J Anaesth 1979;51:1027–1033.
602. Fogdall RP, Miller RD. Prolongation of a pancuronium-induced neuromuscular blockade by clindamycin. Anesthesiology 1974;41:407–408.
603. Regli F, Guggenheim P. [Myasthenic syndrome as a rare complication of hydantoin treatment]. Nervenarzt 1965;36:315–318.
604. Wand M, Mather JA. Diphenylhydantoin intoxication mimicking botulism. N Engl J Med 1972;286:88.
605. Brumlik J, Jacobs RS. Myasthenia gravis associated with diphenylhydantoin therapy for epilepsy. Can J Neurol Sci 1974;1:127–129.
606. Coppeto JR. Timolol-associated myasthenia gravis. Am J Ophthalmol 1984;98:244–245.
607. Wislicki L, Rosenblum I. Effects of propranolol on the action of neuromuscular blocking drugs. Br J Anaesth 1967;39:939–942.
608. Jui-Yen T. Clinical and experimental studies on mechanism of neuromuscular blockade by chloroquine diorotate. Jpn J Anesthesiol 1971;20:491–503.
609. Schumm F, Wietholter H, Fateh-Moghadam A. [Myasthenia syndrome during chloroquine treatment]. Dtsch Med Wochenschr 1981;106(51–52):1745–1747.
610. Pichon P, Soichot P, Loche D, Chapelon M. [Myasthenic syndrome induced by chloroquine poisoning: an unusual clinical form confirmed by ocular involvement]. Bull Soc Ophtalmol Fr 1984;84:219–225.
611. Sghirlanzoni A, Mantegazza R, Mora M, et al. Chloroquine myopathy and myasthenia-like syndrome. Muscle Nerve 1988;11:114–119.
612. Robberecht W, Bednarik J, Bourgeois P, et al. Myasthenic syndrome caused by direct effect of chloroquine on neuromuscular junction. Arch Neurol 1989;46:464–468.
613. De Bleecker J, De Reuck J, Quatacker J, Meire F. Persisting chloroquine-induced myasthenia? Acta Clin Belg 1991;46:401–406.
614. Klimek A. [The myasthenic syndrome after chloroquine]. Neurol Neurochir Pol 1999;33:951–954.
615. Wright DE, Drouin P. Cisplatin-induced myasthenic syndrome. Clin Pharm 1982;1:76–78.
616. Neil JF, Himmelhoch JM, Licata SM. Emergence of myasthenia gravis during treatment with lithium carbonate. Arch Gen Psychiatry 1976;33:1090–1092.
617. Granacher RP Jr. Neuromuscular problems associated with lithium. Am J Psychiatry 1977;134:702.
618. Lipton ID. Myasthenia gravis unmasked by lithium carbonate. J Clin Psychopharmacol 1987;7:57.
619. Dilsaver SC. Lithium down-regulates nicotinic receptors in skeletal muscle: Cause of lithium associated myasthenic syndrome? J Clin Psychopharmacol 1987;7:369–370.
620. Cohen BA, London RS, Goldstein PJ. Myasthenia gravis and preeclampsia. Obstet Gynecol 1976;48(1 Suppl):35S–37S.
621. Catanzarite VA, McHargue AM, Sandberg EC, Dyson DC. Respiratory arrest during therapy for premature labor in a patient with myasthenia gravis. Obstet Gynecol 1984;64:819–822.
622. Bashuk RG, Krendel DA. Myasthenia gravis presenting as weakness after magnesium administration. Muscle Nerve 1990;13:708–712.
623. Chagnac Y, Hadani M, Goldhammer Y. Myasthenic crisis after intravenous administration of iodinated contrast agent. Neurology 1985;35:1219–1220.
624. Anzola GP, Capra R, Magoni M, Vignolo LA. Myasthenic crisis during intravenous iodinated contrast medium injection. Ital J Neurol Sci 1986;7:273.
625. Frank JH, Cooper GW, Black WC, Phillips LH II. Iodinated contrast agents in myasthenia gravis. Neurology 1987;37:1400–1402.
626. Konen E, Konen O, Katz M, et al. Are referring clinicians aware of patients at risk from intravenous injection of iodinated contrast media? Clin Radiol 2002;57:132–135.
627. Gilbert EW, Stewart CM. Effective treatment of arachnoidism by calcium salts. Am J Med Sci 1935;189:532–536.
628. Nicholson GM, Graudins A. Spiders of medical importance in the Asia-Pacific: Atracotoxin, latrotoxin and related spider neurotoxins. Clin Exp Pharmacol Physiol 2002;29:785–794.
629. Rosenthal G, Marcus M, Bakalash S, Lifshitz T. Late Horner's syndrome following the bite of a black widow spider. Int Ophthalmol 1999;23:115–116.
630. Howard BD, Gundersen CB. Effects and mechanisms of polypeptide neurotoxins that act presynaptically. Annu Rev Pharmacol Toxicol 1980;20:307–336.
631. DelCastillo J, Pumplin DW. Discrete and discontinuous action of brown widow

spider venom on the presynaptic nerve terminals of frog muscle. J Physiol 1975; 252:491–508.

632. Gotlieb A. Spider bites. Lancet 1970;1:246.

633. Cherington M, Snyder R. Tick paralysis, neurophysiologic studies. N Engl J Med 1968;278:95–97.

634. Swift TR, Ignacio OJ. Tick paralysis: Electrophysiologic studies. Neurology 1975;25:1130–1133.

635. Greenstein P. Tick-borne diseases: Tick paralysis. Med Clin North Am 2002; 86:441–446.

636. Vedanarayanan VV, Evans OB, Subramony SH. Tick paralysis in children: Electrophysiology and possibility of misdiagnosis. Neurology 2002;59:1088–1090.

637. McLennan H, Oikawa I. Changes in function of the neuromuscular junction occurring in tick paralysis. Can J Physiol Pharmacol 1972;50:53–58.

638. Cooper BJ, Spence I. Temperature-dependent inhibition of evoked acetylcholine release in tick paralysis. Nature 1976;263:693–695.

639. Warnick JE, Albuquerque EK, Diniz CR. Electrophysiological observations on the action of purified scorpion venom, *Tityustoxin*, on nerve and skeletal muscle of the rat. J Pharmacol Exp Ther 1976;198:155–167.

640. Massensini AR, Romano-Silva MA, Gomez MV. Sodium channel toxins and neurotransmitter release. Neurochem Res 2003;28:1607–1611.

641. Gateau T, Bloom M, Clark R. Response to specific *Centruroides sculpturatus* antivenom in 151 cases of scorpion stings. J Toxicol Clin Toxicol 1994;32: 165–171.

642. Curry SC, Vance MV, Ryan PJ, et al. Envenomation by the scorpion *Centruroides sculpturatus*. J Toxicol Clin Toxicol 1984;21:417–449.

643. Clark RF, Selden BS, Kunkel DB, et al. Abnormal eye movements encountered following severe envenomations by *Centruroides sculpturatus*. Neurology 1991; 41:604.

644. Bergman NJ. Clinical description of *Parabuthus transvaalicus* scorpionism in Zimbabwe. Toxicon 1997;35:759–771.

645. Brumlik J. Myasthenia gravis associated with wasp sting. JAMA 1976;235: 2120–2121.

646. Singh RD, Bhagat A, Pandey AK. Bilateral ptosis following wasp sting. J Assoc Physicians India 2003;51:828–829.

647. Cherington M. Botulism. Ten-year experience. Arch Neurol 1974;30:432–437.

648. Cherington M, Ginsburg S. Wound botulism. Arch Surg 1975;110:436–438.

649. Donadio JA, Gangarosa EJ, Faich GA. Diagnosis and treatment of botulism. J Infect Dis 1971;124:108–112.

650. Merson MH, Dowell VR Jr. Epidemiologic, clinical and laboratory aspects of wound botulism. N Engl J Med 1973;289:1105–1110.

651. Pickett J, Berg B, Chaplin E, Brunstetter-Shafer MA. Syndrome of botulism in infancy: clinical and electrophysiologic study. N Engl J Med 1976;295:770–772.

652. Arnon SS, Midura TF, Damus K, et al. Intestinal infection and toxin production by *Clostridium botulinum* as one cause of sudden infant death syndrome. Lancet 1978;1:1273–1277.

653. Johnson RO, Clay SA, Arnon SS. Diagnosis and management of infant botulism. Am J Dis Child 1979;133:586–593.

654. Koenig MG, Drutz DJ, Mushlin AI, et al. Type B botulism in man. Am J Med 1967;42:208–219.

655. Ryan DW, Cherington M. Human type A botulism. JAMA 1971;216:513–514.

656. Merson MH, Hughes JM, Dowell VR, et al. Current trends in botulism in the United States. JAMA 1974;229:1305–1308.

657. Eisenberg MS, Bender TR. Botulism in Alaska, 1947 through 1974. Early detection of cases and investigation of outbreaks as a means of reducing mortality. JAMA 1976;235:35–38.

658. Lambert EH, Engel AG, Cherington M. End-plate potentials in human botulism. In Bradley WG, ed. Third International Congress on Muscle Disease, Series 334. Amsterdam, Excerpta Medica, 1974:65.

659. Maselli RA, Burnett ME, Tonsgard JH. In vitro microelectrode study of neuromuscular transmission in a case of botulism. Muscle Nerve 1992;15:273–276.

660. Duchen LW. An electron microscopic study of the changes induced by botulinum toxin in the motor end-plates of slow and fast skeletal muscle fibers of the mouse. J Neurol Sci 1971;14:47–60.

661. Jenzer G, Mumenthaler M, Ludin HP, Robert F. Autonomic dysfunction in botulism B: A clinical report. Neurology 1975;25:150–153.

662. Konig H, Gassman HB, Jenzer G. Ocular involvement in benign botulism B. Am J Ophthalmol 1975;80(3 Pt 1):430–432.

663. Miller NR, Moses H. Ocular involvement in wound botulism. Arch Ophthalmol 1977;95:1788–1789.

664. Terranova W, Palumbo JN, Breman JG. Ocular findings in botulism type B. JAMA 1979;241:475–477.

665. Hedges TR 3rd, Jones A, Stark L, Hoyt WF. Botulin ophthalmoplegia. Clinical and oculographic observations. Arch Ophthalmol 1983;101:211–213.

666. Caya JG. *Clostridium botulinum* and the ophthalmologist: A review of botulism, including biological warfare ramifications of botulinum toxin. Surv Ophthalmol 2001;46:25–34.

667. Aghdassi A, Teasdall RD. Acute onset of bulbar and ocular paralysis: An isolated case, with differential diagnosis. Henry Ford Hosp Med J 1977;25:119–123.

668. Ehrenreich H, Garner CG, Witt TN. Complete bilateral internal ophthalmoplegia as sole clinical sign of botulism: Confirmation of diagnosis by single fibre electromyography. J Neurol 1989;236:243–245.

669. Friedman DI, Fortanasce VN, Sadun AA. Tonic pupils as a result of botulism. Am J Ophthalmol 1990;109:236–237.

670. Monaco S, Freddi N, Francavilla E, et al. Transient tonic pupils in botulism type B. J Neurol Sci 1998;156:96–98.

671. de Jesus PV Jr, Slater R, Spitz LK, Penn AS. Neuromuscular physiology of wound botulism. Arch Neurol 1973;29:425–431.

672. Gutmann L, Pratt L. Pathophysiologic aspects of human botulism. Arch Neurol 1976;33:175–179.

673. Puggiari M, Cherington M. Botulism and guanidine. Ten years later. JAMA 1978;240:2276–2277.

674. Schiller HH, Stalberg E. Human botulism studied with single-fiber electromyography. Arch Neurol 1978;35:346–349.

675. Chang GY, Ganguly G. Early antitoxin treatment in wound botulism results in better outcome. Eur Neurol 2003;49:151–153.

676. Oh SJ, Halsey JH Jr, Briggs DD Jr. Guanidine in type B botulism. Arch Intern Med 1975;135:726–728.

677. Faich GA, Graebner RW, Sato S. Failure of guanidine therapy in botulism A. N Engl J Med 1971;285:773–776.

678. Kaplan JE, Davis LE, Narayan V, et al. Botulism, type A, and treatment with guanidine. Ann Neurol 1979;6:69–71.

679. Ball AP, Hopkinson RB, Farrell ID, et al. Human botulism caused by *Clostridium botulinum* type E: The Birmingham outbreak. Q J Med 1979;48:473–491.

680. Siegel LS, Price JI. Ineffectiveness of 3,4-diaminopyridine as a therapy for type C botulism. Toxicon 1987;25:1015–1018.

681. Davis LE, Johnson JK, Bicknell JM, et al. Human type A botulism and treatment with 3,4-diaminopyridine. Electromyogr Clin Neurophysiol 1992;32(7–8): 379–383.

682. Dock M, Ben Ali A, Karras A, et al. [Treatment of severe botulism with 3,4-diaminopyridine]. Presse Med 2002;31:601–602.

683. Lee CY. Elapid neurotoxins and their mode of action. Clin Toxicol 1970;3: 457–472.

684. Vital-Brazil O. Venoms: Their inhibitory action on neuromuscular transmission. In Cheymol J, ed. Neuromuscular Blocking and Stimulating Agents. New York, Pergamon Press, 1972:145–167.

685. Ahuja ML, Singh G. Snakebite in India. In Buckley EE, Porges N, eds. Venoms. Washington DC, AAAS, 1956:341–351.

686. Reid HA. Cobra bites. Br Med J 1964;2:540–545.

687. Pettigrew LC, Glass JP. Neurologic complications of a coral snake bite. Neurology 1984;34:S1–226.

688. Connolly S, Trevett AJ, Nwokolo NC, et al. Neuromuscular effects of Papuan Taipan snake venom. Ann Neurol 1995;38:916–920.

689. Fry BG. Structure-function properties of venom components from Australian elapids. Toxicon 1999;37:11–32.

690. Fohlman J, Eaker D. Isolation and characterization of a lethal myotoxic phopholipase A from the venom of the common sea snake *Enhydrina schistosa* causing myoglobinuria in mice. Toxicon 1977;15:385–393.

691. Naphade RW, Shetti RN. Use of neostigmine after snakebite. Br J Anaesth 1977; 49:1065–1068.

CHAPTER 22

Myopathies Affecting the Extraocular Muscles

Paul N. Hoffman

In this chapter, we consider disorders that produce ocular motor dysfunction from involvement of the extraocular muscles. Some of these disorders affect only the extraocular muscles, whereas others are multisystem disorders in which various organ systems are also affected. The classification that is used is modified from Walton et al. (1), which should be consulted by readers interested in pursuing the subject of muscle disorders.

DEVELOPMENTAL DISORDERS OF EXTRAOCULAR MUSCLE

Anomalous development of extraocular muscles is probably more common than the literature would indicate. Many of these anomalies are recognized only during surgical procedures or at autopsy. The most common congenital anomalies of the extraocular muscles are agenesis, anomalous insertions or origins, and the adherence and fibrosis syndromes.

AGENESIS OF THE EXTRAOCULAR MUSCLES

Most cases of agenesis of the extraocular muscles involve only a single muscle. Isolated agenesis of the lateral rectus muscle (2), medial rectus muscle (2,3), inferior rectus muscle (4–7), superior rectus muscle (8), and superior oblique muscle (2,9) are all well described, particularly in children with craniostenosis (10–12). In some patients, agenesis of more than one muscle occurs (5,6).

ANOMALIES OF EXTRAOCULAR MUSCLE LOCATION

An abnormal insertion of an extraocular muscle is occasionally responsible for ocular motor dysfunction. In its mildest form, this may simply occur as a bifid insertion of the medial (13), lateral (14), or superior rectus (15) muscles. The insertions of the superior and inferior oblique muscles vary widely (16), so it is often difficult to state when they are truly abnormal. Nevertheless, in some patients, the insertions of one or the other of these muscles are clearly abnormal. For example, the superior oblique tendon may insert on the undersurface of the superior rectus muscle, or the inferior oblique tendon may be attached to the lateral rectus muscle. The insertions of the four rectus muscles are much less variable, and thus abnormal insertions are more easily recognized (Fig. 22.1) (14,17). Strebel described monozygotic twins with fusion of the tendons of the superior and medial recti (18). Abnormal insertions of extraocular muscles, like agenesis of the muscles, often occur in children with craniostenosis (19).

Abnormal **origins** of extraocular muscles are quite rare. They appear to affect the inferior oblique muscle more than any of the other extraocular muscles (20).

Occasionally, an extraocular muscle shows underaction because of an abnormally increased length (21). In other instances, an anomalous muscle slip or fibrous band may be present (22) (Fig. 22.2). This phenomenon may be responsible for some cases of the superior oblique tendon sheath syndrome described by Brown (23). Patients with this syndrome show absence of elevation in adduction, improvement of elevation in the primary position, and normal or near-normal elevation in abduction (Fig. 22.3). Forced duction testing (see Chapter 18) shows mechanical limitation of motion upward and inward in the involved eye, but upward saccadic velocities are normal (24). Electromyographic (EMG) studies show no evidence of neuropathic abnormalities (25).

The cause of the congenital form of the superior oblique tendon sheath syndrome is unknown. The initial theory ad-

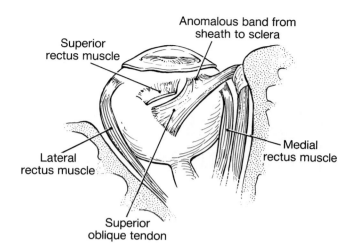

Figure 22.2. Anomalous tendon sheath resulting in tethering of the superior rectus and preventing normal vertical gaze. (Redrawn from Raab EL. Superior oblique tendon sheath syndrome: An unusual case. Ann Ophthalmol 1976;8:345–347.)

vanced by Brown (23)—that a short anterior sheath was caused by congenital paralysis of the inferior oblique muscle—is not supported by EMG studies, saccadic velocity studies, or findings at surgery (26). A restrictive band posterior and inferior to the globe may be responsible for Brown's syndrome in most patients.

CONGENITAL ADHERENCE AND FIBROSIS SYNDROMES

Johnson (27) described two types of adherence syndromes associated with defective eye movements. In one type, there were adhesions between the sheaths of the lateral rectus and inferior oblique muscles that made it impossible to abduct the eye. The disorder was usually bilateral. The second type was characterized by adherence between the sheaths of the superior rectus and superior oblique muscles, preventing elevation of the affected eye.

Congenital fibrosis of the extraocular muscles (CFEOM) is quite rare (28–30). It is characterized by (*a*) ophthalmoplegia, (*b*) blepharoptosis, (c) fibrosis of all the extraocular muscles, (*d*) fibrosis of Tenon's capsule, (*e*) adhesions between muscles, Tenon's capsule, and globe, and (*f*) inelasticity and fragility of the conjunctiva. CFEOM is associated with mutations at three distinct loci, FEOM1, FEOM2, and FEOM3, located on chromosomes 12, 11, and 16, respectively (31–34).

Autosomal-dominant CFEOM is associated with heterozygous mutations of the FEOM1 or FEOM3 locus (31–33). The proteins encoded by the FEOM1 and FEOM3 genes have not been identified (31,33). FEOM1 mutations are associated with the CFEOM1 phenotype, which is characterized by (*a*) ptosis, (*b*) eyes fixed 20°–30° below the horizontal (infraduction), (*c*) absence of elevation or depression of the eyes, (*d*) little or no horizontal movement with an eso- or

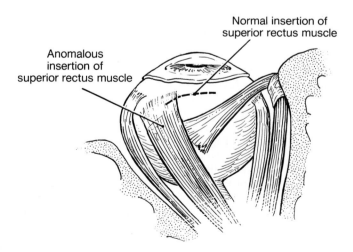

Figure 22.1. Anomalous insertion of the superior rectus muscle in a patient with strabismus. The superior rectus muscle inserts just superior to the lateral rectus muscle. (Redrawn from Rosenbaum AL, Jampolsky A. Pseudoparalysis caused by anomalous insertion of superior rectus muscle. Arch Ophthalmol 1975;93:535–537.)

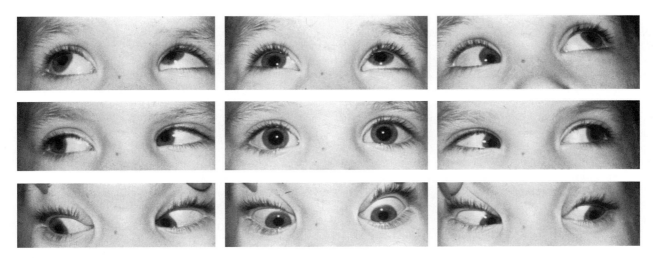

Figure 22.3. Four-year-old child with congenital Brown's superior oblique tendon sheath syndrome. Note marked limitation of upward movement of the right eye when the eye is adducted, compared to mild limitation of upward movement of the eye when it is abducted. The patient was able to fuse in the primary position. (Courtesy of Jacqueline E. Morris, C.O.)

exo-deviation, and (*e*) chin elevation (32,33,35) (Fig. 22.4; Table 22.1). FEOM3 mutations are most frequently associated with the less severe CFEOM3 phenotype, with either bilateral or unilateral involvement of the eyes (31,36). Less commonly, FEOM3 mutations are associated with the CFEOM1 phenotype (33) (Table 22.1).

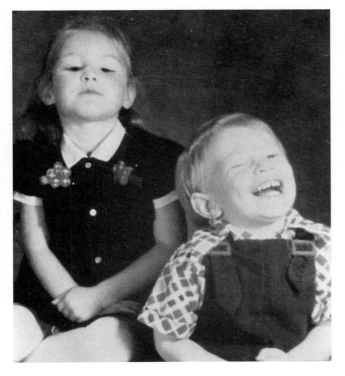

Figure 22.4. Congenital fibrosis syndrome in a brother and sister. Because of the bilateral ptosis and ophthalmoplegia, both children have adopted a head posture with the chin elevated. (Courtesy of Dr. Stewart M. Wolff.)

Autosomal-recessive CFEOM is associated with homozygous mutations of the FEOM2 locus, which encodes ARIX (34,37), a homeodomain transcription factor protein necessary for the formation of cranial nerve III (oculomotor) and IV (trochlear) motor neurons in zebrafish and mouse (38,39). ARIX mutations result in a distinct phenotype (CFEOM2) in which the eyes are primarily exotrophic (maximally abducted) and may be mildly hypo- or hypertrophic (37) (Table 22.1). This pattern of deviation reflects the loss of cranial nerve III and IV motor neurons (34). ARIX mutations are not associated with either the CFEOM1 or CFEOM3 phenotype (33), suggesting that the FEOM1 and FEOM3 genes act downstream to ARIX.

In nearly all patients, CFEOM excludes systemic neuropathic or myopathic abnormalities, but some patients have facial diparesis (40), and individual patients have inguinal hernias and cryptorchidism (41) or a cleft palate (40).

Histopathologic findings in some patients with CFEOM include replacement of muscle tissue with fibrous tissue and degenerative changes in the muscles (30,41,42). In other patients, however, the muscles are normal or show minimal pathologic changes (43). Electron microscopic evaluation in some cases reveals active fibrocyte proliferation and absence of striated muscle tissue (44). Extensive neuropathologic examination of a single case of CFEOM 1 (40) showed absence of the superior division of the oculomotor nerve and its corresponding motor neurons, atrophy and fibrotic replacement of the levator palpebrae superioris and superior rectus, and abnormalities in all of the extraocular muscles, not just those innervated by the superior division of the oculomotor nerve. This is consistent with the view that CFEOM is actually caused by the maldevelopment of cranial nerve III and/or IV motor neurons (40,43), similar to Duane's syndrome, a congenital fibrosis syndrome presumably resulting from impaired development of cranial nerve VI (abducens) motor neurons (45,46) (see Chapter 20).

Table 22.1
Congenital Fibrosis of the Extraocular Muscles Syndromes

Phenotype	Inheritance	Locus (Chromosome)	Gene	Clinical Presentation
CFEOM1	AD	FEOM1 (12cen)	Unknown	Bilateral ptosis, ophthalmoplegia, eye is primarily hypotrophic, may also be eso- or exotrophic, inability to elevate globe above midline, absence of superior division of cranial nerve III with loss of corresponding oculomotor subnuclei
CFEOM2	AR	FEOM2 (11q13)	ARIX	Bilateral ptosis, ophthalmoplegia, eye is primarily exotrophic, may also be mildly hypo-or hypertrophic
CFEOM3	AD	FEOM3 (16qter)	Unknown	Unilateral or bilateral, ptosis and motility defects range from severe (with eye primarily hypotrophic and exotrophic) to mild and asymmetric, phenotypes overlap with CFEOM1 and CFEOM2

AD, autosomal dominant; AR, autosomal recessive.

CONGENITAL MYOPATHIES

BACKGROUND AND CLASSIFICATION

Some congenital, primarily nonprogressive myopathies affect the extraocular muscles. Although the disorders in this group are similar to one another clinically and are called collectively **structurally defined congenital myopathies**, they have distinctive morphologic features. The primary congenital myopathies are (*a*) central core myopathy (47), (*b*) nemaline myopathy (48), (*c*) centronuclear (or myotubular) myopathy (49), (*d*) multicore disease (50), and (*e*) congenital fiber-type disproportion (51).

A second group of congenital myopathies remains to be characterized fully. These disorders generally present with congenital hypotonia or with early onset generalized weakness that does not progress. Some have ocular features; others do not (52). Skeletal deformities, such as high-arched palate, scoliosis, and a slender body habitus often mark these myopathies as beginning in utero; however, disparate phenotypes, in which symptoms appear and even progress in adult life, without dysmorphic features to mark a developmental onset, also occur in nemaline, centronuclear, and multicore myopathies (53,54).

Most congenital myopathies are mild and nonprogressive or slowly progressive. Some cases, however, are severe, relentlessly progressive, or both, resulting in substantial debilitation (55–57).

Congenital myopathies must be differentiated by the neuro-ophthalmologist from other causes of congenital hypotonic weakness. For example, Werdnig-Hoffman disease (acute or type I spinal muscular atrophy), a point mutation or short deletion at 5q11–q13 involving survival motor neuron protein (SMN) (58), is neurogenic, uniformly fatal, and rarely if ever affects extraocular muscles (59). In fact, ptosis or external ophthalmoplegia probably indicates that a congenital hypotonic disorder is a myopathy (60). More chronic forms of spinal muscular atrophy also spare extraocular muscles. Congenital myotonic dystrophy, neonatal myasthenia gravis, and infant botulism commonly cause hypotonia, weakness, facial paresis, and ophthalmoparesis.

Central Core Myopathy

In 1956, Shy and Magee reported a new muscular disorder in which Gomori trichrome and oxidative enzyme staining showed that almost every muscle fiber exhibited a well-defined, round, central core that lacked mitochondria (47). The term ''central core disease'' was later coined by Greenfield et al. (61), the first time that a structural abnormality of the muscle fiber was considered to be ''primary'' in skeletal muscle pathology. The disorder was congenital and nonprogressive and affected five persons in the same family over three generations, indicating autosomal-dominant inheritance.

Most cases of central core disease exhibit a clinical pattern similar to that of the original cases identified by Shy and Magee (47). The muscular weakness appears in early childhood. Marked hypotonia is rarely noted, but motor milestones are usually slightly delayed. The lower extremities are most severely affected, particularly proximally. The facial, sternocleidomastoid, and trapezius muscles may be slightly affected. Extraocular muscles are occasionally involved (52). Central core disease is caused by a mutation in the ryanodine receptor calcium channel (chromosome 19q13.1) (62,63). Patients with this condition are also at risk for malignant hyperthermia, with which central core disease is allelic (64).

Nemaline Myopathy

In nemaline myopathy (also called ''rod myopathy''), myriads of minute rod-shaped granules are present in most of the muscle fibers (48,65) (Fig. 22.5). In most cases, inheritance is autosomal dominant and associated with mutations of nebulin, a protein associated with thin filaments in skeletal muscle (66). Patients with this condition typically have a dysmorphic, elongated, weak face and a high-arched palate (52). Ptosis and ophthalmoparesis occasionally occur and may be severe (67,68) (Fig. 22.6).

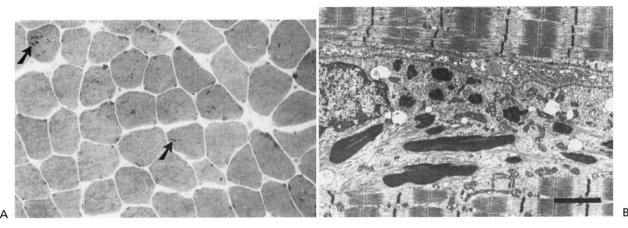

Figure 22.5. Histopathology of nemaline myopathy. *A,* Muscle biopsy shows small collections of rod-like structures (*arrows*). Modified Gomori trichrome stain. Scale = 100 μm. *B,* Electron micrograph of the biopsy specimen shows a cluster of rod bodies adjacent to a nucleus at the periphery of a fiber in longitudinal section. Scale = 2 μm. (From Wright RA, Plant GT, Landon DN, et al. Nemaline myopathy: An unusual cause of ophthalmoparesis. J Neuroophthalmol 1997;17:39–43.)

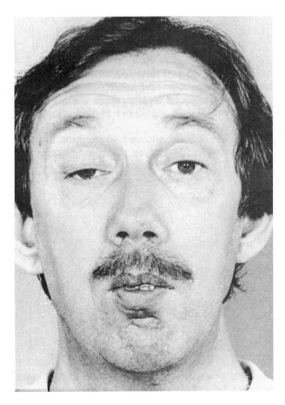

Figure 22.6. Appearance of a 45-year-old man with nemaline myopathy. Note bilateral asymmetric ptosis. The patient must use the frontalis muscle to help raise the eyelids. (From Wright RA, Plant GT, Landon DN, et al. Nemaline myopathy: An unusual cause of ophthalmoparesis. J Neuroophthalmol 1997;17:39–43.)

Centronuclear (Myotubular) Myopathy

In centronuclear myopathy, most muscle fibers show centrally located nuclei around which there is a small area devoid of enzymatic activity (Fig. 22.7). Because there are wide differences among patients with this disease with respect to mode of inheritance, age of onset, clinical severity, presence or absence of ocular signs, and histochemical abnormalities, this morphologic syndrome must subsume several different disorders.

In some cases of centronuclear myopathy, selective involvement of type 1 fibers is so striking that such cases are considered a specific form of the disorder (55). Although most of these patients show no evidence of extraocular muscle involvement, Radu et al. described a patient with limitation of ocular movement (69).

Centronuclear myopathy with type 1 fiber atrophy may be familial. A dominant mode of transmission was suggested in a family reported by Karpati et al. (70), whereas an autosomal-recessive mode of expression was postulated by Radu et al. (69) to explain the transmission of the disease in the pedigree that they studied. The heterogeneity of findings and genetic transmission in these cases argues against their being a single entity, and they will probably be reclassified in the future.

Early onset centronuclear myopathy, the most common variety, is characterized clinically by severe neonatal hypotonia, relatively slight delay in motor development, diffuse muscle weakness with easy fatigability, scapular winging and waddling gait, and severe dysfunction of the flexors of the feet (49). In addition, patients with this disorder have bilateral facial and masticatory weakness as well as ptosis and external ophthalmoplegia (71) (Fig. 22.8). There is generalized areflexia without myotonia or fasciculation. A few patients have cataracts (72). The course of the disease is generally slowly progressive, with some patients becoming severely disabled by the fourth decade of life (73). The disor-

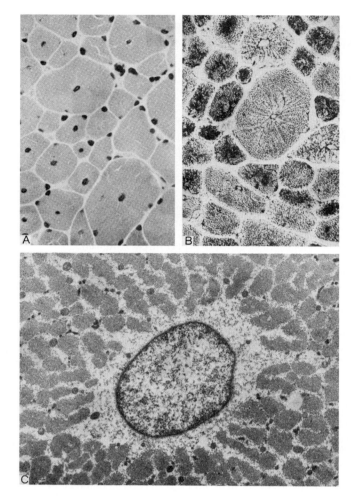

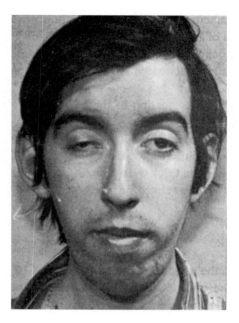

Figure 22.8. Centronuclear myopathy in a 20-year-old man with generalized muscular weakness, a high-arched palate, moderate scoliosis, and winged scapulae. (From Jadros-Santel D, Grcevic N, Dogan S, et al. Centronuclear myopathy with type 1 fiber hypotrophy and "fingerprint" inclusions associated with Marfan's syndrome. J Neurol Sci 1980;45:43–46.)

Figure 22.7. Histopathology of centronuclear myopathy. *A*, Note centrally located nuclei in most of the fibers; hematoxylin and eosin stain, ×160. *B*, Radial disposition of the intermyofibrillary network in the large fibers can be seen with NADH-tetrazolium reductase stain; ×160. *C*, Electron micrograph of a single fiber shows a small area devoid of organelles surrounding the centrally located nucleus; ×14,000. (From Fardeau M. Congenital myopathies. In: Mastaglia FL, Walton J, eds. Skeletal Muscle Pathology. Edinburgh: Churchill Livingstone, 1982:161.)

der causes death in some persons (74). On the other hand, in some patients who are severely affected in early childhood the disease may nevertheless remain stable or progress slowly (75). An autosomal-recessive transmission pattern was initially proposed by Sher et al. (76). The number of apparently sporadic cases may indirectly support this hypothesis; however, an alternative possibility is an autosomal-dominant gene with variable expression (77).

In some cases of centronuclear myopathy, muscle weakness does not appear until adulthood (70,78). Most patients with this **late-onset** form of centronuclear myopathy have muscle wasting and weakness, mainly of the trunk and limb-girdle muscles. Unlike the early onset form of centronuclear myopathy, extraocular muscle involvement (69,78) and ptosis (79) are rare. No clear-cut morphologic differences dis-

tinguish the early onset and late-onset types of centronuclear myopathy. In the latter, however, a dominant mode of inheritance is more often demonstrated (79,80).

A severe **neonatal** form of centronuclear myopathy occurs only in males and is linked to chromosome Xq28 (81,82,83). The responsible gene, MTM1, encodes myotubularin, a highly conserved phosphatase (84). Mortality of affected male children was 25% in one reported family (57) and 100% in a second (85). Diminution of fetal movement and polyhydramnios are often noted in affected infants, and death from respiratory failure usually occurs in the first few hours or days of life. Only a few affected children can overcome these neonatal difficulties. These children show a slow improvement in their motor condition but manifest ptosis and external ophthalmoplegia (86).

Multicore Disease

The term "multicore disease" was proposed by Engel et al. to denote a congenital, nonprogressive myopathy in which the primary histopathologic change is multiple, focal loss of normal sarcomeric cross-striations (50). These foci of myofibrillar disruption are devoid of mitochondria (Fig. 22.9), giving affected muscle fibers a punched-out appearance like central core disease on oxidative enzyme histochemical staining, but the lesions are smaller and multiple. The disorder is not linked to central core disease or to malignant hyperthermia. Most cases of multicore disease are sporadic, but inheritance in some families seems to be autosomal dominant (50,87) or autosomal recessive (60,88,89).

Clinically, most cases of multicore disease share the usual

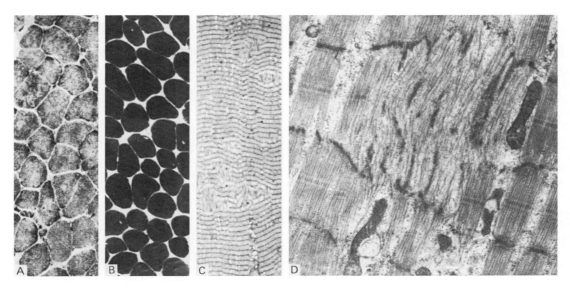

Figure 22.9. Histopathology of multicore disease. *A,* Small defects and irregularities are present in the intermyofibrillar network of involved skeletal muscle fibers; NADH-tetrazolium reaction; ×135. *B,* Myofibrillar ATPase reaction after preincubation at pH 4.35 showing type 1 fiber uniformity; ×135. *C,* A thick section of epoxy-embedded skeletal muscle shows several foci of disrupted myofibrillar striations; ×340. *D,* Electron micrograph of an involved skeletal muscle fiber shows a small focus of sarcomeric disorganization. (From Fardeau M. Congenital myopathies. In: Mastaglia FL, Walton J, eds. Skeletal Muscle Pathology. Edinburgh: Churchill Livingstone, 1982:161.)

pattern of a benign congenital myopathy: floppiness at birth, delayed motor development, and a generalized reduction in muscle bulk. Facial weakness may be present. Ocular involvement includes isolated, bilateral ptosis (50,60,90), mild limitation of ocular movement (89,91), and complete external ophthalmoplegia (60,92). Cardiac abnormalities are sometimes present and include congenital defects (50) or cardiac hypertrophy (93). Most patients have a nonprogressive course, but mild worsening of signs may occur both in early onset and late-onset cases.

Congenital Fiber-Type Disproportion

This entity was recognized as a result of a review by Brooke and Engel (51) of a series of children's muscle biopsies that were grouped according to changes in fiber size. One group, comprising 10 children with nonprogressive weakness, had type 1 fibers that were significantly smaller than type 2 fibers (Fig. 22.10). After studying 12 additional cases, Brooke (94) proposed the term "congenital fiber-type disproportion" (CFTD) for this group, based on a fairly uniform clinical picture, a possible familial incidence, and a relatively good prognosis.

Children with this disorder are hypotonic at birth. Other features include a long thin face, open mouth, and a high-arched palate. Muscle weakness is diffuse. Affected persons are generally of short stature and low body weight, and they frequently have skeletal abnormalities, particularly congenital hip dislocation. Deep tendon reflexes are weak or absent. Respiratory problems may occur within the first 2 years of life, after which patients generally slowly improve.

Owen et al. (95) described a patient with bilateral ptosis and ophthalmoplegia in the setting of CFTD. The patient was an 8-year-old girl whose ophthalmologic findings were present when she was first examined at 2 years of age; the findings did not change over the following 6 years (Fig. 22.11).

Whether CFTD is a true entity is unclear. It may better be considered a sign pinpointing the onset of a disorder during fetal development of fiber types. A similar disproportion in fiber size may be encountered in most of the other congenital myopathies, in congenital myotonic dystrophy (96), in the infantile variety of fascioscapulohumeral dystrophy (71), and in some neurogenic disorders (51). In fact, one of the original cases of CFTD was subsequently shown to be a muscular dystrophy (97). It therefore may be that the histologic picture of CFTD represents more than one disorder and that it is not in itself a sufficient criterion to characterize a subgroup of congenital myopathies. Nevertheless, it is clear that a "pure" size disproportion of muscle fibers is highly suggestive of a congenital myopathy and that there are numerous cases of congenital hypotonia in which CFTD is the only histologic abnormality.

Congenital Myopathies with Intracytoplasmic Inclusion Bodies

Some congenital myopathies are characterized histologically primarily by intracytoplasmic inclusion bodies within affected muscle fibers (71). These myopathies include fingerprint body myopathy (98), reducing body myopathy (56), and congenital (neuro)myopathy with cytoplasmic bodies (99). One of the patients with reducing body myopathy had mild bilateral ptosis and diffuse muscle weakness.

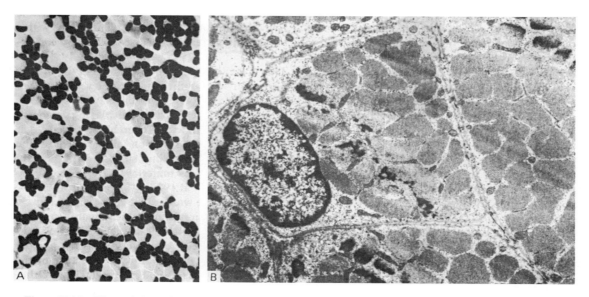

Figure 22.10. Histopathology of congenital fiber type disproportion. *A,* Myofibrillar ATPase reaction after preincubation at pH 4.65 shows that all type 1 fibers are small; ×135. *B,* Electron micrograph shows normal appearance of small, type 1 fibers; ×5,850. (From Fardeau M. Congenital myopathies. In: Mastaglia FL, Walton J, eds. Skeletal Muscle Pathology. Edinburgh: Churchill Livingstone, 1982:161.)

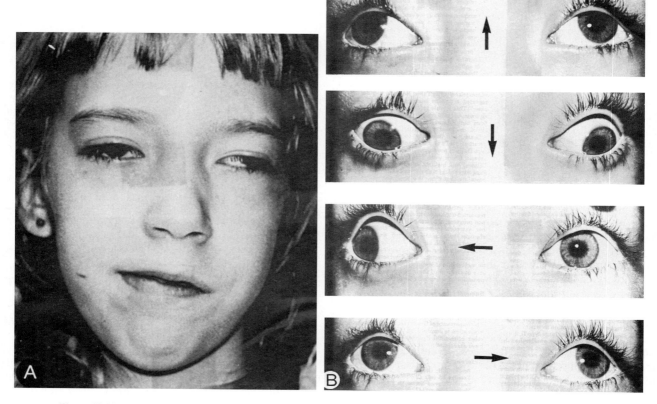

Figure 22.11. Clinical appearance of an 8-year-old girl with congenital fiber-type disproportion. *A,* The patient has myopathic facies, bilateral ptosis, and exotropia. *B,* The patient has profound ophthalmoparesis. Only abduction of the right eye is normal. (From Owen JS, Kline LB, Oh SJ, et al. Ophthalmoplegia and ptosis in congenital fiber-type disproportion. J Pediatr Ophthalmol Strabis 1981;18:55–60.)

Miscellaneous Congenital Myopathies

The morphologically defined congenital myopathies described above have withstood the test of time in numerous patients and separate families. Several other congenital myopathies, although morphologically distinct, are dubious entities because clinical or genetic heterogeneity does not justify their recognition as distinct entities. These include familial myopathy with probable lysis of myofibrils in type 1 fibers (100), sarcotubular myopathy (101), cytoplasmic body myopathy (102), zebra body myopathy (103), tubular aggregate myopathy (104), and trilaminar muscle fiber disease (105). Patients with these disorders do not have ptosis or clinical evidence of extraocular muscle involvement. Reducing body myopathy is in the same rare but dubious category (56,106) but, as noted above, may be associated with ptosis.

Mace et al. reported a pedigree in which seven members had congenital ptosis, myopia, and varying degrees of ophthalmoplegia (107). The transmission was thought to be autosomal dominant. The disorder remained static throughout life and was not associated with either a generalized muscular disorder or neurologic deterioration. A biopsy from the medial rectus muscle of an affected family member showed nonspecific changes. The etiology of this disorder is unclear.

RELATIONSHIP AMONG THE DIFFERENT CONGENITAL MYOPATHIES

It is clear that individual patients may show structural alterations of muscle fibers that are ''characteristic'' of more than one type of congenital myopathy (108). The frequency with which such associations are encountered suggests some relationship among the different structural congenital myopathies. It is therefore likely that either the structural alterations are, in fact, insufficient to permit an exact classification of these disorders or that the production of structural abnormalities occurs as a continuum during muscle development and thus allows multiple patterns to emerge. Theoretical constructs view the congenital myopathies as errors in developmental stages of muscle embryogenesis—fusion of myoblasts into multinuclear myotubes, nuclear migration, nerve-controlled differentiation of muscle fiber types, and growth (71,109). Although ''myopathic,'' they may have some neurogenic bases, given the determinant developmental roles that innervation and firing patterns have on muscle development, histochemistry, and trophism.

To further confuse the issue, Berard-Badier et al. (110) described abnormalities similar to those observed in the congenital myopathies in patients with congenital strabismus, Duane's retraction syndrome, and ocular motor paralysis. These changes include disorganization of myofilaments, double Z-disks, rods, curving arrays of myofibrils, concentrically disposed electron-dense sarcotubules, and subsarcolemmal inclusions, such as dense bodies, laminated bodies, lipofuscin granules, and lipid droplets. Because Duane's retraction syndrome and ocular motor nerve paralysis are clearly neurogenic disorders, the electron microscopic changes described above may be much more nonspecific than previously suspected, simply representing the limited repertoire of muscle to neurogenic, other secondary, or primary myogenic influences.

MUSCULAR DYSTROPHIES

The term ''muscular dystrophy'' covers a group of genetically determined disorders that cause **progressive** weakness and wasting of the skeletal muscles and that are assumed to affect the muscle cell directly (111). Some forms cause death after 15–20 years, whereas others are compatible with a normal life expectancy. The distinction between the terms ''myopathy'' and ''dystrophy'' breaks down, however, when it is realized that some glycogenolytic myopathies, like acid maltase deficiency, can progress inexorably like dystrophies, and some dystrophies, like Becker dystrophy, may hardly progress at all. Nevertheless, the diagnostic category is a tradition. Although the diagnosis of this group of disorders cannot be established by morphology alone, histologic examination of an affected muscle can exclude other myopathies (e.g., the congenital myopathies and the mitochondrial myopathies). In others, molecular genetic testing can provide the correct diagnosis.

Muscular dystrophies are historically subdivided on the basis of age of onset, mode of inheritance, and clinical features:

1. The dystrophin-deficient dystrophies, including the severe X-linked pseudohypertrophic muscular dystrophy of Duchenne (112), with its more benign ''Becker'' variant (113)

2. The dystrophin-associated glycoprotein disorders that may resemble Duchenne or Becker dystrophy, including mutations of merosin and the α-, β-, γ-, or δ-sarcoglycans (114–116)
3. Various limb-girdle dystrophies, including severe childhood-onset autosomal recessive (chromosome 13) muscular dystrophy, juvenile scapulohumeral dystrophy of Erb, pelvifemoral dystrophy of Leyden and Möbius (117,118), and adult-onset autosomal-dominant limb-girdle dystrophy
4. The fascioscapulohumeral dystrophy of Landouzy and Déjérine (119)
5. Distal dystrophies (myopathies) of Welander (120), Miyoshi (121), and others
6. Various congenital muscular dystrophies, including Fukuyama dystrophy (122,123), muscle-eye-brain disease (124,125), and Walker-Warburg syndrome (126)
7. Myotonic muscular dystrophy (127)
8. Proximal myotonic myopathy (128,129)
9. Oculopharyngeal muscular dystrophy (130,131).

Only the last four of these disorders are of neuro-ophthalmologic importance and are discussed in detail below. The reader interested in obtaining more information regarding the muscular dystrophies in general should consult the authoritative texts of Mastaglia and Walton (132), Brooke (133), Swash and Schwartz (134), Engel and Franzini-Armstrong (90), Walton et al. (1,135), and Griggs et al. (104).

CONGENITAL MUSCULAR DYSTROPHIES

A number of patients have dystrophic muscle pathology associated with symptoms that are present at birth and a variable clinical course. These patients are said to have congenital muscular dystrophy (CMD) (136). CMD is by no means rare. Rospide et al. (137) believed that it represented 16% of childhood muscular dystrophies, and Donner et al. (138) estimated that it represented 9% of all neuromuscular disorders seen in a pediatric hospital.

Patients with CMD show generalized muscle involvement at birth. Muscle atrophy and weakness are symmetric and predominate in proximal muscles. Neither ptosis nor ophthalmoplegia is present in patients with the most common forms of simple CMD confined to skeletal muscle, such as merosin-deficient CMD (139,116), the sarcoglycanopathies (115), and the mutations in other dystrophin-associated glycoproteins (114,140). However, non-muscular ocular involvement is common in three congenital dystrophy syndromes that are really multisystemic disorders of eye, brain, and skeletal muscle. These three, the Fukuyama type of CMD (122,141), so-called muscle-eye-brain disease (122,124,125,142), and the Walker-Warburg syndrome (143), are associated with mutations that result in protein glycosylation defects (144–146). The reader interested in learning more about these disorders should consult Haltia et al. (147) for a review and comparison of their ocular findings.

Fukuyama Congenital Muscular Dystrophy

The Fukuyama type of CMD is transmitted as an autosomal-recessive trait with no sex predilection, a high incidence of consanguinity, and a high frequency of affected siblings. The mutant gene, located on chromosome 9q31, encodes fukutin, a putative glycosyltransferase (144,148,149).

Patients with Fukuyama dystrophy have CMD associated with central nervous system (CNS) involvement, including mental retardation and convulsions. Children are severely weak from birth, and only a few children can walk without assistance. Most survive beyond infancy to remain relatively stable (150), but the average life span is only 8–10 years (141). Serum levels of creatinine kinase (CK) are elevated, and the muscle biopsy shows myopathic and fibrotic changes. Ventricular enlargement and hypoplasia of the cerebellar vermis are seen with computed tomographic (CT) scanning, and magnetic resonance (MR) imaging shows severe signal abnormalities in white matter.

The neuropathologic findings include polymicrogyria of the cerebrum and cerebellum, loss of cerebral cytoarchitecture with demyelination and proliferation of interstitial tissue, occasionally absent or hypoplastic corpus callosum, and brain stem pyramidal tract abnormalities (141). Chronic meningeal thickening, lymphocytic infiltration of intracranial tissues, and proliferation of meningeal tissue and blood vessels are less common.

Ocular involvement in Fukuyama CMD is inconsistent, but it is milder than that in muscle-eye-brain disease and Walker-Warburg syndrome (147) (discussed later). Ocular findings include occasional optic nerve hypoplasia and optic atrophy, as well as pathologic high myopia, cataracts, retinal abnormalities, and weakness of the orbicularis oculi muscles (141,151). Chijiiwa et al. (152) described gross mottling of retinal pigment epithelium and abnormal retinal vessels in two patients with this disorder. Weinstein et al. (153) performed a complete autopsy on a 1-year-old child with Fukuyama CMD and found numerous ocular abnormalities, including a small anterior polar cataract, anomalous ciliary processes, absence of vitreous, and optic nerve hypoplasia. In addition, these authors reported that the retinas of both eyes were extremely dysplastic, with a glial or glial-vascular membrane involving the inner retinal layers in most areas. Incomplete retinal vascularization, temporally displaced foveas, and irregularities of the retinal pigment epithelium were also present.

Muscle-Eye-Brain Disease

This autosomal-recessive disorder is associated with homozygous mutations in O-mannose beta-1,2–N-acetylglucosaminyltransferase (POMGnT1), an enzyme that participates in O-mannosyl glycan synthesis (145). It is characterized by severe congenital hypotonic weakness from both progressive CNS disease and CMD. Though the cerebral and visual abnormalities are severe, most patients reach adulthood (average age of death, 18). As in Fukuyama dystrophy, levels of serum CK are elevated, and muscle biopsy shows mild myopathy with fibrosis.

Ocular abnormalities are more consistent and severe in muscle-eye-brain disease than in Fukuyama dystrophy, but they are less uniform than in Walker-Warburg syndrome (147,142). High myopia is common. Haltia et al. (147) reported the first two postmortem studies of brain and eye pathology. Ocular findings in these cases included severe generalized loss of retinal ganglion cells, retinochoroidal scars, a pronounced preretinal membrane and gliosis, mottled retinal pigment epithelium, and mild optic nerve and chiasm atrophy with reactive gliosis. The microscopic and macroscopic features of the cortex were highly abnormal. Apart from argyric areas limited to the occipital cortex, the brain looked "cobblestoned" by coarse and nodular gyri (pachy/polymicrogyria). The cerebral and cerebellar cortices were totally disorganized, lacked horizontal lamination, and contained haphazard islands of cortical neurons separated by pial gliovascular strands. Likewise, the cerebellar vermis, the pons, and the pyramids were hypoplastic. White matter was less affected. Spinal cord was thin, but spinal roots were spared.

Walker-Warburg Syndrome

The Walker-Warburg syndrome is an autosomal-recessive disorder with more severe findings than either Fukuyama dystrophy or muscle-eye-brain disease (154). The Walker-Warburg syndrome is associated with homozygous mutations in the gene encoding O-mannosyltransferase 1

(POMT1), which like POMGnT1 (the mutant protein in muscle-eye-brain disease) participates in O-mannosyl glycan synthesis (146). Although the neuropathologic features of Walker-Warburg syndrome are the same as those of muscle-eye-brain disease, they are more extensive and include the macroscopic features of arrhinencephaly: cephalocele, hemispheric fusion, agenesis of the corpus callosum, or a combination of these manifestations (155).

The ocular malformations in Walker-Warburg syndrome are also more severe than in muscle-eye-brain disease. Typical ocular features include retinal dysplasia and nonattachment, persistent hyperplastic primary vitreous, optic nerve atrophy, microphthalmia, corneal opacities, congenital cataract, and congenital glaucoma (156).

The skeletal muscle biopsy changes in Walker-Warburg syndrome are similar to those of muscle-eye-brain disease and less severe than those in Fukuyama dystrophy. Levels of serum CK are elevated in this disorder as it is in the other two.

Nosologic Relations of Congenital Muscular Dystrophies

The genetics and immunohistochemistry of the simple congenital dystrophies of skeletal muscle that resemble dystrophinopathies are still being defined. Laminin and α-sarcoglycan deficiency may be common to several diseases because of the interdependent linkages of all the cytoskeletal proteins of the sarcolemma (157,115). Few congenital dystrophic disorders of merosin-, laminin-, sarcoglycan-, and dystrophin-associated proteins affect the eye or extraocular muscles. It is the dramatic white matter signal change on MR imaging that links merosin-deficient CMD to the three congenital dystrophies with ocular and brain malformations.

MYOTONIC MUSCULAR DYSTROPHIES

Myotonic dystrophy (dystrophia myotonica 1 [DM1]) and the less severe proximal myotonic myopathy (PROMM [DM2]) are autosomal-dominant disorders associated with nucleotide repeat expansions in untranslated regions of the respective target genes. The genetic defect in DM1 is amplification of an unstable trinucleotide CTG repeat located in the 3′ untranslated region of the gene that encodes dystrophia myotonica protein kinase (DMPK) on chromosome 19 (158,159). DM1 is highly variable in severity and age of onset, and it exhibits "anticipation," the phenomenon of increasing severity of inherited disease in successive generations of an affected family. The number of CTG repeats ranges from about 50 in patients who are mildly affected to thousands in severely affected patients (160–162). Amplification of the CTG repeat is the molecular basis for genetic anticipation. Although the mutation does not alter the protein-coding region of the DMPK gene, the CTG repeats can disrupt RNA splicing and cellular metabolism by interacting with RNA-binding proteins (163).

PROMM/DM2 is caused by a CCTG expansion (approximately 5,000 repeats) in intron 1 of the gene encoding zinc finger protein 9 (ZNF9) (163). Like the CTG expansion of the DMPK gene in DM1, the CCTG expansion does not alter the protein-coding region of the ZNF9 gene. However, the CCTG repeats can also disrupt RNA splicing and cellular metabolism by interacting with RNA-binding proteins (163).

Myotonic Dystrophy (DM1)

Myotonic dystrophy (DM1) is the most common inherited neuromuscular disease in adults, with a prevalence of approximately 5 per 100,000 (164,165). DM1 is a multisystem disorder characterized by progressive wasting and weakness of distal muscles and myotonia (166). Many patients are recognized instantly by their characteristic frontal balding, long face, ptosis, hollowing of the masseter and temporalis muscles, slackened mouth, facial weakness, and thin neck and limbs. Other features include intellectual impairment, testicular atrophy, excessive daytime somnolence, insulin resistance, and cardiac conduction defects. The most important finding on physical examination is myotonia—involuntary delayed relaxation following a contraction, such as after sustained handgrip. However, most patients with DM1 complain of weakness, not the myotonia. The phenomenon of myotonia in ion channelopathy is discussed later.

Men and women are equally at risk, with one exception. When DM1 presents at birth (i.e., congenital DM1), weakness is severe and mental retardation is the rule (167). Paternal inheritance of very large CTG repeats is genetically inhibited, accounting for maternal inheritance of the congenital form.

Clinical Manifestations

The clinical features of DM1 were described in the classic monograph by Harper (168) and subsequently by Harper and Rüdel (169) and by Moxley (166).

SYSTEMIC MANIFESTATIONS

Myotonia is distinctive diagnostically but is often inconstant. It is almost always present electromyographically after the age of 5 years, but it may vary clinically from inapparent to severe. Severity may vary during the day, usually being most severe early in the morning or during rest after exercise. It may be increased by excitement and by cold. It can often be brought out by asking the patient to shake hands. In affected persons, the handclasp is continued after an attempt is made to release the grasp. In some instances, it may be impossible to open the eyelids after they are forcibly closed. Tapping the muscles with a hammer or finger is often sufficient to induce a prolonged contraction. Repetition of a movement eventually abolishes the myotonia. From the patient's perspective, however, myotonia is eclipsed in importance by weakness.

Weakness and **wasting** of the muscles of the jaw and face cause the temples to appear sunken and the face to become narrowed, appear lengthened, and lose its expression (Fig. 22.12). The voice becomes monotonous and frequently has a nasal twang, either through atrophy or myotonia of the palatal muscles. It may be impossible for the patient to hold the head up for any length of time because of weakness of

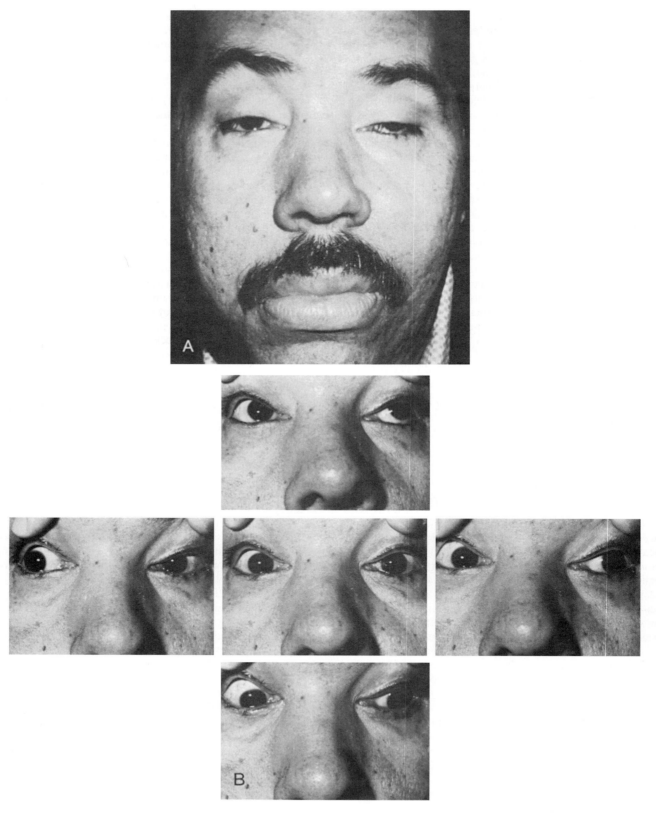

Figure 22.12.   Severe ptosis (*A*) and ophthalmoplegia (*B*) in a 49-year-old man with myotonic dystrophy (DM1). (Courtesy of Dr. Thomas L. Slamovits.)

the paraspinal muscles, and the sternocleidomastoid muscles and other neck flexors are often wasted until they become mere cords.

Muscle wasting is often most apparent distally in the forearms and hands, ankle dorsiflexors, and quadriceps, leading to the erroneous diagnosis of neuropathy. In congenital or early onset severe disease, weakness and hypotonia may be more proximal or universal (167).

Cardiac conduction defects occur in 90% of patients with DM1 and include first-degree heart, left anterior hemiblock, right bundle branch block, and complete heart block (170). These defects can cause syncope or sudden death (171). Mitral valve prolapse occurs with a higher prevalence than in the normal population, but it is seldom clinically significant and does not require antibiotic prophylaxis. Fatal cases of congestive failure were reported by Fisch and Evans (172) but are rare except for cor pulmonale.

Weakness of the respiratory muscles of the chest and diaphragm produces **hypoventilation**, especially nocturnally, leading to disordered sleep and daytime hypersomnolence. Central respiratory drive may also be decreased in patients with DM1. Aspiration and pneumonia frequently complicate the lives of affected patients and may cause death.

Prominent structural changes in the brain are infrequent in patients with DM1. Adie and Greenfield (173) did not find any pathologic changes in the CNS of affected patients, but Refsum et al. demonstrated enlargement of the third ventricle and basal cisterns that was most pronounced in patients with severe mental retardation (174). MR imaging reveals nonspecific abnormalities in a significant percentage of patients with DM1 (175,176). For example, Miaux et al. performed MR imaging on 13 patients with DM1 (177) and found some degree of cerebral atrophy in all of the patients with DM1 and high-signal areas on T2-weighted images in the subcortical white matter in 9 of the patients (70%).

Many but not all patients with DM1 have mild **mental retardation** (178), although it may require as many as three or four generations before mental retardation becomes evident in the pedigree of a family with this disorder. Bird et al. (179) tested cognitive and personality function in 29 patients with DM1; about one third of the patients had low scores on tests of cognitive function. The weakest cognitive functions were immediate recall, abstraction, and spatial manipulation and orientation; the strongest were verbal and informational. Of 25 patients for whom personality profiles were constructed, 56% had personality abnormalities, with serious personality defects being present most often in patients with low cognitive ability and advanced physical handicap. Patients with DM1 are often described as having an apathetic, indifferent, even paranoid style, and as having an odd sense of humor. There was no ''typical'' personality pattern representative of the entire group of patients evaluated by Bird et al. (179), however, leading these investigators to suggest that many of the personality abnormalities observed in patients with DM1 are secondary, the result of persons with limited resources attempting to cope with a physically deforming and debilitating disorder.

Patients with DM1 may have **frontal bossing**, hyperostosis interna, or diffuse thickening of the calvaria that, with cranial muscle wasting, contributes to the V-shaped or ''hatchet-faced'' appearance. Other common deformities include high-arched palate, prognathism or micrognathism, small sella turcica, scoliosis, kyphosis, and pectus excavatum (180).

Gastrointestinal symptoms occur in three of every four patients with DM1 and may be caused by striated or smooth muscle involvement. Evaluation of dysphagia by cine-esophagography can demonstrate aspiration from impaired cricopharyngeal coordination or relaxation, diminished esophageal motility, cardiospasm, or esophageal dilation (181,182). Other gastrointestinal symptoms include constipation, fecal incontinence, intermittent diarrhea, urinary retention, and epigastric pain (183). Uterine inertia produces prolonged labor, and there is a high rate of fetal loss (184). Impaired colonic motility is associated with fecal impaction and megacolon. Prolonged relaxation of the anal sphincters is caused by reflex-induced myotonia.

As DM1 progresses, diminished 17-ketosteroid levels and **infertility** occur in both men and women. This is associated with testicular atrophy in men (185) and fetal wastage in women. Gonadal insufficiency ranged from 100% of a series of 700 patients (186) to 80% of affected males (187). Androgen-responsive impotence occurs in some men. Insulin resistance is common, but overt diabetes mellitus is not.

OCULAR MANIFESTATIONS

The ocular changes in DM1 were described in detail by Babel (188). **Ptosis** is frequently present and may be mild or profound (Fig. 22.12). In addition, there may be **weakness of the orbicularis oculi muscles**, producing infrequent blinking and difficulty closing the eyes. When the orbicularis is affected, there may be bilateral lower lid retraction (189) or delayed opening of the eyes after forceful closure. The combination of ptosis and orbicularis weakness, particularly when combined with ophthalmoparesis, may suggest a diagnosis of myasthenia gravis or chronic progressive external ophthalmoplegia (CPEO).

Abnormal eye movements are present in many patients with DM1 (180,190–192). In its mildest form, the ocular motor involvement consists of slowed saccades in patients who have a full range of eye movements and no visual complaints (193,194). In other patients, however, there are varying degrees of ophthalmoparesis (195,196) (Fig. 22.12). Although some investigators suggest a neurogenic basis for this progressive external ophthalmoplegia, pathologic examination of extraocular muscles from affected patients suggests that the ophthalmoplegia is caused by primary muscle involvement similar to that found in other voluntary muscles in the body (see below).

Cataract is the most common ocular abnormality in patients with DM1, occurring in nearly 100% of patients with the disease. The severity of the cataract is not related to the severity of the disease (197). Even if lens changes are not visible by ophthalmoscope, slit-lamp biomicroscopy will usually reveal some lens opacification, although Dr. Frank Walsh observed a patient with severe DM1 who had clear lenses (198).

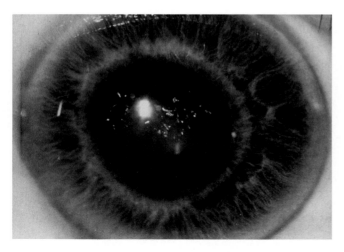

Figure 22.13. Cataract in a patient with myotonic dystrophy (DM1) consists of numerous dot opacities, each having a different color. The opacities were located primarily in the posterior subcortical region of the lens.

Myotonic cataracts have two major features. The first was described as "iridescent dust" by Vogt (199) and as "fine points mixed with colored crystals" by Burian and Burns (191). These abnormal areas are located in a thin band of anterior and posterior cortex just beneath the lens capsule (Fig. 22.13). The crystals may be opaque and white, but they are more often red, green, or blue. They are often globular, but they may be quite irregular. The second characteristic feature of myotonic cataracts is a stellate grouping of opacities at the posterior pole along the posterior suture lines (200) (Fig. 22.14). The stellate configuration was considered

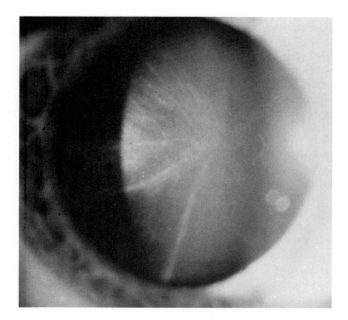

Figure 22.14. Cataract in a patient with myotonic dystrophy (DM1) consists of spoke-like opacities of the posterior subcortical region of the lens.

by Vos to be a later stage than that of the colored crystals (197).

Nonspecific corneal changes occur in some patients with DM1. Birnbacher (201) described a patient with DM1 for about 15 years in whom there was reduced vision in both eyes from corneal epithelial dystrophy. Maillard reported similar findings in a patient in whom the dystrophy worsened after cataract extraction (202).

Verbiest first described sluggish pupillary responses in a patient who also had slow and limited eye movements (203). Thompson et al. reviewed the literature on pupillary abnormalities in patients with DM1 and concluded that the pupils in such patients (*a*) tend to be miotic, (*b*) react sluggishly and incompletely to both light and near stimuli, (*c*) react normally to psychosensory stimuli, and (*d*) do not tend to fatigue on repeated stimuli any more than normal pupils (204). Although changes in pupillary reaction may be detected with pupillographic techniques (see Chapter 15), most patients with DM1 appear clinically to have normally reactive pupils.

Vascular abnormalities of the iris occur in many patients with DM1 (205,206,207). These iris neovascular tufts can usually be identified by slit-lamp biomicroscopy. They show leakage of dye after intravenous injection of fluorescein. In most cases, they are of no consequence, but they can bleed spontaneously or after mild ocular trauma, resulting in a hyphema. The iris neovascular tufts observed in patients with DM1 may be related to the insulin insensitivity and possible defective hormone-receptor interactions that may be present in patients with DM1 (207,208), even though such patients do not have other evidence of diabetic vasculopathy.

The ciliary processes may be short and depigmented in patients with DM1 (209). These abnormalities may explain the finding of ocular hypotony in many patients with this disorder.

Retinal abnormalities occur in patients with DM1. The involvement ranges from abnormalities of dark adaptation and electroretinography in patients with no visual complaints and normal-appearing fundi to decreased vision with pigmentary retinopathy involving the macula, peripheral retina, or both (188,191,209–212) (Fig. 22.15). Regardless of the degree of retinopathy, it is not as severe as retinitis pigmentosa and does not cause blindness. In fact, several investigators (188,213) expressed the opinion that the retinopathies observed in patients with DM1 as well as in patients with mitochondrial disorders (e.g., the Kearns-Sayre syndrome; see below) are similar in appearance, electrophysiologic dysfunction, and visual prognosis. DM1 patients with retinopathy may have altered retinal pigment epithelial and retinal membrane function that results in degenerative or "senescent" retinal and choroidal changes (214,215); however, Stanescu-Segal believed that the electroretinographic pattern is not that of a simple retinal degeneration and that the retinopathy is related to more complicated metabolic abnormalities (213).

Abnormal visual evoked potentials may be found in patients with DM1 who have no visible retinal abnormalities and a normal electroretinogram (ERG). Gott et al. (216) recorded pattern-reversal visual evoked potentials in 17 pa-

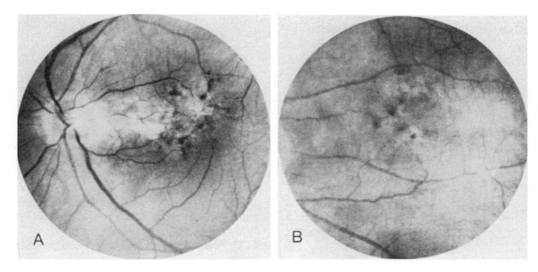

Figure 22.15. Chorioretinopathy in myotonic dystrophy (DM1). *A,* Posterior pole of the left eye in a 50-year-old man. Note the streak-like arrangement of the pigment clumps radiating from the fovea as well as the white streak extending between the disc and the macula. *B,* Posterior pole of the left eye in a 36-year-old woman. Note pigment clumps and surrounding white streaks in the macula. (From Burian HM, Burns CA. Ocular changes in myotonic dystrophy. Am J Ophthalmol 1967;63:22–24.)

tients with DM1 and found abnormalities of latency or amplitude in 10 (59%), all of whom had visual acuity of 20/30 or better without any evidence of retinal abnormality. Although such patients may have had subclinical retinal dysfunction altering the ERG and thus affecting the visual evoked potentials, Kirkham and Coupland found similar abnormalities in 10 members of a family, all of whom had normal ERGs (217). The results of these studies suggest that at least some patients with DM1 have dysfunction in the visual sensory conducting system other than at the retinal level.

Brand (218) was one of the first investigators to report ocular hypotony in patients with DM1. Similar findings were described by Van Dyk and Swan (219) and by Burian and Burns (191). Raitta and Karli studied 33 patients with DM1 and found pressures of 10 mm Hg or less in 19 of 66 eyes (212).

Muscle Pathology

Nearly every pathologic change possible in skeletal muscle occurs in DM1. In the earliest stages of the disease, a muscle biopsy may appear completely normal or may show only a slight excess of central nuclei. As the disease progresses, nuclei appear increased in number, located centrally, and arranged in long rows. These changes, although prominent (Fig. 22.16), are not pathognomonic; they indicate only chronicity. What is characteristic is the abundance and variety of other pathologic abnormalities, including variation in the caliber of the fibers, myofiber degeneration and regeneration, ringed fibers ("ringbinden") or myofibrils with an aberrant course, sarcoplasmic masses of tightly packed disordered myofilaments, focal areas of myofibrillar disruption and Z-band streaming, and associated secondary changes in mitochondria or the sarcotubular system. In the advanced

stages of the disease, a large proportion of the total fiber population is lost and is replaced by connective tissue and fat cells. This pathologic end stage is indistinguishable from the advanced stage of other muscular dystrophies, except that the residual fibers may continue to show prominent "nuclear rowing" described above. The nonspecificity of muscle pathology is less an issue now with highly specific and sensitive molecular genetic testing.

Ocular Pathology

The extraocular muscles may undergo changes similar to those described above (220–223). Kuwabara and Lessell examined specimens from two patients and observed multifocal loss of myofilaments, myofibrillar fragments of short size and irregular orientation, focal increases in mitochondria, sarcoplasmic reticular changes, and convoluted T tubules (223). They also noted nonspecific changes, including an increase in lipofuscin granules and the presence of lipid droplets. The final stage of disease was characterized by extraocular muscle atrophy. Similar changes were reported by Ginsberg et al. (221), who also noted proliferation of mitochondria in the extraocular muscles.

Eshaghian et al. (224) studied four lenses from patients with DM1 by transmission electron microscopy. These investigators found that the iridescent "crystals" seen in myotonic cataract are not crystals at all but represent whorls of lens fiber plasma membrane.

Pathologic changes in the iris and ciliary body in patients with DM1 are nonspecific and consist of hyalinization, vacuole degeneration, and interstitial proliferation (221,225). Whether these changes are responsible for the pupillary abnormalities observed in patients with DM1 is unclear.

The retinal lesions observed in patients with DM1 are

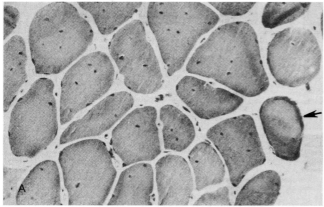

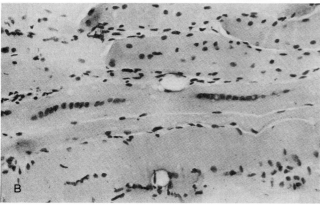

Figure 22.16. Histopathology of skeletal muscle fibers in myotonic dystrophy (DM1). *A*, Cross-section of involved muscle shows variation in both diameter and shape of fibers. Sarcolemmal nuclei are increased in number, and many have a central location. The *arrow* shows "ringbinden"; ×340. *B*, One fiber in longitudinal section contains rows of central sarcolemmal nuclei; ×340. (From Aström KE, Adams RD. Myotonic disorders. In: Mastaglia FL, Walton JN, eds. Skeletal Muscle Pathology. Edinburgh: Churchill Livingstone, 1982:266.)

many and varied. Atrophy of the inner retinal layers with preservation of photoreceptors occurs (215), particularly in the peripheral retina. In the macula, increased pigmentation with a granular (214), striate (211,214), or stellate (222) pattern may occur. Foci of pigmented cells in the outer plexiform layer (211) and macular edema over subretinal fluid (226) are also observed. The macular changes reported by Ginsberg et al. (221) consisted of an organizing serous retinopathy with early pigment epithelial atrophy consistent with idiopathic involutional degeneration. Nonspecific changes similar to those of age-related macular degeneration can also occur in young patients with DM1 (227,215).

Diagnosis and Treatment

The patient's presentation for cataract extraction may be the family's initial presentation, and it is therefore incumbent on the neuro-ophthalmologist to recognize the syndrome. The diagnosis is supported by findings of myotonia on EMG and multihued speckled cataracts on slit-lamp examination.

Testing of DNA for the CTG repeat can be performed when the diagnosis is not clinically obvious, thus eliminating the need for a muscle biopsy (228).

When troublesome, myotonia can be treated with phenytoin or other drugs, but few patients request this therapy. Distal weakness causing footdrop is treated with ankle-foot orthoses. Cardiac conduction defects may require pacemakers.

Treatment of ophthalmoparesis is usually unnecessary because the limitation of eye movement in patients with DM1 is usually symmetric. Thus, such patients do not commonly report diplopia. Prisms can be used to treat patients with diplopia in primary position. Surgery is unwarranted.

Treatment of ptosis is somewhat problematic in patients with DM1 because of the commonly associated orbicularis weakness. If the eyelids are raised to a "normal" level, such patients may develop severe tearing and irritation from exposure keratopathy, and some patients may even develop corneal ulceration, leading to blindness. Thus, the eyelids should be raised only when ptosis is interfering with function and only as high as needed to improve vision.

Proximal Myotonic Myopathy (PROMM/DM2)

Proximal myotonic myopathy (PROMM/DM2) has certain features in common with DM1 but has a different clinical presentation. The clinical features of PROMM/DM2 are muscle stiffness, myotonia, weakness, muscle pain, and cataracts. These problems can occur singly or in various combinations. Initial symptoms usually develop between 20 and 60 years of age. Many patients first complain of intermittent stiffness in the thigh muscles of one or both legs and of intermittent grip myotonia. In other patients, cataracts are the first manifestation of the disorder. These may appear in late childhood or early adolescence and are indistinguishable from those in DM1, being posterior subcapsular, iridescent, multicolored opacities. Cardiac arrhythmias occur in some patients.

EMG usually reveals myotonic discharges in affected patients, including those without obvious clinical myotonia. However, these discharges are scarce and difficult to detect (166). Muscle biopsy usually reveals a nonspecific myopathy. In contrast to DM1, there are no ringbinden or subsarcolemmal masses, and there is no evidence of selective type 1 fiber atrophy.

The prognosis of PROMM/DM2 is more favorable than that of DM1. Most patients do not show any deterioration of mental status, dysarthria, dysphagia, or respiratory failure. Nonsteroidal anti-inflammatory drugs and muscle relaxants can be used to treat the muscle pain experienced by these patients, and antimyotonia therapy, including mexiletine, phenytoin, and acetazolamide, can be used in patients with severe myotonic stiffness and grip myotonia. Cataract surgery is warranted in some patients.

OCULOPHARYNGEAL MUSCULAR DYSTROPHY

In 1915, Taylor described a hereditary condition characterized by "progressive vagus-glossopharyngeal paralysis with ptosis," stating that the disorder progressed slowly and eventually caused death by starvation (130). Subsequently, Victor et al. called the syndrome "oculopharyngeal muscular dystrophy" (OPMD) (131). Many affected families are of French-Canadian heritage (130,229). OPMD is generally inherited as an autosomal-dominant trait, but rare autosomal-recessive cases have been reported (see below).

The two essential clinical characteristics of OPMD are ptosis and dysphagia (230) (Fig. 22.17). Although neither symptom usually presents until late in life (231), mild ptosis usually precedes any significant dysphagia, often by several years. The best way to assess the onset and familial occurrence is by examining old family photographs for ptosis. The ptosis in patients with OPMD is eventually always bilateral, rarely complete, and usually symmetric, although one eyelid may become ptotic weeks or months before the other. External ophthalmoplegia is present in most patients; however, in the series reported by Johnson and Kuwabara, only three patients had limitation of ocular motility (232). By comparison, limb muscle weakness is mild and proximal, if present at all. This is not a rare condition: patients with OPMD represented 33% of patients with acquired ptosis in the series reported by Johnson and Kuwabara (232).

Dysphagia may be disabling. At first there is difficulty only in swallowing solid foods, but eventually swallowing liquids also becomes difficult, and several attempts at swallowing may be necessary to empty the upper pharynx. Examination of the swallowing mechanisms in affected patients usually reveals weak movements in the pharynx and larynx. The pharyngeal musculature cannot propel the bolus of food into the upper esophagus, partly because of dysfunction of the pharyngeal musculature and partly because of the absence of reflex relaxation of the cricopharyngeal muscle. Degeneration of the pharyngeal striated musculature evidently results in uncoordinated activity, with material pooling in the pyriform sinuses and regurgitating into the nasopharynx rather than passing into the esophagus. Ingested material may thus be aspirated, resulting in recurrent pneumonitis. Some patients with severe dysphagia are treated successfully with cricopharyngeal myotomy (233), but a percutaneous feeding gastrostomy is a more practical treatment and is more commonly used.

The mutation in OPMD, which is located on chromosome 14q11, increases the length of a polyalanine sequence located at the N terminus of the polyadenylate binding protein nuclear 1 (PABPN1) (formerly called polyadenylate binding protein 2, PABP2) (234,235). This polyalanine sequence is

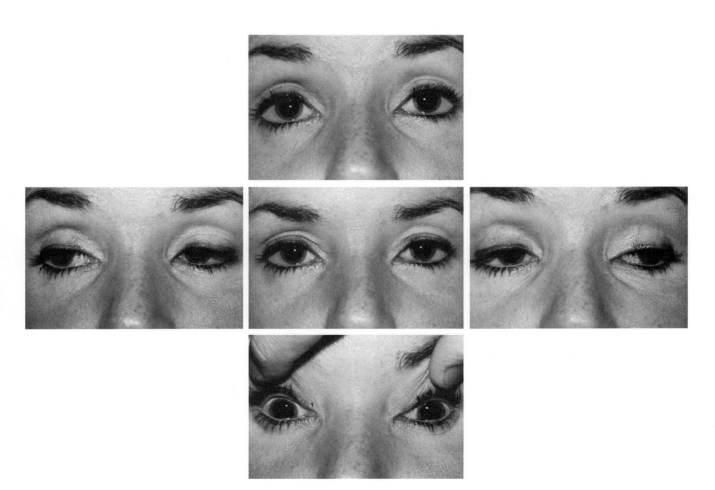

Figure 22.17. Ptosis and ophthalmoplegia in a patient with oculopharyngeal dystrophy (OPMD).

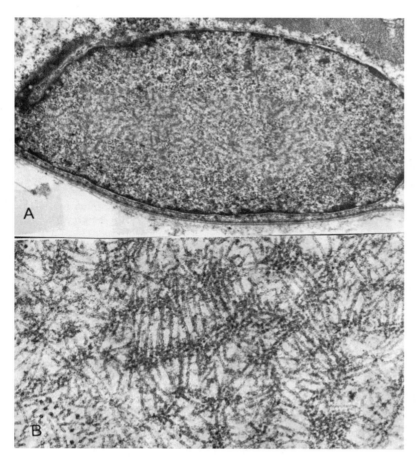

Figure 22.18. Nuclear inclusions in skeletal muscle of patients with oculopharyngeal dystrophy (OPMD). *A*, Transverse electron microscope section of a muscle fiber shows a subsarcolemmal nucleus that contains abundant filamentary inclusions arranged in palisades; ×13,000. *B*, At higher magnification, the intranuclear inclusions can be seen to consist of tubular filaments that do not have any specific orientation. (From Tomé FMS, Fardeau M. Nuclear inclusions in oculopharyngeal dystrophy. Acta Neuropathol 1980; 49:85–87.)

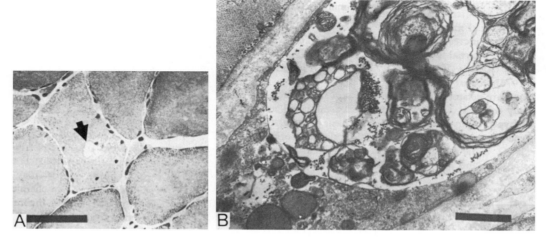

Figure 22.19. Vacuoles within an affected muscle in a patient with oculopharyngeal dystrophy (OPMD). The rimmed vacuole (*arrow*) in *A* corresponds to an autophagic vacuole within a muscle fiber (*B*). *A*, Gomori trichrome stain; bar = 50 μm. *B*, Electron micrograph; bar = 1 μm. (From Schmalbruch H. The muscular dystrophies. In: Mastaglia FL, Walton J, eds. Skeletal Muscle Pathology. Edinburgh: Churchill Livingstone, 1982:235.)

normally encoded by a (GCG)6 repeat that expands to (GCG)8–13 in affected families. The most severely affected patients are heterozygotic for (GCG)9 and a (GCG)7 allele that also occurs in unaffected individuals. However, homozygosity for the (GCG)7 allele results in autosomal-recessive disease (235).

PABPN1 mutations are associated with the morphologic hallmark of OPMD, intranuclear filamentous inclusions comprising PABPN1, sequestered polyadenylated RNA, and ubiquitin (236) (Fig. 22.18) (237). These intranuclear inclusions are confined to muscle cells, where PABPN1 plays a specific role in differentiation (237,238). The association of several neurodegenerative disorders with the intracellular aggregation of mutant proteins (e.g., tau in the case of Alzheimer's disease) (239) suggests that the reduced solubility of mutant PABPN1 and its tendency to form intranuclear aggregates play a direct role in the pathogenesis of OPMD (237).

Rimmed autophagic vacuoles are generally seen in OPMD (240) (Fig. 22.19). Unlike the filaments associated with intranuclear inclusions, which are 8.5 nm in diameter and can be detected only using electron microscopy (Fig. 22.18), the vacuoles are readily detectable using light microscopy (Fig. 22.19). Although Dubowitz and Brooke considered the vacuoles to be a prerequisite for the diagnosis of OPMD (241),

only intranuclear inclusions were present in all cases of OPMD reviewed by Tome et al. (238).

As in other dystrophies, biopsies from affected muscles show advanced degenerative changes, fibrosis, abundant central nuclei, altered myofibrils and Z-bands, and other nonspecific changes. "Ragged red" fibers with mitochondrial proliferation and other mitochondrial abnormalities are sometimes found, but these are probably the result of age-related mitochondrial DNA mutations (see below), phenomena unrelated to the pathogenesis of OPMD.

Satoyoshi and Kinoshita described a single family in which two generations were affected by an autosomal-dominantly inherited myopathy characterized by slowly progressive ptosis; external ophthalmoplegia; weakness of the masseter, facial, and bulbar muscles; and distal (rather than proximal) involvement of the limbs (242). The condition began around 40 years of age or later. Muscle biopsies from all affected family members showed myopathic changes, and in one case autopsy disclosed no pathologic changes in the peripheral or central nervous systems. Satoyoshi and Kinoshita used the term "oculopharyngodistal myopathy" to separate this condition from typical oculopharyngeal muscular dystrophy (242). This syndrome may be identical to that described by Schotland and Rowland (243).

ION CHANNEL DISORDERS

MYOTONIA

Myotonia is a phenomenon in which muscle fibers have a pathologically persistent activity after a strong contraction or are continuously active when they should be relaxed. Myotonia is identified physiologically as a delay in muscle relaxation after percussion or electric stimulation of a muscle, or after a voluntary contraction. The phenomenon is caused by mutations affecting chloride, sodium, and calcium ion channels in surface membranes (see below). It persists after blockage of either the peripheral nerve or the neuromuscular junction. In patients with myotonia, the spontaneous action potentials as recorded in the EMG are high-frequency discharges of single muscle fibers that wax and wane in both amplitude and frequency. When translated into sound, these discharges produce a noise resembling that of a dive-bomber or a motorcycle engine.

Clinical myotonia is a common feature of a number of different genetically determined, primary muscle diseases, including autosomal-dominant myotonia congenita (244), autosomal-recessive myotonia (245,246), paramyotonia congenital (247), the familial periodic paralyses (248,249), myotonic muscular dystrophy (127,250) (see above), and chondrodystrophic myotonia (251,252).

Myotonia Congenita

Autosomal-dominant (244) and autosomal-recessive myotonia congenita (245,246) result from allelic mutations of the chloride channel gene encoded on chromosome 7q35 (253,254,166). Myotonic symptoms, noted in the first years

of life and often worse in males than females, frequently lessen by the 20s or 30s. Myotonia of limb muscles is more likely to occur when strenuous exertion is initiated after a period of rest; myotonia is then followed by transient weakness. Unlike paramyotonia, the myotonia is not aggravated by cooling, and long-lasting paralysis does not occur (255). This is one of a few neuromuscular disorders in which prominent hypertrophy can occur, particularly in the masseter, proximal arms, thighs, calves, and extensor digitorum brevis.

Patients with myotonia congenita often have eyelid myotonia. At the very least, lid lag is usually present, and frank blepharospasm may occur in some patients after forced closure of the eyelids. Strabismus is said to occur in some patients, but not ptosis or generalized ophthalmoplegia. Swallowing and voice are spared, but chewing is sometimes affected.

Needle EMG shows typical myotonic runs. Muscle biopsy is nonspecific. Specific genetic diagnosis is possible.

The pathophysiology of the myotonia is thought to be caused by both low chloride channel conductance and abnormal reopening of sodium channels. Treatment, which is most often successful with mexiletine or quinine, and less so with procainamide or phenytoin, is best undertaken several days before vigorous activity rather than on a regular basis (255).

Paramyotonia Congenita

In 1886, Eulenburg described paramyotonia congenita, a condition characterized by autosomal-dominant inheritance, paradoxic myotonia (i.e., myotonia that worsens with exercise), exacerbation of myotonia by cold, and periodic attacks of weakness (247). The disorder is caused by mutations in the sodium channel gene and is allelic to hyperkalemic periodic paralysis, accounting for the great overlap between the two syndromes (256,257). Neither ptosis nor ophthalmoplegia occurs in patients with this disease; however, some patients show myotonic lid lag similar to that observed in other myotonic disorders, including myotonia congenita (258). Paramyotonia may be induced by placing ice cubes over the eyelids. Specific genetic diagnosis is available. Paramyotonia often responds to mexiletine and acetazolamide, but not usually to drugs like quinine or phenytoin, which are used to treat other myotonias.

Periodic Paralysis

Familial Periodic Paralysis

Familial periodic paralysis is a rare syndrome characterized by abnormal flux of potassium across muscle membranes and by spells of severe flaccid weakness in the limb muscles. The spells last minutes to hours and are provoked by rest following exercise. Bulbar and ocular muscles are rarely affected; thus, patients with this disorder do not often present to the ophthalmologist (but see below). Respiratory muscles are almost never affected. The syndrome is subdivided into hyper-, hypo-, and normokalemic types, but all three types share onset by the third decade of life, greater severity in males, autosomal-dominant inheritance, and oliguria preceding attacks. In rare patients, hypo- or hyperkalemia causes a complicating cardiac arrhythmia. Examination shows normal strength between attacks, but if the attacks are frequent and not treated, mild fixed proximal weakness may develop. Myotonia, especially eyelid myotonia, may be seen. During paralytic attacks, muscles are inexcitable and deep tendon reflexes are hypoactive or absent. The histologic hallmark is a vacuolar myopathy most consistently associated with the permanent myopathy that develops after repeated attacks (259). The vacuoles are typically large, central, loculated, and limited by a delicate membrane. They are derived from dilated proteins of sarcoplasmic reticulum and transverse tubules (259,260).

Hypokalemic periodic paralysis is caused by mutations in the dihydropyridine receptor calcium channel encoded at chromosome 1q31–q32 (261,262), but the pathophysiologic mechanism by which these mutations alter potassium flux across muscle membrane is incompletely known. The age of onset is from about 5 years to the 30s (263). Attack frequency is highly variable, but attacks are often more severe and longer-lasting (up to 24 hours) than the spells in hyperkalemic periodic paralysis. Attacks can be precipitated by carbohydrate loading and rest before exercise (e.g., the classic Sunday-morning athlete after a night of pizza and beer). Weakness of extraocular muscles or ptosis rarely occurs, but eyelid myotonia is common, causing lid lag (260,264) (Fig. 22.20). The myotonia in hypokalemic periodic paralysis is confined to lid muscles. Thus, EMG evidence of myotonia in limb muscles makes other forms of periodic paralysis more likely (264).

The diagnosis of hypokalemic periodic paralysis is made by serial electrolyte determinations, electrocardiogram

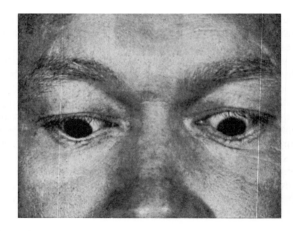

Figure 22.20. Lid lag in hypokalemic familial periodic paralysis. The upper lids floated down about 20 seconds after the photograph was taken. (From Resnick JS, Engel WK. Myotonic lid lag in hypokalemic periodic paralysis. J Neurol Neurosurg Psychiatry 1967;30:47–51.)

(ECG), exclusion of thyrotoxicosis (an important acquired cause of hypokalemic periodic paralysis in young Hispanic and Asian men), EMG, the McManis exercise test (265), and insulin/glucose provocative testing if necessary (104).

Acute treatment is with oral intake of potassium chloride

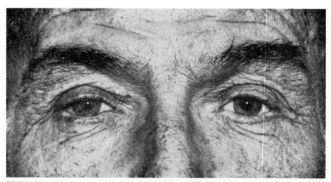
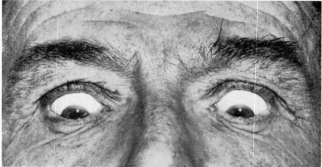

Figure 22.21. Lid retraction and lag in hyperkalemic familial periodic paralysis. *Top,* The eyelids are in normal position when the patient is looking straight ahead. *Bottom,* When the patient looks down, there are marked lid retraction and lid lag that disappear within 1 minute. (From McArdle B. Adynamia episodica hereditaria and its treatment. Brain 1962; 85:121–148.)

and gentle exercise. Acetazolamide can help prevent further attacks. Thyrotoxic periodic paralysis requires specific anti-thyroid therapy.

Hyperkalemic periodic paralysis is caused by mutations in the sodium channel α-subunit gene at 17q13.1–q13.3, causing defective sodium channel inactivation (266,267). Attacks of paralysis usually present before 10 years of age and are often milder and shorter than those in patients with hypokalemic periodic paralysis. They occur after fasting or during rest following exercise. Cranial muscles are affected in about half the cases. Myotonia may be prominent by both examination and EMG studies. Muscle hypertrophy may be present. Sensory symptoms occur, but without sensory signs.

Eyelid abnormalities may be significant in patients with hyperkalemic periodic paralysis. McArdle observed transient attacks of "staring" in affected young children (268). In adults, the sclera above the cornea is visible when the patient looks down after looking upward (Fig. 22.21). Lid lag is commonly present during attacks but may disappear after repeated up-and-down movements of the eyes (268). It may be brought on by placing an ice cube against the eyelids for several minutes.

Diagnosis is made by serial electrolyte determinations, ECG, EMG studies, and exercise testing (265). Provocative testing with potassium loading is rarely indicated (104). Specific molecular diagnosis is possible.

Acute attacks are not often severe enough to require treatment other than ingestion of simple carbohydrates. Prophylaxis against further attacks, to forestall any permanent weakness, requires thiazide diuretics.

Normokalemic periodic paralysis is rare. Its nosologic distinction from hyperkalemic periodic paralysis is unclear because serum potassium levels may be normal in some patients with hyperkalemic periodic paralysis, normokalemic patients may have potassium-sensitive periodic paralysis, and at least one family with normokalemic periodic paralysis displayed the common sodium channel mutation associated with hyperkalemic periodic paralysis.

Schwartz-Jampel Syndrome (Chondrodystrophic Myotonia)

Schwartz and Jampel first described a rare syndrome of dwarfism, abnormalities of long bones and the face, blepharospasm, and myotonic symptoms (251). The facial appearance of blepharospasm, puckered lips, myokymic twitching of the chin, low-set ears, receding chin, a high-pitched forced voice, and high-arched palate is distinctive. Frequent ophthalmologic features include myopia, cataract, strabismus, and nystagmus (255). Serum CK levels are usually normal. Although muscle biopsies show many changes, none are specific. Most early case series suggested that the typical EMG discharges are true myotonic potentials generated in muscle. However, Fowler et al. demonstrated that this condition is not a true myotonia, because EMG discharges from affected muscles are abolished by d-tubocurarine (269). The mutant gene, which is located on chromosome 1p34–36.1 (270), encodes perlecan, a heparan sulfate proteoglycan component of the basement membrane that is responsible for the localization of acetylcholinesterase in the postsynaptic clefts of the neuromuscular junction (271,272,273). Thus, the abnormal activity of affected muscles appears to reflect prolonged activation of postsynaptic receptors resulting from the impaired degradation of acetylcholine at the neuromuscular junction (272).

MITOCHONDRIAL MYOPATHIES (MITOCHONDRIAL ENCEPHALOMYOPATHIES)

BACKGROUND

The mitochondrial encephalomyopathies are a genetically and biochemically diverse set of disorders that are defined by structural abnormalities of mitochondria on muscle biopsy (274–276). The histologic hallmark of these disorders is the abnormal accumulation of increased numbers of enlarged mitochondria beneath the sarcolemma of affected muscle fibers. Because of their irregular appearance and their strikingly dark-red color when stained with the modified Gomori trichrome stain (277), these abnormal muscle fibers are called **ragged-red fibers** (RRF) (278) (Fig. 22.22). In patients with ophthalmoplegia, RRFs are usually present in skeletal muscles (275,276,279–283). They are also found in the orbicularis oculi muscle (284) and in the extraocular muscles (285) of affected patients (Fig. 22.23). Affected muscle fibers are irregularly distributed and often arranged in small groups.

When viewed with the electron microscope, the mitochondria in affected muscle fibers appear more numerous and more variable in size than in normal muscle fibers. The mitochondria are often enlarged, with distorted or disorganized cristae that are sometimes arranged concentrically. Paracrystalline inclusions are invariably present within the cristae, and similar inclusions may also be observed outside the cristae (Fig. 22.24). Similar mitochondrial inclusions may be observed in liver cells (286), in sweat glands (280), and in the granular and Purkinje cells of the cerebellum (287) of affected patients.

In most cases, RRFs reflect the presence of mutations in mitochondrial DNA (mtDNA) that are capable of reducing the synthesis and abundance of respiratory chain proteins encoded by the mitochondrial genome. Before considering the nature of these mutations and the mechanisms by which they may impair mitochondrial protein synthesis, we will describe the clinical features of the two most common syndromes in which ophthalmoplegia is a prominent feature, chronic progressive external ophthalmoplegia (CPEO) and the Kearns-Sayre syndrome (KSS).

MITOCHONDRIAL DISORDERS ASSOCIATED WITH EXTERNAL OPHTHALMOPLEGIA

Chronic Progressive External Ophthalmoplegia

CPEO is the most frequent manifestation of mitochondrial myopathies. Harding et al. reviewed the records of 60 patients with mitochondrial myopathy examined at the National Hospital, Queen Square, and found that 54 of the pa-

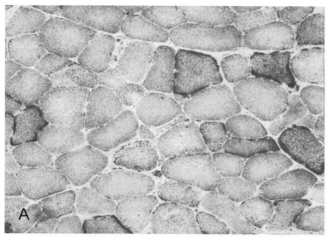

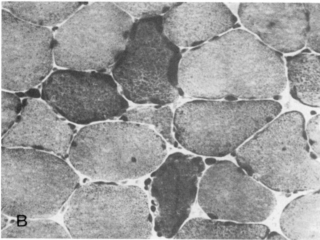

Figure 22.22. "Ragged red" fibers in chronic progressive external ophthalmoplegia. *A,* Succinate dehydrogenase reaction shows increased activity at the periphery of some muscle fibers in a patient with chronic progressive external ophthalmoplegia. Although mitochondrial protein synthesis is reduced in affected fibers, the activity of this enzyme is preserved since the protein subunits of complex II (succinate dehydrogenase-ubiquinone reductase) are encoded exclusively by the nuclear genome. *B,* A group of three "ragged red" fibers surround an atrophic, angulated muscle fiber. Modified Gomori trichrome stain. (From Morgan-Hughes JA. Mitochondrial myopathies. In: Mastaglia FL, Walton J, eds. Skeletal Muscle Pathology. Edinburgh: Churchill Livingstone, 1982:309.)

tients (90%) had ocular or oculomotor abnormalities and that CPEO was the presenting feature in about two thirds of the patients (288). CPEO may occur in association with a variety of myopathic and other disorders (e.g., Graves' disease, myasthenia gravis, and brain stem glioma) (289,290); this is simply a clinical sign and not a nosologic entity.

Generalized skeletal muscle weakness is present in most patients with CPEO (291). Among 52 patients with CPEO evaluated by Petty et al., weakness of other muscles was absent in only three patients, facial weakness alone was present in two patients, and weakness of the limbs was present in 47 patients (274). Nevertheless, because ptosis and ophthalmoplegia can occur in the absence of weakness in other muscles (292), these abnormalities are discussed separately.

In patients who are not born with obvious external ophthalmoplegia, **ptosis** is usually the first evidence of involvement and may precede ophthalmoparesis by months to years (293) (Fig. 22.25). The ptosis is slowly progressive and tends to become complete in most cases. Characteristically, it is bilateral, but unilateral ptosis can be present for years before the opposite side becomes involved or ophthalmoparesis is observed. In a patient described by Walsh and Hoyt, there was an interval of 8 years before involvement of the other eye (294). Petty et al. found that the ptosis was unilateral in 4 of 52 patients (8%) with mitochondrial myopathy (274). As the ptosis progresses, it eventually interferes with vision, and the patient must tilt the head backward and use the frontalis muscles to elevate the eyelids (Fig. 22.26). In patients with mitochondrial encephalomyopathies, the ptosis is fixed, unlike the variable, fatigable ptosis in myasthenia gravis.

Although most investigators describe ptosis as the earliest sign of CPEO, Bing and Haymaker suggested that in some patients it was the last sign to develop (295). Miller observed a patient with complete ophthalmoplegia who had no significant ptosis (295), and Walsh and Hoyt observed absence of ptosis with almost total external ophthalmoplegia in a brother and sister whose father had profound ptosis as well as an inability to move the eyes (294). Petty et al. reported that ptosis was absent in only 1 of 52 patients with ophthalmoplegia (274).

Because **limitation of ocular movements** is generally symmetric, most patients with CPEO do not report diplopia and are not aware of a problem with ocular motility until it is of such severity that it limits peripheral vision or until someone points it out to them. For this reason, immobility of the eyes is usually severe when such patients are first

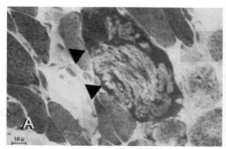

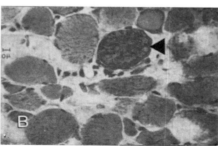

Figure 22.23. Histopathology of orbicularis oculi muscle in chronic progressive external ophthalmoplegia. "Ragged red" muscle fibers can be identified by a number of stains, including modified trichrome (*A*) and hematoxylin and eosin (*B*). The *arrows* identify the abnormal muscle fibers. (From Eshaghian J, Anderson RL, Weingeist TA, et al. Orbicularis oculi muscle in chronic progressive external ophthalmoplegia. Arch Ophthalmol 1980;98:1070–1073.)

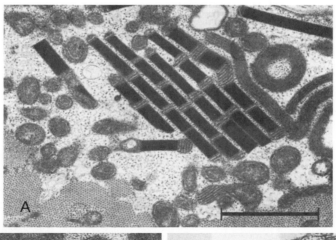

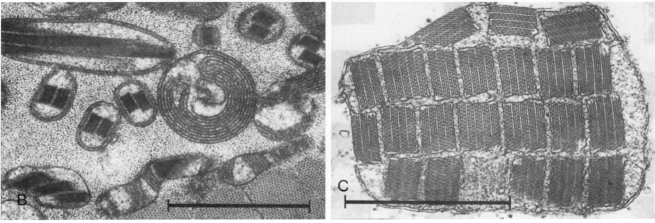

Figure 22.24. Mitochondrial inclusions in chronic progressive external ophthalmoplegia. *A*, Intramembrane crystals arranged in chains separated by transverse mitochondrial cristae. *B*, Mitochondria contain "parking lot" inclusions or multiple concentric cristae embedded in glycogen. Bars = 2 μm. *C*, An enlarged mitochondrion contains 22 intracrystal paracrystalline inclusions. Bar = 1 μm. (From Morgan-Hughes JA. Mitochondrial myopathies. In: Mastaglia FL, Walton J, eds. Skeletal Muscle Pathology. Edinburgh: Churchill Livingstone, 1982:309.)

examined (Fig. 22.25). In many cases, downward movements are relatively intact compared with upward and horizontal movements.

Blodi et al. first reported the ocular EMG findings in several patients with CPEO (296,297). These investigators found frequent co-contraction (co-innervation of agonist-antagonist muscles at the same time) of the extraocular muscles. Other investigators performed similar studies and found both normal and co-contraction firing patterns in patients with CPEO (298,299). The reason that such patients should show co-contraction firing patterns is unclear.

Both ultrasonography and CT scanning in patients with CPEO show thin, presumably atrophic, extraocular muscles (Fig. 22.27). The thinning is usually symmetric.

Most patients with CPEO have generalized, symmetric limitation of eye movement. Thus, they do not report diplopia. In the rare patients who have asymmetric limitation of movement and complain of double vision, prism therapy or surgery may be used to improve ocular alignment

(300–302), at least temporarily. Surgery to raise the eyelids can be performed in patients with severe ptosis that prevents them from functioning normally, but because such patients may also have weakness of the orbicularis oculi muscles, care must be taken to avoid raising the eyelids so much that the patient develops exposure keratopathy from inability to close the eyes (303,304).

Kearns-Sayre Syndrome

Kearns and Sayre reported two patients with CPEO, "retinitis pigmentosa," and complete heart block (305). Subsequently, many similar cases were described (306–310). KSS is defined by the combination of CPEO and pigmentary retinopathy before the age of 20 years, together with one or more of the following: complete heart block, cerebrospinal fluid (CSF) protein more than 1 mg/mL, cerebellar ataxia, short stature, deafness, dementia, and endocrine abnormalities (307,311). The occurrence of similar mutations of mtDNA in CPEO and KSS supports the view that these dis-

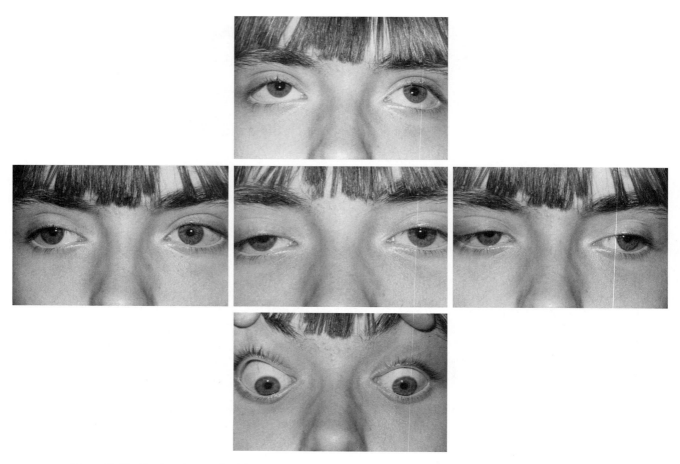

Figure 22.25.   Ptosis and external ophthalmoplegia in a patient with mitochondrial cytopathy. The patient had no evidence of retinopathy or cardiac disease.

orders are part of a continuous spectrum of the same disease (275,311).

In most instances, the retinopathy that occurs in patients with KSS is different from that seen in patients with the group of hereditary retinal disorders collectively known as retinitis pigmentosa. Kearns and Sayre originally called the retinopathy seen in their two patients ''atypical retinitis pigmentosa'' (305), but subsequent reports employed the term ''pigmentary retinopathy'' to emphasize the distinction. Although cases of CPEO associated with what appears to be typical retinitis pigmentosa probably occur (298), the pigmentary retinopathy of the Kearns-Sayre syndrome generally can be differentiated from retinitis pigmentosa by both clinical and electrophysiologic criteria.

The pattern of retinal involvement is particularly important. In contrast to retinitis pigmentosa, which usually affects the peripheral and midperipheral retina, at least initially (312,313), the retinopathy of KSS usually occurs initially in the posterior fundus (Fig. 22.28). Severe involvement of the peripapillary zone is typical. In this region, retinal epithelial atrophy frequently results in increased visibility of the choroidal vessels and the appearance of ''choroidal sclerosis'' (306,305), although rare cases occur in which a pattern of

choroideremia is present (314). In advanced cases, a metallic sheen or mottled fluorescent appearance surrounds the optic nerve. ''Bone spicule'' pigment formation, a common feature of retinitis pigmentosa, rarely occurs. Examination of affected fundi usually shows diffuse depigmentation of the retinal pigment epithelium with a characteristic mottled ''salt-and-pepper'' pattern of pigment clumping similar to that seen in patients with congenital rubella. This appearance may be most marked around the macula (315). Pallor of the optic disc, attenuation of retinal vessels, visual field defects, and posterior cataracts—all common in patients with retinitis pigmentosa—rarely if ever occur. As might be expected, visual symptoms such as night blindness or diminished visual acuity are generally mild and occur in only about 40–50% of patients (307,316). However, there are rare cases of KSS with CNS involvement in which bone spicule formation and pigment clumping in the macula are associated with profound loss of visual acuity (316).

The results of electrophysiologic tests performed on patients with KSS also differ from those in patients with retinitis pigmentosa (317). Although exceptional cases exist (318), dark adaptometry and electroretinography are usually normal or only mildly abnormal (281,298). In most cases in

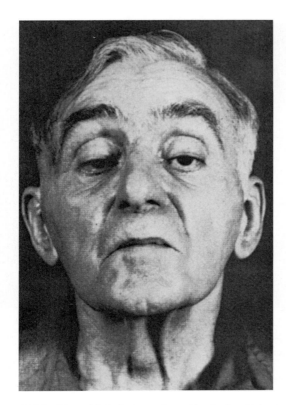

Figure 22.26. Myopathic facies in a patient with mitochondrial cytopathy and chronic progressive external ophthalmoplegia. Note flat, expressionless facial features associated with continuous wrinkling of the frontalis muscles and a posterior head tilt in order to compensate for bilateral ptosis. (Courtesy of Dr. I. Lewis and the Canadian Medical Association Journal.)

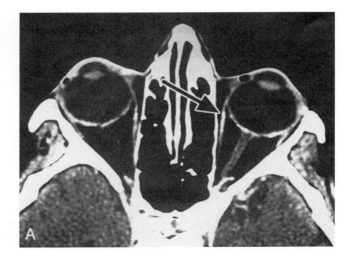

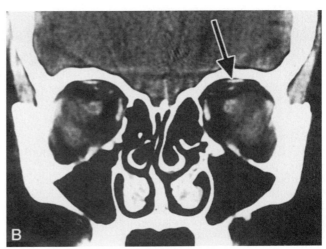

Figure 22.27. Computed tomographic scanning of extraocular muscles in a patient with chronic progressive external ophthalmoplegia. *A*, Axial view shows marked thinning of left medial rectus muscle (*arrow*). *B*, Coronal view shows similar thinning of left superior rectus muscle (*arrow*). (From Wallace DK, Sprunger DT, Helveston EM, et al. Surgical management of strabismus associated with chronic progressive external ophthalmoplegia. Ophthalmology 1997;104:695–700.)

which there are abnormal electrophysiologic studies, observable retinal abnormalities are present. In one patient followed for 8 years, however, a diminished b-wave amplitude preceded the widespread appearance of a retinal pigmentary disturbance (319). In addition, Drachman reported a case of CPEO with a subnormal ERG in the absence of observable retinopathy (320), and Trobe and Watson described a patient with CPEO, visual field defects, and normal-appearing retinas on both clinical and fluorescein angiographic examinations in whom ERG showed b-wave amplitudes that were one-tenth normal in each eye in both light- and dark-adapted states (321).

Histopathologic studies performed on the eyes of patients with KSS generally reveal distortion and atrophy of the photoreceptors accompanied by aberrant pigment in all layers of the sensory retina (305,306,322–324). In the study performed by Newell and Polascik, the retinal pigment epithelium contained focal areas of macrophages ingesting pigment (324). Although postmortem autolysis destroyed much of the internal structure of the mitochondria, transmission electron microscopy revealed enlarged mitochondria, many of which contained paracrystalline inclusions, in the choroid, retinal pigment epithelium, and all layers of the sensory retina. The largest number of abnormal mitochondria were in the inner segments of the retinal photoreceptors, in the outer

plexiform layer of the retina, and in the nonpigmented epithelium of the ciliary body.

In the two eyes studied histopathologically by Eagle et al., there was atrophy of the retinal pigment epithelium that was most marked posteriorly (322,323). The preservation of peripheral rods and cones appeared to mirror the health of the underlying peripheral retinal pigment epithelium. This pattern of photoreceptor degeneration led Eagle et al. (322,323) as well as other investigators (325) to postulate that the primary defect producing the retinopathy of KSS is in the retinal pigment epithelium.

Patients with KSS typically have cardiac conduction disturbances (305,306). The actual time of onset and the frequency of cardiac involvement in patients with KSS are vari-

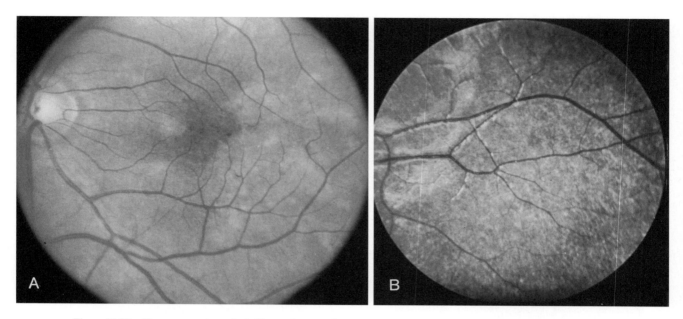

Figure 22.28. Pigmentary retinopathy in Kearns-Sayre syndrome. *A*, Posterior pole of a 17-year-old male shows mild pigmentary disturbance with pigment clumping overlying white streaks. Note resemblance to retinopathy of myotonic dystrophy (Fig. 22.15). *B*, Stippled retinal pigmentary disturbance in a 35-year-old woman with Kearns-Sayre syndrome.

able. Two of the patients described by Darsee et al. had the onset of heart block 8 and 6 years, respectively, after the onset of ptosis (326). Daniele and Corea reported the onset of cardiac involvement in a patient more than 15 years following the onset of other clinical symptoms and signs of KSS (325). The patient was followed closely with periodic examinations that were normal until shortly after two brief and ill-defined episodes of palpitations.

Patients with KSS may develop primary cardiac dysfunction at any time, leading to stroke or death from the direct effects of an arrhythmia or from a cardiac embolus (327,328). Thus, any patient with CPEO and a pigmentary retinopathy or neurologic dysfunction but with a normal ECG should be warned of the possibility of future cardiac disease, and the symptoms of such disease should be explained. In addition, such patients should undergo cardiac examinations at regular intervals, regardless of their age.

Although the cardiac dysfunction that occurs in patients with KSS can often be managed effectively with an artificial pacemaker (320), patients may die suddenly, even after insertion of a pacemaker (329), because of a decreased ventilatory response to hypoxia and hypercarbia caused by deficient brain stem respiratory control mechanisms (330). Cardiac failure in patients with KSS can be successfully treated with cardiac transplantation. Tranchant et al. reported stable cardiac function 18 months after transplantation in a 38-year-old man with KSS (331).

Cardiac abnormalities other than conduction defects occur less commonly. Two patients studied by Leveille and Newell also had echocardiographic evidence of intraventricular septal hypertrophy of the idiopathic hypertrophic subaortic stenosis type (281). Darsee et al. reported mitral valve prolapse

with mitral regurgitation in seven patients with CPEO and ataxia (326). In all patients, cardiac symptoms worsened as the ophthalmoparesis progressed.

One of the two patients originally described by Kearns and Sayre had **weakness of skeletal muscles** in addition to ophthalmoplegia (305). Kearns later described limb and trunk weakness in six of nine patients with KSS (306). Kiloh and Nevin reported involvement of nonocular muscle groups in 25% of patients with CPEO (332). Facial muscles, particularly the orbicularis oculi muscles, may be affected. Such patients may thus be unable not only to open the eyelids but also to close them tightly. With involvement of the frontalis muscle, there is an increasing inability to wrinkle the forehead and use the frontalis to help open the eyelids. This results in an apparent worsening of ptosis. All muscles of the face may eventually become affected, and the face thus becomes thin and expressionless. In some patients, the muscles of mastication become involved, and the patients report difficulty chewing.

With progression of the disease, there is often weakness and wasting of the neck and shoulder muscles. Although the muscles of the extremities may be involved, the weakness is often mild. One of the patients examined by Leveille and Newell was unaware that he had weakness of his arms, and another denied weakness but was noted by her family to lift a coffee cup with two hands to avoid spilling (281).

Patients with KSS usually have evidence of **neurologic dysfunction**. Abnormalities include cerebellar ataxia, pendular nystagmus, vestibular dysfunction, hearing loss, impaired intellectual function, and peripheral neuropathy. In addition, in many patients there is elevation of CSF protein content. Spongiform changes in the brain are present in al-

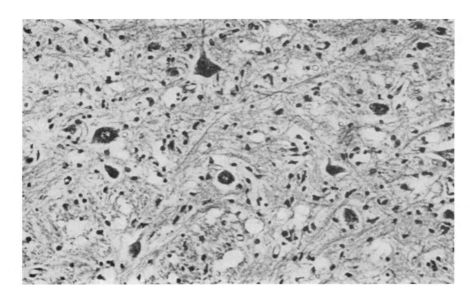

Figure 22.29. Spongiform degeneration and astrocytic gliosis in the cerebral cortex of a patient with Kearns-Sayre syndrome. (From Castaigne P, Laplane D, Escourolle R, et al. Ophthalmoplegie externe progressive avec spongiose des moyaux du tronc cérébral. Rev Neurol (Paris) 1971; 124:454–466.)

most every patient in whom an autopsy is performed (305,333,334) (Fig. 22.29).

CNS involvement in KSS is reflected in MR imaging abnormalities with high signal intensity for proton density, T2-weighted, and T2-weighted fluid attenuated inversion recovery (FLAIR) sequences. These abnormalities are present in the brain stem, globus pallidus, thalamus, and white matter of the cerebrum and cerebellum (335). In addition, regional abnormalities of brain metabolism are demonstrated in patients with KSS using MR spectroscopy (MRS). These changes include an increase in the lactate/creatine resonance intensity ratio (an index of impairment of oxidative metabolism) in resting occipital cortex, as well as a significant decrease in N-acetylaspartate/creatine (a measure of neuron loss or dysfunction) in cerebral cortex (336,337).

Endocrine dysfunction is common in patients with KSS. In addition to short stature, hypoparathyroidism with low or absent parathyroid hormone levels is well documented, and tetany may be a presenting symptom (338). A survey of the literature by Harvey and Barnett revealed that short stature was present in 38% of cases, gonadal dysfunction after puberty affecting both sexes in 20% of cases, and diabetes mellitus in 13% of patients, half of whom required insulin (339). Dysthyroidism, hyperaldosteronism, and hypomagnesemia were uncommon. Bone or tooth abnormalities and calcification of the basal ganglia were found both in those with and without hypoparathyroidism (339).

There is no adequate treatment for KSS. Berio and Piazzi reported a response to controlled carbohydrate intake and coenzyme Q10 therapy (340), but their experience is unique. As is the case with CPEO, some patients with diplopia benefit from treatment with prisms or strabismus surgery. Ptosis may also be treated surgically.

MITOCHONDRIAL GENETICS

Mitochondria are the only cellular organelles, aside from the nucleus, containing DNA (275,276). The mtDNA is a 16,569 base pair circle of double-stranded DNA. The majority of the 67 or so mitochondrial proteins are encoded by the nuclear genome, translated on cytoplasmic ribosomes, and transported into mitochondria. Mitochondrial DNA encodes 13 mitochondrial proteins as well as the two ribosomal RNAs (rRNAs) and 22 transfer RNAs (tRNAs) required to translate these proteins (341). Oxidative phosphorylation is carried out by the four multiprotein complexes of the respiratory chain and adenosine triphosphate (ATP) synthetase (complex V). The mtDNA encodes seven subunits of complex I (NADH-ubiquinone reductase), one subunit of complex III (ubiquinol-cytochrome c reductase), three subunits of complex IV (cytochrome c oxidase), and two subunits of ATP synthetase. Because the protein subunits of complex II (succinate dehydrogenase-ubiquinone reductase) are encoded exclusively by the nuclear genome, complex II activity is not impaired by mutations of the mitochondrial genome (342).

Mitochondria lack efficient mechanisms for DNA repair, and mutations of mtDNA (i.e., point mutations and deletions) increase with age (343). Because individual mitochondria typically contain 10–100 copies of mtDNA, such mutations produce a mixture of mutant and normal mtDNA, a condition called heteroplasmy. The shorter length of deleted genomes allows them to replicate faster than full-length mtDNA, resulting in an age-related increase in the proportion of deleted genomes within individual mitochondria. The random segregation of these molecules as cells divide during development can produce populations of cells highly enriched in either mutant or normal mtDNA, depending when in the course of development these mutations occur (301).

Mitochondrial protein synthesis depends exclusively on mitochondrial-encoded tRNAs, which use a genetic code different from that of nuclear-encoded tRNAs (344). Because the genes encoding mitochondrial tRNAs are distributed along the entire length of the mtDNA (341), large deletions of mtDNA invariably result in the loss of several tRNAs. Deletions of mtDNA are associated with an overall reduction in the translation of mitochondrial mRNAs, including those located outside the deleted region (345,346). For example, in a patient with a deletion of mtDNA that did not include the gene encoding subunit II of cytochrome c oxidase (COX), COX deficiency in affected muscle fibers was associated with reduced levels of all three mitochondrial-encoded subunits, including subunit II (345). Levels of nuclear-encoded COX subunits were unaltered in this patient.

Mutation in nuclear-encoded proteins that decrease mitochondrial DNA copy number can also reduce mitochondrial protein synthesis. For example, in the mitochondrial DNA depletion syndrome, an autosomal recessive disorder of infancy or childhood, mutations in two genes involved in deoxyribonucleotide metabolism, the deoxyguanosine kinase gene (DGK) and the thymidine kinase 2 gene (TK2), markedly reduce mitochondrial DNA copy number (347).

The severity of oxidative dysfunction within an affected cell appears to correlate with the proportion of deleted mtDNA. In somatic cell hybrids containing both wild-type mtDNA and deleted mtDNA from KSS patients, cells with 70% deleted mtDNAs had normal oxidative function, whereas cells with more than 99% deleted mtDNAs had severely compromised oxidative function and abnormal morphology (348). Oxidative capacity in patients with point mutations or large deletions correlates even more closely with the mutation load (349).

RRFs are the morphologic correlates of impaired mitochondrial protein synthesis in muscle fibers (350). The morphologic changes associated with RRFs are segmental (350) and related to local variations in the proportion of deleted mtDNA along individual muscle fibers (351,352).

The function of mitochondrial tRNAs can also be impaired by point mutations in highly conserved regions of tRNA genes. Mitochondrial protein synthesis cannot be maintained in the presence of homoplasmic mutations that result in the inactivation of essential tRNAs (353,354). In contrast, heteroplasmic mutations can be complemented by tRNAs encoded by normal mtDNA within the same mitochondrion, assuming that the amount of tRNA transcribed from the normal genomes exceeds the threshold required to maintain adequate levels of translation (355,356). In the case of a point mutation in tRNA$^{Leu(UUR)}$ (i.e., the A3243G transition), this threshold was examined using two criteria: the appearance of RRF and the loss of COX immunoreactivity. The COX holoenzyme comprises three structural proteins encoded by the mitochondrial genome and 10 nuclear-encoded regulatory subunits (357). COX-positive muscle fibers with normal morphology contained up to 50% mutant mtDNA, COX-positive RRF contained 90% mutant mtDNA, and COX-negative RRF contained more than 95% mutant mtDNA (358).

POINT MUTATIONS OF MITOCHONDRIAL tRNAS IN MATERNALLY INHERITED OPHTHALMOPLEGIA

Although most cases of CPEO are sporadic, some are hereditary (275,276,359). Because nearly all mtDNA is maternally transmitted (360), point mutations in mtDNA show a maternal pattern of inheritance. Mothers pass these mutations to offspring of both sexes, but the mutations are passed to subsequent generations only through the female line. Maternal inheritance of CPEO is associated with point mutations in highly conserved regions of mitochondrial tRNAs (361,362). The best characterized of these mutations is the A→G transition of nucleotide-3243 of tRNA$^{Leu(UUR)}$ (i.e., the A3243G transition) (362). This mutation is most often associated with the clinical phenotype called MELAS syndrome (mitochondrial encephalomyopathy, lactic acidosis, and stroke-like episodes). MELAS syndrome is characterized by (a) stroke before the age of 40 years, (b) encephalopathy characterized by seizures, dementia, or both, and (c) evidence of mitochondrial dysfunction characterized by lactic acidosis, RRFs in skeletal muscle, or both (363). This illustrates a recurring theme in mitochondrial diseases: a given mutation of mtDNA can be associated with more than one disease phenotype, in this case CPEO and MELAS.

This diversity of clinical presentation can be explained, at least in part, by heteroplasmy and the random segregation of mtDNA during cell division. The proportion of mutant mtDNA required to produce a mutant phenotype depends on the ATP requirements of the tissue, which are especially high in muscle and brain. In the case of the A3243G transition, one would expect a high proportion of mutant mtDNA in the extraocular muscles in patients with CPEO, and in brain and skeletal muscles in patients with MELAS. Additional genetic factors may also influence the phenotypic expression of mitochondrial mutations (364).

SINGLE DELETIONS OF mtDNA IN SPORADIC OPHTHALMOPLEGIA

Most cases of CPEO and KSS are sporadic (275,276,365, 366) and associated with single deletions of mtDNA (275,367,368). Deleted mtDNAs appear to be distributed to a wider variety of tissues in KSS than CPEO (369), and duplications of mtDNA appear to be present in all cases of KSS but are absent in CPEO (370). Duplications of mtDNA are also found in patients with either diabetes mellitus or Pearson's syndrome, a mitochondrial disease characterized by infantile sideroblastic pancytopenia, insufficiency of the pancreas, and hepatic dysfunction (371).

In sporadic cases of KSS and CPEO, all the mutant mtDNAs within an individual have the same deletion. These deletions differ among patients in both size and location, except for one, 4,977 base pairs long, that is found in more than one third of all patients with deletions (i.e., the so-called common deletion). The common deletion was found to be flanked by a perfect 13-base pair direct repeat in the normal mitochondrial genome, suggesting that homologous recombination may play a role in this deletion (372). The common deletion has also been detected in the peripheral blood, but not skeletal muscle, of patients with Pearson's syndrome (373). Using polymerase chain reaction (PCR), measurable levels of the common deletion can also be detected in some human oocytes, indicating that it can be transmitted in the female germ line (374).

Deletions of mtDNA impair mitochondrial protein synthesis; the severity of dysfunction within an affected cell correlates with the proportion of deleted mtDNA. The close association between deletions of mtDNA and dysfunction of the extraocular muscles may be related to the relatively high metabolic activity of these muscles, which are tonically active while the eyes are maintained in primary position. Experimental studies show that the replication of mtDNA is stimulated by the tonic activation of muscle fibers (375,376). As mentioned above, the shorter length of deleted mtDNAs allows them to replicate faster than normal, full-length mtDNA. This could cause an age-related increase in the proportion of deleted mtDNA in tonically active muscles, eventually resulting in impaired mitochondrial protein synthesis.

MULTIPLE DELETIONS OF mtDNA IN AUTOSOMAL-DOMINANT AND AUTOSOMAL-RECESSIVE OPHTHALMOPLEGIA

Autosomal-dominant and autosomal-recessive ophthalmoplegias are associated with multiple deletions of mtDNA (275,276,377). These deletions occur at multiple sites, involving a large portion of mtDNA, and most of them seem to be flanked by direct sequence repeats, shown to be ''hot spots'' in the case of single large deletions (378,379). The mutations map to sites on the nuclear genome that influence mtDNA replication or the size of nucleotide pools that support replication. Dominant mutations have been identified in genes encoding (a) mtDNA polymerase gamma (POLG), the sole polymerase responsible for mtDNA replication (380), (b) Twinkle, a putative helicase protein that may unwind mtDNA during replication (381), and (c) adenine nucleotide translocator (ANT1), which influences the size of ATP and ADP pools within mitochondria by controlling the transport of these nucleotides across the inner mitochondrial membrane (382). An autosomal-recessive mutation is associated with the gene encoding thymidine phosphorylase (TP), which is responsible for the thymidine salvage pathway in mitochondria, which are incapable of de novo thymidine synthesis (383).

A number of different clinical phenotypes are associated with autosomal-dominant ophthalmoplegia. In one lineage, they included dysphagia, exercise intolerance, lactic acidosis, cataract formation, and early death (384). In seven Japanese families, autosomal-dominant ophthalmoplegia was associated with muscle atrophy, proximal muscle weakness, hearing loss, and ataxia (385). In another series, it was associated with muscle weakness and recurrent myoglobinuria (386). Peripheral neuropathy was present in several pedigrees of autosomal-dominant ophthalmoplegia associated with multiple deletions of mtDNA (387). Some affected members of a Swedish pedigree evaluated by Moslemi et al. had cataracts, ataxia, tremor, peripheral neuropathy, mental retardation, or a combination of these manifestations (379).

Autosomal-recessive ophthalmoplegia is associated with the **MNGIE syndrome** (mitochondrial neurogastrointestinal encephalomyopathy) (388,389). Patients with the MNGIE syndrome also have mild peripheral neuropathy, leukoencephalopathy, and gastrointestinal symptoms (recurrent nausea, vomiting, or diarrhea) with intestinal dysmotility. By contrast, a disablingly severe sensory ataxic neuropathy with dysarthria and ophthalmoplegia (SANDO) occurs as a sporadic disorder in association with multiple mitochondrial DNA deletions (390).

DIAGNOSIS OF MITOCHONDRIAL MYOPATHY IN PATIENTS WITH OPHTHALMOPLEGIA

It is important to distinguish the mitochondrial myopathies from autosomal-dominant oculopharyngeal muscular dystrophy (see above) and myasthenia gravis, because these disorders have distinct therapeutic and genetic implications. Muscle biopsy is the single most useful diagnostic tool for evaluating patients with suspected mitochondrial disease. The presence of RRFs on muscle biopsy, in excess of what can be accounted for by age, establishes the diagnosis of mitochondrial myopathy (274,282,391).

Mutations of mtDNA (both deletions and point mutations) can be detected in muscle, blood, and other biopsied tissue using PCR (392,393). It is clear, however, that a single mutation of mtDNA may be associated with more than one phenotype. For example, the A3242G transition in tRNA$^{Leu(UUR)}$ is associated with both MELAS and CPEO, and the common deletion of mtDNA is associated with Pearson's syndrome as well as KSS (394). In both of these examples, the different clinical phenotypes correlate with distinct distributions of mutant mtDNAs in various tissues (i.e., CNS, skeletal muscle, and blood).

The diagnosis of KSS is aided by the finding of elevated levels of lactic acid in blood or CSF and by low-density lesions in the basal ganglia on MR imaging (391). MRS is a valuable tool for diagnosing abnormalities of energy metabolism in brain and other tissues (336,337), but it is not available for generalized screening of patients with suspected mitochondrial mutations.

All patients with known or presumed CPEO should undergo a careful ophthalmologic assessment, including a dilated ophthalmoscopic examination to determine whether a pigmentary retinopathy is present. In addition, patients with CPEO with pigmentary retinopathy or neurologic dysfunction should undergo an immediate assessment of cardiac function, and patients in whom no disturbances are found should nevertheless be monitored with periodic ECGs.

ENCEPHALOMYOPATHY WITH OPHTHALMOPLEGIA FROM VITAMIN E DEFICIENCY

In 1950, Bassen and Kornzweig described a condition characterized by acanthocytosis, pigmentary retinopathy, progressive ataxia, and neuropathy (395). The disorder results from the lack of apolipoprotein B, which is essential to the transport of fat-soluble vitamins, and is called **abetalipoproteinemia** or the **Bassen-Kornzweig syndrome**. The syndrome is caused by lack of vitamin E because of impaired intestinal absorption of lipids and lipid-soluble vitamins

(334,396). In fact, the neurologic disorder of abetalipoproteinemia is identical to that observed in other forms of human vitamin E deficiency, whether caused by malabsorption, cholestatic liver disease with impaired secretion of bile salts, bowel resection, or cystic fibrosis (397–401). The neurologic signs in patients with vitamin E deficiency include ataxia, areflexia, and loss of vibratory sensation due both to demyelinating neuropathy and neuronal degeneration of the cerebellum. The ocular motor abnormalities in patients with this disorder include abnormally slow voluntary saccades, slow or absent fast components of vestibular and optokinetic nystagmus, strabismus, pseudointernuclear ophthalmoplegia with dissociated nystagmus in the adducting eye on attempted horizontal gaze, and moderate to severe progressive external ophthalmoplegia (400–404). Kommerell described an ''internuclear ophthalmoplegia of abduction'' (e.g., posterior internuclear ophthalmoplegia of Lutz) in a 5-year-old girl with severe cholestatic liver disease (405). He postulated that the patient had some type of ''hepatotoxic encephalopathy,'' and in fact it seems likely that the patient had a vitamin E deficiency syndrome. Cremer and Halmagyi reported a similar case (406).

Two patients with abetalipoproteinemia described by Behrens et al. (404) developed unilateral ptosis when they looked to the right or left. The ptosis was always on the side of the abducting eye. One of the patients described by Yee et al. also had a similar appearance (403). The etiology of this ''alternating ptosis'' is unclear, but it may represent development of, or unmasking of, a pre-existing, ocular motor-levator synkinesis. Many patients with vitamin E deficiency syndromes develop pigmentary retinopathy in addition to ocular motor abnormalities (407). This retinopathy is similar in appearance and visual outcome to the retinopathies observed in patients with mitochondrial cytopathies (see previous discussion).

Vitamin E deficiency produces a true multisystem disorder. The disease appeared initially to be a pure myopathy, because biopsy specimens from affected patients showed distinctive autofluorescent inclusions in muscle fibers (398,399). However, there is also extensive involvement of peripheral and central nerve tissue, including dystrophic changes in the brain, spinal cord, and dorsal roots. Werlin et al. performed biopsies of peripheral nerve and striated muscle in two children with chronic cholestasis and vitamin E deficiency (401). These investigators found ultrastructural evidence of damage to peripheral nerve, including disruption of the myelin sheath. Although electron-dense deposits and autofluorescent inclusions (398,399) accumulate in striated muscle, the myopathy is trivial clinically. In the patient described by Hoogenraad et al., a biopsy specimen from the inferior oblique muscle showed only minimal abnormalities (400). In some fibers, glycogen was absent.

In patients with the vitamin E deficiency syndrome, the neurologic defects, including the ocular motor disturbances, can be improved if the serum vitamin E level is restored to normal with supplemental vitamin E therapy, administered via either an oral or parenteral route (334,399,400). Other fat-soluble vitamins should also be administered.

INFLAMMATORY MYOPATHIES

The term ''myositis'' can be used for any disorder in which inflammation affects muscle. The inflammation may be confined to a single muscle or may be diffuse. Inflammatory myopathies may be separated into two major categories: myopathies caused by an identified infective agent and idiopathic inflammatory myopathies (408,409).

INFECTIVE MYOSITIS

Infective myositis may be caused by bacteria, viruses, parasites, or fungi. These organisms and the diseases they produce are discussed in detail in other chapters. It suffices here to describe their effects on the extraocular muscles.

Bacteria that produce pyomyositis are commonly *Staphylococcus aureus, Streptococcus pyogenes,* and *Clostridium welchii.* These and other bacteria usually produce ophthalmoparesis indirectly when there is a generalized, suppurative orbital inflammation with swelling of soft tissues. On rare occasions, however, true extraocular myositis occurs from direct muscle invasion by bacteria. The bacteria usually gain entrance to the orbit from infected paranasal sinuses, often after trauma. Recognition is important because of the immediate need for antibiotics.

Viruses associated with an infective myopathy include the influenza virus and the Coxsackie A and B viruses. The extraocular muscles are not involved in most cases.

Although many **parasites** can theoretically involve the extraocular muscles, the most frequent and best-known form of parasitic infestation of muscle in general and extraocular muscle in particular is **trichinosis**. The causative agent, *Trichinella spiralis,* is a nematode that is usually acquired in humans as the result of ingesting raw or incompletely cooked pork, bear meat, or horse meat (410). After penetration of the small intestine, the larvae enter the lymphatic system and the bloodstream and are disseminated widely throughout the body. According to Adams, involvement of the extraocular muscles is common (Fig. 22.30), occurring second in frequency after involvement of the diaphragm (411). The clinical course has three stages. The first, the invasion period or intestinal stage, commences with the liberation of encysted larvae from the infected meat. It is characterized by diarrhea, vomiting, fever, and weakness. This stage persists for about 7 days. The second phase begins about 1 week after ingestion of tainted meat and is the period during which the disease is disseminated throughout the body. It is characterized by fever, peripheral leukocytosis and eosinophilia, headache, urticaria, muscle pain, weakness, edema of the eyelids and face, conjunctivitis, and headache. It is during this period that myocardial and skeletal muscle involvement become evident, and in some cases there is severe kidney involvement. Convalescence, the third stage, begins about 5–8 weeks after the onset of symptoms.

Patients with trichinosis often develop ocular signs early in the course of the disease. Chemosis of the conjunctiva is characteristic and primarily occurs over the extraocular

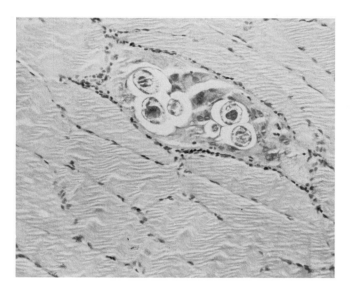

Figure 22.30. Trichinosis involving the extraocular muscles. Several cysts are present within a single extraocular muscle fiber, surrounded by chronic inflammatory mononuclear cells. (Courtesy of Dr. W. Richard Green.)

muscles. There is a varying degree of ophthalmoparesis from muscle involvement, and movement of the eyes is painful. Other ocular signs include proptosis, optic neuritis, and retinal ischemia (412).

Other parasites that produce infective myopathies include *Cysticercus* (413), *Echinococcus, Toxoplasma gondii, Sarcocystis,* and *Trypanosoma* (414). These parasites produce ophthalmoparesis by direct invasion of the extraocular muscles (413,414).

A variety of **fungi** can produce orbital inflammation with limitation of ocular motility. As with other infective agents, the inflammatory response may be granulomatous or nongranulomatous and may produce ophthalmoplegia through inflammation of ocular motor nerves, extraocular muscles, or soft tissue. The fungi most commonly responsible for orbital inflammation include organisms from the class Phycomycetes (mucormycosis) and *Aspergillus.*

Neither tuberculosis nor syphilis commonly involves the orbit. Nevertheless, tubercles and syphilitic gummas may occur in the orbital nerves, the optic nerve, and the extraocular muscles (415).

IDIOPATHIC MYOSITIS

Idiopathic myositis affecting the extraocular muscles usually occurs as an isolated phenomenon unassociated with systemic disease. In some cases, however, **orbital myositis** is part of a systemic process.

Myositis Limited to the Orbit

Local inflammatory conditions may produce limitation of ocular motility. Such conditions may be focal, as in the acquired form of Brown's superior oblique tendon sheath syn-

drome (416). The acquired form of this syndrome differs from its congenital counterpart in that it is often intermittent and is associated with inflammation and scarring, either within the superior oblique tendon or next to the anterior sheath (417,418) (Fig. 22.31). It may occur following superior oblique surgery, retinal detachment surgery, or trauma; in association with paranasal sinus disease; or with either the adult or juvenile forms of rheumatoid arthritis (26,416). Most cases of acquired Brown's syndrome are intermittent (416). Although persistent cases imply predominant scarring and contracture rather than inflammation, some respond to local injections of corticosteroids (419).

More diffuse involvement of one or more extraocular muscles occurs in the condition that is called **orbital myositis** or the myositic form of idiopathic inflammatory orbital pseudotumor (414,420,421). Patients with this condition usually experience sudden diplopia associated with orbital pain that ranges from mild to excruciating, conjunctival chemosis and injection, and occasionally proptosis (Fig. 22.32). Ultrasonography, CT scanning, and MR imaging show enlargement of one or more extraocular muscles (422), and biopsies of involved muscles show infiltration with chronic inflammatory cells (Fig. 22.33). Orbital myositis may occur not only as an isolated phenomenon but also in association with systemic disorders characterized by vasculitis or granulomatous inflammation, including systemic lupus erythematosus, rheumatoid arthritis, sarcoidosis, and Wegener's granulomatosis (423,424).

Systemic Myositis

Dermatomyositis

Dermatomyositis should not be considered polymyositis with a rash. Rather, it is a systemic vasculopathic autoim-

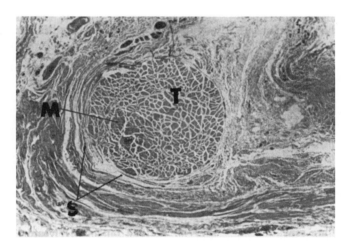

Figure 22.31. Pathology of acquired Brown's superior oblique tendon sheath syndrome. Note dense connective tissue surrounding tendon sheath, which may represent perisheath scarring. M, superior oblique muscle; S, superior oblique sheath; T, superior oblique tendon. (From Wright KW, Silverstein D, Marrone AC, et al. Acquired inflammatory superior oblique tendon sheath syndrome: A clinicopathologic study. Arch Ophthalmol 1982;100:1752–1754.)

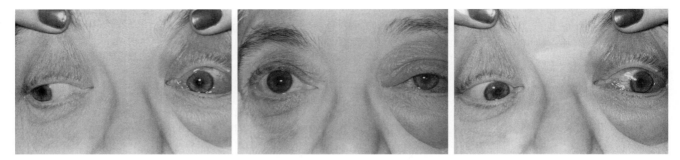

Figure 22.32. Orbital myositis affecting several extraocular muscles of the left eye in a 54-year-old woman. The patient shows proptosis, diffuse eyelid edema, conjunctival chemosis, and ophthalmoparesis.

mune disorder with histopathologic abnormalities and disease mechanisms distinct from polymyositis (425). Fever, skin lesions, arthritis, Raynaud's phenomenon, gastrointestinal manifestations, and even cardiac dysfunction may occur in this disease, but weakness of proximal limb-girdle muscles is most often the dominant feature (426). The skin signs are distinctive—heliotrope orbital/malar rash, Gottron's nodules and periungual erythema, and extensor surface rash. When skin manifestations are transient or slight, the diagnosis may be missed. The distinctive skeletal muscle pathology indicates the diagnosis: perifascicular myofiber necrosis or atrophy; deposition of complement-mediated immune complexes on capillary endothelium, resulting in capillary destruction (427); primary inflammation surrounding nonnecrotic myofibers; and sometimes perivascular inflammation.

Although ophthalmoplegia is documented so infrequently in patients with dermatomyositis that "it may be stated not to occur" (428), Susac et al. described a 47-year-old woman

with ptosis, external ophthalmoplegia, and limb weakness as the first signs of dermatomyositis (429). In this patient, the diagnosis was made by elevated levels of serum enzymes and their response to systemic corticosteroid administration, muscle and skin biopsies, and EMG evidence of myopathic potentials. Tonali et al. also described a patient with external ophthalmoplegia who was initially thought to have myasthenia gravis but in whom a diagnosis of dermatomyositis was eventually made (430).

Treatment begins with corticosteroids. Second-line therapies are methotrexate, azathioprine, and cyclosporine. Temporary improvement can be obtained with intravenous human immunoglobulin.

Polymyositis

In polymyositis, signs are limited to the skeletal muscle, and proximal weakness predominates in the legs over the

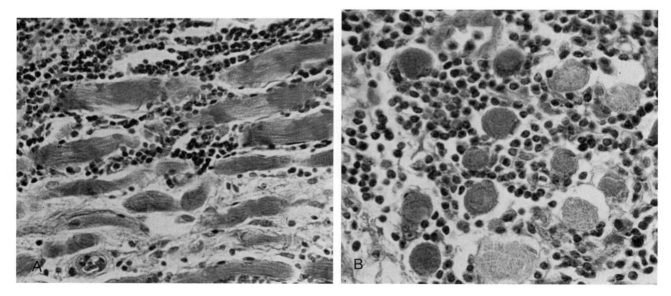

Figure 22.33. Pathology of extraocular muscle in orbital myositis. Longitudinal sections (*A*) and cross-sections (*B*) of involved extraocular muscle show muscle fibers separated by numerous chronic inflammatory cells and interstitial edema. (Courtesy of Dr. W. Richard Green.)

arms. Less than 25% of patients have either muscle pain or dysphagia. Although the face and jaw may be weak, ptosis and ophthalmoplegia are uncommon. If they occur, one should consider myasthenia gravis as an overlapping second autoimmune disease. The muscle biopsy in polymyositis shows myofiber necrosis, regeneration, and primary inflammation but none of the perifascicular or vascular changes of dermatomyositis.

ENDOCRINE MYOPATHIES

GRAVES' DISEASE

Perhaps the most common systemic disorder associated with diplopia, ophthalmoparesis, and infiltration of extraocular muscles is Graves' disease (431—433) (Fig. 22.34). Graves' orbitopathy often occurs in the context of mild hyperthyroid myopathy, producing mild proximal limb muscle weakness. Serum CK activity is normal in hyperthyroid myopathy. The incidence of myasthenia gravis is also increased in frequency in patients with Graves' disease, potentially producing diagnostic confusion about the pathophysiology of the ophthalmoparesis. Jacobson measured the titer of acetylcholine (ACh) receptor antibodies in 50 consecutive patients with Graves' ophthalmopathy and compared the clinical and biochemical features of those who had positive titers to those who did not (434). Four of the patients (8%) had positive titers. No clinical or serologic distinguishing features were identified, and none of these patients developed clinical features of myasthenia during a median follow-up period of 4.5 years (434). Graves' orbitopathy may occur months or years before there is any clinical or laboratory evidence of thyroid dysfunction (435). Such persons are said to have "euthyroid Graves' disease."

The extraocular muscles are the primary focus of thyroid disease within the orbit (436). In a retrospective study, De Waard et al. found motility disturbances in 83% of patients with Graves' disease (437). Both imaging studies (i.e., ultrasonography, CT scanning, MR imaging) and pathologic examination of affected muscles demonstrate involvement of the muscle tissue itself, with sparing of the muscle tendons (Fig. 22.35). This finding is in contrast to involvement of the muscles by idiopathic inflammatory pseudotumor or orbital myositis, which tend to involve the tendon as well as the muscle.

Ultrasonography, CT scanning, and MR imaging can all be used to diagnose dysthyroid ophthalmopathy (420,438). For ultrasonography to be useful, the test must be performed by an experienced ultrasonographer who can perform the scan in both B- and standardized A-modes. CT scanning must include axial and direct coronal views of the extraocular muscles. MR imaging must concentrate on the orbit.

Pathologic examination of extraocular muscles in patients with Graves' disease reveals lymphocyte and plasma cell infiltration along with edema within the endomysium of the extraocular muscles (439). Although there is controversy, the primary autoimmune target in Graves' ophthalmopathy appears to be orbital fibroblasts rather than muscle cells (440,441). The nature of the orbital antigen recognized by the infiltrating T lymphocytes is unknown (442). Cytokines (i.e., interleukin-1α, transforming growth factor β, and interferon-γ) released by T lymphocytes appear to stimulate the proliferation of orbital fibroblasts and increase their synthesis of glycosaminoglycans (441). Although the muscles are enlarged, the muscle cells are morphologically intact (Fig. 22.36). In addition to diplopia, involvement of extraocular muscles may produce proptosis, swelling of the conjunctiva and eyelid, and compression optic neuropathy.

In the early stages of extraocular muscle involvement, the muscles become enlarged, resulting in limitation of ocular motility. If this limitation is symmetric among the muscles of both eyes, patients will not report diplopia even though they may have severe limitation of ocular motility. In most cases, however, asymmetric involvement of the two eyes or of the extraocular muscles in one eye causes diplopia that may be vertical, horizontal, or oblique (443,444) (Fig.

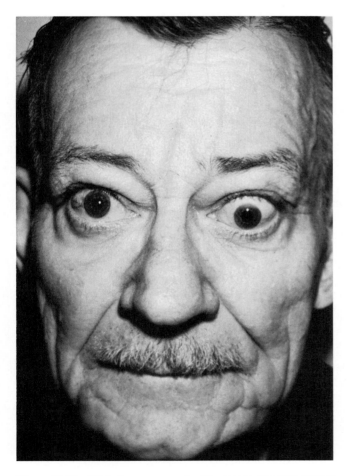

Figure 22.34. Clinical appearance of a 65-year-old man with Graves' ophthalmopathy. Note marked upper and lower eyelid retraction, bilateral proptosis, and marked left hypotropia.

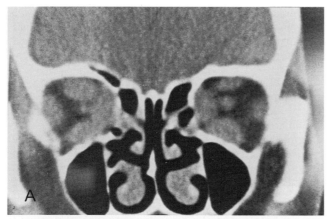

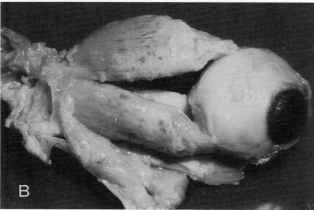

Figure 22.35. Appearance of the extraocular muscles in Graves' ophthalmopathy. *A,* Computed tomographic scan, coronal view, shows generalized enlargement of all extraocular muscles, worse on the right side. *B,* Pathologic specimen from a patient with Graves' ophthalmopathy shows marked enlargement of all extraocular muscles. (*B,* Courtesy of Drs. Ralph C. Eagle, Jr., and W. Richard Green.)

22.37). Hermann described two patients with Graves' disease who developed diplopia. Forced duction testing showed no mechanical limitation of motion, whereas saccadic velocity tests using electro-oculography suggested paresis of the inferior rectus muscle from muscle fiber weakness (445). Despite this report, it is clear that the diplopia that occurs in all patients with thyroid eye disease is associated with characteristic saccadic velocity measurements (446) and is caused by mechanical restriction of the affected muscles.

As thyroid eye disease progresses, the infiltration and edema of the extraocular muscles produce loss of muscle tissue, and the muscles become fibrotic. In such cases, proptosis may be minimal despite severe diplopia. Ultrasonography, CT scanning, and MR imaging may show normal or thinned extraocular muscles, and only a fibrous band may be found at surgery.

In patients suspected of having Graves' disease as the cause of their diplopia, ultrasonography, CT scanning, and MR imaging are the most important tests to obtain (438). Diseases such as inflammatory orbital pseudotumor, tumor

infiltration, orbital venous congestion, and trichinosis may all produce large extraocular muscles (447,448), and scanning artifacts occasionally result in confusion regarding diagnosis (449). Nevertheless, these studies, when combined with a careful history and clinical examination and when performed in the appropriate manner and interpreted correctly, will usually differentiate among these conditions without difficulty (447,436).

Patients with clinical and imaging evidence of thyroid eye disease should undergo appropriate tests of thyroid function to determine the state of the thyroid and pituitary glands and the need for therapy (450,451). The two thyroid hormones, thyroxine (T4) and triiodothyronine (T3), can be measured directly in serum by radioimmunoassay (RIA). Most serum T4 and T3 circulates bound to specific serum-binding proteins, but the unbound fraction, free T4, correlates best with hormone activity and can be measured directly or can be estimated from the T3-resin uptake as the free T4 index. Although hyperthyroidism is usually associated with increased levels of serum T4 and T3 and free T4 index, about 5% of patients have a normal serum T4 and free T4 associ-

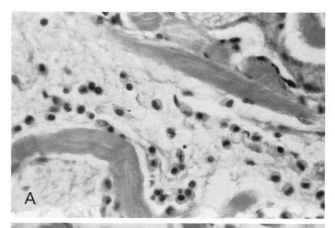

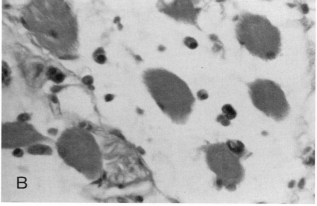

Figure 22.36. Pathology of extraocular muscles in Graves' ophthalmopathy. Longitudinal section (*A*) and cross-sections (*B*) through involved extraocular muscle show muscle fibers separated by acute and chronic inflammatory cells, primarily plasma cells and lymphocytes, and interstitial fluid. (Courtesy of Dr. W. Richard Green.)

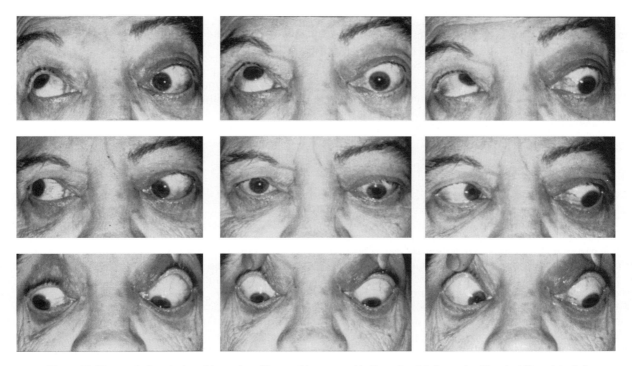

Figure 22.37. Marked vertical strabismus in a 63-year-old woman with Graves' ophthalmopathy. Note inability of the left eye to elevate above the midline. Despite the marked extraocular muscle involvement, the patient showed almost no proptosis. (Courtesy of Jacqueline E. Morris, C.O.)

ated with a selective increase in T3 secretion (452). Patients with T3-toxicosis are clinically indistinguishable from other patients with hyperthyroidism and have identical ocular symptoms and signs (453). Thyroid-stimulating hormone (TSH) and thyroid-stimulating antibody levels should also be measured (454).

Patients with systemic evidence of dysthyroidism who have evidence of orbitopathy should have an aggressive approach to normalization of their systemic disease (455). Patients who are hypothyroid should be treated with replacement therapy. Although there is controversy regarding the potential for radioablation of the thyroid gland to produce or exacerbate the ocular manifestations in patients with hyperthyroidism (432,456,457), we and others believe that this therapy is the best method of rendering patients permanently euthyroid (455). The major risk of radioablation of the thyroid gland is the sudden change from hyperthyroidism to hypothyroidism that occurs in patients treated in this manner. It is this sudden change that, in our experience, often triggers the development or exacerbation of the orbitopathy. Accordingly, we recommend that patients with Graves' disease who are treated with radioablation be followed carefully after treatment so that they can be treated with replacement therapy as soon as they become hypothyroid.

Treatment of the orbitopathy associated with Graves' disease is extremely successful. Irritation and swelling can be treated with a short (1–2 months) course of systemic corticosteroids or with low-dose (2,000 cGy) orbital radiation therapy (458), although the latter treatment is controversial

(459). Proptosis can be treated with orbital decompression using a variety of techniques (460,461). Strabismus can be treated in several ways. Some patients can be treated with prisms, others with surgery. In some cases, a combination of these treatments is needed.

OTHER ENDOCRINE MYOPATHIES

Cushing's Syndrome

Proximal muscle weakness is a common finding in patients with Cushing's syndrome and can be caused both by hypokalemia and by a direct effect of cortisol on muscle cell protein turnover, producing atrophy (462). The diagnosis rests on the typical cushingoid habitus, normal serum CK levels, and elevated urinary 24-hour free cortisol levels. It remits with successful treatment of the underlying condition (463).

Some patients with Cushing's syndrome develop ophthalmoparesis and mild exophthalmos. Because most of these patients harbor microadenomas that are too small to damage the intracranial portions of the ocular motor nerves, it is likely that the limitation of ocular motility is caused by direct involvement of the extraocular muscles; indeed, ultrasonography and other imaging studies in such patients often show enlargement of the extraocular muscles.

Pathologic studies of skeletal muscle in patients with Cushing's syndrome show a consistent increase in the number of lipid droplets in type 1 fibers (464). This may be a reflection of the known capacity for cortisol to liberate free fatty acids from neutral fat stored in adipose tissue. Myosin is preferentially depleted in type II fibers, especially if there is coexistent denervation or malnutrition (462).

Corticosteroids

Slansky et al. described proptosis and limitation of ocular motility in patients on long-term systemic corticosteroid therapy (465). It is possible that the orbital tissue changes in these patients represent a local toxic myopathy similar to

that observed in Cushing's syndrome. Eye signs are extraordinarily rare in this condition.

Other

Endocrine myopathies occur with hyperparathyroidism, hypoparathyroidism, acquired hypothyroidism, adrenal insufficiency, and acromegaly. The myopathic features tend to be mild and similar in all cases. Extraocular muscle involvement is rare.

TRAUMATIC MYOPATHIES

Trauma is probably the most common cause of isolated extraocular muscle damage (466). When the injury is not associated with orbital fracture, ocular motor dysfunction may be caused by intramuscular edema and hemorrhage, by muscle laceration (467), or by avulsion of the muscle origin or insertion (468–470). When there is associated orbital fracture, the same mechanisms of injury may occur. In addition, however, the extraocular muscles and surrounding tissue may be injured by bone fragments or become entrapped within the fracture site (471), producing restriction of ocular motility (Figs. 22.38 and 22.39).

Iatrogenic trauma to the orbit may also produce ocular motor dysfunction by direct muscle injury. Extraocular muscle imbalance occurs occasionally after retinal detachment surgery (472), usually related to the size and location of the silicone material used during a scleral buckling procedure. Inadvertent injury to the extraocular muscles may occur dur-

ing both cataract and glaucoma surgery. The superior rectus muscle may be injured by a bridle suture placed to stabilize the eye during surgery; however, the most common injury is damage to the inferior rectus muscle, inferior oblique muscle, or both from the toxic effects of the local anesthetic (usually lidocaine or Marcaine) (473). Both transient and permanent extraocular muscle imbalance after blepharoplasty are well recognized (474), and several investigators documented injury to the superior oblique tendon during this procedure (475,476). The mechanism of such damage is thought to be edema and hemorrhage into and around the extraocular muscles with secondary muscle contracture. Injury to the extraocular muscles may occur during surgery on the paranasal sinuses, particularly during ethmoidectomy, because both the medial rectus and superior oblique muscles are adjacent to the medial orbital wall (477). Raab described a patient who developed acute limitation of ocular motility

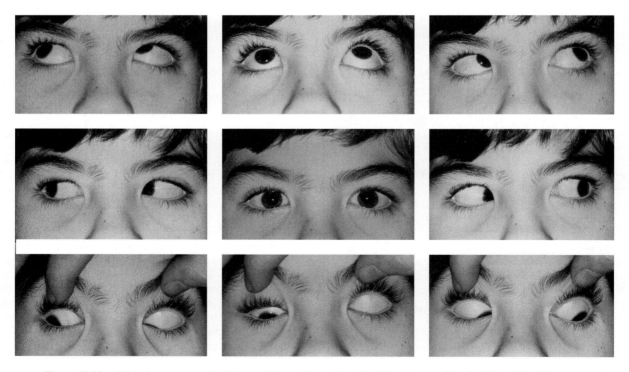

Figure 22.38. Clinical appearance of a 10-year-old boy with a right orbital floor fracture. Note inability of the right eye to fully elevate or depress.

after a periocular corticosteroid injection for uveitis (478). Surgical exploration performed 7 months after the onset of diplopia demonstrated a thinned, atrophic superior rectus muscle. Because the corticosteroid injection was delivered in the superior fornix at the 12 o'clock position, Raab postulated that injury to the superior rectus muscle or its nerve was the most likely explanation for the ocular motor dysfunction in this patient (478).

OTHER MYOPATHIES

Acute necrotizing myopathy in association with carcinoma is so rare that it is best considered an uncertain entity. Paraneoplastic neuropathies are common, and most patients with subacute proximal weakness and wasting occurring with cancer have neurogenic disease or paraneoplastic myositis. The paucity of clinical, neurophysiologic, and pathologic details in single case reports of paraneoplastic myopathy makes pathophysiologic correlations difficult (479,480). Nevertheless, Swash described a patient with bladder carcinoma who developed rapidly progressive, painless, muscular weakness associated with external ophthalmoplegia (480).

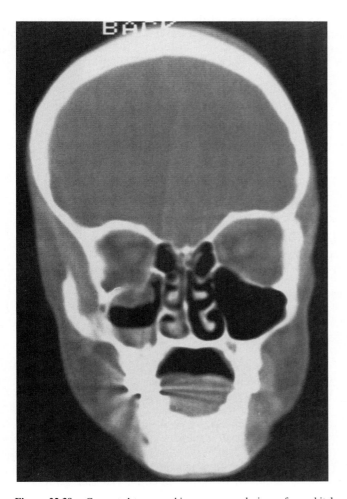

Figure 22.39. Computed tomographic scan, coronal view, of an orbital floor fracture. The scan shows a dehiscence in the floor of the right orbit with prolapse of tissue into the maxillary sinus. There is a soft tissue density in the floor of the sinus, indicating either swollen mucosa or blood. (Courtesy of Dr. Nicholas T. Iliff.)

The patient died 5 weeks after the onset of symptoms, and postmortem examination of skeletal muscles, including the extraocular muscles, showed variable fiber size, endomysial edema, and scattered fibers undergoing hyaline necrosis or phagocytosis; however, vacuolar changes appeared to predominate over necrosis. Although the patient also had evidence of an acute carcinomatous neuropathy at autopsy, with few motor end-plates being identified even in the extraocular muscles, it was thought that the acute neuropathy supervened during the last 3 weeks of the patient's life and that the initial paralysis, including the ophthalmoplegia, was probably caused by the necrotizing myopathy.

Any local orbital process that acts as a space-occupying lesion can cause limitation of ocular motility simply by its mass effect. **Tumors** within the muscle cone typically produce limitation of motion in this manner. In addition, rhabdomyosarcoma occasionally arises in one or more of the extraocular muscles, producing limitation of motion; however, because such patients typically present in childhood or adolescence with rapidly progressive proptosis, the diagnosis is rarely in question (481).

Discrete and diffuse metastases of carcinomas and lymphomas to the extraocular muscles are common (448, 482,483) (Fig. 22.40). In such cases, CT scanning and MR imaging may show focal or generalized enlargement of the infiltrated extraocular muscle or muscles.

Infiltration of extraocular muscles can occur in patients with **amyloidosis**. Amyloid is a homogeneous, eosinophilic, extracellular protein that may be demonstrated with light microscopy by its characteristic staining properties with metachromatic dyes and Congo red, and with electron microscopy by its composition of fine, rigid, nonbranching fibrils (484,485). Amyloidosis is classified on the basis of its clinical features into three general categories (486): (*a*) primary (systemic or localized; familial or sporadic), (*b*) secondary, and (*c*) amyloidosis associated with multiple myeloma. Amyloidosis is considered primary when no underlying disease is present, and the amyloid affects only mesodermal tissue. Primary amyloidosis usually involves cardiovascular, smooth, and skeletal muscle, but in rare cases it is localized to the orbit. Both systemic and orbital primary amyloidosis may occur as familial or sporadic entities. Secondary amyloidosis occurs in association with systemic diseases, including tuberculosis, rheumatoid arthritis, and leprosy, and involves the kidneys, liver, spleen, and adrenal glands. Finally, some amyloid deposits are shown to be homologous with portions of immunoglobulin light chains in patients with multiple myeloma. This association is thus considered a separate category of disease.

Although only small, clinically insignificant deposits of

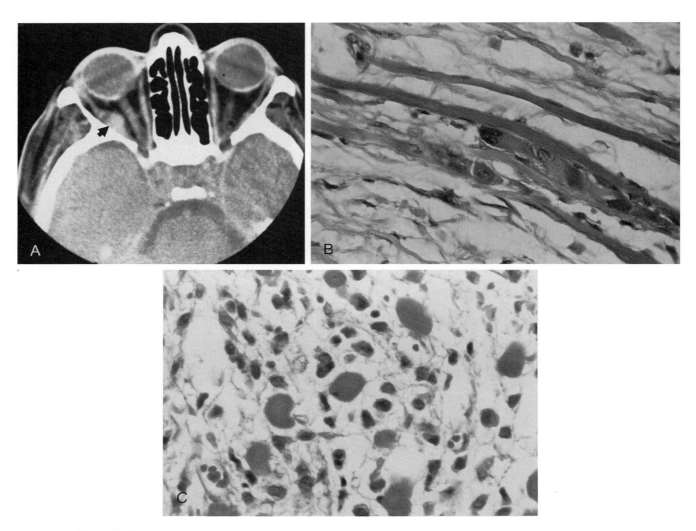

Figure 22.40. Metastatic carcinoma involving the extraocular muscles. *A*, Computed tomographic scan from a patient with metastatic breast carcinoma shows a focal enlargement of the right lateral rectus muscle (*arrow*) in a woman reporting painless diplopia. She had no proptosis. Although a needle biopsy of the muscle was nondiagnostic, the patient had resolution of diplopia and improvement in the appearance of the muscle following orbital irradiation. *B*, Longitudinal section of an extraocular muscle in a patient with metastatic carcinoma shows malignant cells between muscle fibers. *C*, Cross-section of an extraocular muscle in a patient with metastatic carcinoma and proptosis shows that individual muscle fibers are separated by tumor cells and interstitial edema. (*A*, Courtesy of Drs. C. Citrin and B. Brown. *C*, Courtesy of Dr. W. Richard Green.)

amyloid in the eye occur in secondary amyloidosis (487,488), extraocular muscle infiltration is common in primary amyloidosis (489–490) and also occurs in patients with amyloidosis associated with multiple myeloma (491). In some patients, the involvement is subclinical, producing no ocular motor dysfunction (490), whereas in other cases, varying degrees of proptosis and ophthalmoparesis are present, depending on the extent of extraocular muscle load (489) (Fig. 22.41).

Patients with high-flow carotid-cavernous sinus fistulas or arteriovenous malformations often develop enlargement of the extraocular muscles because of the greatly **increased venous pressure** within the orbit (448) (see Chapter 42). Similarly, in rare patients, tumors or aneurysms in the ante-

rior temporal fossa may compress draining orbital veins and produce a similar picture. Patients with such lesions may thus have diplopia from both ocular motor nerve palsies and from swelling of the extraocular muscles themselves. The diagnosis is established by neuroimaging studies, including ultrasonography, CT scanning, MR imaging, and selective arteriography.

Localized **ischemia of extraocular muscles** can produce clinical limitation of ocular motility. Barricks et al. performed a histologic examination on the brain stem, ocular motor nerves, and extraocular muscles of an 80-year-old man who died shortly after developing complete bilateral blindness, ptosis, and ophthalmoparesis in the setting of giant cell arteritis (492). These investigators found no evi-

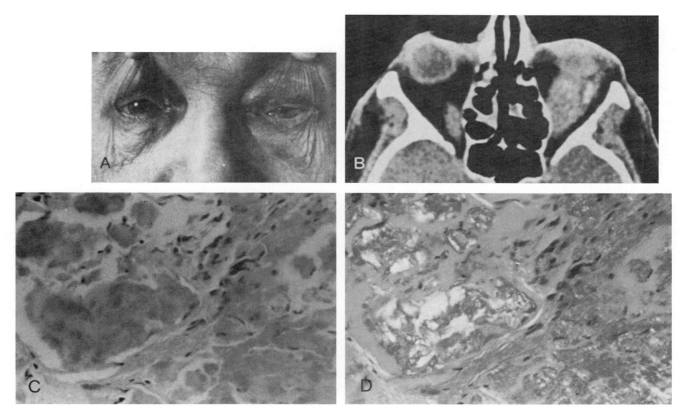

Figure 22.41. Orbital amyloidosis. *A*, A patient with multiple myeloma has complete ptosis and ophthalmoplegia. *B*, In another patient with proptosis and ophthalmoparesis, the left inferior rectus muscle is markedly enlarged. *C*, Biopsy of this muscle shows large amounts of amorphous material that stain positively for amyloid. *D*, A phase contrast photomicrograph of the field shown in *C* reveals that the amorphous material is birefringent, a characteristic of amyloid. (*A*, From Raflo GT, Farrell TA, Sioussat RS. Complete ophthalmoplegia secondary to amyloidosis associated with multiple myeloma. Am J Ophthalmol 1981;92:221–224. *D*, Courtesy of Dr. Thomas C. Spoor.)

dence of ischemia in the brain stem or throughout the length of the ocular motor nerves. The orbital arteries, however, were involved by arteritis, and all extraocular muscles showed patchy, variable changes consistent with ischemia. The study performed by Barricks et al. proved that at least some patients with giant cell arteritis who develop diplopia and ophthalmoplegia do so from ischemic extraocular myopathy rather than from ischemia of the ocular motor nerves or brain stem (492). A similar patient with giant cell arteritis and fluctuating paresis of multiple extraocular muscles was reported by Goldberg (493). Although it seems likely that this patient also had ophthalmoparesis caused by extraocular muscle ischemia, no pathologic examination was performed. Ischemia of the extraocular muscles is probably responsible for at least some cases of ophthalmoparesis that occur in association with systemic vascular diseases, particularly those characterized by vasculitis (e.g., periarteritis nodosa, systemic lupus erythematosus). In most cases, however, histologic proof of such a mechanism is lacking.

Sandyk and Brennan described a 12-year-old girl who developed diplopia on lateral gaze (494). A complete evaluation that included a jejunal biopsy demonstrated evidence of **celiac disease** (nontropical sprue). A biopsy of the right medial rectus showed atrophic muscle fibers with hyaline changes and fatty infiltration. Treatment with a gluten-free diet, vitamin B12, iron, and multivitamins was associated with compete return of normal ocular motility and alignment. Although skeletal myopathy is occasionally a presenting feature of adult celiac disease (495), this case is the only one in which ocular myopathy was the presenting feature of the disease in a child.

Patients with **skeletal muscle storage diseases** usually present in one of two ways. First, there may be pain, weakness, and rhabdomyolysis that are induced by exercise or fasting. This presentation occurs in patients with impaired metabolism of glycogen (symptoms after brief exercise) or of fatty acids (symptoms after extended exercise or fasting) that reduces the rate at which skeletal muscle can generate high-energy phosphate bonds. Plasma membrane integrity is thus compromised, and rhabdomyolysis occurs. Patients with myophosphorylase deficiency (McArdle's disease) (496), muscle phosphofructokinase deficiency (Tarui's disease) (497), and carnitine palmityl acyltransferase deficiency (498) present with exercise-induced weakness. Most patients with these disorders have no disturbances of ocular motility or alignment (499).

A second presentation in patients with skeletal muscle storage diseases is fixed muscle weakness. In these patients, excess glycogen or triglyceride causes disruption of myofibrillar architecture. Patients with acid maltase deficiency (Pompe's disease) (500), brancher enzyme deficiency (Andersen's disease) (501,502), debrancher enzyme deficiency (503), and carnitine deficiency (504) have fixed muscle weakness. Extensive deposits of free and lysosomal glycogen were found by Smith and Reinecke in the inferior oblique muscle of a 3-year-old boy with acid maltase deficiency who underwent strabismus surgery for a V-pattern esotropia (505). Whether these deposits were responsible for the strabismus is unclear, although Toussaint and Danis described complete disappearance of normal extraocular muscle fibers associated with large intramuscular glycogen-containing vacuoles in a 5-month-old infant (506).

Drug-induced toxic myopathies are rare without the superimposition of another risk factor, such as renal insufficiency, hepatic insufficiency, malnutrition, or a concomitant drug interaction, that elevates levels of the offending drug (507). Biologic toxins affect muscles through direct, cell-specific interactions. Drugs and toxins can cause muscle weakness by affecting muscle fibers or their neuromuscular junctions. Direct effects on muscle include (a) myonecrosis with or without myoglobinuria (e.g., ethanol in the malnourished, lovastatin or its analogs taken concomitantly with cyclosporine), and (b) excessive autophagy (e.g., chloroquine, colchicine, amphiphilic drugs). Undoubtedly, myotoxic reactions also occur in extraocular muscles, but there are few well-documented cases.

The **venom of the common sea snake,** *Enhydrina schistosa,* produces an unusual myotoxic reaction that apparently can involve the extraocular muscles. According to Reid, the primary clinical manifestations of this type of poisoning are trismus, flaccid paresis of the extremities, and myoglobinuria (508). In severe poisoning, there may be ptosis and limitation of ocular motility. Fohlman and Eaker isolated and characterized a lethal myotoxic phospholipase A from the venom of the sea snake (509). Thus, it is likely, although not proven histologically, that the ocular motor weakness is myopathic in origin and not caused by damage to ocular motor nuclei or nerves.

REFERENCES

1. Walton J, Karpati G, Hilton-Jones D. Disorders of Voluntary Muscle. New York: Churchhill Livingstone, 1994.
2. Duke-Elder S. System of Ophthalmology. Vol 3, Part 2. St Louis: CV Mosby, 1973:736.
3. Girard J, Neely RA. Agenesis of the medial rectus muscle: Correction of a case by transplantation of slips from the vertical recti. Arch Ophthalmol 1958;59:337–341.
4. Stieren E. Congenital absence of both inferior recti muscles. Am Med 1903;5:581.
5. Posey WC. Anomalies of eye muscles. Trans Am Acad Ophthalmol Otolaryngol 1921;26:83–89.
6. Casten VG. Isolated congenital absence of the inferior rectus muscle. Arch Ophthalmol 1940;24:55–61.
7. Taylor RH, Kraft SP. Aplasia of the inferior rectus muscle: A case report and review of the literature. Ophthalmology 1997;104:415–418.
8. Steinheim A. Blepharoptosis congenita und defect der musculi recti superioris. Klin Monatsbl Augenheilkd 1877;15:99–102.
9. Kaufmann H, Kluxen M. Ein fall von aplasie des musculus obliqus superior. Klin Monatsbl Augenheilkd 1972;160:710–713.
10. Diamond GR, Katowitz JA, Whitaker LA. Variations in extraocular muscle and structure in craniofacial dysostosis. Am J Ophthalmol 1980;90:416–418.
11. Robb RM, Boger WP III. Vertical strabismus associated with plagiocephaly. J Pediatr Ophthalmol Strabis 1983;20:58–62.
12. Miller NR. Walsh and Hoyt's Clinical Neuro-Ophthalmology. 4th ed. Baltimore: Williams & Wilkins, 1985:785.
13. Apple C. Congenital abducens paralysis. Am J Ophthalmol 1939;22:169–173.
14. Natale A. Congenital ptosis and muscle anomalies of the eye. Arch Oftalmol B Aires 1929;4:14.
15. Scassellati-Sforzolini G. Una sindrome molto rara: Difetto congenito monolaterale della elevazione con retrazione del globo. Riv Otoneurooftalmol 1958;33:431–439.
16. Fink WH. A study of the anatomical variations in the attachment of the oblique muscles of the eyeball. Trans Am Acad Ophthalmol Otolaryngol 1947;52:500–513.
17. Axenfeld T, Schürenberg E. Beiträge zur kenntniss der angeborenen beweglichkensdefekte der augen: I. Angeborene cyclische oculomotoriuserkrankung einseitiger accommodationskrampf. Klin Monatsbl Augenheilkd 1901;39:64–73.
18. Strebel J. Esophorie und anaphorie bei gleichgeschlechtigen zwillingen. Klin Monatsbl Augenheilkd 1937;98:788–789.
19. Denis D, Genitori L, Conrath J, et al. Ocular findings in children operated on for plagiocephaly and trigonocephaly. Childs Nerv System 1996;12:683–689.
20. Whitnall SE. An Anatomy of the Human Orbit and Accessory Organs of Vision. 2nd ed. London: Oxford University Press, 1932.
21. White JW. Paralysis of the superior rectus and inferior oblique muscle of the same eye. Arch Ophthalmol 1942;27:366–371.
22. Lyle DJ, McGavic JS. The cause of voluntary forward luxation of the eyeball: A case report with anatomical findings at necropsy. Am J Ophthalmol 1936;19:316–320.
23. Brown HW. Congenital structural muscle anomalies. In: Allen JH, ed. Strabismus Ophthalmic Symposium. St Louis: CV Mosby, 1950:205.
24. Metz HS. Saccadic velocity measurements in Brown's syndrome. Ann Ophthalmol 1979;11:636–638.
25. Breinin GM. New aspects of ophthalmoneurologic diagnosis. Arch Ophthalmol 1959;58:375.
26. Parks MM, Brown M. Superior oblique tendon sheath syndrome of Brown. Am J Ophthalmol 1975;79:82–86.
27. Johnson LV. Adherence syndrome (pseudoparalysis lateral or superior rectus muscles). Arch Ophthalmol 1950;44:870–888.
28. Heuck G. Über angeborenen vererbten beweglichkeitsdefekts der augen. Klin Monatsbl Augenheilkd 1879;17:253–278.
29. Brown HW. Congenital structural muscle anomalies. In: Allen JH, ed. Strabismus Ophthalmic Symposium. St Louis: CV Mosby, 1950:229.
30. Laughlin RC. Congenital fibrosis of the extraocular muscles. Am J Ophthalmol 1956;41:432–438.
31. Doherty EJ, Macy ME, Wang SM, et al. CFEOM3; a new extraocular congenital fibrosis syndrome that maps to 16q24.2–q24.3. Invest Ophthalmol Vis Sci 1999;40:1687–1694.
32. Engle EC, Kunkel LM, Specht LA, et al. Mapping a gene for congenital fibrosis of the extraocular muscles to the centromeric region of chromosome 12. Nat Genet 1994;7:69–73.
33. Engle EC, McIntosh N, Yamada K, et al. CFEOM1, the classic familial form of congenital fibrosis of the extraocular muscles, is genetically heterogeneous but does not result from mutations in ARIX. BMC Genet 2002;3:3.
34. Nakano M, Yamada K, Fain J, et al. Homozygous mutations in ARIX(PHOX2A) result in congenital fibrosis of the extraocular muscles type 2. Nat Genet 2001;29:315–320.
35. Gillies WE, Brooks AMV, et al. Congenital fibrosis of the extraocular muscles: A new group of dominantly inherited ocular fibrosis with radiologic findings. Ophthalmology 1995;102:607–612.
36. von Noorden GK. Congenital hereditary ptosis with inferior rectus fibrosis. Arch Ophthalmol 1970;83:378–380.
37. Wang SM, Zwaan J, Mullaney PB, et al. Congenital fibrosis of the extraocular muscles type 2, an inherited exotropic strabismus fixus, maps to distal 11q13. Am J Hum Genet 1998;63:517–525.
38. Guo S, Brush J, Teraoka H, et al. Development of noradrenergic neurons in the zebrafish hindbrain requires BMP, FGF8, and the homeodomain protein soulless/Phox2a. Neuron 1999;24:555–566.
39. Pattyn A, Morin X, Cremer H, et al. Expression and interactions of the two closely related homeobox genes Phox2a and Phox2b during neurogenesis. Development 1997;124:4065–4075.
40. Engle EC, Goumnerov BC, McKeown CA, et al. Oculomotor nerve and muscle abnormalities in congenital fibrosis of the extraocular muscles. Ann Neurol 1997;41:314–325.
41. Apt L, Axelrod RN. Generalized fibrosis of the extraocular muscles. Am J Ophthalmol 1978;85:822–829.
42. Holmes WJ. Hereditary congenital ophthalmoplegia. Trans Am Ophthalmol Soc 1956;53:245–253.

43. Assaf AA. Bilateral congenital vertical gaze disorders: Congenital muscle fibrosis or congenital central nervous system abnormality? Neuroophthalmology 1997;17:23–30.

44. Harley RD, Rodrigues M. Congenital fibrosis of ocular muscles. Presented before the American Association of Pediatric Ophthalmology, San Francisco, April 4, 1977.

45. Hotchkiss M, Miller NR, Clark AW, et al. Bilateral Duane's retraction syndrome: A clinicopathologic case report. Arch Ophthalmol 1980;98:870–874.

46. Miller NR, Kiel SM, Green WR, et al. Unilateral Duane's retraction syndrome (type 1). Arch Ophthalmol 1982;100:1468–1472.

47. Shy GM, Magee KR. A new congenital nonprogressive myopathy. Brain 1956; 79:610–621.

48. Shy GM, Engel WK, Somers JE, et al. Nemaline myopathy: A new congenital myopathy. Brain 1963;86:793–810.

49. Spiro AJ, Shy GM, Gonatas NK. Myotubular myopathy: Persistence of fetal muscle in an adolescent boy. Arch Neurol 1966;14:1–14.

50. Engel AG, Gomez MR, Groover RV. Multicore disease: A recently recognized congenital myopathy associated with multifocal degeneration of muscle fibers. Mayo Clin Proc 1971;46:666–681.

51. Brooke MH, Engel WK. The histographic analysis of human muscle biopsies with regard to fiber types IV: Children's biopsies. Neurology 1969;19:591–605.

52. Bodensteiner JB. Congenital myopathies. Muscle Nerve 1994;17:131–144.

53. Bonnette H, Roelofs R, Olson WH. Multicore disease: Report of a case with onset in middle age. Neurology 1974;24:1039–1044.

54. Brooke MH. A Clinician's View of Neuromuscular Disease. Baltimore: Williams & Wilkins, 1977.

55. Engel WK, Gold GN, Karpati G. Type 1 fiber hypotrophy and central nuclei: A rare congenital muscle abnormality with a possible experimental model. Arch Neurol 1968;18:435–444.

56. Brooke MH, Neville HE. Reducing body myopathy. Neurology 1972;22: 829–840.

57. Van Wijngaarden GK, Fleury P, Bethlem J, et al. Familial "myotubular" myopathy. Neurology 1969;19:901–908.

58. Lefebvre S, Burglen L, Reboullet S, et al. Identification and characterization of a spinal muscular atrophy-determining gene. Cell 1995;80:155–165.

59. Brandt S. Werdnig-Hoffman's Infantile Progressive Muscular Dystrophy. Copenhagen: Munksgaard, 1950.

60. Gordon PH, Hays AP, Rowland LP, et al. Erroneous diagnosis corrected after 28 years: Not spinal muscular atrophy with ophthalmoplegia but minicore myopathy. Arch Neurol 1996;53:1194–1196.

61. Greenfield JG, Cornman T, Shy GM. The prognostic value of the muscle biopsy in the floppy infant. Brain 1958;81:461–484.

62. Quane KA, Healy JM, Keating KE, et al. Mutations in the ryanodine receptor gene in central core disease and malignant hyperthermia. Nat Genet 1993:5: 51–55.

63. Zhang Y, Chen HS, Khanna VK, et al. A mutation in the human ryanodine receptor gene associated with central core disease. Nat Genet 1993;5:46–50.

64. Quane KA, Keating KE, Manning BM, et al. Detection of a novel common mutation in the ryanodine gene in malignant hyperthermia: Implications for diagnosis and heterogeneity studies. Hum Mol Genet 1994;3:471–476.

65. Engel WK, Resnick JS. Lateonset rod myopathy: A newly recognized, acquired and progressive disease. Neurology 1966;16:308–309.

66. Pelin K, Hilpela P, Donner K, et al. Mutations in the nebulin gene associated with autosomal recessive nemaline myopathy. Proc Natl Acad Sci USA 1999; 96:2305–2310.

67. Hopkins IJ, Lindsey JR, Ford FR. Nemaline myopathy: A long-term clinicopathologic study of affected mother and daughter. Brain 1966;89:299–310.

68. Wright RA, Plant GT, Landon DN, et al. Nemaline myopathy: An unusual cause of ophthalmoparesis. J Neuroophthalmol 1997;17:39–43.

69. Radu H, Ionescu V, Radu A, et al. Hypotrophic type 1 muscle fibers with central nuclei, and central myofibrillar lysis preferentially involving type 2 fibers. Eur Neurol 1974;11:108–127.

70. Karpati G, Carpenter S, Nelson RF. Type 1 muscle fiber atrophy and central nuclei: A rare familial neuromuscular disease. J Neurol Sci 1970;10:489–500.

71. Fardeau M. Congenital myopathies. In: Mastaglia FL, Walton J, eds. Skeletal Muscle Pathology. Edinburgh: Churchill Livingstone, 1982:161.

72. Hawkes CH, Absolon MJ. Myotubular myopathy associated with cataract and electrical myotonia. J Neurol Neurosurg Psychiatry 1975;38:761–764.

73. Palmucci L, Bertolotto A, Monga G, et al. Histochemical and ultrastructural findings in a case of centronuclear myopathy. Eur Neurol 1978;17:327–332.

74. Bradley WG, Price DLK, Watanabe CK. Familial centronuclear myopathy. J Neurol Neurosurg Psychiatry 1970;33:687–693.

75. Bill PLA, Cole G, Proctor NSF. Centronuclear myopathy. J Neurol Neurosurg Psychiatry 1979;42:548–556.

76. Sher JH, Rimalovski AB, Athanassiades TJ, et al. Familial centronuclear myopathy: A clinical and pathological study. Neurology 1967;17:727.

77. Dubowitz V. The floppy infant. Clinics in Developmental Medicine, No 76. Philadelphia: Lippincott, 1980.

78. Bergen BJ, Carry MP, Wilson WB, et al. Centronuclear myopathy: Extraocular- and limb-muscle findings in an adult. Muscle Nerve 1980;3:165–171.

79. McLeod JG, Baker W, Lethlean AK, et al. Centronuclear myopathy with autosomal dominant inheritance. J Neurol Sci 1972;15:375–387.

80. Pepin B, Mikol J, Goldstein B, et al. Forme familiale de myopathie centronucléaire de l'adulte. Rev Neurol 1976;132:845–857.

81. Thomas N, Sarfarzai M, Roberts K, et al. X-linked myotubular myopathy (MTM1): Evidence for linkage to Xa28 DNA markers. Cytogenet Cell Genet 1987;46:704.

82. Laporte J, Hu LJ, Kretz C, et al. 1 A gene mutated in X-linked myotubular myopathy defines a new putative tyrosine phosphatase family conserved in yeast. Nat Genet 1996;13:175–182.

83. Thomas N, Wallgren-Pettersson C. X-linked myotubular myopathy. Neuromusc Disord 1996;6:129–132.

84. Buj-Bello A, Biancalana V, Moutou C, et al. Identification of novel mutations in the MTM1 gene causing severe and mild forms of X-linked myotubular myopathy. Hum Mutat 1999;14:320–325.

85. Barth PG, Van Wijngaarden GK, Bethlem J. X-linked myotubular myopathy with fatal neonatal asphyxia. Neurology 1975;25:531–536.

86. Fardeau M, Godet-Guillain J, Tomé FMS, et al. Congenital neuromuscular disorders: A critical review. In: Aguayo AJ, Karpati G, eds. Current Topics in Nerve and Muscle Research. Amsterdam: Excerpta Medica, 1978:164.

87. Paljarvi L, Kalimo H, Lang H, et al. Minicore myopathy with dominant inheritance. J Neurol Sci 1987;77:11–22.

88. Heffner R, Cohen M, Duffner P, et al. Multicore disease in twins. J Neurol Neurosurg Psychiatry 1976;39:602–606.

89. Van Wijngaarden GK, Bethlem J, Dingemans KP, et al. Familial focal loss of striations. J Neurol 1977;216:163–172.

90. Engel AG, Franzini-Armstrong C. Myology: Basic and Clinical. 2nd ed. New York: McGraw Hill, 1994.

91. Schotland DL. An electron microscopic study of target fibers, targetlike fibers and related abnormalities in human muscle. J Neuropathol Exp Neurol 1969; 28:214–228.

92. Mukoyama M, Matsuoka Y, Kato H, et al. Multicore disease. Clin Neurol 1973; 13:221–227.

93. de Lumley L, Vallat JM, Catanzano G. Etude clinique et ultrastructurale d'un cas de myopathie congénitale à foyers multiles. Sem Hop Paris 1976;52:733–736.

94. Brooke MH. Congenital fiber type disproportion. In: Kakulas BA, ed. Clinical Studies in Myology. Amsterdam: Excerpta Medica, 1973:147.

95. Owen JS, Kline LB, Oh SJ, et al. Ophthalmoplegia and ptosis in congenital fiber type disproportion. J Pediatr Ophthalmol Strabis 1981;18:55–60.

96. Farkas-Bargeton E, Tomé FMS, Fardeau M, et al. Histochemical and ultrastructural study of muscle biopsies in three cases of dystrophica myotonica in the newborn child. J Neurol Sci 1974;21:273.

97. Brooke MH, Carroll JE, Ringel SP. Congenital hypotonia revisited. Muscle Nerve 1979;2:84–100.

98. Engel AG, Angelini C, Gomez MR. Fingerprint body myopathy. Mayo Clin Proc 1972;47:377–388.

99. Kinoshita M, Satoyoshi E, Kumagai M. Familial type 1 fiber atrophy. J Neurol Sci 1975;25:11.

100. Cancilla PA, Kalyanaraman K, Verity MA, et al. Familial myopathy with probable lysis of myofibrils of type I fibers. Neurology 1971;21:579–585.

101. Jerusalem F, Engel AG, Gomez MR. Sarcotubular myopathy: A newly recognized, benign, congenital, familial muscle disease. Neurology 1973;23:897–906.

102. Engel WK. The essentiality of histo- and cytochemical studies of skeletal muscle in the investigation of neuromuscular disease. Neurology 1962;12:778–794.

103. Lake BD, Wilson J. Zebra body myopathy: Clinical, histochemical and ultrastructural studies. J Neurol Sci 1975;24:437–446.

104. Griggs RC, Mendell JR, Miller RG. Evaluation and Treatment of Myopathies. Philadelphia: FA Davis, 1995.

105. Ringel SP, Neville HE, Duster MC, et al. A new congenital neuromuscular disease with trilaminar fibers. Neurology 1978;28:282–289.

106. Tomé FMS, Fardeau M. Congenital myopathy with "reducing bodies" in muscle fibers. Acta Neuropathol 1975;31:207–217.

107. Mace JW, Sponaugle HD, Mitsunaga RY, et al. Congenital hereditary nonprogressive external ophthalmoplegia. Am J Dis Child 1971;122:261–263.

108. Karpati G, Carpenter S, Andermann F. A new concept of childhood nemaline myopathy. Arch Neurol 1971;24:291–304.

109. Sarnat HB. Developmental disorders of muscle. In: Mastaglia FL, Walton J, eds. Skeletal Muscle Pathology. Edinburgh: Churchill Livingstone, 1982:140.

110. Berard-Badier M, Pellissier JF, Toga M, et al. Ultrastructural studies of extraocular muscles in ocular motility disorders. II. Morphological analysis of 38 biopsies. Graefes Arch Klin Exp Ophthalmol 1978;208:193–205.

111. Dubowitz V. The muscular dystrophies: Clarity or chaos? N Engl J Med 1997; 336:650–651.

112. Duchenne GB. Recherches sur la paralysie musculaire pseudohypertrophique ou paralysie myosclésée. Arch Gen Med 1868;11:5, 178, 305, 421, 552.

113. Becker PE, Kiener F. Eine neue X-chromosomale muskeldystrophie. Arch Psychiatr Nervenkr 1955;193:427–448.

114. Matsumura K, Campbell KP. Dystrophinglycoprotein complex: Its role in the molecular pathogenesis of muscular dystrophies. Muscle Nerve 1994;17:2–15.

115. Duggan DJ, Gorospe JR, Fanin M, et al. Mutations in the sarcoglycan genes in patients with myopathy. N Engl J Med 1997;336:618–624.

116. Philpot J, Sewry C, Pennock J, et al. Clinical phenotype in congenital muscular dystrophy: Correlation with expression of merosin in skeletal muscle. Neuromusc Disord 1995;5:301–305.
117. Leyden E. Klinik der Rückenmarks Krankheiten. Berlin: Hirchwald, 1876.
118. Möbius PJ. Über die hereditaren nervenkrankheiten. Samm Klin Vort 1879;171:1505.
119. Landouzy L, Déjérine J. De la myopathie atrophique progressive (myopathie hereditaire), débutant, dans l'enfance, par le face, sans alteration du système nerveux. Comptes Rendus Hebd Seances Acad Sci 1884;98:53–55.
120. Welander L. Myopathia distalis tarda hereditaria. Acta Med Scand 1951;141(Suppl 264):1–124.
121. Miyoshi K, Iwasa M, Kawa H, et al. Autosomalrecessive distal muscular dystrophy: A new type of distal muscular dystrophy observed characteristically in Japan. Nippon Rinsho 1977;35:3922–3928.
122. Fukuyama Y, Kawazura M, Haruna H. A peculiar form of congenital progressive muscular dystrophy: Report of 15 cases. Paediatr Univers Tokyo 1960;4:5.
123. Yoshioka M, Kuroki S, Kondo T. Ocular manifestations in Fukuyama-type congenital muscular dystrophy. Brain Dev 1990;12:423–426.
124. Santavuori P, Leisti J, Kruus S. Muscle, eye and brain disease: A new syndrome. Neuropadiatrie 1977;8(Suppl):553–558.
125. Santavuori P, Somer H, Sainio K, et al. Muscle eye brain disease (MEB). Brain Dev 1989;11:147–153.
126. Walker AE. Lissencephaly. Arch Neurol Psychiatr 1942;48:13–29.
127. Steinert H. Über das klinische und anatomische bild des muskelschwundes der myotoniker. Dtsch Z Nervenheilkd 1909;37:38–104.
128. Ricker K, Koch MC, Lehmann-Horn F, et al. Proximal myotonic myopathy: A new dominant disorder with myotonia, muscle weakness, and cataracts. Neurology 1994;44:1448–1452.
129. Thornton CA, Griggs RC, Moxley RT III. Myotonic dystrophy with no trinucleotide repeat expansion. Ann Neurol 1994;35:269–272.
130. Taylor EW. Progressive vagus-glossopharyngeal paralysis with ptosis: Contribution to group of family diseases. J Nerv Ment Dis 1915;42:129–139.
131. Victor M, Hayes R, Adams RD. Oculopharyngeal muscular dystrophy: A familial disease of late life characterized by dysphagia and progressive ptosis of the eyelids. N Engl J Med 1962;267:1267–1273.
132. Mastaglia FL, Walton J. Skeletal Muscle Pathology. Edinburgh: Churchill Livingstone, 1982.
133. Brooke MH. A Clinician's View of Neuromuscular Diseases. 2nd ed. Baltimore: Williams & Wilkins, 1986.
134. Swash M, Schwartz MS. Neuromuscular Diseases: A Practical Approach to Diagnosis and Management. 2nd ed. New York: Springer Verlag, 1988.
135. Dubowitz V. Muscle Disorders in Childhood. Philadelphia: WB Saunders, 1995.
136. Howard R. A case of congenital defect of the muscular system (dystrophica muscularis congenita) and its association with congenital talipes equinovarus. Proc R Soc Med 1908;1:157–166.
137. Rospide HAD, Vincent O, Gaudin ES, et al. Distrofia muscular congenita pura. Acta Neurol Latinoam 1972;18:20.
138. Donner M, Rapola J, Somer H. Congenital muscular dystrophy: A clinicopathological and followup study of 15 patients. Neuropaediatrie 1975;6:239–258.
139. Helbling-Leclerc A, Zhang X, Topaloglu H, et al. Mutations in the laminin 2 chain gene (LAMA2) cause merosin-deficient congenital muscular dystrophy. Nat Genet 1995;11:216–218.
140. Campbell KP. Three muscular dystrophies: Loss of cytoskeleton-extracellular matrix linkage. Cell 1995;80:675–679.
141. Fukuyama Y, Osawa M, Suzuki H. Congenital progressive muscular dystrophy of Fukuyama type: Clinical, genetic and pathological considerations. Brain Dev 1981;3:1–29.
142. Pihko H, Lappi M, Raitta C, et al. Ocular findings in muscle eye brain disease: A follow-up study. Brain Dev 1995;17:57–61.
143. Warburg M. The heterogeneity of microphthalmia in the mentally retarded. Birth Defects 1971;7:136–154.
144. Kobayashi K, Nakahori Y, Miyake M, et al. An ancient retrotransposal insertion causes Fukuyama-type congenital muscular dystrophy. Nature 1998;394:388–392.
145. Yoshida A, Kobayashi K, Manya H, et al. Muscular dystrophy and neuronal migration disorder caused by mutations in a glycosyltransferase, POMGnT1. Dev Cell 2001;1:717–724.
146. Beltran-Valero dB, Currier S, Steinbrecher A, et al. Mutations in the O-mannosyltransferase gene POMT1 give rise to the severe neuronal migration disorder Walker-Warburg syndrome. Am J Hum Genet 2002;71:1033–1043.
147. Haltia M, Leivo I, Somer H, et al. Muscle-eye-brain disease: A neuropathological study. Ann Neurol 1997;41:173–180.
148. Aravind L, Koonin EV. The fukutin protein family—predicted enzymes modifying cell-surface molecules. Curr Biol 1999;9:R836–R837.
149. Toda T, Segawa M, Nomura Y, et al. Localization of the gene for Fukuyama-type congenital muscular dystrophy to chromosome 9q3133. Nat Genet 1994;5:283–286.
150. Dubowitz V. Workshop report: 22nd ENMC-Sponsored Workshop on Congenital Muscular Dystrophy held in Baarn, The Netherlands, May 14–16, 1993. Neuromuscul Disord 1993;4:75–81.
151. Honda Y, Yoshioka M. Ophthalmological findings of muscular dystrophies: A survey of 53 cases. J Pediatr Ophthalmol Strabismus 1978;15:236–238.
152. Chijiiwa T, Nishimura M, Inomata H, et al. Ocular manifestations of congenital muscular dystrophy (Fukuyama type). Ann Ophthalmol 1983;15:921–928.
153. Weinstein JM, Sassani JW, Towfigi J. A floppy infant with ocular abnormalities. Presented at the 16th Annual Frank B. Walsh Society Meeting, Cleveland, Feb. 24, 1984.
154. Williams RS, Swishet CN, Jennings M, et al. Cerebro-ocular dysgenesis (Walker-Warburg Syndrome): Neuropathological and etiological analysis. Neurology 1984;34:1531–1541.
155. Dobyns W, Kirkpatrick JB, Hittner HM, et al. Syndromes with lissencephaly II. Walker-Warburg and cerebro-oculo-muscular syndromes and a new syndrome with type II lissencephaly. Am J Med Genet 1985;22:157–195.
156. Warburg M. Ocular malformations and lissencephaly. Eur J Pediatr 1987;146:450–452.
157. Hayashi YK, Koga R, Tsukahara T, et al. Deficiency of laminin alpha 2 chain mRNA in muscle in a patient with merosin-negative congenital muscular dystrophy. Muscle Nerve 1995;18:1027–1030.
158. Brook JD, McCurrach ME, Harley HG, et al. Molecular basis of myotonic dystrophy: Expansion of a trinucleotide (CTG) repeat at the 3′ end of a transcript encoding a protein kinase family member. Cell 1992;68:799–808.
159. Fu YH, Pizzuti A, Fenwick RJ Jr. An unstable triplet repeat in a gene related to myotonic muscular dystrophy. Science 1992;255:1256–1258.
160. Tsilfidis C, MacKenzie AE, Mettler G, et al. Correlation between CTG trinucleotide repeat length and frequency of severe congenital myotonic dystrophy. Nat Genet 1992;1:192–195.
161. Harley HG, Rundle SA, MacMillan JC, et al. Size of the unstable CTG repeat sequence in relation to phenotype and parental transmission in myotonic dystrophy. Am J Hum Genet 1993;52:1164–1174.
162. Redman JB, Fenwick RG, Fu YH, et al. Relationship between parental trinucleotide CTG repeat length and severity of myotonic dystrophy in offspring. JAMA 1993;269:1960–1965.
163. Liquori CL, Ricker K, Moseley ML, et al. Myotonic dystrophy type 2 caused by a CCTG expansion in intron 1 of ZNF9. Science 2001;293:864–867.
164. Klein D. La dystrophie myotonique (Steinert) et la myotonie congénitale (Thomsen) en Suisse: Etude clinique, génétique et démographique. J Genet Hum 1958;7(Suppl):1.
165. Grimm T. The ages at onset and at death in dystrophia myotonica. J Genet Hum 1975;23(Suppl):172.
166. Moxley RT III. Myotonic disorders in childhood: Diagnosis and treatment. J Child Neurol 1997;12:116–129.
167. Dodge PR, Gamstorp I, Byers RK, et al. Myotonic dystrophy in infancy and childhood. Pediatrics 1965;35:3–19.
168. Harper PS. Myotonic Dystrophy. Philadelphia: WB Saunders, 1979.
169. Harper PS, Rüdel R. Myotonic dystrophy. In: Engel AG, Franzini-Armstrong C, eds. Myology. 2nd ed. New York: McGraw-Hill, 1994:1192.
170. Motta J, Guilleminault C, Billingham M, et al. Cardiac abnormalities in myotonic dystrophy: Electrophysiologic and histopathologic studies. Am J Med 1979;67:467–473.
171. Griggs RC. Cardiac conduction in myotonic dystrophy. Am J Med 1975;59:37–42.
172. Fisch C, Evans PV. The heart in dystrophia myotonica: Report of an autopsied case. N Engl J Med 1954;251:527–529.
173. Adie WJ, Greenfield JG. Dystrophica myotonica (myotonia atrophica). Brain 1923;46:73–127.
174. Refsum S, Engeset A, Lönnum A. Pneumoencephalographic changes in dystrophia myotonica. Acta Neurol Psychiatr Scand 1959;137(Suppl):98–99.
175. Damian MS, Bachmann G, Herrmann D, et al. Magnetic resonance imaging of muscle and brain in myotonic dystrophy. J Neurol 1993;240:8–12.
176. Abe K, Fujimora H, Toyooka K, et al. Involvement of the central nervous system in myotonic dystrophy. J Neurol Sci 1994;127:179–185.
177. Miaux Y, Chiras J, Eymard B, et al. Cranial MRI findings in myotonic dystrophy. Neuroradiology 1997;39:166–170.
178. Batten FE, Gibb HP. Myotonia atrophica. Brain 1909;32:187–205.
179. Bird TD, Follett C, Griep E. Cognitive and personality function in myotonic muscular dystrophy. J Neurol Neurosurg Psychiatry 1983;46:971–980.
180. Caughey JE, Myrianthopoulos NC. Dystrophia Myotonica and Related Disorders. Springfield, IL: Charles C Thomas, 1963.
181. Hughes DTD, Swann J, Gleeson JA, et al. Abnormalities in swallowing associated with dystrophia myotonica. Brain 1965;88:1037–1042.
182. Siegel CI, Hendrix TR, Harvey JC. The swallowing disorder in myotonic dystrophy. Gastroenterology 1966;50:541–550.
183. Harvey JC, Sherbourne DH, Siegel CI. Smooth muscle involvement in myotonic dystrophy. Am J Med 1965;39:81–90.
184. Shore RN. Myotonic dystrophy: Hazards of pregnancy and infancy. Dev Med Child Neurol 1975;17:356–361.
185. Clarke BG, Shapiro S, Monroe RG. Myotonia atrophica with testicular atrophy: Urinary excretion of interstitial cellstimulating (luteinizing) hormone, androgens and 17-ketosteroids. J Clin Endocrinol 1956;16:1235–1244.
186. Buscaino GA, Sanna G. Ghiandole endocrine e distrofia miotonica: Revisione critica su oltre 700 casi. Acta Neurol 1963;18:357–372.

187. Drucker WD, Rowland LP, Sterling K, et al. On the function of the endocrine glands in myotonic muscular dystrophy. Am J Med 1961;31:941–950.

188. Babel J. Ophthalmological Aspects of Myotonic Dystrophy. Neuro-genetics and Neuro-ophthalmology. Amsterdam: Elsevier/North Holland, 1981:19.

189. Cohen MM, Lessell S. Retraction of the lower eyelid. Neurology 1979;29: 386–389.

190. Verrey F. Myotonie dystrophique (maladie de Steinert) avec altèration maculaire dègenèrative. Ophthalmologica 1947;114:281–284.

191. Burian HM, Burns CA. Ocular changes in myotonic dystrophy. Am J Ophthalmol 1967;63:22–24.

192. Walsh FB, Hoyt WF. Clinical Neuro-Ophthalmology. 3rd ed. Baltimore: Williams & Wilkins, 1969:1273.

193. Baloh RW, Konrad HR, Sills AW, et al. The saccade velocity test. Neurology 1975;25:1071–1076.

194. Verhagen WIM, Ter Bruggen JP, Huygen PLM. Oculomotor, auditory, and vestibular responses in myotonic dystrophy. Arch Neurol 1992;49:954–969.

195. AzuaraBlanco A, Katz LJ, Arkfeld DF, et al. Myotonic dystrophy mimicking bilateral internuclear ophthalmoplegia. Neuroophthalmology 1997;17:11–14.

196. Miller NR. Walsh and Hoyt's Clinical Neuro-Ophthalmology. 4th ed. Baltimore: Williams & Wilkins, 1985:797.

197. Vos TA. Twenty-five years of dystrophia myotonica. Ophthalmologica 1961; 141:37–45.

198. Walsh FB, Hoyt WF. Clinical Neuro-Ophthalmology. 3rd ed. Baltimore: Williams & Wilkins, 1969:1271.

199. Vogt A. Die cataract bei myotonischer dystrophie. Schweiz Med Wochenschr 1921;2:669–674.

200. Fleischer B. Über myotonische dystrophy mit katarakt. Albrecht von Graefes Arch Klin Exp Ophthalmol 1918;96:91–133.

201. Birnbacher T. Hornhautepithelveränderungen bei einem fall von myotoner dystrophie. Z Augenheilkd 1927;62:44–48.

202. Maillard S. Ein fall von degenerativer hornhautveränderung bei myotoniekatarakt. Klin Monatsbl Augenheilkd 1926;77:647–649.

203. Verbiest H. Observation sur le mécanism de la convergence myotonique dans un cas de la maladie de Steinert. Rev Neurol (Paris) 1937;67:387–390.

204. Thompson HS, van Allen MW, von Noorden GK. The pupil in myotonic dystrophy. Invest Ophthalmol 1964;3:325–338.

205. Cobb B. Vascular tufts at the pupillary margin: A preliminary report on 44 patients. Trans Ophthalmol Soc UK 1968;88:211–221.

206. Stern LZ, Cross HE, Crebo AR. Abnormal iris vasculature in myotonic dystrophy: An anterior segment angiographic study. Arch Neurol 1978;35:224–227.

207. Mason GI. Iris neovascular tufts: Relationship to rubeosis, insulin, and hypotony. Arch Ophthalmol 1979;97:2346–2352.

208. Moxley RT, Corbett AJ, Minaker KL, et al. Whole body insulin resistance in myotonic dystrophy. Ann Neurol 1984;15:157–162.

209. Hayasaka S, Kiyosawa M, Katsumata S, et al. Ciliary and retinal changes in myotonic dystrophy. Arch Ophthalmol 1984;102:88–93.

210. Slatt B. Myotonia dystrophia: A review of 17 cases. Can Med Assoc J 1961; 85:250–261.

211. Betten MG, Bilchik RC, Smith ME. Pigmentary retinopathy of myotonic dystrophy. Am J Ophthalmol 1971;72:720–723.

212. Raitta C, Karli P. Ocular findings in myotonic dystrophy. Ann Ophthalmol 1982; 14:647–650.

213. Stanescu-Segal B. Rétinopathie de l'ophtalmoplégie plus. J Fr Ophtalmol 1983; 6:537.

214. Babel J, Tsacopoulos M. Les lésions rétiniennes de la dystrophie myotonique: Étude histologique. Ann Ocul 1970;203:1049–1065.

215. Houber JP, Babel J. Les lésions uvéorétiniennes de la dystrophie myotonique: Étude histologique. Ann Oculist 1970;203:1067–1076.

216. Gott PS, Karnaze DS, Keane JR. Abnormal visual evoked potentials in myotonic dystrophy. Neurology 1983;33:1622–1625.

217. Kirkham TH, Coupland SG. Myotonic dystrophy: Normal electroretinal function associated with visual-evoked potential abnormalities. In: Huber A, Klein D, eds. Neuro-genetics and Neuro-ophthalmology. Amsterdam: Elsevier/North-Holland, 1981:51.

218. Brand I. Intraokuläre hypotonie bei myotonikern. Ophthalmologica 1955;129: 81–88.

219. Van Dyk HJL, Swan KC. The cataract patient with myotonic dystrophy. Trans Am Acad Ophthalmol Otolaryngol 1967;71:838–846.

220. Junge J. Ocular changes in dystrophia myotonica, paramyotonia and myotonia congenita. Doc Ophthalmol 1966;21:1–115.

221. Ginsberg J, Hamblet J, Menefee M. Ocular abnormality in myotonic dystrophy. Ann Ophthalmol 1978;10:1021–1028.

222. Ketelsen UP, Schmidt D, Beckmann R, et al. Kearns-Sayre syndrome: Primarily a mitochondriopathy? Dev Ophthalmol 1982;6:118–137.

223. Kuwabara T, Lessell S. Electron microscopic study of extraocular muscles in myotonic dystrophy. Am J Ophthalmol 1976;82:303–309.

224. Eshaghian J, March WF, Goossens W, et al. Ultrastructure of cataract in myotonic dystrophy. Invest Ophthalmol Vis Sci 1978;17:289–293.

225. Trelles JO, Gutierrez C, Aranibar A, et al. Estudio anatomoclinico de la enfermedad de Steinert. Rev Neuropsiquiatr 1956;19:139–204.

226. Burns CA. Ocular histopathology of myotonic dystrophy. Am J Ophthalmol 1969;68:416–422.

227. Manschot WA. Histological findings in a case of dystrophica myotonica. Ophthalmologica 1968;155:294–296.

228. Shelbourne P, Davies J, Buxton J, et al. Direct diagnosis of myotonic dystrophy with a disease-specific DNA marker. N Engl J Med 1993;328:471–475.

229. Murphy SF, Drachman DB. The oculopharyngeal syndrome. JAMA 1968;203: 1003–1008.

230. Hayes R, London W, Seidman J, et al. Oculopharyngeal muscular dystrophy. N Engl J Med 1963;268:163.

231. Bray GM, Kaarsoo M, Ross RT. Ocular myopathy with dysphagia. Neurology 1965;15:678–684.

232. Johnson CC, Kuwabara T. Oculopharyngeal muscular dystrophy. Am J Ophthalmol 1974;77:872–879.

233. Montgomery WW, Lynch JP. Oculopharyngeal muscular dystrophy treated by inferior constrictor myotomy. Trans Am Acad Ophthalmol Otolaryngol 1971; 75:986–993.

234. Brais B, Xie YG, Sanson M, et al. The oculopharyngeal muscular dystrophy locus maps to the region of the cardiac c and b myosin heavy chain genes on chromosome 14q11.2q13. Hum Mol Genet 1995;4:429–434.

235. Brais B, Bouchard JP, Xie YG, et al. Short GCG expansions in the PABP2 gene cause oculopharyngeal muscular dystrophy. Nat Genet 1998;18:164–167.

236. Tomé FMS, Fardeau M. Nuclear inclusions in oculopharyngeal dystrophy. Acta Neuropathol 1980;49:85–87.

237. Calado A, Tome FM, Brais B, et al. Nuclear inclusions in oculopharyngeal muscular dystrophy consist of poly(A) binding protein 2 aggregates which sequester poly(A) RNA. Hum Mol Genet 2000;9:2321–2328.

238. Tomé FMS, Chateau D, Helbling-Leclerc A, et al. Morphological changes in muscle fibers in oculopharyngeal muscular dystrophy. Neuromuscul Disord 1997;7(Suppl 1):S63–S69.

239. Trojanowski JQ, Lee VM. The role of tau in Alzheimer's disease. Med Clin North Am 2002;86:615–627.

240. Little BW, Perl DP. Oculopharyngeal muscular dystrophy: An autopsied case from French-Canadian kindred. J Neurol Sci 1982;53:145–158.

241. Dubowitz V, Brooke MH. Muscle biopsy: A modern approach. Major Problems in Neurology. Vol 2. Philadelphia: WB Saunders, 1973:231.

242. Satoyoshi E, Kinoshita M. Oculopharyngodistal myopathy: Report of four families. Arch Neurol 1977;34:89–92.

243. Schotland DL, Rowland LP. Muscular dystrophy. Arch Neurol 1964;10: 433–445.

244. Thomsen J. Tonische krämpfe in willkürlich beweglichen muskeln in folgre von vererbter psychischer disposition (ataxia muscularis). Arch Psychiatr 1876;6: 702–718.

245. Becker PE. Die Heterogenei der Myotonien. Amsterdam: Excerpta Medica, 1961:1547.

246. Becker PE. Genetic approaches to the nosology of muscle disease: Myotonias and similar diseases. In: Bergsma D, ed. The Clinical Delineation of Birth Defects—Part VII, Muscle. Baltimore: Williams & Wilkins, 1971:52.

247. Eulenburg A. Über eine familiare, durch 6 generationen verfolgbare form congenitaler paramyotonie. Neurol Zentralbl 1886;5:265–272.

248. Holtzapple GE. Periodic paralysis. JAMA 1905;45:1224–1231.

249. Gamstorp I. Adynamia episodica hereditaria. Acta Paediatr Scand 1956;45(Suppl 108):1–126.

250. Curschmann H. Über familiäre atrophische myotonie. Dtsch Z Nervenheilkd 1912;45:161–202.

251. Schwartz O, Jampel RS. Congenital blepharophimosis associated with a unique generalized myopathy. Arch Ophthalmol 1962;68:52–57.

252. Aberfeld DC, Hinterbuchner LP, Schneider M. Myotonia, dwarfism, diffuse bone disease and unusual ocular and facial abnormalities (a new syndrome). Brain 1965;88:313–322.

253. Koch M, Steinmeyer K, Lorenz C, et al. The skeletal muscle chloride channel in dominant and recessive human myotonia. Science 1992;257:797–800.

254. George AL, Crackower MA, Abdalla JA, et al. Molecular basis of Thomsen's disease (autosomal dominant myotonia congenita). Nature Gen 1993;3:305–310.

255. Rüdel R, Lehmann-Horn F, Ricker K. Altered excitability of the muscle cell membrane. In: Engel AL, FranziniArmstrong C, eds. Myology. 2nd ed. McGraw-Hill, 1994:1291.

256. Ptacek LJ, Trimmer JS, Agnew WS, et al. Paramyotonia congenita and hyperkalemic periodic paralysis map to the same sodium channel gene locus. Am J Hum Genet 1991;49:851–854.

257. McClatchey AI, MckennaYasek D, Cros D, et al. Novel mutations in families with unusual and variable disorders of the skeletal muscle sodium channel. Nat Genet 1992;2:148–152.

258. Riggs JE, Schochet SS, Fakadej AV, et al. Mitochondrial encephalomyopathy with decreased succinate/cytochrome c reductase activity. Neurology 1984;34: 48.

259. Tomé FMS. Periodic paralysis and electrolyte disorders. In: Mastaglia FL, Walton J, eds. Skeletal Muscle Pathology. Edinburgh: Churchill Livingstone, 1982: 287.

260. Odor DL, Patel AN, Pearce LA. Familial hypokalemic periodic paralysis with

permanent myopathy: A clinical and ultrastructural study. J Neuropathol Exp Neurol 1967;26:98–114.

261. Jurkat-Rott K, Lehmann-Horn F, Elbaz A, et al. A calcium channel mutation causing hypokalemic periodic paralysis. Hum Mol Genet 1994;3:1415–1419.

262. Ptacek LJ, Tawil R, Griggs RC, et al. Dihydropyridine receptor mutations cause hypokalemic periodic paralysis. Cell 1994;77:863–868.

263. Pearson CM. The periodic paralyses: Differential features and pathological observations in permanent myopathic weakness. Brain 1964;87:341–354.

264. Resnick JS, Engel WK. Myotonic lid lag in hypokalemic periodic paralysis. J Neurol Neurosurg Psychiatry 1967;30:47–51.

265. McManis PG, Lambert EH, Daube JR. The exercise test in periodic paralysis. Muscle Nerve 1986;9:704–710.

266. Fontaine B, Khurana TS, Hoffman EP, et al. Hyperkalemic periodic paralysis and the adult muscle sodium channel asubunit gene. Science 1990;250:1000–1002.

267. Ptacek LJ, George AL, Griggs RC, et al. Identification of a mutation in the gene causing hyperkalemic periodic paralysis. Cell 1991;67:1021–1027.

268. McArdle B. Adynamia episodica hereditaria and its treatment. Brain 1962;85:121–148.

269. Fowler WM, Layzer RB, Taylor RG, et al. The Schwartz-Jampel syndrome: Its clinical, physiological and histologic expression. J Neurol Sci 1974;22:127–146.

270. Nicole S, Ben Hamida C, Beighton P, et al. Localization of the Schwartz-Jampel syndrome (SJS) locus to chromosome 1p34–p36.1 by homozygosity. Hum Mol Genet 1995;4:1633–1636.

271. Arikawa-Hirasawa E, Le AH, Nishino I, et al. Structural and functional mutations of the perlecan gene cause Schwartz-Jampel syndrome, with myotonic myopathy and chondrodysplasia. Am J Hum Genet 2002;70:1368–1375.

272. Arikawa-Hirasawa E, Rossi SG, Rotundo RL, et al. Absence of acetylcholinesterase at the neuromuscular junctions of perlecan-null mice. Nat Neurosci 2002;5:119–123.

273. Salpeter MM. Electron microscope radioautography as a quantitative tool in enzyme cytochemistry. I. The distribution of acetylcholinesterase at motor end plates of a vertebrate twitch muscle. J Cell Biol 1967;32:379–389.

274. Petty RK, Harding AE, Morgan-Hughes JA. The clinical features of mitochondrial myopathy. Brain 1986;109:915–938.

275. DiMauro, S. Lessons from mitochondrial DNA mutations. Cell Dev Biol 2001:9:397–405.

276. DiMauro S, Schon EA. Mitochondrial respiratory-chain diseases. N Engl J Med 2003;348:2656–2668.

277. Engel WK, Cunningham GG. Rapid examination of muscle tissue: An improved trichrome method for rapid diagnosis of muscle biopsy fresh frozen section. Neurology 1963;13:919–923.

278. Engel WK. Muscle biopsies in neuromuscular diseases. Pediatr Clin North Am 1967;14:963–995.

279. Mölbert E, Doden W. Chronisch progressive oculäre muskeldystrophie im elektronenmikroskopischen. Ber Dtsch Ophthalmol Ges 1959;62:392–397.

280. Karpati G, Carpenter S, Larbrisseau, et al. The Kearns-Sayre syndrome: A multisystem disease with mitochondrial abnormality demonstrated in skeletal muscle and skin. J Neurol Sci 1973;19:133–151.

281. Leveille AS, Newell FW. Autosomal dominant Kearns-Sayre syndrome. Ophthalmology 1980;87:99–108.

282. Rowland LP, Blake DM, Hirano M, et al. Clinical syndromes associated with ragged red fibers. Rev Neurol (Paris) 1991;147:467–473.

283. Schotland DL, DiMauro S, Bonilla E, et al. Neuromuscular disorder associated with a defect in mitochondrial energy supply. Arch Neurol 1976;33:475–479.

284. Eshaghian J, Anderson RL, Weingeist TA, et al. Orbicularis oculi muscle in chronic progressive external ophthalmoplegia. Arch Ophthalmol 1980;98:1070–1073.

285. Ringel SP, Wilson WB, Barden MT. Extraocular muscle biopsy in chronic progressive external ophthalmoplegia. Ann Neurol 1979;6:326–339.

286. Gonatas NK, Evangelista I, Martin J. A generalised disorder of nervous system, skeletal muscle and heart resembling Refsum's disease and Hurler's syndrome. II. Ultrastructure. Am J Med 1967;42:169–178.

287. Schneck L, Adachi M, Briet P, et al. Ophthalmoplegia plus with morphological and chemical studies of cerebellar and muscle tissue. J Neurol Sci 1973;19:37–44.

288. Harding AE, Sanders MD, Petty RKH, et al. The neuro-ophthalmological features of mitochondrial myopathy. Presented at the Fifth Meeting of the International Neuro-Ophthalmology Society, Antwerp, Belgium, May 14–18, 1984.

289. Drachman DA. Ophthalmoplegia plus: A classification of the disorders associated with progressive external ophthalmoplegia. In: Vinken PJ, Bruyn GW, eds. Handbook of Clinical Neurology. Vol 22. New York: American Elsevier, 1975:203.

290. Rowland LP. Progressive external ophthalmoplegia. In: Vinken PJ, Bruyn GW, eds. Handbook of Clinical Neurology, Vol 22. New York: American Elsevier, 1975:177.

291. Danta G, Hilton RC, Lynch PG. Chronic progressive external ophthalmoplegia. Brain 1975;98:473–492.

292. Kamieniecka Z, Sjo O. Mitochondrial myopathy as a cause of ptosis and ophthalmoplegia in elderly females. Acta Ophthalmol 1984;62:401–412.

293. Kosmorsky G, Johns DR. Neuroophthalmologic manifestations of mitochondrial DNA disorders: Chronic progressive external ophthalmoplegia, Kearns-Sayre syndrome, and Leber's hereditary optic neuropathy. Neurol Clin 1991;9:147–161.

294. Walsh FB, Hoyt WF. Clinical Neuro-Ophthalmology. 3rd ed. Baltimore: Williams & Wilkins, 1969:1256.

295. Bing R, Haymaker W. Compendium of Regional Diagnosis in Lesions of the Brain and Spinal Cord. 11th ed. St Louis: Mosby, 1940.

296. Blodi FC, van Allen MW. Electromyographic studies in some neuro-ophthalmologic disorders. XVIII Concil Ophthalmol Belg 1958;1:1621–1627.

297. Blodi FC. Electromyographic evidence for supranuclear gaze palsies. Trans Ophthalmol Soc UK 1970;90:451–469.

298. Koerner F, Schlote W. Chronic progressive external ophthalmoplegia: Association with retinal pigmentary changes and evidence in favor of ocular myopathy. Arch Ophthalmol 1972;88:155–166.

299. Metz HS, Meshel L. Ocular saccades in progressive external ophthalmoplegia. Ann Neurol 1974;6:623–628.

300. Sorkin JA, Shoffner JM, Grossniklaus HE, et al. Strabismus and mitochondrial defects in chronic progressive external ophthalmoplegia. Am J Ophthalmol 1997;123:235–242.

301. Brown MD, Wallace DC. Molecular basis of mitochondrial DNA disease. J Bioenerg Biomembr 1994;26:273–289.

302. Wallace DK, Sprunger DT, Helveston EM, et al. Surgical management of strabismus associated with chronic progressive external ophthalmoplegia. Ophthalmology 1997;104:695–700.

303. Lane CM, Collin JRO. Treatment of ptosis in chronic progressive external ophthalmoplegia. Br J Ophthalmol 1987;71:290–294.

304. Shorr N, Goldberg RA. Management of ptosis in chronic progressive external ophthalmoplegia. Ophthalmic Plast Reconstr Surg 1987;3:141–145.

305. Kearns TP, Sayre GP. Retinitis pigmentosa, external ophthalmoplegia, and complete heart block. Arch Ophthalmol 1958;60:280–289.

306. Kearns TP. External ophthalmoplegia, pigmentary degeneration of the retina, and cardiomyopathy: A newly recognized syndrome. Trans Am Ophthalmol Soc 1965;63:559–625.

307. Berenberg RA, Pellock JM, DiMauro S, et al. Lumping or splitting? ''Ophthalmoplegia plus'' or Kearns-Sayre syndrome? Ann Neurol 1977;1:37–54.

308. Bastiaensen LAK. Chronic Progressive External Ophthalmoplegia. Winchester, MA: Sijthoff-Noordoff, 1978.

309. Bastiaensen LAK, Frenken CWGM, ter Laak HJ, et al. Kearns syndrome: A heterogeneous group of disorders with CPEO, or a nosological entity? Doc Ophthalmol 1982;52:207–225.

310. Bastiaensen LAK, Notermans SLH, Ramaekers CH, et al. Kearns syndrome or Kearns disease: Further evidence of a genuine entity in a case with uncommon features. Ophthalmologica 1982;184:40–50.

311. Reichmann H, Degoul F, Gold R, et al. Histological, enzymatic and mitochondrial DNA studies in patients with Kearns-Sayre syndrome and chronic progressive external ophthalmoplegia. Eur Neurol 1991;31:108–113.

312. Deutman AF. Rod-cone dystrophy: Primary, hereditary pigmentary retinopathy, retinitis pigmentosa. In: Krill AE, Archer DB, eds. Krill's Hereditary Retinal and Choroidal Diseases. Vol 2. Hagerstown, MD: Harper & Row, 1977:479.

313. Carr RE. Primary retinal degenerations. In: Duane TD, ed. Clinical Ophthalmology. Vol 3, Chap 24. Hagerstown, MD: Harper & Row, 1980.

314. Herzberg NH, van Schooneveld MJ, Bleeker-Wagemakers EM, et al. Kearns Sayre syndrome with a phenocopy of choroideremia instead of pigmentary retinopathy. Neurology 1993;43:218–221.

315. Metz HS, Cohen M. Progressive external ophthalmoplegia. Ann Ophthalmol 1973;5:775–778.

316. Mullie MA, Harding AE, Petty RK, et al. The retinal manifestations of mitochondrial myopathy. A study of 22 cases. Arch Ophthalmol 1985;103:1825–1830.

317. Seah ABH, Newman, NJ. Mitochondrial Diseases. In: Heckenlively JR, Arden GB, eds. Principles and Practice of Clinical Electrophysiology of Vision. 2nd ed. Boston: MIT Press.

318. Thorson JC, Bell WE. Progressive dystrophic external ophthalmoplegia with abiotrophic fundus changes. Arch Ophthalmol 1959;62:833–838.

319. Jampel RS. Ophthalmoplegia and retinal degeneration associated with spinocerebellar ataxia. Arch Ophthalmol 1961;66:247–259.

320. Drachman DA. Ophthalmoplegia plus: The neurodegenerative disorders associated with progressive external ophthalmoplegia. Arch Neurol 1968;18:654–674.

321. Trobe JD, Watson RT. Retinal degeneration without pigment alterations in progressive external ophthalmoplegia. Am J Ophthalmol 1977;83:372–376.

322. Eagle RC Jr, Hedges TR, Yanoff M. The atypical pigmentary retinopathy of Kearns-Sayre syndrome: A light and electron microscopic study. Ophthalmology 1982;89:1433–1440.

323. Eagle RC Jr, Hedges TR, Yanoff M. The Kearns-Sayre syndrome: A light and electron microscopic study. Trans Am Ophthalmol Soc 1982;80:218–234.

324. Newell FW, Polascik MA. Mitochondrial disease and retinal pigmentary degeneration. Council Ophthalmol 1979;1:615–617.

325. Daniele S, Corea L. The cardiac involvement in chronic progressive external ophthalmoplegia: Consideration on the Kearns-Sayre syndrome. Albrecht von Graefes Arch Klin Exp Ophthalmol 1981;216:129–133.

326. Darsee JR, Miklozek CL, Heymsfield SB, et al. Mitral valve prolapse and ophthalmoplegia: A progressive, cardioneurologic syndrome. Ann Intern Med 1980;92:735–741.

327. Butler IJ, Gadoth N. Kearns-Sayre syndrome. Arch Intern Med 1976;136:1290–1293.
328. Kosinski C, Mull M, Lethen H, et al. Evidence for cardioembolic stroke in a case of Kearns-Sayre syndrome. Stroke 1995;26:1950–1952.
329. Clark DS, Myerburg RJ, Morales AR, et al. Heart block in Kearns Sayre syndrome. Chest 1975;68:727–730.
330. Carroll JE, Zwillich C, Weil JV, et al. Depressed ventilatory response in oculocraniosomatic neuromuscular disease. Neurology 1976;26:140–146.
331. Tranchant C, Mousson B, Mohr M, et al. Cardiac transplantation in an incomplete Kearns-Sayre syndrome with mitochondrial DNA deletion. Neuromuscul Disord 1993;3:561–566.
332. Kiloh LG, Nevin S. Progressive dystrophy of external ocular muscles (ocular myopathy). Brain 1951;74:115–143.
333. Drachman DA. Ophthalmoplegia plus: The neurodegenerative disorders associated with progressive external ophthalmoplegia. Arch Neurol 1968;18:654–674.
334. Rowland LP. Molecular genetics, pseudogenetics, and clinical neurology. Neurology 1983;33;1179–1195.
335. Nakagawa E, Hirano S, Yamanouchi H, et al. Progressive brainstem and white matter lesions in Kearns-Sayre syndrome: A case report. Brain Dev 1994;16:416–418.
336. Mathews PM, Andermann F, Silver K, et al. Proton MR spectroscopic characterization of differences in regional brain metabolic abnormalities in mitochondrial encephalomyopathies. Neurology 1993;43:2484–2490.
337. Kuwabara T, Watanabe H, Tanaka K, et al. Mitochondrial encephalomyopathy: Elevated visual cortex lactate unresponsive to photic stimulation: A localized 1H-MRS study. Neurology 1994;44:557.
338. Toppet M, Telerman-Toppet N, Szliwowski HB, et al. Oculo-cranio-somatic neuromuscular disease with hypoparathyroidism. Am J Dis Child 1977;131:437–441.
339. Harvey JN, Barnett D. Endocrine dysfunction in Kearns-Sayre syndrome. Clin Endocrinol 1992;37:97–104.
340. Berio A, Piazzi A. Improvement of Kearns-Sayre syndrome with controlled carbohydrate intake and coenzyme Q10 therapy. Ophthalmologica 1994;208:342–343.
341. Anderson S, Bankier AT, Barrell BG, et al. Sequence and organization of the human mitochondrial genome. Nature 1981;290:457–465.
342. Rivner MH, Shamsnia M, Swift TR, et al. Kearns-Sayre syndrome and complex II deficiency. Neurology 1989;39:693–696.
343. Harding AE. Growing old: The most common mitochondrial disease of all? Nat Genet 1992;2:251–252.
344. Barrell BG, Anderson S, Bankier AT, et al. Different pattern of codon recognition by mammalian mitochondrial tRNAs. Proc Natl Acad Sci USA 1980;77:3164–3166.
345. Mita S, Schmidt B, Schon EA, et al. Detection of "deleted" mitochondrial genomes in cytochrome-c oxidase-deficient muscle fibers of a patient with Kearns-Sayre syndrome. Proc Natl Acad Sci USA 1989;86:9509–9513.
346. Nakase H, Moraes CT, Rizzuto R, et al. Transcription and translation of deleted mitochondrial genomes in Kearns-Sayre syndrome: Implications for pathogenesis. Am J Hum Genet 1990;46:418–427.
347. Mancuso M, Filosto M, Bonilla E, et al. Mitochondrial myopathy of childhood associated with mitochondrial DNA depletion and a homozygous mutation (T77M) in the TK2 gene. Arch Neurol 2003;60:1007–1009.
348. Sancho S, Moraes CT, Tanji K, et al. Structural and functional mitochondrial abnormalities associated with high levels of partially deleted mitochondrial DNAs in somatic cell hybrids. Somat Cell Mol Genet 1992;18:431–442.
349. Jeppesen TD, Schwartz M, Olsen DB, et al. Oxidative capacity correlates with muscle mutation load in mitochondrial myopathy. Ann Neurol 2003;54:86–92.
350. Reichmann H. Enzyme activity analyses along ragged-red and normal single muscle fibres. Histochemistry 1992;98:131–134.
351. Collins S, Rudduck C, Marzuki S, et al. Mitochondrial genome distribution in histochemically cytochrome c oxidase-negative muscle fibres in patients with a mixture of deleted and wild-type mitochondrial DNA. Biochim Biophys Acta 1991;1097:309–317.
352. Moraes CT, Sciacco M, Ricci E, et al. Mitochondrial myopathy, mtDNA deletion, Kearns-Sayre syndrome and progressive external ophthalmoplegia. Phenotype-genotype correlations in skeletal muscle of patients with mtDNA deletions. Muscle Nerve 1995;3(Suppl):150–153.
353. Shoubridge EA. Segregation of mitochondrial DNAs carrying a pathogenic point mutation tRNA (leu3243) in cybrid cells. Biochem Biophys Res Commun 1995;213:189–195.
354. Matthews PM, Brown RM, Morten K, et al. Intracellular heteroplasmy for disease-associated point mutations in mtDNA: Implications for disease expression and evidence for mitotic segregation of heteroplasmic units of mtDNA. Hum Genet 1995;96:261–268.
355. Nonaka I. Mitochondrial diseases. Curr Opin Neurol Neurosurg 1992;5:622–632.
356. Shoubridge EA. Mitochondrial DNA diseases: histological and cellular studies. J Bioenerg Biomembr 1994;26:301–310.
357. Kadenbach B, Jarausch J, Hartmann R, et al. Separation of mammalian cytochrome c oxidase into 13 polypeptides by a sodium dodecyl sulfate-gel electrophoretic procedure. Anal Biochem 1983;129:517–521.
358. Petruzzella V, Moraes CT, Sano MC, et al. Extremely high levels of mutant mtDNAs co-localize with cytochrome c oxidase-negative ragged-red fibers in patients harboring a point mutation at nt 3243. Hum Mol Genet 1994;3:449–454.
359. Harding AE, Petty RK, Morgan-Hughes JA. Mitochondrial myopathy: a genetic study of 71 cases. J Med Genet 1988;25:528–535.
360. Giles RE, Blanc H, Cann HM, et al. Maternal inheritance of human mitochondrial DNA. Proc Natl Acad Sci USA 1980;77:6715–6719.
361. Lauber J, Marsac C, Kadenbach B, et al. Mutations in mitochondrial tRNA genes: A frequent cause of neuromuscular diseases. Nucleic Acids Res 1991;19:1393–1397.
362. Zupanc ML, Moraes CT, Shanske S, et al. Deletion of mitochondrial DNA in patients with combined features of Kearns-Sayre and MELAS syndromes. Ann Neurol 1991;29:680–683.
363. Hirano M, Ricci E, Koenigsberger MR, et al. Melas: An original case and clinical criteria for diagnosis. Neuromuscul Disord 1992;2:125–135.
364. Morgan-Hughes JA, Sweeney MG, Cooper JM, et al. Mitochondrial DNA (mtDNA) diseases: Correlation of genotype to phenotype. Biochim Biophys Acta 1995;1271:135–140.
365. Holt IJ, Harding AE, Morgan-Hughes JA. Deletions of muscle mitochondrial DNA in mitochondrial myopathies: Sequence analysis and possible mechanisms. Nucleic Acids Res 1989;17:4465–4469.
366. Harding AE, Hammans SR. Deletions of the mitochondrial genome. J Inherit Metab Dis 1992;15:480–486.
367. Holt IJ, Harding AE, Morgan-Hughes JA. Deletions of muscle mitochondrial DNA in patients with mitochondrial myopathies. Nature 1988;331:717–719.
368. Zeviani M, Moraes CT, DiMauro S, et al. Deletions of mitochondrial DNA in Kearns-Sayre syndrome. Neurology 1988;38:1339–1346.
369. Ponzetto C, Bresolin N, Bordoni A, et al. Kearns-Sayre syndrome: Different amounts of deleted mitochondrial DNA are present in several autoptic tissues. J Neurol Sci 1990;96:207–210.
370. Poulton J, Morten KJ, Weber K, et al. Are duplications of mitochondrial DNA characteristic of Kearns-Sayre syndrome? Hum Mol Genet 1994;3:947–951.
371. Poulton J, Morten KJ, Marchington D, et al. Duplications of mitochondrial DNA in Kearns-Sayre syndrome. Muscle Nerve 1995;3(Suppl):S154–S158.
372. Schon EA, Rizzuto R, Moraes CT, et al. A direct repeat is a hotspot for large-scale deletion of human mitochondrial DNA . Science 1989;244:346–349.
373. Bernes SM, Bacino C, Prezant TR, et al. Identical mitochondrial DNA deletion in mother with progressive external ophthalmoplegia and son with Pearson marrow-pancreas syndrome. J Pediatr 1993;123:598–602.
374. Chen X, Prosser R, Simonetti S, et al. Rearranged mitochondrial genomes are present in human oocytes. Am J Hum Genet 1995;57:239–247.
375. Williams RS. Mitochondrial gene expression in mammalian striated muscle. Evidence that variation in gene dosage is the major regulatory event. J Biol Chem 1986;261:12390–12394.
376. Williams RS, Salmons S, Newsholme EA, et al. Regulation of nuclear and mitochondrial gene expression by contractile activity in skeletal muscle. J Biol Chem 1986;261:376–380.
377. Shoubridge EA. Autosomal dominant chronic progressive external ophthalmoplegia: A tale of two genomes. Ann Neurol 1996;40:693–694.
378. Haltia M, Suomalainen A, Majander A, et al. Disorders associated with multiple deletions of mitochondrial DNA. Brain Pathol 1992;2:133–139.
379. Moslemi AR, Melberg A, Holme E, et al. Clonal expression of mitochondrial DNA with multiple deletions in autosomal dominant progressive external ophthalmoplegia. Ann Neurol 1996;40:707–713.
380. Van Goethem G, Dermaut B, Lofgren A, et al. Mutation of POLG is associated with progressive external ophthalmoplegia characterized by mtDNA deletions. Nat Genet 2001;28:211–212.
381. Spelbrink JN, Li FY, Tiranti V, et al. Human mitochondrial DNA deletions associated with mutations in the gene encoding Twinkle, a phage T7 gene 4–like protein localized in mitochondria. Nat Genet 2001;28:223–231.
382. Kaukonen J, Juselius JK, Tiranti V, et al. Role of adenine nucleotide translocator 1 in mtDNA maintenance. Science 2000;289:782–785.
383. Nishino I, Spinazzola A, Hirano M. Thymidine phosphorylase gene mutations in MNGIE, a human mitochondrial disorder. Science 1999;283:689–692.
384. Servidei S, Zeviani M, Manfredi G, et al. Dominantly inherited mitochondrial myopathy with multiple deletions of mitochondrial DNA: Clinical, morphologic, and biochemical studies. Neurology 1991;41:1053–1059.
385. Kawai H, Akaike M, Yokoi K, et al. Mitochondrial encephalomyopathy with autosomal-dominant inheritance: A clinical and genetic entity of mitochondrial diseases. Muscle Nerve 1995;18:753–760.
386. Suomalainen A, Majander A, Haltia M, et al. Multiple deletions of mitochondrial DNA in several tissues of a patient with severe retarded depression and familial progressive external ophthalmoplegia. J Clin Invest 1992;90:61–66.
387. Torbergsen T, Stalberg E, Bless JK. Nerve-muscle involvement in a large family with mitochondrial cytopathy: Electrophysiological studies. Muscle Nerve 1991;14:35–41.
388. Bardosi A, Creutzfeldt W, DiMauro S, et al. Myo-, neuro-, gastrointestinal encephalopathy (MNGIE syndrome) due to partial deficiency of cytochrome-c-oxidase. A new mitochondrial multisystem disorder. Acta Neuropathol (Berl) 1987;74:248–258.
389. Threlkeld AB, Miller NR, Golnik K, et al. Ophthalmologic involvement in the

myoneurogastrointestinal encephalomyopathy (MNGIE) syndrome. Am J Ophthalmol 1992;114:322–328.

390. Fadic R, Russell JA, et al. Sensory ataxic neuropathy as the presenting feature of a novel mitochondrial disease. Neurology 1997;49:239–245.

391. Jackson MJ, Schaefer JA, Johnson MA, et al. Presentation and clinical investigation of mitochondrial respiratory chain disease. A study of 51 patients. Brain 1995;118:339–357.

392. Ernst BP, Wilichowski E, Wagner M, et al. Deletion screening of mitochondrial DNA via multiprimer DNA amplification. Mol Cell Probes 1994;8:45–49.

393. Wang H, Fliegel L, Cass CE, et al. Quantification of mitochondrial DNA in heteroplasmic fibroblasts with competitive PCR. Biotechniques 1994;17:76–78.

394. Simonsz HJ, Bärlocher K, Rötig A. Kearns-Sayre syndrome developing in a boy who survived Pearson's syndrome caused by mitochondrial DNA deletion. Doc Ophthalmol 1992;82:73–79.

395. Bassen FA, Kornzweig AL. Malformation of erythrocytes in a case of atypical retinitis pigmentosa. Blood 1950;5:381–387.

396. Muller DPR, Lloyd JK, Wolff OH. Vitamin E and neurological function. Lancet 1983;1:225–228.

397. Tomasi LG. Reversibility of human myopathy caused by vitamin E deficiency. Neurology 1979;29:1182–1186.

398. Rosenblum JL, Keating JP, Prensky AL, et al. A progressive neurologic syndrome in children with chronic liver disease. N Engl J Med 1981;304:503–508.

399. Guggenheim MA, Ringel SP, Silverman A, et al. Progressive neuromuscular disease in children with chronic cholestasis and vitamin E deficiency: Diagnosis and treatment with tocopherol. J Pediatr 1982;100:51–58.

400. Hoogenraad TU, Jennekens FGI, Van Ketel BA, et al. External eye muscle palsies and atypical retinitis pigmentosa in an adult with cystic fibrosis. Neuro-ophthalmology 1982;2:267–273.

401. Werlin SL, Harb JM, Swick H, et al. Neuromuscular dysfunction and ultrastructural pathology in children with chronic cholestasis and vitamin E deficiency. Ann Neurol 1983;13:291–296.

402. Jampel RS, Falls HF. Atypical retinitis pigmentosa, acanthocytosis and heredodegenerative neuromuscular disease. Arch Ophthalmol 1958;59:818–820.

403. Yee RD, Cogan DG, Zee DS. Ophthalmoplegia and dissociated nystagmus in abetalipoproteinemia. Arch Ophthalmol 1976;94:571–575.

404. Behrens M, Leavitt J, Brin M. Ophthalmoparesis in abetalipoproteinemia. Presented at the Fifth Meeting of the International Neuro-Ophthalmology Society. Antwerp, Belgium, May 14–18, 1984.

405. Kommerell G. Internuclear ophthalmoplegia of abduction: Isolated impairment of phasic ocular motor activity in supranuclear lesions. Arch Ophthalmol 1975;93:531–534.

406. Cremer PD, Halmagyi GM. Eye movement disorders in a patient with liver disease. Neuroophthalmology 1996;16(Suppl):276.

407. Cogan DG, Rodrigues M, Chu FC, et al. Ocular abnormalities in abetalipoproteinemia: A clinicopathologic correlation. Ophthalmology 1984;91:991–998.

408. Dalakas MC. Polymyositis and Dermatomyositis. Boston: Butterworth, 1988.

409. Dalakas MC. Polymyositis, dermatomyositis and inclusion-body myositis. N Engl J Med 1991;325:1487–1498.

410. Bouree P, Bouvier JB, Passeron J, et al. Outbreak of trichinosis near Paris. Br Med J 1979;1:1047–1049.

411. Adams RD. Diseases of Muscle: A Study in Pathology. Hagerstown, MD: Harper & Row, 1975.

412. Croll M, Croll LJ. Ocular manifestations of trichinosis. Am J Ophthalmol 1952;35:985–992.

413. Rusin A. Cysticercosis of the superior rectus muscle. Klin Oczna 1973;43:207–210.

414. Jakobiec FA, Jones IS. Orbital inflammations. In: Jones IS, Jakobiec FA, eds. Diseases of the Orbit. Hagerstown, MD: Harper & Row, 1979:187–256.

415. Whitfield R, Wirostko E. Ocular syphilis. In: Locatcher-Khorazo D, Seegal B, eds. Microbiology of the Eye. St Louis: CV Mosby, 1972:322.

416. Brown HW. True and simulated superior oblique tendon sheath syndrome. Doc Ophthalmol 1973;34:123–136.

417. Sandford-Smith JH. Superior oblique tendon sheath syndrome and its relation to stenosing tenosynovitis. Br J Ophthalmol 1973;59:859–865.

418. Wright KW, Silverstein D, Marrone AC, et al. Acquired inflammatory superior oblique tendon sheath syndrome: A clinicopathologic study. Arch Ophthalmol 1982;100:1752–1754.

419. Hermann JS. Acquired Brown's syndrome of inflammatory origin. Response to locally injected steroids. Arch Ophthalmol 1978;96:1228–1232.

420. Nugent RA, Belkin RI, Neigel JM, et al. Graves orbitopathy: Correlation of CT and clinical findings. Radiology 1990;177:675–682.

421. Rootman J, Nugent R. The classification and management of acute orbital pseudotumors. Ophthalmology 1982;89:1040–1048.

422. Siatkowski RM, Capo H, Byrne SF, et al. Clinical and echographic findings in idiopathic orbital myositis. Am J Ophthalmol 1994;118:343–350.

423. Drachman DA. Neurological complications of Wegener's granulomatosis. Arch Neurol 1963;8:145–153.

424. Pinchoff BS, Spahlinger DA, Bergstrom TJ, et al. Extraocular muscle involvement in Wegener's granulomatosis. J Clin Neuroophthalmol 1983;3:163–168.

425. Banker BQ, Victor M. Dermatomyositis (systemic angiopathy) of childhood. Medicine 1966;45:261–289.

426. Barwick DD, Walton JN. Polymyositis. Am J Med 1963;35:646–660.

427. Kissel JT, Mendell JR, Rammohan KW. Microvascular deposition of complement membrane attack complex in dermatomyositis. N Engl J Med 1986;314:329–334.

428. Rowland LP, Schotland DL. Neoplasms and muscle disease. In: Brain L, Norris F, eds. The Remote Effects of Cancer on the Nervous System. New York: Grune & Stratton, 1965:84.

429. Susac JO, Garcia-Mullin R, Glaser JS. Ophthalmoplegia in dermatomyositis. Neurology 1973;23:305–310.

430. Tonali P, Garcovich A, Scoppetta C, et al. Oftalmoplegia in dermatomiosite. Minerva Med 1975;66:309–317.

431. Hall R, Boniach D, Kirkham K, et al. Ophthalmic Graves' disease: Diagnosis and pathogenesis. Lancet 1970;1:375–378.

432. Tallstedt L, Lundell G, Torring O, et al. Occurrence of ophthalmopathy after treatment for Graves' hypothyroidism. N Engl J Med 1992;326:1733–1738.

433. Bahn RS, Heufelder AE. Pathogenesis of Graves' ophthalmopathy. N Engl J Med 1993;329:1468–1475.

434. Jacobson DM. Acetylcholine receptor antibodies in patients with Graves' ophthalmopathy. J Neuroophthalmol 1995;15:166–170.

435. Solomon DH, Chopra IJ, Chopra U, et al. Identification of subgroups of euthyroid Graves' ophthalmopathy. N Engl J Med 1977;296:181–186.

436. Trokel SL, Jakobiec FA. Correlation of CT scanning and pathologic features of ophthalmic Graves' disease. Ophthalmology 1981;88:553–564.

437. De Waard R, Koornneef L, Verbeeten B Jr. Motility disturbances in Graves' ophthalmopathy. Doc Ophthalmol 1983;56:41–47.

438. Prummel MF, Suttorp-Schulten MSA, Wiersinga WM, et al. A new ultrasonographic method to detect disease activity and predict response to immunosuppressive treatment in Graves ophthalmopathy. Ophthalmology 1993;100:556–561.

439. Miller JE, van Heuven W, Ward R. Surgical correction of hypotropia associated with thyroid dysfunction. Arch Ophthalmol 1965;74:509–515.

440. Metcalfe RA, Davies R, Weetman AP. Analysis of fibroblast-stimulating activity in IgG from patients with Graves' dermopathy. Thyroid 1993;3:207.

441. Bahn RS. The fibroblast is the target cell in the connective tissue manifestations of Graves' disease. Int Arch Allergy Immunol 1995;106:213–218.

442. Arnold K, Tandon N, McIntosh RS, et al. T cell responses to orbital antigens in thyroid-associated ophthalmopathy. Clin Exp Immunol 1994;96:329–334.

443. Caygill WM. Excyclotropia in dysthyroid ophthalmopathy. Am J Ophthalmol 1972;73:437–441.

444. Apers RC, Bierlaagh JJM. Indications and results of eye muscle surgery in thyroid ophthalmopathy. Ophthalmologica 1976;173:171–179.

445. Hermann JS. Paretic thyroid myopathy. Ophthalmology 1982;89:473–478.

446. Metz HS. Saccadic velocity studies in patients with endocrine ocular disease. Am J Ophthalmol 1977;84:695–699.

447. Alper MG. Computerized tomography (CT) in diagnosis of inflammatory orbital pseudotumor and Graves' disease. In: Thompson HS, Daroff R, Frisén L, et al., eds. Topics in Neuro-Ophthalmology. Baltimore: Williams & Wilkins, 1979:347.

448. Trokel SL, Hilal SK. Recognition and differential diagnosis of enlarged extraocular muscles in computed tomography. Am J Ophthalmol 1979;87:503–512.

449. Susac JO, Martins AN, Robinson B, et al. False diagnosis of orbital apex tumor by CAT scan in thyroid eye disease. Ann Neurol 1977;1:397–398.

450. Riddick FA Jr. Update on thyroid diseases. Ophthalmology 1981;88:467–470.

451. Surks MI. Assessment of thyroid function. Ophthalmology 1981;88:476–478.

452. Hollander CS. On the nature of the circulating thyroid hormone: Clinical studies of T3 and T4 in serum using gas chromatographic methods. Trans Assoc Am Physicians 1968;81:76–91.

453. Hornblass A, Yagoda A. Thyroid ophthalmopathy related to T3-toxicosis: A variant of classical Graves' disease. Ann Ophthalmol 1980;12:49.

454. Kazuo K, Fujikado T, Ohmi G, et al. Value of thyroid stimulating antibody in the diagnosis of thyroid-associated ophthalmopathy of euthyroid patients. Br J Ophthalmol 1997;81:1080–1083.

455. Marcocci C, Bartalena L, Bogazzi F, et al. Radioiodine and thyroid associated ophthalmopathy. Orbit 1996;15:197–203.

456. Bartley GB, Fatourechi V, Kadrmas EF, et al. Chronology of Graves' ophthalmopathy in an incidence cohort. Am J Ophthalmol 1996;121:426–434.

457. DeGroot LJ, Benjasuratwong Y. Evaluation of thyroid ablative therapy for ophthalmopathy of Graves' disease. Orbit 1996;15:187–196.

458. Wiersinga WM. Advances in medical therapy of thyroid-associated ophthalmopathy. Orbit 1996;15:177–186.

459. Gorman CA, Garrity JA, Fatourechi V, et al. The aftermath of orbital radiotherapy for Graves' ophthalmopathy. Ophthalmology 2002:109:2100–2107.

460. Kennedy DW, Goodstein MI, Miller NR, et al. Transnasal endoscopic orbital decompression. Arch Otolaryngol Head Neck Surg 1990;116:275–282.

461. Lee AG, McKenzie BA, Miller NR, et al. Long-term results of orbital decompression in thyroid eye disease. Orbit 1995;14:59–70.

462. Goldberg AL, Goldspink DF. Influence of food deprivation and adrenal steroids on DNA synthesis in various mammalian tissues. Am J Physiol 1975;228:310–317.

463. Müller R, Kugelberg E. Myopathy in Cushing's syndrome. J Neurol Neurosurg Psychiatry 1959;22:314–319.

464. Harriman DGF, Reed L. The incidence of lipid droplets in human muscle in neuromuscular disorders. J Pathol 1972;106:1–24.

465. Slansky HH, Kolbert G, Gartner S. Exophthalmos induced by steroids. Arch Ophthalmol 1967;77:579–580.

466. Krarup J, de Decker W. Kompendium der direkten augenmuskelverletzungen. Klin Monatsbl Augenheilkd 1982;181:437–443.

467. Duke-Elder S, MacFaul PA. Mechanical injuries. In: Duke-Elder S, ed. System of Ophthalmology. Vol 14, Part 1. St Louis: CV Mosby, 1972:441.

468. Berlin R. In: Graefe A, Saemisch T, eds. Handbuch der Gesammten Augenheilkunde. Vol 6, Part 4. Leipzig: Verlag Wilhelm Engelmann, 1880:644.

469. Dimmer F. Zur lehre von den traumatischen augennusellähmungen aus orbitaler ursache. Z Augenheilkd 1903;9:337–353.

470. Corrado L. Lacerzione del muscolo retto inferiore da cornata. Rass Ital Ottal 1951;20:185–198.

471. Smith B, Regan WF. Blowout fracture of the floor of the orbit: Mechanism and correction of internal orbital fracture. Am J Ophthalmol 1957;44:733–739.

472. Frey RG. Über augenmuskelstörungen nach chirurgischer behandlung der netzhautabheburg. Albrecht von Graefes Arch Klin Exp Ophthalmol 1955;156:561–565.

473. Hunter DG, Lam GC, Guyton DL. Inferior oblique muscle injury from local anesthesia for cataract surgery. Ophthalmology 1995;102:501–509.

474. Smith B. Postsurgical complications of cosmetic blepharoplasty. Trans Am Acad Ophthalmolic Otolaryngol 1969;73:1162–1164.

475. Levine MR, Boynton J, Tenzel RR, et al. Complications of blepharoplasty. Ophthalmolic Surg 1975;6:53–57.

476. Wesley RE, Pollard ZF, McCord CD Jr. Superior oblique paresis after blepharoplasty. Plast Reconstr Surg 1980;66:283–286.

477. Mark LE, Kennerdell JS. Medial rectus injury from intranasal surgery. Arch Ophthalmolic 1979;97:459–461.

478. Raab EL. Limitation of motility after periocular corticosteroid injection. Am J Ophthalmol 1974;78:996–998.

479. Urich H, Wilkinson M. Necrosis of muscle with carcinoma: Myositis or myopathy? J Neurol Neurosurg Psychiatry 1970;33:398–407.

480. Swash M. Acute fatal carcinomatous neuromyopathy. Arch Neurol 1974;30:324–326.

481. Knowles DM II, Jakobiec FA, Jones IS. Rhabdomyosarcoma. In: Jones IS, Jakobiec FA, eds. Diseases of the Orbit. Hagerstown, MD: Harper & Row, 1979:435.

482. Horner F. Carcinoma der duramater. Klin Monatsbl Augenheilkd 1864;2:186–190.

483. Wintersteiner H. Ein fall von augenmuskelmetastaseh nach carcinoma mammae. Klin Monatsbl Augenheilkd 1899;37:331–338.

484. Cohen AS. Amyloidosis. N Engl J Med 1967;277:522–530.

485. Lampert PW. Amyloid and amyloid-like deposits. In: Minckler J, ed. Pathology of the Nervous System. Vol 1. New York: McGraw-Hill, 1968:1121.

486. Reimann HA, Koucky RF, Eklund CM. Primary amyloidosis limited to tissue of mesodermal origin. Am J Pathol 1935;11:977–988.

487. Schmidt MB. Über die beteiligung des auges an der allgemeinen amyloid degeneration. Zentralbl Allg Pathol Pathol Anat 1905;16:49–51.

488. Brownstein MH, Elliott R, Helwig EB. Ophthalmologic aspects of amyloidosis. Am J Ophthalmol 1970;69:423–430.

489. Macoul KL, Winter FC. External ophthalmoplegia: Secondary to systemic amyloidosis. Arch Ophthalmol 1968;79:182–184.

490. Goebel HH, Friedman AH. Extraocular muscle involvement in idiopathic primary amyloidosis. Am J Ophthalmol 1971;71:1121–1127.

491. Rodman HI, Ford RL. Orbital involvement in multiple myeloma: Review of the literature and report of three cases. Arch Ophthalmol 1972;87:30–35.

492. Barricks ME, Traviesa DB, Glaser JS, et al. Ophthalmoplegia in cranial arteritis. Brain 1977;100:209–221.

493. Goldberg RT. Ocular muscle paresis and cranial arteritis: An unusual case. Ann Ophthalmol 1983;15:240–243.

494. Sandyk R, Brennan MJW. Isolated ocular myopathy and celiac disease in childhood. Neurology 1983;33:792.

495. Hardoff D, Sharf B, Berger A. Myopathy as a presentation of coeliac disease. Dev Med Child Neurol 1980;22:781–783.

496. McArdle B. Myopathy due to a defect in muscle glycogen breakdown. Clin Sci 1951;10:13.

497. Tarui S, Okuno G, Ikura Y, et al. Phosphofructokinase deficiency in skeletal muscle: A new type of glycogenosis. Biochem Biophys Res Commun 1965;19:517–523.

498. McGarry JD, Foster DW. The metabolism of octanoyl carnitine in perfused livers from fed and fasted rats: Evidence for a possible regulatory role of carnitine acyltransferase in the control of ketogenesis. J Biol Chem 1974;249:7984–7990.

499. Pleasure D, Bonilla E. Skeletal muscle storage diseases: Myopathies resulting from errors in carbohydrate and fatty acid metabolism. In: Mastaglia FL, Walton J, eds. Skeletal Muscle Pathology. Edinburgh: Churchill Livingstone, 1982:340.

500. Pompe JC. Hypertrophie idiopatique de coeur. Ann Anat Pathol 1933;10:23–35.

501. Andersen DH. Familial cirrhosis of the liver with storage of abnormal glycogen. Lab Invest 1956;5:11–20.

502. DiMauro S, Eastwood AB. Disorders of glycogen and lipid metabolism. Adv Neurol 1977;17:123–142.

503. DiMauro S, Hartwig GB, Hays A, et al. Debrancher deficiency: Neuromuscular disorder in five adults. Ann Neurol 1979;5:422–436.

504. Engel AG, Angelini C. Carnitine deficiency of human skeletal muscle with associated lipid storage myopathy: A new syndrome. Science 1973;179:899–902.

505. Smith RR, Reinecke RD. Electron microscopy of ocular muscle in type II glycogenosis (Pompe's disease). Am J Ophthalmol 1972;73:965–970.

506. Toussaint D, Danis P. Ocular histopathology in generalized glycogenosis (Pompe's disease). Arch Ophthalmol 1965;73:342–349.

507. Kuncl RW, Wiggins WW. Toxic myopathies. Neurol Clin 1988;6:593–619.

508. Reid HA. Myoglobinuria and sea snakebite poisoning. Br Med J 1961;1:1284–1289.

509. Fohlman J, Eaker D. Isolation and characterization of a lethal myotoxic phospholipase A from the venom of the common sea snake Enhydrina schistosa causing myoglobinuria in mice. Toxicon 1977;15:385–393.

510. Rosenbaum AL, Jampolsky A. Pseudoparalysis caused by anomalous insertion of superior rectus muscle. Arch Ophthalmol 1975;93:535–537.

511. Raab EL. Superior oblique tendon sheath syndrome: An unusual case. Ann Ophthalmol 1976;8:345–347.

512. Jadros-Santel D, Grcevic N, Dogan S, et al. Centronuclear myopathy with type 1 fiber hypotrophy and "fingerprint" inclusions associated with Marfan's syndrome. J Neurol Sci 1980;45:43–46.

513. Aström KE, Adams RD. Myotonic disorders. In: Mastaglia FL, Walton JN, eds. Skeletal Muscle Pathology. Edinburgh: Churchill Livingstone, 1982:266.

514. Schmalbruch H. The muscular dystrophies. In: Mastaglia FL, Walton J, eds. Skeletal Muscle Pathology. Edinburgh: Churchill Livingstone, 1982:235.

515. Morgan-Hughes JA. Mitochondrial myopathies. In: Mastaglia FL, Walton J, eds. Skeletal Muscle Pathology. Edinburgh: Churchill Livingstone, 1982:309.

516. Castaigne P, Laplane D, Escourolle R, et al. Ophthalmoplegie externe progressive avec spongiose des moyaux du tronc cérébral. Rev Neurol (Paris) 1971;124:454–466.

517. Raflo GT, Farrell TA, Sioussat RS. Complete ophthalmoplegia secondary to amyloidosis associated with multiple myeloma. Am J Ophthalmol 1981;92:221–224.

CHAPTER 23

Nystagmus and Related Ocular Motility Disorders

R. John Leigh and Janet C. Rucker

GENERAL CONCEPTS AND CLINICAL APPROACH

This chapter concerns abnormal eye movements that disrupt steady fixation and thereby degrade vision. We now know a good deal about the normal anatomy, physiology, and pharmacology of ocular motor control (1). Our approach is to apply this knowledge to nystagmus and other ocular oscillations, since pathophysiology provides a sounder conceptual framework than a system based solely on phenomenology.

We first summarize the mechanisms by which gaze is normally held steady to achieve clear and stable vision (2). We then discuss the pathogenesis and clinical features of each of the disorders that disrupt steady gaze, including the various forms of pathologic nystagmus and saccadic intrusions. Finally, we summarize currently available treatments for these abnormal eye movements and their visual consequences.

1133

NORMAL MECHANISMS FOR GAZE STABILITY

In order for us to see an object best, its image must be held steady over the foveal region of the retina. Although the visual system can tolerate some motion of images on the retina (3), if this motion becomes excessive (more than about 5°/second for Snellen optotypes), vision declines. Furthermore, if the image is moved from the fovea to peripheral retina, it will be seen less clearly.

In healthy persons, three separate mechanisms work together to prevent deviation of the line of sight from the object of regard. The first is fixation, which has two distinct components: (*a*) the visual system's ability to detect retinal image drift and program corrective eye movements; and (*b*) the suppression of unwanted saccades that would take the eye off target. The second mechanism is the vestibulo-ocular reflex, by which eye movements compensate for head perturbations at short latency and thus maintain clear vision during natural activities, especially locomotion. The third mechanism is the ability of the brain to hold the eye at an eccentric position in the orbit against the elastic pull of the suspensory ligaments and extraocular muscles, which tend to return it toward central position. For all three gaze-holding mechanisms to work effectively, their performance must be tuned by adaptive mechanisms that monitor the visual consequences of eye movements.

TYPES OF ABNORMAL EYE MOVEMENTS THAT DISRUPT STEADY FIXATION: NYSTAGMUS AND SACCADIC INTRUSIONS

The essential difference between nystagmus and saccadic intrusions lies in the **initial** eye movement that takes the line of sight off the object of regard. For nystagmus, it is a slow drift (or "slow phase"), as opposed to an inappropriate saccadic movement that intrudes on steady fixation. After the initial movement, corrective or other abnormal eye movements may follow. Thus, nystagmus may be defined as a repetitive, to-and-fro movement of the eyes that is initiated by a slow phase (drift). Saccadic intrusions, on the other hand, are rapid eye movements that take the eye off target. They include a spectrum of abnormal movements, ranging from single saccades to sustained saccadic oscillations.

DIFFERENCES BETWEEN PHYSIOLOGIC AND PATHOLOGIC NYSTAGMUS

It is important to realize that not all nystagmus is pathologic. **Physiologic nystagmus** preserves clear vision during self-rotation. Under most circumstances, for example during locomotion, head movements are small and the vestibulo-ocular reflex is able to generate eye movements that compensate for them. Consequently, the line of sight remains pointed at the object of regard. In response to large head or body rotations, however, the vestibulo-ocular reflex alone cannot preserve clear vision because the eyes are limited in their range of rotation. Thus, during sustained rotations, quick phases occur to reset the eyes into their working range: **vestibular nystagmus**. If rotation is sustained for several seconds, the vestibular afferents no longer accurately signal head rotation, and visually driven or **optokinetic nystagmus** takes over to stop excessive slip of stationary retinal images. Additional examples of physiologic nystagmus are **arthrokinetic** and **audiokinetic nystagmus** (discussion following). In contrast to vestibular and optokinetic nystagmus, **pathologic nystagmus** causes excessive drift of stationary retinal images that degrades vision and may produce illusory motion of the seen world: **oscillopsia** (4–7). An exception is congenital nystagmus, which may be associated with normal visual acuity and which seldom causes oscillopsia (8).

Nystagmus, both physiologic and pathologic, may consist of alternating slow drifts (slow phases) in one direction and corrective, resetting saccades (quick phases) in the other: **jerk nystagmus** (Fig. 23.1A). Pathologic nystagmus may,

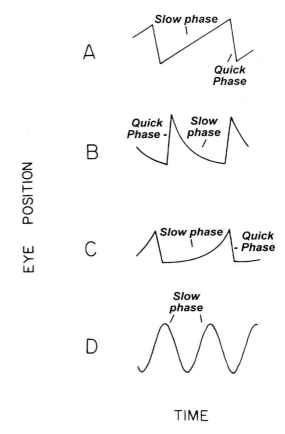

Figure 23.1. Four common slow-phase waveforms of nystagmus. *A*, Constant velocity drift of the eyes. This occurs in nystagmus caused by peripheral or central vestibular disease and also with lesions of the cerebral hemisphere. The added quick-phases give a "saw-toothed" appearance. *B*, Drift of the eyes back from an eccentric orbital position toward the midline (gaze-evoked nystagmus). The drift shows a negative exponential time course, with decreasing velocity. This waveform reflects an unsustained eye position signal caused by a "leaky" neural integrator. *C*, Drift of the eyes away from the central position with a positive exponential time course (increasing velocity). This waveform suggests an unstable neural integrator and is usually encountered in congenital nystagmus. *D*, Pendular nystagmus, which is encountered as a type of congenital nystagmus and with acquired brainstem disease. (From Leigh RJ, Zee DS. The Neurology of Eye Movements. Ed 3. New York, Oxford University Press, 1999.)

however, also consist of smooth to-and-fro oscillations: **pendular nystagmus** (Fig. 23.1*D*). Conventionally, jerk nystagmus is described according to the direction of the quick phase. Thus, if the slow movement is drifting up, the nystagmus is called "downbeating"; if the slow movement is to the right, the nystagmus is "left-beating." Although it is convenient to describe the frequency, amplitude, and direction of the quick phases of the nystagmus, it should be remembered that it is the slow phase that reflects the underlying abnormality.

Nystagmus may occur in any plane, although it is often predominantly horizontal, vertical, or torsional. Physiologic nystagmus is essentially conjugate. Pathologic nystagmus, on the other hand, may have different amplitudes in the two eyes (dissociated nystagmus); it may go in different directions leading to different trajectories of nystagmus in the two eyes; or may have different temporal properties, i.e., phase shift between the two eyes, leading to movements that are sometimes in opposite directions (disconjugate nystagmus).

METHODS OF OBSERVING, ELICITING, AND RECORDING NYSTAGMUS

It is often possible to diagnose the cause of nystagmus through careful history and systematic examination of the patient (9,10). History should include duration of nystagmus, whether it interferes with vision and causes oscillopsia, and accompanying neurological symptoms. The physician should also determine if nystagmus and attendant visual symptoms are worse with viewing far or near objects, with patient motion, or with different gaze angles (e.g., worse on right gaze). If the patient habitually tilts or turns the head, the physician should determine whether or not these features are evident on old photographs.

Before assessing eye movements, the physician must examine the visual system, looking for signs of optic nerve demyelination or malformation, or ocular albinism which often suggests the diagnosis. The stability of fixation should be assessed with the eyes close to central position, viewing near and far targets, and at eccentric gaze angles. It is often useful to record the direction and amplitude of nystagmus for each of the cardinal gaze positions. If the patient has a head turn or tilt, the eyes should be observed in various directions of gaze when the head is in that position as well as when the head is held straight. During fixation, each eye should be occluded in turn to check for latent nystagmus. The presence of pseudonystagmus and oscillopsia in patients with head tremor who have lost their vestibulo-ocular reflex must be differentiated from true nystagmus.

Subtle forms of nystagmus, due to low amplitude or inconstant presence, require prolonged observation over 2–3 minutes. Low amplitude nystagmus may be detected only by viewing the patient's retina with an ophthalmoscope (11). (Note, however, that the direction of horizontal or vertical nystagmus is inverted when viewed through the ophthalmoscope.) The effect of **removal of fixation** should always be determined. Nystagmus caused by peripheral vestibular imbalance may be apparent **only** under these circumstances.

Removal of fixation is often achieved by eyelid closure; nystagmus is then evaluated by recording eye movements, by palpating the globes, or by auscultation with a stethoscope. Lid closure itself may affect nystagmus, however, and it is better to evaluate the effects of removing fixation with the eyelids open. Several clinical methods are available, such as Frenzel goggles which consist of 10- to 20-diopter spherical convex lenses placed in a frame that has its own light source. The goggles defocus the patient's vision, thus preventing fixation of objects, and also provide the examiner with a magnified, illuminated view of the patient's eyes. An alternative is to use two high-plus spherical lenses from a trial case, or to determine the effect of transiently covering the viewing eye during ophthalmoscopy in an otherwise dark room.

Evaluation of nystagmus is incomplete without a systematic examination of each functional class of eye movements (vestibular, optokinetic, smooth-pursuit, saccades, vergence) and their effect on the nystagmus, since different forms of nystagmus can be directly attributed to abnormalities of some of these movements. Physiological optokinetic nystagmus occurs during self-rotation, but it can be elicited at the bedside using a small drum or tape with alternating black and white lines, although larger displays are more effective in patients with voluntary gaze palsies. The slow phases represent visual tracking, including smooth pursuit; the resetting quick phases are saccadic in origin (12). In children and patients with impaired voluntary gaze, an optokinetic stimulus often provides useful information about both pursuit and saccadic systems (13–17). Vestibular nystagmus can be conveniently induced by rotating the patient in a swivel office chair for 30 seconds and then stopping: postrotational nystagmus and vertigo are induced, which may help patients identify the nature of any paroxysmal attacks of dizziness. Caloric and other forms of induced vestibular nystagmus are described below.

It is often helpful to **measure the nystagmus waveform** because the shape of the slow phase often provides a pathophysiological signature of the underlying disorder (18,19). To properly characterize nystagmus, it is important to measure eye position and velocity, as well as target position, during attempted fixation at different gaze angles, in darkness, and during vestibular, optokinetic, saccadic, pursuit, and vergence movements. Common slow-phase waveforms of nystagmus are shown in Figure 23.1.

Conventionally, nystagmus is measured in terms of its amplitude, frequency, and their product: intensity. However, visual symptoms caused by nystagmus usually correlate best with the speed of the slow phase and displacement of the image of the object of regard from the fovea (7).

There are many different methods now available for recording eye movements, and these are discussed more fully elsewhere (20,21). Because many patients with nystagmus cannot accurately point their eyes at visual targets, precise measurement is best achieved with the magnetic search coil technique (Fig. 23.2), since the contact lens that the patient wears can be precalibrated on a protractor-gimbal device. In addition, this is the only technique that permits precise measurement of horizontal, vertical, and torsional oscilla-

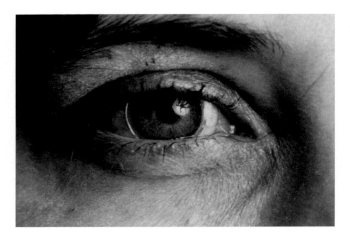

Figure 23.2. A method for precise measurement of horizontal, vertical, and torsional eye rotations. The subject is wearing a Silastic © annulus embedded in which are two coils of wire, one wound in the frontal plane (to sense horizontal and vertical movements) and the other effectively in the sagittal plane (to sense torsional eye movements). When the subject sits in a magnetic field, voltages are induced in these search coils that can be used to measure eye position. (From Leigh RJ, Zee DS. The Neurology of Eye Movements. Ed 3. New York, Oxford University Press, 1999.)

tions over an extended range of amplitudes and frequencies. Although originally introduced as a research tool, the technique is now widely used to evaluate clinical disorders of eye movements, and is well tolerated (22). We have studied over 500 patients with this method.

CLASSIFICATION OF NYSTAGMUS BASED ON PATHOGENESIS

Our classification of nystagmus starts by relating the various forms of nystagmus to disorders of visual fixation, the vestibulo-ocular reflex, or the mechanism for eccentric gaze-holding. In addition, the adaptive processes that optimize these eye movements may be affected by disease, and we discuss these recalibration mechanisms as we deal with each class of nystagmus. Some forms of nystagmus can be better explained than others by this scheme. Nonetheless, our goal is to provide current hypotheses for nystagmus and saccadic intrusions whenever possible. Some hypotheses are backed by substantial evidence, whereas others are more tentative. The justification for this approach is that it provides explanations for clinical findings when knowledge allows, but also provides provisional hypotheses for other disorders that can be tested in future studies.

NYSTAGMUS ASSOCIATED WITH DISEASE OF THE VISUAL SYSTEM AND ITS PROJECTIONS TO BRAINSTEM AND CEREBELLUM

ORIGIN AND NATURE OF NYSTAGMUS ASSOCIATED WITH DISEASE OF THE VISUAL PATHWAYS

Disorders of the visual pathways are often associated with nystagmus. The most obvious example is the nystagmus that invariably accompanies blindness (23,24). How does this arise? At least two separate mechanisms can be identified: the visual fixation mechanism itself and the visually mediated calibration mechanism that optimizes its action.

The smooth visual fixation mechanism stops the eyes from drifting away from a stationary object of regard (25,26). For example, if a normal subject attempts to fixate on the remembered location of a target while in darkness, the eye drifts off target several times faster than if the subject fixates the visible target (27). Uncorrected drifts are eventually remedied by a saccade that places the image back on the fovea. This fixation mechanism depends upon the motion detection (magnocellular) portion of the visual system (28) which is inherently slow, with a response time of about 100 milliseconds that encumbers all visually mediated eye movements, including fixation, smooth pursuit, and optokinetic responses. If the response time is delayed further by disease of the visual system, then the attempts by the brain to correct eye drifts may actually add to the retinal error rather than reduce it, and may lead to ocular oscillations (29).

Vision is also needed for recalibrating and optimizing all types of eye movements. These functions depend on visual projections to the cerebellum, the structure called by Robinson "the ocular motor repair shop" (30). Thus, signals from secondary visual areas concerned with motion-vision project

to the cerebellum via the pontine nuclei and middle cerebellar peduncle (see Chapter 17). For example, neurons in the dorsolateral pontine nuclei and Purkinje cells in the cerebellar flocculus both encode visual-motion signals (31,32). Visual signals for recalibration may also pass via the inferior olive, which sends climbing fibers to the cerebellum (33,34). If the ocular motor system is to be recalibrated, visual signals need to be compared with eye movement commands. At present, it is not certain how or where this function is performed. One possibility is a group of cells in the paramedian tracts (PMT) in the lower pons, which receive inputs from almost all ocular motor structures and which project to the cerebellar flocculus (35). Lesions at any part of this visual-motor recalibration pathway can deprive the brain of signals that hold each of the eyes on the object of regard, the result being drifts of the eyes off target, leading to nystagmus.

Disease affecting any part of the visual system, from retina to cortical visual areas, or interrupting visual projections to pons and cerebellum, may be associated with nystagmus. In this section, we first catalogue the features of nystagmus reported with disease localized to the different sites in this pathway. We then describe features of acquired pendular nystagmus, one of the most common forms of nystagmus associated with disease affecting the visual system or its brainstem-cerebellar projections.

CLINICAL FEATURES OF NYSTAGMUS WITH LESIONS AFFECTING THE VISUAL PATHWAYS

Disease of the Retina

Congenital or acquired retinal disorders causing blindness, such as Leber's congenital amaurosis, lead to continuous jerk nystagmus with components in all three planes, which changes direction over the course of seconds or minutes (Fig. 23.3*A*). The drifting ''null point''—the eye position at which nystagmus changes direction—probably reflects inability to calibrate the ocular motor system, and it has also been reported after experimental cerebellectomy (36). This nystagmus often shows the increasing-velocity waveform (Fig. 23.1*C*) that was once thought to be specific for congenital nystagmus (discussion following). Recent developments in gene therapy for retinal disorders suggest that if vision can be restored, nystagmus will be suppressed (37,38).

Disease Affecting the Optic Nerves

Optic nerve disease is commonly associated with pendular nystagmus. With unilateral disease of the optic nerve, nystagmus largely affects the abnormal eye (monocular nystag-

mus), with prominent, vertical, low-frequency, bidirectional drifts (Fig. 23.3*B*); horizontal drifts are generally unidirectional with corrective quick-phases (24,39). When disease affects both optic nerves, the amplitude of nystagmus is often greater in the eye with poorer vision (the Heimann-Bielschowsky phenomenon) (40). This phenomenon is not confined to primary optic nerve disease, however, and also occurs in patients with profound amblyopia, dense cataract, and high myopia (24,39,41). Oscillations may disappear when vision is restored or they may persist (42), leading to oscillopsia. The former findings support the contention that these ocular oscillations are primarily caused by loss of vision rather than by any primary disorder of the ocular motor system. The origin of vertical drifts that occur in a blind eye is unknown but has been attributed to disturbance of either the vertical vergence mechanism (41), or to a monocular visual stabilization system (24).

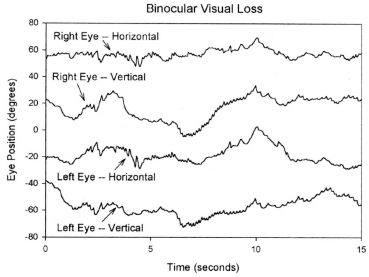

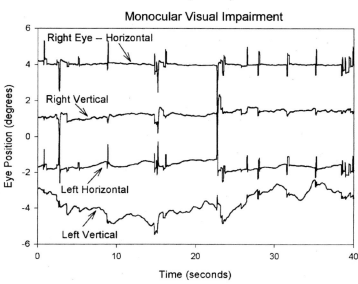

Figure 23.3. Nystagmus and gaze instability associated with visual loss. *A*, Binocular blindness since birth due to Leber's congenital amaurosis. In the horizontal plane, nystagmus changes direction (evident in velocity channels) and there is a ''wandering null point.'' Slow-phase waveforms are variably linear decreasing velocity or, especially in the vertical plane, increasing velocity. *B*, Patient who had defocused vision since childhood following eye trauma and removal of his left lens. Following implantation of an artificial lens at age 35 years, his corrected visual acuity was 20/20 OD and 20/25 OS, but he was unable to maintain steady fixation with the left eye and suffered from variable diplopia and abnormal motion of vision in his left eye that he could not control. His left eye shows the Heimann-Bielschowsky phenomenon, vertical instability of fixation with slow drifts (17).

In infants, the appearance of monocular, vertical pendular nystagmus raises the possibility of optic nerve tumor and neuroimaging studies are indicated (43,44). However, monocular oscillations in children are sometimes due to spasmus nutans (45,46); this condition is discussed below. Monocular visual impairment, such as amblyopia, also leads to horizontal nystagmus and, if present from birth, the features are those of latent nystagmus, which is discussed in a later section.

Disease Affecting the Optic Chiasm

Parasellar lesions such as pituitary tumors have traditionally, albeit rarely, been associated with **seesaw nystagmus,** which is discussed in detail in a later section. Seesaw nystagmus also occurs in patients and in a mutant strain of dogs that lack an optic chiasm (47–49). It remains possible that visual inputs, especially crossed inputs, are important for optimizing vertical-torsional eye movements and if interrupted, might lead to seesaw oscillations (50,51).

Disease Affecting the Postchiasmal Visual System

Horizontal nystagmus is a documented finding in patients with unilateral disease of the cerebral hemispheres, especially when the lesion is large and posterior (52). Such patients show a constant-velocity drift of the eyes toward the intact hemisphere (i.e., quick phases directed toward the side of the lesion, which are often low amplitude). Such patients usually also show asymmetry of horizontal smooth pursuit, brought out at the bedside using an optokinetic tape or drum (53,54); the response is reduced when the stripes move, or the drum is rotated, toward the side of the lesion. This asymmetry of visual tracking has led to the suggestion that nystagmus in such patients reflects an imbalance of pursuit tone as the cause (52). Whether this asymmetry occurs primarily from impairment of parietal cortex necessary for directing visual attention (55), or from disruption of cortical areas important for processing motion-vision (28,56,57), remains unclear.

ACQUIRED PENDULAR NYSTAGMUS AND ITS RELATIONSHIP TO DISEASE OF THE VISUAL PATHWAYS

Acquired pendular nystagmus (Fig. 23.4) is one of the more common types of nystagmus and is associated with the most distressing visual symptoms. Its pathogenesis remains undefined, and more than one mechanism may be responsible. It is encountered in a variety of conditions (Table 23.1).

Acquired pendular nystagmus usually has horizontal, vertical, and torsional components with the same frequency, although one component may predominate. (In congenital pendular nystagmus, however, the oscillation usually is predominantly horizontal, with a small torsional and negligible vertical component.) If the horizontal and vertical oscillatory components are in phase, the trajectory of the nystagmus is oblique. If the horizontal and vertical oscillatory components are out of phase, the trajectory is elliptical (Fig. 23.4*B*). A special case is a phase difference of 90° and equal amplitude

Table 23.1
Etiology of Pendular Nystagmus

Visual loss (including unilateral disease of the optic nerve)
Disorders of central myelin
    Multiple sclerosis
    Pelizaeus-Merzbacher disease
    Peroxisomal assembly disorders
    Cockayne's syndrome
    Toluene abuse
Oculopalatal myoclonus
Acute brainstem stroke
Whipple's disease
Spinocerebellar degenerations
Congenital nystagmus

of the horizontal and vertical components, when the trajectory is circular. When the oscillations of each eye are compared, the nystagmus may be conjugate, but often the trajectories are dissimilar, and the size of oscillations is different (sometimes appearing monocular), and there may be an asynchrony of timing (phase shift). The latter may reach 180°, in which case the oscillations are convergent-divergent (29).

The temporal waveform usually approximates a sine wave, but more complex oscillations have been noted (29). The frequency of oscillations ranges from 1–8 Hz, with a typical value of 3.5 Hz (58). For any particular patient, the frequency tends to remain fairly constant; only rarely is the frequency of oscillations different in the two eyes (59). In some patients, the nystagmus stops momentarily after a saccade. This phenomenon is called postsaccadic suppression (60). A more common feature is that the oscillations are ''reset'' or phase-shifted by saccades (61). Acquired pendular nystagmus may be suppressed or brought out by eyelid closure (62,63) or evoked by convergence (64). In some patients with this condition, smooth pursuit may be intact, so that despite the oscillations, tracking eye movements occur with nystagmus superimposed (58).

Acquired Pendular Nystagmus with Demyelinating Disease

Acquired pendular nystagmus is a common feature of acquired and congenital disorders of central myelin, such as multiple sclerosis (MS) (64), toluene abuse (65), Pelizaeus-Merzbacher disease (66), and peroxisomal disorders (67). Since optic neuritis often coexists in patients with MS who have pendular nystagmus, prolonged response time of the visual processing might be responsible for the ocular oscillations. However, the nystagmus often remains unchanged in darkness, when visual inputs should have no influence on eye movements. In normal subjects, it is possible to induce spontaneous ocular oscillations by experimentally delaying the latency of visual feedback during fixation (Fig. 23.4*C*); however, the frequency of these induced oscillations is less than 2.5 Hz, which is lower than in most patients with pendular nystagmus (29). When this experimental technique is applied to patients with acquired pendular nystagmus, it does not change the characteristics of the nystagmus, but instead

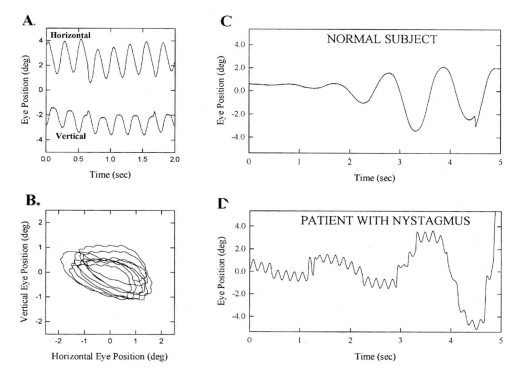

Figure 23.4. Acquired pendular nystagmus. *A*, Time plots of nystagmus of the patient's right eye while fixating a central visual target. The horizontal and vertical records have been offset from zero eye position for convenience of display. Upward deflections correspond to rightward or upward eye rotations. *B*, Nystagmus trajectory seen as a scan path of eye movements in the horizontal and vertical planes corresponding to the time plot in *A*. The scan path corresponded to the direction of oscillopsia that the patient reported. *C and D,* Examples of ocular oscillations induced by imposing an effective delay in visual feedback. *C*, Normal subject. An effective delay in visual feedback of 480 msec was imposed at time zero. The subject developed ocular oscillations at about 1.0 Hz. *D*, Patient with multiple sclerosis and acquired pendular nystagmus. The effects of imposing an electronic delay of 480 msec. The oscillations of her nystagmus (unchanged at 6.5 Hz) were superimposed upon growing 0.67 Hz oscillations induced by the electronic manipulation. (Panels *C* and *D* adapted from Averbuch-Heller L, Zivotofsky AZ, Das VE, et al. Investigations of the pathogenesis of acquired pendular nystagmus. Brain 1995;188:369–378.)

superimposes lower-frequency oscillations similar to those induced in normal subjects (Fig. 23.4*D*). Thus, disturbance of visual fixation from visual delays can not be held accountable for the high-frequency oscillations that often characterize acquired pendular nystagmus.

A more likely possibility is that visual projections to the cerebellum are impaired, leading to instability in the reciprocal connections between brainstem nuclei and cerebellum that are important for recalibration. The high prevalence of internuclear ophthalmoplegia (INO) in these patients, suggests involvement of paramedian brainstem regions, including the cell groups of the paramedian tracts (PMT) (35,68–70). PMT cell groups send a neural copy of ocular motor signals to the cerebellum, and seem important for the integration and calibration of eye movement commands. The observation that acquired pendular nystagmus is "reset" or phase-shifted after saccades (more so with large saccades) suggested that the oscillations arise in the brainstem-cerebellar gaze-holding network (the neural integrator for eye movements—which is discussed in the section "Nystagmus Due to Abnormalities of the Mechanism for Holding Eccentric Gaze") (61).

Oculopalatal Myoclonus (Oculopalatal Tremor)

Acquired pendular nystagmus may be one component of the syndrome of oculopalatal (pharyngo-laryngo-diaphragmatic) myoclonus (71–73). This condition usually develops several months after brainstem or cerebellar infarction, although it may not be recognized until years later. Oculopalatal myoclonus also occurs with degenerative conditions (74). The term "myoclonus" is misleading, since the movements of affected muscles are to and fro and are approximately synchronized, typically at a rate of about 2 cycles per second. The palatal movements may be termed "tremor," rather than myoclonus, and the eye movements are really a form of pendular nystagmus (75). Although the palate is most often affected, movements of the eyes, facial muscles, pharynx, tongue, larynx, diaphragm, mouth of the eustachian tube, neck, trunk, and extremities may occur.

The ocular movements typically consist of to-and-fro oscillations, less sinusoidal than with demyelinating disease, and often with a large vertical component, although they may also have small horizontal or torsional components. The movements may be somewhat disconjugate (both horizon-

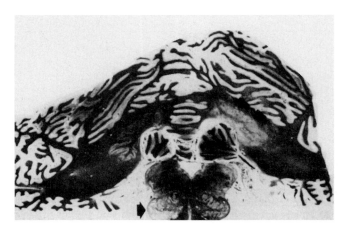

Figure 23.5. Pathology of oculopalatal myoclonus. A section through the cerebellum and medulla shows marked demyelination of the right dentate nucleus and restiform body (*double arrows*). The left inferior olive is hypertrophic and shows mild demyelination (*arrow*). (From Nathanson M. Arch Neurol Psychiatr 1956;75:285–296.)

tally and vertically) (58), with some orbital position dependency (72), and some patients show cyclovergence (torsional vergence) oscillations. Occasionally, patients develop the eye oscillations without movements of the palate, especially following brainstem infarction. Eyelid closure may bring out the vertical ocular oscillations (62). The nystagmus sometimes disappears with sleep, but the palatal movements usually persist. The condition is usually intractable, and spontaneous remission is uncommon (76). Vertical pendular oscillations sometimes occur in the acute period following pontine infarction (77), but the pathogenesis of these movements is probably different than that of oculopalatal myoclonus, since they often resolve spontaneously.

The main pathologic finding with palatal myoclonus is hypertrophy of the inferior olivary nucleus (Fig. 23.5), which may be seen during life using magnetic resonance (MR) imaging (74). There may also be destruction of the contralateral dentate nucleus (71). Histologically, the olivary nucleus has enlarged, vacuolated neurons with enlarged astrocytes. Functional scanning demonstrates increased glucose metabolism (78). Guillain and Mollaret proposed that disruption of connections between the dentate nucleus and the contralateral inferior olivary nucleus, which run via the red nucleus and central tegmental tract, is responsible for the syndrome (71). However, neither the dentate nucleus nor the red nucleus has been shown to have a specific role in ocular motor control. Thus, it has thus been postulated that the nystagmus results from instability in the projection from the inferior olive to the cerebellar flocculus, a structure thought to be important in the adaptive control of the vestibulo-ocular reflex (69,72). It is also possible that disruption of projections from the cell groups of the paramedian tracts (PMT) (35) to the cerebellum leads to the ocular oscillations.

Whipple's Disease and Other Predominantly Convergent-Divergent Pendular Oscillations

Comparatively little has been written about vergence pendular oscillations, which are often small in amplitude, and there is some evidence that they are often overlooked by clinicians. More widespread use of the magnetic search coil technique has made it easier to identify the convergent-divergent components of this form of nystagmus. Averbuch-Heller and colleagues reported three patients with pendular oscillations that were about 180° out of phase in the horizontal and torsional planes but had conjugate vertical components (29). In one of these patients, the torsional component of the oscillations had the largest amplitude. Thus, the patient actually had a cyclovergence nystagmus.

Vergence pendular oscillations occur in patients with MS (79), brainstem stroke (58), and cerebral Whipple's disease (80). In Whipple's disease, the oscillations typically have a frequency of about 1.0 Hz and are accompanied by concurrent contractions of the masticatory muscles, a phenomenon called oculomasticatory myorhythmia. Supranuclear paralysis of vertical gaze also occurs in this setting and is similar to that encountered in progressive supranuclear palsy (81).

At least two possible explanations have been offered to account for the convergent-divergent nature of vergence pendular oscillations: a phase shift between the eyes, produced by dysfunction in the normal yoking mechanisms, or an oscillation affecting the vergence system itself (79). The latter explanation is more likely, because patients who have been studied show no phase shift (i.e., are conjugate) vertically, and because the relationship between the horizontal and torsional components is similar to that occurring during normal vergence movements (excyclovergence with horizontal convergence) (29). Under experimental conditions, the vergence system can be made to oscillate at frequencies up to 2.5 Hz—lower than that reported in patients with conditions other than Whipple's disease (30,80). To account for these higher-frequency oscillations, it seems necessary to postulate instability within the brainstem-cerebellar connections of the vergence system, for example, between the nucleus reticularis tegmenti pontis and cerebellar nucleus interpositus, which may help hold vergence angle steady (29,82).

NYSTAGMUS CAUSED BY VESTIBULAR IMBALANCE

Nystagmus related to imbalance in the vestibular pathway can be caused by damage to peripheral or central structures. Because the nystagmus varies, it usually is possible to distinguish nystagmus caused by peripheral vestibular imbalance from nystagmus caused by central vestibular imbalance.

NYSTAGMUS CAUSED BY PERIPHERAL VESTIBULAR IMBALANCE

Clinical Features of Peripheral Vestibular Nystagmus

Disease affecting the peripheral vestibular pathway (i.e., the labyrinth, vestibular nerve, and its root entry zone) causes nystagmus with linear slow phases (Fig. 23.1*A*). Such unidirectional slow-phase drifts reflect an imbalance in the level of tonic neural activity in the vestibular nuclei. If disease leads to reduced activity, for example, in the vestibular nuclei on the left side, then the vestibular nuclei on the right side will drive the eyes in a slow phase to the left. In this example, quick phases will be directed to the right—away from the side of the lesion. Paradoxically, some patients show nystagmus with a horizontal component that beats toward the side of the lesion. Such cases may be "recovery nystagmus" (83), which represents the effects of a central adaptation process. An imbalance of vestibular tone usually also causes vertigo and a tendency to fall toward the side of the lesion. Apart from these attendant symptoms, two features of the nystagmus itself are useful in identifying the vestibular periphery as the culprit: its trajectory (direction) and whether it is suppressed by visual fixation.

The trajectory of nystagmus can often be related to the geometric relationships of the semicircular canals and to the finding that experimental stimulation of an individual canal produces nystagmus in the plane of that canal. Thus, complete unilateral labyrinthine destruction leads to a mixed horizontal-torsional nystagmus (the sum of canal directions from one ear), whereas in benign paroxysmal positional vertigo (BPPV), a mixed upbeat-torsional nystagmus reflects posterior semicircular canal stimulation. Pure vertical or pure torsional nystagmus almost never occurs with peripheral vestibular disease, because this would require selective lesions of individual canals from one or both ears, an unlikely event.

Nystagmus caused by disease of the vestibular periphery often is more prominent, or may only become apparent, when **visual fixation is prevented**. The reason for this is that when visually generated eye movements are working normally, as they usually are in patients with peripheral vestibular disease, they will slow or stop the eyes from drifting.

Another common, but not specific, feature of nystagmus caused by peripheral vestibular disease is that its intensity increases when the eyes are turned in the direction of the quick phase—**Alexander's law** (84). This probably reflects an adaptive strategy developed to counteract the drift of the vestibular nystagmus and so establish an orbital position (i.e., in the direction of the slow phases) in which the eyes are quiet and vision is clear. This phenomenon forms the basis for a common classification of unidirectional nystagmus. Nystagmus is called "first degree" if it is present only on looking in the direction of the quick phases, "second degree" if it is also present in the central position, and "third degree" if it is present on looking in all directions of gaze.

Although these clinical features help make the diagnosis of peripheral vestibular disease, it is important to realize that brainstem and cerebellar disorders may sometimes mimic peripheral disease and, especially in elderly patients or those with risk factors for vascular disease, careful observation is the prudent course.

Nystagmus Induced by Change of Head Position

Vestibular nystagmus is often influenced by changes in head position. This feature can be used to aid in diagnosis, especially of **benign paroxysmal positional vertigo** (BPPV). Patients with BPPV complain of brief episodes of vertigo precipitated by change of head position, such as when they turn over in bed or look up to a high shelf. The condition may follow head injury or viral neurolabyrinthitis (85).

To test for nystagmus and vertigo in a patient with possible BPPV, the examiner should turn the patient's head toward one shoulder and then quickly move the head and neck together into a head-hanging (down 30–45°) position. About 2–5 seconds after the affected ear is moved to this dependent position, a patient with BPPV will report the onset of vertigo, and a mixed upbeat-torsional nystagmus, best viewed with Frenzel goggles, will develop. The direction of the nystagmus changes with the direction of gaze. Upon looking toward the dependent ear, it becomes more torsional; on looking toward the higher ear, it becomes more vertical. This pattern of nystagmus corresponds closely to stimulation of the posterior semicircular canal of the dependent ear (which causes slow phases mainly by activating the ipsilateral superior oblique and contralateral inferior rectus muscles). The nystagmus increases for up to 10 seconds, but it then fatigues and is usually gone by 40 seconds. When the patient sits back up, a similar but milder recurrence of these symptoms occurs, with the nystagmus being directed opposite to the initial nystagmus. Repeating this procedure several times will decrease the symptoms and make the signs more difficult to elicit. This habituation of the response is of diagnostic value, since a clinical picture similar to that of BPPV can be caused by cerebellar tumors, MS, or posterior circulation infarction. With such central processes, however, there is no latency to onset of nystagmus and no habituation of the response with repetitive testing. Some patients present with the lateral canal variant of BPPV (86,87); sudden horizontal head turns as the patient lies supine may induce a paroxysm of horizontal nystagmus beating toward the ground and vertigo.

Studies show that otolithic debris in the respective canals (canalolithiasis) interferes with the flow of endolymph or movement of the cupula and is probably responsible for BPPV and its variants (88,89). Neck movement causing vertebrobasilar kinking and vertigo as an isolated manifestation of transient brainstem ischemia is an uncommon mechanism; in such cases, associated neurologic symptoms are usually present (90).

Nystagmus that persists after a horizontal change in head position (e.g., with the subject supine and the head turned to the right or left) is less specific than transient nystagmus induced by changes in head position. Indeed, some otherwise normal subjects develop nystagmus that is horizontal with respect to the head and becomes evident behind Frenzel goggles during static, horizontal positional testing. Such positional nystagmus may remain beating in the same direction whether the head is turned to the right or left, or it may change direction with lateral head turn such that it is either always beating toward the earth (geotropic) or away from the earth (ageotropic or apogeotropic). Sustained geotropic and ageotropic nystagmus probably reflect the effects of changing otolithic influences and may be encountered with either peripheral, or central vestibular lesions (90,91). Only if such nystagmus is present during visual fixation does it suggest the possibility of central disease. Occasionally, disease affecting central vestibular connections, such as a cerebellar tumor (92), infarction (93,94), or MS may produce nystagmus associated with postural vertigo and severe nausea with vomiting. These manifestations may suggest a peripheral lesion; however, the characteristics of the nystagmus are usually central, rather than peripheral. Alcohol is well know to cause positional nystagmus, and both central and peripheral mechanisms contribute (95).

In patients who have symptomatically recovered from a unilateral, peripheral vestibulopathy, nystagmus can often be induced following vigorous head shaking in the horizontal or the vertical plane for 10–15 seconds (96–98). After horizontal head shaking, patients may show horizontal nystagmus with quick phases directed away from the side of the lesion. Vertical nystagmus following horizontal head shaking (an example of "perverted nystagmus") often implies central vestibular disease (99,100). After vertical head shaking, patients with unilateral peripheral vestibular lesions may show less prominent nystagmus with horizontal quick phases directed toward the side of the lesion. Hyperventilation-induced nystagmus occurs in patients with schwannoma and other tumors of the 8th cranial nerve (9,101). Indeed, hyperventilating 25 deep breaths is useful in the evaluation of the dizzy patient. Patients with cerebellar disease may show transient downbeating nystagmus after horizontal head shaking or hyperventilation (102).

Nystagmus Induced by Proprioceptive and Auditory Stimuli

It is uncertain whether or not an imbalance of cervical inputs can produce a nystagmus similar to that caused by peripheral vestibular disease. In normal human subjects, eye movements generated from cervical proprioception—the cervico-ocular reflex (COR)—play little role in the stabilization of gaze (103), although the COR does increase in responsiveness in individuals who have lost vestibular function (104,105), and in certain patients with cerebellar disease (106).

The perception of passive body motion relies primarily on vestibular and visual information. However, an illusion of body rotation accompanied by a conjugate, horizontal, jerk nystagmus—**arthrokinetic nystagmus**—can be induced when the horizontally extended arm of a normal, stationary subject is passively rotated about a vertical axis in the shoulder joint (107). The slow phase of the nystagmus is in a direction opposite to that of the arm movement. The mean slow-phase velocity increases with increasing arm velocity, and the nystagmus continues for a short time following cessation of arm movement (arthrokinetic after-nystagmus). The existence of arthrokinetic circularvection and nystagmus suggests that there exists in normal humans a functionally significant somatosensory-vestibular interaction within the central vestibular system, at least for afferent pathways carrying position and kinesthetic information from the joints.

Normal stationary subjects in darkness may experience illusory self-rotation when exposed to a rotating sound field (108,109). This illusion is generally accompanied by **audio-kinetic nystagmus**, which is conjugate and horizontal, with the slow phase in the direction opposite to that of the experienced self-rotation (110). This nystagmus indicates that apparent, as well as actual, body orientation can influence ocular motor control. Neither the illusory self-rotation nor the nystagmus occurs when the subject is exposed to a rotating sound field in the light, i.e., when a stable visual environment is present, suggesting that visual information must dominate auditory information in determining apparent body orientation and sensory localization (110). Patients who develop vestibular symptoms and nystagmus when exposed to certain sounds—**Tullio's phenomenon**—often have dehiscence of the superior semicircular canal or pathologic stimulation of otolithic organs (111–116).

Peripheral Vestibular Nystagmus Induced by Caloric or Galvanic Stimulation

Nystagmus induced by caloric stimulation of one ear has all the features of that caused by unilateral or asymmetric peripheral vestibular disease. During caloric stimulation, a temperature gradient across the temporal bone induces a convection current in the endolymph of a semicircular canal if it is orientated vertical to the earth (117). A second mechanism, which probably involves the effects of cooling the vestibular nerve, is less important (118,119). Before attempting to induce caloric nystagmus, the physician must first check that the tympanic membrane is visible and intact. The subject is then placed supine and the neck is flexed 30°. A cold stimulus (30°C) induces horizontal slow-phase components directed toward the stimulated ear (quick phases in the opposite direction). With a warm stimulus (44°C) and the same head orientation, quick phases are toward the stimulated ear (hence the mnemonic, **COWS**: cold-opposite, warm-same).

Caloric stimulation is an important way to test each peripheral labyrinth; details of quantitative testing are summarized elsewhere (91). Bedside testing with ice-cold water is especially useful in the evaluation of the unconscious patient (120,121). In this setting, tonic eye deviation indicates preservation of pontine function. Induction of caloric nystagmus is also a useful way to confirm preservation of consciousness in patients feigning coma. Suppression of caloric nystagmus by visual fixation depends on pathways important for visually mediated eye movements. For example, caloric nystagmus is impaired in patients with lesions of the cerebellar flocculus (122). Galvanic stimulation of the peripheral labyrinth also induces nystagmus but, at present, this is largely used as a research tool (91,123,124).

NYSTAGMUS CAUSED BY CENTRAL VESTIBULAR IMBALANCE

Clinical Features of Central Vestibular Nystagmus

In this section, we describe the clinical features of three common forms of nystagmus thought to be caused by imbal-

Table 23.2
Etiology of Downbeat Nystagmus

Cerebellar degeneration, including familial episodic ataxia, and
   paraneoplastic degeneration
Craniocervical anomalies, including Arnold-Chiari malformation
Infarction of brainstem or cerebellum
Dolichoectasia of the vertebrobasilar artery
Multiple sclerosis
Cerebellar tumor, including hemangioblastoma
Syringobulbia
Encephalitis
Head trauma
Toxic-metabolic
Anticonvulsant medication
Lithium intoxication
Alcohol
Wernicke's encephalopathy
Magnesium depletion
Vitamin B_{12} deficiency
Toluene abuse
Congenital
Transient finding in otherwise normal infants

---

ance of central vestibular connections: downbeat, upbeat, and torsional nystagmus. We also discuss the less common phenomenon of horizontal nystagmus caused by central vestibular imbalance. Finally, we offer a pathophysiologic scheme to account for these forms of central vestibular nystagmus.

Downbeat nystagmus occurs in a variety of disorders (Table 23.2), but it is most commonly associated with disease affecting the cerebellum, the craniocervical junction, or the blood vessels in these regions (125–128). It may also be a manifestation of drug intoxication, notably by lithium (129–133). Downbeat nystagmus is usually present with the eyes in central position, but its amplitude may be so small that it can only be detected by viewing the ocular fundus with an ophthalmoscope. In addition, it may occur intermittently (134). Generally, Alexander's law is obeyed: nystagmus intensity is greatest in downgaze and least in upgaze. Usually the waveform is linear, but it may be increasing in velocity (Fig. 23.1C). The latter is usually the case if Alexander's law is violated (i.e., when the nystagmus increases in upgaze). This phenomenon may reflect instability of the mechanism for eccentric gaze-holding. Most often, it is enhanced by having the patient look down and to one side. Downbeat nystagmus may also be evoked by placing the patient in a head-hanging position (135–137). Some normal subjects may show ''chin-beating'' nystagmus when they are placed upside down in darkness (or wear Frenzel goggles) (137,138); such nystagmus is usually absent in normal eyes during fixation (136). Convergence may influence the amplitude and frequency of the nystagmus or convert it to upbeat nystagmus. Some patients show combined divergent and downbeat nystagmus (139). In most patients, removal of fixation (e.g., with Frenzel goggles) does not substantially influence slow-phase velocity, although the frequency of quick phases may diminish.

A variety of ocular motor abnormalities often accompany downbeat nystagmus and reflect coincident cerebellar involvement. Vertical smooth pursuit and the vertical vestibulo-ocular reflex are abnormal because of impaired ability to generate smooth downward eye movements; such asymmetries cannot simply be attributed to superimposed nystagmus (126). Sometimes, the vestibulo-ocular reflex for upward eye movements is hyperactive, with a gain exceeding 1.0 (140). Impairment of eccentric horizontal gaze-holding, smooth pursuit, and combined eye-head tracking also commonly coexist. Vertical diplopia usually reflects associated skew deviation (126). The visual consequences of downbeat nystagmus are oscillopsia and postural instability (141).

Upbeat nystagmus that is present with the eyes close to central position occurs in many clinical conditions (Table 23.3). Nystagmus intensity is usually greatest in upgaze, and it usually does not increase on right or left gaze (126). As with downbeat nystagmus, slow phases are often increasing in velocity if Alexander's law is violated (Fig. 23.1C). Removal of visual fixation has little influence on slow-phase velocity. Convergence is variously reported to enhance, suppress, or convert upbeat nystagmus to downbeat (126, 142,143). Placing the patient in a head-hanging position increases the nystagmus in some individuals. It should be noted that the nystagmus in many patients with benign paroxysmal positional vertigo is upbeating. However, this is a transient phenomenon brought on by quickly placing the patient with the affected side down. Furthermore, the nystagmus of BPPV has a torsional component, and its direction depends upon the direction of gaze. As is the case with downbeat nystagmus, patients with upbeat nystagmus often show asymmetries of vertical vestibular and smooth pursuit eye movements, as well as associated cerebellar eye movement findings.

Torsional nystagmus is a less commonly recognized form of central vestibular nystagmus than downbeat or upbeat nystagmus. It is often difficult to detect except by careful observation of conjunctival vessels or by noting the direction of retinal movement on either side of the fovea, using

Table 23.3
Etiology of Upbeat Nystagmus

Cerebellar degenerations, including familial episodic ataxia
Multiple sclerosis
Infarction of medulla, midbrain, or cerebellum
Tumors of the medulla, midbrain, or cerebellum
Wernicke's encephalopathy
Brainstem encephalitis
Behçet's syndrome
Meningitis
Leber's congenital amaurosis or other congenital disorder of the anterior
   visual pathways
Thalamic arteriovenous malformation
Organophosphate poisoning
Tobacco
Associated with middle ear disease
Congenital
Transient finding in otherwise normal infants

Table 23.4
Etiology of Torsional Nystagmus

Syringobulbia, with or without syringomyelia and
    Chiari malformation
Brainstem stroke (Wallenberg's syndrome) or
    arteriovenous malformation
Brainstem tumor
Multiple sclerosis
Oculopalatal myoclonus
Head trauma
Congenital
Associated with the ocular tilt reaction

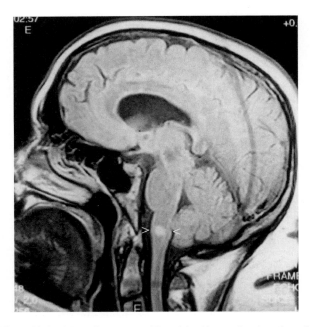

Figure 23.6. Magnetic resonance T2-weighted image showing a hyperintense signal in the medulla of a patient with upbeat nystagmus and multiple sclerosis (99). After horizontal head-shaking, she developed downbeating nystagmus (perverted head-shaking nystagmus) and tumbling vertigo.

an ophthalmoscope or contact lens. Although both peripheral vestibular and congenital nystagmus may have torsional components, purely torsional nystagmus, like purely vertical nystagmus, indicates disease affecting central vestibular connections (see Table 23.4) (144–147). Torsional nystagmus shares many of the features of downbeat and upbeat nystagmus, including modulation by head rotations, variable slow-phase waveforms, and suppression by convergence (146). It is also probably a common finding in patients with the ocular tilt reaction (148). Nonrhythmic but continuous torsional eye movements may be a feature of paraneoplastic encephalopathy (149).

Horizontal nystagmus in central position from central vestibular imbalance is an uncommon but well-documented phenomenon. The underlying disorder usually is an Arnold-Chiari malformation (9,150). The slow-phase waveform in this form of nystagmus may be of the increasing-velocity type, making distinction from congenital nystagmus potentially difficult. However, patients with acquired central vestibular horizontal nystagmus typically report recent onset of visual symptoms, such as oscillopsia, and measurements usually demonstrate an associated vertical component that is absent in congenital nystagmus. Patients with horizontal nystagmus that is present in the central position always should be observed continuously for 2–3 minutes to exclude the possibility that the nystagmus is actually periodic alternating nystagmus (PAN, discussion following).

Pathogenesis of Central Vestibular Nystagmus

Our understanding of the pathogenesis of central forms of vestibular nystagmus has increased because of more cases with clinicopathologic correlation, the development of animal and mathematic models, and the application of modern anatomy and physiology. Downbeat nystagmus is usually associated with lesions of the vestibulocerebellum flocculus, paraflocculus, nodulus, and uvula and the underlying medulla (126,151). Upbeat nystagmus is most commonly reported in patients with medullary lesions (Fig. 23.6) (152–156). These lesions variably affect the perihypoglossal nuclei and adjacent medial vestibular nucleus (structures important for gaze-holding), and the ventral tegmentum, which contains projections from the vestibular nuclei that receive inputs from the anterior semicircular canals (157). Upbeat nystagmus occurs in patients with lesions affecting the cau-

dal medulla (158), anterior vermis of the cerebellum (152), or the adjacent brachium conjunctivum and midbrain (159–161). These cases suggest that lesions at several distinct sites can cause both upbeat and downbeat nystagmus. However, it is possible to account for these findings by considering the fundamental anatomic fact that, unlike the horizontal vestibular system which is right-left symmetric, the connections for vertical vestibular responses are dissimilar for upward or downward eye movements, both anatomically and pharmacologically. These up-down asymmetries involve connections subserving: (a) the vertical vestibulo-ocular reflex; (b) the otolith-ocular reflexes; (c) the vestibulocerebellum; (d) the network for eccentric gaze-holding (neural integrator); and (e) the smooth pursuit system.

Excitatory projections for the vertical vestibulo-ocular reflex from the posterior semicircular canals, which mediate downward eye movements, synapse in the medial vestibular nucleus and then cross dorsally in the medulla beneath the nucleus prepositus hypoglossi to reach the contralateral medial longitudinal fasciculus (MLF). Experimental lesions that damage this pathway cause upward eye drifts and downbeat nystagmus (162). On the other hand, it appears that excitatory connections from the anterior semicircular canals, which mediate upward eye movements, take different routes; more than one pathway may contribute (163). In addition, a central imbalance of otolithic inputs may contribute to vertical nystagmus (164), and account for "chin-beating" nystagmus when normal subjects are positioned upside down in darkness (137,138). The case for the cerebellar flocculus being an important structure in the production of downbeat nystagmus rests on the finding that Purkinje cells send inhibitory projections to the central connections of the anterior semicircular canal but not to the posterior canal (Fig. 23.7) (165–167). This asymmetry of inhibitory projections accounts for the finding that experimental flocculectomy causes downbeat nystagmus (168). This lesion disinhibits the projections to the anterior canal but not to the posterior canal, causing the eyes to drift up and producing downbeat nystagmus (167). A neural network that includes the vestibulocerebellum and the nucleus prepositus hypoglossi and adjacent medial vestibular nucleus is also thought to be important for the eccentric gaze-holding mechanism. Consistent with this hypothesis is the report of a patient with lithium intoxication, who had downbeat nystagmus and a complete failure of gaze-holding, and showed lesions in the nucleus prepositus hypoglossi (130). (However, a range of disorders of eye movements are reported with lithium [131,169–172], so more than one mechanism may be disrupted by it.) Lesions of the vestibulocerebellum may cause instability of this network, making the eyes drift at increasing velocity away from central position in the vertical or horizontal planes (150,173–175). It has also been suggested that the characteristics of downbeat nystagmus could be explained by a central imbalance in smooth pursuit with cerebellar lesions (140). Resolution of upbeat or downbeat nystagmus after the first few months of life in otherwise normal infants (176,177) may reflect calibration of pursuit or gaze-holding mechanisms as the visual system becomes fully myelinated.

PERIODIC ALTERNATING NYSTAGMUS

Periodic alternating nystagmus is a spontaneous horizontal nystagmus, present in central gaze, that reverses direction approximately every 90–120 seconds (Fig. 23.8). Because the period of oscillation is about 4 minutes, the disorder may be missed unless the examiner observes the nystagmus for several minutes. As the nystagmus finishes one half-cycle (e.g., of right-beating nystagmus), a brief transition period occurs during which there may be upbeating or downbeating nystagmus or saccadic movements before the next half-cycle (e.g., of left-beating nystagmus) starts. A congenital form of PAN also exists (discussed in the section ''Congenital Nystagmus''), but this is usually much less regular in the timing of reversal of direction and shows slow-phase waveforms typical of congenital nystagmus. PAN must also be differentiated from ''ping-pong gaze,'' an ocular deviation that reverses direction not over several minutes but every few seconds and that is encountered in unconscious patients with large bihemispheric lesions (178).

In most patients with acquired PAN, the nystagmus has the same characteristics in light or in darkness. Smooth pursuit and optokinetic nystagmus are usually impaired (179). Vestibular stimuli are able to reset the oscillations, and critically timed rotational stimuli can stop PAN for several minutes (179,180).

Acquired PAN occurs in association with a number of

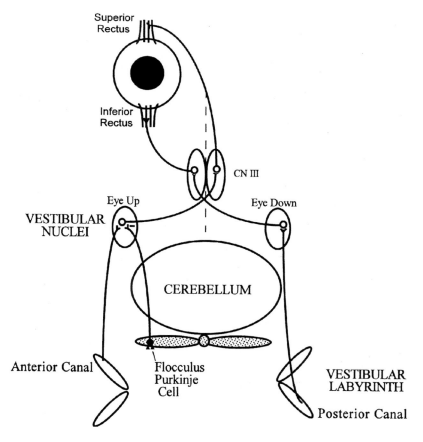

Figure 23.7. Schematic hypothesis for downbeat nystagmus. Inputs from the anterior semicircular canals of the vestibular labyrinth evoke upward eye movements via projections through the superior vestibular nuclei to motoneurons supplying elevator muscles, including the superior rectus (CN III is oculomotor nucleus). Inputs from the posterior semicircular canals evoke downward eye movements via projections through the medial vestibular nuclei to motoneurons supplying depressor muscles, including the inferior rectus. The flocculus of the cerebellum inhibits anterior but not posterior canal projections in the vestibular nuclei. If inhibition from the flocculus is impaired, the eyes will drift upward causing downbeat nystagmus. (Schematic based on Ito M, Nisimaru N, Yamamoto M. Specific patterns of neuronal connexions involved in the control of the rabbit's vestibulo-ocular reflexes by the cerebellar flocculus. J Physiol (Lond) 1977; 265:833–854; Baloh RW, Spooner JW. Downbeat nystagmus: A type of central vestibular nystagmus. Neurology 1981;31:304–310.)

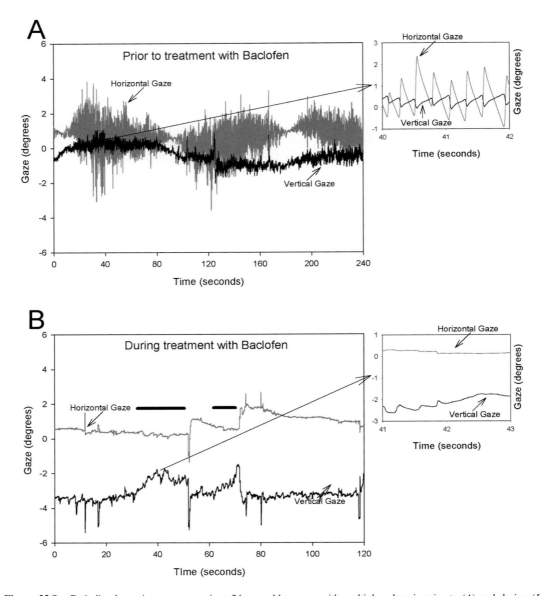

Figure 23.8. Periodic alternating nystagmus in a 24-year-old woman with multiple sclerosis prior to (*A*) and during (*B*) treatment with baclofen. Before treatment, PAN reverses direction approximately every 90 seconds; there is an associated downbeat nystagmus (evident in the *inset at right*, which has a magnified time scale). During treatment with baclofen, PAN is essentially abolished, even when the room was switched to complete darkness (indicated by horizontal bars in *B*, and shown in more detail in inset at right). Upward deflections indicate rightward or upward eye movements. (From Garbutt S, Thakore N, Rucker JC, Han Y, Kumar AN, Leigh RJ. Effects of visual fixation and convergence on periodic alternating nystagmus due to multiple sclerosis. Neuro-Ophthalmology, in press.)

conditions (Table 23.5), many of which affect the cerebellum. Experimental ablation of the nodulus and uvula of the cerebellum in monkeys causes PAN when the animals are placed in a dark room. Baclofen abolishes this nystagmus (181). One function of the nodulus and uvula is to control the time course of rotationally induced nystagmus—so-called ''velocity storage'' (182). Following ablation of the nodulus and uvula, the duration (velocity storage) of rotationally induced nystagmus is prolonged excessively. It is postulated

that normal vestibular repair mechanisms reverse the direction of this nystagmus, thus producing the oscillations of PAN (179,181,182). These oscillations would ordinarily be blocked by visual stabilization mechanisms that tend to suppress nystagmus, but disease of the cerebellum that causes PAN usually also impairs these mechanisms.

Two other unusual disorders may be related to PAN. The first is a variation of PAN, in which oscillations occurred in both the horizontal and vertical planes, 90° out of phase,

Table 23.5
Etiology of Periodic Alternating Nystagmus

Chiari malformations and other hindbrain anomalies
Multiple sclerosis
Cerebellar degenerations
Cerebellar tumor, abscess, cyst, and other mass lesion
Creutzfeldt-Jakob disease
Ataxia telangiectasia
Brainstem infarction
Anticonvulsant medications
Lithium intoxication
Infections affecting cerebellum, including syphilis
Hepatic encephalopathy
Trauma
Following visual loss (from vitreous hemorrhage or cataract)
Congenital nystagmus

and has been called **periodic alternating windmill nystagmus** (183). This phenomenon occurred in a blind patient. The second is the report of a patient with paroxysms of mixed torsional-horizontal-vertical nystagmus that occurred every 2 minutes in association with nausea (184). In this patient, the initial mechanism was probably caused by paroxysmal hyperactivity in one vestibular nucleus complex, unlike PAN, in which prolongation of the vestibular response is the initial mechanism. However, in both entities, an adaptive mechanism appears to influence the nystagmus every 2 minutes. This is perhaps the most direct evidence that dysfunction of an ocular motor recalibration mechanism can lead to nystagmus.

SEESAW AND HEMI-SEESAW NYSTAGMUS

In seesaw and hemi-seesaw nystagmus, one half-cycle consists of elevation and intorsion of one eye and synchronous depression and extorsion of the other eye; during the next half-cycle, the vertical and torsional movements reverse. The waveform may be pendular (185–188) or jerk. In the latter case, the slow phase corresponds to one half-cycle (189). A seesaw component is present in many central forms of nystagmus. Seesaw nystagmus may be congenital (185,190), or acquired (Table 23.6). Quantitative studies have done

Table 23.6
Etiology of Seesaw Nystagmus

Meso-diencephalic disease*a*
Parasellar masses
Brainstem stroke
Septo-optic dysplasia
Chiari malformation
Syringobulbia
Retinitis pigmentosa
Head trauma
Congenital form, including agenesis of optic
    chiasm, and as a transient finding in albinism

a Includes hemi-seesaw nystagmus.

much to clarify the characteristics and pathogenesis of seesaw nystagmus. It has been proposed that jerk seesaw nystagmus (hemi-seesaw nystagmus) occurs in patients with lesions in the region of the interstitial nucleus of Cajal (INC) (189), although experimental inactivation of this structure has not produced this nystagmus (191). Such patients often have a contralateral **ocular tilt reaction**. With a right INC lesion, the reaction consists of a left head tilt, a skew deviation with a right hypertopia, tonic intorsion of the right eye and extorsion of the left eye, and misperception that earth-vertical is tilted to the left (189,192). Rarely, the ocular tilt reaction is paroxysmal in form, in which case it is ipsilateral to the INC lesion; however paroxysmal skew deviation is also reported with lesions of the cerebellar uvula (193). Some patients with this condition also show corresponding paroxysms of jerk seesaw nystagmus (189). The ocular tilt reaction is believed to be caused by an imbalance of central otolithic projections from vestibular nuclei to the INC. Stimulation in the region of INC in monkeys, for example, produces an ocular tilt reaction consisting of extorsion and depression of the eye on the stimulated side and intorsion and elevation of the other eye (194); somewhat similar results have been reported in humans (195,196). Thus, the various forms of the ocular tilt reaction are similar to the slow phase of jerk seesaw nystagmus. Isolated INC lesions may be characterized by ipsilesional torsional nystagmus and a restricted range of vertical saccades that are not slowed (197). If the adjacent rostral interstitial nucleus of the MLF (riMLF) is also damaged, however, either no quick phases (189), or contralesional quick phases (198), may be observed. (As discussed in Chapter 17, each riMLF contributes to upward and downward saccades but only to ipsilaterally directed torsional quick phases.)

Pendular seesaw nystagmus has most often been reported in patients with large tumors in the region of the optic chiasm and diencephalon (Fig. 23.9), and thus these oscillations

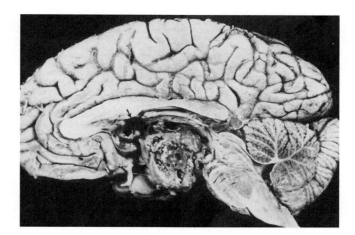

Figure 23.9. Pathology of seesaw nystagmus. A 47-year-old woman developed progressive visual loss and was noted to have bitemporal hemianopia and seesaw nystagmus. The patient died 8 months later, following subtotal removal of a craniopharyngioma. Note that the diencephalon and rostral mesencephalon are compressed and partially destroyed by the tumor that did not, however, obstruct the foramina of Monro (*arrow*).

have been attributed to either compression of the diencephalon or to the effects of chiasmal visual field defects. One aspect of the vestibular responses concerns movements to compensate for head roll motion if the subject looks at an object located off the midsagittal plane; in this case a seesaw rotation of the eyes is the geometrically appropriate compensation (199). Normal calibration of this response, which would require that motion-visual information be sent to the cerebellum could be impaired with large suprasellar lesions, leading to the pendular variant of seesaw nystagmus (188). Thus, both the jerk and pendular variants of seesaw nystagmus probably arise from imbalance or miscalibration of vestibular responses that normally function to optimize gaze during head rotations in roll.

NYSTAGMUS DUE TO ABNORMALITIES OF THE MECHANISM FOR HOLDING ECCENTRIC GAZE

GAZE-EVOKED NYSTAGMUS

Nystagmus that is induced by turning the eye to an eccentric position in the orbit is called **gaze-evoked nystagmus**. It is the most common form of nystagmus encountered in clinical practice. Although the terms gaze-evoked nystagmus, end-point nystagmus, and gaze-paretic nystagmus are often used synonymously, gaze-evoked nystagmus is a general term that includes both physiologic and pathologic nystagmus. When the nystagmus is physiologic, the term end-point nystagmus is appropriate (see below). When the nystagmus is associated with a paresis of gaze, as in patients with ocular motor nerve palsies or weakness of the extraocular muscles, the term gaze-paretic nystagmus is appropriate.

Gaze-evoked nystagmus usually occurs on lateral or upward gaze, seldom on looking down. If fixation is impaired or prevented (e.g., in darkness), the slow phases consist of centripetal drifts that may have an exponentially decaying waveform (Fig. 23.1B). If visual fixation is possible, however, the slow phases have a more linear profile.

In order to understand how gaze-evoked nystagmus arises, one must consider the neural command required to hold the eye steadily at an eccentric position in the orbit. When the eye is turned toward a corner of the orbit, the fascia and ligaments that suspend the eye exert an elastic force to return toward central position. Overcoming this elastic restoring force requires a tonic contraction of the extraocular muscles. This is achieved by an eye position signal to the ocular motoneurons, called a step, that is generated by the gaze-holding network, also called the neural integrator. This network includes the vestibulocerebellum, the medial vestibular nucleus and adjacent nucleus prepositus hypoglossi in the medulla, and the interstitial nucleus of Cajal (INC) in the midbrain.

Gaze-evoked nystagmus is caused by a deficient step, such that the eyes cannot be maintained at an eccentric orbital position and are pulled back toward central position by the elastic forces of the orbital fascia. Corrective quick phases then move the eyes back toward the desired position in the orbit. Frequently, lesions that produce gaze-evoked nystagmus also impair visual fixation and smooth pursuit.

Gaze-evoked nystagmus may be caused by a variety of medications, including alcohol, anticonvulsants, and sedatives. Gaze-evoked nystagmus may also be caused by structural lesions that damage the gaze-holding neural network. Experimental lesions of the nucleus prepositus hypoglossi/medial vestibular nucleus region effectively abolish horizontal gaze-holding function (200–202), and also partially impair vertical gaze-holding. Inactivation of INC abolishes vertical gaze-holding function (203). Experimental flocculectomy greatly, but not completely, impairs horizontal gaze holding (168) in addition to causing downbeat nystagmus.

Rarely, cerebellar lesions cause the gaze-holding mechanism to become unstable, so that the eyes drift with increasing velocity away from central position in either the vertical (173) or the horizontal plane (150). This "gaze-instability nystagmus" often violates Alexander's law.

Another cause of gaze-evoked nystagmus is familial episodic ataxia type 2 (EA-2), which is characterized by attacks of ataxia and vertigo lasting hours, with interictal nystagmus. They nystagmus is typically gaze-evoked with a vertical component that can be downbeat or upbeat. Pursuit and optokinetic responses may be impaired, whereas vestibular responses may be normal or increased (204).

Differences between Physiologic End-Point Nystagmus and Pathologic Gaze-Evoked Nystagmus

Gaze-evoked nystagmus is commonly encountered in normal subjects, in which cases it is often called end-point nystagmus (205–207). It typically occurs on looking far laterally and is poorly sustained. The nystagmus is primarily horizontal. It is usually symmetric, but it may be asymmetric, being more prominent on looking to one side than to the other (207). In some normal persons, the nystagmus is sustained, occurs with less than full deviations of the eye, and may be slightly dissociated or have a torsional component. In addition, some normals show pendular oscillations in far eccentric gaze (208). In such individuals, this physiologic form of gaze-evoked nystagmus can usually be differentiated from that caused by disease, since the former has lower intensity (i.e., slower drift) and, most importantly, is not accompanied by other ocular motor abnormalities. Pathologic gaze-evoked nystagmus, in contrast, is accompanied by other defects of eye movements, such as impaired smooth pursuit (209).

Dissociated Nystagmus

A special type of pathologic gaze-evoked nystagmus is dissociated or "ataxic" nystagmus. This type of nystagmus is most commonly encountered with an **internuclear ophthalmoplegia** (INO). Dissociated nystagmus is, in fact, a series of saccades followed by postsaccadic drift that occurs when the patient attempts to look laterally away from the side of the lesion. Since the saccades initiate the oscillations, this ocular motor abnormality is not a true nystagmus, but rather a series of saccadic pulses. Consider, for example, a

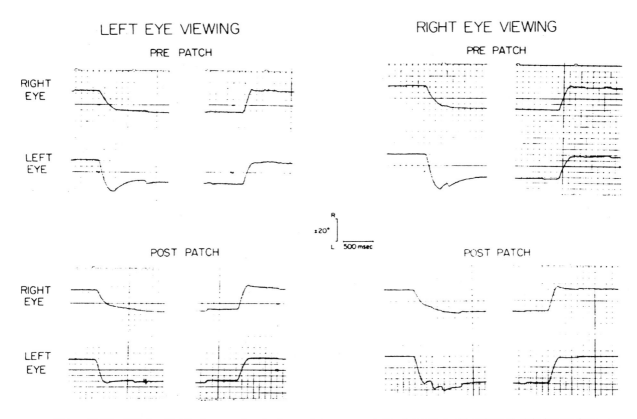

Figure 23.10. Effects of habitual monocular viewing on the eye movements of a patient with unilateral, right internuclear ophthalmoplegia. Pre-patch data were obtained after habitual binocular viewing, but the patient preferred to fixate with the right eye. Post-patch data were obtained after 5 days of patching of the right eye to ensure habitual left eye viewing. Left and right eye viewing refer to the viewing conditions at the time the eye movements were recorded. *Post-patch*: Note the decrease in the abduction nystagmus of the left eye (decrease in the size of the abduction saccadic pulse and of the backward postsaccadic drift), with a commensurate decrease in the size of the saccadic pulse and increase of the onward postsaccadic drift for the adduction saccades made by the right eye. These changes were independent of which eye was viewing during the recording session. Patching led to little change in the adducting saccades made by the left eye or abducting saccades made by the right eye (vertical bar indicates +20°; horizontal bar, 500 msec). (From Zee DS, Hain TC, Carl JR. Abduction nystagmus in internuclear ophthalmoplegia. Ann Neurol 1987;21:383–388.)

patient with a right-sided INO (Fig. 23.10, *top*). When the patient attempts to look to the left, the adducting saccades of the right eye are slow and hypometric. Each consists of a hypometric pulse, followed by a glissadic drift of the eye toward the target. Abducting saccades in the left eye are hypermetric, overshooting the target, and are followed by a glissadic backward drift of the eye. A series of such small saccades and drifts gives the appearance of dissociated nystagmus. Because of the difference in the velocity of the adducting saccades in the eye on the side of the lesion and the abducting saccades in the contralateral eye, comparison of horizontal saccades made by each eye is most useful in making the diagnosis of an INO. When the INO is subtle, moving an optokinetic tape or rotating an optokinetic drum toward the side of the affected medial rectus muscle induces asymmetric quick phases, with smaller-sized movements in the affected eye. Some caution is required in interpreting this sign, however, since abducting saccades are normally slightly faster than adducting saccades (210). In addition,

there are settings other than an INO in which patients may show an asymmetry of saccadic velocities, with the adducting eye moving more slowly than the abducting eye (discussion following). Nevertheless, when one observes slowed adducting saccades in one eye and normal abducting saccades in the opposite eye in a patient with no previous history of strabismus surgery, a diagnosis of INO is likely. Quantitative comparison of the velocity of the two eyes may be required to make the diagnosis of INO in subtle cases (211).

Several explanations have been offered to account for dissociated nystagmus in INO (9,212), but the most plausible suggestion is that it represents an attempt by the brain to adaptively correct hypometric saccades due to the weak medial rectus muscle. Acute experimental INO by local anesthetic blockade of the medial longitudinal fasciculus (MLF), produces paresis of the ipsilateral medial rectus, but does not produce abducting nystagmus in the contralateral eye (213). To compensate for the weakness of the medial rectus, there may be an adaptive increase in innervation to the adducting eye and, because of Hering's law of equal innervation, a commensurate increase in the innervation to the normal, abducting eye results. Although this adaptive change may help get the paretic eye on target, it leads to overshooting saccades and postsaccadic drift of the abducting eye if the patient attempts to fixate with the ipsilesional eye. Support for this interpretation comes from the observation that patching the eye with the adduction weakness for several days almost abolishes the overshoot and pulse-step mismatch of the abducting eye when the latter eye fixates (Fig. 23.10, *bottom left*) (212). Additional support for the view that the abduction nystagmus of an INO is a compensatory response to a "peripheral" weakness comes from the observation that surgically caused medial rectus weakness leads to a similar nystagmus, which resolves if the eye with the weak medial rectus is patched for several days (214). In addition to previous extraocular muscle surgery, both myasthenia gravis (215) and the Miller Fisher syndrome (216) may produce a dissociated nystagmus similar to that seen in an INO.

Dissociated nystagmus characterized by larger movements in the **adducting** eye occurs when some patients with abducens nerve palsy look into the paretic field (9). Indeed, whenever a patient habitually prefers to fixate with a paretic eye, the normal eye will show a dissociated nystagmus while looking in the direction of action of the paretic muscle, regardless of the pathogenesis of the weakness.

Bruns' Nystagmus

Tumors in the cerebellopontine angle, such as meningiomas or schwannomas of the vestibulocochlear nerve, may produce a low-frequency, large-amplitude nystagmus when the patient looks toward the side of the lesion, and a high-frequency, small-amplitude nystagmus when the patient looks toward the side opposite the lesion. The nystagmus that occurs on gaze toward the side of the lesion is gaze-evoked nystagmus caused by defective gaze holding, whereas the nystagmus that occurs during gaze toward the side opposite the lesion is caused by vestibular imbalance. This special nystagmus is called **Bruns' nystagmus** (217,218).

CONVERGENCE-RETRACTION NYSTAGMUS

So-called convergence-retraction nystagmus is characterized by quick phases that converge or retract the eyes on attempts to look up. It is elicited either by asking the patient to make an upward saccade or by using a handheld optokinetic drum or tape and moving the stripes or figures down. This maneuver produces slow, downward, pursuit eye movements, but upward quick phases are replaced by rapid convergent movements, retractory movements, or both. Affected patients usually have impaired or absent upward gaze for both pursuit and saccadic eye movements; however, in some cases upward pursuit appears normal, whereas upward saccades are obviously abnormal. Convergence-retraction nystagmus is commonly produced by lesions of the mesen-

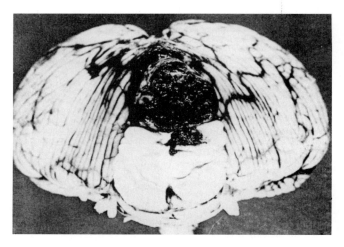

Figure 23.11. Pathology of convergence-retraction nystagmus. A pinealoma is compressing the dorsal midbrain of a 13-year-old boy who also had inability to elevate the eyes above the horizontal midline, limitation of downward gaze, and anisocoria.

cephalon that damage the posterior commissure, such as pineal tumors (219–221); an example is shown in Figure 23.11. It has been proposed that convergence-retraction nystagmus is, in fact, a saccadic disorder rather than nystagmus because the primary adductive movements are asynchronous adducting saccades (222). However, other studies have indicated that the movements may be vergence in origin (223); more studies are needed to resolve this issue. During horizontal saccades, the abnormal pattern of convergent innervation manifests itself as slowing of the abducting eye: "pseudo-abducens palsy" (219,221). Convergence-retraction nystagmus may also occur with a Chiari malformation or epileptic seizures (224,225). Convergence-retraction nystagmus is usually intermittent, being determined by saccadic activity, and it thus can be differentiated from other more continuous forms of disjunctive nystagmus, such as convergent-divergent pendular nystagmus (29,79) and the oculomasticatory myorhythmia characteristic of Whipple's disease (80).

Jerk-waveform **divergence nystagmus** is diagnosed infrequently, but it may occur in patients with cerebellar disease, such as the Chiari malformation. In such cases, combined divergent and downbeat nystagmus produces slow phases that are directed upward and inward (139).

CENTRIPETAL AND REBOUND NYSTAGMUS

If a patient with gaze-evoked nystagmus attempts to look eccentrically for a sustained period, the nystagmus may begin to decrease in amplitude and may even reverse direction, so that the eye begins to drift centrifugally ("centripetal nystagmus") (226). If the eyes are then returned to the central position, a short-lived nystagmus with slow drifts in the direction of the prior eccentric gaze occurs. This is called **rebound nystagmus** (227,228). Both centripetal and rebound nystagmus may reflect an attempt by brainstem or cerebellar mechanisms to correct for the centripetal drift of gaze-evoked nystagmus. Rebound nystagmus typically occurs in patients with cerebellar disease, but it has been reported following experimental lesions in the region of the nucleus prepositus hypoglossi and medial vestibular nucleus (200), and in normal subjects with typical gaze-evoked nystagmus (207). Extreme gaze deviation away from the side of the lesion in one patient with a lateral medullary infarction was reported to cause this type of paroxysmal nystagmus and vertigo lasting about 1 minute (229). Such a phenomenon could be explained by a sustained eye position signal causing an imbalance of central vestibular mechanisms. Rebound nystagmus has been reported in a patient with a tumor confined to the flocculus (230); other ocular motor abnormalities, including impaired smooth pursuit and gaze-evoked nystagmus persisted after the tumor invaded the vestibular nuclei, but the rebound nystagmus disappeared. Such findings have suggested that rebound is due to a the development of a bias within the vestibular nuclei.

CONGENITAL FORMS OF NYSTAGMUS

NATURE AND FORMS OF CONGENITAL OCULAR OSCILLATIONS

In this section, we review those forms of nystagmus that develop during infancy (231). Advances have been made with the identification of congenital forms of nystagmus in mutant dogs with abnormal anatomy of the visual system (47), and in normal monkeys that are deprived of binocular vision during early life (232). However, although some patients with congenital nystagmus show visual abnormalities, others with similar ocular oscillations do not. Furthermore, the characteristic waveforms, e.g., pendular (Fig. 23.1D) or jerk (Fig. 23.1A), do not specify pathogenesis or indicate whether the congenital nystagmus is associated with visual system anomalies (18). Thus, the underlying mechanisms are not fully understood. Three distinct syndromes are currently recognized: congenital nystagmus, latent nystagmus, and spasmus nutans.

Although there is no widely accepted classification of nystagmus in infancy, the Classification of Eye Movement Abnormalities and Strabismus (CEMAS) Working Group (233) has proposed that the term infantile nystagmus syndrome (INS) be used to encompass what has previously been called congenital nystagmus, including motor or sensory varieties. The main criteria for defining INS are infantile onset and accelerating slow-phase waveforms (Fig. 23.1C). However, a potential problem posed by the CEMAS classification for some ophthalmologists is that measurement of eye movements, which is necessary to characterize the waveforms, may not be available. In additional, CEMAS has called latent nystagmus Fusional Maldevelopment Nystagmus Syndrome (FMNS). In this chapter, we will continue to use the terms "congenital nystagmus" and "latent nystagmus" but the reader should note that a transition of terminology may occur in the neuro-ophthalmological community over the next few years.

CONGENITAL NYSTAGMUS

Clinical Features

Congenital nystagmus is usually diagnosed during infancy, but occasionally presents during adult life (234,235) when it may create a diagnostic problem, especially if the patient has other symptoms, such as headaches or dizziness. Certain clinical features usually differentiate congenital nystagmus from other ocular oscillations. It is almost always conjugate and horizontal, even on up or down gaze. A small torsional component to the nystagmus is probably common (236), but is difficult to identify clinically. Only rarely is congenital nystagmus purely vertical (237–239). Congenital nystagmus is usually accentuated by the attempt to visually fixate an object and by attention or anxiety. Eyelid closure (240) and convergence usually suppress it (241–243), but occasionally congenital nystagmus is evoked by viewing a near target (79,244). Its intensity may also be influenced by viewing the vertical lines of an optokinetic tape (245). Congenital nystagmus often decreases when the eyes are moved into a particular position in the orbit, called the "null" region. In some patients, the direction of the nystagmus spontaneously reverses direction during sustained viewing of a fixation point (18,246,247). The direction of the nystagmus may also be influenced by which eye is viewing, with the nystagmus beating away from the covered eye; this is similar to latent nystagmus (see below).

The most distinctive feature of congenital nystagmus is its waveforms, the most common of which are increasing-velocity (Fig. 23.1C) and pendular (Fig. 23.1D). Frequently superimposed on these waveforms, which may be combined, are **foveation periods**—the hallmark of congenital nystagmus (18,248,249). During each cycle, usually after a quick phase, there is a brief period when the eye is still and is pointed at the object of regard. With jerk waveforms, the quick phases (saccades) may brake the oscillation (250) or bring the eye to the target. With pendular waveforms, the oscillation is flattened by a foveation period when the eye is closest to the target (Fig. 23.12). The particular waveform that is seen in a patient with congenital nystagmus depends in part upon the patient's age. Most infants show large-amplitude "triangular" waveforms. Shortly thereafter, the waveform becomes pendular, but it changes again to a jerk type as the patient reaches about one year of age (251,252). These waveforms are so characteristic of congenital nystagmus that reliable records of eye position and velocity will often secure the diagnosis.

In those individuals with congenital nystagmus that spontaneously changes direction, the timings of reversal tend to be this irregular. This aperiodic alternating congenital nystagmus appears to have a different pathogenesis than acquired periodic alternating nystagmus (247,253,254).

Foveation periods are only rarely reported in acquired forms of nystagmus (255). They are probably one reason (along with elevated thresholds for motion detection) why most patients with congenital nystagmus do not complain of oscillopsia, despite otherwise nearly continuous move-

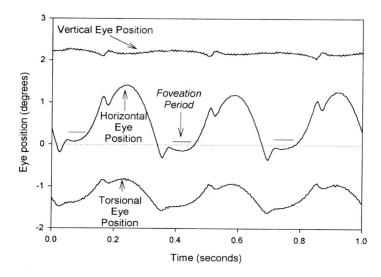

Figure 23.12. A pendular type of congenital nystagmus waveform with superimposed quick phases, showing the large horizontal component, smaller torsional component, and almost absent vertical component. Note that vertical and torsional channels have been offset to aid clarity of display. Foveation periods follow quick phases (when eye position is close to zero) and are indicated by horizontal bars. Upward deflections indicate rightward (horizontal), upward (vertical), or clockwise (torsional) eye rotations, with respect to the patient.

ment of their eyes (8,256–262), and why many have normal visual acuity (263,264). However, foveation periods are not invariably present in congenital nystagmus. When they are absent or poorly developed, vision is usually impaired (265).

Up to 30% of patients with congenital nystagmus also have strabismus (266). A commonly described associated finding in such patients is ''inverted pursuit'' or ''reversed optokinetic nystagmus'' (267). With a handheld optokinetic drum or tape, quick phases are directed in the same direction as the drum rotates or the tape moves. In fact, based on measurements made of tracking during the foveation period, it has been shown that both smooth pursuit and optokinetic eye movements are preserved in at least some individuals with congenital nystagmus (268,269). Similarly, vestibular responses are generally normal in patients with congenital nystagmus if judged by retinal image stability during foveation periods (270,271). Thus, their view of the world is similar whether they are stationary or in motion (272). In those patients with associated visual disorders such as albinism, however, vestibular responses to lower frequencies of head rotations and optokinetic responses may be impaired (273,274).

Occasional patients exhibit congenital nystagmus only during attempted smooth tracking (275), and others can voluntarily release or inhibit their congenital nystagmus, suggesting that fixation plays some role in the oscillations (276). Congenital nystagmus associated with congenital gaze-holding failure (i.e., leaky neural integrator) has been reported in a kindred (277) suggesting that, at least in this family, instability of the gaze-holding mechanism (neural integrator) is unlikely to have been the primary cause of the nystagmus.

Head turns are common in patients with congenital nystagmus and are an adaptive strategy to bring the eyes close to the null position in the orbit, where nystagmus is reduced (278). The observation of such a head turn in childhood photographs is often helpful in diagnosing congenital nystagmus. Another strategy used by patients with either congenital or latent nystagmus (discussion following) is to pur-

posely induce an esotropia to suppress the nystagmus. Such an esotropia requires a head turn to direct the viewing eye at the object of interest. This phenomenon is called the nystagmus blockage syndrome (279,280).

Some patients with congenital nystagmus also show head oscillations (271,281,282). Such head movements cannot act as an adaptive strategy to improve vision, however, unless the vestibulo-ocular reflex is negated. In fact, head movements are not compensatory in most patients with congenital nystagmus and tend to increase when the individual attends to an object, an effort that also increases the nystagmus. It seems possible, therefore, that the head tremor and ocular oscillations represent the output of a common disordered neural mechanism (282).

Pathogenesis of Congenital Nystagmus

As noted earlier, nystagmus developing early in life and showing some of the waveform characteristics of congenital nystagmus in humans also occurs in mutant dogs who lack the normal hemidecussation of fibers in the optic chiasm (47), and in normal monkeys who are subjected to monocular visual deprivation in infancy (232). It is also associated with a variety of visual system disorders, including ocular and oculocutaneous albinism (283–286), achromatopsia, retinal cone dystrophy, optic nerve hypoplasia, Leber's congenital amaurosis, retinal coloboma, aniridia, corectopia, congenital stationary night blindness, Chédiak-Higashi syndrome, Joubert syndrome, and peroxisomal disorders (287). Because of the many diagnostic possibilities, a complete ophthalmologic evaluation and an electroretinogram must be performed in patients with congenital nystagmus associated with decreased visual acuity or visual dysfunction (287–289). Congenital nystagmus, both with and without associated visual system abnormalities, may be familial (290). Several modes of inheritance have been reported (231,291–293); in X-linked forms (292), the mothers may show subtle ocular motor abnormalities. Congenital nystagmus, with some similarities of waveform, has been reported in monozygotic twins (294). However, there may be considerable differences in waveforms among members of a single family with hereditary congenital nystagmus (290).

The known anatomic variations of the anterior visual system in individuals with congenital nystagmus, such as excessive crossing at the chiasm in association with albinism (295–297), or absent crossing of nasal fibers in achiasmatic subjects with congenital seesaw nystagmus (47–49), have led to the development of models for congenital nystagmus based on "miswiring" of visual pathways (276,298). A model postulating that maladaptation to early visual deprivation leads to instability of the gaze-holding mechanisms has also been proposed (299). Further work is required to validate these models.

LATENT (OCCLUSION) NYSTAGMUS

Clinical Features

True **latent nystagmus** is a horizontal jerk nystagmus that is absent when both eyes are viewing but appears when one eye is covered. This conjugate nystagmus is characterized by quick phases of both eyes that beat toward the side of the fixating eye. In most patients, a low-amplitude nystagmus is also present when both eyes are viewing, and is called "manifest latent nystagmus" (300). It apparently occurs because only one eye is fixating, and vision from the other deviated eye is suppressed (301,302). Latent nystagmus usually reverses direction upon covering of either eye. In some patients, however, it is present when one eye is covered but is absent when the other is covered. Occasional patients can control their latent nystagmus at will (303). Latent nystagmus is usually associated with strabismus, typically esotropia (304). Amblyopia is frequent, whereas binocular vision with normal stereopsis is rare. Latent nystagmus has been described in identical twins (305).

The slow phase of latent nystagmus usually shows a decaying velocity waveform when the eyes are close to central position (Fig. 23.1*B*), in contrast to the increasing velocity waveform of congenital nystagmus. A number of studies suggest that foveation may occur during the slowest part of the drift if the amplitude of the nystagmus is large, and immediately after the quick phase if the amplitude is small (306). Latent nystagmus usually follows Alexander's law, with the nystagmus being greatest on looking in the direction of the quick phases, away from the covered eye. Some patients turn the head to keep the viewing eye in an adducted position, where nystagmus is minimal. Occasionally, congenital and latent nystagmus coexist, in which case the waveforms may be quite complex. Rarely, in such patients, if vision is clearer with the latent nystagmus waveforms than with the congenital nystagmus waveforms, the patients switch from congenital to latent nystagmus as one eye becomes esotropic and the other takes up fixation (279). In addition to strabismus, patients with latent nystagmus frequently show an upward deviation of the covered eye (alternating sursumduction or dissociated vertical deviation) (307). In such patients, the nystagmus often has a torsional component (307). Latent nystagmus is quite common, and accurate diagnosis is important to avoid inappropriate investigations. It should be differentiated from gaze-evoked nystagmus in association with strabismus, especially abducting nystagmus occurring with INO, in which an exotropia may be present.

Pathogenesis of Latent Nystagmus

Latent nystagmus is thought to be caused by a defect in cortical motion processing that results from lack of development of binocular vision (308). It is a common feature of Down's syndrome (309). Individuals with latent nystagmus often show impaired initiation of smooth pursuit in a specific pattern: nasal target motion evokes more vigorous pursuit than temporal motion, and vertical optokinetic motion evokes responses with horizontal components (17). A related theory is that latent nystagmus is caused by an imbalance in the subcortical optokinetic system (308), perhaps secondary to a loss of cortical motion detectors. This would account for the temporal-nasal directional predominance of monocular optokinetic responses shown by some patients with latent nystagmus and of normal infants prior to maturation of cortical vision (310). Animal models of monocular deprivation support this view (311). Another proposal is that latent nystagmus is caused by a defect in the influence of the internal representation of egocentric coordinates upon the direction of gaze. Support for this hypothesis comes from the observation that a patient with lifelong monocular blindness was able to reverse the direction of his latent nystagmus by attempting to view from his blind eye (312). It is also possible that an abnormality of extraocular proprioception predisposes to latent nystagmus (313), since extraocular proprioception is important for the normal development of binocularity (314). These proposed mechanisms may not be mutually exclusive, and their relative importance is unclear.

SPASMUS NUTANS

Spasmus nutans is characterized by the triad of nystagmus, head nodding, and an anomalous head position, such as torticollis (315). It usually begins in the first year of life, although it may not be detected until the child is 3 or 4 years old. Neurologic abnormalities are absent, although strabismus or amblyopia may coexist. The syndrome is sometimes familial and has been reported in monozygotic twins (316). Spasmus nutans spontaneously remits, usually within 1 to 2 years after onset, although it may last for over 8 years (317).

The most consistent feature of spasmus nutans is the nystagmus, although head nodding may be the first abnormality to be noticed (45,317–319). Because the nystagmus is usually intermittent and has a small-amplitude, high-frequency (3–11 Hz) pendular waveform, it can easily be overlooked. When recognized, however, it has a "shimmering" quality.

The nystagmus of spasmus nutans almost always differs in the two eyes, and it may even be uniocular (Fig. 23.13). Other distinguishing features are the variability of the amplitude of nystagmus in each eye and the difference in the phase relationship between the two eyes. Even over the course of a few seconds or minutes, the oscillations may variably be conjugate, disconjugate, dissociated, or purely monocular (Fig. 23.13). The plane of the nystagmus is predominantly

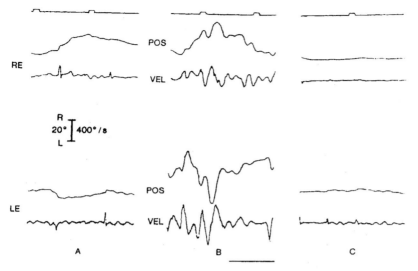

Figure 23.13. Examples of nystagmus of spasmus nutans from one child during a single recording session. *A*, There are binocular oscillations with no phase difference between the eyes. *B*, There are binocular oscillations with an approximately 180° phase difference between the eyes. *C*, There are uniocular oscillations of the left eye. LE, left eye; RE, right eye; POS, position; VEL, velocity; timing marks at top of records indicate 1-second intervals. (From Weissman BM, Dell'Osso LF, Abel LA et al. Spasmus nutans: A quantitative prospective study. Arch Ophthalmol 1987;105:525–528.)

horizontal, but it may have vertical or torsional components. It may sometimes be brought out by evoking the near response (320).

The head nodding of spasmus nutans is irregular, with horizontal or vertical components. It is usually more prominent when the child attempts to inspect something of interest. About two-thirds of the patients have an additional head tilt or turn. In some patients, the head nodding appears to turn off the nystagmus (318,319); however, it is unclear whether head nodding, turning, or tilting are always adaptive strategies adopted to reduce the nystagmus or if they are simply another manifestation of the underlying abnormality in the central nervous system.

Two main clinical decisions must be made by the physician who sees a child with eye and head oscillations. The first is to determine if the nystagmus is associated with reti-

nal disease or a tumor of the visual pathway, particularly an optic chiasmal glioma (43,44,321). A careful ophthalmologic evaluation must be performed in all children, with particular emphasis on the anterior visual system. If there is any suggestion that the child has optic nerve or chiasmal dysfunction, neuroimaging studies should be performed. Some experts recommend that neuroimaging be performed on all children, given the difficulties inherent in eliciting a history of visual loss, and ophthalmoscopy, in small children. The second decision is to determine whether the ocular motor disturbance is actually spasmus nutans, which will resolve over time, or congenital nystagmus, which probably will not. Spasmus nutans usually can be differentiated from congenital and latent nystagmus by its intermittency, high frequency, and dissociated characteristics. If the child will cooperate, eye movement recordings often help differentiate between these two entities (45).

EYE MOVEMENTS DURING EPILEPTIC SEIZURES

Several forms of nystagmus occur as manifestations of epileptic seizures (322–326). Although such **epileptic nystagmus** is probably quite common, only rarely have eye movements been reliably measured during seizures.

Patients with epileptic foci affecting portions of the cortex concerned with the programming of smooth pursuit and saccades (see Chapter 17) may show either ipsiversive or contraversive eye deviation and nystagmus. In patients with epileptic saccadic activity, the underlying focus usually affects the occipito-temporo-parietal junction (322). In one such patient who had a right temporo-occipital focus, the seizure began with a contraversive (leftward) gaze deviation due to a staircase of small saccades (324). After a few seconds, left-beating nystagmus commenced, with slow phases that showed a decreasing-velocity waveform. The nystagmus was accompanied by high-voltage spike activity of 11–14 Hz that did not spread to the frontal cortex. At the end of the seizure, the eyes returned to central position. This patient was unresponsive, partly from a metabolic encephalopathy.

Her gaze deviation was initiated by saccades, and the subsequent nystagmus was probably caused by an impaired gaze-holding mechanism (i.e., a deficient neural integrator).

In another patient, who also had a seizure focus in the right temporo-occipital cortex, the initial eye movement was an ipsiversive gaze deviation, followed by a left-beating nystagmus that had linear slow phases (326). During the nystagmus, sharp wave activity of 12–14 Hz occurred. The patient with the ipsiversive deviation was conscious throughout the entire attack. His gaze deviation may have been a smooth pursuit movement, with the resetting leftward-beating quick phases of nystagmus triggered by the eccentric eye position and ipsilateral rightward drift of the eyes.

Thus, contraversive quick phases in epileptic patients may result from two different mechanisms. First, they may be primary, contraversive saccades that are caused by epileptic activity in the saccadic regions, and that are followed by centripetal drift from impaired gaze-holding. Such drifts are often seen in patients taking antiepileptic medications. Second, they may be secondary, reflexive contraversive saccades that are correcting a slow ipsiversive deviation across the midline that is caused by epileptic activation of either the smooth pursuit or optokinetic regions. The second mechanism produces true nystagmus, whereas the first is actually a saccadic disorder. Experimental studies in awake monkeys indicate that the threshold for stimulating pursuit eye movements is lower than that for stimulating saccades (327).

To induce epileptic nystagmus in awake patients, the frequency of discharge must be high (above 10 spikes per second) and must affect the temporo-parieto-occipital junction area (322). In patients with coexistent brainstem lesions, the only manifestation of such activity may be rapid, small-amplitude, vertical eye movements (328). The absence of horizontal movements in such patients reflects dysfunction of the paramedian pontine reticular formation (PPRF).

EYELID NYSTAGMUS

Several studies have defined the anatomic and physiologic links between eye and eyelid movements (329–332), and have evaluated the common effects of disease on both (330). Upward movements of the eyelids frequently accompany upward movements of vertical nystagmus. In fact, the absence of lid nystagmus in a patient with upbeat nystagmus may suggest disconnection between the premotor signals for the superior rectus and levator palpebrae superioris, implicating the region between the riMLF and the oculomotor nucleus. For the same reasons, lid nystagmus unaccompanied by vertical eye nystagmus may reflect midbrain lesions (333,334). In patients with long-standing compression of the central caudal nucleus, ''midbrain ptosis'' may occur (see Chapter 24), and this may lead to lid nystagmus (334).

Occasionally, twitches of the eyelid accompany horizontal nystagmus. This phenomenon was described in a patient with Wallenberg's lateral medullary syndrome (335), in whom lid nystagmus was inhibited by convergence. In other patients, eyelid nystagmus may be induced by convergence. This is called Pick's sign (336–338). In both cases, lesions are often present in the medulla, cerebellum, or both structures (336,337). The curious association of eyelid nystagmus with convergence may occur because the eyelid normally retracts with near effort. Therefore, any compromise of lid function will become more evident on attempt to converge. Eyelid nystagmus has been likened to the pathologic form of gaze-evoked nystagmus that occurs in patients with cerebellar disease and that is often associated with downward drifts of the eyelids, followed by corrective rapid upward movements (337).

SACCADIC INTRUSIONS

COMMON FEATURES OF SACCADIC INTRUSIONS

Several types of inappropriate saccadic eye movements may intrude upon steady fixation. These are schematized in Figure 23.14, and actual recorded examples are shown in Figure 23.15. Saccadic intrusions must be differentiated from nystagmus, in which a drift of the eyes from the desired position of gaze is the primary abnormality, and from saccadic dysmetria (Fig. 23.14A), in which the eye over- or under-shoots a target, sometimes several times, before achieving stable fixation (339,340). Because all of these movements are often rapid and brief, it may be necessary to measure eye and target position, as well as eye velocity, in order to identify accurately the saccadic abnormality. In this section, we first describe the characteristics of each type of saccadic intrusion and then review possible mechanisms of pathogenesis.

SQUARE-WAVE JERKS

Square-wave jerks, also called Gegenrucke, are a common finding in healthy persons, particularly the elderly (341–344). They have a typical profile on eye movement records, and it is this profile from which their name is derived. They are small, conjugate saccades, ranging from 0.5 to 5.0° in size, that take the eye away from the fixation position and return it after about 200 milliseconds (Figs. 23.14C and 23.15A). They are often more prominent during smooth pursuit, are most easily detected during ophthalmoscopy, and are also present in darkness.

Square-wave jerks with an increased frequency (up to 2 Hz) occur in certain cerebellar syndromes (345,346), in progressive supranuclear palsy (347,348), and in cerebral hemispheric disease (349). When very frequent, they are called square-wave oscillations (350). These movements may be mistaken for nystagmus. Cigarette smoking increases the frequency of square-wave jerks (351,352).

MACROSQUARE-WAVE JERKS (SQUARE-WAVE PULSES)

Macrosquare-wave jerks are large eye movements, typically greater than 5°, that occur at a frequency of about 2–3 Hz. After taking the eye off the target, they return it after a latency of about 80 milliseconds (Fig. 23.14D) (353). These eye movements occur in light or darkness, and they occasionally are suppressed during monocular fixation (354). Macrosquare-wave jerks occur in bursts and vary in amplitude. They are encountered in disease states that disrupt cerebellar outflow, such as MS.

MACROSACCADIC OSCILLATIONS

Macrosaccadic oscillations usually consist of horizontal saccades that occur in bursts, initially building up and then decreasing in amplitude, with intersaccadic intervals of about 200 milliseconds (Figs. 23.14B and 23.15C). Described originally in cerebellar patients, macrosaccadic oscillations are thought to be an extreme form of saccadic dysmetria, in which the patient's saccades are so hypermetric that they overshoot the target continuously in both directions and thus oscillate around the fixation point (355,356). They

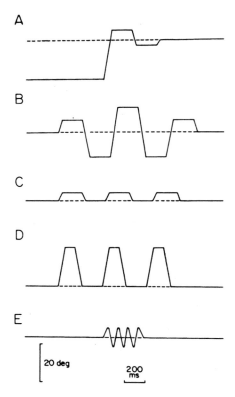

Figure 23.14. Schematic drawings of various saccadic oscillations. *A*, Saccadic dysmetria: Saccades with inappropriate amplitudes that occur in response to target jumps. *B*, Macrosaccadic oscillations: Hypermetric saccades about the position of the target. *C*, Square-wave jerks: Small, inappropriately occurring saccades away from and back to the position of the target. *D*, Macrosquare-wave jerks: Large, uncalled-for saccades away from and back to the position of the target. *E*, Ocular flutter: To-and-fro back-to-back saccades without an intersaccadic interval. (From Leigh RJ, Zee DS. The Neurology of Eye Movements. Ed 3. Philadelphia, FA Davis, 1991.)

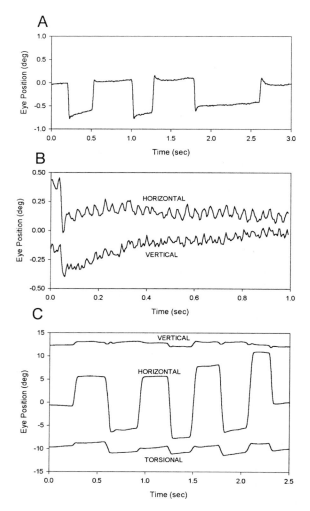

Figure 23.15. Actual recordings of saccadic oscillations. *A*, Horizontal saccadic intrusions (square-wave jerks) that repeatedly move the image of regard off the fovea. The patient had progressive supranuclear palsy. *B*, Diagonal microsaccadic flutter that was detectable only with an ophthalmoscope, but because of its high frequency it caused oscillopsia and impaired vision in this patient, who was otherwise well. *C*, Macrosaccadic oscillations from the right eye of a patient with a pontine infarction (357). Fixation is interrupted by bursts of saccadic intrusions that are time-locked in the horizontal, vertical, and torsional planes. The return saccade usually overshoots the central fixation point. Torsional and vertical tracings have been offset for convenience of display. Upward deflections correspond to rightward, upward, or clockwise eye rotations, with respect to the patient.

are usually induced by a gaze shift, but they may also occur during attempted fixation or even in darkness (357). They are often visually disabling (358). They may have vertical or torsional components and, occasionally, the former may be quite prominent clinically (359). Macrosaccadic oscillations are occasionally encountered in patients with myasthenia gravis after administration of edrophonium (360). In such patients who have severe ophthalmoparesis, suddenly reversing the neuromuscular block with edrophonium reveals the adaptive efforts that the brain has been making—increasing innervation (gain) especially for saccades. Consequently, for a short period, saccadic gain is too high and the eyes oscillate either side of a visual target.

SACCADIC PULSES, OCULAR FLUTTER, AND OPSOCLONUS

Saccadic pulses are brief intrusions upon steady fixation. They are produced when a saccadic pulse is unaccompanied by a step command. The eye movement thus consists of a saccade away from the fixation position, with a rapid drift

back. Saccadic pulses may occur in series or as doublets. They are encountered in some normal subjects and in patients with MS (361). Saccadic pulses may occur in other disorders (362). Their pathophysiology is not well understood.

There is a continuum between saccadic pulses and saccadic oscillations without an intersaccadic interval (363, 364). The latter may occur in one direction, usually the horizontal plane, in which case they are called **ocular flutter** (Fig. 23.14*E*), or they may be multivectorial, in which case they are termed **opsoclonus** or **saccadomania**. The frequency of oscillations is usually high, typically 10–15 cycles per second, being higher with smaller-sized movements. Ocular flutter may be intermittent and mainly associated with voluntary saccades (flutter dysmetria) or convergence movements (365). Occasionally, the amplitude of the oscillations is very small (''microflutter'') (366). In such cases, the movements may be detected only with a slit lamp or an ophthalmoscope or by using eye movement recordings, even though they are producing oscillopsia or other visual symptoms. Sometimes such microflutter has components in all three planes (Fig. 23.15B).

Sustained opsoclonus is a striking finding, in which multidirectional conjugate saccades, usually of large amplitude, interfere with steady fixation, smooth pursuit, or convergence. These movements may persist during sleep. Opsoclonus is often accompanied by myoclonus—brief jerky involuntary limb movements—hence the term ''opsoclonus-myoclonus.'' In children, this syndrome is called ''dancing eyes and dancing feet'' (367). Ataxia and encephalopathy may also accompany opsoclonus.

The reported causes of ocular flutter and opsoclonus are summarized in Table 23.7. In about 50% of cases, the etiology remains obscure. In children, about half the cases of opsoclonus are associated with tumors of neural crest origin, such as neuroblastoma. In adults, opsoclonus occurs most often in association with small-cell lung, breast, and other cancers (368). Low CSF concentrations of 5-hydroxyindolacetic acid (5-HIAA) and homovanillic acid (HVA) can often be demonstrated in children with the opsoclonus-myoclonus syndrome (369). However, CSF abnormalities may occur in opsoclonus associated with both tumor and encephalitis (370) and, therefore, do not help to distinguish between the infectious and paraneoplastic etiologies.

Various autoantibodies can be detected in sera of some

Table 23.7
Etiology of Ocular Flutter and Opsoclonus[a]

Viral encephalitis
As a component of the syndrome of myoclonic encephalopathy of infants ("dancing eyes and dancing feet")
Paraneoplastic (occult tumor, especially small-cell lung and breast cancers)
Neuroblastoma
Other tumors
Trauma (in association with hypoxia and sepsis)
Meningitis
Intracranial tumors
Hydrocephalus
Thalamic hemorrhage
Multiple sclerosis
Hyperosmolar coma
Associated with systemic disease; e.g., viral hepatitis, sarcoid, AIDS
Side effects of drugs: lithium, amitriptyline, phenytoin, and diazepam
Toxins: chlordecone, thallium, strychnine, toluene, and organophosphates
Transient phenomenon of healthy neonates
Voluntary "nystagmus" or psychogenic flutter

[a] Not all case reports have documented the abnormality with eye movement recordings.

patients with opsoclonus. Of these, anti-Ri antibody is the most common (371–373), but various other antibodies have been demonstrated (374). Anti-Ri is reported in association with cancer of the breast or pelvic organs and, less commonly, in patients with small-cell lung or bladder cancer. Sometimes, however, no tumor can be found (375–377). A second antibody, anti-Hu, has been reported with opsoclonus in two children with neuroblastoma and in an adult with small-cell lung cancer (372,378). This is an antineuronal antibody that binds nuclear RNA and is usually associated with paraneoplastic sensory neuronopathy, cerebellar degeneration, and limbic encephalitis. A third type of antibody, directed against neurofilaments, was found in a child with paraneoplastic opsoclonus (379). Recent studies have emphasized the diversity of immunity to neuronal autoantigens (374), with only a minority of patients showing immunoreactivity to specific antineuronal antibodies (368).

The prognosis of idiopathic opsoclonus (including patients with manifestations of brainstem encephalitis) is generally good (368). Some patients with paraneoplastic opsoclonus myoclonus show spontaneous remissions, irrespective of the underlying tumor (372). Patients whose tumor can be identified and treated may recover neurologically; those who are not treated have a more severe course (368).

VOLUNTARY SACCADIC OSCILLATIONS OR VOLUNTARY NYSTAGMUS

Some normal subjects can voluntarily induce saccadic oscillations, usually by converging; this party trick has been called voluntary nystagmus but is really psychogenic flutter (380–382). Voluntary nystagmus is found in about 5–8% of the population and may occur as a familial trait (381). The oscillations are conjugate, with frequency and amplitude similar to those encountered in ocular flutter and opsoclonus. Although usually confined to the horizontal plane, voluntary nystagmus can occasionally be vertical or torsional (383), and may be accompanied by a head tremor (384). Voluntary nystagmus can be produced in the light or dark and with the eyes open or closed. It causes oscillopsia and reduced visual acuity and is often accompanied by eyelid flutter, a strained facial expression, and convergence. Individuals who are able to produce voluntary nystagmus may also be able to superimpose voluntary saccades on smooth movements during tracking of a target (385). The clinical challenge is to be able to distinguish voluntary forms of saccadic oscillations, which have no pathologic significance, from disorders such as ocular flutter and opsoclonus, which require a complete evaluation.

PATHOGENESIS OF SACCADIC INTRUSIONS

Neural Substrate

As discussed in Chapter 17, the brainstem circuits responsible for generating saccades are well worked out and provide a means for testing brainstem and cerebellar function (386). Thus, the saccadic command is generated by burst neurons of the brainstem reticular formation that project monosynaptically to ocular motoneurons The burst neurons for horizontal saccades are located in the PPRF (387), whereas the burst neurons for vertical and torsional saccades are located in the riMLF (388). Burst neurons discharge only during saccadic eye movements. The activity of all saccadic burst neurons is gated by omnipause neurons, which are crucial for suppressing unwanted saccades during fixation and slow eye movements. The omnipause neurons are located in the caudal pons within the raphe interpositus nucleus (RIP), adjacent to the abducens nucleus (389,390). Inputs into omnipause neurons arise in the superior colliculus, frontal eye fields, and mesencephalic reticular formation.

Square-Wave Jerks

During steady fixation, the threshold for electrical stimulation of saccades in either the frontal eye fields or the superior colliculus is elevated (391,392), which is probably mediated through the projections of these structures to the omnipause neurons. In the rostral superior colliculus, a distinct population of "fixation neurons" has been identified (393), whereas in the frontal eye fields, neurons active during suppression of saccades have been identified (391). Pharmacologic inactivation at both sites leads to disruption of fixation by saccadic intrusions, but not by flutter or opsoclonus (394,395). Furthermore, inactivation of the mesencephalic reticular formation may cause saccadic intrusions (396). Thus, impairment of any of these projections to the omnipause neurons can lead to saccadic intrusions, possibly explaining the increased incidence of square-wave jerks with cerebral hemispheric disease (349), and in progressive supranuclear palsy, in which the mesencephalic reticular formation and superior colliculus are both affected (397). We have also noted the development, and subsequent disappearance, of saccadic intrusions during recovery from peripheral extraocular muscle weakness, e.g., in the Miller Fisher syndrome or bilateral abducens palsy. It seems possible that this reflects central adaptation of saccadic commands in response to peripheral weakness.

Ocular Flutter and Opsoclonus

The pathogenesis of saccadic oscillations without an intersaccadic interval, e.g., ocular flutter and opsoclonus, seems closely related to the properties of the burst neurons themselves. Burst neurons have very high discharge rates (up to 1,000 spikes per second), and they discharge vigorously even for small saccades (398). The anatomical connections between burst neurons in the brainstem and their high discharge rates ("gain") predisposes to oscillations if the omnipause neurons are not actively inhibiting them and no specific saccadic command has been issued. Thus, normal subjects may show transient saccadic oscillations when, for example, they make a saccade in combination with a vergence movements (399). In this case, the saccade shifts the direction of gaze quickly, but the vergence movement takes much longer to align both eyes. While the vergence component is being completed, small conjugate horizontal oscillations are evident, indicating that the omnipause neurons are unable to

selectively shut off the saccadic burst neurons when their job is done (399). Theoretically, therefore, disease affecting omnipause neurons, or their afferents, might be expected to lead to saccadic oscillations such as ocular flutter and opsoclonus (363), especially if the membrane properties of the burst neurons became more excitable. Some experimental data are in conflict with this hypothesis, however, since chemical lesions of the omnipause neurons are reported to cause slowing of both horizontal and vertical saccades (400). Attempts to demonstrate histopathologic changes in omnipause neurons in some patients with paraneoplastic saccadic oscillations have usually failed to show any changes (401,402), although one study demonstrated complete absence of cells in the omnipause region of a patient with paraneoplastic saccadic oscillations (377). In this patient, intracellular deposits of anti-Ri IgG were discovered predominantly in the brainstem, especially in the reticular formation of pons and midbrain. Posner has suggested that, in paraneoplastic opsoclonus, the tumor and certain CNS structures share an epitope (372). This common epitope elicits an efficient immune response against the tumor, thus conferring a more indolent oncologic course, but it also elicits an immune response against normal neural tissue, causing the neurologic syndrome (see Chapter 36). One patient developed ocular flutter in association with an MS lesion in the PPRF region; as the lesion resolved, so did the oscillations (403). Furthermore, in two patients with presumed viral opsoclonus-myoclonus, MR imaging demonstrated lesions involving the pontine tegmentum (404).

There is some evidence that impaired glycinergic transmission may play a role in the pathogenesis of both ocular flutter and opsoclonus (405). First, poisoning with a glycinergic antagonist, strychnine, can produce both myoclonus and opsoclonus (406). Second, in generalized myoclonic conditions, such as hyperekplexia, abnormal receptors to glycine are found (407). The concurrent appearance of opsoclonus with myoclonus may suggest a similar mechanism. Third, glycine is identified as the neurotransmitter of the omnipause neurons (390). Since the latter are often implicated in the pathogenesis of saccadic intrusions, glycinergic dysfunction, presumably caused by autoantibodies, might be responsible for the opsoclonus-myoclonus syndrome.

Cerebellum and Saccadic Oscillations

Cerebellar dysfunction has traditionally been blamed for ocular flutter and opsoclonus (402,408,409). Functional imaging in patients with opsoclonus has shown activation of deep cerebellar nuclei (410). However, experimental lesions of the cerebellum do not produce these oscillations, even though striking saccadic dysmetria can be produced, especially when the caudal fastigial nuclei of the cerebellum are inactivated (411,412). Reliable measurements of eye movements are often necessary to make the distinction between severe forms of saccadic dysmetria and saccadic oscillations without an intersaccadic interval, such as ocular flutter and opsoclonus; such records are often absent from clinical reports.

OSCILLATIONS WITH DISEASE AFFECTING OCULAR MOTONEURONS AND EXTRAOCULAR MUSCLE

SUPERIOR OBLIQUE MYOKYMIA (SUPERIOR OBLIQUE MICROTREMOR)

Superior oblique myokymia (SOM) was first described by Duane in 1906 (413), but clinicians became generally aware of the disorder following the description by Hoyt and Keane in 1970 (414). Typical symptoms include monocular blurring of vision, tremulous sensations in the eye (414–417), brief episodes of vertical or torsional diplopia, and vertical or torsional oscillopsia. Attacks last less than 10 seconds and may occur many times per day; they may be elicited on by looking downward, by tilting the head toward the side of the affected eye, and by blinking. The majority of patients with SOM have no underlying disease, although cases have been reported following trochlear nerve palsy, after mild head trauma, in the setting of MS, after brainstem stroke, and in patients with cerebellar tumor (414–420).

The eye movements of SOM are often difficult to appreciate on gross examination, although they are usually apparent during examination with the ophthalmoscope or slit-lamp biomicroscope. They consist of spasms of cyclotorsional and vertical movements. Measurement of the movements of SOM using the magnetic search coil technique reveals an initial intorsion and depression of the affected eye, followed by irregular oscillations of small amplitude and variable frequency (418–421). Some resemble jerk nystagmus, with frequencies of 2–6 Hz, but superimposed upon these oscillations are low-amplitude, irregular oscillations with frequencies ranging up to 50 Hz.

Electromyographic recordings from superior oblique muscles affected by SOM reveal some fibers that discharge either spontaneously or following contraction of the muscle (414,422,423). These muscle potentials are abnormal, with increased duration (greater than 2 milliseconds) and amplitude, and they are polyphasic, with a spontaneous discharge rate of approximately 45 Hz. Spontaneous activity is absent only with large saccades in the "off" (upward) direction and is less affected by vestibular eye movements. Some firing units show an irregular discharge following muscle contraction before subsiding to a regular discharge of 35 Hz. These findings suggest that the etiology of SOM is neuronal damage and subsequent regeneration, leading to desynchronized contraction of muscle fibers. Indeed, experimental le-

sions of the trochlear nerve demonstrate regenerative capacities such that the remaining motor neurons increase their number of axons to hold the total constant (424). Superior oblique myokymia only rarely is preceded by an ipsilateral trochlear nerve palsy (414,425), but the possibility remains that mild damage to the trochlear nerve could trigger the regeneration mechanism for maintaining a constant number of axons in the nerve. Some of these cases might be predisposed to develop SOM.

OCULAR NEUROMYOTONIA

This rare disorder is characterized by episodes of diplopia that are usually precipitated by holding the eyes in eccentric gaze, often sustained adduction (426–431). Most reported patients have undergone radiation to the parasellar region, but idiopathic cases have been reported (432).

The episodic nature of the diplopia associated with ocular neuromyotonia often suggests myasthenia gravis, but anticholinergic medicines are ineffective in this condition. Other conditions that may mimic ocular neuromyotonia include superior oblique myokymia, thyroid eye disease, and cyclic oculomotor palsy.

The symptoms of ocular neuromyotonia are caused by involuntary, and at times painful, contraction of the lateral rectus muscle, the superior oblique muscle, or one or more extraocular muscles innervated by the oculomotor nerve (the latter case is particularly common). Extraocular muscles innervated by more than one ocular motor nerve may occasionally be affected, and rare patients with bilateral ocular neuromyotonia have been reported (433). Comparing symptoms with attempts at eccentric gaze-holding may aid in making the diagnosis, as symptoms may be absent in primary position but evoked by sustained eccentric gaze.

The mechanism responsible for ocular neuromyotonia is unknown, although both ephaptic neural transmission and changes in the pattern of neuronal transmission following denervation have been suggested, since spontaneous activity is seen in the ocular electromyogram of some affected patients (427,428). Axonal hyperexcitability caused by dysfunction of potassium channels has also been implicated in the production of neuromyotonia by analogy with systemic neuromyotonia (434).

SPONTANEOUS EYE MOVEMENTS IN UNCONSCIOUS PATIENTS

The examination of eye movements often provides important diagnostic information in unconscious patients (121,435,436). Deviations of one or both eyes and vestibular eye movements (induced by head rotation or caloric stimulation) are discussed in Chapters 17 and 18. In this section, we summarize spontaneous eye movements. Although some of these eye movements have been regarded as saccadic intrusions, this issue remains unclear because, for example, it is not possible to elicit quick phases of nystagmus with caloric stimulation in unconscious patients. There is a

great need for investigation of the pathogenesis of these disorders.

Slow conjugate or disconjugate roving eye movements are similar to the eye movements of light sleep, but they are slower than the rapid movements of paradoxic or rapid eye movement (REM) sleep. The presence of these eye movements suggests that the brainstem gaze mechanisms are intact (435).

Ocular bobbing consists of intermittent, usually conjugate, rapid downward movement of the eyes followed by a

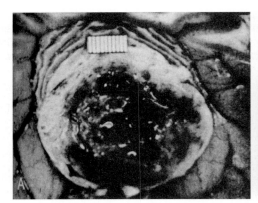
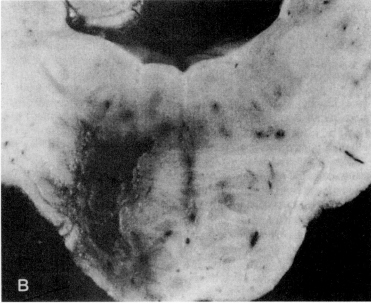

Figure 23.16. Pathology of ocular bobbing. *A,* Section through the midpons demonstrating a massive area of hemorrhage and necrosis in a 2-year-old girl with a pontine glioblastoma who developed a left hemiparesis, obtundation, seizures, and ocular bobbing. *B,* Organizing hematoma in the caudal portion of the basis pontis on the right side in a 57-year-old woman who developed a right gaze palsy, right facial palsy, and obtundation. (*A,* From Daroff RB, Waldman J. J Neurol Neurosurg Psychiatry 1965;28:375–377. *B,* From Katz B, Hoyt WF, Townsend J. J Clin Neuroophthalmol 1982;2:193–195.)

slower return to central position. Reflex-induced horizontal eye movements are usually absent. Classic ocular bobbing is a sign of intrinsic pontine lesions, usually hemorrhage (Fig. 23.16), but it has also been reported in patients with cerebellar lesions that compress the pons.(437–446) and in patients with metabolic and toxic encephalopathies (447,448). An inverse form of ocular bobbing is characterized by a slow downward movement and rapid return to midposition: "ocular dipping" (449–455). "Reverse bobbing" is characterized by a rapid deviation of the eyes upward and a slow return to the horizontal (456), whereas the terms "reverse dipping" or "converse bobbing" describe a slow upward drift of the eyes followed by a rapid return to central position (457,458). In general, the variants of ocular bobbing are less reliable for localization than is the classic form. Nevertheless, because some patients show several types of bobbing, a common underlying pathophysiology is possibly responsible (459,460). Since the pathways that mediate upward and downward eye movements differ anatomically and pharmacologically, it seems possible that these movements represent a varying imbalance of mechanisms

for vertical gaze. Repetitive vertical eye movements, including variants of ocular bobbing, that contain convergent-divergent components may indicate disease affecting the dorsal midbrain (461,462).

Ping-pong gaze consists of slow, horizontal, conjugate deviations of the eyes alternating every few seconds (178). Ping-pong gaze usually occurs with bilateral infarction of the cerebral hemispheres or of the cerebral peduncles (463). Transient oscillations with a similar periodicity to ping-pong gaze can sometimes be induced by a rapid horizontal head rotation in patients with bilateral hemispheric disease (464).

Periodic alternating gaze deviation, in which conjugate gaze deviations change direction every 2 minutes, occurs in some patients with hepatic encephalopathy (465). This phenomenon is related to PAN, which is discussed above.

Rapid, small-amplitude, vertical eye movements may be the only manifestation of epileptic seizures in patients with coexistent brainstem injury (328). Rapid monocular eye movements with horizontal, vertical, or torsional components may also indicate brainstem dysfunction.

TREATMENTS FOR NYSTAGMUS AND SACCADIC INTRUSIONS

RATIONAL BASIS FOR TREATMENT

Ideally, knowledge of the pathogenesis of a form of nystagmus should suggest the treatment. Perhaps the best example for this is the acquired form of PAN, for which an animal model exists, pharmacologic mechanisms have been established, and drug treatment (baclofen) is usually effective.

Although such knowledge is still lacking for many forms of nystagmus and saccadic intrusions, headway has been made. In this section, we summarize current concepts of relevant pharmacology and the best therapies for the various disorders. It should be noted that although a number of drugs have been reported to improve nystagmus in individual patients, few have been subjected to controlled clinical trials. When drug treatments fail or effective drugs cannot be tolerated by the patient, certain optical devices may be used to either suppress the nystagmus or negate its visual consequences. Finally, surgery can be performed to either weaken the extraocular muscles or reattach them to the globe in such a way that the resting position of the eyes is at the null position.

It is essential to carefully evaluate patients before and during therapy for abnormal eye movements. In the case of new treatments, it is best to carry out a controlled, masked evaluation. Careful measurements of visual acuity using near and far test charts and systematic eye movement examination are essential. It is also very useful to record the oscillations. This can be achieved semiquantitatively by video, but it is best performed using one of several recording techniques, ideally the magnetic search coil method (Fig. 23.2).

PHARMACOLOGIC TREATMENTS (466,467)

Nystagmus from Vestibular Imbalance

Peripheral Vestibular Imbalance

Nystagmus caused by peripheral vestibular lesions usually resolves spontaneously over the course of a few days. Present approaches use vestibular suppressants for 24–48 hours, primarily for severe vertigo and nausea. If the nystagmus persists after this time, exercises are used to accelerate the brain's ability to redress the imbalance (468). In the case of BPPV, maneuvers to displace otolithic debris from the affected semicircular canal and exercises to sustain recovery are usually effective (90,469–472).

Central Vestibular Mechanisms—Pharmacologic Basis

The technique of pharmacologic inactivation by microinjection of drugs into the brainstem and cerebellum has provided some useful insights and clues to clinicians interested in treating abnormal eye movements. Thus, unilateral microinjection of the $GABA_A$ agonist muscimol into the medial vestibular nucleus and nucleus prepositus hypoglossi of the monkey and cat produces bilateral gaze-evoked nystagmus (201,473,474). In addition, there is evidence that prolongation of the peripheral vestibular signal by central mechanisms, called velocity storage, by the nodulus and uvula of the cerebellum is regulated by inhibitory pathways that use $GABA_B$ (475). The velocity-storage phenomenon in normal monkeys is suppressed by the $GABA_B$ agonist baclofen (475), and mildly enhanced by both diazepam (476) and picrotoxin (477). Acquired PAN, which is thought to be partly caused by abnormal prolongation of velocity storage, is abolished by baclofen, and this response occurs with both experimental and clinical lesions of the nodulus and uvula (181,478). Microinjection of drugs with effects on glutamate receptors into medial vestibular nucleus/nucleus prepositus hypoglossi also effects gaze-holding ability (474). There is also evidence that nicotinic acetylcholinergic mechanisms play a role in vestibular-mediated vertical eye movements. Nicotine can produce upbeat nystagmus in normal subjects in darkness (479,480) and intravenous physostigmine may

increase the intensity of downbeat nystagmus (481) In addition, intravenous opioids have been reported to induce downbeat nystagmus (482,483).

Downbeat and Upbeat Nystagmus

The $GABA_A$ agonist clonazepam is reported to be effective in reducing downbeat nystagmus (484). A single dose of 1–2 mg of clonazepam was administered to determine whether long-term therapy was likely to be effective. Baclofen may reduce the velocity of both upbeat and downbeat nystagmus and reduce associated oscillopsia (481). Barton and colleagues performed a double-blind study in which two patients with downbeat nystagmus experienced reduction in nystagmus after intravenous scopolamine (485). Improvement of occasional patients with downbeat nystagmus with trihexyphenidyl has been reported (486). However, all of these therapies are ineffective in many patients with downbeat nystagmus.

A new approach to the treatment of downbeat nystagmus arose out of the seminal observation by Griggs that nystagmus occurring in episodic ataxia type 2 responds to acetazolamide (487); this disorder is now known to be a calcium channelopathy (488,489). This led to a study of 3,4-diaminopyridine, a potassium channel blocker, as a treatment for downbeat nystagmus. Strupp and colleagues studied 17 patients with downbeat nystagmus due to a range of disorders (490). Ten of the patients showed a decrease of more than 50% in their nystagmus 30 minutes after ingesting 20 mg of 3,4-diaminopyridine. This medication was generally well tolerated, although it is known to induce seizures in some subjects. The possible mechanism of action of 3,4-diaminopyridine relates to one hypothesis for downbeat nystagmus described earlier in this chapter (167).

The cerebellum inhibits vestibular circuits mediating upward, but not downward, eye movements (Fig. 23.7) (165,166). Consequently, impaired cerebellar inhibition could cause uninhibited upward drifts of the eyes, which evoke corrective rapid downward movements: downbeat nystagmus. Potassium channels are abundant on cerebellar Purkinje cells—the output neurons from cerebellar cortex—and a related agent, 4-aminopyridine, is reported to increase the discharge of these neurons by affecting the slowly depolarizing potential. Enhancement of Purkinje cell activity due to 3,4-diaminopyridine could restore to normal levels the inhibitory influence of the cerebellar cortex upon vertical vestibular eye movements. Studies are under way to determine the long-term effects of these drugs on nystagmus and its visual consequences, and to compare 3,4-diaminopyridine and 4-aminopyridine; the latter penetrates the blood-brain barrier better, has a longer half-life, and is generally better tolerated.

The recent demonstration that a patient with downbeat nystagmus showed antiglutamic acid decarboxylase antibodies in the vestibular complex raises the possibility of evaluating drugs with glutamate effects in patients with downbeat nystagmus (491).

Periodic Alternating Nystagmus

As noted before, this is the best example of a form of nystagmus for which drug treatment is based on known pathophysiology and pharmacology. Most cases of acquired PAN respond to baclofen (180,478). The congenital form of PAN, which probably has a different pathogenesis than the acquired form, only occasionally responds to baclofen (492), but one child did show a response to dextroamphetamine (493).

Acquired Pendular Nystagmus

The neuropharmacology of acquired pendular nystagmus is unknown, and more than one mechanism may be involved. This type of nystagmus used to be treated with barbiturates (73), but sedative side effects limit the use of this class of drugs.

In the case of oculopalatal myoclonus, increased acetylcholine esterase activity and cholinergic denervation supersensitivity has been reported in hypertrophied inferior olivary nucleus (494,495), prompting trials of anticholinergic agents for acquired pendular nystagmus. Initial studies showed that individual patients may be helped by trihexyphenidyl (496,497). One double-blind crossover trial compared trihexyphenidyl with tridihexethyl chloride (a quaternary anticholinergic that does not cross the blood-brain barrier) in 10 patients, 5 of whom had acquired pendular nystagmus. Of these five, only two showed a decrease in nystagmus and an improvement of visual acuity when given tridihexethyl chloride. Trihexyphenidyl had no effect on the nystagmus in any patient. Significantly, neither of the two patients whose nystagmus improved with medication elected to continue the drug because of anticholinergic side effects. In another masked study, scopolamine, benztropine, and glycopyrrolate (a quaternary agent devoid of central nervous activity) were administered intravenously to five patients with acquired pendular nystagmus (485). The results, confirming an earlier report (58), demonstrated a single dose of scopolamine effectively reduced nystagmus and improved vision in all five patients, whereas benztropine was less effective, and glycopyrrolate had no significant effect.

Why did intravenous scopolamine suppress acquired pendular nystagmus, but oral trihexyphenidyl did not? One possibility is that trihexyphenidyl selectively antagonizes only the *m1* muscarinic receptors, whereas scopolamine probably affects all five subtypes of muscarinic receptors (498). However, this is not the whole story, because in an open trial of transdermal scopolamine, which included four patients with acquired pendular nystagmus, two showed a decrease, one showed no effect, and one showed an increase of nystagmus (499). Thus, scopolamine does not appear to be a promising treatment for acquired pendular nystagmus. Intravenous administration is not a practical therapy, and clouds the sensorium. Occasional patients show some improvement with transdermal scopolamine, but this is often not sustained (499), and prolonged use of this mode of therapy is also not without risk.

Reports that the neurotransmitter GABA contributed to the normal function of the gaze-holding mechanism (201,473,474) focused attention on drugs with GABAergic effects. Valproate is reported to help some patients with acquired pendular nystagmus (500). Isoniazid has also been studied as treatment for acquired pendular nystagmus in three patients with MS, and reduced nystagmus and relieved oscillopsia in two (501). However, isoniazid has potential side effects, and better-tolerated drugs have become available, notably **gabapentin**, which has been evaluated in controlled trials (75). Of 15 patients with acquired pendular nystagmus studied in a double-blind comparison with baclofen, visual acuity improved with gabapentin, but not with baclofen; an example is shown in Figure 23.17. Gabapentin significantly reduced nystagmus in all three planes, but baclofen did so only in the vertical plane. In 10 of the 15 patients, reduction of nystagmus was substantial, and 8 elected to continue taking the medication. The main side effect of gabapentin was increased ataxia and unsteadiness. However, the demonstration that the more purely GABAergic agent vigabatrin failed to suppress nystagmus led to the

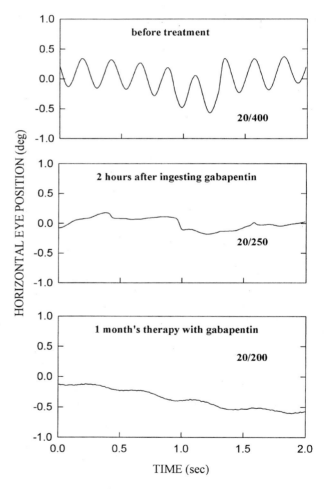

Figure 23.17. Effects of gabapentin on the horizontal component of pendular nystagmus in a 41-year-old woman with multiple sclerosis. After the initial recording (*top*), the patient was given 300 mg of gabapentin, which reduced her oscillations and improved her vision (*middle*). The effect was sustained two months later, when she was taking a dose of 300 mg three times per day. Visual acuity measurements of the recorded eye are shown at the *right* in each panel.

suggestion that gabapentin was probably working through a different transmitter mechanism, such as glutamate (502).

One agent with effects on gluatamate receptors is memantine, which has recently received approval from the U.S. Food and Drug Administration for treatment of Alzheimer's disease. Memantine has been in use in Germany for over 20 years, and is known to be a safe and well-tolerated drug. It is a low-to-moderate uncompetitive (open channel) N-methyl-D-aspartate (NMDA) receptor antagonist. A study from the University of Munich reported that it suppressed acquired pendular nystagmus in patients with multiple sclerosis (503). There is need for a controlled study comparing memantine with gabapentin. At present, gabapentin has been shown to be effective in some patients with pendular nystagmus as part of the syndrome of oculopalatal tremor (75), but memantine has not been studied in this disorder. Palatal tremor may respond to carbamazepine in some patients (504,505). Occasional patients with acquired pendular nystagmus benefit from both gabapentin and surgical recession of muscles (506); the effects of surgery are described below.

Alcohol has been reported to suppress acquired pendular nystagmus (507). Smoking cannabis has been reported to suppress both acquired pendular nystagmus (508), and congenital nystagmus (509), but formal evaluations of this potential therapy are hindered at present by current social views on cannabis.

Seesaw Nystagmus

Improvement in seesaw nystagmus has been reported in some patients treated with alcohol (510,511). Clonazepam has reduced the nystagmus and associated oscillopsia in occasional patients (512). Two patients with pendular seesaw nystagmus showed reduction of their nystagmus with gabapentin, but more studies are needed to confirm this (75).

Familial Episodic Ataxia with Nystagmus

The attacks of episodic ataxia type 2 (EA-2), which is a calcium channelopathy, respond well to treatment with acetazolamide (489). However, the interictal nystagmus and ataxia (which in some patients is progressive) usually do respond. The briefer attacks of episodic ataxia type 1 (EA-1), which is a potassium channelopathy, respond to acetazolamide in some patients. The attacks of EA-1 spontaneously improve with time in some patients (489).

Saccadic Intrusions: Square-Wave Jerks

Both the frontal eye fields and the superior colliculus send brainstem projections that influence the omnipause neurons that gate saccades (discussed earlier). Experimental studies have elucidated the pharmacology of one part of this descending pathway (513). The nondopaminergic portion of the substantia nigra, the pars reticulata (SNpr), receives inputs from the caudate nucleus and selectively gates reflexive or voluntary saccades via the superior colliculus. This is accomplished, in part, by a phasic modulation of tonic inhibitory influence of the SNpr upon the superior colliculus. The caudate nucleus appears to facilitate the initiation of voluntary self-generated types of saccades and to aid steady fixation by preventing unwanted reflexive saccades to stimuli. The nigrotectal pathway is GABAergic, and injection of bicuculline into the superior colliculus increases the frequency and amplitude of the saccades, which take the form of square-wave intrusions (514). Furthermore, pharmacologic inactivation of the frontal eye fields with bicuculline causes saccadic intrusions (395). This experimental evidence suggests that treatment with GABA agonists might prevent inappropriate saccades. In fact, several benzodiazepines (diazepam, clonazepam) and the barbiturate phenobarbital were effective in abolishing high-amplitude square-wave jerks and macrosaccadic oscillations in one patient (515). There is also some evidence that amphetamines can suppress square-wave jerks in some patients (516). On the other hand, both nicotine (479) and opiates (483) are reported to induce square-wave jerks. Thus, more work is needed to better understand the pharmacology of saccadic intrusions and how they can be treated.

Ocular Flutter and Opsoclonus

Patients with parainfectious opsoclonus-myoclonus often improve spontaneously, but intravenous immunoglobulin may speed recovery (517). Similarly, although propranolol, verapamil, clonazepam, gabapentin, and thiamine have all been reported to diminish microsaccadic ocular flutter in individual patients (366,518,519), the effect may have been due to spontaneous remission. Opsoclonus associated with neural crest tumors in children usually responds to corticosteroid treatment (520); however, up to 50% of such children have persistent neurological disabilities, including ataxia, poor speech, and cognitive problems (372,518). Similar responses to steroids may occur in children with parainfectious or idiopathic opsoclonus (518). Treatment with steroids has not been uniformly successful in such cases, although plasmapheresis, intravenous immunoglobulin, and immunoadsorption therapy have occasionally proved effective (370,521,522).

Superior Oblique Myokymia and Ocular Neuromyotonia

Superior oblique myokymia spontaneously resolves in some patients (417), and others are not sufficiently bothered by their symptoms that they request treatment. Individual patients have responded to carbamazepine, baclofen, b-adrenergic blocking agents, or gabapentin given systemically or topically (415,416,419). Patients who do not respond to drug therapy, who develop side effects from the drugs, or who do not wish to take drugs for their condition, may experience complete relief of symptoms after extraocular muscle surgery (discussion following).

Ocular neuromyotonia is usually responsive to carbamazepine (432,433).

OPTICAL TREATMENTS

Convergence prisms provide one optical approach for patients with congenital or acquired nystagmus whose nystagmus dampens when they view a near target (242,523); a useful starting point is 7.00-diopter base-out prisms combined with −1.00-diopter spheres to compensate for accommodation (although the spherical correction may not be needed in presbyopic individuals). In some patients with congenital nystagmus, the resultant improvement of vision is sufficient for them to qualify for a driver's license. Patients whose nystagmus is worse during near viewing may benefit from wearing base-in (divergence) prisms (64).

Theoretically, it should be possible to use prisms to help patients whose nystagmus is reduced or absent when the eyes are moved into a particular position in the orbit: the null region. For patients with congenital nystagmus, there is usually some horizontal eye position in which the nystagmus is minimized, whereas downbeat nystagmus may decrease or disappear in upgaze. In practice, patients use head turns to bring their eyes to the optimum position, and only rarely are prisms that produce a conjugate shift helpful.

A different approach to the treatment of nystagmus has been the use of an optical system that stabilizes images on the retina (524). This system consists of a high-plus spectacle lens worn in combination with a high-minus contact lens. The system is designed on the principle that stabilization of images on the retina could be achieved if the power of the spectacle lens focused the primary image close to the center of rotation of the eye. However, such images are then defocused, and a contact lens is required to extend the clear image back onto the retina. Since the contact lens moves with the eye, it does not negate the effect of retinal image stabilization produced by the spectacle lens. With such a system, it is possible to achieve up to about 90% stabilization of images upon the retina. There are several limitations to the system, however. One is that it disables all eye movements (including the vestibulo-ocular reflex and vergence) and thus is useful only when the patient is stationary and is viewing monocularly. Another limitation is that with the highest-power components (contact lens of −58.00 diopters and spectacle lens of +32diopters), the field of view is limited. Some patients with ataxia or tremor (such as those with MS) have difficulty inserting the contact lens. However, initial problems posed by rigid polymethyl methacrylate contact lenses can be overcome by using gas-permeable, or even soft contact lenses (525). Most patients do not need the highest power components for oscillopsia to be abolished, and vision to be improved. We have found that in selected patients the device may prove useful for limited periods of time, for example, if the patient wishes to watch a television program (526).

Contact lenses alone sometimes suppress congenital nystagmus (527). This effect is not from the mass of the lenses but is probably mediated via trigeminal afferents (528); this issue is discussed further below.

A more recent innovation has been to use an electronic circuit to distinguish between the nystagmus oscillations and normal eye movements (529). This approach is most applicable in patients with pendular nystagmus. Eye movements are measured using an infrared sensor and, after filtering, fed to a phase-locked loop that generates a signal similar to the nystagmus but is insensitive to other eye movements, such as saccades. This electronic signal is then used to rotate Risley prisms, through which the patient views the environment. When the Risley prisms rotate in synchrony with the patients nystagmus, they negate the visual effects of the ocular oscillations. Improvement and miniaturization of a prototype device may eventually lead to a spectacle-mounted device that selectively cancels out the visual effects of pathological nystagmus (529,530).

The main therapy for latent nystagmus consists of measures to improve vision, particularly patching for amblyopia in children (531).

BOTULINUM TOXIN TREATMENT OF NYSTAGMUS

An approach to treatment of nystagmus that has gained some popularity is injection of botulinum toxin into either the extraocular muscles or the retrobulbar space (532,533). Using both techniques, Ruben and colleagues reported improvement of vision in most of their 12 patients with a variety of diagnoses (534). The major side effect was ptosis. However, eye movements were not systematically measured and compared before and after injection. Repka and colleagues also described improvement of vision following retrobulbar injection of botulinum toxin in six patients and documented the effects on eye movements (535). The main reservation expressed by these authors was the temporary nature of the treatment and the necessity for repeated injections, with their attendant risks. We measured binocular eye rotations in three planes before and after monocular injection of botulinum toxin either into the horizontal recti (536), or into the retrobulbar space (537). Nystagmus was abolished or reduced in the treated eye for about 2–3 months, but no patient was pleased with the results because of ptosis, diplopia, increase of nystagmus in the noninjected eye or, in one patient, filamentary keratitis. No patient that we studied elected to repeat the procedure.

SURGICAL PROCEDURES FOR NYSTAGMUS

Two surgical procedures may be effective for certain patients with congenital nystagmus. One is the Anderson-Kestenbaum operation (538–540). This procedure is designed to move the attachments of the extraocular muscles so that the new central position of the eyes is at the null position. It is performed after first making careful eye movement measurements of nystagmus intensity with the eyes in various positions of gaze and determining the approximate null position. The appropriate extraocular muscles are then weakened or strengthened as necessary to achieve the required shift in the position of the null (541–543). The Anderson-Kestenbaum procedure not only shifts and broadens the null region, but also results in decreased nystagmus outside the region. It is of uncertain value in the treatment of acquired forms of nystagmus.

The second procedure is an artificial divergence operation (544,545). It may be helpful in patients with congenital nystagmus that dampens or is suppressed during near viewing and who have stereopsis. Studies comparing these two methods indicate that the artificial divergence operation generally results in a better visual outcome than the Anderson-Kestenbaum procedure alone (543,545–547).

Several authors have recommended performing large recessions of all of the horizontal rectus muscles for treatment of patients with congenital nystagmus (548,549). Based on a long experience, Dell'Osso noted that any surgical procedure that detached and reattached the extraocular muscles tended to suppress congenital nystagmus. This led him to suggest that simply dissecting the perimuscular fascia and then reattaching the muscles at the same site on the globe might prove effective, especially in cases when convergence does not dampen the nystagmus. Results of this procedure on a canine model for congenital nystagmus supported this hypothesis (550). Reported lack of effect in monkeys concerns *latent nystagmus,* not typical congenital nystagmus (551,552). Preliminary results of a large, controlled clinical trial suggest that the operation is effective in some patients (242,553).

How could such a procedure damp congenital nystagmus? Recent studies by Büttner-Ennever and colleagues have indicated that the terminal portion of the extraocular muscles, near their site of their attachment, contains multiply-innervated muscle fibers (554). Using rabies toxin as an anatomic tracer, it has been possible to show that a separate group of ocular motor neurons (distinct from the classic oculomotor, trochlear, and abducens nuclei, and surrounding each of them) innervates these multiply-innervated fibers.

Finally, it is known that ocular proprioceptors (the pallisade organs) lie at the insertion site of the extraocular muscles (554). Thus, procedures similar to those proposed by Dell'Osso may work by disrupting a proprioceptive feedback pathway that normally sets the tone of the extraocular muscles.

There is also some evidence that the tendino-scleral junction may contain neurovascular abnormalities in the eyes of patients with congenital nystagmus (555). This suggestion, and the ''orbital revolution'' set in motion by the discovery of pulleys for the extraocular muscles by Miller and Demer, promise the development of new therapies for congenital nystagmus (556).

The role of surgery in the treatment of acquired nystagmus is not well established, although individual patients may benefit from recession operations (506,557). However, it is clear that suboccipital decompression improves downbeat nystagmus in Chiari syndromes and also prevents progression of other neurologic deficits (558–560).

As noted above, SOM that does not respond to treatment with medication may respond to extraocular muscle surgery. The procedure used by most surgeons is a superior oblique tenectomy combined with myectomy of the ipsilateral inferior oblique muscle (414,415,417,422,561). However, Kosmorsky and colleagues reported successful treatment of a patient with SOM by performing a nasal transposition of the anterior portion of the affected superior oblique tendon, thereby weakening cyclorotation (562).

OTHER FORMS OF TREATMENT

A variety of methods other than those described above have been used to treat nystagmus, principally the congenital variety. Electrical stimulation or vibration over the forehead may suppress congenital nystagmus (264). The mechanism of vibration on eye movements is uncertain, since vibration over the mastoid in patients who have lost vestibular function induces ocular torsion (563). However, it is postulated that the suppressive effect on congenital nystagmus, as well as suppression induced by wearing contact lenses (528), may be exerted via the trigeminal system, which receives extraocular proprioception (264,554).

Acupuncture administered to the neck muscles may suppress congenital nystagmus in some patients via a similar mechanism (564,565). Biofeedback has also been reported to help some patients with congenital nystagmus (566,567). The role of any of these treatments in clinical practice has yet to be demonstrated.

REFERENCES

1. Kaminski HJ, Leigh RJ. Neurobiology of eye movements: From molecules to behavior. Ann New York Acad Sci 2002;1:619.
2. Leigh RJ, Das VE, Seidman SH. A neurobiological approach to acquired nystagmus. Ann NY Acad Sci 2002;956:380–390.
3. Carpenter RHS. The visual origins of ocular motility. In Carpenter RHS, ed. Eye Movements. Vol 8. London: MacMillan Press, 1991:1–10.
4. Bender MB. Oscillopsia. Arch Neurol 1965;13:204–213.
5. Wist ER, Brandt T, Krafczyk S. Oscillopsia and retinal slip: Evidence supporting a clinical test. Brain 1983;106:153–168.
6. Stahl JS, Averbuch-Heller L, Leigh RJ. Acquired nystagmus. Arch Ophthalmol 2000;118:544–549.
7. Leigh RJ, Averbuch-Heller L, Tomsak RL, Remler BF, Yaniglos SS, Dell'Osso LF. Treatment of abnormal eye movements that impair vision: Strategies based on current concepts of physiology and pharmacology. Ann Neurol 1994;36:129–141.
8. Abadi RV, Whittle JP, Worfolk R. Oscillopsia and tolerance to retinal image movement in congenital nystagmus. Invest Ophthalmol Vis Sci 1999;40:339–345.
9. Leigh R, Zee D. The Neurology of Eye Movements. Ed 3. New York, Oxford University Press, 1999.
10. Serra A, Leigh RJ. Diagnostic value of nystagmus: Spontaneous and induced ocular oscillations. J Neurol Neurosurg Psychiatry 2002;73:615–618.
11. Zee DS. Ophthalmoscopy in examination of patients with vestibular disorders. Ann Neurol 1978;3:373–374.
12. Trillenberg P, Zee DS, Shelhamer M. On the distribution of fast-phase intervals in optokinetic and vestibular nystagmus. Biol Cybern 2002;87:68–78.
13. Garbutt S, Harris CM. Abnormal vertical optokinetic nystagmus in infants and children. Br J Ophthalmol 2000;84:451–455.
14. Garbutt S, Harwood MR, Harris CM. Comparison of the main sequence of reflexive saccades and the quick phases of optokinetic nystagmus. Br J Ophthalmol 2001;85:1477–1483.
15. Garbutt S, Harwood MR, Harris CM. Anticompensatory eye position (''contraversion'') in optokinetic nystagmus. Ann NY Acad Sci 2002;956:445–448.
16. Garbutt S, Han Y, Kumar AN, et al. Vertical optokinetic nystagmus and saccades in normal human subjects. Invest Ophthalmol Vis Sci 2003;44:3833–3841.
17. Garbutt S, Han Y, Kumar AN, et al. Disorders of vertical optokinetic nystagmus in patients with ocular misalignment. Vision Res 2003;43:347–357.
18. Dell'Osso LF, Daroff RB. Congenital nystagmus waveforms and foveation strategy. Documenta Ophthalmologica 1975;39:155–182.
19. Abadi RV, Dickinson CM. Waveform characteristics in congenital nystagmus. Documenta Ophthalmologica 1986;64:153–167.
20. Carpenter RHS. Movements of the Eyes. Ed 2. London: Pion, 1988.
21. DiScenna AO, Das VE, Zivotofsky AZ, Seidman SH, Leigh RJ. Evaluation of a video tracking device for measurement of horizontal and vertical eye rotations during locomotion. J Neurosci Methods 1995;58:89–94.
22. Murphy P, Duncan A, Glennie A, Knox P. The effect of sceral search coil lens wear on the eye. Br J Ophthalmol 2001;85:332–335.
23. Leigh RJ, Zee DS. Eye movements of the blind. Invest Ophthalmol Vis Sci 1980;19:328–331.
24. Leigh RJ, Thurston SE, Tomsak RL, Grossman GE, Lanska DJ. Effect of monocular visual loss upon stability of gaze. Invest Ophthalmol Vis Sci 1989;30:288–292.
25. Luebke AE, Robinson DA. Transition dynamics between pursuit and fixation suggest different systems. Vision Res 1988;28:941–946.
26. Leigh RJ, Huebner WP, Gordon JL. Supplementation of the human vestibulo-

ocular reflex by visual fixation and smooth pursuit. J Vestibular Res 1994;4: 347–353.

27. Steinman RM, Haddad GM, Skavenski AA, Wyman D. Miniature eye movement. Science 1973;181:810–819.

28. Zeki S. A Vision of the Brain. London: Blackwell Scientific, 1993.

29. Averbuch-Heller L, Zivotofsky AZ, Remler BF, Das VE, Dell'Osso LF, Leigh RJ. Convergent-divergent pendular nystagmus: possible role of the vergence system. Neurology 1995;45:509–515.

30. Robinson DA. The control of eye movements. In Handbook of Physiology: The Nervous System. Vol 2, Part 2. Bethesda, American Physiological Society, 1981.

31. Belton T, McCrea RA. Role of the cerebellar flocculus region in the coordination of eye and head movements during gaze pursuit. J Neurophysiol 2000;84: 1614–1626.

32. Suzuki DA, May JG, Keller EL, Yee RD. Visual motion response properties of neurons in dorsolateral pontine nucleus of alert monkey. J Neurophysiol 1990; 63:37–59.

33. Ito M. Cerebellar flocculus hypothesis. Nature 1993;363:24–25.

34. Luebke AE, Robinson DA. Gain changes of the cat's vestibulo-ocular reflex after flocculus deactivation. Exp Brain Res 1994;98:379–390.

35. Büttner-Enever JA, Horn AK. Pathways from cell groups of the paramedian tracts to the floccular region. Ann NY Acad Sci 1996;781:532–540.

36. Robinson DA. The effect of cerebellectomy on the cat's vestibulo-ocular integrator. Brain Res 1974;71:195–207.

37. Narfstrom K, Katz ML, Bragadottir R, et al. Functional and structural recovery of the retina after gene therapy in the RPE65 null mutation dog. Invest Ophthalmol Vis Sci 2003;44:1663–1672.

38. Acland G, Aguirre G, Ray J, et al. Gene therapy restores vision in a canine model of childhood blindness. Nature Genetics 2001;28:92–95.

39. Pritchard C, Flynn JT, Smith JL. Wave form characteristics of vertical oscillations in long-standing vision loss. J Pediatr Ophthalmol Strabismus 1988;25: 233–236.

40. Barton JJS, Cox TA. Acquired pendular nystagmus in multiple sclerosis: Clinical observations and the role of optic neuropathy. J Neurol Neurosurg Psychiatry 1993;56:262–267.

41. Yee RD, Jelks GW, Baloh RW, Honrubia V. Uniocular nystagmus in monocular visual loss. Ophthalmology 1979;86:511–518.

42. Pratt-Johnson JA, Tillson G. Intractable diplopia after vision restoration in unilateral cataract. Am J Ophthalmol 1989;107:23–26.

43. Farmer J, Hoyt CS. Monocular nystagmus in infancy and early childhood. Am J Ophthalmol 1984;98:504–509.

44. Lavery MA, O'Neill JF, Chu FC, Martyn LJ. Acquired nystagmus in early childhood: A presenting sign of intracranial tumor. Ophthalmology 1984;91: 425–435.

45. Weissman BM, Dell'Osso LF, Abel LA, Leigh RJ. Spasmus nutans: A quantitative prospective study. Arch Ophthalmol 1987;105:525–528.

46. Gottlob I, Zubcov AA, Catalano RA, et al. Signs distinguishing spasmus nutans (with and without central nervous system lesions) from infantile nystagmus. Ophthalmology 1990;97:1166–1175.

47. Dell'Osso LF, Williams RW. Ocular motor abnormalities in achiasmatic mutant Belgian sheepdogs: Unyoked eye movements in a mammal. Vision Res 1995; 35:109–116.

48. Apkarian P, Bour LJ, Barth PG, et al. Non-decussating retinal-fugal fibre syndrome: An inborn achiasmatic malformation associated with visuotopic misrouting, visual evoked potential ipsilateral asymmetry and nystagmus. Brain 1995; 118:1195–1216.

49. Apkarian P, Bour LJ. See-saw nystagmus and congenital nystagmus identified in the non-decussating retinal-fugal fiber syndrome. Strabismus 2001;9:143–163.

50. Barton JJS. Blink- and saccade-induced seesaw nystagmus. Neurology 1995; 45:831–833.

51. Averbuch-Heller L, Leigh RJ. Saccade-induced nystagmus. Neurology 1996;46: 289.

52. Sharpe JA, Lo AW, Rabinovitch HE. Control of the saccadic and smooth pursuit systems after cerebral hemidecortication. Brain 1979;102:387–403.

53. Cogan DG, Loeb DR. Optokinetic response and intracranial lesions. Arch Neurol Psychiatry 1949;61:183–187.

54. Kömpf D. The significance of optokinetic nystagmus asymmetry in hemispheric lesions. Neuroophthalmology 1986;6:61–64.

55. Morrow MJ. Craniotopic defects of smooth pursuit and saccadic eye movement. Neurology 1996;46:514–521.

56. Thurston SE, Leigh RJ, Crawford TJ, et al. Two distinct deficits of visual tracking caused by unilateral lesions of cerebral cortex in humans. Ann Neurol 1988; 23:266–273.

57. Dieterich M, Bense S, Stephan T, et al. fMRI signal increases and decreases in cortical areas during small-field optokinetic stimulation and central fixation. Exp Brain Res 2003;148:117–127.

58. Gresty MA, Ell JJ, Findley LJ. Acquired pendular nystagmus: Its characteristics, localising value and pathophysiology. J Neurol Neurosurg Psychiatry 1982;45: 431–439.

59. Barton JJS. Is acquired pendular nystagmus always phase locked? J Neurol Neurosurg Psychiatry 1994;57:1263–1264.

60. Aschoff JC, Conrad B, Kornhuber HH. Acquired pendular nystagmus with oscil-

61. Das VE, Oruganti P, Kramer PD, Leigh RJ. Experimental tests of a neural-network model for ocular oscillations caused by disease of central myelin. Exp Brain Res 2000;133:189–197.

62. Jacobs L, Bender MB. Palato-ocular synchrony during eyelid closure. Arch Neurol 1976;33:289–291.

63. Fukushima M, Enomoto H, Tsutsui J. Visually suppressed acquired pendular nystagmus in four cases with spinocerebellar degeneration. Neuroophthalmol Jpn 1984;1:54–59.

64. Barton JJ, Cox TA, Digre KB. Acquired convergence-evoked pendular nystagmus in multiple sclerosis. J Neuroophthalmol 1999;19:34–38.

65. Maas EF, Ashe J, Spiegel P, Zee DS, Leigh RJ. Acquired pendular nystagmus in toluene addiction. Neurology 1991;41:282–285.

66. Trobe JD, Sharpe JA, Hirsh DK, Gebarski SS. Nystagmus of Pelizaeus-Merzbacher disease. Arch Neurol 1991;48:87–91.

67. Kori AA, Robin NH, Jacobs JB, et al. Pendular nystagmus in patients with peroxisomal assembly disorder. Arch Neurol 1998;55:554–558.

68. Büttner U, Helmchen C, Büttner-Ennever JA. The localizing value of nystagmus in brainstem disorders. Neuroophthalmology 1995;15:283–290.

69. Lopez LI, Bronstein AM, Gresty MA, DuBoulay EP, Rudge P. Clinical and MRI correlates in 27 patients with acquired pendular nystagmus. Brain 1996; 119:465–472.

70. Nakamagoe K, Iwamoto Y, Yoshida K. Evidence for brainstem structures participating in oculomotor integration. Science 2000;288:857–859.

71. Guillain G, Mollaret P. Deux cas myoclonies synchrones et rhythmées vélopharyngo-laryngo-oculodiaphragmatiques: Le problèm anatomique et physiolopathologique de ce syndrome. Rev Neurol (Paris) 1931;2:545–566.

72. Nakada T, Kwee IL. Oculopalatal myoclonus. Brain 1986;109:431–441.

73. Nathanson M. Palatal myoclonus: Further clinical and pathophysiological observations. Arch Neurol Psychiatr 1956;75:285–296.

74. Sperling MR, Herrmann J. Syndrome of palatal myoclonus and progressive ataxia: Two cases with magnetic resonance imaging. Neurology 1985;35: 1212–1214.

75. Averbuch-Heller L, Tusa RJ, Fuhry L, Rottach KG, Ganser GL, Heide W et al. A double-blind controlled study of gabapentin and baclofen as treatment for acquired nystagmus. Ann Neurol 1997;41:818–825.

76. Jacobs L, Newman RP, Bozian D. Disappearing palatal myoclonus. Neurology 1981;31:748–751.

77. Keane JR. Acute vertical ocular myoclonus. Neurology 1986;36:86–89.

78. Dubinsky RM, Hallet M, DiChiro G, Fulham M, Schwankhaus J. Increased glucose metabolism in the medulla of patients with palatal myoclonus. Neurology 1991;41:557–562.

79. Sharpe JA, Hoyt WF, Rosenberg MA. Convergence-evoked nystagmus: Congenital and acquired forms. Arch Neurol 1975;32:191–194.

80. Schwartz MA, Selhorst JB, Ochs AL, et al. Oculomasticatory myorhythmia: A unique movement disorder occurring in Whipple's disease. Ann Neurol 1986; 20:677–683.

81. Averbuch-Heller L, Paulson G, Daroff R, Leigh R. Whipple's disease mimicking progressive supranuclear palsy: The diagnostic value of eye movement recording. J Neurol Neurosurg Psychiatry 1999;66:532–535.

82. Gamlin PD, Clarke RJ. Single-unit activity in the primate nucleus reticularis tegmenti pontis related to vergence and ocular accommodation. J Neurophysiol 1995;73:2115–2119.

83. McClure JA, Copp CC, Lycett P. Recovery nystagmus in Meniere's disease. Laryngoscope 1981;91:1727–1737.

84. Robinson DA, Zee DS, Hain TC, et al. Alexander's law: Its behavior and origin in the human vestibulo-ocular reflex. Ann Neurol 1984;16:714–722.

85. Baloh RW. Clinical practice. Vestibular neuritis. N Engl J Med 2003;348: 1027–1032.

86. Baloh RW, Jacobson K, Honrubia V. Horizontal semicircular canal variant of benign positional vertigo. Neurology 1993;43:2542–2549.

87. Bisdorff AR, Debatisse D. Localizing signs in positional vertigo due to lateral canal cupulolithiasis. Neurology 2001;57:1085–1088.

88. Parnes LS, McClure JA. Free floating endolymph particles: A new operative finding during posterior semicircular canal occlusion. Laryngoscope 1992;102: 988–992.

89. Brandt T, Steddin S. Current view of the mechanism of benign paroxysmal positioning vertigo: Cupulolithiasis or canalolithiasis? J Vestibular Res 1993;3: 373–382.

90. Brandt T. Vertigo. Its Multisensory Syndromes. Ed 2. London, Springer-Verlag, 1999.

91. Baloh RW, Halmagyi GM. Disorders of the Vestibular System. Oxford, Oxford University Press, 1996.

92. Drachman DA, Diamond ER, Hart CW. Postural-evoked vomiting associated with posterior fossa lesions. Ann Otol Rhinol Laryngol 1977;86:97–101.

93. Duncan GW, Parker SW, Fisher CM. Acute cerebellar infarction in the PICA territory. Arch Neurol 1975;32:364–368.

94. Lee H, Yi HA, Cho YW, et al. Nodulus infarction mimicking acute peripheral vestibulopathy. Neurology 2003;60:1700–1702.

95. Fetter M, Haslwanter T, Bork M, Dichgans J. New insights into positional alcohol nystagmus using three-dimensional eye-movement analysis. Ann Neurol 1999;45:216–223.

96. Hain TC, Spindler J. Head-shaking nystagmus. In: Sharpe JA, Barber HO, eds. The Vestibulo-Ocular Reflex and Vertigo. New York: Raven Press, 1993: 217–228.

97. Zee DS. Afternystagmus and headshaking nystagmus. Equilibrium Res 1993; 52:442–447.

98. Katsarkas A, Smith H, Galiana H. Head-shaking nystagmus (HSN): Theoretical explanation and the experimental proof. Acta Otolaryngol 2000;120:177–181.

99. Minagar A, Sheremata WA, Tusa RJ. Perverted head-shaking nystagmus: A possible mechanism. Neurology 2001;57:887–889.

100. Strupp M. Perverted head-shaking nystagmus: Two possible mechanisms. J Neurol 2002;249:118–119.

101. Minor LB, Haslwanter T, Straumann D, Zee DS. Hyperventilation-induced nystagmus in patients with vestibular schwannoma. Neurology 1999;53:2158–2168.

102. Walker MF, Zee DS. The effect of hyperventilation on downbeat nystagmus in cerebellar disorders. Neurology 1999;53:1576–1579.

103. Sawyer RN, Thurston SE, Becker KR, et al. The cervico-ocular reflex of normal human subjects in response to transient and sinusoidal trunk rotations. J Vestibular Res 1994;4:245–249.

104. Kasai T, Zee DS. Eye-head coordination in labyrinthine-defective human beings. Brain Research 1978;144:123–141.

105. Bronstein AM, Hood JD. Oscillopsia of peripheral vestibular origin. Central and cervical compensatory mechanisms. Acta Otolaryngol (Stockh) 1987;104:1987.

106. Bronstein AM, Hood JD. Cervical nystagmus due to loss of cerebellar inhibition on the cervico-ocular reflex: A case report. J Neurol Neurosurg Psychiatry 1985; 48:128–131.

107. Brandt T, Büchele W, Arnold F. Arthrokinetic nystagmus and egomotion sensation. Exp Brain Res 1977;30:331–338.

108. Dodge R. Thresholds of rotation. J Exp Psychol 1923;6:107–137.

109. Graybiel A. The oculogravic illusion. Arch Ophthalmol 1952;48:605–615.

110. Lackner J. Induction of illusory self-rotation and nystagmus by a rotating soundfield. Aviat Space Environ Med 1977;48:129–131.

111. Dieterich M, Brandt T, Fries W. Otolith function in man: results from a case of otolith Tullio phenomenon. Brain 1989;112:1377–1392.

112. Rottach KG, von Maydell RD, DiScenna AO, Zivotofsky AZ, Averbuch-Heller L, Leigh RJ. Quantitative measurements of eye movements in a patient with Tullio phenomenon. J Vestibular Res 1996;6:255–259.

113. Halmagyi GM, Aw ST, McGarvie LA, et al. Superior semicircular canal dehiscence simulating otosclerosis. J Laryngol Otol 2003;117:553–557.

114. Halmagyi GM, McGarvie LA, Aw ST, Yavor RA, Todd MJ. The click-evoked vestibulo-ocular reflex in superior semicircular canal dehiscence. Neurology 2003;60:1172–1175.

115. Ostrowski VB, Byskosh A, Hain TC. Tullio phenomenon with dehiscence of the superior semicircular canal. Otol Neurotol 2001;22:61–65.

116. Cremer PD, Minor LB, Carey JP, Della Santina CC. Eye movements in patients with superior canal dehiscence syndrome align with the abnormal canal. Neurology 2000;55:1833–1841.

117. Baloh RW. Robert Barany and the controversy surrounding his discovery of the caloric reaction. Neurology 2002;58:1094–1099.

118. Paige GD. Caloric responses after horizontal canal inactivation. Acta Otolaryngol (Stockh) 1981;100:321–327.

119. Arai Y, Yakushin SB, Cohen B, Suzuki J, Raphan T. Spatial orientation of caloric nystagmus in semicircular canal-plugged monkeys. J Neurophysiol 2002; 88:914–928.

120. Nathanson M, Bergman PS, Anderson PJ. Significance of oculocephalic and caloric responses in the unconscious patient. Neurology 1957;7:829–832.

121. Plum F, Posner JB. The Diagnosis of Stupor and Coma. Ed 3. Philadelphia: F.A. Davis, 1981.

122. Takemori S, Cohen B. Loss of visual suppression of vestibular nystagmus after flocculus lesions. Brain Res 1974;72:213–224.

123. Schneider E, Glasauer S, Dieterich M. Comparison of human ocular torsion patterns during natural and galvanic vestibular stimulation. J Neurophysiol 2002; 87:2064–2073.

124. Jahn K, Naessl A, Schneider E, et al. Inverse U-shaped curve for age dependency of torsional eye movement responses to galvanic vestibular stimulation. Brain 2003;126:1579–1589.

125. Halmagyi GM, Rudge P, Gresty MA, Sanders MD. Downbeating nystagmus: A review of 62 cases. Arch Neurol 1983;40:777–784.

126. Baloh RW, Yee RD. Spontaneous vertical nystagmus. Rev Neurol (Paris) 1989; 145:527–532.

127. Jacobson DM, Corbett JJ. Downbeat nystagmus and dolichoectasia of the vertebrobasilar artery. J Neuroophthalmol 2002;22:150–151.

128. Lee AG. Downbeat nystagmus associated with caudal brainstem compression by the vertebral artery. J Neuroophthalmol 2001;21:219–220.

129. Apte SN, Langston JW. Permanent neurological deficits due to lithium toxicity. Ann Neurol 1983;13:453–455.

130. Corbett JJ, Jacobson DM, Thompson HS, et al. Downbeating nystagmus and other ocular motor defects caused by lithium toxicity. Neurology 1989;39: 481–487.

131. Halmagyi GM, Lessell I, Curthoys IS, et al. Lithium-induced downbeat nystagmus. Am J Ophthalmol 1989;107:664–670.

132. Williams DP, Troost BT, Rogers J. Lithium-induced downbeat nystagmus. Arch Neurol 1988;45:1022–1023.

133. Remler BF, Leigh RJ, Osorio I, Tomsak RL. The characteristics and mechanisms of visual disturbance associated with anticonvulsant therapy. Neurology 1990; 40:791–796.

134. Yee RD, Baloh RW, Honrubia V. Episodic vertical oscillopsia and downbeat nystagmus in a Chiari malformation. Arch Ophthalmol 1984;102:723–725.

135. Bertholon P, Bronstein AM, Davies RA, et al. Positional down beating nystagmus in 50 patients: cerebellar disorders and possible anterior semicircular canalithiasis. J Neurol Neurosurg Psychiatry 2002;72:366–372.

136. Leigh RJ. Clinical significance of positionally induced downbeat nystagmus. Ann Neurol 2003;53:688.

137. Marti S, Palla A, Straumann D. Gravity dependence of ocular drift in patients with cerebellar downbeat nystagmus. Ann Neurol 2002;52:712–721.

138. Kim JI, Somers JT, Stahl JS, et al. Vertical nystagmus in normal subjects: Effects of head position, nicotine and scopolamine. J Vestib Res 2000;10:291–300.

139. Yee RD, Baloh RW, Honrubia V, et al. Slow build-up of optokinetic nystagmus associated with downbeat nystagmus. Invest Ophthalmol Vis Sci 1979;18: 622–629.

140. Zee DS, Friendlich AR, Robinson DA. The mechanism of downbeat nystagmus. Arch Neurol 1974;30:227–237.

141. Büchele W, Brandt T, Degner D. Ataxia and oscillopsia in downbeat-nystagmus vertigo syndrome. Adv Oto-Rhino-Laryngol 1983;30:291–297.

142. Cox TA, Corbett JJ, Thompson HS, Lennarson L. Upbeat nystagmus changing to downbeat nystagmus with convergence. Neurology 1981;31:891–892.

143. Fetter M, Dichgans J. Upbeat nystagmus changing to downbeat nystagmus with convergence in a patient with a lower medullary lesion. Neuroophthalmology 1990;10:89–95.

144. Morrow MJ, Sharpe JA. Torsional nystagmus in the lateral medullary syndrome. Ann Neurol 1988;24:390–398.

145. Weissman JD, Seidman SH, Dell'Osso LF, et al. Torsional, see-saw, "bowtie" nystagmus in association with brain stem anomalies. Neuro-ophthalmology 1990;10:315–318.

146. Noseworthy JH, Ebers GC, Leigh RJ, Dell'Osso LF. Torsional nystagmus: Quantitative features and possible pathogenesis. Neurology 1988;38:992–994.

147. Lopez L, Bronstein AM, Gresty MA, Rudge P, DuBoulay EP. Torsional nystagmus. A neuro-otological and MRI study of 35 cases. Brain 1992;115:1107–1124.

148. Averbuch-Heller L, Rottach KG, Zivotofsky AZ, et al. Torsional eye movements in patients with skew deviation and spasmodic torticollis: Responses to static and dynamic head roll. Neurology 1997;48:506–514.

149. Rosenthal JG, Selhorst JB. Continuous non-rhythmic cycloversion: A possible paraneoplastic disorder. Neuroophthalmology 1987;7:291–295.

150. Barton JJS, Sharpe JA. Oscillopsia and horizontal nystagmus with accelerating slow phases following lumbar puncture in the Arnold-Chiari malformation. Ann Neurol 1993;33:418–421.

151. Durig JS, Jen JC, Demer JL. Ocular motility in genetically defined autosomal dominant cerebellar ataxia. Am J Ophthalmol 2002;133:718–721.

152. Daroff RB, Troost BT. Upbeat nystagmus. JAMA 1973;225:312.

153. Gilman N, Baloh RW. Primary position upbeat nystagmus. Neurology 1977;27: 294–297.

154. Fisher A, Gresty M, Chambers B, Rudge P. Primary position upbeating nystagmus: A variety of central positional nystagmus. Brain 1983;106:949–964.

155. Keane JR, Itabashi HH. Upbeat nystagmus: Clinicopathologic study of two patients. Neurology 1987;37:491–494.

156. Munro NA, Gaymard B, Rivaud S, et al. Upbeat nystagmus in a patient with a small medullary infarct. J Neurol Neurosurg Psychiatry 1993;56:1126–1128.

157. Ranalli PJ, Sharpe JA. Upbeat nystagmus and the ventral tegmental pathway of the upward vestibulo-ocular reflex. Neurology 1988;38:1329–1330.

158. Tilikete C, Hermier M, Pelisson D, Vighetto A. Saccadic lateropulsion and upbeat nystagmus: Disorders of caudal medulla. Ann Neurol 2002;52:658–662.

159. Nakada T, Remler MP. Primary position upbeat nystagmus: Another central vestibular nystagmus? J Clin Neuroophthalmol 1981;1:181–185.

160. Kattah JC, Dagli TF. Compensatory head tilt in upbeating nystagmus. J Clin Neuro-ophthalmol 1990;10:27–31.

161. Benjamin EE, Zimmerman CF, Troost BT. Lateropulsion and upbeat nystagmus are manifestations of central vestibular dysfunction. Arch Neurol 1986;43: 962–964.

162. de Jong JM, Cohen B, Matsuo V, Uemura T. Midsagittal pontomedullary brainstem section: Effects on ocular adduction and nystagmus. Exp Neurol 1980;68: 420–428.

163. McCrea R, Strassman A, Highstein S. Anatomical and physiological characteristics of vestibular neurons mediating the vertical vestibulo-ocular reflexes of the squirrel monkey. J Comp Neurol 1987;264:571–594.

164. Gresty MA, Barratt HJ, Rudge P, Page N. Analysis of downbeat nystagmus. Otolithic vs semicircular canal influences. Arch Neurol 1986;43:52–55.

165. Ito M, Nisimaru N, Yamamoto M. Specific patterns of neuronal connexions involved in the control of the rabbit's vestibulo-ocular reflexes by the cerebellar flocculus. J Physiol (Lond) 1977;265:833–854.

166. Baloh RW, Spooner JW. Downbeat nystagmus: A type of central vestibular nystagmus. Neurology 1981;31:304–310.

167. Leigh RJ. Potassium channels, the cerebellum, and treatment for downbeat nystagmus. Neurology 2003;61:158–159.

168. Zee DS, Yamazaki A, Butler PH, Gücer G. Effects of ablation of flocculus and paraflocculus on eye movements in primate. J Neurophysiol 1981;46:878–899.

169. Deleu D, Ebinger G. Lithium-induced internuclear ophthalmoplegia. Clinical Neuropharmacology 1989;12:244–226.

170. Flechtner K-M, Mackert A, Thies K, et al. Lithium effect on smooth pursuit eye movements of healthy volunteers. Biol Psychiatr 1992;32:932–938.

171. Lee MS, Lessell S. Lithium-induced periodic alternating nystagmus. Neurology 2003;60:344.

172. Sandyk R. Oculogyric crisis induced by lithium carbonate. Eur Neurol 1984;23:92–94.

173. Zee DS, Leigh RJ, Mathieu-Millaire F. Cerebellar control of ocular gaze stability. Ann Neurol 1980;7:37–40.

174. Abel LA, Traccis S, Dell'Osso LF, Ansevin CF. Variable waveforms in downbeat nystagmus imply short-term gain changes. Ann Neurol 1983;13:616–620.

175. Glasauer S, Hoshi M, Kempermann U, Eggert T, Buttner U. Three-dimensional eye position and slow phase velocity in humans with downbeat nystagmus. J Neurophysiol 2003;89:338–354.

176. Hoyt CS. Nystagmus and other abnormal ocular movements in children. Ped Clin North Amer 1987;34:1415–1423.

177. Good WV, Hou C, Carden SM. Transient, idiopathic nystagmus in infants. Dev Med Child Neurol 2003;45:304–307.

178. Ishikawa H, Ishikawa S, Mukuno K. Short-cycle periodic (ping-pong) gaze. Neurology 1993;43:1067–1070.

179. Leigh RJ, Robinson DA, Zee DS. A hypothetical explanation for periodic alternating nystagmus: Instability in the optokinetic-vestibular system. Ann NY Acad Sci 1981;374:619–635.

180. Furman JM, Wall C III, Pang D. Vestibular function in periodic alternating nystagmus. Brain 1990;113:1425–1439.

181. Waespe W, Cohen B, Raphan T. Dynamic modification of the vestibulo-ocular reflex by the nodulus and uvula. Science 1985;228:199–202.

182. Cohen B, Henn V, Raphan T, Dennett D. Velocity storage, nystagmus, and visual-vestibular interactions in humans. Ann NY Acad Sci 1981;374:421–433.

183. Sanders MD, Glaser JS. Alternating windmill nystagmus. In: Smith JL, ed. Neuro-Ophthalmology. Vol 7. St. Louis: CV Mosby, 1973:133–136.

184. Lawden MC, Bronstein AM, Kennard C. Repetitive paroxysmal nystagmus and vertigo. Neurology 1995;45:276–280.

185. Daroff RB. See-saw nystagmus. Neurology 1965;15:874–877.

186. Drachman DA. See-saw nystagmus. J Neurol Neurosurg Psychiatry 1966;29:356–361.

187. Druckman R, Ellis P, Kleinfeld J, Waldman M. See-saw nystagmus. Arch Ophthalmol 1966;76:668–675.

188. Nakada T, Kwee IL. Seesaw nystagmus. Role of visuovestibular interaction in its pathogenesis. J Clin Neuroophthalmol 1988;8:171–177.

189. Halmagyi GM, Aw ST, Dehaene I, et al. Jerk-waveform see-saw nystagmus due to unilateral meso-diencephalic lesion. Brain 1994;117:775–788.

190. Schmidt D, Kommerell G. Congenitaler Schaukel-nystagmus (seesaw nystagmus): Ein fall mit erhaltenen gesichtsfeldern, vertikaler blickparese und kopftremor. Graefes Arch Klin Exp Ophthalmol 1974;191:265–272.

191. Rambold H, Helmchen C, Buttner U. Unilateral muscimol inactivations of the interstitial nucleus of Cajal in the alert rhesus monkey do not elicit seesaw nystagmus. Neurosci Lett 1999;272:75–78.

192. Brandt T, Dieterich M. Vestibular syndromes in the roll plane: topographic diagnosis from brain stem to cortex. Ann Neurol 1994;36:337–347.

193. Radtke A, Bronstein AM, Gresty MA, et al. Paroxysmal alternating skew deviation and nystagmus after partial destruction of the uvula. J Neurol Neurosurg Psychiatry 2001;70:790–793.

194. Westheimer G, Blair SM. The ocular tilt reaction: A brainstem oculomotor routine. Invest Ophthalmol 1975;14:833–839.

195. Sano K, Sekino H, Tsukamoto N, Yoshimasu N, Ishijima B. Stimulation and destruction of the region of the interstitial nucleus in cases of torticollis and see-saw nystagmus. Confin Neurol 1972;34:331–338.

196. Lueck CJ, Hamlyn P, Crawford TJ, et al. A case of ocular tilt reaction and torsional nystagmus due to direct stimulation of the midbrain in man. Brain 1991;114:2069–2079.

197. Helmchen C, Rambold H, Kempermann U, et al. Localizing value of torsional nystagmus in small midbrain lesions. Neurology 2002;59:1956–1964.

198. Helmchen C, Glasauer S, Bartl K. Contralesionally beating torsional nystagmus in a unilateral rostral midbrain lesion. Neurology 1996;47:482–486.

199. Seidman SH, Telford L, Paige GD. Vertical, torsional and horizontal eye movement responses to head roll in the squirrel monkey. Exp Brain Res 1995;104:218–226.

200. Cannon SC, Robinson DA. Loss of the neural integrator of the oculomotor system from brain stem lesions in monkey. J Neurophysiol 1987;57:1383–1409.

201. Mettens P, Godaux E, Cheron G, Galiana HL. Effect of muscimol microinjections into the prepositus hypoglossi and the medial vestibular nuclei on cat eye movements. J Neurophysiol 1994;72:785–802.

202. Kaneko CR. Eye movement deficits following ibotenic acid lesions of the nucleus prepositus hypoglossi in monkeys. II. Pursuit, vestibular, and optokinetic responses. J Neurophysiol 1999;81:668–681.

203. Crawford JD, Cadera W, Vilis T. Generation of torsional and vertical eye position signals by the interstitial nucleus of Cajal. Science 1991;252:1551–1553.

204. Baloh RW, Yue Q, Furman JM, Nelson SF. Familial episodic ataxia: Clinical heterogeneity in four families linked to chromosome 19p. Ann Neurol 1997;41:8–16.

205. Abel LA, Parker L, Daroff RB, Dell'Osso LF. End-point nystagmus. Invest Ophthalmol Vis Sci 1978;17:539–544.

206. Eizenman M, Cheng P, Sharpe JA, Frecker RC. End-point nystagmus and ocular drift: An experimental and theoretical study. Vision Res 1990;30:863–877.

207. Shallo-Hoffmann J, Schwarze H, Simonsz H, Muhlendyck H. A reexamination of end-point and rebound nystagmus in normals. Invest Ophthalmol Vis Sci 1990;31:388–392.

208. Abadi RV, Scallan CJ. Ocular oscillations on eccentric gaze. Vision Res 2001;41:2895–2907.

209. Büttner U, Grundei T. Gaze-evoked nystagmus and smooth pursuit deficits: their relationship studied in 52 patients. J Neurol 1995;242:384–389.

210. Collewijn H, Erkelens CJ, Steinman RM. Binocular coordination of human horizontal saccadic eye movements. J Physiol (Lond) 1988;40:157–182.

211. Frohman TC, Frohman EM, O'Suilleabhain P, et al. Accuracy of clinical detection of INO in MS: Corroboration with quantitative infrared oculography. Neurology 2003;61:848–850.

212. Zee DS, Hain TC, Carl JR. Abduction nystagmus in internuclear ophthalmoplegia. Ann Neurol 1987;21:383–388.

213. Gamlin PD, Gnadt JW, Mays LE. Lidocaine-induced unilateral internuclear ophthalmoplegia: Effects on convergence and conjugate eye movements. J Neurophysiol 1989;62:82–95.

214. von Noorden GK, Tredici TD, Ruttum M. Pseudo-internuclear ophthalmoplegia after surgical paresis of the medial rectus muscle. Am J Ophthalmol 1984;98:602–608.

215. Glaser JS. Myasthenic pseudo-internuclear ophthalmoplegia. Arch Ophthalmol 1966;75:363–366.

216. Swick HM. Pseudointernuclear ophthalmoplegia in acute idiopathic polyneuritis (Fisher's syndrome). Am J Ophthalmol 1974;77:725–728.

217. Bruns L. Die Geschwulste des Nervensystems. Berlin: S. Karger, 1908.

218. Nedzelski JM. Cerebellopontine angle tumors: bilateral flocculus compression as a cause of associated oculomotor abnormalities. Laryngoscope 1983;93:1251–1260.

219. Daroff RB, Hoyt WF. Supranuclear disorders of ocular control systems in man: Clinical, anatomical and physiological correlations 1969. In: Bach-y-Rita P, Collins CC, Hyde JE, eds. The Control of Eye Movements. New York: Academic Press, 1971:175–235.

220. Keane JR. The pretectal syndrome. Neurology 1990;40:684–690.

221. Pullicino P, Lincoff N, Truax BT. Abnormal vergence with upper brainstem infarcts: pseudoabducens palsy. Neurology 2000;55:352–358.

222. Ochs AL, Stark L, Hoyt WF, D'Amico D. Opposed adducting saccades in convergence-retraction nystagmus. A patient with sylvian aqueduct syndrome. Brain 1979;102:479–508.

223. Rambold H, Kompf D, Helmchen C. Convergence retraction nystagmus: A disorder of vergence? Ann Neurol 2001;50:677–681.

224. Young GB, Brown JD, Boltin CF, Sibbald WM. Periodic lateralized epileptiform discharges (PLEDs) and nystagmus retractorius. Ann Neurol 1977;2:61–62.

225. Brenner RP, Carlow TJ. PLEDs and nystagmus retractorius. Ann Neurol 1979;5:403.

226. Leech J, Gresty M, Hess K, Rudge P. Gaze failure, drifting eye movements, and centripetal nystagmus in cerebellar disease. Brit J Ophthalmol 1977;61:774–781.

227. Hood JD, Kayan A, Leech J. Rebound nystagmus. Brain 1973;96:507–526.

228. Bondar RL, Sharpe JA, Lewis AJ. Rebound nystagmus in olivocerebellar atrophy: A clinicopathological correlation. Ann Neurol 1984;15:474–477.

229. Büttner U, Straube A, Brandt T. Paroxysmal spontaneous nystagmus and vertigo evoked by lateral eye position. Neurology 1987;37:1553–1555.

230. Yamazaki A, Zee DS. Rebound nystagmus: EOG analysis of a case with a floccular tumor. Brit J Ophthalmol 1979;63:782–786.

231. Abadi RV, Bjerre A. Motor and sensory characteristics of infantile nystagmus. Br J Ophthalmol 2002;86:1152–1160.

232. Tusa RJ, Mustari MJ, Das VE, Boothe RG. Animal models for visual deprivation-induced strabismus and nystagmus. Ann NY Acad Sci 2002;956:346–360.

233. Classification of Eye Movement Abnormalities and Strabismus (CEMAS) Working Group. *http://www.nei.nih.gov/news/statements/cemas* 2003, Ref Type: Electronic Citation.

234. Gresty MA, Bronstein AM, Page NG, Rudge P. Congenital-type nystagmus emerging in later life. Neurology 1991;41:653–656.

235. Friedman DI, Dell'Osso LF. "Reappearance" of congenital nystagmus after minor head trauma. Neurology 1993;43:2414–2416.

236. Averbuch-Heller L, Dell'Osso LF, Leigh RJ, Jacobs JB, Stahl JS. The torsional component of "horizontal" congenital nystagmus. J Neuroophthalmol 2002;22: 22–32.

237. Sogg RL, Hoyt WF. Intermittent vertical nystagmus in a father and son. Arch Ophthalmol 1962;68:515–517.

238. Marmor MF. Hereditary vertical nystagmus. Arch Ophthalmol 1973;90: 107–111.

239. Bixenman WW. Congenital hereditary downbeat nystagmus. Can J Ophthalmol 1983;18:344–348.

240. Shibasaki H, Motomura S. Suppression of congenital nystagmus. J Neurol Neurosurg Psychiatry 1978;41:1078–1083.

241. Dickinson CM. The elucidation and use of the effect of near fixation in congenital nystagmus. Ophthal Physiol Opt 1986;6:303–311.

242. Dell'Osso LF. Development of new treatments for congenital nystagmus. Ann NY Acad Sci 2002;956:361–379.

243. Shawkat FS, Kriss A, Thompson D, et al. Vertical or asymmetric nystagmus need not imply neurological disease. Br J Ophthalmol 2000;84:175–180.

244. Zak TA. Infantile convergence-evoked nystagmus. Ann Ophthalmol 1983;15: 368–369.

245. Daroff RB, Hoyt WF, Bettman JW Jr, Lessell S. Suppression and facilitation of congenital nystagmus by vertical lines. Neurology 1973;23:530–533.

246. Abadi RV, Pascal E. Periodic alternating nystagmus in humans with albinism. Invest Ophthalmol Vis Sci 1994;35:4080–4086.

247. Shallo-Hoffmann J, Riordan-Eva P. Recognizing periodic alternating nystagmus. Strabismus 2001;9:203–215.

248. Bedell HE, White JW, Abplanalp PL. Variability of foveations in congenital nystagmus. Clinical Vision Science 1989;4:247–252.

249. Dell'Osso LF, Van der Steen J, Steinman RM, Collewijn H. Foveation dynamics in congenital nystagmus. I. Fixation. Documenta Ophthlamologica 1992;79: 1–23.

250. Dell'Osso LF, Daroff RB. Braking saccade: A new fast eye movement. Aviat Space Environ Med 1976;47:435–437.

251. Reinecke RD, Guo S, Goldstein HP. Waveform evolution in infantile nystagmus: An electro-oculo-graphic study of 35 cases. Binocular Vis 1988;31:191–202.

252. Hertle RW, Maldanado VK, Maybodi M, Yang D. Clinical and ocular motor analysis of the infantile nystagmus syndrome in the first 6 months of life. Br J Ophthalmol 2002;86:670–675.

253. Shallo-Hoffmann J, Faldon M, Tusa RJ. The incidence and waveform characteristics of periodic alternating nystagmus in congenital nystagmus. Invest Ophthalmol Vis Sci 1999;40:2546–2553.

254. Gradstein L, Reinecke RD, Wizov SS, Goldstein HP. Congenital periodic alternating nystagmus. Diagnosis and management. Ophthalmology 1997;104: 918–928.

255. Stahl JS, Rottach KG, Averbuch-Heller L, et al. A pilot study of gabapentin as treatment for acquired nystagmus. Neuroophthalmology 1996;16:107–113.

256. Dell'Osso LF, Averbuch-Heller L, Leigh RJ. Oscillopsia suppression and foveation-period variation in congenital, latent, and acquired nystagmus. Neuroophthalmology 1997;18:163–183.

257. Goldstein HP, Gottlob I, Fendick MG. Visual remapping in infantile nystagmus. Vision Res 1992;32:1115–1124.

258. Hertle RW, FitzGibbon EJ, Avallone JM, Cheeseman E, Tsilou EK. Onset of oscillopsia after visual maturation in patients with congenital nystagmus. Ophthalmology 2001;108:2301–2307.

259. Tkalcevic LA, Abel LA. Effects of stimulus size and luminance on oscillopsia in congenital nystagmus. Vision Res 2003;43:2697–2705.

260. Dell'Osso LF, Jacobs JB. An expanded nystagmus acuity function: Intra- and intersubject prediction of best-corrected visual acuity. Doc Ophthalmol 2002; 104:249–276.

261. Cesarelli M, Bifulco P, Loffredo L, Bracale M. Relationship between visual acuity and eye position variability during foveations in congenital nystagmus. Doc Ophthalmol 2000;101:59–72.

262. Ukwade MT, Bedell HE. Stereothresholds in persons wtih congenital nystagmus and in normal observers during comparable retinal image motion. Vision Res 1999;39:2963–2973.

263. Dell'Osso LF. Congenital and latent/manifest latent nystagmus: Diagnosis, treatment, foveation, oscillopsia and acuity. Jpn J Ophthalmol 1994;38:329–336.

264. Sheth NV, Dell'Osso LF, Leigh RJ, Peckham HP. The effects of afferent stimulation on congenital nystagmus foveation periods. Vision Res 1995;35:2371–2382.

265. Bedell HE, Bollenbacher MA. Perception of motion smear in normal observers and in persons with congenital nystagmus. Invest Ophthalmol Vis Sci 1996;37: 188–195.

266. Hertle RW, Dell'Osso LF. Clinical and ocular motor analysis of congenital nystagmus in infancy. J AAPOS 1999;3:70–79.

267. Halmagyi GM, Gresty MA, Leech J. Reversed optokinetic nystagmus (OKN): Mechanism and clinical significance. Ann Neurol 1980;7:429–435.

268. Kurzan R, Büttner U. Smooth pursuit mechanisms in congenital nystagmus. Neuroophthalmology 1989;9:313–325.

269. Dell'Osso LF, Van der Steen J, Steinman RM, Collewijn H. Foveation dynamics in congenital nystagmus. II. Smooth pursuit. Documenta Ophthlamologica 1992; 79:25–49.

270. Yee RD, Baloh RW, Honrubia V, Kim YS. A study of congenital nystagmus: Vestibular aspects. J Otolaryngol 1981;10:89–98.

271. Carl JR, Optican LM, Chu FC, Zee DS. Head shaking and vestibulo-ocular reflex in congenital nystagmus. Invest Ophthalmol Vis Sci 1985;26:1043–1050.

272. Dell'Osso LF, Van der Steen J, Steinman RM, Collewijn H. Foveation dynamics in congenital nystagmus. III. Vestibulo-ocular reflex. Documenta Ophthlamologica 1992;79:51–70.

273. Demer JL, Zee DS. Vestibulo-ocular and optokinetic deficits in albinos with congenital nystagmus. Invest Ophthalmol Vis Sci 1984;25:74–78.

274. Gresty MA, Barratt HJ, Page NG, Ell JJ. Assessment of vestibulo-ocular reflexes in congenital nystagmus. Ann Neurol 1985;17:129–136.

275. Kelly BJ, Rosenberg ML, Zee DS, Optican LM. Unilateral pursuit-induced congenital nystagmus. Neurology 1989;39:414–416.

276. Tusa RJ, Zee DS, Hain TC, Simonsz HJ. Voluntary control of congenital nystagmus. Clinical Vision Sci 1992;7:195–210.

277. Dell'Osso LF, Weisman BM, Leigh RJ, Abel RJ, Sheth NV. Hereditary congenital nystagmus and gaze-holding failure: The role of the neural integrator. Neurology 1993;43:1741–1749.

278. Stevens DJ, Hertle RW. Relationships between visual acuity and anomalous head posture in patients with congenital nystagmus. J Pediatr Ophthalmol Strabismus 2003;40:259–264.

279. Dell'Osso LF, Ellenberger C Jr, Abel LA, Flynn JT. The nystagmus blockage syndrome: Congenital nystagmus, manifest latent nystagmus, or both? Invest Ophthalmol Vis Sci 1983;24:1580–1587.

280. von Noorden GK, Avilla C, Sidokaro Y, LaRoche R. Latent nystagmus and strabismic amblyopia. Am J Ophthalmol 1987;103:87–89.

281. Gresty MA, Halmagyi GM. Head nodding associated with idiopathic childhood nystagmus. Ann NY Acad Sci 1981;374:614–618.

282. Dell'Osso LF, Daroff RB. Abnormal head positions and head motion associated with nystagmus. In Keller EL, Zee DS, eds. Adaptive Processes in Visual and Oculomotor Systems. Oxford, Pergamon Press, 1986:473–478.

283. Simon JW, Kandel GL, Krohel GB, Nelsen PT. Albinotic characteristics in congenital nystagmus. Am J Ophthalmol 1984;97:320–327.

284. Collewijn H, Apkarian P, Spekreijse H. The oculomotor behavior of human albinos. Brain 1985;108:1–28.

285. Abadi RV, Pascal E. The recognition and management of albinism. Ophthal Physiol Opt 1989;9:3–15.

286. Faugere V, Tuffery-Giraud S, Hamel C, Claustres M. Identification of three novel OA1 gene mutations identified in three families misdiagnosed with congenital nystagmus and carrier status determination by real-time quantitative PCR assay. BMC Genet 2003;4:1.

287. Weiss AH, Biersdorf WR. Visual sensory disorders in congenital nystagmus. Ophthalomology 1989;96:517–523.

288. Good PA, Searle AE, Campbell S, Crews SJ. Value of the ERG in congenital nystagmus. Br J Ophthalmol 1989;73:512–515.

289. Lambert SR, Taylor D, Kriss A. The infant with nystagmus: Normal appearing fundi, but an abnormal ERG. Ophthalmology 1989;34:173–186.

290. Dell'Osso LF, Flynn JT, Daroff RB. Hereditary congenital nystagmus: An intrafamilial study. Arch Ophthalmol 1974;92:366–374.

291. Oetting WS, Armstrong CM, Holleschau AM, et al. Evidence for genetic heterogeneity in families with congenital motor nystagmus (CN). Ophthalmic Genet 2000;21:227–233.

292. Kerrison JB, Vagefi MR, Barmada MM, Maumenee IH. Congenital motor nystagmus linked to Xq26-q27. Am J Hum Genet 1999;64:600–607.

293. Kerrison JB, Koenekoop RK, Arnould VJ, et al. Clinical features of autosomal dominant congenital nystagmus linked to chromosome 6P12. Am J Ophthalmol 1998;125:64–70.

294. Abadi RV, Dickinson CM, Lomas MS, Ackerley R. Congenital idiopathic nystagmus in identical twins. Br J Ophthalmol 1983;67:693–695.

295. Guillery RW, Okoro AN, Witkop CJ Jr. Abnormal visual pathways in the brain of a human albino. Brain Res 1975;96:373–377.

296. Creel D, O'Donnell FE Jr, Witkop CJ. Visual system anomalies in human ocular albinos. Science 1978;201:931–933.

297. McCarty JW, Demer JL, Hovis LA, Nuwer MR. Ocular motility anomalies in developmental misdirection of the optic chiasm. Am J Ophthalmol 1992;113: 86–95.

298. Optican LM, Zee DS. A hypothetical explanation of congenital nystagmus. Biol Cyber 1984;50:119–134.

299. Harris C. Problems in modelling congenital nystagmus: Towards a new model. In: Findlay JM, Walker R, Kentridge RW, eds. Eye Movement Research: Mechanisms, Processes and Applications. Amsterdam: Elsevier; 1995:239–253.

300. Abadi RV, Scallan CJ. Waveform characteristics of manifest latent nystagmus. Invest Ophthalmol Vis Sci 2000;41:3805–3817.

301. Dell'Osso LF, Schmidt D, Daroff RB. Latent, manifest latent, and congenital nystagmus. Arch Ophthalmol 1979;97:1877–1885.

302. Gresty MA, Metcalfe T, Timms C, et al. Neurology of latent nystagmus. Brain 1992;115:1303–1321.
303. Kommerell G, Zee DS. Latent nystagmus. Release and suppression at will. Invest Ophthalmol Vis Sci 1993;34:1785–1792.
304. Dell'Osso LF, Traccis S, Abel LA. Strabismus: A necessary condition for latent and manifest latent nystagmus. Neuroophthalmology 1983;3:247–257.
305. Abramson D. Latent nystagmus in identical twins. Arch Ophthalmol 1973;89:256–257.
306. Dell'Osso LF, Leigh RJ, Sheth NV, Daroff RB. Two types of foveation strategy in "latent" nystagmus: Visual acuity and stability. Neuroophthalmology 1995;15:1–20.
307. Anderson JR. Latent nystagmus and alternating hyperphoria. Br J Ophthalmol 1954;38:217–231.
308. Tychsen L, Lisberger SG. Maldevelopment of visual motion processing in humans who had strabismus with onset in infancy. J Neurosci 1986;6:2495–2508.
309. Averbuch-Heller L, Dell'Osso LF, Remler BF, et al. Latent nystagmus in Down's syndrome. Neurology 1997;48(Suppl 2):A133.
310. Hainline L, Abramov I. Saccades and small-field optokinetic nystagmus in infants. J Am Optom Assoc 1985;56:620–626.
311. Tusa RJ, Mustari MJ, Burrows AF, Fuchs AF. Gaze-stabilizing deficits and latent nystagmus in monkeys with brief, early-onset visual deprivation: Eye movement recordings. J Neurophysiol 2001;86:651–661.
312. Dell'Osso LF, Abel LA, Daroff RB. Latent/manifest latent nystagmus reversal using an ocular prosthesis: Implications for vision and ocular dominance. Invest Ophthalmol Vis Sci 1987;28:1873–1876.
313. Ishikawa S. Latent nystagmus and its etiology. In: Reinecke RD, ed. Third Meeting of the International Strabismological Association, Kyoto. New York: Grune & Stratton, 1979:203–214.
314. Buisseret P. Influence of extraocular muscle proprioception on vision. Physiol Rev 1995;75:323.
315. Norton EW, Cogan DG. Spasmus nutans: A clinical study of 20 cases followed 2 years or more since onset. Arch Ophthalmol 1954;52:442–446.
316. Hoyt CS, Aicardi E. Acquired monocular nystagmus in monozygous twins. J Pediatr Ophthalmol Strabismus 1979;16:115–118.
317. Gottlob I, Wizov SS, Reinecke RD. Spasmus nutans: A long-term follow-up. Invest Ophthalmol Vis Sci 1995;36:2768–2771.
318. Gresty M, Leech J, Sanders M, Eggars H. A study of head and eye movement in spasmus nutans. Br J Ophthalmol 1976;60:652–654.
319. Gresty MA, Ell JJ. Spasmus nutans or congenital nystagmus? Classification according to objective criteria. Br J Ophthalmol 1981;65:510–511.
320. Chrousos GA, Ballen AE, Matsuo V, Cogan DG. Near-evoked nystagmus in spasmus nutans. J Pediatr Ophthalmol Strabismus 1986;23:141–143.
321. Lambert SR, Newman NJ. Retinal disease masquerading as spasmus nutans. Neurology 1993;43:1607–1609.
322. Kaplan PW, Tusa RJ. Neurophysiologic and clinical correlations of epileptic nystagmus. Neurology 1993;43:2508–2514.
323. Jacome DE, FitzGerald R. Monocular ictal nystagmus. Arch Neurol 1982;39:653–656.
324. Thurston SE, Leigh RJ, Osorio I. Epileptic gaze deviation and nystagmus. Neurology 1985;35:1518–1521.
325. Kaplan PW, Lesser RP. Vertical and horizontal epileptic gaze deviation and nystagmus. Neurology 1989;39:1391–1393.
326. Tusa RJ, Kaplan PW, Hain TC, Naidu S. Ipsiversive eye deviation and epileptic nystagmus. Neurology 1990;40:662–665.
327. Komatsu H, Wurtz RH. Modulation of pursuit eye movements by stimulation of cortical areas MT and MST. J Neurophysiol 1989;62:31–47.
328. Simon RP, Aminoff MJ. Electrographic status epilepticus in fatal anoxic coma. Ann Neurol 1986;20:351–355.
329. Schmidtke K, Büttner-Ennever JA. Nervous control of eyelid function: A review of clinical, experimental and pathological data. Brain 1992;115:227–247.
330. Averbuch-Heller L. Neurology of the eyelids. Curr Opin Ophthalmol 1997;8:27–34.
331. Guitton D, Simard R, Codère F. Upper eyelid movements measured with a search coil during blinks and vertical saccades. Invest Ophthalmol Vis Sci 1991;32:3298–3305.
332. Evinger LC, Manning KA, Sibony PA. Eyelid movements: Mechanisms and normal data. Invest Ophthalmol Vis Sci 1991;32:387–400.
333. Brusa A, Massa S, Piccardo A, Stoehr R, Bronzini E. Le nystagmus palpebral. Rev Neurol (Paris) 1984;140:288–292.
334. Brodsky MC, Boop FA. Lid nystagmus as a sign of intrinsic midbrain disease. J Neuroophthalmol 1995;15:236–240.
335. Daroff RB, Hoyt WF, Sanders MD, Nelson LR. Gaze-evoked eyelid and ocular nystagmus inhibited by the near reflex: Unusual ocular motor phenomena in a lateral medullary syndrome. J Neurol Neurosurg Psychiatry 1968;31:362–367.
336. Sanders MD, Hoyt WF, Daroff RB. Lid nystagmus evoked by ocular convergence: An ocular electromyographic study. J Neurol Neurosurg Psychiatry 1968;31:368–371.

337. Safran AB, Berney J, Safran E. Convergence-evoked eyelid nystagmus. Am J Ophthalmol 1982;93:48.
338. Howard RS. A case of convergence evoked eyelid nystagmus. J Clin Neuroophthalmol 1986;6:169–171.
339. Selhorst JB, Stark L, Ochs AL, Hoyt WF. Disorders in cerebellar ocular motor control. I. Saccadic overshoot dysmetria, an oculographic, control system and clinico-anatomic analysis. Brain 1976;99:497–508.
340. Bötzel K, Rottach K, Buttner U. Normal and pathological saccadic dysmetria. Brain 1993;116:337–353.
341. Herishanu Y, Sharpe JA. Normal square wave jerks. Invest Ophthalmol Vis Sci 1981;20:268–272.
342. Elidan J, Gay Y, Lev S. Square wave jerks: Incidence, characteristic, and significance. J Otolaryngol 1984;13:375–381.
343. Shallo-Hoffmann J, Petersen J, Mühlendyck H. How normal are "normal" square wave jerks? Invest Ophthalmol Vis Sci 1989;30:1009–1011.
344. Shallo-Hoffmann J, Sendler B, Mühlendyck H. Normal square wave jerks in differing age groups. Invest Ophthalmol Vis Sci 1990;31:1649–1652.
345. Dale R, Kirby A, Jampel RS. Square wave jerks in Friedreich's ataxia. Am J Ophthalmol 1978;85:400–406.
346. Sharpe JA, Fletcher WA. Saccadic intrusions and oscillations. Can J Neurol Sci 1984;11:426–433.
347. Troost BT, Daroff RB. The ocular motor defects in progressive supranuclear palsy. Ann Neurol 1977;2:397–403.
348. Rascol O, Sabatini U, Simonetta-Moreau M, et al. Square wave jerks in Parkinsonian syndromes. J Neurol Neurosurg Psychiatry 1991;54:599–602.
349. Sharpe JA, Herishanu YO, White OB. Cerebral square wave jerks. Neurology 1982;37:1389–1392.
350. Abel LA, Traccis S, Dell'Osso LF, et al. Square wave oscillation: The relationship of saccadic intrusions and oscillations. Neuroophthalmology 1984;4:21–25.
351. Sibony PA, Evinger C, Manning K. Tobacco-induced primary-position upbeat nystagmus. Ann Neurol 1987;21:53–58.
352. Sibony PA, Evinger C, Manning KA. The effects of tobacco smoking on smooth pursuit eye movements. Ann Neurol 1988;23:238–241.
353. Dell'Osso LF, Troost BT, Daroff RB. Macro square wave jerks. Neurology 1975;25:975–979.
354. Dell'Osso LF, Abel LA, Daroff RB. "Inverse latent" macro square-wave jerks and macro saccadic oscillations. Ann Neurol 1977;2:57–60.
355. Selhorst JB, Stark L, Ochs AL, Hoyt WF. Disorders in cerebellar ocular motor control. II. Macrosaccadic oscillation: An oculographic, control system and clinico-anatomical analysis. Brain 1976;99:509–522.
356. Kase M, Nagata R, Arikado T. Macrosaccadic oscillation, saccadic dysmetria and motor error in spinocerebellar degeneration. Jpn J Ophthalmol 1985;29:369–377.
357. Averbuch-Heller L, Kori AA, Rottach K, Dell'Osso LF, Remler BF, Leigh RJ. Dysfunction of pontine omnipause neurons causes impaired fixation: macrosaccadic oscillations with a unilateral pontine lesion. Neuroophthalmology 1996;16:99–106.
358. Swartz B, Li S, Bespalova I, et al. Pathogenesis of clincial signs in recessive cerebellar ataxia with saccadic intrusions and neuropathy. Ann Neurol 2003;54:xx.
359. Fukazawa T, Tashiro K, Hamada T, Kase M. Multisystem degeneration: drugs and square wave jerks. Neurology 1986;36:1230–1233.
360. Komiyama A, Toda H, Johkura K. Edrophonium-induced macrosaccadic oscillations in myasthenia gravis. Ann Neurol 1999;45:522–525.
361. Herishanu YO, Sharpe JA. Saccadic intrusions in internuclear ophthalmoplegia. Ann Neurol 1983;14:67–72.
362. Selhorst JB. Myoclonic ocular jerks. Ann Neurol 1983;13:212–213.
363. Zee DS, Robinson DA. A hypothetical explanation of saccadic oscillations. Ann Neurol 1979;5:405–414.
364. Bergenius J. Saccade abnormalities in patients with ocular flutter. Acta Otolaryngol 1986;102:228–233.
365. Bhidayasiri R, Somers JT, Kim JI, et al. Ocular oscillations induced by shifts of the direction and depth of visual fixation. Ann Neurol 2001;49:24–28.
366. Ashe J, Hain TC, Zee DS, Schatz NJ. Microsaccadic flutter. Brain 1991;114:461–472.
367. Dyken P, Kolar O. Dancing eye, dancing feet: Infantile polymyoclonia. Brain 1968;91:305–320.
368. Bataller L, Graus F, Saiz A, Vilchez J. Clinical outcome in adult onset idiopathic or paraneoplastic opsoclonus-myoclonus. Brain 2001;124:437–443.
369. Pranzatelli MR, Huang Y, Tate E, et al. Cerebrospinal fluid 5-hydroxyindoleacetic acid and homovanillic acid in the pediatric opsoclonus-myoclonus syndrome. Ann Neurol 1995;37:189–197.
370. Engle EC, Hedley-White T. A 29-month-old girl with worsening ataxia, nystagmus, and subsequent opsoclonus and myoclonus. Case records of the Massachusetts General Hospital. N Engl J Med 1995;333:1995.
371. Luque FA, Furneaux HM, Ferziger R, et al. Anti-Ri: An antibody associated with paraneoplastic opsoclonus and breast cancer. Ann Neurol 1991;29:241–251.
372. Posner JB. Neurological Complications of Cancer. Philadelphia: F.A. Davis, 1995.

373. Shams'ili S, Grefkens J, de Leeuw B, et al. Paraneoplastic cerebellar degeneration associated with antineuronal antibodies: Analysis of 50 patients. Brain 2003; 126:1409–1418.

374. Bataller L, Rosenfeld MR, Graus F, et al. Autoantigen diversity in the opsoclonus-myoclonus syndrome. Ann Neurol 2003;53:347–353.

375. Dropcho EJ, Kline LB, Riser J. Antineuronal (anti-Ri) antibodies in a patient with steroid-responsive opsoclonus-myoclonus. Neurology 1993;43:207–211.

376. Casado JL, Gil-Peralta A, Graus F, et al. Anti-ri antibodies associated with opsoclonus and progressive encephalomyelitis with rigidity. Neurology 1994; 44:1521–1522.

377. Hormigo A, Rosenblum MK, River ME, Posner JB. Immunological and pathological study of anti-Ri-associated encephalopathy. Ann Neurol 1994;36: 896–902.

378. Hersh B, Dalmau J, Dangond F, et al. Paraneoplastic opsoclonus-myoclonus associated with anti-Hu antibody. Neurology 1994;44:1754–1755.

379. Noetzel MJ, Cawley LP, James VL, et al. Anti-neurofilament protein antibodies in opsoclonus-myoclonus. J Neuroimmunol 1987;15:137–145.

380. Shults W, Stark L, Hoyt W, Ochs A. Normal saccadic structure of voluntary nystagmus. Arch Ophthalmol 1977;95:1399–1404.

381. Zahn JR. Incidence and characteristics of voluntary nystagmus. J Neurol Neurosurg Psychiatry 1978;41:617–623.

382. Hotson JR. Convergence-initiated voluntary flutter: A normal intrinsic capability in man. Brain Res 1984;294:299–304.

383. Krohel G, Griffin JF. Voluntary vertical nystagmus. Neurology 1979;29: 1153–1154.

384. Lee J, Gresty M. A case of voluntary nystagmus and head tremor. J Neurol Neurosurg Psychiatry 1993;56:1321–1322.

385. Ciuffreda KJ. Voluntary nystagmus: New findings and clinical implications. Am J Optom Physiol Opt 1980;57:795–800.

386. Leigh RJ, Kennard C. Using saccades as a research tool in the clinical neurosciences. Brain 2003;127:1–18.

387. Horn AKE, Büttner-Ennever JA, Suzuki Y, Henn V. Histological identification of premotor neurons for horizontal saccades in monkey and man by parvalbumin immunostaining. J Comp Neurol 1997;359:350–363.

388. Horn AKE, Büttner-Ennever JA. Premotor neurons for vertical eye-movements in the rostral mesencephalon of monkey and man: Histological idnetification by parvalbumin immunostaining. J Compar Neurol 1998 (In press).

389. Büttner-Ennever JA, Cohen B, Pause M, Fries W. Raphe nucleus of pons containing omnipause neurons of the oculomotor system in the monkey, and its homologue in man. J Compar Neurol 1988;267:307–321.

390. Horn AKE, Büttner-Ennever JA, Wahle P, Reichenberger I. Neurotransmitter profile of saccadic omnipause neurons in nucleus raphe interpositus. J Neuroscience 1994;14:2032–2046.

391. Goldberg ME, Bushnell MC, Bruce CJ. The effect of attentive fixation on eye movements evoked by electrical stimulation of the frontal eye fields. Exp Brain Res 1986;61:579–584.

392. Sparks DL, Mays LE. Spatial localization of saccade targets. I. Compensation for stimulation-induced perturbations in eye position. J Neurophysiol 1983;49: 45–63.

393. Munoz DP, Wurtz RH. Fixation cells in monkey superior colliculus. I. Characteristics of cell discharge. J Neurophysiol 1993;70:559–575.

394. Munoz DP, Wurtz RH. Fixation cells in monkey superior colliculus. II. Reversible activation and deactivation. J Neurophysiol 1993;70:576–589.

395. Dias EC, Kiesau M, Segraves MA. Acute activation and inactivation of macaque frontal eye field with GABA-related drugs. J Neurophysiol 1995;74:2744–2748.

396. Waitzman DM, Silakov VL. Effects of reversible lesions of the central mesencephalic reticular formation (cMRF) on primate saccadic eye movements. Soc Neurosci Abstr 1994;20:1399.

397. Steele JC, Richardson JC, Olszewski J. Progressive supranuclear palsy: A heterogeneous degeneration involving the brain stem, basal ganglia and cerebellum with vertical gaze and pseudobulbar palsy, nuchal dystonia and dementia. Arch Neurol 1964;10:333–359.

398. van Gisbergen JAM, Robinson DA, Gielen S. A quantitative analysis of generation of saccadic eye movements by burst neurons. J Neurophysiol 1981;45: 417–442.

399. Ramat S, Somers JT, Das VE, Leigh RJ. Conjugate ocular oscillations during shifts of the direction and depth of visual fixation. Invest Ophthalmol Vis Sci 1999;40:1681–1686.

400. Kaneko CRS. Effect of ibotenic acid lesions of the omnipause neurons on saccadic eye movements in Rhesus macaques. J Neurophysiol 1996;75:2229–2242.

401. Ridley A, Kennard C, Scholtz CL, et al. Omnipause neurons in two cases of opsoclonus associated with oat cell carcinoma of the lung. Brain 1987;110: 1699–1709.

402. Wong AM, Musallam S, Tomlinson RD, Shannon P, Sharpe JA. Opsoclonus in three dimensions: oculographic, neuropathologic and modelling correlates. J Neurol Sci 2001;189:71–81.

403. Schon F, Hodgson TL, Mort D, Kennard C. Ocular flutter associated with a localized lesion in the paramedian pontine reticular formation. Ann Neurol 2001; 50:413–416.

404. Hattori T, Hirayama K, Imai T, et al. Pontine lesions in opsoclonus-myoclonus syndrome shown by MRI. J Neurol Neurosurg Psychiatry 1988;51:1572–1575.

405. Averbuch-Heller L, Remler B. Opsoclonus. Semin Neurol 1996;16:21–26.

406. Blain PG, Nightingale S, Stoddart JC. Strychnine poisoning: Abnormal eye movements. J Toxicol Clin Toxicol 1982;19:215–217.

407. Rajendra S, Schofield P. Molecular mechanisms of inherited startle syndromes. Trends Neurosci 1995;18:80–82.

408. Cogan DG. Opsoclonus, body tremulousness, and benign encephalitis. Arch Ophthalmol 1968;79:545–551.

409. Ellenberger C Jr, Campa JF, Netsky MG. Opsoclonus and parenchymatous degeneration of the cerebellum: Cerebellar origin of an abnormal eye movement. Neurology 1968;18:1041–1046.

410. Helmchen C, Rambold H, Sprenger A, et al. Cerebellar activation in opsoclonus: An fMRI study. Neurology 2003;61:412–415.

411. Optican LM, Robinson DA. Cerebellar-dependent adaptive control of primate saccadic system. J Neurophysiol 1980;44:1058–1076.

412. Robinson FR, Straube A, Fuchs AF. Role of the caudal fastigial nucleus in saccade generation. II. Effects of muscimol inactivation. J Neurophysiol 1993; 70:1741–1758.

413. Duane A. Unilateral rotary nystagmus. Trans Am Ophthalmol Soc 1906;11: 63–67.

414. Hoyt WF, Keane JR. Superior oblique myokymia: Report and discussion on five cases of benign intermittent uniocular microtremor. Arch Ophthal 1970;84: 461–467.

415. Susac J, Smith J, Schatz N. Superior oblique myokymia. Arch Neurol 1973;29: 432–434.

416. Rosenberg M, Glaser J. Superior oblique myokymia. Ann Neurol 1983;13: 667–669.

417. Brazis PW, Miller NR, Henderer JD, Lee AG. The natural history and results of treatment of superior oblique myokymia. Neuroophthalmology 1994;12: 1063–1067.

418. Morrow MJ, Sharpe JA, Ranalli PJ. Superior oblique myokymia associated with a posterior fossa tumor: oculographic correlation with an idiopathic case. Neurology 1990;40:367–370.

419. Leigh RJ, Tomsak RL, Seidman SH, Dell'Osso LF. Superior oblique myokymia: Quantitative characteristics of the eye movements in three patients. Arch Ophthalmol 1991;109:1710–1713.

420. Thurston SE, Saul RF. Superior oblique myokymia: Quantitative description of the eye movement. Neurology 1991;35:1518–1521.

421. Tomsak RL, Kosmorsky GA, Leigh RJ. Gabapentin attenuates superior oblique myokymia. Am J Ophthalmol 2002;133:721–723.

422. Kommerell G, Schaubele G. Superior oblique myokymia. An electromyographical analysis. Trans Ophthal Soc UK 1980;100:504–506.

423. Komai K, Mimura O, Uyama J, et al. Neuro-ophthalmological evaluation of superior oblique myokymia. Neuroophthalmology 1992;12:135–140.

424. Murphy E, Brown J, Iannuzzelli PG, Baker RS. Regeneration and soma size changes following axotomy of the trochlear nerve. J Comp Neurol 1990;292: 524–536.

425. Lee JP. Superior oblique myokymia: A possible etiologic factor. Arch Ophthalmol 1984;102:1178–1179.

426. Clark E. A case of apparent intermittent overaction of the left superior oblique. Br Orthop J 1966;23:116–117.

427. Ricker VK, Mertens HG. Okuläre Neuromyotonie. Klin Monatsbl Augenheilkd 1970;156:837–842.

428. Papst W. Zur Differentialdiagnose der okulären Neuromyotonie. Ophthalmologica 1972;164:252–263.

429. Lessell S, Lessell IM, Rizzo JFI. Ocular neuromyotonia after radiation therapy. Am J Ophthalmol 1986;102:766–770.

430. Shults W, Hoyt W, Behrens M, et al. Ocular neuromyotonia: A clinical description of six patients. Arch Ophthalmol 1986;104:1028–1034.

431. Newman SA. Gaze-induced strabismus. Surv Ophthalmol 1993;38:303–309.

432. Frohman EM, Zee DS. Ocular neuromyotonia: Clinical features, physiological mechanisms, and response to therapy. Ann Neurol 1995;37:620–626.

433. Morrow MJ, Kao GW, Arnold AC. Bilateral ocular neuromyotonia: Oculographic correlations. Neurology 1996;46:264–266.

434. Newsom-Davis J, Mills KR. Immunological associations of acquired neuromyotonia (Isaac's syndrome). Brain 1993;116:453–469.

435. Fisher CM. Neurological examination of the comatose patient. Acta Neurol Scand 1969;45(Suppl 36):1–56.

436. Buettner UW, Zee DS. Vestibular testing in comatose patients. Arch Neurol 1989;46:561–563.

437. Fisher CM. Ocular bobbing. Arch Neurol 1964;11:543–546.

438. Daroff RB, Waldman AL. Ocular bobbing. J Neurol Neurosurg Psychiatry 1965; 28:375–377.

439. Susac JO, Hoyt WF, Daroff RB, Lawrence W. Clinical spectrum of ocular bobbing. J Neurol Neurosurg Psychiatry 1970;33:771–775.

440. Bosch EP, Kennedy SS, Aschenbrener CA. Ocular bobbing: Myth of its localizing value. Neurology 1975;25:949–953.

441. Katz B, Hoyt WF, Townsend J. Ocular bobbing and unilateral pontine hemorrhage. J Clin Neuroophthalmol 1982;2:193–195.

442. Larmande P, Limodin J, Henin D, Lapierre F. Ocular bobbing: Abnormal eye movement or eye movement's abnormality? Ophthalmologica 1983;187: 161–165.

443. Zegers de Beyl D, Flament-Durand J, Borenstein S, Brunko E. Ocular bobbing and myoclonus in central pontine myelinolysis. J Neurol Neurosurg Psychiatry 1983;46:564–565.

444. Tijssen CC, Ter Bruggen JP. Locked-in syndrome associated with ocular bobbing. Acta Neurol Scand 1986;73:444–446.

445. Rosa A, Masmoudi K, Mizon JP. Typical and atypical ocular bobbing: Pathology through five case reports. Neuroophthalmology 1987;7:285–290.

446. Gaymard B. Disconjugate ocular bobbing. Neurology 1993;43:2151.

447. Drake ME Jr, Erwin CW, Massey EW. Ocular bobbing in metabolic encephalopathy: Clinical, pathologic, and electrophysiologic study. Neurology 1982;32:1029–1031.

448. Hata S, Bernstein E, Davis LE. Atypical ocular bobbing in acute organophosphate poisoning. Arch Neurol 1986;43:185–186.

449. Knobler RL, Somasundaram M, Schutta HS. Inverse ocular bobbing. Ann Neurol 1981;9:194–197.

450. Ropper AH. Ocular dipping in anoxic coma. Arch Neurol 1981;38:297–299.

451. Ropper AH. Atypical ocular bobbing. Ann Neurol 1981;10:400.

452. Luda E. Ocular dipping. Arch Neurol 1982;39:67.

453. van Weerden TW, van Woerkom TC. Ocular dipping. Neurology 1985;35:135.

454. Safran AB, Berney J. Synchronism of reverse ocular bobbing and blinking. Am J Ophthalmol 1983;95:863–864.

455. Stark SR, Masucci EF, Kurtzke JF. Ocular dipping. Neurology 1984;34:391–393.

456. Titer EM, Laureno R. Inverse/reverse ocular bobbing. Ann Neurol 1988;23:103–104.

457. Goldschmidt TJ, Wall M. Slow-upward ocular bobbing. J Clin Neuroophthalmol 1987;7:241–243.

458. Mehler MF. The clinical spectrum of ocular bobbing and ocular dipping. J Neurol Neurosurg Psychiatry 1988;51:725–727.

459. Brusa A, Firpo MP, Massa S, Piccardo A, Bronzini E. Typical and reverse bobbing: a case with localizing value. European Neurol 1984;23:151–155.

460. Rosenberg ML. Spontaneous vertical eye movements in coma. Ann Neurol 1986;20:635–637.

461. Keane JR. Pretectal pseudobobbing. Five patients with 'V'-pattern convergence nystagmus. Arch Neurol 1985;42:592–594.

462. Rosenberg ML, Calvert PC. Ocular bobbing in association with other signs of midbrain dysfunction. Arch Neurol 1986;43:314–315.

463. Larmande P, Dongmo L, Limodin J, Ruchoux M. Periodic alternating gaze: A case without any hemispheric lesion. Neurosurgery 1987;20:481–483.

464. Leigh RJ, Hanley DF, Munschauer FEI, Lasker AG. Eye movements induced by head rotations in unresponsive patients. Ann Neurol 1983;15:465–473.

465. Averbuch-Heller L, Meiner Z. Reversible periodic alternating gaze deviation in hepatic encephalopathy. Neurology 1995;45:191–192.

466. Buttner U, Fuhry L. Drug therapy of nystagmus and saccadic intrusions. Adv Otorhinolaryngol 1999;55:195–227.

467. Leigh RJ, Tomsak R. Drug treatments for eye movement disorders. J Neurol Neurosurg Psychiatry 2003;74:1–4.

468. Herdman SJ. Vestibular Rehabilitation. Ed 2. Philadelphia, F.A. Davis, 1998.

469. Brandt T, Steddin S, Daroff RB. Therapy for benign paroxysmal positioning vertigo, revisited. Neurology 1994;44:796–800.

470. Epley JM. Human experience with canalith repositioning maneuvers. Ann NY Acad Sci 2001;942:179–191.

471. Asprella LG, Gagliardi G, Cifarelli D, Larotonda G. "Step by step" treatment of lateral semicircular canal canalolithiasis under videonystagmoscopic examination. Acta Otorhinolaryngol Ital 2003;23:10–15.

472. Froehling DA, Bowen JM, Mohr DN, et al. The canalith repositioning procedure for the treatment of benign paroxysmal positional vertigo: Randomized controlled trial. Mayo Clin Proc 2000;75:695–700.

473. Straube A, Kurzan R, Büttner U. Differential effects of bicuculline and muscimol microinjections into the vestibular nuclei on simian eye movements. Exp Brain Res 1991;86:347–358.

474. Arnold DB, Robinson DA, Leigh RJ. Nystagmus induced by pharmacological inactivation of the brainstem ocular motor integrator in monkey. Vision Res 1999;39:4286–4295.

475. Cohen B, Helwig D, Raphan T. Baclofen and velocity storage: A model of the effects of the drug on the vestibulo-ocular reflex in the rhesus monkey. J Physiol (Lond) 1987;393:703–725.

476. Blair SM, Gavin M. Modifications of vestibulo-ocular reflex induced by diazepam. Arch Otolaryngol 1979;105:698–701.

477. Gavin M, Blair S. Modification of the Macaque's vestibulo-ocular reflex by picrotoxin. Arch Otolaryngol 1981;107:372–376.

478. Halmagyi GM, Rudge P, Gresty MA, Leigh RJ, Zee DS. Treatment of periodic alternating nystagmus. Ann Neurol 1980;8:609–611.

479. Sibony PA, Evinger C, Manning K, Pellegrini JJ. Nicotine and tobacco-induced nystagmus. Ann Neurol 1990;28:198.

480. Pereira CB, Strupp M, Eggert T, Straube A, Brandt T. Nicotine-induced nystagmus: three-dimensional analysis and dependence on head position. Neurology 2000;55:1563–1566.

481. Dieterich M, Straube A, Brandt T, Paulus W, Büttner U. The effects of baclofen and cholinergic drugs on upbeat and downbeat nystagmus. J Neurol Neurosurg Psychiatry 1991;54:627–632.

482. Henderson RD, Wijdicks EF. Downbeat nystagmus associated with intravenous patient-controlled administration of morphine. Anesth Analg 2000;91:691–692.

483. Rottach KG, Wohlgemuth WA, Dzaja AE, Eggert T, Straube A. Effects of intravenous opioids on eye movements in humans: possible mechanisms. J Neurol 2002;249:1200–1205.

484. Currie JN, Matsuo V. The use of clonazepam in the treatment of nystagmus-induced oscillopsia. Ophthalmology 1986;93:924–932.

485. Barton JJS, Huaman AG, Sharpe JA. Muscarinic antagonists in the treatment of acquired pendular and downbeat nystagmus: Double-blind, randomized trial of three intravenous drugs. Ann Neurol 1994;35:319–325.

486. Leigh RJ, Burnstine TH, Ruff RL, Kasmer RJ. The effect of anticholinergic agents upon acquired nystagmus: A double-blind study of trihexyphenidyl and tridihexethyl chloride. Neurology 1991;41:1737–1741.

487. Griggs RC, Moxley R, Lafrance R, McQuillen J. Hereditary paroxysmal ataxia: response to acetazolamide. Neurology 1978;28:1259–1264.

488. Griggs RC, Nutt JG. Episodic ataxias as channelopathies. Ann Neurology 1995;37:285–286.

489. Baloh RW, Jen JC. Genetics of familial episodic vertigo and ataxia. Ann NY Acad Sci 2002;956:338–345.

490. Strupp M, Schuler O, Krafczyk S, et al. Treatment of downbeat nystagmus with 3,4-diaminopyridine: A placebo-controlled study. Neurology 2003;61:165–170.

491. Antonini G, Nemni R, Giubilei F, et al. Autoantibodies to glutamic acid decarboxylase in downbeat nystagmus. J Neurol Neurosurg Psychiatry 2003;74:998–999.

492. Solomon D, Shepard N, Mishra A. Congenital periodic alternating nystagmus: response to baclofen. Ann NY Acad Sci 2002;956:611–615.

493. Hertle RW, Maybodi M, Bauer RM, Walker K. Clinical and oculographic response to Dexedrine in a patient with rod-cone dystrophy, exotropia, and congenital aperiodic alternating nystagmus. Binocul Vis Strabismus Q 2001;16:259–264.

494. Matsuo F, Ajax E. Palatal myoclonus and denervation supersensitivity in the central nervous system. Ann Neurol 1979;5:72–78.

495. Koeppen AH. Olivary hypertrophy: Histochemical demonstration of hydrolytic enzymes. Neurology 1980;30:471–480.

496. Herishanu Y, Louzoun Z. Trihexyphenidyl treatment of vertical pendular nystagmus. Neurology 1986;36:82–84.

497. Jabbari B, Rosenberg M, Scherokman B, et al. Effectiveness of trihexyphenidyl against pendular nystagmus and palatal myoclonus: Evidence of cholinergic dysfunction. Movement Disorders 1987;2:93–98.

498. Buckley NJ, Bonner TI, Buckley CM, Brann MR. Antagonist binding properties of five cloned muscarinic receptors expressed in CHO-K1 cells. Mol Pharmacol 1989;35:469–476.

499. Kim JI, Averbuch-Heller L, Leigh RJ. Evaluation of transdermal scopolamine as treatment for acquired nystagmus. J Neuroophthalmol 2001;21:188–192.

500. Lefkowitz D, Harpold G. Treatment of ocular myoclonus with valproic acid. Ann Neurol 1985;17:103–104.

501. Traccis S, Rosati G, Monaco MF, Aiello I, Agnetti V. Successful treatment of acquired pendular elliptical nystagmus in multiple sclerosis with isoniazid and base-out prisms. Neurology 1990;40:492–494.

502. Bandini F, Castello E, Mazzella L, Mancardi GL, Solaro C. Gabapentin but not vigabatrin is effective in the treatment of acquired nystagmus in multiple sclerosis: How valid is the GABAergic hypothesis? J Neurol Neurosurg Psychiatry 2001;71:107–110.

503. Starck M, Albrecht H, Straube A, Dieterich M. Drug therapy for acquired pendular nystagmus in multiple sclerosis. J Neurology 1997;244:9–16.

504. Ferro JM, Castro-Caldas A. Palatal myoclonus and carbamazepine. Ann Neurol 1981;10:402–403.

505. Sakai T, Shiraishi S, Murakami S. Palatal myoclonus responding to carbamazepine. Ann Neurol 1981;9:199–200.

506. Jain S, Proudlock F, Constantinescu CS, Gottlob I. Combined pharmacologic and surgical approach to acquired nystagmus due to multiple sclerosis. Am J Ophthalmol 2002;134:780–782.

507. Mossman S, Bronstein A, Rudge P, Gresty MA. Acquired pendular nystagmus suppressed by alcohol. Neuroophthalmology 1993;13:99–106.

508. Schon F, Hart PE, Hodgson TL, et al. Suppression of pendular nystagmus by smoking cannabis in a patient with multiple sclerosis. Neurology 1999;53:2209–2210.

509. Dell'Osso LF. Suppression of pendular nystagmus by smoking cannabis in a patient with multiple sclerosis. Neurology 2000;54:2190–2191.

510. Frisén L, Wikkelso C. Posttraumatic seesaw nystagmus abolished by ethanol ingestion. Neurology 1986;136:841–844.

511. Lepore FE. Ethanol-induced reduction of pathological nystagmus. Neurology 1987;37:887.

512. Cochin JP, Hannequin D, Domarcolino C, Didier T, Augustin P. Intermittent see-saw nystagmus abolished by clonazepam. Rev Neurol (Paris) 1995;151:60–62.

513. Hikosaka O, Takikawa Y, Kawagoe R. Role of the basal ganglia in the control of purposive saccadic eye movements. Physiol Rev 2000;80:953–978.

514. Hikosaka O, Wurtz RH. Modification of saccadic eye movements by GABA-related substances. I. Effect of muscimol and bicuculline in monkey superior colliculus. J Neurophysiol 1985;53:266–291.

515. Tychsen L, Sitaram N. Catecholamine depletion produces irrepressible saccadic eye movements in normal humans. Ann Neurol 1989;25:444–449.

516. Currie JN, Goldberg ME, Matsuo V, FitzGibbon EJ. Dyslexia with saccadic intrusions: A treatable reading disorder with a characteristic oculomotor sign. Neurology 1986;36(Suppl 10):xx.

517. Pless M, Ronthal M. Treatment of opsoclonus-myoclonus with high-dose intravenous immunoglobulin. Neurology 1996;46:583–584.

518. Pranzatelli MR. The neurobiology of the opsoclonus-myoclonus syndrome. Clin Neuropharmacol 1992;15:186–228.

519. Moretti R, Torre P, Antonello D, Nasuelli D, Cazzato G. Opsoclonus-myoclonus syndrome: Gabapentin as a new therapeutic proposal. Eur J Neurology 2000;7:455–456.

520. Koh PS, Raffensperger JG, Berry S, et al. Long-term outcome in children with opsoclonus-myoclonus and ataxia and coincident neuroblastoma. J Pediatrics 1994;125:712–716.

521. Nitschke M, Hochberg F, Dropcho E. Improvement of paraneoplastic opsoclonus-myoclonus after protein A column therapy. N Engl J Med 1995;332:192.

522. Cher LM, Hochberg FH, Teruya J, et al. Therapy for paraneoplastic neurologic syndromes in six patients with protein A column immunoadsorption. Cancer 1995;75:1678–1683.

523. Hertle RW. Examination and refractive management of patients with nystagmus. Surv Ophthalmol 2000;45:215–222.

524. Rushton D, Cox N. A new optical treatment for oscillopsia. J Neurol Neurosurg Psychiatry 1987;50:411–415.

525. Yaniglos SS, Leigh RJ. Refinement of an optical device that stabilizes vision in patients with nystagmus. Optometry Vis Sci 1992;69:447–450.

526. Yaniglos SS, Stahl JS, Leigh RJ. Evaluation of current optical methods for treating the visual consequences of nystagmus. Ann NY Acad Sci 2002;956:598–600.

527. Biousse V, Tusa R, Russell B, et al. The use of contact lenses to treat visually symptomatic congenital nystagmus. J Neurol Neurosurg Psychiatry 2003.

528. Dell'Osso LF, Traccis S, Erzurum SI. Contact lenses and congenital nystagmus. Clin Vis Sci 1988;3:229–232.

529. Stahl JS, Lehmkuhle M, Wu K, et al. Prospects for treating acquired pendular nystagmus with servo-controlled optics. Invest Ophthalmol Vis Sci 2000;41:1084–1090.

530. Stahl JS, Plant GT, Leigh RJ. Medical treatment of nystagmus and its visual consequences. J R Soc Med 2002;95:235–237.

531. von Noorden GK. Binocular Vision and Ocular Motility. Ed 5. St Louis, CV Mosby; 1996.

532. Crone RA, de Jong PT, Notermans G. Behandlung des Nystagmus durch Injektion von Botulinustoxin in die Augenmuskeln. Klin Mbl Augenheilk 1984;184:216–217.

533. Helveston EM, Pogrebniak AE. Treatment of acquired nystagmus with botulinum A toxin. Am J Ophthalmol 1988;106:584–586.

534. Ruben ST, Lee JP, Oneil D, Dunlop I, Elston JS. The use of botulinum toxin for treatment of acquired nystagmus and oscillopsia. Ophthalmology 1994;101:783–787.

535. Repka MX, Savino PJ, Reinecke RD. Treatment of acquired nystagmus with botulinum neurotoxin A. Arch Ophthalmol 1994;112:1320–1324.

536. Leigh RJ, Tomsak RL, Grant MP, et al. Effectiveness of botulinum toxin administered to abolish acquired nystagmus. Ann Neurol 1992;32:633–642.

537. Tomsak RL, Remler BF, Averbuch-Heller L, Chandran M, Leigh RJ. Unsatisfactory treatment of acquired nystagmus with retrobulbar botulinum toxin. Am J Ophthalmol 1995;119:489–496.

538. Anderson JR. Causes and treatment of congenital eccentric nystagmus. Br J Ophthalmol 1953;37:267–281.

539. Kestenbaum A. Nouvelle operation de nystagmus. Bull Soc Ophtalmol Fr 1953;6:599–602.

540. Lee IS, Lee JB, Kim HS, et al. Modified Kestenbaum surgery for correction of abnormal head posture in infantile nystagmus: Outcome in 63 patients with graded augmentation. Binocul Vis Strabismus Q 2000;15:53–58.

541. Dell'Osso LF, Flynn JT. Congenital nystagmus surgery: A quantitative evaluation of the effects. Arch Ophthalmol 1979;97:462–469.

542. D'Esposito M, Reccia R, Roberti G, Russo P. Amount of surgery in congenital nystagmus. Ophthalmologica 1989;198:145–151.

543. Zubcov AA, Stark N, Weber A, Wizov SS, Reinecke RD. Improvement of visual acuity after surgery for nystagmus. Ophthalmology 1993;100:1488–1497.

544. Cüppers C. Probleme der operativen Therapie des okularen Nystagmus. Klin Mbl Augenheilk 1971;159:145–157.

545. Sendler S, Shallo-Hoffmann J, Mühlendyck H. Die Artifizielle-Divergenz-Operation beim kongenitale Nystagmus. Fortschr Ophthalmol 1990;87:85–89.

546. Kaufmann H, Kolling G. Therapie bei Nystagmuspatienten mit Binokularfunktionen mit und ohne Kopfzwangshaltung. Ber Dtsch Ophthalmol Ges 1981;78:815–819.

547. Graf M. Kestenbaum and artificial divergence surgery for abnormal head turn secondary to nystagmus: Specific and nonspecific effects of artificial divergence. Strabismus 2002;10:69–74.

548. Helveston EM, Ellis FD, Plager DA. Large recession of the horizontal recti for treatment of nystagmus. Ophthalmology 1991;98:1302–1305.

549. von Noorden GK, Sprunger DT. Large rectus muscle recession for the treatment of congenital nystagmus. Arch Ophthalmol 1991;109:221–224.

550. Dell'Osso LF, Hertle RW, Williams RW, Jacobs JB. A new surgery for congenital nystagmus: Effects of tenotomy on an achiasmatic canine and the role of extraocular proprioception. J AAPOS 1999;3:166–182.

551. Wong AM, Tychsen L. Effects of extraocular muscle tenotomy on congenital nystagmus in macaque monkeys. J AAPOS 2002;6:100–107.

552. Dell'Osso LF, Hertle RW. Effects of extraocular muscle tenotomy on congenital nystagmus in macaque monkeys. J AAPOS 2002;6:334–336.

553. Hertle RW, Dell'Osso LF, FitzGibbon EJ, et al. Horizontal rectus tenotomy in patients with congenital nystagmus. Ophthalmology 2003;110:2097–2105.

554. Büttner-Ennever JA, Horn AK, Graf W, Ugolini G. Modern concepts of brainstem anatomy: From extraocular motoneurons to proprioceptive pathways. Ann NY Acad Sci 2002;956:75–84.

555. Hertle RW, Chan CC, Galita DA, Maybodi M, Crawford MA. Neuroanatomy of the extraocular muscle tendon enthesis in macaque, normal human, and patients with congenital nystagmus. J AAPOS 2002;6:319–327.

556. Demer JL. Pivotal role of orbital connective tissues in binocular alignment and strabismus. Invest Ophthalmol Vis Sci 2003.

557. Depalo C, Hertle RW, Yang D. Eight eye muscle surgical treatment in a patient with acquired nystagmus and strabismus: a case report. Binocul Vis Strabismus Q 2003;18:151–158.

558. Pedersen RA, Troost BT, Abel LA, Zorub D. Intermittent downbeat nystagmus and oscillopsia reversed by suboccipital craniectomy. Neurology 1980;30:1239–1242.

559. Dones J, De Jesus O, Colen CB, Toledo MM, Delgado M. Clinical outcomes in patients with Chiari I malformation: A review of 27 cases. Surg Neurol 2003;60:142–147.

560. Spooner JW, Baloh RW. Arnold-Chiari malformation: Improvement in eye movements after surgical treatment. Brain 1981;104:51–60.

561. Palmer EA, Shults WT. Superior oblique myokymia: Preliminary results of surgical treatment. J Pediatric Ophthalmol Strabismus 1984;21:96–101.

562. Kosmorsky GS, Ellis BD, Fogt N, Leigh RJ. The treatment of superior oblique myokymia utilizing the Harada-Ito procedure. J Neuroophthalmol 1995;15:142–146.

563. Karlberg M, Aw ST, Black RA, et al. Vibration-induced ocular torsion and nystagmus after unilateral vestibular deafferentation. Brain 2003;126:956–964.

564. Ishikawa S, Ozawa H, Fujiyama Y. Treatment of nystagmus by acupuncture. Highlights in Neuro-Ophthalmology: Proceedings of the Sixth Meeting of the International Neuro-Ophthalmology Society (INOS). Amsterdam, Aeolus Press, 1987:227–232.

565. Blekher T, Yamada T, Yee RD, Abel LA. Effects of acupuncture on foveation characteristics in congenital nystagmus. Br J Ophthalmol 1998;82:115–120.

566. Abadi RV, Carden D, Simpson J. A new treatment for congenital nystagmus. Br J Ophthalmol 1980;64:2–6.

567. Ciuffreda KJ, Goldrich SG, Neary C. Use of eye movement auditory biofeedback in the control of nystagmus. Am J Optom Physiol Optics 1982:396–409.

568. Averbuch-Heller L, Zivotofsky AZ, Das VE, DiScenna AO, Leigh RJ. Investigations of the pathogenesis of acquired pendular nystagmus. Brain 1995;188:369–378.

SECTION IV:
The Eyelid

Neil R. Miller, section editor

The eyelids contain three main muscles that, under normal circumstances, permit synchronized opening and closing. Each of these muscles and the three separate neural networks that innervate them can be affected-alone or in combination-by congenital and acquired myopathic, neuromuscular, and neurologic disorders. This section consists of a single chapter in which the normal structure and function of the eyelids is discussed as are various pathologic processes of neuro-ophthalmologic importance that prevent normal-or produce inappropriate-eyelid opening or closing.

SECTION IV
The Flaccid

CHAPTER 24

Normal and Abnormal Eyelid Function

Barry Skarf

Disorders of neuro-ophthalmologic significance may affect not only visual sensory, ocular motor, and pupil function but also the function of the eyelids. Indeed, the inability of a patient to fully open or close his or her eyelids may be the first sign of a more extensive process, the early diagnosis and treatment of which may be crucial to the ultimate well being of the patient. This chapter describes the elements that make up a complete assessment of eyelid function, the anatomy of the structures that provide normal eyelid function, and the various pathologic processes that impair eyelid opening and closure.

EXAMINATION OF EYELID FUNCTION

Detailed observation of eyelid position and movement is an important but often neglected part of the neuro-ophthalmologic examination (Table 24.1). In evaluating the eyelids, one should note the resting position of the upper and lower eyelids, assess the ability of the upper eyelid to open and close, and observe the various settings in which eyelid opening and closing occur, including voluntary, reflex, and spontaneous blinking, and lid movements accompanying eye movements.

Patients with eyelid dysfunction often complain of visual problems. Many of these problems are neurologic in origin. For example, laxity of the eyelids from a facial palsy can cause exposure keratopathy with associated blurring of vision, ocular pain, and tearing. However, the same clinical symptoms can also result from involutional changes in the elastic connective tissue supporting the lids. Ptosis, which also can be neurologic and non-neurologic in origin, can produce visual problems, even when incomplete, if the eyelashes or lid margin cover the pupil. When obtaining a history, it is important to inquire about the onset, duration and progression of the problem, and fluctuations of symptoms at different times of the day, in different seasons, and in different environmental conditions. Systemic diseases often affect eyelid function, but patients may have no reason to associate them with their eye problems. Therefore, a thorough medical history with particular attention to thyroid conditions, diabetes mellitus, systemic hypertension, myopathies, myasthenia gravis, sarcoidosis, and facial paresis should be obtained. In many situations, old photographs are useful in establishing the presence of a pre-existing condition such as ptosis or eyelid retraction which may have only recently become symptomatic or noticed by the patient.

The detailed examination of the eyelids should proceed as outlined in Table 24.1, with the examiner noting any abnormalities or asymmetries. In addition, because abnormalities of eyelid position, function, or both often are associated with other neuro-ophthalmic signs, a complete eyelid evaluation must be accompanied by an assessment of visual sensory function, ocular motility and alignment, pupil function, function of the trigeminal and facial nerves, and the status of the orbit, particularly for signs of orbital disease such as proptosis or enophthalmos.

All lid movements result from the interaction of four simple forces: (*a*) an active closing force produced by the orbicularis oculi muscle; (*b*) an active opening force generated by the levator palpebrae superioris muscle (often called the levator muscle or, simply, "the levator"); (*c*) an active opening force generated by a smooth muscle—Müller's muscle

Table 24.1
Examination of the Eyelids

1. General observation of contour, shape, and symmetry of eyelids.
2. Abnormal movements: Involuntary twitches, fasiculations, and synkinesis with other facial muscles.
3. The palpebral fissure (opening) is measured in primary position, and if an abnormality is suspected, in upgaze and downgaze, for each eye. If there is a strabismus or apparent retraction of the eyelid, these measurements are made with the contralateral eye occluded.
4. Upper eyelid position can also be documented and evaluated by measuring the distance between the upper eyelid margin and the corneal light reflex (marginal-reflex distance, or MRD).
5. Levator function is assessed by measuring difference in position of the eyelid margin between downgaze to upgaze while preventing contraction of the frontalis muscle by holding down the eyebrow.
6. Eyelid movement during slow pursuit of a target from upgaze to downgaze is observed for lid retraction or lid lag.
7. Fatigability of the levator is assessed by having the patient maintain maximal upgaze on a target for at least 1 minute. A progressive drooping of the eyelid during this test is a sign of ocular myasthenia gravis.
8. Cogan's lid twitch, which is an upward overshoot of the eyelid on refixation from downgaze to primary position, is also a sign of myasthenia.
9. Synkinesis between the levator and other muscles (especially the ocular motor muscles, but, also occasionally with muscles innervated by cranial nerves V, VII, IX, and XI) is noted.
10. Abnormal spontaneous contractions of the orbicularis oculi, such as twitches, tics, fasciculation, blepharospasm, and synkinesis with other facial muscles and may also be signs of disease.
11. The strength and function of the orbicularis oculi is evaluated by observing normal blinking for frequency (rate) and completeness, and by testing the strength of closure by attempting to pry open the forcibly closed eyes.

(also called the superior tarsal muscle); and (*d*) passive lid-closing forces produced by stretching of ligaments and tendons of the eyelid. For example, normal blinks result from a cessation of the tonically active levator followed by a transient burst of the normally quiescent orbicularis oculi. The active orbicularis oculi force combined with passive lid-closing forces rapidly lower the lid. When the orbicularis oculi activity terminates, the tonic levator activity resumes. This action slowly raises the eyelid until the passive closing forces match the active opening forces generated by the levator. Moving the lid in conjunction with vertical eye movements involves changes only in the activity of the levator. This muscle receives an eye movement input qualitatively identical with that of its developmental progenitor, the superior rectus muscle. As the eye elevates, the tonic activity on the levator increases and raises the eyelid. With decreases in levator activity, the passive downward forces pull the lid down until the passive closing and active opening forces again match. By understanding these forces, it is possible to determine which element or elements of the lid system that are affected by a local, systemic, or neurologic disorder.

ANATOMY OF THE EYELID SYSTEM

The eyelids contain three main muscles innervated by three different neural networks. The oculomotor nerve (see Chapter 17) provides innervation to the levator palpebrae superioris muscle that keeps the eyelids open, a function assisted somewhat by Müller's muscle which is innervated by the sympathetic nervous system (see Chapter 14). Eyelid closure is achieved by contraction of the orbicularis oculi muscle, innervated by the facial nerve (see below).

SURFACE ANATOMY

The palpebral fissure, the opening between the upper and lower eyelids, is the entrance into the conjunctival sac bounded by the margins of the lids (Fig. 24.1). When the lids are open, the palpebral fissure is an asymmetric ellipse 22–30 mm long and 12–15 mm high. In newborn infants, the upper eyelid rises well above the cornea, and the lower eyelid crosses the inferior margin of the cornea. By adulthood, the upper eyelid covers the upper cornea, and the lower lid lies at or slightly below its inferior margin. The lateral extent of the palpebral fissure is at the same level or slightly higher than its medial extent when the eyelids are open, but when they are closed, the outer angle of the fissure is 2–3 mm below the level of the median angle. The eyelids are firmly fixed at the inner angle, and only the position of the outer canthus is changed on opening and closing the lids.

The width of the palpebral fissure often influences judgment regarding the size and prominence of the eye. When one fissure is abnormally wide, as may occur in patients with thyroid orbitopathy or upgaze paresis, the eye may appear

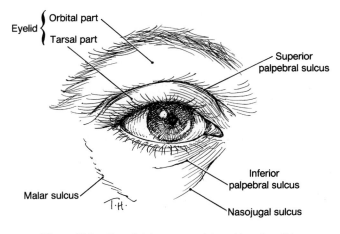

Figure 24.1. Superficial anatomy of the orbit and eyelids.

proptotic or enlarged when, in fact, it is of normal size and is in the same anteroposterior position in the orbit as the opposite eye. When the palpebral fissure is narrowed, as in Horner syndrome, the eye may appear enophthalmic.

The eyelids have several characteristic folds. A well-delineated superior palpebral sulcus, also called the upper eyelid crease, lies 3–4 mm above the lid margin and is the most conspicuous of the eyelid folds (Fig. 24.1). The crease represents the interface where the orbicularis oculi attaches to the tarsus and where the levator aponeurosis attaches to the pretarsal skin. It divides each eyelid into an orbital and a tarsal portion. The orbital portion lies between the margins of the orbit and the globe, whereas the tarsal portion lies in direct relation to the globe.

The upper tarsus extends about 29 mm from medial to lateral and is 10 mm high at the center of the lid. The lower tarsus is 3.5–5 mm high at the center of the lower lid but is the same length as the upper tarsus. The tarsi contain sebaceous glands of the eyelid, called the Meibomian glands. Firmly attached to the posterior aspect of the tarsus is the tarsal conjunctiva.

The orbital septum is a mesodermal layer extending from the bony margin of the orbit toward the upper tarsus. The septum attaches to the levator aponeurosis about 3.4 mm above the upper border of the tarsus. It acts as a barrier for anterior migration of fat pads and as an attachment of the aponeurosis to the overlying skin.

ANATOMY OF THE MUSCLES OF EYELID OPENING AND POSITIONING

The principal muscle involved in opening the upper eyelid and in maintaining normal lid posture is the levator palpebrae superioris. Two accessory muscles of lid opening, Müller's muscle and the frontalis muscle, play only minor roles.

Levator Palpebrae Superioris

The levator palpebrae superioris muscle originates at the annulus of Zinn and courses anteriorly along the superior aspect of the orbit, passing through a suspensory structure, Whitnall's ligament (also called the superior transverse ligament), to which it is attached by bands of connective tissue (Fig. 24.2). This suspensory ligament alters the pulling direction of the levator palpebrae from horizontal to nearly vertical. The attachment of the levator to Whitnall's ligament is an important component of the passive lid-closing forces acting upon the upper eyelid and described above (Fig. 24.3). The levator does not extend all the way from its origin to the superior tarsus. Instead, it begins to gradually transition from muscle to tendon just posterior to Whitnall's ligament, such that anterior to Whitnall's ligament, it exists only as a tendinous aponeurosis. It is this aponeurosis that fuses with the orbital septum and attaches to the superior tarsus.

The levator contains four types of muscles fibers (1). Three are singly innervated fibers similar to those found in other extraocular muscles: red fast-twitch fibers, intermediate fast-twitch fibers, and pale fast-twitch fibers. Fast-twitch fibers, particularly the red type, are highly resistant to fatigue and thus help sustain contraction against the passive down-

ward force produced by various ligaments and gravity. Fast-twitch fibers also probably play an important role in the generation of lid saccades. The fourth type of muscle fiber is found only in the levator: the levator slow-twitch fiber. The slow-twitch fibers of the levator may assist the red fast-twitch fibers in resisting the passive downward forces described above. Thus, the fiber composition of the human levator palpabrae is consistent with its two main roles: sustained contraction against the passive downward forces acting on the upper lid and active upward lid movements accompanying saccadic eye movements (2).

The levator palpebrae superioris is innervated by branches of the superior division of the oculomotor nerve. A detailed description of the anatomy of the nerve is presented in Chapter 17 of this text and is not repeated here.

Müller's Muscle

Müller's muscle is a thin band of smooth muscle about 10 mm in width that inserts on the superior border of the upper tarsus (Figs. 24.2 and 24.4). The muscle originates 10–12 mm above the tarsus from tendons inserted near the origin of the levator aponeurosis. Muller's muscle is innervated by fibers of the oculosympathetic pathway. These are described in detail in Chapter 14 of this text and are not repeated here. The mean total excursion of Müller's muscle is 3 mm, which raises the upper eyelid 1.5 mm (3,4).

Although Müller's muscle is located in the upper eyelid, there is a similar, much smaller, sympathetically innervated muscle located in the lower eyelid. Hypofunction of this

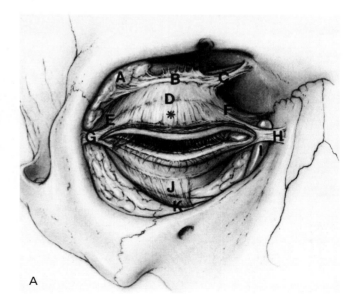

Figure 24.2. Anatomy of the levator palpebrae superioris muscle and its aponeurosis. *A*, Anterior view shows relationship of the levator aponeurosis (D) to the superior tarsus (*) and to Whitnall's ligament (B). A, lacrimal gland; C, superior oblique tendon sheath; E, lateral horn of the levator aponeurosis; F, medial horn of the levator aponeurosis; G, lateral canthal tendon; H, medial canthal tendon; I, lacrimal sac; J, lower eyelid retractors; K, inferior oblique muscle. *(Figure continues.)*

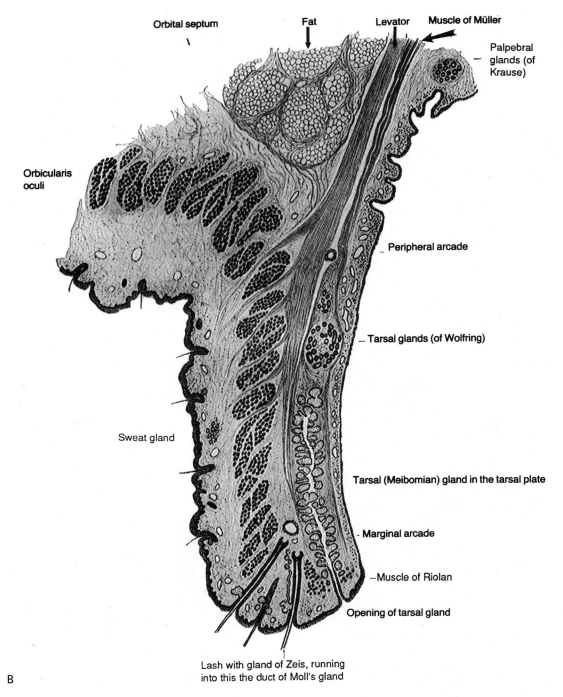

Orbital septum

Fat

Levator

Muscle of Müller

Palpebral glands (of Krause)

Orbicularis oculi

Peripheral arcade

Tarsal glands (of Wolfring)

Sweat gland

Tarsal (Meibomian) gland in the tarsal plate

Marginal arcade

Muscle of Riolan

Opening of tarsal gland

Lash with gland of Zeis, running into this the duct of Moll's gland

B

Figure 24.2.   Continued. *B,* Vertical section through the upper eyelid. Note relationship of the levator to the tarsus, to the orbicularis, and to Müller's muscle, which is located just beneath it. (*A,* From Beard C. Ptosis. Ed 2. St Louis: CV Mosby, 1976. *B,* From Bron AJ, Tripathi RC, Tripathi BJ. Wolff's Anatomy of the Eye and Orbit. Ed 8. London: Chapman & Hall Medical, 1997.)

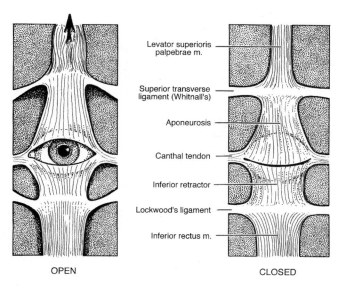

OPEN   CLOSED

Levator superioris palpebrae m.
Superior transverse ligament (Whitnall's)
Aponeurosis
Canthal tendon
Inferior retractor
Lockwood's ligament
Inferior rectus m.

Figure 24.3. Schematic of the elastic structures responsible for the passive forces acting on the upper and lower eyelid. Elevating the lid to the open position or in upward gaze, increases the tension along the orbicularis oculi (not shown), Whitnall's ligament, the canthal-tarsal complex, and Lockwood's ligament. Relaxation of the levator palpebrae releases this stored elastic energy causing the eyelid to close or descend on downgaze. (From Sibony PA, Manning KA, Evinger C. Eyelid movements in facial paralysis. Arch Ophthalmol 1991;109:1555–1561.)

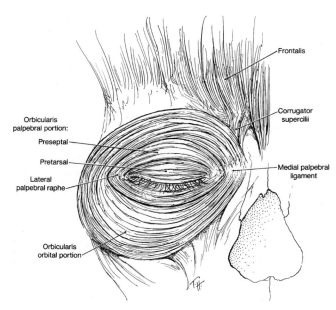

Frontalis
Corrugator supercilii
Medial palpebral ligament
Orbicularis palpebral portion:
Preseptal
Pretarsal
Lateral palpebral raphe
Orbicularis orbital portion

Figure 24.5. Anatomy of the orbicularis oculi muscle and associated muscles. Note that the orbicularis has three separate divisions: pretarsal, preseptal, and palpebral.

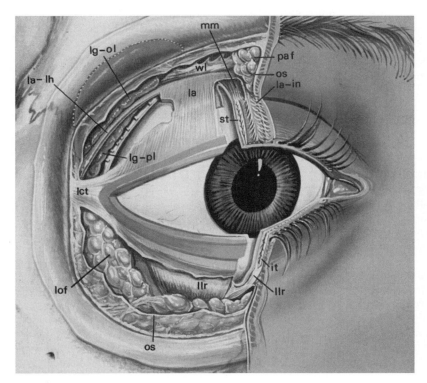

Figure 24.4. Anatomy of Müller's muscle. Anterior view of transected and partially dissected upper and lower eyelids. The lateral portion of the orbital septum and the levator have been excised to demonstrate adjacent relationships. Note that Müller's muscle (mm) is located just underneath the levator aponeurosis (la) and inserts directly into the upper aspect of the superior tarsus (st), whereas the levator aponeurosis inserts into the anterior aspect of the tarsus (la-in). it, inferior tarsus; la-lh, lateral horn of levator aponeurosis; lct, lateral canthal tendon; lg-ol, orbital lobe of lacrimal gland; lg-pl, palpebral lobe of lacrimal gland; llr, lower lid retractors; lof, lateral orbital fat; os, orbital septum (cut edge); paf, preaponeurotic fat; wl, Whitnall's ligament. (From Rootman J, Stewart B, Goldberg RA. Orbital Surgery: A Conceptual Approach. Philadelphia: Lippincott-Raven, 1995.)

muscle (such as occurs in Horner syndrome [discussion following]) results in slight elevation of the lower eyelid (upside-down ptosis).

Frontalis and Associated Muscles

The muscles controlling the eyebrow contribute to the eyelid appearance and, to a lesser extent, its elevation. Control of the eyebrow involves three sets of muscles: frontalis, procerus, and corrugator superciliaris (Fig. 24.5). The frontalis has no bony insertions. It originates as an extension of the anterior belly of the epicranius with connections to the occipital muscle via the galea aponeurotica, and it has cutaneous insertions at the level of the eyebrow. Frontalis fibers also intermingle with peripheral orbicularis oculi muscle fibers. Contraction of the frontalis raises the entire eyebrow and the upper eyelid through its cutaneous and orbicularis oculi connections.

The procerus muscle originates from the medial portion of the lower region of the frontalis muscle and inserts on the nasal bone. Contraction of the procerus pulls the medial portion of the eyebrow downward. The corrugator superciliaris lies beneath the frontalis and orbicularis oculi originating from the medial origin of the frontal bone. The corrugator superciliaris extends 2–3 cm laterally, where it blends with the frontalis and orbicularis oculi fibers. Contraction of the corrugator superciliaris pulls the eyebrow medially and downward.

ANATOMY OF THE MUSCLES OF EYELID CLOSURE

The primary muscle responsible for eyelid closure, the **orbicularis oculi**, is a typical striated muscle. It completely covers the orbital opening, forming concentric rings around the palpebral fissure and surrounding bone (Fig. 24.5). It is responsible not only for active eyelid closure but also for much of the facial expression around the eyes. It can be divided into three parts: orbital, preseptal, and pretarsal (5,6).

The **orbital** part of the orbicularis oculi forms a complete ellipse, overlying the orbital rim and the cheek. This is the thickest portion of the muscle and participates primarily in forceful eyelid closure (7). The **preseptal** orbicularis oculi is formed by two half-ellipses of muscle fibers separated by the medial and lateral canthal tendons. These fibers arise from the lateral aspect of the medial canthal tendon and the underlying bone. They then separate, cross the upper and lower lids, and fuse laterally as the lateral palpebral raphe that overlies the lateral canthal tendon. The **pretarsal** portion of the orbicularis oculi is anterior to the upper and lower tarsal plates. Medially and laterally, the fibers fuse to form the medial and lateral canthal tendons, respectively.

Orbicularis oculi muscle fibers exhibit characteristics typical of other skeletal muscles. The pretarsal region of the orbicularis oculi muscle is predominantly composed of intermediate fast-twitch (type IIa) and pale fast-twitch (type IIb) fibers. A smaller number of slow-twitch (type I) fibers are also present. The presence of fast-twitch fibers capable of rapid, albeit fatigable contractions is consistent with the phasic functions of orbicularis oculi activity during blinks.

ABNORMALITIES OF EYELID OPENING

Abnormalities of eyelid opening include **ptosis**—insufficient opening of the eyelid—which can be caused by a variety of congenital and acquired disorders, many of which are of neuro-ophthalmologic importance, and **retraction**, a very sign of thyroid eye disease and an occasional sign of other neuropathic, neuromuscular, myopathic, and mechanical disorders.

PTOSIS

A deficiency of levator tonus produces the clinical sign called blepharoptosis or ptosis. Ptosis may be produced by damage to the motor system controlling eyelid elevation and position at any point along the pathway, from the cerebral cortex to the levator muscle itself. Topical diagnosis of ptosis depends on the character of the deficiency and on evidence of neuropathic, neuromuscular, aponeurotic, developmental, mechanical, or myopathic disease (8–10).

The degree of ptosis can be quantified clinically by measuring the vertical length of the palpebral fissure—about 9 mm in normal subjects—assuming the lower eyelid is normally positioned. A more useful measure is the distance between the upper lid margin and the midcorneal reflex when the globe is in primary position. This is called the uMRD. Ptosis can be defined as an uMRD less than 2 mm or an asymmetry of more than 2 mm between eyes (11). Using this definition, most patients with ptosis exhibit a contraction of the superior visual field to 30° or less (12).

Neurogenic Ptosis

Neurogenic ptosis may be caused by supranuclear, nuclear, or infranuclear dysfunction. In some cases, associated symptoms and signs make the distinctions among these causes obvious; in other cases, however, neither the location nor the nature of the lesion is clear.

Supranuclear Ptosis

Unilateral ptosis is a rare manifestation of hemisphere dysfunction. This manifestation, called **cortical ptosis**, usually, although not invariably, is contralateral to the lesion. Unilateral ptosis has been described contralateral to lesions of the angular gyrus (13), to seizure foci in the temporal lobe (14), to hemispheric stroke (15,16), and to frontal lobe arteriovenous malformations (AVMs) (17). It also has been described ipsilateral to ischemic hemispheric strokes (15,16) (Fig. 24.6).

Bilateral cortical ptosis can also occur (16,17). It is associated most frequently with extensive nondominant hemisphere lesions. In most instances, the ptosis is accompanied by midline shift, gaze deviation to the right, and other signs of right hemisphere dysfunction, including left hemiparesis.

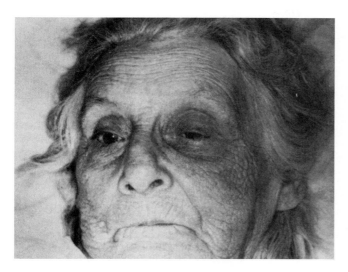

Figure 24.6. Unilateral supranuclear (cortical) ptosis. The patient developed a left ptosis associated with a left hemiparesis from a right hemisphere stroke. The patient also has a pre-existing right ptosis from dehiscence of the levator tendon. (From Caplan LR. Cerebral ptosis. J Neurol Neurosurg Psychiatry 1974;37:1–7.)

The ptosis is often asymmetric, perhaps because of an associated ipsilateral facial weakness or possibly an asymmetric supranuclear input. In the setting of cerebral infarction, the ptosis is transient, lasting from several days to 5 months or more (16,18–21) (Fig. 24.7). On rare occasions, it is accompanied by other supranuclear eyelid disturbances, such as blepharospasm or levator inhibition (18,20). The association of bilateral cerebral ptosis with nondominant hemisphere lesions suggests cortical asymmetry in the control of eyelid position.

The extrapyramidal system primarily affects the eyelids by modifying the excitability of the blink reflex, although it also modulates eyelid position to a limited extent. In one series, for example, 10 of 70 patients with Parkinson disease had ptosis (22). A more common extrapyramidal insuffi-

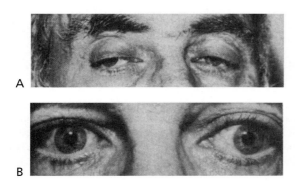

Figure 24.7. Bilateral supranuclear ptosis. *A,* The patient has bilateral severe ptosis that occurred when he experienced acute bilateral frontal lobe infarctions. *B,* Two months later, the patient's ptosis has completely resolved. (From Krohel GB, Griffin JF. Cortical blepharoptosis. Am J Ophthalmol 1978;85:632–634.)

ciency of eyelid opening, however, is **apraxia of eyelid opening** (AEO) (23). The main clinical features of AEO are as follows: (*a*) a transient inability to initiate lid opening; (*b*) the absence of any significant evidence of orbicularis oculi contraction, such as lowering of the brow beneath the orbital rim (Charcot sign); (*c*) frontalis contraction during attempts to open the eyelids; and (*d*) the absence of any other signs of neural or myopathic dysfunction (24,25). Most patients with AEO show a paucity of blinking interrupted by gentle closure of both eyelids that may last up to 30 seconds or longer. AEO occurs most commonly in patients with progressive supranuclear palsy, Parkinson disease, and atypical parkinsonism including that induced by methyl-phenyl-tetrahydropyridine (MPTP) (25–31). AEO has also been reported in single cases of otherwise typical essential blepharospasm (32–34): Shy-Drager syndrome (25), adult-onset Hallervorden-Spatz disease (35), Huntington's chorea, cerebral diplegia with parkinsonism, frontotemporal gunshot injury (24), right hemisphere stroke (36), Wilson disease (37), and amyotrophic lateral sclerosis parkinsonism-dementia complex (38). In rare instances, AEO occurs as an isolated finding (39).

Electromyographic (EMG) studies show that patients with AEO can be separated into several groups related to the activity of their levator and orbicularis oculi muscles. The first group consists of patients who exhibit intermittent variable periods of levator inhibition without any orbicularis oculi activity (Fig.24.8). Such patients may occasionally show typical episodes of blepharospasm (29,40,41). The second group consists of patients in whom blepharospasm involving primarily the pretarsal segment of the orbicularis oculi is prominent (33,40–42) (Fig. 24.9). In this group, the condition often is called **atypical blepharospasm**. The third group of patients with a clinical picture of AEO actually have ''motor persistence'' of the pretarsal segment of the orbicularis oculi; i.e., an inability to inhibit pretarsal orbicularis contractions after voluntary eyelid closure (41). Without EMG, it is impossible to distinguish patients whose AEO is caused by levator inhibition from patients with atypical blepharospasm or motor persistence of the orbicularis oculi.

Treatment of involuntary eyelid closure caused by supranuclear inhibition of levator activity is not particularly successful. Individual case reports suggest that several drugs may be useful, including desipramine (43) and L-dopa (39). Injection of the orbicularis oculi and frontalis muscles with botulinum toxin type A produces variable results, depending on the degree of orbicularis contraction that accompanies the levator inhibition (44,45). However, we believe this treatment is worth trying in patients with AEO, even though the results are less than satisfactory.

Ptosis may develop in certain eccentric positions of gaze from congenital supranuclear inhibition of the levator; i.e., **supranuclear oculopalpebral synkinesia**. In such cases, lid position in primary gaze may be normal, or the lid may be slightly ptotic. When the patient adducts (or occasionally abducts) the eye on the affected side, however, the eyelid drops abruptly because of a loss of levator muscle tone. When the eye returns toward center, or toward the opposite side, the levator contracts and the eyelid returns to a normal

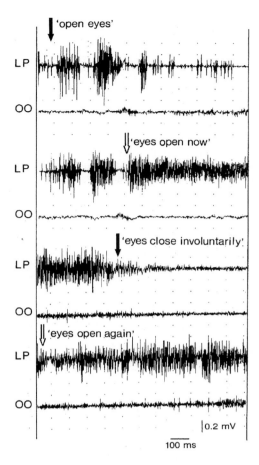

Figure 24.8. Electromyography (EMG) of the levator palpebrae (LP) and orbicularis oculi (OO) muscles in a patient with apraxia of eyelid opening characterized by periods of levator inhibition without activity of the orbicularis oculi. Following the command "open eyes" (*top arrow*), the LP shows intermittent and irregular bursts of action potentials, until a steady activity, causing opening of the eyes, is achieved (*open arrow*). After a short period of involuntary closure of the eyelids due to inhibition of LP, the eyes open again because of the return of LP muscle activity. Note that there is no activity of the OO muscle during this period. (From Aramideh M, Ongerboer deVisser BW, Devriese PP, et al. Electromyographic features of levator palpebrae superioris and orbicularis oculi muscles in blepharospasm. Brain 1994;117:27–38.)

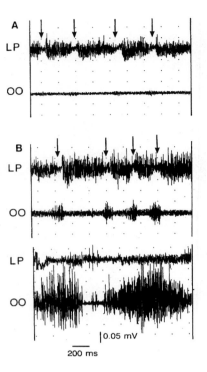

Figure 24.9. Electromyography (EMG) of the levator palpebrae (LP) and orbicularis oculi (OO) muscles in a patient with apraxia of eyelid opening in whom only the pretarsal portion of the OO is active during periods of LP inhibition. *A*, No activity is recorded from the **preseptal** portion of the OO even during brief periods of LP inhibition (*arrows*). *B*, EMG recording from the same patient but with the needle inserted into the **pretarsal** portion of the OO. Note marked activity of the OO during short (*arrows in A*); and long (*B*) periods of LP inhibition (*B*). (From Aramideh M, Ongerboer deVisser BW, Devriese PP, et al. Electromyographic features of levator palpebrae superioris and orbicularis oculi muscles in blepharospasm. Brain 1994;117:27–38.)

position. The synkinesia may be unilateral (Fig. 24.10) or bilateral (Fig. 24.11) (47–49). It may occur as an isolated phenomenon or in association with other congenital syndromes, such as the Duane retraction syndrome (46,48). The causes of supranuclear paradoxical levator inhibition are unclear. They may involve a variety of mechanisms, including ephaptic transmission or disturbances in the supranuclear pathways responsible for levator tonus, excitation, and inhibition.

Ptosis associated with mouth opening—**the inverse Marcus Gunn phenomenon**—is a rare condition in which the ipsilateral eyelid closes when the external pterygoid muscle moves the jaw to the opposite side (Fig. 24.12). Patients with this condition have a mild ptosis of the affected eyelid

when the eyes are in primary position and the mouth is closed. EMG studies confirm that the associated ptosis is consequent to levator inhibition without contraction of the orbicularis oculi (50). This syndrome is an inverse of the Marcus Gunn jaw-winking phenomenon (see below) and probably represents a supranuclear synkinesis affecting the oculomotor and trigeminal nerves.

Ptosis from Lesions of the Oculomotor Nucleus, Fascicle, or Nerve

By far, the most common causes of acquired neurogenic ptosis are related to dysfunction of the oculomotor nucleus, fascicle, or nerve. Because the central caudal subnucleus of the oculomotor nucleus supplies bilateral equal innervation to the levator muscles, ptosis resulting from a nuclear midbrain lesion is invariably bilateral and symmetric, usually complete, or at least very severe (Fig. 24.13). This **midbrain ptosis** is commonly associated with other signs of mesencephalic dysfunction. However, in some cases, only the central caudal subnucleus of the oculomotor nuclear complex is affected (Fig. 24.14) or it is much more severely affected than

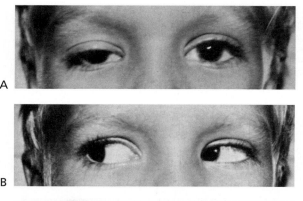

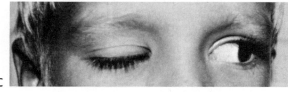

Figure 24.10. Congenital unilateral supranuclear oculopalpebral synkinesia. *A,* This young child has moderate right ptosis when looking straight ahead. *B,* When the patient looks to the right, the position of both upper eyelids is normal. *C,* On left gaze, there is almost complete right ptosis from inhibition of the levator muscle. Note that the left upper eyelid remains in a normal position in all positions of gaze. (Courtesy of Dr. C. Hedges.)

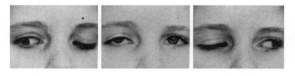

Figure 24.11. Congenital bilateral supranuclear oculopalpebral synkinesia. *Center,* In primary position, the patient has a moderate right ptosis. On right gaze (*right*), the patient develops a marked left ptosis, whereas on left gaze (*left*), the patient develops a marked right ptosis. (Courtesy of Dr. H. Rose.)

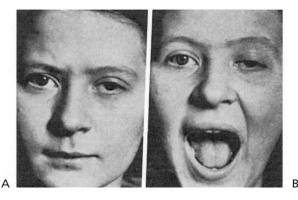

Figure 24.12. The Inverse Marcus Gunn phenomenon. *A,* When the patient looks straight ahead, she has a mild left ptosis. *B,* When the patient opens her mouth, the ptosis increases from inhibition of the left levator muscle.

the other oculomotor subnuclei, and bilateral, severe, symmetric ptosis is the predominant or only manifestation of the nuclear lesion (51–57) (Fig. 24.13). Rarely, mesencephalic ptosis is associated with a Cogan lid-twitch and fatigue, thus mimicking ocular myasthenia gravis (58,59). Midbrain ptosis may be either congenital, occurring as a consequence of dysplasia or aplasia of the oculomotor nucleus, or acquired. Acquired causes include ischemia, inflammation, infiltration, compression, and metabolic and toxic processes (60).

Lesions of the **fascicle of the oculomotor nerve** produce unilateral oculomotor nerve dysfunction that may be mild or severe. The dysfunction may be isolated or associated with a contralateral hemiplegia, cerebellar ataxia, or rubral tremor, depending on whether adjacent structures in the midbrain (e.g., cerebral peduncle, red nucleus) are also affected by the lesion (see Chapter 20). For example, in some cases, the associated signs of midbrain dysfunction are minimal and consist of nothing more than an oculomotor nerve palsy and an abnormal masseter reflex (61). When ptosis occurs in patients with a lesion of the oculomotor fascicle, it is always unilateral, of variable severity, and, in our experience, associated with weakness of one or more of the extraocular muscles innervated by the oculomotor nerve. Pupillary involvement is commonly but not invariably present.

The ptosis that accompanies a lesion of the **peripheral oculomotor nerve** is, like that caused by a fascicular lesion, unilateral and usually accompanied by ophthalmoparesis, pupillary involvement, or both (see Chapter 20). Rarely, however, ptosis precedes the other signs of oculomotor nerve dysfunction by days, weeks, or even months, depending on the location and nature of the lesion. Isolated ptosis caused by peripheral oculomotor nerve dysfunction has been reported in patients with aneurysms (62,63), pituitary adenomas (64,65), meningiomas (66), and meningitis (67). Some of these cases are examples of truly isolated ptosis. Inothers, there are other symptoms, for example, headache, or subtle signs of oculomotor dysfunction, a mildly dilated but reactive pupil, an incomitant phoria, or asymptomatic underaction of the superior rectus that is only evident on extreme upgaze. Recurrent, isolated ptosis lasting 6–8 weeks has been described with ophthalmoplegic migraine (68). Isolated, complete, neurogenic ptosis can also occur from orbital trauma that generates forceful anterior displacement of the upper eyelid with denervation of the levator muscle (69). This form of ptosis usually resolves spontaneously within weeks.

Ptosis from Lesions of the Oculosympathetic Pathways

Lesions of the oculosympathetic pathway produce **Horner syndrome**, a condition that is characterized in part by a partial, unilateral ptosis from hypofunction of Müller's muscle. The ptosis of Horner syndrome usually can be differentiated from the ptosis associated with oculomotor nerve dysfunction by their differing appearance and associated findings (see Chapter 16). The ptosis in Horner syndrome is often mild, variable, and always associated with ipsilateral miosis. Involvement of a sympathetically innervated smooth

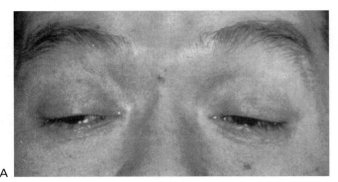

A

Figure 24.13. Isolated, bilateral ptosis in a patient with brainstem encephalitis and discrete inflammatory foci in the caudal mesencephalon. *A,* External appearance of the patient. Note symmetric severe ptosis. *B,* Extraocular movements are normal. (From Conway VH, Rozdilsky B, Schneider RJ, et al. Isolated bilateral complete ptosis. Can J Ophthalmol 1983;18:37–40.)

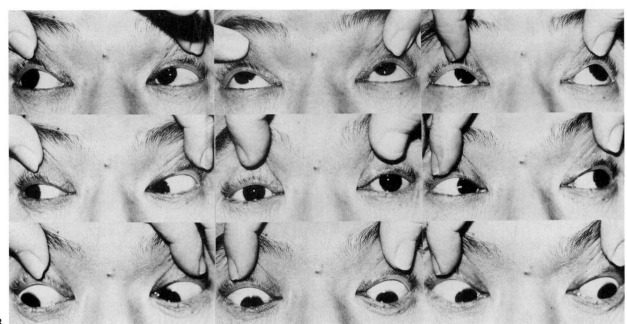

B

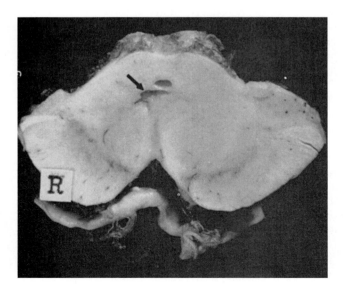

Figure 24.14. Pathology of isolated midbrain ptosis. A discrete area of infarction (*arrow*) is present in the caudal portion of the oculomotor nuclear complex in the region of the central caudal subnucleus. (From Growdon JH, Winkler GF, Wray SH. Midbrain ptosis: A case with clinicopathologic correlation. Arch Neurol 1974;30:179–181.)

muscle in the lower eyelid similar to Müller's muscle in the upper eyelid (see above) results in elevation (''upside-down'' ptosis) of the lower eyelid. The combination of ptosis of the upper eyelid and elevation of the lower eyelid produces the appearance of enophthalmos, although exophthalmometry invariably shows no asymmetry of the two eyes. Other signs of Horner syndrome include ipsilateral facial anhidrosis in patients with first-order or second-order neuron lesions, mildly reduced intraocular pressure in the affected eye, heterochromia in congenital and very long-standing cases, and an increased accommodation amplitude (Fig. 24.15). Horner syndrome is discussed in detail in Chapter 16 of this text.

The ptosis occasionally observed after conjunctival instillation of timolol maleate, a β-adrenergic blocking agent, may be caused by Müller's muscle blockade (70). Similarly, thymoxamine (α-adrenergic blocking agent) may cause ptosis when given topically or parenterally (71,72).

Ptosis from Disinsertion, Dehiscence, or Thinning of the Levator Aponeurosis

The most common cause of acquired ptosis in adults is a dehiscence, disinsertion, or thinning of the levator aponeurosis. Ptosis caused by such defects of the levator tendon may be bilateral or unilateral and can vary in its severity. In the early stages, the ptosis may be barely evident in primary position, but because it typically worsens in downgaze, the eyelid may obstruct the visual axis when the patient attempts to read (73–76). The presence of anisocoria (i.e., physiologic anisocoria that occurs in about 20% of normal individuals [see Chapter 16]) or a mild and asymptomatic heterophoria, or the frequent worsening of symptoms at the end of the day, may lead to the erroneous diagnosis of oculomotor nerve palsy or myasthenia gravis in such patients (77). However, the findings of normal levator excursion, an elevated or absent superior lid crease, a deep superior eyelid sulcus, worsening of ptosis in downgaze, and thinning of the skin above the tarsal plate should distinguish an aponeurotic ptosis from developmental, neurogenic, and myogenic causes (8,73,75,78,79) (Fig. 24.16).

Levator aponeurotic defects commonly occur in the elderly from involutional or degenerative changes that result in disinsertion, dehiscence, or thinning of the aponeurosis (80,81). Among patients between ages 15 and 50, aponeurotic ptosis is most commonly associated with a long history of wearing rigid contact lenses. In such patients, repeated manipulation and traction of the upper eyelid while inserting or removing contact lenses causes disinsertion or thinning of the tendon (82–85).

Damage to the levator aponeurosis other than that associ-

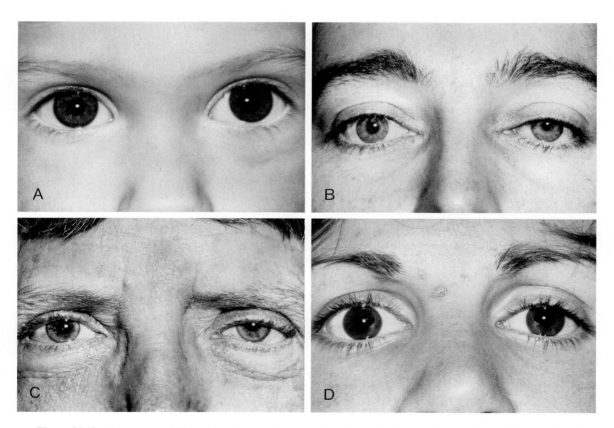

Figure 24.15. Appearance of Horner syndrome in four patients. *A,* Congenital right Horner syndrome. Note associated heterochromia iridis and minimal ptosis. *B,* Left Horner syndrome after neck trauma. *C,* Left Horner syndrome associated with apical lung (Pancoast) tumor. *D,* Left Horner syndrome in a patient with Raeder's paratrigeminal neuralgia.

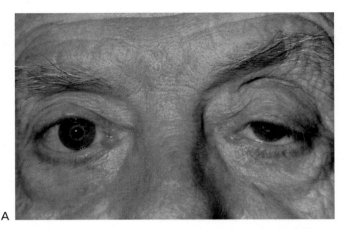

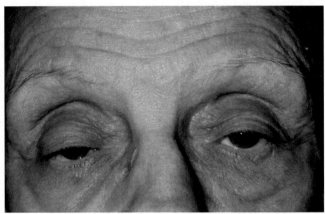

Figure 24.16. Ptosis from levator dehiscence. *A,* Unilateral ptosis. Note the difference in location of the superior lid folds, with the left being much higher than the right. Also note the deepened superior sulcus on the left side. *B,* Bilateral ptosis from levator dehiscence. Both eyelids show high superior lid folds and deep superior sulci. (Courtesy of Dr. Nicholas T. Iliff.)

neurotic defects may also occur after episodes of eyelid edema caused by allergic reactions (81). In rare cases, congenital ptosis is caused by defects of the levator aponeurosis (95).

Myopathic Ptosis

Ptosis that occurs from damage to the levator palpebrae superioris muscle itself (as opposed to its tendon) may be either congenital (i.e., developmental) or acquired.

Congenital Myopathic Ptosis (Developmental Ptosis)

Although congenital ptosis occasionally is neurogenic (e.g., oculomotor nerve palsy, Marcus Gunn jaw-winking phenomenon, Horner syndrome) or traumatic (e.g., from a forceps delivery) in origin, the most common form is caused by a developmental myopathy of the levator palpebrae superioris muscle. A decrease in striated muscle fibers, hyaline degeneration, fatty replacement, an increase in endomysial collagen, and loss of cross-striations characterize this disorder histopathologically (81,96,97). Because developmental ptosis may worsen with age, it may not be noticed until early

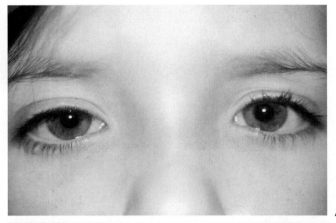

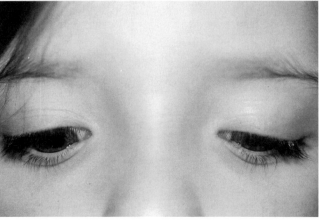

Figure 24.17. Developmental (congenital) ptosis. *A,* When the patient looks straight ahead, she has a very mild right ptosis. *B,* When the patient looks down, there is mild lid lag on the right but not on the left.

ated with contact lens wear can occur from trauma, including that associated with ocular and orbital surgery. Thus, ptosis not infrequently occurs after cataract extraction, glaucoma surgery, radial keratotomy, orbital surgery, conjunctival procedures, enucleations, strabismus surgery, and blepharoplasty. Ptosis following orbital surgery or blepharoplasty in which there is deep orbital fat dissection or supratarsal fixation, is likely a result of direct injury to the levator aponeurosis. The aponeurosis also may be stretched or damaged from postoperative swelling, injection of an anesthetic into the upper eyelid, the use of a rigid lid speculum, ocular compression and massage, or attempts by the patient to open the eyelid against a tight patch. The myotoxic effects of anesthetic injections and trauma to the levator itself from bridle sutures or retrobulbar injections may also play a role in some cases (79,85–93).

In addition to the mechanisms described above, ptosis from damage to or dysfunction of the levator aponeurosis may be associated with blepharochalasis, thyroid orbitopathy, pregnancy, and chronic use of topical steroids (9). Apo-

childhood or even later in life. Childhood photographs are sometimes helpful in establishing onset. In addition, about 15% of the patients have a family history of congenital ptosis, so obtaining a family history is crucial.

Developmental ptosis is characterized by a deficiency in levator excursion (as opposed to ptosis caused by defects in the levator aponeurosis), an elevated or absent superior lid crease, and, most importantly, lid-lag on downgaze (75,81) (Fig. 24.17). The majority of cases are unilateral, but about 20% are bilateral (98). Patients with severe developmental ptosis, particularly that which is bilateral, may exhibit a compensatory chin elevation or frontalis contraction.

Developmental ptosis may exist in isolation, or it may be associated with other ocular findings, including strabismic or occlusion (deprivation) amblyopia, astigmatism, and anisometropia (98–102). Because the levator derives embryo logically from the same anlage as the superior rectus, it is not surprising that underaction of the superior rectus frequently accompanies developmental ptosis (103) (Fig. 24.18).

Developmental ptosis may be associated with a variety of congenital ocular or systemic malformations. In some cases, the association is distinctive enough to constitute a well-defined syndrome, such as the blepharophimosis-epicanthus-ptosis syndrome (104), the congenital fibrosis syndrome (105), and Goldenhar syndrome (106). In other cases, developmental ptosis occurs in association with less clearly defined entities, including anomalies of the brain, heart, urogenital, skeletal, or auditory systems (107–111).

Acquired Myopathic Ptosis

Acquired myopathic ptosis occurs in a number of the mitochondrial cytopathies characterized by chronic progressive external ophthalmoplegia (CPEO) (see Chapter 22). In some patients, the ptosis is the presenting sign and may persist in isolation for months to years before the development of ophthalmoplegia. Ptosis of this type usually is bilateral, relatively symmetric, and very slowly progressive. The superior palpebral lid fold may be completely absent. Excessive wrinkling of the brow and backward head tilting are commonly employed to facilitate vision beneath the drooping lids (Fig. 24.19). Orbicularis oculi function, tested by forced lid closure, is frequently weak, and this combination of weakness of both eyelid opening and eyelid closure serves to distinguish the condition from other causes of ptosis except myasthenia gravis and myotonic dystrophy (discussion following).

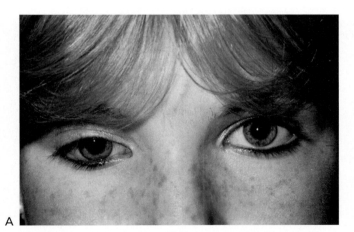
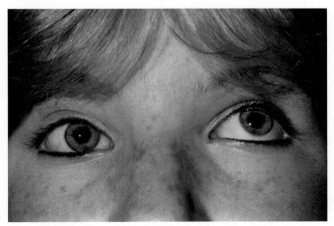

A

B

Figure 24.18. Unilateral congenital ptosis with ipsilateral hypotropia and limitation of upward gaze. *A,* When the patient looks straight ahead, she has a moderate right ptosis and there is a slight right hypotropia. *B,* On attempted upward gaze, the left eye elevates, but the right eye does not. (Courtesy of Dr. Nicholas T. Iliff.)

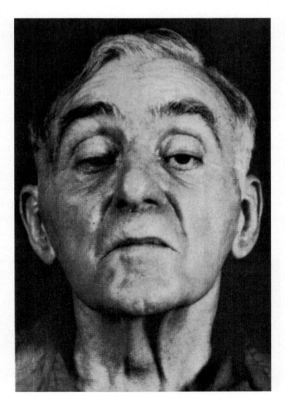

Figure 24.19. Ptosis in chronic progressive external ophthalmoplegia. Note symmetric bilateral ptosis associated with an abnormal head posture characterized by elevation of chin.

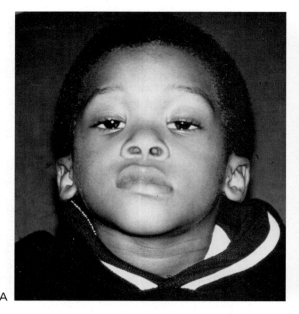
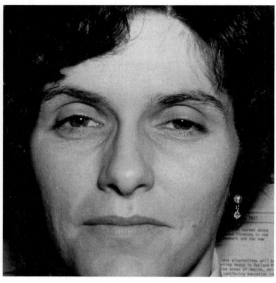

Figure 24.20. Ptosis in myasthenia gravis. *A,* In a 5-year-old boy with symmetric bilateral ptosis, there is an abnormal head posture characterized by elevation of chin similar to that seen in the patient with chronic progressive external ophthalmoplegia seen in Figure 24.19. *B,* In a young woman with bilateral asymmetric ptosis, the head posture is normal.

Because the manifestations of the disease are so slowly progressive and in part because they tend to be symmetric, patients with ptosis associated with CPEO are remarkablytolerant of their symptoms, and thus generally present relatively late in their course.

Bilateral partial ptosis contributes to the characteristic facies of patients with myotonic dystrophy (myotonia dystrophica). It may also occur in the various types of familial periodic paralysis.

The levator palpebrae superioris muscle may be damaged by a variety of inflammatory, ischemic, or infiltrative processes affecting the orbit. Occasionally, ptosis is the most prominent manifestation. For example, lymphoid infiltration, sarcoidosis, amyloidosis, and idiopathic inflammatory disease of the orbit can sometimes selectively affect the levator and spare the extraocular muscles (112,113). Patients with diabetes mellitus also may develop unilateral or bilateral ptosis in association with other evidence of microangiopathic changes elsewhere in the body. Although most of these patients probably have a localized infarction in the midbrain, which affects either the oculomotor nerve nucleus or fascicle, or in the peripheral oculomotor nerve, chronic hypoxia of the levator muscle is responsible for this form of ptosis in some diabetic patients (114).

Neuromuscular Ptosis

Recognition of neuromuscular ptosis depends in part on the absence of clinical signs of an oculomotor or sympathetic lesion and the presence of clinical signs of neuromuscular disease. Ptosis in myasthenia gravis may occur in isolation, but it is more often associated with diplopia, varying degrees of ophthalmoparesis, weakness of the orbicularis oculi, and normal pupillary function by clinical testing (see Chapter

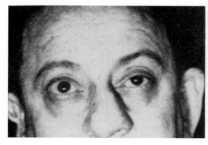
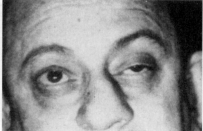
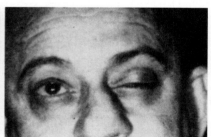

Figure 24.21. Fatigue of ptosis in myasthenia gravis. Increasing ptosis over a 3-minute period during sustained attempted upward gaze in a 58-year-old man with myasthenia gravis. (From Cogan DG. Myasthenia gravis. A review of the disease and a description of lid twitch as a characteristic sign. Arch Ophthalmol 1965;74:217–221.)

21). Ultimately, ptosis occurs in the majority of patients with myasthenia gravis. Regardless of when it develops, the ptosis of myasthenia gravis may be unilateral or bilateral, and when it is bilateral, it may also be symmetric or asymmetric (Fig. 24.20).

The hallmark of myasthenic ptosis is its fatigability and tendency to fluctuate in severity (Fig. 24.21), although this feature is by no means pathognomonic. A similar tendency to fatigue (although not to the same degree) occurs in patients with aponeurotic defects and oculomotor nerve palsies. Patients with ptosis from myasthenia gravis, myasthenic syndromes, botulism, or drugs affecting neuromuscular transmission usually have sufficient signs and symptoms to allow the correct diagnosis to be made, such as Cogan lid-twitch (Fig. 24.22), enhancement of ptosis (Fig. 24.23), and the orbicularis "peek" sign (Fig. 24.24). In addition, unless it is complete, myasthenic ptosis often improves when ice is held to the affected eyelid for 2 minutes (the ice test—see Chapter 21) (Fig. 24.25).

Ptosis may be produced by neuromuscular disorders other than myasthenia gravis, including botulism and certain envenomations. In such cases, the history as well as accompanying signs or symptoms—particularly pupillary involvement—allow the correct diagnosis (Fig. 24.26). Neuromuscular disorders of neuro-ophthalmologic importance are described in detail in Chapter 21 of this text. In addition, botulinum toxins, injected for blepharospasm or for cosmetic reasons, may spread to the levator muscle, producing transient ptosis.

Mechanical Ptosis

Any process that increases the weight of the eyelid or mechanically interferes with the normal excursion of the eyelid can result in ptosis. The most common causes are neoplastic or inflammatory infiltration or mass effect on the eyelid (e.g., neurofibroma, capillary hemangioma, metastatic lesions, basal cell carcinoma, lymphoid lesions, and amyloidosis) (115,116) and edema (e.g., after trauma or from blepharochalasis, inflammatory disease of the lid and orbit, acute thyroid eye disease, or giant papillary conjunctivitis). In contrast to conditions that increase the mass of the eyelid and cause ptosis in both primary and downward gaze, malignant and inflammatory infiltration of the superior orbital tissues may produce ptosis in primary gaze with "hang-up" (i.e., pseudoretraction) of the upper lid on downgaze. This can occur with minimal evidence of orbital disease and can be an important sign of orbital malignancy or inflammation in patients with adult-onset ptosis (117).

Cicatricial changes from trauma and diseases such as trachoma, erythema multiforme, and pemphigoid may also result in an adhesive or restrictive type of ptosis. Entrapment of (e.g., from orbital roof fracture) or encroachment on (e.g., from bony fragments, intraorbital foreign bodies, subperiosteal and intraorbital hematomas, mass lesions) the levator can interfere mechanically with the movement and position of the eyelid. In such cases, the history and associated findings usually are sufficient to make the correct diagnosis.

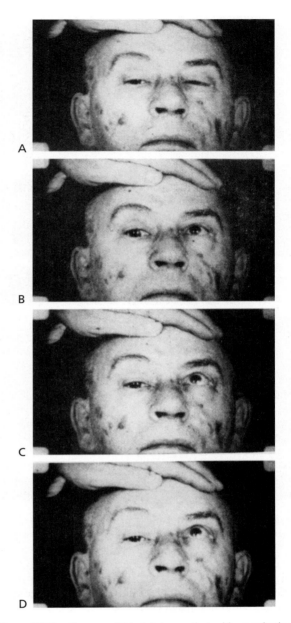

Figure 24.22. Cogan eyelid twitch in a patient with myasthenia gravis shown in successive frames of a movie. *A,* The patient is looking downward and both lids are lowered, left more than right. *B,* The appearance of the patient immediately after making an upward saccade so that he is now looking straight ahead. Note normal elevation of left eyelid but incomplete elevation of left eyelid. *C and D,* Progressive right ptosis as the patient maintains gaze straight ahead. The overall appearance is that of a "twitch" in which the right eyelid raises and then progressively falls. The entire process takes only a few seconds. (From Cogan DG. Myasthenia gravis: A review of the disease and a description of lid twitch as a characteristic sign. Arch Ophthalmol 1965;74:217–221.)

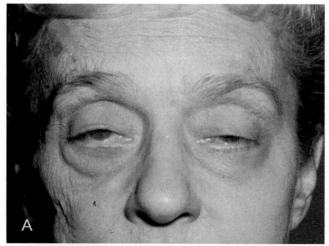

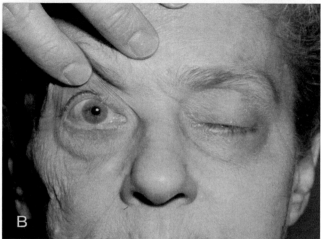

Figure 24.23. Enhancement of ptosis in an elderly woman with myasthenia gravis. *A,* The patient has bilateral asymmetric ptosis. *B,* When the right eyelid is elevated manually, the left ptosis increases.

Cutaneous leishmaniasis of the face can involve the eyelids causing chronic ptosis (118,119).

Pseudoptosis

Pseudoptosis is an apparent ptosis unrelated to defects in the neural, neuromuscular, or myogenic components of eye-

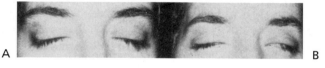

Figure 24.24. Orbicularis ''peek'' sign of myasthenia gravis. The patient initially is able to close the eyes tightly (*A*), but the orbicularis oculi fatigues, and the inferior sclera becomes visible (*B*). (From Osher RH, Griggs RC. Orbicularis fatigue: The ''peek'' sign of myasthenia gravis. Arch Ophthalmol 1979;97:677–679.)

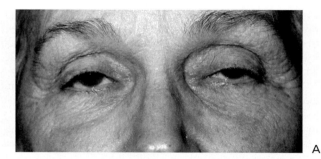

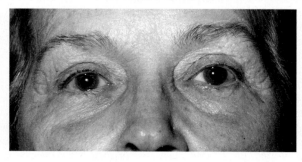

Figure 24.25. Results of ice test in a patient with myasthenia gravis. *A,* Before ice is applied. *B,* After ice has been applied to right upper eyelid for 2 minutes. Note marked elevation of both eyelids.

lid elevation. Pseudoptosis may be present because the eye on the same side is abnormal in size, shape, or position; e.g., in patients with anophthalmos, phthisis bulbi, microphthalmos, or enophthalmos. Conversely, patients who present with isolated unilateral lid retraction and proptosis from thyroid orbitopathy are sometimes mistakenly thought to have ptosis of the other eye. We have examined a young man who was referred to an oculoplastic specialist for repair of unilateral ptosis when, in fact, he had contralateral proptosis caused by an optic nerve glioma. In some persons, excessively loose skin (dermatochalasis) or prolapsed orbital fat (blepharochalasis) causes the skin of the upper eyelid to overhang the lid margin, simulating ptosis (Fig. 24.27).

Pseudoptosis often occurs in patients with a hypertropia who fixate with the higher eye. In such cases, the contralateral eye is hypotropic. Because the position of the upper eyelid on that side is appropriate to the position of the hypotropic eye, that eyelid is lower than the eyelid on the contralateral side (the side of the higher eye that is fixating), and the patient appears to have a ptosis. However, when the hypertropic eye is covered, and the patient fixates with the previously hypotropic eye, the ''ptosis'' disappears (Fig. 24.28).

Pseudoptosis may occur in patients with downgaze paralysis (120,121). When such patients attempt to look downward, their eyes remain in the primary position, but their eyelids lower normally (Fig. 24.29).

Narrowing of the lid fissure from hemifacial contracture, hemifacial spasm, blepharospasm, or a previous facial nerve palsy may mimic ptosis (discussion following). In such patients, the presence of other evidence of abnormal facial movement usually suggests the correct diagnosis.

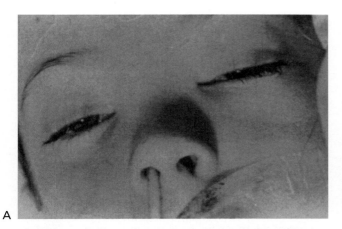

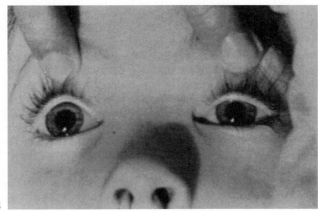

Figure 24.26. Eyelid ptosis in botulism. *A,* The patient has a bilateral severe ptosis. *B,* The pupils are dilated and nonreactive. The patient was also ophthalmoplegic.

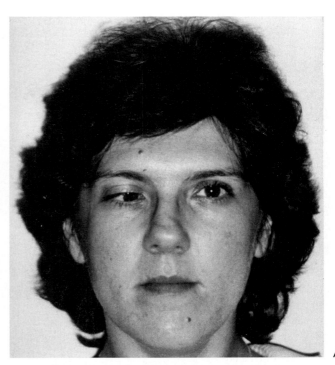

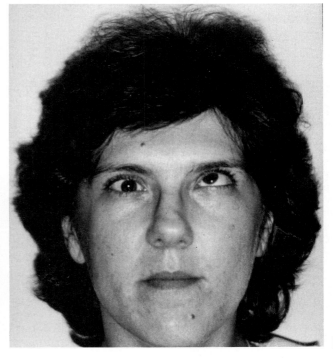

Figure 24.27. Bilateral pseudoptosis from dermatochalasis in an elderly man. Note folds of skin from the superior eyelids that obscure the upper half of both corneas. (Courtesy of Dr. Nicholas T. Iliff.)

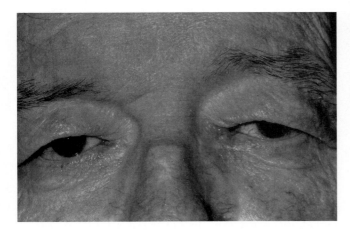

Figure 24.28. Unilateral pseudoptosis from vertical strabismus. *A,* The patient has a marked right hypotropia and is fixating with the left eye. The right upper lid appears ptotic, but in fact, the lid is in a position appropriate to the position of the eye. *B,* When the patient fixates with her right eye, the ''ptosis'' disappears because the right eye is now in normal position. (Courtesy of Jacqueline M. Pappas, C.O.)

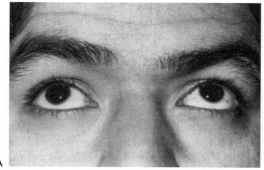

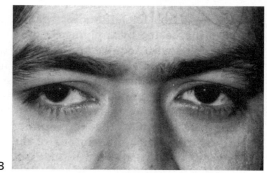

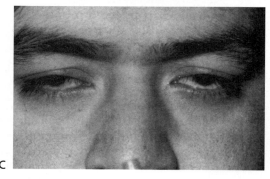

Figure 24.29. Bilateral pseudoptosis from bilateral downgaze paralysis. In primary position (*B*), there appears to be bilateral ptosis; however, the upward movement of the eyelids is normal (*A*), and on downgaze (*C*), the patient's eyes remain looking straight ahead while the eyelids lower normally, resulting in pseudoptosis. (From LoBue TD, Feldon SE. Reverse Collier's sign: Pseudoblepharoptosis associated with downgaze paralysis. Am J Ophthalmol 1983;95:120–121.)

Apparent ptosis can be caused by voluntary stimulation of one or both orbicularis oculi muscles. Patients with nonorganic overactivity of the orbicularis oculi usually show mild or pronounced wrinkling of the eyelids proportional to the amount of narrowing of the fissure and depression of the brow (although occasionally the brow is elevated). Indicative of levator tone, the upper eyelid crease is present in primary gaze and may deepen in upgaze. In addition, one can often see—and always feel—fine tremors of the affected eyelid as the patient attempts to maintain the "ptotic" lid position. Patients with organic ptosis do not show a delay in returning to their baseline lid position after manual elevation of the eyelid. In contrast, patients with nonorganic ptosis may

sometimes exhibit a slight lag before the orbicularis oculi is factitiously reactivated (122). Nonorganic ptosis may occur in isolation or in association with other somatic complaints.

Treatment of Ptosis

A variety of surgical procedures can be used to treat ptosis. The treatment for any individual patient depends on the etiology of the ptosis, the amount of levator function, and the preference of the surgeon (17,123–126).

EYELID RETRACTION

Inappropriate and excessive elevation of the eyelids—eyelid retraction—makes a patient appear to be staring and also produces an illusion of exophthalmos. Mild degrees of lid retraction are frequently difficult to evaluate. The resting position of the upper lid is influenced by many factors, including age, alertness, and direction of gaze. Normal variations in resting lid position, or upper lid posture, are exemplified by the striking difference between infants and adults. The infant's eyelid, which barely touches the upper corneal limbus, may appear normal, whereas a similar lid position in an adult is abnormal and represents excessive lid elevation. In general, upper lid position is abnormal if it exposes sclera between the lid margin and the upper corneal limbus when the patient's head is straight and both of the patient's eyes are directed straight ahead.

Eyelid retraction may be unilateral or bilateral. The levator muscle is unique in being subjected to the influence of **two** yoke muscles—the contralateral levator and the ipsilateral superior rectus. Thus, eyelid retraction can result from inappropriate excitation or hyperactivity of ipsilateral levator neurons directly or indirectly via its yoke muscles, from oculosympathetic excitation or inappropriate hyperactivity, and from contracture or shortening of the levator muscle or its tendon, Müller's muscle, or the superior rectus muscle. Causes of eyelid retraction may be classified as neuropathic, neuromuscular, myopathic, and mechanical (127,128).

Neuropathic Eyelid Retraction

Neuropathic eyelid retraction may be caused by supranuclear, nuclear, or infranuclear mechanisms. In some cases, the pathophysiology is clear; in others, it is either unknown or multifactorial.

Supranuclear Eyelid Retraction

Although true retraction of the eyelids does not usually occur from lesions in the cerebral hemisphere, intermittent or prolonged inappropriate eyelid opening sometimes develops in patients with unilateral nondominant or bilateral cerebral hemisphere disease. Such patients may be unable to close their eyelids on command (i.e., compulsive eye opening) (129), or they may close their eyes only briefly before opening them again (i.e., motor impersistence) (130). These patients have a supranuclear disturbance of orbicularis control and have normal levator relaxation.

Supranuclear bilateral eyelid retraction—**Collier sign**—most commonly occurs with lesions of the dorsal mesen-

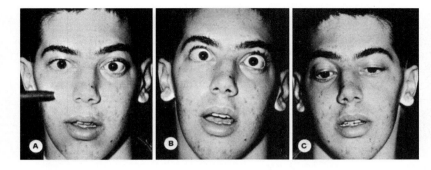

Figure 24.30. Bilateral eyelid retraction in a patient with a dorsal mesencephalic syndrome (Collier sign). *A*, The patient has moderate bilateral eyelid retraction when looking straight ahead. *B*, On attempted upward gaze, the eyes do not elevate, but the eyelids elevate normally, producing marked eyelid retraction and stare. *C*, On attempted downward gaze, the eyelids move normally with the eyes, and the eyelid retraction and stare disappear.

cephalon (131). This type of lid retraction is almost invariably associated with other evidence of dorsal mesencephalic dysfunction, most often a deficiency of upward gaze but also convergence-retraction nystagmus and pupillary light-near dissociation. The dosal mesencephalic syndrome, also called Parinaud syndrome, is discussed in Chapter 19 of this text. It suffices here to emphasize that the eyelid retraction that occurs with lesions of the dorsal mesencephalon is usually symmetric and sustained as long as the patient directs the eyes straight ahead or slightly upward, increases as the patient looks up, and follows the eyes in a normal fashion when the patient looks down (Fig. 24.30). These features distinguish eyelid retraction from lesions of the dorsal mesencephalon from the more common form of lid retraction

seen in thyroid orbitopathy, in which lid lag is invariably present (discussion following).

The nucleus of the posterior commissure (nPC) appears to be the premotor structure responsible for mesencephalic lid retraction. As noted above, lesions that damage this structure in the dorsal mesencephalon generally produce bilateral lid retraction; however, they may also damage the oculomotor nerve fascicle on one side, producing a ptosis on the side of the fascicular damage. This results in a condition characterized by ptosis on one side and primary eyelid retraction (i.e., not secondary to the contralateral ptosis) on the other. This condition is called the "plus-minus syndrome" (132,133) (Fig. 24.31). Imaging studies in patients with this syndrome show unilateral paramedian lesions, usually in-

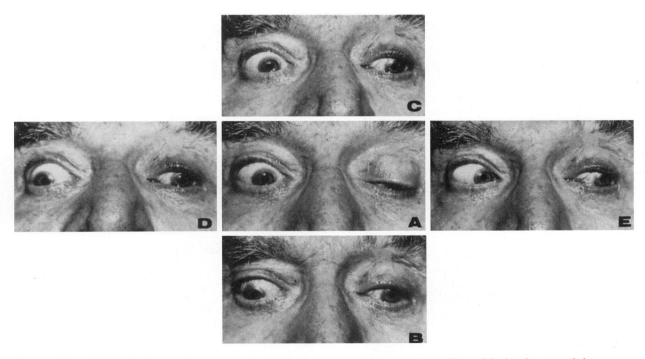

Figure 24.31. Unilateral ptosis associated with contralateral upper eyelid retraction from a lesion of the dorsal mesencephalon that also damages the fascicle of the oculomotor nerve on one side (plus-minus syndrome). *A*, The patient has marked eyelid retraction on the right and marked ptosis on the left. *B–D* show upward gaze paresis, left third nerve palsy, and lid-lag on downgaze. Computed tomographic scanning showed a paramedian midbrain infarct located ventrally and laterally to the aqueduct, extending from the midline to the area of the red nucleus laterally. (From Gaymard B, Lafitte C, Gelot A, et al. Plus-minus syndrome. J Neurol Neurosurg Psychiatry 1992;55:846–848.)

farctions, dorsal and rostral to the red nucleus in the area of the nPC, extending ventrocaudally to the fascicle of the oculomotor nerve on the ptotic side. Thus, damage to the nPC apparently causes bilateral supranuclear lid retraction that may be masked on one side by an associated fascicular oculomotor nerve palsy.

Sustained eyelid retraction may be observed with any of the disorders known to produce a dorsal mesencephalic syndrome. In a series of 206 patients with this condition, 40% of whom had lid retraction, the most common causes were hydrocephalus (39%), stroke (26%), and tumor (22%) (134) (Fig. 24.32). The remaining cases included infection (encephalitis, abscess), tentorial herniation, trauma, AVMs, congenital, Wernicke syndrome, and Bassen-Kornzweig syndrome. Other causes of the dorsal mesencephalic syndrome are multiple sclerosis (MS) and shunt malfunction (134).

Neurodegenerative conditions that cause supranuclear disturbances in upgaze may cause lid retraction. For example, lid retraction is common among patients with progressive supranuclear palsy (135,136), Parkinson disease (22), and Machado-Joseph disease (spinocerebellar ataxia, type 3) (137). In addition, some patients with severe Guillain-Barré syndrome (GBS) demonstrate marked bilateral limitation of upper lid descent during the acute phase of their illness (138–140) (Fig. 24.33).This phenomenon is not explained by associated facial weakness; it may be caused by supranuclear levator dysfunction.

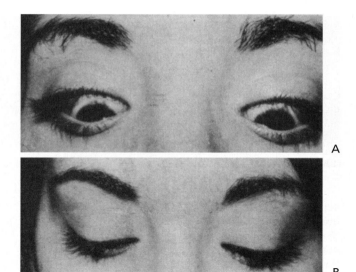

Figure 24.33. Bilateral eyelid lag on downward gaze in a patient with Guillain-Barré syndrome. *A*, Bilateral lid-lag on downward gaze during the acute phase of the disease. *B*, Three months later, there is normal lid relaxation on downward gaze. (From Keane JR. Lid-lag in the Guillain-Barré syndrome. Arch Neurol 1975;32:478–479.)

Lid retraction and slight downward gaze of both eyes in response to a sudden decrease in ambient light is a physiologic reflex seen in infants between 1 and 5 months of age. Sometimes called the "eye-popping reflex" or "nonpathologic lid retraction," it is a useful way of assessing levator function in infants (141) (Fig. 24.34).Transient, clonic, bilateral lid retraction with spastic downward gaze deviation that resolves after several weeks also occurs in otherwise healthy neonates (142). This may be a variant of the benign, transient, supranuclear disturbances of ocular motility that frequently occur in such infants (143).

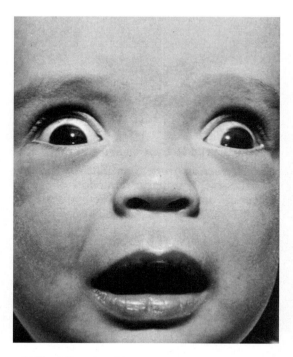

Figure 24.32. Bilateral eyelid retraction in a baby with communicating hydrocephalus. On attempted upgaze, there is no upward movement of the eyes (in fact, the eyes are resting slightly below the horizontal midline), but the eyelids elevate normally. This appeareance is often called (the "setting sun" sign).

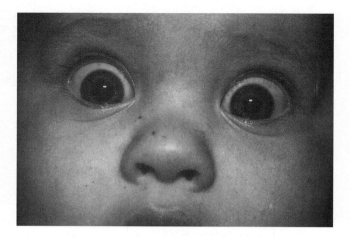

Figure 24.34. Eyelid retraction with a sudden decrease in ambient illumination in an otherwise healthy infant (the eye -popping reflex). Note physiologic anisocoria. (From Bartley GB. The differential diagnosis and classification of eyelid retractions. Ophthalmology 1996;103:168–176.)

Coma and stupor are commonly associated with eyelid closure caused by an absence of levator tonus. Occasionally, however, levator tonus persists and produces the incongruous picture of intermittently open lids in an unresponsive patient (coma vigil). This sign usually indicates disease of the ventral mesencephalon and pons, but it may occur with diffuse hemisphere disease (persistent vegetative state). Comatose patients with Cheyne-Stokes respiration sometimes open their eyes during the rapid-breathing phase and close them during the slow-breathing phase. Phasic lid opening that was synchronous with the inspiratory phase of respiration in comatose patients has been observed (144). Still another interesting reflexive opening of the eyelids may be demonstrated in some comatose patients by raising their head or turning it from side to side (13). Most commonly observed in infants and children, this phenomenon seems analogous to the doll's head movements of the eyes. Rarely, comatose patients maintain constantly open, unblinking eyes caused by a failure of levator inhibition (145).

Some patients with extrapyramidal syndromes (e.g., post-encephalitic parkinsonism, progressive supranuclear palsy) have defective inhibition of their eyelids during downward gaze. Such patients have normal lid position when they look straight ahead; however, the lids lag behind briefly as the eyes follow an object downward (144). Patients with a unilateral midbrain lesion dorsal to the red nucleus may also exhibit lid lag without lid retraction (146). The lesion in these patients is postulated to disrupt the pathways between the rostral interstitial nucleus of the medial longitudinal fasciculus (MLF) and the central caudal subnucleus of the oculomotor nuclear complex while sparing the nPC.

Eyelid Nystagmus

Eyelid nystagmus is a repetitive up and down movement of the upper eyelids in which there is a rapid upward phase, simulating eyelid retraction, followed by a slow downward drift. It usually is induced by convergence or gaze shifts and may be associated with certain types of nystagmus, such as convergence-retraction nystagmus or oculopalatal myoclonus (147). Unlike ocular jerk-type nystagmus, in which the slow phase is pathologic and the quick phase is a physiologic response designed to bring the eyes back to a normal position (see Chapter 23), in eyelid nystagmus, the upward quick movement is pathologic and the downward slow movement restores the eyelids to their normal position.

Convergence-evoked eyelid nystagmus most often occurs in patients with MS (148) or cerebellar tumors invading the 4th ventricle (144,149,150). It has also been reported in patients with Fisher syndrome (151), posttraumatic dorsal midbrain syndrome (152), and pontomedullary angioma (153).

Gaze-evoked eyelid nystagmus is usually associated with damage to the brainstem, cerebellum, or both structures (59,149,150,154). Gaze-evoked eyelid nystagmus that is present only when looking at a distant, eccentrically placed object can occur in patients with the lateral medullary syndrome of Wallenberg (154) (see Chapter 19). The nystagmus stops during eccentric fixation of a near target (154,155).

Horizontal gaze-induced eyelid nystagmus also has been reported in patients with intrinsic midbrain tumors, such as astrocytomas (59).

Eyelid nystagmus may occur synchronously with convergence-retraction nystagmus (156). This type of lid movement may be evoked when a patient with a pretectal or peri-aqueductal lesion (i.e., a dorsal mesencephalic syndrome) attempts to make voluntary upward saccades, or as the patient watches downward-moving optokinetic stimuli. In such patients, upward gaze (particularly saccadic eye movements) is invariably defective. A similar phenomenon occurs in patients with a global paresis of gaze from Fisher syndrome (151).

Eyelid Retraction from Paradoxical Levator Excitation

Eyelid retraction from paradoxical levator excitation may be congenital or acquired. It may occur from lesions of supranuclear, nuclear, or infranuclear pathways.

Eyelid Retraction in Patients with Congenital and Acquired Defects of Horizontal Eye Movements

Elevation of the ipsilateral eyelid may be observed in normal subjects during abduction and, less commonly, on adduction (157) (Fig. 24.35). The lid retraction on attempted abduction in patients with Duane retraction syndrome and in patients with acquired abducens nerve palsies (Fig. 24.36) may represent an exaggerated expression of this physiologic synkinesis.

Eyelid Retraction Evoked by Jaw Movement (Marcus Gunn Jaw-Winking Phenomenon)

The Marcus Gunn jaw-winking phenomenon is a paradoxical elevation of one eyelid that occurs with certain movements of the jaw (158,159). It is caused by a synkinesis between the pterygoid muscles and the levator (160). The associated movements of lid and jaw are termed a "trigemino-oculomotor" synkinesis and are subdivided into an external pterygoid-levator synkinesis and an internal pterygoid-levator synkinesis (160). Stimuli other than movement of the pterygoids can also produce the same kind of eyelid retraction in some of the patients with this condition.

Simultaneous contraction of the levator with the external pterygoid muscle is the most common form of the Marcus Gunn jaw-winking phenomenon. The affected eyelid is usually ptotic when the jaw muscles are at rest; however, when the jaw muscles contract, the eyelid elevates to a normal position or may even retract and will remain in this position as long as the jaw muscles are active. Elevation of the upper lid may occur (*a*) when the mandible is moved to the opposite side (contraction of the ipsilateral external pterygoid muscle); (*b*) when the mandible is projected forward or the tongue is protruded (bilateral contraction of the external pterygoid muscles); or (*c*) on wide opening of the mouth (i.e., strong depression of the mandible) (Fig. 24.37). In all of these settings, the abnormal levator contraction is most evident when the patient is looking downward.

In most instances, external pterygoid-levator synkinesis

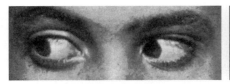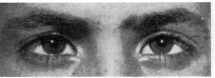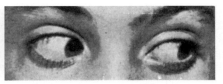

Figure 24.35.   Physiologic synkinesis between normal eye movement and levator muscles. Subject with normal ocular motility shows elevation of both upper eyelids in extreme right and left horizontal gaze. (From Ticho U. Synkinesis of upper lid elevation occurring in horizontal eye movements. Acta Ophthalmol 1971;49:232–238.).

is congenital and is first recognized during the act of sucking soon after birth (161–164). The condition improves with age in some patients (165,166) but not in others (164,167).

Patients with the Marcus Gunn jaw-winking phenomenon may have levator synkinesias that involve cranial nerves in addition to, or other than, the trigeminal nerve. For example, the eyelid may elevate with teeth clenching (160,168), smiling (169), sternocleidomastoid contraction, tongue protrusion (170), inspiration (171), or voluntary nystagmus (172). In some patients, jaw movements may induce not only elevation of the eyelid but also involuntary movements of the eyes (173–176).

Patients with the Marcus Gunn phenomenon commonly have associated ocular abnormalities, including strabismus, amblyopia, anisometropia, and congenital nystagmus (164,167). The most common ocular motor disturbances are

double elevator palsy, unilateral superior rectus palsy, Duane retraction syndrome (177), and adduction palsy with synergistic divergence (178). Rarely, trigemino-oculomotor synkinesis is associated with the triad of ipsilateral facial hemiatrophy, heterochromia, and poliosis.

The cause of the synkinesis between the pterygoid muscles and the levator muscle in the Marcus Gunn jaw-winking phenomenon is unknown. Although the possibility of a supranuclear synkinesis has been suggested, most investigators believe that a branch of the trigeminal nerve has been congenitally misdirected to the levator muscle (158). EMG studies are consistent with this concept (160,168,179) and histopathologic analysis of the levator reveals evidence of neurogenic atrophy with aberrant reinnervation on the affected side and, to a lesser degree, the clinically unaffected side (180).

Treatment of patients with the Marcus Gunn jaw-winking phenomenon depends on their ophthalmologic and cosmetic status. Amblyopia should always be treated aggressively, and vertical strabismus should be corrected before attempting surgical repair of ptosis. Eyelid surgery should only be contemplated after the patient (when age permits), parents, and surgeon agree that the jaw-winking, ptosis, or both, are objectionable. Surgery usually consists of weakening the levator aponeurotic complex combined with a lid elevation procedure (164,166,167,181–185).

Eyelid Retraction with Contralateral Ptosis from Combined Paradoxical Levator Excitation and Contralateral Levator Inhibition

Cases of congenital oculopalpebral synkinesias occur in which horizontal gaze induces reciprocal inhibition of one levator on abduction and excitation of the other on adduction, resulting in a gaze-induced seesaw-like movement of the eyelids, with ptosis on the side of the abducting eye and eyelid retraction on the side of the adducting eye (186,187). This seesaw-like synkinesis of the eyelids may, in rare cases, be induced by movements of the jaw from side to side. When the mouth is opened in such cases, both eyelids retract simultaneously (178,188) (Fig. 24.38). The pathogenesis of this condition is unknown but probably involves anomalous innervation at the level of the peripheral nerves rather than ephaptic transmission between brainstem nuclei.

Eyelid Retraction from Aberrant Regeneration of the Oculomotor Nerve

Eyelid retraction can be caused by aberrant regeneration of the oculomotor nerve and may be congenital or acquired.

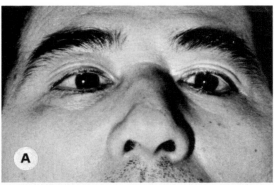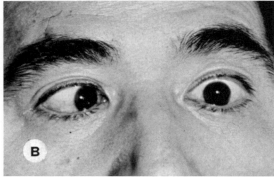

Figure 24.36.   Eyelid retraction associated with left abduction paralysis. *A*, Primary position, the patient's upper eyelids are in normal and equal position. *B*, On attempted gaze left, the left eye abducts only to the midline, and there is elevation of the left upper lid and eyebrow.

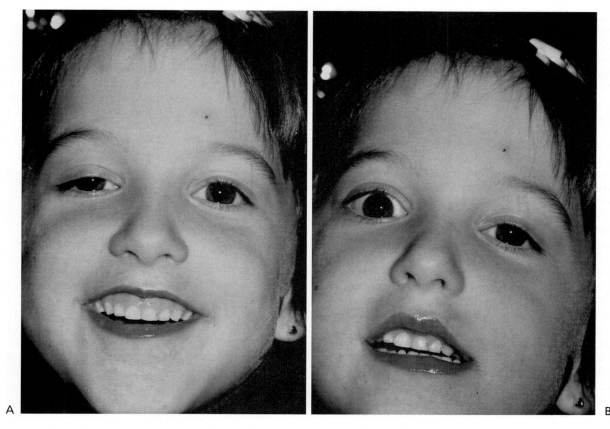

Figure 24.37. The Marcus Gunn jaw-winking phenomenon. *A*, The child has a congenital right ptosis. *B*, When the child moves her jaw to the left, the right eyelid elevates, and the ptosis disappears. (Courtesy of Dr. Nicholas T. Iliff.)

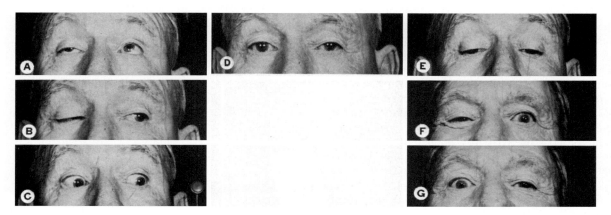

Figure 24.38. Synkinetic levator inhibition during conjugate gaze associated with paradoxic excitation with jaw opening resulting in bilateral jaw winking (''seesaw jaw winking''). *A*, There is inhibition of the right levator in upgaze. *B*, There is inhibition of the right levator in left gaze. *C*, The levator inhibition changes to bilateral levator excitation when the mouth is opened. *D*, During gaze straight ahead, there is no significant ptosis on either side. *E*, Levator inhibition is normal in downward gaze; both eyelids are in normal position. *F*, Elevation of left upper eyelid occurs with jaw thrust to right. *G*, Elevation of right upper eyelid occurs with jaw thrust to left.

It usually occurs during attempted infraduction, adduction, or both. During abduction of the affected eye, the eyelid becomes ptotic. This phenomenon is explained by reciprocal innervation. When the lateral rectus muscle contracts both the ipsilateral medial rectus and the levator are inhibited.

Lid retraction due to aberrant regeneration of the oculomotor nerve usually develops several months after an acute oculomotor nerve palsy, in which case the condition is known as **secondary aberrant regeneration of the oculomotor nerve.** However, when a slowly progressive compressive process (such as an aneurysm, miningioma, or schwannoma that is usually, but not always, located within the cavernous sinus) (see Chapter 20) damages the nerve so insidiously that aberrant regeneration occurs without a period of acute oculomotor dysfunction the condition is called **primary aberrant regeneration of the oculomotor nerve.** Although most cases of secondary aberrant regeneration of the oculomotor nerve occur from non-ischemic damage to the nerve, rare patients have been reported in which the condition occured after an ischemic brainstem lesion, presumably affecting the third nerve fascicle (189).

A patient with bilateral traumatic oculomotor nerve palsies treated surgically subsequently (2 years later) developed bilateral, alternating cyclic eyelid retraction that occurred every 1–2 minutes and lasted 5 seconds in each eye (190). Two other conditions that may cause periodic eyelid retraction are oculomotor palsy with cyclic spasms, a condition that usually is congenital, and ocular neuromyotonia, an acquired condition that usually occurs after radiation therapy for a basal skull mass (see Chapter 20). In both conditions, the eyelid retraction usually is unilateral and associated with pupillary constriction and spasms of one or more of the extraocular muscles innervated by the oculomotor nerve. Isolated eyelid retraction has not been observed in these conditions.

Eyelid Retraction Associated with Contralateral Ptosis

Patients with unilateral ptosis who, for any of a number of reasons (e.g., congenital or acquired strabismus, amblyopia, cataract), fixate with the eye on the side of the ptosis may develop retraction of the eyelid on the opposite side. Depending on the technique used to detect this phenomenon, the frequency of this secondary eyelid retraction varies from 2–66%. The methods include brief or prolonged occlusion of the eye on the side of the ptosis, manual elevation of the ptotic lid, or 2.5% phenylephrine applied to the eye on the side of the ptosis, while carefully observing the position of the contralateral retracted eyelid (191–195). Brief monocular occlusion probably is the least sensitive method, because the retracted eyelid may not reposition immediately. In most cases, secondary retraction of the eyelid in a patient with contralateral ptosis may be most easily detected if the ptotic eyelid is first manually closed and then allowed to open, because release of the manually closed eyelid sometimes causes an obvious upward flick of the contralateral eyelid as the latter resumes its retracted position (193).

The explanation for the phenomenon of unilateral eyelid retraction associated with contralateral ptosis is based on Hering's law. Intended to explain the conjugate movement of both eyes, Hering's law states that yoked extraocular muscles receive equal degrees of innervation. This law also applies to the levator muscles. Thus, in an attempt to maintain the normal position of a ptotic eyelid, the innervational drive to both lids increases, causing the ptotic lid to assume a more normal position, and the unaffected lid to retract. Secondary retraction of the eyelid in patients with contralateral ptosis is most likely to occur when the ptosis is severe, acquired, and ipsilateral to the dominant eye (194,196) (Fig. 24.39).

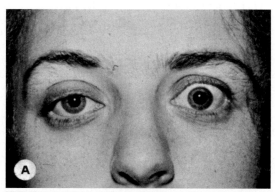
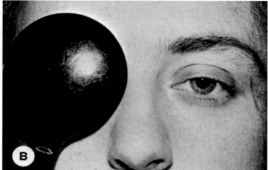
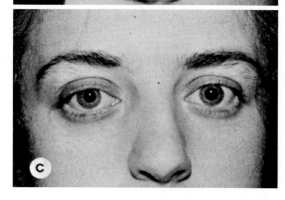

Figure 24.39. Unilateral eyelid retraction secondary to contralateral ptosis (secondary eyelid retraction) in a patient with myasthenia gravis. *A,* The patient has moderate right ptosis and marked left upper eyelid retraction. *B,* When the right eye is covered with an occluder, the left eyelid retraction disappears as levator tonus is reduced bilaterally. *C,* After an intravenous injection of edrophonium chloride (Tensilon), the right eyelid elevates, and the left eyelid retraction disappears. Eyelid retraction occurs in this setting because Hering's law of equal innervation to agonist muscles applies to the levator muscles as well as to the extraocular muscles.

The failure to recognize this phenomenon may lead to the erroneous diagnosis of thyroid orbitopathy.

The sensory stimulus for increasing tone in the contralateral levator muscle in patients with unilateral ptosis is unclear. Some authors believe it is the relative decrease in retinal illumination or the contraction of the superior visual field in the eye on the side of the ptosis (194).

Eyelid Retraction from Sympathetic Hyperfunction

Patients with neck trauma may develop a syndrome of recurrent throbbing headaches and oculosympathetic hyperactivity characterized by ipsilateral lid retraction, hyperhydrosis, and mydriasis—the **Claude-Bernard syndrome**. During the headache-free interval, some of these patients have a Horner syndrome. The syndrome is thought to be caused by sympathetic irritation or hyperactivity (197).

Sympathetic hyperactivity is also thought to be responsible for some cases of lid retraction observed in patients with thyroid orbitopathy (see below). Indeed, dilute solutions of both direct and indirect adrenergic stimulants (e.g., cocaine, hydroxyamphetamine, phenylephrine, apraclonidine, naphazoline) will widen the palpebral fissure in such patients (198–200).

Neuromuscular Eyelid Retraction

Transient, spontaneous eyelid retraction occurs in patients with **myasthenia gravis** without evidence of thyroid dysfunction (201) (Fig. 24.40). This phenomenon, which usually occurs on return of the eyes from upward gaze to primary position, appears to be caused by post-tetanic facilitation of the levator muscle. Like the lid retraction of midbrain disease (i.e., Collier sign), neuromuscular lid retraction may be bilateral and symmetric, bilateral but asymmetric, or completely unilateral. Unlike the eyelid retraction of the dorsal mesencephalic syndrome, however, in patients with neuromuscular eyelid retraction, the levator usually fails to "relax" smoothly and completely, and the lid fold fails to smooth out as the eyes move downward. Momentary lid retraction also may be seen in patients with myasthenia after the patient makes an upward saccade from downgaze to primary position (Cogan lid-twitch) (Fig. 24.22). Finally, patients with myasthenia may develop retraction of the eyelid secondary to ptosis of the contralateral eyelid (191,192)

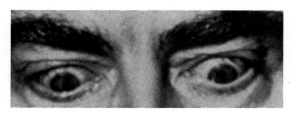

Figure 24.40. Transient, bilateral, asymmetric upper eyelid retraction in a patient with myasthenia gravis. This retraction occurred following prolonged upgaze. It persisted for several seconds and then disappeared. (From Puklin JE, Sacks JG, Boshes B. Transient eyelid retraction in myasthenia gravis. J Neurol Neurosurg Psychiatry 1976;39:44–47.)

(Fig. 24.39). Associated weakness of the orbicularis oculi, disturbances of eye movement or alignment, or both, usually suggests the correct diagnosis; however, in rare instances, the eyelid retraction is the initial sign of the disorder.

Eyelid retraction may result from topical or systemic administration of drugs that affect the neuromuscular junction. The anticholinesterase agents edrophonium chloride (Tensilon) and neostigmine methylsulfate (Prostigmin) produce eyelid retraction in some patients with myasthenia gravis. In addition, subparalytic doses of succinylcholine can produce shortening of the levator muscle fibers associated with the depolarization effect of the drug, resulting in lid retraction (144).

Myopathic Eyelid Retraction

Myopathic eyelid retraction occurs in both children and adults. In children, it is particularly tempting to make the diagnosis of myopathic retraction simply because the patient is a child; however, because eyelid retraction that occurs in childhood may be caused by hyperthyroidism, primary aberrant regeneration of the oculomotor nerve, the dorsal midbrain syndrome, hydrocephalus, or the Marcus Gunn jaw-winking phenomenon (202), the diagnosis of congenital or developmental eyelid retraction should be made only after these and other causes have been excluded.

Congenital myopathic eyelid retraction can be unilateral or bilateral and may be associated with nonspecific strabismus, underaction of the superior rectus on the side of the retraction, or lower lid retraction (202–205). The condition also may be associated with other developmental anomalies, including optic disc hypoplasia, craniosynostosis, and Down syndrome (202). In such cases, levator excursion is normal and there often is lagophthalmos on downgaze, indicating either failure of appropriate inhibition of levator tonus or decreased elasticity of the levator or its suspensory ligaments. Routine histology of the levator muscle typically shows no specific abnormalities (205). In some cases, however, the medial and lateral horns of the levator aponeurosis appear thickened (206,207), and in one case the levator muscle was fibrotic (202).

Thyroid orbitopathy with involvement of the levator muscle on one or both sides is the most common cause of acquired unilateral and bilateral sustained lid retraction in adults (208,209). The eyelid signs of thyroid orbitopathy, which have a variety of names, are produced by pathologic shortening of the levator muscle, resulting in the inability of the muscle fibers to lengthen normally. Thus, patients with dysthyroid disease may show retraction of one or both upper eyelids associated with infrequent or incomplete blinking (Stellwag sign), abnormal widening of the palpebral fissure (Dalrymple sign), lid lag on attempted downward gaze (Graefe sign), or a combination of these signs (Figs. 24.41 and 24.42). In addition, during the examination, the physician may have difficulty everting the patient's upper eyelid (Gifford sign).

Patients with dysthyroid eyelid retraction may be chemically hyperthyroid, hypothyroid, or euthyroid. The retraction itself may be unilateral or bilateral and transient or persistent

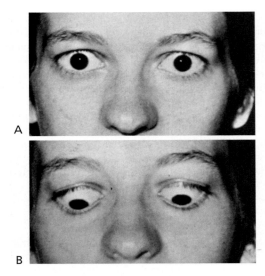

Figure 24.41. Bilateral eyelid retraction (*A*), and lid-lag on downward gaze (*B*), in a patient with thyroid orbitopathy.

(Fig. 24.42). It can occur in isolation, but it is more often associated with other signs of thyroid orbitopathy. If the lid retraction is mild and unassociated with other signs of thyroid orbitopathy, there may be difficulty in distinguishing lid retraction from pseudoptosis on the opposite side (see above). Levator excursion appears to be increased in patients with thyroid orbitopathy (210), and high-resolution sagittal computed tomographic (CT) scans show enlargement of the levator-superior rectus muscle complex in such cases (211). In addition, EMG studies of the levator muscle demonstrate normal levator inhibition during downward gaze in patients with dysthyroid disease (212,213).

Multiple factors are involved in the genesis of dysthyroid lid retraction. Based on the inflammatory and fibrotic

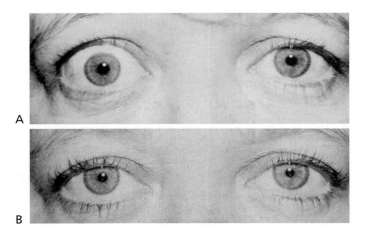

Figure 24.42. Unilateral upper eyelid retraction in a woman with thyroid orbitopathy. Patient was euthyroid at the time of the initial photo (*A*). After more than 4 years of lid retraction, the affected eyelid spontaneously returned to a normal position (*B*).

changes observed in the extraocular muscles, it would seem most likely that contracture or adhesive effects on the levator are the main reasons for persistent thyroid eyelid retraction (214–218); however, in some cases, the levator muscle shows surprisingly little fibrosis or inflammation and is characterized instead by enlargement or hypertrophy of individual muscle fibers (11). Thus, the lid retraction that occurs in some patients with thyroid eye disease may result from some form of levator muscle ''hyperactivity'' (11,217). Indeed, the spontaneous reversibility of lid retraction in some cases (Fig. 24.42) and the development of ptosis after injections of botulinum toxin type A in others would seem to argue against a restrictive fibrosis, in at least some cases.

Sympathetic stimulation induced by thyrotoxicosis or overmedication with thyroid replacement appears to be responsible for eyelid retraction in a minority of cases of thyroid orbitopathy. In such cases, the lid retraction often resolves with improvement in thyroid status, and it responds transiently to topical sympatholytics, such as thymoxamine and guanethidine (71). However, although sympathetic overstimulation may play a role in some cases of dysthyroid eyelid retraction, this mechanism does not explain the often asymmetric or unilateral cases, the absence of pupillary findings, and the fact that in some cases, the retraction persists as the patient becomes euthyroid (219).

Dysthyroid lid retraction results from restriction of the inferior rectus muscle in some cases (220,221). Because the levator receives the same eye-movement signal as the superior rectus (see above), the increased drive on the superior rectus to overcome inferior rectus restriction causes excessive levator tonus. Recession of the inferior rectus in such cases results in a dramatic improvement in lid retraction.

In newborns with myopathic lid retraction, the cause usually is maternal hyperthyroidism. In such cases, the condition is transient and resolves in 2–3 weeks as the infant establishes its own endocrinologic equilibrium (222). There also are rare thyroid patients with ptosis (e.g., from myasthenia gravis, an aponeurotic defect from recurrent lid swelling, overcorrection from previous surgery for lid retraction) who develop secondary retraction of the contralateral eyelid (223,224) (see earlier).

The treatment of eyelid retraction in patients with thyroid orbitopathy is primarily surgical and consists of various levator-lengthening procedures (214,225–227), excision of Müller's muscle (228), and combined procedures on both muscles (229). Although topical sympatholytic agents (e.g., guanethidine, thymoxamine) may be used to reduce the retraction of the levator muscle by producing a sympathetic ptosis (196), these drugs are impractical for constant use. Guanethidine has a delayed effect and produces considerable corneal irritation. Topical thymoxamine, a selective α-adrenergic blocking agent, causes prompt ptosis, but it too causes considerable corneal irritation, and its long-term effects are unknown (73). Injection of botulinum toxin type A into the levator muscle may correct eyelid retraction temporarily (230,231), but the degree of the response and its duration are unpredictable. We thus find this form of treatment impractical for most patients.

Eyelid retraction occurs with increased frequency in pa-

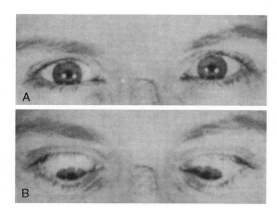

Figure 24.43. Myotonic eyelid retraction and lid lag (levator myotonia) in a patient with hyperkalemic periodic paralysis. *A,* When the patient looks straight ahead, the eyelids are slightly retracted. *B,* On downward gaze, there is marked eyelid lag. (From Layzer RB, Lovelace RE, Rowland LP. Hyperkalemic periodic paralysis. Arch Neurol 1967;16:455–471.)

tients with severe liver disease (Summerskill sign). The appearance is similar to that seen in patients with thyroid orbitopathy (232,233).

Myotonic eyelid retraction and lid lag may be observed in patients with both hyperkalemic and hypokalemic familial periodic paralysis (234–236) (Fig. 24.43). A similar myotonic lid lag may occur in patients with myotonic dystrophy and in patients with congenital myotonia (237).

Mild eyelid retraction can occur in association with an ipsilateral facial nerve palsy because orbicularis oculi tonus contributes to the passive downward forces acting on the upper eyelid (128) (Fig. 24.44). A similar mechanism may explain the lid retraction seen in some patients with ocular myasthenia gravis (see earlier and Chapter 21).

Mechanical Lid Retraction

The upper eyelid ordinarily maintains its position relative to the pupil even when an eye is proptosed by 10 mm or

more (208). Thus, patients who exhibit lid retraction associated with ipsilateral proptosis almost invariably have thyroid orbitopathy and not an orbital mass. Nevertheless, various local processes can damage the eyelid and produce mechanical lid retraction (128).

Cutaneous cicatricial changes of the upper eyelid can produce eyelid retraction. The most common causes are burns and deep lacerations. Less commonly, cicatricial eyelid re-

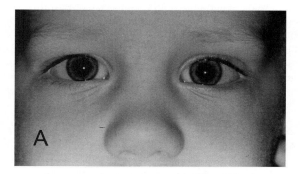

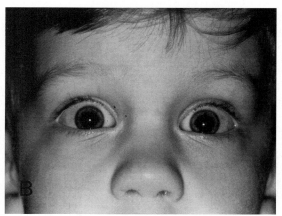

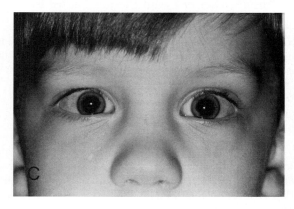

Figure 24.45. Bilateral upper eyelid retraction after surgery on the superior rectus muscles. *A,* Preoperative appearance. The patient has a V-pattern esotropia with bilateral overaction of the inferior oblique muscles. *B,* Immediate postoperative appearance. After bilateral superior rectus recessions and inferior oblique weakening procedures, the patient has bilateral upper eyelid retraction. *C,* Six months after surgery, mild upper eyelid retraction remains. (Courtesy of Dr. David L. Guyton.)

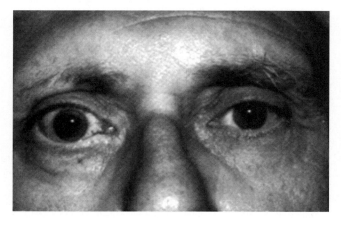

Figure 24.44. Unilateral upper and lower right-sided eyelid retraction in a patient with a right facial nerve palsy. (From Bartley GB. The differential diagnosis and classification of eyelid retractions. Ophthalmology 1996; 103:168–176.)

traction occurs from damage to the eyelid from orbital cellulitis with necrosis (particularly from staphylococci and group A streptococci), herpes zoster, scleroderma, or atopic dermatitis (128).

Eyelid retraction can occasionally be caused by contact lens wear. It resolves when the contact lens is removed (128). In some cases, a contact lens becomes displaced superiorly but is thought by the patient to have been lost. The retained lens causes an inflammatory reaction in the superior fornix and eventually becomes embedded in an inflammatory cyst, the nature of which may not be appreciated until the cyst is opened surgically and the contact lens is found within it (238).

Postsurgical lid retraction is most often seen as an overcorrection after surgery for ptosis, although a variety of procedures, including vertical rectus muscle surgery (Fig. 24.45), trabeculectomy, cataract extraction, scleral buckling, blepharoplasty, myectomy for blepharospasm, orbital floor repair, and maxillectomy can also result in lid retraction. The mechanism is often a consequence of induced underaction of the superior rectus. As a result of the surgical weakening of the superior rectus, the nervous system compensates for its decreased effectiveness by increasing the drive to the superior rectus motoneurons. As emphasized above, the levator motoneurons share the increased motor drive to superior rectus motoneurons, resulting in increased tone in the levator muscle. Other mechanisms causing postsurgical lid retraction include restriction of the inferior rectus muscle, cicatricial adhesion, or damage to the ligaments that create the passive downward eyelid forces (128,239–241).

Blowout fractures of the orbit may cause lid retraction by entrapment of the surrounding connective tissue. Lid retraction can also occur during an effort to elevate or fixate with a hypotropic or restricted eye (239,242).

ABNORMALITIES OF EYELID CLOSURE

As with eyelid opening, abnormalities of eyelid closure may occur from disorders involving any part of the pathway for contracture of the orbicularis oculi, from the cerebral cortex to the muscle itself (Figs. 24.46–24.48). Such disorders may be congenital or acquired and may be caused by either hypofunction or hyperfunction of the orbicularis muscle and, to a lesser extent, by the muscles that assist the orbicularis in eyelid closure (i.e., the frontalis, procerus, and corrugator superciliaris).

INSUFFICIENCY OF EYELID CLOSURE

As with eyelid opening, insufficient eyelid closure can be neuropathic, neuromuscular, or myopathic in origin. Arriving at the correct diagnosis thus requires a careful history and complete examination, sometimes followed by appropriate ancillary studies.

Insufficiency of Eyelid Closure Caused by Neuropathic Disease

Neuropathic causes of insufficient eyelid closure may be supranuclear, nuclear, or infranuclear. In some cases, the cause is clearly neuropathic but the precise mechanism is unknown or multifactorial.

Insufficiency of Eyelid Closure Caused by Supranuclear Disorders

Voluntary eyelid closure is mediated by the pyramidal system (Fig. 24.46). Patients with localized subcortical capsular lesions usually can close both eyes, although the force of closure is diminished, and the ability to wink may be lost on the contralateral paretic side (Revilliod sign) (243). In some cases, paresis is profound and yet spontaneous involuntary or emotional movements of the facial and orbicularis muscles remain undisturbed (automatic-voluntary dissociation) (244) (Fig. 24.49).

Bilateral inability to voluntarily close the eyelids may result from a unilateral lesion, usually in the nondominant frontal lobe, but it more commonly develops with bilateral frontal lobe lesions (129,245). This phenomenon is called **supranuclear paralysis of voluntary lid closure** (246) or compulsive eye opening. Patients with this syndrome are unable to initiate voluntary closure of either eyelid, even though they retain their ability to comprehend the task and have intact reflex eyelid closure (Fig. 24.50). Although some investigators consider this phenomenon to be an apraxia of eyelid closure (247), it actually is caused by true motor dysfunction (248). Supranuclear paralysis of eyelid closure can occur in patients with unilateral or bilateral infarcts or tumors in the frontal lobe (246), Creutzfeldt-Jakob disease (248), progressive supranuclear palsy (31,249), and motor neuron disease (246,250).

Motor **impersistence** of eyelid closure also occurs in patients with bilateral or unilateral hemispheric lesions. When such patients are instructed to close the eyelids and keep them closed, they are unable to obey. The eyelids close, often develop a fine tremor, and then almost immediately reopen (130,251). This phenomenon most frequently is seen in patients with a nondominant hemisphere stroke and is most evident during the first week after the stroke (252). Occasionally, the condition is unilateral.

It is likely that supranuclear paralysis of eyelid closure (i.e., compulsive eye opening) and motor impersistence of eyelid closure have a common origin because they can coexist in the same patient and develop in similar clinical settings. EMG studies, however, have yielded conflicting results. In one patient with progressive supranuclear palsy, EMG showed both inadequate inhibition of the levator and insufficient orbicularis oculi activity (136). In another EMG study, patients with Parkinson disease with motor impersistence showed a supranuclear disturbance of orbicularis control, rather than levator inhibition (253).

Cortical lesions may also affect involuntary lid closure. For example, the blink response to a threatening gesture is absent in patients with homonymous hemianopia when the gesture is presented in the blind field of vision. The blink to threat is also lost in patients with cortical blindness and

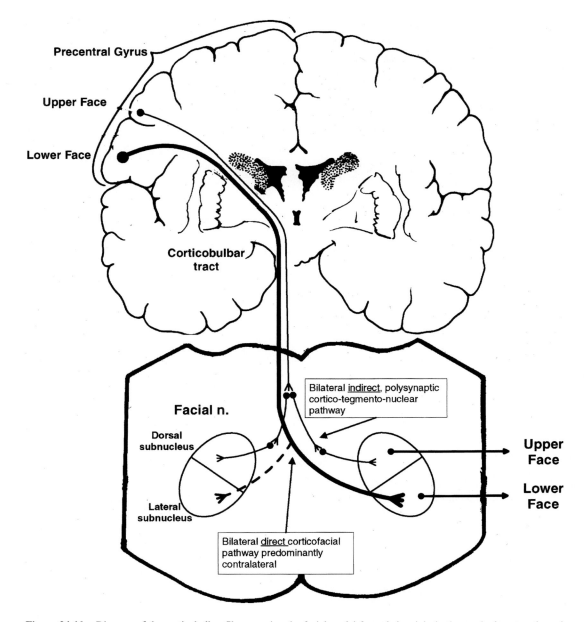

Figure 24.46. Diagram of the corticobulbar fibers serving the facial nuclei from their origin in the cerebral cortex, through the internal capsule into the brainstem at the level of the facial nucleus. Note that projections are bilateral along two pathways: A direct, predominantly contralateral projection to the lateral subnucleus responsible for lower facial muscles, and an indirect pathway through the pontine reticular formation to the dorsal subnucleus that innervates the upper facial muscles.

may be absent in patients with profound visual inattention associated with large parieto-occipital or parietotemporal lesions. Loss of spontaneous blinking was described in a patient with Balint syndrome caused by bilateral parieto-occipital lesions (254).

Insufficiency of Eyelid Closure Caused by Brainstem Disorders

Unilateral weakness of eyelid closure and facial movement may result from unilateral damage to the facial nerve nucleus or fascicle. In such instances, other evidence of brainstem disease is almost always present, including reduction in corneal sensation, ipsilateral abducens nerve paresis or horizontal gaze paralysis, and ipsilateral cerebellar ataxia.

Bilateral weakness of eyelid closure occurs as part of the facial diplegia that is caused by lesions of the pontine tegmentum. Such lesions may be congenital or acquired. Acquired processes include ischemia, inflammation, infiltration, and compression.

When insufficiency of eyelid closure results from damage

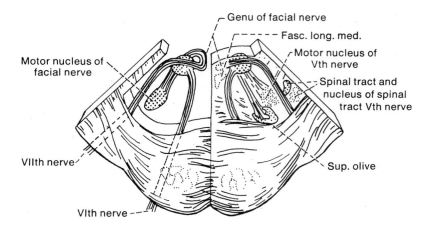

Figure 24.47. Diagram of the anatomy of the facial nerve nuclei and fascicles, showing the intrapontine course of the fascicles and their relationship to surrounding structures. Note proximity of the facial nerve nuclei and fascicles to the abducens nerve nuclei and fascicles (VIth nerve), motor nucleus of the trigeminal (Vth) nerve, spinal tract and nucleus of the spinal tract of the Vth nerve, and the medial longitudinal fasciculus (Fasc. long med). (From Brodal A. Neurological Anatomy in Relation to Clinical Medicine. Ed 3. New York: Oxford Universtiy Press, 1981:495.)

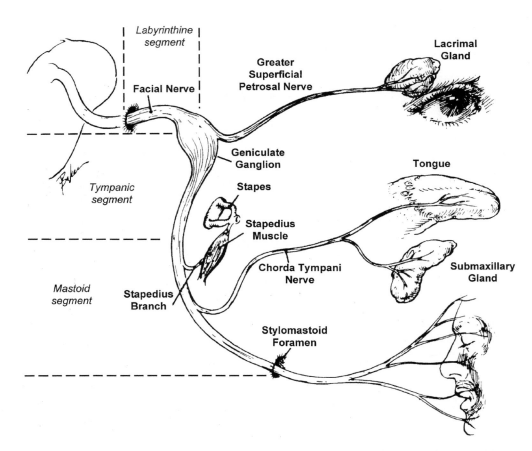

Figure 24.48. Schematic drawing of the branches of the facial nerve showing the different functions of those branches. The branches and their functions include the greater superficial petrosal nerve (reflex tearing), the nerve to the stapedius muscle (stapedius reflex), the chorda tympani nerve (taste on the anterior two -thirds of the tongue and submaxillary gland secretion), and peripheral motor branches to the facial muscles. (From Alford BR, Jerger JF, Coats AC, et al. Neurophysiology of facial nerve testing. Arch Otolaryngol 1973;97:214–219.)

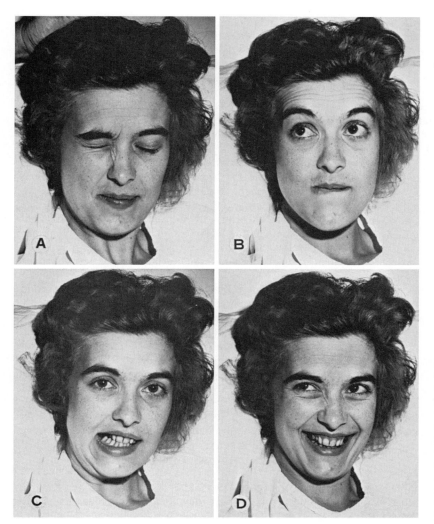

Figure 24.49. Central volitional (supranuclear) paralysis of the orbicularis oculi after a subcortical hematoma that caused a left hemiplegia and a left facial nerve paresis. *A*, When the patient is told to close her eyes tightly, the left orbicularis oculi, left corrugator muscle, and the other muscles of the left lower side of the face fail to respond. *B*, Volitional control of the forehead is normal. *C*, Left lower facial weakness is evident when the patient attempts to show her teeth. *D*, A spontaneous smile (emotional-extrapyramidal-facial innervation) evokes symmetric contraction of all facial muscles, including the orbicularis oculi, indicating that nuclear and infranuclear pathways are intact.

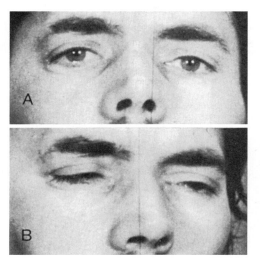

Figure 24.50. Supranuclear paralysis of voluntary eyelid closure (compulsive eyelid opening) in a patient with Creutzfeldt-Jakob disease. *A*, The patient has no movement of the eyelids when told to close his eyes, even though he understands what he is being told to do and is attempting to do it. *B*, The patient shows some ability to blink to a visual threat. (From Russell RW. Supranuclear palsy of eyelid closure. Brain 1980;103:71–82.)

to the facial nerve fascicle within the brainstem, there usually is complete facial paralysis associated with other signs of brainstem dysfunction, such as ipsilateral horizontal gaze palsy from damage to the ipsilateral abducens nucleus or paramedian pontine reticular formation, ipsilateral abduction weakness from damage to the ipsilateral abducens nerve fascicle, and contralateral hemiparesis from damage to the ipsilateral pyramidal tract (Fig. 24.47). The combination of ipsilateral facial nerve palsy, ipsilateral abduction weakness, and contralateral hemiparesis is called the Millard-Gubler syndrome (see Chapter 20).

Insufficiency of Eyelid Closure from Peripheral Facial Nerve Palsy

The insufficiency or weakness of eyelid closure associated with lesions of the facial nerve is usually combined with weakness of other facial muscles supplied by that nerve (255). A standardized clinical method of assessing the degree of facial palsy classifies the severity into six grades—I to VI—based on the residual motion of the forehead, eyelid, and mouth, as well as the appearance of the face at rest (256). Grades I and II indicate minimal or mild paresis, with acceptable appearance and movement, whereas grade VI represents total paralysis. With respect to the eyelid, mild weakness (grade II) of the orbicularis oculi from facial nerve paresis may be characterized by normal symmetry and tone, with only minimal effort being required to completely close the eyelid. The lower eyelid may be slightly retracted in patients with this grade of weakness (257). Patients with moderate paresis (grade III) may close the eyes completely but only with extreme effort. Incomplete reflex and voluntary eyelid closure occurs with moderately severe (grade IV) or severe (grade V) dysfunction. In these severe cases, the lower eyelid sags, whereas the resting position of the upper eyelid remains unchanged or is slightly retracted (Figs. 24.44 and 24.51). Epiphora may occur in these patients from impaired lacrimal drainage and corneal exposure.

Topographic diagnosis of facial nerve paresis may be facilitated by the relationship of the facial nerve to surrounding structures and by the fact that along its course, the nerve gives off various branches that subserve specific functions (255). The facial nerve, in addition to innervating the facial musculature, is also responsible for reflex tearing (via the greater superficial petrosal nerve), hearing (via the nerve to the stapedius muscle), taste on the anterior two-thirds of the tongue (via the chorda tympani), and salivation (via nerve branches to the sublingual and submandibular glands) (Fig. 24.48). Thus, by testing for reflex tearing using a Schirmer test (see Chapter 15), hearing, taste, and ability of an individual with peripheral facial weakness to produce saliva, one often can determine the location of the responsible lesion (discussion following). In addition, various electrodiagnostic tests, including nerve excitability, electromyography, blink reflex, and electroneurography help determine the extent of dysfunction and prognosis for facial nerve recovery (255,258).

Lesions in the cerebellopontine angle (CPA) that produce unilateral facial nerve paresis usually are also characterized by signs and symptoms related to dysfunction of the vestibulocochlear and trigeminal nerves. Common manifestations thus include unilateral sensorineural hearing loss, tinnitus, vertigo, facial pain and numbness, corneal hypesthesia, and unsteadiness of gait. All of the components of the facial nerve may be affected. Less common manifestations include hemifacial spasm, nystagmus, evidence of cerebellar dysfunction (e.g., ataxia and tremor), and hydrocephalus. Nevertheless, although most patients with lesions in the CPA present with multiple neurologic findings, facial nerve paralysis may be the only manifestation, particularly in children (259,260).

Lesions of the CPA that may cause a facial nerve paresis include vestibular and trigeminal schwannomas, meningiomas, epidermoids, lipomas, arachnoid cysts, aneurysms, metastatic lesions, and glomus jugulare tumors. Granulomas

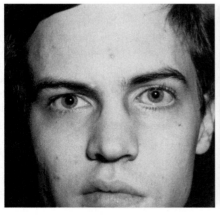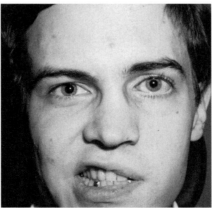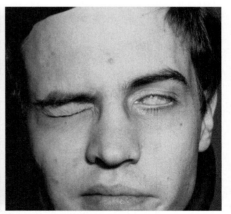

A,B   C

Figure 24.51.   Peripheral facial nerve palsy after removal of a vestibular schwannoma. *A,* The patient has a complete facial nerve palsy. Note the widened left lid fissure and sag of the left lower eyelid. *B,* When the patient attempts to show his teeth, lower facial weakness is evident. This weakness did not improve when extrapyramidal facial innervation was stimulated. *C,* On attempted eyelid closure, there is almost complete paralysis of the left orbicularis oculi muscle. Note intact Bell's phenomenon.

associated with tuberculosis, sarcoid, syphilis, or certain fungal infections can also damage the facial nerve in the CPA.

A facial nerve lesion located within the facial canal between the internal auditory meatus and the geniculate ganglion produces many of the same signs as those encountered with lesions in the CPA, except that brainstem signs are absent, and there is no evidence of dysfunction of the trigeminal nerve. Lesions between the geniculate ganglion and the branch to the stapedius muscle produce similar manifestations except that reflex lacrimation is preserved because the lesion is distal to the superficial petrosal nerve. Damage to the facial nerve between the branch to the stapedius muscle and the chorda tympani produces facial paralysis, loss of taste on the anterior two-thirds of the tongue, and diminution of salivary secretion.

Lesions of the facial nerve distal to the takeoff of the chorda tympani produce only facial motor paralysis. Facial neuropathies that localize to the intratemporal portion of the facial nerve may be caused by fractures of the temporal bone, herpes zoster (Ramsey Hunt syndrome), otitis media, and neoplasms. The condition called ''Bell's palsy'' belongs in this category (discussion following). Lesions distal to the stylomastoid foramen may affect one or more peripheral branches of the facial nerve and are usually caused by facial trauma, facial surgery, or disease of the parotid gland.

Distinguishing central and proximal peripheral lesions of the facial nerve from distal peripheral lesions is critically important. Unfortunately, although topographic analysis of facial nerve function often permits such differentiation, the findings in patients with lesions along the intratemporal segment of the facial nerve are often variable and inconsistent. This is particularly true in cases of Bell's palsy, for which magnetic resonance (MR) imaging can show areas of demyelination anywhere from the brainstem to the periphery (261,262). The usefulness of precise localization along this segment of the facial nerve in diagnosis, management, and prognosis is limited (258,263).

The majority (about 50–70%) of isolated facial nerve palsies are idiopathic and are called Bell's palsy (264,265). The diagnosis of Bell's palsy is based on a constellation of findings and the exclusion of other known causes. The condition usually is unilateral, although bilateral cases occur in 0.1–1.0% of patients (266–268). About 60% of patients with a Bell's palsy have a history of a viral prodrome. The onset of facial motor weakness is acute and frequently accompanied by pain or numbness of the face, neck, or tongue. The pain is characteristically located in the retroauricular area. Hypesthesia or dysesthesia in the distribution of the trigeminal or glossopharyngeal nerve occurs in 25–35% of patients. Sensory findings may precede the onset of facial paresis and usually do not persist beyond 7–10 days. Dysgeusia and dysacusis are fairly common accompaniments. Both subjective and objective signs of dry eye are present in 15–17% of patients. Epiphora from exposure or paralytic ectropion is common (263,269,270). The incidence of Bell's palsy is higher in adults than in children, and the condition occurs in both sexes with equal frequency. Familial cases are extremely unusual (271,272).

Mounting evidence implicates a viral etiology in the pathogenesis of Bell's palsy. First, serologic studies reveal evidence of a variety of infectious agents, particularly the herpes group of viruses, mumps virus, and rubella virus in patients in whom the condition occurs (273–275). Second, evidence of herpes simplex virus is often found in the geniculate ganglion of adults with Bell's palsy using the polymerase chain reaction and *in situ* hybridization (276,277). Third, some investigators have found histopathologic evidence of inflammatory changes within the facial nerve of patients with Bell's palsy (278–280). Fourth, some patients with Bell's palsy can be found to have widespread subclinical disturbances in the peripheral and central nervous systems indicative of a more widespread cranial polyneuropathy (281–285). Finally, epidemiologic studies suggest an infectious process in many cases of Bell's palsy (286). Nevertheless, although it is likely that an immunologic response associated with infection is responsible for many cases, some authors maintain that the crucial factor is swelling of the facial nerve (from inflammation, ischemia, or both) within the facial canal (278,287,288).

In a study based on the untreated natural history of more than 1,000 patients with Bell's palsy (289), Petersen found that among the 30% of patients with incomplete facial paresis, nearly all achieved complete recovery. Among the 70% with complete paralysis, the prognosis was still quite good if signs of recovery began within the first 3 weeks of onset.

Overall, 85% of patients with Bell's palsy eventually recover completely or are left with only slight residual deficits. The remaining 15% require 3–6 months before showing signs of improvement but have permanent deficits consisting of residual weakness, tonic contracture, synkinesis, spasms, or gustatory lacrimation (crocodile tears) (269,290–292). Clinical factors that adversely affect recovery include advanced age (over 60), diabetes mellitus, complete paralysis, decreased tearing, hyperacusis, and delay in the onset of recovery (263,289,293,294). In 7–10% of cases, recurrences occur on the same side or alternate from side to side (295).

The efficacy of systemic corticosteroids in the treatment of Bell's palsy is somewhat controversial. Patients treated with prednisone appear to have less denervation and greater improvement in functional grade at recovery than patients who are not treated in some studies but not in others (294). Although steroids may not entirely prevent partial denervation or contracture, their use may speed recovery and may also reduce the risk of gustatory lacrimation from autonomic synkinesis and of progression from incomplete to complete paralysis. Thus, most physicians treat patients with prednisone in a dose of 1 mg/kg/day for 10–14 days followed by a rapid taper.

Because herpes simplex virus is also implicated in the pathogenesis of Bell's palsy (275) and because herpes zoster oticus can occur without a rash (i.e., zoster sine herpete) (296), some clinicians recommend using acyclovir along with systemic corticosteroids in the treatment of patients with Bell's palsy (269,297). However, there is no difference in the outcome of patients treated with steroids alone compared with patients treated with both steroids and acyclovir (298).

There is strong pathologic, clinical, and neuroimaging evidence that the pathogenesis of facial nerve damage in patients with Bell's palsy is compression of the nerve at the meatal foramen and along its labyrinthine segment. Decompression procedures that expose more distal segments thus have been abandoned in favor of decompression of the meatal foramen and labyrinthine segment of the facial nerve via a middle fossa craniotomy (288). Nonetheless, the effectiveness of canal decompression in the treatment of Bell's palsy is unproven, and enthusiasm for the procedure has waned (269, 299,300).

An isolated facial nerve palsy that may mimic Bell's palsy can occur in a large number of systemic disorders. These include infections and inflammations (herpes zoster oticus, acquired immune deficiency syndrome, otitis media, mastoiditis, Lyme disease, syphilis, sarcoidosis, tetanus), ischemia (diabetes mellitus, hypertension), and immune-mediated inflammatory diseases (periarteritis, GBS, post vaccination demyelination, MS). Neoplastic causes of isolated peripheral facial palsy include vestibular and facial nerve schwannomas, meningiomas, glomus jugulare tumors, lipomas, dermoids, epidermoids, parotid tumors, carcinomatous meningitis, cholesteatomas, metastatic tumors, and lymphoid lesions. Miscellaneous causes include toxic agents (thalidomide, ethylene glycol, organophosphate poisoning), trauma (temporal bone fractures, facial injuries, barotrauma from scuba diving), iatrogenic injuries (from local anesthetic blocks and facial surgery), amyloidosis, Paget disease, and benign intracranial hypertension (265,270,299,301–315).

Because so many conditions can cause an acute, initially isolated, facial nerve paresis, progression of a facial palsy for longer than 3 weeks, lack of recovery after 3–6 months, development of hemifacial spasm, prolonged otalgia or facial pain, or recurrence of paralysis after recovery should prompt closer investigation of a "Bell's palsy" to rule out an underlying systemic inflammatory or infectious etiology or a neoplasm.

In patients with congenital or developmental facial nerve paresis, there may be other evidence of incomplete development (i.e., hypoplasia) or agenesis of the facial nerve. Such patients may have Möbius syndrome, congenital unilateral lower lip paralysis (CULLP), hemifacial microsomia, or other associated developmental defects, such as aural atresia and microtia (316,317). Acquired prenatal causes include birth trauma and exposure to thalidomide or rubella virus (317,318).

Less than 1% of all facial nerve palsies are bilateral and simultaneous. Such cases usually are idiopathic (i.e., Bell's palsy) or caused by Lyme disease, sarcoidosis, GBS, Fisher syndrome, brainstem encephalitis, or neoplasia (e.g., carcinomatous meningitis, glioma). Less common causes include meningitis (e.g., from syphilis, tuberculosis, cryptococcus), diabetes mellitus, head trauma, pontine hemorrhage, systemic lupus erythematosus, ethylene glycol ingestion, benign intracranial hypertension, and Wernicke-Korsakoff syndrome (319–323).

The rehabilitation and supportive management of patients with a facial nerve palsy depends on the stage and severity of facial weakness. During the acute phase, treatment should be directed at preventing the complications of corneal exposure by using topical lubricants and, in some cases, cellophane wrap occlusive dressings or self-adhesive occlusive bubbles. If supportive therapy fails, a temporary or permanent tarsorrhaphy should be performed. When the facial nerve has been severed or severely damaged, and recovery is not likely to occur, procedures that juxtapose the upper and lower eyelids and improve eyelid (and other facial muscle) function should be considered, including permanent tarsorrhaphy, lateral canthoplasty to treat the effects of paralytic ectropion, and insertion of a gold weight or palpebral spring (cerclage) to reanimate the upper eyelid. Facial reanimation can sometimes be accomplished using a variety of techniques, including direct facial nerve repair, autogenous nerve grafts, cross facial nerve grafting, and nerve crossovers using the hypoglossal nerve. In addition, temporalis muscle transfers, free-muscle grafts, and facial suspension with fascia lata, tendon, or alloplastic materials can be used (324–330).

Abnormal Eyelid Closure Associated with Aberrant Regeneration of the Facial Nerve

Aberrant regeneration of the facial nerve (AFR) may occur after damage to the facial nerve, particularly after compression or trauma (331). It develops in 10–20% of patients with Bell's palsy. The previously paralyzed side of the face is invariably weak and may appear contracted (Fig. 24.52). Typically, each closure of the eye occurs simultaneously with a twitch at the corner of the mouth that also may be accompanied by dimpling of the chin and contraction of the platysma. During forced lid closure, there is an exaggerated contraction of all facial muscles on the side of the previously paretic facial nerve. Conversely, both voluntary and involuntary movements of the lips or the corner of the mouth precipitate co-contraction of the orbicularis oculi on the affected side that may superficially resemble hemifacial spasm or the inverse Marcus Gunn jaw-winking phenomenon (see earlier); however, unlike hemifacial spasm, which occurs spontaneously (discussion following), the eyelid and facial spasms that occur in patients with aberrant regeneration of the facial nerve are induced by voluntary or involuntary movements of the eyelid or mouth. Similarly, unlike the inverse Marcus Gunn phenomenon, in which the eyelid closure is caused by levator inhibition (332), narrowing of the lid fissure in aberrant regeneration of the facial nerve is caused by inappropriate contraction of the orbicularis oculi muscle (333).

AFR may present with ptosis on the affected side, without apparent synkinesis, so that the underlying etiology is not recognized, especially if a history of previously facial nerve paralysis is not obtained. In one series, 15 patients with AFR, who presented with ptosis, had decreased palpebral apertures with reduced upper and lower lid MRD, reduced orbicularis strength, but increased muscle tone on the affected side. The diagnosis of AFR is confirmed in this setting by demonstrating increased ptosis during cheek puffing, a finding present in all 15 patients (334).

Insufficiency of Eyelid Closure Caused by Neuromuscular Disease

The orbicularis oculi often is weak in diseases that affect the neuromuscular junction. **Myasthenia gravis** characteris-

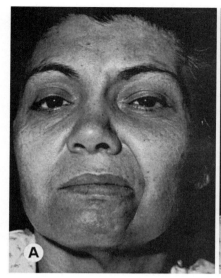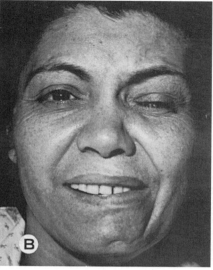

Figure 24.52. Aberrant regeneration of the left facial nerve after an acute peripheral facial nerve paresis producing facial contracture and partial closure of the left eyelid associated with certain movements of the mouth. *A*, The patient has a narrowed left interpalpebral fissure and a deepened left nasolabial groove. *B*, Any spontaneous or voluntary movement of the lower face, such as trying to smile, produces co-movements of all muscles on the left side of the face, resulting in eyelid closure.

tically produces weakness of eyelid closure, usually combined with ptosis. This weakness of orbicularis function is responsible for the "peek phenomenon" (335), in which a patient with myasthenia gravis initially is able to close the eyelids, but as closure is maintained, the orbicularis fatigues and the eyelids separate, exposing the globe. Weakness of the orbicularis oculi in patients with neuromuscular disease also may be characterized by retraction of the lower eyelid (257). Botulism also can cause weakness of the facial muscles, including the eyelids, as can certain envenomations (e.g., snake and spider bites) that affect the neuromuscular junction. The diagnosis of neuromuscular disease, particularly myasthenia gravis, should be considered in any patient with weakness of eyelid closure associated with ptosis, ophthalmoparesis, or both.

Insufficiency of Eyelid Closure Caused by Myopathic Disease

The orbicularis oculi muscle is almost always weakened by any disease that weakens the facial musculature. Weakness of the orbicularis muscle may be characterized not only

by weakness of spontaneous or forced eyelid closure but also by lack of upper facial expression, wasting of eyelid tissue, and fatigue of the eyelids during attempted sustained closure. In addition, there may be retraction of the lower eyelid (257) or paralytic ectropion (Fig. 24.53). Myogenic weakness of the orbicularis oculi is usually bilateral. Weakness in the pretarsal segment impairs blinking but must be significant before blinking is overtly impaired. Because lacrimal drainage depends in part on normal muscle action in the lower eyelid, weakness of contraction may result in epiphora. The most common causes of myopathic insufficiency of eyelid closure are congenital muscular dystrophy, myotonic dystrophy, and the mitochondrial cytopathies associated with CPEO (Fig. 24.54).

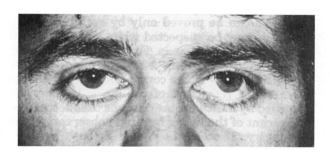

Figure 24.53. Bilateral, symmetric lower eyelid retraction in a patient with myotonic dystrophy and generalized facial weakness. (From Cohen MM, Lessell S. Retraction of the lower eyelid. Neurology 1979; 29:386–389.)

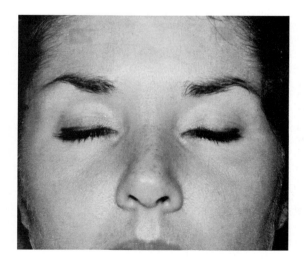

Figure 24.54. Bilateral orbicularis oculi weakness in a patient with chronic progressive external ophthalmoplegia. The patient is attempting to close her eyelids as tightly as possible. Note lack of folds in the upper eyelids and inability to "bury" the lashes.

EXCESSIVE OR ANOMALOUS EYELID CLOSURE

Unlike insufficient eyelid closure, which can be caused by neurologic, neuromuscular, or myopathic causes, excessive or inappropriate eyelid closure usually is neurologic in origin.

Essential Blepharospasm and the Blepharospasm-Oromandibular Dystonia Syndrome (Meige Syndrome; Brueghel Syndrome)

Blepharospasm is an involuntary closure of the eyelids evoked by contraction of the orbicularis oculi. When blepharospasm occurs in isolation without other evidence of neurologic or ocular disease, the condition is called essential blepharospasm (Fig. 24.55). When these focal dystonic eyelid movements spread to other cranial muscles, the syndrome is called blepharospasm-oromandibular dystonia or Meige syndrome (336–342). The disorder occurs most frequently in women over 50 years of age. Initially, there is an increased frequency of blinking, particularly in response to sunlight, wind, noise, movement, or stress. This blinking progresses to involuntary spasms, initially on one side, but inevitably on both. Certain maneuvers like touching the eyelid, coughing, vocalizing, or chewing gum may alleviate the spasms, which increase in frequency and severity as the disease progresses.

Patients with Meige syndrome may experience involuntary chewing movements, lip pursing, trismus, wide opening of the mouth, spasmodic deviations of the jaw, abnormal tongue movements (protrusion, retraction, and writhing), spasmodic dysphonia, and, rarely, difficulty swallowing (343–345). In addition to orofacial spasms, such patients may have oculogyric crises, platysmal contractions, torticollis, retrocollis, or other forms of focal dystonia. Generalized dystonia is rare, however.

Many patients with essential blepharospasm and Meige syndrome stop reading, watching television, and driving;

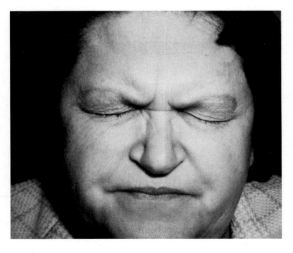

Figure 24.55. Essential blepharospasm. The patient first noted intermittent spasms of lid closure several years earlier. By the time she was examined, she was experiencing almost continuous, bilateral symmetric spasms of the orbicularis oculi muscles.

some become depressed, occupationally disabled and, in some cases, functionally blind. The disorder may plateau at any point along its progression. Remissions are rare but occur in about 11% of patients, almost always within 5 years of the onset of symptoms (340,343,346,347).

Most cases of essential blepharospasm and Meige syndrome are sporadic, although there are familial occurrences (348). In addition, patients with essential blepharospasm and Meige syndrome often have a family history of other movement disorders (e.g., essential tremor, Parkinson disease, oromandibular dystonia, blepharospasm, habit tics) (339, 342,347,349,350), or they may give a past history of tics or excessive blinking, sometimes dating back to childhood (341,352). Thus, familial blepharospasm and craniocervical dystonia may be phenotypically heterogeneous and autosomal-dominantly inherited with incomplete penetrance (349).

Many patients with blepharospasm, whether of the essential variety or part of Meige syndrome, complain of dryness, grittiness, irritation, or photophobia. Such patients typically have evidence of dry eyes or ocular surface disease by slit-lamp biomicroscopy or Schirmer testing (343,347,351,353). Indeed, disturbances of the ocular surface may be a precondition for blepharospasm in certain cases. On the other hand, some patients with blepharospasm have severe photophobia with no evidence of dry eyes or ocular inflammation or with dry eyes out of proportion to their complaints. In such patients, a supranuclear neuropathic mechanism may be responsible.

Although there are scattered reports of an association between blepharospasm and certain autoimmune disorders (e.g., systemic lupus erythematosus, myasthenia gravis, rheumatoid arthritis, thyroid disease) (354–357), there is no convincing evidence that autoimmunity is the underlying mechanism of idiopathic blepharospasm.

EMG studies of the orbicularis oculi in patients with blepharospasm show a variety of patterns. The most common is repetitive bursts that last 100–200 msec, with variable interburst intervals ranging from 200–800 msec. Some patients exhibit tonic spasms lasting 3–4 seconds (358,359) or combinations of tonic and repetitive bursts. The characteristic lowering of the brow (Charcot sign) may be absent among a subgroup of patients with blepharospasm in whom contractions are confined to the pretarsal portion of the orbicularis oculi (42).

The cause of essential blepharospasm and Meige syndrome is uncertain. Although psychologic factors are an important component of this disorder in some patients (342,360–362), there is abundant clinical and neurophysiologic evidence that essential blepharospasm and Meige syndrome are **focal dystonias** caused by dysfunction of the basal ganglia or brainstem (336,363). For example, blepharospasm can be a component of an assortment of extrapyramidal and brainstem disorders, and imaging studies show that focal lesions of the rostral brainstem, diencephalon, and basal ganglia may be associated with blepharospasm (364). In addition, there is clear evidence of brainstem dysfunction in many patients with essential blepharospasm. About 30% of patients with essential blepharospasm exhibit abnormalities of the brainstem auditory-evoked response that localize to the mid to upper brainstem (365). The reciprocal relationship between the orbicularis oculi and levator may be altered in such patients, and there may be inappropriate episodes of levator inhibition or co-contraction (42,359). Although the latency of the blink and corneal reflexes are normal in patients with essential blepharospasm, both amplitude and duration are abnormally increased (358,363). Patients with essential blepharospasm and patients with oromandibular dystonia have a more rapid R2 recovery cycle than normal control subjects, indicating that the brainstem interneurons that mediate the blink reflex are abnormally excitable (358, 366–368). Similar findings can be documented in many patients with other cranial dystonias, even in those without blepharospasm (363,366,367,370–373). The basal ganglia, which play a central role in the genesis of these movement disorders, are probably responsible for this facilitatory effect on brainstem interneurons.

Blepharospasm may be associated with a variety of eye movement disturbances that also occur in other extrapyramidal disorders. Motion-picture or video analysis of eyelid movements in patients with essential blepharospasm reveals impersistence of gaze, eyelid retraction, head tilt, and head jerk (374,375). In addition, some patients experience episodes of prolonged involuntary conjugate spasmodic upward deviations lasting 1–10 seconds (33). These episodes are similar to those seen in patients with oculogyric crises. Abnormalities in saccadic eye movements also occur in patients with essential blepharospasm. They are nonspecific (376,377) but consistent with extrapyramidal dysfunction (378).

The histopathologic findings in patients with essential blepharospasm are variable, although the basal ganglia are often abnormal. Some cases show microscopic abnormalities that consist of neuronal cell loss and severe gliosis in a unique pattern that produces a ''mosaic appearance'' in the dorsal halves of the caudate and putamen (379). In others, there is mild- to- moderate cell loss in the pars compacta of the substantia nigra, the locus ceruleus, and several other areas in the brainstem (380,381). Some cases show no abnormalities or unrelated changes (382,383); however, the lack of morphologic changes does not necessarily imply normal function. For example, neurochemical analysis of the brain from a patient with Meige syndrome who had no significant neuropathologic findings at autopsy nevertheless demonstrated substantial increases in norepinephrine and dopamine in the red nucleus and substantia nigra (384).

Botulinum toxin type A is the primary form of therapy for patients with blepharospasm. Its effects generally last 2–4 months. Other drugs can also be used to treat essential blepharospasm and Meige syndrome, but they are less efficacious. For example, in some patients with mild essential blepharospasm, tranquilizers may be of short-term benefit. For patients with more severe disease, drugs that inhibit catecholamine synthesis (α-methyl-1-tyrosine), block dopamine receptors (phenothiazine, butyrophenones), deplete brain monoamines (reserpine, tetrabenazine), or increase central cholinergic effects (physostigmine, choline, lecithin) may suppress the abnormal movements (340,385–389). Tetrabenazine, clonazepam, trihexyphenidyl, lithium carbonate,

and baclofen are of particular benefit in selected patients (340,342,390,391). In addition, selective inhibitors of serotonin re-uptake, such as fluoxetine (Prozac), may reduce facial and eyelid spasms in patients with severe blepharospasm, Meige syndrome, or both (392). L-dopa occasionally is useful in patients with blepharospasm related to parkinsonism, particularly that form induced by MPTP (393), but this drug is of little or no benefit in the treatment of essential blepharospasm.

Essential blepharospasm can be treated surgically by removing all or part of the orbicularis oculi muscle (394–398) or by avulsing or otherwise destroying branches of the facial nerve (399–403). Complications, variable effectiveness, and frequent recurrence are major limitations of both procedures (403,404); however, comparisons of the two approaches (403,405) indicate that myectomy is preferable because it results in a more prolonged relief of symptoms, fewer recurrences requiring additional surgery, greater patient acceptance, and fewer complications than selective facial nerve avulsion. Nevertheless, complete healing may take 6 months or more after myectomy and may be associated with considerable facial swelling from lymphedema. In addition, subsequent injections of botulinum toxin are associated with increased discomfort in the region of surgery. With facial nerve avulsion, there is a fourfold increase in the need for secondary procedures in addition to the complications associated with facial paresis and particularly insufficient eyelid closure (405,406–408). We believe that surgery should be reserved for patients with disabling blepharospasm that does not respond to botulinum toxin, oral medications, or a combination of these treatments, or for patients who cannot tolerate these treatments.

Patients with essential blepharospasm often have associated dermatochalasis, ptosis, or both. These can be treated with blepharoplasty and ptosis surgery, both of which often reduce the severity of the blepharospasm to some extent. However, these procedures are merely adjuncts to the treatment of blepharospasm and should not be considered as primary treatments for the condition.

Blepharospasm Associated with Lesions of the Brainstem and Basal Ganglia

Blepharospasm may be caused by a variety of lesions and disorders of the basal ganglia and mesodiencephalic region. These include strokes, demyelinating diseases (364,409,410), progressive supranuclear palsy (31,135,136), Parkinson disease (29), MPTP-induced parkinsonism (393), Huntington disease, Wilson disease, Lytico-Bodig syndrome (38), Hallervorden-Spatz syndrome (411,412), olivopontocerebellar atrophy (413), communicating hydrocephalus (249,414), and encephalitis lethargica (415). Calcification of the basal ganglia associated with blepharospasm occurs in some patients with Meige syndrome (416), pseudohypoparathyroidism (417), and ill-defined neurodegenerative disorders of unknown etiology (418).

The blepharospasm that follows a cerebrovascular accident frequently begins months to years after the stroke and is associated with other localizing signs, such as hemiplegia, midbrain ocular motor dysfunction, and extrapyramidal signs (361,409,419–423). The causative lesion may be unilateral or bilateral, but the blepharospasm usually is bilateral and symmetric. Delayed blepharospasm after stroke also may be associated with palatal or oculopalatal myoclonus (27,424,425).

There are several possible explanations for the delay in onset of blepharospasm in patients with lesions of the brainstem and basal ganglia: (*a*) denervation supersensitivity of the facial nuclear complex; (*b*) disinhibition of facial nuclear and brainstem reflexes; and (*c*) delayed-onset dystonia caused by sprouting of surviving axons (409). If one assumes that the basal ganglia facilitate the development of blepharospasm, this delay is not surprising because eyelid spasms would not develop until there was an adaptive increase in blink excitability from chronic trigeminal stimulation.

Blepharoclonus and Reflex Blepharospasm

Typical blepharospasm is characterized by repetitive episodes of tonic contractions of the orbicularis oculi, and EMG studies show that the orbicularis contractions in many such patients consist of rhythmic phasic bursts at a rate of 3–6 Hz. When such contractions result in visible repetitive upward jerks of the eyelids, the term **blepharoclonus** is used (426,427).

Blepharoclonus occurs in patients with brainstem syndromes caused by stroke or trauma (428), hydrocephalus from aqueductal stenosis in the setting of parkinsonism (429), and MS (426). In one case, blepharoclonus was precipitated by eccentric gaze and was not present when the patient looked straight ahead (426).

Reflex blepharospasm is a condition in which eyelid spasms are induced by voluntary lid closure or attempts to manually open the eyelids. It is a well-documented finding in patients with recent, nondominant temporoparietal strokes, in which case it is associated with hemiplegia (430). The lid spasms usually are confined to the nonparalyzed side and are evoked when the examiner attempts to hold the eyelids apart. Some patients with spontaneous blepharospasm from extrapyramidal or brainstem lesions also have reflex blepharospasm during attempts by the examiner to open the eyelids (364,403,419). Likewise, gentle lid closure in some patients with Parkinson disease will evoke a ''lid tremor'' that EMG reveals is a result of reciprocal contractions of the levator and orbicularis oculi muscles (253). Rarely, reflex blepharospasm is hereditary, with onset in early childhood (431).

Blepharoclonus and reflex blepharospasm probably are different manifestations of similar pathophysiologic processes. Although the origin of the primary stimulus may vary (e.g., extrapyramidal dysfunction, hemisphere or brainstem lesions, or stretching of the orbicularis), the final pathway is an increase in blink excitability. Suprasegmental disinhibition or adaptive responses to peripheral lesions enhance the neuronal activity of the blink pathways.

Although blepharoclonus and reflex blepharospasm usually occur in patients with cortical, extrapyramidal, brain-

stem, and trigeminal disturbances, some patients with these conditions have no evidence of neurologic disease (432).

Ocular Blepharospasm

Blepharospasm occasionally is caused by irritative or painful ocular disease. Photophobia and lacrimation are also present in patients with this form of blepharospasm, often called **ocular blepharospasm**. The most common causes of ocular blepharospasm are disturbances of the eyelids (e.g., blepharitis, trichiasis, entropion), disturbances of the corneal epithelium, severe dry eyes, iritis, scleritis, and angle-closure glaucoma. Although less common, patients with ocular albinism, congenital achromatopsia, aniridia, or posterior subcapsular cataracts may experience blepharospasm and photophobia in response to bright light (433). Chemotherapeutic agents such as cyclophosphamide, doxorubicin, fluorouracil, tegafur (furanyl-5-fluorouracil), and mitomycin-C (434–436) may produce ocular irritation and severe blepharospasm, as may a variety of topical medications (437.)

Rarely, patients with strabismus develop what appears to be a unilateral tonic blepharospasm to avoid diplopia. This is particularly common in patients with acquired paralytic strabismus and in patients with intermittent exotropia. It is most obvious in bright light.

In our experience, patients with essential blepharospasm often have ocular surface abnormalities that may contribute to the spasms, but true ocular blepharospasm is rare. Nevertheless, ocular causes of blepharospasm should always be excluded before a search for a neurologic cause of blepharospasm is undertaken or a diagnosis of essential blepharospasm is made.

Blepharospasm Associated with Drug-Induced Tardive Dyskinesia

Patients with tardive dyskinesia have blepharospasm and facial tics similar to those seen in patients with Meige syndrome (see above); however, patients with tardive dyskinesia have choreic movements of the extremities as opposed to the more sustained, dystonic movements observed in patients with Meige syndrome (438–440). The most important distinguishing feature of tardive dyskinesia, however, is that it is always drug-induced, usually developing 1–2 years after starting the medication. In most instances, the responsible agents are antipsychotic or neuroleptic drugs, such as dopamine-blocking or dopamine-stimulating agents (439,441–443). Drug-induced dyskinesia can also occur after the use of antiemetics, anorectics, or nasal decongestants that contain sympathomimetic agents and antihistamines (444–447). Orofacial dyskinesia developed in one patient following an overdose of carbamazepine (448).

From 15–30% of patients on continuous neuroleptic therapy eventually develop tardive dyskinesia (449–452). The risk of acquiring this complication increases with higher doses and prolonged use of the drug, and with increasing age of the patient. Women are more frequently affected than men.

The blepharospasm and facial tics of tardive dyskinesia may improve if the drug responsible is identified and discontinued. If the symptoms persist, or if the drug cannot be stopped for medical reasons, botulinum toxin can be used to control the spasms.

In contrast to tardive dyskinesia, which occurs 1–2 years after initiating drug therapy, some patients develop an acute dystonic reaction after 2–5 days on neuroleptics. The reaction usually consists of abnormal posturing and intermittent or sustained muscle spasms, but some patients develop blepharospasm or oculogyric crises. This reaction is more likely to occur among young patients on high doses of medication (452).

Facial Tics and Tourette Syndrome

In contrast to the sustained, dystonic movements typical of blepharospasm, facial tics are usually brief, clonic, and jerk-like. They tend to be stereotyped and repetitive. They can vary in frequency, increasing when the patient is bored, tired, or anxious. Eye-winking tics are most commonly observed in childhood, tend to be unilateral, and affect boys more often than girls. They resolve spontaneously after months or years (352).

When facial tics begin between 2 and 15 years of age, last more than 1 year, fluctuate in severity, and are associated with tics in multiple other bodily locations, vocalizations (e.g., grunting, sniffing, barking, throat-clearing, utterance of obscenities), obscene gestures, and other aberrancies of behavior, Tourette syndrome (also called Gilles de la Tourette syndrome) is the likely diagnosis (400,453–456). Ocular manifestations are common in this condition and include increased blinking, blepharospasm, forced staring, and involuntary gaze deviation (456,457).

Patients with Tourette syndrome have enhanced recovery cycles (372). In addition, tics and blepharospasm may coexist in the same patient and among other family members. These findings suggest that many of these disorders share common underlying mechanisms.

Nonorganic Blepharospasm

Nonorganic blepharospasm generally has a sudden onset and usually is preceded by an emotionally traumatic event (458,459). Although quite rare, it is more common among children and young adults with serious psychologic problems. The blepharospasm is frequently bilateral and may last for hours, weeks, or even months, at which point it may resolve spontaneously. The eyelids are sometimes gently, sometimes forcibly, closed. In some patients, psychotherapy, behavior therapy, hypnosis, or biofeedback are of benefit (460–462). In others, a single injection of botulinum toxin is sufficient to eliminate the spasms permanently.

Focal Seizures

Several eyelid phenomena are associated with seizures. An adversive (jacksonian) seizure from an irritative focus in the frontal eye fields can evoke contralateral spasmodic eyelid closure, twitching of the face, and "spastic" lateral gaze. Blinking or fluttering of the eyelids also may be observed in psychomotor or absence seizures (463–465).

Blinking is usually bilateral and symmetric, although unilateral blinking ipsilateral to the seizure focus has been described (466).

A form of **photomyoclonic epilepsy** consists of the combination of eyelid "myoclonia" and absence spells. Upon closure of the eyelids, patients with this condition experience marked eyelid spasms, upward deviation of the eyes, and brief periods during which they seem unaware of their surroundings (i.e., absence spells) and electroencephalography shows bilateral 3–5 Hz spike-and-wave discharges (465,467). These seizures are triggered by the elimination of central fixation (i.e., they are fixation-off sensitive) (468). The marked jerking of the lids during eyelid closure and the upward gaze deviation that occur in photomyoclonic epilepsy usually are sufficient to distinguish this condition from the slight flutter of the eyelids unassociated with ocular gaze deviation that is seen in patients with pure absence seizures.

Seizures induced by eyelid closure or blinking represent a rare form of stimulus-sensitive epilepsy (usually absences or myoclonic attacks). The stimulus responsible for inducing the seizure in some cases is presumed to be proprioceptive. In other cases, a loss of central fixation brought on by eyelid closure precipitates the seizure. In addition, a decrease in retinal illumination alone, or with eyelid closure, is sufficient to induce a "scotosensitive" seizure (469–476).

Lid-Triggered Synkinesias

Eyelid closure occasionally triggers movements of muscles that are not innervated by the facial nerve, presumably from a central or supranuclear disturbance (477). In one patient with a progressive neurodegenerative condition of unknown etiology, eyelid closure was associated with mouth opening and fanning of the fingers (478). In another case, eyelid closure was associated with closing of the hand.

In some patients with such eyelid-triggered dyskinesias, firm external stimulation of the cornea elicits a brisk anterolateral jaw movement to the side opposite the stimulus associated with eyelid closure: the **corneomandibular reflex**. In other patients, an acquired **palpebromandibular synkinesia** is present that is similar to the corneomandibular reflex except that the jaw movements that regularly accompany spontaneous eye blinks can occur without an external corneal stimulus (479). The palpebromandibular reflex usually is associated with bihemispheric or upper brainstem pathology.

Facial Myokymia (with and without Spastic Paretic Facial Contracture)

The term facial myokymia refers to involuntary, fine, continuous, undulating contractions that spread across facial muscles. The contractions are usually unilateral. Electrophysiologically, affected muscles show brief tetanic bursts of motor-unit potentials that recur in a rhythmic or semirhythmic fashion several times a second as singlets, doublets, or groups (480–482). These bursts recur at a rate of 3–8 Hz.

The most common type of facial myokymia occurs in otherwise normal persons and affects only the orbicularis oculi of the lower (or, occasionally, the upper) eyelid on one side. This **eyelid myokymia** often begins at times of excessive fatigue or stress. It usually lasts for several days, but it may persist for a few weeks and even for several months. During this time, it is usually intermittent, lasting for several hours at a time. Patients with this condition may become alarmed, particularly because they can feel the eyelid fasciculations. They often believe that their eye is "jumping," and some patients actually experience oscillopsia from the effects of the myokymic eyelid against the globe (483); however, this type of transient eyelid myokymia is almost always benign.

Eyelid myokymia that persists continuously for several months or even years may be an isolated phenomenon of no systemic or neurologic significance; however, it also may be the first sign of MS or an intrinsic lesion near the facial nerve nucleus in the dorsal pons. Thus, we believe that patients in whom isolated eyelid myokymia persists for more than 3 months should undergo MR imaging, as should patients with eyelid myokymia who have or develop other neurologic manifestations.

Many disorders characterized by involuntary movements of the facial muscles can begin with eyelid myokymia, including essential blepharospasm, Meige syndrome, hemifacial spasm, and **spastic-paretic facial contracture**. This last disorder is characterized by myokymia that first begins in the orbicularis oculi muscle and gradually spreads to most of the muscles on one side of the face. At the same time, associated tonic contracture of the affected muscles becomes evident. Over a period of weeks or months, the nasolabial groove slowly deepens, the corner of the mouth is drawn laterally, the palpebral fissure narrows, and all the facial muscles become weak. As the contracture becomes more pronounced, voluntary facial movements on the affected side diminish (Fig. 24.56). Spastic-paretic facial contracture is a sign of pontine dysfunction in the region of the facial nerve nucleus. Disorders that may produce it include MS (484,485), intrinsic brainstem neoplasms (particularly gliomas but also metastatic tumors) (486–489), extra-axial neoplasms compressing the brainstem (e.g., chordomas) (489,490), syringobulbia (491), brainstem vascular lesions (493), GBS (482), obstructive hydrocephalus (493), subarachnoid hemorrhage (494), basilar invagination (495), Machado-Joseph disease (496), brainstem tuberculoma (497), cysticercosis (398), and autosomal-dominant striatonigral degeneration (483). In most instances, the phenomenon and the pathology that causes it are unilateral, but bilateral facial myokymia from bilateral pontine disease may occur in patients with GBS (482,500,501), following cardiopulmonary arrest (502), during the course of a lymphocytic meningoradiculitis (503), and following exposure to a variety of toxins (492,504).

The pathophysiology of transient facial myokymia is unknown. MR imaging in patients with MS who have continuous facial myokymia often shows changes consistent with demyelination in the postgenu portion of the fascicle of the facial nerve in the dorsolateral pontine tegmentum (485). In all autopsy cases in which a brainstem tumor is responsible for the condition, the tumor infiltrates the pontine tegmen-

tum, basis pontis, or both, sparing the facial nerve nucleus and its neurons (486,488,489,505). It has therefore been suggested that the lack of direct damage to the ipsilateral facial nerve nucleus in the presence of more rostrally placed lesions produces a functional deafferentation, possibly of local circuit neurons. This, in turn, results in hyperexcitability of facial nerve neurons, thus causing myokymia or spastic-paretic facial contracture (487,489). When the facial nerve nucleus itself is damaged by the pathologic process, the facial spasm resolves, leaving only facial paralysis and contracture (492,497). This hypothesis explains the phenomenon of facial myokymia and spastic-paretic facial contracture in patients with brainstem lesions but not in patients with peripheral neuropathies (discussion following).

Facial Myokymia with Peripheral Neuropathy

The development of facial myokymia in patients with GBS, poliomyelitis, parotid gland tumor, and some other disorders of the peripheral facial nerve (506–508) indicates that damage to the peripheral facial nerve alone can produce hyperactivity of facial muscles. Other evidence that peripheral nerve injury can produce facial hyperactivity includes EMG studies that reveal that myokymia is common in patients with Bell's palsy (509), and the observation that timber rattlesnake evenomation causes facial myokymia from damage to the peripheral portion of the facial nerve (510). Thus, the occurrence of facial myokymia in a patient with apparent peripheral facial nerve dysfunction does not necessarily indicate an underlying central process (501). Myokymic discharges of peripheral nerve origin are usually attributed to spontaneous ectopic excitation arising in demyelinated fibers.

Hemifacial Spasm

Hemifacial spasm (HFS) is characterized by involuntary paroxysmal bursts of painless, unilateral, tonic or clonic contractions of muscles innervated by the facial nerve (Fig. 24.57). It occurs most commonly in middle-aged adults, but it may develop at any age, including infancy and childhood (511–515). The condition is almost always sporadic, but there are familial cases (516–518). Bilateral cases occur but are exceptionally rare (511,519), and some reported cases may actually be examples of blepharospasm with Meige syndrome.

HFS usually first appears as spasms of the orbicularis oculi and then spreads slowly to the lower facial muscles over months to years. The spasms may occur spontaneously or be triggered by voluntary facial movements or changes in position (520), and they may worsen with fatigue, stress, or anxiety. Long-standing HFS almost always is associated with ipsilateral lower facial weakness (521,522), although this may be hard to detect, either because it usually is fairly mild or because of the constant spasms. In any event, facial movements between spasms usually appear normal. Most patients with HFS have clinical evidence, EMG evidence, or both, of synkinesis between the orbicularis oculi and orbicularis oris muscles (523).

There is considerable evidence, based primarily on direct

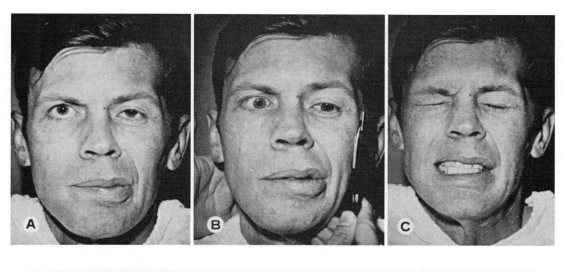

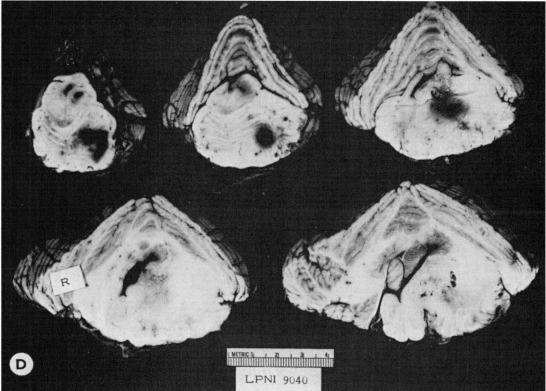

Figure 24.56. Spastic paretic facial contracture associated with a pontine astrocystoma. *A*, The patient's face is at rest. Note deepened nasolabial groove and narrowed palpebral fissure on the left. *B*, On attempted left gaze, the patient shows a horizontal gaze palsy. *C*, Voluntary forced eyelid closure exposes the paresis of the left orbicularis oculi and the left side of the face. The patient subsequently died and an autopsy was performed. *D*, Serial sections through the brainstem of the patient show a left-sided astrocytoma. (From Sogg RL, Hoyt WF, Boldrey E. Spastic paretic facial contracture: A rare sign of brain stem tumor. Neurology 1963;13:607–612.)

observations at surgery, that most cases of HFS are caused by pulsatile compression of the proximal region of the facial nerve at the root entry zone (the transitional zone between central and peripheral myelin) by normal vessels in an aber- rant location (524–530) or by dolichoectatic vessels (528,531). The blood vessels most commonly responsible for the compression are the anterior inferior cerebellar artery, the posterior inferior cerebellar artery, and the vertebral ar-

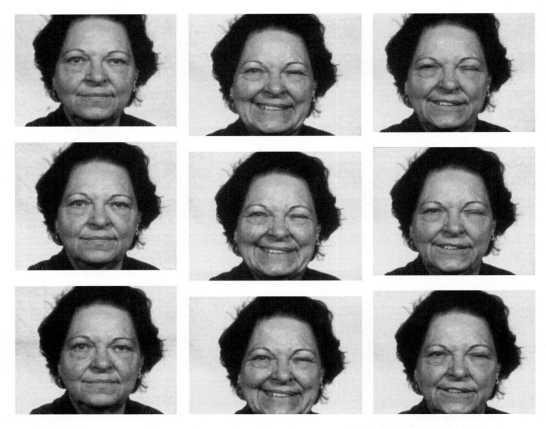

Figure 24.57. Left hemifacial spasm. Photograph is a composite of multiple frames of a video that shows the development of the hemifacial spasm. Note that between spasms, the patient's face appears normal; however, when the spasms occur, the left side of the mouth draws up, the midfacial muscles contract, and the left eyelid closes. (From Garibaldi DC, Miller NR. Tortuous basilar artery as etiology of hemifacial spasm. Arch Neurol 2003;60:626–627.)

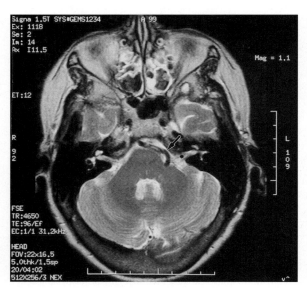

Figure 24.58. Neuroimaging showing vascular compression of the left facial nerve in a the patient with ipsilateral hemifacial spasm shown in Figure 24.57. Proton-density magnetic resonance image, axial view, shows compression of the left facial nerve (*) by a tortuous basilar artery (*arrow*). The patient was treated successfully with botulinum toxin A. (From Garibaldi DC, Miller NR. Tortuous basilar artery as etiology of hemifacial spasm. Arch Neurol 2003;60:626–627.)

tery. Less commonly, one or more veins accompanying these vessels appear to be responsible. A variety of imaging techniques, including CT scanning, MR imaging, MR angiography, and CT angiography may show ipsilateral displacement, tortuosity, or enlargement of the basilar or vertebral arteries in patients with HFS (532–537) (Fig. 24.58).

Although HFS appears to be caused by vascular compression from otherwise normal arteries or veins in over 99% of cases, vascular structures other than normal vessels also can compress the facial nerve at the root entry zone, producing HFS. These lesions include aneurysms (524, 531,538–540), AVMs (524,540), infratemporal hemangiomas (541), and arterial dissections (542) (Fig. 24.59). Extra-axial tumors located in the CPA can produce HFS. These include epidermoids, vestibular schwannomas (acoustic neuromas), meningiomas, cholesteatomas, and lipomas (543–545). Occasionally, HSF is produced by intraparenchymal brainstem lesions, including tumors and granulomas (546,547). Other rare causes include arachnoid cysts (548,549), MS (546), pontine infarction (550), hemosiderosis (551), arachnoiditis (552), and lesions or structural abnormalities of the bone of the skull base (553–557). HFS may occur as a false localizing sign in patients with tumors located in the contralateral CPA (558,559) and in patients with pseudotumor cerebri (560). It may also occur after injury to the peripheral facial nerve (512,561–563). In some cases, HFS is associated with evidence of hyperactivity of other cranial nerves. The most common association is with trigeminal neuralgia (564–566).

Although there is general agreement regarding the importance of facial nerve decompression in the treatment of HFS (discussion following), the underlying neurophysiologic mechanism that produces the condition remains controversial (523,567–569). One theory is that HFS is the result of ephaptic transmission or crosstalk between branches of the facial nerve at the root entry zone; for example, in an area of demyelination (523,526,570–574). Another theory, however, is that the facial motor nucleus changes in response to

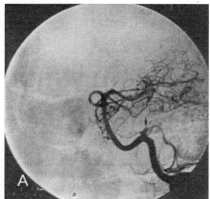

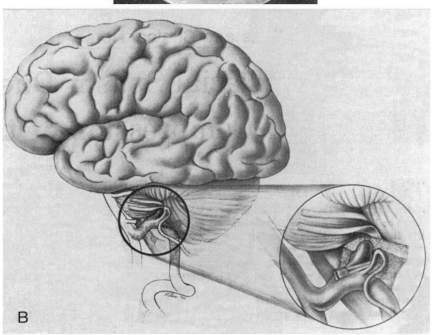

Figure 24.59. Hemifacial spasm caused by an intracranial aneurysm. *A*, In a patient with left-sided hemifacial spasm, a vertebral artery angiogram (oblique projection) shows an aneurysm at the origin of the posterior inferior cerebellar artery (*arrow*). *B*, Schematic representation of the aneurysmal compression of the left facial nerve before and after clipping and mobilization of the aneurysm. (From Maroon JC, Lunsford LD, Deeb ZL. Hemifacial spasm due to aneurysmal compression of the facial nerve. Arch Neurol 1978;35:545–546.)

peripheral nerve injury (546,547,575–579). Central anatomic change in response to peripheral nerve injury is a well-established phenomenon that could theoretically unmask synkinetic facial movements (561). It has also been suggested that chronic pulsatile arterial antidromic stimulation of the facial nerve increases the excitability of facial motor neurons through a phenomenon called ''kindling'' (577–580).

There appears to be a subgroup of patients with HFS who have no obvious vascular compression yet improve after surgery. The improvement in such patients may be consequent to mild operative trauma and manipulation of the nerve since the nerve was not decompressed (581–583). In addition, the severity of vascular compression observed in patients with HFS is extremely variable, ranging from obvious displacement and grooving of the facial nerve, to displacement without grooving, and to touching without either displacement or grooving. That veins and, in some cases, venules, can cause HFS by apparent compression of the facial nerve is also problematic.

The only way to cure HFS is posterior fossa microvascular decompression (524–525,527–529,538,581,584–587). Although this procedure has potential mortality and a well-defined morbidity (discussion following), the results are generally excellent. When performed by an experienced surgeon, the overall cure rate is 85–90%. In most patients who are cured, the HFS disappears within 3–10 days after surgery, although in a smaller group, resolution can take weeks to months. Among patients whose HFS persists or recurs after apparently successful surgery (i.e., the vessel compressing the nerve is identified and moved), 5–10% are cured after a second operation (587).

The complication rate of posterior fossa microvascular decompression for HFS, like the success rate, varies according to the experience of the surgeon performing the operation. In some series, the complication rate is reported to be as high as 25%; in others, it is 1–2% (523,586,587). The most common persistent complications are ipsilateral hearing loss (1–13%) and facial paralysis (1–6%). The mortality with this procedure is exceptionally low; however, death or disabling stroke from brainstem or cerebellar infarction can occur.

The results of medical therapy for HFS are generally disappointing. The most commonly used drugs are carbamazepine (Tegretol) (588,589), diphenylhydantoin (Dilantin), and dimethylaminoethanol (Deanol) (590). Gabapentin (Neurontin) has also been reported to be of value in selected patients.

Surgical procedures other than microvascular decompression, including intracanalicular facial nerve neurotomy (591) and partial avulsion, section, longitudinal splitting, or radiofrequency destruction of the extracranial portion of the facial nerve (592–594), generally produce disappointing results. In some instances, after section of the facial nerve, a hypoglossal-facial anastomosis is performed to relieve the resultant facial paralysis (595). None of these procedures is without complication, and the recurrence rate is considerable.

Intramuscular injections of botulinum toxin can be used to control, but not cure, HFS (596,597). In our opinion, this mode of therapy is the best alternative for patients who are unwilling or unable to undergo posterior fossa microvascular decompression of the facial nerve (see above). Other injectable drugs, particularly doxorubicin (Adriamycin) continue to be investigated (598,599).

Excessive Eyelid Closure of Neuromuscular Origin

Neuromuscular hyperexcitability of the orbicularis oculi usually is part of a generalized disorder. The excitability may be latent, spasmodic, or constant. In hypoparathyroidism or during hyperventilation, a tap over the lateral orbital margin produces contraction of the ipsilateral orbicularis muscles and the surrounding facial muscles (latent hyperexcitability). Strychnine poisoning causes spasmodic hyperexcitability and tetanus causes a constant or sustained neuromuscular hyperexcitability manifested in the facial muscles as **risus sardonicus** (600–602) (Fig. 24.60).

Excessive Eyelid Closure of Myopathic Origin

Myotonia of the orbicularis oculi may occur in association with a number of disorders. For example, patients can develop eyelid myotonia in association with primary hypothyroidism (603,604). The myotonia typically disappears after such patients are treated with replacement thyroid medication (Fig. 24.61).

Patients with both the congenital and adult forms of myotonic dystrophy may show myotonia of the orbicularis oculi.

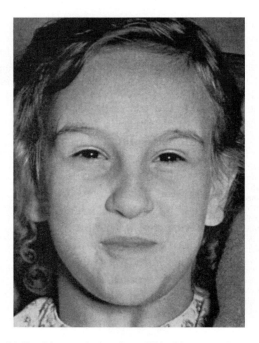

Figure 24.60. Risus sardonicus in a child with tetanus. Increased tone of all facial muscles is evident. Note that the child appears to be smiling. Her apparent bilateral ptosis is caused by myotonia of the orbicularis oculi muscles. (From Ford FR. Diseases of the Nervous System in Infancy, Childhood and Adolescence, 5th Ed 5. Springfield, IL: CC Thomas, 1966:621.)

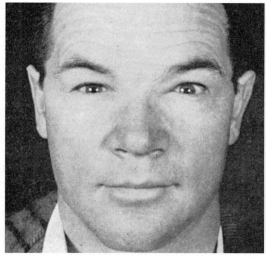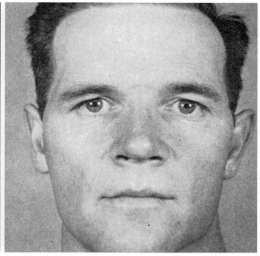

A   B

Figure 24.61. Myotonia of the orbicularis oculi in a patient with hypothyroidism. Both photographs were taken 2 seconds after forceful closure of the patient's eyelids. *A,* The patient has difficulty opening the eyes due to myotonia of the orbicularis oculi muscles. *B,* After thyroid hormone therapy was instituted, the patient's myotonia disappeared. (From Sisson JC, Beierwaltes WH, Koepke GH, et al. "Myotonia" of the orbicularis oculi with myxedema. Arch Intern Med 1962;110:323–327.)

One infant with congenital myotonic dystrophy exhibited a startle response to a loud noise or a bright light that produced tight eye closure followed by slow opening over many seconds (605). In adults with myotonic dystrophy, EMG studies demonstrate evidence of prolonged contraction in the orbicularis oculi following a blink (606) (see Chapter 22).

Myotonia of the orbicularis oculi may occur in patients with hyperkalemic familial periodic paralysis. Slowness of eyelid opening or temporary narrowing of the palpebral fissure may occur following sustained eyelid closure, application of ice to the lids, or administration of potassium salts (235). Eyelid myotonia can also occur in patients with chondrodystrophic myotonia (Schwartz-Jampel syndrome) (607) (see Chapter 22).

REFERENCES

1. Porter JD, Burns LA, May PJ. Morphological substrate for eyelid movements: Innervation and structure of primate levator palpebrae superioris and orbicularis oculi muscles. J Comp Neurol 1989;287:64–81.
2. Evinger C, Manning KA, Pellegrini JJ, et al. Not looking while leaping: the Linkage of blinking and saccadic gaze shifts. Exp Brain Res 1994;100:337–344.
3. Felt DP, Frueh BR. A pharmacologic study of the sympathetic eyelid tarsal muscles. Ophthalmic Plast Reconstruct Surg 1988;4:15–24.
4. Small RG, Sabates NR, Burrows D. The measurement and definition of ptosis. Ophthalmic Plastic and Reconstructive Plast Reconstruct Surg 1989;5:171–175.
5. Doxanas MT, Anderson RL. Clinical Orbital Anatomy. Baltimore: Williams & Wilkins, 1984:57–89.
6. Patrinely JR, Anderson RL. Anatomy of the orbicularis oculi and other facial muscles. In Jankovic J, Tolosa E, eds. Advances in Neurology.Vol 49: Facial Dyskinesias. Vol 49. New York: Raven Press, 1988:15–23.
7. Gordon G. Observations upon the movement of the eyelids. Br J Ophthalmol 1951;35:339–351.
8. Frueh BR. The mechanistic classification of ptosis. Ophthalmology 1980;87:1019–1021.
9. Beard C. Ptosis. Ed 3. St Louis: CV Mosby, 1981.
10. Beard C. A new classification of blepharoptosis. Int Ophthalmol Clin 1989;29:214–216.
11. Small KW, Buckley EG. Recurrent blepharoptosis secondary to a pituitary tumor. Am J Ophthalmol 1988;106:760–761.
12. Meyer DR, Linberg JV, Powell SR, et al. Quantitating the superior visual field loss associated with ptosis. Arch Ophthalmol 1989;107:840–843.
13. Cogan DG. Neurology of the Ocular Muscles. Ed 2. Springfield, IL: CC Thomas, 1956:139–148.
14. Afifi AK, Corbett JJ, Thompson HS, et al. Seizure induced miosis and ptosis: Association with temporal lobe magnetic resonance imaging abnormaltiies. J Child Neurol 1990;5:142–146.
15. Caplan LR. Cerebral ptosis. J Neurol Neurosurg Psychiatry 1974;34:1–7.
16. Averbuch-Heller L, Leigh RJ, Mermelstein V, et al. Ptosis in patients with hemispheric strokes. Neurology 2002;58:620–624.
17. Lowenstein DH, Koch TK, Edwards MS. Cerebral ptosis with contralateral arteriovenous malformation: A report of two cases. Ann Neurol 1987;21:404–407.
18. Nutt JG. Lid abnormalities secondary to cerebral hemisphere lesions. Ann Neurol 1977;1:149–151.
19. Krohel GB, Griffin JF. Cortical blepharoptosis. Am J Ophthalmol 1978;85:632–634.
20. Lepore FE. Bilateral cerebral ptosis. Neurology 1987;37:1043–1046.
21. Kishi M, Kurihara T, Kinoshita M. A case of bilateral ptosis associated with cerebral hemispheric lesions. Jpn J Psychiatry and Neurol 1990;44:585–588.
22. Corin MS, Elizan TS, Bender MB. Oculomotor function in patients with Parkinson's disease. J Neurol Sci 1972;15:251–256.
23. Boghen D. Apraxia of Eyelid Opening: A review. Neurology 1997;48:1491–1494.
24. Goldstein JE, Cogan DG. Apraxia of lid opening. Arch Ophthalmol 1965;73:155–159.
25. Lepore FE, Duvoisin RC. "Apraxia" of eyelid opening: An involuntary levator inhibition. Neurology 1985;35:423–427.
26. Dehaene I. Apraxia of eyelid-opening in progressive supranuclear palsy. [Letter]. Ann Neurol 1984;15:115–116.
27. Jankovic J. Apraxia of eyelid opening in progressive supranuclear palsy. [Reply]. Ann Neurol 1984;15:115–116.
28. Brusa A, Mancardi G, Meneghini S, et al. "Apraxia" of eye opening in idiopathic Parkinson's disease. Neurology 1986;36:134.
29. Esteban A, Gimenez-Roldan S. Involuntary closure of eyelids in parkinsonism: Electrophysiological evidence for prolonged inhibition of the levator palpebrae muscles. J Neurol Sci 1988;85:333–345.
30. Lepore FE. So-called apraxias of lid movement. Adv Neurol 1988;49:85–90.
31. Golbe LI, Davis PH, Lepore FE. Eyelid movement abnormalities in progressive supranuclear palsy. Movement Move Disord 1989;4:297–302.
32. Jordan DR, Anderson RL, Digre K. Apraxia of lid opening in blepharospasm. Ophthalmic Ophthal Surg 1990;21:331–334.
33. Aramideh M, Bour LJ, Koelman HTM, et al. Abnormal eye movements in blepharospasm and involuntary levator palpebrae inhibition: Clinical and pathophysiological considerations. Brain 1994;117:1457–1474.
34. Verghese J, Milling C, Rosenbaum DM. Ptosis, blepharospasm, and apraxia of eyelid opening secondary to putaminal hemorrhage. Neurology 1999;53:652.
35. Jankovic J, Kirkpatrick JB, Blomquist KA, et al. Adult onset Hallervorden Spatz disease presenting as familial parkinsonism. Neurology 1985;35:227–234.

36. Johnston JC, Rosenbaum DM, Piccone CM, et al. Apraxia of eyelid opening secondary to right hemispheric infarction. Ann Neurol 1989;25:622–624.

37. Keane JR. Lid-opening apraxia in Wilson's disease. J Clin Neuroophthalmol 1988;8:31–33.

38. Lepore FE, Steele JC, Cox TA, et al. Supranuclear disturbances of ocular motility in Lytico-Bodig. Neurology 1988;38:1849–1853.

39. Dewey RB Jr, Maraganore DM. Isolated eyelid opening apraxia: Report of a new levodopa-responsive syndrome. Neurology 1994;44:1752–1754.

40. Aramideh M, Ongerboer de Visser BW, Koelman JHTM, et al. Clinical and electromyographic features of levator palpebrae superioris muscle dysfunction in involuntary eyelid closure. Mov Disord 1995;9:395–402.

41. Aramideh M, Ongerboer de Visser BW, Koelman JHTM, et al. Motor persistence of orbicularis oculi muscle in eyelid-opening disorders. Neurology 1995;45:897–902.

42. Elston JS. A new variant of blepharospasm. J Neurol Neurosurg Psychiatry 1992;55:369–371.

43. Newman G. Treatment of progressive supranuclear palsy with tricyclic antidepressants. Neurology 1985;35:1189–1193.

44. Katz B, Rosenberg JH. Botulinum therapy for apraxia of eyelid opening. Am J Ophthalmol 1987;103:718–719.

45. Mauriello JA Jr, Coniaris H, Haupt EJ. Use of botulinum toxin in the treatment of one 100 patients with facial dyskinesias. Ophthalmology 1987;94:976–979.

46. Pham RTH, Levine MR, Marcotty A. Congenital synkinetic movements associated with elevation of the upper eyelid. Ophthalmic Plast Reconstruct Surg 1994; 10:30–33.

47. Walsh FB, Hoyt WF. Clinical Neuro-Ophthalmology. Ed 3, Vol 1. Baltimore, Williams & Wilkins, 1969:315.

48. Rice CD, Weaver RG, Benjamin E, et al. Unilateral blepharoptosis with synkinetic movements of the eyelids on horizontal gaze. J Pediatr Ophthalmol Strabis 1986;23:201–205.

49. Sen DK. Paradoxical movements of the eyelid and eyeball. J Pediatr Ophthalmol Strabis 1979;23:201.

50. Lubkin V. The inverse Marcus Gunn phenomenon: An electromyographic contribution. Arch Neurol 1978;35:249.

51. Barton JJS, Kardon RH, Slagel D, et al. Bilateral central ptosis in acquired immunodeficiency syndrome. Can J Neurol Sci 1995;22:52–55.

52. Martin TJ, Corbett JJ, Babikian PV, et al. Bilateral ptosis due to mesencephalic lesions with relative preservation of ocular motility. J Neuroophthalmol 1996; 16:258–263.

53. Stevenson GC, Hoyt WF. Metastasis to midbrain from mammary carcinoma: Cause of bilateral ptosis and ophthalmoplegia. JAMA 1963;186:514–516.

54. Growdon JH, Winkler GF, Wray SH. Midbrain ptosis: A case with clinicopathologic correlation. Arch Neurol 1974;30:179–181.

55. Meienberg O, Mumenthaler M, Karbowski K. Quadriparesis and nuclear oculomotor palsy with total bilateral ptosis mimicking coma: A mesencephalic "locked-in syndrome"? Arch Neurol 1979;36:708–710.

56. Conway VH, Rozdilsky B, Schneider RJ, et al. Isolated bilateral complete ptosis. Can J Ophthalmol 1983;18:37–40.

57. Saeki N, Yamaura A, Sunami K. Bilateral ptosis with pupil sparing because of a discrete midbrain lesion: magnetic resonance imaging evidence of topographic arrangement within the oculomotor nerve. J Neuroophthalmol 2000;20:130–134.

58. Ragge NK, Hoyt WF. Midbrain myasthenia: fatigable ptosis, lid twitch sign and ophthalmoparesis from a dorsal midbrain glioma. Neurology 1992;42:917–919.

59. Brodsky MC, Boop FA. Lid nystagmus as a sign of intrinsic midbrain disease. J Neuroophthalmol 1995;15:236–240.

60. Parmeggiani A, Posar A, Leonardi M, et al. Neurological imparment in congenital bilateral ptosis with ophthalmolplegia. Brain Dev 1992;14:107–109.

61. Hopfer HC, Gutmann L. Diabetic 3rd neve palsy: Evidence for mesencephalic lesion. Neurology 1990;40:1041–1045.

62. Bartleson JD, Trautmann JC, Sundt TM. Minimal oculomotor nerve paresis secondary to unruptured intracranial aneurysm. Arch Neurol 1986;43:1015–1020.

63. Good EF. Ptosis as the sole manifestation of compression of the oculomotor nerve by an aneurysm of the posterior communication artery. J Clin Neuroophthalmol 1990;10:59–61.

64. Small RG, Fransen SR, Adams R, et al. The effect of phenylephrine on Müller muscle: A blepharogram study of eyelid motion. Ophthalmology 1995;102:599–606.

65. Yen MY, Liu JH, Jaw SJ. Ptosis as the early manifestation of pituitary tumor. Br J Ophthalmol 1990;74:188–191.

66. Miller NR. Walsh and Hoyt's Clinical Neuro-Ophthalmology. Ed 4, Vol 2. Baltimore, Williams & Wilkins, 1985:940.

67. Wand O. Ptosis associated with aseptic meningitis. Arch Ophthalmol 1972;88:334–335.

68. Stidham DB, Butler IJ. Recurrent isolated ptosis in presumed ophthalmoplegic migraine of childhood. Ophthalmology 2000;107:1476–1478.

69. McCulley TJ, Kersten RC, Yip CC, et al. Isolated unilateral neurogenic blepharoptosis secondary to eyelid trauma. Am J Ophthalmol 2002;134:626–627.

70. Berstein LP, Henkind P. Additional information on adverse reactions to timolol. Am J Ophthalmol 1981;92:295–296.

71. Dixon RS, Anderson RL, Hatt MU. The use of thymoxamine in eyelid retraction. Arch Ophthalmol 1979;97:2147–2150.

72. Chitkara DK, Hudson JM. Blepharoptosis caused by systemic thymoxamine. Arch Ophthalmol 1991;111:524–525.

73. Dryden RM, Kahanic DA. Worsening of blepharoptosis in downgaze. Ophthalmic Plast Recontruct Surg 1992;8:126–129.

74. Wojno TH. Downgaze ptosis. Ophthalmic Plastic Reconstruct Surg 1993;9:83–89.

75. Meyer DR, Rheeman CH. Downgaze eyelid position in patients with blepharoptosis. Ophthalmology 1995;102:1517–1523.

76. Olsen JJ, Putterman A. Loss of vertical palpebral fissure height on downgaze in acquired ptosis. Arch Ophthalmol 1996;113:1293–1297.

77. Deady JP, Morell AJ, Sutton GA. Recognizing aponeurotic ptosis. J Neurol Neurosurg Psychiatry 1989;52:996–998.

78. Jones LT, Quickert MD, Wobig JL. The cure of ptosis by aponeurotic repair. Arch Ophthalmol 1975;93:629–634.

79. Paris GL, Quickert MH. Disinsertion of the aponeurosis of the levator palpebrae superioris muscle after cataract extraction. Am J Ophthalmol 1976;81:337–340.

80. Dortzbach RK, Sutula FC. Involutional blepharoptosis: A histopathological study. Arch Ophthalmol 1980;98:2045–2049.

81. Sutula FC. Histological changes in congenital and acquired blepharoptosis. Eye 1988;2:179–184.

82. Epstein G, Putterman AM. Acquired blepharoptosis secondary to contact lens wear. Am J Ophthalmol 1981;91:634.

83. von den Bosch WA, Lemji HG. Blepharoptosis induced by prolonged hard contact lens. Ophthalmology 1992;99:1759–1765.

84. Kersten RC, Conciliis C, Kulwin DR. Acquired ptosis in the young and middle-aged adult population. Ophthalmology 1995;102:924–928.

85. Paris GL, Beard C. Blepharoptosis following dermolipoma surgery. Ann Ophthalmol 1973;5:697–699.

86. Alpar JJ. Acquired ptosis following cataract and glaucoma surgery. Glaucoma 1982;4:66–68.

87. Baylis HI, Sutcliffe T, Fett DR. Levator injury during blepharoplasty. Arch Ophthalmol 1984;102:570–571.

88. Kaplan LJ, Jaffe JS, Clayman JM. Ptosis and cataract surgery: A multivariant computer analysis of a prospective study. Ophthalmology 1985;92:237–242.

89. Linberg JV, McDonald MB, Safir A. Ptosis following radial keratotomy. Ophthalmology 1986;93:1509–1512.

90. Rainin EA, Carlson BM. Postoperative diplopia and ptosis: a clinical hypothesis based on the myotoxicity of local anesthetics. Arch Ophthal 1985;103:1337–1339.

91. Arden RL, Moore GK. Complete post traumatic ptosis: a mechanism of recovery. Laryngoscope 1989;99:1175–1179.

92. Loeffler M, Solomon LD, Renaud M. Postcataract extraction ptosis: Effect of the bridle suture. J Cat Refract Surg 1990;16:501–504.

93. Feibel RM, Custer PL, Gordon MO. Post catarct ptosis: A randomized double masked comparison of peribulbar and retrobulbar anesthesia. Ophthalmology 1993;100:660–665.

94. Older JJ. Levator aponeurosis disinsertion in the young adult: A cause of ptosis. Arch Ophthalmol 1978;96:1857–1858.

95. Anderson RL, Gordy DD. Aponeurotic defects in congenital ptosis. Ophthalmology 1979;86:1493–1499.

96. Berke RN, Wadsworth JAC. Histology of levator muscle in congenital and acquired ptosis. Arch Ophthalmol 1955;53:413–428.

97. Spaeth EB. An analysis of the causes, types, and factors important in the correction of congenital blepharoptosis. Am J Ophthalmol 1971;71:696–717.

98. Harrad RA, Graham CM, Collin JRO. Amblyopia and strabismus in congenital ptosis. Eye 1998;2:625–627.

99. Anderson RL, Baumgartner SA. Strabis in ptosis. Arch Ophthalmol 1980;98:1062–1067.

100. Anderson RL, Baumgartner SA. Amblyopia in ptosis. Arch Ophthalmol 1980;98:1068–1069.

101. Merriam WW, Ellis FD, Helveston EM. Congenital blepharoptosis, anisometropia, and amblyopia. Am J Ophthalmol 1980;89:401–407.

102. Hoyt CS, Stone RD, Fromer D, et al. Monocular axial myopia associated with neonatal eyelid closure in human infants. Am J Ophthalmol 1981;91:197–200.

103. Sevel D. Ptosis and underaction of the superior rectus muscle. Ophthalmology 1984;91:1080–1085.

104. Oley C, Baraitser M. Blepharophimosis, ptosis, epicanthus inversus syndrome (BPES syndrome). J Med Genetics 1988;25:47–51.

105. Hertle RW, Katowitz JA, Young TL, et al. Congenital unilateral fibrosis, blepharoptosis, and enophthalmos syndrome. Ophthalmology 1992;99:347–355.

106. Mansour AM, Wang F, Hekund P, et al. Ocular findings in the facioauriculovertebral sequence (Goldenhar-Gorlin syndrome). Am J Ophthalmol 1985;100:555–559.

107. Duker JS, Weiss JS, Siber M, et al. Ocular findings in a new heritable syndrome of brain, eye and urogenital abnormalties. Am J Ophthalmol 1985;99:51–55.

108. Larned DE, Flanagan JC, Nelson LE, et al. The association of congenital ptosis and congenital heart disease. Ophthalmology 1986;93:492–494.

109. Tsukahara M, Azuno Y, Kajii T. Type A1 brachydactyly, dwarfism, ptosis,

mixed partial hearing loss, microcephaly and mental retardation. Am J Med Genet 1989;33:7–9.

110. Gerates WJ. Ocular Syndromes. Philadelphia, Lea & Febiger, 1969.

111. Jones KL. Smith's Recognizable Patterns of Human Malformation. Ed 3. WB Saunders, Philadelphia, 1982.

112. Snead JW, Seidenstein L, Knific RJ, et al. Isolated orbital sarcoidosis as a cause of blepharoptosis. Am J Ophthalmol 1991;112:739.

113. Gonnering RS, Sonneland PR. Ptosis and dermatochalasis as presenting signs in a case of occult primary systemic amyloidosis (AL). Ophthalmic Surg 1986; 18:495–496.

114. Bastiaensen LAK. Narrowing of the palpebral fissure in diabetes. Doc Ophthalmol 1983;56:5–10.

115. Klapper SR, Jordan DR, Pelletier C, et al. Ptosis in Waldenstrom's macroglobulinemia. Am J Ophthalmol 1998;126:315–317.

116. Hill VE, Brownstein S, Jordan DR. Ptosis secondary to amyloidosis of the tarsal conjunctiva and tarsus. Am J Ophthalmol 1997;123:852–854.

117. Uddin JM, Rose GE. Downgaze :hang: Hang-up'' of the upper eyelid in patients with adult-onset prosis: An important sign of possible orbital malignancy. Ophthalmology 2003;110:1433–6.and Rose, 20031436.

118. Satici A, Gurler B, Gurel MS, et al. Mechanical ptosis and lagophthalmos in cutaneous leishmaniasis. Br J Ophthalmol 1998;82:975.

119. Chaudry IA, Hylton C, DesMarchais B. Bilateral ptosis and lower eyelid ectropion secondary to cutaneous leishmaniasis. Arch Ophthalmol 1998;116: 1244–1245.

120. Cogan DG. Paralysis of down-gaze. Arch Ophthalmol 1974;91:192–199.

121. LoBue TD, Feldon SE. Reverse Collier's sign: Pseudoblepharoptosis associated with downgaze paralysis. Am J Ophthalmol 1983;95:120–121.

122. Safran AB. Clues to the diagnosis of functional unilateral blepharoptosis. Amer J Ophthalmol 1985;99:612–613.

123. Crawford JS, Iliff CE, Stasior OG. Symposium on congenital ptosis. J Pediatr Ophthalmol Strabis 1982;19:245–258.

124. Iliff NT. Surgery of the eyelids and lacrimal drainage apparatus. In: Rice TA, Michels RG, Stark WJ, eds. Ophthalmic Surgery. Ed 4. St Louis, CV Mosby, 1984:30–38.

125. Schaefer AJ, Schaefer DD. Classification and correction of ptosis. In: Stewart WB, ed. Ophthalmology Monographs 8. Surgery of the Eyelid, Orbit and Lacrimal System. Ophthalmology Monographs 8, Vol 2. San Francisco, American Academy of Ophthalmology, 1993:84–133.

126. McCord CD. Eyelid Surgery: Principles and Techniques. Philadelphia, Lippincott-Raven, 1995.

127. Smith JL. Pathologic lid retraction and lid position in neurology. In: Smith JL, ed. Neuro-Ophthalmology Update. New York, Masson, 1977:9–16.

128. Bartley GB. The differential diagnosis and classification of eyelid retractions. Ophthalmology 1996;103:168–176.

129. Berlin L. Compulsive eye opening and associated phenomena. Arch Neurol Psychiatr 1955;73:597–601.

130. Fisher CM. Left hemiplegia and motor impersistence. J Nerv Ment Dis 1956; 123:201–218.

131. Collier J. Nuclear ophthalmoplegia: With especial reference to retraction of lids and ptosis and to lesions of posterior commissure. Brain 1927;50:488–498.

132. Gaymard B, Lafitte C, Gelot A, et al. Plus-minus syndrome. J Neurol Neurosurg Psychiatry 1992;55:846–848.

133. Galetta SL, Gray LG, Raps EC, et al. Unilateral ptosis and contralateral eyelid retraction from a thalamic midbrain infarction. J Clin Neuroophthalmol 1993; 13:221–224.

134. Keane JR. The pretectal syndrome. Neurology 1990;40:684–690.

135. Friedman DI, Jankovic J, McCrary JA. Neuro-ophthalmic findings in progressive supranuclear palsy. J Clin Neuroophthalmol 1992;12:104–109.

136. Grandas F, Esteban A. Eyelid motor abnormalities in progressive supranuclear palsy. J Neural Transm 1994;42 (Suppl):33–41.

137. Sudarsky L, Corwin L, Dawson DM. Machado-Joseph disease in New England: Clinical description and distinction for the olivopontocerebellar atrophies. Mov Disord 1992;7:204–208.

138. Keane JR. Lid-lag in the Guillain-Barré syndrome. Arch Neurol 1975;32: 478–479.

139. Neetens A, Smet H. Lid-lag in Guillain-Barré-Strohl syndrome. Arch Neurol 1988;45:1046–1047.

140. Tan E, Kansu T, Kirkali P, et al. Lid-lag and the Guillain-Barré syndrome. J Clin Neuroophthalmol 1990;10:121–123.

141. Rubin SE, Calhoun JH. Assessing levator palpebrae superioris muscle function in infants. Am J Ophthalmol 1984;98:377–378.

142. Miller NR. Walsh and Hoyt's Clinical Neuro-Ophthalmology Ed 4, Vol 2. Baltimore, Williams & Wilkins, 1985:947.

143. Hoyt CS, Mousel DK, Weber AA. Transient supranuclear disturbances of gaze in healthy neonates. Am J Ophthalmol 1980;89:708–713.

144. Miller NR. Walsh and Hoyt's Clinical Neuro-Ophthalmology Ed 4, Vol 2. Baltimore, Williams & Wilkins, 1985:948–953.

145. Keane JR. Spastic eyelids: Failure of levator inhibition in unconscious states. Arch Neurol 1975;32:695–698.

146. Galetta SL, Gray LG, Raps EC, et al. Pretectal eyelid retraction and lag. Ann Neurol 1993;33:554–557.

147. Cooper JC. Eye movements associated with myoclonus. Am J Ophthalmol 1958; 46:205–210.

148. Pick A. Kleine beiträge zur neurologie des auges. II. Über des nystagmus der bulbi begleitende gleichartige bewegungen des oberen augenlides (nystagmus des oberlides). Arch Augenheilkd 1916;80:36–40.

149. Sanders MD, Hoyt WF, Daroff RB. Lid nystagmus evoked by ocular convergence: An ocular electromyographic study. J Neurol Neurosurg Psychiatry 1968; 31:368–371.

150. Safran AB, Berney J, Safran E. Convergence-evoked eyelid nystagmus. Am J Ophthalmol 1982;93:48–51.

151. Salisachs P, Lapresle J. Upper lid jerks in Fisher syndrome. Eur Neurol 1977; 15:237–240.

152. Rohmer F, Conraux C, Collard M. Nystagmus de convergence et nystamus des paupieres. Rev oto-Neuro-Oto-Neuroophthalmol 1972;44:89–94.

153. Howard RS. A case of convergence evoked eyelid nystagmus. J Clin Neuro-ophthalmol 1986;6:169–171.

154. Daroff RB, Hoyt WF, Sanders MD, et al. Gaze-evoked eyelid and ocular nystagmus inhibited by the near reflex: unusual ocular motor phenomena in a lateral medullary syndrome. J Neurol Neurosurg Psychiatry 1968;31:362–367.

155. Sittig O. Kasuistischer beitrag zur frage des lidnystagmus nebst bemerkungen zu einer eventuellen lokalisatorischen gedeutung. Neurol Zbl 1917;36:72–74.

156. Askenasy H, Wijsenbeek H, Herzberger E. Retraction nystagmus and retraction of eyelids due to arteriovenous aneurysm of midbrain. Arch Neurol Psychiatr 1953;69:236–241.

157. Ticho U. Synkinesis of upper lid elevation occurring in horizontal eye movements. Acta Ophthalmol 1971;49:232–238.

158. Gunn RM. Congenital ptosis with peculiar associated movements of the affected lid. Trans Ophthalmol Soc UK 1883;3:283–287.

159. Sinclair WW. Abnormal associated movements of the lids. Ophthalmol Rev 1895;14:307–319.

160. Sano K. Trigemino-oculomotor synkineses. Neurologia 1959;1:29–51.

161. Kuder GG, Laws HW. Hereditary Marcus Gunn phenomenon. Can J Ophthalmol 1968;3:97–98.

162. Kirkham TH. Familial Marcus Gunn phenomenon. Br J Ophthalmol 1969;53: 282–283.

163. Walsh FB, Hoyt WF. Clinical Neuro-Ophthalmology. Ed 3, Vol 1. Baltimore, Williams & Wilkins, 1969:311–312.

164. Pratt SG, Beyer CK, Johnson CC. The Marcus Gunn phenomenon: A review of 71 cases. Ophthalmology 1984;90:27–30.

165. Duke-Elder S. System of Ophthalmology. Vol 3, Part 2. St Louis, CV Mosby, 1963:900–905.

166. Iliff CE. The optimum time for surgery in the Marcus Gunn phenomenon. Trans Am Acad Ophthalmol Otolaryngol 1970;74:1005–1010.

167. Doucet TW, Crawford JS. The quantification, natural course, and surgical results in 57 eyes with Marcus Gunn (jaw-winking) syndrome. Am J Ophthalmol 1981; 92:702–707.

168. Papst W, Rossmann H. Die ptosis der oberlides: Ihre atiologie und therapie unter besonderer berücksichtigung elektromyographischer befunde. Bibl Ophthalmol 1966;69:1–41.

169. Kirkham TH. Paradoxical elevation of eyelid on smiling. Am J Ophthalmol 1971;72:207–208.

170. Parry R. An unusual case of the Marcus Gunn syndrome. Trans Ophthalmol Soc UK 1957;77:181–185.

171. Brain WR. Diseases of the Nervous System. London, Oxford University Press, 1933:150.

172. Soria F. Fenómeno de Marcus Gunn y nistagmus voluntario. Arch Soc Oftalmol Hisp -Am 1947;7:325–334.

173. Garkal RS. Marcus Gunn phenomenon associated with synkinetic oculo-palpebral movements. Br J Ophthalmol 1961;45:566–567.

174. Oesterle CS, Faulkner WJ, Clay R, et al., Eye bobbing associated with jaw movement. Ophthalmology 1982;89:63–67.

175. Hwang JM, Park SH. A case of Marcus Gunn jaw winking and pseudo inferior oblique overation. Am J Ophthalmol 2001;131:148–150.

176. Kodsi S. Marcus Gunn jaw winking with trigemino-abducens synkinesis. J AAPOS 2000;4:316–317.

177. Isenberg S, Blechman B. Marcus Gunn jaw winking and Duane's retraction syndrome. J Ped Ophthalmol Strabis 1983;20:235–237.

178. Hamed LM, Dennehy PJ, Lingua RW. Synergistic divergence and jaw winking phenomenon. J Ped Ophthalmol Strabis 1990;27:88–90.

179. Hepler RS, Hoyt WF, Loeffler JD. Paradoxical synkinetic levator inhibition and excitation: An electromyographic study of unilateral oculopalpebral and bilateral mandibulopalpebral (Marcus Gunn) synkinesis in a 74-year-old man. Arch Neurol 1968;18:416–424.

180. Lyness RW, Collin JRO, Alexander RA, et al. Histological appearances of the levator palpebrae superioris in the Marcus Gunn phenomenon. Br J Ophthalmol 1988;72:104–109.

181. Putterman AM. Jaw-winking blepharoptosis treated by the Fasanella-Servat procedure. Am J Ophthalmol 1973;75:1016–1022.

182. Callahan MA, Callahan A. Ophthalmic Plastic and Orbital Surgery. Birmingham, AL, Aesculapius Publishing Co, 1979:69.

183. Bullock JD. Marcus Gunn jaw-winking ptosis: Classification and surgical management. J Pediatr Ophthalmol Strabis 1980;17:375–379.
184. Dillman DB, Anderson RL. Levator myectomy in synkinetic ptosis. Arch Ophthalmol 1984;102:422–423.
185. Neuhaus RW. Eyelid suspension with a transposed levator palpebrae superioris muscle. Am J Ophthalmol 1985;100:308–311.
186. Hoyt WF, Daroff RB. Supranuclear disorders of ocular control systems in man: Clinical, anatomical and physiological correlations—1969. In: Bach-y-Rita P, Collins CC, eds. The Control of Eye Movements. New York, Academic Press, 1971:221–222.
187. Pang MP, Zweifach PH, Goodwin J. Inherited levator-medial rectus synkinesis. Arch Ophthalmol 1986;104:1489–1491.
188. Schultz RO, Burian HM. Bilateral jaw winking reflex in association with multiple congenital anomalies. Arch Ophthalmol 1960;64:946–950.
189. Messe SR, Shin RK, Liu GT, et al. Oculomotor synkinesis following a midbrain stroke. Neurology 2001;57:1106–1107.
190. Lam BL, Nerad JA, Thompson HS. Paroxysmal eyelid retractions. Am J Ophthalmol 1992;114:105–107.
191. Kansu T, Subutay N. Lid retraction in myasthenia gravis. J Clin Neuroophthalmol 1987;7:145–148.
192. Lepore FE. Unilateral ptosis and Hering's law. Neurology 1988;38:319–322.
193. Kratky V, Harvey JT. Tests for contralateral pseudoretraction in blepharoptosis. Ophthalmic Plast Reconstruct Surgery 1992;8:22–25.
194. Meyer DR, Wobig JL. Detection of contralateral eyelid retraction associated with blepharoptosis. Ophthalmology 1992;99:366–375.
195. Lyon DB, Gonnering RS, Dortzbach RK, et al. Unilateral ptosis and eye dominance. Ophthalmic Plast Reconstr Surg 1993;9:237–240.
196. Gay AJ, Salmon ML, Windsor CE. Hering's law, the levators, and their relationship in disease states. Arch Ophthalmol 1967;77:157–160.
197. Vijayan N. A new post traumatic headache syndrome: Clinical and therapeutic observations. Headache 1977;17:19–22.
198. Glatt HJ, Fett DR, Putterman AM. Comparison of 2.5% and 10% phenylephrine in the elevation of upper eyelids with ptosis. Ophthalmic Surg 1990;3:173–176.
199. Munden PM, Kardon RH, Denison CE, et al. Palpebral fissure responses to topical adrenergic drugs. Am J Ophthalmol 1991;111:706–710.
200. Uncini A, De Nicola G, Di Muzio A, et al. Topical napazoline in the treatment of myopathic ptosis. Acta Neurol Scand 1993;87:322–324.
201. Puklin JE, Sacks JG, Boshes B. Transient eyelid retraction in myasthenia gravis. J Neurol Neurosurg Psychiatry 1976;39:44–47.
202. Stout AU, Borchert M. Etiology of eyelid retraction in children: A retrospective study. J Pediatr Ophthalmol Strabis 1993;30:96–99.
203. Hiles DA, Wilder LW. Congenital entropion of the upper lids. J Pediatr Ophthalmol 1969;6:157–161.
204. Zak TA. Congenital primary upper eyelid entropion. J Pediatr Ophthalmol Strabis 1984;21:69–73.
205. Collin JRO, Allen L, Castronuovo S. Congenital eyelid retraction. Br J Ophthalmol 1990;74:542–544.
206. Leone CR, Lewis R. Congenital upper eyelid retraction. J Ped Ophthalmol Strabis 1976;13:350–352.
207. Ballen PH, Rochkopf L. Congenital retraction of the upper lid. Ophthalmol Surg 1987;18:689–690.
208. Pochin EE. Unilateral retraction of the upper lid in Graves' disease. Clin Sci 1937;1938;3:197–209.
209. Pochin EE. The mechanism of lid retraction in Graves' disease. Clin Sci 1939;4:91–101.
210. Frueh BR, Garber FW, Musch D. The effects of Graves eye disease on levator muscle function. Ophthalmic Surg 1986;17:142–145.
211. Ohnishi T, Noguchi S, Murakami N, et al. Levator palpebrae superioris muscle: MR evaluation of enlargement as a cause of upper eyelid retraction in Graves' disease. Radiology 1993;188:115–118.
212. Breinin GM. Cited by McLean JM, Norton EWD. Unilateral lid retraction without exophthalmos. Arch Ophthalmol 1959;61:681–686.
213. Papst W, Esslen E. Die bedeutung der elektromyographie für die analyse von motilitätsstörungen der augen. Bibl Ophthalmol 1961;57:132–135.
214. Grove AS. Upper eyelid retraction and Graves disease. Ophthalmology 1981;88:499–506.
215. Trokel SL, Jakobiec FA. Correlation of CT scanning and pathological features of ophthalmic Graves disease. Ophthalmology 1981;88:553–564.
216. Feldon SE, Levin L. Graves Ophthalmology. V. Aetiology of upper eyelid retraction in Graves Ophthalmology. Br J Ophthalmol 1990;74:484–485.
217. Simonsz HJ, Kommerell G. Increased muscle tension and reduced elasticity of affected muscles in recent onset Graves disease caused primarily by active muscle contraction. Doc Ophthalmol 1989;72:215–224.
218. Frueh BR. Eyelid retraction in Graves' eye disease. Ophthalmology 1989;96:1574.
219. McClean JM, Norton EWD. Unilateral lid retraction without exophthalmos. Arch Ophthalmol 1958;61:681–686.
220. Wesley RE, Bond JB. Upper eyelid retraction from inferior rectus restriction in dysthyroid orbit disease. Ann Ophthalmol 1987;19:34–36.
221. Hamed LM, Lessner AM. Fixation duress in the pathogenesis of upper eyelid retraction in thyroid orbitopathy: A prospective study. Ophthalmology 1994;101:1608–1613.
222. Lewis JC, MacGregor AG. Congenital hyperthyroidism. Lancet 1957;1:14–16.
223. Lohman L, Burns JA, Penland WR, et al. Unilateral eyelid retraction secondary to contralateral ptosis in dysthyroid ophthalmopathy. J Clin Neuroophthalmol 1984;4:163–166.
224. Gonnering RS. Pseudoretraction of the eyelid in thyroid-associated orbitopathy. Arch Ophthalmol 1988;106:1078–1080.
225. Chalfin J, Putterman AM. Müller's muscle excision and levator recession in retracted upper lid. Arch Ophthalmol 1979;97:1487–1491.
226. Harvey JT, Anderson RL. The aponeurotic approach to eyelid retraction. Ophthalmology 1981;88:513–524.
227. Leone CR Jr. The management of ophthalmic Graves' disease. Ophthalmology 1984;91:770–779.
228. Dixon RS. The surgical management of thyroid-related upper eyelid retraction. Ophthalmology 1982;89:52–57.
229. Putterman AM. Surgical treatment of thyroid-related upper eyelid retraction: Graded Müller's muscle excision and levator recession. Ophthalmology 1981;88:507–512.
230. Biglan AW. Control of eyelid retraction associated with Graves' disease with botulinum A toxin. Ophthalmic Surg 1994;25:186–188.
231. Ebner R. Botulinum toxin type A in upper lid retraction of Graves' ophthalmopathy. J Clin Neuroophthalmol 1993;13:258–261.
232. Summerskill WHJ, Molnar GD. Eye signs in hepatic cirrhosis. N Engl J Med 1962;266:1244–1248.
233. Miller NR. Hepatic cirrhosis as a cause of eyelid retraction. Am J Ophthalmol 1991;112:94–95.
234. van't Hoff W. Familial myotonic periodic paralysis. Q J Med 1962;31:385–402.
235. Layzer RB, Lovelace RE, Rowland LP. Hyperkalemic periodic paralysis. Arch Neurol 1967;16:455–471.
236. Resnick JS, Engel WK. Myotonic lid-lag in hypokalemic periodic paralysis. J Neurol Neurosurg Psychiatry 1967;30:47–51.
237. Davidson SI. The eye in dystrophia myotonica: With a report on electromyography of the extraocular muscles. Br J Ophthalmol 1961;45:183–196.
238. Weinstein GS, Myers BB. Eyelid retraction as a complication of an embedded hard contact lens. Am J Ophthalmol 1993;116:102–103.
239. Putterman AM, Urist MJ. Upper eyelid retraction after filtering procedures. Ann Ophthalmol 1975;7:263–266.
240. Pacheco EM, Guyton DL, Repka MX. Changes in eyelid position accompanying vertical rectus muscle surgery and prevention of lower lid retraction. J Pediatric Ophthalmol Strabis 1992;29:265–272.
241. Mauriello JA Jr, Palydowycz SB. Upper eyelid retraction after retinal detachment repair. Ophthalmic Surg 1993;24:694–697.
242. Conway ST. Lid retraction following blow-out fracture of the orbit. Ophthalmic Surg 1988;19:279–281.
243. Bazhenov DI. Inability to close one eye at a time. Vestn Oftalmol 1935;6:870–873.
244. Miller NR. Walsh and Hoyt's Clinical Neuro-Ophthalmology, 4th ed. Ed 4 Vol 2. Baltimore, Williams & Wilkins, 1985:968.
245. Lewandowsky M. Ueber apraxie des lidschlusses. Berl Klin Wochenschr 1907;44:921–923.
246. Lessell S. Supranuclear paralysis of voluntary lid closure. Arch Ophthalmol 1972;88:241–244.
247. Hoyt WF, Loeffler JD. Neurology of the orbicularis oculi: Anatomic, physiologic, and clinical aspects of lid closure. In: Smith JL, ed. Neuro-Ophthalmology. Vol 2. St Louis, CV Mosby, 1965:167–205.
248. Ross Russell RW. Supranuclear palsy of eyelid closure. Brain 1980;103:71–82.
249. Jankovic J. Blepharospasm associated with palatal myoclonus and communicating hydrocephalus. Neurology 1984;34:1522–1533.
250. Nishimura M, Tojima M, Suga M, et al. Chronic progressive spinobulbar spasticity with disturbance of voluntary eyelid closure. J Neurol Sci 1990;96:183–190.
251. Joynt RJ, Benton AL, Fogel ML. Behavioral and pathological correlates of motor impersistence. Neurology 1962;12:876–881.
252. De Renzi E, Gentilini M, Bazolli C. Eyelid movement diorders and motor impersistence in acute hemispheric disease. Neurology 1986;365:414–418.
253. Loeffler JD, Slatt B, Hoyt WF. Motor abnormalities of the eyelids in Parkinson's disease. Arch Ophthalmol 1966;76:178–185.
254. Watson RT, Rapcsak SZ. Loss of spontaneous blinking in a patient with Balint's syndrome. Arch Neurol 1989;46:567–570.
255. Podvinec M. Facial nerve disorders: Anatomical, histological and clinical aspects. Adv Otorhinolaryngol 1984;32:124–193.
256. House JW, Brackmann DE. Facial nerve grading system. Otolaryngol Head Neck Surg 1985;93:146–147.
257. Cohen MM, Lessell S. Retraction of the lower eyelid. Neurology 1979;29:386–389.
258. Cramer HB, Kartush JM. Testing facial nerve function. Otolaryngol Clin North Am 1991;24:555–557.
259. Browder JP. Facial paralysis in children. ENT J 1978;57:278–283.
260. May M, Fria TJ, Blumenthal F, et al. Facial paralysis in children: Differential diagnosis. Otolaryngol Head Neck Surg 1981;89:841–848.

261. Jonsson L, Hemmingsson A, Thomander L, et al. Magnetic resonance imaging in patients with Bell's palsy. Acta Otolaryngol (Stockh) suppl 1989;468(Suppl): 403–405.

262. Schwaber MK, Larson TC, Zealear DL, et al. Gadolinium-enhanced magnetic resonance imaging in Bell's palsy. Laryngoscope 1990;100:1264–1269.

264. Adour KK. Bell's palsy: A complete expression of acute benign cranial polyneuritis. Prim Care 1975;2:717–733.

265. Adour KK, Byl FM, Hilsinger RL Jr, et al. The true nature of Bell's palsy: An analysis of 1,000 consecutive patients. Laryngoscope 1978;88:787–801.

266. Adour KK, Swanson PJ Jr. Facial paralysis in 403 consecutive patients: Emphasis on treatment response in patients with Bell's palsy. Trans Am Acad Ophthalmol Otolaryngol 1971;75:1284–1301.

267. Hauser WA. Incidence and prognosis of Bell's palsy in the population of Rochester, Minnesota. Mayo Clin Proc 1971;46:258–264.

268. Goff CW, Cerciello R, Holmes GL. Bilateral Bell's palsy. Am J Dis Child 1983; 137:83.

269. Adour KK. Medical management of idiopathic (Bell's) palsy. Otolaryngol Clin N Am 1991;24:663–673.

270. May M, Klein SR. The differential diagnosis of facial nerve palsy. Otolaryngol Clin North Am 1991;24:613–641.

271. Alter M. Familial aggregation of Bell's palsy. Arch Neurol 1963;8:557–564.

272. Currie S. Familial oculomotor palsy with Bell's palsy. Brain 1970;93:193–198.

273. Smith MD, Scott GM, Rom S. Herpes simplex virus and facial palsy. J Infection 1987;15:259–261.

274. Morgan M, Nathwani D. Facial palsy and infection: the unfolding story. Clin Infect Dis 1992;14:263–271.

275. Spruance S. Bell's palsy and herpes simplex virus. Ann Internal Med 1994;120: 1045–1046.

276. Faruta Y, Takasu T, Sato KC, et al. Latent herpes simplex virus type I in human geniculate ganglia. Acta Neuropathol (Berl) 1992;84:39–44.

277. Takasu T, Faruta Y, Sato KC, et al. Detection of latent herpes simplex virus DNA and RNA in human geniculate ganglia by the polymerase chain reaction. Acta Otolaryngol 1992;112:1004–1011.

278. Ulrich J, Podvinec M, Hofer H. Histological and ultrastructural changes in idiopathic facial palsy. ORL 1978;40:303–311.

279. Matsumoto Y, Pulec JL, Patterson MJ, et al. Facial nerve biopsy for etiologic clarification of Bell's palsy. Ann Otol Rhinol Laryngol 1988;97:22–27.

280. Liston SL, Klied S. Histopathology of Bell's palsy. Laryngoscope 1989;99: 23–26.

281. Adour KK. Cranial polyneuritis and Bell's palsy. Arch Otolarygol 1976;102: 262–264.

282. Nieuwmeyer PA, Visser SL, Feenstra L. Bell's palsy: A polyneuropathy. Am J Otol 1985;6:250–252.

283. Hanner P, Badr G, Rosenhall U, et al. Trigeminal dysfunction in patients with Bell's palsy. Acta Otolaryngol 1986;101:224–230.

284. Uri N, Schuchman G. Vestibular abnormalities in patients with Bell's palsy. J Laryngol Otol 1986;100:1125–1128.

285. Hanner P, Andersen O, Frisen L, et al. Clinical observations of effects on central nervous system in patients with acute facial palsy. Arch Otolaryngol Head Neck Surg 1987;113:516–520.

286. Kaplan JE, Greenspan JR, Bomgaars M, et al. Simultaneous outbreaks of Guillain-Barré syndrome and Bell's palsy in Hawaii in 1981. JAMA 1983;250: 2635–2640.

287. Fisch U, Felix H. On the pathogenesis of Bell's palsy. Acta Otolaryngol 1983; 95:532–538.

288. Marsh MA, Coker NJ. Surgical decompression of idiopathic facial palsy. Otolaryngol Clin North Am 1991;24:675–689.

289. Petersen E. The natural history of Bell's palsy. Am J Otol 1982;4:107–111.

290. Olsen PZ. Prediction of recovery in Bell's palsy. Acta Neurol Scand Suppl 1975; 61(Suppl):1–121.

291. May M, Wette R, Hardin WB Jr, et al. The use of steroids in Bell's palsy: A prospective controlled study. Laryngoscope 1976;86:1111–1122.

292. Wolf SM, Wagner JH Jr, Davidson S, et al. Treatment of Bell's palsy with prednisone: A prospective, randomized study. Neurology 1978;28:158–161.

293. Kerbavaz RJ, Hilsinger RL, Adour KK. The facial paralysis prognostic index. Otolaryngol Head Neck Surg 1983;91:284–289.

294. Austin JR, Peskind SP, Austin SG, et al. Idiopathic facial nerve paralsysis: A randomized double blind controlled study of placebo versus prednisone. Laryngoscope 1993;103:1326–1333.

295. Pitts DB, Adour KK, Hilsinger RL. Recurrent Bell's palsy: Analysis of 140 patients. Laryngoscope 1988;98:535–540.

296. Tomita H, Tanaka M, Kukimoto N, et al. An ELISA study on varicella zoster virus infectionin acute facial palsy. Acta Otolaryngol Suppl (Stockh) 1988;446: 10–16.

297. Dickens JRE, Smith JT, Graham SS. Herpes zoster oticus: Treatment with intravenous acyclovir. Laryngoscope 1988;98:776–779.

298. Ramos Macias A, de Miguel Martinez I, Martin Sanchez AM, et al. The incorporation of acyclovir in the treatment of peripheral facial paralysis: A study of 45 cases. Acta Otorhinolaringol Esp (Spain) 1992;43:117–120.

299. Adour KK, Diamond C. Decompression of the facial nerve in Bell's palsy: A historical review. Otolaryngol Head Neck Surg 1982;90:453–460.

300. May M, Klein SR, Taylor FH. Idiopathic (Bell's) facial palsy: Natural history defies steroid or surgical treatment. Laryngoscope 1985;95:406–409.

301. Park HW, Watkins AL. Facial paralysis: Analysis of 500 cases. Arch Phys Med 1949;30:749–761.

302. Korczyn AD. Bell's palsy and diabetes mellitus. Lancet 1971;1:108–110.

303. Korczyn AD. Prevalence of diabetes mellitus in Bell's palsy. Lancet 1971;1: 862.

304. Brackman DE. Bell's palsy: Incidence, etiology, and results of medical treatment. Otolaryngol Clin N Am 1974;7:357–368.

305. Chutorian AM, Gold AP, Braun CW. Benign intracranial hypertension and Bell's palsy. N Engl J Med 1977;296:1214–1215.

306. Davis LE, Sperry S. Bell's palsy and secondary syphilis: CSF spirochetes detected by immunofluorescence. Ann Neurol 1978;4:378–380.

307. Pecket P, Schattner A. Concurrent Bell's palsy and diabetes mellitus: A diabetic mononeuropathy? J Neurol Neurosurg Psychiatry 1982;45:652–655.

308. Cohen JP, Lachman LJ, Hammerschlag PE. Reversible facial paralysis in sarcoidosis: Confirmation by serum angiotensin-converting enzyme assay. Arch Otolaryngol 1983;109:832–835.

309. Pillsbury HC, Price HC, Gardiner LJ. Primary tumors of the facial nerve: Diagnosis and management. Laryngoscope 1983;93:1045–1048.

310. Wiet RJ, Lotan AN, Monsell EM, et al. Tumor involvement of the facial nerve. Laryngoscope 1983;93:1301–1309.

311. Clark JR, Carlson RD, Sasaki CT, et al. Facial paralysis in Lyme disease. Laryngoscope 1985;95:1341–1345.

312. May M. The Facial Nerve. New York, Thieme Inc, 1986.

313. May M, Hughes GB. Facial nerve disorders: Update. Am J Otology 1987;8: 167–180.

314. Brown MM, Thompson A, Goh BT, et al. Bell's palsy and HIV infection. J Neurol Neurosurg Psychiatry 1988;51:425–426.

315. Thomke F, Urban PP, Marx JJ, et al. Seventh nerve palsies may be the only clinical sign of small pontine infarctions in diabetis and hypertensive patients. J Neurol 2002;249:1556–1562.

316. Bergstrom L, Baker BB. Syndromes associated with congenital facial paralysis. Otolaryngol Head Neck Surg 1981;89:336–342.

317. Orobello P. Congenital and acquired facial nerve paralysis in children. Otolaryngol Clin North Am 1991;24:647–652.

318. Falco NA, Eriksson E. Facial nerve palsy in the newborn: incidence and outcome. Plast Reconstruct Surg 1990;85:1–4.

319. Berger JR, Ayyar DR. Neurological complications of ethylene glycol intoxication: Report of a case. Arch Neurol 1981;38:724–726.

320. Fellman DM. Facial diplegia following ethylene glycol ingestion. Arch Neurol 1982;39:739–740.

321. Kiwak KJ, Levine SE. Benign intracranial hypertension and facial diplegia. Arch Neurol 1984;41:787–788.

322. Rice JP, Horowitz M, Chin D. Wernicke-Korsakoff syndrome with bilateral facial palsy. J Neurol Neurosurg Psychiatry 1984;47:1356–1357.

323. Keane JR. Bilateral 7th nerve palsy: Analysis of 43 cases and review of the literature. Neurology 1994;44:1198–1202.

324. Andersen JG. Surgical treatment of lagophthalmos in leprosy by the Gillies temporalis transfer. Br J Plast Surg 1961;14:339–345.

325. Levine RE, House WF, Hitselberger WE. Ocular complications of VIIth nerve paralysis and management with the palpebral spring. Am J Ophthalmol 1972; 73:219–228.

326. Banuelos A. Combined operation for facial palsy. Arch Ophthalmol 1973;89: 329–331.

327. Rich AM. Surgical management of the paralysed orbicularis oculi. Trans Am Acad Ophthalmol Otolaryngol 1974;78:622–631.

328. Seiff SR, Chang J. Management of ophthalmic complications of facial nerve palsy. Otolaryngol Clin North Am 1992;25:669–690.

329. Jobe RP. The use of gold weights in the upper eyelid. Br J Plastic Surg 1993; 46:343–344.

330. Catalano PJ, Bergstein MJ, Biller HF. Comprehensive management of the eye in facial paralysis. Arch Otolaryngol Head Neck Surg 1995;121:81–86.

331. Baker RS, Stava MW, Nelson KR, et al. Aberrant reinnervation of facial musculature in subhuman primate: A correlative analysis of eyelid kinematics, muscle synkinesis, and motoneuron localization. Neurology 1994;44:2165–2173.

332. Rana PVS, Wadia RS. The Marin-Amat syndrome: An unusual facial synkinesia. J Neurol Neurosurg Psychiatry 1985;48:939–941.

333. Frueh BR. Associated facial contractions after 7th nerve palsy mimicking jaw-winking. Ophthalmology 1983;90:1105–1109.

334. Chen C, Malhotra R, Muecke J, et al. Aberrant facial nerve regeneration (AFR): An under-recognized cause of ptosis. Eye 2004;18:159–162.

335. Osher RH, Griggs RC. Orbicularis fatigue: The "peek" sign of myasthenia gravis. Arch Ophthalmol 1979;97:677–679.

336. Marsden CD. Blepharospasm-oromandibular dystonia syndrome (Brueghels syndrome): A variant of adult onset torsion dystonia. J Neurol Neurosurg Psychiatry 1976;59:1204–1209.

337. Tolosa ES, Klawans HL. Meige's disease: A clinical form of a facial convulsion, bilateral and medial. Arch Neurol 1979;36:635–637.

338. Gollomp S, Ilson J, Burke R, et al. Meige syndrome: A review of 31 cases. Neurology 1981;31 (Suppl):78.

339. Tolosa ES. Clinical features of Meige's disease (idiopathic orofacial dystonia). Arch Neurol 1981;38:147–151.

340. Jankovic J, Havins WE, Wilkins RB. Blinking and blepharospasm: Mechanism, diagnosis, and management. JAMA 1982;248:3160–3164.
341. Tanner CM, Glantz RH, Klawans HL. Meige disease: Acute and chronic cholinergic effects. Neurology 1982;32:783–785.
342. Jankovic J, Ford J. Blepahrospasm and orofacial-cervical dystonia: Clinical and pharmalogical findings in 100 patients. Ann Neurol 1983;13:402–411.
343. Jacome DE, Yanez GF. Spastic dysphonia and Meige disease. Neurology 1980; 30:349.
344. Marsden CD, Sheehy MP. Spastic dysphonia, Meige disease, and torsion dystonia. Neurology 1982;32:1202–1203.
345. Kakigi R, Shibasaki H, Kuroda Y, et al. Meige's syndrome associated with spasmodic dysphagia. J Neurol Neurosurg Psychiatry 1983;46:589–590.
346. Jankovic J, Orman, J. Blepharospasm: Demographic and clinical survey of 250 patients. Ann Ophthalmol 1984;16:371–376.
347. Grandas F, Elston J, Quinn N, et al. Blepharospasm: A review of 264 patients. J Neurol Neurosurg Psychiatry 1988;51:767–772.
348. Nutt JG, Hammerstad JP. Blepharospasm and oromandibular dystonia (Meige's syndrome) in sisters. Ann Neurol 1981;9:189–191.
349. Defazio G, Livrea P, Guanti G, et al. Genetic contribution to idiopathic adult onset blepharospasm and cranial cervical dystonia. Eur Neurol 1993;33: 345–355.
350. Jankovic J, Nutt JG. Blepharospasm and cranial cervical dystonia (Meige's syndrome): Familial occurrence. In: Jankovic J, Tolosa E, eds. Adv Neurology: Facial Dyskineisas. Vol 49. New York, Raven Press, 1988:pp 117–123.
351. Elston JS, Marsden CD, Grandas F, et al. The significance of ophthalmological symptoms in idiopathic blepharospasm. Eye 1988;2:435–439.
352. Elston JS, Cas Granje F, Lees AJ. The relationship betyween eye winking tics, frequent eye blinking and blepharospasm. J Neurol Neurosurg Psychiatry 1989; 52:477–480.
353. Price J, Oday J. A comparative study of tear secretion in blepharospasm and hemifacial spasm patients treated with botulinum toxin. J Clin Neuroophthalmol 1993;13:67–71.
354. Kurlan R, Jankovic J, Rubin A, et al. Coexistent Meiges syndrome and myasthenia gravis: A relationship between blinking and extraocular muscle fatigue. Arch Neurol 1987;44:1057–1060.
355. Nutt JG, Muenter MD, Aronson A, et al. Epidemiology of focal and generalized dystonia in Rochester, Minn. Mov Disord 1988;3:188–194.
356. Rajagopalan N, Humphrey PRD, Bucknall RC. Torticollis and blepharospasm in systemic lupus erythematosus. Mov Disord 1989;4:345–348.
357. Grandas F, Elston J, Quinn N, et al. Letters to the editor. Mov Disord 1990;5: 89.
358. Berardelli A, Rothwell JC, Marsden CD. Pathophysiology of blepharospasm and oromandibular dystonia. Brain 1985;108:593–608.
359. Aramideh M, Ongerboer de Visser BW, Devriese PP, et al. Electromyographic features of levator palpebrae superioris and orbicularis oculi muscles in blepharospasm. Brain 1994;117:27–38.
360. Diamond EL, Trobe JD, Belar CD. Psychological aspects of essential blepharospasm. J Nerv Ment Dis 1984;172:749–756.
361. Keane JR, Young JA. Blepharospasm with bilateral basal ganglia infarction. Arch Neurol 1985;42:1206–1208.
362. Bihari K, Pigott TA, Hill JL. Blepharospasm and obsessive obsessive compulsive disorder. J Nerv Ment Dis 1992;180:130–132.
363. Berardelli A, Rothwell JC, Day BL, et al. The pathophysiology of cranial dystonia. Adv Neurol 1988;50:525–535.
364. Jankovic J. Blepharospasm associated with basal ganglia lesions. Arch Neurol 1986;43:866–868.
365. Creel DJ, Holds JB, Anderson J. Auditory brainstem responses in blepharospasm. Electroencephalography Clin Neurophys 1993;86:138–140.
366. Kimura J. Blink reflex in facial dyskinesia. In: Jankovic J, Tolosa E, eds. Advances in Neurology: Facial Dyskinesias. Vol 49. New York, Raven Press, New York, 1988:39–63.
367. Tolosa ES, Montserrat L, Bayers A. Blink reflex studies in focal dystonias: Enhanced excitability of brainstem interneurons in cranial dystonia and spasmodic torticollis. Mov Disord 1988;3:61–69.
368. Aramideh M, Eekhof JLA, Bour JHT, et al. Electromyography and recovery of the blink reflex in involuntary eyelid colosure: A comparative study. J Neurol Neurosurg Psychiatry 1995;58:692–698.
369. Kimura J. Disorder of interneurons in Parkinsonism. Brain 1973;96:87–96.
370. Cohen LG, Ludlow CL, Warden M, et al. Blink reflex excitability recovery curves in patients with spasmodic dysphonia. Neurology 1989;39:572–577.
371. Iriarte LM, Chacon J, Madrazo J, et al. Blink reflex in dyskinetic and nondyskinetic patients with Parkinsons's disease. Eur Neurol 1989;29:67–70.
372. Smith SJM, Lees AJ. Abnormalities of the blink reflex in Gilles de la Tourette syndrome. J Neurol Neurosurg Psychiatry 1989;52:895–898.
373. Nakashima K, Rothwell JC, Thompson PD, et al. The blink reflex in patients with idiopathic torsion dystonia. Arch Neurol 1990;47:413–416.
374. Coles WH. Signs of essential blepharospasm: A motion-picture analysis. Arch Ophthalmol 1977;95:1006–1009.
375. Elston JS. Long-term results of treatment of idiopathic blepharospasm with botulinum toxin injections. Br J Ophthalmol 1987;71:664–668.
376. Demer JL, Holds JB, Hovis LA. Ocular movements in essential blepharospasm. Am J Ophthalmol 1990;15:674–682.
377. Lueck CJ, Tanyeri S, Crawford TJ, et al. Saccadic eye movements in essential blepharospasm. J Neurol 1990;237:226–229.
378. Hotson JR, Boman DR. Memory-contingent saccades and the substantia nigra postulate for essential blepharospasm. Brain 1991;114:295–307.
379. Altrocchi PH, Forno LS. Spontaneous oral-facial dyskinesia: neuropathology of a case. Neurology 1983;33:802–805.
380. Zweig RM, Jankel WR, Whitehouse PJ, et al. Brainstem pathology in dystonia. Neurology 1986;361(Suppl):74–75.
381. Kulisevsky J, Marti MJ, Ferrer I, et al. Miege syndrome neuropathology of a case. Mov Disord 1988;3:10–175.
382. Garcia-Albea E, Franch O, Munoz D, et al. Brueghel's syndrome: Report of a case with postmortem studies. J Neurol Neurosurg Psychiatry 1981;44:437–440.
383. Gibb WRG, Lees AJ, Marsden CD. Pathological report of four patients presenting with cranial dystonias. Mov Disord 1988;3:211–221.
384. Jankovic J, Svendsen CN, Bird ED. Brain neurotransmitters in dystonia. N Engl J Med 1987;316:278–279.
385. Tolosa ES, Lai C. Meige disease: Striatal dopaminergic preponderance. Neurology 1979;29:1126–1130.
386. Skarf JB, Sharpe JA. Essential blepharospasm: A review of medical management and a therapeutic trial of choline chloride. Am J Ophthalmol 1981;92:742.
387. Micheli F, Fernández Pardel MM, Leiguarda RC. Beneficial effects of lisuride in Meige disease. Neurology 1982;32:432–434.
388. Marsden CD, Lang AE, Sheehy MP. Pharmacology of cranial dystonia. Neurology 1983;33:1100–1101.
389. Nutt JG, Hammerstad JP, deGarmo P, et al. Cranial dystonia: Double-blind crossover study of anticholinergics. Neurology 1984;34:215–217.
390. Merikangas JR, Reynolds CF III. Blepharospasm: Successful treatment with clonazepam. Ann Neurol 1979;5:401–402.
391. Fahn S, Bressman S, Burke R, et al. Treatment of blepharospasm with high dose baclofen. Ann Neurol 1983;14:112.
392. Schrieber S, Pick CG. Fluoxetine for blepharospasm: Interaction of serotonin and dopamine. J Nerv Ment Dis 1995;88:719–721.
393. Hotson JR, Langston EB, Langston JW. Saccade respnses to dopamine in human MPTP-induced parkinsonism. Ann Neurol 1986;20:456–463.
394. Callahan A. Surgical correction of intractable blepharospasm. Am J Ophthalmol 1965;60:788–791.
395. Putterman AM, Urist M. Treatment of essential blepharospasm with a frontalis sling. Arch Ophthalmol 1972;88:278–281.
396. Gillum WN, Anderson RL. Blepharospasm surgery: An anatomical approach. Arch Ophthalmol 1981;99:1056–1062.
397. McCord CD Jr, Shore J, Putnam JR. Treatment of essential blepharospasm. II. A modification of exposure for the muscle stripping technique. Arch Ophthalmol 1984;102:269–273.
398. Anderson RL, Patrinely JR. Surgical management of blepharospasm. Adv Neurol 1988;49:501–520.
399. Frueh BR, Callahan A, Dortzbach RK, et al. A profile of patients with intractable blepharospasm. Trans Am Acad Ophthalmol Otolaryngol 1976;81:591–594.
400. Harrison MS. The facial tics. J Laryngol Otol 1976;90:561–570.
401. Spector GJ, Smith PG, Burde RM. Selective facial neurectomy for essential blepharospasm. Laryngoscope 1981;91:1896–1903.
402. Dobie RA, Fisch U. Primary and revision surgery (selective neurectomy) for facial hyperkinesia. Arch Otolaryngol Head Neck Surg 1986;112:154–163.
403. Bates AK, Halliday BL, Bailey CS, et al. Surgical management of essential blepharospasm. Br J Ophthalmol 1991;75:487–490.
404. Small RG. Essential blepharospasm. Arch Ophthalmol 1984;102:972–973.
405. McCord CD Jr, Coles WH, Shore JW, et al. Treatment of essential blepharospasm. I. Comparison of facial nerve avulsion and eyebrow-eyelid muscle stripping procedure. Arch Ophthalmol 1984;102:266–268.
406. Dortzbach RK. Complications in surgery for blepharospasm. Am J Ophthalmol 1973;5:142–147.
407. Frueh BR, Callahan A, Dortzbach RK, et al. The effects of differential section of the VIIth nerve on patients with intractable blepharospasm. Trans Am Acad Ophthalmol Otolaryngol 1976;81:595–602.
408. Lemagne JM, Gersdorff M. Treatment of benign essential blepharospasm and hemifacial spasm by selective section of the facial nerve: technique and results. Orbit 1988;7:43–46.
409. Jankovic J, Patel SC. Blepharospasm associated with brainstem lesions. Neurology 1983;33:1237–1240.
410. Jankovic J, Shutish PC. Blepharospasm associated with brainstem lesions. Neurology 1983;33:1237–1240.
411. Dooling EC, Schoene WC, Richardson EP. Hallervorden-Spatz syndrome. Arch Neurol 1974;30:70–83.
412. Angelini L, Nardocci N, Rumi V, et al. Hallervorden-Spatz: Clinical and MRI study of 11 cases diagnosied in life. J Neurol 1992;239:417–425.
413. Janati A, Metzer WS, Archer RL, et al. Blepharospasm associated with olivopontocerebellar atrophy. J Clin Neuroophthalmol 1989;1:281–284.
414. Sandyk R, Gillman MA. Blepharospasm associated with palatal myoclonus and communicating hydrocephalus. Neurology 1984;34:1522–1533.

415. Metz LN, Magee KR. Postencephalitic blepharospasm. Arch Ophthalmol 1960; 63:692–697.

416. Herraiz J, Roquer J, Escudero D, et al. Meiges syndrome and bilateral pallidal calcifications. J Neurol 1988;235:384.

417. Björk A, Kugelberg E. The electrical activity of the muscles of the eye and eyelids in various positions and during movement. EEG Clin Neurophysiol 1953; 5:595–602.

418. Leenders KL, Frakowiak RSJ, Quinn N, et al. Ipsilateral blepharospasm and contralateral hemidystonia and parkinsonism in a patient with a unilateral rostral brainstem-thalamic lesion: Structural and functional abnormalities studied with CT, MRI, and PET scanning. Mov Disord 1986;1:51–58.

419. Powers JM. Blepharospasm due to unilateral diencephalan infarction. Neurology 1985;35:283–284.

420. Palakurthy PR, Iyer V. Blepharospasm accompanying hypoxic encephalopathy. Mov Disord 1987;2:131–134.

421. Kulisevsky J, Avila A, Roig C, et al. Unilateral blepharospasm stemming from a thalamomesencephalic lesion. Mov Disord 1993;8:239–240.

422. Barton JJS, Cox TA, Calne DA. Involuntary ocular deviations and generalized dystonia in multiple sclerosis: a case report. J Clin Neuroophthalmol 1994;14: 160–162.

423. Lauterbach EC, Price ST, Spears E, et al. Serotonin responsive and nonresponsive diurnal depressive mood disorders and pathological affect in thalamic infarct associated with myoclonus and blepharospasm. Biol Psychiat 1994;35:488–490.

424. Lange AE, Sharpe JA. Blepharospasm associated with palatal myoclonus and communicating hydrocephalus. Neurology 1984;34:1522–1533.

425. Davis WA. Dyskinesia associated with chronic antihistamine use. N Engl J Med 1976;294:113.

426. Keane JR. Gaze-evoked blepharoclonus. Ann Neurol 1978;3:243–245.

427. Behrman S, Scott DF. Blepharoclonus provoked by voluntary eye closure. Mov Disord 1988;3:326–328.

428. Safran AB, Berney J. Synchronisim of reverse ocular bobbing and blinking. Am J Ophthalmol 1983;95:401.

429. Gatto M, Micheli F, Pardal MF. Blepharoclonus and parkinsonism associated with aqueductal stenosis. Mov Disord 1990;5:310–313.

430. Fisher CM. Reflex blepharospasm. Neurology 1963;13:77–78.

431. Irvine AR, Daroff RB, Sanders MD, et al. Familial reflex blepharospasm. Am J Ophthalmol 1968;65:889–890.

432. Obeso JA, Artieda J, Marsden CD. Stretch reflex blepharospasm. Neurology 1985;35:1378–1380.

433. Salorio DP, Conte RQ. Ophthalmologic causes of blepharospasm. Adv Neurol 1988;49:91–102.

434. Fraunfelder FT. Interim report: National registry of possible drug-induced ocular side effects. Ophthalmology 1980;87:87–90.

435. Griffin JD, Garnick MB. Eye toxicity of cancer chemotherapy: A review of the literature. Cancer 1981;48:1539–1549.

436. Salminen L, Jäntti V, Grönross M. Blepharospasm associated with tegafur combination chemotherapy. Am J Ophthalmol 1984;97:649–650.

437. Smith MB. Handbook of Ocular Toxicity. Littleton, MA, PSG Publishing Co, 1976.

438. Granacher RP. Differential diagnosis of tardive dyskinesia: An overview. Am J Psychiatr 1981;138:1288–1297.

439. Jankovic J. Drug-induced and other orofacial-cervical dyskinesias. Ann Intern Med 1981;94:788–793.

440. Simpson GM, Pi EH, Sramek JJ. Management of tardive dyskinesia: Current update. Drugs 1982;23:381–393.

441. Weiner WJ, Nausieda PA, Glantz RH. Meige syndrome (blepharospasm-oro-mandibular dystonia) after long-term neuroleptic therapy. Neurology 1981;31: 1555–1556.

442. Burke RE, Fahn S, Jankovic J, et al. Tardive dystonia: Late-onset and persistent dystonia caused by antipsychotic drugs. Neurology 1982;32:1335–1346.

443. Weiner WJ, Nausieda PA. Meige's syndrome during long-term dopaminergic therapy in Parkinson's disease. Arch Neurol 1982;39:451–452.

444. Thatch BT, Chase TN, Bosma JF. Oral facial dyskinesia associated with prolonged use of antihistaminic decongestants. N Engl J Med 1975;293:486–487.

445. Davis KD, Dostrovsky JO. Modulatory influences of red nucleus stimulation on the somatosensory responses of cat trigeminal subnucleus oralis neurons. Exp Neurol 1986;91:80–101.

446. Barone DA, Raniolo J. Facial dyskinesia from overdose of an antihistamine. N Engl J Med 1980;303:107.

447. Powers JM. Decongestant-induced blepharospasm and orofacial dystonia. JAMA 1982;247:3244–3245.

448. Joyce RP, Gunderson CH. Carbamazepine-induced orofacial dyskinesia. Neurology 1980;30:1333–1334.

449. Anon. Editorial: Tardive dyskinesia. Br Med J 1979;2:1313.

450. Anon. Editorial: Tardive dyskinesia. Lancet 1979;2:447.

451. Anon. Task Force on Late Neurologic Effects of Antipsychotic Drugs: Tardive dyskinesia: summary of a task force report of the American Psychiatric Association. Am J Psychiatr 1980;137:1163–1172.

452. Koller WC. Movement Disorders. In: Chokroverty S, ed. Chapter 16. PMA Publishing Co, 1990:335–352.

453. Sweet RD, Solomon GE, Wayne H, et al. Neurological features of Gilles de la Tourette's syndrome. J Neurol Neurosurg Psychiatry 1973;36:1–9.

454. Shapiro AK, Shapiro ES, Brunn RD, et al. Gilles de la Tourette syndrome. New York, Raven Press, 1978.

455. Shapiro E, Shapiro AK. Tic disorders. JAMA 1981;245:1583–1585.

456. Frankel M, Cummings JL. Neuro-ophthalmic abnormalities in Tourette's syndrome: Functional and anatomic implications. Neurology 1984;34:359–361.

457. Jankovic J, Stone L. Dystonic tics in patients with Tourette's syndrome. Mov Disord 1991;6:248–252.

458. Assail M. Hysterical blepharospasm. Dis Nerv Syst 1967;28:256–258.

459. Cavenar J, Brantley IJ, Braasch E. Blepharospasm: Organic or functional? Psychosomatics 1978;19:623–628.

460. Reckless JB. Hysterical blepharospasm treated by psychotherapy and conditioning procedures in a group setting. Psychosomatics 1972;13:263–264.

461. Wickramasekera I. Hypnosis and broad-spectrum behavior therapy for blepharospasm: A case study. lnt. J Clin Exp Hypn 1974;22:201–209.

462. Roxanas MR, Thomas MR, Rapp MS. Biofeedback treatment of blepharospasm with spasmodic torticollis. Can Med Assoc J 1978;119:48–49.

463. Bancaud J. Les crisies epileptiques d'origine occipitale (etude stereo-electroencephalographique). Rev Otoneuro-ophthalmol 1969;41:299–315.

464. Panayiotopoulos CP, Obeid T, Waheed G. Differentiation of typical absence seizures in epileptic syndromes. Brain 1989;112:1039–1056.

465. Appleton RE, Panayiotopoulos CP, Acomb BA, et al. Eyelid myoclonia with typical absences: An epilepsy syndrome. J Neurol Neurosurg Psychiatry 1993; 56:1312–1316.

466. Wada JA. Unilateral blinking as a lateralizing sign of partial complex seizure of temporal lobe origin. In: Wada JA, Penry JK, eds. Advances in Epileptology: Xth Epilepsy International Symposium. New York, NY, Raven Press, 1980:533.

467. Jeavons PM. Nosological problems of myoclonic epilepsies in childhood and adolescence. Develop Med Child Neurol 1977;19:3–8.

468. Panayiotopoulos CP. Fixation-off-sensitive epilepsy in eyelid myoclonia with absence seizures. Ann Neurol 1987;22:87–89.

469. Green JB. Seizures on closing the eyes. Electroencephalographic studies. Neurology 1968;18:391–396.

470. Lewis JA. Eye closure as a motor triger for seizures. Neurology 1972;22: 1145–1150.

471. Vignaendra V, Ghee LT, Lee LC, et al. Epileptic discharges triggered by blinking and eye closure. Electroencephalogr Clin Neurophys 1976;40:491–498.

472. Darby CE, Korte RA, Binnie CD, et al. The self induction of epileptic seizures by eye closure. Epilepsia 1980;21:31–42.

473. Lugaresi E, Cirignotta F, Montagna P. Occipital lobe epilepsy with scotosensitive seizures: the role of central vision. Epilepsia 1980;25:115–120.

474. Panayiotopoulos CP. The inhibitory effect of central vision on occipital lobe seizures. Neurology 1981;31:1331–1333.

475. Terzano MG, Parrino L, Manzoni GC, et al. Seizures triggered by blinking when beginning to speak. Arch Neurol 1983;40:103–106.

476. Rafal R, Laxar KD, Janowsky JS. Seizures triggered by blinking in a non-photosensitive epileptic. J Neurol Neurosurg Psychiatry 1986;49:445–447.

477. Shahani BT, Young RR. Human orbicularis oculi reflexes. Neurology 1972;22: 149–154.

478. Chu F, Reingold DB, Cogan DG. Lid triggered synkinesis. Ophthalmology 1981; 88:1019–1023.

479. Pullicino PM, Jacobs L, McCall WD, et al. Spontaneous palpebromandibular synkinesia: A localizing clinical sign. Ann Neurol 1994;35:222–228.

480. Matthews WB. Facial myokymia. J Neurol Neurosurg Psychiatry 1966;29: 35–39.

481. Hjorth RJ, Willison RG. The electromyogram in facial myokymia and hemifacial spasm. J Neurol Sci 1973;20:117–126.

482. Mateer JE, Gutmann L, McComas CF. Myokymia in Guillain-Barré syndrome. Neurology 1983;33:374–376.

483. Reinecke RD. Translated myokymia of the lower eyelid causing uniocular vertical pseudonystagmus. Am J Ophthalmol 1973;75:150–151.

484. Gutmann L, Thompson HG Jr, Martin JD. Transient facial myokymia: An uncommon manifestation of multiple sclerosis. JAMA 1969;209:389–391.

485. Jacobs L, Kaba S, Pullicino P. The lesion causing continuous facial myokymia in multiple sclerosis. Arch Neurol 1994;51:1115–1119.

486. Sethi PK, Smith BH, Kalyanaraman K. Facial myokymia: A clinicopathological study. J Neurol Neurosurg Psychiatry 1974;37:745–749.

487. Tenser RB, Corbett JJ. Myokymia and facial contraction in brain stem glioma: An electromyographic study. Arch Neurol 1974;30:425–427.

488. Negri S, Caraceni T, de Lorenzi L. Facial myokymia and brain-stem tumor. Eur Neurol 1976;14:108–118.

489. Waybright EA, Gutmann L, Chou SM. Facial myokymia: Pathological features. Arch Neurol 1979;36:244–245.

490. Kiriyanthan G, Krauss JK, Glocker FX, et al. Facial myokymia due to acoustic neurinoma. Surgical Surg Neurol 1994;41:498–501.

491. Riaz G, Campbell WW, Carr J, et al. Facial myokymia in syringobulbia. Arch Neurol 1990;47:472–474.

492. Radu EW, Skorpil V, Kaeser HE. Facial myokymia. Eur Neurol 1975;13: 499–512.

493. Sandyk R. Facial myokymia. J Neurosurg 1983;59:1108–1109.

494. Blumenthal DT, Guttman L, Suater K. Subarachnoid hemorrhage induces facial myokymia. Muscle Nerve 1994;17:1484–1485.

495. Chalk CH, Litchy WJ, Ebersold MJ, et al. Facial myokymia and unilateral basilar invagination. Neurology 1988;38:1811–1812.

496. Takiyama Y, Ikemoto S, Tanaka Y, et al. A large Japanese family with Machado-Joseph disease: Clinical and gentetic studies. Acta Neurol Scand 1989;79:214–222.

497. Boghen D, Filiatrault R, Descarries L. Myokymia and facial contracture in brain stem tuberculoma: A clinicopathologic report. Neurology 1977;27:270–272.

498. Keane JR. Cysticercosis: unusual neuroophthalmic signs. J Clin Neuroophthalmol 1993;13:194–199.

499. Rosenberg RN, Nyhan WL, Bay C, et al. Autosomal dominant striatonigral degeneration. Neurology 1976;26:703–714.

500. Daube JR, Kelly JJ, Martin RA. Facial myokymia with polyradiculopathy. Neurology 1979;29:662–669.

501. Van Zandycke M, Martin J-J, Vande Gaer L, et al. Facial myokymia in the Guillain-Barré syndrome: A clinicopathologic study. Neurology 1982;32:744–748.

502. Morris HH III, Estes ML. Bilateral facial myokymia following cardiopulmonary arrest. Arch Neurol 1981;38:393–394.

503. Gemignani F, Juvarra G, Calzetti S. Facial myokymia in the course of lymphocytic meningoradiculitis: Case report. Neurology 1981;31:1177–1180.

504. Feldman RG, White RF, Currie JN, et al. Long-term follow-up after single toxic exposure to trichloroethylene. Am J Ind Med 1985;8:119–126.

505. Cherington M, Sadler KM, Ryan DW. Facial myokymia. Surg Neurol 1979;11:478–480.

506. Wallis WE, van Poznak A, Plum F. Generalized muscular stiffness, fasciculation, and myokymia of peripheral nerve origin. Arch Neurol 1970;22:430–439.

507. Welch LK, Appenzeller O, Bicknell JM. Peripheral neuropathy associated with myokymia, sustained muscular contraction, and continuous motor unit activity. Neurology 1972;22:161–169.

508. Medina JL, Chokroverty S, Reyes M. Localized myokymia caused by peripheral nerve injury. Arch Neurol 1977;33:587–588.

509. Bettoni L, Bortone E, Ghizzoni P, et al. Myokymia in the course of Bell's palsy. J Neurol Sci 1988;84:69–76.

510. Brick JF, Gutmann L, Brick J, et al. Timber rattlesnake venom induced myokymia: Evidence for peripheral nerve origin. Neurology 1987;37:1545–1546.

511. Ehni G, Woltman HW. Hemifacial spasm: Review of one hundred and 106 cases. Arch Neurol Psychiatry 1945;53:205–211.

512. Wartenberg R. Hemifacial Spasm: A Clinical and Pathophysiological Study. New York, Oxford University Press, 1952.

513. Auger RG, Whisnant JP. Hemifacial spasm in Rochester and Olmsted County. Arch Neurol 1990;47:1233–1234.

514. Flueler U, Taylor D, Hing S, et al. Hemifacial spasm in infancy. Arch Ophthalmol 1990;108:812–815.

515. Kobata H, Kondo A, Kinuta Y, et al. Hemifacial spasm in childhood and adolescence. Neurosurgery 1995;36:710–714.

516. Friedman A, Jamrozik Z, Bojakowski J. Familial hemifacial spasm. Mov Disord 1989;4:213–218.

517. Carter JB, Patrinely JR, Jankovic J, et al. Boniuk familial hemifacial spasm. Arch Ophthalmol 1990;108:249–250.

518. Micheli F, Scorticati MC, Gatto E, et al. Familial hemifacial spasm. Mov Disord 1994;9:330–332.

519. Holds JB, Anderson RL, Jordan DR, et al. Bilateral hemifacial spasm. J Clin Neuroophthalmol 1990;10:153–154.

520. Moore AP. Postural fluctuation of hemifacial spasm. J Neurosurg 1984;60:190–191.

521. Frueh BR, Preston RA, Musch DC. Facial nerve injury and hemifacial spasm. Am J Ophthalmol 1990;110:421–423.

522. Manning KA, Evinger C, Sibony PA. Eyelid movement before and after botulinum therapy in patients with lid spasm. Ann Neurol 1990;28:653–660.

523. Kim P, Fukushima T. Observations on synkinesis in patients with hemifacial spasm: Effect of microvascular decompression and etiological considerations. J Neurosurg 1984;60:821–827.

524. Gardner WJ, Sava GA. Hemifacial spasm: A reversible pathophysiologic state. J Neurosurg 1962;19:240–247.

525. Jannetta PJ. Microsurgical exploration and decompression of the facial nerve in hemifacial spasm. Curr Top Surg Res 1970;2:217–220.

526. Jannetta PJ, Hackett E, Ruby JR. Electromyographic and electron microscopic correlates in hemifacial spasm treated by microsurgical relief of neurovascular compression. Surg Forum 1970;21:449–451.

527. Jannetta PJ. The cause of hemifacial spasm: Definitive microsurgical treatment at the brain stem in 31 patients. Trans Am Acad Ophthalmol Otolaryngol 1974;80:319–322.

528. Jannetta PJ, Abbasy M, Maroon JC, et al. Etiology and definitive microsurgical treatment of hemifacial spasm. J Neurosurg 1977;47:321–328.

529. Jannetta PJ. Hemifacial spasm caused by a venule: Case report. Neurosurgery 1984;14:89–92.

530. Jannetta PJ. Observations on the etiology of trigeminal neuralgia, hemifacial spasm, acoustic nerve dysfunction and glossopharyngeal neuralgia: Definitive

531. Neagoy DR, Dohn DF. Hemifacial spasm secondary to vascular compression of the facial nerve. Cleve Clin Q 1974;41:205–214.

532. Tash R, DeMerritt J, Sze G, et al. Hemifacial spasm: MR imaging features. AJNR Am J Neuroradiol 1991;12:839–842.

533. Adler CH, Zimmerman RA, Savino PJ, et al. Hemifacial spasm: evaluation by magnetic resonance imaging. Ann Neurol 1992;32:502–506.

534. Furuya Y, Ryu H, Uemura K, et al. MRI of intracranial neurovascular compression. J Comp Assist Tomogr 1992;16:503–505.

535. Bernardi B, Zimmerman RA, Savino PJ, et al. Magnetic resonance tomographic angiography in the investigation of hemifacial spasm. Neuroradiology 1993;35:606–611.

536. Ushiro K, Yanagida M, Kumazawa T, et al. Imaging of vascular compression in hemifacial spasm. Acta Otolaryngol 1993;500(Suppl):54–57.

537. Garbaldi DC, Miller NR. Tortuous basilar artery as etiology of hemifacial spasm. Arch Neurol 2003;60:626–627.

538. Maroon JC. Hemifacial spasm: A vascular cause. Arch Neurol 1978;35:481–483.

539. Maroon JC, Lunsford LD, Deeb ZL. Hemifacial spasm due to aneurysmal compression of the facial nerve. Arch Neurol 1978;35:545–546.

540. Nagata S, Matsushima T, Fujii K, et al. Hemifacial spasm due to tumor, aneurysm, or arteriovenous. Surg Neurol 1992;38:204–209.

541. Eby TL, Fisch U, Makek MS. Facial nerve management in temporal bone hemangiomas. Am J Otol 1992;13:223–232.

542. Matsumoto K, Saijo T, Kuyama H, et al. Hemifacial spasm caused by a spontaneous dissecting. J Neurosurg 1991;74:650–652.

543. Levin JM, Lee JE. Hemifacial spasm due to cerebellopontine angle lipoma: Case report. Neurology 1987;37:337–339.

544. Digre KB, Corbett JJ. Hemifacial spasm: Differential diagnosis, mechanism and treatment. In: Jankovic J, Tolosa E, eds. Advances in Neurology. Vol 49: Facial Dyskineisas. Vol 49. New York, Raven Press, 1988:117–123.

545. Auger RG, Piepgras DG. Hemifacial spasm associated with epidermoid tumors of the cerebellopontine angle. Neurology 1989;39:577–580.

546. Telischi FF, Grobman LR, Sheremata WA, et al. Hemifacial spasm. Occurrence in multiple sclerosis. Arch Otolaryngol Head Neck Surg 1991;117:554–556.

547. Westra I, Drummond GT. Occult pontine glioma in a patient with hemifacial spasm. Can J Ophthalmol 1991;26:148–151.

548. Altinors N, Kars Z, Cepoglu C. Rare causes of hemifacial spasm: Report of two cases. Clin Neurol Neurosurg 1991;93:155–158.

549. Higashi S, Yamashita J, Yamamoto Y, et al. Hemifacial spasm associated with a cerebellopontine angle. Surg Neurol 1992;37:289–292.

550. Vermersch P, Petit H, Marion MH, et al. Hemifacial spasm due to pontine infarction. J Neurol Neurosurg Psychiatry 1991;54:1018.

551. River Y, Honigman S, Gomori JM, et al. Superficial hemosiderosis of the central nervous system. Mov Disord 1994;9:559–562.

552. Sandyk R. Hemifacial spasm in tuberculous meningitis. Postgrad Med J 1983;59:570–571.

553. Maroun FB, Jacob J, Mangan M. Hemifacial spasm. Neurosurgery 1987;20:994–995.

554. Maroun FB, Jacob JC, Weir BK, et al. Hemifacial spasm and craniovertebral anomaly. Canadian Journal of Neurological Sciences.Can J Neurolog Sci 1990;17:424–426.

555. Fernandez JM, Mederer S, Alvarez-Sabin J, et al. Hemifacial spasm associated with Paget's disease of bone. Neurology 1991;41:1322–1323.

556. Kurimoto M, Ohara S, Takaku A. Basilar impression in osteogenesis imperfecta tarda: Case report. J Neurosurg 1991;74:136–138.

557. Ing EB, Savino PJ, Bosley TM, et al. Hemifacial spasm and osteitis deformans. Am J Ophthalmol 1995;119:376–377.

558. Nishi T, Matsukado Y, Nagahiro S, et al. Hemifacial spasm due to contralateral acoustic neuroma: case report. Neurology 1987;37:339–342.

559. Rhee BA, Kim TS, Kim GK, et al. Hemifacial spasm caused by contralateral cerebellopontine. Neurosurgery 1995;36:393–395.

560. Selky AK, Purvin VA. Hemifacial spasm: An unusual manifestation of idiopathic J Neuroophthalmology 1994;14:196–198.

561. Ferguson JH. Hemifacial spasm and the facial nucleus. Ann Neurol 1978;4:97–103.

562. Martinelli P, Gabellini AS, Lugaresi E. Facial nucleus involvement in postparalytic hemifacial spasm. J Neurol Neurosurg Psychiatry 1983;46:586–587.

563. Martinelli P, Giuliani S, Ippoliti M. Hemifacial spasm due to peripheral injury of facial nerve: a movement disorder. Mov Disord 1992;7:181–184.

564. Eidelman BH, Nielsen VK, Moller M, et al. Vascular compression, hemifacial spasm and multiple cranial neuropathy. Neurology 1985;35:712–716.

565. Ohashi N, Yasumura S, Mizukoshi K, et al. Involvement of the VIIIth cranial nerve and the brainstem. Acta Oto-Laryngologica 1991;111:1060–1064.

566. Ballantyne ES, Page RD, Meaney JF, et al. Coexistent trigeminal neuralgia, hemifacial spasm, and hypertension: preoperative imaging of neurovascular compression: Case report. J Neurosurg 1994;80:559–563.

567. Moller AR, Jannetta PJ. Reply from the authors. Neurology 1986;36:591.

568. Nielsen VK. Indirect and direct evidence of ephaptic transmission in hemifacial spasm. Neurology 1986;36:592.

569. Ravits J, Hallet M. Pathophysiology of hemifacial spasm: Localization of the lesion in hemifacial spasm. Neurology 1986;36:591.

570. Auger RG. Hemifacial spasm: Clinical and electrophysiologic observations. Neurology 1979;29:1261–1272.

571. Hopf HC, Lowitzsch K. Hemifacial spasm: location of the lesion by electrophysiological means. Muscle Nerve 1982;5:S84–S88.

572. Iwakuma T, Matsumoto A, Nakamura N. Hemifacial spasm: Comparison of three different operative procedures in 110 patients. J Neurosurg 1982;57:753–756.

573. Kugmagami H. Neuropathological findings of hemifacial spasm and trigeminal neuralgia. Arch Otolaryngol 1974;99:160–164.

574. Ruby JR, Jannetta PJ. Hemifacial spasm: Ultrastructural changes in the facial nerve induced by neurovascular compression. Surg Neurol 1975;4:369–370.

575. Moller AR, Jannetta PJ. On the origin of synkinesis in hemifacial spasm results of intracranial recordings. J Neurosurg 1984;61:569–576.

576. Moller AR, Jannetta PJ. Hemifacial spasm: Results of electrophysiologic recordings during microvascular decompression operations. Neurology 1985;35:969–974.

577. Moller AR, Jannetta PJ. Microvascular decompression in hemifacial spasm: intraoperative electrophysiological observations. Neurosurgery 1985;16:612–618.

578. Moller AR. The cranial nerve vascular compression syndrome. I. A review. Acta Neurochir 1991;113:18–23.

579. Moller AR. The cranial nerve vascular compression syndrome. II. A review. Acta Neurochir 1991;113:24–30.

580. Sen CN, Moller AR. Signs of hemifacial spasm created by chronic periodic stimulation of the facial nerve in the rat. Exp Neurol 1987;98:336–349.

581. Fabinyi GCA, Adams CBT. Hemifacial spasm: Treatment by posterior fossa surgery. J Neurol Neurosurg Psychiatry 1978;41:829–833.

582. Aoki N, Nagao T. Resolution of hemifacial spasm after posterior fossa exploration without vascular decompression. Neurosurg 1986;18:478–479.

583. Adams CBT. Microvascular compression: an alternative view and hypothesis. J Neurosurg 1989;57:1–12.

584. Jannetta PJ. Neurovascular compression in cranial nerves and systemic disease. Ann Surg 1980;192:518–525.

585. Auger RG, Piepgras DG, Laws ER Jr, et al. Microvascular decompression of the facial nerve for hemifacial spasm: Clinical and electrophysiological observations. Neurology 1981;31:346–350.

586. Loeser JD, Chen J. Hemifacial spasm: Treatment by microsurgical facial nerve decompression. Neurosurgery 1983;13:141–146.

587. Barker FG 2nd, Jannetta PJ, Bissonette DJ, et al. Microvascular decompression for hemifacial spasm. J Neurosurg 1995;82:201–210.

588. Shaywitz BA. Hemifacial spasm in a child treated with carbamazepine. Arch Neurol 1974;31:63.

589. Alexander GE, Moses H. Carbamazepine for hemifacial spasm. Neurology 1982;2:286–287.

590. Hughes EC, Brackmann DE, Weinstein RC. Seventh nerve spasm: Effect of modification of cholinergic balance. Otolaryngol Head Neck Surg 1980;88:491–499.

591. Celis-Blaubach A, Higuera Castillo A. Idiopathic hemifacial spasm. Acta Otolaryngol 1974;77:221–227.

592. Sadé J. Subtotal evulsion of the facial nerve in hemifacial spasm. Acta Otolaryngol 1974;78:410–417.

593. Hori T, Fukushima T, Terao H, et al. Percutaneous radiofrequency facial nerve coagulation in the management of facial spasm. J Neurosurg 1981;54:655–658.

594. Fan Z. Intracranial longitudinal splitting of facial nerve: A new approach. Ann Oto Rhinol Laryngol 1993;102:108–109.

595. Harrison MJG, Andrew J. Recurrence of hemifacial spasm after hypoglossal facial anastomosis. J Neurol Neurosurg Psychiatry 1981;44:558–559.

596. Chen CR, Lu C-S, Tsai C-H. Botulinum toxin A injection in the treatment of hemifacial spasm. Acta Neurol Scand 1996;94:207–211.

597. Mauriello JA Jr, Leone T, Dhillon S, et al. Treatment choices of 119 patients with hemifacial spasm over 11 years. Clin Neurol Neurosurg 1996;98:213–216.

598. Baker L, Wirtschafter JD. Experimental doxorubicin myopathies: A permanent treatment for eyelid spasms? Arch Ophthalmol 1987;105:1265–1268.

599. Wirtschafter JD, Lander T, Kirsch J, et al. Heterogeneous length and in-series arrangement of myofibers do not extend the length of the eyelid. Trans Am Ophthalmol Soc 1994;92:88–90.

600. Ford FR. Diseases of the Nervous System in Infancy, Childhood and Adolescence. Ed 5. Springfield, IL, CC Thomas, 1966:617–625.

601. Weinstein L. Tetanus. N Engl J Med 1973;289:1293–1296.

602. Bratzlavsky M, VanderEecken H. Medullary actions of tetanus toxin: An electrophysiological study in man. Arch Neurol 1976;33:783–785.

603. Goldstone H, Ford FR. Severe myotonia as a complication of postoperative thyroid deficiency: Complete relief of myotonia by thyroid extract: Report of two cases. Bull Johns Hopkins Hosp 1955;97:53–58.

604. Sisson JC, Beierwaltes WH, Koepke GH, et al. "Myotonia" of the orbicularis oculi with myxedema. Arch Intern Med 1962;110:323–327.

605. Dodge PR, Gamstrop I, Byers RK, et al. Myotonic dystrophy in infancy and childhood. Pediatrics 1965;35:3–19.

606. Van Allen MW, Blodi FC. Electromyographic study of reciprocal innervation in blinking. Neurology 1962;12:371–377.

607. Scaff M, Mendonca L, Levy JA, et al. Chondrodystrophic myotonia: Electromyographic and cardiac features of a case. Acta Neurol Scand 1979;60:243–249.

SECTION V:
Facial Pain and Headache

Valérie Biousse, section editor

Somatic sensation in the eye, the face, and the cranium is mediated by a complex system of receptors, afferent neurons, brainstem nuclei, and projections to the thalamus, cerebral cortex, and other brainstem nuclei. The trigeminal nerve, with its three trunks and their branches, gasserian ganglion, and sensory root, is the principle somatic afferent pathway for this system, disorders of which can produce various disturbances, most commonly facial numbness, facial pain, and headache. These subjects are considered in the context of their neuro-ophthalmologic significance in the two chapters that comprise this section.

CHAPTER 25

The Trigeminal Nerve and Its Central Connections

Grant T. Liu

Because the three divisions of the trigeminal nerve run in close proximity to cranial nerves II, III, IV, and VI, sensory dysfunction in the face may be a symptom in neuro-ophthalmic patients with vision loss and eye movement disorders. In addition, the trigeminal nuclei are located at all levels of the brainstem, and subsequent central pathways connect these nuclei with the thalami and sensory cortices. Thus, sensory abnormalities of the face often accompany neurologic syndromes due to lesions throughout the central nervous system.

An understanding of the relevant anatomy, along with accurate sensory and motor testing, enables the clinician to localize the lesion more accurately. This chapter covers trigeminal system anatomy and physiology, the examination of the trigeminal nerve system, and topical diagnosis of disturbances of the trigeminal nerve and its central connections.

ANATOMY AND PHYSIOLOGY OF THE TRIGEMINAL NERVE AND ITS CENTRAL CONNECTIONS

This section discusses the anatomy and physiology of the trigeminal nerve and its central connections centripetally. The branches of the trigeminal nerve are considered first, then the gasserian ganglion and trigeminal roots are reviewed. The central connections are discussed last.

MAJOR DIVISIONS OF THE TRIGEMINAL NERVE

Somatic sensory impulses converge upon the gasserian ganglion from the eye, the deep and superficial structures of the face, and the cranium via three major nerves: the ophthalmic, the maxillary, and the mandibular divisions of the trigeminal nerve (Fig. 25.1). Although these nerve trunks represent an afferent system, we describe their anatomy and that of their branches in a centrifugal sequence, from the gasserian ganglion to their connections in the periphery. The mandibular nerve is the only one of the three divisions that contains axons of the motor division of the trigeminal system. Some peripheral branches of the trigeminal nerve contain pre- or postganglionic parasympathetic fibers or post-

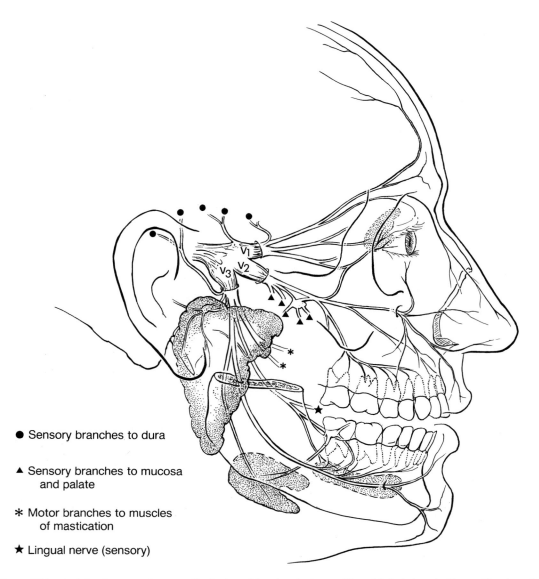

● Sensory branches to dura

▲ Sensory branches to mucosa
  and palate

✴ Motor branches to muscles
  of mastication

★ Lingual nerve (sensory)

Figure 25.1. Peripheral motor and sensory distribution of the trigeminal nerve. V_1, ophthalmic branch; V_2, maxillary branch; V_3, mandibular branch. Details of branches highlighted in Figure 25.5 (V_1), Figure 25.7 (V_2), and Figure 25.8 (V_3).

ganglionic sympathetic fibers to supply salivary, sweat, or other glands of face, eyes, and mouth (1).

Ophthalmic Nerve (V1)

The ophthalmic or first division is purely sensory and is smaller than the other two divisions. It supplies sensation to the entire eyeball, forehead, lacrimal gland, caruncle, and lacrimal sac. It also supplies the upper eyelids, the frontal sinuses, and the side of the nose. Its cutaneous representation is overlapped by that of the maxillary division (Figs. 25.1 and 25.2).

The ophthalmic nerve arises from the anteromedial aspect of the gasserian ganglion (2). It immediately enters the cavernous sinus inferiorly, where it lies embedded in the lateral wall below the trochlear nerve (Fig. 25.3). Umansky and

Nathan (3) studied the cavernous sinus in 70 specimens and found that the lateral wall of the sinus is composed of two layers, a superficial dural layer and a deep layer. The deep layer is formed by the sheaths of the oculomotor (III) and trochlear (IV) nerves, by the sheaths of the ophthalmic and maxillary nerves (V1,2), and by a reticular membrane that extends between the sheaths.

Within the cavernous sinus, the ophthalmic nerve gives off fine twigs to the oculomotor, trochlear, and abducens nerves, thereby supplying sensation to the muscles innervated by these structures. At this level it also gives off recurrent branches that cross, are adherent to the trochlear nerve, and are distributed to the tentorium cerebelli and dura over the posterior pole of the brain (discussion following).

Sympathetic filaments join the ophthalmic nerve from the

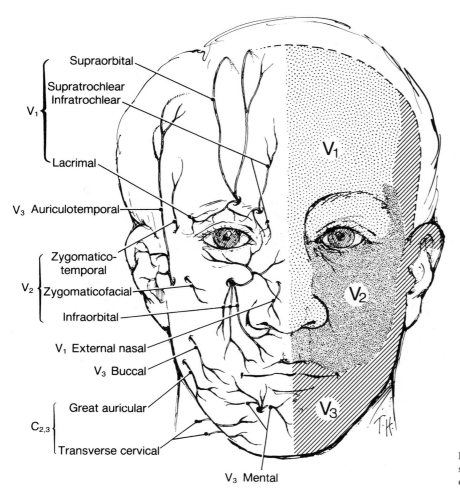

Figure 25.2. Sensory nerves of the face and scalp. Note the distribution of the three divisions of the trigeminal nerve and their areas of overlap.

cavernous plexus situated around the internal carotid artery. According to Parkinson and coworkers (4–6), the sympathetic nerve is a single trunk that runs with the carotid artery. In the cavernous sinus, the trunk joins the abducens nerve briefly before separating and joining the ophthalmic nerve (Fig. 25.4).

Toward the front of the cavernous sinus, and before leaving it, the ophthalmic nerve slopes slightly upward and divides into its three main branches—the lacrimal, frontal, and nasociliary nerves—all of which enter the orbit through the superior orbital fissure (7) (Fig. 25.5).

Trigeminal Innervation of Intracranial Structures

The brain is not innervated by nociceptors. The innervation of the dura of the middle fossa and the middle meningeal vessels is through the maxillary and mandibular (second and third) divisions of the trigeminal nerve, whereas fibers from the ophthalmic (first) division innervate the dura of the anterior fossa (excluding the lateral convexity), the tentorium, and both the falx and the superior sagittal sinus anteriorly and posteriorly.

In monkeys, it has been confirmed that the ophthalmic

division of the trigeminal nerve, with a minor contribution from the maxillary division, innervates the vessels in the circle of Willis (8,9). Within the gasserian ganglion of rats, cells that innervate the forehead tend to be clustered around those that send afferents to the ipsilateral middle cerebral artery (10). Their proximity may provide, in part, the anatomic substrate for referred headache pain. The central connections of these neurons are discussed later in this chapter.

The trigeminal innervation of cerebral blood vessels and dura has important theoretic implications regarding the pathophysiology and treatment of migraine (11–13) (see Chapter 26).

Lacrimal Nerve

This nerve passes through the lateral side of the superior orbital fissure above the lateral rectus muscle to enter the lacrimal gland. It divides into two divisions, either just before entering the gland or within the gland itself. The superior division, which supplies the gland, ends in the conjunctiva and the skin of the upper eyelid, whereas the lower division descends along the orbital wall to anastomose with a branch from the maxillary division.

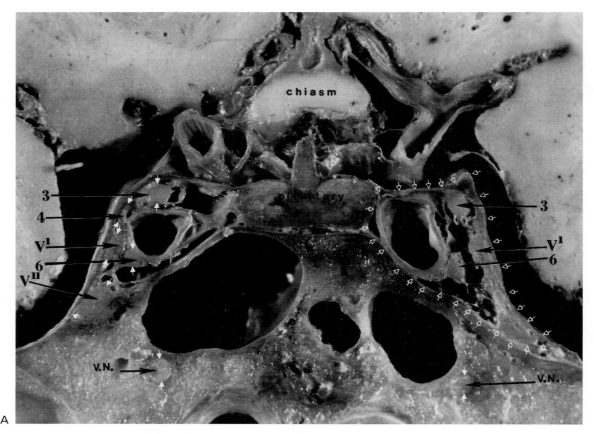

A

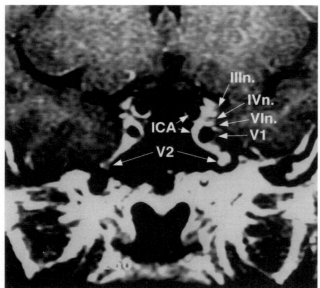

B

Figure 25.3. *A,* Location of the trigeminal trunks in the cavernous sinus. 3, oculomotor nerve; 4, trochlear nerve; V¹, ophthalmic branch of the trigeminal nerve; V², maxillary branch of the trigeminal nerve; 6, abducens nerve; V.N., vidian nerve. On the left side, the location of each nerve is identified by *solid white arrows.* On the right side, the boundaries of the cavernous sinus are identified by *open white arrows. B,* Contrast-enhanced T1-weighted magnetic resonance image, coronal view through the cavernous sinus similar to that in *A.* ICA, internal carotid artery; IIIn., oculomotor nerve; IVn., trochlear nerve; VIn., abducens nerve; V1, ophthalmic branch of the trigeminal nerve; V2, maxillary branch of the trigeminal nerve.

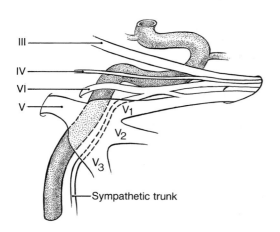

Figure 25.4. Drawing of relationship between the sympathetic fibers, the abducens nerve, and the ophthalmic division of the trigeminal nerve. The sympathetic trunk ascends with the internal carotid artery. It joins briefly with the abducens nerve (VI) then leaves the nerve to join with the ophthalmic branch (V₁) of the trigeminal nerve (V₁).

nasal cavity, breaking up into three terminal branches. Two of these branches, the medial and lateral internal nasal branches, are distributed to the anterior nasal cavity, whereas the third continues anteriorly to the end of the nose as the external nasal nerve.

The branches of the nasociliary nerve are as follows: (*a*) the long or sensory root leaves the nerve either just before it enters the orbit or immediately thereafter and passes to the ciliary ganglion into the short ciliary nerves; (*b*) the long ciliary nerves, usually two but occasionally three, surround the optic nerve and pass forward to the iris, ciliary body, and cornea—these nerves also carry dilator fibers from the cavernous sympathetic plexus to the dilator pupillae; (*c*) the infratrochlear nerve is distributed to the medial canthus, to the skin and conjunctiva of the upper eyelid, and to the root of the nose, lacrimal sac, and caruncle; (*d*) nasal branches, usually three, supply the mucous membrane of the anterior part of the nasal septum, the anterior portion of the lateral nasal wall, and the middle and inferior turbinate bones as well as the skin over the cartilaginous tip of the nose (Figs. 25.1, 25.2, and 25.5).

Frontal Nerve

The frontal nerve enters the orbit above the superior rectus muscle and the levator palpebrae superioris. It hugs the roof of the orbit, and, at about the middle of the orbit, it gives off the supratrochlear nerve, after which point it becomes the supraorbital nerve. The supraorbital nerve supplies the skin of the forehead near the midline, the skin and conjunctiva of the upper eyelid, and the skin on the side of the nose. The supraorbital nerve leaves the orbit by passing through the supraorbital notch in company with the supraorbital artery and proceeds superiorly giving off twigs to the eyelids and frontal sinus. Whitnall (14) noted that neuralgia in the forehead may persist after resection of the supratrochlear nerve and that in such an instance, resection of the frontal nerve may be necessary.

Nasociliary Nerve

The nasociliary nerve is of particular ophthalmic interest because it is the nerve of sensory supply to the eye. Because of its long course through the orbit and cranial cavity and its supply to the nose, it is in contact with many structures. Consequently, neurologic involvement is not uncommon. According to Whitnall (14), this nerve enters the orbit through the annulus of Zinn between the two divisions of the oculomotor nerve and courses obliquely beneath the superior rectus muscle. It then crosses over the optic nerve along with the ophthalmic artery toward the medial orbital wall, where it lies between the superior oblique and medial rectus muscles, still adjacent to the artery. The nasociliary nerve leaves the orbit by traversing the anterior ethmoidal foramen and reenters the cranial vault, where it crosses the anterior portion of the cribriform plate beneath the dura of the anterior cranial fossa, adjacent to the olfactory lobe. It then crosses through a slit, the nasal fissure or anterior nasal canal, at the side of the crista galli and enters the

Maxillary Nerve (V2)

The maxillary division is a purely sensory division of the trigeminal nerve. It supplies the skin of the cheek, part of the temporal region, the lower eyelid, upper lip, side of the nose, part of the mucous membrane of the nose, the teeth of the upper jaw, nasopharynx, maxillary sinus, soft palate, tonsil, and roof of the mouth (Fig. 25.2).

The maxillary nerve arises from the frontal central portion of the gasserian ganglion and is usually described as entering the cavernous sinus to lie beneath the ophthalmic division, where it may be separated from the sphenoid sinus by only a thin layer of bone (Fig. 25.3). Here the maxillary nerve may produce a bulge into the lateral wall of the sphenoid sinus (15,16). Henderson (17) investigated the causes of certain unexpected, and sometimes unsatisfactory, results after gasserian ganglion injections for trigeminal neuralgia and studied the relationship of the human maxillary nerve to the cavernous sinus. He concluded that the greater part of the nerve is embedded in the dura of the middle fossa just lateral to the cavernous sinus, rather than within the wall of the sinus. He also found that the origin of the nerve crosses a separate dural sinus that connects the cavernous sinus and the pterygoid venous plexus. Henderson (17) postulated that injection of this "trigeminal" sinus, rather than the gasserian ganglion, was considered to be responsible for some clinical failures in treatment of trigeminal neuralgia. Umansky and Nathan (3) agreed that there is considerable variation in location of the maxillary nerve within the cavernous sinus. In their specimens, only in some cases were either the maxillary nerve or the gasserian ganglion located partially within the lateral wall of the sinus, although when these structures were present, they were located in the deep layer of the wall.

The most important of the intracranial branches from the maxillary nerve is the middle meningeal nerve that supplies the dura mater of the middle cranial fossa. The maxillary

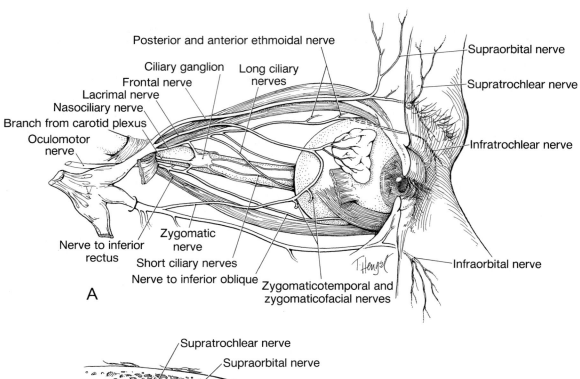

Posterior and anterior ethmoidal nerve

Ciliary ganglion   Long ciliary
Frontal nerve   nerves
Lacrimal nerve
Nasociliary nerve
Branch from carotid plexus
Oculomotor
nerve

Supraorbital nerve

Supratrochlear nerve

Infratrochlear nerve

Nerve to inferior
rectus
Short ciliary nerves
Nerve to inferior oblique

Zygomatic
nerve

Zygomaticotemporal and
zygomaticofacial nerves

Infraorbital nerve

A

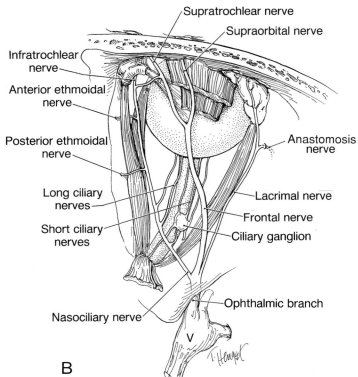

Supratrochlear nerve

Supraorbital nerve

Infratrochlear
nerve
Anterior ethmoidal
nerve
Posterior ethmoidal
nerve
Long ciliary
nerves
Short ciliary
nerves
Nasociliary nerve

Anastomosis
nerve

Lacrimal nerve

Frontal nerve

Ciliary ganglion

Ophthalmic branch

V

B

Figure 25.5. The branches of the ophthalmic (first) division of the trigeminal nerve (V_1) seen from the side (*A*), and from above (*B*). In *A*, orbital portions of the second division (V_2) are also depicted.

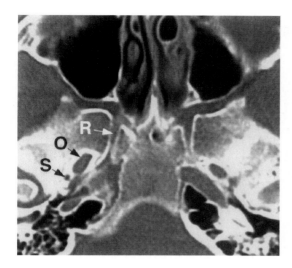

Figure 25.6. Computerized tomography (CT), axial view and bone windows through the skull base demonstrating the foramen rotundum (R), through which the maxillary division (V$_2$) exits the skull; the foramen ovale (O), through which the mandibular division (V$_3$) exits the skull; and the foramen spinosum (S), through which the middle meningeal artery enters the skull.

nerve then passes through the foramen rotundum (Fig. 25.6), which lies in the medial aspect of the greater wing of the sphenoid bone (18) to the pterygopalatine fossa (19), where the nerve gives off: (*a*) two large pterygopalatine nerves, which enter the pterygopalatine ganglion, and then divide into branches that supply portions of the nasopharynx, hard and soft palate, and nasal cavity; (*b*) several posterior superior alveolar nerves that pass through the pterygomaxillary

fissure to provide sensation for the upper gums and molar teeth; and (*c*) the zygomatic nerve, which enters the orbit through the inferior orbital fissure. This nerve in turn divides into two branches: (*a*) the zygomaticofacial branch, which appears on the face after passing through the zygomatic foramen to supply the skin over the zygomatic bone; and (*b*) the zygomaticotemporal branch, which innervates the skin over the temporal side of the zygomatic bone. Within the orbit the zygomatic nerve communicates with the lacrimal nerve (Figs. 25.2, 25.5, and 25.7). This communication is particularly important because the parasympathetic fibers in the facial nerve gain access to the lacrimal gland via this route (see Chapter 24).

Distal to the pterygopalatine fossa, the maxillary nerve travels through the inferior orbital fissure into the orbit, where it becomes the infraorbital nerve (Fig. 25.7). This nerve is the terminal branch of the maxillary nerve. It passes through the orbital floor in either a canal, the infraorbital canal, or simply a shallow depression only partially covered with bone, the infraorbital groove. While in the canal, it supplies branches to the teeth. The infraorbital nerve exits the orbit through the infraorbital foramen to supply the skin and subcutaneous tissue of the face below and nasal to the orbit (Figs. 25.2, 25.5, and 25.7).

Although it is unclear whether or not the maxillary nerve supplies any sensory fibers that innervate the eye in humans, there is some suggestive evidence of this in animals. In cats and monkeys, Morgan et al. (20) and Marfurt et al. (21) found that the maxillary nerve may carry a small percentage of corneal afferents. Ruskell (22) performed careful dissections of 13 rhesus monkeys and 12 cynomolgous monkeys and showed the presence of an orbitociliary branch of the maxillary nerve. Degeneration experiments combined with

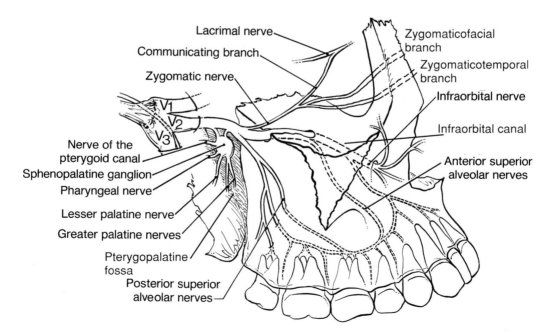

Figure 25.7. The branches of the maxillary (second) division of the trigeminal nerve (V$_2$).

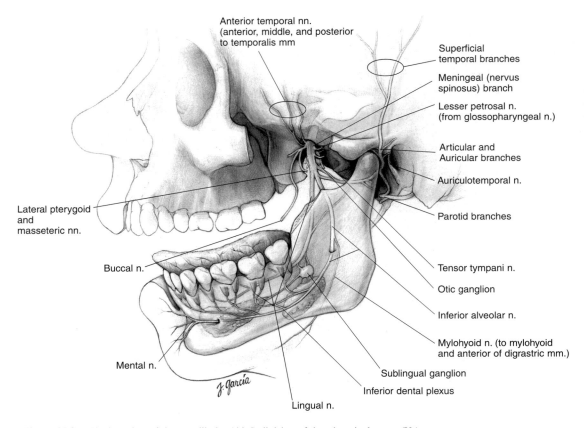

Figure 25.8. The branches of the mandibular (third) division of the trigeminal nerve (V₃).

electron microscopy were used to confirm the pathway and to demonstrate the passage of maxillary fibers through the ciliary ganglion into short ciliary nerves. Whether these nerves serve a sensory function different from that of the nerves that originate from the ophthalmic nerve is not apparent from Ruskell's study. In addition, even though Beauvieux and Dupas (23) observed a ciliary ganglion root of maxillary nerve origin in some of their human preparations, the existence of sensory nerves originating from the maxillary nerve and innervating the eye has not been shown convincingly in humans.

Mandibular Nerve (V3)

The mandibular division, which does not enter the cavernous sinus, contains motor and sensory fibers (Fig. 25.8). The motor portion supplies muscles that derive from the first pharyngeal (branchial) arch of the embryo (1).

The mandibular nerve is formed by a large sensory root from the gasserian ganglion that passes inferiorly together with the motor root of the trigeminal nerve. These two roots lie close together in the middle cranial fossa and pass through the foramen ovale to the infratemporal fossa, where they form a single trunk (Fig. 25.9).The foramen ovale sits in the posteromedial aspect of the greater wing of the sphenoid bone (18) (Fig. 25.6). The undivided trunk lies 3.75 cm medial to the tubercle at the root of the zygoma. This portion

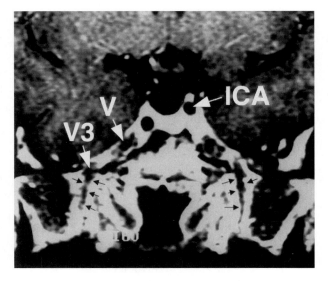

Figure 25.9. Contrast-enhanced T1-weighted magnetic resonance image (MRI), coronal view posterior to that of Figure 25.3*B* (behind the cavernous sinus), demonstrating the gasserian ganglion (V) and the mandibular division (V3) heading caudally through the foramen ovale into the infratemporal fossa, at which point the nerve is highlighted by *white arrows*. ICA, internal carotid artery.

of the nerve gives off: (*a*) a recurrent neural plexus that accompanies the middle meningeal artery through the foramen spinosum (Fig. 25.6) to supply the dura mater on the temporal side of the cranium (24); (*b*) the nerve to the medial pterygoid, which passes through or around the otic ganglion to the tensor tympani and tensor veli palatini muscles (1). The trunk then divides into anterior, principally motor, and posterior, principally sensory, divisions.

The anterior division, containing most of the motor part of the trigeminal nerve, supplies the muscles of mastication. It passes downward and forward, medial to the lateral pterygoid muscle, and separates into the following motor branches: (*a*) a branch to the lateral pterygoid muscle; (*b*) a branch to the masseter muscle that passes over the superior border of the lateral pterygoid muscle and through the mandibular notch of the mandible and gives a filament to the temporomandibular joint; (*c*) two deep temporal branches, anterior and posterior, to the temporal muscle, that also ascend above the lateral pterygoid muscle; and (*d*) the buccinator nerve, which passes obliquely forward between the two heads of the lateral pterygoid muscle to reach the masseter (buccinator) muscle.

Injury to the motor part of the trigeminal nerve results in ipsilateral deviation of the jaw upon protrusion because of paralysis of the ipsilateral lateral pterygoid; upon retraction, the jaw deviates contralaterally as a result of paralysis of the temporalis (discussion following) (1). The sensory portion of the anterior division, the buccal nerve, supplies the skin and mucous membranes of the cheek as well as part of the gums.

The posterior division of the nerve has three major subdivisions, each with mixed functions (1):

1. The auriculotemporal nerve and its branches supply the upper part of the lateral surface of the ear, the upper part of the meatus, the tympanic membrane, the parotid gland, and the skin of the side of the head. Autonomic fibers within the auriculotemporal nerve include secretomotor postganglionic parasympathetic fibers from the otic ganglion destined for the parotid gland and also postganglionic sympathetic fibers from the plexus on the middle meningeal artery. The auriculotemporal nerve lies in close proximity to the temporomandibular joint capsular region, lateral pterygoid muscle, and middle meningeal artery (25,26).
2. The lingual nerve supplies sensation to the the gums and anterior portion of the tongue. The lingual nerve is joined by the chordi tympani of the facial nerve, which contains taste fibers for the anterior two-thirds of the tongue and preganglionic parasympathetic fibers destined for the submandibular ganglion. Postganglionic parasympathetic fibers leave the ganglion and return to the lingual nerve before reaching the salivary glands.
3. The inferior alveolar nerve itself has three branches: the mylohyoid nerve, the motor branch, innervates the mylohyoid muscle and the anterior belly of the digastric muscle; the inferior dental plexus supplies the gums and the teeth of the mandible; and the mental nerve supplies the skin of the chin and the skin and mucous membrane of the lower lip and gums (Figs. 25.1 and 25.2).

Jaw proprioception is mediated by stretch receptors in jaw muscles and mechanoreceptors in the periodontal membrane (27). Afferent axons from these receptors travel primarily within the mandibular nerve, and their cell bodies are located in the mesencephalic nucleus of the trigeminal nerve (discussion following). Collateral branches from the mesencephalic nucleus connect directly to the trigeminal motor nucleus, thereby providing a monosynaptic pathway for the jaw-jerk (masseter) reflex. Interested readers are referred to the electrophysiologic investigations of the trigeminal motor system in humans by Cruccu and colleagues (28,29) and by Türk et al. (30).

GASSERIAN (TRIGEMINAL, SEMILUNAR) GANGLION

The crescent-shaped gasserian ganglion lies on the anterior superior surface of the petrous bone in the middle fossa of the skull (Fig. 25.9). It is an expansion of the proximal sensory root from the brainstem and lies within Meckel's cave, surrounded by arachnoid and dura (31). Meckel's cave is bounded by dura laterally, the ascending precavernous portion of the internal carotid artery medially, and the cavernous sinus anteriorly. Meckel's cave often can be identified on computed tomographic (CT) scanning or magnetic resonance (MR) imaging (32–37).

The fine structure of the gasserian ganglion is essentially similar to that of the spinal root ganglia, although it is significantly larger (38–40). It contains the cells that give rise to the three divisions of the trigeminal nerve. The site of formation of the ophthalmic nerve is widely separated from that of the maxillary and mandibular nerves, which run more closely together.

The gasserian ganglion contains the cells of origin of all the trigeminal sensory axons. These are unipolar cells, whose axons bifurcate into an anterior branch, which proceeds distally in one of the three nerve divisions, and the posterior branch, which extends into the pons. The motor root does not enter the ganglion.

The gasserian ganglion and the proximal portions of the ophthalmic and maxillary divisions receive most of their blood supply from branches of the inferolateral trunk, which itself derives from the intracavernous carotid artery (41,42). Within the cavernous sinus, the distal ophthalmic nerve is supplied by the artery to the superior orbital fissure, whereas the distal maxillary nerve is supplied by the artery to the foramen rotundum. Both of these arteries are distal branches of the inferolateral trunk. The medial third of the gasserian ganglion can also receive blood from the tentorial artery of the meningohypophyseal trunk (also from the intracavernous carotid), while the lateral third can also be fed by the middle meningeal artery.

TRIGEMINAL ROOT

The sensory and motor divisions of the trigeminal nerve exist as separate "roots" from the pons. The exit of the motor root lies immediately cephalad to the point of entrance of the sensory root.

Microvascular relationships of the trigeminal roots have

been described by numerous investigators (2,43–45). Hardy and Rhoton (2) and Hardy et al. (44) reported that approximately half of cadaveric trigeminal roots had some contact with an artery, usually the superior cerebellar artery. Haines et al. (43) found contact between the trigeminal root and the superior cerebellar artery in 35% of 40 autopsy specimens. Klun and Prestor (45) discovered contact with the trigeminal root in 32% of specimens, but actual compression in only another 8% either by the superior cerebellar artery (most commonly), the anterior inferior cerebellar artery, a pontine branch of the basilar artery, or in one instance, a vein. Compression of the trigeminal nerve root by surrounding arterial and venous structures is one cause of trigeminal neuralgia (46–51) (see Chapter 26).

The trigeminal roots are supplied by a group of vessels called the trigeminal arteries, which orginate from the superior cerebellar artery, the posterolateral, superolateral, and inferolateral pontine arteries, the anterior inferior cerebellar artery, the basilar artery trunk, and the trigeminocerebellar artery (52). The superolateral pontine artery, which is a small branch of the basilar artery, and the anterior inferior cerebellar arteries are the most common parent vessels.

Sensory Root

The fibers of the sensory root run parallel and become arranged in separate bundles by the enveloping supporting tissues (31).

In their study of 50 human trigeminal nerves, Gudmundsson et al. (53) found that the length of the sensory root from the pons to the gasserian ganglion varied from 18–26 mm, with the average being 22 mm. In half of the nerves studied, small bundles of sensory fibers arose from the pons outside the main sensory fiber bundle. These aberrant or accessory sensory fibers usually arose around the rostral two-thirds of the pons, and most entered the root within 12 mm of the pons. Of the total of 66 aberrant rootlets observed by Gudmundsson et al. (53), 49 passed into the ophthalmic nerve, 10 into the maxillary nerve, and 7 into the mandibular nerve.

Kerr (39) studied the somatotopic organization of the nonhuman primate sensory root. Ophthalmic division fibers were ventrally placed within the sensory root; mandibular division fibers were dorsally placed; and maxillary fibers occupied the intermediate zone. Mira et al. (54) found a similar disposition of fibers in human sensory roots, whereas Gudmundsson et al. (53) and Stechison et al. (55) found that fibers from the ophthalmic division are usually **rostromedial** and the mandibular fibers are usually **caudolateral**. Pelletier et al. (56) confirmed a somatotopic arrangement of the three divisions within the sensory root. However, these investigators found that sensory modalities were diffusely represented within each division, and they offered this as an explanation why large sections (even 50% or more) of sensory root divisions may be performed without appreciable sensory loss.

The vast majority of corneal afferents travel within the ophthalmic division of the trigeminal sensory root. A small minority course within the maxillary division (20).

Stibbe (57,58) and Mira et al. (54) found nerve cells in the human sensory root of both humans and dogs. The nerve cells appear to be localized to the proximal portion of the sensory root in humans. The presence of these nerve cells far from the gasserian ganglion may indicate an accessory relay station for trigeminal sensory fibers. In fact, it has been suggested that some light touch sensation is carried by this group of fibers (59,60). Supporting this concept is the work of Hussein et al. (61), who treated 25 trigeminal neuralgia patients with fractional section of the trigeminal nerve via a posterior fossa approach. The procedure was effective in relieving pain, while preserving corneal sensation and motor root function. Of the patients who were treated, 19 showed slight loss of light touch sensation. In 15 of these patients, there was dissociation of sensory loss between pinprick (pain) and light touch. The pattern of dissociated sensory loss produced in these patients suggests that fibers carrying light touch sensation tend to collect in the medial part of the main sensory root as it enters the pons.

Motor Root

The motor root emerges from the pons as separate bundles at two major levels, the fibers from the dorsal level originating from the mesencephalic nucleus. Gudmundsson et al. (53) found the human motor root to be composed of as many as 14 separately originating rootlets that usually join about 1 cm from the pons. In addition, Gudmundsson et al. (53) demonstrated anastomoses between the motor and sensory roots in the majority of nerves that they examined. These anastomoses may explain the discovery by Mira et al. (54) of nerve cells in the human motor nerve root similar to cells observed in the sensory root (57,58). The function of these cells is unknown, but they may serve some type of sensory function.

The motor root accompanies the sensory root from the lateral pons through the subarachnoid space, through the dura, and into Meckel's cave, where it is concealed by the overlying gasserian ganglion. As it passes the median surface of the ganglion, it is joined by the peripheral sensory fibers that arise from sensory cells in the maxillary region of the ganglion.

AFFERENT TRIGEMINAL FIBERS IN THE BRAINSTEM

The afferent sensory trigeminal fibers arising from their cell bodies in the gasserian ganglion enter the lateral pons and course in a dorsomedial direction. Some of them dichotomize into a short ascending and a long descending branch. Most fibers run caudally without bifurcating. The mass of descending fibers constitutes the **trigeminal spinal tract**, a distinct fiber bundle that is situated just underneath the lateral surface of the medulla oblongata, and slightly deeper in the lower part of the pons, where it is covered by fibers of the middle cerebellar peduncle. The fibers of this tract continue into the two most rostral segments of the spinal cord in the zona terminalis (Figs. 25.10 and 25.11). The fibers that are found in the spinal tract, as well as numerous collaterals, end in a longitudinal cell column medial to the tract, the **nucleus of the trigeminal spinal tract**. Early in-

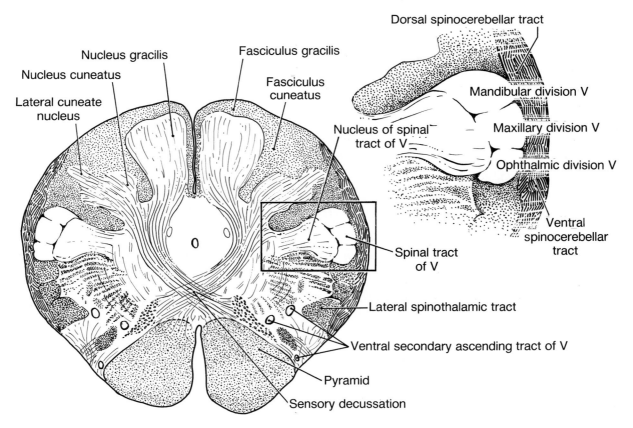

Figure 25.10.   Cross section of medulla 6 mm below the obex. The *box* surrounds fibers traveling in the descending tract of the trigeminal nerve. The *inset* shows the relative positions of the fibers from the ophthalmic, maxillary, and mandibular divisions within the descending tract of the trigeminal nerve. The ophthalmic fibers carry impulses for pain (including the cornea) and temperature sensations to the spinal nucleus of the trigeminal nerve. (Redrawn from Taren JA, Kahn EA. Anatomic pathways related to pain in the face and neck. J Neurosurg 1962;19:116–121.)

vestigations on the trigeminal spinal tract and its nucleus indicated that a divisional lamination exists. The ophthalmic component is situated most ventrally in the tract. Kerr (39) studied this lamination and by the Nauta technique was able to show a very discrete segregation of the ventral ophthalmic portion from the more dorsal maxillary and mandibular portions. He showed that the afferent fibers of all divisions proceed in diminishing numbers caudally to C_2. Similar laminations of the ophthalmic and other divisions of the trigeminal nerve are present in the spinal nucleus and in the main sensory nucleus.

The fibers of the trigeminal spinal tract distribute to the nucleus of the spinal tract in an orderly manner (62). The medullary tractotomy of Sjöqvist (63) for the treatment of trigeminal neuralgia is based on this pattern of distribution of fibers. The procedure consists of transecting the trigeminal spinal tract by a superficial incision in the lowest part of the medulla, thus preventing the impulses in the descending fibers of the tract from reaching the nucleus. The procedure abolishes pain sensibility in the ipsilateral half of the face but has little effect on the sense of touch. Further experience (64) has shown that the incision may be made more caudally.

Thus, only the most caudal part of the spinal nucleus may be involved in the transmission of pain perception (discussion following). The corneal reflex may be completely spared after the Sjöqvist operation.

Although the majority of primary trigeminal afferent fibers project to the trigeminal nuclear complex through the trigeminal spinal tract, those fibers that enter the pons within the motor root, composed of axons with terminals in the oral cavity and the muscles of mastication, bypass the motor nucleus of the trigeminal nerve to collect into a bundle that continues forward along the ventrolateral, and then the lateral, border of the periventricular gray matter to the rostral end of the midbrain. The cells of origin of this group of fibers, the nucleus of the mesencephalic root, are scattered throughout the rostral pontine and mesencephalic tegmentum.

NUCLEI OF THE TRIGEMINAL NERVE

The nuclei of the trigeminal nerve may be considered as three separate units: (*a*) the motor nucleus (special visceral efferent); (*b*) the sensory mesencephalic nucleus (general somatic afferent); and (*c*) the sensory nuclear complex, actu-

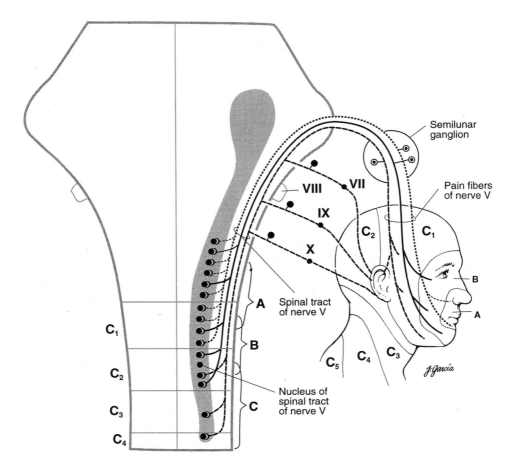

Figure 25.11.   Distribution of pain fibers carried via cranial nerves to the nucleus of the trigeminal spinal tract. Also note the ''onionskin'' distribution of pain fibers on the face (A, B, and C) associated with their rostral to caudal representation in the nucleus of the spinal tract of nerve V. (From Crosby EC, Humphrey T, Lauer EW. Correlative Anatomy of the Nervous System. New York: Macmillan, 1962.)

ally composed of two distinct nuclei—the main sensory nucleus and the nucleus of the spinal tract (general somatic afferent) (65) (Figs. 25.12 and 25.13).

Motor Nucleus

The motor nucleus is situated slightly farther from the ventricular floor than are the nuclei of the oculomotor, trochlear, and abducens nerves. It lies medial to the main sensory nucleus. Fibers from the mesencephalic root are closely associated with fibers from the motor nucleus, and both motor and mesencephalic fibers pass forward in the mandibular section of the nerve (Fig. 25.12*A*).

Mesencephalic Nucleus

Most, if not all, neurons in the trigeminal mesencephalic complex are unipolar, primary afferent cells comparable to sensory ganglion cells (66). Unlike sensory ganglion cells, however, the cell bodies of these neurons have remained within the central nervous system. These are the only primary sensory neuron cell bodies in the central nervous sys-

tem that derive from the neural crest (27). They form a column at the edge of the central gray matter that extends from the posterior commissure rostrally to the level of the trigeminal motor nucleus caudally (Fig. 25.12). Most of these neurons are **proprioceptive** in function (67,68), with receptor terminals responding to stretch in the muscles of mastication. Other mesencephalic neurons innervate the dental supporting tissues (67–69).

Trigeminal Sensory Nuclear Complex

Main Sensory Nucleus

The main sensory nucleus forms the most rostral portion of the trigeminal nuclear complex (excluding the separate mesencephalic nucleus) and is situated lateral to the motor nucleus (70) (Figs. 25.12 and 25.13). Because the sense of touch is mediated by fibers that are somewhat thicker than those mediating pain, and the fibers that end in the main sensory nucleus are, in general, thicker than those to the spinal nucleus, it has generally been proposed that the main sensory nucleus provides the brainstem relay for **tactile** sen-

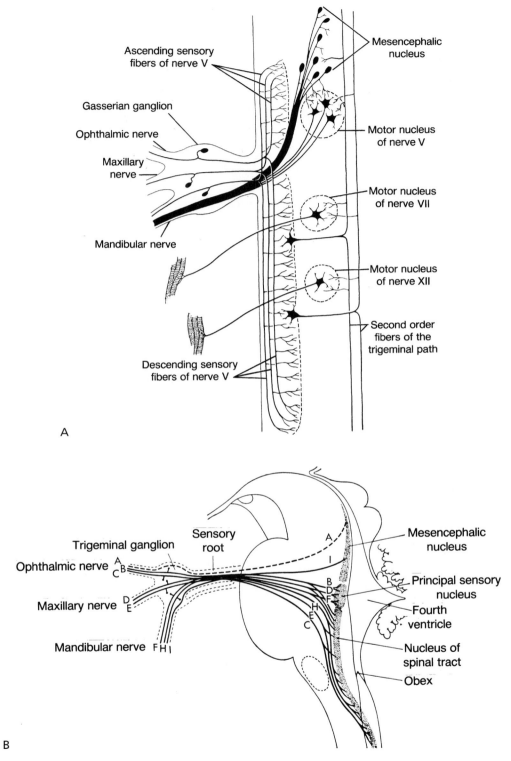

Figure 25.12. *A,* Diagram of nuclei and central connections of the trigeminal nerve. *B,* Nuclei receiving the primary afferent fibers of the trigeminal nerve. A, proprioceptive fibers from the extraocular muscles; B, tactile and pressure fibers from the ophthalmic area; C, pain and temperature fibers from the ophthalmic area; D, tactile and pressure fibers from the maxillary area; E, pain and temperature fibers from the maxillary area; F, tactile and pressure fibers from the mandibular area; H, pain and temperature fibers from the mandibular area; I, proprioceptive fibers from the muscles of mastication. (From Williams PL, Warwick R. Gray's Anatomy. Ed 35. Philadelphia: WB Saunders, 1975.)

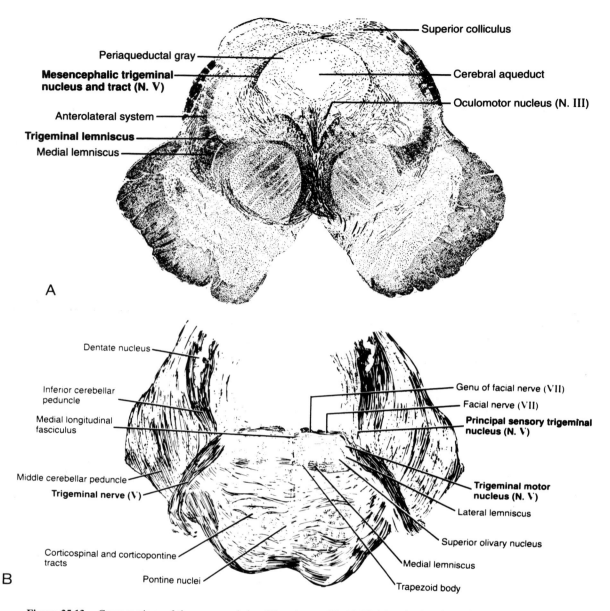

Figure 25.13. Cross sections of the mesencephalon (*A*) and pons (*B*), highlighting the locations of trigeminal structures. Section through the medulla is illustrated in Figure 25.10.

sations from the head, although this is probably an oversimplification.

Most neurons within this nucleus project to the contralateral **nucleus ventralis posteromedialis** (VPM) of the thalamus. These fibers emerge from the ventromedial margin of the main sensory nucleus and pass to the contralateral brainstem to ascend in the trigeminal lemniscus (71) (Fig. 25.14). A smaller population of neurons in the dorsomedial portion of the nucleus, with an input from oral structures, project to the ipsilateral VPM (discussion following). Functionally and anatomically, the main sensory nucleus and its contralateral ascending projections are analogous to the cuneate and grac-

ile nuclei in the medulla and their thalamic connections. The cuneate and gracile nuclei receive tactile information from dorsal horn sensory neurons and then send fibers that decussate and ascend within the medial lemniscus to reach the thalamus (27).

Nucleus of the Spinal Tract

The nucleus of the spinal tract is a long nucleus that extends down the spinal cord as far as the second cervical root and merges with the substantia gelatinosa (70) (Figs. 25.11 and 25.12). In mammals, this nucleus is divisible into three distinct portions: (*a*) the nucleus oralis; (*b*) the nucleus inter-

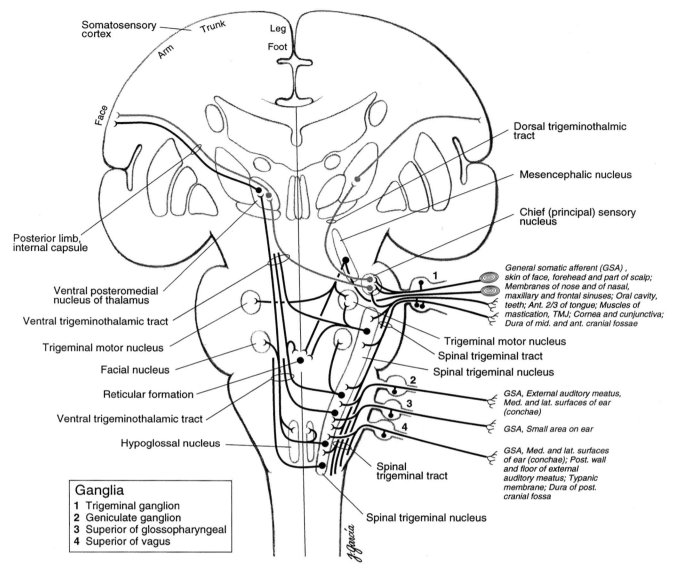

Figure 25.14. Summary of the central connections and ascending projections of the trigeminal system. (From Haines DE. Neuroanatomy. An Atlas of Structures, Sections, and Systems. Ed 4. Baltimore, Williams & Wilkins, 1995:170–171.)

coolers; and (*c*) the nucleus caudalis (65). Each of these nuclei receives input from all the trigeminal roots via the descending spinal trigeminal tract. The fibers from each of the three divisions of the nerve are somatotopically arranged in this tract, with those from the ophthalmic division located most ventrally and those from the mandibular located most dorsally. In humans the ophthalmic division extends farthest caudally. The nucleus of the spinal trigeminal tract is related primarily to the transmission of impulses that are perceived consciously as **pain** and **temperature**. Although the nucleus caudalis is still considered the main termination of trigeminal nociceptive fibers, there is accumulating evidence that the more rostral subnuclei also receive nociceptive information from orofacial structures (72). Readers interested in more

details regarding the processing of nociceptive information in the trigeminal nuclei are referred to the in-depth reviews by Shults (73). Nucleus oralis and interpolaris have important roles in oral and dental sensation (74).

Nucleus (pars) Oralis

This nucleus extends from the rostral pole of the facial nucleus to the rostral third of the inferior olive in the mammal. The axons of most neurons in this nucleus join the contralateral medial lemniscus and project to the VPM (75).

Nucleus (pars) Interpolaris

This nucleus, which is continuous with the nucleus oralis, extends from the rostral third of the inferior olive to the obex. The thalamic projection is entirely to the contralateral VPM (76). Interpolaris neurons can be classified functionally according to their responsiveness to cutaneous stimuli as low-threshold mechanoreceptive or cutaneous nociceptive (77).

Nucleus (pars) Caudalis

This nucleus extends from the obex to the first cervical root and is considered an upward extension of the spinal dorsal horn. The nucleus is organized into three main subnuclei (65) or four laminae (78): (a) subnucleus marginalis (or zonalis) (lamina I of Rexed); (b) subnucleus gelatinosus (laminae II and III of Rexed); and (c) subnuclei magnocellularis (lamina IV of Rexed). The laminar organization is similar to that found in the posterior horn of the spinal cord.

The primary afferent projection to nucleus caudalis includes both myelinated fibers (79) and unmyelinated fibers. Both groups of fibers penetrate the nucleus from the spinal tract in a spatially ordered radial pattern. The larger fibers terminate mainly within the deep zone of subnucleus gelatinosus (lamina III) (80,81) and within subnucleus magnocellularis. A few smaller fibers may be traced to subnucleus marginalis and into the subjacent reticular formation. It is believed that unmyelinated fibers terminate in the superficial zone of subnucleus gelatinosus (lamina II). More extensive description of these regions is found in reviews by Darian-Smith (66) and Bereiter et al. (82).

Afferent fibers from the perioral region synapse rostrally in nucleus caudalis, whereas those from peripheral areas of the face connect to more caudal parts of the nucleus. This creates a concentric, onionskin organization of the face for pain (Fig. 25.11).

Interconnections among the Trigeminal Spinal Nuclei and Subnuclei

Many neurons of the spinal trigeminal tract send their axons into an extensive longitudinal axon plexus consisting of interconnected small bundles of myelinated and unmyelinated axons (the deep bundles). These bundles run through the entire nucleus of the spinal tract and contain both ascending and descending axons. The axons of the bundles give off widely spaced, simple collaterals that effectively link different levels of the nucleus (83). The reader is referred to the detailed review by Ikeda et al. (84) of the various intra- and internuclear connections of the trigeminal brainstem structures.

Location of Corneal Afferents in the Trigeminal Nuclei

The somatotopic localization of the afferent fibers and neurons subserving the corneal reflex are of practical interest in neuro-ophthalmology. Marfurt and Del Toro (85) and Marfurt and Echtenkamp (86) demonstrated that corneal afferents project to multiple levels of the spinal nucleus. In monkeys, connections were mainly to caudal pars interpolaris and rostral pars caudalis, along with less dense projections to pars oralis, caudal pars caudalis, and the trigeminal main sensory nucleus. Sparse projections to C_1 and C_2

were also found. In the rat, fibers relaying nociceptive information from the cornea synapse in the ventrolateral caudal interpolaris and rostral caudalis (87).

Location of Dural and Blood Vessel Afferents in Trigeminal Nuclei

Stimulation experiments in cats demonstrate nociceptive afferents from the middle meningeal artery and sagittal sinus synapse primarily in the nucleus caudalis, with other connections to nucleus oralis and nucleus interpolaris (88,89). Nociceptive afferents from the dura overlying these areas project to the rostral two-thirds of the nucleus caudalis and caudal nucleus interpolaris (90,91). These neurons in turn project to cells in the VPM nucleus of the thalamus (92) (discussion following). These structures are thought to comprise the central anatomic substrate that subserves migraine headache pain (11,93).

SUPRANUCLEAR TRIGEMINAL CONNECTIONS AND PROJECTIONS

Pathways between the Trigeminal Nuclei and Other Brainstem Areas

These pathways, composed of short neurons in the tegmentum, connect the various trigeminal sensory nuclei with motor nuclei of the brainstem, including the ocular motor nuclei, the motor nuclei of the trigeminal nerve, the facial, glossopharyngeal, vagal, and hypoglossal nuclei, and the vestibular nuclei. Ascending components of this diffuse system conduct impulses slowly cephalad by multisynaptic pathways through the dorsal part of the hypothalamus to the ventromedial nuclei of the thalamus, from which they are diffusely distributed to many areas of the cerebral cortex. Cells within the trigeminal nuclei send collateral axons to the superior colliculus, cerebellar cortex, and deep nuclei (94,95).

Pathways from the Trigeminal Nuclei to the Thalamus

The ascending pathways from the main sensory nucleus and the nucleus of the spinal tract of the trigeminal nerve form an important secondary ascending system—the **ventral secondary ascending tract of the trigeminal nerve** (also termed the trigeminothalamic tract, or ventral trigeminal tract) (Fig. 25.14). The fascicles of this tract, transmitting impulses of pain and temperature and arising from all levels of the trigeminal nuclei, turn obliquely forward to cross the midline at a considerable distance in front of the cell bodies of the neurons from which they arise. After crossing, these bundles gradually accumulate in the lateral part of the brainstem so that by the time they reach the pons, they overlie and are intermingled dorsally with the other components of the medial lemniscus. Where the medial lemniscus shifts dorsally at the level of the midbrain, the ventral secondary ascending tract of the trigeminal nerve lies medial to it. The system terminates in the VPM nucleus of the thalamus.

An entirely separate projection system to higher centers passes from the main sensory nucleus of the trigeminal nerve. This is the **dorsal secondary ascending tract of the**

trigeminal nerve (trigeminal lemniscus, or dorsal trigeminal tract) that, after its origin from the main sensory nucleus, swings into the mid-dorsal tegmental region of the pons. Most fibers decussate, but dorsomedial axons remain ipsilateral (Fig. 25.14). In its course, the dorsal secondary ascending tract of the trigeminal nerve lies dorsal to the red nucleus and medial to the medial lemniscus at upper midbrain levels. The partial decussation makes it impossible to lose finer tactile sensibility on one side of the face unless there is damage to the trigeminal peripheral roots or the trigeminal nucleus (in the pons) is damaged. Section of one tract does not eliminate tactile sensibility from either side of the face, whereas bilateral section of the tract produces loss of discriminatory tactile sensibility on both sides of the face. In addition, lesions in the region of the Sylvian aqueduct may also produce bilateral loss of facial tactile sensibility, but only when both tracts are damaged. The dorsal secondary ascending tract of the trigeminal nerve also projects to the VPM nucleus of the thalamus.

Incoming pain stimuli from the face are relayed to the thalamus via the ventral secondary ascending tract of the trigeminal nerve (Fig. 25.14). The caudal portion of this tract and its nucleus extend at least to the level of the second cervical segment. Pain impulses from the neck enter the cord at C1 and C2. Second-order neurons that are in the same area as the spinal nucleus of the trigeminal nerve relay the pain impulses to the thalamus via the lateral spinothalamic tract. Clinically, the sensation of pain in the face may be associated with pain in the neck. Cervical disease may produce face pain, and stimulation of the trigeminal nerve in the face may produce occipital pain. Taren and Kahn (96) concluded from studies of patients with medullary tractotomies that pain stimuli to the face (or cervical region) have two possible anatomic pathways to the thalamus: the lateral spinothalamic tract and the ventral secondary ascending tract of the trigeminal nerve, each ending in definite portions of the posterior ventral thalamus. They also proposed that pain stimuli from either the face or cervical region could ''crosssynapse'' into either ascending cervicothalamic pathway. Kerr (97) in a discussion of the paper by Taren and Kahn (96) noted that these investigators had been able to follow the overlapping zones of the descending trigeminal pathways and the root fibers of C_1, C_2, and C_3 to cervical levels as low as C_6. He found that in identical levels of the dorsal horn in the first and second cervical segments, afferent descending fibers seemed to terminate on the same nuclear groups. To clarify this problem, he carried out a microelectrode study of the area and found that some neurons receive convergent fibers from the trigeminal and cervical systems. Thus, the same neuron could be triggered by stimuli delivered to the peripheral branches of the trigeminal and cervical roots. Kerr (97) estimated that 25–30% of the neurons in this area responded to stimuli from either peripheral sensory region and stated: ''Stimulation of the dorsal root of the first dorsal cervical segment produces referred pain to the back of the eye, the forehead, and, occasionally, to the vertex; rarely is pain evoked in the back of the head.''

Corticofugal Fibers to the Trigeminal Nuclei

Corticofugal fibers project downward to the main sensory nucleus of the trigeminal nerve and to the subdivisions of the nucleus of the spinal tract of the trigeminal nerve. These fibers arise from widespread areas of the cerebral cortex, including frontal, temporal, parietal, and occipital regions. The fibers are both ipsilateral and contralateral, with the crossed bundles predominating. They are likely functionally related to the inhibition of the sensory impulses projected on the primary nuclei.

The motor nucleus of the trigeminal nerve receives fibers from the corticobulbar tracts of each side, although the majority of the fibers reaching the nucleus are crossed.

Thalamus and Thalamocortical Projections

The sensory system of the face and eye projects from the brainstem to the thalamus (Fig. 25.14). The thalamocortical sensory system mediates somesthetic sensation from the periphery through the thalamus to the primary sensory area of the cerebral cortex.

Thalamus

Lying deep between the brainstem and the cortex is the large sensory nucleus, the thalamus. Through this midline cellular mass pass all sensory tracts except that for olfaction, and within it are the relays for all sensory information from the external environment—the head and body relays that modify incoming information and pass it on to the cerebral hemispheres for processing.

The thalamus is a large, ovoid ganglionic mass situated obliquely between the midbrain and hypothalamus below and the corpus striatum above. It is roofed completely by the cerebral hemispheres. It lies along the lateral wall of the third ventricle, which forms its main medial relation. Its anterior extremity bulges into the floor of the lateral ventricle. Its lateral surface is related to the internal capsule that separates it from the lentiform nucleus. Anteriorly, the two thalami are close together. The posterior extremity of each is enlarged and prominent, forming the pulvinar that overhangs the medial and lateral geniculate bodies, also part of the thalamic complex.

The internal structure of the thalamus is composed of an intricate conglomeration of nuclei that act as discrete and separable cellular masses associated with the various thalamic projecting systems. The subdivisions of the various parts of the thalamus have been the object of many investigations. The important work of Walker (98) is the basis for most classifications of this structure; however, certain modifications of this classification have been made since Walker's original description (99,100).

The **nucleus ventralis posterior** (posterior ventral thalamic nucleus) is the largest cell mass in the ventral nuclear group. It occupies the caudal half of the diencephalon. It lies ventral and ventrolateral to the dorsomedial nucleus and the internal medullary lamina, ventral and ventromedial to the lateral nuclear group, dorsal to the zona incerta, and internal to the external medullary lamina and the scattered cells of the reticular nucleus. Lateral to the reticular nucleus lies the posterior limb of the internal capsule. The nucleus ventralis posterior is usually subdivided into a larger lateral and a smaller medial group.

The posterior ventral thalamic nucleus is the site of termination of many of the major ascending sensory systems, including those discussed in this chapter. The lateral part of the posterior ventral nucleus receives the terminal fibers of the gracile and cuneate components of the medial lemniscus. These components of the medial lemniscus carry impulses produced by tactile and proprioceptive stimuli from the body.

From uppermost cord and lower brainstem levels, impulses evoked by painful, thermal, and tactile stimulation of the face are projected contralaterally via the ventral secondary ascending tract of the trigeminal nerve to the nucleus ventralis posteromedialis (posteromedial ventral thalamic nucleus; arcuate nucleus; VPM) (Fig. 25.14). Refined tactile, and perhaps proprioceptive, impulses from the face are probably relayed bilaterally to this nucleus.

The **nucleus ventralis posterolateralis** (posterolateral ventral thalamic nucleus; VPL) is the region of termination not only of the ventral spinothalamic tract but also of the lateral spinothalamic tract. In addition to mediating impulses that are interpreted as pain, some fibers in the lateral spinothalamic tract carry impulses interpreted as itching.

The posterior ventral thalamic nucleus has a well-defined somatotopic organization. The ascending systems from the lower extremity terminate in the most dorsolateral part of the complex; those from the upper extremity end in an intermediate position; and those from the face, ear, and mouth (including taste) distribute most ventromedially in the nucleus.

Cells within the VPM nucleus are likely organized somatotopically into rods (101,102). In turn, the rods project in an organized fashion to columns in the sensory cortex. Sensory information from the rest of the body is probably processed in a similar manner.

Thalamocortical Connections

The outgoing impulses from the posterior ventral nucleus discharge particularly to the cerebral cortex, although this nucleus has other connections, such as those with the basal ganglia. The projection to the cerebral cortex leads to the paracentral and postcentral gyri. Their fibers fan out in broad sweeps into the posterior limb of the internal capsule. From the dorsolateral portion of the nucleus comes the dorsocaudal part of the thalamocortical (or sensory) radiations. Those from the intermediate parts of the nucleus are intermediate in the bundle. Fibers from the most medial part of the nucleus are in the ventrorostral segment of the sensory radiations, as the latter intersects with the internal capsule. As the upper limits of the internal capsule are reached, the bundle fans out with the most ventrorostral fascicles being distributed to the lower part of the postcentral gyrus and the other bundles systematically distributed above them. The face and forehead are represented among the intermediate bundles of the thalamocortical projection.

Corticothalamic Projections

In addition to the connections already discussed, there are also corticofugal connections from the postcentral gyrus to the posterior ventral nucleus of the thalamus. Apparently these also end in accordance with a somatotopic pattern, with those projecting to the medial part of the nucleus having originated from the "face" area of the postcentral cortex.

Primary Somatic Sensory Cortex

A broad band in the anterior part of the parietal cortex forms the area of the primary sensory cortex that represents the cortical end station of the main somatic afferent system. Anteriorly, it reaches into the depths of the central sulcus and extends posteriorly to occupy the entire postcentral gyrus to the postcentral sulcus. On the medial surface, it continues into the paracentral lobule.

Stimulation of primary somatic sensory cortex in animals and humans, as well as data from intraoperative somatory sensory-evoked potential studies (103), reveal that the surface of the opposite side of the body is topographically represented in an orderly sequence. As elsewhere in the sensory system, the arrangement is in the order of spinal innervation, representing the metameric order of the dermatomes ("sensory homunculus"). The face, the occiput, and the upper arm are represented in an intermediate superior segment of the posterior central gyrus. The mouth, tongue, and pharynx are represented most inferiorly in the gyrus near the Sylvian fissure. The degree and extent of the cortical representation of a particular region depend on the richness of the peripheral neural innervation. Thus, the representation of the forefinger and thumb are huge compared with that of the trunk. With regard to structures in the trigeminal sensory system, the lips and other oral structures have the largest representation in primary somatic sensory cortex.

In the monkey, the region of the somatic sensory cortex subserving the eye is located between the areas for the forelimb or the forehead and nose (104). By testing the reactions of human subjects during surgery, Penfield and Rasmussen (105) found that ocular sensation in humans is usually elicited by stimulation of the corresponding area in the precentral gyrus. Just as the motor eye field is displaced anterior to the main motor strip, so is the sensory representation of the eyes. Penfield and Rasmussen (105) found that ocular sensation could be elicited by stimulation of the postcentral gyrus in only one of their eight patients. Stimulation of the sensory field of the eye produced curious sensations described as a "twisting feeling" or "tingling" usually felt in the contralateral eye but sometimes in both eyes.

EXTRAOCULAR MUSCLE AFFERENTS

The trigeminal pathways of the extraocular muscle afferents are becoming more clearly delineated and it is evident that proprioceptive information is important at least in eye movement control and perhaps also in other visual functions. The central nervous system has three possible ways of checking eye movement accuracy: visual feedback, corollary discharge (an internal efference copy of the motor command [106]), and eye muscle proprioception (107,108). The reader is referred to Steinbach's review (107), in which he summarizes the possible role of eye muscle proprioception in (a) maintence of stability in conjugacy and fixation; (b) specification of visual direction; (c) development of some aspects of normal visual function; and (d) depth perception, vergence, and other binocular functions. In the final analysis, it is most likely that the muscle afferents in human extraocular muscles provide no conscious perception of eye position but are certainly involved in subconscious control and monitoring of muscular contractions (109,110).

PRINCIPLES AND TECHNIQUES OF THE EXAMINATION OF THE TRIGEMINAL NERVE SYSTEM

Because the trigeminal nerve is mainly a sensory afferent, sensory testing remains the mainstay of the clinical examination. However, a thorough understanding of the efferent motor pathways and trigeminal reflexes allows the examiner to evaluate the various functions of the trigeminal system more effectively, leading to more accurate neuroanatomic localization. In addition, trigeminal nerve function should be examined within the context of its three divisions.

TESTS OF CUTANEOUS SENSATION

The sense of touch may be easily tested with a small wisp of cotton or the edge of a tissue. One may also use a light brush of the fingertips against the skin of the face. If reliability is in doubt, the patient should be asked to close the eyes and then indicate each touch. Although the most sensitive test is to compare the sense of light touch on one side with the other, this method frequently leads to spurious information. The nasal mucosa is highly sensitive to the lightest touch, and the comparison of the ''nasal tickle'' response may also be useful. Because the gingiva is also innervated by the trigeminal nerve, testing inside the mouth may produce useful information. In particular, patients with nonorganic sensory loss often do not note sensory changes inside the mouth. One may use the sharp end of a broken tongue blade to check gingival sensation, again comparing one side with the other. It is imperative to check all three branches of the trigeminal nerve bilaterally, as they may be differentially affected, depending on the location of the lesion.

Pain sensation is estimated by response to pinpricks. If an area of decreased response or subjectively blunted sensation is found, it can be outlined by proceeding from the region of blunted sensation outward, noting the borders of normal sensation. As is observed in plotting relative defects in the visual field, there is often a graduated cutaneous sensory loss with margins that vary with the degree of stimulation. Consequently, heavier pinpricks are likely to show a smaller field of sensory loss than are light pinpricks. When an area of suspected decreased sensation is found, it should be compared directly with the equivalent area of skin on the other side of the body. The use of the Wartenberg wheel, a pinwheel that applies a constant stimulus by rolling over the skin, can no longer be recommended because of universal precautions that need to be followed to avoid the transmission of blood-borne illness, such as hepatitis C or the acquired immune deficiency syndrome (AIDS). Many clinicians employ a single-use straight pin or safety pin to test pain sensation, but there are disposable plastic-tipped sharp devices designed specifically for this task.

Sensations of heat and cold may be tested with glass tubes containing comfortably hot and cold water. With the patient's eyes closed, the skin is lightly touched by tubes alternately while the patient indicates if the sensation is hot or cold. Another convenient method is to use the coolness of a metal examination tool, such as a tuning fork or ophthalmoscope handle, to compare the sense of cold between the right and left sides.

Vibratory testing is frequently used to detect nonorganic sensory findings. Because vibration sense is carried by bone, there should be very little difference between a stimulus applied to the left of midline and the same stimulus applied to the right of midline, especially over the frontal area. When patients report inability to feel vibration on one side of the forehead, it usually implies a nonorganic component to the exam.

TESTS OF CORNEAL SENSATION

Assessment of response to corneal pain stimulation is made by both subjective report and objective observation. The patient's report of differences in sensation after equal stimulation of the two corneas may indicate unilateral reduction in ophthalmic division sensory function; however, only the alert, relatively intelligent, and comfortable patient can contribute this information reliably. More often, the examiner must rely upon objective signs, such as involuntary blink reflex and head withdrawal. These are of particular value in examination of the obtunded or semicomatose individual. Both depth of coma and difference in corneal sensitivity can be assessed by the patient's involuntary response to corneal stimulation. It should be noted that long-time contact wearers may have a substantial reduction in response to corneal stimulation, but this should be symmetric.

Corneal sensitivity varies widely among normal persons. Clinically, a mild depression in corneal sensitivity must be judged by comparison of sensitivity between the two corneas. Before attributing such a difference to a trigeminal nerve lesion, one must be satisfied that neither unilateral ocular disease (e.g., herpetic keratitis) nor weakness of one orbicularis oculi muscle (e.g., Bell's palsy) is responsible for a difference in response between the two eyes. When testing corneal sensitivity in the presence of unknown or suspected unilateral eyelid weakness, the comparison should be made between blink responses of the normally innervated eyelids when one cornea, then the other, is alternately stimulated.

A small piece of clean cotton or the end of a cotton-tipped applicator drawn to a fine point can serve as a useful corneal stimulator, as can the rolled corner of a piece of facial tissue. After being reassured that the test is not harmful, the patient is directed to stare upward and away from the laterally approaching stimulus. It is preferable first to stimulate the relatively insensitive bulbar conjunctiva in order to evaluate the patient's general tendency to blink. Then the cornea is touched with the cotton tip or tissue without touching the eyelashes or eyelid margins, and the patient's response is observed. When testing the corneas, the same relative quadrants should be stimulated since there are substantial regional differences in corneal sensitivity in normal persons, with sensitivity being greater centrally than peripherally and greater in the horizontal than in the vertical meridian.

When corneal sensitivity needs to be quantified, for study purposes for instance, anesthesiometers can be used. For example, the instrument designed by Cochet and Bonnet (111) has a nylon filament that is 0.12 mm in diameter and can be varied in length so that the pressure applied to the cornea varies from 11–200 mg per 0.0113 mm^2 (scale reading, 6.0–0.5 cm). The end point occurs when the nylon filament becomes bent about 5° from the perpendicular.

TESTS OF MOTOR FUNCTION

Clinical Tests

Strength of the masseter and temporalis muscles is tested by noting their volume and firmness during forceful closure of the jaws. If the patient has dentures or many missing teeth, it is helpful to place a moist towel or another soft cloth between the jaws. Although bilateral lesions of the motor division produce weakness of muscles of jaw closure and chewing, the more common unilateral lesions produce only an asymmetry of muscular contraction on the two sides.

Strength of the pterygoid muscles is estimated by feeling the forcefulness of mouth opening against pressure and the strength of forceful deviation of the opened jaw to either side, recalling that contraction of each muscle causes deviation of the jaw to the opposite side. Therefore, weakness of the right internal and external pterygoid muscles is manifested by a spontaneous deviation of the opened mandible to the right and by weakness of forceful movement toward the left. Deviation is best seen by noting the relationship between the upper and lower incisors when the jaw is opened and closed; not by the position of the lips (112).

Less frequently performed tests of the motor division of the trigeminal nerve include observations of the force of contraction of the muscles in the floor of the mouth upon swallowing (mylohyoid muscle and anterior belly of the digastric), slight tilt of the uvula to the affected side (tensor veli palatini), and subjective or objective dysacousis, especially for high tones (tensor tympani muscle).

Neurophysiologic Tests

Needle electromyographic (EMG) evaluation of the trigeminal nerve is relatively straightforward because only the mandibular division has any motor output. Only two muscles are routinely examined—the masseter and the temporalis—because both muscles are superficial and easily stud-

ied with minimal discomfort. The pterygoid is a much deeper structure and more difficult to assess, and thus it is not routinely evaluated by most electromyographers. Abnormal spontaneous activity, such as fibrillations and positive sharp waves, indicate peripheral denervation. Voluntary units may be examined, but their configuration is quite different from most skeletal muscle, leading to some confusion for the less experienced examiner. It is also hard for many patients to fully relax these muscles, creating further difficulty in the examination. EMG is most useful in peripheral nerve trauma, such as may result from facial fractures. Myokymia may also be detected on EMG.

TRIGEMINAL REFLEXES: PHYSIOLOGY AND NEUROLOGIC SIGNIFICANCE

Afferent trigeminal impulses evoke a number of other motor reflexes that depend on polysynaptic pathways in the brainstem tegmentum (113). Some of these reflexes are proprioceptive or myotactic (with short latency), whereas others are nociceptive (with long latency). Still others are part of complex synkineses.

Trigeminal Blink Reflexes

Stimulation of the ophthalmic division of the trigeminal nerve, by a gentle tap on the forehead, touching the cornea, cutaneous stimulation, or supraorbital nerve stimulation, leads to bilateral reflex contraction of the orbicularis oculi with a latency following stimulation that varies extensively (25–40 msec) (Fig. 25.15). Ongerboer de Visser et al. (114) found latencies ranging from 36–64 msec in normal adults, with a definite increase in latency with increasing age. There appears to be a minimal latency difference between the ipsilateral and contralateral sides, with the ipsilateral response occurring less than 6 msec before the contralateral response. When the blink reflex is elicited by a glabellar tap, blinks cease or markedly diminish in amplitude in normal children and adults after two to five taps delivered at the rate of one per second. Zametkin et al. (115) examined 164 children between the ages of 2 days and 18 years, as well as 18 adults aged 18–50 years. They found that the blink reflex was extinguished promptly in infants and children up to 1 year of age, after which the number of responses elicited before extinction occurred rose steadily during early childhood, remained stable until approximately 6 years of age, and then declined rapidly, reaching the adult level at 12 years of age.

The afferent fibers of the blink reflex are within the ophthalmic branch of the trigeminal nerve and are probably the small myelinated (A delta fibers) that run in the long ciliary branches of the nerve (116). There is at least one synapse in the descending nucleus and possibly one in the main sensory nucleus. From there, secondary and tertiary fibers connect with both facial nuclei to activate the orbicularis oculi on both sides (efferent arm). Other synapses undoubtedly exist between the sensory and motor nuclei, because the central delay for this reflex is about 40 msec. Stimulation of the sclera or eyelashes gives a much more latent reaction than that obtained by direct corneal stimulation, but these sites have the lowest thresholds for activation of the blink reflex.

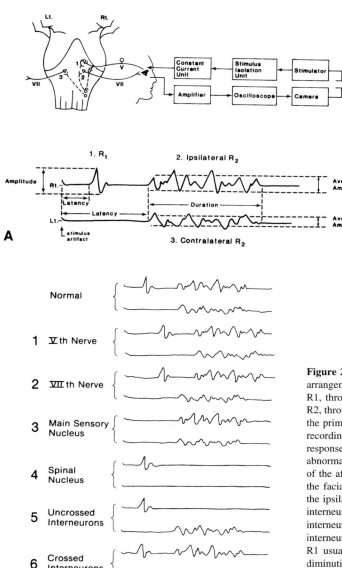

Figure 25.15. Testing the corneal blink reflex. *A, top,* Stimulation and recording arrangement for the blink reflex, with the presumed pathway of the first component, R1, through the pons (1), and the ipsilateral and contralateral second component, R2, through the pons and lateral medulla (2 and 3). The schematic illustration shows the primary afferents of R1 and R2 as one fiber. *A, bottom,* A typical oscilloscope recording of the blink reflex after right-sided stimulation. Note an ipsilateral R1 response and bilateral simultaneous R2 responses. *B,* Five basic types of blink reflex abnormalities. From *top to bottom,* the finding suggests the conduction abnormality of the afferent pathway along the trigeminal nerve (1); the efferent pathway along the facial nerve (2); the main sensory nucleus or pontine interneurons relaying to the ipsilateral facial nucleus (3) (1 in *A*); the spinal tract and nucleus or medullary interneuronal pathways to the facial nuclei on both sides (4); the uncrossed medullary interneurons to the ipsilateral facial nucleus (5) (2 in *A*); and crossed medullary interneurons to the contralateral facial nucleus (6) (3 in *A*). Increased latencies of R1 usually indicate the involvement of the reflex arc itself, whereas the loss or diminution of R1 or R2 may result not only from lesions directly affecting the reflex pathway but also from those indirectly influencing the excitability of the interneurons or motor neurons. (From Kimura J. Electrodiagnosis in Diseases of Nerve and Muscle: Principles and Practice. Ed 2. Philadelphia: FA Davis, 1989:309.)

Kugelberg (117) first described two components in blink reflexes as recorded by EMG from the ipsilateral orbicularis oculi muscle after tapping the glabella or percutaneously stimulating the supraorbital nerve. He concluded that the initial, early component of the blink reflex (R1) had a constant latency (about 12 msec), was relatively constant in size and shape, and was always ipsilateral to the mechanical or electric stimulation. This component was thought to be proprioceptive in nature. The second, late component (R2) had variable latency (20–40 msec), was bilateral, and showed habituation. It was thought to be of polysynaptic origin—a nociceptive reflex evoked by cutaneous stimulation. Subsequent investigations leave little doubt that the second component is a polysynaptic reflex, but the nature of the first component remains somewhat controversial. Kugelberg (117) believed that it was a typical monosynaptic stretch reflex. In contrast, Shahani (118,119) and Shahani and Young (120,121) did not agree with the hypothesis that the first component of the blink reflex is proprioceptive. They postulated that the reflex is instead elicited by stimulating cutaneous afferent nerve fibers.

Alterations in the blink reflex occur in adults with various posterior fossa disorders, including acoustic neuroma, multiple sclerosis, Parkinson disease, trigeminal nerve lesions, and brainstem strokes, tumors, or syrinxes, for instance. Increased latency of the first component of the reflex seems to be a relatively specific sign of a lesion within the pons (122–128). Increased latency of the second component has been reported with lesions of the lateral medulla (129–132). The second component of the blink reflex is likely mediated via medullary pathways that run both ipsilateral and contralateral to the stimulated side before making connections with the ipsilateral and contralateral facial nuclei (133).

Changes in the latency, duration, and amplitude of the second component of the corneal blink reflex also occur in patients with cerebral hemisphere lesions (123,124,131,134, 135). Fisher et al. (136) studied blink reflexes obtained in 34 patients with cerebrovascular lesions, 31 of whom were supratentorial. In 13 patients, the latency of the first component of the reflex on the clinically affected side was significantly delayed acutely but usually resolved within the first week after the event, correlating clinically with the severity of the event. The second component of the reflex was absent in 17 of 34 patients during the early period after the cerebrovascular accident and was associated with decreased corneal sensitivity. Fisher et al. (136) believed that these changes reflect decreased excitability of brainstem structures rather than a lesion within the brainstem in patients with hemisphere dysfunction. Ongerboer de Visser (131) studied corneal reflex latencies in 53 patients with cerebral lesions and identified five distinct types of abnormality in 30 of the individuals. He was in agreement with Fisher et al. (136) that the lower postcentral region has an excitatory influence upon interneurons of the lateral reticular formation of the lower brainstem mediating trigeminofacial connections of the corneal reflex. A decrease in this excitatory influence occurs with postcentral hemisphere lesions and produces an abnormality in corneal reflex latency.

The blink reflex normally habituates (137). Results from functional neuroimaging suggest cerebellar regions may play a role in the modulation of this reflex over time (138).

Loeffler et al. (139) performed an EMG study of the orbicularis muscles in Parkinson disease and noted marked alteration in the latency of the blink reflex in some of their cases. In some patients with advanced disease, the latent period was prolonged to 80–100 msec. Pearce et al. (140) reported that 19 of 20 patients with parkinsonism failed to habituate the blink response to glabellar tap (Myerson's sign) and also reported persistence of the reflex (i.e., decreased habituation) in 13 of 56 patients with parenchymal disease of the brain. Stevens (141) found an increased blink rate or an absent glabellar reflex in nearly one-third of a population of medication-free patients with schizophrenia. Taiminen et al. (142) found reduced habituation of the blink reflex in individuals with schizophrenia and psychotic depression. These findings suggest a possible relationship between the corneal blink rate and central dopamine activity.

Abnormalities of the blink reflex in patients with migraine have lended support to the notion of altered excitability of brainstem trigeminal structures in this condition (143–147).

Trigeminovascular Reflexes

Oculocardiac Reflex

The oculocardiac reflex, also known as Aschner's ocular phenomenon, results in bradycardia in response to mechanical manipulation of the orbit. The afferent pathway of the reflex is the ophthalmic branch of the trigeminal nerve to the brainstem. The sensory impulses pass through polysynaptic pathways in the reticular formation to the visceral motor nuclei of the vagus nerve. There appear to be two distinct types of oculocardiac reflexes: a direct tension dependent pull on extraocular muscles with relatively rapid extinction that may be mediated through stretch receptors, and a prolonged reflex related to diffuse orbital pressure.

Abnormalities of the oculocardiac reflex, particularly of its potentiation or facilitation, are of great importance in ocular surgery. Although the reflex is most frequently encountered during strabismus surgery, cases have been reported in association with laser in situ keratomileusis (LASIK) (148). Vagal reflex activity is increased by many factors. These include drugs such as the phenothiazines, high pCO_2, hypoxia, hyperkalemia, and possibly the direct effect of certain anesthetic agents (149). Preexisting cardiac disease may render the patient abnormally susceptible to the ordinary effects of the oculocardiac reflex, and cardiac arrest may occur.

Diving Reflex

The diving reflex is similar to the oculocardiac reflex, but it is elicited by facial immersion in water. The reflex may be defined as a characteristic pattern of cardiac, respiratory, and vascular responses triggered by immersion of the face. It is a polysynaptic pathway involving trigeminal afferents, brainstem interneurons, and vagal efferents (150). The reflex leads to bradycardia, inhibition of respiration, and peripheral vasoconstriction with increased blood flow to the brain and vital organs.

Corneomandibular Reflex

This reflex is an automatic, involuntary movement of the mandible elicited by corneal stimulation (133). The jaw moves quickly to the opposite side, and at times the mandible moves slightly forward. The mandible moves simultaneously with closure of the eye because of contraction of the ipsilateral external pterygoid. Rarely, both pterygoids contract. The reflex is inconstant and easily fatigued. Any muscular tension interferes with its demonstration. The patient should be relaxed with the mouth opened slightly, allowing the jaw to hang loosely. Mere blinking is not enough to cause the phenomenon, nor is pressure on the globe when the lids are closed. The pathologic corneomandibular reflex indicates bilateral lesions of the corticobulbar tracts to the motor nucleus of the trigeminal nerve, as in amyotrophic lateral sclerosis (151) and strokes (152), for instance. It can be elicited even in comatose patients, in whom the evoked movement of the mandible may be evident even when reflex blinking from corneal stimulation does not occur.

Palpebromandibular Reflex

Pullicino et al. (153) described 14 patients with a reflex characterized by spontaneous anterior or anterolateral movements of the jaw associated with eye blinks. This palpebromandibular reflex is similar to the corneomandibular reflex.

These patients all had either brainstem lesions above the midpons or bilateral cortical disease.

Masseter Reflex (Jaw Jerk)

The jaw jerk is a monosynaptic muscle stretch reflex that is elicited by a brisk tap with the reflex hammer on the front of the chin while the mouth is slightly opened and the jaw is relaxed. The examiner's thumb may be placed on the chin and tapped. The reflex can be reinforced by having the patient bite down lightly on a tongue blade or with Jendrassik's maneuver. The expected response is a contraction of the masseter and temporalis muscles, which causes a sudden closing of the mouth. A unilateral response can occasionally be elicited by tapping the angle of the jaw or tapping a tongue blade placed over the molars of one side. The typical response is usually quite small, and many normal people have no easily elicitable jaw jerk. The masseter reflex can also be exaggerated by anxiety, usually in association with diffuse hyperreflexia.

The reflex is mediated by masseter muscle spindles, whose afferents pass through the trigeminal sensory root and synapse in the mesencephalic trigeminal tract and nucleus (154). A unilateral lesion that destroys the corticobulbar fibers destined to the trigeminal motor nucleus does not alter the functioning of the muscles of mastication, because the motor nucleus of each side receives both crossed and un-crossed fibers. However, when the corticobulbar fibers are bilaterally interrupted in the motor cortex, subcortical regions, internal capsule, or midbrain, there is masticatory paresis that is part of a pseudobulbar palsy. An increased jaw jerk is characteristic of supranuclear involvement of the motor portion of the trigeminal nerve and may be exaggerated to the point of sustained jaw clonus.

Snout and Sucking Reflexes

The **snout reflex**, in which a tap on the upper lip produces lip protrusion or snouting, is one of a group of perioral reflexes whose afferent pathway follows the trigeminal nerve. When the response is increased, tapping the upper or lower lip or philtrum is followed by contraction of the orbicularis oris, as well as the muscles at the base of the nose, leading to closure of the mouth and pursing of the lips as in whistling. In a similar reflex referred to as the **sucking reflex**, stimulation of the lips or skin at the edge of the mouth results in a head turn to that side; the mouth opens, and the patient may suck, bite, or chew. The appearance of these responses is variable in normal persons, and the interpretation of them as pathologic signs is problematic. However, it is clear that the perioral reflexes are more commonly seen, especially in an exaggerated form, in patients with diseases affecting the cortex bilaterally, such as the dementias, Parkinson disease, amyotrophic lateral sclerosis, and bilateral cortical damage from infarct or trauma.

TOPICAL DIAGNOSIS OF DISTURBANCES OF THE TRIGEMINAL NERVE AND ITS CENTRAL CONNECTIONS

Topical diagnosis in the trigeminal somatic sensory system is based on analysis of the pattern and character of various sensory and motor abnormalities. These abnormalities include objective signs (loss or alteration of sensation, muscle weakness, or hyperactivity, as well as changes in trigeminal reflexes) and subjective symptoms (facial pain, neuralgia, headache, and facial paresthesias). The objective trigeminal signs of sensory loss in the face, weakness of jaw muscles, or both, are dependable indicators of the location of the neurologic lesion. On the other hand, topical diagnosis of isolated subjective symptoms of facial pain, neuralgia, or paresthesia is less precise. In either case, an associated neurologic sign (oculomotor nerve palsy, Horner's syndrome, or a brainstem sign) may provide an important clue to the location and nature of the sensory loss or pain.

ALTERATIONS IN CORNEAL SENSATION

For the reader interested in pursuing this topic further, we recommend the comprehensive review of corneal hypesthesia written by Martin and Safran (155).

Physiologic Influences

Alterations in corneal sensitivity occur normally with variations in physiologic and environmental factors. Corneal sensitivity decreases steadily with age (156). In addition, the corneas of brown-eyed individuals are generally less sensitive than those in blue-eyed individuals (157). However, persons with congenital heterochromia have no significant difference in corneal sensitivity between eyes (158), suggesting that the difference in sensitivity between blue eyes and brown eyes may not be related to differences in corneal innervation but rather to inherent differences in a higher sensory mechanism subserving corneal sensation.

Iatrogenic Corneal Hypesthesia

Topical anesthetic agents, such as proparicaine, are commonly used to produce corneal anesthesia. The nonsteroidal anti-inflammatory agents diclofenac and ketorolac also reduce corneal sensitivity when administered topically (159–161) and are used to reduce pain after photorefractive keratectomy. Topical timolol maleate and betaxolol both reduce corneal sensitivity in at least a small proportion of treated subjects (162–166). Elderly patients appear to be particularly susceptible, and affected patients may be at risk of developing keratitis (163,166). The evidence regarding whether or not topical atropine affects corneal sensitivity is conflicting (155).

Ocular surgery, particularly corneal and cataract operations (167,168) but occasionally retinal detachment surgery (169,170), may denervate parts of the cornea, as may panretinal photocoagulation (171). A permanent reduction of corneal sensitivity occurs in 10% of patients who undergo radial keratotomy for myopia and in almost 50% of patients who also receive transverse incisions for astigmatism (172). Photorefractive keratectomy causes a mild decrease in corneal sensitivity that usually resolves within 3 months of surgery (173,174), but corneal hypesthesia may persist after deep stromal ablations (175). Corneal sensitivity may be reduced transiently for months following laser in situ keratomileusis (LASIK) (176,177).

Contact lens wearers typically have reduced corneal sensation (178–181). Millodot (182) showed that both hard and soft contact lenses cause a daily progressive diminution in corneal sensitivity.

Corneal Hypesthesia from Acquired Disease

Isolated corneal hypesthesia may be congenital or heredodegenerative (e.g., corneal dystrophies), but it is usually a result of acquired local disease of the cornea or sclera. Most ocular diseases that cause corneal hypesthesia, such as scleritis (183) or acute angle closure glaucoma (184), are easily recognized and therefore do not cause confusion in neurologic diagnosis. In such circumstances, there is often associated corneal opacity either as a consequence of the primary disease or from secondary traumatic erosion. In most instances, a single eye is affected.

Neurotropic viruses, especially herpes simplex, are a common cause of corneal hypesthesia. Herpes simplex keratitis usually produces a dendritic ulcer but may also cause other corneal lesions such as superficial punctate keratitis (185). Draeger (186) found that corneal sensitivity usually does not recover after interstitial herpetic keratitis and may take more than 2 years to recover after superficial herpetic keratitis.

Subtle unilateral corneal hypesthesia without other changes in facial sensation is often the first objective sign of pressure upon the trigeminal root by a tumor or other lesion in the cerebellopontine angle (CPA). Cushing (187) stated that aside from 8th nerve findings, corneal hypesthesia is the next most frequent early sign of an acoustic neurinoma. This was confirmed in a retrospective study of 126 patients with acoustic neurinomas diagnosed by MR imaging (188). The explanation for the early involvement of corneal sensation is not clear. To explain dysfunction of trigeminal axons in the rostral portion of the nerve from a lesion that encroaches on the nerve caudally, Stechison et al. (55) suggested a ''tenting-up phenomenon of distortion.'' An alternative hypothesis is that the fine-caliber pain fibers (the C fibers) supplying the cornea are particularly vulnerable to stretch or compression.

Unilateral corneal hypesthesia may also occur with various orbital diseases (189), with Adie's tonic pupil (190), with a variety of lower brainstem lesions (191), and with iatrogenic lesions of the trigeminal pathway (rhizotomy for trigeminal neuralgia, for example) (192–195). Bilateral corneal hypesthesia is commonly associated with systemic diseases that cause sensory neuropathies, including diabetes mellitus (196–199), leprosy (200–202), amyloidosis (203), and vitamin A deficiency. In diabetes, the degree of loss of corneal sensation usually parallels the severity of diabetic retinopathy. In addition, corneal sensitivity improves markedly in diabetic patients who are treated topically with an aldose reductase inhibitor (204,205). Nazarian and O'Leary (206) measured corneal touch thresholds in 11 patients with

myasthenia gravis and for unclear reasons found that six had decreased thresholds in one or both eyes.

Toxins that may cause decreased corneal sensation include carbon disulfide (in the rayon industry) and hydrogen sulfide. The associated neurologic or systemic signs and the chief complaints of patients with this type of corneal insensitivity usually preclude any mistaken diagnosis of local ocular disease.

Congenital and Inherited Corneal Hypesthesia

Congenital corneal hypesthesia occurs in a variety of clinical settings—as an isolated finding, as a component of congenital trigeminal anesthesia, in a number of corneal dystrophies, and in association with other developmental anomalies. In addition, Singh and Gibson (207) reported an unusual case of presumed prenatal herpes zoster ophthalmicus that caused permanent corneal anesthesia together with iris heterochromia and atrophy.

Isolated congenital corneal hypesthesia is rare. It is usually bilateral and becomes apparent during infancy or early childhood when painless erosion and opacity of the cornea occur (208,209). Inherited congenital corneal hypesthesia, either unilateral or bilateral, without other findings was reported as an autosomal-dominant condition in two families (210,211). In addition, patients with congenital corneal hypesthesia may have decreased or absent cutaneous sensation in the distribution of the trigeminal nerve, particularly the first division (212–218). This type of congenital trigeminal anesthesia is typically bilateral but may be unilateral. Patients with congenital trigeminal anesthesia usually have normal CT or MR scans. However, there are examples where imaging showed bilateral hypoplasia of trigeminal nerves and gasserian ganglia (215), mild atrophy of cerebellum and brainstem (212), or clinically undetected atrophy of masticator muscles (217).

Isolated corneal hypesthesia and trigeminal hypesthesia occur in association with various congenital anomalies (155,212), including oculoauriculovertebral dysplasia (Goldenhar's syndrome); Möbius syndrome; epidermal nevus syndrome (219); MURCS association (mullarian duct aplasia, renal aplasia, and cervical somite dysplasia) (220); VACTERL (vertebral, anal, cardiovascular, tracheoesophageal, renal, and limb defects) (221); and others (212,222). Decreased corneal sensitivity may also be associated with nephropathic cystinosis (223), abetalipoproteinemia (224), Refsum's syndrome, and progressive hemifacial atrophy (Parry-Romberg syndrome) (225). Because of the potential risk to the cornea in affected persons, many have been treated with either intermittent pressure patching, tarsorrhaphy, or soft contact lenses. In affected infants and young children, recurrent ulcerations of the corneas and erosions of the nasal septum may be caused by self-inflicted injury. Arm splinting may be needed in such persons to allow healing and prevent recurrence (213).

INVOLVEMENT OF THE OPHTHALMIC DIVISION OF THE TRIGEMINAL NERVE

Involvement of the ophthalmic division (V1) by orbital disease is uncommon. Rose and Wright (189) identified periorbital trigeminal sensory loss in 103 (3.3%) of 3,070 patients with orbital disease seen at Moorfields Eye Hospital. Of the 103 patients, 83 had sensory loss in the territory of one or more branches of V1. In almost all patients, the involved cutaneous territory was appropriate to the position of the lesion in the orbit.

In one study (226), cutaneous allodynia (pain induced by normally nonpainful stimuli) and hyperalgesia was found in 22% of patients with trigeminal postherpetic neuralgia.

Nasociliary Branch Lesions

In the series of Rose and Wright (189), only 15 of 103 patients with orbital disease had sensory loss in the infratrochlear territory, and all had additional involvement of other nerves. In contrast, 40 patients had loss of corneal sensation, and this was the only sensory deficit in 15 of these patients. Corneal sensory loss occurred equally often with benign disease and malignancy. Unlike loss of cutaneous sensation, loss of corneal sensation appeared to be unrelated to the position of the lesion in the orbit. Selective involvement of the nasociliary branch may also follow a penetrating orbital injury or extensive orbital surgery.

Frontal Branch Lesions

Hypesthesia in the territory of the supraorbital or supratrochlear nerve is the most common sensory deficit from orbital disease, occurring in 44 patients in the series of Rose and Wright (189). Isolated involvement of one or both nerves was seen in 25 patients. These lesions are very common after contusions, lacerations, surgical incisions, and fractures of the superior orbital rim. In some cases, hypesthesia in this area occurs from pressure on the forehead by an improperly positioned headrest during surgery in the prone position (e.g., during back surgery). Squamous cell carcinoma may also produce supraorbital nerve sensory loss by perineural infiltration (227).

Lacrimal Branch Lesions

Lesions of this branch cause hypesthesia over the lateral bulbar conjunctiva and skin of the lateral canthus. Because sensation in this area is seldom tested, the deficit is probably often overlooked. Of 103 patients with sensory loss from orbital disease (189), 25 had lacrimal branch involvement, and this was the only nerve affected in 10 patients. Lacrimal branch involvement was appropriate to the site of the lesion in the orbit in all but one patient. Rose and Wright (189) did not specifically analyze the causes of lacrimal branch lesions, but 19 patients in their series had lacrimal gland carcinoma, and most of these tumors likely involved the lacrimal branch. Thus, a lacrimal branch sensory deficit should be regarded with some concern, especially if associated with pain. Penetrating lateral orbital injuries and surgical procedures in the region of the lacrimal gland may also involve the sensory lacrimal nerve. A trigeminal neurinoma of the lacrimal nerve has been reported (228).

Syndromes of the Orbital Apex, Superior Orbital Fissure, and Anterior Cavernous Sinus

The ophthalmic division of the trigeminal nerve is usually involved, along with other cranial nerves and sympathetic nerves that travel close to it, in the apex of the orbit and the cavernous sinus (3,7,229–231). In its complete form, the **syndrome of the superior orbital fissure** is characterized by denervation of all branches of the 1st division of the trigeminal nerve, denervation of the sympathetic nerves, paralysis of one or more of the nerves to the ocular muscles (oculomotor, trochlear, and abducens nerves), and, in many cases, proptosis. The complete **syndrome of the orbital apex** is similar to that of the superior orbital fissure except that there is also involvement of the optic nerve. Involvement of the **anterior cavernous sinus** may produce signs that are exactly like those produced by a lesion affecting the superior orbital fissure. Although venous congestion in such cases may suggest that the cavernous sinus rather than the orbital apex is the site of involvement, we prefer to combine the syndromes and refer to them collectively as the **sphenocavernous syndrome**.

Because of the close proximity of the superior orbital fissure, the orbital apex, and the cavernous sinus, any pathologic process (e.g., tumor, inflammation, vascular disease) may begin in one of these regions and rapidly spread to the neighboring regions. Incomplete syndromes are the rule. Lesions that cause these syndromes are discussed in detail in Chapter 20, but pathologic processes include aneurysms, tumors (primary, metastatic, or locally invasive), ischemia, and both septic and aseptic inflammation. Trauma may produce sphenocavernous syndromes by direct damage or indirectly (e.g., carotid-cavernous sinus fistula). Appropriate neuroimaging studies, including CT scanning with both axial and coronal views, MR imaging, and conventional or MR angiography (MRA), usually are sufficient to identify the responsible lesion.

INVOLVEMENT OF THE MAXILLARY DIVISION OF THE TRIGEMINAL NERVE

Damage to the maxillary division (V2) of the trigeminal nerve produces anesthesia or hypesthesia of the skin lateral to the nose, the mucous membrane of the maxillary antrum and lower part of the nose, the upper teeth and gums, the palate anterior to the palatopharyngeal arch, and occasionally the lower part of the cornea (232). As detailed above, the palatine and posterior superior alveolar branches arise in the pterygopalatine fossa before the origin of the infraorbital nerve and supply sensation to the palate and the two posterior upper molars and adjacent gingiva (233). Thus, when a sensory deficit is detected over the cheek, testing sensation in these areas helps to differentiate a lesion of the infraorbital nerve from more proximal pathology (234).

Diseases of the orbit or maxillary sinus may cause hypesthesia in the territory of the infraorbital nerve. Rose and Wright (189) documented infraorbital nerve involvement in 28 of 103 patients who had trigeminal sensory loss caused by orbital disease. Most of the lesions were located along the floor of the orbit. Lesions of the maxillary sinus, including carcinomas (233) and mucoceles (235), may erode the roof of the sinus and compress or infiltrate the infraorbital nerve. Carcinomas arising on the anterior wall of the sinus may invade the alveolar canal and the anterior superior alveolar nerve and produce localized sensory loss of the incisor and canine teeth and adjacent gingiva (233). Anesthesia or hypesthesia of the infraorbital branch is a common consequence of maxillofacial and orbital injuries.

Numbness of the cheek may result from metastatic perineural infiltration of the infraorbital nerve—the numb cheek syndrome (234) (Fig. 25.16). This syndrome may be the presenting feature or the first sign of recurrence of a basal cell or squamous cell carcinoma (232,234,236–238) or the rare amelanotic spindle cell variant of melanoma (desmoplastic malignant melanoma) (239). Brazis et al. (232) coined the term "numb cheek-limp lower lid" syndrome to describe the findings of a patient who developed a numb cheek followed by progressive ipsilateral weakness of lower eyelid closure and upper lip movement. MR imaging showed

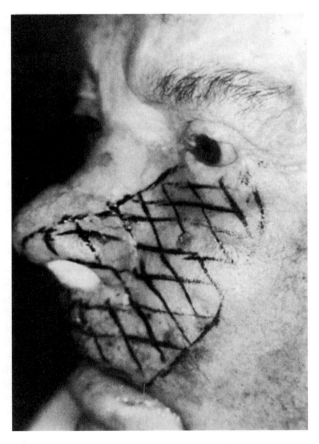

Figure 25.16. Distribution of cutaneous hypesthesia to pin and touch in a patient who developed the "numb cheek" syndrome from infiltrating perineural squamous cell carcinoma. Sensation also was lost over the anterior gingiva but not the posterior gingiva, localizing the lesion to the infraorbital nerve (distal to the pterygopalatine fossa). Note scarring from past surgical procedures, especially about the left eye. (From Campbell WW. The numb cheek syndrome: A sign of infraorbital neuropathy. Neurology 1986;36:421–423.)

a subcutaneous linear band of increased signal intensity over the maxillary sinus; biopsy showed widespread infiltration of infraorbital nerve and facial nerve branches by squamous cell carcinoma.

Other tumors rarely involve V2 in isolation. Erzurum et al. (240) reported a malignant schwannoma of the infraorbital nerve. Isolated maxillary sensory loss also occurs with tumors involving the cavernous sinus or Meckel's cave, including trigeminal schwannoma (241), meningioma (242), and choristoma (243). In such cases, pain in the cheek is usually a prominent symptom.

INVOLVEMENT OF THE MANDIBULAR DIVISION OF THE TRIGEMINAL NERVE

Sensory Abnormalities

Involvement of branches of the mandibular division (V3) of the trigeminal nerve may produce sensory dysfunction, motor dysfunction, or both. Isolated sensory dysfunction can occur in patients with systemic cancer, primarily in the distribution of the inferior alveolar nerve and its terminal cutaneous branch, the mental nerve, producing a numb chin (244–253). The most common neoplasms associated with this **numb chin syndrome** are breast and lymphoproliferative disorders (254–257). Other responsible solid tumors such as prostate cancer (258) have been reported. Lymphoproliferative disorders commonly associated with the numb chin syndrome include Burkitt cell leukemia (L3 ALL) (259,260), Burkitt's lymphoma (261), and lymphoma. When due to cancer, the syndrome may result from metastatic lesions of the jaw, base-of-skull metastases, or leptomeningeal seeding (254). Chin numbness may be the initial sign of cancer, or it may be a late manifestation of malignancy in the setting of stable or progressive systemic disease.

Patients who develop a nontraumatic mental neuropathy should be questioned specifically regarding previous malignancy, including skin lesions of the face, and should undergo contrast-enhanced CT scanning or MR imaging of the head, base of skull, and mandible. Subtle perineural enhancement or effacement of fat planes may provide the only evidence of neoplastic infiltration (262). Lossos and Siegal (254) found that CT scanning and analysis of cerebrospinal fluid (CSF) together provided a diagnosis in 89% of patients. In cases where neuroimaging and CSF results are normal, nuclear bone scanning may provide evidence of bony metastases elsewhere. When the numb chin syndrome is caused by cancer, the prognosis is poor. In the series of Lossos and Siegal (254), median survival after onset of numbness was 5 months for patients with bone metastases and 12 months for those with meningeal disease.

A mental neuropathy is a rare complication of sickle cell disease (263,264). As opposed to the patients with systemic cancer, the patients evaluated by Konotey-Ahulu (263) described a burning sensation of the lower lip, followed later by numbness, and most patients with mental neuropathy in the setting of sickle cell disease also complain of severe bone pain involving the mandible. Bone scans in these patients typically show an area of increased uptake in the mandible, consistent with infarction, and it thus is assumed that the mental neuropathy that occurs in patients with sickle cell disease is caused by infarction of either the inferior alveolar nerve or the mental nerve in their respective canals.

Dental procedures, particularly extractions of the 3rd lower molar teeth (wisdom teeth), may give rise to inferior alveolar or lingual neuropathies (265). Since the lingual nerve is joined by the chorda tympani nerve and passes medial to the roots of the 3rd molar before entering the tongue, damage at this location during extraction or from an injection of an anesthetic agent may cause loss of somatic and taste sensation to the anterior two-thirds of the tongue as well as hypesthesia of the floor of the mouth and inner surface of the lower gums (266). In elderly edentulous patients, a mental neuropathy may be produced by ill-fitting dentures (265) and possibly by age-related mandibular atrophy (267).

Other miscellaneous etiologies of sensory mandibular neuropathy have been described. Krimsky Fischoff et al. (268) reported a patient with systemic sclerosis and CREST syndrome (calcinosis, Raynaud's, esophageal stricture, and telangiectasia) who developed a painful inferior alveolar neuropathy caused by severe mandibular resorption. Perineural spread of tumor has been reported as a cause of auriculotemporal neuropathy (26). Cruccu et al. (269) studied patients with severe diabetic polyneuropathy and chronic inflammatory demyelinating polyneuropathy and found subclinical sensory mandibular nerve abnormalities in over half of them.

Motor Abnormalities

Proximal lesions of V3 may also involve the motor root, resulting in weakness and wasting of the muscles of mastication (Fig. 25.17), deviation of the jaw to that side, flaccidity of half of the floor of the mouth from paralysis of the mylohyoid and anterior belly of the digastric, and dysacusis for low-pitched sounds due to paralysis of the tensor tympani. Isolated involvement of the motor root is extremely rare. Chia (270) reported five young patients who developed unilateral weakness of masticator muscles without sensory loss and who eventually showed wasting and electromyographic evidence of denervation. CT scans were normal. Three of the five patients had acute weakness and in each case, the weakness was preceded by symptoms of the common cold and accompanied by pain in the cheek. Chia (270) suggested that viral infection may play a role in the etiology of this condition. Pure trigeminal motor neuropathy may also caused by blunt head trauma (271), meningiomas (272), and multiple sclerosis (273).

Lesions of the motor root or its branches may produce abnormal or excessive activity of masticator muscles. An example of such a disorder is **hemimasticatory spasm**, a rare idiopathic condition characterized by recurrent spasms of the masseter and temporalis muscles on one side (274–279). Trigeminal nerve function is otherwise normal, and there is no involvement of the facial nerve. It has been suggested that the nerve to the masseter muscle may be entrapped at a point in its course between the lateral pterygoid muscle and the skull, causing focal demyelination and spontaneous neural discharges (277,279).

The mylohyoid muscle and anterior belly of the digastric may also exhibit abnormal spontaneous activity. Hyperexcitability of the mylohyoid branch of the mandibular division was reported by Diaz et al. (280) as a delayed complication of radiotherapy to the base of the skull. These authors described two patients who developed episodic contraction of the muscles in the floor of the mouth on one side.

INVOLVEMENT OF THE GASSERIAN GANGLION OR THE SENSORY ROOT OF THE TRIGEMINAL NERVE

General Considerations

Paralytic lesions of the gasserian ganglion, whether ischemic, inflammatory, compressive, traumatic, toxic, or infiltrative, cannot be differentiated dependably from lesions of the sensory root (281). Involvement of both structures may cause anesthesia in one or more divisions of the trigeminal nerve as well as paralysis of the motor nerve to the muscles of mastication. Certain findings may help, however, to differentiate a lesion in the region of the cavernous sinus, involving the ganglion or root, from focal involvement of the sensory root in the perimesencephalic cistern. A trigeminal deficit associated with ophthalmoplegia usually indicates a lesion of the cavernous sinus or Meckel's cave. In the absence of a more peripheral lesion, sensory loss limited to the ophthalmic distribution signifies a lesion of the cavernous sinus or superior orbital fissure (282), as does the associated finding of paralysis of the ipsilateral oculosympathetic nerve. On the other hand, loss of facial or corneal sensation combined with paralysis of the facial and auditory nerves implies involvement of the sensory root in the basal cistern (e.g., as in the syndrome of the cerebellopontine angle).

Tumors of the middle and posterior fossa are a common cause of trigeminal nerve dysfunction. In a series of 64 patients with facial numbness as an initial or presenting symptom (281), 25% had CPA tumors, and 17% had base-of-skull tumors. Acoustic neuromas are the most common of these tumors and cause trigeminal signs in 9–30% of patients, (188,281,283–286). Hypesthesia from acoustic neuromas may be limited to the cornea but the tumor may also be heralded by hypesthesia in a distribution approximating that of V2 or V3 (287). Puca et al. (285) found masticator weakness in 17% of 30 patients with trigeminal involvement from acoustic neuroma. Acoustic neuromas are discussed further in Chapter 33.

Meningiomas that cause facial numbness arise most often from the cavernous sinus but may also arise from the dura of Meckel's cave, in the CPA (288), or from the inferior aspect of the tentorium. Puca et al. (285) found trigeminal deficits in 10 of 21 patients with "sphenopetrosal" meningiomas; 6 of the 10 patients had trigeminal symptoms in isolation. In the same study, only one of ten CPA meningiomas was associated with facial hypesthesia. In another series of 16 patients with meningiomas of Meckel's cave (242), trigeminal sensory loss was the only sign of disease in 3 of the 8 patients with small tumors (less than 3 cm), and occurred together with ophthalmoplegia in all 8 patients with larger tumors. Trigeminal neuralgia, typical or atypical, was the

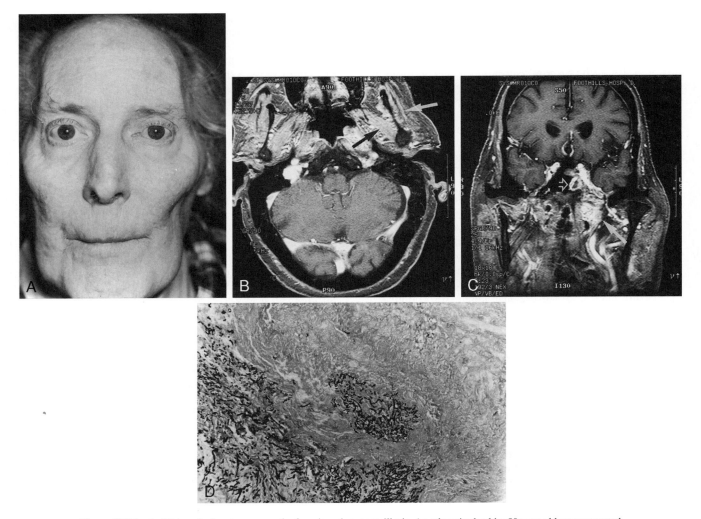

Figure 25.17. Left trigeminal motor neuropathy from invasive aspergillosis. An otherwise healthy 80-year-old man presented with a 6-month history of increasing pain in the left mandibular region. The left masseter and pterygoids were wasted and weak, and there was no sensory deficit. *A*, Photograph showing marked wasting of the left masseter. *B*, Axial MR image illustrating atrophy of the masseter (*white arrow*) and lateral pterygoid muscle (*black arrow*). *C*, Postgadolinium MR image shows irregularly enhancing lesion of infratemporal fossa on the left (*solid arrow*), which extends through the foramen ovale into the cavernous sinus. Also note thickened enhancing mucosa of left sphenoid sinus (*open arrow*). *D*, Photomicrograph of biopsy of infratemporal lesion from left nasopharynx. Multiple fungal organisms with 45° branching hyphae consistent with *Aspergillus* are invading connective tissue. (Grocott, ×40.)

initial symptom in 10 of the 16 patients. Facial pain and numbness also may herald trigeminal root involvement by tentorial meningiomas (289). The mechanism by which meningiomas compromise nerve function is not always simple compression; infiltration of the trigeminal nerve by a benign meningioma of Meckel's cave was demonstrated histologically by Larson et al. (290). Meningiomas are discussed in Chapter 30 of this text.

Schwannomas (neuromas) of the trigeminal nerve are uncommon, but a review by Samii et al. (291) of 190 cases showed that 51% presented with trigeminal symptoms, particularly pain and paresthesia in the V1 and V2 dermatomes. Symptoms often began long before presentation, with a

mean duration of 34 months. The abnormal findings at presentation included facial hypesthesia in 70% of cases, decreased corneal reflex in 56% of cases, and masticator weakness in 34% of cases. Similar results were documented in other series (292–294). Hemorrhage into a schwannoma may produce the acute onset of trigeminal symptoms (295). An unusual symptom of massive trigeminal nerve schwannomas is pathological laughter, attributed in part to seizures or pontine dysfunction (294,296). Schwannomas of the trigeminal nerve are discussed in Chapter 33 of this text.

A variety of other nonmalignant mass lesions may arise from or compress the trigeminal ganglion or root and present with trigeminal symptoms and signs. These include CPA epidermoids (285), intracavernous carotid aneurysms (297), and an assortment of rare lesions, including ependymomas (298), granular cell tumors (299), choristomas (243,300), amyloidomas (301,302), lipomas (303), aspergillomas (304), cavernous hemangiomas of Meckel's cave (305,306), juvenile xanthogranuloma, teratoma (307), and distal aneurysms of the anterior inferior cerebellar artery (308). Chang et al. (309) described a unique intracranial trigeminal lesion in a patient with chronic progressive ophthalmoplegia. MR imaging showed slight enlargement of the cavernous sinus and thickening and contrast-enhancement of the mandibular division of the trigeminal nerve. Biopsy of the lesion (confirmed later by autopsy) disclosed a localized hypertrophic process characterized histologically by periaxonal Schwann cell "onion-bulb" formation.

Trigeminal sensory loss is an underrecognized sign of metastatic perineural spread of orofacial neoplasms to the trigeminal ganglion and root. The development of trigeminal dysfunction often signals the recurrence of a previously treated tumor, particularly a squamous cell carcinoma of the face or oropharyngeal mucosa (237,238,310). Involvement may be limited initially to a single nerve branch, especially the infraorbital nerve (see the section, Involvement of the Maxillary Division of the Trigeminal Nerve in this chapter) (237), but spread of tumor proximally to the cavernous sinus is often present at the time of diagnosis (Fig. 25.18). A similar propensity for producing perineural cavernous sinus invasion is observed with adenoid cystic carcinoma of the lacrimal or salivary glands (311–313) (Fig. 25.19) and nasopharyngeal carcinoma (314). Perineural spread of these neoplasms is best detected by MR imaging with gadolinium enhancement (315). If V3 is involved, the study should extend inferiorly to the lower mandibular margin (282). Ade-

noid cystic carcinoma and nasopharyngeal carcinoma are discussed in Chapter 35 of this text.

MR imaging may also reveal leptomeningeal spread of metastases to trigeminal roots (316) or focal metastatic involvement of the trigeminal ganglion or root by melanoma, lymphoma (317,318), or carcinoma (319,320) (Fig. 25.19). Malignant lesions are suggested by enlarged, enhancing nerves with spiculated margins, whereas benign lesions usually show minimal or no enlargement and smooth margins. Sevick et al. (316) noted that overlap occurs between the MR appearance of benign and malignant lesions and suggested follow-up MR evaluation within several weeks when the diagnosis is not clear clinically. In a review of 17 patients with metastatic lesions of the cavernous sinus, Post et al. (321) noted that 9 had decreased sensation in the distribution of one or more trigeminal divisions, but only 1 had facial numbness as a presenting symptom.

A variety of nonneoplastic disorders may affect the trigeminal ganglion or the sensory or motor roots of the trigeminal nerve. **Gradenigo's syndrome** comprises the triad of trigeminal and abducens nerve palsies and otitis media (322). The trigeminal neuropathy is characterized by excruciating facial pain, and many patients also have ipsilateral facial weakness. Hardjasudarma et al. (323) reported a patient with otitis and ipsilateral facial anesthesia who developed an abducens palsy 3 days later. MR imaging showed swelling and enhancement of the trigeminal root and ganglion and inflammatory changes of the petrous apex. Other inflammatory process that may cause trigeminal neuropathy include sarcoidosis (324,325) and Wegener's granulomatosis (326).

Severe closed head trauma with basal skull fractures may rarely cause unilateral or bilateral injury of the trigeminal ganglion or root (327–330). Typically, other cranial nerves

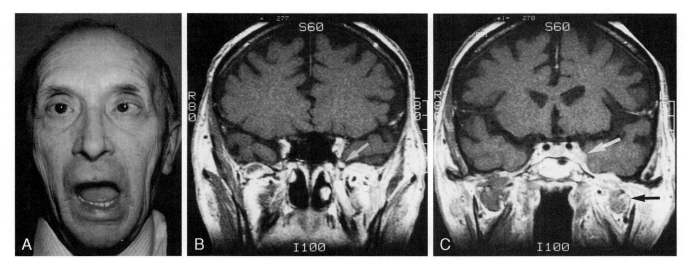

Figure 25.18. Perineural spread of squamous cell carcinoma intracranially along the trigeminal nerve. This 70-year-old man had progressive sensory loss over the left forehead and cheek over a period of 6 months, followed by horizontal diplopia and difficulty chewing. A squamous cell carcinoma was removed from his left temple 2 years earlier. *A,* Photograph showing wasting of left temporalis, deviation of the open jaw to the left, and left esotropia (due to left 6th nerve palsy). *B and C,* Postgadolinium coronal T1-weighted images showing an enlarged enhancing maxillary nerve on the left (*B, arrow*) and posterior extension of tumor into the cavernous sinus (*C, white arrow*) . Note atrophy of left lateral pterygoid muscle (*C, black arrow*).

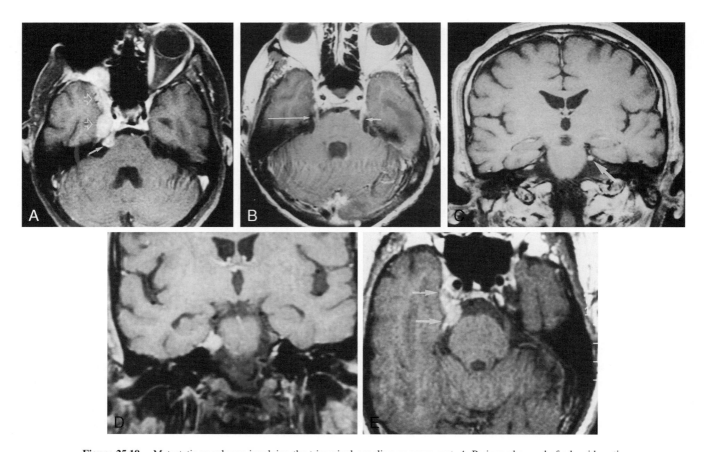

Figure 25.19. Metastatic neoplasms involving the trigeminal ganglion or nerve root. *A*, Perineural spread of adenoid cystic carcinoma originating in the orbit (previous right orbital exenteration). The T1-weighted image postgadolinium shows irregular, enhancing mass extending posteriorly from the right orbit. Mass involves the cisternal (*solid arrow*), as well as the ganglionic and postganglionic (*open arrows*) segments of the 5th nerve; *B*, Leptomeningeal spread of highly anaplastic astrocytoma. Axial T1-weighted MR image shows bilateral enhancement of trigeminal nerve roots with slight enlargement on the left (*short arrow*) and irregular contour on the right (*long arrow*). *C*, Metastatic melanoma (primary tumor involved the left side of face). The T1-weighted coronal image shows smooth contour of left trigeminal nerve root with uniform enhancement and minimal enlargement (*arrow*). *D* and *E*, Lung carcinoma metastatic to trigeminal ganglion and root. *D*, The T1-weighted coronal image shows enlargement of the cisternal portion of the right trigeminal nerve root with uniform enhancement and irregular spiculated margins. *E*, Axial T1-weighted image demonstrates a large, irregular mass involving the cisternal and ganglionic segments of the trigeminal nerve on the right (*arrows*). (From Sevick RJ, Dillon WP, Engstom J, et al. Trigeminal neuropathy: Gd-DTPA enhanced MR imaging. J Comput Assist Tomogr 1991;14:605–611.)

also suffer damage, particularly the abducens nerve. In two cases described by McGovern et al. (328) and Nelson and Kline (329), the sequelae of such an injury included an unusual trigemino-abducens synkinesis, whereby voluntary activation of the masseter or lateral pterygoid triggered abduction of the ipsilateral eye. The postulated explanation for the synkinesis is that regenerating motor fibers of the trigeminal nerve are misdirected along trigeminal channels that normally convey spindle afferent fibers from the lateral rectus. Trigeminal dysfunction may also be a feature of basilar invagination (331).

''False-localizing'' trigeminal symptoms, signs, or both may occur in the presence of an extrinsic, posterior fossa mass (332–335). The mechanism, according to O'Connell (252), is that the mass displaces the brainstem upward or, in

the case of a CPA lesion, to the opposite side. This produces distortion of the sensory root and traction at the dural foramen on one or both sides. O'Connell (252) described four such patients, all of whom had sensory loss on the side opposite a posterior fossa tumor. All four of these patients also had increased intracranial pressure, however, and this may have contributed to the symptoms, because facial hypesthesia occasionally occurs in patients who have non-tumor-induced intracranial hypertension, e.g., communicating hydrocephalus (336) or idiopathic intracranial hypertension (337–339). In these patients, the sensory loss typically resolves when the intracranial pressure is lowered, suggesting that increased intracranial pressure alone may be sufficient to cause false-localizing trigeminal dysfunction. Another mechanism proposed to explain this phenomenon with CPA lesions is that the nerve is pushed against adjacent blood vessels and suffers vascular compression (334).

Isolated trigeminal sensory neuropathy occurs in some patients with various connective tissue diseases, including systemic lupus erythematosus (340), scleroderma (341–346), dermatomyositis (344), Sjögren's syndrome (347), rheumatoid arthritis (348), and mixed connective tissue disease (344,349–351). Hagen et al. (351) found that among patients with trigeminal sensory neuropathy and connective tissue disease, the trigeminal sensory neuropathy developed before general symptoms of connective tissue disease in 7% of the patients and at the same time in 47% of the patients. The pathogenesis of this condition is unknown.

Viral infections such as hepatitis (352) and herpes simplex (353) occasionally produce isolated trigeminal sensory neuropathies.

Several investigators (354–356) have also described patients with an idiopathic acute or subacute, purely sensory, trigeminal neuropathy affecting one or more divisions of the trigeminal nerve. In some cases, there is also an impairment of taste on the affected side. The symptoms typically resolve partially or completely in most of these patients. Blau et al. (354) emphasized that most patients had intact corneal reflexes, normal trigeminal motor function, and absence of pain, although trigeminal neuralgia did develop in one of their patients, and a minority of patients complained of a burning or itching sensation (356).

The diagnosis of idiopathic trigeminal sensory neuropathy is typically one of exclusion following normal MR imaging and serologies to exclude connective tissue disorders (357,358). However, transient MR imaging abnormalities, consisting of enlargement of the trigeminal root and enhancement of the root and ganglion, were described in two patients with this condition by Rorick et al. (359). In both instances, the abnormalities spontaneously disappeared within 4 months. Biopsy-proven cases with nongranulomatous (360,361) and granulomatous (362) inflammatory changes have also been described. These findings suggest that at least some cases of idiopathic trigeminal sensory neuropathy are inflammatory in origin. On the other hand, Jannetta and Robbins (363) performed retromastoid craniectomy on four patients with "idiopathic" trigeminal neuropathy and found that in all cases, the superior or anterior inferior cerebellar arteries were compressing and stretching the trigeminal nerve root. Postoperatively, all patients had pain relief as well as improvement or resolution of their sensory deficit.

Trigeminal sensory neuropathy also occasionally results from ischemia. Miller (364) described an elderly patient with intermittent diplopia from presumed ischemia of the right abducens nerve. The patient later developed a transient right trigeminal sensory neuropathy, which Miller (364) attributed to ischemia of the sensory root. In support of this concept, Mokri et al. (365) described trigeminal nerve palsies in 7 (4%) of 190 patients with spontaneous dissection of the internal carotid artery. Four of the seven patients presented with a syndrome of hemicrania, oculosympathetic palsy, and trigeminal neuropathy. In addition, Rizzo et al. (366) reported ischemia of the trigeminal ganglion in a patient with a dural

external carotid-cavernous sinus fistula. The simultaneous onset of ipsilateral facial and trigeminal sensory neuropathy was described in a patient with diabetes mellitus by Michelucci et al. (367). The sudden onset of a combined palsy in this setting may results from occlusion of the petrosal branch of the middle meningeal artery, and as with most ischemic cranial nerve palsies, partial or complete recovery should be expected. An argument in favor of this mechanism was also made by Lapresle and Lasjaunias (368), who noted that therapeutic embolization of the middle meningeal artery occasionally produces paralysis of both nerves.

Iatrogenic trigeminal neuropathies may occur as a result of trigeminal ablation by surgical means or injection for treatment of trigeminal neuralgia. Rarely, as a result neurotropic ulcers may occur on the face in anesthetic dermatomes (369). A mefloquine-induced trigeminal sensory neuropathy has also been reported (370).

Neuroparalytic (Neurotrophic) Keratitis

This complication of corneal denervation is mentioned here because it most frequently results from lesions (usually surgical) of the trigeminal ganglion, the sensory root, or the descending trigeminal tract in the brainstem. Cases also occur after brainstem injury (371). Magendie (372) first noted that sectioning of the trigeminal nerve causes trophic or degenerative changes in the cornea, clinically referred to as neurotrophic or neuroparalytic keratitis. Neuroparalytic keratitis from damage to the trigeminal sensory nerve root is a potential complication of both radiofrequency trigeminal rhizotomy and retrogasserian glycerol injection for trigeminal neuralgia, and it occasionally complicates operations for large CPA tumors and other posterior fossa lesions.

The earliest sign of neuroparalytic keratopathy is conjunctival hyperemia, often associated with mild corneal haze. These changes may be apparent in severe cases within 24 hours after the operation, at which time the patient may complain of blurred vision in the affected eye. In mild cases, the changes are discernible only with the slit lamp; in such cases, the patient is usually asymptomatic. Very rarely, the earliest changes occur in the iris; there may be iritis with posterior corneal deposits for several days before there is definite evidence of anterior corneal and conjunctival involvement.

In cases of neuroparalytic keratitis in which only the cornea is affected, the appearance of punctate keratitis or of widespread loss of epithelium associated with conjunctival congestion, may not progress further if treatment is instituted immediately. In some cases, secondary infection develops, and the eye is rapidly lost through perforation; however, the disease is essentially a chronic one without acute sensory symptoms because of the patient's inability to perceive pain. Even in severe cases, the institution of proper treatment may serve to retain a useful eye.

Various theories have been advanced regarding the pathogenesis of neuroparalytic keratitis, including trophic disturbances, corneal desiccation, irritative effects, and abnormal cellular metabolism. Although the actual cause probably reflects a combination of factors, it is clear that the trigeminally innervated corneal nerves play an important role in maintaining the anatomical integrity and function of the cornea, particularly the epithelium (373). Diminished secretion of tears likely encourages corneal involvement (374). Reflex tearing is evoked by afferent impulses transmitted through the trigeminal nerve. The same lesions that damage this nerve at the pontine angle, petrous tip, and Meckel's cave frequently affect the efferent nerve of tearing, the nervus intermedius, and the greater superficial petrosal nerve. Heigle and Pflugfelder (374) measured tear production in nine patients with previous herpes zoster ophthalmicus, five of whom had neuroparalytic keratitis. In the latter group they found a tenfold decrease in tear production compared with the group without keratitis. Nasal sensation and the nasal-lacrimal reflex were lost only in the patients with keratitis, and the authors suggested that this finding may portend the development of neuroparalytic keratitis. It is also possible that some humoral agent plays a role in the development of neuroparalytic keratitis.

Lewis et al. (193,194) examined 15 patients with intentional or unintentional V1 lesions 1–5 years after percutaneous radiofrequency trigeminal rhizotomy. Although five patients had a quantitative decrease in sensation in the eye ipsilateral to the rhizotomy compared with the contralateral eye, none had any symptoms or signs of corneal dysfunction. These investigators postulated that intact corneal sensation implies intact axonal mechanisms essential for maintenance of corneal metabolism and function, and that when sensation is absent, these mechanisms may or may not be adequate to preserve corneal integrity. This theory is consistent with the findings in patients with congenital corneal anesthesia or hypesthesia studied by Purcell and Krachmer (210), many of whom had no corneal abnormalities.

Resection of the superior cervical or stellate ganglion may prevent or reduce the risk of the development of neuroparalytic keratitis (375). The exact role of the sympathetic nerves in the production of keratitis is unknown, but sympathectomy may act by eliminating the inhibitory effect of norepenephrine on corneal epithelial mitosis (376).

Treatment of neuroparalytic keratitis is directed toward preventing corneal desiccation and secondary bacterial infection. The use of an airtight shield over the affected eye creates a moist atmosphere over the surface of the cornea and, in our experience, quickly arrests the keratitis. Epithelization of eroded areas usually follows promptly. Tarsorrhaphy has a similar beneficial effect but is often unnecessary if the patient understands that drying of the eye is dangerous and uses a semipressure patch to avoid this complication. Although the use of a topical artificial tear solution or ointment may aid patients with minimal corneal changes, it does not provide adequate protection for patients with severe disease.

INVOLVEMENT OF THE TRIGEMINAL PATHWAYS IN THE BRAINSTEM

The location of a brainstem lesion is usually indicated by distinctive combinations of cranial nerve palsies and long tract signs. We are concerned in this section with the diagnostic features of facial hypalgesia and hypesthesia that ac-

company some of these brainstem syndromes. In most instances, facial sensation is impaired on the side of the lesion, but occasionally, sensory loss is present on the side opposite the lesion. In contrast to peripheral involvement of the trigeminal nerve, sensory loss from brainstem lesions is commonly dissociated. Thus, perception of pain and temperature may be profoundly affected whereas modalities such as light touch and pressure are spared. Sensory defects with peripheral lesions correspond precisely with the distribution of various divisions and branches of the trigeminal nerve, whereas sensory defects from trigeminal lesions in the brainstem may not adhere strictly to these classic subdivisions. Thus, in brainstem lesions, the sensory loss might involve one small area of the mandibular region or extend into an adjacent region subserved by the maxillary nerve. Correlation of these "unorthodox" sensory defects with the size and location of the lesion is far from exact, but certain guidelines have emerged from pathologic studies of acquired disease as well as from tractotomies performed for the relief of facial pain.

Lesions of the Medulla

Lateral Medullary Infarction

Clinically, the classic lesion involving the descending tract and nucleus is a lateral medullary infarct produced by occlusion of a vertebral or posterior inferior cerebellar artery (Wallenberg's syndrome) (377–379). Trigeminal signs include analgesia for pain and temperature on the same side of the face or head and decreased corneal sensation. The modalities of light touch and pressure are usually intact but may be perceived as less intense or having a different quality. In patients with lateral medullary syndrome from vascular lesions, sensory loss is either in a segmental "onionskin" pattern or in a divisional distribution of V1 or both V1 and V2. It should be noted, however, that sparing of intraoral and perioral sensation was described in a patient with Wallenberg's syndrome who otherwise had complete involvement of all three divisions (74). Because intraoral sensation is not often tested routinely, it may be spared more often than is reported with lateral medullary lesions.

Currier et al. (380) noted that the corneal reflex was absent in the lateral medullary syndrome whenever the loss of sensation included the upper face. Corneal sensation may improve following a lateral medullary infarct but always remains defective if careful testing is performed, and neuroparalytic keratitis can occur (364). Chronic facial pain, due to involvement of the lower spinal trigeminal tract, may be a sequela of lateral medullary infarction (381).

Medullary Tractotomy of the Descending Trigeminal Root

In 1938, Sjöquist reported that the descending trigeminal root could be readily cut in the posterolateral aspect of the medulla, with loss of facial pain and thermal anesthesia but with preservation of tactile and position sensibility. This discovery provided a new approach to the problem of intractable facial pain and stimulated further studies of trigeminal pathways in the human brainstem.

As alluded to earlier in this chapter, fibers from the middle of the face and oral mucosa tend to terminate at more rostral brainstem levels than do the fibers from more peripheral areas of the face, even within the same trigeminal region. Thus, medullary tractotomies at or below the level of the obex may fail to produce analgesia of the oral mucosa (96) or teeth (382). Furthermore, although medullary tractotomy initially abolishes trigeminal pain sensation, partial recovery may occur in the perioral and midline regions of the face (382).

Medullary tractotomies, while producing analgesia of the face and cornea, may not produce complete anesthesia. Thus, awareness of the position of the tongue is retained, and food in the mouth is not lost. The corneal sensation of touch is typically preserved. Often in tractotomies at lower medullary levels, the patient may still show a rather slow corneal reflex on stimulation of the cornea although all appreciation of pain stimuli on the face is lost. There are at least two possible explanations for this. The cornea may be stimulated by tactile stimuli that are known to project to the nucleus of the spinal trigeminal tract at upper, as well as lower, brainstem levels. Another possible explanation is that some of the impulses set up by painful stimulation of the cornea project more rostrally on the nucleus of the spinal trigeminal tract, perhaps at or near the level of the motor nucleus of the facial nerve.

Syringobulbia

Syringomyelia, a chronic disease characterized by proliferation of glial tissue and cavity formation in the central portion of the spinal cord, may extend upward to the medulla. Because of the concentric, onionskin organization of the face for pain (Fig. 25.11), involvement of the nucleus of the spinal tract in the lower cervicomedullary area will first cause defective pain and temperature sensation on the outside of the face. As the destructive process ascends in the brainstem **(syringobulbia),** the spared area in the center of the face shrinks in a radial fashion. Herniation of the cerebellar tonsils into or below the foramen magnum (Chiari I malformation) is one of the most common causes of syringomyelia (383).

Lesions of the Pons

Lesions in the lateral tegmentum of the pons may damage any of the brainstem trigeminal nuclei or the nerve fibers entering the brainstem from the trigeminal root, producing signs that are indistinguishable from those caused by damage to the gasserian ganglion or peripheral root, including neuroparalytic keratitis. Involvement of the main sensory nucleus of the trigeminal nerve causes ipsilateral loss of epicritic sensation in the face (two-point discrimination, light touch, etc.). Proper localization of the lesion in such cases is facilitated when there are associated signs of intrinsic pontine disease (e.g., abducens nerve palsy, horizontal gaze palsy, ocular myoclonus, facial myokymia and/or contracture, peripheral facial palsy, ataxia, pyramidal signs). However, small lesions in the lateral pontine tegmentum may present as an isolated trigeminal sensory neuropathy (305,384–388).

In such cases, localization of the lesion may be impossible without neuroimaging, and even thin-section MR imaging may fail to detect the lesion.

Lateral pontine lesions that produce isolated facial numbness include infarction (389,390), demyelination (127, 358,391), infiltration by a neoplasm, and a small hemorrhage, such as that which occurs in patients with a vascular malformation. Holtzman et al. (384), Berlit (385), and Kim et al. (388) each described a young patient who experienced sudden numbness of the face without other symptoms. Each patient was found to have a small hemorrhage in the dorsolateral tegmentum adjacent to the middle cerebellar peduncle. In two of the patients, V2 and V3 dermatomes were preferentially affected, and the third patient later developed masseter weakness.

Like lateral medullary lesions, lateral pontine lesions may interrupt the lateral spinothalamic tract as well as the more medially situated ventral secondary ascending tract of the trigeminal nerve. Such lesions may cause contralateral hemianalgesia of the both the body and face.

Patients with medial pontine lesions may present with prominent trigeminal motor weakness, with or without sensory loss. Three patients with this syndrome were described by three separate groups (392–394). Two patients also exhibited contralateral ataxic hemiparesis. In all three cases, CT scanning showed vascular lesions involving the basis pontis. The mechanism by which basal pontine lesions selectively affect the trigeminal motor nucleus or fascicle is unclear, although the motor nucleus is slightly ventral and medial to the main sensory nucleus.

A unilateral cheiro-oral syndrome, a sensory disturbance involving the contralateral corner of the mouth and palm of the hand, is caused by a lesion either in the paramedian pontine tegmentum, mesencephalon, ventral posterior thalamus, or the postcentral gyrus of the parietal lobe (see below). Matsumoto et al. (395) described two patients with small lesions of who had the bilateral cheiro-oral syndrome, with symptoms on **both** sides of the mouth. The authors suggested that the hand and perioral symptoms on one side were caused by damage to the medial portions of the medial lemniscus and adjacent ventral secondary ascending tract, whereas the perioral symptoms on the other side were related to extension of the lesion across the midline to the medial part of the other ascending tract (395). Pontine lesions are the usual cause of bilateral cheiro-oral syndrome because of the proximity of the both somatic and facial sensory pathways (396). In addition, Yasuda et al. (397) reported a case with numbness in the contralateral foot in addition to the hand and corner of the mouth—the cheiro-oral-pedal syndrome.

Dorsomedial lesions in the lower pons rarely may produce sensory loss only inside the mouth. In such cases, the lesion is thought to damage the spinal trigeminal nucleus while sparing the adjacent trigeminal tract (74) (Fig. 25.20).

Although bilateral facial analgesia or anesthesia is a rare sign, Miller (364) observed it in a 4-month-old infant with congenital facial diplegia, bilateral horizontal gaze palsies, bulbar paralysis, and hypotonia. The infant also had bilateral neuroparalytic keratitis. It was assumed that the child had

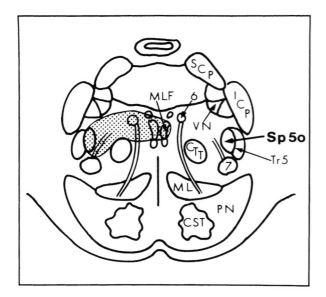

Figure 25.20. Schematic diagram of dorsal lesion (*hatched area*) in lower pons, causing ipsilateral loss of intraoral sensation with intact facial sensation. Note sparing of the descending tract of the trigeminal nerve. The patient also had an ipsilateral facial nerve palsy and one-and-a-half syndrome. SCP, superior cerebellar peduncle; ICP, inferior cerebellar peduncle; VN, vestibular nuclei; Sp5o, spinal nucleus (pars oralis) of trigeminal nerve; Tr5, descending tract of trigeminal nerve; MLF, medial longitudinal fasciculus; CTT, central tegmental tract; ML, medial lemniscus; PN, pontine nuclei; CST, corticospinal tract. (From Graham SH, Sharp FR, Dillon W. Intraoral sensation in patients with brainstem lesions: Role of the rostral spinal trigeminal nuclei in pons. Neurology 1988;38:1529–1533.)

congenital aplasia or hypoplasia of several motor and sensory brainstem nuclei.

Unilateral Spasm and Contracture of the Masseter Muscle: A Sign of Intrinsic Dorsal Pontine Pathology

In Leningrad in 1935, Rasdolsky (398) called attention to a sign of trigeminal involvement that he considered typical of involvement of the dorsal pontine tegmentum by tumor. He reported ipsilateral masseter spasm in five patients with dorsal pontine tumors. All patients had a slowly progressive syndrome characterized by ipsilateral hearing impairment, numbness along the distribution of the trigeminal nerve, loss of the corneal reflex, weakness of the face and forehead, pupillary miosis, ataxia, and progressive spastic contracture of the masseter. His patients were barely able to open their jaws, and their speech was typical in that they were forced to speak "through their teeth." Palpation of the jaw muscles revealed a knotty firmness on the affected side, and the temporalis muscle was obviously wasted as evidenced by concavity of the temporal fossa. Rasdolsky (398) also stressed the peculiar contracted facial musculature on the affected side. Autopsy confirmed that in each case a tumor involved the masticator nucleus, the motor roots of the trigeminal nerve, and all surrounding structures. Many similar cases have been subsequently reported (399–401), although not all of the patients reported have the so-called "masseter sign."

Although neoplasms are the most common cause of spastic paretic facial contracture, this sign also occurs in patients with multiple sclerosis (402), and in patients with other intrinsic lesions of the brainstem, such as tuberculomas (403). Spasms of the masseter muscle also occur in patients with hemimasticatory spasm, but there is no associated contracture of facial muscles and hemimasticatory spasms are paroxysmal (see Involvement of the Mandibular Division of the Trigeminal Nerve in this chapter).

Lesions of the Mesencephalon

Superior lateral lesions of the mesencephalon may involve the trigeminal and spinothalamic pathways (medial lemniscus). For instance, occlusion of the superior cerebellar artery may cause an infarction of the superior lateral portion of the pontomesencephalic tegmentum, resulting in contralateral hemianesthesia of the face and body, cerebellar hypotonia, intention tremor and, occasionally, paresis of vertical gaze (404). Kim (405) described three patients who presented with diplopia and numbness or painful paresthesia on one side of the face. Examination revealed facial hypesthesia on the affected side in two patients and hyperpathia in one. Two patients had contralateral partial oculomotor nerve palsies, and one had an ipsilateral trochlear nerve palsy. MR imaging in each case showed a small lesion involving dorsal midbrain tegmentum, which was postulated to involve the ventral ascending tract and the neighboring oculomotor or trochlear nerve fascicle. One patient also had numbness of the hand on the same side as the facial symptoms, suggesting extension of the lesion laterally to involve the medial lemniscus. Other similar clinical presentations have been described, including a cheiro-oral syndrome without diplopia, resulting from a midbrain hemorrhage (406) or stroke (407), and a cheiro-oral-pedal syndrome with ataxic hemiparesis from a ventrolateral midbrain infarction (408).

INVOLVEMENT OF THE THALAMUS AND THALAMOCORTICAL PROJECTIONS

The thalamogeniculate artery, a proximal branch of the posterior cerebral artery, supplies the posterior part of the lateral nuclear mass of the thalamus. Occlusion of the thalamogeniculate artery produces the classic **thalamic syndrome of Déjerine and Roussy** (409), characterized by complete contralateral hemianesthesia with slight or transient hemiparesis and hemiataxic or choreoathetotic movements of the affected side. The hemianesthesia is usually transitory, but the patient is often left with a "burning" or "ripping" pain and dysesthesia (410). These sensations are often most pronounced in the face. Homonymous hemianopia is commonly associated with the thalamic syndrome and signifies occlusion of the posterior cerebral artery proximal to the thalamogeniculate artery. The Déjerine Roussy syndrome is rarely seen in its complete form in patients with thalamic tumors (411), but it occurs frequently with vascular lesions.

Because the nucleus ventralis posteromedialis (VPM) of the thalamus receives crossed sensory fibers from the opposite side of the face, acute lesions in this nucleus cause analgesia of the face. Touch and vibration sensation may or may not be affected. Iwasaki et al. (412) described a patient with isolated loss of pain and temperature sensation in the left perioral region from a small right thalamic infarction. More commonly, small ventral posterior infarcts cause the cheiro-oral syndrome, characterized by contralateral paresthesia involving the corner of the mouth (especially the upper lip) and the thumb and fingers (especially the index and middle finger). Small hemorrhages may also be responsible (413). The degree of objective sensory loss is variable (414–419). Kim (418) described 10 patients with perioral involvement from thalamic vascular lesions; all 10 had associated paresthesia in the fingers, 4 had numbness in the palm of the hand, and 5 had milder paresthesia in the foot or toes (especially those on the medial side). Two patients developed uncomfortable, often burning, paresthesia in the affected areas.

Autopsy studies of patients with the thalamic cheiro-oral syndrome show localized lesions of the lateral posterior portion of the VPM nucleus and the medial posterior portion of the ventralis postero-lateralis (VPL) nucleus (420,421). Kim (418) and others (415,416) have emphasized that the areas representing the face, hand, and foot, and in particular the upper lip and radial fingers, are contiguous and proceed medially to laterally within the ventral thalamic region. These areas are relatively large compared with the more dorsal projection areas from proximal limbs and trunk. Thus, the pattern of the sensory disturbance in the thalamic cheiro-oral (-pedal) syndrome may be explained by the somatotopic organization of VPL and VPM.

A similar cheiro-oral sensory syndrome, usually associated with a mild hemiparesis, may occur with a lesion of the thalamocortical projections (418,422–424). The typical lesion is an infarction of the posterior limb of the internal capsule at its posterior and superior boundary in the territory of the lateral lenticulostriate arteries. The infarction often extends into the corona radiata and may involve the lenticular nucleus. The sensory disturbance is indistinguishable from that of the thalamic cheiro-oral syndrome, but lesions involving the thalamocortical pathway more often produce hemiparesis and may also affect taste sensation on the opposite side of the tongue (423).

INVOLVEMENT OF THE SENSORY CORTEX (POSTCENTRAL GYRUS)

Although ocular sensation is represented in the midportion of the precentral gyrus, lesions in this area typically do not affect corneal sensitivity. However, as alluded to earlier in this chapter, cerebral lesions in some instances may reduce the contralateral corneal reflex.

Clinically, irritative lesions of the somatic sensory area produce irritative symptoms (numbness, tingling, or a sense of movement) in the corresponding part of the surface of the body, but they rarely cause pain. Focal destruction of cortex leads initially to a localized and complete anesthesia affecting all sensory modalities, but much of this loss is transitory, and a considerable degree of sensibility returns. Complete and lasting anesthesia suggests a lesion at a lower level in the brain. The return of sensation involves those sensations that are most effectively interpreted by the thalamus. It is interesting that in the process of recovery, the most rapid and complete return of sensation occurs in the area supplied by the trigeminal nerve. Pain returns first, the sense of temperature is largely restored, and an appreciation of tactile stimuli is partly regained. The senses of position and discrimination are severely and permanently affected. The greatest loss occurs in the stereognostic sense. It seems, therefore, that the sensory cortex is essential for finer spatial and discriminatory function, whereas the thalamus can analyze and appreciate only the cruder forms of sensation.

Because of the proximity of the face and hand areas in the inferior postcentral gyrus (103), brief episodes of numbness or tingling in the contralateral face and hand often occur together with transient ischemia in the territory of the middle cerebral artery. Migraine sensory auras often are characterized by ipsilateral sensory changes in the face and head. More sustained sensory symptoms in a cheiro-oral distribution occur with parietal lobe tumors (415) and rarely with small infarctions in the parietal operculum (425) or superior postcentral gyrus (426).

CONGENITAL INSENSITIVITY TO PAIN

Most of the patients with congenital insensitivity to pain have a type of hereditary sensory and autonomic neuropathy (HSAN) (427). Some of the HSANs are characterized by distal loss of pain, temperature, light touch, and proprioceptive sensation. However, HSAN III (Riley-Day syndrome, familial dysautonomia) and HSAN IV (congenital pain insensitivity with anhidrosis due to a mutation in the TRK-A gene) have diffuse pain and thermal insensitivity (428). In addition, Donaghy et al. (429) described three members of a consanguinous family who likely had HSAN V (congenital insensitivity to pain with selective loss of small myelinated fibers). A unique feature of this pedigree was that all three affected individuals developed bilateral neurotrophic keratitis in infancy and required corneal transplants. Donaghy et al. (429) pointed out the rarity of corneal opacification in previous reports of hereditary sensory neuropathy, but Miller (364) noted corneal scars in two of five patients with congenital insensitivity to pain, and other authors subsequently described similar patients (430,431).

HYSTERICAL (NONORGANIC) HEMIANESTHESIA

Hysterical hemianesthesia is a conversion reaction that usually involves the entire left side of the body (432,433). It is regularly associated with loss of all types of sensation on the involved side, including the special senses. More important is the characteristic affect on the patient, who invariably displays complete indifference to severe, often absolute, sensory loss. The patient may deny any corneal sensation, even though the corneal blink reflex is normal and symmetric on the two sides. All modalities of sensation are reduced or absent over the side of the face and the corresponding side of the body. The grossness of the sensory loss often helps to distinguish hysterical hemianesthesia from organic disease of the brain.

Two sensory findings that are widely accepted as proof of a hysterical presentation are (*a*) hemianesthesia that splits the midline; and (*b*) unilateral loss of vibratory sensation when the two sides of the forehead are stimulated 1–2 cm from the midline. Both signs, however, are unreliable indicators of hysteria. Rolak (434) tested 100 consecutive patients with hemifacial sensory loss, including 20 patients with psychogenic sensory loss and 80 with structural lesions. Exact splitting of the midline occurred in 20% of those with psychogenic loss and in 8% of those with structural lesions, whereas unilateral loss of vibration sensation was demonstrated in 95% and 86% of patients, respectively. Similarly, Gould et al. (435) found that 21 of 30 patients with acute lesions (mostly strokes) had midline splitting of pain or vibration sensation.

Patients with hysterical hemianesthesia may also claim to have lost one or more of the special senses on the involved side, including hearing, vision, and the sense of smell. Hearing loss is a common finding, but the patient does not complain of it until hearing is tested during the examination. Ipsilateral loss of vision may comprise complete or partial blindness in one eye or a homonymous hemianopia, typically with nonphysiologic features (see Chapter 27). Keane (436) reported ten patients with hysterical hemianopias, eight of whom complained of ipsilateral neurologic symptoms, usually numbness.

REFERENCES

1. Romanes GJ. The peripheral nervous system: Trigeminal nerve. In: Romanes GJ, ed. Cunningham's Textbook of Anatomy. Ed 12. Oxford UK: Oxford University Press, 1981:748–756.
2. Hardy DG, Rhoton AL Jr. Microsurgical relationships of the superior cerebellar artery and the trigeminal nerve. J Neurosurg 1978;49:669–678.
3. Umansky F, Nathan H. The lateral wall of the cavernous sinus: with special reference to the nerves related to it. J Neurosurg 1982;56:228–234.
4. Johnston JA, Parkinson D. Intracranial sympathetic pathways associated with the sixth cranial nerve. J Neurosurg 1974;39:236–243.
5. Parkinson D, Johnston J, Chaudhuri A. Sympathetic connections to the fifth and sixth cranial nerves. Anat Rec 1978;191:221–226.
6. Parkinson D. Sympathetic pathways [letter]. J Neurosurg 1994;81:809–810.
7. Harris FS, Rhoton AL Jr. Anatomy of the cavernous sinus: A microsurgical study. J Neurosurg 1976;45:169–180.
8. Ruskell GL, Simons T. Trigeminal nerve pathways to the cerebral arteries in monkeys. J Anat 1987;155:23–37.
9. Simons T, Ruskell GL. Distribution and termination of trigeminal nerves to the cerebral arteries in monkeys. J Anat 1988;159:57–71.
10. O'Connor TP, van der Kooy D. Pattern of intracranial and extracranial projections of trigeminal ganglion cells. J Neurosci 1986;6:2200–2207.
11. Edvinsson L. Sensory nerves in man and their role in primary headaches. Cephalalgia 2001;21:761–764.
12. Browne PA, Clark GT, Kuboki T, et al. Concurrent cervical and craniofacial pain: A review of empiric and basic science evidence. Oral Surg Oral Med Oral Pathol Oral Radiol Endod 1998;86:633–640.
13. Ramadan NM, Skljarevski V, Phebus LA, et al. 5-HT1F receptor agonists in acute migraine treatment: A hypothesis. Cephalalgia 2003;23:776–785.
14. Whitnall SE. The Anatomy of the Human Orbit and Accessory Organ of Vision. Ed 2. New York: Oxford University Press, 1932:347–372.
15. Fujii K, Chambers SM, Rhoton AL. Neurovascular relationships of the sphenoid sinus: A microsurgical study. J Neurosurg 1979;50:31–39.
16. Alfieri A, Jho H-D. Endoscopic endonasal cavernous sinus surgery: An anatomic study. Neurosurgery 2001;48:827–837.
17. Henderson WR. A note on the relationship of the human maxillary nerve to the cavernous sinus passing through the foramen ovale. J Anat 1966;100:109–115.
18. Ginsberg LE, Pruett SW, Chen MYM, et al. Skull-base foramina of the middle cranial fossa: Reassessment of normal variation with high-resolution CT. Am J Neuroradiol 1994;15:283–291.
19. Moiseiwitsch J, Irvine T. Clinical significance of the length of the pterygopalatine fissue in dental anesthesia. Oral Surg Oral Med Oral Pathol Oral Radiol Endod 2001;92:325–328.
20. Morgan C, Jannetta PJ, deGroat WC. Organization of corneal afferent axons in the trigeminal nerve root entry zone in the cat. Exp Brain Res 1987;68:411–416.
21. Marfurt CF, Kingsley RE, Echtenkamp SE. Sensory and sympathetic innervation of the mammalian cornea: A retrograde tracing study. Invest Ophthalmol Vis Sci 1989;30:461–472.
22. Ruskell GL. Ocular fibers of the maxillary nerves in monkeys. J Anat 1974;118:195–203.
23. Beauvieux J, Dupas J. Étude anatomo-topographique et histologique du ganglion ophtalmique chez l'homme et divers animaux. Arch Ophthalmol 1926;43:641–671.
24. Penfield W, McNaughton F. Dural headache and innervation of the dura mater. Arch Neurol Psychiatr 1940;44:43–75.
25. Schmidt BL, Pogrel MA, Necoechea M, et al. The distribution of the auriculotemporal nerve around the temporomandibular joint. Oral Surg Oral Med Oral Pathol Oral Radiol Endod 1998;86:165–168.
26. Schmalfuss IM, Tart RP, Mukherji S, et al. Perineural tumor spread along the auriculotemporal nerve. Am J Neuroradiol 2002;23:303–311.
27. Dodd J, Kelly JP. Trigeminal system. In: Kandel ER, Schwartz JH, Jessell TM, eds. Principles of Neural Science. East Norwalk: Appleton & Lange, 1991:701–710.
28. Cruccu G, Berardelli A, Inghilleri M, et al. Functional organization of the trigeminal motor system in man: A neurophysiological study. Brain 1989;112:1333–1350.
29. Cruccu G, Agostino R, Inghilleri M, et al. The masseter inhibitory reflex is evoked by innocuous stimuli and mediated by A beta afferent fibres. Exp Brain Res 1989;77:447–450.
30. Türk U, Rosler KM, Mathis J, et al. Assessment of motor pathways to masticatory muscles: An examination technique using electrical and magnetic stimulation. Muscle & Nerve 1994;17:1271–1277.
31. Jannetta PJ. Gross (mesoscopic) description of the human trigeminal ganglion. J Neurosurg 1967;26:109–115.
32. Kapila A, Chakeres DW, Blanco E. The Meckel cave: Computed tomographic study. Part I: Normal anatomy, Part II: Pathology. Radiology 1984;152:425–433.
33. Chui M, Tucker W, Hudson A, et al. High resolution CT of Meckel's cave. Neuroradiology 1985;27:403–409.
34. Daniels DL, Pech P, Pojunas KW, et al. Trigeminal nerve: anatomic correlation with MR imaging. Radiology 1986;159:577–583.
35. Tsuha M, Aoki H, Okamura T. Roentgenological investigation of cavernous sinus structure with special reference to paracavernous cranial nerves. Neuroradiology 1987;29:462–467.
36. Rubinstein D, Stears RL, Stears JC. Trigeminal nerve and ganglion in the Meckel cave: Appearance at CT and MR imaging. Radiology 1994;193:155–159.
37. Williams LS, Schmalfuss IM, Sistrom CL, et al. MR imaging of the trigeminal ganglion, nerve, and the perineural vascular plexus: Normal appearance and variants with correlation to cadaver specimens. Am J Neuroradiol 2003;24:1317–1323.
38. Dixon AD. Fine structure of nerve-cell bodies and satellite cells in the trigeminal ganglion. J Dent Res 1963;42:990–999.
39. Kerr FWL. The divisional organization of afferent fibres of the trigeminal nerve. Brain 1963;86:721–732.
40. Moses HL. Comparative fine structure of the trigeminal ganglion, including autopsy studies. J Neurosurg 1967;26:112–126.
41. Tran-Dinh H. Cavernous branches of the internal carotid artery: anatomy and nomenclature. Neurosurgery 1987;20:205–210.
42. Krisht A, Barnett DW, Barrow DL, et al. The blood supply of the intracavernous cranial nerves: An anatomic study. Neurosurgery 1994;34:275–279.
43. Haines SJ, Jannetta PJ, Zorub DS. Microvascular relations of the trigeminal nerve: An anatomical study with clinical correlation. J Neurosurg 1980;52:381–386.
44. Hardy DG, Peace DA, Rhoton AL Jr. Microsurgical anatomy of the superior cerebellar artery. Neurosurgery 1980;6:10–28.
45. Klun B, Prestor B. Microvascular relations of the trigeminal nerve: An anatomical study. Neurosurgery 1986;19:535–539.
46. Barker FG, Jannetta PJ, Bissonette DJ, et al. The long-term outcome of microvascular decompression for trigeminal neuralgia. N Engl J Med 1996;334:1077–1083.
47. Jawahar A, Kondziolka D, Kanal E, et al. Imaging the trigeminal nerve and pons before and after surgical intervention for trigeminal neuralgia. Neurosurgery 2001;48:101–107.
48. Bakshi R, Lerner A, Fritz JV, et al. Vacular compression in trigeminal neuralgia shown by magnetic resonance imaging and magnetic resonance angiography image registration. Arch Neurol 2001;58:1290–1291.
49. Brisman R, Khandji AG, Mooij RBM. Trigeminal nerve-blood vessel relationship as revealed by high-resolution magnetic resonance imaging and its effect on pain relief after gamma knife radiosurgery for trigeminal neuralgia. Neurosurgery 2002;50:1261–1267.
50. Akimoto H, Nagaoka T, Nariai T, et al. Preoperative evaluation of neurovascular compression in patients with trigeminal neuralgia by use of three-dimentional reconstruction from two types of high-resolution magnetic resonance imaging. Neurosurgery 2002;51:956–962.
51. Tamura Y, Shimano H, Kuroiwa T, et al. Trigeminal neuralgia associated with

a primitive trigeminal artery variant: Case report. Neurosurgery 2003;52: 1217–1220.

52. Marinkovic SV, Gibo H. The blood supply of the trigeminal nerve root, with special reference to the trigeminocerebellar artery. Neurosurgery 1995;37: 309–317.

53. Gudmundsson K, Rhoton AL Jr, Rushton JG. Detailed anatomy of the intracranial portion of the trigeminal nerve. J Neurosurg 1971;35:592–600.

54. Mira KM, Elnaga IA, El-Sherif H. Nerve cells in the intracranial part of the trigeminal nerve of man and dog: Anatomical study of the fifth cranial nerve. J Neurosurg 1971;34:643–646.

55. Stechison MT, Moller A, Lovely TJ. Intraoperative mapping of the trigeminal nerve root: Technique and application in the surgical management of facial pain. Neurosurgery 1996;38:76–82.

56. Pelletier VA, Poulos DA, Lende RA. Functional localization in the trigeminal root. J Neurosurg 1974;40:504–513.

57. Stibbe EP. Some observations on the surgery of trigeminal neuralgia. Br J Surg 1936;24:122–129.

58. Stibbe EP. Surgical anatomy of the subtentorial angle with special reference to the acoustic and trigeminal nerves. Lancet 1939;1:918–921.

59. Dandy WE. The treatment of trigeminal neuralgia by the cerebellar route. Ann Surg 1932;96:787–795.

60. Jannetta PJ. Microsurgical approach to the trigeminal nerve for tic douloureux. In: Krayenbuhl H, Maspes PE, Sweet WH, eds. Progress in Neurological Surgery. Vol. 7. Basel: Karger, 1976:180–200.

61. Hussein M, Wilson LA, Illingworth R. Patterns of sensory loss following fractional posterior fossa Vth nerve section for trigeminal neuralgia. J Neurol Neurosurg Psychiatr 1982;45:786–790.

62. Kerr FWL, Lysak WR. Somatotopic organization of trigeminal-ganglion neurons. Arch Neurol 1964;11:593–602.

63. Sjöqvist O. Studies on Pain Conduction in the Trigeminal Nerve: A Contribution to the Surgical Treatment of Facial Neuralgia. Helsingfors, Mercators Trycheri, 1938.

64. White JC, Sweet WH. Pain, Its Mechanisms and Neurosurgical Control. Springfield IL, Charles C Thomas, 1955.

65. Olszewski J. On the anatomical and functional organization of the spinal trigeminal nucleus. J Comp Neurol 1950;92:401–413.

66. Darian-Smith I. The trigeminal system. In: Iggo A, ed. Handbook of Sensory Physiology. Vol. 2. Berlin: Springer-Verlag, 1973:271–314.

67. Corbin KB, Harrison F. Function of mesencephalic root of fifth cranial nerve. J Neurophysiol 1940;3:423–435.

68. Jerge CR. Organization and function of the trigeminal mesencephalic nucleus. J Neurophysiol 1963;26:379–392.

69. Gabrawi AF, Tarkhan AA. A histological study of the mesencephalic nucleus of the fifth cranial nerve. Acta Anat (Basel) 1967;67:361–368.

70. Afshar F, Dykes E, Watkins ES. Three-dimensional stereotactic anatomy of the human trigeminal nerve nuclear complex. Appl Neurophysiol 1983;46:147–153.

71. Smith RD. Axonal projections and connections of the principal sensory trigeminal nucleus in the monkey. J Comp Neurol 1975;163:347–376.

72. Dallel R, Raboisson P, Auroy P, et al. The rostral part of the trigeminal sensory complex is involved in orofacial nociception. Brain Res 1988;448:7–19.

73. Shults RC. Trigeminal primary afferent receptors. In: Light AR, ed. The Initial Processing of Pain and Its Descending Control: Spinal and Trigeminal Systems. Pain and Headache. Vol. 12. Basel: S Karger AG, 1992:50–74.

74. Graham SH, Sharp FR, Dillon W. Intraoral sensation in patients with brainstem lesions: Role of rostral spinal trigeminal nuclei in pons. Neurology 1988;38: 1529–1533.

75. Rowe MJ, Sessle BJ. Somatic afferent input to posterior thalamic neurones and their axon projection to the cerebral cortex. J Physiol (Lond) 1968;196:19–35.

76. Carpenter MB, Hanna GR. Fiber projections from the spinal trigeminal nucleus in the cat. J Comp Neurol 1961;117:117–132.

77. Hayashi H, Sumino R, Sessle BJ. Functional organization of trigeminal subnucleus interpolaris: Nociceptive and innocuous afferent inputs, projections to thalamus, cerebellum, and spinal cord, and descending modulation from periaqueductal gray. J Neurophysiol 1984;51:890–905.

78. Rexed B. The cytoarchitecture organization of the spinal cord in the cat. J Comp Neurol 1952;96:415–495.

79. Kerr FWL. The ultrastructure of the spinal tract of the trigeminal nerve and the substantia gelatinosa. Exp Neurol 1966;16:359–376.

80. Kerr FWL. Fine structure and functional characteristics of the primary trigeminal neuron. In: Hassler R, Walker AE, eds. Trigeminal Neuralgia. Stuttgart: Verlag, 1970:11–21.

81. Kerr FWL. Electron microscopic observations on degeneration in the subnucleus caudalis of the trigeminal. In: Dubner R, ed. Oro-Facial Sensory and Motor Mechanisms. Vol. 1970. New York: Appleton-Century-Crofts, 1970:11–21.

82. Bereiter DA, Hirata H, Hu JW. Trigeminal subnucleus caudalis: Beyond homologies with the spinal dorsal horn. Pain 2000;88:221–224.

83. Gobel S, Purvis MB. Anatomical studies of the organization of the spinal V nucleus: The deep bundles and the spinal V tract. Brain Res 1972;48:27–44.

84. Ikeda M, Tanami T, Matsushita M. Ascending and descending internuclear connections of the trigeminal sensory nuclei in the cat. A study with the retrograde

and anterograde horseradish peroxidase technique. Neuroscience 1984;12: 1243–1260.

85. Marfurt CF, Del Toro DR. Corneal sensory pathway in the rat: A horseradish peroxidase tracing study. J Comp Neurol 1987;261:450–459.

86. Marfurt CF, Echtenkamp SF. Central projections and trigeminal ganglion location of corneal afferent neurons in the monkey, Macaca fascicularis. J Comp Neurol 1988;272:370–382.

87. Pozo MA, Cervero F. Neurons in the rat spinal trigeminal complex driven by corneal nociceptors: Receptive-field properties and effects of noxious stimulation of the cornea. J Neurophysiol 1993;70:2370–2378.

88. Davis KD, Dostrovsky JO. Responses of feline trigeminal spinal tract nucleus neurons to stimulation of the middle meningeal artery and sagittal sinus. J Neurophysiol 1988;59:648–666.

89. Dostrovsky JO, Davis KD, Kawakita K. Central mechanisms of vascular headaches. Can J Physiol Pharmacol 1991;69:652–658.

90. Strassman A, Mason P, Moskowitz M, et al. Response of brainstem trigeminal neurons to electrical stimulation of the dura. Brain Res 1986;379:242–250.

91. Strassman AM, Potrebic S, Maciewicz RJ. Anatomical properties of brainstem trigeminal neurons that respond to electrical stimulation of dural blood vessels. J Comp Neurol 1994;346:349–365.

92. Zagami AS, Lambert GA. Stimulation of cranial vessels excites nociceptive neurones in several thalamic nuclei of the cat. Exp Brain Res 1990;81:552–566.

93. Goadsby PJ, Zagami AS, Lambert GA. Neural processing of craniovascular pain: A synthesis of the central structures involved in migraine. Headache 1991; 31:365–371.

94. Silverman JD, Kruger L. Projections of the rat trigeminal sensory nuclear complex demonstrated by multiple fluorescent dye retrograde transport. Brain Res 1985;361:383–388.

95. Steindler DA. Trigeminocerebellar, trigeminotectal, and trigeminothalamic projections: A double retrograde axonal tracing study in the mouse. J Comp Neurol 1985;237:155–175.

96. Taren JA, Kahn EA. Anatomic pathways related to pain in the face and neck. J Neurosurg 1962;19:116–121.

97. Kerr FWL. Discussion of Taren JA, Kahn EA. Anatomic pathways related to pain in face and neck. J Neurosurg 1962;19:121.

98. Walker AE. The Primate Thalamus. Chicago: University of Chicago Press, 1938.

99. Eidelberg D, Galaburda AM. Symmetry and asymmetry in the human posterior thalamus. I. Cytoarchitectonic analysis in normal persons. Arch Neurol 1982; 39:325–332.

100. Herrero M-T, Barcia C, Navarro JM. Functional anatomy of the thalamus and basal ganglia. Child's Nerv Syst 2002;18:386–404.

101. Yokota T, Koyama N, Matsumoto N. Somatotopic distribution of trigeminal nociceptive neurons in ventrobasal complex of cat thalamus. J Neurophysiol 1985;53:1387–1400.

102. Jones EG, Hendry SHC, Brandon C. Cytochrome oxidase staining reveals functional organization of monkey somatosensory thalamus. Exp Brain Res 1986; 62:438–442.

103. McCarthy G, Allison T, Spencer DD. Localization of the face area of human sensorimotor cortex by intracranial recording of somatosensory evoked potentials. J Neurosurg 1993;79:874–884.

104. Woolsey CN, Marshall HW, Bard P. Representation of cutaneous tactile sensibility in the cerebral cortex of the monkey as indicated by evoked potentials. Bull Johns Hopkins Hosp 1942;70:399–441.

105. Penfield W, Rasmussen T. The Cerebral Cortex of Man: A Clinical Study of Localization of Function. New York: Macmillan, 1950.

106. Guthrie BL, Porter JD, Sparks DL. Corollary discharge provides accurate eye position information to the oculomotor system. Science 1983;221:1193–1195.

107. Steinbach MJ. Proprioceptive knowledge of eye position. Vision Res 1987;27: 1737–1744.

108. Porter JD, Baker RS, Ragusa RJ, et al. Extraocular muscles: basic and clinical aspects of structure and function. Surv Ophthalmol 1995;39:451–484.

109. Merton PA. Absence of Conscious Position Sense in the Human Eyes. In Bender MB, ed. The Oculomotor System. New York: Harper & Row, 1964:314–320.

110. Skavenski AA. Inflow as a source of extra retinal eye position information. Vision Res 1972;12:221–229.

111. Cochet P, Bonnet R. L'Esthésie Cornéenne. Clinique Ophtalmol 1960;64:2–27.

112. DeJong RN. The Neurologic Examination. Ed 4. Hagerstown: Harper & Row, 1979:163–179.

113. Ongerboer de Visser BW. Anatomical and functional organization of reflexes involving the trigeminal system in man: Jaw reflex, blink reflex, corneal reflex, and exteroceptive suppression. Adv Neurol 1983;39:727–738.

114. Ongerboer de Visser BW, Melchelse K, Megens PHA. Corneal reflex latency in trigeminal nerve lesions. Neurology 1977;27:1164–1167.

115. Zametkin AJ, Stevens JR, Pittman R. Ontogeny of spontaneous blinking and of habituation of the blink reflex. Ann Neurol 1979;5:453–457.

116. Cruccu G, Berardelli A, Manfredi M. Afferents for the human corneal reflex. J Neurol 1987;234:64.

117. Kugelberg E. Facial reflexes. Brain 1952;75:385–396.

118. Shahani B. Effects of sleep on human reflexes with a double component. J Neurol Neurosurg Psychiatr 1968;31:574–579.

119. Shahani B. The human blink reflex. J Neurol Neurosurg Psychiatr 1970;33: 792–800.

120. Shahani B, Young RR. A note on blink reflexes. J Physiol (Lond) 1968;198: 103P–104P.

121. Shahani B, Young RR. Human orbicularis oculi reflexes. Neurology 1972;22: 149–154.

122. Kimura J. The blink reflex as a test for brainstem and higher central nervous system function. In: Desmedt JE, ed. New Developments in Electromyography and Clinical Neurophysiology. Vol. 3. Basel: Karger, 1973:682–691.

123. Kimura J. Effect of hemispheral lesions on the contralateral blink reflex: A clinical study. Neurology 1974;24:168–174.

124. Dehen H, Willer JC, Bathien N. Analyse électrophysiologique du réflexe de clignement (blink reflex) au cours de l'hémiplégie par lésions hémisphériques. Rev Neurol 1975;131:85–94.

125. Kimura J. Electrically elicited blink reflex in diagnosis of multiple sclerosis. Brain 1975;98:413–426.

126. Almárcegui C, Lorente S, Romero MF, et al. Blink reflex in trigeminal hypoesthesia caused by a pontine demyelinating lesion. J Neurol 1999;246:140–141.

127. Pedraza L, Campero M. Trigeminal sensory neuropathy: Anatomico-physiological correlation. J Neurol Neurosurg Psychiatr 2000;68:390.

128. Marx JJ, Thoemke F, Fitzek S, et al. Topodiagnostic value of blink reflex R1 changes: A digital postprocessing MRI correlation study. Muscle Nerve 2001; 24:1327–1331.

129. Kimura J, Lyon LW. Orbicularis oculi reflex in the Wallenberg syndrome: Alteration of the late reflex by lesions of the spinal tract and nucleus of the trigeminal nerve. J Neurol Neurosurg Psychiatr 1972;35:228–233.

130. Ongerboer de Visser BW, Kuypers HGJM. Late blink reflex changes in lateral medullary lesions: An electrophysiological and neuro-anatomical study of Wallenberg's syndrome. Brain 1978;101:285–294.

131. Ongerboer de Visser BW. Comparative study of corneal and blink reflex latencies in patients with segmental or with cerebral lesions. Adv Neurol 1983;39: 757–772.

132. Fitzek S, Fitzek C, Marx J, et al. Blink reflex R2 changes and localisation of lesions in the lower brainstem (Wallenberg's syndrome): An electrophysiological and MRI study. J Neurol Neurosurg Psychiatr 1999;67:630–636.

133. Aramideh M, Ongerboer de Visser BW. Brainstem reflexes: Electrodiagnostic techniques, physiology, normative data, and clinical applications. Muscle Nerve 2002;26:14–30.

134. Ongerboer de Visser BW. Corneal reflex latency in lesions of the lower postcentral region. Neurology 1981;31:701–707.

135. Berardelli A, Accornero N, Cruccu G, et al. The orbicularis oculi response after hemispheral damage. J Neurol Neurosurg Psychiatry 1983;46:837–843.

136. Fisher MA, Shahani B, Young RR. Assessing segmental excitability after acute rostral lesions. II. The blink reflex. Neurology 1979;29:45–50.

137. Schorr A, Ellrich J. Long-term depression of the human blink reflex. Exp Brain Res 2002;147:549–553.

138. Dimitrova A, Weber J, Maschke M, et al. Eyeblink-related areas in human cerebellum as shown by fMRI. Hum Brain Mapping 2002;17:100–115.

139. Loeffler JD, Slatt B, Hoyt WF. Motor abnormalities of the eyelids in Parkinson's disease: Electromyographic observations. Arch Ophthalmol 1966;76:178–185.

140. Pearce J, Aziz H, Gallagher JC. Primitive reflex activity in primary and symptomatic parkinsonism. J Neurol Neurosurg Psychiatr 1968;31:501–508.

141. Stevens JR. Eye-blink and schizophrenia: Psychosis or tardive dyskinesia? Am J Psychiatr 1978;135:223–226.

142. Taiminen T, Jääskeläinen S, Ilonen T, et al. Habituation of the blink reflex in first-episode schizophrenia, psychotic depression and psychotic depression. Schizophrenia Res 2000;44:69–79.

143. Aktekin B, Yaltkaya K, Ozkaynak S, et al. Recovery cycle of the blink reflex and exteroceptive suppression of temporalis muscle activity in migraine and tension-type headache. Headache 2001;41:142–149.

144. de Tommaso M, Murasecco D, Libro G, et al. Modulation of trigeminal reflex excitability in migraine: Effects of attention and habituation on the blink reflex. Int J Psychophysiol 2002;44:239–249.

145. De Marinis M, Pujia A, Natale L, et al. Decreased habituation of the R2 component of the blink reflex in migraine patients. Clin Neurophysiol 2003;114: 889–893.

146. Katsarava Z, Egelhof T, Giffin N, et al. Symptomatic migraine and sensitization of trigeminal nociception associated with contralateral pontine cavernoma. Pain 2003;105:381–384.

147. Katsarava Z, Giffin N, Diener H-C, et al. Abnormal habituation of 'nociceptive' blink reflex in migraine: Evidence for increased excitability of trigeminal nociception. Cephalalgia 2003;23:814–819.

148. Baykara M, Dogru M, Ozmen AT, et al. Oculocardiac reflex in a nonsedated laser in situ keratomileusis patient. J Cataract Refract Surg 2002;28:1698–1699.

149. Hahnenkamp K, Hönemann CW, Fischer LG, et al. Effect of different anaesthetic regimes on the oculocardiac reflex during paediatric strabismus surgery. Paediat Anaesthesia 2000;10:601–608.

150. Hiebert SM, Burch E. Simulated human diving and heart rate: Making the most of the diving response as a laboratory exercise. Adv Physiol Educ 2003;27: 130–145.

151. Okuda B, Kodama N, Kawabata K, et al. Corneomandibular reflex in ALS. Neurology 1999;52:1699.

152. Chang C-W. Electrophysiological assessments of primitive reflexes in stroke patients. Clin Neurophysiol 2001;112:1070–1075.

153. Pullicino PM, Jacobs LM, McCall WD, et al. Spontaneous palpebromandibular synkinesia: A localizing clinical sign. Ann Neurol 1994;35:222–228.

154. Fitzek S, Fitzek C, Hopf HC. The masseter reflex: Postprocessing methods and influence of age and gender. Normative values of the masseter reflex. Eur Neurol 2001;46:202–205.

155. Martin XY, Safran AB. Corneal hypoesthesia. Surv Ophthalmol 1988;33:28–40.

156. Millodot M. The influence of age on the sensitivity of the cornea. Invest Ophthalmol Vis Sci 1977;16:240–242.

157. Millodot M. Do blue-eyed people have more sensitive corneas than brown-eyed people? Nature 1975;255:151–152.

158. Millodot M. Corneal sensitivity in people with the same and with different iris color. Invest Ophthalmol 1976;15:861–862.

159. Szerenyi K, Sorken K, Garbus JJ, et al. Decrease in normal human corneal sensitivity with topical diclofenac sodium. Am J Ophthalmol 1994;118:312–315.

160. Zaidman GW, Amsur K. Diclofenac and its effect on corneal sensation. Arch Ophthalmol 1995;113:262.

161. Seitz B, Sorken K, LaBrie LD, et al. Corneal sensitivity and burning sensation. Comparing topical ketorolac and diclofenac. Arch Ophthalmol 1996;114: 921–924.

162. Katz I. Beta-blockers and the eye: An overview. Ann Ophthalmol 1978;10: 847–850.

163. Van Buskirk EM. Corneal anaesthesia after timolol maleate therapy. Am J Ophthalmol 1979;88:739–743.

164. Calissendorff B. Corneal anesthesia after topical treatment with timolol maleate: A case report. Acta Ophthalmol 1981;59:347–349.

165. Vogel R, Clineschmidt CM, Höeh H, et al. The effect of timolol, betaxolol, and placebo on corneal sensitivity in healthy volunteers. J Ocular Pharmacol 1990; 6:85–90.

166. Weissman SS, Asbell PA. Effects of timolol (0.5%) and betaxolol (0.5%) on corneal sensitivity. Br J Ophthalmol 1990;74:409–412.

167. Schirmer KE, Mellor LD. Corneal sensitivity after cataract extraction. Arch Ophthalmol 1961;65:433–436.

168. John T. Corneal sensation after small incision, sutureless, one-handed phacoemulsification. J Cat Refract Surg 1995;21:425–428.

169. Gibson RA. Reduction of corneal sensation after retinal detachment surgery. Br J Ophthalmol 1981;65:614–617.

170. Hung JY. Corneal sensation in retinal detachment surgery. Ann Ophthalmol 1987;19:313–318.

171. Rogell GD. Corneal hypesthesia and retinopathy in diabetes mellitus. Ophthalmology 1980;87:229–233.

172. Shivitz IA, Arrowsmith PN. Corneal sensitivity after radial keratotomy. Ophthalmology 1988;95:827–832.

173. Eiferman RA, O'Neil KP, Forgey DR, et al. Excimer laser photorefractive keratectomy for myopia: Six-month results. Refract Corneal Surg 1991;7:344–377.

174. Campos M, Hertzog L, Garbus JJ, et al. Corneal sensitivity after photorefractive keratectomy. Am J Ophthalmol 1992;114:51–54.

175. Ishikawa T, Park SB, Cox C, et al. Corneal sensation following excimer laser photorefractive keratectomy in humans. J Refract Corneal Surg 1994;10: 417–422.

176. Toda I, Asano-Kato N, Komai-Hori Y, et al. Dry eye after laser in situ keratomileusis. Am J Ophthalmol 2001;110:497–502.

177. Nassaralla BA, McLeod SD, Nassaralla JJ. Effect of myopic LASIK on human corneal sensitivity. Ophthalmology 2003;110:497–502.

178. Millodot M. Effect of soft lenses on corneal sensitivity. Acta Ophthalmol 1974; 52:603–604.

179. Millodot M. Effect of hard contact lenses on corneal sensitivity and thickness. Acta Ophthalmol 1975;53:576–582.

180. Velasco MJ, Bermudez FJ, Romero J, et al. Variations in corneal sensitivity with hydrogel contact lenses. Acta Ophthalmol 1994;72:53–56.

181. Patel SV, McLaren JW, Hodge DO, et al. Confocal microscopy in vivo in corneas of long-term contact lens wearers. Invest Ophthalmol Vis Sci 2002;43: 995–1003.

182. Millodot M. Effect of length of wear of contact lenses on corneal sensitivity. Acta Ophthalmol 1976;54:721–730.

183. Lyne AJ. Corneal sensation in scleritis and episcleritis. Br J Ophthalmol 1977; 61:650.

184. Patel BCK, Tullo AB. Corneal sensation in acute angle closure glaucoma. Acta Ophthalmol 1988;66:44–46.

185. Kodama T, Hayasaka S, Setogawa T. Immunofluorescent staining and corneal sensitivity in patients suspected of having herpes simplex keratitis. Am J Ophthalmol 1992;113:187–189.

186. Draeger J, Koudelka A, Lubahn E. Zur asthesiometrie der hornhaut. Klin Monatsbl Augenheilkd 1976;169:407–421.

187. Cushing H. Tumors of Nervus Acusticus and Syndrome of Cerebellopontine Angle. Philadelphia, W.B. Saunders, 1916.

188. Selesnick SH, Jackler RK, Pitts LW. The changing clinical presentation of acoustic tumors in the MRI era. Laryngoscope 1993;103:431–436.

189. Rose GE, Wright JE. Trigeminal sensory loss in orbital disease. Br J Ophthalmol 1994;78:427–429.

190. Purcell JJ Jr, Krachmer JH, Thompson HS. Corneal sensation in Adie's syndrome. Am J Ophthalmol 1977;84:496–500.

191. Mensher JH. Corneal nerves. Surv Ophthalmol 1974;19:1–18.

192. Davies MS. Corneal anaesthesia after alcohol injection of the trigeminal sensory root: Examination of 100 anaesthetic corneae. Br J Ophthalmol 1970;54:577–586.

193. Lewis RA, Cobb CA, Keltner JL. Corneal sensitivity after percutaneous radiofrequency trigeminal rhizotomy: A quantitative study. Ann Ophthalmol 1982;14:766–771.

194. Lewis RA, Keltner JL, Cobb CA. Corneal anesthesia after percutaneous radiofrequency trigeminal rhizotomy: A retrospective study. Arch Ophthalmol 1982;100:301–303.

195. Laitinen LV, Brophy BP, Bergenheim AT. Sensory disturbances following retrogasserian glycerol rhizotomy. Br J Neurosurg 1989;3:471–477.

196. Schwartz DE. Corneal sensitivity in diabetes. Arch Ophthalmol 1974;91:174–178.

197. Hyndiuk RA, Kazarian EL, Schultz RD, et al. Neurotrophic corneal ulcers in diabetes mellitus. Arch Ophthalmol 1977;95:2193–2196.

198. Ruben ST. Corneal sensation in insulin-dependent and non-insulin-dependent diabetics with proliferative retinopathy. Acta Ophthalmol 1994;72:576–580.

199. Dogru M, Katakami C, Inoue M. Tear function and ocular surface changes in noninsulin-dependent diabetes mellitus. Ophthalmology 2001;108:586–592.

200. Shields JA, Waring GO, Monte LG. Ocular findings in leprosy. Am J Ophthalmol 1974;77:880–890.

201. Dana MR, Hochman MA, Viana MA, et al. Ocular manifestations of leprosy in a noninstitutionalized community in the U.S. Arch Ophthalmol 1994;112:626–629.

202. Sekhar GC, Vance G, Otton S, et al. Ocular manifestations of Hansen's disease. Doc Ophthalmol 1994;87:211–221.

203. Rosenberg ME, Tervo TMT, Gallar J, et al. Corneal morphology and sensitivity in lattice dystrophy type II (familial amyloidosis, Finnish type). Invest Ophthalmol Vis Sci 2001;42:634–641.

204. Ohashi Y, Matsuda M, Hosotani H, et al. Aldose reductase inhibitor (CT-112) eyedrops for diabetic corneal epitheliopathy. Am J Ophthalmol 1988;105:233–238.

205. Hosotani H, Ohashi Y, Yamada M, et al. Reversal of abnormal corneal epithelial morphologic characteristics and reduced corneal sensitivity in diabetic patients by aldose reductase inhibitor, CT-112. Am J Ophthalmol 1995;119:288–294.

206. Nazarian J, O'Leary DJ. Corneal sensitivity in myasthenia gravis. Br J Ophthalmol 1985;69:519–521.

207. Singh J, Gibson JM. A case of presumed congenital herpes zoster ophthalmicus. Br J Ophthalmol 1993;77:459–461.

208. Carpel EF. Congenital corneal anesthesia. Am J Ophthalmol 1978;85:357–359.

209. Myles WM, LaRoche GR. Congenital corneal anesthesia. Am J Ophthalmol 1994;118:818–820.

210. Purcell JJ Jr, Krachmer JH. Familial corneal hypesthesia. Arch Ophthalmol 1979;97:872–874.

211. Clarke MP, Sullivan TJ, Kobayashi J, et al. Familial congenital corneal anesthesia. Aust NZ J Ophthalmol 1992;20:207–210.

212. Rosenberg ML. Congenital trigeminal anesthesia: A review and classification. Brain 1984;107:1073–1082.

213. Trope GE, Jay JL, Dudgeon J, et al. Self-inflicted corneal injuries in children with congenital corneal anaesthesia. Br J Ophthalmol 1985;69:551–554.

214. Hennis HL, Saunders RA. Unilateral corneal anesthesia. Am J Ophthalmol 1989;108:331–332.

215. Keys CL, Sugar J, Mafee MF. Familial trigeminal anesthesia. Arch Ophthalmol 1990;108:1720–1723.

216. Shorey P, Lobo G. Congenital corneal anesthesia: Problems in diagnosis. J Ped Ophthalmol Strabismus 1990;27:143–147.

217. Heath JD, Long G. Neurotrophic keratitis presenting in infancy with involvement of the motor component of the trigeminal nerve. Br J Ophthalmol 1993;77:679–680.

218. Wong VA, Cline RA, Dubord PJ, et al. Congenital trigeminal anesthesia in two siblings and their long-term follow-up. Am J Ophthalmol 2000;129:96–98.

219. Hirst LW, Farmer ER, Green R, et al. Familial corneal scarring: A new dystrophy? Ophthalmology 1984;91:174–178.

220. Esakowitz L, Yates JRW. Congenital corneal anesthesia and the MURCS association: A case report. Br J Ophthalmol 1988;72:236–238.

221. Cruysberg JRM, Draaijer RW, Pinckers A, et al. Congenital corneal anesthesia in children with the VACTERL association. Am J Ophthalmol 1998;125:96–98.

222. Ramos-Arroya MA, Clark GG, Saksena SS, et al. Congenital corneal anesthesia with retinal abnormalities, deafness, unusual facies, persistent ductus arteriosus, and mental retardation: A new syndrome? Am J Med Genetics 1987;26:345–354.

223. Katz B, Melles RB, Schneider JA. Corneal sensitivity in nephropathic cystinosis. Am J Ophthalmol 1987;104:413–416.

224. Ehlers N, Hansen HJ. A-beta-lipoproteinemia: Ocular involvement in a Danish case. Acta Ophthalmol 1981;59:747–755.

225. Aracena T, Roca FP, Barragan M. Progressive hemifacial atrophy (Parry-Romberg syndrome): Report of two cases. Ann Ophthalmol 1979;11:953–958.

226. Pappagallo M, Oaklander AL, Quatrano-Piacentini AL, et al. Heterogenous patterns of sensory dysfunction in postherpetic neuralgia suggest multiple pathophysiologic mechanisms. Anesthesiology 2000;92:691–698.

227. Csaky KG, Custer P. Perineural invasion of the orbit by squamous cell carcinoma. Ophthalmic Surg 1990;21:218–220.

228. Nadkarni T, Goel A. A trigeminal neurinoma involving the lacrimal nerve: Case report. Br J Neurosurg 1999;13:75–76.

229. Rhoton AL Jr, Hardy DG, Chambers SM. Microsurgical anatomy and dissection of the sphenoid bone, cavernous sinus and sellar region. Surg Neurol 1979;12:63–104.

230. Morard M, Tcherekayev V, de Tribolet N. The superior orbital fissure: A microanatomical study. Neurosurgery 1994;35:1087–1093.

231. Natori Y, Rhoton AL Jr. Microsurgical anatomy of the superior orbital fissure. Neurosurgery 1995;36:762–775.

232. Brazis PW, Vogler JB, Shaw KE. The "numb cheek-limp lower lid" syndrome. Neurology 1991;41:327–328.

233. Liu F-C. A classification system for maxillary sinus carcinoma. Arch Otolaryngol Head Neck Surg 1987;113:409–410.

234. Campbell WW Jr. The numb cheek syndrome: A sign of infraorbital neuropathy. Neurology 1986;36:421–423.

235. Ormerod LD, Weber AL, Rauch SD, et al. Ophthalmic manifestations of maxillary sinus mucoceles. Ophthalmology 1987;94:1013–1019.

236. Eng CT, Vasconez LO. Facial pain due to perineural invasion by basal cell carcinoma. Ann Plastic Surg 1984;12:374–377.

237. Goepfert H, Dichtel WJ, Medina JE, et al. Perineural invasion in squamous cell skin carcinoma of the head and neck. Am J Surg 1984;148:542–547.

238. Clouston PD, Sharpe DM, Corbett AJ, et al. Perineural spread of cutaneous head and neck cancer: Its orbital and central neurologic complications. Arch Neurol 1990;47:73–77.

239. Hughes TAT, Mcqueen INF, Anstey A, et al. Neurotropic malignant melanoma presenting as a trigeminal sensory neuropathy. J Neurol Neurosurg Psychiatry 1995;58:381–382.

240. Erzurum SA, Melen O, Lissner G, et al. Orbital malignant peripheral nerve sheath tumors. Treatment with surgical resection and radiation therapy. J Clin Neuro-ophthalmol 1993;13:1–7.

241. Pollack IF, Sekhar LN, Jannetta PJ, et al. Neurilemmomas of the trigeminal nerve. J Neurosurg 1989;70:737–745.

242. Delfini R, Innocenzi G, Ciappetta P, et al. Meningiomas of Meckel's cave. Neurosurgery 1992;31:1000–1007.

243. Lena G, Dufour T, Gambarelli D, et al. Choristoma of the intracranial maxillary nerve in a child. J Neurosurg 1994;81:788–791.

244. Calverly JR, Mohnac AM. Syndrome of the numb chin. Arch Intern Med 1963;112:57–59.

245. Nobler MP. Mental nerve palsy in malignant lymphoma. Cancer 1969;24:122–127.

246. Rubinstein M. Cranial mononeuropathy as the first sign of intracranial metastases. Ann Intern Med 1969;70:49–54.

247. Horton J, Means ED, Cunningham TJ, et al. The numb chin in breast cancer. J Neurol Neurosurg Psychiatry 1973;36:211–216.

248. Dugan TM, Bernat JL, O'Donnell JF. Lymphoma initially appearing with chin numbness. Arch Neurol 1980;37:327.

249. Massey EW, Moore J, Schold SC Jr. Mental neuropathy from systemic cancer. Neurology 1981;31:1277–1281.

250. Bruyn RPM, Boogerd W. The numb chin. Clin Neurol Neurosurg 1991;93:187–193.

251. Harris CP, Barringer JR. The numb chin in metastatic cancer. West J Med 1991;155:528–531.

252. Kakigi R. Numb chin secondary to Burkitt's cell acute leukemia. Neurology 1991;41:453–454.

253. Burt RK, Sharfman WH, Karp BI, et al. Mental neuropathy (numb chin syndrome). A harbinger of tumor progression or relapse. Cancer 1992;70:877–881.

254. Lossos A, Siegal T. Numb chin syndrome in cancer patients: Etiology, response to treatment and prognostic significance. Neurology 1992;42:1181–1184.

255. Hiraki A, Nakamura S, Abe K, et al. Numb chin syndrome as an initial symptom of acute lymphocytic leukemia: Report of three cases. Oral Surg Oral Med Oral Pathol Oral Radiol Endod 1997;83:555–561.

256. Hogan MC, Lee A, Solberg LA, et al. Unusual presentation of multiple myeloma with unilateral visual loss and numb chin syndrome in young adult. Am J Hematol 2002;70:55–59.

257. Laurencet FM, Anchisi S, Tullen E, et al. Mental neuropathy: Report of five cases and review of the literature. Crit Rev Oncol/Hematol 2000;34:71–79.

258. Halachmi S, Madeb R, Madjar S, et al. Numb chin syndrome as the presenting symptom of metastatic prostate carcinoma. Urology 2000;55:286i–286ii.

259. Fenaux P, Lai JL, Miaux O, et al. Burkitt cell acute leukemia (L3 ALL) in adults: A report of 18 cases. Br J Haematol 1989;71:371–376.

260. Kuroda Y, Fujiyama F, Ohyama T, et al. Numb chin syndrome secondary to Burkitt's cell acute leukemia. Neurology 1991;41:453–454.

261. Sariban E, Donahue A, Magrath IT. Jaw involvement in American Burkitt's lymphoma. Cancer 1984;53:1777–1782.

262. Matzko J, Becker DG, Phillips CD. Obliteration of fat planes by perineural spread of squamous cell carcinoma along the inferior alveolar nerve. Am J Neuroradiol 1994;15:1843–1845.

263. Konotey-Ahulu FID. Mental nerve neuropathy: A complication of sickle cell crisis. Lancet 1972;2:388.

264. Gregory G, Olujohungbe A. Mandibular nerve neuropathy in sickle cell disease: Local factors. Oral Surg Oral Med Oral Pathol 1994;77:66–69.

265. Goldstein NP, Gibilisco JA, Rushton JG. Etiology of trigeminal neuropathy: A study of etiology with emphasis on dental causes. JAMA 1963;184:458–462.

266. Schwankhaus JD. Bilateral anterior lingual hypogeusia and hypesthesia. Neurology 1993;43:2146.

267. Furukawa T. Numb chin syndrome in the elderly. J Neurol Neurosurg Psychiatry 1990;53:173.

268. Krimsky Fischoff D, Sirois D. Painful trigeminal neuropathy caused by severe mandibular resorption and nerve compression in a patient with systemic sclerosis: Case report and literature review. Oral Surg Oral Med Oral Pathol Oral Radiol Endod 2000;90:456–459.

269. Cruccu G, Agostino R, Inghilleri M, et al. Mandibular nerve involvement in diabetic polyneuropathy and chronic inflammatory demyelinating polyneuropathy. Muscle Nerve 1998;21:1673–1679.

270. Chia LG. Pure trigeminal motor neuropathy. Br Med J 1988;296:609–610.

271. Ko KF, Chan KL. A case of isolated pure trigeminal motor neuropathy. Clin Neurol Neurosurg 1995;97:199–200.

272. Palacios E, Valvassori GE. Trigeminal neuropathy secondary to a meningioma. Ear Nose Throat J 2001;80:498.

273. Takamatsu K, Takizawa T, Miyamoto T. A case of pure trigeminal motor neuropathy. Rinsho-Shinkeigaku-Clinical Neurology 1993;33:541–545.

274. Kaufman MD. Masticatory spasm in facial hemiatrophy. Ann Neurol 1980;7:585–587.

275. Thompson PD, Carroll WM. Hemimasticatory spasm: A peripheral paroxysmal cranial neuropathy? J Neurol Neurosurg Psychiatry 1983;46:274–276.

276. Auger RG, Litchy WJ, Cascino TL, et al. Hemimasticatory spasm: Clinical and electrophysiological observations. Neurology 1992;42:2263–2266.

277. Cruccu G, Inghilleri M, Berardelli A, et al. Pathophysiology of hemimasticatory spasm. J Neurol Neurosurg Psychiatry 1994;57:43–50.

278. Ebersbach G, Kabus C, Schelosky L, et al. Hemimasticatory spasm in hemifacial atrophy: Diagnostic and therapeutic aspects in two patients. Mov Disord 1995;10:504–507.

279. Kim JH, Jeon BS, Lee K-W. Hemimasticatory spasm associated with localized scleroderma and facial hemiatrophy. Arch Neurol 2000;57:576–580.

280. Diaz JM, Urban ES, Schiffman JS, et al. Post-irradiation neuromyotonia affecting trigeminal nerve distribution. Neurology 1992;42:1102–1104.

281. Horowitz SH. Isolated facial numbness: Clinical significance and relation to trigeminal neuropathy. Ann Intern Med 1974;80:49–53.

282. Hutchins LG, Harnsberger HR, Hardin CW, et al. The radiologic assessment of trigeminal neuropathy. Am J Neuroradiol 1989;10:1031–1038.

283. Mathew GD, Facer GW, Suh KW, et al. Symptoms, findings, and methods of diagnosis in patients with acoustic neuroma. Larygoscope 1978;88:1893–1903.

284. Harner SG, Laws ER. Diagnosis of acoustic neuroma. Neurosurgery 1981;9:373–379.

285. Puca A, Meglio M, Vari R, et al. Evaluation of fifth nerve dysfunction in 136 patients with middle and posterior cranial fossae tumors. Eur Neurol 1995;35:33–37.

286. Matthies C, Samii M. Management of 1000 vestibular schwannomas (acoustic neuromas): Clinical presentation. Neurosurgery 1997;40:1–10.

287. Pérusse R. Acoustic neuroma presenting as orofacial anesthesia. Int J Oral Maxillofac Surg 1994;23:156–160.

288. Voss NF, Vrionis FD, Heilman CB, et al. Meningiomas of the cerebellopontine angle. Surg Neurol 2000;53:439–447.

289. Burrows HS, Harter DH. Tentorial meningiomas. J Neurol Neurosurg Psychiatry 1962;25:40–44.

290. Larson JJ, Vanloveren HR, Balko MG, et al. Evidence of meningioma infiltration into cranial nerves: Clinical implications for cavernous sinus meningiomas. J Neurosurg 1995;83:596–599.

291. Samii M, Migliori MM, Tatagiba M, et al. Surgical treatment of trigeminal schwannomas. J Neurosurg 1995;82:711–718.

292. Day JD, Fukushima T. The surgical management of trigeminal neuromas. Neurosurgery 1998;42:233–240.

293. Al-Mefty O, Ayoubi S, Gaber E. Trigeminal schwannomas: Removal of dumbbell-shaped tumors through the expanded Meckel cave and outcomes of cranial nerve function. J Neurosurg 2002;96:453–463.

294. Goel A, Muzumdar D, Raman C. Trigeminal neuroma: analysis of surgical experience with 73 cases. Neurosurgery 2003;52:783–790.

295. Asari S, Tsuchida S, Fujiwara A, et al. Trigeminal neuroma presenting with intratumoral hemorrhage: Report of two cases. Clin Neurol Neurosurg 1992;94:219–224.

296. Bhatjiwale M, Nadkarni T, Desai K, et al. Pathological laughter as a presenting symptom of massive trigeminal neuromas: Report of four cases. Neurosurgery 2000;47:469–472.

297. Trobe JD, Glaser JS, Post JD. Meningiomas and aneurysms of the cavernous sinus: Neuro-ophthalmologic features. Arch Ophthalmol 1978;96:457–467.

298. Little NS, Morgan MK, Eckstein RP. Primary ependymoma of a cranial nerve: Case report. J Neurosurg 1994;81:792–794.

299. Carvalho GA, Lindeke A, Tatagiba M, et al. Cranial granular-cell tumor of the trigeminal nerve: Case report. J Neurosurg 1994;81:795–798.

300. Zwick DL, Livingston K, Clapp L, et al. Intracranial trigeminal nerve rhabdomyoma/choristoma in a child: Case report and discussion of possible histogenesis. Hum Pathol 1989;20:390–392.

301. O'Brien TJ, McKelvie PA, Vrodos N. Bilateral trigeminal amyloidoma: An unusual case of trigeminal neuropathy with a review of the literature. J Neurosurg 1994;81:780–783.

302. Matsumoto T, Tani E, Fukami M, et al. Amyloidoma in the gasserian ganglion: Case report. Surg Neurol 1999;52:600–603.

303. Yuh WTC, Barloon TJ, Jacoby CG. Trigeminal nerve lipoma: MR findings. J Comput Assist Tomogr 1987;11:518–521.

304. Wiles CM, Kocen RS, Symon L, et al. Aspergillus granuloma of the trigeminal ganglion. J Neurol Neurosurg Psychiatry 1981;44:451–455.

305. Kuntzer T, Bogousslavsky J, Rilliet B, et al. Herald facial numbness. Eur Neurol 1992;32:297–301.

306. Brazis PW, Sharen RE, Czervionke LF, et al. Hemangioma of the mandibular branch of the trigeminal nerve in the Meckel cave presenting with facial pain and sixth nerve palsy. J Neuroophthalmol 2000;20:14–16.

307. Tobias S, Valarezo J, Meir K, et al. Giant cavernous sinus teratoma: A clinical example of a rare entity, case report. Neurosurgery 2001;48:1367–1371.

308. Zager EL. Isolated trigeminal sensory loss secondary to a distal anterior inferior cerebellar artery aneurysm: Case report. Neurosurgery 1991;28:288–291.

309. Chang Y, Horoupian DS, Jordan J, et al. Localized hypertrophic mononeuropathy of the trigeminal nerve. Arch Pathol Lab Med 1993;117:170–176.

310. Trobe JD, Hood I, Parsons JT, et al. Intracranial spread of squamous cell carcinoma along the trigeminal nerve. Arch Ophthalmol 1982;100:608–611.

311. Laine FJ, Braun IF, Jensen ME, et al. Perineural tumor extension through the foramen ovale: Evaluation with MR imaging. Radiology 1990;174:65–71.

312. Sigal R, Monnet O, De Baere T, et al. Adenoid cystic carcinoma of the head and neck: Evaluation with MR imaging and clinical-pathologic correlation in 27 patients. Radiology 1992;184:95–101.

313. Laccourreye O, Bely N, Halimi P, et al. Cavernous sinus involvement from recurrent adenoid cystic carcinoma. Ann Otol Rhinol Laryngol 1994;103:822–825.

314. Skinner DW, Vanhasselt CA, Tsao SY. Nasopharyngeal carcinoma: Modes of presentation. Ann Otol Rhinol Laryngol 1991;100:544–551.

315. Boerman RH, Maassen EM, Joosten J, et al. Trigeminal neuropathy secondary to perineural invasion of the head and neck. Neurology 1999;53:213–216.

316. Sevick RJ, Dillon WP, Engstom J, et al. Trigeminal neuropathy: Gd-DTPA enhanced MR imaging. J Comput Assist Tomogr 1991;14:605–611.

317. Delpassand ES, Kirkpatrick JB. Cavernous sinus syndrome as the presentation of malignant lymphoma: Case report and review of the literature. Neurosurgery 1988;23:501–504.

318. Abdel Aziz KM, van Loveren HR. Primary lymphoma of Meckel's cave mimicking trigeminal schwannoma: Case report. Neurosurgery 1999;44:859–862.

319. Hirota N, Fujimoto T, Takahashi M, et al. Isolated trigeminal nerve metastases from breast cancer: An unusual cause of trigeminal mononeuropathy. Surg Neurol 1998;49:558–561.

320. Morini A, Manera V, Boninsegna C, et al. Mandibular drop resulting from bilateral metastatic trigeminal neuropathy as the presenting symptom of lung cancer. J Neurol 2000;247:647–649.

321. Post MJD, Glaser JS, Trobe JD. Elusive lesions of the cavernous sinus. In Smith JL, ed. Neuro-Ophthalmology Focus 1980. New York, Masson, 1979:247–260.

322. Marianowski R, Rocton S, Ait-Amer J-L, et al. Conservative management of Gradenigo syndrome in a child. Int J Pediatr Otorhinolaryngol 2001;57:79–83.

323. Hardjasudarma M, Edwards RL, Ganley JP, et al. Magnetic resonance imaging features of Gradenigo's syndrome. Am J Otolaryngol 1995;16:247–250.

324. Quinones-Hinojosa A, Chang EF, Khan SA, et al. Isolated trigeminal nerve sarcoid granuloma mimicking trigeminal schwannoma: Case report. Neurosurgery 2003;52:700–705.

325. Arias M, Iglesisas A, Vila O, et al. MR imaging findings of neurosarcoidosis of the gasserian ganglion: An unusual presentation. Eur Radiol 2002;12:2723–2725.

326. Marsot-Dupuch K, De Givry SC, Ouayoun M. Wegener granulomatosis involving the pterygopalatine fossa: An unusual case of trigeminal neuropathy. Am J Neuroradiol 2002;23:312–315.

327. Summers CG, Wirtschafter JD. Bilateral trigeminal and abducens neuropathies following low-velocity, crushing head injury: Case report. J Neurosurg 1979;50:508–511.

328. McGovern ST, Crompton JL, Ingham P. Trigemino-abducens synkinesis: An unusual case of aberrant regeneration. Aust NZ J Ophthalmol 1986;14:275–279.

329. Nelson SK, Kline L. Acquired trigemino-abducens synkinesis. J Clin Neuro-ophthalmol 1990;10:111–114.

330. Stranjalis G, Sakas DE. Post-traumatic transient bilateral trigeminal neuropathy. Acta Neurochirurg 2002;144:307–308.

331. Hajioff D, Doward N, Wadley J, et al. Precise cannulation of the foramen ovale in trigeminal neuralgia complicating osteogenesis imperfecta with basilar invagination: Technical case report. Neurosurgery 2000;46:1005–1008.

332. O'Connell JEA. Trigeminal false localizing signs and their causation. Brain 1978;101:119–142.

333. Koenig M, Kalyan-Raman K, Sureka ON. Contralateral trigeminal nerve dysfunction as a false localizing sign in acoustic neuroma: A clinical and electrophysiological study. Neurosurgery 1984;14:335–337.

334. Revuelta R, Juambelz P, Balderrama J, et al. Contralateral trigeminal neuralgia. A new clinical manifestation of neurocysticercosis: Case report. Neurosurgery 1995;37:138–139.

335. Ro LS, Chen ST, Tang LM, et al. Concurrent trigeminal, abducens, and facial nerve palsies presenting as false localizing signs: Case report. Neurosurgery 1995;37:322–324.

336. Maurice-Williams RS, Pilling J. Trigeminal sensory symptoms associated with hydrocephalus. J Neurol Neurosurg Psychiatry 1977;40:641–644.

337. Hart RG, Carter JE. Pseudotumor cerebri and facial pain. Arch Neurol 1982; 39:440–442.

338. Davenport RJ, Will RG, Galloway PJ. Isolated intracranial hypertension presenting with trigeminal neuropathy [letter]. J Neurol Neurosurg Psychiatry 1994; 57:381.

339. Arsava EM, Uluc K, Nurlu G, et al. Electrophysiological evidence of trigeminal neuropathy in pseudotumor cerebri. J Neurol 2002;249:1601–1602.

340. Lundberg PO, Werner I. Trigeminal sensory neuropathy in systemic lupus erythematosus. Acta Neurol Scand 1972;48:330–340.

341. Beighton P, Gumpel JM, Cornes NGM. Prodromal trigeminal sensory neuropathy in progressive systemic sclerosis. Ann Rheum Dis 1968;27:367–369.

342. Gumpel JM. Isolated trigeminal neuropathy. Lancet 1970;1:310.

343. Gumpel JM. Trigeminal sensory neuropathy in connective-tissue disease. N Engl J Med 1970;282:514.

344. Ashworth B, Tait GBW. Trigeminal neuropathy in connective tissue disease. Neurology 1971;21:609–614.

345. Teasdall RD, Frayha RA, Shulman LE. Cranial nerve involvement in systemic sclerosis (scleroderma): A report of 10 cases. Medicine 1980;59:149–159.

346. Lecky BRF, Hughes RAC, Murray NMF. Trigeminal sensory neuropathy. Brain 1987;110:1463–1485.

347. Kaltreider HB. The neuropathy of Sjögren's syndrome: Trigeminal nerve involvement. Ann Intern Med 1969;70:751–762.

348. Sokoloff L, Bunim JJ. Vascular lesions in rheumatoid arthritis. J Chronic Dis 1975;5:668–687.

349. Searles RP, Mladinich EK, Messner RP. Isolated trigeminal sensory neuropathy: Early manifestation of mixed connective tissue disease. Neurology 1978;28: 1286–1289.

350. Edmonstone WM, Shepherd TH, Price DK, et al. Mixed connective tissue disease presenting as trigeminal neuropathy. Postgrad Med J 1982;58:237–238.

351. Hagen NA, Stevens JC, Michet CJ. Trigeminal sensory neuropathy associated with connective tissue diseases. Neurology 1990;40:891–896.

352. Mandal BK, Allbeson M. Trigeminal sensory neuropathy and virus hepatitis. Lancet 1972;2:1322.

353. Fisher CM. Trigeminal sensory neuropathy. Arch Neurol 1983;40:591–592.

354. Blau JN, Harris M, Kennett S. Trigeminal sensory neuropathy. N Engl J Med 1969;281:873–876.

355. Eggleston DS, Haskell R. Idiopathic trigeminal sensory neuropathy. Practitioner 1972;208:649–655.

356. Penarrocha M, Alfaro A, Bagan JV, et al. Idiopathic trigeminal sensory neuropathy. J Oral Maxillofac Surg 1992;50:472–476.

357. Shotts RH, Porter SR, Kumar N, et al. Longstanding trigeminal sensory neuropathy of nontraumatic cause. Oral Surg Oral Med Oral Pathol Oral Radiol Endod 1999;87:572–576.

358. Dumas M, Perusse R. Trigeminal sensory neuropathy: A study of 35 cases. Oral Surg Oral Med Oral Pathol Oral Radiol Endod 1999;87:577–582.

359. Rorick MB, Chandar K, Colombi BJ. Inflammatory trigeminal sensory neuropathy mimicking trigeminal neurinoma. Neurology 1996;46:1455–1457.

360. Domínguez J, Lobato RD, Madero S, et al. Surgical findings in idiopathic trigeminal neuropathy mimicking a trigeminal neurinoma. Acta Neurochir (Wien) 1999;141:269–272.

361. Savas A, Deda H, Erden E, et al. Differential diagnosis of idiopathic inflammatory trigeminal snsory neuropathy from neuroma with biopsy: Case report. Neurosurgery 1999;45:1246–1249.

362. Ahn JY, Kwon SO, Shin MS, et al. Chronic granulomatous neuritis in idiopathic trigeminal sensory neuropathy: Report of two cases. J Neurosurg 2002;96: 585–588.

363. Jannetta PJ, Robbins LJ. Trigeminal neuropathy: New observations. Neurosurgery 1980;7:347–351.

364. Miller NR. Walsh and Hoyt's Clinical Neuro-Ophthalmology. Ed 4. Baltimore, William & Wilkins, 1985:1054–1070.

365. Mokri B, Silbert PL, Schievink WI, et al. Cranial nerve palsy in spontaneous dissection of the extracranial internal carotid artery. Neurology 1996;46: 356–359.

366. Rizzo M, Bosch EP, Gross CE. Trigeminal sensory neuropathy due to dural external carotid cavernous sinus fistula. Neurology 1982;32:89–91.

367. Michelucci R, Forti A, de Maria R, et al. Trigeminal and facial nerve involvement from ischemia of the petrosal branch of the middle meningeal artery. J Neurol Neurosurg Psychiatry 1983;46:460–461.

368. Lapresle J, Lasjaunias P. Cranial nerve ischaemic arterial syndromes. Brain 1986;109:207–215.

369. Dicken C. Trigeminal trophic syndrome. Mayo Clin Proc 1997;72:543–545.

370. Watt-Smith S, Mehta K, Scully C. Mefloquine-induced trigeminal sensory neuropathy. Oral Surg Oral Med Oral Pathol Oral Radiol Endod 2001;92:163–165.

371. Davis WG, Drewry RD, Wood TO. Filamentary keratitis and stromal neovascularization associated with brain-stem injury. Am J Ophthalmol 1980;90: 489–491.

372. Magendie M. De l'influence de la cinquième paire de nerfs sur la nutrition et les fonctions de l'oeil. J Physiol (Lond) 1824;4:176–182.

373. Bonini S, Rama P, Olzi D, et al. Neurotrophic keratitis. Eye 2003;17:989–995.

374. Heigle TJ, Pflugfelder SC. Aqueous tear production in patients with neurotrophic keratitis. Cornea 1996;15:135–138.

375. Adams GGW, Cullen JF. Neuroparalytic keratitis and the effect of cervical sympathectomy following operative procedures for trigeminal neuralgia. Scot Med J 1987;32:86–88.

376. Cavanagh HD, Colley AM. The molecular basis of neurotrophic keratitis. Acta Ophthalmol 1989;192(Suppl):115–134.

377. Hörnsten G. Wallenberg's syndrome. Part I. General symptomatology, with special reference to visual disturbances and imbalance. Acta Neurol Scand 1974; 50:434–446.

378. Sacco RL, Freddo L, Bello JA, et al. Wallenberg's lateral medullary syndrome: Clinical-magnetic resonance imaging correlations. Arch Neurol 1993;50: 609–614.

379. Kim JS. Pure lateral medullary infarction: Clinical-radiological correlation of 130 acute, consecutive patients. Brain 2003;126:1864–1872.

380. Currier RD, Giles CL, DeJong RN. Some comments on Wallenberg's lateral medullary syndrome. Neurology 1961;11:778–791.

381. Fitzek S, Baumgärtner U, Fitzek C, et al. Mechanisms and predictors of chronic facial pain in lateral medullary infarction. Ann Neurol 2001;49:493–500.

382. Young RF. Effect of trigeminal tractotomy on dental sensation in humans. J Neurosurg 1982;56:812–818.

383. Klekamp J, Iaconetta G, Samii M. Spontaneous resolution of Chiari I malformation and syringomyelia: Case report and review of the literature. Neurosurgery 2001;48:664–667.

384. Holtzman RNN, Zablonski V, Yang WC, et al. Lateral pontine tegmental hemorrhage presenting as an isolated trigeminal sensory neuropathy. Neurology 1987; 37:704–706.

385. Berlit P. Trigeminal neuropathy in pontine hemorrhage. Eur Neurol 1989;29: 169–170.

386. Veerapen R. Spontaneous lateral pontine hemorrhage with associated trigeminal nerve root hematoma. Neurosurgery 1989;25:451–452.

387. Kiers L, Carroll WM. Blink reflexes and magnetic resonance imaging in focal unilateral central tegmental pathway demyelination. J Neurol Neurosurg Psychiatry 1990;53:526–529.

388. Kim JS, Lee MC, Kim HG, et al. Isolated trigeminal sensory change due to pontine hemorrhage. Clin Neurol Neurosurg 1994;96:168–169.

389. Ishii K, Tamaoka A, Shoji S. Dorsolateral pontine segmental infarction presenting as isolated trigeminal sensory neuropathy. J Neurol Neurosurg Psychiatr 1998;65:702.

390. Fukutake T, Hattori T. Trigeminal root entry zone infarct presenting as isolated trigeminal sensory neuropathy. J Neurol 1999;246:978–979.

391. Nakashima I, Fujihara K, Kimpara T, et al. Linear pontine trigeminal root lesions in multiple sclerosis: Clinical and magnetic resonance imaging studies in 5 cases. Arch Neurol 2001;58:101–104.

392. Sakai T, Murakami S, Ito K. Ataxic hemiparesis with trigeminal weakness. Neurology 1981;31:635–636.

393. Ambrosetto P. Ataxic hemiparesis with contralateral trigeminal nerve impairment due to pontine hemorrhage. Stroke 1987;18:244–245.

394. Oterino A, Berciano J, Calleja J, et al. Tegmental pontine hemorrhage with pure trigeminal motor impairment. Electromyogr Clin Neurophysiol 1994;34: 225–227.

395. Matsumoto S, Kaku S, Yamasaki M, et al. Cheiro-oral syndrome with bilateral oral involvement: A study of pontine lesions by high-resolution magnetic resonance imaging. J Neurol Neurosurg Psychiatry 1989;52:792–794.

396. Chen WH, Lan MY, Chang YY, et al. Bilateral cheiro-oral syndrome. Clin Neurol Neurosurg 1997;99:239–243.

397. Yasuda Y, Morita T, Okada T, et al. Cheiro-oral-pedal syndrome. Eur Neurol 1992;32:106–108.

398. Rasdolsky I. Dorsal-pontines tumor syndrome. Z Gesamte Neurol Psychiatr 1935;152:530–537.

399. Kosary IZ, Shacked IJ, Duaknine G, et al. Continuous facial spasm with tumor of the pons. J Neurosurg 1970;33:212–215.

400. Tenser RB, Corbett JJ. Myokymia and facial contraction in brain stem glioma. Arch Neurol 1974;30:425–427.

401. Krauss JK, Wakhloo AK, Scheremet R, et al. Facial myokymia and spastic paretic facial contracture as the result of anaplastic pontocerebellar glioma. Neurosurgery 1993;32:1031–1034.

402. Jacobs L, Kaba S, Pullicino P. The lesion causing continuous facial myokymia in multiple sclerosis. Arch Neurol 1994;51:1115–1119.

403. Boghen D, Filiatrault R, Descarries L. Myokymia and facial contracture in brain stem tuberculoma. Neurology 1977;27:270–272.

404. Amarenco P, Hauw J-J. Cerebellar infarction in the territory of the superior cerebellar artery: A clinicopathologic study of 33 cases. Neurology 1990;40: 1383–1390.

405. Kim JS. Trigeminal sensory symptoms due to midbrain lesions. Eur Neurol 1993;33:218–220.

406. Ono S, Inoue K. Cheiro-oral syndrome following midbrain hemorrhage. J Neurol 1985;232:304–306.

407. Aizawa H, Makiguchi N, Katayama T, et al. Cheiro-oral syndrome due to a midbrain lesion. Neurology 2002;58:1414.

408. Bogousslavsky J, Maeder P, Regli F, et al. Pure midbrain infarction: Clinical syndromes, MRI, and etiologic patterns. Neurology 1994;44:2032–2040.

409. Déjerine J, Roussy G. Le syndrome thalamique. Rev Neurol (Paris) 1906;14: 521–532.

410. Teasell RW. Thalamic or central pain states poststroke. Pain Res Manage 1996; 1:219–222.

411. Tovi D, Schisano G, Liljeqvist B. Primary tumors of the region of the thalamus. J Neurosurg 1961;18:730–740.

412. Iwasaki Y, Kinoshita M, Ikeda K, et al. Oral Syndrome: An incomplete form of cheiro-oral syndrome? Int J Neurosci 1991;58:271–273.

413. Shintani S, Tsuruoka S, Shiigai T. Pure sensory stroke caused by a cerebral hemorrhage: clinical-radiologic correlations in seven patients. Am J Neuroradiol 2000;21:515–520.

414. Valzelli L. About the cheiro-oral syndrome. Neurology 1987;37:1564–1565.

415. Ten Holter J, Tijssen C. Cheiro-oral syndrome: Does it have a specific localizing value? Eur Neurol 1988;28:326–330.

416. Combarros O, Polo JM, Pascual J, et al. Evidence of somatotopic organization of the sensory thalamus based on infarction in the nucleus ventralis posterior. Stroke 1991;22:1445–1447.

417. Yasuda Y, Matsuda I, Akiguchi I, et al. Cheiro-oral-pedal syndrome in thalamic infarction. Clin Neurol Neurosurg 1993;95:311–314.

418. Kim JS. Restricted acral sensory syndrome following minor stroke. Further observation with special reference to differential severity of symptoms among individual digits. Stroke 1994;25:2497–2502.

419. Kim JS, Lee MC. Stroke and restricted sensory syndromes. Neuroradiology 1994;36:258–263.

420. Garcin R, Lapresle J. Syndrome sensitif de type thalamique et à topographie cheíro-orale par lésion localisée du thalamus. Rev Neurol 1954;90:124–129.

421. Garcin R, Lapresle J. Deuxième observation personelle de syndrome sensitif de type thalamique et à topographie cheíro-orale par lésion localisée du thalamus. Rev Neurol 1960;103:474–481.

422. Omae T, Tsuchiya T, Yamaguchi T. Cheiro-oral syndrome due to lesions of the corona radiata. Stroke 1992;23:599–601.

423. Isono O, Kawamura M, Shiota J, et al. Cheiro-oral topography of sensory disturbances due to lesions of thalamocortical projections. Neurology 1993;43:51–55.

424. Yasuda Y, Watanabe T, Akiguchi I, et al. Cheiro-oral-pedal syndrome in the lesion of thalamocortical projections. Clin Neurol Neurosurg 1994;96:185–187.

425. Bogousslavsky J, Dizerens K, Regli F, et al. Opercular cheiro-oral syndrome. Arch Neurol 1991;48:658–661.

426. Bassetti C, Bogousslavsky J, Regli F. Sensory syndromes in parietal stroke. Neurology 1993;43:1942–1949.

427. Nagasako EM, Oaklander AL, Dworkin RH. Congenital insensitivity to pain: An update. Pain 2003;101:213–219.

428. Shorer Z, Moses SW, Hershkovitz E, et al. Neurophysiologic studies in congenital insensitivity to pain with anhidrosis. Pediatr Neurol 2001;25:397–400.

429. Donaghy M, Hakin RN, Bamford JM, et al. Hereditary sensory neuropathy with neurotrophic keratitis: Description of an autosomal recessive disorder with a selective reduction of small myelinated nerve fibres and a discussion of the classification of the hereditary sensory neuropathies. Brain 1987;110:563–583.

430. Bowe BE, Levartovsky S, Eiferman RA. Neurotrophic corneal ulcers in congenital sensory neuropathy. Am J Ophthalmol 1989;107:303–304.

431. Biedner B, Dagan M, Gedalia A, et al. Congenital insensitivity to pain with neuroparalytic keratitis. Ann Ophthalmol 1990;22:312–313.

432. Magee KR. Hysterical hemiplegia and hemianesthesia. Postgrad Med 1962;31: 339–345.

433. Pascuzzi RM. Nonphysiological (functional) unilateral motor and sensory syndromes involve the left more often than the right body. J Nerv Ment Dis 1994; 182:118–120.

434. Rolak L. Psychogenic sensory loss. J Nerv Ment Dis 1988;176:686–687.

435. Gould R, Miller BL, Goldberg MA, et al. The validity of hysterical signs and symptoms. J Nerv Ment Dis 1986;174:593–597.

436. Keane JR. Hysterical hemianopia: The "missing half" field defect. Arch Ophthalmol 1979;97:865–866.

Headache and Facial Pain

Gregory P. Van Stavern

Headache and facial pain are common complaints and represent a diverse range of etiologies, from benign to life- and vision-threatening. Headache, migraine in particular, has been described in the popular and medical literature for over 3000 years (1). Trepanation, a sign of neurosurgery, has been seen on Neolithic skulls dating from 7000 B.C. (Fig. 26.1). The Ebers papyrus, an ancient Egyptian prescription dating back to 1200 B.C., mentions migraine, neuralgia, and shooting head pains, and is thought to be based on earlier medical documents from 1550 B.C. (2). Indeed, it is estimated that over 90% of individuals have noted at least one headache over their entire life (3). Patients with headache may present initially to a neurologist or ophthalmologist, and are often misdiagnosed initially. Since correct diagnosis facilitates appropriate treatment, it is important for the clinician to be familiar with common causes of head and facial pain. This chapter will focus primarily on those causes of headache and facial pain most relevant to neuro-ophthalmologists.

APPROACH TO HEADACHE AND FACIAL PAIN

Headache and facial pain result from disorders that affect the pain-sensitive structures in the head and neck, such as meninges, blood vessels, and muscles. Pain-sensitive structures responsible for head and facial pain are listed in Table 26.1.

A **history** is the first and most important step in the evaluation of head and facial pain; the examination and any ancillary tests serve to confirm or exclude what is already suspected. In many patients with headache and facial pain, the general neurologic and ophthalmologic examination is normal, and the correct diagnosis rests upon a thorough and accurate history. Most, but by no means all, of the more serious and life-threatening causes of headache present with acute onset of pain: a patient with his or her "first or worst" headache has a greater likelihood of harboring an ominous cause for the head pain than someone with a 10-year history of recurrent, low-grade headache that has not changed in character. Although a chronic and recurrent headache is more likely to represent a benign condition, patients with a headache distinct from previous headaches (in terms of location or quality of pain) are also more likely to harbor a serious underlying illness.

The **location** of the pain may prove helpful. Unilateral headache is an invariable feature of cluster headache and occurs with most migraine attacks. Patients with tension-type headaches generally describe bilateral pain. In patients with ocular pain, a primary ophthalmic etiology should be excluded, while paranasal pain localized to the sinuses might suggest sinus obstruction. A new temporal headache in an elderly patient might raise suspicion of giant cell arteritis (GCA). Figure 26.2 depicts regional pain in common primary headache syndromes. However, since most head and

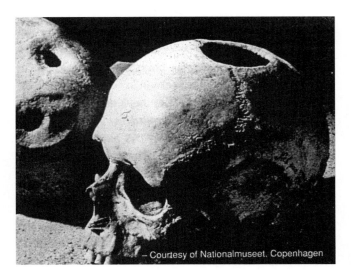

Figure 26.1. Neolithic skull showing trepanation hole (ca. 7000 B.C.) (Courtesy of Nationalmuseet, Copenhagen. From Headache in Clinical Practice. Oxford, UK: Isis Medical Media, 1998.)

Table 26.1
Pain-Sensitive Structures of the Head and Neck

Extracranial

Skin and blood vessels of the scalp
Head and neck muscles
Second and third cervical nerves
Periosteum of the skull
Eyes, ears, teeth, sinuses, oropharynx
Mucous membranes of nasal cavity

Intracranial

Dura mater
Anterior and middle meningeal arteries
Trigeminal (V), glossopharyngeal (IX), and vagus (X) nerves
Proximal portions of internal carotid artery and branches near the circle of
    Willis
Periaqueductal gray matter
Sensory nuclei of the thalamus

facial pain is ultimately mediated by the trigeminal nerve, referred pain may result in false localization.

A complete headache history should include a description of the **quality** of the pain. Migraine headache is typically reported as throbbing; tension-type headache is often de-

scribed as dull and aching, with a band-like sensation around the head. The pain produced by intracranial mass lesions is often dull and steady. A sharp, lancinating quality suggests neuralgic pain. The **tempo** and **evolution** of the pain may suggest a specific diagnosis, since some headache syndromes have fairly characteristic temporal patterns (Fig. 26.3).The onset and duration of the attacks, including time

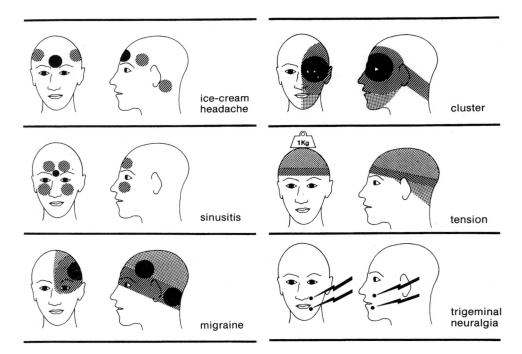

Figure 26.2. Sites of common head and facial pain syndromes. (From Lance JW. Migraine and Other Headaches. New York: Charles Scribner's Sons.)

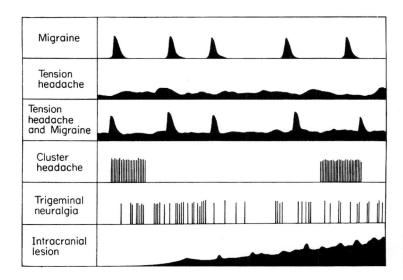

Figure 26.3. Temporal patterns of headache. (From Lance JW. Mechanism and Management of Headache. Ed 5. Oxford, UK: Butterworth-Heinemann, 1993.)

to peak intensity, should be determined. The frequency of attacks should be ascertained; a change in frequency of a preexisting headache raises concern about a secondary headache syndrome superimposed upon previous primary headaches.

Exacerbating and **relieving** factors may provide clues about etiology. Migraine is often provoked by certain foods, worsened by routine physical activity, and may be worse during menses. A positional headache might suggest either increased or decreased intracranial pressure. Pain provoked by chewing or eating might raise suspicion of giant cell arteritis or temporomandibular joint dysfunction. Precipitation of headache with alcohol is common with cluster headache. Migraine headaches are frequently relieved by darkness and sleep.

Associated focal neurologic symptoms which do not meet criteria for migraine with aura might merit further investigation. The general medical history is valuable, as well. Previous head injury might suggest post-traumatic headache. Medical co-morbidities such as hypertension may be relevant when choosing pharmacologic treatments. Family history should be reviewed, as some headache syndromes have a genetic component. A detailed medication history is important, since analgesic overuse may complicate many chronic headaches. Medication history also may help guide future medical treatment.

The **general examination** may help identify an underlying systemic illness. Fever might suggest an intracranial or meningeal infection, but headache can accompany nearly any systemic infectious illness. Inspection of the skin may reveal cutaneous lesions associated with a particular diagnosis (e.g., vesicular lesions in patients with herpes zoster). Blood pressure measurement is important. Although chronic hypertension does not cause headache, an acute rise in arterial pressure might cause sudden head pain. Stroke and subarachnoid hemorrhage (both of which cause headaches) are both associated with an acute rise in blood pressure. Palpa-

tion of the temporal arteries should be performed in all cases where giant cell arteritis is suspected: focal tenderness over the artery, a palpable cord, or obliteration of the pulse increase the likelihood of the disease. Meningeal signs should be sought in patients with an acute onset of headache. Recall that meningeal irritation causes nuchal rigidity in the anterior-posterior rotation, while cervical spine disorders restrict movement in all directions.

The neurologic and neuro-ophthalmic examination is aimed primarily at confirming or excluding a focal deficit, or findings localizable to a specific cranial structure. Such finding would then prompt appropriate further evaluation. The **neuro-ophthalmologic examination** is essential in the evaluation of a patient with headache or facial pain. Funduscopic examination should be performed systematically looking for papilledema; the finding of a Horner syndrome in a patient with unilateral facial or head pain may suggest cluster headache or internal carotid dissection; a 6th nerve palsy or comitant esotropia may raise the possibility of raised intracranial pressure. Finally, ocular causes of facial pain should not be overlooked and a red eye or orbital symptoms should prompt a detailed ophthalmologic examination.

In many patients, the examination is entirely normal, and the physician must decide whether or not to obtain neuroimaging. Since computerized tomography (CT) and magnetic resonance imaging (MRI) are noninvasive and have become widely accessible, many patients with headache will be imaged, whether or not there are clear indications. This is, in part, fostered by the medicolegal climate in the United States. However, neuroimaging is expensive and inconvenient for many patients. In addition, if neuroimaging is required, it is preferable to order the correct study the first time (e.g., MRI or MRA rather than CT). The American Academy of Neurology position paper, based on an analysis of 16 CT and MRI studies, concluded that the routine use of CT or MRI was not warranted in patients whose headaches fit a broad definition of recurrent migraine and who have had no recent change in headache pattern and have no focal neurologic deficits on examination (4). The U.S. Headache Consortium guidelines evaluated the utility of neuroimaging studies in patients with headache. Significant intracranial lesions were found at a rate of only 0.18% in patients with migraine and normal neurologic examinations (5). Some patients with migraine may have non-specific abnormalities on MRI (6,7). Igarashi and colleagues (6) found that 31% of migraineurs had small foci of T2 hyperintensity on MRI; the signal changes were most commonly seen in the centrum semiovale and frontal white matter (Fig. 26.4). A significantly lower number of matched controls without migraine had similar signal changes on brain MRI. There was no correlation between MRI changes and migraine type; ergotamine use; or frequency, duration, or intensity of migraine. These MRI findings are of uncertain clinical significance.

Forsyth and Posner (8) evaluated 111 patients with primary and metastatic brain tumors, and identified headache in 48%. Many of these patients had headaches that were similar to previous headaches, but now were associated with seizures, prolonged nausea, confusion, or other neurologic findings. The authors concluded that a change in headache symptoms is an indication for neuroimaging. In most cases, MRI is superior to CT scan for evaluation. There are a number of disorders causing headache that may be missed by CT scanning, particularly if contrast is not administered (Table 26.2).

There are few published studies evaluating the value of neuroimaging in some of the less common headache disorders. The decision to image in those circumstances should

Table 26.2
Lesions that May Be Missed by CT Scan

Low-grade glial tumors
Vascular malformations (particularly in noncontrast CT)
Venous sinus thrombosis
Cavernous sinus and sellar lesions
Meningeal disease

be made on a case by case basis. Patients with chronic eye pain and a normal neuro-ophthalmic examination are a too-common source of referral to ophthalmologists and neuro-ophthalmologists. These patients are often classified as having "atypical facial pain" and in many cases have a substantial component of analgesic overuse and rebound. The value of imaging in these patients is uncertain. Golnik et al. (9) reviewed 101 patients with unilateral eye and facial pain and noted no findings on examination that would account for the pain. Neuroimaging was normal in 93% of patients; in those with abnormal imaging it was unclear whether the pain was attributable to the lesions found. They concluded that the yield of neuroimaging in a patient with unilateral eye pain and a normal examination is low. The decision to image should be made on a case by case basis. Table 26.3 lists reasonable indications for neuroimaging.

For many patients the etiology of headache and facial pain can usually be ascertained after a careful history and examination. An awareness of relevant neuroanatomy as well as typical presentation for common headache syndromes is essential. If neuroimaging is indicated, the type if image ordered should be the one most likely to confirm or exclude certain diagnoses. For example, CT scanning has high sensitivity for bony lesions and acute hemorrhage and is the test of choice for acute head trauma and neurologic deficits with abrupt onset. MRI has much higher sensitivity

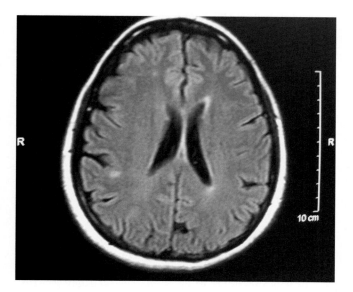

Figure 26.4. MRI of a 53-year-old woman with a long history of migraine. FLAIR sequences. The size and location of the white matter lesions are relatively nonspecific and are atypical for demyelinating disease.

Table 26.3
Indications for Neuroimaging in Patients with Head and Facial Pain

History

The first or worst headache of the patient's life, particularly if abrupt onset
Change in frequency, severity, or clinical features of headache attack
Neurological symptoms that **do not** meet criteria for migraine with aura
Hemicrania that is **always** on the same side and is associated with
    contralateral neurologic symptoms
Positional headache
Lack of improvement with conventional therapy

Examination

Localizable deficits on neurologic or neuro-ophthalmologic exam
Persistent neurologic or neuro-ophthalmologic deficits

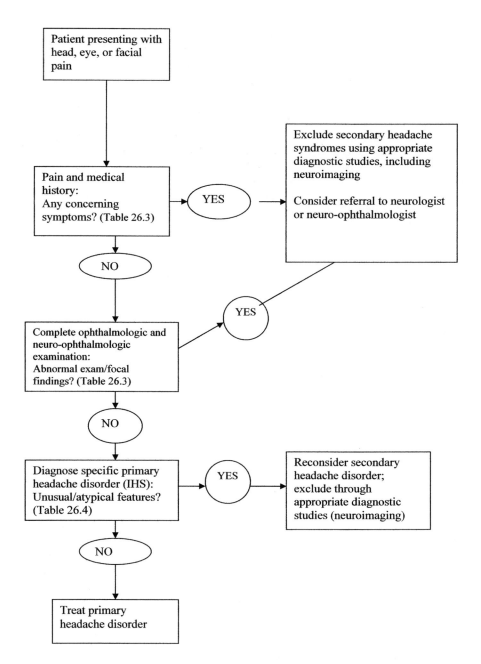

Figure 26.5. Algorithm for management of patients with headache.

for posterior fossa, cavernous sinus, and sella turcica lesions. The MRI may miss orbital pathology unless fat-suppressed orbital sequences (in which the bright T1 signal from orbital fat is eliminated) are specifically ordered. Magnetic resonance angiography and venography are specialized MRI sequences that may be ordered when arterial (e.g., dissection, aneurysm) or venous (e.g., cerebral venous thrombosis) disease is suspected. Figure 26.5 presents a reasonable algorithm for evaluating patients presenting with head and facial pain. It is not intended to be all-inclusive, but rather provide a framework for managing patients with headache.

CLASSIFICATION OF HEADACHE: INTERNATIONAL HEADACHE SOCIETY CRITERIA

Headache may occur in isolation or as part of a symptom complex—the primary headache syndromes, or may be part of an underlying condition, such as brain tumor or stroke —the secondary headache syndromes. Management of secondary headache syndromes is largely determined by the underlying structural or metabolic disorder responsible for the generation of pain. Management of primary headache syndromes, however, is dependent upon accurate diagnosis and classification, which then serves to guide therapy. Prior to 1988, there were no standardized headache classification systems with operational rules and uniform nomenclature. In 1988, the International Headache Society (IHS) instituted a classification system that has become the standard for headache diagnosis (10). The IHS criteria have received broad international support, and the principles of the system have been included in the International Classification of Diseases (ICD). The IHS criteria have established uniform terminology and consistent diagnostic criteria for a range of headache disorders; in turn, this has facilitated epidemiological studies and clinical trials that provide the basis for current research and treatment guidelines. The second edition of the IHS classification was recently completed and follows the same principles as the first edition (11). Several headache syndromes that did not have sufficient valid evidence (e.g., carotidynia) have been eliminated, and new headache syndromes (e.g., hemicrania continua) have been added. As in the first edition, the classification draws upon all forms of available evidence, including clinical description, longitudinal and epidemiological studies, treatment results, genetics, neuroimaging, and pathophysiology. That the classifications remain largely descriptive, in part reflects the subjective nature of pain symptoms. As research identifies more specific, objective markers for pain disorders, the IHS criteria will likely incorporate these findings in future editions. At this point, however, the IHS classification system remains an invaluable source of information and the primary reference for any physician evaluating and managing patients with head and facial pain. Table 26.4 lists the headaches that will be covered in this chapter; they are categorized according to the IHS classification system. The headaches most relevant to neuro-ophthalmologists are highlighted and will be covered in greater detail than the other headaches listed.

IMPACT OF HEADACHE

Headache is a public health problem of tremendous scope and impact. A U.S. survey of 40,000 households (112,000 persons) found that 5.5 days of restricted activity per 100 person-years were due to headache (12). In another study, 8% of males and 14% of females missed all or part of a day at work in the 4-week period prior to the interview (13). Headache also results in frequent utilization of emergency rooms and urgent care centers. Despite this, many headache syndromes (including migraine) remain underdiagnosed.

Data from the American Migraine Study II show that fewer than half (48%) of patients meeting IHS criteria for migraine reported a physician diagnosis of migraine (14). It is therefore important for all physicians encountering patients with headache to be familiar with diagnostic criteria, exclude secondary headache syndromes (through history, exam, diagnostic studies), and either begin management or refer the patient to a physician who can begin appropriate treatment.

NEUROANATOMY AND NEUROPHYSIOLOGY OF PAIN

The International Society for the Study of Pain defines pain as "an unpleasant sensory and emotional experience associated with actual or potential tissue damage" (15). Pain is therefore multidimensional, and may be good or bad, necessary or unnecessary, and is dependent upon self-report of the experience. The relationship between disease (inflammation, tissue damage, nerve damage) and central processing determines a wide range of pain symptoms. Peripheral and central pain pathways have plasticity, and can be modified both functionally and structurally (16). These concepts provide insight both into the underlying mechanisms of pain syndromes, as well as the rationale for therapeutic interventions.

PAIN TERMINOLOGY

Before discussing the pathways involved in processing pain, and the variety of pain syndromes, it is helpful to review some of the terminology used in pain literature. **Referred pain** is pain in an area far removed from the site of tissue injury. **Phantom pain** refers to pain in a part of the body that has been surgically removed or is congenitally absent. **Allodynia** is a nonnoxious stimulus that is perceived as painful (e.g., light touch producing pain). **Sensitization** occurs when a receptor responds to a stimulus in a more intense fashion than expected, or to a stimulus to which it would not normally respond. **Hyperalgesia** is exacerbated pain produced by a noxious stimulus (e.g., mild pinprick causing severe pain out of proportion to the stimulus). **Hyperpathia** refers to intense pain with repetitive stimuli. **Anesthesia** refers to complete loss of sensation. **Paresthesias** are abnormal sensations, such as burning, tingling, or formication, that are not typically painful. A **nociceptor** is a nervous system receptor capable of distinguishing between a noxious and innocuous stimulus.

Head and facial pain may be broadly classified as primary or secondary. **Primary headaches** may be severe and incapacitating but do not cause death or permanent neurologic deficit, and no identifiable etiology is identified. **Secondary headaches** may be caused by a wide range of extracranial and intracranial pathology, and correction of the underlying

Table 26.4
Causes of Head and Facial Pain

PRIMARY HEADACHES
1. Migraine
  a. Migraine without aura
  b. Migraine with aura
    i. **Typical aura with migraine headache**
    ii. **Typical aura without headache**
    iii. Familial hemiplegic migraine
    iv. Basilar type migraine
  c. **Retinal migraine**
  d. **Persistent aura without infarction**
2. Tension-type headache
  a. Frequent episodic tension-type headache
  b. Chronic tension-type headache
3. Cluster headache and other trigeminal-autonomic cephalgias
  a. **Cluster headache**
  b. **Paroxysmal hemicrania**
    i. Episodic paroxysmal hemicrania
    ii. Chronic paroxysmal hemicrania
  c. **Short-lasting unilateral neuralgiform headache with conjunctival injection and tearing (SUNCT)**
4. **Primary stabbing headache**
5. Hemicrania continua
SECONDARY HEADACHES
1. Headaches attributed to head and/or neck trauma
  a. Acute post-traumatic headache
  b. **Chronic post-traumatic headache**
2. Headache attributed to cranial and cervical vascular disorders
  a. Ischemic stroke and transient ischemic attacks
  b. Subarachnoid hemorrhage
  c. Subdural hematoma
  d. Epidural hematoma
  e. Unruptured vascular malformation
  f. **Arterial dissection**
  g. **Pituitary apoplexy**
  h. **Giant cell arteritis**
3. Headache attributed to nonvascular intracranial disorders
  a. High cerebrospinal fluid pressure
    i. **Idiopathic intracranial hypertension**
  b. Low cerebrospinal fluid pressure
  c. Intracranial neoplasm
4. Headache attributed to infection
5. Headache attributed to disorders of homeostasis
  a. Systemic hypertension
  b. High-altitude headache
6. Headache of facial pain attributed to disorders of cranium, neck, eyes, ears, nose, sinuses, teeth, mouth, or other facial or cranial structures
  a. **Acute glaucoma**
  b. **Refractive errors**
  c. **Ocular inflammatory disorders**
7. Headache attributed to a substance or its withdrawal
  a. **Medication overuse headache**
8. Cranial neuralgias and central causes of facial pain
  a. **Trigeminal neuralgia**
  b. Occipital neuralgia
  c. **Supraorbital neuralgia**
  d. Herpes zoster
  e. **Ophthalmoplegic migraine**
  f. Idiopathic facial pain

Disorders most relevant to neuro-ophthalmologists and ophthalmologists are in boldface.

abnormality typically results in relief of pain. All forms of head and facial pain reflect activation of small-caliber nociceptive neurons projecting from the trigeminal and upper cervical dorsal root ganglia to intracranial vascular and meningeal structures. The mechanism by which these nociceptive neurons are initially depolarized is the defining difference between primary and secondary headache syndromes. Once activation has occurred, the underlying principles governing the generation and maintenance of pain is likely to be similar for primary and secondary headaches.

The brain is an insensate organ. During neurosurgical procedures, Penfield (17) demonstrated that stimulation of the brain parenchyma in awake patients caused no pain. The pia, dura, and extracranial blood vessels are innervated by an adventitial plexus comprised of the trigeminal and upper cervical dorsal root ganglia fibers. These pathways mediate all head pain. Pain-sensitive structures of the head and face include the skin and blood vessels of the scalp, the dura, the venous sinuses, the arteries, and the sensory fibers of the fifth, ninth, and tenth nerves (Table 26.1). The primary nociceptive neurons project unmyelinated C fibers which, when activated, transmit nociceptive signals from perivascular terminals through the trigeminal ganglia and synapse centrally on second-order neurons in the trigeminal nucleus caudalis (Table 26.5). The primary afferents are mainly glutamatergic, but they also store substance P, calcitonin G-related peptide (CGRP), and neurokinin A (NKA), all of which may be involved in the modulation of pain (18,19). Trigeminovascular neurons terminate within the trigeminal nucleus caudalis (TNC). Activity within this nucleus is modulated by projections from several sites. Second-order neurons carry nociceptive information from the TNC to numerous subcortical sites, including the cerebellum, the thalamus, as well as other areas of the brain responsible for the emotional response to pain (20,21).

INITIATION PHASE

The initiation of trigeminal and upper cervical nociceptive neurons in secondary headache syndromes is relatively well understood, and may occur by a variety of mechanisms:

1. Mechanical traction (e.g., tumors, vascular malformations).
2. Chemical activation (e.g., subarachnoid hemorrhage, purulent infections).
3. Inflammatory activation (e.g. autoimmune vasculitis).
4. Direct injury (e.g., head trauma, intracranial surgery).

Table 26.5
Processing of Craniovascular Pain

Order	Anatomic Structures	Substructures/Comments
1st	Trigeminal ganglion	Located in middle cranial fossa
2nd	Trigemino-cervical complex	Trigeminal nucleus caudalis and dorsal horns of C1 and C2
3rd	Thalamus	Ventrobasal complex
Final	Cortex	Processing uncertain

5. Exposure to or withdrawal from toxins (e.g., nitroglycerine, caffeine).
6. Metabolic disturbances (e.g., hypoglycemia).

Secondary headache syndromes often have focal neurologic findings that are far more compelling than the headache. Intracranial neoplasms and infectious meningitis frequently present with seizures, and the headache is a minor component of the clinical presentation. However, headache may be the inaugural manifestation of some disorders, such as cerebral venous thrombosis, and focal findings may be delayed for days or weeks (22).

The mechanism of initiation and activation of nociceptive neurons and afferent fibers in primary headache syndromes (e.g., migraine, cluster) remains poorly understood. Since the diagnoses are descriptive, these syndromes may represent final common pathways for a diverse group of processes, some acquired, some genetically determined.

MAINTENANCE OF PAIN

In secondary headache syndromes, the system remains activated by a persistent stimulus, such as traction on pain-sensitive structures by a tumor. In primary headache syndromes such as migraine, the mechanism by which the pain persists and intensifies long after activation has yet to be fully elucidated. There are data suggesting that more than one mechanism may be involved.

Peripheral Sensitization

Sustained peripheral activity can induce significant functional and structural changes in the CNS. Activation of trigeminal nociceptive neurons mediates the central transmission of pain, but also results in the release of vasoactive neuropeptides, including substance P, CGRP, and NKA. These substances induce a sterile inflammatory response, which involves leakage of plasma and plasma protein from small vessels into surrounding tissue, vasodilation, and activation of mast cells (23,24). This process has been termed **neurogenic inflammation**, which under normal conditions minimizes real or threatened tissue injury. This response is felt to be associated with a lowered threshold for subsequent reactivation and may be a method by which headache is amplified and maintained. The release of CGRP from trigeminal sensory afferents causes vasodilation and plasma extravasation from dural vessels. Whether such effects occur in humans during primary headaches (such as migraine) is

uncertain. However, intravenous infusion of CGRP into susceptible individuals elicited migraine-like headaches (25).

Central Sensitization

Recent studies suggests that chemical irritation of the meninges causes the trigeminovascular fibers innervating the dura and central trigeminal neurons to respond to low-intensity stimuli that previously induced minimal or no response (26). This may also reflect structural changes as well. For example, constant firing of A-beta nociceptive fibers may lead to reorganization of A-beta terminals in the dorsal horn of the spinal cord (16). Central sensitization may account for the severe prolonged pain of certain headaches. Burstein and colleagues (26) assessed allodynia during migraine attack and found sensitization of the trigeminal system at a second- or third-order neuron level. The phenomenon of wind-up is well described in animal research and refers to the increase in dorsal horn nociceptive neuron responsiveness (in both magnitude and duration) with each subsequent stimulus above a certain frequency (27). Wind-up is sensitive to N-methyl-D-aspartate (NMDA) receptor antagonists, and a potential mechanism in second-order neuron sensitization may be the removal of magnesium gating at NMDA receptors. This suggests that pharmacologic strategies aimed at NMDA receptors might benefit some primary headache syndromes (2).

The interplay between peripheral and central activation, amplification, and sensitization in primary headache syndromes remains poorly understood. The fact that headache occurs ipsilateral to a dysfunctional hemisphere (as occurs during migraine aura) suggests that the brain can activate or sensitize, directly or indirectly, meningeal nociceptive neurons. Further, limbic prodromal symptoms such as mood change and altered appetite suggest that brain dysfunction may precede and possibly provoke headache in certain settings. Recent observations using positron emission tomography (PET) have implied a primary "generator" role for rostral brainstem structures in patients with migraine (23). The structures that seemed most involved were the periaqueductal gray, the dorsal raphe nucleus, and locus ceruleus. It is also possible that these centers are responsible for modulating the flow of pain impulses, rather than primary generation of pain. It is likely that brainstem centers play a key role in the generation or modulation of pain, and current models of headache and facial pain provide a framework for further investigation. Understanding the pathophysiology may help guide treatments designed to prevent or relieve pain.

PRIMARY HEADACHE SYNDROMES

MIGRAINE

Migraine is derived from the Greek word hemicrania, introduced by Galen in approximately 200 B.C. (2). Over the years, a variety of popular names for this disorder have evolved, including sick headache, blind headache, and bilious headache. Because of his classic descriptions, Aretaeus of Cappadocia (second century A.D.) is credited as the discoverer of migraine headaches. Migraines have appeared in

popular literature for centuries. Shakespeare describes migraine treatment in *Othello* and *King John* (28,29). Lewis Carroll described migrainous phenomena in *Alice in Wonderland* and *Through the Looking Glass*; these included central scotoma, tunnel vision, distortions in body image, and visual hallucinations (30). It is therefore perplexing that, even today, migraine remains underdiagnosed and undertreated (14,31). There are a number of contributing factors. Some health care providers may not devote time and resources to identifying migraine, particularly given the limited time available to evaluate patients in a nonspecialty clinic. Some patients with migraine may fail to seek medical attention. Recent data suggest that the presence of concomitant headache types may interfere with diagnosis as well (14,31).

Epidemiology and Impact of Migraine

Few studies of migraine incidence have been performed, and none has systematically followed a large sample of headache-free individuals across a broad range of ages to ascertain new cases of IHS-defined migraine. Indeed, it is challenging to estimate the incidence of a chronic disorder with episodic manifestations. Stewart (32) estimated migraine incidence using prevalence data. In males, the peak incidence of migraine with aura was 6.6/1000 person-years at 5 years of age; migraine without aura in men peaked at 10/1000 person-years between the ages of 10 and 11 years. In women, the incidence of migraine with aura peaked between ages 12 and 13 (14.1/1000 person-years); migraine without aura peaked between ages 14 and 17 (18.9/1000 person-years).

Migraine prevalence varies by age, gender, race, geography, and socioeconomic status (2). Prior to puberty, migraine prevalence is higher in boys than in girls. As adolescence approaches, prevalence increases more rapidly in girls than boys. Prevalence increases until age 40, after which it declines (Fig. 26.6). Migraine prevalence is highest between the ages 25 and 55 (33). Race and geographic region contribute to migraine prevalence. In one population-based study, prevalence of migraine was lowest in Asian-Americans, intermediate in African-Americans, and highest among Caucasians (34). Several studies have suggested that migraine prevalence is inversely related to socioeconomic status (33,35). This contradicts prior popular beliefs that migraine was more prevalent among those with higher socioeconomic status. However, accurate medical diagnosis of migraine is more common among high-income group, which may have given rise to this misperception.

The economic impact of migraine includes direct costs (the expense of diagnosing and treating a particular disorder) as well as indirect costs (the aggregate economic effects of migraine on productivity at work, at home, and in other roles). It is estimated that migraine headache costs U.S. employers approximately $13 billion per year as a result of missed work and reduced productivity (36).

Genetics of Migraine

Large-scale epidemiologic studies have confirmed the contribution of genetic factors in migraine. In the past, population-based studies were limited by inaccurate diagnosis of migraine in cohorts. The advent of the IHS criteria in 1988 allowed for a more precise definition of migraine. Even so, misdiagnosis and underdiagnosis remain a potential risk, and some patients who do not report migraine at the time of the study may develop symptoms later in life. A study of Danish migraineurs found that first-degree relatives of patients reporting migraine with aura were 3.8 times more likely to experience migraine with aura than the general population (37). A similar but less robust risk was found in first-degree relatives of those patients reporting migraine without aura. Early twin studies had methodologic flaws (38), but more recent reports show a higher concordance rate among monozygotic twins, compared with dizygotic twins, for migraine with and without aura. A large-scale twin survey of the Danish population has estimated that the contribution of genetic effects to susceptibility is 61% for migraine without aura, and 65% for migraine with aura (39).

Recent evidence suggests the involvement in some forms of migraine of the calcium channel gene CACNA1A, which is located on chromosome 19p13. Ophoff (40) identified five unrelated families with familial hemiplegic migraine and mutations in CACNA1A. The gene encodes the alpha-1 subunit for a brain-specific P/Q type calcium channel. The mutations associated with familial hemiplegic migraine, in animal models resulted in the formation of calcium channels with altered biophysical properties (38). A calcium channel defect

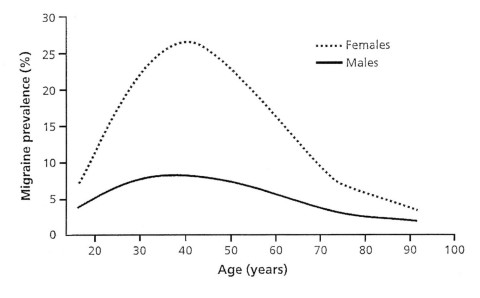

Figure 26.6. Migraine prevalence by age. (From Silberstein SD, Lipton RB. Epidemiology of migraine. Neuroepidemiology 1993; 12:179–194.)

might lead to recurrent headache through several mechanisms, including destabilization of central neuronal control centers involved in the initiation of the attack and disruption of calcium channel functions mediating the release of neurotransmitters (38,40). Mutations of CACNA1A have also been identified in patients with more common forms of migraine. In one family with a history of familial hemiplegic migraine, two individuals who had migraine with aura, but not hemiplegic migraine, had CACNA1A mutations (41). These, and other preliminary data, raise the possibility that migraine is the clinical manifestation of a channel defect. Additional genetic data are needed from other families to determine how widespread CACNA1A mutations are in patients with typical migraine.

It is likely that multiple genes are involved in determining susceptibility to, and clinical expression of, migraine. Although the genes involved in the serotonergic system are good candidates for susceptibility determination, no association with migraine with or without aura has been demonstrated for any of the 5-HT receptor subtype genes evaluated (38). The dopaminergic system may also play a role in migraine susceptibility, and a correlation between migraine and allele distribution for the dopamine D2 receptor gene has been reported (42). The NcoI allele and the C/C genotype for the D2 receptor gene appear significantly more often in migraineurs than in healthy controls. However, this genotype is also more frequently expressed in individuals with psychiatric disorders such as anxiety and depression. Since migraine frequently co-occurs with depression, this might reflect a single locus responsible for multiple conditions; alternatively, these findings may represent a clinical artifact.

Migraine occurs frequently in patients with mitochondrial disorders, such as **m**itochondrial **e**ncephalomyopathy, **l**actic **a**cidosis, and **s**troke-like episodes (MELAS) (43). Since mitochondrial DNA is transmitted maternally, and migraine typically demonstrates maternal inheritance, mitochondrial DNA mutations have been investigated as possible causes of migraine. To date, no association between migraine and known mitochondrial DNA mutations have been established.

Future studies will likely identify additional genes involved in the initiation and maintenance of migraine. This may in turn help clarify the pathophysiology of the disorder and determine appropriate strategies for prevention and treatment.

Migraine and Stroke

The relationship between migraine and stroke is complex. Both are neurological disorders associated with focal neurologic deficits, alterations in cerebral blood flow, and headache. A number of case-control and population-based studies have reported an association between ischemic stroke and migraine. The association is more robust for migraine with aura, which appears to be an independent risk factor for stroke (2,44–46). Migrainous infarction is recognized by the IHS as a distinct entity, and describes a cerebral infarction in which the pathogenesis is directly attributable to migraine. Migrainous infarction occurs during a typical migraine with aura, and is exceedingly rare. However, migraines, with and without aura, are associated with ischemic stroke occurring remote in time from a typical migraine attack. Tzourio et al. (45) found a significant association between migraine and ischemic stroke only in women younger than 45 years of age. The association was greater in those patients who smoked. A follow-up study (46) examined female stroke patients younger than 45 years of age, and found an increased risk for ischemic stroke among women with migraine with and without aura. The risk was increased among women who smoked or were using oral contraceptives (OCs).

The use of OCs and the risk of stroke in migraineurs has long been a source of controversy. Multiple retrospective studies over the past two decades have evaluated the impact of OCs on cerebral ischemic events in patients with migraine; many of these studies were conducted when high-dose estrogen contraceptives were widely used. These data suggest that OCs containing more than 50 mg estrogen are associated with an increased risk of cerebral thrombotic events, while those containing only progestin did not increase risk (47).

Migraine with and without Aura

Migraine may be divided into two major categories: migraine without aura and migraine with aura. Both are clinical syndromes characterized by headache and associated symptoms. Migraine with aura is also characterized by focal neurologic symptoms which typically precede or accompany the headache. Patients with either type may experience a premonitory phase and a resolution phase. These phases may include symptoms such as hyperactivity, hypoactivity, depression, food cravings, and repetitive yawning (48).

Migraine without Aura

Migraine without aura is defined as a recurrent headache disorder manifesting in attacks lasting 4–72 hours. The specific criteria in the IHS second edition (11) are:

A. At least five attacks fulfilling B to D
B. Headache attacks lasting 4–72 hours and occurring less than 15 days/month (untreated or unsuccessfully treated)
C. Headache has at least two of the following characteristics
    1. Unilateral location
    2. Pulsating quality
    3. Moderate or severe pain intensity
    4. Aggravation by, or causing avoidance of, routine physical activity (i.e., walking or climbing stairs)
D. During headache, at least one of the following:
    1. Nausea and/or vomiting
    2. Photophobia and phonophobia
E. Not attributable to another disorder

When eliciting a history, it should be remembered that many patients have more than one primary headache syndrome. Migraine without aura is the disease most likely to accelerate in response to the frequent use of symptomatic medications, resulting in medication overuse headache.

Therefore, a thorough medication history is an indispensable part of the history. Although there is no mention of age in the above criteria, migraine without aura in children is slightly different. The duration is typically 1–72 hours, and the headache is often bilateral; the adult pattern of unilateral headache generally develops in late adolescence or early adult life (49). In young children, photophobia and phonophobia may be inferred from behavior.

Migraine without aura is the most common type of migraine. The average attack frequency is higher than migraine with aura, and the headaches are usually more disabling (2). There is often a strict menstrual relationship. Indeed, pure menstrual migraine and menstrual-related migraine are recognized as distinct subforms of migraine without aura (50).

Migraine with Aura

Migraine with aura is a recurrent disorder manifesting in attacks of reversible focal neurologic symptoms, usually developing gradually over 5–20 minutes and lasting for less than 60 minutes. Headache with the features of migraine without aura usually follows the aura symptoms. Less commonly, the headache may not have migrainous features, or the headache may be completely absent The IHS has described several subforms of migraine with aura (11); included here are those most relevant to neuro-ophthalmology.

Typical Aura with Migraine Headache

This disorder is characterized by a typical aura consisting of visual and/or sensory and/or speech symptoms. Gradual development, duration of less than 1 hour, and complete reversibility define the aura, which is followed by a headache fulfilling criteria for migraine without aura. The specific IHS criteria (11) are:

A. At least two attacks fulfilling criteria B to E.
B. Fully reversible visual and/or sensory and/or speech symptoms but no motor weakness.
C. At least two of the three following:
1. Homonymous visual symptoms including positive features (flickering lights, spots, lines) and/or nega-

tive features (loss of vision) and/or unilateral sensory symptoms.
2. At least one symptom develops gradually within 5 minutes and/or different symptoms occur in succession.
3. Each symptom lasts between 5–60 minutes.
D. Headache that meets criteria for B–D for migraine without aura begins during the aura, or follows the aura within 60 minutes.
E. Not attributed to another disorder.

Migraine Aura

Visual aura is the most common type of aura, and is generally binocular. The classic description is a fortification spectra (2): a zigzag figure that appears near fixation, gradually spreads left or right, and assumes a convex shape with an angulated scintillating edge, leaving variable degrees of absolute or relative scotoma in its wake (Fig. 26.7). However, migraineurs may experience a variety of visual phenomena, including complex disorders of visual perception. Table 26.6 summarizes common and uncommon migrainous visual phenomena, and the characteristics of the visual aura are detailed in Table 27.7 and Figures 26.8 to 26.12. Metamorphopsia refers to distortion of the shapes of images; the patient may perceive objects as being too fat, too thin, or wavy. Some patients with migraine may describe objects appearing too small (micropsia) or too large (macropsia). Metamorphopsia in general is more commonly associated with macular disease than with migraine. Patients with macular edema frequently report micropsia, since the swelling causes increased separation of photoreceptors; macropsia is present with epiretinal membranes but is rarely a macular symptom. Metamorphopsia due to macular disease is generally easily distinguishable from migraine aura: the symptoms are continuous rather than paroxysmal; often unilateral rather than bilateral; and the fundus examination generally shows abnormal macula. Migraineurs may also perceive objects as being too far away (teleopsia).

The Alice in Wonderland syndrome typically refers to

Table 26.6
Visual Phenomena Associated with Migraine

Visual Event	Description	Also Caused by
Fortification spectra	Arc of jagged, serrated, or zigzag lines	Visual seizure, occipital AVM, mass
Scintillating scotoma	Positive fortification spectra on outside and negative scotoma in the middle	Visual seizure, occipital AVM, mass
Micropsia	Objects appear too small	Visual seizure, occipital AVM, mass, macular disease
Macropsia	Objects appear too large	Visual seizure, occipital AVM, mass
Metamorphopsia	Objects appear distorted in shape	Macular disease, visual seizure
"Alice in Wonderland" syndrome	Episodes of distorted body image	Visual seizure, occipital AVM, mass
Palinopsia	Persistence of visual images	Visual seizure; parieto-occipital damage; medications
Cerebral polyopia	Perception of multiple images in both eyes	Visual seizure, right occipital lobe damage
Achromatopsia	Inability to perceive color	Bilateral occipito-temporal damage

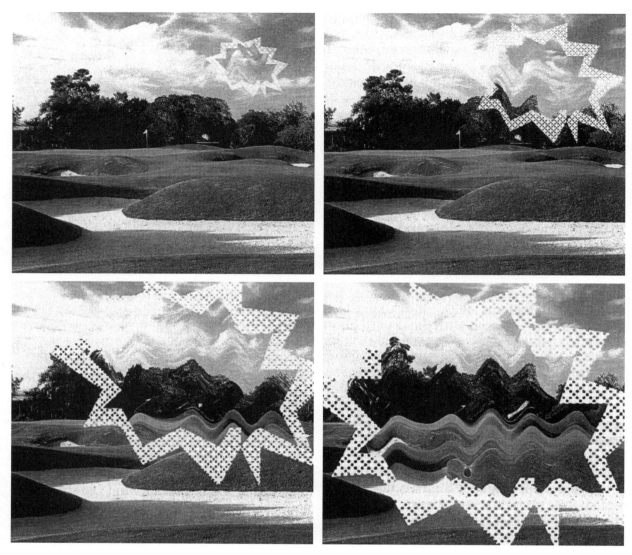

Figure 26.7. Characteristic build-up of a migrainous scintillating scotoma. A small pulsing object is initially noticed in the *upper right* quadrant of both eyes. The object gradually enlarges to consume the homonymous quadrant, and the border consists of colored, shimmering prisms. The visual disturbance eventually consumes the entire visual field before disintegrating.

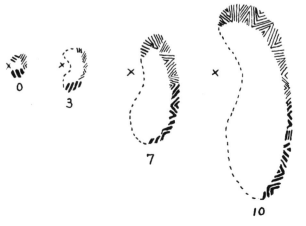

Figure 26.8. Successive maps of a scintillating scotoma showing gradual enlargement of fortification figures and gradual movement away from fixation (x). These drawings were made by Lashley as he observed his own scotomas. (From Lashley KS. Patterns of cerebral integration indicated by the scotomas of migraine. Arch Neurol Psychiatry 1941;46:331–339.)

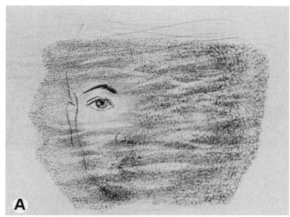

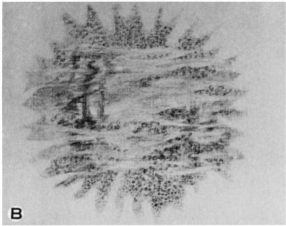

Table 26.7
Characteristics of the Visual Aura in Migraine

Characteristic	Description
Positive or negative phenomena (or both)	Positive phenomena often occur first, and are followed by negative phenomena
Visual field	Scotoma often start centrally and progress peripherally
Shape	Scintillations often C shaped; scotoma may be bean shaped
Motion	Objects may oscillate, rotate, or shimmer
Flicker	Rate usually 10/sec; may change during aura
Color	Any; may have no specific color except bright white
Clarity	May be blurry or hazy
Brightness	Often excessively bright
Evolution/expansion	Buildup occurs in both scotoma and scintillations
Progression	Scintillations may march from center to periphery or vice versa

Figure 26.9. Two examples of the visual aura of migraine drawn by a 50-year-old patient who had suffered from migraine since adolescence. The visual symptoms began following a prodromal period marked by a feeling of apprehension. She first noted horizontal wavering images, as if everything was being observed through a "sheet of water." *A*, This drawing depicts the areas of her son's face that were visible and those that were blurred out. The blurred area included the entire right side of the visual field and the inferior left visual field. She stated that: "Everything looked fluid pinpoint-like globules were present in the area of visual loss . . . it was like snow on a TV screen . . . contours of objects seemed to waver and move like reflections in water . . . there were no zigzags in the periphery . . . it was as if something was wrong with the horizontal adjustment of the TV set . . . all color was gone. The attack lasted about 30 minutes and then I could see again but my face on the right side and my right hand became numb, and then my headache started." *B*, On another occasion, the same patient experienced what she described as a "sunburst attack." It occurred as she was driving down a wooded road. It started as did her usual attacks, and she quickly stopped her car. She remembered that the color green (trees) could be seen only in the central portion of the left field of vision. "Zigzag bright light surrounded the central area, and tiny molecular droplets danced aimlessly through the image. All forms that could be perceived seemed to wobble like reflections in water. Horizontal ripples passed back and forth across the central field of vision. The periphery of vision was blind and seemed like a silvery haze that pulsated in and out at the zigzag zone." This visual aura cleared in 35 minutes and was followed by a right-sided headache and severe nausea.

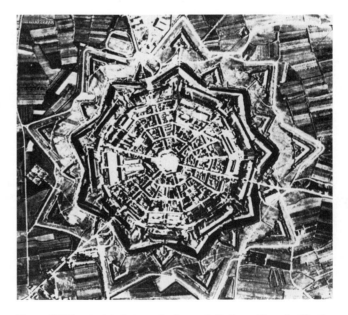

Figure 26.10. Aerial photograph of an early Italian military fortification demonstrating the angulation often seen in the visual aura of migraine with and without headache. (From Hupp SL, Kline LB, Corbett JJ. Visual disturbances of migraine. Surv Ophthalmol 1989;33:221–236.)

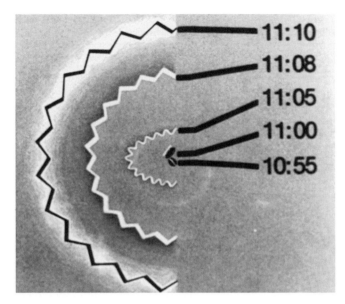

Figure 26.11. Hemianopic nature of a fortification scotoma. Note gradual enlargement of the scotoma over 15 minutes. Also note that the scotoma remains localized to the left homonymous hemifield. (From Hupp SL, Kline LB, Corbett JJ. Visual disturbances of migraine. Surv Ophthalmol 1989; 33:221–236.)

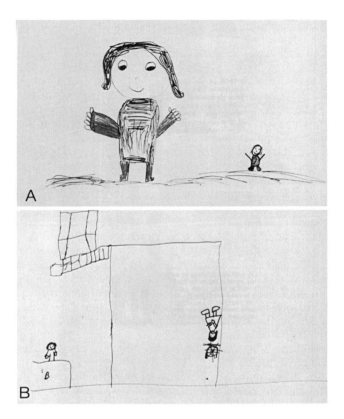

Figure 26.13. Drawings of abnormal visual phenomena observed by children during an attack of migraine. *A,* Drawing of micropsia as observed by a child suffering from migraine with aura. Other children (*right*) appeared unusually small to the patient (*left*) during some of her attacks. *B,* Drawing by a 9-year-old girl who had episodes that began with double vision. Colors of objects then changed, and a bitemporal headache developed. On one occasion before the headache developed, the child saw a picture as being upside down and her mother as walking upside down. In this drawing, a picture in the room (*upper left corner*) is upside down, as is the patient's mother (*right*). (From Hachinski VC, Porchawka J, Steele JC. Visual symptoms in the migraine syndrome. Neurology 1973;23:570–579.)

hallucinations of enlargement, diminution, or distortion of all or part of the body (Fig. 26.13). Lippman (51) originally described seven patients with this syndrome, and recalled that Lewis Carroll (Charles Lutwidge Dodgson), a migraineur himself, also described similar hallucinations in his

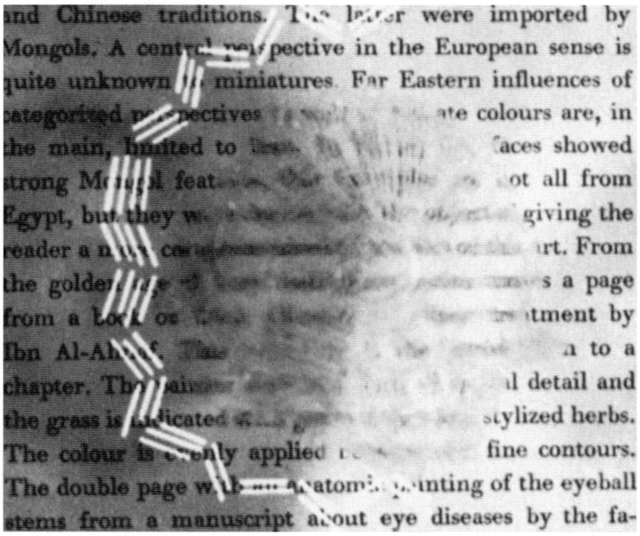

Figure 26.12. Visual aura without headache (acephalgic migraine). Photographic representation of a scintillating scotoma that occurred in a patient without headache. Note darkening of the left homonymous visual field associated with blurring of central vision and a fortification figure in the left hemifield. (From Wiley RG. The scintillating scotoma without headache. Ann Neurol 1979;11:581–585.)

book, *Alice in Wonderland*. Similar patients have been reported, and the syndrome seems to occur primarily in children with migraine (52). Although migraine is the cause in most cases of Alice in Wonderland syndrome, other etiologies such as seizure and encephalitis have been reported (53). These distortions of body image are thought to result from cortical depression in the nondominant parietal lobe (54). Migraine may also result in the perception of multiple images: cerebral polyopia. In such cases, the double vision is present with either eye covered, and does not improve with refraction. Palinopsia refers to a persistent visual afterimage: patients may describe seeing a trail of ghost images while watching an object move across the field of vision. Cerebral polyopia and palinopsia have both been associated with lesions of the nondominant occipital lobe (55,56).

Visual allesthesia, or "upside-down" vision, may also occur during migraine aura (57). The patient may report vertical or horizontal inversion of the visual environment.

Similar phenomena have also been associated with brainstem lesions involving the vestibular nuclei and central vestibular pathways. The time course and the headache following the visual event suggest a migrainous etiology.

Most of the complex visual hallucination and illusions described above can also be caused by visual seizures. This is perhaps not surprising, given the similar phenomenology of migraine and epilepsy. Similar phenomena have been reported to occur in patients with irritative occipital mass lesions, particularly vascular malformations (57). Distinguishing a visual seizure or focal occipital lesion from migraine aura may in most cases be accomplished through a complete history and examination, which must include perimetry. The gradual onset and evolution of symptoms common to migraine aura is not seen with a visual seizure, which is maximal at onset. Visual seizures are generally shorter than migraine auras, lasting 3–5 minutes. In many patients with visual seizures, a visual field defect attributable to a fixed posterior visual pathway lesion may be identified.

Alcohol and illicit drugs may cause visual hallucinations similar to migraine aura. Certain prescription and over-the-counter medications may cause visual phenomena as well; a thorough medication history and a temporal relationship between drug ingestion and visual symptoms suggests the etiology (57).

Regardless of the complexity, a migraine aura should still fulfill the criteria for aura described above; any variation (i.e., rapid onset without gradual evolution, duration too brief or too prolonged) should raise suspicion about an alternate etiology. It bears repeating that complete reversibility is the hallmark of an aura; a focal deficit after the aura has resolved mandates further evaluation, including neuroimaging.

Typical Aura without Headache

This disorder has carried several names over the years, including "acephalgic migraine." The aura fulfills all the criteria detailed above. Patients with typical aura without headache commonly have a history of migraine with aura (2). As patients with typical aura age, the headache may lose migraine characteristics or disappear completely even as auras continue. Some patients, primarily males, will have migraine aura without headache exclusively (58). The differentiation between migraine aura and transient ischemic attack may be difficult in the elderly, but can generally be accomplished with a thorough history and examination. In the Framingham cohort, the incidence of migrainous visual symptoms was 1.33% for women and 1.08% for men. These episodes often occurred after 50 years of age, independent of concurrent headaches and, in some cases, in the absence of a history of recurrent headaches. These episodes did not appear to be associated with an increased incidence of stroke (59).

Fisher described "later life migrainous accompaniments," or migraine aura (often not accompanied by headache) occurring in older patients, some with a previous history of migraine headache (60). He identified a number of clinical features suggestive of migraine accompaniment, including binocular visual symptoms, build-up of scintilla-

Table 26.8
Later-Life Migrainous Accompaniments

The gradual appearance of focal neurologic symptoms, spreading or intensifying over minutes

Positive visual symptoms characteristic of typical migraine aura: Scintillating scotoma, flashing lights, shimmering

Duration of 15–25 minutes

History (may be remote) of similar symptoms associated with migrainous headache

The occurrence of two or more identical spells

"Flurry" of accompaniments (often in the 50–60-year age group)

Generally benign course

(Adapted from Fisher CM. Late-life migraine accompaniments as a cause of unexplained transient ischemic attacks. Can J Neurol Sci 1980;7 : 9–17.)

tions, and duration of 15–20 minutes (Table 26.8). He also reported a midlife "flurry" of identical episodes, and a benign course. Therefore, in patients with typical presentations (binocular symptoms, gradual evolution, duration less than 1 hour) and a normal neurologic and neuro-ophthalmic examination (including visual field testing), extensive diagnostic testing is not routinely indicated. In patients with atypical presentations (brief duration, lack of build-up), noninvasive testing (MR imaging and angiography, echocardiography) is reasonable.

Retinal Migraine

Retinal migraine is defined by repeated attacks of **monocular** visual phenomena including scintillations, scotomata, or blindness associated with typical migraine headache (2). The aura and migraine headache fulfill all the criteria described earlier, with the only distinction being the monocular visual symptoms. Again, history is paramount. Since the visual field is slightly larger temporally than nasally, patients with homonymous visual field defects often report monocular visual loss, localizing it to the eye with the temporal field cut. The patient should be asked specifically whether each eye was alternately covered during the attack. Retinal migraine without headache may occur, but is rare (61). Retinal migraine may be mistaken for an episode of amaurosis fugax, i.e., transient monocular visual loss due to a thromboembolic transient ischemic attack and should only be considered after all other causes of transient monocular loss have been ruled out. The presence of positive visual phenomena is much more suggestive of migraine, although such symptoms have been reported in carotid occlusive disease (62). Duration of 1–10 minutes, sudden rather than gradual onset of symptoms, and lack of typical migraine headache following visual loss would all suggest a thrombo-embolic rather than migrainous etiology.

Persistent Migraine Aura without Infarction

Although migraine aura by IHS criteria lasts less than 60 minutes, persistence of aura for days or years may rarely occur (63), and is included in the second edition of IHS criteria (11). The IHS criteria require previous attacks fulfilling criteria for migraine with aura, similarity of aura symptoms to previous attacks, and exclusion of alternate etiologies, including (as the name implies) migrainous infarction. Indeed, prolonged, continuous photopsias are more suggestive of retinal disease, with involvement of the deep retinal layers. Patients with severe, bilateral visual loss may experience ''release'' hallucinations; these are typically formed (57). Certain medications, most commonly psychoactive drugs, may be associated with positive visual phenomena as well. Occipital seizures typically manifest as paroxysmal rather than continuous photopsias; these photopsias are generally colored, whereas migraine aura is typically achromatic (64). Persistent occipital seizures (''status epilepticus amauroticus'') are rare, but have been reported (65). Therefore, patients presenting with continuous photopsias require a careful headache and medication history, a complete ophthalmic examination (including visual fields and evaluation of the peripheral retina), and in some cases, ancillary testing (such as neuroimaging, EEG, ERG). Treatment of persistent migraine aura is notoriously unsatisfactory, but medications that have been used include amitriptyline and gabapentin.

Familial Hemiplegic Migraine

The IHS defines familial hemiplegic migraine (FHM) as recurrent migraine with aura including motor weakness in which at least one first- or second-degree relative has migraine aura including motor weakness. The disorder has autosomal dominant inheritance, with variable penetrance. The IHS criteria (11) include:

A. At least two attacks fulfilling B–E.
B. Fully reversible motor weakness and at least one of the following other aura symptoms: visual, speech, or sensory disturbance.
C. At least two of the following:
   1. At least one aura symptom develops gradually over more than 5 minutes and/or different symptoms occur in succession.
   2. Each aura symptom lasts less than 24 hours.
   3. Headache that meets criteria for migraine without aura begins during aura or follows aura within 60 minutes.
D. At least one first- or second-degree relative has migraine attacks with aura, including motor weakness.
E. Not attributed to another disorder.

Onset is typically in childhood, and nearly always by the age of 30 years. Onset of FHM after the age of 40 would be extremely atypical, and should prompt consideration of other etiologies. Many patients with FHM may also experience typical migraine with or without aura (2,66).

As noted previously, specific genes have been associated with FHM. Familial hemiplegic migraine type 1 (FHM1) localizes to chromosome 19, and familial hemiplegic migraine type 2 (FHM2) is localized to chromosome 1. Patients with FHM type 1 often have basilar type symptoms in addition to the typical aura, and may experience disturbance of consciousness, fever, CSF pleocytosis, and confusion during

an attack. In most patients the attacks decline in frequency and terminate at between 30–40 years of age. The neurologic signs are always completely reversible, even in patients with prolonged attacks. Brain MRI typically remains normal.

Treatment of FHM differs somewhat from other forms of migraine. Medications with vasoconstrictor effects are best avoided. Severe and persistent hemiplegic migraine has been treated with intravenous dopamine agonists, calcium channel blockers, and acetazolamide (66).

Basilar Type Migraine

Basilar type migraine describes a recurrent attack of migraine with aura in which symptoms clearly originate from the brainstem or both hemispheres, and where no weakness is present. A headache that meets criteria for migraine without aura begins during the aura or follows aura within 60 minutes. This type of migraine is rare and should only be diagnosed after vertebrobasilar ischemia has been ruled out.

Ophthalmoplegic Migraine

Ophthalmoplegic migraine is now classified as a cranial neuralgia by the IHS and is discussed later.

Pathophysiology of Migraine

Migraine may be considered as a sensitivity of neurovascular reactions to certain stimuli or cyclic changes in the central nervous system (2). Any theory of migraine pathogenesis must encompass the initiation, amplification, and maintenance of head pain, as well as the neuroanatomic and neurophysiologic substrates of aura. Traditional theory of migraine pathogenesis has included a **vasogenic** etiology and a **neurogenic** etiology. The vasogenic theory is derived in part from observations made by Wolff and colleagues in the 1930s. Graham and Wolff (67) recorded the pulsations of branches of the superficial temporal artery during migraine headache and observed that the amplitude of the pulse wave diminished as the intensity of the headache was reduced after the injection of ergotamine, a vasoconstrictor. Further, stimulation of intracranial vessels in awake patients during craniotomy caused severe, ipsilateral, throbbing headache. It was felt that intracranial vasoconstriction was responsible for the aura, and the rebound dilation and distension of extracranial vessels resulted in headache. The neurogenic theory holds that the brain is the generator of migraine, and that individual susceptibility reflects differential thresholds. In this model, the vascular changes observed during the headache are the effect rather than the cause. In the past two decades, it has become clear that neither of the traditional theories is adequate to explain all the phenomena that accompany migraine. Over the past decades, advances in neuroimaging have elucidated the mechanism of aura and given insight into potential molecular mediators of headache transduction and generation. In particular, functional imaging modalities, such as positron emission tomography (PET) and functional MRI (fMRI), allow direct observation of physiologic rather than anatomic abnormalities.

Leao (68) originally described a ''spreading depression'' or progressive shutdown in cortical function in animal brain, and felt that this may be related to migraine aura. Cortical stimulation initiates excitation followed by depression of neuronal activity that spreads slowly from the focal site of stimulation at rates ranging from 2–6 mm per minute. Although pial arterial and venous dilation occur simultaneously with the neural activity, spreading depression does not follow vascular boundaries. Functional neuroimaging has allowed detailed investigation of cortical activity during migraine aura. Olesen (69) monitored regional cerebral blood flow (rCBF) in patients with aura-like symptoms undergoing carotid angiography and found a 25–30% decrease in rCBF which began in the occipito-temporal region and spread anteriorly at a rate of 2–3 mm per minute without respecting vascular boundaries. This spreading oligemia has been observed by other investigators using a variety of neuroimaging techniques (70).

The mechanism by which aura transduces headache remains unclear. The trigeminal nucleus caudalis, which is felt to be part of the central pathway mediating migraine pain, is stimulated by spreading depression. Many of the trigeminovascular pathways discussed earlier are likely to be involved in the amplification and maintenance of migraine head pain. Sterile neurogenic inflammation and plasma protein extravasation occurs in response to activation of trigeminal sensory neurons (70,71). This results in meningeal inflammation that persists for minutes to hours. Although neurogenic inflammation is well demonstrated in animals, it is not clear whether this response occurs in humans with migraine. Gene regulation studies in mice have suggested that atrial natriuretic peptide in glia may be an important mediator (72). There may also be molecules that diffuse through the CSF and stimulate the pial vessels that are yet to be identified. The mechanism by which migraine headache is generated without aura is uncertain. However, several investigators have demonstrated cortical events similar to spreading depression in patients with migraine without aura. Woods (73) found bilateral spreading oligemia beginning occipitally in a patient with migraine but no aura. One study using fMRI found spreading depression in the occipital cortex before headache onset in migraine patients with and without aura. This implies that similar primary neuronal and secondary hemodynamic events may precede initiation of headache in all patients. Another mechanism may be the recruitment of cortical-subcortical connections to nociceptive centers via the wave of excitation-suppression invading the cortical components of these networks (70). In this fashion, aura without headache may be an example in which the spreading depression does not involve the cortical-subcortical connections to brainstem nociceptive networks (70,74).

The observation that migraine attacks originate in the brain and can be triggered under certain condition implies the existence of a threshold that governs the incidence of attacks. There is a prevailing theory that migraineurs have transient or persistent hyperexcitability of neurons in the cerebral cortex, particularly the occipital lobe. Although some studies have yielded conflicting results, data have consistently supported cortical hyperexcitability (75,76). Transmagnetic stimulation of the occipital cortex required to produce visual phosphenes is lower in migraine patients with aura than in controls (77). Battelli (78) reported a lower phosphene threshold for transmagnetic stimulation over Brodmann's area V5 in migraineurs, suggesting that hyperexcitability extended beyond the primary visual cortex (V1). Further studies, using magnetoencephalography and fMRI, have confirmed widespread regions of abnormal cortical excitability in patients with migraine (76). Cell membrane excitability appears to be the critical determinant for susceptibility to migraine attacks. There may be multiple factors that increase or decrease neuronal excitability, and modulate the attack threshold.

There is increasing evidence suggesting an important role of serotonin in migraine. In the 1970s, the serotonin receptor mediating constriction of blood vessels was characterized, and shown to correspond to a subtype labeled "5-HT1-like." This led to the development of sumatriptan, a specific agonist of the 5-HT1b, 5-HT1D, and 5-HT1F receptors. Since that time, a large number of serotonin agonists (the triptans) have entered the market, and have revolutioned the abortive treatment of migraine attacks; 5-HT$_{1B/1D}$ receptor agonists block electrical activity in the trigeminocervical region after stimulation of pain-sensitive intracranial structures (2,70). It is uncertain whether these agonists act peripherally, centrally, or both. The blood-brain barrier is relatively impermeable to sumatriptan, a 5-HT$_{1B/1D}$ agonist, which only exerts an inhibitory effect on the trigeminocervical nucleus when the blood-brain barrier has been disrupted. However, there is indirect evidence that the blood-brain barrier may be altered during migraine (2,79). Hoskins and Goadsby (80) have speculated that the antimigraine efficacy of triptans is due to a direct inhibitory effect on second-order trigeminal neurons. 5-HT$_{1F}$ receptors are located on second-order trigeminal neurons, and not on vascular smooth muscle cells. Animal models indicate that selective 5-HT$_{1F}$ agonists might be effective in the treatment of migraine, without the detrimental cardiovascular side effects of the 5-HT$_{1B/1D}$ agonists (76). This has not yet been replicated in human trials. Rostral brainstem structures, such as the periaqueductal gray and locus ceruleus, may also be involved in migraine generation and maintenance (70,76).

A theory of central neuronal hyperexcitability has been proposed, in which common pathways mediating head pain are more easily triggered in patients with episodic migraine. It is clear that migraine pain is the result of a complex interplay between peripheral activation of nociceptors and central modulation. Migraineurs carry a predisposition to activation of these pathways, most likely explainable on a cellular and genetic basis. As functional neuroimaging continues to evolve, and molecular and genetic mediators are more precisely defined, the mechanisms underlying migraine may be further elucidated.

Treatment of Migraine

Effective management of migraine headaches begins with making an accurate diagnosis. Despite the fact that migraine is treatable, many patients find themselves in a paradoxic situation in which they are both undertreated and overmedicated: they take or receive a large number of nonspecific analgesics which are minimally effective for migraine and contribute to analgesic rebound. Treatment of migraine should ideally include nonpharmacologic as well as pharmacologic therapy. Minimizing excessive stress and sleep deprivation, eating regular meals, exercise, and avoidance of common triggers (e.g., wine, chocolate, etc.) are practical measures that should be discussed with any migraine patient. Alternative therapies (biofeedback, relaxation, acupuncture) have been used successfully in conjunction with conventional medical treatment (81). In many patients, a headache diary is invaluable; as it may help the patient and the physician characterize the headaches more clearly. A headache diary may also give patients a sense of control over their illness.

There is an ever-expanding armamentarium of medications available for the treatment of migraine, which can be daunting to practitioners. Treatment of migraine may be divided into acute or abortive treatment, and preventive or prophylactic treatment.

Abortive Treatments

A complete review of all abortive treatments for migraine is beyond the scope of this chapter. A recent review (82) graded the quality of evidence for medications used for acute migraine treatment. The following medications had grade A recommendations, meaning that they were based on multiple, well-designed clinical trials.

Nonsteroidal anti-inflammatory drugs (NSAIDs) are appropriate agents for patients with mild to moderate migraine pain. Specific agents include acetaminophen, ibuprofen, naproxen sodium, and aspirin. Their effect is better when the drug is taken at the beginning of the migraine attack, ideally during the prodromes.

All triptans are **serotonin receptor agonists** with approximately equal affinity for the $5-HT_{1B/1D}$ receptor. They all inhibit the release of vasoactive peptides, promote vasoconstriction, and block pain pathways in the brainstem (70). They are effective and relatively safe for acute therapy of migraine, and are useful choices for patients with moderate to severe migraine. Routes of administration differ among the agents, and intranasal and subcutaneous forms may be beneficial for patients who cannot take oral drugs (secondary to nausea). Although there are pharmacologic differences among the agents, head-to-head efficacy comparison studies are lacking, and there are no clear guidelines in choosing one agent over the other (82). All of the available triptans are contraindicated in patients with cardiovascular disease. Unlike other treatments of acute migraine attack, they may be taken at any time during the migraine; some authors avoid their administration during the aura because of their vasoconstrictive properties.

Ergot alkaloids and derivatives include dihydroergotamine (DHE) and ergotamine as members of the ergot family used in migraine treatment. DHE is recommended for patients with moderate to severe migraine pain. DHE may be delivered subcutaneously, intravenously, intramuscularly, or intranasally. Oral or rectal ergotamine may be useful for certain patients with moderate to severe migraine, but the evidence for efficacy is inconsistent, and side effects are more frequent compared with other abortive agents. They should be taken at the beginning of the migraine attack.

Opioid analgesics must be balanced against the risks of sedation and dependency. Oral opioids may be useful when sedation will not place the patient at risk, and the potential for abuse is discussed in advance. Intranasal butorphanol, a mixed opiate receptor agonist-antagonist, may be useful for some patients, but carries the same risk of dependency.

Antiemetics, are often used as adjuncts to other migraine therapies, but certain drugs in this class may have independent pain-relieving effects. Intravenous metoclopramide and intravenous and intramuscular prochlorperazine may be considered as monotherapy for migraine pain. Oral antiemetics are suggested only for adjunctive use.

Preventive Treatments of Migraine

The main goal of preventive treatment of migraine is to reduce the frequency, severity, and duration of subsequent migraine attacks. Preventive treatment plans often allow for the use of agents for acute attacks. In general, preventive treatment is considered when the frequency of headache is so high that analgesic rebound is likely, when migraine has a substantial impact on a patient's life despite the use of abortive agents, and when contraindications may limit the use and success of acute medications (2). Nonpharmacologic treatments, as discussed above, should be incorporated into the overall management plan. The relative efficacy of pharmacologic versus nonpharmacologic treatment is undetermined (83).

In the United States, only methysergide, propranolol, timolol, and divalproex sodium are approved for the preventive treatment of migraine. However, several other medications have been used, with varying success. The mechanisms of action of the preventive medications are varied, and no single medication had emerged as a clearly dominant treatment. The choice of drugs depends upon the goals of the patient, and may be influenced by patient lifestyle issues, medical co-morbidities, side effect profile, and cost of the drug. The U.S. Headache Consortium has classified migraine prophylactic medications in five groups based on clinical efficacy, adverse effects, safety profile, and expert clinical experience (83). Group 1 drugs have high proven clinical efficacy in migraine treatment, with mild to moderate adverse effects. The use of the medications is supported by Class A scientific evidence, i.e., their efficacy has been shown in multiple, well-designed, randomized trials. **Group 1 drugs** include the anticonvulsant divalproex sodium, the tricyclic antidepressant amitriptyline, and the beta-blockers propranolol and timolol. These are considered first-line treatment in the prophylaxis of migraine. **Group 2 drugs** have lower efficacy than group 1, and mild to moderate side effects. Atenolol, verapamil, aspirin, naproxen, gabapentin, fluoxetine, and magnesium are considered group 2 drugs. **Group 3 drugs** have efficacy based only on clinical experience, but no scientific evidence. This group includes the tricyclic antidepressants nortriptyline and protriptyline, the serotonin-specific reuptake inhibitors sertraline and paroxetine, and the anticonvulsant topiramate. **Group 4 drugs** have medium to high efficacy, but potentially significant side effects. Flunarizine and methysergide are group 4 drugs. **Group 5 drugs** have no evidence showing efficacy over

Table 26.9
Preventive Migraine Medications with Group 1 or Group 2 Level Efficacy

Medication	Class	Dose (mg/day)	Side Effects	Avoid in Patients with	Consider in Patients with
Divalproex sodium	Anticonvulsant	500–1500	Weight gain, tremor, alopecia, elevated liver enzymes	Hepatic disease	Bipolar disorder, seizure disorder
Propranolol	Beta-blocker	80–240	Weight gain, depression, syncope	Asthma, diabetes mellitus, depression	Cardiovascular disease, hypertension
Amitriptyline	Tricyclic antidepressant	50–150	Dry eyes and mouth, drowsiness	Cardiac arrhythmia, elderly patients	Depression, tension-type or chronic daily headache
Gabapentin	Anticonvulsant	900–2400	Drowsiness, dizziness, weight gain	No specific contraindications	Seizure disorder, neuropathic pain
Verapamil	Calcium channel blocker	240	Hypotension, constipation	Orthostatic hypotension	Cardiovascular disease, migraine aura

placebo. This group includes clonidine, carbamazepine, and indomethacin. Table 26.9 shows the common preventive agents used for migraine.

In recent years, botulinum toxin has been reported to be effective in the treatment of migraine (84). The treatment protocol generally involves injections of botulinum toxin into the head, facial, and cervical musculature. The presumed mechanism involves decreasing or eliminating peripheral activation, and thereby reducing central trigeminovascular activation (85). However, to date, there have been no well-designed, randomized, blinded and controlled trials demonstrating efficacy. Further, in many reports, the specific headache types have been inadequately characterized. Therefore, there in no Class A evidence favoring the routine use of botulinum toxin in patients with migraine.

TENSION-TYPE HEADACHE

Tension-type headache (TTH) is the most common form of primary headache, with a lifetime prevalence ranging from 30–78%. However, it remains the least studied of the primary headache syndromes, despite the fact that TTH may have the highest socioeconomic impact (86). Further, migraine headache is often misdiagnosed as TTH. In one study, 37% of patients originally diagnosed with TTH were later found to have migraine (87). The situation is complicated by the fact that migraine and TTH may coexist in the same patient. Indeed, the symptoms of each headache type may overlap. Muscle tension is often considered a unique feature of TTH, while migraine is commonly felt not to be associated with muscle tension or neck pain. Recent studies have suggested that neither of these assumptions may be correct (88). One study demonstrated that of 144 patients meeting IHS criteria for migraine, 75% described neck pain associated with the attacks (89).

The second edition of the IHS criteria (11) divides TTH into episodic and chronic forms. Episodic TTH is further subdivided into frequent and infrequent forms.

Episodic TTH

Episodic TTH is characterized by frequent episodes of headache lasting minutes to days. Patients often describe the pain as pressing or tightening in quality. The head pain is usually bilateral, of mild to moderate intensity, and does not worsen with routine physical activity. Nausea is absent, but photophobia or phonophobia (but not both) may be present. The headaches occur fewer than 15 days a month for at least 3 months. Episodic TTH may be seen in patients with coexisting migraine without aura, and it may be difficult to distinguish between the two. In one population-based study, 83% of individuals with headaches meeting IHS criteria for migraine also had headaches meeting IHS criteria for tension-type headache (90). A headache diary is an important tool to help differentiate between the two headaches, and guide treatment.

Chronic TTH

Chronic TTH is described as daily or very frequent headaches lasting minutes to days. The characteristics of the headache are identical to episodic TTH, but the attacks occur more than 15 days per month for at least 3 months. The patient may have no more than one of the following: photophobia, phonophobia, or mild nausea. The patient must be using analgesics less than 10 days per month; if not, the headache is classified as medication overuse headache.

Pathophysiology of Tension-Type Headache

The exact mechanism of TTH remains undetermined. The traditional theory was that TTH developed due to sustained contraction of pericranial muscles (2). However, muscle contraction may occur to the same degree in migraineurs, and there is no correlation between muscle contraction, tenderness, and the presence of headache (91). It is likely that peripheral pain mechanisms act as a trigger for a central process. Peripheral mechanisms may be most important in episodic TTH, while in chronic TTH, central mechanisms may predominate. Some have argued that TTH and migraine may represent different portions of a distribution of painful, episodic headaches (2, 92). It is not clear whether episodic TTH may be a mild form of migraine without aura.

Treatment of TTH

There are few controlled studies guiding the treatment of TTH. Acute therapy typically involves the structured use of simple analgesics (acetaminophen, aspirin), alone or in combination with NSAIDs. Overuse of these drugs must be limited. Prophylactic therapy should be considered when the frequency, duration, and severity of the headache might lead to disability or the overuse of acute medications. The tricyclic antidepressants are the drugs most commonly used, although with little scientific evidence. Serotonin-specific reuptake agents (SSRIs) may be used as well. Nonpharmacologic treatment, such as biofeedback and relaxation therapy, may be beneficial (2).

TRIGEMINAL AUTONOMIC CEPHALGIAS

This group of headache syndromes shares the clinical features of head and facial pain with prominent cranial autonomic features (11). Although relatively rare, these disorders are important to recognize since they often display an excellent and highly selective response to treatment. In many of these syndromes, the pain is localized to the eye, so the ophthalmologist may be the first health care provider to evaluate the patient, or may see the patient in consultation for unexplained eye pain. Based upon their common clinical phenotype, these headaches have recently been grouped under the term Trigeminal Autonomic Cephalgias (TACs) (11,93). All of these headache types may be associated with structural and vascular lesions, which should be excluded by a combination of careful history and examination, and judiciously chosen ancillary studies.

Pathophysiology of Trigeminal Autonomic Cephalgias: Overview

It is likely that all of the TACs share a similar pathophysiology involving a disturbance in the trigeminal-autonomic reflex. Stimulation of the trigeminal ganglion in animals results in increased extracerebral and cerebral blood flow (93). The major portion of the vasodilator response is mediated via a reflex connection with the facial nerve, the cranial parasympathetic outflow. The parasympathetic arm of this reflex is active in cluster headache (94). Vasoactive intestinal peptide (VIP) and CGRP may be important mediators in this response. Some investigators have suggested that cluster headache originates from the cavernous sinus, based on the intersection of the first division of the trigeminal nerve and the cranial sympathetic and parasympathetic nerves at this location. In one case, cerebral angiography demonstrated narrowing of the cavernous carotid artery during cluster (95). However, some authors have suggested that extreme ophthalmic division pain of many types can result in flow changes in the cavernous sinus, as part of the trigeminal sympathetic reflex (93, 96). Some TACs, such as cluster headache, demonstrate seasonal cycles, implicating the suprachiasmatic nucleus (the so-called hypothalamic pacemaker) and higher, diencephalic centers. Indeed, PET scans obtained in patients with cluster demonstrate unilateral activation in the hypothalamic gray (93). Further investigation, including the use of functional neuroimaging, may yield more insight into the processes driving TACs.

Cluster Headache

Cluster headache has carried a number of names over time, including Horton's headache, petrosal neuralgia, ciliary neuralgia, and others (2). Cluster headache is characterized by recurrent episodes of severe, unilateral orbital or temporal pain. Most patients are restless and agitated during the attack, as opposed to migraine patients, who often prefer to be still. Men are afflicted 3–4 times more frequently than woman. The IHS recognizes both an episodic and chronic cluster headache (11). The chronic form may arise de novo, or may evolve from the episodic form. In the episodic form, the patient must have an attack-free interval of one month. Most individuals with episodic cluster headache experience one or two attack phases per year. Phase duration may range from 4–16 weeks. Each attack phase is followed by a remission period of 6 months to 2 years (2,99). Patients with chronic cluster headache experience attacks for greater than 1 year, with remission periods lasting less than 1 month. The IHS criteria for cluster headache are (11):

A. At least five attacks fulfilling criteria B to D.
B. Severe or very severe unilateral orbital, supraorbital, and/or temporal pain lasting 15–180 minutes, untreated for more than half the period.
C. Headache is accompanied by at least one of the following symptoms or signs, which must be ipsilateral to the pain:
    1. Conjunctival injection.
    2. Nasal congestion, or rhinorrhea, or both.
    3. Eyelid edema.
    4. Forehead and facial sweating.
    5. Miosis, ptosis, or both.
    6. Headache is associated with a sense of restlessness of agitation.
D. Frequency of attacks: From one every other day to 8 per day for more than half the period or time if chronic.
E. Not attributed to another disorder.

The pain is typically excruciating, and has in a few refractory cases resulted in suicide. The attacks are often reliably provoked by alcohol and nitroglycerin.

Cluster headache may occasionally be associated with trigeminal neuralgia: the Cluster-Tic syndrome. Both conditions must be treated for the patient to be headache free. It is important to exclude disorders that mimic cluster headache, including other TACs, carotid artery dissection, pituitary adenoma, cavernous carotid and anterior communicating artery aneurysms, and Tolosa-Hunt syndrome (2,97). The patient's age, gender, the characteristics of the attacks, and the clinical examination usually serve to differentiate secondary causes of cluster-like headaches from primary cluster. For example, a middle-aged man with a long history of paroxysmal attacks fulfilling critertia for cluster headache and a normal interictal examination is unlikely to harbor a secondary cause of headache, and the diagnosis can rest upon clinical criteria. Approximately one-half to two-thirds of patients will develop Horner's syndrome during the attack; after multiple attacks, a permanent Horner's syndrome may result. The mechanism of Horner's syndrome may result from dilation of the internal carotid artery and compression of the sympathetic plexus. (97). Alternatively, dilation and vascular congestion within the cavernous sinus may involve the sympathetic plexus and lead to a transient Horner's syndrome.

Pathophysiology of Cluster Headache

The pathophysiology of cluster headache is unknown. There is growing evidence that the pain and autonomic symptoms result from dual activation of the trigeminal vascular and cranial parasympathetic pathways. Goadsby (94) demonstrated increased levels of CGRP (a marker peptide for the trigeminal vascular system) and VIP (a marker for the cranial parasympathetic system) in the internal jugular vein drainage during attacks. The CGRP levels returned to normal after successful treatment and resolution of the pain. There is evidence that nitric oxide (NO) may play a role in cluster, as well in other TACs and perhaps migraine. NO is increased in patients with cluster headache during and between attacks, and nitroglycerin can consistently provoke attacks in patients with cluster headache (97). These observations, however, do not address the essential feature of the disorder: periodicity. Hypothalamic dysfunction has long been postulated to be a potential cause of the rhythmic nature of cluster, and several studies have reported altered circadian rhythms of hypophysial hormone systems in cluster (98). The suprachiasmatic nucleus (the so-called hypothalamic pacemaker) is regulated by photic stimuli, and governs the synthesis and secretion of melatonin from the pineal gland. A small study demonstrated efficacy of melatonin in cluster headache (99), although the response rate was low. May and colleagues (100) used PET to evaluate variations in regional cerebral blood in nine patients during a cluster attack. These scans were compared with eight patients with chronic cluster headaches who were not in the midst of a cycle. The results suggested that the medial hypothalamus is specifically involved in cluster headache; hypothalamic activation did not occur when nitroglycerin was given outside of an attack, or with experimentally induced first trigeminal division pain. Hypothalamic activation may therefore act in a triggering or permissive manner.

Therefore, dual activation of the trigeminal vascular and cranial parasympathetic system occurs during a "cluster-permissive" period. This period is determined and modulated by dysfunction in the hypothalamus. Activation of the two systems results in the release of marker peptides, which leads to vasodilation, vascular congestion, and possibly neurogenic inflammation. This cascade leads to pain and autonomic symptoms (97).

Treatment of Cluster Headache

As with migraine, treatment of cluster may be either acute or preventive. A limiting factor for acute treatment is that the attacks reach peak intensity very quickly, and are of relatively short duration. Therefore, oral preparations used for migraine attacks may not have a rapid enough onset. Inhalation of 100% oxygen for 15 minutes can arrest an attack (97). The injectable forms of sumatriptan and dihydroergotamine have been shown to be extremely effective for acute treatment of cluster headache (101). Oral triptan preparations have shown modest to no benefit (102). Intranasal lidocaine may be of benefit (2).

Prophylactic treatment is used to shorten attacks and reduce attack frequency. Preventive therapy is frequently required for cluster since the attacks are frequent, severe, and often too short-lived for abortive medications to take effect. Also, overuse of abortive treatments may result in analgesic rebound. A typical regimen involves starting the medication early in the cluster period, continuing the drug until the patient is headache free for 2 weeks, and then tapering the medication. Prednisone is often used as a short-term, transitional therapy, and is the most rapid-acting of the preventive drugs used for cluster headache (101). A typical protocol might be 2–3 weeks of prednisone in tapering doses to break the cycle of headache until other medications become effective. However, steroid-dependence is often seen in these patients who may have rebound cluster headaches. Verapamil, a calcium channel blocker, has proven to be effective for cluster prophylaxis, and is considered by many to be the first-line drug in preventive therapy. Ergotamine tartrate may quickly suppress attacks, but is used less frequently, due to possible physiologic dependence and a contraindication to the concurrent use of sumatriptan for acute treatment. Lithium is highly effective to prevent cluster headaches, and is well tolerated when monitored carefully. Methysergide may also be used for maintenance therapy, but the possible retroperitoneal fibrosis associated with methysergide limit routine use of this medication.

Valproic acid, gabapentin, and topiramate are anticonvulsants that, in open label trials, have been found to be useful for cluster prevention (97). In one open label study, valproic acid produced a response in 73% of subjects with cluster headache (103). Refractory cluster may occur in a small number of patients. In these cases, it may be worthwhile to reevaluate for secondary causes of cluster, such as a compressive or vascular lesion. Combination preventive therapy may occasionally be required, and selected patients may benefit from a short course of intravenous DHE or methylprednisolone. Ablative surgical procedures may be considered in patients who are truly medically refractory, either due to ineffectiveness of medication, or contraindications, or intolerable side effects. The most frequent procedure is radiofrequency trigeminal rhizotomy (97). In a prospective study of 17 patients with chronic, intractable, cluster headache who underwent complete or partial trigeminal root resection, 88% had complete or nearly complete relief of their symptoms after 5 years of follow-up (104). Future surgical treatments may attempt to specifically target the anatomic structures involved in the pathogenesis of cluster. A single case study described the stereotactic implantation of a stimulating electrode into the homolateral posterior hypothalamus of a patient with medically refractory chronic cluster headache. This resulted in complete remission of headache after 6 months of follow up (105). Controlled, randomized trials will be necessary to determine whether these procedures will become part of a routine treatment algorithm for cluster patients.

Chronic Paroxysmal Hemicrania

Chronic paroxysmal hemicrania (CPH) was first described in 1974 (93), and is characterized by frequent, short-lasting attacks of unilateral pain, typically in the orbital, supra-orbital, or temporal region. The IHS criteria are (11) as follows:

A. At least 20 attacks fulfilling B to E.
B. Attacks of severe, unilateral orbital, supraorbital, or temporal pain lasting 2–30 minutes.
C. Attack frequency greater than five per day for more than half the time.
D. Pain is associated with at least one of the following symptoms or signs ipsilateral to the pain:
　1. Conjunctival injection, lacrimation, or both.
　2. Nasal congestion, or rhinorrhea, or both.
　3. Eyelid edema.
　4. Forehead and facial sweating.
　5. Miosis, ptosis, or both.
E. Headache is stopped completely by indomethacin.
F. Not attributable to another disorder.

An episodic form of paroxysmal hemicrania (EPH) has been reported, but is less common; EPH occurs in periods lasting from 7 days to 1 year, and separated by remissions of at least one month. In CPH, the attacks occur for more than 1 year without remission, or with remissions lasting less than 1 month (2,93).

The episodic and chronic forms occur more frequently in women (3:1), with an age range of 6–81 years (mean 34 years). The pain is excruciating, may be throbbing or boring, and builds up rapidly. In contrast to cluster, patients with CPH prefer to be still. CPH and cluster share many characteristics, which may lead to diagnostic uncertainty. Indeed, the final common pathways (activation of trigeminal vascular and cranial parasympathetic outflow systems) are likely similar in both disorders. As with other headache syndromes, secondary causes of CPH should be considered and excluded through history, examination, and selected studies. Secondary CPH has been associated with structural lesions of the frontal lobe and sella turcica (93), cavernous sinus meningioma (106), and collagen vascular disease (107). As with cluster headache, autonomic features are a defining feature of the disorder, and their absence should prompt consideration of another primary or secondary headache syndrome.

Pathophysiology of CPH

Although the pathophysiology of CPH is unknown, available evidence suggests many similarities to cluster headache. Alterations in the cyclic release of catecholamine and beta-endorphins have been observed in CPH, similar to those reported in cluster headache (108). Although studies of autonomic function have been normal, pupillometric studies in CPH have demonstrated miosis ipsilateral to the pain, suggesting a partial Horner's syndrome (109). Increased levels of CGRP and VIP have been found in the cranial venous blood of CPH patients; these levels normalize after treatment (110). Segmental narrowing of the ophthalmic veins on orbital phlebography has been reported, similar to changes seen with cluster (93). It seems that the final pathway involved in CPH is similar to those in cluster. The shorter attack duration, the greater attack frequency, and the selective response to indomethacin may point to differences in the generation of the disorders, perhaps due to differential hypothalamic dysfunction.

Treatment of CPH

Indomethacin is the preferred treatment for CPH. The standard dose is 25 mg three times a day (t.i.d.), increasing to 50 mg t.i.d. after 1 week if there is no response. The response is typically prompt, occurring within one or two days. Other NSAIDs, such as naproxen, have demonstrated some effect on CPH, although less than indomethacin.

Indomethacin is a nonsteroidal indoleacetic acid drug which exerts a selective treatment effect in several headache syndromes, including CPH (2,93). Indomethacin is an inhibitor of cyclooxygenase 1 and 2, and decreases cerebral blood flow and CSF pressure. It had been speculated that the selective effect of indomethacin on certain headaches is related to an effect on nitric oxide synthase (111). Indeed, nitric oxide synthase inhibitors may be effective treatments for CPH (93,111). Although there are clear similarities between cluster and CPH, acute treatments that work quite well for cluster (such as oxygen and sumatriptan) have not been consistently effective for CPH attacks. Hannerz and Jogestrand (112) reported a patient with bilateral CPH who responded to sumatriptan, but others have not found similar results (93). The lack of response may not necessarily imply lack of effect, but rather that the time of onset for such treatments are too long to be of benefit for short-duration headaches. In contrast, verapamil seems to be effective prophylaxis for cluster and CPH.

Short-Lasting Unilateral Neuralgiform Headache with Conjunctival Injection and Tearing (SUNCT)

Short-lasting unilateral neuralgiform headache with conjunctival injection and tearing (SUNCT) was originally described by Sjaastad in 1989. This rare disorder predominately affects men, with a gender ratio of 17:2. Patients experience short-lasting attacks of unilateral pain, most often associated with conjunctival injection and tearing. The attacks are much briefer than in other TACs, with a duration of 5–240 seconds. Paroxysms begin and end abruptly, reaching peak intensity within 2–3 seconds. Attacks may be numerous, with a mean of 28 per day in one study (11,93). In some patients, a dull discomfort persists between attacks. The pain is generally confined to the ocular/periocular region, moderate to severe in intensity, and often described by the patient as burning or electrical. Conjunctival injection and tearing are the most frequent autonomic features. Rhinorrhea, nasal congestion, and forehead sweating occur less commonly. An irregular temporal pattern is the rule, with symptomatic periods alternating with remissions in an unpredictable fashion (114). The tearing and conjunctival injection begins 1–2 seconds after onset of pain. Some patients can precipitate attacks by touching certain trigger zones within the territory of V1–V3. Unlike trigeminal neuralgia, the attacks have no refractory period.

Given the rarity of the disorder, secondary causes of SUNCT should be excluded. The most common lesion mimicking SUNCT is a posterior fossa mass such as a vascular malformation (93,115). Ocular etiologies, such as intermittent angle closure glaucoma, should be considered and excluded with careful slit-lamp and gonioscopic examination. Interestingly, intraocular pressures and corneal temperatures are mildly elevated during the attack, possibly reflecting parasympathetic activation with vasodilation (116). These findings, and others (2), suggest a central pathogenesis for SUNCT as a manifestation of the trigeminal vascular reflex.

It is occasionally difficult to differentiate SUNCT from cluster and CPH. In contrast to cluster headache and CPH, the attacks in SUNCT are shorter and more frequent, and the repertoire of autonomic dysfunction is more limited. Women are more frequently affected in CPH. Both CPH and cluster demonstrate a consistent response to treatment, a feature lacking in SUNCT.

Pathophysiology

The pathophysiology of SUNCT is unknown. As with other TACs, orbital phlebography has been shown to be abnormal in SUNCT, with narrowing of the superior ophthalmic vein ipsilateral to the symptoms (93). Pupillary studies have revealed no abnormalities. Intraocular pressure and corneal temperatures are moderately elevated during attacks, likely reflecting parasympathetic activation and vasodilation (117). There have been few functional neuroimaging studies performed in patients with SUNCT, perhaps due to the relative rarity of the disorder. Functional MRI revealed activation in the region of the ipsilateral posterior hypothalamus in one patient (118). A central triggering mechanism with secondary activation of the trigeminal vascular and cranial parasympathetic pathways seems likely.

Treatment

Unfortunately, no treatments have been shown to be consistently and reproducibly effective for SUNCT. There have been single case reports and small case series describing a response to several agents, including gabapentin, lamotrigine, and sumatriptan (117). Three patients with SUNCT were successfully treated by trigeminal rhizolysis (119). However, two patients were reported to fail several neurosurgical treatments for SUNCT, with residual neurologic deficits (120). Caution is always advised when assessing any therapy for a disorder characterized by an irregular temporal pattern and unpredictable remissions.

Hemicrania Continua

Hemicrania continua (HC) is an uncommon cause of chronic daily headache (121). This disorder is characterized by a continuous, unilateral headache that varies in intensity, without disappearing completely (122). The associated features include autonomic symptoms, "jabs and jolts" (sharp pains lasting less than 1 minute), and migrainous symptoms (nausea, vomiting, photophobia, or phonophobia). As with CPH, HC is exquisitely indomethacin-sensitive, producing a prompt and enduring response in most patients. Some investigators recommend that all patients with chronic, unilateral headache not attributable to other disorders receive an indomethacin trial (121).

OTHER SHORT-LASTING PRIMARY HEADACHES

Primary Stabbing Headache

Primary stabbing headache is defined by the IHS as pain occurring as a single stab or a series of stabs confined to the head and exclusively or predominantly felt in the distribution of the trigeminal nerve (orbit, temple, parietal area). The stabs may last for up to a few seconds and recur with irregular frequency from one to many per day. The stabs may remain localized, or may migrate. The syndrome has carried other names over time, including ice-pick headache, idiopathic jabs and jolts, and ophthalmodynia periodica (123). The duration of the pain ranges from 1–5 seconds, more frequently between 1–2 seconds. The attacks are usually unprovoked. There is tremendous variability in the temporal pattern of the attacks. Some patients may experience a single jab, while others may experience volleys of jabs as often as 50 times per day (2,123). Autonomic symptoms are conspicuously absent. Visual symptoms are generally absent, although there is one report of transient monocular visual loss associated with primary stabbing headache (124). Primary stabbing headache is often associated with other primary headache syndromes, such as migraine. According to some studies, idiopathic stabbing pain may occur in 30–40% of migraineurs (123,125). Peres (126) identified stabbing headache in 41% of patients with hemicrania continua. The absence of autonomic features, as well as the short duration, distinguishes this headache from cluster and CPH. Trigeminal neuralgia may present in a similar fashion, but uncommonly involves V1. Trigeminal neuralgia attacks are usually provoked, and display a consistent response to carbamazepine, features lacking in primary stabbing headache.

The pathogenesis of primary stabbing headache is unknown. Activation of the trigeminal vascular system is the most likely final pathway, but the initial events leading to activation of nociceptive centers is undetermined. It is possible that the stabbing pains may result from spontaneous discharges of trigeminal afferents.

The majority of patients with primary stabbing headache respond quite well to indomethacin, at doses similar to those used for CPH. One report describes resolution of symptoms with melatonin, perhaps implicating the hypothalamic "pacemaker" system in pathogenesis (127). This might suggest similar underlying pathophysiology between primary stabbing headache and cluster headache. The lack of autonomic features in stabbing headache might indicate preferential activation of the trigeminal vascular system with sparing of the cranial parasympathetics. Table 26.10 summarizes the clinical characteristics of short-lasting headaches.

Table 26.10
Clinical Features of Short-Lasting Headaches

Characteristic	Cluster Headache	Chronic Paroxysmal Headache	Episodic Paroxysmal Headache	SUNCT	Idiopathic Stabbing Headache	Trigeminal Neuralgia	Hemicrania Continua
Gender (M:F)	9:1	1:3	1:1	8:1	F>M	F>M	1:1.8
Pain Type	Boring	Throbbing/boring	Throbbing	Stabbing	Stabbing	Stabbing	Steady
Severity	Severe	Severe	Severe	Moderate	Severe	Severe	Moderate
Location	Orbital/temporal	Orbital/temporal	Orbital/temporal	Orbital/temporal	Any	V2/V3 > V1	Unilateral
Attack duration	15–180 min	2–45 min	1–30 min	5–250 sec	<1 sec	<1 sec	Continuous
Attack frequency	1–8/day	1–40/day	3–30/day	1/day to 30/hr	Few to many per day	Few to many per day	May have exacerbations
Autonomic features	Prominent	Prominent	Prominent	Prominent	Absent	Absent	Occasional
Indomethcin-sensitive		Yes	Yes	No	Yes	No	Yes

SECONDARY HEADACHE SYNDROMES

As mentioned earlier, secondary headache syndromes reflect a wide range of intra- and extracranial pathology. In some situations, the diagnosis of secondary headache is straightforward: if a patient develops a new headache at the same time as a brain tumor, it is reasonable to conclude that the headache is secondary to the tumor. However, it is not uncommon for a patient with a primary headache syndrome (such as migraine) to develop worsening of the primary headache in close temporal relationship to a secondary cause of headache (e.g., head trauma). A secondary headache should fulfill the following criteria:

1. Another disorder known to be able to cause headaches has been demonstrated.
2. The headache occurs in close temporal relation to the other disorder and/or there is evidence of a causal relationship.
3. The headache is greatly reduced or disappears within 3 months after successful treatment of spontaneous remission of the causative disorder.

HEAD TRAUMA AND HEADACHE

Headache may occur after injury to the head, neck, or brain. The headache may be related to a structural lesion (e.g., headache attributable to intracranial hematoma), in which case management is directed toward the underlying etiology. A variety of pain patterns that resemble primary headache syndromes may develop after head injury (2). Tension-type headache is the most common pattern, but migraine without aura and a cluster-like pattern have also been described. The role of *litigation* in the development of post-traumatic headache syndromes has been studied, but a conclusive relationship has not been established. A causal relationship between head and/or neck trauma is difficult to establish in patients with very mild head trauma. In such cases, there is often a complex interplay between organic and psychosocial factors.

Post-Traumatic Headache

The IHS recognizes an **acute** and **chronic post-traumatic headache**, with further division into headache associated with mild and moderate or severe head injury. There is no definite relationship between severity of headache and severity of injury, although evidence suggests that post-traumatic headache is less frequent when head injury is more severe (128). The incidence of post-traumatic headache varies widely among studies, ranging from 30–90% of symptomatic patients after head injury (2,129). The headache may be localized or diffuse, episodic or daily. Indeed, the IHS criteria for post-traumatic headache are not primarily concerned with the features of the headache, but with the characteristics of the head injury, and the temporal relationship of the headache to the trauma. By IHS criteria, the headache must occur less than 7 days after head trauma or after regaining consciousness or memory (11). The headache may be accompanied by a multitude of neurological and psychiatric symptoms, most commonly dizziness, irritability, lack of concentration, and intolerance to alcohol. This constellation of features has been called the "post-traumatic syndrome" (2). Less common symptoms include vertigo, tinnitus, insomnia, apathy, easy fatigability, and decreased libido. Nonspecific staring spells, non-vestibular dizziness, and episodic loss of consciousness are rare sequelae of head trauma.

The pathophysiology of post-traumatic headache remains much debated, with advocates for a purely neurogenic mechanism as well as those suggesting a largely psychological etiology (130,131). It is unlikely that a single mechanism or unifying hypothesis can explain all post-traumatic headaches. Late-onset chronic headaches following minor nonconcussive head injury are difficult to explain on a purely neurogenic basis. Conversely, neurobiological factors are likely to play a role in persistent headache beginning hours to days after moderate to severe head trauma. It is probable that a combination of organic and psychosocial factors account for the chronification of post-traumatic symptoms.

Acute pain following head trauma may result from tissue injury to bones, blood vessels, or nerves. Keidel and Ramadan (132) have identified several factors that may contribute to posttraumatic headache:

1. Referred pain from nociceptive input caused by lesions of musculoskeletal, ligamentous, and other soft tissue structures,
2. Activation of meningeal nociceptive afferents due to traumatic epidural, subdural, and subarachnoid bleeding,
3. Stretching of pain-sensitive intracranial structures from increased intracranial pressure,
4. Intracranial hypotension, and
5. Activation of the trigeminovascular system by posttraumatic venous sinus thrombosis.

Diffuse axonal injury may result from angular acceleration of the head, and can occur even in cases of mild head injury. Several researchers have noted that mild head injury patients have more pathologic, radiologic, and electrophysiologic abnormalities than normal controls (130,133). However, many patients with persistent symptoms have no objective findings either on examination, or neuroimaging studies such as CT, MRI, SPECT, or PET.

Multiple studies suggest that compensation issues and malingering are not major factors in post-traumatic headaches (134). However, pre-traumatic psychopathology is more common in chronic post-traumatic headache patients than in patients with chronic TTH and low back pain. A meta-analysis of 2,353 subjects with closed head injury found that more abnormalities and disability were seen in patients with financial incentives (135).

Headache following head injury should always prompt consideration of other secondary trauma-related etiologies, including intracranial hypertension and hypotension, venous sinus thrombosis, carotid or vertebral dissection, intracranial hematoma, and carotid-cavernous fistula. Many of these disorders will be apparent on clinical examination; others may require neurodiagnostic studies, including neuroimaging. Focal deficits on examination, new-onset syncope, impaired arousal and alertness, positional headache, and headache made worse by Valsalva maneuver all require further investigation. As mentioned previously, head injury may trigger or exacerbate a preexisting primary headache syndrome. The mechanism by which this occurs is unknown, although it has been suggested that sensitization may play a role: head trauma may trigger the first attack, initiating the process in predisposed individuals. Indeed, post-traumatic headache is more common in patients with a history of headache (136).

Management of post-traumatic headache is dictated by the clinical syndrome, and by excluding other secondary causes. If a recognizable primary headache syndrome (such as migraine or cluster) has been triggered by head injury, it is treated in the usual manner for that disorder. Coexisting anxiety and depression should be identified and treated. Tricyclic antidepressants are the medications most often used for post-traumatic headache, but few studies have evaluated specific drug regimens. Associated symptoms of irritability, dizziness, depression, and insomnia often respond to tricyclics (2). The SSRIs have been used, with some reports of effectiveness (134). Medication overuse may be a complicating variable that should be addressed if treatment will be successful. Other treatment modalities, including physical therapy, exercise, good sleep hygiene, and psychotherapy, may be of value in certain patients.

HEADACHE ATTRIBUTABLE TO CRANIAL AND CERVICAL VASCULAR DISORDERS

Headache may be associated with vascular disorders. In some of these conditions, such as ischemic or hemorrhagic stroke, the headache is overshadowed by focal neurologic deficits. In others, such as subarachnoid hemorrhage, headache may be the presenting symptom. Headache may be an initial warning symptom in a number of diseases, including carotid artery dissection, giant cell arteritis, and cerebral venous thrombosis. The clinician should therefore be aware of the association of headache with these potentially neurologically and visually devastating diseases. The sudden onset of a new headache should always raise suspicion of a vascular etiology, particularly when the headache is severe ("first and worst headache").

The relationship between headache and cerebral vascular disease was first described by Willis in 1664. Fisher reported the first extensive study of headache and vascular disease in 1968 (137). This study included clinical, arteriographic, and pathologic information as well as detailed descriptions of the headache characteristics. A number of authors have since provided detailed, and often conflicting, information regarding headache and cerebral vascular disease.

Headache and Ischemic Stroke

Headache accompanies stroke in 17–34% of cases (138). It is more frequently associated with strokes in the basilar rather than the carotid territory. The headache onset is usually sudden, moderate in intensity, and has no defining characteristics. It is usually unilateral, and may last more than 24 hours. The presence or absence of head pain is of little practical use regarding stroke etiology, with two exceptions: carotid dissections frequently cause headache, while headache is rare in lacunar infarcts (138). The meninges investing the occipital lobe are innervated by the ophthalmic division of the trigeminal nerve; therefore, posterior circulation strokes may cause ipsilateral eye pain. Since it is not uncommon for patients with homonymous hemianopic defects to localize visual loss to the eye with the temporal field cut, the combination of perceived visual loss and eye pain may lead the physician to assume an ocular cause for the patient's complaints (139). Careful confrontation visual field testing or automated perimetry will clarify the diagnosis.

The mechanism of head pain in stroke is poorly understood. As Fisher has argued (137), the basic atherosclerotic process is nearly always painless. A severe ischemic or hemorrhagic stroke may cause pain by mass effect and stretch of pain-sensitive intracranial structures, but many headache-related strokes are relatively small. The cerebral vessels themselves are pain sensitive, and the pain is likely to be related to activation of perivascular trigeminal afferents. Vasodilation was initially thought to be a potential mechanism for pain (140), but later studies (141,142) suggest that the vasodilation is the result of afferent activation, and the release of vasoactive neuropeptides, are a secondary result, rather than primary cause, of pain.

Transient ischemic attacks (TIAs) may occasionally be associated with headache. Retinal TIAs are less likely to be associated with headache than hemispheric events (143). Since migraine and stroke share similar clinical profiles, it may be difficult to differentiate between migraine with aura and TIA in certain patients (144, 145). The presence of positive visual phenomena such as scintillations suggests migraine as the most likely diagnosis, particularly given a history of episodic headaches with migrainous features. Migraine aura typically lasts 20–30 minutes, in contrast to thrombo-embolic events, which are shorter (1–10 minutes). Migraine visual equivalents have a characteristic build-up or evolution, a feature lacking in TIA. Transient ischemic attacks may rarely cause positive visual phenomena (62, 146), but the duration and lack of build-up help distinguish these episodes from migraine.

Headache and Subarachnoid Hemorrhage

Subarachnoid hemorrhage (SAH) is by far the most common cause of intense and incapacitating headache of abrupt onset, and is associated with high morbidity and mortality (2,147,148). Approximately 15–25% of patients die prior to reaching the hospital, and many survivors are left with varying degrees of neurologic disability. Headache occurs in 85–95% of patients (147). The headache is sudden and explosive in onset, often associated with nausea or vomiting, and is classically described by patients as the "worst headache of my life." The headache is usually followed by pain radiating into the occipital or cervical region. If the headache resolves the patient may not seek medical attention, or may do so and be misdiagnosed as having a migraine or sinus headache. This is referred to as a sentinel headache, or "warning leak," and may occur in 20–60% of patients (148). The headache usually occurs 2–20 days prior to the onset of major subarachnoid hemorrhage and lasts 1–2 days. In two-thirds of patients it is associated with nausea, vomiting, neck pain, or lethargy. In such patients, a high index of suspicion mandates further investigations, including neuroimaging and lumbar puncture. Other presenting symptoms include seizure, lethargy, photophobia, and altered mental status. Terson's syndrome is classically characterized by vitreous hemorrhage associated with subarachnoid hemorrhage secondary to aneurysmal rupture, and may occur in 20–40% of patients with SAH (149). Terson's syndrome has also been reported to occur with epidural and subdural hematomas. The presence of an otherwise unexplained vitreous or preretinal hemorrhage in a patient with new onset headache should raise concern about SAH.

Headache has been reported in approximately 18% of patients with unruptured aneurysms (150). The headache is generally nonspecific, and the relationship with the aneurysm remains debatable. A notable exception is the acute onset of a painful, pupil-involved third nerve palsy, in which case an expanding aneurysm is the default diagnosis until proven otherwise (149).

Headache and Subdural Hematomas

Headaches frequently occur in patients with post-traumatic subdural hematomas (152). In a series reported by McKissock (153), headaches were reported by 11% of patients with acute subdural hematomas, 53% with subacute hematomas, and 81% with chronic subdural hematomas. Because many of the patients with acute subdural hematomas have alterations of consciousness, headaches in this group of patients may be underreported.

Headaches in patients with subdural hematomas vary widely in severity and may be paroxysmal or constant (152). They are usually bilateral; however, when they are unilateral, they are usually on the side of the hematoma.

In most patients, the subdural hematoma occurs after obvious closed head trauma, such as that which occurs in a fall or a severe motor vehicle accident. In other cases, however, exposure to acceleration-deceleration forces, such as those encountered while riding on a roller coaster, can tear bridging cerebral veins, leading to a subdural hematoma (154). The same mechanism may be responsible for subdural hematomas that occur in patients with severe whiplash injuries unassociated with direct head trauma.

Acute subdural hematomas are readily identified by CT scanning. Small, chronic subdural hematomas are occasionally missed on CT; MRI may be more sensitive in such situations.

Headache and Epidural Hamartoma

The classic profile of a patient with an acute epidural hematoma is one who sustains even a minor head injury with or without initial loss of consciousness followed by a lucid interval, but who then deteriorates into coma, usually within 12 hours of the injury (155). Chronic epidural hematomas, however, may produce a persistent headache that is often associated with nausea, vomiting, and memory impairment, suggesting a post-traumatic syndrome. Eventually, however, focal deficits develop, and the correct diagnosis is made (156). As with acute subdural hematomas, CT scan is the initial diagnostic test of choice.

Headache and Intraparenchymal Hemorrhage

Patients with acute intraparenchymal hemorrhage typically experience a sudden severe headache. The hemorrhage may result from a variety of causes, including hypertension, a vascular malformation, a ruptured aneurysm, an infarction, or necrosis within a tumor. In most cases, the headache is generalized, severe, and associated with neurologic deficits that reflect the location and size of the hemorrhage. In some cases, the clinical picture suggests the etiology of the hemorrhage. For instance, the syndrome of occipital apoplexy—sudden headache, stiff neck, and a homonymous visual field defect—is almost pathognomonic for a ruptured occipital lobe arteriovenous malformation (AVM) (157,158).

Headache and Unruptured Vascular Malformation

Unruptured AVMs may produce headache. In a patient with a long history of stereotypic headache that is always unilateral, one should consider the possibility of an AVM rather than migraine with aura (159).

Periodic headaches, sometimes ipsilateral to the lesions, occur in 5–25% of patients with AVMs (160). The headaches may resemble migraine and may be preceded by visual aura. The patient may thus be thought to have migraine with aura. The headaches generally resolve after treatment of the AVM (161). Because the prevalence of migraine in the general population is so high, it is unclear if the headaches associated with intracranial vascular malformations are coincidental or causally related.

Bruyn (161) reviewed epidemiologic data on patients with vascular malformations and migraine-like headaches in the Netherlands. He showed convincingly that the concurrence of the two conditions is probably not fortuitous. Raskin (162) evaluated a large number of such patients whose headaches resolved after the malformations were treated by a variety of methods, including proton beam irradiation, embolization, and surgical extirpation. The head pain gradually diminished in many patients after treatment. Similarly, following embolization, the malformation may dramatically disappear on angiography, and headache may also abruptly subside. Although intracerebral AVMs may generate migraine-like headaches with and without visual aura, some patients continue to experience intractable headaches after treatment has totally eradicated a vascular malformation. Raskin (162) treated 12 patients with cerebral vascular malformations and intractable headaches with repeated doses of intravenous dihydroergotamine (DHE) on an 8-hour schedule. All patients became headache free within 48 hours.

Many of the headaches in these patients are resolved by approaching them therapeutically as having "migraine." Homan and colleagues (163) suggested that perturbation of forebrain projections from the midbrain raphe by the regional ischemia produced by these malformations may underlie the production of migraine-like symptoms by these lesions.

Arterial Dissections

Internal carotid artery dissection is an important cause of head and facial pain. The headache is generally of sudden onset, unilateral, and located in the orbital, periorbital, and frontal region (11,137). Neck pain often accompanies the headache. The pain is moderate to severe, and often throbbing in nature. Biousse et al. (164) studied 67 patients with carotid dissection. Pain was present in 75% of patients; in 60%, pain was the inaugural symptom, while in others the headache followed the onset of other neurological symptoms. Horner's syndrome often accompanies carotid dissection, and reflects disruption of postganglionic sympathetic fibers destined for the eyelid retractors and iris dilator. The incidence of Horner's syndrome in carotid dissection ranges from 31–58% (146,164,165). Some patients may experience transient episodes of visual loss. Other, less common neuro-ophthalmic manifestations of carotid dissection include anterior and posterior ischemic optic neuropathy, central retinal artery occlusion, ocular motor nerve palsies, and ocular ischemic syndrome. Other symptoms include tinnitus, subjective bruit, and hemispheric TIA and stroke (146).

Arterial dissections may occur secondary to head or neck trauma, or spontaneously. It has been reported after relatively minor trauma, such as nose-blowing, sports activities, and high acceleration neck turns during roller coaster rides. Systemic diseases associated with dissection include Marfan's and Ehlers-Danlos' syndromes, syphilis, and fibromuscular dysplasia. Carotid dissection may be diagnosed by MRI and MRA, carotid duplex studies, or conventional cerebral angiography.

Treatment is controversial, but most physicians treat acute, symptomatic dissections with intravenous heparin followed by a 3–6 month course of warfarin. Most patients with spontaneous dissections experience excellent clinical and angiographic recovery, usually within several months. Carotid dissection should always be considered in a patient with a painful Horner's syndrome, head or neck pain preceding an ischemic event, or severe, persistent head or neck pain of sudden onset.

Carotidynia was originally described as neck pain lasting less than 2 weeks with tenderness to palpation over the carotid bifurcation. It has been shown that a number of different distinct diseases (including carotid dissection) may cause pain fulfilling previous IHS criteria (166). Several reports (167,168) have described MRI signal abnormalities in the tissue surrounding the symptomatic artery in patients with symptoms suggesting carotidynia. However, the specificity of these findings, as well as the relationship of the signal changes to the pain, remains unclear. The IHS has therefore removed carotidynia as a separate entity from the second edition (11).

Pituitary Apoplexy

Pituitary apoplexy is an acute, life-threatening condition usually associated with hemorrhagic infarction of the pituitary gland (169). This most frequently occurs with a preexisting pituitary tumor. Sheehan's syndrome refers to ischemic infarction of the pituitary gland after postpartum hemorrhage and hypovolemia. Purely ischemic infarction, with hemorrhagic transformation, of a pituitary macroadenoma may occur as well. The condition is thought to occur due to compression of capillaries or outstripping of vascular supply as the tumor expands. The headache is generally of sudden onset and severe. It is usually retro-orbital, frontal, or diffuse. Neuro-ophthalmic manifestations include unilateral or bilateral visual loss (if there is upward expansion and compression of the chiasm), or ophthalmoplegia (if there is lateral extension into the cavernous sinuses). MRI is the study of choice for diagnosis. Urgent neurosurgical evacuation and management of panhypopituitarism are the mainstays of management (169).

Giant Cell Arteritis

Giant cell arteritis (GCA) is a T-cell-mediated vasculitis with preferential involvement of medium and large cranial arteries. It is primarily a disease of the elderly, with the highest incidence in patients older than 70 years (170). A new headache or dramatic change in previous headache in an elderly patient is the most common presentation of GCA. The incidence of headache in GCA is over 80%. The pain may be localized to the superficial temporal artery, or other branches of the external carotid artery, but is often nonspecific in character and quality. Since the occipital arteries are often involved, pain and localized tenderness in this region is not uncommon, and should be sought by history and examination. The severity of the headache is variable; in one series, headache was the reason for referral in only 41 of 175 patients with GCA (171). Only a few individuals have localized pain, induration, and tenderness over the temporal arteries or erythematous nodules along the vessels, though it is worth looking for these physical signs. In some cases the temporal arteries are palpably indurated and may show a ''ropy'' appearance beneath the skin. Diffuse tenderness of the scalp, face, or oral mucosa results from ischemia secondary to widespread arteritic involvement of extracranial vessels. Some patients describe ''head pains'' rather than headache, indicating the relatively superficial nature of the discomfort. True jaw claudication is nearly pathognomonic for the disease. Vascular jaw claudication results from ischemia to the muscles of mastication, and reflects involvement of both the internal and external carotid artery circulation. Constitutional symptoms, such as fatigue, weight loss, and night sweats, may be present.

Polymyalgia rheumatica (PMR) is also a disease of the elderly, and may coexist with GCA. The clinical picture of PMR consists of pain and stiffness in the shoulder or pelvic girdles. Laboratory studies, including the Westergren sedimentation rate and C-reactive protein, are often abnormal in patients with GCA. Even with a classic clinical picture, the diagnosis still rests upon tissue demonstrating histopathology consistent with GCA (170).

Patients with GCA have a high risk of losing vision, in most cases secondary to arteritic anterior ischemic optic neuropathy. In an elderly patient with new onset headache, the history and examination (including demographic factors) provide the most useful clues regarding the possibility of GCA. In particular, new-onset headache and jaw claudication in an elderly patient should likely be considered GCA until proven otherwise. In most cases, it is the entire clinical picture measured against the practitioner's clinical judgment and level of suspicion which guides management (see Chapter 44).

In most cases, the headache responds dramatically to steroids, often after the first or second dose. Indeed, the IHS criteria for GCA includes major improvement or disappearance of headache within 3 days of treatment (11). It should be noted that many headaches, including migraine, might be steroid responsive. Therefore, improvement of headache after treatment, although expected in GCA, is by no means diagnostic.

HEADACHE ATTRIBUTABLE TO INTRACRANIAL INFECTIONS

Headaches that accompany intracranial infections are usually severe. In patients with brain abscesses, the headache may be related more to the mass than to the infectious process. In such cases, the headache is indistinguishable from that caused by neoplasm except that it tends to be more constant. Bacterial meningitis may present fulminantly, with seizures and altered consciousness. Neuro-ophthalmic find-

ings are often limited to those attributable to elevated intracranial pressure (e.g., papilledema, sixth nerve palsy).

Headaches may occur in any of the various types of meningitis. There is associated cervical rigidity, tenderness of the scalp, and almost always a positive Kernig's sign. The headache itself is continuous and usually nonlocalized. If intracranial pressure is elevated, the headache may be worse when supine.

The pain of inflammation, like the pain provoked by injury or by blood in the subarachnoid space, appears to be caused by the concerted action of neuroactive peptides that are contained in whole blood and are formed from inactive plasma precursors.

HEADACHE ATTRIBUTABLE TO NONVASCULAR INTRACRANIAL DISORDERS

Headache Associated with High and Low Cerebrospinal Fluid (CSF) Pressure

Both increased and decreased intracranial pressure (ICP) can result in headache. Figure 26.14 reviews the pathways of CSF flow. The causes of elevated ICP include intracranial mass lesion causing obstructive hydrocephalus, meningeal processes (meningitis, meningeal carcinomatosis) resulting in impaired absorption at the arachnoid villi, elevated cerebral venous sinus pressure (venous sinus thrombosis, superior vena cava syndrome), overproduction of CSF (from a choroid plexus papilloma), certain toxins and metabolic disturbances, and idiopathic intracranial hypertension (IIH). In many of these conditions, the mechanism of headache is multifactorial, with increased ICP playing a small or large

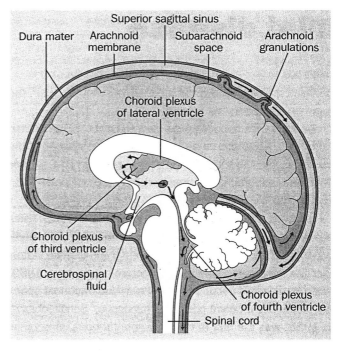

Figure 26.14.   Pathways of CSF flow.

role. In IIH, and similar conditions, the elevated ICP plays a more dominant role in pain generation. Intracranial hypotension results from excessive drainage of CSF; this is due to either an iatrogenic (postlumbar puncture or postneurosurgical) or a spontaneous CSF leak. Patients with headaches related to high or low ICP often describe a positional component: i.e., the headache is worse when erect (low pressure) or supine (high pressure). Although not always present, a positional headache should raise concern about elevated or decreased ICP. Early morning headache, and early morning nausea and emesis, suggest increased ICP. A classic cause of positional headache is a colloid cyst of the third ventricle. The presumed mechanism is a "ball-valve effect"—when the patient suddenly changes position the tumor obstructs the third ventricle and causes a rapid increase in ICP (2). Intracranial masses and meningitis often have accompanying neurologic symptoms, including focal deficits, meningismus, altered level of consciousness, or seizures.

Idiopathic Intracranial Hypertension

The majority of patients with IIH experience headaches, although it is not rare for asymptomatic papilledema to be discovered on routine eye examination. The headache is often retro-orbital, pulsatile, and may be worsened with eye movement (172). Some patients may report worsening of headache upon awakening. The headache may have migrainous features, such as photophobia, nausea, and vomiting. Indeed, migraine and other primary headache syndromes often coexist in these patients. Chronic daily headache secondary to medication overuse is not uncommon in these patients (172). It is therefore critical to be certain the IIH has been securely diagnosed according to the modified Dandy criteria, and that a thorough and complete headache and medication history has been taken. A common situation is a patient with securely diagnosed IIH, normal or stable visual function, and intractable headaches. It is a disservice to the patient to assume that the headache is solely related to elevated ICP and to proceed accordingly (e.g., with increased doses of acetazolamide or CSF diversion procedures). Reviewing medication use and headache history, and a short trial of a broad-spectrum headache agent such as amitriptyline is reasonable in such cases. Repeating a lumbar puncture may be useful, primarily to demonstrate any improvement in headache. In selected cases, when it is clear that elevated ICP is the major cause for headache and the patient is refractory to maximal medical therapy, CSF diversion procedures might be considered. Ventriculoperitoneal and lumboperitoneal shunting are relatively safe, but carry substantial risks of long-term shunt failure, overdrainage, and shunt infection (173).

Intracranial Hypotension

Intracranial hypotension, also called low-pressure syndrome, is due in most cases to a CSF leak. The causes may be divided into symptomatic and spontaneous. The syndrome is characterized by an orthostatic headache (headache worsened when erect) and low CSF volume (2). Indeed, some authors prefer the term CSF hypovolemia, since there are reports of patients with normal CSF pressure presenting with otherwise typical features of the syndrome (174).

Headache is the most common clinical symptom of intracranial hypotension, occurring in nearly all patients. The headache may be frontal, occipital, or diffuse. The headache is worsened in the erect position, and relieved by recumbency. The pain is generally severe, dull or throbbing in nature, and is frequently exacerbated by head-shaking, coughing, sneezing, and Valsalva. The headache of intracranial hypotension may be secondary, in part, to descent of the brain with traction on pain-sensitive intracranial structures. Associated symptoms include nausea, vomiting, and dizziness, and are more likely to occur when the headache is severe.

Lumbar puncture (LP) is the most common cause of symptomatic intracranial hypotension (174). Although headache occurs in 15–30% of patients after LP, whether all such patients have intracranial hypotension is unclear. Onset of headache occurs in most patients within 48 hours, although a delay of 12 days has been reported. In addition to LP, craniotomy and spinal surgery may cause intracranial hypotension as a result of dural tear or avulsion of a nerve root. Spontaneous intracranial hypotension (SIH) was felt to be a rare cause of low CSF pressure, but recent evidence suggests that SIH may be under-recognized. The mechanism of low CSF pressure in SIH in not known, but there are several potential mechanisms (2), including decreased CSF production, increased CSF absorption, and CSF leakage from small, occult, dural tears.

Neuro-ophthalmic manifestations of intracranial hypotension are rare, with the most common being unilateral or bilateral sixth nerve palsies (2,174). The etiology likely involves caudal displacement of the brain with stretch of the nerve. Divergence insufficiency has also been reported. Third nerve palsies may also occur, but such patients have also had large, bilateral, subdural hematomas, with compression of the brainstem and early herniation (175). Superior binasal visual field defects have also been reported, but the mechanism was unclear: the authors postulated that downward prolapse of the optic chiasm may have been responsible (176). Some of the associated neurologic and neuro-ophthalmic features may be due to secondary effects of intracranial hypotension. Subdural fluid collections may occur and cause mass effect, cerebellar tonsillar herniation may cause brainstem compression, and the dilation and engorgement of cortical veins may result in venous sinus thrombosis.

Neuroimaging studies may yield valuable clues suggesting intracranial hypotension. Diffuse, linear, pachymeningeal gadolinium enhancement was noted in 83% of patients in one series (175). The enhancement is frequently thick and uninterrupted. There is no nodularity, and no enhancement of the leptomeninges (i.e., no in-depth enhancement of the cortical sulci), either of which would suggest a primary inflammatory or neoplastic etiology. Subdural fluid collections may occur, and are thought to result from tears in bridging veins. There may be varying degrees of cerebellar tonsillar descent on MRI, resembling Chiari malformation. Other features more easily seen on MRI include reduction in size and effacement of the prepontine cisterns, inferior displacement of the optic chiasm, and reduction and effacement of the perichiasmatic cisterns. Lumbar puncture typically shows opening pressure of 0–70 cm H_2O; however, the opening pressure may be normal. CSF analysis may show mild lymphocytic pleocytosis; this may result from a local inflammatory reaction at the site of CSF leak. Increased red blood cells and xanthochromia may occur, as well as elevated CSF protein. These findings have been attributed to compensatory vasodilation and diapedesis of red blood cells and protein (177). Radionuclide cisternography may demonstrate a dural leak.

Treatment of symptomatic intracranial hypotension is primarily directed toward the underlying etiology. Post-traumatic and postsurgical CSF leaks should be identified and repaired if accessible. The treatment of post-LP headache and SIH are similar. Noninvasive, nonpharmacologic treatments such as bedrest and an abdominal binder are often initially employed, although the effectiveness of these measures is uncertain. Methylxanthines such as caffeine and theophylline decrease cerebral blood flow and increase cerebral vascular resistance; they also increase CSF production by stimulating the sodium-potassium pumps. Caffeine, given either orally or intravenously, is usually the first-line pharmacologic treatment. Well-designed studies (2,174) report a success rate of 70–85%. Oral caffeine dose may be as high as 300 mg. The epidural blood patch is the most commonly used treatment for persistent low-pressure headache, and has the highest success rate (96% in some studies); 10–20 ml of autologous blood is infused into the epidural space under sterile conditions. The presumed mechanism of action involves both volume replacement (immediate effect), and tamponade of the dural leak (latent effect). Some patients, particularly those with SIH, may require repeated blood patches.

Many patients with post-LP headache and SIH have a benign course, with spontaneous resolution in many. Indeed, the rate of spontaneous resolution may be higher than reported, since the syndrome is often under-diagnosed. Poor outcomes have been seen in patients with large subdural fluid collections, and mass effect on the diencephalon (175).

HEADACHE ATTRIBUTABLE TO DISORDERS OF HOMEOSTASIS

Patients with systemic hypertension may develop headaches in the absence of increased intracranial pressure. Although acute paroxysmal hypertension is a well-recognized cause of headache, it is uncertain whether chronic systemic hypertension can result in headache.

The relationship between cerebral blood flow (CBF) and mean arterial pressure is altered in patients with systemic hypertension in that the range of blood pressure over which autoregulatory responses maintains constant CBF is higher (178). There is evidence that this phenomenon occurs primarily at the level of the small-resistance cerebral arteries (179). This shift in cerebral autoregulation may be caused by damaged small arterial walls, or it may be a central response to hypertension. Because the shift is quite variable among hypertensive patients, the compensatory vascular re-

sponse may be causally related to hypertensive headache, although there are no data to support this possibility.

It is estimated that headache occurs in 75% of patients with hypertensive encephalopathy. The headaches associated with hypertensive encephalopathy are similar to those produced by intracranial tumors and may be caused by cerebral edema (180). In this setting, there initially is marked vasoconstriction of cerebral vessels, resulting in ischemia and localized edema. Acute elevation in blood pressure may cause focal cerebral edema or intraparenchymal hemorrhage and produce headache by these mechanisms. In hypertensive encephalopathy, the ophthalmoscopic changes are crucial to the diagnosis; this is further substantiated by neurologic symptoms and signs, urinary changes, and elevation of the serum urea nitrogen. In some instances, hypertensive encephalopathy produces optic disc swelling that is indistinguishable from that produced by an intracranial mass lesion. In most cases, the disc swelling is true papilledema. In other cases, however, it seems to be a local phenomenon. Interestingly, the papilledema of hypertensive encephalopathy is not necessarily associated with the typical ophthalmoscopic findings usually seen in hypertensive retinopathy, such as retinal hemorrhages, cotton wool spots (soft exudates), and narrowing of arteries.

High-Altitude Headache

Experimentally-induced cerebral hypoxemia, especially when coupled with an increase in carbon dioxide tension in the blood, results in the dilation of cerebral vessels, notably the arteries and arterioles (181). These intense, throbbing headaches occur within 24 hours after sudden ascent to altitudes above 9,800 feet (3,000 meters) and are associated with at least one or more symptoms typical of high altitude: Cheyne-Stokes respirations at night, a desire to overbreathe, and dyspnea. Other symptoms of high-altitude sickness include a sensation of fullness of the head, hot flushes of the face, photophobia, injection of the ocular mucosa, and deep cyanosis. Altitude headaches are uncommon below 8,000 feet, appear with increasing frequency at higher elevations, and above 12,000 feet are more or less universal in persons not acclimated to altitude. Headaches similar to those experienced by patients at high altitude may occur in patients with acute mountain sickness, acute pulmonary edema of high altitude, and chronic mountain sickness in otherwise well-acclimated subjects (182).

It is likely that high-altitude headaches are caused by cerebrovascular distention. They can usually be prevented by ingestion of acetazolamide before the ascent to high altitude.

HEADACHE ATTRIBUTABLE TO DISORDERS OF THE EYES

Ocular disease may cause headaches and may be overlooked by the primary care physician and general neurologist. It is important to be aware of these ocular conditions, both to provide accurate and effective management, and to spare the patient unnecessary testing and treatments. Since eye pain is ultimately mediated by the trigeminal nerve, many primary and secondary headache disorders may present with localized eye pain. The history may provide important clues to an ocular etiology. Conjunctival injection, pupillary abnormalities, and corneal edema are common symptoms in eye-related headaches, but are not always present. Visual loss and diplopia associated with head and/or eye pain should suggest an ocular etiology. A complete ophthalmic examination should be performed, with careful inspection of the eyelids, conjunctiva and orbits, biomicroscopic examination of the anterior segment, and measurement of intraocular pressure. Many primary headache syndromes, particularly the trigeminal autonomic cephalgias, may present with pain localized around the eye; in such cases, excluding an ocular etiology allows proper diagnosis and management.

Angle Closure Glaucoma

Primary angle closure glaucoma results when resistance to aqueous flow occurs at the pupillary margin in patients with anatomically shallow anterior chambers: this results in a large force vector posteriorly directed form the iris to the lens. This causes the peripheral iris to billow forward, and obstruct the trabecular meshwork. Common precipitating factors include mydriasis due to stress, medications (including those used for pharmacologic mydriasis), and conditions of dim illumination (183). Acute angle closure presents with cloudy vision and eye pain. The patient may report colored halos around a polychromatic white light. The pain is often severe, and may radiate widely. Nausea and vomiting may accompany the headache. Examination reveals conjunctival injection, and a mid-dilated pupil, as well as clouding of the cornea (due to stromal edema). The globe is hard and tender to palpation, and intraocular pressure (IOP) is usually markedly elevated at the time of the attack (40–80 mm Hg). Subacute angle closure often presents with episodes of conjunctival injection, eye pain, and blurred vision. The symptoms may occur when watching television in a dim room (promoting mydriasis and increasing iris-lens contact). The pain is often mild and dull. In many cases, attacks resolve spontaneously, and IOP is normal on examination. Gonioscopy will often reveal a shallow anterior chamber and peripheral anterior synechiae. The optic disc may be cupped, reflecting previous episodes of prolonged elevation of IOP. Angle closure may be mistaken for cluster headache; however, the autonomic symptoms are more prominent in cluster, the pupil is miotic rather than mid-dilated, and vision and IOP are normal during the attack. A history of recurrent episodes of eye pain, conjunctival injection, and cloudy vision should suggest recurrent angle closure as the diagnosis.

Refractive Errors

"Eyestrain" may cause a mild, persistent brow ache that is aggravated by prolonged visual tasks at the distance where vision is most impaired (183). The pain is mild, and has no associated symptoms such as photophobia, nausea, or vomiting. The IHS criteria (11) require a close temporal relationship between the headache and the visual task, and resolution of the headache within 7 days of correction of refractive error. The visual tasks associated with these headaches are extended and prolonged.

Uveitis

Inflammation of the uveal tract (iris, ciliary body, choroids) is called uveitis. Uveitis may be anterior (iris and/or ciliary body), intermediate (pars plana), or posterior (retina, choroids, vitreous). Uveitis may also be characterized by type of inflammation (granulomatous or nongranulomatous), and course (acute, subacute, chronic). The differential diagnosis of uveitis is broad, and beyond the scope of this section. Patients with anterior uveitis (iritis or iridocyclitis) will typically report photophobia and pain in or around the involved eye. Pain is induced by shining a light in the uninvolved eye (consensual photophobia). Visual acuity is variably affected. Examination may show dilated conjunctival vessels and inflammation in the anterior segment, termed "cell" (white blood cells) and "flare" (proteinaceous debris). These finding are best observed with a biomicroscope (slit lamp); in severe cases of anterior uveitis, a layering of proteinaceous material (pseudohypopyon) may be visible on general inspection. Autonomic symptoms are minimal, distinguishing uveitis from the TACs; IOP is generally normal or low, in contrast to acute angle closure glaucoma. Posterior uveitis may cause minimal conjunctival injection and pain, but often has a more serious visual prognosis. Although both anterior and posterior uveitis may be associated with a diverse group of systemic inflammatory, infectious, and neoplastic diseases, 25–30% of cases are idiopathic. Features more suggestive of an associated systemic disease include bilaterality, granulomatous features, and posterior segment involvement.

The mechanism of the pain of uveitis seems to be related to a breakdown of the blood-aqueous barrier that allows the release of kinins and prostaglandin E1 from polymorphonuclear leukocytes, and the release of substance P and other polypeptides (as well as prostaglandin E2) from the iris itself. These substances are thought to stimulate chemoreceptors in the ciliary body nerve plexus (184).

Optic Neuritis

Pain in or around the eye is present in more than 90% of patients with acute demyelinating optic neuritis. It is usually mild, but it may be severe and may in some cases be more debilitating to the patient than the loss of vision. It may precede or occur concurrently with visual loss, usually is exacerbated by eye movement, and generally lasts no more than a few days. The Optic Neuritis Treatment Trial (ONTT) reported pain in 92% of patients, which was worsened by eye movement in 87% (185). Swartz et al (186) hypothesized that the pain is initiated by inflammation of the optic nerve in the apex of the orbit, where the extraocular muscles are firmly attached to the sheaths of the nerve. In support of this hypothesis, Lepore (187) reported that among 101 eyes with optic neuritis, pain was more commonly present with retrobulbar neuritis than with papillitis; however, in the ONTT, pain was present in 93% of 295 eyes with retrobulbar neuritis and in 90% of 162 eyes with papillitis. Fazzone and Kupersmith (188) found a correlation between pain and length of optic nerve enhancement on MR imaging in patients with optic neuritis. The presence of pain is a helpful differentiating feature from anterior ischemic optic neuropathy, particularly when it is severe and when it occurs or worsens during movement of the eyes. Swartz (186) reported that the incidence of pain in patients with anterior ischemic optic neuropathy (AION) was only 12%. The pain is often described as much more severe by patients with optic neuritis than by patients with AION, and patients with AION rarely experience pain on movement of the eyes.

HEADACHE ATTRIBUTABLE TO A SUBSTANCE OR ITS WITHDRAWAL

Medication Overuse Headache

Medication overuse headache (MOH), also called analgesic rebound headache, was first described in 1951 by Peters and Horton (189). Potentially all analgesic drugs, including over-the-counter agents, may lead to MOH. The most common cause of migraine occurring 15 or more days a month, or a mixed migraine/tension-type headache, is medication overuse. In headache subspecialty practices, medication overuse is the most common cause of intractability (190). The IHS criteria define MOH primarily by treatment days per month (11). The regularity of treatment is important, as well; bunching of treatment days with long periods of no medication intake is less likely to result in MOH. The headache is generally dull, constant, and diffuse. The headache may vary in severity and location. There is evidence of tolerance to analgesics over time, and withdrawal symptoms are observed when medications are discontinued abruptly. Many patients with MOH have a preexisting headache type (usually migraine); their daily headaches may be a mixture of chronic daily headache with superimposed episodic migraine attacks. Recent data suggest that triptans will soon be recognized as the most common group of medications to cause MOH (191). Indeed, the second edition of IHS has a separate entry for triptan overuse (11). Patients with triptan overuse headache typically describe a unilateral, pulsating headache with migrainous qualities.

Chronic daily headache (CDH) accounts for up to 80% of patients seen in headache centers (190). The prevalence of CDH in population-based studies is 4%, with chronic migraine as the most common subtype. Transformed migraine refers to previously episodic migraine headaches that have transformed into a daily or near-daily headache occurring 15 or more day a month. Risk factors for the development of chronic migraine include female gender, high incidence of headaches before transformation, obesity, hypertension, stressful life events, alcohol overuse, and sleep disturbance (192). Recent evidence suggests that medication overuse may be an additional risk factor for the development of CDH. However, while medication overuse is common in patients with frequent headaches, it is unclear whether it is a causal or exacerbating factor. Zwart et al. (193) performed a longitudinal, population-based study spanning 11 years, and found that medication overuse predicted the development of CDH. Since baseline headache status was not collected, the authors could not exclude the possibility that frequent analgesic use was simply a marker for frequent headache; they also could not determine if baseline headache type was a predictor for CDH.

Not all patients who overuse medications develop MOH or CDH. In one study of arthritis clinic patients, all of whom regularly used analgesics, only 8% had CDH. All of these patients had a history of migraine (194). Another study of arthritis clinic patients found no increased incidence of headaches among those consuming large amounts of analgesics (195). It is possible that MOH may be limited to individuals predisposed to suffer headaches.

The mechanisms contributing to chronification of a preexisting headache and MOH are likely multi-factorial. Psychological factors that may play a role include the reinforcing effect of pain relief induced by analgesics. Certain analgesics are physiologically addicting, and may lead to withdrawal headache. This in turn prompts additional self-medication by the patient, contributing to chronification. Barbiturates (present in many prescription drug ''cocktails'' for migraine), opioids, and caffeine are the drugs most likely to result in withdrawal headache. Concomitant medical problems, sleep disturbance, and depression may also play a role.

A careful medication and headache history is critical to identify patients with MOH. In patients with a pre-existing headache syndrome, standard treatments are unlikely to be effective as long as medication overuse persists. Drug withdrawal is the treatment of choice for MOH. The withdrawal may be done as an out-patient or in-patient. A consensus paper from the German Migraine Society recommended out-patient withdrawal for patients who do not take barbiturates or tranquilizers, and are highly motivated. Patient undergoing acute withdrawal should be treated with supportive measures (including fluid replacement), as well as the institution of preventive agents such as amitriptyline or valproate. Some center regularly use intravenous dihydroergotamine for several days to help break the cycle of CDH with medication overuse (196).

CRANIAL NEURALGIAS AND CENTRAL CAUSES OF FACIAL PAIN

Pain in the head and neck is mediated by afferent fibers in the trigeminal nerve, nervus intermedius, glossopharyngeal and vagus nerves, and the upper cervical roots via the occipital nerves. Irritation of the nerves by compression, distortion, or a lesion in the central pathways may give rise to pain experienced in the innervated area. In some cases there is a structural abnormality demonstrated by imaging which is responsible for nerve irritation, but in many cases there is no apparent cause for the pain. Trigeminal neuralgia (tic douloureux), a common cranial neuralgia, is covered in detail in Chapter 25 and will not be discussed further here. One feature common to these disorders is the quality of the pain: neuralgic pain is typically electric or burning in character. Patient may report provocation of symptoms by cold temperature or light touch over the skin of the affected area (allodynia). The attacks are generally brief and the pain is often severe. Autonomic symptoms are uncommon.

Occipital Neuralgia

Occipital neuralgia is a term that is often used broadly (and incorrectly) for any pain in the occipital region. It should be reserved for paroxysmal, unilateral, jabbing, burning, or stabbing pain in the distribution of the greater or lesser occipital nerve. There may be diminished sensation or dysesthesias in the affected area (197), as well as tenderness to palpation of the affected nerve. The pain often radiates to the frontal region. Occipital neuralgia may be caused by any lesion (compressive, traumatic, inflammatory) of the greater occipital nerve anywhere along its course from the C2 dorsal root to the periphery. However, in many cases, a clear-cut etiology is not identified. Myofascial trigger points in the suboccipital muscles may cause referred pain that may be difficult to distinguish from occipital neuralgia. A complete history and physical examination should identify a specific underlying etiology. MRI of the brain and cervical spine may be indicated in cases where a compressive lesion is suspected. Treatment of the neuralgia typically involves medications commonly used in neuralgic pain, including gabapentin, amitriptyline, carbamazepine, and baclofen. Many patients experience relief after local anesthetic injections (197,198); indeed, this may aid the diagnosis of the syndrome. However, section of the nerve rarely results in sustained pain relief (197).

Supraorbital Neuralgia and Other Terminal Branch Neuralgias

Supraorbital neuralgia is an uncommon disorder characterized by pain in the area supplied by the supraorbital nerve. Patients describe paroxysmal or constant pain in the supraorbital notch and the medial forehead. There is often tenderness over the nerve with palpation. Other terminal branch neuralgias, including infraorbital, lingual, alveolar, and mental neuralgia, have also been described, and are included in the second edition of HIS (11). The syndromes may develop secondary to trauma, surgery, or compression, or may be idiopathic. Treatment generally consists of local anesthetic blockade or nerve ablation (199).

Acute Herpes Zoster and Post-Herpetic Neuralgia (PHN)

Herpes zoster occurs due to reactivation of dormant varicella zoster virus within neurons. Herpes zoster affects the trigeminal ganglion in 10–15% of patients, with the ophthalmic division involved in 80% of these patients (200). It is more common in the elderly and the immunocompromised, and such patients are more likely to develop post-herpetic neuralgia.

The pain is typically steady and sustained, and often quite severe. The quality of the pain is generally burning and aching. It may be experienced in the areas innervated by any part of the trigeminal nerve, although the forehead is most common. A characteristic vesicular rash follows the onset of pain by several hours or days. In rare case, the pain may not be followed by a rash (201). Paresthesias, dysesthesias, and electric shock-like pain may be reported. Ophthalmic herpes may be associated with diplopia and strabismus resulting from damage to the third, fourth, or sixth cranial nerves. Rarely, ischemic optic neuropathy may result due to occlusion of the short posterior ciliary arteries (202). A localized, infectious vasculitis is the presumed mechanism. Visual loss more commonly results from corneal involvement. In many patients, the pain persists after the eruption clears. The IHS defines post-herpetic neuralgia in the following manner (11):

1. Pain in the distribution of a nerve or nerve division in the head,
2. Herpetic eruption in the territory of the nerve,
3. Pain precedes herpetic eruption by less than 7 days, and
4. Pain lasts longer than 3 months.

Patients with ophthalmic herpes zoster are more likely to develop post-herpetic neuralgia. Other risk factors include advanced age, immuno-compromised state, and diabetes mellitus (203). The disorder only occurs in 5% of patients under the age of 40 years with acute zoster, but develops in 75% of those over the age of 70 years. The pain is constant, deep, and burning, and may be provoked by light touch. Sleep is often interrupted. The pain may spontaneously remit: after 3 years 56% of patients are free of pain (204). Treatment of acute herpes zoster with antivirals within 72 hours after the onset of rash may reduce the probability of developing post-herpetic neuralgia, or ameliorate the course. Antiviral agents such as famciclovir and valacyclovir have been shown to shorten the duration of post-herpetic neuralgia in patients older than 50 years (205). Oral glucocorticoids may speed the resolution of acute zoster pain, but it is not clear whether they prevent PHN. Once PHN is established, treatment is directed toward symptoms. Tricyclic antidepressants such as amitriptyline are commonly used, although caution must be used in the elderly given the anticholinergic side effects. Gabapentin has proven to be effective in relieving PHN, and is the only systemic medication federally approved for treatment. Topical medications, such as lidocaine, may be effective as well. Capsaicin, a topical agent which depletes substance P, may be helpful, but the burning pain that accompanies its applications limits its usefulness.

Ophthalmoplegic Migraine

Ophthalmoplegic migraine is defined by the IHS as recurrent attacks of headache with migrainous characteristics associated with paralysis of one or more ocular motor nerves (most commonly the oculomotor nerve) (11). Childhood onset is common. The IHS criteria require two attacks, with a migrainous headache overlapping or followed by paresis of one or more ocular motor nerves. The headache typically precedes the oculomotor nerve palsy and is ipsilateral. The pupil is often involved, and the ophthalmoplegia may be permanent. The condition is rare, with a reported incidence of 0.7 per 1,000,000 population (206).

This disorder was considered a variant of migraine and was classified under migraine in the first edition of IHS criteria (10). However, as more information about pathophysiology has arisen, it now seems unlikely that migraine is the underlying etiology. The headache often lasts longer than 1 week, and there may be a delay of up to 4 days from onset of headache to onset of ophthalmoplegia. Further, MRI signal abnormalities within the nerve, typically thickening and enhancement of the nerve as it exits the midbrain, have been described in a number of cases (207–209). The second edition of the IHS now lists ophthalmoplegic migraine among cranial neuralgias rather than migraine (11).

The mechanism of the neuropathy remains unclear. Lance and Zagami (209) suggested that ophthalmoplegic migraine represents a recurrent demyelinating neuropathy. Several patients with clinical evidence of ophthalmoplegic migraine have come to autopsy, but none within the past 50 years. The pathologic specimens were not subjected to detailed microscopic analysis, and several of the patients had neurologic co-morbidities (including tuberculous meningitis), which confounded the pathologic interpretation. Resolution of the oculomotor nerve with standard T2-weighted imaging is suboptimal, and detection of hemosiderin deposition within the nerve (suggesting an intrinsic vascular malformation) is difficult. Higher field strength magnets could potentially improve resolution of the oculomotor nerve and allow more detailed analysis.

There is no well-defined treatment for ophthalmoplegic migraine. Multiple medications, including corticosteroids, have been used to treat or prevent the attacks, with variable to poor results (208).

Persistent Idiopathic Facial Pain

Idiopathic facial pain (IFP), previously called "atypical facial pain," is characterized by the IHS as persistent facial pain that does not have the characteristics of the cranial neuralgias, and is not attributed to another disorder (11). The diagnostic criteria for IFP are as follows:

1. Pain in the face is present daily and persists for all or most of the day. The pain is confined at onset to a limited area on one side of the face–often in the nasolabial fold or side of the chin, may spread to the upper or lower jaw or a wider area of the face or neck, and is deep and poorly localized.
2. The pain is not associated with sensory loss or other physical signs except tenderness of the muscles of mastication.
3. Laboratory investigations, including X-ray of the face and jaws, do not demonstrate relevant abnormalities.

Idiopathic facial pain typically has a steady, diffuse quality. It may be described as deep, aching, pulling, boring, or gnawing in nature. It may develop after a dental procedure or after minor facial trauma. There is a relationship between the severity and frequency of facial pain and the number of traumas. The syndrome is most often seen in patients in their 30s or 40s. Women are affected more frequently than men. As opposed to the cranial neuralgias, the symptoms are not provoked by cold, swallowing, talking, or chewing (210).

The etiology of IFP is unknown. A careful search for local pathology of the eyes, nose, teeth, sinuses, and pharynx should be undertaken. Appropriate imaging studies, including MRI of the brain and face and jaw X-rays should be considered based on each individual case (211). However, in most patients, the work-up fails to reveal relevant imaging or laboratory abnormalities.

In many patients, the pain remains intractable despite multiple inteverntions, including analgesics, nerve blocks, and surgical interventions. A dedicated pain center may be necessary to identify the origins of the pain, and to isolate the factors contributing to the problem. Overuse of analgesics and sleep disturbance may accompany IFP, and should be addressed independently. Psychiatric disorders such as anxiety and depression may be present as well, and appropriate treatment may benefit the facial pain. Multiple modalities are often employed, and may include analgesics, antidepressants, psychotherapy, biofeedback, nerve blocks, and family counseling.

REFERENCES

1. Alvarez WC. Was there sick headache in 3000 B.C.? Gastroenterology 1945;5:524.
2. Silberstein SD, Lipton RB, Goadsby PJ, eds. Headache in Clinical Practice. St Louis, Mosby-Year Book, 1998.
3. Linet MS, Stewart WF, Celentano DD. An epidemiologic study of headache among adolescents and young adults. JAMA 1989;261:2211–2216.
4. Anon. Report of the Quality Standards Subcommittee of the American Academy of Neurology. Practice parameter: The utility of neuroimaging in the evaluation of headache patients with normal neurologic examinations. Neurology 1994;44:1353–1354.
5. Silberstein SD. The U.S. Headache Consortium. Practice parameter: Evidence-based guidelines for migraine headache (and evidence-based review). Report of the Quality Standards Subcommittee of the American Academy of Neurology. Neurology 2000;55:754–763.
6. Igarashi H, Sakai F, Kan S, Okada J et al. Magnetic resonance imaging of the brain in patients with migraine. Cephalalgia 1991;11:69–74.
7. Robbins L, Friedman H. MRI in migraineurs. Headache 1992;32:507–508.
8. Forsyth PA, Posner JB. Headaches in patients with brain tumors: A study of 111 patients. Neurology 1993;43:1678–1683.
9. Golnik K, Harooni H, Lee AG, Eggenberger E. Neuro-imaging in patients with unilateral ocular/facial pain. Poster presentation. American Academy of Ophthalmology Annual Meeting, Anaheim CA, 2003.
10. Anon. Headache Classification Committee of the International Headache Society. Classification and diagnostic criteria for headache disorders, cranial neuralgia, and facial pain. Cephalalgia 1988;8(Suppl 7):1–96.
11. Anon. Headache Classification Committee of the International headache Society. International Classification of Headache Disorders. Ed 2. Cephalagia. 2004;1:1–1600.
12. Black ER. Acute conditions: Incidence and associated disability, United States, July 1976–June 1977. Vital and Health Statistics, Series 10, No. 125, DHEW Publ No. 78-1553. Washington, DC, U.S. Government Printing Office, 1978.
13. Strang PE, Osterhaus JT, Celentano DD, Reed ML. Migraine: patterns of health care use. Neurology 1994;44(Suppl 4):47–55.
14. Lipton RB, Diamond S, Reed ML, Diamond M, Stewart WF. Migraine diagnosis and treatment: Results from the American Migraine Study II. Headache 2001;41:638–645.
15. Anon. IASP Subcommittee on Taxonomy. Pain terms: A list with definitions and notes on usage. Pain 1979;6:247–252.
16. Haigh RC, Blake DR. Understanding pain. Clin Med 2001;1:44–48.
17. Penfield W. A contribution to the mechanism intracranial pain. Assoc Res Nerv Ment Dis 1935;15:399–416.
18. Buzzi MG, Carter WB, Shimizu T, Heath H III, Moskowitz MA. Dihydroergotamine and sumatriptan attenuate levels of CGRP in plasma in rat superior sagittal sinus during electrical stimulation of the trigeminal ganglion. Neuropharmacology 1991;30:1193–2000.
19. Goadsby PJ, Edvinsson L, Ekman R. Release of vasoactive peptides in the extracerebral circulation of man and the cat during activation of the trigeminovascular system. Ann Neurol 1988;23:193–196.
20. Sessle BJ, Hu JW, Dubner R, Lucier GE. Functional properties of neurons in trigeminal subnucleus caudalis of the cat, II. Modulation of responses to noxious and non-noxious stimulation by periaqueductal gray, nucleus raphe magnus, cerebral cortex and afferent influences, and effect of naloxone. J Neurophysiol 1981;45:129–158.

21. Bernard JF, Peschanski M, Besson JM. A possible spino-(trigemino)-ponto-amygdaloid pathway for pain. Neurosci Lett 1989;100:83–88.
22. Biousse V, Bousser MG. Cerebral venous thrombosis. Neurologist 1999;5:326–349.
23. Welch KM, Cutrer FM, Goadsby PJ. Migraine pathogenesis: Neural and vascular mechanisms. Neurology 2003;60(Suppl 2):S9–S14.
24. Dimitriadou V, Buzzi MG, Theoharides TC, Moskowitz MA. Ultrastructural evidence for neurogenically mediated changes in blood vessels of the rat dura mater and tongue following antidromic trigeminal stimulation. Neuroscience 1992;48:187–203.
25. Lassen LH, Jacobsen VB, Pedersen PA, Sperling B et al. Human calcitonin gene-related peptide (hCGRP)-induced headache in migraineurs. Eur J Neurol 1998;5:S3.
26. Burstein R, Yamamura H, Makick A, Strassman AM. J Neurophysiol 1998;79:964–982.
27. Mendell LM. Physiologic properties of unmyelinated fibre projections to the spinal cord. Exp Neurol 1966;16:316–332.
28. Shakespeare W. Othello, The Moor of Venice. In The Complete Works of William Shakespeare. Stamford CT, Longmeadow Press, 1990.
29. Shakespeare W. King John. In The Complete Works of William Shakespeare. Stamford CT, Longmeadow Press, 1990.
30. Carter JL. Visual, somatosensory, olfactory, and gustatory hallucinations. Psychiatr Clin North Am 1992;15:1088–1097.
31. Diamond ML. The role of concomitant headache types and non-headache co-morbidities in the underdiagnosis of migraine. Neurology 2002;58(Suppl 6):S3–S9.
32. Stewart WF, Linet MS, Celentano DD, Van Natta M, Ziegler D. Age and sex-specific incidence rates of migraine with and without visual aura. Am J Epidemiol 1993;34:1111–1120.
33. Stewart WF, Lipton RB, Celentano DD, Reed ML. Prevalence of migraine headache in the United States: Relation to age, income, race, and other sociodemographic factors. JAMA 1992;267:64–69.
34. Stewart WF, Lipton RB, Liberman J. Variation in migraine prevalence by race. Neurology 1996;16:231–238.
35. Kryst S, Scherl E. A population-based survey of the social and personal impact of migraine. Headache 1994;34:344–350.
36. Hu XH, Markson LE, Lipton RB, Stewart WF, Berger ML. Burden of migraine in the United States: Disability and economic costs. Arch Intern Med 1999:159:813–818.
37. Russell M, Oleson J. Increased family risk and evidence of genetic factor in migraine. BMJ 1995;311:541–544.
38. Ferrari MD. Heritability of migraine: Genetic findings. Neurology 2003;60(Suppl 7):S15–S20.
39. Ulrich V, Gervil M, Kyvik KO, Oleson J, Russell MB. The inheritance of migraine with aura estimated by means of structural equation modeling. J Med Gent 1999;36:225–227.
40. Ophoff RA, Terwindt GM, Vergouwe MN et al. Familial hemiplegic migraine and episodic ataxia type 2 are caused by mutations in the Ca^{2+} channel gene. Cell 1996;87:543–552.
41. Terwindt GM, Ophoff RA, Haan J et al. Variable clinical expression of mutations in the P/Q type calcium channel gene in familial hemiplegic migraine: Dutch Migraine Genetics Research Group. Neurology 1998;50:1105–1110.
42. Peroutka SJ, Wilhoit T, Jones K. Clinical susceptibility to migraine is modified by dopamine D2 receptor (DRD2) NcoI alleles. Neurology 1997;49:201–206.
43. Welch KMA, Ramadan NM. Mitochondria, magnesium and migraine. J Neurol Sci 1995;134:9–14.
44. Milahud DM, Bogousslavsky J, van Melle G, Liot P. Ischemic stroke and active migraine. Neurology 2001;57:1805–1811.
45. Tzourio C, Iglesias S, Hubert J-B et al. Migraine and risk of ischaemic stroke: A case-control study. BMJ 1993;307:289–292.
46. Tzourio C, Tehindrazanarivelo A, Iglesias S et al. Case-control study of migraine and risk of ischaemic stroke in young women. BMJ 1995;310:830–833.
47. Breslau N, Rasmussen BK. The impact of migraine: Epidemiology, risk factors, and co-morbidities. Neurology 2001;56:S4–S12.
48. Blau JN. Migraine prodromes separated from the aura: Complete migraine. BMJ 1980;281:658–660.
49. Maytal J, Young M, Shecter A et al. Pediatric migraine and the International Headache Society (IHS) criteria. Neurology 1997;48:602–607.
50. MacGregor EA. ''Menstrual'' migraine: towards a definition. Cephalalgia 1996;16:11–21.
51. Lippman CW. Certain hallucinations peculiar to migraine. J Nerv Ment Dis 1952;116:346–351.
52. Golden GS. The Alice in Wonderland syndrome in juvenile migraine. Pediatrics 1979;63:517–519.
53. Copperman SM. Alice in Wonderland syndrome as a presenting symptom of infectious mononucleosis in children. Clin Pediatr 1977;16:143–146.
54. Rolak LA. Literary neurologic syndromes: Alice in Wonderland. Arch Neurol 1991;48:649–651.
55. Michel EM, Troost BT. Palinopsia: Cerebral localization with computed tomography. Neurology 1980;30:887–889.
56. Jones MR, Waggoner R, Hoyt WF. Cerebral polyopia with extrastriate quad-
57. rantopia: Report of a case with magnetic resonance documentation of V2/V3 cortical infarction. J Neuroophthalmol 1999;19:1–6.
57. Liu GT, Volpe NJ, Galetta SL. Visual hallucinations and Illusions. In Neuro-Ophthalmology. Diagnosis and Management. Ed 1. W.B. Saunders 2001:401–424 .
58. Russell MB, Oleson J. A nosographic analysis of the migraine aura in a general population. Brain 1996;119:355–361.
59. Wijman CAC, Wolf PA, Case CS et al. Migrainous visual accompaniments are not rare in late life: The Framingham Study. Stroke 1998;29:1539–1543.
60. Fisher CM. Late-life migraine accompaniments as a cause of unexplained transient ischemic attacks. Can J Neurol Sci 1980;7:9–17.
61. Chronicle EP, Mulleners WM. Visual system dysfunction in migraine: A review of clinical and psychophysical findings. Cephalalgia 1996;16:252–535.
62. Goodwin JA, Gorelick PB, Helgason CM. Symptoms of amaurosis fugax in atherosclerotic carotid artery disease. Neurology 1987;37:829–835.
63. Liu GT, Schatz NJ, Galetta SK et al. Persistent positive visual phenomena in migraine. Neurology 1995;45:664–668.
64. Hupp S, Kline L, Corbett J. Visual disturbances of migraine. Surv Ophthalmol 1989;33:221–236.
65. Barry E, Sussman NM, Bosley TM, Harner RN. Ictal blindness and status epilepticus amauroticus. Epilepsia 1985;26:577–584.
66. Ducros A, Denier C, Joutel A et al. The clinical spectrum of familial hemiplegic migraine associated with mutations in a neuronal calcium channel. N Engl J Med 2001;345:17–24.
67. Graham JR, Wolff HG. Mechanism of migraine headache and action of ergotamine tartrate. Arch Neurol Psychiatry 1938;39:737–763.
68. Leao AA. Spreading depression of activity in the cerebral cortex. J Neurophysiol 1944;7:359–390.
69. Oleson J, Larsen B, Lauritzen M. Focal hyperemia followed by spreading oligemia and impaired activation of regional cerebral blood flow in classic migraine. Ann Neurol 1981;9:344–352.
70. Welch KM, Cutrer FM, Goadsby PJ. Migraine pathogenesis: Neural and vascular mechanisms. Neurology 2003;7(Suppl 2):S9–S14.
71. Moskowitz MA. Basic mechanisms in vascular headache. Neurol Clin 1990;8:801–815.
72. Choudhuri R, Cui L, Yong C et al. Cortical spreading depression and gene regulation: Relevance to migraine. Ann Neurol 2002;51:499–506.
73. Woods RP, Iacoboni M, Maziotta JC. Brief report: bilateral spreading cerebral hypoperfusion during spontaneous migraine headache. N Engl J Med 1994;331:1689–1692.
74. Cao Y, Welch KMA, Aurora S, Vikingstad EM. Functional MRI-BOLD of visually triggered headache in patients with migraine. Arch Neurol 1999;56:548–554.
75. Welch KMA, D'Andrea G, Tepley N, Barkley GL, Ramadan NM. The concept of migraine as a state of central neuronal hyperexcitability. Headache 1990;8:817–828.
76. Welch KMA. Contemporary concepts of migraine pathogenesis. Neurology 2003;61(Suppl 4):S2–S7.
77. Aurora SK, Ahmad BK, Welch KMA, Bhardwaj P, Ramadan NM. Transcranial magnetic stimulation confirms hyperexcitability of occipital cortex in migraine. Neurology 1998;50:1111–1114.
78. Batelli L, Black KR, Wray SH. Transcranial magnetic stimulation of visual area V5 in migraine. Neurology 2002;58:1066–1069.
79. Bates D, Ashford E, Dawson R et al. Subcutaneous sumatriptan during the migraine aura. Neurology 1994;44:1587–1592.
80. Hoskin KL, Goadsby PJ. Comparison of more and less lipophilic serotonin 5-HT1B1D agonists in a model of trigeminovascular nociception in cat. Exp Neurol 1998;150:45–51.
81. Holroyd KA, Mauskop A. Complementary and alternative treatments. Neurology 2003;60(Suppl 2):S58–S62.
82. Matchar D. Acute management of migraine: Highlights of the US Headache Consortium. Neurology 2003;60(Suppl 2):S21–S23.
83. Silberstein SD, Freitag FG. Preventive treatment of migraine. Neurology 2003;60(Suppl 2):S38–S44.
84. Binder WJ, Brin MF, Blitzer A, Pagoda JM. Botulinum toxin type A (Botox) for treatment of migraine. Dis Mon 2002;48:323–335.
85. Lang AM. Botulinum toxin for myofascial pain disorder. Curr Pain Head Rep 2002;6:355–360.
86. Rasmussen BK, Jensen R, Schroll M, Oleson J. Impact of headache on sickness absence and utilization of medical services: A Danish population study. J Epidemiol Community Health 1992;46:443–446.
87. Diamond ML. The role of concomitant headache types and non-headache co-morbidities in the underdiagnosis of migraine. Neurology 2002;58(Suppl 6):S3–S9.
88. Kaniecki RG. Migraine and tension-type headache. An assessment of challenges in diagnosis. Neurology 2002;58(Suppl 6):S15–S20.
89. Kaniecki RB, Totten J. Cervicalgia in migraine: Prevalence, clinical characteristics, and response to treatment. [Abstr]. Cephalalgia 2001;21:296.
90. Rasmussen BK, Jensen R, Schroll M et al. Interrelations between migraine and tension-type headache in the general population. Arch Neurol 1992;49:914–918.
91. Clark GT, Sakai S, Merrill R, Flack VF, McCreary C. Cross-correlation between

stress, pain, physical activity, and temporalis muscle EMG in tension-type headache. Cephalalgia 1995;15:511–518.
92. Silberstein SD. Chronic daily headache and tension-type headache. Neurology 1993;43:1644–1649.
93. Goadsby PJ, Lipton RB. A review of paroxysmal hemicranias, SUNCT syndrome and other short-lasting headaches with autonomic features, including new cases. Brain 1997;120:193–209.
94. Goadsby PJ, Edvisnnson L. Human in vivo evidence for trigemino-vascular activation in cluster headache. Brain 1994;117:427–434.
95. Ekbom K, Greitz T. Carotid angiography in cluster headache. Acta Radiol 1970; 10:177–186.
96. May A, Kaube H, Buchel C, Rijntjes M, Weiller C, Diener HC. Trigeminal transmitted pain using capsaicin: A PET study. Cephalalgia 1997;17:377.
97. Dodick DW, Saper J. Cluster and chronic daily headache. Neurology 2003; 60(Suppl 2):S31–S37.
98. Leone M, Bussone G. A review of hormonal findings in cluster headache: Evidence for hypothalamic involvement. Cephalalgia 1993;13:309–317.
99. Leone M, D'Amico D, Moschiano F, Fraschini F, Bussone G. Melatonin versus placebo in the prophylaxis of cluster headache: A double blind pilot study with parallel groups. Cephalalgia 1996;16:494–496.
100. May A, Bahra A, Buchel C, Frackowiak RSJ, Goadsby PJ. Hypothalamic activation in cluster headache attacks. Lancet 1998;352:275–278.
101. Anon. The Sumatriptan Cluster Headache Study Group: Treatment of acute cluster headache with sumatriptan. N Engl J Med 1991;325:322–326.
102. Monsatd I, Krabbe A, Micieli G et al. Preemptive oral treatment with sumatriptan during a cluster period. Headache 1995;35:607–613.
103. Hering R, Kuritzky A. Sodium valproate in the treatment of cluster headache: An open clinical trial. Cephalalgia 1989;9:195–198.
104. Jarrar RG, Black DF, Dodick DW et al. Outcome of trigeminal nerve section in the treatment of chronic cluster headache. Neurology 2003;60:1360–1362.
105. Leone M, Franzini A, Broggi G, Bussone G. Hypothalamic deep brain stimulation for intractable chronic cluster headache: A 3-year follow-up. Neurol Sci 2003;24(Suppl 2):S143–145.
106. Sjaastad O, Stovner LJ, Stolt-Nielson A, Antonaci F, Fredrikson TA. CPH and hemicrania continua: Requirements of high indocin doses—an ominous sign? Headache 1995;35:363–367.
107. Medina JL. Organic headaches mimicking chronic paroxysmal hemicrania. Headache 1992;32:73–74.
108. Miciel G, Cavallini A, Facchinetti F, Sances G, Nappi G. Chronic paroxysmal hemicrania: A chronobiological study (case report). Cephalalgia 1989;9: 281–286.
109. Carvalho DSS, Salveson R, Rand T, Smith SE, Sjaastad O. Chronic paroxysmal hemicrania. XIII. The pupillometric pattern. Cephalalgia 1988;8:219–226.
110. Goadsby PJ, Edvinnson L. Neuropeptide changes in a case of chronic paroxysmal hemicrania: Evidence for trigemino-parasympathetic activation. Cephalalgia 1996;16:448–450.
111. Dodick DW. Indomethacin responsive headache syndromes: A hypothesis on the mechanism(s) underlying the efficacy of indomethacin in these disorders. Neurology 1999;52:A210.
112. Hannerz J, Jogestrand T. Intracranial hypertension and sumatriptan efficacy in a case of chronic paroxysmal hemicrania which became bilateral: The mechanism of indomethacin in CPH. Headache 1993;33:320–323.
113. Sjaastad O, Saunte C, Salvesen R, Fredrikson TA, Seim A et al. Short lasting unilateral neuralgiform headache attacks with conjunctival injection, tearing, sweating, and rhinorrhea. Cephalalgia 1989;9:147–156.
114. Pareja JA, Joubert J, Sjaastad O. SUNCT syndrome: Atypical temporal patterns. Headache 1996;36:108–110.
115. Bussone G, Leone M, Dalla Volta G, Strada L et al. Short lasting unilateral neuralgiform headache attacks with tearing and conjunctival injection: First symptomatic case? Cephalalgia 1991;11:123–127.
116. Sjaastad O, Kruszewski P, Fostad K, Elasa T, Qvigstad G. SUNCT syndrome. VII. Ocular and related variables. Headache 1992;32:489–495.
117. Pareja J, Caminero A, Sjaastad O. SUNCT syndrome: diagnosis and treatment. CNS Drugs 2002;16:373–383.
118. May A, Bahra A, Buchel C, Turner R, Goadsby PJ. Functional magnetic resonance imaging in spontaneous attacks of SUNCT: Short lasting neuralgiform headache with conjunctival injection and tearing. Ann Neurol 1999;46:791–794.
119. Hannerz J, Linderoth B. Neurosurgical treatment of short lasting, unilateral, neuralgiform hemicrania with conjunctival injection and tearing. Br J Neurosurg 2002;16:55–58.
120. Black DF, Dodick DW. Two cases of medically and surgically intractable SUNCT: A reason for caution and argument for a central mechanism. Cephalalgia 2002;22:201–204.
121. Spierings EL, Sjaastad O. Hemicrania continua is not that rare. Neurology 2002; 59:476–477.
122. Silberstein SD, Peres MF. Hemicrania continua. Arch Neurol 2002;59: 1029–1030.
123. Pareja JA, Ruiz J, de Isla C, Al-Sabbah H, Espejo J. Idiopathic stabbing headache (jabs and jolts syndrome). Cephalalgia 1996;16:93–96.
124. Ammache M, Graber M, Davis P. Idiopathic stabbing headache associated with monocular visual loss. Arch Neurol 2000;57:745–746.

125. Raskin NH, Schwartz RK. Icepick-like pain. Neurology 1980;30:203–205.
126. Peres MF, Silberstein SD, Nahmias S et al. Hemicrania continua is not that rare. Neurology 2001;57:948–951.
127. Rozen TD. Melatonin as a treatment for idiopathic stabbing headache. Neurology 2003;61:865–866.
128. DeBenedittis G, DeSantis A. Chronic post-traumatic headache: Clinical, psychopathologic features and outcome determinants. J Neurosurg Sci 1983;27: 177–186.
129. Gfeller JD, Chibnall JT, Duckro PN. Postconcussion symptoms and cognitive functioning in posttraumatic headache patients. Headache 1994;34:503–507.
130. Young WB, Packard RC. In Goadsby PJ, Silberstein SD, eds. Posttraumatic Headache and Posttraumatic Syndrome. Boston, Butterworth-Heinemann, 1997; 253–278.
131. Lishman WA. Physiogenesis and psychogenesis in the post-concussional syndrome. Br J Psychiatry 1988;153:460–469.
132. Keidel M, Ramadan NM. Posttraumatic headache. In Oleson J, Tfelt-Hansen P, Welch KMA, eds. The Headaches. Philadelphia, Lippincott Williams & Wilkins, 2000:765–780.
133. Goodman JC. Pathologic changes in mild head injury. Semin Neurol 1994;14: 19–24.
134. Packard RC. Post-traumatic headache: Permanency and relationship to legal settlement. Headache 1992;32:496–500.
135. Binder LM, Rohling ML. Money matters: A meta-analytic review of the effects of financial incentives on recovery after closed-head injury. Am J Psychiatry 1996;153:7–10.
136. Jensen OK, Nielsen FF. The influence of sex and pretraumatic headache on the incidence and severity of headache after head injury. Cephalalgia 1990;10: 285–293.
137. Fisher CM. Headache in cerebrovascular disease. In Vinken PJ, Bryun GW, Eds. Handbook of Clinical Neurology. Headache and Cranial Neuralgias. Vol 5. Amsterdam, North Holland, 1968:124–156.
138. Ferro JM, Melo TP, Oliveira V, Salgado AV et al. A multi-variate study of headache associated with ischemic stroke. Headache 1995;35:315–319.
139. Knox DL, Cogan DG. Eye pain and homonymous hemianopia. Am J Ophthalmol 1962;54:1091–1093.
140. Symonds C. The Circle of Willis. Br Med J 1955;1:119–124.
141. Moskowitz MA. The neurobiology of vascular head pain. Ann Neurol 1984;16: 157–268.
142. Castillo J, Martinez F, Corredera E, Aldrey JM et al. Amino acid transmitters in patients with headache during the acute phase of cerebrovascular ischemic disease. Stroke 1995;26:2035–2039.
143. Ferro JM, Costa I, Melo TP, Canhao P et al. Headache associated with transient ischemic attacks. Headache 1995;35:544–548.
144. Olesen J, Friberg L, Olsen TS, Andersen AR, Lassen NA, Hansen PE, Karle A. Ischaemia-induced (symptomatic) migraine attacks may be more frequent than migraine-induced ischaemic insults. Brain 1993;116:187–202.
145. Edmeads J. Migraine: Disease or syndrome? Path Biol 1992;40:279–283.
146. Biousse V, Touboul PJ, D'Anglejan-Chatillon J et al. Neuro-ophthalmological manifestations of internal carotid artery dissections: A series of 146 patients. Am J Ophthalmol 1998;126:565–577.
147. Adams HP Jr, Jergensen DD, Kassell NF et al. Pitfalls in the recognition of subarachnoid hemorrhage. JAMA 1980;244:794–796.
148. Dodick DW. Thunderclap headache. Headache 2002;42:309–315.
149. Pfausler B, Belcl R, Metzler R et al. Terson's syndrome in spontaneous subarachnoid hemorrhage: A prospective study in 60 consecutive patients. J Neurosurg 1996;85:392–394.
150. Raps EC, Rogers JD, Galetta SL et al. The clinical spectrum of unruptured intracranial aneurysms. Arch Neurol 1993;50:265–268.
151. Lee AG, Hayman LA, Brazis PW. The evaluation of isolated third nerve palsy revisited: An update on the evolving role of magnetic resonance, computed tomography, and catheter angiography. Surv Ophthalmol 2002;41:137–157.
152. Gorelick PB, Hier DB, Caplan LR et al. Headache in acute cerebrovascular disease. Neurology 1986;36:1445–1450.
153. McKissock W. Subdural hamartoma: A review of 389 cases. Lancet 1960;1: 1365–1370.
154. Bo Abbas Y, Bolton CF. Roller coaster headache. N Engl J Med 1995;332: 1585.
155. Lobato RD, Rivas JJ, Gomez PA et al. Head injured patients who talk and deteriorate into coma: Analysis of 211 cases studied with computerized tomography. J Neurosurg 1991;75:256–261.
156. Evans RW. Diagnostic testing for the evaluation of headaches. Neurol Clin 1996; 14:1–26.
157. Troost BT, Newton TH. Occipital lobe arteriovenous malformations: Clinical and radiologic features in 26 cases with comments on the differentiation from migraine. Arch Ophthalmol 1975;93:250–256.
158. Melo TP, Pinto AN, Ferro JM. Headache in intracerebral hematomas. Neurology 1996;47:494–500.
159. Troost BT, Mark LE, Maroon JC. Resolution of classic migraine following removal of an occipital lobe arteriovenous malformation. Ann Neurol 1979;5: 199–201.

160. Aminoff MJ. Management of unruptured cerebral arteriovenous malformations. Clin Neurosurg 1986;33:177–185.

161. Bruyn GW. Intracranial arteriovenous malformation and migraine. Cephalalgia 1984;4:191–207.

162. Raskin NH. Headache. New York, Churchill Livingstone, 1988.

163. Homan RW, Devous MD Sr, Stokely EM et al. Quantification of intracerebral steal in patients with arteriovenous malformation. Arch Neurol 1986;43: 779–785.

164. Biousse V, D'Angelejan Chatillon J, Massiou H et al. Head pain in nontraumatic carotid artery dissection: A series of 65 patients. Cephalalgia 1994;14(1)33–36.

165. Fisher CM, Ojemann RG, Robertson GH. Spontaneous dissection of cervicocerebral arteries. Can J Neurol Sci 1987;5:9–19.

166. Biousse V, Bousser MG. The myth of carotidynia. Neurology 1994;44:993–995.

167. Syms MJ, Burton BS, Burgess LPA. Magnetic resonance imaging in carotidynia. Otolaryngol Head Neck Surg 1997;117(Suppl):156–159.

168. Burton BS, Syms MJ, Petermann GW, Burgess LPA. MR Imaging of patients with carotidynia. Am J Neuroradiol 2000;21:766–769.

169. Biousse V, Newman NJ, Oyesiku NM. Precipitating factors in pituitary apoplexy. J Neurol Neurosurg Psychiatry 2001;71:542–545.

170. Baldursson O, Steinsson K, Bjornsson J, Lie JT. Giant cell arteritis in Iceland: An epidemiologic and histopathologic analysis. Arthritis Rheum 1994;37: 1007–1012.

171. Pauley JW, Hughes JP. Giant cell arteritis, or arteritis of the aged. Br Med J 1960;2:1562–1567.

172. Digre KB. Idiopathic intracranial hypertension headache. Curr Pain Head Rep 2002;6:217–225.

173. Digre KB, Corbett JJ. Idiopathic intracranial hypertension (pseudotumor cerebri): A reappraisal. Neurologist 2002;7:2–67.

174. Mokri B. Spontaneous cerebrospinal fluid leaks, from intracranial hypotension to cerebrospinal fluid hypovolemia: Evolution of a concept. Mayo Clin Proc 1999;74:1113–1123.

175. Chung SJ, Kim SJ, Lee MC. Syndrome of cerebrospinal fluid hypovolemia: Clinical and imaging features and outcome. Neurology 2000;55:1321–1327.

176. Horton JC, Fishman RA. Neurovisual findings in the syndrome of spontaneous intracranial hypotension from dural cerebrospinal fluid leak. Ophthalmology 1994;101:244–251.

177. Fishman RA. Cerebrospinal fluid. In Diseases of the Nervous System. Philadelphia, WB Saunders 1992.

178. Dalessio DJ, Silberstein SD, eds. Wolff's Headache and Other Head Pain. New York, Oxford University Press, 1993.

179. Strandgaard S, Olesen J, Skinhoj E et al. Autoregulation of brain circulation in severe arterial hypertension. Br Med J 1973;1:507–510.

180. Stromberg DD, Fox JR. Pressure in the pial arterial microcirculation of the cat during changes in systemic arterial blood pressure. Circ Res 1972;31:229–239.

181. Dalessio DJ, ed. Wolff's Headache and Other Head Pain. New York, Oxford University Press, 1980.

182. Appenzeller O. Altitude headache. Headache 1972;12:126–130.

183. Carlow TJ. Headaches and the eye. In Dalessio DJ, ed. Wolff's Headache and Other Head Pain. New York, Oxford University Press, 1987:384–400.

184. Unger WG, Perkins ES, Bass MS. The response of the rabbit eye to laser irradiation of the iris. Exp Eye Res 1974;19:367–377.

185. Anopn. Optic Neuritis Study Group. The clinical profile of acute optic neuritis: Experience of the Optic Neuritis Treatment Trial. Arch Ophthalmol 1991;109: 1673–1678.

186. Swartz NG, Beck RW, Savino PJ et al. Pain in anterior ischemic optic neuropathy. J Neuroophthalmol 1995;15:9–10.

187. Lepore FE. The origin of pain in optic neuritis: Determinants of pain in 101 eyes with optic neuritis. Arch Neurol 1991;48:748–749.

188. Fazzone HE, Lefton DR, Kupersmith MJ. Optic neuritis: Correlation of pain and magnetic resonance imaging. Ophthalmology 2003;110:1646–1649.

189. Peters GA, Horton BT. Headache: with special reference to excessive use of ergotamine preparations and withdrawal effects. Mayo Clin Proc 1951;26: 214–226.

190. Lipton RB, Silberstein SD, Saper JR et al. Why headache treatment fails. Neurology 2003;60:1064–1070.

191. Katsarava Z, Fritsche G, Muessig M, Diener HC, Limmroth V. Clinical features of withdrawal headache following overuse of triptans in comparison to other antimigraine drugs. Neurology 2001;56(Suppl 3):A220.

192. Lipton RB, Bigal ME. Chronic daily headache: Is analgesic overuse a cause or a consequence? Neurology 2003;61:154–155.

193. Zwart J-A, Dyb G, Hagen K, Svebak S, Holmen J. Analgesic use: A predictor of chronic daily headache and medication overuse headache. The Head-HUNT Study. Neurology 2003;61:160–164.

194. Bahra A, Walsh M, Menon S, Goadsby PJ. Does chronic daily headache arise de novo in association with regular analgesic use? [abstr]. Cephalalgia 2000; 20:294.

195. Lance F, Parkes C, Wilkinson M. Does analgesic abuse cause headache de novo? Headache 1988;38:61–62.

196. Silberstein SD, Silberstein JR. Chronic daily headache: Long-term prognosis following inpatient treatment with repetitive i.v. DHE. Headache 1992;32: 439–445.

197. Bogduk N. Greater occipital neuralgia. In Long DM, ed. Current Therapy in Neurological Surgery. Toronto, BC Decker Inc 1985:175–180.

198. Ward JB. Greater occipital nerve block. Semin Neurol 2003;23:59–62.

199. Sjaastad O, Stolt-Nielsen A, Pareja JA, Vincent M. Supraorbital neuralgia: The clinical manifestation and a possible therapeutic approach. Headache 1999;39: 204–212.

200. Ragozzino MW, Melton LJ, Kerland LT et al. Population-based study of Herpes Zoster and its sequelae. Medicine 1982;61:310–316.

201. Gilden DH, Wright RR, Schneck SA et al. Zoster sine herpete, a clinical variant. Ann Neurol 1994;35:530–533.

202. Kertes PJ, Baker JD, Noel LP. Neuro-ophthalmic complications of acute varicella. Can J Ophthalmol 1998;33:324–328.

203. Straus SE. Shingles: Sorrows, salves, and solutions. JAMA 1993;269:1836–1839.

204. Kost RG, Straus SE. Postherpetic neuralgia: Pathogenesis, treatment, and prevention. N Engl J Med 1996;335:32–42.

205. Tyring S, Barbarash RA, Nahlik JE et al. Famciclovir for the treatment of acute herpes zoster: Effects on acute disease and post-herpetic neuralgia. Ann Intern Med 1995;123:89–96.

206. Hansen SL, Borelli-Moller L, Strange P et al. Ophthalmoplegic migraine: Diagnostic criteria, incidence of hospitalization, and possible etiology. Acta Neurol Scand 1990;81:54–60.

207. Mark AS, Casselman J, Brown D et al. Ophthalmoplegic migraine: Reversible enhancement and thickening of the cisternal segment of the oculomotor nerve on contrast enhanced MR images. Am J Neuroradiol 1998;19:1887–1891.

208. Carlow TJ. Oculomotor ophthalmoplegic migraine: Is it really migraine? J Neuroophthalmol 2002;22:215–221.

209. Lance JW, Zagami AS. Ophthalmoplegic migraine: A recurrent demyelinating neuropathy? Cephalalgia 2001;21:84–89.

210. Graff-Radford SB. Facial pain. Curr Opin Neurol 2000;13:291–296.

211. Pfaffenrath V, Rath M, Pollmann W, Keeser W. Atypcial facial pain: Application of the IHS criteria in a clinical sample. Cephalalgia 1993;13(Suppl):84–88.

SECTION VI:
Nonorganic Disease

Nancy J. Newman, section editor

Much of the practice of medicine is devoted to the recognition of disorders that simulate organic disease but have no organic basis. This section contains a single chapter that describes various nonorganic disorders of neuro-ophthalmologic significance.

CHAPTER 27

Neuro-Ophthalmologic Manifestations of Nonorganic Disease

Neil R. Miller

Patients who have physical signs and symptoms for which no adequate organic cause can be found may receive any one of a large range of diagnostic labels, including functional illness, functional overlay, hysteria, hysterical overlay, conversion reaction, psychophysiological reaction, somatization reaction, hypochondriasis, invalid reaction, neurasthenia, psychogenic reaction, psychosomatic illness, malingering, and Münchausen's syndrome (1–3). This plethora of labels highlights the confusion that occurs when one tries to fit patients with nonorganic disease into a formal classification.

For instance, it has been stated that *la belle indifférence* is one of the hallmarks of a conversion reaction; however, Chodoff (4) found that most of his "hysterical" patients did not show an indifferent attitude to their illness. Similarly, Stephens and Kamp (5) found indifference in only 32% of their patients, and Ziegler et al. (6) found depression rather than indifference in about one-third of their sample. It seems clear, therefore, that it is difficult to classify various types of nonorganic disease.

GENERAL CONSIDERATIONS

Several issues are addressed in order to better define nonorganic disease. These issues include the nature of the symptom or symptoms, the somatic or physical aspect of the disorder, the ideation and affect of the patient, the patient's attitude toward those trying to diagnose and treat the condition, and the patient's motivation (1).

The **nature of the symptom** and the manner of its communication are crucial in the understanding of a nonorganic disorder. The patient may be stoic and restrained, or histrionic and dramatizing. The symptom may take the form of a physical dysfunction (e.g., strabismus) that is displayed with a minimum of verbal description, or the symptom may be described verbally during the examination. Thus, one must also determine the **nature of the physical dysfunction** and the degree of disability. It is important to determine why the symptoms have focused in a particular area (e.g., the visual system).

Another consideration is the amount of time a patient spends thinking about his or her symptoms and the precise nature of the thoughts in phenomenological terms. This concept is called **ideation**. For example, is the patient phobic or deluded?

A patient's **affect** may tell the physician much about the patient's complaints. Some patients clearly are depressed, whereas others are truly indifferent, and still others are anxious. Of particular interest is a patient's **attitude toward those involved in the diagnosis and treatment of his or her condition**. These are persons with whom one would expect the patient to cooperate in an attempt to get well (7). Is the patient hostile, suspicious, fearful, flirtatious, pleading, aloof, or excessively cooperative and agreeable?

Understanding a patient's **motivation** or incentive for achieving the ''sick role'' and the degree to which he or she is conscious of it may be the most difficult part of the diagnostic process, but it may be the most crucial. The nature of motivation may range from an unconscious seeking of the dependency-gratifying and guilt-allaying aspects of the

''sick role'' to the overtly conscious attempt to obtain attention, sympathy, material gain, or a combination of these (8).

Considering these complicated issues, it is not difficult to classify nonorganic illness clearly and concisely. For this reason, some authors consider all such disorders to be examples of **abnormal illness behavior** (9,10).

TERMINOLOGY

Most nonorganic disturbances are categorized by three types: (*a*) malingering; (*b*) Münchausen syndrome; and (*c*) psychogenic.

MALINGERING

Patients whose symptoms are consciously and voluntarily produced are said to be **malingering**. A symptom reported by a malingerer, such as diplopia, is not psychogenic because the patient is not, in fact, experiencing the symptom. Malingering can be divided into several different categories, including simulation of nonexistent disease, elaboration of preexisting disease, and attribution of a disability to a different cause, usually in the setting of potential compensation (3).

MÜNCHAUSEN SYNDROME

Malingering must be differentiated from **factitious disorder with physical symptoms**, also called the **Münchausen syndrome** (11). Patients with this condition intentionally produce physical symptoms and signs, some of which may be ocular. Symptoms might include swelling and redness of the conjunctiva simulating an orbital cellulitis, scarring of the eyelids and conjunctiva, and even chorioretinal scarring, all of which are then presented to members of the medical profession (12–15). Although the motivation for malingering might be monetary compensation or avoidance of military service, there may be patients with Münchausen syndrome who are thought to harbor a psychological internal need to adopt the role of the sick person.

PSYCHOGENIC DISTURBANCE

Patients whose symptoms seem truly independent of volition are said to have a somatoform disorder or **psychogenic**

disturbance. Examples of psychogenic disturbances include body dysmorphic disorder, conversion disorder (hysteria, conversion reaction), hypochondriasis, and somatization disorder.

A **body dysmorphic disorder** is characterized by a patient's perception of a single physical defect, most often in the facial region, including the eye. The patient is preoccupied with this sign even though it is minimal (e.g., a mild ptosis or anisocoria) or is not present at all.

A **conversion disorder** is diagnosed if alterations or a loss of physical functioning are present that seem to express a psychological conflict or need rather than indicating organic illness. This disorder comprises the clinical syndromes that were previously classified as ''hysteria'' or ''conversion neurosis.'' Patients in whom such disorders occur may subconsciously obtain both primary gain (e.g., protection from trauma or reduction of stress) and secondary gain (e.g., increased attention) (2,3).

Hypochondriasis is the fear of, or strong belief in, specific serious physical conditions accompanied by excessive self-observation and the reporting of numerous physical signs and symptoms. It differs from body dysmorphic disorder in that it includes both symptoms and signs from multiple organ systems throughout the body.

A **somatization disorder** features recurrent and multiple somatic complaints. As in hypochondriasis, multiple organ systems may be mentioned, but the patient's descriptions are vague, and anxiety or depression usually is present.

Unfortunately, there remains a large group of patients in whom a clear distinction between malingering, Münchausen syndrome, and psychogenic or somatoform disturbances simply cannot be made. In such cases, the physician must recognize that there is no organic basis for the patient's symptoms and signs and manage the patient accordingly.

SPECIFIC NONORGANIC NEURO-OPHTHALMOLOGIC DISORDERS

From a neuro-ophthalmologic standpoint, there are five areas that may be affected by nonorganic disease (3,16):

1. Vision, including visual acuity and visual field
2. Ocular motility and alignment
3. Pupillary size and reactivity
4. Eyelid position and function; and
5. Corneal and facial sensation.

The physician faced with a patient complaining of decreased vision or some other disturbance related to the **afferent** or **efferent** visual systems for which there is no apparent

biologic explanation has two responsibilities. First, the physician must ascertain that an organic disorder is not present. This is particularly important as 25–50% of patients with apparent nonorganic visual loss have concomitant organic pathology to explain at least some of the visual deficit (17). Second, the physician should clinically challenge the patient to see or do something that would not be possible if the condition were organic in nature. To best achieve these goals, the physician must adopt an **empathetic** attitude toward the patient regardless of the patient's history, attitude of the patient toward the physician or the disease, or the clinical findings. If the physician has or is perceived to have a cynical, disbelieving, or confrontational attitude, the patient may not cooperate fully during the examination and the results will be unsatisfactory (16).

In the remainder of this chapter we consider the manifestations of nonorganic disease as they pertain to the **afferent** and **efferent** visual systems. Where appropriate, we discuss various methods used to diagnose and treat these manifestations.

NONORGANIC DISEASE AFFECTING THE AFFERENT VISUAL PATHWAY

Nonorganic disease that affects the **afferent** visual system is the most common manifestation of this disorder (16). It may occur as monocular or binocular decreased visual acuity, abnormal visual fields, or both. Color vision often is abnormal in such patients (depending on the manner in which it is tested), but abnormal color vision is rarely a primary complaint (18).

Decreased Visual Acuity

Decreased visual acuity is probably the most common nonorganic disturbance in ophthalmology (3,16,17). It occurs most often in children and young adults (2,19), but it may be observed in patients 60 years of age and older (17,20,21). It may be psychogenic or caused by malingering (22). Nonorganic visual loss that is psychogenic seems to be more common in children, with females being affected much more often than males (19–21,23,24). Malingerers are most often adult males, perhaps because men are more often involved in motor vehicle and work-related accidents than are women.

Patients with nonorganic loss of visual acuity complain of a variable loss of vision in one or both eyes that is not accompanied by a refractive error, a disturbance of the ocular media, or other evidence of retinal or optic nerve dysfunction. Abnormal color perception, an abnormal visual field, or both, may accompany the visual loss.

In many cases, the physician may suspect that the patient's visual loss is nonorganic during the medical history interview which, as noted above, is perhaps the most crucial aspect of the evaluation (3). In addition, the way the patient acts during the history taking may be helpful. Patients who are truly blind in both eyes tend to look directly at the person with whom they are speaking, whereas patients with nonorganic blindness, particularly patients who are malingering, often look in some other direction. Similarly, we have noted that patients claiming complete or nearly complete blindness often wear sunglasses, even though they do not have photophobia, and the external appearance of the eyes is perfectly normal. In any event, the physician who suspects a nonorganic visual process may be able to orient the examination in a way to bring out the nonorganic nature of the visual disturbance (20,25,26).

If a patient claims no perception of light, light perception only, or perception of hand motions by one or both eyes, one can use a rotating optokinetic drum or horizontally moving tape to produce a horizontal jerk nystagmus that indicates

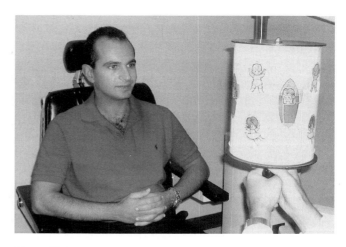

Figure 27.1. Use of the optokinetic drum to detect nonorganic bilateral blindness. The patient is asked to look straight ahead with both eyes open while the drum is rotated, first in one direction, then in the other.

intact vision of at least 20/400 (Fig. 27.1). It is important in this regard that the images on the tape or drum be sufficiently large so that the patient is not able to look around them. When testing a patient who claims complete loss of vision in one eye only, we begin the test by rotating the drum or moving the tape in front of the patient, who has **both** eyes open. Once we elicit good optokinetic nystagmus, we suddenly cover the unaffected eye with the palm of our hand or a handheld occluder (Fig. 27.2). The patient with nonorganic loss of vision in one eye will continue to show a jerk nystagmus. Unlike some authors (27,28), we are not comfortable estimating visual acuity in this setting by using an optokinetic drum with different-sized objects or placing neutral density filters in front of the patient's viewing eye until nystagmus disappears.

A second test that is helpful in detecting visual function in an eye or eyes that are said to have either no perception of light or light perception only is the "mirror test" (29,30). A large mirror is held in front of the patient's face, and the patient is asked to look directly ahead (Fig. 27.3). The mirror is then rotated and twisted back and forth, causing the images in the mirror to move. Patients with vision better than light perception will show a nystagmoid movement of the eyes, since they cannot avoid following the moving reflection in the mirror.

Miller recommended placing an 8-prism diopter loose prism, base in, in front of the affected eye of a patient with presumed monocular blindness and asking the patient to view a distant light or target (31). A report of diplopia indicated that the affected eye was not blind.

An interesting but somewhat extreme course of action, taken in the past by some physicians in the Armed Forces when dealing with persons who claimed to have lost all vision in both eyes but in whom there was no organic evidence of disease, was to place them at "retinal rest" (29). The patients were told that the "retina was fatigued" and that the condition would only respond to rest. The patient would

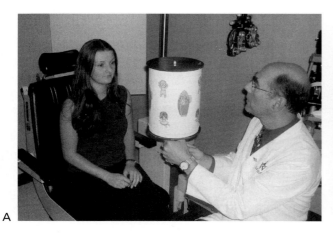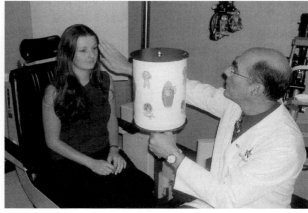

A   B

Figure 27.2. Use of optokinetic drum to detect nonorganic unilateral blindness. *A,* In a patient claiming unilateral blindness, the drum is first rotated while the patient is instructed to look straight ahead with both eyes open. *B,* Once nystagmus is elicited, the examiner continues to rotate the drum and suddenly covers the ''normal'' eye with the palm of the hand and observes the ''blind'' eye for continued nystagmus.

then be hospitalized with light-tight patches over both eyes placed in such a way that it would be immediately obvious if an attempt was made to remove or adjust them. The patient would not be allowed any sensory stimulation such as a radio, television, or compact disc player. No visitors were allowed, and visits by hospital personnel were kept to a minimum. The patient's vision was checked once a day. This procedure invariably resulted in complete return of vision within a very short period of time.

A way to detect nonorganic visual loss in a patient who claims to be unable to see shapes or objects in one or both eyes is to ask the patient to touch the tips of the first fingers of both hands together (3). If the patient claims loss of vision in one eye only, the opposite eye is patched before the test

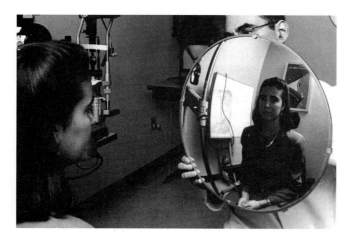

Figure 27.3. Use of a mirror to detect nonorganic blindness. The affected eye is occluded if the patient claims blindness in only one eye; otherwise, both eyes are left open. The patient is instructed to look straight ahead into the mirror, and the mirror is then rotated and turned from side to side. The development of nystagmus or a nystagmoid movement of the eyes indicates that the patient can see moving images in the mirror and thus is not blind.

is performed. As every physician knows, the ability to touch the tips of the fingers of two hands together is based not on vision but on proprioception. Thus, patients with organic blindness can easily bring the tips of the first fingers of both hands together, whereas patients with nonorganic blindness, particularly those who are malingering, will be unable to do so (Fig. 27.4). Similarly, a patient with organic blindness can easily sign his or her name without difficulty, whereas patients with blindness caused by malingering may produce an extremely bizarre signature (32).

Some physicians have tested patients who claim complete or severe loss of vision in one or both eyes by showing them photographs or cards with certain words or phrases that some persons might consider ''objectionable.'' The patient views this series of photographs or cards only with the ''blind'' eye or eyes, and the examiner observes the patient for a response to the content of the material being viewed. Gasps, smiles, or other responses suggest that the patient actually has vision in the affected eye. We are reminded of one young man who claimed to be completely blind in one eye but, after having been shown a series of photographs from a popular men's magazine with no apparent response, then asked if he could see the set of photographs one more time because he thought he ''just might have seen something out of the eye.'' Another patient shown several phrases suggesting actions that were anatomically impossible suddenly began to laugh and admitted that we ''had got'' him. Despite these successes, we consider this test too confrontational to recommend it.

A variety of tests may be performed in patients who claim vision in the range of 20/40 to hand motions in one or both eyes. None of these tests is invariably reliable, but one or more usually is sufficient to provide convincing evidence that visual acuity loss either is nonexistent or not as severe as the patient claims (27). Visual acuity may be tested not by starting from the largest letters or numbers and moving progressively to smaller ones, but by beginning with the

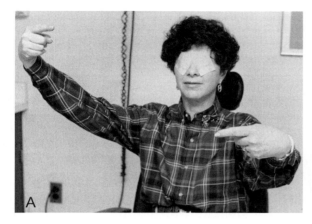

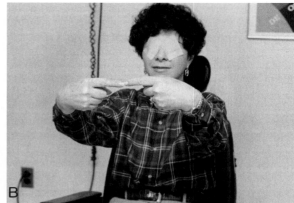

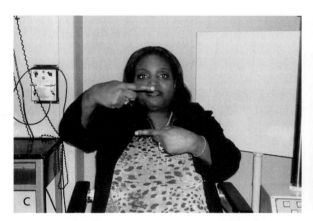

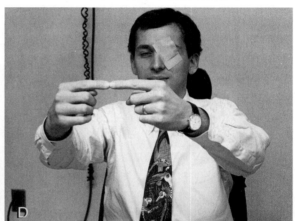

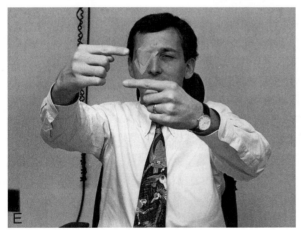

Figure 27.4. Testing nonorganic visual loss by asking a patient who claims monocular or binocular blindness to touch the tips of the first fingers of each hand together. *A and B,* A person who is truly blind can easily touch the tips of the fingers together, using proprioception, as the person in these photographs is doing despite having both eyes occluded. *C,* A woman with nonorganic loss of vision in both eyes is unable to touch the tips of the fingers together, even though she should be able to do so. A person with monocular nonorganic visual loss may touch the tips of the fingers together when viewing with the ''normal'' eye (*D*), but may claim to be unable to do so when viewing with the ''blind'' eye (*E*).

smallest line. Assuming that the patient cannot see this first line after being allowed to concentrate for several minutes, the physician tells the patient that the size of the print is now going to be ''doubled'' in size, and the patient is shown the next larger line and given several minutes to read it. This process is continued until the patient is able to read the line. This method of testing often produces visual acuity better than that initially claimed by the patient. In addition, some projector slides have several 20/20 lines, and these lines may

be shown to the patient in succession as the examiner tells the patient the size of the letters is increasing.

Testing of near vision is also important in patients claiming decreased acuity. A discrepancy in the distance and near-visual acuity that is not attributable to a refractive error or a disturbance of the media, such as an oil drop cataract, usually is evidence of a nonorganic disturbance.

Levi and Feldman reported the use of the Potential Acuity Meter (Mentor, Norwell, Massachusetts) in the diagnosis of nonorganic visual disease (33). First, a determination is made of the patient's best-corrected visual acuity in each eye. The patient's pupils are then dilated, and the patient is told that a test of potential visual function is going to be performed that bypasses or otherwise circumvents the visual problem and that gives the examiner knowledge of what the patient's vision would be if he or she did not have the reported visual problem. A significant improvement in vision in the affected eye or eyes that is unassociated with any abnormality in the ocular media or retina indicates nonorganic visual loss.

Patients claiming decreased vision in one eye only may undergo a "refraction" in which the normal eye is fogged with a high plus lens (e.g., a +5.00 or higher sphere), and a lens with minimal power (e.g., a ±0.50 sphere or cylinder) is placed before the worse eye. The patient is then told to read the chart with "both eyes." A variation of this test is the use of paired cylinders (20,32). A plus cylinder and a minus cylinder of the same power (usually 2–6 diopters) are placed at parallel axes in front of the "normal" eye in a trial frame. The patient's normal correction is placed in front of the affected eye. The patient is asked to read, with both eyes open, a line that previously had been read with the normal eye but not with the affected eye. As the patient begins to read, the axis of one of the cylinders is rotated about 10–15°. The axes of the two cylinders thus will no longer be parallel, blurring vision in the normal eye. If the patient continues to read the line, or can read it again when asked to do so, he or she must be using the affected eye.

Red-green glasses used with a red and green duochrome slide superimposed on the normal vision chart can be used to induce a patient to read with an eye that supposedly cannot see (or cannot see well) by making the patient think that he or she is using both eyes (Fig. 27.5). In this test, the eye

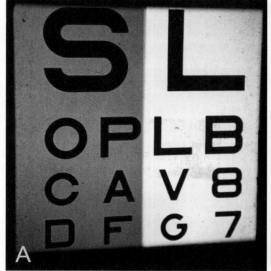

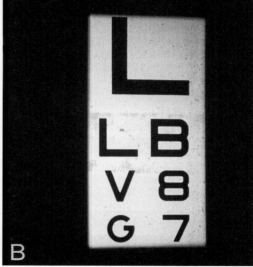

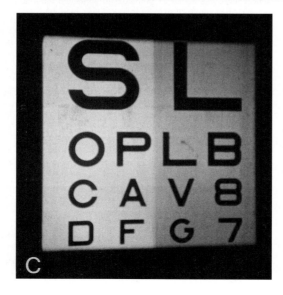

Figure 27.5. Use of red-green glasses with a red-green duochrome slide superimposed on a normal vision chart to detect uniocular nonorganic decreased vision. *A,* Appearance of the chart with superimposed red-green duochrome slide when viewed without red-green lenses. The left side of the chart is seen as red, the right side as green. *B,* The eye viewing through the green lens sees only the letters on the right (green) side of the chart. *C,* The eye viewing through the red lens sees both sets of letters. The lenses are arranged so that the red lens is over the eye with decreased vision, and the patient is asked to read the chart with both eyes open. If the patient reads the letters on both sides of the chart, he or she obviously is using the eye with decreased vision, because the unaffected eye that is viewing through the green lens should only be able to see the letters on one side of the chart.

behind the red lens will see the letters on both sides of the chart, whereas the eye behind the green lens will see only those letters on the green side of the chart. The lenses are arranged so that the red lens is over the eye with decreased vision, and the patient is then asked to read the chart with both eyes open. If the patient reads the entire line, it is obvious that the abnormal eye must be functioning better than the patient claims.

A variant of the red-green glasses/duochrome chart test that employs the red-green glasses and Ishihara color plates can be performed in patients with presumed nonorganic monocular visual loss that is worse than 20/400 (34). The patient should first be tested for ''congenital'' color vision as described below. Once it has been established that color vision is normal, the patient is asked to view the Ishihara color plates while wearing red-green glasses with the red lens over the affected eye. With the exception of plates 1 and 36, the numbers and lines on the Ishihara plates cannot be seen by the eye over which the green filter is placed. Even with visual acuity of 20/400, however, all of the color plates can be seen through a red filter. Thus, a patient who has normal color vision in at least the unaffected eye, who then views the plates through red-green spectacles with the red lens in front of the affected eye, and who correctly identifies the figures on the plates, must have visual acuity of 20/400 or better in the affected eye.

Another use of red-green glasses to detect nonorganic monocular visual loss is to place the glasses on the patient with the red lens in front of the eye with normal sight. The patient is then asked to read small letters on a white sheet of paper that have been written with a red pencil or red felt-tip pen. The patient with organic visual loss will not be able to read the letters, whereas a patient with nonorganic visual loss will be able to do so. The problem with this test is that if the examiner presses too firmly when writing the letters, an impression on the paper will be created that may allow the patient to see the letters through either lens (35). It is for this reason that the author prefers the duochrome test to this variation.

Mojon and Flueckiger developed a near-vision optotype chart with each optotype having a minimum angle of resolution that is independent of the size of the optotype (36). These investigators found that use of this chart correctly identified 100% of patients with organic visual loss and 89% of patients with nonorganic visual loss. This chart can be obtained from Haag-Streit International, Koeniz, Switzerland.

Graf and Roesen described a visual acuity test that consists of 32 white plates with a black Landolt C printed in the center (37). The sequence of the four alternative directions of the C is not predictable, and after plate 21, four plates containing complete circles rather than a C are interspersed among the remaining plates with a C. The test is administered at a distance from which the patient states that he or she is able to recognize the optotypes, and he or she is asked to identify the direction of the C within 2 seconds. The number of correct answers is then compared with the probability of having that number of correct answers by chance given the patient's visual acuity. In addition, the response to the first circle is compared with the responses to the previous

19 Cs. Although the authors were able to detect malingering in 14 of 19 (74%) volunteers and 12 of 15 (80%) patients, we consider this test too complex and time consuming to recommend it.

Polarizing lenses can be used in several ways to detect nonorganic visual loss in a patient with decreased vision in one eye only (Fig. 27.6). In the American Optical Polarizing Test, the patient wears polarizing glasses, and the test object, a Project-O-Chart slide, projects letters alternately so that one letter is seen by both eyes, the next by the right eye, the next by the left eye, etc. Another test uses a polarizing lens

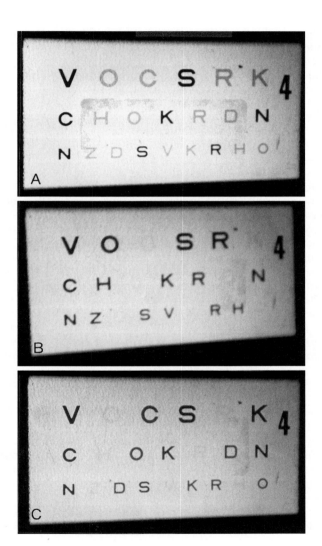

Figure 27.6. Use of polarizing lenses and a Snellen chart with a superimposed polarizing filter to detect uniocular nonorganic decreased vision. The patient wears the polarizing glasses and is asked to view letters, some of which should be seen by both eyes, some only by the right eye, and some only by the left eye. *A,* Appearance of the entire chart when viewed without polarizing lenses. *B,* Appearance of same chart when viewed through one of the polarizing lenses. *C,* Appearance of chart when viewed through the other polarizing lens. Note that certain letters (e.g., V, S, C, K, N, S, and R) can be seen through both lenses, whereas others can be seen through one of the lenses but not the other.

placed before a projector. The patient is asked to read the chart while wearing polarizing lenses, with one eye or the other being allowed to see the whole projected image at a time. Variations of this test have been described by several authors (38).

A prism that is 4 diopters in strength can be used to detect vision in an eye said to have reduced or no vision. The patient is asked to look with both eyes at the vision chart. A 4-prism diopter loose prism is then placed, base-out, over the "affected eye." A patient with normal binocular vision will show a movement of both eyes toward the direction of the apex of the prism followed by a shift of the fellow eye back toward the center. A patient with true decreased or absent vision in the eye over which the prism is placed will show no conjugate movement at all. Similarly, when the prism is placed over the "better eye" of a patient whose other eye truly is blind or has extremely reduced sight, only the first conjugate binocular shift will occur. There will be no compensatory movement of the fellow eye back toward the center.

Several **prism dissociation tests** can be used to detect mild degrees of nonorganic monocular visual loss (39). In this test, the patient is first asked if he or she has experienced double vision in addition to loss of vision in the affected eye. If the answer is negative, the patient is told that the examiner will test the alignment of both eyes and that the test should produce vertical double vision. A 4-prism diopter loose prism is then placed base down in front of the unaffected eye at the same time that a ½-prism diopter prism is simultaneously placed with the base in any direction over the eye with decreased vision. In this way, the patient does not become suspicious that the examiner is paying specific attention to one eye or the other. A 20/20 or larger size Snellen letter is then projected in the distance, and the patient is asked if he or she has double vision. When the patient admits to diplopia, he or she is then asked whether the two letters are of equal quality or sharpness, and an assessment of visual acuity can then be made.

Patients in whom visual acuity is reduced and there is no evidence of a refractive error, disturbance of the ocular media, or a macular abnormality by ophthalmoscopic examination are often assumed to have an underlying optic neuropathy even if the optic disc appears normal. Patients with a true optic neuropathy, however, almost invariably have a disturbance of color vision that can be detected using various types of color plates, such as the Hardy-Rand-Rittler Pseudoisochromatic Plates or the Ishihara Color Plates. We have found it useful to "prepare" the patient suspected of having nonorganic visual loss for the test by asking if he or she was ever diagnosed as having "congenital color blindness." Assuming the patient gives a negative answer, he or she is told that the color vision test the physician is going to perform is a test of congenital color blindness and that the patient should therefore be able to see the figures or numbers.

Testing of stereopsis may be valuable in detecting nonorganic visual loss (30). There is a definite correlation between binocular visual acuity and stereopsis (Table 27.1) (40,41). For instance, a patient with 20/20 vision in one eye and organic visual loss producing visual acuity of 20/200 in the

Table 27.1
Relationship of Visual Acuity and Stereopsis

Visual Acuity	Average Stereopsis[a]
20/20	40
20/25	43
20/30	52
20/40	61
20/50	78
20/70	94
20/100	124
20/200	160

[a] Measured in seconds of image disparity.
(Modified from Levy NS, Glick EB. Stereoscopic perception and Snellen visual acuity. Am J Ophthalmol 1974;78:722–724.)

fellow eye has stereoacuity of only about 180 seconds of arc, whereas a patient with 20/20 visual acuity OU has stereoacuity of 40 seconds of arc. A variety of stereoacuity tests are available, all of which have advantages and disadvantages (Fig. 27.7) (43).

Examination of pupillary responses can be helpful in diagnosing nonorganic visual loss(16). Patients who report complete blindness in both eyes should have pupils that do not react to light stimulation unless the process affects the postgeniculate visual pathways. Thus, the pupils of a patient who cannot perceive light with either eye because of bilateral retinal, optic nerve, or optic tract lesions, or because of damage to the optic chiasm, do not react to light stimulation, whereas the pupils of a patient who is blind from bilateral lesions of the optic radiations or striate cortex will react relatively normally to light. Pupils that react to light stimulation in a patient who claims complete loss of vision in both eyes indicate either that the patient is cerebrally blind (usually from damage to the striate cortex—cortical blindness) or that the patient has nonorganic loss of vision.

Patients with unilateral or asymmetric optic neuropathy invariably have a relative afferent pupillary defect (RAPD) that can easily be detected by performing a swinging flash-

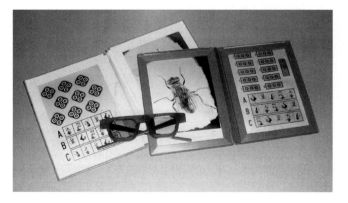

Figure 27.7. Two tests of stereopsis useful in detecting nonorganic visual loss.

light test (see Chapter 15). The absence of an RAPD in a patient with monocular visual loss indicates either that the patient does not have a unilateral optic neuropathy (and thus may support a diagnosis of nonorganic visual loss) or that the patient has a **bilateral** optic neuropathy that is asymmetric. It must be emphasized that patients with electrophysiologic evidence of bilateral optic neuropathy may nevertheless have very asymmetric visual acuity in the two eyes unassociated with a relative afferent pupillary defect. We have seen numerous patients with visual acuity of 10/100–20/400 in one eye and 20/20 in the fellow eye who have had no relative afferent pupillary defect by standard clinical testing, but whose visual evoked responses were bilaterally delayed indicating a bilateral optic neuropathy. Thus, if there is no indication of nonorganic disease in a patient with unexplained, unilateral visual loss without an obvious relative afferent pupillary defect, such a patient should undergo electrophysiologic testing, particularly full-field and multifocal electroretinography and pattern-reversal and flash-evoked visual evoked potentials (44,45).

It must be remembered that although electroretinography is an objective test of overall retinal function, visual evoked responses elicited by pattern reversal may be affected by a variety of factors other than organic disease of the central visual pathways (46). Some of these factors are related to the way the test is performed and include the size and color of the stimuli and the frequency with which they are presented, background illumination, and the state of dark adaptation. Other factors are related to the patient, including age, attention, concentration, pupil size, and fatigue. Indeed, both the amplitude **and** latency of the P100 peak can be consciously or unconsciously altered by a patient who is either not concentrating or not focusing continuously on the target (47).

The management of patients who have nonorganic loss of visual acuity is problematic and often depends on whether the patient is a child or an adult and whether the condition is thought to be psychogenic or caused by malingering. In our experience and in that of others, nonorganic visual loss in children occurs as a situational phenomenon caused by a wide range of academic, social, or familial difficulties (2,19,21). Once we are certain that the condition is nonorganic, we first attempt to ''cure'' the visual loss by informing the child that the only problem is a slight refractive error. A minimal correction is then placed into a trial frame or phoropter, and the patient is told that they ''should see normally'' with this set of glasses. If this is successful, the patient is told not to worry about the visual process and that the refractive error is sufficiently minimal that it probably is not necessary for glasses to be worn. If this maneuver is unsuccessful, we privately inform the parents of our findings so that they will not continue to be concerned about an organic process. We then inform the child that we are happy to report that there is **no irreversible damage to the eyes** and that vision should improve spontaneously with time. We do not specify a particular time frame during which we think this will occur, and we encourage the children to ''do as well as you can'' in school, at home, etc., until vision improves. In our experience and in the experience of others, this approach

is sufficient to solve the problem in the vast majority of cases (20).

Murata and Takahashi evaluated 46 persons under 21 years of age with psychogenic visual loss (48). At final examination, 66 of 78 affected eyes (85%) had visual acuity of 20/20 or better. Dealing with children whose visual loss is associated with complex interpersonal relationships within the family, such as sexual abuse or other social difficulties, is much more difficult and may require the services of a psychotherapist, child psychiatrist, or other specialist (2,49).

The treatment of adults with nonorganic loss of visual acuity is more complicated than the treatment of children, particularly when there is evidence of malingering, and the outcome usually is much less satisfactory (2). As long as there is a motivation for material secondary gain, it may be impossible to ''treat'' such a patient for his or her visual loss. In many cases, the physician must be content that the loss of vision is nonorganic and to record this fact in the patient's chart. We see no purpose in confronting the patient with our belief that the visual loss is nonorganic unless we can convince the patient that ultimately it is not in his or her best interest to continue the charade because we have proof that the visual loss is nonorganic—such proof will eventually cost the patient time, money, or even freedom.

Visual Field Defects

Nonorganic visual field defects can be of several types (16). The most common nonorganic visual field defect is a nonspecifically constricted visual field. When the field is tested kinetically, using either a Goldmann perimeter or a tangent (Bjerrum) screen, the field may have a spiraling nature, becoming smaller and smaller as the test object is moved around the field (Fig. 27.8). Alternatively, the visual field may remain the same size or nearly the same size regardless of the size or brightness of the test stimulus, or it may be inconsistent when tested repeatedly in one or more meridians (50). Other nonorganic visual field defects, however, include unilateral or bilateral central scotomas (51), unilateral hemianopia (52,53), bitemporal hemianopia (54), binasal hemianopia (55), and even homonymous hemianopia (56).

A nonorganically constricted visual field may be diagnosed in a variety of ways. In some cases, the patient can be cajoled into enlarging the field. After completion of perimetry, the patient is told that he or she did fine but that it was clear to the examiner that the patient was responding only when he or she was ''absolutely certain'' that he or she saw the test object. The examiner then explains that the test is to be repeated and encourages the patient to respond at an earlier stage when he or she just barely detects the stimulus (32).

Nonorganic visual field constriction can also be detected by testing the field using a tangent screen with the patient at two different distances from the screen (usually 1 and 2 meters). The size of the test object is varied so that the ratio of the size of the test object and the distance of the patient from the screen remain constant; i.e., a 9-mm-diameter white test object is used when the patient is 1 m from the screen, and an 18-mm-diameter white test object is used when the

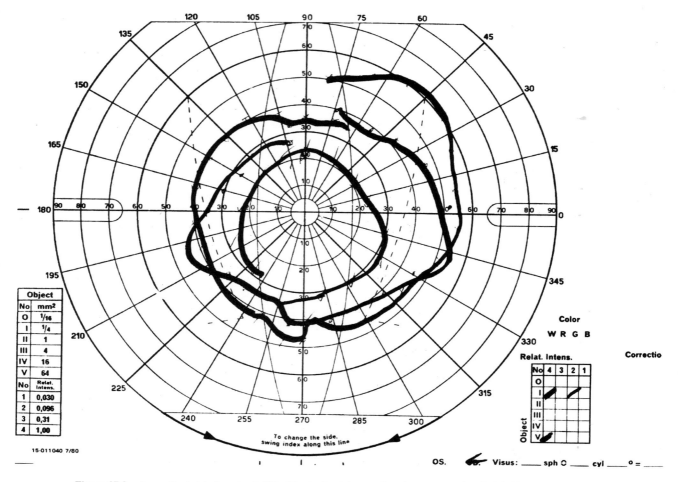

Figure 27.8. In a patient claiming visual difficulties in the right eye, there is a nonorganic spiral field when the eye is tested kinetically using a Goldmann perimeter.

patient is 2 m from the screen. Patients with an organically constricted visual field (e.g., patients with retinitis pigmentosa) will show an increase in the absolute size of the visual field under these conditions when they are moved from 1 m to 2 m away from the screen, whereas patients with nonorganic visual field constriction will maintain the same absolute size of the field constriction. Automated kinetic perimetry can give similar results (56a).

Nonorganic monocular hemianopias and scotomas as well as both binasal and bitemporal hemianopic defects usually can be diagnosed by first performing visual field testing monocularly and then binocularly (Fig. 27.9) (52). If the field defect is present in only one eye when the eyes are tested separately, but is still present when binocular simultaneous field testing is performed, the defect can be assumed to be nonorganic. This method cannot distinguish between organic and nonorganic homonymous hemianopic defects or bilateral central scotomas.

A method for diagnosing nonorganic paracentral visual field defects was reported by Slavin, who used a red Amsler grid with red-green lenses (57). The patient was a 43-year-

old man who had normal visual acuity in both eyes but showed a temporal paracentral scotoma in the visual field of the right eye. When the patient viewed a red Amsler grid with the right eye, he mapped out a discrete temporal scotoma; however, when he again was asked to view the red Amsler grid, this time through red-green lenses with the red lens over the right eye, he noted no scotoma. Since the grid could not be seen with the left eye because it was covered with a green lens, the patient, who thought he was viewing the grid with both eyes, was still viewing it only with the right eye.

A quick method of detecting nonorganic visual field loss of all types is to test saccadic eye movements into the supposedly absent portion of the field (3). The patient assumes that the eye movements and not the visual fields are being tested. This assumption is strengthened by first asking the patient if it hurts to move the eyes. Regardless of the patient's answer (which, interestingly, is often affirmative), the patient is told that the examiner is going to test the eye movements, and the patient is asked to pursue an object in various directions. The patient is then asked to look from the straight

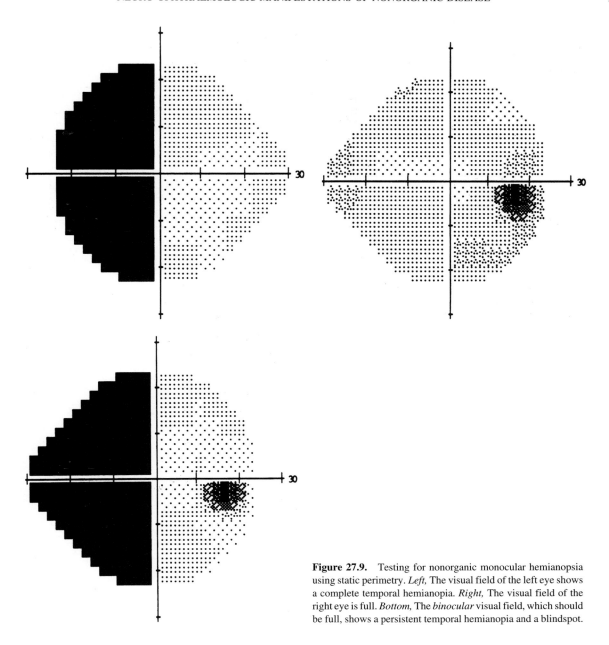

Figure 27.9.   Testing for nonorganic monocular hemianopsia using static perimetry. *Left,* The visual field of the left eye shows a complete temporal hemianopia. *Right,* The visual field of the right eye is full. *Bottom,* The *binocular* visual field, which should be full, shows a persistent temporal hemianopia and a blindspot.

ahead position to an eccentric location where the examiner holds an object. The object is subsequently moved from one location to another with the patient being asked each time to look from the center to the object. If the patient complains that he or she ''cannot see'' that far in the periphery, the examiner explains that he or she understands and that is why the patient should look **directly** at the object rather than to try to see it in the peripheral vision.

It should be noted that patients can create reproducible nonorganic visual field defects not only when tested with kinetic perimetry but also when tested using automated static perimetry (Fig. 27.10) (52,54,58,59). Such patients do not necessarily show an increased number of fixation false-positive, or false-negative errors.

The management of patients with nonorganic visual field constriction is similar to that of patients with nonorganic visual loss. Children and adults who do not seem to be malingering are told that they eventually will improve, and this usually is the case, although we have been impressed that the percentage of patients who can be demonstrated to have normalization of, or significant improvement in, nonorganic visual field defects is substantially less than the percentage who have improvement in nonorganic visual acuity loss (see previous discussion). Kathol et al., for example, examined 42 patients with nonorganic visual loss, of whom 29 (69%) had constricted or spiral fields (20). All patients were then examined 16 to 156 months later. On reexamination, 23 patients (55%) still had constricted or spiral fields. In the same

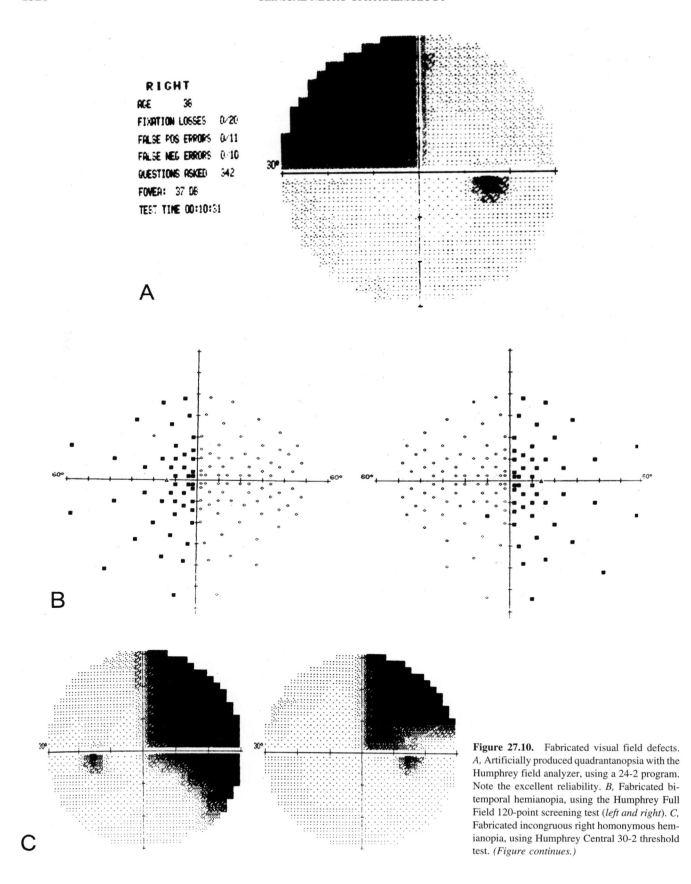

Figure 27.10. Fabricated visual field defects. *A,* Artificially produced quadrantanopsia with the Humphrey field analyzer, using a 24-2 program. Note the excellent reliability. *B,* Fabricated bitemporal hemianopia, using the Humphrey Full Field 120-point screening test (*left and right*). *C,* Fabricated incongruous right homonymous hemianopia, using Humphrey Central 30-2 threshold test. *(Figure continues.)*

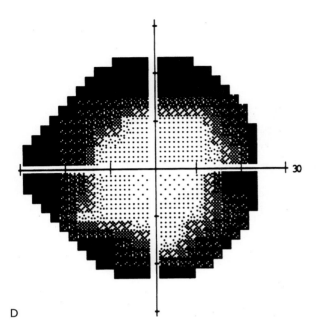

D

Figure 27.10. Continued. *D*, Fabricated constricted visual field in a patient with no clinical or electrophysiologic evidence of retinopathy or optic neuropathy. Note the "squaring" of the field defect, a phenomonen common to nonorganic visual field constriction recorded by automated perimetry. (*A*, From Glovinsky Y, Quigley HA, Bissett RA, et al. Am J Ophthalmol 1990;110:90–91. *B and C*, From MacLeod JDA, Manners RM, Heaven CJ, et al. Visual field defects. Neuroophthalmology 1994;14:185–188.)

study, the number of patients with nonorganic visual acuity defects decreased from 15 to 2.

Murata and Takahashi examined 46 patients less than 21 years old with psychogenic visual loss (48). At final examination, 36 of 50 eyes (72%) showed improvement in visual fields. It is our experience that most patients with nonorganic visual field loss deny that their visual field disturbance significantly limits their daily activities or state that despite their visual difficulties they are able to maintain their normal lifestyle. For this reason, we rarely recommend psychiatric or psychological counseling for these patients, and we generally do not advise confronting adults whose visual field defects are caused by malingering unless it seems likely that one can end the charade with a few well-chosen words.

Monocular Diplopia

Most patients who complain of double vision are suffering from misalignment of the visual axes. In such cases, the diplopia immediately resolves as soon as one eye is covered. Patients in whom diplopia remains despite occlusion of one eye are said to have **monocular diplopia**. This condition is caused most often by a refractive error, particularly by uncorrected or improperly corrected astigmatism; by incorrectly fitted glasses; or by some irregularity of the cornea or lens (60–62). Most patients with this type of organic monocular diplopia will recognize a difference in the intensity of the two images that they see. One image will be fairly clear, but the second image will be perceived as "fuzzy" and

may be described as a "ghost image" that overlaps the clear image. The "diplopia" in such cases usually resolves with a pinhole, a better refraction or fitting of spectacles, or a contact lens. Rare examples of monocular diplopia and, more often, polyopia have been reported in patients with central nervous system (CNS) disease such as migraine, stroke, and brain tumors located in the temporoparietal region (63–65). Patients with cerebral polyopia usually do not complain of overlapping images and generally see each image with equal clarity; however, they complain bitterly of multiple images that may be of different sizes and shapes. Such patients usually have lesions in the parieto-occipital region, and most have obvious CNS disease.

True monocular diplopia (i.e., two separate and equal images of an object seen with one eye only) is almost never caused by organic disease. We and others have seen it most often in children who have found themselves in stressful academic, social, or family situations (25,66). Once both the child and the parents are reassured as to the benign nature of the condition, it usually resolves within a short period of time.

NONORGANIC DISEASE AFFECTING FIXATION, OCULAR MOTILITY, AND ALIGNMENT

Nonorganic disturbances of ocular motor function include disturbances of fixation, ocular motility, and alignment.

Disturbances of Fixation: Voluntary Nystagmus and Voluntary Saccadic Oscillations

Saccadic oscillations in most patients are involuntary eye movements caused by a neurological disease affecting the brainstem, cerebellum, or both. Nevertheless, some persons can produce saccadic oscillations that resemble nystagmus, ocular flutter, or opsoclonus.

Voluntary Nystagmus

Voluntary nystagmus is discussed in Chapter 23 of this text. The condition is characterized by a rapid to-and-fro movement of the eyes that is willfully initiated. It can be sustained for only a few seconds (67). It can be produced by 5–8% of the population (68) and it may occur as a familial trait (67). Voluntary nystagmus consists of rapidly alternating saccades with frequencies that range from 3–42 Hz and amplitudes that range from 0.5–35 (Fig. 27.11) (69,70). There is an inverse relationship between the frequency and the amplitude of the nystagmus (68). Voluntary nystagmus usually is horizontal; however, it can be vertical or torsional (71) and it can be produced in the light or dark and with the eyelids open or closed. It has even been reported as a monocular phenomenon (72), although we have not seen such a case.

Patients with voluntary nystagmus typically complain of oscillopsia and reduced vision (73). Such patients have fluttering of the eyelids and a strained facial expression during the episodes of nystagmus. In addition, the eyes tend to con-

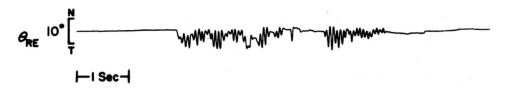

Figure 27.11. Voluntary nystagmus. Ocular motor recordings using a photoelectric method with infrared light. Voluntary nystagmus during binocular fixation. Note bursts of rapidly alternating saccades that vary in frequency and amplitude. RE, eye position of right eye; N, nasal direction; T, temporal direction. (From Ciuffreda KJ. Voluntary nystagmus: New findings and clinical implications. Am J Optom Physiol Optics 1980;57:795–800.)

verge during the nystagmus, since the nystagmus seems to be produced in part by stimulation of normal convergence mechanisms.

Patients who are able to produce voluntary nystagmus are also able to superimpose the nystagmus during normal tracking (74). Such persons often show transient nystagmoid movements associated with oscillopsia after an intense period of nystagmus.

Voluntary nystagmus has no pathologic significance. It may, however, be mistaken for certain pathologic conditions that affect fixation, including acquired nystagmus and saccadic intrusions.

Voluntary Saccadic Oscillations

Yee et al. described two persons who were able to produce large-amplitude to-and-fro saccadic oscillations (75). One of the persons, in fact, was the primary author of the article and clearly produced the oscillations voluntarily. The other man was involved in a motor vehicle accident in which he suffered a whiplash injury when the car he was driving was struck from behind by another car. Neither person had any evidence of neurological dysfunction, and an assessment that included a neurological examination, computed tomographic scanning, magnetic resonance imaging, and lumbar puncture in the person involved in the accident revealed no abnormalities. The authors believed that this person also produced his saccadic oscillations voluntarily.

Eye movement recordings in both patients showed that the movements were bursts of conjugate saccades in opposing directions, with no intersaccadic interval. Unlike the saccades of voluntary nystagmus (see previous discussion), they were multidirectional (horizontal, vertical, or oblique), had amplitudes up to 40, and sometimes had curvilinear trajectories. These characteristics are similar to those of ocular flutter and opsoclonus, involuntary movements that are caused by significant damage to the brainstem, cerebellum, or both (see Chapter 23); however, patients with true ocular flutter or opsoclonus generally have other neurologic manifestations. The findings reported by Yee et al. (75) indicate that when saccadic oscillations that appear to be ocular flutter or opsoclonus are found in patients who do not have other neurologic signs or symptoms, the possibility of a nonorganic cause should be considered.

Disorders of Ocular Motility and Alignment

Several nonorganic disorders of ocular motility and alignment may be observed in patients both with and without visual complaints. These disorders include insufficiency or paralysis of convergence, spasm of the near reflex, supranuclear horizontal and vertical gaze paresis, and forced downward deviation of the eyes.

Convergence Insufficiency or Paralysis

Convergence insufficiency or paralysis may be nonorganic in nature. We have seen several cases, usually in adolescents, but also in adults. Such patients often have associated insufficiency or paralysis of accommodation, although either disturbance may exist independently. Patients with apparent weakness of convergence may nevertheless show normal convergence when asked to read a paragraph at length during which the eyes are alternately covered. Asking the patient to perform other near tasks such as telling time by looking at his or her wristwatch, may also be associated with normal convergence (Fig. 27.12) (76). We examined one woman who claimed to have myasthenia gravis. Indeed, she had been treated with a thymectomy even though she had no serologic or electromyographic evidence of myasthenia. When examined by us, her only findings were variably decreased accommodation and convergence. Her other responses to testing suggested nonorganic illness and, in fact, a discussion with her primary care physician indicated that she had previously been evaluated by a gastrointestinal disease for various complaints for which no organic cause could be identified. The specialist had indicated that he thought the patient had nonorganic disease.

Spasm of the Near Reflex

The most common nonorganic disturbance of ocular motility and alignment is **spasm of the near reflex** (Fig. 27.13) (76,77). The syndrome is characterized by episodes of intermittent convergence, increased accommodation, and miosis. The degree of convergence is variable. Some patients exhibit marked convergence of both eyes, resulting in a marked esotropia. Other patients show a lesser degree of convergence such that one eye remains relatively straight while the other converges. In all cases, however, the patient seems to have unilateral or, more often, bilateral limitation of abduction during testing of versions although not necessarily during testing of ductions (discussion following). The degree of accommodation spasm also is variable. Some patients produce only a few diopters of myopia, whereas others produce 8–10 diopters of myopia. Miosis is invariably significant in patients who exhibit spasm of the near reflex regard-

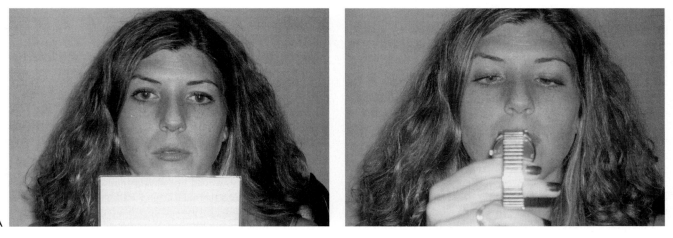

Figure 27.12.   Nonorganic convergence insufficiency. *A,* Inability to converge upon a near target despite encouragement. *B,* Normal near-reflex elicited by asking patient to tell the time by looking at a wristwatch.

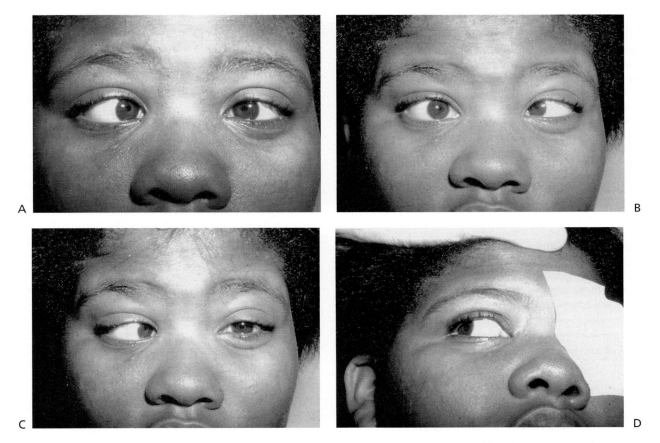

Figure 27.13.   Spasm of the near reflex. The patient is a healthy 15-year-old girl. *A,* In primary position, the eyes are esotropic, and the pupils are constricted. *B,* On attempted right gaze, the right eye does not abduct, even to the midline, and the pupils become more constricted. *C,* On attempted left gaze, the left eye does not abduct beyond the midline, and the pupils become more constricted. *D,* When the left eye is patched and the patient is asked to pursue a target to the right or is asked to fixate a stationary target while the head is rotated to the left, the right eye abducts fully and the pupil becomes less constricted.

less of the degree of accommodation and convergence spasm (77).

Spasm of the near reflex may be mistaken for unilateral or bilateral abducens nerve paresis, divergence insufficiency, horizontal gaze paresis, or even myasthenia gravis. However, the lack of other neurological deficits, the variability of the eye movements, and the constant occurrence of miosis associated with the adductive eye movements generally permit the correct diagnosis to be made (77,78). In addition, despite apparent unilateral or bilateral abduction weakness during testing of versions (with both eyes open), when ductions are tested directly with one eye occluded or indirectly using oculocephalic testing, both eyes invariably have full abduction and the miosis seen when the eyes are in the esotropic position immediately resolves. Covering one eye during a typical spasm also may cause dramatic reversal of the miosis (79). Finally, refraction with and without cycloplegia during a period of spasm establishes the presence of pseudomyopia.

Several organic conditions, in addition to abducens nerve paresis and horizontal gaze paresis, may mimic spasm of the near reflex. Pretectal esotropia, also called pseudo-abducens paresis or pseudo-6th nerve palsy, is a general disordered co-contraction of extraocular muscles and is not related to the near reflex. Convergence nystagmus jerks are not accompanied by miosis in this condition (80). Convergence substitution sometimes occurs when patients with supranuclear horizontal gaze paresis use convergence to move the adducting eye into the limited field of gaze (81). The resulting eye movement may suggest spasm of the near reflex. Finally, there are rare cases of true convergence spasm that have an organic basis. Most of these cases are unassociated with concomitant miosis, but exceptions exist. Kosmorsky et al., for example, observed spasm of the near reflex in a 58-year-old man with **rippling muscle disease** an autosomal-dominant inherited syndrome characterized by muscle stiffness, primarily in the extremities, in which the muscles display an unusual sensitivity to stretch, manifested by rippling waves of muscle contractions (82). Spasm of the near reflex occurred spontaneously when the patient attempted to read, and it could be induced during the neuro-ophthalmologic examination by prolonged near viewing. In addition, several authors have described what seems to be typical spasm of the near reflex in patients with intrinsic lesions of the mesencephalon, or extrinsic lesions compressing the dorsal mesencephalon (80,83). Thus, the examiner who is unsure whether or not spasm of the near reflex is organic must be prepared to give the patient the benefit of the doubt.

Management of persons with nonorganic spasm of the near reflex may consist only of reassurance. Psychiatric counseling may be appropriate in other cases. Schwartze et al. described a patient with spasm of the near reflex who was successfully treated with an amytal interview, during which it was suggested that she was orthophoric (84). In other patients, symptomatic relief may be produced using a cycloplegic drug combined with bifocal spectacles or reading glasses. Manor (85) described the use of special glasses with an opaque inner third of the lens in the treatment of a patient with spasm of the near reflex. These spectacles oc-

clude vision when the eyes are esotropic, thus presumably interrupting the spasm. We have no experience with such glasses.

Spasm of the near reflex should not be treated with strabismus surgery. We examined a patient with spasm of the near reflex who was treated with strabismus surgery after she failed to respond to treatment with topical cycloplegic drugs and bifocals. The patient underwent a recession of the left medial rectus muscle and a resection of the left lateral rectus muscle in an effort to reduce or eliminate the esotropia that occurred during her spasms. After surgery, however, she was still esotropic during spasms and, in addition, was now **exotropic** when she was not experiencing the spasms. She eventually required further surgery to reverse the condition.

Paralysis of Horizontal and Vertical Gaze

We have seen several patients with nonorganic **paralysis of horizontal and vertical eye movements**. The patients would not make voluntary horizontal or vertical saccades or pursuit movements, and they would not fixate on a distant object to allow oculocephalic testing; however, when the patients were observed through a one-way mirror, they could be seen to make absolutely normal pursuit and saccadic eye movements. In addition, measurements of eye movements during chair rotation in light and darkness indicated normal pursuit and saccadic systems.

Forced Downward Deviation of the Eyes in Nonorganic Coma and Seizures

Henry and Woodruff reported that forced deviation of the eyes toward the ground can be used to help differentiate organic from nonorganic coma and seizures (86). Rosenberg (73) emphasized the usefulness of this sign in two patients. The test is performed by moving the patient's head to one side and watching the movement of the patient's eyes. The head is then turned to the opposite side, again while watching the eye position. The typical response of a patient with organic coma is either no movement of the eyes, such as occurs in patients with brainstem disease or drug-induced coma, or a smooth movement of the eyes in the direction **opposite** of the head turn (the normal ''doll's eyes'' response, see Chapter 18). The eyes of a patient feigning a comatose state, however, will be deviated tonically toward the floor as if to avoid looking at the observer (16). On moving the head to the opposite side, the eyes will either saccade directly to the side facing the floor (i.e., in the **same** direction as the head turn) or they occasionally will dart from side to side before coming to rest. Although a true seizure focus may certainly produce a deviation of the eyes to one side, turning the head from side to side in such a setting will not affect this deviation.

NONORGANIC DISORDERS OF PUPILLARY SIZE AND REACTIVITY

A variety of pupillary phenomena have been described in patients with various types of psychiatric and psychogenic diseases. Investigators once hoped that certain disturbances of shape, size, and reactivity of one or both pupils could be used to diagnose specific psychiatric conditions. This has proved not to be the case. Pupillary phenomena associated with psychiatric and psychogenic conditions are considered in detail by Loewenfeld (87), and the interested reader should consult her authoritative text for further information. It suffices here to mention only a few of these phenomena.

Bumke noted that anxious or "neurotic" patients occasionally had widely dilated and poorly reacting pupils (88). The pupils failed to dilate further to a psychosensory stimulus they were already maximally dilated. The pupils of schizophrenic patients are sometimes dilated and unreactive. This phenomenon was described by Westphal who thought it particularly characteristic of the catatonic form of schizophrenia and called the condition "spasmus mobilis" (89,90). This pupillary disturbance seems to be similar to that described by Bumke. Widely dilated pupils during acute attacks of panic also have been described (87). They tend to be associated with generalized autonomic disturbances consistent with sympathetic hyperfunction, including profuse sweating, trembling, tachycardia, and tachypnea. The pupils of such patients appear normal between attacks.

Loewenfeld emphasized the high prevalence of **see-saw anisocoria** in "neurotic" patients (87). She commented that this phenomenon cannot be explained by the emotional or mental state of the patient, because psychosensory dilation is symmetric in such cases. In addition, see-saw anisocoria is transient and often reverses sides from one time to the next, so that it probably results from some type of temporary asymmetry in the central inhibitory neurons located in the mesencephalon. Some patients can voluntarily dilate both pupils. A patient described by Tyrer et al. could dilate both pupils and accelerate his heart rate at will (91).

Perhaps the most common nonorganic pupillary disturbance seen in ophthalmologic practice is a unilateral (and occasionally bilateral) fixed, dilated pupil caused by topical administration of a mydriatic agent (Fig. 27.14). In some cases the topical agent, usually atropine or scopolamine, has been administered by accident. For instance, patients who

have been using a transdermal scopolamine patch to prevent seasickness or postoperative nausea may contaminate their fingertips during placement of the patch. The patients subsequently rub their eyes, and one or both pupils dilate. In addition, atropine and scopolamine are naturally occurring alkaloids produced in certain plants, such as deadly nightshade, henbane, Jimson weed, and moonflower. Topical absorption after ocular contact with these agents in their natural form may occasionally occur, particularly in persons who work outdoors (92,93). Some patients, however, voluntarily place a topical parasympatholytic agent into one or both eyes and then present to a physician complaining of blurred vision.

Pharmacologically dilated pupils are extremely large —larger than the dilated pupils associated with an oculomotor nerve palsy—and usually completely nonreactive to light or near stimulation (Figs. 27.14 and 27.15). They are unassociated with ptosis, diplopia, or strabismus unless there is a preexisting disturbance of eyelid function or ocular motility. The diagnosis of a pharmacologically dilated pupil is made by placing 1–2 drops of 1% pilocarpine in each lower cul-de-sac. A neurologically dilated pupil (i.e., oculomotor nerve paresis, tonic pupil) will constrict maximally within 30 minutes; however, a pharmacologically dilated pupil either is not affected and remains widely dilated (Fig. 27.15) or constricts minimally. Unresponsiveness or even partial responsiveness of a dilated, fixed pupil to a solution of pilocarpine that is of sufficient strength to constrict the opposite, normally reacting pupil is absolute evidence of pharmacologic blockade, regardless of the patient's protestations to the contrary (94).

NONORGANIC DISTURBANCES OF ACCOMMODATION

The role of accommodation spasm in the condition called spasm of the near-reflex is discussed above. In addition, however, nonorganic **weakness or paralysis of accommodation** may occur, primarily in children and young adults. Such patients are unable to read unless provided with an

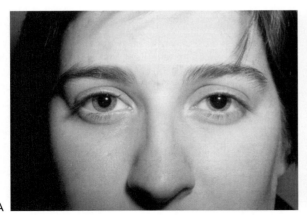 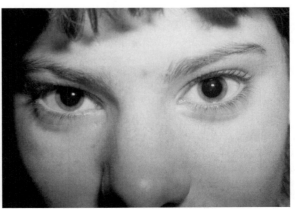

A   B

Figure 27.14. Pupillary dilation caused by voluntary use of a topical paralymphatolytic drug. *A,* Unilateral (left pupil). *B,* Bilateral. Note that in both cases, the affected pupils are extremely large. The size is much greater than that seen in patients with an oculomotor nerve paresis.

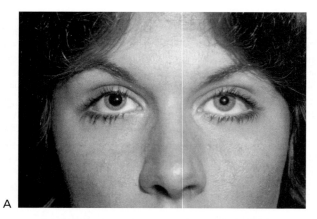

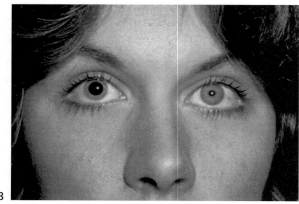

Figure 27.15. Testing for a pharmacologically dilated pupil using a solution of 1% pilocarpine. *A,* Before testing. *B,* The left pupil is markedly constricted, but the right pupil is unchanged in size 45 minutes after placement of two drops of 1% pilocarpine into the lower cul-de-sac of both eyes.

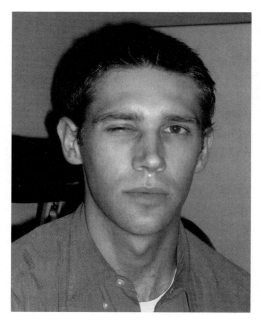

Figure 27.16. Nonorganic (voluntary) unilateral ptosis. Note elevation of the right lower eyelid and slight ptosis of the right eyebrow.

appropriate plus lens, and even then may claim an inability to read clearly. Indeed, it is the failure of a patient with normal distance vision and an inability to read despite an appropriate reading aid that should alert the physician to the possibility that the condition is nonorganic.

NONORGANIC DISTURBANCES OF EYELID FUNCTION

Nonorganic **ptosis** (pseudoptosis) is rare. In most cases, one can see or feel a fine spasm of the supposedly ptotic eyelid. There also tends to be elevation of the lower eyelid and variable relaxation of the elevators of the ipsilateral eyebrow, producing a mild brow ptosis (Fig. 27.16) (73).

Blepharospasm can occur as part of a more extensive neurologic disease, including Huntington's chorea, hepatolenticular degeneration, Hallervorden-Spatz disease, and postencephalitic parkinsonism, and it may also develop after a brainstem stroke or as part of a syndrome of tardive dyskinesia. Other causes of organic blepharospasm include drug toxicity with secondary tardive dyskinesia and ocular surface disease.

Some physicians believe that blepharospasm that is unas-

sociated with overt neurological or ocular disease is always a psychogenic disturbance. Although the condition called "essential blepharospasm" often worsens during periods of stress, it occurs most often in patients who do not have other psychogenic complaints. Interestingly, we have seen two patients with a history of migraine headaches whose migraine attacks stopped coincident with the development of essential blepharospasm, as if the body had substituted one reaction to stress for another.

We have seen several cases of blepharospasm that were clearly psychogenic in nature. One of these patients, a 35-year-old woman, experienced episodes of closure of the eyelids that would last for several hours and that were associated with epiphora. Attempts to open the eyelids during an episode revealed constant spasm of the lids. Pressure over the supraorbital notch is often useful in inducing a person with nonorganic blepharospasm to raise the eyelids. Most cases of psychogenic blepharospasm occur in children and young adults and seem to be triggered by a particular emotionally traumatic event (95).

We have seen no cases of nonorganic eyelid retraction, although patients who are anxious or upset often have variable bilateral eyelid retraction. One patient, referred to us with a diagnosis of presumed psychogenic eyelid retraction because of the variable nature of the condition and the lack of evidence of thyroid eye disease, actually had a mild ptosis on the contralateral side that had not been detected by the referring physician.

NONORGANIC DISTURBANCES OF OCULAR AND FACIAL SENSATION

Anesthesia of the skin of the eyelids and of one or both corneas may be nonorganic, as may hypersensitivity, with the latter being associated with lacrimation, blepharospasm, photophobia, or a combination of these. Sensitive spots along the upper or lower margins of the orbits are common in patients with such complaints.

NONORGANIC DISTURBANCES OF LACRIMATION

Excessive secretion of tears may be nonorganic and may be associated, as noted above, with nonorganic blepharospasm. **Bloody tears** also may be associated with blepharospasm. Walsh observed a patient who produced bloody tears by depositing blood from self-induced nosebleeds into the conjunctival sacs (96).

REFERENCES

1. Pilowsky I. Abnormal illness behaviour. Br J Med Psychol 1969;42:347–351.
2. Rada RT, Meyer GG, Kellner R. Visual conversion reaction in children and adults. J Nerv Ment Dis 1978;166:580–587.
3. Weller M, Wiedemann P. Hysterical symptoms in ophthalmology. Doc Ophthalmol 1989;73:1–33.
4. Chodoff P. A re-examination of some aspects of conversion hysteria. Psychiatry 1954;17:75–81.
5. Stephens JH, Kamp M. On some aspects of hysteria: A clinical study. J Nerv Ment Dis 1962;134:305–315.
6. Ziegler FJ, Imboden JB, Meyer E. Contemporary conversion reactions: A clinical study. Am J Psychiatry 1960;116:901–909.
7. Parsons T. The Social System. New York, Free Press of Glencoe, 1951.
8. Mechanic D. Response factors in illness: The study of illness behaviour. Soc Psychiatr 1966;1:11–20.
9. Mechanic D. The concept of illness behavior. J Chron Dis 1962;15:189–194.
10. Pilowsky I. A general classification of abnormal illness behaviours. Br J Med Psychol 1978;51:131–137.
11. Bursten B. On Münchausen's syndrome. Arch Gen Psychiatry 1965;13:261–267.
12. Smith RE, Conway BP. Alkali retinopathy. Arch Ophthalmol 1976;94:81–84.
13. Rosenberg PN, Krohel GB, Webb RM, Hepler RS. Ocular Münchausen's syndrome. Ophthalmology 1986;93:1120–1123.
14. Voutilainen R, Tuppurainen K. Ocular Münchausen's syndrome induced by incest. Acta Ophthalmol 1989;67:319–321.
15. Anderton LC, Shah P, Doran RM. An unusual case of ocular Münchausen's syndrome. Acta Ophthalmol 1994;72:126–127.
16. Newman NJ. Neuro-ophthalmology and psychiatry. Gen Hosp Psychiatry 1993;15:102–114.
17. Scott JA, Egan RA. Prevalence of organic neuro-ophthalmologic disease in patients with functional visual loss. Am J Ophthalmol 2003;135:670–675.
18. Yamade S, Kono M, Hukami K. Color vision in psychogenic visual disturbance. Folia Ophthalmol Jpn 1989;40:1674–1680.
19. Clarke WN, Noël L P, Bariciak M. Functional visual loss in children: A common problem with an easy solution. Can J Ophthalmol 1996;31:311–313.
20. Kathol RG, Cox TA, Corbett JJ, et al. Functional visual loss: Follow up of 42 cases. Arch Ophthalmol 1983;101:729–735.
21. Keltner JL, May WN, Johnson CA, et al. The California syndrome: Functional visual complaints with potential economic impact. Ophthalmology 1985;92:427–435.
22. Mojon DS, Schlauapfer TE. Nichtorganische Stauorungen in der Ophthalmologie: auUbersicht der Diagnostik und Therapie. Klin Monatsbl Augenheilkd 2001;218:298–304.
23. Mouriaux F, Defoort-Dhellemmes S, Kochman F, et al. Le pithiatisme oculaire chez l'enfant et l'adolescent. J Fr Ophtalmol 1997;20:175–182.
24. Langmann A, Lindner S, Kriechbaum N. Funktionelle Sehstauorung als Konversionssymptom im Kindes- und jugendalter. Klin Monatsbl Augenheilkd 2001;218:677–681.
25. Trauzettel-Klosinski S. Untersuchungsstrategien bei Simulation und funkionellen Sehstauorungen. Klin Monatsbl Augenheilkd 1997;211:73–83.
26. Bienfang DC, Kurtz D. Management of functional visual loss. J Am Optom Assoc 1998;69:12–21.
27. Tsutsui J, Karino T, Kimura H, et al. Evaluation of vision tests in the diagnosis of malingering. Folia Ophthalmol Jpn 1985;36:1159–1164.
28. Miyazaki T, Ueda K, Kurimoto S, et al. Evaluation of psychogenic amblyopia by objective visual acuity and corneal sensation testing. Folia Ophthalmol Jpn 1992;43:434–440.
29. Rieken H. Die Spiegelraumbewegung, eine neue Untersuchungsmethode auf der Grundlage eines "psycho optischen" Reflexes. Graefes Arch Ophthalmol 1943;145:432–453.
30. Kramer KK, La Piana FG, Appleton B. Ocular malingering and hysteria: Diagnosis and management. Surv Ophthalmol 1979;24:89–96.
31. Miller BW. A review of practical tests for ocular malingering and hysteria: Diagnosis and management. Surv Ophthalmol 1973;17:241–246.
32. Thompson HS. Functional visual loss. Am J Ophthalmol 1985;100:209–213.
33. Levi L, Feldman RM. Use of the potential acuity meter in suspected functional visual loss. Am J Ophthalmol 1992;114:502–503.
34. Savir H, Segal M. A simple test for detection of monocular functional visual impairment. Am J Ophthalmol 1988;106:500.
35. Slavin ML. Caution during performance of the red-green glasses test for functional visual loss. J Neuroophthalmol 2000;20:293.
36. Mojon DS, Flueckiger P. A new optotype chart for detection of visual nonorganic visual loss. Ophthalmology 2002;109:810–815.
37. Graf MH, Roesen J. Ocular malingering. A surprising visual acuity test. Arch Ophthalmol 2002;120:756–760.
38. Fahle M, Mohn G. Assessment of visual function in suspected ocular malingering. Br J Ophthalmol 1989;73:651–654.
39. Slavin ML. The prism dissociation test in detecting unilateral functional visual loss. J Clin Neuroophthalmol 1990;10:127–130.
40. Levy NS, Glick EB. Stereoscopic perception and Snellen visual acuity. Am J Ophthalmol 1974;78:722–724.
41. Donzis PB, Rappazzo JA, Burde RM, et al. Effect of binocular variations of Snellen's visual acuity on Titmus stereoacuity. Arch Ophthalmol 1983;101:930–932.
42. Marsh WR, Rawlings SC, Mumma JV. Evaluation of clinical stereoacuity tests. Ophthalmology 1980;87:1265–1272.
43. Simons K. A comparison of the Frisby, Random Dot E, TNO, and Randot Circles stereotests in screening and office use. Arch Ophthalmol 1981;99:446–452.
44. Nakamura A, Akio T, Matsuda E, et al. Pattern visual evoked potentials in malingering. J Neuroophthalmol 2001;21:42–45.
45. Xu S, Meyer D, Yoser S, et al. Pattern visual evoked potential in the diagnosis of functional visual loss. Ophthalmology 2001;108:76–81.
46. Towle VL, Sutcliffe E, Sokol S. Diagnosing functional visual deficits with the P300 component of the visual evoked potential. Arch Ophthalmol 1985;103:47–50.
47. Morgan RK, Nugent B, Harrison JM, et al. Voluntary alteration of pattern visual evoked responses. Ophthalmology 1985;92:1356–1363.
48. Murata M, Takahashi S. Psychogenic visual disturbances in patients under 21 years of age. Folia Ophthalmol Jpn 1993;44:53–58.
49. Koniszewski G, Mösler TA, Barocka A. Psychogen bedingte Sehfunktionsstörungen bei Kindern. Fortschr Ophthalmol 1985;82:457–458.
50. Ohkubo H. Visual field in hysteria: Reliability of visual field by Goldmann perimetry. Doc Ophthalmol 1989;71:61–67.
51. Lincoff HA. Bilateral central scotomas of hysterical origin. Arch Ophthalmol 1959;62:273–279.
52. Gittinger JW Jr. Functional monocular temporal hemianopsia. Am J Ophthalmol 1986;101:226–231.
53. Gittinger JW Jr. Functional hemianopsia: A historical perspective. Surv Ophthalmol 1988;32:427–432.
54. Fish RH, Kline LB, Hanumanthu VK, et al. Hysterical bitemporal hemianopia "cured" with contact lenses. J Clin Neuroophthalmol 1990;10:76–78.
55. Pilley SFJ, Thompson HS. Binasal field loss and prefixation blindness. In Glaser JS and Smith JL, eds. Neuro-Ophthalmology Symposium of the University of Miami and the Bascom Palmer Eye Institute. Vol. 8. St Louis, CV Mosby, 1975:277–284.
56a. Pineless SL, Volpe NJ. Computerized Kinetic perimetry detects tubular visual fields in patients with functional visual loss. Am J Ophthalmol 2004;137:933–935.
56. Garvey JL. Hysteric homonymous hemianopia. Am J Ophthalmol 1922;5:721–722.
57. Slavin ML. The use of red Amsler grid and red green lenses in detecting spurious paracentral visual field defects. Am J Ophthalmol 1987;103:338–339.
58. Thompson JC, Kosmorsky GS, Ellis BD. Fields of dreamers and dreamed up fields: Functional and fake perimetry. Ophthalmology 1996;103:117–125.
59. Martin TJ. Threshold perimetry of each eye with both eyes open in patients with monocular functional (nonorganic) and organic vision loss. Am J Ophthalmol 1998;125:857–865.
60. Amos JF. Diagnosis and management of monocular diplopia. J Am Optom Assoc 1982;53:101–115.
61. Hirst LW, Miller NR, Johnson RT. Monocular polyopia. Arch Neurol 1983;40:756–757.
62. Heher KL, Stark WJ, Miller NR. Oil drop cataracts. J Cataract Refract Surg 1993;19:306–308.
63. Bender MB. Polyopia and monocular diplopia of cerebral origin. Arch Neurol 1945;54:323–338.
64. Meadows JC. Observations on a case of monocular diplopia of cerebral origin. J Neurol Sci 1973;18:249–253.
65. Sinoff SE, Rosenberg M. Permanent cerebral diplopia in a migraineur. Neurology 1990;40:1138–1140.
66. Catalano RA, Simon JA, Krohel GB, et al. Functional visual loss in children. Ophthalmology 1986;93:385–390.
67. Zahn JR. Incidence and characterization of voluntary nystagmus. J Neurol Neurosurg Psychiatry 1978;41:617–623.

68. Stark L, Hoyt WF, Ciuffreda KJ, et al. Voluntary nystagmus consists of overlapping and truncated saccades: An oculographic and control systems analysis. In Zuber BL, ed. Models of Oculomotor Behavior and Control. Boca Raton, FL, CRC Press, 1981:75–89.

69. Shults WT, Stark L, Hoyt WF, et al. Normal saccadic structure of voluntary nystagmus. Arch Ophthalmol 1977;95:1399–1404.

70. Stark L, Shults WT, Ciuffreda KJ, et al. Voluntary nystagmus is saccadic: Evidence from motor and sensory mechanisms. In Proceedings of the Joint Automatic Control Conference, San Francisco. Pittsburgh, Instrument Society of America, 1977:1410–1414.

71. Krohel G, Griffin JF. Voluntary vertical nystagmus. Neurology 1979;29:1153–1154.

72. Blair CJ, Goldberg MF, von Noorden GK. Voluntary nystagmus. Arch Ophthalmol 1967;77:349–354.

73. Rosenberg ML. The eyes in hysterical states of unconsciousness. J Clin Neuroophthalmol 1982;2:259–260.

74. Ciuffreda KJ. Voluntary nystagmus: New findings and clinical implications. Am J Optom Physiol Optics 1980;57:795–800.

75. Yee RD, Spiegel PH, Yamada T, et al. Voluntary saccadic oscillations, resembling ocular flutter and opsoclonus. J Neuroophthalmol 1994;14:95–101.

76. Keane JR. Neuro-ophthalmologic signs and symptoms of hysteria. Neurology 1982;32:757–762.

77. Sarkies NJC, Sanders MD. Convergence spasm. Trans Ophthalmol Soc 1985;104:782–786.

78. Rosenberg ML. Spasm of the near reflex mimicking myasthenia gravis. J Clin Neuroophthalmol 1986;6:106–108.

79. Newman NJ, Lessell S. Pupillary dilatation with monocular occlusion as a sign of nonorganic oculomotor dysfunction. Am J Ophthalmol 1989;108:461–462.

80. Keane JR. Convergence spasm. Neurology 1983;33:1637.

81. Safran AB, Roth A, Gauthier G. Le syndrome des spasmes de convergence (plus): Ou spasmes de convergence symptomatiques. Klin Monatsbl Augenheilkd 1982;180:471–473.

82. Kosmorsky G, Mitsumoto H, Estes M. Double, double, toil and trouble. Presented at the 26th Annual Frank B. Walsh Meeting, Chicago, IL, April 9–10, 1994.

83. Guiloff RJ, Whitely A, Kelly RE. Organic convergence spasm. Acta Neurol Scand 1980;61:252–259.

84. Schwartze GM, McHenry LC Jr, Proctor RC. Convergence spasm treatment by amytal interview: A case report. J Clin Neuroophthalmol 1983;3:123–125.

85. Manor RS. Use of special glasses in treatment of spasm of near reflex. Ann Ophthalmol 1979;11:903–905.

86. Henry JA, Woodruff GHA. A diagnostic sign in states of apparent unconsciousness. Lancet 1978;2:920–921.

87. Loewenfeld IE. The Pupil. Anatomy, Physiology, and Clinical Applications. Vol I. Ames, Iowa State University Press, 1993:1553–1578.

88. Bumke O. Die Pupillenstörungen in Geisteskranken. Vienna, Fischer Verlag, 1904.

89. Westphal A. Über Bisher nicht beschriebene Pupillenerscheinungen in Katatonischen Stupor mit Krankendemonstrationen. Allg Z Psychiatr 1907;64:694–701.

90. Westphal A. Über ein im Katatonischen Stupor beiobachtestes Pupillenphaenomen sowie bemerkungen über die pupillenstarre bei hysterie. Dtsch Med Wochenschr 1907;33:1080–1085.

91. Tyrer JH, Sutherland JM, Eadie MJ. Myosis bilatéral dans les déviations volontaires des yeux dans toutes les directions, dans un syndrome de neuromyélite optique. Rev Neurol 1963;109:72–76.

92. Thompson HS. Cornpicker's pupil: Jimson weed mydriasis. J Iowa Med Soc 1971;61:475–477.

93. Reader AL III. Mydriasis from *Datura wrightii.* Am J Ophthalmol 1977;84:263–264.

94. Thompson HS, Newsom DA, Loewenfeld IE. The fixed dilated pupil: Sudden iridoplegia or mydriatic drops? A simple diagnostic test. Arch Ophthalmol 1971;86:21–27.

95. Cavenar J, Brantley IJ, Braasch E. Blepharospasm: Organic or functional? Psychosomatics 1978;19:623–628.

96. Walsh FB, Hoyt WF. Clinical Neuro-Ophthalmology. Ed 3, Vol 3. Baltimore, Williams & Wilkins, 1969:2530.

Index

Page numbers in *italics* indicate figures. Page numbers followed by *t* indicate tables.